STANDARD
EDITION

2016
ICD-10-CM

INCLUDES
NETTER'S
ANATOMY
ART

Carol J. Buck
MS, CPC, CCS-P

Former Program Director
Medical Secretary Programs
Northwest Technical College
East Grand Forks, Minnesota

ELSEVIER

ELSEVIER

3251 Riverport Lane
St. Louis, Missouri 63043

2016 ICD-10-CM STANDARD EDITION

ISBN: 978-1-4557-7496-8
eISBN: 978-0-323-32062-7

Notice

Knowledge and best practice in this field are constantly changing. As new research and experience broaden our understanding, changes in research methods, professional practices, or medical treatment may become necessary.

Practitioners and researchers must always rely on their own experience and knowledge in evaluating and using any information, methods, compounds, or experiments described herein. In using such information or methods they should be mindful of their own safety and the safety of others, including parties for whom they have a professional responsibility.

With respect to any drug or pharmaceutical products identified, readers are advised to check the most current information provided (i) on procedures featured or (ii) by the manufacturer of each product to be administered, to verify the recommended dose or formula, the method and duration of administration, and contraindications. It is the responsibility of practitioners, relying on their own experience and knowledge of their patients, to make diagnoses, to determine dosages and the best treatment for each individual patient, and to take all appropriate safety precautions.

To the fullest extent of the law, neither the Publisher nor the authors, contributors, or editors, assume any liability for any injury and/or damage to persons or property as a matter of products liability, negligence or otherwise, or from any use or operation of any methods, products, instructions, or ideas contained in the material herein.

Library of Congress Cataloging-in-Publication Data

Buck, Carol J., author.
  2016 ICD-10-CM standard edition / Carol J. Buck.
    p. ; cm.
  ICD-10-CM standard edition
  Includes index.
  ISBN 978-1-4557-7496-8 (pbk. : alk. paper) -- ISBN 978-0-323-32062-7 (eISBN)
  I. Title. II. Title: ICD-10-CM standard edition.
  [DNLM: 1. International statistical classification of diseases and related health problems. 10th revision. Clinical modification. 2. Disease--classification. 3. Clinical Coding--standards. 4. International Classification of Diseases. WB 15]
  RB115
  616.001'2--dc23

2015023082

Director, Private Sector Education & Professional/References: Jeanne R. Olson
Content Development Manager: Luke Held
Publishing Services Manager: Jeffrey Patterson
Project Manager: Lisa A. P. Bushy
Senior Designer: Julia Dummitt

Printed in the United States of America

Last digit is the print number: 9   8   7   6   5   4   3   2   1

Working together
to grow libraries in
developing countries

www.elsevier.com • www.bookaid.org

DEVELOPMENT OF THIS EDITION

Editorial Consultant

Jenna Price
President
Price Editorial Services, LLC
St. Louis, Missouri

Query Team

Patricia Cordy Henricksen, MS, CHCA, CPC-I, CPC, CCP-P, ASC-PM
Auditing and Coding Educator
Soterion Medical Services
Lexington, Kentucky

Jackie L. Grass, CPC
Coding and Reimbursement Specialist
Grand Forks, North Dakota

Kathleen Buchda, CPC, CPMA
Revenue Recognition
New Richmond, Wisconsin

Elsevier/MC Strategies Revenue Cycle, Coding and Compliance Staff

"Experts in providing e-learning on revenue cycle, coding and compliance."

Deborah Neville, RHIA, CCS-P
Director

Lynn-Marie D. Wozniak, MS, RHIT
Content Manager

Sandra L. Macica, MS, RHIA, CCS, ROCC
Product Specialist

Therese M. Jorwic, MPH, RHIA, CCS, CCS-P, FAHIMA
Product Specialist

CONTENTS

GUIDE TO USING THE 2016 ICD-10-CM

Medical coding has long been a part of the health care profession. Through the years medical coding systems have become more complex and extensive. Today, medical coding is an intricate and immense process that is present in every health care setting. The increased use of electronic submissions for health care services only increases the need for coders who understand the coding process.

2016 ICD-10-CM Standard Edition was developed to help meet the needs of coding professionals at all levels by offering a comprehensive coding text at a reasonable price.

All material strictly adheres to the latest government versions available at the time of printing. Updates from the *Definitions of Medicare Code Edits* (MCE) will be posted to the companion website (www. codingupdates.com) when available.

Illustrations and Items

The ICD-10-CM Tabular List contains illustrations, pictures, and items to assist you in understanding difficult terminology, diseases/conditions, or coding in a specific category. Items are always printed in ▆▆▆▆▆ ink so that the added material is not mistaken for official notations or instructions. ▆▆▆▆▆ ink is used for other annotations in the text. Your ideas on what other descriptions or illustrations should be in future editions of this text are always appreciated.

Instructional Notations

Includes Notes

Includes

The word 'Includes' appears immediately under certain categories to further define, or give examples of, the content of the category.

Excludes Notes

The ICD-10-CM has two types of excludes notes. Each note has a different definition for use, but they are both similar in that they indicate that codes excluded from each other are independent of each other.

Excludes1

A type 1 Excludes note is a pure excludes. It means "NOT CODED HERE!" An Excludes1 note indicates that the code excluded should never be used at the same time as the code above the Excludes1 note. An Excludes1 is for use when two conditions cannot occur together, such as a congenital form versus an acquired form of the same condition.

Excludes2

A type 2 Excludes note represents "NOT INCLUDED HERE." An Excludes2 note indicates that the condition excluded is not part of the condition it is excluded from but a patient may have both conditions at the same time. When an Excludes2 note appears under a code, it is acceptable to use both the code and the excluded code together.

Code First/Use Additional Code notes (etiology/manifestation paired codes)

Certain conditions have both an underlying etiology and multiple body system manifestations due to the underlying etiology. For such conditions the ICD-10-CM has a coding convention that requires the underlying condition be sequenced first, followed by the manifestation. Wherever such a combination exists, there is a "use additional code" note at the etiology code, and a "code first" note at the manifestation code. These instructional notes indicate the proper sequencing order of the codes, etiology followed by manifestation.

In most cases the manifestation codes will have in the code title, "in diseases classified elsewhere." Codes with this title are a component of the etiology/manifestation convention. The code title indicates that it is a manifestation code. "In diseases classified elsewhere" codes are never permitted to be used as first-listed or principal diagnosis codes. They must be used in conjunction with an underlying condition code, and they must be listed following the underlying condition.

Use additional

The words indicate an instructional note that another code may be needed.

Code first

The words indicate an instructional note that directs the coder to sequence the underlying condition before the manifestation.

Code also

A "code also" note instructs that two codes may be required to fully describe a condition, but the sequencing of the two codes is discretionary, depending on the severity of the conditions and the reason for the encounter.

Unspecified

The highlight indicates that although the code is valid as a principal (first-listed) diagnosis, it is not as specific as other codes without the highlight.

7th characters and placeholder X

For codes less than 6 characters that require a 7th character a placeholder X should be assigned for all characters less than 6. The 7th character must always be the 7th character of a code.

Annotated

Throughout the manual, revisions, additions, and deleted codes or words are indicated by the following symbols:

    ◄▥▥   **Revised:** Revisions within the line or code from the previous edition are indicated by the arrow.

    ◄   **New:** Additions to the previous edition are indicated by the triangle.

    ~~deleted~~   **Deleted:** Deletions from the previous edition are struck through.

ICD-10-CM Tabular List Symbols

    ●   **Use Additional Character(s):** The red stop sign cautions that the code requires additional character(s) to ensure the greatest specificity.

    X   For codes less than 6 characters that require a 7th character, a placeholder X should be assigned for all characters less than 6. The 7th character must always be the 7th character of a code.

    OGCR   The *Official Guidelines for Coding and Reporting* symbol includes the placement of a portion of a guideline as that guideline pertains to the code by which it is located. The complete OGCR are located in Part I.

SYMBOLS AND CONVENTIONS

ICD-10-CM Tabular

Use Additional Character(s): The red stop sign cautions you that the code requires additional character(s) to ensure greatest specificity.

Volume 1, Tabular List

●K22 **Other diseases of esophagus**

    Excludes2 esophageal varices (I85.-)

X●V00.01 **Pedestrian on foot injured in collision with roller-skater**

A02.20 **Localized salmonella infection, unspecified**

A48.3 **Toxic shock syndrome**

    Use additional code to identify the organism (B95, B96)

B39 **Histoplasmosis**

    Code first associated AIDS (B20)

E34.0 **Carcinoid syndrome**

    Note: May be used as an additional code to identify functional activity associated with a carcinoid tumor.

Placeholder X: The red X reminds you that for codes less than 6 characters that require a 7th character, a placeholder X should be assigned to all characters less than 6.

Unspecified: These codes are for use when the information in the medical record is insufficient to assign a more specific code. For those categories for which an unspecified code is not provided, the "other specified" code may represent both other and unspecified.

Use additional code: Located at the etiology code and directs you to assign a manifestation code.

Code first indicates the etiology code is to be first-listed before the manifestation code.

Notes define terms or give coding instructions.

Codes or index entries are for purposes of illustration only and may not be current.

OGCR Section I.C.6.B.5.

Neoplasm Related Pain Code G89.3 is assigned to pain documented as being related, associated or due to cancer, primary or secondary malignancy, or tumor. This code is assigned regardless of whether the pain is acute or chronic.

OGCR: The *Official Guidelines for Coding and Reporting* are placed near the codes to which they refer and are highlighted.

I70.2   **Atherosclerosis of native arteries of the extremities**
Mönckeberg's (medial) sclerosis

Use additional code, if applicable, to identify chronic total occlusion of artery of extremity (I70.92)

code, if applicable, directs the coder to other conditions that may be appropriate to report.

I74   **Arterial embolism and thrombosis**
Includes   embolic infarction
embolic occlusion
thrombotic infarction
thrombotic occlusion

The word "and" should be interpreted to mean either "and" or "or" when it appears in a statement.

Bold typeface is used on all codes and titles.

I83.001   **Varicose veins of unspecified lower extremity with ulcer of thigh**

"with" should be interpreted to mean "associated with" or "due to."

K73.2   **Chronic active hepatitis, not elsewhere classified**

"not elsewhere classified" or **NEC** identifies a code that is assigned only when the information at hand specifies a condition for which no more specific code is available.

"not otherwise specified" or **NOS** is equivalent to unspecified.

W13.9   **Fall from, out of or through building, not otherwise specified**

Codes or index entries are for purposes of illustration only and may not be current.

Excludes1 means "NOT CODED HERE!" An Excludes1 note indicates that the code excluded should never be assigned at the same time as the code above the Excludes1 note.

M19 Other and unspecified osteoarthritis
    Excludes1   polyarthritis (M15.-)
    Excludes2   arthrosis of spine (M47.-)
                 hallux rigidus (M20.2)
                 osteoarthritis of spine (M47.-)

Excludes2 represents "NOT INCLUDED HERE." An Excludes2 note indicates that the condition excluded is not part of the condition represented by the code, but a patient may have both conditions at the same time and it is acceptable to use both the code and the excluded code together, when appropriate.

Includes: This note appears immediately under a three-character code title to further define, or give examples of, the content.

A06   Amebiasis
    Includes   infection due to Entamoeba histolytica

E26.01   Conn's syndrome
    Code also adrenal adenoma (D35.0)

Code also instructs that two codes may be required to fully describe a condition, but this note does not provide sequencing direction.

Codes titled "other" or "other specified" are for use when the information in the medical record provides detail for which a specific code does not exist.

E25.8   Other adrenogenital disorders

G14   Postpolio syndrome
    Includes   Postpolio myelitic syndrome
    Excludes1   sequelae of poliomyelitis (B91)

Codes or index entries are for purposes of illustration only and may not be current.

Alphabetic Index

Main terms are in **bold** typeface.

Aberrant (congenital) —*see also* Malposition, congenital
    adrenal gland Q89.1

Etiology code first followed by the manifestation code in **brackets**. The code in brackets is always to be sequenced second.

Amyloid heart (disease) E85.4 *[I43]*

Amylophagia —*see* Pica

"see" indicates another term should be referenced.

Angiofibroma —*see also* Neoplasm, benign, by site

"see also" follows a main term and instructs that there is another main term that may also be referenced.

Appendicitis (pneumococcal) (retrocecal) K37
    with
        perforation or rupture K35.2
        peritoneal abscess K35.3

A default code is listed next to the main term and represents that condition most commonly associated with the main term. If a condition is documented in a medical record without any additional information, such as acute or chronic, the default code should be assigned.

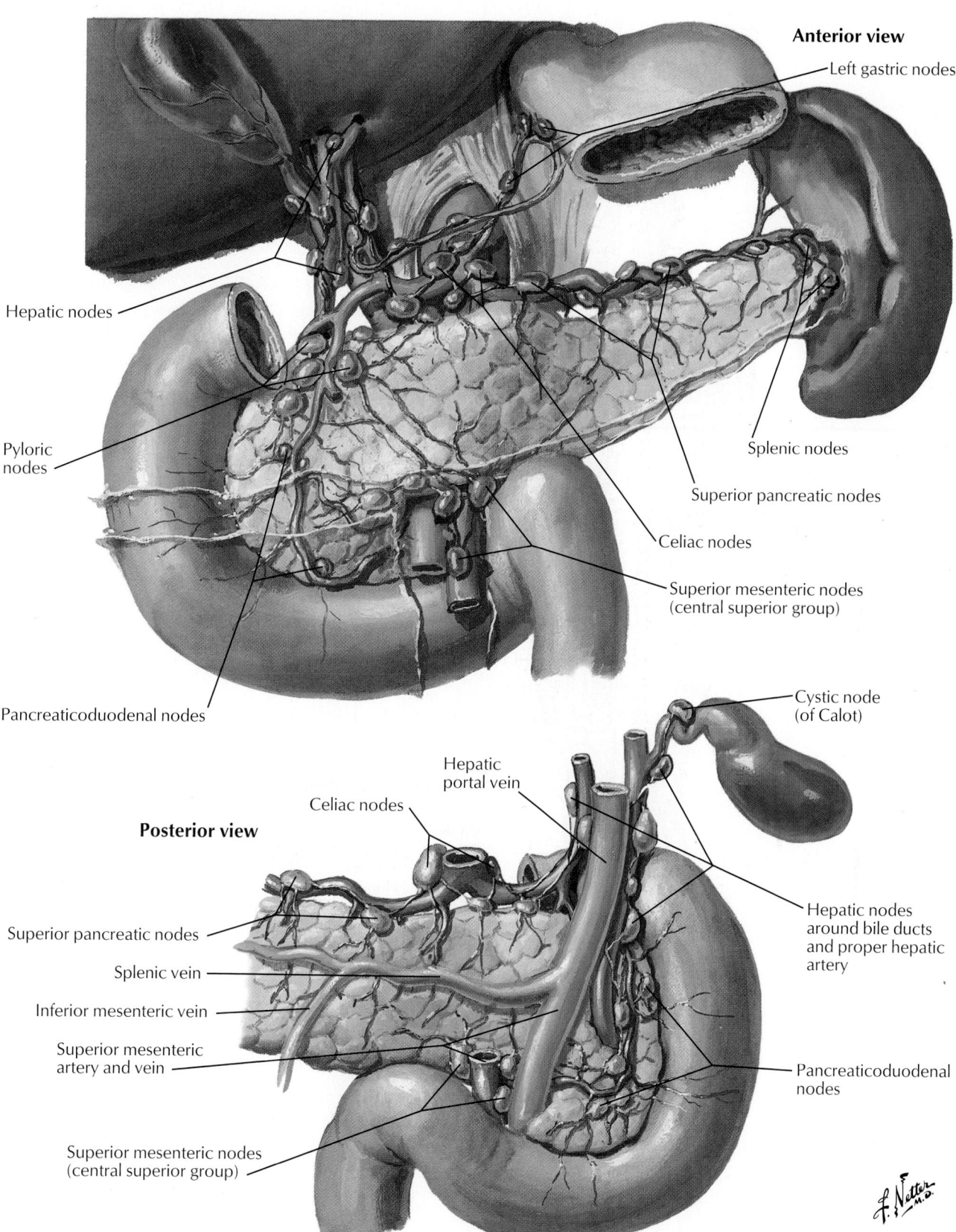

Anterior view

Left gastric nodes

Hepatic nodes

Pyloric nodes

Pancreaticoduodenal nodes

Splenic nodes

Superior pancreatic nodes

Celiac nodes

Superior mesenteric nodes (central superior group)

Cystic node (of Calot)

Posterior view

Hepatic portal vein

Celiac nodes

Superior pancreatic nodes

Splenic vein

Inferior mesenteric vein

Superior mesenteric artery and vein

Superior mesenteric nodes (central superior group)

Hepatic nodes around bile ducts and proper hepatic artery

Pancreaticoduodenal nodes

Plate 315 Lymph Vessels and Nodes of Pancreas. (Netter: Atlas of Human Anatomy, 4 ed, 2006, Saunders.)

Dermatome pattern

Levels of principal dermatomes

C5	Clavicles
C5, 6, 7	Lateral parts of upper limbs
C8; T1	Medial sides of upper limbs
C6	Thumb
C6, 7, 8	Hand
C8	Ring and little fingers
T4	Level of nipples
T10	Level of umbilicus
T12	Inguinal or groin regions
L1, 2, 3, 4	Anterior and inner surfaces of lower limbs
L4, 5; S1	Foot
L4	Medial side of great toe
L5; S1, 2	Outer and posterior sides of lower limbs
S1	Lateral margin of foot and little toe
S2, 3, 4	Perineum

Plate 164 Dermatomes. (Netter: Atlas of Human Anatomy, 4 ed, 2006, Saunders.)

Female: frontal section

Peritoneum
Body of bladder
Fundus of bladder
Interureteric crest
Left ureteric orifice
Trigone of bladder
Neck of bladder
Paravesical endopelvic fascia and vesical venous plexus
Vesical fascia
Tendinous arch of levator ani muscle
Obturator internus muscle
Levator ani muscle

Tendinous arch of pelvic fascia

Urethra
Sphincter urethrae muscle
Perineal membrane
Inferior pubic ramus
Crus of clitoris and ischiocavernosus muscle
Bulb of vestibule and bulbospongiosus muscle
Deep perineal (investing or Gallaudet's) fascia
Superficial perineal (Colles') fascia

Round ligament of uterus

Vagina

Male: frontal section

Peritoneum

Body of bladder
Fundus of bladder
Ductus (vas) deferens
Interureteric crest
Right ureteric orifice
Trigone of bladder
Neck of bladder
Paravesical endopelvic fascia and vesical venous plexus
Tendinous arch of levator ani muscle
Uvula of bladder
Obturator internus muscle
Levator ani muscle
Capsule of prostate
Prostate and prostatic urethra
Seminal colliculus
Bulbourethral (Cowper's) gland
Perineal membrane and sphincter urethrae muscle
Bulbous portion of spongy urethra
Corpus spongiosum and bulbospongiosus muscle
Deep perineal (investing or Gallaudet's) fascia

Internal urethral sphincter
Tendinous arch of pelvic fascia
Anterior recess of ischio-anal fossa
Inferior pubic ramus
Crus of penis and ischiocaver-nosus muscle
Superficial perineal (Colles') fascia

Plate 366   Urinary Bladder: Female and Male. (Netter: Atlas of Human Anatomy, 4 ed, 2006, Saunders.)

NAP-3

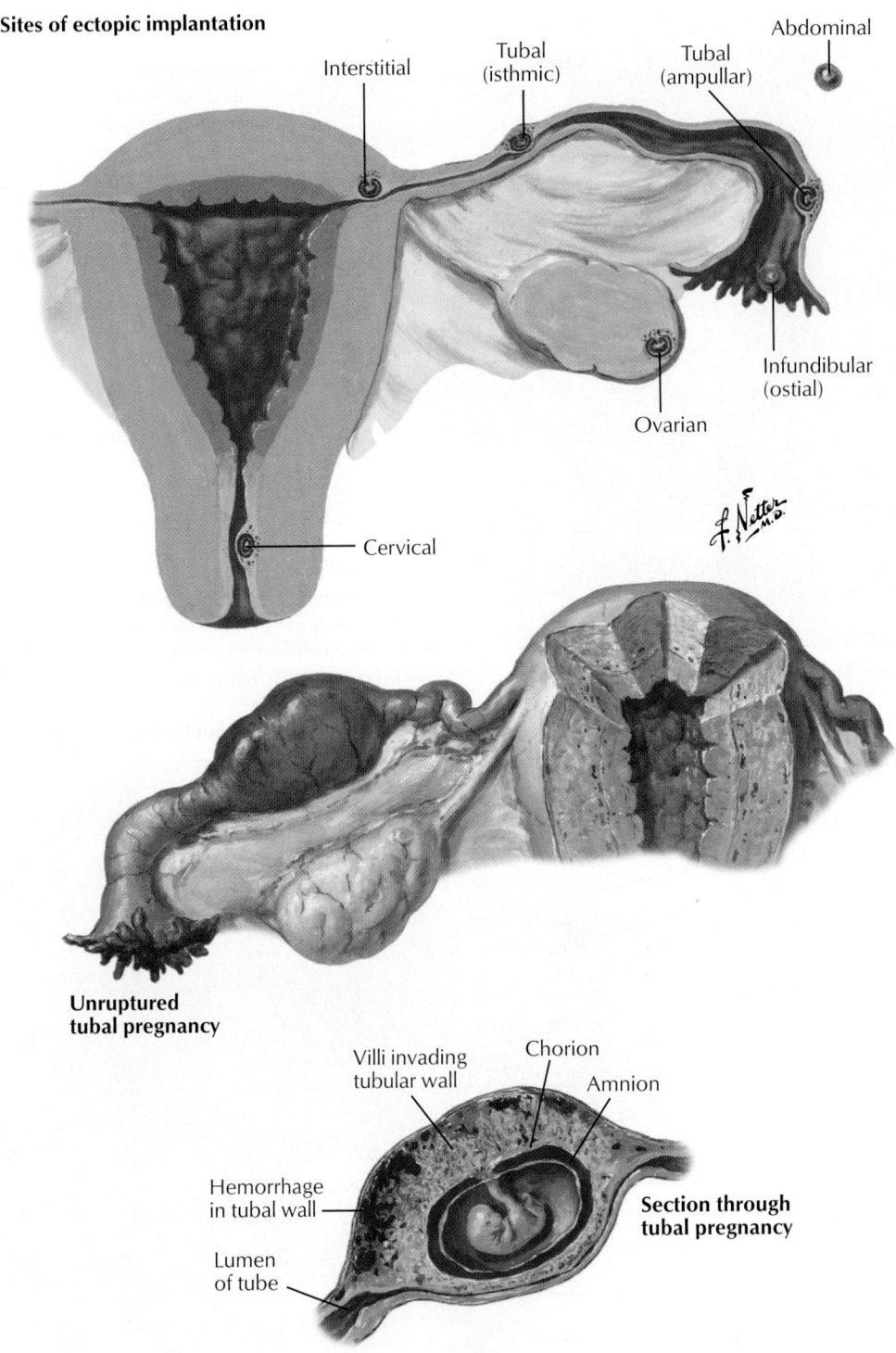

Sites of ectopic implantation

Interstitial

Tubal (isthmic)

Tubal (ampullar)

Abdominal

Infundibular (ostial)

Ovarian

Cervical

Unruptured tubal pregnancy

Villi invading tubular wall

Chorion

Amnion

Hemorrhage in tubal wall

Lumen of tube

Section through tubal pregnancy

Plate 375 Ectopic Pregnancy. (Netter: Atlas of Human Anatomy, 4 ed, 2006, Saunders.)

Superficial inguinal ring

External spermatic fascia

Cremaster muscle and fascia

Septum of scrotum (formed by dartos fascia)

Superficial (dartos) fascia of scrotum

Skin of scrotum

Skin of penis

Superficial fascia of penis (Colles' fascia)

Deep (Buck's) fascia of penis

Testicular artery

Ductus deferens

Artery to ductus deferens

Genital branch of genitofemoral nerve

Pampiniform (venous) plexus

Epididymis

Appendix of epididymis

Appendix of testis

Testis (covered by visceral layer of tunica vaginalis)

Parietal layer of tunica vaginalis

Superficial (dartos) fascia of scrotum

External spermatic fascia

Cremaster muscle and fascia

Internal spermatic fascia

Parietal layer of tunica vaginalis

Epididymis

Testis (covered by visceral layer of tunica vaginalis)

Skin of scrotum

Plate 387   Scrotum and Contents. (Netter: Atlas of Human Anatomy, 4 ed, 2006, Saunders.)

NETTER'S ANATOMY ILLUSTRATIONS

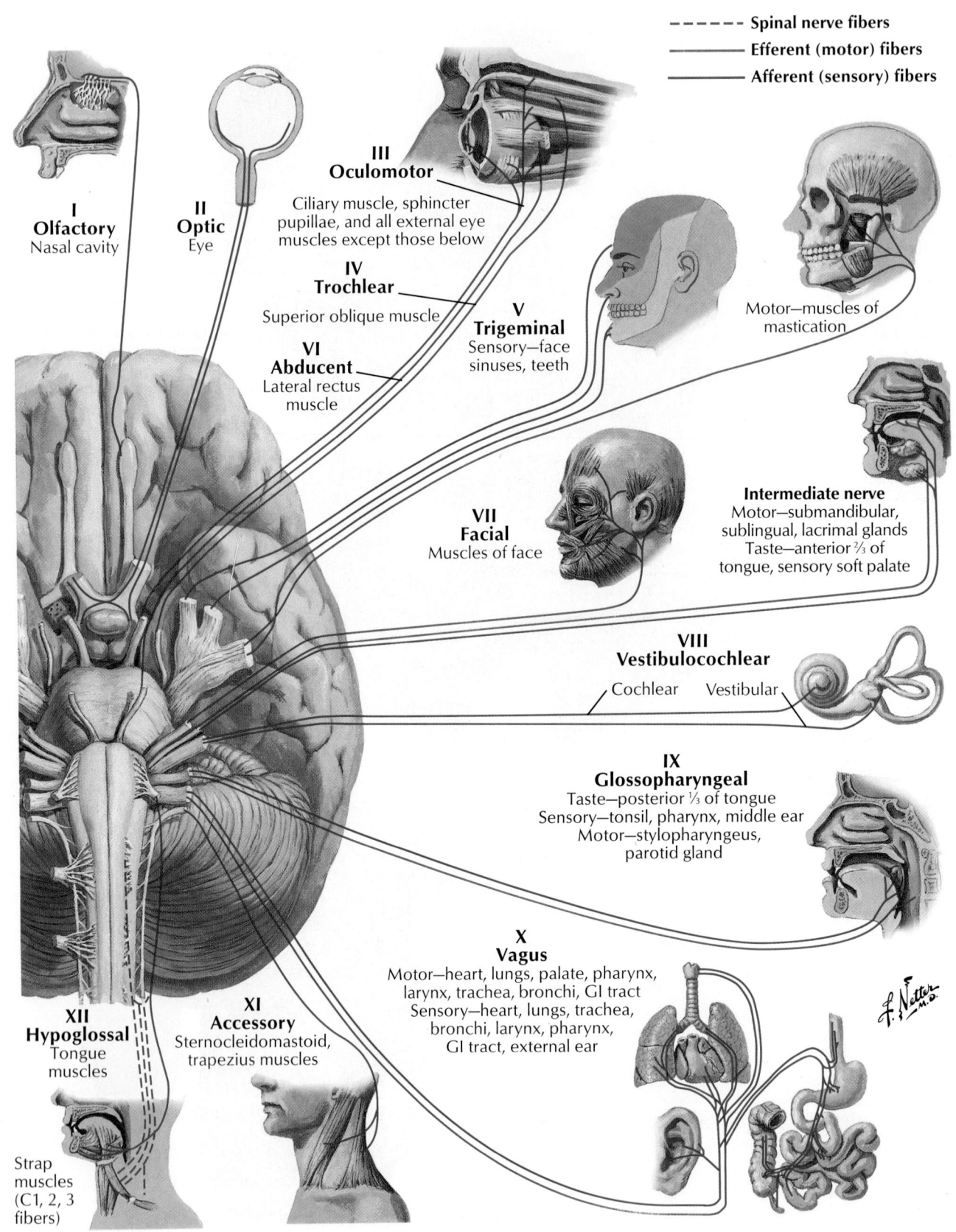

----- Spinal nerve fibers
——— Efferent (motor) fibers
━━━ Afferent (sensory) fibers

I
Olfactory
Nasal cavity

II
Optic
Eye

III
Oculomotor
Ciliary muscle, sphincter
pupillae, and all external eye
muscles except those below

IV
Trochlear
Superior oblique muscle

VI
Abducent
Lateral rectus
muscle

V
Trigeminal
Sensory—face
sinuses, teeth

Motor—muscles of
mastication

VII
Facial
Muscles of face

Intermediate nerve
Motor—submandibular,
sublingual, lacrimal glands
Taste—anterior ⅔ of
tongue, sensory soft palate

VIII
Vestibulocochlear
Cochlear   Vestibular

IX
Glossopharyngeal
Taste—posterior ⅓ of tongue
Sensory—tonsil, pharynx, middle ear
Motor—stylopharyngeus,
parotid gland

X
Vagus
Motor—heart, lungs, palate, pharynx,
larynx, trachea, bronchi, GI tract
Sensory—heart, lungs, trachea,
bronchi, larynx, pharynx,
GI tract, external ear

XII
Hypoglossal
Tongue
muscles

XI
Accessory
Sternocleidomastoid,
trapezius muscles

Strap
muscles
(C1, 2, 3
fibers)

NETTER'S ANATOMY ILLUSTRATIONS

Plate 118   Cranial Nerves (Motor and Sensory Distribution): Schema. (Netter: Atlas of Human Anatomy, 4 ed, 2006, Saunders.)

Superior view

Supratrochlear nerve

Medial rectus muscle

Superior oblique muscle

Infratrochlear nerve

Nasociliary nerve

Trochlear nerve (IV)

Common tendinous ring

Ophthalmic nerve (V₁)

Optic nerve (II)

Internal carotid artery and nerve plexus

Oculomotor nerve (III)

Trochlear nerve (IV)

Abducent nerve (VI)

Tentorium cerebelli

Medial branch } Supraorbital nerve
Lateral branch

Levator palpebrae superioris muscle

Superior rectus muscle

Lacrimal gland

Lacrimal nerve

Lateral rectus muscle

Frontal nerve

Maxillary nerve (V₂)

Meningeal branch of maxillary nerve

Mandibular nerve (V₃)

Lesser petrosal nerve

Meningeal branch of mandibular nerve

Greater petrosal nerve

Trigeminal (semilunar) ganglion

Tentorial (meningeal) branch of ophthalmic nerve

Superior view:
levator palpebrae superioris, superior rectus, and superior oblique muscles partially cut away

Supratrochlear nerve *(cut)*

Supraorbital nerve branches *(cut)*

Infratrochlear nerve

Anterior ethmoidal nerve

Optic nerve (II)

Posterior ethmoidal nerve

Superior branch of oculomotor nerve (III) *(cut)*

Nasociliary nerve

Internal carotid plexus

Trochlear nerve (IV) *(cut)*

Oculomotor nerve (III)

Abducent nerve (VI)

Long ciliary nerves

Short ciliary nerves

Lacrimal nerve

Ciliary ganglion

Parasympathetic root of ciliary ganglion (from inferior branch of oculomotor nerve)

Sympathetic root of ciliary ganglion (from internal carotid plexus)

Sensory root of ciliary ganglion (from nasociliary nerve)

Branches to inferior and medial rectus muscles

Abducent nerve (VI)

Inferior branch of oculomotor nerve (III)

Lacrimal nerve

Frontal nerve *(cut)*

Ophthalmic nerve (V₁)

Plate 86 Nerves of Orbit. (Netter: Atlas of Human Anatomy, 4 ed, 2006, Saunders.)

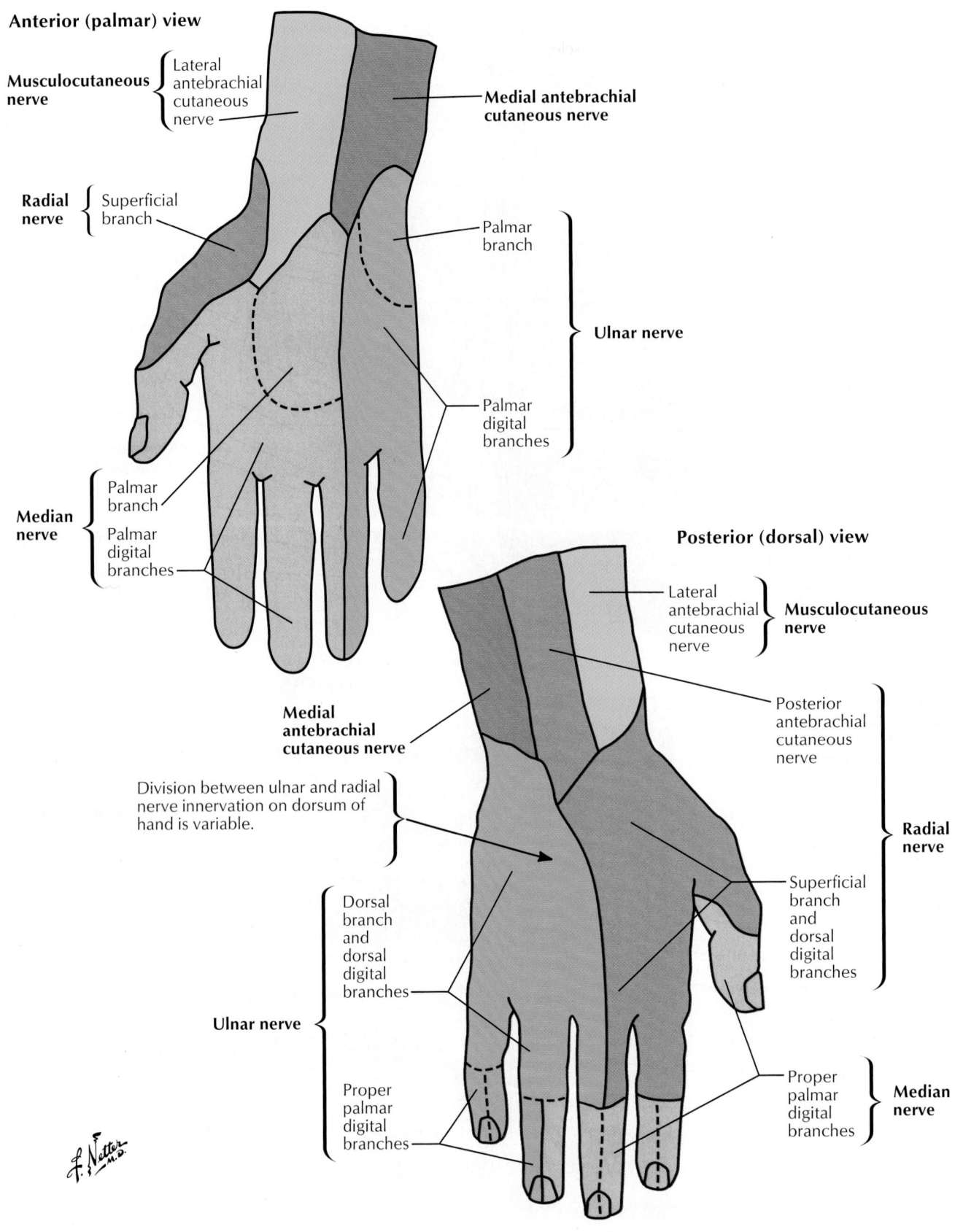

Anterior (palmar) view

Musculocutaneous nerve — Lateral antebrachial cutaneous nerve

Medial antebrachial cutaneous nerve

Radial nerve — Superficial branch

Palmar branch

Ulnar nerve

Palmar digital branches

Median nerve — Palmar branch / Palmar digital branches

Posterior (dorsal) view

Lateral antebrachial cutaneous nerve — **Musculocutaneous nerve**

Medial antebrachial cutaneous nerve

Posterior antebrachial cutaneous nerve

Division between ulnar and radial nerve innervation on dorsum of hand is variable.

Radial nerve

Superficial branch and dorsal digital branches

Ulnar nerve — Dorsal branch and dorsal digital branches

Proper palmar digital branches

Proper palmar digital branches — **Median nerve**

Plate 472   Cutaneous Innervation of Wrist and Hand. (Netter: Atlas of Human Anatomy, 4 ed, 2006, Saunders.)

NETTER'S ANATOMY ILLUSTRATIONS

Anterior view

Deltoid muscle

Coracobrachialis muscle

Biceps brachii muscle { Short head (*cut*)

Long head (*cut*)

Musculocutaneous nerve

Brachialis muscle

Biceps brachii muscle (*cut*) and tendon

Lateral antebrachial cutaneous nerve (from musculocutaneous nerve)

Radial nerve { Deep branch

Superficial branch

Supinator muscle

Brachioradialis muscle

Radial artery

Pronator teres muscle (*partially cut*)

Median nerve

Flexor pollicis longus muscle

Flexor carpi radialis tendon (*cut*)

Flexor retinaculum (transverse carpal ligament)

Superficial branch of radial nerve

Recurrent (motor) branch of median nerve to thenar muscles

Common palmar digital branches of median nerve

Proper palmar digital branches of median nerve

Intercostobrachial nerve

Medial brachial cutaneous nerve

Radial nerve

Ulnar nerve

Medial antebrachial cutaneous nerve

Median nerve

Brachial artery

Bicipital aponeurosis

Humeral head (*cut*) } Pronator teres muscle

Ulnar head

Flexor carpi radialis muscle (*cut*)

Humeroulnar head } Flexor digitorum superficialis muscle (*cut*)

Radial head

Flexor digitorum profundus muscle

Flexor carpi ulnaris muscle

Ulnar artery and nerve

Dorsal branch of ulnar nerve

Flexor digitorum superficialis tendons (*cut*)

Deep palmar branch of ulnar artery and deep branch of ulnar nerve

Superficial branch of ulnar nerve

Superficial palmar arch (*cut*)

Common palmar digital branch of ulnar nerve

Communicating branch of median nerve with ulnar nerve

Proper palmar digital branches of ulnar nerve

Plate 473 Arteries and Nerves of Upper Limb. (Netter: Atlas of Human Anatomy, 4 ed, 2006, Saunders.)

Lateral cutaneous
branch of subcostal nerve

Inguinal ligament (Poupart's)

Superficial circumflex iliac vein

Femoral branches
of genitofemoral nerve

Lateral femoral cutaneous nerve

Saphenous opening (fossa ovalis)

Fascia lata

Anterior cutaneous
branches of femoral nerve

Patellar nerve plexus

Branches of lateral sural cutaneous nerve
(from common fibular [peroneal] nerve)

Deep fascia of leg
(crural fascia)

Superficial fibular (peroneal) nerve
Medial dorsal
cutaneous branch

Intermediate dorsal
cutaneous branch

Small saphenous vein and lateral
dorsal cutaneous nerve (from sural nerve)

Lateral dorsal digital nerve
and vein of 5th toe

Dorsal metatarsal veins

Dorsal digital nerves and veins

Superficial epigastric vein

Ilioinguinal nerve (scrotal branch)
(usually passes through superficial
inguinal ring)

Genital branch of genitofemoral nerve

Femoral vein

Superficial external pudendal vein

Accessory saphenous vein

Great saphenous vein

Cutaneous branches of obturator nerve

Infrapatellar branch of saphenous nerve

Saphenous nerve (terminal branch
of femoral nerve)

Great saphenous vein

Dorsal digital nerves

Dorsal venous arch

Dorsal digital nerve and vein of medial
side of great toe

Dorsal digital branch of deep fibular
(peroneal) nerve

Plate 544 Superficial Nerves and Veins of Lower Limb: Anterior View. (Netter: Atlas of Human Anatomy, 4 ed, 2006, Saunders.)

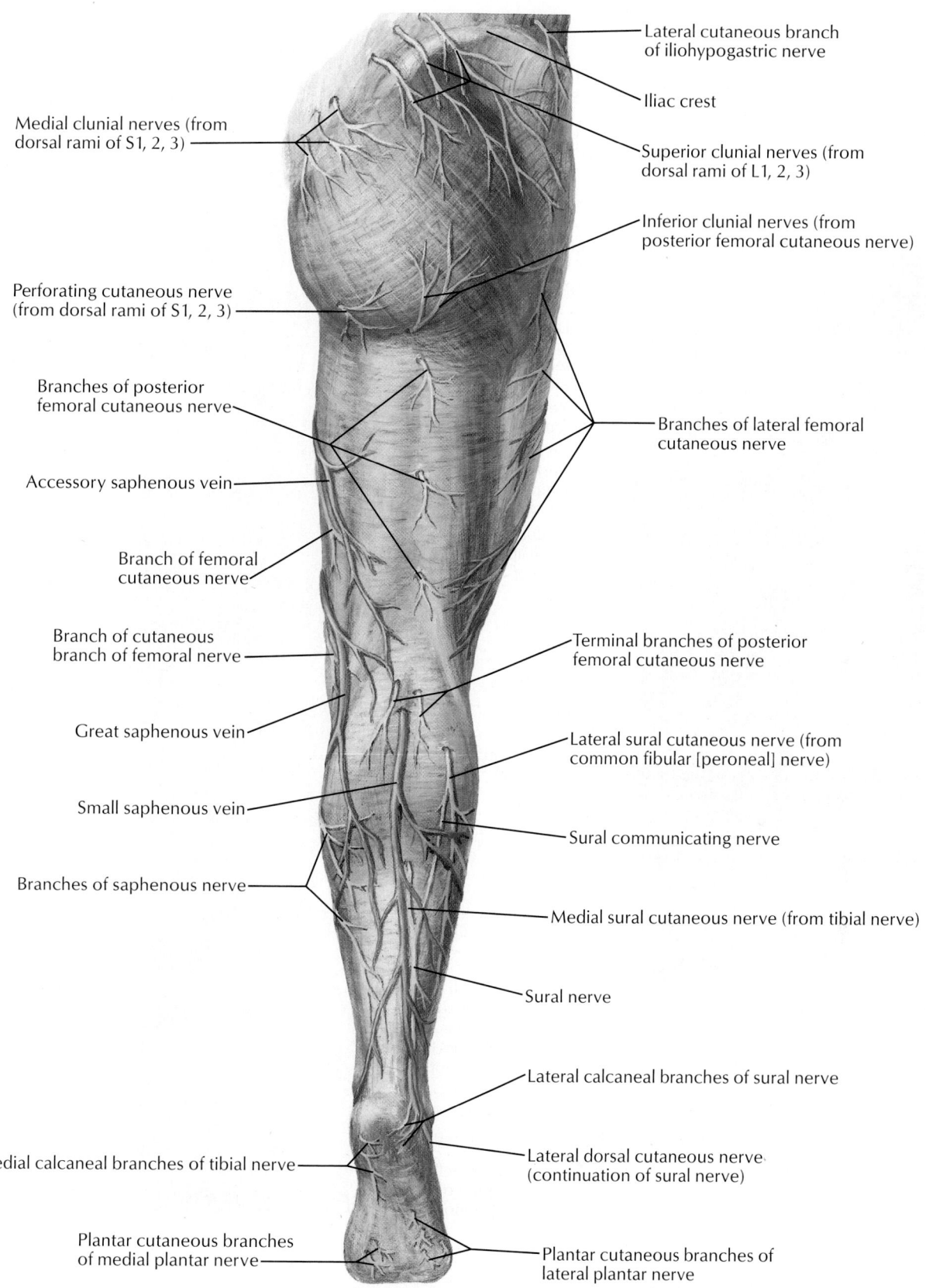

Lateral cutaneous branch
of iliohypogastric nerve

Iliac crest

Medial clunial nerves (from
dorsal rami of S1, 2, 3)

Superior clunial nerves (from
dorsal rami of L1, 2, 3)

Inferior clunial nerves (from
posterior femoral cutaneous nerve)

Perforating cutaneous nerve
(from dorsal rami of S1, 2, 3)

Branches of posterior
femoral cutaneous nerve

Branches of lateral femoral
cutaneous nerve

Accessory saphenous vein

Branch of femoral
cutaneous nerve

Branch of cutaneous
branch of femoral nerve

Terminal branches of posterior
femoral cutaneous nerve

Great saphenous vein

Lateral sural cutaneous nerve (from
common fibular [peroneal] nerve)

Small saphenous vein

Sural communicating nerve

Branches of saphenous nerve

Medial sural cutaneous nerve (from tibial nerve)

Sural nerve

Lateral calcaneal branches of sural nerve

Medial calcaneal branches of tibial nerve

Lateral dorsal cutaneous nerve
(continuation of sural nerve)

Plantar cutaneous branches
of medial plantar nerve

Plantar cutaneous branches of
lateral plantar nerve

Plate 545 Superficial Nerves and Veins of Lower Limb: Posterior View. (Netter: Atlas of Human Anatomy, 4 ed, 2006, Saunders.)

Superficial dissections

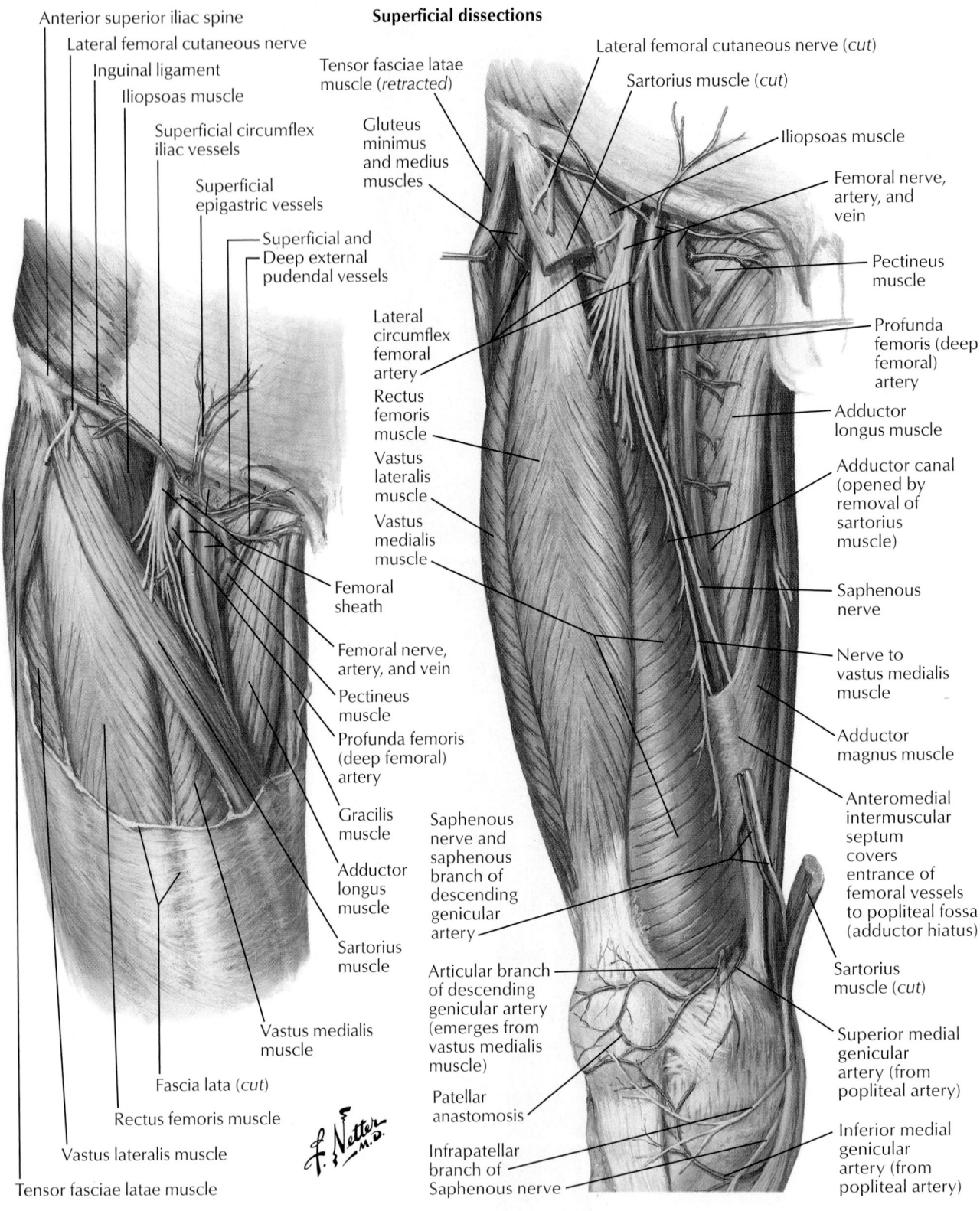

Anterior superior iliac spine

Lateral femoral cutaneous nerve

Inguinal ligament

Iliopsoas muscle

Superficial circumflex iliac vessels

Superficial epigastric vessels

Superficial and Deep external pudendal vessels

Tensor fasciae latae muscle (retracted)

Gluteus minimus and medius muscles

Lateral circumflex femoral artery

Rectus femoris muscle

Vastus lateralis muscle

Vastus medialis muscle

Femoral sheath

Femoral nerve, artery, and vein

Pectineus muscle

Profunda femoris (deep femoral) artery

Gracilis muscle

Adductor longus muscle

Sartorius muscle

Vastus medialis muscle

Fascia lata (cut)

Rectus femoris muscle

Vastus lateralis muscle

Tensor fasciae latae muscle

Saphenous nerve and saphenous branch of descending genicular artery

Articular branch of descending genicular artery (emerges from vastus medialis muscle)

Patellar anastomosis

Infrapatellar branch of Saphenous nerve

Lateral femoral cutaneous nerve (cut)

Sartorius muscle (cut)

Iliopsoas muscle

Femoral nerve, artery, and vein

Pectineus muscle

Profunda femoris (deep femoral) artery

Adductor longus muscle

Adductor canal (opened by removal of sartorius muscle)

Saphenous nerve

Nerve to vastus medialis muscle

Adductor magnus muscle

Anteromedial intermuscular septum covers entrance of femoral vessels to popliteal fossa (adductor hiatus)

Sartorius muscle (cut)

Superior medial genicular artery (from popliteal artery)

Inferior medial genicular artery (from popliteal artery)

F. Netter M.D.

Plate 500   Arteries and Nerves of Thigh: Anterior Views. (Netter: Atlas of Human Anatomy, 4 ed, 2006, Saunders.)

NAP-12

Deep dissection

Deep circumflex iliac artery

Lateral femoral cutaneous nerve

Sartorius muscle (*cut*)

Iliopsoas muscle

Tensor fasciae latae muscle (*retracted*)

Gluteus medius and minimus muscles

Femoral nerve

Rectus femoris muscle (*cut*)

Ascending, transverse and descending branches of Lateral circumflex femoral artery

Medial circumflex femoral artery

Pectineus muscle (*cut*)

Profunda femoris (deep femoral) artery

Perforating branches

Adductor longus muscle (*cut*)

Vastus lateralis muscle

Vastus intermedius muscle

Rectus femoris muscle (*cut*)

Saphenous nerve

Anteromedial intermuscular septum (*opened*)

Vastus medialis muscle

Quadriceps femoris tendon

Patella and patellar anastomosis

Medial patellar retinaculum

Patellar ligament

External iliac artery and vein

Inguinal ligament (Poupart's)

Femoral artery and vein (*cut*)

Pectineus muscle (*cut*)

Obturator canal

Obturator externus muscle

Adductor longus muscle (*cut*)

Anterior branch and Posterior branch of obturator nerve

Quadratus femoris muscle

Adductor brevis muscle

Branches of posterior branch of obturator nerve

Adductor magnus muscle

Gracilis muscle

Cutaneous branch of obturator nerve

Femoral artery and vein (*cut*)

Descending genicular artery
Articular branch
Saphenous branch

Adductor hiatus

Sartorius muscle (*cut*)

Adductor magnus tendon

Adductor tubercle on medial epicondyle of femur

Superior medial genicular artery (from popliteal artery)

Infrapatellar branch of Saphenous nerve

Inferior medial genicular artery (from popliteal artery)

Plate 501   Arteries and Nerves of Thigh: Posterior View. (Netter: Atlas of Human Anatomy, 4 ed, 2006, Saunders.)

Deep dissection

Superior clunial nerves

Gluteus maximus muscle (*cut*)

Medial clunial nerves

Inferior gluteal artery and nerve

Pudendal nerve

Nerve to obturator internus
(and superior gemellus)

Posterior femoral
cutaneous nerve

Sacrotuberous ligament

Ischial tuberosity

Inferior clunial nerves (*cut*)

Adductor magnus muscle

Gracilis muscle

Sciatic nerve

Muscular branches of sciatic nerve

Semitendinosus muscle (*retracted*)

Semimembranosus muscle

Sciatic nerve

Articular branch

Adductor hiatus

Popliteal vein and artery

Superior medial genicular artery

Medial epicondyle of femur

Tibial nerve

Gastrocnemius muscle (medial head)

Medial sural cutaneous nerve

Small saphenous vein

Iliac crest

Gluteal aponeurosis and
gluteus medius muscle (*cut*)

Superior gluteal artery and nerve

Gluteus minimus muscle

Tensor fasciae latae muscle

Piriformis muscle

Gluteus medius muscle (*cut*)

Superior gemellus muscle

Greater trochanter of femur

Obturator internus muscle

Inferior gemellus muscle

Gluteus maximus muscle (*cut*)

Quadratus femoris muscle

Medial circumflex femoral
artery

Vastus lateralis muscle
and iliotibial tract

Adductor minimus part of
adductor magnus muscle

1st perforating artery (from
profunda femoris artery)

Adductor magnus muscle

2nd and 3rd perforating arteries
(from profunda femoris artery)

4th perforating artery (from
profunda femoris artery)

Long head (*retracted*) ⎫ Biceps femoris
Short head ⎭ muscle

Superior lateral genicular artery

Common fibular (peroneal) nerve

Plantaris muscle

Gastrocnemius muscle (lateral head)

Lateral sural cutaneous nerve

F. Netter m.o.

NETTER'S ANATOMY ILLUSTRATIONS

Plate 502 Arteries and Nerves of Thigh: Posterior View. (Netter: Atlas of Human Anatomy, 4 ed, 2006, Saunders.)

Horizontal section

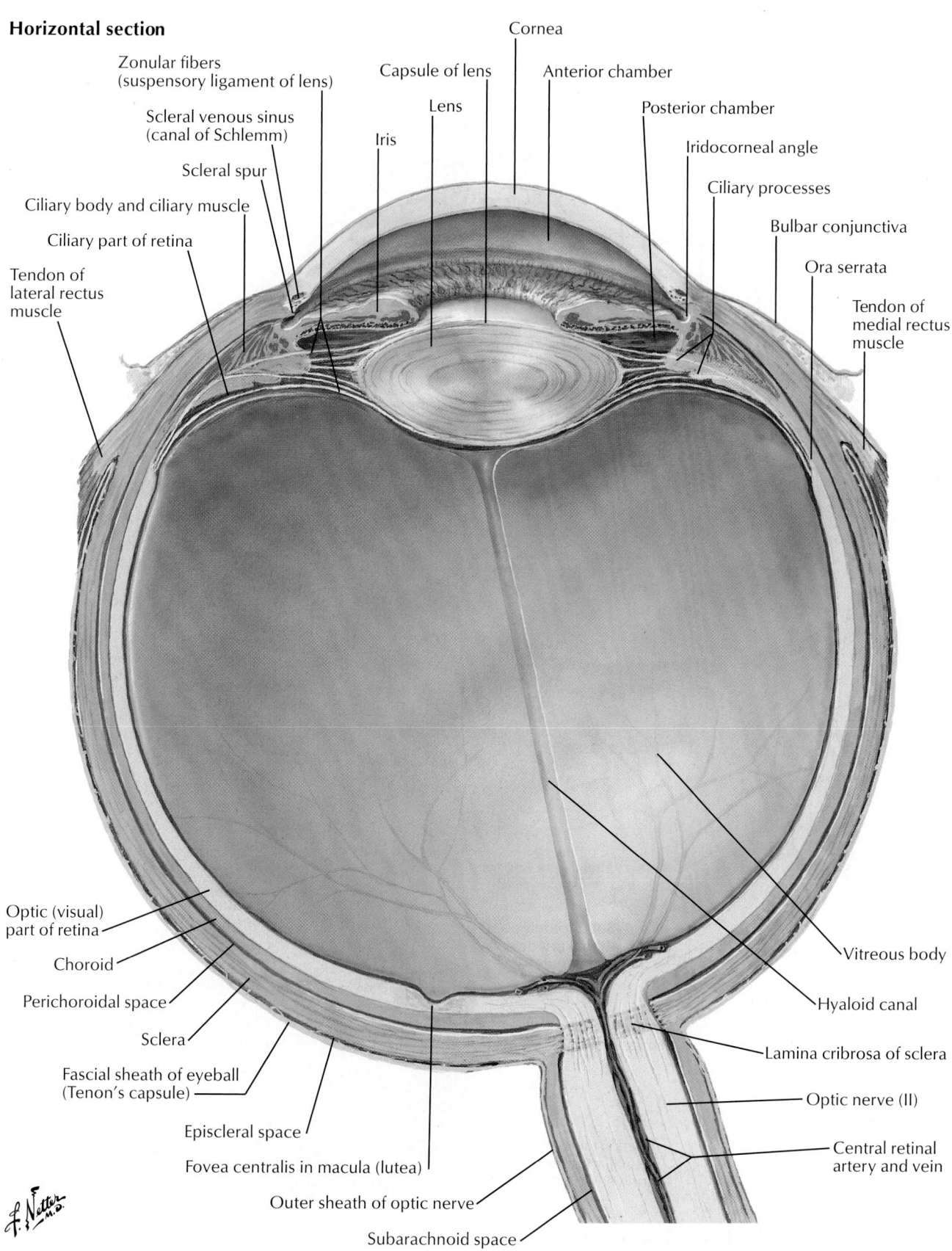

Zonular fibers (suspensory ligament of lens)

Capsule of lens

Cornea

Anterior chamber

Scleral venous sinus (canal of Schlemm)

Lens

Posterior chamber

Scleral spur

Iris

Iridocorneal angle

Ciliary body and ciliary muscle

Ciliary processes

Ciliary part of retina

Bulbar conjunctiva

Tendon of lateral rectus muscle

Ora serrata

Tendon of medial rectus muscle

Optic (visual) part of retina

Choroid

Perichoroidal space

Vitreous body

Sclera

Hyaloid canal

Fascial sheath of eyeball (Tenon's capsule)

Lamina cribrosa of sclera

Episcleral space

Optic nerve (II)

Fovea centralis in macula (lutea)

Central retinal artery and vein

Outer sheath of optic nerve

Subarachnoid space

Plate 87 Eyeball. (Netter: Atlas of Human Anatomy, 4 ed, 2006, Saunders.)

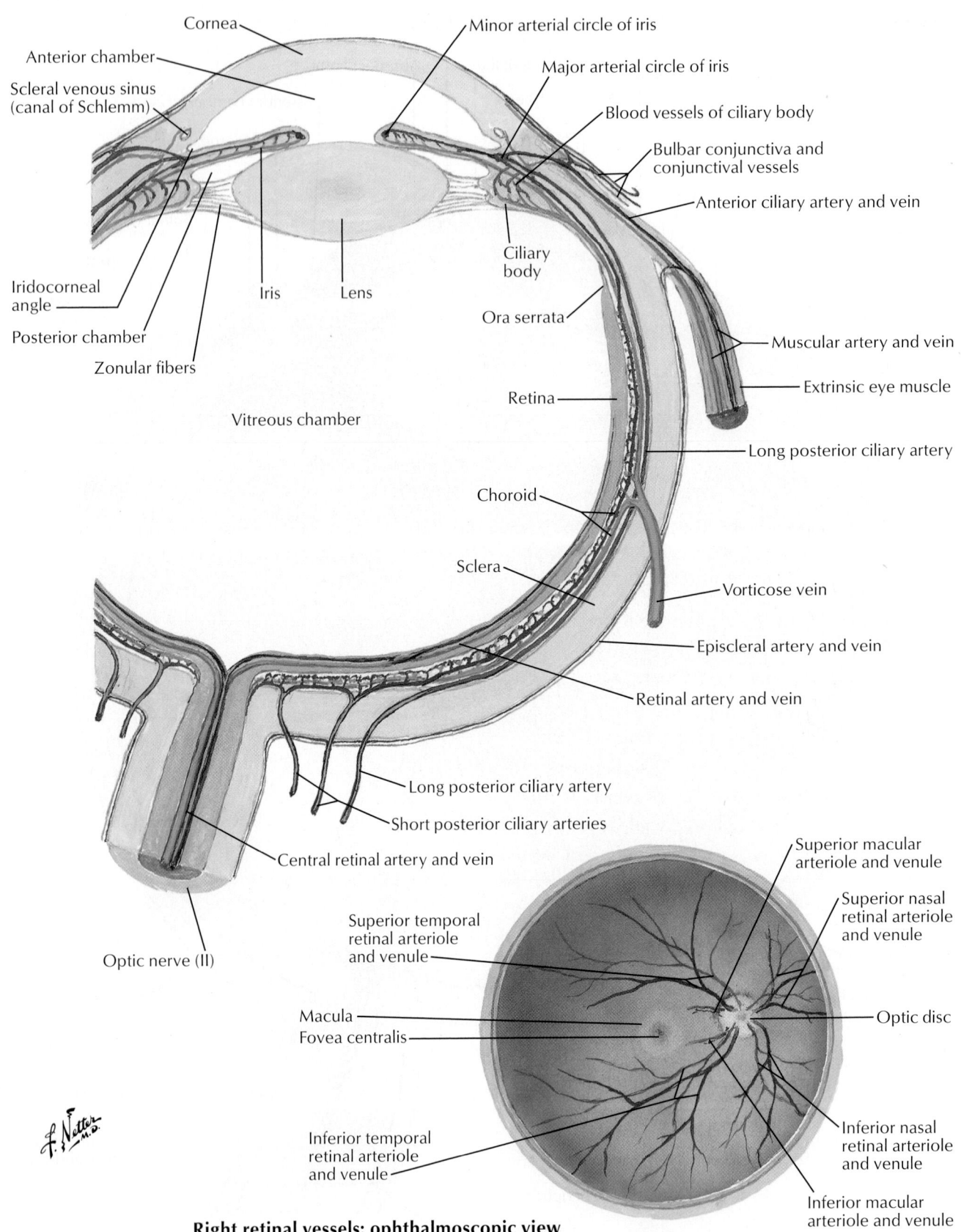

Cornea

Anterior chamber

Scleral venous sinus
(canal of Schlemm)

Iridocorneal
angle

Posterior chamber

Zonular fibers

Iris

Lens

Vitreous chamber

Minor arterial circle of iris

Major arterial circle of iris

Blood vessels of ciliary body

Bulbar conjunctiva and
conjunctival vessels

Anterior ciliary artery and vein

Ciliary
body

Ora serrata

Retina

Choroid

Sclera

Muscular artery and vein

Extrinsic eye muscle

Long posterior ciliary artery

Vorticose vein

Episcleral artery and vein

Retinal artery and vein

Long posterior ciliary artery

Short posterior ciliary arteries

Central retinal artery and vein

Optic nerve (II)

Superior temporal
retinal arteriole
and venule

Macula

Fovea centralis

Inferior temporal
retinal arteriole
and venule

Superior macular
arteriole and venule

Superior nasal
retinal arteriole
and venule

Optic disc

Inferior nasal
retinal arteriole
and venule

Inferior macular
arteriole and venule

Right retinal vessels: ophthalmoscopic view

Plate 90 Intrinsic Arteries and Veins of Eye. (Netter: Atlas of Human Anatomy, 4 ed, 2006, Saunders.)

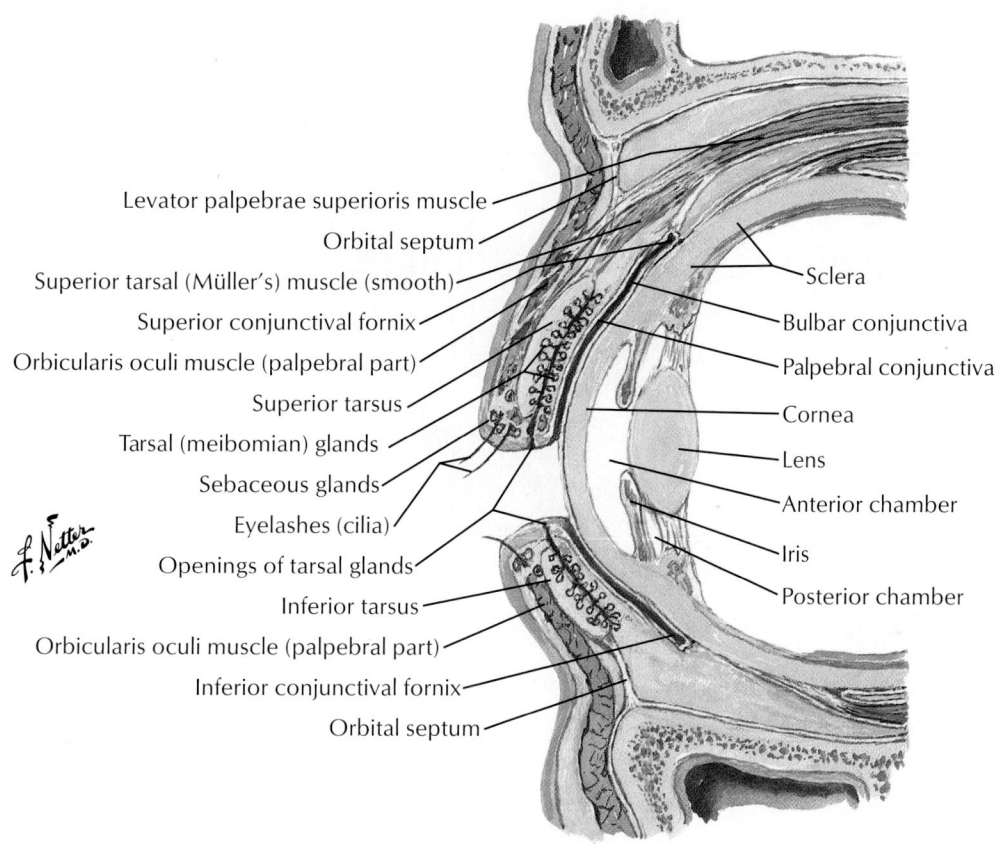

Levator palpebrae superioris muscle
Orbital septum
Superior tarsal (Müller's) muscle (smooth)
Superior conjunctival fornix
Orbicularis oculi muscle (palpebral part)
Superior tarsus
Tarsal (meibomian) glands
Sebaceous glands
Eyelashes (cilia)
Openings of tarsal glands
Inferior tarsus
Orbicularis oculi muscle (palpebral part)
Inferior conjunctival fornix
Orbital septum

Sclera
Bulbar conjunctiva
Palpebral conjunctiva
Cornea
Lens
Anterior chamber
Iris
Posterior chamber

Plate 81, Middle Eyelids. (Netter: Atlas of Human Anatomy, 4 ed, 2006, Saunders.)

Superior palpebral conjunctiva:
tarsal (meibomian) glands
shining through

Superior lacrimal papilla and
punctum

Seen through { Pupil
cornea { Iris

Plica semilunaris

Lacrimal caruncle in
lacrimal lake (lacus lacrimalis)

Corneoscleral junction
(corneal limbus)

Bulbar conjunctiva
over sclera

Inferior lacrimal papilla and
punctum

Inferior conjunctival fornix

Inferior palpebral conjunctiva:
tarsal glands shining through

Plate 81, Upper Eyelid. (Netter: Atlas of Human Anatomy, 4 ed, 2006, Saunders.)

Orbital part of
lacrimal gland

Palpebral part of
lacrimal gland

Excretory ducts of
lacrimal gland

Plica semilunaris

Lacrimal caruncle

Inferior lacrimal papilla and punctum

Superior lacrimal papilla and punctum

Lacrimal canaliculi

Lacrimal sac

Nasolacrimal duct

Opening of
nasolacrimal duct

Frontal bone (*cut away*)

Orbital part of
lacrimal gland

Palpebral part of
lacrimal gland

Excretory ducts of
lacrimal gland

Plica semilunaris
and lacrimal lake

Lacrimal caruncle

Inferior lacrimal papilla and punctum

Opening of nasolacrimal duct

Superior lacrimal papilla and punctum

Lacrimal canaliculi

Lacrimal sac

Nasolacrimal duct

Middle nasal
concha

Nasal cavity

Inferior nasal
concha (*cut*)

Inferior nasal meatus

Plate 82   Lacrimal Apparatus. (Netter: Atlas of Human Anatomy, 4 ed, 2006, Saunders.)

Frontal section

Facial nerve (VII) (*cut*)

Base of stapes in oval (vestibular) window

Limbs of stapes

Vestibule

Prominence of lateral semicircular canal

Semicircular ducts, ampullae, utricle, and saccule

Incus

Facial nerve (VII) (*cut*)

Tegmen tympani

Vestibular nerve

Malleus (head)

Cochlear nerve

Epitympanic recess

Internal acoustic meatus

Auricle

Vestibulocochlear nerve (VIII)

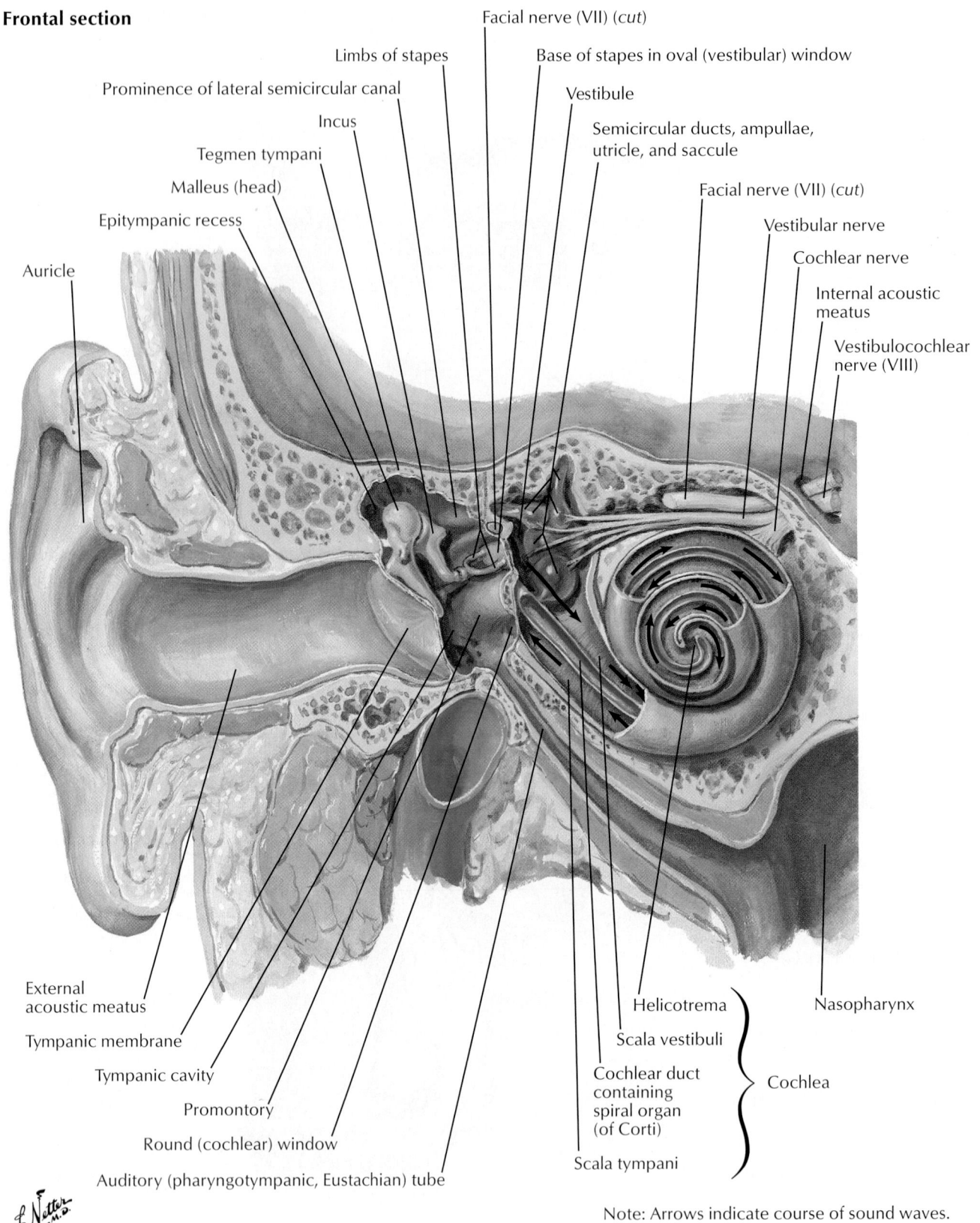

External acoustic meatus

Helicotrema

Nasopharynx

Tympanic membrane

Scala vestibuli

Tympanic cavity

Cochlear duct containing spiral organ (of Corti)

Promontory

Cochlea

Round (cochlear) window

Scala tympani

Auditory (pharyngotympanic, Eustachian) tube

Note: Arrows indicate course of sound waves.

NETTER'S ANATOMY ILLUSTRATIONS

Plate 92   Pathway of Sound Reception. (Netter: Atlas of Human Anatomy, 4 ed, 2006, Saunders.)

NAP-20

Medial wall of tympanic cavity: lateral view

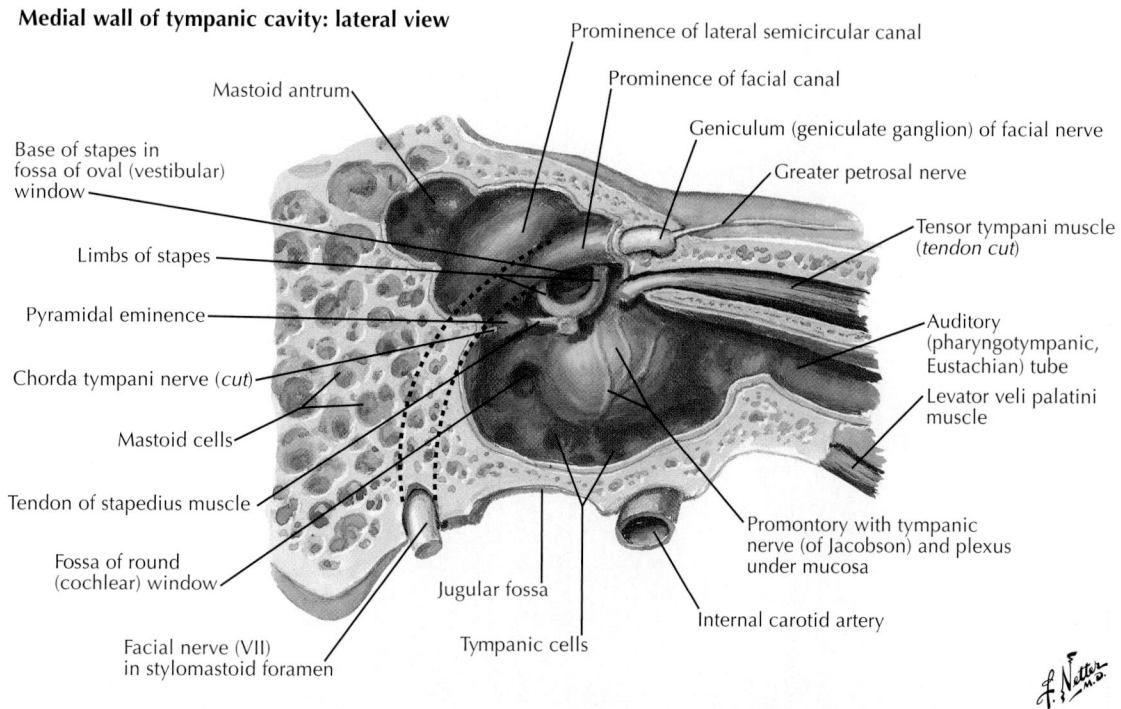

Mastoid antrum

Base of stapes in fossa of oval (vestibular) window

Limbs of stapes

Pyramidal eminence

Chorda tympani nerve (*cut*)

Mastoid cells

Tendon of stapedius muscle

Fossa of round (cochlear) window

Facial nerve (VII) in stylomastoid foramen

Jugular fossa

Tympanic cells

Prominence of lateral semicircular canal

Prominence of facial canal

Geniculum (geniculate ganglion) of facial nerve

Greater petrosal nerve

Tensor tympani muscle (*tendon cut*)

Auditory (pharyngotympanic, Eustachian) tube

Levator veli palatini muscle

Promontory with tympanic nerve (of Jacobson) and plexus under mucosa

Internal carotid artery

Plate 94 Tympanic Cavity. (Netter: Atlas of Human Anatomy, 4 ed, 2006, Saunders.)

Otoscopic view of right tympanic membrane

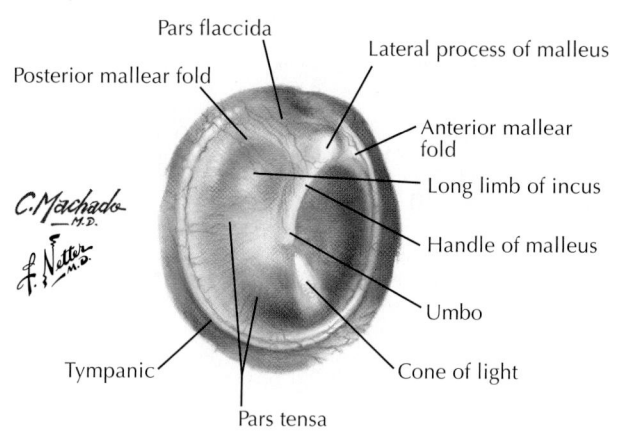

Pars flaccida

Posterior mallear fold

Lateral process of malleus

Anterior mallear fold

Long limb of incus

Handle of malleus

Umbo

Cone of light

Tympanic

Pars tensa

Plate 93 Tympanic Cavity. (Netter: Atlas of Human Anatomy, 4 ed, 2006, Saunders.)

Dissected right bony labyrinth (otic capsule): membranous labyrinth removed

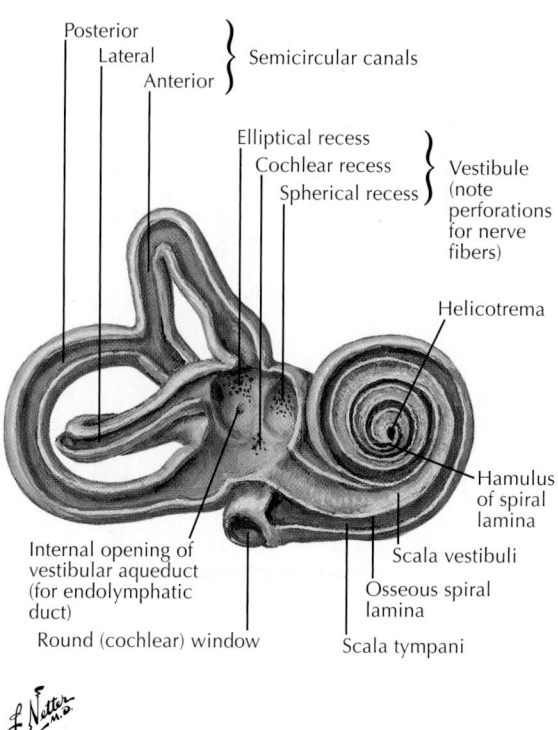

Posterior
Lateral } Semicircular canals
Anterior

Elliptical recess
Cochlear recess } Vestibule
Spherical recess (note perforations for nerve fibers)

Helicotrema

Hamulus of spiral lamina

Scala vestibuli

Osseous spiral lamina

Scala tympani

Internal opening of vestibular aqueduct (for endolymphatic duct)

Round (cochlear) window

Plate 95 Bony Membranous Labyrinth. (Netter: Atlas of Human Anatomy, 4 ed, 2006, Saunders.)

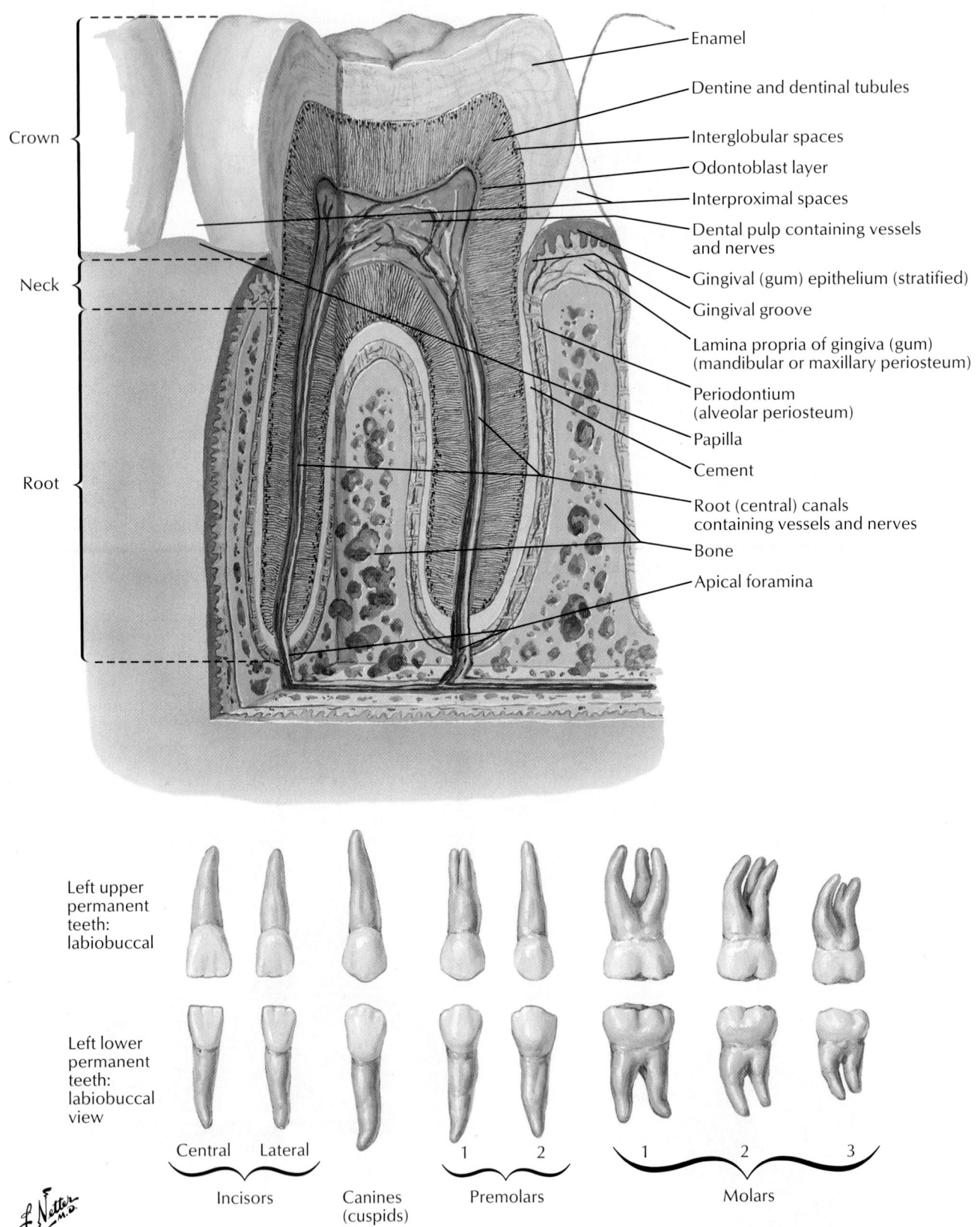

Crown

Neck

Root

Enamel

Dentine and dentinal tubules

Interglobular spaces

Odontoblast layer

Interproximal spaces

Dental pulp containing vessels and nerves

Gingival (gum) epithelium (stratified)

Gingival groove

Lamina propria of gingiva (gum) (mandibular or maxillary periosteum)

Periodontium (alveolar periosteum)

Papilla

Cement

Root (central) canals containing vessels and nerves

Bone

Apical foramina

Left upper permanent teeth: labiobuccal

Left lower permanent teeth: labiobuccal view

Central   Lateral

Incisors

Canines (cuspids)

1   2

Premolars

1   2   3

Molars

Plate 57   Teeth. (Netter: Atlas of Human Anatomy, 4 ed, 2006, Saunders.)

Tongue

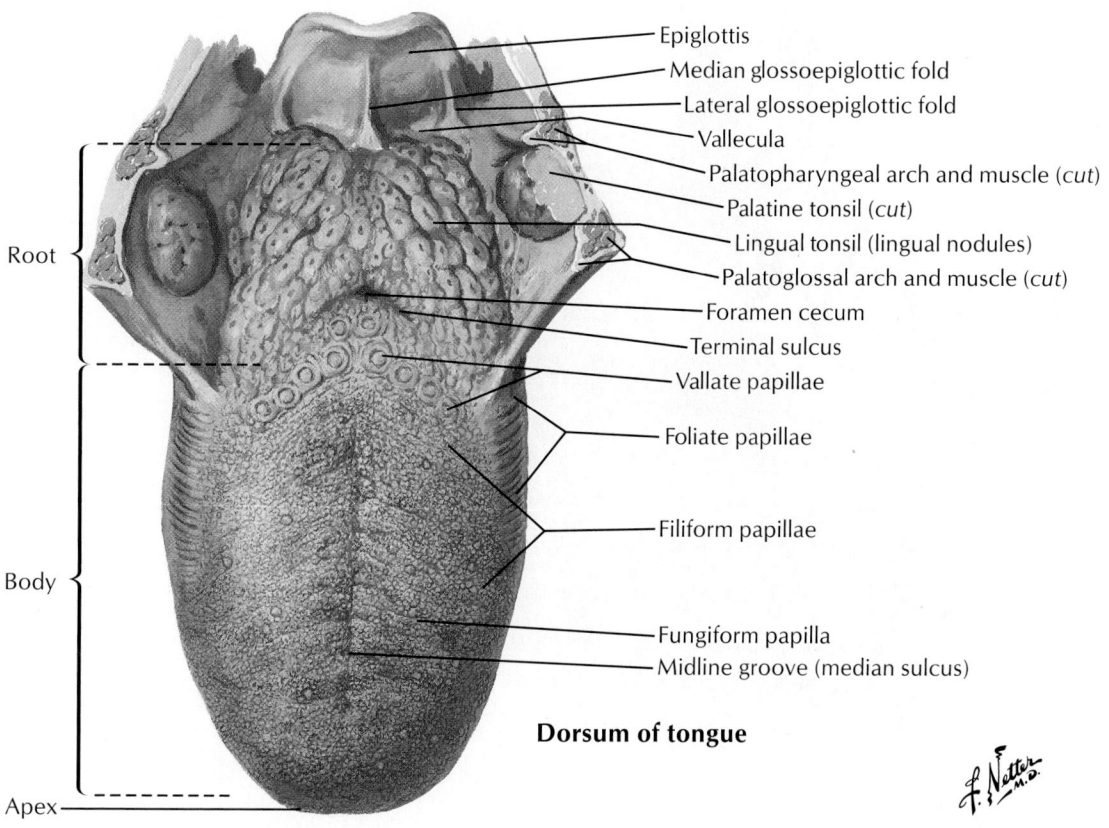

Epiglottis

Median glossoepiglottic fold

Lateral glossoepiglottic fold

Vallecula

Palatopharyngeal arch and muscle (*cut*)

Palatine tonsil (*cut*)

Lingual tonsil (lingual nodules)

Palatoglossal arch and muscle (*cut*)

Foramen cecum

Terminal sulcus

Vallate papillae

Foliate papillae

Filiform papillae

Fungiform papilla

Midline groove (median sulcus)

Root

Body

Apex

Dorsum of tongue

Plate 58 Tongue. (Netter: Atlas of Human Anatomy, 4 ed, 2006, Saunders.)

NAP-23

NETTER'S ANATOMY ILLUSTRATIONS

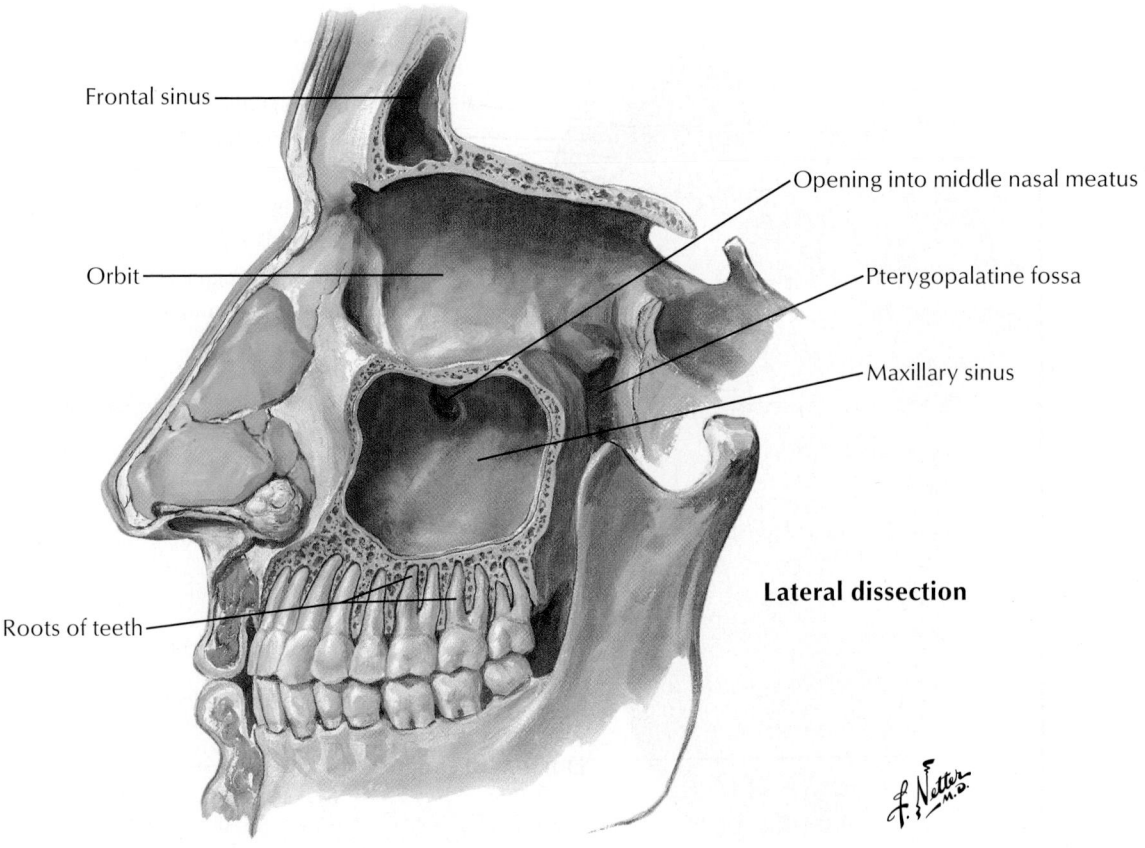

Frontal sinus

Opening into middle nasal meatus

Orbit

Pterygopalatine fossa

Maxillary sinus

Lateral dissection

Roots of teeth

Plate 49 Paranasal Sinuses. (Netter: Atlas of Human Anatomy, 4 ed, 2006, Saunders.)

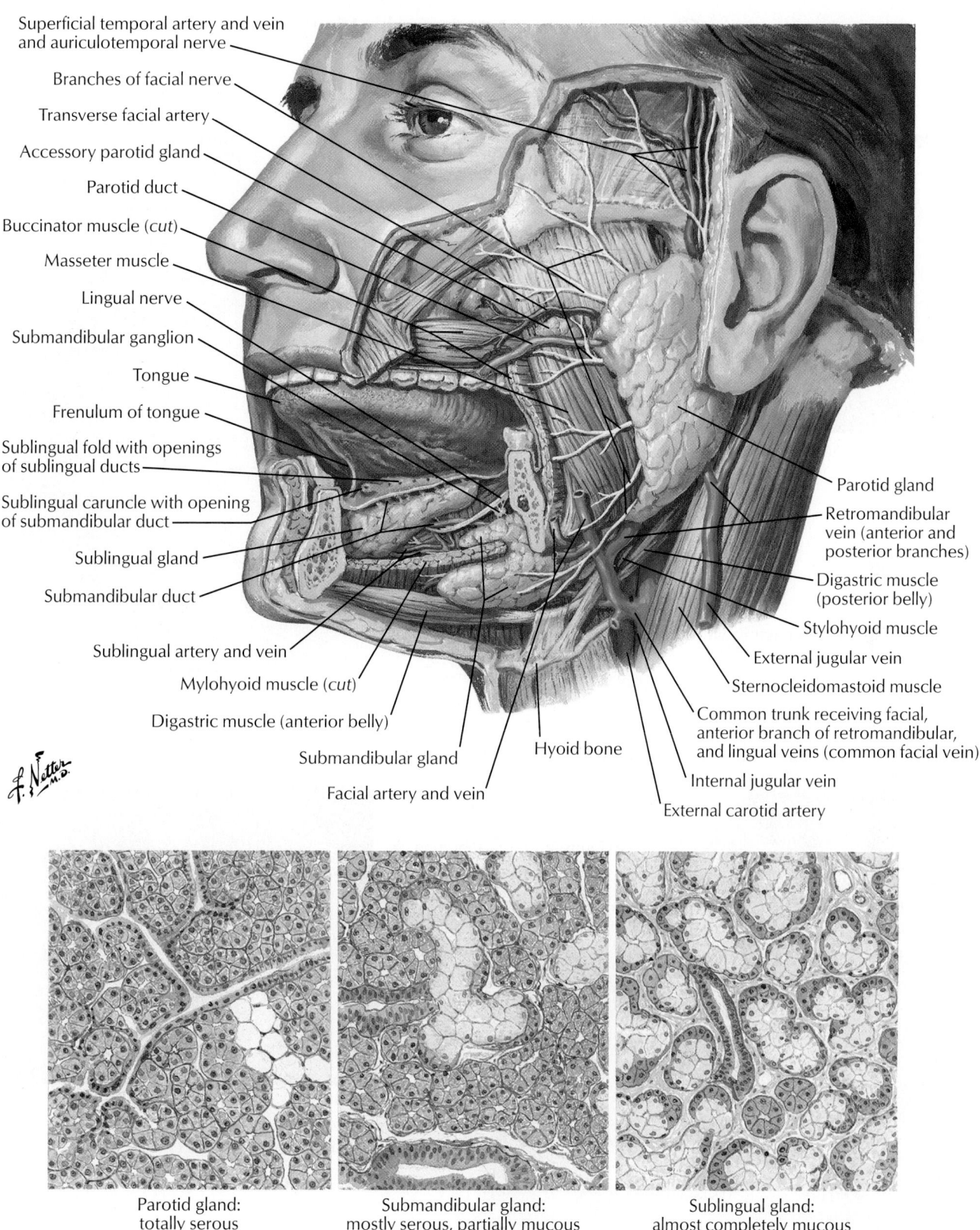

Superficial temporal artery and vein and auriculotemporal nerve

Branches of facial nerve

Transverse facial artery

Accessory parotid gland

Parotid duct

Buccinator muscle (*cut*)

Masseter muscle

Lingual nerve

Submandibular ganglion

Tongue

Frenulum of tongue

Sublingual fold with openings of sublingual ducts

Sublingual caruncle with opening of submandibular duct

Sublingual gland

Submandibular duct

Sublingual artery and vein

Mylohyoid muscle (*cut*)

Digastric muscle (anterior belly)

Submandibular gland

Facial artery and vein

Parotid gland

Retromandibular vein (anterior and posterior branches)

Digastric muscle (posterior belly)

Stylohyoid muscle

External jugular vein

Sternocleidomastoid muscle

Common trunk receiving facial, anterior branch of retromandibular, and lingual veins (common facial vein)

Internal jugular vein

External carotid artery

Hyoid bone

Parotid gland: totally serous

Submandibular gland: mostly serous, partially mucous

Sublingual gland: almost completely mucous

Plate 61 Salivary Glands. (Netter: Atlas of Human Anatomy, 4 ed, 2006, Saunders.)

Coronary Arteries: Arteriographic Views

Right coronary artery: left anterior oblique view

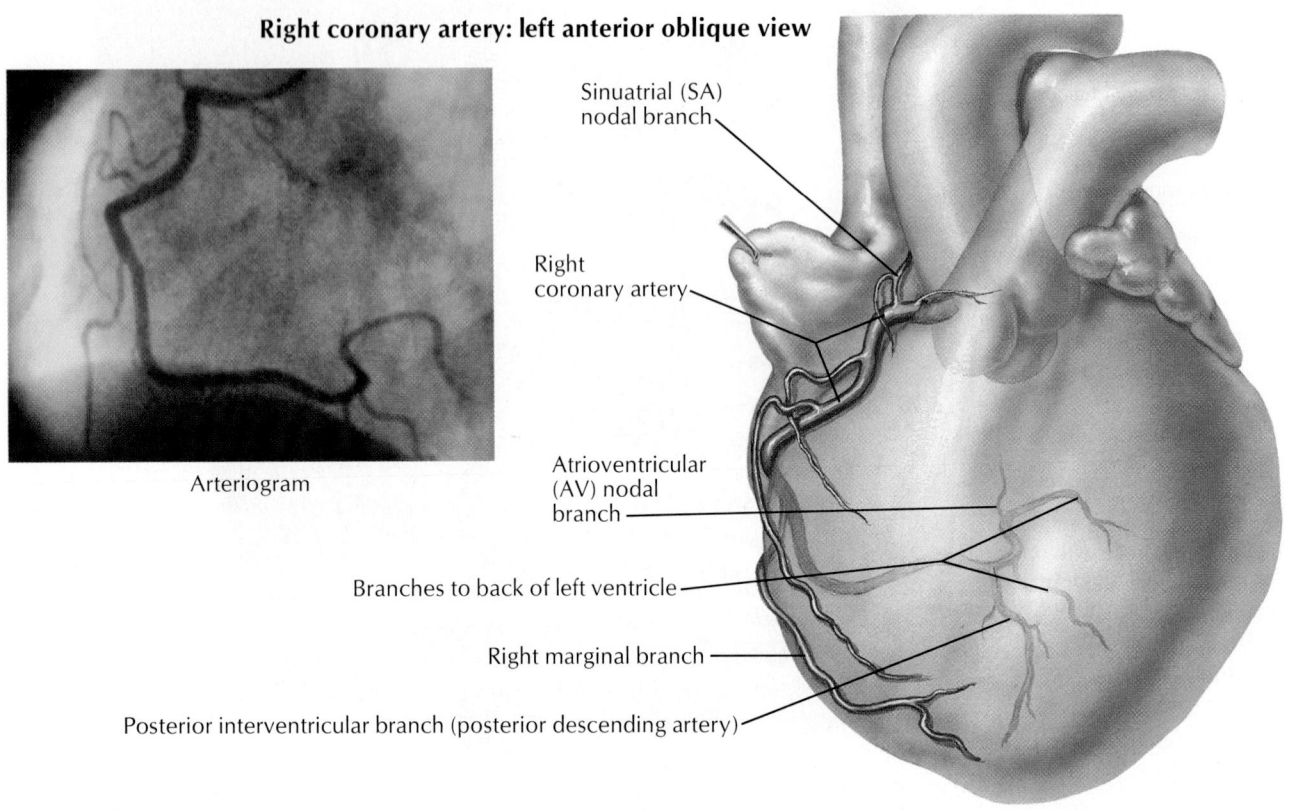

Arteriogram

Sinuatrial (SA) nodal branch

Right coronary artery

Atrioventricular (AV) nodal branch

Branches to back of left ventricle

Right marginal branch

Posterior interventricular branch (posterior descending artery)

Right coronary artery: right anterior oblique view

Sinuatrial (SA) nodal branch

Conus (arteriosus) branch

Right coronary artery

Right marginal branch

Arteriogram

Atrioventricular (AV) nodal branch

Right posterolateral branches (to back of left ventricle)

Posterior interventricular branch (posterior descending artery)

Plate 218 Coronary Arteries: Arteriographic Views. (Netter: Atlas of Human Anatomy, 4 ed, 2006, Saunders.)

Left coronary artery: left anterior oblique view

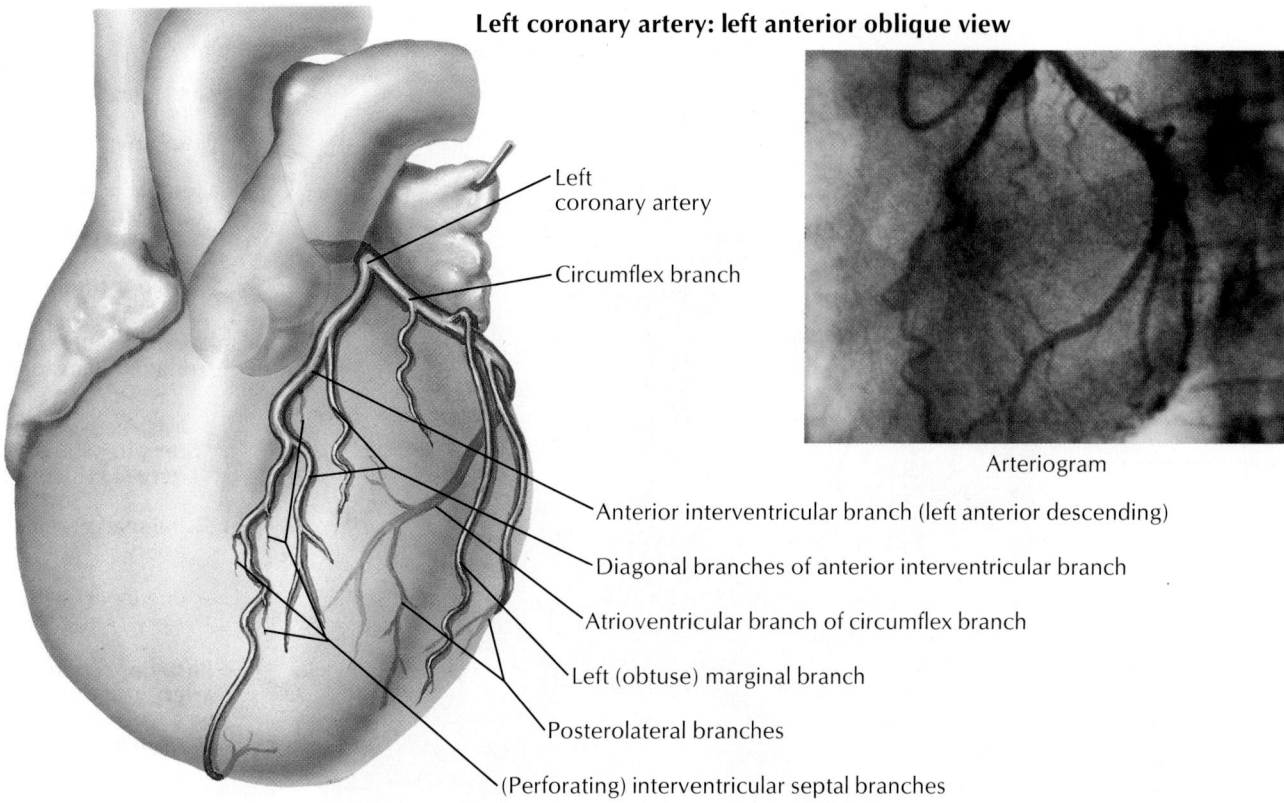

Left coronary artery

Circumflex branch

Arteriogram

Anterior interventricular branch (left anterior descending)

Diagonal branches of anterior interventricular branch

Atrioventricular branch of circumflex branch

Left (obtuse) marginal branch

Posterolateral branches

(Perforating) interventricular septal branches

Left coronary artery: right anterior oblique view

Left coronary artery

Anterior interventricular branch (left anterior descending)

Circumflex branch

(Perforating) interventricular septal branches

Arteriogram

Left (obtuse) marginal branch

Posterolateral branches

Diagonal branch of Anterior interventricular branch

Atrioventricular branch of circumflex branch

Plate 219 Coronary Arteries: Arteriographic Views. (Netter: Atlas of Human Anatomy, 4 ed, 2006, Saunders.)

NAP-27

NETTER'S ANATOMY ILLUSTRATIONS

Corpus callosum

Anterolateral central
(lenticulostriate) arteries

Lateral frontobasal
(orbitofrontal) artery

Prefrontal artery

Precentral (pre-Rolandic)
and central (Rolandic)
sulcal arteries

Anterior parietal
(postcentral sulcal)
artery

Posterior parietal
artery

Branch to
angular gyrus

Temporal branches
(anterior, middle,
and posterior)

Middle cerebral artery
and branches
(deep in lateral cerebral
[Sylvian] sulcus)

Anterior communicating artery

Posterior communicating artery

Anterior inferior cerebellar artery (AICA)

Posterior spinal artery

Paracentral artery

Medial frontal branches

Pericallosal artery

Callosomarginal artery

Polar frontal artery

**Anterior cerebral
arteries**

Medial frontobasal
(orbitofrontal) artery

Distal medial striate
artery (recurrent
artery of Heubner)

Internal carotid
artery

Anterior choroidal
artery

**Posterior cerebral
artery**

Superior cerebellar artery

Basilar and pontine arteries

Labyrinthine (internal
acoustic) artery

Vertebral artery

Posterior inferior cerebellar artery (PICA)

Anterior spinal artery

Corpus striatum
(caudate and lentiform nuclei)

Anterolateral central
(lenticulostriate) arteries

Insula (island of Reil)

Limen of insula

Precentral (pre-Rolandic),
central (Rolandic) sulcal,
and parietal arteries

Lateral cerebral (Sylvian) sulcus

Temporal branches of
middle cerebral artery

Temporal lobe

Middle cerebral artery

Internal carotid artery

Falx cerebri

Callosomarginal arteries
and
Pericallosal arteries
(branches of anterior
cerebral arteries)

Trunk of corpus callosum

Internal capsule

Septum pellucidum

Rostrum of corpus callosum

Anterior cerebral arteries

Distal medial striate artery
(recurrent artery of Heubner)

Anterior communicating artery

Optic chiasm

Plate 141   Arteries of Brain: Frontal View and Section. (Netter: Atlas of Human Anatomy, 4 ed, 2006, Saunders.)

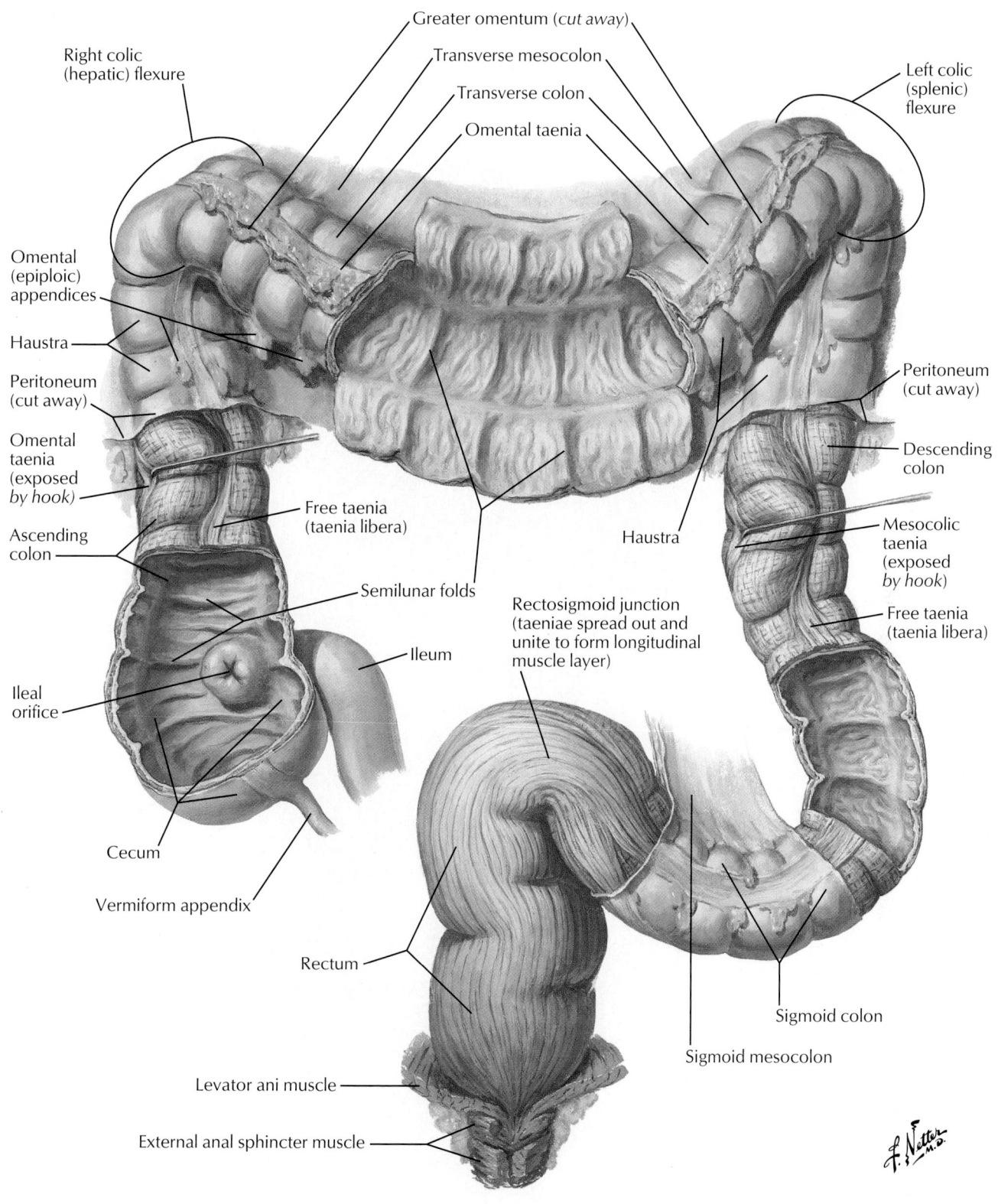

Right colic (hepatic) flexure

Greater omentum (*cut away*)

Transverse mesocolon

Transverse colon

Omental taenia

Left colic (splenic) flexure

Omental (epiploic) appendices

Haustra

Peritoneum (cut away)

Omental taenia (exposed *by hook*)

Ascending colon

Free taenia (taenia libera)

Ileal orifice

Semilunar folds

Cecum

Vermiform appendix

Rectum

Levator ani muscle

External anal sphincter muscle

Ileum

Rectosigmoid junction (taeniae spread out and unite to form longitudinal muscle layer)

Haustra

Peritoneum (cut away)

Descending colon

Mesocolic taenia (exposed *by hook*)

Free taenia (taenia libera)

Sigmoid colon

Sigmoid mesocolon

Plate 284 Mucosa and Musculature of Large Intestine. (Netter: Atlas of Human Anatomy, 4 ed, 2006, Saunders.)

Transverse Section: T3–4 Intervertebral Disc, Manubrium

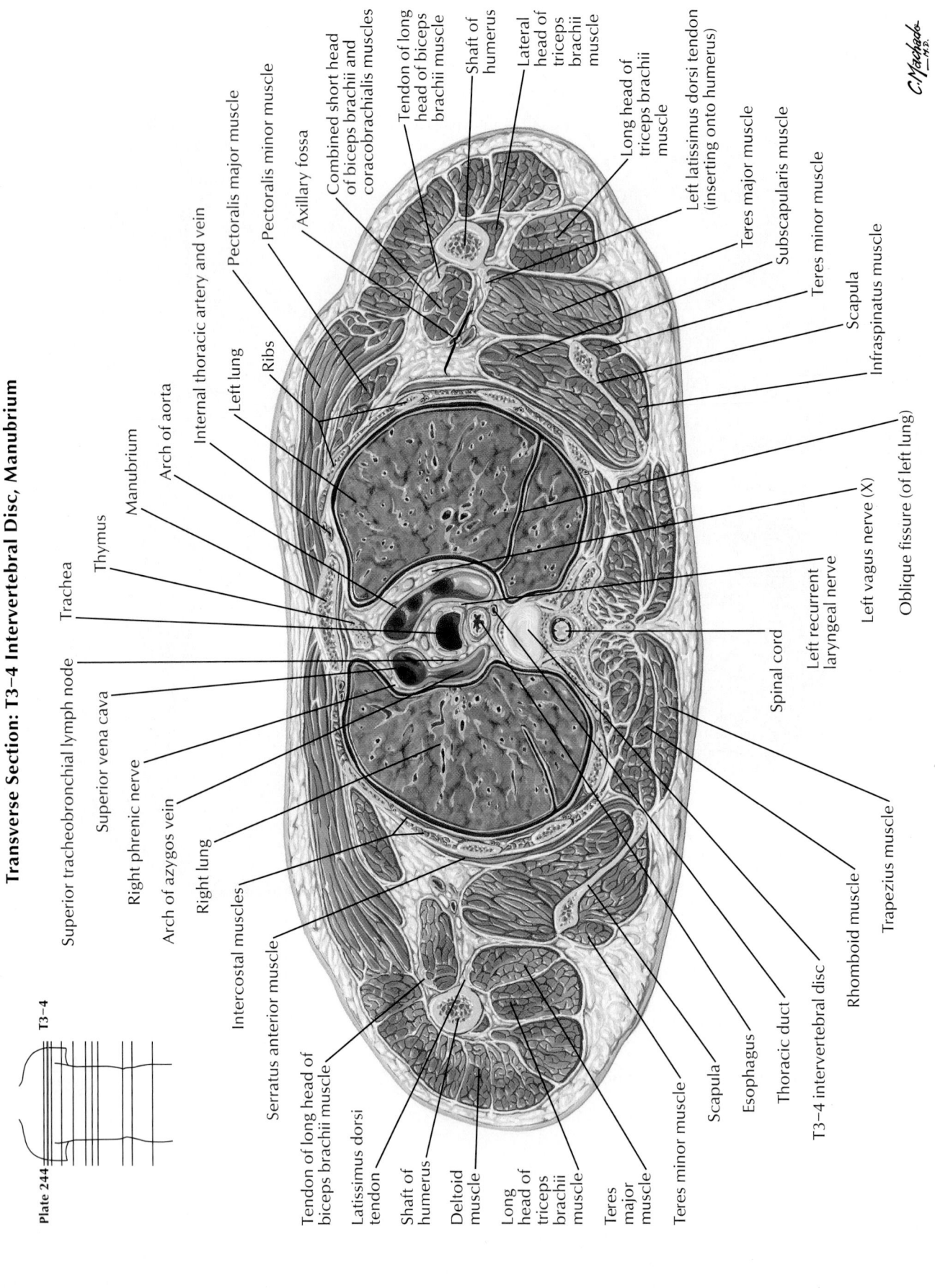

Plate 244 Cross Section of Thorax at T3-4 Disc Level. (Netter: Atlas of Human Anatomy, 4 ed, 2006, Saunders.)

Right knee in extension: posterior view

Posterior cruciate ligament

Anterior cruciate ligament

Posterior meniscofemoral ligament

Lateral condyle of femur (articular surface)

Popliteus tendon

Fibular collateral ligament

Lateral meniscus

Head of fibula

Adductor tubercle on medial epicondyle of femur

Medial condyle of femur (articular surface)

Medial meniscus

Tibial collateral ligament

Medial condyle of tibia

Plate 509 Knee: Cruciate and Collateral Ligaments. (Netter: Atlas of Human Anatomy, 4 ed, 2006, Saunders.)

Paramedian (sagittal) dissection

Ureter

Uterine (fallopian) tube

Ovary

Ligament of ovary

Round ligament of uterus

Broad ligament (*cut*)

Superior pubic ramus (*cut*)

Inferior pubic ramus (*cut*)

Ischiocavernosus muscle

Body of clitoris

Labia minora

Labium majus

Rectouterine pouch (of Douglas)

Peritoneum (*cut edge*)

Vesicouterine pouch

Rectum

Ureter

Urinary bladder

Vagina

Pelvic diaphragm (levator ani muscle)

Deep transverse perineal muscle (*cut*)

External anal sphincter muscle

Median (sagittal) section

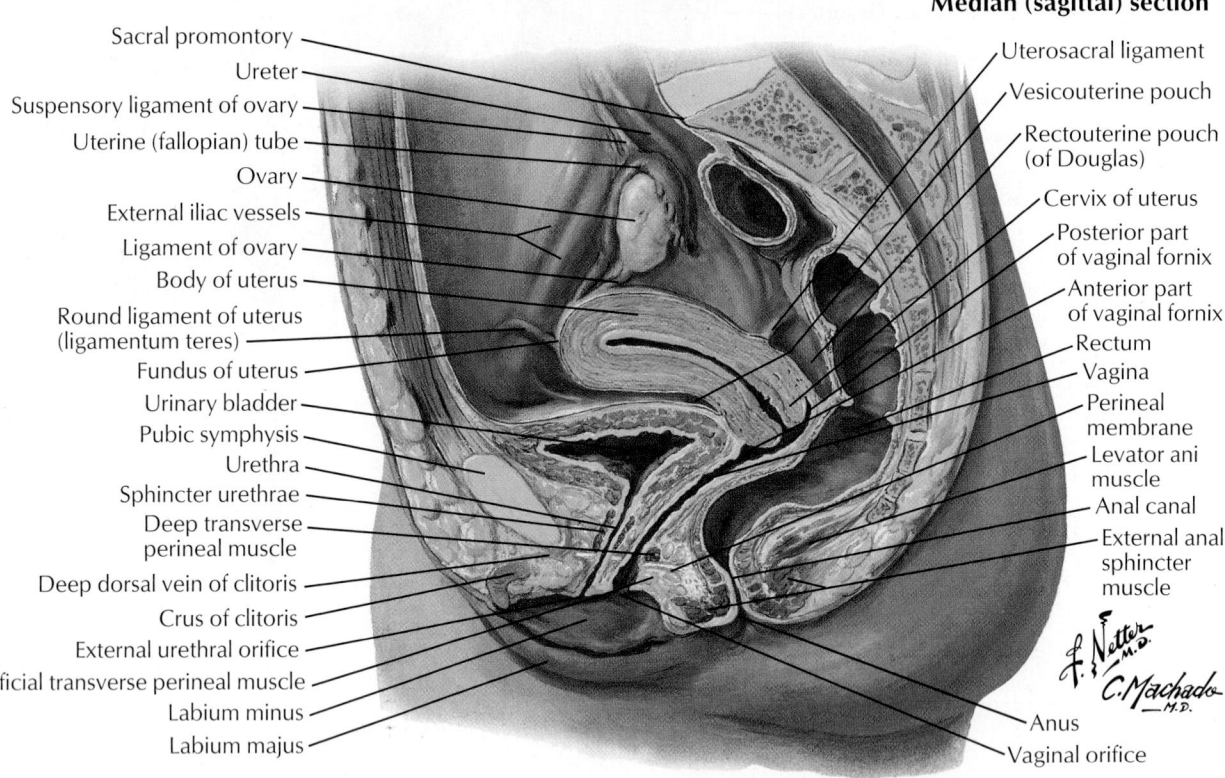

Sacral promontory

Ureter

Suspensory ligament of ovary

Uterine (fallopian) tube

Ovary

External iliac vessels

Ligament of ovary

Body of uterus

Round ligament of uterus (ligamentum teres)

Fundus of uterus

Urinary bladder

Pubic symphysis

Urethra

Sphincter urethrae

Deep transverse perineal muscle

Deep dorsal vein of clitoris

Crus of clitoris

External urethral orifice

Superficial transverse perineal muscle

Labium minus

Labium majus

Uterosacral ligament

Vesicouterine pouch

Rectouterine pouch (of Douglas)

Cervix of uterus

Posterior part of vaginal fornix

Anterior part of vaginal fornix

Rectum

Vagina

Perineal membrane

Levator ani muscle

Anal canal

External anal sphincter muscle

Anus

Vaginal orifice

Plate 360 Pelvic Viscera and Perineum: Female. (Netter: Atlas of Human Anatomy, 4 ed, 2006, Saunders.)

Introduction

ICD-10-CM Official Guidelines for Coding and Reporting 2016
Narrative changes appear in bold text
Items <u>underlined</u> have been moved within the guidelines since the 2014 version
Italics are used to indicate revisions to heading changes

The Centers for Medicare and Medicaid Services (CMS) and the National Center for Health Statistics (NCHS), two departments within the U.S. Federal Government's Department of Health and Human Services (DHHS) provide the following guidelines for coding and reporting using the International Classification of Diseases, 10th Revision, Clinical Modification (ICD-10-CM). These guidelines should be used as a companion document to the official version of the ICD-10-CM as published on the NCHS website. The ICD-10-CM is a morbidity classification published by the United States for classifying diagnoses and reason for visits in all health care settings. The ICD-10-CM is based on the ICD-10, the statistical classification of disease published by the World Health Organization (WHO).

These guidelines have been approved by the four organizations that make up the Cooperating Parties for the ICD-10-CM: the American Hospital Association (AHA), the American Health Information Management Association (AHIMA), CMS, and NCHS.

These guidelines are a set of rules that have been developed to accompany and complement the official conventions and instructions provided within the ICD-10-CM itself. The instructions and conventions of the classification take precedence over guidelines. These guidelines are based on the coding and sequencing instructions in the Tabular List and Alphabetic Index of ICD-10-CM, but provide additional instruction. Adherence to these guidelines when assigning ICD-10-CM diagnosis codes is required under the Health Insurance Portability and Accountability Act (HIPAA). The diagnosis codes (Tabular List and Alphabetic Index)

have been adopted under HIPAA for all healthcare settings. A joint effort between the healthcare provider and the coder is essential to achieve complete and accurate documentation, code assignment, and reporting of diagnoses and procedures. These guidelines have been developed to assist both the healthcare provider and the coder in identifying those diagnoses that are to be reported. The importance of consistent, complete documentation in the medical record cannot be overemphasized. Without such documentation accurate coding cannot be achieved. The entire record should be reviewed to determine the specific reason for the encounter and the conditions treated.

The term encounter is used for all settings, including hospital admissions. In the context of these guidelines, the term provider is used throughout the guidelines to mean physician or any qualified health care practitioner who is legally accountable for establishing the patient's diagnosis. Only this set of guidelines, approved by the Cooperating Parties, is official.

The guidelines are organized into sections. Section I includes the structure and conventions of the classification and general guidelines that apply to the entire classification, and chapter-specific guidelines that correspond to the chapters as they are arranged in the classification. Section II includes guidelines for selection of principal diagnosis for non-outpatient settings. Section III includes guidelines for reporting additional diagnoses in non-outpatient settings. Section IV is for outpatient coding and reporting. It is necessary to review all sections of the guidelines to fully understand all of the rules and instructions needed to code properly.

ICD-10-CM Official Guidelines for Coding and Reporting

Section I. Conventions, general coding guidelines and chapter specific guidelines

A. Conventions for the ICD-10-CM
   1. The Alphabetic Index and Tabular List
   2. Format and Structure:
   3. Use of codes for reporting purposes
   4. Placeholder character
   5. 7th Characters
   6. Abbreviations
      a. Alphabetic Index abbreviations
      b. Tabular List abbreviations
   7. Punctuation
   8. Use of "and"
   9. Other and Unspecified codes
      a. "Other" codes
      b. "Unspecified" codes
   10. Includes Notes
   11. Inclusion terms
   12. Excludes Notes
      a. Excludes1
      b. Excludes2
   13. Etiology/manifestation convention ("code first", "use additional code" and "in diseases classified elsewhere" notes)
   14. "And"
   15. "With"
   16. "See" and "See Also"
   17. "Code also note"
   18. Default codes
B. General Coding Guidelines
   1. Locating a code in the ICD-10-CM
   2. Level of Detail in Coding
   3. Code or codes from A00.0 through T88.9, Z00-Z99.8
   4. Signs and symptoms
   5. Conditions that are an integral part of a disease process
   6. Conditions that are not an integral part of a disease process
   7. Multiple coding for a single condition
   8. Acute and Chronic Conditions
   9. Combination Code
   10. Sequela (Late Effects)
   11. Impending or Threatened Condition
   12. Reporting Same Diagnosis Code More than Once
   13. Laterality
   14. Documentation for BMI, Non-pressure ulcers and Pressure Ulcer Stages
   15. Syndromes
   16. Documentation of Complications of Care
   17. Borderline Diagnosis
   18. Use of Sign/Symptom/Unspecified Codes
C. Chapter-Specific Coding Guidelines
   1. Chapter 1: Certain Infectious and Parasitic Diseases (A00-B99)
      a. Human Immunodeficiency Virus (HIV) Infections
      b. Infectious agents as the cause of diseases classified to other chapters
      c. Infections resistant to antibiotics
      d. Sepsis, Severe Sepsis, and Septic Shock
      e. Methicillin Resistant *Staphylococcus aureus* (MRSA) Conditions
   2. Chapter 2: Neoplasms (C00-D49)
      a. Treatment directed at the malignancy
      b. Treatment of secondary site
      c. Coding and sequencing of complications
      d. Primary malignancy previously excised
      e. Admissions/Encounters involving chemotherapy, immunotherapy and radiation therapy
      f. Admission/encounter to determine extent of malignancy
      g. Symptoms, signs, and abnormal findings listed in Chapter 18 associated with neoplasms
      h. Admission/encounter for pain control/ management
      i. Malignancy in two or more noncontiguous sites
      j. Disseminated malignant neoplasm, unspecified
      k. Malignant neoplasm without specification of site
      l. Sequencing of neoplasm codes
      m. Current malignancy versus personal history of malignancy
      n. Leukemia, Multiple Myeloma, and Malignant Plasma Cell Neoplasms in remission versus personal history
      o. Aftercare following surgery for neoplasm
      p. Follow-up care for completed treatment of a malignancy
      q. Prophylactic organ removal for prevention of malignancy
      r. Malignant neoplasm associated with transplanted organ
   3. Chapter 3: Disease of the blood and blood-forming organs and certain disorders involving the immune mechanism (D50-D89)
   4. Chapter 4: Endocrine, Nutritional, and Metabolic Diseases (E00-E89)
      a. Diabetes mellitus
   5. Chapter 5: Mental, Behavioral and Neurodevelopmental disorders (F01 – F99)
      a. Pain disorders related to psychological factors
      b. Mental and behavioral disorders due to psychoactive substance use
   6. Chapter 6: Diseases of the Nervous System (G00-G99)
      a. Dominant/nondominant side
      b. Pain - Category G89
   7. Chapter 7: Diseases of the Eye and Adnexa (H00-H59)
      a. Glaucoma
   8. Chapter 8: Diseases of the Ear and Mastoid Process (H60-H95)
   9. Chapter 9: Diseases of the Circulatory System (I00-I99)
      a. Hypertension
      b. Atherosclerotic Coronary Artery Disease and Angina
      c. Intraoperative and Postprocedural Cerebrovascular Accident
      d. Sequelae of Cerebrovascular Disease
      e. Acute myocardial infarction (AMI)

Section II. Selection of Principal Diagnosis

Section I. Conventions, general coding guidelines and chapter specific guidelines

The conventions, general guidelines and chapter-specific guidelines are applicable to all health care settings unless otherwise indicated. The conventions and instructions of the classification take precedence over guidelines.

A. Conventions for the ICD-10-CM

The conventions for the ICD-10-CM are the general rules for use of the classification independent of the guidelines. These conventions are incorporated within the Alphabetic Index and Tabular List of the ICD-10-CM as instructional notes.

1. The Alphabetic Index and Tabular List
The ICD-10-CM is divided into the Alphabetic Index, an alphabetical list of terms and their corresponding code, and the Tabular List, a structured list of codes divided into chapters based on body system or condition. The Alphabetic Index consists of the following parts: the Index of Diseases and Injury, the Index of External Causes of Injury, the Table of Neoplasms and the Table of Drugs and Chemicals.

See Section I.C2. General guidelines
See Section I.C.19. Adverse effects, poisoning, underdosing and toxic effects

2. Format and Structure:
The ICD-10-CM Tabular List contains categories, subcategories and codes. Characters for categories, subcategories and codes may be either a letter or a number. All categories are 3 characters. A three-character category that has no further subdivision is equivalent to a code. Subcategories are either 4 or 5 characters. Codes may be 3, 4, 5, 6 or 7 characters. That is, each level of subdivision after a category is a subcategory. The final level of subdivision is a code. Codes that have applicable 7th characters are still referred to as codes, not subcategories. A code that has an applicable 7th character is considered invalid without the 7th character.

The ICD-10-CM uses an indented format for ease in reference

3. Use of codes for reporting purposes
For reporting purposes only codes are permissible, not categories or subcategories, and any applicable 7th character is required.

4. Placeholder character
The ICD-10-CM utilizes a placeholder character "X". The "X" is used as a placeholder at certain codes to allow for future expansion. An example of this is at the poisoning, adverse effect and underdosing codes, categories T36-T50. Where a placeholder exists, the X must be used in order for the code to be considered a valid code.

5. 7th Characters
Certain ICD-10-CM categories have applicable 7th characters. The applicable 7th character is required for all codes within the category, or as the notes in the Tabular List instruct. The 7th character must always be the 7th character in the data field. If a code that requires a 7th character is not 6 characters, a placeholder X must be used to fill in the empty characters.

6. Abbreviations
a. Alphabetic Index abbreviations
NEC "Not elsewhere classifiable"
This abbreviation in the Alphabetic Index represents "other specified". When a specific code is not available for a condition the Alphabetic Index directs the coder to the "other specified" code in the Tabular List.
NOS "Not otherwise specified"
This abbreviation is the equivalent of unspecified.

b. **Tabular List abbreviations**
NEC "Not elsewhere classifiable"
This abbreviation in the Tabular List represents "other specified". When a specific code is not available for a condition the Tabular List includes an NEC entry under a code to identify the code as the "other specified" code.
NOS "Not otherwise specified"
This abbreviation is the equivalent of unspecified.

7. **Punctuation**
[ ] Brackets are used in the Tabular List to enclose synonyms, alternative wording or explanatory phrases. Brackets are used in the Alphabetic Index to identify manifestation codes.
( ) Parentheses are used in both the Alphabetic Index and Tabular List to enclose supplementary words that may be present or absent in the statement of a disease or procedure without affecting the code number to which it is assigned. The terms within the parentheses are referred to as nonessential modifiers. The nonessential modifiers in the Alphabetic Index to Diseases apply to subterms following a main term except when a nonessential modifier and a subentry are mutually exclusive, the subentry takes precedence. For example, in the ICD-10-CM Alphabetic Index under the main term Enteritis, "acute" is a nonessential modifier and "chronic" is a subentry. In this case, the nonessential modifier "acute" does not apply to the subentry "chronic".
: Colons are used in the Tabular List after an incomplete term which needs one or more of the modifiers following the colon to make it assignable to a given category.

8. **Use of "and".**
See Section I.A.14. Use of the term "And"

9. **Other and Unspecified codes**
a. **"Other" codes**
Codes titled "other" or "other specified" are for use when the information in the medical record provides detail for which a specific code does not exist. Alphabetic Index entries with NEC in the line designate "other" codes in the Tabular List. These Alphabetic Index entries represent specific disease entities for which no specific code exists so the term is included within an "other" code.

b. **"Unspecified" codes**
Codes titled "unspecified" are for use when the information in the medical record is insufficient to assign a more specific code. For those categories for which an unspecified code is not provided, the "other specified" code may represent both other and unspecified.
See Section I.B.18 Use of Signs/Symptom/Unspecified Codes

10. **Includes Notes**
This note appears immediately under a three-character code title to further define, or give examples of, the content of the category.

11. **Inclusion terms**
List of terms is included under some codes. These terms are the conditions for which that code is to be used. The terms may be synonyms of the code title, or, in the case of "other specified" codes, the terms are a list of the various conditions assigned to that code. The inclusion terms are not necessarily exhaustive. Additional terms found only in the Alphabetic Index may also be assigned to a code.

12. **Excludes Notes**
The ICD-10-CM has two types of excludes notes. Each type of note has a different definition for use but they are all similar in that they indicate that codes excluded from each other are independent of each other.

a. **Excludes1**
A type 1 Excludes note is a pure excludes note. It means "NOT CODED HERE!" An Excludes1 note indicates that the code excluded should never be used at the same time as the code above the Excludes1 note. An Excludes1 is used when two conditions cannot occur together, such as a congenital form versus an acquired form of the same condition.

b. **Excludes2**
A Type 2 Excludes note represents "Not included here". An excludes2 note indicates that the condition excluded is not part of the condition represented by the code, but a patient may have both conditions at the same time. When an Excludes2 note appears under a code, it is acceptable to use both the code and the excluded code together, when appropriate.

13. **Etiology/manifestation convention ("code first", "use additional code" and "in diseases classified elsewhere" notes)**
Certain conditions have both an underlying etiology and multiple body system manifestations due to the underlying etiology. For such conditions, the ICD-10-CM has a coding convention that requires the underlying condition be sequenced first followed by the manifestation. Wherever such a combination exists, there is a "use additional code" note at the etiology code, and a "code first" note at the manifestation code. These instructional notes indicate the proper sequencing order of the codes, etiology followed by manifestation.

In most cases the manifestation codes will have in the code title, "in diseases classified elsewhere." Codes with this title are a component of the etiology/ manifestation convention. The code title indicates that it is a manifestation code. "In diseases classified elsewhere" codes are never permitted to be used as first-listed or principal diagnosis codes. They must be used in conjunction with an underlying condition code and they must be listed following the underlying condition. See category F02, Dementia in other diseases classified elsewhere, for an example of this convention.

There are manifestation codes that do not have "in diseases classified elsewhere" in the title. For such codes, there is a "use additional code" note at the etiology code and a "code first" note at the manifestation code and the rules for sequencing apply.

In addition to the notes in the Tabular List, these conditions also have a specific Alphabetic Index entry structure. In the Alphabetic Index both conditions are listed together with the etiology code first followed by the manifestation codes in brackets. The code in brackets is always to be sequenced second.

An example of the etiology/manifestation convention is dementia in Parkinson's disease. In the Alphabetic Index, code G20 is listed first, followed by code F02.80 or F02.81 in brackets. Code G20 represents the underlying etiology, Parkinson's disease, and must be sequenced first, whereas codes F02.80 and F02.81 represent the manifestation of dementia in diseases classified elsewhere, with or without behavioral disturbance.

"Code first" and "Use additional code" notes are also used as sequencing rules in the classification for certain codes that are not part of an etiology/manifestation combination.

See Section I.B.7. Multiple coding for a single condition.

14. "And"
The word "and" should be interpreted to mean either "and" or "or" when it appears in a title.

For example, cases of "tuberculosis of bones", "tuberculosis of joints" and "tuberculosis of bones and joints" are classified to subcategory A18.0, Tuberculosis of bones and joints.

15. "With"
The word "with" should be interpreted to mean "associated with" or "due to" when it appears in a code title, the Alphabetic Index, or an instructional note in the Tabular List.

The word "with" in the Alphabetic Index is sequenced immediately following the main term, not in alphabetical order.

16. "See" and "See Also"
The "see" instruction following a main term in the Alphabetic Index indicates that another term should be referenced. It is necessary to go to the main term referenced with the "see" note to locate the correct code.

A "see also" instruction following a main term in the Alphabetic Index instructs that there is another main term that may also be referenced that may provide additional Alphabetic Index entries that may be useful. It is not necessary to follow the "see also" note when the original main term provides the necessary code.

17. "Code also note"
A "code also" note instructs that two codes may be required to fully describe a condition, but this note does not provide sequencing direction.

18. Default codes
A code listed next to a main term in the ICD-10-CM Alphabetic Index is referred to as a default code. The default code represents that condition that is most commonly associated with the main term, or is the unspecified code for the condition. If a condition is documented in a medical record (for example, appendicitis) without any additional information, such as acute or chronic, the default code should be assigned.

B. General Coding Guidelines

1. Locating a code in the ICD-10-CM
To select a code in the classification that corresponds to a diagnosis or reason for visit documented in a medical record, first locate the term in the Alphabetic Index, and then verify the code in the Tabular List. Read and be guided by instructional notations that appear in both the Alphabetic Index and the Tabular List.

It is essential to use both the Alphabetic Index and Tabular List when locating and assigning a code. The Alphabetic Index does not always provide the full code. Selection of the full code, including laterality and any applicable 7th character can only be done in the Tabular List. A dash (-) at the end of an Alphabetic Index entry indicates that additional characters are required. Even if a dash is not included at the Alphabetic Index entry, it is necessary to refer to the Tabular List to verify that no 7th character is required.

2. Level of Detail in Coding
Diagnosis codes are to be used and reported at their highest number of characters available.

ICD-10-CM diagnosis codes are composed of codes with 3, 4, 5, 6 or 7 characters. Codes with three characters are included in ICD-10-CM as the heading of a category of codes that may be further subdivided by the use of fourth and/or fifth characters and/or sixth characters, which provide greater detail.

A three-character code is to be used only if it is not further subdivided. A code is invalid if it has not been coded to the full number of characters required for that code, including the 7th character, if applicable.

3. Code or codes from A00.0 through T88.9, Z00-Z99.8
The appropriate code or codes from A00.0 through T88.9, Z00-Z99.8 must be used to identify diagnoses, symptoms, conditions, problems, complaints or other reason(s) for the encounter/visit.

4. Signs and symptoms
Codes that describe symptoms and signs, as opposed to diagnoses, are acceptable for reporting purposes when a related definitive diagnosis has not been established (confirmed) by the provider.

Chapter 18 of ICD-10-CM, Symptoms, Signs, and Abnormal Clinical and Laboratory Findings, Not Elsewhere Classified (codes R00.0 - R99) contains many, but not all codes for symptoms.
See Section I.B.18 Use of Signs/Symptom/ Unspecified Codes

5. **Conditions that are an integral part of a disease process**
Signs and symptoms that are associated routinely with a disease process should not be assigned as additional codes, unless otherwise instructed by the classification.

6. **Conditions that are not an integral part of a disease process**
Additional signs and symptoms that may not be associated routinely with a disease process should be coded when present.

7. **Multiple coding for a single condition**
In addition to the etiology/manifestation convention that requires two codes to fully describe a single condition that affects multiple body systems, there are other single conditions that also require more than one code. "Use additional code" notes are found in the Tabular List at codes that are not part of an etiology/manifestation pair where a secondary code is useful to fully describe a condition. The sequencing rule is the same as the etiology/manifestation pair, "use additional code" indicates that a secondary code should be added.

For example, for bacterial infections that are not included in chapter 1, a secondary code from category B95, Streptococcus, Staphylococcus, and Enterococcus, as the cause of diseases classified elsewhere, or B96, Other bacterial agents as the cause of diseases classified elsewhere, may be required to identify the bacterial organism causing the infection. A "use additional code" note will normally be found at the infectious disease code, indicating a need for the organism code to be added as a secondary code.

"Code first" notes are also under certain codes that are not specifically manifestation codes but may be due to an underlying cause. When there is a "code first" note and an underlying condition is present, the underlying condition should be sequenced first.

"Code, if applicable, any causal condition first", notes indicate that this code may be assigned as a principal diagnosis when the causal condition is unknown or not applicable. If a causal condition is known, then the code for that condition should be sequenced as the principal or first-listed diagnosis.

Multiple codes may be needed for sequela, complication codes and obstetric codes to more fully describe a condition. See the specific guidelines for these conditions for further instruction.

8. **Acute and Chronic Conditions**
If the same condition is described as both acute (subacute) and chronic, and separate subentries exist in the Alphabetic Index at the same indentation level, code both and sequence the acute (subacute) code first.

9. **Combination Code**
A combination code is a single code used to classify:
Two diagnoses, or
A diagnosis with an associated secondary process (manifestation)
A diagnosis with an associated complication
Combination codes are identified by referring to subterm entries in the Alphabetic Index and by reading the inclusion and exclusion notes in the Tabular List.

Assign only the combination code when that code fully identifies the diagnostic conditions involved or when the Alphabetic Index so directs. Multiple coding should not be used when the classification provides a combination code that clearly identifies all of the elements documented in the diagnosis. When the combination code lacks necessary specificity in describing the manifestation or complication, an additional code should be used as a secondary code.

10. **Sequela (Late Effects)**
A sequela is the residual effect (condition produced) after the acute phase of an illness or injury has terminated. There is no time limit on when a sequela code can be used. The residual may be apparent early, such as in cerebral infarction, or it may occur months or years later, such as that due to a previous injury. **Examples of sequela include: scar formation resulting from a burn, deviated septum due to a nasal fracture, and infertility due to tubal occlusion from old tuberculosis.** Coding of sequela generally requires two codes sequenced in the following order: the condition or nature of the sequela is sequenced first. The sequela code is sequenced second.

An exception to the above guidelines are those instances where the code for the sequela is followed by a manifestation code identified in the Tabular List and title, or the sequela code has been expanded (at the fourth, fifth or sixth character levels) to include the manifestation(s). The code for the acute phase of an illness or injury that led to the sequela is never used with a code for the late effect.
See Section I.C.9. Sequelae of cerebrovascular disease
See Section I.C.15. Sequelae of complication of pregnancy, childbirth and the puerperium
See Section I.C.19. Application of 7th characters for Chapter 19

11. **Impending or Threatened Condition**
Code any condition described at the time of discharge as "impending" or "threatened" as follows:
If it did occur, code as confirmed diagnosis.
If it did not occur, reference the Alphabetic Index to determine if the condition has a subentry term for "impending" or "threatened" and also reference main term entries for "Impending" and for "Threatened."
If the subterms are listed, assign the given code.
If the subterms are not listed, code the existing underlying condition(s) and not the condition described as impending or threatened.

12. **Reporting Same Diagnosis Code More than Once**

Each unique ICD-10-CM diagnosis code may be reported only once for an encounter. This applies to bilateral conditions when there are no distinct codes identifying laterality or two different conditions classified to the same ICD-10-CM diagnosis code.

13. **Laterality**

Some ICD-10-CM codes indicate laterality, specifying whether the condition occurs on the left, right or is bilateral. If no bilateral code is provided and the condition is bilateral, assign separate codes for both the left and right side. If the side is not identified in the medical record, assign the code for the unspecified side.

14. **Documentation for BMI, Non-pressure ulcers and Pressure Ulcer Stages**

For the Body Mass Index (BMI), depth of non-pressure chronic ulcers and pressure ulcer stage codes, code assignment may be based on medical record documentation from clinicians who are not the patient's provider (i.e., physician or other qualified healthcare practitioner legally accountable for establishing the patient's diagnosis), since this information is typically documented by other clinicians involved in the care of the patient (e.g., a dietitian often documents the BMI and nurses often documents the pressure ulcer stages). However, the associated diagnosis (such as overweight, obesity, or pressure ulcer) must be documented by the patient's provider. If there is conflicting medical record documentation, either from the same clinician or different clinicians, the patient's attending provider should be queried for clarification.

The BMI codes should only be reported as secondary diagnoses. As with all other secondary diagnosis codes, the BMI codes should only be assigned when they meet the definition of a reportable additional diagnosis (see Section III, Reporting Additional Diagnoses).

15. **Syndromes**

Follow the Alphabetic Index guidance when coding syndromes. In the absence of Alphabetic Index guidance, assign codes for the documented manifestations of the syndrome. Additional codes for manifestations that are not an integral part of the disease process may also be assigned when the condition does not have a unique code.

16. **Documentation of Complications of Care**

Code assignment is based on the provider's documentation of the relationship between the condition and the care or procedure. The guideline extends to any complications of care, regardless of the chapter the code is located in. It is important to note that not all conditions that occur during or following medical care or surgery are classified as complications. There must be a cause-and-effect relationship between the care provided and the condition, and an indication in the documentation that it is a complication. Query the provider for clarification, if the complication is not clearly documented.

17. **Borderline Diagnosis**

If the provider documents a "borderline" diagnosis at the time of discharge, the diagnosis is coded as confirmed, unless the classification provides a specific entry (e.g., borderline diabetes). If a borderline condition has a specific index entry in ICD-10-CM, it should be coded as such. Since borderline conditions are not uncertain diagnoses, no distinction is made between the care setting (inpatient versus outpatient). Whenever the documentation is unclear regarding a borderline condition, coders are encouraged to query for clarification.

18. **Use of Sign/Symptom/Unspecified Codes**

Sign/symptom and "unspecified" codes have acceptable, even necessary, uses. While specific diagnosis codes should be reported when they are supported by the available medical record documentation and clinical knowledge of the patient's health condition, there are instances when signs/symptoms or unspecified codes are the best choices for accurately reflecting the healthcare encounter. Each healthcare encounter should be coded to the level of certainty known for that encounter.

If a definitive diagnosis has not been established by the end of the encounter, it is appropriate to report codes for sign(s) and/or symptom(s) in lieu of a definitive diagnosis. When sufficient clinical information isn't known or available about a particular health condition to assign a more specific code, it is acceptable to report the appropriate "unspecified" code (e.g., a diagnosis of pneumonia has been determined, but not the specific type). Unspecified codes should be reported when they are the codes that most accurately reflect what is known about the patient's condition at the time of that particular encounter. It would be inappropriate to select a specific code that is not supported by the medical record documentation or conduct medically unnecessary diagnostic testing in order to determine a more specific code.

C. **Chapter-Specific Coding Guidelines**

In addition to general coding guidelines, there are guidelines for specific diagnoses and/or conditions in the classification. Unless otherwise indicated, these guidelines apply to all health care settings. Please refer to Section II for guidelines on the selection of principal diagnosis.

1. **Chapter 1: Certain Infectious and Parasitic Diseases (A00-B99)**

   a. **Human Immunodeficiency Virus (HIV) Infections**

      1) **Code only confirmed cases**

      Code only confirmed cases of HIV infection/illness. This is an exception to the hospital inpatient guideline Section II, H.

In this context, "confirmation" does not require documentation of positive serology or culture for HIV; the provider's diagnostic statement that the patient is HIV positive, or has an HIV-related illness is sufficient.

2) Selection and sequencing of HIV codes

(a) Patient admitted for HIV-related condition

If a patient is admitted for an HIV-related condition, the principal diagnosis should be B20, Human immunodeficiency virus [HIV] disease followed by additional diagnosis codes for all reported HIV-related conditions.

(b) Patient with HIV disease admitted for unrelated condition

If a patient with HIV disease is admitted for an unrelated condition (such as a traumatic injury), the code for the unrelated condition (e.g., the nature of injury code) should be the principal diagnosis. Other diagnoses would be B20 followed by additional diagnosis codes for all reported HIV-related conditions.

(c) Whether the patient is newly diagnosed

Whether the patient is newly diagnosed or has had previous admissions/encounters for HIV conditions is irrelevant to the sequencing decision.

(d) Asymptomatic human immunodeficiency virus

Z21, Asymptomatic human immunodeficiency virus [HIV] infection status, is to be applied when the patient without any documentation of symptoms is listed as being "HIV positive," "known HIV," "HIV test positive," or similar terminology. Do not use this code if the term "AIDS" is used or if the patient is treated for any HIV-related illness or is described as having any condition(s) resulting from his/her HIV positive status; use B20 in these cases.

(e) Patients with inconclusive HIV serology

Patients with inconclusive HIV serology, but no definitive diagnosis or manifestations of the illness, may be assigned code R75, Inconclusive laboratory evidence of human immunodeficiency virus [HIV].

(f) Previously diagnosed HIV-related illness

Patients with any known prior diagnosis of an HIV-related illness should be coded to B20. Once a patient has developed an HIV-related illness, the patient should always be assigned code B20 on every subsequent admission/encounter. Patients previously diagnosed with any HIV illness (B20) should never be assigned to R75 or Z21, Asymptomatic human immunodeficiency virus [HIV] infection status.

(g) HIV Infection in Pregnancy, Childbirth and the Puerperium

During pregnancy, childbirth or the puerperium, a patient admitted (or presenting for a health care encounter) because of an HIV-related illness should receive a principal diagnosis code of O98.7-, Human immunodeficiency [HIV] disease complicating pregnancy, childbirth and the puerperium, followed by B20 and the code(s) for the HIV-related illness(es). Codes from Chapter 15 always take sequencing priority.

Patients with asymptomatic HIV infection status admitted (or presenting for a health care encounter) during pregnancy, childbirth, or the puerperium should receive codes of O98.7- and Z21.

(h) Encounters for testing for HIV

If a patient is being seen to determine his/her HIV status, use code Z11.4, Encounter for screening for human immunodeficiency virus [HIV]. Use additional codes for any associated high risk behavior.

If a patient with signs or symptoms is being seen for HIV testing, code the signs and symptoms. An additional counseling code Z71.7, Human immunodeficiency virus [HIV] counseling, may be used if counseling is provided during the encounter for the test.

When a patient returns to be informed of his/her HIV test results and the test result is negative, use code Z71.7, Human immunodeficiency virus [HIV] counseling.

If the results are positive, see previous guidelines and assign codes as appropriate.

b. Infectious agents as the cause of diseases classified to other chapters

Certain infections are classified in chapters other than Chapter 1 and no organism is identified as part of the infection code. In these instances, it is necessary to use an additional code from Chapter 1 to identify the organism. A code from category B95, Streptococcus, Staphylococcus, and Enterococcus as the cause of diseases classified to other chapters, B96, Other bacterial agents as the cause of diseases classified to other chapters, or B97, Viral agents as the cause of diseases classified to other chapters, is to be used as an additional code to identify the organism. An instructional note will be found at the infection code advising that an additional organism code is required.

c. Infections resistant to antibiotics

Many bacterial infections are resistant to current antibiotics. It is necessary to identify all infections documented as antibiotic resistant. Assign a code from category Z16, Resistance to antimicrobial drugs, following the infection code only if the infection code does not identify drug resistance.

d. Sepsis, Severe Sepsis, and Septic Shock

1) Coding of Sepsis and Severe Sepsis

(a) Sepsis

For a diagnosis of sepsis, assign the appropriate code for the underlying systemic infection. If the type of infection or causal organism is not further specified, assign code A41.9, Sepsis, unspecified organism.

A code from subcategory R65.2, Severe sepsis, should not be assigned unless severe sepsis or an associated acute organ dysfunction is documented.

(i) Negative or inconclusive blood cultures and sepsis
Negative or inconclusive blood cultures do not preclude a diagnosis of sepsis in patients with clinical evidence of the condition, however, the provider should be queried.

(ii) Urosepsis
The term urosepsis is a nonspecific term. It is not to be considered synonymous with sepsis. It has no default code in the Alphabetic Index. Should a provider use this term, he/she must be queried for clarification.

(iii) Sepsis with organ dysfunction
If a patient has sepsis and associated acute organ dysfunction or multiple organ dysfunction (MOD), follow the instructions for coding severe sepsis.

(iv) Acute organ dysfunction that is not clearly associated with the sepsis
If a patient has sepsis and an acute organ dysfunction, but the medical record documentation indicates that the acute organ dysfunction is related to a medical condition other than the sepsis, do not assign a code from subcategory R65.2, Severe sepsis. An acute organ dysfunction must be associated with the sepsis in order to assign the severe sepsis code. If the documentation is not clear as to whether an acute organ dysfunction is related to the sepsis or another medical condition, query the provider.

(b) Severe sepsis
The coding of severe sepsis requires a minimum of 2 codes: first a code for the underlying systemic infection, followed by a code from subcategory R65.2, Severe sepsis. If the causal organism is not documented, assign code A41.9, Sepsis, unspecified organism, for the infection. Additional code(s) for the associated acute organ dysfunction are also required.

Due to the complex nature of severe sepsis, some cases may require querying the provider prior to assignment of the codes.

2) Septic shock

(a) Septic shock generally refers to circulatory failure associated with severe sepsis, and therefore, it represents a type of acute organ dysfunction.

For all cases of septic shock, the code for the systemic infection should be sequenced first, followed by code R65.21, Severe sepsis with septic shock or code T81.12, Postprocedural septic shock. Any additional codes for the other acute organ dysfunctions should also be assigned. As noted in the sequencing instructions in the Tabular List, the code for septic shock cannot be assigned as a principal diagnosis.

3) Sequencing of severe sepsis
If severe sepsis is present on admission, and meets the definition of principal diagnosis, the underlying systemic infection should be assigned as principal diagnosis followed by the appropriate code from subcategory R65.2 as required by the sequencing rules in the Tabular List. A code from subcategory R65.2 can never be assigned as a principal diagnosis.

When severe sepsis develops during an encounter (it was not present on admission) the underlying systemic infection and the appropriate code from subcategory R65.2 should be assigned as secondary diagnoses.

Severe sepsis may be present on admission but the diagnosis may not be confirmed until sometime after admission. If the documentation is not clear whether severe sepsis was present on admission, the provider should be queried.

4) Sepsis and severe sepsis with a localized infection
If the reason for admission is both sepsis or severe sepsis and a localized infection, such as pneumonia or cellulitis, a code(s) for the underlying systemic infection should be assigned first and the code for the localized infection should be assigned as a secondary diagnosis. If the patient has severe sepsis, a code from subcategory R65.2 should also be assigned as a secondary diagnosis. If the patient is admitted with a localized infection, such as pneumonia, and sepsis/severe sepsis doesn't develop until after admission, the localized infection should be assigned first, followed by the appropriate sepsis/severe sepsis codes.

5) Sepsis due to a postprocedural infection

(a) Documentation of causal relationship
As with all postprocedural complications, code assignment is based on the provider's documentation of the relationship between the infection and the procedure.

(b) Sepsis due to a postprocedural infection
For such cases, the postprocedural infection code, such as, T80.2, Infections following infusion, transfusion, and therapeutic injection, T81.4, Infection following a procedure, T88.0, Infection following immunization, or O86.0, Infection of obstetric surgical wound, should be coded first, followed by the code for the specific infection. If the patient has severe sepsis the appropriate code from subcategory R65.2 should also be assigned with the additional code(s) for any acute organ dysfunction.

(c) Postprocedural infection and postprocedural septic shock

In cases where a postprocedural infection has occurred and has resulted in severe sepsis the code for the precipitating complication such as code T81.4, Infection following a procedure, or O86.0, Infection of obstetrical surgical wound should be coded first followed by code R65.**20**, Severe sepsis without septic shock. **A Code for the systemic infection should also be assigned.**

If a postprocedural infection has resulted in postprocedural septic shock, the code for the precipitating complication such as code T81.4, Infection following a procedure, or O86.0, Infection of obstetrical surgical wound should be coded first followed by code T81.12-, Postprocedural septic shock. A code for the systemic infection should also be assigned.

6) Sepsis and severe sepsis associated with a noninfectious process (condition)

In some cases a noninfectious process (condition), such as trauma, may lead to an infection which can result in sepsis or severe sepsis. If sepsis or severe sepsis is documented as associated with a noninfectious condition, such as a burn or serious injury, and this condition meets the definition for principal diagnosis, the code for the noninfectious condition should be sequenced first, followed by the code for the resulting infection. If severe sepsis is present, a code from subcategory R65.2 should also be assigned with any associated organ dysfunction(s) codes. It is not necessary to assign a code from subcategory R65.1, Systemic inflammatory response syndrome (SIRS) of non-infectious origin, for these cases.

If the infection meets the definition of principal diagnosis it should be sequenced before the non-infectious condition. When both the associated non-infectious condition and the infection meet the definition of principal diagnosis either may be assigned as principal diagnosis.

Only one code from category R65, Symptoms and signs specifically associated with systemic inflammation and infection, should be assigned. Therefore, when a non-infectious condition leads to an infection resulting in severe sepsis, assign the appropriate code from subcategory R65.2, Severe sepsis. Do not additionally assign a code from subcategory R65.1, Systemic inflammatory response syndrome (SIRS) of non-infectious origin.

See Section I.C.18. SIRS due to non-infectious process

7) Sepsis and septic shock complicating abortion, pregnancy, childbirth, and the puerperium

See Section I.C.15. Sepsis and septic shock complicating abortion, pregnancy, childbirth and the puerperium

8) Newborn sepsis

See Section I.C.16. f. Bacterial sepsis of Newborn

e. Methicillin Resistant Staphylococcus aureus (MRSA) Conditions

1) Selection and sequencing of MRSA codes

(a) Combination codes for MRSA infection

When a patient is diagnosed with an infection that is due to methicillin resistant *Staphylococcus aureus* (MRSA), and that infection has a combination code that includes the causal organism (e.g., sepsis, pneumonia) assign the appropriate combination code for the condition (e.g., code A41.02, Sepsis due to Methicillin resistant Staphylococcus aureus or code J15.212, Pneumonia due to Methicillin resistant Staphylococcus aureus). Do not assign code B95.62, Methicillin resistant Staphylococcus aureus infection as the cause of diseases classified elsewhere, as an additional code because the combination code includes the type of infection and the MRSA organism. Do not assign a code from subcategory Z16.11, Resistance to penicillins, as an additional diagnosis.

See Section C.1. for instructions on coding and sequencing of sepsis and severe sepsis.

(b) Other codes for MRSA infection

When there is documentation of a current infection (e.g., wound infection, stitch abscess, urinary tract infection) due to MRSA, and that infection does not have a combination code that includes the causal organism, assign the appropriate code to identify the condition along with code B95.62, Methicillin resistant Staphylococcus aureus infection as the cause of diseases classified elsewhere for the MRSA infection. Do not assign a code from subcategory Z16.11, Resistance to penicillins.

(c) Methicillin susceptible Staphylococcus aureus (MSSA) and MRSA colonization

The condition or state of being colonized or carrying MSSA or MRSA is called colonization or carriage, while an individual person is described as being colonized or being a carrier. Colonization means that MSSA or MSRA is present on or in the body without necessarily causing illness. A positive MRSA colonization test might be documented by the provider as "MRSA screen positive" or "MRSA nasal swab positive".

Assign code Z22.322, Carrier or suspected carrier of Methicillin resistant Staphylococcus aureus, for patients documented as having MRSA colonization. Assign code Z22.321, Carrier or suspected carrier of Methicillin susceptible Staphylococcus aureus, for patient documented as having MSSA colonization. Colonization is not necessarily indicative of a disease process or as the cause of a specific condition the patient may have unless documented as such by the provider.

(d) MRSA colonization and infection

If a patient is documented as having both MRSA colonization and infection during a hospital admission, code Z22.322, Carrier or suspected carrier of Methicillin resistant Staphylococcus aureus, and a code for the MRSA infection may both be assigned.

2. Chapter 2: Neoplasms (C00-D49)
General guidelines

Chapter 2 of the ICD-10-CM contains the codes for most benign and all malignant neoplasms. Certain benign neoplasms, such as prostatic adenomas, may be found in the specific body system chapters. To properly code a neoplasm it is necessary to determine from the record if the neoplasm is benign, in-situ, malignant, or of uncertain histologic behavior. If malignant, any secondary (metastatic) sites should also be determined.

Primary malignant neoplasms overlapping site boundaries

A primary malignant neoplasm that overlaps two or more contiguous (next to each other) sites should be classified to the subcategory/code .8 ('overlapping lesion'), unless the combination is specifically indexed elsewhere. For multiple neoplasms of the same site that are not contiguous such as tumors in different quadrants of the same breast, codes for each site should be assigned.

Malignant neoplasm of ectopic tissue

Malignant neoplasms of ectopic tissue are to be coded to the site of origin mentioned, e.g., ectopic pancreatic malignant neoplasms involving the stomach are coded to pancreas, unspecified (C25.9).

The neoplasm table in the Alphabetic Index should be referenced first. However, if the histological term is documented, that term should be referenced first, rather than going immediately to the Neoplasm Table, in order to determine which column in the Neoplasm Table is appropriate. For example, if the documentation indicates "adenoma," refer to the term in the Alphabetic Index to review the entries under this term and the instructional note to "see also neoplasm, by site, benign." The table provides the proper code based on the type of neoplasm and the site. It is important to select the proper column in the table that corresponds to the type of neoplasm. The Tabular List should then be referenced to verify that the correct code has been selected from the table and that a more specific site code does not exist.

See Section I.C.21. Factors influencing health status and contact with health services, Status, for information regarding Z15.0, codes for genetic susceptibility to cancer.

a. Treatment directed at the malignancy

If the treatment is directed at the malignancy, designate the malignancy as the principal diagnosis.

The only exception to this guideline is if a patient admission/encounter is solely for the administration of chemotherapy, immunotherapy or radiation therapy, assign the appropriate Z51.— code as the first-listed or principal diagnosis, and the diagnosis or problem for which the service is being performed as a secondary diagnosis.

b. Treatment of secondary site

When a patient is admitted because of a primary neoplasm with metastasis and treatment is directed toward the secondary site only, the secondary neoplasm is designated as the principal diagnosis even though the primary malignancy is still present.

c. Coding and sequencing of complications

Coding and sequencing of complications associated with the malignancies or with the therapy thereof are subject to the following guidelines:

1) Anemia associated with malignancy

When admission/encounter is for management of an anemia associated with the malignancy, and the treatment is only for anemia, the appropriate code for the malignancy is sequenced as the principal or first-listed diagnosis followed by the appropriate code for the anemia (such as code D63.0, Anemia in neoplastic disease).

2) Anemia associated with chemotherapy, immunotherapy and radiation therapy

When the admission/encounter is for management of an anemia associated with an adverse effect of the administration of chemotherapy or immunotherapy and the only treatment is for the anemia, the anemia code is sequenced first followed by the appropriate codes for the neoplasm and the adverse effect (T45.1X5, Adverse effect of antineoplastic and immunosuppressive drugs).

When the admission/encounter is for management of an anemia associated with an adverse effect of radiotherapy, the anemia code should be sequenced first, followed by the appropriate neoplasm code and code Y84.2, Radiological procedure and radiotherapy as the cause of abnormal reaction of the patient, or of later complication, without mention of misadventure at the time of the procedure.

3) Management of dehydration due to the malignancy

When the admission/encounter is for management of dehydration due to the malignancy and only the dehydration is being treated (intravenous rehydration), the dehydration is sequenced first, followed by the code(s) for the malignancy.

4) Treatment of a complication resulting from a surgical procedure

When the admission/encounter is for treatment of a complication resulting from a surgical procedure, designate the complication as the principal or first-listed diagnosis if treatment is directed at resolving the complication.

d. Primary malignancy previously excised

When a primary malignancy has been previously excised or eradicated from its site and there is no further treatment directed to that site and there is no evidence of any existing primary malignancy, a code from category Z85, Personal history of malignant neoplasm, should be used to indicate the former site of the malignancy. Any mention of extension, invasion, or metastasis to another site is coded as a secondary malignant neoplasm to that site. The secondary site may be the principal or first-listed with the Z85 code used as a secondary code.

e. **Admissions/Encounters involving chemotherapy, immunotherapy and radiation therapy**

   1) **Episode of care involves surgical removal of neoplasm**

   When an episode of care involves the surgical removal of a neoplasm, primary or secondary site, followed by adjunct chemotherapy or radiation treatment during the same episode of care, the code for the neoplasm should be assigned as principal or first-listed diagnosis.

   2) **Patient admission/encounter solely for administration of chemotherapy, immunotherapy and radiation therapy**

   If a patient admission/encounter is solely for the administration of chemotherapy, immunotherapy or radiation therapy assign code Z51.0, Encounter for antineoplastic radiation therapy, or Z51.11, Encounter for antineoplastic chemotherapy, or Z51.12, Encounter for antineoplastic immunotherapy as the first-listed or principal diagnosis. If a patient receives more than one of these therapies during the same admission more than one of these codes may be assigned, in any sequence.

   The malignancy for which the therapy is being administered should be assigned as a secondary diagnosis.

   3) **Patient admitted for radiation therapy, chemotherapy or immunotherapy and develops complications**

   When a patient is admitted for the purpose of radiotherapy, immunotherapy or chemotherapy and develops complications such as uncontrolled nausea and vomiting or dehydration, the principal or first-listed diagnosis is Z51.0, Encounter for antineoplastic radiation therapy, or Z51.11, Encounter for antineoplastic chemotherapy, or Z51.12, Encounter for antineoplastic immunotherapy followed by any codes for the complications.

f. **Admission/encounter to determine extent of malignancy**

   When the reason for admission/encounter is to determine the extent of the malignancy, or for a procedure such as paracentesis or thoracentesis, the primary malignancy or appropriate metastatic site is designated as the principal or first-listed diagnosis, even though chemotherapy or radiotherapy is administered.

g. **Symptoms, signs, and abnormal findings listed in Chapter 18 associated with neoplasms**

   Symptoms, signs, and ill-defined conditions listed in Chapter 18 characteristic of, or associated with, an existing primary or secondary site malignancy cannot be used to replace the malignancy as principal or first-listed diagnosis, regardless of the number of admissions or encounters for treatment and care of the neoplasm.

   See section I.C.21. Factors influencing health status and contact with health services, Encounter for prophylactic organ removal.

h. **Admission/encounter for pain control/management**

   See Section I.C.6. for information on coding admission/encounter for pain control/management.

i. **Malignancy in two or more noncontiguous sites**

   A patient may have more than one malignant tumor in the same organ. These tumors may represent different primaries or metastatic disease, depending on the site. Should the documentation be unclear, the provider should be queried as to the status of each tumor so that the correct codes can be assigned.

j. **Disseminated malignant neoplasm, unspecified**

   Code C80.0, Disseminated malignant neoplasm, unspecified, is for use only in those cases where the patient has advanced metastatic disease and no known primary or secondary sites are specified. It should not be used in place of assigning codes for the primary site and all known secondary sites.

k. **Malignant neoplasm without specification of site**

   Code C80.1, Malignant (primary) neoplasm, unspecified, equates to Cancer, unspecified. This code should only be used when no determination can be made as to the primary site of a malignancy. This code should rarely be used in the inpatient setting.

l. **Sequencing of neoplasm codes**

   1) **Encounter for treatment of primary malignancy**

   If the reason for the encounter is for treatment of a primary malignancy, assign the malignancy as the principal/first-listed diagnosis. The primary site is to be sequenced first, followed by any metastatic sites.

   2) **Encounter for treatment of secondary malignancy**

   When an encounter is for a primary malignancy with metastasis and treatment is directed toward the metastatic (secondary) site(s) only, the metastatic site(s) is designated as the principal/first-listed diagnosis. The primary malignancy is coded as an additional code.

   3) **Malignant neoplasm in a pregnant patient**

   When a pregnant woman has a malignant neoplasm, a code from subcategory O9A.1-, Malignant neoplasm complicating pregnancy, childbirth, and the puerperium, should be sequenced first, followed by the appropriate code from Chapter 2 to indicate the type of neoplasm.

   4) **Encounter for complication associated with a neoplasm**

   When an encounter is for management of a complication associated with a neoplasm, such as dehydration, and the treatment is only for the complication, the complication is coded first, followed by the appropriate code(s) for the neoplasm.

The exception to this guideline is anemia. When the admission/encounter is for management of an anemia associated with the malignancy, and the treatment is only for anemia, the appropriate code for the malignancy is sequenced as the principal or first-listed diagnosis followed by code D63.0, Anemia in neoplastic disease.

5) Complication from surgical procedure for treatment of a neoplasm

When an encounter is for treatment of a complication resulting from a surgical procedure performed for the treatment of the neoplasm, designate the complication as the principal/first-listed diagnosis. See guideline regarding the coding of a current malignancy versus personal history to determine if the code for the neoplasm should also be assigned.

6) Pathologic fracture due to a neoplasm

When an encounter is for a pathological fracture due to a neoplasm, and the focus of treatment is the fracture, a code from subcategory M84.5, Pathological fracture in neoplastic disease, should be sequenced first, followed by the code for the neoplasm.

If the focus of treatment is the neoplasm with an associated pathological fracture, the neoplasm code should be sequenced first, followed by a code from M84.5 for the pathological fracture.

m. Current malignancy versus personal history of malignancy

When a primary malignancy has been excised but further treatment, such as an additional surgery for the malignancy, radiation therapy or chemotherapy is directed to that site, the primary malignancy code should be used until treatment is completed.

When a primary malignancy has been previously excised or eradicated from its site, there is no further treatment (of the malignancy) directed to that site, and there is no evidence of any existing primary malignancy, a code from category Z85, Personal history of malignant neoplasm, should be used to indicate the former site of the malignancy.

See Section I.C.21. Factors influencing health status and contact with health services, History (of)

n. Leukemia, Multiple Myeloma, and Malignant Plasma Cell Neoplasms in remission versus personal history

The categories for leukemia, and category C90, Multiple myeloma and malignant plasma cell neoplasms, have codes indicating whether or not the leukemia has achieved remission. There are also codes Z85.6, Personal history of leukemia, and Z85.79, Personal history of other malignant neoplasms of lymphoid, hematopoietic and related tissues. If the documentation is unclear, as to whether the leukemia has achieved remission, the provider should be queried.

See Section I.C.21. Factors influencing health status and contact with health services, History (of)

o. Aftercare following surgery for neoplasm

See Section I.C.21. Factors influencing health status and contact with health services, Aftercare

p. Follow-up care for completed treatment of a malignancy

See Section I.C.21. Factors influencing health status and contact with health services, Follow-up

q. Prophylactic organ removal for prevention of malignancy

See Section I.C. 21, Factors influencing health status and contact with health services, Prophylactic organ removal

r. Malignant neoplasm associated with transplanted organ

A malignant neoplasm of a transplanted organ should be coded as a transplant complication. Assign first the appropriate code from category T86.-, Complications of transplanted organs and tissue, followed by code C80.2, Malignant neoplasm associated with transplanted organ. Use an additional code for the specific malignancy.

3. Chapter 3: Disease of the blood and blood-forming organs and certain disorders involving the immune mechanism (D50-D89)

Reserved for future guideline expansion

4. Chapter 4: Endocrine, Nutritional, and Metabolic Diseases (E00-E89)

a. Diabetes mellitus

The diabetes mellitus codes are combination codes that include the type of diabetes mellitus, the body system affected, and the complications affecting that body system. As many codes within a particular category as are necessary to describe all of the complications of the disease may be used. They should be sequenced based on the reason for a particular encounter. Assign as many codes from categories E08 – E13 as needed to identify all of the associated conditions that the patient has.

1) Type of diabetes

The age of a patient is not the sole determining factor, though most type 1 diabetics develop the condition before reaching puberty. For this reason type 1 diabetes mellitus is also referred to as juvenile diabetes.

2) Type of diabetes mellitus not documented

If the type of diabetes mellitus is not documented in the medical record the default is E11.-, Type 2 diabetes mellitus.

3) Diabetes mellitus and the use of insulin

If the documentation in a medical record does not indicate the type of diabetes but does indicate that the patient uses insulin, code E11, Type 2 diabetes mellitus, should be assigned. Code Z79.4, Long-term (current) use of insulin, should also be assigned to indicate that the patient uses insulin. Code Z79.4 should not be assigned if insulin is given temporarily to bring a type 2 patient's blood sugar under control during an encounter.

4) Diabetes mellitus in pregnancy and gestational diabetes

See Section I.C.15. Diabetes mellitus in pregnancy.
See Section I.C.15. Gestational (pregnancy induced) diabetes

5) Complications due to insulin pump malfunction

(a) Underdose of insulin due to insulin pump failure

An underdose of insulin due to an insulin pump failure should be assigned to a code from subcategory T85.6, Mechanical complication of other specified internal and external prosthetic devices, implants and grafts, that specifies the type of pump malfunction, as the principal or first-listed code, followed by code T38.3X6-, Underdosing of insulin and oral hypoglycemic [antidiabetic] drugs. Additional codes for the type of diabetes mellitus and any associated complications due to the underdosing should also be assigned.

(b) Overdose of insulin due to insulin pump failure

The principal or first-listed code for an encounter due to an insulin pump malfunction resulting in an overdose of insulin, should also be T85.6-, Mechanical complication of other specified internal and external prosthetic devices, implants and grafts, followed by code T38.3X1-, Poisoning by insulin and oral hypoglycemic [antidiabetic] drugs, accidental (unintentional).

6) Secondary diabetes mellitus

Codes under categories E08, Diabetes mellitus due to underlying condition, E09, Drug or chemical induced diabetes mellitus and E13, Other specified diabetes mellitus, identify complications/ manifestations associated with secondary diabetes mellitus. Secondary diabetes is always caused by another condition or event (e.g., cystic fibrosis, malignant neoplasm of pancreas, pancreatectomy, adverse effect of drug, or poisoning).

(a) Secondary diabetes mellitus and the use of insulin

For patients who routinely use insulin, code Z79.4, Long-term (current) use of insulin, should also be assigned. Code Z79.4 should not be assigned if insulin is given temporarily to bring a patient's blood sugar under control during an encounter.

(b) Assigning and sequencing secondary diabetes codes and its causes

The sequencing of the secondary diabetes codes in relationship to codes for the cause of the diabetes is based on the Tabular List instructions for categories E08, E09 and E13.

(i) Secondary diabetes mellitus due to pancreatectomy For postpancreatectomy diabetes mellitus (lack of insulin due to the surgical removal of all or part of the pancreas), assign code E89.1, Postprocedural hypoinsulinemia. Assign a code from category E13 and a code from subcategory Z90.41-, Acquired absence of pancreas, as additional codes.

(ii) Secondary diabetes due to drugs Secondary diabetes may be caused by an adverse effect of correctly administered medications, poisoning or sequela of poisoning.

See section I.C.19.e for coding of adverse effects and poisoning, and section I.C.20 for external cause code reporting.

5. Chapter 5: Mental, Behavioral and Neurodevelopmental disorders (F01 – F99)

a. Pain disorders related to psychological factors

Assign code F45.41, for pain that is exclusively related to psychological disorders. As indicated by the Excludes 1 note under category G89, a code from category G89 should not be assigned with code F45.41

Code F45.42, Pain disorders with related psychological factors, should be used with a code from category G89, Pain, not elsewhere classified, if there is documentation of a psychological component for a patient with acute or chronic pain.

See Section I.C.6. Pain

c. Mental and behavioral disorders due to psychoactive substance use

1) In Remission

Selection of codes for "in remission" for categories F10-F19, Mental and behavioral disorders due to psychoactive substance use (categories F10-F19 with -.21) requires the provider's clinical judgment. The appropriate codes for "in remission" are assigned only on the basis of provider documentation (as defined in the Official Guidelines for Coding and Reporting).

2) Psychoactive Substance Use, Abuse And Dependence

When the provider documentation refers to use, abuse and dependence of the same substance (e.g. alcohol, opioid, cannabis, etc.), only one code should be assigned to identify the pattern of use based on the following hierarchy:

- If both use and abuse are documented, assign only the code for abuse
- If both abuse and dependence are documented, assign only the code for dependence
- If use, abuse and dependence are all documented, assign only the code for dependence
- If both use and dependence are documented, assign only the code for dependence.

3) Psychoactive Substance Use

As with all other diagnoses, the codes for psychoactive substance use (F10.9-, F11.9-, F12.9-, F13.9-, F14.9-, F15.9-, F16.9-) should only be assigned based on provider documentation and when they meet the definition of a reportable diagnosis (see Section III, Reporting Additional Diagnoses). The codes are to be used only when the psychoactive substance use is associated with a mental or behavioral disorder, and such a relationship is documented by the provider.

6. **Chapter 6: Diseases of the Nervous System (G00-G99)**

   a. Dominant/nondominant side

   Codes from category G81, Hemiplegia and hemiparesis, and subcategories, G83.1, Monoplegia of lower limb, G83.2, Monoplegia of upper limb, and G83.3, Monoplegia, unspecified, identify whether the dominant or nondominant side is affected. Should the affected side be documented, but not specified as dominant or nondominant, and the classification system does not indicate a default, code selection is as follows:

   - For ambidextrous patients, the default should be dominant.
   - If the left side is affected, the default is non-dominant.
   - If the right side is affected, the default is dominant.

   b. Pain - Category G89

   1) General coding information

   Codes in category G89, Pain, not elsewhere classified, may be used in conjunction with codes from other categories and chapters to provide more detail about acute or chronic pain and neoplasm-related pain, unless otherwise indicated below.

   If the pain is not specified as acute or chronic, post-thoracotomy, postprocedural, or neoplasm-related, do not assign codes from category G89.

   A code from category G89 should not be assigned if the underlying (definitive) diagnosis is known, unless the reason for the encounter is pain control/management and not management of the underlying condition.

   When an admission or encounter is for a procedure aimed at treating the underlying condition (e.g., spinal fusion, kyphoplasty), a code for the underlying condition (e.g., vertebral fracture, spinal stenosis) should be assigned as the principal diagnosis. No code from category G89 should be assigned.

   (a) Category G89 Codes as Principal or First-Listed Diagnosis

   Category G89 codes are acceptable as principal diagnosis or the first-listed code:

   - When pain control or pain management is the reason for the admission/encounter (e.g., a patient with displaced intervertebral disc, nerve impingement and severe back pain presents for injection of steroid into the spinal canal). The underlying cause of the pain should be reported as an additional diagnosis, if known.
   - When a patient is admitted for the insertion of a neurostimulator for pain control, assign the appropriate pain code as the principal or first-listed diagnosis. When an admission or encounter is for a procedure aimed at treating the underlying condition and a

neurostimulator is inserted for pain control during the same admission/encounter, a code for the underlying condition should be assigned as the principal diagnosis and the appropriate pain code should be assigned as a secondary diagnosis.

   (b) Use of Category G89 Codes in Conjunction with Site Specific Pain Codes

   (i) Assigning Category G89 and Site-Specific Pain Codes

   Codes from category G89 may be used in conjunction with codes that identify the site of pain (including codes from chapter 18) if the category G89 code provides additional information. For example, if the code describes the site of the pain, but does not fully describe whether the pain is acute or chronic, then both codes should be assigned.

   (ii) Sequencing of Category G89 Codes with Site-Specific Pain Codes

   The sequencing of category G89 codes with site-specific pain codes (including chapter 18 codes), is dependent on the circumstances of the encounter/admission as follows:

   - If the encounter is for pain control or pain management, assign the code from category G89 followed by the code identifying the specific site of pain (e.g., encounter for pain management for acute neck pain from trauma is assigned code G89.11, Acute pain due to trauma, followed by code M54.2, Cervicalgia, to identify the site of pain).
   - If the encounter is for any other reason except pain control or pain management, and a related definitive diagnosis has not been established (confirmed) by the provider, assign the code for the specific site of pain first, followed by the appropriate code from category G89.

   2) Pain due to devices, implants and grafts

   See Section I.C.19. *Pain due to medical devices*

   3) Postoperative Pain

   The provider's documentation should be used to guide the coding of postoperative pain, as well as *Section III. Reporting Additional Diagnoses* and *Section IV. Diagnostic Coding and Reporting in the Outpatient Setting.*

   The default for post-thoracotomy and other postoperative pain not specified as acute or chronic is the code for the acute form.

   Routine or expected postoperative pain immediately after surgery should not be coded.

   (a) Postoperative pain not associated with specific postoperative complication

   Postoperative pain not associated with a specific postoperative complication is assigned to the appropriate postoperative pain code in category G89.

(b) Postoperative pain associated with specific postoperative complication

Postoperative pain associated with a specific postoperative complication (such as painful wire sutures) is assigned to the appropriate code(s) found in Chapter 19, Injury, poisoning, and certain other consequences of external causes. If appropriate, use additional code(s) from category G89 to identify acute or chronic pain (G89.18 or G89.28).

4) Chronic pain

Chronic pain is classified to subcategory G89.2. There is no time frame defining when pain becomes chronic pain. The provider's documentation should be used to guide use of these codes.

5) Neoplasm Related Pain

Code G89.3 is assigned to pain documented as being related, associated or due to cancer, primary or secondary malignancy, or tumor. This code is assigned regardless of whether the pain is acute or chronic.

This code may be assigned as the principal or first-listed code when the stated reason for the admission/encounter is documented as pain control/pain management. The underlying neoplasm should be reported as an additional diagnosis.

When the reason for the admission/encounter is management of the neoplasm and the pain associated with the neoplasm is also documented, code G89.3 may be assigned as an additional diagnosis. It is not necessary to assign an additional code for the site of the pain.

See Section I.C.2 for instructions on the sequencing of neoplasms for all other stated reasons for the admission/ encounter (except for pain control/pain management).

6) Chronic pain syndrome

Central pain syndrome (G89.0) and chronic pain syndrome (G89.4) are different than the term "chronic pain," and therefore codes should only be used when the provider has specifically documented this condition.

See Section I.C.5. Pain disorders related to psychological factors

7. **Chapter 7: Diseases of the Eye and Adnexa (H00-H59)**

a. **Glaucoma**

1) **Assigning Glaucoma Codes**

Assign as many codes from category H40, Glaucoma, as needed to identify the type of glaucoma, the affected eye, and the glaucoma stage.

2) **Bilateral glaucoma with same type and stage**

When a patient has bilateral glaucoma and both eyes are documented as being the same type and stage, and there is a code for bilateral glaucoma, report only the code for the type of glaucoma, bilateral, with the seventh character for the stage.

When a patient has bilateral glaucoma and both eyes are documented as being the same type and stage, and the classification does not provide a code for bilateral glaucoma (i.e. subcategories H40.10, H40.11 and H40.20) report only one code for the type of glaucoma with the appropriate seventh character for the stage.

3) **Bilateral glaucoma stage with different types or stages**

When a patient has bilateral glaucoma and each eye is documented as having a different type or stage, and the classification distinguishes laterality, assign the appropriate code for each eye rather than the code for bilateral glaucoma.

When a patient has bilateral glaucoma and each eye is documented as having a different type, and the classification does not distinguish laterality (i.e. subcategories H40.10, H40.11 and H40.20), assign one code for each type of glaucoma with the appropriate seventh character for the stage.

When a patient has bilateral glaucoma and each eye is documented as having the same type, but different stage, and the classification does not distinguish laterality (i.e. subcategories H40.10, H40.11 and H40.20), assign a code for the type of glaucoma for each eye with the seventh character for the specific glaucoma stage documented for each eye.

4) **Patient admitted with glaucoma and stage evolves during the admission**

If a patient is admitted with glaucoma and the stage progresses during the admission, assign the code for highest stage documented.

5) **Indeterminate stage glaucoma**

Assignment of the seventh character "4" for "indeterminate stage" should be based on the clinical documentation. The seventh character "4" is used for glaucomas whose stage cannot be clinically determined. This seventh character should not be confused with the seventh character "0", unspecified, which should be assigned when there is no documentation regarding the stage of the glaucoma.

8. **Chapter 8: Diseases of the Ear and Mastoid Process (H60-H95)**

Reserved for future guideline expansion

9. **Chapter 9: Diseases of the Circulatory System (I00-I99)**

a. **Hypertension**

1) **Hypertension with Heart Disease**

Heart conditions classified to I50.- or I51.4-I51.9, are assigned to, a code from category I11, Hypertensive heart disease, when a causal relationship is stated (due to hypertension) or implied (hypertensive). Use an additional code from category I50, Heart failure, to identify the type of heart failure in those patients with heart failure.

The same heart conditions (I50.-, I51.4-I51.9) with hypertension, but without a stated causal relationship, are coded separately. Sequence according to the circumstances of the admission/ encounter.

2) Hypertensive Chronic Kidney Disease

Assign codes from category I12, Hypertensive chronic kidney disease, when both hypertension and a condition classifiable to category N18, Chronic kidney disease (CKD), are present. Unlike hypertension with heart disease, ICD-10-CM presumes a cause-and-effect relationship and classifies chronic kidney disease with hypertension as hypertensive chronic kidney disease.

The appropriate code from category N18 should be used as a secondary code with a code from category I12 to identify the stage of chronic kidney disease.

See Section I.C.14. Chronic kidney disease.

If a patient has hypertensive chronic kidney disease and acute renal failure, an additional code for the acute renal failure is required.

3) Hypertensive Heart and Chronic Kidney Disease

Assign codes from combination category I13, Hypertensive heart and chronic kidney disease, when both hypertensive kidney disease and hypertensive heart disease are stated in the diagnosis. Assume a relationship between the hypertension and the chronic kidney disease, whether or not the condition is so designated. If heart failure is present, assign an additional code from category I50 to identify the type of heart failure.

The appropriate code from category N18, Chronic kidney disease, should be used as a secondary code with a code from category I13 to identify the stage of chronic kidney disease.

See Section I.C.14. Chronic kidney disease.

The codes in category I13, Hypertensive heart and chronic kidney disease, are combination codes that include hypertension, heart disease and chronic kidney disease. The Includes note at I13 specifies that the conditions included at I11 and I12 are included together in I13. If a patient has hypertension, heart disease and chronic kidney disease then a code from I13 should be used, not individual codes for hypertension, heart disease and chronic kidney disease, or codes from I11 or I12.

For patients with both acute renal failure and chronic kidney disease an additional code for acute renal failure is required.

4) Hypertensive Cerebrovascular Disease

For hypertensive cerebrovascular disease, first assign the appropriate code from categories I60-I69, followed by the appropriate hypertension code.

5) Hypertensive Retinopathy

Subcategory H35.0, Background retinopathy and retinal vascular changes, should be used with a code from category I10 – I15, Hypertensive disease to include the systemic hypertension. The sequencing is based on the reason for the encounter.

6) Hypertension, Secondary

Secondary hypertension is due to an underlying condition. Two codes are required: one to identify the underlying etiology and one from category I15 to identify the hypertension. Sequencing of codes is determined by the reason for admission/encounter.

7) Hypertension, Transient

Assign code R03.0, Elevated blood pressure reading without diagnosis of hypertension, unless patient has an established diagnosis of hypertension. Assign code O13.-, Gestational [pregnancy-induced] hypertension without significant proteinuria, or O14.-, Pre-eclampsia, for transient hypertension of pregnancy.

8) Hypertension, Controlled

This diagnostic statement usually refers to an existing state of hypertension under control by therapy. Assign the appropriate code from categories I10-I15, Hypertensive diseases.

9) Hypertension, Uncontrolled

Uncontrolled hypertension may refer to untreated hypertension or hypertension not responding to current therapeutic regimen. In either case, assign the appropriate code from categories I10-I15, Hypertensive diseases.

b. Atherosclerotic Coronary Artery Disease and Angina

ICD-10-CM has combination codes for atherosclerotic heart disease with angina pectoris. The subcategories for these codes are I25.11, Atherosclerotic heart disease of native coronary artery with angina pectoris and I25.7, Atherosclerosis of coronary artery bypass graft(s) and coronary artery of transplanted heart with angina pectoris.

When using one of these combination codes it is not necessary to use an additional code for angina pectoris. A causal relationship can be assumed in a patient with both atherosclerosis and angina pectoris, unless the documentation indicates the angina is due to something other than the atherosclerosis.

If a patient with coronary artery disease is admitted due to an acute myocardial infarction (AMI), the AMI should be sequenced before the coronary artery disease.

See Section I.C.9. Acute myocardial infarction (AMI)

c. Intraoperative and Postprocedural Cerebrovascular Accident

Medical record documentation should clearly specify the cause-and-effect relationship between the medical intervention and the cerebrovascular accident in order to assign a code for intraoperative or postprocedural cerebrovascular accident.

Proper code assignment depends on whether it was an infarction or hemorrhage and whether it occurred intraoperatively or postoperatively. If it was a cerebral hemorrhage, code assignment depends on the type of procedure performed.

d. Sequelae of Cerebrovascular Disease
1) Category I69, Sequelae of Cerebrovascular disease

Category I69 is used to indicate conditions classifiable to categories I60-I67 as the causes of sequela (neurologic deficits), themselves classified elsewhere. These "late effects" include neurologic deficits that persist after initial onset of conditions classifiable to categories I60-I67. The neurologic deficits caused by cerebrovascular disease may be present from the onset or may arise at any time after the onset of the condition classifiable to categories I60-I67.

Codes from category I69, Sequelae of cerebrovascular disease, that specify hemiplegia, hemiparesis and monoplegia identify whether the dominant or nondominant side is affected. Should the affected side be documented, but not specified as dominant or nondominant, and the classification system does not indicate a default, code selection is as follows:
- For ambidextrous patients, the default should be dominant.
- If the left side is affected, the default is non-dominant.
- If the right side is affected, the default is dominant.

2) Codes from category I69 with codes from I60-I67

Codes from category I69 may be assigned on a health care record with codes from I60-I67, if the patient has a current cerebrovascular disease and deficits from an old cerebrovascular disease.

3) Codes from category I69 and Personal history of transient ischemic attack (TIA) and cerebral infarction (Z86.73)

Codes from category I69 should not be assigned if the patient does not have neurologic deficits.

See Section I.C.21. 4. History (of) for use of personal history codes

e. Acute myocardial infarction (AMI)
1) ST elevation myocardial infarction (STEMI) and non ST elevation myocardial infarction (NSTEMI)

The ICD-10-CM codes for acute myocardial infarction (AMI) identify the site, such as anterolateral wall or true posterior wall. Subcategories I21.0-I21.2 and code I21.3 are used for ST elevation myocardial infarction (STEMI). Code I21.4, Non-ST elevation (NSTEMI) myocardial infarction, is used for non ST elevation myocardial infarction (NSTEMI) and nontransmural MIs.

If NSTEMI evolves to STEMI, assign the STEMI code. If STEMI converts to NSTEMI due to thrombolytic therapy, it is still coded as STEMI.

For encounters occurring while the myocardial infarction is equal to, or less than, four weeks old, including transfers to another acute setting or a postacute setting, and the patient requires continued care for the myocardial infarction, codes from category I21 may continue to be reported. For encounters after the 4 week time frame and the patient is still receiving care related to the myocardial infarction, the appropriate aftercare code should be assigned, rather than a code from category I21. For old or healed myocardial infarctions not requiring further care, code I25.2, Old myocardial infarction, may be assigned.

2) Acute myocardial infarction, unspecified

Code I21.3, ST elevation (STEMI) myocardial infarction of unspecified site, is the default for unspecified acute myocardial infarction. If only STEMI or transmural MI without the site is documented, assign code I21.3.

3) AMI documented as nontransmural or subendocardial but site provided

If an AMI is documented as nontransmural or subendocardial, but the site is provided, it is still coded as a subendocardial AMI.

See Section I.C.21.3 for information on coding status post administration of tPA in a different facility within the last 24 hours.

4) Subsequent acute myocardial infarction

A code from category I22, Subsequent ST elevation (STEMI) and non ST elevation (NSTEMI) myocardial infarction, is to be used when a patient who has suffered an AMI has a new AMI within the 4 week time frame of the initial AMI. A code from category I22 must be used in conjunction with a code from category I21. The sequencing of the I22 and I21 codes depends on the circumstances of the encounter.

10. Chapter 10: Diseases of the Respiratory System (J00-J99)
a. Chronic Obstructive Pulmonary Disease [COPD] and Asthma
1) Acute exacerbation of chronic obstructive bronchitis and asthma

The codes in categories J44 and J45 distinguish between uncomplicated cases and those in acute exacerbation. An acute exacerbation is a worsening or a decompensation of a chronic condition. An acute exacerbation is not equivalent to an infection superimposed on a chronic condition, though an exacerbation may be triggered by an infection.

b. Acute Respiratory Failure
1) Acute respiratory failure as principal diagnosis

A code from subcategory J96.0, Acute respiratory failure, or subcategory J96.2, Acute and chronic respiratory failure, may be assigned as a principal diagnosis when it is the condition established after study to be chiefly responsible for occasioning the admission to the hospital, and the selection is supported by the Alphabetic Index and Tabular List. However, chapter-specific coding guidelines (such as obstetrics, poisoning, HIV, newborn) that provide sequencing direction take precedence.

2) Acute respiratory failure as secondary diagnosis

Respiratory failure may be listed as a secondary diagnosis if it occurs after admission, or if it is present on admission, but does not meet the definition of principal diagnosis.

3) Sequencing of acute respiratory failure and another acute condition

When a patient is admitted with respiratory failure and another acute condition, (e.g., myocardial infarction, cerebrovascular accident, aspiration pneumonia), the principal diagnosis will not be the same in every situation. This applies whether the other acute condition is a respiratory or nonrespiratory condition. Selection of the principal diagnosis will be dependent on the circumstances of admission. If both the respiratory failure and the other acute condition are equally responsible for occasioning the admission to the hospital, and there are no chapter-specific sequencing rules, the guideline regarding two or more diagnoses that equally meet the definition for principal diagnosis (*Section II, C.*) may be applied in these situations.

If the documentation is not clear as to whether acute respiratory failure and another condition are equally responsible for occasioning the admission, query the provider for clarification.

c. Influenza due to certain identified influenza viruses

Code only confirmed cases of influenza due to certain identified influenza viruses (category J09), and due to other identified influenza virus (category J10). This is an exception to the hospital inpatient guideline Section II, H. (Uncertain Diagnosis).

In this context, "confirmation" does not require documentation of positive laboratory testing specific for avian or other novel influenza A or other identified influenza virus. However, coding should be based on the provider's diagnostic statement that the patient has avian influenza, or other novel influenza A, for category J09, or has another particular identified strain of influenza, such as H1N1 or H3N2, but not identified as novel or variant, for category J10.

If the provider records "suspected" or "possible" or "probable" avian influenza, or novel influenza, or other identified influenza, then the appropriate influenza code from category J11, Influenza due to unidentified influenza virus, should be assigned. A code from category J09, Influenza due to certain identified influenza viruses, should not be assigned nor should a code from category J10, Influenza due to other identified influenza virus.

d. Ventilator associated Pneumonia

1) Documentation of Ventilator associated Pneumonia

As with all procedural or postprocedural complications, code assignment is based on the provider's documentation of the relationship between the condition and the procedure.

Code J95.851, Ventilator associated pneumonia, should be assigned only when the provider has documented ventilator associated pneumonia (VAP). An additional code to identify the organism

(e.g., Pseudomonas aeruginosa, code B96.5) should also be assigned. Do not assign an additional code from categories J12-J18 to identify the type of pneumonia.

Code J95.851 should not be assigned for cases where the patient has pneumonia and is on a mechanical ventilator and the provider has not specifically stated that the pneumonia is ventilator-associated pneumonia. If the documentation is unclear as to whether the patient has a pneumonia that is a complication attributable to the mechanical ventilator, query the provider.

2) Ventilator associated Pneumonia Develops after Admission

A patient may be admitted with one type of pneumonia (e.g., code J13, Pneumonia due to Streptococcus pneumonia) and subsequently develop VAP. In this instance, the principal diagnosis would be the appropriate code from categories J12-J18 for the pneumonia diagnosed at the time of admission. Code J95.851, Ventilator associated pneumonia, would be assigned as an additional diagnosis when the provider has also documented the presence of ventilator associated pneumonia.

11. Chapter 11: Diseases of the Digestive System (K00-K95)
Reserved for future guideline expansion

12. Chapter 12: Diseases of the Skin and Subcutaneous Tissue (L00-L99)

a. Pressure ulcer stage codes

1) Pressure ulcer stages
Codes from category L89, Pressure ulcer, are combination codes that identify the site of the pressure ulcer as well as the stage of the ulcer.

The ICD-10-CM classifies pressure ulcer stages based on severity, which is designated by stages 1-4, unspecified stage and unstageable.

Assign as many codes from category L89 as needed to identify all the pressure ulcers the patient has, if applicable.

2) Unstageable pressure ulcers
Assignment of the code for unstageable pressure ulcer (L89.--0) should be based on the clinical documentation. These codes are used for pressure ulcers whose stage cannot be clinically determined (e.g., the ulcer is covered by eschar or has been treated with a skin or muscle graft) and pressure ulcers that are documented as deep tissue injury but not documented as due to trauma. This code should not be confused with the codes for unspecified stage (L89.--9). When there is no documentation regarding the stage of the pressure ulcer, assign the appropriate code for unspecified stage (L89.--9).

3) Documented pressure ulcer stage
Assignment of the pressure ulcer stage code should be guided by clinical documentation of the stage or documentation of the terms found in the Alphabetic Index. For clinical terms describing the stage that are not found in the Alphabetic Index,

and there is no documentation of the stage, the provider should be queried.

4) Patients admitted with pressure ulcers documented as healed

No code is assigned if the documentation states that the pressure ulcer is completely healed.

5) Patients admitted with pressure ulcers documented as healing

Pressure ulcers described as healing should be assigned the appropriate pressure ulcer stage code based on the documentation in the medical record. If the documentation does not provide information about the stage of the healing pressure ulcer, assign the appropriate code for unspecified stage.

If the documentation is unclear as to whether the patient has a current (new) pressure ulcer or if the patient is being treated for a healing pressure ulcer, query the provider.

6) Patient admitted with pressure ulcer evolving into another stage during the admission

If a patient is admitted with a pressure ulcer at one stage and it progresses to a higher stage, assign the code for the highest stage reported for that site.

13. Chapter 13: Diseases of the Musculoskeletal System and Connective Tissue (M00-M99)

a. Site and laterality

Most of the codes within Chapter 13 have site and laterality designations. The site represents the bone, joint or the muscle involved. For some conditions where more than one bone, joint or muscle is usually involved, such as osteoarthritis, there is a "multiple sites" code available. For categories where no multiple site code is provided and more than one bone, joint or muscle is involved, multiple codes should be used to indicate the different sites involved.

1) Bone versus joint

For certain conditions, the bone may be affected at the upper or lower end, (e.g., avascular necrosis of bone, M87, Osteoporosis, M80, M81). Though the portion of the bone affected may be at the joint, the site designation will be the bone, not the joint.

b. Acute traumatic versus chronic or recurrent musculoskeletal conditions

Many musculoskeletal conditions are a result of previous injury or trauma to a site, or are recurrent conditions. Bone, joint or muscle conditions that are the result of a healed injury are usually found in chapter 13. Recurrent bone, joint or muscle conditions are also usually found in chapter 13. Any current, acute injury should be coded to the appropriate injury code from chapter 19. Chronic or recurrent conditions should generally be coded with a code from chapter 13. If it is difficult to determine from the documentation in the record which code is best to describe a condition, query the provider.

c. Coding of Pathologic Fractures

7th character A is for use as long as the patient is receiving active treatment for the fracture. Examples of active treatment are: surgical treatment,

emergency department encounter, evaluation and **continuing** treatment by **the same or a different physician. While the patient may be seen by a new or different provider over the course of treatment for a pathological fracture, assignment of the 7th character is based on whether the patient is undergoing active treatment and not whether the provider is seeing the patient for the first time.**

7th character, D is to be used for encounters after the patient has completed active treatment. The other 7th characters, listed under each subcategory in the Tabular List, are to be used for subsequent encounters for treatment of problems associated with the healing, such as malunions, nonunions, and sequelae.

Care for complications of surgical treatment for fracture repairs during the healing or recovery phase should be coded with the appropriate complication codes.

See Section I.C.19. Coding of traumatic fractures.

d. Osteoporosis

Osteoporosis is a systemic condition, meaning that all bones of the musculoskeletal system are affected. Therefore, site is not a component of the codes under category M81, Osteoporosis without current pathological fracture. The site codes under category M80, Osteoporosis with current pathological fracture, identify the site of the fracture, not the osteoporosis.

1) Osteoporosis without pathological fracture

Category M81, Osteoporosis without current pathological fracture, is for use for patients with osteoporosis who do not currently have a pathologic fracture due to the osteoporosis, even if they have had a fracture in the past. For patients with a history of osteoporosis fractures, status code Z87.310, Personal history of (healed) osteoporosis fracture, should follow the code from M81.

2) Osteoporosis with current pathological fracture

Category M80, Osteoporosis with current pathological fracture, is for patients who have a current pathologic fracture at the time of an encounter. The codes under M80 identify the site of the fracture. A code from category M80, not a traumatic fracture code, should be used for any patient with known osteoporosis who suffers a fracture, even if the patient had a minor fall or trauma, if that fall or trauma would not usually break a normal, healthy bone.

14. Chapter 14: Diseases of Genitourinary System (N00-N99)

a. Chronic kidney disease

1) Stages of chronic kidney disease (CKD)

The ICD-10-CM classifies CKD based on severity. The severity of CKD is designated by stages 1-5. Stage 2, code N18.2, equates to mild CKD; stage 3, code N18.3, equates to moderate CKD; and stage 4, code N18.4, equates to severe CKD. Code N18.6, End stage renal disease (ESRD), is assigned when the provider has documented end-stage-renal disease (ESRD).

If both a stage of CKD and ESRD are documented, assign code N18.6 only.

2) Chronic kidney disease and kidney transplant status

Patients who have undergone kidney transplant may still have some form of chronic kidney disease CKD because the kidney transplant may not fully restore kidney function. Therefore, the presence of CKD alone does not constitute a transplant complication. Assign the appropriate N18 code for the patient's stage of CKD and code Z94.0, Kidney transplant status. If a transplant complication such as failure or rejection or other transplant complication is documented, see section I.C.19.g for information on coding complications of a kidney transplant. If the documentation is unclear as to whether the patient has a complication of the transplant, query the provider.

3) Chronic kidney disease with other conditions

Patients with CKD may also suffer from other serious conditions, most commonly diabetes mellitus and hypertension. The sequencing of the CKD code in relationship to codes for other contributing conditions is based on the conventions in the Tabular List.

See I.C.9. Hypertensive chronic kidney disease.
See I.C.19. Chronic kidney disease and kidney transplant complications.

15. Chapter 15: Pregnancy, Childbirth, and the Puerperium (O00-O9A)

a. General Rules for Obstetric Cases

1) Codes from chapter 15 and sequencing priority

Obstetric cases require codes from chapter 15, codes in the range O00-O9A, Pregnancy, Childbirth, and the Puerperium. Chapter 15 codes have sequencing priority over codes from other chapters. Additional codes from other chapters may be used in conjunction with chapter 15 codes to further specify conditions. Should the provider document that the pregnancy is incidental to the encounter, then code Z33.1, Pregnant state, incidental, should be used in place of any chapter 15 codes. It is the provider's responsibility to state that the condition being treated is not affecting the pregnancy.

2) Chapter 15 codes used only on the maternal record

Chapter 15 codes are to be used only on the maternal record, never on the record of the newborn.

3) Final character for trimester

The majority of codes in Chapter 15 have a final character indicating the trimester of pregnancy. The timeframes for the trimesters are indicated at the beginning of the chapter. If trimester is not a component of a code it is because the condition always occurs in a specific trimester, or the concept of trimester of pregnancy is not applicable. Certain codes have characters for only certain trimesters because the condition does not occur in all trimesters, but it may occur in more than just one.

Assignment of the final character for trimester should be based on the provider's documentation of the trimester (or number of weeks) for the current admission/encounter. This applies to the assignment of trimester for pre-existing conditions as well as those that develop during or are due to the pregnancy. The provider's documentation of the number of weeks may be used to assign the appropriate code identifying the trimester.

Whenever delivery occurs during the current admission, and there is an "in childbirth" option for the obstetric complication being coded, the "in childbirth" code should be assigned.

4) Selection of trimester for inpatient admissions that encompass more than one trimester

In instances when a patient is admitted to a hospital for complications of pregnancy during one trimester and remains in the hospital into a subsequent trimester, the trimester character for the antepartum complication code should be assigned on the basis of the trimester when the complication developed, not the trimester of the discharge. If the condition developed prior to the current admission/encounter or represents a pre-existing condition, the trimester character for the trimester at the time of the admission/encounter should be assigned.

5) Unspecified trimester

Each category that includes codes for trimester has a code for "unspecified trimester." The "unspecified trimester" code should rarely be used, such as when the documentation in the record is insufficient to determine the trimester and it is not possible to obtain clarification.

6) 7th character for Fetus Identification

Where applicable, a 7th character is to be assigned for certain categories (O31, O32, O33.3 - O33.6, O35, O36, O40, O41, O60.1, O60.2, O64, and O69) to identify the fetus for which the complication code applies.

Assign 7th character "0":
- For single gestations
- When the documentation in the record is insufficient to determine the fetus affected and it is not possible to obtain clarification.
- When it is not possible to clinically determine which fetus is affected.

b. Selection of OB Principal or First-listed Diagnosis

1) Routine outpatient prenatal visits

For routine outpatient prenatal visits when no complications are present, a code from category Z34, Encounter for supervision of normal pregnancy, should be used as the first-listed diagnosis. These codes should not be used in conjunction with chapter 15 codes.

2) Prenatal outpatient visits for high-risk patients

For routine prenatal outpatient visits for patients with high-risk pregnancies, a code from category O09, Supervision of high-risk pregnancy, should be used as the first-listed diagnosis. Secondary chapter 15 codes may be used in conjunction with these codes if appropriate.

3) Episodes when no delivery occurs

In episodes when no delivery occurs, the principal diagnosis should correspond to the principal complication of the pregnancy which necessitated the encounter. Should more than one complication exist, all of which are treated or monitored, any of the complications codes may be sequenced first.

4) When a delivery occurs

When a delivery occurs, the principal diagnosis should correspond to the main circumstances or complication of the delivery. In cases of cesarean delivery, the selection of the principal diagnosis should be the condition established after study that was responsible for the patient's admission. If the patient was admitted with a condition that resulted in the performance of a cesarean procedure, that condition should be selected as the principal diagnosis. If the reason for the admission/encounter was unrelated to the condition resulting in the cesarean delivery, the condition related to the reason for the admission/encounter should be selected as the principal diagnosis.

5) Outcome of delivery

A code from category Z37, Outcome of delivery, should be included on every maternal record when a delivery has occurred. These codes are not to be used on subsequent records or on the newborn record.

c. Pre-existing conditions versus conditions due to the pregnancy

Certain categories in Chapter 15 distinguish between conditions of the mother that existed prior to pregnancy (pre-existing) and those that are a direct result of pregnancy. When assigning codes from Chapter 15, it is important to assess if a condition was pre-existing prior to pregnancy or developed during or due to the pregnancy in order to assign the correct code.

Categories that do not distinguish between pre-existing and pregnancy-related conditions may be used for either. It is acceptable to use codes specifically for the puerperium with codes complicating pregnancy and childbirth if a condition arises postpartum during the delivery encounter.

d. Pre-existing hypertension in pregnancy

Category O10, Pre-existing hypertension complicating pregnancy, childbirth and the puerperium, includes codes for hypertensive heart and hypertensive chronic kidney disease. When assigning one of the O10 codes that includes hypertensive heart disease or hypertensive chronic kidney disease, it is necessary to add a secondary code from the appropriate hypertension category to specify the type of heart failure or chronic kidney disease.

See Section I.C.9. Hypertension.

e. Fetal Conditions Affecting the Management of the Mother

1) Codes from categories O35 and O36

Codes from categories O35, Maternal care for known or suspected fetal abnormality and damage, and O36, Maternal care for other fetal problems, are assigned only when the fetal condition is actually responsible for modifying the management of the mother, i.e., by requiring diagnostic studies, additional observation, special care, or termination of pregnancy. The fact that the fetal condition exists does not justify assigning a code from this series to the mother's record.

2) In utero surgery

In cases when surgery is performed on the fetus, a diagnosis code from category O35, Maternal care for known or suspected fetal abnormality and damage, should be assigned identifying the fetal condition. Assign the appropriate procedure code for the procedure performed.

No code from Chapter 16, the perinatal codes, should be used on the mother's record to identify fetal conditions. Surgery performed in utero on a fetus is still to be coded as an obstetric encounter.

f. HIV Infection in Pregnancy, Childbirth and the Puerperium

During pregnancy, childbirth or the puerperium, a patient admitted because of an HIV-related illness should receive a principal diagnosis from subcategory O98.7-, Human immunodeficiency [HIV] disease complicating pregnancy, childbirth and the puerperium, followed by the code(s) for the HIV-related illness(es).

Patients with asymptomatic HIV infection status admitted during pregnancy, childbirth, or the puerperium should receive codes of O98.7- and Z21, Asymptomatic human immunodeficiency virus [HIV] infection status.

g. Diabetes mellitus in pregnancy

Diabetes mellitus is a significant complicating factor in pregnancy. Pregnant women who are diabetic should be assigned a code from category O24, Diabetes mellitus in pregnancy, childbirth, and the puerperium, first, followed by the appropriate diabetes code(s) (E08-E13) from Chapter 4.

h. Long term use of insulin

Code Z79.4, Long-term (current) use of insulin, should also be assigned if the diabetes mellitus is being treated with insulin.

i. Gestational (pregnancy induced) diabetes

Gestational (pregnancy induced) diabetes can occur during the second and third trimester of pregnancy in women who were not diabetic prior to pregnancy. Gestational diabetes can cause complications in the pregnancy similar to those of pre-existing diabetes mellitus. It also puts the woman at greater risk of developing diabetes after the pregnancy. Codes for gestational diabetes are in subcategory O24.4, Gestational diabetes mellitus. No other code from category O24, Diabetes mellitus in pregnancy, childbirth, and the puerperium, should be used with a code from O24.4.

The codes under subcategory O24.4 include diet controlled and insulin controlled. If a patient with gestational diabetes is treated with both diet and insulin, only the code for insulin-controlled is required.

Code Z79.4, Long-term (current) use of insulin, should not be assigned with codes from subcategory O24.4.

An abnormal glucose tolerance in pregnancy is assigned a code from subcategory O99.81, Abnormal glucose complicating pregnancy, childbirth, and the puerperium.

j. Sepsis and septic shock complicating abortion, pregnancy, childbirth and the puerperium

When assigning a chapter 15 code for sepsis complicating abortion, pregnancy, childbirth, and the puerperium, a code for the specific type of infection should be assigned as an additional diagnosis. If severe sepsis is present, a code from subcategory R65.2, Severe sepsis, and code(s) for associated organ dysfunction(s) should also be assigned as additional diagnoses.

k. Puerperal sepsis

Code O85, Puerperal sepsis, should be assigned with a secondary code to identify the causal organism (e.g., for a bacterial infection, assign a code from category B95-B96, Bacterial infections in conditions classified elsewhere). A code from category A40, Streptococcal sepsis, or A41, Other sepsis, should not be used for puerperal sepsis. If applicable, use additional codes to identify severe sepsis (R65.2-) and any associated acute organ dysfunction.

l. Alcohol and tobacco use during pregnancy, childbirth and the puerperium

1) Alcohol use during pregnancy, childbirth and the puerperium

Codes under subcategory O99.31, Alcohol use complicating pregnancy, childbirth, and the puerperium, should be assigned for any pregnancy case when a mother uses alcohol during the pregnancy or postpartum. A secondary code from category F10, Alcohol related disorders, should also be assigned to identify manifestations of the alcohol use.

2) Tobacco use during pregnancy, childbirth and the puerperium

Codes under subcategory O99.33, Smoking (tobacco) complicating pregnancy, childbirth, and the puerperium, should be assigned for any pregnancy case when a mother uses any type of tobacco product during the pregnancy or postpartum. A secondary code from category F17, Nicotine dependence, should also be assigned to identify the type of nicotine dependence.

m. Poisoning, toxic effects, adverse effects and underdosing in a pregnant patient

A code from subcategory O9A.2, Injury, poisoning and certain other consequences of external causes complicating pregnancy, childbirth, and the puerperium, should be sequenced first, followed by the appropriate injury, poisoning, toxic effect, adverse effect or underdosing code, and then the additional code(s) that specifies the condition caused by the poisoning, toxic effect, adverse effect or underdosing.

See Section I.C.19. Adverse effects, poisoning, underdosing and toxic effects.

n. Normal Delivery, Code O80

1) Encounter for full term uncomplicated delivery

Code O80 should be assigned when a woman is admitted for a full-term normal delivery and delivers a single, healthy infant without any complications antepartum, during the delivery, or postpartum during the delivery episode. Code O80 is always a principal diagnosis. It is not to be used if any other code from chapter 15 is needed to describe a current complication of the antenatal, delivery, or perinatal period. Additional codes from other chapters may be used with code O80 if they are not related to or are in any way complicating the pregnancy.

2) Uncomplicated delivery with resolved antepartum complication

Code O80 may be used if the patient had a complication at some point during the pregnancy, but the complication is not present at the time of the admission for delivery.

3) Outcome of delivery for O80

Z37.0, Single live birth, is the only outcome of delivery code appropriate for use with O80.

o. The Peripartum and Postpartum Periods

1) Peripartum and Postpartum periods

The postpartum period begins immediately after delivery and continues for six weeks following delivery. The peripartum period is defined as the last month of pregnancy to five months postpartum.

2) Peripartum and postpartum complication

A postpartum complication is any complication occurring within the six-week period.

3) Pregnancy-related complications after 6 week period

Chapter 15 codes may also be used to describe pregnancy-related complications after the peripartum or postpartum period if the provider documents that a condition is pregnancy related.

4) Admission for routine postpartum care following delivery outside hospital

When the mother delivers outside the hospital prior to admission and is admitted for routine postpartum care and no complications are noted, code Z39.0, Encounter for care and examination of mother immediately after delivery, should be assigned as the principal diagnosis.

5) Pregnancy associated cardiomyopathy
Pregnancy associated cardiomyopathy, code O90.3, is unique in that it may be diagnosed in the third trimester of pregnancy but may continue to progress months after delivery. For this reason, it is referred to as peripartum cardiomyopathy. Code O90.3 is only for use when the cardiomyopathy develops as a result of pregnancy in a woman who did not have pre-existing heart disease.

p. Code O94, Sequelae of complication of pregnancy, childbirth, and the puerperium

1) Code O94
Code O94, Sequelae of complication of pregnancy, childbirth, and the puerperium, is for use in those cases when an initial complication of a pregnancy develops a sequelae requiring care or treatment at a future date.

2) After the initial postpartum period
This code may be used at any time after the initial postpartum period.

3) Sequencing of Code O94
This code, like all sequela codes, is to be sequenced following the code describing the sequelae of the complication.

q. Termination of Pregnancy and Spontaneous abortions

1) Abortion with Liveborn Fetus
When an attempted termination of pregnancy results in a liveborn fetus assign code Z33.2, Encounter for elective termination of pregnancy and a code from category Z37, Outcome of Delivery.

2) Retained Products of Conception following an abortion
Subsequent encounters for retained products of conception following a spontaneous abortion or elective termination of pregnancy are assigned the appropriate code from category O03, Spontaneous abortion, or codes O07.4, Failed attempted termination of pregnancy without complication and Z33.2, Encounter for elective termination of pregnancy. This advice is appropriate even when the patient was discharged previously with a discharge diagnosis of complete abortion.

3) Complications leading to abortion
Codes from Chapter 15 may be used as additional codes to identify any documented complications of the pregnancy in conjunction with codes in categories in O07 and O08.

r. Abuse in a pregnant patient
For suspected or confirmed cases of abuse of a pregnant patient, a code(s) from subcategories O9A.3, Physical abuse complicating pregnancy, childbirth, and the puerperium, O9A.4, Sexual abuse complicating pregnancy, childbirth, and the puerperium, and O9A.5, Psychological abuse complicating pregnancy, childbirth, and the puerperium, should be sequenced first, followed by the appropriate codes (if applicable) to identify any associated current injury due to physical abuse, sexual abuse, and the perpetrator of abuse.
See Section I.C.19. Adult and child abuse, neglect and other maltreatment.

16. Chapter 16: Certain Conditions Originating in the Perinatal Period (P00-P96)
For coding and reporting purposes the perinatal period is defined as before birth through the 28th day following birth. The following guidelines are provided for reporting purposes

a. General Perinatal Rules

1) Use of Chapter 16 Codes
Codes in this chapter are never for use on the maternal record. Codes from Chapter 15, the obstetric chapter, are never permitted on the newborn record. Chapter 16 codes may be used throughout the life of the patient if the condition is still present.

2) Principal Diagnosis for Birth Record
When coding the birth episode in a newborn record, assign a code from category Z38, Liveborn infants according to place of birth and type of delivery, as the principal diagnosis. A code from category Z38 is assigned only once, to a newborn at the time of birth. If a newborn is transferred to another institution, a code from category Z38 should not be used at the receiving hospital.

A code from category Z38 is used only on the newborn record, not on the mother's record.

3) Use of Codes from other Chapters with Codes from Chapter 16
Codes from other chapters may be used with codes from chapter 16 if the codes from the other chapters provide more specific detail. Codes for signs and symptoms may be assigned when a definitive diagnosis has not been established. If the reason for the encounter is a perinatal condition, the code from chapter 16 should be sequenced first.

4) Use of Chapter 16 Codes after the Perinatal Period
Should a condition originate in the perinatal period, and continue throughout the life of the patient, the perinatal code should continue to be used regardless of the patient's age.

5) Birth process or community acquired conditions
If a newborn has a condition that may be either due to the birth process or community acquired and the documentation does not indicate which it is, the default is due to the birth process and the code from Chapter 16 should be used. If the condition is community-acquired, a code from Chapter 16 should not be assigned.

6) Code all clinically significant conditions
All clinically significant conditions noted on routine newborn examination should be coded. A condition is clinically significant if it requires:
- clinical evaluation; or
- therapeutic treatment; or
- diagnostic procedures; or

- extended length of hospital stay; or
- increased nursing care and/or monitoring; or
- has implications for future health care needs

Note: The perinatal guidelines listed above are the same as the general coding guidelines for "additional diagnoses", except for the final point regarding implications for future health care needs. Codes should be assigned for conditions that have been specified by the provider as having implications for future health care needs.

b. Observation and Evaluation of Newborns for Suspected Conditions not Found

Reserved for future expansion

c. Coding Additional Perinatal Diagnoses

1) Assigning codes for conditions that require treatment

Assign codes for conditions that require treatment or further investigation, prolong the length of stay, or require resource utilization.

2) Codes for conditions specified as having implications for future health care needs

Assign codes for conditions that have been specified by the provider as having implications for future health care needs.

Note: This guideline should not be used for adult patients.

d. Prematurity and Fetal Growth Retardation

Providers utilize different criteria in determining prematurity. A code for prematurity should not be assigned unless it is documented. Assignment of codes in categories P05, Disorders of newborn related to slow fetal growth and fetal malnutrition, and P07, Disorders of newborn related to short gestation and low birth weight, not elsewhere classified, should be based on the recorded birth weight and estimated gestational age. Codes from category P05 should not be assigned with codes from category P07.

When both birth weight and gestational age are available, two codes from category P07 should be assigned, with the code for birth weight sequenced before the code for gestational age.

e. Low birth weight and immaturity status

Codes from category P07, Disorders of newborn related to short gestation and low birth weight, not elsewhere classified, are for use for a child or adult who was premature or had a low birth weight as a newborn and this is affecting the patient's current health status.

See Section I.C.21. Factors influencing health status and contact with health services, Status.

f. Bacterial Sepsis of Newborn

Category P36, Bacterial sepsis of newborn, includes congenital sepsis. If a perinate is documented as having sepsis without documentation of congenital or community acquired, the default is congenital and a code from category P36 should be assigned. If the P36 code includes the causal organism, an additional code from category B95, Streptococcus, Staphylococcus, and Enterococcus as the cause of diseases classified elsewhere, or B96, Other bacterial agents as the cause of diseases classified elsewhere, should not be assigned. If the P36 code does not include the causal organism, assign an additional code from category B96. If applicable, use additional codes to identify severe sepsis (R65.2-) and any associated acute organ dysfunction.

g. Stillbirth

Code P95, Stillbirth, is only for use in institutions that maintain separate records for stillbirths. No other code should be used with P95. Code P95 should not be used on the mother's record.

17. **Chapter 17: Congenital malformations, deformations, and chromosomal abnormalities (Q00-Q99)**

Assign an appropriate code(s) from categories Q00-Q99, Congenital malformations, deformations, and chromosomal abnormalities when a malformation/deformation or chromosomal abnormality is documented. A malformation/deformation/or chromosomal abnormality may be the principal/first-listed diagnosis on a record or a secondary diagnosis.

When a malformation/deformation/or chromosomal abnormality does not have a unique code assignment, assign additional code(s) for any manifestations that may be present.

When the code assignment specifically identifies the malformation/deformation/or chromosomal abnormality, manifestations that are an inherent component of the anomaly should not be coded separately. Additional codes should be assigned for manifestations that are not an inherent component.

Codes from Chapter 17 may be used throughout the life of the patient. If a congenital malformation or deformity has been corrected, a personal history code should be used to identify the history of the malformation or deformity. Although present at birth, malformation/deformation/or chromosomal abnormality may not be identified until later in life. Whenever the condition is diagnosed by the physician, it is appropriate to assign a code from codes Q00-Q99.

For the birth admission, the appropriate code from category Z38, Liveborn infants, according to place of birth and type of delivery, should be sequenced as the principal diagnosis, followed by any congenital anomaly codes, Q00-Q99.

18. **Chapter 18: Symptoms, signs, and abnormal clinical and laboratory findings, not elsewhere classified (R00-R99)**

Chapter 18 includes symptoms, signs, abnormal results of clinical or other investigative procedures, and ill-defined conditions regarding which no diagnosis classifiable elsewhere is recorded. Signs and symptoms that point to a specific diagnosis have been assigned to a category in other chapters of the classification.

a. Use of symptom codes

Codes that describe symptoms and signs are acceptable for reporting purposes when a related definitive diagnosis has not been established (confirmed) by the provider.

b. Use of a symptom code with a definitive diagnosis code

Codes for signs and symptoms may be reported in addition to a related definitive diagnosis when the sign or symptom is not routinely associated with that diagnosis, such as the various signs and symptoms associated with complex syndromes. The definitive diagnosis code should be sequenced before the symptom code.

Signs or symptoms that are associated routinely with a disease process should not be assigned as additional codes, unless otherwise instructed by the classification.

c. Combination codes that include symptoms

ICD-10-CM contains a number of combination codes that identify both the definitive diagnosis and common symptoms of that diagnosis. When using one of these combination codes, an additional code should not be assigned for the symptom.

d. Repeated falls

Code R29.6, Repeated falls, is for use for encounters when a patient has recently fallen and the reason for the fall is being investigated.

Code Z91.81, History of falling, is for use when a patient has fallen in the past and is at risk for future falls. When appropriate, both codes R29.6 and Z91.81 may be assigned together.

e. Coma scale

The coma scale codes (R40.2-) can be used in conjunction with traumatic brain injury codes, acute cerebrovascular disease or sequelae of cerebrovascular disease codes. These codes are primarily for use by trauma registries, but they may be used in any setting where this information is collected. The coma scale codes should be sequenced after the diagnosis code(s).

These codes, one from each subcategory, are needed to complete the scale. The 7th character indicates when the scale was recorded. The 7th character should match for all three codes.

At a minimum, report the initial score documented on presentation at your facility. This may be a score from the emergency medicine technician (EMT) or in the emergency department. If desired, a facility may choose to capture multiple coma scale scores.

Assign code R40.24, Glasgow coma scale, total score, when only the total score is documented in the medical record and not the individual score(s).

f. Functional quadriplegia

Functional quadriplegia (code R53.2) is the lack of ability to use one's limbs or to ambulate due to extreme debility. It is not associated with neurologic deficit or injury, and code R53.2 should not be used for cases of neurologic quadriplegia. It should only be assigned if functional quadriplegia is specifically documented in the medical record.

g. SIRS due to Non-Infectious Process

The systemic inflammatory response syndrome (SIRS) can develop as a result of certain non-infectious disease processes, such as trauma, malignant neoplasm, or pancreatitis. When SIRS is documented with a noninfectious condition, and no subsequent infection is documented, the code for the underlying condition, such as an injury, should be assigned, followed by code R65.10, Systemic inflammatory response syndrome (SIRS) of non-infectious origin without acute organ dysfunction, or code R65.11, Systemic inflammatory response syndrome (SIRS) of non-infectious origin with acute organ dysfunction. If an associated acute organ dysfunction is documented, the appropriate code(s) for the specific type of organ dysfunction(s) should be assigned in addition to code R65.11. If acute organ dysfunction is documented, but it cannot be determined if the acute organ dysfunction is associated with SIRS or due to another condition (e.g., directly due to the trauma), the provider should be queried.

h. Death NOS

Code R99, Ill-defined and unknown cause of mortality, is only for use in the very limited circumstance when a patient who has already died is brought into an emergency department or other healthcare facility and is pronounced dead upon arrival. It does not represent the discharge disposition of death.

19. **Chapter 19: Injury, poisoning, and certain other consequences of external causes (S00-T88)**

a. Application of 7th Characters in Chapter 19

Most categories in chapter 19 have a 7th character requirement for each applicable code. Most categories in this chapter have three 7th character values (with the exception of fractures): A, initial encounter, D, subsequent encounter and S, sequela. Categories for traumatic fractures have additional 7th character values. **While the patient may be seen by a new or different provider over the course of treatment for an injury, assignment of the 7th character is based on whether the patient is undergoing active treatment and not whether the provider is seeing the patient for the first time.**

For complication codes, active treatment refers to treatment for the condition described by the code, even though it may be related to an earlier precipitating problem. For example, code T84.50XA, Infection and inflammatory reaction due to unspecified internal joint prosthesis, initial encounter, is used when active treatment is provided for the infection, even though the condition relates to the prosthetic device, implant or graft that was placed at a previous encounter.

7th character "A", initial encounter is used while the patient is receiving active treatment for the condition. Examples of active treatment are: surgical treatment, emergency department encounter, and evaluation and **continuing** treatment by **the same or a different** physician.

7th character "D" subsequent encounter is used for encounters after the patient has received active treatment of the condition and is receiving routine care for the condition during the healing or recovery phase. Examples of subsequent care are:

cast change or removal, **an x-ray to check healing status of fracture,** removal of external or internal fixation device, medication adjustment, other aftercare and follow up visits following treatment of the injury or condition.

The aftercare Z codes should not be used for aftercare for conditions such as injuries or poisonings, where 7th characters are provided to identify subsequent care. For example, for aftercare of an injury, assign the acute injury code with the 7th character "D" (subsequent encounter).

7th character "S", sequela, is for use for complications or conditions that arise as a direct result of a condition, such as scar formation after a burn. The scars are sequelae of the burn. When using 7th character "S", it is necessary to use both the injury code that precipitated the sequela and the code for the sequela itself. The "S" is added only to the injury code, not the sequela code. The 7th character "S" identifies the injury responsible for the sequela. The specific type of sequela (e.g. scar) is sequenced first, followed by the injury code.

See Section I.B.10. Sequelae, (Late Effects)

b. Coding of Injuries

When coding injuries, assign separate codes for each injury unless a combination code is provided, in which case the combination code is assigned. Code T07, Unspecified multiple injuries should not be assigned in the inpatient setting unless information for a more specific code is not available. Traumatic injury codes (S00-T14.9) are not to be used for normal, healing surgical wounds or to identify complications of surgical wounds.

The code for the most serious injury, as determined by the provider and the focus of treatment, is sequenced first.

1) Superficial injuries

Superficial injuries such as abrasions or contusions are not coded when associated with more severe injuries of the same site.

2) Primary injury with damage to nerves/blood vessels

When a primary injury results in minor damage to peripheral nerves or blood vessels, the primary injury is sequenced first with additional code(s) for injuries to nerves and spinal cord (such as category S04), and/or injury to blood vessels (such as category S15). When the primary injury is to the blood vessels or nerves, that injury should be sequenced first.

c. Coding of Traumatic Fractures

The principles of multiple coding of injuries should be followed in coding fractures. Fractures of specified sites are coded individually by site in accordance with both the provisions within categories S02, S12, S22, S32, S42, S49, S52, S59, S62, S72, S79, S82, S89, S92 and the level of detail furnished by medical record content.

A fracture not indicated as open or closed should be coded to closed. A fracture not indicated whether displaced or not displaced should be coded to displaced.

More specific guidelines are as follows:

1) Initial vs. Subsequent Encounter for Fractures

Traumatic fractures are coded using the appropriate 7th character for initial encounter (A, B, C) while the patient is receiving active treatment for the fracture. Examples of active treatment are: surgical treatment, emergency department encounter, and evaluation and **continuing (ongoing)** treatment by **the same or a different** physician. The appropriate 7th character for initial encounter should also be assigned for a patient who delayed seeking treatment for the fracture or nonunion.

Fractures are coded using the appropriate 7th character for subsequent care for encounters after the patient has completed active treatment of the fracture and is receiving routine care for the fracture during the healing or recovery phase. Examples of fracture aftercare are: cast change or removal, **an x-ray to check healing status of fracture,** removal of external or internal fixation device, medication adjustment, and follow-up visits following fracture treatment.

Care for complications of surgical treatment for fracture repairs during the healing or recovery phase should be coded with the appropriate complication codes.

Care of complications of fractures, such as malunion and nonunion, should be reported with the appropriate 7th character for subsequent care with nonunion (K, M, N,) or subsequent care with malunion (P, Q, R).

Malunion/nonunion: The appropriate 7th character for initial encounter should also be assigned for a patient who delayed seeking treatment for the fracture or nonunion.

A code from category M80, not a traumatic fracture code, should be used for any patient with known osteoporosis who suffers a fracture, even if the patient had a minor fall or trauma, if that fall or trauma would not usually break a normal, healthy bone.

See Section I.C.13. Osteoporosis.

The aftercare Z codes should not be used for aftercare for traumatic fractures. For aftercare of a traumatic fracture, assign the acute fracture code with the appropriate 7th character.

2) Multiple fractures sequencing

Multiple fractures are sequenced in accordance with the severity of the fracture.

d. Coding of Burns and Corrosions

The ICD-10-CM makes a distinction between burns and corrosions. The burn codes are for thermal burns, except sunburns, that come from a heat source, such as a fire or hot appliance. The burn codes are also for burns resulting from electricity and radiation. Corrosions are burns due to chemicals. The guidelines are the same for burns and corrosions.

Current burns (T20-T25) are classified by depth, extent and by agent (X code). Burns are classified by depth as first degree (erythema), second degree (blistering), and third degree (full-thickness involvement). Burns of the eye and internal organs (T26-T28) are classified by site, but not by degree.

1) Sequencing of burn and related condition codes

Sequence first the code that reflects the highest degree of burn when more than one burn is present.

    a. When the reason for the admission or encounter is for treatment of external multiple burns, sequence first the code that reflects the burn of the highest degree.

    b. When a patient has both internal and external burns, the circumstances of admission govern the selection of the principal diagnosis or first-listed diagnosis.

    c. When a patient is admitted for burn injuries and other related conditions such as smoke inhalation and/or respiratory failure, the circumstances of admission govern the selection of the principal or first-listed diagnosis.

2) Burns of the same local site

Classify burns of the same local site (three-character category level, T20-T28) but of different degrees to the subcategory identifying the highest degree recorded in the diagnosis.

3) Non-healing burns

Non-healing burns are coded as acute burns.

Necrosis of burned skin should be coded as a non-healed burn.

4) Infected Burn

For any documented infected burn site, use an additional code for the infection.

5) Assign separate codes for each burn site

When coding burns, assign separate codes for each burn site. Category T30, Burn and corrosion, body region unspecified is extremely vague and should rarely be used.

6) Burns and Corrosions Classified According to Extent of Body Surface Involved

Assign codes from category T31, Burns classified according to extent of body surface involved, or T32, Corrosions classified according to extent of body surface involved, when the site of the burn is not specified or when there is a need for additional data. It is advisable to use category T31 as additional coding when needed to provide data for evaluating burn mortality, such as that needed by burn units. It is also advisable to use category T31 as an additional code for reporting purposes when there is mention of a third-degree burn involving 20 percent or more of the body surface.

Categories T31 and T32 are based on the classic "rule of nines" in estimating body surface involved: head and neck are assigned nine percent, each arm nine percent, each leg 18 percent, the anterior trunk 18 percent, posterior trunk 18 percent, and genitalia one percent. Providers may change these percentage assignments where necessary to accommodate infants and children who have proportionately larger heads than adults, and patients who have large buttocks, thighs, or abdomen that involve burns.

7) Encounters for treatment of sequela of burns

Encounters for the treatment of the late effects of burns or corrosions (i.e., scars or joint contractures) should be coded with a burn or corrosion code with the 7th character "S" for sequela.

8) Sequelae with a late effect code and current burn

When appropriate, both a code for a current burn or corrosion with 7th character "A" or "D" and a burn or corrosion code with 7th character "S" may be assigned on the same record (when both a current burn and sequelae of an old burn exist). Burns and corrosions do not heal at the same rate and a current healing wound may still exist with sequela of a healed burn or corrosion.

See Section I.B.10. Sequela, (Late Effects)

9) Use of an external cause code with burns and corrosions

An external cause code should be used with burns and corrosions to identify the source and intent of the burn, as well as the place where it occurred.

e. Adverse Effects, Poisoning , Underdosing and Toxic Effects

Codes in categories T36-T65 are combination codes that include the substance that was taken as well as the intent. No additional external cause code is required for poisonings, toxic effects, adverse effects and underdosing codes.

1) Do not code directly from the Table of Drugs

Do not code directly from the Table of Drugs and Chemicals. Always refer back to the Tabular List.

2) Use as many codes as necessary to describe

Use as many codes as necessary to describe completely all drugs, medicinal or biological substances.

3) If the same code would describe the causative agent

If the same code would describe the causative agent for more than one adverse reaction, poisoning, toxic effect or underdosing, assign the code only once.

4) If two or more drugs, medicinal or biological substances

If two or more drugs, medicinal or biological substances are reported, code each individually unless a combination code is listed in the Table of Drugs and Chemicals.

5) The occurrence of drug toxicity is classified in ICD-10-CM as follows:

(a) Adverse Effect

When coding an adverse effect of a drug that has been correctly prescribed and properly administered, assign the appropriate code for the nature of the adverse effect followed by the appropriate code for the adverse effect of the drug (T36-T50). The code for the drug should have a 5th or 6th character "5" (for example

T36.0X5-) Examples of the nature of an adverse effect are tachycardia, delirium, gastrointestinal hemorrhaging, vomiting, hypokalemia, hepatitis, renal failure, or respiratory failure.

(b) Poisoning

When coding a poisoning or reaction to the improper use of a medication (e.g., overdose, wrong substance given or taken in error, wrong route of administration), first assign the appropriate code from categories T36-T50. The poisoning codes have an associated intent as their 5th or 6th character (accidental, intentional self-harm, assault and undetermined). Use additional code(s) for all manifestations of poisonings.

If there is also a diagnosis of abuse or dependence of the substance, the abuse or dependence is assigned as an additional code.

Examples of poisoning include:

(i) Error was made in drug prescription Errors made in drug prescription or in the administration of the drug by provider, nurse, patient, or other person.

(ii) Overdose of a drug intentionally taken If an overdose of a drug was intentionally taken or administered and resulted in drug toxicity, it would be coded as a poisoning.

(iii) Nonprescribed drug taken with correctly prescribed and properly administered drug.
If a nonprescribed drug or medicinal agent was taken in combination with a correctly prescribed and properly administered drug, any drug toxicity or other reaction resulting from the interaction of the two drugs would be classified as a poisoning.

(iv) Interaction of drug(s) and alcohol. When a reaction results from the interaction of a drug(s) and alcohol, this would be classified as poisoning.

See Section I.C.4. if poisoning is the result of insulin pump malfunctions.

(c) Underdosing

Underdosing refers to taking less of a medication than is prescribed by a provider or a manufacturer's instruction. For underdosing, assign the code from categories T36-T50 (fifth or sixth character "6").

Codes for underdosing should never be assigned as principal or first-listed codes. If a patient has a relapse or exacerbation of the medical condition for which the drug is prescribed because of the reduction in dose, then the medical condition itself should be coded.

Noncompliance (Z91.12-, Z91.13-) or complication of care (Y63.6-Y63.9) codes are to be used with an underdosing code to indicate intent, if known.

(d) Toxic Effects

When a harmful substance is ingested or comes in contact with a person, this is classified as a toxic effect. The toxic effect codes are in categories T51-T65.

Toxic effect codes have an associated intent: accidental, intentional self-harm, assault and undetermined.

f. Adult and child abuse, neglect and other maltreatment

Sequence first the appropriate code from categories T74.- (Adult and child abuse, neglect and other maltreatment, confirmed) or T76.- (Adult and child abuse, neglect and other maltreatment, suspected) for abuse, neglect and other maltreatment, followed by any accompanying mental health or injury code(s).

If the documentation in the medical record states abuse or neglect it is coded as confirmed (T74.-). It is coded as suspected if it is documented as suspected (T76.-).

For cases of confirmed abuse or neglect an external cause code from the assault section (X92-Y08) should be added to identify the cause of any physical injuries. A perpetrator code (Y07) should be added when the perpetrator of the abuse is known. For suspected cases of abuse or neglect, do not report external cause or perpetrator code.

If a suspected case of abuse, neglect or mistreatment is ruled out during an encounter code Z04.71, Encounter for examination and observation following alleged physical adult abuse, ruled out, or code Z04.72, Encounter for examination and observation following alleged child physical abuse, ruled out, should be used, not a code from T76.

If a suspected case of alleged rape or sexual abuse is ruled out during an encounter code Z04.41, Encounter for examination and observation following alleged physical adult abuse, ruled out, or code Z04.42, Encounter for examination and observation following alleged rape or sexual abuse, ruled out, should be used, not a code from T76.

See Section I.C.15. Abuse in a pregnant patient.

g. Complications of care

1) General guidelines for complications of care

(a) Documentation of complications of care

See Section I.B.16. for information on documentation of complications of care.

2) Pain due to medical devices

Pain associated with devices, implants or grafts left in a surgical site (for example painful hip prosthesis) is assigned to the appropriate code(s) found in Chapter 19, Injury, poisoning, and certain other consequences of external causes. Specific codes for pain due to medical devices are found in the T code section of the ICD-10-CM. Use additional code(s) from category G89 to identify acute or chronic pain due to presence of the device, implant or graft (G89.18 or G89.28).

3) Transplant complications

(a) Transplant complications other than kidney

Codes under category T86, Complications of transplanted organs and tissues, are for use for both complications and rejection of transplanted organs. A transplant complication code is only assigned if the complication affects the function of the transplanted organ. Two codes are required to fully describe a transplant complication: the appropriate code from category T86 and a secondary code that identifies the complication.

Pre-existing conditions or conditions that develop after the transplant are not coded as complications unless they affect the function of the transplanted organs.

See I.C.21. for transplant organ removal status
See I.C.2. for malignant neoplasm associated with transplanted organ.

(b) Kidney transplant complications

Patients who have undergone kidney transplant may still have some form of chronic kidney disease (CKD) because the kidney transplant may not fully restore kidney function. Code T86.1- should be assigned for documented complications of a kidney transplant, such as transplant failure or rejection or other transplant complication. Code T86.1- should not be assigned for post kidney transplant patients who have chronic kidney (CKD) unless a transplant complication such as transplant failure or rejection is documented. If the documentation is unclear as to whether the patient has a complication of the transplant, query the provider.

Conditions that affect the function of the transplanted kidney, other than CKD, should be assigned a code from subcategory T86.1, Complications of transplanted organ, Kidney, and a secondary code that identifies the complication.

For patients with CKD following a kidney transplant, but who do not have a complication such as failure or rejection, *see section I.C.14. Chronic kidney disease and kidney transplant status.*

4) Complication codes that include the external cause

As with certain other T codes, some of the complications of care codes have the external cause included in the code. The code includes the nature of the complication as well as the type of procedure that caused the complication. No external cause code indicating the type of procedure is necessary for these codes.

5) Complications of care codes within the body system chapters

Intraoperative and postprocedural complication codes are found within the body system chapters with codes specific to the organs and structures of that body system. These codes should be sequenced first, followed by a code(s) for the specific complication, if applicable.

20. Chapter 20: External Causes of Morbidity (V00-Y99)

The external causes of morbidity codes should never be sequenced as the first-listed or principal diagnosis.

External cause codes are intended to provide data for injury research and evaluation of injury prevention strategies. These codes capture how the injury or health condition happened (cause), the intent (unintentional or accidental; or intentional, such as suicide or assault), the place where the event occurred the activity of the patient at the time of the event, and the person's status (e.g., civilian, military).

There is no national requirement for mandatory ICD-10-CM external cause code reporting. Unless a provider is subject to a state-based external cause code reporting mandate or these codes are required by a particular payer, reporting of ICD-10-CM codes in Chapter 20, External Causes of Morbidity, is not required. In the absence of a mandatory reporting requirement, providers are encouraged to voluntarily report external cause codes, as they provide valuable data for injury research and evaluation of injury prevention strategies.

a. General External Cause Coding Guidelines

1) Used with any code in the range of A00.0-T88.9, Z00-Z99

An external cause code may be used with any code in the range of A00.0-T88.9, Z00-Z99, classification that is a health condition due to an external cause. Though they are most applicable to injuries, they are also valid for use with such things as infections or diseases due to an external source, and other health conditions, such as a heart attack that occurs during strenuous physical activity.

2) External cause code used for length of treatment

Assign the external cause code, with the appropriate 7th character (initial encounter, subsequent encounter or sequela) for each encounter for which the injury or condition is being treated.

Most categories in chapter 20 have a 7th character requirement for each applicable code. Most categories in this chapter have three 7th character values: A, initial encounter, D, subsequent encounter and S, sequela. While the patient may be seen by a new or different provider over the course of treatment for an injury or condition, assignment of the 7th character for external cause should match the 7th character of the code assigned for the associated injury or condition for the encounter.

3) Use the full range of external cause codes

Use the full range of external cause codes to completely describe the cause, the intent, the place of occurrence and if applicable, the activity of the patient at the time of the event, and the patient's status, for all injuries, and other health conditions due to an external cause.

4) Assign as many external cause codes as necessary

Assign as many external cause codes as necessary to fully explain each cause. If only one external code can be recorded, assign the code most related to the principal diagnosis.

5) The selection of the appropriate external cause code

The selection of the appropriate external cause code is guided by the Alphabetic Index of External Causes and by Inclusion and Exclusion notes in the Tabular List.

6) External cause code can never be a principal diagnosis

An external cause code can never be a principal (first-listed) diagnosis.

7) Combination external cause codes

Certain of the external cause codes are combination codes that identify sequential events that result in an injury, such as a fall which results in striking against an object. The injury may be due to either event or both. The combination external cause code used should correspond to the sequence of events regardless of which caused the most serious injury.

8) No external cause code needed in certain circumstances

No external cause code from Chapter 20 is needed if the external cause and intent are included in a code from another chapter (e.g. T36.0X1- Poisoning by penicillins, accidental (unintentional)).

b. Place of Occurrence Guideline

Codes from category Y92, Place of occurrence of the external cause, are secondary codes for use after other external cause codes to identify the location of the patient at the time of injury or other condition.

Generally, a place of occurrence code is **assigned** only once, at the initial encounter for treatment. **However, in the rare instance that a new injury occurs during hospitalization, an additional place of occurrence code may be assigned.** No 7th characters are used for Y92. Only one code from Y92 should be recorded on a medical record.

Do not use place of occurrence code Y92.9 if the place is not stated or is not applicable.

c. Activity Code

Assign a code from category Y93, Activity code, to describe the activity of the patient at the time the injury or other health condition occurred.

An activity code is used only once, at the initial encounter for treatment. Only one code from Y93 should be recorded on a medical record.

The activity codes are not applicable to poisonings, adverse effects, misadventures or sequela.

Do not assign Y93.9, Unspecified activity, if the activity is not stated.

A code from category Y93 is appropriate for use with external cause and intent codes if identifying the activity provides additional information about the event.

d. Place of Occurrence, Activity, and Status Codes Used with other External Cause Code

When applicable, place of occurrence, activity, and external cause status codes are sequenced after the main external cause code(s). Regardless of the number of external cause codes assigned, there should be only one place of occurrence code, one activity code, and one external cause status code assigned to an encounter.

e. If the Reporting Format Limits the Number of External Cause Codes

If the reporting format limits the number of external cause codes that can be used in reporting clinical data, report the code for the cause/intent most related to the principal diagnosis. If the format permits capture of additional external cause codes, the cause/intent, including medical misadventures, of the additional events should be reported rather than the codes for place, activity, or external status.

f. Multiple External Cause Coding Guidelines

More than one external cause code is required to fully describe the external cause of an illness or injury. The assignment of external cause codes should be sequenced in the following priority:

If two or more events cause separate injuries, an external cause code should be assigned for each cause. The first-listed external cause code will be selected in the following order:

External codes for child and adult abuse take priority over all other external cause codes.
See Section I.C.19., Child and Adult abuse guidelines.

External codes for terrorism events take priority over all other external cause codes except child and adult abuse.

External cause codes for cataclysmic events take priority over all other external cause codes except child and adult abuse and terrorism.

External cause codes for transport accidents take priority over all other external cause codes except cataclysmic events, child and adult abuse and terrorism.

Activity and external cause status codes are assigned following all causal (intent) external cause codes.

The first-listed external cause code should correspond to the cause of the most serious diagnosis due to an assault, accident, or self-harm, following the order of hierarchy listed above.

g. Child and Adult Abuse Guideline

Adult and child abuse, neglect and maltreatment are classified as assault. Any of the assault codes may be used to indicate the external cause of any injury resulting from the confirmed abuse.

For confirmed cases of abuse, neglect and maltreatment, when the perpetrator is known, a code from Y07, Perpetrator of maltreatment and neglect, should accompany any other assault codes.
See Section I.C.19. Adult and child abuse, neglect and other maltreatment

h. Unknown or Undetermined Intent Guideline

If the intent (accident, self-harm, assault) of the cause of an injury or other condition is unknown or unspecified, code the intent as accidental intent. All transport accident categories assume accidental intent.

    1) Use of undetermined intent

External cause codes for events of undetermined intent are only for use if the documentation in the record specifies that the intent cannot be determined.

i. Sequelae (Late Effects) of External Cause Guidelines

    1) Sequelae external cause codes

Sequela are reported using the external cause code with the 7th character "S" for sequela. These codes should be used with any report of a late effect or sequela resulting from a previous injury.

    See Section I.B.10. Sequela, (Late Effects)

    2) Sequela external cause code with a related current injury

A sequela external cause code should never be used with a related current nature of injury code.

    3) Use of sequela external cause codes for subsequent visits

Use a late effect external cause code for subsequent visits when a late effect of the initial injury is being treated. Do not use a late effect external cause code for subsequent visits for follow-up care (e.g., to assess healing, to receive rehabilitative therapy) of the injury when no late effect of the injury has been documented.

j. Terrorism Guidelines

    1) Cause of injury identified by the Federal Government (FBI) as terrorism

When the cause of an injury is identified by the Federal Government (FBI) as terrorism, the first-listed external cause code should be a code from category Y38, Terrorism. The definition of terrorism employed by the FBI is found at the inclusion note at the beginning of category Y38. Use additional code for place of occurrence (Y92.-). More than one Y38 code may be assigned if the injury is the result of more than one mechanism of terrorism.

    2) Cause of an injury is suspected to be the result of terrorism

When the cause of an injury is suspected to be the result of terrorism a code from category Y38 should not be assigned. Suspected cases should be classified as assault.

    3) Code Y38.9, Terrorism, secondary effects

Assign code Y38.9, Terrorism, secondary effects, for conditions occurring subsequent to the terrorist event. This code should not be assigned for conditions that are due to the initial terrorist act.

It is acceptable to assign code Y38.9 with another code from Y38 if there is an injury due to the initial terrorist event and an injury that is a subsequent result of the terrorist event.

k. External cause status

A code from category Y99, External cause status, should be assigned whenever any other external cause code is assigned for an encounter, including an Activity code, except for the events noted below. Assign a code from category Y99, External cause status, to indicate the work status of the person at the time the event occurred. The status code indicates whether the event occurred during military activity, whether a non-military person was at work, whether an individual including a student or volunteer was involved in a non-work activity at the time of the causal event.

A code from Y99, External cause status, should be assigned, when applicable, with other external cause codes, such as transport accidents and falls. The external cause status codes are not applicable to poisonings, adverse effects, misadventures or late effects.

Do not assign a code from category Y99 if no other external cause codes (cause, activity) are applicable for the encounter.

An external cause status code is used only once, at the initial encounter for treatment. Only one code from Y99 should be recorded on a medical record.

Do not assign code Y99.9, Unspecified external cause status, if the status is not stated.

21. **Chapter 21: Factors influencing health status and contact with health services (Z00-Z99)**

Note: The chapter specific guidelines provide additional information about the use of Z codes for specified encounters.

a. Use of Z codes in any healthcare setting

Z codes are for use in any healthcare setting. Z codes may be used as either a first-listed (principal diagnosis code in the inpatient setting) or secondary code, depending on the circumstances of the encounter. Certain Z codes may only be used as first-listed or principal diagnosis.

b. Z Codes indicate a reason for an encounter

Z codes are not procedure codes. A corresponding procedure code must accompany a Z code to describe any procedure performed.

c. Categories of Z Codes

    1) Contact/Exposure

Category Z20 indicates contact with, and suspected exposure to, communicable diseases. These codes are for patients who do not show any sign or symptom of a disease but are suspected to have been exposed to it by close personal contact with an infected individual or are in an area where a disease is epidemic.

Category Z77, **Other contact with and (suspected) exposures hazardous to health,** indicates contact with and suspected exposures hazardous to health.

Contact/exposure codes may be used as a first-listed code to explain an encounter for testing, or, more commonly, as a secondary code to identify a potential risk.

2) Inoculations and vaccinations

Code Z23 is for encounters for inoculations and vaccinations. It indicates that a patient is being seen to receive a prophylactic inoculation against a disease. Procedure codes are required to identify the actual administration of the injection and the type(s) of immunizations given. Code Z23 may be used as a secondary code if the inoculation is given as a routine part of preventive health care, such as a well-baby visit.

3) Status

Status codes indicate that a patient is either a carrier of a disease or has the sequelae or residual of a past disease or condition. This includes such things as the presence of prosthetic or mechanical devices resulting from past treatment. A status code is informative, because the status may affect the course of treatment and its outcome. A status code is distinct from a history code. The history code indicates that the patient no longer has the condition.

A status code should not be used with a diagnosis code from one of the body system chapters, if the diagnosis code includes the information provided by the status code. For example, code Z94.1, Heart transplant status, should not be used with a code from subcategory T86.2, Complications of heart transplant. The status code does not provide additional information. The complication code indicates that the patient is a heart transplant patient.

For encounters for weaning from a mechanical ventilator, assign a code from subcategory J96.1, Chronic respiratory failure, followed by code Z99.11, Dependence on respirator [ventilator] status.

The status Z codes/categories are:

Z14   Genetic carrier
Genetic carrier status indicates that a person carries a gene, associated with a particular disease, which may be passed to offspring who may develop that disease. The person does not have the disease and is not at risk of developing the disease.

Z15   Genetic susceptibility to disease Genetic susceptibility indicates that a person has a gene that increases the risk of that person developing the disease.

Codes from category Z15 should not be used as principal or first-listed codes. If the patient has the condition to which he/she is susceptible, and that condition is the reason for the encounter, the code for the current condition should be sequenced first. If the patient is being seen for follow-up after completed treatment for this condition, and the condition no longer exists, a follow-up code should be sequenced first, followed by the appropriate personal history and genetic susceptibility codes. If the purpose of the encounter is genetic counseling associated with procreative management, code Z31.5, Encounter for genetic counseling, should be assigned as the first-listed code, followed by a code from category Z15. Additional codes should be assigned for any applicable family or personal history.

Z16   Resistance to antimicrobial drugs
This code indicates that a patient has a condition that is resistant to antimicrobial drug treatment. Sequence the infection code first.

Z17   Estrogen receptor status
Z18   Retained foreign body fragments
Z21   Asymptomatic HIV infection status This code indicates that a patient has tested positive for HIV but has manifested no signs or symptoms of the disease.
Z22   Carrier of infectious disease Carrier status indicates that a person harbors the specific organisms of a disease without manifest symptoms and is capable of transmitting the infection.
Z28.3   Underimmunization status
Z33.1   Pregnant state, incidental This code is a secondary code only for use when the pregnancy is in no way complicating the reason for visit. Otherwise, a code from the obstetric chapter is required.
Z66   Do not resuscitate
This code may be used when it is documented by the provider that a patient is on do not resuscitate status at any time during the stay.
Z67   Blood type
Z68   Body mass index (BMI)
Z74.01   Bed confinement status
Z76.82   Awaiting organ transplant status
Z78   Other specified health status
Code Z78.1, Physical restraint status, may be used when it is documented by the provider that a patient has been put in restraints during the current encounter. Please note that this code should not be reported when it is documented by the provider that a patient is temporarily restrained during a procedure.
Z79   Long-term (current) drug therapy
Codes from this category indicate a patient's continuous use of a prescribed drug (including such things as aspirin therapy) for the long-term treatment of a condition or for prophylactic use. It is not for use for patients who have addictions to drugs. This subcategory is not for use of medications for detoxification or maintenance programs to prevent withdrawal symptoms in patients with drug dependence (e.g., methadone maintenance for opiate dependence). Assign the appropriate code for the drug dependence instead.

Assign a code from Z79 if the patient is receiving a medication for an extended period as a prophylactic measure (such as for the prevention of deep vein thrombosis) or as treatment of a chronic condition (such as arthritis) or a disease requiring a lengthy course of treatment (such as cancer). Do not assign a code from category Z79 for medication being administered for a brief period of time to treat an acute illness or injury (such as a course of antibiotics to treat acute bronchitis).

Z88   Allergy status to drugs, medicaments and biological substances Except: Z88.9, Allergy status to unspecified drugs, medicaments and biological substances status

Z89   Acquired absence of limb

Z90   Acquired absence of organs, not elsewhere classified

Z91.0- Allergy status, other than to drugs and biological substances

Z92.82 Status post administration of tPA (rtPA) in a different facility within the last 24 hours prior to admission to a current facility Assign code Z92.82, Status post administration of tPA (rtPA) in a different facility within the last 24 hours prior to admission to current facility, as a secondary diagnosis when a patient is received by transfer into a facility and documentation indicates they were administered tissue plasminogen activator (tPA) within the last 24 hours prior to admission to the current facility. This guideline applies even if the patient is still receiving the tPA at the time they are received into the current facility. The appropriate code for the condition for which the tPA was administered (such as cerebrovascular disease or myocardial infarction) should be assigned first. Code Z92.82 is only applicable to the receiving facility record and not to the transferring facility record.

Z93   Artificial opening status

Z94   Transplanted organ and tissue status

Z95   Presence of cardiac and vascular implants and grafts

Z96   Presence of other functional implants

Z97   Presence of other devices

Z98   Other postprocedural states

Assign code Z98.85, Transplanted organ removal status, to indicate that a transplanted organ has been previously removed. This code should not be assigned for the encounter in which the transplanted organ is removed. The complication necessitating removal of the transplant organ should be assigned for that encounter.

See section I.C.19. for information on the coding of organ transplant complications.

Z99   Dependence on enabling machines and devices, not elsewhere classified

Note: Categories Z89-Z90 and Z93-Z99 are for use only if there are no complications or malfunctions of the organ or tissue replaced, the amputation site or the equipment on which the patient is dependent.

4) History (of)

There are two types of history Z codes, personal and family. Personal history codes explain a patient's past medical condition that no longer exists and is not receiving any treatment, but that has the potential for recurrence, and therefore may require continued monitoring.

Family history codes are for use when a patient has a family member(s) who has had a particular disease that causes the patient to be at higher risk of also contracting the disease.

Personal history codes may be used in conjunction with follow-up codes and family history codes may be used in conjunction with screening codes to explain the need for a test or procedure. History codes are also acceptable on any medical record regardless of the reason for visit. A history of an illness, even if no longer present, is important information that may alter the type of treatment ordered.

The history Z code categories are:

Z80   Family history of primary malignant neoplasm

Z81   Family history of mental and behavioral disorders

Z82   Family history of certain disabilities and chronic diseases (leading to disablement)

Z83   Family history of other specific disorders

Z84   Family history of other conditions

Z85   Personal history of malignant neoplasm

Z86   Personal history of certain other diseases

Z87   Personal history of other diseases and conditions

Z91.4- Personal history of psychological trauma, not elsewhere classified

Z91.5   Personal history of self-harm

Z91.8- Other specified personal risk factors, not elsewhere classified
        Exception:
        Z91.83, Wandering in diseases classified elsewhere

Z92   Personal history of medical treatment Except: Z92.0, Personal history of contraception Except: Z92.82, Status post administration of tPA (rtPA) in a different facility within the last 24 hours prior to admission to a current facility

5) Screening

Screening is the testing for disease or disease precursors in seemingly well individuals so that early detection and treatment can be provided for those who test positive for the disease (e.g., screening mammogram).

The testing of a person to rule out or confirm a suspected diagnosis because the patient has some sign or symptom is a diagnostic examination, not a screening. In these cases, the sign or symptom is used to explain the reason for the test.

A screening code may be a first-listed code if the reason for the visit is specifically the screening exam. It may also be used as an additional code if the screening is done during an office visit for other health problems. A screening code is not necessary if the screening is inherent to a routine examination, such as a pap smear done during a routine pelvic examination.

Should a condition be discovered during the screening then the code for the condition may be assigned as an additional diagnosis.

The Z code indicates that a screening exam is planned. A procedure code is required to confirm that the screening was performed.

The screening Z codes/categories:

Z11   Encounter for screening for infectious and parasitic diseases

Z12   Encounter for screening for malignant neoplasms

Z13   Encounter for screening for other diseases and disorders Except: Z13.9, Encounter for screening, unspecified

Z36   Encounter for antenatal screening for mother

6) Observation

There are two observation Z code categories. They are for use in very limited circumstances when a person is being observed for a suspected condition that is ruled out. The observation codes are not for use if an injury or illness or any signs or symptoms related to the suspected condition are present. In such cases the diagnosis/symptom code is used with the corresponding external cause code.

The observation codes are to be used as principal diagnosis only. Additional codes may be used in addition to the observation code but only if they are unrelated to the suspected condition being observed.

Codes from subcategory Z03.7 Encounter for suspected maternal and fetal conditions ruled out, may either be used as a first-listed or as an additional code assignment depending on the case. They are for use in very limited circumstances on a maternal record when an encounter is for a suspected maternal or fetal condition that is ruled out during that encounter (for example, a maternal or fetal condition may be suspected due to an abnormal test result). These codes should not be used when the condition is confirmed. In those cases, the confirmed condition should be coded. In addition, these codes are not for use if an illness or any signs or symptoms related to the suspected condition or problem are present. In such cases the diagnosis/symptom code is used.

Additional codes may be used in addition to the code from subcategory Z03.7, but only if they are unrelated to the suspected condition being evaluated.

Codes from subcategory Z03.7 may not be used for encounters for antenatal screening of mother. *See Section I.C.21. Screening.*

For encounters for suspected fetal condition that are inconclusive following testing and evaluation, assign the appropriate code from category O35, O36, O40 or O41.

The observation Z code categories:

Z03   Encounter for medical observation for suspected diseases and conditions ruled out

Z04   Encounter for examination and observation for other reasons Except: Z04.9, Encounter for examination and observation for unspecified reason

7) Aftercare

Aftercare visit codes cover situations when the initial treatment of a disease has been performed and the patient requires continued care during the healing or recovery phase, or for the long-term consequences of the disease. The aftercare Z code should not be used if treatment is directed at a current, acute disease. The diagnosis code is to be used in these cases.

Exceptions to this rule are codes Z51.0, Encounter for antineoplastic radiation therapy, and codes from subcategory Z51.1, Encounter for antineoplastic chemotherapy and immunotherapy. These codes are to be first-listed, followed by the diagnosis code when a patient's encounter is solely to receive radiation therapy, chemotherapy, or immunotherapy for the treatment of a neoplasm. If the reason for the encounter is more than one type of antineoplastic therapy, code Z51.0 and a code from subcategory Z51.1 may be assigned together, in which case one of these codes would be reported as a secondary diagnosis.

The aftercare Z codes should also not be used for aftercare for injuries. For aftercare of an injury, assign the acute injury code with the appropriate 7th character (for subsequent encounter).

The aftercare codes are generally first-listed to explain the specific reason for the encounter. An aftercare code may be used as an additional code when some type of aftercare is provided in addition to the reason for admission and no diagnosis code is applicable. An example of this would be the closure of a colostomy during an encounter for treatment of another condition.

Aftercare codes should be used in conjunction with other aftercare codes or diagnosis codes to provide better detail on the specifics of an aftercare encounter visit, unless otherwise directed by the classification. Should a patient receive multiple types of antineoplastic therapy during the same encounter, code Z51.0, Encounter for antineoplastic radiation therapy, and codes from subcategory Z51.1, Encounter for antineoplastic chemotherapy and immunotherapy, may be used together on a record. The sequencing of multiple aftercare codes depends on the circumstances of the encounter.

Certain aftercare Z code categories need a secondary diagnosis code to describe the resolving condition or sequelae. For others, the condition is included in the code title.

Additional Z code aftercare category terms include fitting and adjustment, and attention to artificial openings.

Status Z codes may be used with aftercare Z codes to indicate the nature of the aftercare. For example code Z95.1, Presence of aortocoronary bypass graft, may be used with code Z48.812, Encounter for surgical aftercare following surgery on the circulatory system, to indicate the surgery for which the aftercare is being performed. A status code should not be used when the aftercare code indicates the type of status, such as using Z43.0, Encounter for attention to tracheostomy, with Z93.0, Tracheostomy status.

The aftercare Z category/codes:

Z42	Encounter for plastic and reconstructive surgery following medical procedure or healed injury
Z43	Encounter for attention to artificial openings
Z44	Encounter for fitting and adjustment of external prosthetic device
Z45	Encounter for adjustment and management of implanted device
Z46	Encounter for fitting and adjustment of other devices
Z47	Orthopedic aftercare
Z48	Encounter for other postprocedural aftercare
Z49	Encounter for care involving renal dialysis
Z51	Encounter for other aftercare

8) Follow-up

The follow-up codes are used to explain continuing surveillance following completed treatment of a disease, condition, or injury. They imply that the condition has been fully treated and no longer exists. They should not be confused with aftercare codes, or injury codes with a 7th character for subsequent encounter, that explain ongoing care of a healing condition or its sequelae. Follow-up codes may be used in conjunction with history codes to provide the full picture of the healed condition and its treatment. The follow-up code is sequenced first, followed by the history code.

A follow-up code may be used to explain multiple visits. Should a condition be found to have recurred on the follow-up visit, then the diagnosis code for the condition should be assigned in place of the follow-up code.

The follow-up Z code categories:

Z08	Encounter for follow-up examination after completed treatment for malignant neoplasm
Z09	Encounter for follow-up examination after completed treatment for conditions other than malignant neoplasm
Z39	Encounter for maternal postpartum care and examination

9) Donor

Codes in category Z52, Donors of organs and tissues, are used for living individuals who are donating blood or other body tissue. These codes are only for individuals donating for others, not for self-donations. They are not used to identify cadaveric donations.

10) Counseling

Counseling Z codes are used when a patient or family member receives assistance in the aftermath of an illness or injury, or when support is required in coping with family or social problems. They are not used in conjunction with a diagnosis code when the counseling component of care is considered integral to standard treatment.

The counseling Z codes/categories:

Z30.0-	Encounter for general counseling and advice on contraception
Z31.5	Encounter for genetic counseling
Z31.6-	Encounter for general counseling and advice on procreation
Z32.2	Encounter for childbirth instruction
Z32.3	Encounter for childcare instruction
Z69	Encounter for mental health services for victim and perpetrator of abuse
Z70	Counseling related to sexual attitude, behavior and orientation
Z71	Persons encountering health services for other counseling and medical advice, not elsewhere classified
Z76.81	Expectant mother prebirth pediatrician visit

11) Encounters for Obstetrical and Reproductive Services

See Section I.C.15. Pregnancy, Childbirth, and the Puerperium, for further instruction on the use of these codes.

Z codes for pregnancy are for use in those circumstances when none of the problems or complications included in the codes from the Obstetrics chapter exist (a routine prenatal visit or postpartum care). Codes in category Z34, Encounter for supervision of normal pregnancy, are always first listed and are not to be used with any other code from the OB chapter.

Codes in category Z3A, Weeks of gestation, may be assigned to provide additional information about the pregnancy.

The date of the admission should be used to determine weeks of gestation for inpatient admissions that encompass more than one gestational week.

The outcome of delivery, category Z37, should be included on all maternal delivery records. It is always a secondary code. Codes in category Z37 should not be used on the newborn record.

Z codes for family planning (contraceptive) or procreative management and counseling should be included on an obstetric record either during the pregnancy or the postpartum stage, if applicable.

Z codes/categories for obstetrical and reproductive services:

Z30	Encounter for contraceptive management
Z31	Encounter for procreative management
Z32.2	Encounter for childbirth instruction
Z32.3	Encounter for childcare instruction
Z33	Pregnant state
Z34	Encounter for supervision of normal pregnancy

Z36	Encounter for antenatal screening of mother
Z3A	Weeks of gestation
Z37	Outcome of delivery
Z39	Encounter for maternal postpartum care and examination
Z76.81	Expectant mother prebirth pediatrician visit

12) Newborns and Infants

See Section I.C.16. Newborn (Perinatal) Guidelines, for further instruction on the use of these codes.

Newborn Z codes/categories:

Z76.1	Encounter for health supervision and care of foundling
Z00.1-	Encounter for routine child health examination
Z38	Liveborn infants according to place of birth and type of delivery

13) Routine and administrative examinations

The Z codes allow for the description of encounters for routine examinations, such as, a general check-up, or, examinations for administrative purposes, such as, a pre-employment physical. The codes are not to be used if the examination is for diagnosis of a suspected condition or for treatment purposes. In such cases the diagnosis code is used. During a routine exam, should a diagnosis or condition be discovered, it should be coded as an additional code. Pre-existing and chronic conditions and history codes may also be included as additional codes as long as the examination is for administrative purposes and not focused on any particular condition.

Some of the codes for routine health examinations distinguish between "with" and "without" abnormal findings. Code assignment depends on the information that is known at the time the encounter is being coded. For example, if no abnormal findings were found during the examination, but the encounter is being coded before test results are back, it is acceptable to assign the code for "without abnormal findings." When assigning a code for "with abnormal findings," additional code(s) should be assigned to identify the specific abnormal finding(s).

Pre-operative examination and pre-procedural laboratory examination Z codes are for use only in those situations when a patient is being cleared for a procedure or surgery and no treatment is given.

The Z codes/categories for routine and administrative examinations:

Z00	Encounter for general examination without complaint, suspected or reported diagnosis
Z01	Encounter for other special examination without complaint, suspected or reported diagnosis
Z02	Encounter for administrative examination Except: Z02.9, Encounter for administrative examinations, unspecified
Z32.0-	Encounter for pregnancy test

14) Miscellaneous Z codes

The miscellaneous Z codes capture a number of other health care encounters that do not fall into one of the other categories. Certain of these codes identify the reason for the encounter; others are for use as additional codes that provide useful information on circumstances that may affect a patient's care and treatment.

Prophylactic Organ Removal

For encounters specifically for prophylactic removal of an organ (such as prophylactic removal of breasts due to a genetic susceptibility to cancer or a family history of cancer), the principal or first-listed code should be a code from category Z40, Encounter for prophylactic surgery, followed by the appropriate codes to identify the associated risk factor (such as genetic susceptibility or family history).

If the patient has a malignancy of one site and is having prophylactic removal at another site to prevent either a new primary malignancy or metastatic disease, a code for the malignancy should also be assigned in addition to a code from subcategory Z40.0, Encounter for prophylactic surgery for risk factors related to malignant neoplasms. A Z40.0 code should not be assigned if the patient is having organ removal for treatment of a malignancy, such as the removal of the testes for the treatment of prostate cancer.

Miscellaneous Z codes/categories:

Z28	Immunization not carried out Except: Z28.3, Underimmunization status
Z40	Encounter for prophylactic surgery
Z41	Encounter for procedures for purposes other than remedying health state Except: Z41.9, Encounter for procedure for purposes other than remedying health state, unspecified
Z53	Persons encountering health services for specific procedures and treatment, not carried out
Z55	Problems related to education and literacy
Z56	Problems related to employment and unemployment
Z57	Occupational exposure to risk factors
Z58	Problems related to physical environment
Z59	Problems related to housing and economic circumstances
Z60	Problems related to social environment
Z62	Problems related to upbringing
Z63	Other problems related to primary support group, including family circumstances
Z64	Problems related to certain psychosocial circumstances
Z65	Problems related to other psychosocial circumstances
Z72	Problems related to lifestyle
Z73	Problems related to life management difficulty

Z74   Problems related to care provider dependency Except: Z74.01, Bed confinement status

Z75   Problems related to medical facilities and other health care

Z76.0   Encounter for issue of repeat prescription

Z76.3   Healthy person accompanying sick person

Z76.4   Other boarder to healthcare facility

Z76.5   Malingerer [conscious simulation]

Z91.1-   Patient's noncompliance with medical treatment and regimen

Z91.83   Wandering in diseases classified elsewhere

Z91.89   Other specified personal risk factors, not elsewhere classified

15) Nonspecific Z codes

Certain Z codes are so non-specific, or potentially redundant with other codes in the classification, that there can be little justification for their use in the inpatient setting. Their use in the outpatient setting should be limited to those instances when there is no further documentation to permit more precise coding. Otherwise, any sign or symptom or any other reason for visit that is captured in another code should be used.

Nonspecific Z codes/categories:

Z02.9   Encounter for administrative examinations, unspecified

Z04.9   Encounter for examination and observation for unspecified reason

Z13.9   Encounter for screening, unspecified

Z41.9   Encounter for procedure for purposes other than remedying health state, unspecified

Z52.9   Donor of unspecified organ or tissue

Z86.59   Personal history of other mental and behavioral disorders

Z88.9   Allergy status to unspecified drugs, medicaments and biological substances status

Z92.0   Personal history of contraception

16) Z Codes That May Only be Principal/First-Listed Diagnosis

The following Z codes/categories may only be reported as the principal/first-listed diagnosis, except when there are multiple encounters on the same day and the medical records for the encounters are combined:

Z00   Encounter for general examination without complaint, suspected or reported diagnosis

Z01   Encounter for other special examination without complaint, suspected or reported diagnosis

Z02   Encounter for administrative examination

Z03   Encounter for medical observation for suspected diseases and conditions ruled out

Z04   Encounter for examination and observation for other reasons

Z33.2   Encounter for elective termination of pregnancy

Z31.81   Encounter for male factor infertility in female patient

Z31.82   Encounter for Rh incompatibility status

Z31.83   Encounter for assisted reproductive fertility procedure cycle

Z31.84   Encounter for fertility preservation procedure

Z34   Encounter for supervision of normal pregnancy

Z39   Encounter for maternal postpartum care and examination

Z38   Liveborn infants according to place of birth and type of delivery

Z42   Encounter for plastic and reconstructive surgery following medical procedure or healed injury

Z51.0   Encounter for antineoplastic radiation therapy

Z51.1-   Encounter for antineoplastic chemotherapy and immunotherapy

Z52   Donors of organs and tissues Except: Z52.9, Donor of unspecified organ or tissue

Z76.1   Encounter for health supervision and care of foundling

Z76.2   Encounter for health supervision and care of other healthy infant and child

Z99.12   Encounter for respirator [ventilator] dependence during power failure

Section II. Selection of Principal Diagnosis

The circumstances of inpatient admission always govern the selection of principal diagnosis. The principal diagnosis is defined in the Uniform Hospital Discharge Data Set (UHDDS) as "that condition established after study to be chiefly responsible for occasioning the admission of the patient to the hospital for care."

The UHDDS definitions are used by hospitals to report inpatient data elements in a standardized manner. These data elements and their definitions can be found in the July 31, 1985, Federal Register (Vol. 50, No, 147), pp. 31038-40.

Since that time the application of the UHDDS definitions has been expanded to include all nonoutpatient settings (acute care, short term, long term care and psychiatric hospitals; home health agencies; rehab facilities; nursing homes, etc).

In determining principal diagnosis, coding conventions in the ICD-10-CM, the Tabular List and Alphabetic Index take precedence over these official coding guidelines. (See Section I.A., Conventions for the ICD-10-CM)

The importance of consistent, complete documentation in the medical record cannot be overemphasized. Without such documentation the application of all coding guidelines is a difficult, if not impossible, task.

A. Codes for symptoms, signs, and ill-defined conditions

Codes for symptoms, signs, and ill-defined conditions from Chapter 18 are not to be used as principal diagnosis when a related definitive diagnosis has been established.

B. Two or more interrelated conditions, each potentially meeting the definition for principal diagnosis.

When there are two or more interrelated conditions (such as diseases in the same ICD-10-CM chapter or manifestations characteristically associated with a certain disease) potentially meeting the definition of principal diagnosis, either condition may be sequenced first, unless the circumstances of the admission, the therapy provided, the Tabular List, or the Alphabetic Index indicate otherwise.

C. Two or more diagnoses that equally meet the definition for principal diagnosis

In the unusual instance when two or more diagnoses equally meet the criteria for principal diagnosis as determined by the circumstances of admission, diagnostic workup and/or therapy provided, and the Alphabetic Index, Tabular List, or another coding guidelines does not provide sequencing direction, any one of the diagnoses may be sequenced first.

D. Two or more comparative or contrasting conditions.

In those rare instances when two or more contrasting or comparative diagnoses are documented as "either/or" (or similar terminology), they are coded as if the diagnoses were confirmed and the diagnoses are sequenced according to the circumstances of the admission. If no further determination can be made as to which diagnosis should be principal, either diagnosis may be sequenced first.

E. A symptom(s) followed by contrasting/comparative diagnoses
GUIDELINE HAS BEEN DELETED EFFECTIVE OCTOBER 1, 2014

F. Original treatment plan not carried out

Sequence as the principal diagnosis the condition, which after study occasioned the admission to the hospital, even though treatment may not have been carried out due to unforeseen circumstances.

G. Complications of surgery and other medical care

When the admission is for treatment of a complication resulting from surgery or other medical care, the complication code is sequenced as the principal diagnosis. If the complication is classified to the T80-T88 series and the code lacks the necessary specificity in describing the complication, an additional code for the specific complication should be assigned.

H. Uncertain Diagnosis

If the diagnosis documented at the time of discharge is qualified as "probable", "suspected", "likely", "questionable", "possible", or "still to be ruled out", or other similar terms indicating uncertainty, code the condition as if it existed or was established. The bases for these guidelines are

the diagnostic workup, arrangements for further workup or observation, and initial therapeutic approach that correspond most closely with the established diagnosis.

Note: This guideline is applicable only to inpatient admissions to short-term, acute, long-term care and psychiatric hospitals.

I. Admission from Observation Unit

1. Admission Following Medical Observation

When a patient is admitted to an observation unit for a medical condition, which either worsens or does not improve, and is subsequently admitted as an inpatient of the same hospital for this same medical condition, the principal diagnosis would be the medical condition which led to the hospital admission.

2. Admission Following Post-Operative Observation

When a patient is admitted to an observation unit to monitor a condition (or complication) that develops following outpatient surgery, and then is subsequently admitted as an inpatient of the same hospital, hospitals should apply the Uniform Hospital Discharge Data Set (UHDDS) definition of principal diagnosis as "that condition established after study to be chiefly responsible for occasioning the admission of the patient to the hospital for care."

J. Admission from Outpatient Surgery

When a patient receives surgery in the hospital's outpatient surgery department and is subsequently admitted for continuing inpatient care at the same hospital, the following guidelines should be followed in selecting the principal diagnosis for the inpatient admission:

- If the reason for the inpatient admission is a complication, assign the complication as the principal diagnosis.
- If no complication, or other condition, is documented as the reason for the inpatient admission, assign the reason for the outpatient surgery as the principal diagnosis.
- If the reason for the inpatient admission is another condition unrelated to the surgery, assign the unrelated condition as the principal diagnosis.

K. Admissions/Encounters for Rehabilitation

When the purpose for the admission/encounter is rehabilitation, sequence first the code for the condition for which the service is being performed. For example, for an admission/encounter for rehabilitation for right-sided dominant hemiplegia following a cerebrovascular infarction, report code I69.351, Hemiplegia and hemiparesis following cerebral infarction affecting right dominant side, as the first-listed or principal diagnosis.

If the condition for which the rehabilitation service is no longer present, report the appropriate aftercare code as the first-listed or principal diagnosis. For example, if a patient with severe degenerative osteoarthritis of the hip, underwent hip replacement and the current encounter/admission is for rehabilitation, report code Z47.1, Aftercare following joint replacement surgery, as the first-listed or principal diagnosis.

See Section I.C.21.c.7, Factors influencing health states and contact with health services, Aftercare.

Section III. Reporting Additional Diagnoses

GENERAL RULES FOR OTHER (ADDITIONAL) DIAGNOSES

For reporting purposes the definition for "other diagnoses" is interpreted as additional conditions that affect patient care in terms of requiring:

clinical evaluation; or
therapeutic treatment; or
diagnostic procedures; or
extended length of hospital stay; or
increased nursing care and/or monitoring.

The UHDDS item #11-b defines Other Diagnoses as "all conditions that coexist at the time of admission, that develop subsequently, or that affect the treatment received and/or the length of stay. Diagnoses that relate to an earlier episode which have no bearing on the current hospital stay are to be excluded." UHDDS definitions apply to inpatients in acute care, short-term, long term care and psychiatric hospital setting. The UHDDS definitions are used by acute care short-term hospitals to report inpatient data elements in a standardized manner. These data elements and their definitions can be found in the July 31, 1985, Federal Register (Vol. 50, No, 147), pp. 31038-40.

Since that time the application of the UHDDS definitions has been expanded to include all nonoutpatient settings (acute care, short term, long term care and psychiatric hospitals; home health agencies; rehab facilities; nursing homes, etc). The following guidelines are to be applied in designating "other diagnoses" when neither the Alphabetic Index nor the Tabular List in ICD-10-CM provide direction. The listing of the diagnoses in the patient record is the responsibility of the attending provider.

A. Previous conditions

If the provider has included a diagnosis in the final diagnostic statement, such as the discharge summary or the face sheet, it should ordinarily be coded. Some providers include in the diagnostic statement resolved conditions or diagnoses and status-post procedures from previous admission that have no bearing on the current stay. Such conditions are not to be reported and are coded only if required by hospital policy.

However, history codes (categories Z80-Z87) may be used as secondary codes if the historical condition or family history has an impact on current care or influences treatment.

B. Abnormal findings

Abnormal findings (laboratory, x-ray, pathologic, and other diagnostic results) are not coded and reported unless the provider indicates their clinical significance. If the findings are outside the normal range and the attending provider has ordered other tests to evaluate the condition or prescribed treatment, it is appropriate to ask the provider whether the abnormal finding should be added.

Please note: This differs from the coding practices in the outpatient setting for coding encounters for diagnostic tests that have been interpreted by a provider.

C. Uncertain Diagnosis

If the diagnosis documented at the time of discharge is qualified as "probable", "suspected", "likely", "questionable", "possible", or "still to be ruled out" or other similar terms indicating uncertainty, code the condition as if it existed or was established. The bases for these guidelines are the diagnostic workup, arrangements for further workup or observation, and initial therapeutic approach that correspond most closely with the established diagnosis.

Note: This guideline is applicable only to inpatient admissions to short-term, acute, long-term care and psychiatric hospitals.

Section IV. Diagnostic Coding and Reporting Guidelines for Outpatient Services

These coding guidelines for outpatient diagnoses have been approved for use by hospitals/ providers in coding and reporting hospital-based outpatient services and provider-based office visits.

Information about the use of certain abbreviations, punctuation, symbols, and other conventions used in the ICD-10-CM Tabular List (code numbers and titles), can be found in Section IA of these guidelines, under "Conventions Used in the Tabular List." Section I.B. contains general guidelines that apply to the entire classification. Section I.C. contains chapter-specific guidelines that correspond to the chapters as they are arranged in the classification. Information about the correct sequence to use in finding a code is also described in Section I.

The terms encounter and visit are often used interchangeably in describing outpatient service contacts and, therefore, appear together in these guidelines without distinguishing one from the other.

Though the conventions and general guidelines apply to all settings, coding guidelines for outpatient and provider reporting of diagnoses will vary in a number of instances from those for inpatient diagnoses, recognizing that:

The Uniform Hospital Discharge Data Set (UHDDS) definition of principal diagnosis applies only to inpatients in acute, short-term, long-term care and psychiatric hospitals.

Coding guidelines for inconclusive diagnoses (probable, suspected, rule out, etc.) were developed for inpatient reporting and do not apply to outpatients.

A. Selection of first-listed condition

In the outpatient setting, the term first-listed diagnosis is used in lieu of principal diagnosis.

In determining the first-listed diagnosis the coding conventions of ICD-10-CM, as well as the general and disease specific guidelines take precedence over the outpatient guidelines.

Diagnoses often are not established at the time of the initial encounter/visit. It may take two or more visits before the diagnosis is confirmed.

The most critical rule involves beginning the search for the correct code assignment through the Alphabetic Index. Never begin searching initially in the Tabular List as this will lead to coding errors.

1. Outpatient Surgery

When a patient presents for outpatient surgery (same day surgery), code the reason for the surgery as the first-listed diagnosis (reason for the encounter), even if the surgery is not performed due to a contraindication.

2. Observation Stay

When a patient is admitted for observation for a medical condition, assign a code for the medical condition as the first-listed diagnosis.

When a patient presents for outpatient surgery and develops complications requiring admission to observation, code the reason for the surgery as the first reported diagnosis (reason for the encounter), followed by codes for the complications as secondary diagnoses.

B. Codes from A00.0 through T88.9, Z00-Z99

The appropriate code(s) from A00.0 through T88.9, Z00-Z99 must be used to identify diagnoses, symptoms, conditions, problems, complaints, or other reason(s) for the encounter/visit.

C. Accurate reporting of ICD-10-CM diagnosis codes

For accurate reporting of ICD-10-CM diagnosis codes, the documentation should describe the patient's condition, using terminology which includes specific diagnoses as well as symptoms, problems, or reasons for the encounter. There are ICD-10-CM codes to describe all of these.

D. Codes that describe symptoms and signs

Codes that describe symptoms and signs, as opposed to diagnoses, are acceptable for reporting purposes when a diagnosis has not been established (confirmed) by the provider. Chapter 18 of ICD-10-CM, Symptoms, Signs, and Abnormal Clinical and Laboratory Findings Not Elsewhere Classified (codes R00-R99) contain many, but not all codes for symptoms.

E. Encounters for circumstances other than a disease or injury

ICD-10-CM provides codes to deal with encounters for circumstances other than a disease or injury. The Factors Influencing Health Status and Contact with Health Services codes (Z00-Z99) are provided to deal with occasions when circumstances other than a disease or injury are recorded as diagnosis or problems.

See Section I.C.21. Factors influencing health status and contact with health services.

F. Level of Detail in Coding

1. ICD-10-CM codes with 3, 4, 5, 6 or 7 characters

ICD-10-CM is composed of codes with 3, 4, 5, 6 or 7 characters. Codes with three characters are included in ICD-10-CM as the heading of a category of codes that may be further subdivided by the use of fourth, fifth, sixth or seventh characters to provide greater specificity.

2. Use of full number of characters required for a code

A three-character code is to be used only if it is not further subdivided. A code is invalid if it has not been coded to the full number of characters required for that code, including the 7th character, if applicable.

G. ICD-10-CM code for the diagnosis, condition, problem, or other reason for encounter/visit

List first the ICD-10-CM code for the diagnosis, condition, problem, or other reason for encounter/visit shown in the medical record to be chiefly responsible for the services provided. List additional codes that describe any coexisting conditions. In some cases the first-listed diagnosis may be a symptom when a diagnosis has not been established (confirmed) by the physician.

H. Uncertain diagnosis

Do not code diagnoses documented as "probable", "suspected," "questionable," "rule out," or "working diagnosis" or other similar terms indicating uncertainty. Rather, code the condition(s) to the highest degree of certainty for that encounter/visit, such as symptoms, signs, abnormal test results, or other reason for the visit.

Please note: This differs from the coding practices used by short-term, acute care, long-term care and psychiatric hospitals.

I. Chronic diseases

Chronic diseases treated on an ongoing basis may be coded and reported as many times as the patient receives treatment and care for the condition(s)

J. Code all documented conditions that coexist

Code all documented conditions that coexist at the time of the encounter/visit, and require or affect patient care treatment or management. Do not code conditions that were previously treated and no longer exist. However, history codes (categories Z80-Z87) may be used as secondary codes if the historical condition or family history has an impact on current care or influences treatment.

K. Patients receiving diagnostic services only

For patients receiving diagnostic services only during an encounter/visit, sequence first the diagnosis, condition, problem, or other reason for encounter/visit shown in the medical record to be chiefly responsible for the outpatient services provided during the encounter/visit. Codes for other diagnoses (e.g., chronic conditions) may be sequenced as additional diagnoses.

For encounters for routine laboratory/radiology testing in the absence of any signs, symptoms, or associated diagnosis, assign Z01.89, Encounter for other specified special examinations. If routine testing is performed during the same encounter as a test to evaluate a sign, symptom, or diagnosis, it is appropriate to assign both the Z code and the code describing the reason for the non-routine test.

For outpatient encounters for diagnostic tests that have been interpreted by a physician, and the final report is available at the time of coding, code any confirmed or definitive diagnosis(es) documented in the interpretation. Do not code related signs and symptoms as additional diagnoses.

Please note: This differs from the coding practice in the hospital inpatient setting regarding abnormal findings on test results.

L. **Patients receiving therapeutic services only**
For patients receiving therapeutic services only during an encounter/visit, sequence first the diagnosis, condition, problem, or other reason for encounter/visit shown in the medical record to be chiefly responsible for the outpatient services provided during the encounter/visit. Codes for other diagnoses (e.g., chronic conditions) may be sequenced as additional diagnoses.

The only exception to this rule is that when the primary reason for the admission/encounter is chemotherapy or radiation therapy, the appropriate Z code for the service is listed first, and the diagnosis or problem for which the service is being performed listed second.

M. **Patients receiving preoperative evaluations only**
For patients receiving preoperative evaluations only, sequence first a code from subcategory Z01.81, Encounter for pre-procedural examinations, to describe the pre-op consultations. Assign a code for the condition to describe the reason for the surgery as an additional diagnosis. Code also any findings related to the pre-op evaluation.

N. **Ambulatory surgery**
For ambulatory surgery, code the diagnosis for which the surgery was performed. If the postoperative diagnosis is known to be different from the preoperative diagnosis at the time the diagnosis is confirmed, select the postoperative diagnosis for coding, since it is the most definitive.

O. **Routine outpatient prenatal visits**
See Section I.C.15. Routine outpatient prenatal visits.

P. **Encounters for general medical examinations with abnormal findings**
The subcategories for encounters for general medical examinations, Z00.0-, provide codes for with and without abnormal findings. Should a general medical examination result in an abnormal finding, the code for general medical examination with abnormal finding should be assigned as the first-listed diagnosis. A secondary code for the abnormal finding should also be coded.

Q. **Encounters for routine health screenings**
See Section I.C.21. Factors influencing health status and contact with health services, Screening

Appendix I
Present on Admission Reporting Guidelines

Introduction

These guidelines are to be used as a supplement to the *ICD-10-CM Official Guidelines for Coding and Reporting* to facilitate the assignment of the Present on Admission (POA) indicator for each diagnosis and external cause of injury code reported on claim forms (UB-04 and 837 Institutional).

These guidelines are not intended to replace any guidelines in the main body of the *ICD-10-CM Official Guidelines for Coding and Reporting*. The POA guidelines are not intended to provide guidance on when a condition should be coded, but rather, how to apply the POA indicator to the final set of diagnosis codes that have been assigned in accordance with Sections I, II, and III of the official coding guidelines. Subsequent to the assignment of the ICD-10-CM codes, the POA indicator should then be assigned to those conditions that have been coded.

As stated in the Introduction to the ICD-10-CM Official Guidelines for Coding and Reporting, a joint effort between the healthcare provider and the coder is essential to achieve complete and accurate documentation, code assignment, and reporting of diagnoses and procedures. The importance of consistent, complete documentation in the medical record cannot be overemphasized. Medical record documentation from any provider involved in the care and treatment of the patient may be used to support the determination of whether a condition was present on admission or not. In the context of the official coding guidelines, the term "provider" means a physician or any qualified healthcare practitioner who is legally accountable for establishing the patient's diagnosis.

These guidelines are not a substitute for the provider's clinical judgment as to the determination of whether a condition was/was not present on admission. The provider should be queried regarding issues related to the linking of signs/symptoms, timing of test results, and the timing of findings.

General Reporting Requirements

All claims involving inpatient admissions to general acute care hospitals or other facilities that are subject to a law or regulation mandating collection of present on admission information.

Present on admission is defined as present at the time the order for inpatient admission occurs—conditions that develop during an outpatient encounter, including emergency department, observation, or outpatient surgery, are considered as present on admission.

POA indicator is assigned to principal and secondary diagnoses (as defined in Section II of the Official Guidelines for Coding and Reporting) and the external cause of injury codes.

Issues related to inconsistent, missing, conflicting or unclear documentation must still be resolved by the provider.

If a condition would not be coded and reported based on UHDDS definitions and current official coding guidelines, then the POA indicator would not be reported.

Reporting Options

Y - Yes

N - No

U - Unknown

W - Clinically undetermined

Unreported/Not used - (Exempt from POA reporting)

Reporting Definitions

Y = present at the time of inpatient admission

N = not present at the time of inpatient admission

U = documentation is insufficient to determine if condition is present on admission

W = provider is unable to clinically determine whether condition was present on admission or not

Timeframe for POA Identification and Documentation

There is no required timeframe as to when a provider (per the definition of "provider" used in these guidelines) must identify or document a condition to be present on admission. In some clinical situations, it may not be possible for a provider to make a definitive diagnosis (or a condition may not be recognized or reported by the patient) for a period of time after admission. In some cases it may be several days before the provider arrives at a definitive diagnosis. This does not mean that the condition was not present on admission. Determination of whether the condition was present on admission or not will be based on the applicable POA guideline as identified in this document, or on the provider's best clinical judgment.

If at the time of code assignment the documentation is unclear as to whether a condition was present on admission or not, it is appropriate to query the provider for clarification.

Assigning the POA Indicator

Condition is on the "Exempt from Reporting" list

Leave the "present on admission" field blank if the condition is on the list of ICD-10-CM codes for which this field is not applicable. This is the only circumstance in which the field may be left blank.

POA Explicitly Documented

Assign Y for any condition the provider explicitly documents as being present on admission.

Assign N for any condition the provider explicitly documents as not present at the time of admission.

Conditions diagnosed prior to inpatient admission

Assign "Y" for conditions that were diagnosed prior to admission (example: hypertension, diabetes mellitus, asthma)

Conditions diagnosed during the admission but clearly present before admission

Assign "Y" for conditions diagnosed during the admission that were clearly present but not diagnosed until after admission occurred.

Diagnoses subsequently confirmed after admission are considered present on admission if at the time of admission they are documented as suspected, possible, rule out, differential diagnosis, or constitute an underlying cause of a symptom that is present at the time of admission.

Condition develops during outpatient encounter prior to inpatient admission

Assign Y for any condition that develops during an outpatient encounter prior to a written order for inpatient admission.

Documentation does not indicate whether condition was present on admission

Assign "U" when the medical record documentation is unclear as to whether the condition was present on admission. "U" should not be routinely assigned and used only in very limited circumstances. Coders are encouraged to query the providers when the documentation is unclear.

Documentation states that it cannot be determined whether the condition was or was not present on admission

Assign "W" when the medical record documentation indicates that it cannot be clinically determined whether or not the condition was present on admission.

Chronic condition with acute exacerbation during the admission

If a single code identifies both the chronic condition and the acute exacerbation, see POA guidelines pertaining to combination codes.

If a single code only identifies the chronic condition and not the acute exacerbation (e.g., acute exacerbation of chronic leukemia), assign "Y."

Conditions documented as possible, probable, suspected, or rule out at the time of discharge

If the final diagnosis contains a possible, probable, suspected, or rule out diagnosis, and this diagnosis was based on signs, symptoms or clinical findings suspected at the time of inpatient admission, assign "Y."

If the final diagnosis contains a possible, probable, suspected, or rule out diagnosis, and this diagnosis was based on signs, symptoms or clinical findings that were not present on admission, assign "N".

Conditions documented as impending or threatened at the time of discharge

If the final diagnosis contains an impending or threatened diagnosis, and this diagnosis is based on symptoms or clinical findings that were present on admission, assign "Y".

If the final diagnosis contains an impending or threatened diagnosis, and this diagnosis is based on symptoms or clinical findings that were not present on admission, assign "N".

Acute and Chronic Conditions

Assign "Y" for acute conditions that are present at time of admission and N for acute conditions that are not present at time of admission.

Assign "Y" for chronic conditions, even though the condition may not be diagnosed until after admission.

If a single code identifies both an acute and chronic condition, see the POA guidelines for combination codes.

Combination Codes

Assign "N" if any part of the combination code was not present on admission (e.g., COPD with acute exacerbation and the exacerbation was not present on admission; gastric ulcer that does not start bleeding until after admission; asthma patient develops status asthmaticus after admission).

Assign "Y" if all parts of the combination code were present on admission (e.g., patient with acute prostatitis admitted with hematuria).

If the final diagnosis includes comparative or contrasting diagnoses, and both were present, or suspected, at the time of admission, assign "Y".

For infection codes that include the causal organism, assign "Y" if the infection (or signs of the infection) was present on admission, even though the culture results may not be known until after admission (e.g., patient is admitted with pneumonia and the provider documents pseudomonas as the causal organism a few days later).

Same Diagnosis Code for Two or More Conditions

When the same ICD-10-CM diagnosis code applies to two or more conditions during the same encounter (e.g. two separate conditions classified to the same ICD-10-CM diagnosis code):

Assign "Y" if all conditions represented by the single ICD-10-CM code were present on admission (e.g. bilateral unspecified age-related cataracts).

Assign "N" if any of the conditions represented by the single ICD-10-CM code was not present on admission (e.g. traumatic secondary and recurrent hemorrhage and seroma is assigned to a single code T79.2, but only one of the conditions was present on admission).

Obstetrical conditions

Whether or not the patient delivers during the current hospitalization does not affect assignment of the POA indicator. The determining factor for POA assignment is whether the pregnancy complication or obstetrical condition described by the code was present at the time of admission or not.

If the pregnancy complication or obstetrical condition was present on admission (e.g., patient admitted in preterm labor), assign "Y".

If the pregnancy complication or obstetrical condition was not present on admission (e.g., 2nd degree laceration during delivery, postpartum hemorrhage that occurred during current hospitalization, fetal distress develops after admission), assign "N".

If the obstetrical code includes more than one diagnosis and any of the diagnoses identified by the code were not present on admission assign "N".

(e.g., Category O11, Pre-existing hypertension with pre-eclampsia)

GUIDELINES (ICD-10-CM)

Perinatal conditions

Newborns are not considered to be admitted until after birth. Therefore, any condition present at birth or that developed in utero is considered present at admission and should be assigned "Y". This includes conditions that occur during delivery (e.g., injury during delivery, meconium aspiration, exposure to streptococcus B in the vaginal canal).

Congenital conditions and anomalies

Assign "Y" for congenital conditions and anomalies except for categories Q00-Q99, Congenital anomalies, which are on the exempt list. Congenital conditions are always considered present on admission.

External cause of injury codes

Assign "Y" for any external cause code representing an external cause of morbidity that occurred prior to inpatient admission (e.g., patient fell out of bed at home, patient fell out of bed in emergency room prior to admission).

Assign "N" for any external cause code representing an external cause of morbidity that occurred during inpatient hospitalization (e.g., patient fell out of hospital bed during hospital stay, patient experienced an adverse reaction to a medication administered after inpatient admission).

Categories and Codes
Exempt from Diagnosis Present on Admission
Requirement

Note: "Diagnosis present on admission" for these code categories are exempt because they represent circumstances regarding the healthcare encounter or factors influencing health status that do not represent a current disease or injury or are always present on admission

B90-B94, Sequelae of infectious and parasitic diseases

E64, Sequelae of malnutrition and other nutritional deficiencies

I25.2, Old myocardial infarction

I69, Sequelae of cerebrovascular disease

O09, Supervision of high risk pregnancy

O66.5, Attempted application of vacuum extractor and forceps

O80, Encounter for full-term uncomplicated delivery

O94, Sequelae of complication of pregnancy, childbirth, and the puerperium

P00, Newborn (suspected to be) affected by maternal conditions that may be unrelated to present pregnancy

Q00 - Q99, Congenital malformations, deformations and chromosomal abnormalities

S00-T88.9, Injury, poisoning and certain other consequences of external causes with 7th character representing subsequent encounter or sequela

V00-V09, Pedestrian injured in transport accident

Except V00.81-, Accident with wheelchair (powered)

V00.83-, Accident with motorized mobility scooter

V10-V19, Pedal cycle rider injured in transport accident

V20-V29, Motorcycle rider injured in transport accident

V30-V39, Occupant of three-wheeled motor vehicle injured in transport accident

V40-V49, Car occupant injured in transport accident

V50-V59, Occupant of pick-up truck or van injured in transport accident

V60-V69, Occupant of heavy transport vehicle injured in transport accident

V70-V79, Bus occupant injured in transport accident

V80-V89, Other land transport accidents

V90-V94, Water transport accidents

V95-V97, Air and space transport accidents

V98-V99, Other and unspecified transport accidents

W09, Fall on and from playground equipment

W14, Fall from tree

W15, Fall from cliff

W17.0, Fall into well

W17.1, Fall into storm drain or manhole

W18.01, Striking against sports equipment with subsequent fall

W21, Striking against or struck by sports equipment

W30, Contact with agricultural machinery

W31, Contact with other and unspecified machinery

W32-W34, Accidental handgun discharge and malfunction

W35- W40, Exposure to inanimate mechanical forces

W52, Crushed, pushed or stepped on by crowd or human stampede

W56, Contact with nonvenomous marine animal

W58, Contact with crocodile or alligator

W61, Contact with birds (domestic) (wild)

W62, Contact with nonvenomous amphibians

W89, Exposure to man-made visible and ultraviolet light

X02, Exposure to controlled fire in building or structure

X03, Exposure to controlled fire, not in building or structure

X04, Exposure to ignition of highly flammable material

X52, Prolonged stay in weightless environment

X71, Intentional self-harm by drowning and submersion

Except X71.0-, Intentional self-harm by drowning and submersion while in bath tub

X72, Intentional self-harm by handgun discharge

X73, Intentional self-harm by rifle, shotgun and larger firearm discharge

X74, Intentional self-harm by other and unspecified firearm and gun discharge

X75, Intentional self-harm by explosive material

X76, Intentional self-harm by smoke, fire and flames

X77, Intentional self-harm by steam, hot vapors and hot objects

X81, Intentional self-harm by jumping or lying in front of moving object

X82, Intentional self-harm by crashing of motor vehicle

X83, Intentional self-harm by other specified means

Y03, Assault by crashing of motor vehicle

Y07, Perpetrator of assault, maltreatment and neglect

Y08.8, Assault by strike by sports equipment

Y21, Drowning and submersion, undetermined intent

Y22, Handgun discharge, undetermined intent

Y23, Rifle, shotgun and larger firearm discharge, undetermined intent

Y24, Other and unspecified firearm discharge, undetermined intent

Y30, Falling, jumping or pushed from a high place, undetermined intent

Y32, Assault by crashing of motor vehicle, undetermined intent

Y37, Military operations

Y36, Operations of war

Y92, Place of occurrence of the external cause

Y93, Activity code

Y99, External cause status

Z00, Encounter for general examination without complaint, suspected or reported diagnosis

Z01, Encounter for other special examination without complaint, suspected or reported diagnosis

Z02, Encounter for administrative examination

Z03, Encounter for medical observation for suspected diseases and conditions ruled out

Z08, Encounter for follow-up examination following completed treatment for malignant neoplasm

Z09, Encounter for follow-up examination after completed treatment for conditions other than malignant neoplasm

Z11, Encounter for screening for infectious and parasitic diseases

Z11.8, Encounter for screening for other infectious and parasitic diseases

Z12, Encounter for screening for malignant neoplasms

Z13, Encounter for screening for other diseases and disorders

Z13.4, Encounter for screening for certain developmental disorders in childhood

Z13.5, Encounter for screening for eye and ear disorders

Z13.6, Encounter for screening for cardiovascular disorders

Z13.83, Encounter for screening for respiratory disorder NEC

Z13.89, Encounter for screening for other disorder

Z13.89, Encounter for screening for other disorder

Z14, Genetic carrier

Z15, Genetic susceptibility to disease

Z17, Estrogen receptor status

Z18, Retained foreign body fragments

Z22, Carrier of infectious disease

Z23, Encounter for immunization

Z28, Immunization not carried out and underimmunization status

Z28.3, Underimmunization status

Z30, Encounter for contraceptive management

Z31, Encounter for procreative management

Z34, Encounter for supervision of normal pregnancy

Z36, Encounter for antenatal screening of mother

Z37, Outcome of delivery

Z38, Liveborn infants according to place of birth and type of delivery

Z39, Encounter for maternal postpartum care and examination

Z41, Encounter for procedures for purposes other than remedying health state

Z42, Encounter for plastic and reconstructive surgery following medical procedure or healed injury

Z43, Encounter for attention to artificial openings

Z44, Encounter for fitting and adjustment of external prosthetic device

Z45, Encounter for adjustment and management of implanted device

Z46, Encounter for fitting and adjustment of other devices

Z47.8, Encounter for other orthopedic aftercare

Z49, Encounter for care involving renal dialysis

Z51, Encounter for other aftercare

Z51.5, Encounter for palliative care

Z51.8, Encounter for other specified aftercare

Z52, Donors of organs and tissues

Z59, Problems related to housing and economic circumstances

Z63, Other problems related to primary support group, including family circumstances

Z65, Problems related to other psychosocial circumstances

Z65.8, Other specified problems related to psychosocial circumstances

Z67.1 - Z67.9, Blood type

Z68, Body mass index (BMI)

Z72, Problems related to lifestyle

Z74.01, Bed confinement status

Z76, Persons encountering health services in other circumstances

Z77.110- Z77.128, Environmental pollution and hazards in the physical environment

Z78, Other specified health status

Z79, Long term (current) drug therapy

Z80, Family history of primary malignant neoplasm

Z81, Family history of mental and behavioral disorders

Z82, Family history of certain disabilities and chronic diseases (leading to disablement)

Z83, Family history of other specific disorders

Z84, Family history of other conditions

Z85, Personal history of primary malignant neoplasm

Z86, Personal history of certain other diseases

Z87, Personal history of other diseases and conditions

Z87.828, Personal history of other (healed) physical injury and trauma

Z87.891, Personal history of nicotine dependence

Z88, Allergy status to drugs, medicaments and biological substances

Z89, Acquired absence of limb

Z90.710, Acquired absence of both cervix and uterus

Z91.0, Allergy status, other than to drugs and biological substances

Z91.4, Personal history of psychological trauma, not elsewhere classified

Z91.5, Personal history of self-harm

Z91.8, Other specified risk factors, not elsewhere classified

Z92, Personal history of medical treatment

Z93, Artificial opening status

Z94, Transplanted organ and tissue status

Z95, Presence of cardiac and vascular implants and grafts

Z97, Presence of other devices

Z98, Other postprocedural states

Z99, Dependence on enabling machines and devices, not elsewhere classified

Alphabetic Index

A

Aarskog's syndrome Q87.1
Abandonment —see Maltreatment
Abasia (-astasia) (hysterical) F44.4
Abderhalden-Kaufmann-Lignac syndrome (cystinosis) E72.04
Abdomen, abdominal —see also condition
  acute R10.0
  angina K55.1
  muscle deficiency syndrome Q79.4
Abdominalgia —see Pain, abdominal
Abduction contracture, hip or other joint —see Contraction, joint
Aberrant (congenital) —see also Malposition, congenital
  adrenal gland Q89.1
  artery (peripheral) Q27.8
    basilar NEC Q28.1
    cerebral Q28.3
    coronary Q24.5
    digestive system Q27.8
    eye Q15.8
    lower limb Q27.8
    precerebral Q28.1
    pulmonary Q25.79
    renal Q27.2
    retina Q14.1
    specified site NEC Q27.8
    subclavian Q27.8
    upper limb Q27.8
    vertebral Q28.1
  breast Q83.8
  endocrine gland NEC Q89.2
  hepatic duct Q44.5
  pancreas Q45.3
  parathyroid gland Q89.2
  pituitary gland Q89.2
  sebaceous glands, mucous membrane, mouth, congenital Q38.6
  spleen Q89.09
  subclavian artery Q27.8
  thymus (gland) Q89.2
  thyroid gland Q89.2
  vein (peripheral) NEC Q27.8
    cerebral Q28.3
    digestive system Q27.8
    lower limb Q27.8
    precerebral Q28.1
    specified site NEC Q27.8
    upper limb Q27.8
Aberration
  distantial —see Disturbance, visual
  mental F99
Abetalipoproteinemia E78.6
Abiotrophy R68.89
Ablatio, ablation
  retinae —see Detachment, retina
Ablepharia, ablepharon Q10.3
Abnormal, abnormality, abnormalities —see also Anomaly
  acid-base balance (mixed) E87.4
  albumin R77.0
  alphafetoprotein R77.2
  alveolar ridge K08.9
  anatomical relationship Q89.9
  apertures, congenital, diaphragm Q79.1
  auditory perception H93.29-
    diplacusis —see Diplacusis
    hyperacusis —see Hyperacusis
    recruitment —see Recruitment, auditory
    threshold shift —see Shift, auditory threshold
  autosomes Q99.9
    fragile site Q95.5
  basal metabolic rate R94.8
  biosynthesis, testicular androgen E29.1
  bleeding time R79.1

Abnormal, abnormality, abnormalities — (Continued)
  blood level (of)
    cobalt R79.0
    copper R79.0
    iron R79.0
    lithium R78.89
    magnesium R79.0
    mineral NEC R79.0
    zinc R79.0
  blood pressure
    elevated R03.0
    low reading (nonspecific) R03.1
  blood sugar R73.09
  blood-gas level R79.81
  bowel sounds R19.15
    absent R19.11
    hyperactive R19.12
  brain scan R94.02
  breathing R06.9
  caloric test R94.138
  cerebrospinal fluid R83.9
    cytology R83.6
    drug level R83.2
    enzyme level R83.0
    hormones R83.1
    immunology R83.4
    microbiology R83.5
    nonmedicinal level R83.3
    specified type NEC R83.8
  chemistry, blood R79.9
    C-reactive protein R79.82
    drugs —see Findings, abnormal, in blood
    gas level R79.81
    minerals R79.0
    pancytopenia D61.818
    PTT R79.1
    specified NEC R79.89
    toxins —see Findings, abnormal, in blood
  chest sounds (friction) (rales) R09.89
  chromosome, chromosomal Q99.9
    with more than three X chromosomes, female Q97.1
    analysis result R89.8
      bronchial washings R84.8
      cerebrospinal fluid R83.8
      cervix uteri NEC R87.89
      nasal secretions R84.8
      nipple discharge R89.8
      peritoneal fluid R85.89
      pleural fluid R84.8
      prostatic secretions R86.8
      saliva R85.89
      seminal fluid R86.8
      sputum R84.8
      synovial fluid R89.8
      throat scrapings R84.8
      vagina R87.89
      vulva R87.89
      wound secretions R89.8
    dicentric replacement Q93.2
    ring replacement Q93.2
    sex Q99.8
      female phenotype Q97.9
        specified NEC Q97.8
      male phenotype Q98.9
        specified NEC Q98.8
      structural male Q98.6
    specified NEC Q99.8
  clinical findings NEC R68.89
  coagulation D68.9
    newborn, transient P61.6
    profile R79.1
    time R79.1
  communication —see Fistula
  conjunctiva, vascular H11.41-
  coronary artery Q24.5
  cortisol-binding globulin E27.8

Abnormal, abnormality, abnormalities — (Continued)
  course, eustachian tube Q17.8
  creatinine clearance R94.4
  cytology
    anus R85.619
      atypical squamous cells cannot exclude high grade squamous intraepithelial lesion (ASC-H) R85.611
      atypical squamous cells of undetermined significance (ASC-US) R85.610
      cytologic evidence of malignancy R85.614
      high grade squamous intraepithelial lesion (HGSIL) R85.613
      human papillomavirus (HPV) DNA test
        high risk positive R85.81
        low risk postive R85.82
      inadequate smear R85.615
      low grade squamous intraepithelial lesion (LGSIL) R85.612
      satisfactory anal smear but lacking transformation zone R85.616
      specified NEC R85.618
      unsatisfactory smear R85.615
    female genital organs —see Abnormal, Papanicolaou (smear)
  dark adaptation curve H53.61
  dentofacial NEC —see Anomaly, dentofacial
  development, developmental Q89.9
    central nervous system Q07.9
  diagnostic imaging
    abdomen, abdominal region NEC R93.5
    biliary tract R93.2
    breast R92.8
    central nervous system NEC R90.89
    cerebrovascular NEC R90.89
    coronary circulation R93.1
    digestive tract NEC R93.3
    gastrointestinal (tract) R93.3
    genitourinary organs R93.8
    head R93.0
    heart R93.1
    intrathoracic organ NEC R93.8
    limbs R93.6
    liver R93.2
    lung (field) R91.8
    musculoskeletal system NEC R93.7
    retroperitoneum R93.5
    site specified NEC R93.8
    skin and subcutaneous tissue R93.8
    skull R93.0
    urinary organs R93.4
  direction, teeth, fully erupted M26.30
  ear ossicles, acquired NEC H74.39-
    ankylosis —see Ankylosis, ear ossicles
    discontinuity —see Discontinuity, ossicles, ear
    partial loss —see Loss, ossicles, ear (partial)
  Ebstein Q22.5
  echocardiogram R93.1
  echoencephalogram R90.81
  echogram —see Abnormal, diagnostic imaging
  electrocardiogram [ECG] [EKG] R94.31
  electroencephalogram [EEG] R94.01
  electrolyte —see Imbalance, electrolyte
  electromyogram [EMG] R94.131
  electro-oculogram [EOG] R94.110
  electrophysiological intracardiac studies R94.39
  electroretinogram [ERG] R94.111
  erythrocytes
    congenital, with perinatal jaundice D58.9
  feces (color) (contents) (mucus) R19.5

◀ New   ◀⁕ Revised   ~~deleted~~ Deleted

Abnormal, abnormality, abnormalities —
      (Continued)
   finding —see Findings, abnormal, without
         diagnosis
   fluid
      amniotic —see Abnormal, specimen,
            specified
      cerebrospinal —see Abnormal,
            cerebrospinal fluid
      peritoneal —see Abnormal, specimen,
            digestive organs
      pleural —see Abnormal, specimen,
            respiratory organs
      synovial —see Abnormal, specimen,
            specified
      thorax (bronchial washings) (pleural
            fluid) —see Abnormal, specimen,
            respiratory organs
      vaginal —see Abnormal, specimen, female
            genital organs
   form
      teeth K00.2
      uterus —see Anomaly, uterus
   function studies
      auditory R94.120
      bladder R94.8
      brain R94.09
      cardiovascular R94.30
      ear R94.128
      endocrine NEC R94.7
      eye NEC R94.118
      kidney R94.4
      liver R94.5
      nervous system
         central NEC R94.09
         peripheral NEC R94.138
      pancreas R94.8
      placenta R94.8
      pulmonary R94.2
      special senses NEC R94.128
      spleen R94.8
      thyroid R94.6
      vestibular R94.121
   gait —see Gait
      hysterical F44.4
   gastrin secretion E16.4
   globulin R77.1
      cortisol-binding E27.8
      thyroid-binding E07.89
   glomerular, minor (see also N00-N07 with
         fourth character .0) N05.0
   glucagon secretion E16.3
   glucose tolerance (test) (non-fasting)
         R73.09
   gravitational (G) forces or states (effect of)
         T75.81
   hair (color) (shaft) L67.9
      specified NEC L67.8
   hard tissue formation in pulp (dental)
         K04.3
   head movement R25.0
   heart
      rate R00.9
         specified NEC R00.8
      shadow R93.1
      sounds NEC R01.2
   hemoglobin (disease) (see also Disease,
         hemoglobin) D58.2
      trait —see Trait, hemoglobin, abnormal
   histology NEC R89.7
   immunological findings R89.4
      in serum R76.9
         specified NEC R76.8
   increase in appetite R63.2
   involuntary movement —see Abnormal,
         movement, involuntary
   jaw closure M26.51
   karyotype R89.8
   kidney function test R94.4
   knee jerk R29.2
   leukocyte (cell) (differential) NEC D72.9

Abnormal, abnormality, abnormalities —
      (Continued)
   liver
   loss of
      height R29.890
      weight R63.4
   mammogram NEC R92.8
      calcification (calculus) R92.1
      microcalcification R92.0
   Mantoux test R76.11
   movement (disorder) —see also Disorder,
         movement
      head R25.0
      involuntary R25.9
         fasciculation R25.3
         of head R25.0
         spasm R25.2
         specified type NEC R25.8
         tremor R25.1
   myoglobin (Aberdeen) (Annapolis) R89.7
   neonatal screening P09
   oculomotor study R94.113
   palmar creases Q82.8
   Papanicolaou (smear)
      anus R85.619
         atypical squamous cells cannot
               exclude high grade squamous
               intraepithelial lesion (ASC-H)
               R85.611
         atypical squamous cells of undetermined
               significance (ASC-US) R85.610
         cytologic evidence of malignancy
               R85.614
         high grade squamous intraepithelial
               lesion (HGSIL) R85.613
         human papillomavirus (HPV)
               DNA test
            high risk positive R85.81
            low risk postive R85.82
         inadequate smear R85.615
         low grade squamous intraepithelial
               lesion (LGSIL) R85.612
         satisfactory anal smear but lacking
               transformation zone R85.616
         specified NEC R85.618
         unsatisfactory smear R85.615
      bronchial washings R84.6
      cerebrospinal fluid R83.6
      cervix R87.619
         atypical squamous cells cannot
               exclude high grade squamous
               intraepithelial lesion (ASC-H)
               R87.611
         atypical squamous cells of undetermined
               significance (ASC-US) R87.610
         cytologic evidence of malignancy
               R87.614
         high grade squamous intraepithelial
               lesion (HGSIL) R87.613
         inadequate smear R87.615
         low grade squamous intraepithelial
               lesion (LGSIL) R87.612
         non-atypical endometrial cells
               R87.618
         satisfactory cervical smear but
               lacking transformation zone
               R87.616
         specified NEC R87.618
         thin preparaton R87.619
         unsatisfactory smear R87.615
      nasal secretions R84.6
      nipple discharge R89.6
      peritoneal fluid R85.69
      pleural fluid R84.6
      prostatic secretions R86.6
      saliva R85.69
      seminal fluid R86.6
      sites NEC R89.6
      sputum R84.6
      synovial fluid R89.6
      throat scrapings R84.6

Abnormal, abnormality, abnormalities —
      (Continued)
   Papanicolaou (smear) (Continued)
      vagina R87.629
         atypical squamous cells cannot
               exclude high grade squamous
               intraepithelial lesion (ASC-H)
               R87.621
         atypical squamous cells of
               undetermined significance
               (ASC-US) R87.620
         cytologic evidence of malignancy
               R87.624
         high grade squamous intraepithelial
               lesion (HGSIL) R87.623
         inadequate smear R87.625
         low grade squamous intraepithelial
               lesion (LGSIL) R87.622
         specified NEC R87.628
         thin preparation R87.629
         unsatisfactory smear R87.625
      vulva R87.69
      wound secretions R89.6
   partial thromboplastin time (PTT) R79.1
   pelvis (bony) —see Deformity, pelvis
   percussion, chest (tympany) R09.89
   periods (grossly) —see Menstruation
   phonocardiogram R94.39
   plantar reflex R29.2
   plasma
      protein R77.9
         specified NEC R77.8
      viscosity R70.1
   pleural (folds) Q34.0
   posture R29.3
   product of conception O02.9
      specified type NEC O02.89
   prothrombin time (PT) R79.1
   pulmonary
      artery, congenital Q25.79
      function, newborn P28.89
      test results R94.2
   pulsations in neck R00.2
   pupillary H21.56-
      function (reaction) (reflex) —see Anomaly,
            pupil, function
   radiological examination —see Abnormal,
         diagnostic imaging
   red blood cell (s) (morphology) (volume)
         R71.8
   reflex —see Reflex
   renal function test R94.4
   response to nerve stimulation R94.130
   retinal correspondence H53.31
   retinal function study R94.111
   rhythm, heart —see also Arrhythmia
   saliva —see Abnormal, specimen, digestive
         organs
   scan
      kidney R94.4
      liver R93.2
      thyroid R94.6
   secretion
      gastrin E16.4
      glucagon E16.3
   semen, seminal fluid —see Abnormal,
         specimen, male genital organs
   serum level (of)
      acid phosphatase R74.8
      alkaline phosphatase R74.8
      amylase R74.8
      enzymes R74.9
         specified NEC R74.8
      lipase R74.8
      triacylglycerol lipase R74.8
   shape
      gravid uterus —see Anomaly, uterus
   sinus venosus Q21.1
   size, tooth, teeth K00.2
   spacing, tooth, teeth, fully erupted
         M26.30

Abnormal, abnormality, abnormalities —
(Continued)
specimen
digestive organs (peritoneal fluid) (saliva)
R85.9
cytology R85.69
drug level R85.2
enzyme level R85.0
histology R85.7
hormones R85.1
immunology R85.4
microbiology R85.5
nonmedicinal level R85.3
specified type NEC R85.89
female genital organs (secretions) (smears)
R87.9
cytology R87.69
cervix R87.619
human papillomavirus (HPV) DNA
test
high risk positive R87.810
low risk positive R87.820
inadequate (unsatisfactory) smear
R87.615
non-atypical endometrial cells
R87.618
specified NEC R87.618
vagina R87.629
human papillomavirus (HPV) DNA
test
high risk positive R87.811
low risk positive R87.821
inadequate (unsatisfactory) smear
R87.625
vulva R87.69
drug level R87.2
enzyme level R87.0
histological R87.7
hormones R87.1
immunology R87.4
microbiology R87.5
nonmedicinal level R87.3
specified type NEC R87.89
male genital organs (prostatic secretions)
(semen) R86.9
cytology R86.6
drug level R86.2
enzyme level R86.0
histological R86.7
hormones R86.1
immunology R86.4
microbiology R86.5
nonmedicinal level R86.3
specified type NEC R86.8
nipple discharge —see Abnormal,
specimen, specified
respiratory organs (bronchial washings)
(nasal secretions) (pleural fluid)
(sputum) R84.9
cytology R84.6
drug level R84.2
enzyme level R84.0
histology R84.7
hormones R84.1
immunology R84.4
microbiology R84.5
nonmedicinal level R84.3
specified type NEC R84.8
specified organ, system and tissue NOS
R89.9
cytology R89.6
drug level R89.2
enzyme level R89.0
histology R89.7
hormones R89.1
immunology R89.4
microbiology R89.5
nonmedicinal level R89.3
specified type NEC R89.8
synovial fluid —see Abnormal, specimen,
specified

Abnormal, abnormality, abnormalities —
(Continued)
specimen (Continued)
thorax (bronchial washings) (pleural
fluids) —see Abnormal, specimen,
respiratory organs
vagina (secretion) (smear) R87.629
vulva (secretion) (smear) R87.69
wound secretion —see Abnormal,
specimen, specified
spermatozoa —see Abnormal, specimen, male
genital organs
sputum (amount) (color) (odor) R09.3
stool (color) (contents) (mucus) R19.5
bloody K92.1
guaiac positive R19.5
synchondrosis Q78.8
thermography (see also Abnormal, diagnostic
imaging) R93.8
thyroid-binding globulin E07.89
tooth, teeth (form) (size) K00.2
toxicology (findings) R78.9
transport protein E88.09
tumor marker NEC R97.8
ultrasound results —see Abnormal, diagnostic
imaging
umbilical cord complicating delivery O69.9
urination NEC R39.19
urine (constituents) R82.90
bile R82.2
cytological examination R82.8
drugs R82.5
fat R82.0
glucose R81
heavy metals R82.6
hemoglobin R82.3
histological examination R82.8
ketones R82.4
microbiological examination (culture) R82.7
myoglobin R82.1
positive culture R82.7
protein —see Proteinuria
specified substance NEC R82.99
chromoabnormality NEC R82.91
substances nonmedical R82.6
uterine hemorrhage —see Hemorrhage,
uterus
vectorcardiogram R94.39
visually evoked potential (VEP) R94.112
white blood cells D72.9
specified NEC D72.89
X-ray examination —see Abnormal,
diagnostic imaging
Abnormity (any organ or part) —see Anomaly
Abocclusion M26.29
hemolytic disease (newborn) P55.1
incompatibility reaction ABO —see
Complication (s), transfusion,
incompatibility reaction, ABO
Abolition, language R48.8
Aborter, habitual or recurrent —see Loss (of),
pregnancy, recurrent
Abortion (complete) (spontaneous)
O03.9
with
retained products of conception - see
Abortion, incomplete
attempted (elective) (failed) O07.4
complicated by O07.30
afibrinogenemia O07.1
cardiac arrest O07.36
chemical damage of pelvic organ (s)
O07.34
circulatory collapse O07.31
cystitis O07.38
defibrination syndrome O07.1
electrolyte imbalance O07.33
embolism (air) (amniotic fluid) (blood
clot) (fat) (pulmonary) (septic)
(soap) O07.2
endometritis O07.0

Abortion (Continued)
attempted (Continued)
complicated by (Continued)
genital tract and pelvic infection O07.0
hemolysis O07.1
hemorrhage (delayed) (excessive) O07.1
infection
genital tract or pelvic O07.0
urinary tract tract O07.38
intravascular coagulation O07.1
laceration of pelvic organ (s) O07.34
metabolic disorder O07.33
oliguria O07.32
oophoritis O07.0
parametritis O07.0
pelvic peritonitis O07.0
perforation of pelvic organ (s) O07.34
renal failure or shutdown O07.32
salpingitis or salpingo-oophoritis O07.0
sepsis O07.37
shock O07.31
specified condition NEC O07.39
tubular necrosis (renal) O07.32
uremia O07.32
urinary tract infection O07.38
venous complication NEC O07.35
embolism (air) (amniotic fluid) (blood
clot) (fat) (pulmonary) (septic)
(soap) O07.2
complicated (by) (following) O03.80
afibrinogenemia O03.6
cardiac arrest O03.86
chemical damage of pelvic organ (s) O03.84
circulatory collapse O03.81
cystitis O03.88
defibrination syndrome O03.6
electrolyte imbalance O03.83
embolism (air) (amniotic fluid) (blood
clot) (fat) (pulmonary) (septic) (soap)
O03.7
endometritis O03.5
genital tract and pelvic infection O03.5
hemolysis O03.6
hemorrhage (delayed) (excessive) O03.6
infection
genital tract or pelvic O03.5
urinary tract O03.88
intravascular coagulation O03.6
laceration of pelvic organ (s) O03.84
metabolic disorder O03.83
oliguria O03.82
oophoritis O03.5
parametritis O03.5
pelvic peritonitis O03.5
perforation of pelvic organ (s) O03.84
renal failure or shutdown O03.82
salpingitis or salpingo-oophoritis O03.5
sepsis O03.87
shock O03.81
specified condition NEC O03.89
tubular necrosis (renal) O03.82
uremia O03.82
urinary tract infection O03.88
venous complication NEC O03.85
embolism (air) (amniotic fluid) (blood
clot) (fat) (pulmonary) (septic)
(soap) O03.7
failed —see Abortion, attempted
habitual or recurrent N96
with current abortion —see categories
O03-O06
without current pregnancy N96
care in current pregnancy O26.2-
incomplete (spontaneous) O03.4
complicated (by) (following) O03.30
afibrinogenemia O03.1
cardiac arrest O03.36
chemical damage of pelvic organ (s)
O03.34
circulatory collapse O03.31
cystitis O03.38

◀ New ◀▥ Revised ~~deleted~~ Deleted

Abortion *(Continued)*
  incomplete *(Continued)*
    complicated *(Continued)*
      defibrination syndrome O03.1
      electrolyte imbalance O03.33
      embolism (air) (amniotic fluid) (blood
        clot) (fat) (pulmonary) (septic)
        (soap) O03.2
      endometritis O03.0
      genital tract and pelvic infection O03.0
      hemolysis O03.1
      hemorrhage (delayed) (excessive)
        O03.1
      infection
        genital tract or pelvic O03.0
        urinary tract O03.38
      intravascular coagulation O03.1
      laceration of pelvic organ (s) O03.34
      metabolic disorder O03.33
      oliguria O03.32
      oophoritis O03.0
      parametritis O03.0
      pelvic peritonitis O03.0
      perforation of pelvic organ (s) O03.34
      renal failure or shutdown O03.32
      salpingitis or salpingo-oophoritis O03.0
      sepsis O03.37
      shock O03.31
      specified condition NEC O03.39
      tubular necrosis (renal) O03.32
      uremia O03.32
      urinary infection O03.38
      venous complication NEC O03.35
        embolism (air) (amniotic fluid) (blood
          clot) (fat) (pulmonary) (septic)
          (soap) O03.2
  induced (encounter for) Z33.2
    complicated by O04.80
      afibrinogenemia O04.6
      cardiac arrest O04.86
      chemical damage of pelvic organ (s)
        O04.84
      circulatory collapse O04.81
      cystitis O04.88
      defibrination syndrome O04.6
      electrolyte imbalance O04.83
      embolism (air) (amniotic fluid) (blood
        clot) (fat) (pulmonary) (septic)
        (soap) O04.7
      endometritis O04.5
      genital tract and pelvic infection O04.5
      hemolysis O04.6
      hemorrhage (delayed) (excessive)
        O04.6
      infection
        genital tract or pelvic O04.5
        urinary tract O04.88
      intravascular coagulation O04.6
      laceration of pelvic organ (s) O04.84
      metabolic disorder O04.83
      oliguria O04.82
      oophoritis O04.5
      parametritis O04.5
      pelvic peritonitis O04.5
      perforation of pelvic organ (s) O04.84
      renal failure or shutdown O04.82
      salpingitis or salpingo-oophoritis O04.5
      sepsis O04.87
      shock O04.81
      specified condition NEC O04.89
      tubular necrosis (renal) O04.82
      uremia O04.82
      urinary tract infection O04.88
      venous complication NEC O04.85
        embolism (air) (amniotic fluid) (blood
          clot) (fat) (pulmonary) (septic)
          (soap) O04.7
  missed O02.1
  spontaneous —*see* Abortion (complete)
    (spontaneous)
    threatened O20.0

Abortion *(Continued)*
  threatened (spontaneous) O20.0
  tubal O00.1
Abortus fever A23.1
Aboulomania F60.7
Abrami's disease D59.8
Abramov-Fiedler myocarditis (acute isolated
  myocarditis) I40.1
Abrasion T14.8
  abdomen, abdominal (wall) S30.811
  alveolar process S00.512
  ankle S90.51-
  antecubital space —*see* Abrasion, elbow
  anus S30.817
  arm (upper) S40.81-
  auditory canal —*see* Abrasion, ear
  auricle —*see* Abrasion, ear
  axilla —*see* Abrasion, arm
  back, lower S30.810
  breast S20.11-
  brow S00.81
  buttock S30.810
  calf —*see* Abrasion, leg
  canthus —*see* Abrasion, eyelid
  cheek S00.81
    internal S00.512
  chest wall —*see* Abrasion, thorax
  chin S00.81
  clitoris S30.814
  cornea S05.0-
  costal region —*see* Abrasion, thorax
  dental K03.1
  digit (s)
    foot —*see* Abrasion, toe
    hand —*see* Abrasion, finger
  ear S00.41-
  elbow S50.31-
  epididymis S30.813
  epigastric region S30.811
  epiglottis S10.11
  esophagus (thoracic) S27.818
    cervical S10.11
  eyebrow —*see* Abrasion, eyelid
  eyelid S00.21-
  face S00.81
  finger (s) S60.41-
    index S60.41-
    little S60.41-
    middle S60.41-
    ring S60.41-
  flank S30.811
  foot (except toe (s) alone) S90.81-
    toe —*see* Abrasion, toe
  forearm S50.81-
    elbow only —*see* Abrasion, elbow
  forehead S00.81
  genital organs, external
    female S30.816
    male S30.815
  groin S30.811
  gum S00.512
  hand S60.51-
  head S00.91
    ear —*see* Abrasion, ear
    eyelid —*see* Abrasion, eyelid
    lip S00.511
    nose S00.31
    oral cavity S00.512
    scalp S00.01
    specified site NEC S00.81
  heel —*see* Abrasion, foot
  hip S70.21-
  inguinal region S30.811
  interscapular region S20.419
  jaw S00.81
  knee S80.21-
  labium (majus) (minus) S30.814
  larynx S10.11
  leg (lower) S80.81-
    knee —*see* Abrasion, knee
    upper —*see* Abrasion, thigh

Abrasion *(Continued)*
  lip S00.511
  lower back S30.810
  lumbar region S30.810
  malar region S00.81
  mammary —*see* Abrasion, breast
  mastoid region S00.81
  mouth S00.512
  nail
    finger —*see* Abrasion, finger
    toe —*see* Abrasion, toe
  nape S10.81
  nasal S00.31
  neck S10.91
    specified site NEC S10.81
    throat S10.11
  nose S00.31
  occipital region S00.01
  oral cavity S00.512
  orbital region —*see* Abrasion, eyelid
  palate S00.512
  palm —*see* Abrasion, hand
  parietal region S00.01
  pelvis S30.810
  penis S30.812
  perineum
    female S30.814
    male S30.810
  periocular area —*see* Abrasion, eyelid
  phalanges
    finger —*see* Abrasion, finger
    toe —*see* Abrasion, toe
  pharynx S10.11
  pinna —*see* Abrasion, ear
  popliteal space —*see* Abrasion, knee
  prepuce S30.812
  pubic region S30.810
  pudendum
    female S30.816
    male S30.815
  sacral region S30.810
  scalp S00.01
  scapular region —*see* Abrasion, shoulder
  scrotum S30.813
  shin —*see* Abrasion, leg
  shoulder S40.21-
  skin NEC T14.8
  sternal region S20.319
  submaxillary region S00.81
  submental region S00.81
  subungual
    finger (s) —*see* Abrasion, finger
    toe (s) —*see* Abrasion, toe
  supraclavicular fossa S10.81
  supraorbital S00.81
  temple S00.81
  temporal region S00.81
  testis S30.813
  thigh S70.31-
  thorax, thoracic (wall) S20.91
    back S20.41-
    front S20.31-
  throat S10.11
  thumb S60.31-
  toe (s) (lesser) S90.416
    great S90.41-
  tongue S00.512
  tooth, teeth (dentifrice) (habitual) (hard
    tissues) (occupational) (ritual)
    (traditional) K03.1
  trachea S10.11
  tunica vaginalis S30.813
  tympanum, tympanic membrane —*see*
    Abrasion, ear
  uvula S00.512
  vagina S30.814
  vocal cords S10.11
  vulva S30.814
  wrist S60.81-
Abrism —*see* Poisoning, food, [
  plant

Abscess *(Continued)*
   intramammary —*see* Abscess, breast
   intraorbital —*see* Abscess, orbit
   intraperitoneal K65.1
   intrasphincteric (anus) K61.4
   intraspinal G06.1
   intratonsillar J36
   ischiorectal (fossa) K61.3
   jaw (bone) (lower) (upper) M27.2
   joint —*see* Arthritis, pyogenic or pyemic
      spine (tuberculous) A18.01
         nontuberculous —*see* Spondylopathy,
            infective
   kidney N15.1
      with calculus N20.0
         with hydronephrosis N13.6
      puerperal (postpartum) O86.21
   knee —*see also* Abscess, lower limb
      joint M00.9
   labium (majus) (minus) N76.4
   lacrimal
      caruncle —*see* Inflammation, lacrimal,
         passages, acute
      gland —*see* Dacryoadenitis
      passages (duct) (sac) —*see* Inflammation,
         lacrimal, passages, acute
   lacunar N34.0
   larynx J38.7
   lateral (alveolar) K04.7
      with sinus K04.6
   leg (any part) —*see* Abscess, lower limb
   lens H27.8
   lingual K14.0
      tonsil J36
   lip K13.0
   Littre's gland N34.0
   liver (cholangitic) (hematogenic)
      (lymphogenic) (pylephlebitic)
      (pyogenic) K75.0
      amebic (due to Entamoeba histolytica)
         (dysenteric) (tropical) A06.4
         with
            brain abscess (and liver or lung
               abscess) A06.6
            lung abscess A06.5
   loin (region) L02.211
   lower limb L02.41-
   lumbar (tuberculous) A18.01
      nontuberculous L02.212
   lung (miliary) (putrid) J85.2
      with pneumonia J85.1
         due to specified organism *(see*
            Pneumonia, in (due to))*
      amebic (with liver abscess) A06.5
         with
            brain abscess A06.6
            pneumonia A06.5
   lymph, lymphatic, gland or node (acute) —*see*
      also Lymphadenitis, acute
      mesentery I88.0
   malar M27.2
   mammary gland —*see* Abscess, breast
   marginal, anus K61.0
   mastoid —*see* Mastoiditis, acute
   maxilla, maxillary M27.2
      molar (tooth) K04.7
         with sinus K04.6
      premolar K04.7
      sinus (chronic) J32.0
   mediastinum J85.3
   meibomian gland —*see* Hordeolum
   meninges G06.2
   mesentery, mesenteric K65.1
   mesosalpinx —*see* Salpingitis
   mons pubis L02.215
   mouth (floor) K12.2
   muscle —*see* Myositis, infective
   myocardium I40.0
   nabothian (follicle) —*see* Cervicitis
   nasal J32.9
   nasopharyngeal J39.1

Abscess *(Continued)*
   navel L02.216
      newborn P38.9
         with mild hemorrhage P38.1
         without hemorrhage P38.9
   neck (region) L02.11
      lymph gland or node L04.0
   nephritic —*see* Abscess, kidney
   nipple N61
      associated with
         lactation —*see* Pregnancy, complicated
            by,
         pregnancy —*see* Pregnancy, complicated
            by
   nose (external) (fossa) (septum) J34.0
      sinus (chronic) —*see* Sinusitis
   omentum K65.1
   operative wound T81.4
   orbit, orbital —*see* Cellulitis, orbit
   otogenic G06.0
   ovary, ovarian (corpus luteum) —*see*
      Oophoritis
   oviduct —*see* Oophoritis
   palate (soft) K12.2
      hard M27.2
   palmar (space) —*see* Abscess, hand
   pancreas (duct) —*see* Pancreatitis, acute
   parafrenal N48.21
   parametric, parametrium N73.2
      acute N73.0
      chronic N73.1
   paranephric N15.1
   parapancreatic —*see* Pancreatitis, acute
   parapharyngeal J39.0
   pararectal K61.1
   parasinus —*see* Sinusitis
   parauterine *(see also* Disease, pelvis,
      inflammatory) N73.2
   paravaginal —*see* Vaginitis
   parietal region (scalp) L02.811
   parodontal K05.21
   parotid (duct) (gland) K11.3
      region K12.2
   pectoral (region) L02.213
   pelvis, pelvic
      female —*see* Disease, pelvis, inflammatory
      male, peritoneal K65.1
   penis N48.21
      gonococcal (accessory gland) (periurethral)
         A54.1
   perianal K61.0
   periapical K04.7
      with sinus (alveolar) K04.6
   periappendicular K35.3
   pericardial I30.1
   pericecal K35.3
   pericemental K05.21
   pericholecystic —*see* Cholecystitis, acute
   pericoronal K05.21
   peridental K05.21
   perimetric *(see also* Disease, pelvis,
      inflammatory) N73.2
   perinephric, perinephritic —*see* Abscess,
      kidney
   perineum, perineal (superficial) L02.215
      urethra N34.0
   periodontal (parietal) K05.21
      apical K04.7
   periosteum, periosteal —*see also*
      Osteomyelitis, specified type NEC
      with osteomyelitis —*see also* Osteomyelitis,
         specified type NEC
         acute —*see* Osteomyelitis, acute
         chronic —*see* Osteomyelitis, chronic
   peripharyngeal J39.0
   peripleuritic J86.9
      with fistula J86.0
   periprostatic N41.2
   perirectal K61.1
   perirenal (tissue) —*see* Abscess, kidney
   perisinuous (nose) —*see* Sinusitis

Abscess *(Continued)*
   peritoneum, peritoneal (perforated)
      (ruptured) K65.1
      with appendicitis K35.3
      pelvic
         female —*see* Peritonitis, pelvic, female
         male K65.1
      postoperative T81.4
      puerperal, postpartum, childbirth O85
      tuberculous A18.31
   peritonsillar J36
   perityphlic K35.3
   periureteral N28.89
   periurethral N34.0
      gonococcal (accessory gland) (periurethral)
         A54.1
   periuterine *(see also* Disease, pelvis,
      inflammatory) N73.2
   perivesical —*see* Cystitis, specified type NEC
   petrous bone —*see* Petrositis
   phagedenic NOS L02.91
      chancroid A57
   pharynx, pharyngeal (lateral) J39.1
   pilonidal L05.01
   pituitary (gland) E23.6
   pleura J86.9
      with fistula J86.0
   popliteal —*see* Abscess, lower limb
   postcecal K35.3
   postlaryngeal J38.7
   postnasal J34.0
   postoperative (any site) T81.4
      retroperitoneal K68.11
   postpharyngeal J39.0
   posttonsillar J36
   post-typhoid A01.09
   pouch of Douglas —*see* Peritonitis, pelvic,
      female
   premammary —*see* Abscess, breast
   prepatellar —*see* Abscess, lower limb
   prostate N41.2
      gonococcal (acute) (chronic) A54.22
   psoas muscle K68.12
   puerperal - code by site under Puerperal,
      abscess
   pulmonary —*see* Abscess, lung
   pulp, pulpal (dental) K04.0
   rectovaginal septum K63.0
   rectovesical —*see* Cystitis, specified type NEC
   rectum K61.1
   renal —*see* Abscess, kidney
   retina —*see* Inflammation, chorioretinal
   retrobulbar —*see* Abscess, orbit
   retrocecal K65.1
   retrolaryngeal J38.7
   retromammary —*see* Abscess, breast
   retroperitoneal NEC K68.19
      postprocedural K68.11
   retropharyngeal J39.0
   retrouterine —*see* Peritonitis, pelvic, female
   retrovesical —*see* Cystitis, specified type NEC
   root, tooth K04.7
      with sinus (alveolar) K04.6
   round ligament *(see also* Disease, pelvis,
      inflammatory) N73.2
   rupture (spontaneous) NOS L02.91
   sacrum (tuberculous) A18.01
      nontuberculous M46.28
   salivary (duct) (gland) K11.3
   scalp (any part) L02.811
   scapular —*see* Osteomyelitis, specified type
      NEC
   sclera —*see* Scleritis
   scrofulous (tuberculous) A18.2
   scrotum N49.2
   seminal vesicle N49.0
   septal, dental K04.7
      with sinus (alveolar) K04.6
   serous —*see* Periostitis
   shoulder (region) —*see* Abscess, upper lim
   sigmoid K63.0

Abscess *(Continued)*
  sinus (accessory) (chronic) (nasal) —*see also*
    Sinusitis
    intracranial venous (any) G06.0
  Skene's duct or gland N34.0
  skin —*see* Abscess, by site
  specified site NEC L02.818
  spermatic cord N49.1
  sphenoidal (sinus) (chronic) J32.3
  spinal cord (any part) (staphylococcal) G06.1
    tuberculous A17.81
  spine (column) (tuberculous) A18.01
    epidural G06.1
    nontuberculous —*see* Osteomyelitis,
      vertebra
  spleen D73.3
    amebic A06.89
  stitch T81.4
  subarachnoid G06.2
    brain G06.0
    spinal cord G06.1
  subareolar —*see* Abscess, breast
  subcecal K35.3
  subcutaneous —*see also* Abscess, by site
    pheomycotic (chromomycotic) B43.2
  subdiaphragmatic K65.1
  subdural G06.2
    brain G06.0
      sequelae G09
    spinal cord G06.1
  subgaleal L02.811
  subhepatic K65.1
  sublingual K12.2
    gland K11.3
  submammary —*see* Abscess, breast
  submandibular (region) (space) (triangle)
    K12.2
    gland K11.3
  submaxillary (region) L02.01
    gland K11.3
  submental L02.01
    gland K11.3
  subperiosteal —*see* Osteomyelitis, specified
    type NEC
  subphrenic K65.1
    postoperative T81.4
  suburethral N34.0
  sudoriparous L75.8
  supraclavicular (fossa) —*see* Abscess, upper
    limb
  suprapelvic, acute N73.0
  suprarenal (capsule) (gland) E27.8
  sweat gland L74.8
  tear duct —*see* Inflammation, lacrimal,
    passages, acute
  temple L02.01
  temporal region L02.01
  temporosphenoidal G06.0
  tendon (sheath) M65.00
    ankle M65.07-
    foot M65.07-
    forearm M65.03-
    hand M65.04-
    lower leg M65.06-
    pelvic region M65.05-
    shoulder region M65.01-
    specified site NEC M65.08
    thigh M65.05-
    upper arm M65.02-
  testis N45.4
  thigh —*see* Abscess, lower limb
  thorax J86.9
    with fistula J86.0
  throat J39.1
  thumb —*see also* Abscess, hand
    nail —*see* Cellulitis, finger
  thymus (gland) E32.1
  thyroid (gland) E06.0
  toe (any) —*see also* Abscess, foot
    nail —*see* Cellulitis, toe
  tongue (staphylococcal) K14.0

Abscess *(Continued)*
  tonsil (s) (lingual) J36
  tonsillopharyngeal J36
  tooth, teeth (root) K04.7
    with sinus (alveolar) K04.6
    supporting structures NEC K05.21
  trachea J39.8
  trunk L02.219
    abdominal wall L02.211
    back L02.212
    chest wall L02.213
    groin L02.214
    perineum L02.215
    umbilicus L02.216
  tubal —*see* Salpingitis
  tuberculous —*see* Tuberculosis, abscess
  tubo-ovarian —*see* Salpingo-oophoritis
  tunica vaginalis N49.1
  umbilicus L02.216
  upper
    limb L02.41-
    respiratory J39.8
  urethral (gland) N34.0
  urinary N34.0
  uterus, uterine (wall) —*see also* Endometritis
    ligament (*see also* Disease, pelvis,
      inflammatory) N73.2
    neck —*see* Cervicitis
  uvula K12.2
  vagina (wall) —*see* Vaginitis
  vaginorectal —*see* Vaginitis
  vas deferens N49.1
  vermiform appendix K35.3
  vertebra (column) (tuberculous) A18.01
    nontuberculous —*see* Osteomyelitis,
      vertebra
  vesical —*see* Cystitis, specified type NEC
  vesico-uterine pouch —*see* Peritonitis, pelvic,
    female
  vitreous (humor) —*see* Endophthalmitis,
    purulent
  vocal cord J38.3
  von Bezold's —*see* Mastoiditis, acute
  vulva N76.4
  vulvovaginal gland N75.1
  web space —*see* Abscess, hand
  wound T81.4
  wrist —*see* Abscess, upper limb
Absence (of) (organ or part) (complete or
  partial)
  adrenal (gland) (congenital) Q89.1
    acquired E89.6
  albumin in blood E88.09
  alimentary tract (congenital) Q45.8
    upper Q40.8
  alveolar process (acquired) —*see* Anomaly,
    alveolar
  ankle (acquired) Z89.44-
  anus (congenital) Q42.3
    with fistula Q42.2
  aorta (congenital) Q25.4
  appendix, congenital Q42.8
  arm (acquired) Z89.20-
    above elbow Z89.22-
      congenital (with hand present) —*see*
        Agenesis, arm, with hand present
        and hand —*see* Agenesis, forearm,
        and hand
    below elbow Z89.21-
      congenital (with hand present) —*see*
        Agenesis, arm, with hand present
        and hand —*see* Agenesis, forearm,
        and hand
    congenital —*see* Defect, reduction, upper
      limb
    shoulder (following explantation of
      shoulder joint prosthesis) (joint) (with
      or without presence of antibiotic-
      impregnated cement spacer) Z89.23-
    congenital (with hand present) —*see*
      Agenesis, arm, with hand present

Absence *(Continued)*
  artery (congenital) (peripheral) Q27.8
    brain Q28.3
    coronary Q24.5
    pulmonary Q25.79
    specified NEC Q27.8
    umbilical Q27.0
  atrial septum (congenital) Q21.1
  auditory canal (congenital) (external) Q16.1
  auricle (ear), congenital Q16.0
  bile, biliary duct, congenital Q44.5
  bladder (acquired) Z90.6
    congenital Q64.5
  bowel sounds R19.11
  brain Q00.0
    part of Q04.3
  breast (s) (and nipple (s)) (acquired) Z90.1-
    congenital Q83.8
  broad ligament Q50.6
  bronchus (congenital) Q32.4
  canaliculus lacrimalis, congenital Q10.4
  cerebellum (vermis) Q04.3
  cervix (acquired) (with uterus) Z90.710
    with remaining uterus Z90.712
    congenital Q51.5
  chin, congenital Q18.8
  cilia (congenital) Q10.3
    acquired —*see* Madarosis
  clitoris (congenital) Q52.6
  coccyx, congenital Q76.49
  cold sense R20.8
  congenital
    lumen —*see* Atresia
    organ or site NEC —*see* Agenesis
    septum —*see* Imperfect, closure
  corpus callosum Q04.0
  cricoid cartilage, congenital Q31.8
  diaphragm (with hernia), congenital Q79.1
  digestive organ (s) or tract, congenital
    Q45.8
    acquired NEC Z90.49
    upper Q40.8
  ductus arteriosus Q28.8
  duodenum (acquired) Z90.49
    congenital Q41.0
  ear, congenital Q16.9
    acquired H93.8-
    auricle Q16.0
    external Q16.0
    inner Q16.5
    lobe, lobule Q17.8
    middle, except ossicles Q16.4
      ossicles Q16.3
    ossicles Q16.3
  ejaculatory duct (congenital) Q55.4
  endocrine gland (congenital) NEC Q89.2
    acquired E89.89
  epididymis (congenital) Q55.4
    acquired Z90.79
  epiglottis, congenital Q31.8
  esophagus (congenital) Q39.8
    acquired (partial) Z90.49
  eustachian tube (congenital) Q16.2
  extremity (acquired) Z89.9
    congenital Q73.0
    knee (following explantation of knee joint
      prosthesis) (joint) (with or without
      presence of antibiotic-impregnated
      cement spacer) Z89.52-
    lower (above knee) Z89.619
      below knee Z89.51-
    upper —*see* Absence, arm
  eye (acquired) Z90.01
    congenital Q11.1
    muscle (congenital) Q10.3
  eyeball (acquired) Z90.01
  eyelid (fold) (congenital) Q10.3
    acquired Z90.01
  face, specified part NEC Q18.8
  fallopian tube (s) (acquired) Z90.79
    congenital Q50.6

Absence *(Continued)*
  family member (causing problem in home)
    NEC *(see also* Disruption, family)
    Z63.32
  femur, congenital —*see* Defect, reduction,
    lower limb, longitudinal, femur
  fibrinogen (congenital) D68.2
    acquired D65
  finger (s) (acquired) Z89.02-
    congenital —*see* Agenesis, hand
  foot (acquired) Z89.43-
    congenital —*see* Agenesis, foot
  forearm (acquired) —*see* Absence, arm, below
    elbow
  gallbladder (acquired) Z90.49
    congenital Q44.0
  gamma globulin in blood D80.1
    hereditary D80.0
  genital organs
    acquired (female) (male) Z90.79
    female, congenital Q52.8
      external Q52.71
      internal NEC Q52.8
    male, congenital Q55.8
  genitourinary organs, congenital NEC
    female Q52.8
    male Q55.8
  globe (acquired) Z90.01
    congenital Q11.1
  glottis, congenital Q31.8
  hand and wrist (acquired) Z89.11-
    congenital —*see* Agenesis, hand
  head, part (acquired) NEC Z90.09
  heat sense R20.8
  hip (following explantation of hip joint
    prosthesis) (joint) (with or without
    presence of antibiotic-impregnated
    cement spacer) Z89.62-
  hymen (congenital) Q52.4
  ileum (acquired) Z90.49
    congenital Q41.2
  immunoglobulin, isolated NEC D80.3
    IgA D80.2
    IgG D80.3
    IgM D80.4
  incus (acquired) —*see* Loss, ossicles, ear
    congenital Q16.3
  inner ear, congenital Q16.5
  intestine (acquired) (small) Z90.49
    congenital Q41.9
      specified NEC Q41.8
    large Z90.49
      congenital Q42.9
        specified NEC Q42.8
  iris, congenital Q13.1
  jejunum (acquired) Z90.49
    congenital Q41.1
  joint
    acquired
      hip (following explantation of hip
        joint prosthesis) (with or without
        presence of antibiotic-impregnated
        cement spacer) Z89.62-
      knee (following explantation of knee
        joint prosthesis) (with or without
        presence of antibiotic-impregnated
        cement spacer) Z89.52-
      shoulder (following explantation of
        shoulder joint prosthesis) (with
        or without presence of antibiotic-
        impregnated cement spacer)
        Z89.23-
    congenital NEC Q74.8
  kidney (s) (acquired) Z90.5
    congenital Q60.2
      bilateral Q60.1
      unilateral Q60.0
  knee (following explantation of knee joint
    prosthesis) (joint) (with or without
    presence of antibiotic-impregnated
    cement spacer) Z89.52-

Absence *(Continued)*
  labyrinth, membranous Q16.5
  larynx (congenital) Q31.8
    acquired Z90.02
  leg (acquired) (above knee) Z89.61-
    below knee (acquired) Z89.51-
    congenital —*see* Defect, reduction, lower
      limb
  lens (acquired) —*see also* Aphakia
    congenital Q12.3
    post cataract extraction Z98.4-
  limb (acquired) —*see* Absence, extremity
  lip Q38.6
  liver (congenital) Q44.7
  lung (fissure) (lobe) (bilateral) (unilateral)
    (congenital) Q33.3
    acquired (any part) Z90.2
  menstruation —*see* Amenorrhea
  muscle (congenital) (pectoral) Q79.8
    ocular Q10.3
  neck, part Q18.8
  neutrophil —*see* Agranulocytosis
  nipple (s) (with breast (s)) (acquired)
    Z90.1-
    congenital Q83.2
  nose (congenital) Q30.1
    acquired Z90.09
  organ
    of Corti, congenital Q16.5
    or site, congenital NEC Q89.8
      acquired NEC Z90.89
  osseous meatus (ear) Q16.4
  ovary (acquired)
    bilateral Z90.722
    congenital
      bilateral Q50.02
      unilateral Q50.01
    unilateral Z90.721
  oviduct (acquired)
    bilateral Z90.722
    congenital Q50.6
    unilateral Z90.721
  pancreas (congenital) Q45.0
    acquired Z90.410
      complete Z90.410
      partial Z90.411
      total Z90.410
  parathyroid gland (acquired)
    E89.2
    congenital Q89.2
  patella, congenital Q74.1
  penis (congenital) Q55.5
    acquired Z90.79
  pericardium (congenital) Q24.8
  pituitary gland (congenital) Q89.2
    acquired E89.3
  prostate (acquired) Z90.79
    congenital Q55.4
  pulmonary valve Q22.0
  punctum lacrimale (congenital) Q10.4
  radius, congenital —*see* Defect, reduction,
    upper limb, longitudinal, radius
  rectum (congenital) Q42.1
    with fistula Q42.0
    acquired Z90.49
  respiratory organ NOS Q34.9
  rib (acquired) Z90.89
    congenital Q76.6
  sacrum, congenital Q76.49
  salivary gland (s), congenital Q38.4
  scrotum, congenital Q55.29
  seminal vesicles (congenital) Q55.4
    acquired Z90.79
  septum
    atrial (congenital) Q21.1
    between aorta and pulmonary artery
      Q21.4
    ventricular (congenital) Q20.4
  sex chromosome
    female phenotype Q97.8
    male phenotype Q98.8

Absence *(Continued)*
  skull bone (congenital) Q75.8
    with
      anencephaly Q00.0
      encephalocele —*see* Encephalocele
      hydrocephalus Q03.9
        with spina bifida —*see* Spina
          bifida, by site, with
          hydrocephalus
      microcephaly Q02
  spermatic cord, congenital Q55.4
  spine, congenital Q76.49
  spleen (congenital) Q89.01
    acquired Z90.81
  sternum, congenital Q76.7
  stomach (acquired) (partial) Z90.3
    congenital Q40.2
  superior vena cava, congenital
    Q26.8
  teeth, tooth (congenital) K00.0
    acquired (complete) K08.109
      class I K08.101
      class II K08.102
      class III K08.103
      class IV K08.104
      due to
        caries K08.139
          class I K08.131
          class II K08.132
          class III K08.133
          class IV K08.134
        periodontal disease K08.129
          class I K08.121
          class II K08.122
          class III K08.123
          class IV K08.124
      specified NEC K08.199
        class I K08.191
        class II K08.192
        class III K08.193
        class IV K08.194
      trauma K08.119
        class I K08.111
        class II K08.112
        class III K08.113
        class IV K08.114
    partial K08.409
      class I K08.401
      class II K08.402
      class III K08.403
      class IV K08.404
      due to
        caries K08.439
          class I K08.431
          class II K08.432
          class III K08.433
          class IV K08.434
        periodontal disease K08.429
          class I K08.421
          class II K08.422
          class III K08.423
          class IV K08.424
        specified NEC K08.499
        class I K08.491
        class II K08.492
        class III K08.493
        class IV K08.494
      trauma K08.419
        class I K08.411
        class II K08.412
        class III K08.413
        class IV K08.414
  tendon (congenital) Q79.8
  testis (congenital) Q55.0
    acquired Z90.79
  thumb (acquired) Z89.01-
    congenital —*see* Agenesis, hand
  thymus gland Q89.2
  thyroid (gland) (acquired) E89.0
    cartilage, congenital Q31.8
    congenital E03.1

Absence *(Continued)*
  toe (s) (acquired) Z89.42-
    with foot —*see* Absence, foot and
        ankle
    congenital —*see* Agenesis, foot
    great Z89.41-
  tongue, congenital Q38.3
  trachea (cartilage), congenital Q32.1
  transverse aortic arch, congenital
      Q25.4
  tricuspid valve Q22.4
  umbilical artery, congenital Q27.0
  upper arm and forearm with hand present,
      congenital —*see* Agenesis, arm, with
      hand present
  ureter (congenital) Q62.4
    acquired Z90.6
  urethra, congenital Q64.5
  uterus (acquired) Z90.710
    with cervix Z90.710
    with remaining cervical stump
        Z90.711
    congenital Q51.0
  uvula, congenital Q38.5
  vagina, congenital Q52.0
  vas deferens (congenital) Q55.4
    acquired Z90.79
  vein (peripheral) congenital NEC
      Q27.8
    cerebral Q28.3
    digestive system Q27.8
    great Q26.8
    lower limb Q27.8
    portal Q26.5
    precerebral Q28.1
    specified site NEC Q27.8
    upper limb Q27.8
  vena cava (inferior) (superior), congenital
      Q26.8
  ventricular septum Q20.4
  vertebra, congenital Q76.49
  vulva, congenital Q52.71
  wrist (acquired) Z89.12-
Absorbent system disease I87.8
Absorption
  carbohydrate, disturbance K90.4
  chemical —*see* Table of Drugs and
      Chemicals
    through placenta (newborn) P04.9
      environmental substance P04.6
      nutritional substance P04.5
      obstetric anesthetic or analgesic drug
          P04.0
  drug NEC —*see* Table of Drugs and
      Chemicals
    addictive
      through placenta (newborn) P04.49
        cocaine P04.41
    medicinal
      through placenta (newborn) P04.1
    through placenta (newborn) P04.1
      obstetric anesthetic or analgesic drug
          P04.0
  fat, disturbance K90.4
    pancreatic K90.3
  noxious substance —*see* Table of Drugs and
      Chemicals
  protein, disturbance K90.4
  starch, disturbance K90.4
  toxic substance —*see* Table of Drugs and
      Chemicals
  uremic —*see* Uremia
Abstinence symptoms, syndrome
  alcohol F10.239
    with delirium F10.231
  cocaine F14.23
  neonatal P96.1
  nicotine —*see* Dependence, drug, nicotine,
      with, withdrawal
  opioid F11.93
    with dependence F11.23

Abstinence symptoms, syndrome *(Continued)*
  psychoactive NEC F19.939
    with
      delirium F19.931
      dependence F19.239
        with
          delirium F19.231
          perceptual disturbance F19.232
        uncomplicated F19.230
      perceptual disturbance F19.932
    uncomplicated F19.930
  sedative F13.939
    with
      delirium F13.931
      dependence F13.239
        with
          delirium F13.231
          perceptual disturbance F13.232
        uncomplicated F13.230
      perceptual disturbance F13.932
    uncomplicated F13.930
  stimulant NEC F15.93
    with dependence F15.23
Abulia R68.89
Abulomania F60.7
Abuse
  adult —*see* Maltreatment, adult
    as reason for
      couple seeking advice (including
          offender) Z63.0
  alcohol (non-dependent) F10.10
    with
      anxiety disorder F10.180
      intoxication F10.129
        with delirium F10.121
        uncomplicated F10.120
      mood disorder F10.14
      other specified disorder F10.188
      psychosis F10.159
        delusions F10.150
        hallucinations F10.151
      sexual dysfunction F10.181
      sleep disorder F10.182
      unspecified disorder F10.19
    counseling and surveillance Z71.41
  amphetamine (or related substance) —*see*
      Abuse, drug, stimulant NEC
  analgesics (non-prescribed) (over the counter)
      F55.8
  antacids F55.0
  antidepressants —*see* Abuse, drug,
      psychoactive NEC
  anxiolytic —*see* Abuse, drug, sedative
  barbiturates —*see* Abuse, drug, sedative
  caffeine —*see* Abuse, drug, stimulant NEC
  cannabis, cannabinoids —*see* Abuse, drug,
      cannabis
  child —*see* Maltreatment, child
  cocaine —*see* Abuse, drug, cocaine
  drug NEC (non-dependent) F19.10
    with sleep disorder F19.182
    amphetamine type —*see* Abuse, drug,
        stimulant NEC
    analgesics (non-prescribed) (over the
        counter) F55.8
    antacids F55.0
    antidepressants —*see* Abuse, drug,
        psychoactive NEC
    anxiolytics —*see* Abuse, drug, sedative
    barbiturates —*see* Abuse, drug, sedative
    caffeine —*see* Abuse, drug, stimulant NEC
    cannabis F12.10
      with
        anxiety disorder F12.180
        intoxication F12.129
          with
            delirium F12.121
            perceptual disturbance
                F12.122
          uncomplicated F12.120
        other specified disorder F12.188

Abuse *(Continued)*
  drug NEC *(Continued)*
    cannabis *(Continued)*
      with *(Continued)*
        psychosis F12.159
          delusions F12.150
          hallucinations F12.151
        unspecified disorder F12.19
    cocaine F14.10
      with
        anxiety disorder F14.180
        intoxication F14.129
          with
            delirium F14.121
            perceptual disturbance F14.122
          uncomplicated F14.120
        mood disorder F14.14
        other specified disorder F14.188
        psychosis F14.159
          delusions F14.150
          hallucinations F14.151
        sexual dysfunction F14.181
        sleep disorder F14.182
        unspecified disorder F14.19
    counseling and surveillance Z71.51
    hallucinogen F16.10
      with
        anxiety disorder F16.180
        flashbacks F16.183
        intoxication F16.129
          with
            delirium F16.121
            perceptual disturbance F16.122
          uncomplicated F16.120
        mood disorder F16.14
        other specified disorder F16.188
        perception disorder, persisting F16.183
        psychosis F16.159
          delusions F16.150
          hallucinations F16.151
        unspecified disorder F16.19
    hashish —*see* Abuse, drug, cannabis
    herbal or folk remedies F55.1
    hormones F55.3
    hypnotics —*see* Abuse, drug, sedative
    inhalant F18.10
      with
        anxiety disorder F18.180
        dementia, persisting F18.17
        intoxication F18.129
          with delirium F18.121
          uncomplicated F18.120
        mood disorder F18.14
        other specified disorder F18.188
        psychosis F18.159
          delusions F18.150
          hallucinations F18.151
        unspecified disorder F18.19
    laxatives F55.2
    LSD —*see* Abuse, drug, hallucinogen
    marihuana —*see* Abuse, drug, cannabis
    morphine type (opioids) —*see* Abuse, drug,
        opioid
    opioid F11.10
      with
        intoxication F11.129
          with
            delirium F11.121
            perceptual disturbance F11.122
          uncomplicated F11.120
        mood disorder F11.14
        other specified disorder F11.188
        psychosis F11.159
          delusions F11.150
          hallucinations F11.151
        sexual dysfunction F11.181
        sleep disorder F11.182
        unspecified disorder F11.19
    PCP (phencyclidine) (or related
        substance) —*see* Abuse, drug,
        hallucinogen

◀ New   ◀▦ Revised   ~~deleted~~ Deleted

Abuse *(Continued)*
  drug NEC *(Continued)*
    psychoactive NEC F19.10
      with
        amnestic disorder F19.16
        anxiety disorder F19.180
        dementia F19.17
        intoxication F19.129
          with
            delirium F19.121
            perceptual disturbance F19.122
          uncomplicated F19.120
        mood disorder F19.14
        other specified disorder F19.188
        psychosis F19.159
          delusions F19.150
          hallucinations F19.151
        sexual dysfunction F19.181
        sleep disorder F19.182
        unspecified disorder F19.19
    sedative, hypnotic or anxiolytic F13.10
      with
        anxiety disorder F13.180
        intoxication F13.129
          with delirium F13.121
          uncomplicated F13.120
        mood disorder F13.14
        other specified disorder F13.188
        psychosis F13.159
          delusions F13.150
          hallucinations F13.151
        sexual dysfunction F13.181
        sleep disorder F13.182
        unspecified disorder F13.19
    solvent —*see* Abuse, drug, inhalant
    steroids F55.3
    stimulant NEC F15.10
      with
        anxiety disorder F15.180
        intoxication F15.129
          with
            delirium F15.121
            perceptual disturbance F15.122
          uncomplicated F15.120
        mood disorder F15.14
        other specified disorder F15.188
        psychosis F15.159
          delusions F15.150
          hallucinations F15.151
        sexual dysfunction F15.181
        sleep disorder F15.182
        unspecified disorder F15.19
    tranquilizers —*see* Abuse, drug, sedative
    vitamins F55.4
  hallucinogens —*see* Abuse, drug, hallucinogen
  hashish —*see* Abuse, drug, cannabis
  herbal or folk remedies F55.1
  hormones F55.3
  hypnotic —*see* Abuse, drug, sedative
  inhalant —*see* Abuse, drug, inhalant
  laxatives F55.2
  LSD —*see* Abuse, drug, hallucinogen
  marihuana —*see* Abuse, drug, cannabis
  morphine type (opioids) —*see* Abuse, drug, opioid
  non-psychoactive substance NEC F55.8
    antacids F55.0
    folk remedies F55.1
    herbal remedies F55.1
    hormones F55.3
    laxatives F55.2
    steroids F55.3
    vitamins F55.4
  opioids —*see* Abuse, drug, opioid
  PCP (phencyclidine) (or related substance) —*see* Abuse, drug, hallucinogen
  physical (adult) (child) —*see* Maltreatment
  psychoactive substance —*see* Abuse, drug, psychoactive NEC

Abuse *(Continued)*
  psychological (adult) (child) —*see* Maltreatment
  sedative —*see* Abuse, drug, sedative
  sexual —*see* Maltreatment
  solvent —*see* Abuse, drug, inhalant
  steroids F55.3
  vitamins F55.4
Acalculia R48.8
  developmental F81.2
Acanthamebiasis (with) B60.10
  conjunctiva B60.12
  keratoconjunctivitis B60.13
  meningoencephalitis B60.11
  other specified B60.19
Acanthocephaliasis B83.8
Acanthocheilonemiasis B74.4
Acanthocytosis E78.6
Acantholysis L11.9
Acanthosis (acquired) (nigricans) L83
  benign Q82.8
  congenital Q82.8
  seborrheic L82.1
    inflamed L82.0
  tongue K14.3
Acapnia E87.3
Acarbia E87.2
Acardia, acardius Q89.8
Acardiacus amorphus Q89.8
Acardiotrophia I51.4
Acariasis B88.0
  scabies B86
Acarodermatitis (urticarioides) B88.0
Acarophobia F40.218
Acatalasemia, acatalasia E80.3
Acathisia (drug induced) G25.71
Accelerated atrioventricular conduction I45.6
Accentuation of personality traits (type A) Z73.1
Accessory (congenital)
  adrenal gland Q89.1
  anus Q43.4
  appendix Q43.4
  atrioventricular conduction I45.6
  auditory ossicles Q16.3
  auricle (ear) Q17.0
  biliary duct or passage Q44.5
  bladder Q64.79
  blood vessels NEC Q27.9
    coronary Q24.5
  bone NEC Q79.8
  breast tissue, axilla Q83.1
  carpal bones Q74.0
  cecum Q43.4
  chromosome (s) NEC (nonsex) Q92.9
    with complex rearrangements NEC Q92.5
      seen only at prometaphase Q92.8
    13 —*see* Trisomy, 13
    18 —*see* Trisomy, 18
    21 —*see* Trisomy, 21
    partial Q92.9
    sex
      female phenotype Q97.8
  coronary artery Q24.5
  cusp (s), heart valve NEC Q24.8
    pulmonary Q22.3
  cystic duct Q44.5
  digit (s) Q69.9
  ear (auricle) (lobe) Q17.0
  endocrine gland NEC Q89.2
  eye muscle Q10.3
  eyelid Q10.3
  face bone (s) Q75.8
  fallopian tube (fimbria) (ostium) Q50.6
  finger (s) Q69.0
  foreskin N47.8
  frontonasal process Q75.8

Accessory *(Continued)*
  gallbladder Q44.1
  genital organ (s)
    female Q52.8
      external Q52.79
      internal NEC Q52.8
    male Q55.8
  genitourinary organs NEC Q89.8
    female Q52.8
    male Q55.8
  hallux Q69.2
  heart Q24.8
    valve NEC Q24.8
      pulmonary Q22.3
  hepatic ducts Q44.5
  hymen Q52.4
  intestine (large) (small) Q43.4
  kidney Q63.0
  lacrimal canal Q10.6
  leaflet, heart valve NEC Q24.8
  ligament, broad Q50.6
  liver Q44.7
    duct Q44.5
  lobule (ear) Q17.0
  lung (lobe) Q33.1
  muscle Q79.8
  navicular of carpus Q74.0
  nervous system, part NEC Q07.8
  nipple Q83.3
  nose Q30.8
  organ or site not listed —*see* Anomaly, by site
  ovary Q50.31
  oviduct Q50.6
  pancreas Q45.3
  parathyroid gland Q89.2
  parotid gland (and duct) Q38.4
  pituitary gland Q89.2
  preauricular appendage Q17.0
  prepuce N47.8
  renal arteries (multiple) Q27.2
  rib Q76.6
    cervical Q76.5
  roots (teeth) K00.2
  salivary gland Q38.4
  sesamoid bones Q74.8
    foot Q74.2
    hand Q74.0
  skin tags Q82.8
  spleen Q89.09
  sternum Q76.7
  submaxillary gland Q38.4
  tarsal bones Q74.2
  teeth, tooth K00.1
  tendon Q79.8
  thumb Q69.1
  thymus gland Q89.2
  thyroid gland Q89.2
  toes Q69.2
  tongue Q38.3
  tooth, teeth K00.1
  tragus Q17.0
  ureter Q62.5
  urethra Q64.79
  urinary organ or tract NEC Q64.8
  uterus Q51.2
  vagina Q52.10
  valve, heart NEC Q24.8
    pulmonary Q22.3
  vertebra Q76.49
  vocal cords Q31.8
  vulva Q52.79
Accident
  birth —*see* Birth, injury
  cardiac —*see* Infarct, myocardium
  cerebral I63.9
  cerebrovascular (embolic) (ischemic) (thrombotic) I63.9
    aborted I63.9
    hemorrhagic —*see* Hemorrhage, intracranial, intracerebral

Accident *(Continued)*
  cerebrovascular *(Continued)*
    old (without sequelae) Z86.73
      with sequelae (of) —*see* Sequelae,
        infarction, cerebral
    coronary —*see* Infarct, myocardium
    craniovascular I63.9
    vascular, brain I63.9
Accidental —*see* condition
Accommodation (disorder) —*see also* condition
  hysterical paralysis of F44.89
  insufficiency of H52.4
  paresis —*see* Paresis, of accommodation
  spasm —*see* Spasm, of accommodation
Accouchement —*see* Delivery
Accreta placenta O43.21-
Accretio cordis (nonrheumatic) I31.0
Accretions, tooth, teeth K03.6
Acculturation difficulty Z60.3
Accumulation secretion, prostate N42.89
Acephalia, acephalism, acephalus, acephaly
  Q00.0
Acephalobrachia monster Q89.8
Acephalochirus monster Q89.8
Acephalogaster Q89.8
Acephalostomus monster Q89.8
Acephalothorax Q89.8
Acerophobia F40.298
Acetonemia R79.89
  in Type 1 diabetes E10.10
    with coma E10.11
Acetonuria R82.4
Achalasia (cardia) (esophagus) K22.0
  congenital Q39.5
  pylorus Q40.0
  sphincteral NEC K59.8
Ache (s) —*see* Pain
Acheilia Q38.6
Achilloburitis —*see* Tendinitis, Achilles
Achillodynia —*see* Tendinitis, Achilles
Achlorhydria, achlorhydric (neurogenic)
  K31.83
  anemia D50.8
  diarrhea K31.83
  psychogenic F45.8
  secondary to vagotomy K91.1
Achluophobia F40.228
Acholia K82.8
Acholuric jaundice (familial)
  (splenomegalic) —*see also* Spherocytosis
  acquired D59.8
Achondrogenesis Q77.0
Achondroplasia (osteosclerosis congenita)
  Q77.4
Achroma, cutis L80
Achromat (ism), achromatopsia (acquired)
  (congenital) H53.51
Achromia, congenital —*see* Albinism
Achromia parasitica B36.0
Achylia gastrica K31.89
  psychogenic F45.8
Acid
  burn —*see* Corrosion
  deficiency
    amide nicotinic E52
    ascorbic E54
    folic E53.8
    nicotinic E52
    pantothenic E53.8
  intoxication E87.2
  peptic disease K30
  phosphatase deficiency E83.39
  stomach K30
    psychogenic F45.8
Acidemia E87.2
  argininosuccinic E72.22
  isovaleric E71.110
  metabolic (newborn) P19.9
    first noted before onset of labor P19.0
    first noted during labor P19.1
    noted at birth P19.2

Acidemia *(Continued)*
  methylmalonic E71.120
  pipecolic E72.3
  propionic E71.121
Acidity, gastric (high) K30
  psychogenic F45.8
Acidocytopenia —*see* Agranulocytosis
Acidocytosis D72.1
Acidopenia —*see* Agranulocytosis
Acidosis (lactic) (respiratory) E87.2
  in Type 1 diabetes E10.10
    with coma E10.11
  kidney, tubular N25.89
  lactic E87.2
  metabolic NEC E87.2
    with respiratory acidosis E87.4
    late, of newborn P74.0
  mixed metabolic and respiratory,
    newborn P84
  newborn P84
  renal (hyperchloremic) (tubular)
    N25.89
  respiratory E87.2
    complicated by
      metabolic
        acidosis E87.4
        alkalosis E87.4
Aciduria
  argininosuccinic E72.22
  glutaric (type I) E72.3
    type II E71.313
    type III E71.5-
  orotic (congenital) (hereditary) (pyrimidine
    deficiency) E79.8
    anemia D53.0
Acladiosis (skin) B36.0
Aclasis, diaphyseal Q78.6
Acleistocardia Q21.1
Aclusion —*see* Anomaly, dentofacial,
  malocclusion
Acne L70.9
  artificialis L70.8
  atrophica L70.2
  cachecticorum (Hebra) L70.8
  conglobata L70.1
  cystic L70.0
  decalvans L66.2
  excoriée des jeunes filles L70.5
  frontalis L70.2
  indurata L70.0
  infantile L70.4
  keloid L73.0
  lupoid L70.2
  necrotic, necrotica (miliaris) L70.2
  neonatal L70.4
  nodular L70.0
  occupational L70.8
  picker's L70.5
  pustular L70.0
  rodens L70.0
  rosacea L71.9
  specified NEC L70.8
  tropica L70.3
  varioliformis L70.2
  vulgaris L70.0
Acnitis (primary) A18.4
Acosta's disease T70.29
Acoustic —*see* condition
Acousticophobia F40.298
Acquired —*see also* condition
  immunodeficiency syndrome
    (AIDS) B20
Acrania Q00.0
Acroangiodermatitis I78.9
Acroasphyxia, chronic I73.89
Acrobystitis N47.7
Acrocephalopolysyndactyly Q87.0
Acrocephalosyndactyly Q87.0
Acrocephaly Q75.0
Acrochondrohyperplasia —*see* Syndrome,
  Marfan's

Acrocyanosis I73.8
  newborn P28.2
    meaning transient blue hands and feet -
      omit code
Acrodermatitis L30.8
  atrophicans (chronica) L90.4
  continua (Hallopeau) L40.2
  enteropathica (hereditary) E83.2
  Hallopeau's L40.2
  infantile papular L44.4
  perstans L40.2
  pustulosa continua L40.2
  recalcitrant pustular L40.2
Acrodynia —*see* Poisoning, mercury
Acromegaly, acromegalia E22.0
Acromelalgia I73.81
Acromicria, acromikria Q79.8
Acronyx L60.0
Acropachy, thyroid —*see* Thyrotoxicosis
Acroparesthesia (simple) (vasomotor)
  I73.89
Acropathy, thyroid —*see* Thyrotoxicosis
Acrophobia F40.241
Acroposthitis N47.7
Acroscleriasis, acroscleroderma,
  acrosclerosis —*see* Sclerosis, systemic
Acrosphacelus I96
Acrospiroma, eccrine —*see* Neoplasm, skin,
  benign
Acrostealgia —*see* Osteochondropathy
Acrotrophodynia —*see* Immersion
ACTH ectopic syndrome E24.3
Actinic —*see* condition
Actinobacillosis, actinobacillus A28.8
  mallei A24.0
  muris A25.1
Actinomyces israelii (infection) —*see*
  Actinomycosis
Actinomycetoma (foot) B47.1
Actinomycosis, actinomycotic A42.9
  with pneumonia A42.0
  abdominal A42.1
  cervicofacial A42.2
  cutaneous A42.89
  gastrointestinal A42.1
  pulmonary A42.0
  sepsis A42.7
  specified site NEC A42.89
Actinoneuritis G62.82
Action, heart
  disorder I49.9
  irregular I49.9
    psychogenic F45.8
Activated protein C resistance D68.51
Active —*see* condition
Acute —*see also* condition
  abdomen R10.0
  gallbladder —*see* Cholecystitis, acute
Acyanotic heart disease (congenital) Q24.9
Acystia Q64.5
Adair-Dighton syndrome (brittle bones and
  blue sclera, deafness) Q78.0
Adamantinoblastoma —*see* Ameloblastoma
Adamantinoma —*see also* Cyst, calcifying
  odontogenic
  long bones C40.90
    lower limb C40.2-
    upper limb C40.0-
  malignant C41.1
    jaw (bone) (lower) C41.1
      upper C41.0
    tibial C40.2-
Adamantoblastoma —*see* Ameloblastoma
Adams-Stokes (-Morgagni) disease or
  syndrome I45.9
Adaption reaction —*see* Disorder, adjustment
Addiction (*see also* Dependence) F19.20
  alcohol, alcoholic (ethyl) (methyl) (wood)
    (without remission) F10.20
    with remission F10.21
  drug —*see* Dependence, drug

Addiction (Continued)
ethyl alcohol (without remission) F10.20
with remission F10.21
heroin —see Dependence, drug, opioid
methyl alcohol (without remission) F10.20
with remission F10.21
methylated spirit (without remission) F10.20
with remission F10.21
morphine(-like substances) —see
Dependence, drug, opioid
nicotine —see Dependence, drug, nicotine
opium and opioids —see Dependence, drug,
opioid
tobacco —see Dependence, drug, nicotine
Addisonian crisis E27.2
Addison's
anemia (pernicious) D51.0
disease (bronze) or syndrome E27.1
tuberculous A18.7
keloid L94.0
Addison-Biermer anemia (pernicious) D51.0
Addison-Schilder complex E71.528
Additional —see also Accessory
chromosome (s) Q99.8
21 —see Trisomy, 21
sex —see Abnormal, chromosome, sex
Adduction contracture, hip or other joint —see
Contraction, joint
Adenitis —see also Lymphadenitis
acute, unspecified site L04.9
axillary I88.9
acute L04.2
chronic or subacute I88.1
Bartholin's gland N75.8
bulbourethral gland —see Urethritis
cervical I88.9
acute L04.0
chronic or subacute I88.1
chancroid (Hemophilus ducreyi) A57
chronic, unspecified site I88.1
Cowper's gland —see Urethritis
due to Pasteurella multocida (p. septica)
A28.0
epidemic, acute B27.09
gangrenous L04.9
gonorrheal NEC A54.89
groin I88.9
acute L04.1
chronic or subacute I88.1
infectious (acute) (epidemic) B27.09
inguinal I88.9
acute L04.1
chronic or subacute I88.1
lymph gland or node, except mesenteric
I88.9
acute —see Lymphadenitis, acute
chronic or subacute I88.1
mesenteric (acute) (chronic) (nonspecific)
(subacute) I88.0
parotid gland (suppurative) —see
Sialoadenitis
salivary gland (any) (suppurative) —see
Sialoadenitis
scrofulous (tuberculous) A18.2
Skene's duct or gland —see Urethritis
strumous, tuberculous A18.2
subacute, unspecified site I88.1
sublingual gland (suppurative) —see
Sialoadenitis
submandibular gland (suppurative) —see
Sialoadenitis
submaxillary gland (suppurative) —see
Sialoadenitis
tuberculous —see Tuberculosis, lymph gland
urethral gland —see Urethritis
Wharton's duct (suppurative) —see
Sialoadenitis
Adenoacanthoma —see Neoplasm, malignant,
by site
Adenoameloblastoma —see Cyst, calcifying
odontogenic

Adenocarcinoid (tumor) —see Neoplasm,
malignant, by site
Adenocarcinoma —see also Neoplasm,
malignant, by site
acidophil
specified site —see Neoplasm, malignant,
by site
unspecified site C75.1
adrenal cortical C74.0-
alveolar —see Neoplasm, lung, malignant
apocrine
breast —see Neoplasm, breast, malignant
in situ
breast D05.8-
specified site NEC —see Neoplasm, skin,
in situ
unspecified site D04.9
specified site NEC —see Neoplasm, skin,
malignant
unspecified site C44.99
basal cell
specified site —see Neoplasm, skin,
malignant
unspecified site C08.9
basophil
specified site —see Neoplasm, malignant,
by site
unspecified site C75.1
bile duct type C22.1
liver C22.1
specified site NEC —see Neoplasm,
malignant, by site
unspecified site C22.1
bronchiolar —see Neoplasm, lung, malignant
bronchioloalveolar —see Neoplasm, lung,
malignant
ceruminous C44.29-
cervix, in situ (see also Carcinoma, cervix
uteri, in situ) D06.9
chromophobe
specified site —see Neoplasm, malignant,
by site
unspecified site C75.1
diffuse type
specified site —see Neoplasm, malignant,
by site
unspecified site C16.9
duct
infiltrating
with Paget's disease —see Neoplasm,
breast, malignant
specified site —see Neoplasm,
malignant, by site
unspecified site (female) C50.91-
male C50.92-
specified site —see Neoplasm, malignant,
by site
unspecified site
female C56.9
male C61
eosinophil
specified site —see Neoplasm, malignant,
by site
unspecified site C75.1
follicular
with papillary C73
moderately differentiated C73
specified site —see Neoplasm, malignant,
by site
trabecular C73
unspecified site C73
well differentiated C73
Hurthle cell C73
in
adenomatous
polyposis coli C18.9
infiltrating duct
with Paget's disease —see Neoplasm,
breast, malignant
specified site —see Neoplasm, malignant,
by site

Adenocarcinoma (Continued)
infiltrating duct (Continued)
unspecified site (female) C50.91-
male C50.92-
inflammatory
specified site —see Neoplasm, malignant,
by site
unspecified site (female) C50.91-
male C50.92-
intestinal type
specified site —see Neoplasm, malignant,
by site
unspecified site C16.9
intracystic papillary
intraductal
breast D05.1-
noninfiltrating
breast D05.1-
papillary
with invasion
specified site —see Neoplasm,
malignant, by site
unspecified site (female)
C50.91-
male C50.92-
breast D05.1-
specified site NEC —see Neoplasm, in
situ, by site
unspecified site D05.1-
specified site NEC —see Neoplasm, in
situ, by site
unspecified site D05.1-
papillary
with invasion
specified site —see Neoplasm,
malignant, by site
unspecified site (female) C50.91-
male C50.92-
breast D05.1-
specified site —see Neoplasm, in situ,
by site
unspecified site D05.1-
specified site NEC —see Neoplasm, in situ,
by site
unspecified site D05.1-
islet cell
with exocrine, mixed
specified site —see Neoplasm,
malignant, by site
unspecified site C25.9
pancreas C25.4
specified site NEC —see Neoplasm,
malignant, by site
unspecified site C25.4
lobular
in situ
breast D05.0-
specified site NEC —see Neoplasm, in
situ, by site
unspecified site D05.0-
specified site —see Neoplasm, malignant,
by site
unspecified site (female) C50.91-
male C50.92-
mucoid —see also Neoplasm, malignant, by
site
cell
specified site —see Neoplasm,
malignant, by site
unspecified site C75.1
nonencapsulated sclerosing C73
papillary
with follicular C73
follicular variant C73
intraductal (noninfiltrating)
with invasion
specified site —see Neoplasm,
malignant, by site
unspecified site (female) C50.91-
male C50.92-
breast D05.1-

Adenocarcinoma (Continued)
  papillary (Continued)
    intraductal (Continued)
      specified site NEC —see Neoplasm, in situ, by site
      unspecified site D05.1-
    serous
      specified site —see Neoplasm, malignant, by site
      unspecified site C56.9
  papillocystic
    specified site —see Neoplasm, malignant, by site
    unspecified site C56.9
  pseudomucinous
    specified site —see Neoplasm, malignant, by site
    unspecified site C56.9
  renal cell C64-
  sebaceous —see Neoplasm, skin, malignant, by site
  serous —see also Neoplasm, malignant, by site
    papillary
      specified site —see Neoplasm, malignant, by site
      unspecified site C56.9
  sweat gland —see Neoplasm, skin, malignant
  water-clear cell C75.0
Adenocarcinoma-in-situ —see also Neoplasm, in situ, by site
  breast D05.9-
Adenofibroma
  clear cell —see Neoplasm, benign, by site
  endometrioid D27.9
    borderline malignancy D39.10
    malignant C56-
  mucinous
    specified site —see Neoplasm, benign, by site
    unspecified site D27.9
  papillary
    specified site —see Neoplasm, benign, by site
    unspecified site D27.9
  prostate —see Enlargement, enlarged, prostate
  serous
    specified site —see Neoplasm, benign, by site
    unspecified site D27.9
  specified site —see Neoplasm, benign, by site
  unspecified site D27.9
Adenofibrosis
  breast —see Fibroadenosis, breast
  endometrioid N80.0
Adenoiditis (chronic) J35.02
  with tonsillitis J35.03
  acute J03.90
    recurrent J03.91
    specified organism NEC J03.80
      recurrent J03.81
    staphylococcal J03.80
      recurrent J03.81
    streptococcal J03.00
      recurrent J03.01
Adenoids —see condition
Adenolipoma —see Neoplasm, benign, by site
Adenolipomatosis, Launois-Bensaude E88.89
Adenolymphoma
  specified site —see Neoplasm, benign, by site
  unspecified site D11.9
Adenoma —see also Neoplasm, benign, by site
  acidophil
    specified site —see Neoplasm, benign, by site
    unspecified site D35.2
  acidophil-basophil, mixed
    specified site —see Neoplasm, benign, by site
    unspecified site D35.2

Adenoma (Continued)
  adrenal (cortical) D35.00
    clear cell D35.00
    compact cell D35.00
    glomerulosa cell D35.00
    heavily pigmented variant D35.00
    mixed cell D35.00
  alpha-cell
    pancreas D13.7
    specified site NEC —see Neoplasm, benign, by site
    unspecified site D13.7
  alveolar D14.30
  apocrine
    breast D24-
    specified site NEC —see Neoplasm, skin, benign, by site
    unspecified site D23.9
  basal cell D11.9
  basophil
    specified site —see Neoplasm, benign, by site
    unspecified site D35.2
  basophil-acidophil, mixed
    specified site —see Neoplasm, benign, by site
    unspecified site D35.2
  beta-cell
    pancreas D13.7
    specified site NEC —see Neoplasm, benign, by site
    unspecified site D13.7
  bile duct D13.4
    common D13.5
    extrahepatic D13.5
    intrahepatic D13.4
    specified site NEC —see Neoplasm, benign, by site
    unspecified site D13.4
  black D35.00
  bronchial D38.1
    cylindroid type —see Neoplasm, lung, malignant
  ceruminous D23.2-
  chief cell D35.1
  chromophobe
    specified site —see Neoplasm, benign, by site
    unspecified site D35.2
  colloid
    specified site —see Neoplasm, benign, by site
    unspecified site D34
  duct
  eccrine, papillary —see Neoplasm, skin, benign
  endocrine, multiple
    single specified site —see Neoplasm, uncertain behavior, by site
    two or more specified sites D44-
    unspecified site D44.9
  endometrioid —see also Neoplasm, benign
    borderline malignancy —see Neoplasm, uncertain behavior, by site
  eosinophil
    unspecified site D35.2
  fetal
    specified site —see Neoplasm, benign, by site
    unspecified site D34
  follicular
    specified site —see Neoplasm, benign, by site
    unspecified site D34
  hepatocellular D13.4
  Hurthle cell D34
  islet cell
    pancreas D13.7
    specified site NEC —see Neoplasm, benign, by site
    unspecified site D13.7

Adenoma (Continued)
  liver cell D13.4
  macrofollicular
    specified site —see Neoplasm, benign, by site
    unspecified site D34
  malignant, malignum —see Neoplasm, malignant, by site
  microcystic
    pancreas D13.7
    specified site NEC —see Neoplasm, benign, by site
    unspecified site D13.7
  microfollicular
    specified site —see Neoplasm, benign, by site
    unspecified site D34
  mucoid cell
    specified site —see Neoplasm, benign, by site
    unspecified site D35.2
  multiple endocrine
    single specified site —see Neoplasm, uncertain behavior, by site
    two or more specified sites D44-
    unspecified site D44.9
  nipple D24-
  papillary —see also Neoplasm, benign, by site
    eccrine —see Neoplasm, skin, benign, by site
  Pick's tubular
    specified site —see Neoplasm, benign, by site
    unspecified site
      female D27.9
      male D29.20
  pleomorphic
    carcinoma in —see Neoplasm, salivary gland, malignant
    specified site —see Neoplasm, malignant, by site
    unspecified site C08.9
  polypoid —see also Neoplasm, benign
    adenocarcinoma in —see Neoplasm, malignant, by site
    adenocarcinoma in situ —see Neoplasm, in situ, by site
  prostate —see Neoplasm, benign, prostate
  rete cell D29.20
  sebaceous —see Neoplasm, skin, benign
  Sertoli cell
    specified site —see Neoplasm, benign, by site
    unspecified site
      female D27.9
      male D29.20
  skin appendage —see Neoplasm, skin, benign
  sudoriferous gland —see Neoplasm, skin, benign
  sweat gland —see Neoplasm, skin, benign
  testicular
    unspecified site
      female D27.9
      male D29.20
  tubular —see also Neoplasm, benign, by site
    adenocarcinoma in —see Neoplasm, malignant, by site
    adenocarcinoma in situ —see Neoplasm, in situ, by site
    Pick's
      specified site —see Neoplasm, benign
      unspecified site
        female D27.9
        male D29.20
  tubulovillous —see also Neoplasm, benign, by site
    adenocarcinoma in —see Neoplasm, malignant, by site
    adenocarcinoma in situ —see Neoplasm, in situ, by site

Adenoma (Continued)
  villous —see Neoplasm, uncertain behavior, by site
    adenocarcinoma in —see Neoplasm, malignant, by site
    adenocarcinoma in situ —see Neoplasm, in situ, by site
  water-clear cell D35.1
Adenomatosis
  endocrine (multiple) E31.20
    single specified site —see Neoplasm, uncertain behavior, by site
  erosive of nipple D24-
  pluriendocrine —see Adenomatosis, endocrine
  pulmonary D38.1
    malignant —see Neoplasm, lung, malignant
  specified site —see Neoplasm, benign, by site
  unspecified site D12.6
Adenomatous
  goiter (nontoxic) E04.9
    with hyperthyroidism —see Hyper-thyroidism, with, goiter, nodular
    toxic —see Hyperthyroidism, with, goiter, nodular
Adenomyoma —see also Neoplasm, benign, by site
  prostate —see Enlarged, prostate
Adenomyometritis N80.0
Adenomyosis N80.0
Adenopathy (lymph gland) R59.9
  generalized R59.1
  inguinal R59.0
  localized R59.0
  mediastinal R59.0
  mesentery R59.0
  syphilitic (secondary) A51.49
  tracheobronchial R59.0
    tuberculous A15.4
      primary (progressive) A15.7
  tuberculous —see also Tuberculosis, lymph gland
    tracheobronchial A15.4
      primary (progressive) A15.7
Adenosalpingitis —see Salpingitis
Adenosarcoma —see Neoplasm, malignant, by site
Adenosclerosis I88.8
Adenosis (sclerosing) breast —see Fibroadenosis, breast
Adenovirus, as cause of disease classified elsewhere B97.0
Adentia (complete) (partial) —see Absence, teeth
Adherent —see also Adhesions
  labia (minora) N90.89
  pericardium (nonrheumatic) I31.0
    rheumatic I09.2
  placenta (with hemorrhage) O72.0
    without hemorrhage O73.0
  prepuce, newborn N47.0
  scar (skin) L90.5
  tendon in scar L90.5
Adhesions, adhesive (postinfective) K66.0
  with intestinal obstruction K56.5
  abdominal (wall) —see Adhesions, peritoneum
  appendix K38.8
  bile duct (common) (hepatic) K83.8
  bladder (sphincter) N32.89
  bowel —see Adhesions, peritoneum
  cardiac I31.0
    rheumatic I09.2
  cecum —see Adhesions, peritoneum
  cervicovaginal N88.1
    congenital Q52.8
    postpartal O90.89
    old N88.1
  cervix N88.1
  ciliary body NEC —see Adhesions, iris

Adhesions, adhesive (Continued)
  clitoris N90.89
  colon —see Adhesions, peritoneum
  common duct K83.8
  congenital —see also Anomaly, by site
    fingers —see Syndactylism, complex, fingers
    omental, anomalous Q43.3
    peritoneal Q43.3
    tongue (to gum or roof of mouth) Q38.3
  conjunctiva (acquired) H11.21-
    congenital Q15.8
  cystic duct K82.8
  diaphragm —see Adhesions, peritoneum
  due to foreign body —see Foreign body
  duodenum —see Adhesions, peritoneum
  ear
    middle H74.1-
  epididymis N50.8
  epidural —see Adhesions, meninges
  epiglottis J38.7
  eyelid H02.59
  female pelvis N73.6
  gallbladder K82.8
  globe H44.89
  heart I31.0
    rheumatic I09.2
  ileocecal (coil) —see Adhesions, peritoneum
  ileum —see Adhesions, peritoneum
  intestine —see also Adhesions, peritoneum
    with obstruction K56.5
  intra-abdominal —see Adhesions, peritoneum
  iris H21.50-
    anterior H21.51-
    goniosynechiae H21.52-
    posterior H21.54-
    to corneal graft T85.89
  joint —see Ankylosis
    knee M23.8X
    temporomandibular M26.61
  labium (majus) (minus), congenital Q52.5
  liver —see Adhesions, peritoneum
  lung J98.4
  mediastinum J98.5
  meninges (cerebral) (spinal) G96.12
    congenital Q07.8
    tuberculous (cerebral) (spinal) A17.0
  mesenteric —see Adhesions, peritoneum
  nasal (septum) (to turbinates) J34.89
  ocular muscle —see Strabismus, mechanical
  omentum —see Adhesions, peritoneum
  ovary N73.6
    congenital (to cecum, kidney or omentum) Q50.39
  paraovarian N73.6
  pelvic (peritoneal)
    female N73.6
      postprocedural N99.4
    male —see Adhesions, peritoneum
    postpartal (old) N73.6
    tuberculous A18.17
  penis to scrotum (congenital) Q55.8
  periappendiceal —see also Adhesions, peritoneum
  pericardium (nonrheumatic) I31.0
    focal I31.8
    rheumatic I09.2
    tuberculous A18.84
  pericholecystic K82.8
  perigastric —see Adhesions, peritoneum
  periovarian N73.6
  periprostatic N42.89
  perirectal —see Adhesions, peritoneum
  perirenal N28.89
  peritoneum, peritoneal (postinfective) (postprocedural) K66.0
    with obstruction (intestinal) K56.5
    congenital Q43.3
    pelvic, female N73.6
      postprocedural N99.4

Adhesions, adhesive (Continued)
  peritoneum, peritoneal (Continued)
    postpartal, pelvic N73.6
      to uterus N73.6
    peritubal N73.6
    periureteral N28.89
    periuterine N73.6
    perivesical N32.89
    perivesicular (seminal vesicle) N50.8
    pleura, pleuritic J94.8
      tuberculous NEC A15.6
    pleuropericardial J94.8
    postoperative (gastrointestinal tract) K66.0
      with obstruction K91.3
      due to foreign body accidentally left in wound —see Foreign body, accidentally left during a procedure
    pelvic peritoneal N99.4
    urethra —see Stricture, urethra, postprocedural
    vagina N99.2
  postpartal, old (vulva or perineum) N90.89
  preputial, prepuce N47.5
  pulmonary J98.4
  pylorus —see Adhesions, peritoneum
  sciatic nerve —see Lesion, nerve, sciatic
  seminal vesicle N50.8
  shoulder (joint) —see Capsulitis, adhesive
  sigmoid flexure —see Adhesions, peritoneum
  spermatic cord (acquired) N50.8
    congenital Q55.4
  spinal canal G96.12
  stomach —see Adhesions, peritoneum
  subscapular —see Capsulitis, adhesive
  temporomandibular M26.61
  tendinitis —see also Tenosynovitis, specified type NEC
    shoulder —see Capsulitis, adhesive
  testis N44.8
  tongue, congenital (to gum or roof of mouth) Q38.3
    acquired K14.8
  trachea J39.8
  tubo-ovarian N73.6
  tunica vaginalis N44.8
  uterus N73.6
    internal N85.6
    to abdominal wall N73.6
  vagina (chronic) N89.5
    postoperative N99.2
  vitreomacular H43.82-
  vitreous H43.89
  vulva N90.89
Adiaspiromycosis B48.8
Adie (-Holmes) pupil or syndrome —see Anomaly, pupil, function, tonic pupil
Adiponecrosis neonatorum P83.8
Adiposis —see also Obesity
  cerebralis E23.6
  dolorosa E88.2
Adiposity —see also Obesity
  heart —see Degeneration, myocardial
  localized E65
Adiposogenital dystrophy E23.6
Adjustment
  disorder —see Disorder, adjustment
  implanted device —see Encounter (for), adjustment (of)
  prosthesis, external —see Fitting
  reaction —see Disorder, adjustment
Administration of tPA (rtPA) in a different facility within the last 24 hours prior to admission to current facility Z92.82
Admission (for) —see also Encounter (for)
  adjustment (of)
    artificial
      arm Z44.00-
        complete Z44.01-
        partial Z44.02-
      eye Z44.2

Admission *(Continued)*
  adjustment *(Continued)*
    artificial *(Continued)*
      leg Z44.10-
        complete Z44.11-
        partial Z44.12-
    brain neuropacemaker Z46.2
      implanted Z45.42
    breast
      implant Z45.81
      prosthesis (external) Z44.3
    colostomy belt Z46.89
    contact lenses Z46.0
    cystostomy device Z46.6
    dental prosthesis Z46.3
    device NEC
      abdominal Z46.89
      implanted Z45.89
        cardiac Z45.09
          defibrillator (with synchronous
            cardiace pacemaker) Z45.02
          pacemaker Z45.018
            pulse generator Z45.010
        hearing device Z45.328
          bone conduction Z45.320
          cochlear Z45.321
        infusion pump Z45.1
        nervous system Z45.49
          CSF drainage Z45.41
          hearing device —*see* Admission,
            adjustment, device, implanted,
            hearing device
          neuropacemaker Z45.42
          visual substitution Z45.31
        specified NEC Z45.89
        vascular access Z45.2
        visual substitution Z45.31
      nervous system Z46.2
        implanted —*see* Admission,
          adjustment, device, implanted,
          nervous system
    orthodontic Z46.4
    prosthetic Z44.9
      arm —*see* Admission, adjustment,
        artificial, arm
      breast Z44.3
      dental Z46.3
      eye Z44.2
      leg —*see* Admission, adjustment,
        artificial, leg
      specified type NEC Z44.8
    substitution
      auditory Z46.2
        implanted —*see* Admission,
          adjustment, device, implanted,
          hearing device
      nervous system Z46.2
        implanted —*see* Admission,
          adjustment, device, implanted,
          nervous system
      visual Z46.2
        implanted Z45.31
    urinary Z46.6
    hearing aid Z46.1
      implanted —*see* Admission, adjustment,
        device, implanted, hearing device
    ileostomy device Z46.89
    intestinal appliance or device NEC
      Z46.89
    neuropacemaker (brain) (peripheral nerve)
      (spinal cord) Z46.2
      implanted Z45.42
    orthodontic device Z46.4
    orthopedic (brace) (cast) (device) (shoes)
      Z46.89
    pacemaker
      cardiac Z45.018
        pulse generator Z45.010
      nervous system Z46.2
        implanted Z45.42
    portacath (port-a-cath) Z45.2

Admission *(Continued)*
  adjustment *(Continued)*
    prosthesis Z44.9
      arm —*see* Admission, adjustment,
        artificial, arm
      breast Z44.3
      dental Z46.3
      eye Z44.2
      leg —*see* Admission, adjustment,
        artificial, leg
      specified NEC Z44.8
      spectacles Z46.0
  aftercare (*see also* Aftercare) Z51.89
    postpartum
      immediately after delivery Z39.0
      routine follow-up Z39.2
    radiation therapy (antineoplastic) Z51.0
  attention to artificial opening (of) Z43.9
    artificial vagina Z43.7
    colostomy Z43.3
    cystostomy Z43.5
    enterostomy Z43.4
    gastrostomy Z43.1
    ileostomy Z43.2
    jejunostomy Z43.4
    nephrostomy Z43.6
    specified site NEC Z43.8
      intestinal tract Z43.4
      urinary tract Z43.6
    tracheostomy Z43.0
    ureterostomy Z43.6
    urethrostomy Z43.6
  breast augmentation or reduction Z41.1
  breast reconstruction following mastectomy
    Z42.1
  change of
    dressing (nonsurgical) Z48.00
    neuropacemaker device (brain) (peripheral
      nerve) (spinal cord) Z46.2
      implanted Z45.42
    surgical dressing Z48.01
  circumcision, ritual or routine (in absence of
    diagnosis) Z41.2
  clinical research investigation (control)
    (normal comparison) (participant)
    Z00.6
  contraceptive management Z30.9
  cosmetic surgery NEC Z41.1
  counseling (*see also* Counseling)
    dietary Z71.3
    HIV Z71.7
    human immunodeficiency virus Z71.7
    nonattending third party Z71.0
    procreative management NEC Z31.69
  delivery, full-term, uncomplicated O80
    cesarean, without indication O82
  dietary surveillance and counseling Z71.3
  ear piercing Z41.3
  examination at health care facility (adult) (*see*
    also Examination) Z00.00
    with abnormal findings Z00.01
    clinical research investigation (control)
      (normal comparison) (participant)
      Z00.6
    dental Z01.20
      with abnormal findings Z01.21
    donor (potential) Z00.5
    ear Z01.10
      with abnormal findings NEC
        Z01.118
    eye Z01.00
      with abnormal findings Z01.01
    general, specified reason NEC Z00.8
    hearing Z01.10
      with abnormal findings NEC
        Z01.118
    postpartum checkup Z39.2
    psychiatric (general) Z00.8
      requested by authority Z04.6
    vision Z01.00
      with abnormal findings Z01.01

Admission *(Continued)*
  fitting (of)
    artificial
      arm —*see* Admission, adjustment,
        artificial, arm
      eye Z44.2
      leg —*see* Admission, adjustment,
        artificial, leg
    brain neuropacemaker Z46.2
      implanted Z45.42
    breast prosthesis (external) Z44.3
    colostomy belt Z46.89
    contact lenses Z46.0
    cystostomy device Z46.6
    dental prosthesis Z46.3
    dentures Z46.3
    device NEC
      abdominal Z46.89
      nervous system Z46.2
        implanted —*see* Admission,
          adjustment, device, implanted,
          nervous system
      orthodontic Z46.4
      prosthetic Z44.9
        breast Z44.3
        dental Z46.3
        eye Z44.2
      substitution
        auditory Z46.2
          implanted —*see* Admission,
            adjustment, device, implanted,
            hearing device
        nervous system Z46.2
          implanted —*see* Admission,
            adjustment, device, implanted,
            nervous system
        visual Z46.2
          implanted Z45.31
    hearing aid Z46.1
    ileostomy device Z46.89
    intestinal appliance or device NEC
      Z46.89
    neuropacemaker (brain) (peripheral nerve)
      (spinal cord) Z46.2
      implanted Z45.42
    orthodontic device Z46.4
    orthopedic device (brace) (cast) (shoes)
      Z46.89
    prosthesis Z44.9
      arm —*see* Admission, adjustment,
        artificial, arm
      breast Z44.3
      dental Z46.3
      eye Z44.2
      leg —*see* Admission, adjustment,
        artificial, leg
      specified type NEC Z44.8
    spectacles Z46.0
  follow-up examination Z09
  intrauterine device management Z30.431
    initial prescription Z30.014
  mental health evaluation Z00.8
    requested by authority Z04.6
  observation —*see* Observation
  Papanicolaou smear, cervix Z12.4
    for suspected malignant neoplasm
      Z12.4
  plastic and reconstructive surgery following
    medical procedure or healed injury
    NEC Z42.8
  plastic surgery, cosmetic NEC Z41.1
  postpartum observation
    immediately after delivery Z39.0
    routine follow-up Z39.2
  poststerilization (for restoration) Z31.0
    aftercare Z31.42
  procreative management Z31.9
  prophylactic (measure)
    organ removal Z40.00
      breast Z40.01
      ovary Z40.02

◀ New   ◀╎╎╎ Revised   ~~deleted~~ Deleted

Admission (Continued)
  prophylactic (Continued)
    organ removal (Continued)
      specified organ NEC Z40.09
      testes Z40.09
    vaccination Z23
  psychiatric examination (general) Z00.8
    requested by authority Z04.6
  radiation therapy (antineoplastic) Z51.0
  reconstructive surgery following medical
    procedure or healed injury NEC
    Z42.8
  removal of
    cystostomy catheter Z43.5
    drains Z48.03
    dressing (nonsurgical) Z48.00
    intrauterine contraceptive device Z30.432
    neuropacemaker (brain) (peripheral nerve)
      (spinal cord) Z46.2
      implanted Z45.42
    staples Z48.02
    surgical dressing Z48.01
    sutures Z48.02
    ureteral stent Z46.6
  respirator [ventilator] use during power
    failure Z99.12
  restoration of organ continuity
    (poststerilization) Z31.0
    aftercare Z31.42
  sensitivity test —see also Test, skin
    allergy NEC Z01.82
    Mantoux Z11.1
  tuboplasty following previous sterilization
    Z31.0
    aftercare Z31.42
  vasoplasty following previous sterilization
    Z31.0
    aftercare Z31.42
  vision examination Z01.00
    with abnormal findings Z01.01
  waiting period for admission to other facility
    Z75.1
Adnexitis (suppurative) —see
  Salpingo-oophoritis
Adolescent X-linked adrenoleukodystrophy
  E71.521
Adrenal (gland) —see condition
Adrenalism, tuberculous A18.7
Adrenalitis, adrenitis E27.8
  autoimmune E27.1
  meningococcal, hemorrhagic A39.1
Adrenarche, premature E27.0
Adrenocortical syndrome —see Cushing's,
  syndrome
Adrenogenital syndrome E25.9
  acquired E25.8
  congenital E25.0
  salt loss E25.0
Adrenogenitalism, congenital E25.0
Adrenoleukodystrophy E71.529
  neonatal E71.511
  X-linked E71.529
    Addison only phenotype E71.528
    Addison-Schilder E71.528
    adolescent E71.521
    adrenomyeloneuropathy E71.522
    childhood cerebral E71.520
    other specified E71.528
Adrenomyeloneuropathy E71.522
Adventitious bursa —see Bursopathy, specified
  type NEC
Adverse effect —see Table of Drugs and
  Chemicals, categories T36-T50, with 6th
  character 5
Advice —see Counseling
Adynamia (episodica) (hereditary) (periodic)
  G72.3
Aeration lung imperfect, newborn —see
  Atelectasis
Aerobullosis T70.3
Aerocele —see Embolism, air

Aerodermectasia
  subcutaneous (traumatic) T79.7
Aerodontalgia T70.29
Aeroembolism T70.3
Aerogenes capsulatus infection A48.0
Aero-otitis media T70.0
Aerophagy, aerophagia (psychogenic) F45.8
Aerophobia F40.228
Aerosinusitis T70.1
Aerotitis T70.0
Affection —see Disease
Afibrinogenemia (see also Defect, coagulation)
  D68.8
  acquired D65
  congenital D68.2
  following ectopic or molar pregnancy O08.1
  in abortion —see Abortion, by type,
    complicated by, afibrinogenemia
  puerperal O72.3
African
  sleeping sickness B56.9
  tick fever A68.1
  trypanosomiasis B56.9
    gambian B56.0
    rhodesian B56.1
Aftercare (see also Care) Z51.89
  following surgery (for) (on)
    amputation Z47.81
    attention to
      drains Z48.03
      dressings (nonsurgical) Z48.00
        surgical Z48.01
      sutures Z48.02
    circulatory system Z48.812
    delayed (planned) wound closure Z48.1
    digestive system Z48.815
    explantation of joint prosthesis (staged
      procedure)
      hip Z47.32
      knee Z47.33
      shoulder Z47.31
    genitourinary system Z48.816
    joint replacement Z47.1
    neoplasm Z48.3
    nervous system Z48.811
    oral cavity Z48.814
    organ transplant
      bone marrow Z48.290
      heart Z48.21
      heart-lung Z48.280
      kidney Z48.22
      liver Z48.23
      lung Z48.24
      multiple organs NEC Z48.288
      specified NEC Z48.298
    orthopedic NEC Z47.89
    planned wound closure Z48.1
    removal of internal fixation device Z47.2
    respiratory system Z48.813
    scoliosis Z47.82
    sense organs Z48.810
    skin and subcutaneous tissue Z48.817
    specified body system
      circulatory Z48.812
      digestive Z48.815
      genitourinary Z48.816
      nervous Z48.811
      oral cavity Z48.814
      respiratory Z48.813
      sense organs Z48.810
      skin and subcutaneous tissue Z48.817
      teeth Z48.814
    specified NEC Z48.89
    spinal Z48.89
    teeth Z48.814
  fracture — code to fracture with seventh
    character D
  involving
    removal of
      drains Z48.03
      dressings (nonsurgical) Z48.00

Aftercare (Continued)
  involving (Continued)
    removal of (Continued)
      staples Z48.02
      surgical dressings Z48.01
      sutures Z48.02
    neuropacemaker (brain) (peripheral nerve)
      (spinal cord) Z46.2
      implanted Z45.42
    orthopedic NEC Z47.89
    postprocedural —see Aftercare, following
      surgery
After-cataract —see Cataract, secondary
Agalactia (primary) O92.3
  elective, secondary or therapeutic O92.5
Agammaglobulinemia (acquired (secondary))
    (nonfamilial) D80.1
  with
    immunoglobulin-bearing B-lymphocytes
      D80.1
    lymphopenia D81.9
  autosomal recessive (Swiss type) D80.0
  Bruton's X-linked D80.0
  common variable (CVAgamma) D80.1
  congenital sex-linked D80.0
  hereditary D80.0
  lymphopenic D81.9
  Swiss type (autosomal recessive) D80.0
  X-linked (with growth hormone deficiency)
    (Bruton) D80.0
Aganglionosis (bowel) (colon) Q43.1
Age (old) —see Senility
Agenesis
  adrenal (gland) Q89.1
  alimentary tract (complete) (partial) NEC
    Q45.8
    upper Q40.8
  anus, anal (canal) Q42.3
    with fistula Q42.2
  aorta Q25.4
  appendix Q42.8
  arm (complete) Q71.0-
    with hand present Q71.1-
  artery (peripheral) Q27.9
    brain Q28.3
    coronary Q24.5
    pulmonary Q25.79
    specified NEC Q27.8
    umbilical Q27.0
  auditory (canal) (external) Q16.1
  auricle (ear) Q16.0
  bile duct or passage Q44.5
  bladder Q64.5
  bone Q79.9
  brain Q00.0
    part of Q04.3
  breast (with nipple present) Q83.8
    with absent nipple Q83.0
  bronchus Q32.4
  canaliculus lacrimalis Q10.4
  carpus —see Agenesis, hand
  cartilage Q79.9
  cecum Q42.8
  cerebellum Q04.3
  cervix Q51.5
  chin Q18.8
  cilia Q10.3
  circulatory system, part NOS Q28.9
  clavicle Q74.0
  clitoris Q52.6
  coccyx Q76.49
  colon Q42.9
    specified NEC Q42.8
  corpus callosum Q04.0
  cricoid cartilage Q31.8
  diaphragm (with hernia) Q79.1
  digestive organ (s) or tract (complete)
    (partial) NEC Q45.8
    upper Q40.8
  ductus arteriosus Q28.8
  duodenum Q41.0

Agenesis *(Continued)*
  ear Q16.9
    auricle Q16.0
    lobe Q17.8
  ejaculatory duct Q55.4
  endocrine (gland) NEC Q89.2
  epiglottis Q31.8
  esophagus Q39.8
  eustachian tube Q16.2
  eye Q11.1
    adnexa Q15.8
  eyelid (fold) Q10.3
  face
    bones NEC Q75.8
    specified part NEC Q18.8
  fallopian tube Q50.6
  femur —*see* Defect, reduction, lower limb,
      longitudinal, femur
  fibula —*see* Defect, reduction, lower limb,
      longitudinal, fibula
  finger (complete) (partial) —*see* Agenesis,
      hand
  foot (and toes) (complete) (partial) Q72.3-
  forearm (with hand present) —*see* Agenesis,
      arm, with hand present
      and hand Q71.2-
  gallbladder Q44.0
  gastric Q40.2
  genitalia, genital (organ (s))
    female Q52.8
      external Q52.71
      internal NEC Q52.8
    male Q55.8
  glottis Q31.8
  hair Q84.0
  hand (and fingers) (complete) (partial) Q71.3-
  heart Q24.8
    valve NEC Q24.8
      pulmonary Q22.0
  hepatic Q44.7
  humerus —*see* Defect, reduction, upper limb
  hymen Q52.4
  ileum Q41.2
  incus Q16.3
  intestine (small) Q41.9
    large Q42.9
      specified NEC Q42.8
  iris (dilator fibers) Q13.1
  jaw M26.09
  jejunum Q41.1
  kidney (s) (partial) Q60.2
    bilateral Q60.1
    unilateral Q60.0
  labium (majus) (minus) Q52.71
  labyrinth, membranous Q16.5
  lacrimal apparatus Q10.4
  larynx Q31.8
  leg (complete) Q72.0-
    with foot present Q72.1-
    lower leg (with foot present) —*see*
        Agenesis, leg, with foot present
        and foot Q72.2-
  lens Q12.3
  limb (complete) Q73.0
    lower —*see* Agenesis, leg
    upper —*see* Agenesis, arm
  lip Q38.0
  liver Q44.7
  lung (fissure) (lobe) (bilateral) (unilateral)
      Q33.3
  mandible, maxilla M26.09
  metacarpus —*see* Agenesis, hand
  metatarsus —*see* Agenesis, foot
  muscle Q79.8
    eyelid Q10.3
    ocular Q15.8
  musculoskeletal system NEC Q79.8
  nail (s) Q84.3
  neck, part Q18.8
  nerve Q07.8
  nervous system, part NEC Q07.8

Agenesis *(Continued)*
  nipple Q83.2
  nose Q30.1
  nuclear Q07.8
  organ
    of Corti Q16.5
    or site not listed —*see* Anomaly, by site
  osseous meatus (ear) Q16.1
  ovary
    bilateral Q50.02
    unilateral Q50.01
  oviduct Q50.6
  pancreas Q45.0
  parathyroid (gland) Q89.2
  parotid gland (s) Q38.4
  patella Q74.1
  pelvic girdle (complete) (partial) Q74.2
  penis Q55.5
  pericardium Q24.8
  pituitary (gland) Q89.2
  prostate Q55.4
  punctum lacrimale Q10.4
  radioulnar —*see* Defect, reduction, upper
      limb
  radius —*see* Defect, reduction, upper limb,
      longitudinal, radius
  rectum Q42.1
    with fistula Q42.0
  renal Q60.2
    bilateral Q60.1
    unilateral Q60.0
  respiratory organ NEC Q34.8
  rib Q76.6
  roof of orbit Q75.8
  round ligament Q52.8
  sacrum Q76.49
  salivary gland Q38.4
  scapula Q74.0
  scrotum Q55.29
  seminal vesicles Q55.4
  septum
    atrial Q21.1
    between aorta and pulmonary artery
        Q21.4
    ventricular Q20.4
  shoulder girdle (complete) (partial) Q74.0
  skull (bone) Q75.8
    with
      anencephaly Q00.0
      encephalocele —*see* Encephalocele
      hydrocephalus Q03.9
        with spina bifida —*see* Spina bifida, by
            site, with hydrocephalus
      microcephaly Q02
  spermatic cord Q55.4
  spinal cord Q06.0
  spine Q76.49
  spleen Q89.01
  sternum Q76.7
  stomach Q40.2
  submaxillary gland (s) (congenital) Q38.4
  tarsus —*see* Agenesis, foot
  tendon Q79.8
  testicle Q55.0
  thymus (gland) Q89.2
  thyroid (gland) E03.1
    cartilage Q31.8
  tibia —*see* Defect, reduction, lower limb,
      longitudinal, tibia
  tibiofibular —*see* Defect, reduction, lower
      limb, specified type NEC
  toe (and foot) (complete) (partial) —*see*
      Agenesis, foot
  tongue Q38.3
  trachea (cartilage) Q32.1
  ulna —*see* Defect, reduction, upper limb,
      longitudinal, ulna
  upper limb —*see* Agenesis, arm
  ureter Q62.4
  urethra Q64.5
  urinary tract NEC Q64.8

Agenesis *(Continued)*
  uterus Q51.0
  uvula Q38.5
  vagina Q52.0
  vas deferens Q55.4
  vein (s) (peripheral) Q27.9
    brain Q28.3
    great NEC Q26.8
    portal Q26.5
  vena cava (inferior) (superior) Q26.8
  vermis of cerebellum Q04.3
  vertebra Q76.49
  vulva Q52.71
Ageusia R43.2
Agitated —*see* condition
Agitation R45.1
Aglossia (congenital) Q38.3
Aglossia-adactylia syndrome Q87.0
Aglycogenosis E74.00
Agnosia (body image) (other senses) (tactile)
    R48.1
  developmental F88
  verbal R48.1
    auditory R48.1
      developmental F80.2
    developmental F80.2
  visual (object) R48.3
Agoraphobia F40.00
  with panic disorder F40.01
  without panic disorder F40.02
Agrammatism R48.8
Agranulocytopenia —*see* Agranulocytosis
Agranulocytosis (chronic) (cyclical) (genetic)
    (infantile) (periodic) (pernicious) (*see also*
    Neutropenia) D70.9
  congenital D70.0
  cytoreductive cancer chemotherapy sequela
      D70.1
  drug-induced D70.2
    due to cytoreductive cancer chemotherapy
        D70.1
  due to infection D70.3
  secondary D70.4
    drug-induced D70.2
      due to cytoreductive cancer
          chemotherapy D70.1
Agraphia (absolute) R48.8
  with alexia R48.0
  developmental F81.81
Ague (dumb) —*see* Malaria
Agyria Q04.3
Ahumada-del Castillo syndrome E23.0
Aichomophobia F40.298
AIDS (related complex) B20
Ailment heart —*see* Disease, heart
Ailurophobia F40.218
Ainhum (disease) L94.6
AIPHI (acute idiopathic pulmonary hemorrhage
    in infants (over 28 days old)) R04.81
Air
  anterior mediastinum J98.2
  compressed, disease T70.3
  conditioner lung or pneumonitis J67.7
  embolism (artery) (cerebral) (any site) T79.0
    with ectopic or molar pregnancy O08.2
    due to implanted device NEC —*see*
        Complications, by site and type,
        specified NEC
    following
      abortion —*see* Abortion by type,
          complicated by, embolism
      ectopic or molar pregnancy O08.2
      infusion, therapeutic injection or
          transfusion T80.0
    in pregnancy, childbirth or puerperium —
        see Embolism, obstetric
    traumatic T79.0
  hunger, psychogenic F45.8
  rarefied, effects of —*see* Effect, adverse, high
      altitude
  sickness T75.3

◀ New   ◀ Revised   ~~deleted~~ Deleted

Airplane sickness T75.3
Akathisia (drug-induced) (treatment- induced)
  G25.71
  neuroleptic induced (acute) G25.71
Akinesia R29.898
Akinetic mutism R41.89
Akureyri's disease G93.3
Alactasia, congenital E73.0
Alagille's syndrome Q44.7
Alastrim B03
Albers-Schönberg syndrome Q78.2
Albert's syndrome —see Tendinitis, Achilles
Albinism, albino E70.30
  with hematologic abnormality E70.339
    Chédiak-Higashi syndrome E70.330
    Hermansky-Pudlak syndrome E70.331
    other specified E70.338
  I E70.320
  II E70.321
  ocular E70.319
    autosomal recessive E70.311
    other specified E70.318
    X-linked E70.310
  oculocutaneous E70.329
    other specified E70.328
    tyrosinase (ty) negative E70.320
    tyrosinase (ty) positive E70.321
  other specified E70.39
Albinismus E70.30
Albright (-McCune)(-Sternberg) syndrome
  Q78.1
Albuminous —see condition
Albuminuria, albuminuric (acute) (chronic)
  (subacute) (see also Proteinuria) R80.9
  complicating pregnancy —see Proteinuria,
    gestational
  with
    gestational hypertension —see
      Pre-eclampsia
    pre-existing hypertension —see
      Hypertension, complicating
      pregnancy, pre-existing, with,
      pre-eclampsia
  gestational —see Proteinuria, gestational
  with
    gestational hypertension —see
      Pre-eclampsia
    pre-existing hypertension —see
      Hypertension, complicating
      pregnancy, pre-existing, with,
      pre-eclampsia
  orthostatic R80.2
  postural R80.2
  pre-eclamptic —see Pre-eclampsia
  scarlatinal A38.8
Albuminurophobia F40.298
Alcaptonuria E70.29
Alcohol, alcoholic, alcohol-induced
  addiction (without remission) F10.20
    with remission F10.21
  amnestic disorder, persisting F10.96
    with dependence F10.26
  brain syndrome, chronic F10.97
    with dependence F10.27
  cardiopathy I42.6
  counseling and surveillance Z71.41
    family member Z71.42
  delirium (acute) (tremens) (withdrawal)
    F10.231
    with intoxication F10.921
    in
      abuse F10.121
      dependence F10.221
  dementia F10.97
    with dependence F10.27
  deterioration F10.97
    with dependence F10.27
  hallucinosis (acute) F10.951
    in
      abuse F10.151
      dependence F10.251

Alcohol, alcoholic, alcohol-induced (Continued)
  insanity F10.959
  intoxication (acute) (without dependence)
    F10.129
    with
      delirium F10.121
      dependence F10.229
        with delirium F10.221
        uncomplicated F10.220
      uncomplicated F10.120
  jealousy F10.988
  Korsakoff's, Korsakov's, Korsakow's
    F10.26
  liver K70.9
    acute —see Disease, liver, alcoholic,
      hepatitis
  mania (acute) (chronic) F10.959
  paranoia, paranoid (type) psychosis F10.950
  pellagra E52
  poisoning, accidental (acute) NEC —see
    Table of Drugs and Chemicals, alcohol,
    poisoning
  psychosis —see Psychosis, alcoholic
  withdrawal (without convulsions) F10.239
    with delirium F10.231
Alcoholism (chronic) (without remission)
  F10.20
  with
    psychosis —see Psychosis, alcoholic
    remission F10.21
  Korsakov's F10.96
    with dependence F10.26
Alder (-Reilly) anomaly or syndrome
  (leukocyte granulation) D72.0
Aldosteronism E26.9
  familial (type I) E26.02
  glucocorticoid-remediable E26.02
  primary (due to (bilateral) adrenal
    hyperplasia) E26.09
  primary NEC E26.09
  secondary E26.1
  specified NEC E26.89
Aldosteronoma D44.10
Aldrich(-Wiskott) syndrome (eczema-
  thrombocytopenia) D82.0
Alektorophobia F40.218
Aleppo boil B55.1
Aleukemic —see condition Aleukia
  congenital D70.0
  hemorrhagica D61.9
    congenital D61.09
  splenica D73.1
Alexia R48.0
  developmental F81.0
  secondary to organic lesion R48.0
Algoneurodystrophy M89.00
  ankle M89.07-
  foot M89.07-
  forearm M89.03-
  hand M89.04-
  lower leg M89.06-
  multiple sites M89.0-
  shoulder M89.01-
  specified site NEC M89.08
  thigh M89.05-
  upper arm M89.02-
Algophobia F40.298
Alienation, mental —see Psychosis
Alkalemia E87.3
Alkalosis E87.3
  metabolic E87.3
    with respiratory acidosis E87.4
  respiratory E87.3
Alkaptonuria E70.29
Allen-Masters syndrome N83.8
Allergy, allergic (reaction) (to) T78.40
  air-borne substance NEC (rhinitis) J30.89
  alveolitis (extrinsic) J67.9
    due to
      Aspergillus clavatus J67.4
      Cryptostroma corticale J67.6

Allergy, allergic (Continued)
  alveolitis (Continued)
    due to (Continued)
      organisms (fungal, thermophilic
        actinomycete) growing in
        ventilation (air conditioning)
        systems J67.7
    specified type NEC J67.8
  anaphylactic reaction or shock T78.2
  angioneurotic edema T78.3
  animal (dander) (epidermal) (hair) (rhinitis)
    J30.81
  bee sting (anaphylactic shock) —see Toxicity,
    venom, arthropod, bee
  biological —see Allergy, drug
  colitis K52.2
  dander (animal) (rhinitis) J30.81
  dandruff (rhinitis) J30.81
  dental restorative material (existing) K08.55
  dermatitis —see Dermatitis, contact, allergic
  diathesis —see History, allergy
  drug, medicament & biological (any)
    (external) (internal) T78.40
    correct substance properly administered —
      see Table of Drugs and Chemicals, by
      drug, adverse effect
    wrong substance given or taken NEC (by
      accident) —see Table of Drugs and
      Chemicals, by drug, poisoning
  due to pollen J30.1
  dust (house) (stock) (rhinitis) J30.89
    with asthma —see Asthma, allergic
      extrinsic
  eczema —see Dermatitis, contact, allergic
  epidermal (animal) (rhinitis) J30.81
  feathers (rhinitis) J30.89
  food (any) (ingested) NEC T78.1
    anaphylactic shock —see Shock,
      anaphylactic, due to food
    dermatitis —see Dermatitis, due to,
      food
    dietary counseling and surveillance
      Z71.3
    in contact with skin L23.6
    rhinitis J30.5
    status (without reaction) Z91.018
      eggs Z91.012
      milk products Z91.011
      peanuts Z91.010
      seafood Z91.013
      specified NEC Z91.018
  gastrointestinal K52.2
  grain J30.1
  grass (hay fever) (pollen) J30.1
    asthma —see Asthma, allergic extrinsic
  hair (animal) (rhinitis) J30.81
  history (of) —see History, allergy
  horse serum —see Allergy, serum
  inhalant (rhinitis) J30.89
    pollen J30.1
  kapok (rhinitis) J30.89
  medicine —see Allergy, drug
  milk protein K52.2
  nasal, seasonal due to pollen J30.1
  pneumonia J82
  pollen (any) (hay fever) J30.1
    asthma —see Asthma, allergic extrinsic
  primrose J30.1
  primula J30.1
  purpura D69.0
  ragweed (hay fever) (pollen) J30.1
    asthma —see Asthma, allergic extrinsic
  rose (pollen) J30.1
  seasonal NEC J30.2
  Senecio jacobae (pollen) J30.1
  serum (see also Reaction, serum) T80.69
    anaphylactic shock T80.59
  shock (anaphylactic) T78.2
    due to
      administration of blood and blood
        products T80.51

Allergy, allergic (Continued)
  shock (Continued)
    due to (Continued)
      adverse effect of correct medicinal
          substance properly administered
          T88.6
      immunization T80.52
      serum NEC T80.59
      vaccination T80.52
  specific NEC T78.49
  tree (any) (hay fever) (pollen) J30.1
    asthma —see Asthma, allergic extrinsic
  upper respiratory J30.9
  urticaria L50.0
  vaccine —see Allergy, serum
  wheat —see Allergy, food
Allescheriasis B48.2
Alligator skin disease Q80.9
Allocheiria, allochiria R20.8
Almeida's disease —see
    Paracoccidioidomycosis
Alopecia (hereditaria) (seborrheica) L65.9
  androgenic L64.9
    drug-induced L64.0
    specified NEC L64.8
  areata L63.9
    ophiasis L63.2
    specified NEC L63.8
    totalis L63.0
    universalis L63.1
  cicatricial L66.9
    specified NEC L66.8
  circumscripta L63.9
  congenital, congenitalis Q84.0
  due to cytotoxic drugs NEC L65.8
  mucinosa L65.2
  postinfective NEC L65.8
  postpartum L65.0
  premature L64.8
  specific (syphilitic) A51.32
  specified NEC L65.8
  syphilitic (secondary) A51.32
  totalis (capitis) L63.0
  universalis (entire body) L63.1
  X-ray L58.1
Alpers' disease G31.81
Alpine sickness T70.29
Alport syndrome Q87.81
ALTE (apparent life threatening event) in
    newborn and infant R68.13
Alteration (of), Altered
  awareness, transient R40.4
  mental status R41.82
  pattern of family relationships affecting child
      Z62.898
  sensation
    following
      cerebrovascular disease I69.998
        cerebral infarction I69.398
        intracerebral hemorrhage I69.198
        nontraumatic intracranial hemorrhage
            NEC I69.298
        specified disease NEC I69.898
        subarachnoid hemorrhage I69.098
Alternating —see condition
Altitude, high (effects) —see Effect, adverse,
    high altitude
Aluminosis (of lung) J63.0
Alveolitis
  allergic (extrinsic) —see Pneumonitis,
      hypersensitivity
  due to
    Aspergillus clavatus J67.4
    Cryptostroma corticale J67.6
  fibrosing (cryptogenic) (idiopathic) J84.112
  jaw M27.3
  sicca dolorosa M27.3
Alveolus, alveolar —see condition
Alymphocytosis D72.810
  thymic (with immunodeficiency) D82.1
Alymphoplasia, thymic D82.1

Alzheimer's disease or sclerosis —see Disease,
    Alzheimer's
Amastia (with nipple present) Q83.8
  with absent nipple Q83.0
Amathophobia F40.228
Amaurosis (acquired) (congenital) —see also
    Blindness
  fugax G45.3
  hysterical F44.6
  Leber's congenital H35.50
  uremic —see Uremia
Amaurotic idiocy (infantile) (juvenile) (late) E75.4
Amaxophobia F40.248
Ambiguous genitalia Q56.4
Amblyopia (congenital) (ex anopsia) (partial)
    (suppression) H53.00-
  anisometropic —see Amblyopia, refractive
  deprivation H53.01-
  hysterical F44.6
  nocturnal —see also Blindness, night
    vitamin A deficiency E50.5
  refractive H53.02-
  strabismic H53.03-
  tobacco H53.8
  toxic NEC H53.8
  uremic —see Uremia
Ameba, amebic (histolytica) —see also
    Amebiasis
  abscess (liver) A06.4
Amebiasis A06.9
  with abscess —see Abscess, amebic
  acute A06.0
  chronic (intestine) A06.1
    with abscess —see Abscess, amebic
  cutaneous A06.7
  cutis A06.7
  cystitis A06.81
  genitourinary tract NEC A06.82
  hepatic —see Abscess, liver, amebic
  intestine A06.0
  nondysenteric colitis A06.2
  skin A06.7
  specified site NEC A06.89
Ameboma (of intestine) A06.3
Amelia Q73.0
  lower limb —see Agenesis, leg
  upper limb —see Agenesis, arm
Ameloblastoma —see also Cyst, calcifying
    odontogenic
  long bones C40.9-
    lower limb C40.2-
    upper limb C40.0-
  malignant C41.1
    jaw (bone) (lower) C41.1
      upper C41.0
  tibial C40.2-
Amelogenesis imperfecta K00.5
  nonhereditaria (segmentalis) K00.4
Amenorrhea N91.2
  hyperhormonal E28.8
  primary N91.0
  secondary N91.1
Amentia —see Disability, intellectual
  Meynert's (nonalcoholic) F04
American
  leishmaniasis B55.2
  mountain tick fever A93.2
Ametropia —see Disorder, refraction
Amianthosis J61
Amimia R48.8
Amino-acid disorder E72.9
  anemia D53.0
Aminoacidopathy E72.9
Aminoaciduria E72.9
Amnes (t)ic syndrome (post-traumatic) F04
  induced by
    alcohol F10.96
      with dependence F10.26
    psychoactive NEC F19.96
      with
        abuse F19.16
        dependence F19.26

Amnes (t)ic syndrome (Continued)
  induced by (Continued)
    sedative F13.96
      with dependence F13.26
Amnesia R41.3
  anterograde R41.1
  auditory R48.8
  dissociative F44.0
  hysterical F44.0
  postictal in epilepsy —see Epilepsy
  psychogenic F44.0
  retrograde R41.2
  transient global G45.4
Amnion, amniotic —see condition
Amnionitis —see Pregnancy, complicated by
Amok F68.8
Amoral traits F60.89
Ampulla
  lower esophagus K22.8
  phrenic K22.8
Amputation —see also Absence, by site,
    acquired
  neuroma (postoperative) (traumatic) —see
      Complications, amputation stump,
      neuroma
  stump (surgical)
    abnormal, painful, or with complication
        (late) —see Complications,
        amputation stump
    healed or old NOS Z89.9
  traumatic (complete) (partial)
    arm (upper) (complete) S48.91-
      at
        elbow S58.01-
          partial S58.02-
        shoulder joint (complete) S48.01-
          partial S48.02-
      between
        elbow and wrist (complete) S58.11-
          partial S58.12-
        shoulder and elbow (complete) S48.11-
          partial S48.12-
      partial S48.92-
    breast (complete) S28.21-
      partial S28.22-
    clitoris (complete) S38.211
      partial S38.212
    ear (complete) S08.11-
      partial S08.12-
    finger (complete) (metacarpophalangeal)
        S68.11-
      index S68.11-
      little S68.11-
      middle S68.11-
      partial S68.12-
        index S68.12-
        little S68.12-
        middle S68.12-
        ring S68.12-
      ring S68.11-
      thumb —see Amputation, traumatic,
          thumb
      transphalangeal (complete) S68.61-
        index S68.61-
        little S68.61-
        middle S68.61-
        partial S68.62-
          index S68.62-
          little S68.62-
          middle S68.62-
          ring S68.62-
        ring S68.61-
    foot (complete) S98.91-
      at ankle level S98.01-
        partial S98.02-
      midfoot S98.31-
        partial S98.32-
      partial S98.92-
    forearm (complete) S58.91-
      at elbow level (complete) S58.01-
        partial S58.02-

◀ New   ◀═ Revised   ~~deleted~~ Deleted

Amputation (Continued)
　traumatic (Continued)
　　forearm (Continued)
　　　between elbow and wrist (complete)
　　　　S58.11-
　　　　　partial S58.12-
　　　　partial S58.92-
　　　genital organ (s) (external)
　　　　female (complete) S38.211
　　　　　partial S38.212
　　　　male
　　　　　penis (complete) S38.221
　　　　　　partial S38.222
　　　　　scrotum (complete) S38.231
　　　　　　partial S38.232
　　　　　testes (complete) S38.231
　　　　　　partial S38.232
　　　hand (complete) (wrist level) S68.41-
　　　　finger (s) alone —see Amputation,
　　　　　traumatic, finger
　　　　partial S68.42-
　　　　thumb alone —see Amputation,
　　　　　traumatic, thumb
　　　　transmetacarpal (complete) S68.71-
　　　　　partial S68.72-
　　　head
　　　　ear —see Amputation, traumatic, ear
　　　　nose (partial) S08.812
　　　　　complete S08.811
　　　　part S08.89
　　　　　scalp S08.0
　　　hip (and thigh) (complete) S78.91-
　　　　at hip joint (complete) S78.01-
　　　　　partial S78.02-
　　　　between hip and knee (complete) S78.11-
　　　　　partial S78.12-
　　　　partial S78.92-
　　　labium (majus) (minus) (complete) S38.21-
　　　　partial S38.21-
　　　leg (lower) S88.91-
　　　　at knee level S88.01-
　　　　　partial S88.02-
　　　　between knee and ankle S88.11-
　　　　　partial S88.12-
　　　　partial S88.92-
　　　nose (partial) S08.812
　　　　complete S08.811
　　　penis (complete) S38.221
　　　　partial S38.222
　　　scrotum (complete) S38.231
　　　　partial S38.232
　　　shoulder —see Amputation, traumatic, arm
　　　　at shoulder joint —see Amputation,
　　　　　traumatic, arm, at shoulder joint
　　　testes (complete) S38.231
　　　　partial S38.232
　　　thigh —see Amputation, traumatic, hip
　　　thorax, part of S28.1
　　　　breast —see Amputation, traumatic,
　　　　　breast
　　　thumb (complete) (metacarpophalangeal)
　　　　S68.01-
　　　　partial S68.02-
　　　　transphalangeal (complete) S68.51-
　　　　　partial S68.52-
　　　toe (lesser) S98.13-
　　　　great S98.11-
　　　　　partial S98.12-
　　　　more than one S98.21-
　　　　　partial S98.22-
　　　　partial S98.14-
　　　vulva (complete) S38.211
　　　　partial S38.212
Amputee (bilateral) (old) Z89.9
Amsterdam dwarfism Q87.1
Amusia R48.8
　developmental F80.89
Amyelencephalus, amyelencephaly Q00.0
Amyelia Q06.0
Amygdalitis —see Tonsillitis
Amygdalolith J35.8

Amyloid heart (disease) E85.4 [I43]
Amyloidosis (generalized) (primary) E85.9
　with lung involvement E85.4 [J99]
　familial E85.2
　genetic E85.2
　heart E85.4 [I43]
　hemodialysis-associated E85.3
　liver E85.4 [K77]
　localized E85.4
　neuropathic heredofamilial E85.1
　non-neuropathic heredofamilial E85.0
　organ limited E85.4
　Portuguese E85.1
　pulmonary E85.4 [J99]
　secondary systemic E85.3
　skin (lichen) (macular) E85.4 [L99]
　specified NEC E85.8
　subglottic E85.4 [J99]
Amylopectinosis (brancher enzyme deficiency)
　E74.03
Amylophagia —see Pica
Amyoplasia congenita Q79.8
Amyotonia M62.89
　congenita G70.2
Amyotrophia, amyotrophy, amyotrophic
　G71.8
　congenita Q79.8
　diabetic —see Diabetes, amyotrophy
　lateral sclerosis G12.21
　neuralgic G54.5
　spinal progressive G12.21
Anacidity, gastric K31.83
　psychogenic F45.8
Anaerosis of newborn P28.89
Analbuminemia E88.09
Analgesia —see Anesthesia
Analphalipoproteinemia E78.6
Anaphylactic
　purpura D69.0
　shock or reaction —see Shock, anaphylactic
Anaphylactoid shock or reaction —see Shock,
　anaphylactic
Anaphylactoid syndrome of pregnancy
　O88.01-
Anaphylaxis —see Shock, anaphylactic
Anaplasia cervix (see also Dysplasia, cervix)
　N87.9
Anaplasmosis, human A77.49
Anarthria R47.1
Anasarca R60.1
　cardiac —see Failure, heart, congestive
　lung J18.2
　newborn P83.2
　nutritional E43
　pulmonary J18.2
　renal N04.9
Anastomosis
　aneurysmal —see Aneurysm
　arteriovenous ruptured brain I60.8
　intestinal K63.89
　　complicated NEC K91.89
　　　involving urinary tract N99.89
　retinal and choroidal vessels (congenital)
　　Q14.8
Anatomical narrow angle H40.03-
Ancylostoma, ancylostomiasis (braziliense)
　(caninum) (ceylanicum) (duodenale)
　B76.0
　Necator americanus B76.1
Andersen's disease (glycogen storage)
　E74.09
Anderson-Fabry disease E75.21
Andes disease T70.29
Andrews' disease (bacterid) L08.89
Androblastoma
　benign
　　specified site —see Neoplasm, benign, by
　　　site
　　unspecified site
　　　female D27.9
　　　male D29.20

Androblastoma (Continued)
　malignant
　　specified site —see Neoplasm, malignant,
　　　by site
　　unspecified site
　　　female C56.9
　　　male C62.90
　specified site —see Neoplasm, uncertain
　　behavior, by site
　tubular
　　with lipid storage
　　　specified site —see Neoplasm, benign,
　　　　by site
　　　unspecified site
　　　　female D27.9
　　　　male D29.20
　　specified site —see Neoplasm, benign, by site
　　unspecified site
　　　female D27.9
　　　male D29.20
　unspecified site
　　female D39.10
　　male D40.10
Androgen insensitivity syndrome (see also
　Syndrome, androgen insensitivity) E34.50
Androgen resistance syndrome (see also
　Syndrome, androgen insensitivity) E34.50
Android pelvis Q74.2
　with disproportion (fetopelvic) O33.3
　　causing obstructed labor O65.3
Androphobia F40.290
Anectasis, pulmonary (newborn) —see
　Atelectasis
Anemia (essential) (general) (hemoglobin
　deficiency) (infantile) (primary)
　(profound) D64.9
　with (due to) (in)
　　disorder of
　　　anaerobic glycolysis D55.2
　　　pentose phosphate pathway D55.1
　　koilonychia D50.9
　achlorhydric D50.8
　achrestic D53.1
　Addison (-Biermer) (pernicious) D51.0
　agranulocytic —see Agranulocytosis
　amino-acid-deficiency D53.0
　aplastic D61.9
　　congenital D61.09
　　drug-induced D61.1
　　due to
　　　drugs D61.1
　　　external agents NEC D61.2
　　　infection D61.2
　　　radiation D61.2
　　idiopathic D61.3
　　red cell (pure) D60.9
　　　chronic D60.0
　　　congenital D61.01
　　　specified type NEC D60.8
　　　transient D60.1
　　specified type NEC D61.89
　　toxic D61.2
　aregenerative
　　congenital D61.09
　asiderotic D50.9
　atypical (primary) D64.9
　Baghdad spring D55.0
　Balantidium coli A07.0
　Biermer's (pernicious) D51.0
　blood loss (chronic) D50.0
　　acute D62
　bothriocephalus B70.0 [D63.8]
　brickmaker's B76.9 [D63.8]
　cerebral I67.89
　childhood D58.9
　chlorotic D50.8
　chronic
　　blood loss D50.0
　　hemolytic D58.9
　　　idiopathic D59.9
　　simple D53.9

Anemia (Continued)
  chronica congenita aregenerativa D61.09
  combined system disease NEC D51.0 [G32.0]
    due to dietary vitamin B12 deficiency
      D51.3 [G32.0]
  complicating pregnancy, childbirth
    or puerperium —see Pregnancy,
    complicated by (management affected
    by), anemia
  congenital P61.4
    aplastic D61.09
    due to isoimmunization NOS P55.9
    dyserythropoietic, dyshematopoietic
      D64.4
    following fetal blood loss P61.3
    Heinz body D58.2
    hereditary hemolytic NOS D58.9
    pernicious D51.0
    spherocytic D58.0
  Cooley's (erythroblastic) D56.1
  cytogenic D51.0
  deficiency D53.9
    2, 3 diphosphoglycurate mutase D55.2
    2, 3 PG D55.2
    6 phosphogluconate dehydrogenase
      D55.1
    6-PGD D55.1
    amino-acid D53.0
    combined B12 and folate D53.1
    enzyme D55.9
      drug-induced (hemolytic) D59.2
      glucose-6-phosphate dehydrogenase
        (G6PD) D55.0
      glycolytic D55.2
      nucleotide metabolism D55.3
      related to hexose monophosphate
        (HMP) shunt pathway NEC D55.1
      specified type NEC D55.8
    erythrocytic glutathione D55.1
    folate D52.9
      dietary D52.0
      drug-induced D52.1
    folic acid D52.9
      dietary D52.0
      drug-induced D52.1
    G SH D55.1
    G6PD D55.0
    GGS-R D55.1
    glucose-6-phosphate dehydrogenase D55.0
    glutathione reductase D55.1
    glyceraldehyde phosphate dehydrogenase
      D55.2
    hexokinase D55.2
    iron D50.9
      secondary to blood loss (chronic) D50.0
    nutritional D53.9
      with
        poor iron absorption D50.8
        specified deficiency NEC D53.8
    phosphofructo-aldolase D55.2
    phosphoglycerate kinase D55.2
    PK D55.2
    protein D53.0
    pyruvate kinase D55.2
    transcobalamin II D51.2
    triose-phosphate isomerase D55.2
    vitamin B12 NOS D51.9
      dietary D51.3
      due to
        intrinsic factor deficiency D51.0
        selective vitamin B12 malabsorption
          with proteinuria D51.1
      pernicious D51.0
      specified type NEC D51.8
  Diamond-Blackfan (congenital hypoplastic)
    D61.01
  dibothriocephalus B70.0 [D63.8]
  dimorphic D53.1
  diphasic D53.1
  Diphyllobothrium (Dibothriocephalus) B70.0
    [D63.8]

Anemia (Continued)
  due to (in) (with)
    antineoplastic chemotherapy D64.81
    blood loss (chronic) D50.0
      acute D62
    chemotherapy, antineoplastic D64.81
    chronic disease classified elsewhere NEC
      D63.8
    chronic kidney disease D63.1
    deficiency
      amino-acid D53.0
      copper D53.8
      folate (folic acid) D52.9
        dietary D52.0
        drug-induced D52.1
      molybdenum D53.8
      protein D53.0
      zinc D53.8
    dietary vitamin B12 deficiency D51.3
    disorder of
      glutathione metabolism D55.1
      nucleotide metabolism D55.3
    drug —see Anemia, by type —see also Table
      of Drugs and Chemicals
    end stage renal disease D63.1
    enzyme disorder D55.9
    fetal blood loss P61.3
    fish tapeworm (D latum) infestation B70.0
      [D63.8]
    hemorrhage (chronic) D50.0
      acute D62
    impaired absorption D50.9
    loss of blood (chronic) D50.0
      acute D62
    myxedema E03.9 [D63.8]
    Necator americanus B76.1 [D63.8]
    prematurity P61.2
    selective vitamin B12 malabsorption with
      proteinuria D51.1
    transcobalamin II deficiency D51.2
  Dyke-Young type (secondary) (symptomatic)
    D59.1
  dyserythropoietic (congenital) D64.4
  dyshematopoietic (congenital) D64.4
  Egyptian B76.9 [D63.8]
  elliptocytosis —see Elliptocytosis
  enzyme-deficiency, drug-induced D59.2
  epidemic (see also Ancylostomiasis) B76.9
    [D63.8]
  erythroblastic
    familial D56.1
    newborn (see also Disease, hemolytic) P55.9
    of childhood D56.1
  erythrocytic glutathione deficiency D55.1
  erythropoietin-resistant anemia (EPO
    resistant anemia) D63.1
  Faber's (achlorhydric anemia) D50.9
  factitious (self-induced blood letting) D50.0
  familial erythroblastic D56.1
  Fanconi's (congenital pancytopenia) D61.09
  favism D55.0
  fish tapeworm (D. latum) infestation B70.0
    [D63.8]
  folate (folic acid) deficiency D52.9
  glucose-6-phosphate dehydrogenase (G6PD)
    deficiency D55.0
  glutathione-reductase deficiency D55.1
  goat's milk D52.0
  granulocytic —see Agranulocytosis
  Heinz body, congenital D58.2
  hemolytic D58.9
    acquired D59.9
      with hemoglobinuria NEC D59.6
      autoimmune NEC D59.1
      infectious D59.4
      specified type NEC D59.8
      toxic D59.4
    acute D59.9
      due to enzyme deficiency specified type
        NEC D55.8
    Lederer's D59.1

Anemia (Continued)
  hemolytic (Continued)
    autoimmune D59.1
      drug-induced D59.0
    chronic D58.9
      idiopathic D59.9
    cold type (secondary) (symptomatic) D59.1
    congenital (spherocytic) —see
      Spherocytosis
    due to
      cardiac conditions D59.4
      drugs (nonautoimmune) D59.2
        autoimmune D59.1
      enzyme disorder D55.9
        drug-induced D59.2
      presence of shunt or other internal
        prosthetic device D59.4
    familial D58.9
    hereditary D58.9
      due to enzyme disorder D55.9
        specified type NEC D55.8
      specified type NEC D58.8
    idiopathic (chronic) D59.9
    mechanical D59.4
    microangiopathic D59.4
    nonautoimmune D59.4
      drug-induced D59.2
    nonspherocytic
      congenital or hereditary NEC D55.8
        glucose-6-phosphate dehydrogenase
          deficiency D55.0
        pyruvate kinase deficiency D55.2
        type
          I D55.1
          II D55.2
      type
        I D55.1
        II D55.2
    secondary D59.4
      autoimmune D59.1
    specified (hereditary) type NEC D58.8
    Stransky-Regala type (see also
      Hemoglobinopathy) D58.8
    symptomatic D59.4
      autoimmune D59.1
    toxic D59.4
    warm type (secondary) (symptomatic)
      D59.1
  hemorrhagic (chronic) D50.0
    acute D62
  Herrick's D57.1
  hexokinase deficiency D55.2
  hookworm B76.9 [D63.8]
  hypochromic (idiopathic) (microcytic)
    (normoblastic) D50.9
    due to blood loss (chronic) D50.0
      acute D62
    familial sex-linked D64.0
    pyridoxine-responsive D64.3
    sideroblastic, sex-linked D64.0
  hypoplasia, red blood cells D61.9
    congenital or familial D61.01
  hypoplastic (idiopathic) D61.9
    congenital or familial (of childhood)
      D61.01
  hypoproliferative (refractive) D61.9
  idiopathic D64.9
    aplastic D61.3
    hemolytic, chronic D59.9
  in (due to) (with)
    chronic kidney disease D63.1
    end stage renal disease D63.1
    failure, kidney (renal) D63.1
    neoplastic disease (see also Neoplasm)
      D63.0
  intertropical (see also Ancylostomiasis)
    D63.8
  iron deficiency D50.9
    secondary to blood loss (chronic) D50.0
      acute D62
    specified type NEC D50.8

◀ New   ◀◀ Revised   ~~deleted~~ Deleted

Anemia (Continued)
Joseph-Diamond-Blackfan (congenital
    hypoplastic) D61.01
Lederer's (hemolytic) D59.1
leukoerythroblastic D61.82
macrocytic D53.9
    nutritional D52.0
    tropical D52.8
malarial (see also Malaria) B54 [D63.8]
malignant (progressive) D51.0
malnutrition D53.9
marsh (see also Malaria) B54 [D63.8]
Mediterranean (with other
    hemoglobinopathy) D56.9
megaloblastic D53.1
    combined B12 and folate deficiency
        D53.1
    hereditary D51.1
    nutritional D52.0
    orotic aciduria D53.0
    refractory D53.1
    specified type NEC D53.1
megalocytic D53.1
microcytic (hypochromic) D50.9
    due to blood loss (chronic) D50.0
        acute D62
    familial D56.8
microdrepanocytosis D57.40
microelliptopoikilocytic (Rietti-Greppi-
    Micheli) D56.9
miner's B76.9 [D63.8]
myelodysplastic D46.9
myelofibrosis D75.81
myelogenous D64.89
myelopathic D64.89
myelophthisic D61.82
myeloproliferative D47.Z9
newborn P61.4
    due to
        ABO (antibodies, isoimmunization,
            maternal/fetal incompatibility)
            P55.1
        Rh (antibodies, isoimmunization,
            maternal/fetal incompatibility)
            P55.0
    following fetal blood loss P61.3
    posthemorrhagic (fetal) P61.3
nonspherocytic hemolytic —see Anemia,
    hemolytic, nonspherocytic
normocytic (infectional) D64.9
    due to blood loss (chronic) D50.0
        acute D62
    myelophthisic D61.82
nutritional (deficiency) D53.9
    with
        poor iron absorption D50.8
        specified deficiency NEC D53.8
    megaloblastic D52.0
of prematurity P61.2
orotaciduric (congenital) (hereditary) D53.0
osteosclerotic D64.89
ovalocytosis (hereditary) —see Elliptocytosis
paludal (see also Malaria) B54 [D63.8]
pernicious (congenital) (malignant)
    (progressive) D51.0
pleochromic D64.89
    of sprue D52.8
posthemorrhagic (chronic) D50.0
    acute D62
    newborn P61.3
postoperative (postprocedural)
    due to (acute) blood loss D62
        chronic blood loss D50.0
    specified NEC D64.9
postpartum O90.81
pressure D64.89
progressive D64.9
    malignant D51.0
    pernicious D51.0
protein-deficiency D53.0
pseudoleukemica infantum D64.89

Anemia (Continued)
pure red cell D60.9
    congenital D61.01
pyridoxine-responsive D64.3
pyruvate kinase deficiency D55.2
refractory D46.4
    with
        excess of blasts D46.20
            1 (RAEB 1) D46.21
            2 (RAEB 2) D46.22
            in transformation (RAEB T) —see
                Leukemia, acute myeloblastic
        hemochromatosis D46.1
        sideroblasts (ring) (RARS) D46.1
    without ring sideroblasts, so stated D46.0
    without sideroblasts without excess of
        blasts D46.0
    megaloblastic D53.1
    sideroblastic D46.1
    sideropenic D50.9
Rietti-Greppi-Micheli D56.9
scorbutic D53.2
secondary to
    blood loss (chronic) D50.0
        acute D62
    hemorrhage (chronic) D50.0
        acute D62
semiplastic D61.89
sickle-cell —see Disease, sickle-cell
sideroblastic D64.3
    hereditary D64.0
    hypochromic, sex-linked D64.0
    pyridoxine-responsive NEC D64.3
    refractory D46.1
    secondary (due to)
        disease D64.1
        drugs and toxins D64.2
    specified type NEC D64.3
sideropenic (refractory) D50.9
    due to blood loss (chronic) D50.0
        acute D62
simple chronic D53.9
specified type NEC D64.89
spherocytic (hereditary) —see Spherocytosis
splenic D64.89
splenomegalic D64.89
stomatocytosis D58.8
syphilitic (acquired) (late) A52.79 [D63.8]
target cell D64.89
thalassemia D56.9
thrombocytopenic —see Thrombocytopenia
toxic D61.2
tropical B76.9 [D63.8]
    macrocytic D52.8
tuberculous A18.89 [D63.8]
vegan D51.3
vitamin
    B6-responsive D64.3
    B12 deficiency (dietary) pernicious D51.0
von Jaksch's D64.89
Witts' (achlorhydric anemia) D50.8
Anemophobia F40.228
Anencephalus, anencephaly Q00.0
Anergasia —see Psychosis, organic
Anesthesia, anesthetic R20.0
complication or reaction NEC (see also
    Complications, anesthesia) T88.59
    due to
        correct substance properly
            administered —see Table of Drugs
            and Chemicals, by drug, adverse
            effect
        overdose or wrong substance given —see
            Table of Drugs and Chemicals, by
            drug, poisoning
cornea H18.81-
dissociative F44.6
functional (hysterical) F44.6
hyperesthetic, thalamic G89.0
hysterical F44.6
local skin lesion R20.0

Anesthesia, anesthetic (Continued)
sexual (psychogenic) F52.1
shock (due to) T88.2
skin R20.0
testicular N50.9
Anetoderma (maculosum) (of) L90.8
Jadassohn-Pellizzari L90.2
Schweniger-Buzzi L90.1
Aneurin deficiency E51.9
Aneurysm (anastomotic) (artery) (cirsoid)
    (diffuse) (false) (fusiform) (multiple)
    (saccular) I72.9
abdominal (aorta) I71.4
    ruptured I71.3
    syphilitic A52.01
aorta, aortic (nonsyphilitic) I71.9
    abdominal I71.4
        ruptured I71.3
    arch I71.2
        ruptured I71.1
    arteriosclerotic I71.9
        ruptured I71.8
    ascending I71.2
        ruptured I71.1
    congenital Q25.4
    descending I71.9
        abdominal I71.4
            ruptured I71.3
        ruptured I71.8
        thoracic I71.2
            ruptured I71.1
    ruptured I71.8
    sinus, congenital Q25.4
    syphilitic A52.01
    thoracic I71.2
        ruptured I71.1
    thoracoabdominal I71.6
        ruptured I71.5
    thorax, thoracic (arch) I71.2
        ruptured I71.1
    transverse I71.2
        ruptured I71.1
    valve (heart) (see also Endocarditis, aortic)
        I35.8
arteriosclerotic I72.9
    cerebral I67.1
        ruptured —see Hemorrhage, intracranial,
            subarachnoid
arteriovenous (congenital) —see also
    Malformation, arteriovenous
    acquired I77.0
        brain I67.1
        coronary I25.41
        pulmonary I28.0
    brain Q28.2
        ruptured I60.8
    peripheral —see Malformation,
        arteriovenous, peripheral
    precerebral vessels Q28.0
    specified site NEC —see also Malformation,
        arteriovenous
        acquired I77.0
basal —see Aneurysm, brain
berry (congenital) (nonruptured) I67.1
    ruptured I60.7
brain I67.1
    arteriosclerotic I67.1
        ruptured —see Hemorrhage, intracranial,
            subarachnoid
    arteriovenous (congenital) (nonruptured)
        Q28.2
        acquired I67.1
            ruptured I60.8
        ruptured I60.8
    berry (congenital) (nonruptured) I67.1
        ruptured (see also Hemorrhage,
            intracranial, subarachnoid) I60.7
    congenital Q28.3
        ruptured I60.7
    meninges I67.1
        ruptured I60.8

Aneurysm *(Continued)*
  brain *(Continued)*
    miliary (congenital) (nonruptured) I67.1
      ruptured (*see also* Hemorrhage,
          intracranial, subarachnoid) I60.7
    mycotic I33.0
      ruptured —*see* Hemorrhage, intracranial,
          subarachnoid
    syphilitic (hemorrhage) A52.05
  cardiac (false) (*see also* Aneurysm, heart)
      I25.3
  carotid artery (common) (external) I72.0
    internal (intracranial) I67.1
      extracranial portion I72.0
    ruptured into brain I60.0-
    syphilitic A52.09
      intracranial A52.05
  cavernous sinus I67.1
    arteriovenous (congenital) (nonruptured)
        Q28.3
      ruptured I60.8
  celiac I72.8
  central nervous system, syphilitic A52.05
  cerebral —*see* Aneurysm, brain
  chest —*see* Aneurysm, thorax
  circle of Willis I67.1
    congenital Q28.3
      ruptured I60.6
    ruptured I60.6
  common iliac artery I72.3
  congenital (peripheral) Q27.8
    brain Q28.3
      ruptured I60.7
    coronary Q24.5
    digestive system Q27.8
    lower limb Q27.8
    pulmonary Q25.79
    retina Q14.1
    specified site NEC Q27.8
    upper limb Q27.8
  conjunctiva —*see* Abnormality, conjunctiva,
      vascular
  conus arteriosus —*see* Aneurysm, heart
  coronary (arteriosclerotic) (artery) I25.41
    arteriovenous, congenital Q24.5
    congenital Q24.5
    ruptured —*see* Infarct, myocardium
    syphilitic A52.06
    vein I25.89
  cylindroid (aorta) I71.9
    ruptured I71.8
    syphilitic A52.01
  ductus arteriosus Q25.0
  endocardial, infective (any valve) I33.0
  femoral (artery) (ruptured) I72.4
  gastroduodenal I72.8
  gastroepiploic I72.8
  heart (wall) (chronic or with a stated duration
      of over 4 weeks) I25.3
    valve —*see* Endocarditis
  hepatic I72.8
  iliac (common) (artery) (ruptured) I72.3
  infective I72.9
    endocardial (any valve) I33.0
  innominate (nonsyphilitic) I72.8
    syphilitic A52.09
  interauricular septum —*see* Aneurysm, heart
  interventricular septum —*see* Aneurysm,
      heart
  intrathoracic (nonsyphilitic) I71.2
    ruptured I71.1
    syphilitic A52.01
  lower limb I72.4
  lung (pulmonary artery) I28.1
  mediastinal (nonsyphilitic) I72.8
    syphilitic A52.09
  miliary (congenital) I67.1
    ruptured —*see* Hemorrhage, intracerebral,
        subarachnoid, intracranial
  mitral (heart) (valve) I34.8
  mural —*see* Aneurysm, heart

Aneurysm *(Continued)*
  mycotic I72.9
    endocardial (any valve) I33.0
      ruptured, brain —*see* Hemorrhage,
          intracerebral, subarachnoid
  myocardium —*see* Aneurysm, heart
  neck I72.0
  pancreaticoduodenal I72.8
  patent ductus arteriosus Q25.0
  peripheral NEC I72.8
    congenital Q27.8
      digestive system Q27.8
      lower limb Q27.8
      specified site NEC Q27.8
      upper limb Q27.8
  popliteal (artery) (ruptured) I72.4
  precerebral, congenital (nonruptured)
      Q28.1
  pulmonary I28.1
    arteriovenous Q25.72
      acquired I28.0
    syphilitic A52.09
    valve (heart) —*see* Endocarditis,
        pulmonary
  racemose (peripheral) I72.9
    congenital —*see* Aneurysm,
        congenital
  radial I72.1
  Rasmussen NEC A15.0
  renal (artery) I72.2
  retina —*see also* Disorder, retina,
      microaneurysms
    congenital Q14.1
    diabetic —*see* Diabetes, microaneurysms,
        retinal
  sinus of Valsalva Q25.4
  specified NEC I72.8
  spinal (cord) I72.8
    syphilitic (hemorrhage) A52.09
  splenic I72.8
  subclavian (artery) (ruptured)
      I72.8
    syphilitic A52.09
  superior mesenteric I72.8
  syphilitic (aorta) A52.01
    central nervous system A52.05
    congenital (late) A50.54 *[I79.0]*
    spine, spinal A52.09
  thoracoabdominal (aorta) I71.6
    ruptured I71.5
    syphilitic A52.01
  thorax, thoracic (aorta) (arch) (nonsyphilitic)
      I71.2
    ruptured I71.1
    syphilitic A52.01
  traumatic (complication) (early),
      specified site —*see* Injury,
      blood vessel
  tricuspid (heart) (valve) I07.8
  ulnar I72.1
  upper limb (ruptured) I72.1
  valve, valvular —*see* Endocarditis
  visceral NEC I72.8
  venous (*see also* Varix) I86.8
    congenital Q27.8
      digestive system Q27.8
      lower limb Q27.8
      specified site NEC Q27.8
      upper limb Q27.8
  ventricle —*see* Aneurysm, heart
  visceral NEC I72.8
Angelman syndrome Q93.5
Anger R45.4
Angiectasis, angiectopia I99.8
Angiitis I77.6
  allergic granulomatous M30.1
  hypersensitivity M31.0
  necrotizing M31.9
    specified NEC M31.8
  nervous system, granulomatous
      I67.7

Angina (attack) (cardiac) (chest) (heart)
    (pectoris) (syndrome) (vasomotor)
    I20.9
  with
    atherosclerotic heart disease —*see*
        Arteriosclerosis, coronary
        (artery)
    documented spasm I20.1
  abdominal K55.1
  accelerated —*see* Angina, unstable
  agranulocytic —*see* Agranulocytosis
  angiospastic —*see* Angina, with documented
      spasm
  aphthous B08.5
  crescendo —*see* Angina, unstable
  croupous J05.0
  cruris I73.9
  de novo effort —*see* Angina, unstable
  diphtheritic, membranous A36.0
  equivalent I20.8
  exudative, chronic J37.0
  following acute myocardial infarction
      I23.7
  gangrenous diphtheritic A36.0
  intestinal K55.1
  Ludovici K12.2
  Ludwig's K12.2
  malignant diphtheritic A36.0
  membranous J05.0
    diphtheritic A36.0
    Vincent's A69.1
  mesenteric K55.1
  monocytic —*see* Mononucleosis, infectious
  of effort —*see* Angina, specified NEC
  phlegmonous J36
    diphtheritic A36.0
  post-infarctional I23.7
  pre-infarctional —*see* Angina, unstable
  Prinzmetal —*see* Angina, with documented
      spasm
  progressive —*see* Angina, unstable
  pseudomembranous A69.1
  pultaceous, diphtheritic A36.0
  spasm-induced —*see* Angina, with
      documented spasm
  specified NEC I20.8
  stable I20.9
  stenocardia —*see* Angina, specified NEC
  stridulous, diphtheritic A36.2
  tonsil J36
  trachealis J05.0
  unstable I20.0
  variant —*see* Angina, with documented
      spasm
  Vincent's A69.1
  worsening effort —*see* Angina, unstable
Angioblastoma —*see* Neoplasm, connective
    tissue, uncertain behavior
Angiocholecystitis —*see* Cholecystitis, acute
Angiocholitis (*see also* Cholecystitis, acute)
    K83.0
Angiodysgenesis spinalis G95.19
Angiodysplasia (cecum) (colon) K55.20
  with bleeding K55.21
  duodenum (and stomach) K31.819
    with bleeding K31.811
  stomach (and duodenum) K31.819
    with bleeding K31.811
Angioedema (allergic) (any site) (with urticaria)
    T78.3
  hereditary D84.1
Angioendothelioma —*see* Neoplasm, uncertain
    behavior, by site
  benign D18.00
    intra-abdominal D18.03
    intracranial D18.02
    skin D18.01
    specified site NEC D18.09
  bone —*see* Neoplasm, bone, malignant
  Ewing's —*see* Neoplasm, bone, malignant
Angioendotheliomatosis C85.8-

◀ New   ◀▥ Revised   ~~deleted~~ Deleted

Angiofibroma —see also Neoplasm, benign, by site
  juvenile
    specified site —see Neoplasm, benign, by site
    unspecified site D10.6
Angiohemophilia (A) (B) D68.0
Angioid streaks (choroid) (macula) (retina) H35.33
Angiokeratoma —see Neoplasm, skin, benign
  corporis diffusum E75.21
Angioleiomyoma —see Neoplasm, connective tissue, benign
Angiolipoma —see also Lipoma
  infiltrating —see Lipoma
Angioma —see also Hemangioma, by site
  capillary I78.1
  hemorrhagicum hereditaria I78.0
  intra-abdominal D18.03
  intracranial D18.02
  malignant —see Neoplasm, connective tissue, malignant
  plexiform D18.00
    intra-abdominal D18.03
    intracranial D18.02
    skin D18.01
    specified site NEC D18.09
  senile I78.1
  serpiginosum L81.7
  skin D18.01
  specified site NEC D18.09
  spider I78.1
  stellate I78.1
  venous Q28.3
Angiomatosis Q82.8
  bacillary A79.89
  encephalotrigeminal Q85.8
  hemorrhagic familial I78.0
  hereditary familial I78.0
  liver K76.4
Angiomyolipoma —see Lipoma
Angiomyoliposarcoma —see Neoplasm, connective tissue, malignant
Angiomyoma —see Neoplasm, connective tissue, benign
Angiomyosarcoma —see Neoplasm, connective tissue, malignant
Angiomyxoma —see Neoplasm, connective tissue, uncertain behavior
Angioneurosis F45.8
Angioneurotic edema (allergic) (any site) (with urticaria) T78.3
  hereditary D84.1
Angiopathia, angiopathy I99.9
  cerebral I67.9
    amyloid E85.4 [I68.0]
  diabetic (peripheral) —see Diabetes, angiopathy
  peripheral I73.9
    diabetic —see Diabetes, angiopathy
    specified type NEC I73.89
  retinae syphilitica A52.05
  retinalis (juvenilis)
    diabetic —see Diabetes, retinopathy
    proliferative —see Retinopathy, proliferative
Angiosarcoma —see also Neoplasm, connective tissue, malignant
  liver C22.3
Angiosclerosis —see Arteriosclerosis
Angiospasm (peripheral) (traumatic) (vessel) I73.9
  brachial plexus G54.0
  cerebral G45.9
  cervical plexus G54.2
  nerve
    arm —see Mononeuropathy, upper limb
      axillary G54.0
      median —see Lesion, nerve, median
      ulnar —see Lesion, nerve, ulnar
    axillary G54.0

Angiospasm (Continued)
  nerve (Continued)
    leg —see Mononeuropathy, lower limb
    median —see Lesion, nerve, median
    plantar —see Lesion, nerve, plantar
    ulnar —see Lesion, nerve, ulnar
Angiospastic disease or edema I73.9
Angiostrongyliasis
  due to
    Parastrongylus
      cantonensis B83.2
      costaricensis B81.3
  intestinal B81.3
Anguillulosis —see Strongyloidiasis
Angulation
  cecum —see Obstruction, intestine
  coccyx (acquired) (see also subcategory) M43.8
    congenital NEC Q76.49
  femur (acquired) —see also Deformity, limb, specified type NEC, thigh
    congenital Q74.2
  intestine (large) (small) —see Obstruction, intestine
  sacrum (acquired) (see also subcategory) M43.8
    congenital NEC Q76.49
  sigmoid (flexure) —see Obstruction, intestine
  spine —see Dorsopathy, deforming, specified NEC
  tibia (acquired) —see also Deformity, limb, specified type NEC, lower leg
    congenital Q74.2
  ureter N13.5
    with infection N13.6
  wrist (acquired) —see also Deformity, limb, specified type NEC, forearm
    congenital Q74.0
Angulus infectiosus (lips) K13.0
Anhedonia R45.84
Anhidrosis L74.4
Anhydration, anhydremia E86.0
  with
    hypernatremia E87.0
    hyponatremia E87.1
Anhydremia E86.0
  with
    hypernatremia E87.0
    hyponatremia E87.1
Anidrosis L74.4
Aniridia (congenital) Q13.1
Anisakiasis (infection) (infestation) B81.0
Anisakis larvae infestation B81.0
Aniseikonia H52.32
Anisocoria (pupil) H57.02
  congenital Q13.2
Anisocytosis R71.8
Anisometropia (congenital) H52.31
Ankle —see condition
Ankyloblepharon (eyelid) (acquired) —see also Blepharophimosis
  filiforme (adnatum) (congenital) Q10.3
  total Q10.3
Ankyloglossia Q38.1
Ankylosis (fibrous) (osseous) (joint) M24.60
  ankle M24.67-
  arthrodesis status Z98.1
  cricoarytenoid (cartilage) (joint) (larynx) J38.7
  dental K03.5
  ear ossicles H74.31-
  elbow M24.62-
  foot M24.67-
  hand M24.64-
  hip M24.65-
  incostapedial joint (infectional) —see Ankylosis, ear ossicles
  jaw (temporomandibular) M26.61
  knee M24.66-
  lumbosacral (joint) M43.27
  postoperative (status) Z98.1
  produced by surgical fusion, status Z98.1
  sacro-iliac (joint) M43.28

Ankylosis (Continued)
  shoulder M24.61-
  spine (joint) —see also Fusion, spine
    spondylitic —see Spondylitis, ankylosing
  surgical Z98.1
  temporomandibular M26.61
  tooth, teeth (hard tissues) K03.5
  wrist M24.63-
Ankylostoma —see Ancylostoma
Ankylostomiasis —see Ancylostomiasis
Ankylurethria —see Stricture, urethra
Annular —see also condition
  detachment, cervix N88.8
  organ or site, congenital NEC —see Distortion
  pancreas (congenital) Q45.1
Anodontia (complete) (partial) (vera) K00.0
  acquired K08.10
Anomaly, anomalous (congenital) (unspecified type) Q89.9
  abdominal wall NEC Q79.59
  acoustic nerve Q07.8
  adrenal (gland) Q89.1
  Alder (-Reilly) (leukocyte granulation) D72.0
  alimentary tract Q45.9
    upper Q40.9
  alveolar M26.70
    hyperplasia M26.79
      mandibular M26.72
      maxillary M26.71
    hypoplasia M26.79
      mandibular M26.74
      maxillary M26.73
    ridge (process) M26.79
    specified NEC M26.79
  ankle (joint) Q74.2
  anus Q43.9
  aorta (arch) NEC Q25.4
    coarctation (preductal) (postductal) Q25.1
  aortic cusp or valve Q23.9
  appendix Q43.8
  apple peel syndrome Q41.1
  aqueduct of Sylvius Q03.0
    with spina bifida —see Spina bifida, with hydrocephalus
  arm Q74.0
  arteriovenous NEC
    coronary Q24.5
    gastrointestinal Q27.33
      acquired —see Angiodysplasia
  artery (peripheral) Q27.9
    basilar NEC Q28.1
    cerebral Q28.3
    coronary Q24.5
    digestive system Q27.8
    eye Q15.8
    great Q25.9
      specified NEC Q25.8
    lower limb Q27.8
    peripheral Q27.9
      specified NEC Q27.8
    pulmonary NEC Q25.79
    renal Q27.2
    retina Q14.1
    specified site NEC Q27.8
    subclavian Q27.8
    umbilical Q27.0
    upper limb Q27.8
    vertebral NEC Q28.1
  aryteno-epiglottic folds Q31.8
  atrial
    bands or folds Q20.8
    septa Q21.1
  atrioventricular
    excitation I45.6
    septum Q21.0
  auditory canal Q17.8
  auricle
    ear Q17.8
      causing impairment of hearing Q16.9
    heart Q20.8
  Axenfeld's Q15.0

Anomaly, anomalous *(Continued)*
  back Q89.9
  band
    atrial Q20.8
    heart Q24.8
    ventricular Q24.8
  Bartholin's duct Q38.4
  biliary duct or passage Q44.5
  bladder Q64.70
    absence Q64.5
    diverticulum Q64.6
    exstrophy Q64.10
      cloacal Q64.12
      extroversion Q64.19
      specified type NEC Q64.19
      supravesical fissure Q64.11
    neck obstruction Q64.31
    specified type NEC Q64.79
  bone Q79.9
    arm Q74.0
    face Q75.9
    leg Q74.2
    pelvic girdle Q74.2
    shoulder girdle Q74.0
    skull Q75.9
      with
        anencephaly Q00.0
        encephalocele —*see* Encephalocele
        hydrocephalus Q03.9
          with spina bifida —*see* Spina bifida,
            by site, with hydrocephalus
        microcephaly Q02
  brain (multiple) Q04.9
    vessel Q28.3
  breast Q83.9
  broad ligament Q50.6
  bronchus Q32.4
  bulbus cordis Q21.9
  bursa Q79.9
  canal of Nuck Q52.4
  canthus Q10.3
  capillary Q27.9
  cardiac Q24.9
    chambers Q20.9
      specified NEC Q20.8
    septal closure Q21.9
      specified NEC Q21.8
    valve NEC Q24.8
      pulmonary Q22.3
  cardiovascular system Q28.8
  carpus Q74.0
  caruncle, lacrimal Q10.6
  cascade stomach Q40.2
  cauda equina Q06.3
  cecum Q43.9
  cerebral Q04.9
    vessels Q28.3
  cervix Q51.9
  Chédiak-Higashi(-Steinbrinck) (congenital
    gigantism of peroxidase granules)
    E70.330
  cheek Q18.9
  chest wall Q67.8
    bones Q76.9
  chin Q18.9
  chordae tendineae Q24.8
  choroid Q14.3
    plexus Q07.8
  chromosomes, chromosomal Q99.9
    D (1) —*see* condition, chromosome 13
    E (3) —*see* condition, chromosome 18
    G —*see* condition, chromosome 21
    sex
      female phenotype Q97.8
      gonadal dysgenesis (pure) Q99.1
      Klinefelter's Q98.4
      male phenotype Q98.9
      Turner's Q96.9
    specified NEC Q99.8
  cilia Q10.3
  circulatory system Q28.9

Anomaly, anomalous *(Continued)*
  clavicle Q74.0
  clitoris Q52.6
  coccyx Q76.49
  colon Q43.9
  common duct Q44.5
  communication
    coronary artery Q24.5
    left ventricle with right atrium Q21.0
  concha (ear) Q17.3
  connection
    portal vein Q26.5
    pulmonary venous Q26.4
      partial Q26.3
      total Q26.2
    renal artery with kidney Q27.2
  cornea (shape) Q13.4
  coronary artery or vein Q24.5
  cranium —*see* Anomaly, skull
  cricoid cartilage Q31.8
  cystic duct Q44.5
  dental
    alveolar —*see* Anomaly, alveolar
    arch relationship M26.20
      specified NEC M26.29
  dentofacial M26.9
    alveolar —*see* Anomaly, alveolar
    dental arch relationship M26.20
      specified NEC M26.29
    functional M26.50
      specified NEC M26.59
    jaw-cranial base relationship M26.10
      asymmetry M26.12
        maxillary M26.11
      specified type NEC M26.19
    jaw size M26.00
      macrogenia M26.05
      mandibular
        hyperplasia M26.03
        hypoplasia M26.04
      maxillary
        hyperplasia M26.01
        hypoplasia M26.02
      microgenia M26.06
      specified type NEC M26.09
    malocclusion M26.4
      dental arch relationship NEC M26.29
      jaw-cranial base relationship —*see*
        Anomaly, dentofacial, jaw-cranial
        base relationship
      jaw size —*see* Anomaly, dentofacial, jaw
        size
      specified type NEC M26.89
    temporomandibular joint M26.60
      adhesions M26.61
      ankylosis M26.61
      arthralgia M26.62
      articular disc M26.63
      specified type NEC M26.69
    tooth position, fully erupted M26.30
      specified NEC M26.39
  dermatoglyphic Q82.8
  diaphragm (apertures) NEC Q79.1
  digestive organ (s) or tract Q45.9
    lower Q43.9
    upper Q40.9
  distance, interarch (excessive) (inadequate)
    M26.25
  distribution, coronary artery Q24.5
  ductus
    arteriosus Q25.0
    botalli Q25.0
  duodenum Q43.9
  dura (brain) Q04.9
    spinal cord Q06.9
  ear (external) Q17.9
    causing impairment of hearing Q16.9
    inner Q16.5
    middle (causing impairment of hearing)
      Q16.4
    ossicles Q16.3

Anomaly, anomalous *(Continued)*
  Ebstein's (heart) (tricuspid valve) Q22.5
  ectodermal Q82.9
  Eisenmenger's (ventricular septal defect)
    Q21.8
  ejaculatory duct Q55.4
  elbow Q74.0
  endocrine gland NEC Q89.2
  epididymis Q55.4
  epiglottis Q31.8
  esophagus Q39.9
  eustachian tube Q17.8
  eye Q15.9
    anterior segment Q13.9
      specified NEC Q13.89
    posterior segment Q14.9
      specified NEC Q14.8
    ptosis (eyelid) Q10.0
    specified NEC Q15.8
  eyebrow Q18.8
  eyelid Q10.3
    ptosis Q10.0
  face Q18.9
    bone (s) Q75.9
  fallopian tube Q50.6
  fascia Q79.9
  femur NEC Q74.2
  fibula NEC Q74.2
  finger Q74.0
  fixation, intestine Q43.3
  flexion (joint) NOS Q74.9
    hip or thigh Q65.89
  foot NEC Q74.2
    varus (congenital) Q66.3
  foramen
    Botalli Q21.1
    ovale Q21.1
  forearm Q74.0
  forehead Q75.8
  form, teeth K00.2
  fovea centralis Q14.1
  frontal bone —*see* Anomaly, skull
  gallbladder (position) (shape) (size)
    Q44.1
  Gartner's duct Q52.4
  gastrointestinal tract Q45.9
  genitalia, genital organ (s) or system
    female Q52.9
      external Q52.70
      internal NOS Q52.9
    male Q55.9
      hydrocele P83.5
      specified NEC Q55.8
  genitourinary NEC
    female Q52.9
    male Q55.9
  Gerbode Q21.0
  glottis Q31.8
  granulation or granulocyte, genetic
    (constitutional) (leukocyte) D72.0
  gum Q38.6
  gyri Q07.9
  hair Q84.2
  hand Q74.0
  hard tissue formation in pulp K04.3
  head —*see* Anomaly, skull
  heart Q24.9
    auricle Q20.8
    bands or folds Q24.8
    fibroelastosis cordis I42.4
    obstructive NEC Q22.6
    patent ductus arteriosus (Botalli) Q25.0
    septum Q21.9
      auricular Q21.1
      interatrial Q21.1
      interventricular Q21.0
        with pulmonary stenosis or atresia,
          dextraposition of aorta and
          hypertrophy of right ventricle
          Q21.3
      specified NEC Q21.8

◀ New   ◀▥ Revised   ~~deleted~~ Deleted

Anomaly, anomalous *(Continued)*
  heart *(Continued)*
    septum *(Continued)*
      ventricular Q21.0
        with pulmonary stenosis or atresia, dextraposition of aorta and hypertrophy of right ventricle Q21.3
      tetralogy of Fallot Q21.3
    valve NEC Q24.8
      aortic
        bicuspid valve Q23.1
        insufficiency Q23.1
        stenosis Q23.0
          subaortic Q24.4
      mitral
        insufficiency Q23.3
        stenosis Q23.2
      pulmonary Q22.3
        atresia Q22.0
        insufficiency Q22.2
        stenosis Q22.1
          infundibular Q24.3
          subvalvular Q24.3
      tricuspid
        atresia Q22.4
        stenosis Q22.4
    ventricle Q20.8
  heel NEC Q74.2
  Hegglin's D72.0
  hemianencephaly Q00.0
  hemicephaly Q00.0
  hemicrania Q00.0
  hepatic duct Q44.5
  hip NEC Q74.2
  hourglass stomach Q40.2
  humerus Q74.0
  hydatid of Morgagni
    female Q50.5
    male (epididymal) Q55.4
      testicular Q55.29
  hymen Q52.4
  hypersegmentation of neutrophils, hereditary D72.0
  hypophyseal Q89.2
  ileocecal (coil) (valve) Q43.9
  ileum Q43.9
  ilium NEC Q74.2
  integument Q84.9
    specified NEC Q84.8
  interarch distance (excessive) (inadequate) M26.25
  intervertebral cartilage or disc Q76.49
  intestine (large) (small) Q43.9
    with anomalous adhesions, fixation or malrotation Q43.3
  iris Q13.2
  ischium NEC Q74.2
  jaw —*see* Anomaly, dentofacial
    alveolar —*see* Anomaly, alveolar
  jaw-cranial base relationship —*see* Anomaly, dentofacial, jaw-cranial base relationship
  jejunum Q43.8
  joint Q74.9
    specified NEC Q74.8
  Jordan's D72.0
  kidney (s) (calyx) (pelvis) Q63.9
    artery Q27.2
    specified NEC Q63.8
  Klippel-Feil (brevicollis) Q76.1
  knee Q74.1
  labium (majus) (minus) Q52.70
  labyrinth, membranous Q16.5
  lacrimal apparatus or duct Q10.6
  larynx, laryngeal (muscle) Q31.9
    web (bed) Q31.0
  lens Q12.9
  leukocytes, genetic D72.0
    granulation (constitutional) D72.0
  lid (fold) Q10.3

Anomaly, anomalous *(Continued)*
  ligament Q79.9
    broad Q50.6
    round Q52.8
  limb Q74.9
    lower NEC Q74.2
      reduction deformity —*see* Defect, reduction, lower limb
    upper Q74.0
  lip Q38.0
  liver Q44.7
    duct Q44.5
  lower limb NEC Q74.2
  lumbosacral (joint) (region) Q76.49
    kyphosis —*see* Kyphosis, congenital
    lordosis —*see* Lordosis, congenital
  lung (fissure) (lobe) Q33.9
  mandible —*see* Anomaly, dentofacial
  maxilla —*see* Anomaly, dentofacial
  May (-Hegglin) D72.0
  meatus urinarius NEC Q64.79
  meningeal bands or folds Q07.9
    constriction of Q07.8
    spinal Q06.9
  meninges Q07.9
    cerebral Q04.8
    spinal Q06.9
  meningocele Q05.9
  mesentery Q45.9
  metacarpus Q74.0
  metatarsus NEC Q74.2
  middle ear Q16.4
    ossicles Q16.3
  mitral (leaflets) (valve) Q23.9
    insufficiency Q23.3
    specified NEC Q23.8
    stenosis Q23.2
  mouth Q38.6
  Müllerian —*see also* Anomaly, by site
    uterus NEC Q51.818
  multiple NEC Q89.7
  muscle Q79.9
    eyelid Q10.3
  musculoskeletal system, except limbs Q79.9
  myocardium Q24.8
  nail Q84.6
  narrowness, eyelid Q10.3
  nasal sinus (wall) Q30.8
  neck (any part) Q18.9
  nerve Q07.9
    acoustic Q07.8
    optic Q07.8
  nervous system (central) Q07.9
  nipple Q83.9
  nose, nasal (bones) (cartilage) (septum) (sinus) Q30.9
    specified NEC Q30.8
  ocular muscle Q15.8
  omphalomesenteric duct Q43.0
  opening, pulmonary veins Q26.4
  optic
    disc Q14.2
    nerve Q07.8
  opticociliary vessels Q13.2
  orbit (eye) Q10.7
  organ Q89.9
    of Corti Q16.5
  origin
    artery
      innominate Q25.8
      pulmonary Q25.79
      renal Q27.2
      subclavian Q25.8
  osseous meatus (ear) Q16.1
  ovary Q50.39
  oviduct Q50.6
  palate (hard) (soft) NEC Q38.5
  pancreas or pancreatic duct Q45.3
  papillary muscles Q24.8
  parathyroid gland Q89.2
  paraurethral ducts Q64.79

Anomaly, anomalous *(Continued)*
  parotid (gland) Q38.4
  patella Q74.1
  Pelger-Huët (hereditary hyposegmentation) D72.0
  pelvic girdle NEC Q74.2
  pelvis (bony) NEC Q74.2
    rachitic E64.3
  penis (glans) Q55.69
  pericardium Q24.8
  peripheral vascular system Q27.9
  Peter's Q13.4
  pharynx Q38.8
  pigmentation L81.9
    congenital Q82.8
  pituitary (gland) Q89.2
  pleural (folds) Q34.0
  portal vein Q26.5
    connection Q26.5
  position, tooth, teeth, fully erupted M26.30
    specified NEC M26.39
  precerebral vessel Q28.1
  prepuce Q55.69
  prostate Q55.4
  pulmonary Q33.9
    artery NEC Q25.79
    valve Q22.3
      atresia Q22.0
      insufficiency Q22.2
      specified type NEC Q22.3
      stenosis Q22.1
        infundibular Q24.3
        subvalvular Q24.3
    venous connection Q26.4
      partial Q26.3
      total Q26.2
  pupil Q13.2
    function H57.00
      anisocoria H57.02
      Argyll Robertson pupil H57.01
      miosis H57.03
      mydriasis H57.04
      specified type NEC H57.09
      tonic pupil H57.05-
  pylorus Q40.3
  radius Q74.0
  rectum Q43.9
  reduction (extremity) (limb)
    femur (longitudinal) —*see* Defect, reduction, lower limb, longitudinal, femur
    fibula (longitudinal) —*see* Defect, reduction, lower limb, longitudinal, fibula
    lower limb —*see* Defect, reduction, lower limb
    radius (longitudinal) —*see* Defect, reduction, upper limb, longitudinal, radius
    tibia (longitudinal) —*see* Defect, reduction, lower limb, longitudinal, tibia
    ulna (longitudinal) —*see* Defect, reduction, upper limb, longitudinal, ulna
    upper limb —*see* Defect, reduction, upper limb
  refraction —*see* Disorder, refraction
  renal Q63.9
    artery Q27.2
    pelvis Q63.9
      specified NEC Q63.8
  respiratory system Q34.9
    specified NEC Q34.8
  retina Q14.1
  rib Q76.6
    cervical Q76.5
  Rieger's Q13.81
  rotation —*see* Malrotation
    hip or thigh Q65.89
  round ligament Q52.8
  sacroiliac (joint) NEC Q74.2

Anomaly, anomalous *(Continued)*
  sacrum NEC Q76.49
    kyphosis —*see* Kyphosis, congenital
    lordosis —*see* Lordosis, congenital
  saddle nose, syphilitic A50.57
  salivary duct or gland Q38.4
  scapula Q74.0
  scrotum —*see* Malformation, testis and
      scrotum
  sebaceous gland Q82.9
  seminal vesicles Q55.4
  sense organs NEC Q07.8
  sex chromosomes NEC —*see also* Anomaly,
      chromosomes
    female phenotype Q97.8
    male phenotype Q98.9
  shoulder (girdle) (joint) Q74.0
  sigmoid (flexure) Q43.9
  simian crease Q82.8
  sinus of Valsalva Q25.4
  skeleton generalized Q78.9
  skin (appendage) Q82.9
  skull Q75.9
    with
      anencephaly Q00.0
      encephalocele —*see* Encephalocele
      hydrocephalus Q03.9
        with spina bifida —*see* Spina bifida, by
          site, with hydrocephalus
      microcephaly Q02
  specified organ or site NEC Q89.8
  spermatic cord Q55.4
  spine, spinal NEC Q76.49
    column NEC Q76.49
      kyphosis —*see* Kyphosis, congenital
      lordosis —*see* Lordosis, congenital
    cord Q06.9
    nerve root Q07.8
  spleen Q89.09
    agenesis Q89.01
  stenonian duct Q38.4
  sternum NEC Q76.7
  stomach Q40.3
  submaxillary gland Q38.4
  tarsus NEC Q74.2
  tendon Q79.9
  testis —*see* Malformation, testis and
      scrotum
  thigh NEC Q74.2
  thorax (wall) Q67.8
    bony Q76.9
  throat Q38.8
  thumb Q74.0
  thymus gland Q89.2
  thyroid (gland) Q89.2
    cartilage Q31.8
  tibia NEC Q74.2
    saber A50.56
  toe Q74.2
  tongue Q38.3
  tooth, teeth K00.9
    eruption K00.6
    position, fully erupted M26.30
    spacing, fully erupted M26.30
  trachea (cartilage) Q32.1
  tragus Q17.9
  tricuspid (leaflet) (valve) Q22.9
    atresia or stenosis Q22.4
    Ebstein's Q22.5
  Uhl's (hypoplasia of myocardium, right
      ventricle) Q24.8
  ulna Q74.0
  umbilical artery Q27.0
  union
    cricoid cartilage and thyroid cartilage
        Q31.8
    thyroid cartilage and hyoid bone
        Q31.8
    trachea with larynx Q31.8
  upper limb Q74.0
  urachus Q64.4

Anomaly, anomalous *(Continued)*
  ureter Q62.8
    obstructive NEC Q62.39
      cecoureterocele Q62.32
      orthotopic ureterocele Q62.31
  urethra Q64.70
    absence Q64.5
    double Q64.74
    fistula to rectum Q64.73
    obstructive Q64.39
      stricture Q64.32
    prolapse Q64.71
    specified type NEC Q64.79
  urinary tract Q64.9
  uterus Q51.9
    with only one functioning horn
        Q51.4
  uvula Q38.5
  vagina Q52.4
  valleculae Q31.8
  valve (heart) NEC Q24.8
    coronary sinus Q24.5
    inferior vena cava Q24.8
    pulmonary Q22.3
    sinus coronario Q24.5
    venae cavae inferioris Q24.8
  vas deferens Q55.4
  vascular Q27.9
    brain Q28.3
    ring Q25.4
  vein (s) (peripheral) Q27.9
    brain Q28.3
    cerebral Q28.3
    coronary Q24.5
    developmental Q28.3
    great Q26.9
      specified NEC Q26.8
  vena cava (inferior) (superior) Q26.9
  venous —*see* Anomaly, vein (s)
  venous return Q26.8
  ventricular
    bands or folds Q24.8
    septa Q21.0
  vertebra Q76.49
    kyphosis —*see* Kyphosis, congenital
    lordosis —*see* Lordosis, congenital
  vesicourethral orifice Q64.79
  vessel (s) Q27.9
    optic papilla Q14.2
    precerebral Q28.1
  vitelline duct Q43.0
  vitreous body or humor Q14.0
  vulva Q52.70
  wrist (joint) Q74.0
Anomia R48.8
Anonychia (congenital) Q84.3
  acquired L60.8
Anophthalmos, anophthalmus (congenital)
    (globe) Q11.1
  acquired Z90.01
Anopia, anopsia H53.46-
  quadrant H53.46-
Anorchia, anorchism, anorchidism Q55.0
Anorexia R63.0
  hysterical F44.89
  nervosa F50.00
    atypical F50.9
    binge-eating type F50.2
      with purging F50.02
    restricting type F50.01
Anorgasmy, psychogenic (female)
    F52.31
  male F52.32
Anosmia R43.0
  hysterical F44.6
  postinfectional J39.8
Anosognosia R41.89
Anosteoplasia Q78.9
Anovulatory cycle N97.0
Anoxemia R09.02
  newborn P84

Anoxia (pathological) R09.02
  altitude T70.29
  cerebral G93.1
    complicating
      anesthesia (general) (local) or other
          sedation T88.59
        in labor and delivery O74.3
        in pregnancy O29.21-
        postpartum, puerperal O89.2
      delivery (cesarean) (instrumental)
          O75.4
    during a procedure G97.81
    newborn P84
    resulting from a procedure G97.82
  due to
    drowning T75.1
    high altitude T70.29
  heart —*see* Insufficiency, coronary
  intrauterine P84
  myocardial —*see* Insufficiency, coronary
  newborn P84
  spinal cord G95.11
  systemic (by suffocation) (low content in
      atmosphere) —*see* Asphyxia,
      traumatic
Anteflexion —*see* Anteversion
Antenatal
  care (normal pregnancy) Z34.90
  screening (encounter for) of mother
      Z36
Antepartum —*see* condition
Anterior —*see* condition
Antero-occlusion M26.220
Anteversion
  cervix —*see* Anteversion, uterus
  femur (neck), congenital Q65.89
  uterus, uterine (cervix) (postinfectional)
      (postpartal, old) N85.4
    congenital Q51.818
    in pregnancy or childbirth —*see* Pregnancy,
        complicated by
Anthophobia F40.228
Anthracosilicosis J60
Anthracosis (lung) (occupational) J60
  lingua K14.3
Anthrax A22.9
  with pneumonia A22.1
  cerebral A22.8
  colitis A22.2
  cutaneous A22.0
  gastrointestinal A22.2
  inhalation A22.1
  intestinal A22.2
  meningitis A22.8
  pulmonary A22.1
  respiratory A22.1
  sepsis A22.7
  specified manifestation NEC A22.8
Anthropoid pelvis Q74.2
  with disproportion (fetopelvic) O33.0
Anthropophobia F40.10
  generalized F40.11
Antibodies, maternal (blood group) —*see*
    Isoimmunization, affecting management
    of pregnancy
  anti-D —*see* Isoimmunization, affecting
    management of pregnancy, Rh
    newborn P55.0
Antibody
  anticardiolipin R76.0
    with
      hemorrhagic disorder D68.312
      hypercoagulable state D68.61
  antiphosphatidylglycerol R76.0
    with
      hemorrhagic disorder D68.312
      hypercoagulable state D68.61
  antiphosphatidylinositol R76.0
    with
      hemorrhagic disorder D68.312
      hypercoagulable state D68.61

◀ New   ⬅ Revised   ~~deleted~~ Deleted

Antibody (Continued)
  antiphosphatidylserine R76.0
    with
      hemorrhagic disorder D68.312
      hypercoagulable state D68.61
    antiphospholipid R76.0
    with
      hemorrhagic disorder D68.312
      hypercoagulable state D68.61
Anticardiolipin syndrome D68.61
Anticoagulant, circulating (intrinsic) (see also -
    Disorder, hemorrhagic) D68.318
  drug-induced (extrinsic) (see also - Disorder,
    hemorrhagic) D68.32
Antidiuretic hormone syndrome E22.2
Antimonial cholera —see Poisoning,
    antimony
Antiphospholipid
  antibody
    with hemorrhagic disorder D68.312
  syndrome D68.61
Antisocial personality F60.2
Antithrombinemia —see Circulating
    anticoagulants
Antithromboplastinemia D68.318
Antithromboplastinogenemia D68.318
Antitoxin complication or reaction —see
    Complications, vaccination
Antlophobia F40.228
Antritis J32.0
  maxilla J32.0
    acute J01.00
      recurrent J01.01
  stomach K29.60
    with bleeding K29.61
Antrum, antral —see condition
Anuria R34
  calculus (impacted) (recurrent) (see also
    Calculus, urinary) N20.9
  following
    abortion —see Abortion by type
      complicated by, renal failure
    ectopic or molar pregnancy O08.4
  newborn P96.0
  postprocedural N99.0
  postrenal N13.8
  traumatic (following crushing) T79.5
Anus, anal —see condition
Anusitis K62.89
Anxiety F41.9
  depression F41.8
  episodic paroxysmal F41.0
  generalized F41.1
  hysteria F41.8
  neurosis F41.1
  panic type F41.0
  reaction F41.1
  separation, abnormal (of childhood) F93.0
  specified NEC F41.8
  state F41.1
Aorta, aortic —see condition
Aortectasia —see Ectasia, aorta
  with aneurysm —see Aneurysm, aorta
Aortitis (nonsyphilitic) (calcific) I77.6
  arteriosclerotic I70.0
  Doehle-Heller A52.02
  luetic A52.02
  rheumatic —see Endocarditis, acute,
    rheumatic
  specific (syphilitic) A52.02
  syphilitic A52.02
    congenital A50.54 [I79.1]
Apathetic thyroid storm —see Thyrotoxicosis
Apathy R45.3
Apeirophobia F40.228
Apepsia K30
  psychogenic F45.8
Aperistalsis, esophagus K22.0
Apertognathia M26.29
Apert's syndrome Q87.0
Aphagia R13.0
  psychogenic F50.9

Aphakia (acquired) (postoperative) H27.0-
  congenital Q12.3
Aphasia (amnestic) (global) (nominal)
    (semantic) (syntactic) R47.01
  acquired, with epilepsy (Landau-Kleffner
    syndrome) —see Epilepsy, specified
    NEC
  auditory (developmental) F80.2
  developmental (receptive type) F80.2
    expressive type F80.1
    Wernicke's F80.2
  following
    cerebrovascular disease I69.920
      cerebral infarction I69.320
      intracerebral hemorrhage I69.120
      nontraumatic intracranial hemorrhage
        NEC I69.220
      specified disease NEC I69.820
      subarachnoid hemorrhage I69.020
  primary progressive G31.01 [F02.80]
    with behavioral disturbance G31.01
      [F02.81]
  progressive isolated G31.01 [F02.80]
    with behavioral disturbance G31.01
      [F02.81]
  sensory F80.2
  syphilis, tertiary A52.19
  Wernicke's (developmental) F80.2
Aphonia (organic) R49.1
  hysterical F44.4
  psychogenic F44.4
Aphthae, aphthous —see also condition
  Bednar's K12.0
  cachectic K14.0
  epizootic B08.8
  fever B08.8
  oral (recurrent) K12.0
  stomatitis (major) (minor) K12.0
  thrush B37.0
  ulcer (oral) (recurrent) K12.0
    genital organ (s) NEC
      female N76.6
      male N50.8
    larynx J38.7
Apical —see condition
Apiphobia F40.218
Aplasia —see also Agenesis
  abdominal muscle syndrome Q79.4
  alveolar process (acquired) —see Anomaly,
    alveolar
    congenital Q38.6
  aorta (congenital) Q25.4
  axialis extracorticalis (congenita) E75.29
  bone marrow (myeloid) D61.9
    congenital D61.01
  brain Q00.0
    part of Q04.3
  bronchus Q32.4
  cementum K00.4
  cerebellum Q04.3
  cervix (congenital) Q51.5
  congenital pure red cell D61.01
  corpus callosum Q04.0
  cutis congenita Q84.8
  erythrocyte congenital D61.01
  extracortical axial E75.29
  eye Q11.1
  fovea centralis (congenital) Q14.1
  gallbladder, congenital Q44.0
  iris Q13.1
  labyrinth, membranous Q16.5
  limb (congenital) Q73.8
    lower —see Defect, reduction, lower
      limb
    upper —see Agenesis, arm
  lung, congenital (bilateral) (unilateral)
    Q33.3
  pancreas Q45.0
  parathyroid-thymic D82.1
  Pelizaeus-Merzbacher E75.29
  penis Q55.5
  prostate Q55.4

Aplasia (Continued)
  red cell (with thymoma) D60.9
    acquired D60.9
      due to drugs D60.9
    adult D60.9
    chronic D60.0
    congenital D61.01
    constitutional D61.01
    due to drugs D60.9
    hereditary D61.01
    of infants D61.01
    primary D61.01
    pure D61.01
      due to drugs D60.9
    specified type NEC D60.8
    transient D60.1
  round ligament Q52.8
  skin Q84.8
  spermatic cord Q55.4
  spleen Q89.01
  testicle Q55.0
  thymic, with immunodeficiency D82.1
  thyroid (congenital) (with myxedema)
    E03.1
  uterus Q51.0
  ventral horn cell Q06.1
Apnea, apneic (of) (spells) R06.81
  newborn NEC P28.4
    obstructive P28.4
    sleep (central) (obstructive) (primary)
      P28.3
  prematurity P28.4
  sleep G47.30
    central (primary) G47.31
      in conditions classified elsewhere
        G47.37
    obstructive (adult) (pediatric) G47.33
    primary central G47.31
    specified NEC G47.39
Apneumatosis, newborn P28.0
Apocrine metaplasia (breast) —see Dysplasia,
    mammary, specified type NEC
Apophysitis (bone) —see also
    Osteochondropathy
  calcaneus M92.8
  juvenile M92.9
Apoplectiform convulsions (cerebral ischemia)
    I67.82
Apoplexia, apoplexy, apoplectic
  adrenal A39.1
  heart (auricle) (ventricle) —see Infarct,
    myocardium
  heat T67.0
  hemorrhagic (stroke) —see Hemorrhage,
    intracranial
  meninges, hemorrhagic —see Hemorrhage,
    intracranial, subarachnoid
  uremic N18.9 [I68.8]
Appearance
  bizarre R46.1
  specified NEC R46.89
  very low level of personal hygiene R46.0
Appendage
  epididymal (organ of Morgagni) Q55.4
  intestine (epiploic) Q43.8
  preauricular Q17.0
  testicular (organ of Morgagni) Q55.29
Appendicitis (pneumococcal) (retrocecal) K37
  with
    perforation or rupture K35.2
    peritoneal abscess K35.3
    peritonitis NEC K35.3
      generalized (with perforation or
        rupture) K35.2
      localized (with perforation or rupture)
        K35.3
  acute (catarrhal) (fulminating) (gangrenous)
    (obstructive) (retrocecal) (suppurative)
    K35.80
    with
      peritoneal abscess K35.3

Appendicitis *(Continued)*
  acute *(Continued)*
    with *(Continued)*
      peritonitis NEC K35.3
        generalized (with perforation or rupture) K35.2
        localized (with perforation or rupture) K35.3
      specified NEC K35.89
  amebic A06.89
  chronic (recurrent) K36
  exacerbation —*see* Appendicitis, acute
  gangrenous —*see* Appendicitis, acute
  healed (obliterative) K36
  interval K36
  neurogenic K36
  obstructive K36
  recurrent K36
  relapsing K36
  subacute (adhesive) K36
  subsiding K36
  suppurative —*see* Appendicitis, acute
  tuberculous A18.32
Appendicopathia oxyurica B80
Appendix, appendicular —*see also* condition
  epididymis Q55.4
  Morgagni
    female Q50.5
    male (epididymal) Q55.4
      testicular Q55.29
  testis Q55.29
Appetite
  depraved —*see* Pica
  excessive R63.2
  lack or loss (*see also* Anorexia) R63.0
    nonorganic origin F50.8
    psychogenic F50.8
  perverted (hysterical) —*see* Pica
Apple peel syndrome Q41.1
Apprehension state F41.1
Apprehensiveness, abnormal F41.9
Approximal wear K03.0
Apraxia (classic) (ideational) (ideokinetic) (ideomotor) (motor) (verbal) R48.2
  following
    cerebrovascular disease I69.990
      cerebral infarction I69.390
      intracerebral hemorrhage I69.190
      nontraumatic intracranial hemorrhage NEC I69.290
      specified disease NEC I69.890
      subarachnoid hemorrhage I69.090
  oculomotor, congenital H51.8
Aptyalism K11.7
Apudoma —*see* Neoplasm, uncertain behavior, by site
Aqueous misdirection H40.83-
Arabicum elephantiasis —*see* Infestation, filarial
Arachnitis —*see* Meningitis
Arachnodactyly —*see* Syndrome, Marfan's
Arachnoiditis (acute) (adhesive) (basal) (brain) (cerebrospinal) —*see* Meningitis
Arachnophobia F40.210
Arboencephalitis, Australian A83.4
Arborization block (heart) I45.5
ARC (AIDS-related complex) B20
Arches —*see* condition
Arcuate uterus Q51.810
Arcuatus uterus Q51.810
Arcus (cornea) senilis —*see* Degeneration, cornea, senile
Arc-welder's lung J63.4
Areflexia R29.2
Areola —*see* condition
Argentaffinoma —*see also* Neoplasm, uncertain behavior, by site
  malignant —*see* Neoplasm, malignant, by site
  syndrome E34.0
Argininemia E72.21

Arginosuccinic aciduria E72.22
Argyll Robertson phenomenon, pupil or syndrome (syphilitic) A52.19
  atypical H57.09
  nonsyphilitic H57.09
Argyria, argyriasis
  conjunctival H11.13-
  from drug or medicament —*see* Table of Drugs and Chemicals, by substance
Argyrosis, conjunctival H11.13-
Arhinencephaly Q04.1
Ariboflavinosis E53.0
Arm —*see* condition
Arnold-Chiari disease, obstruction or syndrome (type II) Q07.00
  with
    hydrocephalus Q07.02
      with spina bifida Q07.03
    spina bifida Q07.01
      with hydrocephalus Q07.03
  type III —*see* Encephalocele
  type IV Q04.8
Aromatic amino-acid metabolism disorder E70.9
  specified NEC E70.8
Arousals, confusional G47.51
Arrest, arrested
  cardiac I46.9
    complicating
      abortion —*see* Abortion, by type, complicated by, cardiac arrest
      anesthesia (general) (local) or other sedation —*see* Table of Drugs and Chemicals, by drug
      in labor and delivery O74.2
      in pregnancy O29.11-
        postpartum, puerperal O89.1
      delivery (cesarean) (instrumental) O75.4
    due to
      cardiac condition I46.2
      specified condition NEC I46.8
    intraoperative I97.71-
    newborn P29.81
    postprocedural I97.12-
      obstetric procedure O75.4
  cardiorespiratory —*see* Arrest, cardiac
  circulatory —*see* Arrest, cardiac
  deep transverse O64.0
  development or growth
    bone —*see* Disorder, bone, development or growth
    child R62.50
    tracheal rings Q32.1
  epiphyseal
    complete
      femur M89.15-
      humerus M89.12-
      tibia M89.16-
      ulna M89.13-
      forearm M89.13-
        specified NEC M89.13-
        ulna —*see* Arrest, epiphyseal, by type, ulna
      lower leg M89.16-
        specified NEC M89.168
        tibia —*see* Arrest, epiphyseal, by type, tibia
    partial
      femur M89.15-
      humerus M89.12-
      tibia M89.16-
      ulna M89.13-
      specified NEC M89.18
  granulopoiesis —*see* Agranulocytosis
  growth plate —*see* Arrest, epiphyseal
  heart —*see* Arrest, cardiac
  legal, anxiety concerning Z65.3
  physeal —*see* Arrest, epiphyseal
  respiratory R09.2
    newborn P28.81
  sinus I45.5

Arrest, arrested *(Continued)*
  spermatogenesis (complete) —*see* Azoospermia
    incomplete —*see* Oligospermia
  transverse (deep) O64.0
Arrhenoblastoma
  benign
    specified site —*see* Neoplasm, benign, by site
    unspecified site
      female D27.9
      male D29.20
  malignant
    specified site —*see* Neoplasm, malignant, by site
    unspecified site
      female C56.9
      male C62.90
  specified site —*see* Neoplasm, uncertain behavior, by site
  unspecified site
    female D39.10
    male D40.10
Arrhythmia (auricle)(cardiac) (juvenile) (nodal) (reflex)(sinus)(supraventricular) (transitory)(ventricle) I49.9
  block I45.9
  extrasystolic I49.49
  newborn
    bradycardia P29.12
    occurring before birth P03.819
      before onset of labor P03.810
      during labor P03.811
    tachycardia P29.11
  psychogenic F45.8
  specified NEC I49.8
  vagal R55
  ventricular re-entry I47.0
Arrillaga-Ayerza syndrome (pulmonary sclerosis with pulmonary hypertension) I27.0
Arsenical pigmentation L81.8
  from drug or medicament —*see* Table of Drugs and Chemicals
Arsenism —*see* Poisoning, arsenic
Arterial —*see* condition
Arteriofibrosis —*see* Arteriosclerosis
Arteriolar sclerosis —*see* Arteriosclerosis
Arteriolith —*see* Arteriosclerosis
Arteriolitis I77.6
  necrotizing, kidney I77.5
  renal —*see* Hypertension, kidney
Arteriolosclerosis —*see* Arteriosclerosis
Arterionephrosclerosis —*see* Hypertension, kidney
Arteriopathy I77.9
Arteriosclerosis, arteriosclerotic (diffuse) (obliterans) (of) (senile) (with calcification) I70.90
  aorta I70.0
  arteries of extremities —*see* Arteriosclerosis, extremities
  brain I67.2
  bypass graft
    coronary —*see* Arteriosclerosis, coronary, bypass graft
    extremities —*see* Arteriosclerosis, extremities, bypass graft
  cardiac —*see* Disease, heart, ischemic, atherosclerotic
  cardiopathy —*see* Disease, heart, ischemic, atherosclerotic
  cardiorenal —*see* Hypertension, cardiorenal
  cardiovascular —*see* Disease, heart, ischemic, atherosclerotic
  carotid (*see also* Occlusion, artery, carotid) I65.2-
  central nervous system I67.2
  cerebral I67.2
  cerebrovascular I67.2

◀ New   ◀ Revised   ~~deleted~~ Deleted

Arteriosclerosis, arteriosclerotic *(Continued)*
  coronary (artery) I25.10
    bypass graft I25.810
      with
        angina pectoris I25.709
          with documented spasm I25.701
          specified type NEC I25.708
          unstable I25.700
        ischemic chest pain I25.709
      autologous artery I25.810
        with
          angina pectoris I25.729
            with documented spasm I25.721
            specified type I25.728
            unstable I25.720
          ischemic chest pain I25.729
      autologous vein I25.810
        with
          angina pectoris I25.719
            with documented spasm I25.711
            specified type I25.718
            unstable I25.710
          ischemic chest pain I25.719
      nonautologous biological I25.810
        with
          angina pectoris I25.739
            with documented spasm I25.731
            specified type I25.738
            unstable I25.730
          ischemic chest pain I25.739
      specified type NEC I25.810
        with
          angina pectoris I25.799
            with documented spasm I25.791
            specified type I25.798
            unstable I25.790
          ischemic chest pain I25.799
    due to
      calcified coronary lesion (severely) I25.84
      lipid rich plaque I25.83
    native vessel
      with
        angina pectoris I25.119
          with documented spasm I25.111
          specified type NEC I25.118
          unstable I25.110
        ischemic chest pain I25.119
    transplanted heart I25.811
      bypass graft I25.812
        with
          angina pectoris I25.769
            with documented spasm I25.761
            specified type I25.768
            unstable I25.760
          ischemic chest pain I25.769
      native coronary artery I25.811
        with
          angina pectoris I25.759
            with documented spasm I25.751
            specified type I25.758
            unstable I25.750
          ischemic chest pain I25.759
  extremities (native arteries) I70.209
    bypass graft I70.309
      autologous vein graft I70.409
        leg I70.409
          with
            gangrene (and intermittent claudication, rest pain and ulcer) I70.469
            intermittent claudication I70.419
            rest pain (and intermittent claudication) I70.429

Arteriosclerosis, arteriosclerotic *(Continued)*
  extremities *(Continued)*
    bypass graft *(Continued)*
      autologous vein graft *(Continued)*
        leg *(Continued)*
          bilateral I70.403
            with
              gangrene (and intermittent claudication, rest pain and ulcer) I70.463
              intermittent claudication I70.413
              rest pain (and intermittent claudication) I70.423
              specified type NEC I70.493
          left I70.402
            with
              gangrene (and intermittent claudication, rest pain and ulcer) I70.462
              intermittent claudication I70.412
              rest pain (and intermittent claudication) I70.422
              ulceration (and intermittent claudication and rest pain) I70.449
                ankle I70.443
                calf I70.442
                foot site NEC I70.445
                heel I70.444
                lower leg NEC I70.448
                midfoot I70.444
                thigh I70.441
              specified type NEC I70.492
          right I70.401
            with
              gangrene (and intermittent claudication, rest pain and ulcer) I70.461
              intermittent claudication I70.411
              rest pain (and intermittent claudication) I70.421
              ulceration (and intermittent claudication and rest pain) I70.439
                ankle I70.433
                calf I70.432
                foot site NEC I70.435
                heel I70.434
                lower leg NEC I70.438
                midfoot I70.434
                thigh I70.431
              specified type NEC I70.491
          specified type NEC I70.499
        specified NEC I70.408
          with
            gangrene (and intermittent claudication, rest pain and ulcer) I70.468
            intermittent claudication I70.418
            rest pain (and intermittent claudication) I70.428
            ulceration (and intermittent claudication and rest pain) I70.45
            specified type NEC I70.498
      leg I70.309
        with
          gangrene (and intermittent claudication, rest pain and ulcer) I70.369
          intermittent claudication I70.319
          rest pain (and intermittent claudication) I70.329
        bilateral I70.303
          with
            gangrene (and intermittent claudication, rest pain and ulcer) I70.363

Arteriosclerosis, arteriosclerotic *(Continued)*
  extremities *(Continued)*
    bypass graft *(Continued)*
      leg *(Continued)*
        bilateral *(Continued)*
          with *(Continued)*
            intermittent claudication I70.313
            rest pain (and intermittent claudication) I70.323
            specified type NEC I70.393
        left I70.302
          with
            gangrene (and intermittent claudication, rest pain and ulcer) I70.362
            intermittent claudication I70.312
            rest pain (and intermittent claudication) I70.322
            ulceration (and intermittent claudication and rest pain) I70.349
              ankle I70.343
              calf I70.342
              foot site NEC I70.345
              heel I70.344
              lower leg NEC I70.348
              midfoot I70.344
              thigh I70.341
            specified type NEC I70.392
        right I70.301
          with
            gangrene (and intermittent claudication, rest pain and ulcer) I70.361
            intermittent claudication I70.311
            rest pain (and intermittent claudication) I70.321
            ulceration (and intermittent claudication and rest pain) I70.339
              ankle I70.333
              calf I70.332
              foot site NEC I70.335
              heel I70.334
              lower leg NEC I70.338
              midfoot I70.334
              thigh I70.331
            specified type NEC I70.391
        specified type NEC I70.399
      nonautologous biological graft I70.509
        leg I70.509
          with
            gangrene (and intermittent claudication, rest pain and ulcer) I70.569
            intermittent claudication I70.519
            rest pain (and intermittent claudication) I70.529
          bilateral I70.503
            with
              gangrene (and intermittent claudication, rest pain and ulcer) I70.563
              intermittent claudication I70.513
              rest pain (and intermittent claudication) I70.523
              specified type NEC I70.593
          left I70.502
            with
              gangrene (and intermittent claudication, rest pain and ulcer) I70.562
              intermittent claudication I70.512
              rest pain (and intermittent claudication) I70.522

Arteriosclerosis, arteriosclerotic *(Continued)*
  extremities *(Continued)*
    bypass graft *(Continued)*
      nonautologous biological graft
        (Continued)
        leg *(Continued)*
          left *(Continued)*
            with *(Continued)*
              ulceration (and intermittent
                claudication and rest
                pain) I70.549
              ankle I70.543
              calf I70.542
              foot site NEC I70.545
              heel I70.544
              lower leg NEC I70.548
              midfoot I70.544
              thigh I70.541
            specified type NEC I70.592
          right I70.501
            with
              gangrene (and intermittent
                claudication, rest pain
                and ulcer) I70.561
              intermittent claudication
                I70.511
              rest pain (and intermittent
                claudication) I70.521
              ulceration (and intermittent
                claudication and rest
                pain) I70.539
              ankle I70.533
              calf I70.532
              foot site NEC I70.535
               heel I70.534
              lower leg NEC I70.538
               midfoot I70.534
              thigh I70.531
            specified type NEC I70.591
          specified type NEC I70.599
        specified NEC I70.508
          with
            gangrene (and intermittent
              claudication, rest pain and
              ulcer) I70.568
            intermittent claudication I70.518
            rest pain (and intermittent
              claudication) I70.528
            ulceration (and intermittent
              claudication and rest pain)
              I70.55
            specified type NEC I70.598
      nonbiological graft I70.609
        leg I70.609
          with
            gangrene (and intermittent
              claudication, rest pain and
              ulcer) I70.669
            intermittent claudication
              I70.619
            rest pain (and intermittent
              claudication) I70.629
          bilateral I70.603
            with
              gangrene (and intermittent
                claudication, rest pain
                and ulcer) I70.663
              intermittent claudication
                I70.613
              rest pain (and intermittent
                claudication) I70.623
            specified type NEC I70.693
          left I70.602
            with
              gangrene (and intermittent
                claudication, rest pain
                and ulcer) I70.662
              intermittent claudication
                I70.612
              rest pain (and intermittent
                claudication) I70.622

Arteriosclerosis, arteriosclerotic *(Continued)*
  extremities *(Continued)*
    bypass graft *(Continued)*
      nonbiological graft *(Continued)*
        leg *(Continued)*
          left *(Continued)*
            with *(Continued)*
              ulceration (and intermittent
                claudication and rest
                pain) I70.649
              ankle I70.643
              calf I70.642
              foot site NEC I70.645
              heel I70.644
              lower leg NEC I70.648
              midfoot I70.644
              thigh I70.641
            specified type NEC I70.692
          right I70.601
            with
              gangrene (and intermittent
                claudication, rest pain
                and ulcer) I70.661
              intermittent claudication
                I70.611
              rest pain (and intermittent
                claudication) I70.621
              ulceration (and intermittent
                claudication and rest
                pain) I70.639
              ankle I70.633
              calf I70.632
              foot site NEC I70.635
              heel I70.634
              lower leg NEC I70.638
              midfoot I70.634
              thigh I70.631
            specified type NEC I70.691
          specified type NEC I70.699
        specified NEC I70.608
          with
            gangrene (and intermittent
              claudication, rest pain and
              ulcer) I70.668
            intermittent claudication
              I70.618
            rest pain (and intermittent
              claudication) I70.628
            ulceration (and intermittent
              claudication and rest pain)
              I70.65
            specified type NEC I70.698
      specified graft NEC I70.709
        leg I70.709
          with
            gangrene (and intermittent
              claudication, rest pain and
              ulcer) I70.769
            intermittent claudication
              I70.719
            rest pain (and intermittent
              claudication) I70.729
          bilateral I70.703
            with
              gangrene (and intermittent
                claudication, rest pain
                and ulcer) I70.763
              intermittent claudication
                I70.713
              rest pain (and intermittent
                claudication) I70.723
            specified type NEC I70.793
          left I70.702
            with
              gangrene (and intermittent
                claudication, rest pain
                and ulcer) I70.762
              intermittent claudication
                I70.712
              rest pain (and intermittent
                claudication) I70.722

Arteriosclerosis, arteriosclerotic *(Continued)*
  extremities *(Continued)*
    bypass graft *(Continued)*
      specified graft NEC *(Continued)*
        leg *(Continued)*
          left *(Continued)*
            with *(Continued)*
              ulceration (and intermittent
                claudication and rest
                pain) I70.749
              ankle I70.743
              calf I70.742
              foot site NEC I70.745
              heel I70.744
              lower leg NEC I70.748
              midfoot I70.744
              thigh I70.741
            specified type NEC I70.792
          right I70.701
            with
              gangrene (and intermittent
                claudication, rest pain
                and ulcer) I70.761
              intermittent claudication
                I70.711
              rest pain (and intermittent
                claudication) I70.721
              ulceration (and intermittent
                claudication and rest
                pain) I70.739
              ankle I70.733
              calf I70.732
              foot site NEC I70.735
              heel I70.734
              lower leg NEC I70.738
              midfoot I70.734
              thigh I70.731
            specified type NEC I70.791
          specified type NEC I70.799
        specified NEC I70.708
          with
            gangrene (and intermittent
              claudication, rest pain and
              ulcer) I70.768
            intermittent claudication
              I70.718
            rest pain (and intermittent
              claudication) I70.728
            ulceration (and intermittent
              claudication and rest pain)
              I70.75
            specified type NEC I70.798
        specified NEC I70.308
          with
            gangrene (and intermittent
              claudication, rest pain and
              ulcer) I70.368
            intermittent claudication I70.318
            rest pain (and intermittent
              claudication) I70.328
            ulceration (and intermittent
              claudication and rest pain)
              I70.35
            specified type NEC I70.398
        leg I70.209
          with
            gangrene (and intermittent
              claudication, rest pain and ulcer)
              I70.269
            intermittent claudication I70.219
            rest pain (and intermittent
              claudication) I70.229
          bilateral I70.203
            with
              gangrene (and intermittent
                claudication, rest pain and
                ulcer) I70.263
              intermittent claudication I70.213
              rest pain (and intermittent
                claudication) I70.223
            specified type NEC I70.293

◀ New   ⬅ Revised   ~~deleted~~ Deleted

Arteriosclerosis, arteriosclerotic *(Continued)*
  extremities *(Continued)*
    leg *(Continued)*
      left I70.202
        with
          gangrene (and intermittent
            claudication, rest pain and
            ulcer) I70.262
          intermittent claudication I70.212
          rest pain (and intermittent
            claudication) I70.222
          ulceration (and intermittent
            claudication and rest pain)
            I70.249
            ankle I70.243
            calf I70.242
            foot site NEC I70.245
            heel I70.244
            lower leg NEC I70.248
            midfoot I70.244
            thigh I70.241
        specified type NEC I70.292
      right I70.201
        with
          gangrene (and intermittent
            claudication, rest pain and
            ulcer) I70.261
          intermittent claudication I70.211
          rest pain (and intermittent
            claudication) I70.221
          ulceration (and intermittent
            claudication and rest pain)
            I70.239
            ankle I70.233
            calf I70.232
            foot site NEC I70.235
            heel I70.234
            lower leg NEC I70.238
            midfoot I70.234
            thigh I70.231
        specified type NEC I70.291
      specified type NEC I70.299
    specified site NEC I70.208
      with
        gangrene (and intermittent
          claudication, rest pain and ulcer)
          I70.268
        intermittent claudication I70.218
        rest pain (and intermittent
          claudication) I70.228
        ulceration (and intermittent
          claudication and rest pain)
          I70.25
      specified type NEC I70.298
  generalized I70.91
  heart (disease) —*see* Arteriosclerosis,
    coronary (artery)
  kidney —*see* Hypertension, kidney
  medial —*see* Arteriosclerosis, extremities
  mesenteric (artery) K55.1
  Mönckeberg's —*see* Arteriosclerosis,
    extremities
  myocarditis I51.4
  peripheral (of extremities) —*see*
    Arteriosclerosis, extremities
  pulmonary (idiopathic) I27.0
  renal (arterioles) —*see also* Hypertension,
    kidney
    artery I70.1
  retina (vascular) I70.8 *[H35.0-]*
  specified artery NEC I70.8
  spinal (cord) G95.19
  vertebral (artery) I67.2
Arteriospasm I73.9
Arteriovenous —*see* condition
Arteritis I77.6
  allergic M31.0
  aorta (nonsyphilitic) I77.6
    syphilitic A52.02
  aortic arch M31.4
  brachiocephalic M31.4

Arteritis *(Continued)*
  brain I67.7
    syphilitic A52.04
  cerebral I67.7
    in
      diseases classified elsewhere I68.2
      systemic lupus erythematosus M32.19
    listerial A32.89
    syphilitic A52.04
    tuberculous A18.89
  coronary (artery) I25.89
    rheumatic I01.8
      chronic I09.89
    syphilitic A52.06
  cranial (left) (right), giant cell M31.6
  deformans —*see* Arteriosclerosis
  giant cell NEC M31.6
    with polymyalgia rheumatica M31.5
  necrosing or necrotizing M31.9
    specified NEC M31.8
  nodosa M30.0
  obliterans —*see* Arteriosclerosis
  pulmonary I28.8
  rheumatic —*see* Fever, rheumatic
  senile —*see* Arteriosclerosis
  suppurative I77.2
  syphilitic (general) A52.09
    brain A52.04
    coronary A52.06
    spinal A52.09
  temporal, giant cell M31.6
  young female aortic arch syndrome M31.4
Artery, arterial —*see also* condition
  abscess I77.89
  single umbilical Q27.0
Arthralgia (allergic) —*see also* Pain, joint
  in caisson disease T70.3
  temporomandibular M26.62
Arthritis, arthritic (acute) (chronic)
    (nonpyogenic) (subacute) M19.90
  allergic —*see* Arthritis, specified form NEC
  ankylosing (crippling) (spine) —*see also*
    Spondylitis, ankylosing
    sites other than spine —*see* Arthritis,
      specified form NEC
  atrophic —*see* Osteoarthritis
    spine —*see* Spondylitis, ankylosing
  back —*see* Spondylopathy, inflammatory
  blennorrhagic (gonococcal) A54.42
  Charcot's —*see* Arthropathy, neuropathic
    diabetic —*see* Diabetes, arthropathy,
      neuropathic
    syringomyelic G95.0
  chylous (filarial) (*see also* category M01) B74.9
  climacteric (any site) NEC —*see* Arthritis,
    specified form NEC
  crystal (-induced) —*see* Arthritis, in, crystals
  deformans —*see* Osteoarthritis
  degenerative —*see* Osteoarthritis
  due to or associated with
    acromegaly E22.0
    brucellosis —*see* Brucellosis
    caisson disease T70.3
    diabetes —*see* Diabetes, arthropathy
    dracontiasis (*see also* category M01) B72
    enteritis NEC
      regional —*see* Enteritis, regional
    erysipelas (*see also* category M01) A46
    erythema
      epidemic A25.1
      nodosum L52
    filariasis NOS B74.9
    glanders A24.0
    helminthiasis (*see also* category M01) B83.9
    hemophilia D66 *[M36.2]*
    Henoch-(Schönlein) purpura D69.0 *[M36.4]*
    human parvovirus (*see also* category M01)
      B97.6
    infectious disease NEC —*see* category M01
    leprosy (*see also* category M01) (*see also*
      Leprosy) A30.9

Arthritis, arthritic *(Continued)*
  due to or associated with *(Continued)*
    Lyme disease A69.23
    mycobacteria (*see also* category M01)
      A31.8
    parasitic disease NEC (*see also* category
      M01) B89
    paratyphoid fever (*see also* category M01)
      (*see also* Fever, paratyphoid) A01.4
    rat bite fever (*see also* category M01)
      A25.1
    regional enteritis —*see* Enteritis, regional
    respiratory disorder NOS J98.9
    serum sickness (*see also* Reaction, serum)
      T80.69
    syringomyelia G95.0
    typhoid fever A01.04
  epidemic erythema A25.1
  febrile —*see* Fever, rheumatic
  gonococcal A54.42
  gouty (acute) —*see* Gout, idiopathic
  in (due to)
    acromegaly (*see also* subcategory M14.8-)
      E22.0
    amyloidosis (*see also* subcategory M14.8-)
      E85.4
    bacterial disease (*see also* subcategory M01)
      A49.9
    Behçet's syndrome M35.2
    caisson disease (*see also* subcategory
      M14.8-) T70.3
    coliform bacilli (Escherichia coli) —*see*
      Arthritis, in, pyogenic organism NEC
    crystals M11.9
      dicalcium phosphate —*see* Arthritis, in,
        crystals, specified type NEC
      hydroxyapatite M11.0-
      pyrophosphate —*see* Arthritis, in,
        crystals, specified type NEC
      specified type NEC M11.80
        ankle M11.87-
        elbow M11.82-
        foot joint M11.87-
        hand joint M11.84-
        hip M11.85-
        knee M11.86-
        multiple sites M11.8-
        shoulder M11.81-
        vertebrae M11.88
        wrist M11.83-
    dermatoarthritis, lipoid E78.81
    dracontiasis (dracunculiasis) (*see also*
      category M01) B72
    endocrine disorder NEC (*see also*
      subcategory M14.8-) E34.9
    enteritis, infectious NEC (*see also* category
      M01) A09
      specified organism NEC (*see also*
        category M01) A08.8
    erythema
      multiforme (*see also* subcategory M14.8-)
        L51.9
      nodosum (*see also* subcategory M14.8-)
        L52
    gout —*see* Gout, idiopathic
    helminthiasis NEC (*see also* category M01)
      B83.9
    hemochromatosis (*see also* subcategory
      M14.8-) E83.118
    hemoglobinopathy NEC D58.2 *[M36.3]*
    hemophilia NEC D66 *[M36.2]*
    Hemophilus influenzae M00.8- *[B96.3]*
    Henoch(-Schönlein) purpura D69.0 *[M36.4]*
    hyperparathyroidism NEC (*see also*
      subcategory M14.8-) E21.3
    hypersensitivity reaction NEC T78.49
      [M36.4]
    hypogammaglobulinemia (*see also*
      subcategory M14.8-) D80.1
    hypothyroidism NEC (*see also* subcategory
      M14.8-) E03.9

Arthritis, arthritic *(Continued)*
  in *(Continued)*
    infection —*see* Arthritis, pyogenic or
        pyemic
      spine —*see* Spondylopathy, infective
    infectious disease NEC —*see* category
        M01
    leprosy *(see also* category M01) A30.9
    leukemia NEC C95.9- *[M36.1]*
    lipoid dermatoarthritis E78.81
    Lyme disease A69.23
    Mediterranean fever, familial *(see also*
        subcategory M14.8-) E85.0
    Meningococcus A39.83
    metabolic disorder NEC *(see also*
        subcategory M14.8-) E88.9
    multiple myelomatosis C90.0- *[M36.1]*
    mumps B26.85
    mycosis NEC *(see also* category M01)
        B49
    myelomatosis (multiple) C90.0- *[M36.1]*
    neurological disorder NEC G98.0
    ochronosis *(see also* subcategory M14.8-)
        E70.29
    O'nyong-nyong *(see also* category M01)
        A92.1
    parasitic disease NEC *(see also* category
        M01) B89
    paratyphoid fever *(see also* category M01)
        A01.4
    Pseudomonas —*see* Arthritis, pyogenic,
        bacterial NEC
    psoriasis L40.50
    pyogenic organism NEC —*see* Arthritis,
        pyogenic, bacterial NEC
    Reiter's disease —*see* Reiter's disease
    respiratory disorder NEC *(see also*
        subcategory M14.8-) J98.9
    reticulosis, malignant *(see also* subcategory
        M14.8-) C86.0
    rubella B06.82
    Salmonella (arizonae) (cholerae-suis)
        (enteritidis) (typhimurium)
        A02.23
    sarcoidosis D86.86
    specified bacteria NEC —*see* Arthritis,
        pyogenic, bacterial NEC
    sporotrichosis B42.82
    syringomyelia G95.0
    thalassemia NEC D56.9 *[M36.3]*
    tuberculosis —*see* Tuberculosis, arthritis
    typhoid fever A01.04
    urethritis, Reiter's —*see* Reiter's disease
    viral disease NEC *(see also* category M01)
        B34.9
  infectious or infective —*see also* Arthritis,
      pyogenic or pyemic
    spine —*see* Spondylopathy, infective
  juvenile M08.90
    with systemic onset —*see* Still's disease
    ankle M08.97-
    elbow M08.92-
    foot joint M08.97-
    hand joint M08.94-
    hip M08.95-
    knee M08.96-
    multiple site M08.99
    pauciarticular M08.40
      ankle M08.47-
      elbow M08.42-
      foot joint M08.47-
      hand joint M08.44-
      hip M08.45-
      knee M08.46-
      shoulder M08.41-
      vertebrae M08.48
      wrist M08.43-
    psoriatic L40.54
    rheumatoid —*see* Arthritis, rheumatoid,
        juvenile
    shoulder M08.91-

Arthritis, arthritic *(Continued)*
  juvenile *(Continued)*
    specified type NEC M08.80
      ankle M08.87-
      elbow M08.82-
      foot joint M08.87-
      hand joint M08.84-
      hip M08.85-
      knee M08.86-
      multiple site M08.89
      shoulder M08.81-
      specified joint NEC M08.88
      vertebrae M08.88
      wrist M08.83-
    vertebra M08.98
    wrist M08.93-
  meaning osteoarthritis —*see* Osteoarthritis
  meningococcal A39.83
  menopausal (any site) NEC —*see* Arthritis,
      specified form NEC
  mutilans (psoriatic) L40.52
  mycotic NEC *(see also* category M01) B49
  neuropathic (Charcot) —*see* Arthropathy,
      neuropathic
    diabetic —*see* Diabetes, arthropathy,
        neuropathic
    nonsyphilitic NEC G98.0
    syringomyelic G95.0
  ochronotic *(see also* subcategory M14.8-) E70.29
  palindromic (any site) —*see* Rheumatism,
      palindromic
  pneumococcal M00.10
    ankle M00.17-
    elbow M00.12-
    foot joint —*see* Arthritis, pneumococcal,
        ankle
    hand joint M00.14-
    hip M00.15-
    knee M00.16-
    multiple site M00.19
    shoulder M00.11-
    vertebra M00.18
    wrist M00.13-
  postdysenteric —*see* Arthropathy,
      postdysenteric
  postmeningococcal A39.84
  postrheumatic, chronic —*see* Arthropathy,
      postrheumatic, chronic
  primary progressive —*see also* Arthritis,
      specified form NEC
    spine —*see* Spondylitis, ankylosing
  psoriatic L40.50
  purulent (any site except spine) —*see*
      Arthritis, pyogenic or pyemic
    spine —*see* Spondylopathy, infective
  pyogenic or pyemic (any site except spine)
      M00.9
    bacterial NEC M00.80
      ankle M00.87-
      elbow M00.82-
      foot joint —*see* Arthritis, pyogenic,
          bacterial NEC, ankle
      hand joint M00.84-
      hip M00.85-
      knee M00.86-
      multiple site M00.89
      shoulder M00.81-
      vertebra M00.88
      wrist M00.83-
    pneumococcal —*see* Arthritis,
        pneumococcal
    spine —*see* Spondylopathy, infective
    staphylococcal —*see* Arthritis,
        staphylococcal
    streptococcal —*see* Arthritis, streptococcal
        NEC
      pneumococcal —*see* Arthritis,
          pneumococcal
  reactive —*see* Reiter's disease
  rheumatic —*see also* Arthritis, rheumatoid
    acute or subacute —*see* Fever, rheumatic

Arthritis, arthritic *(Continued)*
  rheumatoid M06.9
    with
      carditis —*see* Rheumatoid, carditis
      endocarditis —*see* Rheumatoid, carditis
      heart involvement NEC —*see*
          Rheumatoid, carditis
      lung involvement —*see* Rheumatoid,
          lung
      myocarditis —*see* Rheumatoid, carditis
      myopathy —*see* Rheumatoid, myopathy
      pericarditis —*see* Rheumatoid, carditis
      polyneuropathy —*see* Rheumatoid,
          polyneuropathy
      rheumatoid factor —*see* Arthritis,
          rheumatoid, seropositive
      splenoadenomegaly and leukopenia —
          see Felty's syndrome
      vasculitis —*see* Rheumatoid, vasculitis
      visceral involvement NEC —*see*
          Rheumatoid, arthritis, with
          involvement of organs NEC
    juvenile (with or without rheumatoid
        factor) M08.00
      ankle M08.07-
      elbow M08.02-
      foot joint M08.07-
      hand joint M08.04-
      hip M08.05-
      knee M08.06-
      multiple site M08.09
      shoulder M08.01-
      vertebra M08.08
      wrist M08.03-
    seronegative M06.00
      ankle M06.07-
      elbow M06.02-
      foot joint M06.07-
      hand joint M06.04-
      hip M06.05-
      knee M06.06-
      multiple sites M06.09
      shoulder M06.01-
      vertebra M06.08
      wrist M06.03-
    seropositive M05.9
      without organ involvement M05.70
        ankle M05.77-
        elbow M05.72-
        foot joint M05.77-
        hand joint M05.74-
        hip M05.75-
        knee M05.76-
        multiple sites M05.79
        shoulder M05.71-
        vertebra —*see* Spondylitis, ankylosing
        wrist M05.73-
      specified NEC M05.80
        ankle M05.87-
        elbow M05.82-
        foot joint M05.87-
        hand joint M05.84-
        hip M05.85-
        knee M05.86-
        multiple sites M05.89
        shoulder M05.81-
        vertebra —*see* Spondylitis, ankylosing
        wrist M05.83-
    specified type NEC M06.80
      ankle M06.87-
      elbow M06.82-
      foot joint M06.87-
      hand joint M06.84-
      hip M06.85-
      knee M06.86-
      multiple site M06.89
      shoulder M06.81-
      vertebra M06.88
      wrist M06.83-
    spine —*see* Spondylitis, ankylosing
  rubella B06.82

◀ New   ◀▦ Revised   ~~deleted~~ Deleted

Arthritis, arthritic *(Continued)*
scorbutic *(see also* subcategory M14.8-) E54
senile or senescent —*see* Osteoarthritis
septic (any site except spine) —*see* Arthritis,
    pyogenic or pyemic
  spine —*see* Spondylopathy, infective
serum (nontherapeutic) (therapeutic) —*see*
    Arthropathy, postimmunization
specified form NEC M13.80
  ankle M13.87-
  elbow M13.82-
  foot joint M13.87-
  hand joint M13.84-
  hip M13.85-
  knee M13.86-
  multiple site M13.89
  shoulder M13.81-
  specified joint NEC M13.88
  wrist M13.83-
spine —*see also* Spondylopathy,
    inflammatory
  infectious or infective NEC —*see*
      Spondylopathy, infective
  Marie-Strümpell —*see* Spondylitis,
      ankylosing
  pyogenic —*see* Spondylopathy, infective
  rheumatoid —*see* Spondylitis, ankylosing
  traumatic (old) —*see* Spondylopathy,
      traumatic
tuberculous A18.01
staphylococcal M00.00
  ankle M00.07-
  elbow M00.02-
  foot joint —*see* Arthritis, staphylococcal,
      ankle
  hand joint M00.04-
  hip M00.05-
  knee M00.06-
  multiple site M00.09
  shoulder M00.01-
  vertebra M00.08
  wrist M00.03-
streptococcal NEC M00.20
  ankle M00.27-
  elbow M00.22-
  foot joint —*see* Arthritis, streptococcal,
      ankle
  hand joint M00.24-
  hip M00.25-
  knee M00.26-
  multiple site M00.29
  shoulder M00.21-
  vertebra M00.28
  wrist M00.23-
suppurative —*see* Arthritis, pyogenic or
    pyemic
syphilitic (late) A52.16
  congenital A50.55 *[M12.80]*
syphilitica deformans (Charcot) A52.16
temporomandibular M26.69
toxic of menopause (any site) —*see* Arthritis,
    specified form NEC
transient —*see* Arthropathy, specified form
    NEC
traumatic (chronic) —*see* Arthropathy,
    traumatic
tuberculous A18.02
  spine A18.01
uratic —*see* Gout, idiopathic
urethritica (Reiter's) —*see* Reiter's disease
vertebral —*see* Spondylopathy, inflammatory
villous (any site) —*see* Arthropathy, specified
    form NEC
Arthrocele —*see* Effusion, joint
Arthrodesis status Z98.1
Arthrodynia —*see also* Pain, joint
Arthrodysplasia Q74.9
Arthrofibrosis, joint —*see* Ankylosis
Arthrogryposis (congenital) Q68.8
  multiplex congenita Q74.3
Arthrokatadysis M24.7

Arthropathy *(see also* Arthritis) M12.9
Charcot's —*see* Arthropathy, neuropathic
  diabetic —*see* Diabetes, arthropathy,
      neuropathic
  syringomyelic G95.0
cricoarytenoid J38.7
crystal(-induced) —*see* Arthritis, in, crystals
diabetic NEC —*see* Diabetes, arthropathy
distal interphalangeal, psoriatic L40.51
enteropathic M07.60
  ankle M07.67-
  elbow M07.62-
  foot joint M07.67-
  hand joint M07.64-
  hip M07.65-
  knee M07.66-
  multiple site M07.69
  shoulder M07.61-
  vertebra M07.68
  wrist M07.63-
following intestinal bypass M02.00
  ankle M02.07-
  elbow M02.02-
  foot joint M02.07-
  hand joint M02.04-
  hip M02.05-
  knee M02.06-
  multiple site M02.09
  shoulder M02.01-
  vertebra M02.08
  wrist M02.03-
gouty —*see also* Gout, idiopathic
  in (due to)
    Lesch-Nyhan syndrome E79.1 *[M14.8-]*
    sickle-cell disorders D57- *[M14.8-]*
hemophilic NEC D66 *[M36.2]*
  in (due to)
    hyperparathyroidism NEC E21.3
        [M14.8-]
    metabolic disease NOS E88.9 *[M14.8-]*
in (due to)
  acromegaly E22.0 *[M14.8-]*
  amyloidosis E85.4 *[M14.8-]*
  blood disorder NOS D75.9 *[M36.3]*
  diabetes —*see* Diabetes, arthropathy
  endocrine disease NOS E34.9 *[M14.8-]*
  erythema
    multiforme L51.9 *[M14.8-]*
    nodosum L52 *[M14.8-]*
  hemochromatosis E83.118 *[M14.8-]*
  hemoglobinopathy NEC D58.2 *[M36.3]*
  hemophilia NEC D66 *[M36.2]*
  Henoch-Schönlein purpura D69.0
      [M36.4]
  hyperthyroidism E05.90 *[M14.8-]*
  hypothyroidism E03.9 *[M14.8-]*
  infective endocarditis I33.0 *[M12.80]*
  leukemia NEC C95.9- *[M12.80]*
  malignant histiocytosis C96.A *[M36.1]*
  metabolic disease NOS E88.9 *[M14.8-]*
  multiple myeloma C90.0- *[M36.1]*
  neoplastic disease NOS *(see also* Neoplasm)
      D49.9 *[M36.1]*
  nutritional deficiency *(see also* subcategory
      M14.8-) E63.9
  psoriasis NOS L40.50
  sarcoidosis D86.86
  syphilis (late) A52.77
    congenital A50.55 *[M12.80]*
  thyrotoxicosis *(see also* subcategory M14.8-)
      E05.90
  ulcerative colitis K51.90 *[M07.60]*
  viral hepatitis (postinfectious) NEC B19.9
      [M12.80]
  Whipple's disease *(see also* subcategory
      M14.8-) K90.81
Jaccoud —*see* Arthropathy, postrheumatic,
    chronic
juvenile —*see* Arthritis, juvenile
  psoriatic L40.54
mutilans (psoriatic) L40.52

Arthropathy *(Continued)*
neuropathic (Charcot) M14.60
  ankle M14.67-
  diabetic —*see* Diabetes, arthropathy,
      neuropathic
  elbow M14.62-
  foot joint M14.67-
  hand joint M14.64-
  hip M14.65-
  knee M14.66-
  multiple site M14.69
  nonsyphilitic NEC G98.0
  shoulder M14.61-
  syringomyelic G95.0
  vertebra M14.68
  wrist M14.63-
osteopulmonary —*see* Osteoarthropathy,
    hypertrophic, specified NEC
postdysenteric M02.10
  ankle M02.17-
  elbow M02.12-
  foot joint M02.17-
  hand joint M02.14-
  hip M02.15-
  knee M02.16-
  multiple site M02.19
  shoulder M02.11-
  vertebra M02.18
  wrist M02.13-
postimmunization M02.20
  ankle M02.27-
  elbow M02.22-
  foot joint M02.27-
  hand joint M02.24-
  hip M02.25-
  knee M02.26-
  multiple site M02.29
  shoulder M02.21-
  vertebra M02.28
  wrist M02.23-
postinfectious NEC B99 *[M12.80]*
  in (due to)
    enteritis due to Yersinia enterocolitica
        A04.6 *[M12.80]*
    syphilis A52.77
    viral hepatitis NEC B19.9 *[M12.80]*
postrheumatic, chronic (Jaccoud) M12.00
  ankle M12.07-
  elbow M12.02-
  foot joint M12.07-
  hand joint M12.04-
  hip M12.05-
  knee M12.06-
  multiple site M12.09
  shoulder M12.01-
  specified joint NEC M12.08
  vertebrae M12.08
  wrist M12.03-
psoriatic NEC L40.59
  interphalangeal, distal L40.51
reactive M02.9
  in (due to)
    infective endocarditis I33.0 *[M02.9]*
  specified type NEC M02.80
    ankle M02.87-
    elbow M02.82-
    foot joint M02.87-
    hand joint M02.84-
    hip M02.85-
    knee M02.86-
    multiple site M02.89
    shoulder M02.81-
    vertebra M02.88
    wrist M02.83-
specified form NEC M12.80
  ankle M12.87-
  elbow M12.82-
  foot joint M12.87-
  hand joint M12.84-
  hip M12.85-
  knee M12.86-
  multiple site M12.89

Arthropathy *(Continued)*
  specified form NEC *(Continued)*
    shoulder M12.81-
    specified joint NEC M12.88
    vertebrae M12.88
    wrist M12.83-
  syringomyelic G95.0
  tabes dorsalis A52.16
  tabetic A52.16
  transient —*see* Arthropathy, specified form
      NEC
  traumatic M12.50
    ankle M12.57-
    elbow M12.52-
    foot joint M12.57-
    hand joint M12.54-
    hip M12.55-
    knee M12.56-
    multiple site M12.59
    shoulder M12.51-
    specified joint NEC M12.58
    vertebrae M12.58
    wrist M12.53-
Arthropyosis —*see* Arthritis, pyogenic or pyemic
Arthrosis (deformans) (degenerative) (localized)
    (*see also* Osteoarthritis) M19.90
  spine —*see* Spondylosis
Arthus' phenomenon or reaction T78.41
  due to
    drug —*see* Table of Drugs and Chemicals,
        by drug
Articular —*see* condition
Articulation, reverse (teeth) M26.24
Artificial
  insemination complication —*see*
      Complications, artificial, fertilization
  opening status (functioning) (without
      complication) Z93.9
    anus (colostomy) Z93.3
    colostomy Z93.3
    cystostomy Z93.50
      appendico-vesicostomy Z93.52
      cutaneous Z93.51
      specified NEC Z93.59
    enterostomy Z93.4
    gastrostomy Z93.1
    ileostomy Z93.2
    intestinal tract NEC Z93.4
    jejunostomy Z93.4
    nephrostomy Z93.6
    specified site NEC Z93.8
    tracheostomy Z93.0
    ureterostomy Z93.6
    urethrostomy Z93.6
    urinary tract NEC Z93.6
    vagina Z93.8
  vagina status Z93.8
Arytenoid —*see* condition
Asbestosis (occupational) J61
ASC-H (atypical squamous cells cannot exclude
    high grade squamous intraepithelial lesion
    on cytologic smear)
  anus R85.611
  cervix R87.611
  vagina R87.621
ASC-US (atypical squamous cells of
    undetermined significance on cytologic
    smear)
  anus R85.610
  cervix R87.610
  vagina R87.620
Ascariasis B77.9
  with
    complications NEC B77.89
    intestinal complications B77.0
    pneumonia, pneumonitis B77.81
Ascaridosis, ascaridiasis —*see* Ascariasis
Ascaris (infection) (infestation)
    (lumbricoides) —*see* Ascariasis
Ascending —*see* condition
Aschoff's bodies —*see* Myocarditis, rheumatic

Ascites (abdominal) R18.8
  cardiac I50.9
  chylous (nonfilarial) I89.8
    filarial —*see* Infestation, filarial
  due to
    cirrhosis, alcoholic K70.31
    hepatitis
      alcoholic K70.11
      chronic active K71.51
      S. japonicum B65.2
    heart I50.9
  malignant R18.0
  pseudochylous R18.8
  syphilitic A52.74
  tuberculous A18.31
Aseptic —*see* condition
Asherman's syndrome N85.6
Asialia K11.7
Asiatic cholera —*see* Cholera
Asimultagnosia (simultanagnosia) R48.3
Askin's tumor —*see* Neoplasm, connective
    tissue, malignant
Asocial personality F60.2
Asomatognosia R41.4
Aspartylglucosaminuria E77.1
Asperger's disease or syndrome F84.5
Aspergilloma —*see* Aspergillosis
Aspergillosis (with pneumonia) B44.9
  bronchopulmonary, allergic B44.81
  disseminated B44.7
  generalized B44.7
  pulmonary NEC B44.1
    allergic B44.81
    invasive B44.0
  specified NEC B44.89
  tonsillar B44.2
Aspergillus (flavus) (fumigatus) (infection)
    (terreus) —*see* Aspergillosis
Aspermatogenesis —*see* Azoospermia
Aspermia (testis) —*see* Azoospermia
Asphyxia, asphyxiation (by) R09.01
  antenatal P84
  birth P84
  bunny bag —*see* Asphyxia, due to,
      mechanical threat to breathing, trapped
      in bed clothes
  crushing S28.0
  drowning T75.1
  gas, fumes, or vapor —*see* Table of Drugs and
      Chemicals
  inhalation —*see* Inhalation
  intrauterine P84
  local I73.00
    with gangrene I73.01
  mucus —*see also* Foreign body, respiratory
      tract, causing asphyxia
  newborn P84
  pathological R09.01
  postnatal P84
    mechanical —*see* Asphyxia, due to,
        mechanical threat to breathing
  prenatal P84
  reticularis R23.1
  strangulation —*see* Asphyxia, due to,
      mechanical threat to breathing
  submersion T75.1
  traumatic T71.9
    due to
      crushed chest S28.0
      foreign body (in) —*see* Foreign body,
          respiratory tract, causing asphyxia
      low oxygen content of ambient air T71.20
        due to
          being trapped in
            low oxygen environment T71.29
              in car trunk T71.221
                circumstances undetermined
                    T71.224
                done with intent to harm by
                    another person T71.223
                self T71.222

Asphyxia, asphyxiation *(Continued)*
  traumatic *(Continued)*
    due to *(Continued)*
      low oxygen content of ambient air
          (Continued)
        due to *(Continued)*
          being trapped in *(Continued)*
            low oxygen environment
                (Continued)
              in refrigerator T71.231
                circumstances undetermined
                    T71.234
                done with intent to harm by
                    another person T71.233
                self T71.232
            cave-in T71.21
      mechanical threat to breathing
          (accidental) T71.191
        circumstances undetermined T71.194
        done with intent to harm by
            another person T71.193
        self T71.192
        hanging T71.161
          circumstances undetermined
              T71.164
          done with intent to harm by
              another person T71.163
          self T71.162
        plastic bag T71.121
          circumstances undetermined
              T71.124
          done with intent to harm by
              another person T71.123
          self T71.122
        smothering
          in furniture T71.151
            circumstances undetermined
                T71.154
            done with intent to harm by
                another person T71.153
            self T71.152
          under
            another person's body T71.141
              circumstances undetermined
                  T71.144
              done with intent to harm
                  T71.143
            pillow T71.111
              circumstances undetermined
                  T71.114
              done with intent to harm by
                  another person T71.113
              self T71.112
        trapped in bed clothes T71.131
          circumstances undetermined
              T71.134
          done with intent to harm by
              another person T71.133
          self T71.132
      vomiting, vomitus —*see* Foreign body,
          respiratory tract, causing asphyxia
Aspiration
  amniotic (clear) fluid (newborn) P24.10
    with
      pneumonia (pneumonitis) P24.11
      respiratory symptoms P24.11
  blood
    newborn (without respiratory symptoms)
        P24.20
      with
        pneumonia (pneumonitis) P24.21
        respiratory symptoms P24.21
    specified age NEC —*see* Foreign body,
        respiratory tract
  bronchitis J69.0
  food or foreign body (with asphyxiation) —
      see Asphyxia, food
  liquor (amnii) (newborn) P24.10
    with
      pneumonia (pneumonitis) P24.11
      respiratory symptoms P24.11

◀ New   ◀▦ Revised   ~~deleted~~ Deleted

Aspiration *(Continued)*
 meconium (newborn) (without respiratory
  symptoms) P24.00
  with
   pneumonitis (pneumonitis) P24.01
   respiratory symptoms P24.01
 milk (newborn) (without respiratory
  symptoms) P24.30
  with
   pneumonia (pneumonitis) P24.31
   respiratory symptoms P24.31
  specified age NEC —*see* Foreign body,
   respiratory tract
 mucus —*see also* Foreign body, by site,
  causing asphyxia
  newborn P24.10
   with
    pneumonia (pneumonitis) P24.11
    respiratory symptoms P24.11
 neonatal P24.9
  specific NEC (without respiratory
   symptoms) P24.80
   with
    pneumonia (pneumonitis) P24.81
    respiratory symptoms P24.81
 newborn P24.9
  specific NEC (without respiratory
   symptoms) P24.80
   with
    pneumonia (pneumonitis) P24.81
    respiratory symptoms P24.81
 pneumonia J69.0
 pneumonitis J69.0
 syndrome of newborn —*see* Aspiration, by
  substance, with pneumonia
 vernix caseosa (newborn) P24.80
  with
   pneumonia (pneumonitis) P24.81
   respiratory symptoms P24.81
 vomitus —*see also* Foreign body, respiratory
  tract
  newborn (without respiratory symptoms)
   P24.30
   with
    pneumonia (pneumonitis)
     P24.31
    respiratory symptoms P24.31
Asplenia (congenital) Q89.01
 postsurgical Z90.81
Assam fever B55.0
Assault, sexual —*see* Maltreatment
Assmann's focus NEC A15.0
Astasia (-abasia) (hysterical) F44.4
Asteatosis cutis L85.3
Astereognosia, astereognosis R48.1
Asterixis R27.8
 in liver disease K71.3
Asteroid hyalitis —*see* Deposit, crystalline
Asthenia, asthenic R53.1
 cardiac *(see also* Failure, heart) I50.9
  psychogenic F45.8
 cardiovascular *(see also* Failure, heart)
  I50.9
  psychogenic F45.8
 heart *(see also* Failure, heart) I50.9
  psychogenic F45.8
 hysterical F44.4
 myocardial *(see also* Failure, heart)
  I50.9
  psychogenic F45.8
 nervous F48.8
 neurocirculatory F45.8
 neurotic F48.8
 psychogenic F48.8
 psychoneurotic F48.8
 psychophysiologic F48.8
 reaction (psychophysiologic) F48.8
 senile R54
Asthenopia —*see also* Discomfort, visual
 hysterical F44.6
 psychogenic F44.6

Asthenospermia —*see* Abnormal, specimen,
 male genital organs
Asthma, asthmatic (bronchial) (catarrh)
 (spasmodic) J45.909
 with
  chronic obstructive bronchitis
   J44.9
   with
    acute lower respiratory infection
     J44.0
    exacerbation (acute) J44.1
  chronic obstructive pulmonary disease
   J44.9
   with
    acute lower respiratory infection
     J44.0
    exacerbation (acute) J44.1
  exacerbation (acute) J45.901
  hay fever —*see* Asthma, allergic extrinsic
  rhinitis, allergic —*see* Asthma, allergic
   extrinsic
  status asthmaticus J45.902
 allergic extrinsic J45.909
  with
   exacerbation (acute) J45.901
   status asthmaticus J45.902
 atopic —*see* Asthma, allergic extrinsic
 cardiac —*see* Failure, ventricular, left
 cardiobronchial I50.1
 childhood J45.909
  with
   exacerbation (acute) J45.901
   status asthmaticus J45.902
 chronic obstructive J44.9
  with
   acute lower respiratory infection
    J44.0
   exacerbation (acute) J44.1
 collier's J60
 cough variant J45.991
 detergent J69.8
 due to
  detergent J69.8
  inhalation of fumes J68.3
 eosinophilic J82
 extrinsic, allergic —*see* Asthma, allergic
  extrinsic
 grinder's J62.8
 hay —*see* Asthma, allergic extrinsic
 heart I50.1
 idiosyncratic —*see* Asthma, nonallergic
 intermittent (mild) J45.20
  with
   exacerbation (acute) J45.21
   status asthmaticus J45.22
 intrinsic, nonallergic —*see* Asthma,
  nonallergic
 Kopp's E32.8
 late-onset J45.909
  with
   exacerbation (acute) J45.901
   status asthmaticus J45.902
 mild intermittent J45.20
  with
   exacerbation (acute) J45.21
   status asthmaticus J45.22
 mild persistent J45.30
  with
   exacerbation (acute) J45.31
   status asthmaticus J45.32
 Millar's (laryngismus stridulus)
  J38.5
 miner's J60
 mixed J45.909
  with
   exacerbation (acute) J45.901
   status asthmaticus J45.902
 moderate persistent J45.40
  with
   exacerbation (acute) J45.41
   status asthmaticus J45.42

Asthma, asthmatic *(Continued)*
 nervous —*see* Asthma, nonallergic
 nonallergic (intrinsic) J45.909
  with
   exacerbation (acute) J45.901
   status asthmaticus J45.902
  persistent
   mild J45.30
    with
     exacerbation (acute) J45.31
     status asthmaticus J45.32
   moderate J45.40
    with
     exacerbation (acute) J45.41
     status asthmaticus J45.42
   severe J45.50
    with
     exacerbation (acute) J45.51
     status asthmaticus J45.52
 platinum J45.998
 pneumoconiotic NEC J64
 potter's J62.8
 predominantly allergic J45.909
 psychogenic F54
 pulmonary eosinophilic J82
 red cedar J67.8
 Rostan's I50.1
 sandblaster's J62.8
 sequoiosis J67.8
 severe persistent J45.50
  with
   exacerbation (acute) J45.51
   status asthmaticus J45.52
 specified NEC J45.998
 stonemason's J62.8
 thymic E32.8
 tuberculous —*see* Tuberculosis, pulmonary
 Wichmann's (laryngismus stridulus) J38.5
 wood J67.8
Astigmatism (compound) (congenital)
 H52.20-
 irregular H52.21-
 regular H52.22-
Astraphobia F40.220
Astroblastoma
 specified site —*see* Neoplasm, malignant, by
  site
 unspecified site C71.9
Astrocytoma (cystic)
 anaplastic
  specified site —*see* Neoplasm, malignant,
   by site
  unspecified site C71.9
 fibrillary
  specified site —*see* Neoplasm, malignant,
   by site
  unspecified site C71.9
 fibrous
  specified site —*see* Neoplasm, malignant,
   by site
  unspecified site C71.9
 gemistocytic
  specified site —*see* Neoplasm, malignant,
   by site
  unspecified site C71.9
 juvenile
  specified site —*see* Neoplasm, malignant,
   by site
  unspecified site C71.9
 pilocytic
  specified site —*see* Neoplasm, malignant,
   by site
  unspecified site C71.9
 piloid
  specified site —*see* Neoplasm, malignant,
   by site
  unspecified site C71.9
 protoplasmic
  specified site —*see* Neoplasm, malignant,
   by site
  unspecified site C71.9

Astrocytoma (Continued)
  specified site NEC —see Neoplasm,
    malignant, by site
  subependymal D43.2
    giant cell
      specified site —see Neoplasm, uncertain
        behavior, by site
      unspecified site D43.2
    specified site —see Neoplasm, uncertain
      behavior, by site
    unspecified site D43.2
  unspecified site C71.9
Astroglioma
  specified site —see Neoplasm, malignant, by
    site
  unspecified site C71.9
Asymbolia R48.8
Asymmetry —see also Distortion
  between native and reconstructed breast N65.1
  face Q67.0
  jaw (lower) —see Anomaly, dentofacial, jaw-
    cranial base relationship, asymmetry
Asynergia, asynergy R27.8
  ventricular I51.89
Asystole (heart) —see Arrest, cardiac
At risk
  for falling Z91.81
Ataxia, ataxy, ataxic R27.0
  acute R27.8
  brain (hereditary) G11.9
  cerebellar (hereditary) G11.9
    with defective DNA repair G11.3
    alcoholic G31.2
    early-onset G11.1
    in
      alcoholism G31.2
      myxedema E03.9 [G13.2]
      neoplastic disease (see also Neoplasm)
        D49.9 [G13.1]
      specified disease NEC G32.81
    late-onset (Marie's) G11.2
  cerebral (hereditary) G11.9
  congenital nonprogressive G11.0
  family, familial —see Ataxia, hereditary
  following
    cerebrovascular disease I69.993
      cerebral infarction I69.393
      intracerebral hemorrhage I69.193
      nontraumatic intracranial hemorrhage
        NEC I69.293
      specified disease NEC I69.893
      subarachnoid hemorrhage I69.093
  Friedreich's (heredofamilial) (cerebellar)
    (spinal) G11.1
  gait R26.0
    hysterical F44.4
  general R27.8
  gluten M35.9 [G32.81]
    with celiac disease K90.0 [G32.81]
  hereditary G11.9
    with neuropathy G60.2
    cerebellar —see Ataxia, cerebellar
    spastic G11.4
    specified NEC G11.8
    spinal (Friedreich's) G11.1
  heredofamilial —see Ataxia, hereditary
  Hunt's G11.1
  hysterical F44.4
  locomotor (progressive) (syphilitic) (partial)
    (spastic) A52.11
    diabetic —see Diabetes, ataxia
  Marie's (cerebellar) (heredofamilial) (late-
    onset) G11.2
  nonorganic origin F44.4
  nonprogressive, congenital G11.0
  psychogenic F44.4
  Roussy-Lévy G60.0
  Sanger-Brown's (hereditary) G11.2
  spastic hereditary G11.4
  spinal
    hereditary (Friedreich's) G11.1
    progressive (syphilitic) A52.11

Ataxia, ataxy, ataxic (Continued)
  spinocerebellar, X-linked recessive G11.1
  telangiectasia (Louis-Bar) G11.3
Ataxia-telangiectasia (Louis-Bar) G11.3
Atelectasis (massive) (partial) (pressure)
    (pulmonary) J98.11
  newborn P28.10
    due to resorption P28.11
    partial P28.19
    primary P28.0
    secondary P28.19
  primary (newborn) P28.0
  tuberculous —see Tuberculosis, pulmonary
Atelocardia Q24.9
Atelomyelia Q06.1
Atheroembolism
  of
    extremities
      lower I75.02-
      upper I75.01-
    kidney I75.81
    specified NEC I75.89
Atheroma, atheromatous (see also
    Arteriosclerosis) I70.90
  aorta, aortic I70.0
    valve (see also Endocarditis, aortic) I35.8
  aorto-iliac I70.0
  artery —see Arteriosclerosis
  basilar (artery) I67.2
  carotid (artery) (common) (internal) I67.2
  cerebral (arteries) I67.2
  coronary (artery) I25.10
    with angina pectoris —see Arteriosclerosis,
      coronary (artery)
  degeneration —see Arteriosclerosis
  heart, cardiac —see Disease, heart, ischemic,
    atherosclerotic
  mitral (valve) I34.8
  myocardium, myocardial —see Disease, heart,
    ischemic, atherosclerotic
  pulmonary valve (heart) (see also
    Endocarditis, pulmonary) I37.8
  tricuspid (heart) (valve) I36.8
  valve, valvular —see Endocarditis
  vertebral (artery) I67.2
Atheromatosis —see Arteriosclerosis
Atherosclerosis —see also Arteriosclerosis
  coronary
    artery I25.10
      with angina pectoris —see
        Arteriosclerosis, coronary (artery),
      due to
        calcified coronary lesion (severely)
          I25.84
        lipid rich plaque I25.83
    transplanted heart I25.811
      bypass graft I25.812
        with angina pectoris —see
          Arteriosclerosis, coronary (artery)
      native coronary artery I25.811
        with angina pectoris —see
          Arteriosclerosis, coronary (artery)
Athetosis (acquired) R25.8
  bilateral (congenital) G80.3
  congenital (bilateral) (double) G80.3
  double (congenital) G80.3
  unilateral R25.8
Athlete's
  foot B35.3
  heart I51.7
Athrepsia E41
Athyrea (acquired) —see also Hypothyroidism
  congenital E03.1
Atonia, atony, atonic
  bladder (sphincter) (neurogenic) N31.2
  capillary I78.8
  cecum K59.8
    psychogenic F45.8
  colon —see Atony, intestine
  congenital P94.2
  esophagus K22.8

Atonia, atony, atonic (Continued)
  intestine K59.8
    psychogenic F45.8
  stomach K31.89
    neurotic or psychogenic F45.8
  uterus (during labor) O62.2
    with hemorrhage (postpartum) O72.1
    postpartum (with hemorrhage) O72.1
      without hemorrhage O75.89
Atopy —see History, allergy
Atransferrinemia, congenital E88.09
Atresia, atretic
  alimentary organ or tract NEC Q45.8
    upper Q40.8
  ani, anus, anal (canal) Q42.3
    with fistula Q42.2
  aorta (arch) (ring) Q25.2
  aortic (orifice) (valve) Q23.0
    arch Q25.2
    congenital with hypoplasia of ascending
      aorta and defective development of
      left ventricle (with mitral stenosis)
      Q23.4
    in hypoplastic left heart syndrome Q23.4
  aqueduct of Sylvius Q03.0
    with spina bifida —see Spina bifida, with
      hydrocephalus
  artery NEC Q27.8
    cerebral Q28.3
    coronary Q24.5
    digestive system Q27.8
    eye Q15.8
    lower limb Q27.8
    pulmonary Q25.5
    specified site NEC Q27.8
    umbilical Q27.0
    upper limb Q27.8
  auditory canal (external) Q16.1
  bile duct (common) (congenital) (hepatic)
    Q44.2
    acquired —see Obstruction, bile duct
  bladder (neck) Q64.39
    obstruction Q64.31
  bronchus Q32.4
  cecum Q42.8
  cervix (acquired) N88.2
    congenital Q51.828
    in pregnancy or childbirth —see Anomaly,
      cervix, in pregnancy or childbirth
      causing obstructed labor O65.5
  choana Q30.0
  colon Q42.9
    specified NEC Q42.8
  common duct Q44.2
  cricoid cartilage Q31.8
  cystic duct Q44.2
    acquired K82.8
      with obstruction K82.0
  digestive organs NEC Q45.8
  duodenum Q41.0
  ear canal Q16.1
  ejaculatory duct Q55.4
  epiglottis Q31.8
  esophagus Q39.0
    with tracheoesophageal fistula Q39.1
  eustachian tube Q17.8
  fallopian tube (congenital) Q50.6
    acquired N97.1
  follicular cyst N83.0
  foramen of
    Luschka Q03.1
      with spina bifida —see Spina bifida, with
        hydrocephalus
    Magendie Q03.1
      with spina bifida —see Spina bifida, with
        hydrocephalus
  gallbladder Q44.1
  genital organ
    external
      female Q52.79
      male Q55.8

Atresia, atretic *(Continued)*
  genital organ *(Continued)*
    internal
      female Q52.8
      male Q55.8
  glottis Q31.8
  gullet Q39.0
    with tracheoesophageal fistula Q39.1
  heart valve NEC Q24.8
    pulmonary Q22.0
    tricuspid Q22.4
  hymen Q52.3
    acquired (postinfective) N89.6
  ileum Q41.2
  intestine (small) Q41.9
    large Q42.9
      specified NEC Q42.8
  iris, filtration angle Q15.0
  jejunum Q41.1
  lacrimal apparatus Q10.4
  larynx Q31.8
  meatus urinarius Q64.33
  mitral valve Q23.2
    in hypoplastic left heart syndrome Q23.4
  nares (anterior) (posterior) Q30.0
  nasopharynx Q34.8
  nose, nostril Q30.0
    acquired J34.89
  organ or site NEC Q89.8
  osseous meatus (ear) Q16.1
  oviduct (congenital) Q50.6
    acquired N97.1
  parotid duct Q38.4
    acquired K11.8
  pulmonary (artery) Q25.5
    valve Q22.0
  pulmonic Q22.0
  pupil Q13.2
  rectum Q42.1
    with fistula Q42.0
  salivary duct Q38.4
    acquired K11.8
  sublingual duct Q38.4
    acquired K11.8
  submandibular duct Q38.4
    acquired K11.8
  submaxillary duct Q38.4
    acquired K11.8
  thyroid cartilage Q31.8
  trachea Q32.1
  tricuspid valve Q22.4
  ureter Q62.10
    pelvic junction Q62.11
    vesical orifice Q62.12
  ureteropelvic junction Q62.11
  ureterovesical orifice Q62.12
  urethra (valvular) Q64.39
    stricture Q64.32
  urinary tract NEC Q64.8
  uterus Q51.818
    acquired N85.8
  vagina (congenital) Q52.4
    acquired (postinfectional) (senile) N89.5
  vas deferens Q55.3
  vascular NEC Q27.8
    cerebral Q28.3
    digestive system Q27.8
    lower limb Q27.8
    specified site NEC Q27.8
    upper limb Q27.8
  vein NEC Q27.8
    digestive system Q27.8
    great Q26.8
    lower limb Q27.8
    portal Q26.5
    pulmonary Q26.3
    specified site NEC Q27.8
    upper limb Q27.8
  vena cava (inferior) (superior) Q26.8

Atresia, atretic *(Continued)*
  vesicourethral orifice Q64.31
  vulva Q52.79
    acquired N90.5
Atrichia, atrichosis —*see* Alopecia
Atrophia —*see also* Atrophy
  cutis senilis L90.8
    due to radiation L57.8
  gyrata of choroid and retina H31.23
  senilis R54
    dermatological L90.8
      due to radiation (nonionizing) (solar) L57.8
  unguium L60.3
    congenita Q84.6
Atrophie blanche (en plaque) (de Milian) L95.0
Atrophoderma, atrophodermia (of) L90.9
  diffusum (idiopathic) L90.4
  maculatum L90.8
    et striatum L90.8
      due to syphilis A52.79
    syphilitic A51.39
  neuriticum L90.8
  Pasini and Pierini L90.3
  pigmentosum Q82.1
  reticulatum symmetricum faciei L66.4
  senile L90.8
    due to radiation (nonionizing) (solar) L57.8
  vermiculata (cheeks) L66.4
Atrophy, atrophic (of)
  adrenal (capsule) (gland) E27.49
    primary (autoimmune) E27.1
  alveolar process or ridge (edentulous) K08.20
  anal sphincter (disuse) N81.84
  appendix K38.8
  arteriosclerotic —*see* Arteriosclerosis
  bile duct (common) (hepatic) K83.8
  bladder N32.89
    neurogenic N31.8
  blanche (en plaque) (of Milian) L95.0
  bone (senile) NEC —*see also* Disorder, bone, specified type NEC
    due to
      tabes dorsalis (neurogenic) A52.11
  brain (cortex) (progressive) G31.9
    frontotemporal circumscribed G31.01
      [F02.80]
      with behavioral disturbance G31.01
        [F02.81]
    senile NEC G31.1
  breast N64.2
    obstetric —*see* Disorder, breast, specified type NEC
  buccal cavity K13.79
  cardiac —*see* Degeneration, myocardial
  cartilage (infectional) (joint) —*see* Disorder, cartilage, specified NEC
  cerebellar —*see* Atrophy, brain
  cerebral —*see* Atrophy, brain
  cervix (mucosa) (senile) (uteri) N88.8
    menopausal N95.8
  Charcot-Marie-Tooth G60.0
  choroid (central) (macular) (myopic) (retina) H31.10-
    diffuse secondary H31.12-
    gyrate H31.23
    senile H31.11-
  ciliary body —*see* Atrophy, iris
  conjunctiva (senile) H11.89
  corpus cavernosum N48.89
  cortical —*see* Atrophy, brain
  cystic duct K82.8
  Déjérine-Thomas G23.8
  disuse NEC —*see* Atrophy, muscle
  Duchenne-Aran G12.21
  ear H93.8-
  edentulous alveolar ridge K08.20
  endometrium (senile) N85.8
    cervix N88.8
  enteric K63.89
  epididymis N50.8

Atrophy, atrophic *(Continued)*
  eyeball —*see* Disorder, globe, degenerated condition, atrophy
  eyelid (senile) —*see* Disorder, eyelid, degenerative
  facial (skin) L90.9
  fallopian tube (senile) N83.32
    with ovary N83.33
  fascioscapulohumeral (Landouzy- Déjérine) G71.0
  fatty, thymus (gland) E32.8
  gallbladder K82.8
  gastric K29.40
    with bleeding K29.41
  gastrointestinal K63.89
  glandular I89.8
  globe H44.52-
  gum K06.0
  hair L67.8
  heart (brown) —*see* Degeneration, myocardial
  hemifacial Q67.4
    Romberg G51.8
  infantile E41
    paralysis, acute —*see* Poliomyelitis, paralytic
  intestine K63.89
  iris (essential) (progressive) H21.26-
    specified NEC H21.29
  kidney (senile) (terminal) (*see also* Sclerosis, renal) N26.1
    congenital or infantile Q60.5
      bilateral Q60.4
      unilateral Q60.3
    hydronephrotic —*see* Hydronephrosis
  lacrimal gland (primary) H04.14-
    secondary H04.15-
  Landouzy-Déjérine G71.0
  laryngitis, infective J37.0
  larynx J38.7
  Leber's optic (hereditary) H47.22
  lip K13.0
  liver (yellow) K72.90
    with coma K72.91
    acute, subacute K72.00
      with coma K72.01
    chronic K72.10
      with coma K72.11
  lung (senile) J98.4
  macular (dermatological) L90.8
    syphilitic, skin A51.39
      striated A52.79
  mandible (edentulous) K08.20
    minimal K08.21
    moderate K08.22
    severe K08.23
  maxilla K08.20
    minimal K08.24
    moderate K08.25
    severe K08.26
  muscle, muscular (diffuse) (general) (idiopathic) (primary) M62.50
    ankle M62.57-
    Duchenne-Aran G12.21
    foot M62.57-
    forearm M62.53-
    hand M62.54-
    infantile spinal G12.0
    lower leg M62.56-
    multiple sites M62.59
    myelopathic —*see* Atrophy, muscle, spinal
    myotonic G71.11
    neuritic G58.9
    neuropathic (peroneal) (progressive) G60.0
    pelvic (disuse) N81.84
    peroneal G60.0
    progressive (bulbar) G12.21
      adult G12.1
      infantile (spinal) G12.0
      spinal G12.9
        adult G12.1
        infantile G12.0

Atrophy, atrophic *(Continued)*
  muscle, muscular *(Continued)*
    pseudohypertrophic G71.0
    shoulder region M62.51-
    specified site NEC M62.58
    spinal G12.9
      adult form G12.1
      Aran-Duchenne G12.21
      childhood form, type II G12.1
      distal G12.1
      hereditary NEC G12.1
      infantile, type I (Werdnig- Hoffmann)
        G12.0
      juvenile form, type III (Kugelberg-
        Welander) G12.1
      progressive G12.21
      scapuloperoneal form G12.1
      specified NEC G12.8
    syphilitic A52.78
    thigh M62.55-
    upper arm M62.52-
  myocardium —*see* Degeneration, myocardial
  myometrium (senile) N85.8
    cervix N88.8
  myopathic NEC —*see* Atrophy, muscle
  myotonia G71.11
  nail L60.3
  nasopharynx J31.1
  nerve —*see also* Disorder, nerve
    abducens —*see* Strabismus, paralytic, sixth
      nerve
    accessory G52.8
    acoustic or auditory —*see* subcategory
      H93.3
    cranial G52.9
      eighth (auditory) —*see* subcategory
        H93.3
      eleventh (accessory) G52.8
      fifth (trigeminal) G50.8
      first (olfactory) G52.0
      fourth (trochlear) —*see* Strabismus,
        paralytic, fourth nerve
      second (optic) H47.20
      sixth (abducens) —*see* Strabismus,
        paralytic, sixth nerve
      tenth (pneumogastric) (vagus) G52.2
      third (oculomotor) —*see* Strabismus,
        paralytic, third nerve
      twelfth (hypoglossal) G52.3
    hypoglossal G52.3
    oculomotor —*see* Strabismus, paralytic,
      third nerve
    olfactory G52.0
    optic (papillomacular bundle)
      syphilitic (late) A52.15
        congenital A50.44
    pneumogastric G52.2
    trigeminal G50.8
    trochlear —*see* Strabismus, paralytic,
      fourth nerve
    vagus (pneumogastric) G52.2
  neurogenic, bone, tabetic A52.11
  nutritional E41
  old age R54
  olivopontocerebellar G23.8
  optic (nerve) H47.20
    glaucomatous H47.23-
    hereditary H47.22
    primary H47.21-
    specified type NEC H47.29-
    syphilitic (late) A52.15
      congenital A50.44
  orbit H05.31-
  ovary (senile) N83.31
    with fallopian tube N83.33
  oviduct (senile) —*see* Atrophy, fallopian tube
  palsy, diffuse (progressive) G12.22
  pancreas (duct) (senile) K86.8
  parotid gland K11.0
  pelvic muscle N81.84
  penis N48.89

Atrophy, atrophic *(Continued)*
  pharynx J39.2
  pluriglandular E31.8
    autoimmune E31.0
  polyarthritis M15.9
  prostate N42.89
  pseudohypertrophic (muscle) G71.0
  renal *(see also* Sclerosis, renal) N26.1
  retina, retinal (postinfectional) H35.89
  rhinitis J31.0
  salivary gland K11.0
  scar L90.5
  sclerosis, lobar (of brain) G31.09 *[F02.80]*
    with behavioral disturbance G31.09
      [F02.81]
  scrotum N50.8
  seminal vesicle N50.8
  senile R54
    due to radiation (nonionizing) (solar)
      L57.8
  skin (patches) (spots) L90.9
    degenerative (senile) L90.8
    due to radiation (nonionizing) (solar)
      L57.8
    senile L90.8
  spermatic cord N50.8
  spinal (acute) (cord) G95.89
    muscular —*see* Atrophy, muscle, spinal
    paralysis G12.20
      acute —*see* Poliomyelitis, paralytic
      meaning progressive muscular atrophy
        G12.21
  spine (column) —*see* Spondylopathy,
    specified NEC
  spleen (senile) D73.0
  stomach K29.40
    with bleeding K29.41
  striate (skin) L90.6
    syphilitic A52.79
  subcutaneous L90.9
  sublingual gland K11.0
  submandibular gland K11.0
  submaxillary gland K11.0
  Sudeck's —*see* Algoneurodystrophy
  suprarenal (capsule) (gland) E27.49
    primary E27.1
  systemic affecting central nervous system
    in
      myxedema E03.9 *[G13.2]*
      neoplastic disease *(see also* Neoplasm)
        D49.9 *[G13.1]*
      specified disease NEC G13.8
  tarso-orbital fascia, congenital Q10.3
  testis N50.0
  thenar, partial —*see* Syndrome, carpal tunnel
  thymus (fatty) E32.8
  thyroid (gland) (acquired) E03.4
    with cretinism E03.1
    congenital (with myxedema) E03.1
  tongue (senile) K14.8
    papillae K14.4
  trachea J39.8
  tunica vaginalis N50.8
  turbinate J34.89
  tympanic membrane (nonflaccid) H73.82-
    flaccid H73.81-
  upper respiratory tract J39.8
  uterus, uterine (senile) N85.8
    cervix N88.8
    due to radiation (intended effect)
      N85.8
      adverse effect or misadventure
        N99.89
  vagina (senile) N95.2
  vas deferens N50.8
  vascular I99.8
  vertebra (senile) —*see* Spondylopathy,
    specified NEC
  vulva (senile) N90.5
  Werdnig-Hoffmann G12.0
  yellow —*see* Failure, hepatic

Attack, attacks
  with alteration of consciousness (with
    automatisms) —*see* Epilepsy,
    localization-related, symptomatic, with
    complex partial seizures
  without alteration of consciousness —
    see Epilepsy, localization-related,
    symptomatic, with simple partial seizures
  Adams-Stokes I45.9
  akinetic —*see* Epilepsy, generalized, specified
    NEC
  angina —*see* Angina
  atonic —*see* Epilepsy, generalized, specified
    NEC
  benign shuddering G25.83
  cataleptic —*see* Catalepsy
  coronary —*see* Infarct, myocardium
  cyanotic, newborn P28.2
  drop NEC R55
  epileptic —*see* Epilepsy
  heart —*see* infarct, myocardium
  hysterical F44.9
  jacksonian —*see* Epilepsy, localization-
    related, symptomatic, with simple
    partial seizures
  myocardium, myocardial —*see* Infarct,
    myocardium
  myoclonic —*see* Epilepsy, generalized,
    specified NEC
  panic F41.0
  psychomotor —*see* Epilepsy, localization-
    related, symptomatic, with complex
    partial seizures
  salaam —*see* Epilepsy, spasms
  schizophreniform, brief F23
  shuddering, benign G25.83
  Stokes-Adams I45.9
  syncope R55
  transient ischemic (TIA) G45.9
    specified NEC G45.8
  unconsciousness R55
    hysterical F44.89
  vasomotor R55
  vasovagal (paroxysmal) (idiopathic) R55
Attention (to)
  artificial
    opening (of) Z43.9
      digestive tract NEC Z43.4
        colon Z43.3
        ilium Z43.2
        stomach Z43.1
      specified NEC Z43.8
      trachea Z43.0
      urinary tract NEC Z43.6
        cystostomy Z43.5
        nephrostomy Z43.6
        ureterostomy Z43.6
        urethrostomy Z43.6
      vagina Z43.7
  colostomy Z43.3
  cystostomy Z43.5
  deficit disorder or syndrome F98.8
    with hyperactivity —*see* Disorder,
      attention-deficit hyperactivity
  gastrostomy Z43.1
  ileostomy Z43.2
  jejunostomy Z43.4
  nephrostomy Z43.6
  surgical dressings Z48.01
  sutures Z48.02
  tracheostomy Z43.0
  ureterostomy Z43.6
  urethrostomy Z43.6
Attrition
  gum K06.0
  tooth, teeth (excessive) (hard tissues) K03.0
Atypical, atypism —*see also* condition
  cells (on cytolgocial smear) (endocervical)
    (endometrial) (glandular)
    cervix R87.619
    vagina R87.629

◀ New   ◀▥ Revised   ~~deleted~~ Deleted

Atypical, atypism (Continued)
  cervical N87.9
  endometrium N85.9
    hyperplasia N85.00
  parenting situation Z62.9
Auditory —see condition
Aujeszky's disease B33.8
Aurantiasis, cutis E67.1
Auricle, auricular —see also condition
  cervical Q18.2
Auriculotemporal syndrome G50.8
Austin Flint murmur (aortic insufficiency) I35.1
Australian
  Q fever A78
  X disease A83.4
Autism, autistic (childhood) (infantile) F84.0
  atypical F84.9
Autodigestion R68.89
Autoerythrocyte sensitization (syndrome)
  D69.2
Autographism L50.3
Autoimmune
  disease (systemic) M35.9
  inhibitors to clotting factors D68.311
  lymphoproliferative syndrome [ALPS]
    D89.82
  thyroiditis E06.3
Autointoxication R68.89
Automatism G93.89
  with temporal sclerosis G93.81
  epileptic —see Epilepsy, localization- related,
    symptomatic, with complex partial
    seizures
  paroxysmal, idiopathic —see Epilepsy,
    localization-related, symptomatic, with
    complex partial seizures
Autonomic, autonomous
  bladder (neurogenic) N31.2
  hysteria seizure F44.5
Autosensitivity, erythrocyte D69.2
Autosensitization, cutaneous L30.2
Autosome —see condition by chromosome
  involved

Autotopagnosia R48.1
Autotoxemia R68.89
Autumn —see condition
Avellis' syndrome G46.8
Aversion
  oral R63.3
    newborn P92.-
    nonorganic origin F98.2
  sexual F52.1
Aviator's
  disease or sickness —see Effect, adverse, high
    altitude
  ear T70.0
Avitaminosis (multiple) (see also Deficiency,
    vitamin) E56.9
  B E53.9
    with
      beriberi E51.11
      pellagra E52
  B2 E53.0
  B6 E53.1
  B12 E53.8
  D E55.9
    with rickets E55.0
  G E53.0
  K E56.1
  nicotinic acid E52
AVNRT (atrioventricular nodal re-entrant
    tachycardia) I47.1
AVRT (atrioventricular nodal re-entrant
    tachycardia) I47.1
Avulsion (traumatic)
  blood vessel —see Injury, blood vessel
  bone —see Fracture, by site
  cartilage —see also Dislocation, by site
    symphyseal (inner), complicating delivery
      O71.6
  external site other than limb —see Wound,
    open, by site
  eye S05.7-
  head (intracranial)
    external site NEC S08.89
    scalp S08.0

Avulsion (Continued)
  internal organ or site —see Injury, by site
  joint —see also Dislocation, by site
    capsule —see Sprain, by site
  kidney S37.06-
  ligament —see Sprain, by site
  limb —see also Amputation, traumatic, by site
    skin and subcutaneous tissue —see Wound,
      open, by site
  muscle —see Injury, muscle
  nerve (root) —see Injury, nerve
  scalp S08.0
  skin and subcutaneous tissue —see Wound,
    open, by site
  spleen S36.032
  symphyseal cartilage (inner), complicating
    delivery O71.6
  tendon —see Injury, muscle
  tooth S03.2
Awareness of heart beat R00.2
Axenfeld's
  anomaly or syndrome Q15.0
  degeneration (calcareous) Q13.4
Axilla, axillary —see also condition
  breast Q83.1
Axonotmesis —see Injury, nerve
Ayerza's disease or syndrome (pulmonary
    artery sclerosis with pulmonary
    hypertension) I27.0
Azoospermia (organic) N46.01
  due to
    drug therapy N46.021
    efferent duct obstruction N46.023
    infection N46.022
    radiation N46.024
    specified cause NEC N46.029
    systemic disease N46.025
Azotemia R79.89
  meaning uremia N19
Aztec ear Q17.3
Azygos
  continuation inferior vena cava Q26.8
  lobe (lung) Q33.1

B

Baastrup's disease —see Kissing spine
Babesiosis B60.0
Babington's disease (familial hemorrhagic telangiectasia) I78.0
Babinski's syndrome A52.79
Baby
  crying constantly R68.11
  floppy (syndrome) P94.2
Bacillary —see condition
Bacilluria N39.0
Bacillus —see also Infection, bacillus
  abortus infection A23.1
  anthracis infection A22.9
  coli infection (see also Escherichia coli) B96.20
  Flexner's A03.1
  mallei infection A24.0
  Shiga's A03.0
  suipestifer infection —see Infection, salmonella
Back —see condition
Backache (postural) M54.9
  sacroiliac M53.3
  specified NEC M54.89
Backflow —see Reflux
Backward reading (dyslexia) F81.0
Bacteremia R78.81
  with sepsis —see Sepsis
Bactericholia —see Cholecystitis, acute
Bacterid, bacteride (pustular) L40.3
Bacterium, bacteria, bacterial
  agent NEC, as cause of disease classified elsewhere B96.89
  in blood —see Bacteremia
  in urine —see Bacteriuria
Bacteriuria, bacteruria N39.0
  asymptomatic N39.0
Bacteroides
  fragilis, as cause of disease classified elsewhere B96.6
Bad
  heart —see Disease, heart
  trip
    due to drug abuse —see Abuse, drug, hallucinogen
    due to drug dependence —see Dependence, drug, hallucinogen
Baelz's disease (cheilitis glandularis apostematosa) K13.0
Baerensprung's disease (eczema marginatum) B35.6
Bagasse disease or pneumonitis J67.1
Bagassosis J67.1
Baker's cyst —see Cyst, Baker's
Bakwin-Krida syndrome (craniometaphyseal dysplasia) Q78.5
Balancing side interference M26.56
Balanitis (circinata) (erosiva) (gangrenosa) (phagedenic) (vulgaris) N48.1
  amebic A06.82
  candidal B37.42
  due to Haemophilus ducreyi A57
  gonococcal (acute) (chronic) A54.09
  xerotica obliterans N48.0
Balanoposthitis N47.6
  gonococcal (acute) (chronic) A54.09
  ulcerative (specific) A63.8
Balanorrhagia —see Balanitis
Balantidiasis, balantidiosis A07.0
Bald tongue K14.4
Baldness —see also Alopecia
  male-pattern —see Alopecia, androgenic
Balkan grippe A78
Balloon disease —see Effect, adverse, high altitude
Balo's disease (concentric sclerosis) G37.5
Bamberger-Marie disease —see Osteoarthropathy, hypertrophic, specified type NEC
Bancroft's filariasis B74.0

Band (s)
  adhesive —see Adhesions, peritoneum
  anomalous or congenital —see also Anomaly, by site
    heart (atrial) (ventricular) Q24.8
    intestine Q43.3
    omentum Q43.3
  cervix N88.1
  constricting, congenital Q79.8
  gallbladder (congenital) Q44.1
  intestinal (adhesive) —see Adhesions, peritoneum
  obstructive
    intestine K56.5
    peritoneum K56.5
  periappendiceal, congenital Q43.3
  peritoneal (adhesive) —see Adhesions, peritoneum
  uterus N73.6
    internal N85.6
  vagina N89.5
Bandemia D72.825
Bandl's ring (contraction), complicating delivery O62.4
Bangkok hemorrhagic fever A91
Bang's disease (brucella abortus) A23.1
Bankruptcy, anxiety concerning Z59.8
Bannister's disease T78.3
  hereditary D84.1
Banti's disease or syndrome (with cirrhosis) (with portal hypertension) K76.6
Bar, median, prostate —see Enlargement, enlarged, prostate
Barcoo disease or rot —see Ulcer, skin
Barlow's disease E54
Barodontalgia T70.29
Baron Münchausen syndrome —see Disorder, factitious
Barosinusitis T70.1
Barotitis T70.0
Barotrauma T70.29
  odontalgia T70.29
  otitic T70.0
  sinus T70.1
Barraquer (-Simons) disease or syndrome (progressive lipodystrophy) E88.1
Barré-Guillain disease or syndrome G61.0
Barré-Liéou syndrome (posterior cervical sympathetic) M53.0
Barrel chest M95.4
Barrett's
  disease —see Barrett's, esophagus
  esophagus K22.70
    with dysplasia K22.719
      high grade K22.711
      low grade K22.710
    without dysplasia K22.70
  syndrome —see Barrett's, esophagus
  ulcer K22.10
    with bleeding K22.11
    without bleeding K22.10
Barth syndrome E78.71
Bársony (-Polgár) (-Teschendorf) syndrome (corkscrew esophagus) K22.4
Bartholinitis (suppurating) N75.8
  gonococcal (acute) (chronic) (with abscess) A54.1
Bartonellosis A44.9
  cutaneous A44.1
  mucocutaneous A44.1
  specified NEC A44.8
  systemic A44.0
Barton's fracture S52.56-
Bartter's syndrome E26.81
Basal —see condition
Basan's (hidrotic) ectodermal dysplasia Q82.4
Baseball finger —see Dislocation, finger
Basedow's disease (exophthalmic goiter) —see Hyperthyroidism, with, goiter
Basic —see condition
Basilar —see condition

Bason's (hidrotic) ectodermal dysplasia Q82.4
Basopenia —see Agranulocytosis
Basophilia D72.824
Basophilism (cortico-adrenal) (Cushing's) (pituitary) E24.0
Bassen-Kornzweig disease or syndrome E78.6
Bat ear Q17.5
Bateman's
  disease B08.1
  purpura (senile) D69.2
Bathing cramp T75.1
Bathophobia F40.248
Batten (-Mayou) disease E75.4
  retina E75.4 [H36]
Batten-Steinert syndrome G71.11
Battered —see Maltreatment
Battey Mycobacterium infection A31.0
Battle exhaustion F43.0
Battledore placenta O43.19-
Baumgarten-Cruveilhier cirrhosis, disease or syndrome K74.69
Bauxite fibrosis (of lung) J63.1
Bayle's disease (general paresis) A52.17
Bazin's disease (primary) (tuberculous) A18.4
Beach ear —see Swimmer's, ear
Beaded hair (congenital) Q84.1
Béal conjunctivitis or syndrome B30.2
Beard's disease (neurasthenia) F48.8
Beat (s)
  atrial, premature I49.1
  ectopic I49.49
  elbow —see Bursitis, elbow
  escaped, heart I49.49
  hand —see Bursitis, hand
  knee —see Bursitis, knee
  premature I49.40
    atrial I49.1
    auricular I49.1
    supraventricular I49.1
Beau's
  disease or syndrome —see Degeneration, myocardial
  lines (transverse furrows on fingernails) L60.4
Bechterev's syndrome —see Spondylitis, ankylosing
Beck's syndrome (anterior spinal artery occlusion) I65.8
Becker's
  cardiomyopathy I42.8
  disease
    idiopathic mural endomyocardial disease I42.3
    myotonia congenita, recessive form G71.12
  dystrophy G71.0
  pigmented hairy nevus D22.5
Beckwith-Wiedemann syndrome Q87.3
Bed confinement status Z74.01
Bed sore —see Ulcer, pressure, by site
Bedbug bite (s) —see Bite (s), by site, superficial, insect
Bedclothes, asphyxiation or suffocation by —see Asphyxia, traumatic, due to, mechanical, trapped
Bednar's
  aphthae K12.0
  tumor —see Neoplasm, malignant, by site
Bedridden Z74.01
Bedsore —see Ulcer, pressure, by site
Bedwetting —see Enuresis
Bee sting (with allergic or anaphylactic shock) —see Toxicity, venom, arthropod, bee
Beer drinker's heart (disease) I42.6
Begbie's disease (exophthalmic goiter) —see Hyperthyroidism, with, goiter
Behavior
  antisocial
    adult Z72.811
    child or adolescent Z72.810
  disorder, disturbance —see Disorder, conduct
  disruptive —see Disorder, conduct

◀ New   ◀░ Revised   ~~deleted~~ Deleted

Behavior *(Continued)*
  drug seeking Z72.89
  inexplicable R46.2
  marked evasiveness R46.5
  obsessive-compulsive R46.81
  overactivity R46.3
  poor responsiveness R46.4
  self-damaging (life-style) Z72.89
  sleep-incompatible Z72.821
  slowness R46.4
  specified NEC R46.89
  strange (and inexplicable) R46.2
  suspiciousness R46.5
  type A pattern Z73.1
  undue concern or preoccupation with stressful events R46.6
  verbosity and circumstantial detail obscuring reason for contact R46.7
Behcet's disease or syndrome M35.2
Behr's disease —*see* Degeneration, macula
Beigel's disease or morbus (white piedra) B36.2
Bejel A65
Bekhterev's syndrome —*see* Spondylitis, ankylosing
Belching —*see* Eructation
Bell's
  mania F30.8
  palsy, paralysis G51.0
    infant or newborn P11.3
  spasm G51.3
Bence Jones albuminuria or proteinuria NEC R80.3
Bends T70.3
Benedikt's paralysis or syndrome G46.3
Benign *(see also* condition)
  prostatic hyperplasia —*see* Hyperplasia, prostate
Bennett's fracture (displaced) S62.21-
Benson's disease —*see* Deposit, crystalline
Bent
  back (hysterical) F44.4
  nose M95.0
    congenital Q67.4
Bereavement (uncomplicated) Z63.4
Bergeron's disease (hysterical chorea) F44.4
Berger's disease —*see* Nephropathy, IgA
Beriberi (dry) E51.11
  heart (disease) E51.12
  polyneuropathy E51.11
  wet E51.12
    involving circulatory system E51.11
Berlin's disease or edema (traumatic) S05.8X-
Berlock (berloque) dermatitis L56.2
Bernard-Horner syndrome G90.2
Bernard-Soulier disease or thrombopathia D69.1
Bernhardt (-Roth) disease —*see* Mononeuropathy, lower limb, meralgia paresthetica
Bernheim's syndrome —*see* Failure, heart, congestive
Bertielliasis B71.8
Berylliosis (lung) J63.2
Besnier-Boeck (-Schaumann) disease —*see* Sarcoidosis
Besnier's
  lupus pernio D86.3
  prurigo L20.0
Bestiality F65.89
Best's disease H35.50
Beta-mercaptolactate-cysteine disulfiduria E72.09
Betalipoproteinemia, broad or floating E78.2
Betting and gambling Z72.6
  pathological (compulsive) F63.0
Bezoar T18.9
  intestine T18.3
  stomach T18.2
Bezold's abscess —*see* Mastoiditis, acute
Bianchi's syndrome R48.8

Bicornate or bicornis uterus Q51.3
  in pregnancy or childbirth O34.59-
    causing obstructed labor O65.5
Bicuspid aortic valve Q23.1
Biedl-Bardet syndrome Q87.89
Bielschowsky (-Jansky) disease E75.4
Biermer's (pernicious) anemia or disease D51.0
Biett's disease L93.0
Bifid (congenital)
  apex, heart Q24.8
  clitoris Q52.6
  kidney Q63.8
  nose Q30.2
  patella Q74.1
  scrotum Q55.29
  toe NEC Q74.2
  tongue Q38.3
  ureter Q62.8
  uterus Q51.3
  uvula Q35.7
Biforis uterus (suprasimplex) Q51.3
Bifurcation (congenital)
  gallbladder Q44.1
  kidney pelvis Q63.8
  renal pelvis Q63.8
  rib Q76.6
  tongue, congenital Q38.3
  trachea Q32.1
  ureter Q62.8
  urethra Q64.74
  vertebra Q76.49
Big spleen syndrome D73.1
Bigeminal pulse R00.8
Bilateral —*see* condition
Bile
  duct —*see* condition
  pigments in urine R82.2
Bilharziasis —*see also* Schistosomiasis
  chyluria B65.0
  cutaneous B65.3
  galacturia B65.0
  hematochyluria B65.0
  intestinal B65.1
  lipemia B65.9
  lipuria B65.0
  oriental B65.2
  piarhemia B65.9
  pulmonary NOS B65.9 *[J99]*
    pneumonia B65.9 *[J17]*
  tropical hematuria B65.0
  vesical B65.0
Biliary —*see* condition
Bilirubin metabolism disorder E80.7
  specified NEC E80.6
Bilirubinemia, familial nonhemolytic E80.4
Bilirubinuria R82.2
Biliuria R82.2
Bilocular stomach K31.2
Binswanger's disease I67.3
Biparta, bipartite
  carpal scaphoid Q74.0
  patella Q74.1
  vagina Q52.10
Bird
  face Q75.8
  fancier's disease or lung J67.2
Birt-Hogg-Dube syndrome Q87.89
Birth
  complications in mother —*see* Delivery, complicated
  compression during NOS P15.9
  defect —*see* Anomaly
  immature (less than 37 completed weeks) —*see* Preterm, newborn
    extremely (less than 28 completed weeks) —*see* Immaturity, extreme
  inattention, at or after —*see* Maltreatment, child, neglect
  injury NOS P15.9
    basal ganglia P11.1
    brachial plexus NEC P14.3

Birth *(Continued)*
  injury NOS *(Continued)*
    brain (compression) (pressure) P11.2
    central nervous system NOS P11.9
    cerebellum P11.1
    cerebral hemorrhage P10.1
    external genitalia P15.5
    eye P15.3
    face P15.4
    fracture
      bone P13.9
        specified NEC P13.8
      clavicle P13.4
      femur P13.2
      humerus P13.3
      long bone, except femur P13.3
      radius and ulna P13.3
      skull P13.0
      spine P11.5
      tibia and fibula P13.3
    intracranial P11.2
      laceration or hemorrhage P10.9
        specified NEC P10.8
    intraventricular hemorrhage P10.2
    laceration
      brain P10.1
      by scalpel P15.8
      peripheral nerve P14.9
    liver P15.0
    meninges
      brain P11.1
      spinal cord P11.5
    nerve
      brachial plexus P14.3
      cranial NEC (except facial) P11.4
      facial P11.3
      peripheral P14.9
      phrenic (paralysis) P14.2
    paralysis
      facial nerve P11.3
      spinal P11.5
    penis P15.5
    rupture
      spinal cord P11.5
    scalp P12.9
    scalpel wound P15.8
    scrotum P15.5
    skull NEC P13.1
      fracture P13.0
    specified type NEC P15.8
    spinal cord P11.5
    spine P11.5
    spleen P15.1
    sternomastoid (hematoma) P15.2
    subarachnoid hemorrhage P10.3
    subcutaneous fat necrosis P15.6
    subdural hemorrhage P10.0
    tentorial tear P10.4
    testes P15.5
    vulva P15.5
  lack of care, at or after —*see* Maltreatment, child, neglect
  neglect, at or after —*see* Maltreatment, child, neglect
  palsy or paralysis, newborn, NOS (birth injury) P14.9
  premature (infant) —*see* Preterm, newborn
  shock, newborn P96.89
  trauma —*see* Birth, injury
  weight
    4000 grams to 4499 grams P08.1
    4500 grams or more P08.0
    low (2499 grams or less) —*see* Low, birthweight
      extremely (999 grams or less) —*see* Low, birthweight, extreme
Birthmark Q82.5
Bisalbuminemia E88.09
Biskra's button B55.1

Bite (s) (animal) (human)
abdomen, abdominal
  wall S31.159
    with penetration into peritoneal cavity
      S31.659
    epigastric region S31.152
      with penetration into peritoneal cavity
        S31.652
    left
      lower quadrant S31.154
        with penetration into peritoneal
          cavity S31.654
      upper quadrant S31.151
        with penetration into peritoneal
          cavity S31.651
    periumbilic region S31.155
      with penetration into peritoneal cavity
        S31.655
    right
      lower quadrant S31.153
        with penetration into peritoneal
          cavity S31.653
      upper quadrant S31.150
        with penetration into peritoneal
          cavity S31.650
    superficial NEC S30.871
      insect S30.861
alveolar (process) —see Bite, oral cavity
amphibian (venomous) —see Venom, bite,
  amphibian
animal —see also Bite, by site
  venomous —see Venom
ankle S91.05-
  superficial NEC S90.57-
    insect S90.56-
antecubital space —see Bite, elbow
anus S31.835
  superficial NEC S30.877
    insect S30.867
arm (upper) S41.15-
  lower —see Bite, forearm
  superficial NEC S40.87-
    insect S40.86-
arthropod NEC —see Venom, bite,
  arthropod
auditory canal (external) (meatus) —
  see Bite, ear
auricle, ear —see Bite, ear
axilla —see Bite, arm
back —see also Bite, thorax, back
  lower S31.050
    with penetration into retroperitoneal
      space S31.051
    superficial NEC S30.870
      insect S30.860
bedbug —see Bite (s), by site, superficial,
  insect
breast S21.05-
  superficial NEC S20.17-
    insect S20.16-
brow —see Bite, head, specified site NEC
buttock S31.805
  left S31.825
  right S31.815
  superficial NEC S30.870
    insect S30.860
calf —see Bite, leg
canaliculus lacrimalis —see Bite, eyelid
canthus, eye —see Bite, eyelid
centipede —see Toxicity, venom, arthropod,
  centipede
cheek (external) S01.45-
  internal —see Bite, oral cavity
  superficial NEC S00.87
    insect S00.86
chest wall —see Bite, thorax
chigger B88.0
chin —see Bite, head, specified site
  NEC
clitoris —see Bite, vulva
costal region —see Bite, thorax

Bite (Continued)
digit (s)
  hand —see Bite, finger
  toe —see Bite, toe
ear (canal) (external) S01.35-
  superficial NEC S00.47-
    insect S00.46-
elbow S51.05-
  superficial NEC S50.37-
    insect S50.36-
epididymis —see Bite, testis
epigastric region —see Bite, abdomen
epiglottis —see Bite, neck, specified site
  NEC
esophagus, cervical S11.25
  superficial NEC S10.17
    insect S10.16
eyebrow —see Bite, eyelid
eyelid S01.15-
  superficial NEC S00.27-
    insect S00.26-
face NEC —see Bite, head, specified site
  NEC
finger (s) S61.259
  with
    damage to nail S61.359
  index S61.258
    with
      damage to nail S61.358
    left S61.251
      with
        damage to nail S61.351
    right S61.250
      with
        damage to nail S61.350
    superficial NEC S60.478
      insect S60.46-
  little S61.25-
    with
      damage to nail S61.35-
    superficial NEC S60.47-
      insect S60.46-
  middle S61.25-
    with
      damage to nail S61.35-
    superficial NEC S60.47-
      insect S60.46-
  ring S61.25-
    with
      damage to nail S61.35-
    superficial NEC S60.47-
      insect S60.46-
  superficial NEC S60.479
    insect S60.469
  thumb —see Bite, thumb
flank —see Bite, abdomen, wall
flea —see Bite, by site, superficial,
  insect
foot (except toe (s) alone) S91.35-
  superficial NEC S90.87-
    insect S90.86-
  toe —see Bite, toe
forearm S51.85-
  elbow only —see Bite, elbow
  superficial NEC S50.87-
    insect S50.86-
forehead —see Bite, head, specified site
  NEC
genital organs, external
  female S31.552
    superficial NEC S30.876
      insect S30.866
    vagina and vulva —see Bite, vulva
  male S31.551
    penis —see Bite, penis
    scrotum —see Bite, scrotum
    superficial NEC S30.875
      insect S30.865
    testes —see Bite, testis
groin —see Bite, abdomen, wall
gum —see Bite, oral cavity

Bite (Continued)
hand S61.45-
  finger —see Bite, finger
  superficial NEC S60.57-
    insect S60.56-
  thumb —see Bite, thumb
head S01.95
  cheek —see Bite, cheek
  ear —see Bite, ear
  eyelid —see Bite, eyelid
  lip —see Bite, lip
  nose —see Bite, nose
  oral cavity —see Bite, oral cavity
  scalp —see Bite, scalp
  specified site NEC S01.85
    superficial NEC S00.87
      insect S00.86
  superficial NEC S00.97
    insect S00.96
  temporomandibular area —see Bite, cheek
heel —see Bite, foot
hip S71.05-
  superficial NEC S70.27-
    insect S70.26-
hymen S31.45
hypochondrium —see Bite, abdomen, wall
hypogastric region —see Bite, abdomen, wall
inguinal region —see Bite, abdomen, wall
insect —see Bite, by site, superficial, insect
instep —see Bite, foot
interscapular region —see Bite, thorax, back
jaw —see Bite, head, specified site NEC
knee S81.05-
  superficial NEC S80.27-
    insect S80.26-
labium (majus) (minus) —see Bite, vulva
lacrimal duct —see Bite, eyelid
larynx S11.015
  superficial NEC S10.17
    insect S10.16
leg (lower) S81.85-
  ankle —see Bite, ankle
  foot —see Bite, foot
  knee —see Bite, knee
  superficial NEC S80.87-
    insect S80.86-
  toe —see Bite, toe
  upper —see Bite, thigh
lip S01.551
  superficial NEC S00.571
    insect S00.561
lizard (venomous) —see Venom, bite, reptile
loin —see Bite, abdomen, wall
lower back —see Bite, back, lower
lumbar region —see Bite, back, lower
malar region —see Bite, head, specified site
  NEC
mammary —see Bite, breast
marine animals (venomous) —see Toxicity,
  venom, marine animal
mastoid region —see Bite, head, specified site
  NEC
mouth —see Bite, oral cavity
nail
  finger —see Bite, finger
  toe —see Bite, toe
nape —see Bite, neck, specified site NEC
nasal (septum) (sinus) —see Bite, nose
nasopharynx —see Bite, head, specified site
  NEC
neck S11.95
  involving
    cervical esophagus —see Bite,
      esophagus, cervical
    larynx —see Bite, larynx
    pharynx —see Bite, pharynx
    thyroid gland S11.15
    trachea —see Bite, trachea
  specified site NEC S11.85
    superficial NEC S10.87
      insect S10.86

◀ New   ⫸ Revised   ~~deleted~~ Deleted

Bite *(Continued)*
neck *(Continued)*
superficial NEC S10.97
insect S10.96
throat S11.85
superficial NEC S10.17
insect S10.16
nose (septum) (sinus) S01.25
superficial NEC S00.37
insect S00.36
occipital region —*see* Bite, scalp
oral cavity S01.552
superficial NEC S00.572
insect S00.562
orbital region —*see* Bite, eyelid
palate —*see* Bite, oral cavity
palm —*see* Bite, hand
parietal region —*see* Bite, scalp
pelvis S31.050
with penetration into retroperitoneal space S31.051
superficial NEC S30.870
insect S30.860
penis S31.25
superficial NEC S30.872
insect S30.862
perineum
female —*see* Bite, vulva
male —*see* Bite, pelvis
periocular area (with or without lacrimal passages) —*see* Bite, eyelid
phalanges
finger —*see* Bite, finger
toe —*see* Bite, toe
pharynx S11.25
superficial NEC S10.17
insect S10.16
pinna —*see* Bite, ear
poisonous —*see* Venom
popliteal space —*see* Bite, knee
prepuce —*see* Bite, penis
pubic region —*see* Bite, abdomen, wall
rectovaginal septum —*see* Bite, vulva
red bug B88.0
reptile NEC —*see also* Venom, bite, reptile
nonvenomous —*see* Bite, by site
snake —*see* Venom, bite, snake
sacral region —*see* Bite, back, lower
sacroiliac region —*see* Bite, back, lower
salivary gland —*see* Bite, oral cavity
scalp S01.05
superficial NEC S00.07
insect S00.06
scapular region —*see* Bite, shoulder
scrotum S31.35
superficial NEC S30.873
insect S30.863
sea-snake (venomous) —*see* Toxicity, venom, snake, sea snake
shin —*see* Bite, leg
shoulder S41.05-
superficial NEC S40.27-
insect S40.26-
snake —*see also* Venom, bite, snake
nonvenomous —*see* Bite, by site
spermatic cord —*see* Bite, testis
spider (venomous) —*see* Toxicity, venom, spider
nonvenomous —*see* Bite, by site, superficial, insect
sternal region —*see* Bite, thorax, front
submaxillary region —*see* Bite, head, specified site NEC
submental region —*see* Bite, head, specified site NEC
subungual
finger (s) —*see* Bite, finger
toe —*see* Bite, toe
superficial —*see* Bite, by site, superficial
supraclavicular fossa S11.85

Bite *(Continued)*
supraorbital —*see* Bite, head, specified site NEC
temple, temporal region —*see* Bite, head, specified site NEC
temporomandibular area —*see* Bite, cheek
testis S31.35
superficial NEC S30.873
insect S30.863
thigh S71.15-
superficial NEC S70.37-
insect S70.36-
thorax, thoracic (wall) S21.95
back S21.25-
with penetration into thoracic cavity S21.45-
breast —*see* Bite, breast
front S21.15-
with penetration into thoracic cavity S21.35-
superficial NEC S20.97
back S20.47-
front S20.37-
insect S20.96
back S20.46-
front S20.36-
throat —*see* Bite, neck, throat
thumb S61.05-
with
damage to nail S61.15-
superficial NEC S60.37-
insect S60.36-
thyroid S11.15
superficial NEC S10.87
insect S10.86
toe (s) S91.15-
with
damage to nail S91.25-
great S91.15-
with
damage to nail S91.25-
lesser S91.15-
with
damage to nail S91.25-
superficial NEC S90.47-
great S90.47-
insect S90.46-
great S90.46-
tongue S01.552
trachea S11.025
superficial NEC S10.17
insect S10.16
tunica vaginalis —*see* Bite, testis
tympanum, tympanic membrane —*see* Bite, ear
umbilical region S31.155
uvula —*see* Bite, oral cavity
vagina —*see* Bite, vulva
venomous —*see* Venom
vocal cords S11.035
superficial NEC S10.17
insect S10.16
vulva S31.45
superficial NEC S30.874
insect S30.864
wrist S61.55-
superficial NEC S60.87-
insect S60.86-
Biting, cheek or lip K13.1
Biventricular failure (heart) I50.9
Björck (-Thorson) syndrome (malignant carcinoid) E34.0
Black
death A20.9
eye S00.1-
hairy tongue K14.3
heel (foot) S90.3-
lung (disease) J60
palm (hand) S60.22-
Blackfan-Diamond anemia or syndrome (congenital hypoplastic anemia) D61.01

Blackhead L70.0
Blackout R55
Bladder —*see* condition
Blast (air) (hydraulic) (immersion) (underwater)
blindness S05.8X-
injury
abdomen or thorax —*see* Injury, by site
ear (acoustic nerve trauma) —*see* Injury, nerve, acoustic, specified type NEC
syndrome NEC T70.8
Blastoma —*see* Neoplasm, malignant, by site
pulmonary —*see* Neoplasm, lung, malignant
Blastomycosis, blastomycotic B40.9
Brazilian —*see* Paracoccidioidomycosis
cutaneous B40.3
disseminated B40.7
European —*see* Cryptococcosis
generalized B40.7
keloidal B48.0
North American B40.9
primary pulmonary B40.0
pulmonary B40.2
acute B40.0
chronic B40.1
skin B40.3
South American —*see* Paracoccidioidomycosis
specified NEC B40.89
Bleb (s) R23.8
emphysematous (lung) (solitary) J43.9
endophthalmitis H59.43
filtering (vitreous), after glaucoma surgery Z98.83
inflamed (infected), postprocedural H59.40
stage 1 H59.41
stage 2 H59.42
stage 3 H59.43
lung (ruptured) J43.9
congenital —*see* Atelectasis
newborn P25.8
subpleural (emphysematous) J43.9
Blebitis, postprocedural H59.40
stage 1 H59.41
stage 2 H59.42
stage 3 H59.43
Bleeder (familial) (hereditary) —*see* Hemophilia
Bleeding —*see also* Hemorrhage
anal K62.5
anovulatory N97.0
atonic, following delivery O72.1
capillary I78.8
puerperal O72.2
contact (postcoital) N93.0
due to uterine subinvolution N85.3
ear —*see* Otorrhagia
excessive, associated with menopausal onset N92.4
familial —*see* Defect, coagulation
following intercourse N93.0
gastrointestinal K92.2
hemorrhoids —*see* Hemorrhoids
intermenstrual (regular) N92.3
irregular N92.1
intraoperative —*see* Complication, intraoperative, hemorrhage
irregular N92.6
menopausal N92.4
newborn, intraventricular —*see* Newborn, affected by, hemorrhage, intraventricular
nipple N64.59
nose R04.0
ovulation N92.3
postclimacteric N95.0
postcoital N93.0
postmenopausal N95.0
postoperative —*see* Complication, postprocedural, hemorrhage
preclimacteric N92.4
puberty (excessive, with onset of menstrual periods) N92.2

Bleeding *(Continued)*
rectum, rectal K62.5
  newborn P54.2
tendencies —*see* Defect, coagulation
throat R04.1
tooth socket (post-extraction) K91.840
umbilical stump P51.9
uterus, uterine NEC N93.9
  climacteric N92.4
  dysfunctional of functional N93.8
  menopausal N92.4
  preclimacteric or premenopausal
    N92.4
  unrelated to menstrual cycle N93.9
vagina, vaginal (abnormal) N93.9
  dysfunctional or functional N93.8
  newborn P54.6
vicarious N94.89
Blennorrhagia, blennorrhagic —*see* Gonorrhea
Blennorrhea (acute) (chronic) —*see also*
  Gonorrhea
inclusion (neonatal) (newborn) P39.1
lower genitourinary tract (gonococcal)
  A54.00
neonatorum (gonococcal ophthalmia)
  A54.31
Blepharelosis —*see* Entropion
Blepharitis (angularis) (ciliaris) (eyelid)
  (marginal) (nonulcerative) H01.009
herpes zoster B02.39
left H01.006
  lower H01.005
  upper H01.004
right H01.003
  lower H01.002
  upper H01.001
squamous H01.029
  left H01.026
    lower H01.025
    upper H01.024
  right H01.023
    lower H01.022
    upper H01.021
ulcerative H01.019
  left H01.016
    lower H01.015
    upper H01.014
  right H01.013
    lower H01.012
    upper H01.011
Blepharochalasis H02.30
congenital Q10.0
left H02.36
  lower H02.35
  upper H02.34
right H02.33
  lower H02.32
  upper H02.31
Blepharoclonus H02.59
Blepharoconjunctivitis H10.50-
angular H10.52-
contact H10.53-
ligneous H10.51-
Blepharophimosis (eyelid) H02.529
congenital Q10.3
left H02.526
  lower H02.525
  upper H02.524
right H02.523
  lower H02.522
  upper H02.521
Blepharoptosis H02.40-
congenital Q10.0
mechanical H02.41-
myogenic H02.42-
neurogenic H02.43-
paralytic H02.43-
Blepharopyorrhea, gonococcal A54.39
Blepharospasm G24.5
drug induced G24.01
Blighted ovum O02.0

Blind —*see also* Blindness
bronchus (congenital) Q32.4
loop syndrome K90.2
  congenital Q43.8
sac, fallopian tube (congenital) Q50.6
spot, enlarged —*see* Defect, visual field,
  localized, scotoma, blind spot area
tract or tube, congenital NEC —*see* Atresia,
  by site
Blindness (acquired) (congenital) (both eyes)
  H54.0
blast S05.8X-
color —*see* Deficiency, color vision
concussion S05.8X-
cortical H47.619
  left brain H47.612
  right brain H47.611
day H53.11
due to injury (current episode) S05.9-
  sequelae — code to injury with seventh
    character S
eclipse (total) —*see* Retinopathy, solar
emotional (hysterical) F44.6
face H53.16
hysterical F44.6
legal (both eyes) (USA definition) H54.8
mind R48.8
night H53.60
  abnormal dark adaptation curve H53.61
  acquired H53.62
  congenital H53.63
  specified type NEC H53.69
  vitamin A deficiency E50.5
one eye (other eye normal) H54.40
  left (normal vision on right) H54.42
    low vision on right H54.12
  low vision, other eye H54.10
  right (normal vision on left) H54.41
    low vision on left H54.11
psychic R48.8
river B73.01
snow —*see* Photokeratitis
sun, solar —*see* Retinopathy, solar
transient —*see* Disturbance, vision, subjective,
  loss, transient
traumatic (current episode) S05.9-
word (developmental) F81.0
  acquired R48.0
  secondary to organic lesion R48.0
Blister (nonthermal)
abdominal wall S30.821
alveolar process S00.522
ankle S90.52-
antecubital space —*see* Blister, elbow
anus S30.827
arm (upper) S40.82-
auditory canal —*see* Blister, ear
auricle —*see* Blister, ear
axilla —*see* Blister, arm
back, lower S30.820
beetle dermatitis L24.89
breast S20.12-
brow S00.82
calf —*see* Blister, leg
canthus —*see* Blister, eyelid
cheek S00.82
  internal S00.522
chest wall —*see* Blister, thorax
chin S00.82
costal region —*see* Blister, thorax
digit (s)
  foot —*see* Blister, toe
  hand —*see* Blister, finger
due to burn —*see* Burn, by site, second degree
ear S00.42-
elbow S50.32-
epiglottis S10.12
esophagus, cervical S10.12
eyebrow —*see* Blister, eyelid
eyelid S00.22-
face S00.82

Blister *(Continued)*
fever B00.1
finger (s) S60.429
  index S60.42-
  little S60.42-
  middle S60.42-
  ring S60.42-
foot (except toe (s) alone) S90.82-
  toe —*see* Blister, toe
forearm S50.82-
  elbow only —*see* Blister, elbow
forehead S00.82
fracture - omit code
genital organ
  female S30.826
  male S30.825
gum S00.522
hand S60.52-
head S00.92
  ear —*see* Blister, ear
  eyelid —*see* Blister, eyelid
  lip S00.521
  nose S00.32
  oral cavity S00.522
  scalp S00.02
  specified site NEC S00.82
heel —*see* Blister, foot
hip S70.22-
interscapular region S20.429
jaw S00.82
knee S80.22-
larynx S10.12
leg (lower) S80.82-
  knee —*see* Blister, knee
  upper —*see* Blister, thigh
lip S00.521
malar region S00.82
mammary —*see* Blister, breast
mastoid region S00.82
mouth S00.522
multiple, skin, nontraumatic R23.8
nail
  finger —*see* Blister, finger
  toe —*see* Blister, toe
nasal S00.32
neck S10.92
  specified site NEC S10.82
  throat S10.12
nose S00.32
occipital region S00.02
oral cavity S00.522
orbital region —*see* Blister, eyelid
palate S00.522
palm —*see* Blister, hand
parietal region S00.02
pelvis S30.820
penis S30.822
periocular area —*see* Blister, eyelid
phalanges
  finger —*see* Blister, finger
  toe —*see* Blister, toe
pharynx S10.12
pinna —*see* Blister, ear
popliteal space —*see* Blister, knee
scalp S00.02
scapular region —*see* Blister, shoulder
scrotum S30.823
shin —*see* Blister, leg
shoulder S40.22-
sternal region S20.329
submaxillary region S00.82
submental region S00.82
subungual
  finger (s) —*see* Blister, finger
  toe (s) —*see* Blister, toe
supraclavicular fossa S10.82
supraorbital S00.82
temple S00.82
temporal region S00.82
testis S30.823
thermal —*see* Burn, second degree, by site

◀ New   ◀◀ Revised   ~~deleted~~ Deleted

Blister *(Continued)*
　thigh S70.32-
　thorax, thoracic (wall) S20.92
　　back S20.42-
　　front S20.32-
　throat S10.12
　thumb S60.32-
　toe (s) S90.42-
　　great S90.42-
　tongue S00.522
　trachea S10.12
　tympanum, tympanic membrane —*see* Blister,
　　ear
　upper arm —*see* Blister, arm (upper)
　uvula S00.522
　vagina S30.824
　vocal cords S10.12
　vulva S30.824
　wrist S60.82-
Bloating R14.0
Bloch-Sulzberger disease or syndrome Q82.3
Block, blocked
　alveolocapillary J84.10
　arborization (heart) I45.5
　arrhythmic I45.9
　atrioventricular (incomplete) (partial) I44.30
　　with atrioventricular dissociation I44.2
　　complete I44.2
　　　congenital Q24.6
　　congenital Q24.6
　　first degree I44.0
　　second degree (types I and II) I44.1
　　specified NEC I44.39
　　third degree I44.2
　　types I and II I44.1
　auriculoventricular —*see* Block,
　　atrioventricular
　bifascicular (cardiac) I45.2
　bundle-branch (complete) (false) (incomplete)
　　I45.4
　　bilateral I45.2
　　left I44.7
　　　with right bundle branch block I45.2
　　　hemiblock I44.60
　　　　anterior I44.4
　　　　posterior I44.5
　　　incomplete I44.7
　　　　with right bundle branch block I45.2
　　right I45.10
　　　with
　　　　left bundle branch block I45.2
　　　　left fascicular block I45.2
　　　specified NEC I45.19
　　Wilson's type I45.19
　cardiac I45.9
　conduction I45.9
　　complete I44.2
　fascicular (left) I44.60
　　anterior I44.4
　　posterior I44.5
　　right I45.0
　　specified NEC I44.69
　foramen Magendie (acquired) G91.1
　　congenital Q03.1
　　　with spina bifida —*see* Spina bifida, by
　　　　site, with hydrocephalus
　heart I45.9
　　bundle branch I45.4
　　　bilateral I45.2
　　complete (atrioventricular) I44.2
　　congenital Q24.6
　　first degree (atrioventricular) I44.0
　　second degree (atrioventricular) I44.1
　　specified type NEC I45.5
　　third degree (atrioventricular) I44.2
　hepatic vein I82.0
　intraventricular (nonspecific) I45.4
　　bundle branch
　　　bilateral I45.2
　kidney N28.9
　　postcystoscopic or postprocedural N99.0

Block, blocked *(Continued)*
　Mobitz (types I and II) I44.1
　myocardial —*see* Block, heart
　nodal I45.5
　organ or site, congenital NEC —*see* Atresia,
　　by site
　portal (vein) I81
　second degree (types I and II) I44.1
　sinoatrial I45.5
　sinoauricular I45.5
　third degree I44.2
　trifascicular I45.3
　tubal N97.1
　vein NOS I82.90
　Wenckebach (types I and II) I44.1
Blockage —*see* Obstruction
Blocq's disease F44.4
Blood
　constituents, abnormal R78.9
　disease D75.9
　donor —*see* Donor, blood
　dyscrasia D75.9
　　with
　　　abortion —*see* Abortion, by type,
　　　　complicated by, hemorrhage
　　　ectopic pregnancy O08.1
　　　molar pregnancy O08.1
　　following ectopic or molar pregnancy
　　　O08.1
　　newborn P61.9
　　puerperal, postpartum O72.3
　flukes NEC —*see* Schistosomiasis
　in
　　feces K92.1
　　　occult R19.5
　　urine —*see* Hematuria
　mole O02.0
　occult in feces R19.5
　pressure
　　decreased, due to shock following injury
　　　T79.4
　　examination only Z01.30
　　fluctuating I99.8
　　high —*see* Hypertension
　　　borderline R03.0
　　　incidental reading, without diagnosis of
　　　　hypertension R03.0
　　low —*see also* Hypotension
　　　incidental reading, without diagnosis of
　　　　hypotension R03.1
　spitting —*see* Hemoptysis
　staining cornea —*see* Pigmentation, cornea,
　　stromal
　transfusion
　　reaction or complication —*see*
　　　Complications, transfusion
　type
　　A (Rh positive) Z67.10
　　　Rh negative Z67.11
　　AB (Rh positive) Z67.30
　　　Rh negative Z67.31
　　B (Rh positive) Z67.20
　　　Rh negative Z67.21
　　O (Rh positive) Z67.40
　　　Rh negative Z67.41
　　Rh (positive) Z67.90
　　　negative Z67.91
　vessel rupture —*see* Hemorrhage
　vomiting —*see* Hematemesis
Blood-forming organs, disease D75.9
Bloodgood's disease —*see* Mastopathy,
　cystic
Bloom (-Machacek)(-Torre) syndrome
　Q82.8
Blount's disease or osteochondrosis —*see*
　Osteochondrosis, juvenile, tibia
Blue
　baby Q24.9
　diaper syndrome E72.09
　dome cyst (breast) —*see* Cyst, breast
　dot cataract Q12.0

Blue *(Continued)*
　nevus D22.9
　sclera Q13.5
　　with fragility of bone and deafness Q78.0
　toe syndrome I75.02-
Blueness —*see* Cyanosis
Blues, postpartal O90.6
　baby O90.6
Blurring, visual H53.8
Blushing (abnormal) (excessive) R23.2
BMI —*see* Body, mass index
Boarder, hospital NEC Z76.4
　accompanying sick person Z76.3
　healthy infant or child Z76.2
　　foundling Z76.1
Bockhart's impetigo L01.02
Bodechtel-Guttman disease (subacute
　sclerosing panencephalitis) A81.1
Boder-Sedgwick syndrome (ataxia-
　telangiectasia) G11.3
Body, bodies
　Aschoff's —*see* Myocarditis, rheumatic
　asteroid, vitreous —*see* Deposit, crystalline
　cytoid (retina) —*see* Occlusion, artery, retina
　drusen (degenerative) (macula) (retinal) —*see
　　also* Degeneration, macula, drusen
　optic disc —*see* Drusen, optic disc
　foreign —*see* Foreign body
　loose
　　joint, except knee —*see* Loose, body, joint
　　　knee M23.4-
　　sheath, tendon —*see* Disorder, tendon,
　　　specified type NEC
　mass index (BMI)
　　adult
　　　19 or less Z68.1
　　　20.0-20.9 Z68.20
　　　21.0-21.9 Z68.21
　　　22.0-22.9 Z68.22
　　　23.0-23.9 Z68.23
　　　24.0-24.9 Z68.24
　　　25.0-25.9 Z68.25
　　　26.0-26.9 Z68.26
　　　27.0-27.9 Z68.27
　　　28.0-28.9 Z68.28
　　　29.0-29.9 Z68.29
　　　30.0-30.9 Z68.30
　　　31.0-31.9 Z68.31
　　　32.0-32.9 Z68.32
　　　33.0-33.9 Z68.33
　　　34.0-34.9 Z68.34
　　　35.0-35.9 Z68.35
　　　36.0-36.9 Z68.36
　　　37.0-37.9 Z68.37
　　　38.0-38.9 Z68.38
　　　39.0-39.9 Z68.39
　　　40.0-44.9 Z68.41
　　　45.0-49.9 Z68.42
　　　50.0-59.9 Z68.43
　　　60.0-69.9 Z68.44
　　　70 and over Z68.45
　　pediatric
　　　5th percentile to less than 85th percentile
　　　　for age Z68.52
　　　85th percentile to less than 95th
　　　　percentile for age Z68.53
　　　greater than or equal to ninety-fifth
　　　　percentile for age Z68.54
　　　less than fifth percentile for age Z68.51
　Mooser's A75.2
　rice —*see also* Loose, body, joint
　　knee M23.4-
　rocking F98.4
Boeck's
　disease or sarcoid —*see* Sarcoidosis
　lupoid (miliary) D86.3
Boerhaave's syndrome (spontaneous
　esophageal rupture) K22.3
Boggy
　cervix N88.8
　uterus N85.8

◀ New　◀ Revised　~~deleted~~ Deleted

Boil —see also Furuncle, by site
　Aleppo B55.1
　Baghdad B55.1
　Delhi B55.1
　lacrimal
　　gland —see Dacryoadenitis
　　passages (duct) (sac) —see Inflammation,
　　　lacrimal, passages, acute
　Natal B55.1
　orbit, orbital —see Abscess, orbit
　tropical B55.1
Bold hives —see Urticaria
Bombé, iris —see Membrane, pupillary
Bone —see condition
Bonnevie-Ullrich syndrome Q87.1
Bonnier's syndrome —see subcategory
　H81.8
Bonvale dam fever T73.3
Bony block of joint —see Ankylosis
BOOP (bronchiolitis obliterans organized
　pneumonia) J84.89
Borderline
　diabetes mellitus R73.09
　hypertension R03.0
　osteopenia M85.8-
　pelvis, with obstruction during labor
　　O65.1
　personality F60.3
Borna disease A83.9
Bornholm disease B33.0
Boston exanthem A88.0
Botalli, ductus (patent) (persistent) Q25.0
Bothriocephalus latus infestation B70.0
Botulism (foodborne intoxication) A05.1
　infant A48.51
　non-foodborne A48.52
　wound A48.52
Bouba —see Yaws
Bouchard's nodes (with arthropathy) M15.2
Bouffée délirante F23
Bouillaud's disease or syndrome (rheumatic
　heart disease) I01.9
Bourneville's disease Q85.1
Boutonniere deformity (finger) —see
　Deformity, finger, boutonniere
Bouveret (-Hoffmann) syndrome (paroxysmal
　tachycardia) I47.9
Bovine heart —see Hypertrophy, cardiac
Bowel —see condition
Bowen's
　dermatosis (precancerous) —see Neoplasm,
　　skin, in situ
　disease —see Neoplasm, skin, in situ
　epithelioma —see Neoplasm, skin, in situ
　type
　　epidermoid carcinoma-in-situ —see
　　　Neoplasm, skin, in situ
　　intraepidermal squamous cell carcinoma —
　　　see Neoplasm, skin, in situ
Bowing
　femur —see also Deformity, limb, specified
　　type NEC, thigh
　　congenital Q68.3
　fibula —see also Deformity, limb, specified
　　type NEC, lower leg
　　congenital Q68.4
　forearm —see Deformity, limb, specified type
　　NEC, forearm
　leg (s), long bones, congenital Q68.5
　radius —see Deformity, limb, specified type
　　NEC, forearm
　tibia —see also Deformity, limb, specified type
　　NEC, lower leg
　　congenital Q68.4
Bowleg (s) (acquired) M21.16-
　congenital Q68.5
　rachitic E64.3
Boyd's dysentery A03.2
Brachial —see condition
Brachycardia R00.1
Brachycephaly Q75.0

Bradley's disease A08.19
Bradyarrhythmia, cardiac I49.8
Bradycardia (sinoatrial) (sinus) (vagal) R00.1
　neonatal P29.12
　reflex G90.09
　tachycardia syndrome I49.5
Bradykinesia R25.8
Bradypnea R06.89
Bradytachycardia I49.5
Brailsford's disease or osteochondrosis —see
　Osteochondrosis, juvenile, radius
Brain —see also condition
　death G93.82
　syndrome —see Syndrome, brain
Branched-chain amino-acid disorder E71.2
Branchial —see condition
　cartilage, congenital Q18.2
Branchiogenic remnant (in neck) Q18.0
Brandt's syndrome (acrodermatitis
　enteropathica) E83.2
Brash (water) R12
Bravais-jacksonian epilepsy —see Epilepsy,
　localization-related, symptomatic, with
　simple partial seizures
Braxton Hicks contractions —see False, labor
Brazilian leishmaniasis B55.2
BRBPR K62.5
Break, retina (without detachment) H33.30-
　with retinal detachment —see Detachment,
　　retina
　horseshoe tear H33.31-
　multiple H33.33-
　round hole H33.32-
Breakdown
　device, graft or implant (see also
　　Complications, by site and type,
　　mechanical) T85.618
　arterial graft NEC —see Complication,
　　cardiovascular device, mechanical,
　　vascular
　breast (implant) T85.41
　catheter NEC T85.618
　　cystostomy T83.010
　　dialysis (renal) T82.41
　　　intraperitoneal T85.611
　　infusion NEC T82.514
　　　spinal (epidural) (subdural) T85.610
　　urinary (indwelling) T83.018
　electronic (electrode) (pulse generator)
　　(stimulator)
　　bone T84.310
　　cardiac T82.119
　　　electrode T82.110
　　　pulse generator T82.111
　　　specified type NEC T82.118
　　nervous system —see Complication,
　　　prosthetic device, mechanical,
　　　electronic nervous system
　　　stimulator
　　urinary —see Complication,
　　　genitourinary, device, urinary,
　　　mechanical
　fixation, internal (orthopedic) NEC —see
　　Complication, fixation device,
　　mechanical
　gastrointestinal —see Complications,
　　prosthetic device, mechanical,
　　gastrointestinal device
　genital NEC T83.418
　　intrauterine contraceptive device T83.31
　　penile prosthesis T83.410
　heart NEC —see Complication,
　　cardiovascular device, mechanical
　joint prosthesis —see Complications...,
　　joint prosthesis,internal, mechanical,
　　by site
　ocular NEC —see Complications, prosthetic
　　device, mechanical, ocular device
　orthopedic NEC —see Complication,
　　orthopedic, device, mechanical
　specified NEC T85.618

Breakdown (Continued)
　device, graft or implant (Continued)
　　sutures, permanent T85.612
　　　used in bone repair —see Complications,
　　　　fixation device, internal
　　　　(orthopedic)
　　urinary NEC —see also Complication,
　　　genitourinary, device, urinary,
　　　mechanical
　　　graft T83.21
　　vascular NEC —see Complication,
　　　cardiovascular device, mechanical
　　ventricular intracranial shunt T85.01
　nervous F48.8
　perineum O90.1
　respirator J95.850
　　specified NEC J95.859
　ventilator J95.850
　　specified NEC J95.859
Breast —see also condition
　buds E30.1
　　in newborn P96.89
　dense R92.2
　nodule N63
Breath
　foul R19.6
　holder, child R06.89
　holding spell R06.89
　shortness R06.02
Breathing
　labored —see Hyperventilation
　mouth R06.5
　　causing malocclusion M26.5
　periodic R06.3
　　high altitude G47.32
Breathlessness R06.81
Breda's disease —see Yaws
Breech presentation (mother) O32.1
　causing obstructed labor O64.1
　footling O32.8
　　causing obstructed labor O64.8
　incomplete O32.8
　　causing obstructed labor O64.8
Breisky's disease N90.4
Brennemann's syndrome I88.0
Brenner
　tumor (benign) D27.9
　　borderline malignancy D39.1-
　　malignant C56
　　proliferating D39.1
Bretonneau's disease or angina A36.0
Breus' mole O02.0
Brevicollis Q76.49
Brickmakers' anemia B76.9 [D63.8]
Bridge, myocardial Q24.5
Bright red blood per rectum (BRBPR) K62.5
Bright's disease —see also Nephritis
　arteriosclerotic —see Hypertension, kidney
Brill (-Zinsser) disease (recrudescent typhus)
　A75.1
　flea-borne A75.2
　louse-borne A75.1
Brill-Symmers' disease C82.90
Brion-Kayser disease —see Fever, parathyroid
Briquet's disorder or syndrome F45.0
Brissaud's
　infantilism or dwarfism E23.0
　motor-verbal tic F95.2
Brittle
　bones disease Q78.0
　nails L60.3
　　congenital Q84.6
Broad —see also condition
　beta disease E78.2
　ligament laceration syndrome N83.8
Broad- or floating-betalipoproteinemia
　E78.2
Brock's syndrome (atelectasis due to enlarged
　lymph nodes) J98.19
Brocq-Duhring disease (dermatitis
　herpetiformis) L13.0

Brodie's abscess or disease M86.8X-
Broken
  arches —see also Deformity, limb, flat foot
  arm (meaning upper limb) —see Fracture,
    arm
  back —see Fracture, vertebra
  bone —see Fracture
  implant or internal device —see
    Complications, by site and type,
    mechanical
  leg (meaning lower limb) —see Fracture, leg
  nose S02.2
  tooth, teeth —see Fracture, tooth
Bromhidrosis, bromidrosis L75.0
Bromidism, bromism G92
  chronic (dependence) F13.20
  due to
    correct substance properly administered —
      see Table of Drugs and Chemicals, by
      drug, adverse effect
    overdose or wrong substance given or
      taken —see Table of Drugs and
      Chemicals, by drug, poisoning
Bromidrosiphobia F40.298
Bronchi, bronchial —see condition
Bronchiectasis (cylindrical) (diffuse) (fusiform)
  (localized) (saccular) J47.9
  with
    acute
      bronchitis J47.0
      lower respiratory infection J47.0
    exacerbation (acute) J47.1
  congenital Q33.4
  tuberculous NEC —see Tuberculosis,
    pulmonary
Bronchiolectasis —see Bronchiectasis
Bronchiolitis (acute) (infective) (subacute)
  J21.9
  with
    bronchospasm or obstruction J21.9
    influenza, flu or grippe —see Influenza,
      with, respiratory manifestations
      NEC
  chemical (chronic) J68.4
    acute J68.0
  chronic (fibrosing) (obliterative) J44.9
  due to
    external agent —see Bronchitis, acute, due
      to
    human metapneumovirus J21.1
    respiratory syncytial virus J21.0
    specified organism NEC J21.8
  fibrosa obliterans J44.9
  influenzal —see Influenza, with, respiratory
    manifestations NEC
  obliterans J42
    with organizing pneumonia (BOOP)
      J84.89
  obliterative (chronic) (subacute) J44.9
    due to chemicals, gases, fumes or vapors
      (inhalation) J68.4
    due to fumes or vapors J68.4
  respiratory, interstitial lung disease J84.115
Bronchitis (diffuse) (fibrinous) (hypostatic)
  (infective) (membranous) J40
  with
    influenza, flu or grippe —see Influenza,
      with, respiratory manifestations NEC
    obstruction (airway) (lung) J44.9
    tracheitis (15 years of age and above) J40
      acute or subacute J20.9
      chronic J42
      under 15 years of age J20.9
  acute or subacute (with bronchospasm or
    obstruction) J20.9
    with
      bronchiectasis J47.0
      chronic obstructive pulmonary disease
        J44.0
      chemical (due to gases, fumes or vapors)
        J68.0

Bronchitis (Continued)
  acute or subacute (Continued)
    due to
      fumes or vapors J68.0
      Haemophilus influenzae J20.1
      Mycoplasma pneumoniae J20.0
      radiation J70.0
      specified organism NEC J20.8
      Streptococcus J20.2
      virus
        coxsackie J20.3
        echovirus J20.7
        parainfluenzae J20.4
        respiratory syncytial J20.5
        rhinovirus J20.6
    viral NEC J20.8
  allergic (acute) J45.909
    with
      exacerbation (acute) J45.901
      status asthmaticus J45.902
  arachidic T17.528
  aspiration (due to fumes or vapors) J68.0
  asthmatic J45.9
    chronic J44.9
      with
        acute lower respiratory infection J44.0
        exacerbation (acute) J44.1
  capillary —see Pneumonia, broncho
  caseous (tuberculous) A15.5
  Castellani's A69.8
  catarrhal (15 years of age and above) J40
    acute —see Bronchitis, acute
    chronic J41.0
    under 15 years of age J20.9
  chemical (acute) (subacute) J68.0
    chronic J68.4
    due to fumes or vapors J68.0
      chronic J68.4
  chronic J42
    with
      airways obstruction J44.9
      tracheitis (chronic) J42
      asthmatic (obstructive) J44.9
    catarrhal J41.0
    chemical (due to fumes or vapors) J68.4
    due to
      chemicals, gases, fumes or vapors
        (inhalation) J68.4
      radiation J70.1
      tobacco smoking J41.0
    emphysematous J44.9
    mucopurulent J41.1
    non-obstructive J41.0
    obliterans J44.9
    obstructive J44.9
    purulent J41.1
    simple J41.0
  croupous —see Bronchitis, acute
  due to gases, fumes or vapors (chemical)
    J68.0
  emphysematous (obstructive) J44.9
  exudative —see Bronchitis, acute
  fetid J41.1
  grippal —see Influenza, with, respiratory
    manifestations NEC
  in those under 15 years age —see Bronchitis,
    acute
    chronic —see Bronchitis, chronic
  influenzal —see Influenza, with, respiratory
    manifestations NEC
  mixed simple and mucopurulent J41.8
  moulder's J62.8
  mucopurulent (chronic) (recurrent) J41.1
    acute or subacute J20.9
    simple (mixed) J41.8
  obliterans (chronic) J44.9
  obstructive (chronic) (diffuse) J44.9
  pituitous J41.1
  pneumococcal, acute or subacute J20.2
  pseudomembranous, acute or subacute —see
    Bronchitis, acute

Bronchitis (Continued)
  purulent (chronic) (recurrent) J41.1
    acute or subacute —see Bronchitis, acute
  putrid J41.1
  senile (chronic) J42
  simple and mucopurulent (mixed) J41.8
  smokers' J41.0
  spirochetal NEC A69.8
  subacute —see Bronchitis, acute
  suppurative (chronic) J41.1
    acute or subacute —see Bronchitis, acute
  tuberculous A15.5
  under 15 years of age —see Bronchitis, acute
    chronic —see Bronchitis, chronic
  viral NEC, acute or subacute (see also
    Bronchitis, acute) J20.8
Bronchoalveolitis J18.0
Bronchoaspergillosis B44.1
Bronchocele meaning goiter E04.0
Broncholithiasis J98.09
  tuberculous NEC A15.5
Bronchomalacia J98.09
  congenital Q32.2
Bronchomycosis NOS B49 [J99]
  candidal B37.1
Bronchopleuropneumonia —see Pneumonia,
  broncho
Bronchopneumonia —see Pneumonia, broncho
Bronchopneumonitis —see Pneumonia,
  broncho
Bronchopulmonary —see condition
Bronchopulmonitis —see Pneumonia, broncho
Bronchorrhagia (see Hemoptysis)
Bronchorrhea J98.09
  acute J20.9
  chronic (infective) (purulent) J42
Bronchospasm (acute) J98.01
  with
    bronchiolitis, acute J21.9
    bronchitis, acute (conditions in J20) —see
      Bronchitis, acute
  due to external agent —see condition,
    respiratory, acute, due to
  exercise induced J45.990
Bronchospirochetosis A69.8
  Castellani A69.8
Bronchostenosis J98.09
Bronchus —see condition
Brontophobia F40.220
Bronze baby syndrome P83.8
Brooke's tumor —see Neoplasm, skin, benign
Brown enamel of teeth (hereditary) K00.5
Brown's sheath syndrome H50.61-
Brown-Séquard disease, paralysis or
  syndrome G83.81
Bruce sepsis A23.0
Brucellosis (infection) A23.9
  abortus A23.1
  canis A23.3
  dermatitis A23.9
  melitensis A23.0
  mixed A23.8
  sepsis A23.9
    melitensis A23.0
    specified NEC A23.8
  suis A23.2
Bruck-de Lange disease Q87.1
Bruck's disease —see Deformity, limb
Brugsch's syndrome Q82.8
Bruise (skin surface intact) —see also Contusion
  with
    open wound —see Wound, open
  internal organ —see Injury, by site
  newborn P54.5
  scalp, due to birth injury, newborn P12.3
  umbilical cord O69.5
Bruit (arterial) R09.89
  cardiac R01.1
Brush burn —see Abrasion, by site
Bruton's X-linked agammaglobulinemia
  D80.0

Bruxism
  psychogenic F45.8
  sleep related G47.63
Bubbly lung syndrome P27.0
Bubo I88.8
  blennorrhagic (gonococcal) A54.89
  chancroidal A57
  climatic A55
  due to Haemophilus ducreyi A57
  gonococcal A54.89
  indolent (nonspecific) I88.8
  inguinal (nonspecific) I88.8
    chancroidal A57
    climatic A55
    due to H. ducreyi A57
    infective I88.8
  scrofulous (tuberculous) A18.2
  soft chancre A57
  suppurating —see Lymphadenitis, acute
  syphilitic (primary) A51.0
    congenital A50.07
  tropical A55
  virulent (chancroidal) A57
Bubonic plague A20.0
Bubonocele —see Hernia, inguinal
Buccal —see condition
Buchanan's disease or osteochondrosis
  M91.0
Buchem's syndrome (hyperostosis corticalis)
  M85.2
Bucket-handle fracture or tear (semilunar
  cartilage) —see Tear, meniscus
Budd-Chiari syndrome (hepatic vein
  thrombosis) I82.0
Budgerigar fancier's disease or lung
  J67.2
Buds
  breast E30.1
    in newborn P96.89
Buerger's disease (thromboangiitis obliterans)
  I73.1
Bulbar —see condition
Bulbus cordis (left ventricle) (persistent)
  Q21.8
Bulimia (nervosa) F50.2
  atypical F50.9
  normal weight F50.9
Bulky
  stools R19.5
  uterus N85.2
Bulla (e) R23.8
  lung (emphysematous) (solitary) J43.9
    newborn P25.8
Bullet wound —see also Wound, open
  fracture - code as Fracture, by site
  internal organ —see Injury, by site
Bundle
  branch block (complete) (false)
    (incomplete) —see Block, bundle-branch
  of His —see condition
Bunion —see Deformity, toe, hallux valgus
Buphthalmia, buphthalmos (congenital)
  Q15.0
Burdwan fever B55.0
Bürger-Grütz disease or syndrome
  E78.3
Buried
  penis (congenital) Q55.64
    acquired N48.83
  roots K08.3
Burke's syndrome K86.8
Burkitt
  cell leukemia C91.0-
  lymphoma (malignant) C83.7-
    small noncleaved, diffuse C83.7-
    spleen C83.77
    undifferentiated C83.7-
  tumor C83.7-
  type
    acute lymphoblastic leukemia C91.0-
    undifferentiated C83.7-

Burn (electricity) (flame) (hot gas, liquid or hot
    object) (radiation) (steam) (thermal) T30.0
  abdomen, abdominal (muscle) (wall) T21.02
    first degree T21.12
    second degree T21.22
    third degree T21.32
  above elbow T22.039
    first degree T22.139
    left T22.032
      first degree T22.132
      second degree T22.232
      third degree T22.332
    right T22.031
      first degree T22.131
      second degree T22.231
      third degree T22.331
    second degree T22.239
    third degree T22.339
  acid (caustic) (external) (internal) —see
    Corrosion, by site
  alimentary tract NEC T28.2
    esophagus T28.1
    mouth T28.0
    pharynx T28.0
  alkaline (caustic) (external) (internal) —see
    Corrosion, by site
  ankle T25.019
    first degree T25.119
    left T25.012
      first degree T25.112
      second degree T25.212
      third degree T25.312
    multiple with foot —see Burn, lower, limb,
      multiple, ankle and foot
    right T25.011
      first degree T25.111
      second degree T25.211
      third degree T25.311
    second degree T25.219
    third degree T25.319
  anus —see Burn, buttock
  arm (lower) (upper) —see Burn, upper, limb
  axilla T22.049
    first degree T22.149
    left T22.042
      first degree T22.142
      second degree T22.242
      third degree T22.342
    right T22.041
      first degree T22.141
      second degree T22.241
      third degree T22.341
    second degree T22.249
    third degree T22.349
  back (lower) T21.04
    first degree T21.14
    second degree T21.24
    third degree T21.34
    upper T21.03
      first degree T21.13
      second degree T21.23
      third degree T21.33
  blisters - code as Burn, second degree, by site
  breast (s) —see Burn, chest wall
  buttock (s) T21.05
    first degree T21.15
    second degree T21.25
    third degree T21.35
  calf T24.039
    first degree T24.139
    left T24.032
      first degree T24.132
      second degree T24.232
      third degree T24.332
    right T24.031
      first degree T24.131
      second degree T24.231
      third degree T24.331
    second degree T24.239
    third degree T24.339
  canthus (eye) —see Burn, eyelid

Burn (Continued)
  caustic acid or alkaline —see Corrosion, by
    site
  cervix T28.3
  cheek T20.06
    first degree T20.16
    second degree T20.26
    third degree T20.36
  chemical (acids) (alkalines) (caustics)
    (external) (internal) —see Corrosion,
    by site
  chest wall T21.01
    first degree T21.11
    second degree T21.21
    third degree T21.31
  chin T20.03
    first degree T20.13
    second degree T20.23
    third degree T20.33
  colon T28.2
  conjunctiva (and cornea) —see Burn, cornea
  cornea (and conjunctiva) T26.1-
    chemical —see Corrosion, cornea
  corrosion (external) (internal) —see
    Corrosion, by site
  deep necrosis of underlying tissue - code as
    Burn, third degree, by site
  dorsum of hand T23.069
    first degree T23.169
    left T23.062
      first degree T23.162
      second degree T23.262
      third degree T23.362
    right T23.061
      first degree T23.161
      second degree T23.261
      third degree T23.361
    second degree T23.269
    third degree T23.369
  due to ingested chemical agent —see
    Corrosion, by site
  ear (auricle) (external) (canal) T20.01
    first degree T20.11
    second degree T20.21
    third degree T20.31
  elbow T22.029
    first degree T22.129
    left T22.022
      first degree T22.122
      second degree T22.222
      third degree T22.322
    right T22.021
      first degree T22.121
      second degree T22.221
      third degree T22.321
    second degree T22.229
    third degree T22.329
  epidermal loss - code as Burn, second degree,
    by site
  erythema, erythematous - code as Burn, first
    degree, by site
  esophagus T28.1
  extent (percentage of body surface)
    less than 10 percent T31.0
    10-19 percent T31.10
      with 0-9 percent third degree burns
        T31.10
      with 10-19 percent third degree burns
        T31.11
    20-29 percent T31.20
      with 0-9 percent third degree burns
        T31.20
      with 10-19 percent third degree burns
        T31.21
      with 20-29 percent third degree burns
        T31.22
    30-39 percent T31.30
      with 0-9 percent third degree burns
        T31.30
      with 10-19 percent third degree burns
        T31.31

◀ New   ◀▥ Revised   ~~deleted~~ Deleted

Burn *(Continued)*
  extent *(Continued)*
    30-39 percent *(Continued)*
      with 20-29 percent third degree burns T31.32
      with 30-39 percent third degree burns T31.33
    40-49 percent T31.40
      with 0-9 percent third degree burns T31.40
      with 10-19 percent third degree burns T31.41
      with 20-29 percent third degree burns T31.42
      with 30-39 percent third degree burns T31.43
      with 40-49 percent third degree burns T31.44
    50-59 percent T31.50
      with 0-9 percent third degree burns T31.50
      with 10-19 percent third degree burns T31.51
      with 20-29 percent third degree burns T31.52
      with 30-39 percent third degree burns T31.53
      with 40-49 percent third degree burns T31.54
      with 50-59 percent third degree burns T31.55
    60-69 percent T31.60
      with 0-9 percent third degree burns T31.60
      with 10-19 percent third degree burns T31.61
      with 20-29 percent third degree burns T31.62
      with 30-39 percent third degree burns T31.63
      with 40-49 percent third degree burns T31.64
      with 50-59 percent third degree burns T31.65
      with 60-69 percent third degree burns T31.66
    70-79 percent T31.70
      with 0-9 percent third degree burns T31.70
      with 10-19 percent third degree burns T31.71
      with 20-29 percent third degree burns T31.72
      with 30-39 percent third degree burns T31.73
      with 40-49 percent third degree burns T31.74
      with 50-59 percent third degree burns T31.75
      with 60-69 percent third degree burns T31.76
      with 70-79 percent third degree burns T31.77
    80-89 percent T31.80
      with 0-9 percent third degree burns T31.80
      with 10-19 percent third degree burns T31.81
      with 20-29 percent third degree burns T31.82
      with 30-39 percent third degree burns T31.83
      with 40-49 percent third degree burns T31.84
      with 50-59 percent third degree burns T31.85
      with 60-69 percent third degree burns T31.86
      with 70-79 percent third degree burns T31.87
      with 80-89 percent third degree burns T31.88
    90 percent or more T31.90
      with 0-9 percent third degree burns T31.90
      with 10-19 percent third degree burns T31.91

Burn *(Continued)*
  extent *(Continued)*
    90 percent or more *(Continued)*
      with 20-29 percent third degree burns T31.92
      with 30-39 percent third degree burns T31.93
      with 40-49 percent third degree burns T31.94
      with 50-59 percent third degree burns T31.95
      with 60-69 percent third degree burns T31.96
      with 70-79 percent third degree burns T31.97
      with 80-89 percent third degree burns T31.98
      with 90 percent or more third degree burns T31.99
  extremity —*see* Burn, limb
  eye (s) and adnexa T26.4-
    with resulting rupture and destruction of eyeball T26.2-
    conjunctival sac —*see* Burn, cornea
    cornea —*see* Burn, cornea
    lid —*see* Burn, eyelid
    periocular area —*see* Burn, eyelid
    specified site NEC T26.3-
  eyeball —*see* Burn, eye
  eyelid (s) T26.0-
    chemical —*see* Corrosion, eyelid
  face —*see* Burn, head
  finger T23.029
    first degree T23.129
    left T23.022
      first degree T23.122
      second degree T23.222
      third degree T23.322
    multiple sites (without thumb) T23.039
      with thumb T23.049
        first degree T23.149
        left T23.042
          first degree T23.142
          second degree T23.242
          third degree T23.342
        right T23.041
          first degree T23.141
          second degree T23.241
          third degree T23.341
      second degree T23.249
      third degree T23.349
    first degree T23.139
    left T23.032
      first degree T23.132
      second degree T23.232
      third degree T23.332
    right T23.031
      first degree T23.131
      second degree T23.231
      third degree T23.331
    second degree T23.239
    third degree T23.339
    right T23.021
      first degree T23.121
      second degree T23.221
      third degree T23.321
    second degree T23.229
    third degree T23.329
  flank —*see* Burn, abdominal wall
  foot T25.029
    first degree T25.129
    left T25.022
      first degree T25.122
      second degree T25.222
      third degree T25.322
    multiple with ankle —*see* Burn, lower, limb, multiple, ankle and foot
    right T25.021
      first degree T25.121
      second degree T25.221
      third degree T25.321

Burn *(Continued)*
  foot *(Continued)*
      second degree T25.229
      third degree T25.329
  forearm T22.019
    first degree T22.119
    left T22.012
      first degree T22.112
      second degree T22.212
      third degree T22.312
    right T22.011
      first degree T22.111
      second degree T22.211
      third degree T22.311
    second degree T22.219
    third degree T22.319
  forehead T20.06
    first degree T20.16
    second degree T20.26
    third degree T20.36
  fourth degree - code as Burn, third degree, by site
  friction —*see* Burn, by site
  from swallowing caustic or corrosive substance NEC —*see* Corrosion, by site
  full thickness skin loss - code as Burn, third degree, by site
  gastrointestinal tract NEC T28.2
    from swallowing caustic or corrosive substance T28.7
  genital organs
    external
      female T21.07
        first degree T21.17
        second degree T21.27
        third degree T21.37
      male T21.06
        first degree T21.16
        second degree T21.26
        third degree T21.36
    internal T28.3
      from caustic or corrosive substance T28.8
  groin —*see* Burn, abdominal wall
  hand (s) T23.009
    back —*see* Burn, dorsum of hand
    finger —*see* Burn, finger
    first degree T23.109
    left T23.002
      first degree T23.102
      second degree T23.202
      third degree T23.302
    multiple sites with wrist T23.099
      first degree T23.199
      left T23.092
        first degree T23.192
        second degree T23.292
        third degree T23.392
      right T23.091
        first degree T23.191
        second degree T23.291
        third degree T23.391
      second degree T23.299
      third degree T23.399
    palm —*see* Burn, palm
    right T23.001
      first degree T23.101
      second degree T23.201
      third degree T23.301
    second degree T23.209
    third degree T23.309
    thumb —*see* Burn, thumb
  head (and face) (and neck) T20.00
    cheek —*see* Burn, cheek
    chin —*see* Burn, chin
    ear —*see* Burn, ear
    eye (s) only —*see* Burn, eye
    first degree T20.10
    forehead —*see* Burn, forehead
    lip —*see* Burn, lip

Burn (Continued)

head (Continued)

multiple sites T20.09

first degree T20.19

second degree T20.29

third degree T20.39

neck —see Burn, neck

nose —see Burn, nose

scalp —see Burn, scalp

second degree T20.20

third degree T20.30

hip (s) —see Burn, lower, limb

inhalation —see Burn, respiratory tract

caustic or corrosive substance (fumes) —see
Corrosion, respiratory tract

internal organ (s) T28.40

alimentary tract T28.2

esophagus T28.1

eardrum T28.41

esophagus T28.1

from caustic or corrosive substance
(swallowing) NEC —see Corrosion,
by site

genitourinary T28.3

mouth T28.0

pharynx T28.0

respiratory tract —see Burn, respiratory
tract

specified organ NEC T28.49

interscapular region —see Burn, back, upper

intestine (large) (small) T28.2

knee T24.029

first degree T24.129

left T24.022

first degree T24.122

second degree T24.222

third degree T24.322

right T24.021

first degree T24.121

second degree T24.221

third degree T24.321

second degree T24.229

third degree T24.329

labium (majus) (minus) —see Burn, genital
organs, external, female

lacrimal apparatus, duct, gland or sac —see
Burn, eye, specified site NEC

larynx T27.0

with lung T27.1

leg (s) (lower) (upper) —see Burn, lower,
limb

lightning —see Burn, by site

limb (s)

lower (except ankle or foot alone) —see
Burn, lower, limb

upper —see Burn, upper limb

lip (s) T20.02

first degree T20.12

second degree T20.22

third degree T20.32

lower

back —see Burn, back

limb T24.009

ankle —see Burn, ankle

calf —see Burn, calf

first degree T24.109

foot —see Burn, foot

hip —see Burn, thigh

knee —see Burn, knee

left T24.002

first degree T24.102

second degree T24.202

third degree T24.302

multiple sites, except ankle and foot
T24.099

ankle and foot T25.099

first degree T25.199

left T25.092

first degree T25.192

second degree T25.292

third degree T25.392

Burn (Continued)

lower (Continued)

limb (Continued)

multiple sites, except ankle and foot
(Continued)

ankle and foot (Continued)

right T25.091

first degree T25.191

second degree
T25.291

third degree T25.391

second degree T25.299

third degree T25.399

first degree T24.199

left T24.092

first degree T24.192

second degree T24.292

third degree T24.392

right T24.091

first degree T24.191

second degree
T24.291

third degree T24.391

second degree T24.299

third degree T24.399

right T24.001

first degree T24.101

second degree T24.201

third degree T24.301

second degree T24.209

thigh —see Burn, thigh

third degree T24.309

toe —see Burn, toe

lung (with larynx and trachea)
T27.1

mouth T28.0

neck T20.07

first degree T20.17

second degree T20.27

third degree T20.37

nose (septum) T20.04

first degree T20.14

second degree T20.24

third degree T20.34

ocular adnexa —see Burn, eye

orbit region —see Burn, eyelid

palm T23.059

first degree T23.159

left T23.052

first degree T23.152

second degree T23.252

third degree T23.352

right T23.051

first degree T23.151

second degree T23.251

third degree T23.351

second degree T23.259

third degree T23.359

partial thickness - code as Burn,
unspecified degree, by site

pelvis —see Burn, trunk

penis —see Burn, genital organs,
external, male

perineum

female —see Burn, genital organs,
external, female

male —see Burn, genital organs,
external, male

periocular area —see Burn, eyelid

pharynx T28.0

rectum T28.2

respiratory tract T27.3

larynx —see Burn, larynx

specified part NEC T27.2

trachea —see Burn, trachea

sac, lacrimal —see Burn, eye, specified site
NEC

scalp T20.05

first degree T20.15

second degree T20.25

third degree T20.35

Burn (Continued)

scapular region T22.069

first degree T22.169

left T22.062

first degree T22.162

second degree T22.262

third degree T22.362

right T22.061

first degree T22.161

second degree T22.261

third degree T22.361

second degree T22.269

third degree T22.369

sclera —see Burn, eye, specified site NEC

scrotum —see Burn, genital organs, external,
male

shoulder T22.059

first degree T22.159

left T22.052

first degree T22.152

second degree T22.252

third degree T22.352

right T22.051

first degree T22.151

second degree T22.251

third degree T22.351

second degree T22.259

third degree T22.359

stomach T28.2

temple —see Burn, head

testis —see Burn, genital organs, external, male

thigh T24.019

first degree T24.119

left T24.012

first degree T24.112

second degree T24.212

third degree T24.312

right T24.011

first degree T24.111

second degree T24.211

third degree T24.311

second degree T24.219

third degree T24.319

thorax (external) —see Burn, trunk

throat (meaning pharynx) T28.0

thumb (s) T23.019

first degree T23.119

left T23.012

first degree T23.112

second degree T23.212

third degree T23.312

multiple sites with fingers T23.049

first degree T23.149

left T23.042

first degree T23.142

second degree T23.242

third degree T23.342

right T23.041

first degree T23.141

second degree T23.241

third degree T23.341

second degree T23.249

third degree T23.349

right T23.011

first degree T23.111

second degree T23.211

third degree T23.311

second degree T23.219

third degree T23.319

toe T25.039

first degree T25.139

left T25.032

first degree T25.132

second degree T25.232

third degree T25.332

right T25.031

first degree T25.131

second degree T25.231

third degree T25.331

second degree T25.239

third degree T25.339

◀ New ◀ Revised ~~deleted~~ Deleted

Burn (Continued)
  tongue T28.0
  tonsil (s) T28.0
  trachea T27.0
    with lung T27.1
  trunk T21.00
    abdominal wall —see Burn, abdominal
      wall
    anus —see Burn, buttock
    axilla —see Burn, upper limb
    back —see Burn, back
    breast —see Burn, chest wall
    buttock —see Burn, buttock
    chest wall —see Burn, chest wall
    first degree T21.10
    flank —see Burn, abdominal wall
    genital
      female —see Burn, genital organs,
        external, female
      male —see Burn, genital organs, external,
        male
    groin —see Burn, abdominal wall
    interscapular region —see Burn, back,
      upper
    labia —see Burn, genital organs, external,
      female
    lower back —see Burn, back
    penis —see Burn, genital organs, external,
      male
    perineum
      female —see Burn, genital organs,
        external, female
      male —see Burn, genital organs, external,
        male
    scapula region —see Burn, scapular
      region
    scrotum —see Burn, genital organs,
      external, male
    second degree T21.20
    specified site NEC T21.09
      first degree T21.19
      second degree T21.29
      third degree T21.39
    testes —see Burn, genital organs, external,
      male
    third degree T21.30
    upper back —see Burn, back, upper
    vulva —see Burn, genital organs, external,
      female
  unspecified site with extent of body surface
    involved specified
    less than 10 percent T31.0
    10-19 percent (0-9 percent third degree)
      T31.10
      with 10-19 percent third degree T31.11
    20-29 percent (0-9 percent third degree)
      T31.20
      with
        10-19 percent third degree T31.21
        20-29 percent third degree T31.22
    30-39 percent (0-9 percent third degree)
      T31.30
      with
        10-19 percent third degree T31.31
        20-29 percent third degree T31.32
        30-39 percent third degree T31.33
    40-49 percent (0-9 percent third degree)
      T31.40
      with
        10-19 percent third degree T31.41
        20-29 percent third degree T31.42
        30-39 percent third degree T31.43
        40-49 percent third degree T31.44
    50-59 percent (0-9 percent third degree)
      T31.50
      with
        10-19 percent third degree T31.51
        20-29 percent third degree T31.52
        30-39 percent third degree T31.53
        40-49 percent third degree T31.54
        50-59 percent third degree T31.55

Burn (Continued)
  unspecified site with extent of body surface
    involved specified (Continued)
    60-69 percent (0-9 percent third degree)
      T31.60
      with
        10-19 percent third degree T31.61
        20-29 percent third degree T31.62
        30-39 percent third degree T31.63
        40-49 percent third degree T31.64
        50-59 percent third degree T31.65
        60-69 percent third degree T31.66
    70-79 percent (0-9 percent third degree)
      T31.70
      with
        10-19 percent third degree T31.71
        20-29 percent third degree T31.72
        30-39 percent third degree T31.73
        40-49 percent third degree T31.74
        50-59 percent third degree T31.75
        60-69 percent third degree T31.76
        70-79 percent third degree T31.77
    80-89 percent (0-9 percent third degree)
      T31.80
      with
        10-19 percent third degree T31.81
        20-29 percent third degree T31.82
        30-39 percent third degree T31.83
        40-49 percent third degree T31.84
        50-59 percent third degree T31.85
        60-69 percent third degree T31.86
        70-79 percent third degree T31.87
        80-89 percent third degree T31.88
    90 percent or more (0-9 percent third
      degree) T31.90
      with
        10-19 percent third degree T31.91
        20-29 percent third degree T31.92
        30-39 percent third degree T31.93
        40-49 percent third degree T31.94
        50-59 percent third degree T31.95
        60-69 percent third degree T31.96
        70-79 percent third degree T31.97
        80-89 percent third degree T31.98
        90-99 percent third degree T31.99
  upper limb T22.00
    above elbow —see Burn, above elbow
    axilla —see Burn, axilla
    elbow —see Burn, elbow
    first degree T22.10
    forearm —see Burn, forearm
    hand —see Burn, hand
    interscapular region —see Burn, back,
      upper
    multiple sites T22.099
      first degree T22.199
      left T22.092
        first degree T22.192
        second degree T22.292
        third degree T22.392
      right T22.091
        first degree T22.191
        second degree T22.291
        third degree T22.391
      second degree T22.299
      third degree T22.399
    scapular region —see Burn, scapular region
    second degree T22.20
    shoulder —see Burn, shoulder
    third degree T22.30
    wrist —see Burn, wrist
  uterus T28.3
  vagina T28.3
  vulva —see Burn, genital organs, external,
    female
  wrist T23.079
    first degree T23.179
    left T23.072
      first degree T23.172
      second degree T23.272
      third degree T23.372

Burn (Continued)
  wrist (Continued)
    multiple sites with hand T23.099
      first degree T23.199
      left T23.092
        first degree T23.192
        second degree T23.292
        third degree T23.392
      right T23.091
        first degree T23.191
        second degree T23.291
        third degree T23.391
      second degree T23.299
      third degree T23.399
    right T23.071
      first degree T23.171
      second degree T23.271
      third degree T23.371
    second degree T23.279
    third degree T23.379
Burnett's syndrome E83.52
Burning
  feet syndrome E53.9
  sensation R20.8
  tongue K14.6
Burn-out (state) Z73.0
Burns' disease or osteochondrosis —see
  Osteochondrosis, juvenile, ulna
Bursa —see condition
Bursitis M71.9
  Achilles —see Tendinitis, Achilles
  adhesive —see Bursitis, specified NEC
  ankle —see Enthesopathy, lower limb, ankle,
    specified type NEC
  calcaneal —see Enthesopathy, foot, specified
    type NEC
  collateral ligament, tibial —see Bursitis, tibial
    collateral
  due to use, overuse, pressure —see also
    Disorder, soft tissue, due to use,
    specified type NEC
    specified NEC —see Disorder, soft tissue,
      due to use, specified NEC
  Duplay's M75.0
  elbow NEC M70.3-
    olecranon M70.2-
  finger —see Disorder, soft tissue, due to use,
    specified type NEC, hand
  foot —see Enthesopathy, foot, specified type
    NEC
  gonococcal A54.49
  gouty —see Gout, idiopathic
  hand M70.1-
  hip NEC M70.7-
    trochanteric M70.6-
  infective NEC M71.10
    abscess —see Abscess, bursa
    ankle M71.17-
    elbow M71.12-
    foot M71.17-
    hand M71.14-
    hip M71.15-
    knee M71.16-
    multiple sites M71.19
    shoulder M71.11-
    specified site NEC M71.18
    wrist M71.13-
  ischial —see Bursitis, hip
  knee NEC M70.5-
    prepatellar M70.4-
  occupational NEC —see also Disorder, soft
    tissue, due to, use
  olecranon —see Bursitis, elbow, olecranon
  pharyngeal J39.1
  popliteal —see Bursitis, knee
  prepatellar M70.4-
  radiohumeral M77.8
  rheumatoid M06.20
    ankle M06.27-
    elbow M06.22-
    foot joint M06.27-

Bursitis *(Continued)*
  rheumatoid *(Continued)*
    hand joint M06.24-
    hip M06.25-
    knee M06.26-
    multiple site M06.29
    shoulder M06.21-
    vertebra M06.28
    wrist M06.23-
  scapulohumeral —*see* Bursitis, shoulder
  semimembranous muscle (knee) —*see*
      Bursitis, knee
  shoulder M75.5-
    adhesive —*see* Capsulitis, adhesive
  specified NEC M71.50
    ankle M71.57-
    due to use, overuse or pressure —*see*
        Disorder, soft tissue, due to, use
    elbow M71.52-
    foot M71.57-
    hand M71.54-
    hip M71.55-
    knee M71.56-
    shoulder —*see* Bursitis, shoulder
    specified site NEC M71.58

Bursitis *(Continued)*
  specified NEC *(Continued)*
    tibial collateral M76.4-
    wrist M71.53-
  subacromial —*see* Bursitis, shoulder
  subcoracoid —*see* Bursitis, shoulder
  subdeltoid —*see* Bursitis, shoulder
  syphilitic A52.78
  Thornwaldt, Tornwaldt J39.2
  tibial collateral —*see* Bursitis, tibial collateral
  toe —*see* Enthesopathy, foot, specified type
      NEC
  trochanteric (area) —*see* Bursitis, hip,
      trochanteric
  wrist —*see* Bursitis, hand
Bursopathy M71.9
  specified type NEC M71.80
    ankle M71.87-
    elbow M71.82-
    foot M71.87-
    hand M71.84-
    hip M71.85-
    knee M71.86-
    multiple sites M71.89
    shoulder M71.81-

Bursopathy *(Continued)*
  specified type NEC *(Continued)*
    specified site NEC M71.88
    wrist M71.83-
Burst stitches or sutures (complication of
    surgery) T81.31
  external operation wound T81.31
  internal operation wound T81.32
Buruli ulcer A31.1
Bury's disease L95.1
Buschke's
  disease B45.3
  scleredema —*see* Sclerosis, systemic
Busse-Buschke disease B45.3
Buttock —*see* condition
Button
  Biskra B55.1
  Delhi B55.1
  oriental B55.1
Buttonhole deformity (finger) —*see* Deformity,
    finger, boutonniere
Bwamba fever A92.8
Byssinosis J66.0
Bywaters' syndrome T79.5

C

Cachexia R64
 cancerous R64
 cardiac —see Disease, heart
 dehydration E86.0
  with
   hypernatremia E87.0
   hyponatremia E87.1
  due to malnutrition R64
 exophthalmic —see Hyperthyroidism
 heart —see Disease, heart
 hypophyseal E23.0
 hypopituitary E23.0
 lead —see Poisoning, lead
 malignant R64
 marsh —see Malaria
 nervous F48.8
 old age R54
 paludal —see Malaria
 pituitary E23.0
 renal N28.9
 saturnine —see Poisoning, lead
 senile R54
 Simmonds' E23.0
 splenica D73.0
 strumipriva E03.4
 tuberculous NEC —see Tuberculosis
Café au lait spots L81.3
Caffey's syndrome Q78.8
Caisson disease T70.3
Cake kidney Q63.1
Caked breast (puerperal, postpartum)
  O92.79
Calabar swelling B74.3
Calcaneal spur —see Spur, bone, calcaneal
Calcaneo-apophysitis M92.8
Calcareous —see condition
Calcicosis J62.8
Calciferol (vitamin D) deficiency E55.9
 with rickets E55.0
Calcification
 adrenal (capsule) (gland) E27.49
  tuberculous E35 [B90.8]
 aorta I70.0
 artery (annular) —see Arteriosclerosis
 auricle (ear) —see Disorder, pinna, specified
  type NEC
 basal ganglia G23.8
 bladder N32.89
  due to Schistosoma hematobium B65.0
 brain (cortex) —see Calcification, cerebral
 bronchus J98.09
 bursa M71.40
  ankle M71.47-
  elbow M71.42-
  foot M71.47-
  hand M71.44-
  hip M71.45-
  knee M71.46-
  multiple sites M71.49
  shoulder M75.3-
  specified site NEC M71.48
  wrist M71.43-
 cardiac —see Degeneration, myocardial
 cerebral (cortex) G93.89
  artery I67.2
 cervix (uteri) N88.8
 choroid plexus G93.89
 conjunctiva —see Concretion, conjunctiva
 corpora cavernosa (penis) N48.89
 cortex (brain) —see Calcification, cerebral
 dental pulp (nodular) K04.2
 dentinal papilla K00.4
 fallopian tube N83.8
 falx cerebri G96.19
 gallbladder K82.8
 general E83.59
 heart —see also Degeneration, myocardial
  valve —see Endocarditis
 idiopathic infantile arterial (IIAC) Q28.8

Calcification (Continued)
 intervertebral cartilage or disc
  (postinfective) —see Disorder, disc,
  specified NEC
 intracranial —see Calcification, cerebral
 joint —see Disorder, joint, specified type
  NEC
 kidney N28.89
  tuberculous N29 [B90.1]
 larynx (senile) J38.7
 lens —see Cataract, specified NEC
 lung (active) (postinfectional) J98.4
  tuberculous B90.9
 lymph gland or node (postinfectional) I89.8
  tuberculous (see also Tuberculosis, lymph
  gland) B90.8
 mammographic R92.1
 massive (paraplegic) —see Myositis,
  ossificans, in, quadriplegia
 medial —see Arteriosclerosis, extremities
 meninges (cerebral) (spinal) G96.19
 metastatic E83.59
 Mönckeberg's —see Arteriosclerosis,
  extremities
 muscle M61.9
  due to burns —see Myositis, ossificans, in,
  burns
  paralytic —see Myositis, ossificans, in,
  quadriplegia
  specified type NEC M61.40
   ankle M61.47-
   foot M61.47-
   forearm M61.43-
   hand M61.44-
   lower leg M61.46-
   multiple sites M61.49
   pelvic region M61.45-
   shoulder region M61.41-
   specified site NEC M61.48
   thigh M61.45-
   upper arm M61.42-
 myocardium, myocardial —see Degeneration,
  myocardial
 ovary N83.8
 pancreas K86.8
 penis N48.89
 periarticular —see Disorder, joint, specified
  type NEC
 pericardium (see also Pericarditis) I31.1
 pineal gland E34.8
 pleura J94.8
  postinfectional J94.8
  tuberculous NEC B90.9
 pulpal (dental) (nodular) K04.2
 sclera H15.89
 spleen D73.89
 subcutaneous L94.2
 suprarenal (capsule) (gland) E27.49
 tendon (sheath) —see also Tenosynovitis,
  specified type NEC
  with bursitis, synovitis or tenosynovitis —
  see Tendinitis, calcific
 trachea J39.8
 ureter N28.89
 vitreous —see Deposit, crystalline
Calcified —see Calcification
Calcinosis (interstitial) (tumoral) (universalis)
  E83.59
 with Raynaud's phenomenon, esophageal
  dysfunction, sclerodactyly,
  telangiectasia (CREST syndrome)
  M34.1
 circumscripta (skin) L94.2
 cutis L94.2
Calciphylaxis (see also Calcification, by site)
  E83.59
Calcium
 deposits —see Calcification, by site
 metabolism disorder E83.50
 salts or soaps in vitreous —see Deposit,
  crystalline

Calciuria R82.99
Calculi —see Calculus
Calculosis, intrahepatic —see Calculus, bile
  duct
Calculus, calculi, calculous
 ampulla of Vater —see Calculus, bile duct
 anuria (impacted) (recurrent) (see also
  Calculus, urinary) N20.9
 appendix K38.1
 bile duct (common) (hepatic) K80.50
  with
   calculus of gallbladder —see Calculus,
   gallbladder and bile duct
   cholangitis K80.30
    with
     cholecystitis —see Calculus, bile
     duct, with cholecystitis
     obstruction K80.31
    acute K80.32
     with
      chronic cholangitis K80.36
       with obstruction K80.37
      obstruction K80.33
    chronic K80.34
     with
      acute cholangitis K80.36
       with obstruction K80.37
      obstruction K80.35
   cholecystitis (with cholangitis) K80.40
    with obstruction K80.41
    acute K80.42
     with
      chronic cholecystitis K80.46
       with obstruction K80.47
      obstruction K80.43
    chronic K80.44
     with
      acute cholecystitis K80.46
       with obstruction K80.47
      obstruction K80.45
   obstruction K80.51
  biliary —see also Calculus, gallbladder
   specified NEC K80.80
    with obstruction K80.81
  bilirubin, multiple —see Calculus,
   gallbladder
  bladder (encysted) (impacted) (urinary)
   (diverticulum) N21.0
  bronchus J98.09
  calyx (kidney) (renal) —see Calculus, kidney
  cholesterol (pure) (solitary) —see Calculus,
   gallbladder
  common duct (bile) —see Calculus, bile duct
  conjunctiva —see Concretion, conjunctiva
  cystic N21.0
   duct —see Calculus, gallbladder
  dental (subgingival) (supragingival)
   K03.6
  diverticulum
   bladder N21.0
   kidney N20.0
  epididymis N50.8
  gallbladder K80.20
   with
    bile duct calculus —see Calculus,
    gallbladder and bile duct
    cholecystitis K80.10
     with obstruction K80.11
     acute K80.00
      with
       chronic cholecystitis K80.12
        with obstruction K80.13
       obstruction K80.01
     chronic K80.10
      with
       acute cholecystitis K80.12
        with obstruction K80.13
       obstruction K80.11
     specified NEC K80.18
      with obstruction K80.19
     obstruction K80.21

Calculus, calculi, calculous *(Continued)*
  gallbladder and bile duct K80.70
    with
      cholecystitis K80.60
        with obstruction K80.61
        acute K80.62
          with
            chronic cholecystitis K80.66
              with obstruction K80.67
            obstruction K80.63
          chronic K80.64
            with
              acute cholecystitis K80.66
                with obstruction K80.67
              obstruction K80.65
      obstruction K80.71
  hepatic (duct) —*see* Calculus, bile duct
  hepatobiliary K80.80
    with obstruction K80.81
  ileal conduit N21.8
  intestinal (impaction) (obstruction) K56.49
  kidney (impacted) (multiple) (pelvis)
      (recurrent) (staghorn) N20.0
    with calculus, ureter N20.2
    congenital Q63.8
  lacrimal passages —*see* Dacryolith
  liver (impacted) —*see* Calculus, bile duct
  lung J98.4
  mammographic R92.1
  nephritic (impacted) (recurrent) —*see*
      Calculus, kidney
  nose J34.89
  pancreas (duct) K86.8
  parotid duct or gland K11.5
  pelvis, encysted —*see* Calculus, kidney
  prostate N42.0
  pulmonary J98.4
  pyelitis (impacted) (recurrent) N20.0
    with hydronephrosis N13.2
  pyelonephritis (impacted) (recurrent) —*see*
      category N20
    with hydronephrosis N13.2
  renal (impacted) (recurrent) —*see* Calculus,
      kidney
  salivary (duct) (gland) K11.5
  seminal vesicle N50.8
  staghorn —*see* Calculus, kidney
  Stensen's duct K11.5
  stomach K31.89
  sublingual duct or gland K11.5
    congenital Q38.4
  submandibular duct, gland or region K11.5
  submaxillary duct, gland or region K11.5
  suburethral N21.8
  tonsil J35.8
  tooth, teeth (subgingival) (supragingival)
      K03.6
  tunica vaginalis N50.8
  ureter (impacted) (recurrent) N20.1
    with calculus, kidney N20.2
      with hydronephrosis N13.2
        with infection N13.6
  urethra (impacted) N21.1
  urinary (duct) (impacted) (passage) (tract)
      N20.9
    with hydronephrosis N13.2
      with infection N13.6
    in (due to)
      lower N21.9
        specified NEC N21.8
  vagina N89.8
  vesical (impacted) N21.0
  Wharton's duct K11.5
  xanthine E79.8 *[N22]*
Calicectasis N28.89
Caliectasis N28.89
California
  disease B38.9
  encephalitis A83.5
Caligo cornea —*see* Opacity, cornea, central
Callositas, callosity (infected) L84

Callus (infected) L84
  bone —*see* Osteophyte
    excessive, following fracture - code as
        Sequelae of fracture
Calorie deficiency or malnutrition *(see also*
    Malnutrition) E46
Calvé-Perthes disease —*see* Legg-Calve-Perthes
    disease
Calvé's disease —*see* Osteochondrosis, juvenile,
    spine
Calvities —*see* Alopecia, androgenic
Cameroon fever —*see* Malaria
Camptocormia (hysterical) F44.4
Camurati-Engelmann syndrome Q78.3
Canal —*see also* condition
  atrioventricular common Q21.2
Canaliculitis (lacrimal) (acute) (subacute)
    H04.33-
  Actinomyces A42.89
  chronic H04.42-
Canavan's disease E75.29
Canceled procedure (surgical) Z53.9
  because of
    contraindication Z53.09
      smoking Z53.01
    left against medical advice (AMA) Z53.21
    patient's decision Z53.20
      for reasons of belief or group pressure
          Z53.1
      specified reason NEC Z53.29
    specified reason NEC Z53.8
Cancer —*see also* Neoplasm, by site, malignant
  bile duct type, liver C22.1
  blood —*see* Leukemia
  breast *(see also* Neoplasm, breast, malignant)
      C50.91-
  hepatocellular C22.0
  lung *(see also* Neoplasm, lung, malignant)
      C34.90-
  ovarian *(see also* Neoplasm, ovary, malignant)
      C56.9-
  unspecified site (primary) C80.1
Cancer (o)phobia F45.29
Cancerous —*see* Neoplasm, malignant, by site
Cancrum oris A69.0
Candidiasis, candidal B37.9
  balanitis B37.42
  bronchitis B37.1
  cheilitis B37.83
  congenital P37.5
  cystitis B37.41
  disseminated B37.7
  endocarditis B37.6
  enteritis B37.82
  esophagitis B37.81
  intertrigo B37.2
  lung B37.1
  meningitis B37.5
  mouth B37.0
  nails B37.2
  neonatal P37.5
  onychia B37.2
  oral B37.0
  osteomyelitis B37.89
  otitis externa B37.84
  paronychia B37.2
  perionyxis B37.2
  pneumonia B37.1
  proctitis B37.82
  pulmonary B37.1
  pyelonephritis B37.49
  sepsis B37.7
  skin B37.2
  specified site NEC B37.89
  stomatitis B37.0
  systemic B37.7
  urethritis B37.41
  urogenital site NEC B37.49
  vagina B37.3
  vulva B37.3
  vulvovaginitis B37.3

Candidid L30.2
Candidosis —*see* Candidiasis
Candiru infection or infestation B88.8
Canities (premature) L67.1
  congenital Q84.2
Canker (mouth) (sore) K12.0
  rash A38.9
Cannabinosis J66.2
Canton fever A75.9
Cantrell's syndrome Q87.89
Capillariasis (intestinal) B81.1
  hepatic B83.8
Capillary —*see* condition
Caplan's syndrome —*see* Rheumatoid, lung
Capsule —*see* condition
Capsulitis (joint) —*see also* Enthesopathy
  adhesive (shoulder) M75.0-
  hepatic K65.8
  labyrinthine —*see* Otosclerosis, specified NEC
  thyroid E06.9
Caput
  crepitus Q75.8
  medusae I86.8
  succedaneum P12.81
Car sickness T75.3
Carapata (disease) A68.0
Carate —*see* Pinta
Carbon lung J60
Carbuncle L02.93
  abdominal wall L02.231
  anus K61.0
  auditory canal, external —*see* Abscess, ear,
      external
  auricle ear —*see* Abscess, ear, external
  axilla L02.43-
  back (any part) L02.232
  breast N61
  buttock L02.33
  cheek (external) L02.03
  chest wall L02.233
  chin L02.03
  corpus cavernosum N48.21
  ear (any part) (external) (middle) —*see*
      Abscess, ear, external
  external auditory canal —*see* Abscess, ear,
      external
  eyelid —*see* Abscess, eyelid
  face NEC L02.03
  femoral (region) —*see* Carbuncle, lower limb
  finger —*see* Carbuncle, hand
  flank L02.231
  foot L02.63-
  forehead L02.03
  genital —*see* Abscess, genital
  gluteal (region) L02.33
  groin L02.234
  hand L02.53-
  head NEC L02.831
  heel —*see* Carbuncle, foot
  hip —*see* Carbuncle, lower limb
  kidney —*see* Abscess, kidney
  knee —*see* Carbuncle, lower limb
  labium (majus) (minus) N76.4
  lacrimal
    gland —*see* Dacryoadenitis
    passages (duct) (sac) —*see* Inflammation,
        lacrimal, passages, acute
  leg —*see* Carbuncle, lower limb
  lower limb L02.43-
  malignant A22.0
  navel L02.236
  neck L02.13
  nose (external) (septum) J34.0
  orbit, orbital —*see* Abscess, orbit
  palmar (space) —*see* Carbuncle, hand
  partes posteriores L02.33
  pectoral region L02.233
  penis N48.21
  perineum L02.235
  pinna —*see* Abscess, ear, external
  popliteal —*see* Carbuncle, lower limb

◀ New   ◀▥ Revised   ~~deleted~~ Deleted

Carbuncle *(Continued)*
  scalp L02.831
  seminal vesicle N49.0
  shoulder —*see* Carbuncle, upper limb
  specified site NEC L02.838
  temple (region) L02.03
  thumb —*see* Carbuncle, hand
  toe —*see* Carbuncle, foot
  trunk L02.239
    abdominal wall L02.231
    back L02.232
    chest wall L02.233
    groin L02.234
    perineum L02.235
    umbilicus L02.236
  umbilicus L02.236
  upper limb L02.43-
  urethra N34.0
  vulva N76.4
Carbunculus —*see* Carbuncle
Carcinoid (tumor) —*see* Tumor, carcinoid
Carcinoidosis E34.0
Carcinoma (malignant) —*see also* Neoplasm, by
    site, malignant
  acidophil
    specified site —*see* Neoplasm, malignant,
      by site
    unspecified site C75.1
  acidophil-basophil, mixed
    specified site —*see* Neoplasm, malignant,
      by site
    unspecified site C75.1
  adnexal (skin) —*see* Neoplasm, skin,
    malignant
  adrenal cortical C74.0-
  alveolar —*see* Neoplasm, lung, malignant
    cell —*see* Neoplasm, lung, malignant
  ameloblastic C41.1
    upper jaw (bone) C41.0
  apocrine
    breast —*see* Neoplasm, breast, malignant
    specified site NEC —*see* Neoplasm, skin,
      malignant
    unspecified site C44.99
  basal cell (pigmented) (*see also* Neoplasm,
    skin, malignant) C44.91
    fibro-epithelial —*see* Neoplasm, skin,
      malignant
    morphea —*see* Neoplasm, skin, malignant
    multicentric —*see* Neoplasm, skin,
      malignant
  basaloid
  basal-squamous cell, mixed —*see* Neoplasm,
    skin, malignant
  basophil
    specified site —*see* Neoplasm, malignant,
      by site
    unspecified site C75.1
  basophil-acidophil, mixed
    specified site —*see* Neoplasm, malignant,
      by site
    unspecified site C75.1
  basosquamous —*see* Neoplasm, skin,
    malignant
  bile duct
    with hepatocellular, mixed C22.0
    liver C22.1
    specified site NEC —*see* Neoplasm,
      malignant, by site
    unspecified site C22.1
  branchial or branchiogenic C10.4
  bronchial or bronchogenic —*see* Neoplasm,
    lung, malignant
  bronchiolar —*see* Neoplasm, lung, malignant
  bronchioloalveolar —*see* Neoplasm, lung,
    malignant
  C cell
    specified site —*see* Neoplasm, malignant,
      by site
    unspecified site C73
  ceruminous C44.29-

Carcinoma *(Continued)*
  cervix uteri
    in situ D06.9
      endocervix D06.0
      exocervix D06.1
      specified site NEC D06.7
  chorionic
    specified site —*see* Neoplasm, malignant,
      by site
    unspecified site
      female C58
      male C62.90
  chromophobe
    specified site —*see* Neoplasm, malignant,
      by site
    unspecified site C75.1
  cloacogenic
    specified site —*see* Neoplasm, malignant,
      by site
    unspecified site C21.2
  diffuse type
    specified site —*see* Neoplasm, malignant,
      by site
    unspecified site C16.9
  duct (cell)
    with Paget's disease —*see* Neoplasm,
      breast, malignant
    infiltrating
      with lobular carcinoma (in situ)
        specified site —*see* Neoplasm,
          malignant, by site
        unspecified site (female) C50.91-
          male C50.92-
      specified site —*see* Neoplasm,
        malignant, by site
      unspecified site (female) C50.91-
        male C50.92-
  ductal
    with lobular
      specified site —*see* Neoplasm,
        malignant, by site
      unspecified site (female) C50.91-
        male C50.92-
  ductular, infiltrating
    specified site —*see* Neoplasm, malignant,
      by site
    unspecified site (female) C50.91-
      male C50.92-
  embryonal
    liver C22.7
  endometrioid
    specified site —*see* Neoplasm, malignant,
      by site
    unspecified site
      female C56.9
      male C61
  eosinophil
    specified site —*see* Neoplasm, malignant,
      by site
    unspecified site C75.1
  epidermoid —*see also* Neoplasm, skin
      malignant
    in situ, Bowen's type —*see* Neoplasm, skin,
      in situ
  fibroepithelial, basal cell —*see* Neoplasm,
    skin, malignant
  follicular
    with papillary (mixed) C73
    moderately differentiated C73
    pure follicle C73
    specified site —*see* Neoplasm, malignant,
      by site
    trabecular C73
    unspecified site C73
    well differentiated C73
  generalized, with unspecified primary site
    C80.0
  glycogen-rich —*see* Neoplasm, breast,
    malignant
  granulosa cell C56-
  hepatic cell C22.0

Carcinoma *(Continued)*
  hepatocellular C22.0
    with bile duct, mixed C22.0
    fibrolamellar C22.0
  hepatocholangiolitic C22.0
  Hurthle cell C73
  in
    adenomatous
      polyposis coli C18.9
    pleomorphic adenoma —*see* Neoplasm,
      salivary glands, malignant
    situ —*see* Carcinoma-in-situ
  infiltrating
    duct
      with lobular
        specified site —*see* Neoplasm,
          malignant, by site
        unspecified site (female) C50.91-
          male C50.92-
      with Paget's disease —*see* Neoplasm,
        breast, malignant
      specified site —*see* Neoplasm,
        malignant
      unspecified site (female) C50.91-
        male C50.92-
    ductular
      specified site —*see* Neoplasm,
        malignant
      unspecified site (female) C50.91-
        male C50.92-
    lobular
      specified site —*see* Neoplasm,
        malignant
      unspecified site (female) C50.91-
        male C50.92-
  inflammatory
    specified site —*see* Neoplasm, malignant
    unspecified site (female) C50.91-
      male C50.92-
  intestinal type
    specified site —*see* Neoplasm, malignant,
      by site
    unspecified site C16.9
  intracystic
    noninfiltrating —*see* Neoplasm, in situ,
      by site
  intraductal (noninfiltrating)
    with Paget's disease —*see* Neoplasm,
      breast, malignant
    breast D05.1-
    papillary
      with invasion
        specified site —*see* Neoplasm,
          malignant, by site
        unspecified site (female) C50.91-
          male C50.92-
      breast D05.1-
      specified site NEC —*see* Neoplasm,
        in situ, by site
      unspecified site (female) D05.1-
    specified site NEC —*see* Neoplasm,
      in situ, by site
    unspecified site (female) D05.1-
  intraepidermal —*see* Neoplasm, in situ
    squamous cell, Bowen's type —*see*
      Neoplasm, skin, in situ
  intraepithelial —*see* Neoplasm, in situ,
      by site
    squamous cell —*see* Neoplasm, in situ,
      by site
  intraosseous C41.1
    upper jaw (bone) C41.0
  islet cell
    with exocrine, mixed
      specified site —*see* Neoplasm,
        malignant, by site
      unspecified site C25.9
    pancreas C25.4
    specified site NEC —*see* Neoplasm,
      malignant, by site
    unspecified site C25.4

Carcinoma (Continued)
  juvenile, breast —see Neoplasm, breast,
      malignant
  large cell
    small cell
      specified site —see Neoplasm,
          malignant, by site
      unspecified site C34.90
  Leydig cell (testis)
    specified site —see Neoplasm, malignant,
        by site
    unspecified site
      female C56.9
      male C62.90
  lipid-rich (female) C50.91-
      male C50.92-
  liver cell C22.0
  liver NEC C22.7
  lobular (infiltrating)
    with intraductal
      specified site —see Neoplasm,
          malignant, by site
      unspecified site (female) C50.91-
          male C50.92-
    noninfiltrating
      breast D05.0-
      specified site NEC —see Neoplasm, in
          situ, by site
      unspecified site D05.0-
    specified site —see Neoplasm, malignant,
        by site
    unspecified site (female) C50.91-
        male C50.92-
  medullary
    with
      amyloid stroma
        specified site —see Neoplasm,
            malignant, by site
        unspecified site C73
      lymphoid stroma
        specified site —see Neoplasm,
            malignant, by site
        unspecified site (female) C50.91-
            male C50.92-
  Merkel cell C4A.9
    anal margin C4A.51
    anal skin C4A.51
    canthus C4A.1-
    ear and external auricular canal C4A.2-
    external auricular canal C4A.2-
    eyelid, including canthus C4A.1-
    face C4A.30
      specified NEC C4A.39
    hip C4A.7-
    lip C4A.0
    lower limb, including hip C4A.7-
    neck C4A.4
    nodal presentation C7B.1
    nose C4A.31
    overlapping sites C4A.8
    perianal skin C4A.51
    scalp C4A.4
    secondary C7B.1
    shoulder C4A.6-
    skin of breast C4A.52
    trunk NEC C4A.59
    upper limb, including shoulder C4A.6-
    visceral metastatic C7B.1
  metastatic —see Neoplasm, secondary
  metatypical —see Neoplasm, skin, malignant
  morphea, basal cell —see Neoplasm, skin,
      malignant
  mucoid
    cell
      specified site —see Neoplasm,
          malignant, by site
      unspecified site C75.1
  neuroendocrine —see also Tumor,
      neuroendocrine
    high grade, any site C7A.1
    poorly differentiated, any site C7A.1

Carcinoma (Continued)
  nonencapsulated sclerosing C73
  noninfiltrating
    intracystic —see Neoplasm, in situ, by site
    intraductal
      breast D05.1-
      papillary
        breast D05.1-
        specified site NEC —see Neoplasm, in
            situ, by site
        unspecified site D05.1-
      specified site —see Neoplasm, in situ,
          by site
      unspecified site D05.1-
    lobular
      breast D05.0-
      specified site NEC —see Neoplasm, in
          situ, by site
      unspecified site (female) D05.0-
  oat cell
    specified site —see Neoplasm, malignant,
        by site
    unspecified site C34.90
  odontogenic C41.1
    upper jaw (bone) C41.0
  papillary
    with follicular (mixed) C73
    follicular variant C73
    intraductal (noninfiltrating)
      with invasion
        specified site —see Neoplasm,
            malignant, by site
        unspecified site (female) C50.91-
            male C50.92-
      breast D05.1-
      specified site NEC —see Neoplasm, in
          situ, by site
      unspecified site D05.1-
    serous
      specified site —see Neoplasm,
          malignant, by site
      surface
        specified site —see Neoplasm,
            malignant, by site
        unspecified site C56.9
      unspecified site C56.9
  papillocystic
    specified site —see Neoplasm, malignant,
        by site
    unspecified site C56.9
  parafollicular cell
    specified site —see Neoplasm, malignant,
        by site
    unspecified site C73
  pilomatrix —see Neoplasm, skin, malignant
  pseudomucinous
    specified site —see Neoplasm, malignant,
        by site
    unspecified site C56.9
  renal cell C64-
  Schmincke —see Neoplasm, nasopharynx,
      malignant
  Schneiderian
    specified site —see Neoplasm, malignant,
        by site
    unspecified site C30.0
  sebaceous —see Neoplasm, skin, malignant
  secondary —see also Neoplasm, secondary,
      by site
    Merkel cell C7B.1
  secretory, breast —see Neoplasm, breast,
      malignant
  serous
    papillary
      specified site —see Neoplasm,
          malignant, by site
      unspecified site C56.9
    surface, papillary
      specified site —see Neoplasm,
          malignant, by site
      unspecified site C56.9

Carcinoma (Continued)
  Sertoli cell
    specified site —see Neoplasm, malignant,
        by site
    unspecified site C62.90
      female C56.9
      male C62.90
  skin appendage —see Neoplasm, skin,
      malignant
  small cell
    fusiform cell
      specified site —see Neoplasm,
          malignant, by site
      unspecified site C34.90
    intermediate cell
      specified site —see Neoplasm,
          malignant, by site
      unspecified site C34.90
    large cell
      specified site —see Neoplasm,
          malignant, by site
      unspecified site C34.90
  solid
    with amyloid stroma
      specified site —see Neoplasm,
          malignant, by site
      unspecified site C73
    microinvasive
      specified site —see Neoplasm,
          malignant, by site
      unspecified site C53.9
  sweat gland —see Neoplasm, skin,
      malignant
  theca cell C56.-
  thymic C37
  unspecified site (primary) C80.1
  water-clear cell C75.0
Carcinoma-in-situ —see also Neoplasm, in situ,
    by site
  breast NOS D05.9-
    specified type NEC D05.8-
  epidermoid —see also Neoplasm, in situ, by
      site
    with questionable stromal invasion
      cervix D06.9
      specified site NEC —see Neoplasm, in
          situ, by site
      unspecified site D06.9
    Bowen's type —see Neoplasm, skin,
        in situ
  intraductal
    breast D05.1-
    specified site NEC —see Neoplasm, in situ,
        by site
    unspecified site D05.1-
  lobular
    with
      infiltrating duct
        breast (female) C50.91-
            male C50.92-
        specified site NEC —see Neoplasm,
            malignant
        unspecified site (female) C50.91-
            male C50.92-
      intraductal
        breast D05.8-
        specified site NEC —see Neoplasm, in
            situ, by site
        unspecified site (female) D05.8-
    breast D05.0-
    specified site NEC —see Neoplasm, in situ,
        by site
    unspecified site D05.0-
  squamous cell —see also Neoplasm, in situ,
      by site
    with questionable stromal invasion
      cervix D06.9
      specified site NEC —see Neoplasm, in
          situ, by site
      unspecified site D06.9
Carcinomaphobia F45.29

Carcinomatosis C80.0
  peritonei C78.6
  unspecified site (primary) (secondary) C80.0
Carcinosarcoma —see Neoplasm, malignant,
    by site
  embryonal —see Neoplasm, malignant, by
    site
Cardia, cardial —see condition
Cardiac —see also condition
  death, sudden —see Arrest, cardiac
  pacemaker
    in situ Z95.0
      management or adjustment Z45.018
  tamponade I31.4
Cardialgia —see Pain, precordial
Cardiectasis —see Hypertrophy, cardiac
Cardiochalasia K21.9
Cardiomalacia I51.5
Cardiomegalia glycogenica diffusa E74.02 [I43]
Cardiomegaly —see also Hypertrophy, cardiac
  congenital Q24.8
  glycogen E74.02 [I43]
  idiopathic I51.7
Cardiomyoliposis I51.5
Cardiomyopathy (familial) (idiopathic) I42.9
  alcoholic I42.6
  amyloid E85.4 [I43]
  arteriosclerotic —see Disease, heart, ischemic,
    atherosclerotic
  beriberi E51.12
  cobalt-beer I42.6
  congenital I42.4
  congestive I42.0
  constrictive NOS I42.5
  dilated I42.0
  due to
    alcohol I42.6
    beriberi E51.12
    cardiac glycogenosis E74.02 [I43]
    drugs I42.7
    external agents NEC I42.7
    Friedreich's ataxia G11.1
    myotonia atrophica G71.11 [I43]
    progressive muscular dystrophy G71.0
  glycogen storage E74.02 [I43]
  hypertensive —see Hypertension, heart
  hypertrophic (nonobstructive) I42.2
    obstructive I42.1
      congenital Q24.8
  in
    Chagas' disease (chronic) B57.2
      acute B57.0
    sarcoidosis D86.85
  ischemic I25.5
  metabolic E88.9 [I43]
    thyrotoxic E05.90 [I43]
      with thyroid storm E05.91 [I43]
  newborn I42.8
    congenital I42.4
  nutritional E63.9 [I43]
    beriberi E51.12
  obscure of Africa I42.8
  peripartum O90.3
  postpartum O90.3
  restrictive NEC I42.5
  rheumatic I09.0
  secondary I42.9
  stress induced I51.81
  takotsubo I51.81
  thyrotoxic E05.90 [I43]
    with thyroid storm E05.91 [I43]
  toxic NEC I42.7
  tuberculous A18.84
  viral B33.24
Cardionephritis —see Hypertension,
    cardiorenal
Cardionephropathy —see Hypertension,
    cardiorenal
Cardionephrosis —see Hypertension,
    cardiorenal
Cardiopathia nigra I27.0

Cardiopathy (see also Disease, heart) I51.9
  idiopathic I42.9
  mucopolysaccharidosis E76.3 [I52]
Cardiopericarditis —see Pericarditis
Cardiophobia F45.29
Cardiorenal —see condition
Cardiorrhexis —see Infarct, myocardium
Cardiosclerosis —see Disease, heart, ischemic,
    atherosclerotic
Cardiosis —see Disease, heart
Cardiospasm (esophagus) (reflex) (stomach)
    K22.0
  congenital Q39.5
    with megaesophagus Q39.5
Cardiostenosis —see Disease, heart
Cardiosymphysis I31.0
Cardiovascular —see condition
Carditis (acute) (bacterial) (chronic) (subacute)
    I51.89
  meningococcal A39.50
  rheumatic —see Disease, heart, rheumatic
  rheumatoid —see Rheumatoid, carditis
  viral B33.20
Care (of) (for) (following)
  child (routine) Z76.2
  family member (handicapped) (sick)
    creating problem for family Z63.6
    provided away from home for holiday
      relief Z75.5
    unavailable, due to
      absence (person rendering care)
        (sufferer) Z74.2
      inability (any reason) of person
        rendering care Z74.2
  foundling Z76.1
  holiday relief Z75.5
  improper —see Maltreatment
  lack of (at or after birth) (infant) —see
    Maltreatment, child, neglect
  lactating mother Z39.1
  palliative Z51.5
  postpartum
    immediately after delivery Z39.0
    routine follow-up Z39.2
  respite Z75.5
  unavailable, due to
    absence of person rendering care
      Z74.2
    inability (any reason) of person
      rendering care Z74.2
  well-baby Z76.2
Caries
  bone NEC A18.03
  dental K02.9
    arrested (coronal) (root) K02.3
    chewing surface
      limited to enamel K02.51
        penetrating into dentin K02.52
        penetrating into pulp K02.53
    coronal surface
      chewing surface
        limited to enamel K02.51
          penetrating into dentin K02.52
          penetrating into pulp K02.53
      pit and fissure surface
        limited to enamel K02.51
          penetrating into dentin K02.52
          penetrating into pulp K02.53
      smooth surface
        limited to enamel K02.61
          penetrating into dentin K02.62
          penetrating into pulp K02.63
    pit and fissure surface
      limited to enamel K02.51
        penetrating into dentin K02.52
        penetrating into pulp K02.53
    root K02.7
    smooth surface
      limited to enamel K02.61
        penetrating into dentin K02.62
        penetrating into pulp K02.63

Caries (Continued)
  external meatus —see Disorder, ear, external,
    specified type NEC
  hip (tuberculous) A18.02
  initial (tooth)
    chewing surface K02.51
    pit and fissure surface K02.51
    smooth surface K02.61
  knee (tuberculous) A18.02
  labyrinth —see subcategory H83.8
  limb NEC (tuberculous) A18.03
  mastoid process (chronic) —see Mastoiditis,
    chronic
    tuberculous A18.03
  middle ear —see subcategory H74.8
  nose (tuberculous) A18.03
  orbit (tuberculous) A18.03
  ossicles, ear —see Abnormal, ear ossicles
  petrous bone —see Petrositis
  root (dental) (tooth) K02.7
  sacrum (tuberculous) A18.01
  spine, spinal (column) (tuberculous) A18.01
  syphilitic A52.77
    congenital (early) A50.02 [M90.80]
  tooth, teeth —see Caries, dental
  tuberculous A18.03
  vertebra (column) (tuberculous) A18.01
Carious teeth —see Caries, dental
Carneous mole O02.0
Carnitine insufficiency E71.40
Carotid body or sinus syndrome G90.01
Carotidynia G90.01
Carotinemia (dietary) E67.1
Carotinosis (cutis) (skin) E67.1
Carpal tunnel syndrome —see Syndrome,
    carpal tunnel
Carpenter's syndrome Q87.0
Carpopedal spasm —see Tetany
Carr-Barr-Plunkett syndrome Q97.1
Carrier (suspected) of
  amebiasis Z22.1
  bacterial disease NEC Z22.39
    diphtheria Z22.2
    intestinal infectious NEC Z22.1
      typhoid Z22.0
    meningococcal Z22.31
    sexually transmitted Z22.4
    specified NEC Z22.39
    staphylococcal (Methicillin susceptible)
      Z22.321
        Methicillin resistant Z22.322
    streptococcal Z22.338
      group B Z22.330
    typhoid Z22.0
  cholera Z22.1
  diphtheria Z22.2
  gastrointestinal pathogens NEC Z22.1
  genetic Z14.8
    cystic fibrosis Z14.1
    hemophilia A (asymptomatic) Z14.01
      symptomatic Z14.02
  gonorrhea Z22.4
  HAA (hepatitis Australian-antigen) Z22.59
  HB (c)(s)-AG Z22.51
  hepatitis (viral) Z22.50
    Australia-antigen (HAA) Z22.59
    B surface antigen (HBsAg) Z22.51
      with acute delta- (super)infection
        B17.0
    C Z22.52
    specified NEC Z22.59
  human T-cell lymphotropic virus type-1
    (HTLV-1) infection Z22.6
  infectious organism Z22.9
    specified NEC Z22.8
  meningococci Z22.31
  Salmonella typhosa Z22.0
  serum hepatitis —see Carrier, hepatitis
  staphylococci (Methicillin susceptible)
    Z22.321
      Methicillin resistant Z22.322

Carrier of *(Continued)*
  streptococci Z22.338
    group B Z22.330
  syphilis Z22.4
  typhoid Z22.0
  venereal disease NEC Z22.4
Carrion's disease A44.0
Carter's relapsing fever (Asiatic) A68.1
Cartilage —*see* condition
Caruncle (inflamed)
  conjunctiva (acute) —*see* Conjunctivitis, acute
  labium (majus) (minus) N90.89
  lacrimal —*see* Inflammation, lacrimal,
    passages
  myrtiform N89.8
  urethral (benign) N36.2
Cascade stomach K31.2
Caseation lymphatic gland (tuberculous) A18.2
Cassidy (-Scholte) syndrome (malignant
    carcinoid) E34.0
Castellani's disease A69.8
Castration, traumatic, male S38.231
Casts in urine R82.99
Cat
  cry syndrome Q93.4
  ear Q17.3
  eye syndrome Q92.8
Catabolism, senile R54
Catalepsy (hysterical) F44.2
  schizophrenic F20.2
Cataplexy (idiopathic) —*see* - Narcolepsy
Cataract (cortical) (immature) (incipient) H26.9
  with
    neovascularization —*see* Cataract,
      complicated
  age-related —*see* Cataract, senile
  anterior
    and posterior axial embryonal Q12.0
    pyramidal Q12.0
  associated with
    galactosemia E74.21 [H28]
    myotonic disorders G71.19 [H28]
  blue Q12.0
  central Q12.0
  cerulean Q12.0
  complicated H26.20
    with
      neovascularization H26.21-
      ocular disorder H26.22-
      glaucomatous flecks H26.23-
  congenital Q12.0
  coraliform Q12.0
  coronary Q12.0
  crystalline Q12.0
  diabetic —*see* Diabetes, cataract
  drug-induced H26.3-
  due to
    ocular disorder —*see* Cataract, complicated
    radiation H26.8
  electric H26.8
  extraction status Z98.4-
  glass-blower's H26.8
  heat ray H26.8
  heterochromic —*see* Cataract, complicated
  hypermature —*see* Cataract, senile,
    morgagnian type
  in (due to)
    chronic iridocyclitis —*see* Cataract,
      complicated
    diabetes —*see* Diabetes, cataract
    endocrine disease E34.9 [H28]
    eye disease —*see* Cataract, complicated
    hypoparathyroidism E20.9 [H28]
    malnutrition-dehydration E46 [H28]
    metabolic disease E88.9 [H28]
    myotonic disorders G71.19 [H28]
    nutritional disease E63.9 [H28]
  infantile —*see* Cataract, presenile
  irradiational —*see* Cataract, specified NEC
  juvenile —*see* Cataract, presenile
  malnutrition-dehydration E46 [H28]

Cataract *(Continued)*
  morgagnian —*see* Cataract, senile,
    morgagnian type
  myotonic G71.19 [H28]
  myxedema E03.9 [H28]
  nuclear
    embryonal Q12.0
    sclerosis —*see* Cataract, senile, nuclear
  presenile H26.00-
    combined forms H26.06-
    cortical H26.01-
      lamellar —*see* Cataract, presenile, cortical
    nuclear H26.03-
    specified NEC H26.09
    subcapsular polar (anterior) H26.04-
      posterior H26.05-
    zonular —*see* Cataract, presenile, cortical
  secondary H26.40
    Soemmering's ring H26.41-
    specified NEC H26.49-
    to eye disease —*see* Cataract, complicated
  senile H25.9
    brunescens —*see* Cataract, senile, nuclear
    combined forms H25.81-
    coronary —*see* Cataract, senile, incipient
    cortical H25.01-
    hypermature —*see* Cataract, senile,
      morgagnian type
    incipient (mature) (total) H25.09-
      cortical —*see* Cataract, senile, cortical
      subcapsular —*see* Cataract, senile,
        subcapsular
    morgagnian type (hypermature) H25.2-
    nuclear (sclerosis) H25.1-
    polar subcapsular (anterior) (posterior) —
      see Cataract, senile, incipient
    punctate —*see* Cataract, senile, incipient
    specified NEC H25.89
    subcapsular polar (anterior) H25.03-
      posterior H25.04-
  snowflake —*see* Diabetes, cataract
  specified NEC H26.8
  toxic —*see* Cataract, drug-induced
  traumatic H26.10-
    localized H26.11-
    partially resolved H26.12-
    total H26.13-
  zonular (perinuclear) Q12.0
Cataracta —*see also* Cataract
  brunescens —*see* Cataract, senile, nuclear
  centralis pulverulenta Q12.0
  cerulea Q12.0
  complicata —*see* Cataract, complicated
  congenita Q12.0
  coralliformis Q12.0
  coronaria Q12.0
  diabetic —*see* Diabetes, cataract
  membranacea
    accreta —*see* Cataract, secondary
    congenita Q12.0
  nigra —*see* Cataract, senile, nuclear
  sunflower —*see* Cataract, complicated
Catarrh, catarrhal (acute) (febrile) (infectious)
    (inflammation) (*see also* condition) J00
  bronchial —*see* Bronchitis
  chest —*see* Bronchitis
  chronic J31.0
  due to congenital syphilis A50.03
  enteric —*see* Enteritis
  eustachian H68.009
  fauces —*see* Pharyngitis
  gastrointestinal —*see* Enteritis
  gingivitis K05.00
    nonplaque induced K05.01
    plaque induced K05.00
  hay —*see* Fever, hay
  intestinal —*see* Enteritis
  larynx, chronic J37.0
  liver B15.9
    with hepatic coma B15.0
  lung —*see* Bronchitis

Catarrh, catarrhal *(Continued)*
  middle ear, chronic —*see* Otitis, media,
    nonsuppurative, chronic, serous
  mouth K12.1
  nasal (chronic) —*see* Rhinitis
  nasobronchial J31.1
  nasopharyngeal (chronic) J31.1
    acute J00
  pulmonary —*see* Bronchitis
  spring (eye) (vernal) —*see* Conjunctivitis,
    acute, atopic
  summer (hay) —*see* Fever, hay
  throat J31.2
  tubotympanal —*see also* Otitis, media,
    nonsuppurative
    chronic —*see* Otitis, media,
      nonsuppurative, chronic, serous
Catatonia (schizophrenic) F20.2
Catatonic
  disorder due to known physiologic condition
    F06.1
  schizophrenia F20.2
  stupor R40.1
Cat-scratch —*see also* Abrasion
  disease or fever A28.1
Cauda equina —*see* condition
Cauliflower ear M95.1-
Causalgia (upper limb) G56.4-
  lower limb G57.7-
Cause
  external, general effects T75.89
Caustic burn —*see* Corrosion, by site
Cavare's disease (familial periodic paralysis)
    G72.3
Cave-in, injury
  crushing (severe) —*see* Crush
  suffocation —*see* Asphyxia, traumatic, due to
    low oxygen, due to cave-in
Cavernitis (penis) N48.29
Cavernositis N48.29
Cavernous —*see* condition
Cavitation of lung —*see also* Tuberculosis,
    pulmonary
  nontuberculous J98.4
Cavities, dental —*see* Caries, dental
Cavity
  lung —*see* Cavitation of lung
  optic papilla Q14.2
  pulmonary —*see* Cavitation of lung
Cavovarus foot, congenital Q66.1
Cavus foot (congenital) Q66.7
  acquired —*see* Deformity, limb, foot, specified
    NEC
Cazenave's disease L10.2
Cecitis K52.9
  with perforation, peritonitis, or rupture K65.8
Cecum —*see* condition
Celiac
  artery compression syndrome I77.4
  disease K90.0
  infantilism K90.0
Cell (s), cellular —*see also* condition
  in urine R82.99
Cellulitis (diffuse) (phlegmonous) (septic)
    (suppurative) L03.90
  abdominal wall L03.311
  anaerobic A48.0
  ankle —*see* Cellulitis, lower limb
  anus K61.0
  arm —*see* Cellulitis, upper limb
  auricle (ear) —*see* Cellulitis, ear
  axilla L03.11-
  back (any part) L03.312
  broad ligament
    acute N73.0
  buttock L03.317
  cervical (meaning neck) L03.221
  cervix (uteri) —*see* Cervicitis
  cheek (external) L03.211
    internal K12.2
  chest wall L03.313

◀ New   ◀▥ Revised   ~~deleted~~ Deleted

Cellulitis *(Continued)*
  chronic L03.90
  clostridial A48.0
  corpus cavernosum N48.22
  digit
    finger —*see* Cellulitis, finger
    toe —*see* Cellulitis, toe
  Douglas' cul-de-sac or pouch
    acute N73.0
  drainage site (following operation) T81.4
  ear (external) H60.1-
  eosinophilic (granulomatous) L98.3
  erysipelatous —*see* Erysipelas
  external auditory canal —*see* Cellulitis, ear
  eyelid —*see* Abscess, eyelid
  face NEC L03.211
  finger (intrathecal) (periosteal)
      (subcutaneous) (subcuticular) L03.01-
  foot —*see* Cellulitis, lower limb
  gangrenous —*see* Gangrene
  genital organ NEC
    female (external) N76.4
    male N49.9
      multiple sites N49.8
      specified NEC N49.8
  gluteal (region) L03.317
  gonococcal A54.89
  groin L03.314
  hand —*see* Cellulitis, upper limb
  head NEC L03.811
    face (any part, except ear, eye and nose)
        L03.211
  heel —*see* Cellulitis, lower limb
  hip —*see* Cellulitis, lower limb
  jaw (region) L03.211
  knee —*see* Cellulitis, lower limb
  labium (majus) (minus) —*see* Vulvitis
  lacrimal passages —*see* Inflammation,
      lacrimal, passages
  larynx J38.7
  leg —*see* Cellulitis, lower limb
  lip K13.0
  lower limb L03.11-
    toe —*see* Cellulitis, toe
  mouth (floor) K12.2
  multiple sites, so stated L03.90
  nasopharynx J39.1
  navel L03.316
    newborn P38.9
      with mild hemorrhage P38.1
      without hemorrhage P38.9
  neck (region) L03.221
  nose (septum) (external) J34.0
  orbit, orbital H05.01-
  palate (soft) K12.2
  pectoral (region) L03.313
  pelvis, pelvic (chronic)
    female (*see also* Disease, pelvis,
        inflammatory) N73.2
      acute N73.0
    following ectopic or molar pregnancy
        O08.0
    male K65.0
  penis N48.22
  perineal, perineum L03.315
  perirectal K61.1
  peritonsillar J36
  periurethral N34.0
  periuterine (*see also* Disease, pelvis,
      inflammatory) N73.2
    acute N73.0
  pharynx J39.1
  rectum K61.1
  retroperitoneal K68.9
  round ligament
    acute N73.0
  scalp (any part) L03.811
  scrotum N49.2
  seminal vesicle N49.0
  shoulder —*see* Cellulitis, upper limb
  specified site NEC L03.818

Cellulitis *(Continued)*
  submandibular (region) (space) (triangle)
      K12.2
    gland K11.3
  submaxillary (region) K12.2
    gland K11.3
  thigh —*see* Cellulitis, lower limb
  thumb (intrathecal) (periosteal)
      (subcutaneous) (subcuticular) —*see*
      Cellulitis, finger
  toe (intrathecal) (periosteal) (subcutaneous)
      (subcuticular) L03.03-
  tonsil J36
  trunk L03.319
    abdominal wall L03.311
    back (any part) L03.312
    buttock L03.317
    chest wall L03.313
    groin L03.314
    perineal, perineum L03.315
    umbilicus L03.316
    tuberculous (primary) A18.4
    umbilicus L03.316
  upper limb L03.11-
    axilla —*see* Cellulitis, axilla
    finger —*see* Cellulitis, finger
    thumb —*see* Cellulitis, finger
  vaccinal T88.0
  vocal cord J38.3
  vulva —*see* Vulvitis
  wrist —*see* Cellulitis, upper limb
Cementoblastoma, benign —*see* Cyst,
    calcifying odontogenic
Cementoma —*see* Cyst, calcifying odontogenic
Cementoperiostitis —*see* Periodontitis
Cementosis K03.4
Central auditory processing disorder H93.25
Central pain syndrome G89.0
Cephalematocele, cephal (o)hematocele
  newborn P52.8
    birth injury P10.8
  traumatic —*see* Hematoma, brain
Cephalematoma, cephalhematoma (calcified)
  newborn (birth injury) P12.0
  traumatic —*see* Hematoma, brain
Cephalgia, cephalalgia —*see also* Headache
  histamine G44.009
    intractable G44.001
    not intractable G44.009
  trigeminal autonomic (TAC) NEC G44.099
    intractable G44.091
    not intractable G44.099
Cephalic —*see* condition
Cephalitis —*see* Encephalitis
Cephalocele —*see* Encephalocele
Cephalomenia N94.89
Cephalopelvic —*see* condition
Cerclage (with cervical incompetence) in
    pregnancy —*see* Incompetence, cervix, in
    pregnancy
Cerebellitis —*see* Encephalitis
Cerebellum, cerebellar —*see* condition
Cerebral —*see* condition
Cerebritis —*see* Encephalitis
Cerebro-hepato-renal syndrome Q87.89
Cerebromalacia —*see* Softening, brain
  sequelae of cerebrovascular disease I69.398
Cerebroside lipidosis E75.22
Cerebrospasticity (congenital) G80.1
Cerebrospinal —*see* condition
Cerebrum —*see* condition
Ceroid-lipofuscinosis, neuronal E75.4
Cerumen (accumulation) (impacted) H61.2-
Cervical —*see also* condition
  auricle Q18.2
  dysplasia in pregnancy —*see* Abnormal,
      cervix, in pregnancy or childbirth
  erosion in pregnancy —*see* Abnormal, cervix,
      in pregnancy or childbirth
  fibrosis in pregnancy —*see* Abnormal, cervix,
      in pregnancy or childbirth

Cervical *(Continued)*
  fusion syndrome Q76.1
  rib Q76.5
  shortening (complicating pregnancy)
      O26.87-
Cervicalgia M54.2
Cervicitis (acute) (chronic) (nonvenereal)
    (senile (atrophic)) (subacute) (with
    ulceration) N72
  with
    abortion —*see* Abortion, by type
      complicated by genital tract and
          pelvic infection
    ectopic pregnancy O08.0
    molar pregnancy O08.0
  chlamydial A56.09
  gonococcal A54.03
  herpesviral A60.03
  puerperal (postpartum) O86.11
  syphilitic A52.76
  trichomonal A59.09
  tuberculous A18.16
Cervicocolpitis (emphysematosa) (*see also*
    Cervicitis) N72
Cervix —*see* condition
Cesarean delivery, previous, affecting
    management of pregnancy O34.21
Céstan (-Chenais) paralysis or syndrome
    G46.3
Céstan-Raymond syndrome I65.8
Cestode infestation B71.9
  specified type NEC B71.8
Cestodiasis B71.9
Chabert's disease A22.9
Chacaleh E53.8
Chafing L30.4
Chagas' (-Mazza) disease (chronic) B57.2
  with
    cardiovascular involvement NEC B57.2
    digestive system involvement B57.30
      megacolon B57.32
      megaesophagus B57.31
      other specified B57.39
    megacolon B57.32
    megaesophagus B57.31
    myocarditis B57.2
    nervous system involvement B57.40
      meningitis B57.41
      meningoencephalitis B57.42
      other specified B57.49
    specified organ involvement NEC B57.5
  acute (with) B57.1
    cardiovascular NEC B57.0
    myocarditis B57.0
Chagres fever B50.9
Chairridden Z74.09
Chalasia (cardiac sphincter) K21.9
Chalazion H00.19
  left H00.16
    lower H00.15
    upper H00.14
  right H00.13
    lower H00.12
    upper H00.11
Chalcosis —*see also* Disorder, globe,
    degenerative, chalcosis
  cornea —*see* Deposit, cornea
  crystalline lens —*see* Cataract, complicated
  retina H35.89
Chalicosis (pulmonum) J62.8
Chancre (any genital site) (hard) (hunterian)
    (mixed) (primary) (seronegative)
    (seropositive) (syphilitic) A51.0
  congenital A50.07
  conjunctiva NEC A51.2
  Ducrey's A57
  extragenital A51.2
  eyelid A51.2
  lip A51.2
  nipple A51.2
  Nisbet's A57

Chancre (Continued)
 of
  carate A67.0
  pinta A67.0
  yaws A66.0
 palate, soft A51.2
 phagedenic A57
 simple A57
 soft A57
  bubo A57
  palate A51.2
 urethra A51.0
 yaws A66.0
Chancroid (anus) (genital) (penis) (perineum)
  (rectum) (urethra) (vulva) A57
Chandler's disease (osteochondritis dissecans,
  hip) —see Osteochondritis, dissecans, hip
Change (s) (in) (of) —see also Removal
 arteriosclerotic —see Arteriosclerosis
 bone —see also Disorder, bone
  diabetic —see Diabetes, bone change
 bowel habit R19.4
 cardiorenal (vascular) —see Hypertension,
  cardiorenal
 cardiovascular —see Disease, cardiovascular
 circulatory I99.9
 cognitive (mild) (organic) R41.89
 color, tooth, teeth
  during formation K00.8
  posteruptive K03.7
 contraceptive device Z30.433
 corneal membrane H18.30
  Bowman's membrane fold or rupture
   H18.31-
  Descemet's membrane
   fold H18.32-
   rupture H18.33-
 coronary —see Disease, heart, ischemic
 degenerative, spine or vertebra —see
   Spondylosis
 dental pulp, regressive K04.2
 dressing (nonsurgical) Z48.00
  surgical Z48.01
 heart —see Disease, heart
 hip joint —see Derangement, joint, hip
 hyperplastic larynx J38.7
 hypertrophic
  nasal sinus J34.89
  turbinate, nasal J34.3
  upper respiratory tract J39.8
 indwelling catheter Z46.6
 inflammatory —see also Inflammation
  sacroiliac M46.1
 job, anxiety concerning Z56.1
 joint —see Derangement, joint
 life —see Menopause
 mental status R41.82
 minimal (glomerular) (see also N00-N07 with
  fourth character .0) N05.0
 myocardium, myocardial —see Degeneration,
  myocardial - of life —see Menopause
 pacemaker Z45.018
  pulse generator Z45.010
 personality (enduring) F68.8
  due to (secondary to)
   general medical condition F07.0
  secondary (nonspecific) F60.89
 regressive, dental pulp K04.2
 renal —see Disease, renal
 retina H35.9
  myopic H44.2-
 sacroiliac joint M53.3
 senile (see also condition) R54
 sensory R20.8
 skin R23.9
  acute, due to ultraviolet radiation L56.9
   specified NEC L56.8
  chronic, due to nonionizing radiation L57.9
   specified NEC L57.8
  cyanosis R23.0
  flushing R23.2

Change (Continued)
 skin (Continued)
  pallor R23.1
  petechiae R23.3
  specified change NEC R23.8
  swelling —see Mass, localized
  texture R23.4
 trophic
  arm —see Mononeuropathy, upper limb
  leg —see Mononeuropathy, lower limb
 vascular I99.9
 vasomotor I73.9
 voice R49.9
  psychogenic F44.4
  specified NEC R49.8
Changing sleep-work schedule, affecting sleep
  G47.26
Changuinola fever A93.1
Chapping skin T69.8
Charcot-Marie-Tooth disease, paralysis or
  syndrome G60.0
Charcot's
 arthropathy —see Arthropathy, neuropathic
 cirrhosis K74.3
 disease (tabetic arthropathy) A52.16
 joint (disease) (tabetic) A52.16
  diabetic —see Diabetes, with, arthropathy
  syringomyelic G95.0
 syndrome (intermittent claudication) I73.9
CHARGE association Q89.8
Charley-horse (quadriceps) M62.831
 traumatic (quadriceps) S76.11-
Charlouis' disease —see Yaws
Cheadle's disease E54
Checking (of)
 cardiac pacemaker (battery) (electrode (s))
  Z45.018
  pulse generator Z45.010
 intrauterine contraceptive device Z30.431
Check-up —see Examination
Chédiak-Higashi (-Steinbrinck) syndrome
  (congenital gigantism of peroxidase
  granules) E70.330
Cheek —see condition
Cheese itch B88.0
Cheese-washer's lung J67.8
Cheese-worker's lung J67.8
Cheilitis (acute) (angular) (catarrhal) (chronic)
  (exfoliative) (gangrenous) (glandular)
  (infectional) (suppurative) (ulcerative)
  (vesicular) K13.0
 actinic (due to sun) L56.8
  other than from sun L59.8
 candidal B37.83
Cheilodynia K13.0
Cheiloschisis —see Cleft, lip
Cheilosis (angular) K13.0
 with pellagra E52
 due to
  vitamin B2 (riboflavin) deficiency E53.0
Cheiromegaly M79.89
Cheiropompholyx L30.1
Cheloid —see Keloid
Chemical burn —see Corrosion, by site
Chemodectoma —see Paraganglioma,
  nonchromaffin
Chemosis, conjunctiva —see Edema,
  conjunctiva
Chemotherapy (session) (for)
 cancer Z51.11
 neoplasm Z51.11
Cherubism M27.8
Chest —see condition
Cheyne-Stokes breathing (respiration) R06.3
Chiari's
 disease or syndrome (hepatic vein
  thrombosis) I82.0
 malformation
  type I G93.5
  type II —see Spina bifida
 net Q24.8

Chicago disease B40.9
Chickenpox —see Varicella
Chiclero ulcer or sore B55.1
Chigger (infestation) B88.0
Chignon (disease) B36.8
 newborn (from vacuum extraction) (birth
  injury) P12.1
Chilaiditi's syndrome (subphrenic
  displacement, colon) Q43.3
Chilblain (s) (lupus) T69.1
Child
 custody dispute Z65.3
Childbirth —see Delivery
Childhood
 cerebral X-linked adrenoleukodystrophy
  E71.520
 period of rapid growth Z00.2
Chill (s) R68.83
 with fever R50.9
 without fever R68.83
 congestive in malarial regions B54
Chilomastigiasis A07.8
Chimera 46,XX/46,XY Q99.0
Chin —see condition
Chinese dysentery A03.9
Chionophobia F40.228
Chitral fever A93.1
Chlamydia, chlamydial A74.9
 cervicitis A56.09
 conjunctivitis A74.0
 cystitis A56.01
 endometritis A56.11
 epididymitis A56.19
 female
  pelvic inflammatory disease A56.11
  pelviperitonitis A56.11
 orchitis A56.19
 peritonitis A74.81
 pharyngitis A56.4
 proctitis A56.3
 psittaci (infection) A70
 salpingitis A56.11
 sexually-transmitted infection NEC
  A56.8
 specified NEC A74.89
 urethritis A56.01
 vulvovaginitis A56.02
Chlamydiosis —see Chlamydia
Chloasma (skin) (idiopathic) (symptomatic)
  L81.1
 eyelid H02.719
  hyperthyroid E05.90 [H02.719]
   with thyroid storm E05.91 [H02.719]
  left H02.716
   lower H02.715
   upper H02.714
  right H02.713
   lower H02.712
   upper H02.711
Chloroma C92.3-
Chlorosis D50.9
 Egyptian B76.9 [D63.8]
 miner's B76.9 [D63.8]
Chlorotic anemia D50.8
Chocolate cyst (ovary) N80.1
Choked
 disc or disk —see Papilledema
 on food, phlegm, or vomitus NOS —see
  Foreign body, by site
 while vomiting NOS —see Foreign body, by
  site
Chokes (resulting from bends) T70.3
Choking sensation R09.89
Cholangiectasis K83.8
Cholangiocarcinoma
 with hepatocellular carcinoma, combined
  C22.0
 liver C22.1
 specified site NEC —see Neoplasm,
  malignant, by site
 unspecified site C22.1

◀ New   ◀ Revised   ~~deleted~~ Deleted

Cholangiohepatitis K83.8
  due to fluke infestation B66.1
Cholangiohepatoma C22.0
Cholangiolitis (acute) (chronic) (extrahepatic)
    (gangrenous) (intrahepatic) K83.0
  paratyphoidal —see Fever, paratyphoid
  typhoidal A01.09
Cholangioma D13.4
  malignant —see Cholangiocarcinoma
Cholangitis (ascending) (primary) (recurrent)
    (sclerosing) (secondary) (stenosing)
    (suppurative) K83.0
  with calculus, bile duct —see Calculus, bile
      duct, with cholangitis
  chronic nonsuppurative destructive K74.3
Cholecystectasia K82.8
Cholecystitis K81.9
  with
    calculus, stones in
      bile duct (common) (hepatic) —
          see Calculus, bile duct, with
          cholecystitis
      cystic duct —see Calculus, gallbladder,
          with cholecystitis
      gallbladder —see Calculus, gallbladder,
          with cholecystitis
      choledocholithiasis —see Calculus, bile
          duct, with cholecystitis
      cholelithiasis —see Calculus, gallbladder,
          with cholecystitis
  acute (emphysematous) (gangrenous)
      (suppurative) K81.0
    with
      calculus, stones in
        cystic duct —see Calculus,
            gallbladder, with cholecystitis,
            acute
        gallbladder —see Calculus,
            gallbladder, with cholecystitis,
            acute
        choledocholithiasis —see Calculus, bile
            duct, with cholecystitis, acute
        cholelithiasis —see Calculus,
            gallbladder, with cholecystitis,
            acute
    chronic cholecystitis K81.2
      with gallbladder calculus K80.12
        with obstruction K80.13
  chronic K81.1
    with acute cholecystitis K81.2
      with gallbladder calculus K80.12
        with obstruction K80.13
  emphysematous (acute) —see Cholecystitis,
      acute
  gangrenous —see Cholecystitis, acute
  paratyphoidal, current A01.4
  suppurative —see Cholecystitis, acute
  typhoidal A01.09
Cholecystolithiasis —see Calculus, gallbladder
Choledochitis (suppurative) K83.0
Choledocholith —see Calculus, bile duct
Choledocholithiasis (common duct) (hepatic
    duct) —see Calculus, bile duct
  cystic —see Calculus, gallbladder
  typhoidal A01.09
Cholelithiasis (cystic duct) (gallbladder)
    (impacted) (multiple) —see Calculus,
    gallbladder
  bile duct (common) (hepatic) —see Calculus,
      bile duct
  hepatic duct —see Calculus, bile duct
  specified NEC K80.80
    with obstruction K80.81
Cholemia —see also Jaundice
  familial (simple) (congenital) E80.4
  Gilbert's E80.4
Choleperitoneum, choleperitonitis K65.3
Cholera (Asiatic) (epidemic) (malignant)
    A00.9
  antimonial —see Poisoning, antimony
  classical A00.0

Cholera (Continued)
  due to Vibrio cholerae 01 A00.9
    biovar cholerae A00.0
    biovar eltor A00.1
    el tor A00.1
  el tor A00.1
Cholerine —see Cholera
Cholestasis NEC K83.1
  with hepatocyte injury K71.0
  due to total parenteral nutrition (TPN) K76.89
  pure K71.0
Cholesteatoma (ear) (middle) (with reaction)
    H71.9-
  attic H71.0-
  external ear (canal) H60.4-
  mastoid H71.2-
  postmastoidectomy cavity (recurrent) —see
      Complications, postmastoidectomy,
      recurrent cholesteatoma
  recurrent (postmastoidectomy) —see
      Complications, postmastoidectomy,
      recurrent cholesteatoma
  tympanum H71.1-
Cholesteatosis, diffuse H71.3-
Cholesteremia E78.0
Cholesterin in vitreous —see Deposit,
    crystalline
Cholesterol
  deposit
    retina H35.89
    vitreous —see Deposit, crystalline
  elevated (high) E78.0
    with elevated (high) triglycerides E78.2
    screening for Z13.220
  imbibition of gallbladder K82.4
Cholesterolemia (essential) (familial)
    (hereditary) (pure) E78.0
Cholesterolosis, cholesterosis (gallbladder)
    K82.4
  cerebrotendinous E75.5
Cholocolic fistula K82.3
Choluria R82.2
Chondritis M94.8X9
  aurical H61.03-
  costal (Tietze's) M94.0
  external ear H61.03-
  patella, posttraumatic —see Chondromalacia,
      patella
  pinna H61.03-
  purulent M94.8X-
  tuberculous NEC A18.02
    intervertebral A18.01
Chondroblastoma —see also Neoplasm, bone,
    benign
  malignant —see Neoplasm, bone, malignant
Chondrocalcinosis M11.20
  ankle M11.27-
  elbow M11.22-
  familial M11.10
    ankle M11.17-
    elbow M11.12-
    foot joint M11.17-
    hand joint M11.14-
    hip M11.15-
    knee M11.16-
    multiple site M11.19
    shoulder M11.11-
    vertebrae M11.18
    wrist M11.13-
  foot joint M11.27-
  hand joint M11.24-
  hip M11.25-
  knee M11.26-
  multiple site M11.29
  shoulder M11.21-
  specified type NEC M11.20
    ankle M11.27-
    elbow M11.22-
    foot joint M11.27-
    hand joint M11.24-
    hip M11.25-

Chondrocalcinosis (Continued)
  specified type NEC (Continued)
    knee M11.26-
    multiple site M11.29
    shoulder M11.21-
    vertebrae M11.28
    wrist M11.23-
  vertebrae M11.28
  wrist M11.23-
Chondrodermatitis nodularis helicis or
    anthelicis —see Perichondritis, ear
Chondrodysplasia Q78.9
  with hemangioma Q78.4
  calcificans congenita Q77.3
  fetalis Q77.4
  metaphyseal (Jansen's) (McKusick's)
      (Schmid's) Q78.5
  punctata Q77.3
Chondrodystrophy, chondrodystrophia
    (familial) (fetalis) (hypoplastic) Q78.9
  calcificans congenita Q77.3
  myotonic (congenital) G71.13
  punctata Q77.3
Chondroectodermal dysplasia Q77.6
Chondrogenesis imperfecta Q77.4
Chondrolysis M94.35-
Chondroma —see also Neoplasm, cartilage,
    benign
  juxtacortical —see Neoplasm, bone, benign
  periosteal —see Neoplasm, bone, benign
Chondromalacia (systemic) M94.20
  acromioclavicular joint M94.21-
  ankle M94.27-
  elbow M94.22-
  foot joint M94.27-
  glenohumeral joint M94.21-
  hand joint M94.24-
  hip M94.25-
  knee M94.26-
    patella M22.4-
  multiple sites M94.29
  patella M22.4-
  rib M94.28
  sacroiliac joint M94.259
  shoulder M94.21-
  sternoclavicular joint M94.21-
  vertebral joint M94.28
  wrist M94.23-
Chondromatosis —see also Neoplasm, cartilage,
    uncertain behavior
  internal Q78.4
Chondromyxosarcoma —see Neoplasm,
    cartilage, malignant
Chondro-osteodysplasia (Morquio-Brailsford
    type) E76.219
Chondro-osteodystrophy E76.29
Chondro-osteoma —see Neoplasm, bone,
    benign
Chondropathia tuberosa M94.0
Chondrosarcoma —see Neoplasm, cartilage,
    malignant
  juxtacortical —see Neoplasm, bone, malignant
  mesenchymal —see Neoplasm, connective
      tissue, malignant
  myxoid —see Neoplasm, cartilage, malignant
Chordee (nonvenereal) N48.89
  congenital Q54.4
  gonococcal A54.09
Chorditis (fibrinous) (nodosa) (tuberosa) J38.2
Chordoma —see Neoplasm, vertebral (column),
    malignant
Chorea (chronic) (gravis) (posthemiplegic)
    (senile) (spasmodic) G25.5
  with
    heart involvement I02.0
      active or acute (conditions in I01-) I02.0
      rheumatic I02.9
        with valvular disorder I02.0
    rheumatic heart disease (chronic) (inactive)
        (quiescent) — code to rheumatic heart
        condition involved

Chorea (Continued)
  drug-induced G25.4
  habit F95.8
  hereditary G10
  Huntington's G10
  hysterical F44.4
  minor I02.9
    with heart involvement I02.0
  progressive G25.5
    hereditary G10
  rheumatic (chronic) I02.9
    with heart involvement I02.0
  Sydenham's I02.9
    with heart involvement —see Chorea, with
      rheumatic heart disease
    nonrheumatic G25.5
Choreoathetosis (paroxysmal) G25.5
Chorioadenoma (destruens) D39.2
Chorioamnionitis O41.12-
Chorioangioma D26.7
Choriocarcinoma —see Neoplasm, malignant,
  by site
  combined with
    embryonal carcinoma —see Neoplasm,
      malignant, by site
    other germ cell elements —see Neoplasm,
      malignant, by site
    teratoma —see Neoplasm, malignant, by
      site
  specified site —see Neoplasm, malignant, by
    site
  unspecified site
    female C58
    male C62.90
Chorioencephalitis (acute) (lymphocytic)
  (serous) A87.2
Chorioepithelioma —see Choriocarcinoma
Choriomeningitis (acute) (lymphocytic)
  (serous) A87.2
Chorionepithelioma —see Choriocarcinoma
Chorioretinitis —see also Inflammation,
  chorioretinal
  disseminated —see also Inflammation,
    chorioretinal, disseminated
    in neurosyphilis A52.19
  Egyptian B76.9 [D63.8]
  focal —see also Inflammation, chorioretinal,
    focal
  histoplasmic B39.9 [H32]
  in (due to)
    histoplasmosis B39.9 [H32]
    syphilis (secondary) A51.43
      late A52.71
    toxoplasmosis (acquired) B58.01
      congenital (active) P37.1 [H32]
    tuberculosis A18.53
  juxtapapillary, juxtapapillaris —see
    Inflammation, chorioretinal, focal,
    juxtapapillary
  leprous A30.9 [H32]
  miner's B76.9 [D63.8]
  progressive myopia (degeneration) H44.2-
  syphilitic (secondary) A51.43
    congenital (early) A50.01 [H32]
      late A50.32
    late A52.71
  tuberculous A18.53
Chorioretinopathy, central serous H35.71-
Choroid —see condition
Choroideremia H31.21
Choroiditis —see Chorioretinitis
Choroidopathy —see Disorder, choroid
Choroidoretinitis —see Chorioretinitis
Choroidoretinopathy, central serous —see
  Chorioretinopathy, central serous
Christian-Weber disease M35.6
Christmas disease D67
Chromaffinoma —see also Neoplasm, benign,
  by site
  malignant —see Neoplasm, malignant, by site
Chromatopsia —see Deficiency, color vision

Chromhidrosis, chromidrosis L75.1
Chromoblastomycosis —see Chromomycosis
Chromoconversion R82.91
Chromomycosis B43.9
  brain abscess B43.1
  cerebral B43.1
  cutaneous B43.0
  skin B43.0
  specified NEC B43.8
  subcutaneous abscess or cyst B43.2
Chromophytosis B36.0
Chromosome —see condition by chromosome
  involved
  D (1) —see condition, chromosome 13
  E (3) —see condition, chromosome 18
  G —see condition, chromosome 21
Chromotrichomycosis B36.8
Chronic —see condition
  fracture —see Fracture, pathological
Churg-Strauss syndrome M30.1
Chyle cyst, mesentery I89.8
Chylocele (nonfilarial) I89.8
  filarial (see also Infestation, filarial) B74.9
    [N51]
  tunica vaginalis N50.8
    filarial (see also Infestation, filarial) B74.9
      [N51]
Chylomicronemia (fasting) (with
  hyperprebetalipoproteinemia) E78.3
Chylopericardium I31.3
  acute I30.9
Chylothorax (nonfilarial) I89.8
  filarial (see also Infestation, filarial) B74.9
    [J91.8]
Chylous —see condition
Chyluria (nonfilarial) R82.0
  due to
    bilharziasis B65.0
    Brugia (malayi) B74.1
      timori B74.2
    schistosomiasis (bilharziasis) B65.0
    Wuchereria (bancrofti) B74.0
  filarial —see Infestation, filarial
Cicatricial (deformity) —see Cicatrix
Cicatrix (adherent) (contracted) (painful)
  (vicious) (see also Scar) L90.5
  adenoid (and tonsil) J35.8
  alveolar process M26.79
  anus K62.89
  auricle —see Disorder, pinna, specified type
    NEC
  bile duct (common) (hepatic) K83.8
  bladder N32.89
  bone —see Disorder, bone, specified type
    NEC
  brain G93.89
  cervix (postoperative) (postpartal) N88.1
  common duct K83.8
  cornea H17.9
    tuberculous A18.59
  duodenum (bulb), obstructive K31.5
  esophagus K22.2
  eyelid —see Disorder, eyelid function
  hypopharynx J39.2
  lacrimal passages —see Obstruction, lacrimal
  larynx J38.7
  lung J98.4
  middle ear —see subcategory H74.8
  mouth K13.79
  muscle M62.89
    with contracture —see Contraction, muscle
    NEC
  nasopharynx J39.2
  palate (soft) K13.79
  penis N48.89
  pharynx J39.2
  prostate N42.89
  rectum K62.89
  retina —see Scar, chorioretinal
  semilunar cartilage —see Derangement,
    meniscus

Cicatrix (Continued)
  seminal vesicle N50.8
  skin L90.5
    infected L08.89
    postinfective L90.5
    tuberculous B90.8
  specified site NEC L90.5
  throat J39.2
  tongue K14.8
  tonsil (and adenoid) J35.8
  trachea J39.8
  tuberculous NEC B90.9
  urethra N36.8
  uterus N85.8
  vagina N89.8
    postoperative N99.2
  vocal cord J38.3
  wrist, constricting (annular) L90.5
CIDP (chronic inflammatory demyelinating
  polyneuropathy) G61.81
CIN —see Neoplasia, intraepithelial, cervix
Cinchonism —see Deafness, ototoxic
  correct substance properly administered —see
    Table of Drugs and Chemicals, by drug,
    adverse effect
  overdose or wrong substance given or
    taken —see Table of Drugs and
    Chemicals, by drug, poisoning
Circle of Willis —see condition
Circular —see condition
Circulating anticoagulants (see also - Disorder,
  hemorrhagic) D68.318
  due to drugs (see also - Disorder,
    hemorrhagic) D68.32
  following childbirth O72.3
Circulation
  collateral, any site I99.8
  defective (lower extremity) I99.8
    congenital Q28.9
  embryonic Q28.9
  failure (peripheral) R57.9
    newborn P29.89
  fetal, persistent P29.3
  heart, incomplete Q28.9
Circulatory system —see condition
Circulus senilis (cornea) —see Degeneration,
  cornea, senile
Circumcision (in absence of medical indication)
  (ritual) (routine) Z41.2
Circumscribed —see condition
Circumvallate placenta O43.11-
Cirrhosis, cirrhotic (hepatic) (liver) K74.60
  alcoholic K70.30
    with ascites K70.31
  atrophic —see Cirrhosis, liver
  Baumgarten-Cruveilhier K74.69
  biliary (cholangiolitic) (cholangitic)
    (hypertrophic) (obstructive)
    (pericholangiolitic) K74.5
    due to
      Clonorchiasis B66.1
      flukes B66.3
    primary K74.3
    secondary K74.4
  cardiac (of liver) K76.1
  Charcot's K74.3
  cholangiolitic, cholangitic, cholostatic
    (primary) K74.3
  congestive K76.1
  Cruveilhier-Baumgarten K74.69
  cryptogenic (liver) K74.69
  due to
    hepatolenticular degeneration E83.01
    Wilson's disease E83.01
    xanthomatosis E78.2
  fatty K76.0
    alcoholic K70.0
  Hanot's (hypertrophic) K74.3
  hepatic —see Cirrhosis, liver
  hypertrophic K74.3
  Indian childhood K74.69

◀ New   ◀‖‖ Revised   ~~deleted~~ Deleted

Cirrhosis, cirrhotic *(Continued)*
  kidney —*see* Sclerosis, renal
  Laennec's K70.30
    with ascites K70.31
    alcoholic K70.30
      with ascites K70.31
    nonalcoholic K74.69
  liver K74.60
    alcoholic K70.30
      with ascites K70.31
      fatty K70.0
    congenital P78.81
    syphilitic A52.74
  lung (chronic) J84.10
  macronodular K74.69
    alcoholic K70.30
      with ascites K70.31
  micronodular K74.69
    alcoholic K70.30
      with ascites K70.31
  mixed type K74.69
  monolobular K74.3
  nephritis —*see* Sclerosis, renal
  nutritional K74.69
    alcoholic K70.30
      with ascites K70.31
  obstructive —*see* Cirrhosis, biliary
  ovarian N83.8
  pancreas (duct) K86.8
  pigmentary E83.110
  portal K74.69
    alcoholic K70.30
      with ascites K70.31
  postnecrotic K74.69
    alcoholic K70.30
      with ascites K70.31
  pulmonary J84.10
  renal —*see* Sclerosis, renal
  spleen D73.2
  stasis K76.1
  Todd's K74.3
  unilobar K74.3
  xanthomatous (biliary) K74.5
    due to xanthomatosis (familial) (metabolic) (primary) E78.2
Cistern, subarachnoid R93.0
Citrullinemia E72.23
Citrullinuria E72.23
Civatte's disease or poikiloderma L57.3
Clam digger's itch B65.3
Clammy skin R23.1
Clap —*see* Gonorrhea
Clarke-Hadfield syndrome (pancreatic infantilism) K86.8
Clark's paralysis G80.9
Clastothrix L67.8
Claude Bernard-Horner syndrome G90.2
  traumatic —*see* Injury, nerve, cervical sympathetic
Claude's disease or syndrome G46.3
Claudicatio venosa intermittens I87.8
Claudication, intermittent I73.9
  cerebral (artery) G45.9
  spinal cord (arteriosclerotic) G95.19
    syphilitic A52.09
  venous (axillary) I87.8
Claustrophobia F40.240
Clavus (infected) L84
Clawfoot (congenital) Q66.89
  acquired —*see* Deformity, limb, clawfoot
Clawhand (acquired) —*see also* Deformity, limb, clawhand
  congenital Q68.1
Clawtoe (congenital) Q66.89
  acquired —*see* Deformity, toe, specified NEC
Clay eating —*see* Pica
Cleansing of artificial opening —*see* Attention to, artificial, opening

Cleft (congenital) —*see also* Imperfect, closure
  alveolar process M26.79
  branchial (cyst) (persistent) Q18.2
  cricoid cartilage, posterior Q31.8
  lip (unilateral) Q36.9
    with cleft palate Q37.9
      hard Q37.1
        with soft Q37.5
      soft Q37.3
        with hard Q37.5
    bilateral Q36.0
      with cleft palate Q37.8
        hard Q37.0
          with soft Q37.4
        soft Q37.2
          with hard Q37.4
    median Q36.1
  nose Q30.2
  palate Q35.9
    with cleft lip (unilateral) Q37.9
      bilateral Q37.8
    hard Q35.1
      with
        cleft lip (unilateral) Q37.1
          bilateral Q37.0
        soft Q35.5
          with cleft lip (unilateral) Q37.5
            bilateral Q37.4
    medial Q35.5
    soft Q35.3
      with
        cleft lip (unilateral) Q37.3
          bilateral Q37.2
        hard Q35.5
          with cleft lip (unilateral) Q37.5
            bilateral Q37.4
  penis Q55.69
  scrotum Q55.29
  thyroid cartilage Q31.8
  uvula Q35.7
Cleidocranial dysostosis Q74.0
Cleptomania F63.2
Clicking hip (newborn) R29.4
Climacteric (female) —*see also* Menopause
  arthritis (any site) NEC —*see* Arthritis, specified form NEC
  depression (single episode) F32.8
  male (symptoms) (syndrome) NEC N50.8
  paranoid state F22
  polyarthritis NEC —*see* Arthritis, specified form NEC
  symptoms (female) N95.1
Clinical research investigation (clinical trial) (control subject) (normal comparison) (participant) Z00.6
Clitoris —*see* condition Cloaca (persistent) Q43.7
Clonorchiasis, clonorchis infection (liver) B66.1
Clonus R25.8
Closed bite M26.29
Clostridium (C.) perfringens, as cause of disease classified elsewhere B96.7
Closure
  congenital, nose Q30.0
  cranial sutures, premature Q75.0
  defective or imperfect NEC —*see* Imperfect, closure
  fistula, delayed —*see* Fistula
  foramen ovale, imperfect Q21.1
  hymen N89.6
  interauricular septum, defective Q21.1
  interventricular septum, defective Q21.0
  lacrimal duct —*see also* Stenosis, lacrimal, duct
    congenital Q10.5
  nose (congenital) Q30.0
    acquired M95.0
  of artificial opening —*see* Attention to, artificial, opening

Closure *(Continued)*
  primary angle, without glaucoma damage H40.06-
  vagina N89.5
  valve —*see* Endocarditis
  vulva N90.5
Clot (blood) —*see also* Embolism
  artery (obstruction) (occlusion) —*see* Embolism
  bladder N32.89
  brain (intradural or extradural) —*see* Occlusion, artery, cerebral
  circulation I74.9
  heart —*see also* Infarct, myocardium
    not resulting in infarction I24.0
  vein —*see* Thrombosis
Clouded state R40.1
  epileptic —*see* Epilepsy, specified NEC
  paroxysmal —*see* Epilepsy, specified NEC
Cloudy antrum, antra J32.0
Clouston's (hidrotic) ectodermal dysplasia Q82.4
Clubbed nail pachydermoperiostosis M89.40 [L62]
Clubbing of finger (s) (nails) R68.3
Clubfinger R68.3
  congenital Q68.1
Clubfoot (congenital) Q66.89
  acquired —*see* Deformity, limb, clubfoot
  equinovarus Q66.0
  paralytic —*see* Deformity, limb, clubfoot
Clubhand (congenital) (radial) Q71.4-
  acquired —*see* Deformity, limb, clubhand
Clubnail R68.3
  congenital Q84.6
Clump, kidney Q63.1
Clumsiness, clumsy child syndrome F82
Cluttering F98.81
Clutton's joints A50.51 [M12.80]
Coagulation, intravascular (diffuse) (disseminated) —*see also* Defibrination syndrome
  complicating abortion —*see* Abortion, by type, complicated by, intravascular coagulation
  following ectopic or molar pregnancy O08.1
Coagulopathy —*see also* Defect, coagulation
  consumption D65
  intravascular D65
  newborn P60
Coalition
  calcaneo-scaphoid Q66.89
  tarsal Q66.89
Coalminer's
  elbow —*see* Bursitis, elbow, olecranon
  lung or pneumoconiosis J60
Coalworker's lung or pneumoconiosis J60
Coarctation
  aorta (preductal) (postductal) Q25.1
  pulmonary artery Q25.71
Coated tongue K14.3
Coats' disease (exudative retinopathy) —*see* Retinopathy, exudative
Cocainism —*see* Dependence, drug, cocaine
Coccidioidomycosis B38.9
  cutaneous B38.3
  disseminated B38.7
  generalized B38.7
  meninges B38.4
  prostate B38.81
  pulmonary B38.2
    acute B38.0
    chronic B38.1
  skin B38.3
  specified NEC B38.89
Coccidioidosis —*see* Coccidioidomycosis
Coccidiosis (intestinal) A07.3
Coccydynia, coccygodynia M53.3
Coccyx —*see* condition
Cochin-China diarrhea K90.1
Cockayne's syndrome Q87.1

Cocked up toe —*see* Deformity, toe, specified NEC
Cock's peculiar tumor L72.3
Codman's tumor —*see* Neoplasm, bone, benign
Coenurosis B71.8
Coffee-worker's lung J67.8
Cogan's syndrome H16.32-
  oculomotor apraxia H51.8
Coitus, painful (female) N94.1
  male N53.12
  psychogenic F52.6
Cold J00
  with influenza, flu, or grippe —*see* Influenza, with, respiratory manifestations NEC
  agglutinin disease or hemoglobinuria (chronic) D59.1
  bronchial —*see* Bronchitis
  chest —*see* Bronchitis
  common (head) J00
  effects of T69.9
    specified effect NEC T69.8
  excessive, effects of T69.9
    specified effect NEC T69.8
  exhaustion from T69.8
  exposure to T69.9
    specified effect NEC T69.8
  head J00
  injury syndrome (newborn) P80.0
  on lung —*see* Bronchitis
  rose J30.1
  sensitivity, auto-immune D59.1
  virus J00
Coldsore B00.1
Colibacillosis A49.8
  as the cause of other disease (*see also* Escherichia coli) B96.20
  generalized A41.50
Colic (bilious) (infantile) (intestinal) (recurrent) (spasmodic) R10.83
  abdomen R10.83
    psychogenic F45.8
  appendix, appendicular K38.8
  bile duct —*see* Calculus, bile duct
  biliary —*see* Calculus, bile duct
  common duct —*see* Calculus, bile duct
  cystic duct —*see* Calculus, gallbladder
  Devonshire NEC —*see* Poisoning, lead
  gallbladder —*see* Calculus, gallbladder
  gallstone —*see* Calculus, gallbladder
    gallbladder or cystic duct —*see* Calculus, gallbladder
  hepatic (duct) —*see* Calculus, bile duct
  hysterical F45.8
  kidney N23
  lead NEC —*see* Poisoning, lead
  mucous K58.9
    with diarrhea K58.0
    psychogenic F54
  nephritic N23
  painter's NEC —*see* Poisoning, lead
  pancreas K86.8
  psychogenic F45.8
  renal N23
  saturnine NEC —*see* Poisoning, lead
  ureter N23
  urethral N36.8
    due to calculus N21.1
  uterus NEC N94.89
    menstrual —*see* Dysmenorrhea
  worm NOS B83.9
Colicystitis —*see* Cystitis
Colitis (acute) (catarrhal) (chronic) (noninfective) (hemorrhagic) (*see also* Enteritis) K52.9
  allergic K52.2
  amebic (acute) (*see also* Amebiasis) A06.0
    nondysenteric A06.2
  anthrax A22.2
  bacillary —*see* Infection, Shigella
  balantidial A07.0
  Clostridium difficile A04.7

Colitis (*Continued*)
  coccidial A07.3
  collagenous K52.89
  cystica superficialis K52.89
  dietary counseling and surveillance (for) Z71.3
  dietetic K52.2
  drug-induced K52.1
  due to radiation K52.0
  eosinophilic K52.82
  food hypersensitivity K52.2
  giardial A07.1
  granulomatous —*see* Enteritis, regional, large intestine
  infectious —*see* Enteritis, infectious
  ischemic K55.9
    acute (fulminant) (subacute) K55.0
    chronic K55.1
    due to mesenteric artery insufficiency K55.1
    fulminant (acute) K55.0
  left sided K51.50
    with
      abscess K51.514
      complication K51.519
        specified NEC K51.518
      fistula K51.513
      obstruction K51.512
      rectal bleeding K51.511
  lymphocytic K52.89
  membranous
    psychogenic F54
  microscopic (collagenous) (lymphocytic) K52.89
  mucous —*see* Syndrome, irritable, bowel
    psychogenic F54
  noninfective K52.9
    specified NEC K52.89
  polyposa —*see* Polyp, colon, inflammatory
  protozoal A07.9
  pseudomembranous A04.7
  pseudomucinous —*see* Syndrome, irritable, bowel
  regional —*see* Enteritis, regional, large intestine
  segmental —*see* Enteritis, regional, large intestine
  septic —*see* Enteritis, infectious
  spastic K58.9
    with diarrhea K58.0
    psychogenic F54
  staphylococcal A04.8
    foodborne A05.0
  subacute ischemic K55.0
  thromboulcerative K55.0
  toxic NEC K52.1
    due to Clostridium difficile A04.7
  transmural —*see* Enteritis, regional, large intestine
  trichomonal A07.8
  tuberculous (ulcerative) A18.32
  ulcerative (chronic) K51.90
    with
      complication K51.919
        abscess K51.914
        fistula K51.913
        obstruction K51.912
        rectal bleeding K51.911
        specified complication NEC K51.918
    enterocolitis —*see* Enterocolitis, ulcerative
    ileocolitis —*see* Ileocolitis, ulcerative
    mucosal proctocolitis —*see* Proctocolitis, mucosal
    proctitis —*see* Proctitis, ulcerative
    pseudopolyposis —*see* Polyp, colon, inflammatory
    psychogenic F54
    rectosigmoiditis —*see* Rectosigmoiditis, ulcerative

Colitis (*Continued*)
  ulcerative (*Continued*)
    specified type NEC K51.80
      with
        complication K51.819
          abscess K51.814
          fistula K51.813
          obstruction K51.812
          rectal bleeding K51.811
          specified complication NEC K51.818
Collagenosis, collagen disease (nonvascular) (vascular) M35.9
  cardiovascular I42.8
  reactive perforating L87.1
  specified NEC M35.8
Collapse R55
  adrenal E27.2
  cardiorespiratory R57.0
  cardiovascular R57.0
    newborn P29.89
  circulatory (peripheral) R57.9
    during or after labor and delivery O75.1
    following ectopic or molar pregnancy O08.3
    newborn P29.89
  during or
    after labor and delivery O75.1
    resulting from a procedure, not elsewhere classified T81.10
  external ear canal —*see* Stenosis, external ear canal
  general R55
  heart —*see* Disease, heart
  heat T67.1
  hysterical F44.89
  labyrinth, membranous (congenital) Q16.5
  lung (massive) (*see also* Atelectasis) J98.19
    pressure due to anesthesia (general) (local) or other sedation T88.2
      during labor and delivery O74.1
      in pregnancy O29.02-
      postpartum, puerperal O89.09
  myocardial —*see* Disease, heart
  nervous F48.8
  neurocirculatory F45.8
  nose M95.0
  postoperative T81.10
  pulmonary (*see also* Atelectasis) J98.19
    newborn —*see* Atelectasis
  trachea J39.8
  tracheobronchial J98.09
  valvular —*see* Endocarditis
  vascular (peripheral) R57.9
    during or after labor and delivery O75.1
    following ectopic or molar pregnancy O08.3
    newborn P29.89
  vertebra M48.50-
    cervical region M48.52-
    cervicothoracic region M48.53-
    in (due to)
      metastasis —*see* Collapse, vertebra, in, specified disease NEC
      osteoporosis (*see also* Osteoporosis) M80.88
        cervical region M80.88
        cervicothoracic region M80.88
        lumbar region M80.88
        lumbosacral region M80.88
        multiple sites M80.88
        occipito-atlanto-axial region M80.88
        sacrococcygeal region M80.88
        thoracic region M80.88
        thoracolumbar region M80.88
      specified disease NEC M48.50-
        cervical region M48.52-
        cervicothoracic region M48.53-
        lumbar region M48.56-
        lumbosacral region M48.57-
        occipito-atlanto-axial region M48.51-

Collapse *(Continued)*
  vertebra *(Continued)*
    in *(Continued)*
      specified disease NEC *(Continued)*
        sacrococcygeal region M48.58-
        thoracic region M48.54-
        thoracolumbar region M48.55-
      lumbar region M48.56-
      lumbosacral region M48.57-
      occipito-atlanto-axial region M48.51-
      sacrococcygeal region M48.58-
      thoracic region M48.54-
      thoracolumbar region M48.55-
Collateral —*see also* condition
  circulation (venous) I87.8
  dilation, veins I87.8
Colles' fracture S52.53-
Collet (-Sicard) syndrome G52.7
Collier's asthma or lung J60
Collodion baby Q80.2
Colloid nodule (of thyroid) (cystic) E04.1
Coloboma (iris) Q13.0
  eyelid Q10.3
  fundus Q14.8
  lens Q12.2
  optic disc (congenital) Q14.2
    acquired H47.31-
Coloenteritis —*see* Enteritis
Colon —*see* condition
Colonization
  MRSA (Methicillin resistant Staphylococcus aureus) Z22.322
  MSSA (Methicillin susceptible Staphylococcus aureus) Z22.321
  status —*see* Carrier (suspected) of
Coloptosis K63.4
Color blindness —*see* Deficiency, color vision
Colostomy
  attention to Z43.3
  fitting or adjustment Z46.89
  malfunctioning K94.03
  status Z93.3
Colpitis (acute) —*see* Vaginitis
Colpocele N81.5
Colpocystitis —*see* Vaginitis
Colpospasm N94.2
Column, spinal, vertebral —*see* condition
Coma R40.20
  with
    motor response (none) R40.231
      abnormal R40.233
      extension R40.232
      flexion withdrawal R40.234
      localizes pain R40.235
      obeys commands R40.236
    opening of eyes (never) R40.211
      in response to
        pain R40.212
        sound R40.213
      spontaneous R40.214
    verbal response (none) R40.221
      confused conversation R40.224
      inappropriate words R40.223
      incomprehensible words R40.222
      oriented R40.225
  eclamptic —*see* Eclampsia
  epileptic —*see* Epilepsy
  Glasgow, scale score —*see* Glasgow coma scale
  hepatic —*see* Failure, hepatic, by type, with coma
  hyperglycemic (diabetic) —*see* Diabetes, coma
  hyperosmolar (diabetic) —*see* Diabetes, coma
  hypoglycemic (diabetic) —*see* Diabetes, coma, hypoglycemic
    nondiabetic E15
  in diabetes —*see* Diabetes, coma
  insulin-induced —*see* Coma, hypoglycemic
  myxedematous E03.5
  newborn P91.5
  persistent vegetative state R40.3

Coma *(Continued)*
  specified NEC, without documented Glasgow coma scale score, or with partial Glasgow coma scale score reported R40.244
Comatose —*see* Coma
Combat fatigue F43.0
Combined —*see* condition
Comedo, comedones (giant) L70.0
Comedocarcinoma —*see also* Neoplasm, breast, malignant
  noninfiltrating
    breast D05.8-
    specified site —*see* Neoplasm, in situ, by site
    unspecified site D05.8-
Comedomastitis —*see* Ectasia, mammary duct
Comminuted fracture - code as Fracture, closed
Common
  arterial trunk Q20.0
  atrioventricular canal Q21.2
  atrium Q21.1
  cold (head) J00
  truncus (arteriosus) Q20.0
  variable immunodeficiency —*see* Immunodeficiency, common variable
  ventricle Q20.4
Commotio, commotion (current)
  brain —*see* Injury, intracranial, concussion
  cerebri —*see* Injury, intracranial, concussion
  retinae S05.8X-
  spinal cord —*see* Injury, spinal cord, by region
  spinalis —*see* Injury, spinal cord, by region
Communication
  between
    base of aorta and pulmonary artery Q21.4
    left ventricle and right atrium Q20.5
    pericardial sac and pleural sac Q34.8
    pulmonary artery and pulmonary vein, congenital Q25.72
  congenital between uterus and digestive or urinary tract Q51.7
Compartment syndrome (deep) (posterior) (traumatic) T79.A0
  abdomen T79.A3
  lower extremity (hip, buttock, thigh, leg, foot, toes) T79.A2
  nontraumatic
    abdomen M79.A3
    lower extremity (hip, buttock, thigh, leg, foot, toes) M79.A2-
    specified site NEC M79.A9
    upper extremity (shoulder, arm, forearm, wrist, hand, fingers) M79.A1-
  specified site NEC T79.A9
  upper extremity (shoulder, arm, forearm, wrist, hand, fingers) T79.A1
Compensation
  failure —*see* Disease, heart
  neurosis, psychoneurosis —*see* Disorder, factitious
Complaint —*see also* Disease
  bowel, functional K59.9
    psychogenic F45.8
  intestine, functional K59.9
    psychogenic F45.8
  kidney —*see* Disease, renal
  miners' J60
Complete —*see* condition
Complex
  Addison-Schilder E71.528
  cardiorenal —*see* Hypertension, cardiorenal
  Costen's M26.69
  disseminated mycobacterium avium-intracellulare (DMAC) A31.2
  Eisenmenger's (ventricular septal defect) I27.89
  hypersexual F52.8
  jumped process, spine —*see* Dislocation, vertebra

Complex *(Continued)*
  primary, tuberculous A15.7
  Schilder-Addison E71.528
  subluxation (vertebral) M99.19
    abdomen M99.19
    acromioclavicular M99.17
    cervical region M99.11
    cervicothoracic M99.11
    costochondral M99.18
    costovertebral M99.18
    head region M99.10
    hip M99.15
    lower extremity M99.16
    lumbar region M99.13
    lumbosacral M99.13
    occipitocervical M99.10
    pelvic region M99.15
    pubic M99.15
    rib cage M99.18
    sacral region M99.14
    sacrococcygeal M99.14
    sacroiliac M99.14
    specified NEC M99.19
    sternochondral M99.18
    sternoclavicular M99.17
    thoracic region M99.12
    thoracolumbar M99.12
    upper extremity M99.17
  Taussig-Bing (transposition, aorta and overriding pulmonary artery) Q20.1
Complication (s) (from) (of)
  accidental puncture or laceration during a procedure (of) —*see* Complications, intraoperative (intraprocedural), puncture or laceration
  amputation stump (surgical) (late) NEC T87.9
    dehiscence T87.81
    infection or inflammation T87.40
      lower limb T87.4-
      upper limb T87.4-
    necrosis T87.50
      lower limb T87.5-
      upper limb T87.5-
    neuroma T87.30
      lower limb T87.3-
      upper limb T87.3-
    specified type NEC T87.89
  anastomosis (and bypass) —*see also* Complications, prosthetic device or implant
    intestinal (internal) NEC K91.89
      involving urinary tract N99.89
    urinary tract (involving intestinal tract) N99.89
    vascular —*see* Complications, cardiovascular device or implant
  anesthesia, anesthetic (*see also* Anesthesia, complication) T88.59
    brain, postpartum, puerperal O89.2
    cardiac
      in
        labor and delivery O74.2
        pregnancy O29.19-
      postpartum, puerperal O89.1
    central nervous system
      in
        labor and delivery O74.3
        pregnancy O29.29-
      postpartum, puerperal O89.2
    difficult or failed intubation T88.4
      in pregnancy O29.6-
    failed sedation (conscious) (moderate) during procedure T88.52
    hyperthermia, malignant T88.3
    hypothermia T88.51
    intubation failure T88.4
    malignant hyperthermia T88.3

Complication (*Continued*)
  anesthesia, anesthetic (*Continued*)
    pulmonary
      in
        labor and delivery O74.1
        pregnancy NEC O29.09-
      postpartum, puerperal O89.09
    shock T88.2
    spinal and epidural
      in
        labor and delivery NEC O74.6
          headache O74.5
        pregnancy NEC O29.5X-
      postpartum, puerperal NEC O89.5
        headache O89.4
  anti-reflux device —*see* Complications,
      esophageal anti-reflux device
  aortic (bifurcation) graft —*see* Complications,
      graft, vascular
  aortocoronary (bypass) graft —*see*
      Complications, coronary artery (bypass)
      graft
  aortofemoral (bypass) graft —*see*
      Complications, extremity artery
      (bypass) graft
  arteriovenous
    fistula, surgically created T82.9
      embolism T82.818
      fibrosis T82.828
      hemorrhage T82.838
      infection or inflammation T82.7
      mechanical
        breakdown T82.510
        displacement T82.520
        leakage T82.530
        malposition T82.520
        obstruction T82.590
        perforation T82.590
        protrusion T82.590
      pain T82.848
      specified type NEC T82.898
      stenosis T82.858
      thrombosis T82.868
    shunt, surgically created T82.9
      embolism T82.818
      fibrosis T82.828
      hemorrhage T82.838
      infection or inflammation T82.7
      mechanical
        breakdown T82.511
        displacement T82.521
        leakage T82.531
        malposition T82.521
        obstruction T82.591
        perforation T82.591
        protrusion T82.591
      pain T82.848
      specified type NEC T82.898
      stenosis T82.858
      thrombosis T82.868
  arthroplasty —*see* Complications, joint
      prosthesis
  artificial
    fertilization or insemination N98.9
      attempted introduction (of)
        embryo in embryo transfer N98.3
        ovum following in vitro fertilization
          N98.2
      hyperstimulation of ovaries N98.1
      infection N98.0
      specified NEC N98.8
    heart T82.9
      embolism T82.817
      fibrosis T82.827
      hemorrhage T82.837
      infection or inflammation T82.7
      mechanical
        breakdown T82.512
        displacement T82.522
        leakage T82.532
        malposition T82.522

Complication (*Continued*)
  artificial (*Continued*)
    heart (*Continued*)
      mechanical (*Continued*)
        obstruction T82.592
        perforation T82.592
        protrusion T82.592
      pain T82.847
      specified type NEC T82.897
      stenosis T82.857
      thrombosis T82.867
    opening
      cecostomy —*see* Complications,
        colostomy
      colostomy —*see* Complications,
        colostomy
      cystostomy —*see* Complications,
        cystostomy
      enterostomy —*see* Complications,
        enterostomy
      gastrostomy —*see* Complications,
        gastrostomy
      ileostomy —*see* Complications,
        enterostomy
      jejunostomy —*see* Complications,
        enterostomy
      nephrostomy —*see* Complications,
        stoma, urinary tract
      tracheostomy —*see* Complications,
        tracheostomy
      ureterostomy —*see* Complications,
        stoma, urinary tract
      urethrostomy —*see* Complications,
        stoma, urinary tract
    balloon implant or device
      gastrointestinal T85.9
        embolism T85.81
        fibrosis T85.82
        hemorrhage T85.83
        infection and inflammation
          T85.79
        pain T85.84
        specified type NEC T85.89
        stenosis T85.85
        thrombosis T85.86
      vascular (counterpulsation) T82.9
        embolism T82.818
        fibrosis T82.828
        hemorrhage T82.838
        infection or inflammation T82.7
        mechanical
          breakdown T82.513
          displacement T82.523
          leakage T82.533
          malposition T82.523
          obstruction T82.593
          perforation T82.593
          protrusion T82.593
        pain T82.848
        specified type NEC T82.898
        stenosis T82.858
        thrombosis T82.868
    bariatric procedure
      gastric band procedure K95.09
        infection K95.01
      specified procedure NEC K95.89
        infection K95.81
    bile duct implant (prosthetic) T85.9
      embolism T85.81
      fibrosis T85.82
      hemorrhage T85.83
      infection and inflammation T85.79
      mechanical
        breakdown T85.510
        displacement T85.520
        malfunction T85.510
        malposition T85.520
        obstruction T85.590
        perforation T85.590
        protrusion T85.590
        specified NEC T85.590

Complication (*Continued*)
  bile duct implant (*Continued*)
    pain T85.84
    specified type NEC T85.89
    stenosis T85.85
    thrombosis T85.86
  bladder device (auxiliary) —*see*
      Complications, genitourinary, device or
      implant, urinary system
  bleeding (postoperative) —*see* Complication,
      postoperative, hemorrhage
    intraoperative —*see* Complication,
      intraoperative, hemorrhage
  blood vessel graft —*see* Complications, graft,
      vascular
  bone
    device NEC T84.9
      embolism T84.81
      fibrosis T84.82
      hemorrhage T84.83
      infection or inflammation T84.7
      mechanical
        breakdown T84.318
        displacement T84.328
        malposition T84.328
        obstruction T84.398
        perforation T84.398
        protrusion T84.398
      pain T84.84
      specified type NEC T84.89
      stenosis T84.85
      thrombosis T84.86
    graft —*see* Complications, graft, bone
    growth stimulator (electrode) —*see*
      Complications, electronic stimulator
      device, bone
    marrow transplant —*see* Complications,
      transplant, bone, marrow
  brain neurostimulator (electrode) —*see*
      Complications, electronic stimulator
      device, brain
  breast implant (prosthetic) T85.9
    capsular contracture T85.44
    embolism T85.81
    fibrosis T85.82
    hemorrhage T85.83
    infection and inflammation
      T85.79
    mechanical
      breakdown T85.41
      displacement T85.42
      leakage T85.43
      malposition T85.42
      obstruction T85.49
      perforation T85.49
      protrusion T85.49
      specified NEC T85.49
    pain T85.84
    specified type NEC T85.89
    stenosis T85.85
    thrombosis T85.86
  bypass —*see also* Complications, prosthetic
      device or implant
    aortocoronary —*see* Complications,
      coronary artery (bypass) graft
    arterial —*see also* Complications, graft,
      vascular
      extremity —*see* Complications, extremity
        artery (bypass) graft
  cardiac —*see also* Disease, heart
    device, implant or graft T82.9
      embolism T82.817
      fibrosis T82.827
      hemorrhage T82.837
      infection or inflammation T82.7
      valve prosthesis T82.6
      mechanical
        breakdown T82.519
          specified device NEC T82.518
        displacement T82.529
          specified device NEC T82.528

Complication (Continued)
  cardiac (Continued)
    device, implant or graft (Continued)
      mechanical (Continued)
        leakage T82.539
          specified device NEC T82.538
        malposition T82.529
          specified device NEC T82.528
        obstruction T82.599
          specified device NEC T82.598
        perforation T82.599
          specified device NEC T82.598
        protrusion T82.599
          specified device NEC T82.598
        pain T82.847
        specified type NEC T82.897
        stenosis T82.857
        thrombosis T82.867
  cardiovascular device, graft or implant
    T82.9
    aortic graft —see Complications, graft,
      vascular
    arteriovenous
      fistula, artificial —see Complication,
        arteriovenous, fistula, surgically
        created
      shunt —see Complication, arteriovenous,
        shunt, surgically created
    artificial heart —see Complication,
      artificial, heart
    balloon (counterpulsation) device —see
      Complication, balloon implant,
      vascular
    carotid artery graft —see Complications,
      graft, vascular
    coronary bypass graft —see Complication,
      coronary artery (bypass) graft
    dialysis catheter (vascular) —see
      Complication, catheter, dialysis
    electronic T82.9
      electrode T82.9
        embolism T82.817
        fibrosis T82.827
        hemorrhage T82.837
        infection T82.7
        mechanical
          breakdown T82.110
          displacement T82.120
          leakage T82.190
          obstruction T82.190
          perforation T82.190
          protrusion T82.190
          specified type NEC T82.190
        pain T82.847
        specified NEC T82.897
        stenosis T82.857
        thrombosis T82.867
      embolism T82.817
      fibrosis T82.827
      hemorrhage T82.837
      infection T82.7
      mechanical
        breakdown T82.119
        displacement T82.129
        leakage T82.199
        obstruction T82.199
        perforation T82.199
        protrusion T82.199
        specified type NEC T82.199
      pain T82.847
      pulse generator T82.9
        embolism T82.817
        fibrosis T82.827
        hemorrhage T82.837
        infection T82.7
        mechanical
          breakdown T82.111
          displacement T82.121
          leakage T82.191
          obstruction T82.191
          perforation T82.191

Complication (Continued)
  cardiovascular device, graft or implant
    (Continued)
    electronic (Continued)
      pulse generator (Continued)
        mechanical (Continued)
          protrusion T82.191
          specified type NEC T82.191
        pain T82.847
        specified NEC T82.897
        stenosis T82.857
        thrombosis T82.867
      specified condition NEC T82.897
      specified device NEC T82.9
        embolism T82.817
        fibrosis T82.827
        hemorrhage T82.837
        infection T82.7
        mechanical
          breakdown T82.118
          displacement T82.128
          leakage T82.198
          obstruction T82.198
          perforation T82.198
          protrusion T82.198
          specified type NEC T82.198
        pain T82.847
        specified NEC T82.897
        stenosis T82.857
        thrombosis T82.867
      stenosis T82.857
      thrombosis T82.867
    extremity artery graft —see Complication,
      extremity artery (bypass) graft
    femoral artery graft —see Complication,
      extremity artery (bypass) graft
    heart
      transplant —see Complication,
        transplant, heart
      valve —see Complication, prosthetic
        device, heart valve
      graft —see Complication, heart, valve,
        graft
    heart-lung transplant —see Complication,
      transplant, heart, with lung
    infection or inflammation T82.7
    umbrella device —see Complication,
      umbrella device, vascular
    vascular graft (or anastomosis) —see
      Complication, graft, vascular
  carotid artery (bypass) graft —see
    Complications, graft, vascular
  catheter (device) NEC —see also
    Complications, prosthetic device or
    implant
    cystostomy T83.9
      embolism T83.81
      fibrosis T83.82
      hemorrhage T83.83
      infection and inflammation
        T83.59
      mechanical
        breakdown T83.010
        displacement T83.020
        leakage T83.030
        malposition T83.020
        obstruction T83.090
        perforation T83.090
        protrusion T83.090
        specified NEC T83.090
      pain T83.84
      specified type NEC T83.89
      stenosis T83.85
      thrombosis T83.86
    dialysis (vascular) T82.9
      embolism T82.818
      fibrosis T82.828
      hemorrhage T82.838
      infection and inflammation T82.7
      intraperitoneal —see Complications,
        catheter, intraperitoneal

Complication (Continued)
  catheter NEC (Continued)
    dialysis (Continued)
      mechanical
        breakdown T82.41
        displacement T82.42
        leakage T82.43
        malposition T82.42
        obstruction T82.49
        perforation T82.49
        protrusion T82.49
      pain T82.848
      specified type NEC T82.898
      stenosis T82.858
      thrombosis T82.868
    epidural infusion T85.9
      embolism T85.81
      fibrosis T85.82
      hemorrhage T85.83
      infection and inflammation T85.79
      mechanical
        breakdown T85.610
        displacement T85.620
        leakage T85.630
        malfunction T85.610
        malposition T85.620
        obstruction T85.690
        perforation T85.690
        protrusion T85.690
        specified NEC T85.690
      pain T85.84
      specified type NEC T85.89
      stenosis T85.85
      thrombosis T85.86
    intraperitoneal dialysis T85.9
      embolism T85.81
      fibrosis T85.82
      hemorrhage T85.83
      infection and inflammation T85.71
      mechanical
        breakdown T85.611
        displacement T85.621
        leakage T85.631
        malfunction T85.611
        malposition T85.621
        obstruction T85.691
        perforation T85.691
        protrusion T85.691
        specified NEC T85.691
      pain T85.84
      specified type NEC T85.89
      stenosis T85.85
      thrombosis T85.86
    intravenous infusion T82.9
      embolism T82.818
      fibrosis T82.828
      hemorrhage T82.838
      infection or inflammation T82.7
      mechanical
        breakdown T82.514
        displacement T82.524
        leakage T82.534
        malposition T82.524
        obstruction T82.594
        perforation T82.594
        protrusion T82.594
      pain T82.848
      specified type NEC T82.898
      stenosis T82.858
      thrombosis T82.868
    subdural infusion T85.9
      embolism T85.81
      fibrosis T85.82
      hemorrhage T85.83
      infection and inflammation T85.79
      mechanical
        breakdown T85.610
        displacement T85.620
        leakage T85.630
        malfunction T85.610
        malposition T85.620

◀ New   ◀▥ Revised   ~~deleted~~ Deleted

Complication *(Continued)*
  electronic stimulator device *(Continued)*
    spinal cord T85.9
      embolism T85.81
      fibrosis T85.82
      hemorrhage T85.83
      infection and inflammation
        T85.79
      mechanical
        breakdown T85.112
        displacement T85.122
        leakage T85.192
        malposition T85.122
        obstruction T85.192
        perforation T85.192
        protrusion T85.192
        specified NEC T85.192
      pain T85.84
      specified type NEC T85.89
      stenosis T85.85
      thrombosis T85.86
    urinary T83.9
      embolism T83.81
      fibrosis T83.82
      hemorrhage T83.83
      infection and inflammation T83.59
      mechanical
        breakdown T83.110
        displacement T83.120
        malposition T83.120
        perforation T83.190
        protrusion T83.190
        specified NEC T83.190
      pain T83.84
      specified type NEC T83.89
      stenosis T83.85
      thrombosis T83.86
  electroshock therapy T88.9
    specified NEC T88.8
  endocrine E34.9
    postprocedural
      adrenal hypofunction E89.6
      hypoinsulinemia E89.1
      hypoparathyroidism E89.2
      hypopituitarism E89.3
      hypothyroidism E89.0
      ovarian failure E89.40
        asymptomatic E89.40
        symptomatic E89.41
      specified NEC E89.89
      testicular hypofunction E89.5
  endodontic treatment NEC M27.59
  enterostomy (stoma) K94.10
    hemorrhage K94.11
    infection K94.12
    malfunction K94.13
    mechanical K94.13
    specified complication NEC K94.19
  episiotomy, disruption O90.1
  esophageal anti-reflux device T85.9
    embolism T85.81
    fibrosis T85.82
    hemorrhage T85.83
    infection and inflammation T85.79
    mechanical
      breakdown T85.511
      displacement T85.521
      malfunction T85.511
      malposition T85.521
      obstruction T85.591
      perforation T85.591
      protrusion T85.591
      specified NEC T85.591
    pain T85.84
    specified type NEC T85.89
    stenosis T85.85
    thrombosis T85.86
  esophagostomy K94.30
    hemorrhage K94.31
    infection K94.32
    malfunction K94.33

Complication *(Continued)*
  esophagostomy *(Continued)*
    mechanical K94.33
    specified complication NEC K94.39
  extracorporeal circulation T80.90
  extremity artery (bypass) graft T82.9
    arteriosclerosis —*see* Arteriosclerosis,
      extremities, bypass graft
    embolism T82.818
    fibrosis T82.828
    hemorrhage T82.838
    infection and inflammation T82.7
    mechanical
      breakdown T82.318
        femoral artery T82.312
      displacement T82.328
        femoral artery T82.322
      leakage T82.338
        femoral artery T82.332
      malposition T82.328
        femoral artery T82.322
      obstruction T82.398
        femoral artery T82.392
      perforation T82.398
        femoral artery T82.392
      protrusion T82.398
        femoral artery T82.392
    pain T82.848
    specified type NEC T82.898
    stenosis T82.858
    thrombosis T82.868
  eye H57.9
    corneal graft —*see* Complications, graft,
      cornea
    implant (prosthetic) T85.9
      embolism T85.81
      fibrosis T85.82
      hemorrhage T85.83
      infection and inflammation T85.79
      mechanical
        breakdown T85.318
        displacement T85.328
        leakage T85.398
        malposition T85.328
        obstruction T85.398
        perforation T85.398
        protrusion T85.398
        specified NEC T85.398
      pain T85.84
      specified type NEC T85.89
      stenosis T85.85
      thrombosis T85.86
    intraocular lens —*see* Complications,
      intraocular lens
    orbital prosthesis —*see* Complications,
      orbital prosthesis
  female genital N94.9
    device, implant or graft NEC —*see*
      Complications, genitourinary, device
      or implant, genital tract
  femoral artery (bypass) graft —*see*
    Complication, extremity artery (bypass)
    graft
  fixation device, internal (orthopedic) T84.9
    infection and inflammation T84.60
      arm T84.61-
        humerus T84.61-
        radius T84.61-
        ulna T84.61-
      leg T84.629
        femur T84.62-
        fibula T84.62-
        tibia T84.62-
      specified site NEC T84.69
      spine T84.63
    mechanical
      breakdown
        limb T84.119
          carpal T84.210
          femur T84.11-
          fibula T84.11-

Complication *(Continued)*
  fixation device, internal *(Continued)*
    mechanical *(Continued)*
      breakdown *(Continued)*
        limb *(Continued)*
          humerus T84.11-
          metacarpal T84.210
          metatarsal T84.213
          phalanx
            foot T84.213
            hand T84.210
          radius T84.11-
          tarsal T84.213
          tibia T84.11-
          ulna T84.11-
        specified bone NEC T84.218
        spine T84.216
      displacement
        limb T84.129
          carpal T84.220
          femur T84.12-
          fibula T84.12-
          humerus T84.12-
          metacarpal T84.220
          metatarsal T84.223
          phalanx
            foot T84.223
            hand T84.220
          radius T84.12-
          tarsal T84.223
          tibia T84.12-
          ulna T84.12-
        specified bone NEC T84.228
        spine T84.226
      malposition —*see* Complications,
        fixation device, internal,
        mechanical, displacement
      obstruction —*see* Complications, fixation
        device, internal, mechanical,
        specified type NEC
      perforation —*see* Complications, fixation
        device, internal, mechanical,
        specified type NEC
      protrusion —*see* Complications, fixation
        device, internal, mechanical,
        specified type NEC
      specified type NEC
        limb T84.199
          carpal T84.290
          femur T84.19-
          fibula T84.19-
          humerus T84.19-
          metacarpal T84.290
          metatarsal T84.293
          phalanx
            foot T84.293
            hand T84.290
          radius T84.19-
          tarsal T84.293
          tibia T84.19-
          ulna T84.19-
        specified bone NEC T84.298
        vertebra T84.296
    specified type NEC T84.89
      embolism T84.81
      fibrosis T84.82
      hemorrhage T84.83
      pain T84.84
      specified complication NEC T84.89
      stenosis T84.85
      thrombosis T84.86
  following
    acute myocardial infarction NEC I23.8
    aneurysm (false) (of cardiac wall) (of
      heart wall) (ruptured) I23.3
    angina I23.7
    atrial
      septal defect I23.1
      thrombosis I23.6
    cardiac wall rupture I23.3
    chordae tendinae rupture I23.4

Complication (Continued)
  following (Continued)
    acute myocardial infarction NEC
      (Continued)
      defect
        septal
          atrial (heart) I23.1
          ventricular (heart) I23.2
      hemopericardium I23.0
      papillary muscle rupture I23.5
      rupture
        cardiac wall I23.3
          with hemopericardium
            I23.0
        chordae tendineae I23.4
        papillary muscle I23.5
      specified NEC I23.8
      thrombosis
        atrium I23.6
        auricular appendage I23.6
        ventricle (heart) I23.6
      ventricular
        septal defect I23.2
        thrombosis I23.6
    ectopic or molar pregnancy O08.9
      cardiac arrest O08.81
      sepsis O08.82
      specified type NEC O08.89
      urinary tract infection O08.83
    termination of pregnancy —see Abortion
  gastrointestinal K92.9
    bile duct prosthesis —see Complications,
      bile duct implant
    esophageal anti-reflux device —see
      Complications, esophageal
      anti-reflux device
    postoperative
      colostomy —see Complications,
        colostomy
      dumping syndrome K91.1
      enterostomy —see Complications,
        enterostomy
      gastrostomy —see Complications,
        gastrostomy
      malabsorption NEC K91.2
      obstruction K91.3
      postcholecystectomy syndrome
        K91.5
      specified NEC K91.89
      vomiting after GI surgery K91.0
    prosthetic device or implant
      bile duct prosthesis —see Complications,
        bile duct implant
      esophageal anti-reflux device —see
        Complications, esophageal anti-
        reflux device
      specified type NEC
        embolism T85.81
        fibrosis T85.82
        hemorrhage T85.83
        mechanical
          breakdown T85.518
          displacement T85.528
          malfunction T85.518
          malposition T85.528
          obstruction T85.598
          perforation T85.598
          protrusion T85.598
          specified NEC T85.598
        pain T85.84
        specified complication NEC
          T85.89
        stenosis T85.85
        thrombosis T85.86
  gastrostomy (stoma) K94.20
    hemorrhage K94.21
    infection K94.22
    malfunction K94.23
    mechanical K94.23
    specified complication NEC
      K94.29

Complication (Continued)
  genitourinary
    device or implant T83.9
      genital tract T83.9
        infection or inflammation T83.6
        intrauterine contraceptive device —see
          Complications, intrauterine,
          contraceptive device
        mechanical —see Complications, by
          device, mechanical
        mesh —see Complications, mesh
        penile prosthesis —see Complications,
          prosthetic device, penile
        specified type NEC T83.89
          embolism T83.81
          fibrosis T83.82
          hemorrhage T83.83
          pain T83.84
          specified complication NEC T83.89
          stenosis T83.85
          thrombosis T83.86
        vaginal mesh —see Complications,
          mesh
      urinary system T83.9
        cystostomy catheter —see
          Complication, catheter,
          cystostomy
        electronic stimulator —see
          Complications, electronic
          stimulator device, urinary
        indwelling urethral catheter —see
          Complications, catheter, urethral,
          indwelling
        infection or inflammation T83.59
          indwelling urinary catheter T83.51
        kidney transplant —see Complication,
          transplant, kidney
        organ graft —see Complication, graft,
          urinary organ
        specified type NEC T83.89
          embolism T83.81
          fibrosis T83.82
          hemorrhage T83.83
          mechanical T83.198
            breakdown T83.118
            displacement T83.128
            malfunction T83.118
            malposition T83.128
            obstruction T83.198
            perforation T83.198
            protrusion T83.198
            specified NEC T83.198
          pain T83.84
          specified complication NEC
            T83.89
          stenosis T83.85
          thrombosis T83.86
        sphincter implant —see
          Complications, implant, urinary
          sphincter
    postprocedural
      pelvic peritoneal adhesions N99.4
      renal failure N99.0
      specified NEC N99.89
      stoma —see Complications, stoma,
        urinary tract
      urethral stricture —see Stricture, urethra,
        postprocedural
      vaginal
        adhesions N99.2
        vault prolapse N99.3
  graft (bypass) (patch) —see also
    Complications, prosthetic device or
    implant
    aorta —see Complications, graft,
      vascular
    arterial —see Complication, graft,
      vascular
    bone T86.839
      failure T86.831
      infection T86.832

Complication (Continued)
  graft (Continued)
    bone (Continued)
      mechanical T84.318
        breakdown T84.318
        displacement T84.328
        protrusion T84.398
        specified type NEC T84.398
      rejection T86.830
      specified type NEC T86.838
    carotid artery —see Complications, graft,
      vascular
    cornea T86.849
      failure T86.841
      infection T86.842
      mechanical T85.398
        breakdown T85.318
        displacement T85.328
        protrusion T85.398
        specified type NEC T85.398
      rejection T86.840
      retroprosthetic membrane T85.398
      specified type NEC T86.848
    femoral artery (bypass) —see Complication,
      extremity artery (bypass) graft
    genital organ or tract —see Complications,
      genitourinary, device or implant,
      genital tract
    muscle T84.9
      breakdown T84.410
      displacement T84.420
      embolism T84.81
      fibrosis T84.82
      hemorrhage T84.83
      infection and inflammation T84.7
      mechanical NEC T84.490
      pain T84.84
      specified type NEC T84.89
      stenosis T84.85
      thrombosis T84.86
    nerve —see Complication, prosthetic device
      or implant, specified NEC
    skin —see Complications, prosthetic device
      or implant, skin graft
    tendon T84.9
      breakdown T84.410
      displacement T84.420
      embolism T84.81
      fibrosis T84.82
      hemorrhage T84.83
      infection and inflammation T84.7
      mechanical NEC T84.490
      pain T84.84
      specified type NEC T84.89
      stenosis T84.85
      thrombosis T84.86
    urinary organ T83.9
      embolism T83.81
      fibrosis T83.82
      hemorrhage T83.83
      infection and inflammation T83.59
        indwelling urinary catheter T83.51
      mechanical
        breakdown T83.21
        displacement T83.22
        leakage T83.23
        malposition T83.22
        obstruction T83.29
        perforation T83.29
        protrusion T83.29
        specified NEC T83.29
      pain T83.84
      specified type NEC T83.89
      stenosis T83.85
      thrombosis T83.86
    vascular T82.9
      embolism T82.818
      femoral artery —see Complication,
        extremity artery (bypass) graft
      fibrosis T82.828
      hemorrhage T82.838

◀ New   ◀▥ Revised   ~~deleted~~ Deleted

Complication *(Continued)*
 graft *(Continued)*
  vascular *(Continued)*
   mechanical
    breakdown T82.319
     aorta (bifurcation) T82.310
     carotid artery T82.311
     specified vessel NEC T82.318
    displacement T82.329
     aorta (bifurcation) T82.320
     carotid artery T82.321
     specified vessel NEC T82.328
    leakage T82.339
     aorta (bifurcation) T82.330
     carotid artery T82.331
     specified vessel NEC T82.338
    malposition T82.329
     aorta (bifurcation) T82.320
     carotid artery T82.321
     specified vessel NEC T82.328
    obstruction T82.399
     aorta (bifurcation) T82.390
     carotid artery T82.391
     specified vessel NEC T82.398
    perforation T82.399
     aorta (bifurcation) T82.390
     carotid artery T82.391
     specified vessel NEC T82.398
    protrusion T82.399
     aorta (bifurcation) T82.390
     carotid artery T82.391
     specified vessel NEC T82.398
   pain T82.848
   specified complication NEC
    T82.898
   stenosis T82.858
   thrombosis T82.868
 heart I51.9
  assist device
   infection and inflammation T82.7
  following acute myocardial infarction —
    see Complications, following, acute
    myocardial infarction
  postoperative —*see* Complications,
    circulatory system
  transplant —*see* Complication, transplant,
    heart
   and lung (s) —*see* Complications,
    transplant, heart, with lung
  valve
   graft (biological) T82.9
    embolism T82.817
    fibrosis T82.827
    hemorrhage T82.837
    infection and inflammation
     T82.7
    mechanical T82.228
     breakdown T82.221
     displacement T82.222
     leakage T82.223
     malposition T82.222
     obstruction T82.228
     perforation T82:228
     protrusion T82.228
    pain T82.847
    specified type NEC T82.897
    stenosis T82.857
    thrombosis T82.867
   prosthesis T82.9
    embolism T82.817
    fibrosis T82.827
    hemorrhage T82.837
    infection or inflammation T82.6
    mechanical T82.09
     breakdown T82.01
     displacement T82.02
     leakage T82.03
     malposition T82.02
     obstruction T82.09
     perforation T82.09
     protrusion T82.09

Complication *(Continued)*
 heart *(Continued)*
  valve *(Continued)*
   prosthesis *(Continued)*
    pain T82.847
    specified type NEC T82.897
     mechanical T82.09
    stenosis T82.857
    thrombosis T82.867
 hematoma
  intraoperative —*see* Complication,
    intraoperative, hemorrhage
  postprocedural —*see* Complication,
    postprocedural, hemorrhage
 hemodialysis —*see* Complications,
    dialysis
 hemorrhage
  intraoperative —*see* Complication,
    intraoperative, hemorrhage
  postprocedural —*see* Complication,
    postprocedural, hemorrhage
 ileostomy (stoma) —*see* Complications,
    enterostomy
 immunization (procedure) —*see*
    Complications, vaccination
 implant —*see also* Complications, by site and
    type
  urinary sphincter T83.9
   embolism T83.81
   fibrosis T83.82
   hemorrhage T83.83
   infection and inflammation T83.59
   mechanical
    breakdown T83.111
    displacement T83.121
    leakage T83.191
    malposition T83.121
    obstruction T83.191
    perforation T83.191
    protrusion T83.191
    specified NEC T83.191
   pain T83.84
   specified type NEC T83.89
   stenosis T83.85
   thrombosis T83.86
 infusion (procedure) T80.90
  air embolism T80.0
  blood —*see* Complications, transfusion
  catheter —*see* Complications, catheter
  infection T80.29
  pump —*see* Complications, cardiovascular,
    device or implant
  sepsis T80.29
  serum reaction (*see also* Reaction, serum)
    T80.69
   anaphylactic shock (*see also* Shock,
    anaphylactic) T80.59
  specified type NEC T80.89
 inhalation therapy NEC T81.81
 injection (procedure) T80.90
  drug reaction —*see* Reaction, drug
  infection T80.29
  sepsis T80.29
  serum (prophylactic) (therapeutic) —*see*
    Complications, vaccination
  specified type NEC T80.89
  vaccine (any) —*see* Complications,
    vaccination
 inoculation (any) —*see* Complications,
    vaccination
 insulin pump
  infection and inflammation T85.72
  mechanical
   breakdown T85.614
   displacement T85.624
   leakage T85.633
   malposition T85.624
   obstruction T85.694
   perforation T85.694
   protrusion T85.694
   specified NEC T85.694

Complication *(Continued)*
 intestinal pouch NEC K91.858
 intraocular lens (prosthetic) T85.9
  embolism T85.81
  fibrosis T85.82
  hemorrhage T85.83
  infection and inflammation T85.79
  mechanical
   breakdown T85.21
   displacement T85.22
   malposition T85.22
   obstruction T85.29
   perforation T85.29
   protrusion T85.29
   specified NEC T85.29
  pain T85.84
  specified type NEC T85.89
  stenosis T85.85
  thrombosis T85.86
 intraoperative (intraprocedural)
  cardiac arrest
   during cardiac surgery I97.710
   during other surgery I97.711
  cardiac functional disturbance NEC
   during cardiac surgery I97.790
   during other surgery I97.791
  hemorrhage (hematoma) (of)
   circulatory system organ or structure
    during cardiac bypass I97.411
    during cardiac catheterization I97.410
    during other circulatory system
     procedure I97.418
    during other procedure I97.42
   digestive system organ
    during procedure on digestive system
     K91.61
    during procedure on other organ
     K91.62
   ear
    during procedure on ear and mastoid
     process H95.21
    during procedure on other organ
     H95.22
   endocrine system organ or structure
    during procedure on endocrine
     system organ or structure E36.01
    during procedure on other organ
     E36.02
   eye and adnexa
    during ophthalmic procedure H59.11-
    during other procedure H59.12-
   genitourinary organ or structure
    during procedure on genitourinary
     organ or structure N99.61
    during procedure on other organ
     N99.62
   mastoid process
    during procedure on ear and mastoid
     process H95.21
    during procedure on other organ
     H95.22
   musculoskeletal structure
    during musculoskeletal surgery
     M96.810
    during non-orthopedic surgery
     M96.811
    during orthopedic surgery M96.810
   nervous system
    during a nervous system procedure
     G97.31
    during other procedure G97.32
   respiratory system
    during other procedure J95.62
    during procedure on respiratory
     system organ or structure
     J95.61
   skin and subcutaneous tissue
    during a dermatologic procedure
     L76.01
    during a procedure on other organ
     L76.02

Complication *(Continued)*
  intraoperative *(Continued)*
    hemorrhage *(Continued)*
      spleen
        during a procedure on other organ
          D78.02
        during a procedure on the spleen
          D78.01
    puncture or laceration (accidental)
        (unintentional) (of)
      brain
        during a nervous system procedure
          G97.48
        during other procedure G97.49
      circulatory system organ or structure
        during circulatory system procedure
          I97.51
        during other procedure I97.52
      digestive system
        during procedure on digestive system
          K91.71
        during procedure on other organ
          K91.72
      ear
        during procedure on ear and mastoid
          process H95.31
        during procedure on other organ
          H95.32
      endocrine system organ or structure
        during procedure on endocrine
          system organ or structure E36.11
        during procedure on other organ
          E36.12
      eye and adnexa
        during ophthalmic procedure H59.21-
        during other procedure H59.22-
      genitourinary organ or structure
        during procedure on genitourinary
          organ or structure N99.71
        during procedure on other organ
          N99.72
      mastoid process
        during procedure on ear and mastoid
          process H95.31
        during procedure on other organ
          H95.32
      musculoskeletal structure
        during musculoskeletal surgery
          M96.820
        during non-orthopedic surgery
          M96.821
        during orthopedic surgery M96.820
      nervous system
        during a nervous system procedure
          G97.48
        during other procedure G97.49
      respiratory system
        during other procedure J95.72
        during procedure on respiratory
          system organ or structure J95.71
      skin and subcutaneous tissue
        during a dermatologic procedure
          L76.11
        during a procedure on other organ
          L76.12
      spleen
        during a procedure on other organ
          D78.12
        during a procedure on the spleen
          D78.11
    specified NEC
      circulatory system I97.88
      digestive system K91.81
      ear H95.88
      endocrine system E36.8
      eye and adnexa H59.88
      genitourinary system N99.81
      mastoid process H95.88
      musculoskeletal structure M96.89
      nervous system G97.81
      respiratory system J95.88

Complication *(Continued)*
  intraoperative *(Continued)*
    specified NEC *(Continued)*
      skin and subcutaneous tissue L76.81
      spleen D78.81
  intraperitoneal catheter (dialysis)
      (infusion) —*see* Complications, catheter,
      intraperitoneal
  intrauterine
    contraceptive device
      embolism T83.81
      fibrosis T83.82
      hemorrhage T83.83
      infection and inflammation T83.6
      mechanical
        breakdown T83.31
        displacement T83.32
        malposition T83.32
        obstruction T83.39
        perforation T83.39
        protrusion T83.39
        specified NEC T83.39
      pain T83.84
      specified type NEC T83.89
      stenosis T83.85
      thrombosis T83.86
    procedure (fetal), to newborn P96.5
  jejunostomy (stoma) —*see* Complications,
      enterostomy
  joint prosthesis, internal T84.9
    breakage (fracture) T84.01-
    dislocation T84.02-
    fracture T84.01-
    infection or inflammation T84.50
      hip T84.5-
      knee T84.5-
      specified joint NEC T84.59
    instability T84.02-
    malposition —*see* Complications, joint
        prosthesis, mechanical,
        displacement
    mechanical
      breakage, broken T84.01-
      dislocation T84.02-
      fracture T84.01-
      instability T84.02-
      leakage —*see* Complications, joint
          prosthesis, mechanical, specified
          NEC
      loosening T84.039
        hip T84.03-
        knee T84.03-
        specified joint NEC T84.038
      obstruction —*see* Complications, joint
          prosthesis, mechanical, specified
          NEC
      perforation —*see* Complications, joint
          prosthesis, mechanical, specified
          NEC
      periprosthetic
        fracture T84.049
          hip T84.04-
          knee T84.04-
          other specified joint T84.048
        osteolysis T84.059
          hip T84.05-
          knee T84.05-
          other specified joint T84.058
      protrusion —*see* Complications, joint
          prosthesis, mechanical, specified
          NEC
      specified complication NEC T84.099
        hip T84.09-
        knee T84.09-
        other specified joint T84.098
      subluxation T84.02-
      wear of articular bearing surface
          T84.069
        hip T84.06-
        knee T84.06-
        other specified joint T84.068

Complication *(Continued)*
  joint prosthesis, internal *(Continued)*
    specified joint NEC T84.89
      embolism T84.81
      fibrosis T84.82
      hemorrhage T84.83
      pain T84.84
      specified complication NEC T84.89
      stenosis T84.85
      thrombosis T84.86
    subluxation T84.02-
  kidney transplant —*see* Complications,
      transplant, kidney
  labor O75.9
    specified NEC O75.89
  liver transplant (immune or nonimmune) —
      see Complications, transplant, liver
  lumbar puncture G97.1
    cerebrospinal fluid leak G97.0
    headache or reaction G97.1
  lung transplant —*see* Complications,
      transplant, lung
    and heart —*see* Complications, transplant,
        lung, with heart
  male genital N50.9
    device, implant or graft —*see*
        Complications, genitourinary, device
        or implant, genital tract
    postprocedural or postoperative —*see*
        Complications, genitourinary,
        postprocedural
    specified NEC N99.89
  mastoid (process) procedure
    intraoperative H95.88-
      hematoma —*see* Complications,
          intraoperative, hemorrhage
          (hematoma) (of), mastoid
          process
      hemorrhage —*see* Complications,
          intraoperative, hemorrhage
          (hematoma) (of), mastoid
          process
      laceration —*see* Complications,
          intraoperative, puncture or
          laceration..., mastoid process
      specified NEC H95.88-
    postmastoidectomy —*see* Complications,
        postmastoidectomy
    postoperative H95.89-
      external ear canal stenosis H95.81-
      hematoma —*see* Complications...,
          postprocedural, hemorrhage
          (hematoma) (of), mastoid
          process
      hemorrhage —*see* Complications...,
          postprocedural, hemorrhage
          (hematoma) (of), mastoid
          process
      postmastoidectomy —*see* Complications,
          postmastoidectomy
      specified NEC H95.89-
  mastoidectomy cavity —*see* Complications,
      postmastoidectomy
  mechanical —*see* Complications, by site and
      type, mechanical
  medical procedures (*see also* Complication(s),
      intraoperative) T88.9
  metabolic E88.9
    postoperative E89.89
      specified NEC E89.89
  molar pregnancy NOS O08.9
    damage to pelvic organs O08.6
    embolism O08.2
    genital infection O08.0
    hemorrhage (delayed) (excessive)
        O08.1
    metabolic disorder O08.5
    renal failure O08.4
    shock O08.3
    specified type NEC O08.0
    venous complication NEC O08.7

◀ New   ◀▥ Revised   ~~deleted~~ Deleted

Complication (Continued)
    musculoskeletal system —see also
        Complication, intraoperative
        (intraprocedural), by site
    device, implant or graft NEC —see
        Complications, orthopedic, device or
        implant
    internal fixation (nail) (plate) (rod) —see
        Complications, fixation device,
        internal
    joint prosthesis —see Complications, joint
        prosthesis
    postoperative (postprocedural) M96.89
        with osteoporosis —see Osteoporosis
        fracture following insertion of device —
            see Fracture, following insertion of
            orthopedic implant, joint prosthesis
            or bone plate
        joint instability after prosthesis removal
            M96.89
        lordosis M96.4
        postlaminectomy syndrome NEC
            M96.1
            kyphosis M96.3
        pseudarthrosis M96.0
        specified complication NEC M96.89
    post radiation M96.89
        kyphosis M96.3
        scoliosis M96.5
        specified complication NEC M96.89
    nephrostomy (stoma) —see Complications,
        stoma, urinary tract, external NEC
    nervous system G98.8
        central G96.9
        device, implant or graft —see also
            Complication, prosthetic device or
            implant, specified NEC
            electronic stimulator (electrode (s)) —
                see Complications, electronic
                stimulator device
            ventricular shunt —see Complications,
                ventricular shunt
        electronic stimulator (electrode (s)) —see
            Complications, electronic stimulator
            device
        postprocedural G97.82
            intracranial hypotension G97.2
            specified NEC G97.82
            spinal fluid leak G97.0
    newborn, due to intrauterine (fetal)
        procedure P96.5
    nonabsorbable (permanent) sutures —see
        Complication, sutures, permanent
    obstetric O75.9
        procedure (instrumental) (manual)
            (surgical) specified NEC O75.4
        specified NEC O75.89
        surgical wound NEC O90.89
            hematoma O90.2
            infection O86.0
    ocular lens implant —see Complications,
        intraocular lens
    ophthalmologic
        postprocedural bleb —see Blebitis
    orbital prosthesis T85.9
        embolism T85.81
        fibrosis T85.82
        hemorrhage T85.83
        infection and inflammation T85.79
        mechanical
            breakdown T85.31-
            displacement T85.32-
            malposition T85.32-
            obstruction T85.39-
            perforation T85.39-
            protrusion T85.39-
            specified NEC T85.39-
        pain T85.84
        specified type NEC T85.89
        stenosis T85.85
        thrombosis T85.86

Complication (Continued)
    organ or tissue transplant (partial) (total) —
        see Complications, transplant
    orthopedic —see also Disorder, soft tissue
        device or implant T84.9
            bone
                device or implant —see Complication,
                    bone, device NEC
                graft —see Complication, graft, bone
            breakdown T84.418
            displacement T84.428
            electronic bone stimulator —see
                Complications, electronic
                stimulator device, bone
            embolism T84.81
            fibrosis T84.82
            fixation device —see Complication,
                fixation device, internal
            hemorrhage T84.83
            infection or inflammation T84.7
            joint prosthesis —see Complication, joint
                prosthesis, internal
            malfunction T84.418
            malposition T84.428
            mechanical NEC T84.498
            muscle graft —see Complications, graft,
                muscle
            obstruction T84.498
            pain T84.84
            perforation T84.498
            protrusion T84.498
            specified complication NEC T84.89
            stenosis T84.85
            tendon graft —see Complications, graft,
                tendon
            thrombosis T84.86
        fracture (following insertion of device) —
            see Fracture, following insertion of
            orthopedic implant, joint prosthesis
            or bone plate
        postprocedural M96.89
            fracture —see Fracture, following
                insertion of orthopedic implant,
                joint prosthesis or bone plate
            postlaminectomy syndrome NEC
                M96.1
                kyphosis M96.3
                lordosis M96.4
            postradiation
                kyphosis M96.2
                scoliosis M96.5
            pseudarthrosis post-fusion M96.0
            specified type NEC M96.89
    pacemaker (cardiac) —see Complications,
        cardiovascular device or implant,
        electronic
    pancreas transplant —see Complications,
        transplant, pancreas
    penile prosthesis (implant) —see
        Complications, prosthetic device,
        penile
    perfusion NEC T80.90
    perineal repair (obstetrical) NEC O90.89
        disruption O90.1
        hematoma O90.2
        infection (following delivery) O86.0
    phototherapy T88.9
        specified NEC T88.8
    postmastoidectomy NEC H95.19-
        cyst, mucosal H95.13-
        granulation H95.12-
        inflammation, chronic H95.11-
        recurrent cholesteatoma H95.0-
    postoperative —see Complications,
        postprocedural
        circulatory —see Complications, circulatory
            system
        ear —see Complications, ear
        endocrine —see Complications,
            endocrine
        eye —see Complications, eye

Complication (Continued)
    postoperative (Continued)
        lumbar puncture G97.1
            cerebrospinal fluid leak G97.0
        nervous system (central) (peripheral) —see
            Complications, nervous system
        respiratory system —see Complications,
            respiratory system
    postprocedural —see also Complications,
        surgical procedure
        cardiac arrest
            following cardiac surgery I97.120
            following other surgery I97.121
        cardiac functional disturbance NEC
            following cardiac surgery I97.190
            following other surgery I97.191
        cardiac insufficiency
            following cardiac surgery I97.110
            following other surgery I97.111
        chorioretinal scars following retinal
            surgery H59.81-
        following cataract surgery
            cataract (lens) fragments H59.02-
            cystoid macular edema H59.03-
            specified NEC H59.09-
            vitreous (touch) syndrome H59.01-
        heart failure
            following cardiac surgery I97.130
            following other surgery I97.131
        hemorrhage (hematoma) (of)
            circulatory system organ or structure
                following a cardiac bypass I97.611
                following a cardiac catheterization
                    I97.610
                following other circulatory system
                    procedure I97.618
                following other procedure I97.62
            digestive system
                following procedure on digestive
                    system K91.840
                following procedure on other organ
                    K91.841
            ear
                following other procedure H95.42
                following procedure on ear and
                    mastoid process H95.41
            endocrine system
                following endocrine system
                    procedure E89.810
                following other procedure
                    E89.811
            eye and adnexa
                following ophthalmic procedure
                    H59.31-
                following other procedure H59.32-
            genitourinary organ or structure
                following procedure on
                    genitourinary organ or
                    structure N99.820
                following procedure on other organ
                    N99.821
            mastoid process
                following other procedure H95.42
                following procedure on ear and
                    mastoid process H95.41
            musculoskeletal structure
                following musculoskeletal surgery
                    M96.830
                following non-orthopedic surgery
                    M96.831
                following orthopedic surgery
                    M96.830
            nervous system
                following a nervous system procedure
                    G97.51
                following other procedure G97.52
            respiratory system
                following other procedure J95.831
                following procedure on respiratory
                    system organ or structure
                    J95.830

Complication *(Continued)*
  postprocedural *(Continued)*
    hemorrhage *(Continued)*
      skin and subcutaneous tissue
        following a dermatologic procedure
          L76.21
        following a procedure on other organ
          L76.22
      spleen
        following procedure on other organ
          D78.22
        following procedure on the spleen
          D78.21
    specified NEC
      circulatory system I97.89
      digestive K91.89
      ear H95.89
      endocrine E89.89
      eye and adnexa H59.89
      genitourinary N99.89
      mastoid process H95.89
      metabolic E89.89
      musculoskeletal structure M96.89
      nervous system G97.82
      respiratory system J95.89
      skin and subcutaneous tissue L76.82
      spleen D78.89
  pregnancy NEC —*see* Pregnancy,
    complicated by
  prosthetic device or implant T85.9
    bile duct —*see* Complications, bile duct
      implant
    breast —*see* Complications, breast implant
    cardiac and vascular NEC —*see*
      Complications, cardiovascular
      device or implant
    corneal transplant —*see* Complications,
      graft, cornea
    electronic nervous system stimulator —*see*
      Complications, electronic stimulator
      device
    epidural infusion catheter —*see*
      Complications, catheter, epidural
    esophageal anti-reflux device —*see*
      Complications, esophageal anti-reflux
      device
    genital organ or tract —*see* Complications,
      genitourinary, device or implant,
      genital tract
    heart valve —*see* Complications, heart,
      valve, prosthesis
    infection or inflammation T85.79
      intestine transplant T86.892
      liver transplant T86.43
      lung transplant T86.812
      pancreas transplant T86.892
      skin graft T86.822
    intraocular lens —*see* Complications,
      intraocular lens
    intraperitoneal (dialysis) catheter —
      see Complications, catheter,
      intraperitoneal
    joint —*see* Complications, joint prosthesis,
      internal
    mechanical NEC T85.698
      dialysis catheter (vascular) —*see also*
        Complication, catheter, dialysis,
        mechanical
        peritoneal —*see* Complication,
          catheter, intraperitoneal,
          mechanical
      gastrointestinal device T85.598
      ocular device T85.398
      subdural (infusion) catheter T85.690
      suture, permanent T85.692
        that for bone repair —*see*
          Complications, fixation device,
          internal (orthopedic), mechanical
      ventricular shunt
        breakdown T85.01
        displacement T85.02
        leakage T85.03

Complication *(Continued)*
  prosthetic device or implant *(Continued)*
    mechanical NEC *(Continued)*
      ventricular shunt *(Continued)*
        malposition T85.02
        obstruction T85.09
        perforation T85.09
        protrusion T85.09
        specified NEC T85.09
    mesh
      erosion (to surrounding organ or tissue)
        T83.718
        vaginal (into pelvic floor muscles)
          T83.711
      exposure (into surrounding organ or
        tissue) T83.728
        vaginal (into vagina) (through vaginal
          wall) T83.721
    orbital —*see* Complications, orbital
      prosthesis
    penile T83.9
      embolism T83.81
      fibrosis T83.82
      hemorrhage T83.83
      infection and inflammation T83.6
      mechanical
        breakdown T83.410
        displacement T83.420
        leakage T83.490
        malposition T83.420
        obstruction T83.490
        perforation T83.490
        protrusion T83.490
        specified NEC T83.490
      pain T83.84
      specified type NEC T83.89
      stenosis T83.85
      thrombosis T83.86
    prosthetic materials NEC
      erosion (to surrounding organ or tissue)
        T83.718
        vaginal (into pelvic floor muscles)
          T83.711
      exposure (into surrounding organ or
        tissue) T83.728
        vaginal (into vagina) (through vaginal
          wall) T83.721
    skin graft T86.829
      artificial skin or decellularized
        allodermis
        embolism T85.81
        fibrosis T85.82
        hemorrhage T85.83
        infection and inflammation T85.79
        mechanical
          breakdown T85.613
          displacement T85.623
          malfunction T85.613
          malposition T85.623
          obstruction T85.693
          perforation T85.693
          protrusion T85.693
          specified NEC T85.693
        pain T85.84
        specified type NEC T85.89
        stenosis T85.85
        thrombosis T85.86
      failure T86.821
      infection T86.822
      rejection T86.820
      specified NEC T86.828
    specified NEC T85.9
      embolism T85.81
      fibrosis T85.82
      hemorrhage T85.83
      infection and inflammation T85.79
      mechanical
        breakdown T85.618
        displacement T85.628
        leakage T85.638
        malfunction T85.618
        malposition T85.628

Complication *(Continued)*
  prosthetic device or implant *(Continued)*
    specified NEC *(Continued)*
      mechanical *(Continued)*
        obstruction T85.698
        perforation T85.698
        protrusion T85.698
        specified NEC T85.698
      pain T85.84
      specified type NEC T85.89
      stenosis T85.85
      thrombosis T85.86
    subdural infusion catheter —*see*
      Complications, catheter, subdural
    sutures —*see* Complications, sutures
    urinary organ or tract NEC —*see*
      Complications, genitourinary, device
      or implant, urinary system
    vascular —*see* Complications,
      cardiovascular device or implant
    ventricular shunt —*see* Complications,
      ventricular shunt (device)
  puerperium —*see* Puerperal
  puncture, spinal G97.1
    cerebrospinal fluid leak G97.0
    headache or reaction G97.1
  pyelogram N99.89
  radiation
    kyphosis M96.2
    scoliosis M96.5
  reattached
    extremity (infection) (rejection)
      lower T87.1X-
      upper T87.0X-
    specified body part NEC T87.2
  reconstructed breast
    asymmetry between native and
      reconstructed breast N65.1
    deformity N65.0
    disproportion between native and
      reconstructed breast N65.1
    excess tissue N65.0
    misshappen N65.0
  reimplant NEC —*see also* Complications,
    prosthetic device or implant
    limb (infection) (rejection) —*see*
      Complications, reattached,
      extremity
    organ (partial) (total) —*see* Complications,
      transplant
    prosthetic device NEC —*see* Complications,
      prosthetic device
  renal N28.9
    allograft —*see* Complications, transplant,
      kidney
    dialysis —*see* Complications, dialysis
  respirator
    mechanical J95.850
      specified NEC J95.859
  respiratory system J98.9
    device, implant or graft —*see*
      Complication, prosthetic device or
      implant, specified NEC
    lung transplant —*see* Complications,
      prosthetic device or implant, lung
      transplant
    postoperative J95.89
      air leak J95.812
      Mendelson's syndrome (chemical
        pneumonitis) J95.4
      pneumothorax J95.811
      pulmonary insufficiency (acute) (after
        nonthoracic surgery) J95.2
      chronic J95.3
      following thoracic surgery J95.1
      respiratory failure (acute) J95.821
      acute and chronic J95.822
      specified NEC J95.89
      subglottic stenosis J95.5
      tracheostomy complication —*see*
        Complications, tracheostomy
  therapy T81.89

◀ New   ◀▥ Revised   ~~deleted~~ Deleted

Complication *(Continued)*
  sedation during labor and delivery
    O74.9
    cardiac O74.2
    central nervous system O74.3
    pulmonary NEC O74.1
  shunt —*see also* Complications, prosthetic
    device or implant
    arteriovenous —*see* Complications,
      arteriovenous, shunt
    ventricular (communicating) —*see*
      Complications, ventricular shunt
  skin
    graft T86.829
      failure T86.821
      infection T86.822
      rejection T86.820
      specified type NEC T86.828
  spinal
    anesthesia —*see* Complications, anesthesia,
      spinal
    catheter (epidural) (subdural) —*see*
      Complications, catheter
    puncture or tap G97.1
      cerebrospinal fluid leak G97.0
      headache or reaction G97.1
  stent
    bile duct —*see* Complications, bile duct
      prosthesis
    urinary T83.9
      embolism T83.81
      fibrosis T83.82
      hemorrhage T83.83
      infection and inflammation T83.59
      mechanical
        breakdown T83.112
        displacement T83.122
        leakage T83.192
        malposition T83.122
        obstruction T83.192
        perforation T83.192
        protrusion T83.192
        specified NEC T83.192
      pain T83.84
      specified type NEC T83.89
      stenosis T83.85
      thrombosis T83.86
  stoma
    digestive tract
      colostomy —*see* Complications,
        colostomy
      enterostomy —*see* Complications,
        enterostomy
      esophagostomy —*see* Complications,
        esophagostomy
      gastrostomy —*see* Complications,
        gastrostomy
    urinary tract N99.538
      cystostomy —*see* Complications,
        cystostomy
      external NOS N99.528
        hemorrhage N99.520
        infection N99.521
        malfunction N99.522
        specified type NEC N99.528
      hemorrhage N99.530
      infection N99.531
      malfunction N99.532
      specified type NEC N99.538
  stomach banding —*see* Complication (s),
    bariatric procedure
  stomach stapling —*see* Complication (s),
    bariatric procedure
  surgical material, nonabsorbable —*see*
    Complication, suture, permanent
  surgical procedure (on) T81.9
    amputation stump (late) —*see*
      Complications, amputation
      stump
    cardiac —*see* Complications, circulatory
      system

Complication *(Continued)*
  surgical procedure *(Continued)*
    cholesteatoma, recurrent —*see*
      Complications, postmastoidectomy,
      recurrent cholesteatoma
    circulatory (early) —*see* Complications,
      circulatory system
    digestive system —*see* Complications,
      gastrointestinal
    dumping syndrome (postgastrectomy)
      K91.1
    ear —*see* Complications, ear
    elephantiasis or lymphedema I97.89
      postmastectomy I97.2
    emphysema (surgical) T81.82
    endocrine —*see* Complications, endocrine
    eye —*see* Complications, eye
    fistula (persistent postoperative) T81.83
    foreign body inadvertently left in wound
      (sponge) (suture) (swab) —*see*
      Foreign body, accidentally left during
      a procedure
    gastrointestinal —*see* Complications,
      gastrointestinal
    genitourinary NEC N99.89
    hematoma
      intraoperative —*see* Complication,
        intraoperative, hemorrhage
      postprocedural —*see* Complication,
        postprocedural, hemorrhage
    hemorrhage
      intraoperative —*see* Complication,
        intraoperative, hemorrhage
      postprocedural —*see* Complication,
        postprocedural, hemorrhage
    hepatic failure K91.82
    hyperglycemia (postpancreatectomy) E89.1
    hypoinsulinemia (postpancreatectomy)
      E89.1
    hypoparathyroidism
      (postparathyroidectomy) E89.2
    hypopituitarism (posthypophysectomy)
      E89.3
    hypothyroidism (post-thyroidectomy)
      E89.0
    intestinal obstruction K91.3
    intracranial hypotension following
      ventricular shunting
      (ventriculostomy) G97.2
    lymphedema I97.89
      postmastectomy I97.2
    malabsorption (postsurgical) NEC K91.2
      osteoporosis —*see* Osteoporosis,
        postsurgical malabsorption
    mastoidectomy cavity NEC —*see*
      Complications, postmastoidectomy
    metabolic E89.89
      specified NEC E89.89
    musculoskeletal —*see* Complications,
      musculoskeletal system
    nervous system (central) (peripheral) —*see*
      Complications, nervous system
    ovarian failure E89.40
      asymptomatic E89.40
      symptomatic E89.41
    peripheral vascular —*see* Complications,
      surgical procedure, vascular
    postcardiotomy syndrome I97.0
    postcholecystectomy syndrome K91.5
    postcommissurotomy syndrome I97.0
    postgastrectomy dumping syndrome
      K91.1
    postlaminectomy syndrome NEC M96.1
      kyphosis M96.3
    postmastectomy lymphedema syndrome
      I97.2
    postmastoidectomy cholesteatoma —*see*
      Complications, postmastoidectomy,
      recurrent cholesteatoma
    postvagotomy syndrome K91.1
    postvalvulotomy syndrome I97.0

Complication *(Continued)*
  surgical procedure *(Continued)*
    pulmonary insufficiency (acute) J95.2
      chronic J95.3
      following thoracic surgery J95.1
    reattached body part —*see* Complications,
      reattached
    respiratory —*see* Complications,
      respiratory system
    shock (hypovolemic) T81.19
    spleen (postoperative) D78.89
      intraoperative D78.81
    stitch abscess T81.4
    subglottic stenosis (postsurgical) J95.5
    testicular hypofunction E89.5
    transplant —*see* Complications, organ or
      tissue transplant
    urinary NEC N99.89
    vaginal vault prolapse (posthysterectomy)
      N99.3
    vascular (peripheral)
      artery T81.719
        mesenteric T81.710
        renal T81.711
        specified NEC T81.718
      vein T81.72
    wound infection T81.4
  suture, permanent (wire) NEC T85.9
    with repair of bone —*see* Complications,
      fixation device, internal
    embolism T85.81
    fibrosis T85.82
    hemorrhage T85.83
    infection and inflammation T85.79
    mechanical
      breakdown T85.612
      displacement T85.622
      malfunction T85.612
      malposition T85.622
      obstruction T85.692
      perforation T85.692
      protrusion T85.692
      specified NEC T85.692
    pain T85.84
    specified type NEC T85.89
    stenosis T85.85
    thrombosis T85.86
  tracheostomy J95.00
    granuloma J95.09
    hemorrhage J95.01
    infection J95.02
    malfunction J95.03
    mechanical J95.03
    obstruction J95.03
    specified type NEC J95.09
    tracheo-esophageal fistula J95.04
  transfusion (blood) (lymphocytes) (plasma)
    T80.92
    air embolism T80.0
    circulatory overload E87.71
    febrile nonhemolytic transfusion reaction
      R50.84
    hemochromatosis E83.111
    hemolysis T80.89
    hemolytic reaction (antigen unspecified)
      T80.919
    incompatibility reaction (antigen
      unspecified) T80.919
      ABO T80.30
        delayed serologic (DSTR) T80.39
        hemolytic transfusion reaction
          (HTR) (unspecified time after
          transfusion) T80.319
          acute (AHTR) (less than 24 hours
            after transfusion) T80.310
          delayed (DHTR) (24 hours or more
            after transfusion) T80.311
        specified NEC T80.39
      acute (antigen unspecified) T80.910
      delayed (antigen unspecified) T80.911
      delayed serologic (DSTR) T80.89

Complication *(Continued)*
  transfusion *(Continued)*
    incompatibility reaction *(Continued)*
      Non-ABO (minor antigens (Duffy) (Kell) (Kidd) (Lewis) (M) (N) (P) (S)) T80.A0
        delayed serologic (DSTR) T80.A9
        hemolytic transfusion reaction (HTR) (unspecified time after transfusion) T80.A19
          acute (AHTR) (less than 24 hours after transfusion) T80.A10
          delayed (DHTR) (24 hours or more after transfusion) T80.A11
        specified NEC T80.A9
      Rh (antigens (C) (c) (D) (E) (e)) (factor) T80.40
        delayed serologic (DSTR) T80.49
        hemolytic transfusion reaction (HTR) (unspecified time after transfusion) T80.419
          acute (AHTR) (less than 24 hours after transfusion) T80.410
          delayed (DHTR) (24 hours or more after transfusion) T80.411
        specified NEC T80.49
      infection T80.29
        acute T80.22
      reaction NEC T80.89
      sepsis T80.29
      shock T80.89
  transplant T86.90
    bone T86.839
      failure T86.831
      infection T86.832
      rejection T86.830
      specified type NEC T86.838
    bone marrow T86.00
      failure T86.02
      infection T86.03
      rejection T86.01
      specified type NEC T86.09
    cornea T86.849
      failure T86.841
      infection T86.842
      rejection T86.840
      specified type NEC T86.848
    failure T86.92
    heart T86.20
      with lung T86.30
      cardiac allograft vasculopathy T86.290
        failure T86.32
        infection T86.33
        rejection T86.31
        specified type NEC T86.39
      failure T86.22
      infection T86.23
      rejection T86.21
      specified type NEC T86.298
    infection T86.93
    intestine T86.859
      failure T86.851
      infection T86.852
      rejection T86.850
      specified type NEC T86.858
    kidney T86.10
      failure T86.12
      infection T86.13
      rejection T86.11
      specified type NEC T86.19
    liver T86.40
      failure T86.42
      infection T86.43
      rejection T86.41
      specified type NEC T86.49
    lung T86.819
      with heart T86.30
        failure T86.32
        infection T86.33
        rejection T86.31
        specified type NEC T86.39

Complication *(Continued)*
  transplant *(Continued)*
    lung *(Continued)*
      failure T86.811
      infection T86.812
      rejection T86.810
      specified type NEC T86.818
    malignant neoplasm C80.2
    pancreas T86.899
      failure T86.891
      infection T86.892
      rejection T86.890
      specified type NEC T86.898
    peripheral blood stem cells T86.5
    post-transplant lymphoproliferative disorder (PTLD) D47.Z1
    rejection T86.91
    skin T86.829
      failure T86.821
      infection T86.822
      rejection T86.820
      specified type NEC T86.828
    specified
      tissue T86.899
        failure T86.891
        infection T86.892
        rejection T86.890
        specified type NEC T86.898
      type NEC T86.99
    stem cell (from peripheral blood) (from umbilical cord) T86.5
    umbilical cord stem cells T86.5
  trauma (early) T79.9
    specified NEC T79.8
  ultrasound therapy NEC T88.9
  umbilical cord NEC
    complicating delivery O69.9
      specified NEC O69.89
  umbrella device, vascular T82.9
    embolism T82.818
    fibrosis T82.828
    hemorrhage T82.838
    infection or inflammation T82.7
    mechanical
      breakdown T82.515
      displacement T82.525
      leakage T82.535
      malposition T82.525
      obstruction T82.595
      perforation T82.595
      protrusion T82.595
    pain T82.848
    specified type NEC T82.898
    stenosis T82.858
    thrombosis T82.868
  urethral catheter —*see* Complications, catheter, urethral, indwelling
  vaccination T88.1
    anaphylaxis NEC T80.52
    arthropathy —*see* Arthropathy, postimmunization
    cellulitis T88.0
    encephalitis or encephalomyelitis G04.02
    infection (general) (local) NEC T88.0
    meningitis G03.8
    myelitis G04.89
    protein sickness T80.62
    rash T88.1
    reaction (allergic) T88.1
      serum T80.62
    sepsis T88.0
    serum intoxication, sickness, rash, or other serum reaction NEC T80.62
    anaphylactic shock T80.52
    shock (allergic) (anaphylactic) T80.52
    vaccinia (generalized) (localized) T88.1
  vas deferens device or implant —*see* Complications, genitourinary, device or implant, genital tract

Complication *(Continued)*
  vascular I99.9
    device or implant T82.9
      embolism T82.818
      fibrosis T82.828
      hemorrhage T82.838
      infection or inflammation T82.7
      mechanical
        breakdown T82.519
          specified device NEC T82.518
        displacement T82.529
          specified device NEC T82.528
        leakage T82.539
          specified device NEC T82.538
        malposition T82.529
          specified device NEC T82.528
        obstruction T82.599
          specified device NEC T82.598
        perforation T82.599
          specified device NEC T82.598
        protrusion T82.599
          specified device NEC T82.598
      pain T82.848
      specified type NEC T82.898
      stenosis T82.858
      thrombosis T82.868
    dialysis catheter —*see* Complication, catheter, dialysis
    following infusion, therapeutic injection or transfusion T80.1
    graft T82.9
      embolism T82.818
      fibrosis T82.828
      hemorrhage T82.838
      mechanical
        breakdown T82.319
          aorta (bifurcation) T82.310
          carotid artery T82.311
          specified vessel NEC T82.318
        displacement T82.329
          aorta (bifurcation) T82.320
          carotid artery T82.321
          specified vessel NEC T82.328
        leakage T82.339
          aorta (bifurcation) T82.330
          carotid artery T82.331
          specified vessel NEC T82.338
        malposition T82.329
          aorta (bifurcation) T82.320
          carotid artery T82.321
          specified vessel NEC T82.328
        obstruction T82.399
          aorta (bifurcation) T82.390
          carotid artery T82.391
          specified vessel NEC T82.398
        perforation T82.399
          aorta (bifurcation) T82.390
          carotid artery T82.391
          specified vessel NEC T82.398
        protrusion T82.399
          aorta (bifurcation) T82.390
          carotid artery T82.391
          specified vessel NEC T82.398
      pain T82.848
      specified complication NEC T82.898
      stenosis T82.858
      thrombosis T82.868
    postoperative —*see* Complications, postoperative, circulatory
    vena cava device (filter) (sieve) (umbrella) —*see* Complications, umbrella device, vascular
  ventilation therapy NEC T81.81
  ventilator
    mechanical J95.850
      specified NEC J95.859
  ventricular (communicating) shunt (device) T85.9
    embolism T85.81
    fibrosis T85.82
    hemorrhage T85.83

◀ New   ◀◁ Revised   ~~deleted~~ Deleted

Congestion, congestive (*Continued*)
  hepatic K76.1
  hypostatic (lung) —*see* Edema, lung
  intestine K63.89
  kidney N28.89
  labyrinth —*see* subcategory H83.8
  larynx J37.0
  liver K76.1
  lung R09.89
    active or acute —*see* Pneumonia
  malaria, malarial —*see* Malaria
  nasal R09.81
  nose R09.81
  orbit, orbital —*see also* Exophthalmos
    inflammatory (chronic) —*see* Inflammation,
      orbit
  ovary N83.8
  pancreas K86.8
  pelvic, female N94.89
  pleural J94.8
  prostate (active) N42.1
  pulmonary —*see* Congestion, lung
  renal N28.89
  retina H35.81
  seminal vesicle N50.1
  spinal cord G95.19
  spleen (chronic) D73.2
  stomach K31.89
  trachea —*see* Tracheitis
  urethra N36.8
  uterus N85.8
    with subinvolution N85.3
  venous (passive) I87.8
  viscera R68.89
Congestive —*see* Congestion
Conical
  cervix (hypertrophic elongation) N88.4
  cornea —*see* Keratoconus
  teeth K00.2
Conjoined twins Q89.4
Conjugal maladjustment Z63.0
  involving divorce or estrangement Z63.5
Conjunctiva —*see* condition
Conjunctivitis (staphylococcal) (streptococcal)
    NOS H10.9
  Acanthamoeba B60.12
  acute H10.3-
    atopic H10.1-
    chemical (*see also* Corrosion, cornea) H10.21-
    mucopurulent H10.02-
      follicular H10.01-
    pseudomembranous H10.22-
    serous except viral H10.23-
      viral —*see* Conjunctivitis, viral
    toxic H10.21-
  adenoviral (acute) (follicular) B30.1
  allergic (acute) —*see* Conjunctivitis, acute,
      atopic
    chronic H10.45
      vernal H10.44
  anaphylactic —*see* Conjunctivitis, acute,
      atopic
  Apollo B30.3
  atopic (acute) —*see* Conjunctivitis, acute,
      atopic
  Béal's B30.2
  blennorrhagic (gonococcal) (neonatorum)
      A54.31
  chemical (acute) (*see also* Corrosion, cornea)
      H10.21-
  chlamydial A74.0
    due to trachoma A71.1
    neonatal P39.1
  chronic (nodosa) (petrificans) (phlyctenular)
      H10.40-
    allergic H10.45
      vernal H10.44
    follicular H10.43-
    giant papillary H10.41-
    simple H10.42-
    vernal H10.44

Conjunctivitis (*Continued*)
  coxsackievirus 24 B30.3
  diphtheritic A36.86
  due to
    dust —*see* Conjunctivitis, acute, atopic
    filariasis B74.9
    mucocutaneous leishmaniasis B55.2
  enterovirus type 70 (hemorrhagic) B30.3
  epidemic (viral) B30.9
    hemorrhagic B30.3
  gonococcal (neonatorum) A54.31
  granular (trachomatous) A71.1
    sequelae (late effect) B94.0
  hemorrhagic (acute) (epidemic) B30.3
  herpes zoster B02.31
  in (due to)
    Acanthamoeba B60.12
    adenovirus (acute) (follicular) B30.1
    Chlamydia A74.0
    coxsackievirus 24 B30.3
    diphtheria A36.86
    enterovirus type 70 (hemorrhagic) B30.3
    filariasis B74.9
    gonococci A54.31
    herpes (simplex) virus B00.53
      zoster B02.31
    infectious disease NEC B99
    meningococci A39.89
    mucocutaneous leishmaniasis B55.2
    rosacea L71.9
    syphilis (late) A52.71
    zoster B02.31
  inclusion A74.0
  infantile P39.1
    gonococcal A54.31
  Koch-Weeks' —*see* Conjunctivitis, acute,
      mucopurulent
  light —*see* Conjunctivitis, acute, atopic
  ligneous —*see* Blepharoconjunctivitis,
      ligneous
  meningococcal A39.89
  mucopurulent —*see* Conjunctivitis, acute,
      mucopurulent
  neonatal P39.1
    gonococcal A54.31
  Newcastle B30.8
  of Béal B30.2
  parasitic
    filariasis B74.9
    mucocutaneous leishmaniasis B55.2
  Parinaud's H10.89
  petrificans H10.89
  rosacea L71.9
  specified NEC H10.89
  swimming-pool B30.1
  trachomatous A71.1
    acute A71.0
    sequelae (late effect) B94.0
  traumatic NEC H10.89
  tuberculous A18.59
  tularemic A21.1
  tularensis A21.1
  viral B30.9
    due to
      adenovirus B30.1
      enterovirus B30.3
    specified NEC B30.8
Conjunctivochalasis H11.82-
Connective tissue —*see* condition
Conn's syndrome E26.01
Conradi (-Hunermann) disease Q77.3
Consanguinity Z84.3
  counseling Z71.89
Conscious simulation (of illness) Z76.5
Consecutive —*see* condition
Consolidation lung (base) —*see* Pneumonia,
    lobar
Constipation (atonic) (neurogenic) (simple)
    (spastic) K59.00
  drug-induced —*see* Table of Drugs and
    Chemicals

Constipation (*Continued*)
  outlet dysfunction K59.02
  psychogenic F45.8
  slow transit K59.01
  specified NEC K59.09
Constitutional —*see also* condition
  substandard F60.7
Constitutionally substandard F60.7
Constriction —*see also* Stricture
  auditory canal —*see* Stenosis, external ear
    canal
  bronchial J98.09
  duodenum K31.5
  esophagus K22.2
  external
    abdomen, abdominal (wall) S30.841
    alveolar process S00.542
    ankle S90.54-
    antecubital space —*see* Constriction,
      external, forearm
    arm (upper) S40.84-
    auricle —*see* Constriction, external, ear
    axilla —*see* Constriction, external, arm
    back, lower S30.840
    breast S20.14-
    brow S00.84
    buttock S30.840
    calf —*see* Constriction, external, leg
    canthus —*see* Constriction, external, eyelid
    cheek S00.84
      internal S00.542
    chest wall —*see* Constriction, external,
      thorax
    chin S00.84
    clitoris S30.844
    costal region —*see* Constriction, external,
      thorax
    digit (s)
      foot —*see* Constriction, external, toe
      hand —*see* Constriction, external, finger
    ear S00.44-
    elbow S50.34-
    epididymis S30.843
    epigastric region S30.841
    esophagus, cervical S10.14
    eyebrow —*see* Constriction, external, eyelid
    eyelid S00.24-
    face S00.84
    finger (s) S60.44-
      index S60.44-
      little S60.44-
      middle S60.44-
      ring S60.44-
    flank S30.841
    foot (except toe (s) alone) S90.84-
      toe —*see* Constriction, external, toe
    forearm S50.84-
      elbow only —*see* Constriction, external,
        elbow
    forehead S00.84
    genital organs, external
      female S30.846
      male S30.845
    groin S30.841
    gum S00.542
    hand S60.54-
    head S00.94
      ear —*see* Constriction, external, ear
      eyelid —*see* Constriction, external, eyelid
      lip S00.541
      nose S00.34
      oral cavity S00.542
      scalp S00.04
      specified site NEC S00.84
    heel —*see* Constriction, external, foot
    hip S70.24-
    inguinal region S30.841
    interscapular region S20.449
    jaw S00.84
    knee S80.24-
    labium (majus) (minus) S30.844

◀ New   ◀≡ Revised   ~~deleted~~ Deleted

Constriction (*Continued*)
  external (*Continued*)
    larynx S10.14
    leg (lower) S80.84-
      knee —*see* Constriction, external, knee
      upper —*see* Constriction, external, thigh
    lip S00.541
    lower back S30.840
    lumbar region S30.840
    malar region S00.84
    mammary —*see* Constriction, external, breast
    mastoid region S00.84
    mouth S00.542
    nail
      finger —*see* Constriction, external, finger
      toe —*see* Constriction, external, toe
    nasal S00.34
    neck S10.94
      specified site NEC S10.84
      throat S10.14
    nose S00.34
    occipital region S00.04
    oral cavity S00.542
    orbital region —*see* Constriction, external, eyelid
    palate S00.542
    palm —*see* Constriction, external, hand
    parietal region S00.04
    pelvis S30.840
    penis S30.842
    perineum
      female S30.844
      male S30.840
    periocular area —*see* Constriction, external, eyelid
    phalanges
      finger —*see* Constriction, external, finger
      toe —*see* Constriction, external, toe
    pharynx S10.14
    pinna —*see* Constriction, external, ear
    popliteal space —*see* Constriction, external, knee
    prepuce S30.842
    pubic region S30.840
    pudendum
      female S30.846
      male S30.845
    sacral region S30.840
    scalp S00.04
    scapular region —*see* Constriction, external, shoulder
    scrotum S30.843
    shin —*see* Constriction, external, leg
    shoulder S40.24-
    sternal region S20.349
    submaxillary region S00.84
    submental region S00.84
    subungual
      finger (s) —*see* Constriction, external, finger
      toe (s) —*see* Constriction, external, toe
    supraclavicular fossa S10.84
    supraorbital S00.84
    temple S00.84
    temporal region S00.84
    testis S30.843
    thigh S70.34-
    thorax, thoracic (wall) S20.94
      back S20.44-
      front S20.34-
    throat S10.14
    thumb S60.34-
    toe (s) (lesser) S90.44-
      great S90.44-
    tongue S00.542
    trachea S10.14
    tunica vaginalis S30.843
    uvula S00.542

Constriction (*Continued*)
  external (*Continued*)
    vagina S30.844
    vulva S30.844
    wrist S60.84-
  gallbladder —*see* Obstruction, gallbladder
  intestine —*see* Obstruction, intestine
  larynx J38.6
    congenital Q31.8
      specified NEC Q31.8
      subglottic Q31.1
  organ or site, congenital NEC —*see* Atresia, by site
  prepuce (acquired) (congenital) N47.1
  pylorus (adult hypertrophic) K31.1
    congenital or infantile Q40.0
    newborn Q40.0
  ring dystocia (uterus) O62.4
  spastic —*see also* Spasm
    ureter N13.5
  ureter N13.5
    with infection N13.6
  urethra —*see* Stricture, urethra
  visual field (peripheral) (functional) —*see* Defect, visual field
Constrictive —*see* condition
Consultation
  without complaint or sickness Z71.9
    feared complaint unfounded Z71.1
    specified reason NEC Z71.89
  medical —*see* Counseling, medical
  religious Z71.81
  specified reason NEC Z71.89
  spiritual Z71.81
Consumption —*see* Tuberculosis
Contact (with) —*see also* Exposure (to)
  acariasis Z20.7
  AIDS virus Z20.6
  air pollution Z77.110
  algae and algae toxins Z77.121
  algae bloom Z77.121
  anthrax Z20.810
  aromatic (hazardous) compounds NEC Z77.028
  aromatic amines Z77.020
  aromatic dyes NOS Z77.028
  arsenic Z77.010
  asbestos Z77.090
  bacterial disease NEC Z20.818
  benzene Z77.021
  blue-green algae bloom Z77.121
  body fluids (potentially hazardous) Z77.21
  brown tide Z77.121
  chemicals (chiefly nonmedicinal) (hazardous) NEC Z77.098
  cholera Z20.09
  chromium compounds Z77.018
  communicable disease Z20.9
    bacterial NEC Z20.818
    specified NEC Z20.89
    viral NEC Z20.828
  cyanobacteria bloom Z77.121
  dyes Z77.098
  Escherichia coli (E. coli) Z20.01
  fiberglass —*see* Table of Drugs and Chemicals, fiberglass
  German measles Z20.4
  gonorrhea Z20.2
  hazardous metals NEC Z77.018
  hazardous substances NEC Z77.29
  hazards in the physical environment NEC Z77.128
  hazards to health NEC Z77.9
  HIV Z20.6
  HTLV-III/LAV Z20.6
  human immunodeficiency virus (HIV) Z20.6
  infection Z20.9
    specified NEC Z20.89
  infestation (parasitic) NEC Z20.7
  intestinal infectious disease NEC Z20.09
    Escherichia coli (E. coli) Z20.01

Contact (*Continued*)
  lead Z77.011
  meningococcus Z20.811
  mold (toxic) Z77.120
  nickel dust Z77.018
  noise Z77.122
  parasitic disease Z20.7
  pediculosis Z20.7
  pfiesteria piscicida Z77.121
  poliomyelitis Z20.89
  pollution
    air Z77.110
    environmental NEC Z77.118
    soil Z77.112
    water Z77.111
  polycyclic aromatic hydrocarbons Z77.028
  rabies Z20.3
  radiation, naturally occurring NEC Z77.123
  radon Z77.123
  red tide (Florida) Z77.121
  rubella Z20.4
  sexually-transmitted disease Z20.2
  smallpox (laboratory) Z20.89
  syphilis Z20.2
  tuberculosis Z20.1
  uranium Z77.012
  varicella Z20.820
  venereal disease Z20.2
  viral disease NEC Z20.828
  viral hepatitis Z20.5
  water pollution Z77.111
Contamination, food —*see* Intoxication, foodborne
Contraception, contraceptive
  advice Z30.09
  counseling Z30.09
  device (intrauterine) (in situ) Z97.5
    causing menorrhagia T83.83
    checking Z30.431
    complications —*see* Complications, intrauterine, contraceptive device
    in place Z97.5
    initial prescription Z30.014
    reinsertion Z30.433
    removal Z30.432
    replacement Z30.433
  emergency (postcoital) Z30.012
  initial prescription Z30.019
    injectable Z30.013
    intrauterine device Z30.014
    pills Z30.011
    postcoital (emergency) Z30.012
    specified type NEC Z30.018
    subdermal implantable Z30.019
  maintenance Z30.40
    examination Z30.8
    injectable Z30.42
    intrauterine device Z30.431
    pills Z30.41
    specified type NEC Z30.49
    subdermal implantable Z30.49
  management Z30.9
    specified NEC Z30.8
  postcoital (emergency) Z30.012
  prescription Z30.019
    repeat Z30.40
  sterilization Z30.2
  surveillance (drug) —*see* Contraception, maintenance
Contraction (s), contracture, contracted
  Achilles tendon —*see also* Short, tendon, Achilles
    congenital Q66.89
  amputation stump (surgical) (flexion) (late) next proximal joint T87.89
  anus K59.8
  bile duct (common) (hepatic) K83.8
  bladder N32.89
    neck or sphincter N32.0
  bowel, cecum, colon or intestine, any part —*see* Obstruction, intestine

Contraction, contracture, contracted
(Continued)
Braxton Hicks —see False, labor
breast implant, capsular T85.44
bronchial J98.09
burn (old) —see Cicatrix
cervix —see Stricture, cervix
cicatricial —see Cicatrix
conjunctiva, trachomatous, active A71.1
    sequelae (late effect) B94.0
Dupuytren's M72.0
eyelid —see Disorder, eyelid function
fascia (lata) (postural) M72.8
    Dupuytren's M72.0
    palmar M72.0
    plantar M72.2
finger NEC —see also Deformity, finger
    congenital Q68.1
    joint —see Contraction, joint, hand
flaccid —see Contraction, paralytic
gallbladder K82.0
heart valve —see Endocarditis
hip —see Contraction, joint, hip
hourglass
    bladder N32.89
        congenital Q64.79
    gallbladder K82.0
        congenital Q44.1
    stomach K31.89
        congenital Q40.2
        psychogenic F45.8
    uterus (complicating delivery) O62.4
hysterical F44.4
internal os —see Stricture, cervix
joint (abduction) (acquired) (adduction)
        (flexion) (rotation) M24.50
    ankle M24.57-
    congenital NEC Q68.8
        hip Q65.89
    elbow M24.52-
    foot joint M24.57-
    hand joint M24.54-
    hip M24.55-
        congenital Q65.89
    hysterical F44.4
    knee M24.56-
    shoulder M24.51-
    wrist M24.53-
kidney (granular) (secondary) N26.9
    congenital Q63.8
    hydronephritic —see Hydronephrosis
    Page N26.2
    pyelonephritic —see Pyelitis, chronic
    tuberculous A18.11
ligament —see also Disorder, ligament
    congenital Q79.8
muscle (postinfective) (postural) NEC M62.40
    with contracture of joint —see Contraction,
        joint
    ankle M62.47-
    congenital Q79.8
        sternocleidomastoid Q68.0
    extraocular —see Strabismus
    eye (extrinsic) —see Strabismus
    foot M62.47-
    forearm M62.43-
    hand M62.44-
    hysterical F44.4
    ischemic (Volkmann's) T79.6
    lower leg M62.46-
    multiple sites M62.49
    pelvic region M62.45-
    posttraumatic —see Strabismus, paralytic
    psychogenic F45.8
        conversion reaction F44.4
    shoulder region M62.41-
    specified site NEC M62.48
    thigh M62.45-
    upper arm M62.42-
    neck —see Torticollis
    ocular muscle —see Strabismus

Contraction, contracture, contracted
(Continued)
organ or site, congenital NEC —see Atresia,
    by site
outlet (pelvis) —see Contraction, pelvis
palmar fascia M72.0
paralytic
    joint —see Contraction, joint
    muscle —see also Contraction, muscle NEC
        ocular —see Strabismus, paralytic
pelvis (acquired) (general) M95.5
    with disproportion (fetopelvic) O33.1
        causing obstructed labor O65.1
        inlet O33.2
        mid-cavity O33.3
        outlet O33.3
plantar fascia M72.2
premature
    atrium I49.1
    auriculoventricular I49.49
    heart I49.49
    junctional I49.2
    supraventricular I49.1
    ventricular I49.3
prostate N42.89
pylorus NEC —see also Pylorospasm
    psychogenic F45.8
rectum, rectal (sphincter) K59.8
ring (Bandl's) (complicating delivery) O62.4
scar —see Cicatrix
spine —see Dorsopathy, deforming
sternocleidomastoid (muscle), congenital
    Q68.0
stomach K31.89
    hourglass K31.89
        congenital Q40.2
        psychogenic F45.8
    psychogenic F45.8
tendon (sheath) M62.40
    with contracture of joint —see Contraction,
        joint
    Achilles —see Short, tendon, Achilles
    ankle M62.47-
        Achilles —see Short, tendon, Achilles
    foot M62.47-
    forearm M62.43-
    hand M62.44-
    lower leg M62.46-
    multiple sites M62.49
    neck M62.48
    pelvic region M62.45-
    shoulder region M62.41-
    specified site NEC M62.48
    thigh M62.45-
    thorax M62.48
    trunk M62.48
    upper arm M62.42-
toe —see Deformity, toe, specified NEC
ureterovesical orifice (postinfectional) N13.5
    with infection N13.6
urethra —see also Stricture, urethra
    orifice N32.0
uterus N85.8
    abnormal NEC O62.9
    clonic (complicating delivery) O62.4
    dyscoordinate (complicating delivery) O62.4
    hourglass (complicating delivery) O62.4
    hypertonic O62.4
    hypotonic NEC O62.2
    inadequate
        primary O62.0
        secondary O62.1
    incoordinate (complicating delivery) O62.4
    poor O62.2
    tetanic (complicating delivery) O62.4
vagina (outlet) N89.5
vesical N32.89
    neck or urethral orifice N32.0
visual field —see Defect, visual field,
    generalized
Volkmann's (ischemic) T79.6

Contusion (skin surface intact) T14.8
abdomen, abdominal (muscle) (wall) S30.1
adnexa, eye NEC S05.8X-
adrenal gland S37.812
alveolar process S00.532
ankle S90.0-
antecubital space —see Contusion, forearm
anus S30.3
arm (upper) S40.02-
    lower (with elbow) —see Contusion,
        forearm
auditory canal —see Contusion, ear
auricle —see Contusion, ear
axilla —see Contusion, arm, upper
back —see also Contusion, thorax, back
    lower S30.0
bile duct S36.13
bladder S37.22
bone NEC T14.8
brain (diffuse) —see Injury, intracranial, diffuse
    focal —see Injury, intracranial, focal
brainstem S06.38-
breast S20.0-
broad ligament S37.892
brow S00.83
buttock S30.0
canthus, eye S00.1-
cauda equina S34.3
cerebellar, traumatic S06.37-
cerebral S06.33-
    left side S06.32-
    right side S06.31-
cheek S00.83
    internal S00.532
chest (wall) —see Contusion, thorax
chin S00.83
clitoris S30.23
colon —see Injury, intestine, large, contusion
common bile duct S36.13
conjunctiva S05.1-
    with foreign body (in conjunctival sac) —
        see Foreign body, conjunctival sac
conus medullaris (spine) S34.139
cornea —see Contusion, eyeball
    with foreign body —see Foreign body,
        cornea
corpus cavernosum S30.21
cortex (brain) (cerebral) —see Injury,
    intracranial, diffuse
    focal —see Injury, intracranial, focal
costal region —see Contusion, thorax
cystic duct S36.13
diaphragm S27.802
duodenum S36.420
ear S00.43-
elbow S50.0-
    with forearm —see Contusion, forearm
epididymis S30.22
epigastric region S30.1
epiglottis S10.0
esophagus (thoracic) S27.812
    cervical S10.0
eyeball S05.1-
eyebrow S00.1-
eyelid (and periocular area) S00.1-
face NEC S00.83
fallopian tube S37.529
    bilateral S37.522
    unilateral S37.521
femoral triangle S30.1
finger (s) S60.00
    with damage to nail (matrix) S60.10
    index S60.02-
        with damage to nail S60.12-
    little S60.05-
        with damage to nail S60.15-
    middle S60.03-
        with damage to nail S60.13-
    ring S60.04-
        with damage to nail S60.14-
    thumb —see Contusion, thumb

◀ New   ◀▦ Revised   ~~deleted~~ Deleted

Contusion (Continued)
  flank S30.1
  foot (except toe (s) alone) S90.3-
    toe —see Contusion, toe
  forearm S50.1-
    elbow only —see Contusion, elbow
  forehead S00.83
  gallbladder S36.122
  genital organs, external
    female S30.202
    male S30.201
  globe (eye) —see Contusion, eyeball
  groin S30.1
  gum S00.532
  hand S60.22-
    finger (s) —see Contusion, finger
    wrist —see Contusion, wrist
  head S00.93
    ear —see Contusion, ear
    eyelid —see Contusion, eyelid
    lip S00.531
    nose S00.33
    oral cavity S00.532
    scalp S00.03
    specified part NEC S00.83
  heel —see Contusion, foot
  hepatic duct S36.13
  hip S70.0-
  ileum S36.428
  iliac region S30.1
  inguinal region S30.1
  interscapular region S20.229
  intra-abdominal organ S36.92
    colon —see Injury, intestine, large,
      contusion
    liver S36.112
    pancreas —see Contusion, pancreas
    rectum S36.62
    small intestine —see Injury, intestine, small,
      contusion
    specified organ NEC S36.892
    spleen —see Contusion, spleen
    stomach S36.32
  iris (eye) —see Contusion, eyeball
  jaw S00.83
  jejunum S36.428
  kidney S37.01-
    major (greater than 2 cm) S37.02-
    minor (less than 2 cm) S37.01-
  knee S80.0-
  labium (majus) (minus) S30.23
  lacrimal apparatus, gland or sac S05.8X-
  larynx S10.0
  leg (lower) S80.1-
    knee —see Contusion, knee
  lens —see Contusion, eyeball
  lip S00.531
  liver S36.112
  lower back S30.0
  lumbar region S30.0
  lung S27.329
    bilateral S27.322
    unilateral S27.321
  malar region S00.83
  mastoid region S00.83
  membrane, brain —see Injury, intracranial,
    diffuse
    focal —see Injury, intracranial, focal
  mesentery S36.892
  mesosalpinx S37.892
  mouth S00.532
  muscle —see Contusion, by site
  nail
    finger —see Contusion, finger, with
      damage to nail
    toe —see Contusion, toe, with damage to
      nail
  nasal S00.33
  neck S10.93
    specified site NEC S10.83
    throat S10.0

Contusion (Continued)
  nerve —see Injury, nerve
  newborn P54.5
  nose S00.33
  occipital
    lobe (brain) —see Injury, intracranial,
      diffuse
      focal —see Injury, intracranial,
        focal
    region (scalp) S00.03
  orbit (region) (tissues) S05.1-
  ovary S37.429
    bilateral S37.422
    unilateral S37.421
  palate S00.532
  pancreas S36.229
    body S36.221
    head S36.220
    tail S36.222
  parietal
    lobe (brain) —see Injury, intracranial,
      diffuse
      focal —see Injury, intracranial, focal
    region (scalp) S00.03
  pelvic organ S37.92
    adrenal gland S37.812
    bladder S37.22
    fallopian tube —see Contusion, fallopian
      tube
    kidney —see Contusion, kidney
    ovary —see Contusion, ovary
    prostate S37.822
    specified organ NEC S37.892
    ureter S37.12
    urethra S37.32
    uterus S37.62
  pelvis S30.0
  penis S30.21
  perineum
    female S30.23
    male S30.0
  periocular area S00.1-
  peritoneum S36.81
  periurethral tissue —see Contusion,
    urethra
  pharynx S10.0
  pinna —see Contusion, ear
  popliteal space —see Contusion, knee
  prepuce S30.21
  prostate S37.822
  pubic region S30.1
  pudendum
    female S30.202
    male S30.201
  quadriceps femoris —see Contusion, thigh
  rectum S36.62
  retroperitoneum S36.892
  round ligament S37.892
  sacral region S30.0
  scalp S00.03
    due to birth injury P12.3
  scapular region —see Contusion, shoulder
  sclera —see Contusion, eyeball
  scrotum S30.22
  seminal vesicle S37.892
  shoulder S40.01-
  skin NEC T14.8
  small intestine —see Injury, intestine, small,
    contusion
  spermatic cord S30.22
  spinal cord —see Injury, spinal cord,
    by region
      cauda equina S34.3
      conus medullaris S34.139
  spleen S36.029
    major S36.021
    minor S36.020
  sternal region S20.219
  stomach S36.32
  subconjunctival S05.1-
  subcutaneous NEC T14.8

Contusion (Continued)
  submaxillary region S00.83
  submental region S00.83
  subperiosteal NEC T14.8
  subungual
    finger —see Contusion, finger, with
      damage to nail
    toe —see Contusion, toe, with damage to
      nail
  supraclavicular fossa S10.83
  supraorbital S00.83
  suprarenal gland S37.812
  temple (region) S00.83
  temporal
    lobe (brain) —see Injury, intracranial,
      diffuse
      focal —see Injury, intracranial, focal
    region S00.83
  testis S30.22
  thigh S70.1-
  thorax (wall) S20.20
    back S20.22-
    front S20.21-
  throat S10.0
  thumb S60.01-
    with damage to nail S60.11-
  toe (s) (lesser) S90.12-
    with damage to nail S90.22-
    great S90.11-
      with damage to nail S90.21-
      specified type NEC S90.221
  tongue S00.532
  trachea (cervical) S10.0
    thoracic S27.52
  tunica vaginalis S30.22
  tympanum, tympanic membrane —see
    Contusion, ear
  ureter S37.12
  urethra S37.32
  urinary organ NEC S37.892
  uterus S37.62
  uvula S00.532
  vagina S30.23
  vas deferens S37.892
  vesical S37.22
  vocal cord (s) S10.0
  vulva S30.23
  wrist S60.21-
Conus (congenital) (any type) Q14.8
  cornea —see Keratoconus
  medullaris syndrome G95.81
Conversion hysteria, neurosis or reaction F44.9
Converter, tuberculosis (test reaction) R76.11
Conviction (legal), anxiety concerning Z65.0
  with imprisonment Z65.1
Convulsions (idiopathic) (see also Seizure (s))
    R56.9
  apoplectiform (cerebral ischemia) I67.82
  benign neonatal (familial) —see Epilepsy,
    generalized, idiopathic
  dissociative F44.5
  epileptic —see Epilepsy
  epileptiform, epileptoid —see Seizure,
    epileptiform
  ether (anesthetic) —see Table of Drugs and
    Chemicals, by drug
  febrile R56.00
    with status epilepticus G40.901
    complex R56.01
      with status epilepticus G40.901
    simple R56.00
  hysterical F44.5
  infantile P90
    epilepsy —see Epilepsy
  jacksonian —see Epilepsy, localization-
    related, symptomatic, with simple
    partial seizures
  myoclonic G25.3
  neonatal, benign (familial) —see Epilepsy,
    generalized, idiopathic
  newborn P90

Convulsions *(Continued)*
  obstetrical (nephritic) (uremic) —*see*
      Eclampsia
  paretic A52.17
  post traumatic R56.1
  psychomotor —*see* Epilepsy, localization-
      related, symptomatic, with complex
      partial seizures
  recurrent R56.9
  reflex R25.8
  scarlatinal A38.8
  tetanus, tetanic —*see* Tetanus
  thymic E32.8
Convulsive —*see also* Convulsions
Cooley's anemia D56.1
Coolie itch B76.9
Cooper's
  disease —*see* Mastopathy, cystic
  hernia —*see* Hernia, abdomen, specified site
      NEC
Copra itch B88.0
Coprophagy F50.8
Coprophobia F40.298
Coproporphyria, hereditary E80.29
Cor
  biloculare Q20.8
  bovis, bovinum —*see* Hypertrophy, cardiac
  pulmonale (chronic) I27.81
      acute I26.09
  triatriatum, triatrium Q24.2
  triloculare Q20.8
      biatrium Q20.4
      biventriculare Q21.1
Corbus' disease (gangrenous balanitis) N48.1
Cord —*see also* condition
  around neck (tightly) (with compression)
      complicating delivery O69.1
  bladder G95.89
      tabetic A52.19
Cordis ectopia Q24.8
Corditis (spermatic) N49.1
Corectopia Q13.2
Cori's disease (glycogen storage) E74.03
Corkhandler's disease or lung J67.3
Corkscrew esophagus K22.4
Corkworker's disease or lung J67.3
Corn (infected) L84
Cornea —*see also* condition
  donor Z52.5
  plana Q13.4
Cornelia de Lange syndrome Q87.1
Cornu cutaneum L85.8
Cornual gestation or pregnancy O00.8
Coronary (artery) —*see* condition
Coronavirus, as cause of disease classified
      elsewhere B97.29
  SARS-associated B97.21
Corpora —*see also* condition
  amylacea, prostate N42.89
  cavernosa —*see* condition
Corpulence —*see* Obesity
Corpus —*see* condition
Corrected transposition Q20.5
Corrosion (injury) (acid) (caustic) (chemical)
      (lime) (external) (internal) T30.4
  abdomen, abdominal (muscle) (wall) T21.42
      first degree T21.52
      second degree T21.62
      third degree T21.72
  above elbow T22.439
      first degree T22.539
      left T22.432
          first degree T22.532
          second degree T22.632
          third degree T22.732
      right T22.431
          first degree T22.531
          second degree T22.631
          third degree T22.731
      second degree T22.639
      third degree T22.739

Corrosion *(Continued)*
  alimentary tract NEC T28.7
  ankle T25.419
      first degree T25.519
      left T25.412
          first degree T25.512
          second degree T25.612
          third degree T25.712
      multiple with foot —*see* Corrosion,
          lower, limb, multiple, ankle
          and foot
      →right T25.411
          first degree T25.511
          second degree T25.611
      →third degree T25.711
      second degree T25.619
      third degree T25.719
  anus —*see* Corrosion, buttock
  arm (s) (meaning upper limb (s)) —*see*
      Corrosion, upper limb
  axilla T22.449
      first degree T22.549
      left T22.442
          first degree T22.542
          second degree T22.642
          third degree T22.742
      right T22.441
          first degree T22.541
          second degree T22.641
          third degree T22.741
      second degree T22.649
      third degree T22.749
  back (lower) T21.44
      first degree T21.54
      second degree T21.64
      third degree T21.74
      upper T21.43
          first degree T21.53
          second degree T21.63
          third degree T21.73
  blisters - code as Corrosion, second degree,
      by site
  breast (s) —*see* Corrosion, chest wall
  buttock (s) T21.45
      first degree T21.55
      second degree T21.65
      third degree T21.75
  calf T24.439
      first degree T24.539
      left T24.432
          first degree T24.532
          second degree T24.632
          third degree T24.732
      right T24.431
          first degree T24.531
          second degree T24.631
          third degree T24.731
      second degree T24.639
      third degree T24.739
  canthus (eye) —*see* Corrosion,
      eyelid
  cervix T28.8
  cheek T20.46
      first degree T20.56
      second degree T20.66
      third degree T20.76
  chest wall T21.41
      first degree T21.51
      second degree T21.61
      third degree T21.71
  chin T20.43
      first degree T20.53
      second degree T20.63
      third degree T20.73
  colon T28.7
  conjunctiva (and cornea) —*see* Corrosion,
      cornea
  cornea (and conjunctiva) T26.6-
  deep necrosis of underlying tissue -
      code as Corrosion, third degree,
      by site

Corrosion *(Continued)*
  dorsum of hand T23.469
      first degree T23.569
      left T23.462
          first degree T23.562
          second degree T23.662
          third degree T23.762
      right T23.461
          first degree T23.561
          second degree T23.661
          third degree T23.761
      second degree T23.669
      third degree T23.769
  ear (auricle) (external) (canal)
      T20.41
      drum T28.91
      first degree T20.51
      second degree T20.61
      third degree T20.71
  elbow T22.429
      first degree T22.529
      left T22.422
          first degree T22.522
          second degree T22.622
          third degree T22.722
      right T22.421
          first degree T22.521
          second degree T22.621
          third degree T22.721
      second degree T22.629
      third degree T22.729
  entire body —*see* Corrosion, multiple
      body regions
  epidermal loss - code as Corrosion,
      second degree, by site
  epiglottis T27.4
  erythema, erythematous - code
      as Corrosion, first degree,
      by site
  esophagus T28.6
  extent (percentage of body surface)
      less than 10 percent T32.0
      10-19 percent (0-9 percent third degree)
          T32.10
          with 10-19 percent third degree
              T32.11
      20-29 percent (0-9 percent third degree)
          T32.20
          with
              10-19 percent third degree T32.21
              20-29 percent third degree T32.22
      30-39 percent (0-9 percent third degree)
          T32.30
          with
              10-19 percent third degree T32.31
              20-29 percent third degree T32.32
              30-39 percent third degree T32.33
      40-49 percent (0-9 percent third degree)
          T32.40
          with
              10-19 percent third degree T32.41
              20-29 percent third degree T32.42
              30-39 percent third degree T32.43
              40-49 percent third degree T32.44
      50-59 percent (0-9 percent third degree)
          T32.50
          with
              10-19 percent third degree T32.51
              20-29 percent third degree T32.52
              30-39 percent third degree T32.53
              40-49 percent third degree T32.54
              50-59 percent third degree T32.55
      60-69 percent (0-9 percent third degree)
          T32.60
          with
              10-19 percent third degree T32.61
              20-29 percent third degree T32.62
              30-39 percent third degree T32.63
              40-49 percent third degree T32.64
              50-59 percent third degree T32.65
              60-69 percent third degree T32.66

◀ New   ◀▥ Revised   ~~deleted~~ Deleted

Corrosion (Continued)

extent (Continued)

70-79 percent (0-9 percent third degree) T32.70

with

10-19 percent third degree T32.71
20-29 percent third degree T32.72
30-39 percent third degree T32.73
40-49 percent third degree T32.74
50-59 percent third degree T32.75
60-69 percent third degree T32.76
70-79 percent third degree T32.77

80-89 percent (0-9 percent third degree) T32.80

with

10-19 percent third degree T32.81
20-29 percent third degree T32.82
30-39 percent third degree T32.83
40-49 percent third degree T32.84
50-59 percent third degree T32.85
60-69 percent third degree T32.86
70-79 percent third degree T32.87
80-89 percent third degree T32.88

90 percent or more (0-9 percent third degree) T32.90

with

10-19 percent third degree T32.91
20-29 percent third degree T32.92
30-39 percent third degree T32.93
40-49 percent third degree T32.94
50-59 percent third degree T32.95
60-69 percent third degree T32.96
70-79 percent third degree T32.97
80-89 percent third degree T32.98
90-99 percent third degree T32.99

extremity —see Corrosion, limb
eye (s) and adnexa T26.9-

with resulting rupture and destruction of eyeball T26.7-
conjunctival sac —see Corrosion, cornea
cornea —see Corrosion, cornea
lid —see Corrosion, eyelid
periocular area —see Corrosion eyelid
specified site NEC T26.8-

eyeball —see Corrosion, eye
eyelid (s) T26.5-
face —see Corrosion, head
finger T23.429

first degree T23.529
left T23.422

first degree T23.522
second degree T23.622
third degree T23.722

multiple sites (without thumb) T23.439

with thumb T23.449

first degree T23.549
left T23.442

first degree T23.542
second degree T23.642
third degree T23.742

right T23.441

first degree T23.541
second degree T23.641
third degree T23.741

second degree T23.649
third degree T23.749

first degree T23.539
left T23.432

first degree T23.532
second degree T23.632
third degree T23.732

right T23.431

first degree T23.531
second degree T23.631
third degree T23.731

second degree T23.639
third degree T23.739

right T23.421

first degree T23.521
second degree T23.621
third degree T23.721

Corrosion (Continued)

finger (Continued)

second degree T23.629
third degree T23.729

flank —see Corrosion, abdomen
foot T25.429

first degree T25.529
left T25.422

first degree T25.522
second degree T25.622
third degree T25.722

multiple with ankle —see Corrosion, lower, limb, multiple, ankle and foot

right T25.421

first degree T25.521
second degree T25.621
third degree T25.721

second degree T25.629
third degree T25.729

forearm T22.419

first degree T22.519
left T22.412

first degree T22.512
second degree T22.612
third degree T22.712

right T22.411

first degree T22.511
second degree T22.611
third degree T22.711

second degree T22.619
third degree T22.719

forehead T20.46

first degree T20.56
second degree T20.66
third degree T20.76

fourth degree - code as Corrosion, third degree, by site
full thickness skin loss - code as Corrosion, third degree, by site
gastrointestinal tract NEC T28.7
genital organs

external

female T21.47

first degree T21.57
second degree T21.67
third degree T21.77

male T21.46

first degree T21.56
second degree T21.66
third degree T21.76

internal T28.8

groin —see Corrosion, abdominal wall
hand (s) T23.409

back —see Corrosion, dorsum of hand
finger —see Corrosion, finger
first degree T23.509
left T23.402

first degree T23.502
second degree T23.602
third degree T23.702

multiple sites with wrist T23.499

first degree T23.599
left T23.492

first degree T23.592
second degree T23.692
third degree T23.792

right T23.491

first degree T23.591
second degree T23.691
third degree T23.791

second degree T23.699
third degree T23.799

palm —see Corrosion, palm
right T23.401

first degree T23.501
second degree T23.601
third degree T23.701

second degree T23.609
third degree T23.709

thumb —see Corrosion, thumb

Corrosion (Continued)

head (and face) (and neck) T20.40

cheek —see Corrosion, cheek
chin —see Corrosion, chin
ear —see Corrosion, ear
eye (s) only —see Corrosion, eye
first degree T20.50
forehead —see Corrosion, forehead
lip —see Corrosion, lip
multiple sites T20.49

first degree T20.59
second degree T20.69
third degree T20.79

neck —see Corrosion, neck
nose —see Corrosion, nose
scalp —see Corrosion, scalp
second degree T20.60
third degree T20.70

hip (s) —see Corrosion, lower, limb
inhalation —see Corrosion, respiratory tract
internal organ (s) (see also Corrosion, by site) T28.90

alimentary tract T28.7
esophagus T28.6
esophagus T28.6
genitourinary T28.8
mouth T28.5
pharynx T28.5
specified organ NEC T28.99

interscapular region —see Corrosion, back, upper
intestine (large) (small) T28.7
knee T24.429

first degree T24.529
left T24.422

first degree T24.522
second degree T24.622
third degree T24.722

right T24.421

first degree T24.521
second degree T24.621
third degree T24.721

second degree T24.629
third degree T24.729

labium (majus) (minus) —see Corrosion, genital organs, external, female
lacrimal apparatus, duct, gland or sac —see Corrosion, eye, specified site NEC
larynx T27.4

with lung T27.5

leg (s) (meaning lower limb (s)) —see Corrosion, lower limb
limb (s)

lower —see Corrosion, lower, limb
upper —see Corrosion, upper limb

lip (s) T20.42

first degree T20.52
second degree T20.62
third degree T20.72

lower

back —see Corrosion, back
limb T24.409

ankle —see Corrosion, ankle
calf —see Corrosion, calf
first degree T24.509
foot —see Corrosion, foot
hip —see Corrosion, thigh
knee —see Corrosion, knee
left T24.402

first degree T24.502
second degree T24.602
third degree T24.702

multiple sites, except ankle and foot T24.499

ankle and foot T25.499

first degree T25.599
left T25.492

first degree T25.592
second degree T25.692
third degree T25.792

Corrosion (*Continued*)
  lower (*Continued*)
    limb (*Continued*)
      multiple sites, except ankle and foot (*Continued*)
        ankle and foot (*Continued*)
          right T25.491
            first degree T25.591
            second degree T25.691
            third degree T25.791
          second degree T25.699
          third degree T25.799
        first degree T24.599
        left T24.492
          first degree T24.592
          second degree T24.692
          third degree T24.792
        right T24.491
          first degree T24.591
          second degree T24.691
          third degree T24.791
        second degree T24.699
        third degree T24.799
      right T24.401
        first degree T24.501
        second degree T24.601
        third degree T24.701
      second degree T24.609
      thigh —*see* Corrosion, thigh
      third degree T24.709
  lung (with larynx and trachea) T27.5
  mouth T28.5
  neck T20.47
    first degree T20.57
    second degree T20.67
    third degree T20.77
  nose (septum) T20.44
    first degree T20.54
    second degree T20.64
    third degree T20.74
  ocular adnexa —*see* Corrosion, eye
  orbit region —*see* Corrosion, eyelid
  palm T23.459
    first degree T23.559
    left T23.452
      first degree T23.552
      second degree T23.652
      third degree T23.752
    right T23.451
      first degree T23.551
      second degree T23.651
      third degree T23.751
    second degree T23.659
    third degree T23.759
  partial thickness - code as Corrosion, unspecified degree, by site
  pelvis —*see* Corrosion, trunk
  penis —*see* Corrosion, genital organs, external, male
  perineum
    female —*see* Corrosion, genital organs, external, female
    male —*see* Corrosion, genital organs, external, male
  periocular area —*see* Corrosion, eyelid
  pharynx T28.5
  rectum T28.7
  respiratory tract T27.7
    larynx —*see* Corrosion, larynx
    specified part NEC T27.6
    trachea —*see* Corrosion, larynx
  sac, lacrimal —*see* Corrosion, eye, specified site NEC
  scalp T20.45
    first degree T20.55
    second degree T20.65
    third degree T20.75

Corrosion (*Continued*)
  scapular region T22.469
    first degree T22.569
    left T22.462
      first degree T22.562
      second degree T22.662
      third degree T22.762
    right T22.461
      first degree T22.561
      second degree T22.661
      third degree T22.761
    second degree T22.669
    third degree T22.769
  sclera —*see* Corrosion, eye, specified site NEC
  scrotum —*see* Corrosion, genital organs, external, male
  shoulder T22.459
    first degree T22.559
    left T22.452
      first degree T22.552
      second degree T22.652
      third degree T22.752
    right T22.451
      first degree T22.551
      second degree T22.651
      third degree T22.751
    second degree T22.659
    third degree T22.759
  stomach T28.7
  temple —*see* Corrosion, head
  testis —*see* Corrosion, genital organs, external, male
  thigh T24.419
    first degree T24.519
    left T24.412
      first degree T24.512
      second degree T24.612
      third degree T24.712
    right T24.411
      first degree T24.511
      second degree T24.611
      third degree T24.711
    second degree T24.619
    third degree T24.719
  thorax (external) —*see* Corrosion, trunk
  throat (meaning pharynx) T28.5
  thumb (s) T23.419
    first degree T23.519
    left T23.412
      first degree T23.512
      second degree T23.612
      third degree T23.712
    multiple sites with fingers T23.449
      first degree T23.549
      left T23.442
        first degree T23.542
        second degree T23.642
        third degree T23.742
      right T23.441
        first degree T23.541
        second degree T23.641
        third degree T23.741
      second degree T23.649
      third degree T23.749
    right T23.411
      first degree T23.511
      second degree T23.611
      third degree T23.711
    second degree T23.619
    third degree T23.719
  toe T25.439
    first degree T25.539
    left T25.432
      first degree T25.532
      second degree T25.632
      third degree T25.732
    right T25.431
      first degree T25.531
      second degree T25.631
      third degree T25.731

Corrosion (*Continued*)
  toe (*Continued*)
    second degree T25.639
    third degree T25.739
  tongue T28.5
  tonsil (s) T28.5
  total body —*see* Corrosion, multiple body regions
  trachea T27.4
    with lung T27.5
  trunk T21.40
    abdominal wall —*see* Corrosion, abdominal wall
    anus —*see* Corrosion, buttock
    axilla —*see* Corrosion, upper limb
    back —*see* Corrosion, back
    breast —*see* Corrosion, chest wall
    buttock —*see* Corrosion, buttock
    chest wall —*see* Corrosion, chest wall
    first degree T21.50
    flank —*see* Corrosion, abdominal wall
    genital
      female —*see* Corrosion, genital organs, external, female
      male —*see* Corrosion, genital organs, external, male
    groin —*see* Corrosion, abdominal wall
    interscapular region —*see* Corrosion, back, upper
    labia —*see* Corrosion, genital organs, external, female
    lower back —*see* Corrosion, back
    penis —*see* Corrosion, genital organs, external, male
    perineum
      female —*see* Corrosion, genital organs, external, female
      male —*see* Corrosion, genital organs, external, male
    scapular region —*see* Corrosion, upper limb
    scrotum —*see* Corrosion, genital organs, external, male
    second degree T21.60
    shoulder —*see* Corrosion, upper limb
    specified site NEC T21.49
      first degree T21.59
      second degree T21.69
      third degree T21.79
    testes —*see* Corrosion, genital organs, external, male
    third degree T21.70
    upper back —*see* Corrosion, back, upper
    vagina T28.8
    vulva —*see* Corrosion, genital organs, external, female
  unspecified site with extent of body surface involved specified
    less than 10 percent T32.0
    10-19 percent (0-9 percent third degree) T32.10
      with 10-19 percent third degree T32.11
    20-29 percent (0-9 percent third degree) T32.20
      with
        10-19 percent third degree T32.21
        20-29 percent third degree T32.22
    30-39 percent (0-9 percent third degree) T32.30
      with
        10-19 percent third degree T32.31
        20-29 percent third degree T32.32
        30-39 percent third degree T32.33
    40-49 percent (0-9 percent third degree) T32.40
      with
        10-19 percent third degree T32.41
        20-29 percent third degree T32.42
        30-39 percent third degree T32.43
        40-49 percent third degree T32.44

Corrosion *(Continued)*
unspecified site with extent of body surface
involved specified *(Continued)*
50-59 percent (0-9 percent third degree)
T32.50
with
10-19 percent third degree T32.51
20-29 percent third degree T32.52
30-39 percent third degree T32.53
40-49 percent third degree T32.54
50-59 percent third degree T32.55
60-69 percent (0-9 percent third degree)
T32.60
with
10-19 percent third degree T32.61
20-29 percent third degree T32.62
30-39 percent third degree T32.63
40-49 percent third degree T32.64
50-59 percent third degree T32.65
60-69 percent third degree T32.66
70-79 percent (0-9 percent third degree)
T32.70
with
10-19 percent third degree T32.71
20-29 percent third degree T32.72
30-39 percent third degree T32.73
40-49 percent third degree T32.74
50-59 percent third degree T32.75
60-69 percent third degree T32.76
70-79 percent third degree T32.77
80-89 percent (0-9 percent third degree)
T32.80
with
10-19 percent third degree T32.81
20-29 percent third degree T32.82
30-39 percent third degree T32.83
40-49 percent third degree T32.84
50-59 percent third degree T32.85
60-69 percent third degree T32.86
70-79 percent third degree T32.87
80-89 percent third degree T32.88
90 percent or more (0-9 percent third
degree) T32.90
with
10-19 percent third degree T32.91
20-29 percent third degree T32.92
30-39 percent third degree T32.93
40-49 percent third degree T32.94
50-59 percent third degree T32.95
60-69 percent third degree T32.96
70-79 percent third degree T32.97
80-89 percent third degree T32.98
90-99 percent third degree T32.99
upper limb (axilla) (scapular region) T22.40
above elbow —*see* Corrosion, above
elbow
axilla —*see* Corrosion, axilla
elbow —*see* Corrosion, elbow
first degree T22.50
forearm —*see* Corrosion, forearm
hand —*see* Corrosion, hand
interscapular region —*see* Corrosion, back,
upper
multiple sites T22.499
first degree T22.599
left T22.492
first degree T22.592
second degree T22.692
third degree T22.792
right T22.491
first degree T22.591
second degree T22.691
third degree T22.791
second degree T22.699
third degree T22.799
scapular region —*see* Corrosion, scapular
region
second degree T22.60
shoulder —*see* Corrosion, shoulder
third degree T22.70
wrist —*see* Corrosion, hand

Corrosion *(Continued)*
uterus T28.8
vagina T28.8
vulva —*see* Corrosion, genital organs,
external, female
wrist T23.479
first degree T23.579
left T23.472
first degree T23.572
second degree T23.672
third degree T23.772
multiple sites with hand T23.499
first degree T23.599
left T23.492
first degree T23.592
second degree T23.692
third degree T23.792
right T23.491
first degree T23.591
second degree T23.691
third degree T23.791
second degree T23.699
third degree T23.799
right T23.471
first degree T23.571
second degree T23.671
third degree T23.771
second degree T23.679
third degree T23.779
Corrosive burn —*see* Corrosion
Corsican fever —*see* Malaria
Cortical —*see* condition
Cortico-adrenal —*see* condition
Coryza (acute) J00
with grippe or influenza —*see* Influenza,
with, respiratory manifestations
NEC
syphilitic
congenital (chronic) A50.05
Costen's syndrome or complex M26.69
Costiveness —*see* Constipation
Costochondritis M94.0
Cot death R99
Cotard's syndrome F22
Cotia virus B08.8
Cotton wool spots (retinal) H35.81
Cotungo's disease —*see* Sciatica
Cough (affected) (chronic) (epidemic) (nervous)
R05
with hemorrhage —*see* Hemoptysis
bronchial R05
with grippe or influenza —*see* Influenza,
with, respiratory manifestations
NEC
functional F45.8
hysterical F45.8
laryngeal, spasmodic R05
psychogenic F45.8
smokers' J41.0
tea taster's B49
Counseling (for) Z71.9
abuse NEC
perpetrator Z69.82
victim Z69.81
alcohol abuser Z71.41
family Z71.42
child abuse
nonparental
perpetrator Z69.021
victim Z69.020
parental
perpetrator Z69.011
victim Z69.010
consanguinity Z71.89
contraceptive Z30.09
dietary Z71.3
drug abuser Z71.51
family member Z71.52
family Z71.89
fertility preservation (prior to cancer therapy)
(prior to removal of gonads) Z31.62

Counseling *(Continued)*
for non-attending third party Z71.0
related to sexual behavior or orientation
Z70.2
genetic NEC Z31.5
health (advice) (education) (instruction) —*see*
Counseling, medical
human immunodeficiency virus (HIV)
Z71.7
impotence Z70.1
insulin pump use Z46.81
medical (for) Z71.9
boarding school resident Z59.3
consanguinity Z71.89
feared complaint and no disease found
Z71.1
human immunodeficiency virus (HIV)
Z71.7
institutional resident Z59.3
on behalf of another Z71.0
related to sexual behavior or orientation
Z70.2
person living alone Z60.2
specified reason NEC Z71.89
natural family planning
procreative Z31.61
to avoid pregnancy Z30.02
perpetrator (of)
abuse NEC Z69.82
child abuse
non-parental Z69.021
parental Z69.011
rape NEC Z69.82
spousal abuse Z69.12
procreative NEC Z31.69
fertility preservation (prior to cancer
therapy) (prior to removal of
gonads) Z31.62
using natural family planning
Z31.61
promiscuity Z70.1
rape victim Z69.81
religious Z71.81
sex, sexual (related to) Z70.9
attitude (s) Z70.0
behavior or orientation Z70.1
combined concerns Z70.3
non-responsiveness Z70.1
on behalf of third party Z70.2
specified reason NEC Z70.8
specified reason NEC Z71.89
spiritual Z71.81
spousal abuse (perpetrator) Z69.12
victim Z69.11
substance abuse Z71.89
alcohol Z71.41
drug Z71.51
tobacco Z71.6
tobacco use Z71.6
use (of)
insulin pump Z46.81
victim (of)
abuse Z69.81
child abuse
by parent Z69.010
non-parental Z69.020
rape NEC Z69.81
Coupled rhythm R00.8
Couvelaire syndrome or uterus (complicating
delivery) O45.8X-
Cowperitis —*see* Urethritis
Cowper's gland —*see* condition
Cowpox B08.010
due to vaccination T88.1
Coxa
magna M91.4-
plana M91.2-
valga (acquired) —*see also* Deformity, limb,
specified type NEC, thigh
congenital Q65.81
sequelae (late effect) of rickets E64.3

Coxa (Continued)
  vara (acquired) —see also Deformity, limb,
      specified type NEC, thigh
    congenital Q65.82
    sequelae (late effect) of rickets E64.3
Coxalgia, coxalgic (nontuberculous) —see also
    Pain, joint, hip
  tuberculous A18.02
Coxitis —see Monoarthritis, hip
Coxsackie (virus) (infection) B34.1
  as cause of disease classified elsewhere B97.11
  carditis B33.20
  central nervous system NEC A88.8
  endocarditis B33.21
  enteritis A08.39
  meningitis (aseptic) A87.0
  myocarditis B33.22
  pericarditis B33.23
  pharyngitis B08.5
  pleurodynia B33.0
  specific disease NEC B33.8
Crabs, meaning pubic lice B85.3
Crack baby P04.41
Cracked nipple N64.0
  associated with
    lactation O92.13
    pregnancy O92.11-
    puerperium O92.12
Cracked tooth K03.81
Cradle cap L21.0
Craft neurosis F48.8
Cramp (s) R25.2
  abdominal —see Pain, abdominal
  bathing T75.1
  colic R10.83
    psychogenic F45.8
  due to immersion T75.1
  fireman T67.2
  heat T67.2
  immersion T75.1
  intestinal —see Pain, abdominal
    psychogenic F45.8
  leg, sleep related G47.62
  limb (lower) (upper) NEC R25.2
    sleep related G47.62
  linotypist's F48.8
    organic G25.89
  muscle (limb) (general) R25.2
    due to immersion T75.1
    psychogenic F45.8
  occupational (hand) F48.8
    organic G25.89
  salt-depletion E87.1
  sleep related, leg G47.62
  stoker's T67.2
  swimmer's T75.1
  telegrapher's F48.8
    organic G25.89
  typist's F48.8
    organic G25.89
  uterus N94.89
    menstrual —see Dysmenorrhea
  writer's F48.8
    organic G25.89
Cranial —see condition
Craniocleidodysostosis Q74.0
Craniofenestria (skull) Q75.8
Craniolacunia (skull) Q75.8
Craniopagus Q89.4
Craniopathy, metabolic M85.2
Craniopharyngeal —see condition
Craniopharyngioma D44.4
Craniorachischisis (totalis) Q00.1
Cranioschisis Q75.8
Craniostenosis Q75.0
Craniosynostosis Q75.0
Craniotabes (cause unknown) M83.8
  neonatal P96.3
  rachitic E64.3
  syphilitic A50.56
Cranium —see condition

Craw-craw —see Onchocerciasis
Creaking joint —see Derangement, joint,
    specified type NEC
Creeping
  eruption B76.9
  palsy or paralysis G12.22
Crenated tongue K14.8
Creotoxism A05.9
Crepitus
  caput Q75.8
  joint —see Derangement, joint, specified type
    NEC
Crescent or conus choroid, congenital Q14.3
CREST syndrome M34.1
Cretin, cretinism (congenital) (endemic)
    (nongoitrous) (sporadic) E00.9
  pelvis
    with disproportion (fetopelvic) O33.0
      causing obstructed labor O65.0
  type
    hypothyroid E00.1
    mixed E00.2
    myxedematous E00.1
    neurological E00.0
Creutzfeldt-Jakob disease or syndrome (with
    dementia) A81.00
  familial A81.09
  iatrogenic A81.09
  specified NEC A81.09
  sporadic A81.09
  variant (vCJD) A81.01
Crib death R99
Cribriform hymen Q52.3
Cri-du-chat syndrome Q93.4
Crigler-Najjar disease or syndrome E80.5
Crime, victim of Z65.4
Crimean hemorrhagic fever A98.0
Criminalism F60.2
Crisis
  abdomen R10.0
  acute reaction F43.0
  addisonian E27.2
  adrenal (cortical) E27.2
  celiac K90.0
  Dietl's N13.8
  emotional —see also Disorder, adjustment
    acute reaction to stress F43.0
    specific to childhood and adolescence
      F93.8
  glaucomatocyclitic —see Glaucoma,
      secondary, inflammation
  heart —see Failure, heart
  nitritoid I95.2
    correct substance properly administered —
        see Table of Drugs and Chemicals, by
        drug, adverse effect
    overdose or wrong substance given or
        taken —see Table of Drugs and
        Chemicals, by drug, poisoning
  oculogyric H51.8
    psychogenic F45.8
  Pel's (tabetic) A52.11
  psychosexual identity F64.2
  renal N28.0
  sickle-cell D57.00
    with
      acute chest syndrome D57.01
      splenic sequestration D57.02
    state (acute reaction) F43.0
  tabetic A52.11
  thyroid —see Thyrotoxicosis with thyroid
      storm
  thyrotoxic —see Thyrotoxicosis with thyroid
      storm
Crocq's disease (acrocyanosis) I73.89
Crohn's disease —see Enteritis, regional
Crooked septum, nasal J34.2
Cross syndrome E70.328
Crossbite (anterior) (posterior) M26.24
Cross-eye —see Strabismus, convergent
    concomitant

Croup, croupous (catarrhal) (infectious)
    (inflammatory) (nondiphtheritic) J05.0
  bronchial J20.9
  diphtheritic A36.2
  false J38.5
  spasmodic J38.5
    diphtheritic A36.2
  stridulous J38.5
    diphtheritic A36.2
Crouzon's disease Q75.1
Crowding, tooth, teeth, fully erupted M26.31
CRST syndrome M34.1
Cruchet's disease A85.8
Cruelty in children —see also Disorder,
    conduct
Crural ulcer —see Ulcer, lower limb
Crush, crushed, crushing T14.8
  abdomen S38.1
  ankle S97.0-
  arm (upper) (and shoulder) S47.-
  axilla —see Crush, arm
  back, lower S38.1
  buttock S38.1
  cheek S07.0
  chest S28.0
  cranium S07.1
  ear S07.0
  elbow S57.0-
  extremity
    lower
      ankle —see Crush, ankle
      below knee —see Crush, leg
      foot —see Crush, foot
      hip —see Crush, hip
      knee —see Crush, knee
      thigh —see Crush, thigh
      toe —see Crush, toe
    upper
      below elbow S67.9-
      elbow —see Crush, elbow
      finger —see Crush, finger
      forearm —see Crush, forearm
      hand —see Crush, hand
      thumb —see Crush, thumb
      upper arm —see Crush, arm
      wrist —see Crush, wrist
  face S07.0
  finger (s) S67.1-
    with hand (and wrist) —see Crush, hand,
        specified site NEC
    index S67.19-
    little S67.19-
    middle S67.19-
    ring S67.19-
    thumb —see Crush, thumb
  foot S97.8-
    toe —see Crush, toe
  forearm S57.8-
  genitalia, external
    female S38.002
      vagina S38.03
      vulva S38.03
    male S38.001
      penis S38.01
      scrotum S38.02
      testis S38.02
  hand (except fingers alone) S67.2-
    with wrist S67.4-
  head S07.9
    specified NEC S07.8
  heel —see Crush, foot
  hip S77.0-
    with thigh S77.2-
  internal organ (abdomen, chest, or pelvis)
      NEC T14.8
  knee S87.0-
  labium (majus) (minus) S38.03
  larynx S17.0
  leg (lower) S87.8-
    knee —see Crush, knee
  lip S07.0

◀ New   ◀||| Revised   ~~deleted~~ Deleted

Crush, crushed, crushing (Continued)
lower
back S38.1
leg —see Crush, leg
neck S17.9
nerve —see Injury, nerve
nose S07.0
pelvis S38.1
penis S38.01
scalp S07.8
scapular region —see Crush, arm
scrotum S38.02
severe, unspecified site T14.8
shoulder (and upper arm) —see Crush, arm
skull S07.1
syndrome (complication of trauma) T79.5
testis S38.02
thigh S77.1-
with hip S77.2-
throat S17.8
thumb S67.0-
with hand (and wrist) —see Crush, hand, specified site NEC
toe (s) S97.10-
great S97.11-
lesser S97.12-
trachea S17.0
vagina S38.03
vulva S38.03
wrist S67.3-
with hand S67.4-
Crusta lactea L21.0
Crusts R23.4
Crutch paralysis —see Injury, brachial plexus
Cruveilhier-Baumgarten cirrhosis, disease or syndrome K74.69
Cruveilhier's atrophy or disease G12.8
Crying (constant) (continuous) (excessive)
child, adolescent, or adult R45.83
infant (baby) (newborn) R68.11
Cryofibrinogenemia D89.2
Cryoglobulinemia (essential) (idiopathic) (mixed) (primary) (purpura) (secondary) (vasculitis) D89.1
with lung involvement D89.1 [J99]
Cryptitis (anal) (rectal) K62.89
Cryptococcosis, cryptococcus (infection) (neoformans) B45.9
bone B45.3
cerebral B45.1
cutaneous B45.2
disseminated B45.7
generalized B45.7
meningitis B45.1
meningocerebralis B45.1
osseous B45.3
pulmonary B45.0
skin B45.2
specified NEC B45.8
Cryptopapillitis (anus) K62.89
Cryptophthalmos Q11.2
syndrome Q87.0
Cryptorchid, cryptorchism, cryptorchidism Q53.9
bilateral Q53.20
abdominal Q53.21
perineal Q53.22
unilateral Q53.10
abdominal Q53.11
perineal Q53.12
Cryptosporidiosis A07.2
hepatobiliary B88.8
respiratory B88.8
Cryptostromosis J67.6
Crystalluria R82.99
Cubitus
congenital Q68.8
valgus (acquired) M21.0-
congenital Q68.8
sequelae (late effect) of rickets E64.3

Cubitus (Continued)
varus (acquired) M21.1-
congenital Q68.8
sequelae (late effect) of rickets E64.3
Cultural deprivation or shock Z60.3
Curling esophagus K22.4
Curling's ulcer —see Ulcer, peptic, acute
Curschmann (-Batten) (-Steinert) **disease or syndrome** G71.11
Curse, Ondine's —see Apnea, sleep
Curvature
organ or site, congenital NEC —see Distortion
penis (lateral) Q55.61
Pott's (spinal) A18.01
radius, idiopathic, progressive (congenital) Q74.0
spine (acquired) (angular) (idiopathic) (incorrect) (postural) —see Dorsopathy, deforming
congenital Q67.5
due to or associated with
Charcot-Marie-Tooth disease (see also subcategory M49.8) G60.0
osteitis
deformans M88.88
fibrosa cystica (see also subcategory M49.8) E21.0
tuberculosis (Pott's curvature) A18.01
sequelae (late effect) of rickets E64.3
tuberculous A18.01
Cushingoid due to steroid therapy E24.2
correct substance properly administered —see Table of Drugs and Chemicals, by drug, adverse effect
overdose or wrong substance given or taken —see Table of Drugs and Chemicals, by drug, poisoning
Cushing's
syndrome or disease E24.9
drug-induced E24.2
iatrogenic E24.2
pituitary-dependent E24.0
specified NEC E24.8
ulcer —see Ulcer, peptic, acute
Cusp, Carabelli - omit code
Cut (external) —see also Laceration
muscle —see Injury, muscle
Cutaneous —see also condition
hemorrhage R23.3
larva migrans B76.9
Cutis —see also condition
hyperelastica Q82.8
acquired L57.4
laxa (hyperelastica) —see Dermatolysis
marmorata R23.8
osteosis L94.2
pendula —see Dermatolysis
rhomboidalis nuchae L57.2
verticis gyrata Q82.8
acquired L91.8
Cyanosis R23.0
due to
patent foramen botalli Q21.1
persistent foramen ovale Q21.1
enterogenous D74.8
paroxysmal digital —see Raynaud's disease
with gangrene I73.01
retina, retinal H35.89
Cyanotic heart disease I24.9
congenital Q24.9
Cycle
anovulatory N97.0
menstrual, irregular N92.6
Cyclencephaly Q04.9
Cyclical vomiting (see also Vomiting, cyclical) G43.A0
psychogenic F50.8
Cyclitis (see also Iridocyclitis) H20.9
chronic —see Iridocyclitis, chronic
Fuchs' heterochromic H20.81-
granulomatous —see Iridocyclitis, chronic

Cyclitis (Continued)
lens-induced —see Iridocyclitis, lens-induced
posterior H30.2-
Cycloid personality F34.0
Cyclophoria H50.54
Cyclopia, cyclops Q87.0
Cyclopism Q87.0
Cyclosporiasis A07.4
Cyclothymia F34.0
Cyclothymic personality F34.0
Cyclotropia H50.41-
Cylindroma —see also Neoplasm, malignant, by site
eccrine dermal —see Neoplasm, skin, benign
skin —see Neoplasm, skin, benign
Cylindruria R82.99
Cynanche
diphtheritic A36.2
tonsillaris J36
Cynophobia F40.218
Cynorexia R63.2
Cyphosis —see Kyphosis
Cyprus fever —see Brucellosis
Cyst (colloid) (mucous) (simple) (retention)
adenoid (infected) J35.8
adrenal gland E27.8
congenital Q89.1
air, lung J98.4
allantoic Q64.4
alveolar process (jaw bone) M27.40
amnion, amniotic O41.8X-
anterior
chamber (eye) —see Cyst, iris
nasopalatine K09.1
antrum J34.1
anus K62.89
apical (tooth) (periodontal) K04.8
appendix K38.8
arachnoid, brain (acquired) G93.0
congenital Q04.6
arytenoid J38.7
Baker's M71.2-
ruptured M66.0
tuberculous A18.02
Bartholin's gland N75.0
bile duct (common) (hepatic) K83.5
bladder (multiple) (trigone) N32.89
blue dome (breast) —see Cyst, breast
bone (local) NEC M85.60
aneurysmal M85.50
ankle M85.57-
foot M85.57-
forearm M85.53-
hand M85.54-
jaw M27.49
lower leg M85.56-
multiple site M85.59
neck M85.58
rib M85.58
shoulder M85.51-
skull M85.58
specified site NEC M85.58
thigh M85.55-
toe M85.57-
upper arm M85.52-
vertebra M85.58
solitary M85.40
ankle M85.47-
fibula M85.46-
foot M85.47-
hand M85.44-
humerus M85.42-
jaw M27.49
neck M85.48
pelvis M85.45-
radius M85.43-
rib M85.48
shoulder M85.41-
skull M85.48
specified site NEC M85.48

Cyst *(Continued)*
  bone NEC *(Continued)*
    solitary *(Continued)*
      tibia M85.46-
      toe M85.47-
      ulna M85.43-
      vertebra M85.48
    specified type NEC M85.60
      ankle M85.67-
      foot M85.67-
      forearm M85.63-
      hand M85.64-
      jaw M27.40
        developmental (nonodontogenic)
          K09.1
          odontogenic K09.0
        latent M27.0
      lower leg M85.66-
      multiple site M85.69
      neck M85.68
      rib M85.68
      shoulder M85.61-
      skull M85.68
      specified site NEC M85.68
      thigh M85.65-
      toe M85.67-
      upper arm M85.62-
      vertebra M85.68
  brain (acquired) G93.0
    congenital Q04.6
    hydatid B67.99 *[G94]*
    third ventricle (colloid), congenital Q04.6
  branchial (cleft) Q18.0
  branchiogenic Q18.0
  breast (benign) (blue dome) (pedunculated)
    (solitary) N60.0-
    involution —*see* Dysplasia, mammary,
      specified type NEC
    sebaceous —*see* Dysplasia, mammary,
      specified type NEC
  broad ligament (benign) N83.8
  bronchogenic (mediastinal) (sequestration)
    J98.4
    congenital Q33.0
  buccal K09.8
  bulbourethral gland N36.8
  bursa, bursal NEC M71.30
    with rupture —*see* Rupture, synovium
    ankle M71.37-
    elbow M71.32-
    foot M71.37-
    hand M71.34-
    hip M71.35-
    multiple sites M71.39
    pharyngeal J39.2
    popliteal space —*see* Cyst, Baker's
    shoulder M71.31-
    specified site NEC M71.38
    wrist M71.33-
  calcifying odontogenic D16.5
    upper jaw (bone) (maxilla) D16.4
  canal of Nuck (female) N94.89
    congenital Q52.4
  canthus —*see* Cyst, conjunctiva
  carcinomatous —*see* Neoplasm, malignant,
    by site
  cauda equina G95.89
  cavum septi pellucidi —*see* Cyst, brain
  celomic (pericardium) Q24.8
  cerebellopontine (angle) —*see* Cyst, brain
  cerebellum —*see* Cyst, brain
  cerebral —*see* Cyst, brain
  cervical lateral Q18.1
  cervix NEC N88.8
    embryonic Q51.6
    nabothian N88.8
  chiasmal optic NEC —*see* Disorder, optic,
    chiasm
  chocolate (ovary) N80.1
  choledochus, congenital Q44.4
  chorion O41.8X-

Cyst *(Continued)*
  choroid plexus G93.0
  ciliary body —*see* Cyst, iris
  clitoris N90.7
  colon K63.89
  common (bile) duct K83.5
  congenital NEC Q89.8
    adrenal gland Q89.1
    epiglottis Q31.8
    esophagus Q39.8
    fallopian tube Q50.4
    kidney Q61.00
      more than one (multiple) Q61.02
      specified as polycystic Q61.3
        adult type Q61.2
        infantile type NEC Q61.19
          collecting duct dilation Q61.11
      solitary Q61.01
    larynx Q31.8
    liver Q44.6
    lung Q33.0
    mediastinum Q34.1
    ovary Q50.1
    oviduct Q50.4
    periurethral (tissue) Q64.79
    prepuce Q55.69
    salivary gland (any) Q38.4
    sublingual Q38.6
    submaxillary gland Q38.6
    thymus (gland) Q89.2
    tongue Q38.3
    ureterovesical orifice Q62.8
    vulva Q52.79
  conjunctiva H11.44-
  cornea H18.89-
  corpora quadrigemina G93.0
  corpus
    albicans N83.29
    luteum (hemorrhagic) (ruptured) N83.1
  Cowper's gland (benign) (infected) N36.8
  cranial meninges G93.0
  craniobuccal pouch E23.6
  craniopharyngeal pouch E23.6
  cystic duct K82.8
  Cysticercus —*see* Cysticercosis
  Dandy-Walker Q03.1
    with spina bifida —*see* Spina bifida
  dental (root) K04.8
    developmental K09.0
    eruption K09.0
    primordial K09.0
  dentigerous (mandible) (maxilla) K09.0
  dermoid —*see* Neoplasm, benign, by site
    with malignant transformation C56.-
    implantation
      external area or site (skin) NEC L72.0
      iris —*see* Cyst, iris, implantation
      vagina N89.8
      vulva N90.7
    mouth K09.8
    oral soft tissue K09.8
    sacrococcygeal —*see* Cyst, pilonidal
  developmental K09.1
    odontogenic K09.0
    oral region (nonodontogenic) K09.1
    ovary, ovarian Q50.1
  dura (cerebral) G93.0
    spinal G96.19
  ear (external) Q18.1
  echinococcal —*see* Echinococcus
  embryonic
    cervix uteri Q51.6
    fallopian tube Q50.4
    vagina Q51.6
  endometrium, endometrial (uterus) N85.8
    ectopic —*see* Endometriosis
  enterogenous Q43.8
  epidermal, epidermoid (inclusion) *(see also*
    Cyst, skin) L72.0
    mouth K09.8
    oral soft tissue K09.8

Cyst *(Continued)*
  epididymis N50.3
  epiglottis J38.7
  epiphysis cerebri E34.8
  epithelial (inclusion) L72.0
  epoophoron Q50.5
  eruption K09.0
  esophagus K22.8
  ethmoid sinus J34.1
  external female genital organs NEC
    N90.7
  eye NEC H57.8
    congenital Q15.8
  eyelid (sebaceous) H02.829
    infected —*see* Hordeolum
    left H02.826
      lower H02.825
      upper H02.824
    right H02.823
      lower H02.822
      upper H02.821
  fallopian tube N83.8
    congenital Q50.4
  fimbrial (twisted) Q50.4
  fissural (oral region) K09.1
  follicle (graafian) (hemorrhagic) N83.0
    nabothian N88.8
  follicular (atretic) (hemorrhagic) (ovarian)
    N83.0
    dentigerous K09.0
    odontogenic K09.0
    skin L72.9
      specified NEC L72.8
  frontal sinus J34.1
  gallbladder K82.8
  ganglion —*see* Ganglion
  Gartner's duct Q52.4
  gingiva K09.0
  gland of Moll —*see* Cyst, eyelid
  globulomaxillary K09.1
  graafian follicle (hemorrhagic) N83.0
  granulosal lutein (hemorrhagic) N83.1
  hemangiomatous D18.00
    intra-abdominal D18.03
    intracranial D18.02
    skin D18.01
    specified site NEC D18.09
  hydatid *(see also* Echinococcus) B67.90
    brain B67.99 *[G94]*
    liver *(see also* Cyst, liver, hydatid) B67.8
    lung NEC B67.99 *[J99]*
    Morgagni
      female Q50.5
      male (epididymal) Q55.4
        testicular Q55.29
    specified site NEC B67.99
  hymen N89.8
    embryonic Q52.4
  hypopharynx J39.2
  hypophysis, hypophyseal (duct) (recurrent)
    E23.6
    cerebri E23.6
  implantation (dermoid)
    external area or site (skin) NEC L72.0
    iris —*see* Cyst, iris, implantation
    vagina N89.8
    vulva N90.7
  incisive canal K09.1
  inclusion (epidermal) (epithelial)
    (epidermoid) (squamous) L72.0
    not of skin - code under Cyst, by site
  intestine (large) (small) K63.89
  intracranial —*see* Cyst, brain
  intraligamentous —*see also* Disorder,
    ligament
    knee —*see* Derangement, knee
  intrasellar E23.6
  iris H21.309
    exudative H21.31-
    idiopathic H21.30-
    implantation H21.32-

◀ New   ◀|||| Revised   ~~deleted~~ Deleted

Cyst *(Continued)*
  iris *(Continued)*
    parasitic H21.33-
    pars plana (primary) H21.34-
      exudative H21.35-
  jaw (bone) M27.40
    aneurysmal M27.49
    developmental (odontogenic) K09.0
    fissural K09.1
    hemorrhagic M27.49
    traumatic M27.49
  joint NEC —*see* Disorder, joint, specified type
      NEC
  kidney (acquired) N28.1
    calyceal —*see* Hydronephrosis
    congenital Q61.00
    more than one (multiple) Q61.02
      specified as polycystic Q61.3
        adult type (autosomal dominant)
          Q61.2
        infantile type (autosomal recessive)
          NEC Q61.19
            collecting duct dilation Q61.11
    pyelogenic —*see* Hydronephrosis
    simple N28.1
    solitary (single) Q61.01
      acquired N28.1
  labium (majus) (minus) N90.7
    sebaceous N90.7
  lacrimal —*see also* Disorder, lacrimal system,
      specified NEC
    gland H04.13-
    passages or sac —*see* Disorder, lacrimal
      system, specified NEC
  larynx J38.7
  lateral periodontal K09.0
  lens H27.8
    congenital Q12.8
  lip (gland) K13.0
  liver (idiopathic) (simple) K76.89
    congenital Q44.6
    hydatid B67.8
      granulosus B67.0
      multilocularis B67.5
  lung J98.4
    congenital Q33.0
    giant bullous J43.9
  lutein N83.1
  lymphangiomatous D18.1
  lymphoepithelial, oral soft tissue K09.8
  macula —*see* Degeneration, macula, hole
  malignant —*see* Neoplasm, malignant, by site
  mammary gland —*see* Cyst, breast
  mandible M27.40
    dentigerous K09.0
    radicular K04.8
  maxilla M27.40
    dentigerous K09.0
    radicular K04.8
  medial, face and neck Q18.8
  median
    anterior maxillary K09.1
    palatal K09.1
  mediastinum, congenital Q34.1
  meibomian (gland) —*see* Chalazion
    infected —*see* Hordeolum
  membrane, brain G93.0
  meninges (cerebral) G93.0
    spinal G96.19
  meniscus, knee —*see* Derangement, knee,
      meniscus, cystic
  mesentery, mesenteric K66.8
    chyle I89.8
  mesonephric duct
    female Q50.5
    male Q55.4
  milk N64.89
  Morgagni (hydatid)
    female Q50.5
    male (epididymal) Q55.4
      testicular Q55.29
  mouth K09.8

Cyst *(Continued)*
  Müllerian duct Q50.4
    appendix testis Q55.29
    cervix Q51.6
    fallopian tube Q50.4
    female Q50.4
    male Q55.29
    prostatic utricle Q55.4
    vagina (embryonal) Q52.4
  multilocular (ovary) D39.10
    benign —*see* Neoplasm, benign, by site
  myometrium N85.8
  nabothian (follicle) (ruptured) N88.8
  nasoalveolar K09.1
  nasolabial K09.1
  nasopalatine (anterior) (duct) K09.1
  nasopharynx J39.2
  neoplastic —*see* Neoplasm, uncertain
      behavior, by site
    benign —*see* Neoplasm, benign, by site
  nervous system NEC G96.8
  neuroenteric (congenital) Q06.8
  nipple —*see* Cyst, breast
  nose (turbinates) J34.1
    sinus J34.1
  odontogenic, developmental K09.0
  omentum (lesser) K66.8
    congenital Q45.8
  ora serrata —*see* Cyst, retina, ora serrata
  oral
    region K09.9
      developmental (nonodontogenic) K09.1
        specified NEC K09.8
    soft tissue K09.9
      specified NEC K09.8
  orbit H05.81-
  ovary, ovarian (twisted) N83.20
    adherent N83.20
    chocolate N80.1
    corpus
      albicans N83.29
      luteum (hemorrhagic) N83.1
    dermoid D27.9
    developmental Q50.1
    due to failure of involution NEC N83.20
    endometrial N80.1
    follicular (graafian) (hemorrhagic) N83.0
    hemorrhagic N83.20
    in pregnancy or childbirth O34.8-
      with obstructed labor O65.5
    multilocular D39.10
    pseudomucinous D27.9
    retention N83.29
    serous N83.20
    specified NEC N83.29
    theca lutein (hemorrhagic) N83.1
    tuberculous A18.18
  oviduct N83.8
  palate (median) (fissural) K09.1
  palatine papilla (jaw) K09.1
  pancreas, pancreatic (hemorrhagic) (true) K86.2
    congenital Q45.2
    false K86.3
  paralabral
    hip M24.85-
    shoulder S43.43-
  paramesonephric duct Q50.4
    female Q50.4
    male Q55.29
  paranephric N28.1
  paraphysis, cerebri, congenital Q04.6
  parasitic B89
  parathyroid (gland) E21.4
  paratubal N83.8
  paraurethral duct N36.8
  paroophoron Q50.5
  parotid gland K11.6
  parovarian Q50.5
  pelvis, female N94.89
    in pregnancy or childbirth O34.8-
      causing obstructed labor O65.5

Cyst *(Continued)*
  penis (sebaceous) N48.89
  periapical K04.8
  pericardial (congenital) Q24.8
    acquired (secondary) I31.8
  pericoronal K09.0
  periodontal K04.8
    lateral K09.0
  peripelvic (lymphatic) N28.1
  peritoneum K66.8
    chylous I89.8
  periventricular, acquired, newborn P91.1
  pharynx (wall) J39.2
  pilar L72.11
  pilonidal (infected) (rectum) L05.91
    with abscess L05.01
    malignant C44.59-
  pituitary (duct) (gland) E23.6
  placenta O43.19-
  pleura J94.8
  popliteal —*see* Cyst, Baker's
  porencephalic Q04.6
    acquired G93.0
  postanal (infected) —*see* Cyst, pilonidal
  postmastoidectomy cavity (mucosal) —*see*
      Complications, postmastoidectomy, cyst
  preauricular Q18.1
  prepuce N47.4
    congenital Q55.69
  primordial (jaw) K09.0
  prostate N42.83
  pseudomucinous (ovary) D27.9
  pupillary, miotic H21.27-
  radicular (residual) K04.8
  radiculodental K04.8
  ranular K11.8
  Rathke's pouch E23.6
  rectum (epithelium) (mucous) K62.89
  renal —*see* Cyst, kidney
  residual (radicular) K04.8
  retention (ovary) N83.29
    salivary gland K11.6
  retina H33.19-
    ora serrata H33.11-
    parasitic H33.12-
  retroperitoneal K68.9
  sacrococcygeal (dermoid) —*see* Cyst,
      pilonidal
  salivary gland or duct (mucous extravasation
      or retention) K11.6
  Sampson's N80.1
  sclera H15.89
  scrotum L72.9
    sebaceous L72.3
  sebaceous (duct) (gland) L72.3
    breast —*see* Dysplasia, mammary, specified
      type NEC
    eyelid —*see* Cyst, eyelid
    genital organ NEC
      female N94.89
      male N50.8
    scrotum L72.3
  semilunar cartilage (knee) (multiple) —*see*
      Derangement, knee, meniscus, cystic
  seminal vesicle N50.8
  serous (ovary) N83.20
  sinus (accessory) (nasal) J34.1
  Skene's gland N36.8
  skin L72.9
    breast —*see* Dysplasia, mammary, specified
      type NEC
    epidermal, epidermoid L72.0
    epithelial L72.0
    eyelid —*see* Cyst, eyelid
    genital organ NEC
      female N90.7
      male N50.8
    inclusion L72.0
    scrotum L72.9
    sebaceous L72.3
    sweat gland or duct L74.8

Cyst *(Continued)*
  solitary
    bone —*see* Cyst, bone, solitary
    jaw M27.40
    kidney N28.1
  spermatic cord N50.8
  sphenoid sinus J34.1
  spinal meninges G96.19
  spleen NEC D73.4
    congenital Q89.09
    hydatid (*see also* Echinococcus) B67.99
      [D77]
  Stafne's M27.0
  subarachnoid intrasellar R93.0
  subcutaneous, pheomycotic (chromomycotic)
    B43.2
  subdural (cerebral) G93.0
    spinal cord G96.19
  sublingual gland K11.6
  submandibular gland K11.6
  submaxillary gland K11.6
  suburethral N36.8
  suprarenal gland E27.8
  suprasellar —*see* Cyst, brain
  sweat gland or duct L74.8
  synovial —*see also* Cyst, bursa
    ruptured —*see* Rupture, synovium
  tarsal —*see* Chalazion
  tendon (sheath) —*see* Disorder, tendon,
    specified type NEC
  testis N44.2
    tunica albuginea N44.1
  theca lutein (ovary) N83.1
  Thornwaldt's J39.2
  thymus (gland) E32.8
  thyroglossal duct (infected) (persistent) Q89.2
  thyroid (gland) E04.1
  thyrolingual duct (infected) (persistent) Q89.2
  tongue K14.8
  tonsil J35.8
  tooth —*see* Cyst, dental
  Tornwaldt's J39.2
  trichilemmal (proliferating) L72.12
  trichodermal L72.12
  tubal (fallopian) N83.8
    inflammatory —*see* Salpingitis, chronic
  tubo-ovarian N83.8
    inflammatory N70.13
  tunica
    albuginea testis N44.1
    vaginalis N50.8
  turbinate (nose) J34.1
  Tyson's gland N48.89
  urachus, congenital Q64.4
  ureter N28.89
  ureterovesical orifice N28.89
  urethra, urethral (gland) N36.8
  uterine ligament N83.8
  uterus (body) (corpus) (recurrent) N85.8
    embryonic Q51.818
      cervix Q51.6
  vagina, vaginal (implantation) (inclusion)
    (squamous cell) (wall) N89.8
    embryonic Q52.4
  vallecula, vallecular (epiglottis) J38.7
  vesical (orifice) N32.89
  vitreous body H43.89
  vulva (implantation) (inclusion) N90.7
    congenital Q52.79
    sebaceous gland N90.7
  vulvovaginal gland N90.7
  wolffian
    female Q50.5
    male Q55.4
Cystadenocarcinoma —*see* Neoplasm,
  malignant, by site
  bile duct C22.1
  endometrioid —*see* Neoplasm, malignant,
    by site
    specified site —*see* Neoplasm, malignant,
      by site

Cystadenocarcinoma *(Continued)*
  endometrioid *(Continued)*
    unspecified site
      female C56.9
      male C61
  mucinous
    papillary
      specified site —*see* Neoplasm,
        malignant, by site
      unspecified site C56.9
    specified site —*see* Neoplasm, malignant,
      by site
    unspecified site C56.9
  papillary
    mucinous
      specified site —*see* Neoplasm,
        malignant, by site
      unspecified site C56.9
    pseudomucinous
      specified site —*see* Neoplasm,
        malignant, by site
      unspecified site C56.9
    serous
      specified site —*see* Neoplasm,
        malignant, by site
      unspecified site C56.9
    specified site —*see* Neoplasm, malignant,
      by site
    unspecified site C56.9
  pseudomucinous
    papillary
      specified site —*see* Neoplasm,
        malignant, by site
      unspecified site C56.9
    specified site —*see* Neoplasm, malignant,
      by site
    unspecified site C56.9
  serous
    papillary
      specified site —*see* Neoplasm,
        malignant, by site
      unspecified site C56.9
    specified site —*see* Neoplasm, malignant,
      by site
    unspecified site C56.9
Cystadenofibroma
  clear cell —*see* Neoplasm, benign, by site
  endometrioid D27.9
    borderline malignancy D39.1-
    malignant C56.-
  mucinous
    specified site —*see* Neoplasm, benign, by site
    unspecified site D27.9
  serous
    specified site —*see* Neoplasm, benign, by site
    unspecified site D27.9
  specified site —*see* Neoplasm, benign, by site
  unspecified site D27.9
Cystadenoma —*see also* Neoplasm, benign, by
  site
  bile duct D13.4
  endometrioid —*see* Neoplasm, benign, by site
    borderline malignancy —*see* Neoplasm,
      uncertain behavior, by site
  malignant —*see* Neoplasm, malignant,
    by site
  mucinous
    borderline malignancy
      ovary C56.-
      specified site NEC —*see* Neoplasm,
        uncertain behavior, by site
      unspecified site C56.9
    papillary
      borderline malignancy
        ovary C56.-
        specified site NEC —*see* Neoplasm,
          uncertain behavior, by site
        unspecified site C56.9
      specified site —*see* Neoplasm, benign,
        by site
      unspecified site D27.9

Cystadenoma *(Continued)*
  mucinous *(Continued)*
    specified site —*see* Neoplasm, benign, by
      site
    unspecified site D27.9
  papillary
    borderline malignancy
      ovary C56-
      specified site NEC —*see* Neoplasm,
        uncertain behavior, by site
      unspecified site C56.9
    lymphomatosum
      specified site —*see* Neoplasm, benign,
        by site
      unspecified site D11.9
    mucinous
      borderline malignancy
        ovary C56.-
        specified site NEC —*see* Neoplasm,
          uncertain behavior, by site
        unspecified site C56.9
      specified site —*see* Neoplasm, benign,
        by site
      unspecified site D27.9
    pseudomucinous
      borderline malignancy
        ovary C56.-
        specified site NEC —*see* Neoplasm,
          uncertain behavior, by site
        unspecified site C56.9
      specified site —*see* Neoplasm, benign,
        by site
      unspecified site D27.9
    serous
      borderline malignancy
        ovary C56.-
        specified site NEC —*see* Neoplasm,
          uncertain behavior, by site
        unspecified site C56.9
      specified site —*see* Neoplasm, benign,
        by site
      unspecified site D27.9
    specified site —*see* Neoplasm, benign, by
      site
    unspecified site D27.9
  pseudomucinous
    borderline malignancy
      ovary C56.-
      specified site NEC —*see* Neoplasm,
        uncertain behavior, by site
      unspecified site C56.9
    papillary
      borderline malignancy
        ovary C56.-
        specified site NEC —*see* Neoplasm,
          uncertain behavior, by site
        unspecified site C56.9
      specified site —*see* Neoplasm, benign,
        by site
      unspecified site D27.9
    specified site —*see* Neoplasm, benign, by
      site
    unspecified site D27.9
  serous
    borderline malignancy
      ovary C56.-
      specified site NEC —*see* Neoplasm,
        uncertain behavior, by site
      unspecified site C56.9
    papillary
      borderline malignancy
        ovary C56.-
        specified site NEC —*see* Neoplasm,
          uncertain behavior, by site
        unspecified site C56.9
      specified site —*see* Neoplasm, benign,
        by site
      unspecified site D27.9
    specified site —*see* Neoplasm, benign, by
      site
    unspecified site D27.9

◄ New   ◄▥ Revised   ~~deleted~~ Deleted

Cystathionine synthase deficiency E72.11
Cystathioninemia E72.19
Cystathioninuria E72.19
Cystic —see also condition
  breast (chronic) —see Mastopathy, cystic
  corpora lutea (hemorrhagic) N83.1
  duct —see condition
  eyeball (congenital) Q11.0
  fibrosis —see Fibrosis, cystic
  kidney (congenital) Q61.9
    adult type Q61.2
    infantile type NEC Q61.19
      collecting duct dilatation Q61.11
    medullary Q61.5
  liver, congenital Q44.6
  lung disease J98.4
    congenital Q33.0
  mastitis, chronic —see Mastopathy, cystic
  medullary, kidney Q61.5
  meniscus —see Derangement, knee,
    meniscus, cystic
  ovary N83.20
Cysticercosis, cysticerciasis B69.9
  with
    epileptiform fits B69.0
    myositis B69.81
  brain B69.0
  central nervous system B69.0
  cerebral B69.0
  ocular B69.1
  specified NEC B69.89
Cysticercus cellulose infestation —see
    Cysticercosis
Cystinosis (malignant) E72.04
Cystinuria E72.01
Cystitis (exudative) (hemorrhagic) (septic)
    (suppurative) N30.90
  with
    fibrosis —see Cystitis, chronic, interstitial
    hematuria N30.91
    leukoplakia —see Cystitis, chronic,
      interstitial
    malakoplakia —see Cystitis, chronic,
      interstitial
    metaplasia —see Cystitis, chronic,
      interstitial
    prostatitis N41.3
  acute N30.00
    with hematuria N30.01
    of trigone N30.30
      with hematuria N30.31
  allergic —see Cystitis, specified type NEC
  amebic A06.81
  bilharzial B65.9 [N33]

Cystitis (Continued)
  blennorrhagic (gonococcal) A54.01
  bullous —see Cystitis, specified type NEC
  calculous N21.0
  chlamydial A56.01
  chronic N30.20
    with hematuria N30.21
    interstitial N30.10
      with hematuria N30.11
    of trigone N30.30
      with hematuria N30.31
    specified NEC N30.20
      with hematuria N30.21
  cystic (a) —see Cystitis, specified type NEC
  diphtheritic A36.85
  echinococcal
    granulosus B67.39
    multilocularis B67.69
  emphysematous —see Cystitis, specified type
    NEC
  encysted —see Cystitis, specified type NEC
  eosinophilic —see Cystitis, specified type
    NEC
  follicular —see Cystitis, of trigone
  gangrenous —see Cystitis, specified type NEC
  glandularis —see Cystitis, specified type NEC
  gonococcal A54.01
  incrusted —see Cystitis, specified type NEC
  interstitial (chronic) —see Cystitis, chronic,
    interstitial
  irradiation N30.40
    with hematuria N30.41
  irritation —see Cystitis, specified type NEC
  malignant —see Cystitis, specified type NEC
  of trigone N30.30
    with hematuria N30.31
  panmural —see Cystitis, chronic, interstitial
  polyposa —see Cystitis, specified type NEC
  prostatic N41.3
  puerperal (postpartum) O86.22
  radiation —see Cystitis, irradiation
  specified type NEC N30.80
    with hematuria N30.81
  subacute —see Cystitis, chronic
  submucous —see Cystitis, chronic, interstitial
  syphilitic (late) A52.76
  trichomonal A59.03
  tuberculous A18.12
  ulcerative —see Cystitis, chronic, interstitial
Cystocele (-urethrocele)
  female N81.10
    with prolapse of uterus —see Prolapse,
      uterus
    lateral N81.12

Cystocele (Continued)
  female (Continued)
    midline N81.11
    paravaginal N81.12
  in pregnancy or childbirth O34.8-
    causing obstructed labor O65.5
  male N32.89
Cystolithiasis N21.0
Cystoma —see also Neoplasm, benign, by site
  endometrial, ovary N80.1
  mucinous
    specified site —see Neoplasm, benign, by
      site
    unspecified site D27.9
  serous
    specified site —see Neoplasm, benign, by
      site
    unspecified site D27.9
  simple (ovary) N83.29
Cystoplegia N31.2
Cystoptosis N32.89
Cystopyelitis —see Pyelonephritis
Cystorrhagia N32.89
Cystosarcoma phyllodes D48.6-
  benign D24-
  malignant —see Neoplasm, breast, malignant
Cystostomy
  attention to Z43.5
  complication —see Complications,
    cystostomy
  status Z93.50
    appendico-vesicostomy Z93.52
    cutaneous Z93.51
    specified NEC Z93.59
Cystourethritis —see Urethritis
Cystourethrocele —see also Cystocele
  female N81.10
    with uterine prolapse —see Prolapse,
      uterus
    lateral N81.12
    midline N81.11
    paravaginal N81.12
  male N32.89
Cytomegalic inclusion disease
  congenital P35.1
Cytomegalovirus infection B25.9
Cytomycosis (reticuloendothelial) B39.4
Cytopenia D75.9
  refractory
    with multilineage dysplasia D46.A
      and ring sideroblasts (RCMD RS) D46.B
Czerny's disease (periodic hydrarthrosis of the
    knee) —see Effusion, joint, knee

D

Daae (-Finsen) disease (epidemic pleurodynia) B33.0
Dabney's grip B33.0
Da Costa's syndrome F45.8
Dacryoadenitis, dacryadenitis H04.00-
　acute H04.01-
　chronic H04.02-
Dacryocystitis H04.30-
　acute H04.32-
　chronic H04.41-
　neonatal P39.1
　phlegmonous H04.31-
　syphilitic A52.71
　　congenital (early) A50.01
　trachomatous, active A71.1
　　sequelae (late effect) B94.0
Dacryocystoblenorrhea —see Inflammation, lacrimal, passages, chronic
Dacryocystocele —see Disorder, lacrimal system, changes
Dacryolith, dacryolithiasis H04.51-
Dacryoma —see Disorder, lacrimal system, changes
Dacryopericystitis —see Dacryocystitis
Dacryops H04.11-
Dacryostenosis —see also Stenosis, lacrimal
　congenital Q10.5
Dactylitis
　bone —see Osteomyelitis
　sickle-cell D57.00
　　Hb C D57.219
　　Hb SS D57.00
　　specified NEC D57.819
　skin L08.9
　syphilitic A52.77
　tuberculous A18.03
Dactylolysis spontanea (ainhum) L94.6
Dactylosymphysis Q70.9
　fingers —see Syndactylism, complex, fingers
　toes —see Syndactylism, complex, toes
Damage
　arteriosclerotic —see Arteriosclerosis
　brain (nontraumatic) G93.9
　　anoxic, hypoxic G93.1
　　　resulting from a procedure G97.82
　　child NEC G80.9
　　due to birth injury P11.2
　cardiorenal (vascular) —see Hypertension, cardiorenal
　cerebral NEC —see Damage, brain
　coccyx, complicating delivery O71.6
　coronary —see Disease, heart, ischemic
　eye, birth injury P15.3
　liver (nontraumatic) K76.9
　　alcoholic K70.9
　　due to drugs —see Disease, liver, toxic
　　toxic —see Disease, liver, toxic
　medication T88.7
　pelvic
　　joint or ligament, during delivery O71.6
　　organ NEC
　　　during delivery O71.5
　　　following ectopic or molar pregnancy O08.6
　renal —see Disease, renal
　subendocardium, subendocardial —see Degeneration, myocardial
　vascular I99.9
Dana-Putnam syndrome (subacute combined sclerosis with pernicious anemia) —see Degeneration, combined
Danbolt (-Cross) syndrome (acrodermatitis enteropathica) E83.2
Dandruff L21.0
Dandy-Walker syndrome Q03.1
　with spina bifida —see Spina bifida
Danlos' syndrome Q79.6

Darier (-White) disease (congenital) Q82.8
　meaning erythema annulare centrifugum L53.1
Darier-Roussy sarcoid D86.3
Darling's disease or histoplasmosis B39.4
Darwin's tubercle Q17.8
Dawson's (inclusion body) encephalitis A81.1
De Beurmann (-Gougerot) disease B42.1
De la Tourette's syndrome F95.2
De Lange's syndrome Q87.1
De Morgan's spots (senile angiomas) I78.1
De Quervain's
　disease (tendon sheath) M65.4
　syndrome E34.51
　thyroiditis (subacute granulomatous thyroiditis) E06.1
De Toni-Fanconi (-Debré) syndrome E72.09
　with cystinosis E72.04
Dead
　fetus, retained (mother) O36.4
　　early pregnancy O02.1
　labyrinth —see subcategory H83.2
　ovum, retained O02.0
Deaf nonspeaking NEC H91.3
Deafmutism (acquired) (congenital) NEC H91.3
　hysterical F44.6
　syphilitic, congenital (see also subcategory H94.8) A50.09
Deafness (acquired) (complete) (hereditary) (partial) H91.9-
　with blue sclera and fragility of bone Q78.0
　auditory fatigue —see Deafness, specified type NEC
　aviation T70.0
　　nerve injury —see Injury, nerve, acoustic, specified type NEC
　boilermaker's —see subcategory H83.3
　central —see Deafness, sensorineural
　conductive H90.2
　　and sensorineural, mixed H90.8
　　　bilateral H90.6
　　bilateral H90.0
　　unilateral H90.1-
　congenital H90.5
　　with blue sclera and fragility of bone Q78.0
　due to toxic agents —see Deafness, ototoxic
　emotional (hysterical) F44.6
　functional (hysterical) F44.6
　high frequency H91.9-
　hysterical F44.6
　low frequency H91.9-
　mental R48.8
　mixed conductive and sensorineural H90.8
　　bilateral H90.6
　　unilateral H90.7-
　nerve —see Deafness, sensorineural
　neural —see Deafness, sensorineural
　noise-induced —see also subcategory H83.3
　　nerve injury —see Injury, nerve, acoustic, specified type NEC
　nonspeaking H91.3
　ototoxic —see subcategory H91.0
　perceptive —see Deafness, sensorineural
　psychogenic (hysterical) F44.6
　sensorineural H90.5
　　and conductive, mixed H90.8
　　　bilateral H90.6
　　bilateral H90.3
　　unilateral H90.4-
　sensory —see Deafness, sensorineural
　specified type NEC —see subcategory H91.8
　sudden (idiopathic) H91.2-
　syphilitic A52.15
　transient ischemic H93.01-
　traumatic —see Injury, nerve, acoustic, specified type NEC
　word (developmental) H93.25

Death (cause unknown) (of) (unexplained) (unspecified cause) R99
　brain G93.82
　cardiac (sudden) (with successful resuscitation) — code to underlying disease
　　family history of Z82.41
　　personal history of Z86.74
　family member (assumed) Z63.4
Debility (chronic) (general) (nervous) R53.81
　congenital or neonatal NOS P96.9
　nervous R53.81
　old age R54
　senile R54
Débove's disease (splenomegaly) R16.1
Decalcification
　bone —see Osteoporosis
　teeth K03.89
Decapsulation, kidney N28.89
Decay
　dental —see Caries, dental
　senile R54
　tooth, teeth —see Caries, dental
Deciduitis (acute)
　following ectopic or molar pregnancy O08.0
Decline (general) —see Debility
　cognitive, age-associated R41.81
Decompensation
　cardiac (acute) (chronic) —see Disease, heart
　cardiovascular —see Disease, cardiovascular
　heart —see Disease, heart
　hepatic —see Failure, hepatic
　myocardial (acute) (chronic) —see Disease, heart
　respiratory J98.8
Decompression sickness T70.3
Decrease (d)
　absolute neutrophile count —see Neutropenia
　blood
　　platelets —see Thrombocytopenia
　　pressure R03.1
　　　due to shock following injury T79.4
　　　operation T81.19
　estrogen E28.39
　　postablative E89.40
　　　asymptomatic E89.40
　　　symptomatic E89.41
　fragility of erythrocytes D58.8
　function
　　lipase (pancreatic) K90.3
　　ovary in hypopituitarism E23.0
　　parenchyma of pancreas K86.8
　　pituitary (gland) (anterior) (lobe) E23.0
　　　posterior (lobe) E23.0
　functional activity R68.89
　glucose R73.09
　hematocrit R71.0
　hemoglobin R71.0
　leukocytes D72.819
　　specified NEC D72.818
　libido R68.82
　lymphocytes D72.810
　platelets D69.6
　respiration, due to shock following injury T79.4
　sexual desire R68.82
　tear secretion NEC —see Syndrome, dry eye
　tolerance
　　fat K90.4
　　glucose R73.09
　　pancreatic K90.3
　　salt and water E87.8
　vision NEC H54.7
　white blood cell count D72.819
　　specified NEC D72.818
Decubitus (ulcer) —see Ulcer, pressure, by site
　cervix N86
Deepening acetabulum —see Derangement, joint, specified type NEC, hip

◀ New　◀▥ Revised　deleted Deleted

Defect, defective Q89.9
  3-beta-hydroxysteroid dehydrogenase E25.0
  11-hydroxylase E25.0
  21-hydroxylase E25.0
  abdominal wall, congenital Q79.59
  antibody immunodeficiency D80.9
  aorticopulmonary septum Q21.4
  atrial septal (ostium secundum type) Q21.1
    following acute myocardial infarction
      (current complication) I23.1
    ostium primum type Q21.2
  atrioventricular
    canal Q21.2
    septum Q21.2
  auricular septal Q21.1
  bilirubin excretion NEC E80.6
  biosynthesis, androgen (testicular) E29.1
  bulbar septum Q21.0
  catalase E80.3
  cell membrane receptor complex (CR3) D71
  circulation I99.9
    congenital Q28.9
    newborn Q28.9
  coagulation (factor) (see also Deficiency,
    factor) D68.9
    with
      ectopic pregnancy O08.1
      molar pregnancy O08.1
    acquired D68.4
    antepartum with hemorrhage —see
      Hemorrhage, antepartum, with
      coagulation defect
    due to
      liver disease D68.4
      vitamin K deficiency D68.4
    hereditary NEC D68.2
    intrapartum O67.0
    newborn, transient P61.6
    postpartum O72.3
    specified type NEC D68.8
  complement system D84.1
  conduction (heart) I45.9
    bone —see Deafness, conductive
  congenital, organ or site not listed —see
    Anomaly, by site
  coronary sinus Q21.1
  cushion, endocardial Q21.2
  degradation, glycoprotein E77.1
  dental bridge, crown, fillings —see Defect,
    dental restoration
  dental restoration K08.50
    specified NEC K08.59
  dentin (hereditary) K00.5
  Descemet's membrane, congenital Q13.89
  developmental —see also Anomaly
    cauda equina Q06.3
  diaphragm
    with elevation, eventration or hernia —see
      Hernia, diaphragm
    congenital Q79.1
      with hernia Q79.0
      gross (with hernia) Q79.0
  ectodermal, congenital Q82.9
  Eisenmenger's Q21.8
  enzyme
    catalase E80.3
    peroxidase E80.3
  esophagus, congenital Q39.9
  extensor retinaculum M62.89
  fibrin polymerization D68.2
  filling
    bladder R93.4
    kidney R93.4
    stomach R93.3
    ureter R93.4
  Gerbode Q21.0
  glycoprotein degradation E77.1
  Hageman (factor) D68.2
  hearing —see Deafness
  high grade F70
  interatrial septal Q21.1

Defect, defective (Continued)
  interauricular septal Q21.1
  interventricular septal Q21.0
    with dextroposition of aorta, pulmonary
      stenosis and hypertrophy of right
      ventricle Q21.3
    in tetralogy of Fallot Q21.3
  learning (specific) —see Disorder, learning
  lymphocyte function antigen-1 (LFA-1) D84.0
  lysosomal enzyme, post-translational
    modification E77.0
  major osseous M89.70
    ankle M89.77-
    carpus M89.74-
    clavicle M89.71-
    femur M89.75-
    fibula M89.76-
    fingers M89.74-
    foot M89.77-
    forearm M89.73-
    hand M89.74-
    humerus M89.72-
    lower leg M89.76-
    metacarpus M89.74-
    metatarsus M89.77-
    multiple sites M89.79
    pelvic region M89.75-
    pelvis M89.75-
    radius M89.73-
    scapula M89.71-
    shoulder region M89.71-
    specified NEC M89.78
    tarsus M89.77-
    thigh M89.75-
    tibia M89.76-
    toes M89.77-
    ulna M89.73-
  mental —see Disability, intellectual
  modification, lysosomal enzymes, post-
    translational E77.0
  obstructive, congenital
    renal pelvis Q62.39
    ureter Q62.39
      atresia —see Atresia, ureter
      cecoureterocele Q62.32
      megaureter Q62.2
      orthotopic ureterocele Q62.31
  osseous, major M89.70
    ankle M89.77-
    carpus M89.74-
    clavicle M89.71-
    femur M89.75-
    fibula M89.76-
    fingers M89.74-
    foot M89.77-
    forearm M89.73-
    hand M89.74-
    humerus M89.72-
    lower leg M89.76-
    metacarpus M89.74-
    metatarsus M89.77-
    multiple sites M89.9
    pelvic region M89.75-
    pelvis M89.75-
    radius M89.73-
    scapula M89.71-
    shoulder region M89.71-
    specified NEC M89.78
    tarsus M89.77-
    thigh M89.75-
    tibia M89.76-
    toes M89.77-
    ulna M89.73-
  osteochondral NEC (see also Deformity)
    M95.8-
  ostium
    primum Q21.2
    secundum Q21.1
  peroxidase E80.3
  placental blood supply —see Insufficiency,
    placental

Defect, defective (Continued)
  platelets, qualitative D69.1
    constitutional D68.0
  postural NEC, spine —see Dorsopathy,
    deforming
  reduction
    limb Q73.8
      lower Q72.9-
        absence —see Agenesis, leg
        foot —see Agenesis, foot
        longitudinal
          femur Q72.4-
          fibula Q72.6-
          tibia Q72.5-
        specified type NEC Q72.89-
        split foot Q72.7-
      specified type NEC Q73.8
      upper Q71.9-
        absence —see Agenesis, arm
        forearm —see Agenesis, forearm
        hand —see Agenesis, hand
        lobster-claw hand Q71.6-
        longitudinal
          radius Q71.4-
          ulna Q71.5-
        specified type NEC Q71.89-
  renal pelvis Q63.8
    obstructive Q62.39
  respiratory system, congenital Q34.9
  restoration, dental K08.50
    specified NEC K08.59
  retinal nerve bundle fibers H35.89
  septal (heart) NOS Q21.9
    acquired (atrial) (auricular) (ventricular)
      (old) I51.0
    atrial Q21.1
      concurrent with acute myocardial
        infarction —see Infarct,
        myocardium
      following acute myocardial infarction
        (current complication) I23.1
    ventricular (see also Defect, ventricular
      septal) Q21.0
  sinus venosus Q21.1
  speech R47.9
    developmental F80.9
    specified NEC R47.89
  Taussig-Bing (aortic transposition and
    overriding pulmonary artery) Q20.1
  teeth, wedge K03.1
  vascular (local) I99.9
    congenital Q27.9
  ventricular septal Q21.0
    concurrent with acute myocardial
      infarction —see Infarct, myocardium
    following acute myocardial infarction
      (current complication) I23.2
    in tetralogy of Fallot Q21.3
  vision NEC H54.7
  visual field H53.40
    bilateral
      heteronymous H53.47
      homonymous H53.46-
    generalized contraction H53.48-
    localized
      arcuate H53.43-
      scotoma (central area) H53.41-
        blind spot area H53.42-
      sector H53.43-
      specified type NEC H53.45-
  voice R49.9
    specified NEC R49.8
  wedge, tooth, teeth (abrasion) K03.1
Deferentitis N49.1
  gonorrheal (acute) (chronic) A54.23
Defibrination (syndrome) D65
  antepartum —see Hemorrhage, antepartum,
    with coagulation defect, disseminated
    intravascular coagulation
  following ectopic or molar pregnancy O08.1
  intrapartum O67.0

Defibrination (Continued)
  newborn P60
  postpartum O72.3
Deficiency, deficient
  3-beta hydroxysteroid dehydrogenase E25.0
  11-hydroxylase E25.0
  21-hydroxylase E25.0
  5-alpha reductase (with male
      pseudohermaphroditism) E29.1
  abdominal muscle syndrome Q79.4
  AC globulin (congenital) (hereditary) D68.2
    acquired D68.4
  accelerator globulin (Ac G) (blood) D68.2
  acid phosphatase E83.39
  activating factor (blood) D68.2
  adenosine deaminase (ADA) D81.3
  aldolase (hereditary) E74.19
  alpha-1-antitrypsin E88.01
  amino-acids E72.9
  anemia —see Anemia
  aneurin E51.9
  antibody with
    hyperimmunoglobulinemia D80.6
    near-normal immunoglobins D80.6
  antidiuretic hormone E23.2
  anti-hemophilic
    factor (A) D66
      B D67
      C D68.1
    globulin (AHG) NEC D66
  antithrombin (antithrombin III) D68.59
  ascorbic acid E54
  attention (disorder) (syndrome) F98.8
    with hyperactivity —see Disorder,
        attention-deficit hyperactivity
  autoprothrombin
    I D68.2
    II D67
    C D68.2
  beta-glucuronidase E76.29
  biotin E53.8
  biotin-dependent carboxylase D81.819
  biotinidase D81.810
  brancher enzyme (amylopectinosis) E74.03
  C1 esterase inhibitor (C1-INH) D84.1
  calciferol E55.9
    with
      adult osteomalacia M83.8
      rickets —see Rickets
  calcium (dietary) E58
  calorie, severe E43
    with marasmus E41
      and kwashiorkor E42
  cardiac —see Insufficiency, myocardial
  carnitine E71.40
    due to
      hemodialysis E71.43
      inborn errors of metabolism E71.42
      Valproic acid therapy E71.43
    iatrogenic E71.43
    muscle palmityltransferase E71.314
    primary E71.41
    secondary E71.448
  carotene E50.9
  central nervous system G96.8
  ceruloplasmin (Wilson) E83.01
  choline E53.8
  Christmas factor D67
  chromium E61.4
  clotting (blood) (see also Deficiency,
      coagulation factor) D68.9
  clotting factor NEC (hereditary) (see also
      Deficiency, factor) D68.2
  coagulation NOS D68.9
    with
      ectopic pregnancy O08.1
      molar pregnancy O08.1
    acquired (any) D68.4
    antepartum hemorrhage —see
        Hemorrhage, antepartum, with
        coagulation defect

Deficiency, deficient (Continued)
  coagulation NOS (Continued)
    clotting factor NEC (see also Deficiency,
        factor) D68.2
    due to
      hyperprothrombinemia D68.4
      liver disease D68.4
      vitamin K deficiency D68.4
    newborn, transient P61.6
    postpartum O72.3
    specified NEC D68.8
  cognitive F09
  color vision H53.50
    achromatopsia H53.51
    acquired H53.52
    deuteranomaly H53.53
    protanomaly H53.54
    specified type NEC H53.59
    tritanomaly H53.55
  combined glucocorticoid and
      mineralocorticoid E27.49
  contact factor D68.2
  copper (nutritional) E61.0
  corticoadrenal E27.40
    primary E27.1
  craniofacial axis Q75.0
  cyanocobalamin E53.8
  debrancher enzyme (limit dextrinosis) E74.03
  dehydrogenase
    long chain/very long chain acyl CoA
        E71.310
    medium chain acyl CoA E71.311
    short chain acyl CoA E71.312
  diet E63.9
  dihydropyrimidine dehydrogenase (DPD)
      E88.89
  disaccharidase E73.9
  edema —see Malnutrition, severe
  endocrine E34.9
  energy-supply —see Malnutrition
  enzymes, circulating NEC E88.09
  ergosterol E55.9
    with
      adult osteomalacia M83.8
      rickets —see Rickets
  essential fatty acid (EFA) E63.0
  factor —see also Deficiency, coagulation
    Hageman D68.2
    I (congenital) (hereditary) D68.2
    II (congenital) (hereditary) D68.2
    IX (congenital) (functional) (hereditary)
        (with functional defect) D67
    multiple (congenital) D68.8
      acquired D68.4
    V (congenital) (hereditary) D68.2
    VII (congenital) (hereditary) D68.2
    VIII (congenital) (functional) (hereditary)
        (with functional defect) D66
      with vascular defect D68.0
    X (congenital) (hereditary) D68.2
    XI (congenital) (hereditary) D68.1
    XII (congenital) (hereditary) D68.2
    XIII (congenital) (hereditary) D68.2
  femoral, proximal focal (congenital) —
      see Defect, reduction, lower limb,
      longitudinal, femur
  fibrin-stabilizing factor (congenital)
      (hereditary) D68.2
    acquired D68.4
  fibrinase D68.2
  fibrinogen (congenital) (hereditary) D68.2
    acquired D65
  folate E53.8
  folic acid E53.8
  foreskin N47.3
  fructokinase E74.11
  fructose 1,6-diphosphatase E74.19
  fructose-1-phosphate aldolase E74.19
  galactokinase E74.29
  galactose-1-phosphate uridyl transferase
      E74.29

Deficiency, deficient (Continued)
  gammaglobulin in blood D80.1
    hereditary D80.0
  glass factor D68.2
  glucocorticoid E27.49
    mineralocorticoid E27.49
  glucose-6-phosphatase E74.01
  glucose-6-phosphate dehydrogenase anemia
      D55.0
  glucuronyl transferase E80.5
  glycogen synthetase E74.09
  gonadotropin (isolated) E23.0
  growth hormone (idiopathic) (isolated) E23.0
  Hageman factor D68.2
  hemoglobin D64.9
  hepatophosphorylase E74.09
  homogentisate 1,2-dioxygenase E70.29
  hormone
    anterior pituitary (partial) NEC E23.0
      growth E23.0
    growth (isolated) E23.0
    pituitary E23.0
    testicular E29.1
  hypoxanthine-(guanine)-
      phosphoribosyltransferase (HG-PRT)
      (total HG-PRT) E79.1
  immunity D84.9
    cell-mediated D84.8
      with thrombocytopenia and eczema
          D82.0
    combined D81.9
    humoral D80.9
    IgA (secretory) D80.2
    IgG D80.3
    IgM D80.4
  immuno —see Immunodeficiency
  immunoglobulin, selective
    A (IgA) D80.2
    G (IgG) (subclasses) D80.3
    M (IgM) D80.4
  inositol (B complex) E53.8
  intrinsic
    factor (congenital) D51.0
    sphincter N36.42
      with urethral hypermobility N36.43
  iodine E61.8
    congenital syndrome —see Syndrome,
        iodine-deficiency, congenital
  iron E61.1
    anemia D50.9
  kalium E87.6
  kappa-light chain D80.8
  labile factor (congenital) (hereditary) D68.2
    acquired D68.4
  lacrimal fluid (acquired) —see also Syndrome,
      dry eye
    congenital Q10.6
  lactase
    congenital E73.0
    secondary E73.1
  Laki-Lorand factor D68.2
  lecithin cholesterol acyltransferase E78.6
  lipocaic K86.8
  lipoprotein (familial) (high density) E78.6
  liver phosphorylase E74.09
  lysosomal alpha-1, 4 glucosidase E74.02
  magnesium E61.2
  major histocompatibility complex
    class I D81.6
    class II D81.7
  manganese E61.3
  menadione (vitamin K) E56.1
    newborn P53
  mental (familial) (hereditary) —see Disability,
      intellectual
  methylenetetrahydrofolate reductase
      (MTHFR) E72.12
  mineral NEC E61.8
  mineralocorticoid E27.49
    with glucocorticoid E27.49
  molybdenum (nutritional) E61.5

◄ New   ◄▦ Revised   deleted Deleted

Deficiency, deficient *(Continued)*
  moral F60.2
  multiple nutrient elements E61.7
  muscle
    carnitine (palmityltransferase) E71.314
    phosphofructokinase E74.09
  myoadenylate deaminase E79.2
  myocardial —*see* Insufficiency, myocardial
  myophosphorylase E74.04
  NADH diaphorase or reductase (congenital) D74.0
  NADH-methemoglobin reductase (congenital) D74.0
  natrium E87.1
  niacin (amide) (-tryptophan) E52
  nicotinamide E52
  nicotinic acid E52
  number of teeth —*see* Anodontia
  nutrient element E61.9
    multiple E61.7
    specified NEC E61.8
  nutrition, nutritional E63.9
    sequelae —*see* Sequelae, nutritional deficiency
    specified NEC E63.8
  ornithine transcarbamylase E72.4
  ovarian E28.39
  oxygen —*see* Anoxia
  pantothenic acid E53.8
  parathyroid (gland) E20.9
  perineum (female) N81.89
  phenylalanine hydroxylase E70.1
  phosphoenolpyruvate carboxykinase E74.4
  phosphofructokinase E74.19
  phosphomannomutuse E74.8
  phosphomannose isomerase E74.8
  phosphomannosyl mutase E74.8
  phosphorylase kinase, liver E74.09
  pituitary hormone (isolated) E23.0
  plasma thromboplastin
    antecedent (PTA) D68.1
    component (PTC) D67
  platelet NEC D69.1
    constitutional D68.0
  polyglandular E31.8
    autoimmune E31.0
  potassium (K) E87.6
  prepuce N47.3
  proaccelerin (congenital) (hereditary) D68.2
    acquired D68.4
  proconvertin factor (congenital) (hereditary) D68.2
    acquired D68.4
  protein *(see also* Malnutrition) E46
    anemia D53.0
    C D68.59
    S D68.59
  prothrombin (congenital) (heredItary) D68.2
    acquired D68.4
  Prower factor D68.2
  pseudocholinesterase E88.09
  PTA (plasma thromboplastin antecedent) D68.1
  PTC (plasma thromboplastin component) D67
  purine nucleoside phosphorylase (PNP) D81.5
  pyracin (alpha) (beta) E53.1
  pyridoxal E53.1
  pyridoxamine E53.1
  pyridoxine (derivatives) E53.1
  pyruvate
    carboxylase E74.4
    dehydrogenase E74.4
  riboflavin (vitamin B2) E53.0
  salt E87.1
  secretion
    ovary E28.39
    salivary gland (any) K11.7
    urine R34
  selenium (dietary) E59
  serum antitrypsin, familial E88.01

Deficiency, deficient *(Continued)*
  short stature homeobox gene (SHOX)
    with
      dyschondrosteosis Q78.8
      short stature (idiopathic) E34.3
      Turner's syndrome Q96.9
  sodium (Na) E87.1
  SPCA (factor VII) D68.2
  sphincter, intrinsic N36.42
    with urethral hypermobility N36.43
  stable factor (congenital) (hereditary) D68.2
    acquired D68.4
  Stuart-Prower (factor X) D68.2
  sucrase E74.39
  sulfatase E75.29
  sulfite oxidase E72.19
  thiamin, thiaminic (chloride) E51.9
    beriberi (dry) E51.11
      wet E51.12
  thrombokinase D68.2
    newborn P53
  thyroid (gland) —*see* Hypothyroidism
  tocopherol E56.0
  tooth bud K00.0
  transcobalamine II (anemia) D51.2
  vanadium E61.6
  vascular I99.9
  vasopressin E23.2
  viosterol —*see* Deficiency, calciferol
  vitamin (multiple) NOS E56.9
    A E50.9
      with
        Bitot's spot (corneal) E50.1
        follicular keratosis E50.8
        keratomalacia E50.4
        manifestations NEC E50.8
        night blindness E50.5
        scar of cornea, xerophthalmic E50.6
        xeroderma E50.8
        xerophthalmia E50.7
        xerosis
          conjunctival E50.0
            and Bitot's spot E50.1
          cornea E50.2
            and ulceration E50.3
      sequelae E64.1
    B (complex) NOS E53.9
      with
        beriberi (dry) E51.11
          wet E51.12
        pellagra E52
    B1 NOS E51.9
      beriberi (dry) E51.11
        with circulatory system manifestations E51.11
        wet E51.12
    B12 E53.8 —
    B2 (riboflavin) E53.0
    B6 E53.1
    C E54
      sequelae E64.2
    D E55.9
      with
        adult osteomalacia M83.8
        rickets —*see* Rickets
      25-hydroxylase E83.32
    E E56.0
    folic acid E53.8
    G E53.0
    group B E53.9
      specified NEC E53.8
    H (biotin) E53.8
    K E56.1
      of newborn P53
    nicotinic E52
    P E56.8
    PP (pellagra-preventing) E52
    specified NEC E56.8
    thiamin E51.9
      beriberi —*see* Beriberi
  zinc, dietary E60

Deficit —*see also* Deficiency
  attention and concentration R41.840
    disorder —*see* Attention, deficit
  cognitive communication R41.841
  cognitive NEC R41.89
    following
      cerebral infarction I69.31
      cerebrovascular disease I69.91
        specified disease NEC I69.81
      intracerebral hemorrhage I69.11
      nontraumatic intracranial hemorrhage NEC I69.21
      subarachnoid hemorrhage I69.01
  concentration R41.840
  executive function R41.844
  frontal lobe R41.844
  neurologic NEC R29.818
    ischemic
      reversible (RIND) I63.9
        prolonged (PRIND) I63.9
  oxygen R09.02
  prolonged reversible ischemic neurologic (PRIND) I63.9
  psychomotor R41.843
  visuospatial R41.842
Deflection
  radius —*see* Deformity, limb, specified type NEC, forearm
  septum (acquired) (nasal) (nose) J34.2
  spine —*see* Curvature, spine
  turbinate (nose) J34.2
Defluvium
  capillorum —*see* Alopecia
  ciliorum —*see* Madarosis
  unguium L60.8
Deformity Q89.9
  abdomen, congenital Q89.9
  abdominal wall
    acquired M95.8
    congenital Q79.59
  acquired (unspecified site) M95.9
  adrenal gland Q89.1
  alimentary tract, congenital Q45.9
    upper Q40.9
  ankle (joint) (acquired) —*see also* Deformity, limb, lower leg
    abduction —*see* Contraction, joint, ankle
    congenital Q68.8
    contraction —*see* Contraction, joint, ankle
    specified type NEC —*see* Deformity, limb, foot, specified NEC
  anus (acquired) K62.89
    congenital Q43.9
  aorta (arch) (congenital) Q25.4
    acquired I77.89
  aortic
    arch, acquired I77.89
    cusp or valve (congenital) Q23.8
      acquired *(see also* Endocarditis, aortic) I35.8
  arm (acquired) (upper) —*see also* Deformity, limb, upper arm
    congenital Q68.8
    forearm —*see* Deformity, limb, forearm
  artery (congenital) (peripheral) NOS Q27.9
    acquired I77.89
    coronary (acquired) I25.9
      congenital Q24.5
    umbilical Q27.0
  atrial septal Q21.1
  auditory canal (external) (congenital) —*see also* Malformation, ear, external
    acquired —*see* Disorder, ear, external, specified type NEC
  auricle
    ear (congenital) —*see also* Malformation, ear, external
      acquired —*see* Disorder, pinna, deformity
  back —*see* Dorsopathy, deforming

Deformity *(Continued)*
  bile duct (common) (congenital) (hepatic)
      Q44.5
    acquired K83.8
  biliary duct or passage (congenital) Q44.5
    acquired K83.8
  bladder (neck) (trigone) (sphincter)
      (acquired) N32.89
    congenital Q64.79
  bone (acquired) NOS M95.9
    congenital Q79.9
    turbinate M95.0
  brain (congenital) Q04.9
    acquired G93.89
    reduction Q04.3
  breast (acquired) N64.89
    congenital Q83.9
    reconstructed N65.0
  bronchus (congenital) Q32.4
    acquired NEC J98.09
  bursa, congenital Q79.9
  canaliculi (lacrimalis) (acquired) —*see also*
      Disorder, lacrimal system, changes
    congenital Q10.6
  canthus, acquired —*see* Disorder, eyelid,
      specified type NEC
  capillary (acquired) I78.8
  cardiovascular system, congenital Q28.9
  caruncle, lacrimal (acquired) —*see also*
      Disorder, lacrimal system, changes
    congenital Q10.6
  cascade, stomach K31.2
  cecum (congenital) Q43.9
    acquired K63.89
  cerebral, acquired G93.89
    congenital Q04.9
  cervix (uterus) (acquired) NEC N88.8
    congenital Q51.9
  cheek (acquired) M95.2
    congenital Q18.9
  chest (acquired) (wall) M95.4
    congenital Q67.8
    sequelae (late effect) of rickets E64.3
  chin (acquired) M95.2
    congenital Q18.9
  choroid (congenital) Q14.3
    acquired H31.8
    plexus Q07.8
      acquired G96.19
  cicatricial —*see* Cicatrix
  cilia, acquired —*see* Disorder, eyelid,
      specified type NEC
  clavicle (acquired) M95.8
    congenital Q68.8
  clitoris (congenital) Q52.6
    acquired N90.89
  clubfoot —*see* Clubfoot
  coccyx (acquired) —*see* subcategory M43.8
  colon (congenital) Q43.9
    acquired K63.89
  concha (ear), congenital —*see also*
      Malformation, ear, external
    acquired —*see* Disorder, pinna, deformity
  cornea (acquired) H18.70
    congenital Q13.4
    descemetocele —*see* Descemetocele
    ectasia —*see* Ectasia, cornea
    specified NEC H18.79-
    staphyloma —*see* Staphyloma, cornea
  coronary artery (acquired) I25.9
    congenital Q24.5
  cranium (acquired) —*see* Deformity, skull
  cricoid cartilage (congenital) Q31.8
    acquired J38.7
  cystic duct (congenital) Q44.5
    acquired K82.8
  Dandy-Walker Q03.1
    with spina bifida —*see* Spina bifida
  diaphragm (congenital) Q79.1
    acquired J98.6
  digestive organ NOS Q45.9

Deformity *(Continued)*
  ductus arteriosus Q25.0
  duodenal bulb K31.89
  duodenum (congenital) Q43.9
    acquired K31.89
  dura —*see* Deformity, meninges
  ear (acquired) —*see also* Disorder, pinna,
      deformity
    congenital (external) Q17.9
      internal Q16.5
      middle Q16.4
        ossicles Q16.3
      ossicles Q16.3
  ectodermal (congenital) NEC Q84.9
  ejaculatory duct (congenital) Q55.4
    acquired N50.8
  elbow (joint) (acquired) —*see also* Deformity,
      limb, upper arm
    congenital Q68.8
    contraction —*see* Contraction, joint, elbow
  endocrine gland NEC Q89.2
  epididymis (congenital) Q55.4
    acquired N50.8
  epiglottis (congenital) Q31.8
    acquired J38.7
  esophagus (congenital) Q39.9
    acquired K22.8
  eustachian tube (congenital) NEC Q17.8
  eye, congenital Q15.9
  eyebrow (congenital) Q18.8
  eyelid (acquired) —*see also* Disorder, eyelid,
      specified type NEC
    congenital Q10.3
  face (acquired) M95.2
    congenital Q18.9
  fallopian tube, acquired N83.8
  femur (acquired) —*see* Deformity, limb,
      specified type NEC, thigh
  fetal
    with fetopelvic disproportion O33.7
    causing obstructed labor O66.3
  finger (acquired) M20.00-
    boutonniere M20.02-
    congenital Q68.1
    flexion contracture —*see* Contraction, joint,
        hand
    mallet finger M20.01-
    specified NEC M20.09-
    swan-neck M20.03-
  flexion (joint) (acquired) (*see also* Deformity,
      limb, flexion) M21.20
    congenital NOS Q74.9
      hip Q65.89
  foot (acquired) —*see also* Deformity, limb,
      lower leg
    cavovarus (congenital) Q66.1
    congenital NOS Q66.9
      specified type NEC Q66.89
    specified type NEC —*see* Deformity, limb,
        foot, specified NEC
    valgus (congenital) Q66.6
      acquired —*see* Deformity, valgus, ankle
    varus (congenital) NEC Q66.3
      acquired —*see* Deformity, varus, ankle
  forearm (acquired) —*see also* Deformity, limb,
      forearm
    congenital Q68.8
  forehead (acquired) M95.2
    congenital Q75.8
  frontal bone (acquired) M95.2
    congenital Q75.8
  gallbladder (congenital) Q44.1
    acquired K82.8
  gastrointestinal tract (congenital) NOS Q45.9
    acquired K63.89
  genitalia, genital organ (s) or system NEC
    female (congenital) Q52.9
      acquired N94.89
      external Q52.70
    male (congenital) Q55.9
      acquired N50.8

Deformity *(Continued)*
  globe (eye) (congenital) Q15.8
    acquired H44.89
  gum, acquired NEC K06.8
  hand (acquired) —*see* Deformity, limb, hand
    congenital Q68.1
  head (acquired) M95.2
    congenital Q75.8
  heart (congenital) Q24.9
    septum Q21.9
      auricular Q21.1
      ventricular Q21.0
    valve (congenital) NEC Q24.8
      acquired —*see* Endocarditis
  heel (acquired) —*see* Deformity, foot
  hepatic duct (congenital) Q44.5
    acquired K83.8
  hip (joint) (acquired) —*see also* Deformity,
      limb, thigh
    congenital Q65.9
    due to (previous) juvenile
        osteochondrosis —*see* Coxa, plana
    flexion —*see* Contraction, joint, hip
  hourglass —*see* Contraction, hourglass
  humerus (acquired) M21.82-
    congenital Q74.0
  hypophyseal (congenital) Q89.2
  ileocecal (coil) (valve) (acquired) K63.89
    congenital Q43.9
  ileum (congenital) Q43.9
    acquired K63.89
  ilium (acquired) M95.5
    congenital Q74.2
  integument (congenital) Q84.9
  intervertebral cartilage or disc (acquired) —
      see Disorder, disc, specified NEC
  intestine (large) (small) (congenital) NOS
      Q43.9
    acquired K63.89
  intrinsic minus or plus (hand) —*see*
      Deformity, limb, specified type NEC,
      forearm
  iris (acquired) H21.89
    congenital Q13.2
  ischium (acquired) M95.5
    congenital Q74.2
  jaw (acquired) (congenital) M26.9
  joint (acquired) NEC M21.90
    congenital Q68.8
    elbow M21.92-
    hand M21.94-
    hip M21.95-
    knee M21.96-
    shoulder M21.92-
    wrist M21.93-
  kidney (s) (calyx) (pelvis) (congenital) Q63.9
    acquired N28.89
    artery (congenital) Q27.2
      acquired I77.89
  Klippel-Feil (brevicollis) Q76.1
  knee (acquired) NEC —*see also* Deformity,
      limb, lower leg
    congenital Q68.2
  labium (majus) (minus) (congenital) Q52.79
    acquired N90.89
  lacrimal passages or duct (congenital) NEC
      Q10.6
    acquired —*see* Disorder, lacrimal system,
        changes
  larynx (muscle) (congenital) Q31.8
    acquired J38.7
    web (glottic) Q31.0
  leg (upper) (acquired) NEC —*see also*
      Deformity, limb, thigh
    congenital Q68.8
    lower leg —*see* Deformity, limb, lower leg
  lens (acquired) H27.8
    congenital Q12.9
  lid (fold) (acquired) —*see also* Disorder,
      eyelid, specified type NEC
    congenital Q10.3

◀ New   ◀▥ Revised   ~~deleted~~ Deleted

Deformity *(Continued)*
- ligament (acquired) —*see* Disorder, ligament
  - congenital Q79.9
- limb (acquired) M21.90
  - clawfoot M21.53-
  - clawhand M21.51-
  - clubfoot M21.54-
  - clubhand M21.52-
  - congenital, except reduction deformity Q74.9
  - flat foot M21.4-
  - flexion M21.20
    - ankle M21.27-
    - elbow M21.22-
    - finger M21.24-
    - hip M21.25-
    - knee M21.26-
    - shoulder M21.21-
    - toe M21.27-
    - wrist M21.23-
  - foot
    - claw —*see* Deformity, limb, clawfoot
    - club —*see* Deformity, limb, clubfoot
    - drop M21.37-
    - flat —*see* Deformity, limb, flat foot
    - specified NEC M21.6X-
  - forearm M21.93-
  - hand M21.94-
  - lower leg M21.96-
  - specified type NEC M21.80
    - forearm M21.83-
    - lower leg M21.86-
    - thigh M21.85-
    - upper arm M21.82-
  - thigh M21.95-
  - unequal length M21.70
    - short site is
      - femur M21.75-
      - fibula M21.76-
      - humerus M21.72-
      - radius M21.73-
      - tibia M21.76-
      - ulna M21.73-
  - upper arm M21.92-
  - valgus —*see* Deformity, valgus
  - varus —*see* Deformity, varus
  - wrist drop M21.33-
- lip (acquired) NEC K13.0
  - congenital Q38.0
- liver (congenital) Q44.7
  - acquired K76.89
- lumbosacral (congenital) (joint) (region) Q76.49
  - acquired —*see* subcategory M43.8
  - kyphosis —*see* Kyphosis, congenital
  - lordosis —*see* Lordosis, congenital
- lung (congenital) Q33.9
  - acquired J98.4
- lymphatic system, congenital Q89.9
- Madelung's (radius) Q74.0
- mandible (acquired) (congenital) M26.9
- maxilla (acquired) (congenital) M26.9
- meninges or membrane (congenital) Q07.9
  - cerebral Q04.8
    - acquired G96.19
  - spinal cord (congenital) G96.19
    - acquired G96.19
- metacarpus (acquired) —*see* Deformity, limb, forearm
  - congenital Q74.0
- metatarsus (acquired) —*see* Deformity, foot
  - congenital Q66.9
- middle ear (congenital) Q16.4
  - ossicles Q16.3
- mitral (leaflets) (valve) I05.8
  - parachute Q23.2
  - stenosis, congenital Q23.2
- mouth (acquired) K13.79
  - congenital Q38.6
- multiple, congenital NEC Q89.7

Deformity *(Continued)*
- muscle (acquired) M62.89
  - congenital Q79.9
    - sternocleidomastoid Q68.0
- musculoskeletal system (acquired) M95.9
  - congenital Q79.9
  - specified NEC M95.8
- nail (acquired) L60.8
  - congenital Q84.6
- nasal —*see* Deformity, nose
- neck (acquired) M95.3
  - congenital Q18.9
    - sternocleidomastoid Q68.0
- nervous system (congenital) Q07.9
- nipple (congenital) Q83.9
  - acquired N64.89
- nose (acquired) (cartilage) M95.0
  - bone (turbinate) M95.0
  - congenital Q30.9
    - bent or squashed Q67.4
  - saddle M95.0
    - syphilitic A50.57
  - septum (acquired) J34.2
    - congenital Q30.8
  - sinus (wall) (congenital) Q30.8
    - acquired M95.0
  - syphilitic (congenital) A50.57
    - late A52.73
- ocular muscle (congenital) Q10.3
  - acquired —*see* Strabismus, mechanical
- opticociliary vessels (congenital) Q13.2
- orbit (eye) (congenital) H05.30
  - atrophy —*see* Atrophy, orbit
  - congenital Q10.7
  - due to
    - bone disease NEC H05.32-
    - trauma or surgery H05.33-
  - enlargement —*see* Enlargement, orbit
  - exostosis —*see* Exostosis, orbit
- organ of Corti (congenital) Q16.5
- ovary (congenital) Q50.39
  - acquired N83.8
- oviduct, acquired N83.8
- palate (congenital) Q38.5
  - acquired M27.8
  - cleft (congenital) —*see* Cleft, palate
- pancreas (congenital) Q45.3
  - acquired K86.8
- parathyroid (gland) Q89.2
- parotid (gland) (congenital) Q38.4
  - acquired K11.8
- patella (acquired) —*see* Disorder, patella, specified NEC
- pelvis, pelvic (acquired) (bony) M95.5
  - with disproportion (fetopelvic) O33.0
    - causing obstructed labor O65.0
  - congenital Q74.2
  - rachitic sequelae (late effect) E64.3
- penis (glans) (congenital) Q55.69
  - acquired N48.89
- pericardium (congenital) Q24.8
  - acquired —*see* Pericarditis
- pharynx (congenital) Q38.8
  - acquired J39.2
- pinna, acquired —*see also* Disorder, pinna, deformity
  - congenital Q17.9
- pituitary (congenital) Q89.2
- posture —*see* Dorsopathy, deforming
- prepuce (congenital) Q55.69
  - acquired N47.8
- prostate (congenital) Q55.4
  - acquired N42.89
- pupil (congenital) Q13.2
  - acquired —*see* Abnormality, pupillary
- pylorus (congenital) Q40.3
  - acquired K31.89
- rachitic (acquired), old or healed E64.3
- radius (acquired) —*see also* Deformity, limb, forearm
  - congenital Q68.8

Deformity *(Continued)*
- rectum (congenital) Q43.9
  - acquired K62.89
- reduction (extremity) (limb), congenital *(see also* condition and site) Q73.8
  - brain Q04.3
  - lower —*see* Defect, reduction, lower limb
  - upper —*see* Defect, reduction, upper limb
- renal —*see* Deformity, kidney
- respiratory system (congenital) Q34.9
- rib (acquired) M95.4
  - congenital Q76.6
  - cervical Q76.5
- rotation (joint) (acquired) —*see* Deformity, limb, specified site NEC
  - congenital Q74.9
  - hip —*see* Deformity, limb, specified type NEC, thigh
    - congenital Q65.89
- sacroiliac joint (congenital) Q74.2
  - acquired —*see* subcategory M43.8
- sacrum (acquired) —*see* subcategory M43.8
- saddle
  - back —*see* Lordosis
  - nose M95.0
    - syphilitic A50.57
- salivary gland or duct (congenital) Q38.4
  - acquired K11.8
- scapula (acquired) M95.8
  - congenital Q68.8
- scrotum (congenital) —*see also* Malformation, testis and scrotum
  - acquired N50.8
- seminal vesicles (congenital) Q55.4
  - acquired N50.8
- septum, nasal (acquired) J34.2
- shoulder (joint) (acquired) —*see* Deformity, limb, upper arm
  - congenital Q74.0
  - contraction —*see* Contraction, joint, shoulder
- sigmoid (flexure) (congenital) Q43.9
  - acquired K63.89
- skin (congenital) Q82.9
- skull (acquired) M95.2
  - congenital Q75.8
    - with
      - anencephaly Q00.0
      - encephalocele —*see* Encephalocele
      - hydrocephalus Q03.9
        - with spina bifida —*see* Spina bifida, by site, with hydrocephalus
      - microcephaly Q02
- soft parts, organs or tissues (of pelvis)
  - in pregnancy or childbirth NEC O34.8-
    - causing obstructed labor O65.5
- spermatic cord (congenital) Q55.4
  - acquired N50.8
  - torsion —*see* Torsion, spermatic cord
- spinal —*see* Dorsopathy, deforming
  - column (acquired) —*see* Dorsopathy, deforming
  - congenital Q67.5
  - cord (congenital) Q06.9
    - acquired G95.89
  - nerve root (congenital) Q07.9
- spine (acquired) —*see also* Dorsopathy, deforming
  - congenital Q67.5
  - rachitic E64.3
  - specified NEC —*see* Dorsopathy, deforming, specified NEC
- spleen
  - acquired D73.89
  - congenital Q89.09
- Sprengel's (congenital) Q74.0
- sternocleidomastoid (muscle), congenital Q68.0
- sternum (acquired) M95.4
  - congenital NEC Q76.7

Deformity *(Continued)*
- stomach (congenital) Q40.3
  - acquired K31.89
- submandibular gland (congenital) Q38.4
- submaxillary gland (congenital) Q38.4
  - acquired K11.8
- talipes —*see* Talipes
- testis (congenital) —*see also* Malformation, testis and scrotum
  - acquired N44.8
    - torsion —*see* Torsion, testis
- thigh (acquired) —*see also* Deformity, limb, thigh
  - congenital NEC Q68.8
- thorax (acquired) (wall) M95.4
  - congenital Q67.8
  - sequelae of rickets E64.3
- thumb (acquired) —*see also* Deformity, finger
  - congenital NEC Q68.1
- thymus (tissue) (congenital) Q89.2
- thyroid (gland) (congenital) Q89.2
  - cartilage Q31.8
    - acquired J38.7
- tibia (acquired) —*see also* Deformity, limb, specified type NEC, lower leg
  - congenital NEC Q68.8
  - saber (syphilitic) A50.56
- toe (acquired) M20.6-
  - congenital Q66.9
  - hallux rigidus M20.2-
  - hallux valgus M20.1-
  - hallux varus M20.3-
  - hammer toe M20.4-
  - specified NEC M20.5X-
- tongue (congenital) Q38.3
  - acquired K14.8
- tooth, teeth K00.2
- trachea (rings) (congenital) Q32.1
  - acquired J39.8
- transverse aortic arch (congenital) Q25.4
- tricuspid (leaflets) (valve) I07.8
  - atresia or stenosis Q22.4
  - Ebstein's Q22.5
- trunk (acquired) M95.8
  - congenital Q89.9
- ulna (acquired) —*see also* Deformity, limb, forearm
  - congenital NEC Q68.8
- urachus, congenital Q64.4
- ureter (opening) (congenital) Q62.8
  - acquired N28.89
- urethra (congenital) Q64.79
  - acquired N36.8
- urinary tract (congenital) Q64.9
  - urachus Q64.4
- uterus (congenital) Q51.9
  - acquired N85.8
- uvula (congenital) Q38.5
- vagina (acquired) N89.8
  - congenital Q52.4
- valgus NEC M21.00
  - ankle M21.07-
  - elbow M21.02-
  - hip M21.05-
  - knee M21.06-
- valve, valvular (congenital) (heart) Q24.8
  - acquired —*see* Endocarditis
- varus NEC M21.10
  - ankle M21.17-
  - elbow M21.12-
  - hip M21.15
  - knee M21.16-
  - tibia —*see* Osteochondrosis, juvenile, tibia
- vas deferens (congenital) Q55.4
  - acquired N50.8
- vein (congenital) Q27.9
  - great Q26.9
- vertebra —*see* Dorsopathy, deforming
- vertical talus (congenital) Q66.80
  - left foot Q66.82
  - right foot Q66.81

Deformity *(Continued)*
- vesicourethral orifice (acquired) N32.89
  - congenital NEC Q64.79
- vessels of optic papilla (congenital) Q14.2
- visual field (contraction) —*see* Defect, visual field
- vitreous body, acquired H43.89
- vulva (congenital) Q52.79
  - acquired N90.89
- wrist (joint) (acquired) —*see also* Deformity, limb, forearm
  - congenital Q68.8
  - contraction —*see* Contraction, joint, wrist

Degeneration, degenerative
- adrenal (capsule) (fatty) (gland) (hyaline) (infectional) E27.8
- amyloid (*see also* Amyloidosis) E85.9
- anterior cornua, spinal cord G12.29
- anterior labral S43.49-
- aorta, aortic I70.0
  - fatty I77.89
- aortic valve (heart) —*see* Endocarditis, aortic
- arteriovascular —*see* Arteriosclerosis
- artery, arterial (atheromatous) (calcareous) — *see also* Arteriosclerosis
  - cerebral, amyloid E85.4 *[I68.0]*
  - medial —*see* Arteriosclerosis, extremities
- articular cartilage NEC —*see* Derangement, joint, articular cartilage, by site
- atheromatous —*see* Arteriosclerosis
- basal nuclei or ganglia G23.9
  - specified NEC G23.8
- bone NEC —*see* Disorder, bone, specified type NEC
- brachial plexus G54.0
- brain (cortical) (progressive) G31.9
  - alcoholic G31.2
  - arteriosclerotic I67.2
  - childhood G31.9
    - specified NEC G31.89
  - cystic G31.89
    - congenital Q04.6
  - in
    - alcoholism G31.2
    - beriberi E51.2
    - cerebrovascular disease I67.9
    - congenital hydrocephalus Q03.9
      - with spina bifida —*see also* Spina bifida
    - Fabry-Anderson disease E75.21
    - Gaucher's disease E75.22
    - Hunter's syndrome E76.1
    - lipidosis
      - cerebral E75.4
      - generalized E75.6
    - mucopolysaccharidosis —*see* Mucopolysaccharidosis
    - myxedema E03.9 *[G32.89]*
    - neoplastic disease (*see also* Neoplasm) D49.6 *[G32.89]*
    - Niemann-Pick disease E75.249 *[G32.89]*
    - sphingolipidosis E75.3 *[G32.89]*
    - vitamin B12 deficiency E53.8 *[G32.89]*
  - senile NEC G31.1
- breast N64.89
- Bruch's membrane —*see* Degeneration, choroid
- capillaries (fatty) I78.8
  - amyloid E85.8 *[I79.8]*
- cardiac —*see also* Degeneration, myocardial
  - valve, valvular —*see* Endocarditis
- cardiorenal —*see* Hypertension, cardiorenal
- cardiovascular —*see also* Disease, cardiovascular
  - renal —*see* Hypertension, cardiorenal
- cerebellar NOS G31.9
  - alcoholic G31.2
  - primary (hereditary) (sporadic) G11.9
- cerebral —*see* Degeneration, brain
- cerebrovascular I67.9
  - due to hypertension I67.4

Degeneration, degenerative *(Continued)*
- cervical plexus G54.2
- cervix N88.8
  - due to radiation (intended effect) N88.8
    - adverse effect or misadventure N99.89
- chamber angle H21.21-
- changes, spine or vertebra —*see* Spondylosis
- chorioretinal —*see also* Degeneration, choroid
  - hereditary H31.20
- choroid (colloid) (drusen) H31.10-
  - atrophy —*see* Atrophy, choroidal
  - hereditary —*see* Dystrophy, choroidal, hereditary
- ciliary body H21.22-
- cochlear —*see* subcategory H83.8
- combined (spinal cord) (subacute) E53.8 *[G32.0]*
  - with anemia (pernicious) D51.0 *[G32.0]*
    - due to dietary vitamin B12 deficiency D51.3 *[G32.0]*
  - in (due to)
    - vitamin B12 deficiency E53.8 *[G32.0]*
      - anemia D51.9 *[G32.0]*
- conjunctiva H11.10
  - concretions —*see* Concretion, conjunctiva
  - deposits —*see* Deposit, conjunctiva
  - pigmentations —*see* Pigmentation, conjunctiva
  - pinguecula —*see* Pinguecula
  - xerosis —*see* Xerosis, conjunctiva
- cornea H18.40
  - calcerous H18.43
    - band keratopathy H18.42-
  - familial, hereditary —*see* Dystrophy, cornea
  - hyaline (of old scars) H18.49
  - keratomalacia —*see* Keratomalacia
  - nodular H18.45-
  - peripheral H18.46-
  - senile H18.41-
  - specified type NEC H18.49
- cortical (cerebellar) (parenchymatous) G31.89
  - alcoholic G31.2
  - diffuse, due to arteriopathy I67.2
- corticobasal G31.85
- cutis L98.8
  - amyloid E85.4 *[L99]*
- dental pulp K04.2
- disc disease —*see* Degeneration, intervertebral disc NEC
- dorsolateral (spinal cord) —*see* Degeneration, combined
- extrapyramidal G25.9
- eye, macular —*see also* Degeneration, macula
  - congenital or hereditary —*see* Dystrophy, retina
- facet joints —*see* Spondylosis
- fatty
  - liver NEC K76.0
    - alcoholic K70.0
- grey matter (brain) (Alpers') G31.81
- heart —*see also* Degeneration, myocardial
  - amyloid E85.4 *[I43]*
  - atheromatous —*see* Disease, heart, ischemic, atherosclerotic
  - ischemic —*see* Disease, heart, ischemic
- hepatolenticular (Wilson's) E83.01
- hepatorenal K76.7
- hyaline (diffuse) (generalized)
  - localized —*see* Degeneration, by site
- infrapatellar fat pad M79.4
- intervertebral disc NOS
  - with
    - myelopathy —*see* Disorder, disc, with, myelopathy
    - radiculitis or radiculopathy —*see* Disorder, disc, with, radiculopathy
  - cervical, cervicothoracic —*see* Disorder, disc, cervical, degeneration
    - with
      - myelopathy —*see* Disorder, disc, cervical, with myelopathy

Degeneration, degenerative *(Continued)*
 intervertebral disc NOS *(Continued)*
  cervical, cervicothoracic *(Continued)*
   with *(Continued)*
    neuritis, radiculitis or
     radiculopathy —*see* Disorder,
     disc, cervical, with neuritis
   lumbar region M51.36
    with
     myelopathy M51.06
     neuritis, radiculitis, radiculopathy or
      sciatica M51.16
   lumbosacral region M51.37
    with
     neuritis, radiculitis, radiculopathy or
      sciatica M51.17
   sacrococcygeal region M53.3
   thoracic region M51.34
    with
     myelopathy M51.04
     neuritis, radiculitis, radiculopathy
      M51.14
   thoracolumbar region M51.35
    with
     myelopathy M51.05
     neuritis, radiculitis, radiculopathy
      M51.15
  intestine, amyloid E85.4
  iris (pigmentary) H21.23-
  ischemic —*see* Ischemia
  joint disease —*see* Osteoarthritis
  kidney N28.89
   amyloid E85.4 *[N29]*
   cystic, congenital Q61.9
   fatty N28.89
   polycystic Q61.3
    adult type (autosomal dominant) Q61.2
    infantile type (autosomal recessive) NEC
     Q61.19
     collecting duct dilatation Q61.11
  Kuhnt-Junius *(see also* Degeneration, macula)
   H35.32
  lens —*see* Cataract
  lenticular (familial) (progressive) (Wilson's)
   (with cirrhosis of liver) E83.01
  liver (diffuse) NEC K76.89
   amyloid E85.4 *[K77]*
   cystic K76.89
    congenital Q44.6
   fatty NEC K76.0
    alcoholic K70.0
   hypertrophic K76.89
   parenchymatous, acute or subacute
    K72.00
    with coma K72.01
   pigmentary K76.89
   toxic (acute) K71.9
  lung J98.4
  lymph gland I89.8
   hyaline I89.8
  macula, macular (acquired) (age-related)
   (senile) H35.30
   angioid streaks H35.33
   atrophic age-related H35.31
   congenital or hereditary —*see* Dystrophy,
    retina
   cystoid H35.35-
   drusen H35.36-
   exudative H35.32
   hole H35.34-
   nonexudative H35.31
   puckering H35.37-
   toxic H35.38-
  membranous labyrinth, congenital (causing
   impairment of hearing) Q16.5
  meniscus —*see* Derangement, meniscus
  mitral —*see* Insufficiency, mitral
  Mönckeberg's —*see* Arteriosclerosis,
   extremities
  motor centers, senile G31.1
  multi-system G90.3

Degeneration, degenerative *(Continued)*
 mural —*see* Degeneration, myocardial
 muscle (fatty) (fibrous) (hyaline)
  (progressive) M62.89
  heart —*see* Degeneration, myocardial
 myelin, central nervous system G37.9
 myocardial, myocardium (fatty) (hyaline)
  (senile) I51.5
  with rheumatic fever (conditions in I00)
   I09.0
   active, acute or subacute I01.2
    with chorea I02.0
   inactive or quiescent (with chorea)
    I09.0
  hypertensive —*see* Hypertension, heart
  rheumatic —*see* Degeneration, myocardial,
   with rheumatic fever
  syphilitic A52.06
 nasal sinus (mucosa) J32.9
  frontal J32.1
  maxillary J32.0
 nerve —*see* Disorder, nerve
 nervous system G31.9
  alcoholic G31.2
  amyloid E85.4 *[G99.8]*
  autonomic G90.9
  fatty G31.89
  specified NEC G31.89
 nipple N64.89
 olivopontocerebellar (hereditary) (familial)
  G23.8
 osseous labyrinth —*see* subcategory H83.8
 ovary N83.8
  cystic N83.20
  microcystic N83.20
 pallidal pigmentary (progressive) G23.0
 pancreas K86.8
  tuberculous A18.83
 penis N48.89
 pigmentary (diffuse) (general)
  localized —*see* Degeneration, by site
  pallidal (progressive) G23.0
 pineal gland E34.8
 pituitary (gland) E23.6
 popliteal fat pad M79.4
 posterolateral (spinal cord) —*see*
  Degeneration, combined
 pulmonary valve (heart) I37.8
 pulp (tooth) K04.2
 pupillary margin H21.24-
 renal —*see* Degeneration, kidney
 retina H35.9
  hereditary (cerebroretinal) (congenital)
   (juvenile) (macula) (peripheral)
   (pigmentary) —*see* Dystrophy, retina
  Kuhnt-Junius *(see also* Degeneration,
   macula) H35.32
  macula (cystic) (exudative) (hole)
   (nonexudative) (pseudohole) (senile)
   (toxic) —*see* Degeneration, macula
  peripheral H35.40
   lattice H35.41-
   microcystoid H35.42-
   paving stone H35.43-
   secondary
    pigmentary H35.45-
    vitreoretinal H35.46-
   senile reticular H35.44-
  pigmentary (primary) —*see also* Dystrophy,
   retina
  secondary —*see* Degeneration, retina,
   peripheral, secondary
  posterior pole —*see* Degeneration, macula
 saccule, congenital (causing impairment of
  hearing) Q16.5
 senile R54
  brain G31.1
  cardiac, heart or myocardium —*see*
   Degeneration, myocardial
  motor centers G31.1
  vascular —*see* Arteriosclerosis

Degeneration, degenerative *(Continued)*
 sinus (cystic) —*see also* Sinusitis
  polypoid J33.1
 skin L98.8
  amyloid E85.4 *[L99]*
  colloid L98.8
 spinal (cord) G31.89
  amyloid E85.4 *[G32.89]*
  combined (subacute) —*see* Degeneration,
   combined
  dorsolateral —*see* Degeneration, combined
  familial NEC G31.89
  fatty G31.89
  funicular —*see* Degeneration, combined
  posterolateral —*see* Degeneration,
   combined
  subacute combined —*see* Degeneration,
   combined
  tuberculous A17.81
 spleen D73.0
  amyloid E85.4 *[D77]*
 stomach K31.89
 striatonigral G23.2
 suprarenal (capsule) (gland) E27.8
 synovial membrane (pulpy) —*see* Disorder,
  synovium, specified type NEC
 tapetoretinal —*see* Dystrophy, retina
 thymus (gland) E32.8
  fatty E32.8
 thyroid (gland) E07.89
 tricuspid (heart) (valve) I07.9
 tuberculous NEC —*see* Tuberculosis
 turbinate J34.89
 uterus (cystic) N85.8
 vascular (senile) —*see* Arteriosclerosis
  hypertensive —*see* Hypertension
 vitreoretinal, secondary —*see* Degeneration,
  retina, peripheral, secondary,
  vitreoretinal
 vitreous (body) H43.81-
 Wallerian —*see* Disorder, nerve
 Wilson's hepatolenticular E83.01
Deglutition
 paralysis R13.0
  hysterical F44.4
 pneumonia J69.0
Degos' disease I77.89
Dehiscence (of)
 amputation stump T87.81
 cesarean wound O90.0
 closure of
  cornea T81.31
  craniotomy T81.32
  fascia (muscular) (superficial) T81.32
  internal organ or tissue T81.32
  laceration (external) (internal) T81.33
  ligament T81.32
  mucosa T81.31
  muscle or muscle flap T81.32
  ribs or rib cage T81.32
  skin and subcutaneous tissue (full-
   thickness) (superficial) T81.31
  skull T81.32
  sternum (sternotomy) T81.32
  tendon T81.32
  traumatic laceration (external) (internal)
   T81.33
 episiotomy O90.1
 operation wound NEC T81.31
  external operation wound (superficial)
   T81.31
  internal operation wound (deep)
   T81.32
 perineal wound (postpartum) O90.1
 traumatic injury wound repair T81.33
 wound T81.30
  traumatic repair T81.33
Dehydration E86.0
 hypertonic E87.0
 hypotonic E87.1
 newborn P74.1

Déjérine-Roussy syndrome G93.89
Déjérine-Sottas disease or neuropathy
  (hypertrophic) G60.0
Déjérine-Thomas atrophy G23.8
Delay, delayed
  any plane in pelvis
    complicating delivery O66.9
  birth or delivery NOS O63.9
  closure, ductus arteriosus (Botalli) P29.3
  coagulation —see Defect, coagulation
  conduction (cardiac) (ventricular) I45.9
  delivery, second twin, triplet, etc O63.2
  development R62.50
    global F88
    intellectual (specific) F81.9
    language F80.9
      due to hearing loss F80.4
    learning F81.9
    pervasive F84.9
    physiological R62.50
      specified stage NEC R62.0
    reading F81.0
    sexual E30.0
    speech F80.9
      due to hearing loss F80.4
    spelling F81.81
  gastric emptying K30
  menarche E30.0
  menstruation (cause unknown) N91.0
  milestone R62.0
  passage of meconium (newborn) P76.0
  primary respiration P28.9
  puberty (constitutional) E30.0
  separation of umbilical cord P96.82
  sexual maturation, female E30.0
  sleep phase syndrome G47.21
  union, fracture —see Fracture, by site
  vaccination Z28.9
Deletion (s)
  autosome Q93.9
    identified by fluorescence in situ
      hybridization (FISH) Q93.89
    identified by in situ hybridization (ISH)
      Q93.89
  chromosome
    with complex rearrangements NEC Q93.7
    part of NEC Q93.5
    seen only at prometaphase Q93.89
    short arm
      4 Q93.3
      5p Q93.4
      22q11.2 Q93.81
    specified NEC Q93.89
  long arm chromosome 18 or 21 Q93.89
    with complex rearrangements NEC
      Q93.7
  microdeletions NEC Q93.88
Delhi boil or button B55.1
Delinquency (juvenile) (neurotic) F91.8
  group Z72.810
Delinquent immunization status Z28.3
Delirium, delirious (acute or subacute) (not
    alcohol or drug-induced) (with dementia)
    R41.0
  alcoholic (acute) (tremens) (withdrawal)
    F10.921
    with intoxication F10.921
      in
        abuse F10.121
        dependence F10.221
  due to (secondary to)
    alcohol
      intoxication F10.921
        in
          abuse F10.121
          dependence F10.221
      withdrawal F10.231
    amphetamine intoxication F15.921
      in
        abuse F15.121
        dependence F15.221

Delirium, delirious (Continued)
  due to (Continued)
    anxiolytic
      intoxication F13.921
        in
          abuse F13.121
          dependence F13.221
      withdrawal F13.231
    cannabis intoxication (acute) F12.921
      in
        abuse F12.121
        dependence F12.221
    cocaine intoxication (acute) F14.921
      in
        abuse F14.121
        dependence F14.221
    general medical condition F05
    hallucinogen intoxication F16.921
      in
        abuse F16.121
        dependence F16.221
    hypnotic
      intoxication F13.921
        in
          abuse F13.121
          dependence F13.221
      withdrawal F13.231
    inhalant intoxication (acute) F18.921
      in
        abuse F18.121
        dependence F18.221
    multiple etiologies F05
    opioid intoxication (acute) F11.921
      in
        abuse F11.121
        dependence F11.221
    phencyclidine intoxication (acute) F16.921
      in
        abuse F16.121
        dependence F16.221
    psychoactive substance NEC intoxication
      (acute) F19.921
      in
        abuse F19.121
        dependence F19.221
    sedative
      intoxication F13.921
        in
          abuse F13.121
          dependence F13.221
      withdrawal F13.231
    unknown etiology F05
  exhaustion F43.0
  hysterical F44.89
  postprocedural (postoperative) F05
  puerperal F05
  thyroid —see Thyrotoxicosis with thyroid
    storm
  traumatic —see Injury, intracranial
  tremens (alcohol-induced) F10.231
    sedative-induced F13.231
Delivery (childbirth) (labor)
  arrested active phase O62.1
  cesarean (for)
    without indication O82
    abnormal
      pelvis (bony) (deformity) (major) NEC
        with disproportion (fetopelvic)
        O33.0
      with obstructed labor O65.0
      presentation or position O32.9
    abruptio placentae (see also Abruptio
      placentae) 045.9-
    acromion presentation O32.2
    atony, uterus O62.2
    breech presentation O32.1
      incomplete O32.8
    brow presentation O32.3
    cephalopelvic disproportion O33.9
    cerclage O34.3-
    chin presentation O32.3

Delivery (Continued)
  cesarean (Continued)
    cicatrix of cervix O34.4-
    contracted pelvis (general)
      inlet O33.2
      outlet O33.3
    cord presentation or prolapse O69.0
    cystocele O34.8-
    deformity (acquired) (congenital)
      pelvic organs or tissues NEC O34.8-
      pelvis (bony) NEC O33.0
    disproportion NOS O33.9
    eclampsia —see Eclampsia
    face presentation O32.3
    failed
      forceps O66.5
      induction of labor O61.9
        instrumental O61.1
        mechanical O61.1
        medical O61.0
        specified NEC O61.8
        surgical O61.1
      trial of labor NOS O66.40
        following previous cesarean delivery
          O66.41
      vacuum extraction O66.5
      ventouse O66.5
    fetal-maternal hemorrhage O43.01-
    hemorrhage (intrapartum) O67.9
      with coagulation defect O67.0
      specified cause NEC O67.8
    high head at term O32.4
    hydrocephalic fetus O33.6
    incarceration of uterus O34.51-
    incoordinate uterine action O62.4
    increased size, fetus O33.5
    inertia, uterus O62.2
      primary O62.0
      secondary O62.1
    lateroversion, uterus O34.59-
    mal lie O32.9
    malposition
      fetus O32.9
      pelvic organs or tissues NEC O34.8-
      uterus NEC O34.59-
    malpresentation NOS O32.9
    oblique presentation O32.2
    occurring after 37 completed weeks of
      gestation but before 39 completed
      weeks gestation due to (spontaneous)
      onset of labor O75.82
    oversize fetus O33.5
    pelvic tumor NEC O34.8-
    placenta previa O44.1-
      without hemorrhage O44.0-
    placental insufficiency O36.51-
    planned, occurring after 37 completed
      weeks of gestation but before 39
      completed weeks gestation due to
      (spontaneous) onset of labor O75.82
    polyp, cervix O34.4-
      causing obstructed labor O65.5
    poor dilatation, cervix O62.0
    pre-eclampsia O14.9-
      mild O14.0-
      moderate O14.0-
      severe
        with hemolysis, elevated liver
          enzymes and low platelet count
          (HELLP) O14.2-
    previous
      cesarean delivery O34.21
      surgery (to)
        cervix O34.4-
        gynecological NEC O34.8-
        rectum O34.7-
        uterus O34.29
        vagina O34.6-
    prolapse
      arm or hand O32.2
      uterus O34.52-

◀ New   ◀▦ Revised   ~~deleted~~ Deleted

Delivery *(Continued)*
  cesarean *(Continued)*
    prolonged labor NOS O63.9
    rectocele O34.8-
    retroversion
      uterus O34.53-
    rigid
      cervix O34.4-
      pelvic floor O34.8-
      perineum O34.7-
      vagina O34.6-
      vulva O34.7-
    sacculation, pregnant uterus O34.59-
    scar (s)
      cervix O34.4-
      cesarean delivery O34.21
      uterus O34.29
    Shirodkar suture in situ O34.3-
    shoulder presentation O32.2
    stenosis or stricture, cervix O34.4-
    streptococcus B carrier state O99.824
    transverse presentation or lie O32.2
    tumor, pelvic organs or tissues NEC
      O34.8-
      cervix O34.4-
    umbilical cord presentation or prolapse
      O69.0
  completely normal case O80
  complicated O75.9
    by
      abnormal, abnormality (of)
        forces of labor O62.9
          specified type NEC O62.8
        glucose O99.814
        uterine contractions NOS O62.9
      abruptio placentae *(see also* Abruptio
        placentae) O45.9-
      abuse
        physical O9A.32
        psychological O9A.52
        sexual O9A.42
      adherent placenta O72.0
        without hemorrhage O73.0
      alcohol use O99.314
      anemia (pre-existing) O99.02
      anesthetic death O74.8
      annular detachment of cervix O71.3
      atony, uterus O62.2
      attempted vacuum extraction and
        forceps O66.5
      Bandl's ring O62.4
      bariatric surgery status O99.844
      biliary tract disorder O26.62
      bleeding —*see* Delivery, complicated by,
        hemorrhage
      blood disorder NEC O99.12
      cervical dystocia (hypotonic) O62.2
        primary O62.0
        secondary O62.1
      circulatory system disorder O99.42
      compression of cord (umbilical) NEC
        O69.2
      condition NEC O99.89
      contraction, contracted ring O62.4
      cord (umbilical)
        around neck
          with compression O69.1
          without compression O69.81
        bruising O69.5
        complication O69.9
          specified NEC O69.89
        compression NEC O69.2
        entanglement O69.2
          without compression O69.82
        hematoma O69.5
        presentation O69.0
        prolapse O69.0
        short O69.3
        thrombosis (vessels) O69.5
        vascular lesion O69.5
      Couvelaire uterus O45.8X-

Delivery *(Continued)*
  complicated *(Continued)*
    by *(Continued)*
      damage to (injury to) NEC
        perineum O71.82
        periurethral tissue O71.82
        vulva O71.82
      delay following rupture of membranes
        (spontaneous) —*see* Pregnancy,
        complicated by, premature rupture
        of membranes
      depressed fetal heart tones O76
      diabetes O24.92
        gestational O24.429
          diet controlled O24.420
          insulin controlled O24.424
        pre-existing O24.32
          specified NEC O24.82
          type 1 O24.02
          type 2 O24.12
      diastasis recti (abdominis) O71.89
      dilatation
        bladder O66.8
        cervix incomplete, poor or slow O62.0
      disease NEC O99.89
      disruptio uteri —*see* Delivery,
        complicated by, rupture, uterus
      drug use O99.324
      dysfunction, uterus NOS O62.9
        hypertonic O62.4
        hypotonic O62.2
          primary O62.0
          secondary O62.1
        incoordinate O62.4
      eclampsia O15.1
      embolism (pulmonary) —*see* Embolism,
        obstetric
      endocrine, nutritional or metabolic
        disease NEC O99.284
      failed
        attempted vaginal birth after previous
          cesarean delivery O66.41
        induction of labor O61.9
          instrumental O61.1
          mechanical O61.1
          medical O61.0
          specified NEC O61.8
          surgical O61.1
        trial of labor O66.40
      female genital mutilation O65.5
      fetal
        abnormal acid-base balance O68
        acidemia O68
        acidosis O68
        alkalosis O68
        death, early O02.1
        deformity O66.3
        heart rate or rhythm (abnormal) (non-
          reassuring) O76
        hypoxia O77.8
        stress O77.9
          due to drug administration O77.1
          electrocardiographic evidence of
            O77.8
          specified NEC O77.8
          ultrasound evidence of O77.8
      fever during labor O75.2
      gastric banding status O99.844
      gastric bypass status O99.844
      gastrointestinal disease NEC
        O99.62
      gestational diabetes O24.429
        diet controlled O24.420
        insulin (and diet) controlled
          O24.424
      gonorrhea O98.22
      hematoma O71.7
        ischial spine O71.7
        pelvic O71.7
        vagina O71.7
        vulva or perineum O71.7

Delivery *(Continued)*
  complicated *(Continued)*
    by *(Continued)*
      hemorrhage (uterine) O67.9
        associated with
          afibrinogenemia O67.0
          coagulation defect O67.0
          hyperfibrinolysis O67.0
          hypofibrinogenemia O67.0
        due to
          low-lying placenta O44.1-
          placenta previa O44.1-
          premature separation of placenta
            (normally implanted) *(see also*
            Abruptio placentae) O45.9-
          retained placenta O72.0
          uterine leiomyoma O67.8
        placenta NEC O67.8
        postpartum NEC (atonic) (immediate)
          O72.1
          with retained or trapped placenta
            O72.0
          delayed O72.2
          secondary O72.2
          third stage O72.0
      hourglass contraction, uterus O62.4
      hypertension, hypertensive (pre-
        existing) —*see* Hypertension,
        complicated by, childbirth (labor)
      hypotension O26.5-
      incomplete dilatation (cervix) O62.0
      incoordinate uterus contractions
        O62.4
      inertia, uterus O62.2
        during latent phase of labor O62.0
        primary O62.0
        secondary O62.1
      infection (maternal) O98.92
        carrier state NEC O99.834
        gonorrhea O98.22
        human immunodeficiency virus (HIV)
          O98.72
        sexually transmitted NEC O98.32
        specified NEC O98.82
        syphilis O98.12
        tuberculosis O98.02
        viral hepatitis O98.42
        viral NEC O98.52
      injury (to mother) *(see also* Delivery,
        complicated, by, damage to)
        O71.9
        nonobstetric O9A.22
        caused by abuse —*see* Delivery,
          complicated by, abuse
      intrauterine fetal death, early O02.1
      inversion, uterus O71.2
      laceration (perineal) O70.9
        anus (sphincter) O70.4
          with third degree laceration
            O70.2
            with mucosa O70.3
          without third degree laceration
            O70.4
        bladder (urinary) O71.5
        bowel O71.5
        cervix (uteri) O71.3
        fourchette O70.0
        hymen O70.0
        labia O70.0
        pelvic
          floor O70.1
          organ NEC O71.5
        perineum, perineal O70.9
          first degree O70.0
          fourth degree O70.3
          muscles O70.1
          second degree O70.1
          skin O70.0
          slight O70.0
          third degree O70.2
        peritoneum (pelvic) O71.5

Delivery *(Continued)*
  complicated *(Continued)*
    by *(Continued)*
      laceration *(Continued)*
        rectovaginal (septum) (without
            perineal laceration) O71.4
          with perineum O70.2
            with anal or rectal mucosa
              O70.3
        specified NEC O71.89
        sphincter ani —*see* Delivery,
            complicated, by, laceration, anus
            (sphincter)
        urethra O71.5
        uterus O71.81
          before labor O71.81
        vagina, vaginal (deep) (high) (without
            perineal laceration) O71.4
          with perineum O70.0
            muscles, with perineum O70.1
        vulva O70.0
      liver disorder O26.62
      malignancy O9A.12
      malnutrition O25.2
      malposition, malpresentation
        without obstruction O32.9 —*see
            also* Delivery, complicated by,
            obstruction
          breech O32.1
          compound O32.6
          face (brow) (chin) O32.3
          footling O38.8
          high head O32.4
          oblique O32.2
          specified NEC O32.8
          transverse O32.2
          unstable lie O32.0
        placenta (with hemorrhage) O44.1-
          without hemorrhage O44.0-
        uterus or cervix O65.5
      meconium in amniotic fluid O77.0
      mental disorder NEC O99.344
      metrorrhexis —*see* Delivery, complicated
          by, rupture, uterus
      nervous system disorder O99.354
      obesity (pre-existing) O99.214
      obesity surgery status O99.844
      obstetric trauma O71.9
        specified NEC O71.89
      obstructed labor
        due to
          breech (complete) (frank)
              presentation O64.1
            incomplete O64.8
          brow presenation O64.3
          buttock presentation O64.1
          chin presentation O64.2
          compound presentation O64.5
          contracted pelvis O65.1
          deep transverse arrest O64.0
          deformed pelvis O65.0
          dystocia (fetal) O66.9
            due to
              conjoined twins O66.3
              fetal
                abnormality NEC O66.3
                ascites O66.3
                hydrops O66.3
                meningomyelocele O66.3
                sacral teratoma O66.3
                tumor O66.3
              hydrocephalic fetus O66.3
              shoulder O66.0
          face presentation O64.2
          fetopelvic disproportion O65.4
          footling presentation O64.8
          impacted shoulders O66.0
          incomplete rotation of fetal head
              O64.0
          large fetus O66.2
          locked twins O66.1

Delivery *(Continued)*
  complicated *(Continued)*
    by *(Continued)*
      obstructed labor *(Continued)*
        due to *(Continued)*
          malposition O64.9
            specified NEC O64.8
          malpresentation O64.9
            specified NEC O64.8
          multiple fetuses NEC O66.6
          pelvic
            abnormality (maternal) O65.9
              organ O65.5
                specified NEC O65.8
            contraction
              inlet O65.2
              mid-cavity O65.3
              outlet O65.3
          persistent (position)
            occipitoiliac O64.0
            occipitoposterior O64.0
            occipitosacral O64.0
            occipitotransverse O64.0
          prolapsed arm O64.4
          shoulder presentation O64.4
        specified NEC O66.8
      pathological retraction ring, uterus
          O62.4
      penetration, pregnant uterus by
          instrument O71.1
      perforation —*see* Delivery, complicated
          by, laceration
      placenta, placental
        ablatio (*see also* Abruptio placentae)
            O45.9-
        abnormality O43.9-
          specified NEC O43.89-
        abruptio (*see also* Abruptio placentae)
            O45.9-
        accreta O43.21-
        adherent (with hemorrhage) O72.0
          without hemorrhage O73.0
        detachment (premature) (*see also*
            Abruptio placentae) O45.9-
        disorder O43.9-
          specified NEC O43.89-
        hemorrhage NEC O67.8
        increta O43.22-
        low (implantation) O44.1-
          without hemorrhage O44.0-
        malformation O43.10-
        malposition O44.1-
          without hemorrhage O44.0-
        percreta O43.23-
        previa (central) (lateral) (low)
            (marginal) (partial) (total) O44.1-
          without hemorrhage O44.0-
        retained (with hemorrhage) O72.0
          without hemorrhage O73.0
        separation (premature) O45.9-
          specified NEC O45.8X-
        vicious insertion O44.1-
      precipitate labor O62.3
      premature rupture, membranes (*see
          also* Pregnancy, complicated by,
          premature rupture of membranes)
          O42.90
      prolapse
        arm or hand O32.2
        cord (umbilical) O69.0
        foot or leg O32.8
        uterus O34.52-
      prolonged labor O63.9
        first stage O63.0
        second stage O63.1
      protozoal disease (maternal) O98.62
      respiratory disease NEC O99.52
      retained membranes or portions of
          placenta O72.2
        without hemorrhage O73.1
      retarded birth O63.9

Delivery *(Continued)*
  complicated *(Continued)*
    by *(Continued)*
      retention of secundines (with
          hemorrhage) O72.0
        without hemorrhage O73.0
        partial O72.2
          without hemorrhage O73.1
      rupture
        bladder (urinary) O71.5
        cervix O71.3
        pelvic organ NEC O71.5
        urethra O71.5
        uterus (during or after labor) O71.1
          before labor O71.0-
      separation, pubic bone (symphysis
          pubis) O71.6
      shock O75.1
      shoulder presentation O64.4
      skin disorder NEC O99.72
      spasm, cervix O62.4
      stenosis or stricture, cervix O65.5
      streptococcus B carrier state O99.824
      subluxation of symphysis (pubis) O26.72
      syphilis (maternal) O98.12
      tear —*see* Delivery, complicated by,
          laceration
      tetanic uterus O62.4
      trauma (obstetrical) (*see also* Delivery,
          complicated, by, damage to) O71.9
        non-obstetric O9A.22
        periurethral O71.82
        specified NEC O71.89
      tuberculosis (maternal) O98.02
      tumor, pelvic organs or tissues NEC
          O65.5
      umbilical cord around neck
        with compression O69.1
        without compression O69.81
      uterine inertia O62.2
        during latent phase of labor O62.0
        primary O62.0
        secondary O62.1
      vasa previa O69.4
      velamentous insertion of cord O43.12-
    specified complication NEC O75.89
  delayed NOS O63.9
    following rupture of membranes
      artificial O75.5
    second twin, triplet, etc. O63.2
  forceps, low following failed vacuum
      extraction O66.5
  missed (at or near term) O36.4
  normal O80
  obstructed —*see* Delivery, complicated by,
      obstruction
  precipitate O62.3
  preterm (*see also* Pregnancy, complicated by,
      preterm labor) O60.10
  spontaneous O80
  term pregnancy NOS O80
  uncomplicated O80
  vaginal, following previous cesarean delivery
      O34.21
Delusions (paranoid) —*see* Disorder, delusional
Dementia (degenerative (primary)) (old age)
    (persisting) F03.90
  with
    aggressive behavior F03.91
    behavioral disturbance F03.91
    combative behavior F03.91
    Lewy bodies G31.83 *[F02.80]*
      with behavioral disturbance G31.83
          [F02.81]
    Parkinson's disease G20 *[F02.80]*
      with behavioral disturbance G20
          [F02.81]
    Parkinsonism G31.83 *[F02.80]*
      with behavioral disturbance G31.83
          [F02.81]
    violent behavior F03.91

◀ New ◀▥▥ Revised ~~deleted~~ Deleted

Dementia *(Continued)*
alcoholic F10.97
with dependence F10.27
Alzheimer's type —*see* Disease, Alzheimer's
arteriosclerotic —*see* Dementia, vascular
atypical, Alzheimer's type —*see* Disease, Alzheimer's, specified NEC
congenital —*see* Disability, intellectual
frontal (lobe) G31.09 *[F02.80]*
with behavioral disturbance G31.09 *[F02.81]*
frontotemporal G31.09 *[F02.80]*
with behavioral disturbance G31.09 *[F02.81]*
specified NEC G31.09 *[F02.80]*
with behavioral disturbance G31.09 *[F02.81]*
in (due to)
alcohol F10.97
with dependence F10.27
Alzheimer's disease —*see* Disease, Alzheimer's
arteriosclerotic brain disease —*see* Dementia, vascular
cerebral lipidoses E75.- *[F02.80]*
with behavioral disturbance E75.- *[F02.81]*
Creutzfeldt-Jakob disease *(see also* Creutzfeldt-Jakob disease or syndrome (with dementia)) A81.00
epilepsy G40.- *[F02.80]*
with behavioral disturbance G40.- *[F02.81]*
hepatolenticular degeneration E83.01 *[F02.80]*
with behavioral disturbance E83.01 *[F02.81]*
human immunodeficiency virus (HIV) disease B20 *[F02.80]*
with behavioral disturbance B20 *[F02.81]*
Huntington's disease or chorea G10
hypercalcemia E83.52 *[F02.80]*
with behavioral disturbance E83.52 *[F02.81]*
hypothyroidism, acquired E03.9 *[F02.80]*
with behavioral disturbance E03.9 *[F02.81]*
due to iodine deficiency E01.8 *[F02.80]*
with behavioral disturbance E01.8 *[F02.81]*
inhalants F18.97
with dependence F18.27
multiple
etiologies F03
sclerosis G35 *[F02.80]*
with behavioral disturbance G35 *[F02.81]*
neurosyphilis A52.17 *[F02.80]*
with behavioral disturbance A52.17 *[F02.81]*
juvenile A50.49 *[F02.80]*
with behavioral disturbance A50.49 *[F02.81]*
niacin deficiency E52 *[F02.80]*
with behavioral disturbance E52 *[F02.81]*
paralysis agitans G20 *[F02.80]*
with behavioral disturbance G20 *[F02.81]*
Parkinson's disease G20 *[F02.80]*
pellagra E52 *[F02.80]*
with behavioral disturbance E52 *[F02.81]*
Pick's G31.01 *[F02.80]*
with behavioral disturbance G31.01 *[F02.81]*
polyarteritis nodosa M30.0 *[F02.80]*
with behavioral disturbance M30.0 *[F02.81]*

Dementia *(Continued)*
in *(Continued)*
psychoactive drug F19.97
with dependence F19.27
inhalants F18.97
with dependence F18.27
sedatives, hypnotics or anxiolytics F13.97
with dependence F13.27
sedatives, hypnotics or anxiolytics F13.97
with dependence F13.27
systemic lupus erythematosus M32.- *[F02.80]*
with behavioral disturbance M32.- *[F02.81]*
trypanosomiasis
African B56.9 *[F02.80]*
with behavioral disturbance B56.9 *[F02.81]*
unknown etiology F03
vitamin B12 deficiency E53.8 *[F02.80]*
with behavioral disturbance E53.8 *[F02.81]*
volatile solvents F18.97
with dependence F18.27
infantile, infantilis F84.3
Lewy body G31.83 *[F02.80]*
with behavioral disturbance G31.83 *[F02.81]*
multi-infarct —*see* Dementia, vascular
paralytica, paralytic (syphilitic) A52.17 *[F02.80]*
with behavioral disturbance A52.17 *[F02.81]*
juvenilis A50.45
paretic A52.17
praecox —*see* Schizophrenia
presenile F03
Alzheimer's type —*see* Disease, Alzheimer's, early onset
primary degenerative F03
progressive, syphilitic A52.17
senile F03
with acute confusional state F05
Alzheimer's type —*see* Disease, Alzheimer's, late onset
depressed or paranoid type F03
vascular (acute onset) (mixed) (multi-infarct) (subcortical) F01.50
with behavioral disturbance F01.51
Demineralization, bone —*see* Osteoporosis
Demodex folliculorum (infestation) B88.0
Demophobia F40.248
Demoralization R45.3
Demyelination, demyelinization
central nervous system G37.9
specified NEC G37.8
corpus callosum (central) G37.1
disseminated, acute G36.9
specified NEC G36.8
global G35
in optic neuritis G36.0
Dengue (classical) (fever) A90
hemorrhagic A91
sandfly A93.1
Dennie-Marfan syphilitic syndrome A50.45
Dens evaginatus, in dente or invaginatus K00.2
Dense breasts R92.2
Density
increased, bone (disseminated) (generalized) (spotted) —*see* Disorder, bone, density and structure, specified type NEC
lung (nodular) J98.4
Dental —*see also* condition
examination Z01.20
with abnormal findings Z01.21
restoration
aesthetically inadequate or displeasing K08.56

Dental *(Continued)*
restoration *(Continued)*
defective K08.50
specified NEC K08.59
failure of marginal integrity K08.51
failure of periodontal anatomical integrity K08.54
Dentia praecox K00.6
Denticles (pulp) K04.2
Dentigerous cyst K09.0
Dentin
irregular (in pulp) K04.3
opalescent K00.5
secondary (in pulp) K04.3
sensitive K03.89
Dentinogenesis imperfecta K00.5
Dentinoma —*see* Cyst, calcifying odontogenic
Dentition (syndrome) K00.7
delayed K00.6
difficult K00.7
precocious K00.6
premature K00.6
retarded K00.6
Dependence (on) (syndrome) F19.20
with remission F19.21
alcohol (ethyl) (methyl) (without remission) F10.20
with
amnestic disorder, persisting F10.26
anxiety disorder F10.280
dementia, persisting F10.27
intoxication F10.229
with delirium F10.221
uncomplicated F10.220
mood disorder F10.24
psychotic disorder F10.259
with
delusions F10.250
hallucinations F10.251
remission F10.21
sexual dysfunction F10.281
sleep disorder F10.282
specified disorder NEC F10.288
withdrawal F10.239
with
delirium F10.231
perceptual disturbance F10.232
uncomplicated F10.230
counseling and surveillance Z71.41
amobarbital —*see* Dependence, drug, sedative
amphetamine (s) (type) —*see* Dependence, drug, stimulant NEC
amytal (sodium) —*see* Dependence, drug, sedative
analgesic NEC F55.8
anesthetic (agent) (gas) (general) (local) NEC —*see* Dependence, drug, psychoactive NEC
anxiolytic NEC —*see* Dependence, drug, sedative
barbital (s) —*see* Dependence, drug, sedative
barbiturate (s) (compounds) (drugs classifiable to T42) —*see* Dependence, drug, sedative
benzedrine —*see* Dependence, drug, stimulant NEC
bhang —*see* Dependence, drug, cannabis
bromide (s) NEC —*see* Dependence, drug, sedative
caffeine —*see* Dependence, drug, stimulant NEC
cannabis (sativa) (indica) (resin) (derivatives) (type) —*see* Dependence, drug, cannabis
chloral (betaine) (hydrate) —*see* Dependence, drug, sedative
chlordiazepoxide —*see* Dependence, drug, sedative
coca (leaf) (derivatives) —*see* Dependence, drug, cocaine
cocaine —*see* Dependence, drug, cocaine

Dependence *(Continued)*
codeine —*see* Dependence, drug, opioid
combinations of drugs F19.20
dagga —*see* Dependence, drug, cannabis
demerol —*see* Dependence, drug, opioid
dexamphetamine —*see* Dependence, drug, stimulant NEC
dexedrine —*see* Dependence, drug, stimulant NEC
dextromethorphan —*see* Dependence, drug, opioid
dextromoramide —*see* Dependence, drug, opioid
dextro-nor-pseudo-ephedrine —*see* Dependence, drug, stimulant NEC
dextrorphan —*see* Dependence, drug, opioid
diazepam —*see* Dependence, drug, sedative
dilaudid —*see* Dependence, drug, opioid
D-lysergic acid diethylamide —*see* Dependence, drug, hallucinogen
drug NEC F19.20
  with sleep disorder F19.282
  cannabis F12.20
    with
      anxiety disorder F12.280
      intoxication F12.229
        with
          delirium F12.221
          perceptual disturbance F12.222
        uncomplicated F12.220
      other specified disorder F12.288
      psychosis F12.259
        delusions F12.250
        hallucinations F12.251
      unspecified disorder F12.29
    in remission F12.21
  cocaine F14.20
    with
      anxiety disorder F14.280
      intoxication F14.229
        with
          delirium F14.221
          perceptual disturbance F14.222
        uncomplicated F14.220
      mood disorder F14.24
      other specified disorder F14.288
      psychosis F14.259
        delusions F14.250
        hallucinations F14.251
      sexual dysfunction F14.281
      sleep disorder F14.282
      unspecified disorder F14.29
      withdrawal F14.23
    in remission F14.21
    withdrawal symptoms in newborn P96.1
  counseling and surveillance Z71.51
  hallucinogen F16.20
    with
      anxiety disorder F16.280
      flashbacks F16.283
      intoxication F16.229
        with delirium F16.221
        uncomplicated F16.220
      mood disorder F16.24
      other specified disorder F16.288
      perception disorder, persisting F16.283
      psychosis F16.259
        delusions F16.250
        hallucinations F16.251
      unspecified disorder F16.29
    in remission F16.21
  in remission F19.21
  inhalant F18.20
    with
      anxiety disorder F18.280
      dementia, persisting F18.27
      intoxication F18.229
        with delirium F18.221
        uncomplicated F18.220
      mood disorder F18.24
      other specified disorder F18.288

Dependence *(Continued)*
drug NEC *(Continued)*
  inhalant *(Continued)*
    with *(Continued)*
      psychosis F18.259
        delusions F18.250
        hallucinations F18.251
      unspecified disorder F18.29
    in remission F18.21
  nicotine F17.200
    with disorder F17.209
      remission F17.201
      specified disorder NEC F17.208
      withdrawal F17.203
    chewing tobacco F17.220
      with disorder F17.229
        remission F17.221
        specified disorder NEC F17.228
        withdrawal F17.223
    cigarettes F17.210
      with disorder F17.219
        remission F17.211
        specified disorder NEC F17.218
        withdrawal F17.213
    specified product NEC F17.290
      with disorder F17.299
        remission F17.291
        specified disorder NEC F17.298
        withdrawal F17.293
  opioid F11.20
    with
      intoxication F11.229
        with
          delirium F11.221
          perceptual disturbance F11.222
        uncomplicated F11.220
      mood disorder F11.24
      other specified disorder F11.288
      psychosis F11.259
        delusions F11.250
        hallucinations F11.251
      sexual dysfunction F11.281
      sleep disorder F11.282
      unspecified disorder F11.29
      withdrawal F11.23
    in remission F11.21
  psychoactive NEC F19.20
    with
      amnestic disorder F19.26
      anxiety disorder F19.280
      dementia F19.27
      intoxication F19.229
        with
          delirium F19.221
          perceptual disturbance F19.222
        uncomplicated F19.220
      mood disorder F19.24
      other specified disorder F19.288
      psychosis F19.259
        delusions F19.250
        hallucinations F19.251
      sexual dysfunction F19.281
      sleep disorder F19.282
      unspecified disorder F19.29
      withdrawal F19.239
        with
          delirium F19.231
          perceptual disturbance F19.232
        uncomplicated F19.230
  sedative, hypnotic or anxiolytic F13.20
    with
      amnestic disorder F13.26
      anxiety disorder F13.280
      dementia, persisting F13.27
      intoxication F13.229
        with delirium F13.221
        uncomplicated F13.220
      mood disorder F13.24
      other specified disorder F13.288

Dependence *(Continued)*
drug NEC *(Continued)*
  sedative, hypnotic or anxiolytic *(Continued)*
    with *(Continued)*
      psychosis F13.259
        delusions F13.250
        hallucinations F13.251
      sexual dysfunction F13.281
      sleep disorder F13.282
      unspecified disorder F13.29
      withdrawal F13.239
        with
          delirium F13.231
          perceptual disturbance F13.232
        uncomplicated F13.230
    in remission F13.21
  stimulant NEC F15.20
    with
      anxiety disorder F15.280
      intoxication F15.229
        with
          delirium F15.221
          perceptual disturbance F15.222
        uncomplicated F15.220
      mood disorder F15.24
      other specified disorder F15.288
      psychosis F15.259
        delusions F15.250
        hallucinations F15.251
      sexual dysfunction F15.281
      sleep disorder F15.282
      unspecified disorder F15.29
      withdrawal F15.23
    in remission F15.21
  ethyl
    alcohol (without remission) F10.20
      with remission F10.21
    bromide —*see* Dependence, drug, sedative
    carbamate F19.20
    chloride F19.20
    morphine —*see* Dependence, drug, opioid
  ganja —*see* Dependence, drug, cannabis
  glue (airplane) (sniffing) —*see* Dependence, drug, inhalant
  glutethimide —*see* Dependence, drug, sedative
  hallucinogenics —*see* Dependence, drug, hallucinogen
  hashish —*see* Dependence, drug, cannabis
  hemp —*see* Dependence, drug, cannabis
  heroin (salt) (any) —*see* Dependence, drug, opioid
  hypnotic NEC —*see* Dependence, drug, sedative
  Indian hemp —*see* Dependence, drug, cannabis
  inhalants —*see* Dependence, drug, inhalant
  khat —*see* Dependence, drug, stimulant NEC
  laudanum —*see* Dependence, drug, opioid
  LSD (-25) (derivatives) —*see* Dependence, drug, hallucinogen
  luminal —*see* Dependence, drug, sedative
  lysergic acid —*see* Dependence, drug, hallucinogen
  maconha —*see* Dependence, drug, cannabis
  marihuana —*see* Dependence, drug, cannabis
  meprobamate —*see* Dependence, drug, sedative
  mescaline —*see* Dependence, drug, hallucinogen
  methadone —*see* Dependence, drug, opioid
  methamphetamine (s) —*see* Dependence, drug, stimulant NEC
  methaqualone —*see* Dependence, drug, sedative
  methyl
    alcohol (without remission) F10.20
      with remission F10.21
    bromide —*see* Dependence, drug, sedative
    morphine —*see* Dependence, drug, opioid

◀ New   ◀▥ Revised   ~~deleted~~ Deleted

Dependence *(Continued)*
 methyl *(Continued)*
  phenidate —*see* Dependence, drug,
   stimulant NEC
  sulfonal —*see* Dependence, drug, sedative
 morphine (sulfate) (sulfite) (type) —*see*
  Dependence, drug, opioid
 narcotic (drug) NEC —*see* Dependence, drug,
  opioid
 nembutal —*see* Dependence, drug, sedative
 neraval —*see* Dependence, drug, sedative
 neravan —*see* Dependence, drug, sedative
 neurobarb —*see* Dependence, drug, sedative
 nicotine —*see* Dependence, drug, nicotine
 nitrous oxide F19.20
 nonbarbiturate sedatives and tranquilizers
  with similar effect —*see* Dependence,
  drug, sedative
 on
  artificial heart (fully implantable)
   (mechanical) Z95.812
  aspirator Z99.0
  care provider (because of) Z74.9
   impaired mobility Z74.09
   need for
    assistance with personal care Z74.1
    continuous supervision Z74.3
    no other household member able to
     render care Z74.2
    specified reason NEC Z74.8
  machine Z99.89
   enabling NEC Z99.89
   specified type NEC Z99.89
  renal dialysis (hemodialysis) (peritoneal)
   Z99.2
  respirator Z99.11
  ventilator Z99.11
  wheelchair Z99.3
 opiate —*see* Dependence, drug, opioid
 opioids —*see* Dependence, drug, opioid
 opium (alkaloids) (derivatives) (tincture) —
  see Dependence, drug, opioid
 oxygen (long-term) (supplemental) Z99.81
 paraldehyde —*see* Dependence, drug,
  sedative
 paregoric —*see* Dependence, drug, opioid
 PCP (phencyclidine) (*see also* Abuse, drug,
  hallucinogen) F16.20
 pentobarbital —*see* Dependence, drug,
  sedative
 pentobarbitone (sodium) —*see* Dependence,
  drug, sedative
 pentothal —*see* Dependence, drug, sedative
 peyote —*see* Dependence, drug, hallucinogen
 phencyclidine (PCP) (and related substances)
  (*see also* Abuse, drug, hallucinogen) F16.20
 phenmetrazine —*see* Dependence, drug,
  stimulant NEC
 phenobarbital —*see* Dependence, drug,
  sedative
 polysubstance F19.20
 psilocibin, psilocin, psilocyn, psilocyline —*see*
  Dependence, drug, hallucinogen
 psychostimulant NEC —*see* Dependence,
  drug, stimulant NEC
 secobarbital —*see* Dependence, drug, sedative
 seconal —*see* Dependence, drug, sedative
 sedative NEC —*see* Dependence, drug,
  sedative
 specified drug NEC —*see* Dependence, drug
 stimulant NEC —*see* Dependence, drug,
  stimulant NEC
 substance NEC —*see* Dependence, drug
 supplemental oxygen Z99.81
 tobacco —*see* Dependence, drug, nicotine
  counseling and surveillance Z71.6
 tranquilizer NEC —*see* Dependence, drug,
  sedative
 vitamin B6 E53.1
 volatile solvents —*see* Dependence, drug,
  inhalant

Dependency
 care-provider Z74.9
 passive F60.7
 reactions (persistent) F60.7
Depersonalization (in neurotic state) (neurotic)
 (syndrome) F48.1
Depletion
 extracellular fluid E86.9
 plasma E86.1
 potassium E87.6
  nephropathy N25.89
 salt or sodium E87.1
  causing heat exhaustion or prostration
   T67.4
  nephropathy N28.9
 volume NOS E86.9
Deployment (current) (military) status Z56.82
 in theater or in support of military war,
  peacekeeping and humanitarian
  operations Z56.82
 personal history of Z91.82
  military war, peacekeeping and
   humanitarian deployment (current or
   past conflict) Z91.82
 returned from Z91.82
Depolarization, premature I49.40
 atrial I49.1
 junctional I49.2
 specified NEC I49.49
 ventricular I49.3
Deposit
 bone in Boeck's sarcoid D86.89
 calcareous, calcium —*see* Calcification
 cholesterol
  retina H35.89
  vitreous (body) (humor) —*see* Deposit,
   crystalline
 conjunctiva H11.11-
 cornea H18.00-
  argentous H18.02-
  due to metabolic disorder H18.03-
  Kayser-Fleischer ring H18.04-
  pigmentation —*see* Pigmentation, cornea
 crystalline, vitreous (body) (humor) H43.2-
 hemosiderin in old scars of cornea —*see*
  Pigmentation, cornea, stromal
 metallic in lens —*see* Cataract, specified NEC
 skin R23.8
 tooth, teeth (betel) (black) (green) (materia
  alba) (orange) (tobacco) K03.6
 urate, kidney —*see* Calculus, kidney
Depraved appetite —*see* Pica
Depressed
 HDL cholesterol E78.6
Depression (acute) (mental) F32.9
 agitated (single episode) F32.2
 anaclitic —*see* Disorder, adjustment
 anxiety F41.8
  persistent F34.1
 arches —*see also* Deformity, limb, flat foot
 atypical (single episode) F32.8
 basal metabolic rate R94.8
 bone marrow D75.89
 central nervous system R09.2
 cerebral R29.818
  newborn P91.4
 cerebrovascular I67.9
 chest wall M95.4
 climacteric (single episode) F32.8
 endogenous (without psychotic symptoms)
  F33.2
  with psychotic symptoms F33.3
 functional activity R68.89
 hysterical F44.89
 involutional (single episode) F32.8
 major F32.9
  with psychotic symptoms F32.3
  recurrent —*see* Disorder, depressive,
   recurrent
 manic-depressive —*see* Disorder, depressive,
  recurrent

Depression *(Continued)*
 masked (single episode) F32.8
 medullary G93.89
 menopausal (single episode) F32.8
 metatarsus —*see* Depression, arches
 monopolar F33.9
 nervous F34.1
 neurotic F34.1
 nose M95.0
 postnatal F53
 postpartum F53
 post-psychotic of schizophrenia F32.8
 post-schizophrenic F32.8
 psychogenic (reactive) (single episode)
  F32.9
 psychoneurotic F34.1
 psychotic (single episode) F32.3
  recurrent F33.3
 reactive (psychogenic) (single episode)
  F32.9
  psychotic (single episode) F32.3
 recurrent —*see* Disorder, depressive,
  recurrent
 respiratory center G93.89
 seasonal —*see* Disorder, depressive, recurrent
 senile F03
 severe, single episode F32.2
 situational F43.21
 skull Q67.4
 specified NEC (single episode) F32.8
 sternum M95.4
 visual field —*see* Defect, visual field
 vital (recurrent) (without psychotic
  symptoms) F33.2
  with psychotic symptoms F33.3
  single episode F32.2
Deprivation
 cultural Z60.3
 effects NOS T73.9
  specified NEC T73.8
 emotional NEC Z65.8
  affecting infant or child —*see*
   Maltreatment, child, psychological
 food T73.0
 protein —*see* Malnutrition
 sleep Z72.820
 social Z60.4
  affecting infant or child —*see*
   Maltreatment, child, psychological
 specified NEC T73.8
 vitamins —*see* Deficiency, vitamin
 water T73.1
Derangement
 ankle (internal) —*see* Derangement, joint,
  ankle
 cartilage (articular) NEC —*see* Derangement,
  joint, articular cartilage, by site
  recurrent —*see* Dislocation, recurrent
 cruciate ligament, anterior, current injury —
  see Sprain, knee, cruciate, anterior
 elbow (internal) —*see* Derangement, joint,
  elbow
 hip (joint) (internal) (old) —*see* Derangement,
  joint, hip
 joint (internal) M24.9
  ankylosis —*see* Ankylosis
  articular cartilage M24.10
   ankle M24.17-
   elbow M24.12-
   foot M24.17-
   hand M24.14-
   hip M24.15-
   knee NEC M23.9-
   loose body —*see* Loose, body
   shoulder M24.11-
   wrist M24.13-
  contracture —*see* Contraction, joint
  current injury —*see also* Dislocation
   knee, meniscus or cartilage —*see* Tear,
    meniscus

Derangement *(Continued)*
  joint *(Continued)*
    dislocation
      pathological —*see* Dislocation,
        pathological
      recurrent —*see* Dislocation, recurrent
    knee —*see* Derangement, knee
    ligament —*see* Disorder, ligament
    loose body —*see* Loose, body
    recurrent —*see* Dislocation, recurrent
    specified type NEC M24.80
      ankle M24.87-
      elbow M24.82-
      foot joint M24.87-
      hand joint M24.84-
      hip M24.85-
      shoulder M24.81-
      wrist M24.83-
    temporomandibular M26.69
  knee (recurrent) M23.9-
    ligament disruption, spontaneous
      M23.60-
      anterior cruciate M23.61-
      capsular M23.67-
      instability, chronic M23.5-
      lateral collateral M23.64-
      medial collateral M23.63-
      posterior cruciate M23.62-
    loose body M23.4-
    meniscus M23.30-
      cystic M23.00-
        lateral M23.002
          anterior horn M23.04-
          posterior horn M23.05-
          specified NEC M23.06-
        medial M23.005
          anterior horn M23.01-
          posterior horn M23.02-
          specified NEC M23.03-
      degenerate —*see* Derangement, knee,
        meniscus, specified NEC
      detached —*see* Derangement, knee,
        meniscus, specified NEC
      due to old tear or injury M23.20-
        lateral M23.20-
          anterior horn M23.24-
          posterior horn M23.25-
          specified NEC M23.26-
        medial M23.20-
          anterior horn M23.21-
          posterior horn M23.22-
          specified NEC M23.23-
      retained —*see* Derangement, knee,
        meniscus, specified NEC
      specified NEC M23.30-
        lateral M23.30-
          anterior horn M23.34-
          posterior horn M23.35-
          specified NEC M23.36-
        medial M23.30-
          anterior horn M23.31-
          posterior horn M23.32-
          specified NEC M23.33-
    old M23.8X-
    specified NEC —*see* subcategory M23.8
  low back NEC —*see* Dorsopathy, specified
    NEC
  meniscus —*see* Derangement, knee,
    meniscus
  mental —*see* Psychosis
  patella, specified NEC —*see* Disorder,
    patella, derangement NEC
  semilunar cartilage (knee) —*see*
    Derangement, knee, meniscus,
    specified NEC
  shoulder (internal) —*see* Derangement,
    joint, shoulder
Dercum's disease E88.2
Derealization (neurotic) F48.1
Dermal —*see* condition
Dermaphytid —*see* Dermatophytosis

Dermatitis (eczematous) L30.9
  ab igne L59.0
  acarine B88.0
  actinic (due to sun) L57.8
    other than from sun L59.8
  allergic —*see* Dermatitis, contact, allergic
  ambustionis, due to burn or scald —*see* Burn
  amebic A06.7
  ammonia L22
  arsenical (ingested) L27.8
  artefacta L98.1
    psychogenic F54
  atopic L20.9
    psychogenic F54
    specified NEC L20.89
  autoimmune progesterone L30.8
  berlock, berloque L56.2
  blastomycotic B40.3
  blister beetle L24.89
  bullous, bullosa L13.9
    mucosynechial, atrophic L12.1
    seasonal L30.8
    specified NEC L13.8
  calorica L59.0
    due to burn or scald —*see* Burn
  caterpillar L24.89
  cercarial B65.3
  combustionis L59.0
    due to burn or scald —*see* Burn
  congelationis T69.1
  contact (occupational) L25.9
    allergic L23.9
      due to
        adhesives L23.1
        cement L23.5
        chemical products NEC L23.5
        chromium L23.0
        cosmetics L23.2
        dander (cat) (dog) L23.81
        drugs in contact with skin L23.3
        dyes L23.4
        food in contact with skin L23.6
        hair (cat) (dog) L23.81
        insecticide L23.5
        metals L23.0
        nickel L23.0
        plants, non-food L23.7
        plastic L23.5
        rubber L23.5
        specified agent NEC L23.89
      due to
        cement L25.3
        chemical products NEC L25.3
        cosmetics L25.0
        dander (cat) (dog) L23.81
        drugs in contact with skin L25.1
        dyes L25.2
        food in contact with skin L25.4
        hair (cat) (dog) L23.81
        plants, non-food L25.5
        specified agent NEC L25.8
    irritant L24.9
      due to
        cement L25.3
        chemical products NEC L24.5
        cosmetics L24.3
        detergents L24.0
        drugs in contact with skin L24.4
        food in contact with skin L24.6
        oils and greases L24.1
        plants, non-food L24.7
        solvents L24.2
        specified agent NEC L24.89
  contusiformis L52
  diabetic —*see* E08-E13 with .620
  diaper L22
  diphtheritica A36.3
  dry skin L85.3
  due to
    acetone (contact) (irritant) L24.2
    acids (contact) (irritant) L24.5

Dermatitis *(Continued)*
  due to *(Continued)*
    adhesive (s) (allergic) (contact) (plaster)
      L23.1
      irritant L24.5
    alcohol (irritant) (skin contact) (substances in
      category T51) L24.2
      taken internally L27.8
    alkalis (contact) (irritant) L24.5
    arsenic (ingested) L27.8
    carbon disulfide (contact) (irritant) L24.2
    caustics (contact) (irritant) L24.5
    cement (contact) L25.3
    cereal (ingested) L27.2
    chemical (s) NEC L25.3
      taken internally L27.8
    chlorocompounds L24.2
    chromium (contact) (irritant) L24.81
    coffee (ingested) L27.2
    cold weather L30.8
    cosmetics (contact) L25.0
      allergic L23.2
      irritant L24.3
    cyclohexanes L24.2
    dander (cat) (dog) L23.81
    Demodex species B88.0
    Dermanyssus gallinae B88.0
    detergents (contact) (irritant) L24.0
    dichromate L24.81
    drugs and medicaments (generalized)
      (internal use) L27.0
      external —*see* Dermatitis, due to, drugs,
        in contact with skin
      in contact with skin L25.1
        allergic L23.3
        irritant L24.4
      localized skin eruption L27.1
      specified substance —*see* Table of Drugs
        and Chemicals
    dyes (contact) L25.2
      allergic L23.4
      irritant L24.89
    epidermophytosis —*see* Dermatophytosis
    esters L24.2
    external irritant NEC L24.9
    fish (ingested) L27.2
    flour (ingested) L27.2
    food (ingested) L27.2
      in contact with skin L25.4
    fruit (ingested) L27.2
    furs (allergic) (contact) L23.81
    glues —*see* Dermatitis, due to, adhesives
    glycols L24.2
    greases NEC (contact) (irritant) L24.1
    hair (cat) (dog) L23.81
    hot
      objects and materials —*see* Burn
      weather or places L59.0
    hydrocarbons L24.2
    infrared rays L59.8
    ingestion, ingested substance L27.9
      chemical NEC L27.8
      drugs and medicaments —*see*
        Dermatitis, due to, drugs
      food L27.2
      specified NEC L27.8
    insecticide in contact with skin L24.5
    internal agent L27.9
      drugs and medicaments (generalized) —
        see Dermatitis, due to, drugs
      food L27.2
    irradiation —*see* Dermatitis, due to,
      radioactive substance
    ketones L24.2
    lacquer tree (allergic) (contact) L23.7
    light (sun) NEC L57.8
      acute L56.8
      other L59.8
    Liponyssoides sanguineus B88.0
    low temperature L30.8
    meat (ingested) L27.2

Dermatitis *(Continued)*
  due to *(Continued)*
    metals, metal salts (contact) (irritant)
      L24.81
    milk (ingested) L27.2
    nickel (contact) (irritant) L24.81
    nylon (contact) (irritant) L24.5
    oils NEC (contact) (irritant) L24.1
    paint solvent (contact) (irritant) L24.2
    petroleum products (contact) (irritant)
      (substances in T52) L24.2
    plants NEC (contact) L25.5
      allergic L23.7
      irritant L24.7
    plasters (adhesive) (any) (allergic) (contact)
      L23.1
      irritant L24.5
    plastic (contact) L25.3
    preservatives (contact) —*see* Dermatitis,
      due to, chemical, in contact with
      skin
    primrose (allergic) (contact) L23.7
    primula (allergic) (contact) L23.7
    radiation L59.8
      nonionizing (chronic exposure) L57.8
      sun NEC L57.8
        acute L56.8
    radioactive substance L58.9
      acute L58.0
      chronic L58.1
    radium L58.9
      acute L58.0
      chronic L58.1
    ragweed (allergic) (contact) L23.7
    Rhus (allergic) (contact) (diversiloba)
      (radicans) (toxicodendron) (venenata)
      (verniciflua) L23.7
    rubber (contact) L24.5
    Senecio jacobaea (allergic) (contact)
      L23.7
    solvents (contact) (irritant) (substances in
      categories T52) L24.2
    specified agent NEC (contact) L25.8
      allergic L23.89
      irritant L24.89
    sunshine NEC L57.8
      acute L56.8
    tetrachlorethylene (contact) (irritant)
      L24.2
    toluene (contact) (irritant) L24.2
    turpentine (contact) L24.2
    ultraviolet rays (sun NEC) (chronic
      exposure) L57.8
      acute L56.8
    vaccine or vaccination L27.0
      specified substance —*see* Table of Drugs
        and Chemicals
    varicose veins —*see* Varix, leg, with,
      inflammation
    X-rays L58.9
      acute L58.0
      chronic L58.1
  dyshydrotic L30.1
  dysmenorrheica N94.6
  escharotica —*see* Burn
  exfoliative, exfoliativa (generalized) L26
    neonatorum L00
  eyelid —*see also* Dermatosis, eyelid
    allergic H01.119
      left H01.116
        lower H01.115
        upper H01.114
      right H01.113
        lower H01.112
        upper H01.111
    contact —*see* Dermatitis, eyelid,
      allergic
    due to
      Demodex species B88.0
      herpes (zoster) B02.39
        simplex B00.59

Dermatitis *(Continued)*
  eyelid *(Continued)*
    eczematous H01.139
      left H01.136
        lower H01.135
        upper H01.134
      right H01.133
        lower H01.132
        upper H01.131
  facta, factitia, factitial L98.1
    psychogenic F54
  flexural NEC L20.82
  friction L30.4
  fungus B36.9
    specified type NEC B36.8
  gangrenosa, gangrenous infantum
    L08.0
  harvest mite B88.0
  heat L59.0
  herpesviral, vesicular (ear) (lip) B00.1
  herpetiformis (bullous) (erythematous)
    (pustular) (vesicular) L13.0
    juvenile L12.2
    senile L12.0
  hiemalis L30.8
  hypostatic, hypostatica —*see* Varix, leg, with,
    inflammation
  infectious eczematoid L30.3
  infective L30.3
  irritant —*see* Dermatitis, contact, irritant
  Jacquet's (diaper dermatitis) L22
  Leptus B88.0
  lichenified NEC L28.0
  medicamentosa (generalized) (internal
    use) —*see* Dermatitis, due to drugs
  mite B88.0
  multiformis L13.0
    juvenile L12.2
  napkin L22
  neurotica L13.0
  nummular L30.0
  papillaris capillitii L73.0
  pellagrous E52
  perioral L71.0
  photocontact L56.2
  polymorpha dolorosa L13.0
  pruriginosa L13.0
  pruritic NEC L30.8
  psychogenic F54
  purulent L08.0
  pustular
    contagious B08.02
    subcorneal L13.1
  pyococcal L08.0
  pyogenica L08.0
  repens L40.2
  Ritter's (exfoliativa) L00
  Schamberg's L81.7
  schistosome B65.3
  seasonal bullous L30.8
  seborrheic L21.9
    infantile L21.1
    specified NEC L21.8
  sensitization NOS L23.9
  septic L08.0
  solare L57.8
  specified NEC L30.8
  stasis I87.2
    with varicose ulcer —*see* Varix, leg, with
      ulcer, with inflammation
    due to postthrombotic syndrome —*see*
      Syndrome, postthrombotic
  suppurative L08.0
  traumatic NEC L30.4
  trophoneurotica L13.0
  ultraviolet (sun) (chronic exposure) L57.8
    acute L56.8
  varicose —*see* Varix, leg, with, inflammation
  vegetans L10.1
  verrucosa B43.0
  vesicular, herpesviral B00.1

Dermatoarthritis, lipoid E78.81
Dermatochalasis, eyelid H02.839
  left H02.836
    lower H02.835
    upper H02.834
  right H02.833
    lower H02.832
    upper H02.831
Dermatofibroma (lenticulare) —*see* Neoplasm,
  skin, benign
  protuberans —*see* Neoplasm, skin, uncertain
    behavior
Dermatofibrosarcoma (pigmented)
  (protuberans) —*see* Neoplasm, skin,
  malignant
Dermatographia L50.3
Dermatolysis (exfoliativa) (congenital)
  Q82.8
  acquired L57.4
  eyelids —*see* Blepharochalasis
  palpebrarum —*see* Blepharochalasis
  senile L57.4
Dermatomegaly NEC Q82.8
Dermatomucosomyositis M33.10
  with
    myopathy M33.12
    respiratory involvement M33.11
    specified organ involvement NEC
      M33.19
Dermatomycosis B36.9
  furfuracea B36.0
  specified type NEC B36.8
Dermatomyositis (acute) (chronic) —*see also*
  Dermatopolymyositis
  in (due to) neoplastic disease (*see also*
    Neoplasm) D49.9 *[M36.0]*
Dermatoneuritis of children —*see* Poisoning,
  mercury
Dermatophilosis A48.8
Dermatophytid L30.2
Dermatophytide —*see* Dermatophytosis
Dermatophytosis (epidermophyton) (infection)
  (Microsporum) (tinea) (Trichophyton)
  B35.9
  beard B35.0
  body B35.4
  capitis B35.0
  corporis B35.4
  deep-seated B35.8
  disseminated B35.8
  foot B35.3
  granulomatous B35.8
  groin B35.6
  hand B35.2
  nail B35.1
  perianal (area) B35.6
  scalp B35.0
  specified NEC B35.8
Dermatopolymyositis M33.90
  with
    myopathy M33.92
    respiratory involvement M33.91
    specified organ involvement NEC
      M33.99
  in neoplastic disease (*see also* Neoplasm)
    D49.9 *[M36.0]*
  juvenile M33.00
    with
      myopathy M33.02
      respiratory involvement M33.01
      specified organ involvement NEC
        M33.09
  specified NEC M33.10
    myopathy M33.12
    respiratory involvement M33.11
    specified organ involvement NEC M33.19
Dermatopolyneuritis —*see* Poisoning, mercury
Dermatorrhexis Q79.6
  acquired L57.4
Dermatosclerosis —*see also* Scleroderma
  localized L94.0

Dermatosis L98.9
  Andrews' L08.89
  Bowen's —see Neoplasm, skin, in situ
  bullous L13.9
    specified NEC L13.8
  exfoliativa L26
  eyelid (noninfectious)
    dermatitis —see Dermatitis, eyelid
    discoid lupus erythematosus —see Lupus,
      erythematosus, eyelid
    xeroderma —see Xeroderma, acquired,
      eyelid
  factitial L98.1
  febrile neutrophilic L98.2
  gonococcal A54.89
  herpetiformis L13.0
    juvenile L12.2
  linear IgA L13.8
  menstrual NEC L98.8
  neutrophilic, febrile L98.2
  occupational —see Dermatitis, contact
  papulosa nigra L82.1
  pigmentary L81.9
    progressive L81.7
    Schamberg's L81.7
  psychogenic F54
  purpuric, pigmented L81.7
  pustular, subcorneal L13.1
  transient acantholytic L11.1
Dermographia, dermographism L50.3
Dermoid (cyst) —see also Neoplasm, benign,
  by site
  with malignant transformation C56-
  due to radiation (nonionizing) L57.8
Dermopathy
  infiltrative with thyrotoxicosis —see
    Thyrotoxicosis
  nephrogenic fibrosing L90.8
Dermophytosis —see Dermatophytosis
Descemetocele H18.73-
Descemet's membrane —see condition
Descending —see condition
Descensus uteri —see Prolapse, uterus
Desert
  rheumatism B38.0
  sore —see Ulcer, skin
Desertion (newborn) —see Maltreatment
Desmoid (extra-abdominal) (tumor) —see
  Neoplasm, connective tissue, uncertain
  behavior
  abdominal D48.1
Despondency F32.9
Desquamation, skin R23.4
Destruction, destructive —see also Damage
  articular facet —see also Derangement, joint,
    specified type NEC
    knee M23.8X-
    vertebra —see Spondylosis
  bone —see also Disorder, bone, specified type
    NEC
    syphilitic A52.77
  joint —see also Derangement, joint, specified
    type NEC
    sacroiliac M53.3
  rectal sphincter K62.89
  septum (nasal) J34.89
  tuberculous NEC —see Tuberculosis
  tympanum, tympanic membrane
    (nontraumatic) —see Disorder,
    tympanic membrane, specified
    NEC
  vertebral disc —see Degeneration,
    intervertebral disc
Destructiveness —see also Disorder, conduct
  adjustment reaction —see Disorder,
    adjustment
Desultory labor O62.2
Detachment
  cartilage —see Sprain
  cervix, annular N88.8
    complicating delivery O71.3

Detachment (Continued)
  choroid (old) (postinfectional) (simple)
    (spontaneous) H31.40-
    hemorrhagic H31.41-
    serous H31.42-
  ligament —see Sprain
  meniscus (knee) —see also Derangement,
    knee, meniscus, specified NEC
    current injury —see Tear, meniscus
    due to old tear or injury —see
      Derangement, knee, meniscus, due
      to old tear
  retina (without retinal break) (serous) H33.2-
    with retinal:
      break H33.00-
        giant H33.03-
        multiple H33.02-
        single H33.01-
      dialysis H33.04-
    pigment epithelium —see Degeneration,
      retina, separation of layers, pigment
      epithelium detachment
    rhegmatogenous —see Detachment, retina,
      with retinal, break
    specified NEC H33.8
    total H33.05-
    traction H33.4-
  vitreous (body) H43.81
Detergent asthma J69.8
Deterioration
  epileptic F06.8
  general physical R53.81
  heart, cardiac —see Degeneration, myocardial
  mental —see Psychosis
  myocardial, myocardium —see Degeneration,
    myocardial
  senile (simple) R54
Deuteranomaly (anomalous trichromat) H53.53
Deuteranopia (complete) (incomplete) H53.53
Development
  abnormal, bone Q79.9
  arrested R62.50
    bone —see Arrest, development or growth,
      bone
    child R62.50
    due to malnutrition E45
  defective, congenital —see also Anomaly, by
    site
    cauda equina Q06.3
    left ventricle Q24.8
      in hypoplastic left heart syndrome
        Q23.4
      valve Q24.8
        pulmonary Q22.3
  delayed (see also Delay, development) R62.50
    arithmetical skills F81.2
    language (skills) (expressive) F80.1
    learning skill F81.9
    mixed skills F88
    motor coordination F82
    reading F81.0
    specified learning skill NEC F81.89
    speech F80.9
    spelling F81.81
    written expression F81.81
  imperfect, congenital —see also Anomaly, by
    site
    heart Q24.9
    lungs Q33.6
  incomplete
    bronchial tree Q32.4
    organ or site not listed —see Hypoplasia,
      by site
    respiratory system Q34.9
  sexual, precocious NEC E30.1
  tardy, mental (see also Disability, intellectual)
    F79
Developmental —see condition
  testing, child —see Examination, child
Devergie's disease (pityriasis rubra pilaris)
  L44.0

Deviation (in)
  conjugate palsy (eye) (spastic) H51.0
  esophagus (acquired) K22.8
  eye, skew H51.8
  midline (jaw) (teeth) (dental arch) M26.29
    specified site NEC —see Malposition
  nasal septum J34.2
    congenital Q67.4
  opening and closing of the mandible M26.53
  organ or site, congenital NEC —see
    Malposition, congenital
  septum (nasal) (acquired) J34.2
    congenital Q67.4
  sexual F65.9
    bestiality F65.89
    erotomania F52.8
    exhibitionism F65.2
    fetishism, fetishistic F65.0
      transvestism F65.1
    frotteurism F65.81
    masochism F65.51
    multiple F65.89
    necrophilia F65.89
    nymphomania F52.8
    pederosis F65.4
    pedophilia F65.4
    sadism, sadomasochism F65.52
    satyriasis F52.8
    specified type NEC F65.89
    transvestism F64.1
    voyeurism F65.3
  teeth, midline M26.29
  trachea J39.8
  ureter, congenital Q62.61
Device
  cerebral ventricle (communicating) in situ
    Z98.2
  contraceptive —see Contraceptive, device
  drainage, cerebrospinal fluid, in situ Z98.2
Devic's disease G36.0
Devil's
  grip B33.0
  pinches (purpura simplex) D69.2
Devitalized tooth K04.99
Devonshire colic —see Poisoning, lead
Dextraposition, aorta Q20.3
  in tetralogy of Fallot Q21.3
Dextrinosis, limit (debrancher enzyme
  deficiency) E74.03
Dextrocardia (true) Q24.0
  with
    complete transposition of viscera Q89.3
    situs inversus Q89.3
Dextrotransposition, aorta Q20.3
d-glycericacidemia E72.59
Dhat syndrome F48.8
Dhobi itch B35.6
Di George's syndrome D82.1
Di Guglielmo's disease C94.0-
Diabetes, diabetic (mellitus) (sugar) E11.9
  with
    amyotrophy E11.44
    arthropathy NEC E11.618
    autonomic (poly)neuropathy E11.43
    cataract E11.36
    Charcot's joints E11.610
    chronic kidney disease E11.22
    circulatory complication NEC E11.59
    complication E11.8
      specified NEC E11.69
    dermatitis E11.620
    foot ulcer E11.621
    gangrene E11.52
    gastroparesis E11.43
    glomerulonephrosis, intracapillary E11.21
    glomerulosclerosis, intercapillary E11.21
    hyperglycemia E11.65
    hyperosmolarity E11.00
      with coma E11.01
    hypoglycemia E11.649
      with coma E11.641

Diabetes, diabetic *(Continued)*
  with *(Continued)*
    kidney complications NEC E11.29
    Kimmelsteil-Wilson disease E11.21
    loss of protective sensation (LOPS) —*see*
        Diabetes, by type, with neuropathy
    mononeuropathy E11.41
    myasthenia E11.44
    necrobiosis lipoidica E11.620
    nephropathy E11.21
    neuralgia E11.42
    neurologic complication NEC E11.49
    neuropathic arthropathy E11.610
    neuropathy E11.40
    ophthalmic complication NEC E11.39
    oral complication NEC E11.638
    periodontal disease E11.630
    peripheral angiopathy E11.51
      with gangrene E11.52
    polyneuropathy E11.42
    renal complication NEC E11.29
    renal tubular degeneration E11.29
    retinopathy E11.319
      with macular edema E11.311
      nonproliferative E11.329
        with macular edema E11.321
        mild E11.329
          with macular edema E11.321
        moderate E11.339
          with macular edema E11.331
        severe E11.349
          with macular edema E11.341
      proliferative E11.359
        with macular edema E11.351
    skin complication NEC E11.628
    skin ulcer NEC E11.622
  bronzed E83.110
  complicating pregnancy —*see* Pregnancy,
    complicated by, diabetes
  dietary counseling and surveillance Z71.3
  due to drug or chemical E09.9
    with
      amyotrophy E09.44
      arthropathy NEC E09.618
      autonomic (poly)neuropathy E09.43
      cataract E09.36
      Charcot's joints E09.610
      chronic kidney disease E09.22
      circulatory complication NEC E09.59
      complication E09.8
        specified NEC E09.69
      dermatitis E09.620
      foot ulcer E09.621
      gangrene E09.52
      gastroparesis E09.43
      glomerulonephrosis, intracapillary
        E09.21
      glomerulosclerosis, intercapillary E09.21
      hyperglycemia E09.65
      hyperosmolarity E09.00
        with coma E09.01
      hypoglycemia E09.649
        with coma E09.641
      ketoacidosis E09.10
        with coma E09.11
      kidney complications NEC E09.29
      Kimmelsteil-Wilson disease E09.21
      mononeuropathy E09.41
      myasthenia E09.44
      necrobiosis lipoidica E09.620
      nephropathy E09.21
      neuralgia E09.42
      neurologic complication NEC E09.49
      neuropathic arthropathy E09.610
      neuropathy E09.40
      ophthalmic complication NEC E09.39
      oral complication NEC E09.638
      periodontal disease E09.630
      peripheral angiopathy E09.51
        with gangrene E09.52
      polyneuropathy E09.42

Diabetes, diabetic *(Continued)*
  due to drug or chemical *(Continued)*
    with *(Continued)*
      renal complication NEC E09.29
      renal tubular degeneration E09.29
      retinopathy E09.319
        with macular edema E09.311
        nonproliferative E09.329
          with macular edema E09.321
          mild E09.329
            with macular edema E09.321
          moderate E09.339
            with macular edema E09.331
          severe E09.349
            with macular edema E09.341
        proliferative E09.359
          with macular edema E09.351
      skin complication NEC E09.628
      skin ulcer NEC E09.622
  due to underlying condition E08.9
    with
      amyotrophy E08.44
      arthropathy NEC E08.618
      autonomic (poly)neuropathy E08.43
      cataract E08.36
      Charcot's joints E08.610
      chronic kidney disease E08.22
      circulatory complication NEC E08.59
      complication E08.8
        specified NEC E08.69
      dermatitis E08.620
      foot ulcer E08.621
      gangrene E08.52
      gastroparesis E08.43
      glomerulonephrosis, intracapillary
        E08.21
      glomerulosclerosis, intercapillary
        E08.21
      hyperglycemia E08.69
      hyperosmolarity E08.00
        with coma E08.01
      hypoglycemia E08.649
        with coma E08.641
      ketoacidosis E08.10
        with coma E08.11
      kidney complications NEC E08.29
      Kimmelsteil-WIlson disease E08.21
      mononeuropathy E08.41
      myasthenia E08.44
      necrobiosis lipoidica E08.620
      nephropathy E08.21
      neuralgia E08.42
      neurologic complication NEC E08.49
      neuropathic arthropathy E08.610
      neuropathy E08.40
      ophthalmic complication NEC
        E08.39
      oral complication NEC E08.638
      periodontal disease E08.630
      peripheral angiopathy E08.51
        with gangrene E08.52
      polyneuropathy E08.42
      renal complication NEC E08.29
      renal tubular degeneration E08.29
      retinopathy E08.319
        with macular edema E08.311
        nonproliferative E08.329
          with macular edema E08.321
          mild E08.329
            with macular edema E08.321
          moderate E08.339
            with macular edema E08.331
          severe E08.349
            with macular edema E08.341
        proliferative E08.359
          with macular edema E08.351
      skin complication NEC E08.628
      skin ulcer NEC E08.622
  gestational (in pregnancy) O24.419
    affecting newborn P70.0
    diet-controlled O24.410

Diabetes, diabetic *(Continued)*
  gestational *(Continued)*
    in childbirth O24.429
      diet-controlled O24.420
      insulin (and diet) controlled
        O24.424
    insulin (and diet) controlled
      O24.414
    puerperal O24.439
      diet-controlled O24.430
      insulin (and diet) controlled O24.434
  hepatogenous E13.9
  inadequately controlled — code to Diabetes,
    by type, with hyperglycemia
  insipidus E23.2
    nephrogenic N25.1
    pituitary E23.2
    vasopressin resistant N25.1
  insulin dependent — code to type of
    diabetes
  juvenile-onset —*see* Diabetes, type 1
  ketosis-prone —*see* Diabetes, type 1
  latent R73.09
  neonatal (transient) P70.2
  non-insulin dependent — code to type of
    diabetes
  out of control — code to Diabetes, by type,
    with hyperglycemia
  phosphate E83.39
  poorly controlled — code to Diabetes, by
    type, with hyperglycemia
  postpancreatectomy —*see* Diabetes, specified
    type NEC
  postprocedural —*see* Diabetes, specified type
    NEC
  secondary diabetes mellitus NEC —*see*
    Diabetes, specified type NEC
  specified type NEC E13.9
    with
      amyotrophy E13.44
      arthropathy NEC E13.618
      autonomic (poly)neuropathy E13.43
      cataract E13.36
      Charcot's joints E13.610
      chronic kidney disease E13.22
      circulatory complication NEC E13.59
      complication E13.8
        specified NEC E13.69
      dermatitis E13.620
      foot ulcer E13.621
      gangrene E13.52
      gastroparesis E13.43
      glomerulonephrosis, intracapillary
        E13.21
      glomerulosclerosis, intercapillary
        E13.21
      hyperglycemia E13.65
      hyperosmolarity E13.00
        with coma E13.01
      hypoglycemia E13.649
        with coma E13.641
      ketoacidosis E13.10
        with coma E13.11
      kidney complications NEC E13.29
      Kimmelsteil-Wilson disease E13.21
      mononeuropathy E13.41
      myasthenia E13.44
      necrobiosis lipoidica E13.620
      nephropathy E13.21
      neuralgia E13.42
      neurologic complication NEC E13.49
      neuropathic arthropathy E13.610
      neuropathy E13.40
      ophthalmic complication NEC E13.39
      oral complication NEC E13.638
      periodontal disease E13.630
      peripheral angiopathy E13.51
        with gangrene E13.52
      polyneuropathy E13.42
      renal complication NEC E13.29
      renal tubular degeneration E13.29

Diabetes, diabetic (*Continued*)
  specified type NEC (*Continued*)
    with (*Continued*)
      retinopathy E13.319
        with macular edema E13.311
        nonproliferative E13.329
          with macular edema E13.321
          mild E13.329
            with macular edema E13.321
          moderate E13.339
            with macular edema E13.331
          severe E13.349
            with macular edema E13.341
        proliferative E13.359
          with macular edema E13.351
      skin complication NEC E13.628
      skin ulcer NEC E13.622
  steroid-induced —*see* Diabetes, due to, drug or chemical
  type 1 E10.9
    with
      amyotrophy E10.44
      arthropathy NEC E10.618
      autonomic (poly)neuropathy E10.43
      cataract E10.36
      Charcot's joints E10.610
      chronic kidney disease E10.22
      circulatory complication NEC E10.59
      complication E10.8
        specified NEC E10.69
      dermatitis E10.620
      foot ulcer E10.621
      gangrene E10.52
      gastroparesis E10.43
      glomerulonephrosis, intracapillary E10.21
      glomerulosclerosis, intercapillary E10.21
      hyperglycemia E10.65
      hypoglycemia E10.649
        with coma E10.641
      ketoacidosis E10.10
        with coma E10.11
      kidney complications NEC E10.29
      Kimmelstiel-Wilson disease E10.21
      mononeuropathy E10.41
      myasthenia E10.44
      necrobiosis lipoidica E10.620
      nephropathy E10.21
      neuralgia E10.42
      neurologic complication NEC E10.49
      neuropathic arthropathy E10.610
      neuropathy E10.40
      ophthalmic complication NEC E10.39
      oral complication NEC E10.638
      periodontal disease E10.630
      peripheral angiopathy E10.51
        with gangrene E10.52
      polyneuropathy E10.42
      renal complication NEC E10.29
      renal tubular degeneration E10.29
      retinopathy E10.319
        with macular edema E10.311
        nonproliferative E10.329
          with macular edema E10.321
          mild E10.329
            with macular edema E10.321
          moderate E10.339
            with macular edema E10.331
          severe E10.349
            with macular edema E10.341
        proliferative E10.359
          with macular edema E10.351
      skin complication NEC E10.628
      skin ulcer NEC E10.622
  type 2 E11.9
    with
      amyotrophy E11.44
      arthropathy NEC E11.618
      autonomic (poly)neuropathy E11.43
      cataract E11.36
      Charcot's joints E11.610

Diabetes, diabetic (*Continued*)
  type 2 (*Continued*)
    with (*Continued*)
      chronic kidney disease E11.22
      circulatory complication NEC E11.59
      complication E11.8
        specified NEC E11.69
      dermatitis E11.620
      foot ulcer E11.621
      gangrene E11.52
      gastroparesis E11.43
      glomerulonephrosis, intracapillary E11.21
      glomerulosclerosis, intercapillary E11.21
      hyperglycemia E11.65
      hyperosmolarity E11.00
        with coma E11.01
      hypoglycemia E11.649
        with coma E11.641
      kidney complications NEC E11.29
      Kimmelstiel-Wilson disease E11.21
      mononeuropathy E11.41
      myasthenia E11.44
      necrobiosis lipoidica E11.620
      nephropathy E11.21
      neuralgia E11.42
      neurologic complication NEC E11.49
      neuropathic arthropathy E11.610
      neuropathy E11.40
      ophthalmic complication NEC E11.39
      oral complication NEC E11.638
      periodontal disease E11.630
      peripheral angiopathy E11.51
        with gangrene E11.52
      polyneuropathy E11.42
      renal complication NEC E11.29
      renal tubular degeneration E11.29
      retinopathy E11.319
        with macular edema E11.311
        nonproliferative E11.329
          with macular edema E11.321
          mild E11.329
            with macular edema E11.321
          moderate E11.339
            with macular edema E11.331
          severe E11.349
            with macular edema E11.341
        proliferative E11.359
          with macular edema E11.351
      skin complication NEC E11.628
      skin ulcer NEC E11.622
Diacyclothrombopathia D69.1
Diagnosis deferred R69
Dialysis (intermittent) (treatment)
  noncompliance (with) Z91.15
  renal (hemodialysis) (peritoneal), status Z99.2
  retina, retinal —*see* Detachment, retina, with retinal, dialysis
Diamond-Blackfan anemia (congenital hypoplastic) D61.01
Diamond-Gardener syndrome (autoerythrocyte sensitization) D69.2
Diaper rash L22
Diaphoresis (excessive) R61
Diaphragm —*see* condition
Diaphragmalgia R07.1
Diaphragmatitis, diaphragmitis J98.6
Diaphysial aclasis Q78.6
Diaphysitis —*see* Osteomyelitis, specified type NEC
Diarrhea, diarrheal (disease) (infantile) (inflammatory) R19.7
  achlorhydric K31.83
  allergic K52.2
  amebic (*see also* Amebiasis) A06.0
    with abscess —*see* Abscess, amebic
    acute A06.0
    chronic A06.1
    nondysenteric A06.2
  bacillary —*see* Dysentery, bacillary
  balantidial A07.0

Diarrhea, diarrheal (*Continued*)
  cachectic NEC K52.89
  Chilomastix A07.8
  choleriformis A00.1
  chronic (noninfectious) K52.9
  coccidial A07.3
  Cochin-China K90.1
    strongyloidiasis B78.0
  Dientamoeba A07.8
  dietetic K52.2
  drug-induced K52.1
  due to
    bacteria A04.9
      specified NEC A04.8
    Campylobacter A04.5
    Capillaria philippinensis B81.1
    Clostridium difficile A04.7
    Clostridium perfringens (C) (F) A04.8
    Cryptosporidium A07.2
    drugs K52.1
    Escherichia coli A04.4
      enteroaggregative A04.4
      enterohemorrhagic A04.3
      enteroinvasive A04.2
      enteropathogenic A04.0
      enterotoxigenic A04.1
      specified NEC A04.4
    food hypersensitivity K52.2
    Necator americanus B76.1
    S. japonicum B65.2
    specified organism NEC A08.8
      bacterial A04.8
      viral A08.39
    Staphylococcus A04.8
    Trichuris trichiuria B79
    virus —*see* Enteritis, viral
    Yersinia enterocolitica A04.6
  dysenteric A09
  endemic A09
  epidemic A09
  flagellate A07.9
  Flexner's (ulcerative) A03.1
  functional K59.1
    following gastrointestinal surgery K91.89
    psychogenic F45.8
  Giardia lamblia A07.1
  giardial A07.1
  hill K90.1
  infectious A09
  malarial —*see* Malaria
  mite B88.0
  mycotic NEC B49
  neonatal (noninfectious) P78.3
  nervous F45.8
  neurogenic K59.1
  noninfectious K52.9
  postgastrectomy K91.1
  postvagotomy K91.1
  protozoal A07.9
    specified NEC A07.8
  psychogenic F45.8
  specified
    bacterium NEC A04.8
    virus NEC A08.39
  strongyloidiasis B78.0
  toxic K52.1
  trichomonal A07.8
  tropical K90.1
  tuberculous A18.32
  viral —*see* Enteritis, viral
Diastasis
  cranial bones M84.88
    congenital NEC Q75.8
  joint (traumatic) —*see* Dislocation
  muscle M62.00
    ankle M62.07-
    congenital Q79.8
    foot M62.07-
    forearm M62.03-
    hand M62.04-
    lower leg M62.06-

◀ New   ⬅ Revised   ~~deleted~~ Deleted

Diastasis *(Continued)*
  muscle *(Continued)*
    pelvic region M62.05-
    shoulder region M62.01-
    specified site NEC M62.08
    thigh M62.05-
    upper arm M62.02-
  recti (abdomen)
    complicating delivery O71.89
    congenital Q79.59
Diastema, tooth, teeth, fully erupted M26.32
Diastematomyelia Q06.2
Diataxia, cerebral G80.4
Diathesis
  allergic —*see* History, allergy
  bleeding (familial) D69.9
  cystine (familial) E72.00
  gouty —*see* Gout
  hemorrhagic (familial) D69.9
    newborn NEC P53
  spasmophilic R29.0
Diaz's disease or osteochondrosis (juvenile)
    (talus) —*see* Osteochondrosis, juvenile,
    tarsus
Dibothriocephalus, dibothriocephaliasis
    (latus) (infection) (infestation) B70.0
  larval B70.1
Dicephalus, dicephaly Q89.4
Dichotomy, teeth K00.2
Dichromat, dichromatopsia (congenital) —*see*
    Deficiency, color vision
Dichuchwa A65
Dicroceliasis B66.2
Didelphia, didelphys —*see* Double uterus
Didymytis N45.1
  with orchitis N45.3
Dietary
  inadequacy or deficiency E63.9
  surveillance and counseling Z71.3
Dietl's crisis N13.8
Dieulafoy lesion (hemorrhagic)
  duodenum K31.82
  esophagus K22.8
  intestine (colon) K63.81
  stomach K31.82
Difficult, difficulty (in)
  acculturation Z60.3
  feeding R63.3
    newborn P92.9
      breast P92.5
      specified NEC P92.8
    nonorganic (infant or child) F98.29
  intubation, in anesthesia T88.4
  mechanical, gastroduodenal stoma K91.89
    causing obstruction K91.3
  reading (developmental) F81.0
    secondary to emotional disorders F93.9
  spelling (specific) F81.81
    with reading disorder F81.89
    due to inadequate teaching Z55.8
  swallowing —*see* Dysphagia
  walking R26.2
  work
    conditions NEC Z56.5
    schedule Z56.3
Diffuse —*see* condition
DiGeorge's syndrome (thymic hypoplasia)
    D82.1
Digestive —*see* condition
Dihydropyrimidine dehydrogenase disease
    (DPD) E88.89
Diktyoma —*see* Neoplasm, malignant, by site
Dilaceration, tooth K00.4
Dilatation
  anus K59.8
    venule —*see* Hemorrhoids
  aorta (focal) (general) —*see* Ectasia, aorta
    with aneurysm —*see* Aneurysm, aorta
  artery —*see* Aneurysm
  bladder (sphincter) N32.89
    congenital Q64.79

Dilatation *(Continued)*
  blood vessel I99.8
  bronchial J47.9
    with
      exacerbation (acute) J47.1
      lower respiratory infection J47.0
  calyx (due to obstruction) —*see*
      Hydronephrosis
  capillaries I78.8
  cardiac (acute) (chronic) —*see also*
      Hypertrophy, cardiac
    congenital Q24.8
    valve NEC Q24.8
      pulmonary Q22.3
    valve —*see* Endocarditis
  cavum septi pellucidi Q06.8
  cervix (uteri) —*see also* Incompetency,
      cervix
    incomplete, poor, slow complicating
        delivery O62.0
  colon K59.3
    congenital Q43.1
    psychogenic F45.8
  common duct (acquired) K83.8
    congenital Q44.5
  cystic duct (acquired) K82.8
    congenital Q44.5
  duct, mammary —*see* Ectasia, mammary
      duct
  duodenum K59.8
  esophagus K22.8
    congenital Q39.5
    due to achalasia K22.0
  eustachian tube, congenital Q17.8
  gallbladder K82.8
  gastric —*see* Dilatation, stomach
  heart (acute) (chronic) —*see also* Hypertrophy,
      cardiac
    congenital Q24.8
    valve —*see* Endocarditis
  ileum K59.8
    psychogenic F45.8
  jejunum K59.8
    psychogenic F45.8
  kidney (calyx) (collecting structures) (cystic)
      (parenchyma) (pelvis) (idiopathic)
      N28.89
  lacrimal passages or duct —*see* Disorder,
      lacrimal system, changes
  lymphatic vessel I89.0
  mammary duct —*see* Ectasia, mammary
      duct
  Meckel's diverticulum (congenital) Q43.0
    malignant —*see* Table of Neoplasms, small
        intestine, malignant
  myocardium (acute) (chronic) —*see*
      Hypertrophy, cardiac organ or site,
      congenital NEC —*see* Distortion
  pancreatic duct K86.8
  pericardium —*see* Pericarditis
  pharynx J39.2
  prostate N42.89
  pulmonary
    artery (idiopathic) I28.8
    valve, congenital Q22.3
  pupil H57.04
  rectum K59.3
  saccule, congenital Q16.5
  salivary gland (duct) K11.8
  sphincter ani K62.89
  stomach K31.89
    acute K31.0
    psychogenic F45.8
  submaxillary duct K11.8
  trachea, congenital Q32.1
  ureter (idiopathic) N28.82
    congenital Q62.2
    due to obstruction N13.4
  urethra (acquired) N36.8
  vasomotor I73.9
  vein I86.8

Dilatation *(Continued)*
  ventricular, ventricle (acute) (chronic) —*see
      also* Hypertrophy, cardiac
    cerebral, congenital Q04.8
  venule NEC I86.8
  vesical orifice N32.89
Dilated, dilation —*see* Dilatation
Diminished, diminution
  hearing (acuity) —*see* Deafness
  sense or sensation (cold) (heat) (tactile)
      (vibratory) R20.8
  vision NEC H54.7
  vital capacity R94.2
Diminuta taenia B71.0
Dimitri-Sturge-Weber disease Q85.8
Dimple
  parasacral, pilonidal or postanal —*see* Cyst,
      pilonidal
Dioctophyme renalis (infection) (infestation)
    B83.8
Dipetalonemiasis B74.4
Diphallus Q55.69
Diphtheria, diphtheritic (gangrenous)
    (hemorrhagic) A36.9
  carrier (suspected) Z22.2
  cutaneous A36.3
  faucial A36.0
  infection of wound A36.3
  laryngeal A36.2
  myocarditis A36.81
  nasal, anterior A36.89
  nasopharyngeal A36.1
  neurological complication A36.89
  pharyngeal A36.0
  specified site NEC A36.89
  tonsillar A36.0
Diphyllobothriasis (intestine) B70.0
  larval B70.1
Diplacusis H93.22-
Diplegia (upper limbs) G83.0
  congenital (cerebral) G80.8
  facial G51.0
  lower limbs G82.20
  spastic G80.1
Diplococcus, diplococcal —*see* condition
Diplopia H53.2
Dipsomania F10.20
  with
    psychosis —*see* Psychosis, alcoholic
    remission F10.21
Dipylidiasis B71.1
Direction, teeth, abnormal, fully erupted
    M26.30
Dirofilariasis B74.8
Dirt-eating child F98.3
Disability, disabilities
  heart —*see* Disease, heart
  intellectual F79
    with
      autistic features F84.9
    mild (I.Q. 50-69) F70
    moderate (I.Q. 35-49) F71
    profound (I.Q. under 20) F73
    severe (I.Q. 20-34) F72
    specified level NEC F78
  knowledge acquisition F81.9
  learning F81.9
  limiting activities Z73.6
  spelling, specific F81.81
Disappearance of family member Z63.4
Disarticulation —*see* Amputation
  meaning traumatic amputation —*see*
      Amputation, traumatic
Discharge (from)
  abnormal finding in —*see* Abnormal,
      specimen
  breast (female) (male) N64.52
  diencephalic autonomic idiopathic —*see*
      Epilepsy, specified NEC
  ear —*see also* Otorrhea
    blood —*see* Otorrhagia

Discharge *(Continued)*
excessive urine R35.8
nipple N64.52
penile R36.9
postnasal R09.82
prison, anxiety concerning Z65.2
urethral R36.9
without blood R36.0
hematospermia R36.1
vaginal N89.8
Discitis, diskitis M46.40
cervical region M46.42
cervicothoracic region M46.43
lumbar region M46.46
lumbosacral region M46.47
multiple sites M46.49
occipito-atlanto-axial region M46.41
pyogenic —*see* Infection, intervertebral
disc, pyogenic
sacrococcygeal region M46.48
thoracic region M46.44
thoracolumbar region M46.45
Discoid
meniscus (congenital) Q68.6
semilunar cartilage (congenital) —*see*
Derangement, knee, meniscus,
specified NEC
Discoloration
nails L60.8
teeth (posteruptive) K03.7
during formation K00.8
Discomfort
chest R07.89
visual H53.14-
Discontinuity, ossicles, ear
H74.2-
Discord (with)
boss Z56.4
classmates Z55.4
counselor Z64.4
employer Z56.4
family Z63.8
fellow employees Z56.4
in-laws Z63.1
landlord Z59.2
lodgers Z59.2
neighbors Z59.2
probation officer Z64.4
social worker Z64.4
teachers Z55.4
workmates Z56.4
Discordant connection
atrioventricular (congenital) Q20.5
ventriculoarterial Q20.3
Discrepancy
centric occlusion maximum intercuspation
M26.55
leg length (acquired) —*see* Deformity, limb,
unequal length
congenital —*see* Defect, reduction, lower
limb
uterine size date O26.84-
Discrimination
ethnic Z60.5
political Z60.5
racial Z60.5
religious Z60.5
sex Z60.5
Disease, diseased —*see also* Syndrome
absorbent system I87.8
acid-peptic K30
Acosta's T70.29
Adams-Stokes (-Morgagni) (syncope with
heart block) I45.9
Addison's anemia (pernicious) D51.0
adenoids (and tonsils) J35.9
adrenal (capsule) (cortex) (gland) (medullary)
E27.9
hyperfunction E27.0
specified NEC E27.8
ainhum L94.6

Disease, diseased *(Continued)*
airway
obstructive, chronic J44.9
due to
cotton dust J66.0
specific organic dusts NEC J66.8
reactive —*see* Asthma
akamushi (scrub typhus) A75.3
Albers-Schönberg (marble bones) Q78.2
Albert's —*see* Tendinitis, Achilles
alimentary canal K63.9
alligator-skin Q80.9
acquired L85.0
alpha heavy chain C88.3
alpine T70.29
altitude T70.20
alveolar ridge
edentulous K06.9
specified NEC K06.8
alveoli, teeth K08.9
Alzheimer's G30.9 *[F02.80]*
with behavioral disturbance G30.9
[F02.81]
early onset G30.0 *[F02.80]*
with behavioral disturbance G30.0
[F02.81]
late onset G30.1 *[F02.80]*
with behavioral disturbance G30.1
[F02.81]
specified NEC G30.8 *[F02.80]*
with behavioral disturbance G30.8
[F02.81]
amyloid —*see* Amyloidosis
Andersen's (glycogenosis IV) E74.09
Andes T70.29
Andrews' (bacterid) L08.89
angiospastic I73.9
cerebral G45.9
vein I87.8
anterior
chamber H21.9
horn cell G12.29
antiglomerular basement membrane
(anti-GBM) antibody M31.0
tubulo-interstitial nephritis N12
antral —*see* Sinusitis, maxillary
anus K62.9
specified NEC K62.89
aorta (nonsyphilitic) I77.9
syphilitic NEC A52.02
aortic (heart) (valve) I35.9
rheumatic I06.9
Apollo B30.3
aponeuroses —*see* Enthesopathy
appendix K38.9
specified NEC K38.8
aqueous (chamber) H21.9
Arnold-Chiari —*see* Arnold-Chiari disease
arterial I77.9
occlusive —*see* Occlusion, by site
due to stricture or stenosis I77.1
arteriocardiorenal —*see* Hypertension,
cardiorenal
arteriolar (generalized) (obliterative)
I77.9
arteriorenal —*see* Hypertension, kidney
arteriosclerotic —*see also* Arteriosclerosis
cardiovascular —*see* Disease, heart,
ischemic, atherosclerotic
coronary (artery) —*see* Disease, heart,
ischemic, atherosclerotic
heart —*see* Disease, heart, ischemic,
atherosclerotic
artery I77.9
cerebral I67.9
coronary I25.10
with angina pectoris —*see*
Arteriosclerosis, coronary
(artery),
arthropod-borne NOS (viral) A94
specified type NEC A93.8

Disease, diseased *(Continued)*
atticoantral, chronic H66.20
left H66.22
with right H66.23
right H66.21
with left H66.23
auditory canal —*see* Disorder, ear, external
auricle, ear NEC —*see* Disorder, pinna
Australian X A83.4
autoimmune (systemic) NOS M35.9
hemolytic (cold type) (warm type) D59.1
drug-induced D59.0
thyroid E06.3
aviator's —*see* Effect, adverse, high altitude
Ayala's Q78.5
Ayerza's (pulmonary artery sclerosis with
pulmonary hypertension) I27.0
Babington's (familial hemorrhagic
telangiectasia) I78.0
bacterial A49.9
specified NEC A48.8
zoonotic A28.9
specified type NEC A28.8
Baelz's (cheilitis glandularis apostematosa)
K13.0
bagasse J67.1
balloon —*see* Effect, adverse, high altitude
Bang's (brucella abortus) A23.1
Bannister's T78.3
barometer makers' —*see* Poisoning, mercury
Barraquer (-Simons') (progressive
lipodystrophy) E88.1
Barrett's —*see* Barrett's, esophagus
Bartholin's gland N75.9
basal ganglia G25.9
degenerative G23.9
specified NEC G23.8
specified NEC G25.89
Basedow's (exophthalmic goiter) —*see*
Hyperthyroidism, with, goiter (diffuse)
Bateman's B08.1
Batten-Steinert G71.11
Battey A31.0
Beard's (neurasthenia) F48.8
Becker
idiopathic mural endomyocardial I42.3
myotonia congenita G71.12
Begbie's (exophthalmic goiter) —*see*
Hyperthyroidism, with, goiter (diffuse)
behavioral, organic F07.9
Beigel's (white piedra) B36.2
Benson's —*see* Deposit, crystalline
Bernard-Soulier (thrombopathy) D69.1
Bernhardt (-Roth) —*see* Mononeuropathy,
lower limb, meralgia paresthetica
Biermer's (pernicious anemia) D51.0
bile duct (common) (hepatic) K83.9
with calculus, stones —*see* Calculus, bile
duct
specified NEC K83.8
biliary (tract) K83.9
specified NEC K83.8
Billroth's —*see* Spina bifida
bird fancier's J67.2
black lung J60
bladder N32.9
in (due to)
schistosomiasis (bilharziasis) B65.0 *[N33]*
specified NEC N32.89
bleeder's D66
blood D75.9
forming organs D75.9
vessel I99.9
Bloodgood's —*see* Mastopathy, cystic
Bodechtel-Guttmann (subacute sclerosing
panencephalitis) A81.1
bone —*see also* Disorder, bone
aluminum M83.4
fibrocystic NEC
jaw M27.49
bone-marrow D75.9

◀ New   ◀▦ Revised   ~~deleted~~ Deleted

Disease, diseased *(Continued)*
  Borna A83.9
  Bornholm (epidemic pleurodynia) B33.0
  Bouchard's (myopathic dilatation of the
      stomach) K31.0
  Bouillaud's (rheumatic heart disease) I01.9
  Bourneville (-Brissaud) (tuberous sclerosis)
      Q85.1
  Bouveret (-Hoffmann) (paroxysmal
      tachycardia) I47.9
  bowel K63.9
    functional K59.9
      psychogenic F45.8
  brain G93.9
    arterial, artery I67.9
    arteriosclerotic I67.2
    congenital Q04.9
    degenerative —*see* Degeneration, brain
    inflammatory —*see* Encephalitis
    organic G93.9
      arteriosclerotic I67.2
    parasitic NEC B71.9 *[G94]*
    senile NEC G31.1
    specified NEC G93.89
  breast *(see also* Disorder, breast*)* N64.9
    cystic (chronic) —*see* Mastopathy, cystic
    fibrocystic —*see* Mastopathy, cystic
    Paget's
      female, unspecified side C50.91-
      male, unspecified side C50.92-
    specified NEC N64.89
  Breda's —*see* Yaws
  Bretonneau's (diphtheritic malignant angina)
      A36.0
  Bright's —*see* Nephritis
    arteriosclerotic —*see* Hypertension, kidney
  Brill's (recrudescent typhus) A75.1
  Brill-Zinsser (recrudescent typhus) A75.1
  Brion-Kayser —*see* Fever, paratyphoid
  broad
    beta E78.2
    ligament (noninflammatory) N83.9
      inflammatory —*see* Disease, pelvis,
          inflammatory
      specified NEC N83.8
  Brocq-Duhring (dermatitis herpetiformis)
      L13.0
  Brocq's
    meaning
      dermatitis herpetiformis L13.0
      prurigo L28.2
  bronchopulmonary J98.4
  bronchus NEC J98.09
  bronze Addison's E27.1
    tuberculous A18.7
  budgerigar fancier's J67.2
  Buerger's (thromboangiitis obliterans)
      I73.1
  bullous L13.9
    chronic of childhood L12.2
    specified NEC L13.8
  Bürger-Grütz (essential familial
      hyperlipemia) E78.3
  bursa —*see* Bursopathy
  caisson T70.3
  California —*see* Coccidioidomycosis
  capillaries I78.9
    specified NEC I78.8
  Carapata A68.0
  cardiac —*see* Disease, heart
  cardiopulmonary, chronic I27.9
  cardiorenal (hepatic) (hypertensive)
      (vascular) —*see* Hypertension,
      cardiorenal
  cardiovascular (atherosclerotic) I25.10
    with angina pectoris —*see* Arteriosclerosis,
        coronary (artery),
    congenital Q28.9
    hypertensive —*see* Hypertension, heart
    newborn P29.9
      specified NEC P29.89

Disease, diseased *(Continued)*
  cardiovascular *(Continued)*
    renal (hypertensive) —*see* Hypertension,
        cardiorenal
    syphilitic (asymptomatic) A52.00
  cartilage —*see* Disorder, cartilage
  Castellani's A69.8
  cat-scratch A28.1
  Cavare's (familial periodic paralysis)
      G72.3
  cecum K63.9
  celiac (adult) (infantile) K90.0
  cellular tissue L98.9
  central core G71.2
  cerebellar, cerebellum —*see* Disease, brain
  cerebral —*see also* Disease, brain
    degenerative —*see* Degeneration, brain
  cerebrospinal G96.9
  cerebrovascular I67.9
    acute I67.89
      embolic I63.4-
      thrombotic I63.3-
    arteriosclerotic I67.2
    specified NEC I67.89
  cervix (uteri) (noninflammatory) N88.9
    inflammatory —*see* Cervicitis
    specified NEC N88.8
  Chabert's A22.9
  Chandler's (osteochondritis dissecans, hip) —
      see Osteochondritis, dissecans, hip
  Charlouis —*see* Yaws
  Chédiak-Steinbrinck (-Higashi) (congenital
      gigantism of peroxidase granules)
      E70.330
  chest J98.9
  Chiari's (hepatic vein thrombosis) I82.0
  Chicago B40.9
  Chignon B36.8
  chigo, chigoe B88.1
  childhood granulomatous D71
  Chinese liver fluke B66.1
  chlamydial A74.9
    specified NEC A74.89
  cholecystic K82.9
  choroid H31.9
    specified NEC H31.8
  Christmas D67
  chronic bullous of childhood L12.2
  chylomicron retention E78.3
  ciliary body H21.9
    specified NEC H21.89
  circulatory (system) NEC I99.8
    newborn P29.9
    syphilitic A52.00
      congenital A50.54
  coagulation factor deficiency (congenital) —
      see Defect, coagulation
  coccidioidal —*see* Coccidioidomycosis
  cold
    agglutinin or hemoglobinuria D59.1
      paroxysmal D59.6
    hemagglutinin (chronic) D59.1
  collagen NOS (nonvascular) (vascular)
      M35.9
    specified NEC M35.8
  colon K63.9
    functional K59.9
      congenital Q43.2
    ischemic K55.0
  combined system —*see* Degeneration,
      combined
  compressed air T70.3
  Concato's (pericardial polyserositis)
      A19.9
    nontubercular I31.1
    pleural —*see* Pleurisy, with effusion
  conjunctiva H11.9
    chlamydial A74.0
    specified NEC H11.89
    viral B30.9
      specified NEC B30.8

Disease, diseased *(Continued)*
  connective tissue, systemic (diffuse) M35.9
    in (due to)
      hypogammaglobulinemia D80.1 *[M36.8]*
      ochronosis E70.29 *[M36.8]*
    specified NEC M35.8
  Conor and Bruch's (boutonneuse fever) A77.1
  Cooper's —*see* Mastopathy, cystic
  Cori's (glycogenosis III) E74.03
  corkhandler's or corkworker's J67.3
  cornea H18.9
    specified NEC H18.89-
  coronary (artery) —*see* Disease, heart,
      ischemic, atherosclerotic
    congenital Q24.5
    ostial, syphilitic (aortic) (mitral)
        (pulmonary) A52.03
  corpus cavernosum N48.9
    specified NEC N48.89
  Cotugno's —*see* Sciatica
  coxsackie (virus) NEC B34.1
  cranial nerve NOS G52.9
  Creutzfeldt-Jakob —*see* Creutzfeldt- Jakob
      disease or syndrome
  Crocq's (acrocyanosis) I73.89
  Crohn's —*see* Enteritis, regional
  Curschmann G71.11
  cystic
    breast (chronic) —*see* Mastopathy, cystic
    kidney, congenital Q61.9
    liver, congenital Q44.6
    lung J98.4
      congenital Q33.0
  cytomegalic inclusion (generalized) B25.9
    with pneumonia B25.0
    congenital P35.1
  cytomegaloviral B25.9
    specified NEC B25.8
  Czerny's (periodic hydrarthrosis of the
      knee) —*see* Effusion, joint, knee
  Daae (-Finsen) (epidemic pleurodynia) B33.0
  Darling's —*see* Histoplasmosis capsulati
  Débove's (splenomegaly) R16.1
  deer fly —*see* Tularemia
  Degos' I77.8
  demyelinating, demyelinizating (nervous
      system) G37.9
    multiple sclerosis G35
    specified NEC G37.8
  dense deposit *(see also* N00-N07 with fourth
      character .6) N05.6
  deposition, hydroxyapatite —*see* Disease,
      hydroxyapatite deposition
  de Quervain's (tendon sheath) M65.4
    thyroid (subacute granulomatous
        thyroiditis) E06.1
  Devergie's (pityriasis rubra pilaris) L44.0
  Devic's G36.0
  diaphorase deficiency D74.0
  diaphragm J98.6
  diarrheal, infectious NEC A09
  digestive system K92.9
    specified NEC K92.89
  disc, degenerative —*see* Degeneration,
      intervertebral disc
  discogenic —*see also* Displacement,
      intervertebral disc NEC
    with myelopathy —*see* Disorder, disc, with,
        myelopathy
  diverticular —*see* Diverticula
  Dubois (thymus) A50.59 *[E35]*
  Duchenne-Griesinger G71.0
  Duchenne's
    muscular dystrophy G71.0
    pseudohypertrophy, muscles G71.0
  ductless glands E34.9
  Duhring's (dermatitis herpetiformis) L13.0
  duodenum K31.9
    specified NEC K31.89
  Dupré's (meningism) R29.1
  Dupuytren's (muscle contracture) M72.0

Disease, diseased *(Continued)*
Durand-Nicholas-Favre (climatic bubo) A55
Duroziez's (congenital mitral stenosis) Q23.2
ear —*see* Disorder, ear
Eberth's —*see* Fever, typhoid
Ebola (virus) A98.4
Ebstein's heart Q22.5
Echinococcus —*see* Echinococcus
echovirus NEC B34.1
Eddowes' (brittle bones and blue sclera) Q78.0
edentulous (alveolar) ridge K06.9
  specified NEC K06.8
Edsall's T67.2
Eichstedt's (pityriasis versicolor) B36.0
Ellis-van Creveld (chondroectodermal dysplasia) Q77.6
end stage renal (ESRD) N18.6
  due to hypertension I12.0
endocrine glands or system NEC E34.9
endomyocardial (eosinophilic) I42.3
English (rickets) E55.0
enteroviral, enterovirus NEC B34.1
  central nervous system NEC A88.8
epidemic B99.9
  specified NEC B99.8
epididymis N50.9
Erb (-Landouzy) G71.0
Erdheim-Chester (ECD) E88.89
esophagus K22.9
  functional K22.4
  psychogenic F45.8
  specified NEC K22.8
Eulenburg's (congenital paramyotonia) G71.19
eustachian tube —*see* Disorder, eustachian tube
external
  auditory canal —*see* Disorder, ear, external
  ear —*see* Disorder, ear, external
extrapyramidal G25.9
  specified NEC G25.89
eye H57.9
  anterior chamber H21.9
  inflammatory NEC H57.8
  muscle (external) —*see* Strabismus
  specified NEC H57.8
  syphilitic —*see* Oculopathy, syphilitic
eyeball H44.9
  specified NEC H44.89
eyelid —*see* Disorder, eyelid
  specified NEC —*see* Disorder, eyelid, specified type NEC
eyeworm of Africa B74.3
facial nerve (seventh) G51.9
  newborn (birth injury) P11.3
Fahr (of brain) G23.8
Fahr Volhard (of kidney) I12.-
fallopian tube (noninflammatory) N83.9
  inflammatory —*see* Salpingo-oophoritis
  specified NEC N83.8
familial periodic paralysis G72.3
Fanconi's (congenital pancytopenia) D61.09
fascia NEC —*see also* Disorder, muscle
  inflammatory —*see* Myositis
  specified NEC M62.89
Fauchard's (periodontitis) —*see* Periodontitis
Favre-Durand-Nicolas (climatic bubo) A55
Fede's K14.0
Feer's —*see* Poisoning, mercury
female pelvic inflammatory (*see also* Disease, pelvis, inflammatory) N73.9
  syphilitic (secondary) A51.42
  tuberculous A18.17
Fernels' (aortic aneurysm) I71.9
fibrocaseous of lung —*see* Tuberculosis, pulmonary
fibrocystic —*see* Fibrocystic disease
Fiedler's (leptospiral jaundice) A27.0
fifth B08.3
file-cutter's —*see* Poisoning, lead

Disease, diseased *(Continued)*
fish-skin Q80.9
  acquired L85.0
Flajani (-Basedow) (exophthalmic goiter) — *see* Hyperthyroidism, with, goiter (diffuse)
flax-dresser's J66.1
fluke —*see* Infestation, fluke
foot and mouth B08.8
foot process N04.9
Forbes' (glycogenosis III) E74.03
Fordyce-Fox (apocrine miliaria) L75.2
Fordyce's (ectopic sebaceous glands) (mouth) Q38.6
Forestier's (rhizomelic pseudopolyarthritis) M35.3
  meaning ankylosing hyperostosis —*see* Hyperostosis, ankylosing
Fothergill's
  neuralgia —*see* Neuralgia, trigeminal
  scarlatina anginosa A38.9
Fournier (gangrene) N49.3
  female N76.89
fourth B08.8
Fox (-Fordyce) (apocrine miliaria) L75.2
Francis' —*see* Tularemia
Franklin C88.2
Frei's (climatic bubo) A55
Friedreich's
  combined systemic or ataxia G11.1
  myoclonia G25.3
frontal sinus —*see* Sinusitis, frontal
fungus NEC B49
Gaisböck's (polycythemia hypertonica) D75.1
gallbladder K82.9
  calculus —*see* Calculus, gallbladder
  cholecystitis —*see* Cholecystitis
  cholesterolosis K82.4
  fistula —*see* Fistula, gallbladder
  hydrops K82.1
  obstruction —*see* Obstruction, gallbladder
  perforation K82.2
  specified NEC K82.8
gamma heavy chain C88.2
Gamna's (siderotic splenomegaly) D73.2
Gamstorp's (adynamia episodica hereditaria) G72.3
Gandy-Nanta (siderotic splenomegaly) D73.2
ganister J62.8
gastric —*see* Disease, stomach
gastroesophageal reflux (GERD) K21.9
  with esophagitis K21.0
gastrointestinal (tract) K92.9
  amyloid E85.4
  functional K59.9
    psychogenic F45.8
  specified NEC K92.89
Gee (-Herter) (-Heubner) (-Thaysen) (nontropical sprue) K90.0
genital organs
  female N94.9
  male N50.9
Gerhardt's (erythromelalgia) I73.81
Gibert's (pityriasis rosea) L42
Gierke's (glycogenosis I) E74.01
Gilles de la Tourette's (motor-verbal tic) F95.2
gingiva K06.9
  specified NEC K06.8
gland (lymph) I89.9
Glanzmann's (hereditary hemorrhagic thrombasthenia) D69.1
glass-blower's (cataract) —*see* Cataract, specified NEC
salivary gland hypertrophy K11.1
Glisson's —*see* Rickets
globe H44.9
  specified NEC H44.89
glomerular —*see also* Glomerulonephritis
  with edema —*see* Nephrosis
  acute —*see* Nephritis, acute
  chronic —*see* Nephritis, chronic

Disease, diseased *(Continued)*
glomerular *(Continued)*
  minimal change N05.0
  rapidly progressive N01.9
glycogen storage E74.00
  Andersen's E74.09
  Cori's E74.03
  Forbes' E74.03
  generalized E74.00
  glucose-6-phosphatase deficiency E74.01
  heart E74.02 *[143]*
  hepatorenal E74.09
  Hers' E74.09
  liver and kidney E74.09
  McArdle's E74.04
  muscle phosphofructokinase E74.09
  myocardium E74.02 *[143]*
  Pompe's E74.02
  Tauri's E74.09
  type 0 E74.09
  type I E74.01
  type II E74.02
  type III E74.03
  type IV E74.09
  type V E74.04
  type VI-XI E74.09
  Von Gierke's E74.01
Goldstein's (familial hemorrhagic telangiectasia) I78.0
gonococcal NOS A54.9
graft-versus-host (GVH) D89.813
  acute D89.810
  acute on chronic D89.812
  chronic D89.811
grainhandler's J67.8
granulomatous (childhood) (chronic) D71
Graves' (exophthalmic goiter) —*see* Hyperthyroidism, with, goiter (diffuse)
Griesinger's —*see* Ancylostomiasis
Grisel's M43.6
Gruby's (tinea tonsurans) B35.0
Guillain-Barré G61.0
Guinon's (motor-verbal tic) F95.2
gum K06.9
gynecological N94.9
H (Hartnup's) E72.02
Haff —*see* Poisoning, mercury
Hageman (congenital factor XII deficiency) D68.2
hair (color) (shaft) L67.9
  follicles L73.9
  specified NEC L73.8
Hamman's (spontaneous mediastinal emphysema) J98.2
hand, foot and mouth B08.4
Hansen's —*see* Leprosy
Hantavirus, with pulmonary manifestations B33.4
  with renal manifestations A98.5
Harada's H30.81-
Hartnup (pellagra-cerebellar ataxia-renal aminoaciduria) E72.02
Hart's (pellagra-cerebellar ataxia-renal aminoaciduria) E72.02
Hashimoto's (struma lymphomatosa) E06.3
Hb —*see* Disease, hemoglobin
heart (organic) I51.9
  with
    pulmonary edema (acute) (*see also* Failure, ventricular, left) I50.1
    rheumatic fever (conditions in I00)
      active I01.9
        with chorea I02.0
        specified NEC I01.8
      inactive or quiescent (with chorea) I09.9
        specified NEC I09.89
  amyloid E85.4 *[143]*
  aortic (valve) I35.9

◀ New   ◀▥ Revised   ~~deleted~~ Deleted

Disease, diseased (Continued)
  heart (Continued)
    arteriosclerotic or sclerotic (senile) —
        see Disease, heart, ischemic,
        atherosclerotic
    artery, arterial —see Disease, heart,
        ischemic, atherosclerotic
    beer drinkers' I42.6
    beriberi (wet) E51.12
    black I27.0
    congenital Q24.9
      cyanotic Q24.9
      specified NEC Q24.8
    coronary —see Disease, heart, ischemic
    cryptogenic I51.9
    fibroid —see Myocarditis
    functional I51.89
      psychogenic F45.8
    glycogen storage E74.02 [I43]
    gonococcal A54.83
    hypertensive —see Hypertension, heart
    hyperthyroid (see also Hyperthyroidism)
        E05.90 [I43]
      with thyroid storm E05.91 [I43]
    ischemic (chronic or with a stated duration
        of over 4 weeks) I25.9
      atherosclerotic (of) I25.10
        with angina pectoris —see
            Arteriosclerosis, coronary
            (artery)
        coronary artery bypass graft —see
            Arteriosclerosis, coronary
            (artery),
      cardiomyopathy I25.5
      diagnosed on ECG or other special
          investigation, but currently
          presenting no symptoms I25.6
      silent I25.6
      specified form NEC I25.89
    kyphoscoliotic I27.1
    meningococcal A39.50
      endocarditis A39.51
      myocarditis A39.52
      pericarditis A39.53
    mitral I05.9
      specified NEC I05.8
    muscular —see Degeneration,
        myocardial
    psychogenic (functional) F45.8
    pulmonary (chronic) I27.9
      in schistosomiasis B65.9 [I52]
      specified NEC I27.89
    rheumatic (chronic) (inactive) (old)
        (quiescent) (with chorea) I09.9
      active or acute I01.9
        with chorea (acute) (rheumatic)
            (Sydenham's) I02.0
      specified NEC I09.89
    senile —see Myocarditis
    syphilitic A52.06
      aortic A52.03
        aneurysm A52.01
      congenital A50.54 [I52]
    thyrotoxic (see also Thyrotoxicosis) E05.90
        [I43]
      with thyroid storm E05.91 [I43]
    valve, valvular (obstructive)
        (regurgitant) —see also Endocarditis
      congenital NEC Q24.8
        pulmonary Q22.3
    vascular —see Disease, cardiovascular
  heavy chain NEC C88.2
    alpha C88.3
    gamma C88.2
    mu C88.2
  Hebra's
    pityriasis
      maculata et circinata L42
      rubra pilaris L44.0
    prurigo L28.2
  hematopoietic organs D75.9

Disease, diseased (Continued)
  hemoglobin or Hb
    abnormal (mixed) NEC D58.2
      with thalassemia D56.9
    AS genotype D57.3
    Bart's D56.0
    C (Hb-C) D58.2
      with other abnormal hemoglobin NEC
          D58.2
      elliptocytosis D58.1
      Hb-S D57.2-
      sickle-cell D57.2-
      thalassemia D56.8
    Constant Spring D58.2
    D (Hb-D) D58.2
    E (Hb-E) D58.2
    E-beta thalassemia D56.5
    elliptocytosis D58.1
    H (Hb-H) (thalassemia) D56.0
      with other abnormal hemoglobin NEC
          D56.9
      Constant Spring D56.0
    I thalassemia D56.9
    M D74.0
    S or SS D57.1
    SC D57.2-
    SD D57.8-
    SE D57.8-
    spherocytosis D58.0
    unstable, hemolytic D58.2
  hemolytic (newborn) P55.9
    autoimmune (cold type) (warm type) D59.1
    drug-induced D59.0
    due to or with
      incompatibility
        ABO (blood group) P55.1
        blood (group) (Duffy) (K(ell)) (Kidd)
            (Lewis) (M) (S) NEC P55.8
        Rh (blood group) (factor) P55.0
        Rh negative mother P55.0
      specified type NEC P55.8
    unstable hemoglobin D58.2
  hemorrhagic D69.9
    newborn P53
  Henoch (-Schönlein) (purpura nervosa)
      D69.0
  hepatic —see Disease, liver
  hepatobiliary K83.9
    toxic K71.9
  hepatolenticular E83.01
  heredodegenerative NEC
    spinal cord G95.89
  herpesviral, disseminated B00.7
  Hers' (glycogenosis VI) E74.09
  Herter (-Gee) (-Heubner) (nontropical sprue)
      K90.0
  Heubner-Herter (nontropical sprue) K90.0
  high fetal gene or hemoglobin thalassemia
      D56.9
  Hildenbrand's —see Typhus
  hip (joint) M25.9
    congenital Q65.89
    suppurative M00.9
    tuberculous A18.02
  His (-Werner) (trench fever) A79.0
  Hodgson's I71.2
    ruptured I71.1
  Holla —see Spherocytosis
  hookworm B76.9
    specified NEC B76.8
  host-versus-graft D89.813
    acute D89.810
    acute on chronic D89.812
    chronic D89.811
  human immunodeficiency virus (HIV) B20
  Huntington's G10
  Hutchinson's (cheiropompholyx) —see
      Hutchinson's disease
  hyaline (diffuse) (generalized)
    membrane (lung) (newborn) P22.0
    adult J80

Disease, diseased (Continued)
  hydatid —see Echinococcus
  hydroxyapatite deposition M11.00
    ankle M11.07-
    elbow M11.02-
    foot joint M11.07-
    hand joint M11.04-
    hip M11.05-
    knee M11.06-
    multiple site M11.09
    shoulder M11.01-
    vertebra M11.08
    wrist M11.03-
  hyperkinetic —see Hyperkinesia
  hypertensive —see Hypertension
  hypophysis E23.7
  Iceland G93.3
  I-cell E77.0
  immune D89.9
  immunoproliferative (malignant) C88.9
    small intestinal C88.3
    specified NEC C88.8
  inclusion B25.9
    salivary gland B25.9
  infectious, infective B99.9
    congenital P37.9
      specified NEC P37.8
      viral P35.9
        specified type NEC P35.8
    specified NEC B99.8
  inflammatory
    penis N48.29
      abscess N48.21
      cellulitis N48.22
    prepuce N47.7
      balanoposthitis N47.6
    tubo-ovarian —see Salpingo-oophoritis
  intervertebral disc —see also Disorder, disc
    with myelopathy —see Disorder, disc, with,
        myelopathy
    cervical, cervicothoracic —see Disorder,
        disc, cervical
    with
      myelopathy —see Disorder, disc,
          cervical, with myelopathy
      neuritis, radiculitis or
          radiculopathy —see Disorder,
          disc, cervical, with neuritis
      specified NEC —see Disorder, disc,
          cervical, specified type NEC
    lumbar (with)
      myelopathy M51.06
      neuritis, radiculitis, radiculopathy or
          sciatica M51.16
      specified NEC M51.86
    lumbosacral (with)
      neuritis, radiculitis, radiculopathy or
          sciatica M51.17
      specified NEC M51.87
    specified NEC —see Disorder, disc,
        specified NEC
    thoracic (with)
      myelopathy M51.04
      neuritis, radiculitis or radiculopathy
          M51.14
      specified NEC M51.84
    thoracolumbar (with)
      myelopathy M51.05
      neuritis, radiculitis or radiculopathy
          M51.15
      specified NEC M51.85
  intestine K63.9
    functional K59.9
      psychogenic F45.8
      specified NEC K59.8
    organic K63.9
    protozoal A07.9
    specified NEC K63.89
  iris H21.9
    specified NEC H21.89
  iron metabolism or storage E83.10

Disease, diseased *(Continued)*
island (scrub typhus) A75.3
itai-itai —*see* Poisoning, cadmium
Jakob-Creutzfeldt —*see* Creutzfeldt- Jakob
    disease or syndrome
jaw M27.9
    fibrocystic M27.49
    specified NEC M27.8
jigger B88.1
joint —*see also* Disorder, joint
    Charcot's —*see* Arthropathy, neuropathic
      (Charcot)
    degenerative —*see* Osteoarthritis
      multiple M15.9
      spine —*see* Spondylosis
    hypertrophic —*see* Osteoarthritis
    sacroiliac M53.3
    specified NEC —*see* Disorder, joint,
      specified type NEC
    spine NEC —*see* Dorsopathy
    suppurative —*see* Arthritis, pyogenic or
      pyemic
Jourdain's (acute gingivitis) K05.00
    nonplaque induced K05.01
    plaque induced K05.00
Kaschin-Beck (endemic polyarthritis) M12.10
    ankle M12.17-
    elbow M12.12-
    foot joint M12.17-
    hand joint M12.14-
    hip M12.15-
    knee M12.16-
    multiple site M12.19
    shoulder M12.11-
    vertebra M12.18
    wrist M12.13-
Katayama B65.2
Kedani (scrub typhus) A75.3
Keshan E59
kidney (functional) (pelvis) N28.9
    chronic N18.9
      hypertensive —*see* Hypertension, kidney
      stage 1 N18.1
      stage 2 (mild) N18.2
      stage 3 (moderate) N18.3
      stage 4 (severe) N18.4
      stage 5 N18.5
    complicating pregnancy —*see* Pregnancy,
      complicated by, renal disease
    cystic (congenital) Q61.9
    diabetic - see E08-E13 with .22
    fibrocystic (congenital) Q61.8
    hypertensive —*see* Hypertension, kidney
    in (due to)
      schistosomiasis (bilharziasis) B65.9 [N29]
    multicystic Q61.4
    polycystic Q61.3
      adult type Q61.2
      childhood type NEC Q61.19
        collecting duct dilatation Q61.11
    Kimmelstiel (-Wilson) (intercapillary polycystic
      (congenital) glomerulosclerosis) —*see*
      E08-E13 with .21
Kimura D21.9
    specified site (see Neoplasm, connective
      tissue benign)
Kinnier Wilson's (hepatolenticular
    degeneration) E83.01
kissing —*see* Mononucleosis, infectious
Klebs' (*see also* Glomerulonephritis) N05.-
Klippel-Feil (brevicollis) Q76.1
Köhler-Pellegrini-Stieda (calcification, knee
    joint) —*see* Bursitis, tibial collateral
Kok Q89.8
König's (osteochondritis dissecans) —*see*
    Osteochondritis, dissecans
Korsakoff's (nonalcoholic) F04
    alcoholic F10.96
      with dependence F10.26
Kostmann's (infantile genetic
    agranulocytosis) D70.0

Disease, diseased *(Continued)*
kuru A81.81
Kyasanur Forest A98.2
labyrinth, ear —*see* Disorder, ear, inner
lacrimal system —*see* Disorder, lacrimal
    system
Lafora's —*see* Epilepsy, generalized,
    idiopathic
Lancereaux-Mathieu (leptospiral jaundice)
    A27.0
Landry's G61.0
Larrey-Weil (leptospiral jaundice) A27.0
larynx J38.7
legionnaires' A48.1
    nonpneumonic A48.2
Lenegre's I44.2
lens H27.9
    specified NEC H27.8
Lev's (acquired complete heart block) I44.2
Lewy body (dementia) G31.83 *[F02.80]*
    with behavioral disturbance G31.83
      [F02.81]
Lichtheim's (subacute combined sclerosis
    with pernicious anemia) D51.0
Lightwood's (renal tubular acidosis) N25.89
Lignac's (cystinosis) E72.04
lip K13.0
lipid-storage E75.6
    specified NEC E75.5
Lipschütz's N76.6
liver (chronic) (organic) K76.9
    alcoholic (chronic) K70.9
      acute —*see* Disease, liver, alcoholic,
        hepatitis
      cirrhosis K70.30
        with ascites K70.31
      failure K70.40
        with coma K70.41
      fatty liver K70.0
      fibrosis K70.2
      hepatitis K70.10
        with ascites K70.11
      sclerosis K70.2
    cystic, congenital Q44.6
    drug-induced (idiosyncratic) (toxic)
      (predictable) (unpredictable) —*see*
      Disease, liver, toxic
    end stage K72.90
      due to hepatitis —*see* Hepatitis
    fatty, nonalcoholic (NAFLD) K76.0
      alcoholic K70.0
    fibrocystic (congenital) Q44.6
    fluke
      Chinese B66.1
      oriental B66.1
      sheep B66.3
    glycogen storage E74.09 *[K77]*
    in (due to)
      schistosomiasis (bilharziasis) B65.9 *[K77]*
    inflammatory K75.9
      alcoholic K70.1
      specified NEC K75.89
    polycystic (congenital) Q44.6
    toxic K71.9
      with
        cholestasis K71.0
        cirrhosis (liver) K71.7
        fibrosis (liver) K71.7
        focal nodular hyperplasia K71.8
        hepatic granuloma K71.8
        hepatic necrosis K71.10
          with coma K71.11
        hepatitis NEC K71.6
          acute K71.2
          chronic
            active K71.50
              with ascites K71.51
            lobular K71.4
            persistent K71.3
          lupoid K71.50
            with ascites K71.51

Disease, diseased *(Continued)*
liver *(Continued)*
    toxic *(Continued)*
      with *(Continued)*
        peliosis hepatis K71.8
        veno-occlusive disease (VOD) of liver
          K71.8
    veno-occlusive K76.5
Lobo's (keloid blastomycosis) B48.0
Lobstein's (brittle bones and blue sclera)
    Q78.0
Ludwig's (submaxillary cellulitis) K12.2
lumbosacral region M53.87
lung J98.4
    black J60
    congenital Q33.9
    cystic J98.4
      congenital Q33.0
    fibroid (chronic) —*see* Fibrosis, lung
    fluke B66.4
      oriental B66.4
    in
      amyloidosis E85.4 *[J99]*
      sarcoidosis D86.0
      Sjögren's syndrome M35.02
      systemic
        lupus erythematosus M32.13
        sclerosis M34.81
    interstitial J84.9
      of childhood, specified NEC J84.848
      respiratory bronchiolitis J84.115
      specified NEC J84.89
    obstructive (chronic) J44.9
      with
        acute
          bronchitis J44.0
          exacerbation NEC J44.1
          lower respiratory infection J44.0
        alveolitis, allergic J67.9
        asthma J44.9
        bronchiectasis J47.9
          with
            exacerbation (acute) J47.1
            lower respiratory infection J47.0
        bronchitis J44.9
          with
            exacerbation (acute) J44.1
            lower respiratory infection J44.0
        emphysema J44.9
        hypersensitivity pneumonitis J67.9
      decompensated J44.1
        with
          exacerbation (acute) J44.1
    polycystic J98.4
      congenital Q33.0
    rheumatoid (diffuse) (interstitial) —*see*
      Rheumatoid, lung
Lutembacher's (atrial septal defect with
    mitral stenosis) Q21.1
Lyme A69.20
lymphatic (gland) (system) (channel) (vessel)
    I89.9
lymphoproliferative D47.9
    specified NEC D47.Z9
    T-gamma D47.Z9
    X-linked D82.3
Magitot's M27.2
malarial —*see* Malaria
malignant —*see also* Neoplasm, malignant,
    by site
Manson's B65.1
maple bark J67.6
maple-syrup-urine E71.0
Marburg (virus) A98.3
Marion's (bladder neck obstruction) N32.0
Marsh's (exophthalmic goiter) —*see*
    Hyperthyroidism, with, goiter (diffuse)
mastoid (process) —*see* Disorder, ear,
    middle
Mathieu's (leptospiral jaundice) A27.0
Maxcy's A75.2

◀ New   ◀▥ Revised   ~~deleted~~ Deleted

Disease, diseased (Continued)

McArdle (-Schmid-Pearson) (glycogenosis V) E74.04
mediastinum J98.5
medullary center (idiopathic) (respiratory) G93.89
Meige's (chronic hereditary edema) Q82.0
meningococcal —see Infection, meningococcal
mental F99
  organic F09
mesenchymal M35.9
mesenteric embolic K55.0
metabolic, metabolism E88.9
  bilirubin E80.7
metal-polisher's J62.8
metastatic (see also Neoplasm, secondary, by site) C79.9
microvascular — code to condition
microvillus
  atrophy Q43.8
  inclusion (MVD) Q43.8
middle ear —see Disorder, ear, middle
Mikulicz' (dryness of mouth, absent or decreased lacrimation) K11.8
Milroy's (chronic hereditary edema) Q82.0
Minamata —see Poisoning, mercury
minicore G71.2
Minor's G95.19
Minot's (hemorrhagic disease, newborn) P53
Minot-von Willebrand-Jürgens (angiohemophilia) D68.0
Mitchell's (erythromelalgia) I73.81
mitral (valve) I05.9
  nonrheumatic I34.9
mixed connective tissue M35.1
moldy hay J67.0
Monge's T70.29
Morgagni-Adams-Stokes (syncope with heart block) I45.9
Morgagni's (syndrome) (hyperostosis frontalis interna) M85.2
Morton's (with metatarsalgia) —see Lesion, nerve, plantar
Morvan's G60.8
motor neuron (bulbar) (familial) (mixed type) (spinal) G12.20
  amyotrophic lateral sclerosis G12.21
  progressive bulbar palsy G12.22
  specified NEC G12.29
moyamoya I67.5
mu heavy chain disease C88.2
multicore G71.2
muscle —see also Disorder, muscle
  inflammatory —see Myositis
  ocular (external) —see Strabismus
musculoskeletal system, soft tissue —see also Disorder, soft tissue
  specified NEC —see Disorder, soft tissue, specified type NEC
mushroom workers' J67.5
mycotic B49
myelodysplastic, not classified C94.6
myeloproliferative, not classified C94.6
  chronic D47.1
myocardium, myocardial (see also Degeneration, myocardial) I51.5
  primary (idiopathic) I42.9
myoneural G70.9
Naegeli's D69.1
nails L60.9
  specified NEC L60.8
Nairobi (sheep virus) A93.8
nasal J34.9
nemaline body G71.2
nerve —see Disorder, nerve
nervous system G98.8
  autonomic G90.9
  central G96.9
    specified NEC G96.8
  congenital Q07.9
  parasympathetic G90.9

Disease, diseased (Continued)

nervous system (Continued)
  specified NEC G98.8
  sympathetic G90.9
  vegetative G90.9
neuromuscular system G70.9
Newcastle B30.8
Nicolas (-Durand)-Favre (climatic bubo) A55
nipple N64.9
  Paget's C50.01-
    female C50.01-
    male C50.02-
Nishimoto (-Takeuchi) I67.5
nonarthropod-borne NOS (viral) B34.9
  enterovirus NEC B34.1
nonautoimmune hemolytic D59.4
  drug-induced D59.2
Nonne-Milroy-Meige (chronic hereditary edema) Q82.0
nose J34.9
nucleus pulposus —see Disorder, disc
nutritional E63.9
oast-house-urine E72.19
ocular
  herpesviral B00.50
  zoster B02.30
obliterative vascular I77.1
Ohara's —see Tularemia
Opitz's (congenital splenomegaly) D73.2
Oppenheim-Urbach (necrobiosis lipoidica diabeticorum) —see E08-E13 with .620
optic nerve NEC —see Disorder, nerve, optic
  orbit —see Disorder, orbit
Oriental liver fluke B66.1
Oriental lung fluke B66.4
Ormond's N13.5
Oropouche virus A93.0
Osler-Rendu (familial hemorrhagic telangiectasia) I78.0
osteofibrocystic E21.0
Otto's M24.7
outer ear —see Disorder, ear, external
ovary (noninflammatory) N83.9
  cystic N83.20
  inflammatory —see Salpingo-oophoritis
  polycystic E28.2
  specified NEC N83.8
Owren's (congenital) —see Defect, coagulation
pancreas K86.9
  cystic K86.2
  fibrocystic E84.9
  specified NEC K86.8
panvalvular I08.9
  specified NEC I08.8
parametrium (noninflammatory) N83.9
parasitic B89
  cerebral NEC B71.9 [G94]
  intestinal NOS B82.9
  mouth B37.0
  skin NOS B88.9
  specified type —see Infestation
  tongue B37.0
parathyroid (gland) E21.5
  specified NEC E21.4
Parkinson's G20
parodontal K05.6
Parrot's (syphilitic osteochondritis) A50.02
Parry's (exophthalmic goiter) —see Hyperthyroidism, with, goiter (diffuse)
Parson's (exophthalmic goiter) —see Hyperthyroidism, with, goiter (diffuse)
Paxton's (white piedra) B36.2
pearl-worker's —see Osteomyelitis, specified type NEC
Pellegrini-Stieda (calcification, knee joint) — see Bursitis, tibial collateral
pelvis, pelvic
  female NOS N94.9
    specified NEC N94.89
  gonococcal (acute) (chronic) A54.24

Disease, diseased (Continued)

pelvis, pelvic (Continued)
  inflammatory (female) N73.9
    acute N73.0
    chronic N73.1
    specified NEC N73.8
    syphilitic (secondary) A51.42
      late A52.76
    tuberculous A18.17
  organ, female N94.9
  peritoneum, female NEC N94.89
penis N48.9
  inflammatory N48.29
    abscess N48.21
    cellulitis N48.22
  specified NEC N48.89
periapical tissues NOS K04.90
periodontal K05.6
  specified NEC K05.5
periosteum —see Disorder, bone, specified type NEC
peripheral
  arterial I73.9
  autonomic nervous system G90.9
  nerves —see Polyneuropathy
  vascular NOS I73.9
peritoneum K66.9
  pelvic, female NEC N94.89
  specified NEC K66.8
persistent mucosal (middle ear) H66.20
  left H66.22
    with right H66.23
  right H66.21
    with left H66.23
Petit's —see Hernia, abdomen, specified site NEC
pharynx J39.2
  specified NEC J39.2
Phocas' —see Mastopathy, cystic
photochromogenic (acid-fast bacilli) (pulmonary) A31.0
  nonpulmonary A31.9
Pick's G31.01 [F02.80]
  with behavioral disturbance G31.01 [F02.81]
pigeon fancier's J67.2
pineal gland E34.8
pink —see Poisoning, mercury
Pinkus' (lichen nitidus) L44.1
pinworm B80
Piry virus A93.8
pituitary (gland) E23.7
pituitary-snuff-taker's J67.8
pleura (cavity) J94.9
  specified NEC J94.8
pneumatic drill (hammer) T75.21
Pollitzer's (hidradenitis suppurativa) L73.2
polycystic
  kidney or renal Q61.3
    adult type Q61.2
    childhood type NEC Q61.19
      collecting duct dilatation Q61.11
  liver or hepatic Q44.6
  lung or pulmonary J98.4
    congenital Q33.0
  ovary, ovaries E28.2
  spleen Q89.09
polyethylene T84.05-
Pompe's (glycogenosis II) E74.02
Posadas-Wernicke B38.9
Potain's (pulmonary edema) —see Edema, lung
prepuce N47.8
  inflammatory N47.7
  balanoposthitis N47.6
Pringle's (tuberous sclerosis) Q85.1
prion, central nervous system A81.9
  specified NEC A81.89
prostate N42.9
  specified NEC N42.89

Disease, diseased *(Continued)*
  protozoal B64
    acanthamebiasis —*see* Acanthamebiasis
    African trypanosomiasis —*see* African
      trypanosomiasis
    babesiosis B60.0
    Chagas disease —*see* Chagas disease
    intestine, intestinal A07.9
    leishmaniasis —*see* Leishmaniasis
    malaria —*see* Malaria
    naegleriasis B60.2
    pneumocystosis B59
    specified organism NEC B60.8
    toxoplasmosis —*see* Toxoplasmosis
  pseudo-Hurler's E77.0
  psychiatric F99
  psychotic —*see* Psychosis
  Puente's (simple glandular cheilitis)
    K13.0
  puerperal (*see also* Puerperal) O90.89
  pulmonary —*see also* Disease, lung
    artery I28.9
    chronic obstructive J44.9
      with
        acute bronchitis J44.0
        exacerbation (acute) J44.1
        lower respiratory infection (acute)
          J44.0
      decompensated J44.1
        with
          exacerbation (acute) J44.1
    heart I27.9
      specified NEC I27.89
    hypertensive (vascular) I27.0
    valve I37.9
      rheumatic I09.89
  pulp (dental) NOS K04.90
  pulseless M31.4
  Putnam's (subacute combined sclerosis with
    pernicious anemia) D51.0
  Pyle (-Cohn) (craniometaphyseal dysplasia)
    Q78.5
  ragpicker's or ragsorter's A22.1
  Raynaud's —*see* Raynaud's disease
  reactive airway —*see* Asthma
  Reclus' (cystic) —*see* Mastopathy,
    cystic
  rectum K62.9
    specified NEC K62.89
  Refsum's (heredopathia atactica
    polyneuritiformis) G60.1
  renal (functional) (pelvis) (*see also* Disease,
    kidney) N28.9
    with
      edema —*see* Nephrosis
      glomerular lesion —*see*
        Glomerulonephritis
        with edema —*see* Nephrosis
      interstitial nephritis N12
    acute N28.9
    chronic (*see also* Disease, kidney, chronic)
      N18.9
    cystic, congenital Q61.9
    diabetic —*see* E08-E13 with .22
    end-stage (failure) N18.6
      due to hypertension I12.0
    fibrocystic (congenital) Q61.8
    hypertensive —*see* Hypertension,
      kidney
    lupus M32.14
    phosphate-losing (tubular) N25.0
    polycystic (congenital) Q61.3
      adult type Q61.2
      childhood type NEC Q61.19
        collecting duct dilatation Q61.11
    rapidly progressive N01.9
    subacute N01.9
  Rendu-Osler-Weber (familial hemorrhagic
    telangiectasia) I78.0
  renovascular (arteriosclerotic) —*see*
    Hypertension, kidney

Disease, diseased *(Continued)*
  respiratory (tract) J98.9
    acute or subacute NOS J06.9
      due to
        chemicals, gases, fumes or vapors
          (inhalation) J68.3
        external agent J70.9
          specified NEC J70.8
        radiation J70.0
        smoke inhalation J70.5
      noninfectious J39.8
    chronic NOS J98.9
      due to
        chemicals, gases, fumes or vapors
          J68.4
        external agent J70.9
          specified NEC J70.8
        radiation J70.1
    newborn P27.9
      specified NEC P27.8
    due to
      chemicals, gases, fumes or vapors J68.9
        acute or subacute NEC J68.3
        chronic J68.4
      external agent J70.9
        specified NEC J70.8
    newborn P28.9
      specified type NEC P28.89
    upper J39.9
      acute or subacute J06.9
      noninfectious NEC J39.8
      specified NEC J39.8
      streptococcal J06.9
  retina, retinal H35.9
    Batten's or Batten-Mayou E75.4 *[H36]*
    specified NEC H35.89
  rheumatoid —*see* Arthritis, rheumatoid
  rickettsial NOS A79.9
    specified type NEC A79.89
  Riga (-Fede) (cachectic aphthae) K14.0
  Riggs' (compound periodontitis) —*see*
    Periodontitis
  Ritter's L00
  Rivalta's (cervicofacial actinomycosis)
    A42.2
  Robles' (onchocerciasis) B73.01
  Roger's (congenital interventricular septal
    defect) Q21.0
  Rosenthal's (factor XI deficiency) D68.1
  Ross River B33.1
  Rossbach's (hyperchlorhydria) K30
  Rotes Quérol —*see* Hyperostosis, ankylosing
  Roth (-Bernhardt) —*see* Mononeuropathy,
    lower limb, meralgia paresthetica
  Runeberg's (progressive pernicious anemia)
    D51.0
  sacroiliac NEC M53.3
  salivary gland or duct K11.9
    inclusion B25.9
    specified NEC K11.8
    virus B25.9
  sandworm B76.9
  Schimmelbusch's —*see* Mastopathy, cystic
  Schmorl's —*see* Schmorl's disease or nodes
  Schönlein (-Henoch) (purpura rheumatica)
    D69.0
  Schottmüller's —*see* Fever, paratyphoid
  Schultz's (agranulocytosis) —*see*
    Agranulocytosis
  Schwalbe-Ziehen-Oppenheim G24.1
  Schwartz-Jampel G71.13
  sclera H15.9
    specified NEC H15.89
  scrofulous (tuberculous) A18.2
  scrotum N50.9
  sebaceous glands L73.9
  semilunar cartilage, cystic —*see also*
    Derangement, knee, meniscus, cystic
  seminal vesicle N50.9
  serum NEC (*see also* Reaction, serum)
    T80.69

Disease, diseased *(Continued)*
  sexually transmitted A64
    anogenital
      herpesviral infection —*see* Herpes,
        anogenital
      warts A63.0
    chancroid A57
    chlamydial infection —*see* Chlamydia
    gonorrhea —*see* Gonorrhea
    granuloma inguinale A58
    specified organism NEC A63.8
    syphilis —*see* Syphilis
    trichomoniasis —*see* Trichomoniasis
  Sézary C84.1-
  shimamushi (scrub typhus) A75.3
  shipyard B30.0
  sickle-cell D57.1
    with crisis (vasoocclusive pain) D57.00
      with
        acute chest syndrome D57.01
        splenic sequestration D57.02
    elliptocytosis D57.8-
    Hb-C D57.20
      with crisis (vasoocclusive pain) D57.219
        with
          acute chest syndrome D57.211
          splenic sequestration D57.212
      without crisis D57.20
    Hb-SD D57.80
      with crisis D57.819
        with
          acute chest syndrome D57.811
          splenic sequestration D57.812
    Hb-SE D57.80
      with crisis D57.819
        with
          acute chest syndrome D57.811
          splenic sequestration D57.812
    specified NEC D57.80
      with crisis D57.819
        with
          acute chest syndrome D57.811
          splenic sequestration D57.812
    spherocytosis D57.80
      with crisis D57.819
        with
          acute chest syndrome D57.811
          splenic sequestration D57.812
    thalassemia D57.40
      with crisis (vasoocclusive pain) D57.419
        with
          acute chest syndrome D57.411
          splenic sequestration D57.412
      without crisis D57.40
  silo-filler's J68.8
    bronchitis J68.0
    pneumonitis J68.0
    pulmonary edema J68.1
  simian B B00.4
  Simons' (progressive lipodystrophy) E88.1
  sin nombre virus B33.4
  sinus —*see* Sinusitis
  Sirkari's B55.0
  sixth B08.20
    due to human herpesvirus 6 B08.21
    due to human herpesvirus 7 B08.22
  skin L98.9
    due to metabolic disorder NEC E88.9
      [L99]
    specified NEC L98.8
  slim (HIV) B20
  small vessel I73.9
  Sneddon-Wilkinson (subcorneal pustular
    dermatosis) L13.1
  South African creeping B88.0
  spinal (cord) G95.9
    congenital Q06.9
    specified NEC G95.89
  spine —*see also* Spondylopathy
    joint —*see* Dorsopathy
    tuberculous A18.01

◀ New   ◀▥ Revised   ~~deleted~~ Deleted

Disease, diseased (Continued)
    spinocerebellar (hereditary) G11.9
        specified NEC G11.8
    spleen D73.9
        amyloid E85.4 [D77]
        organic D73.9
        polycystic Q89.09
        postinfectional D73.89
    sponge-diver's —see Toxicity, venom, marine
        animal, sea anemone
    Startle Q89.8
    Steinert's G71.11
    Sticker's (erythema infectiosum) B08.3
    Stieda's (calcification, knee joint) —see
        Bursitis, tibial collateral
    Stokes' (exophthalmic goiter) —see
        Hyperthyroidism, with, goiter (diffuse)
    Stokes-Adams (syncope with heart block)
        I45.9
    stomach K31.9
        functional, psychogenic F45.8
        specified NEC K31.89
    stonemason's J62.8
    storage
        glycogen —see Disease, glycogen storage
        mucopolysaccharide —see
            Mucopolysaccharidosis
    striatopallidal system NEC G25.89
    Stuart-Prower (congenital factor X deficiency)
        D68.2
    Stuart's (congenital factor X deficiency) D68.2
    subcutaneous tissue —see Disease, skin
    supporting structures of teeth K08.9
        specified NEC K08.8
    suprarenal (capsule) (gland) E27.9
        hyperfunction E27.0
        specified NEC E27.8
    sweat glands L74.9
        specified NEC L74.8
    Sweeley-Klionsky E75.21
    Swift (-Feer) —see Poisoning, mercury
    swimming-pool granuloma A31.1
    Sylvest's (epidemic pleurodynia) B33.0
    sympathetic nervous system G90.9
    synovium —see Disorder, synovium
    syphilitic —see Syphilis
    systemic tissue mast cell C96.2
    tanapox (virus) B08.71
    Tangier E78.6
    Tarral-Besnier (pityriasis rubra pilaris) L44.0
    Tauri E74.09
    tear duct —see Disorder, lacrimal system
    tendon, tendinous —see also Disorder, tendon
        nodular —see Trigger finger
    terminal vessel I73.9
    testis N50.9
    thalassemia Hb-S —see Disease, sickle-cell,
        thalassemia
    Thaysen-Gee (nontropical sprue) K90.0
    Thomsen G71.12
    throat J39.2
        septic J02.0
    thromboembolic —see Embolism
    thymus (gland) E32.9
        specified NEC E32.8
    thyroid (gland) E07.9
        heart (see also Hyperthyroidism) E05.90
            [I43]
            with thyroid storm E05.91 [I43]
        specified NEC E07.89
    Tietze's M94.0
    tongue K14.9
        specified NEC K14.8
    tonsils, tonsillar (and adenoids) J35.9
    tooth, teeth K08.9
        hard tissues K03.9
            specified NEC K03.89
        pulp NEC K04.99
        specified NEC K08.8
    Tourette's F95.2
    trachea NEC J39.8

Disease, diseased (Continued)
    tricuspid I07.9
        nonrheumatic I36.9
    triglyceride-storage E75.5
    trophoblastic —see Mole, hydatidiform
    tsutsugamushi A75.3
    tube (fallopian) (noninflammatory) N83.9
        inflammatory —see Salpingitis
        specified NEC N83.8
    tuberculous NEC —see Tuberculosis
    tubo-ovarian (noninflammatory) N83.9
        inflammatory —see Salpingo-oophoritis
        specified NEC N83.8
    tubotympanic, chronic —see Otitis, media,
        suppurative, chronic, tubotympanic
    tubulo-interstitial N15.9
        specified NEC N15.8
    tympanum —see Disorder, tympanic
        membrane
    Uhl's Q24.8
    Underwood's (sclerema neonatorum)
        P83.0
    Unverricht (-Lundborg) —see Epilepsy,
        generalized, idiopathic
    Urbach-Oppenheim (necrobiosis lipoidica
        diabeticorum) —see E08-E13 with
        .620
    ureter N28.9
        in (due to)
            schistosomiasis (bilharziasis) B65.0
            [N29]
    urethra N36.9
        specified NEC N36.8
    urinary (tract) N39.9
        bladder N32.9
            specified NEC N32.89
        specified NEC N39.8
    uterus (noninflammatory) N85.9
        infective —see Endometritis
        inflammatory —see Endometritis
        specified NEC N85.8
    uveal tract (anterior) H21.9
        posterior H31.9
    vagabond's B85.1
    vagina, vaginal (noninflammatory) N89.9
        inflammatory NEC N76.89
        specified NEC N89.8
    valve, valvular I38
        multiple I08.9
            specified NEC I08.8
    van Creveld-von Gierke (glycogenosis I)
        E74.01
    vas deferens N50.9
    vascular I99.9
        arteriosclerotic —see Arteriosclerosis
        ciliary body NEC —see Disorder, iris,
            vascular
        hypertensive —see Hypertension
        iris NEC —see Disorder, iris, vascular
        obliterative I77.1
            peripheral I73.9
        occlusive I99.8
        peripheral (occlusive) I73.9
            in diabetes mellitus —see E08-E13 with
            .51
    vasomotor I73.9
    vasospastic I73.9
    vein I87.9
    venereal (see also Disease, sexually
        transmitted) A64
        chlamydial NEC A56.8
            anus A56.3
            genitourinary NOS A56.2
            pharynx A56.4
            rectum A56.3
        fifth A55
        sixth A55
        specified nature or type NEC A63.8
    vertebra, vertebral —see also Spondylopathy
        disc —see Disorder, disc
    vibration —see Vibration, adverse effects

Disease, diseased (Continued)
    viral, virus (see also Disease, by type of virus)
        B34.9
        arbovirus NOS A94
        arthropod-borne NOS A94
        congenital P35.9
            specified NEC P35.8
        Hanta (with renal manifestations)
            (Dobrava) (Puumala) (Seoul) A98.5
            with pulmonary manifestations (Andes)
                (Bayou) (Bermejo) (Black Creek
                Canal) (Choclo) (Juquitiba)
                (Laguna negra) (Lechiguanas)
                (New York) (Oran) (Sin nombre)
                B33.4
        Hantaan (Korean hemorrhagic fever) A98.5
        human immunodeficiency (HIV) B20
        Kunjin A83.4
        nonarthropod-borne NOS B34.9
        Powassan A84.8
        Rocio (encephalitis) A83.6
        Sin nombre (Hantavirus) (cardio)-
            pulmonary syndrome B33.4
        Tahyna B33.8
        vesicular stomatitis A93.8
    vitreous H43.9
        specified NEC H43.89
    vocal cord J38.3
    Volkmann's, acquired T79.6
    von Eulenburg's (congenital paramyotonia)
        G71.19
    von Gierke's (glycogenosis I) E74.01
    von Graefe's —see Strabismus, paralytic,
        ophthalmoplegia, progressive
    von Willebrand (-Jürgens) (angiohemophilia)
        D68.0
    Vrolik's (osteogenesis imperfecta) Q78.0
    vulva (noninflammatory) N90.9
        inflammatory NEC N76.89
        specified NEC N90.89
    Wallgren's (obstruction of splenic vein with
        collateral circulation) I87.8
    Wassilieff's (leptospiral jaundice) A27.0
    wasting NEC R64
        due to malnutrition E41
    Waterhouse-Friderichsen A39.1
    Wegner's (syphilitic osteochondritis) A50.02
    Weil's (leptospiral jaundice of lung) A27.0
    Weir Mitchell's (erythromelalgia) I73.81
    Werdnig-Hoffmann G12.0
    Wermer's E31.21
    Werner-His (trench fever) A79.0
    Werner-Schultz (neutropenic splenomegaly)
        D73.81
    Wernicke-Posadas B38.9
    whipworm B79
    white blood cells D72.9
        specified NEC D72.89
    white matter R90.82
    white-spot, meaning lichen sclerosus et
        atrophicus L90.0
        penis N48.0
        vulva N90.4
    Wilkie's K55.1
    Wilkinson-Sneddon (subcorneal pustular
        dermatosis) L13.1
    Willis' —see Diabetes
    Wilson's (hepatolenticular degeneration)
        E83.01
    woolsorter's A22.1
    yaba monkey tumor B08.72
    yaba pox (virus) B08.72
    zoonotic, bacterial A28.9
        specified type NEC A28.8
Disfigurement (due to scar) L90.5
Disgerminoma —see Dysgerminoma
DISH (diffuse idiopathic skeletal
    hyperostosis) —see Hyperostosis,
    ankylosing
Disinsertion, retina —see Detachment, retina
Dislocatable hip, congenital Q65.6

Dislocation (articular)
  with fracture —see Fracture
  acromioclavicular (joint) S43.10-
    with displacement
        100%-200% S43.12-
        more than 200% S43.13-
    inferior S43.14-
    posterior S43.15-
  ankle S93.0-
  astragalus —see Dislocation, ankle
  atlantoaxial S13.121
  atlantooccipital S13.111
  atloidooccipital S13.111
  breast bone S23.29
  capsule, joint code by site under Dislocation
  carpal (bone) —see Dislocation, wrist
  carpometacarpal (joint) NEC S63.05-
    thumb S63.04-
  cartilage (joint) - code by site under
      Dislocation
  cervical spine (vertebra) —see Dislocation,
      vertebra, cervical
  chronic —see Dislocation, recurrent
  clavicle —see Dislocation, acromioclavicular
      joint
  coccyx S33.2
  congenital NEC Q68.8
  coracoid —see Dislocation, shoulder
  costal cartilage S23.29
  costochondral S23.29
  cricoarytenoid articulation S13.29
  cricothyroid articulation S13.29
  dorsal vertebra —see Dislocation, vertebra,
      thoracic
  ear ossicle —see Discontinuity, ossicles, ear
  elbow S53.10-
    congenital Q68.8
    pathological —see Dislocation, pathological
        NEC, elbow
    radial head alone —see Dislocation, radial
        head
    recurrent —see Dislocation, recurrent,
        elbow
    traumatic S53.10-
        anterior S53.11-
        lateral S53.14-
        medial S53.13-
        posterior S53.12-
        specified type NEC S53.19-
  eye, nontraumatic —see Luxation, globe
  eyeball, nontraumatic —see Luxation, globe
  femur
    distal end —see Dislocation, knee
    proximal end —see Dislocation, hip
  fibula
    distal end —see Dislocation, ankle
    proximal end —see Dislocation, knee
  finger S63.25-
    index S63.25-
    interphalangeal S63.27-
        distal S63.29-
            index S63.29-
            little S63.29-
            middle S63.29-
            ring S63.29-
        index S63.27-
        little S63.27-
        middle S63.27-
        proximal S63.28-
            index S63.28-
            little S63.28-
            middle S63.28-
            ring S63.28-
        ring S63.27-
    little S63.25-
    metacarpophalangeal S63.26-
        index S63.26-
        little S63.26-
        middle S63.26-
        ring S63.26-
    middle S63.25-

Dislocation (Continued)
  finger (Continued)
    recurrent —see Dislocation, recurrent,
        finger
    ring S63.25-
    thumb —see Dislocation, thumb
  foot S93.30-
    recurrent —see Dislocation, recurrent,
        foot
    specified site NEC S93.33-
    tarsal joint S93.31-
    tarsometatarsal joint S93.32-
    toe —see Dislocation, toe
  fracture —see Fracture
  glenohumeral (joint) —see Dislocation,
      shoulder
  glenoid —see Dislocation, shoulder
  habitual —see Dislocation, recurrent
  hip S73.00-
    anterior S73.03-
        obturator S73.02-
    central S73.04-
    congenital (total) Q65.2
        bilateral Q65.1
        partial Q65.5
            bilateral Q65.4
            unilateral Q65.3-
        unilateral Q65.0-
    developmental M24.85-
    pathological —see Dislocation, pathological
        NEC, hip
    posterior S73.01-
    recurrent —see Dislocation, recurrent, hip
  humerus, proximal end —see Dislocation,
      shoulder
  incomplete —see Subluxation, by site
  incus —see Discontinuity, ossicles, ear
  infracoracoid —see Dislocation, shoulder
  innominate (pubic junction) (sacral junction)
      S33.39
    acetabulum —see Dislocation, hip
  interphalangeal (joint (s))
    finger S63.279
        distal S63.29-
            index S63.29-
            little S63.29-
            middle S63.29-
            ring S63.29-
        index S63.27-
        little S63.27-
        middle S63.27-
        proximal S63.28-
            index S63.28-
            little S63.28-
            middle S63.28-
            ring S63.28-
        ring S63.27-
    foot or toe —see Dislocation, toe
    thumb S63.12-
        distal joint S63.14-
        proximal joint S63.13-
  jaw (cartilage) (meniscus) S03.0
  joint prosthesis —see Complications, joint
      prosthesis, mechanical, displacement,
      by site
  knee S83.106
    cap —see Dislocation, patella
    congenital Q68.2
    old M23.8X-
    patella —see Dislocation, patella
    pathological —see Dislocation, pathological
        NEC, knee
    proximal tibia
        anteriorly S83.11-
        laterally S83.14-
        medially S83.13-
        posteriorly S83.12-
    recurrent —see also Derangement, knee,
        specified NEC
    specified type NEC S83.19-
  lacrimal gland H04.16-

Dislocation (Continued)
  lens (complete) H27.10-
    anterior H27.12-
    congenital Q12.1
    ocular implant —see Complications,
        intraocular lens
    partial H27.11-
    posterior H27.13-
    traumatic S05.8X-
  ligament code by site under Dislocation
  lumbar (vertebra) —see Dislocation, vertebra,
      lumbar
  lumbosacral (vertebra) —see also Dislocation,
      vertebra, lumbar
    congenital Q76.49
  mandible S03.0
  meniscus (knee) —see Tear, meniscus
    other sites code by site under Dislocation
  metacarpal (bone)
    distal end —see Dislocation, finger
    proximal end S63.06-
  metacarpophalangeal (joint)
    finger S63.26-
        index S63.26-
        little S63.26-
        middle S63.26-
        ring S63.26-
    thumb S63.11-
  metatarsal (bone) —see Dislocation, foot
  metatarsophalangeal (joint (s)) —see
      Dislocation, toe
  midcarpal (joint) S63.03-
  midtarsal (joint) —see Dislocation, foot
  neck S13.20
    specified site NEC S13.29
    vertebra —see Dislocation, vertebra,
        cervical
  nose (septal cartilage) S03.1
  occipitoatloid S13.111
  old —see Derangement, joint, specified type
      NEC
  ossicles, ear —see Discontinuity, ossicles,
      ear
  partial —see Subluxation, by site
  patella S83.006
    congenital Q74.1
    lateral S83.01-
    recurrent (nontraumatic) M22.0-
        incomplete M22.1-
    specified type NEC S83.09-
  pathological NEC M24.30
    ankle M24.37-
    elbow M24.32-
    foot joint M24.37-
    hand joint M24.34-
    hip M24.35-
    knee M24.36-
    lumbosacral joint —see subcategory
        M53.2
    pelvic region —see Dislocation,
        pathological, hip
    sacroiliac —see subcategory M53.2
    shoulder M24.31-
    wrist M24.33-
  pelvis NEC S33.30
    specified NEC S33.39
  phalanx
    finger or hand —see Dislocation, finger
    foot or toe —see Dislocation, toe
  prosthesis, internal —see Complications,
      prosthetic device, by site, mechanical
  radial head S53.006
    anterior S53.01-
    posterior S53.02-
    specified type NEC S53.09-
  radiocarpal (joint) S63.02-
  radiohumeral (joint) —see Dislocation, radial
      head
  radioulnar (joint)
    distal S63.01-
    proximal —see Dislocation, elbow

◀ New   ◀▥ Revised   ~~deleted~~ Deleted

Dislocation (Continued)
   radius
      distal end —see Dislocation, wrist
      proximal end —see Dislocation, radial
         head
      recurrent M24.40
         ankle M24.47-
         elbow M24.42-
         finger M24.44-
         foot joint M24.47-
         hand joint M24.44-
         hip M24.45-
         knee M24.46-
            patella —see Dislocation, patella,
               recurrent
         patella —see Dislocation, patella, recurrent
         sacroiliac —see subcategory M53.2
         shoulder M24.41-
         toe M24.47-
         vertebra (see also subcategory) M43.5
            atlantoaxial M43.4
               with myelopathy M43.3
         wrist M24.43-
   rib (cartilage) S23.29
   sacrococcygeal S33.2
   sacroiliac (joint) (ligament) S33.2
      congenital Q74.2
      recurrent —see subcategory M53.2
   sacrum S33.2
   scaphoid (bone) (hand) (wrist) —see
      Dislocation, wrist
      foot —see Dislocation, foot
   scapula —see Dislocation, shoulder, girdle,
      scapula
   semilunar cartilage, knee —see Tear, meniscus
   septal cartilage (nose) S03.1
   septum (nasal) (old) J34.2
   sesamoid bone code by site under Dislocation
   shoulder (blade) (ligament) (joint) (traumatic)
      S43.006
      acromioclavicular —see Dislocation,
         acromioclavicular
      chronic —see Dislocation, recurrent,
         shoulder
      congenital Q68.8
      girdle S43.30-
         scapula S43.31-
         specified site NEC S43.39-
      humerus S43.00-
         anterior S43.01-
         inferior S43.03-
         posterior S43.02-
      pathological —see Dislocation, pathological
         NEC, shoulder
      recurrent —see Dislocation, recurrent,
         shoulder
      specified type NEC S43.08-
   spine
      cervical —see Dislocation, vertebra, cervical
      congenital Q76.49
      due to birth trauma P11.5
      lumbar —see Dislocation, vertebra, lumbar
      thoracic —see Dislocation, vertebra,
         thoracic
   spontaneous —see Dislocation, pathological
   sternoclavicular (joint) S43.206
      anterior S43.21-
      posterior S43.22-
   sternum S23.29
   subglenoid —see Dislocation, shoulder
   symphysis pubis S33.4
   talus —see Dislocation, ankle
   tarsal (bone (s)) (joint (s)) —see Dislocation,
      foot
   tarsometatarsal (joint (s)) —see Dislocation,
      foot
   temporomandibular (joint) S03.0
   thigh, proximal end —see Dislocation, hip
   thorax S23.20
      specified site NEC S23.29
      vertebra —see Dislocation, vertebra

Dislocation (Continued)
   thumb S63.10-
      interphalangeal joint —see Dislocation,
         interphalangeal (joint), thumb
      metacarpophalangeal joint —see
         Dislocation, metacarpophalangeal
         (joint), thumb
   thyroid cartilage S13.29
   tibia
      distal end —see Dislocation, ankle
      proximal end —see Dislocation, knee
   tibiofibular (joint)
      distal —see Dislocation, ankle
      superior —see Dislocation, knee
   toe (s) S93.106
      great S93.10-
         interphalangeal joint S93.11-
         metatarsophalangeal joint S93.12-
      interphalangeal joint S93.119
      lesser S93.106
         interphalangeal joint S93.11-
         metatarsophalangeal joint S93.12-
      metatarsophalangeal joint S93.12-
   tooth S03.2
   trachea S23.29
   ulna
      distal end S63.07-
      proximal end —see Dislocation, elbow
   ulnohumeral (joint) —see Dislocation, elbow
   vertebra (articular process) (body)
      (traumatic)
      cervical S13.101
         atlantoaxial joint S13.121
         atlantooccipital joint S13.111
         atloidooccipital joint S13.111
         joint between
            C0 and C1 S13.111
            C1 and C2 S13.121
            C2 and C3 S13.131
            C3 and C4 S13.141
            C4 and C5 S13.151
            C5 and C6 S13.161
            C6 and C7 S13.171
            C7 and T1 S13.181
         occipitoatloid joint S13.111
      congenital Q76.49
      lumbar S33.101
         joint between
            L1 and L2 S33.111
            L2 and L3 S33.121
            L3 and L4 S33.131
            L4 and L5 S33.141
      nontraumatic —see Displacement,
         intervertebral disc
      partial —see Subluxation, by site
      recurrent NEC —see subcategory
         M43.5
      thoracic S23.101
         joint between
            T1 and T2 S23.111
            T2 and T3 S23.121
            T3 and T4 S23.123
            T4 and T5 S23.131
            T5 and T6 S23.133
            T6 and T7 S23.141
            T7 and T8 S23.143
            T8 and T9 S23.151
            T9 and T10 S23.153
            T10 and T11 S23.161
            T11 and T12 S23.163
            T12 and L1 S23.171
   wrist (carpal bone) S63.006
      carpometacarpal joint —see Dislocation,
         carpometacarpal (joint)
      distal radioulnar joint —see Dislocation,
         radioulnar (joint), distal
      metacarpal bone, proximal —see
         Dislocation, metacarpal (bone),
         proximal end
      midcarpal —see Dislocation, midcarpal
         (joint)

Dislocation (Continued)
   wrist (Continued)
      radiocarpal joint —see Dislocation,
         radiocarpal (joint)
      recurrent —see Dislocation, recurrent,
         wrist
      specified site NEC S63.09-
      ulna —see Dislocation, ulna, distal end
   xiphoid cartilage S23.29
Disorder (of) —see also Disease
   acantholytic L11.9
      specified NEC L11.8
   acute
      psychotic —see Psychosis, acute
      stress F43.0
   adjustment (grief) F43.20
      with
         anxiety F43.22
            with depressed mood F43.23
         conduct disturbance F43.24
            with emotional disturbance
               F43.25
         depressed mood F43.21
            with anxiety F43.23
         other specified symptom F43.29
   adrenal (capsule) (gland) (medullary)
      E27.9
      specified NEC E27.8
   adrenogenital E25.9
      drug-induced E25.8
      iatrogenic E25.8
      idiopathic E25.8
   adult personality (and behavior) F69
      specified NEC F68.8
   affective (mood) —see Disorder, mood
   aggressive, unsocialized F91.1
   alcohol-related F10.99
      with
         amnestic disorder, persisting
            F10.96
         anxiety disorder F10.980
         dementia, persisting F10.97
         intoxication F10.929
            with delirium F10.921
            uncomplicated F10.920
         mood disorder F10.94
         other specified F10.988
         psychotic disorder F10.959
            with
               delusions F10.950
               hallucinations F10.951
         sexual dysfunction F10.981
         sleep disorder F10.982
   allergic —see Allergy
   alveolar NEC J84.09
   amino-acid
      cystathioninuria E72.19
      cystinosis E72.04
      cystinuria E72.01
      glycinuria E72.09
      homocystinuria E72.11
      metabolism —see Disturbance,
         metabolism, amino-acid
      specified NEC E72.8
      neonatal, transitory P74.8
      renal transport NEC E72.09
      transport NEC E72.09
   amnesic, amnestic
      alcohol-induced F10.96
         with dependence F10.26
      due to (secondary to) general medical
         condition F04
      psychoactive NEC-induced F19.96
         with
            abuse F19.16
            dependence F19.26
      sedative, hypnotic or anxiolytic-
         induced F13.96
         with dependence F13.26
   anaerobic glycolysis with anemia
      D55.2

Disorder *(Continued)*
  anxiety F41.9
    due to (secondary to)
      alcohol F10.980
      amphetamine F15.980
        in
          abuse F15.180
          dependence F15.280
      anxiolytic F13.980
        in
          abuse F13.180
          dependence F13.280
      caffeine F15.980
        in
          abuse F15.180
          dependence F15.280
      cannabis F12.980
        in
          abuse F12.180
          dependence F12.280
      cocaine F14.980
        in
          abuse F14.180
          dependence F14.180
      general medical condition F06.4
      hallucinogen F16.980
        in
          abuse F16.180
          dependence F16.280
      hypnotic F13.980
        in
          abuse F13.180
          dependence F13.280
      inhalant F18.980
        in
          abuse F18.180
          dependence F18.280
      phencyclidine F16.980
        in
          abuse F16.180
          dependence F16.280
      psychoactive substance NEC
        F19.980
        in
          abuse F19.180
          dependence F19.280
      sedative F13.980
        in
          abuse F13.180
          dependence F13.280
      volatile solvents F18.980
        in
          abuse F18.180
          dependence F18.280
    generalized F41.1
    mixed
      with depression (mild) F41.8
      specified NEC F41.3
    organic F06.4
    phobic F40.9
      of childhood F40.8
    specified NEC F41.8
  aortic valve —*see* Endocarditis, aortic
  aromatic amino-acid metabolism E70.9
    specified NEC E70.8
  arteriole NEC I77.89
  artery NEC I77.89
  articulation —*see* Disorder, joint
  attachment (childhood)
    disinhibited F94.2
    reactive F94.1
  attention-deficit hyperactivity (adolescent)
    (adult) (child) F90.9
    combined type F90.2
    hyperactive type F90.1
    inattentive type F90.0
    specified type NEC F90.8
  attention-deficit without hyperactivity
    (adolescent) (adult) (child) F90.0
  auditory processing (central) H93.25
  autistic F84.0

Disorder *(Continued)*
  autonomic nervous system G90.9
    specified NEC G90.8
  avoidant, child or adolescent F40.10
  balance
    acid-base E87.8
      mixed E87.4
    electrolyte E87.8
    fluid NEC E87.8
  behavioral (disruptive) —*see* Disorder,
    conduct
  beta-amino-acid metabolism E72.8
  bile acid and cholesterol metabolism
    E78.70
    Barth syndrome E78.71
    other specified E78.79
    Smith-Lemli-Opitz syndrome E78.72
  bilirubin excretion E80.6
  binocular
    movement H51.9
      convergence
        excess H51.12
        insufficiency H51.11
      internuclear ophthalmoplegia —*see*
        Ophthalmoplegia, internuclear
      palsy of conjugate gaze H51.0
      specified type NEC H51.8
    vision NEC —*see* Disorder, vision,
      binocular
  bipolar (I) F31.9
    current episode
      depressed F31.9
        with psychotic features F31.5
        without psychotic features
          F31.30
        mild F31.31
        moderate F31.32
        severe (without psychotic features)
          F31.4
        with psychotic features
          F31.5
      hypomanic F31.0
      manic F31.9
        with psychotic features F31.2
        without psychotic features F31.10
        mild F31.11
        moderate F31.12
        severe (without psychotic features)
          F31.13
        with psychotic features F31.2
      mixed F31.60
        mild F31.61
        moderate F31.62
        severe (without psychotic features)
          F31.63
        with psychotic features F31.64
      severe depression (without psychotic
        features) F31.4
        with psychotic features F31.5
    II F31.81
    in remission (currently) F31.70
      in full remission
        most recent episode
          depressed F31.76
          hypomanic F31.72
          manic F31.74
          mixed F31.78
      in partial remission
        most recent episode
          depressed F31.75
          hypomanic F31.71
          manic F31.73
          mixed F31.77
    organic F06.30
    single manic episode F30.9
      mild F30.11
      moderate F30.12
      severe (without psychotic symptoms)
        F30.13
      with psychotic symptoms F30.2
    specified NEC F31.89

Disorder *(Continued)*
  bladder N32.9
    functional NEC N31.9
    in schistosomiasis B65.0 *[N33]*
    specified NEC N32.89
  bleeding D68.9
  blood D75.9
    in congenital early syphilis A50.09 *[D77]*
  body dysmorphic F45.22
  bone M89.9
    continuity M84.9
      specified type NEC M84.80
        ankle M84.87-
        fibula M84.86-
        foot M84.87-
        hand M84.84-
        humerus M84.82-
        neck M84.88
        pelvis M84.859
        radius M84.83-
        rib M84.88
        shoulder M84.81-
        skull M84.88
        thigh M84.85-
        tibia M84.86-
        ulna M84.83-
        vertebra M84.88
    density and structure M85.9
      cyst —*see also* Cyst, bone, specified type
        NEC
        aneurysmal —*see* Cyst, bone,
          aneurysmal
        solitary —*see* Cyst, bone, solitary
      diffuse idiopathic skeletal
        hyperostosis —*see* Hyperostosis,
        ankylosing
      fibrous dysplasia (monostotic) —*see*
        Dysplasia, fibrous, bone
      fluorosis —*see* Fluorosis, skeletal
      hyperostosis of skull M85.2
      osteitis condensans —*see* Osteitis,
        condensans
      specified type NEC M85.8-
        ankle M85.87-
        foot M85.87-
        forearm M85.83-
        hand M85.84-
        lower leg M85.86-
        multiple sites M85.89
        neck M85.88
        rib M85.88
        shoulder M85.81-
        skull M85.88
        thigh M85.85-
        upper arm M85.82-
        vertebra M85.88
    development and growth NEC
      M89.20
      carpus M89.24-
      clavicle M89.21-
      femur M89.25-
      fibula M89.26-
      finger M89.24-
      humerus M89.22-
      ilium M89.259
      ischium M89.259
      metacarpus M89.24-
      metatarsus M89.27-
      multiple sites M89.29
      neck M89.28
      radius M89.23-
      rib M89.28
      scapula M89.21-
      skull M89.28
      tarsus M89.27-
      tibia M89.26-
      toe M89.27-
      ulna M89.23-
      vertebra M89.28
    specified type NEC M89.8X-
  brachial plexus G54.0

◀ New   ◀▥ Revised   ~~deleted~~ Deleted

Disorder *(Continued)*
  branched-chain amino-acid metabolism
    E71.2
    specified NEC E71.19
  breast N64.9
    agalactia —*see* Agalactia
    associated with
      lactation O92.70
        specified NEC O92.79
      pregnancy O92.20
        specified NEC O92.29
      puerperium O92.20
        specified NEC O92.29
    cracked nipple —*see* Cracked nipple
    galactorrhea —*see* Galactorrhea
    hypogalactia O92.4
    lactation disorder NEC O92.79
    mastitis —*see* Mastitis
    nipple infection —*see* Infection, nipple
    retracted nipple —*see* Retraction, nipple
    specified type NEC N64.89
  Briquet's F45.0
  bullous, in diseases classified elsewhere L14
  cannabis use
    due to drug abuse —*see* Abuse, drug,
      cannabis
    due to drug dependence —*see* Dependence,
      drug, cannabis
  carbohydrate
    absorption, intestinal NEC E74.39
    metabolism (congenital) E74.9
      specified NEC E74.8
  cardiac, functional I51.89
  carnitine metabolism E71.40
  cartilage M94.9
    articular NEC —*see* Derangement, joint,
      articular cartilage
    chondrocalcinosis —*see*
      Chondrocalcinosis
    specified type NEC M94.8X-
      articular —*see* Derangement, joint,
        articular cartilage
      multiple sites M94.8X0
  catatonic
    due to (secondary to) known physiological
      condition F06.1
    organic F06.1
  central auditory processing H93.25
  cervical
    region NEC M53.82
    root (nerve) NEC G54.2
  character NOS F60.9
  childhood disintegrative NEC F84.3
  cholesterol and bile acid metabolism E78.70
    Barth syndrome E78.71
    other specified E78.79
    Smith-Lemli-Opitz syndrome E78.72
  choroid H31.9
    atrophy —*see* Atrophy, choroid
    degeneration —*see* Degeneration, choroid
    detachment —*see* Detachment, choroid
    dystrophy —*see* Dystrophy, choroid
    hemorrhage —*see* Hemorrhage, choroid
    rupture —*see* Rupture, choroid
    scar —*see* Scar, chorioretinal
    solar retinopathy —*see* Retinopathy, solar
    specified type NEC H31.8
  ciliary body —*see* Disorder, iris
    degeneration —*see* Degeneration, ciliary
      body
  coagulation (factor) (*see also* Defect,
    coagulation) D68.9
    newborn, transient P61.6
  coccyx NEC M53.3
  cognitive F09
    due to (secondary to) general medical
      condition F09
    persisting R41.89
      due to
        alcohol F10.97
          with dependence F10.27

Disorder *(Continued)*
  cognitive *(Continued)*
    persisting *(Continued)*
      due to *(Continued)*
        anxiolytics F13.97
          with dependence F13.27
        hypnotics F13.97
          with dependence F13.27
        sedatives F13.97
          with dependence F13.27
        specified substance NEC F19.97
          with
            abuse F19.17
            dependence F19.27
  communication F80.9
  conduct (childhood) F91.9
    adjustment reaction —*see* Disorder,
      adjustment
    adolescent onset type F91.2
    childhood onset type F91.1
    compulsive F63.9
    confined to family context F91.0
    depressive F91.8
    group type F91.2
    hyperkinetic —*see* Disorder, attention-
      deficit hyperactivity
    oppositional defiance F91.3
    socialized F91.2
    solitary aggressive type F91.1
    specified NEC F91.8
    unsocialized (aggressive) F91.1
  conduction, heart I45.9
  congenital glycosylation (CDG)
    E74.8
  conjunctiva H11.9
    infection —*see* Conjunctivitis
  connective tissue, localized L94.9
    specified NEC L94.8
  conversion —*see* Disorder, dissociative
  convulsive (secondary) —*see* Convulsions
  cornea H18.9
    deformity —*see* Deformity, cornea
    degeneration —*see* Degeneration,
      cornea
    deposits —*see* Deposit, cornea
    due to contact lens H18.82-
      specified as edema —*see* Edema,
        cornea
    edema —*see* Edema, cornea
    keratitis —*see* Keratitis
    keratoconjunctivitis —*see*
      Keratoconjunctivitis
    membrane change —*see* Change, corneal
      membrane
    neovascularization —*see*
      Neovascularization, cornea
    scar —*see* Opacity, cornea
    specified type NEC H18.89-
    ulcer —*see* Ulcer, cornea
  corpus cavernosum N48.9
  cranial nerve —*see* Disorder, nerve, cranial
  cyclothymic F34.0
  defiant oppositional F91.3
  delusional (persistent) (systematized)
    F22
    induced F24
  depersonalization F48.1
  depressive F32.9
    major F32.9
      with psychotic symptoms F32.3
      in remission (full) F32.5
        partial F32.4
      recurrent F33.9
      single episode F32.9
        mild F32.0
        moderate F32.1
        severe (without psychotic symptoms)
          F32.2
          with psychotic symptoms
            F32.3
    organic F06.31

Disorder *(Continued)*
  depressive *(Continued)*
    recurrent F33.9
      current episode
        mild F33.0
        moderate F33.1
        severe (without psychotic symptoms)
          F33.2
          with psychotic symptoms F33.3
      in remission F33.40
        full F33.42
        partial F33.41
      specified NEC F33.8
    single episode —*see* Episode, depressive
  developmental F89
    arithmetical skills F81.2
    coordination (motor) F82
    expressive writing F81.81
    language F80.9
      expressive F80.1
      mixed receptive and expressive
        F80.2
      receptive type F80.2
      specified NEC F80.89
    learning F81.9
      arithmetical F81.2
      reading F81.0
    mixed F88
    motor coordination or function F82
    pervasive F84.9
      specified NEC F84.8
    phonological F80.0
    reading F81.0
    scholastic skills —*see also* Disorder,
      learning
      mixed F81.89
    specified NEC F88
    speech F80.9
      articulation F80.0
      specified NEC F80.89
    written expression F81.81
  diaphragm J98.6
  digestive (system) K92.9
    newborn P78.9
      specified NEC P78.89
    postprocedural —*see* Complication,
      gastrointestinal
    psychogenic F45.8
  disc (intervertebral) M51.9
    with
      myelopathy
        cervical region M50.00
        cervicothoracic region M50.03
        high cervical region M50.01
        lumbar region M51.06
        mid-cervical region M50.02
        sacrococcygeal region M53.3
        thoracic region M51.04
        thoracolumbar region M51.05
      radiculopathy
        cervical region M50.10
        cervicothoracic region M50.13
        high cervical region M50.11
        lumbar region M51.16
        lumbosacral region M51.17
        mid-cervical region M50.12
        sacrococcygeal region M53.3
        thoracic region M51.14
        thoracolumbar region M51.15
    cervical M50.90
      with
        myelopathy M50.00
          C2-C3 M50.01
          C3-C4 M50.01
          C4-C5 M50.02
          C5-C6 M50.02
          C6-C7 M50.02
          C7-T1 M50.03
          cervicothoracic region M50.03
          high cervical region M50.01
          mid-cervical region M50.02

Disorder (*Continued*)
  disc (*Continued*)
    cervical (*Continued*)
      with (*Continued*)
        neuritis, radiculitis or radiculopathy
          M50.10
          C2-C3 M50.11
          C3-C4 M50.11
          C4-C5 M50.12
          C5-C6 M50.12
          C6-C7 M50.12
          C7-T1 M50.13
          cervicothoracic region M50.13
          high cervical region M50.11
          mid-cervical region M50.12
        C2-C3 M50.91
        C3-C4 M50.91
        C4-C5 M50.92
        C5-C6 M50.92
        C6-C7 M50.92
        C7-T1 M50.93
        cervicothoracic region M50.93
        degeneration M50.30
          C2-C3 M50.31
          C3-C4 M50.31
          C4-C5 M50.32
          C5-C6 M50.32
          C6-C7 M50.32
          C7-T1 M50.33
          cervicothoracic region M50.33
          high cervical region M50.31
          mid-cervical region M50.32
        displacement M50.20
          C2-C3 M50.21
          C3-C4 M50.21
          C4-C5 M50.22
          C5-C6 M50.22
          C6-C7 M50.22
          C7-T1 M50.23
          cervicothoracic region M50.23
          high cervical region M50.21
          mid-cervical region M50.22
        high cervical region M50.91
        mid-cervical region M50.92
        specified type NEC M50.80
          C2-C3 M50.81
          C3-C4 M50.81
          C4-C5 M50.82
          C5-C6 M50.82
          C6-C7 M50.82
          C7-T1 M50.83
          cervicothoracic region M50.83
          high cervical region M50.81
          mid-cervical region M50.82
    specified NEC
      lumbar region M51.86
      lumbosacral region M51.87
      sacrococcygeal region M53.3
      thoracic region M51.84
      thoracolumbar region M51.85
  disinhibited attachment (childhood)
    F94.2
  disintegrative, childhood NEC F84.3
  disruptive behavior F98.9
  dissocial personality F60.2
  dissociative F44.9
    affecting
      motor function F44.4
        and sensation F44.7
      sensation F44.6
        and motor function F44.7
    brief reactive F43.0
    due to (secondary to) general medical
      condition F06.8
    mixed F44.7
    organic F06.8
    other specified NEC F44.89
  double heterozygous sickling —*see* Disease,
    sickle-cell
  dream anxiety F51.5
  drug induced hemorrhagic D68.32

Disorder (*Continued*)
  drug related F19.99
    abuse —*see* Abuse, drug
    dependence —*see* Dependence,
      drug
  dysmorphic body F45.1
  dysthymic F34.1
  ear H93.9-
    bleeding —*see* Otorrhagia
    deafness —*see* Deafness
    degenerative H93.09-
    discharge —*see* Otorrhea
    external H61.9-
      auditory canal stenosis —*see* Stenosis,
        external ear canal
      exostosis —*see* Exostosis, external ear
        canal
      impacted cerumen —*see* Impaction,
        cerumen
      otitis —*see* Otitis, externa
      perichondritis —*see* Perichondritis,
        ear
      pinna —*see* Disorder, pinna
      specified type NEC H61.89-
        in diseases classified elsewhere
          H62.8X-
    inner H83.9-
      vestibular dysfunction —*see* Disorder,
        vestibular function
    middle H74.9-
      adhesive H74.1-
      ossicle —*see* Abnormal, ear ossicles
      polyp —*see* Polyp, ear (middle)
      specified NEC, in diseases classified
        elsewhere H75.8-
    postprocedural —*see* Complications, ear,
      procedure
    specified NEC, in diseases classified
      elsewhere H94.8-
  eating (adult) (psychogenic) F50.9
    anorexia —*see* Anorexia
    bulimia F50.2
    child F98.29
      pica F98.3
      rumination disorder F98.21
    pica F50.8
      childhood F98.3
  electrolyte (balance) NEC E87.8
    with
      abortion —*see* Abortion by type
        complicated by specified condition
          NEC
      ectopic pregnancy O08.5
      molar pregnancy O08.5
      acidosis (metabolic) (respiratory)
        E87.2
      alkalosis (metabolic) (respiratory)
        E87.3
  elimination, transepidermal L87.9
    specified NEC L87.8
  emotional (persistent) F34.9
    of childhood F93.9
      specified NEC F93.8
  endocrine E34.9
    postprocedural E89.89
    specified NEC E89.89
  erectile (male) (organic) (*see also*
    Dysfunction, sexual, male, erectile)
    N52.9
    nonorganic F52.21
  erythematous —*see* Erythema
  esophagus K22.9
    functional K22.4
    psychogenic F45.8
  eustachian tube H69.9-
    infection —*see* Salpingitis, eustachian
    obstruction —*see* Obstruction, eustachian
      tube
    patulous —*see* Patulous, eustachian
      tube
    specified NEC H69.8-

Disorder (*Continued*)
  extrapyramidal G25.9
    in diseases classified elsewhere —*see*
      category G26
    specified type NEC G25.89
  eye H57.9
    postprocedural —*see* Complication,
      postprocedural, eye
  eyelid H02.9
    cyst —*see* Cyst, eyelid
    degenerative H02.70
      chloasma —*see* Chloasma, eyelid
      madarosis —*see* Madarosis
      specified type NEC H02.79
      vitiligo —*see* Vitiligo, eyelid
      xanthelasma —*see* Xanthelasma
    dermatochalasis —*see* Dermato-chalasis
    edema —*see* Edema, eyelid
    elephantiasis —*see* Elephantiasis, eyelid
    foreign body, retained —*see* Foreign body,
      retained, eyelid
    function H02.59
      abnormal innervation syndrome —*see*
        Syndrome, abnormal innervation
      blepharochalasis —*see* Blepharochalasis
      blepharoclonus —*see* Blepharoclonus
      blepharophimosis —*see*
        Blepharophimosis
      blepharoptosis —*see* Blepharoptosis
      lagophthalmos —*see* Lagophthalmos
      lid retraction —*see* Retraction, lid
    hypertrichosis —*see* Hypertrichosis, eyelid
    specified type NEC H02.89
    vascular H02.879
      left H02.876
        lower H02.875
        upper H02.874
      right H02.873
        lower H02.872
        upper H02.871
  factitious F68.10
    with predominantly
      physical symptoms F68.12
        with psychological symptoms F68.13
      psychological symptoms F68.11
        with physical symptoms F68.13
  factor, coagulation —*see* Defect, coagulation
  fatty acid
    metabolism E71.30
      specified NEC E71.39
    oxidation
      LCAD E71.310
      MCAD E71.311
      SCAD E71.312
      specified deficiency NEC E71.318
  feeding (infant or child) (*see also* Disorder,
    eating) R63.3-
  feigned (with obvious motivation) Z76.5
    without obvious motivation —*see* Disorder,
      factitious
  female
    hypoactive sexual desire F52.0
    orgasmic F52.31
    sexual arousal F52.22
  fibroblastic M72.9
    specified NEC M72.8
  fluency
    adult onset F98.5
    childhood onset F80.81
    following
      cerebral infarction I69.323
      cerebrovascular disease I69.923
        specified disease NEC I69.823
      intracerebral hemorrhage I69.123
      nontraumatic intracranial hemorrhage
        NEC I69.223
      subarachnoid hemorrhage I69.023
    in conditions classified elsewhere R47.82
  fluid balance E87.8
  follicular (skin) L73.9
    specified NEC L73.8

◀ New   ◀▦ Revised   ~~deleted~~ Deleted

Disorder (Continued)
  fructose metabolism E74.10
    essential fructosuria E74.11
    fructokinase deficiency E74.11
    fructose-1, 6-diphosphatase deficiency
        E74.19
    hereditary fructose intolerance E74.12
    other specified E74.19
  functional polymorphonuclear neutrophils
      D71
  gallbladder, biliary tract and pancreas in
      diseases classified elsewhere K87
  gamma-glutamyl cycle E72.8
  gastric (functional) K31.9
    motility K30
    psychogenic F45.8
    secretion K30
  gastrointestinal (functional) NOS K92.9
    newborn P78.9
    psychogenic F45.8
  gender-identity or -role F64.9
    childhood F64.2
    effect on relationship F66
    of adolescence or adulthood
        (nontranssexual) F64.1
    specified NEC F64.8
    uncertainty F66
  genitourinary system
    female N94.9
    male N50.9
    psychogenic F45.8
  globe H44.9
    degenerated condition H44.50
      absolute glaucoma H44.51-
      atrophy H44.52-
      leucocoria H44.53-
    degenerative H44.30
      chalcosis H44.31-
      myopia H44.2-
      siderosis H44.32-
      specified type NEC H44.39-
    endophthalmitis —see Endophthalmitis
    foreign body, retained —see Foreign body,
        intraocular, old, retained
    hemophthalmos —see Hemophthalmos
    hypotony H44.40
      due to
        ocular fistula H44.42-
        specified disorder NEC H44.43-
      flat anterior chamber H44.41-
      primary H44.44-
    luxation —see Luxation, globe
    specified type NEC H44.89
  glomerular (in) N05.9
    amyloidosis E85.4 [N08]
    cryoglobulinemia D89.1 [N08]
    disseminated intravascular coagulation
        D65 [N08]
    Fabry's disease E75.21 [N08]
    familial lecithin cholesterol acyltransferase
        deficiency E78.6 [N08]
    Goodpasture's syndrome M31.0
    hemolytic-uremic syndrome D59.3
    Henoch (-Schönlein) purpura D69.0 [N08]
    malariae malaria B52.0
    microscopic polyangiitis M31.7 [N08]
    multiple myeloma C90.0- [N08]
    mumps B26.83
    schistosomiasis B65.9 [N08]
    sepsis NEC A41.- [N08]
      streptococcal A40.- [N08]
    sickle-cell disorders D57.- [N08]
    strongyloidiasis B78.9 [N08]
    subacute bacterial endocarditis I33.0 [N08]
    syphilis A52.75
    systemic lupus erythematosus M32.14
    thrombotic thrombocytopenic purpura
        M31.1 [N08]
    Waldenström macroglobulinemia C88.0
        [N08]
    Wegener's granulomatosis M31.31

Disorder (Continued)
  gluconeogenesis E74.4
  glucosaminoglycan metabolism —
      see Disorder, metabolism,
      glucosaminoglycan
  glycine metabolism E72.50
    d-glycericacidemia E72.59
    hyperhydroxyprolinemia E72.59
    hyperoxaluria E72.53
    hyperprolinemia E72.59
    non-ketotic hyperglycinemia E72.51
    oxalosis E72.53
    oxaluria E72.53
    sarcosinemia E72.59
    trimethylaminuria E72.52
  glycoprotein metabolism E77.9
    specified NEC E77.8
  habit (and impulse) F63.9
    involving sexual behavior NEC F65.9
    specified NEC F63.89
  heart action I49.9
  hematological D75.9
    newborn (transient) P61.9
      specified NEC P61.8
  hematopoietic organs D75.9
  hemorrhagic NEC D69.9
    drug-induced D68.32
    due to
      extrinsic circulating anticoagulants D68.32
      increase in
        anti-IIa D68.32
        anti-Xa D68.32
      intrinsic
        circulating anticoagulants D68.318
        increase in
          antithrombin D68.318
          anti-VIIIa D68.318
          anti-IXa D68.318
          anti-XIa D68.318
    following childbirth O72.3
  hemostasis —see Defect, coagulation
  histidine metabolism E70.40
    histidinemia E70.41
    other specified E70.49
  hyperkinetic —see Disorder, attention-deficit
      hyperactivity
  hyperleucine-isoleucinemia E71.19
  hypervalinemia E71.19
  hypoactive sexual desire F52.0
  hypochondriacal F45.20
    body dysmorphic F45.22
    neurosis F45.21
    other specified F45.29
  identity
    dissociative F44.81
    of childhood F93.8
  immune mechanism (immunity) D89.9
    specified type NEC D89.89
  impaired renal tubular function N25.9
    specified NEC N25.89
  impulse (control) F63.9
  inflammatory
    pelvic, in diseases classified elsewhere —
        see category N74
    penis N48.29
      abscess N48.21
      cellulitis N48.22
  integument, newborn P83.9
    specified NEC P83.8
  intermittent explosive F63.81
  internal secretion pancreas —see Increased,
      secretion, pancreas, endocrine
  intestine, intestinal
    carbohydrate absorption NEC E74.39
      postoperative K91.2
    functional NEC K59.9
      postoperative K91.89
    psychogenic F45.8
    vascular K55.9
      chronic K55.1
      specified NEC K55.8

Disorder (Continued)
  intraoperative (intraprocedural) —see
      Complications, intraoperative
  involuntary emotional expression (IEED)
      F48.2
  iris H21.9
    adhesions —see Adhesions, iris
    atrophy —see Atrophy, iris
    chamber angle recession —see Recession,
        chamber angle
    cyst —see Cyst, iris
    degeneration —see Degeneration, iris
    in diseases classified elsewhere H22
    iridodialysis —see Iridodialysis
    iridoschisis —see Iridoschisis
    miotic pupillary cyst —see Cyst, pupillary
    pupillary
      abnormality —see Abnormality,
          pupillary
      membrane —see Membrane, pupillary
    specified type NEC H21.89
    vascular NEC H21.1X-
  iron metabolism E83.10
    specified NEC E83.19
  isovaleric acidemia E71.110
  jaw, developmental M27.0
    temporomandibular —see Anomaly,
        dentofacial, temporomandibular joint
  joint M25.9
    derangement —see Derangement, joint
    effusion —see Effusion, joint
    fistula —see Fistula, joint
    hemarthrosis —see Hemarthrosis
    instability —see Instability, joint
    osteophyte —see Osteophyte
    pain —see Pain, joint
    psychogenic F45.8
    specified type NEC M25.80
      ankle M25.87-
      elbow M25.82-
      foot joint M25.87-
      hand joint M25.84-
      hip M25.85-
      knee M25.86-
      shoulder M25.81-
      wrist M25.83-
    stiffness —see Stiffness, joint
  ketone metabolism E71.32
  kidney N28.9
    functional (tubular) N25.9
    in
      schistosomiasis B65.9 [N29]
    tubular function N25.9
      specified NEC N25.89
  lacrimal system H04.9
    changes H04.69
      fistula —see Fistula, lacrimal
    gland H04.19
      atrophy —see Atrophy, lacrimal gland
      cyst —see Cyst, lacrimal, gland
      dacryops —see Dacryops
      dislocation —see Dislocation, lacrimal
          gland
      dry eye syndrome —see Syndrome, dry
          eye
      infection —see Dacryoadenitis
      granuloma —see Granuloma, lacrimal
      inflammation —see Inflammation, lacrimal
      obstruction —see Obstruction, lacrimal
      specified NEC H04.89
  lactation NEC O92.79
  language (developmental) F80.9
    expressive F80.1
    mixed receptive and expressive F80.2
    receptive F80.2
  late luteal phase dysphoric N94.89
  learning (specific) F81.9
    acalculia R48.8
    alexia R48.0
    mathematics F81.2
    reading F81.0

Disorder *(Continued)*
  learning *(Continued)*
    specified NEC F81.89
    spelling F81.81
    written expression F81.81
  lens H27.9
    aphakia —*see* Aphakia
    cataract —*see* Cataract
    dislocation —*see* Dislocation, lens
    specified type NEC H27.8
  ligament M24.20
    ankle M24.27-
    attachment, spine —*see* Enthesopathy, spinal
    elbow M24.22-
    foot joint M24.27-
    hand joint M24.24-
    hip M24.25-
    knee —*see* Derangement, knee, specified NEC
    shoulder M24.21-
    vertebra M24.28
    wrist M24.23-
  ligamentous attachments —*see also* Enthesopathy
    spine —*see* Enthesopathy, spinal
  lipid
    metabolism, congenital E78.9
    storage E75.6
      specified NEC E75.5
  lipoprotein
    deficiency (familial) E78.6
    metabolism E78.9
      specified NEC E78.89
  liver K76.9
    malarial B54 *[K77]*
  low back —*see also* Dorsopathy, specified NEC
  lumbosacral
    plexus G54.1
    root (nerve) NEC G54.4
  lung, interstitial, drug-induced J70.4
    acute J70.2
    chronic J70.3
  lymphoproliferative, post-transplant (PTLD) D47.Z1
  lysine and hydroxylysine metabolism E72.3
  male
    erectile (organic) *(see also* Dysfunction, sexual, male, erectile) N52.9
      nonorganic F52.21
    hypoactive sexual desire F52.0
    orgasmic F52.32
  manic F30.9
    organic F06.33
  mastoid —*see also* Disorder, ear, middle
    postprocedural —*see* Complications, ear, procedure
  meniscus —*see* Derangement, knee, meniscus
  menopausal N95.9
    specified NEC N95.8
  menstrual N92.6
    psychogenic F45.8
    specified NEC N92.5
  mental (or behavioral) (nonpsychotic) F99
    due to (secondary to)
      amphetamine
        due to drug abuse —*see* Abuse, drug, stimulant
        due to drug dependence —*see* Dependence, drug, stimulant
      brain disease, damage and dysfunction F09
      caffeine use
        due to drug abuse —*see* Abuse, drug, stimulant
        due to drug dependence —*see* Dependence, drug, stimulant
      cannabis use
        due to drug abuse —*see* Abuse, drug, cannabis
        due to drug dependence —*see* Dependence, drug, cannabis

Disorder *(Continued)*
  mental *(Continued)*
    due to *(Continued)*
      general medical condition F09
      sedative or hypnotic use
        due to drug abuse —*see* Abuse, drug, sedative
        due to drug dependence —*see* Dependence, drug, sedative
      tobacco (nicotine) use —*see* Dependence, drug, nicotine
    following organic brain damage F07.9
      frontal lobe syndrome F07.0
      personality change F07.0
      postconcussional syndrome F07.81
      specified NEC F07.89
    infancy, childhood or adolescence F98.9
    neurotic —*see* Neurosis
    organic or symptomatic F09
    presenile, psychotic F03
    problem NEC
    psychoneurotic —*see* Neurosis
    psychotic —*see* Psychosis
    puerperal F53
    senile, psychotic NEC F03
  metabolic, amino acid, transitory, newborn P74.8
  metabolism NOS E88.9
    amino-acid E72.9
      aromatic E70.9
        albinism —*see* Albinism
        histidine E70.40
          histidinemia E70.41
          other specified E70.49
        hyperphenylalaninemia E70.1
          classical phenylketonuria E70.0
        other specified E70.8
        tryptophan E70.5
        tyrosine E70.20
          hypertyrosinemia E70.21
          other specified E70.29
      branched chain E71.2
        3-methylglutaconic aciduria E71.111
        hyperleucine-isoleucinemia E71.19
        hypervalinemia E71.19
        isovaleric acidemia E71.110
        maple syrup urine disease E71.0
        methylmalonic acidemia E71.120
        organic aciduria NEC E71.118
        other specified E71.19
        proprionate NEC E71.128
        proprionic acidemia E71.121
      glycine E72.50
        d-glycericacidemia E72.59
        hyperhydroxyprolinemia E72.59
        hyperoxaluria E72.53
        hyperprolinemia E72.59
        non-ketotic hyperglycinemia E72.51
        other specified E72.59
        sarcosinemia E72.59
        trimethylaminuria E72.52
      hydroxylysine E72.3
      lysine E72.3
      ornithine E72.4
      other specified E72.8
        beta-amino acid E72.8
        gamma-glutamyl cycle E72.8
      straight-chain E72.8
      sulfur-bearing E72.10
        homocystinuria E72.11
        methylenetetrahydrofolate reductase deficiency E72.12
        other specified E72.19
    bile acid and cholesterol metabolism E78.70
    bilirubin E80.7
      specified NEC E80.6
    calcium E83.50
      hypercalcemia E83.52
      hypocalcemia E83.51
      other specified E83.59

Disorder *(Continued)*
  metabolism NOS *(Continued)*
    carbohydrate E74.9
      specified NEC E74.8
    cholesterol and bile acid metabolism E78.70
    congenital E88.9
    copper E83.00
      specified type NEC E83.09
      Wilson's disease E83.01
    cystinuria E72.01
    fructose E74.10
    galactose E74.20
    glucosaminoglycan E76.9
      mucopolysaccharidosis —*see* Mucopolysaccharidosis
      specified NEC E76.8
    glutamine E72.8
    glycine E72.50
    glycogen storage (hepatorenal) E74.09
    glycoprotein E77.9
      specified NEC E77.8
    glycosaminoglycan E76.9
      specified NEC E76.8
    in labor and delivery O75.89
    iron E83.10
    isoleucine E71.19
    leucine E71.19
    lipoid E78.9
    lipoprotein E78.9
      specified NEC E78.89
    magnesium E83.40
      hypermagnesemia E83.41
      hypomagnesemia E83.42
      other specified E83.49
    mineral E83.9
      specified NEC E83.89
    mitochondrial E88.40
      MELAS syndrome E88.41
      MERRF syndrome (myoclonic epilepsy associated with ragged-red fibers) E88.42
      other specified E88.49
    ornithine E72.4
    phosphatases E83.30
    phosphorus E83.30
      acid phosphatase deficiency E83.39
      hypophosphatasia E83.39
      hypophosphatemia E83.39
        familial E83.31
      other specified E83.39
      pseudovitamin D deficiency E83.32
    plasma protein NEC E88.09
    porphyrin —*see* Porphyria
    postprocedural E89.89
      specified NEC E89.89
    purine E79.9
      specified NEC E79.8
    pyrimidine E79.9
      specified NEC E79.8
    pyruvate E74.4
    serine E72.8
    sodium E87.8
    specified NEC E88.89
    threonine E72.8
    valine E71.19
    zinc E83.2
  methylmalonic acidemia E71.120
  micturition NEC R39.19
    feeling of incomplete emptying R39.14
    hesitancy R39.11
    poor stream R39.12
    psychogenic F45.8
    split stream R39.13
    straining R39.16
    urgency R39.15
  mitochondrial metabolism E88.40
  mitral (valve) —*see* Endocarditis, mitral

◀ New   ◀▦ Revised   ~~deleted~~ Deleted

Disorder *(Continued)*
  mixed
    anxiety and depressive F41.8
    of scholastic skills (developmental)
        F81.89
    receptive expressive language F80.2
  mood F39
    bipolar —*see* Disorder, bipolar
    depressive —*see* Disorder, depressive
    due to (secondary to)
      alcohol F10.94
      amphetamine F15.94
        in
          abuse F15.14
          dependence F15.24
      anxiolytic F13.94
        in
          abuse F13.14
          dependence F13.24
      cocaine F14.94
        in
          abuse F14.14
          dependence F14.24
      general medical condition F06.30
      hallucinogen F16.94
        in
          abuse F16.14
          dependence F16.24
      hypnotic F13.94
        in
          abuse F13.14
          dependence F13.24
      inhalant F18.94
        in
          abuse F18.14
          dependence F18.24
      opioid F11.94
        in
          abuse F11.14
          dependence F11.24
      phencyclidine (PCP) F16.94
        in
          abuse F16.14
          dependence F16.24
      physiological condition F06.30
        with
          depressive features F06.31
          major depressive-like episode
              F06.32
          manic features F06.33
          mixed features F06.34
      psychoactive substance NEC F19.94
        in
          abuse F19.14
          dependence F19.24
      sedative F13.94
        in
          abuse F13.14
          dependence F13.24
      volatile solvents F18.94
        in
          abuse F18.14
          dependence F18.24
  manic episode F30.9
    with psychotic symptoms F30.2
    without psychotic symptoms
        F30.10
      mild F30.11
      moderate F30.12
      severe F30.13
    in remission (full) F30.4
      partial F30.3
    specified type NEC F30.8
  organic F06.30
    right hemisphere F07.89
  persistent F34.9
    cyclothymia F34.0
    dysthymia F34.1
    specified type NEC F34.8
  recurrent F39
  right hemisphere organic F07.89

Disorder *(Continued)*
  movement G25.9
    drug-induced G25.70
      akathisia G25.71
      specified NEC G25.79
    hysterical F44.4
    in diseases classified elsewhere —*see*
        category G26
    periodic limb G47.61
      sleep related G47.61
    sleep related NEC G47.69
    specified NEC G25.89
    stereotyped F98.4
    treatment-induced G25.9
  multiple personality F44.81
  muscle M62.9
    attachment, spine —*see* Enthesopathy,
        spinal
    in trichinellosis —*see* Trichinellosis, with
        muscle disorder
    psychogenic F45.8
    specified type NEC M62.89
    tone, newborn P94.9
      specified NEC P94.8
  muscular
    attachments —*see also* Enthesopathy
      spine —*see* Enthesopathy, spinal
    urethra N36.44
  musculoskeletal system, soft tissue —*see*
        Disorder, soft tissue
    postprocedural M96.89
    psychogenic F45.8
  myoneural G70.9
    due to lead G70.1
    specified NEC G70.89
    toxic G70.1
  myotonic NEC G71.19
  nail, in diseases classified elsewhere L62
  neck region NEC —*see* Dorsopathy, specified
        NEC
  nerve G58.9
    abducent NEC —*see* Strabismus, paralytic,
        sixth nerve
    accessory G52.8
    acoustic —*see* subcategory H93.3
    auditory —*see* subcategory H93.3
    auriculotemporal G50.8
    axillary G54.0
    cerebral —*see* Disorder, nerve, cranial
    cranial G52.9
      eighth —*see* subcategory H93.3
      eleventh G52.8
      fifth G50.9
      first G52.0
      fourth NEC —*see* Strabismus, paralytic,
          fourth nerve
      multiple G52.7
      ninth G52.1
      second NEC —*see* Disorder, nerve, optic
      seventh NEC G51.8
      sixth NEC —*see* Strabismus, paralytic,
          sixth nerve
      specified NEC G52.8
      tenth G52.2
      third NEC —*see* Strabismus, paralytic,
          third nerve
      twelfth G52.3
    entrapment —*see* Neuropathy, entrapment
    facial G51.9
      specified NEC G51.8
    femoral —*see* Lesion, nerve, femoral
    glossopharyngeal NEC G52.1
    hypoglossal G52.3
    intercostal G58.0
    lateral
      cutaneous of thigh —*see*
          Mononeuropathy, lower limb,
          meralgia paresthetica
    popliteal —*see* Lesion, nerve, popliteal
    lower limb —*see* Mononeuropathy, lower
        limb

Disorder *(Continued)*
  nerve *(Continued)*
    medial popliteal —*see* Lesion, nerve,
        popliteal, medial
    median NEC —*see* Lesion, nerve,
        median
    multiple G58.7
    oculomotor NEC —*see* Strabismus,
        paralytic, third nerve
    olfactory G52.0
    optic NEC H47.09-
      hemorrhage into sheath —*see*
          Hemorrhage, optic nerve
      ischemic H47.01-
    peroneal —*see* Lesion, nerve, popliteal
    phrenic G58.8
    plantar —*see* Lesion, nerve, plantar
    pneumogastric G52.2
    posterior tibial —*see* Syndrome, tarsal
        tunnel
    radial —*see* Lesion, nerve, radial
    recurrent laryngeal G52.2
    root G54.9
      cervical G54.2
      lumbosacral G54.1
      specified NEC G54.8
      thoracic G54.3
    sciatic NEC —*see* Lesion, nerve, sciatic
    specified NEC G58.8
      lower limb —*see* Mononeuropathy,
          lower limb, specified NEC
      upper limb —*see* Mononeuropathy,
          upper limb, specified NEC
    sympathetic G90.9
    tibial —*see* Lesion, nerve, popliteal,
        medial
    trigeminal G50.9
      specified NEC G50.8
    trochlear NEC —*see* Strabismus, paralytic,
        fourth nerve
    ulnar —*see* Lesion, nerve, ulnar
    upper limb —*see* Mononeuropathy, upper
        limb
    vagus G52.2
  nervous system G98.8
    autonomic (peripheral) G90.9
      specified NEC G90.8
    central G96.9
      specified NEC G96.8
    parasympathetic G90.9
    specified NEC G98.8
    sympathetic G90.9
    vegetative G90.9
  neurohypophysis NEC E23.3
  neurological NEC R29.818
  neuromuscular G70.9
    hereditary NEC G71.9
    specified NEC G70.89
    toxic G70.1
  neurotic F48.9
    specified NEC F48.8
  neutrophil, polymorphonuclear D71
  nicotine use —*see* Dependence, drug,
      nicotine
  nightmare F51.5
  nose J34.9
    specified NEC J34.89
  obsessive-compulsive F42
  odontogenesis NOS K00.9
  opioid use
    with
      opioid-induced psychotic disorder
          F11.959
        with
          delusions F11.950
          hallucinations F11.951
    due to drug abuse —*see* Abuse, drug,
        opioid
    due to drug dependence —*see* Dependence,
        drug, opioid
  oppositional defiant F91.3

Disorder (Continued)
  optic
    chiasm H47.49
      due to
        inflammatory disorder H47.41
        neoplasm H47.42
        vascular disorder H47.43
    disc H47.39-
      coloboma —see Coloboma, optic disc
      drusen —see Drusen, optic disc
      pseudopapilledema —see
          Pseudopapilledema
    radiations —see Disorder, visual, pathway
    tracts —see Disorder, visual, pathway
  orbit H05.9
    cyst —see Cyst, orbit
    deformity —see Deformity, orbit
    edema —see Edema, orbit
    enophthalmos —see Enophthalmos
    exophthalmos —see Exophthalmos
    hemorrhage —see Hemorrhage, orbit
    inflammation —see Inflammation, orbit
    myopathy —see Myopathy, extraocular
        muscles
    retained foreign body —see Foreign body,
        orbit, old
    specified type NEC H05.89
  organic
    anxiety F06.4
    catatonic F06.1
    delusional F06.2
    dissociative F06.8
    emotionally labile (asthenic) F06.8
    mood (affective) F06.30
    schizophrenia-like F06.2
  orgasmic (female) F52.31
    male F52.32
  ornithine metabolism E72.4
  overanxious F41.1
    of childhood F93.8
  pain
    with related psychological factors F45.42
    exclusively related to psychological factors
        F45.41
  pancreatic internal secretion E16.9
    specified NEC E16.8
  panic F41.0
    with agoraphobia F40.01
  papulosquamous L44.9
    in diseases classified elsewhere L45
    specified NEC L44.8
  paranoid F22
    induced F24
    shared F24
  parathyroid (gland) E21.5
    specified NEC E21.4
  parietoalveolar NEC J84.09
  paroxysmal, mixed R56.9
  patella M22.9-
    chondromalacia —see Chondromalacia,
        patella
    derangement NEC M22.3X-
    recurrent
      dislocation —see Dislocation, patella,
          recurrent
      subluxation —see Dislocation, patella,
          recurrent, incomplete
    specified NEC M22.8X-
  patellofemoral M22.2X-
  pentose phosphate pathway with anemia
      D55.1
  perception, due to hallucinogens F16.983
    in
      abuse F16.183
      dependence F16.283
  peripheral nervous system NEC G64
  peroxisomal E71.50
    biogenesis
      neonatal adrenoleukodystrophy E71.511
      specified disorder NEC E71.518
      Zellweger syndrome E71.510

Disorder (Continued)
  peroxisomal (Continued)
    rhizomelic chondrodysplasia punctata
        E71.540
    specified form NEC E71.548
      group 1 E71.518
      group 2 E71.53
      group 3 E71.542
    X-linked adrenoleukodystrophy
        E71.529
      adolescent E71.521
      adrenomyeloneuropathy E71.522
      childhood E71.520
      specified form NEC E71.528
    Zellweger-like syndrome E71.541
  persistent
    (somatoform) pain F45.41
    affective (mood) F34.9
  personality (see also Personality) F60.9
    affective F34.0
    aggressive F60.3
    amoral F60.2
    anankastic F60.5
    antisocial F60.2
    anxious F60.6
    asocial F60.2
    asthenic F60.7
    avoidant F60.6
    borderline F60.3
    change (secondary) due to general medical
        condition F07.0
    compulsive F60.5
    cyclothymic F34.0
    dependent (passive) F60.7
    depressive F34.1
    dissocial F60.2
    emotional instability F60.3
    expansive paranoid F60.0
    explosive F60.3
    following organic brain damage
        F07.9
    histrionic F60.4
    hyperthymic F34.0
    hypothymic F34.1
    hysterical F60.4
    immature F60.89
    inadequate F60.7
    labile F60.3
    mixed (nonspecific) F60.89
    moral deficiency F60.2
    narcissistic F60.81
    negativistic F60.89
    obsessional F60.5
    obsessive (-compulsive) F60.5
    organic F07.9
    overconscientious F60.5
    paranoid F60.0
    passive (-dependent) F60.7
    passive-aggressive F60.89
    pathological NEC F60.9
    pseudosocial F60.2
    psychopathic F60.2
    schizoid F60.1
    schizotypal F21
    self-defeating F60.7
    specified NEC F60.89
    type A F60.5
    unstable (emotional) F60.3
  pervasive, developmental F84.9
  phobic anxiety, childhood F40.8
  phosphate-losing tubular N25.0
  pigmentation L81.9
    choroid, congenital Q14.3
    diminished melanin formation L81.6
    iron L81.8
    specified NEC L81.8
  pinna (noninfective) H61.10-
    deformity, acquired H61.11-
    hematoma H61.12-
    perichondritis —see Perichondritis, ear
    specified type NEC H61.19-

Disorder (Continued)
  pituitary gland E23.7
    iatrogenic (postprocedural) E89.3
    specified NEC E23.6
  platelets D69.1
  plexus G54.9
    specified NEC G54.8
  polymorphonuclear neutrophils D71
  porphyrin metabolism —see Porphyria
  postconcussional F07.81
  posthallucinogen perception F16.983
    in
      abuse F16.183
      dependence F16.283
  postmenopausal N95.9
    specified NEC N95.8
  postprocedural (postoperative) —see
      Complications, postprocedural
  post-transplant lymphoproliferative D47.z1
  post-traumatic stress (PTSD) F43.10
    acute F43.11
    chronic F43.12
  premenstrual dysphoric (PMDD) N94.3
  prepuce N47.8
  propionic acidemia E71.121
  prostate N42.9
    specified NEC N42.89
  psychogenic NOS (see also condition) F45.9
    anxiety F41.8
    appetite F50.9
    asthenic F48.8
    cardiovascular (system) F45.8
    compulsive F42
    cutaneous F54
    depressive F32.9
    digestive (system) F45.8
    dysmenorrheic F45.8
    dyspneic F45.8
    endocrine (system) F54
    eye NEC F45.8
    feeding —see Disorder, eating
    functional NEC F45.8
    gastric F45.8
    gastrointestinal (system) F45.8
    genitourinary (system) F45.8
    heart (function) (rhythm) F45.8
    hyperventilatory F45.8
    hypochondriacal —see Disorder,
        hypochondriacal
    intestinal F45.8
    joint F45.8
    learning F81.9
    limb F45.8
    lymphatic (system) F45.8
    menstrual F45.8
    micturition F45.8
    monoplegic NEC F44.4
    motor F44.4
    muscle F45.8
    musculoskeletal F45.8
    neurocirculatory F45.8
    obsessive F42
    occupational F48.8
    organ or part of body NEC F45.8
    paralytic NEC F44.4
    phobic F40.9
    physical NEC F45.8
    rectal F45.8
    respiratory (system) F45.8
    rheumatic F45.8
    sexual (function) F52.9
    skin (allergic) (eczematous) F54
    sleep F51.9
    specified part of body NEC F45.8
    stomach F45.8
  psychological F99
    associated with
      disease classified elsewhere F54
      sexual
        development F66
        relationship F66
        uncertainty about gender identity F66

◀ New   ◀▥ Revised   ~~deleted~~ Deleted

Disorder (Continued)
  psychomotor NEC F44.4
    hysterical F44.4
  psychoneurotic —see also Neurosis
    mixed NEC F48.8
  psychophysiologic —see Disorder,
      somatoform
  psychosexual F65.9
    development F66
    identity of childhood F64.2
  psychosomatic NOS —see Disorder,
      somatoform
    multiple F45.0
    undifferentiated F45.1
  psychotic —see Psychosis
    transient (acute) F23
  puberty E30.9
    specified NEC E30.8
  pulmonary (valve) —see Endocarditis,
      pulmonary
  purine metabolism E79.9
  pyrimidine metabolism E79.9
  pyruvate metabolism E74.4
  reactive attachment (childhood) F94.1
  reading R48.0
    developmental (specific) F81.0
  receptive language F80.2
  receptor, hormonal, peripheral (see also
      Syndrome, androgen insensitivity)
      E34.50
  recurrent brief depressive F33.8
  reflex R29.2
  refraction H52.7
    aniseikonia H52.32
    anisometropia H52.31
    astigmatism —see Astigmatism
    hypermetropia —see Hypermetropia
    myopia —see Myopia
    presbyopia H52.4
    specified NEC H52.6
  relationship F68.8
    due to sexual orientation F66
  REM sleep behavior G47.52
  renal function, impaired (tubular) N25.9
  resonance R49.9
    specified NEC R49.8
  respiratory function, impaired —see also
      Failure, respiration
    postprocedural —see Complication,
        postoperative, respiratory system
    psychogenic F45.8
  retina H35.9
    angioid streaks H35.33
    changes in vascular appearance H35.01-
    degeneration —see Degeneration, retina
    dystrophy (hereditary) —see Dystrophy,
        retina
    edema H35.81
    hemorrhage —see Hemorrhage, retina
    ischemia H35.82
    macular degeneration —see Degeneration,
        macula
    microaneurysms H35.04-
    microvascular abnormality NEC
        H35.09
    neovascularization —see
        Neovascularization, retina
    retinopathy —see Retinopathy
    separation of layers H35.70
      central serous chorioretinopathy
          H35.71-
      pigment epithelium detachment (serous)
          H35.72-
        hemorrhagic H35.73-
    specified type NEC H35.89
    telangiectasis —see Telangiectasis, retina
    vasculitis —see Vasculitis, retina
  retroperitoneal K68.9
  right hemisphere organic affective F07.89
  rumination (infant or child) F98.21
  sacrum, sacrococcygeal NEC M53.3

Disorder (Continued)
  schizoaffective F25.9
    bipolar type F25.0
    depressive type F25.1
    manic type F25.0
    mixed type F25.0
    specified NEC F25.8
  schizoid of childhood F84.5
  schizophreniform F20.81
    brief F23
  schizotypal (personality) F21
  secretion, thyrocalcitonin E07.0
  seizure (see also Epilepsy) G40.909
    intractable G40.919
      with status epilepticus G40.911
  semantic pragmatic F80.89
    with autism F84.0
  sense of smell R43.1
    psychogenic F45.8
  separation anxiety, of childhood F93.0
  sexual
    arousal, female F52.22
    aversion F52.1
    function, psychogenic F52.9
    maturation F66
    nonorganic F52.9
    preference (see also Deviation, sexual) F65.9
      fetishistic transvestism F65.1
    relationship F66
  shyness, of childhood and adolescence
      F40.10
  sibling rivalry F93.8
  sickle-cell (sickling) (homozygous) —see
      Disease, sickle-cell
    heterozygous D57.3
    specified type NEC D57.8-
    trait D57.3
  sinus (nasal) J34.9
    specified NEC J34.89
  skin L98.9
    atrophic L90.9
      specified NEC L90.8
    granulomatous L92.9
      specified NEC L92.8
    hypertrophic L91.9
      specified NEC L91.8
    infiltrative NEC L98.6
    newborn P83.9
      specified NEC P83.8
    psychogenic (allergic) (eczematous)
        F54
  sleep G47.9
    breathing-related —see Apnea, sleep
    circadian rhythm G47.20
      advance sleep phase type G47.22
      delayed sleep phase type G47.21
      due to
        alcohol
          abuse F10.182
          dependence F10.282
          use F10.982
        amphetamines
          abuse F15.182
          dependence F15.282
          use F15.982
        caffeine
          abuse F15.182
          dependence F15.282
          use F15.982
        cocaine
          abuse F14.182
          dependence F14.282
          use F14.982
        drug NEC
          abuse F19.182
          dependence F19.282
          use F19.982
        opioid
          abuse F11.182
          dependence F11.282
          use F11.982

Disorder (Continued)
  sleep (Continued)
    circadian rhythm (Continued)
      due to (Continued)
        psychoactive substance NEC
          abuse F19.182
          dependence F19.282
          use F19.982
        sedative, hypnotic, or anxiolytic
          abuse F13.182
          dependence F13.282
          use F13.982
        stimulant NEC
          abuse F15.182
          dependence F15.282
          use F15.982
      free running type G47.24
      in conditions classified elsewhere
          G47.27
      irregular sleep wake type G47.23
      jet lag type G47.25
      shift work type G47.26
      specified NEC G47.29
    due to
      alcohol
        abuse F10.182
        dependence F10.282
        use F10.982
      amphetamine
        abuse F15.182
        dependence F15.282
        use F15.982
      anxiolytic
        abuse F13.182
        dependence F13.282
        use F13.982
      caffeine
        abuse F15.182
        dependence F15.282
        use F15.982
      cocaine
        abuse F14.182
        dependence F14.282
        use F14.982
      drug NEC
        abuse F19.182
        dependence F19.282
        use F19.982
      hypnotic
        abuse F13.182
        dependence F13.282
        use F13.982
      opioid
        abuse F11.182
        dependence F11.282
        use F11.982
      psychoactive substance NEC
        abuse F19.182
        dependence F19.282
        use F19.982
      sedative
        abuse F13.182
        dependence F13.282
        use F13.982
      stimulant NEC
        abuse F15.182
        dependence F15.282
        use F15.982
    emotional F51.9
    excessive somnolence —see Hypersomnia
    hypersomnia type —see Hypersomnia
    initiating or maintaining —see Insomnia
    nightmares F51.5
    nonorganic F51.9
      specified NEC F51.8
    parasomnia type G47.50
    specified NEC G47.8
    terrors F51.4
    walking F51.3
  sleep-wake pattern or schedule —see
      Disorder, sleep, circadian rhythm

Disorder *(Continued)*
  social
    anxiety of childhood F40.10
    functioning in childhood F94.9
      specified NEC F94.8
  soft tissue M79.9
    ankle M79.9
    due to use, overuse and pressure
        M70.90
      ankle M70.97-
      bursitis —*see* Bursitis
      foot M70.97-
      forearm M70.93-
      hand M70.94-
      lower leg M70.96-
      multiple sites M70.99
      pelvic region M70.95-
      shoulder region M70.91-
      specified site NEC M70.98
      specified type NEC M70.80
        ankle M70.87-
        foot M70.87-
        forearm M70.83-
        hand M70.84-
        lower leg M70.86-
        multiple sites M70.89
        pelvic region M70.85-
        shoulder region M70.81-
        specified site NEC M70.88
        thigh M70.85-
        upper arm M70.82-
      thigh M70.95-
      upper arm M70.92-
    foot M79.9
    forearm M79.9
    hand M79.9
    lower leg M79.9
    multiple sites M79.9
    occupational —*see* Disorder, soft tissue,
        due to use, overuse and pressure
    pelvic region M79.9
    shoulder region M79.9
    specified type NEC M79.89
    thigh M79.9
    upper arm M79.9
  somatization F45.0
  somatoform F45.9
    pain (persistent) F45.41
    somatization (multiple) (long-lasting) F45.0
    specified NEC F45.8
    undifferentiated F45.1
  somnolence, excessive —*see* Hypersomnia
  specific
    arithmetical F81.2
    developmental, of motor F82
    reading F81.0
    speech and language F80.9
    spelling F81.81
    written expression F81.81
  speech R47.9
    articulation (functional) (specific) F80.0
    developmental F80.9
    specified NEC R47.89
  spelling (specific) F81.81
  spine —*see also* Dorsopathy
    ligamentous or muscular attachments,
        peripheral —*see* Enthesopathy, spinal
    specified NEC —*see* Dorsopathy, specified
        NEC
  stereotyped, habit or movement F98.4
  stomach (functional) —*see* Disorder, gastric
  stress F43.9
    post-traumatic F43.10
      acute F43.11
      chronic F43.12
  sulfur-bearing amino-acid metabolism
      E72.10
  sweat gland (eccrine) L74.9
    apocrine L75.9
      specified NEC L75.8
    specified NEC L74.8

Disorder *(Continued)*
  synovium M67.90
    acromioclavicular M67.91-
    ankle M67.97-
    elbow M67.92-
    foot M67.97-
    forearm M67.93-
    hand M67.94-
    hip M67.95-
    knee M67.96-
    multiple sites M67.99
    rupture —*see* Rupture, synovium
    shoulder M67.91-
    specified type NEC M67.80
      acromioclavicular M67.81-
      ankle M67.87-
      elbow M67.82-
      foot M67.87-
      hand M67.84-
      hip M67.85-
      knee M67.86-
      multiple sites M67.89
      wrist M67.83-
    synovitis —*see* Synovitis
    upper arm M67.92-
    wrist M67.93-
  temperature regulation, newborn P81.9
    specified NEC P81.8
  temporomandibular joint —*see* Anomaly,
      dentofacial, temporomandibular joint
  tendon M67.90
    acromioclavicular M67.91-
    ankle M67.97-
    contracture —*see* Contracture, tendon
    elbow M67.92-
    foot M67.97-
    forearm M67.93-
    hand M67.94-
    hip M67.95-
    knee M67.96-
    multiple sites M67.99
    rupture —*see* Rupture, tendon
    shoulder M67.91-
    specified type NEC M67.80
      acromioclavicular M67.81-
      ankle M67.87-
      elbow M67.82-
      foot M67.87-
      hand M67.84-
      hip M67.85-
      knee M67.86-
      multiple sites M67.89
      trunk M67.88
      wrist M67.83-
    synovitis —*see* Synovitis
    tendinitis —*see* Tendinitis
    tenosynovitis —*see* Tenosynovitis
    trunk M67.98
    upper arm M67.92-
    wrist M67.93-
  thoracic root (nerve) NEC G54.3
  thyrocalcitonin hypersecretion E07.0
  thyroid (gland) E07.9
    function NEC, neonatal, transitory P72.2
    iodine-deficiency related E01.8
    specified NEC E07.89
  tic —*see* Tic
  tooth K08.9
    development K00.9
      specified NEC K00.8
    eruption K00.6
  Tourette's F95.2
  trance and possession F44.89
  tricuspid (valve) —*see* Endocarditis,
      tricuspid
  tryptophan metabolism E70.5
  tubular, phosphate-losing N25.0
  tubulo-interstitial (in)
    brucellosis A23.9 *[N16]*
    cystinosis E72.04
    diphtheria A36.84

Disorder *(Continued)*
  tubulo-interstitial *(Continued)*
    glycogen storage disease E74.00 *[N16]*
    leukemia NEC C95.9- *[N16]*
    lymphoma NEC C85.9- *[N16]*
    mixed cryoglobulinemia D89.1 *[N16]*
    multiple myeloma C90.0- *[N16]*
    Salmonella infection A02.25
    sarcoidosis D86.84
    sepsis A41.9 *[N16]*
      streptococcal A40.9 *[N16]*
    systemic lupus erythematosus M32.15
    toxoplasmosis B58.83
    transplant rejection T86.91 *[N16]*
    Wilson's disease E83.01 *[N16]*
  tubulo-renal function, impaired N25.9
    specified NEC N25.89
  tympanic membrane H73.9-
    atrophy —*see* Atrophy, tympanic
        membrane
    infection —*see* Myringitis
    perforation —*see* Perforation, tympanum
    specified NEC H73.89-
  unsocialized aggressive F91.1
  urea cycle metabolism E72.20
    argininemia E72.21
    arginosuccinic aciduria E72.22
    citrullinemia E72.23
    ornithine transcarbamylase deficiency
        E72.4
    other specified E72.29
  ureter (in) N28.9
    schistosomiasis B65.0 *[N29]*
    tuberculosis A18.11
  urethra N36.9
    specified NEC N36.8
  urinary system N39.9
    specified NEC N39.8
  valve, heart
    aortic —*see* Endocarditis, aortic
    mitral —*see* Endocarditis, mitral
    pulmonary —*see* Endocarditis, pulmonary
    rheumatic
      aortic —*see* Endocarditis, aortic,
          rheumatic
      mitral —*see* Endocarditis, mitral
      pulmonary —*see* Endocarditis,
          pulmonary, rheumatic
      tricuspid —*see* Endocarditis, tricuspid
    tricuspid —*see* Endocarditis, tricuspid
  vestibular function H81.9-
    specified NEC —*see* subcategory H81.8
    in diseases classified elsewhere H82.-
    vertigo —*see* Vertigo
  vision, binocular H53.30
    abnormal retinal correspondence H53.31
    diplopia H53.2
    fusion with defective stereopsis H53.32
    simultaneous perception H53.33
    suppression H53.34
  visual
    cortex
      blindness H47.619
        left brain H47.612
        right brain H47.611
      due to
        inflammatory disorder H47.629
          left brain H47.622
          right brain H47.621
        neoplasm H47.639
          left brain H47.632
          right brain H47.631
        vascular disorder H47.649
          left brain H47.642
          right brain H47.641
    pathway H47.9
      due to
        inflammatory disorder H47.51-
        neoplasm H47.52-
        vascular disorder H47.53-
      optic chiasm —*see* Disorder, optic, chiasm

◀ New   ◀━ Revised   ~~deleted~~ Deleted

Disorder *(Continued)*
  vitreous body H43.9
    crystalline deposits —*see* Deposit,
      crystalline
    degeneration —*see* Degeneration, vitreous
    hemorrhage —*see* Hemorrhage, vitreous
    opacities —*see* Opacity, vitreous
    prolapse —*see* Prolapse, vitreous
    specified type NEC H43.89
  voice R49.9
    specified type NEC R49.8
  volatile solvent use
    due to drug abuse —*see* Abuse, drug,
      inhalant
    due to drug dependence —*see* Dependence,
      drug, inhalant
  white blood cells D72.9
    specified NEC D72.89
  withdrawing, child or adolescent F40.10
Disorientation R41.0
Displacement, displaced
  acquired traumatic of bone, cartilage, joint,
    tendon NEC —*see* Dislocation
  adrenal gland (congenital) Q89.1
  appendix, retrocecal (congenital) Q43.8
  auricle (congenital) Q17.4
  bladder (acquired) N32.89
    congenital Q64.19
  brachial plexus (congenital) Q07.8
  brain stem, caudal (congenital) Q04.8
  canaliculus (lacrimalis), congenital Q10.6
  cardia through esophageal hiatus (congenital)
    Q40.1
  cerebellum, caudal (congenital) Q04.8
  cervix —*see* Malposition, uterus
  colon (congenital) Q43.3
  device, implant or graft (*see also*
    Complications, by site and type,
    mechanical) T85.628
    arterial graft NEC —*see* Complication,
      cardiovascular device, mechanical,
      vascular
    breast (implant) T85.42
    catheter NEC T85.628
      dialysis (renal) T82.42
        intraperitoneal T85.621
      infusion NEC T82.524
        spinal (epidural) (subdural)
          T85.620
      urinary (indwelling) T83.028
        cystostomy T83.020
    electronic (electrode) (pulse generator)
      (stimulator) —*see* Complication,
      electronic stimulator
    fixation, internal (orthopedic) NEC —*see*
      Complication, fixation device,
      mechanical
    gastrointestinal —*see* Complications,
      prosthetic device, mechanical,
      gastrointestinal device
    genital NEC T83.428
      intrauterine contraceptive device
        T83.32
      penile prosthesis T83.420
    heart NEC —*see* Complication,
      cardiovascular device, mechanical
    joint prosthesis —*see* Complications, joint
      prosthesis, mechanical
    ocular —*see* Complications, prosthetic
      device, mechanical, ocular device
    orthopedic NEC —*see* Complication,
      orthopedic, device or graft,
      mechanical
    specified NEC T85.628
    urinary NEC —*see also* Complication,
      genitourinary, device, urinary,
      mechanical
      graft T83.22
    vascular NEC —*see* Complication,
      cardiovascular device, mechanical
  ventricular intracranial shunt T85.02

Displacement, displaced *(Continued)*
  electronic stimulator
    bone T84.320
    cardiac —*see* Complications, cardiac
      device, electronic
    nervous system —*see* Complication,
      prosthetic device, mechanical,
      electronic nervous system
      stimulator
    urinary —*see* Complications, electronic
      stimulator, urinary
  esophageal mucosa into cardia of stomach,
    congenital Q39.8
  esophagus (acquired) K22.8
    congenital Q39.8
  eyeball (acquired) (lateral) (old) —*see*
    Displacement, globe
    congenital Q15.8
    current —*see* Avulsion, eye
  fallopian tube (acquired) N83.4
    congenital Q50.6
    opening (congenital) Q50.6
  gallbladder (congenital) Q44.1
  gastric mucosa (congenital) Q40.2
  globe (acquired) (old) (lateral) H05.21-
    current —*see* Avulsion, eye
  heart (congenital) Q24.8
    acquired I51.89
  hymen (upward) (congenital) Q52.4
  intervertebral disc NEC
    with myelopathy —*see* Disorder, disc, with,
      myelopathy
    cervical, cervicothoracic (with)
      M50.20
      myelopathy —*see* Disorder, disc,
        cervical, with myelopathy
      neuritis, radiculitis or radiculopathy —
        see Disorder, disc, cervical, with
        neuritis
    due to trauma —*see* Dislocation, vertebra
    lumbar region M51.26
      with
        neuritis, radiculitis, radiculopathy or
          sciatica M51.16
    lumbosacral region M51.27
      with
        myelopathy M51.07
        neuritis, radiculitis, radiculopathy or
          sciatica M51.17
    sacrococcygeal region M53.3
    thoracic region M51.24
      with
        myelopathy M51.04
        neuritis, radiculitis, radiculopathy
          M51.14
    thoracolumbar region M51.25
      with
        myelopathy M51.05
        neuritis, radiculitis, radiculopathy
          M51.15
  intrauterine device T83.32
  kidney (acquired) N28.83
    congenital Q63.2
  lachrymal, lacrimal apparatus or duct
    (congenital) Q10.6
  lens, congenital Q12.1
  macula (congenital) Q14.1
  Meckel's diverticulum Q43.0
    malignant —*see* Table of Neoplasms, small
      intestine, malignant
  nail (congenital) Q84.6
    acquired L60.8
  opening of Wharton's duct in mouth
    Q38.4
  organ or site, congenital NEC —*see*
    Malposition, congenital
  ovary (acquired) N83.4
    congenital Q50.39
    free in peritoneal cavity (congenital)
      Q50.39
    into hernial sac N83.4

Displacement, displaced *(Continued)*
  oviduct (acquired) N83.4
    congenital Q50.6
  parathyroid (gland) E21.4
  parotid gland (congenital) Q38.4
  punctum lacrimale (congenital) Q10.6
  sacro-iliac (joint) (congenital) Q74.2
    current injury S33.2
    old —*see* subcategory M53.2
  salivary gland (any) (congenital) Q38.4
  spleen (congenital) Q89.09
  stomach, congenital Q40.2
  sublingual duct Q38.4
  tongue (downward) (congenital) Q38.3
  tooth, teeth, fully erupted M26.30
    horizontal M26.33
    vertical M26.34
  trachea (congenital) Q32.1
  ureter or ureteric opening or orifice
    (congenital) Q62.62
  uterine opening of oviducts or fallopian tubes
    Q50.6
  uterus, uterine —*see* Malposition, uterus
  ventricular septum Q21.0
    with rudimentary ventricle Q20.4
Disproportion
  between native and reconstructed breast
    N65.1
  fiber-type G71.2
Disruptio uteri —*see* Rupture, uterus
Disruption (of)
  ciliary body NEC H21.89
  closure of
    cornea T81.31
    craniotomy T81.32
    fascia (muscular) (superficial) T81.32
    internal organ or tissue T81.32
    laceration (external) (internal) T81.33
    ligament T81.32
    mucosa T81.31
    muscle or muscle flap T81.32
    ribs or rib cage T81.32
    skin and subcutaneous tissue (full-
      thickness) (superficial) T81.31
    skull T81.32
    sternum (sternotomy) T81.32
    tendon T81.32
    traumatic laceration (external) (internal)
      T81.33
  family Z63.8
    due to
      absence of family member due to
        military deployment Z63.31
      absence of family member NEC
        Z63.32
      alcoholism and drug addiction in
        family Z63.72
      bereavement Z63.4
      death (assumed) or disappearance of
        family member Z63.4
      divorce or separation Z63.5
      drug addiction in family Z63.72
      return of family member from military
        deployment (current or past
        conflict) Z63.71
      stressful life events NEC Z63.79
  iris NEC H21.89
  ligament (s) —*see also* Sprain
    knee
      current injury —*see* Dislocation,
        knee
      old (chronic) —*see* Derangement,
        knee, ligament, instability,
        chronic
      spontaneous NEC —*see* Derangement,
        knee, disruption ligament
  ossicular chain —*see* Discontinuity, ossicles,
    ear
  pelvic ring (stable) S32.810
    unstable S32.811
  traumatic injury wound repair T81.33

Disruption *(Continued)*
wound T81.30
  episiotomy O90.1
  operation T81.31
    cesarean O90.0
    external operation wound (superficial)
      T81.31
    internal operation wound (deep)
      T81.32
  perineal (obstetric) O90.1
  traumatic injury repair T81.33
Dissatisfaction with
  employment Z56.9
  school environment Z55.4
Dissecting —*see* condition
Dissection
  aorta I71.00
    abdominal I71.02
    thoracic I71.01
    thoracoabdominal I71.03
  artery
    carotid I77.71
    cerebral (nonruptured) I67.0
      ruptured —*see* Hemorrhage, intracranial,
        subarachnoid
    coronary I25.42
    iliac I77.72
    renal I77.73
    specified NEC I77.79
    vertebral I77.74
  traumatic —*see* Wound, open, by site
  vascular I99.8
  wound —*see* Wound, open
Disseminated —*see* condition
Dissociation
  auriculoventricular or atrioventricular (AV)
      (any degree) (isorhythmic) I45.89
    with heart block I44.2
    interference I45.89
Dissociative reaction, state F44.9
Dissolution, vertebra —*see* Osteoporosis
Distension, distention
  abdomen R14.0
  bladder N32.89
  cecum K63.89
  colon K63.89
  gallbladder K82.8
  intestine K63.89
  kidney N28.89
  liver K76.89
  seminal vesicle N50.8
  stomach K31.89
    acute K31.0
    psychogenic F45.8
  ureter —*see* Dilatation, ureter
  uterus N85.8
Distoma hepaticum infestation B66.3
Distomiasis B66.9
  bile passages B66.3
  hemic B65.9
  hepatic B66.3
    due to Clonorchis sinensis B66.1
  intestinal B66.5
  liver B66.3
    due to Clonorchis sinensis B66.1
  lung B66.4
  pulmonary B66.4
Distomolar (fourth molar) K00.1
Disto-occlusion (Division I) (Division II)
  M26.212
Distortion (s) (congenital)
  adrenal (gland) Q89.1
  arm NEC Q68.8
  bile duct or passage Q44.5
  bladder Q64.79
  brain Q04.9
  cervix (uteri) Q51.9
  chest (wall) Q67.8
    bones Q76.8
  clavicle Q74.0
  clitoris Q52.6

Distortion *(Continued)*
  coccyx Q76.49
  common duct Q44.5
  coronary Q24.5
  cystic duct Q44.5
  ear (auricle) (external) Q17.3
    inner Q16.5
    middle Q16.4
      ossicles Q16.3
  endocrine NEC Q89.2
  eustachian tube Q17.8
  eye (adnexa) Q15.8
  face bone (s) NEC Q75.8
  fallopian tube Q50.6
  femur NEC Q68.8
  fibula NEC Q68.8
  finger (s) Q68.1
  foot Q66.9
  genitalia, genital organ (s)
    female Q52.8
      external Q52.79
      internal NEC Q52.8
  gyri Q04.8
  hand bone (s) Q68.1
  heart (auricle) (ventricle) Q24.8
    valve (cusp) Q24.8
  hepatic duct Q44.5
  humerus NEC Q68.8
  hymen Q52.4
  intrafamilial communications
    Z63.8
  jaw NEC M26.89
  labium (majus) (minus) Q52.79
  leg NEC Q68.8
  lens Q12.8
  liver Q44.7
  lumbar spine Q76.49
    with disproportion O33.8
      causing obstructed labor O65.0
  lumbosacral (joint) (region) Q76.49
    kyphosis —*see* Kyphosis, congenital
    lordosis —*see* Lordosis, congenital
  nerve Q07.8
  nose Q30.8
  organ
    of Corti Q16.5
    or site not listed —*see* Anomaly, by site
      ossicles, ear Q16.3
  oviduct Q50.6
  pancreas Q45.3
  parathyroid (gland) Q89.2
  pituitary (gland) Q89.2
  radius NEC Q68.8
  sacroiliac joint Q74.2
  sacrum Q76.49
  scapula Q74.0
  shoulder girdle Q74.0
  skull bone (s) NEC Q75.8
    with
      anencephalus Q00.0
      encephalocele —*see* Encephalocele
      hydrocephalus Q03.9
        with spina bifida —*see* Spina bifida,
          with hydrocephalus
      microcephaly Q02
  spinal cord Q06.8
  spine Q76.49
    kyphosis —*see* Kyphosis, congenital
    lordosis —*see* Lordosis, congenital
  spleen Q89.09
  sternum NEC Q76.7
  thorax (wall) Q67.8
    bony Q76.8
  thymus (gland) Q89.2
  thyroid (gland) Q89.2
  tibia NEC Q68.8
  toe (s) Q66.9
  tongue Q38.3
  trachea (cartilage) Q32.1
  ulna NEC Q68.8
  ureter Q62.8

Distortion *(Continued)*
  urethra Q64.79
    causing obstruction Q64.39
  uterus Q51.9
  vagina Q52.4
  vertebra Q76.49
    kyphosis —*see* Kyphosis, congenital
    lordosis —*see* Lordosis, congenital
  visual —*see also* Disturbance, vision
    shape and size H53.15
  vulva Q52.79
  wrist (bones) (joint) Q68.8
Distress
  abdomen —*see* Pain, abdominal
  acute respiratory (adult) (child) J80
  epigastric R10.13
  fetal P84
    complicating pregnancy —*see* Stress, fetal
  gastrointestinal (functional) K30
    psychogenic F45.8
  intestinal (functional) NOS K59.9
    psychogenic F45.8
  maternal, during labor and delivery
    O75.0
  respiratory R06.00
    adult J80
    child J80
    newborn P22.9
      specified NEC P22.8
    orthopnea R06.01
    psychogenic F45.8
    shortness of breath R06.02
    specified type NEC R06.09
Distribution vessel, atypical Q27.9
  coronary artery Q24.5
  precerebral Q28.1
Districhiasis L68.8
Disturbance (s) —*see also* Disease
  absorption K90.9
    calcium E58
    carbohydrate K90.4
    fat K90.4
      pancreatic K90.3
    protein K90.4
    starch K90.4
    vitamin —*see* Deficiency, vitamin
  acid-base equilibrium E87.8
    mixed E87.4
  activity and attention (with hyperkinesis) —
    see Disorder, attention-deficit
    hyperactivity
  amino acid transport E72.00
  assimilation, food K90.9
  auditory nerve, except deafness —*see*
    subcategory H93.3
  behavior —*see* Disorder, conduct
  blood clotting (mechanism) (*see also* Defect,
    coagulation) D68.9
  cerebral
    nerve —*see* Disorder, nerve, cranial
    status, newborn P91.9
      specified NEC P91.8
  circulatory I99.9
  conduct (*see also* Disorder, conduct)
    F91.9
    adjustment reaction —*see* Disorder,
      adjustment
    compulsive F63.9
    disruptive F91.9
    hyperkinetic —*see* Disorder, attention-
      deficit hyperactivity
    socialized F91.2
    specified NEC F91.8
    unsocialized F91.1
  coordination R27.8
  cranial nerve —*see* Disorder, nerve,
    cranial
  deep sensibility —*see* Disturbance,
    sensation
  digestive K30
    psychogenic F45.8

◀ New ◀▥ Revised ~~deleted~~ Deleted

Disturbance *(Continued)*
electrolyte —*see also* Imbalance, electrolyte
  newborn, transitory P74.4
    hyperammonemia P74.6
    potassium balance P74.3
    sodium balance P74.2
    specified type NEC P74.4
emotions specific to childhood and
  adolescence F93.9
  with
    anxiety and fearfulness NEC F93.8
    elective mutism F94.0
    oppositional disorder F91.3
    sensitivity (withdrawal) F40.10
    shyness F40.10
    social withdrawal F40.10
  involving relationship problems F93.8
  mixed F93.8
  specified NEC F93.8
endocrine (gland) E34.9
  neonatal, transitory P72.9
  specified NEC P72.8
equilibrium R42
fructose metabolism E74.10
gait —*see* Gait
  hysterical F44.4
  psychogenic F44.4
gastrointestinal (functional) K30
  psychogenic F45.8
habit, child F98.9
hearing, except deafness and tinnitus —*see*
  Abnormal, auditory perception
heart, functional (conditions in I44-I50)
  due to presence of (cardiac) prosthesis
    I97.19-
  postoperative I97.89
    cardiac surgery I97.19-
hormones E34.9
innervation uterus (parasympathetic)
  (sympathetic) N85.8
keratinization NEC
  gingiva K05.10
    nonplaque induced K05.11
    plaque induced K05.10
  lip K13.0
  oral (mucosa) (soft tissue) K13.29
  tongue K13.29
learning (specific) —*see* Disorder,
  learning
memory —*see* Amnesia
  mild, following organic brain damage
    F06.8
mental F99
  associated with diseases classified
    elsewhere F54
metabolism E88.9
  with
    abortion —*see* Abortion, by type with
      other specified complication
    ectopic pregnancy O08.5
    molar pregnancy O08.5
  amino-acid E72.9
    aromatic E70.9
    branched-chain E71.2
    straight-chain E72.8
    sulfur-bearing E72.10
  ammonia E72.20
  arginine E72.21
  arginosuccinic acid E72.22
  carbohydrate E74.9
  cholesterol E78.9
  citrulline E72.23
  cystathionine E72.19
  general E88.9
  glutamine E72.8
  histidine E70.40
  homocystine E72.19
  hydroxylysine E72.3
  in labor or delivery O75.89
  iron E83.10
  lipoid E78.9

Disturbance *(Continued)*
metabolism *(Continued)*
  lysine E72.3
  methionine E72.19
  neonatal, transitory P74.9
    calcium and magnesium P71.9
      specified type NEC P71.8
    carbohydrate metabolism P70.9
      specified type NEC P70.8
    specified NEC P74.8
  ornithine E72.4
  phosphate E83.39
  sodium NEC E87.8
  threonine E72.8
  tryptophan E70.5
  tyrosine E70.20
  urea cycle E72.20
motor R29.2
nervous, functional R45.0
neuromuscular mechanism (eye), due to
  syphilis A52.15
nutritional E63.9
  nail L60.3
ocular motion H51.9
  psychogenic F45.8
oculogyric H51.8
  psychogenic F45.8
oculomotor H51.9
  psychogenic F45.8
olfactory nerve R43.1
optic nerve NEC —*see* Disorder, nerve,
  optic
oral epithelium, including tongue NEC
  K13.29
perceptual due to
  alcohol withdrawal F10.232
  amphetamine intoxication F15.922
    in
      abuse F15.122
      dependence F15.222
  anxiolytic withdrawal F13.232
  cannabis intoxication (acute) F12.922
    in
      abuse F12.122
      dependence F12.222
  cocaine intoxication (acute) F14.922
    in
      abuse F14.122
      dependence F14.222
  hypnotic withdrawal F13.232
  opioid intoxication (acute) F11.922
    in
      abuse F11.122
      dependence F11.222
  phencyclidine intoxication (acute)
    F19.922
    in
      abuse F19.122
      dependence F19.222
  sedative withdrawal F13.232
personality (pattern) (trait) (*see also* Disorder,
  personality) F60.9
  following organic brain damage
    F07.9
polyglandular E31.9
  specified NEC E31.8
potassium balance, newborn P74.3
psychogenic F45.9
psychomotor F44.4
psychophysical visual H53.16
pupillary —*see* Anomaly, pupil, function
reflex R29.2
rhythm, heart I49.9
salivary secretion K11.7
sensation (cold) (heat) (localization) (tactile
  discrimination) (texture) (vibratory)
  NEC R20.9
  hysterical F44.6
  skin R20.9
    anesthesia R20.0
    hyperesthesia R20.3

Disturbance *(Continued)*
sensation *(Continued)*
  skin *(Continued)*
    hypoesthesia R20.1
    paresthesia R20.2
    specified type NEC R20.8
  smell R43.9
    and taste (mixed) R43.8
    anosmia R43.0
    parosmia R43.1
    specified NEC R43.8
  taste R43.9
    and smell (mixed) R43.8
    parageusia R43.2
    specified NEC R43.8
sensory —*see* Disturbance, sensation
situational (transient) —*see also* Disorder,
  adjustment
  acute F43.0
sleep G47.9
  nonorganic origin F51.9
smell —*see* Disturbance, sensation,
  smell
sociopathic F60.2
sodium balance, newborn P74.2
speech R47.9
  developmental F80.9
  specified NEC R47.89
stomach (functional) K31.9
sympathetic (nerve) G90.9
taste —*see* Disturbance, sensation,
  taste
temperature
  regulation, newborn P81.9
    specified NEC P81.8
  sense R20.8
    hysterical F44.6
tooth
  eruption K00.6
  formation K00.4
  structure, hereditary NEC K00.5
touch —*see* Disturbance, sensation
vascular I99.9
  arteriosclerotic —*see* Arteriosclerosis
vasomotor I73.9
vasospastic I73.9
vision, visual H53.9
  following
    cerebral infarction I69.398
    cerebrovascular disease I69.998
      specified NEC I69.898
    intracerebral hemorrhage I69.198
    nontraumatic intracranial hemorrhage
      NEC I69.298
    specified disease NEC I69.898
    subarachnoid hemorrhage I69.098
  psychophysical H53.16
  specified NEC H53.8
  subjective H53.10
    day blindness H53.11
    discomfort H53.14-
    distortions of shape and size H53.15
    loss
      sudden H53.13-
      transient H53.12-
    specified type NEC H53.19
voice R49.9
  psychogenic F44.4
  specified NEC R49.8
Diuresis R35.8
Diver's palsy, paralysis or squeeze T70.3
Diverticulitis (acute) K57.92
  bladder —*see* Cystitis
  ileum —*see* Diverticulitis, intestine, small
  intestine K57.92
    with
      abscess, perforation or peritonitis
        K57.80
        with bleeding K57.81
      bleeding K57.93
    congenital Q43.8

Diverticulitis *(Continued)*
  intestine *(Continued)*
    large K57.32
      with
        abscess, perforation or peritonitis
          K57.20
          with bleeding K57.21
        bleeding K57.33
        small intestine K57.52
          with
            abscess, perforation or peritonitis
              K57.40
              with bleeding K57.41
            bleeding K57.53
    small K57.12
      with
        abscess, perforation or peritonitis
          K57.00
          with bleeding K57.01
        bleeding K57.13
        large intestine K57.52
          with
            abscess, perforation or peritonitis
              K57.40
              with bleeding K57.41
            bleeding K57.53
Diverticulosis K57.90
  with bleeding K57.91
  large intestine K57.30
    with
      bleeding K57.31
      small intestine K57.50
        with bleeding K57.51
  small intestine K57.10
    with
      bleeding K57.11
      large intestine K57.50
        with bleeding K57.51
Diverticulum, diverticula (multiple) K57.90
  appendix (noninflammatory) K38.2
  bladder (sphincter) N32.3
    congenital Q64.6
  bronchus (congenital) Q32.4
    acquired J98.09
  calyx, calyceal (kidney) N28.89
  cardia (stomach) K31.4
  cecum —*see* Diverticulosis, intestine, large
    congenital Q43.8
  colon —*see* Diverticulosis, intestine, large
    congenital Q43.8
  duodenum —*see* Diverticulosis, intestine,
    small
    congenital Q43.8
  epiphrenic (esophagus) K22.5
  esophagus (congenital) Q39.6
    acquired (epiphrenic) (pulsion) (traction)
      K22.5
  eustachian tube —*see* Disorder, eustachian
    tube, specified NEC
  fallopian tube N83.8
  gastric K31.4
  heart (congenital) Q24.8
  ileum —*see* Diverticulosis, intestine, small
  jejunum —*see* Diverticulosis, intestine, small
  kidney (pelvis) (calyces) N28.89
    with calculus —*see* Calculus, kidney
  Meckel's (displaced) (hypertrophic) Q43.0
    malignant —*see* Table of Neoplasms; small
      intestine, malignant
  midthoracic K22.5
  organ or site, congenital NEC —*see* Distortion
  pericardium (congenital) (cyst) Q24.8
    acquired I31.8
  pharyngoesophageal (congenital) Q39.6
    acquired K22.5
  pharynx (congenital) Q38.7
  rectosigmoid —*see* Diverticulosis, intestine,
    large
    congenital Q43.8
  rectum —*see* Diverticulosis, intestine, large
  Rokitansky's K22.5

Diverticulum, diverticula *(Continued)*
  seminal vesicle N50.8
  sigmoid —*see* Diverticulosis, intestine, large
    congenital Q43.8
  stomach (acquired) K31.4
    congenital Q40.2
  trachea (acquired) J39.8
  ureter (acquired) N28.89
    congenital Q62.8
  ureterovesical orifice N28.89
  urethra (acquired) N36.1
    congenital Q64.79
  ventricle, left (congenital) Q24.8
  vesical N32.3
    congenital Q64.6
  Zenker's (esophagus) K22.5
Division
  cervix uteri (acquired) N88.8
  glans penis Q55.69
  labia minora (congenital) Q52.79
  ligament (partial or complete) (current) —*see*
    also Sprain
    with open wound —*see* Wound, open
  muscle (partial or complete) (current) —*see*
    also Injury, muscle
    with open wound —*see* Wound, open
  nerve (traumatic) —*see* Injury, nerve
  spinal cord —*see* Injury, spinal cord,
    by region
  vein I87.8
Divorce, causing family disruption Z63.5
Dix-Hallpike neurolabyrinthitis —*see*
  Neuronitis, vestibular
Dizziness R42
  hysterical F44.89
  psychogenic F45.8
DMAC (disseminated mycobacterium avium-
  intracellulare complex) A31.2
DNR (do not resuscitate) Z66
Doan-Wiseman syndrome (primary splenic
  neutropenia) —*see* Agranulocytosis
Doehle-Heller aortitis A52.02
Dog bite —*see* Bite
Dohle body panmyelopathic syndrome
  D72.0
Dolichocephaly Q67.2
Dolichocolon Q43.8
Dolichostenomelia —*see* Syndrome, Marfan's
Donohue's syndrome E34.8
Donor (organ or tissue) Z52.9
  blood (whole) Z52.000
    autologous Z52.010
    specified component (lymphocytes)
      (platelets) NEC Z52.008
      autologous Z52.018
      specified donor NEC Z52.098
    specified donor NEC Z52.090
    stem cells Z52.001
      autologous Z52.011
      specified donor NEC Z52.091
  bone Z52.20
    autologous Z52.21
    marrow Z52.3
    specified type NEC Z52.29
  cornea Z52.5
  egg (Oocyte) Z52.819
    age 35 and over Z52.812
      anonymous recipient Z52.812
      designated recipient Z52.813
    under age 35 Z52.810
      anonymous recipient Z52.810
      designated recipient Z52.811
  kidney Z52.4
  liver Z52.6
  lung Z52.89
  lymphocyte —*see* Donor, blood, specified
    components NEC
  Oocyte —*see* Donor, egg
  platelets Z52.008
  potential, examination of Z00.5
  semen Z52.89

Donor *(Continued)*
  skin Z52.10
    autologous Z52.11
    specified type NEC Z52.19
  specified organ or tissue NEC Z52.89
  sperm Z52.89
Donovanosis A58
Dorsalgia M54.9
  psychogenic F45.41
  specified NEC M54.89
Dorsopathy M53.9
  deforming M43.9
    specified NEC —*see* subcategory M43.8
  specified NEC M53.80
    cervical region M53.82
    cervicothoracic region M53.83
    lumbar region M53.86
    lumbosacral region M53.87
    occipito-atlanto-axial region M53.81
    sacrococcygeal region M53.88
    thoracic region M53.84
    thoracolumbar region M53.85
Double
  albumin E88.09
  aortic arch Q25.4
  auditory canal Q17.8
  auricle (heart) Q20.8
  bladder Q64.79
  cervix Q51.820
    with doubling of uterus (and vagina)
      Q51.10
      with obstruction Q51.11
  inlet ventricle Q20.4
  kidney with double pelvis (renal) Q63.0
  meatus urinarius Q64.75
  monster Q89.4
  outlet
    left ventricle Q20.2
    right ventricle Q20.1
  pelvis (renal) with double ureter Q62.5
  tongue Q38.3
  ureter (one or both sides) Q62.5
    with double pelvis (renal) Q62.5
  urethra Q64.74
  urinary meatus Q64.75
  uterus Q51.2
    with
      doubling of cervix (and vagina)
        Q51.10
        with obstruction Q51.11
      in pregnancy or childbirth O34.59-
        causing obstructed labor O65.5
  vagina Q52.10
    with doubling of uterus (and cervix)
      Q51.10
      with obstruction Q51.11
  vision H53.2
  vulva Q52.79
Douglas' pouch, cul-de-sac —*see* condition
Down syndrome Q90.9
  meiotic nondisjunction Q90.0
  mitotic nondisjunction Q90.1
  mosaicism Q90.1
  translocation Q90.2
DPD (dihydropyrimidine dehydrogenase
  deficiency) E88.89
Dracontiasis B72
Dracunculiasis, dracunculosis B72
Dream state, hysterical F44.89
Drepanocytic anemia —*see* Disease, sickle-cell
Dresbach's syndrome (elliptocytosis) D58.1
Dreschlera (hawaiiensis) (infection) B43.8
Dressler's syndrome I24.1
Drift, ulnar —*see* Deformity, limb, specified
  type NEC, forearm
Drinking (alcohol)
  excessive, to excess NEC (without
    dependence) F10.10
    habitual (continual) (without remission)
      F10.20
      with remission F10.21

◀ New ⏴ Revised ~~deleted~~ Deleted

Drip, postnasal (chronic) R09.82
  due to
    allergic rhinitis —*see* Rhinitis, allergic
    common cold J00
    gastroesophageal reflux —*see* Reflux,
      gastroesophageal
    nasopharyngitis —*see* Nasopharyngitis
    other known condition — code to
      condition
    sinusitis —*see* Sinusitis
Droop
  facial R29.810
    cerebrovascular disease I69.992
      cerebral infarction I69.392
      intracerebral hemorrhage I69.192
      nontraumatic intracranial hemorrhage
        NEC I69.292
      specified disease NEC I69.892
      subarachnoid hemorrhage I69.092
Drop (in)
  attack NEC R55
  finger —*see* Deformity, finger
  foot —*see* Deformity, limb, foot, drop
  hematocrit (precipitous) R71.0
  hemoglobin R71.0
  toe —*see* Deformity, toe, specified NEC
  wrist —*see* Deformity, limb, wrist drop
Dropped heart beats I45.9
Dropsy, dropsical —*see also* Hydrops
  abdomen R18.8
  brain —*see* Hydrocephalus
  cardiac, heart —*see* Failure, heart, congestive
  gangrenous —*see* Gangrene
  heart —*see* Failure, heart, congestive
  kidney —*see* Nephrosis
  lung —*see* Edema, lung
  newborn due to isoimmunization P56.0
  pericardium —*see* Pericarditis
Drowned, drowning (near) T75.1
Drowsiness R40.0
Drug
  abuse counseling and surveillance Z71.51
  addiction —*see* Dependence
  dependence —*see* Dependence
  habit —*see* Dependence
  harmful use —*see* Abuse, drug
  induced fever R50.2
  overdose —*see* Table of Drugs and Chemicals,
    by drug, poisoning
  poisoning —*see* Table of Drugs and
    Chemicals, by drug, poisoning
  resistant organism infection (*see also*
    Resistant, organism, to, drug) Z16.30
  therapy
    long term (current) (prophylactic) —*see*
      Therapy, drug long-term (current)
      (prophylactic)
    short term - omit code
  wrong substance given or taken in error —*see*
    Table of Drugs and Chemicals, by drug,
    poisoning
Drunkenness (without dependence) F10.129
  acute in alcoholism F10.229
  chronic (without remission) F10.20
    with remission F10.21
  pathological (without dependence) F10.129
    with dependence F10.229
  sleep F51.9
Drusen
  macula (degenerative) (retina) —*see*
    Degeneration, macula, drusen
  optic disc H47.32-
Dry, dryness —*see also* condition
  larynx J38.7
  mouth R68.2
    due to dehydration E86.0
  nose J34.89
  socket (teeth) M27.3
  throat J39.2
DSAP L56.5
Duane's syndrome H50.81-

Dubin-Johnson disease or syndrome E80.6
Dubois' disease (thymus gland) A50.59 *[E35]*
Dubowitz' syndrome Q87.1
Duchenne-Aran muscular atrophy G12.21
Duchenne-Griesinger disease G71.0
Duchenne's
  disease or syndrome
    motor neuron disease G12.22
    muscular dystrophy G71.0
  locomotor ataxia (syphilitic) A52.11
  paralysis
    birth injury P14.0
    due to or associated with
      motor neuron disease G12.22
      muscular dystrophy G71.0
Ducrey's chancre A57
Duct, ductus —*see* condition
Duhring's disease (dermatitis herpetiformis)
  L13.0
Dullness, cardiac (decreased) (increased) R01.2
Dumb ague —*see* Malaria
Dumbness —*see* Aphasia
Dumdum fever B55.0
Dumping syndrome (postgastrectomy) K91.1
Duodenitis (nonspecific) (peptic) K29.80
  with bleeding K29.81
Duodenocholangitis —*see* Cholangitis
Duodenum, duodenal —*see* condition
Duplay's bursitis or periarthritis —*see*
  Tendinitis, calcific, shoulder
Duplication, duplex —*see also* Accessory
  alimentary tract Q45.8
  anus Q43.4
  appendix (and cecum) Q43.4
  biliary duct (any) Q44.5
  bladder Q64.79
  cecum (and appendix) Q43.4
  cervix Q51.820
  chromosome NEC
    with complex rearrangements NEC
      Q92.5
    seen only at prometaphase Q92.8
  cystic duct Q44.5
  digestive organs Q45.8
  esophagus Q39.8
  frontonasal process Q75.8
  intestine (large) (small) Q43.4
  kidney Q63.0
  liver Q44.7
  pancreas Q45.3
  penis Q55.69
  respiratory organs NEC Q34.8
  salivary duct Q38.4
  spinal cord (incomplete) Q06.2
  stomach Q40.2
Dupré's disease (meningism) R29.1
Dupuytren's contraction or disease M72.0
Durand-Nicolas-Favre disease A55
Durotomy (inadvertent) (incidental) G97.41
Duroziez's disease (congenital mitral stenosis)
  Q23.2
Dutton's relapsing fever (West African) A68.1
Dwarfism E34.3
  achondroplastic Q77.4
  congenital E34.3
  constitutional E34.3
  hypochondroplastic Q77.4
  hypophyseal E23.0
  infantile E34.3
  Laron-type E34.3
  Lorain (-Levi) type E23.0
  metatropic Q77.8
  nephrotic-glycosuric (with
    hypophosphatemic rickets) E72.09
  nutritional E45
  pancreatic K86.8
  pituitary E23.0
  renal N25.0
  thanatophoric Q77.1
Dyke-Young anemia (secondary)
  (symptomatic) D59.1

Dysacusis —*see* Abnormal, auditory
  perception
Dysadrenocortism E27.9
  hyperfunction E27.0
Dysarthria R47.1
  following
    cerebral infarction I69.322
    cerebrovascular disease I69.922
      specified disease NEC I69.822
    intracerebral hemorrhage I69.122
    nontraumatic intracranial hemorrhage
      NEC I69.222
    subarachnoid hemorrhage I69.022
Dysautonomia (familial) G90.1
Dysbarism T70.3
Dysbasia R26.2
  angiosclerotica intermittens I73.9
  hysterical F44.4
  lordotica (progressiva) G24.1
  nonorganic origin F44.4
  psychogenic F44.4
Dysbetalipoproteinemia (familial) E78.2
Dyscalculia R48.8
  developmental F81.2
Dyschezia K59.00
Dyschondroplasia (with hemangiomata)
  Q78.4
Dyschromia (skin) L81.9
Dyscollagenosis M35.9
Dyscranio-pygo-phalangy Q87.0
Dyscrasia
  blood (with) D75.9
    antepartum hemorrhage —*see*
      Hemorrhage, antepartum, with
      coagulation defect
    intrapartum hemorrhage O67.0
    newborn P61.9
      specified type NEC P61.8
    puerperal, postpartum O72.3
    polyglandular, pluriglandular E31.9
Dysendocrinism E34.9
Dysentery, dysenteric (catarrhal) (diarrhea)
  (epidemic) (hemorrhagic) (infectious)
  (sporadic) (tropical) A09
  abscess, liver A06.4
  amebic (*see also* Amebiasis) A06.0
    with abscess —*see* Abscess, amebic
    acute A06.0
    chronic A06.1
  arthritis (*see also* category M01) A09
    bacillary (*see also* category M01) A03.9
  bacillary A03.9
    arthritis (*see also* category M01)
      A03.9
    Boyd A03.2
    Flexner A03.1
    Schmitz (-Stutzer) A03.0
    Shiga (-Kruse) A03.0
    Shigella A03.9
      boydii A03.2
      dysenteriae A03.0
      flexneri A03.1
      group A A03.0
      group B A03.1
      group C A03.2
      group D A03.3
      sonnei A03.3
      specified type NEC A03.8
    Sonne A03.3
    specified type NEC A03.8
  balantidial A07.0
  Balantidium coli A07.0
  Boyd's A03.2
  candidal B37.82
  Chilomastix A07.8
  Chinese A03.9
  coccidial A07.3
  Dientamoeba (fragilis) A07.8
  Embadomonas A07.8
  Entamoeba, entamebic —*see* Dysentery,
    amebic

Dysentery, dysenteric *(Continued)*
Flexner-Boyd A03.2
Flexner's A03.1
Giardia lamblia A07.1
Hiss-Russell A03.1
Lamblia A07.1
leishmanial B55.0
malarial —*see* Malaria
metazoal B82.0
monilial B37.82
protozoal A07.9
Salmonella A02.0
schistosomal B65.1
Schmitz (-Stutzer) A03.0
Shiga (-Kruse) A03.0
Shigella NOS —*see* Dysentery, bacillary
Sonne A03.3
strongyloidiasis B78.0
trichomonal A07.8
viral (*see also* Enteritis, viral) A08.4
Dysequilibrium R42
Dysesthesia R20.8
hysterical F44.6
Dysfibrinogenemia (congenital) D68.2
Dysfunction
adrenal E27.9
hyperfunction E27.0
autonomic
due to alcohol G31.2
somatoform F45.8
bladder N31.9
neurogenic NOS —*see* Dysfunction,
bladder, neuromuscular
neuromuscular NOS N31.9
atonic (motor) (sensory) N31.2
autonomous N31.2
flaccid N31.2
nonreflex N31.2
reflex N31.1
specified NEC N31.8
uninhibited N31.0
bleeding, uterus N93.8
cerebral G93.89
colon K59.9
psychogenic F45.8
colostomy K94.03
cystic duct K82.8
cystostomy (stoma) —*see* Complications,
cystostomy
ejaculatory N53.19
anejaculatory orgasm N53.13
painful N53.12
premature F52.4
retarded N53.11
endocrine NOS E34.9
endometrium N85.8
enterostomy K94.13
gallbladder K82.8
gastrostomy (stoma) K94.23
gland, glandular NOS E34.9
heart I51.89
hemoglobin D75.89
hepatic K76.89
hypophysis E23.7
hypothalamic NEC E23.3
ileostomy (stoma) K94.13
jejunostomy (stoma) K94.13
kidney —*see* Disease, renal
labyrinthine —*see* subcategory H83.2
left ventricular, following sudden emotional
stress I51.81
liver K76.89
male —*see* Dysfunction, sexual, male
orgasmic (female) F52.31
male F52.32
ovary E28.9
specified NEC E28.8
papillary muscle I51.89
parathyroid E21.4
physiological NEC R68.89
psychogenic F59

Dysfunction *(Continued)*
pineal gland E34.8
pituitary (gland) E23.3
platelets D69.1
polyglandular E31.9
specified NEC E31.8
psychophysiologic F59
psychosexual F52.9
with
dyspareunia F52.6
premature ejaculation F52.4
vaginismus F52.5
pylorus K31.9
rectum K59.9
psychogenic F45.8
reflex (sympathetic) —*see* Syndrome, pain,
complex regional I
segmental —*see* Dysfunction, somatic
senile R54
sexual (due to) R37
alcohol F10.981
amphetamine F15.981
in
abuse F15.181
dependence F15.281
anxiolytic F13.981
in
abuse F13.181
dependence F13.281
cocaine F14.981
in
abuse F14.181
dependence F14.281
excessive sexual drive F52.8
failure of genital response (male)
F52.21
female F52.22
female N94.9
aversion F52.1
dyspareunia N94.1
psychogenic F52.6
frigidity F52.22
nymphomania F52.8
orgasmic F52.31
psychogenic F52.9
aversion F52.1
dyspareunia F52.6
frigidity F52.22
nymphomania F52.8
orgasmic F52.31
vaginismus F52.5
vaginismus N94.2
psychogenic F52.5
hypnotic F13.981
in
abuse F13.181
dependence F13.281
inhibited orgasm (female) F52.31
male F52.32
lack
of sexual enjoyment F52.1
or loss of sexual desire F52.0
male N53.9
anejaculatory orgasm N53.13
ejaculatory N53.19
painful N53.12
premature F52.4
retarded N53.11
erectile N52.9
drug induced N52.2
due to
disease classified elsewhere N52.1
drug N52.2
postoperative (postprocedural) N52.39
following
prostatectomy N52.34
radical N52.31
radical cystectomy N52.32
urethral surgery N52.33
psychogenic F52.21
specified cause NEC N52.8

Dysfunction *(Continued)*
sexual *(Continued)*
male *(Continued)*
erectile *(Continued)*
vasculogenic
arterial insufficiency N52.01
with corporo-venous occlusive
N52.03
corporo-venous occlusive N52.02
with arterial insufficiency
N52.03
impotence —*see* Dysfunction, sexual,
male, erectile
psychogenic F52.9
aversion F52.1
erectile F52.21
orgasmic F52.32
premature ejaculation F52.4
satyriasis F52.8
specified type NEC F52.8
specified type NEC N53.8
nonorganic F52.9
specified NEC F52.8
opioid F11.981
in
abuse F11.181
dependence F11.281
orgasmic dysfunction (female) F52.31
male F52.32
premature ejaculation F52.4
psychoactive substances NEC F19.981
in
abuse F19.181
dependence F19.281
psychogenic F52.9
sedative F13.981
in
abuse F13.181
dependence F13.281
sexual aversion F52.1
vaginismus (nonorganic) (psychogenic)
F52.5
sinoatrial node I49.5
somatic M99.09
abdomen M99.09
acromioclavicular M99.07
cervical region M99.01
cervicothoracic M99.01
costochondral M99.08
costovertebral M99.08
head region M99.00
hip M99.05
lower extremity M99.06
lumbar region M99.03
lumbosacral M99.03
occipitocervical M99.00
pelvic region M99.05
pubic M99.05
rib cage M99.08
sacral region M99.04
sacrococcygeal M99.04
sacroiliac M99.04
specified NEC M99.09
sternochondral M99.08
sternoclavicular M99.07
thoracic region M99.02
thoracolumbar M99.02
upper extremity M99.07
somatoform autonomic F45.8
stomach K31.89
psychogenic F45.8
suprarenal E27.9
hyperfunction E27.0
symbolic R48.9
specified type NEC R48.8
temporomandibular (joint) M26.69
joint-pain syndrome M26.62
testicular (endocrine) E29.9
specified NEC E29.8
thymus E32.9
thyroid E07.9

◀ New   ◀▦ Revised   ~~deleted~~ Deleted

Dysfunction (Continued)
 ureterostomy (stoma) —see Complications,
  stoma, urinary tract
 urethrostomy (stoma) —see Complications,
  stoma, urinary tract
 uterus, complicating delivery O62.9
  hypertonic O62.4
  hypotonic O62.2
   primary O62.0
   secondary O62.1
 ventricular I51.9
  with congestive heart failure I50.9-
   left, reversible, following sudden
    emotional stress I51.81
Dysgenesis
 gonadal (due to chromosomal anomaly)
  Q96.9
  pure Q99.1
 renal Q60.5
  bilateral Q60.4
  unilateral Q60.3
 reticular D72.0
 tidal platelet D69.3
Dysgerminoma
 specified site —see Neoplasm, malignant,
  by site
 unspecified site
  female C56.9
  male C62.90
Dysgeusia R43.2
Dysgraphia R27.8
Dyshidrosis, dysidrosis L30.1
Dyskaryotic cervical smear R87.619
Dyskeratosis L85.8
 cervix —see Dysplasia, cervix
 congenital Q82.8
 uterus NEC N85.8
Dyskinesia G24.9
 biliary (cystic duct or gallbladder)
  K82.8
 drug induced
  orofacial G24.01
 esophagus K22.4
 hysterical F44.4
 intestinal K59.8
 nonorganic origin F44.4
 orofacial (idiopathic) G24.4
  drug induced G24.01
 psychogenic F44.4
 subacute, drug induced G24.01
 tardive G24.01
  neuroleptic induced G24.01
 trachea J39.8
 tracheobronchial J98.09
Dyslalia (developmental) F80.0
Dyslexia R48.0
 developmental F81.0
Dyslipidemia E78.5
 depressed HDL cholesterol E78.6
 elevated fasting triglycerides E78.1
Dysmaturity —see also Light for dates
 pulmonary (newborn) (Wilson-Mikity)
  P27.0
Dysmenorrhea (essential) (exfoliative)
  N94.6
 congestive (syndrome) N94.6
 primary N94.4
 psychogenic F45.8
 secondary N94.5
Dysmetabolic syndrome X E88.81
Dysmetria R27.8
Dysmorphism (due to)
 alcohol Q86.0
 exogenous cause NEC Q86.8
 hydantoin Q86.1
 warfarin Q86.2
Dysmorphophobia (nondelusional) F45.22
 delusional F22
Dysnomia R47.01
Dysorexia R63.0
 psychogenic F50.8

Dysostosis
 cleidocranial, cleidocranialis Q74.0
 craniofacial Q75.1
 Fairbank's (idiopathic familial generalized
  osteophytosis) Q78.9
 mandibulofacial (incomplete) Q75.4
 multiplex E76.01
 oculomandibular Q75.5
Dyspareunia (female) N94.1
 male N53.12
 nonorganic F52.6
 psychogenic F52.6
 secondary N94.1
Dyspepsia R10.13
 atonic K30
 functional (allergic) (congenital)
  (gastrointestinal) (occupational) (reflex)
  K30
 intestinal K59.8
 nervous F45.8
 neurotic F45.8
 psychogenic F45.8
Dysphagia R13.10
 cervical R13.19
 following
  cerebral infarction I69.391
  cerebrovascular disease I69.991
   specified NEC I69.891
  intracerebral hemorrhage I69.191
  nontraumatic intracranial hemorrhage
   NEC I69.291
  specified disease NEC I69.891
  subarachnoid hemorrhage I69.091
 functional (hysterical) F45.8
 hysterical F45.8
 nervous (hysterical) F45.8
 neurogenic R13.19
 oral phase R13.11
 oropharyngeal phase R13.12
 pharyneal phase R13.13
 pharyngoesophageal phase R13.14
 psychogenic F45.8
 sideropenic D50.1
 spastica K22.4
 specified NEC R13.19
Dysphagocytosis, congenital D71
Dysphasia R47.02
 developmental
  expressive type F80.1
  receptive type F80.2
 following
  cerebrovascular disease I69.921
   cerebral infarction I69.321
   intracerebral hemorrhage I69.121
  nontraumatic intracranial hemorrhage NEC
   I69.221
   specified disease NEC I69.821
   subarachnoid hemorrhage I69.021
Dysphonia R49.0
 functional F44.4
 hysterical F44.4
 psychogenic F44.4
 spastica J38.3
Dysphoria, postpartal O90.6
Dyspituitarism E23.3
Dysplasia —see also Anomaly
 acetabular, congenital Q65.89
 alveolar capillary, with vein misalignment
  J84.843
 anus (histologically confirmed) (mild)
  (moderate) K62.82
  severe D01.3
 arrhythmogenic right ventricular I42.8
 arterial, fibromuscular I77.3
 asphyxiating thoracic (congenital) Q77.2
 brain Q07.9
 bronchopulmonary, perinatal P27.1
 cervix (uteri) N87.9
  mild N87.0
  moderate N87.1
  severe D06.9

Dysplasia (Continued)
 chondroectodermal Q77.6
 colon D12.6
 craniometaphyseal Q78.5
 dentinal K00.5
 diaphyseal, progressive Q78.3
 dystrophic Q77.5
 ectodermal (anhidrotic) (congenital)
  (hereditary) Q82.4
  hydrotic Q82.8
 epithelial, uterine cervix —see Dysplasia,
  cervix
 eye (congenital) Q11.2
 fibrous
  bone NEC (monostotic) M85.00
   ankle M85.07-
   foot M85.07-
   forearm M85.03-
   hand M85.04-
   lower leg M85.06-
   multiple site M85.09
   neck M85.08
   rib M85.08
   shoulder M85.01-
   skull M85.08
   specified site NEC M85.08
   thigh M85.05-
   toe M85.07-
   upper arm M85.02-
   vertebra M85.08
  diaphyseal, progressive Q78.3
  jaw M27.8
  polyostotic Q78.1
 florid osseous —see also Cyst, calcifying
  odontogenic
 high grade, focal D12.6
 hip, congenital Q65.89
 joint, congenital Q74.8
 kidney Q61.4
  multicystic Q61.4
 leg Q74.2
 lung, congenital (not associated with short
  gestation) Q33.6
 mammary (gland) (benign) N60.9-
  cyst (solitary) —see Cyst, breast
  cystic —see Mastopathy, cystic
  duct ectasia —see Ectasia, mammary
   duct
  fibroadenosis —see Fibroadenosis, breast
  fibrosclerosis —see Fibrosclerosis, breast
  specified type NEC N60.8-
 metaphyseal (Jansen's) (McKusick's)
  (Schmid's) Q78.5
 muscle Q79.8
 oculodentodigital Q87.0
 periapical (cemental) (cemento-osseous) —see
  Cyst, calcifying odontogenic
 periosteum —see Disorder, bone, specified
  type NEC
 polyostotic fibrous Q78.1
 prostate (see also Neoplasia, intraepithelial,
  prostate) N42.3
  severe D07.5
 renal Q61.4
  multicystic Q61.4
 retinal, congenital Q14.1
 right ventricular, arrhythmogenic I42.8
 septo-optic Q04.4
 skin L98.8
 spinal cord Q06.1
 spondyloepiphyseal Q77.7
 thymic, with immunodeficiency
  D82.1
 vagina N89.3
  mild N89.0
  moderate N89.1
  severe NEC D07.2
 vulva N90.3
  mild N90.0
  moderate N90.1
  severe NEC D07.1

Dyspnea (nocturnal) (paroxysmal) R06.00
  asthmatic (bronchial) J45.909
    with
      bronchitis J45.909
        with
          exacerbation (acute) J45.901
          status asthmaticus J45.902
        chronic J44.9
      exacerbation (acute) J45.901
      status asthmaticus J45.902
    cardiac —see Failure, ventricular, left
  cardiac —see Failure, ventricular, left
  functional F45.8
  hyperventilation R06.4
  hysterical F45.8
  newborn P28.89
  psychogenic F45.8
  shortness of breath R06.02
  specified type NEC R06.09
Dyspraxia R27.8
  developmental (syndrome) F82
Dysproteinemia E88.09
Dysreflexia, autonomic G90.4
Dysrhythmia
  cardiac I49.9
    newborn
      bradycardia P29.12
        occurring before birth P03.819
          before onset of labor P03.810
          during labor P03.811
      tachycardia P29.11
    postoperative I97.89
  cerebral or cortical —see Epilepsy
Dyssomnia —see Disorder, sleep
Dyssynergia
  biliary K83.8
  bladder sphincter N36.44
  cerebellaris myoclonica (Hunt's ataxia)
    G11.1
Dysthymia F34.1
Dysthyroidism E07.9
Dystocia O66.9
  affecting newborn P03.1
  cervical (hypotonic) O62.2
    affecting newborn P03.6
    primary O62.0
    secondary O62.1
  contraction ring O62.4
  fetal O66.9
    abnormality NEC O66.3
    conjoined twins O66.3
    oversize O66.2
  maternal O66.9
  positional O64.9
  shoulder (girdle) O66.0
    causing obstructed labor O66.0
  uterine NEC O62.4

Dystonia G24.9
  deformans progressiva G24.1
  drug induced NEC G24.09
    acute G24.02
    specified NEC G24.09
  familial G24.1
  idiopathic G24.1
    familial G24.1
    nonfamilial G24.2
    orofacial G24.4
  lenticularis G24.8
  musculorum deformans G24.1
  neuroleptic induced (acute) G24.02
  orofacial (idiopathic) G24.4
  oromandibular G24.4
    due to drug G24.01
  specified NEC G24.8
  torsion (familial) (idiopathic) G24.1
    acquired G24.8
    genetic G24.1
    symptomatic (nonfamilial) G24.2
Dystonic movements R25.8
Dystrophy, dystrophia
  adiposogenital E23.6
  Becker's type G71.0
  cervical sympathetic G90.2
  choroid (hereditary) H31.20
    central areolar H31.22
    choroideremia H31.21
    gyrate atrophy H31.23
    specified type NEC H31.29
  cornea (hereditary) H18.50
    endothelial H18.51
    epithelial H18.52
    granular H18.53
    lattice H18.54
    macular H18.55
    specified type NEC H18.59
  Duchenne's type G71.0
  due to malnutrition E45
  Erb's G71.0
  Fuchs' H18.51
  Gower's muscular G71.0
  hair L67.8
  infantile neuraxonal G31.89
  Landouzy-Déjérine G71.0
  Leyden-Möbius G71.0
  muscular G71.0
    benign (Becker type) G71.0
    congenital (hereditary) (progressive)
      (with specific morphological
      abnormalities of the muscle fiber)
      G71.0
      myotonic G71.11
    distal G71.0
    Duchenne type G71.0
    Emery-Dreifuss G71.0

Dystrophy, dystrophia (Continued)
  muscular (Continued)
    Erb type G71.0
    facioscapulohumeral G71.0
    Gower's G71.0
    hereditary (progressive) G71.0
    Landouzy-Déjérine type G71.0
    limb-girdle G71.0
    myotonic G71.11
    progressive (hereditary) G71.0
      Charcot-Marie (-Tooth) type
      G60.0
    pseudohypertrophic (infantile)
      G71.0
    severe (Duchenne type) G71.0
  myocardium, myocardial —see
    Degeneration, myocardial
  nail L60.3
    congenital Q84.6
  nutritional E45
  ocular G71.0
  oculocerebrorenal E72.03
  oculopharyngeal G71.0
  ovarian N83.8
  polyglandular E31.8
  reflex (neuromuscular) (sympathetic) —
    see Syndrome, pain, complex
    regional I
  retinal (hereditary) H35.50
    in
      lipid storage disorders E75.6
        [H36]
      systemic lipidoses E75.6 [H36]
    involving
      pigment epithelium H35.54
      sensory area H35.53
    pigmentary H35.52
    vitreoretinal H35.51
  Salzmann's nodular —see Degeneration,
    cornea, nodular
  scapuloperoneal G71.0
  skin NEC L98.8
  sympathetic (reflex) —see Syndrome, pain,
    complex regional I
    cervical G90.2
  tapetoretinal H35.54
  thoracic, asphyxiating Q77.2
  unguium L60.3
    congenital Q84.6
  vitreoretinal H35.51
  vulva N90.4
  yellow (liver) —see Failure, hepatic
Dysuria R30.0
  psychogenic F45.8

◀ New   ◀ Revised   deleted Deleted

E

Eales' disease H35.06-
Ear —*see also* condition
  piercing Z41.3
  tropical B36.8
  wax (impacted) H61.20
    left H61.22
      with right H61.23
    right H61.21
      with left H61.23
Earache —*see* subcategory H92.0
Early satiety R68.81
Eaton-Lambert syndrome—*see* Syndrome,
    Lambert-Eaton
Eberth's disease (typhoid fever) A01.00
Ebola virus disease A98.4
Ebstein's anomaly or syndrome (heart) Q22.5
Eccentro-osteochondrodysplasia E76.29
Ecchondroma —*see* Neoplasm, bone, benign
Ecchondrosis D48.0
Ecchymosis R58
  conjunctiva —*see* Hemorrhage, conjunctiva
  eye (traumatic) —*see* Contusion, eyeball
  eyelid (traumatic) —*see* Contusion, eyelid
  newborn P54.5
  spontaneous R23.3
  traumatic —*see* Contusion
Echinococciasis —*see* Echinococcus
Echinococcosis —*see* Echinococcus
Echinococcus (infection) B67.90
  granulosus B67.4
    bone B67.2
    liver B67.0
    lung B67.1
    multiple sites B67.32
    specified site NEC B67.39
    thyroid B67.31 [E35]
  liver NOS B67.8
    granulosus B67.0
    multilocularis B67.5
  lung NEC B67.99
    granulosus B67.1
    multilocularis B67.69
  multilocularis B67.7
    liver B67.5
    multiple sites B67.61
    specified site NEC B67.69
  specified site NEC B67.99
    granulosus B67.39
    multilocularis B67.69
  thyroid NEC B67.99
    granulosus B67.31 [E35]
    multilocularis B67.69 [E35]
Echinorhynchiasis B83.8
Echinostomiasis B66.8
Echolalia R48.8
Echovirus, as cause of disease classified
    elsewhere B97.12
Eclampsia, eclamptic (coma) (convulsions)
    (delirium) (with hypertension) NEC O15.9
  during labor and delivery O15.1
  postpartum O15.2
  pregnancy O15.0-
  puerperal O15.2
Economic circumstances affecting care Z59.9
Economo's disease A85.8
Ectasia, ectasis
  annuloaortic I35.8
  aorta I77.819
    with aneurysm —*see* Aneurysm, aorta
    abdominal I77.811
    thoracic I77.810
    thoracoabdominal I77.812
  breast —*see* Ectasia, mammary duct
  capillary I78.8
  cornea H18.71-
  gastric antral vascular (GAVE) K31.819
    with hemorrhage K31.811
    without hemorrhage K31.819
  mammary duct N60.4-

Ectasia, ectasis (*Continued*)
  salivary gland (duct) K11.8
  sclera —*see* Sclerectasia
Ecthyma L08.0
  contagiosum B08.02
  gangrenosum L08.0
  infectiosum B08.02
Ectocardia Q24.8
Ectodermal dysplasia (anhidrotic) Q82.4
Ectodermosis erosiva pluriorificialis
    L51.1
Ectopic, ectopia (congenital)
  abdominal viscera Q45.8
    due to defect in anterior abdominal wall
      Q79.59
  ACTH syndrome E24.3
  adrenal gland Q89.1
  anus Q43.5
  atrial beats I49.1
  beats I49.49
    atrial I49.1
    ventricular I49.3
  bladder Q64.10
  bone and cartilage in lung Q33.5
  brain Q04.8
  breast tissue Q83.8
  cardiac Q24.8
  cerebral Q04.8
  cordis Q24.8
  endometrium —*see* Endometriosis
  gastric mucosa Q40.2
  gestation —*see* Pregnancy, by site
  heart Q24.8
  hormone secretion NEC E34.2
  kidney (crossed) (pelvis) Q63.2
  lens, lentis Q12.1
  mole —*see* Pregnancy, by site
  organ or site NEC —*see* Malposition,
    congenital
  pancreas Q45.3
  pregnancy —*see* Pregnancy, ectopic
  pupil —*see* Abnormality, pupillary
  renal Q63.2
  sebaceous glands of mouth Q38.6
  spleen Q89.09
  testis Q53.00
    bilateral Q53.02
    unilateral Q53.01
  thyroid Q89.2
  tissue in lung Q33.5
  ureter Q62.63
  ventricular beats I49.3
  vesicae Q64.10
Ectromelia Q73.8
  lower limb —*see* Defect, reduction, limb,
    lower, specified type NEC
  upper limb —*see* Defect, reduction, limb,
    upper, specified type NEC
Ectropion H02.109
  cervix N86
    with cervicitis N72
  congenital Q10.1
  eyelid (paralytic) H02.109
    cicatricial H02.119
      left H02.116
        lower H02.115
        upper H02.114
      right H02.113
        lower H02.112
        upper H02.111
    congenital Q10.1
    left H02.106
      lower H02.105
      upper H02.104
    mechanical H02.129
      left H02.126
        lower H02.125
        upper H02.124
      right H02.123
        lower H02.122
        upper H02.121

Ectropion (*Continued*)
  eyelid (*Continued*)
    right H02.103
      lower H02.102
      upper H02.101
    senile H02.139
      left H02.136
        lower H02.135
        upper H02.134
      right H02.133
        lower H02.132
        upper H02.131
    spastic H02.149
      left H02.146
        lower H02.145
        upper H02.144
      right H02.143
        lower H02.142
        upper H02.141
  iris H21.89
  lip (acquired) K13.0
    congenital Q38.0
  urethra N36.8
  uvea H21.89
Eczema (acute) (chronic) (erythematous)
    (fissum) (rubrum) (squamous) (*see also*
    Dermatitis) L30.9
  contact —*see* Dermatitis, contact
  dyshydrotic L30.1
  external ear —*see* Otitis, externa, acute,
    eczematoid
  flexural L20.82
  herpeticum B00.0
  hypertrophicum L28.0
  hypostatic —*see* Varix, leg, with,
    inflammation
  impetiginous L01.1
  infantile (due to any substance)
    L20.83
    intertriginous L21.1
    seborrheic L21.1
  intertriginous NEC L30.4
    infantile L21.1
  intrinsic (allergic) L20.84
  lichenified NEC L28.0
  marginatum (hebrae) B35.6
  pustular L30.3
  stasis —*see* Varix, leg, with, inflammation
  vaccination, vaccinatum T88.1
  varicose —*see* Varix, leg, with,
    inflammation
Eczematid L30.2
Eddowes (-Spurway) syndrome Q78.0
Edema, edematous (infectious) (pitting)
    (toxic) R60.9
  with nephritis —*see* Nephrosis
  allergic T78.3
  amputation stump (surgical) (sequelae
    (late effect)) T87.89
  angioneurotic (allergic) (any site) (with
    urticaria) T78.3
    hereditary D84.1
  angiospastic I73.9
  Berlin's (traumatic) S05.8X-
  brain (cytotoxic) (vasogenic) G93.6
    due to birth injury P11.0
    newborn (anoxia or hypoxia) P52.4
      birth injury P11.0
    traumatic —*see* Injury, intracranial,
      cerebral edema
  cardiac —*see* Failure, heart, congestive
  cardiovascular —*see* Failure, heart,
    congestive
  cerebral —*see* Edema, brain
  cerebrospinal —*see* Edema, brain
  cervix (uteri) (acute) N88.8
    puerperal, postpartum O90.89
  chronic hereditary Q82.0
  circumscribed, acute T78.3
    hereditary D84.1
  conjunctiva H11.42-

Edema, edematous (*Continued*)
  cornea H18.2-
    idiopathic H18.22-
    secondary H18.23-
      due to contact lens H18.21-
  due to
    lymphatic obstruction I89.0
    salt retention E87.0
  epiglottis —*see* Edema, glottis
  essential, acute T78.3
    hereditary D84.1
  extremities, lower —*see* Edema, legs
  eyelid NEC H02.849
    left H02.846
      lower H02.845
      upper H02.844
    right H02.843
      lower H02.842
      upper H02.841
  familial, hereditary Q82.0
  famine —*see* Malnutrition, severe
  generalized R60.1
  glottis, glottic, glottidis (obstructive) (passive)
      J38.4
    allergic T78.3
      hereditary D84.1
  heart —*see* Failure, heart, congestive
  heat T67.7
  hereditary Q82.0
  inanition —*see* Malnutrition, severe
  intracranial G93.6
  iris H21.89
  joint —*see* Effusion, joint
  larynx —*see* Edema, glottis
  legs R60.0
    due to venous obstruction I87.1
    hereditary Q82.0
  localized R60.0
    due to venous obstruction I87.1
  lower limbs —*see* Edema, legs
  lung J81.1
    with heart condition or failure —*see*
        Failure, ventricular, left
    acute J81.0
    chemical (acute) J68.1
      chronic J68.1
    chronic J81.1
      due to
        chemicals, gases, fumes or vapors
            (inhalation) J68.1
        external agent J70.9
          specified NEC J70.8
        radiation J70.1
    due to
      chemicals, fumes or vapors (inhalation)
          J68.1
      external agent J70.9
        specified NEC J70.8
      high altitude T70.29
      near drowning T75.1
      radiation J70.0
    meaning failure, left ventricle I50.1
  lymphatic I89.0
    due to mastectomy I97.2
  macula H35.81
    cystoid, following cataract surgery —*see*
        Complications, postprocedural,
        following cataract surgery
    diabetic —*see* Diabetes, by type, with,
        retinopathy, with macular edema
  malignant —*see* Gangrene, gas
  Milroy's Q82.0
  nasopharynx J39.2
  newborn P83.30
    hydrops fetalis —*see* Hydrops, fetalis
    specified NEC P83.39
  nutritional —*see also* Malnutrition, severe
    with dyspigmentation, skin and hair E40
  optic disc or nerve —*see* Papilledema
  orbit H05.22-
  pancreas K86.8

Edema, edematous (*Continued*)
  papilla, optic —*see* Papilledema
  penis N48.89
  periodic T78.3
    hereditary D84.1
  pharynx J39.2
  pulmonary —*see* Edema, lung
  Quincke's T78.3
    hereditary D84.1
  renal —*see* Nephrosis
  retina H35.81
    diabetic —*see* Diabetes, by type, with,
        retinopathy, with macular edema
  salt E87.0
  scrotum N50.8
  seminal vesicle N50.8
  spermatic cord N50.8
  spinal (cord) (vascular) (nontraumatic) G95.19
  starvation —*see* Malnutrition, severe
  stasis —*see* Hypertension, venous, (chronic)
  subglottic —*see* Edema, glottis
  supraglottic —*see* Edema, glottis
  testis N44.8
  tunica vaginalis N50.8
  vas deferens N50.8
  vulva (acute) N90.89
Edentulism —*see* Absence, teeth, acquired
Edsall's disease T67.2
Educational handicap Z55.9
  specified NEC Z55.8
Edward's syndrome —*see* Trisomy, 18
Effect, adverse
  abnormal gravitational (G) forces or states
      T75.81
  abuse —*see* Maltreatment
  air pressure T70.9
    specified NEC T70.8
  altitude (high) —*see* Effect, adverse, high
      altitude
  anesthesia (*see also* Anesthesia) T88.59
    in labor and delivery O74.9
    in pregnancy NEC O29.3-
    local, toxic
      in labor and delivery O74.4-
      postpartum, puerperal O89.3
    postpartum, puerperal O89.9
    specified NEC T88.59
      in labor and delivery O74.8
      postpartum, puerperal O89.8
    spinal and epidural T88.59
      headache T88.59
        in labor and delivery O74.5
        postpartum, puerperal O89.4
      specified NEC
        in labor and delivery O74.6
        postpartum, puerperal O89.5
  antitoxin —*see* Complications, vaccination
  atmospheric pressure T70.9
    due to explosion T70.8
    high T70.3
    low —*see* Effect, adverse, high altitude
    specified effect NEC T70.8
  biological, correct substance properly
      administered —*see* Effect, adverse, drug
  blood (derivatives) (serum) (transfusion) —
      see Complications, transfusion
  chemical substance —*see* Table of Drugs and
      Chemicals
  cold (temperature) (weather) T69.9
    chilblains T69.1
    frostbite —*see* Frostbite
    specified effect NEC T69.8
  drugs and medicaments T88.7
    specified drug —*see* Table of Drugs and
        Chemicals, by drug, adverse effect
    specified effect — code to condition
  electric current, electricity (shock) T75.4
    burn —*see* Burn
  exertion (excessive) T73.3
  exposure —*see* Exposure
    external cause NEC T75.89

Effect, adverse (*Continued*)
  foodstuffs T78.1
    allergic reaction —*see* Allergy, food
      causing anaphylaxis —*see* Shock,
          anaphylactic, due to food
    noxious —*see* Poisoning, food, noxious
  gases, fumes, or vapors T59.9-
    specified agent —*see* Table of Drugs and
        Chemicals
  glue (airplane) sniffing
    due to drug abuse —*see* Abuse, drug,
        inhalant
    due to drug dependence —*see* Dependence,
        drug, inhalant
  heat —*see* Heat
  high altitude NEC T70.29
    anoxia T70.29
    on
      ears T70.0
      sinuses T70.1
    polycythemia D75.1
  high pressure fluids T70.4
  hot weather —*see* Heat
  hunger T73.0
  immersion, foot —*see* Immersion
  immunization —*see* Complications,
      vaccination
  immunological agents —*see* Complications,
      vaccination
  infrared (radiation) (rays) NOS T66
    dermatitis or eczema L59.8
  infusion —*see* Complications, infusion
  lack of care of infants —*see* Maltreatment,
      child
  lightning —*see* Lightning
  medical care T88.9
    specified NEC T88.8
  medicinal substance, correct, properly
      administered —*see* Effect, adverse, drug
  motion T75.3
  noise, on inner ear —*see* subcategory H83.3
  overheated places —*see* Heat
  psychosocial, of work environment Z56.5
  radiation (diagnostic) (infrared) (natural
      source) (therapeutic) (ultraviolet)
      (X-ray) NOS T66
    dermatitis or eczema —*see* Dermatitis, due
        to, radiation
    fibrosis of lung J70.1
    pneumonitis J70.0
    pulmonary manifestations
      acute J70.0
      chronic J70.1
    skin L59.9
  radioactive substance NOS
    dermatitis or eczema —*see* Radiodermatitis
  reduced temperature T69.9
    immersion foot or hand —*see* Immersion
    specified effect NEC T69.8
  serum NEC (*see also* Reaction, serum)
      T80.69
  specified NEC T78.8
    external cause NEC T75.89
  strangulation —*see* Asphyxia, traumatic
  submersion T75.1
  thirst T73.1
  toxic —*see* Toxicity
  transfusion —*see* Complications, transfusion
  ultraviolet (radiation) (rays) NOS T66
    burn —*see* Burn
    dermatitis or eczema —*see* Dermatitis, due
        to, ultraviolet rays
      acute L56.8
  vaccine (any) —*see* Complications,
      vaccination
  vibration —*see* Vibration, adverse effects
  water pressure NEC T70.9
    specified NEC T70.8
  weightlessness T75.82
  whole blood —*see* Complications, transfusion
  work environment Z56.5

◀ New　◀◀ Revised　~~deleted~~ Deleted

Effect (s) (of) (from) —*see* Effect, adverse NEC
Effects, late —*see* Sequelae
Effluvium
    anagen L65.1
    telogen L65.0
Effort syndrome (psychogenic) F45.8
Effusion
    amniotic fluid —*see* Pregnancy, complicated
        by, prematue rupture of membranes
    brain (serous) G93.6
    bronchial —*see* Bronchitis
    cerebral G93.6
    cerebrospinal —*see also* Meningitis
        vessel G93.6
    chest —*see* Effusion, pleura
    chylous, chyliform (pleura) J94.0
    intracranial G93.6
    joint M25.40
        ankle M25.47-
        elbow M25.42-
        foot joint M25.47-
        hand joint M25.44-
        hip M25.45-
        knee M25.46-
        shoulder M25.41-
        specified joint NEC M25.48
        wrist M25.43-
    malignant pleural J91.0
    meninges —*see* Meningitis
    pericardium, pericardial (noninflammatory)
        I31.3
        acute —*see* Pericarditis, acute
    peritoneal (chronic) R18.8
    pleura, pleurisy, pleuritic, pleuropericardial
        J90
        chylous, chyliform J94.0
        due to systemic lupus erythematosis
            M32.13
        influenzal —*see* Influenza, with, respiratory
            manifestations NEC
        malignant J91.0
        newborn P28.89
        tuberculous NEC A15.6
            primary (progressive) A15.7
    spinal —*see* Meningitis
    thorax, thoracic —*see* Effusion, pleura
Egg shell nails L60.3
    congenital Q84.6
Egyptian splenomegaly B65.1
Ehlers-Danlos syndrome Q79.6
Ehrlichiosis A77.40
    due to
        E. chafeensis A77.41
        E. sennetsu A79.81
        specified organism NEC A77.49
Eichstedt's disease B36.0
Eisenmenger's
    complex or syndrome I27.89
    defect Q21.8
Ejaculation
    painful N53.12
    premature F52.4
    retarded N53.11
    retrograde N53.14
    semen, painful N53.12
        psychogenic F52.6
Ekbom's syndrome (restless legs) G25.81
Ekman's syndrome (brittle bones and blue
    sclera) Q78.0
Elastic skin Q82.8
    acquired L57.4
Elastofibroma —*see* Neoplasm, connective
    tissue, benign
Elastoma (juvenile) Q82.8
    Miescher's L87.2
Elastomyofibrosis I42.4
Elastosis
    actinic, solar L57.8
    atrophicans (senile) L57.4
    perforans serpiginosa L87.2
    senilis L57.4

Elbow —*see* condition
Electric current, electricity, effects (concussion)
    (fatal) (nonfatal) (shock) T75.4
    burn —*see* Burn
Electric feet syndrome E53.8
Electrocution T75.4
    from electroshock gun (taser) T75.4
Electrolyte imbalance E87.8
    with
        abortion —*see* Abortion by type,
            complicated by, electrolyte imbalance
        ectopic pregnancy O08.5
        molar pregnancy O08.5
Elephantiasis (nonfilarial) I89.0
    arabicum —*see* Infestation, filarial
    bancroftian B74.0
    congenital (any site) (hereditary) Q82.0
    due to
        Brugia (malayi) B74.1
            timori B74.2
        mastectomy I97.2
        Wuchereria (bancrofti) B74.0
    eyelid H02.859
        left H02.856
            lower H02.855
            upper H02.854
        right H02.853
            lower H02.852
            upper H02.851
    filarial, filariensis —*see* Infestation, filarial
    glandular I89.0
    graecorum A30.9
    lymphangiectatic I89.0
    lymphatic vessel I89.0
        due to mastectomy I97.2
    scrotum (nonfilarial) I89.0
    streptococcal I89.0
    surgical I97.89
        postmastectomy I97.2
    telangiectodes I89.0
    vulva (nonfilarial) N90.89
Elevated, elevation
    antibody titer R76.0
    basal metabolic rate R94.8
    blood pressure —*see also* Hypertension
        reading (incidental) (isolated) (nonspecific),
            no diagnosis of hypertension R03.0
    blood sugar R73.9
    body temperature (of unknown origin) R50.9
    C-reactive protein (CRP) R79.82
    cancer antigen 125 [CA 125] R97.1
    carcinoembryonic antigen [CEA] R97.0
    cholesterol E78.0
        with high triglycerides E78.2
    conjugate, eye H51.0
    diaphragm, congenital Q79.1
    erythrocyte sedimentation rate R70.0
    fasting glucose R73.01
    fasting triglycerides E78.1
    finding on laboratory examination —*see*
        Findings, abnormal, inconclusive,
        without diagnosis, by type of exam
    GFR (glomerular filtration rate) —*see*
        Findings, abnormal, inconclusive,
        without diagnosis, by type of exam
    glucose tolerance (oral) R73.02
    immunoglobulin level R76.8
    indoleacetic acid R82.5
    lactic acid dehydrogenase (LDH) level R74.0
    leukocytes D72.829
    lipoprotein a level E78.8
    liver function
        study R94.5
        test R79.89
            alkaline phosphatase R74.8
            aminotransferase R74.0
            bilirubin R17
            hepatic enzyme R74.8
            lactate dehydrogenase R74.0
    lymphocytes D72.820
    prostate specific antigen [PSA] R97.2

Elevated, elevation (Continued)
    Rh titer —*see* Complication (s), transfusion,
        incompatibility reaction, Rh (factor)
    scapula, congenital Q74.0
    sedimentation rate R70.0
    SGOT R74.0
    SGPT R74.0
    transaminase level R74.0
    triglycerides E78.1
        with high cholesterol E78.2
    tumor associated antigens [TAA] NEC
        R97.8
    tumor specific antigens [TSA] NEC R97.8
    urine level of
        17-ketosteroids R82.5
        catecholamine R82.5
        indoleacetic acid R82.5
        steroids R82.5
        vanillylmandelic acid (VMA) R82.5
    venous pressure I87.8
    white blood cell count D72.829
        specified NEC D72.828
Elliptocytosis (congenital) (hereditary) D58.1
    Hb C (disease) D58.1
    hemoglobin disease D58.1
    sickle-cell (disease) D57.8-
        trait D57.3
Ellison-Zollinger syndrome E16.4
Ellis-van Creveld syndrome
    (chondroectodermal dysplasia) Q77.6
Elongated, elongation (congenital) —*see also*
    Distortion
    bone Q79.9
    cervix (uteri) Q51.828
        acquired N88.4
        hypertrophic N88.4
    colon Q43.8
    common bile duct Q44.5
    cystic duct Q44.5
    frenulum, penis Q55.69
    labia minora (acquired) N90.6
    ligamentum patellae Q74.1
    petiolus (epiglottidis) Q31.8
    tooth, teeth K00.2
    uvula Q38.6
Eltor cholera A00.1
Emaciation (due to malnutrition) E41
Embadomoniasis A07.8
Embedded tooth, teeth K01.0
    root only K08.3
Embolic —*see* condition
Embolism (multiple) (paradoxical) I74.9
    air (any site) (traumatic) T79.0
        following
            abortion —*see* Abortion by type
                complicated by embolism
            ectopic pregnancy O08.2
            infusion, therapeutic injection or
                transfusion T80.0
            molar pregnancy O08.2
            procedure NEC
                artery T81.719
                    mesenteric T81.710
                    renal T81.711
                    specified NEC T81.718
                vein T81.72
        in pregnancy, childbirth or puerperium —
            see Embolism, obstetric
    amniotic fluid (pulmonary) —*see also*
        Embolism, obstetric
        following
            abortion —*see* Abortion by type
                complicated by embolism
            ectopic pregnancy O08.2
            molar pregnancy O08.2
    aorta, aortic I74.10
        abdominal I74.09
            saddle I74.01
        bifurcation I74.09
            saddle I74.01
        thoracic I74.11

Embolism *(Continued)*
  artery I74.9
    auditory, internal I65.8
    basilar —*see* Occlusion, artery, basilar
    carotid (common) (internal) —*see*
      Occlusion, artery, carotid
    cerebellar (anterior inferior) (posterior
      inferior) (superior) I66.3
    cerebral —*see* Occlusion, artery, cerebral
    choroidal (anterior) I66.8
    communicating posterior I66.8
    coronary —*see also* Infarct, myocardium
      not resulting in infarction I24.0
    extremity I74.4
      lower I74.3
      upper I74.2
    hypophyseal I66.8
    iliac I74.5
    limb I74.4
      lower I74.3
      upper I74.2
    mesenteric (with gangrene) K55.0
    ophthalmic —*see* Occlusion, artery, retina
    peripheral I74.4
    pontine I66.8
    precerebral —*see* Occlusion, artery,
      precerebral
    pulmonary —*see* Embolism, pulmonary
    renal N28.0
    retinal —*see* Occlusion, artery, retina
    septic I76
    specified NEC I74.8
    vertebral —*see* Occlusion, artery, vertebral
  basilar (artery) I65.1
  blood clot
    following
      abortion —*see* Abortion by type
        complicated by embolism
      ectopic or molar pregnancy O08.2
    in pregnancy, childbirth or puerperium —
      see Embolism, obstetric
  brain —*see also* Occlusion, artery, cerebral
    following
      abortion —*see* Abortion by type
        complicated by embolism
      ectopic or molar pregnancy O08.2
    puerperal, postpartum, childbirth —*see*
      Embolism, obstetric
  capillary I78.8
  cardiac —*see also* Infarct, myocardium
    not resulting in infarction I24.0
  carotid (artery) (common) (internal) —*see*
    Occlusion, artery, carotid
  cavernous sinus (venous) —*see* Embolism,
    intracranial venous sinus
  cerebral —*see* Occlusion, artery, cerebral
  cholesterol —*see* Atheroembolism
  coronary (artery or vein) (systemic) —*see*
    Occlusion, coronary
  due to device, implant or graft —*see also*
    Complications, by site and type,
    specified NEC
    arterial graft NEC T82.818
    breast (implant) T85.81
    catheter NEC T85.81
      dialysis (renal) T82.818
        intraperitoneal T85.81
      infusion NEC T82.818
        spinal (epidural) (subdural) T85.81
      urinary (indwelling) T83.81
    electronic (electrode) (pulse generator)
      (stimulator)
      bone T84.81
      cardiac T82.817
      nervous system (brain) (peripheral
        nerve) (spinal) T85.81
      urinary T83.81
    fixation, internal (orthopedic) NEC T84.81
    gastrointestinal (bile duct) (esophagus)
      T85.81
    genital NEC T83.81

Embolism *(Continued)*
  due to device, implant or graft *(Continued)*
    heart (graft) (valve) T82.817
    joint prosthesis T84.81
    ocular (corneal graft) (orbital implant)
      T85.81
    orthopedic (bone graft) NEC T86.838
    specified NEC T85.81
    urinary (graft) NEC T83.81
    vascular NEC T82.818
    ventricular intracranial shunt T85.81
  extremities
    lower —*see* Embolism, vein, lower
      extremity
      arterial I74.3
    upper I74.2
  eye H34.9
  fat (cerebral) (pulmonary) (systemic) T79.1
    complicating delivery —*see* Embolism,
      obstetric
    following
      abortion —*see* Abortion by type
        complicated by embolism
      ectopic or molar pregnancy O08.2
  following
    abortion —*see* Abortion by type
      complicated by embolism
    ectopic or molar pregnancy O08.2
    infusion, therapeutic injection or
      transfusion
      air T80.0
  heart (fatty) —*see also* Infarct, myocardium
    not resulting in infarction I24.0
  hepatic (vein) I82.0
  in pregnancy, childbirth or puerperium —*see*
    Embolism, obstetric
  intestine (artery) (vein) (with gangrene) K55.0
  intracranial —*see also* Occlusion, artery,
    cerebral
    venous sinus (any) G08
      nonpyogenic I67.6
  intraspinal venous sinuses or veins G08
    nonpyogenic G95.19
  kidney (artery) N28.0
  lateral sinus (venous) —*see* Embolism,
    intracranial, venous sinus
  leg —*see* Embolism, vein, lower extremity
    arterial I74.3
  longitudinal sinus (venous) —*see* Embolism,
    intracranial, venous sinus
  lung (massive) —*see* Embolism, pulmonary
  meninges I66.8
  mesenteric (artery) (vein) (with gangrene)
    K55.0
  obstetric (in) (pulmonary)
    childbirth O88.82
      air O88.02
      amniotic fluid O88.12
      blood clot O88.22
      fat O88.82
      pyemic O88.32
      septic O88.32
      specified type NEC O88.82
    pregnancy O88.81-
      air O88.01-
      amniotic fluid O88.11-
      blood clot O88.21-
      fat O88.81-
      pyemic O88.31-
      septic O88.31-
      specified type NEC O88.81-
    puerperal O88.83
      air O88.03
      amniotic fluid O88.13
      blood clot O88.23
      fat O88.83
      pyemic O88.33
      septic O88.33
      specified type NEC O88.83
  ophthalmic —*see* Occlusion, artery, retina
  penis N48.81

Embolism *(Continued)*
  peripheral artery NOS I74.4
  pituitary E23.6
  popliteal (artery) I74.3
  portal (vein) I81
  postoperative, postprocedural
    artery T81.719
      mesenteric T81.710
      renal T81.711
      specified NEC T81.718
    vein T81.72
  precerebral artery —*see* Occlusion, artery,
    precerebral
  puerperal —*see* Embolism, obstetric
  pulmonary (acute) (artery) (vein) I26.99
    with acute cor pulmonale I26.09
    chronic I27.82
    following
      abortion —*see* Abortion by type
        complicated by embolism
      ectopic or molar pregnancy O08.2
    healed or old Z86.711
    in pregnancy, childbirth or puerperium —
      see Embolism, obstetric
    personal history of Z86.711
    saddle I26.92
      with acute cor pulmonale I26.02
    septic I26.90
      with acute cor pulmonale I26.01
  pyemic (multiple) I76
    following
      abortion —*see* Abortion by type
        complicated by embolism
      ectopic or molar pregnancy O08.2
    Hemophilus influenzae A41.3
    pneumococcal A40.3
      with pneumonia J13
    puerperal, postpartum, childbirth (any
      organism) —*see* Embolism, obstetric
    specified organism NEC A41.89
    staphylococcal A41.2
    streptococcal A40.9
  renal (artery) N28.0
    vein I82.3
  retina, retinal —*see* Occlusion, artery, retina
  saddle
    abdominal aorta I74.01
    pulmonary artery I26.92
      with acute cor pulmonale I26.02
  septic (arterial) I76
    complicating abortion —*see* Abortion, by
      type, complicated by, embolism
  sinus —*see* Embolism, intracranial, venous
    sinus
  soap complicating abortion —*see* Abortion,
    by type, complicated by, embolism
  spinal cord G95.19
    pyogenic origin G06.1
  spleen, splenic (artery) I74.8
  upper extremity I74.2
  vein (acute) I82.90
    antecubital I82.61-
      chronic I82.71-
    axillary I82.A1-
      chronic I82.A2-
    basilic I82.61-
      chronic I82.71-
    brachial I82.62-
      chronic I82.72-
    brachiocephalic (innominate) I82.290
      chronic I82.291
    cephalic I82.61-
      chronic I82.71-
    chronic I82.91
    deep (DVT) I82.40-
      calf I82.4Z-
        chronic I82.5Z-
      lower leg I82.4Z-
        chronic I82.5Z-
      thigh I82.4Y-
        chronic I82.5Y-

◀ New   ◀▥▥ Revised   ~~deleted~~ Deleted

Embolism (Continued)
  vein (Continued)
    deep (Continued)
      upper leg I82.4Y
        chronic I82.5y--
      femoral I82.41-
        chronic I82.51-
      iliac (iliofemoral) I82.42-
        chronic I82.52-
      innominate I82.290
        chronic I82.291
      internal jugular I82.C1-
        chronic I82.C2-
      lower extremity
        deep I82.40-
          chronic I82.50-
            specified NEC I82.49-
              chronic NEC I82.59-
        distal
          deep I82.4Z-
        proximal
          deep I82.4Y-
            chronic I82.5Y-
        superficial I82.81-
      popliteal I82.43-
        chronic I82.53-
      radial I82.62-
        chronic I82.72-
      renal I82.3
      saphenous (greater) (lesser) I82.81-
      specified NEC I82.890
        chronic NEC I82.891
      subclavian I82.B1-
        chronic I82.B2-
      thoracic NEC I82.290
        chronic I82.291
      tibial I82.44-
        chronic I82.54-
      ulnar I82.62-
        chronic I82.72-
      upper extremity I82.60-
        chronic I82.70-
        deep I82.62-
          chronic I82.72-
        superficial I82.61-
          chronic I82.71-
    vena cava
      inferior (acute) I82.220
        chronic I82.221
      superior (acute) I82.210
        chronic I82.211
    venous sinus G08
    vessels of brain —see Occlusion, artery,
      cerebral
Embolus —see Embolism
Embryoma —see also Neoplasm, uncertain
    behavior, by site
  benign —see Neoplasm, benign, by site
  kidney C64.-
  liver C22.0
  malignant —see also Neoplasm, malignant,
      by site
    kidney C64.-
    liver C22.0
    testis C62.9-
      descended (scrotal) C62.1-
      undescended C62.0-
  testis C62.9-
    descended (scrotal) C62.1-
    undescended C62.0-
Embryonic
  circulation Q28.9
  heart Q28.9
  vas deferens Q55.4
Embryopathia NOS Q89.9
Embryotoxon Q13.4
Emesis —see Vomiting
Emotional lability R45.86
Emotionality, pathological F60.3
Emotogenic disease —see Disorder,
    psychogenic

Emphysema (atrophic) (bullous) (chronic)
    (interlobular) (lung) (obstructive)
    (pulmonary) (senile) (vesicular)
    J43.9
  cellular tissue (traumatic) T79.7
    surgical T81.82
  centrilobular J43.2
  compensatory J98.3
  congenital (interstitial) P25.0
  conjunctiva H11.89
  connective tissue (traumatic) T79.7
    surgical T81.82
  due to chemicals, gases, fumes or vapors
      J68.4
  eyelid (s) —see Disorder, eyelid, specified
      type NEC
    surgical T81.82
    traumatic T79.7
  interstitial J98.2
    congenital P25.0
    perinatal period P25.0
  laminated tissue T79.7
    surgical T81.82
  mediastinal J98.2
    newborn P25.2
  orbit, orbital —see Disorder, orbit, specified
      type NEC
  panacinar J43.1
  panlobular J43.1
  specified NEC J43.8
  subcutaneous (traumatic) T79.7
    nontraumatic J98.2
    postprocedural T81.82
    surgical T81.82
  surgical T81.82
  thymus (gland) (congenital) E32.8
  traumatic (subcutaneous) T79.7
  unilateral J43.0
Empty nest syndrome Z60.0
Empyema (acute) (chest) (double) (pleura)
    (supradiaphragmatic) (thorax) J86.9
  with fistula J86.0
  accessory sinus (chronic) —see Sinusitis
  antrum (chronic) —see Sinusitis, maxillary
  brain (any part) —see Abscess, brain
  ethmoidal (chronic) (sinus) —see Sinusitis,
      ethmoidal
  extradural —see Abscess, extradural
  frontal (chronic) (sinus) —see Sinusitis,
      frontal
  gallbladder K81.0
  mastoid (process) (acute) —see Mastoiditis,
      acute
  maxilla, maxillary M27.2
    sinus (chronic) —see Sinusitis,
        maxillary
  nasal sinus (chronic) —see Sinusitis
  sinus (accessory) (chronic) (nasal) —see
      Sinusitis
  sphenoidal (sinus) (chronic) —see Sinusitis,
      sphenoidal
  subarachnoid —see Abscess, extradural
  subdural —see Abscess, subdural
  tuberculous A15.6
  ureter —see Ureteritis
  ventricular —see Abscess, brain
En coup de sabre lesion L94.1
Enamel pearls K00.2
Enameloma K00.2
Enanthema, viral B09
Encephalitis (chronic) (hemorrhagic)
    (idiopathic) (nonepidemic) (spurious)
    (subacute) G04.90
  acute (see also Encephalitis, viral) A86
    disseminated G04.00
      infectious G04.01
      noninfectious G04.81
      postimmunization (postvaccination)
          G04.02
      postinfectious G04.01
    inclusion body A85.8

Encephalitis (Continued)
  acute (Continued)
    necrotizing hemorrhagic G04.30
      postimmunization G04.32
      postinfectious G04.31
      specified NEC G04.39
  arboviral, arbovirus NEC A85.2
  arthropod-borne NEC (viral) A85.2
  Australian A83.4
  California (virus) A83.5
  Central European (tick-borne) A84.1
  Czechoslovakian A84.1
  Dawson's (inclusion body) A81.1
  diffuse sclerosing A81.1
  disseminated, acute G04.00
  due to
    cat scratch disease A28.1
    human immunodeficiency virus (HIV)
        disease B20 [G05.3]
    malaria —see Malaria
    rickettsiosis —see Rickettsiosis
    smallpox inoculation G04.02
    typhus —see Typhus
  Eastern equine A83.2
  endemic (viral) A86
  epidemic NEC (viral) A86
  equine (acute) (infectious) (viral) A83.9
    Eastern A83.2
    Venezuelan A92.2
    Western A83.1
  Far Eastern (tick-borne) A84.0
  following vaccination or other immunization
      procedure G04.02
  herpes zoster B02.0
  herpesviral B00.4
    due to herpesvirus 6 B10.01
    due to herpesvirus 7 B10.09
    specified NEC B10.09
  Ilheus (virus) A83.8
  in (due to)
    actinomycosis A42.82
    adenovirus A85.1
    African trypanosomiasis B56.9 [G05.3]
    Chagas' disease (chronic) B57.42
    cytomegalovirus B25.8
    enterovirus A85.0
    herpes (simplex) virus B00.4
      due to herpesvirus 6 B10.01
      due to herpesvirus 7 B10.09
      specified NEC B10.09
    infectious disease NEC B99 [G05.3]
    influenza —see Influenza, with,
        encephalopathy
    listeriosis A32.12
    measles B05.0
    mumps B26.2
    naegleriasis B60.2
    parasitic disease NEC B89 [G05.3]
    poliovirus A80.9 [G05.3]
    rubella B06.01
    syphilis
      congenital A50.42
      late A52.14
    systemic lupus erythematosus M32.19
    toxoplasmosis (acquired) B58.2
      congenital P37.1
    tuberculosis A17.82
    zoster B02.0
  inclusion body A81.1
  infectious (acute) (virus) NEC A86
  Japanese (B type) A83.0
  La Crosse A83.5
  lead —see Poisoning, lead
  lethargica (acute) (infectious) A85.8
  louping ill A84.8
  lupus erythematosus, systemic M32.19
  lymphatica A87.2
  Mengo A85.8
  meningococcal A39.81
  Murray Valley A83.4
  otitic NEC H66.40 [G05.3]

Encephalitis *(Continued)*
  parasitic NOS B71.9
  periaxial G37.0
  periaxialis (concentrica) (diffuse) G37.5
  postchickenpox B01.11
  postexanthematous NEC B09
  postimmunization G04.02
  postinfectious NEC G04.01
  postmeasles B05.0
  postvaccinal G04.02
  postvaricella B01.11
  postviral NEC A86
  Powassan A84.8
  Rasmussen G04.81
  Rio Bravo A85.8
  Russian
    autumnal A83.0
    spring-summer (taiga) A84.0
  saturnine —*see* Poisoning, lead
  specified NEC G04.81
  St. Louis A83.3
  subacute sclerosing A81.1
  summer A83.0
  suppurative G04.81
  tick-borne A84.9
  Torula, torular (cryptococcal) B45.1
  toxic NEC G92
  trichinosis B75 *[G05.3]*
  type
    B A83.0
    C A83.3
  van Bogaert's A81.1
  Venezuelan equine A92.2
  Vienna A85.8
  viral, virus A86
    arthropod-borne NEC A85.2
      mosquito-borne A83.9
        Australian X disease A83.4
        California virus A83.5
        Eastern equine A83.2
        Japanese (B type) A83.0
        Murray Valley A83.4
        specified NEC A83.8
        St. Louis A83.3
        type B A83.0
        type C A83.3
        Western equine A83.1
      tick-borne A84.9
        biundulant A84.1
        central European A84.1
        Czechoslovakian A84.1
        diphasic meningoencephalitis A84.1
        Far Eastern A84.0
        Russian spring-summer (taiga) A84.0
        specified NEC A84.8
      specified type NEC A85.8
    Western equine A83.1
Encephalocele Q01.9
  frontal Q01.0
  nasofrontal Q01.1
  occipital Q01.2
  specified NEC Q01.8
Encephalocystocele —*see* Encephalocele
Encephaloduroarteriomyosynangiosis (EDAMS) I67.5
Encephalomalacia (brain) (cerebellar) (cerebral) —*see* Softening, brain
Encephalomeningitis —*see* Meningoencephalitis
Encephalomeningocele —*see* Encephalocele
Encephalomeningomyelitis —*see* Meningoencephalitis
Encephalomyelitis *(see also* Encephalitis) G04.90
  acute disseminated G04.00
    infectious G04.01
    noninfectious G04.81
    postimmunization G04.02
    postinfectious G04.01

Encephalomyelitis *(Continued)*
  acute necrotizing hemorrhagic G04.30
    postimmunization G04.32
    postinfectious G04.31
    specified NEC G04.39
  benign myalgic G93.3
  equine A83.9
    Eastern A83.2
    Venezuelan A92.2
    Western A83.1
  in diseases classified elsewhere G05.3
  myalgic, benign G93.3
  postchickenpox B01.11
  postinfectious NEC G04.01
  postmeasles B05.0
  postvaccinal G04.02
  postvaricella B01.11
  rubella B06.01
  specified NEC G04.81
  Venezuelan equine A92.2
Encephalomyelocele —*see* Encephalocele
Encephalomyelomeningitis —*see* Meningoencephalitis
Encephalomyelopathy G96.9
Encephalomyeloradiculitis (acute) G61.0
Encephalomyeloradiculoneuritis (acute) (Guillain-Barré) G61.0
Encephalomyeloradiculopathy G96.9
Encephalopathia hyperbilirubinemica, newborn P57.9
  due to isoimmunization (conditions in P55) P57.0
Encephalopathy (acute) G93.40
  acute necrotizing hemorrhagic G04.30
    postimmunization G04.32
    postinfectious G04.31
    specified NEC G04.39
  alcoholic G31.2
  anoxic —*see* Damage, brain, anoxic
  arteriosclerotic I67.2
  centrolobar progressive (Schilder) G37.0
  congenital Q07.9
  degenerative, in specified disease NEC G32.89
  due to
    drugs *(see also* Table of Drugs and Chemicals) G92
  demyelinating callosal G37.1
  hepatic —*see* Failure, hepatic
  hyperbilirubinemic, newborn P57.9
    due to isoimmunization (conditions in P55) P57.0
  hypertensive I67.4
  hypoglycemic E16.2
  hypoxic —*see* Damage, brain, anoxic
  hypoxic ischemic P91.60
    mild P91.61
    moderate P91.62
    severe P91.63
  in (due to) (with)
    birth injury P11.1
    hyperinsulinism E16.1 *[G94]*
    influenza —*see* Influenza, with, encephalopathy
    lack of vitamin *(see also* Deficiency, vitamin) E56.9 *[G32.89]*
    neoplastic disease *(see also* Neoplasm) D49.9 *[G13.1]*
    serum *(see also* Reaction, serum) T80.69
    syphilis A52.17
    trauma (postconcussional) F07.81
      current injury —*see* Injury, intracranial
    vaccination G04.02
  lead —*see* Poisoning, lead
  metabolic G93.41
    drug induced G92
    toxic G92
  myoclonic, early, symptomatic —*see* Epilepsy, generalized, specified NEC
  necrotizing, subacute (Leigh) G31.82
  pellagrous E52 *[G32.89]*

Encephalopathy *(Continued)*
  portosystemic —*see* Failure, hepatic
  postcontusional F07.81
    current injury —*see* Injury, intracranial, diffuse
  posthypoglycemic (coma) E16.1 *[G94]*
  postradiation G93.89
  saturnine —*see* Poisoning, lead
  septic G93.41
  specified NEC G93.49
  spongiform, subacute (viral) A81.09
  toxic G92
    metabolic G92
  traumatic (postconcussional) F07.81
    current injury —*see* Injury, intracranial
  vitamin B deficiency NEC E53.9 *[G32.89]*
    vitamin B1 E51.2
  Wernicke's E51.2
Encephalorrhagia —*see* Hemorrhage, intracranial, intracerebral
Encephalosis, posttraumatic F07.81
Enchondroma —*see also* Neoplasm, bone, benign
Enchondromatosis (cartilaginous) (multiple) Q78.4
Encopresis R15.9
  functional F98.1
  nonorganic origin F98.1
  psychogenic F98.1
Encounter (with health service) (for) Z76.89
  adjustment and management (of)
    breast implant Z45.81
    implanted device NEC Z45.89
    myringotomy device (stent) (tube) Z45.82
  administrative purpose only Z02.9
    examination for
      adoption Z02.82
      armed forces Z02.3
      disability determination Z02.71
      driving license Z02.4
      employment Z02.1
      insurance Z02.6
      medical certificate NEC Z02.79
      paternity testing Z02.81
      residential institution admission Z02.2
      school admission Z02.0
      sports Z02.5
      specified reason NEC Z02.89
  aftercare —*see* Aftercare
  antenatal screening Z36
  assisted reproductive fertility procedure cycle Z31.83
  blood typing Z01.83
    Rh typing Z01.83
  breast augmentation or reduction Z41.1
  breast implant exchange (different material) (different size) Z45.81
  breast reconstruction following mastectomy Z42.1
  check-up —*see* Examination
  chemotherapy for neoplasm Z51.11
  colonoscopy, screening Z12.11
  counseling —*see* Counseling
  delivery, full-term, uncomplicated O80
    cesarean, without indication O82
  ear piercing Z41.3
  examination —*see* Examination
  expectant parent (s) (adoptive) pre-birth pediatrician visit Z76.81
  fertility preservation procedure (prior to cancer therapy) (prior to removal of gonads) Z31.84
  fitting (of) —*see* Fitting (and adjustment) (of)
  genetic
    counseling Z31.5
    testing —*see* Test, genetic
  hearing conservation and treatment Z01.12
  immunotherapy for neoplasm Z51.12
  in vitro fertilization cycle Z31.83

◀ New   ◀▥ Revised   ~~deleted~~ Deleted

Encounter *(Continued)*
  instruction (in)
    child care (postpartal) (prenatal) Z32.3
    childbirth Z32.2
    natural family planning
      procreative Z31.61
      to avoid pregnancy Z30.02
    insulin pump titration Z46.81
    joint prosthesis insertion following prior
      explantation of joint prosthesis (staged
      procedure)
      hip Z47.32
      knee Z47.33
      shoulder Z47.31
  laboratory (as part of a general medical
    examination) Z00.00
    with abnormal findings Z00.01
  mental health services (for)
    abuse NEC
      perpetrator Z69.82
      victim Z69.81
    child abuse
      nonparental
        perpetrator Z69.021
        victim Z69.020
      parental
        perpetrator Z69.011
        victim Z69.010
    spousal or partner abuse
      perpetrator Z69.12
      victim Z69.11
  observation (for) (ruled out)
    exposure to (suspected)
      anthrax Z03.810
      biological agent NEC Z03.818
  pediatrician visit, by expectant parent (s)
    (adoptive) Z76.81
  plastic and reconstructive surgery following
    medical procedure or healed injury
    NEC Z42.8
  pregnancy
    supervision of —*see* Pregnancy,
      supervision of
    test Z32.00
      result negative Z32.02
      result positive Z32.01
  radiation therapy (antineoplastic) Z51.0
  radiological (as part of a general medical
    examination) Z00.00
    with abnormal findings Z00.01
  reconstructive surgery following medical
    procedure or healed injury NEC Z42.8
  removal (of) —*see also* Removal
    artificial
      arm Z44.00-
        complete Z44.01-
        partial Z44.02-
      eye Z44.2-
      leg Z44.10-
        complete Z44.11-
        partial Z44.12-
    breast implant Z45.81
      tissue expander (without synchronous
        insertion of permanent implant)
        Z45.81
    device Z46.9
      specified NEC Z46.89
    external
      fixation device — code to fracture with
        seventh character D
      prosthesis, prosthetic device Z44.9
        breast Z44.3-
        specified NEC Z44.8
    implanted device NEC Z45.89
    insulin pump Z46.81
    internal fixation device Z47.2
    myringotomy device (stent) (tube) Z45.82
    nervous system device NEC Z46.2
      brain neuropacemaker Z46.2
      visual substitution device Z46.2
        implanted Z45.31

Encounter *(Continued)*
  removal *(Continued)*
    non-vascular catheter Z46.82
    orthodontic device Z46.4
    stent
      ureteral Z46.6
    urinary device Z46.6
  repeat cervical smear to confirm findings of
    recent normal smear following initial
    abnormal smear Z01.42
  respirator [ventilator] use during power
    failure (Z99.12)
  Rh typing Z01.83
  screening —*see* Screening
  specified NEC Z76.89
  sterilization Z30.2
  suspected condition, ruled out
    amniotic cavity and membrane Z03.71
    cervical shortening Z03.75
    fetal anomaly Z03.73
    fetal growth Z03.74
    maternal and fetal conditions NEC Z03.79
    oligohydramnios Z03.71
    placental problem Z03.72
    polyhydramnios Z03.71
  suspected exposure (to), ruled out
    anthrax Z03.810
    biological agents NEC Z03.818
  termination of pregnancy, elective Z33.2
  testing —*see* Test
  therapeutic drug level monitoring Z51.81
  titration, insulin pump Z46.81
  to determine fetal viability of pregnancy
    O36.80
  training
    insulin pump Z46.81
  X-ray of chest (as part of a general medical
    examination Z00.00)
    with abnormal findings Z00.01
Encystment —*see* Cyst
Endarteritis (bacterial, subacute) (infective)
    I77.6
  brain I67.7
  cerebral or cerebrospinal I67.7
  deformans —*see* Arteriosclerosis
  embolic —*see* Embolism
  obliterans —*see also* Arteriosclerosis
    pulmonary I28.8
  pulmonary I28.8
  retina —*see* Vasculitis, retina
  senile —*see* Arteriosclerosis
  syphilitic A52.09
    brain or cerebral A52.04
    congenital A50.54 *[I79.8]*
  tuberculous A18.89
Endemic —*see* condition
Endocarditis (chronic) (marantic) (nonbacterial)
    (thrombotic) (valvular) I38
  with rheumatic fever (conditions in I00)
    active —*see* Endocarditis, acute, rheumatic
    inactive or quiescent (with chorea) I09.1
  acute or subacute I33.9
    infective I33.0
    rheumatic (aortic) (mitral) (pulmonary)
      (tricuspid) I01.1
      with chorea (acute) (rheumatic)
        (Sydenham's) I02.0
  aortic (heart) (nonrheumatic) (valve) I35.8
    with
      mitral disease I08.0
        with tricuspid (valve) disease I08.3
        active or acute I01.1
          with chorea (acute) (rheumatic)
            (Sydenham's) I02.0
      rheumatic fever (conditions in I00)
        active —*see* Endocarditis, acute,
          rheumatic
        inactive or quiescent (with chorea)
          I06.9
      tricuspid (valve) disease I08.2
        with mitral (valve) disease I08.3

Endocarditis *(Continued)*
  aortic *(Continued)*
    acute or subacute I33.9
    arteriosclerotic I35.8
    rheumatic I06.9
      with mitral disease I08.0
        with tricuspid (valve) disease I08.3
        active or acute I01.1
          with chorea (acute) (rheumatic)
            (Sydenham's) I02.0
        active or acute I01.1
          with chorea (acute) (rheumatic)
            (Sydenham's) I02.0
        specified NEC I06.8
      specified cause NEC I35.8
      syphilitic A52.03
    arteriosclerotic I38
    atypical verrucous (Libman-Sacks) M32.11
    bacterial (acute) (any valve) (subacute) I33.0
    candidal B37.6
    congenital Q24.8
    constrictive I33.0
    Coxiella burnetii A78 *[I39]*
    Coxsackie B33.21
    due to
      prosthetic cardiac valve T82.6
      Q fever A78 *[I39]*
      Serratia marcescens I33.0
      typhoid (fever) A01.02
    gonococcal A54.83
    infectious or infective (acute) (any valve)
      (subacute) I33.0
    lenta (acute) (any valve) (subacute) I33.0
    Libman-Sacks M32.11
    listerial A32.82
    Löffler's I42.3
    malignant (acute) (any valve) (subacute) I33.0
    meningococcal A39.51
    mitral (chronic) (double) (fibroid) (heart)
      (inactive) (valve) (with chorea) I05.9
      with
        aortic (valve) disease I08.0
          with tricuspid (valve) disease I08.3
          active or acute I01.1
            with chorea (acute) (rheumatic)
              (Sydenham's) I02.0
        rheumatic fever (conditions in I00)
          active —*see* Endocarditis, acute,
            rheumatic
          inactive or quiescent (with chorea)
            I05.9
        tricuspid (valve) disease I08.1
          with aortic (valve) disease I08.3
      active or acute I01.1
        with chorea (acute) (rheumatic)
          (Sydenham's) I02.0
      bacterial I33.0
      arteriosclerotic I34.8
      nonrheumatic I34.8
        acute or subacute I33.9
      specified NEC I05.8
    monilial B37.6
    multiple valves I08.9
      specified disorders I08.8
    mycotic (acute) (any valve) (subacute) I33.0
    pneumococcal (acute) (any valve) (subacute)
      I33.0
    pulmonary (chronic) (heart) (valve) I37.8
      with rheumatic fever (conditions in I00)
        active —*see* Endocarditis, acute,
          rheumatic
        inactive or quiescent (with chorea)
          I09.89
          with aortic, mitral or tricuspid disease
            I08.8
      acute or subacute I33.9
        rheumatic I01.1
          with chorea (acute) (rheumatic)
            (Sydenham's) I02.0
      arteriosclerotic I37.8
      congenital Q22.2

Endocarditis *(Continued)*
  pulmonary *(Continued)*
    rheumatic (chronic) (inactive) (with chorea)
      I09.89
      active or acute I01.1
        with chorea (acute) (rheumatic)
          (Sydenham's) I02.0
    syphilitic A52.03
  purulent (acute) (any valve) (subacute) I33.0
  Q fever A78 *[I39]*
  rheumatic (chronic) (inactive) (with chorea)
    I09.1
    active or acute (aortic) (mitral)
      (pulmonary) (tricuspid) I01.1
      with chorea (acute) (rheumatic)
        (Sydenham's) I02.0
  rheumatoid —*see* Rheumatoid, carditis
  septic (acute) (any valve) (subacute) I33.0
  streptococcal (acute) (any valve) (subacute)
    I33.0
  subacute —*see* Endocarditis, acute
  suppurative (acute) (any valve) (subacute)
    I33.0
  syphilitic A52.03
  toxic I33.9
  tricuspid (chronic) (heart) (inactive)
    (rheumatic) (valve) (with chorea) I07.9
    with
      aortic (valve) disease I08.2
        mitral (valve) disease I08.3
      mitral (valve) disease I08.1
        aortic (valve) disease I08.3
      rheumatic fever (conditions in I00)
        active —*see* Endocarditis, acute,
          rheumatic
        inactive or quiescent (with chorea)
          I07.8
    active or acute I01.1
      with chorea (acute) (rheumatic)
        (Sydenham's) I02.0
    arteriosclerotic I36.8
    nonrheumatic I36.8
      acute or subacute I33.9
    specified cause, except rheumatic I36.8
  tuberculous —*see* Tuberculosis, endocarditis
  typhoid A01.02
  ulcerative (acute) (any valve) (subacute) I33.0
  vegetative (acute) (any valve) (subacute) I33.0
  verrucous (atypical) (nonbacterial)
    (nonrheumatic) M32.11
Endocardium, endocardial —*see also* condition
  cushion defect Q21.2
Endocervicitis —*see also* Cervicitis
  due to intrauterine (contraceptive) device
    T83.6
  hyperplastic N72
Endocrine —*see* condition
Endocrinopathy, pluriglandular E31.9
Endodontic
  overfill M27.52
  underfill M27.53
Endodontitis K04.0
Endomastoiditis —*see* Mastoiditis
Endometrioma N80.9
Endometriosis N80.9
  appendix N80.5
  bladder N80.8
  bowel N80.5
  broad ligament N80.3
  cervix N80.0
  colon N80.5
  cul-de-sac (Douglas') N80.3
  exocervix N80.0
  fallopian tube N80.2
  female genital organ NEC N80.8
  gallbladder N80.8
  in scar of skin N80.6
  internal N80.0
  intestine N80.5
  lung N80.8
  myometrium N80.0

Endometriosis *(Continued)*
  ovary N80.1
  parametrium N80.3
  pelvic peritoneum N80.3
  peritoneal (pelvic) N80.3
  rectovaginal septum N80.4
  rectum N80.5
  round ligament N80.3
  skin (scar) N80.6
  specified site NEC N80.8
  stromal D39.0
  umbilicus N80.8
  uterus (internal) N80.0
  vagina N80.4
  vulva N80.8
Endometritis (decidual) (nonspecific)
  (purulent) (senile (atrophic) (suppurative)
  N71.9
  with ectopic pregnancy O08.0
  acute N71.0
  blenorrhagic (gonococcal) (acute) (chronic)
    A54.24
  cervix, cervical (with erosion or ectropion) —
    see also Cervicitis
    hyperplastic N72
  chlamydial A56.11
  chronic N71.1
  following
    abortion —*see* Abortion by type
      complicated by genital infection
    ectopic or molar pregnancy O08.0
  gonococcal, gonorrheal (acute) (chronic)
    A54.24
  hyperplastic (*see also* Hyperplasia,
    endometrial) N85.00-
    cervix N72
  puerperal, postpartum, childbirth O86.12
  subacute N71.0
  tuberculous A18.17
Endometrium —*see* condition
Endomyocardiopathy, South African I42.3
Endomyocarditis —*see* Endocarditis
Endomyofibrosis I42.3
Endomyometritis —*see* Endometritis
Endopericarditis —*see* Endocarditis
Endoperineuritis —*see* Disorder, nerve
Endophlebitis —*see* Phlebitis
Endophthalmia —*see* Endophthalmitis,
  purulent
Endophthalmitis (acute) (infective) (metastatic)
  (subacute) H44.009
  bleb associated H59.4 —*see also* Bleb,
    inflamed (infected), postprocedural
  gonorrheal A54.39
  in (due to)
    cysticercosis B69.1
    onchocerciasis B73.01
    toxocariasis B83.0
  panuveitis —*see* Panuveitis
  parasitic H44.12-
  purulent H44.00-
    panophthalmitis —*see* Panophthalmitis
    vitreous abscess H44.02-
  specified NEC H44.19
  sympathetic —*see* Uveitis, sympathetic
Endosalpingioma D28.2
Endosalpingiosis N94.89
Endosteitis —*see* Osteomyelitis
Endothelioma, bone —*see* Neoplasm, bone,
  malignant
Endotheliosis (hemorrhagic infectional) D69.8
Endotoxemia — code to condition
Endotrachelitis —*see* Cervicitis
Engelmann (-Camurati) syndrome Q78.3
English disease —*see* Rickets
Engman's disease L30.3
Engorgement
  breast N64.59
    newborn P83.4
    puerperal, postpartum O92.79
  lung (passive) —*see* Edema, lung

Engorgement *(Continued)*
  pulmonary (passive) —*see* Edema, lung
  stomach K31.89
  venous, retina —*see* Occlusion, retina, vein,
    engorgement
Enlargement, enlarged —*see also* Hypertrophy
  adenoids J35.2
    with tonsils J35.3
  alveolar ridge K08.8
    congenital —*see* Anomaly, alveolar
  apertures of diaphragm (congenital) Q79.1
  gingival K06.1
  heart, cardiac —*see* Hypertrophy, cardiac
  lacrimal gland, chronic H04.03-
  liver —*see* Hypertrophy, liver
  lymph gland or node R59.9
    generalized R59.1
    localized R59.0
  orbit H05.34-
  organ or site, congenital NEC —*see* Anomaly,
    by site
  parathyroid (gland) E21.0
  pituitary fossa R93.0
  prostate N40.0
    with lower urinary tract symptoms (LUTS)
      N40.1
    without lower urinary tract symptoms
      (LUTS) N40.0
  sella turcica R93.0
  spleen —*see* Splenomegaly
  thymus (gland) (congenital) E32.0
  thyroid (gland) —*see* Goiter
  tongue K14.8
  tonsils J35.1
    with adenoids J35.3
  uterus N85.2
Enophthalmos H05.40-
  due to
    orbital tissue atrophy H05.41-
    trauma or surgery H05.42-
Enostosis M27.8
Entamebic, entamebiasis —*see* Amebiasis
Entanglement
  umbilical cord (s) O69.2
    with compression O69.2
      without compression O69.82
    around neck (with compression) O69.1
      without compression O69.81
    of twins in monoamniotic sac O69.2
Enteralgia —*see* Pain, abdominal
Enteric —*see* condition
Enteritis (acute) (diarrheal) (hemorrhagic)
  (noninfective) (septic) K52.9
  adenovirus A08.2
  aertrycke infection A02.0
  allergic K52.2
  amebic (acute) A06.0
    with abscess —*see* Abscess, amebic
    chronic A06.1
      with abscess —*see* Abscess, amebic
      nondysenteric A06.2
    nondysenteric A06.2
  astrovirus A08.32
  bacillary NOS A03.9
  bacterial A04.9
    specified NEC A04.8
  calicivirus A08.31
  candidal B37.82
  Chilomastix A07.8
  choleriformis A00.1
  chronic (noninfectious) K52.9
    ulcerative —*see* Colitis, ulcerative
  cicatrizing (chronic) —*see* Enteritis, regional,
    small intestine
  Clostridium
    botulinum (food poisoning) A05.1
    difficile A04.7
  coccidial A07.3
  coxsackie virus A08.39
  dietetic K52.2
  drug-induced K52.1

◀ New   ◀ Revised   ~~deleted~~ Deleted

Enteritis *(Continued)*
  due to
    astrovirus A08.32
    calicivirus A08.31
    coxsackie virus A08.39
    drugs K52.1
    echovirus A08.39
    enterovirus NEC A08.39
    food hypersensitivity K52.2
    infectious organism (bacterial) (viral) —*see*
      Enteritis, infectious
    torovirus A08.39
    Yersinia enterocolitica A04.6
  echovirus A08.39
  eltor A00.1
  enterovirus NEC A08.39
  eosinophilic K52.81
  epidemic (infectious) A09
  fulminant K55.0
  gangrenous —*see* Enteritis, infectious
  giardial A07.1
  infectious NOS A09
    due to
      adenovirus A08.2
      Aerobacter aerogenes A04.8
      Arizona (bacillus) A02.0
      bacteria NOS A04.9
        specified NEC A04.8
      Campylobacter A04.5
      Clostridium difficile A04.7
      Clostridium perfringens A04.8
      Enterobacter aerogenes A04.8
      enterovirus A08.39
      Escherichia coli A04.4
        enteroaggregative A04.4
        enterohemorrhagic A04.3
        enteroinvasive A04.2
        enteropathogenic A04.0
        enterotoxigenic A04.1
        specified NEC A04.4
      specified
        bacteria NEC A04.8
        virus NEC A08.39
      Staphylococcus A04.8
      virus NEC A08.4
        specified type NEC A08.39
      Yersinia enterocolitica A04.6
    specified organism NEC A08.8
  influenzal —*see* Influenza, with, digestive
    manifestations
  ischemic K55.9
    acute K55.0
    chronic K55.1
  microsporidial A07.8
  mucomembranous, myxomembranous —*see*
    Syndrome, irritable bowel
  mucous —*see* Syndrome, irritable bowel
  necroticans A05.2
  necrotizing of newborn —*see* Enterocolitis,
    necrotizing, in newborn
  neurogenic —*see* Syndrome, irritable
    bowel
  newborn necrotizing —*see* Enterocolitis,
    necrotizing, in newborn
  noninfectious K52.9
  norovirus A08.11
  parasitic NEC B82.9
  paratyphoid (fever) —*see* Fever, paratyphoid
  protozoal A07.9
    specified NEC A07.8
  radiation K52.0
  regional (of) K50.90
    with
      complication K50.919
        abscess K50.914
        fistula K50.913
        intestinal obstruction K50.912
        rectal bleeding K50.911
        specified complication NEC K50.918
    colon —*see* Enteritis, regional, large
      intestine

Enteritis *(Continued)*
  regional *(Continued)*
    duodenum —*see* Enteritis, regional, small
      intestine
    ileum —*see* Enteritis, regional, small
      intestine
    jejunum —*see* Enteritis, regional, small
      intestine
    large bowel —*see* Enteritis, regional, large
      intestine
    large intestine (colon) (rectum) K50.10
      with
        complication K50.119
          abscess K50.114
          fistula K50.113
          intestinal obstruction K50.112
          rectal bleeding K50.111
          small intestine (duodenum) (ileum)
            (jejunum) involvement K50.80
            with
              complication K50.819
                abscess K50.814
                fistula K50.813
                intestinal obstruction
                  K50.812
                rectal bleeding K50.811
                specified complication NEC
                  K50.818
          specified complication NEC K50.118
    rectum —*see* Enteritis, regional, large
      intestine
    small intestine (duodenum) (ileum)
      (jejunum) K50.00
      with
        complication K50.019
          abscess K50.014
          fistula K50.013
          intestinal obstruction K50.012
          large intestine (colon) (rectum)
            involvement K50.80
            with
              complication K50.819
                abscess K50.814
                fistula K50.813
                intestinal obstruction
                  K50.812
                rectal bleeding K50.811
                specified complication NEC
                  K50.818
          rectal bleeding K50.011
          specified complication NEC
            K50.018
  rotaviral A08.0
  Salmonella, salmonellosis (arizonae)
    (cholerae-suis) (enteritidis)
    (typhimurium) A02.0
  segmental —*see* Enteritis, regional
  septic A09
  Shigella —*see* Infection, Shigella
  small round structured NEC A08.19
  spasmodic, spastic —*see* Syndrome, irritable
    bowel
  staphylococcal A04.8
    due to food A05.0
  torovirus A08.39
  toxic NEC K52.1
    due to Clostridium difficile A04.7
  trichomonal A07.8
  tuberculous A18.32
  typhosa A01.00
  ulcerative (chronic) —*see* Colitis, ulcerative
  viral A08.4
    adenovirus A08.2
    enterovirus A08.39
    Rotavirus A08.0
    small round structured NEC A08.19
    specified NEC A08.39
    virus specified NEC A08.39
Enterobiasis B80
Enterobius vermicularis (infection) (infestation)
  B80

Enterocele —*see also* Hernia, abdomen
  pelvic, pelvis (acquired) (congenital)
    N81.5
  vagina, vaginal (acquired) (congenital)
    NEC N81.5
Enterocolitis *(see also* Enteritis) K52.9
  due to Clostridium difficile A04.7
  fulminant ischemic K55.0
  granulomatous —*see* Enteritis, regional
  hemorrhagic (acute) K55.0
    chronic K55.1
  infectious NEC A09
  ischemic K55.9
  necrotizing
    due to Clostridium difficile A04.7
    in newborn P77.9
      stage 1 (without pneumatosis, without
        perforation) P77.1
      stage 2 (with pneumatosis, without
        perforation) P77.2
      stage 3 (with pneumatosis, with
        perforation) P77.3
    noninfectious K52.9
    newborn —*see* Enterocolitis, necrotizing, in
      newborn
  pseudomembranous (newborn) A04.7
  radiation K52.0
    newborn —*see* Enterocolitis, necrotizing, in
      newborn
  ulcerative (chronic) —*see* Pancolitis,
    ulcerative (chronic)
Enterogastritis —*see* Enteritis
Enteropathy K63.9
  gluten-sensitive K90.0
  hemorrhagic, terminal K55.0
  protein-losing K90.4
Enteroperitonitis —*see* Peritonitis
Enteroptosis K63.4
Enterorrhagia K92.2
Enterospasm —*see also* Syndrome, irritable,
  bowel
  psychogenic F45.8
Enterostenosis —*see also* Obstruction, intestine
  K56.69
Enterostomy
  complication —*see* Complication,
    enterostomy
  status Z93.4
Enterovirus, as cause of disease classified
  elsewhere B97.10
  coxsackievirus B97.11
  echovirus B97.12
  other specified B97.19
Enthesopathy (peripheral) M77.9
  Achilles tendinitis —*see* Tendinitis,
    Achilles
  ankle and tarsus M77.9
    specified type NEC —*see* Enthesopathy,
      foot, specified type NEC
  anterior tibial syndrome M76.81-
  calcaneal spur —*see* Spur, bone, calcaneal
  elbow region M77.8
    lateral epicondylitis —*see* Epicondylitis,
      lateral
    medial epicondylitis —*see* Epicondylitis,
      medial
  foot NEC M77.9
    metatarsalgia —*see* Metatarsalgia
    specified type NEC M77.5-
  forearm M77.9
  gluteal tendinitis —*see* Tendinitis, gluteal
  hand M77.9
  hip —*see* Enthesopathy, lower limb, specified
    type NEC
  iliac crest spur —*see* Spur, bone, iliac crest
  iliotibial band syndrome —*see* Syndrome,
    iliotibial band
  knee —*see* Enthesopathy, lower limb, lower
    leg, specified type NEC
  lateral epicondylitis —*see* Epicondylitis,
    lateral

Enthesopathy (Continued)
  lower limb (excluding foot) M76.9
    Achilles tendinitis —see Tendinitis, Achilles
    anterior tibial syndrome M76.81-
    gluteal tendinitis —see Tendinitis, gluteal
    iliac crest spur —see Spur, bone, iliac crest
    iliotibial band syndrome —see Syndrome,
      iliotibial band
    patellar tendinitis —see Tendinitis, patellar
    pelvic region —see Enthesopathy, lower
      limb, specified type NEC
    peroneal tendinitis —see Tendinitis,
      peroneal
    posterior tibial syndrome M76.82-
    psoas tendinitis —see Tendinitis, psoas
    shoulder M77.9
    specified type NEC M76.89-
    tibial collateral bursitis —see Bursitis, tibial
      collateral
  medial epicondylitis —see Epicondylitis,
    medial
  multiple sites M77.9
  patellar tendinitis —see Tendinitis, patellar
  pelvis M77.9
  periarthritis of wrist —see Periarthritis,
    wrist
  peroneal tendinitis —see Tendinitis,
    peroneal
  posterior tibial syndrome M76.82-
  psoas tendinitis —see Tendinitis, psoas
  shoulder region —see Lesion, shoulder
  specified site NEC M77.9
  specified type NEC M77.8
  spinal M46.00
    cervical region M46.02
    cervicothoracic region M46.03
    lumbar region M46.06
    lumbosacral region M46.07
    multiple sites M46.09
    occipito-atlanto-axial region M46.01
    sacrococcygeal region M46.08
    thoracic region M46.04
    thoracolumbar region M46.05
  tibial collateral bursitis —see Bursitis, tibial
    collateral
  upper arm M77.9
  wrist and carpus NEC M77.8
    calcaneal spur —see Spur, bone, calcaneal
    periarthritis of wrist —see Periarthritis,
      wrist
Entomophobia F40.218
Entomophthoromycosis B46.8
Entrance, air into vein —see Embolism, air
Entrapment, nerve —see Neuropathy,
  entrapment
Entropion (eyelid) (paralytic) H02.009
  cicatricial H02.019
    left H02.016
      lower H02.015
      upper H02.014
    right H02.013
      lower H02.012
      upper H02.011
  congenital Q10.2
  left H02.006
    lower H02.005
    upper H02.004
  mechanical H02.029
    left H02.026
      lower H02.025
      upper H02.024
    right H02.023
      lower H02.022
      upper H02.021
  right H02.003
    lower H02.002
    upper H02.001
  senile H02.039
    left H02.036
      lower H02.035
      upper H02.034

Entropion (Continued)
  senile (Continued)
    right H02.033
      lower H02.032
      upper H02.031
    spastic H02.049
      left H02.046
        lower H02.045
        upper H02.044
      right H02.043
        lower H02.042
        upper H02.041
Enucleated eye (traumatic, current) S05.7-
Enuresis R32
  functional F98.0
  habit disturbance F98.0
  nocturnal N39.44
    psychogenic F98.0
  nonorganic origin F98.0
  psychogenic F98.0
Eosinopenia —see Agranulocytosis
Eosinophilia (allergic) (hereditary) (idiopathic)
  (secondary) D72.1
  with
    angiolymphoid hyperplasia (ALHE)
      D18.01
    infiltrative J82
    Löffler's J82
    peritoneal —see Peritonitis, eosinophilic
    pulmonary NEC J82
    tropical (pulmonary) J82
Eosinophilia-myalgia syndrome M35.8
Ependymitis (acute) (cerebral) (chronic)
  (granular) —see Encephalomyelitis
Ependymoblastoma
  specified site —see Neoplasm, malignant, by
    site
  unspecified site C71.9
Ependymoma (epithelial) (malignant)
  anaplastic
    specified site —see Neoplasm, malignant,
      by site
    unspecified site C71.9
  benign
    specified site —see Neoplasm, benign, by
      site
    unspecified site D33.2
  myxopapillary D43.2
    specified site —see Neoplasm, uncertain
      behavior, by site
    unspecified site D43.2
  papillary D43.2
    specified site —see Neoplasm, uncertain
      behavior, by site
    unspecified site D43.2
  specified site —see Neoplasm, malignant, by
    site
  unspecified site C71.9
Ependymopathy G93.89
Ephelis, ephelides L81.2
Epiblepharon (congenital) Q10.3
Epicanthus, epicanthic fold (eyelid)
  (congenital) Q10.3
Epicondylitis (elbow)
  lateral M77.1-
  medial M77.0-
Epicystitis —see Cystitis
Epidemic —see condition
Epidermidalization, cervix —see Dysplasia,
  cervix
Epidermis, epidermal —see condition
Epidermodysplasia verruciformis B07.8
Epidermolysis
  bullosa (congenital) Q81.9
    acquired L12.30
      drug-induced L12.31
      specified cause NEC L12.35
    dystrophica Q81.2
    letalis Q81.1
    simplex Q81.0
    specified NEC Q81.8

Epidermolysis (Continued)
  necroticans combustiformis L51.2
  due to drug —see Table of Drugs and
    Chemicals, by drug
Epidermophytid —see Dermatophytosis
Epidermophytosis (infected) —see
  Dermatophytosis
Epididymis —see condition
Epididymitis (acute) (nonvenereal) (recurrent)
  (residual) N45.1
  with orchitis N45.3
  blennorrhagic (gonococcal) A54.23
  caseous (tuberculous) A18.15
  chlamydial A56.19
  filarial (see also Infestation, filarial) B74.9
    [N51]
  gonococcal A54.23
  syphilitic A52.76
  tuberculous A18.15
Epididymo-orchitis (see also Epididymitis)
  N45.3
Epidural —see condition
Epigastrium, epigastric —see condition
Epigastrocele —see Hernia, ventral
Epiglottis —see condition
Epiglottitis, epiglottiditis (acute) J05.10
  with obstruction J05.11
  chronic J37.0
Epignathus Q89.4
Epilepsia partialis continua (see also
  Kozhevnikof's epilepsy) G40.1-
Epilepsy, epileptic, epilepsia (attack)
  (cerebral) (convulsion) (fit) (seizure)
  G40.909

> Note: the following terms are to be
> considered equivalent to intractable:
> pharmacoresistant (pharmacologically
> resistant), treatment resistant, refractory
> (medically) and poorly controlled

  with
    complex partial seizures —see Epilepsy,
      localization-related, symptomatic,
      with complex partial seizures
    grand mal seizures on awakening —
      see Epilepsy, generalized, specified
      NEC
    myoclonic absences —see Epilepsy,
      generalized, specified NEC
    myoclonic-astatic seizures —see Epilepsy,
      generalized, specified NEC
    simple partial seizures —see Epilepsy,
      localization-related, symptomatic,
      with simple partial seizures
  akinetic —see Epilepsy, generalized, specified
    NEC
  benign childhood with centrotemporal EEG
    spikes —see Epilepsy, localization-
    related, idiopathic
  benign myoclonic in infancy G40.80-
  Bravais-jacksonian —see Epilepsy,
    localization-related, symptomatic,
    with simple partial seizures
  childhood
    with occipital EEG paroxysms —see
      Epilepsy, localization-related,
      idiopathic
    absence G40.A09
      intractable G40.A19
        with status epilepticus G40.A11
        without status epilepticus
          G40.A19
      not intractable G40.A09
        with status epilepticus G40.A01
        without status epilepticus
          G40.A09
  climacteric —see Epilepsy, specified NEC
  cysticercosis B69.0
  deterioration (mental) F06.8
  due to syphilis A52.19

◄ New   ◄▥ Revised   ~~deleted~~ Deleted

Epilepsy, epileptic, epilepsia *(Continued)*
  focal —*see* Epilepsy, localization-related,
    symptomatic, with simple partial
    seizures
  generalized
    idiopathic G40.309
      intractable G40.319
        with status epilepticus G40.311
        without status epilepticus G40.319
      not intractable G40.309
        with status epilepticus G40.301
        without status epilepticus G40.309
    specified NEC G40.409
      intractable G40.419
        with status epilepticus G40.411
        without status epilepticus G40.419
      not intractable G40.409
        with status epilepticus G40.401
        without status epilepticus G40.409
  impulsive petit mal —*see* Epilepsy, juvenile
    myoclonic
  intractable G40.919
    with status epilepticus G40.911
    without status epilepticus G40.919
  juvenile absence G40.A09
    intractable G40.A19
      with status epilepticus G40.A11
      without status epilepticus G40.A19
    not intractable G40.A09
      with status epilepticus G40.A01
      without status epilepticus G40.A09
  juvenile myoclonic G40.B11
    intractable G40.B19
      with status epilepticus G40.B11
      without status epilepticus G40.B19
    not intractable G40.B09
      with status epilepticus G40.B01
      without status epilepticus G40.B09
  localization-related (focal) (partial)
    idiopathic G40.009
      with seizures of localized onset G40.009
        intractable G40.019
          with status epilepticus G40.011
          without status epilepticus G40.019
        not intractable G40.009
          with status epilepticus G40.001
          without status epilepticus G40.009
    symptomatic
      with complex partial seizures G40.209
        intractable G40.219
          with status epilepticus G40.211
          without status epilepticus G40.219
        not intractable G40.209
          with status epilepticus G40.201
          without status epilepticus
            G40.209
      with simple partial seizures G40.109
        intractable G40.119
          with status epilepticus G40.111
          without status epilepticus
            G40.119
        not intractable G40.109
          with status epilepticus G40.101
          without status epilepticus
            G40.109
  myoclonus, myoclonic (progressive) —*see*
    Epilepsy, generalized, specified NEC
  not intractable G40.909
    with status epilepticus G40.901
    without status epilepticus G40.909
  on awakening —*see* Epilepsy, generalized,
    specified NEC
  parasitic NOS B71.9 *[G94]*
  partialis continua *(see also* Kozhevnikof's
    epilepsy) G40.1-
  peripheral —*see* Epilepsy, specified NEC
  procursiva —*see* Epilepsy, localization-
    related, symptomatic, with simple
    partial seizures
  progressive (familial) myoclonic —*see*
    Epilepsy, generalized, idiopathic

Epilepsy, epileptic, epilepsia *(Continued)*
  reflex —*see* Epilepsy, specified NEC
  related to
    alcohol G40.509
      not intractable G40.509
        with status epilepticus G40.501
        without status epliepticus G40.509
    drugs G40.509
      not intractable G40.509
        with status epilepticus G40.501
        without status epliepticus G40.509
    external causes G40.509
      not intractable G40.509
        with status epilepticus G40.501
        without status epilepticus G40.509
    hormonal changes G40.509
      not intractable G40.509
        with status epilepticus G40.501
        without status epilepticus G40.509
    sleep deprivation G40.509
      not intractable G40.509
        with status epilepticus G40.501
        without status epilepticus G40.509
    stress G40.509
      not intractable G40.509
        with status epilepticus G40.501
        without status epilepticus G40.509
  somatomotor —*see* Epilepsy, localization-
    related, symptomatic, with simple
    partial seizures
  somatosensory —*see* Epilepsy, localization-
    related, symptomatic, with simple
    partial seizures
  spasms G40.822
    intractable G40.824
      with status epilepticus G40.823
      without status epilepticus G40.824
    not intractable G40.822
      with status epilepticus G40.821
      without status epilepticus G40.822
  specified NEC G40.802
    intractable G40.804
      with status epilepticus G40.803
      without status epilepticus G40.804
    not intractable G40.802
      with status epilepticus G40.801
      without status epilepticus G40.802
  syndromes
    generalized
      idiopathic G40.309
        intractable G40.319
          with status epilepticus G40.311
          without status epilepticus G40.319
        not intractable G40.309
          with status epilepticus G40.301
          without status epilepticus G40.309
      specified NEC G40.409
        intractable G40.419
          with status epilepticus G40.411
          without status epilepticus G40.419
        not intractable G40.409
          with status epilepticus G40.401
          without status epilepticus G40.409
    localization-related (focal) (partial)
      idiopathic G40.009
        with seizures of localized onset
          G40.009
          intractable G40.019
            with status epilepticus G40.011
            without status epilepticus
              G40.019
          not intractable G40.009
            with status epilepticus G40.001
            without status epilepticus G40.009
      symptomatic
        with complex partial seizures
          G40.209
          intractable G40.219
            with status epilepticus G40.211
            without status epilepticus
              G40.219

Epilepsy, epileptic, epilepsia *(Continued)*
  syndromes *(Continued)*
    localization-related *(Continued)*
      symptomatic *(Continued)*
        with complex partial seizures
          (Continued)
          not intractable G40.209
            with status epilepticus G40.201
            without status epilepticus G40.209
        with simple partial seizures G40.109
          intractable G40.119
            with status epilepticus G40.111
            without status epilepticus G40.119
          not intractable G40.109
            with status epilepticus G40.101
            without status epilepticus G40.109
    specified NEC G40.802
      intractable G40.804
        with status epilepticus G40.803
        without status epilepticus G40.804
      not intractable G40.802
        with status epilepticus G40.801
        without status epilepticus G40.802
  tonic (-clonic) —*see* Epilepsy, generalized,
    specified NEC
  twilight F05
  uncinate (gyrus) —*see* Epilepsy, localization-
    related, symptomatic, with complex
    partial seizures
  Unverricht (-Lundborg) (familial
    myoclonic) —*see* Epilepsy, generalized,
    idiopathic
  visceral —*see* Epilepsy, specified NEC
  visual —*see* Epilepsy, specified NEC
Epiloia Q85.1
Epimenorrhea N92.0
Epipharyngitis —*see* Nasopharyngitis
Epiphora H04.20-
  due to
    excess lacrimation H04.21-
    insufficient drainage H04.22-
Epiphyseal arrest —*see* Arrest, epiphyseal
Epiphyseolysis, epiphysiolysis —*see*
  Osteochondropathy
Epiphysitis —*see also* Osteochondropathy
  juvenile M92.9
  syphilitic (congenital) A50.02
Epiplocele —*see* Hernia, abdomen
Epiploitis —*see* Peritonitis
Epiplosarcomphalocele —*see* Hernia, umbilicus
Episcleritis (suppurative) H15.10-
  in (due to)
    syphilis A52.71
    tuberculosis A18.51
  nodular H15.12-
  periodica fugax H15.11-
    angioneurotic —*see* Edema, angioneurotic
  syphilitic (late) A52.71
  tuberculous A18.51
Episode
  affective, mixed F39
  depersonalization (in neurotic state) F48.1
  depressive F32.9
    major F32.9
      mild F32.0
      moderate F32.1
      severe (without psychotic symptoms)
        F32.2
        with psychotic symptoms F32.3
    recurrent F33.9
      brief F33.8
    specified NEC F32.8
  hypomanic F30.8
  manic F30.9
    with
      psychotic symptoms F30.2
      remission (full) F30.4
        partial F30.3
    without psychotic symptoms F30.10
      mild F30.11
      moderate F30.12

Episode *(Continued)*
  manic *(Continued)*
    without psychotic symptoms *(Continued)*
      severe (without psychotic symptoms) F30.13
        with psychotic symptoms F30.2
    other specified F30.8
    recurrent F31.89
    psychotic F23
      organic F06.8
    schizophrenic (acute) NEC, brief F23
Epispadias (female) (male) Q64.0
Episplenitis D73.89
Epistaxis (multiple) R04.0
  hereditary I78.0
  vicarious menstruation N94.89
Epithelioma (malignant) —*see also* Neoplasm, malignant, by site
  adenoides cysticum —*see* Neoplasm, skin, benign
  basal cell —*see* Neoplasm, skin, malignant
  benign —*see* Neoplasm, benign, by site
  Bowen's —*see* Neoplasm, skin, in situ
  calcifying, of Malherbe —*see* Neoplasm, skin, benign
  external site —*see* Neoplasm, skin, malignant
  intraepidermal, Jadassohn —*see* Neoplasm, skin, benign
  squamous cell —*see* Neoplasm, malignant, by site
Epitheliomatosis pigmented Q82.1
Epitheliopathy, multifocal placoid pigment H30.14-
Epithelium, epithelial —*see* condition
Epituberculosis (with atelectasis) (allergic) A15.7
Eponychia Q84.6
Epstein's
  nephrosis or syndrome —*see* Nephrosis
  pearl K09.8
Epulis (gingiva) (fibrous) (giant cell) K06.8
Equinia A24.0
Equinovarus (congenital) (talipes) Q66.0
  acquired —*see* Deformity, limb, clubfoot
Equivalent
  convulsive (abdominal) —*see* Epilepsy, specified NEC
  epileptic (psychic) —*see* Epilepsy, localization-related, symptomatic, with complex partial seizures
Erb (-Duchenne) paralysis (birth injury) (newborn) P14.0
Erb's
  disease G71.0
  palsy, paralysis (brachial) (birth) (newborn) P14.0
  spinal (spastic) syphilitic A52.17
  pseudohypertrophic muscular dystrophy G71.0
Erb-Goldflam disease or syndrome G70.00
  with exacerbation (acute) G70.01
  in crisis G70.01
Erdheim's syndrome (acromegalic macrospondylitis) E22.0
Erection, painful (persistent) —*see* Priapism
Ergosterol deficiency (vitamin D) E55.9
  with
    adult osteomalacia M83.8
    rickets —*see* Rickets
Ergotism —*see also* Poisoning, food, noxious, plant
  from ergot used as drug (migraine therapy) —*see* Table of Drugs and Chemicals
Erosio interdigitalis blastomycetica B37.2
Erosion
  artery I77.2
    without rupture I77.89
  bone —*see* Disorder, bone, density and structure, specified NEC
  bronchus J98.09

Erosion *(Continued)*
  cartilage (joint) —*see* Disorder, cartilage, specified type NEC
  cervix (uteri) (acquired) (chronic) (congenital) N86
    with cervicitis N72
  cornea (nontraumatic) —*see* Ulcer, cornea
    recurrent H18.83-
    traumatic —*see* Abrasion, cornea
  dental (idiopathic) (occupational) (due to diet, drugs or vomiting) K03.2
  duodenum, postpyloric —*see* Ulcer, duodenum
  esophagus K22.10
    with bleeding K22.11
  gastric —*see* Ulcer, stomach
  gastrojejunal —*see* Ulcer, gastrojejunal
  implanted mesh —*see* Complications, mesh
  intestine K63.3
  lymphatic vessel I89.8
  pylorus, pyloric (ulcer) —*see* Ulcer, stomach
  spine, aneurysmal A52.09
  stomach —*see* Ulcer, stomach
  teeth (idiopathic) (occupational) (due to diet, drugs or vomiting) K03.2
  urethra N36.8
  uterus N85.8
Erotomania F52.8
Error
  metabolism, inborn —*see* Disorder, metabolism
  refractive —*see* Disorder, refraction
Eructation R14.2
  nervous or psychogenic F45.8
Eruption
  creeping B76.9
  drug (generalized) (taken internally) L27.0
    fixed L27.1
    in contact with skin —*see* Dermatitis, due to drugs
    localized L27.1
  Hutchinson, summer L56.4
  Kaposi's varicelliform B00.0
  napkin L22
  polymorphous light (sun) L56.4
  recalcitrant pustular L13.8
  ringed R23.8
  skin (nonspecific) R21
    creeping (meaning hookworm) B76.9
    due to inoculation/vaccination (generalized) *(see also* Dermatitis, due to, vaccine) L27.0
      localized L27.1
    erysipeloid A26.0
    feigned L98.1
    Kaposi's varicelliform B00.0
    lichenoid L28.0
    meaning dermatitis —*see* Dermatitis
    toxic NEC L53.0
  tooth, teeth, abnormal (incomplete) (late) (premature) (sequence) K00.6
  vesicular R23.8
Erysipelas (gangrenous) (infantile) (newborn) (phlegmonous) (suppurative) A46
  external ear A46 [H62.40]
  puerperal, postpartum O86.89
Erysipeloid A26.9
  cutaneous (Rosenbach's) A26.0
  disseminated A26.8
  sepsis A26.7
  specified NEC A26.8
Erythema, erythematous (infectional) (inflammation) L53.9
  ab igne L59.0
  annulare (centrifugum) (rheumaticum) L53.1
  arthriticum epidemicum A25.1
  brucellum —*see* Brucellosis
  chronic figurate NEC L53.3
  chronicum migrans (Borrelia burgdorferi) A69.20
  diaper L22

Erythema, erythematous *(Continued)*
  due to
    chemical NEC L53.0
      in contact with skin L24.5
    drug (internal use) —*see* Dermatitis, due to, drugs
  elevatum diutinum L95.1
  endemic E52
  epidemic, arthritic A25.1
  figuratum perstans L53.3
  gluteal L22
  heat - code by site under Burn, first degree
  ichthyosiforme congenitum bullous Q80.3
  in diseases classified elsewhere L54
  induratum (nontuberculous) L52
    tuberculous A18.4
  infectiosum B08.3
  intertrigo L30.4
  iris L51.9
  marginatum L53.2
    in (due to) acute rheumatic fever I00
  medicamentosum —*see* Dermatitis, due to, drugs
  migrans A26.0
    chronicum A69.20
    tongue K14.1
  multiforme (major) (minor) L51.9
    bullous, bullosum L51.1
    conjunctiva L51.1
    nonbullous L51.0
    pemphigoides L12.0
    specified NEC L51.8
  napkin L22
  neonatorum P83.8
    toxic P83.1
  nodosum L52
    tuberculous A18.4
  palmar L53.8
  pernio T69.1
  rash, newborn P83.8
  scarlatiniform (recurrent) (exfoliative) L53.8
  solare L55.0
  specified NEC L53.8
  toxic, toxicum NEC L53.0
    newborn P83.1
  tuberculous (primary) A18.4
Erythematous, erythematosus —*see* condition
Erythermalgia (primary) I73.81
Erythralgia I73.81
Erythrasma L08.1
Erythredema (polyneuropathy) —*see* Poisoning, mercury
Erythremia (acute) C94.0-
  chronic D45
  secondary D75.1
Erythroblastopenia *(see also* Aplasia, red cell) D60.9
  congenital D61.01
Erythroblastophthisis D61.09
Erythroblastosis (fetalis) (newborn) P55.9
  due to
    ABO (antibodies) (incompatibility) (isoimmunization) P55.1
    Rh (antibodies) (incompatibility) (isoimmunization) P55.0
Erythrocyanosis (crurum) I73.89
Erythrocythemia —*see* Erythremia
Erythrocytosis (megalosplenic) (secondary) D75.1
  familial D75.0
  oval, hereditary —*see* Elliptocytosis
  secondary D75.1
  stress D75.1
Erythroderma (secondary) *(see also* Erythema) L53.9
  bullous ichthyosiform, congenital Q80.3
  desquamativum L21.1
  ichthyosiform, congenital (bullous) Q80.3
  neonatorum P83.8
  psoriaticum L40.8

Erythrodysesthesia, palmar plantar (PPE)
  L27.1
Erythrogenesis imperfecta D61.09
Erythroleukemia C94.0-
Erythromelalgia I73.81
Erythrophagocytosis D75.89
Erythrophobia F40.298
Erythroplakia, oral epithelium, and tongue
  K13.29
Erythroplasia (Queyrat) D07.4
  specified site —see Neoplasm, skin, in situ
  unspecified site D07.4
Escherichia coli (E. coli), as cause of disease
    classified elsewhere B96.20
  non-O157 Shiga toxin-producing (with
    known O group) B96.22
  non-Shiga toxin-producing B96.29
  O157 with confirmation of Shiga toxin when
    H antigen is unknown, or is not H7
    B96.21
  O157:H- (nonmotile) with confirmation of
    Shiga toxin B96.21
  O157:H7 with or without confirmation of
    Shiga toxin-production B96.21
  Shiga toxin-producing (with unspecified O
    group) (STEC) B96.23
  O157 B96.21
  O157:H7 with or without confirmation of
    Shiga toxin-production B96.21
    specified NEC B96.22
  specified NEC B96.29
Esophagismus K22.4
Esophagitis (acute) (alkaline) (chemical)
    (chronic) (infectional) (necrotic) (peptic)
    (postoperative) K20.9
  candidal B37.81
  due to gastrointestinal reflux disease K21.0
  eosinophilic K20.0
  reflux K21.0
  specified NEC K20.8
  tuberculous A18.83
  ulcerative K22.10
    with bleeding K22.11
Esophagocele K22.5
Esophagomalacia K22.8
Esophagospasm K22.4
Esophagostenosis K22.2
Esophagostomiasis B81.8
Esophagotracheal —see condition
Esophagus —see condition
Esophoria H50.51
  convergence, excess H51.12
  divergence, insufficiency H51.8
Esotropia —see Strabismus, convergent
    concomitant
Espundia B55.2
Essential —see condition
Esthesioneuroblastoma C30.0
Esthesioneurocytoma C30.0
Esthesioneuroepithelioma C30.0
Esthiomene A55
Estivo-autumnal malaria (fever) B50.9
Estrangement (marital) Z63.5
  parent-child NEC Z62.890
Estriasis —see Myiasis
Ethanolism —see Alcoholism
Etherism —see Dependence, drug, inhalant
Ethmoid, ethmoidal —see condition
Ethmoiditis (chronic) (nonpurulent)
    (purulent) —see also Sinusitis, ethmoidal
  influenzal —see Influenza, with, respiratory
    manifestations NEC
  Woakes' J33.1
Ethylism —see Alcoholism
Eulenburg's disease (congenital paramyotonia)
  G71.19
Eumycetoma B47.0
Eunuchoidism E29.1
  hypogonadotropic E23.0
European blastomycosis —see Cryptococcosis
Eustachian —see condition

Evaluation (for) (of)
  development state
    adolescent Z00.3
    period of
      delayed growth in childhood Z00.70
        with abnormal findings Z00.71
      rapid growth in childhood Z00.2
    puberty Z00.3
  growth and developmental state (period of
    rapid growth) Z00.2
    delayed growth Z00.70
      with abnormal findings Z00.71
  mental health (status) Z00.8
    requested by authority Z04.6
  period of
    delayed growth in childhood Z00.70
      with abnormal findings Z00.71
    rapid growth in childhood Z00.2
  suspected condition —see Observation
Evans syndrome D69.41
Event, apparent life threatening in newborn
    and infant (ALTE) R68.13
Eventration —see also Hernia, ventral
  colon into chest —see Hernia, diaphragm
  diaphragm (congenital) Q79.1
Eversion
  bladder N32.89
  cervix (uteri) N86
    with cervicitis N72
  foot NEC —see also Deformity, valgus, ankle
    congenital Q66.6
  punctum lacrimale (postinfectional) (senile)
    H04.52-
  ureter (meatus) N28.89
  urethra (meatus) N36.8
  uterus N81.4
Evidence
  cytologic
    of malignancy on anal smear R85.614
    of malignancy on cervical smear R87.614
    of malignancy on vaginal smear R87.624
Evisceration
  birth injury P15.8
  traumatic NEC
    eye —see Enucleated eye
Evulsion —see Avulsion
Ewing's sarcoma or tumor —see Neoplasm,
    bone, malignant
Examination (for) (following) (general) (of)
    (routine) Z00.00
  with abnormal findings Z00.01
  abuse, physical (alleged), ruled out
    adult Z04.71
    child Z04.72
  adolescent (development state) Z00.3
  alleged rape or sexual assault (victim), ruled
    out
    adult Z04.41
    child Z04.42
  allergy Z01.82
  annual (adult) (periodic) (physical) Z00.00
    with abnormal findings Z00.01
    gynecological Z01.419
      with abnormal findings Z01.411
  antibody response Z01.84
  blood —see Examination, laboratory
  blood pressure Z01.30
    with abnormal findings Z01.31
  cancer staging —see Neoplasm, malignant,
    by site
  cervical Papanicolaou smear Z12.4
    as part of routine gynecological
      examination Z01.419
      with abnormal findings Z01.411
  child (over 28 days old) Z00.129
    with abnormal findings Z00.121
    under 28 days old —see Newborn,
      examination
  clinical research control or normal
    comparison (control) (participant)
    Z00.6

Examination (Continued)
  contraceptive (drug) maintenance (routine)
    Z30.8
    device (intrauterine) Z30.431
  dental Z01.20
    with abnormal findings Z01.21
  developmental —see Examination, child
  donor (potential) Z00.5
  ear Z01.10
    with abnormal findings NEC Z01.118
  eye Z01.00
    with abnormal findings Z01.01
  following
    accident NEC Z04.3
      transport Z04.1
      work Z04.2
    assault, alleged, ruled out
      adult Z04.71
      child Z04.72
    motor vehicle accident Z04.1
    treatment (for) Z09
      combined NEC Z09
        fracture Z09
        malignant neoplasm Z08
      malignant neoplasm Z08
      mental disorder Z09
      specified condition NEC Z09
  follow-up (routine) (following) Z09
    chemotherapy NEC Z09
      malignant neoplasm Z08
    fracture Z09
    malignant neoplasm Z08
    postpartum Z39.2
    psychotherapy Z09
    radiotherapy NEC Z09
      malignant neoplasm Z08
    surgery NEC Z09
      malignant neoplasm Z08
  gynecological Z01.419
    with abnormal findings Z01.411
    for contraceptive maintenance Z30.8
  health —see Examination, medical
  hearing Z01.10
    with abnormal findings NEC Z01.118
    following failed hearing screening Z01.110
  immunity status testing Z01.84
  laboratory (as part of a general medical
      examination) Z00.00
    with abnormal findings Z00.01
    preprocedural Z01.812
  lactating mother Z39.1
  medical (adult) (for) (of) Z00.00
    with abnormal findings Z00.01
    administrative purpose only Z02.9
      specified NEC Z02.89
    admission to
      armed forces Z02.3
      old age home Z02.2
      prison Z02.89
      residential institution Z02.2
      school Z02.0
        following illness or medical treatment
          Z02.0
      summer camp Z02.89
    adoption Z02.82
    blood alcohol or drug level Z02.83
    camp (summer) Z02.89
    clinical research, normal subject (control)
      (participant) Z00.6
    control subject in clinical research (normal
      comparison) (participant) Z00.6
    donor (potential) Z00.5
    driving license Z02.4
    general (adult) Z00.00
      with abnormal findings Z00.01
    immigration Z02.89
    insurance purposes Z02.6
    marriage Z02.89
    medicolegal reasons NEC Z04.8
    naturalization Z02.89
    participation in sport Z02.5

Examination (Continued)
  medical (Continued)
    paternity testing Z02.81
    population survey Z00.8
    pre-employment Z02.1
    pre-operative —see Examination,
        pre-procedural
    pre-procedural
      cardiovascular Z01.810
      respiratory Z01.811
      specified NEC Z01.818
    preschool children
      for admission to school Z02.0
    prisoners
      for entrance into prison Z02.89
    recruitment for armed forces Z02.3
    specified NEC Z00.8
    sport competition Z02.5
  medicolegal reason NEC Z04.8
  newborn —see Newborn, examination
  pelvic (annual) (periodic) Z01.419
    with abnormal findings Z01.411
  period of rapid growth in childhood Z00.2
  periodic (adult) (annual) (routine) Z00.00
    with abnormal findings Z00.01
  physical (adult) —see also Examination,
      medical Z00.00
    sports Z02.5
  postpartum
    immediately after delivery Z39.0
    routine follow-up Z39.2
  pre-chemotherapy (antineoplastic) Z01.818
  prenatal (normal pregnancy) (see also
      Pregnancy, normal) Z34.9-
  pre-procedural (pre-operative)
    cardiovascular Z01.810
    laboratory Z01.812
    respiratory Z01.811
    specified NEC Z01.818
  prior to chemotherapy (antineoplastic)
      Z01.818
  psychiatric NEC Z00.8
    follow-up not needing further care Z09
    requested by authority Z04.6
  radiological (as part of a general medical
      examination) Z00.00
    with abnormal findings Z00.01
  repeat cervical smear to confirm findings of
      recent normal smear following initial
      abnormal smear Z01.42
  skin (hypersensitivity) Z01.82
  special (see also Examination, by type) Z01.89
    specified type NEC Z01.89
  specified type or reason NEC Z04.8
  teeth Z01.20
    with abnormal findings Z01.21
  urine —see Examination, laboratory
  vision Z01.00
    with abnormal findings Z01.01
Exanthem, exanthema —see also Rash
  with enteroviral vesicular stomatitis B08.4
  Boston A88.0
  epidemic with meningitis A88.0 [G02]
  subitum B08.20
    due to human herpesvirus 6 B08.21
    due to human herpesvirus 7 B08.22
  viral, virus B09
    specified type NEC B08.8
Excess, excessive, excessively
  alcohol level in blood R78.0
  androgen (ovarian) E28.1
  attrition, tooth, teeth K03.0
  carotene, carotin (dietary) E67.1
  cold, effects of T69.9
    specified effect NEC T69.8
  convergence H51.12
  crying
    in child, adolescent, or adult R45.83
    in infant R68.11
  development, breast N62
  divergence H51.8

Excess, excessive, excessively (Continued)
  drinking (alcohol) NEC (without
      dependence) F10.10
    habitual (continual) (without remission)
        F10.20
  eating R63.2
  estrogen E28.0
  fat —see also Obesity
    in heart —see Degeneration, myocardial
    localized E65
  foreskin N47.8
  gas R14.0
  glucagon E16.3
  heat —see Heat
  intermaxillary vertical dimension of fully
      erupted teeth M26.37
  interocclusal distance of fully erupted teeth
      M26.37
  kalium E87.5
  large
    colon K59.3
      congenital Q43.8
    infant P08.0
    organ or site, congenital NEC —see
        Anomaly, by site
  long
    organ or site, congenital NEC —see
        Anomaly, by site
  menstruation (with regular cycle) N92.0
    with irregular cycle N92.1
  napping Z72.821
  natrium E87.0
  number of teeth K00.1
  nutrient (dietary) NEC R63.2
  potassium (K) E87.5
  salivation K11.7
  secretion —see also Hypersecretion
    milk O92.6
    sputum R09.3
    sweat R61
  sexual drive F52.8
  short
    organ or site, congenital NEC —see
        Anomaly, by site
    umbilical cord in labor or delivery O69.3
  skin, eyelid (acquired) —see Blepharochalasis
    congenital Q10.3
  sodium (Na) E87.0
  spacing of fully erupted teeth M26.32
  sputum R09.3
  sweating R61
  thirst R63.1
    due to deprivation of water T73.1
  tuberosity of jaw M26.07
  vitamin
    A (dietary) E67.0
      administered as drug (prolonged
          intake) —see Table of Drugs and
          Chemicals, vitamins, adverse
          effect
      overdose or wrong substance given or
          taken —see Table of Drugs and
          Chemicals, vitamins, poisoning
    D (dietary) E67.3
      administered as drug (prolonged
          intake) —see Table of Drugs and
          Chemicals, vitamins, adverse
          effect
      overdose or wrong substance given or
          taken —see Table of Drugs and
          Chemicals, vitamins, poisoning
  weight
    gain R63.5
    loss R63.4
Excitability, abnormal, under minor stress
    (personality disorder) F60.3
Excitation
  anomalous atrioventricular I45.6
  psychogenic F30.8
  reactive (from emotional stress, psychological
      trauma) F30.8

Excitement
  hypomanic F30.8
  manic F30.9
  mental, reactive (from emotional stress,
      psychological trauma) F30.8
  state, reactive (from emotional stress,
      psychological trauma) F30.8
Excoriation (traumatic) —see also Abrasion
  neurotic L98.1
Exfoliation
  due to erythematous conditions according to
      extent of body surface involved L49.0
    10-19 percent of body surface L49.1
    20-29 percent of body surface L49.2
    30-39 percent of body surface L49.3
    40-49 percent of body surface L49.4
    50-59 percent of body surface L49.5
    60-69 percent of body surface L49.6
    70-79 percent of body surface L49.7
    80-89 percent of body surface L49.8
    90-99 percent of body surface L49.9
    less than 10 percent of body surface L49.0
  teeth, due to systemic causes K08.0
Exfoliative —see condition
Exhaustion, exhaustive (physical NEC) R53.83
  battle F43.0
  cardiac —see Failure, heart
  delirium F43.0
  due to
    cold T69.8
    excessive exertion T73.3
    exposure T73.2
    neurasthenia F48.8
  heart —see Failure, heart
  heat (see also Heat, exhaustion) T67.5
    due to
      salt depletion T67.4
      water depletion T67.3
  maternal, complicating delivery O75.81
  mental F48.8
  myocardium, myocardial —see Failure, heart
  nervous F48.8
  old age R54
  psychogenic F48.8
  psychosis F43.0
  senile R54
  vital NEC Z73.0
Exhibitionism F65.2
Exocervicitis —see Cervicitis
Exomphalos Q79.2
  meaning hernia —see Hernia, umbilicus
Exophoria H50.52
  convergence, insufficiency H51.11
  divergence, excess H51.8
Exophthalmos H05.2-
  congenital Q15.8
  constant NEC H05.24-
  displacement, globe —see Displacement,
      globe
  due to thyrotoxicosis (hyperthyroidism) —see
      Hyperthyroidism, with, goiter (diffuse)
  dysthyroid —see Hyperthyroidism, with,
      goiter (diffuse)
  goiter —see Hyperthyroidism, with, goiter
      (diffuse)
  intermittent NEC H05.25-
  malignant —see Hyperthyroidism, with,
      goiter (diffuse)
  orbital
    edema —see Edema, orbit
    hemorrhage —see Hemorrhage, orbit
  pulsating NEC H05.26-
  thyrotoxic, thyrotropic —see
      Hyperthyroidism, with, goiter (diffuse)
Exostosis —see also Disorder, bone
  cartilaginous —see Neoplasm, bone, benign
  congenital (multiple) Q78.6
  external ear canal H61.81-
  gonococcal A54.49
  jaw (bone) M27.8
  multiple, congenital Q78.6

◀ New   ◀▥ Revised   ~~deleted~~ Deleted

Exostosis (Continued)
  orbit H05.35-
  osteocartilaginous —see Neoplasm, bone, benign
  syphilitic A52.77
Exotropia —see Strabismus, divergent concomitant
Explanation of
  investigation finding Z71.2
  medication Z71.89
Exposure (to) (see also Contact, with) T75.89
  acariasis Z20.7
  AIDS virus Z20.6
  air pollution Z77.110
  algae and algae toxins Z77.121
  algae bloom Z77.121
  anthrax Z20.810
  aromatic amines Z77.020
  aromatic (hazardous) compounds NEC Z77.028
  aromatic dyes NOS Z77.028
  arsenic Z77.010
  asbestos Z77.090
  bacterial disease NEC Z20.818
  benzene Z77.021
  blue-green algae bloom Z77.121
  body fluids (potentially hazardous) Z77.21
  brown tide Z77.121
  chemicals (chiefly nonmedicinal) (hazardous) NEC Z77.098
  cholera Z20.09
  chromium compounds Z77.018
  cold, effects of T69.9
    specified effect NEC T69.8
  communicable disease Z20.9
    bacterial NEC Z20.818
    specified NEC Z20.89
    viral NEC Z20.828
  cyanobacteria bloom Z77.121
  disaster Z65.5
  discrimination Z60.5
  dyes Z77.098
  effects of T73.9
  environmental tobacco smoke (acute) (chronic) Z77.22
  Escherichia coli (E. coli) Z20.01
  exhaustion due to T73.2
  fiberglass —see Table of Drugs and Chemicals, fiberglass
  German measles Z20.4
  gonorrhea Z20.2
  hazardous metals NEC Z77.018
  hazardous substances NEC Z77.29
  hazards in the physical environment NEC Z77.128
  hazards to health NEC Z77.9
  human immunodeficiency virus (HIV) Z20.6
  human T-lymphotropic virus type-1 (HTLV-1) Z20.89

Exposure (Continued)
  implanted
    mesh —see Complications, mesh
    prosthetic materials NEC —see Complications, prosthetic materials NEC
  infestation (parasitic) NEC Z20.7
  intestinal infectious disease NEC Z20.09
    Escherichia coli (E. coli) Z20.01
  lead Z77.011
  meningococcus Z20.811
  mold (toxic) Z77.120
  nickel dust Z77.018
  noise Z77.122
  occupational
    air contaminants NEC Z57.39
    dust Z57.2
    environmental tobacco smoke Z57.31
    extreme temperature Z57.6
    noise Z57.0
    radiation Z57.1
    risk factors Z57.9
      specified NEC Z57.8
    toxic agents (gases) (liquids) (solids) (vapors) in agriculture Z57.4
    toxic agents (gases) (liquids) (solids) (vapors) in industry NEC Z57.5
    vibration Z57.7
  parasitic disease NEC Z20.7
  pediculosis Z20.7
  persecution Z60.5
  pfiesteria piscicida Z77.121
  poliomyelitis Z20.89
  pollution
    air Z77.110
    environmental NEC Z77.118
    soil Z77.112
    water Z77.111
  polycyclic aromatic hydrocarbons Z77.028
  prenatal (drugs) (toxic chemicals) —see Newborn, affected by (suspected to be), noxious substances transmitted via placenta or breast milk
  rabies Z20.3
  radiation, naturally occurring NEC Z77.123
  radon Z77.123
  red tide (Florida) Z77.121
  rubella Z20.4
  second hand tobacco smoke (acute) (chronic) Z77.22
    in the perinatal period P96.81
  sexually-transmitted disease Z20.2
  smallpox (laboratory) Z20.89
  syphilis Z20.2
  terrorism Z65.4
  torture Z65.4
  tuberculosis Z20.1
  uranium Z77.012
  varicella Z20.820

Exposure (Continued)
  venereal disease Z20.2
  viral disease NEC Z20.828
  war Z65.5
  water pollution Z77.111
Exsanguination —see Hemorrhage
Exstrophy
  abdominal contents Q45.8
  bladder Q64.10
    cloacal Q64.12
    specified type NEC Q64.19
    supravesical fissure Q64.11
Extensive —see condition
Extra —see also Accessory
  marker chromosomes (normal individual) Q92.61
    in abnormal individual Q92.62
  rib Q76.6
    cervical Q76.5
Extrasystoles (supraventricular) I49.49
  atrial I49.1
  auricular I49.1
  junctional I49.2
  ventricular I49.3
Extrauterine gestation or pregnancy —see Pregnancy, by site
Extravasation
  blood R58
  chyle into mesentery I89.8
  pelvicalyceal N13.8
  pyelosinus N13.8
  urine (from ureter) R39.0
  vesicant agent
    antineoplastic chemotherapy T80.810
    other agent NEC T80.818
Extremity —see condition, limb
Extrophy —see Exstrophy
Extroversion
  bladder Q64.19
  uterus N81.4
    complicating delivery O71.2
    postpartal (old) N81.4
Extruded tooth (teeth) M26.34
Extrusion
  breast implant (prosthetic) T85.42
  eye implant (globe) (ball) T85.328
  intervertebral disc —see Displacement, intervertebral disc
  ocular lens implant (prosthetic) —see Complications, intraocular lens
  vitreous —see Prolapse, vitreous
Exudate
  pleural —see Effusion, pleura
  retina H35.89
Exudative —see condition
Eye, eyeball, eyelid —see condition
Eyestrain —see Disturbance, vision, subjective
Eyeworm disease of Africa B74.3

F

Faber's syndrome (achlorhydric anemia) D50.9
Fabry (-Anderson) disease E75.21
Faciocephalalgia, autonomic (see also
    Neuropathy, peripheral, autonomic)
    G90.09
Factor (s)
    psychic, associated with diseases classified
        elsewhere F54
    psychological
        affecting physical conditions F54
        or behavioral
            affecting general medical condition F54
            associated with disorders or diseases
                classified elsewhere F54
Fahr disease (of brain) G23.8
Fahr Volhard disease (of kidney) I12.-
Failure, failed
    abortion —see Abortion, attempted
    aortic (valve) I35.8
        rheumatic I06.8
    attempted abortion —see Abortion, attempted
    biventricular I50.9
    bone marrow —see Anemia, aplastic
    cardiac —see Failure, heart
    cardiorenal (chronic) I50.9
        hypertensive I13.2
    cardiorespiratory (see also Failure, heart)
        R09.2
    cardiovascular (chronic) —see Failure, heart
    cerebrovascular I67.9
    cervical dilatation in labor O62.0
    circulation, circulatory (peripheral) R57.9
        newborn P29.89
    compensation —see Disease, heart
    compliance with medical treatment or
        regimen —see Noncompliance
    congestive —see Failure, heart, congestive
    dental implant (endosseous) M27.69
        due to
            failure of dental prosthesis M27.63
            lack of attached gingiva M27.62
            occlusal trauma (poor prosthetic design)
                M27.62
            parafunctional habits M27.62
            periodontal infection (peri-implantitis)
                M27.62
            poor oral hygiene M27.62
        osseointegration M27.61
            due to
                complications of systemic disease
                    M27.61
                poor bone quality M27.61
            iatrogenic M27.61
            post-osseointegration
                biological M27.62
                due to complications of systemic disease
                    M27.62
                iatrogenic M27.62
                mechanical M27.63
            pre-integration M27.61
            pre-osseointegration M27.61
        specified NEC M27.69
    descent of head (at term) of pregnancy
        (mother) O32.4
    endosseous dental implant —see Failure,
        dental implant
    engagement of head (term of pregnancy)
        (mother) O32.4
    erection (penile) (see also Dysfunction, sexual,
        male, erectile) N52.9
        nonorgqanic F52.21
    examination (s), anxiety concerning Z55.2
    expansion terminal respiratory units
        (newborn) (primary) P28.0
    forceps NOS (with subsequent cesarean
        delivery) O66.5
    gain weight (child over 28 days old) R62.51
        adult R62.7
        newborn P92.6

Failure, failed (Continued)
    genital response (male) F52.21
        female F52.22
    heart (acute) (senile) (sudden) I50.9
        with
            acute pulmonary edema —see Failure,
                ventricular, left
            decompensation —see Failure, heart,
                congestive
            dilatation —see Disease, heart
        arteriosclerotic I70.90
        biventricular I50.9
        combined left-right sided I50.9
        compensated I50.9
        complicating
            anesthesia (general) (local) or other
                sedation
                in labor and delivery O74.2
                in pregnancy O29.12-
                postpartum, puerperal O89.1
            delivery (cesarean) (instrumental) O75.4
        congestive (compensated)
            (decompensated) I50.9
            with rheumatic fever (conditions in I00)
                active I01.8
                inactive or quiescent (with chorea)
                    I09.81
            newborn P29.0
            rheumatic (chronic) (inactive) (with
                chorea) I09.81
                active or acute I01.8
                with chorea I02.0
        decompensated I50.9
        degenerative —see Degeneration,
            myocardial
        diastolic (congestive) I50.30
            acute (congestive) I50.31
                and (on) chronic (congestive) I50.33
            chronic (congestive) I50.32
                and (on) acute (congestive) I50.33
            combined with systolic (congestive)
                I50.40
                acute (congestive) I50.41
                    and (on) chronic (congestive)
                        I50.43
                chronic (congestive) I50.42
                    and (on) acute (congestive) I50.43
        due to presence of cardiac prosthesis
            I97.13-
        following cardiac surgery I97.13-
        high output NOS I50.9
        hypertensive —see Hypertension, heart
        left (ventricular) —see Failure, ventricular,
            left
        low output (syndrome) NOS I50.9
        newborn P29.0
        organic —see Disease, heart
        peripartum O90.3
        postprocedural I97.13-
        rheumatic (chronic) (inactive) I09.9
        right (ventricular) (secondary to left
            heart failure) —see Failure, heart,
            congestive
        systolic (congestive) I50.20
            acute (congestive) I50.21
                and (on) chronic (congestive)
                    I50.23
            chronic (congestive) I50.22
                and (on) acute (congestive) I50.23
            combined with diastolic (congestive)
                I50.40
                acute (congestive) I50.41
                    and (on) chronic (congestive)
                        I50.43
                chronic (congestive) I50.42
                    and (on) acute (congestive)
                        I50.43
        thyrotoxic (see also Thyrotoxicosis)
            E05.90 [143]
            with thyroid storm E05.91 [143]
        valvular —see Endocarditis

Failure, failed (Continued)
    hepatic K72.90
        with coma K72.91
        acute or subacute K72.00
            with coma K72.01
            due to drugs K71.10
                with coma K71.11
        alcoholic (acute) (chronic) (subacute)
            K70.40
            with coma K70.41
        chronic K72.10
            with coma K72.11
            due to drugs (acute) (subacute) (chronic)
                K71.10
                with coma K71.11
        due to drugs (acute) (subacute) (chronic)
            K71.10
            with coma K71.11
        postprocedural K91.82
    hepatorenal K76.7
    induction (of labor) O61.9
        abortion —see Abortion, attempted
        by
            oxytocic drugs O61.0
            prostaglandins O61.0
        instrumental O61.1
        mechanical O61.1
        medical O61.0
        specified NEC O61.8
        surgical O61.1
    intubation during anesthesia T88.4
        in pregnancy O29.6-
        labor and delivery O74.7
        postpartum, puerperal O89.6
    involution, thymus (gland) E32.0
    kidney (see also Disease, kidney, chronic) N19
        acute (see also Failure, renal, acute) N17.9-
        diabetic - see E08-E13 with .22
    lactation (complete) O92.3
        partial O92.4
    Leydig's cell, adult E29.1
    liver —see Failure, hepatic
    menstruation at puberty N91.0
    mitral I05.8
    myocardial, myocardium (see also Failure,
        heart) I50.9
        chronic (see also Failure, heart, congestive)
            I50.9
        congestive (see also Failure, heart,
            congestive) I50.9
    orgasm (female) (psychogenic) F52.31
        male F52.32
    ovarian (primary) E28.39
        iatrogenic E89.40
            asymptomatic E89.40
            symptomatic E89.41
        postprocedural (postablative)
            (postirradiation) (postsurgical)
            E89.40
            asymptomatic E89.40
            symptomatic E89.41
    ovulation causing infertility N97.0
    polyglandular, autoimmune E31.0
    prosthetic joint implant —see Complications,
        joint prosthesis, mechanical,
        breakdown, by site
    renal N19
        with
            tubular necrosis (acute) N17.0
        acute N17.9
            with
                cortical necrosis N17.1
                medullary necrosis N17.2
                tubular necrosis N17.0
            specified NEC N17.8
        chronic N18.9
            hypertensive —see Hypertension,
                kidney
        congenital P96.0
        end stage (chronic) N18.6
            due to hypertension I12.0

◀ New   ◀▥ Revised   ~~deleted~~ Deleted

Failure, failed *(Continued)*
  renal *(Continued)*
    following
      abortion —*see* Abortion by type
      complicated by specified
        condition NEC
      crushing T79.5
      ectopic or molar pregnancy O08.4
      labor and delivery (acute) O90.4
    hypertensive —*see* Hypertension,
      kidney
    postprocedural N99.0
  respiration, respiratory J96.9
    with
      hypercapnia J96.92
      hypoxia J96.91
    acute J96.00
      with
        hypercapnia J96.02
        hypoxia J96.01
    acute and (on) chronic J96.20
      with
        hypercapnia J96.22
        hypoxia J96.21
    center G93.89
    chronic J96.10
      with
        hypercapnia J96.12
        hypoxia J96.11
    newborn P28.5
    postprocedural (acute) J95.821
      acute and chronic J95.822
  rotation
    cecum Q43.3
    colon Q43.3
    intestine Q43.3
    kidney Q63.2
  sedation (conscious) (moderate) during
    procedure T88.52
    history of Z92.83
  segmentation —*see also* Fusion
    fingers —*see* Syndactylism, complex,
      fingers
    vertebra Q76.49
      with scoliosis Q76.3
  seminiferous tubule, adult E29.1
  senile (general) R54
  sexual arousal (male) F52.21
    female F52.22
  testicular endocrine function E29.1
  to thrive (child over 28 days old)
    R62.51
    adult R62.7
    newborn P92.6
  transplant T86.92
    bone T86.831
      marrow T86.02
    cornea T86.841
    heart T86.22
      with lung (s) T86.32
    intestine T86.851
    kidney T86.12
    liver T86.42
    lung (s) T86.811
      with heart T86.32
    pancreas T86.891
    skin (allograft) (autograft) T86.821
    specified organ or tissue NEC T86.891
    stem cell (peripheral blood) (umbilical
      cord) T86.5
  trial of labor (with subsequent cesarean
    delivery) O66.40
    following previous cesarean delivery
      O66.41
  tubal ligation N99.89
  urinary —*see* Disease, kidney, chronic
  vacuum extraction NOS (with subsequent
    cesarean delivery) O66.5
  vasectomy N99.89
  ventouse NOS (with subsequent cesarean
    delivery) O66.5

Failure, failed *(Continued)*
  ventricular (*see also* Failure, heart) I50.9
    left I50.1
      with rheumatic fever (conditions in I00)
        active I01.8
          with chorea I02.0
        inactive or quiescent (with chorea)
          I09.81
      rheumatic (chronic) (inactive) (with
        chorea) I09.81
        active or acute I01.8
          with chorea I02.0
    right (*see also* Failure, heart, congestive)
      I50.9
  vital centers, newborn P91.8
Fainting (fit) R55
Fallen arches —*see* Deformity, limb, flat foot
Falling, falls (repeated) R29.6
  any organ or part —*see* Prolapse
Fallopian
  insufflation Z31.41
  tube —*see* condition
Fallot's
  pentalogy Q21.8
  tetrad or tetralogy Q21.3
  triad or trilogy Q22.3
False —*see also* condition
  croup J38.5
  joint —*see* Nonunion, fracture
  labor (pains) O47.9
    at or after 37 completed weeks of gestation
      O47.1
    before 37 completed weeks of gestation
      O47.0-
  passage, urethra (prostatic) N36.5
  pregnancy F45.8
Family, familial —*see also* condition
  disruption Z63.8
    involving divorce or separation Z63.5
  Li-Fraumeni (syndrome) Z15.01
  planning advice Z30.09
  problem Z63.9
    specified NEC Z63.8
  retinoblastoma C69.2-
Famine (effects of) T73.0
  edema —*see* Malnutrition, severe
Fanconi (-de Toni)(-Debré) syndrome E72.09
  with cystinosis E72.04
Fanconi's anemia (congenital pancytopenia)
  D61.09
Farber's disease or syndrome E75.29
Farcy A24.0
Farmer's
  lung J67.0
  skin L57.8
Farsightedness —*see* Hypermetropia
Fascia —*see* condition
Fasciculation R25.3
Fasciitis M72.9
  diffuse (eosinophilic) M35.4
  infective M72.8
    necrotizing M72.6
  necrotizing M72.6
  nodular M72.4
  perirenal (with ureteral obstruction)
    N13.5
    with infection N13.6
  plantar M72.2
  specified NEC M72.8
  traumatic (old) M72.8
  current - code by site under Sprain
Fascioliasis B66.3
Fasciolopsis, fasciolopsiasis (intestinal)
  B66.5
Fascioscapulohumeral myopathy G71.0
Fast pulse R00.0
Fat
  embolism —*see* Embolism, fat
  excessive —*see also* Obesity
    in heart —*see* Degeneration, myocardial
  in stool R19.5

Fat *(Continued)*
  localized (pad) E65
    heart —*see* Degeneration, myocardial
    knee M79.4
    retropatellar M79.4
  necrosis
    breast N64.1
    mesentery K65.4
    omentum K65.4
  pad E65
    knee M79.4
Fatigue R53.83
  auditory deafness —*see* Deafness
  chronic R53.82
  combat F43.0
  general R53.83
    psychogenic F48.8
  heat (transient) T67.6
  muscle M62.89
  myocardium —*see* Failure, heart
  neoplasm-related R53.0
  nervous, neurosis F48.8
  operational F48.8
  psychogenic (general) F48.8
  senile R54
  voice R49.8
Fatness —*see* Obesity
Fatty —*see also* condition
  apron E65
  degeneration —*see* Degeneration, fatty
  heart (enlarged) —*see* Degeneration,
    myocardial
  liver NEC K76.0
    alcoholic K70.0
    nonalcoholic K76.0
  necrosis —*see* Degeneration, fatty
Fauces —*see* condition
Fauchard's disease (periodontitis) —*see*
  Periodontitis
Faucitis J02.9
Favism (anemia) D55.0
Favus —*see* Dermatophytosis
Fazio-Londe disease or syndrome
  G12.1
Fear complex or reaction F40.9
Fear of —*see* Phobia
Feared complaint unfounded Z71.1
Febris, febrile —*see also* Fever
  flava (*see also* Fever, yellow) A95.9
  melitensis A23.0
  pestis —*see* Plague
  recurrens —*see* Fever, relapsing
  rubra A38.9
Fecal
  incontinence R15.9
  smearing R15.1
  soiling R15.1
  urgency R15.2
Fecalith (impaction) K56.41
  appendix K38.1
  congenital P76.8
Fede's disease K14.0
Feeble rapid pulse due to shock following
  injury T79.4
Feeble-minded F70
Feeding
  difficulties R63.3
  problem R63.3
    newborn P92.9
      specified NEC P92.8
    nonorganic (adult) —*see* Disorder,
      eating
Feeling (of)
  foreign body in throat R09.89
Feer's disease —*see* Poisoning, mercury
Feet —*see* condition
Feigned illness Z76.5
Feil-Klippel syndrome (brevicollis) Q76.1
Feinmesser's (hidrotic) ectodermal dysplasia
  Q82.4
Felinophobia F40.218

Felon —see also Cellulitis, digit
  with lymphangitis —see Lymphangitis, acute,
    digit
Felty's syndrome M05.00
  ankle M05.07-
  elbow M05.02-
  foot joint M05.07-
  hand joint M05.04-
  hip M05.05-
  knee M05.06-
  multiple site M05.09
  shoulder M05.01-
  vertebra —see Spondylitis, ankylosing
  wrist M05.03-
Female genital cutting status —see Female
  genital mutilation status (FGM)
Female genital mutilation status (FGM) N90.810
  specified NEC N90.818
  type I (clitorectomy status) N90.811
  type II (clitorectomy with excision of labia
    minora status) N90.812
  type III (infibulation status) N90.813
  type IV N90.818
Femur, femoral —see condition
Fenestration, fenestrated —see also Imperfect,
  closure
  aortico-pulmonary Q21.4
  cusps, heart valve NEC Q24.8
    pulmonary Q22.3
  pulmonic cusps Q22.3
Fernell's disease (aortic aneurysm) I71.9
Fertile eunuch syndrome E23.0
Fetid
  breath R19.6
  sweat L75.0
Fetishism F65.0
  transvestic F65.1
Fetus, fetal —see also condition
  alcohol syndrome (dysmorphic) Q86.0
  compressus O31.0-
  hydantoin syndrome Q86.1
  lung tissue P28.0
  papyraceous O31.0-
Fever (inanition) (of unknown origin)
    (persistent) (with chills) (with rigor) R50.9
  abortus A23.1
  Aden (dengue) A90
  African tick-borne A68.1
  American
    mountain (tick) A93.2
    spotted A77.0
  aphthous B08.8
  arbovirus, arboviral A94
    hemorrhagic A94
    specified NEC A93.8
  Argentinian hemorrhagic A96.0
  Assam B55.0
  Australian Q A78
  Bangkok hemorrhagic A91
  Barmah forest A92.8
  Bartonella A44.0
  bilious, hemoglobinuric B50.8
  blackwater B50.8
  blister B00.1
  Bolivian hemorrhagic A96.1
  Bonvale dam T73.3
  boutonneuse A77.1
  brain —see Encephalitis
  Brazilian purpuric A48.4
  breakbone A90
  Bullis A77.0
  Bunyamwera A92.8
  Burdwan B55.0
  Bwamba A92.8
  Cameroon —see Malaria
  Canton A75.9
  catarrhal (acute) J00
    chronic J31.0
  cat-scratch A28.1
  Central Asian hemorrhagic A98.0
  cerebral —see Encephalitis

Fever (Continued)
  cerebrospinal meningococcal A39.0
  Chagres B50.9
  Chandipura A92.8
  Changuinola A93.1
  Charcot's (biliary) (hepatic) (intermittent) —
    see Calculus, bile duct
  Chikungunya (viral) (hemorrhagic)
    A92.0
  Chitral A93.1
  Colombo —see Fever, paratyphoid
  Colorado tick (virus) A93.2
  congestive (remittent) —see Malaria
  Congo virus A98.0
  continued malarial B50.9
  Corsican —see Malaria
  Crimean-Congo hemorrhagic A98.0
  Cyprus —see Brucellosis
  dandy A90
  deer fly —see Tularemia
  dengue (virus) A90
    hemorrhagic A91
    sandfly A93.1
  desert B38.0
  drug induced R50.2
  due to
    conditions classified elsewhere
      R50.81
    heat T67.0
  enteric A01.00
  enteroviral exanthematous (Boston
    exanthem) A88.0
  ephemeral (of unknown origin) R50.9
  epidemic hemorrhagic A98.5
  erysipelatous —see Erysipelas
  estivo-autumnal (malarial) B50.9
  famine A75.0
  five day A79.0
  following delivery O86.4
  Fort Bragg A27.89
  gastroenteric A01.00
  gastromalarial —see Malaria
  Gibraltar —see Brucellosis
  glandular —see Mononucleosis, infectious
  Guama (viral) A92.8
  Haverhill A25.1
  hay (allergic) J30.1
    with asthma (bronchial) J45.909
      with
        exacerbation (acute) J45.901
        status asthmaticus J45.902
    due to
      allergen other than pollen J30.89
      pollen, any plant or tree J30.1
  heat (effects) T67.0
  hematuric, bilious B50.8
  hemoglobinuric (malarial) (bilious) B50.8
  hemorrhagic (arthropod-borne) NOS A94
    with renal syndrome A98.5
    arenaviral A96.9
      specified NEC A96.8
    Argentinian A96.0
    Bangkok A91
    Bolivian A96.1
    Central Asian A98.0
    Chikungunya A92.0
    Crimean-Congo A98.0
    dengue (virus) A91
    epidemic A98.5
    Junin (virus) A96.0
    Korean A98.5
    Kyasanur forest A98.2
    Machupo (virus) A96.1
    mite-borne A93.8
    mosquito-borne A92.8
    Omsk A98.1
    Philippine A91
    Russian A98.5
    Singapore A91
    Southeast Asia A91
    Thailand A91

Fever (Continued)
  hemorrhagic NOS (Continued)
    tick-borne NEC A93.8
    viral A99
      specified NEC A98.8
  hepatic —see Cholecystitis
  herpetic —see Herpes
  icterohemorrhagic A27.0
  Indiana A93.8
  infective B99.9
    specified NEC B99.8
  intermittent (bilious) —see also Malaria
    of unknown origin R50.9
    pernicious B50.9
  iodide R50.2
  Japanese river A75.3
  jungle —see also Malaria
    yellow A95.0
  Junin (virus) hemorrhagic A96.0
  Katayama B65.2
  kedani A75.3
  Kenya (tick) A77.1
  Kew Garden A79.1
  Korean hemorrhagic A98.5
  Lassa A96.2
  Lone Star A77.0
  Machupo (virus) hemorrhagic A96.1
  malaria, malarial —see Malaria
  Malta A23.9
  Marseilles A77.1
  marsh —see Malaria
  Mayaro (viral) A92.8
  Mediterranean (see also Brucellosis) A23.9
    familial E85.0
    tick A77.1
  meningeal —see Meningitis
  Meuse A79.0
  Mexican A75.2
  mianeh A68.1
  miasmatic —see Malaria
  mosquito-borne (viral) A92.9
    hemorrhagic A92.8
  mountain —see also Brucellosis
    meaning Rocky Mountain spotted fever
      A77.0
    tick (American) (Colorado) (viral) A93.2
  Mucambo (viral) A92.8
  mud A27.9
  Neapolitan —see Brucellosis
  neutropenic D70.9
  newborn P81.9
    environmental P81.0
  Nine-Mile A78
  non-exanthematous tick A93.2
  North Asian tick-borne A77.2
  Omsk hemorrhagic A98.1
  O'nyong-nyong (viral) A92.1
  Oropouche (viral) A93.0
  Oroya A44.0
  paludal —see Malaria
  Panama (malarial) B50.9
  Pappataci A93.1
  paratyphoid A01.4
    A A01.1
    B A01.2
    C A01.3
  parrot A70
  periodic (Mediterranean) E85.0
  persistent (of unknown origin) R50.9
  petechial A39.0
  pharyngoconjunctival B30.2
  Philippine hemorrhagic A91
  phlebotomus A93.1
  Piry (virus) A93.8
  Pixuna (viral) A92.8
  Plasmodium ovale B53.0
  polioviral (nonparalytic) A80.4
  Pontiac A48.2
  postimmunization R50.83
  postoperative R50.82
    due to infection T81.4

◀ New   ◀▥ Revised   ~~deleted~~ Deleted

Fever *(Continued)*
  posttransfusion R50.84
  postvaccination R50.83
  presenting with conditions classified
      elsewhere R50.81
  pretibial A27.89
  puerperal O86.4
  Q A78
  quadrilateral A78
  quartan (malaria) B52.9
  Queensland (coastal) (tick) A77.3
  quintan A79.0
  rabbit —*see* Tularemia
  rat-bite A25.9
    due to
      Spirillum A25.0
      Streptobacillus moniliformis A25.1
  recurrent —*see* Fever, relapsing
  relapsing (Borrelia) A68.9
    Carter's (Asiatic) A68.1
    Dutton's (West African) A68.1
    Koch's A68.9
    louse-borne A68.0
    Novy's
      louse-borne A68.0
      tick-borne A68.1
    Obermeyer's (European) A68.0
    tick-borne A68.1
  remittent (bilious) (congestive) (gastric) —*see*
      Malaria
  rheumatic (active) (acute) (chronic) (subacute)
      I00
    with central nervous system involvement
        I02.9
    active with heart involvement (*see*
        category) I01
    inactive or quiescent with
      cardiac hypertrophy I09.89
      carditis I09.9
      endocarditis I09.1
        aortic (valve) I06.9
          with mitral (valve) disease I08.0
        mitral (valve) I05.9
          with aortic (valve) disease I08.0
        pulmonary (valve) I09.89
        tricuspid (valve) I07.8
      heart disease NEC I09.89
      heart failure (congestive) (conditions in
          I50.9) I09.81
      left ventricular failure (conditions in
          I50.1) I09.81
      myocarditis, myocardial degeneration
          (conditions in I51.4) I09.0
      pancarditis I09.9
      pericarditis I09.2
  Rift Valley (viral) A92.4
  Rocky Mountain spotted A77.0
  rose J30.1
  Ross River B33.1
  Russian hemorrhagic A98.5
  San Joaquin (Valley) B38.0
  sandfly A93.1
  Sao Paulo A77.0
  scarlet A38.9
  seven day (leptospirosis) (autumnal)
      (Japanese) A27.89
    dengue A90
  shin-bone A79.0
  Singapore hemorrhagic A91
  solar A90
  Songo A98.5
  sore B00.1
  South African tick-bite A68.1
  Southeast Asia hemorrhagic A91
  spinal —*see* Meningitis
  spirillary A25.0
  splenic —*see* Anthrax
  spotted A77.9
    American A77.0
    Brazilian A77.0
    cerebrospinal meningitis A39.0

Fever *(Continued)*
  spotted *(Continued)*
    Colombian A77.0
    due to Rickettsia
      australis A77.3
      conorii A77.1
      rickettsii A77.0
      sibirica A77.2
      specified type NEC A77.8
    Ehrlichiosis A77.40
      due to
        E. chafeensis A77.41
        specified organism NEC A77.49
    Rocky Mountain A77.0
  steroid R50.2
  streptobacillary A25.1
  subtertian B50.9
  Sumatran mite A75.3
  sun A90
  swamp A27.9
  swine A02.8
  sylvatic, yellow A95.0
  Tahyna B33.8
  tertian —*see* Malaria, tertian
  Thailand hemorrhagic A91
  thermic T67.0
  three-day A93.1
  tick
    American mountain A93.2
    Colorado A93.2
    Kemerovo A93.8
    Mediterranean A77.1
    mountain A93.2
    nonexanthematous A93.2
    Quaranfil A93.8
  tick-bite NEC A93.8
  tick-borne (hemorrhagic) NEC A93.8
  trench A79.0
  tsutsugamushi A75.3
  typhogastric A01.00
  typhoid (abortive) (hemorrhagic)
      (intermittent) (malignant) A01.00
    complicated by
      arthritis A01.04
      heart involvement A01.02
      meningitis A01.01
      osteomyelitis A01.05
      pneumonia A01.03
      specified NEC A01.09
  typhomalarial —*see* Malaria
  typhus —*see* Typhus (fever)
  undulant —*see* Brucellosis
  unknown origin R50.9
  uveoparotid D86.89
  valley B38.0
  Venezuelan equine A92.2
  vesicular stomatitis A93.8
  viral hemorrhagic —*see* Fever, hemorrhagic,
      by type of virus
  Volhynian A79.0
  Wesselsbron (viral) A92.8
  West
    African B50.8
    Nile (viral) A92.30
      with
        complications NEC A92.39
        cranial nerve disorders A92.32
        encephalitis A92.31
        encephalomyelitis A92.31
        neurologic manifestation NEC
            A92.32
        optic neuritis A92.32
        polyradiculitis A92.32
  Whitmore's —*see* Melioidosis
  Wolhynian A79.0
  worm B83.9
  yellow A95.9
    jungle A95.0
    sylvatic A95.0
    urban A95.1
  Zika (viral) A92.8

Fibrillation
  atrial or auricular (established) I48.91
    chronic I48.2
    paroxysmal I48.0
    permanent I48.2
    persistent I48.1
  cardiac I49.8
  heart I49.8
  muscular M62.89
  ventricular I49.01
Fibrin
  ball or bodies, pleural (sac) J94.1
  chamber, anterior (eye) (gelatinous
      exudate) —*see* Iridocyclitis, acute
Fibrinogenolysis —*see* Fibrinolysis
Fibrinogenopenia D68.8
  acquired D65
  congenital D68.2
Fibrinolysis (hemorrhagic) (acquired) D65
  antepartum hemorrhage —*see* Hemorrhage,
      antepartum, with coagulation defect
  following
    abortion —*see* Abortion by type
        complicated by hemorrhage
    ectopic or molar pregnancy O08.1
  intrapartum O67.0
  newborn, transient P60
  postpartum O72.3
Fibrinopenia (hereditary) D68.2
  acquired D68.4
Fibrinopurulent —*see* condition
Fibrinous —*see* condition
Fibroadenoma
  cellular intracanalicular D24-
  giant D24-
  intracanalicular
    cellular D24-
    giant D24-
    specified site —*see* Neoplasm, benign, by
        site
    unspecified site D24-
  juvenile D24-
  pericanalicular
    specified site —*see* Neoplasm, benign, by
        site
    unspecified site D24-
  phyllodes D24-
  prostate D29.1
  specified site NEC —*see* Neoplasm, benign,
      by site
  unspecified site D24-
Fibroadenosis, breast (chronic) (cystic) (diffuse)
    (periodic) (segmental) N60.2-
Fibroangioma —*see also* Neoplasm, benign, by
    site
  juvenile
    specified site —*see* Neoplasm, benign, by
        site
    unspecified site D10.6
Fibrochondrosarcoma —*see* Neoplasm,
    cartilage, malignant
Fibrocystic
  disease —*see also* Fibrosis, cystic
    breast —*see* Mastopathy, cystic
    jaw M27.49
    kidney (congenital) Q61.8
    liver Q44.6
    pancreas E84.9
  kidney (congenital) Q61.8
Fibrodysplasia ossificans progressiva —*see*
    Myositis, ossificans, progressiva
Fibroelastosis (cordis) (endocardial)
    (endomyocardial) I42.4
Fibroid (tumor) —*see also* Neoplasm, connective
    tissue, benign
  disease, lung (chronic) —*see* Fibrosis, lung
  heart (disease) —*see* Myocarditis
  in pregnancy or childbirth O34.1-
    causing obstructed labor O65.5
  induration, lung (chronic) —*see* Fibrosis, lung
  lung —*see* Fibrosis, lung

Fibroid (*Continued*)
　pneumonia (chronic) —*see* Fibrosis, lung
　uterus D25.9
Fibrolipoma —*see* Lipoma
Fibroliposarcoma —*see* Neoplasm, connective
　　tissue, malignant
Fibroma —*see also* Neoplasm, connective tissue,
　　benign
　ameloblastic —*see* Cyst, calcifying
　　odontogenic
　bone (nonossifying) —*see* Disorder, bone,
　　specified type NEC
　　ossifying —*see* Neoplasm, bone,
　　　benign
　cementifying —*see* Neoplasm, bone,
　　benign
　chondromyxoid —*see* Neoplasm, bone,
　　benign
　desmoplastic —*see* Neoplasm, connective
　　tissue, uncertain behavior
　durum —*see* Neoplasm, connective tissue,
　　benign
　fascial —*see* Neoplasm, connective tissue,
　　benign
　invasive —*see* Neoplasm, connective tissue,
　　uncertain behavior
　molle —*see* Lipoma
　myxoid —*see* Neoplasm, connective tissue,
　　benign
　nasopharynx, nasopharyngeal (juvenile)
　　D10.6
　nonosteogenic (nonossifying) —*see* Dysplasia,
　　fibrous
　odontogenic (central) —*see* Cyst, calcifying
　　odontogenic
　ossifying —*see* Neoplasm, bone, benign
　periosteal —*see* Neoplasm, bone, benign
　soft —*see* Lipoma
Fibromatosis M72.9
　abdominal —*see* Neoplasm, connective tissue,
　　uncertain behavior
　aggressive —*see* Neoplasm, connective tissue,
　　uncertain behavior
　congenital generalized —*see* Neoplasm,
　　connective tissue, uncertain behavior
　Dupuytren's M72.0
　gingival K06.1
　palmar (fascial) M72.0
　plantar (fascial) M72.2
　pseudosarcomatous (proliferative)
　　(subcutaneous) M72.4
　retroperitoneal D48.3
　specified NEC M72.8
Fibromyalgia M79.7
Fibromyoma —*see also* Neoplasm, connective
　　tissue, benign
　uterus (corpus) —*see also* Leiomyoma, uterus
　　in pregnancy or childbirth —*see* Fibroid, in
　　　pregnancy or childbirth
　　　causing obstructed labor O65.5
Fibromyositis M79.7
Fibromyxolipoma D17.9
Fibromyxoma —*see* Neoplasm, connective
　　tissue, benign
Fibromyxosarcoma —*see* Neoplasm, connective
　　tissue, malignant
Fibro-odontoma, ameloblastic —*see* Cyst,
　　calcifying odontogenic
Fibro-osteoma —*see* Neoplasm, bone, benign
Fibroplasia, retrolental H35.17
Fibropurulent —*see* condition
Fibrosarcoma —*see also* Neoplasm, connective
　　tissue, malignant
　ameloblastic C41.1
　　upper jaw (bone) C41.0
　congenital —*see* Neoplasm, connective tissue,
　　malignant
　fascial —*see* Neoplasm, connective tissue,
　　malignant
　infantile —*see* Neoplasm, connective tissue,
　　malignant

Fibrosarcoma (*Continued*)
　odontogenic C41.1
　　upper jaw (bone) C41.0
　periosteal —*see* Neoplasm, bone, malignant
Fibrosclerosis
　breast N60.3-
　multifocal M35.5
　penis (corpora cavernosa) N48.6
Fibrosis, fibrotic
　adrenal (gland) E27.8
　amnion O41.8X-
　anal papillae K62.89
　arteriocapillary —*see* Arteriosclerosis
　bladder N32.89
　　interstitial —*see* Cystitis, chronic,
　　　interstitial
　　localized submucosal —*see* Cystitis,
　　　chronic, interstitial
　　panmural —*see* Cystitis, chronic,
　　　interstitial
　breast —*see* Fibrosclerosis, breast
　capillary (*see also* Arteriosclerosis) I70.90
　　lung (chronic) —*see* Fibrosis, lung
　cardiac —*see* Myocarditis
　cervix N88.8
　chorion O41.8X-
　corpus cavernosum (sclerosing) N48.6
　cystic (of pancreas) E84.9
　　with
　　　distal intestinal obstruction syndrome
　　　　E84.19
　　　fecal impaction E84.19
　　　intestinal manifestations NEC E84.19
　　　pulmonary manifestations E84.0
　　　specified manifestations NEC E84.8
　due to device, implant or graft (*see also*
　　Complications, by site and type,
　　specified NEC) T85.82
　　arterial graft NEC T82.828
　　breast (implant) T85.82
　　catheter NEC T85.82
　　　dialysis (renal) T82.828
　　　　intraperitoneal T85.82
　　　infusion NEC T82.828
　　　　spinal (epidural) (subdural) T85.82
　　　urinary (indwelling) T83.82
　　electronic (electrode) (pulse generator)
　　　(stimulator)
　　　bone T84.82
　　　cardiac T82.827
　　　nervous system (brain) (peripheral
　　　　nerve) (spinal) T85.82
　　　urinary T83.82
　　fixation, internal (orthopedic) NEC T84.82
　　gastrointestinal (bile duct) (esophagus)
　　　T85.82
　　genital NEC T83.82
　　heart NEC T82.827
　　joint prosthesis T84.82
　　ocular (corneal graft) (orbital implant)
　　　NEC T85.82
　　orthopedic NEC T84.82
　　specified NEC T85.82
　　urinary NEC T83.82
　　vascular NEC T82.828
　　ventricular intracranial shunt T85.82
　ejaculatory duct N50.8
　endocardium —*see* Endocarditis
　endomyocardial (tropical) I42.3
　epididymis N50.8
　eye muscle —*see* Strabismus, mechanical
　heart —*see* Myocarditis
　hepatic —*see* Fibrosis, liver
　hepatolienal (portal hypertension) K76.6
　hepatosplenic (portal hypertension) K76.6
　infrapatellar fat pad M79.4
　intrascrotal N50.8
　kidney N26.9
　liver K74.0
　　with sclerosis K74.2
　　alcoholic K70.2

Fibrosis, fibrotic (*Continued*)
　lung (atrophic) (chronic) (confluent)
　　(massive) (perialveolar) (peribronchial)
　　J84.10
　　with
　　　anthracosilicosis J60
　　　anthracosis J60
　　　asbestosis J61
　　　bagassosis J67.1
　　　bauxite J63.1
　　　berylliosis J63.2
　　　byssinosis J66.0
　　　calcicosis J62.8
　　　chalicosis J62.8
　　　dust reticulation J64
　　　farmer's lung J67.0
　　　ganister disease J62.8
　　　graphite J63.3
　　　pneumoconiosis NOS J64
　　　siderosis J63.4
　　　silicosis J62.8
　　capillary J84.10
　　congenital P27.8
　　diffuse (idiopathic) J84.10
　　　chemicals, gases, fumes or vapors
　　　　(inhalation) J68.4
　　　interstitial J84.10
　　　　acute J84.114
　　　　talc J62.0
　　following radiation J70.1
　　idiopathic J84.112
　　postinflammatory J84.10
　　silicotic J62.8
　　tuberculous —*see* Tuberculosis, pulmonary
　lymphatic gland I89.8
　median bar —*see* Hyperplasia, prostate
　mediastinum (idiopathic) J98.5
　meninges G96.19
　myocardium, myocardial —*see* Myocarditis
　ovary N83.8
　oviduct N83.8
　pancreas K86.8
　penis NEC N48.6
　pericardium I31.0
　perineum, in pregnancy or childbirth O34.7-
　　causing obstructed labor O65.5
　pleura J94.1
　popliteal fat pad M79.4
　prostate (chronic) —*see* Hyperplasia, prostate
　pulmonary (*see also* Fibrosis, lung) J84.10
　　congenital P27.8
　　idiopathic J84.112
　rectal sphincter K62.89
　retroperitoneal, idiopathic (with ureteral
　　obstruction) N13.5
　　with infection N13.6
　sclerosing mesenteric (idiopathic) K65.4
　scrotum N50.8
　seminal vesicle N50.8
　senile R54
　skin L90.5
　spermatic cord N50.8
　spleen D73.89
　　in schistosomiasis (bilharziasis) B65.9
　　　[D77]
　subepidermal nodular —*see* Neoplasm, skin,
　　benign
　submucous (oral) (tongue) K13.5
　testis N44.8
　　chronic, due to syphilis A52.76
　thymus (gland) E32.8
　tongue, submucous K13.5
　tunica vaginalis N50.8
　uterus (non-neoplastic) N85.8
　vagina N89.8
　valve, heart —*see* Endocarditis
　vas deferens N50.8
　vein I87.8
Fibrositis (periarticular) M79.7
　nodular, chronic (Jaccoud's) (rheumatoid) —
　　see Arthropathy, postrheumatic, chronic

Fibrothorax J94.1
Fibrotic —*see* Fibrosis
Fibrous —*see* condition
Fibroxanthoma —*see also* Neoplasm, connective
tissue, benign
  atypical —*see* Neoplasm, connective tissue,
    uncertain behavior
  malignant —*see* Neoplasm, connective tissue,
    malignant
Fibroxanthosarcoma —*see* Neoplasm,
  connective tissue, malignant
Fiedler's
  disease (icterohemorrhagic leptospirosis)
    A27.0
  myocarditis (acute) I40.1
Fifth disease B08.3
  venereal A55
Filaria, filarial, filariasis —*see* Infestation,
  filarial
Filatov's disease —*see* Mononucleosis,
  infectious
File-cutter's disease —*see* Poisoning, lead
Filling defect
  biliary tract R93.2
  bladder R93.4
  duodenum R93.3
  gallbladder R93.2
  gastrointestinal tract R93.3
  intestine R93.3
  kidney R93.4
  stomach R93.3
  ureter R93.4
Fimbrial cyst Q50.4
Financial problem affecting care NOS Z59.9
  bankruptcy Z59.8
  foreclosure on loan Z59.8
Findings, abnormal, inconclusive, without
  diagnosis —*see also* Abnormal
  17-ketosteroids, elevated R82.5
  acetonuria R82.4
  alcohol in blood R78.0
  anisocytosis R71.8
  antenatal screening of mother O28.9
    biochemical O28.1
    chromosomal O28.5
    cytological O28.2
    genetic O28.5
    hematological O28.0
    radiological O28.4
    specified NEC O28.8
    ultrasonic O28.3
  antibody titer, elevated R76.0
  anticardiolipin antibody R76.0
  antiphosphatidylglycerol antibody R76.0
  antiphosphatidylinositol antibody R76.0
  antiphosphatidylserine antibody R76.0
  antiphospholipid antibody R76.0
  bacteriuria N39.0
  bicarbonate E87.8
  bile in urine R82.2
  blood sugar R73.09
    high R73.9
    low (transient) E16.2
  body fluid or substance, specified NEC R88.8
  casts, urine R82.99
  catecholamines R82.5
  cells, urine R82.99
  chloride E87.8
  cholesterol E78.9
    high E78.0
      with high triglycerides E78.2
  chyluria R82.0
  cloudy
    dialysis effluent R88.0
    urine R82.90
  creatinine clearance R94.4
  crystals, urine R82.99
  culture
    blood R78.81
    positive —*see* Positive, culture
  echocardiogram R93.1

Findings, abnormal, inconclusive, without
  diagnosis (*Continued*)
  electrolyte level, urinary R82.99
  function study NEC R94.8
    bladder R94.8
    endocrine NEC R94.7
      thyroid R94.6
    kidney R94.4
    liver R94.5
    pancreas R94.8
    placenta R94.8
    pulmonary R94.2
    spleen R94.8
  gallbladder, nonvisualization R93.2
  glucose (tolerance test) (non-fasting)
    R73.09
  glycosuria R81
  heart
    shadow R93.1
    sounds R01.2
  hematinuria R82.3
  hematocrit drop (precipitous) R71.0
  hemoglobinuria R82.3
  human papillomavirus (HPV) DNA test
    positive
    cervix
      high risk R87.810
      low risk R87.820
    vagina
      high risk R87.811
      low risk R87.821
  in blood (of substance not normally found in
    blood) R78.9
    addictive drug NEC R78.4
    alcohol (excessive level) R78.0
    cocaine R78.2
    hallucinogen R78.3
    heavy metals (abnormal level) R78.79
    lead R78.71
    lithium (abnormal level) R78.89
    opiate drug R78.1
    psychotropic drug R78.5
    specified substance NEC R78.89
    steroid agent R78.6
  indoleacetic acid, elevated R82.5
  ketonuria R82.4
  lactic acid dehydrogenase (LDH) R74.0
  liver function test R79.89
  mammogram NEC R92.8
    calcification (calculus) R92.1
    inconclusive result (due to dense breasts)
      R92.2
    microcalcification R92.0
  mediastinal shift R93.8
  melanin, urine R82.99
  myoglobinuria R82.1
  neonatal screening P09
  nonvisualization of gallbladder R93.2
  odor of urine NOS R82.90
  Papanicolaou cervix R87.619
    non-atypical endometrial cells R87.618
  pneumoencephalogram R93.0
  poikilocytosis R71.8
  potassium (deficiency) E87.6
    excess E87.5
  PPD R76.11
  radiologic (X-ray) R93.8
    abdomen R93.5
    biliary tract R93.2
    breast R92.8
    gastrointestinal tract R93.3
    genitourinary organs R93.8
    head R93.0
    inconclusive due to excess body fat of
      patient R93.9
    intrathoracic organs NEC R93.1
    placenta R93.8
    retroperitoneum R93.5
    skin R93.8
    skull R93.0
    subcutaneous tissue R93.8

Findings, abnormal, inconclusive, without
  diagnosis (*Continued*)
  red blood cell (count) (morphology) (sickling)
    (volume) R71.8
  scan NEC R94.8
    bladder R94.8
    bone R94.8
    kidney R94.4
    liver R93.2
    lung R94.2
    pancreas R94.8
    placental R94.8
    spleen R94.8
    thyroid R94.6
  sedimentation rate, elevated R70.0
  SGOT R74.0
  SGPT R74.0
  sodium (deficiency) E87.1
    excess E87.0
  specified body fluid NEC R88.8
  stress test R94.39
  thyroid (function) (metabolic rate) (scan)
    (uptake) R94.6
  transaminase (level) R74.0
  triglycerides E78.9
    high E78.1
      with high cholesterol E78.2
  tuberculin skin test (without active
    tuberculosis) R76.11
  urine R82.90
    acetone R82.4
    bacteria N39.0
    bile R82.2
    casts or cells R82.99
    chyle R82.0
    culture positive R82.7
    glucose R81
    hemoglobin R82.3
    ketone R82.4
    sugar R81
  vanillylmandelic acid (VMA), elevated
    R82.5
  vectorcardiogram (VCG) R94.39
  ventriculogram R93.0
  white blood cell (count) (differential)
    (morphology) D72.9
  xerography R92.8
Finger —*see* condition
Fire, Saint Anthony's —*see* Erysipelas
Fire-setting
  pathological (compulsive) F63.1
Fish hook stomach K31.89
Fishmeal-worker's lung J67.8
Fissure, fissured
  anus, anal K60.2
    acute K60.0
    chronic K60.1
    congenital Q43.8
  ear, lobule, congenital Q17.8
  epiglottis (congenital) Q31.8
  larynx J38.7
    congenital Q31.8
  lip K13.0
    congenital —*see* Cleft, lip
  nipple N64.0
    associated with
      lactation O92.13
      pregnancy O92.11-
      puerperium O92.12
  nose Q30.2
  palate (congenital) —*see* Cleft, palate
  skin R23.4
  spine (congenital) —*see also* Spina bifida
    with hydrocephalus —*see* Spina bifida, by
      site, with hydrocephalus
  tongue (acquired) K14.5
    congenital Q38.3
Fistula (cutaneous) L98.8
  abdomen (wall) K63.2
    bladder N32.2
    intestine NEC K63.2

Fistula *(Continued)*
  abdomen *(Continued)*
    ureter N28.89
    uterus N82.5
  abdominorectal K63.2
  abdominosigmoidal K63.2
  abdominothoracic J86.0
  abdominouterine N82.5
    congenital Q51.7
  abdominovesical N32.2
  accessory sinuses —*see* Sinusitis
  actinomycotic —*see* Actinomycosis
  alveolar antrum —*see* Sinusitis, maxillary
  alveolar process K04.6
  anorectal K60.5
  antrobuccal —*see* Sinusitis, maxillary
  antrum —*see* Sinusitis, maxillary
  anus, anal (recurrent) (infectional) K60.3
    congenital Q43.6
      with absence, atresia and stenosis Q42.2
    tuberculous A18.32
  aorta-duodenal I77.2
  appendix, appendicular K38.3
  arteriovenous (acquired) (nonruptured) I77.0
    brain I67.1
      congenital Q28.2
        ruptured I60.8
      ruptured I60.8
    cerebral —*see* Fistula, arteriovenous, brain
    congenital (peripheral) —*see also*
      Malformation, arteriovenous
      brain Q28.2
        ruptured I60.8
      coronary Q24.5
      pulmonary Q25.72
    coronary I25.41
      congenital Q24.5
    pulmonary I28.0
      congenital Q25.72
    surgically created (for dialysis) Z99.2
      complication —*see* Complication,
        arteriovenous, fistula, surgically
        created
    traumatic —*see* Injury, blood vessel
  artery I77.2
  aural (mastoid) —*see* Mastoiditis, chronic
  auricle —*see also* Disorder, pinna, specified
    type NEC
    congenital Q18.1
  Bartholin's gland N82.8
  bile duct (common) (hepatic) K83.3
    with calculus, stones —*see* Calculus, bile
      duct
  biliary (tract) —*see* Fistula, bile duct
  bladder (sphincter) NEC (*see also* Fistula,
    vesico-) N32.2
    into seminal vesicle N32.2
  bone —*see also* Disorder, bone, specified type
    NEC
    with osteomyelitis, chronic —*see*
      Osteomyelitis, chronic, with draining
      sinus
  brain G93.89
    arteriovenous (acquired) I67.1
      congenital Q28.2
  branchial (cleft) Q18.0
  branchiogenous Q18.0
  breast N61
    puerperal, postpartum or gestational, due
      to mastitis (purulent) —*see* Mastitis,
      obstetric, purulent
  bronchial J86.0
  bronchocutaneous, bronchomediastinal,
    bronchopleural,
    bronchopleuromediastinal (infective)
    J86.0
    tuberculous NEC A15.5
  bronchoesophageal J86.0
    congenital Q39.2
      with atresia of esophagus Q39.1
  bronchovisceral J86.0

  buccal cavity (infective) K12.2
  cecosigmoidal K63.2
  cecum K63.2
  cerebrospinal (fluid) G96.0
  cervical, lateral Q18.1
  cervicoaural Q18.1
  cervicosigmoidal N82.4
  cervicovesical N82.1
  cervix N82.8
  chest (wall) J86.0
  cholecystenteric —*see* Fistula, gallbladder
  cholecystocolic —*see* Fistula, gallbladder
  cholecystocolonic —*see* Fistula, gallbladder
  cholecystoduodenal —*see* Fistula,
    gallbladder
  cholecystogastric —*see* Fistula, gallbladder
  cholecystointestinal —*see* Fistula,
    gallbladder
  choledochoduodenal —*see* Fistula,
    bile duct
  cholocolic K82.3
  coccyx —*see* Sinus, pilonidal
  colon K63.2
  colostomy K94.09
  common duct —*see* Fistula, bile duct
  congenital, site not listed —*see* Anomaly, by
    site
  coronary, arteriovenous I25.41
    congenital Q24.5
  costal region J86.0
  cul-de-sac, Douglas' N82.8
  cystic duct —*see also* Fistula, gallbladder
    congenital Q44.5
  dental K04.6
  diaphragm J86.0
  duodenum K31.6
  ear (external) (canal) —*see* Disorder, ear,
    external, specified type NEC
  enterocolic K63.2
  enterocutaneous K63.2
  enterouterine N82.4
    congenital Q51.7
  enterovaginal N82.4
    congenital Q52.2
    large intestine N82.3
    small intestine N82.2
  enterovesical N32.1
  epididymis N50.8
    tuberculous A18.15
  esophagobronchial J86.0
    congenital Q39.2
      with atresia of esophagus Q39.1
  esophagocutaneous K22.8
  esophagopleural-cutaneous J86.0
  esophagotracheal J86.0
    congenital Q39.2
      with atresia of esophagus Q39.1
  esophagus K22.8
    congenital Q39.2
      with atresia of esophagus Q39.1
  ethmoid —*see* Sinusitis, ethmoidal
  eyeball (cornea) (sclera) —*see* Disorder, globe,
    hypotony
  eyelid H01.8
  fallopian tube, external N82.5
  fecal K63.2
    congenital Q43.6
  from periapical abscess K04.6
  frontal sinus —*see* Sinusitis, frontal
  gallbladder K82.3
    with calculus, cholelithiasis, stones —*see*
      Calculus, gallbladder
  gastric K31.6
  gastrocolic K31.6
    congenital Q40.2
    tuberculous A18.32
  gastroenterocolic K31.6
  gastroesophageal K31.6
  gastrojejunal K31.6
  gastrojejunocolic K31.6

  genital tract (female) N82.9
    specified NEC N82.8
    to intestine NEC N82.4
    to skin N82.5
  hepatic artery-portal vein, congenital Q26.6
  hepatopleural J86.0
  hepatopulmonary J86.0
  ileorectal or ileosigmoidal K63.2
  ileovaginal N82.2
  ileovesical N32.1
  ileum K63.2
  in ano K60.3
    tuberculous A18.32
  inner ear (labyrinth) —*see* subcategory H83.1
  intestine NEC K63.2
  intestinocolonic (abdominal) K63.2
  intestinoureteral N28.89
  intestinouterine N82.4
  intestinovaginal N82.4
    large intestine N82.3
    small intestine N82.2
  intestinovesical N32.1
  ischiorectal (fossa) K61.3
  jejunum K63.2
  joint M25.10
    ankle M25.17-
    elbow M25.12-
    foot joint M25.17-
    hand joint M25.14-
    hip M25.15-
    knee M25.16-
    shoulder M25.11-
    specified joint NEC M25.18
    tuberculous —*see* Tuberculosis, joint
    vertebrae M25.18
    wrist M25.13-
  kidney N28.89
  labium (majus) (minus) N82.8
  labyrinth —*see* subcategory H83.1
  lacrimal (gland) (sac) H04.61-
  lacrimonasal duct —*see* Fistula, lacrimal
  laryngotracheal, congenital Q34.8
  larynx J38.7
  lip K13.0
    congenital Q38.0
  lumbar, tuberculous A18.01
  lung J86.0
  lymphatic I89.8
  mammary (gland) N61
  mastoid (process) (region) —*see* Mastoiditis,
    chronic
  maxillary J32.0
  medial, face and neck Q18.8
  mediastinal J86.0
  mediastinobronchial J86.0
  mediastinocutaneous J86.0
  middle ear —*see* subcategory H74.8
  mouth K12.2
  nasal J34.89
    sinus —*see* Sinusitis
  nasopharynx J39.2
  nipple N64.0
  nose J34.89
  oral (cutaneous) K12.2
    maxillary J32.0
    nasal (with cleft palate) —*see* Cleft, palate
  orbit, orbital —*see* Disorder, orbit, specified
    type NEC
  oroantral J32.0
  oviduct, external N82.5
  palate (hard) M27.8
  pancreatic K86.8
  pancreaticoduodenal K86.8
  parotid (gland) K11.4
    region K12.2
  penis N48.89
  perianal K60.3
  pericardium (pleura) (sac) —*see* Pericarditis
  pericecal K63.2
  perineorectal K60.4
  perineosigmoidal K63.2

Fistula (*Continued*)
  perineum, perineal (with urethral
      involvement) NEC N36.0
    tuberculous A18.13
    ureter N28.89
  perirectal K60.4
    tuberculous A18.32
  peritoneum K65.9
  pharyngoesophageal J39.2
  pharynx J39.2
    branchial cleft (congenital) Q18.0
  pilonidal (infected) (rectum) —*see* Sinus,
      pilonidal
  pleura, pleural, pleurocutaneous,
      pleuroperitoneal J86.0
    tuberculous NEC A15.6
  pleuropericardial I31.8
  portal vein-hepatic artery, congenital Q26.6
  postauricular H70.81-
  postoperative, persistent T81.83
    specified site —*see* Fistula, by site
  preauricular (congenital) Q18.1
  prostate N42.89
  pulmonary J86.0
    arteriovenous I28.0
      congenital Q25.72
    tuberculous —*see* Tuberculosis, pulmonary
  pulmonoperitoneal J86.0
  rectolabial N82.4
  rectosigmoid (intercommunicating) K63.2
  rectoureteral N28.89
  rectourethral N36.0
    congenital Q64.73
  rectouterine N82.4
    congenital Q51.7
  rectovaginal N82.3
    congenital Q52.2
    tuberculous A18.18
  rectovesical N32.1
    congenital Q64.79
  rectovesicovaginal N82.3
  rectovulval N82.4
    congenital Q52.79
  rectum (to skin) K60.4
    congenital Q43.6
      with absence, atresia and stenosis Q42.0
    tuberculous A18.32
  renal N28.89
  retroauricular —*see* Fistula, postauricular
  salivary duct or gland (any) K11.4
    congenital Q38.4
  scrotum (urinary) N50.8
    tuberculous A18.15
  semicircular canals —*see* subcategory H83.1
  sigmoid K63.2
    to bladder N32.1
  sinus —*see* Sinusitis
  skin L98.8
    to genital tract (female) N82.5
  splenocolic D73.89
  stercoral K63.2
  stomach K31.6
  sublingual gland K11.4
  submandibular gland K11.4
  submaxillary (gland) K11.4
    region K12.2
  thoracic J86.0
    duct I89.8
  thoracoabdominal J86.0
  thoracogastric J86.0
  thoracointestinal J86.0
  thorax J86.0
  thyroglossal duct Q89.2
  thyroid E07.89
  trachea, congenital (external) (internal) Q32.1
  tracheoesophageal J86.0
    congenital Q39.2
      with atresia of esophagus Q39.1
    following tracheostomy J95.04
  traumatic arteriovenous —*see* Injury, blood
      vessel, by site

Fistula (*Continued*)
  tuberculous - code by site under
      Tuberculosis
  typhoid A01.09
  umbilicourinary Q64.8
  urachus, congenital Q64.4
  ureter (persistent) N28.89
  ureteroabdominal N28.89
  ureterorectal N28.89
  ureterosigmoido-abdominal N28.89
  ureterovaginal N82.1
  ureterovesical N32.2
  urethra N36.0
    congenital Q64.79
    tuberculous A18.13
  urethroperineal N36.0
  urethroperineovesical N32.2
  urethrorectal N36.0
    congenital Q64.73
  urethroscrotal N50.8
  urethrovaginal N82.1
  urethrovesical N32.2
  urinary (tract) (persistent) (recurrent)
      N36.0
  uteroabdominal N82.5
    congenital Q51.7
  uteroenteric, uterointestinal N82.4
    congenital Q51.7
  uterorectal N82.4
    congenital Q51.7
  uteroureteric N82.1
  uterourethral Q51.7
  uterovaginal N82.8
  uterovesical N82.1
    congenital Q51.7
  uterus N82.8
  vagina (postpartal) (wall) N82.8
  vaginocutaneous (postpartal) N82.5
  vaginointestinal NEC N82.4
    large intestine N82.3
    small intestine N82.2
  vaginoperineal N82.5
  vasocutaneous, congenital Q55.7
  vesical NEC N32.2
  vesicoabdominal N32.2
  vesicocervicovaginal N82.1
  vesicocolic N32.1
  vesicocutaneous N32.2
  vesicoenteric N32.1
  vesicointestinal N32.1
  vesicometrorectal N82.4
  vesicoperineal N32.2
  vesicorectal N32.1
    congenital Q64.79
  vesicosigmoidal N32.1
  vesicosigmoidovaginal N82.3
  vesicoureteral N32.2
  vesicoureterovaginal N82.1
  vesicourethral N32.2
  vesicourethrorectal N32.1
  vesicouterine N82.1
    congenital Q51.7
  vesicovaginal N82.0
  vulvorectal N82.4
    congenital Q52.79
Fit R56.9
  epileptic —*see* Epilepsy
  fainting R55
  hysterical F44.5
  newborn P90
Fitting (and adjustment) (of)
  artificial
    arm —*see* Admission, adjustment, artificial,
        arm
    breast Z44.3
    eye Z44.2
    leg —*see* Admission, adjustment, artificial,
        leg
  automatic implantable cardiac defibrillator
      (with synchronous cardiac pacemaker)
      Z45.02

Fitting (*Continued*)
  brain neuropacemaker Z46.2
    implanted Z45.42
  cardiac defibrillator —*see* Fitting (and
      adjustment) (of), automatic implantable
      cardiac defibrillator
  catheter, non-vascular Z46.82
  colostomy belt Z46.89
  contact lenses Z46.0
  cystostomy device Z46.6
  defibrillator, cardiac —*see* Fitting (and
      adjustment) (of), automatic implantable
      cardiac defibrillator
  dentures Z46.3
  device NOS Z46.9
    abdominal Z46.89
    gastrointestinal NEC Z46.59
    implanted NEC Z45.89
    nervous system Z46.2
      implanted —*see* Admission, adjustment,
          device, implanted, nervous
          system
    orthodontic Z46.4
    orthoptic Z46.0
    orthotic Z46.89
    prosthetic (external) Z44.9
      breast Z44.3
      dental Z46.3
      eye Z44.2
      specified NEC Z44.8
    specified NEC Z46.89
    substitution
      auditory Z46.2
        implanted —*see* Admission,
            adjustment, device, implanted,
            hearing device
      nervous system Z46.2
        implanted —*see* Admission,
            adjustment, device, implanted,
            nervous system
      visual Z46.2
        implanted Z45.31
      urinary Z46.6
  gastric lap band Z46.51
  gastrointestinal appliance NEC Z46.59
  glasses (reading) Z46.0
  hearing aid Z46.1
  ileostomy device Z46.89
  insulin pump Z46.81
  intestinal appliance NEC Z46.89
  myringotomy device (stent) (tube) Z45.82
  neuropacemaker Z46.2
    implanted Z45.42
  non-vascular catheter Z46.82
  orthodontic device Z46.4
  orthopedic device (brace) (cast) (corset)
      (shoes) Z46.89
  pacemaker (cardiac) Z45.018
    nervous system (brain) (peripheral nerve)
        (spinal cord) Z46.2
      implanted Z45.42
    pulse generator Z45.010
  portacath (port-a-cath) Z45.2
  prosthesis (external) Z44.9
    arm —*see* Admission, adjustment, artificial,
        arm
    breast Z44.3
    dental Z46.3
    eye Z44.2
    leg —*see* Admission, adjustment, artificial,
        leg
    specified NEC Z44.8
  spectacles Z46.0
  wheelchair Z46.89
Fitzhugh-Curtis syndrome
  due to
    Chlamydia trachomatis A74.81
    Neisseria gonorrhorea (gonococcal
        peritonitis) A54.85
Fitz's syndrome (acute hemorrhagic
    pancreatitis) K85.8

Fixation
joint —*see* Ankylosis
larynx J38.7
stapes —*see* Ankylosis, ear ossicles
deafness —*see* Deafness, conductive
uterus (acquired) —*see* Malposition, uterus
vocal cord J38.3
Flabby ridge K06.8
Flaccid —*see also* condition
palate, congenital Q38.5
Flail
chest S22.5-
newborn (birth injury) P13.8
joint (paralytic) M25.20
ankle M25.27-
elbow M25.22-
foot joint M25.27-
hand joint M25.24-
hip M25.25-
knee M25.26-
shoulder M25.21-
specified joint NEC M25.28
wrist M25.23-
Flajani's disease —*see* Hyperthyroidism, with, goiter (diffuse)
Flap, liver K71.3
Flashbacks (residual to hallucinogen use) F16.283
Flat
chamber (eye) —*see* Disorder, globe, hypotony, flat anterior chamber
chest, congenital Q67.8
foot (acquired) (fixed type) (painful) (postural) —*see also* Deformity, limb, flat foot
congenital (rigid) (spastic (everted)) Q66.5-
rachitic sequelae (late effect) E64.3
organ or site, congenital NEC —*see* Anomaly, by site
pelvis M95.5
with disproportion (fetopelvic) O33.0
causing obstructed labor O65.0
congenital Q74.2
Flatau-Schilder disease G37.0
Flatback syndrome M40.30
lumbar region M40.36
lumbosacral region M40.37
thoracolumbar region M40.35
Flattening
head, femur M89.8X5
hip —*see* Coxa, plana
lip (congenital) Q18.8
nose (congenital) Q67.4
acquired M95.0
Flatulence R14.3
psychogenic F45.8
Flatus R14.3
vaginalis N89.8
Flax-dresser's disease J66.1
Flea bite —*see* Injury, bite, by site, superficial, insect
Flecks, glaucomatous (subcapsular) —*see* Cataract, complicated
Fleischer (-Kayser) ring (cornea) H18.04-
Fleshy mole O02.0
Flexibilitas cerea —*see* Catalepsy
Flexion
amputation stump (surgical) T87.89
cervix —*see* Malposition, uterus
contracture, joint —*see* Contraction, joint
deformity, joint (*see also* Deformity, limb, flexion) M21.20
hip, congenital Q65.89
uterus —*see also* Malposition, uterus
lateral —*see* Lateroversion, uterus
Flexner-Boyd dysentery A03.2
Flexner's dysentery A03.1
Flexure —*see* Flexion
Flint murmur (aortic insufficiency) I35.1
Floater, vitreous —*see* Opacity, vitreous

Floating
cartilage (joint) —*see also* Loose, body, joint
knee —*see* Derangement, knee, loose body
gallbladder, congenital Q44.1
kidney N28.89
congenital Q63.8
spleen D73.89
Flooding N92.0
Floor —*see* condition
Floppy
baby syndrome (nonspecific) P94.2
iris syndrome (intraoperative) (IFIS) H21.81
nonrheumatic mitral valve syndrome I34.1
Flu —*see also* Influenza
avian (*see also* Influenza, due to, identified novel influenza A virus) J09.X2
bird (*see also* Influenza, due to, identified novel influenza A virus) J09.X2
intestinal NEC A08.4
swine (viruses that normally cause infections in pigs) (*see also* Influenza, due to, identified novel influenza A virus) J09.X2
Fluctuating blood pressure I99.8
Fluid
abdomen R18.8
chest J94.8
heart —*see* Failure, heart, congestive
joint —*see* Effusion, joint
loss (acute) E86.9
with
hypernatremia E87.0
hyponatremia E87.1
lung —*see* Edema, lung
overload E87.70
specified NEC E87.79
peritoneal cavity R18.8
pleural cavity J94.8
retention R60.9
Flukes NEC —*see also* Infestation, fluke
blood NEC —*see* Schistosomiasis
liver B66.3
Fluor (vaginalis) N89.8
trichomonal or due to Trichomonas (vaginalis) A59.00
Fluorosis
dental K00.3
skeletal M85.10
ankle M85.17-
foot M85.17-
forearm M85.13-
hand M85.14-
lower leg M85.16-
multiple site M85.19
neck M85.18
rib M85.18
shoulder M85.11-
skull M85.18
specified site NEC M85.18
thigh M85.15-
toe M85.17-
upper arm M85.12-
vertebra M85.18
Flush syndrome E34.0
Flushing R23.2
menopausal N95.1
Flutter
atrial or auricular I48.92
atypical I48.4
type I I48.3
type II I48.4
typical I48.3
heart I49.8
atrial or auricular I48.92
atypical I48.4
type I I48.3
type II I48.4
typical I48.3
ventricular I49.02
ventricular I49.02

FNHTR (febrile nonhemolytic transfusion reaction) R50.84
Fochier's abscess - code by site under Abscess
Focus, Assmann's —*see* Tuberculosis, pulmonary
Fogo selvagem L10.3
Foix-Alajouanine syndrome G95.19
Fold, folds (anomalous) —*see also* Anomaly, by site
Descemet's membrane —*see* Change, corneal membrane, Descemet's, fold
epicanthic Q10.3
heart Q24.8
Folie à deux F24
Follicle
cervix (nabothian) (ruptured) N88.8
graafian, ruptured, with hemorrhage N83.0
nabothian N88.8
Follicular —*see* condition
Folliculitis (superficial) L73.9
abscedens et suffodiens L66.3
cyst N83.0
decalvans L66.2
deep —*see* Furuncle, by site
gonococcal (acute) (chronic) A54.01
keloid, keloidalis L73.0
pustular L01.02
ulerythematosa reticulata L66.4
Folliculome lipidique
specified site —*see* Neoplasm, benign, by site
unspecified site
female D27.9
male D29.20
Følling's disease E70.0
Follow-up —*see* Examination, follow-up
Fong's syndrome (hereditary osteo-onychodysplasia) Q78.5
Food
allergy L27.2
asphyxia (from aspiration or inhalation) —*see* Foreign body, by site
choked on —*see* Foreign body, by site
deprivation T73.0
specified kind of food NEC E63.8
intoxication —*see* Poisoning, food
lack of T73.0
poisoning —*see* Poisoning, food
rejection NEC —*see* Disorder, eating
strangulation or suffocation —*see* Foreign body, by site
toxemia —*see* Poisoning, food
Foot —*see* condition
Foramen ovale (nonclosure) (patent) (persistent) Q21.1
Forbes' glycogen storage disease E74.03
Fordyce-Fox disease L75.2
Fordyce's disease (mouth) Q38.6
Forearm —*see* condition
Foreign body
with
laceration —*see* Laceration, by site, with foreign body
puncture wound —*see* Puncture, by site, with foreign body
accidentally left following a procedure T81.509
aspiration T81.506
resulting in
adhesions T81.516
obstruction T81.526
perforation T81.536
specified complication NEC T81.596
cardiac catheterization T81.505
resulting in
acute reaction T81.60
aseptic peritonitis T81.61
specified NEC T81.69
adhesions T81.515
obstruction T81.525
perforation T81.535
specified complication NEC T81.595

Foreign body *(Continued)*
  accidentally left following a procedure
    (Continued)
    causing
      acute reaction T81.60
        aseptic peritonitis T81.61
        specified complication NEC T81.69
      adhesions T81.519
      aseptic peritonitis T81.61
      obstruction T81.529
      perforation T81.539
      specified complication NEC T81.599
    endoscopy T81.504
      resulting in
        adhesions T81.514
        obstruction T81.524
        perforation T81.534
        specified complication NEC T81.594
    immunization T81.503
      resulting in
        adhesions T81.513
        obstruction T81.523
        perforation T81.533
        specified complication NEC T81.593
    infusion T81.501
      resulting in
        adhesions T81.511
        obstruction T81.521
        perforation T81.531
        specified complication NEC T81.591
    injection T81.503
      resulting in
        adhesions T81.513
        obstruction T81.523
        perforation T81.533
        specified complication NEC T81.593
    kidney dialysis T81.502
      resulting in
        adhesions T81.512
        obstruction T81.522
        perforation T81.532
        specified complication NEC T81.592
    packing removal T81.507
      resulting in
        acute reaction T81.60
          aseptic peritonitis T81.61
          specified NEC T81.69
        adhesions T81.517
        obstruction T81.527
        perforation T81.537
        specified complication NEC T81.597
    puncture T81.506
      resulting in
        adhesions T81.516
        obstruction T81.526
        perforation T81.536
        specified complication NEC T81.596
    specified procedure NEC T81.508
      resulting in
        acute reaction T81.60
          aseptic peritonitis T81.61
          specified NEC T81.69
        adhesions T81.518
        obstruction T81.528
        perforation T81.538
        specified complication NEC T81.598
    surgical operation T81.500
      resulting in
        acute reaction T81.60
          aseptic peritonitis T81.61
          specified NEC T81.69
        adhesions T81.510
        obstruction T81.520
        perforation T81.530
        specified complication NEC T81.590
    transfusion T81.501
      resulting in
        adhesions T81.511
        obstruction T81.521
        perforation T81.531
        specified complication NEC T81.591

Foreign body *(Continued)*
  alimentary tract T18.9
    anus T18.5
    colon T18.4
    esophagus —*see* Foreign body, esophagus
    mouth T18.0
    multiple sites T18.8
    rectosigmoid (junction) T18.5
    rectum T18.5
    small intestine T18.3
    specified site NEC T18.8
    stomach T18.2
  anterior chamber (eye) S05.5-
  auditory canal —*see* Foreign body, entering
    through orifice, ear
  bronchus T17.508
    causing
      asphyxiation T17.500
        food (bone) (seed) T17.520
        gastric contents (vomitus) T17.510
        specified type NEC T17.590
      injury NEC T17.508
        food (bone) (seed) T17.528
        gastric contents (vomitus) T17.518
        specified type NEC T17.598
  canthus —*see* Foreign body, conjunctival sac
  ciliary body (eye) S05.5-
  conjunctival sac T15.1-
  cornea T15.0-
  entering through orifice
    accessory sinus T17.0
    alimentary canal T18.9
      multiple parts T18.8
      specified part NEC T18.8
    alveolar process T18.0
    antrum (Highmore's) T17.0
    anus T18.5
    appendix T18.4
    auditory canal —*see* Foreign body, entering
      through orifice, ear
    auricle —*see* Foreign body, entering
      through orifice, ear
    bladder T19.1
    bronchioles —*see* Foreign body, respiratory
      tract, specified site NEC
    bronchus (main) —*see* Foreign body,
      bronchus
    buccal cavity T18.0
    canthus (inner) —*see* Foreign body,
      conjunctival sac
    cecum T18.4
    cervix (canal) (uteri) T19.3
    colon T18.4
    conjunctival sac —*see* Foreign body,
      conjunctival sac
    cornea —*see* Foreign body, cornea
    digestive organ or tract NOS T18.9
      multiple parts T18.8
      specified part NEC T18.8
    duodenum T18.3
    ear (external) T16.-
    esophagus —*see* Foreign body, esophagus
    eye (external) NOS T15.9-
      conjunctival sac —*see* Foreign body,
        conjunctival sac
      cornea —*see* Foreign body, cornea
      specified part NEC T15.8-
    eyeball —*see also* Foreign body, entering
      through orifice, eye, specified part
      NEC
      with penetrating wound —*see* Puncture,
        eyeball
    eyelid —*see also* Foreign body, conjunctival
      sac
      with
        laceration —*see* Laceration, eyelid,
          with foreign body
        puncture —*see* Puncture, eyelid, with
          foreign body
        superficial injury —*see* Foreign body,
          superficial, eyelid

Foreign body *(Continued)*
  entering through orifice *(Continued)*
    gastrointestinal tract T18.9
      multiple parts T18.8
      specified part NEC T18.8
    genitourinary tract T19.9
      multiple parts T19.8
      specified part NEC T19.8
    globe —*see* Foreign body, entering through
      orifice, eyeball
    gum T18.0
    Highmore's antrum T17.0
    hypopharynx —*see* Foreign body, pharynx
    ileum T18.3
    intestine (small) T18.3
      large T18.4
    lacrimal apparatus (punctum) —*see*
      Foreign body, entering through
      orifice, eye, specified part NEC
    large intestine T18.4
    larynx —*see* Foreign body, larynx
    lung —*see* Foreign body, respiratory tract,
      specified site NEC
    maxillary sinus T17.0
    mouth T18.0
    nasal sinus T17.0
    nasopharynx —*see* Foreign body, pharynx
    nose (passage) T17.1
    nostril T17.1
    oral cavity T18.0
    palate T18.0
    penis T19.4
    pharynx —*see* Foreign body, pharynx
    piriform sinus —*see* Foreign body, pharynx
    rectosigmoid (junction) T18.5
    rectum T18.5
    respiratory tract —*see* Foreign body,
      respiratory tract
    sinus (accessory) (frontal) (maxillary)
      (nasal) T17.0
      piriform —*see* Foreign body, pharynx
    small intestine T18.3
    stomach T18.2
    suffocation by —*see* Foreign body, by site
    tear ducts or glands —*see* Foreign body,
      entering through orifice, eye,
      specified part NEC
    throat —*see* Foreign body, pharynx
    tongue T18.0
    tonsil, tonsillar (fossa) —*see* Foreign body,
      pharynx
    trachea —*see* Foreign body, trachea
    ureter T19.8
    urethra T19.0
    uterus (any part) T19.3
    vagina T19.2
    vulva T19.2
  esophagus T18.108
    causing
      injury NEC T18.108
        food (bone) (seed) T18.128
        gastric contents (vomitus) T18.118
        specified type NEC T18.198
      tracheal compression T18.100
        food (bone) (seed) T18.120
        gastric contents (vomitus) T18.110
        specified type NEC T18.190
  felling of, in throat R09.89
  fragment —*see* Retained, foreign body
    fragments (type of)
  genitourinary tract T19.9
    bladder T19.1
    multiple parts T19.8
    penis T19.4
    specified site NEC T19.8
    urethra T19.0
    uterus T19.3
      IUD Z97.5
    vagina T19.2
      contraceptive device Z97.5
    vulva T19.2

◀ New   ◀▥ Revised   ~~deleted~~ Deleted

Foreign body (Continued)
  granuloma (old) (soft tissue) —see also
    Granuloma, foreign body
    skin L92.3
  in
    laceration —see Laceration, by site, with
      foreign body
    puncture wound —see Puncture, by site,
      with foreign body
    soft tissue (residual) M79.5
  inadvertently left in operation wound —see
    Foreign body, accidentally left during a
    procedure
  ingestion, ingested NOS T18.9
  inhalation or inspiration —see Foreign body,
    by site
  internal organ, not entering through a natural
    orifice - code as specific injury with
    foreign body
  intraocular S05.5-
    old, retained (nonmagnetic) H44.70-
      anterior chamber H44.71-
      ciliary body H44.72-
      iris H44.72-
      lens H44.73-
      magnetic H44.60-
        anterior chamber H44.61-
        ciliary body H44.62-
        iris H44.62-
        lens H44.63-
        posterior wall H44.64-
        specified site NEC H44.69-
        vitreous body H44.65-
      posterior wall H44.74-
      specified site NEC H44.79-
      vitreous body H44.75-
    iris —see Foreign body, intraocular
  lacrimal punctum —see Foreign body,
    entering through orifice, eye, specified
    part NEC
  larynx T17.308
    causing
      asphyxiation T17.300
        food (bone) (seed) T17.320
        gastric contents (vomitus) T17.310
        specified type NEC T17.390
      injury NEC T17.308
        food (bone) (seed) T17.328
        gastric contents (vomitus) T17.318
        specified type NEC T17.398
  lens —see Foreign body, intraocular
  ocular muscle S05.4-
    old, retained —see Foreign body, orbit, old
  old or residual
    soft tissue (residual) M79.5
  operation wound, left accidentally —see
    Foreign body, accidentally left during a
    procedure
  orbit S05.4-
    old, retained H05.5-
  pharynx T17.208
    causing
      asphyxiation T17.200
        food (bone) (seed) T17.220
        gastric contents (vomitus)
          T17.210
        specified type NEC T17.290
      injury NEC T17.208
        food (bone) (seed) T17.228
        gastric contents (vomitus)
          T17.218
        specified type NEC T17.298
  respiratory tract T17.908
    bronchioles —see Foreign body, respiratory
      tract, specified site NEC
    bronchus —see Foreign body, bronchus
    causing
      asphyxiation T17.900
        food (bone) (seed) T17.920
        gastric contents (vomitus) T17.910
        specified type NEC T17.990

Foreign body (Continued)
  respiratory tract (Continued)
    causing (Continued)
      injury NEC T17.908
        food (bone) (seed) T17.928
        gastric contents (vomitus) T17.918
        specified type NEC T17.998
    larynx —see Foreign body, larynx
    lung —see Foreign body, respiratory tract,
      specified site NEC
    multiple parts —see Foreign body,
      respiratory tract, specified site NEC
    nasal sinus T17.0
    nasopharynx —see Foreign body, pharynx
    nose T17.1
    nostril T17.1
    pharynx —see Foreign body, pharynx
    specified site NEC T17.808
      causing
        asphyxiation T17.800
          food (bone) (seed) T17.820
          gastric contents (vomitus)
            T17.810
          specified type NEC T17.890
        injury NEC T17.808
          food (bone) (seed) T17.828
          gastric contents (vomitus)
            T17.818
          specified type NEC T17.898
    throat —see Foreign body, pharynx
    trachea —see Foreign body, trachea
  retained (old) (nonmagnetic) (in)
    anterior chamber (eye) —see Foreign body,
      intraocular, old, retained, anterior
      chamber
      magnetic —see Foreign body, intraocular,
        old, retained, magnetic, anterior
        chamber
    ciliary body —see Foreign body,
      intraocular, old, retained, ciliary
      body
      magnetic —see Foreign body, intraocular,
        old, retained, magnetic, ciliary
        body
    eyelid H02.819
      left H02.816
        lower H02.815
        upper H02.814
      right H02.813
        lower H02.812
        upper H02.811
    fragments —see Retained, foreign body
      fragments (type of)
    globe —see Foreign body, intraocular, old,
      retained
      magnetic —see Foreign body, intraocular,
        old, retained, magnetic
    intraocular —see Foreign body, intraocular,
      old, retained
      magnetic —see Foreign body, intraocular,
        old, retained, magnetic
    iris —see Foreign body, intraocular, old,
      retained, iris
      magnetic —see Foreign body, intraocular,
        old, retained, magnetic, iris
    lens —see Foreign body, intraocular, old,
      retained, lens
      magnetic —see Foreign body, intraocular,
        old, retained, magnetic, lens
    muscle —see Foreign body, retained, soft
      tissue
    orbit —see Foreign body, orbit, old
    posterior wall of globe —see Foreign body,
      intraocular, old, retained, posterior
      wall
      magnetic —see Foreign body, intraocular,
        old, retained, magnetic, posterior
        wall
    retrobulbar —see Foreign body, orbit, old,
      retrobulbar
    soft tissue M79.5

Foreign body (Continued)
  retained (Continued)
    vitreous —see Foreign body, intraocular,
      old, retained, vitreous body
      magnetic —see Foreign body, intraocular,
        old, retained, magnetic, vitreous
        body
  retina S05.5-
  superficial, without open wound
    abdomen, abdominal (wall) S30.851
    alveolar process S00.552
    ankle S90.55-
    antecubital space —see Foreign body,
      superficial, forearm
    anus S30.857
    arm (upper) S40.85-
    auditory canal —see Foreign body,
      superficial, ear
    auricle —see Foreign body, superficial, ear
    axilla —see Foreign body, superficial, arm
    back, lower S30.850
    breast S20.15-
    brow S00.85
    buttock S30.850
    calf —see Foreign body, superficial, leg
    canthus —see Foreign body, superficial,
      eyelid
    cheek S00.85
      internal S00.552
    chest wall —see Foreign body, superficial,
      thorax
    chin S00.85
    clitoris S30.854
    costal region —see Foreign body,
      superficial, thorax
    digit (s)
      foot —see Foreign body, superficial, toe
      hand —see Foreign body, superficial,
        finger
    ear S00.45-
    elbow S50.35-
    epididymis S30.853
    epigastric region S30.851
    epiglottis S10.15
    esophagus, cervical S10.15
    eyebrow —see Foreign body, superficial,
      eyelid
    eyelid S00.25-
    face S00.85
    finger (s) S60.459
      index S60.45-
      little S60.45-
      middle S60.45-
      ring S60.45-
    flank S30.851
    foot (except toe (s) alone) S90.85-
      toe —see Foreign body, superficial, toe
    forearm S50.85-
      elbow only —see Foreign body,
        superficial, elbow
    forehead S00.85
    genital organs, external
      female S30.856
      male S30.855
    groin S30.851
    gum S00.552
    hand S60.55-
    head S00.95
      ear —see Foreign body, superficial, ear
      eyelid —see Foreign body, superficial,
        eyelid
      lip S00.551
      nose S00.35
      oral cavity S00.552
      scalp S00.05
      specified site NEC S00.85
    heel —see Foreign body, superficial, foot
    hip S70.25-
    inguinal region S30.851
    interscapular region S20.459
    jaw S00.85

◀ New   ◀‖‖ Revised   ~~deleted~~ Deleted

Foreign body *(Continued)*
  superficial, without open wound *(Continued)*
    knee S80.25-
    labium (majus) (minus) S30.854
    larynx S10.15
    leg (lower) S80.85-
      knee —*see* Foreign body, superficial, knee
      upper —*see* Foreign body, superficial, thigh
    lip S00.551
    lower back S30.850
    lumbar region S30.850
    malar region S00.85
    mammary —*see* Foreign body, superficial, breast
    mastoid region S00.85
    mouth S00.552
    nail
      finger —*see* Foreign body, superficial, finger
      toe —*see* Foreign body, superficial, toe
    nape S10.85
    nasal S00.35
    neck S10.95
      specified site NEC S10.85
      throat S10.15
    nose S00.35
    occipital region S00.05
    oral cavity S00.552
    orbital region —*see* Foreign body, superficial, eyelid
    palate S00.552
    palm —*see* Foreign body, superficial, hand
    parietal region S00.05
    pelvis S30.850
    penis S30.852
    perineum
      female S30.854
      male S30.850
    periocular area —*see* Foreign body, superficial, eyelid
    phalanges
      finger —*see* Foreign body, superficial, finger
      toe —*see* Foreign body, superficial, toe
    pharynx S10.15
    pinna —*see* Foreign body, superficial, ear
    popliteal space —*see* Foreign body, superficial, knee
    prepuce S30.852
    pubic region S30.850
    pudendum
      female S30.856
      male S30.855
    sacral region S30.850
    scalp S00.05
    scapular region —*see* Foreign body, superficial, shoulder
    scrotum S30.853
    shin —*see* Foreign body, superficial, leg
    shoulder S40.25-
    sternal region S20.359
    submaxillary region S00.85
    submental region S00.85
    subungual
      finger (s) —*see* Foreign body, superficial, finger
      toe (s) —*see* Foreign body, superficial, toe
    supraclavicular fossa S10.85
    supraorbital S00.85
    temple S00.85
    temporal region S00.85
    testis S30.853
    thigh S70.35-
    thorax, thoracic (wall) S20.95
      back S20.45-
      front S20.35-
    throat S10.15
    thumb S60.35-

Foreign body *(Continued)*
  superficial, without open wound *(Continued)*
    toe (s) (lesser) S90.456
      great S90.45-
    tongue S00.552
    trachea S10.15
    tunica vaginalis S30.853
    tympanum, tympanic membrane —*see* Foreign body, superficial, ear
    uvula S00.552
    vagina S30.854
    vocal cords S10.15
    vulva S30.854
    wrist S60.85-
  swallowed T18.9
  trachea T17.408
    causing
      asphyxiation T17.400
        food (bone) (seed) T17.420
        gastric contents (vomitus) T17.410
        specified type NEC T17.490
      injury NEC T17.408
        food (bone) (seed) T17.428
        gastric contents (vomitus) T17.418
        specified type NEC T17.498
  type of fragment —*see* Retained, foreign body fragments (type of)
  vitreous (humor) S05.5-
Forestier's disease (rhizomelic pseudopolyarthritis) M35.3-
  meaning ankylosing hyperostosis —*see* Hyperostosis, ankylosing
Formation
  hyalin in cornea —*see* Degeneration, cornea
  sequestrum in bone (due to infection) —*see* Osteomyelitis, chronic
  valve
    colon, congenital Q43.8
    ureter (congenital) Q62.39
Formication R20.2
Fort Bragg fever A27.89
Fossa —*see also* condition
  pyriform —*see* condition
Foster-Kennedy syndrome H47.14-
Fothergill's
  disease (trigeminal neuralgia) —*see also* Neuralgia, trigeminal
    scarlatina anginosa A38.9
Foul breath R19.6
Foundling Z76.1
Fournier disease or gangrene N49.3
  female N76.89
Fourth
  cranial nerve —*see* condition
  molar K00.1
Foville's (peduncular) disease or syndrome G46.3
Fox (-Fordyce) disease (apocrine miliaria) L75.2
Fracture, burst —*see* Fracture, traumatic, by site
Fracture, chronic —*see* Fracture, pathological
Fracture, insufficiency —*see* Fracture, pathologic, by site
Fracture, pathological (pathologic) —*see also* Fracture, traumatic M84.40
  ankle M84.47-
  carpus M84.44-
  clavicle M84.41-
  dental implant M27.63
  dental restorative material K08.539
    with loss of material K08.531
    without loss of material K08.530
  due to
    neoplastic disease NEC (*see also* Neoplasm) M84.50
      ankle M84.57-
      carpus M84.54-
      clavicle M84.51-
      femur M84.55-
      fibula M84.56-
      finger M84.54-
      hip M84.559

Fracture, pathological *(Continued)*
  due to *(Continued)*
    neoplastic disease NEC *(Continued)*
      humerus M84.52-
      ilium M84.550
      ischium M84.550
      metacarpus M84.54-
      metatarsus M84.57-
      neck M84.58
      pelvis M84.550
      radius M84.53-
      rib M84.58
      scapula M84.51-
      skull M84.58
      specified site NEC M84.58
      tarsus M84.57-
      tibia M84.56-
      toe M84.57-
      ulna M84.53-
      vertebra M84.58
    osteoporosis M80.80
      disuse —*see* Osteoporosis, specified type NEC, with pathological fracture
      drug-induced —*see* Osteoporosis, drug induced, with pathological fracture
      idiopathic —*see* Osteoporosis, specified type NEC, with pathological fracture
      postmenopausal —*see* Osteoporosis, postmenopausal, with pathological fracture
      postoophorectomy —*see* Osteoporosis, postoophorectomy, with pathological fracture
      postsurgical malabsorption —*see* Osteoporosis, specified type NEC, with pathological fracture
      specified cause NEC —*see* Osteoporosis, specified type NEC, with pathological fracture
    specified disease NEC M84.60
      ankle M84.67-
      carpus M84.64-
      clavicle M84.61-
      femur M84.65-
      fibula M84.66-
      finger M84.64-
      hip M84.65-
      humerus M84.62-
      ilium M84.650
      ischium M84.650
      metacarpus M84.64-
      metatarsus M84.67-
      neck M84.68
      radius M84.63-
      rib M84.68
      scapula M84.61-
      skull M84.68
      tarsus M84.67-
      tibia M84.66-
      toe M84.67-
      ulna M84.63-
      vertebra M84.68
  femur M84.45-
  fibula M84.46-
  finger M84.44-
  hip M84.459
  humerus M84.42-
  ilium M84.454
  ischium M84.454
  joint prosthesis —*see* Complications, joint prosthesis, mechanical, breakdown, by site
  periprosthetic —*see* Complications, joint prosthesis, mechanical, periprosthesis, fracture, by site
  metacarpus M84.44-
  metatarsus M84.47-
  neck M84.48
  pelvis M84.454
  radius M84.43-

Fracture, pathological *(Continued)*
  restorative material (dental) K08.539
    with loss of material K08.531
    without loss of material K08.530
  rib M84.48
  scapula M84.41-
  skull M84.48
  tarsus M84.47-
  tibia M84.46-
  toe M84.47-
  ulna M84.43-
  vertebra M84.48
Fracture, traumatic (abduction) (adduction)
    (separation) *(see also* Fracture,
    pathological) T14.8
  acetabulum S32.40-
    column
      anterior (displaced) (iliopubic) S32.43-
        nondisplaced S32.436
      posterior (displaced) (ilioischial) S32.443
        nondisplaced S32.44-
    dome (displaced) S32.48-
      nondisplaced S32.48
    specified NEC S32.49-
    transverse (displaced) S32.45-
      with associated posterior wall fracture
        (displaced) S32.46-
        nondisplaced S32.46-
      nondisplaced S32.45-
    wall
      anterior (displaced) S32.41-
        nondisplaced S32.41-
      medial (displaced) S32.47-
        nondisplaced S32.47-
      posterior (displaced) S32.42-
        with associated transverse fracture
          (displaced) S32.46-
          nondisplaced S32.46-
        nondisplaced S32.42-
  acromion *—see* Fracture, scapula, acromial
      process
  ankle S82.899
    bimalleolar (displaced) S82.84-
      nondisplaced S82.84-
    lateral malleolus only (displaced) S82.6-
      nondisplaced S82.6-
    medial malleolus (displaced) S82.5-
      associated with Maisonneuve's
        fracture *—see* Fracture,
        Maisonneuve's
      nondisplaced S82.5-
    talus *—see* Fracture, tarsal, talus
    trimalleolar (displaced) S82.85-
      nondisplaced S82.85-
  arm (upper) *—see also* Fracture, humerus,
      shaft
    humerus *—see* Fracture, humerus
    radius *—see* Fracture, radius
    ulna *—see* Fracture, ulna
  astragalus *—see* Fracture, tarsal, talus
  atlas *—see* Fracture, neck, cervical vertebra,
      first
  axis *—see* Fracture, neck, cervical vertebra,
      second
  back *—see* Fracture, vertebra
  Barton's *—see* Barton's fracture
  base of skull *—see* Fracture, skull, base
  basicervical (basal) (femoral) S72.0
  Bennett's *—see* Bennett's fracture
  bimalleolar *—see* Fracture, ankle, bimalleolar
  blow-out S02.3
  bone NEC T14.8
    birth injury P13.9
    following insertion of orthopedic implant,
        joint prosthesis or bone plate *—see*
        Fracture, following insertion of
        orthopedic implant, joint prosthesis
        or bone plate
    in (due to) neoplastic disease NEC *—see*
        Fracture, pathological, due to,
        neoplastic disease

Fracture, traumatic *(Continued)*
  bone NEC *(Continued)*
    pathological (cause unknown) *—see*
        Fracture, pathological
  breast bone *—see* Fracture, sternum
  bucket handle (semilunar cartilage) *—see*
      Tear, meniscus
  burst *—see* Fracture, traumatic, by site
  calcaneus *—see* Fracture, tarsal, calcaneus
  carpal bone (s) S62.10-
    capitate (displaced) S62.13-
      nondisplaced S62.13-
    cuneiform *—see* Fracture, carpal bone,
        triquetrum
    hamate (body) (displaced) S62.143
      hook process (displaced) S62.15-
        nondisplaced S62.15-
      nondisplaced S62.14-
    larger multangular *—see* Fracture, carpal
        bones, trapezium
    lunate (displaced) S62.12-
      nondisplaced S62.12-
    navicular S62.00-
      distal pole (displaced) S62.01-
        nondisplaced S62.01-
      middle third (displaced) S62.02-
        nondisplaced S62.02-
      proximal third (displaced) S62.03-
        nondisplaced S62.03-
      volar tuberosity *—see* Fracture, carpal
          bones, navicular, distal pole
    os magnum *—see* Fracture, carpal bones,
        capitate
    pisiform (displaced) S62.16-
      nondisplaced S62.16-
    semilunar *—see* Fracture, carpal bones,
        lunate
    smaller multangular *—see* Fracture, carpal
        bones, trapezoid
    trapezium (displaced) S62.17-
      nondisplaced S62.17-
    trapezoid (displaced) S62.18-
      nondisplaced S62.18-
    triquetrum (displaced) S62.11-
      nondisplaced S62.11-
    unciform *—see* Fracture, carpal bones,
        hamate
  cervical *—see* Fracture, vertebra, cervical
  clavicle S42.00-
    acromial end (displaced) S42.03-
      nondisplaced S42.03-
    birth injury P13.4
    lateral end *—see* Fracture, clavicle, acromial
        end
    shaft (displaced) S42.02-
      nondisplaced S42.02-
    sternal end (anterior) (displaced) S42.01-
      nondisplaced S42.01-
      posterior S42.01-
  coccyx S32.2
  collapsed *—see* Collapse, vertebra
  collar bone *—see* Fracture, clavicle
  Colles' *—see* Colles' fracture
  compression, not due to trauma *—see*
      Collapse, vertebra
  coronoid process *—see* Fracture, ulna, upper
      end, coronoid process
  corpus cavernosum penis S39.840
  costochondral cartilage S23.41
  costochondral, costosternal junction *—see*
      Fracture, rib
  cranium *—see* Fracture, skull
  cricoid cartilage S12.8
  cuboid (ankle) *—see* Fracture, tarsal, cuboid
  cuneiform
    foot *—see* Fracture, tarsal, cuneiform
    wrist *—see* Fracture, carpal, triquetrum
  delayed union *—see* Delay, union, fracture
  dental restorative material K08.539
    with loss of material K08.531
    without loss of material K08.530

Fracture, traumatic *(Continued)*
  due to
    birth injury *—see* Birth, injury,
        fracture
    osteoporosis *—see* Osteoporosis,
        with fracture
  Dupuytren's *—see* Fracture, ankle, lateral
      malleolus
  elbow S42.40-
  ethmoid (bone) (sinus) *—see* Fracture, skull,
      base
  face bone S02.92
  fatigue *—see also* Fracture, stress
    vertebra M48.40
      cervical region M48.42
      cervicothoracic region M48.43
      lumbar region M48.46
      lumbosacral region M48.47
      occipito-atlanto-axial region M48.41
      sacrococcygeal region M48.48
      thoracic region M48.44
      thoracolumbar region M48.45
  femur, femoral S72.9-
    basicervical (basal) S72.0
    birth injury P13.2
    capital epiphyseal S79.01-
    condyles, epicondyles *—see* Fracture,
        femur, lower end
    distal end *—see* Fracture, femur,
        lower end
    epiphysis
      head *—see* Fracture, femur, upper end,
          epiphysis
      lower *—see* Fracture, femur, lower end,
          epiphysis
      upper *—see* Fracture, femur, upper end,
          epiphysis
    following insertion of implant, prosthesis
        or plate M96.66-
    head *—see* Fracture, femur, upper end,
        head
    intertrochanteric *—see* Fracture, femur,
        trochanteric
    intratrochanteric *—see* Fracture, femur,
        trochanteric
    lower end S72.40-
      condyle (displaced) S72.41-
        lateral (displaced) S72.42-
          nondisplaced S72.42-
        medial (displaced) S72.43-
          nondisplaced S72.43-
        nondisplaced S72.41-
      epiphysis (displaced) S72.44-
        nondisplaced S72.44-
      physeal S79.10-
        Salter-Harris
          Type I S79.11-
          Type II S79.12-
          Type III S79.13-
          Type IV S79.14-
        specified NEC S79.19-
      specified NEC S72.49-
      supracondylar (displaced) S72.45-
        with intracondylar extension
            (displaced) S72.46-
          nondisplaced S72.46-
        nondisplaced S72.45-
      torus S72.47-
    neck *—see* Fracture, femur, upper end,
        neck
    pertrochanteric *—see* Fracture, femur,
        trochanteric
    shaft (lower third) (middle third) (upper
        third) S72.30-
      comminuted (displaced) S72.35-
        nondisplaced S72.35-
      oblique (displaced) S72.33-
        nondisplaced S72.33-
      segmental (displaced) S72.36-
        nondisplaced S72.36-
      specified NEC S72.39-

◀ New   ◀▥ Revised   ~~deleted~~ Deleted

Fracture, traumatic *(Continued)*
femur, femoral *(Continued)*
shaft *(Continued)*
spiral (displaced) S72.34-
nondisplaced S72.34-
transverse (displaced) S72.32-
nondisplaced S72.32-
specified site NEC —*see* subcategory S72.8
subcapital (displaced) S72.01-
subtrochanteric (region) (section)
(displaced) S72.2-
nondisplaced S72.2-
transcervical —*see* Fracture, femur, upper
end, neck
transtrochanteric —*see* Fracture, femur,
trochanteric
trochanteric S72.10-
apophyseal (displaced) S72.13-
nondisplaced S72.13-
greater trochanter (displaced) S72.11-
nondisplaced S72.11-
intertrochanteric (displaced) S72.14-
nondisplaced S72.14-
lesser trochanter (displaced) S72.12-
nondisplaced S72.12-
upper end S72.00-
apophyseal (displaced) S72.13-
nondisplaced S72.13-
cervicotrochanteric —*see* Fracture,
femur, upper end, neck, base
epiphysis (displaced) S72.02-
nondisplaced S72.02-
head S72.05-
articular (displaced) S72.06-
nondisplaced S72.06-
specified NEC S72.09-
intertrochanteric (displaced) S72.14-
nondisplaced S72.14-
intracapsular S72.01-
midcervical (displaced) S72.03-
nondisplaced S72.03-
neck S72.00-
base (displaced) S72.04-
nondisplaced S72.04-
specified NEC S72.09-
pertrochanteric —*see* Fracture, femur,
upper end, trochanteric
physeal S79.00-
Salter-Harris type I S79.01-
specified NEC S79.09-
subcapital (displaced) S72.01-
subtrochanteric (displaced) S72.2-
nondisplaced S72.2-
transcervical —*see* Fracture, femur,
upper end, midcervical
trochanteric S72.10-
greater (displaced) S72.11-
nondisplaced S72.11-
lesser (displaced) S72.12-
nondisplaced S72.12-
fibula (shaft) (styloid) S82.40-
comminuted (displaced) S82.45-
nondisplaced S82.45-
following insertion of implant, prosthesis
or plate M96.67-
involving ankle or malleolus —*see*
Fracture, fibula, lateral malleolus
lateral malleolus (displaced) S82.6-
nondisplaced S82.6-
lower end
physeal S89.30-
Salter-Harris
Type I S89.31-
Type II S89.32-
specified NEC S89.39-
specified NEC S82.83-
torus S82.82-
oblique (displaced) S82.43-
nondisplaced S82.43-
segmental (displaced) S82.46-
nondisplaced S82.46-

Fracture, traumatic *(Continued)*
fibula *(Continued)*
specified NEC S82.49-
spiral (displaced) S82.44-
nondisplaced S82.44-
transverse (displaced) S82.42-
nondisplaced S82.42-
upper end
physeal S89.20-
Salter-Harris
Type I S89.21-
Type II S89.22-
specified NEC S89.29-
specified NEC S82.83-
torus S82.81-
finger (except thumb) S62.60-
distal phalanx (displaced) S62.63-
nondisplaced S62.66-
index S62.60-
distal phalanx (displaced) S62.63-
nondisplaced S62.66-
medial phalanx (displaced) S62.62-
nondisplaced S62.65-
proximal phalanx (displaced) S62.61-
nondisplaced S62.64-
little S62.60-
distal phalanx (displaced) S62.63-
nondisplaced S62.66-
medial phalanx (displaced) S62.62-
nondisplaced S62.65-
proximal phalanx (displaced) S62.61-
nondisplaced S62.64-
medial phalanx (displaced) S62.62-
nondisplaced S62.65-
middle S62.60-
distal phalanx (displaced) S62.63-
nondisplaced S62.66-
medial phalanx (displaced) S62.62-
nondisplaced S62.65-
proximal phalanx (displaced) S62.61-
nondisplaced S62.64-
proximal phalanx (displaced) S62.61-
nondisplaced S62.64-
ring S62.60-
distal phalanx (displaced) S62.63-
nondisplaced S62.66-
medial phalanx (displaced) S62.62-
nondisplaced S62.65-
proximal phalanx (displaced) S62.61-
nondisplaced S62.64-
thumb —*see* Fracture, thumb
following insertion (intraoperative)
(postoperative) of orthopedic implant,
joint prosthesis or bone plate M96.69
femur M96.66-
fibula M96.67-
humerus M96.62-
pelvis M96.65
radius M96.63-
specified bone NEC M96.69
tibia M96.67-
ulna M96.63-
foot S92.90-
astragalus —*see* Fracture, tarsal, talus
calcaneus —*see* Fracture, tarsal, calcaneus
cuboid —*see* Fracture, tarsal, cuboid
cuneiform —*see* Fracture, tarsal, cuneiform
metatarsal —*see* Fracture, metatarsal
navicular —*see* Fracture, tarsal, navicular
talus —*see* Fracture, tarsal, talus
tarsal —*see* Fracture, tarsal
toe —*see* Fracture, toe
forearm S52.9-
radius —*see* Fracture, radius
ulna —*see* Fracture, ulna
fossa (anterior) (middle) (posterior) S02.19
frontal (bone) (skull) S02.0
sinus S02.19
glenoid (cavity) (scapula) —*see* Fracture,
scapula, glenoid cavity
greenstick —*see* Fracture, by site

Fracture, traumatic *(Continued)*
hallux —*see* Fracture, toe, great
hand S62.9-
carpal —*see* Fracture, carpal bone
finger (except thumb) —*see* Fracture, finger
metacarpal —*see* Fracture, metacarpal
navicular (scaphoid) (hand) —*see* Fracture,
carpal bone, navicular
thumb —*see* Fracture, thumb
healed or old
with complications - code by Nature of the
complication
heel bone —*see* Fracture, tarsal, calcaneus
Hill-Sachs S42.29-
hip —*see* Fracture, femur, neck
humerus S42.30-
anatomical neck —*see* Fracture, humerus,
upper end
articular process —*see* Fracture, humerus,
lower end
capitellum —*see* Fracture, humerus, lower
end, condyle, lateral
distal end —*see* Fracture, humerus, lower
end
epiphysis
lower —*see* Fracture, humerus, lower
end, physeal
upper —*see* Fracture, humerus, upper
end, physeal
external condyle —*see* Fracture, humerus,
lower end, condyle, lateral
following insertion of implant, prosthesis
or plate M96.62-
great tuberosity —*see* Fracture, humerus,
upper end, greater tuberosity
intercondylar —*see* Fracture, humerus,
lower end
internal epicondyle —*see* Fracture,
humerus, lower end, epicondyle,
medial
lesser tuberosity —*see* Fracture, humerus,
upper end, lesser tuberosity
lower end S42.40-
condyle
lateral (displaced) S42.45-
nondisplaced S42.45-
medial (displaced) S42.46-
nondisplaced S42.46-
epicondyle
lateral (displaced) S42.43-
nondisplaced S42.43-
medial (displaced) S42.44-
incarcerated S42.44-
nondisplaced S42.44-
physeal S49.10-
Salter-Harris
Type I S49.11-
Type II S49.12-
Type III S49.13-
Type IV S49.14-
specified NEC S49.19-
specified NEC (displaced) S42.49-
nondisplaced S42.49-
supracondylar (simple) (displaced)
S42.41-
comminuted (displaced) S42.42-
nondisplaced S42.42-
nondisplaced S42.41-
torus S42.48-
transcondylar (displaced) S42.47-
nondisplaced S42.47-
proximal end —*see* Fracture, humerus,
upper end
shaft S42.30-
comminuted (displaced) S42.35-
nondisplaced S42.35-
greenstick S42.31-
oblique (displaced) S42.33-
nondisplaced S42.33-
segmental (displaced) S42.36-
nondisplaced S42.36-

Fracture, traumatic (Continued)
humerus (Continued)
shaft (Continued)
specified NEC S42.39-
spiral (displaced) S42.34-
nondisplaced S42.34-
transverse (displaced) S42.32-
nondisplaced S42.32-
supracondylar —see Fracture, humerus,
lower end
surgical neck —see Fracture, humerus,
upper end, surgical neck
trochlea —see Fracture, humerus, lower
end, condyle, medial
tuberosity —see Fracture, humerus, upper
end
upper end S42.20-
anatomical neck —see Fracture, humerus,
upper end, specified NEC
articular head —see Fracture, humerus,
upper end, specified NEC
epiphysis —see Fracture, humerus,
upper end, physeal
greater tuberosity (displaced) S42.25-
nondisplaced S42.25-
lesser tuberosity (displaced) S42.26-
nondisplaced S42.26-
physeal S49.00-
Salter-Harris
Type I S49.01-
Type II S49.02-
Type III S49.03-
Type IV S49.04-
specified NEC S49.09-
specified NEC (displaced) S42.29-
nondisplaced S42.29-
surgical neck (displaced) S42.21-
four-part S42.24-
nondisplaced S42.21-
three-part S42.23-
two-part (displaced) S42.22-
nondisplaced S42.22-
torus S42.27-
transepiphyseal —see Fracture, humerus,
upper end, physeal
hyoid bone S12.8
ilium S32.30-
with disruption of pelvic ring —see
Disruption, pelvic ring
avulsion (displaced) S32.31-
nondisplaced S32.31-
specified NEC S32.39-
impaction, impacted - code as Fracture, by
site
innominate bone —see Fracture, ilium
instep —see Fracture, foot
ischium S32.60-
with disruption of pelvic ring —see
Disruption, pelvic ring
avulsion (displaced) S32.61-
nondisplaced S32.61-
specified NEC S32.69-
jaw (bone) (lower) —see Fracture, mandible
upper —see Fracture, maxilla
joint prosthesis —see Complications, joint
prosthesis, mechanical, breakdown, by
site
periprosthetic —see Complications,
joint prosthesis, mechanical,
periprosthesis, fracture, by site
knee cap —see Fracture, patella
larynx S12.8
late effects —see Sequelae, fracture
leg (lower) S82.9-
ankle —see Fracture, ankle
femur —see Fracture, femur
fibula —see Fracture, fibula
malleolus —see Fracture, ankle
patella —see Fracture, patella
specified site NEC S82.89-
tibia —see Fracture, tibia

Fracture, traumatic (Continued)
lumbar spine —see Fracture, vertebra, lumbar
lumbosacral spine S32.9
Maisonneuve's (displaced) S82.86-
nondisplaced S82.86-
malar bone (see also Fracture, maxilla) S02.400
malleolus —see Fracture, ankle
malunion —see Fracture, by site
mandible (lower jawbone) S02.609
alveolus S02.67
angle (of jaw) S02.65
body, unspecified S02.600
condylar process S02.61
coronoid process S02.63
ramus, unspecified S02.64
specified site NEC S02.69
subcondylar process S02.62
symphysis S02.66
manubrium (sterni) S22.21
dissociation from sternum S22.23
march —see Fracture, traumatic, stress, by site
maxilla, maxillary (bone) (sinus) (superior)
(upper jaw) S02.401
alveolus S02.42
inferior —see Fracture, mandible
LeFort I S02.411
LeFort II S02.412
LeFort III S02.413
metacarpal S62.309
base (displaced) S62.319
nondisplaced S62.349
fifth S62.30-
base (displaced) S62.31-
nondisplaced S62.34-
neck (displaced) S62.33-
nondisplaced S62.36-
shaft (displaced) S62.32-
nondisplaced S62.35-
specified NEC S62.398
first S62.20-
base NEC (displaced) S62.23-
nondisplaced S62.23-
Bennett's —see Bennett's fracture
neck (displaced) S62.25-
nondisplaced S62.25-
shaft (displaced) S62.24-
nondisplaced S62.24-
specified NEC S62.29-
fourth S62.30-
base (displaced) S62.31-
nondisplaced S62.34-
neck (displaced) S62.33-
nondisplaced S62.36-
shaft (displaced) S62.32-
nondisplaced S62.35-
specified NEC S62.39-
neck (displaced) S62.33-
nondisplaced S62.36-
Rolando's —see Rolando's fracture
second S62.30-
base (displaced) S62.31-
nondisplaced S62.34-
neck (displaced) S62.33-
nondisplaced S62.36-
shaft (displaced) S62.32-
nondisplaced S62.35-
specified NEC S62.39-
shaft (displaced) S62.32-
nondisplaced S62.35-
specified NEC S62.399
third S62.30-
base (displaced) S62.31-
nondisplaced S62.34-
neck (displaced) S62.33-
nondisplaced S62.36-
shaft (displaced) S62.32-
nondisplaced S62.35-
specified NEC S62.39-
metastatic —see Fracture, pathological,
due to, neoplastic disease —see also
Neoplasm

Fracture, traumatic (Continued)
metatarsal bone S92.30-
fifth (displaced) S92.35-
nondisplaced S92.35-
first (displaced) S92.31-
nondisplaced S92.31-
fourth (displaced) S92.34-
nondisplaced S92.34-
second (displaced) S92.32-
nondisplaced S92.32-
third (displaced) S92.33-
nondisplaced S92.33-
Monteggia's —see Monteggia's fracture
multiple
hand (and wrist) NEC —see Fracture, by
site
ribs —see Fracture, rib, multiple
nasal (bone (s)) S02.2
navicular (scaphoid) (foot) —see also Fracture,
tarsal, navicular
hand —see Fracture, carpal, navicular
neck S12.9
cervical vertebra S12.9
fifth (displaced) S12.400
nondisplaced S12.401
specified type NEC (displaced)
S12.490
nondisplaced S12.491
first (displaced) S12.000
burst (stable) S12.01
unstable S12.02
lateral mass (displaced) S12.040
nondisplaced S12.041
nondisplaced S12.001
posterior arch (displaced) S12.030
nondisplaced S12.031
specified type NEC (displaced)
S12.090
nondisplaced S12.091
fourth (displaced) S12.300
nondisplaced S12.301
specified type NEC (displaced)
S12.390
nondisplaced S12.391
second (displaced) S12.100
dens (anterior) (displaced) (type II)
S12.110
nondisplaced S12.112
posterior S12.111
specified type NEC (displaced)
S12.120
nondisplaced S12.121
nondisplaced S12.101
specified type NEC (displaced)
S12.190
nondisplaced S12.191
seventh (displaced) S12.600
nondisplaced S12.601
specified type NEC (displaced)
S12.690
displaced S12.691
sixth (displaced) S12.500
nondisplaced S12.501
specified type NEC (displaced)
S12.590
displaced S12.591
third (displaced) S12.200
nondisplaced S12.201
specified type NEC (displaced)
S12.290
displaced S12.291
hyoid bone S12.8
larynx S12.8
specified site NEC S12.8
thyroid cartilage S12.8
trachea S12.8
neoplastic NEC —see Fracture, pathological,
due to, neoplastic disease
neural arch —see Fracture, vertebra
newborn —see Birth, injury, fracture
nontraumatic —see Fracture, pathological

◀ New   ◀━━ Revised   ~~deleted~~ Deleted

Fracture, traumatic *(Continued)*
  nonunion —*see* Nonunion, fracture
  nose, nasal (bone) (septum) S02.2
  occiput —*see* Fracture, skull, base, occiput
  odontoid process —*see* Fracture, neck,
    cervical vertebra, second
  olecranon (process) (ulna) —*see* Fracture,
    ulna, upper end, olecranon process
  orbit, orbital (bone) (region) S02.8
    floor (blow-out) S02.3
    roof S02.19
  os
    calcis —*see* Fracture, tarsal, calcaneus
    magnum —*see* Fracture, carpal, capitate
    pubis —*see* Fracture, pubis
  palate S02.8
  parietal bone (skull) S02.0
  patella S82.00-
    comminuted (displaced) S82.04-
      nondisplaced S82.04-
    longitudinal (displaced) S82.02-
      nondisplaced S82.02-
    osteochondral (displaced) S82.01-
      nondisplaced S82.01-
    specified NEC S82.09-
    transverse (displaced) S82.03-
      nondisplaced S82.03-
  pedicle (of vertebral arch) —*see* Fracture,
    vertebra
  pelvis, pelvic (bone) S32.9
    acetabulum —*see* Fracture, acetabulum
    circle —*see* Disruption, pelvic ring
    following insertion of implant, prosthesis
      or plate M96.65
    ilium —*see* Fracture, ilium
    ischium —*see* Fracture, ischium
    multiple
      with disruption of pelvic ring (circle) —
        see Disruption, pelvic ring
      without disruption of pelvic ring (circle)
        S32.82
    pubis —*see* Fracture, pubis
    sacrum —*see* Fracture, sacrum
    specified site NEC S32.89
  phalanx
    foot —*see* Fracture, toe
    hand —*see* Fracture, finger
  pisiform —*see* Fracture, carpal, pisiform
  pond —*see* Fracture, skull
  prosthetic device, internal —*see*
    Complications, prosthetic device, by
    site, mechanical
  pubis S32.50-
    with disruption of pelvic ring —*see*
      Disruption, pelvic ring
    specified site NEC S32.59-
    superior rim S32.59-
  radius S52.9-
    distal end —*see* Fracture, radius,
      lower end
    following insertion of implant, prosthesis
      or plate M96.63-
    head —*see* Fracture, radius, upper end,
      head
    lower end S52.50-
      Barton's —*see* Barton's fracture
      Colles' —*see* Colles' fracture
      extraarticular NEC S52.55-
      intraarticular NEC S52.57-
      physeal S59.20-
        Salter-Harris
          Type I S59.21-
          Type II S59.22-
          Type III S59.23-
          Type IV S59.24-
        specified NEC S59.29-
      Smith's —*see* Smith's fracture
      specified NEC S52.59-
      styloid process (displaced) S52.51-
        nondisplaced S52.51-
      torus S52.52-

Fracture, traumatic *(Continued)*
  radius *(Continued)*
    neck —*see* Fracture, radius, upper end
    proximal end —*see* Fracture, radius, upper
      end
    shaft S52.30-
      bent bone S52.38-
      comminuted (displaced) S52.35-
        nondisplaced S52.35-
      Galeazzi's —*see* Galeazzi's fracture
      greenstick S52.31-
      oblique (displaced) S52.33-
        nondisplaced S52.33-
      segmental (displaced) S52.36-
        nondisplaced S52.36-
      specified NEC S52.39-
      spiral (displaced) S52.34-
        nondisplaced S52.34-
      transverse (displaced) S52.32-
        nondisplaced S52.32-
    upper end S52.10-
      head (displaced) S52.12-
        nondisplaced S52.12-
      neck (displaced) S52.13-
        nondisplaced S52.13-
      physeal S59.10-
        Salter-Harris
          Type I S59.11-
          Type II S59.12-
          Type III S59.13-
          Type IV S59.14-
        specified NEC S59.19-
      specified NEC S52.18-
      torus S52.11-
  ramus
    inferior or superior, pubis —*see* Fracture,
      pubis
    mandible —*see* Fracture, mandible
  restorative material (dental) K08.539
    with loss of material K08.531
    without loss of material K08.530
  rib S22.3-
    with flail chest —*see* Flail, chest
    multiple S22.4-
      with flail chest —*see* Flail, chest
  root, tooth —*see* Fracture, tooth
  sacrum S32.10
    specified NEC S32.19
    Type
      1 S32.14
      2 S32.15
      3 S32.16
      4 S32.17
    Zone
      I S32.119
        displaced (minimally) S32.111
          severely S32.112
        nondisplaced S32.110
      II S32.129
        displaced (minimally) S32.121
          severely S32.122
        nondisplaced S32.120
      III S32.139
        displaced (minimally) S32.131
          severely S32.132
        nondisplaced S32.130
  scaphoid (hand) —*see also* Fracture, carpal,
    navicular
    foot —*see* Fracture, tarsal, navicular
  scapula S42.10-
    acromial process (displaced) S42.12-
      nondisplaced S42.12-
    body (displaced) S42.11-
      nondisplaced S42.11-
    coracoid process (displaced) S42.13-
      nondisplaced S42.13-
    glenoid cavity (displaced) S42.14-
      nondisplaced S42.14-
    neck (displaced) S42.15-
      nondisplaced S42.15-
    specified NEC S42.19-

Fracture, traumatic *(Continued)*
  semilunar bone, wrist —*see* Fracture, carpal,
    lunate
  sequelae —*see* Sequelae, fracture
  sesamoid bone
    hand —*see* Fracture, carpal
    other - code by site under Fracture
  shepherd's —*see* Fracture, tarsal, talus
  shoulder (girdle) S42.9-
    blade —*see* Fracture, scapula
  sinus (ethmoid) (frontal) S02.19
  skull S02.91
    base S02.10
      occiput S02.119
        condyle S02.113
          type I S02.110
          type II S02.111
          type III S02.112
          specified NEC S02.118
        specified NEC S02.19
    birth injury P13.0
    frontal bone S02.0
    parietal bone S02.0
    specified site NEC S02.8
    temporal bone S02.19
    vault S02.0
  Smith's —*see* Smith's fracture
  sphenoid (bone) (sinus) S02.19
  spine —*see* Fracture, vertebra
  spinous process —*see* Fracture, vertebra
  spontaneous (cause unknown) —*see* Fracture,
    pathological
  stave (of thumb) —*see* Fracture, metacarpal,
    first
  sternum S22.20
    with flail chest —*see* Flail, chest
    body S22.22
    manubrium S22.21
    xiphoid (process) S22.24
  stress M84.30
    ankle M84.37-
    carpus M84.34-
    clavicle M84.31-
    femoral neck M84.359
    femur M84.35-
    fibula M84.36-
    finger M84.34-
    hip M84.359
    humerus M84.32-
    ilium M84.350
    ischium M84.350
    metacarpus M84.34-
    metatarsus M84.37-
    neck —*see* Fracture, fatigue, vertebra
    pelvis M84.350
    radius M84.33-
    rib M84.38
    scapula M84.31-
    skull M84.38
    tarsus M84.37-
    tibia M84.36-
    toe M84.37-
    ulna M84.33-
    vertebra —*see* Fracture, fatigue, vertebra
  supracondylar, elbow —*see* Fracture,
    humerus, lower end, supracondylar
  symphysis pubis —*see* Fracture, pubis
  talus (ankle bone) —*see* Fracture, tarsal,
    talus
  tarsal bone (s) S92.20-
    astragalus —*see* Fracture, tarsal, talus
    calcaneus S92.00-
      anterior process (displaced) S92.02-
        nondisplaced S92.02-
      body (displaced) S92.01-
        nondisplaced S92.01-
      extraarticular NEC (displaced)
        S92.05-
        nondisplaced S92.05-
      intraarticular (displaced) S92.06-
        nondisplaced S92.06-

Fracture, traumatic *(Continued)*
 tarsal bone *(Continued)*
  calcaneus *(Continued)*
   tuberosity (displaced) S92.04-
    avulsion (displaced) S92.03-
     nondisplaced S92.03-
    nondisplaced S92.04-
  cuboid (displaced) S92.21-
   nondisplaced S92.21-
  cuneiform
   intermediate (displaced) S92.23-
    nondisplaced S92.23-
   lateral (displaced) S92.22-
    nondisplaced S92.22-
   medial (displaced) S92.24-
    nondisplaced S92.24-
  navicular (displaced) S92.25-
   nondisplaced S92.25-
  scaphoid —*see* Fracture, tarsal,
     navicular
  talus S92.10-
   avulsion (displaced) S92.15-
    nondisplaced S92.15-
   body (displaced) S92.12-
    nondisplaced S92.12-
   dome (displaced) S92.14-
    nondisplaced S92.14-
   head (displaced) S92.12-
    nondisplaced S92.12-
   lateral process (displaced) S92.14-
    nondisplaced S92.14-
   neck (displaced) S92.11-
    nondisplaced S92.11-
   posterior process (displaced)
      S92.13-
    nondisplaced S92.13-
   specified NEC S92.19-
 temporal bone (styloid) S02.19
 thorax (bony) S22.9
  with flail chest —*see* Flail, chest
  rib S22.3-
   multiple S22.4-
    with flail chest —*see* Flail, chest
  sternum S22.20
   body S22.22
   manubrium S22.21
   xiphoid process S22.24
  vertebra (displaced) S22.009
   burst (stable) S22.001
    unstable S22.002
   eighth S22.069
    burst (stable) S22.061
     unstable S22.062
    specified type NEC S22.068
    wedge compression S22.060
   eleventh S22.089
    burst (stable) S22.081
     unstable S22.082
    specified type NEC S22.088
    wedge compression S22.080
   fifth S22.059
    burst (stable) S22.051
     unstable S22.052
    specified type NEC S22.058
    wedge compression S22.050
   first S22.019
    burst (stable) S22.011
     unstable S22.012
    specified type NEC S22.018
    wedge compression S22.010
   fourth S22.049
    burst (stable) S22.041
     unstable S22.042
    specified type NEC S22.048
    wedge compression S22.040
   ninth S22.079
    burst (stable) S22.071
     unstable S22.072
    specified type NEC S22.078
    wedge compression S22.070
   nondisplaced S22.001

Fracture, traumatic *(Continued)*
 thorax *(Continued)*
  vertebra *(Continued)*
   second S22.029
    burst (stable) S22.021
     unstable S22.022
    specified type NEC S22.028
    wedge compression S22.020
   seventh S22.069
    burst (stable) S22.061
     unstable S22.062
    specified type NEC S22.068
    wedge compression S22.060
   sixth S22.059
    burst (stable) S22.051
     unstable S22.052
    specified type NEC S22.058
    wedge compression S22.050
   specified type NEC S22.008
   tenth S22.079
    burst (stable) S22.071
     unstable S22.072
    specified type NEC S22.078
    wedge compression S22.070
   third S22.039
    burst (stable) S22.031
     unstable S22.032
    specified type NEC S22.038
    wedge compression S22.030
   twelfth S22.089
    burst (stable) S22.081
     unstable S22.082
    specified type NEC S22.088
    wedge compression S22.080
   wedge compression S22.000
 thumb S62.50-
  distal phalanx (displaced) S62.52-
   nondisplaced S62.52-
  proximal phalanx (displaced) S62.51-
   nondisplaced S62.51-
 thyroid cartilage S12.8
 tibia (shaft) S82.20-
  comminuted (displaced) S82.25-
   nondisplaced S82.25-
  condyles —*see* Fracture, tibia, upper end
  distal end —*see* Fracture, tibia, lower end
  epiphysis
   lower —*see* Fracture, tibia, lower end
   upper —*see* Fracture, tibia, upper end
  following insertion of implant, prosthesis
     or plate M96.67-
  head (involving knee joint) —*see* Fracture,
     tibia, upper end
  intercondyloid eminence —*see* Fracture,
     tibia, upper end
  involving ankle or malleolus —*see*
     Fracture, ankle, medial malleolus
  lower end S82.30-
   physeal S89.10-
    Salter-Harris
     Type I S89.11-
     Type II S89.12-
     Type III S89.13-
     Type IV S89.14-
    specified NEC S89.19-
   pilon (displaced) S82.87-
    nondisplaced S82.87-
   specified NEC S82.39-
   torus S82.31-
  malleolus —*see* Fracture, ankle, medial
     malleolus
  oblique (displaced) S82.23-
   nondisplaced S82.23-
  pilon —*see* Fracture, tibia, lower end,
     pilon
  proximal end —*see* Fracture, tibia, upper
     end
  segmental (displaced) S82.26-
   nondisplaced S82.26-
  specified NEC S82.29-
  spine —*see* Fracture, upper end, spine

Fracture, traumatic *(Continued)*
 tibia *(Continued)*
  spiral (displaced) S82.24-
   nondisplaced S82.24-
  transverse (displaced) S82.22-
   nondisplaced S82.22-
  tuberosity —*see* Fracture, tibia, upper end,
     tuberosity
  upper end S82.10-
   bicondylar (displaced) S82.14-
    nondisplaced S82.14-
   lateral condyle (displaced) S82.12-
    nondisplaced S82.12-
   medial condyle (displaced) S82.13-
    nondisplaced S82.13-
   physeal S89.00-
    Salter-Harris
     Type I S89.01-
     Type II S89.02-
     Type III S89.03-
     Type IV S89.04-
    specified NEC S89.09-
   plateau —*see* Fracture, tibia, upper end,
      bicondylar
   specified NEC S82.19-
   spine (displaced) S82.11-
    nondisplaced S82.11-
   torus S82.16-
   tuberosity (displaced) S82.15-
    nondisplaced S82.15-
 toe S92.91-
  great (displaced) S92.40-
   distal phalanx (displaced) S92.42-
    nondisplaced S92.42-
   nondisplaced S92.40-
   proximal phalanx (displaced) S92.41-
    nondisplaced S92.41-
   specified NEC S92.49-
  lesser (displaced) S92.50-
   distal phalanx (displaced) S92.53-
    nondisplaced S92.53-
   medial phalanx (displaced) S92.52-
    nondisplaced S92.52-
   nondisplaced S92.50-
   proximal phalanx (displaced) S92.51-
    nondisplaced S92.51-
   specified NEC S92.59-
 tooth (root) S02.5
 trachea (cartilage) S12.8
 transverse process —*see* Fracture, vertebra
 trapezium or trapezoid bone —*see* Fracture,
    carpal
 trimalleolar —*see* Fracture, ankle, trimalleolar
 triquetrum (cuneiform of carpus) —*see*
    Fracture, carpal, triquetrum
 trochanter —*see* Fracture, femur,
    trochanteric
 tuberosity (external) - code by site under
    Fracture
 ulna (shaft) S52.20-
  bent bone S52.28-
  coronoid process —*see* Fracture, ulna,
     upper end, coronoid process
  distal end —*see* Fracture, ulna, lower end
  following insertion of implant, prosthesis
     or plate M96.63-
  head S52.00-
  lower end S52.60-
   physeal S59.00-
    Salter-Harris
     Type I S59.01-
     Type II S59.02-
     Type III S59.03-
     Type IV S59.04-
    specified NEC S59.09-
   specified NEC S52.69-
   styloid process (displaced) S52.61-
    nondisplaced S52.61-
   torus S52.62-
  proximal end —*see* Fracture, ulna, upper
     end

◀ New   ◀▥ Revised   ~~deleted~~ Deleted

Fracture, traumatic *(Continued)*
  ulna *(Continued)*
    shaft S52.20-
      comminuted (displaced) S52.25-
        nondisplaced S52.25-
      greenstick S52.21-
      Monteggia's —*see* Monteggia's fracture
      oblique (displaced) S52.23-
        nondisplaced S52.23-
      segmental (displaced) S52.26-
        nondisplaced S52.26-
      specified NEC S52.29-
      spiral (displaced) S52.24-
        nondisplaced S52.24-
      transverse (displaced) S52.22-
        nondisplaced S52.22-
    upper end S52.00-
      coronoid process (displaced) S52.04-
        nondisplaced S52.04-
      olecranon process (displaced)
          S52.02-
        with intraarticular extension
            S52.03-
        nondisplaced S52.02-
          with intraarticular extension
              S52.03-
      specified NEC S52.09-
      torus S52.01-
  unciform —*see* Fracture, carpal, hamate
  vault of skull S02.0
  vertebra, vertebral (arch) (body) (column)
        (neural arch) (pedicle) (spinous process)
        (transverse process)
    atlas —*see* Fracture, neck, cervical vertebra,
        first
    axis —*see* Fracture, neck, cervical vertebra,
        second
    cervical (teardrop) S12.9
      axis —*see* Fracture, neck, cervical
          vertebra, second
      first (atlas) —*see* Fracture, neck, cervical
          vertebra, first
      second (axis) —*see* Fracture, neck,
          cervical vertebra, second
    chronic M84.48
    coccyx S32.2
    dorsal —*see* Fracture, thorax, vertebra
    lumbar S32.009
      burst (stable) S32.001
        unstable S32.002
      fifth S32.059
        burst (stable) S32.051
          unstable S32.052
        specified type NEC S32.058
        wedge compression S32.050
      first S32.019
        burst (stable) S32.011
          unstable S32.012
        specified type NEC S32.018
        wedge compression S32.010
      fourth S32.049
        burst (stable) S32.041
          unstable S32.042
        specified type NEC S32.048
        wedge compression S32.040
      second S32.029
        burst (stable) S32.021
          unstable S32.022
        specified type NEC S32.028
        wedge compression S32.020
      specified type NEC S32.008
      third S32.039
        burst (stable) S32.031
          unstable S32.032
        specified type NEC S32.038
        wedge compression S32.030
      wedge compression S32.000
    metastatic —*see* Collapse, vertebra, in,
        specified disease NEC —*see also*
        Neoplasm
    newborn (birth injury) P11.5

Fracture, traumatic *(Continued)*
  vertebra, vertebral *(Continued)*
    sacrum S32.10
      specified NEC S32.19
      Type
        1 S32.14
        2 S32.15
        3 S32.16
        4 S32.17
      Zone
        I S32.119
          displaced (minimally) S32.111
            severely S32.112
          nondisplaced S32.110
        II S32.129
          displaced (minimally) S32.121
            severely S32.122
          nondisplaced S32.120
        III S32.139
          displaced (minimally) S32.131
            severely S32.132
          nondisplaced S32.130
    thoracic —*see* Fracture, thorax, vertebra
  vertex S02.0
  vomer (bone) S02.2
  wrist S62.10-
    carpal —*see* Fracture, carpal bone
    navicular (scaphoid) (hand) —*see* Fracture,
        carpal, navicular
  xiphisternum, xiphoid (process) S22.24
  zygoma S02.442
Fragile, fragility
  autosomal site Q95.5
  bone, congenital (with blue sclera) Q78.0
  capillary (hereditary) D69.8
  hair L67.8
  nails L60.3
  non-sex chromosome site Q95.5
  X chromosome Q99.2
Fragilitas
  crinium L67.8
  ossium (with blue sclerae) (hereditary)
      Q78.0
  unguium L60.3
    congenital Q84.6
Fragments, cataract (lens), following cataract
    surgery H59.02-
  retained foreign body —*see* Retained, foreign
      body fragments (type of)
Frailty (frail) R54
  mental R41.81
Frambesia, frambesial (tropica) —*see also* Yaws
  initial lesion or ulcer A66.0
  primary A66.0
Frambeside
  gummatous A66.4
  of early yaws A66.2
Frambesioma A66.1
Franceschetti-Klein (-Wildervanck) disease or
    syndrome Q75.4
Francis' disease —*see* Tularemia
Franklin disease C88.2
Frank's essential thrombocytopenia D69.3
Fraser's syndrome Q87.0
Freckle (s) L81.2
  malignant melanoma in —*see* Melanoma
  melanotic (Hutchinson's) —*see* Melanoma,
      in situ
  retinal D49.81
Frederickson's hyperlipoproteinemia, type
  I and V E78.3
  IIA E78.0
  IIB and III E78.2
  IV E78.1
Freeman Sheldon syndrome Q87.0
Freezing —*see also* Effect, adverse, cold T69.9
Freiberg's disease (infraction of metatarsal
      head or osteochondrosis) —*see*
      Osteochondrosis, juvenile, metatarsus
Frei's disease A55
Fremitus, friction, cardiac R01.2

Frenum, frenulum
  external os Q51.828
  tongue (shortening) (congenital) Q38.1
Frequency micturition (nocturnal) R35.0
  psychogenic F45.8
Frey's syndrome
  auriculotemporal G50.8
  hyperhidrosis L74.52
Friction
  burn —*see* Burn, by site
  fremitus, cardiac R01.2
  precordial R01.2
  sounds, chest R09.89
Friderichsen-Waterhouse syndrome or disease
    A39.1
Friedländer's B (bacillus) NEC *(see also*
    condition) A49.8
Friedreich's
  ataxia G11.1
  combined systemic disease G11.1
  facial hemihypertrophy Q67.4
  sclerosis (cerebellum) (spinal cord)
      G11.1
Frigidity F52.22
Fröhlich's syndrome E23.6
Frontal —*see also* condition
  lobe syndrome F07.0
Frostbite (superficial) T33.90
  with
    partial thickness skin loss —*see* Frostbite
        (superficial), by site
    tissue necrosis T34.90
  abdominal wall T33.3
    with tissue necrosis T34.3
  ankle T33.81-
    with tissue necrosis T34.81-
  arm T33.4-
    with tissue necrosis T34.4-
    finger (s) —*see* Frostbite, finger
    hand —*see* Frostbite, hand
    wrist —*see* Frostbite, wrist
  ear T33.01-
    with tissue necrosis T34.01-
  face T33.09
    with tissue necrosis T34.09
  finger T33.53-
    with tissue necrosis T34.53-
  foot T33.82-
    with tissue necrosis T34.82-
  hand T33.52-
    with tissue necrosis T34.52-
  head T33.09
    with tissue necrosis T34.09
    ear —*see* Frostbite, ear
    nose —*see* Frostbite, nose
  hip (and thigh) T33.6-
    with tissue necrosis T34.6-
  knee T33.7-
    with tissue necrosis T34.7-
  leg T33.9-
    with tissue necrosis T34.9-
    ankle —*see* Frostbite, ankle
    foot —*see* Frostbite, foot
    knee —*see* Frostbite, knee
    lower T33.9-
      with tissue necrosis T34.7-
    thigh —*see* Frostbite, hip
    toe —*see* Frostbite, toe
  limb
    lower T33.99
      with tissue necrosis T34.99
    upper —*see* Frostbite, arm
  neck T33.1
    with tissue necrosis T34.1
  nose T33.02
    with tissue necrosis T34.02
  pelvis T33.3
    with tissue necrosis T34.3
  specified site NEC T33.99
    with tissue necrosis T34.99
  thigh —*see* Frostbite, hip

Frostbite *(Continued)*
  thorax T33.2
    with tissue necrosis T34.2
  toes T33.83-
    with tissue necrosis T34.83-
  trunk T33.99
    with tissue necrosis T34.99
  wrist T33.51-
    with tissue necrosis T34.51-
Frotteurism F65.81
Frozen *(see also* Effect, adverse, cold) T69.9
  pelvis (female) N94.89
    male K66.8
  shoulder —*see* Capsulitis, adhesive
Fructokinase deficiency E74.11
Fructose 1,6 diphosphatase deficiency E74.19
Fructosemia (benign) (essential) E74.12
Fructosuria (benign) (essential) E74.11
Fuchs'
  black spot (myopic) H44.2-
  dystrophy (corneal endothelium) H18.51
  heterochromic cyclitis —*see* Cyclitis, Fuchs'
    heterochromic
Fucosidosis E77.1
Fugue R68.89
  dissociative F44.1
  hysterical (dissociative) F44.1
  postictal in epilepsy —*see* Epilepsy
  reaction to exceptional stress (transient)
    F43.0
Fulminant, fulminating —*see* condition
Functional —*see also* condition
  bleeding (uterus) N93.8
Functioning, intellectual, borderline R41.83
Fundus —*see* condition
Fungemia NOS B49
Fungus, fungous
  cerebral G93.89
  disease NOS B49
  infection —*see* Infection, fungus
Funiculitis (acute) (chronic) (endemic) N49.1
  gonococcal (acute) (chronic) A54.23
  tuberculous A18.15
Funnel
  breast (acquired) M95.4
    congenital Q67.6
    sequelae (late effect) of rickets E64.3
  chest (acquired) M95.4
    congenital Q67.6
    sequelae (late effect) of rickets E64.3
  pelvis (acquired) M95.5
    with disproportion (fetopelvic) O33.3
      causing obstructed labor O65.3
    congenital Q74.2
FUO (fever of unknown origin) R50.9
Furfur L21.0
  microsporon B36.0
Furrier's lung J67.8
Furrowed K14.5
  nail (s) (transverse) L60.4
    congenital Q84.6
  tongue K14.5
    congenital Q38.3
Furuncle L02.92
  abdominal wall L02.221
  ankle —*see* Furuncle, lower limb
  antecubital space —*see* Furuncle, upper limb
  anus K61.0
  arm —*see* Furuncle, upper limb

Furuncle *(Continued)*
  auditory canal, external —*see* Abscess, ear,
    external
  auricle (ear) —*see* Abscess, ear, external
  axilla (region) L02.42-
  back (any part) L02.222
  breast N61
  buttock L02.32
  cheek (external) L02.02
  chest wall L02.223
  chin L02.02
  corpus cavernosum N48.21
  ear, external —*see* Abscess, ear, external
  external auditory canal —*see* Abscess, ear,
    external
  eyelid —*see* Abscess, eyelid
  face L02.02
  femoral (region) —*see* Furuncle, lower limb
  finger —*see* Furuncle, hand
  flank L02.221
  foot L02.62-
  forehead L02.02
  gluteal (region) L02.32
  groin L02.224
  hand L02.52-
  head L02.821
    face L02.02
  hip —*see* Furuncle, lower limb
  kidney —*see* Abscess, kidney
  knee —*see* Furuncle, lower limb
  labium (majus) (minus) N76.4
  lacrimal
    gland —*see* Dacryoadenitis
    passages (duct) (sac) —*see* Inflammation,
      lacrimal, passages, acute
  leg (any part) —*see* Furuncle, lower limb
  lower limb L02.42-
  malignant A22.0
  mouth K12.2
  navel L02.226
  neck L02.12
  nose J34.0
  orbit, orbital —*see* Abscess, orbit
  palmar (space) —*see* Furuncle, hand
  partes posteriores L02.32
  pectoral region L02.223
  penis N48.21
  perineum L02.225
  pinna —*see* Abscess, ear, external
  popliteal —*see* Furuncle, lower limb
  prepatellar —*see* Furuncle, lower limb
  scalp L02.821
  seminal vesicle N49.0
  shoulder —*see* Furuncle, upper limb
  specified site NEC L02.828
  submandibular K12.2
  temple (region) L02.02
  thumb —*see* Furuncle, hand
  toe —*see* Furuncle, foot
  trunk L02.229
    abdominal wall L02.221
    back L02.222
    chest wall L02.223
    groin L02.224
    perineum L02.225
    umbilicus L02.226
  umbilicus L02.226
  upper limb L02.42-
  vulva N76.4

Furunculosis —*see* Furuncle
Fused —*see* Fusion, fused
Fusion, fused (congenital)
  astragaloscaphoid Q74.2
  atria Q21.1
  auditory canal Q16.1
  auricles, heart Q21.1
  binocular with defective stereopsis H53.32
  bone Q79.8
  cervical spine M43.22
  choanal Q30.0
  commissure, mitral valve Q23.2
  cusps, heart valve NEC Q24.8
    mitral Q23.2
    pulmonary Q22.1
    tricuspid Q22.4
  ear ossicles Q16.3
  fingers Q70.0-
  hymen Q52.3
  joint (acquired) —*see also* Ankylosis
    congenital Q74.8
  kidneys (incomplete) Q63.1
  labium (majus) (minus) Q52.5
  larynx and trachea Q34.8
  limb, congenital Q74.8
    lower Q74.2
    upper Q74.0
  lobes, lung Q33.8
  lumbosacral (acquired) M43.27
    arthrodesis status Z98.1
    congenital Q76.49
    postprocedural status Z98.1
  nares, nose, nasal, nostril (s) Q30.0
  organ or site not listed —*see* Anomaly,
    by site
  ossicles Q79.9
    auditory Q16.3
  pulmonic cusps Q22.1
  ribs Q76.6
  sacroiliac (joint) (acquired) M43.28
    arthrodesis status Z98.1
    congenital Q74.2
    postprocedural status Z98.1
  spine (acquired) NEC M43.20
    arthrodesis status Z98.1
    cervical region M43.22
    cervicothoracic region M43.23
    congenital Q76.49
    lumbar M43.26
    lumbosacral region M43.27
    occipito-atlanto-axial region M43.21
    postoperative status Z98.1
    sacrococcygeal region M43.28
    thoracic region M43.24
    thoracolumbar region M43.25
  sublingual duct with submaxillary duct at
    opening in mouth Q38.4
  testes Q55.1
  toes Q70.2
  tooth, teeth K00.2
  trachea and esophagus Q39.8
  twins Q89.4
  vagina Q52.4
  ventricles, heart Q21.0
  vertebra (arch) —*see* Fusion, spine
  vulva Q52.5
Fusospirillosis (mouth) (tongue) (tonsil)
  A69.1
Fussy baby R68.12

◀ New   ◀▥ Revised   ~~deleted~~ Deleted

G

Gain in weight (abnormal) (excessive) —*see also* Weight, gain
Gaisböck's disease (polycythemia hypertonica) D75.1
Gait abnormality R26.9
　ataxic R26.0
　falling R29.6
　hysterical (ataxic) (staggering) F44.4
　paralytic R26.1
　spastic R26.1
　specified type NEC R26.89
　staggering R26.0
　unsteadiness R26.81
　walking difficulty NEC R26.2
Galactocele (breast) N64.89
　puerperal, postpartum O92.79
Galactokinase deficiency E74.29
Galactophoritis N61
　gestational, puerperal, postpartum O91.2-
Galactorrhea O92.6
　not associated with childbirth N64.3
Galactosemia (classic) (congenital) E74.21
Galactosuria E74.29
Galacturia R82.0
　schistosomiasis (bilharziasis) B65.0
Galeazzi's fracture S52.37-
Galen's vein —*see* condition
Galeophobia F40.218
Gall duct —*see* condition
Gallbladder —*see also* condition
　acute K81.0
Gallop rhythm R00.8
Gallstone (colic) (cystic duct) (gallbladder) (impacted) (multiple) —*see also* Calculus, gallbladder
　with
　　cholecystitis —*see* Calculus, gallbladder, with cholecystitis
　　bile duct (common) (hepatic) —*see* Calculus, bile duct
　causing intestinal obstruction K56.3
　specified NEC K80.80
　　with obstruction K80.81
Gambling Z72.6
　pathological (compulsive) F63.0
Gammopathy (of undetermined significance [MGUS]) D47.2
　associated with lymphoplasmacytic dyscrasia D47.2
　monoclonal D47.2
　polyclonal D89.0
Gamna's disease (siderotic splenomegaly) D73.1
Gamophobia F40.298
Gampsodactylia (congenital) Q66.7
Gamstorp's disease (adynamia episodica hereditaria) G72.3
Gandy-Nanta disease (siderotic splenomegaly) D73.1
Gang
　membership offenses Z72.810
Gangliocytoma D36.10
Ganglioglioma —*see* Neoplasm, uncertain behavior, by site
Ganglion (compound) (diffuse) (joint) (tendon (sheath)) M67.40
　ankle M67.47-
　foot M67.47-
　forearm M67.43-
　hand M67.44-
　lower leg M67.46-
　multiple sites M67.49
　of yaws (early) (late) A66.6
　pelvic region M67.45-
　periosteal —*see* Periostitis
　shoulder region M67.41-
　specified site NEC M67.48
　thigh region M67.45-
　tuberculous A18.09
　upper arm M67.42-
　wrist M67.43-

Ganglioneuroblastoma —*see* Neoplasm, nerve, malignant
Ganglioneuroma D36.10
　malignant —*see* Neoplasm, nerve, malignant
Ganglioneuromatosis D36.10
Ganglionitis
　fifth nerve —*see* Neuralgia, trigeminal
　gasserian (postherpetic) (postzoster) B02.21
　geniculate G51.1
　　newborn (birth injury) P11.3
　　postherpetic, postzoster B02.21
　herpes zoster B02.21
　postherpetic geniculate B02.21
Gangliosidosis E75.10
　GM1 E75.19
　GM2 E75.00
　　other specified E75.09
　　Sandhoff disease E75.01
　　Tay-Sachs disease E75.02
　GM3 E75.19
　mucolipidosis IV E75.11
Gangosa A66.5
Gangrene, gangrenous (connective tissue) (dropsical) (dry) (moist) (skin) (ulcer) (*see also* Necrosis) I96
　with diabetes (mellitus) —*see* Diabetes, gangrene
　abdomen (wall) I96
　alveolar M27.3
　appendix K35.80
　　with
　　　perforation or rupture K35.2
　　　peritoneal abscess K35.3
　　　peritonitis NEC K35.3
　　　　generalized (with perforation or rupture) K35.2
　　　　localized (with perforation or rupture) K35.3
　arteriosclerotic (general) (senile) —*see* Arteriosclerosis, extremities, with, gangrene
　auricle I96
　Bacillus welchii A48.0
　bladder (infectious) —*see* Cystitis, specified type NEC
　bowel, cecum, or colon —*see* Gangrene, intestine
　Clostridium perfringens or welchii A48.0
　cornea H18.89-
　corpora cavernosa N48.29
　　noninfective N48.89
　cutaneous, spreading I96
　decubital —*see* Ulcer, pressure, by site
　diabetic (any site) —*see* Diabetes, gangrene
　emphysematous —*see* Gangrene, gas
　epidemic —*see* Poisoning, food, noxious, plant
　epididymis (infectional) N45.1
　erysipelas —*see* Erysipelas
　extremity (lower) (upper) I96
　Fournier N49.3
　　female N76.89
　fusospirochetal A69.0
　gallbladder —*see* Cholecystitis, acute
　gas (bacillus) A48.0
　　following
　　　abortion —*see* Abortion by type complicated by infection
　　　ectopic or molar pregnancy O08.0
　glossitis K14.0
　hernia —*see* Hernia, by site, with gangrene
　intestine, intestinal (hemorrhagic) (massive) K55.0
　　with
　　　mesenteric embolism K55.0
　　　obstruction —*see* Obstruction, intestine
　laryngitis J04.0

Gangrene, gangrenous (Continued)
　limb (lower) (upper) I96
　lung J85.0
　　spirochetal A69.8
　lymphangitis I89.1
　Meleney's (synergistic) —*see* Ulcer, skin
　mesentery K55.0
　　with
　　　embolism K55.0
　　　intestinal obstruction —*see* Obstruction, intestine
　mouth A69.0
　ovary —*see* Oophoritis
　pancreas K85.9
　penis N48.29
　　noninfective N48.89
　perineum I96
　pharynx —*see also* Pharyngitis
　　Vincent's A69.1
　presenile I73.1
　progressive synergistic —*see* Ulcer, skin
　pulmonary J85.0
　pulpal (dental) K04.1
　quinsy J36
　Raynaud's (symmetric gangrene) I73.01
　retropharyngeal J39.2
　scrotum N49.3
　　noninfective N50.8
　senile (atherosclerotic) —*see* Arteriosclerosis, extremities, with, gangrene
　spermatic cord N49.1
　　noninfective N50.8
　spine I96
　spirochetal NEC A69.8
　spreading cutaneous I96
　stomatitis A69.0
　symmetrical I73.01
　testis (infectional) N45.2
　　noninfective N44.8
　throat —*see also* Pharyngitis
　　diphtheritic A36.0
　　Vincent's A69.1
　thyroid (gland) E07.89
　tooth (pulp) K04.1
　tuberculous NEC —*see* Tuberculosis
　tunica vaginalis N49.1
　　noninfective N50.8
　umbilicus I96
　uterus —*see* Endometritis
　uvulitis K12.2
　vas deferens N49.1
　　noninfective N50.8
　vulva N76.89
Ganister disease J62.8
Ganser's syndrome (hysterical) F44.89
Gardner-Diamond syndrome (autoerythrocyte sensitization) D69.2
Gargoylism E76.01
Garré's disease, osteitis (sclerosing), osteomyelitis —*see* Osteomyelitis, specified type NEC
Garrod's pad, knuckle M72.1
Gartner's duct
　cyst Q52.4
　persistent Q50.6
Gas R14.3
　asphyxiation, inhalation, poisoning, suffocation NEC —*see* Table of Drugs and Chemicals
　excessive R14.0
　gangrene A48.0
　　following
　　　abortion —*see* Abortion by type complicated by infection
　　　ectopic or molar pregnancy O08.0
　on stomach R14.0
　pains R14.1
Gastralgia —*see also* Pain, abdominal
Gastrectasis K31.0
　psychogenic F45.8
Gastric —*see* condition

Gastrinoma
  malignant
    pancreas C25.4
    specified site NEC —see Neoplasm,
      malignant, by site
    unspecified site C25.4
  specified site —see Neoplasm, uncertain
    behavior
  unspecified site D37.9
Gastritis (simple) K29.70
  with bleeding K29.71
  acute (erosive) K29.00
    with bleeding K29.01
  alcoholic K29.20
    with bleeding K29.21
  allergic K29.60
    with bleeding K29.61
  atrophic (chronic) K29.40
    with bleeding K29.41
  chronic (antral) (fundal) K29.50
    with bleeding K29.51
    atrophic K29.40
      with bleeding K29.41
    superficial K29.30
      with bleeding K29.31
  dietary counseling and surveillance Z71.3
  due to diet deficiency E63.9
  eosinophilic K52.81
  giant hypertrophic K29.60
    with bleeding K29.61
  granulomatous K29.60
    with bleeding K29.61
  hypertrophic (mucosa) K29.60
    with bleeding K29.61
  nervous F54
  spastic K29.60
    with bleeding K29.61
  specified NEC K29.60
    with bleeding K29.61
  superficial chronic K29.30
    with bleeding K29.31
  tuberculous A18.83
  viral NEC A08.4
Gastrocarcinoma —see Neoplasm, malignant,
  stomach
Gastrocolic —see condition
Gastrodisciasis, gastrodiscoidiasis B66.8
Gastroduodenitis K29.90
  with bleeding K29.91
  virus, viral A08.4
    specified type NEC A08.39
Gastrodynia —see Pain, abdominal
Gastroenteritis (acute) (chronic) (noninfectious)
  (see also Enteritis) K52.9
  allergic K52.2
  dietetic K52.2
  drug-induced K52.1
  due to
    Cryptosporidium A07.2
    drugs K52.1
    food poisoning —see Intoxication, foodborne
    radiation K52.0
  eosinophilic K52.81
  epidemic (infectious) A09
  food hypersensitivity K52.2
  infectious —see Enteritis, infectious
  influenzal —see Influenza, with
    gastroenteritis
  noninfectious K52.9
    specified NEC K52.89
  rotaviral A08.0
  Salmonella A02.0
  toxic K52.1
  viral NEC A08.4
    acute infectious A08.39
      type Norwalk A08.11
    infantile (acute) A08.39
    Norwalk agent A08.11
    rotaviral A08.0
    severe of infants A08.39
    specified type NEC A08.39

Gastroenteropathy (see also Gastroenteritis)
  K52.9
  acute, due to Norovirus A08.11
  acute, due to Norwalk agent A08.11
  infectious A09
Gastroenteroptosis K63.4
Gastroesophageal laceration-hemorrhage
  syndrome K22.6
Gastrointestinal —see condition
Gastrojejunal —see condition
Gastrojejunitis (see also Enteritis) K52.9
Gastrojejunocolic —see condition
Gastroliths K31.89
Gastromalacia K31.89
Gastroparalysis K31.84
  diabetic —see Diabetes, gastroparalysis
Gastroparesis K31.84
  diabetic —see Diabetes, by type, with
    gastroparesis
Gastropathy K31.9
  congestive portal K31.89
  erythematous K29.70
  exudative K90.89
  portal hypertensive K31.89
Gastroptosis K31.89
Gastrorrhagia K92.2
  psychogenic F45.8
Gastroschisis (congenital) Q79.3
Gastrospasm (neurogenic) (reflex) K31.89
  neurotic F45.8
  psychogenic F45.8
Gastrostaxis —see Gastritis, with bleeding
Gastrostenosis K31.89
Gastrostomy
  attention to Z43.1
  status Z93.1
Gastrosuccorrhea (continuous) (intermittent)
  K31.89
  neurotic F45.8
  psychogenic F45.8
Gatophobia F40.218
Gaucher's disease or splenomegaly (adult)
  (infantile) E75.22
Gee (-Herter)(-Thaysen) disease (nontropical
  sprue) K90.0
Gélineau's syndrome G47.419
  with cataplexy G47.411
Gemination, tooth, teeth K00.2
Gemistocytoma
  specified site —see Neoplasm, malignant, by
    site
  unspecified site C71.9
General, generalized —see condition
Genetic
  carrier (status)
    cystic fibrosis Z14.1
    hemophilia A (asymptomatic) Z14.01
      symptomatic Z14.02
    specified NEC Z14.8
  susceptibility to disease NEC Z15.89
    malignant neoplasm Z15.09
      breast Z15.01
      endometrium Z15.04
      ovary Z15.02
      prostate Z15.03
      specified NEC Z15.09
    multiple endocrine neoplasia Z15.81
Genital —see condition
Genito-anorectal syndrome A55
Genitourinary system —see condition
Genu
  congenital Q74.1
  extrorsum (acquired) —see also Deformity,
    varus, knee
    congenital Q74.1
    sequelae (late effect) of rickets E64.3
  introrsum (acquired) —see also Deformity,
    valgus, knee
    congenital Q74.1
    sequelae (late effect) of rickets E64.3
  rachitic (old) E64.3

Genu (Continued)
  recurvatum (acquired) —see also Deformity,
    limb, specified type NEC, lower leg
    congenital Q68.2
    sequelae (late effect) of rickets E64.3
  valgum (acquired) (knock-knee) M21.06-
    congenital Q74.1
    sequelae (late effect) of rickets E64.3
  varum (acquired) (bowleg) M21.16-
    congenital Q74.1
    sequelae (late effect) of rickets E64.3
Geographic tongue K14.1
Geophagia —see Pica
Geotrichosis B48.3
  stomatitis B48.3
Gephyrophobia F40.242
Gerbode defect Q21.0
GERD (gastroesophageal reflux disease)
  K21.9
Gerhardt's
  disease (erythromelalgia) I73.81
  syndrome (vocal cord paralysis)
    J38.00
    bilateral J38.02
    unilateral J38.01
German measles —see also Rubella
  exposure to Z20.4
Germinoblastoma (diffuse) C85.9-
  follicular C82.9-
Germinoma —see Neoplasm, malignant,
  by site
Gerontoxon —see Degeneration, cornea,
  senile
Gerstmann-Sträussler-Scheinker syndrome
  (GSS) A81.82
Gerstmann's syndrome R48.8
  developmental F81.2
Gestation (period) —see also Pregnancy
  ectopic —see Pregnancy, by site
  multiple O30.9-
    greater than quadruplets —see Pregnancy,
      multiple (gestation), specified NEC
    specified NEC —see Pregnancy, multiple
      (gestation), specified NEC
Gestational
  mammary abscess O91.11-
  purulent mastitis O91.11-
  subareolar abscess O91.11-
Ghon tubercle, primary infection A15.7
Ghost
  teeth K00.4
  vessels (cornea) H16.41-
Ghoul hand A66.3
Gianotti-Crosti disease L44.4
Giant
  cell
    epulis K06.8
    peripheral granuloma K06.8
  esophagus, congenital Q39.5
  kidney, congenital Q63.3
  urticaria T78.3
    hereditary D84.1
Giardiasis A07.1
Gibert's disease or pityriasis L42
Giddiness R42
  hysterical F44.89
  psychogenic F45.8
Gierke's disease (glycogenosis I) E74.01
Gigantism (cerebral) (hypophyseal) (pituitary)
  E22.0
  constitutional E34.4
Gilbert's disease or syndrome E80.4
Gilchrist's disease B40.9
Gilford-Hutchinson disease E34.8
Gilles de la Tourette's disease or syndrome
  (motor-verbal tic) F95.2
Gingivitis K05.10
  acute (catarrhal) K05.00
    necrotizing A69.1
    nonplaque induced K05.01
    plaque induced K05.00

◀ New   ◀▥ Revised   ~~deleted~~ Deleted

Gingivitis (Continued)
  chronic (desquamative) (hyperplastic)
    (simple marginal) (ulcerative) K05.10
    nonplaque induced K05.11
    plaque induced K05.10
  expulsiva —see Periodontitis
  necrotizing ulcerative (acute) A69.1
  pellagrous E52
    acute necrotizing A69.1
  Vincent's A69.1
Gingivoglossitis K14.0
Gingivopericementitis —see Periodontitis
Gingivosis —see Gingivitis, chronic
Gingivostomatitis K05.10
  herpesviral B00.2
  necrotizing ulcerative (acute) A69.1
Gland, glandular —see condition
Glanders A24.0
Glanzmann (-Naegeli) disease or
  thrombasthenia D69.1
Glasgow coma scale
  total score
    3-8 R40.243
    9-12 R40.242
    13-15 R40.241
Glass-blower's disease (cataract) —see
  Cataract, specified NEC
Glaucoma H40.9
  with
    increased episcleral venous pressure
      H40.81-
    pseudoexfoliation of lens —see Glaucoma,
      open angle, primary, capsular
  absolute H44.51-
  angle-closure (primary) H40.20-
    acute (attack) (crisis) H40.21-
    chronic H40.22-
    intermittent H40.23-
    residual stage H40.24-
  borderline H40.00-
  capsular (with pseudoexfoliation of lens) —
    see Glaucoma, open angle, primary,
    capsular
  childhood Q15.0
  closed angle —see Glaucoma, angle-closure
  congenital Q15.0
  corticosteroid-induced —see Glaucoma,
    secondary, drugs
  hypersecretion H40.82-
  in (due to)
    amyloidosis E85.4 [H42]
    aniridia Q13.1 [H42]
    concussion of globe —see Glaucoma,
      secondary, trauma
    dislocation of lens —see Glaucoma,
      secondary
    disorder of lens NEC —see Glaucoma,
      secondary
    drugs —see Glaucoma, secondary, drugs
    endocrine disease NOS E34.9 [H42]
    eye
      inflammation —see Glaucoma,
        secondary, inflammation
      trauma —see Glaucoma, secondary,
        trauma
    hypermature cataract —see Glaucoma,
      secondary
    iridocyclitis —see Glaucoma, secondary,
      inflammation
    lens disorder —see Glaucoma, secondary,
    Lowe's syndrome E72.03 [H42]
    metabolic disease NOS E88.9 [H42]
    ocular disorders NEC —see Glaucoma,
      secondary
    onchocerciasis B73.02
    pupillary block —see Glaucoma, secondary
    retinal vein occlusion —see Glaucoma,
      secondary
    Rieger's anomaly Q13.81 [H42]
    rubeosis of iris —see Glaucoma, secondary
    tumor of globe —see Glaucoma, secondary

Glaucoma (Continued)
  infantile Q15.0
  low tension —see Glaucoma, open angle,
    primary, low-tension
  malignant H40.83-
  narrow angle —see Glaucoma, angle-closure
  newborn Q15.0
  noncongestive (chronic) —see Glaucoma,
    open angle
  nonobstructive —see Glaucoma, open
    angle
  obstructive —see also Glaucoma,
    angle-closure
    due to lens changes —see Glaucoma,
      secondary
  open angle H40.10-
    primary H40.11-
      capsular (with pseudoexfoliation of lens)
        H40.14-
      low-tension H40.12-
      pigmentary H40.13-
      residual stage H40.15-
  phacolytic —see Glaucoma, secondary
  pigmentary —see Glaucoma, open angle,
    primary, pigmentary
  postinfectious —see Glaucoma, secondary,
    inflammation
  secondary (to) H40.5-
    drugs H40.6-
    inflammation H40.4-
    trauma H40.3-
  simple (chronic) H40.11
  simplex H40.11
  specified type NEC H40.89
  suspect H40.00-
  syphilitic A52.71
  traumatic —see also Glaucoma, secondary,
    trauma
    newborn (birth injury) P15.3
  tuberculous A18.59
Glaucomatous flecks (subcapsular) —see
  Cataract, complicated
Glazed tongue K14.4
Gleet (gonococcal) A54.01
Glénard's disease K63.4
Glioblastoma (multiforme)
  with sarcomatous component
    specified site —see Neoplasm, malignant,
      by site
    unspecified site C71.9
  giant cell
    specified site —see Neoplasm, malignant,
      by site
    unspecified site C71.9
  specified site —see Neoplasm, malignant, by
    site
  unspecified site C71.9
Glioma (malignant)
  astrocytic
    specified site —see Neoplasm, malignant,
      by site
    unspecified site C71.9
  mixed
    specified site —see Neoplasm, malignant,
      by site
    unspecified site C71.9
  nose Q30.8
  specified site NEC —see Neoplasm,
    malignant, by site
  subependymal D43.2
    specified site —see Neoplasm, uncertain
      behavior, by site
    unspecified site D43.2
  unspecified site C71.9
Gliomatosis cerebri C71.0
Glioneuroma —see Neoplasm, uncertain
  behavior, by site
Gliosarcoma
  specified site —see Neoplasm, malignant, by
    site
  unspecified site C71.9

Gliosis (cerebral) G93.89
  spinal G95.89
Glisson's disease —see Rickets
Globinuria R82.3
Globus (hystericus) F45.8
Glomangioma D18.00
  intra-abdominal D18.03
  intracranial D18.02
  skin D18.01
  specified site NEC D18.09
Glomangiomyoma D18.00
  intra-abdominal D18.03
  intracranial D18.02
  skin D18.01
  specified site NEC D18.09
Glomangiosarcoma —see Neoplasm, connective
  tissue, malignant
Glomerular
  disease in syphilis A52.75
  nephritis —see Glomerulonephritis
Glomerulitis —see Glomerulonephritis
Glomerulonephritis (see also Nephritis)
  N05.9
  with
    edema —see Nephrosis
    minimal change N05.0
    minor glomerular abnormality N05.0
  acute N00.9
  chronic N03.9
  crescentic (diffuse) NEC (see also N00-N07
    with fourth character .7) N05.7
  dense deposit (see also N00-N07 with fourth
    character .6) N05.6
  diffuse
    crescentic (see also N00-N07 with fourth
      character .7) N05.7
    endocapillary proliferative (see also
      N00N07 with fourth character .4)
      N05.4
    membranous (see also N00-N07 with fourth
      character .2) N05.2
    mesangial proliferative (see also N00N07
      with fourth character .3) N05.3
    mesangiocapillary (see also N00-N07 with
      fourth character .5) N05.5
    sclerosing N05.8
  endocapillary proliferative (diffuse) NEC (see
    also N00-N07 with fourth character .4)
    N05.4
  extracapillary NEC (see also N00-N07 with
    fourth character .7) N05.7
  focal (and segmental) (see also N00-N07 with
    fourth character .1) N05.1
  hypocomplementemic —see
    Glomerulonephritis,
    membranoproliferative
  IgA —see Nephropathy, IgA
  immune complex (circulating) NEC
    N05.8
  in (due to)
    amyloidosis E85.4 [N08]
    bilharziasis B65.9 [N08]
    cryoglobulinemia D89.1 [N08]
    defibrination syndrome D65 [N08]
    diabetes mellitus —see Diabetes,
      glomerulosclerosis
    disseminated intravascular coagulation
      D65 [N08]
    Fabry (-Anderson) disease E75.21 [N08]
    Goodpasture's syndrome M31.0
    hemolytic-uremic syndrome D59.3
    Henoch (-Schönlein) purpura D69.0
      [N08]
    lecithin cholesterol acyltransferase
      deficiency E78.6 [N08]
    microscopic polyangiitis M31.7 [N08]
    multiple myeloma C90.0- [N08]
    Plasmodium malariae B52.0
    schistosomiasis B65.9 [N08]
    sepsis A41.9- [N08]
      streptococcal A40- [N08]

◄ New   ⬅ Revised   ~~deleted~~ Deleted

Glomerulonephritis (Continued)
in (Continued)
  sickle-cell disorders D57.- [N08]
  strongyloidiasis B78.9 [N08]
  subacute bacterial endocarditis I33.0
    [N08]
  syphilis (late) congenital A50.59 [N08]
  systemic lupus erythematosus M32.14
  thrombotic thrombocytopenic purpura
    M31.1 [N08]
  typhoid fever A01.09
  Waldenström macroglobulinemia C88.0
    [N08]
  Wegener's granulomatosis M31.31
latent or quiescent N03.9
lobular, lobulonodular —see
    Glomerulonephritis,
    membranoproliferative
membranoproliferative (diffuse) (type 1
    or 3) (see also N00-N07 with fourth
    character .5) N05.5
  dense deposit (type 2) NEC (see also
    N00-N07 with fourth character .6)
    N05.6
membranous (diffuse) NEC (see also N00-N07
    with fourth character .2) N05.2
mesangial
  IgA/IgG —see Nephropathy, IgA
  proliferative (diffuse) NEC (see also
    N00-N07 with fourth character .3)
    N05.3
mesangiocapillary (diffuse) NEC (see also
    N00-N07 with fourth character .5)
    N05.5
necrotic, necrotizing NEC (see also N00-N07
    with fourth character .8) N05.8
nodular —see Glomerulonephritis,
    membranoproliferative
poststreptococcal NEC N05.9
  acute N00.9
  chronic N03.9
  rapidly progressive N01.9
proliferative NEC (see also N00-N07 with
    fourth character .8) N05.8
  diffuse (lupus) M32.14
rapidly progressive N01.9
sclerosing, diffuse N05.8
specified pathology NEC (see also N00-N07
    with fourth character .8) N05.8
subacute N01.9
Glomerulopathy —see Glomerulonephritis
Glomerulosclerosis —see also Sclerosis,
    renal
  intercapillary (nodular) (with diabetes) —see
    Diabetes, glomerulosclerosis
  intracapillary —see Diabetes,
    glomerulosclerosis
Glossagra K14.6
Glossalgia K14.6
Glossitis (chronic superficial) (gangrenous)
    (Moeller's) K14.0
  areata exfoliativa K14.1
  atrophic K14.4
  benign migratory K14.1
  cortical superficial, sclerotic K14.0
  Hunter's D51.0
  interstitial, sclerous K14.0
  median rhomboid K14.2
  pellagrous E52
  superficial, chronic K14.0
Glossocele K14.8
Glossodynia K14.6
  exfoliativa K14.4
Glossoncus K14.8
Glossopathy K14.9
Glossophytia K14.3
Glossoplegia K14.8
Glossoptosis K14.8
Glossopyrosis K14.6
Glossotrichia K14.3
Glossy skin L90.8

Glottis —see condition
Glottitis (see also Laryngitis) J04.0
Glucagonoma
  pancreas
    benign D13.7
    malignant C25.4
    uncertain behavior D37.8
  specified site NEC
    benign —see Neoplasm, benign, by site
    malignant —see Neoplasm, malignant, by
      site
    uncertain behavior —see Neoplasm,
      uncertain behavior, by site
  unspecified site
    benign D13.7
    malignant C25.4
    uncertain behavior D37.8
Glucoglycinuria E72.51
Glucose-galactose malabsorption E74.39
Glue
  ear —see Otitis, media, nonsuppurative,
    chronic, mucoid
  sniffing (airplane) —see Abuse, drug,
    inhalant
    dependence —see Dependence, drug,
      inhalant
Glutaric aciduria E72.3
Glycinemia E72.51
Glycinuria (renal) (with ketosis) E72.09
Glycogen
  infiltration —see Disease, glycogen storage
  storage disease —see Disease, glycogen
    storage
Glycogenosis (diffuse) (generalized) —see also
    Disease, glycogen storage
  cardiac E74.02 [I43]
  diabetic, secondary —see Diabetes,
    glycogenosis, secondary
  pulmonary interstitial J84.842
Glycopenia E16.2
Glycosuria R81
  renal E74.8
Gnathostoma spinigerum (infection)
    (infestation), gnathostomiasis (wandering
    swelling) B83.1
Goiter (plunging) (substernal) E04.9
  with
    hyperthyroidism (recurrent) —see
      Hyperthyroidism, with, goiter
    thyrotoxicosis —see Hyperthyroidism,
      with, goiter
  adenomatous —see Goiter, nodular
  cancerous C73
  congenital (nontoxic) E03.0
    diffuse E03.0
    parenchymatous E03.0
    transitory, with normal functioning
      P72.0
  cystic E04.2
    due to iodine-deficiency E01.1
  due to
    enzyme defect in synthesis of thyroid
      hormone E07.1
    iodine-deficiency (endemic) E01.2
  dyshormonogenetic (familial) E07.1
  endemic (iodine-deficiency) E01.2
    diffuse E01.0
    multinodular E01.1
  exophthalmic —see Hyperthyroidism, with,
    goiter
  iodine-deficiency (endemic) E01.2
    diffuse E01.0
    multinodular E01.1
    nodular E01.1
  lingual Q89.2
  lymphadenoid E06.3
  malignant C73
  multinodular (cystic) (nontoxic) E04.2
    toxic or with hyperthyroidism E05.20
      with thyroid storm E05.21
  neonatal NEC P72.0

Goiter (Continued)
  nodular (nontoxic) (due to) E04.9
    with
      hyperthyroidism E05.20
        with thyroid storm E05.21
      thyrotoxicosis E05.20
        with thyroid storm E05.21
    endemic E01.1
    iodine-deficiency E01.1
    sporadic E04.9
    toxic E05.20
      with thyroid storm E05.21
  nontoxic E04.9
    diffuse (colloid) E04.0
    multinodular E04.2
    simple E04.0
    specified NEC E04.8
    uninodular E04.1
  simple E04.0
  toxic —see Hyperthyroidism, with, goiter
  uninodular (nontoxic) E04.1
    toxic or with hyperthyroidism E05.10
      with thyroid storm E05.11
Goiter-deafness syndrome E07.1
Goldberg syndrome Q89.8
Goldberg-Maxwell syndrome E34.51
Goldblatt's hypertension or kidney I70.1
Goldenhar (-Gorlin) syndrome Q87.0
Goldflam-Erb disease or syndrome G70.00
  with exacerbation (acute) G70.01
  in crisis G70.01
Goldscheider's disease Q81.8
Goldstein's disease (familial hemorrhagic
    telangiectasia) I78.0
Golfer's elbow —see Epicondylitis, medial
Gonadoblastoma
  specified site —see Neoplasm, uncertain
    behavior, by site
  unspecified site
    female D39.10
    male D40.10
Gonecystitis —see Vesiculitis
Gongylonemiasis B83.8
Goniosynechiae —see Adhesions, iris,
    goniosynechiae
Gonococcemia A54.86
Gonococcus, gonococcal (disease) (infection)
    (see also condition) A54.9
  anus A54.6
  bursa, bursitis A54.49
  conjunctiva, conjunctivitis (neonatorum)
    A54.31
  endocardium A54.83
  eye A54.30
    conjunctivitis A54.31
    iridocyclitis A54.32
    keratitis A54.33
    newborn A54.31
    other specified A54.39
  fallopian tubes (acute) (chronic) A54.24
  genitourinary (organ) (system) (tract) (acute)
    lower A54.00
      with abscess (accessory gland)
        (periurethral) A54.1
    upper (see also condition) A54.29
  heart A54.83
  iridocyclitis A54.32
  joint A54.42
  lymphatic (gland) (node) A54.89
  meninges, meningitis A54.81
  musculoskeletal A54.40
    arthritis A54.42
    osteomyelitis A54.43
    other specified A54.49
    spondylopathy A54.41
  pelviperitonitis A54.24
  pelvis (acute) (chronic) A54.24
  pharynx A54.5
  proctitis A54.6
  pyosalpinx (acute) (chronic) A54.24
  rectum A54.6

◀ New   ◀▥ Revised   ~~deleted~~ Deleted

Gonococcus, gonococcal (Continued)
  skin A54.89
  specified site NEC A54.89
  tendon sheath A54.49
  throat A54.5
  urethra (acute) (chronic) A54.01
    with abscess (accessory gland)
        (periurethral) A54.1
  vulva (acute) (chronic) A54.02
Gonocytoma
  specified site —see Neoplasm, uncertain
        behavior, by site
  unspecified site
    female D39.10
    male D40.10
Gonorrhea (acute) (chronic) A54.9
  Bartholin's gland (acute) (chronic) (purulent)
      A54.02
    with abscess (accessory gland)
        (periurethral) A54.1
  bladder A54.01
  cervix A54.03
  conjunctiva, conjunctivitis (neonatorum)
      A54.31
  contact Z20.2
  Cowper's gland (with abscess) A54.1
  exposure to Z20.2
  fallopian tube (acute) (chronic) A54.24
  kidney (acute) (chronic) A54.21
  lower genitourinary tract A54.00
    with abscess (accessory gland)
        (periurethral) A54.1
  ovary (acute) (chronic) A54.24
  pelvis (acute) (chronic) A54.24
    female pelvic inflammatory disease A54.24
  penis A54.09
  prostate (acute) (chronic) A54.22
  seminal vesicle (acute) (chronic) A54.23
  specified site not listed (see also Gonococcus)
      A54.89
  spermatic cord (acute) (chronic) A54.23
  urethra A54.01
    with abscess (accessory gland)
        (periurethral) A54.1
  vagina A54.02
  vas deferens (acute) (chronic) A54.23
  vulva A54.02
Goodall's disease A08.19
Goodpasture's syndrome M31.0
Gopalan's syndrome (burning feet) E53.0
Gorlin-Chaudry-Moss syndrome Q87.0
Gottron's papules L94.4
Gougerot's syndrome (trisymptomatic) L81.7
Gougerot-Blum syndrome (pigmented
      purpuric lichenoid dermatitis) L81.7
Gougerot-Carteaud disease or syndrome
      (confluent reticulate papillomatosis) L83
Gouley's syndrome (constrictive pericarditis)
      I31.1
Goundou A66.6
Gout, chronic (see also Gout, gouty) M1A.9-
  drug-induced M1A.20
    ankle M1A.27-
    elbow M1A.22-
    foot joint M1A.27-
    hand joint M1A.24-
    hip M1A.25-
    knee M1A.26-
    multiple site M1A.29-
    shoulder M1A.21-
    vertebrae M1A.28
    wrist M1A.23-
  idiopathic M1A.00
    ankle M1A.07-
    elbow M1A.02-
    foot joint M1A.07-
    hand joint M1A.04-
    hip M1A.05-
    knee M1A.06-
    multiple site M1A.09
    shoulder M1A.01-

Gout, chronic (Continued)
  idiopathic (Continued)
    vertebrae M1A.08
    wrist M1A.03-
  in (due to) renal impairment M1A.30
    ankle M1A.37-
    elbow M1A.32-
    foot joint M1A.37-
    hand joint M1A.34-
    hip M1A.35-
    knee M1A.36-
    multiple site M1A.39
    shoulder M1A.31-
    vertebrae M1A.38
    wrist M1A.33-
  lead-induced M1A.10
    ankle M1A.17-
    elbow M1A.12-
    foot joint M1A.17-
    hand joint M1A.14-
    hip M1A.15-
    knee M1A.16-
    multiple site M1A.19
    shoulder M1A.11-
    vertebrae M1A.18
    wrist M1A.13-
  primary —see Gout, chronic, idiopathic
  saturnine —see Gout, chronic, lead-induced
  secondary NEC M1A.40
    ankle M1A.47-
    elbow M1A.42-
    foot joint M1A.47-
    hand joint M1A.44-
    hip M1A.45-
    knee M1A.46-
    multiple site M1A.49
    shoulder M1A.41-
    vertebrae M1A.48
    wrist M1A.43-
  syphilitic (see also subcategory M14.8-) A52.77
  tophi M1A.9
Gout, gouty (acute) (attack) (flare) (see also
      Gout, chronic) M10.9-
  drug-induced M10.20
    ankle M10.27-
    elbow M10.22-
    foot joint M10.27-
    hand joint M10.24-
    hip M10.25-
    knee M10.26-
    multiple site M10.29
    shoulder M10.21-
    vertebrae M10.28
    wrist M10.23-
  idiopathic M10.00
    ankle M10.07-
    elbow M10.02-
    foot joint M10.07-
    hand joint M10.04-
    hip M10.05-
    knee M10.06-
    multiple site M10.09
    shoulder M10.01-
    vertebrae M10.08
    wrist M10.03-
  in (due to) renal impairment M10.30
    ankle M10.37-
    elbow M10.32-
    foot joint M10.37-
    hand joint M10.34-
    hip M10.35-
    knee M10.36-
    multiple site M10.39
    shoulder M10.31-
    vertebrae M10.38
    wrist M10.33-
  lead-induced M10.10
    ankle M10.17-
    elbow M10.12-
    foot joint M10.17-
    hand joint M10.14-

Gout, gouty (Continued)
  lead-induced (Continued)
    hip M10.15-
    knee M10.16-
    multiple site M10.19
    shoulder M10.11-
    vertebrae M10.18
    wrist M10.13-
  primary —see Gout, idiopathic
  saturnine —see Gout, lead-induced
  secondary NEC M10.40
    ankle M10.47-
    elbow M10.42-
    foot joint M10.47-
    hand joint M10.44-
    hip M10.45-
    knee M10.46-
    multiple site M10.49
    shoulder M10.41-
    vertebrae M10.48
    wrist M10.43-
  syphilitic (see also subcategory M14.8-) A52.77
  tophi NEC —see Gout, chronic
Gower's
  muscular dystrophy G71.0
  syndrome (vasovagal attack) R55
Gradenigo's syndrome —see Otitis, media,
      suppurative, acute
Graefe's disease —see Strabismus, paralytic,
      ophthalmoplegia, progressive
Graft-versus-host disease D89.813
  acute D89.810
  acute on chronic D89.812
  chronic D89.811
Grain mite (itch) B88.0
Grainhandler's disease or lung J67.8
Grand mal —see Epilepsy, generalized,
      specified NEC
Grand multipara status only (not pregnant)
      Z64.1
  pregnant —see Pregnancy, complicated by,
      grand multiparity
Granite worker's lung J62.8
Granular —see also condition
  inflammation, pharynx J31.2
  kidney (contracting) —see Sclerosis, renal
  liver K74.69
Granulation tissue (abnormal) (excessive)
      L92.9
  postmastoidectomy cavity —see
      Complications, postmastoidectomy,
      granulation
Granulocytopenia (primary) (malignant) —see
      Agranulocytosis
Granuloma L92.9
  abdomen K66.8
    from residual foreign body L92.3
    pyogenicum L98.0
  actinic L57.5
  annulare (perforating) L92.0
  apical K04.5
  aural —see Otitis, externa, specified NEC
  beryllium (skin) L92.3
  bone
    eosinophilic C96.6
    from residual foreign body —see
        Osteomyelitis, specified type NEC
    lung C96.6
  brain (any site) G06.0
    schistosomiasis B65.9 [G07]
  canaliculus lacrimalis —see Granuloma,
      lacrimal
  candidal (cutaneous) B37.2
  cerebral (any site) G06.0
  coccidioidal (primary) (progressive) B38.7
    lung B38.1
    meninges B38.4
  colon K63.89
  conjunctiva H11.22-
  dental K04.5
  ear, middle —see Cholesteatoma

Granuloma *(Continued)*
 eosinophilic C96.6
  bone C96.6
  lung C96.6
  oral mucosa K13.4
  skin L92.2
 eyelid H01.8
 facial (e) L92.2
 foreign body (in soft tissue) NEC M60.20
  ankle M60.27-
  foot M60.27-
  forearm M60.23-
  hand M60.24-
  in operation wound —*see* Foreign body, accidentally left during a procedure
  lower leg M60.26-
  pelvic region M60.25-
  shoulder region M60.21-
  skin L92.3
  specified site NEC M60.28
  subcutaneous tissue L92.3
  thigh M60.25-
  upper arm M60.22-
 gangraenescens M31.2
 genito-inguinale A58
 giant cell (central) (reparative) (jaw) M27.1
  gingiva (peripheral) K06.8
 gland (lymph) I88.8
 hepatic NEC K75.3
  in (due to)
   berylliosis J63.2 [K77]
   sarcoidosis D86.89
 Hodgkin C81.9
 ileum K63.89
 infectious B99.9
  specified NEC B99.8
 inguinale (Donovan) (venereal) A58
 intestine NEC K63.89
 intracranial (any site) G06.0
 intraspinal (any part) G06.1
 iridocyclitis —*see* Iridocyclitis, chronic
 jaw (bone) (central) M27.1
  reparative giant cell M27.1
 kidney (*see also* Infection, kidney) N15.8
 lacrimal H04.81-
 larynx J38.7
 lethal midline (faciale) (e)) M31.2
 liver NEC —*see* Granuloma, hepatic
 lung (infectious) —*see also* Fibrosis, lung
  coccidioidal B38.1
  eosinophilic C96.6
 Majocchi's B35.8
 malignant (facial (e)) M31.2
 mandible (central) M27.1
 midline (lethal) M31.2
 monilial (cutaneous) B37.2
 nasal sinus —*see* Sinusitis
 operation wound T81.89
  foreign body —*see* Foreign body, accidentally left during a procedure
  stitch T81.89
  talc —*see* Foreign body, accidentally left during a procedure
 oral mucosa K13.4
 orbit, orbital H05.11-
 paracoccidioidal B41.8
 penis, venereal A58
 periapical K04.5
 peritoneum K66.8
  due to ova of helminths NOS (*see also* Helminthiasis) B83.9 [K67]
 postmastoidectomy cavity —*see* Complications, postmastoidectomy, recurrent cholesteatoma
 prostate N42.89
 pudendi (ulcerating) A58
 pulp, internal (tooth) K03.3
 pyogenic, pyogenicum (of) (skin) L98.0
  gingiva K06.8
  maxillary alveolar ridge K04.5
  oral mucosa K13.4

Granuloma *(Continued)*
 rectum K62.89
 reticulohistiocytic D76.3
 rubrum nasi L74.8
 Schistosoma —*see* Schistosomiasis
 septic (skin) L98.0
 silica (skin) L92.3
 sinus (accessory) (infective) (nasal) —*see* Sinusitis
 skin L92.9
  from residual foreign body L92.3
  pyogenicum L98.0
 spine
  syphilitic (epidural) A52.19
  tuberculous A18.01
 stitch (postoperative) T81.89
 suppurative (skin) L98.0
 swimming pool A31.1
 talc —*see also* Granuloma, foreign body
  in operation wound —*see* Foreign body, accidentally left during a procedure
 telangiectaticum (skin) L98.0
 tracheostomy J95.09
 trichophyticum B35.8
 tropicum A66.4
 umbilicus L92.9
 urethra N36.8
 uveitis —*see* Iridocyclitis, chronic
 vagina A58
 venereum A58
 vocal cord J38.3
Granulomatosis L92.9
 lymphoid C83.8-
 miliary (listerial) A32.89
 necrotizing, respiratory M31.30
 progressive septic D71
 specified NEC L92.8
 Wegener's M31.30
  with renal involvement M31.31
Granulomatous tissue (abnormal) (excessive) L92.9
Granulosis rubra nasi L74.8
Graphite fibrosis (of lung) J63.3
Graphospasm F48.8
 organic G25.89
Grating scapula M89.8X1
Gravel (urinary) —*see* Calculus, urinary
Graves' disease —*see* Hyperthyroidism, with, goiter
Gravis —*see* condition
Grawitz tumor C64.-
Gray syndrome (newborn) P93.0
Grayness, hair (premature) L67.1
 congenital Q84.2
Green sickness D50.8
Greenfield's disease
 meaning
  concentric sclerosis (encephalitis periaxialis concentrica) G37.5
  metachromatic leukodystrophy E75.25
Greenstick fracture - code as Fracture, by site
Grey syndrome (newborn) P93.0
Grief F43.21
 prolonged F43.29
 reaction (*see also* Disorder, adjustment) F43.20
Griesinger's disease B76.9
Grinder's lung or pneumoconiosis J62.8
Grinding, teeth
 psychogenic F45.8
 sleep related G47.63
Grip
 Dabney's B33.0
 devil's B33.0
Grippe, grippal —*see also* Influenza
 Balkan A78
 summer, of Italy A93.1
Grisel's disease M43.6
Groin —*see* condition
Grooved tongue K14.5

Ground itch B76.9
Grover's disease or syndrome L11.1
Growing pains, children R29.898
Growth (fungoid) (neoplastic) (new) —*see also* Neoplasm
 adenoid (vegetative) J35.8
 benign —*see* Neoplasm, benign, by site
 malignant —*see* Neoplasm, malignant, by site
 rapid, childhood Z00.2
 secondary —*see* Neoplasm, secondary, by site
Gruby's disease B35.0
Gubler-Millard paralysis or syndrome G46.3
Guerin-Stern syndrome Q74.3
Guidance, insufficient anterior (occlusal) M26.54
Guillain-Barré disease or syndrome G61.0
 sequelae G65.0
Guinea worms (infection) (infestation) B72
Guinon's disease (motor-verbal tic) F95.2
Gull's disease E03.4
Gum —*see* condition
Gumboil K04.7
 with sinus K04.6
Gumma (syphilitic) A52.79
 artery A52.09
  cerebral A52.04
 bone A52.77
  of yaws (late) A66.6
 brain A52.19
 cauda equina A52.19
 central nervous system A52.3
 ciliary body A52.71
 congenital A50.59
 eyelid A52.71
 heart A52.06
 intracranial A52.19
 iris A52.71
 kidney A52.75
 larynx A52.73
 leptomeninges A52.19
 liver A52.74
 meninges A52.19
 myocardium A52.06
 nasopharynx A52.73
 neurosyphilitic A52.3
 nose A52.73
 orbit A52.71
 palate (soft) A52.79
 penis A52.76
 pericardium A52.06
 pharynx A52.73
 pituitary A52.79
 scrofulous (tuberculous) A18.4
 skin A52.79
 specified site NEC A52.79
 spinal cord A52.19
 tongue A52.79
 tonsil A52.73
 trachea A52.73
 tuberculous A18.4
 ulcerative due to yaws A66.4
 ureter A52.75
 yaws A66.4
  bone A66.6
Gunn's syndrome Q07.8
Gunshot wound —*see also* Wound, open
 fracture - code as Fracture, by site
 internal organs —*see* Injury, by site
Gynandrism Q56.0
Gynandroblastoma
 specified site —*see* Neoplasm, uncertain behavior, by site
 unspecified site
  female D39.10
  male D40.10
Gynecological examination (periodic) (routine) Z01.419
 with abnormal findings Z01.411
Gynecomastia N62
Gynephobia F40.291
Gyrate scalp Q82.8

◀ New   ◀▥ Revised   ~~deleted~~ Deleted

H

H (Hartnup's) disease E72.02
Haas' disease or osteochondrosis (juvenile)
  (head of humerus) —see Osteochondrosis,
  juvenile, humerus
Habit, habituation
  bad sleep Z72.821
  chorea F95.8
  disturbance, child F98.9
  drug —see Dependence, drug
  irregular sleep Z72.821
  laxative F55.2
  spasm —see Tic
  tic —see Tic
Haemophilus (H.) influenzae, as cause of
  disease classified elsewhere B96.3
Haff disease —see Poisoning, mercury
Hageman's factor defect, deficiency or disease
  D68.2
Haglund's disease or osteochondrosis
  (juvenile) (os tibiale externum) —see
  Osteochondrosis, juvenile, tarsus
Hailey-Hailey disease Q82.8
Hair —see also condition
  plucking F63.3
    in stereotyped movement disorder F98.4
  tourniquet syndrome —see also Constriction,
    external, by site
    finger S60.44-
    penis S30.842
    thumb S60.34-
    toe S90.44-
Hairball in stomach T18.2
Hair-pulling, pathological (compulsive) F63.3
Hairy black tongue K14.3
Half vertebra Q76.49
Halitosis R19.6
Hallerman-Streiff syndrome Q87.0
Hallervorden-Spatz disease G23.0
Hallopeau's acrodermatitis or disease L40.2
Hallucination R44.3
  auditory R44.0
  gustatory R44.2
  olfactory R44.2
  specified NEC R44.2
  tactile R44.2
  visual R44.1
Hallucinosis (chronic) F28
  alcoholic (acute) F10.951
    in
      abuse F10.151
      dependence F10.251
  drug-induced F19.951
    cannabis F12.951
    cocaine F14.951
    hallucinogen F16.151
    in
      abuse F19.151
        cannabis F12.151
        cocaine F14.151
        hallucinogen F16.151
        inhalant F18.151
        opioid F11.151
        sedative, anxiolytic or hypnotic
          F13.151
        stimulant NEC F15.151
      dependence F19.251
        cannabis F12.251
        cocaine F14.251
        hallucinogen F16.251
        inhalant F18.251
        opioid F11.251
        sedative, anxiolytic or hypnotic
          F13.251
        stimulant NEC F15.251
    inhalant F18.951
    opioid F11.951
    sedative, anxiolytic or hypnotic F13.951
    stimulant NEC F15.951
  organic F06.0

Hallux
  deformity (acquired) NEC M20.5X-
  limitus M20.5X-
  malleus (acquired) NEC M20.3-
  rigidus (acquired) M20.2-
    congenital Q74.2
    sequelae (late effect) of rickets E64.3
  valgus (acquired) M20.1-
    congenital Q66.6
  varus (acquired) M20.3-
    congenital Q66.3
Halo, visual H53.19
Hamartoma, hamartoblastoma Q85.9
  epithelial (gingival), odontogenic, central
    or peripheral —see Cyst, calcifying
    odontogenic
Hamartosis Q85.9
Hamman-Rich syndrome J84.114
Hammer toe (acquired) NEC —see also
  Deformity, toe, hammer toe
  congenital Q66.89
  sequelae (late effect) of rickets E64.3
Hand —see condition
Hand-foot syndrome L27.1
Handicap, handicapped
  educational Z55.9
    specified NEC Z55.8
Hand-Schüller-Christian disease or syndrome
  C96.5
Hanging (asphyxia) (strangulation)
  (suffocation) —see Asphyxia, traumatic,
  due to mechanical threat
Hangnail —see also Cellulitis, digit
  with lymphangitis —see Lymphangitis, acute,
    digit
Hangover (alcohol) F10.129
Hanhart's syndrome Q87.0
Hanot-Chauffard (-Troisier) syndrome E83.19
Hanot's cirrhosis or disease K74.3
Hansen's disease —see Leprosy
Hantaan virus disease (Korean hemorrhagic
  fever) A98.5
Hantavirus disease (with renal manifestations)
  (Dobrava) (Puumala) (Seoul) A98.5
  with pulmonary manifestations (Andes)
    (Bayou) (Bermejo) (Black Creek Canal)
    (Choclo) (Juquitiba) (Laguna negra)
    (Lechiguanas) (New York) (Oran) (Sin
    nombre) B33.4
Happy puppet syndrome Q93.5
Harada's disease or syndrome H30.81-
Hardening
  artery —see Arteriosclerosis
  brain G93.89
Harelip (complete) (incomplete) —see Cleft, lip
Harlequin (newborn) Q80.4
Harley's disease D59.6
Harmful use (of)
  alcohol F10.10
  anxiolytics —see Abuse, drug, sedative
  cannabinoids —see Abuse, drug, cannabis
  cocaine —see Abuse, drug, cocaine
  drug —see Abuse, drug
  hallucinogens —see Abuse, drug,
    hallucinogen
  hypnotics —see Abuse, drug, sedative -
    opioids —see Abuse, drug, opioid
  PCP (phencyclidine) —see Abuse, drug,
    hallucinogen
  sedatives —see Abuse, drug, sedative
  stimulants NEC —see Abuse, drug, stimulant
Harris' lines —see Arrest, epiphyseal
Hartnup's disease E72.02
Harvester's lung J67.0
Harvesting ovum for in vitro fertilization
  Z31.83
Hashimoto's disease or thyroiditis E06.3
Hashitoxicosis (transient) E06.3
Hassal-Henle bodies or warts (cornea) H18.49
Haut mal —see Epilepsy, generalized, specified
  NEC

Haverhill fever A25.1
Hay fever (see also Fever, hay) J30.1
Hayem-Widal syndrome D59.8
Haygarth's nodes M15.8
Haymaker's lung J67.0
Hb (abnormal)
  Bart's disease D56.0
  disease —see Disease, hemoglobin
  trait —see Trait
Head —see condition
Headache R51
  allergic NEC G44.89
  associated with sexual activity
    G44.82
  chronic daily R51
  cluster G44.009
    chronic G44.029
      intractable G44.021
      not intractable G44.029
    episodic G44.019
      intractable G44.011
      not intractable G44.019
    intractable G44.001
    not intractable G44.009
  cough (primary) G44.83
  daily chronic R51
  drug-induced NEC G44.40
    intractable G44.41
    not intractable G44.40
  exertional (primary) G44.84
  histamine G44.009
    intractable G44.001
    not intractable G44.009
  hypnic G44.81
  lumbar puncture G97.1
  medication overuse G44.40
    intractable G44.41
    not intractable G44.40
  menstrual —see Migraine, menstrual
  migraine (type) (see also Migraine)
    G43.909
  nasal septum R51
  neuralgiform, short lasting unilateral, with
    conjunctival injection and tearing
    (SUNCT) G44.059
    intractable G44.051
    not intractable G44.059
  new daily persistent (NDPH) G44.52
  orgasmic G44.82
  periodic syndromes in adults and children
    G43.C0
    with refractory migraine G43.C1
    intractable G43.C1
    not intractable G43.C0
    without refractory migraine G43.C0
  postspinal puncture G97.1
  post-traumatic G44.309
    acute G44.319
      intractable G44.311
      not intractable G44.319
    chronic G44.329
      intractable G44.321
      not intractable G44.329
    intractable G44.301
    not intractable G44.309
  pre-menstrual —see Migraine, menstrual
  preorgasmic G44.82
  primary
    cough G44.83
    exertional G44.84
    stabbing G44.85
    thunderclap G44.53
  rebound G44.40
    intractable G44.41
    not intractable G44.40
  short lasting unilateral neuralgiform, with
    conjunctival injection and tearing
    (SUNCT) G44.059
    intractable G44.051
    not intractable G44.059
  specified syndrome NEC G44.89

Headache (Continued)
  spinal and epidural anesthesia - induced
      T88.59
    in labor and delivery O74.5
    in pregnancy O29.4-
    postpartum, puerperal O89.4
  spinal fluid loss (from puncture) G97.1
  stabbing (primary) G44.85
  tension (-type) G44.209
    chronic G44.229
      intractable G44.221
      not intractable G44.229
    episodic G44.219
      intractable G44.211
      not intractable G44.219
    intractable G44.201
    not intractable G44.209
  thunderclap (primary) G44.53
  vascular NEC G44.1
Healthy
  infant
    accompanying sick mother Z76.3
    receiving care Z76.2
  person accompanying sick person Z76.3
Hearing examination Z01.10
  with abnormal findings NEC Z01.118
  following failed hearing screening Z01.110
  for hearing conservation and treatment
      Z01.12
Heart —see condition
Heart beat
  abnormality R00.9
    specified NEC R00.8
  awareness R00.2
  rapid R00.0
  slow R00.1
Heartburn R12
  psychogenic F45.8
Heat (effects) T67.9
  apoplexy T67.0
  burn (see also Burn) L55.9
  collapse T67.1
  cramps T67.2
  dermatitis or eczema L59.0
  edema T67.7
  erythema - code by site under Burn, first
      degree
  excessive T67.9
    specified effect NEC T67.8
  exhaustion T67.5
    anhydrotic T67.3
    due to
      salt (and water) depletion T67.4
      water depletion T67.3
        with salt depletion T67.4
  fatigue (transient) T67.6
  fever T67.0
  hyperpyrexia T67.0
  prickly L74.0
  prostration —see Heat, exhaustion
  pyrexia T67.0
  rash L74.0
  specified effect NEC T67.8
  stroke T67.0
  sunburn —see Sunburn
  syncope T67.1
Heavy-for-dates NEC (infant) (4000g to 4499g)
      P08.1
  exceptionally (4500g or more) P08.0
Hebephrenia, hebephrenic (schizophrenia)
      F20.1
Heberden's disease or nodes (with
      arthropathy) M15.1
Hebra's
  pityriasis L26
  prurigo L28.2
Heel —see condition
Heerfordt's disease D86.89
Hegglin's anomaly or syndrome D72.0
Heilmeyer-Schoner disease D45
Heine-Medin disease A80.9

Heinz body anemia, congenital D58.2
Heliophobia F40.228
Heller's disease or syndrome F84.3
HELLP syndrome (hemolysis, elevated liver
      enzymes and low platelet count) O14.2-
Helminthiasis —see also Infestation, helminth
  Ancylostoma B76.0
  intestinal B82.0
    mixed types (types classifiable to more
        than one of the titles B65.0-B81.3 and
        B81.8) B81.4
    specified type NEC B81.8
  mixed types (intestinal) (types classifiable to
      more than one of the titles B65.0-B81.3
      and B81.8) B81.4
  Necator (americanus) B76.1
  specified type NEC B83.8
Heloma L84
Hemangioblastoma —see Neoplasm,
      connective tissue, uncertain behavior
  malignant —see Neoplasm, connective tissue,
      malignant
Hemangioendothelioma —see also Neoplasm,
      uncertain behavior, by site
  benign D18.00
    intra-abdominal D18.03
    intracranial D18.02
    skin D18.01
    specified site NEC D18.09
  bone (diffuse) —see Neoplasm, bone,
      malignant
  epithelioid —see also Neoplasm, uncertain
      behavior, by site
    malignant —see Neoplasm, malignant, by
        site
  malignant —see Neoplasm, connective tissue,
      malignant
Hemangiofibroma —see Neoplasm, benign,
      by site
Hemangiolipoma —see Lipoma
Hemangioma D18.00
  arteriovenous D18.00
    intra-abdominal D18.03
    intracranial D18.02
    skin D18.01
    specified site NEC D18.09
  capillary D18.00
    intra-abdominal D18.03
    intracranial D18.02
    skin D18.01
    specified site NEC D18.09
  cavernous D18.00
    intra-abdominal D18.03
    intracranial D18.02
    skin D18.01
    specified site NEC D18.09
  epithelioid D18.00
    intra-abdominal D18.03
    intracranial D18.02
    skin D18.01
    specified site NEC D18.09
  histiocytoid D18.00
    intra-abdominal D18.03
    intracranial D18.02
    skin D18.01
    specified site NEC D18.09
  infantile D18.00
    intra-abdominal D18.03
    intracranial D18.02
    skin D18.01
    specified site NEC D18.09
  intra-abdominal D18.03
  intracranial D18.02
  intramuscular D18.00
    intra-abdominal D18.03
    intracranial D18.02
    skin D18.01
    specified site NEC D18.09
  juvenile D18.00
  malignant —see Neoplasm, connective tissue,
      malignant

Hemangioma (Continued)
  plexiform D18.00
    intra-abdominal D18.03
    intracranial D18.02
    skin D18.01
    specified site NEC D18.09
  racemose D18.00
    intra-abdominal D18.03
    intracranial D18.02
    skin D18.01
    specified site NEC D18.09
  sclerosing —see Neoplasm, skin, benign
  simplex D18.00
    intra-abdominal D18.03
    intracranial D18.02
    skin D18.01
    specified site NEC D18.09
  skin D18.01
  specified site NEC D18.09
  venous D18.00
    intra-abdominal D18.03
    intracranial D18.02
    skin D18.01
    specified site NEC D18.09
  verrucous keratotic D18.00
    intra-abdominal D18.03
    intracranial D18.02
    skin D18.01
    specified site NEC D18.09
Hemangiomatosis (systemic) I78.8
  involving single site —see Hemangioma
Hemangiopericytoma —see also Neoplasm,
      connective tissue, uncertain behavior
  benign —see Neoplasm, connective tissue,
      benign
  malignant —see Neoplasm, connective tissue,
      malignant
Hemangiosarcoma —see Neoplasm, connective
      tissue, malignant
Hemarthrosis (nontraumatic) M25.00
  ankle M25.07-
  elbow M25.02-
  foot joint M25.07-
  hand joint M25.04-
  hip M25.05-
  in hemophilic arthropathy —see Arthropathy,
      hemophilic
  knee M25.06-
  shoulder M25.01-
  specified joint NEC M25.08
  traumatic —see Sprain, by site
  vertebrae M25.08
  wrist M25.03-
Hematemesis K92.0
  with ulcer - code by site under Ulcer, with
      hemorrhage K27.4
  newborn, neonatal P54.0
    due to swallowed maternal blood P78.2
Hematidrosis L74.8
Hematinuria —see also Hemoglobinuria
  malarial B50.8
Hematobilia K83.8
Hematocele
  female NEC N94.89
    with ectopic pregnancy O00.9
    ovary N83.8
  male N50.1
Hematochezia (see also Melena) K92.1
Hematochyluria —see also Infestation, filarial
  schistosomiasis (bilharziasis) B65.0
Hematocolpos (with hematometra or
      hematosalpinx) N89.7
Hematocornea —see Pigmentation, cornea,
      stromal
Hematogenous —see condition
Hematoma (traumatic) (skin surface intact) —
      see also Contusion
  with
    injury of internal organs —see Injury, by site
    open wound —see Wound, open
  amputation stump (surgical) (late) T87.89

◀ New   ◀▥ Revised   ~~deleted~~ Deleted

Hematoma *(Continued)*
aorta, dissecting I71.00
abdominal I71.02
thoracic I71.01
thoracoabdominal I71.03
aortic intramural —*see* Dissection, aorta
arterial (complicating trauma) —*see* Injury,
blood vessel, by site
auricle —*see* Contusion, ear
nontraumatic —*see* Disorder, pinna,
hematoma
birth injury NEC P15.8
brain (traumatic)
with
cerebral laceration or contusion
(diffuse) —*see* Injury, intracranial,
diffuse
focal —*see* Injury, intracranial,
focal
cerebellar, traumatic S06.37-
intracerebral, traumatic —*see* Injury,
intracranial, intracerebral
hemorrhage
newborn NEC P52.4
birth injury P10.1
nontraumatic —*see* Hemorrhage,
intracranial
subarachnoid, arachnoid, traumatic —*see*
Injury, intracranial, subarachnoid
hemorrhage
subdural, traumatic —*see* Injury,
intracranial, subdural hemorrhage
breast (nontraumatic) N64.89
broad ligament (nontraumatic) N83.7
traumatic S37.892
cerebellar, traumatic S06.37-
cerebral —*see* Hematoma, brain
cerebrum S06.36-
left S06.35-
right S06.34-
cesarean delivery wound O90.2
complicating delivery (perineal) (pelvic)
(vagina) (vulva) O71.7
corpus cavernosum (nontraumatic) N48.89
epididymis (nontraumatic) N50.1
epidural (traumatic) —*see* Injury, intracranial,
epidural hemorrhage
spinal —*see* Injury, spinal cord, by region
episiotomy O90.2
face, birth injury P15.4
genital organ NEC (nontraumatic)
female (nonobstetric) N94.89
traumatic S30.202
male N50.1
traumatic S30.201
internal organs —*see* Injury, by site
intracerebral, traumatic —*see* Injury,
intracranial, intracerebral hemorrhage
intraoperative —*see* Complications,
intraoperative, hemorrhage
labia (nontraumatic) (nonobstetric) N90.8
liver (subcapsular) (nontraumatic) K76.89
birth injury P15.0
mediastinum —*see* Injury, intrathoracic
mesosalpinx (nontraumatic) N83.7
traumatic S37.898
muscle - code by site under Contusion
nontraumatic
muscle M79.81
soft tissue M79.81
obstetrical surgical wound O90.2
orbit, orbital (nontraumatic) —*see also*
Hemorrhage, orbit
traumatic —*see* Contusion, orbit
pelvis (female) (nontraumatic) (nonobstetric)
N94.89
obstetric O71.7
traumatic —*see* Injury, by site
penis (nontraumatic) N48.89
birth injury P15.5
perianal (nontraumatic) K64.5

Hematoma *(Continued)*
perineal S30.23
complicating delivery O71.7
perirenal —*see* Injury, kidney
pinna —*see* Contusion, ear
nontraumatic —*see* Disorder, pinna,
hematoma
placenta O43.89-
postoperative (postprocedural) —*see*
Complication, postprocedural,
hemorrhage
retroperitoneal (nontraumatic) K66.1
traumatic S36.892
scrotum, superficial S30.22
birth injury P15.5
seminal vesicle (nontraumatic) N50.1
traumatic S37.892
spermatic cord (traumatic) S37.892
nontraumatic N50.1
spinal (cord) (meninges) —*see also* Injury,
spinal cord, by region
newborn (birth injury) P11.5
spleen D73.5
intraoperative —*see* Complications,
intraoperative, hemorrhage, spleen
postprocedural (postoperative) —*see*
Complications, postprocedural,
hemorrhage, spleen
sternocleidomastoid, birth injury P15.2
sternomastoid, birth injury P15.2
subarachnoid (traumatic) —*see* Injury,
intracranial, subarachnoid hemorrhage
newborn (nontraumatic) P52.5
due to birth injury P10.3
nontraumatic —*see* Hemorrhage,
intracranial, subarachnoid
subdural (traumatic) —*see* Injury, intracranial,
subdural hemorrhage
newborn (localized) P52.8
birth injury P10.0
nontraumatic —*see* Hemorrhage,
intracranial, subdural
superficial, newborn P54.5
testis (nontraumatic) N50.1
birth injury P15.5
tunica vaginalis (nontraumatic) N50.1
umbilical cord, complicating delivery
O69.5
uterine ligament (broad) (nontraumatic)
N83.7
traumatic S37.892
vagina (ruptured) (nontraumatic) N89.8
complicating delivery O71.7
vas deferens (nontraumatic) N50.1
traumatic S37.892
vitreous —*see* Hemorrhage, vitreous
vulva (nontraumatic) (nonobstetric)
N90.89
complicating delivery O71.7
newborn (birth injury) P15.5
Hematometra N85.7
with hematocolpos N89.7
Hematomyelia (central) G95.19
newborn (birth injury) P11.5
traumatic T14.8
Hematomyelitis G04.90
Hematoperitoneum —*see* Hemoperitoneum
Hematophobia F40.230
Hematopneumothorax (*see* Hemothorax)
Hematopoiesis, cyclic D70.4
Hematoporphyria —*see* Porphyria
Hematorachis, hematorrhachis G95.19
newborn (birth injury) P11.5
Hematosalpinx N83.6
with
hematocolpos N89.7
hematometra N85.7
with hematocolpos N89.7
infectional —*see* Salpingitis
Hematospermia R36.1
Hematothorax (*see* Hemothorax)

Hematuria R31.9
benign (familial) (of childhood) —*see also*
Hematuria, idiopathic
essential microscopic R31.1
due to sulphonamide, sulfonamide —*see* Table
of Drugs and Chemicals, by drug
endemic (*see also* Schistosomiasis) B65.0
gross R31.0
idiopathic N02.9
with glomerular lesion
crescentic (diffuse) glomerulonephritis
N02.7
dense deposit disease N02.6
endocapillary proliferative
glomerulonephritis N02.4
focal and segmental hyalinosis or
sclerosis N02.1
membranoproliferative (diffuse) N02.5
membranous (diffuse) N02.2
mesangial proliferative (diffuse) N02.3
mesangiocapillary (diffuse) N02.5
minor abnormality N02.0
proliferative NEC N02.8
specified pathology NEC N02.8
intermittent —*see* Hematuria, idiopathic
malarial B50.8
microscopic NEC R31.2
benign essential R31.1
paroxysmal —*see also* Hematuria, idiopathic
nocturnal D59.5
persistent —*see* Hematuria, idiopathic
recurrent —*see* Hematuria, idiopathic
tropical (*see also* Schistosomiasis) B65.0
tuberculous A18.13
Hemeralopia (day blindness) H53.11
vitamin A deficiency E50.5
Hemi-akinesia R41.4
Hemianalgesia R20.0
Hemianencephaly Q00.0
Hemianesthesia R20.0
Hemianopia, hemianopsia (heteronymous)
H53.47
homonymous H53.46-
syphilitic A52.71
Hemiathetosis R25.8
Hemiatrophy R68.89
cerebellar G31.9
face, facial, progressive (Romberg) G51.8
tongue K14.8
Hemiballism (us) G25.5
Hemicardia Q24.8
Hemicephalus, hemicephaly Q00.0
Hemichorea G25.5
Hemicolitis, left —*see* Colitis, left sided
Hemicrania
congenital malformation Q00.0
continua G44.51
meaning migraine (*see also* Migraine) G43.909
paroxysmal G44.039
chronic G44.049
intractable G44.041
not intractable G44.049
episodic G44.039
intractable G44.031
not intractable G44.039
intractable G44.031
not intractable G44.039
Hemidystrophy —*see* Hemiatrophy
Hemiectromelia Q73.8
Hemihypalgesia R20.8
Hemihypesthesia R20.1
Hemi-inattention R41.4
Hemimelia Q73.8
lower limb —*see* Defect, reduction, lower
limb, specified type NEC
upper limb —*see* Defect, reduction, upper
limb, specified type NEC
Hemiparalysis —*see* Hemiplegia
Hemiparesis —*see* Hemiplegia
Hemiparesthesia R20.2
Hemiparkinsonism G20

Hemiplegia G81.9-
  alternans facialis G83.89
  ascending NEC G81.90
    spinal G95.89
  congenital (cerebral) G80.8
    spastic G80.2
  embolic (current episode) I63.4-
  flaccid G81.0-
  following
    cerebrovascular disease I69.959
      cerebral infarction I69.35-
      intracerebral hemorrhage I69.15-
      nontraumatic intracranial hemorrhage
        NEC I69.25-
      specified disease NEC I69.85-
      stroke NOS I69.35-
      subarachnoid hemorrhage I69.05-
  hysterical F44.4
  newborn NEC P91.8
    birth injury P11.9
  spastic G81.1-
    congenital G80.2
  thrombotic (current episode) I63.3
Hemisection, spinal cord —see Injury, spinal
    cord, by region
Hemispasm (facial) R25.2
Hemisporosis B48.8
Hemitremor R25.1
Hemivertebra Q76.49
  failure of segmentation with scoliosis Q76.3
  fusion with scoliosis Q76.3
Hemochromatosis E83.119
  with refractory anemia D46.1
  due to repeated red blood cell transfusion
    E83.111
  hereditary (primary) E83.110
  primary E83.110
  specified NEC E83.118
Hemoglobin —see also condition
  abnormal (disease) —see Disease,
    hemoglobin
  AS genotype D57.3
  Constant Spring D58.2
  E-beta thalassemia D56.5
  fetal, hereditary persistence (HPFH) D56.4
  H Constant Spring D56.0
  low NOS D64.9
  S (Hb S), heterozygous D57.3
Hemoglobinemia D59.9
  due to blood transfusion T80.89
  paroxysmal D59.6
    nocturnal D59.5
Hemoglobinopathy (mixed) D58.2
  with thalassemia D56.8
  sickle-cell D57.1
    with thalassemia D57.40
      with crisis (vasoocclusive pain)
        D57.419
        with
          acute chest syndrome D57.411
          splenic sequestration D57.412
      without crisis D57.40
Hemoglobinuria R82.3
  with anemia, hemolytic, acquired (chronic)
    NEC D59.6
  cold (agglutinin) (paroxysmal) (with
    Raynaud's syndrome) D59.6
  due to exertion or hemolysis NEC D59.6
  intermittent D59.6
  malarial B50.8
  march D59.6
  nocturnal (paroxysmal) D59.5
  paroxysmal (cold) D59.6
    nocturnal D59.5
Hemolymphangioma D18.1
Hemolysis
  intravascular
    with
      abortion —see Abortion, by type,
        complicated by, hemorrhage
      ectopic or molar pregnancy O08.1

Hemolysis (Continued)
  intravascular (Continued)
    with (Continued)
      hemorrhage
        antepartum —see Hemorrhage,
          antepartum, with coagulation
          defect
        intrapartum (see also Hemorrhage,
          complicating, delivery) O67.0
      postpartum O72.3
  neonatal (excessive) P58.9
    specified NEC P58.8
Hemolytic —see condition
Hemopericardium I31.2
  following acute myocardial infarction
    (current complication) I23.0
  newborn P54.8
  traumatic —see Injury, heart, with
    hemopericardium
Hemoperitoneum K66.1
  infectional K65.9
  traumatic S36.899
    with open wound —see Wound, open, with
      penetration into peritoneal cavity
Hemophilia (classical) (familial) (hereditary)
    D66
  A D66
  B D67
  C D68.1
  acquired D68.311
  autoimmune D68.311
  calcipriva (see also Defect, coagulation) D68.4
  nonfamilial (see also Defect, coagulation)
    D68.4
  secondary D68.311
  vascular D68.0
Hemophthalmos H44.81-
Hemopneumothorax —see also Hemothorax
  traumatic S27.2
Hemoptysis R04.2
  newborn P26.9
  tuberculous —see Tuberculosis, pulmonary
Hemorrhage, hemorrhagic (concealed) R58
  abdomen R58
  accidental antepartum —see Hemorrhage,
    antepartum
  acute idiopathic pulmonary, in infants
    R04.81
  adenoid J35.8
  adrenal (capsule) (gland) E27.49
    medulla E27.8
    newborn P54.4
  after delivery —see Hemorrhage, postpartum
  alveolar
    lung, newborn P26.8
    process K08.8
  alveolus K08.8
  amputation stump (surgical) T87.89
  anemia (chronic) D50.0
    acute D62
  antepartum (with) O46.90
    with coagulation defect O46.00-
      afibrinogenemia O46.01-
      disseminated intravascular coagulation
        O46.02-
      hypofibrinogenemia O46.01-
      specified defect NEC O46.09-
    before 20 weeks gestation O20.9
      specified type NEC O20.8
      threatened abortion O20.0
    due to
      abruptio placenta (see also Abruptio
        placentae) O45.9-
      leiomyoma, uterus —see Hemorrhage,
        antepartum, specified cause NEC
      placenta previa O44.1-
    specified cause NEC —see subcategory
      O46.8X-
  anus (sphincter) K62.5
  apoplexy (stroke) —see Hemorrhage,
    intracranial, intracerebral

Hemorrhage, hemorrhagic (Continued)
  arachnoid —see Hemorrhage, intracranial,
    subarachnoid
  artery R58
    brain —see Hemorrhage, intracranial,
      intracerebral
  basilar (ganglion) I61.0
  bladder N32.89
  bowel K92.2
    newborn P54.3
  brain (miliary) (nontraumatic) —see
    Hemorrhage, intracranial, intracerebral
    due to
      birth injury P10.1
      syphilis A52.05
    epidural or extradural (traumatic) —
      see Injury, intracranial, epidural
      hemorrhage
    newborn P52.4
      birth injury P10.1
    subarachnoid —see Hemorrhage,
      intracranial, subarachnoid
    subdural —see Hemorrhage, intracranial,
      subdural
  brainstem (nontraumatic) I61.3
    traumatic S06.38-
  breast N64.59
  bronchial tube —see Hemorrhage, lung
  bronchopulmonary —see Hemorrhage, lung
  bronchus —see Hemorrhage, lung
  bulbar I61.5
  capillary I78.8
    primary D69.8
  cecum K92.2
  cerebellar, cerebellum (nontraumatic) I61.4
    newborn P52.6
    traumatic S06.37-
  cerebral, cerebrum —see also Hemorrhage,
    intracranial, intracerebral
    lobe I61.1
    newborn (anoxic) P52.4
      birth injury P10.1
  cerebromeningeal I61.8
  cerebrospinal —see Hemorrhage, intracranial,
    intracerebral
  cervix (uteri) (stump) NEC N88.8
  chamber, anterior (eye) —see Hyphema
  childbirth —see Hemorrhage, complicating,
    delivery
  choroid H31.30-
    expulsive H31.31-
  ciliary body —see Hyphema
  cochlea —see subcategory H83.8
  colon K92.2
  complicating
    abortion —see Abortion, by type,
      complicated by, hemorrhage
    delivery O67.9
      associated with coagulation defect
        (afibrinogenemia) (DIC)
        (hyperfibrinolysis) O67.0
      specified cause NEC O67.8
    surgical procedure —see Hemorrhage,
      intraoperative
  conjunctiva H11.3-
    newborn P54.8
  cord, newborn (stump) P51.9
  corpus luteum (ruptured) cyst N83.1
  cortical (brain) I61.1
  cranial —see Hemorrhage, intracranial
  cutaneous R23.3
    due to autosensitivity, erythrocyte D69.2
    newborn P54.5
  delayed
    following ectopic or molar pregnancy
      O08.1
    postpartum O72.2
  diathesis (familial) D69.9
  disease D69.9
    newborn P53
    specified type NEC D69.8

◀ New   ◀═ Revised   ~~deleted~~ Deleted

Hemorrhage, hemorrhagic (Continued)
  due to or associated with
    afibrinogenemia or other coagulation
      defect (conditions in categories
      D65-D69)
      antepartum —see Hemorrhage,
        antepartum, with coagulation
        defect
      intrapartum O67.0
    dental implant M27.61
    device, implant or graft (see also
      Complications, by site and type,
      specified NEC) T85.83
      arterial graft NEC T82.838
      breast T85.83
      catheter NEC T85.83
        dialysis (renal) T82.838
          intraperitoneal T85.83
        infusion NEC T82.838
          spinal (epidural) (subdural) T85.83
        urinary (indwelling) T83.83
      electronic (electrode) (pulse generator)
        (stimulator)
        bone T84.83
        cardiac T82.837
        nervous system (brain) (peripheral
          nerve) (spinal) T85.83
        urinary T83.83
      fixation, internal (orthopedic) NEC T84.83
      gastrointestinal (bile duct) (esophagus)
        T85.83
      genital NEC T83.83
      heart NEC T82.837
      joint prosthesis T84.83
      ocular (corneal graft) (orbital implant)
        NEC T85.83
      orthopedic NEC T84.83
        bone graft T86.838
      specified NEC T85.83
      urinary NEC T83.83
      vascular NEC T82.838
      ventricular intracranial shunt T85.83
  duodenum, duodenal K92.2
    ulcer —see Ulcer, duodenum, with
      hemorrhage
  dura mater —see Hemorrhage, intracranial,
    subdural
  endotracheal —see Hemorrhage, lung
  epicranial subaponeurotic (massive), birth
    injury P12.2
  epidural (traumatic) —see also Injury,
    intracranial, epidural hemorrhage
    nontraumatic I62.1
  esophagus K22.8
    varix I85.01
      secondary I85.11
  excessive, following ectopic gestation
    (subsequent episode) O08.1
  extradural (traumatic) —see Injury,
    intracranial, epidural hemorrhage
    birth injury P10.8
    newborn (anoxic) (nontraumatic) P52.8
    nontraumatic I62.1
  eye NEC H57.8
    fundus —see Hemorrhage, retina
    lid —see Disorder, eyelid, specified type
      NEC
  fallopian tube N83.6
  fibrinogenolysis —see Fibrinolysis
  fibrinolytic (acquired) —see Fibrinolysis
  from
    ear (nontraumatic) —see Otorrhagia
    tracheostomy stoma J95.01
  fundus, eye —see Hemorrhage, retina
  funis —see Hemorrhage, umbilicus, cord
  gastric —see Hemorrhage, stomach
  gastroenteric K92.2
    newborn P54.3
  gastrointestinal (tract) K92.2
    newborn P54.3
  genital organ, male N50.1

Hemorrhage, hemorrhagic (Continued)
  genitourinary (tract) NOS R31.9
  gingiva K06.8
  globe (eye) —see Hemophthalmos
  graafian follicle cyst (ruptured) N83.0
  gum K06.8
  heart I51.89
  hypopharyngeal (throat) R04.1
  intermenstrual (regular) N92.3
    irregular N92.1
  internal (organs) NEC R58
    capsule I61.0
    ear —see subcategory H83.8
    newborn P54.8
  intestine K92.2
    newborn P54.3
  intra-abdominal R58
  intra-alveolar (lung), newborn P26.8
  intracerebral (nontraumatic) —see
    Hemorrhage, intracranial,
    intracerebral
  intracranial (nontraumatic) I62.9
    birth injury P10.9
    epidural, nontraumatic I62.1
    extradural, nontraumatic I62.1
    intracerebral (nontraumatic) (in) I61.9
      brain stem I61.3
      cerebellum I61.4
      hemisphere I61.2
        cortical (superficial) I61.1
        subcortical (deep) I61.0
      intraoperative
        during a nervous system procedure
          G97.31
        during other procedure G97.32
      intraventricular I61.5
      multiple localized I61.6
      newborn P52.4
        birth injury P10.1
      postprocedural
        following a nervous system procedure
          G97.51
        following other procedure
          G97.52
      specified NEC I61.8
      superficial I61.1
      traumatic (diffuse) —see Injury,
        intracranial, diffuse
        focal —see Injury, intracranial, focal
    newborn P52.9
      specified NEC P52.8
    subarachnoid (nontraumatic) (from)
      I60.9
      intracranial (cerebral) artery I60.7
        anterior communicating I60.2-
        basilar I60.4
        carotid siphon and bifurcation
          I60.0-
        communicating I60.7
          anterior I60.2-
          posterior I60.3-
        middle cerebral I60.1-
        posterior communicating I60.3-
        specified artery NEC I60.6
        vertebral I60.5-
      newborn P52.5
        birth injury P10.3
      specified NEC I60.8
      traumatic S06.6X-
    subdural (nontraumatic) I62.00
      acute I62.01
      birth injury P10.0
      chronic I62.03
      newborn (anoxic) (hypoxic) P52.8
        birth injury P10.0
      spinal G95.19
      subacute I62.02
      traumatic —see Injury, intracranial,
        subdural hemorrhage
    traumatic —see Injury, intracranial, focal
      brain injury

Hemorrhage, hemorrhagic (Continued)
  intramedullary NEC G95.19
  intraocular —see Hemophthalmos
  intraoperative, intraprocedural —see
    Complication, hemorrhage (hematoma),
    intraoperative (intraprocedural), by site
  intrapartum —see Hemorrhage, complicating,
    delivery
  intrapelvic
    female N94.89
    male K66.1
  intraperitoneal K66.1
  intrapontine I61.3
  intraprocedural —see Complication,
    hemorrhage (hematoma), intraoperative
    (intraprocedural), by site
  intrauterine N85.7
    complicating delivery (see also Hemorrhage,
      complicating, delivery) O67.9
    postpartum —see Hemorrhage, postpartum
  intraventricular I61.5
    newborn (nontraumatic) (see also Newborn,
      affected by, hemorrhage) P52.3
      due to birth injury P10.2
      grade
        1 P52.0
        2 P52.1
        3 P52.21
        4 P52.22
  intravesical N32.89
  iris (postinfectional) (postinflammatory)
    (toxic) —see Hyphema
  joint (nontraumatic) —see Hemarthrosis
  kidney N28.89
  knee (joint) (nontraumatic) —see
    Hemarthrosis, knee
  labyrinth —see subcategory H83.8
  lenticular striate artery I61.0
  ligature, vessel —see Hemorrhage,
    postoperative
  liver K76.89
  lung R04.89
    newborn P26.9
      massive P26.1
      specified NEC P26.8
    tuberculous —see Tuberculosis, pulmonary
  massive umbilical, newborn P51.0
  mediastinum —see Hemorrhage, lung
  medulla I61.3
  membrane (brain) I60.8
    spinal cord —see Hemorrhage, spinal cord
  meninges, meningeal (brain) (middle) I60.8
    spinal cord —see Hemorrhage, spinal cord
  mesentery K66.1
  metritis —see Endometritis
  mouth K13.79
  mucous membrane NEC R58
    newborn P54.8
  muscle M62.89
  nail (subungual) L60.8
  nasal turbinate R04.0
    newborn P54.8
  navel, newborn P51.9
  newborn P54.9
    specified NEC P54.8
  nipple N64.59
  nose R04.0
    newborn P54.8
  omentum K66.1
  optic nerve (sheath) H47.02-
  orbit, orbital H05.23-
  ovary NEC N83.8
  oviduct N83.6
  pancreas K86.8
  parathyroid (gland) (spontaneous) E21.4
  parturition —see Hemorrhage, complicating,
    delivery
  penis N48.89
  pericardium, pericarditis I31.2
  peritoneum, peritoneal K66.1
  peritonsillar tissue J35.8
    due to infection J36

Hemorrhage, hemorrhagic *(Continued)*
  petechial R23.3
    due to autosensitivity, erythrocyte D69.2
  pituitary (gland) E23.6
  pleura —*see* Hemorrhage, lung
  polioencephalitis, superior E51.2
  polymyositis —*see* Polymyositis
  pons, pontine I61.3
  posterior fossa (nontraumatic) I61.8
    newborn P52.6
  postmenopausal N95.0
  postnasal R04.0
  postoperative —*see* Complications,
      postprocedural, hemorrhage, by site
  postpartum NEC (following delivery of
      placenta) O72.1
    delayed or secondary O72.2
    retained placenta O72.0
    third stage O72.0
  pregnancy —*see* Hemorrhage, antepartum
  preretinal —*see* Hemorrhage, retina
  prostate N42.1
  puerperal —*see* Hemorrhage, postpartum
    delayed or secondary O72.2
  pulmonary R04.89
    newborn P26.9
      massive P26.1
      specified NEC P26.8
    tuberculous —*see* Tuberculosis, pulmonary
  purpura (primary) D69.3
  rectum (sphincter) K62.5
    newborn P54.2
  recurring, following initial hemorrhage at
      time of injury T79.2
  renal N28.89
  respiratory passage or tract R04.9
    specified NEC R04.89
  retina, retinal (vessels) H35.6-
    diabetic —*see* Diabetes, retinal, hemorrhage
  retroperitoneal R58
  scalp R58
  scrotum N50.1
  secondary (nontraumatic) R58
    following initial hemorrhage at time of
        injury T79.2
  seminal vesicle N50.1
  skin R23.3
    newborn P54.5
  slipped umbilical ligature P51.8
  spermatic cord N50.1
  spinal (cord) G95.19
    newborn (birth injury) P11.5
  spleen D73.5
    intraoperative —*see* Complications,
        intraoperative, hemorrhage, spleen
    postprocedural —*see* Complications,
        postprocedural, hemorrhage, spleen
  stomach K92.2
    newborn P54.3
    ulcer —*see* Ulcer, stomach, with
        hemorrhage
  subarachnoid (nontraumatic) —*see*
      Hemorrhage, intracranial, subarachnoid
  subconjunctival —*see also* Hemorrhage,
      conjunctiva
    birth injury P15.3
  subcortical (brain) I61.0
  subcutaneous R23.3
  subdiaphragmatic R58
  subdural (acute) (nontraumatic) —*see*
      Hemorrhage, intracranial, subdural
  subependymal
    newborn P52.0
      with intraventricular extension P52.1
          and intracerebral extension P52.22
  subgaleal P12.1
  subhyaloid —*see* Hemorrhage, retina
  subperiosteal —*see* Disorder, bone, specified
      type NEC
  subretinal —*see* Hemorrhage, retina
  subtentorial —*see* Hemorrhage, intracranial,
      subdural

Hemorrhage, hemorrhagic *(Continued)*
  subungual L60.8
  suprarenal (capsule) (gland) E27.49
    newborn P54.4
  tentorium (traumatic) NEC —*see*
      Hemorrhage, brain
    newborn (birth injury) P10.4
  testis N50.1
  third stage (postpartum) O72.0
  thorax —*see* Hemorrhage, lung
  throat R04.1
  thymus (gland) E32.8
  thyroid (cyst) (gland) E07.89
  tongue K14.8
  tonsil J35.8
  trachea —*see* Hemorrhage, lung
  tracheobronchial R04.89
    newborn P26.0
  traumatic — code to specific injury
    cerebellar —*see* Hemorrhage, brain
    intracranial —*see* Hemorrhage, brain
    recurring or secondary (following initial
        hemorrhage at time of injury)
        T79.2
  tuberculous NEC (*see also* Tuberculosis,
      pulmonary) A15.0
  tunica vaginalis N50.1
  ulcer - code by site under Ulcer, with
      hemorrhage K27.4
  umbilicus, umbilical
    cord
      after birth, newborn P51.9
      complicating delivery O69.5
    newborn P51.9
      massive P51.0
      slipped ligature P51.8
    stump P51.9
  urethra (idiopathic) N36.8
  uterus, uterine (abnormal) N93.9
    climacteric N92.4
    complicating delivery —*see* Hemorrhage,
        complicating, delivery
    dysfunctional or functional N93.8
    intermenstrual (regular) N92.3
      irregular N92.1
    postmenopausal N95.0
    postpartum —*see* Hemorrhage,
        postpartum
    preclimacteric or premenopausal N92.4
    prepubertal N93.8
    pubertal N92.2
  vagina (abnormal) N93.9
    newborn P54.6
  vas deferens N50.1
  vasa previa O69.4
  ventricular I61.5
  vesical N32.89
  viscera NEC R58
    newborn P54.8
  vitreous (humor) (intraocular) H43.1-
  vulva N90.89
Hemorrhoids (bleeding) (without mention of
    degree) K64.9
  1st degree (grade/stage I) (without prolapse
      outside of anal canal) K64.0
  2nd degree (grade/stage II) (that
      prolapse with straining but retract
      spontaneously) K64.1
  3rd degree (grade/stage III) (that prolapse
      with straining and require manual
      replacement back inside anal canal)
      K64.2
  4th degree (grade/stage IV) (with prolapsed
      tissue that cannot be manually replaced)
      K64.3
  complicating
    pregnancy O22.4
    puerperium O87.2
  external K64.4
    with
      thrombosis K64.5

Hemorrhage, hemorrhagic *(Continued)*
  internal (without mention of degree) K64.8
  prolapsed K64.8
  skin tags
    anus K64.4
    residual K64.4
  specified NEC K64.8
  strangulated (*see also* Hemorrhoids, by
      degree) K64.8
  thrombosed (*see also* Hemorrhoids, by degree)
      K64.5
  ulcerated (*see also* Hemorrhoids, by degree)
      K64.8
Hemosalpinx N83.6
  with
    hematocolpos N89.7
    hematometra N85.7
      with hematocolpos N89.7
Hemosiderosis (dietary) E83.19
  pulmonary, idiopathic E83.1 *[J84.03]*
  transfusion T80.89
Hemothorax (bacterial) (nontuberculous)
    J94.2
  newborn P54.8
  traumatic S27.1
    with pneumothorax S27.2
  tuberculous NEC A15.6
Henoch (-Schönlein) disease or syndrome
    (purpura) D69.0
Henpue, henpuye A66.6
Hepar lobatum (syphilitic) A52.74
Hepatalgia K76.89
Hepatitis K75.9
  acute B17.9
    with coma K72.01
    with hepatic failure —*see* Failure, hepatic
    alcoholic —*see* Hepatitis, alcoholic
    infectious B15.9
      with hepatic coma B15.0
    viral B17.9
  alcoholic (acute) (chronic) K70.10
    with ascites K70.11
  amebic —*see* Abscess, liver, amebic
  anicteric (viral) —*see* Hepatitis, viral
  antigen-associated (HAA) —*see* Hepatitis, B
  Australia-antigen (positive) —*see* Hepatitis, B
  autoimmune K75.4
  B B19.10
    with hepatic coma B19.11
    acute B16.9
      with
        delta-agent (coinfection) (without
            hepatic coma) B16.1
          with hepatic coma B16.0
        hepatic coma (without delta-agent
            coinfection) B16.2
    chronic B18.1
      with delta-agent B18.0
  bacterial NEC K75.89
  C (viral) B19.20
    with hepatic coma B19.21
    acute B17.10
      with hepatic coma B17.11
    chronic B18.2
  catarrhal (acute) B15.9
    with hepatic coma B15.0
  cholangiolitic K75.89
  cholestatic K75.89
  chronic K73.9
    active NEC K73.2
    lobular NEC K73.1
    persistent NEC K73.0
    specified NEC K73.8
  cytomegaloviral B25.1
  due to ethanol (acute) (chronic) —*see*
      Hepatitis, alcoholic
  epidemic B15.9
    with hepatic coma B15.0
  fulminant NEC (viral) —*see* Hepatitis, viral
  granulomatous NEC K75.3
  herpesviral B00.81

◀ New   ◀▥ Revised   ~~deleted~~ Deleted

Hepatitis *(Continued)*
history of
B Z86.19
C Z86.19
homologous serum —*see* Hepatitis, viral,
type B
in (due to)
mumps B26.81
toxoplasmosis (acquired) B58.1
congenital (active) P37.1 *[K77]*
infectious, infective (acute) (chronic)
(subacute) B15.9
with hepatic coma B15.0
inoculation —*see* Hepatitis, viral, type B
interstitial (chronic) K74.69
lupoid NEC K75.2
malignant NEC (with hepatic failure)
K72.90
with coma K72.91
neonatal giant cell P59.29
neonatal (idiopathic) (toxic) P59.29
newborn P59.29
postimmunization —*see* Hepatitis, viral,
type B
post-transfusion —*see* Hepatitis, viral, type B
reactive, nonspecific K75.2
serum —*see* Hepatitis, viral, type B
specified type NEC
with hepatic failure —*see* Failure, hepatic
syphilitic (late) A52.74
congenital (early) A50.08 *[K77]*
late A50.59 *[K77]*
secondary A51.45
toxic (*see also* Disease, liver, toxic) K71.6
tuberculous A18.83
viral, virus B19.9
with hepatic coma B19.0
acute B17.9
chronic B18.9
specified NEC B18.8
type
B B18.1
with delta-agent B18.0
C B18.2
congenital P35.3
coxsackie B33.8 *[K77]*
cytomegalic inclusion B25.1
in remission, any type — code to Hepatitis,
chronic, by type
non-A, non-B B17.8
specified type NEC (with or without coma)
B17.8
type
A B15.9
with hepatic coma B15.0
B B19.10
with hepatic coma B19.11
acute B16.9
with
delta-agent (coinfection) (without
hepatic coma) B16.1
with hepatic coma B16.0
hepatic coma (without delta-
agent coinfection) B16.2
chronic B18.1
with delta-agent B18.0
C B19.20
with hepatic coma B19.21
acute B17.10
with hepatic coma B17.11
chronic B18.2
E B17.2
non-A, non-B B17.8
Hepatization lung (acute) —*see* Pneumonia,
lobar
Hepatoblastoma C22.2
Hepatocarcinoma C22.0
Hepatocholangiocarcinoma C22.0
Hepatocholangioma, benign D13.4
Hepatocholangitis K75.89
Hepatolenticular degeneration E83.01

Hepatoma (malignant) C22.0
benign D13.4
embryonal C22.0
Hepatomegaly —*see also* Hypertrophy, liver
with splenomegaly R16.2
congenital Q44.7
in mononucleosis
gammaherpesviral B27.09
infectious specified NEC B27.89
Hepatoptosis K76.89
Hepatorenal syndrome following labor and
delivery O90.4
Hepatosis K76.89
Hepatosplenomegaly R16.2
hyperlipemic (Bürger-Grütz type) E78.3 *[K77]*
Hereditary —*see* condition
Heredodegeneration, macular —*see* Dystrophy,
retina
Heredopathia atactica polyneuritiformis G60.1
Heredosyphilis —*see* Syphilis, congenital
Herlitz' syndrome Q81.1
Hermansky-Pudlak syndrome E70.331
Hermaphrodite, hermaphroditism (true) Q56.0
46,XX with streak gonads Q99.1
46,XX/46,XY Q99.0
46,XY with streak gonads Q99.1
chimera 46,XX/46,XY Q99.0
Hernia, hernial (acquired) (recurrent) K46.9
with
gangrene —*see* Hernia, by site, with,
gangrene
incarceration —*see* Hernia, by site, with,
obstruction
irreducible —*see* Hernia, by site, with,
obstruction
obstruction —*see* Hernia, by site, with,
obstruction
strangulation —*see* Hernia, by site, with,
obstruction
abdomen, abdominal K46.9
with
gangrene (and obstruction) K46.1
obstruction K46.0
femoral —*see* Hernia, femoral
incisional —*see* Hernia, incisional
inguinal —*see* Hernia, inguinal
specified site NEC K45.8
with
gangrene (and obstruction) K45.1
obstruction K45.0
umbilical —*see* Hernia, umbilical
wall —*see* Hernia, ventral
appendix —*see* Hernia, abdomen
bladder (mucosa) (sphincter)
congenital (female) (male) Q79.51
female —*see* Cystocele
male N32.89
brain, congenital —*see* Encephalocele
cartilage, vertebra —*see* Displacement,
intervertebral disc
cerebral, congenital —*see also* Encephalocele
endaural Q01.8
ciliary body (traumatic) S05.2-
colon —*see* Hernia, abdomen
Cooper's —*see* Hernia, abdomen, specified
site NEC
crural —*see* Hernia, femoral
diaphragm, diaphragmatic K44.9
with
gangrene (and obstruction) K44.1
obstruction K44.0
congenital Q79.0
direct (inguinal) —*see* Hernia, inguinal
diverticulum, intestine —*see* Hernia,
abdomen
double (inguinal) —*see* Hernia, inguinal,
bilateral
due to adhesions (with obstruction) K56.5
epigastric (*see also* Hernia, ventral) K43.9
esophageal hiatus —*see* Hernia, hiatal
external (inguinal) —*see* Hernia, inguinal

Hernia, hernial *(Continued)*
fallopian tube N83.4
fascia M62.89
femoral K41.90
with
gangrene (and obstruction) K41.40
not specified as recurrent K41.40
recurrent K41.41
obstruction K41.30
not specified as recurrent K41.30
recurrent K41.31
bilateral K41.20
with
gangrene (and obstruction) K41.10
not specified as recurrent K41.10
recurrent K41.11
obstruction K41.00
not specified as recurrent K41.00
recurrent K41.01
not specified as recurrent K41.20
recurrent K41.21
not specified as recurrent K41.90
recurrent K41.91
unilateral K41.90
with
gangrene (and obstruction) K41.40
not specified as recurrent K41.40
recurrent K41.41
obstruction K41.30
not specified as recurrent K41.30
recurrent K41.31
not specified as recurrent K41.90
recurrent K41.91
foramen magnum G93.5
congenital Q01.8
funicular (umbilical) —*see also* Hernia,
umbilicus
spermatic (cord) —*see* Hernia, inguinal
gastrointestinal tract —*see* Hernia, abdomen
Hesselbach's —*see* Hernia, femoral, specified
site NEC
hiatal (esophageal) (sliding) K44.9
with
gangrene (and obstruction) K44.1
obstruction K44.0
congenital Q40.1
hypogastric —*see* Hernia, ventral
incarcerated —*see also* Hernia, by site, with
obstruction
with gangrene —*see* Hernia, by site, with
gangrene
incisional K43.92
with
gangrene (and obstruction) K43.1
obstruction K43.0
indirect (inguinal) —*see* Hernia, inguinal
inguinal (direct) (external) (funicular)
(indirect) (internal) (oblique) (scrotal)
(sliding) K40.90
with
gangrene (and obstruction) K40.40
not specified as recurrent K40.40
recurrent K40.41
obstruction K40.30
not specified as recurrent K40.30
recurrent K40.31
bilateral K40.20
with
gangrene (and obstruction)
K40.10
not specified as recurrent
K40.10
recurrent K40.11
obstruction K40.00
not specified as recurrent
K40.00
recurrent K40.01
not specified as recurrent K40.20
recurrent K40.21
not specified as recurrent K40.90
recurrent K40.91

◀ New   ◀═ Revised   ~~deleted~~ Deleted

Herpes, herpesvirus, herpetic (Continued)
  zoster (Continued)
    polyneuropathy B02.23
    specified complication NEC B02.8
    trigeminal neuralgia B02.22
Herpesvirus (human) —see Herpes
Herpetophobia F40.218
Herrick's anemia —see Disease, sickle-cell
Hers' disease E74.09
Herter-Gee syndrome K90.0
Herxheimer's reaction R68.89
Hesitancy
  of micturition R39.11
  urinary R39.11
Hesselbach's hernia —see Hernia, femoral,
  specified site NEC
Heterochromia (congenital) Q13.2
  cataract —see Cataract, complicated
  cyclitis (Fuchs) —see Cyclitis, Fuchs'
    heterochromic
  hair L67.1
  iritis —see Cyclitis, Fuchs' heterochromic
  retained metallic foreign body
    (nonmagnetic) —see Foreign body,
    intraocular, old, retained
    magnetic —see Foreign body, intraocular,
    old, retained, magnetic
  uveitis —see Cyclitis, Fuchs' heterochromic
Heterophoria —see Strabismus, heterophoria
Heterophyes, heterophyiasis (small intestine)
  B66.8
Heterotopia, heterotopic —see also Malposition,
  congenital
  cerebralis Q04.8
Heterotropia —see Strabismus
Heubner-Herter disease K90.0
Hexadactylism Q69.9
HGSIL (cytology finding) (high grade
  squamous intraepithelial lesion on
  cytologic smear) (Pap smear finding)
  anus R85.613
  cervix R87.613
    biopsy (histology) finding — code to CIN
      II or CIN III
  vagina R87.623
    biopsy (histology) finding — code to VAIN
      II or VAIN III
Hibernoma —see Lipoma
Hiccup, hiccough R06.6
  epidemic B33.0
  psychogenic F45.8
Hidden penis (congenital) Q55.64
  acquired N48.83
Hidradenitis (axillaris) (suppurative) L73.2
Hidradenoma (nodular) —see also Neoplasm,
  skin, benign
  clear cell —see Neoplasm, skin, benign
  papillary —see Neoplasm, skin, benign
Hidrocystoma —see Neoplasm, skin, benign
High
  altitude effects T70.20
    anoxia T70.29
    on
      ears T70.0
      sinuses T70.1
    polycythemia D75.1
  arch
    foot Q66.7
    palate, congenital Q38.5
  arterial tension —see Hypertension
  basal metabolic rate R94.8
  blood pressure —see also Hypertension
    borderline R03.0
    reading (incidental) (isolated)
      (nonspecific), without diagnosis of
      hypertension R03.0
  cholesterol E78.0
    with high triglycerides E78.2
  diaphragm (congenital) Q79.1
  expressed emotional level within family Z63.8
  head at term O32.4

High (Continued)
  palate, congenital Q38.5
  risk
    infant NEC Z76.2
    sexual behavior (heterosexual) Z72.51
      bisexual Z72.53
      homosexual Z72.52
  temperature (of unknown origin) R50.9
  thoracic rib Q76.6
  triglycerides E78.1
    with high cholesterol E78.2
Hildenbrand's disease A75.0
Hilum —see condition
Hip —see condition
Hippel's disease Q85.8
Hippophobia F40.218
Hippus H57.09
Hirschsprung's disease or megacolon Q43.1
Hirsutism, hirsuties L68.0
Hirudiniasis
  external B88.3
  internal B83.4
Hiss-Russell dysentery A03.1
Histidinemia, histidinuria E70.41
Histiocytoma —see also Neoplasm, skin, benign
  fibrous —see also Neoplasm, skin, benign
    atypical —see Neoplasm, connective tissue,
      uncertain behavior
    malignant —see Neoplasm, connective
      tissue, malignant
Histiocytosis D76.3
  acute differentiated progressive C96.0
  Langerhans' cell NEC C96.6
    multifocal X
      multisystemic (disseminated) C96.0
      unisystemic C96.5
    pulmonary, adult (adult PLCH) J84.82
    unifocal (X) C96.6
  lipid, lipoid D76.3
    essential E75.29
  malignant C96.A
  mononuclear phagocytes NEC D76.1
    Langerhans' cells C96.6
  non-Langerhans cell D76.3
  polyostotic sclerosing D76.3
  sinus, with massive lymphadenopathy D76.3
  syndrome NEC D76.3
  X NEC C96.6
    acute (progressive) C96.0
    chronic C96.6
    multifocal C96.5
    multisystemic C96.0
    unifocal C96.6
Histoplasmosis B39.9
  with pneumonia NEC B39.2
  African B39.5
  American —see Histoplasmosis, capsulati
  capsulati B39.4
    disseminated B39.3
    generalized B39.3
    pulmonary B39.2
      acute B39.0
      chronic B39.1
  Darling's B39.4
  duboisii B39.5
  lung NEC B39.2
History
  family (of) —see also History, personal (of)
    alcohol abuse Z81.1
    allergy NEC Z84.89
    anemia Z83.2
    arthritis Z82.61
    asthma Z82.5
    blindness Z82.1
    cardiac death (sudden) Z82.41
    carrier of genetic disease Z84.81
    chromosomal anomaly Z82.79
    chronic
      disabling disease NEC Z82.8
      lower respiratory disease Z82.5
    colonic polyps Z83.71

History (Continued)
  family (Continued)
    congenital malformations and
      deformations Z82.79
      polycystic kidney Z82.71
    consanguinity Z84.3
    deafness Z82.2
    diabetes mellitus Z83.3
    disability NEC Z82.8
    disease or disorder (of)
      allergic NEC Z84.89
      behavioral NEC Z81.8
      blood and blood-forming organs Z83.2
      cardiovascular NEC Z82.49
      chronic disabling NEC Z82.8
      digestive Z83.79
      ear NEC Z83.52
      endocrine NEC Z83.49
      eye NEC Z83.518
        glaucoma Z83.511
      genitourinary NEC Z84.2
      glaucoma Z83.511
      hematological Z83.2
      immune mechanism Z83.2
      infectious NEC Z83.1
      ischemic heart Z82.49
      kidney Z84.1
      mental NEC Z81.8
      metabolic Z83.49
      musculoskeletal NEC Z82.69
      neurological NEC Z82.0
      nutritional Z83.49
      parasitic NEC Z83.1
      psychiatric NEC Z81.8
      respiratory NEC Z83.6
      skin and subcutaneous tissue NEC Z84.0
      specified NEC Z84.89
    drug abuse NEC Z81.3
    epilepsy Z82.0
    genetic disease carrier Z84.81
    glaucoma Z83.511
    hearing loss Z82.2
    human immunodeficiency virus (HIV)
      infection Z83.0
    Huntington's chorea Z82.0
    intellectual disability Z81.0
    leukemia Z80.6
    malignant neoplasm (of) NOS Z80.9
      bladder Z80.52
      breast Z80.3
      bronchus Z80.1
      digestive organ Z80.0
      gastrointestinal tract Z80.0
      genital organ Z80.49
        ovary Z80.41
        prostate Z80.42
        specified organ NEC Z80.49
        testis Z80.43
      hematopoietic NEC Z80.7
      intrathoracic organ NEC Z80.2
      kidney Z80.51
      lung Z80.1
      lymphatic NEC Z80.7
      ovary Z80.41
      prostate Z80.42
      respiratory organ NEC Z80.2
      specified site NEC Z80.8
      testis Z80.43
      trachea Z80.1
      urinary organ or tract Z80.59
        bladder Z80.52
        kidney Z80.51
    mental
      disorder NEC Z81.8
    multiple endocrine neoplasia (MEN)
      syndrome Z83.41
    osteoporosis Z82.62
    polycystic kidney Z82.71
    polyps (colon) Z83.71
    psychiatric disorder Z81.8
    psychoactive substance abuse NEC Z81.3

History *(Continued)*
  family *(Continued)*
    respiratory condition NEC Z83.6
      asthma and other lower respiratory
        conditions Z82.5
    self-harmful behavior Z81.8
    skin condition Z84.0
    specified condition NEC Z84.89
    stroke (cerebrovascular) Z82.3
    substance abuse NEC Z81.4
      alcohol Z81.1
      drug NEC Z81.3
      psychoactive NEC Z81.3
      tobacco Z81.2
    sudden cardiac death Z82.41
    tobacco abuse Z81.2
    violence, violent behavior Z81.8
    visual loss Z82.1
  personal (of) *—see also* History,
    family (of)
    abuse
      adult Z91.419
        physical and sexual Z91.410
        psychological Z91.411
      childhood Z62.819
        physical Z62.810
        psychological Z62.811
        sexual Z62.810
    alcohol dependence F10.21
    allergy (to) Z88.9
      analgesic agent NEC Z88.6
      anesthetic Z88.4
      antibiotic agent NEC Z88.1
      anti-infective agent NEC Z88.3
      contrast media Z91.041
      drugs, medicaments and biological
        substances Z88.9
        specified NEC Z88.8
      food Z91.018
        additives Z91.02
        eggs Z91.012
        milk products Z91.011
        peanuts Z91.010
        seafood Z91.013
        specified food NEC Z91.018
      insect Z91.038
        bee Z91.030
      latex Z91.040
      medicinal agents Z88.9
        specified NEC Z88.8
      narcotic agent NEC Z88.5
      nonmedicinal agents Z91.048
      penicillin Z88.0
      serum Z88.7
      specified NEC Z91.09
      sulfonamides Z88.2
      vaccine Z88.7
    anaphylactic shock Z87.892
    anaphylaxis Z87.892
    behavioral disorders Z86.59
    benign carcinoid tumor Z86.012
    benign neoplasm Z86.018
      brain Z86.011
      carcinoid Z86.012
      colonic polyps Z86.010
    brain injury (traumatic) Z87.820
    breast implant removal Z98.86
    calculi, renal Z87.442
    cancer *—see* History, personal (of),
      malignant neoplasm (of)
    cardiac arrest (death), successfully
      resuscitated Z86.74
    cerebral infarction without residual deficit
      Z86.73
    cervical dysplasia Z87.410
    chemotherapy for neoplastic condition
      Z92.21
    childhood abuse *—see* History, personal
      (of), abuse
    cleft lip (corrected) Z87.730
    cleft palate (corrected) Z87.730

History *(Continued)*
  personal *(Continued)*
    collapsed vertebra (healed) Z87.311
      due to osteoporosis Z87.310
    combat and operational stress reaction
      Z86.51
    congenital malformation (corrected)
      Z87.798
      circulatory system (corrected) Z87.74
      digestive system (corrected) NEC
        Z87.738
      ear (corrected) Z87.720
      eye (corrected) Z87.721
      face and neck (corrected) Z87.790
      genitourinary system (corrected) NEC
        Z87.718
      heart (corrected) Z87.74
      integument (corrected) Z87.76
      limb (s) (corrected) Z87.76
      musculoskeletal system (corrected)
        Z87.76
      neck (corrected) Z87.790
      nervous system (corrected) NEC
        Z87.728
      respiratory system (corrected) Z87.75
      sense organs (corrected) NEC Z87.728
      specified NEC Z87.798
    contraception Z92.0
    deployment (military) Z91.82
    diabetic foot ulcer Z86.31
    disease or disorder (of) Z87.898
      blood and blood-forming organs Z86.2
      circulatory system Z86.79
        specified condition NEC Z86.79
      connective tissue NEC Z87.39
      digestive system Z87.19
        colonic polyp Z86.010
        peptic ulcer disease Z87.11
        specified condition NEC Z87.19
      ear Z86.69
      endocrine Z86.39
        diabetic foot ulcer Z86.31
        gestational diabetes Z86.32
        specified type NEC Z86.39
      eye Z86.69
      genital (track) system NEC
        female Z87.42
        male Z87.438
      hematological Z86.2
      Hodgkin Z85.71
      immune mechanism Z86.2
      infectious Z86.19
        malaria Z86.13
        Methicillin resistant Staphylococcus
          aureus (MRSA) Z86.14
        poliomyelitis Z86.12
        specified NEC Z86.19
        tuberculosis Z86.11
      mental NEC Z86.59
      metabolic Z86.39
        diabetic foot ulcer Z86.31
        gestational diabetes Z86.32
        specified type NEC Z86.39
      musculoskeletal NEC Z87.39
      nervous system Z86.69
      nutritional Z86.39
      parasitic Z86.19
      respiratory system NEC Z87.09
      sense organs Z86.69
      skin Z87.2
      specified site or type NEC Z87.898
      subcutaneous tissue Z87.2
      trophoblastic Z87.59
      urinary system NEC Z87.448
    drug dependence *—see* Dependence, drug,
      by type, in remission
    drug therapy
      antineoplastic chemotherapy Z92.21
      estrogen Z92.23
      immunosupression Z92.25
      inhaled steroids Z92.240

History *(Continued)*
  personal *(Continued)*
    drug therapy *(Continued)*
      monoclonal drug Z92.22
      specified NEC Z92.29
      steroid Z92.241
      systemic steroids Z92.241
    dysplasia
      cervical Z87.410
      prostatic Z87.430
      vaginal Z87.411
      vulvar Z87.412
    embolism (venous) Z86.718
      pulmonary Z86.711
    encephalitis Z86.61
    estrogen therapy Z92.23
    extracorporeal membrane oxygenation
      (ECMO) Z92.81
    failed conscious sedation Z92.83
    failed moderate sedation Z92.83
    fall, falling Z91.81
    fracture (healed)
      fatigue Z87.312
      fragility Z87.310
      osteoporosis Z87.310
      pathological NEC Z87.311
      stress Z87.312
      traumatic Z87.81
    gestational diabetes Z86.32
    hepatitis
      B Z86.19
      C Z86.19
    Hodgkin disease Z85.71
    hyperthermia, malignant Z88.4
    hypospadias (corrected) Z87.710
    hysterectomy Z90.710
    immunosuppression therapy Z92.25
    in situ neoplasm
      breast Z86.000
      cervix uteri Z86.001
      specified NEC Z86.008
    infection NEC Z86.19
      central nervous system Z86.61
      Methicillin resistant Staphylococcus
        aureus (MRSA) Z86.14
      urinary (tract) Z87.41
    injury NEC Z87.828
    in utero procedure during pregnancy
      Z98.870
    in utero procedure while a fetus
      Z98.871
    irradiation Z92.3
    kidney stones Z87.442
    leukemia Z85.6
    lymphoma (non-Hodgkin) Z85.72
    malignant melanoma (skin) Z85.820
    malignant neoplasm (of) Z85.9
      accessory sinuses Z85.22
      anus NEC Z85.048
        carcinoid Z85.040
      bladder Z85.51
      bone Z85.830
      brain Z85.841
      breast Z85.3
      bronchus NEC Z85.118
        carcinoid Z85.110
      carcinoid *—see* History, personal (of),
        malignant neoplasm, by site,
        carcinoid
      cervix Z85.41
      colon NEC Z85.038
        carcinoid Z85.030
      digestive organ Z85.00
        specified NEC Z85.09
      endocrine gland NEC Z85.858
      epididymis Z85.48
      esophagus Z85.01
      eye Z85.840
      gastrointestinal tract *—see* History,
        malignant neoplasm, digestive
        organ

◀ New   ⬅ Revised   ~~deleted~~ Deleted

History *(Continued)*
  personal *(Continued)*
    malignant neoplasm *(Continued)*
      genital organ
        female Z85.40
          specified NEC Z85.44
        male Z85.45
          specified NEC Z85.49
      hematopoietic NEC Z85.79
      intrathoracic organ Z85.20-
      kidney NEC Z85.528
        carcinoid Z85.520
      large intestine NEC Z85.038
        carcinoid Z85.030
      larynx Z85.21
      liver Z85.05
      lung NEC Z85.118
        carcinoid Z85.110
      mediastinum Z85.29
      Merkel cell Z85.821
      middle ear Z85.22
      nasal cavities Z85.22
      nervous system NEC Z85.848
      oral cavity Z85.819
        specified site NEC Z85.818
      ovary Z85.43
      pancreas Z85.07
      pelvis Z85.53
      pharynx Z85.819
        specified site NEC Z85.818
      pleura Z85.29
      prostate Z85.46
      rectosigmoid junction NEC Z85.048
        carcinoid Z85.040
      rectum NEC Z85.048
        carcinoid Z85.040
      respiratory organ Z85.20
      sinuses, accessory Z85.22
      skin NEC Z85.828
        melanoma Z85.820
        Merkel cell Z85.821
      small intestine NEC Z85.068
        carcinoid Z85.060
      soft tissue Z85.831
      specified site NEC Z85.89
      stomach NEC Z85.028
        carcinoid Z85.020
      testis Z85.47
      thymus NEC Z85.238
        carcinoid Z85.230
      thyroid Z85.850
      tongue Z85.810
      trachea Z85.12
      ureter Z85.54
      urinary organ or tract Z85.50
        specified NEC Z85.59
      uterus Z85.42
    maltreatment Z91.89
    medical treatment NEC Z92.89
    melanoma (malignant) (skin) Z85.820
    meningitis Z86.61
    mental disorder Z86.59
    Merkel cell carcinoma (skin) Z85.821
    Methicillin resistant Staphylococcus aureus
        (MRSA) Z86.14
    military deployment Z91.82
    military war, peacekeeping and
        humanitarian deployment (current or
        past conflict) Z91.82
    myocardial infarction (old) I25.2
    neglect (in)
      adult Z91.412
      childhood Z62.812
    neoplasm
      benign Z86.018
        brain Z86.011
        colon polyp Z86.010
      in situ
        breast Z86.000
        cervix uteri Z86.001
        specified NEC Z86.008

History *(Continued)*
  personal *(Continued)*
    neoplasm *(Continued)*
      malignant —*see* History of, malignant
          neoplasm
      uncertain behavior Z86.03
    nephrotic syndrome Z87.441
    nicotine dependence Z87.891
    noncompliance with medical treatment or
        regimen —*see* Noncompliance
    nutritional deficiency Z86.39
    obstetric complications Z87.59
      childbirth Z87.59
      pregnancy Z87.59
      pre-term labor Z87.51
      puerperium Z87.59
    osteoporosis fractures Z87.31
    parasuicide (attempt) Z91.5
    physical trauma NEC Z87.828
      self-harm or suicide attempt Z91.5
    pneumonia (recurrent) Z87.01
    poisoning NEC Z91.89
      self-harm or suicide attempt Z91.5
    poor personal hygiene Z91.89
    preterm labor Z87.51
    procedure during pregnancy Z98.870
    procedure while a fetus Z98.871
    prolonged reversible ischemic neurologic
        deficit (PRINO) Z86.73
    prostatic dysplasia Z87.430
    psychiatric disorder NEC Z87.89
    psychological
      abuse
        adult Z91.411
        child Z62.811
      trauma, specified NEC Z91.49
    radiation therapy Z92.3
    removal
      implant
        breast Z98.86
    renal calculi Z87.442
    respiratory condition NEC Z87.09
    retained foreign body fully removed
        Z87.821
    risk factors NEC Z91.89
    self-harm Z91.5
    self-poisoning attempt Z91.5
    sex reassignment Z87.890
    sleep-wake cycle problem Z72.821
    specified NEC Z87.898
    steroid therapy (systemic) Z92.241
      inhaled Z92.240
    stroke without residual deficits
        Z86.73
    substance abuse NEC F10-F19 with
        fifth character 1
    sudden cardiac arrest Z86.74
    sudden cardiac death successfully
        resuscitated Z86.74
    suicide attempt Z91.5
    surgery NEC Z98.89
      sex reassignment Z87.890
      transplant —*see* Transplant
    thrombophlebitis Z86.72
    thrombosis (venous) Z86.718
      pulmonary Z86.711
    tobacco dependence Z87.891
    transient ischemic attack (TIA) without
        residual deficits Z86.73
    trauma (physical) NEC Z87.828
      psychological NEC Z91.49
      self-harm Z91.5
    traumatic brain injury Z87.820
    unhealthy sleep-wake cycle Z72.821
    urinary (recurrent) (tract) infection (s)
        Z87.440
    urinary calculi Z87.42
    vaginal dysplasia Z87.411
    venous thrombosis or embolism Z86.718
      pulmonary Z86.711
    vulvar dysplasia Z87.412

His-Werner disease A79.0
HIV (*see also* Human, immunodeficiency virus)
    B20
  laboratory evidence (nonconclusive) R75
  nonconclusive test (in infants) R75
  positive, seropositive Z21
Hives (bold) —*see* Urticaria
Hoarseness R49.0
Hobo Z59.0
Hodgkin disease —*see* Lymphoma,
    Hodgkin
Hodgson's disease I71.2
  ruptured I71.1
Hoffa-Kastert disease E88.89
Hoffa's disease E88.89
Hoffmann-Bouveret syndrome I47.9
Hoffmann's syndrome E03.9 *[G73.7]*
Hole (round)
  macula H35.34-
  retina (without detachment) —*see* Break,
      retina, round hole
    with detachment —*see* Detachment, retina,
        with retinal, break
Holiday relief care Z75.5
Hollenhorst's plaque —*see* Occlusion, artery,
    retina
Hollow foot (congenital) Q66.7
  acquired —*see* Deformity, limb, foot, specified
      NEC
Holoprosencephaly Q04.2
Holt-Oram syndrome Q87.2
Homelessness Z59.0
Homesickness —*see* Disorder, adjustment
Homocystinemia, homocystinuria E72.11
Homogentisate 1,2-dioxygenase deficiency
    E70.29
Homologous serum hepatitis (prophylactic)
    (therapeutic) —*see* Hepatitis, viral,
    type B
Honeycomb lung J98.4
  congenital Q33.0
Hooded
  clitoris Q52.6
  penis Q55.69
Hookworm (anemia) (disease) (infection)
    (infestation) B76.9
  specified NEC B76.8
Hordeolum (eyelid) (externum) (recurrent)
    H00.019
  internum H00.029
    left H00.026
      lower H00.025
      upper H00.024
    right H00.023
      lower H00.022
      upper H00.021
  left H00.016
    lower H00.015
    upper H00.014
  right H00.013
    lower H00.012
    upper H00.011
Horn
  cutaneous L85.8
  nail L60.2
    congenital Q84.6
Horner (-Claude Bernard) syndrome G90.2
  traumatic —*see* Injury, nerve, cervical
      sympathetic
Horseshoe kidney (congenital) Q63.1
Horton's headache or neuralgia G44.099
  intractable G44.091
  not intractable G44.099
Hospital hopper syndrome —*see* Disorder,
    factitious
Hospitalism in children —*see* Disorder,
    adjustment
Hostility R45.5
  towards child Z62.3
Hot flashes
  menopausal N95.1

Hourglass (contracture) —see also Contraction, hourglass
  stomach K31.89
    congenital Q40.2
    stricture K31.2
Household, housing circumstance affecting care Z59.9
  specified NEC Z59.8
Housemaid's knee —see Bursitis, prepatellar
Hudson (-Stähli) line (cornea) —see Pigmentation, cornea, anterior
Human
  bite (open wound) —see also Bite
    intact skin surface —see Bite, superficial
  herpesvirus —see Herpes
  immunodeficiency virus (HIV) disease (infection) B20
    asymptomatic status Z21
    contact Z20.6
    counseling Z71.7
    dementia B20 [F02.80]
      with behavioral disturbance B20 [F02.81]
    exposure to Z20.6
    laboratory evidence R75
    type-2 (HIV 2) as cause of disease classified elsewhere B97.35
  papillomavirus (HPV)
    DNA test positive
      high risk
        cervix R87.810
        vagina R87.811
      low risk
        cervix R87.820
        vagina R87.821
    screening for Z11.51
  T-cell lymphotropic virus
    type-1 (HTLV-I) infection B33.3
      as cause of disease classified elsewhere B97.33
      carrier Z22.6
    type-2 (HTLV-II) as cause of disease classified elsewhere B97.34
Humidifier lung or pneumonitis J67.7
Humiliation (experience) in childhood Z62.898
Humpback (acquired) —see Kyphosis
Hunchback (acquired) —see Kyphosis
Hunger T73.0
  air, psychogenic F45.8
Hungry bone syndrome E83.81
Hunner's ulcer —see Cystitis, chronic, interstitial
Hunter's
  glossitis D51.0
  syndrome E76.1
Huntington's disease or chorea G10
  with dementia G10 [F02.80]
    with behavioral disturbance G10 [F02.81]
Hunt's
  disease or syndrome (herpetic geniculate ganglionitis) B02.21
    dyssynergia cerebellaris myoclonica G11.1
  neuralgia B02.21
Hurler (-Scheie) disease or syndrome E76.02
Hurst's disease G36.1
Hurthle cell
  adenocarcinoma C73
  adenoma D34
  carcinoma C73
  tumor D34
Hutchinson-Boeck disease or syndrome —see Sarcoidosis
Hutchinson-Gilford disease or syndrome E34.8
Hutchinson's
  disease, meaning
    angioma serpiginosum L81.7
    pompholyx (cheiropompholyx) L30.1
    prurigo estivalis L56.4
    summer eruption or summer prurigo L56.4
  melanotic freckle —see Melanoma, in situ
    malignant melanoma in —see Melanoma

Hutchinson's (Continued)
  teeth or incisors (congenital syphilis) A50.52
  triad (congenital syphilis) A50.53
Hyalin plaque, sclera, senile H15.89
Hyaline membrane (disease) (lung) (pulmonary) (newborn) P22.0
Hyalinosis
  cutis (et mucosae) E78.89
  focal and segmental (glomerular) (see also N00-N07 with fourth character .1) N05.1
Hyalitis, hyalosis, asteroid —see also Deposit, crystalline
  syphilitic (late) A52.71
Hydatid
  cyst or tumor —see Echinococcus
  mole —see Hydatidiform mole
  Morgagni
    female Q50.5
    male (epididymal) Q55.4
      testicular Q55.29
Hydatidiform mole (benign) (complicating pregnancy) (delivered) (undelivered) O01.9
  classical O01.0
  complete O01.0
  incomplete O01.1
  invasive D39.2
  malignant D39.2
  partial O01.1
Hydatidosis —see Echinococcus
Hydradenitis (axillaris) (suppurative) L73.2
Hydradenoma —see Hidradenoma
Hydramnios O40.-
Hydrancephaly, hydranencephaly Q04.3
  with spina bifida —see Spina bifida, with hydrocephalus
Hydrargyrism NEC —see Poisoning, mercury
Hydrarthrosis —see also Effusion, joint
  gonococcal A54.42
  intermittent M12.40
    ankle M12.47-
    elbow M12.42-
    foot joint M12.47-
    hand joint M12.44-
    hip M12.45-
    knee M12.46-
    multiple site M12.49
    shoulder M12.41-
    specified joint NEC M12.48
    wrist M12.43-
  of yaws (early) (late) (see also subcategory M14.8-) A66.6
  syphilitic (late) A52.77
    congenital A50.55 [M12.80]
Hydremia D64.89
Hydrencephalocele (congenital) —see Encephalocele
Hydrencephalomeningocele (congenital) —see Encephalocele
Hydroa R23.8
  aestivale L56.4
  vacciniforme L56.4
Hydroadenitis (axillaris) (suppurative) L73.2
Hydrocalycosis —see Hydronephrosis
Hydrocele (spermatic cord) (testis) (tunica vaginalis) N43.3
  canal of Nuck N94.89
  communicating N43.2
    congenital P83.5
  congenital P83.5
  encysted N43.0
  female NEC N94.89
  infected N43.1
  newborn P83.5
  round ligament N94.89
  specified NEC N43.2
  spinalis —see Spina bifida
  vulva N90.89

Hydrocephalus (acquired) (external) (internal) (malignant) (recurrent) G91.9
  aqueduct Sylvius stricture Q03.0
  causing disproportion O33.6
    with obstructed labor O66.3
  communicating G91.0
  congenital (external) (internal) Q03.9
    with spina bifida Q05.4
      cervical Q05.0
      dorsal Q05.1
      lumbar Q05.2
      lumbosacral Q05.2
      sacral Q05.3
      thoracic Q05.1
      thoracolumbar Q05.1
    specified NEC Q03.8
  due to toxoplasmosis (congenital) P37.1
  foramen Magendie block (acquired) G91.1
    congenital (see also Hydrocephalus, congenital) Q03.1
  in (due to)
    infectious disease NEC B89 [G91.4]
    neoplastic disease NEC (see also Neoplasm) G91.4
    parasitic disease B89 [G91.4]
  newborn Q03.9
    with spina bifida —see Spina bifida, with hydrocephalus
  noncommunicating G91.1
  normal pressure G91.2
    secondary G91.0
  obstructive G91.1
  otitic G93.2
  post-traumatic NEC G91.3
  secondary G91.4
    post-traumatic G91.3
  specified NEC G91.8
  syphilitic, congenital A50.49
Hydrocolpos (congenital) N89.8
Hydrocystoma —see Neoplasm, skin, benign
Hydroencephalocele (congenital) —see Encephalocele
Hydroencephalomeningocele (congenital) —see Encephalocele
Hydrohematopneumothorax —see Hemothorax
Hydromeningitis —see Meningitis
Hydromeningocele (spinal) —see also Spina bifida
  cranial —see Encephalocele
Hydrometra N85.8
Hydrometrocolpos N89.8
Hydromicrocephaly Q02
Hydromphalos (since birth) Q45.8
Hydromyelia Q06.4
Hydromyelocele —see Spina bifida
Hydronephrosis (atrophic) (early) (functionless) (intermittent) (primary) (secondary) NEC N13.30
  with
    infection N13.6
    obstruction (by) (of)
      renal calculus N13.2
        with infection N13.6
      ureteral NEC N13.1
        with infection N13.6
        calculus N13.2
          with infection N13.6
      ureteropelvic junction (congenital) Q62.0
        with infection N13.6
      ureteral stricture NEC N13.1
        with infection N13.6
  congenital Q62.0
  specified type NEC N13.39
  tuberculous A18.11
Hydropericarditis —see Pericarditis
Hydropericardium —see Pericarditis
Hydroperitoneum R18.8
Hydrophobia —see Rabies
Hydrophthalmos Q15.0
Hydropneumohemothorax —see Hemothorax
Hydropneumopericarditis —see Pericarditis

◀ New   ◀▬ Revised   ~~deleted~~ Deleted

Hydropneumopericardium —*see* Pericarditis
Hydropneumothorax J94.8
  traumatic —*see* Injury, intrathoracic, lung
  tuberculous NEC A15.6
Hydrops R60.9
  abdominis R18.8
  articulorum intermittens —*see* Hydrarthrosis,
    intermittent
  cardiac —*see* Failure, heart, congestive
  causing obstructed labor (mother) O66.3
  endolymphatic H81.0-
  fetal —*see* Pregnancy, complicated by,
    hydrops, fetalis
  fetalis P83.2
    due to
      ABO isoimmunization P56.0
      alpha thalassemia D56.0
      hemolytic disease P56.90
        specified NEC P56.99
      isoimmunization (ABO) (Rh) P56.0
      other specified nonhemolytic disease
        NEC P83.2
      Rh incompatibility P56.0
    during pregnancy —*see* Pregnancy,
      complicated by, hydrops, fetalis
  gallbladder K82.1
  joint —*see* Effusion, joint
  labyrinth H81.0
  newborn (idiopathic) P83.2
    due to
      ABO isoimmunization P56.0
      alpha thalassemia D56.0
      hemolytic disease P56.90
        specified NEC P56.99
      isoimmunization (ABO) (Rh) P56.0
      Rh incompatibility P56.0
  nutritional —*see* Malnutrition, severe
  pericardium —*see* Pericarditis
  pleura —*see* Hydrothorax
  spermatic cord —*see* Hydrocele
Hydropyonephrosis N13.6
Hydrorachis Q06.4
Hydrorrhea (nasal) J34.89
  pregnancy —*see* Rupture, membranes,
    premature
Hydrosadenitis (axillaris) (suppurative) L73.2
Hydrosalpinx (fallopian tube) (follicularis)
  N70.11
Hydrothorax (double) (pleura) J94.8
  chylous (nonfilarial) I89.8
    filarial (*see also* Infestation, filarial) B74.9
      [J91.8]
  traumatic —*see* Injury, intrathoracic
  tuberculous NEC (non primary) A15.6
Hydroureter (*see also* Hydronephrosis) N13.4
  with infection N13.6
  congenital Q62.39
Hydroureteronephrosis —*see* Hydronephrosis
Hydrourethra N36.8
Hydroxykynureninuria E70.8
Hydroxylysinemia E72.3
Hydroxyprolinemia E72.59
Hygiene, sleep
  abuse Z72.821
  inadequate Z72.821
  poor Z72.821
Hygroma (congenital) (cystic) D18.1
  praepatellare, prepatellar —*see* Bursitis,
    prepatellar
Hymen —*see* condition
Hymenolepis, hymenolepiasis (diminuta)
  (infection) (infestation) (nana) B71.0
Hypalgesia R20.8
Hyperacidity (gastric) K31.89
  psychogenic F45.8
Hyperactive, hyperactivity F90.9
  basal cell, uterine cervix —*see* Dysplasia,
    cervix
  bowel sounds R19.12
  cervix epithelial (basal) —*see* Dysplasia,
    cervix

Hyperactive, hyperactivity (*Continued*)
  child F90.9
    attention deficit —*see* Disorder, attention-
      deficit hyperactivity
  detrusor muscle N32.81
  gastrointestinal K31.89
    psychogenic F45.8
  nasal mucous membrane J34.3
  stomach K31.89
  thyroid (gland) —*see* Hyperthyroidism
Hyperacusis H93.23-
Hyperadrenalism E27.5
Hyperadrenocorticism E24.9
  congenital E25.0
  iatrogenic E24.2
    correct substance properly administered —
      see Table of Drugs and Chemicals, by
      drug, adverse effect
    overdose or wrong substance given or
      taken —*see* Table of Drugs and
      Chemicals, by drug, poisoning
  not associated with Cushing's syndrome
    E27.0
  pituitary-dependent E24.0
Hyperaldosteronism E26.9
  familial (type I) E26.02
  glucocorticoid-remediable E26.02
  primary (due to (bilateral) adrenal
    hyperplasia) E26.09
  primary NEC E26.09
  secondary E26.1
  specified NEC E26.89
Hyperalgesia R20.8
Hyperalimentation R63.2
  carotene, carotin E67.1
  specified NEC E67.8
  vitamin
    A E67.0
    D E67.3
Hyperaminoaciduria
  arginine E72.21
  cystine E72.01
  lysine E72.3
  ornithine E72.4
Hyperammonemia (congenital) E72.20
Hyperazotemia —*see* Uremia
Hyperbetalipoproteinemia (familial) E78.0
  with prebetalipoproteinemia E78.2
Hyperbilirubinemia
  constitutional E80.6
  familial conjugated E80.6
  neonatal (transient) —*see* Jaundice, newborn
Hypercalcemia, hypocalciuric, familial E83.52
Hypercalciuria, idiopathic E83.52
Hypercapnia R06.89
  newborn P84
Hypercarotenemia, hypercarotinemia (dietary)
  E67.1
Hypercementosis K03.4
Hyperchloremia E87.8
Hyperchlorhydria K31.89
  neurotic F45.8
  psychogenic F45.8
Hypercholesterinemia —*see*
  Hypercholesterolemia
Hypercholesterolemia (essential) (familial)
  (hereditary) (primary) (pure) E78.0
  with hyperglyceridemia, endogenous E78.2
  dietary counseling and surveillance Z71.3
Hyperchylia gastrica, psychogenic F45.8
Hyperchylomicronemia (familial) (primary)
  E78.3
  with hyperbetalipoproteinemia E78.3
Hypercoagulable (state) D68.59
  activated protein C resistance D68.51
  antithrombin (III) deficiency D68.59
  factor V Leiden mutation D68.51
  primary NEC D68.59
  protein C deficiency D68.59
  protein S deficiency D68.59
  prothrombin gene mutation D68.52

Hypercoagulable (*Continued*)
  secondary D68.69
  specified NEC D68.69
Hypercoagulation (state) D68.59
Hypercorticalism, pituitary-dependent E24.0
Hypercorticosolism —*see* Cushing's, syndrome
Hypercorticosteronism E24.2
  correct substance properly administered —*see*
    Table of Drugs and Chemicals, by drug,
    adverse effect
  overdose or wrong substance given or
    taken —*see* Table of Drugs and
    Chemicals, by drug, poisoning
Hypercortisonism E24.2
  correct substance properly administered —*see*
    Table of Drugs and Chemicals, by drug,
    adverse effect
  overdose or wrong substance given or
    taken —*see* Table of Drugs and
    Chemicals, by drug, poisoning
Hyperekplexia Q89.8
Hyperelectrolytemia E87.8
Hyperemesis R11.10
  with nausea R11.2
  gravidarum (mild) O21.0
    with
      carbohydrate depletion O21.1
      dehydration O21.1
      electrolyte imbalance O21.1
      metabolic disturbance O21.1
      severe (with metabolic disturbance) O21.1
  projectile R11.12
  psychogenic F45.8
Hyperemia (acute) (passive) R68.89
  anal mucosa K62.89
  bladder N32.89
  cerebral I67.89
  conjunctiva H11.43-
  ear internal, acute —*see* subcategory
    H83.0
  enteric K59.8
  eye —*see* Hyperemia, conjunctiva
  eyelid (active) (passive) —*see* Disorder,
    eyelid, specified type NEC
  intestine K59.8
  iris —*see* Disorder, iris, vascular
  kidney N28.89
  labyrinth —*see* subcategory H83.0
  liver (active) K76.89
  lung (passive) —*see* Edema, lung
  pulmonary (passive) —*see* Edema, lung
  renal N28.89
  retina H35.89
  stomach K31.89
Hyperesthesia (body surface) R20.3
  larynx (reflex) J38.7
    hysterical F44.89
  pharynx (reflex) J39.2
    hysterical F44.89
Hyperestrogenism (drug-induced) (iatrogenic)
  E28.0
Hyperexplexia Q89.8
Hyperfibrinolysis —*see* Fibrinolysis
Hyperfructosemia E74.19
Hyperfunction
  adrenal cortex, not associated with Cushing's
    syndrome E27.0
    medulla E27.5
      adrenomedullary E27.5
    virilism E25.9
      congenital E25.0
  ovarian E28.8
  pancreas K86.8
  parathyroid (gland) E21.3
  pituitary (gland) (anterior) E22.9
    specified NEC E22.8
  polyglandular E31.1
  testicular E29.0
Hypergammaglobulinemia D89.2
  polyclonal D89.0
  Waldenström D89.0

Hypergastrinemia E16.4
Hyperglobulinemia R77.1
Hyperglycemia, hyperglycemic (transient)
    R73.9
  coma —see Diabetes, by type, with coma
  postpancreatectomy E89.1
Hyperglyceridemia (endogenous) (essential)
    (familial) (hereditary) (pure) E78.1
  mixed E78.3
Hyperglycinemia (non-ketotic) E72.51
Hypergonadism
  ovarian E28.8
  testicular (primary) (infantile) E29.0
Hyperheparinemia D68.32
Hyperhidrosis, hyperidrosis R61
  focal
    primary L74.519
      axilla L74.510
      face L74.511
      palms L74.512
      soles L74.513
    secondary L74.52
  generalized R61
  localized
    primary L74.519
      axilla L74.510
      face L74.511
      palms L74.512
      soles L74.513
    secondary L74.52
  psychogenic F45.8
  secondary R61
    focal L74.52
Hyperhistidinemia E70.41
Hyperhomocysteinemia E72.11
Hyperhydroxyprolinemia E72.59
Hyperinsulinism (functional) E16.1
  with
    coma (hypoglycemic) E15
    encephalopathy E16.1 [G94]
  ectopic E16.1
  therapeutic misadventure (from
      administration of insulin) —see
      subcategory T38.3
Hyperkalemia E87.5
Hyperkeratosis (see also Keratosis) L85.9
  cervix N88.0
  due to yaws (early) (late) (palmar or plantar)
      A66.3
  follicularis Q82.8
    penetrans (in cutem) L87.0
  palmoplantaris climacterica L85.1
  pinta A67.1
  senile (with pruritus) L57.0
  universalis congenita Q80.8
  vocal cord J38.3
  vulva N90.4
Hyperkinesia, hyperkinetic (disease) (reaction)
    (syndrome) (childhood) (adolescence) —
    see also Disorder, attention-deficit
    hyperactivity
  heart I51.89
Hyperleucine-isoleucinemia E71.19
Hyperlipemia, hyperlipidemia E78.5
  combined E78.2
    familial E78.4
  group
    A E78.0
    B E78.1
    C E78.2
    D E78.3
  mixed E78.2
  specified NEC E78.4
Hyperlipidosis E75.6
  hereditary NEC E75.5
Hyperlipoproteinemia E78.5
  Fredrickson's type
    I E78.3
    IIa E78.0
    IIb E78.2
    III E78.2

Hyperlipoproteinemia (Continued)
  Fredrickson's type (Continued)
    IV E78.1
    V E78.3
  low-density-lipoprotein-type (LDL) E78.0
  very-low-density-lipoprotein-type (VLDL)
      E78.1
Hyperlucent lung, unilateral J43.0
Hyperlysinemia E72.3
Hypermagnesemia E83.41
  neonatal P71.8
Hypermenorrhea N92.0
Hypermethioninemia E72.19
Hypermetropia (congenital) H52.0-
Hypermobility, hypermotility
  cecum —see Syndrome, irritable bowel
  coccyx —see subcategory M53.2
  colon —see Syndrome, irritable bowel
    psychogenic F45.8
  ileum K58.9
  intestine (see also Syndrome, irritable bowel)
      K58.9
    psychogenic F45.8
  meniscus (knee) —see Derangement, knee,
      meniscus
  scapula —see Instability, joint, shoulder
  stomach K31.89
    psychogenic F45.8
  syndrome M35.7
  urethra N36.41
    with intrinsic sphincter deficiency N36.43
Hypernasality R49.21
Hypernatremia E87.0
Hypernephroma C64.-
Hyperopia —see Hypermetropia
Hyperorexia nervosa F50.2
Hyperornithinemia E72.4
Hyperosmia R43.1
Hyperosmolality E87.0
Hyperostosis (monomelic) —see also Disorder,
      bone, density and structure, specified NEC
  ankylosing (spine) M48.10
    cervical region M48.12
    cervicothoracic region M48.13
    lumbar region M48.16
    lumbosacral region M48.17
    multiple sites M48.19
    occipito-atlanto-axial region M48.11
    sacrococcygeal region M48.18
    thoracic region M48.14
    thoracolumbar region M48.15
  cortical (skull) M85.2
    infantile M89.8X-
  frontal, internal of skull M85.2
  interna frontalis M85.2
  skeletal, diffuse idiopathic —see
      Hyperostosis, ankylosing
  skull M85.2
    congenital Q75.8
  vertebral, ankylosing —see Hyperostosis,
      ankylosing
Hyperovarism E28.8
Hyperoxaluria (primary) E72.53
Hyperparathyroidism E21.3
  primary E21.0
  secondary (renal) N25.81
    non-renal E21.1
  specified NEC E21.2
  tertiary E21.2
Hyperpathia R20.8
Hyperperistalsis R19.2
  psychogenic F45.8
Hyperpermeability, capillary I78.8
Hyperphagia R63.2
Hyperphenylalaninemia NEC E70.1
Hyperphoria (alternating) H50.53
Hyperphosphatemia E83.39
Hyperpiesis, hyperpiesia —see Hypertension
Hyperpigmentation —see also Pigmentation
  melanin NEC L81.4
  postinflammatory L81.0

Hyperpinealism E34.8
Hyperpituitarism E22.9
Hyperplasia, hyperplastic
  adenoids J35.2
  adrenal (capsule) (cortex) (gland) E27.8
    with
      sexual precocity (male) E25.9
        congenital E25.0
      virilism, adrenal E25.9
        congenital E25.0
      virilization (female) E25.9
        congenital E25.0
    congenital E25.0
    salt-losing E25.0
  adrenomedullary E27.5
  angiolymphoid, eosinophilia (ALHE) D18.01
  appendix (lymphoid) K38.0
  artery, fibromuscular I77.3
  bone —see also Hypertrophy, bone
    marrow D75.89
  breast —see also Hypertrophy, breast
    ductal (atypical) N60.9-
  C-cell, thyroid E07.0
  cementation (tooth) (teeth) K03.4
  cervical gland R59.0
  cervix (uteri) (basal cell) (endometrium)
      (polypoid) —see also Dysplasia, cervix
    congenital Q51.828
  clitoris, congenital Q52.6
  denture K06.2
  endocervicitis N72
  endometrium, endometrial (adenomatous)
      (benign) (cystic) (glandular) (glandular-
      cystic) (polypoid) N85.00
    with atypia N85.02
    cervix —see Dysplasia, cervix
    complex (without atypia) N85.01
    simple (without atypia) N85.01
  epithelial L85.9
    focal, oral, including tongue K13.29
    nipple N62
    skin L85.9
    tongue K13.29
    vaginal wall N89.3
  erythroid D75.89
  fibromuscular of artery (carotid) (renal) I77.3
  genital
    female NEC N94.89
    male N50.8
  gingiva K06.1
  glandularis cystica uteri (interstitialis) (see also
      Hyperplasia, endometrial) N85.00-
  gum K06.1
  hymen, congenital Q52.4
  irritative, edentulous (alveolar) K06.2
  jaw M26.09
    alveolar M26.79
    lower M26.03
      alveolar M26.72
    upper M26.01
      alveolar M26.71
  kidney (congenital) Q63.3
  labia N90.6
    epithelial N90.3
  liver (congenital) Q44.7
    nodular, focal K76.89
  lymph gland or node R59.9
  mandible, mandibular M26.03
    alveolar M26.72
    unilateral condylar M27.8
  maxilla, maxillary M26.01
    alveolar M26.71
  myometrium, myometrial N85.2
  neuroendocrine cell, of infancy J84.841
  nose
    lymphoid J34.89
    polypoid J33.9
  oral mucosa (irritative) K13.6
  organ or site, congenital NEC —see Anomaly,
      by site
  ovary N83.8

Hyperplasia, hyperplastic *(Continued)*
 palate, papillary (irritative) K13.6
 pancreatic islet cells E16.9
  alpha E16.8
   with excess
    gastrin E16.4
    glucagon E16.3
  beta E16.1
 parathyroid (gland) E21.0
 pharynx (lymphoid) J39.2
 prostate (adenofibromatous) (nodular)
   N40.0
  with lower urinary tract symptoms (LUTS)
    N40.1
  without lower urinary tract symptoms
    (LUTS) N40.0
 renal artery I77.89
 reticulo-endothelial (cell) D75.89
 salivary gland (any) K11.1
 Schimmelbusch's —*see* Mastopathy,
   cystic
 suprarenal capsule (gland) E27.8
 thymus (gland) (persistent) E32.0
 thyroid (gland) —*see* Goiter
 tonsils (faucial) (infective) (lingual)
   (lymphoid) J35.1
  with adenoids J35.3
 unilateral condylar M27.8
 uterus, uterine N85.2
  endometrium (glandular) (*see also*
    Hyperplasia, endometrial)
    N85.00-
 vulva N90.6
  epithelial N90.3
Hyperpnea —*see* Hyperventilation
Hyperpotassemia E87.5
Hyperprebetalipoproteinemia (familial)
  E78.1
Hyperprolactinemia E22.1
Hyperprolinemia (type I) (type II) E72.59
Hyperproteinemia E88.09
Hyperprothrombinemia, causing coagulation
  factor deficiency D68.4
Hyperpyrexia R50.9
 heat (effects) T67.0
 malignant, due to anesthetic T88.3
 rheumatic —*see* Fever, rheumatic
 unknown origin R50.9
Hyper-reflexia R29.2
Hypersalivation K11.7
Hypersecretion
 ACTH (not associated with Cushing's
   syndrome) E27.0
  pituitary E24.0
 adrenaline E27.5
 adrenomedullary E27.5
 androgen (testicular) E29.0
  ovarian (drug-induced) (iatrogenic)
    E28.1
 calcitonin E07.0
 catecholamine E27.5
 corticoadrenal E24.9
 cortisol E24.9
 epinephrine E27.5
 estrogen E28.0
 gastric K31.89
  psychogenic F45.8
 gastrin E16.4
 glucagon E16.3
 hormone (s)
  ACTH (not associated with Cushing's
    syndrome) E27.0
   pituitary E24.0
  antidiuretic E22.2
  growth E22.0
  intestinal NEC E34.1
  ovarian androgen E28.1
  pituitary E22.9
  testicular E29.0
  thyroid stimulating E05.80
   with thyroid storm E05.81

Hypersecretion *(Continued)*
 insulin —*see* Hyperinsulinism
 lacrimal glands —*see* Epiphora
 medulloadrenal E27.5
 milk O92.6
 ovarian androgens E28.1
 salivary gland (any) K11.7
 thyrocalcitonin E07.0
 upper respiratory J39.8
Hypersegmentation, leukocytic, hereditary
  D72.0
Hypersensitive, hypersensitiveness,
  hypersensitivity —*see also* Allergy
 carotid sinus G90.01
 colon —*see* Irritable, colon
 drug T88.7
 gastrointestinal K52.2
  psychogenic F45.8
 labyrinth —*see* subcategory H83.2
 pain R20.8
 pneumonitis —*see* Pneumonitis,
   allergic
 reaction T78.40
  upper respiratory tract NEC J39.3
Hypersomnia (organic) G47.10
 due to
  alcohol
   abuse F10.182
   dependence F10.282
   use F10.982
  amphetamines
   abuse F15.182
   dependence F15.282
   use F15.982
  caffeine
   abuse F15.182
   dependence F15.282
   use F15.982
  cocaine
   abuse F14.182
   dependence F14.282
   use F14.982
  drug NEC
   abuse F19.182
   dependence F19.282
   use F19.982
  medical condition G47.14
  mental disorder F51.13
  opioid
   abuse F11.182
   dependence F11.282
   use F11.982
  psychoactive substance NEC
   abuse F19.182
   dependence F19.282
   use F19.982
  sedative, hypnotic, or anxiolytic
   abuse F13.182
   dependence F13.282
   use F13.982
  stimulant NEC
   abuse F15.182
   dependence F15.282
   use F15.982
 idiopathic G47.11
  with long sleep time G47.11
  without long sleep time G47.12
 menstrual related G47.13
 nonorganic origin F51.11
  specified NEC F51.19
 not due to a substance or known
   physiological condition F51.11
  specified NEC F51.19
 primary F51.11
 recurrent G47.13
 specified NEC G47.19
Hypersplenia, hypersplenism D73.1
Hyperstimulation, ovaries (associated with
  induced ovulation) N98.1
Hypersusceptibility —*see* Allergy
Hypertelorism (ocular) (orbital) Q75.2

Hypertension, hypertensive (accelerated)
  (benign) (essential) (idiopathic)
  (malignant) (systemic) I10
 with
  heart involvement (conditions in
    I51.4-I51.9 due to hypertension) —*see*
    Hypertension, heart
  kidney involvement —*see* Hypertension,
    kidney
 benign, intracranial G93.2
 borderline R03.0
 cardiorenal (disease) I13.10
  with heart failure I13.0
   with stage 1 through stage 4 chronic
     kidney disease I13.0
   with stage 5 or end stage renal disease
     I13.2
  without heart failure I13.10
   with stage 1 through stage 4 chronic
     kidney disease I13.10
   with stage 5 or end stage renal disease
     I13.11
 cardiovascular
  disease (arteriosclerotic) (sclerotic) —*see*
    Hypertension, heart
  renal (disease) —*see* Hypertension,
    cardiorenal
 chronic venous —*see* Hypertension, venous
   (chronic)
 complicating
  childbirth (labor) O10.92
   with
    heart disease O10.12
     with renal disease O10.32
    renal disease O10.22
     with heart disease O10.32
   essential O10.02
   secondary O10.42
  pregnancy O16.-
   with edema (*see also* Pre-eclampsia) O14.9-
   gestational (pregnancy induced)
     (transient) (without proteinuria)
     O13.-
   with proteinuria O14.9-
    mild pre-eclampsia O14.0-
    moderate pre-eclampsia O14.0-
    severe pre-eclampsia O14.1-
     with hemolysis, elevated liver
       enzymes and low platelet
       count (HELLP) O14.2-
   pre-existing O10.91-
    with
     heart disease O10.11-
      with renal disease O10.31-
     pre-eclampsia O11.-
     renal disease O10.21-
      with heart disease O10.31-
    essential O10.01-
    secondary O10.41-
  puerperium pre-existing O10.93
   with
    heart disease O10.13
     with renal disease O10.33
    renal disease O10.23
     with heart disease O10.33
   essential O10.03
   pregnancy-induced O13.9
   secondary O10.43
 due to
  endocrine disorders I15.2
  pheochromocytoma I15.2
  renal disorders NEC I15.1
   arterial I15.0
  renovascular disorders I15.0
  specified disease NEC I15.8
 encephalopathy I67.4
 gestational (without significant proteinuria)
   (pregnancy-induced) (transient) O13.-
  with significant proteinuria —*see*
    Pre-eclampsia
 Goldblatt's I70.1

Hypertension, hypertensive (*Continued*)
heart (disease) (conditions in I51.4-I51.9 due to hypertension) I11.9
  with
    heart failure (congestive) I11.0
    kidney disease (chronic) —*see*
      Hypertension, cardiorenal
intracranial (benign) G93.2
kidney I12.9
  with
    heart disease —*see* Hypertension, cardiorenal
    stage 1 through stage 4 chronic kidney disease I12.9
    stage 5 chronic kidney disease (CKD) or end stage renal disease (ESRD) I12.0
lesser circulation I27.0
newborn P29.2
  pulmonary (persistent) P29.3
ocular H40.05-
pancreatic duct — code to underlying condition
  with chronic pancreatitis K86.1
portal (due to chronic liver disease) (idiopathic) K76.6
  gastropathy K31.89
in (due to) schistosomiasis (bilharziasis) B65.9 [*K77*]
postoperative I97.3
psychogenic F45.8
pulmonary (artery) (secondary) NEC I27.2
  with
    cor pulmonale (chronic) I27.2
      acute I26.09
    right heart ventricular strain/failure I27.2
      acute I26.09
  of newborn (persistent) P29.3
  primary (idiopathic) I27.0
renal —*see* Hypertension, kidney
renovascular I15.0
secondary NEC I15.9
  due to
    endocrine disorders I15.2
    pheochromocytoma I15.2
    renal disorders NEC I15.1
      arterial I15.0
    renovascular disorders I15.0
  specified NEC I15.8
venous (chronic)
  due to
    deep vein thrombosis —*see* Syndrome, postthrombotic
  idiopathic I87.309
    with
      inflammation I87.32-
        with ulcer I87.33-
      specified complication NEC I87.39-
      ulcer I87.31-
        with inflammation I87.33-
    asymptomatic I87.30-
Hypertensive urgency —*see* Hypertension
Hyperthecosis ovary E28.8
Hyperthermia (of unknown origin) —*see also* Hyperpyrexia
malignant, due to anesthesia T88.3
newborn P81.9
  environmental P81.0
Hyperthyroid (recurrent) —*see* Hyperthyroidism
Hyperthyroidism (latent) (pre-adult) (recurrent) E05.90
with
  goiter (diffuse) E05.00
    with thyroid storm E05.01
    nodular (multinodular) E05.20
      with thyroid storm E05.21
      uninodular E05.10
        with thyroid storm E05.11
  storm E05.91

Hyperthyroidism (*Continued*)
due to ectopic thyroid tissue E05.30
  with thyroid storm E05.31
neonatal, transitory P72.1
specified NEC E05.80
  with thyroid storm E05.81
Hypertony, hypertonia, hypertonicity
bladder N31.8
congenital P94.1
stomach K31.89
  psychogenic F45.8
uterus, uterine (contractions) (complicating delivery) O62.4
Hypertrichosis L68.9
congenital Q84.2
eyelid H02.869
  left H02.866
    lower H02.865
    upper H02.864
  right H02.863
    lower H02.862
    upper H02.861
lanuginosa Q84.2
  acquired L68.1
localized L68.2
specified NEC L68.8
Hypertriglyceridemia, essential E78.1
Hypertrophy, hypertrophic
adenofibromatous, prostate —*see* Enlargement, enlarged, prostate
adenoids (infective) J35.2
  with tonsils J35.3
adrenal cortex E27.8
alveolar process or ridge —*see* Anomaly, alveolar
anal papillae K62.89
artery I77.89
  congenital NEC Q27.8
    digestive system Q27.8
    lower limb Q27.8
    specified site NEC Q27.8
    upper limb Q27.8
auricular —*see* Hypertrophy, cardiac
Bartholin's gland N75.8
bile duct (common) (hepatic) K83.8
bladder (sphincter) (trigone) N32.89
bone M89.30
  carpus M89.34-
  clavicle M89.31-
  femur M89.35-
  fibula M89.36-
  finger M89.34-
  humerus M89.32-
  ilium M89.359
  ischium M89.359
  metacarpus M89.34-
  metatarsus M89.37-
  multiple sites M89.39
  neck M89.38
  radius M89.33-
  rib M89.38
  scapula M89.31-
  skull M89.38
  tarsus M89.37-
  tibia M89.36-
  toe M89.37-
  ulna M89.33-
  vertebra M89.38
brain G93.89
breast N62
  cystic —*see* Mastopathy, cystic
  newborn P83.4
  pubertal, massive N62
  puerperal, postpartum —*see* Disorder, breast, specified type NEC
  senile (parenchymatous) N62
cardiac (chronic) (idiopathic) I51.7
  with rheumatic fever (conditions in I00)
    active I01.8
    inactive or quiescent (with chorea) I09.89
  congenital NEC Q24.8

Hypertrophy, hypertrophic (*Continued*)
cardiac (*Continued*)
  fatty —*see* Degeneration, myocardial
  hypertensive —*see* Hypertension, heart
  rheumatic (with chorea) I09.89
    active or acute I01.8
      with chorea I02.0
  valve —*see* Endocarditis
cartilage —*see* Disorder, cartilage, specified type NEC
cecum —*see* Megacolon
cervix (uteri) N88.8
  congenital Q51.828
  elongation N88.4
clitoris (cirrhotic) N90.89
  congenital Q52.6
colon —*see also* Megacolon
  congenital Q43.2
conjunctiva, lymphoid H11.89
corpora cavernosa N48.89
cystic duct K82.8
duodenum K31.89
endometrium (glandular) (*see also* Hyperplasia, endometrial) N85.00-
  cervix N88.8
epididymis N50.8
esophageal hiatus (congenital) Q79.1
  with hernia —*see* Hernia, hiatal
eyelid —*see* Disorder, eyelid, specified type NEC
fat pad E65
  knee (infrapatellar) (popliteal) (prepatellar) (retropatellar) M79.4
foot (congenital) Q74.2
frenulum, frenum (tongue) K14.8
  lip K13.0
gallbladder K82.8
gastric mucosa K29.60
  with bleeding K29.61
gland, glandular R59.9
  generalized R59.1
  localized R59.0
gum (mucous membrane) K06.1
heart (idiopathic) —*see also* Hypertrophy, cardiac
  valve (*see also* Endocarditis) I38
hemifacial Q67.4
hepatic —*see* Hypertrophy, liver
hiatus (esophageal) Q79.1
hilus gland R59.0
hymen, congenital Q52.4
ileum K63.89
intestine NEC K63.89
jejunum K63.89
kidney (compensatory) N28.81
  congenital Q63.3
labium (majus) (minus) N90.6
ligament —*see* Disorder, ligament
lingual tonsil (infective) J35.1
  with adenoids J35.3
lip K13.0
  congenital Q18.6
liver R16.0
  acute K76.89
  cirrhotic —*see* Cirrhosis, liver
  congenital Q44.7
  fatty —*see* Fatty, liver
lymph, lymphatic gland R59.9
  generalized R59.1
  localized R59.0
  tuberculous —*see* Tuberculosis, lymph gland
mammary gland —*see* Hypertrophy, breast
Meckel's diverticulum (congenital) Q43.0
  malignant —*see* Table of Neoplasms, small intestine, malignant
median bar —*see* Hyperplasia, prostate
meibomian gland —*see* Chalazion
meniscus, knee, congenital Q74.1
metatarsal head —*see* Hypertrophy, bone, metatarsus

◄ New ◄═ Revised ~~deleted~~ Deleted

Hypertrophy, hypertrophic *(Continued)*
  metatarsus —*see* Hypertrophy, bone,
    metatarsus
  mucous membrane
    alveolar ridge K06.2
    gum K06.1
    nose (turbinate) J34.3
  muscle M62.89
  muscular coat, artery I77.89
  myocardium —*see also* Hypertrophy, cardiac
    idiopathic I42.2
  myometrium N85.2
  nail L60.2
    congenital Q84.5
  nasal J34.89
    alae J34.89
    bone J34.89
    cartilage J34.89
    mucous membrane (septum) J34.3
    sinus J34.89
    turbinate J34.3
  nasopharynx, lymphoid (infectional) (tissue)
    (wall) J35.2
  nipple N62
  organ or site, congenital NEC —*see* Anomaly,
    by site - ovary N83.8
  palate (hard) M27.8
    soft K13.79
  pancreas, congenital Q45.3
  parathyroid (gland) E21.0
  parotid gland K11.1
  penis N48.89
  pharyngeal tonsil J35.2
  pharynx J39.2
    lymphoid (infectional) (tissue) (wall)
      J35.2
  pituitary (anterior) (fossa) (gland) E23.6
  prepuce (congenital) N47.8
    female N90.89
  prostate —*see* Enlargement, enlarged,
    prostate
    congenital Q55.4
  pseudomuscular G71.0
  pylorus (adult) (muscle) (sphincter) K31.1
    congenital or infantile Q40.0
  rectal, rectum (sphincter) K62.89
  rhinitis (turbinate) J31.0
  salivary gland (any) K11.1
    congenital Q38.4
  scaphoid (tarsal) —*see* Hypertrophy, bone,
    tarsus
  scar L91.0
  scrotum N50.8
  seminal vesicle N50.8
  sigmoid —*see* Megacolon
  skin L91.9
    specified NEC L91.8
  spermatic cord N50.8
  spleen —*see* Splenomegaly
  spondylitis —*see* Spondylosis
  stomach K31.89
  sublingual gland K11.1
  submandibular gland K11.1
  suprarenal cortex (gland) E27.8
  synovial NEC M67.20
    acromioclavicular M67.21-
    ankle M67.27-
    elbow M67.22-
    foot M67.27-
    hand M67.24-
    hip M67.25-
    knee M67.26-
    multiple sites M67.29
    specified site NEC M67.28
    wrist M67.23-
  tendon —*see* Disorder, tendon, specified type
    NEC
  testis N44.8
    congenital Q55.29
  thymic, thymus (gland) (congenital)
    E32.0

Hypertrophy, hypertrophic *(Continued)*
  thyroid (gland) —*see* Goiter
  toe (congenital) Q74.2
    acquired —*see also* Deformity, toe, specified
      NEC
  tongue K14.8
    congenital Q38.2
    papillae (foliate) K14.3
  tonsils (faucial) (infective) (lingual)
    (lymphoid) J35.1
    with adenoids J35.3
  tunica vaginalis N50.8
  ureter N28.89
  urethra N36.8
  uterus N85.2
    neck (with elongation) N88.4
    puerperal O90.89
  uvula K13.79
  vagina N89.8
  vas deferens N50.8
  vein I87.8
  ventricle, ventricular (heart) —*see also*
    Hypertrophy, cardiac
    congenital Q24.8
    in tetralogy of Fallot Q21.3
  verumontanum N36.8
  vocal cord J38.3
  vulva N90.6
    stasis (nonfilarial) N90.6
Hypertropia H50.2-
Hypertyrosinemia E70.21
Hyperuricemia (asymptomatic) E79.0
Hypervalinemia E71.19
Hyperventilation (tetany) R06.4
  hysterical F45.8
  psychogenic F45.8
  syndrome F45.8
Hypervitaminosis (dietary) NEC E67.8
  A E67.0
    administered as drug (prolonged intake) —
      see Table of Drugs and Chemicals,
      vitamins, adverse effect
    overdose or wrong substance given or
      taken —*see* Table of Drugs and
      Chemicals, vitamins, poisoning
  B6 E67.2
  D E67.3
    administered as drug (prolonged intake) —
      see Table of Drugs and Chemicals,
      vitamins, adverse effect
    overdose or wrong substance given or
      taken —*see* Table of Drugs and
      Chemicals, vitamins, poisoning
  K E67.8
    administered as drug (prolonged intake) —
      see Table of Drugs and Chemicals,
      vitamins, adverse effect
    overdose or wrong substance given or
      taken —*see* Table of Drugs and
      Chemicals, vitamins, poisoning
Hypervolemia E87.70
  specified NEC E87.79
Hypesthesia R20.1
  cornea —*see* Anesthesia, cornea
Hyphema H21.0-
  traumatic S05.1-
Hypoacidity, gastric K31.89
  psychogenic F45.8
Hypoadrenalism, hypoadrenia E27.40
  primary E27.1
  tuberculous A18.7
Hypoadrenocorticism E27.40
  pituitary E23.0
  primary E27.1
Hypoalbuminemia E88.09
Hypoaldosteronism E27.40
Hypoalphalipoproteinemia E78.6
Hypobarism T70.29
Hypobaropathy T70.29
Hypobetalipoproteinemia (familial)
  E78.6

Hypocalcemia E83.51
  dietary E58
  neonatal P71.1
    due to cow's milk P71.0
  phosphate-loading (newborn) P71.1
Hypochloremia E87.8
Hypochlorhydria K31.89
  neurotic F45.8
  psychogenic F45.8
Hypochondria, hypochondriac,
  hypochondriasis (reaction) F45.21
  sleep F51.03
Hypochondrogenesis Q77.0
Hypochondroplasia Q77.4
Hypochromasia, blood cells D50.8
Hypodontia —*see* Anodontia
Hypoeosinophilia D72.89
Hypoesthesia R20.1
Hypofibrinogenemia D68.8
  acquired D65
  congenital (hereditary) D68.2
Hypofunction
  adrenocortical E27.40
    drug-induced E27.3
    postprocedural E89.6
    primary E27.1
  adrenomedullary, postprocedural E89.6
  cerebral R29.818
  corticoadrenal NEC E27.40
  intestinal K59.8
  labyrinth —*see* subcategory H83.2
  ovary E28.39
  pituitary (gland) (anterior) E23.0
  testicular E29.1
    postprocedural (postsurgical)
      (postirradiation) (iatrogenic) E89.5
Hypogalactia O92.4
Hypogammaglobulinemia (*see also*
  Agammaglobulinemia) D80.1
  hereditary D80.0
  nonfamilial D80.1
  transient, of infancy D80.7
Hypogenitalism (congenital) —*see*
  Hypogonadism
Hypoglossia Q38.3
Hypoglycemia (spontaneous) E16.2
  coma E15
  diabetic —*see* Diabetes, coma
  diabetic —*see* Diabetes, hypoglycemia
  dietary counseling and surveillance Z71.3
  drug-induced E16.0
    with coma (nondiabetic) E15
  due to insulin E16.0
    with coma (nondiabetic) E15
    therapeutic misadventure —*see*
      subcategory T38.3
  functional, nonhyperinsulinemic E16.1
  iatrogenic E16.0
    with coma (nondiabetic) E15
  in infant of diabetic mother P70.1
    gestational diabetes P70.0
  infantile E16.1
  leucine-induced E71.19
  neonatal (transitory) P70.4
    iatrogenic P70.3
  reactive (not drug-induced) E16.1
  transitory neonatal P70.4
Hypogonadism
  female E28.39
  hypogonadotropic E23.0
  male E29.1
  ovarian (primary) E28.39
  pituitary E23.0
  testicular (primary) E29.1
Hypohidrosis, hypoidrosis L74.4
Hypoinsulinemia, postprocedural E89.1
Hypokalemia E87.6
Hypoleukocytosis —*see* Agranulocytosis
Hypolipoproteinemia (alpha) (beta) E78.6
Hypomagnesemia E83.42
  neonatal P71.2

Hypomania, hypomanic reaction F30.8
Hypomenorrhea —see Oligomenorrhea
Hypometabolism R63.8
Hypomotility
    gastrointestinal (tract) K31.89
        psychogenic F45.8
    intestine K59.8
        psychogenic F45.8
    stomach K31.89
        psychogenic F45.8
Hyponasality R49.22
Hyponatremia E87.1
Hypo-osmolality E87.1
Hypo-ovarianism, hypo-ovarism E28.39
Hypoparathyroidism E20.9
    familial E20.8
    idiopathic E20.0
    neonatal, transitory P71.4
    postprocedural E89.2
    specified NEC E20.8
Hypoperfusion (in)
    newborn P96.89
Hypopharyngitis —see Laryngopharyngitis
Hypophoria H50.53
Hypophosphatemia, hypophosphatasia
        (acquired) (congenital) (renal) E83.39
    familial E83.31
Hypophyseal, hypophysis —see also condition
    dwarfism E23.0
    gigantism E22.0
Hypopiesis —see Hypotension
Hypopinealism E34.8
Hypopituitarism (juvenile) E23.0
    drug-induced E23.1
    due to
        hypophysectomy E89.3
        radiotherapy E89.3
    iatrogenic NEC E23.1
    postirradiation E89.3
    postpartum E23.0
    postprocedural E89.3
Hypoplasia, hypoplastic
    adrenal (gland), congenital Q89.1
    alimentary tract, congenital Q45.8
        upper Q40.8
    anus, anal (canal) Q42.3
        with fistula Q42.2
    aorta, aortic Q25.4
        ascending, in hypoplastic left heart
            syndrome Q23.4
        valve Q23.1
            in hypoplastic left heart syndrome
                Q23.4
    areola, congenital Q83.8
    arm (congenital) —see Defect, reduction,
        upper limb
    artery (peripheral) Q27.8
        brain (congenital) Q28.3
        coronary Q24.5
        digestive system Q27.8
        lower limb Q27.8
        pulmonary Q25.79
            functional, unilateral J43.0
        retinal (congenital) Q14.1
        specified site NEC Q27.8
        umbilical Q27.0
        upper limb Q27.8
    auditory canal Q17.8
        causing impairment of hearing Q16.9
    biliary duct or passage Q44.5
    bone NOS Q79.9
        face Q75.8
        marrow D61.9
            megakaryocytic D69.49
        skull —see Hypoplasia, skull
    brain Q02
        gyri Q04.3
        part of Q04.3
    breast (areola) N64.82
    bronchus Q32.4
    cardiac Q24.8

Hypoplasia, hypoplastic (Continued)
    carpus —see Defect, reduction, upper limb,
        specified type NEC
    cartilage hair Q78.5
    cecum Q42.8
    cementum K00.4
    cephalic Q02
    cerebellum Q04.3
    cervix (uteri), congenital Q51.821
    clavicle (congenital) Q74.0
    coccyx Q76.49
    colon Q42.9
        specified NEC Q42.8
    corpus callosum Q04.0
    cricoid cartilage Q31.2
    digestive organ (s) or tract NEC Q45.8
        upper (congenital) Q40.8
    ear (auricle) (lobe) Q17.2
        middle Q16.4
    enamel of teeth (neonatal) (postnatal)
        (prenatal) K00.4
    endocrine (gland) NEC Q89.2
    endometrium N85.8
    epididymis (congenital) Q55.4
    epiglottis Q31.2
    erythroid, congenital D61.01
    esophagus (congenital) Q39.8
    eustachian tube Q17.8
    eye Q11.2
    eyelid (congenital) Q10.3
    face Q18.8
        bone (s) Q75.8
    femur (congenital) —see Defect,
        reduction, lower limb, specified
        type NEC
    fibula (congenital) —see Defect,
        reduction, lower limb, specified
        type NEC
    finger (congenital) —see Defect,
        reduction, upper limb, specified
        type NEC
    focal dermal Q82.8
    foot —see Defect, reduction, lower limb,
        specified type NEC
    gallbladder Q44.0
    genitalia, genital organ (s)
        female, congenital Q52.8
            external Q52.79
            internal NEC Q52.8
        in adiposogenital dystrophy E23.6
    glottis Q31.2
    hair Q84.2
    hand (congenital) —see Defect, reduction,
        upper limb, specified type NEC
    heart Q24.8
    humerus (congenital) —see Defect,
        reduction, upper limb, specified
        type NEC
    intestine (small) Q41.9
        large Q42.9
            specified NEC Q42.8
    jaw M26.09
        alveolar M26.79
        lower M26.04
            alveolar M26.74
        upper M26.02
            alveolar M26.73
    kidney (s) Q60.5
        bilateral Q60.4
        unilateral Q60.3
    labium (majus) (minus), congenital Q52.79
    larynx Q31.2
    left heart syndrome Q23.4
    leg (congenital) —see Defect, reduction, lower
        limb
    limb Q73.8
        lower (congenital) —see Defect, reduction,
            lower limb
        upper (congenital) —see Defect, reduction,
            upper limb
    liver Q44.7

Hypoplasia, hypoplastic (Continued)
    lung (lobe) (not associated with short
        gestation) Q33.6
        associated with immaturity, low birth
            weight, prematurity, or short
            gestation P28.0
    mammary (areola), congenital Q83.8
    mandible, mandibular M26.04
        alveolar M26.74
        unilateral condylar M27.8
    maxillary M26.02
        alveolar M26.73
    medullary D61.9
    megakaryocytic D69.49
    metacarpus —see Defect, reduction, upper
        limb, specified type NEC
    metatarsus —see Defect, reduction, lower
        limb, specified type NEC
    muscle Q79.8
    nail (s) Q84.6
    nose, nasal Q30.1
    optic nerve H47.03-
    osseous meatus (ear) Q17.8
    ovary, congenital Q50.39
    pancreas Q45.0
    parathyroid (gland) Q89.2
    parotid gland Q38.4
    patella Q74.1
    pelvis, pelvic girdle Q74.2
    penis (congenital) Q55.62
    peripheral vascular system Q27.8
        digestive system Q27.8
        lower limb Q27.8
        specified site NEC Q27.8
        upper limb Q27.8
    pituitary (gland) (congenital) Q89.2
    pulmonary (not associated with short
        gestation) Q33.6
        artery, functional J43.0
        associated with short gestation P28.0
    radioulnar —see Defect, reduction, upper
        limb, specified type NEC
    radius —see Defect, reduction, upper limb
    rectum Q42.1
        with fistula Q42.0
    respiratory system NEC Q34.8
    rib Q76.6
    right heart syndrome Q22.6
    sacrum Q76.49
    scapula Q74.0
    scrotum Q55.1
    shoulder girdle Q74.0
    skin Q82.8
    skull (bone) Q75.8
        with
            anencephaly Q00.0
            encephalocele —see Encephalocele
            hydrocephalus Q03.9
                with spina bifida —see Spina bifida, by
                    site, with hydrocephalus
            microcephaly Q02
    spinal (cord) (ventral horn cell) Q06.1
    spine Q76.49
    sternum Q76.7
    tarsus —see Defect, reduction, lower limb,
        specified type NEC
    testis Q55.1
    thymic, with immunodeficiency D82.1
    thymus (gland) Q89.2
        with immunodeficiency D82.1
    thyroid (gland) E03.1
        cartilage Q31.2
    tibiofibular (congenital) —see Defect,
        reduction, lower limb, specified type
        NEC
    toe —see Defect, reduction, lower limb,
        specified type NEC
    tongue Q38.3
    Turner's K00.4
    ulna (congenital) —see Defect, reduction,
        upper limb

◀ New   ◀▦ Revised   deleted Deleted

Hypoplasia, hypoplastic *(Continued)*
  umbilical artery Q27.0
  unilateral condylar M27.8
  ureter Q62.8
  uterus, congenital Q51.811
  vagina Q52.4
  vascular NEC peripheral Q27.8
    brain Q28.3
    digestive system Q27.8
    lower limb Q27.8
    specified site NEC Q27.8
    upper limb Q27.8
  vein (s) (peripheral) Q27.8
    brain Q28.3
    digestive system Q27.8
    great Q26.8
    lower limb Q27.8
    specified site NEC Q27.8
    upper limb Q27.8
  vena cava (inferior) (superior) Q26.8
  vertebra Q76.49
  vulva, congenital Q52.79
  zonule (ciliary) Q12.8
Hypopotassemia E87.6
Hypoproconvertinemia, congenital
    (hereditary) D68.2
Hypoproteinemia E77.8
Hypoprothrombinemia (congenital)
    (hereditary) (idiopathic) D68.2
  acquired D68.4
  newborn, transient P61.6
Hypoptyalism K11.7
Hypopyon (eye) (anterior chamber) —*see*
    Iridocyclitis, acute, hypopyon
Hypopyrexia R68.0
Hyporeflexia R29.2
Hyposecretion
  ACTH E23.0
  antidiuretic hormone E23.2
  ovary E28.39
  salivary gland (any) K11.7
  vasopressin E23.2
Hyposegmentation, leukocytic, hereditary
    D72.0
Hyposiderinemia D50.9
Hypospadias Q54.9
  balanic Q54.0
  coronal Q54.0
  glandular Q54.0
  penile Q54.1
  penoscrotal Q54.2

Hypospadias *(Continued)*
  perineal Q54.3
  specified NEC Q54.8
Hypospermatogenesis —*see* Oligospermia
Hyposplenism D73.0
Hypostasis pulmonary, passive —*see* Edema,
    lung
Hypostatic —*see* condition
Hyposthenuria N28.89
Hypotension (arterial) (constitutional) I95.9
  chronic I95.89
  drug-induced I95.2
  due to (of) hemodialysis I95.3
  iatrogenic I95.89
  idiopathic (permanent) I95.0
  intracranial, following ventricular shunting
      (ventriculostomy) G97.2
  intra-dialytic I95.3
  maternal, syndrome (following labor and
      delivery) O26.5-
  neurogenic, orthostatic G90.3
  orthostatic (chronic) I95.1
    due to drugs I95.2
    neurogenic G90.3
  postoperative I95.81
  postural I95.1
  specified NEC I95.89
Hypothermia (accidental) T68
  due to anesthesia, anesthetic T88.51
  low environmental temperature T68
  neonatal P80.9
    environmental (mild) NEC P80.8
    mild P80.8
    severe (chronic) (cold injury syndrome)
        P80.0
    specified NEC P80.8
  not associated with low environmental
      temperature R68.0
Hypothyroidism (acquired) E03.9
  congenital (without goiter) E03.1
    with goiter (diffuse) E03.0
  due to
    exogenous substance NEC E03.2
    iodine-deficiency, acquired E01.8
      subclinical E02
    irradiation therapy E89.0
    medicament NEC E03.2
    P-aminosalicylic acid (PAS) E03.2
    phenylbutazone E03.2
    resorcinol E03.2
    sulfonamide E03.2

Hypothyroidism *(Continued)*
  due to *(Continued)*
    surgery E89.0
    thiourea group drugs E03.2
  iatrogenic NEC E03.2
  iodine-deficiency (acquired) E01.8
    congenital —*see* Syndrome, iodine-
        deficiency, congenital
    subclinical E02
  neonatal, transitory P72.2
  postinfectious E03.3
  postirradiation E89.0
  postprocedural E89.0
  postsurgical E89.0
  specified NEC E03.8
  subclinical, iodine-deficiency related E02
Hypotonia, hypotonicity, hypotony
  bladder N31.2
  congenital (benign) P94.2
  eye —*see* Disorder, globe, hypotony
Hypotrichosis —*see* Alopecia
Hypotropia H50.2-
Hypoventilation R06.89
  congenital central alveolar G47.35
  sleep related
    idiopathic nonobstructive alveolar G47.34
    in conditions classified elsewhere G47.36
Hypovitaminosis —*see* Deficiency, vitamin
Hypovolemia E86.1
  surgical shock T81.19
  traumatic (shock) T79.4
Hypoxemia R09.02
  newborn P84
  sleep related, in conditions classified
      elsewhere G47.36
Hypoxia (*see also* Anoxia) R09.02
  cerebral, during a procedure NEC G97.81
    postprocedural NEC G97.82
  intrauterine P84
  myocardial —*see* Insufficiency, coronary
  newborn P84
  sleep-related G47.34
Hypsarhythmia —*see* Epilepsy, generalized,
    specified NEC
Hysteralgia, pregnant uterus O26.89-
Hysteria, hysterical (conversion) (dissociative
    state) F44.9
  anxiety F41.8
  convulsions F44.5
  psychosis, acute F44.9
Hysteroepilepsy F44.5

I

Ichthyoparasitism due to Vandellia cirrhosa
B88.8
Ichthyosis (congenital) Q80.9
  acquired L85.0
  fetalis Q80.4
  hystrix Q80.8
  lamellar Q80.2
  lingual K13.29
  palmaris and plantaris Q82.8
  simplex Q80.0
  vera Q80.8
  vulgaris Q80.0
  X-linked Q80.1
Ichthyotoxism —*see* Poisoning, fish
  bacterial —*see* Intoxication, foodborne
Icteroanemia, hemolytic (acquired) D59.9
  congenital —*see* Spherocytosis
Icterus —*see also* Jaundice
  conjunctiva R17
  gravis, newborn P55.0
  hematogenous (acquired) D59.9
  hemolytic (acquired) D59.9
    congenital —*see* Spherocytosis
  hemorrhagic (acute) (leptospiral)
      (spirochetal) A27.0
    newborn P53
  infectious B15.9
    with hepatic coma B15.0
    leptospiral A27.0
    spirochetal A27.0
  neonatorum —*see* Jaundice, newborn
  newborn P59.9
  spirochetal A27.0
Ictus solaris, solis T67.0
Ideation
  homicidal R45.850
  suicidal R45.851
Identity disorder (child) F64.9
  gender role F64.2
  psychosexual F64.2
Idioglossia F80.0
Idiopathic —*see* condition
Idiot, idiocy (congenital) F73
  amaurotic (Bielschowsky(-Jansky)) (family)
      (infantile (late)) (juvenile (late)) (Vogt-
      Spielmeyer) E75.4
  microcephalic Q02
Id reaction (due to bacteria) L30.2
IgE asthma J45.909
IIAC (idiopathic infantile arterial calcification)
    Q28.8
Ileitis (chronic) (noninfectious) (*see also*
    Enteritis) K52.9
  backwash —*see* Pancolitis, ulcerative
      (chronic)
  infectious A09
  regional (ulcerative) —*see* Enteritis, regional,
      small intestine
  segmental —*see* Enteritis, regional
  terminal (ulcerative) —*see* Enteritis, regional,
      small intestine
Ileocolitis (*see also* Enteritis) K52.9
  infectious A09
  regional —*see* Enteritis, regional
Ileostomy
  attention to Z43.2
  malfunctioning K94.13
  status Z93.2
    with complication —*see* Complications,
        enterostomy
Ileotyphus —*see* Typhoid
Ileum —*see* condition
Ileus (bowel) (colon) (inhibitory) (intestine)
    K56.7
  adynamic K56.0
  due to gallstone (in intestine) K56.3
  duodenal (chronic) K31.5
  gallstone K56.3
  mechanical NEC K56.69

Ileus (*Continued*)
  meconium P76.0
    in cystic fibrosis E84.11
    meaning meconium plug (without cystic
        fibrosis) P76.0
  myxedema K59.8
  neurogenic K56.0
    Hirschsprung's disease or megacolon
        Q43.1
  newborn
    due to meconium P76.0
      in cystic fibrosis E84.11
      meaning meconium plug (without cystic
          fibrosis) P76.0
    transitory P76.1
  obstructive K56.69
  paralytic K56.0
Iliac —*see* condition
Iliotibial band syndrome M76.3-
Illiteracy Z55.0
Illness (*see also* Disease) R69
  manic-depressive —*see* Disorder, bipolar
Imbalance R26.89
  autonomic G90.8
  constituents of food intake E63.1
  electrolyte E87.8
    with
      abortion —*see* Abortion by type,
          complicated by, electrolyte
          imbalance
      molar pregnancy O08.5
    due to hyperemesis gravidarum O21.1
    following ectopic or molar pregnancy
        O08.5
    neonatal, transitory NEC P74.4
      potassium P74.3
      sodium P74.2
  endocrine E34.9
  eye muscle NOS H50.9
  hormone E34.9
  hysterical F44.4
  labyrinth —*see* subcategory H83.2
  posture R29.3
  protein-energy —*see* Malnutrition
  sympathetic G90.8
Imbecile, imbecility (I.Q. 35-49) F71
Imbedding, intrauterine device T83.39
Imbibition, cholesterol (gallbladder) K82.4
Imbrication, teeth, fully erupted M26.30
Imerslund (-Gräsbeck) **syndrome** D51.1
Immature —*see also* Immaturity
  birth (less than 37 completed weeks) —*see*
      Preterm, newborn
  extremely (less than 28 completed
      weeks) —*see* Immaturity, extreme
  personality F60.89
Immaturity (less than 37 completed weeks) —
    see also Preterm, newborn
  extreme of newborn (less than 28 completed
      weeks of gestation) (less than
      196 completed days of gestation)
      (unspecified weeks of gestation) P07.20
    gestational age
      23 completed weeks (23 weeks, 0 days
          through 23 weeks, 6 days) P07.22
      24 completed weeks (24 weeks, 0 days
          through 24 weeks, 6 days) P07.23
      25 completed weeks (25 weeks, 0 days
          through 25 weeks, 6 days) P07.24
      26 completed weeks (26 weeks, 0 days
          through 26 weeks, 6 days) P07.25
      27 completed weeks (27 weeks, 0 days
          through 27 weeks, 6 days) P07.26
      less than 23 completed weeks P07.21
  fetus or infant light-for-dates —*see*
      Light-for-dates
  lung, newborn P28.0
  organ or site NEC —*see* Hypoplasia
  pulmonary, newborn P28.0
  reaction F60.89
  sexual (female) (male), after puberty E30.0

Immersion T75.1
  foot T69.02-
  hand T69.01-
Immobile, immobility
  complete, due to severe physical disability or
      frailty R53.2
  intestine K59.8
  syndrome (paraplegic) M62.3
Immune reconstitution (inflammatory)
    syndrome [IRIS] D89.3
Immunization —*see also* Vaccination
  ABO —*see* Incompatibility, ABO
    in newborn P55.1
  complication —*see* Complications,
      vaccination
  encounter for Z23
  not done (not carried out) Z28.9
    because (of)
      acute illness of patient Z28.01
      allergy to vaccine (or component) Z28.04
      caregiver refusal Z28.82
      chronic illness of patient Z28.02
      contraindication NEC Z28.09
      group pressure Z28.1
      guardian refusal Z28.82
      immune compromised state of patient
          Z28.03
      parent refusal Z28.82
      patient's belief Z28.1
      patient had disease being vaccinated
          against Z28.81
      patient refusal Z28.21
      religious beliefs of patient Z28.1
      specified reason NEC Z28.89
        of patient Z28.29
      unspecified patient reason Z28.20
  Rh factor
    affecting management of pregnancy NEC
        O36.09-
      anti-D antibody O36.01-
    from transfusion —*see* Complication (s),
        transfusion, incompatibility reaction,
        Rh (factor)
Immunocytoma C83.0-
Immunodeficiency D84.9
  with
    adenosine-deaminase deficiency D81.3
    antibody defects D80.9
      specified type NEC D80.8
    hyperimmunoglobulinemia D80.6
    increased immunoglobulin M (IgM) D80.5
    major defect D82.9
      specified type NEC D82.8
    partial albinism D82.8
    short-limbed stature D82.2
    thrombocytopenia and eczema D82.0
  antibody with
    hyperimmunoglobulinemia D80.6
    near-normal immunoglobulins D80.6
  autosomal recessive, Swiss type D80.0
  combined D81.9
    biotin-dependent carboxylase D81.819
      biotinidase D81.810
      holocarboxylase synthetase D81.818
      specified type NEC D81.818
    severe (SCID) D81.9
      with
        low or normal B-cell numbers D81.2
        low T- and B-cell numbers D81.1
        reticular dysgenesis D81.0
    specified type NEC D81.89
  common variable D83.9
    with
      abnormalities of B-cell numbers and
          function D83.0
      autoantibodies to B- or T-cells D83.2
      immunoregulatory T-cell disorders
          D83.1
    specified type NEC D83.8
  following hereditary defective response to
      Epstein-Barr virus (EBV) D82.3

◀ New   ◀◀ Revised   ~~deleted~~ Deleted

Immunodeficiency *(Continued)*
   selective, immunoglobulin
      A (IgA) D80.2
      G (IgG) (subclasses) D80.3
      M (IgM) D80.4
   severe combined (SCID) D81.9
   specified type NEC D84.8
   X-linked, with increased IgM D80.5
Immunotherapy (encounter for)
   antineoplastic Z51.12
Impaction, impacted
   bowel, colon, rectum *(see also* Impaction, fecal) K56.49
      by gallstone K56.3
   calculus —*see* Calculus
   cerumen (ear) (external) H61.2-
   cuspid —*see* Impaction, tooth
   dental (same or adjacent tooth) K01.1
   fecal, feces K56.41
   fracture —*see* Fracture, by site
   gallbladder —*see* Calculus, gallbladder
   gallstone (s) —*see* Calculus, gallbladder
      bile duct (common) (hepatic) —*see* Calculus, bile duct
      cystic duct —*see* Calculus, gallbladder
      in intestine, with obstruction (any part) K56.3
   intestine (calculous) NEC *(see also* Impaction, fecal) K56.49
      gallstone, with ileus K56.3
   intrauterine device (IUD) T83.39
   molar —*see* Impaction, tooth
   shoulder, causing obstructed labor O66.0
   tooth, teeth K01.1
   turbinate J34.89
Impaired, impairment (function)
   auditory discrimination —*see* Abnormal, auditory perception
   cognitive, mild, so stated G31.84
   dual sensory Z73.82
   fasting glucose R73.01
   glucose tolerance (oral) R73.02
   hearing —*see* Deafness
   heart —*see* Disease, heart
   kidney N28.9
      disorder resulting from N25.9
         specified NEC N25.89
   liver K72.90
      with coma K72.91
   mastication K08.8
   mild cognitive, so stated G31.84
   mobility
      ear ossicles —*see* Ankylosis, ear ossicles
      requiring care provider Z74.09
   myocardium, myocardial —*see* Insufficiency, myocardial
   rectal sphincter R19.8
   renal (acute) (chronic) N28.9
      disorder resulting from N25.9
         specified NEC N25.89
   vision NEC H54.7
      both eyes H54.3
Impediment, speech R47.9
   psychogenic (childhood) F98.8
   slurring R47.81
   specified NEC R47.89
Impending
   coronary syndrome I20.0
   delirium tremens F10.239
   myocardial infarction I20.0
Imperception auditory (acquired) —*see also* Deafness
   congenital H93.25
Imperfect
   aeration, lung (newborn) NEC —*see* Atelectasis
   closure (congenital)
      alimentary tract NEC Q45.8
         lower Q43.8
         upper Q40.8
      atrioventricular ostium Q21.2

Imperfect *(Continued)*
   closure *(Continued)*
      atrium (secundum) Q21.1
      branchial cleft or sinus Q18.0
      choroid Q14.3
      cricoid cartilage Q31.8
      cusps, heart valve NEC Q24.8
         pulmonary Q22.3
      ductus
         arteriosus Q25.0
         Botalli Q25.0
      ear drum (causing impairment of hearing) Q16.4
      esophagus with communication to bronchus or trachea Q39.1
      eyelid Q10.3
      foramen
         botalli Q21.1
         ovale Q21.1
      genitalia, genital organ (s) or system
         female Q52.8
            external Q52.79
            internal NEC Q52.8
         male Q55.8
      glottis Q31.8
      interatrial ostium or septum Q21.1
      interauricular ostium or septum Q21.1
      interventricular ostium or septum Q21.0
      larynx Q31.8
      lip —*see* Cleft, lip
      nasal septum Q30.3
      nose Q30.2
      omphalomesenteric duct Q43.0
      optic nerve entry Q14.2
      organ or site not listed —*see* Anomaly, by site
      ostium
         interatrial Q21.1
         interauricular Q21.1
         interventricular Q21.0
      palate —*see* Cleft, palate
      preauricular sinus Q18.1
      retina Q14.1
      roof of orbit Q75.8
      sclera Q13.5
      septum
         aorticopulmonary Q21.4
         atrial (secundum) Q21.1
         between aorta and pulmonary artery Q21.4
         heart Q21.9
         interatrial (secundum) Q21.1
         interauricular (secundum) Q21.1
         interventricular Q21.0
            in tetralogy of Fallot Q21.3
         nasal Q30.3
         ventricular Q21.0
            with pulmonary stenosis or atresia, dextraposition of aorta, and hypertrophy of right ventricle Q21.3
            in tetralogy of Fallot Q21.3
      skull Q75.0
         with
            anencephaly Q00.0
            encephalocele —*see* Encephalocele
            hydrocephalus Q03.9
               with spina bifida —*see* Spina bifida, by site, with hydrocephalus
            microcephaly Q02
      spine (with meningocele) —*see* Spina bifida
      trachea Q32.1
      tympanic membrane (causing impairment of hearing) Q16.4
      uterus Q51.818
      vitelline duct Q43.0
   erection —*see* Dysfunction, sexual, male, erectile
   fusion —*see* Imperfect, closure
   inflation, lung (newborn) —*see* Atelectasis

Imperfect *(Continued)*
   posture R29.3
   rotation, intestine Q43.3
   septum, ventricular Q21.0
Imperfectly descended testis —*see* Cryptorchid
Imperforate (congenital) —*see also* Atresia
   anus Q42.3
      with fistula Q42.2
   cervix (uteri) Q51.828
   esophagus Q39.0
      with tracheoesophageal fistula Q39.1
   hymen Q52.3
   jejunum Q41.1
   pharynx Q38.8
   rectum Q42.1
      with fistula Q42.0
   urethra Q64.39
   vagina Q52.4
Impervious (congenital) —*see also* Atresia
   anus Q42.3
      with fistula Q42.2
   bile duct Q44.2
   esophagus Q39.0
      with tracheoesophageal fistula Q39.1
   intestine (small) Q41.9
      large Q42.9
         specified NEC Q42.8
   rectum Q42.1
      with fistula Q42.0
   ureter —*see* Atresia, ureter
   urethra Q64.39
Impetiginization of dermatoses L01.1
Impetigo (any organism) (any site) (circinate) (contagiosa) (simplex) (vulgaris) L01.00
   Bockhart's L01.02
   bullous, bullosa L01.03
   external ear L01.00 *[H62.40]*
   follicularis L01.02
   furfuracea L30.5
   herpetiformis L40.1
      nonobstetrical L40.1
   neonatorum L01.03
   nonbullous L01.01
   specified type NEC L01.09
   ulcerative L01.09
Impingement (on teeth)
   soft tissue
      anterior M26.81
      posterior M26.82
Implant, endometrial N80.9
Implantation
   anomalous —*see* Anomaly, by site
      ureter Q62.63
   cyst
      external area or site (skin) NEC L72.0
      iris —*see* Cyst, iris, implantation
      vagina N89.8
      vulva N90.7
   dermoid (cyst) —*see* Implantation, cyst
Impotence (sexual) N52.9
   counseling Z70.1
   organic origin *(see also* Dysfunction, sexual, male, erectile) N52.9
   psychogenic F52.21
Impression, basilar Q75.8
Imprisonment, anxiety concerning Z65.1
Improper care (child) (newborn) —*see* Maltreatment
Improperly tied umbilical cord (causing hemorrhage) P51.8
Impulsiveness (impulsive) R45.87
Inability to swallow —*see* Aphagia
Inaccessible, inaccessibility
   health care NEC Z75.3
      due to
         waiting period Z75.2
            for admission to facility elsewhere Z75.1
      other helping agencies Z75.4
Inactive —*see* condition

Inadequate, inadequacy
- aesthetics of dental restoration K08.56
- biologic, constitutional, functional, or social F60.7
- development
  - child R62.50
  - genitalia
    - after puberty NEC E30.0
    - congenital
      - female Q52.8
        - external Q52.79
        - internal Q52.8
      - male Q55.8
  - lungs Q33.6
    - associated with short gestation P28.0
  - organ or site not listed —see Anomaly, by site
- diet (causing nutritional deficiency) E63.9
- eating habits Z72.4
- environment, household Z59.1
- family support Z63.8
- food (supply) NEC Z59.4
  - hunger effects T73.0
- functional F60.7
- household care, due to
  - family member
    - handicapped or ill Z74.2
    - on vacation Z75.5
    - temporarily away from home Z74.2
  - technical defects in home Z59.1
  - temporary absence from home of person rendering care Z74.2
- housing (heating) (space) Z59.1
- income (financial) Z59.6
- intrafamilial communication Z63.8
- material resources Z59.9
- mental —see Disability, intellectual
- parental supervision or control of child Z62.0
- personality F60.7
- pulmonary
  - function R06.89
    - newborn P28.5
  - ventilation, newborn P28.5
- sample of cytologic smear
  - anus R85.615
  - cervix R87.615
  - vagina R87.625
- social F60.7
  - insurance Z59.7
  - skills NEC Z73.4
- supervision of child by parent Z62.0
- teaching affecting education Z55.8
- welfare support Z59.7

Inanition R64
- with edema —see Malnutrition, severe
- due to
  - deprivation of food T73.0
  - malnutrition —see Malnutrition
- fever R50.9

Inappropriate
- change in quantitative human chorionic gonadotropin (hCG) in early pregnancy O02.81
- diet or eating habits Z72.4
- level of quantitative human chorionic gonadotropin (hCG) for gestational age in early pregnancy O02.81
- secretion
  - antidiuretic hormone (ADH) (excessive) E22.2
  - deficiency E23.2
  - pituitary (posterior) E22.2

Inattention at or after birth —see Neglect

Incarceration, incarcerated
- enterocele K46.0
  - gangrenous K46.1
- epiplocele K46.0
  - gangrenous K46.1
- exophthalmos K42.0
  - gangrenous K42.1

Incarceration, incarcerated *(Continued)*
- hernia —see also Hernia, by site, with obstruction
  - with gangrene —see Hernia, by site, with gangrene
  - iris, in wound —see Injury, eye, laceration, with prolapse
  - lens, in wound —see Injury, eye, laceration, with prolapse
  - omphalocele K42.0
  - prison, anxiety concerning Z65.1
  - rupture —see Hernia, by site
  - sarcoepiplocele K46.0
    - gangrenous K46.1
  - sarcoepiplomphalocele K42.0
    - with gangrene K42.1
  - uterus N85.8
    - gravid O34.51-
      - causing obstructed labor O65.5

Incised wound
- external —see Laceration
- internal organs —see Injury, by site

Incision, incisional
- hernia K43.2
  - with
    - gangrene (and obstruction) K43.1
    - obstruction K43.0
- surgical, complication —see Complications, surgical procedure
- traumatic
  - external —see Laceration
  - internal organs —see Injury, by site

Inclusion
- azurophilic leukocytic D72.0
- blennorrhea (neonatal) (newborn) P39.1
- gallbladder in liver (congenital) Q44.1

Incompatibility
- ABO
  - affecting management of pregnancy O36.11-
    - anti-A sensitization O36.11-
    - anti-B sensitization O36.19-
    - specified NEC O36.19-
  - infusion or transfusion reaction —see Complication (s), transfusion, incompatibility reaction, ABO
  - newborn P55.1
- blood (group) (Duffy) (K(ell)) (Kidd) (Lewis) (M) (S) NEC
  - affecting management of pregnancy O36.11-
    - anti-A sensitization O36.11-
    - anti-B sensitization O36.19-
  - infusion or transfusion reaction T80.89
  - newborn P55.8
- divorce or estrangement Z63.5
- Rh (blood group) (factor) Z31.82
  - affecting management of pregnancy NEC O36.09-
    - anti-D antibody O36.01-
  - infusion or transfusion reaction —see Complication (s), transfusion, incompatibility reaction, Rh (factor)
  - newborn P55.0
- rhesus —see Incompatibility, Rh

Incompetency, incompetent, incompetence
- annular
  - aortic (valve) —see Insufficiency, aortic
  - mitral (valve) I34.0
  - pulmonary valve (heart) I37.1
- aortic (valve) —see Insufficiency, aortic
- cardiac valve —see Endocarditis
- cervix, cervical (os) N88.3
  - in pregnancy O34.3-
- chronotropic I45.89
  - with
    - autonomic dysfunction G90.8
    - ischemic heart disease I25.89
    - left ventricular dysfunction I51.89
    - sinus node dysfunction I49.8
- esophagogastric (junction) (sphincter) K22.0

Incompetency, incompetent, incompetence *(Continued)*
- mitral (valve) —see Insufficiency, mitral
- pelvic fundus N81.89
- pubocervical tissue N81.82
- pulmonary valve (heart) I37.1
  - congenital Q22.3
- rectovaginal tissue N81.83
- tricuspid (annular) (valve) —see Insufficiency, tricuspid
- valvular —see Endocarditis
  - congenital Q24.8
- vein, venous (saphenous) (varicose) —see Varix, leg

Incomplete —see also condition
- bladder, emptying R33.9
- defecation R15.0
- expansion lungs (newborn) NEC —see Atelectasis
- rotation, intestine Q43.3

Inconclusive
- diagnostic imaging due to excess body fat of patient R93.9
- findings on diagnostic imaging of breast NEC R92.8
- mammogram (due to dense breasts) R92.2

Incontinence R32
- anal sphincter R15.9
- feces R15.9
  - nonorganic origin F98.1
- overflow N39.490
- psychogenic F45.8
- rectal R15.9
- reflex N39.498
- stress (female) (male) N39.3
  - and urge N39.46
- urethral sphincter R32
- urge N39.41
  - and stress (female) (male) N39.46
- urine (urinary) R32
  - continuous N39.45
  - due to cognitive impairment, or severe physical disability or immobility R39.81
  - functional R39.81
  - mixed (stress and urge) N39.46
  - nocturnal N39.44
  - nonorganic origin F98.0
  - overflow N39.490
  - post dribbling N39.43
  - reflex N39.498
  - specified NEC N39.498
  - stress (female) (male) N39.3
    - and urge N39.46
  - total N39.498
  - unaware N39.42
  - urge N39.41
    - and stress (female) (male) N39.46

Incontinentia pigmenti Q82.3

Incoordinate, incoordination
- esophageal-pharyngeal (newborn) —see Dysphagia
- muscular R27.8
- uterus (action) (contractions) (complicating delivery) O62.4

Increase, increased
- abnormal, in development R63.8
- androgens (ovarian) E28.1
- anticoagulants (antithrombin) (anti-VIIIa) (anti-IXa) (anti-Xa) (anti-XIa) —see Circulating anticoagulants)
- cold sense R20.8
- estrogen E28.0
- function
  - adrenal
    - cortex —see Cushing's, syndrome
    - medulla E27.5
  - pituitary (gland) (anterior) (lobe) E22.9
    - posterior E22.2
- heat sense R20.8
- intracranial pressure (benign) G93.2

◄ New ◄◄◄ Revised ~~deleted~~ Deleted

Increase, increased (Continued)
permeability, capillaries I78.8
pressure, intracranial G93.2
secretion
gastrin E16.4
glucagon E16.3
pancreas, endocrine E16.9
growth hormone-releasing hormone E16.8
pancreatic polypeptide E16.8
somatostatin E16.8
vasoactive-intestinal polypeptide E16.8
sphericity, lens Q12.4
splenic activity D73.1
venous pressure I87.8
portal K76.6
Increta placenta O43.22-
Incrustation, cornea, foreign body (lead) (zinc) —see Foreign body, cornea
Incyclophoria H50.54
Incyclotropia —see Cyclotropia
Indeterminate sex Q56.4
India rubber skin Q82.8
Indigestion (acid) (bilious) (functional) K30
catarrhal K31.89
due to decomposed food NOS A05.9
nervous F45.8
psychogenic F45.8
Indirect —see condition
Induratio penis plastica N48.6
Induration, indurated
brain G93.89
breast (fibrous) N64.51
puerperal, postpartum O92.29
broad ligament N83.8
chancre
anus A51.1
congenital A50.07
extragenital NEC A51.2
corpora cavernosa (penis) (plastic) N48.6
liver (chronic) K76.89
lung (black) (chronic) (fibroid) (see also Fibrosis, lung) J84.10
essential brown J84.03
penile (plastic) N48.6
phlebitic —see Phlebitis
skin R23.4
Inebriety (without dependence) —see Alcohol, intoxication
Inefficiency, kidney N28.9
Inelasticity, skin R23.4
Inequality, leg (length) (acquired) —see also Deformity, limb, unequal length
congenital —see Defect, reduction, lower limb
lower leg —see Deformity, limb, unequal length
Inertia
bladder (neurogenic) N31.2
stomach K31.89
psychogenic F45.8
uterus, uterine during labor O62.2
during latent phase of labor O62.0
primary O62.0
secondary O62.1
vesical (neurogenic) N31.2
Infancy, infantile, infantilism —see also condition
celiac K90.0
genitalia, genitals (after puberty) E30.0
Herter's (nontropical sprue) K90.0
intestinal K90.0
Lorain E23.0
pancreatic K86.8
pelvis M95.5
with disproportion (fetopelvic) O33.1
causing obstructed labor O65.1
pituitary E23.0
renal N25.0
uterus —see Infantile, genitalia

Infant (s) —see also Infancy
excessive crying R68.11
irritable child R68.12
lack of care —see Neglect
liveborn (singleton) Z38.2
born in hospital Z38.00
by cesarean Z38.01
born outside hospital Z38.1
multiple NEC Z38.8
born in hospital Z38.68
by cesarean Z38.69
born outside hospital Z38.7
quadruplet Z38.8
born in hospital Z38.63
by cesarean Z38.64
born outside hospital Z38.7
quintuplet Z38.8
born in hospital Z38.65
by cesarean Z38.66
born outside hospital Z38.7
triplet Z38.8
born in hospital Z38.61
by cesarean Z38.62
born outside hospital Z38.7
twin Z38.5
born in hospital Z38.30
by cesarean Z38.31
born outside hospital Z38.4
of diabetic mother (syndrome of) P70.1
gestational diabetes P70.0
Infantile —see also condition
genitalia, genitals E30.0
os, uterine E30.0
penis E30.0
testis E29.1
uterus E30.0
Infantilism —see Infancy
Infarct, infarction
adrenal (capsule) (gland) E27.49
appendices epiploicae K55.0
bowel K55.0
brain (stem) —see Infarct, cerebral
breast N64.89
brewer's (kidney) N28.0
cardiac —see Infarct, myocardium
cerebellar —see Infarct, cerebral
cerebral (see also Occlusion, artery cerebral or precerebral, with infarction) I63.9-
aborted I63.9
cortical I63.9
due to
cerebral venous thrombosis, nonpyogenic I63.6
embolism
cerebral arteries I63.4-
precerebral arteries I63.1-
occlusion NEC
cerebral arteries I63.5-
precerebral arteries I63.2-
stenosis NEC
cerebral arteries I63.5-
precerebral arteries I63.2-
thrombosis
cerebral artery I63.3-
precerebral artery I63.0-
intraoperative
during cardiac surgery I97.810
during other surgery I97.811
postprocedural
following cardiac surgery I97.820
following other surgery I97.821
specified NEC I63.8
colon (acute) (agnogenic) (embolic) (hemorrhagic) (nonocclusive) (nonthrombotic) (occlusive) (segmental) (thrombotic) (with gangrene) K55.0
coronary artery —see Infarct, myocardium
embolic —see Embolism
fallopian tube N83.8
gallbladder K82.8
heart —see Infarct, myocardium

Infarct, infarction (Continued)
hepatic K76.3
hypophysis (anterior lobe) E23.6
impending (myocardium) I20.0
intestine (acute) (agnogenic) (embolic) (hemorrhagic) (nonocclusive) (nonthrombotic) (occlusive) (thrombotic) (with gangrene) K55.0
kidney N28.0
liver K76.3
lung (embolic) (thrombotic) —see Embolism, pulmonary
lymph node I89.8
mesentery, mesenteric (embolic) (thrombotic) (with gangrene) K55.0
muscle (ischemic) M62.20
ankle M62.27-
foot M62.27-
forearm M62.23-
hand M62.24-
lower leg M62.26-
pelvic region M62.25-
shoulder region M62.21-
specified site NEC M62.28
thigh M62.25-
upper arm M62.22-
myocardium, myocardial (acute) (with stated duration of 4 weeks or less) I21.3
diagnosed on ECG, but presenting no symptoms I25.2
healed or old I25.2
intraoperative
during cardiac surgery I97.790
during other surgery I97.791
non-Q wave I21.4
non-ST elevation (NSTEMI) I21.4
subsequent I22.2
nontransmural I21.4
past (diagnosed on ECG or other investigation, but currently presenting no symptoms) I25.2
postprocedural
following cardiac surgery I97.190
following other surgery I97.191
Q wave (see also, Infarct, myocardium, by site) I21.3
ST elevation (STEMI) I21.3
anterior (anteroapical) (anterolateral) (anteroseptal) (Q wave) (wall) I21.09
subsequent I22.0
inferior (diaphragmatic) (inferolateral) (inferoposterior) (wall) NEC I21.19
subsequent I22.1
inferoposterior transmural (Q wave) I21.11
involving
coronary artery of anterior wall NEC I21.09
coronary artery of inferior wall NEC I21.19
diagonal coronary artery I21.02
left anterior descending coronary artery I21.02
left circumflex coronary artery I21.21
left main coronary artery I21.01
oblique marginal coronary artery I21.21
right coronary artery I21.11
lateral (apical-lateral) (basal-lateral) (high) I21.29
subsequent I22.8
posterior (posterobasal) (posterolateral) (posteroseptal) (true) I21.29
subsequent I22.8
septal I21.29
subsequent I22.8
specified NEC I21.29
subsequent I22.8
subsequent I22.9

Infarct, infarction (Continued)
  myocardium, myocardial (Continued)
    subsequent (recurrent) (reinfarction) I22.9
      anterior (anteroapical) (anterolateral)
          (anteroseptal) (wall) I22.0
      diaphragmatic (wall) I22.1
      inferior (diaphragmatic) (inferolateral)
          (inferoposterior) (wall) I22.1
      lateral (apical-lateral) (basal-lateral)
          (high) I22.8
      non-ST elevation (NSTEMI) I22.2
      posterior (posterobasal) (posterolateral)
          (posteroseptal) (true) I22.8
      septal I22.8
      specified NEC I22.8
      ST elevation I22.9
        anterior (anteroapical) (anterolateral)
            (anteroseptal) (wall) I22.0
        inferior (diaphragmatic) (inferolateral)
            (inferoposterior) (wall) I22.1
        specified NEC I22.8
      subendocardial I22.2
      transmural I22.9
        anterior (anteroapical) (anterolateral)
            (anteroseptal) (wall) I22.0
        diaphragmatic (wall) I22.1
        inferior (diaphragmatic) (inferolateral)
            (inferoposterior) (wall) I22.1
        lateral (apical-lateral) (basal-lateral)
            (high) I22.8
        posterior (posterobasal)
            (posterolateral) (posteroseptal)
            (true) I22.8
        specified NEC I22.8
    syphilitic A52.06
    transmural I21.3
      anterior (anteroapical) (anterolateral)
          (anteroseptal) (Q wave) (wall) NEC
          I21.09
      inferior (diaphragmatic) (inferolateral)
          (inferoposterior) (Q wave) (wall)
          NEC I21.19
      inferoposterior (Q wave) I21.11
      lateral (apical-lateral) (basal-lateral)
          (high) NEC I21.29
      posterior (posterobasal) (posterolateral)
          (posteroseptal) (true) NEC I21.29
      septal NEC I21.29
      specified NEC I21.29
  nontransmural I21.4
  omentum K55.0
  ovary N83.8
  pancreas K86.8
  papillary muscle —see Infarct, myocardium
  parathyroid gland E21.4
  pituitary (gland) E23.6
  placenta O43.81-
  prostate N42.89
  pulmonary (artery) (vein) (hemorrhagic) —
      see Embolism, pulmonary
  renal (embolic) (thrombotic) N28.0
  retina, retinal (artery) —see Occlusion, artery,
      retina
  spinal (cord) (acute) (embolic) (nonembolic)
      G95.11
  spleen D73.5
    embolic or thrombotic I74.8
  subendocardial (acute) (nontransmural) I21.4
  suprarenal (capsule) (gland) E27.49
  testis N50.1
  thrombotic —see also Thrombosis
    artery, arterial —see Embolism
  thyroid (gland) E07.89
  ventricle (heart) —see Infarct, myocardium
Infecting —see condition
Infection, infected, infective (opportunistic)
    B99.9
  with
    drug resistant organism —see Resistance
        (to), drug —see also specific organism
    lymphangitis —see Lymphangitis

Infection, infected, infective (Continued)
  with (Continued)
    organ dysfunction (acute) R65.20
      with septic shock R65.21
  abscess (skin) - code by site under Abscess
  Absidia —see Mucormycosis
  Acanthamoeba —see Acanthamebiasis
  Acanthocheilonema (perstans) (streptocerca)
      B74.4
  accessory sinus (chronic) —see Sinusitis
  achorion —see Dermatophytosis
  Acremonium falciforme B47.0
  acromioclavicular M00.9
  Actinobacillus (actinomycetem-comitans)
      A28.8
    mallei A24.0
    muris A25.1
  Actinomadura B47.1
  Actinomyces (israelii) (see also Actinomycosis)
      A42.9
  Actinomycetales —see Actinomycosis
  actinomycotic NOS —see Actinomycosis
  adenoid (and tonsil) J03.90
    chronic J35.02
  adenovirus NEC
    as cause of disease classified elsewhere
        B97.0
    unspecified nature or site B34.0
  aerogenes capsulatus A48.0
  aertrycke —see Infection, salmonella
  alimentary canal NOS —see Enteritis,
      infectious
  Allescheria boydii B48.2
  Alternaria B48.8
  alveolus, alveolar (process) K04.7
  Ameba, amebic (histolytica) —see Amebiasis
  amniotic fluid, sac or cavity O41.10-
    chorioamnionitis O41.12-
    placentitis O41.14-
  amputation stump (surgical) —see
      Complication, amputation stump,
      infection
  Ancylostoma (duodenalis) B76.0
  Anisakiasis, Anisakis larvae B81.0
  anthrax —see Anthrax
  antrum (chronic) —see Sinusitis, maxillary
  anus, anal (papillae) (sphincter) K62.89
  arbovirus (arbor virus) A94
    specified type NEC A93.8
  artificial insemination N98.0
  Ascaris lumbricoides —see Ascariasis
  Ascomycetes B47.0
  Aspergillus (flavus) (fumigatus) (terreus) —
      see Aspergillosis
  atypical
    acid-fast (bacilli) —see Mycobacterium,
        atypical
    mycobacteria —see Mycobacterium,
        atypical
    virus A81.9
      specified type NEC A81.89
  auditory meatus (external) —see Otitis,
      externa, infective
  auricle (ear) —see Otitis, externa, infective
  axillary gland (lymph) L04.2
  Bacillus A49.9
    abortus A23.1
    anthracis —see Anthrax
    Ducrey's (any location) A57
    Flexner's A03.1
    Friedländer's NEC A49.8
    gas (gangrene) A48.0
    mallei A24.0
    melitensis A23.0
    paratyphoid, paratyphosus A01.4
      A A01.1
      B A01.2
      C A01.3
    Shiga (-Kruse) A03.0
    suipestifer —see Infection, salmonella
    swimming pool A31.1

Infection, infected, infective (Continued)
  Bacillus (Continued)
    typhosa A01.00
    welchii —see Gangrene, gas
  bacterial NOS A49.9
    as cause of disease classified elsewhere
        B96.89
      Bacteroides fragilis [B. fragilis] B96.6
      Clostridium perfringens [C. perfringens]
          B96.7
      Enterobacter sakazakii B96.89
      Enterococcus B95.2
      Escherichia coli [E. coli] (see also
          Escherichia coli) B96.20
      Helicobacter pylori [H.pylori] B96.81
      Hemophilus influenzae [H. influenzae]
          B96.3
      Klebsiella pneumoniae [K. pneumoniae]
          B96.1
      Mycoplasma pneumoniae [M.
          pneumoniae] B96.0
      Proteus (mirabilis) (morganii) B96.4
      Pseudomonas (aeruginosa) (mallei)
          (pseudomallei) B96.5
      Staphylococcus B95.8
        aureus (methicillin susceptible)
            (MSSA) B95.61
          methicillin resistant (MRSA) B95.62
        specified NEC B95.7
      Streptococcus B95.5
        group A B95.0
        group B B95.1
        pneumoniae B95.3
        specified NEC B95.4
      Vibrio vulnificus B96.82
    specified NEC A48.8
  Bacterium
    paratyphosum A01.4
      A A01.1
      B A01.2
      C A01.3
    typhosum A01.00
  Bacteroides NEC A49.8
    fragilis, as cause of disease classified
        elsewhere B96.6
  Balantidium coli A07.0
  Bartholin's gland N75.8
  Basidiobolus B46.8
  bile duct (common) (hepatic) —see
      Cholangitis
  bladder —see Cystitis
  Blastomyces, blastomycotic —see also
      Blastomycosis
    brasiliensis —see Paracoccidioidomycosis
    dermatitidis —see Blastomycosis
    European —see Cryptococcosis
    Loboi B48.0
    North American B40.9
    South American —see
        Paracoccidioidomycosis
  bleb, postprocedure —see Blebitis
  bone —see Osteomyelitis
  Bordetella —see Whooping cough
  Borrelia bergdorfi A69.20
  brain (see also Encephalitis) G04.90
    membranes —see Meningitis
    septic G06.0
    meninges —see Meningitis, bacterial
  branchial cyst Q18.0
  breast —see Mastitis
  bronchus —see Bronchitis
  Brucella A23.9
    abortus A23.1
    canis A23.3
    melitensis A23.0
    mixed A23.8
    specified NEC A23.8
    suis A23.2
  Brugia (malayi) B74.1
    timori B74.2
  bursa —see Bursitis, infective

◀ New ◀▥ Revised ~~deleted~~ Deleted

Infection, infected, infective *(Continued)*
  enterovirus B34.1
    as cause of disease classified elsewhere
        B97.10
      coxsackievirus B97.11
      echovirus B97.12
      specified NEC B97.19
  Entomophthora B46.8
  Epidermophyton —*see* Dermatophytosis
  epididymis —*see* Epididymitis
  episiotomy (puerperal) O86.0
  Erysipelothrix (insidiosa) (rhusiopathiae) —
      see Erysipeloid
  erythema infectiosum B08.3
  Escherichia (E.) coli NEC A49.8
    as cause of disease classified elsewhere (*see
        also* Escherichia coli) B96.20
      congenital P39.8
        sepsis P36.4
      generalized A41.51
      intestinal —*see* Enteritis, infectious, due to,
          Escherichia coli
  ethmoidal (chronic) (sinus) —*see* Sinusitis,
      ethmoidal
  eustachian tube (ear) —*see* Salpingitis,
      eustachian
  external auditory canal (meatus) NEC —*see*
      Otitis, externa, infective
  eye (purulent) —*see* Endophthalmitis,
      purulent
  eyelid —*see* Inflammation, eyelid
  fallopian tube —*see* Salpingo-oophoritis
  Fasciola (gigantica) (hepatica) (indica)
      B66.3
  Fasciolopsis (buski) B66.5
  filarial —*see* Infestation, filarial
  finger (skin) L08.9
    nail L03.01-
      fungus B35.1
  fish tapeworm B70.0
    larval B70.1
  flagellate, intestinal A07.9
  fluke —*see* Infestation, fluke
  focal
    teeth (pulpal origin) K04.7
    tonsils J35.01
  Fonsecaea (compactum) (pedrosoi) B43.0
  food —*see* Intoxication, foodborne
  foot (skin) L08.9
    dermatophytic fungus B35.3
  Francisella tularensis —*see* Tularemia
  frontal (sinus) (chronic) —*see* Sinusitis,
      frontal
  fungus NOS B49
    beard B35.0
    dermatophytic —*see* Dermatophytosis
    foot B35.3
    groin B35.6
    hand B35.2
    nail B35.1
    pathogenic to compromised host only
        B48.8
    perianal (area) B35.6
    scalp B35.0
    skin B36.9
      foot B35.3
      hand B35.2
      toenails B35.1
  Fusarium B48.8
  gallbladder —*see* Cholecystitis
  gas bacillus —*see* Gangrene, gas
  gastrointestinal —*see* Enteritis, infectious
  generalized NEC —*see* Sepsis
  genital organ or tract
    female —*see* Disease, pelvis,
        inflammatory
    male N49.9
      multiple sites N49.8
      specified NEC N49.8
  Ghon tubercle, primary A15.7
  Giardia lamblia A07.1

Infection, infected, infective *(Continued)*
  gingiva (chronic) K05.10
    acute K05.00
      nonplaque induced K05.01
      plaque induced K05.00
    nonplaque induced K05.11
    plaque induced K05.10
  glanders A24.0
  glenosporopsis B48.0
  Gnathostoma (spinigerum) B83.1
  Gongylonema B83.8
  gonococcal —*see* Gonococcus
  gram-negative bacilli NOS A49.9
  guinea worm B72
  gum (chronic) K05.10
    acute K05.00
      nonplaque induced K05.01
      plaque induced K05.00
    nonplaque induced K05.11
    plaque induced K05.10
  Haemophilus —*see* Infection, Hemophilus
  heart —*see* Carditis
  Helicobacter pylori A04.8
    as cause of disease classified elsewhere
        B96.81
  helminths B83.9
    intestinal B82.0
      mixed (types classifiable to more than
          one of the titles B65.0-B81.3 and
          B81.8) B81.4
      specified type NEC B81.8
    specified type NEC B83.8
  Hemophilus
    aegyptius, systemic A48.4
    ducrey (any location) A57
    generalized A41.3
    influenzae NEC A49.2
      as cause of disease classified elsewhere
          B96.3
  herpes (simplex) —*see also* Herpes
    congenital P35.2
    disseminated B00.7
    zoster B02.9
  herpesvirus, herpesviral —*see* Herpes
  Heterophyes (heterophyes) B66.8
  hip (joint) NEC M00.9
    due to internal joint prosthesis
      left T84.52
      right T84.51
    skin NEC L08.9
  Histoplasma —*see* Histoplasmosis
    American B39.4
    capsulatum B39.4
  hookworm B76.9
  human
    papilloma virus A63.0
    T-cell lymphotropic virus type-1 (HTLV-1)
        B33.3
  hydrocele N43.0
  Hymenolepis B71.0
  hypopharynx —*see* Pharyngitis
  inguinal (lymph) glands L04.1
    due to soft chancre A57
  intervertebral disc, pyogenic M46.30
    cervical region M46.32
    cervicothoracic region M46.33
    lumbar region M46.36
    lumbosacral region M46.37
    multiple sites M46.39
    occipito-atlanto-axial region M46.31
    sacrococcygeal region M46.38
    thoracic region M46.34
    thoracolumbar region M46.35
  intestine, intestinal —*see* Enteritis, infectious
    specified NEC A08.8
  intra-amniotic affecting newborn NEC P39.2
  Isospora belli or hominis A07.3
  Japanese B encephalitis A83.0
  jaw (bone) (lower) (upper) M27.2
  joint NEC M00.9
    due to internal joint prosthesis T84.50

Infection, infected, infective *(Continued)*
  kidney (cortex) (hematogenous) N15.9
    with calculus N20.0
      with hydronephrosis N13.6
    following ectopic gestation O08.83
    pelvis and ureter (cystic) N28.85
    puerperal (postpartum) O86.21
    specified NEC N15.8
  Klebsiella (K.) pneumoniae NEC A49.8
    as cause of disease classified elsewhere
        B96.1
  knee (joint) NEC M00.9
    due to internal joint prosthesis
      left T84.54
      right T84.53
    joint M00.9
    skin L08.9
  Koch's —*see* Tuberculosis
  labia (majora) (minora) (acute) —*see* Vulvitis
  lacrimal
    gland —*see* Dacryoadenitis
    passages (duct) (sac) —*see* Inflammation,
        lacrimal, passages
  lancet fluke B66.2
  larynx NEC J38.7
  leg (skin) NOS L08.9
  Legionella pneumophila A48.1
    nonpneumonic A48.2
  Leishmania —*see also* Leishmaniasis
    aethiopica B55.1
    braziliensis B55.2
    chagasi B55.0
    donovani B55.0
    infantum B55.0
    major B55.1
    mexicana B55.1
    tropica B55.1
  lentivirus, as cause of disease classified
      elsewhere B97.31
  Leptosphaeria senegalensis B47.0
  Leptospira interrogans A27.9
    autumnalis A27.89
    canicola A27.89
    hebdomadis A27.89
    icterohaemorrhagiae A27.0
    pomona A27.89
    specified type NEC A27.89
  leptospirochetal NEC —*see* Leptospirosis
  Listeria monocytogenes —*see also* Listeriosis
    congenital P37.2
  Loa loa B74.3
    with conjunctival infestation B74.3
    eyelid B74.3
  Loboa loboi B48.0
  local, skin (staphylococcal) (streptococcal)
      L08.9
    abscess - code by site under Abscess
    cellulitis - code by site under Cellulitis
    specified NEC L08.89
    ulcer —*see* Ulcer, skin
  Loefflerella mallei A24.0
  lung (*see also* Pneumonia) J18.9
    atypical Mycobacterium A31.0
    spirochetal A69.8
    tuberculous —*see* Tuberculosis,
        pulmonary
    virus —*see* Pneumonia, viral
  lymph gland —*see also* Lymphadenitis,
      acute
    mesenteric I88.0
  lymphoid tissue, base of tongue or posterior
      pharynx, NEC (chronic) J35.03
  Madurella (grisea) (mycetomii) B47.0
  major
    following ectopic or molar pregnancy
        O08.0
    puerperal, postpartum, childbirth O85
  Malassezia furfur B36.0
  Malleomyces
    mallei A24.0
    pseudomallei (whitmori) —*see* Melioidosis

◀ New   ◀◀◀ Revised   ~~deleted~~ Deleted

Infection, infected, infective *(Continued)*
  mammary gland N61
  Mansonella (ozzardi) (perstans) (streptocerca)
      B74.4
  mastoid —*see* Mastoiditis
  maxilla, maxillary M27.2
      sinus (chronic) —*see* Sinusitis,
          maxillary
  mediastinum J98.5
  Medina (worm) B72
  meibomian cyst or gland —*see* Hordeolum
  meninges —*see* Meningitis, bacterial
  meningococcal *(see also* condition)
      A39.9
      adrenals A39.1
      brain A39.81
      cerebrospinal A39.0
      conjunctiva A39.89
      endocardium A39.51
      heart A39.50
          endocardium A39.51
          myocardium A39.52
          pericardium A39.53
      joint A39.83
      meninges A39.0
      meningococcemia A39.4
          acute A39.2
          chronic A39.3
      myocardium A39.52
      pericardium A39.53
      retrobulbar neuritis A39.82
      specified site NEC A39.89
  mesenteric lymph nodes or glands NEC
      I88.0
  Metagonimus B66.8
  metatarsophalangeal M00.9
  methicillin
      resistant Staphylococcus aureus (MRSA)
          A49.02
      susceptible Staphylococcus aureus (MSSA)
          A49.01
  Microsporum, microsporic —*see*
      Dermatophytosis
  mixed flora (bacterial) NEC A49.8
  Monilia —*see* Candidiasis
  Monosporium apiospermum B48.2
  mouth, parasitic B37.0
  Mucor —*see* Mucormycosis
  muscle NEC —*see* Myositis, infective
  mycelium NOS B49
  mycetoma B47.9
      actinomycotic NEC B47.1
      mycotic NEC B47.0
  Mycobacterium, mycobacterial —*see*
      Mycobacterium
  Mycoplasma NEC A49.3
      pneumoniae, as cause of disease classified
          elsewhere B96.0
  mycotic NOS B49
      pathogenic to compromised host only
          B48.8
      skin NOS B36.9
  myocardium NEC I40.0
  nail (chronic)
      with lymphangitis —*see* Lymphangitis,
          acute, digit
      finger L03.01-
          fungus B35.1
      ingrowing L60.0
      toe L03.03-
          fungus B35.1
  nasal sinus (chronic) —*see* Sinusitis
  nasopharynx —*see* Nasopharyngitis
  navel L08.82
  Necator americanus B76.1
  Neisseria —*see* Gonococcus
  Neotestudina rosatii B47.0
  newborn P39.9
      intra-amniotic NEC P39.2
      skin P39.4
      specified type NEC P39.8

Infection, infected, infective *(Continued)*
  nipple N61
      associated with
          lactation O91.03
          pregnancy O91.01-
          puerperium O91.02
  Nocardia —*see* Nocardiosis
  obstetrical surgical wound (puerperal)
      O86.0
  Oesophagostomum (apiostomum)
      B81.8
  Oestrus ovis —*see* Myiasis
  Oidium albicans B37.9
  Onchocerca (volvulus) —*see* Onchocerciasis -
      oncovirus, as cause of disease classified
          elsewhere B97.32
  operation wound T81.4
  Opisthorchis (felineus) (viverrini) B66.0
  orbit, orbital —*see* Inflammation, orbit
  orthopoxvirus NEC B08.09
  ovary —*see* Salpingo-oophoritis
  Oxyuris vermicularis B80
  pancreas (acute) K85.9
      abscess —*see* Pancreatitis, acute
      specified NEC K85.8
  papillomavirus, as cause of disease classified
      elsewhere B97.7
  papovavirus NEC B34.4
  Paracoccidioides brasiliensis —*see*
      Paracoccidioidomycosis
  Paragonimus (westermani) B66.4
  parainfluenza virus B34.8
  parameningococcus NOS A39.9
  parapoxvirus B08.60
      specified NEC B08.69
  parasitic B89
  Parastrongylus
      cantonensis B83.2
      costaricensis B81.3
  paratyphoid A01.4
      Type A A01.1
      Type B A01.2
      Type C A01.3
  paraurethral ducts N34.2
  parotid gland —*see* Sialoadenitis
  parvovirus NEC B34.3
      as cause of disease classified elsewhere
          B97.6
  Pasteurella NEC A28.0
      multocida A28.0
      pestis —*see* Plague
      pseudotuberculosis A28.0
      septica (cat bite) (dog bite) A28.0
      tularensis —*see* Tularemia
  pelvic, female —*see* Disease, pelvis,
      inflammatory
  Penicillium (marneffei) B48.4
  penis (glans) (retention) NEC N48.29
  periapical K04.5
  peridental, periodontal K05.20
      generalized K05.22
      localized K05.21
  perinatal period P39.9
      specified type NEC P39.8
  perineal repair (puerperal) O86.0
  periorbital —*see* Inflammation, orbit
  perirectal K62.89
  perirenal —*see* Infection, kidney
  peritoneal —*see* Peritonitis
  periureteral N28.89
  Petriellidium boydii B48.2
  pharynx —*see also* Pharyngitis
      coxsackievirus B08.5
      posterior, lymphoid (chronic) J35.03
  Phialophora
      gougerotii (subcutaneous abscess or cyst)
          B43.2
      jeanselmei (subcutaneous abscess or cyst)
          B43.2
      verrucosa (skin) B43.0
  Piedraia hortae B36.3

Infection, infected, infective *(Continued)*
  pinta A67.9
      intermediate A67.1
      late A67.2
      mixed A67.3
      primary A67.0
  pinworm B80
  pityrosporum furfur B36.0
  pleuro-pneumonia-like organism (PPLO)
      NEC A49.3
      as cause of disease classified elsewhere
          B96.0
  pneumococcus, pneumococcal NEC
      A49.1
      as cause of disease classified elsewhere
          B95.3
      generalized (purulent) A40.3
          with pneumonia J13
  Pneumocystis carinii (pneumonia)
      B59
  Pneumocystis jiroveci (pneumonia)
      B59
  port or reservoir T80.212
  postoperative T81.4
  postoperative wound T81.4
  postprocedural T81.4
  postvaccinal T88.0
  prepuce NEC N47.7
      with penile inflammation N47.6
  prion —*see* Disease, prion, central nervous
      system
  prostate (capsule) —*see* Prostatitis
  Proteus (mirabilis) (morganii) (vulgaris) NEC
      A49.8
      as cause of disease classified elsewhere
          B96.4
  protozoal NEC B64
      intestinal A07.9
          specified NEC A07.8
      specified NEC B60.8
  Pseudoallescheria boydii B48.2
  Pseudomonas NEC A49.8
      as cause of disease classified elsewhere
          B96.5
      mallei A24.0
      pneumonia J15.1
      pseudomallei —*see* Melioidosis
  puerperal O86.4
      genitourinary tract NEC O86.89
      major or generalized O85
      minor O86.4
      specified NEC O86.89
  pulmonary —*see* Infection, lung
  purulent —*see* Abscess
  Pyrenochaeta romeroi B47.0
  Q fever A78
  rectum (sphincter) K62.89
  renal —*see also* Infection, kidney
      pelvis and ureter (cystic) N28.85
  reovirus, as cause of disease classified
      elsewhere B97.5
  respiratory (tract) NEC J98.8
      acute J22
      chronic J98.8
      influenzal (upper) (acute) —*see* Influenza,
          with, respiratory manifestations NEC
      lower (acute) J22
          chronic —*see* Bronchitis, chronic
      rhinovirus J00
      syncytial virus, as cause of disease
          classified elsewhere B97.4
      upper (acute) NOS J06.9
          chronic J39.8
          streptococcal J06.9
          viral NOS J06.9
  resulting from
      presence of internal prosthesis, implant,
          graft —*see* Complications, by site and
          type, infection
  retortamoniasis A07.8
  retroperitoneal NEC K68.9

Infection, infected, infective (Continued)
retrovirus B33.3
  as cause of disease classified elsewhere
    B97.30
    human
      immunodeficiency, type 2 (HIV 2)
        B97.35
      T-cell lymphotropic
        type I (HTLV-I) B97.33
        type II (HTLV-II) B97.34
    lentivirus B97.31
    oncovirus B97.32
    specified NEC B97.39
Rhinosporidium (seeberi) B48.1
rhinovirus
  as cause of disease classified elsewhere
    B97.89
  unspecified nature or site B34.8
Rhizopus —see Mucormycosis
rickettsial NOS A79.9
roundworm (large) NEC B82.0
  Ascariasis (see also Ascariasis) B77.9
rubella —see Rubella
Saccharomyces —see Candidiasis
salivary duct or gland (any) —see
  Sialoadenitis
Salmonella (aertrycke) (arizonae)
  (callinarum) (cholerae-suis) (enteritidis)
  (suipestifer) (typhimurium) A02.9
  with
    (gastro) enteritis A02.0
    sepsis A02.1
    specified manifestation NEC A02.8
  due to food (poisoning) A02.9
  hirschfeldii A01.3
  localized A02.20
    arthritis A02.23
    meningitis A02.21
    osteomyelitis A02.24
    pneumonia A02.22
    pyelonephritis A02.25
    specified NEC A02.29
  paratyphi A01.4
    A A01.1
    B A01.2
    C A01.3
  schottmuelleri A01.2
  typhi, typhosa —see Typhoid
Sarcocystis A07.8
scabies B86
Schistosoma —see Infestation, Schistosoma
scrotum (acute) NEC N49.2
seminal vesicle —see Vesiculitis
septic
  localized, skin —see Abscess
sheep liver fluke B66.3
Shigella A03.9
  boydii A03.2
  dysenteriae A03.0
  flexneri A03.1
  group
    A A03.0
    B A03.1
    C A03.2
    D A03.3
  Schmitz (-Stutzer) A03.0
  schmitzii A03.0
  shigae A03.0
  sonnei A03.3
  specified NEC A03.8
shoulder (joint) NEC M00.9
  due to internal joint prosthesis T84.59
  skin NEC L08.9
sinus (accessory) (chronic) (nasal) —see also
  Sinusitis
  pilonidal —see Sinus, pilonidal
  skin NEC L08.89
Skene's duct or gland —see Urethritis
skin (local) (staphylococcal) (streptococcal)
  L08.9
  abscess - code by site under Abscess

Infection, infected, infective (Continued)
skin (Continued)
  cellulitis - code by site under Cellulitis
  due to fungus B36.9
    specified type NEC B36.8
  mycotic B36.9
    specified type NEC B36.8
  newborn P39.4
  ulcer —see Ulcer, skin
slow virus A81.9
  specified NEC A81.89
Sparganum (mansoni) (proliferum) (baxteri)
  B70.1
specific —see also Syphilis
  to perinatal period —see Infection,
    congenital
specified NEC B99.8
spermatic cord NEC N49.1
sphenoidal (sinus) —see Sinusitis,
  sphenoidal
spinal cord NOS (see also Myelitis)
  G04.91
  abscess G06.1
  meninges —see Meningitis
  streptococcal G04.89
Spirillum A25.0
spirochetal NOS A69.9
  lung A69.8
  specified NEC A69.8
Spirometra larvae B70.1
spleen D73.89
Sporotrichum, Sporothrix (schenckii) —see
  Sporotrichosis
staphylococcal, unspecified site
  aureus (methicillin susceptible) (MSSA)
    A49.01
    methicillin resistant (MRSA) A49.02
  as cause of disease classified elsewhere
    B95.8
    aureus (methicillin susceptible) (MSSA)
      B95.61
      methicillin resistant (MRSA)
        B95.62
    specified NEC B95.7
  food poisoning A05.0
  generalized (purulent) A41.2
  pneumonia —see Pneumonia,
    staphylococcal
Stellantchasmus falcatus B66.8
streptobacillus moniliformis A25.1
streptococcal NEC A49.1
  as cause of disease classified elsewhere
    B95.5
  B genitourinary complicating
    childbirth O98.82
    pregnancy O98.81-
    puerperium O98.83
  congenital
    sepsis P36.10
      group B P36.0
      specified NEC P36.19
  generalized (purulent) A40.9
Streptomyces B47.1
Strongyloides (stercoralis) —see
  Strongyloidiasis
stump (amputation) (surgical) —see
  Complication, amputation stump,
  infection
subcutaneous tissue, local L08.9
suipestifer —see Infection, salmonella
swimming pool bacillus A31.1
Taenia —see Infestation, Taenia
Taeniarhynchus saginatus B68.1
tapeworm —see Infestation, tapeworm
tendon (sheath) —see Tenosynovitis, infective
  NEC
Ternidens diminutus B81.8
testis —see Orchitis
threadworm B80
throat —see Pharyngitis
thyroglossal duct K14.8

Infection, infected, infective (Continued)
toe (skin) L08.9
  cellulitis L03.03-
    fungus B35.1
  nail L03.03-
    fungus B35.1
tongue NEC K14.0
  parasitic B37.0
tonsil (and adenoid) (faucial) (lingual)
  (pharyngeal) —see Tonsillitis
tooth, teeth K04.7
  periapical K04.7
  peridental, periodontal K05.20
    generalized K05.22
    localized K05.21
  pulp K04.0
  socket M27.3
TORCH —see Infection, congenital
  without active infection P00.2
Torula histolytica —see Cryptococcosis
Toxocara (canis) (cati) (felis) B83.0
Toxoplasma gondii —see Toxoplasma
trachea, chronic J42
trematode NEC —see Infestation, fluke
trench fever A79.0
Treponema pallidum —see Syphilis
Trichinella (spiralis) B75
Trichomonas A59.9
  cervix A59.09
  intestine A07.8
  prostate A59.02
  specified site NEC A59.8
  urethra A59.03
  urogenitalis A59.00
  vagina A59.01
  vulva A59.01
Trichophyton, trichophytic —see
  Dermatophytosis
Trichosporon (beigelii) cutaneum B36.2
Trichostrongylus B81.2
Trichuris (trichiura) B79
Trombicula (irritans) B88.0
Trypanosoma
  brucei
    gambiense B56.0
    rhodesiense B56.1
  cruzi —see Chagas' disease
tubal —see Salpingo-oophoritis
tuberculous NEC —see Tuberculosis
tubo-ovarian —see Salpingo-oophoritis
tunica vaginalis N49.1
tunnel T80.212
tympanic membrane NEC —see Myringitis
typhoid (abortive) (ambulant) (bacillus) —see
  Typhoid
typhus A75.9
  flea-borne A75.2
  mite-borne A75.3
  recrudescent A75.1
  tick-borne A77.9
    African A77.1
    North Asian A77.2
umbilicus L08.82
ureter N28.86
urethra —see Urethritis
urinary (tract) N39.0
  bladder —see Cystitis
  complicating
    pregnancy O23.4-
      specified type NEC O23.3-
  kidney —see Infection, kidney
  newborn P39.3
  puerperal (postpartum) O86.20
  tuberculous A18.13
  urethra —see Urethritis
uterus, uterine —see Endometritis
vaccination T88.0
vaccinia not from vaccination B08.011
vagina (acute) —see Vaginitis
varicella B01.9
varicose veins —see Varix

◄ New   ◄◄ Revised   ~~deleted~~ Deleted

Infection, infected, infective *(Continued)*
vas deferens NEC N49.1
vesical —*see* Cystitis
Vibrio
  cholerae A00.0
    El Tor A00.1
  parahaemolyticus (food poisoning) A05.3
  vulnificus
    as cause of disease classified elsewhere B96.82
    foodborne intoxication A05.5
Vincent's (gum) (mouth) (tonsil) A69.1
virus, viral NOS B34.9
  adenovirus
    as cause of disease classified elsewhere B97.0
    unspecified nature or site B34.0
  arborvirus, arbovirus arthropod-borne A94
  as cause of disease classified elsewhere B97.89
    adenovirus B97.0
    coronavirus B97.29
      SARS-associated B97.21
    coxsackievirus B97.11
    echovirus B97.12
    enterovirus B97.10
      coxsackievirus B97.11
      echovirus B97.12
      specified NEC B97.19
    human
      immunodeficiency, type 2 (HIV 2) B97.35
      metapneumovirus B97.81
      T-cell lymphotropic,
        type I (HTLV-I) B97.33
        type II (HTLV-II) B97.34
    papillomavirus B97.7
    parvovirus B97.6
    reovirus B97.5
    respiratory syncytial B97.4
    retrovirus B97.30
      human
        immunodeficiency, type 2 (HIV 2) B97.35
        T-cell lymphotropic,
          type I (HTLV-I) B97.33
          type II (HTLV-II) B97.34
      lentivirus B97.31
      oncovirus B97.32
      specified NEC B97.39
    specified NEC B97.89
  central nervous system A89
    atypical A81.9
      specified NEC A81.89
    enterovirus NEC A88.8
      meningitis A87.0
    slow virus A81.9
      specified NEC A81.89
    specified NEC A88.8
  chest J98.8
  cotia B08.8
  coxsackie *(see also* Infection, coxsackie) B34.1
    as cause of disease classified elsewhere B97.11
  ECHO
    as cause of disease classified elsewhere B97.12
    unspecified nature or site B34.1
  encephalitis, tick-borne A84.9
  enterovirus, as cause of disease classified elsewhere B97.10
    coxsackievirus B97.11
    echovirus B97.12
    specified NEC B97.19
  exanthem NOS B09
  human metapneumovirus as cause of disease classified elsewhere B97.81
  human papilloma as cause of disease classified elsewhere B97.7
  intestine —*see* Enteritis, viral

Infection, infected, infective *(Continued)*
virus, viral NOS *(Continued)*
  respiratory syncytial
    as cause of disease classified elsewhere B97.4
    bronchopneumonia J12.1
    common cold syndrome J00
    nasopharyngitis (acute) J00
  rhinovirus
    as cause of disease classified elsewhere B97.89
    unspecified nature or site B34.8
  slow A81.9
    specified NEC A81.89
  specified type NEC B33.8
    as cause of disease classified elsewhere B97.89
    unspecified nature or site B34.8
  unspecified nature or site B34.9
  West Nile —*see* Virus, West Nile
  vulva (acute) —*see* Vulvitis
West Nile —*see* Virus, West Nile
whipworm B79
worms B83.9
  specified type NEC B83.8
Wuchereria (bancrofti) B74.0
  malayi B74.1
  yatapoxvirus B08.70
    specified NEC B08.79
yeast *(see also* Candidiasis) B37.9
yellow fever —*see* Fever, yellow
Yersinia
  enterocolitica (intestinal) A04.6
  pestis —*see* Plague
  pseudotuberculosis A28.2
Zeis' gland —*see* Hordeolum
zoonotic bacterial NOS A28.9
Zopfia senegalensis B47.0
Infective, infectious —*see* condition
Infertility
female N97.9
  age-related N97.8
  associated with
    anovulation N97.0
    cervical (mucus) disease or anomaly N88.3
    congenital anomaly
      cervix N88.3
      fallopian tube N97.1
      uterus N97.2
      vagina N97.8
    dysmucorrhea N88.3
    fallopian tube disease or anomaly N97.1
    pituitary-hypothalamic origin E23.0
    specified origin NEC N97.8
    Stein-Leventhal syndrome E28.2
    uterine disease or anomaly N97.2
    vaginal disease or anomaly N97.8
  due to
    cervical anomaly N88.3
    fallopian tube anomaly N97.1
    ovarian failure E28.39
    Stein-Leventhal syndrome E28.2
    uterine anomaly N97.2
    vaginal anomaly N97.8
  nonimplantation N97.2
  origin
    cervical N88.3
    tubal (block) (occlusion) (stenosis) N97.1
    uterine N97.2
    vaginal N97.8
male N46.9
  azoospermia N46.01
    extratesticular cause N46.029
      drug therapy N46.021
      efferent duct obstruction N46.023
      infection N46.022
      radiation N46.024
      specified cause NEC N46.029
      systemic disease N46.025

Infertility *(Continued)*
male *(Continued)*
  oligospermia N46.11
    extratesticular cause N46.129
      drug therapy N46.121
      efferent duct obstruction N46.123
      infection N46.122
      radiation N46.124
      specified cause NEC N46.129
      systemic disease N46.125
  specified type NEC N46.8
Infestation B88.9
Acanthocheilonema (perstans) (streptocerca) B74.4
Acariasis B88.0
  demodex folliculorum B88.0
  sarcoptes scabiei B86
  trombiculae B88.0
Agamofilaria streptocerca B74.4
Ancylostoma, ankylostoma (braziliense) (caninum) (ceylanicum) (duodenale) B76.0
  americanum B76.1
  new world B76.1
Anisakis larvae, anisakiasis B81.0
arthropod NEC B88.2
Ascaris lumbricoides —*see* Ascariasis
Balantidium coli A07.0
beef tapeworm B68.1
Bothriocephalus (latus) B70.0
  larval B70.1
broad tapeworm B70.0
  larval B70.1
Brugia (malayi) B74.1
  timori B74.2
candiru B88.8
Capillaria
  hepatica B83.8
  philippinensis B81.1
cat liver fluke B66.0
cestodes B71.9
  diphyllobothrium —*see* Infestation, diphyllobothrium
  dipylidiasis B71.1
  hymenolepiasis B71.0
  specified type NEC B71.8
chigger B88.0
chigo, chigoe B88.1
Clonorchis (sinensis) (liver) B66.1
coccidial A07.3
crab-lice B85.3
Cysticercus cellulosae —*see* Cysticercosis
Demodex (folliculorum) B88.0
Dermanyssus gallinae B88.0
Dermatobia (hominis) —*see* Myiasis
Dibothriocephalus (latus) B70.0
  larval B70.1
Dicrocoelium dendriticum B66.2
Diphyllobothrium (adult) (latum) (intestinal) (pacificum) B70.0
  larval B70.1
Diplogonoporus (grandis) B71.8
Dipylidium caninum B67.4
Distoma hepaticum B66.3
dog tapeworm B67.4
Dracunculus medinensis B72
dragon worm B72
dwarf tapeworm B71.0
Echinococcus —*see* Echinococcus
Echinostomum ilocanum B66.8
Entamoeba (histolytica) —*see* Infection, Ameba
Enterobius vermicularis B80
eyelid
  in (due to)
    leishmaniasis B55.1
    loiasis B74.3
    onchocerciasis B73.09
    phthiriasis B85.3
    parasitic NOS B89
eyeworm B74.3

Infiltrate, infiltration (Continued)
  liver K76.89
    fatty —see Fatty, liver NEC
    glycogen (see also Disease, glycogen
        storage) E74.03 [K77]
  lung R91.8
    eosinophilic J82
  lymphatic (see also Leukemia, lymphatic)
      C91.9-
    gland I88.9
  muscle, fatty M62.89
  myocardium, myocardial
    fatty —see Degeneration, myocardial
    glycogenic E74.02 [143]
  on chest x-ray R91.8
  pulmonary R91.8
    with eosinophilia J82
  skin (lymphocytic) L98.6
  thymus (gland) (fatty) E32.8
  urine R39.0
  vesicant agent
    antineoplastic chemotherapy T80.810
    other agent NEC T80.818
  vitreous body H43.89
Infirmity R68.89
  senile R54
Inflammation, inflamed, inflammatory (with
    exudation)
  abducent (nerve) —see Strabismus, paralytic,
      sixth nerve
  accessory sinus (chronic) —see Sinusitis
  adrenal (gland) E27.8
  alveoli, teeth M27.3
    scorbutic E54
  anal canal, anus K62.89
  antrum (chronic) —see Sinusitis, maxillary
  appendix —see Appendicitis
  arachnoid —see Meningitis
  areola N61
    puerperal, postpartum or gestational —see
        Infection, nipple
  areolar tissue NOS L08.9
  artery —see Arteritis
  auditory meatus (external) —see Otitis,
      externa
  Bartholin's gland N75.8
  bile duct (common) (hepatic) or passage —see
      Cholangitis
  bladder —see Cystitis
  bone —see Osteomyelitis
  brain —see also Encephalitis
    membrane —see Meningitis
  breast N61
    puerperal, postpartum, gestational —see
        Mastitis, obstetric
  broad ligament —see Disease, pelvis,
      inflammatory
  bronchi —see Bronchitis
  catarrhal J00
  cecum —see Appendicitis
  cerebral —see also Encephalitis
    membrane —see Meningitis
  cerebrospinal
    meningococcal A39.0
  cervix (uteri) —see Cervicitis
  chest J98.8
  chorioretinal H30.9-
    cyclitis —see Cyclitis
    disseminated H30.10-
      generalized H30.13-
      peripheral H30.12-
      posterior pole H30.11-
    epitheliopathy —see Epitheliopathy
    focal H30.00-
      juxtapapillary H30.01-
      macular H30.04-
      paramacular —see Inflammation,
          chorioretinal, focal, macular
      peripheral H30.03-
      posterior pole H30.02-
    specified type NEC H30.89-

Inflammation, inflamed, inflammatory
    (Continued)
  choroid —see Inflammation, chorioretinal
  chronic, postmastoidectomy cavity —see
      Complications, postmastoidectomy,
      inflammation
  colon —see Enteritis
  connective tissue (diffuse) NEC —see
      Disorder, soft tissue, specified type NEC
  cornea —see Keratitis
  corpora cavernosa N48.29
  cranial nerve —see Disorder, nerve, cranial
  Douglas' cul-de-sac or pouch (chronic) N73.0
  due to device, implant or graft —see also
      Complications, by site and type,
      infection or inflammation
    arterial graft T82.7
    breast (implant) T85.79
    catheter T85.79
      dialysis (renal) T82.7
        intraperitoneal T85.71
      infusion T82.7
        spinal (epidural) (subdural) T85.79
      urinary (indwelling) T83.51
    electronic (electrode) (pulse generator)
        (stimulator)
      bone T84.7
      cardiac T82.7
      nervous system (brain) (peripheral
          nerve) (spinal) T85.79
      urinary T83.59
    fixation, internal (orthopedic) NEC —see
        Complication, fixation device,
        infection
    gastrointestinal (bile duct) (esophagus)
        T85.79
    genital NEC T83.6
    heart NEC T82.7
      valve (prosthesis) T82.6
        graft T82.7
    joint prosthesis —see Complication, joint
        prosthesis, infection
    ocular (corneal graft) (orbital implant)
        NEC T85.79
    orthopedic NEC T84.7
    specified NEC T85.79
    urinary NEC T83.59
    vascular NEC T82.7
    ventricular intracranial shunt T85.79
  duodenum K29.80
    with bleeding K29.81
  dura mater —see Meningitis
  ear (middle) —see also Otitis, media
    external —see Otitis, externa
    inner —see subcategory H83.0
  epididymis —see Epididymitis
  esophagus K20.9
  ethmoidal (sinus) (chronic) —see Sinusitis,
      ethmoidal
  eustachian tube (catarrhal) —see Salpingitis,
      eustachian
  eyelid H01.9
    abscess —see Abscess, eyelid
    blepharitis —see Blepharitis
    chalazion —see Chalazion
    dermatosis (noninfectious) —see
        Dermatosis, eyelid
    hordeolum —see Hordeolum
    specified NEC H01.8
  fallopian tube —see Salpingo-oophoritis
  fascia —see Myositis
  follicular, pharynx J31.2
  frontal (sinus) (chronic) —see Sinusitis, frontal
  gallbladder —see Cholecystitis
  gastric —see Gastritis
  gastrointestinal —see Enteritis
  genital organ (internal) (diffuse)
    female —see Disease, pelvis, inflammatory
    male N49.9
      multiple sites N49.8
      specified NEC N49.8

Inflammation, inflamed, inflammatory
    (Continued)
  gland (lymph) —see Lymphadenitis
  glottis —see Laryngitis
  granular, pharynx J31.2
  gum K05.10
    nonplaque induced K05.11
    plaque induced K05.10
  heart —see Carditis
  hepatic duct —see Cholangitis
  ileoanal (internal) pouch K91.850
  ileum —see also Enteritis
    regional or terminal —see Enteritis,
        regional
  intestinal pouch K91.850
  intestine (any part) —see Enteritis
  jaw (acute) (bone) (chronic) (lower)
      (suppurative) (upper) M27.2
  joint NEC —see Arthritis
    sacroiliac M46.1
  kidney —see Nephritis
  knee (joint) M13.169
    tuberculous A18.02
  labium (majus) (minus) —see Vulvitis
  lacrimal
    gland —see Dacryoadenitis
    passages (duct) (sac) —see also
        Dacryocystitis
      canaliculitis —see Canaliculitis, lacrimal
  larynx —see Laryngitis
  leg NOS L08.9
  lip K13.0
  liver (capsule) —see also Hepatitis
    chronic K73.9
    suppurative K75.0
  lung (acute) —see also Pneumonia
    chronic J98.4
  lymphatic vessel —see Lymphangitis
  lymph gland or node —see Lymphadenitis
  maxilla, maxillary M27.2
    sinus (chronic) —see Sinusitis, maxillary
  membranes of brain or spinal cord —see
      Meningitis
  meninges —see Meningitis
  mouth K12.1
  muscle —see Myositis
  myocardium —see Myocarditis
  nasal sinus (chronic) —see Sinusitis
  nasopharynx —see Nasopharyngitis
  navel L08.82
  nerve NEC —see Neuralgia
  nipple N61
    puerperal, postpartum or gestational —see
        Infection, nipple
  nose —see Rhinitis
  oculomotor (nerve) —see Strabismus,
      paralytic, third nerve
  optic nerve —see Neuritis, optic
  orbit (chronic) H05.10
    acute H05.00
      abscess —see Abscess, orbit
      cellulitis —see Cellulitis, orbit
      osteomyelitis —see Osteomyelitis,
          orbit
      periostitis —see Periostitis, orbital
      tenonitis —see Tenonitis, eye
    granuloma —see Granuloma, orbit
    myositis —see Myositis, orbital
  ovary —see Salpingo-oophoritis
  oviduct —see Salpingo-oophoritis
  pancreas (acute) —see Pancreatitis
  parametrium N73.0
  parotid region L08.9
  pelvis, female —see Disease, pelvis,
      inflammatory
  penis (corpora cavernosa) N48.29
  perianal K62.89
  pericardium —see Pericarditis
  perineum (female) (male) L08.9
  perirectal K62.89
  peritoneum —see Peritonitis

Inflammation, inflamed, inflammatory
  (Continued)
  periuterine —see Disease, pelvis,
    inflammatory
  perivesical —see Cystitis
  petrous bone (acute) (chronic) —see Petrositis
  pharynx (acute) —see Pharyngitis
  pia mater —see Meningitis
  pleura —see Pleurisy
  polyp, colon (see also Polyp, colon,
    inflammatory) K51.40
  prostate —see also Prostatitis
    specified type NEC N41.8
  rectosigmoid —see Rectosigmoiditis
  rectum (see also Proctitis) K62.89
  respiratory, upper (see also Infection,
    respiratory, upper) J06.9
    acute, due to radiation J70.0
    chronic, due to external agent —see
        condition, respiratory, chronic, due to
    due to
        chemicals, gases, fumes or vapors
          (inhalation) J68.2
        radiation J70.1
  retina —see Chorioretinitis
  retrocecal —see Appendicitis
  retroperitoneal —see Peritonitis
  salivary duct or gland (any) (suppurative) —
    see Sialoadenitis
  scorbutic, alveoli, teeth E54
  scrotum N49.2
  seminal vesicle —see Vesiculitis
  sigmoid —see Enteritis
  sinus —see Sinusitis
  Skene's duct or gland —see Urethritis
  skin L08.9
  spermatic cord N49.1
  sphenoidal (sinus) —see Sinusitis, sphenoidal
  spinal
    cord —see Encephalitis
    membrane —see Meningitis
    nerve —see Disorder, nerve
  spine —see Spondylopathy, inflammatory
  spleen (capsule) D73.89
  stomach —see Gastritis
  subcutaneous tissue L08.9
  suprarenal (gland) E27.8
  synovial —see Tenosynovitis
  tendon (sheath) NEC —see Tenosynovitis
  testis —see Orchitis
  throat (acute) —see Pharyngitis
  thymus (gland) E32.8
  thyroid (gland) —see Thyroiditis
  tongue K14.0
  tonsil —see Tonsillitis
  trachea —see Tracheitis
  trochlear (nerve) —see Strabismus, paralytic,
    fourth nerve
  tubal —see Salpingo-oophoritis
  tuberculous NEC —see Tuberculosis
  tubo-ovarian —see Salpingo-oophoritis
  tunica vaginalis N49.1
  tympanic membrane —see Tympanitis
  umbilicus, umbilical L08.82
  uterine ligament —see Disease, pelvis,
    inflammatory
  uterus (catarrhal) —see Endometritis
  uveal tract (anterior) NOS —see also
        Iridocyclitis
    posterior —see Chorioretinitis
  vagina —see Vaginitis
  vas deferens N49.1
  vein —see also Phlebitis
    intracranial or intraspinal (septic) G08
    thrombotic I80.9
        leg —see Phlebitis, leg
        lower extremity —see Phlebitis, leg
  vocal cord J38.3
  vulva —see Vulvitis
  Wharton's duct (suppurative) —see
        Sialoadenitis

Inflation, lung, imperfect (newborn) —see
    Atelectasis
Influenza (bronchial) (epidemic) (respiratory
    (upper)) (unidentified influenza virus)
    J11.1
  with
    digestive manifestations J11.2
    encephalopathy J11.81
    enteritis J11.2
    gastroenteritis J11.2
    gastrointestinal manifestations J11.2
    laryngitis J11.1
    myocarditis J11.82
    otitis media J11.83
    pharyngitis J11.1
    pneumonia J11.00
        specified type J11.08
    respiratory manifestations NEC J11.1
    specified manifestation NEC J11.89
  A/H5N1 —see also Influenza, due to,
        identified novel influenza A virus J09.X2
  avian —see also Influenza, due to, identified
        novel influenza A virus J09.X2
  bird (see also Influenza, due to, identified
        novel influenza A virus) J09.X2
  novel (2009) H1N1 influenza (see also
        Influenza, due to, identified influenza
        virus NEC) J10.1
  novel influenza A/H1N1 (see also Influenza,
        due to, identified influenza virus NEC)
        J10.1
  due to
    avian (see also Influenza, due to, identified
        novel influenza A virus) J09.X2
    identified influenza virus NEC J10.1
      with
        digestive manifestations J10.2
        encephalopathy J10.81
        enteritis J10.2
        gastroenteritis J10.2
        gastrointestinal manifestations J10.2
        laryngitis J10.1
        myocarditis J10.82
        otitis media J10.83
        pharyngitis J10.1
        pneumonia (unspecified type) J10.00
          with same identified influenza virus
            J10.01
          specified type NEC J10.08
        respiratory manifestations NEC J10.1
        specified manifestation NEC J10.89
    identified novel influenza A virus J09.X2
      with
        digestive manifestations J09.X3
        encephalopathy J09.X9
        enteritis J09.X3
        gastroenteritis J09.X3
        gastrointestinal manifestations
            J09.X3
        laryngitis J09.X2
        myocarditis J09.X9
        otitis media J09.X9
        pharyngitis J09.X2
        pneumonia J09.X1
        respiratory manifestations NEC J09.X2
        specified manifestation NEC J09.X9
        upper respiratory symptoms J09.X2
    of other animal origin, not bird or swine (see
        also Influenza, due to, identified novel
        influenza A virus) J09.X2
    swine (viruses that normally cause infections
        in pigs) (see also Influenza, due to,
        identified novel influenza A virus) J09.
        X2
Influenza-like disease —see Influenza
Influenzal —see Influenza
Infraction, Freiberg's (metatarsal head) —see
    Osteochondrosis, juvenile, metatarsus
Infraeruption of tooth (teeth) M26.34
Infusion complication, misadventure, or
    reaction —see Complications, infusion

Ingestion
  chemical —see Table of Drugs and Chemicals,
    by substance, poisoning
  drug or medicament
    correct substance properly administered —
        see Table of Drugs and Chemicals, by
        drug, adverse effect
    overdose or wrong substance given or
        taken —see Table of Drugs and
        Chemicals, by drug, poisoning
  foreign body —see Foreign body, alimentary
    tract
  tularemia A21.3
Ingrowing
  hair (beard) L73.1
  nail (finger) (toe) L60.0
Inguinal —see also condition
  testicle Q53.9
    bilateral Q53.21
    unilateral Q53.11
Inhalation
  anthrax A22.1
  flame T27.3
  food or foreign body —see Foreign body, by
    site
  gases, fumes, or vapors NEC T59.9-
    specified agent —see Table of Drugs and
        Chemicals, by substance
  liquid or vomitus —see Asphyxia
  meconium (newborn) P24.00
    with
        with respiratory symptoms P24.01
        pneumonia (pneumonitis) P24.01
  mucus —see Asphyxia, mucus
  oil or gasoline (causing suffocation) —see
        Foreign body, by site
  smoke J70.5
    due to chemicals, gases, fumes and vapors
        J68.9
  steam —see Toxicity, vapors
  stomach contents or secretions —see Foreign
        body, by site
    due to anesthesia (general) (local) or other
        sedation T88.59
    in labor and delivery O74.0
    in pregnancy O29.01-
    postpartum, puerperal O89.01
Inhibition, orgasm
  female F52.31
  male F52.32
Inhibitor, systemic lupus erythematosus
    (presence of) D68.62
Iniencephalus, iniencephaly Q00.2
Injection, traumatic jet (air) (industrial) (water)
    (paint or dye) T70.4
Injury (see also specified injury type)
    T14.90
  abdomen, abdominal S39.91
    blood vessel —see Injury, blood vessel,
        abdomen
    cavity —see Injury, intra-abdominal
    contusion S30.1
    internal —see Injury, intra-abdominal
    intra-abdominal organ —see Injury,
        intra-abdominal
    nerve —see Injury, nerve, abdomen
    open —see Wound, open, abdomen
    specified NEC S39.81
    superficial —see Injury, superficial,
        abdomen
  Achilles tendon S86.00-
    laceration S86.02-
    specified type NEC S86.09-
    strain S86.01-
  acoustic, resulting in deafness —see Injury,
    nerve, acoustic
  adrenal (gland) S37.819
    contusion S37.812
    laceration S37.813
    specified type NEC S37.818
  alveolar (process) S09.93

◀ New   ◀◀ Revised   ~~deleted~~ Deleted

Injury *(Continued)*
  ankle S99.91-
    contusion —*see* Contusion, ankle
    dislocation —*see* Dislocation, ankle
    fracture —*see* Fracture, ankle
    nerve —*see* Injury, nerve, ankle
    open —*see* Wound, open, ankle
    specified type NEC S99.81-
    sprain —*see* Sprain, ankle
    superficial —*see* Injury, superficial,
      ankle
  anterior chamber, eye —*see* Injury, eye,
    specified site NEC
  anus —*see* Injury, abdomen
  aorta (thoracic) S25.00
    abdominal S35.00
      laceration (minor) (superficial)
        S35.01
        major S35.02
      specified type NEC S35.09
    laceration (minor) (superficial)
      S25.01
      major S25.02
    specified type NEC S25.09
  arm (upper) S49.9-
    blood vessel —*see* Injury, blood vessel,
      arm
    contusion —*see* Contusion, arm, upper
    fracture —*see* Fracture, humerus
    lower —*see* Injury, forearm
    muscle —*see* Injury, muscle, shoulder
    nerve —*see* Injury, nerve, arm
    open —*see* Wound, open, arm
    specified type NEC S49.8-
    superficial —*see* Injury, superficial, arm
  artery (complicating trauma) —*see also* Injury,
    blood vessel, by site
    cerebral or meningeal —*see* Injury,
      intracranial
  auditory canal (external) (meatus) S09.91
  auricle, auris, ear S09.91
  axilla —*see* Injury, shoulder
  back —*see* Injury, back, lower
  bile duct S36.13
  birth —*see also* Birth, injury P15.9
  bladder (sphincter) S37.20
    at delivery O71.5
    contusion S37.22
    laceration S37.23
    obstetrical trauma O71.5
    specified type NEC S37.29
  blast (air) (hydraulic) (immersion)
    (underwater) NEC T14.8
    acoustic nerve trauma —*see* Injury, nerve,
      acoustic
    bladder —*see* Injury, bladder
    brain —*see* Concussion
    colon —*see* Injury, intestine, large, blast
      injury
    ear (primary) S09.31-
      secondary S09.39-
    generalized T70.8
    lung —*see* Injury, intrathoracic, lung, blast
      injury
    multiple body organs T70.8
    peritoneum S36.81
    rectum S36.61
    retroperitoneum S36.898
    small intestine S36.419
      duodenum S36.410
      specified site NEC S36.418
    specified
      intra-abdominal organ NEC S36.898
      pelvic organ NEC S37.899
  blood vessel NEC T14.8
    abdomen S35.9-
      aorta —*see* Injury, aorta, abdominal
      celiac artery —*see* Injury, blood vessel,
        celiac artery
      iliac vessel —*see* Injury, blood vessel,
        iliac

Injury *(Continued)*
  blood vessel NEC *(Continued)*
    abdomen *(Continued)*
      laceration S35.91
      mesenteric vessel —*see* Injury,
        mesenteric
      portal vein —*see* Injury, blood vessel,
        portal vein
      renal vessel —*see* Injury, blood vessel,
        renal
      specified vessel NEC S35.8X-
      splenic vessel —*see* Injury, blood vessel,
        splenic
      vena cava —*see* Injury, vena cava,
        inferior
    ankle —*see* Injury, blood vessel, foot
    aorta (abdominal) (thoracic) —*see* Injury,
      aorta
    arm (upper) NEC S45.90-
      forearm —*see* Injury, blood vessel,
        forearm
      laceration S45.91-
      specified
        site NEC S45.80-
          laceration S45.81-
          specified type NEC S45.89-
        type NEC S45.99-
      superficial vein S45.30-
        laceration S45.31-
        specified type NEC S45.39-
    axillary
      artery S45.00-
        laceration S45.01-
        specified type NEC S45.09-
      vein S45.20-
        laceration S45.21-
        specified type NEC S45.29-
    azygos vein —*see* Injury, blood vessel,
      thoracic, specified site NEC
    brachial
      artery S45.10-
        laceration S45.11-
        specified type NEC S45.19-
      vein S45.20-
        laceration S45.219
        specified type NEC S45.29-
    carotid artery (common) (external)
      (internal, extracranial) S15.00-
      internal, intracranial S06.8-
      laceration (minor) (superficial) S15.01-
        major S15.02-
      specified type NEC S15.09-
    celiac artery S35.219
      branch S35.299
        laceration (minor) (superficial) S35.291
          major S35.292
        specified NEC S35.298
      laceration (minor) (superficial) S35.211
        major S35.212
      specified type NEC S35.218
    cerebral —*see* Injury, intracranial
    deep plantar —*see* Injury, blood vessel,
      plantar artery
    digital (hand) —*see* Injury, blood vessel,
      finger
    dorsal
      artery (foot) S95.00-
        laceration S95.01-
        specified type NEC S95.09-
      vein (foot) S95.20-
        laceration S95.21-
        specified type NEC S95.29-
    due to accidental laceration during
      procedure —*see* Laceration, accidental
      complicating surgery
    extremity —*see* Injury, blood vessel, limb
    femoral
      artery (common) (superficial) S75.00-
        laceration (minor) (superficial) S75.01-
          major S75.02-
        specified type NEC S75.09-

Injury *(Continued)*
  blood vessel NEC *(Continued)*
    femoral *(Continued)*
      vein (hip level) (thigh level) S75.10-
        laceration (minor) (superficial) S75.11-
          major S75.12-
        specified type NEC S75.19-
    finger S65.50-
      index S65.50-
        laceration S65.51-
        specified type NEC S65.59-
      laceration S65.51-
      little S65.50-
        laceration S65.51-
        specified type NEC S65.59-
      middle S65.50-
        laceration S65.51-
        specified type NEC S65.59-
      specified type NEC S65.59-
      thumb —*see* Injury, blood vessel, thumb
    foot S95.90-
      dorsal
        artery —*see* Injury, blood vessel,
          dorsal, artery
        vein —*see* Injury, blood vessel, dorsal,
          vein
      laceration S95.91-
      plantar artery —*see* Injury, blood vessel,
        plantar artery
      specified
        site NEC S95.80-
          laceration S95.81-
          specified type NEC S95.89-
        specified type NEC S95.99-
    forearm S55.90-
      laceration S55.91-
      radial artery —*see* Injury, blood vessel,
        radial artery
      specified
        site NEC S55.80-
          laceration S55.81-
          specified type NEC S55.89-
        type NEC S55.99-
      ulnar artery —*see* Injury, blood vessel,
        ulnar artery
      vein S55.20-
        laceration S55.21-
        specified type NEC S55.29-
    gastric
      artery —*see* Injury, mesenteric, artery,
        branch
      vein —*see* Injury, blood vessel, abdomen
    gastroduodenal artery —*see* Injury,
      mesenteric, artery, branch
    greater saphenous vein (lower leg level)
      S85.30-
      hip (and thigh) level S75.20-
        laceration (minor) (superficial) S75.21-
          major S75.22-
        specified type NEC S75.29-
      laceration S85.31-
      specified type NEC S85.39-
    hand (level) S65.90-
      finger —*see* Injury, blood vessel, finger
      laceration S65.91-
      palmar arch —*see* Injury, blood vessel,
        palmar arch
      radial artery —*see* Injury, blood vessel,
        radial artery, hand
      specified
        site NEC S65.80-
          laceration S65.81-
          specified type NEC S65.89-
        type NEC S65.99-
      thumb —*see* Injury, blood vessel,
        thumb
      ulnar artery —*see* Injury, blood vessel,
        ulnar artery, hand
    head S09.0
      intracranial —*see* Injury, intracranial
      multiple S09.0

◀ New　◀◀ Revised　~~deleted~~ Deleted

Injury (Continued)
cecum —see Injury, colon
celiac ganglion or plexus —see Injury, nerve, lumbosacral, sympathetic
cerebellum —see Injury, intracranial
cerebral —see Injury, intracranial
cervix (uteri) —see Injury, uterus
cheek (wall) S09.93
chest —see Injury, thorax
childbirth (newborn) —see also Birth, injury
    maternal NEC O71.9
chin S09.93
choroid (eye) —see Injury, eye, specified site NEC
clitoris S39.94
coccyx —see also Injury, back, lower
    complicating delivery O71.6
colon —see Injury, intestine, large
common bile duct —see Injury, liver
conjunctiva (superficial) —see Injury, eye, conjunctiva
conus medullaris —see Injury, spinal, sacral
cord
    spermatic (pelvic region) S37.898
        scrotal region S39.848
    spinal —see Injury, spinal cord, by region
cornea —see Injury, eye, specified site NEC
    abrasion —see Injury, eye, cornea, abrasion
cortex (cerebral) —see also Injury, intracranial
    visual —see Injury, nerve, optic
costal region NEC S29.9
costochondral NEC S29.9
cranial
    cavity —see Injury, intracranial
    nerve —see Injury, nerve, cranial
crushing —see Crush
cutaneous sensory nerve
cystic duct —see Injury, liver
deep tissue —see Contusion, by site
    meaning pressure ulcer —see Ulcer, pressure, unstageable, by site
delivery (newborn) P15.9
    maternal NEC O71.9
Descemet's membrane —see Injury, eyeball, penetrating
diaphragm —see Injury, intrathoracic, diaphragm
duodenum —see Injury, intestine, small, duodenum
ear (auricle) (external) (canal) S09.91
    abrasion —see Abrasion, ear
    bite —see Bite, ear
    blister —see Blister, ear
    bruise —see Contusion, ear
    contusion —see Contusion, ear
    external constriction —see Constriction, external, ear
    hematoma —see Hematoma, ear
    inner —see Injury, ear, middle
    laceration —see Laceration, ear
    middle S09.30-
        blast —see Injury, blast, ear
        specified NEC S09.39-
    puncture —see Puncture, ear
    superficial —see Injury, superficial, ear
eighth cranial nerve (acoustic or auditory) —
    see Injury, nerve, acoustic
elbow S59.90-
    contusion —see Contusion, elbow
    dislocation —see Dislocation, elbow
    fracture —see Fracture, ulna, upper end
    open —see Wound, open, elbow
    specified NEC S59.80-
    sprain —see Sprain, elbow
    superficial —see Injury, superficial, elbow
eleventh cranial nerve (accessory) —see
    Injury, nerve, accessory
epididymis S39.94
epigastric region S39.91
epiglottis NEC S19.89

Injury (Continued)
esophageal plexus —see Injury, nerve, thorax, sympathetic
esophagus (thoracic part) —see also Injury, intrathoracic, esophagus
    cervical NEC S19.85
eustachian tube S09.30-
eye S05.9-
    avulsion S05.7-
    ball —see Injury, eyeball
    conjunctiva S05.0-
    cornea
        abrasion S05.0-
    laceration S05.3-
        with prolapse S05.2-
    lacrimal apparatus S05.8X-
    orbit penetration S05.4-
    specified site NEC S05.8X-
eyeball S05.8X-
    contusion S05.1-
    penetrating S05.6-
        with
            foreign body S05.5-
            prolapse or loss of intraocular tissue S05.2-
        without prolapse or loss of intraocular tissue S05.3-
    specified type NEC S05.8-
eyebrow S09.93
eyelid S09.93
    abrasion —see Abrasion, eyelid
    contusion —see Contusion, eyelid
    open —see Wound, open, eyelid
face S09.93
fallopian tube S37.509
    bilateral S37.502
        blast injury S37.512
        contusion S37.522
        laceration S37.532
        specified type NEC S37.592
    blast injury (primary) S37.519
        bilateral S37.512
        secondary —see Injury, fallopian tube, specified type NEC
        unilateral S37.511
    contusion S37.529
        bilateral S37.522
        unilateral S37.521
    laceration S37.539
        bilateral S37.532
        unilateral S37.531
    specified type NEC S37.599
        bilateral S37.592
        unilateral S37.591
    unilateral S37.501
        blast injury S37.511
        contusion S37.521
        laceration S37.531
        specified type NEC S37.591
fascia —see Injury, muscle
fifth cranial nerve (trigeminal) —see Injury, nerve, trigeminal
finger (nail) S69.9-
    blood vessel —see Injury, blood vessel, finger
    contusion —see Contusion, finger
    dislocation —see Dislocation, finger
    fracture —see Fracture, finger
    muscle —see Injury, muscle, finger
    nerve —see Injury, nerve, digital, finger
    open —see Wound, open, finger
    specified NEC S69.8-
    sprain —see Sprain, finger
    superficial —see Injury, superficial, finger
first cranial nerve (olfactory) —see Injury, nerve, olfactory
flank —see Injury, abdomen
foot S99.92-
    blood vessel —see Injury, blood vessel, foot
    contusion —see Contusion, foot
    dislocation —see Dislocation, foot

Injury (Continued)
    foot (Continued)
        fracture —see Fracture, foot
        muscle —see Injury, muscle, foot
        open —see Wound, open, foot
        specified type NEC S99.82-
        sprain —see Sprain, foot
        superficial —see Injury, superficial, foot
    forceps NOS P15.9
    forearm S59.91-
        blood vessel —see Injury, blood vessel, forearm
        contusion —see Contusion, forearm
        fracture —see Fracture, forearm
        muscle —see Injury, muscle, forearm
        nerve —see Injury, nerve, forearm
        open —see Wound, open, forearm
        specified NEC S59.81-
        superficial —see Injury, superficial, forearm
    forehead S09.90
    fourth cranial nerve (trochlear) —see Injury, nerve, trochlear
    gallbladder S36.129
        contusion S36.122
        laceration S36.123
        specified NEC S36.128
    ganglion
        celiac, coeliac —see Injury, nerve, lumbosacral, sympathetic
        gasserian —see Injury, nerve, trigeminal
        stellate —see Injury, nerve, thorax, sympathetic
        thoracic sympathetic —see Injury, nerve, thorax, sympathetic
    gasserian ganglion —see Injury, nerve, trigeminal
    gastric artery —see Injury, blood vessel, celiac artery, branch
    gastroduodenal artery —see Injury, blood vessel, celiac artery, branch
    gastrointestinal tract —see Injury, intra-abdominal
        with open wound into abdominal cavity —
            see Wound, open, with penetration into peritoneal cavity
        colon —see Injury, intestine, large
        rectum —see Injury, intestine, large, rectum
            with open wound into abdominal cavity S36.61
        small intestine —see Injury, intestine, small
        specified site NEC —see Injury, intra-abdominal, specified, site NEC
        stomach —see Injury, stomach
    genital organ (s)
        external S39.94
            specified NEC S39.848
        internal S37.90
            fallopian tube —see Injury, fallopian tube
            ovary —see Injury, ovary
            prostate —see Injury, prostate
            seminal vesicle —see Injury, pelvis, organ, specified site NEC
            uterus —see Injury, uterus
            vas deferens —see Injury, pelvis, organ, specified site NEC
        obstetrical trauma O71.9
    gland
        lacrimal laceration —see Injury, eye, specified site NEC
        salivary S09.90
        thyroid NEC S19.84
    globe (eye) S05.90
        specified NEC S05.8X-
    groin —see Injury, abdomen
    gum S09.90
    hand S69.9-
        blood vessel —see Injury, blood vessel, hand
        contusion —see Contusion, hand
        fracture —see Fracture, hand
        muscle —see Injury, muscle, hand

Injury *(Continued)*
  hand *(Continued)*
    nerve —*see* Injury, nerve, hand
    open —*see* Wound, open, hand
    specified NEC S69.8-
    sprain —*see* Sprain, hand
    superficial —*see* Injury, superficial, hand
  head S09.90
    with loss of consciousness S06.9-
    specified NEC S09.8-
  heart S26.90
    with hemopericardium S26.00
      contusion S26.01
      laceration (mild) S26.020
        major S26.022
        moderate S26.021
      specified type NEC S26.09
    without hemopericardium S26.10
      contusion S26.11
      laceration S26.12
      specified type NEC S26.19
    contusion S26.91
    laceration S26.92
    specified type NEC S26.99
  heel —*see* Injury, foot
  hepatic
    artery —*see* Injury, blood vessel, celiac
        artery, branch
    duct —*see* Injury, liver
    vein —*see* Injury, vena cava, inferior
  hip S79.91-
    blood vessel —*see* Injury, blood vessel, hip
    contusion —*see* Contusion, hip
    dislocation —*see* Dislocation, hip
    fracture —*see* Fracture, femur, neck
    muscle —*see* Injury, muscle, hip
    nerve —*see* Injury, nerve, hip
    open —*see* Wound, open, hip
    specified NEC S79.81-
    sprain —*see* Sprain, hip
    superficial —*see* Injury, superficial, hip
  hymen S39.94
  hypogastric
    blood vessel —*see* Injury, blood vessel, iliac
    plexus —*see* Injury, nerve, lumbosacral,
        sympathetic
  ileum —*see* Injury, intestine, small
  iliac region S39.91
  instrumental (during surgery) —*see*
        Laceration, accidental complicating
        surgery
    birth injury —*see* Birth, injury
    nonsurgical —*see* Injury, by site
  obstetrical O71.9
    bladder O71.5
    cervix O71.3
    high vaginal O71.4
    perineal NOS O70.9
    urethra O71.5
    uterus O71.5
      with rupture or perforation O71.1
  internal T14.8
    aorta —*see* Injury, aorta
    bladder (sphincter) —*see* Injury, bladder
      with
        ectopic or molar pregnancy O08.6
        following ectopic or molar pregnancy
            O08.6
        obstetrical trauma O71.5
    bronchus, bronchi —*see* Injury,
        intrathoracic, bronchus
    cecum —*see* Injury, intestine, large
    cervix (uteri) —*see also* Injury, uterus
      with ectopic or molar pregnancy O08.6
      following ectopic or molar pregnancy
          O08.6
      obstetrical trauma O71.3
    chest —*see* Injury, intrathoracic
    gastrointestinal tract —*see* Injury,
        intra-abdominal
    heart —*see* Injury, heart

Injury *(Continued)*
  internal *(Continued)*
    intestine NEC —*see* Injury, intestine
    intrauterine —*see* Injury, uterus
    mesentery —*see* Injury, intra-abdominal,
        specified, site NEC
    pelvis, pelvic (organ) S37.90
      following ectopic or molar pregnancy
          (subsequent episode) O08.6
      obstetrical trauma NEC O71.5
        rupture or perforation O71.1
      specified NEC S39.83
    rectum —*see* Injury, intestine, large,
        rectum
    stomach —*see* Injury, stomach
    ureter —*see* Injury, ureter
    urethra (sphincter) following ectopic or
        molar pregnancy O08.6
    uterus —*see* Injury, uterus
  interscapular area —*see* Injury, thorax
  intestine
    large S36.509
      ascending (right) S36.500
        blast injury (primary) S36.510
          secondary S36.590
        contusion S36.520
        laceration S36.530
        specified type NEC S36.590
      blast injury (primary) S36.519
        ascending (right) S36.510
        descending (left) S36.512
        rectum S36.61
        sigmoid S36.513
        specified site NEC S36.518
        transverse S36.511
      contusion S36.529
        ascending (right) S36.520
        descending (left) S36.522
        rectum S36.62
        sigmoid S36.523
        specified site NEC S36.528
        transverse S36.521
      descending (left) S36.502
        blast injury (primary) S36.512
          secondary S36.592
        contusion S36.522
        laceration S36.532
        specified type NEC S36.592
      laceration S36.539
        ascending (right) S36.530
        descending (left) S36.532
        rectum S36.63
        sigmoid S36.533
        specified site NEC S36.538
        transverse S36.531
      rectum S36.60
        blast injury (primary) S36.61
          secondary S36.69
        contusion S36.62
        laceration S36.63
        specified type NEC S36.69
      sigmoid S36.503
        blast injury (primary) S36.513
          secondary S36.593
        contusion S36.523
        laceration S36.533
        specified type NEC S36.593
      specified
        site NEC S36.508
          blast injury (primary) S36.518
            secondary S36.598
          contusion S36.528
          laceration S36.538
          specified type NEC S36.598
        type NEC S36.599
          ascending (right) S36.590
          descending (left) S36.592
          rectum S36.69
          sigmoid S36.593
          specified site NEC S36.598
          transverse S36.591

Injury *(Continued)*
  intestine *(Continued)*
    large *(Continued)*
      transverse S36.501
        blast injury (primary) S36.511
          secondary S36.591
        contusion S36.521
        laceration S36.531
        specified type NEC S36.591
    small S36.409
      blast injury (primary) S36.419
        duodenum S36.410
        secondary S36.499
          duodenum S36.490
          specified site NEC S36.498
        specified site NEC S36.418
      contusion S36.429
        duodenum S36.420
        specified site NEC S36.428
      duodenum S36.400
        blast injury (primary) S36.410
          secondary S36.490
        contusion S36.420
        laceration S36.430
        specified NEC S36.490
      laceration S36.439
        duodenum S36.430
        specified site NEC S36.438
      specified
        site NEC S36.408
        type NEC S36.499
          duodenum S36.490
          specified site NEC S36.498
  intra-abdominal S36.90
    adrenal gland —*see* Injury, adrenal gland
    bladder —*see* Injury, bladder
    colon —*see* Injury, intestine, large
    contusion S36.92
    fallopian tube —*see* Injury, fallopian tube
    gallbladder —*see* Injury, gallbladder
    intestine —*see* Injury, intestine
    kidney —*see* Injury, kidney
    laceration S36.93
    liver —*see* Injury, liver
    ovary —*see* Injury, ovary
    pancreas —*see* Injury, pancreas
    pelvic NOS S37.90
    peritoneum —*see* Injury, intra-abdominal,
        specified, site NEC
    prostate —*see* Injury, prostate
    rectum —*see* Injury, intestine, large, rectum
    retroperitoneum —*see* Injury, intra-
        abdominal, specified, site NEC
    seminal vesicle —*see* Injury, pelvis, organ,
        specified site NEC
    small intestine —*see* Injury, intestine, small
    specified
      pelvic S37.90
        specified
          site NEC S37.899
            specified type NEC S37.898
            type NEC S37.99
      site NEC S36.899
        contusion S36.892
        laceration S36.893
        specified type NEC S36.898
        type NEC S36.99
    spleen —*see* Injury, spleen
    stomach —*see* Injury, stomach
    ureter —*see* Injury, ureter
    urethra —*see* Injury, urethra
    uterus —*see* Injury, uterus
    vas deferens —*see* Injury, pelvis, organ,
        specified site NEC
  intracranial (traumatic) S06.9-
    cerebellar hemorrhage, traumatic —*see*
        Injury, intracranial, focal
    cerebral edema, traumatic S06.1X-
      diffuse S06.1X-
      focal S06.1X-
    diffuse (axonal) S06.2X-

◀ New   ◀◀ Revised   ~~deleted~~ Deleted

Injury *(Continued)*
  intracranial *(Continued)*
    epidural hemorrhage (traumatic) S06.4X-
    focal brain injury S06.30-
      contusion —*see* Contusion, cerebral
      laceration —*see* Laceration, cerebral
    intracerebral hemorrhage, traumatic
      S06.36-
      left side S06.35-
      right side S06.34-
    subarachnoid hemorrhage, traumatic
      S06.6X-
    subdural hemorrhage, traumatic S06.5X-
  intraocular —*see* Injury, eyeball, penetrating
  intrathoracic S27.9
    bronchus S27.409
      bilateral S27.402
      blast injury (primary) S27.419
        bilateral S27.412
        secondary —*see* Injury, intrathoracic,
          bronchus, specified type NEC
        unilateral S27.411
      contusion S27.429
        bilateral S27.422
        unilateral S27.421
      laceration S27.439
        bilateral S27.432
        unilateral S27.431
      specified type NEC S27.499
        bilateral S27.492
        unilateral S27.491
      unilateral S27.401
    diaphragm S27.809
      contusion S27.802
      laceration S27.803
      specified type NEC S27.808
    esophagus (thoracic) S27.819
      contusion S27.812
      laceration S27.813
      specified type NEC S27.818
    heart —*see* Injury, heart
    hemopneumothorax S27.2
    hemothorax S27.1
    lung S27.309
      aspiration J69.0
      bilateral S27.302
      blast injury (primary) S27.319
        bilateral S27.312
        secondary —*see* Injury, intrathoracic,
          lung, specified type NEC
        unilateral S27.311
      contusion S27.329
        bilateral S27.322
        unilateral S27.321
      laceration S27.339
        bilateral S27.332
        unilateral S27.331
      specified type NEC S27.399
        bilateral S27.392
        unilateral S27.391
      unilateral S27.301
    pleura S27.60
      laceration S27.63
      specified type NEC S27.69
    pneumothorax S27.0
    specified organ NEC S27.899
      contusion S27.892
      laceration S27.893
      specified type NEC S27.898
    thoracic duct —*see* Injury, intrathoracic,
      specified organ NEC
    thymus gland —*see* Injury, intrathoracic,
      specified organ NEC
    trachea, thoracic S27.50
      blast (primary) S27.51
      contusion S27.52
      laceration S27.53
      specified type NEC S27.59
  iris —*see* Injury, eye, specified site NEC
  penetrating —*see* Injury, eyeball,
    penetrating

Injury *(Continued)*
  jaw S09.93
  jejunum —*see* Injury, intestine, small
  joint NOS T14.8
    old or residual —*see* Disorder, joint,
      specified type NEC
  kidney S37.00-
    acute (nontraumatic) N17.9
    contusion —*see* Contusion, kidney
    laceration —*see* Laceration, kidney
    specified NEC S37.09-
  knee S89.9-
    contusion —*see* Contusion, knee
    dislocation —*see* Dislocation, knee
    meniscus (lateral) (medial) —*see* Sprain,
      knee, specified site NEC
      old injury or tear —*see* Derangement,
        knee, meniscus, due to old injury
    open —*see* Wound, open, knee
    specified NEC S89.8-
    sprain —*see* Sprain, knee
    superficial —*see* Injury, superficial, knee
  labium (majus) (minus) S39.94
  labyrinth, ear S09.30-
  lacrimal apparatus, duct, gland, or sac —*see*
    Injury, eye, specified site NEC
  larynx NEC S19.81
  leg (lower) S89.9-
    blood vessel —*see* Injury, blood vessel, leg
    contusion —*see* Contusion, leg
    fracture —*see* Fracture, leg
    muscle —*see* Injury, muscle, leg
    nerve —*see* Injury, nerve, leg
    open —*see* Wound, open, leg
    specified NEC S89.8-
    superficial —*see* Injury, superficial, leg
  lens, eye —*see* Injury, eye, specified site NEC
    penetrating —*see* Injury, eyeball,
      penetrating
  limb NEC T14.8
  lip S09.93
  liver S36.119
    contusion S36.112
    laceration S36.113
      major (stellate) S36.116
      minor S36.114
      moderate S36.115
    specified NEC S36.118
  lower back S39.92
    specified NEC S39.82
  lumbar, lumbosacral (region) S39.92
    plexus —*see* Injury, lumbosacral plexus
  lumbosacral plexus S34.4
  lung —*see also* Injury, intrathoracic, lung
    aspiration J69.0
    transfusion-related (TRALI) J95.84
  lymphatic thoracic duct —*see* Injury,
    intrathoracic, specified organ NEC
  malar region S09.93
  mastoid region S09.90
  maxilla S09.93
  mediastinum —*see* Injury, intrathoracic,
    specified organ NEC
  membrane, brain —*see* Injury, intracranial
  meningeal artery —*see* Injury, intracranial,
    subdural hemorrhage
  meninges (cerebral) —*see* Injury, intracranial
  mesenteric
    artery
      branch S35.299
        laceration (minor) (superficial) S35.291
          major S35.292
        specified NEC S35.298
      inferior S35.239
        laceration (minor) (superficial) S35.231
          major S35.232
        specified NEC S35.238
      superior S35.229
        laceration (minor) (superficial) S35.221
          major S35.222
        specified NEC S35.228

Injury *(Continued)*
  mesenteric *(Continued)*
    plexus (inferior) (superior) —*see* Injury,
      nerve, lumbosacral, sympathetic
    vein
      inferior S35.349
        laceration S35.341
        specified NEC S35.348
      superior S35.339
        laceration S35.331
        specified NEC S35.338
  mesentery —*see* Injury, intra-abdominal,
    specified site NEC
  mesosalpinx —*see* Injury, pelvic organ,
    specified site NEC
  middle ear S09.30-
  midthoracic region NOS S29.9
  mouth S09.93
  multiple NOS T07
  muscle (and fascia) (and tendon)
    abdomen S39.001
      laceration S39.021
      specified type NEC S39.091
      strain S39.011
    abductor
      thumb, forearm level —*see* Injury,
        muscle, thumb, abductor
    adductor
      thigh S76.20-
        laceration S76.22-
        specified type NEC S76.29-
        strain S76.21-
    ankle —*see* Injury, muscle, foot
    anterior muscle group, at leg level (lower)
      S86.20-
      laceration S86.22-
      specified type NEC S86.29-
      strain S86.21-
    arm (upper) —*see* Injury, muscle,
      shoulder
    biceps (parts NEC) S46.20-
      laceration S46.22-
      long head S46.10-
        laceration S46.12-
        specified type NEC S46.19-
        strain S46.11-
      specified type NEC S46.29-
      strain S46.21-
    extensor
      finger (s) (other than thumb) —*see* Injury,
        muscle, finger by site, extensor
      forearm level, specified NEC —*see*
        Injury, muscle, forearm, extensor
      thumb —*see* Injury, muscle, thumb,
        extensor
      toe (large) (ankle level) (foot level) —*see*
        Injury, muscle, toe, extensor
    finger
      extensor (forearm level) S56.40-
        hand level S66.309
          laceration S66.329
          specified type NEC S66.399
          strain S66.319
        laceration S56.429
        specified type NEC S56.499
        strain S56.419
      flexor (forearm level) S56.10-
        hand level S66.109
          laceration S66.129
          specified type NEC S66.199
          strain S66.119
        laceration S56.129
        specified type NEC S56.199
        strain S56.119
      index
        extensor (forearm level)
          hand level S66.308
            laceration S66.32-
            specified type NEC S66.39-
            strain S66.31-
          specified type NEC S56.492-

Injury *(Continued)*
  muscle *(Continued)*
    finger *(Continued)*
      index *(Continued)*
        flexor (forearm level)
          hand level S66.108
            laceration S66.12-
            specified type NEC
              S66.19-
            strain S66.11-
          specified type NEC S56.19-
          strain S56.11-
        intrinsic S66.50-
          laceration S66.52-
          specified type NEC S66.59-
          strain S66.51-
      intrinsic S66.509
        laceration S66.529
        specified type NEC S66.599
        strain S66.519
      little
        extensor (forearm level)
          hand level S66.30-
            laceration S66.32-
            specified type NEC S66.39-
            strain S66.31-
          laceration S56.42-
          specified type NEC S56.49-
          strain S56.41-
        flexor (forearm level)
          hand level S66.10-
            laceration S66.12-
            specified type NEC S66.19-
            strain S66.11-
          laceration S56.12-
          specified type NEC S56.19-
          strain S56.11-
        intrinsic S66.50-
          laceration S66.52-
          specified type NEC S66.59-
          strain S66.51-
      middle
        extensor (forearm level)
          hand level S66.30-
            laceration S66.32-
            specified type NEC
              S66.39-
            strain S66.31-
          laceration S56.42-
          specified type NEC S56.49-
          strain S56.41-
        flexor (forearm level)
          hand level S66.10-
            laceration S66.12-
            specified type NEC
              S66.19-
            strain S66.11-
          laceration S56.12-
          specified type NEC S56.19-
          strain S56.11-
        intrinsic S66.50-
          laceration S66.52-
          specified type NEC S66.59-
          strain S66.51-
      ring
        extensor (forearm level)
          hand level S66.30-
            laceration S66.32-
            specified type NEC S66.39-
            strain S66.31-
          laceration S56.42-
          specified type NEC S56.49-
          strain S56.41-
        flexor (forearm level)
          hand level S66.10-
            laceration S66.12-
            specified type NEC S66.19-
            strain S66.11-
          laceration S56.12-
          specified type NEC S56.19-
          strain S56.11-

Injury *(Continued)*
  muscle *(Continued)*
    finger *(Continued)*
      ring *(Continued)*
        intrinsic S66.50-
          laceration S66.52-
          specified type NEC S66.59-
          strain S66.51-
    flexor
      finger (s) (other than thumb) — *see*
        Injury, muscle, finger
      forearm level, specified NEC — *see*
        Injury, muscle, forearm, flexor
      thumb —*see* Injury, muscle, thumb,
        flexor
      toe (long) (ankle level) (foot level) —*see*
        Injury, muscle, toe, flexor
    foot S96.90-
      intrinsic S96.20-
        laceration S96.22-
        specified type NEC S96.29-
        strain S96.21-
      laceration S96.92-
      long extensor, toe —*see* Injury, muscle,
        toe, extensor
      long flexor, toe —*see* Injury, muscle, toe,
        flexor
      specified
        site NEC S96.80-
          laceration S96.82-
          specified type NEC S96.89-
          strain S96.81-
          type NEC S96.99-
      strain S96.91-
    forearm (level) S56.90-
      extensor S56.50-
        laceration S56.52-
        specified type NEC S56.59-
        strain S56.51-
      flexor S56.20-
        laceration S56.22-
        specified type NEC S56.29-
        strain S56.21-
      laceration S56.92-
      specified S56.99-
        site NEC S56.80-
          laceration S56.82-
          strain S56.81-
          type NEC S56.89-
        strain S56.91-
    hand (level) S66.90-
      laceration S66.92-
      specified
        site NEC S66.80-
          laceration S66.82-
          specified type NEC S66.89-
          strain S66.81-
          type NEC S66.99-
        strain S66.91-
    head S09.10
      laceration S09.12
      specified type NEC S09.19
      strain S09.11
    hip NEC S76.00-
      laceration S76.02-
      specified type NEC S76.09-
      strain S76.01-
    intrinsic
      ankle and foot level —*see* Injury, muscle,
        foot, intrinsic
      finger (other than thumb) —*see* Injury,
        muscle, finger by site, intrinsic
      foot (level) —*see* Injury, muscle, foot,
        intrinsic
      thumb —*see* Injury, muscle, thumb,
        intrinsic
    leg (level) (lower) S86.90-
      Achilles tendon —*see* Injury, Achilles
        tendon
      anterior muscle group —*see* Injury,
        muscle, anterior muscle group

Injury *(Continued)*
  muscle *(Continued)*
    leg *(Continued)*
      laceration S86.92-
      peroneal muscle group —*see* Injury,
        muscle, peroneal muscle group
      posterior muscle group —*see* Injury,
        muscle, posterior muscle group,
        leg level
      specified
        site NEC S86.80-
          laceration S86.82-
          specified type NEC S86.89-
          strain S86.81-
          type NEC S86.99-
      strain S86.91-
    long
      extensor toe, at ankle and foot level —*see*
        Injury, muscle, toe, extensor
      flexor, toe, at ankle and foot level —*see*
        Injury, muscle, toe, flexor
      head, biceps —*see* Injury, muscle, biceps,
        long head
    lower back S39.002
      laceration S39.022
      specified type NEC S39.092
      strain S39.012
    neck (level) S16.9
      laceration S16.2
      specified type NEC S16.8
      strain S16.1
    pelvis S39.003
      laceration S39.023
      specified type NEC S39.093
      strain S39.013
    peroneal muscle group, at leg level (lower)
      S86.30-
      laceration S86.32-
      specified type NEC S86.39-
      strain S86.31-
    posterior muscle (group)
      leg level (lower) S86.10-
        laceration S86.12-
        specified type NEC S86.19-
        strain S86.11-
      thigh level S76.30-
        laceration S76.32-
        specified type NEC S76.39-
        strain S76.31-
    quadriceps (thigh) S76.10-
      laceration S76.12-
      specified type NEC S76.19-
      strain S76.11-
    shoulder S46.90-
      laceration S46.92-
      rotator cuff —*see* Injury, rotator cuff
      specified site NEC S46.80-
        laceration S46.82-
        specified type NEC S46.89-
        strain S46.81-
      specified type NEC S46.99-
      strain S46.91-
    thigh NEC (level) S76.90-
      adductor —*see* Injury, muscle, adductor,
        thigh
      laceration S76.92-
      posterior muscle (group) —*see* Injury,
        muscle, posterior muscle, thigh
        level
      quadriceps —*see* Injury, muscle,
        quadriceps
      specified
        site NEC S76.80-
          laceration S76.82-
          specified type NEC S76.89-
          strain S76.81-
          type NEC S76.99-
      strain S76.91-
    thorax (level) S29.009
      back wall S29.002
      front wall S29.001

◀ New   ◀||||| Revised   ~~deleted~~ Deleted

Injury *(Continued)*
  muscle *(Continued)*
    thorax *(Continued)*
      laceration S29.029
        back wall S29.022
        front wall S29.021
      specified type NEC S29.099
        back wall S29.092
        front wall S29.091
      strain S29.019
        back wall S29.012
        front wall S29.011
    thumb
      abductor (forearm level) S56.30-
        laceration S56.32-
        specified type NEC S56.39-
        strain S56.31-
      extensor (forearm level) S56.30-
        hand level S66.20-
          laceration S66.22-
          specified type NEC S66.29-
          strain S66.21-
        laceration S56.32-
        specified type NEC S56.39-
        strain S56.31-
      flexor (forearm level) S56.00-
        hand level S66.00-
          laceration S66.02-
          specified type NEC S66.09-
          strain S66.01-
        laceration S56.02-
        specified type NEC S56.09-
        strain S56.01-
        wrist level —*see* Injury, muscle,
          thumb, flexor, hand level
      intrinsic S66.40-
        laceration S66.42-
        specified type NEC S66.49-
        strain S66.41-
    toe —*see also* Injury, muscle, foot
      extensor, long S96.10-
        laceration S96.12-
        specified type NEC S96.19-
        strain S96.11-
      flexor, long S96.00-
        laceration S96.02-
        specified type NEC S96.09-
        strain S96.01-
    triceps S46.30-
      laceration S46.32-
      specified type NEC S46.39-
      strain S46.31-
    wrist (and hand) level —*see* Injury, muscle,
      hand
  musculocutaneous nerve —*see* Injury, nerve,
    musculocutaneous
  myocardium —*see* Injury, heart
  nape —*see* Injury, neck
  nasal (septum) (sinus) S09.92
  nasopharynx S09.92
  neck S19.9
    specified NEC S19.80
      specified site NEC S19.89
  nerve NEC T14.8
    abdomen S34.9
      peripheral S34.6
      specified site NEC S34.8
    abducens S04.4-
      contusion S04.4-
      laceration S04.4-
      specified type NEC S04.4-
    abducent —*see* Injury, nerve,
      abducens
    accessory S04.7-
      contusion S04.7-
      laceration S04.7-
      specified type NEC S04.7-
    acoustic S04.6-
      contusion S04.6-
      laceration S04.6-
      specified type NEC S04.6-

Injury *(Continued)*
  nerve NEC *(Continued)*
    ankle S94.9-
      cutaneous sensory S94.3-
      specified site NEC —*see* subcategory
        S94.8
    anterior crural, femoral —*see* Injury, nerve,
      femoral
    arm (upper) S44.9-
      axillary —*see* Injury, nerve, axillary
      cutaneous —*see* Injury, nerve, cutaneous,
        arm
      median —*see* Injury, nerve, median,
        upper arm
      musculocutaneous —*see* Injury, nerve,
        musculocutaneous
      radial —*see* Injury, nerve, radial, upper
        arm
      specified site NEC —*see* subcategory
        S44.8
      ulnar —*see* Injury, nerve, ulnar, arm
    auditory —*see* Injury, nerve, acoustic
    axillary S44.3-
    brachial plexus —*see* Injury, brachial plexus
    cervical sympathetic S14.5
    cranial S04.9
      contusion S04.9
      eighth (acoustic or auditory) —*see* Injury,
        nerve, acoustic
      eleventh (accessory) —*see* Injury, nerve,
        accessory
      fifth (trigeminal) —*see* Injury, nerve,
        trigeminal
      first (olfactory) —*see* Injury, nerve,
        olfactory
      fourth (trochlear) —*see* Injury, nerve,
        trochlear
      laceration S04.9
      ninth (glossopharyngeal) —*see* Injury,
        nerve, glossopharyngeal
      second (optic) —*see* Injury, nerve, optic
      seventh (facial) —*see* Injury, nerve, facial
      sixth (abducent) —*see* Injury, nerve,
        abducens
      specified
        nerve NEC S04.89-
          contusion S04.89-
          laceration S04.89-
          specified type NEC S04.89-
        type NEC S04.9
      tenth (pneumogastric or vagus) —*see*
        Injury, nerve, vagus
      third (oculomotor) —*see* Injury, nerve,
        oculomotor
      twelfth (hypoglossal) —*see* Injury, nerve,
        hypoglossal
    cutaneous sensory
      ankle (level) S94.3-
      arm (upper) (level) S44.5-
      foot (level) —*see* Injury, nerve, cutaneous
        sensory, ankle
      forearm (level) S54.3-
      hip (level) S74.2-
      leg (lower level) S84.2-
      shoulder (level) —*see* Injury, nerve,
        cutaneous sensory, arm
      thigh (level) —*see* Injury, nerve,
        cutaneous sensory, hip
    deep peroneal —*see* Injury, nerve, peroneal,
      foot
    digital
      finger S64.4-
        index S64.49-
        little S64.49-
        middle S64.49-
        ring S64.49-
      thumb S64.3-
      toe —*see* Injury, nerve, ankle, specified
        site NEC
    eighth cranial (acoustic or auditory) —*see*
      Injury, nerve, acoustic

Injury *(Continued)*
  nerve NEC *(Continued)*
    eleventh cranial (accessory) —*see* Injury,
      nerve, accessory
    facial S04.5-
      contusion S04.5-
      laceration S04.5-
      newborn P11.3
      specified type NEC S04.5-
    femoral (hip level) (thigh level) S74.1-
    fifth cranial (trigeminal) —*see* Injury, nerve,
      trigeminal
    finger (digital) —*see* Injury, nerve, digital,
      finger
    first cranial (olfactory) —*see* Injury, nerve,
      olfactory
    foot S94.9-
      cutaneous sensory S94.3-
      deep peroneal S94.2-
      lateral plantar S94.0-
      medial plantar S94.1-
      specified site NEC —*see* subcategory
        S94.8
    forearm (level) S54.9-
      cutaneous sensory —*see* Injury, nerve,
        cutaneous sensory, forearm
      median —*see* Injury, nerve, median
      radial —*see* Injury, nerve, radial
      specified site NEC —*see* subcategory
        S54.8
      ulnar —*see* Injury, nerve, ulnar
    fourth cranial (trochlear) —*see* Injury,
      nerve, trochlear
    glossopharyngeal S04.89-
      specified type NEC S04.89-
    hand S64.9-
      median —*see* Injury, nerve, median,
        hand
      radial —*see* Injury, nerve, radial, hand
      specified NEC —*see* subcategory
        S64.8
      ulnar —*see* Injury, nerve, ulnar, hand
    hip (level) S74.9-
      cutaneous sensory —*see* Injury, nerve,
        cutaneous sensory, hip
      femoral —*see* Injury, nerve, femoral
      sciatic —*see* Injury, nerve, sciatic
      specified site NEC —*see* subcategory
        S74.8
    hypoglossal S04.89-
      specified type NEC S04.89-
    lateral plantar S94.0-
    leg (lower) S84.9-
      cutaneous sensory —*see* Injury, nerve,
        cutaneous sensory, leg
      peroneal —*see* Injury, nerve, peroneal
      specified site NEC —*see* subcategory
        S84.8
      tibial —*see* Injury, nerve, tibial
      upper —*see* Injury, nerve, thigh
    lower
      back —*see* Injury, nerve, abdomen,
        specified site NEC
        peripheral —*see* Injury, nerve,
          abdomen, peripheral
      limb —*see* Injury, nerve, leg
    lumbar plexus —*see* Injury, nerve,
      lumbosacral, sympathetic
    lumbar spinal —*see* Injury, nerve, spinal,
      lumbar
    lumbosacral
      plexus —*see* Injury, nerve, lumbosacral,
        sympathetic
      sympathetic S34.5
    medial plantar S94.1-
    median (forearm level) S54.1-
      hand (level) S64.1-
      upper arm (level) S44.1-
      wrist (level) —*see* Injury, nerve, median,
        hand
    musculocutaneous S44.4-

Injury (Continued)
  nerve NEC (Continued)
    musculospiral (upper arm level) —see
      Injury, nerve, radial, upper arm
    neck S14.9
      peripheral S14.4
      specified site NEC S14.8
      sympathetic S14.5
    ninth cranial (glossopharyngeal) —see
      Injury, nerve, glossopharyngeal
    oculomotor S04.1-
      contusion S04.1-
      laceration S04.1-
      specified type NEC S04.1-
    olfactory S04.81-
      specified type NEC S04.81-
    optic S04.01-
      contusion S04.01-
      laceration S04.01-
      specified type NEC S04.01-
    pelvic girdle —see Injury, nerve, hip
    pelvis —see Injury, nerve, abdomen,
      specified site NEC
    peripheral —see Injury, nerve, abdomen,
      peripheral
    peripheral NEC T14.8
      abdomen —see Injury, nerve, abdomen,
        peripheral
      lower back —see Injury, nerve, abdomen,
        peripheral
      neck —see Injury, nerve, neck,
        peripheral
      pelvis —see Injury, nerve, abdomen,
        peripheral
      specified NEC T14.8
    peroneal (lower leg level) S84.1-
      foot S94.2-
    plexus
      brachial —see Injury, brachial
        plexus
      celiac, coeliac —see Injury, nerve,
        lumbosacral, sympathetic
      mesenteric, inferior —see Injury, nerve,
        lumbosacral, sympathetic
      sacral —see Injury, lumbosacral
        plexus
      spinal
        brachial —see Injury, brachial
          plexus
        lumbosacral —see Injury, lumbosacral
          plexus
    pneumogastric —see Injury, nerve,
      vagus
    radial (forearm level) S54.2-
      hand (level) S64.2-
      upper arm (level) S44.2-
      wrist (level) —see Injury, nerve, radial,
        hand
    root —see Injury, nerve, spinal, root
    sacral plexus —see Injury, lumbosacral
      plexus
    sacral spinal —see Injury, nerve, spinal,
      sacral
    sciatic (hip level) (thigh level) S74.0-
    second cranial (optic) —see Injury, nerve,
      optic
    seventh cranial (facial) —see Injury, nerve,
      facial
    shoulder —see Injury, nerve, arm
    sixth cranial (abducent) —see Injury, nerve,
      abducens
    spinal
      plexus —see Injury, nerve, plexus,
        spinal
      root
        cervical S14.2
        dorsal S24.2
        lumbar S34.21
        sacral S34.22
        thoracic —see Injury, nerve, spinal,
          root, dorsal

Injury (Continued)
  nerve NEC (Continued)
    splanchnic —see Injury, nerve, lumbosacral,
      sympathetic
    sympathetic NEC —see Injury, nerve,
      lumbosacral, sympathetic
      cervical —see Injury, nerve, cervical
        sympathetic
    tenth cranial (pneumogastric or vagus) —
      see Injury, nerve, vagus
    thigh (level) —see Injury, nerve, hip
      cutaneous sensory —see Injury, nerve,
        cutaneous sensory, hip
      femoral —see Injury, nerve, femoral
      sciatic —see Injury, nerve, sciatic
      specified NEC —see Injury, nerve, hip
    third cranial (oculomotor) —see Injury,
      nerve, oculomotor
    thorax S24.9
      peripheral S24.3
      specified site NEC S24.8
      sympathetic S24.4
    thumb, digital —see Injury, nerve, digital,
      thumb
    tibial (lower leg level) (posterior)
      S84.0-
    toe —see Injury, nerve, ankle
    trigeminal S04.3-
      contusion S04.3-
      laceration S04.3-
      specified type NEC S04.3-
    trochlear S04.2-
      contusion S04.2-
      laceration S04.2-
      specified type NEC S04.2-
    twelfth cranial (hypoglossal) —see Injury,
      nerve, hypoglossal
    ulnar (forearm level) S54.0-
      arm (upper) (level) S44.0-
      hand (level) S64.0-
      wrist (level) —see Injury, nerve, ulnar,
        hand
    vagus S04.89-
      specified type NEC S04.89-
    wrist (level) —see Injury, nerve, hand
  ninth cranial nerve (glossopharyngeal) —see
    Injury, nerve, glossopharyngeal
  nose (septum) S09.92
  obstetrical O71.9
    specified NEC O71.89
  occipital (region) (scalp) S09.90
    lobe —see Injury, intracranial
  optic chiasm S04.02
  optic radiation S04.03-
  optic tract and pathways S04.03-
  orbit, orbital (region) —see Injury, eye
    penetrating (with foreign body) —see
      Injury, eye, orbit, penetrating
    specified NEC —see Injury, eye, specified
      site NEC
  ovary, ovarian S37.409
    bilateral S37.402
      contusion S37.422
      laceration S37.432
      specified type NEC S37.492
    blood vessel —see Injury, blood vessel,
      ovarian
    contusion S37.429
      bilateral S37.422
      unilateral S37.421
    laceration S37.439
      bilateral S37.432
      unilateral S37.431
    specified type NEC S37.499
      bilateral S37.492
      unilateral S37.491
    unilateral S37.401
      contusion S37.421
      laceration S37.431
      specified type NEC S37.491
  palate (hard) (soft) S09.93

Injury (Continued)
  pancreas S36.209
    body S36.201
      contusion S36.221
      laceration S36.231
        major S36.261
        minor S36.241
        moderate S36.251
      specified type NEC S36.291
    contusion S36.229
    head S36.200
      contusion S36.220
      laceration S36.230
        major S36.260
        minor S36.240
        moderate S36.250
      specified type NEC S36.290
    laceration S36.239
      major S36.269
      minor S36.249
      moderate S36.259
      specified type NEC S36.299
    tail S36.202
      contusion S36.222
      laceration S36.232
        major S36.262
        minor S36.242
        moderate S36.252
      specified type NEC S36.292
  parietal (region) (scalp) S09.90
    lobe —see Injury, intracranial
  patellar ligament (tendon) S76.10-
    laceration S76.12-
    specified NEC S76.19-
    strain S76.11-
  pelvis, pelvic (floor) S39.93
    complicating delivery O70.1
    joint or ligament, complicating delivery
      O71.6
    organ S37.90
      with ectopic or molar pregnancy O08.6
      complication of abortion —see Abortion
      contusion S37.92
      following ectopic or molar pregnancy
        O08.6
      laceration S37.93
      obstetrical trauma NEC O71.5
      specified
        site NEC S37.899
          contusion S37.892
          laceration S37.893
          specified type NEC S37.898
        type NEC S37.99
    specified NEC S39.83
  penis S39.94
  perineum S39.94
  peritoneum S36.81
    laceration S36.893
  periurethral tissue —see Injury, urethra
    complicating delivery O71.82
  phalanges
    foot —see Injury, foot
    hand —see Injury, hand
  pharynx NEC S19.85
  pleura —see Injury, intrathoracic, pleura
  plexus
    brachial —see Injury, brachial plexus
    cardiac —see Injury, nerve, thorax,
      sympathetic
    celiac, coeliac —see Injury, nerve,
      lumbosacral, sympathetic
    esophageal —see Injury, nerve, thorax,
      sympathetic
    hypogastric —see Injury, nerve,
      lumbosacral, sympathetic
    lumbar, lumbosacral —see Injury,
      lumbosacral plexus
    mesenteric —see Injury, nerve, lumbosacral,
      sympathetic
    pulmonary —see Injury, nerve, thorax,
      sympathetic

◄ New   ◄ Revised   ~~deleted~~ Deleted

Injury *(Continued)*
postcardiac surgery (syndrome) I97.0
prepuce S39.94
prostate S37.829
    contusion S37.822
    laceration S37.823
    specified type NEC S37.828
pubic region S39.94
pudendum S39.94
pulmonary plexus —*see* Injury, nerve, thorax,
    sympathetic
rectovaginal septum NEC S39.83
rectum —*see* Injury, intestine, large, rectum
retina —*see* Injury, eye, specified site NEC
    penetrating —*see* Injury, eyeball,
        penetrating
retroperitoneal —*see* Injury, intra-abdominal,
    specified site NEC
rotator cuff (muscle (s)) (tendon (s)) S46.00-
    laceration S46.02-
    specified type NEC S46.09-
    strain S46.01-
round ligament —*see* Injury, pelvic organ,
    specified site NEC
sacral plexus —*see* Injury, lumbosacral
    plexus
salivary duct or gland S09.93
scalp S09.90
    newborn (birth injury) P12.9
        due to monitoring (electrode) (sampling
            incision) P12.4
        specified NEC P12.89
            caput succedaneum P12.81
scapular region —*see* Injury, shoulder
sclera —*see* Injury, eye, specified site NEC
    penetrating —*see* Injury, eyeball,
        penetrating
scrotum S39.94
second cranial nerve (optic) —*see* Injury,
    nerve, optic
seminal vesicle —*see* Injury, pelvic organ,
    specified site NEC
seventh cranial nerve (facial) —*see* Injury,
    nerve, facial
shoulder S49.9-
    blood vessel —*see* Injury, blood vessel,
        arm
    contusion —*see* Contusion, shoulder
    dislocation —*see* Dislocation, shoulder
    fracture —*see* Fracture, shoulder
    muscle —*see* Injury, muscle, shoulder
    nerve —*see* Injury, nerve, shoulder
    open —*see* Wound, open, shoulder
    specified type NEC S49.8-
    sprain —*see* Sprain, shoulder girdle
    superficial —*see* Injury, superficial,
        shoulder
sinus
    cavernous —*see* Injury, intracranial
    nasal S09.92
sixth cranial nerve (abducent) —*see* Injury,
    nerve, abducens
skeleton, birth injury P13.9
    specified part NEC P13.8
skin NEC T14.8
    surface intact —*see* Injury, superficial
skull NEC S09.90
specified NEC T14.8
spermatic cord (pelvic region) S37.898
    scrotal region S39.848
spinal (cord)
    cervical (neck) S14.109
        anterior cord syndrome S14.139
            C1 level S14.131
            C2 level S14.132
            C3 level S14.133
            C4 level S14.134
            C5 level S14.135
            C6 level S14.136
            C7 level S14.137
            C8 level S14.138

Injury *(Continued)*
spinal *(Continued)*
    cervical *(Continued)*
        Brown-Séquard syndrome
            S14.149
            C1 level S14.141
            C2 level S14.142
            C3 level S14.143
            C4 level S14.144
            C5 level S14.145
            C6 level S14.146
            C7 level S14.147
            C8 level S14.148
        C1 level S14.101
        C2 level S14.102
        C3 level S14.103
        C4 level S14.104
        C5 level S14.105
        C6 level S14.106
        C7 level S14.107
        C8 level S14.108
        central cord syndrome S14.129
            C1 level S14.121
            C2 level S14.122
            C3 level S14.123
            C4 level S14.124
            C5 level S14.125
            C6 level S14.126
            C7 level S14.127
            C8 level S14.128
        complete lesion S14.119
            C1 level S14.111
            C2 level S14.112
            C3 level S14.113
            C4 level S14.114
            C5 level S14.115
            C6 level S14.116
            C7 level S14.117
            C8 level S14.118
        concussion S14.0
        edema S14.0
        incomplete lesion specified NEC
            S14.159
            C1 level S14.151
            C2 level S14.152
            C3 level S14.153
            C4 level S14.154
            C5 level S14.155
            C6 level S14.156
            C7 level S14.157
            C8 level S14.158
        posterior cord syndrome S14.159
            C1 level S14.151
            C2 level S14.152
            C3 level S14.153
            C4 level S14.154
            C5 level S14.155
            C6 level S14.156
            C7 level S14.157
            C8 level S14.158
    dorsal —*see* Injury, spinal, thoracic
    lumbar S34.109
        complete lesion S34.119
            L1 level S34.111
            L2 level S34.112
            L3 level S34.113
            L4 level S34.114
            L5 level S34.115
        concussion S34.01
        edema S34.01
        incomplete lesion S34.129
            L1 level S34.121
            L2 level S34.122
            L3 level S34.123
            L4 level S34.124
            L5 level S34.125
        L1 level S34.101
        L2 level S34.102
        L3 level S34.103
        L4 level S34.104
        L5 level S34.105

Injury *(Continued)*
spinal *(Continued)*
    nerve root NEC
        cervical —*see* Injury, nerve, spinal, root,
            cervical
        dorsal —*see* Injury, nerve, spinal, root,
            dorsal
        lumbar S34.21
        sacral S34.22
        thoracic —*see* Injury, nerve, spinal, root,
            dorsal
    plexus
        brachial —*see* Injury, brachial plexus
        lumbosacral —*see* Injury, lumbosacral
            plexus
    sacral S34.139
        complete lesion S34.131
        incomplete lesion S34.132
    thoracic S24.109
        anterior cord syndrome S24.139
            T1 level S24.131
            T2-T6 level S24.132
            T7-T10 level S24.133
            T11-T12 level S24.134
        Brown-Séquard syndrome
            S24.149
            T1 level S24.141
            T2-T6 level S24.142
            T7-T10 level S24.143
            T11-T12 level S24.144
        complete lesion S24.119
            T1 level S24.111
            T2-T6 level S24.112
            T7-T10 level S24.113
            T11-T12 level S24.114
        concussion S24.0
        edema S24.0
        incomplete lesion specified NEC
            S24.159
            T1 level S24.151
            T2-T6 level S24.152
            T7-T10 level S24.153
            T11-T12 level S24.154
        posterior cord syndrome S24.159
            T1 level S24.151
            T2-T6 level S24.152
            T7-T10 level S24.153
            T11-T12 level S24.154
        T1 level S24.101
        T2-T6 level S24.102
        T7-T10 level S24.103
        T11-T12 level S24.104
    splanchnic nerve —*see* Injury, nerve,
        lumbosacral, sympathetic
    spleen S36.00
        contusion S36.029
            major S36.021
            minor S36.020
        laceration S36.039
            major (massive) (stellate) S36.032
            moderate S36.031
            superficial (capsular) (minor)
                S36.030
        specified type NEC S36.09
    splenic artery —*see* Injury, blood vessel,
        celiac artery, branch
    stellate ganglion —*see* Injury, nerve,
        thorax, sympathetic
    sternal region S29.9
    stomach S36.30
        contusion S36.32
        laceration S36.33
        specified type NEC S36.39
    subconjunctival —*see* Injury, eye,
        conjunctiva
    subcutaneous NEC T14.8
    submaxillary region S09.93
    submental region S09.93
    subungual
        fingers —*see* Injury, hand
        toes —*see* Injury, foot

Injury (Continued)
  superficial NEC T14.8
    abdomen, abdominal (wall) S30.92
      abrasion S30.811
      bite S30.871
        insect S30.861
      contusion S30.1
      external constriction S30.841
      foreign body S30.851
    abrasion —see Abrasion, by site
    adnexa, eye NEC —see Injury, eye,
      specified site NEC
    alveolar process —see Injury, superficial,
      oral cavity
    ankle S90.91-
      abrasion —see Abrasion, ankle
      bite —see Bite, ankle
      blister —see Blister, ankle
      contusion —see Contusion, ankle
      external constriction —see Constriction,
        external, ankle
      foreign body —see Foreign body,
        superficial, ankle
    anus S30.98
    arm (upper) S40.92-
      abrasion —see Abrasion, arm
      bite —see Bite, superficial, arm
      blister —see Blister, arm (upper)
      contusion —see Contusion, arm
      external constriction —see Constriction,
        external, arm
      foreign body —see Foreign body,
        superficial, arm
    auditory canal (external) (meatus) —see
      Injury, superficial, ear
    auricle —see Injury, superficial, ear
    axilla —see Injury, superficial, arm
    back —see also Injury, superficial, thorax,
      back
      lower S30.91
        abrasion S30.810
        contusion S30.0
        external constriction S30.840
        superficial
          bite NEC S30.870
            insect S30.860
          foreign body S30.850
    bite NEC —see Bite, superficial NEC, by
      site
    blister —see Blister, by site
    breast S20.10-
      abrasion —see Abrasion, breast
      bite —see Bite, superficial, breast
      contusion —see Contusion, breast
      external constriction —see Constriction,
        external, breast
      foreign body —see Foreign body,
        superficial, breast
    brow —see Injury, superficial, head,
      specified NEC
    buttock S30.91
    calf —see Injury, superficial, leg
    canthus, eye —see Injury, superficial,
      periocular area
    cheek (external) —see Injury, superficial,
      head, specified NEC
      internal —see Injury, superficial, oral
        cavity
    chest wall —see Injury, superficial,
      thorax
    chin —see Injury, superficial, head NEC
    clitoris S30.95
    conjunctiva —see Injury, eye, conjunctiva
      with foreign body (in conjunctival
        sac) —see Foreign body,
        conjunctival sac
    contusion —see Contusion, by site
    costal region —see Injury, superficial,
      thorax
    digit (s)
      hand —see Injury, superficial, finger

Injury (Continued)
  superficial NEC (Continued)
    ear (auricle) (canal) (external) S00.40-
      abrasion —see Abrasion, ear
      bite —see Bite, superficial, ear
      contusion —see Contusion, ear
      external constriction —see Constriction,
        external, ear
      foreign body —see Foreign body,
        superficial, ear
    elbow S50.90-
      abrasion —see Abrasion, elbow
      bite —see Bite, superficial, elbow
      blister —see Blister, elbow
      contusion —see Contusion, elbow
      external constriction —see Constriction,
        external, elbow
      foreign body —see Foreign body,
        superficial, elbow
    epididymis S30.94
    epigastric region S30.92
    epiglottis —see Injury, superficial, throat
    esophagus
      cervical —see Injury, superficial, throat
    external constriction —see Constriction,
      external, by site
    extremity NEC T14.8
    eyeball NEC —see Injury, eye, specified
      site NEC
    eyebrow —see Injury, superficial,
      periocular area
    eyelid S00.20-
      abrasion —see Abrasion, eyelid
      bite —see Bite, superficial, eyelid
      contusion —see Contusion, eyelid
      external constriction —see Constriction,
        external, eyelid
      foreign body —see Foreign body,
        superficial, eyelid
    face NEC —see Injury, superficial, head,
      specified NEC
    finger (s) S60.949
      abrasion —see Abrasion, finger
      bite —see Bite, superficial, finger
      blister —see Blister, finger
      contusion —see Contusion, finger
      external constriction —see Constriction,
        external, finger
      foreign body —see Foreign body,
        superficial, finger
      index S60.94-
      insect bite —see Bite, by site, superficial,
        insect
      little S60.94-
      middle S60.94-
      ring S60.94-
    flank S30.92
    foot S90.92-
      abrasion —see Abrasion, foot
      bite —see Bite, foot
      blister —see Blister, foot
      contusion —see Contusion, foot
      external constriction —see Constriction,
        external, foot
      foreign body —see Foreign body,
        superficial, foot
    forearm S50.91-
      abrasion —see Abrasion, forearm
      bite —see Bite, forearm, superficial
      blister —see Blister, forearm
      contusion —see Contusion, forearm
      elbow only —see Injury, superficial,
        elbow
      external constriction —see Constriction,
        external, forearm
      foreign body —see Foreign body,
        superficial, forearm
    forehead —see Injury, superficial, head
      NEC
    foreign body —see Foreign body,
      superficial

Injury (Continued)
  superficial NEC (Continued)
    genital organs, external
      female S30.97
      male S30.96
    globe (eye) —see Injury, eye, specified site
      NEC
    groin S30.92
    gum —see Injury, superficial, oral cavity
    hand S60.92-
      abrasion —see Abrasion, hand
      bite —see Bite, superficial, hand
      contusion —see Contusion, hand
      external constriction —see Constriction,
        external, hand
      foreign body —see Foreign body,
        superficial, hand
    head S00.90
      ear —see Injury, superficial, ear
      eyelid —see Injury, superficial, eyelid
      nose S00.30
      oral cavity S00.502
      scalp S00.00
      specified site NEC S00.80
    heel —see Injury, superficial, foot
    hip S70.91-
      abrasion —see Abrasion, hip
      bite —see Bite, superficial, hip
      blister —see Blister, hip
      contusion —see Contusion, hip
      external constriction —see Constriction,
        external, hip
      foreign body —see Foreign body,
        superficial, hip
    iliac region —see Injury, superficial,
      abdomen
    inguinal region —see Injury, superficial,
      abdomen
    insect bite —see Bite, by site, superficial,
      insect
    interscapular region —see Injury,
      superficial, thorax, back
    jaw —see Injury, superficial, head, specified
      NEC
    knee S80.91-
      abrasion —see Abrasion, knee
      bite —see Bite, superficial, knee
      blister —see Blister, knee
      contusion —see Contusion, knee
      external constriction —see Constriction,
        external, knee
      foreign body —see Foreign body,
        superficial, knee
    labium (majus) (minus) S30.95
    lacrimal (apparatus) (gland) (sac) —see
      Injury, eye, specified site NEC
    larynx —see Injury, superficial, throat
    leg (lower) S80.92-
      abrasion —see Abrasion, leg
      bite —see Bite, superficial, leg
      contusion —see Contusion, leg
      external constriction —see Constriction,
        external, leg
      foreign body —see Foreign body,
        superficial, leg
      knee —see Injury, superficial, knee
    limb NEC T14.8
    lip S00.501
    lower back S30.91
    lumbar region S30.91
    malar region —see Injury, superficial, head,
      specified NEC
    mammary —see Injury, superficial, breast
    mastoid region —see Injury, superficial,
      head, specified NEC
    mouth —see Injury, superficial, oral
      cavity
    muscle NEC T14.8
    nail NEC T14.8
      finger —see Injury, superficial, finger
      toe —see Injury, superficial, toe

◀ New   ◀▥ Revised   ~~deleted~~ Deleted

Injury *(Continued)*
  superficial NEC *(Continued)*
    nasal (septum) —*see* Injury, superficial, nose
    neck S10.90
      specified site NEC S10.80
    nose (septum) S00.30
    occipital region —*see* Injury, superficial, scalp
    oral cavity S00.502
    orbital region —*see* Injury, superficial, periocular area
    palate —*see* Injury, superficial, oral cavity
    palm —*see* Injury, superficial, hand
    parietal region —*see* Injury, superficial, scalp
    pelvis S30.91
      girdle —*see* Injury, superficial, hip
    penis S30.93
    perineum
      female S30.95
      male S30.91
    periocular area S00.20-
      abrasion —*see* Abrasion, eyelid
      bite —*see* Bite, superficial, eyelid
      contusion —*see* Contusion, eyelid
      external constriction —*see* Constriction, external, eyelid
      foreign body —*see* Foreign body, superficial, eyelid
    phalanges
      finger —*see* Injury, superficial, finger
      toe —*see* Injury, superficial, toe
    pharynx —*see* Injury, superficial, throat
    pinna —*see* Injury, superficial, ear
    popliteal space —*see* Injury, superficial, knee
    prepuce S30.93
    pubic region S30.91
    pudendum
      female S30.97
      male S30.96
    sacral region S30.91
    scalp S00.00
    scapular region —*see* Injury, superficial, shoulder
    sclera —*see* Injury, eye, specified site NEC
    scrotum S30.94
    shin —*see* Injury, superficial, leg
    shoulder S40.91-
      abrasion —*see* Abrasion, shoulder
      bite —*see* Bite, superficial, shoulder
      blister —*see* Blister, shoulder
      contusion —*see* Contusion, shoulder
      external constriction —*see* Constriction, external, shoulder
      foreign body —*see* Foreign body, superficial, shoulder
    skin NEC T14.8
    sternal region —*see* Injury, superficial, thorax, front
    subconjunctival —*see* Injury, eye, specified site NEC
    subcutaneous NEC T14.8
    submaxillary region —*see* Injury, superficial, head, specified NEC
    submental region —*see* Injury, superficial, head, specified NEC
    subungual
      finger (s) —*see* Injury, superficial, finger
      toe (s) —*see* Injury, superficial, toe
    supraclavicular fossa —*see* Injury, superficial, neck
    supraorbital —*see* Injury, superficial, head, specified NEC
    temple —*see* Injury, superficial, head, specified NEC
    temporal region —*see* Injury, superficial, head, specified NEC
    testis S30.94

Injury *(Continued)*
  superficial NEC *(Continued)*
    thigh S70.92-
      abrasion —*see* Abrasion, thigh
      bite —*see* Bite, superficial, thigh
      blister —*see* Blister, thigh
      contusion —*see* Contusion, thigh
      external constriction —*see* Constriction, external, thigh
      foreign body —*see* Foreign body, superficial, thigh
    thorax, thoracic (wall) S20.90
      abrasion —*see* Abrasion, thorax
      back S20.40-
      bite —*see* Bite, thorax, superficial
      blister —*see* Blister, thorax
      contusion —*see* Contusion, thorax
      external constriction —*see* Constriction, external, thorax
      foreign body —*see* Foreign body, superficial, thorax
      front S20.30-
    throat S10.10
      abrasion S10.11
      bite S10.17
        insect S10.16
      blister S10.12
      contusion S10.0
      external constriction S10.14
      foreign body S10.15
    thumb S60.93-
      abrasion —*see* Abrasion, thumb
      bite —*see* Bite, superficial, thumb
      blister —*see* Blister, thumb
      contusion —*see* Contusion, thumb
      external constriction —*see* Constriction, external, thumb
      foreign body —*see* Foreign body, superficial, thumb
      insect bite —*see* Bite, by site, superficial, insect
      specified type NEC S60.39-
    toe (s) S90.93-
      abrasion —*see* Abrasion, toe
      bite —*see* Bite, toe
      blister —*see* Blister, toe
      contusion —*see* Contusion, toe
      external constriction —*see* Constriction, external, toe
      foreign body —*see* Foreign body, superficial, toe
      great S90.93-
    tongue —*see* Injury, superficial, oral cavity
    tooth, teeth —*see* Injury, superficial, oral cavity
    trachea S10.10
    tunica vaginalis S30.94
    tympanum, tympanic membrane —*see* Injury, superficial, ear
    uvula —*see* Injury, superficial, oral cavity
    vagina S30.95
    vocal cords —*see* Injury, superficial, throat
    vulva S30.95
    wrist S60.91-
  supraclavicular region —*see* Injury, neck
  supraorbital S09.93
  suprarenal gland (multiple) —*see* Injury, adrenal
  surgical complication (external or internal site) —*see* Laceration, accidental complicating surgery
  temple S09.90
  temporal region S09.90
  tendon —*see also* Injury, muscle, by site
    abdomen —*see* Injury, muscle, abdomen
    Achilles —*see* Injury, Achilles tendon
    lower back —*see* Injury, muscle, lower back
    pelvic organs —*see* Injury, muscle, pelvis

Injury *(Continued)*
  tenth cranial nerve (pneumogastric or vagus) —*see* Injury, nerve, vagus
  testis S39.94
  thigh S79.92-
    blood vessel —*see* Injury, blood vessel, hip
    contusion —*see* Contusion, thigh
    fracture —*see* Fracture, femur
    muscle —*see* Injury, muscle, thigh
    nerve —*see* Injury, nerve, thigh
    open —*see* Wound, open, thigh
    specified NEC S79.82-
    superficial —*see* Injury, superficial, thigh
  third cranial nerve (oculomotor) —*see* Injury, nerve, oculomotor
  thorax, thoracic S29.9
    blood vessel —*see* Injury, blood vessel, thorax
    cavity —*see* Injury, intrathoracic
    dislocation —*see* Dislocation, thorax
    external (wall) S29.9
      contusion —*see* Contusion, thorax
      nerve —*see* Injury, nerve, thorax
      open —*see* Wound, open, thorax
      specified NEC S29.8
      sprain —*see* Sprain, thorax
      superficial —*see* Injury, superficial, thorax
    fracture —*see* Fracture, thorax
    internal —*see* Injury, intrathoracic
    intrathoracic organ —*see* Injury, intrathoracic
    sympathetic ganglion —*see* Injury, nerve, thorax, sympathetic
  throat (*see also* Injury, neck) S19.9
  thumb S69.9-
    blood vessel —*see* Injury, blood vessel, thumb
    contusion —*see* Contusion, thumb
    dislocation —*see* Dislocation, thumb
    fracture —*see* Fracture, thumb
    muscle —*see* Injury, muscle, thumb
    nerve —*see* Injury, nerve, digital, thumb
    open —*see* Wound, open, thumb
    specified NEC S69.8-
    sprain —*see* Sprain, thumb
    superficial —*see* Injury, superficial, thumb
  thymus (gland) —*see* Injury, intrathoracic, specified organ NEC
  thyroid (gland) NEC S19.84
  toe S99.92-
    contusion —*see* Contusion, toe
    dislocation —*see* Dislocation, toe
    fracture —*see* Fracture, toe
    muscle —*see* Injury, muscle, toe
    open —*see* Wound, open, toe
    specified type NEC S99.82-
    sprain —*see* Sprain, toe
    superficial —*see* Injury, superficial, toe
  tongue S09.93
  tonsil S09.93
  tooth S09.93
  trachea (cervical) NEC S19.82
    thoracic —*see* Injury, intrathoracic, trachea, thoracic
  transfusion-related acute lung (TRALI) J95.84
  tunica vaginalis S39.94
  twelfth cranial nerve (hypoglossal) —*see* Injury, nerve, hypoglossal
  ureter S37.10
    contusion S37.12
    laceration S37.13
    specified type NEC S37.19
  urethra (sphincter) S37.30
    at delivery O71.5
    contusion S37.32
    laceration S37.33
    specified type NEC S37.38

◀ New ◀▦ Revised ~~deleted~~ Deleted

Insufficiency, insufficient *(Continued)*
  aortic *(Continued)*
    rheumatic I06.1
      with
        mitral (valve) disease I08.0
          with tricuspid (valve) disease
            I08.3
        stenosis I06.2
          with mitral (valve) disease I08.0
            with tricuspid (valve) disease
              I08.3
        tricuspid (valve) disease I08.2
          with mitral (valve) disease I08.3
    specified cause NEC I35.1
    syphilitic A52.03
  arterial I77.1
    basilar G45.0
    carotid (hemispheric) G45.1
    cerebral I67.81
    coronary (acute or subacute) I24.8
    mesenteric K55.1
    peripheral I73.9
    precerebral (multiple) (bilateral) G45.2
    vertebral G45.0
  arteriovenous I99.8
  biliary K83.8
  cardiac —*see also* Insufficiency, myocardial
    due to presence of (cardiac) prosthesis
      I97.11-
    postprocedural I97.11-
  cardiorenal, hypertensive I13.2
  cardiovascular —*see* Disease, cardiovascular
  cerebrovascular (acute) I67.81
    with transient focal neurological signs and
      symptoms G45.8
  circulatory NEC I99.8
    newborn P29.89
  convergence H51.11
  coronary (acute or subacute) I24.8
    chronic or with a stated duration of over 4
      weeks I25.89
  corticoadrenal E27.40
    primary E27.1
  dietary E63.9
  divergence H51.8
  food T73.0
  gastroesophageal K22.8
  gonadal
    ovary E28.39
    testis E29.1
  heart —*see also* Insufficiency, myocardial
    newborn P29.0
    valve —*see* Endocarditis
  hepatic —*see* Failure, hepatic
  idiopathic autonomic G90.09
  interocclusal distance of fully erupted teeth
    (ridge) M26.36
  kidney N28.9
    acute N28.9
    chronic N18.9
  lacrimal (secretion) H04.12-
    passages —*see* Stenosis, lacrimal
  liver —*see* Failure, hepatic
  lung —*see* Insufficiency, pulmonary
  mental (congenital) —*see* Disability,
    intellectual
  mesenteric K55.1
  mitral (valve) I34.0
    with
      aortic valve disease I08.0
        with tricuspid (valve) disease
          I08.3
      obstruction or stenosis I05.2
        with aortic valve disease I08.0
      tricuspid (valve) disease I08.1
        with aortic (valve) disease I08.3
    congenital Q23.3
    rheumatic I05.1
      with
        aortic valve disease I08.0
          with tricuspid (valve) disease I08.3

Insufficiency, insufficient *(Continued)*
  mitral *(Continued)*
    rheumatic *(Continued)*
      with *(Continued)*
        obstruction or stenosis I05.2
          with aortic valve disease I08.0
            with tricuspid (valve) disease
              I08.3
        tricuspid (valve) disease I08.1
          with aortic (valve) disease I08.3
      active or acute I01.1
        with chorea, rheumatic (Sydenham's)
          I02.0
    specified cause, except rheumatic
      I34.0
  muscle —*see also* Disease, muscle
    heart —*see* Insufficiency, myocardial
  ocular NEC H50.9
  myocardial, myocardium (with
    arteriosclerosis) I50.9
    with
      rheumatic fever (conditions in I00)
        I09.9
        active, acute or subacute I01.2
          with chorea I02.0
        inactive or quiescent (with chorea)
          I09.0
    congenital Q24.8
    hypertensive —*see* Hypertension, heart
    newborn P29.0
    rheumatic I09.0
      active, acute, or subacute I01.2
    syphilitic A52.06
  nourishment T73.0
  pancreatic K86.8
  parathyroid (gland) E20.9
  peripheral vascular (arterial) I73.9
  pituitary E23.0
  placental (mother) O36.51-
  platelets D69.6
  prenatal care affecting management of
    pregnancy O09.3-
  progressive pluriglandular E31.0
  pulmonary J98.4
    acute, following surgery (nonthoracic)
      J95.2
      thoracic J95.1
    chronic, following surgery J95.3
    following
      shock J98.4
      trauma J98.4
    newborn P28.5
    valve I37.1
      with stenosis I37.2
      congenital Q22.2
      rheumatic I09.89
        with aortic, mitral or tricuspid (valve)
          disease I08.8
  pyloric K31.89
  renal (acute) N28.9
    chronic N18.9
  respiratory R06.89
    newborn P28.5
  rotation —*see* Malrotation
  sleep syndrome F51.12
  social insurance Z59.7
  suprarenal E27.40
    primary E27.1
  tarso-orbital fascia, congenital Q10.3
  testis E29.1
  thyroid (gland) (acquired) E03.9
    congenital E03.1
  tricuspid (valve) (rheumatic) I07.1
    with
      aortic (valve) disease I08.2
        with mitral (valve) disease I08.3
      mitral (valve) disease I08.1
        with aortic (valve) disease I08.3
      obstruction or stenosis I07.2
        with aortic (valve) disease I08.2
        with mitral (valve) disease I08.3

Insufficiency, insufficient *(Continued)*
  tricuspid *(Continued)*
    congenital Q22.8
    nonrheumatic I36.1
      with stenosis I36.2
  urethral sphincter R32
  valve, valvular (heart) —*see* Endocarditis
    congenital Q24.8
  vascular I99.8
    intestine K55.9
      acute K55.0
      mesenteric K55.1
      peripheral I73.9
    renal —*see* Hypertension, kidney
  velopharyngeal
    acquired K13.79
    congenital Q38.8
  venous (chronic) (peripheral) I87.2
  ventricular —*see* Insufficiency, myocardial
  welfare support Z59.7
Insufflation, fallopian Z31.41
Insular —*see* condition
Insulinoma
  pancreas
    benign D13.7
    malignant C25.4
    uncertain behavior D37.8
  specified site
    benign —*see* Neoplasm, by site, benign
    malignant —*see* Neoplasm, by site,
      malignant
    uncertain behavior —*see* Neoplasm, by site,
      uncertain behavior
  unspecified site
    benign D13.7
    malignant C25.4
    uncertain behavior D37.8
Insuloma —*see* Insulinoma
Interference
  balancing side M26.56
  non-working side M26.56
Intermenstrual —*see* condition
Intermittent —*see* condition
Internal —*see* condition
Interrogation
  cardiac defibrillator (automatic) (implantable)
    Z45.02
  cardiac pacemaker Z45.018
  cardiac (event) (loop) recorder Z45.09
  infusion pump (implanted) (intrathecal)
    Z45.1
  neurostimulator Z46.2
Interruption
  phase-shift, sleep cycle —*see* Disorder, sleep,
    circadian rhythm
  sleep phase-shift, or 24 hour sleep-wake
    cycle —*see* Disorder, sleep, circadian
    rhythm
Interstitial —*see* condition
Intertrigo L30.4
  labialis K13.0
Intervertebral disc —*see* condition
Intestine, intestinal —*see* condition
Intolerance
  carbohydrate K90.4
  disaccharide, hereditary E73.0
  fat NEC K90.4
    pancreatic K90.3
  food K90.4
    dietary counseling and surveillance
      Z71.3
  fructose E74.10
    hereditary E74.12
  glucose(-galactose) E74.39
  gluten K90.0
  lactose E73.9
    specified NEC E73.8
  lysine E72.3
  milk NEC K90.4
    lactose E73.9
  protein K90.4

Intolerance *(Continued)*
starch NEC K90.4
sucrose (-isomaltose) E74.31
Intoxicated NEC (without dependence) —*see*
Alcohol, intoxication
Intoxication
acid E87.2
alcoholic (acute) (without dependence) —*see*
Alcohol, intoxication
alimentary canal K52.1
amphetamine (without dependence) —
see Abuse, drug, stimulant, with
intoxication
with dependence —*see* Dependence, drug,
stimulant, with intoxication
anxiolytic (acute) (without dependence) —*see*
Abuse, drug, sedative, with intoxication
with dependence —*see* Dependence, drug,
sedative, with intoxication
caffeine (acute) (without dependence) —
see Abuse, drug, stimulant, with
intoxication
with dependence —*see* Dependence, drug,
stimulant, with intoxication
cannabinoids (acute) (without dependence) —
see Abuse, drug, cannabis, with
intoxication
with dependence —*see* Dependence, drug,
cannabis, with intoxication
chemical —*see* Table of Drugs and
Chemicals
via placenta or breast milk —*see* -
Absorption, chemical, through
placenta
cocaine (acute) (without dependence) —*see*
Abuse, drug, cocaine, with intoxication
with dependence —*see* Dependence, drug,
cocaine, with intoxication
drug
acute (without dependence) —*see* Abuse,
drug, by type with intoxication
with dependence —*see* Dependence,
drug, by type with intoxication
addictive
via placenta or breast milk —*see*
Absorption, drug, addictive,
through placenta
newborn P93.8
gray baby syndrome P93.0
overdose or wrong substance given or
taken —*see* Table of Drugs and
Chemicals, by drug, poisoning
enteric K52.1
foodborne A05.9
bacterial A05.9
classical (Clostridium botulinum) A05.1
due to
Bacillus cereus A05.4
bacterium A05.9
specified NEC A05.8
Clostridium
botulinum A05.1
perfringens A05.2
welchii A05.2
Salmonella A02.9
with
(gastro) enteritis A02.0
localized infection (s) A02.20
arthritis A02.23
meningitis A02.21
osteomyelitis A02.24
pneumonia A02.22
pyelonephritis A02.25
specified NEC A02.29
sepsis A02.1
specified manifestation NEC A02.8
Staphylococcus A05.0
Vibrio
parahaemolyticus A05.3
vulnificus A05.5
enterotoxin, staphylococcal A05.0
noxious —*see* Poisoning, food, noxious

Intoxication *(Continued)*
gastrointestinal K52.1
hallucinogenic (without dependence) —*see*
Abuse, drug, hallucinogen, with
intoxication
with dependence —*see* Dependence, drug,
hallucinogen, with intoxication
hypnotic (acute) (without dependence) —*see*
Abuse, drug, sedative, with intoxication
with dependence —*see* Dependence, drug,
sedative, with intoxication
inhalant (acute) (without dependence) —*see*
Abuse, drug, inhalant, with intoxication
with dependence —*see* Dependence, drug,
inhalant, with intoxication
meaning
inebriation —*see* category F10
poisoning —*see* Table of Drugs and
Chemicals
methyl alcohol (acute) (without
dependence) —*see* Alcohol, intoxication
opioid (acute) (without dependence) —*see*
Abuse, drug, opioid, with intoxication
with dependence —*see* Dependence, drug,
opioid, with intoxication
pathologic NEC (without dependence) —*see*
Alcohol, intoxication
phencyclidine (without dependence) —*see*
Abuse, drug, psychoactive NEC, with
intoxication
with dependence —*see* Dependence, drug,
psychoactive NEC, with intoxication
potassium (K) E87.5
psychoactive substance NEC (without
dependence) —*see* Abuse, drug,
psychoactive NEC, with intoxication
with dependence —*see* Dependence, drug,
psychoactive NEC, with intoxication
sedative (acute) (without dependence) —*see*
Abuse, drug, sedative, with intoxication
with dependence —*see* Dependence, drug,
sedative, with intoxication
serum (*see also* Reaction, serum) T80.69
uremic —*see* Uremia
volatile solvents (acute) (without
dependence) —*see* Abuse, drug, inhalant,
with intoxication
with dependence —*see* Dependence, drug,
inhalant, with intoxication
water E87.79
Intracranial —*see* condition
Intrahepatic gallbladder Q44.1
Intraligamentous —*see* condition
Intrathoracic —*see also* condition
kidney Q63.2
Intrauterine contraceptive device
checking Z30.431
in situ Z97.5
insertion Z30.430
immediately following removal Z30.433
management Z30.431
reinsertion Z30.433
removal Z30.432
replacement Z30.433
retention in pregnancy O26.3-
Intraventricular —*see* condition
Intrinsic deformity —*see* Deformity
Intubation, difficult or failed T88.4
Intumescence, lens (eye) (cataract) —*see* Cataract
Intussusception (bowel) (colon) (enteric)
(ileocecal) (ileocolic) (intestine) (rectum)
K56.1
appendix K38.8
congenital Q43.8
ureter (with obstruction) N13.5
Invagination (bowel, colon, intestine or rectum)
K56.1
Inversion
albumin-globulin (A-G) ratio E88.09
bladder N32.89
cecum —*see* Intussusception
cervix N88.8

Inversion *(Continued)*
chromosome in normal individual Q95.1
circadian rhythm —*see* Disorder, sleep,
circadian rhythm
nipple N64.59
congenital Q83.8
gestational —*see* Retraction, nipple
puerperal, postpartum —*see* Retraction,
nipple
nyctohemeral rhythm —*see* Disorder, sleep,
circadian rhythm
optic papilla Q14.2
organ or site, congenital NEC —*see* Anomaly,
by site
sleep rhythm —*see* Disorder, sleep, circadian
rhythm
testis (congenital) Q55.29
uterus (chronic) (postinfectional) (postpartal,
old) N85.5
postpartum O71.2
vagina (posthysterectomy) N99.3
ventricular Q20.5
Investigation (*see also* Examination) Z04.9
clinical research subject (control) (normal
comparison) (participant) Z00.6
Involuntary movement, abnormal R25.9
Involution, involutional —*see also* condition
breast, cystic —*see* Dysplasia, mammary,
specified type NEC
depression (single episode) F32.8
recurrent episode F33.9
melancholia (recurrent episode) (single
episode) F32.8
ovary, senile —*see* Atrophy, ovary
thymus failure E32.8
I.Q.
under 20 F73
20-34 F72
35-49 F71
50-69 F70
IRDS (type I) P22.0
type II P22.1
Irideremia Q13.1
Iridis rubeosis —*see* Disorder, iris, vascular
Iridochoroiditis (panuveitis) —*see* Panuveitis
Iridocyclitis H20.9-
acute H20.0-
hypopyon H20.05-
primary H20.01-
recurrent H20.02-
secondary (noninfectious) H20.04-
infectious H20.03-
chronic H20.1-
due to allergy —*see* Iridocyclitis, acute,
secondary
endogenous —*see* Iridocyclitis, acute, primary
Fuchs' —*see* Cyclitis, Fuchs' heterochromic
gonococcal A54.32
granulomatous —*see* Iridocyclitis, chronic
herpes, herpetic (simplex) B00.51
zoster B02.32
hypopyon —*see* Iridocyclitis, acute, hypopyon
in (due to)
ankylosing spondylitis M45.9
gonococcal infection A54.32
herpes (simplex) virus B00.51
zoster B02.32
infectious disease NOS B99
parasitic disease NOS B89 *[H22]*
sarcoidosis D86.83
syphilis A51.43
tuberculosis A18.54
zoster B02.32
lens-induced H20.2-
nongranulomatous —*see* Iridocyclitis, acute
recurrent —*see* Iridocyclitis, acute, recurrent
rheumatic —*see* Iridocyclitis, chronic
subacute —*see* Iridocyclitis, acute
sympathetic —*see* Uveitis, sympathetic
syphilitic (secondary) A51.43
tuberculous (chronic) A18.54
Vogt-Koyanagi H20.82-

◄ New ◀▥▥ Revised ~~deleted~~ Deleted

Iridocyclochoroiditis (panuveitis) —see Panuveitis
Iridodialysis H21.53-
Iridodonesis H21.89
Iridoplegia (complete) (partial) (reflex) H57.09
Iridoschisis H21.25-
Iris —see also condition
  bombé —see Membrane, pupillary
Iritis —see also Iridocyclitis
  chronic —see Iridocyclitis, chronic
  diabetic —see E08-E13 with .39
  due to
    herpes simplex B00.51
    leprosy A30.9 [H22]
  gonococcal A54.32
  gouty M10.9
  granulomatous —see Iridocyclitis, chronic
  lens induced —see Iridocyclitis, lens-induced
  papulosa (syphilitic) A52.71
  rheumatic —see Iridocyclitis, chronic
  syphilitic (secondary) A51.43
    congenital (early) A50.01
    late A52.71
  tuberculous A18.54
Iron —see condition
Iron-miner's lung J63.4
Irradiated enamel (tooth, teeth) K03.89
Irradiation effects, adverse T66
Irreducible, irreducibility —see condition
Irregular, irregularity
  action, heart I49.9
  alveolar process K08.8
  bleeding N92.6
  breathing R06.89
  contour of cornea (acquired) —see Deformity, cornea
    congenital Q13.4
  contour, reconstructed breast N65.0
  dentin (in pulp) K04.3
  eye movements H55.89
    nystagmus —see Nystagmus
    saccadic H55.81
  labor O62.2
  menstruation (cause unknown) N92.6
  periods N92.6
  prostate N42.9
  pupil —see Abnormality, pupillary
  reconstructed breast N65.0
  respiratory R06.89
  septum (nasal) J34.2
  shape, organ or site, congenital NEC —see Distortion
  sleep-wake pattern (rhythm) G47.23
Irritable, irritability R45.4
  bladder N32.89
  bowel (syndrome) K58.9
    with diarrhea K58.0
    psychogenic F45.8
  bronchial —see Bronchitis
  cerebral, in newborn P91.3
  colon K58.9
    with diarrhea K58.0
    psychogenic F45.8
  duodenum K59.8
  heart (psychogenic) F45.8
  hip —see Derangement, joint, specified type NEC, hip
  ileum K59.8
  infant R68.12
  jejunum K59.8
  rectum K59.8
  stomach K31.89
    psychogenic F45.8
  sympathetic G90.8
  urethra N36.8
Irritation
  anus K62.89
  axillary nerve G54.0
  bladder N32.89
  brachial plexus G54.0
  bronchial —see Bronchitis
  cervical plexus G54.2

Irritation (Continued)
  cervix —see Cervicitis
  choroid, sympathetic —see Endophthalmitis
  cranial nerve —see Disorder, nerve, cranial
  gastric K31.89
    psychogenic F45.8
  globe, sympathetic —see Uveitis, sympathetic
  labyrinth —see subcategory H83.2
  lumbosacral plexus G54.1
  meninges (traumatic) —see Injury, intracranial
    nontraumatic —see Meningismus
  nerve —see Disorder, nerve
  nervous R45.0
  penis N48.89
  perineum NEC L29.3
  peripheral autonomic nervous system G90.8
  peritoneum —see Peritonitis
  pharynx J39.2
  plantar nerve —see Lesion, nerve, plantar
  spinal (cord) (traumatic) —see also Injury, spinal cord, by region
    nerve G58.9
      root NEC —see Radiculopathy
    nontraumatic —see Myelopathy
  stomach K31.89
    psychogenic F45.8
  sympathetic nerve NEC G90.8
  ulnar nerve —see Lesion, nerve, ulnar
  vagina N89.8
Ischemia, ischemic I99.8
  bowel (transient)
    acute K55.0
    chronic K55.1
    due to mesenteric artery insufficiency K55.1
  brain —see Ischemia, cerebral
  cardiac (see Disease, heart, ischemic)
  cardiomyopathy I25.5
  cerebral (chronic) (generalized) I67.82
    arteriosclerotic I67.2
    intermittent G45.9
    newborn P91.0
    recurrent focal G45.8
    transient G45.9
  colon chronic (due to mesenteric artery insufficiency) K55.1
  coronary —see Disease, heart, ischemic
  demand (coronary) (see also Angina) I24.8
  heart (chronic or with a stated duration of over 4 weeks) I25.9
    acute or with a stated duration of 4 weeks or less I24.9
    subacute I24.9
  infarction, muscle —see Infarct, muscle
  intestine (large) (small) (transient) K55.9
    acute K55.0
    chronic K55.1
    due to mesenteric artery insufficiency K55.1
  kidney N28.0
  mesenteric, acute K55.0
  muscle, traumatic T79.6
  myocardium, myocardial (chronic or with a stated duration of over 4 weeks) I25.9
    acute, without myocardial infarction I24.0
    silent (asymptomatic) I25.6
    transient of newborn P29.4
  renal N28.0
  retina, retinal —see Occlusion, artery, retina
  small bowel
    acute K55.0
    chronic K55.1
    due to mesenteric artery insufficiency K55.1
  spinal cord G95.11
  subendocardial —see Insufficiency, coronary
  supply (coronary) (see also Angina) I25.9
    due to vasospasm I20.1
Ischial spine —see condition
Ischialgia —see Sciatica
Ischiopagus Q89.4
Ischium, ischial —see condition

Ischuria R34
Iselin's disease or osteochondrosis —see Osteochondrosis, juvenile, metatarsus
Islands of
  parotid tissue in
    lymph nodes Q38.6
    neck structures Q38.6
  submaxillary glands in
    fascia Q38.6
    lymph nodes Q38.6
    neck muscles Q38.6
Islet cell tumor, pancreas D13.7
Isoimmunization NEC —see also Incompatibility
  affecting management of pregnancy (ABO) (with hydrops fetalis) O36.11-
    anti-A sensitization O36.11-
    anti-B sensitization O36.19-
    anti-c sensitization O36.09-
    anti-C sensitization O36.09-
    anti-e sensitization O36.09-
    anti-E sensitization O36.09-
    Rh NEC O36.09-
      anti-D antibody O36.01-
    specified NEC O36.19-
  newborn P55.9
    with
      hydrops fetalis P56.0
      kernicterus P57.0
    ABO (blood groups) P55.1
    Rhesus (Rh) factor P55.0
    specified type NEC P55.8
Isolation, isolated
  dwelling Z59.8
  family Z63.79
  social Z60.4
Isoleucinosis E71.19
Isomerism atrial appendages (with asplenia or polysplenia) Q20.6
Isosporiasis, isosporosis A07.3
Isovaleric acidemia E71.110
Issue of
  medical certificate Z02.79
    for disability determination Z02.71
  repeat prescription (appliance) (glasses) (medicinal substance, medicament, medicine) Z76.0
  contraception —see Contraception
Itch, itching —see also Pruritus
  baker's L23.6
  barber's B35.0
  bricklayer's L24.5
  cheese B88.0
  clam digger's B65.3
  coolie B76.9
  copra B88.0
  dew B76.9
  dhobi B35.6
  filarial —see Infestation, filarial
  grain B88.0
  grocer's B88.0
  ground B76.9
  harvest B88.0
  jock B35.6
  Malabar B35.5
    beard B35.0
    foot B35.3
    scalp B35.0
  meaning scabies B86
  Norwegian B86
  perianal L29.0
  poultrymen's B88.0
  sarcoptic B86
  scabies B86
  scrub B88.0
  straw B88.0
  swimmer's B65.3
  water B76.9
  winter L29.8
Ivemark's syndrome (asplenia with congenital heart disease) Q89.01
Ivory bones Q78.2
Ixodiasis NEC B88.8

J

Jaccoud's syndrome —see Arthropathy, postrheumatic, chronic
Jackson's
    membrane Q43.3
    paralysis or syndrome G83.89
    veil Q43.3
Jacquet's dermatitis (diaper dermatitis) L22
Jadassohn-Pellizari's disease or anetoderma L90.2
Jadassohn's
    blue nevus —see Nevus
    intraepidermal epithelioma —see Neoplasm, skin, benign
Jaffe-Lichtenstein (-Uehlinger) syndrome —see Dysplasia, fibrous, bone NEC
Jakob-Creutzfeldt disease or syndrome —see Creutzfeldt-Jakob disease or syndrome
Jaksch-Luzet disease D64.89
Jamaican
    neuropathy G92
    paraplegic tropical ataxic-spastic syndrome G92
Janet's disease F48.8
Janiceps Q89.4
Jansky-Bielschowsky amaurotic idiocy E75.4
Japanese
    B-type encephalitis A83.0
    river fever A75.3
Jaundice (yellow) R17
    acholuric (familial) (splenomegalic) —see also Spherocytosis
        acquired D59.8
    breast-milk (inhibitor) P59.3
    catarrhal (acute) B15.9
        with hepatic coma B15.0
    cholestatic (benign) R17
    due to or associated with
        delayed conjugation P59.8
            associated with (due to) preterm delivery P59.0
        preterm delivery P59.0
    epidemic (catarrhal) B15.9
        with hepatic coma B15.0
        leptospiral A27.0
        spirochetal A27.0
    familial nonhemolytic (congenital) (Gilbert) E80.4
        Crigler-Najjar E80.5
    febrile (acute) B15.9
        with hepatic coma B15.0
        leptospiral A27.0
        spirochetal A27.0
    hematogenous D59.9
    hemolytic (acquired) D59.9
        congenital —see Spherocytosis

Jaundice (Continued)
    hemorrhagic (acute) (leptospiral) (spirochetal) A27.0
    infectious (acute) (subacute) B15.9
        with hepatic coma B15.0
        leptospiral A27.0
        spirochetal A27.0
    leptospiral (hemorrhagic) A27.0
    malignant (without coma) K72.90
        with coma K72.91
    neonatal —see Jaundice, newborn
    newborn P59.9
        due to or associated with
            ABO
                antibodies P55.1
                incompatibility, maternal/fetal P55.1
                isoimmunization P55.1
            absence or deficiency of enzyme system for bilirubin conjugation (congenital) P59.8
            bleeding P58.1
            breast milk inhibitors to conjugation P59.3
                associated with preterm delivery P59.0
            bruising P58.0
            Crigler-Najjar syndrome E80.5
            delayed conjugation P59.8
                associated with preterm delivery P59.0
            drugs or toxins
                given to newborn P58.42
                transmitted from mother P58.41
            excessive hemolysis P58.9
                due to
                    bleeding P58.1
                    bruising P58.0
                    drugs or toxins
                        given to newborn P58.42
                        transmitted from mother P58.41
                    infection P58.2
                    polycythemia P58.3
                    swallowed maternal blood P58.5
                specified type NEC P58.8
            galactosemia E74.21
            Gilbert syndrome E80.4
            hemolytic disease P55.9
                ABO isoimmunization P55.1
                Rh isoimmunization P55.0
                specified NEC P55.8
            hepatocellular damage P59.20
                specified NEC P59.29
            hereditary hemolytic anemia P58.8
            hypothyroidism, congenital E03.1
            incompatibility, maternal/fetal NOS P55.9
            infection P58.2

Jaundice (Continued)
    newborn (Continued)
        due to or associated with (Continued)
            inspissated bile syndrome P59.1
            isoimmunization NOS P55.9
            mucoviscidosis E84.9
            polycythemia P58.3
            preterm delivery P59.0
            Rh
                antibodies P55.0
                incompatibility, maternal/fetal P55.0
                isoimmunization P55.0
            specified cause NEC P59.8
            swallowed maternal blood P58.5
        spherocytosis (congenital) D58.0
    nonhemolytic congenital familial (Gilbert) E80.4
    nuclear, newborn (see also Kernicterus of newborn) P57.9
    obstructive (see also Obstruction, bile duct) K83.1
    post-immunization —see Hepatitis, viral, type, B
    post-transfusion —see Hepatitis, viral, type, B
    regurgitation (see also Obstruction, bile duct) K83.1
    serum (homologous) (prophylactic) (therapeutic) —see Hepatitis, viral, type, B
    spirochetal (hemorrhagic) A27.0
    symptomatic R17
        newborn P59.9
Jaw —see condition
Jaw-winking phenomenon or syndrome Q07.8
Jealousy
    alcoholic F10.988
    childhood F93.8
    sibling F93.8
Jejunitis —see Enteritis
Jejunostomy status Z93.4
Jejunum, jejunal —see condition
Jensen's disease —see Inflammation, chorioretinal, focal, juxtapapillary
Jerks, myoclonic G25.3
Jervell-Lange-Nielsen syndrome I45.81
Jeune's disease Q77.2
Jigger disease B88.1
Job's syndrome (chronic granulomatous disease) D71
Joint —see also condition
    mice —see Loose, body, joint
        knee M23.4-
Jordan's anomaly or syndrome D72.0
Joseph-Diamond-Blackfan anemia (congenital hypoplastic) D61.01
Jungle yellow fever A95.0
Jüngling's disease —see Sarcoidosis
Juvenile —see condition

◀ New   ◀▥ Revised   ~~deleted~~ Deleted

K

Kahler's disease C90.0-
Kakke E51.11
Kala-azar B55.0
Kallmann's syndrome E23.0
Kanner's syndrome (autism) —*see* Psychosis, childhood
Kaposi's
  dermatosis (xeroderma pigmentosum) Q82.1
  lichen ruber L44.0
    acuminatus L44.0
  sarcoma
    colon C46.4
    connective tissue C46.1
    gastrointestinal organ C46.4
    lung C46.5-
    lymph node (multiple) C46.3
    palate (hard) (soft) C46.2
    rectum C46.4
    skin (multiple sites) C46.0
    specified site NEC C46.7
    stomach C46.4
    unspecified site C46.9
  varicelliform eruption B00.0
    vaccinia T88.1
Kartagener's syndrome or triad (sinusitis, bronchiectasis, situs inversus) Q89.3
Karyotype
  with abnormality except iso (Xq) Q96.2
  45,X Q96.0
  46,X
    iso (Xq) Q96.1
  46,XX Q98.3
    with streak gonads Q50.32
    hermaphrodite (true) Q99.1
    male Q98.3
  46,XY
    with streak gonads Q56.1
    female Q97.3
    hermaphrodite (true) Q99.1
  47,XXX Q97.0
  47,XXY Q98.0
  47,XYY Q98.5
Kaschin-Beck disease —*see* Disease, Kaschin-Beck
Katayama's disease or fever B65.2
Kawasaki's syndrome M30.3
Kayser-Fleischer ring (cornea) (pseudosclerosis) H18.04-
Kaznelson's syndrome (congenital hypoplastic anemia) D61.01
Kearns-Sayre syndrome H49.81-
Kedani fever A75.3
Kelis L91.0
Kelly (-Patterson) syndrome (sideropenic dysphagia) D50.1
Keloid, cheloid L91.0
  acne L73.0
  Addison's L94.0
  cornea —*see* Opacity, cornea
  Hawkin's L91.0
  scar L91.0
Keloma L91.0
Kenya fever A77.1
Keratectasia —*see also* Ectasia, cornea
  congenital Q13.4
Keratinization of alveolar ridge mucosa
  excessive K13.23
  minimal K13.22
Keratinized residual ridge mucosa
  excessive K13.23
  minimal K13.22
Keratitis (nodular) (nonulcerative) (simple) (zonular) H16.9
  with ulceration (central) (marginal) (perforated) (ring) —*see* Ulcer, cornea
  actinic —*see* Photokeratitis
  arborescens (herpes simplex) B00.52
  areolar H16.11-
  bullosa H16.8

Keratitis *(Continued)*
  deep H16.309
    specified type NEC H16.399
  dendritic (a) (herpes simplex) B00.52
  disciform (is) (herpes simplex) B00.52
    varicella B01.81
  filamentary H16.12-
  gonococcal (congenital or prenatal) A54.33
  herpes, herpetic (simplex) B00.52
    zoster B02.33
  in (due to)
    acanthamebiasis B60.13
    adenovirus B30.0
    exanthema (*see also* Exanthem) B09
    herpes (simplex) virus B00.52
    measles B05.81
    syphilis A50.31
    tuberculosis A18.52
    zoster B02.33
  interstitial (nonsyphilitic) H16.30-
    diffuse H16.32-
    herpes, herpetic (simplex) B00.52
      zoster B02.33
    sclerosing H16.33-
    specified type NEC H16.39-
    syphilitic (congenital) (late) A50.31
    tuberculous A18.52
  macular H16.11-
  nummular H16.11-
  oyster shuckers' H16.8
  parenchymatous —*see* Keratitis, interstitial
  petrificans H16.8
  postmeasles B05.81
  punctata
    leprosa A30.9 [H16.14-]
    syphilitic (profunda) A50.31
  punctate H16.14-
  purulent H16.8
  rosacea L71.8
  sclerosing H16.33-
  specified type NEC H16.8
  stellate H16.11-
  striate H16.11-
  superficial H16.10-
    with conjunctivitis —*see* Keratoconjunctivitis
    due to light —*see* Photokeratitis
  suppurative H16.8
  syphilitic (congenital) (prenatal) A50.31
  trachomatous A71.1
    sequelae B94.0
  tuberculous A18.52
  vesicular H16.8
  xerotic (*see also* Keratomalacia) H16.8
    vitamin A deficiency E50.4
Keratoacanthoma L85.8
Keratocele —*see* Descemetocele
Keratoconjunctivitis H16.20-
  Acanthamoeba B60.13
  adenoviral B30.0
  epidemic B30.0
  exposure H16.21-
  herpes, herpetic (simplex) B00.52
    zoster B02.33
  in exanthema (*see also* Exanthem) B09
  infectious B30.0
  lagophthalmic —*see* Keratoconjunctivitis, specified type NEC
  neurotrophic H16.23-
  phlyctenular H16.25-
  postmeasles B05.81
  shipyard B30.0
  sicca (Sjogren's) M35.0-
    not Sjogren's H16.22-
  specified type NEC H16.29-
  tuberculous (phlyctenular) A18.52
  vernal H16.26-
Keratoconus H18.60-
  congenital Q13.4
  stable H18.61-
  unstable H18.62-

Keratocyst (dental) (odontogenic) —*see* Cyst, calcifying odontogenic
Keratoderma, keratodermia (congenital) (palmaris et plantaris) (symmetrical) Q82.8
  acquired L85.1
    in diseases classified elsewhere L86
  climactericum L85.1
  gonococcal A54.89
  gonorrheal A54.89
  punctata L85.2
  Reiter's —*see* Reiter's disease
Keratodermatocele —*see* Descemetocele
Keratoglobus H18.79
  congenital Q15.8
    with glaucoma Q15.0
Keratohemia —*see* Pigmentation, cornea, stromal
Keratoiritis —*see also* Iridocyclitis
  syphilitic A50.39
  tuberculous A18.54
Keratoma L57.0
  palmaris and plantaris hereditarium Q82.8
  senile L57.0
Keratomalacia H18.44-
  vitamin A deficiency E50.4
Keratomegaly Q13.4
Keratomycosis B49
  nigrans, nigricans (palmaris) B36.1
Keratopathy H18.9
  band H18.42-
  bullous H18.1-
  bullous (aphakic), following cataract surgery H59.01-
Keratoscleritis, tuberculous A18.52
Keratosis L57.0
  actinic L57.0
  arsenical L85.8
  congenital, specified NEC Q80.8
  female genital NEC N94.89
  follicularis Q82.8
    acquired L11.0
    congenita Q82.8
    et parafollicularis in cutem penetrans L87.0
    spinulosa (decalvans) Q82.8
    vitamin A deficiency E50.8
  gonococcal A54.89
  male genital (external) N50.8
  nigricans L83
  obturans, external ear (canal) —*see* Cholesteatoma, external ear
  palmaris et plantaris (inherited) (symmetrical) Q82.8
    acquired L85.1
  penile N48.89
  pharynx J39.2
  pilaris, acquired L85.8
  punctata (palmaris et plantaris) L85.2
  scrotal N50.8
  seborrheic L82.1
    inflamed L82.0
  senile L57.0
  solar L57.0
  tonsillaris J35.8
  vagina N89.4
  vegetans Q82.8
  vitamin A deficiency E50.8
  vocal cord J38.3
Kerato-uveitis —*see* Iridocyclitis
Kerion (celsi) B35.0
Kernicterus of newborn (not due to isoimmunization) P57.9
  due to isoimmunization (conditions in P55.0-P55.9) P57.0
  specified type NEC P57.8
Kerunoparalysis T75.09
Keshan disease E59
Ketoacidosis E87.2
  diabetic —*see* Diabetes, by type, with ketoacidosis
Ketonuria R82.4

Ketosis NEC E88.89
  diabetic —*see* Diabetes, by type, with
    ketoacidosis
Kew Garden fever A79.1
Kidney —*see* condition
Kienböck's disease —*see also* Osteochondrosis,
  juvenile, hand, carpal lunate
  adult M93.1
Kimmelstiel (-Wilson) disease —*see* Diabetes,
  Kimmelstiel (-Wilson) disease
Kimura disease D21.9
  specified site (see Neoplasm, connective
    tissue benign)
Kink, kinking
  artery I77.1
  hair (acquired) L67.8
  ileum or intestine —*see* Obstruction,
    intestine
  Lane's —*see* Obstruction, intestine
  organ or site, congenital NEC —*see* Anomaly,
    by site
  ureter (pelvic junction) N13.5
    with
      hydronephrosis N13.1
        with infection N13.6
      pyelonephritis (chronic) N11.1
    congenital Q62.39
  vein (s) I87.8
    caval I87.1
    peripheral I87.1
Kinnier Wilson's disease (hepatolenticular
  degeneration) E83.01
Kissing spine M48.20
  cervical region M48.22
  cervicothoracic region M48.23
  lumbar region M48.26
  lumbosacral region M48.27
  occipito-atlanto-axial region M48.21
  thoracic region M48.24
  thoracolumbar region M48.25
Klatskin's tumor C24.0
Klauder's disease A26.8
Klebs' disease (*see also* Glomerulonephritis)
  N05.-
Klebsiella (K.) pneumoniae, as cause of
  disease classified elsewhere B96.1
Klein (e)-Levin syndrome G47.13
Kleptomania F63.2
Klinefelter's syndrome Q98.4
  karyotype 47,XXY Q98.0
  male with more than two X chromosomes
    Q98.1
Klippel-Feil deficiency, disease, or syndrome
  (brevicollis) Q76.1
Klippel's disease I67.2
Klippel-Trenaunay (-Weber) syndrome
  Q87.2
Klumpke (-Déjerine) palsy, paralysis (birth)
  (newborn) P14.1
Knee —*see* condition
Knock knee (acquired) M21.06-
  congenital Q74.1

Knot (s)
  intestinal, syndrome (volvulus) K56.2
  surfer S89.8-
  umbilical cord (true) O69.2
Knotting (of)
  hair L67.8
  intestine K56.2
Knuckle pad (Garrod's) M72.1
Koch's
  infection —*see* Tuberculosis
  relapsing fever A68.9
Koch-Weeks' conjunctivitis —*see*
    Conjunctivitis, acute, mucopurulent
Köebner's syndrome Q81.8
Köenig's disease (osteochondritis dissecans) —
  see Osteochondritis, dissecans
Köhler-Pellegrini-Steida disease or syndrome
  (calcification, knee joint) —*see* Bursitis,
  tibial collateral
Köhler's disease
  patellar —*see* Osteochondrosis, juvenile,
    patella
  tarsal navicular —*see* Osteochondrosis,
    juvenile, tarsus
Koilonychia L60.3
  congenital Q84.6
Kojevnikov's, epilepsy —*see* Kozhevnikof's
  epilepsy
Koplik's spots B05.9
Kopp's asthma E32.8
Korsakoff's (Wernicke) disease, psychosis or
  syndrome (alcoholic) F10.96
  with dependence F10.26
  drug-induced
    due to drug abuse —*see* Abuse, drug, by
      type, with amnestic disorder
    due to drug dependence —*see* Dependence,
      drug, by type, with amnestic disorder
  nonalcoholic F04
Korsakov's disease, psychosis or syndrome —
  see Korsakoff's disease
Korsakow's disease, psychosis or syndrome —
  see Korsakoff's disease
Kostmann's disease or syndrome (infantile
  genetic agranulocytosis) —*see*
  Agranulocytosis
Kozhevnikof's epilepsy G40.109
  intractable G40.119
    with status epilepticus G40.111
    without status epilepticus G40.119
  not intractable G40.109
    with status epilepticus G40.101
    without status epilepticus G40.109
Krabbe's
  disease E75.23
  syndrome, congenital muscle hypoplasia
    Q79.8
Kraepelin-Morel disease —*see* Schizophrenia
Kraft-Weber-Dimitri disease Q85.8
Kraurosis
  ani K62.89
  penis N48.0

Kraurosis *(Continued)*
  vagina N89.8
  vulva N90.4
Kreotoxism A05.9
Krukenberg's
  spindle —*see* Pigmentation, cornea, posterior
  tumor C79.6-
Kufs' disease E75.4
Kugelberg-Welander disease G12.1
Kuhnt-Junius degeneration (see also
  Degeneration, macula) H35.32
Kümmell's disease or spondylitis —*see*
  Spondylopathy, traumatic
Kupffer cell sarcoma C22.3
Kuru A81.81
Kussmaul's
  disease M30.0
  respiration E87.2
    in diabetic acidosis —*see* Diabetes, by type,
      with ketoacidosis
Kwashiorkor E40
  marasmic, marasmus type E42
Kyasanur Forest disease A98.2
Kyphoscoliosis, kyphoscoliotic (acquired) (see
  also Scoliosis) M41.9
  congenital Q67.5
  heart (disease) I27.1
  sequelae of rickets E64.3
  tuberculous A18.01
Kyphosis, kyphotic (acquired) M40.209
  cervical region M40.202
  cervicothoracic region M40.203
  congenital Q76.419
    cervical region Q76.412
    cervicothoracic region Q76.413
    occipito-atlanto-axial region Q76.411
    thoracic region Q76.414
    thoracolumbar region Q76.415
  Morquio-Brailsford type (spinal) (see also
    subcategory M49.8) E76.219
  postlaminectomy M96.3
  postradiation therapy M96.2
  postural (adolescent) M40.00
    cervicothoracic region M40.03
    thoracic region M40.04
    thoracolumbar region M40.05
  secondary NEC M40.10
    cervical region M40.12
    cervicothoracic region M40.13
    thoracic region M40.14
    thoracolumbar region M40.15
  sequelae of rickets E64.3
  specified type NEC M40.299
    cervical region M40.292
    cervicothoracic region M40.293
    thoracic region M40.294
    thoracolumbar region M40.295
  syphilitic, congenital A50.56
  thoracic region M40.204
  thoracolumbar region M40.205
  tuberculous A18.01
Kyrle disease L87.0

L

Labia, labium —*see* condition
Labile
  blood pressure R09.89
  vasomotor system I73.9
Labioglossal paralysis G12.29
Labium leporinum —*see* Cleft, lip
Labor —*see* Delivery
Labored breathing —*see* Hyperventilation
Labyrinthitis (circumscribed) (destructive)
  (diffuse) (inner ear) (latent) (purulent)
  (suppurative) (*see also* subcategory)
  H83.0
  syphilitic A52.79
Laceration
  with abortion —*see* Abortion, by type,
    complicated by laceration of pelvic
    organs
  abdomen, abdominal
    wall S31.119
      with
        foreign body S31.129
        penetration into peritoneal cavity
          S31.619
          with foreign body S31.629
      epigastric region S31.112
        with
          foreign body S31.122
          penetration into peritoneal cavity
            S31.612
            with foreign body S31.622
      left
        lower quadrant S31.114
          with
            foreign body S31.124
            penetration into peritoneal cavity
              S31.614
              with foreign body S31.624
        upper quadrant S31.111
          with
            foreign body S31.121
            penetration into peritoneal cavity
              S31.611
              with foreign body S31.621
      periumbilic region S31.115
        with
          foreign body S31.125
          penetration into peritoneal cavity
            S31.615
            with foreign body S31.625
      right
        lower quadrant S31.113
          with
            foreign body S31.123
            penetration into peritoneal cavity
              S31.613
              with foreign body S31.623
        upper quadrant S31.110
          with
            foreign body S31.120
           penetration into peritoneal cavity
            S31.610
            with foreign body S31.620
  accidental, complicating surgery —*see*
    Complications, surgical, accidental
    puncture or laceration
  Achilles tendon S86.02-
  adrenal gland S37.813
  alveolar (process) —*see* Laceration, oral cavity
  ankle S91.01-
    with
      foreign body S91.02-
  antecubital space —*see* Laceration, elbow
  anus (sphincter) S31.831
    with
      ectopic or molar pregnancy O08.6
      foreign body S31.832
    complicating delivery —*see* Delivery,
      complicated, by, laceration, anus
      (sphincter)

Laceration (*Continued*)
  anus (*Continued*)
    following ectopic or molar pregnancy
      O08.6
    nontraumatic, nonpuerperal —*see* Fissure,
      anus
  arm (upper) S41.11-
    with foreign body S41.12-
    lower —*see* Laceration, forearm
  auditory canal (external) (meatus) —*see*
    Laceration, ear
  auricle, ear —*see* Laceration, ear
  axilla —*see* Laceration, arm
  back —*see also* Laceration, thorax, back
    lower S31.010
      with
        foreign body S31.020
          with penetration into
            retroperitoneal space S31.021
        penetration into retroperitoneal space
          S31.011
  bile duct S36.13
  bladder S37.23
    with ectopic or molar pregnancy O08.6
    following ectopic or molar pregnancy
      O08.6
    obstetrical trauma O71.5
  blood vessel —*see* Injury, blood vessel
  bowel —*see also* Laceration, intestine
    with ectopic or molar pregnancy O08.6
    complicating abortion —*see* Abortion,
      by type, complicated by, specified
      condition NEC
    following ectopic or molar pregnancy
      O08.6
    obstetrical trauma O71.5
  brain (any part) (cortex) (diffuse)
    (membrane) —*see also* Injury,
    intracranial, diffuse
    during birth P10.8
      with hemorrhage P10.1
    focal —*see* Injury, intracranial, focal brain
      injury
  brainstem S06.38-
  breast S21.01-
    with foreign body S21.02-
  broad ligament S37.893
    with ectopic or molar pregnancy O08.6
    following ectopic or molar pregnancy
      O08.6
    laceration syndrome N83.8
    obstetrical trauma O71.6
    syndrome (laceration) N83.8
  buttock S31.801
    with foreign body S31.802
    left S31.821
      with foreign body S31.822
    right S31.811
      with foreign body S31.812
  calf —*see* Laceration, leg
  canaliculus lacrimalis —*see* Laceration,
    eyelid
  canthus, eye —*see* Laceration, eyelid
  capsule, joint —*see* Sprain
  causing eversion of cervix uteri (old) N86
  central (perineal), complicating delivery
    O70.9
  cerebellum, traumatic S06.37-
  cerebral S06.33-
    during birth P10.8
      with hemorrhage P10.1
    left side S06.32-
    right side S06.31-
  cervix (uteri)
    with ectopic or molar pregnancy O08.6
    following ectopic or molar pregnancy
      O08.6
    nonpuerperal, nontraumatic N88.1
    obstetrical trauma (current) O71.3
    old (postpartal) N88.1
    traumatic S37.63

Laceration (*Continued*)
  cheek (external) S01.41-
    with foreign body S01.42-
    internal —*see* Laceration, oral cavity
  chest wall —*see* Laceration, thorax
  chin —*see* Laceration, head, specified site
    NEC
  chordae tendinae NEC I51.1
    concurrent with acute myocardial
      infarction —*see* Infarct, myocardium
    following acute myocardial infarction
      (current complication) I23.4
  clitoris —*see* Laceration, vulva
  colon —*see* Laceration, intestine, large,
    colon
  common bile duct S36.13
  cortex (cerebral) —*see* Injury, intracranial,
    diffuse
  costal region —*see* Laceration, thorax
  cystic duct S36.13
  diaphragm S27.803
  digit (s)
    foot —*see* Laceration, toe
    hand —*see* Laceration, finger
  duodenum S36.430
  ear (canal) (external) S01.31-
    with foreign body S01.32-
    drum S09.2-
  elbow S51.01-
    with
      foreign body S51.02-
  epididymis —*see* Laceration, testis
  epigastric region —*see* Laceration, abdomen,
    wall, epigastric region
  esophagus K22.8
    traumatic
      cervical S11.21
        with foreign body S11.22
      thoracic S27.813
  eye (ball) S05.3-
    with prolapse or loss of intraocular tissue
      S05.2-
    penetrating S05.6-
  eyebrow —*see* Laceration, eyelid
  eyelid S01.11-
    with foreign body S01.12-
  face NEC —*see* Laceration, head, specified
    site NEC
  fallopian tube S37.539
    bilateral S37.532
    unilateral S37.531
  finger (s) S61.219
    with
      damage to nail S61.319
        with
          foreign body S61.329
      foreign body S61.229
    index S61.218
      with
        damage to nail S61.318
          with
            foreign body S61.328
        foreign body S61.228
    left S61.211
      with
        damage to nail S61.311
          with
            foreign body S61.321
        foreign body S61.221
    right S61.210
      with
        damage to nail S61.310
          with
            foreign body S61.320
        foreign body S61.220
    little S61.218
      with
        damage to nail S61.318
          with
            foreign body S61.328
        foreign body S61.228

Laceration (Continued)
    finger (Continued)
        little (Continued)
            left S61.217
                with
                    damage to nail S61.317
                        with
                            foreign body S61.327
                    foreign body S61.227
            right S61.216
                with
                    damage to nail S61.316
                        with
                            foreign body S61.326
                    foreign body S61.226
        middle S61.218
            with
                damage to nail S61.318
                    with
                        foreign body S61.328
                foreign body S61.228
            left S61.213
                with
                    damage to nail S61.313
                        with
                            foreign body S61.323
                    foreign body S61.223
            right S61.212
                with
                    damage to nail S61.312
                        with
                            foreign body S61.322
                    foreign body S61.222
        ring S61.218
            with
                damage to nail S61.318
                    with
                        foreign body S61.328
                foreign body S61.228
            left S61.215
                with
                    damage to nail S61.315
                        with
                            foreign body S61.325
                    foreign body S61.225
            right S61.214
                with
                    damage to nail S61.314
                        with
                            foreign body S61.324
                    foreign body S61.224
    flank S31.119
        with foreign body S31.129
    foot (except toe (s) alone) S91.319
        with foreign body S91.329
        left S91.312
            with foreign body S91.322
        right S91.311
            with foreign body S91.321
        toe —see Laceration, toe
    forearm S51.819
        with
            foreign body S51.829
        elbow only —see Laceration,
            elbow
        left S51.812
            with
                foreign body S51.822
        right S51.811
            with
                foreign body S51.821
    forehead S01.81
        with foreign body S01.82
    fourchette O70.0
        with ectopic or molar pregnancy
            O08.6
        complicating delivery O70.0
        following ectopic or molar pregnancy
            O08.6
    gallbladder S36.123

Laceration (Continued)
    genital organs, external
        female S31.512
            with foreign body S31.522
            vagina —see Laceration, vagina
            vulva —see Laceration, vulva
        male S31.511
            with foreign body S31.521
            penis —see Laceration, penis
            scrotum —see Laceration, scrotum
            testis —see Laceration, testis
    groin —see Laceration, abdomen, wall
    gum —see Laceration, oral cavity
    hand S61.419
        with
            foreign body S61.429
        finger —see Laceration, finger
        left S61.412
            with
                foreign body S61.422
        right S61.411
            with
                foreign body S61.421
        thumb —see Laceration, thumb
    head S01.91
        with foreign body S01.92
        cheek —see Laceration, cheek
        ear —see Laceration, ear
        eyelid —see Laceration, eyelid
        lip —see Laceration, lip
        nose —see Laceration, nose
        oral cavity —see Laceration, oral
            cavity
        scalp S01.01
            with foreign body S01.02
        specified site NEC S01.81
            with foreign body S01.82
        temporomandibular area —see Laceration,
            cheek
    heart —see Injury, heart, laceration
    heel —see Laceration, foot
    hepatic duct S36.13
    hip S71.019
        with foreign body S71.029
        left S71.012
            with foreign body S71.022
        right S71.011
            with foreign body S71.021
    hymen —see Laceration, vagina
    hypochondrium —see Laceration, abdomen,
        wall
    hypogastric region —see Laceration,
        abdomen, wall
    ileum S36.438
    inguinal region —see Laceration, abdomen,
        wall
    instep —see Laceration, foot
    internal organ —see Injury, by site
    interscapular region —see Laceration, thorax,
        back
    intestine
        large
            colon S36.539
                ascending S36.530
                descending S36.532
                sigmoid S36.533
                specified site NEC S36.538
            rectum S36.63
                transverse S36.531
        small S36.439
            duodenum S36.430
            specified site NEC S36.438
    intra-abdominal organ S36.93
        intestine —see Laceration, intestine
        liver —see Laceration, liver
        pancreas —see Laceration, pancreas
        peritoneum S36.81
        specified site NEC S36.893
        spleen —see Laceration, spleen
        stomach —see Laceration, stomach

Laceration (Continued)
    intracranial NEC —see also Injury,
        intracranial, diffuse
        birth injury P10.9
    jaw —see Laceration, head, specified site NEC
    jejunum S36.438
    joint capsule —see Sprain, by site
    kidney S37.03-
        major (greater than 3 cm) (massive)
            (stellate) S37.06-
        minor (less than 1 cm) S37.04-
        moderate (1 to 3 cm) S37.05-
        multiple S37.06-
    knee S81.01-
        with foreign body S81.02-
    labium (majus) (minus) —see Laceration,
        vulva
    lacrimal duct —see Laceration, eyelid
    large intestine —see Laceration, intestine,
        large
    larynx S11.011
        with foreign body S11.012
    leg (lower) S81.819
        with foreign body S81.829
        foot —see Laceration, foot
        knee —see Laceration, knee
        left S81.812
            with foreign body S81.822
        right S81.811
            with foreign body S81.821
        upper —see Laceration, thigh
    ligament —see Sprain
    lip S01.511
        with foreign body S01.521
    liver S36.113
        major (stellate) S36.116
        minor S36.114
        moderate S36.115
    loin —see Laceration, abdomen, wall
    lower back —see Laceration, back, lower
    lumbar region —see Laceration, back, lower
    lung S27.339
        bilateral S27.332
        unilateral S27.331
    malar region —see Laceration, head, specified
        site NEC
    mammary —see Laceration, breast
    mastoid region —see Laceration, head,
        specified site NEC
    meninges —see Injury, intracranial, diffuse
    meniscus —see Tear, meniscus
    mesentery S36.893
    mesosalpinx S37.893
    mouth —see Laceration, oral cavity
    muscle —see Injury, muscle, by site,
        laceration
    nail
        finger —see Laceration, finger, with
            damage to nail
        toe —see Laceration, toe, with damage to
            nail
    nasal (septum) (sinus) —see Laceration,
        nose
    nasopharynx —see Laceration, head, specified
        site NEC
    neck S11.91
        with foreign body S11.92
        involving
            cervical esophagus S11.21
                with foreign body S11.22
            larynx —see Laceration, larynx
            pharynx —see Laceration, pharynx
            thyroid gland —see Laceration, thyroid
                gland
            trachea —see Laceration, trachea
        specified site NEC S11.81
            with foreign body S11.82
    nerve —see Injury, nerve
    nose (septum) (sinus) S01.21
        with foreign body S01.22

◀ New   ◀▥ Revised   ~~deleted~~ Deleted

Laceration *(Continued)*
ocular NOS S05.3-
  adnexa NOS S01.11-
oral cavity S01.512
  with foreign body S01.522
orbit (eye) —*see* Wound, open, ocular, orbit
ovary S37.439
  bilateral S37.432
  unilateral S37.431
palate —*see* Laceration, oral cavity
palm —*see* Laceration, hand
pancreas S36.239
  body S36.231
    major S36.261
    minor S36.241
    moderate S36.251
  head S36.230
    major S36.260
    minor S36.240
    moderate S36.250
  major S36.269
  minor S36.249
  moderate S36.259
  tail S36.232
    major S36.262
    minor S36.242
    moderate S36.252
pelvic S31.010
  with
    foreign body S31.020
      penetration into retroperitoneal cavity S31.021
    penetration into retroperitoneal cavity S31.011
  floor —*see also* Laceration, back, lower
    with ectopic or molar pregnancy O08.6
    complicating delivery O70.1
    following ectopic or molar pregnancy O08.6
    old (postpartal) N81.89
  organ S37.93
    with ectopic or molar pregnancy O08.6
    adrenal gland S37.813
    bladder S37.23
    fallopian tube —*see* Laceration, fallopian tube
    following ectopic or molar pregnancy O08.6
    kidney —*see* Laceration, kidney
    obstetrical trauma O71.5
    ovary —*see* Laceration, ovary
    prostate S37.823
    specified site NEC S37.893
    ureter S37.13
    urethra S37.33
    uterus S37.63
penis S31.21
  with foreign body S31.22
perineum
  female S31.41
    with
      ectopic or molar pregnancy O08.6
      foreign body S31.42
    during delivery O70.9
      first degree O70.0
      fourth degree O70.3
      second degree O70.1
      third degree O70.2
    old (postpartal) N81.89
    postpartal N81.89
    secondary (postpartal) O90.1
  male S31.119
    with foreign body S31.129
periocular area (with or without lacrimal passages) —*see* Laceration, eyelid
peritoneum S36.893
periumbilic region —*see* Laceration, abdomen, wall, periumbilic
periurethral tissue —*see* Laceration, urethra

Laceration *(Continued)*
phalanges
  finger —*see* Laceration, finger
  toe —*see* Laceration, toe
pharynx S11.21
  with foreign body S11.22
pinna —*see* Laceration, ear
popliteal space —*see* Laceration, knee
prepuce —*see* Laceration, penis
prostate S37.823
pubic region S31.119
  with foreign body S31.129
pudendum —*see* Laceration, genital organs, external
rectovaginal septum —*see* Laceration, vagina
rectum S36.63
retroperitoneum S36.893
round ligament S37.893
sacral region —*see* Laceration, back, lower
sacroiliac region —*see* Laceration, back, lower
salivary gland —*see* Laceration, oral cavity
scalp S01.01
  with foreign body S01.02
scapular region —*see* Laceration, shoulder
scrotum S31.31
  with foreign body S31.32
seminal vesicle S37.893
shin —*see* Laceration, leg
shoulder S41.019
  with foreign body S41.029
  left S41.012
    with foreign body S41.022
  right S41.011
    with foreign body S41.021
small intestine —*see* Laceration, intestine, small
spermatic cord —*see* Laceration, testis
spinal cord (meninges) —*see also* Injury, spinal cord, by region
  due to injury at birth P11.5
  newborn (birth injury) P11.5
spleen S36.039
  major (massive) (stellate) S36.032
  moderate S36.031
  superficial (minor) S36.030
sternal region —*see* Laceration, thorax, front
stomach S36.33
submaxillary region —*see* Laceration, head, specified site NEC
submental region —*see* Laceration, head, specified site NEC
subungual
  finger (s) —*see* Laceration, finger, with damage to nail
  toe (s) —*see* Laceration, toe, with damage to nail
suprarenal gland —*see* Laceration, adrenal gland
temple, temporal region —*see* Laceration, head, specified site NEC
temporomandibular area —*see* Laceration, cheek
tendon —*see* Injury, muscle, by site, laceration
  Achilles S86.02-
tentorium cerebelli —*see* Injury, intracranial, diffuse
testis S31.31
  with foreign body S31.32
thigh S71.11-
  with foreign body S71.12-
thorax, thoracic (wall) S21.91
  with foreign body S21.92
  back S21.22-
    with penetration into thoracic cavity S21.42-
  front S21.12-
    with penetration into thoracic cavity S21.32-

Laceration *(Continued)*
thorax, thoracic *(Continued)*
  back S21.21-
    with
      foreign body S21.22-
        with penetration into thoracic cavity S21.42-
      penetration into thoracic cavity S21.41-
  breast —*see* Laceration, breast
  front S21.11-
    with
      foreign body S21.12-
        with penetration into thoracic cavity S21.32-
      penetration into thoracic cavity S21.31-
thumb S61.019
  with
    damage to nail S61.119
      with
        foreign body S61.129
    foreign body S61.029
  left S61.012
    with
      damage to nail S61.112
        with
          foreign body S61.122
      foreign body S61.022
  right S61.011
    with
      damage to nail S61.111
        with
          foreign body S61.121
      foreign body S61.021
thyroid gland S11.11
  with foreign body S11.12
toe (s) S91.119
  with
    damage to nail S91.219
      with
        foreign body S91.229
    foreign body S91.129
  great S91.113
    with
      damage to nail S91.213
        with
          foreign body S91.223
      foreign body S91.123
    left S91.112
      with
        damage to nail S91.212
          with
            foreign body S91.222
        foreign body S91.122
    right S91.111
      with
        damage to nail S91.211
          with
            foreign body S91.221
        foreign body S91.121
  lesser S91.116
    with
      damage to nail S91.216
        with
          foreign body S91.226
      foreign body S91.126
    left S91.115
      with
        damage to nail S91.215
          with
            foreign body S91.225
        foreign body S91.125
    right S91.114
      with
        damage to nail S91.214
          with
            foreign body S91.224
        foreign body S91.124
tongue —*see* Laceration, oral cavity

Laceration *(Continued)*
  trachea S11.021
    with foreign body S11.022
  tunica vaginalis —*see* Laceration, testis
  tympanum, tympanic membrane —*see*
        Laceration, ear, drum
  umbilical region S31.115
    with foreign body S31.125
  ureter S37.13
  urethra S37.33
    with or following ectopic or molar
        pregnancy O08.6
    obstetrical trauma O71.5
  urinary organ NEC S37.893
  uterus S37.63
    with ectopic or molar pregnancy O08.6
    following ectopic or molar pregnancy
        O08.6
    nonpuerperal, nontraumatic N85.8
    obstetrical trauma NEC O71.81
    old (postpartal) N85.8
  uvula —*see* Laceration, oral cavity
  vagina S31.41
    with
        ectopic or molar pregnancy O08.6
        foreign body S31.42
    during delivery O71.4
        with perineal laceration —*see* Laceration,
            perineum, female, during delivery
    following ectopic or molar pregnancy
        O08.6
    nonpuerperal, nontraumatic N89.8
    old (postpartal) N89.8
  vas deferens S37.893
  vesical —*see* Laceration, bladder
  vocal cords S11.031
    with foreign body S11.032
  vulva S31.41
    with
        ectopic or molar pregnancy O08.6
        foreign body S31.42
    complicating delivery O70.0
    following ectopic or molar pregnancy
        O08.6
    nonpuerperal, nontraumatic N90.89
    old (postpartal) N90.89
  wrist S61.519
    with
        foreign body S61.529
    left S61.512
        with
            foreign body S61.522
    right S61.511
        with
            foreign body S61.521
Lack of
  achievement in school Z55.3
  adequate
    food Z59.4
    intermaxillary vertical dimension of fully
        erupted teeth M26.36
    sleep Z72.820
  appetite (*see* Anorexia) R63.0
  awareness R41.9
  care
    in home Z74.2
    of infant (at or after birth) T76.02
        confirmed T74.02
  cognitive functions R41.9
  coordination R27.9
    ataxia R27.0
    specified type NEC R27.8
  development (physiological) R62.50
    failure to thrive (child over 28 days old)
        R62.51
        adult R62.7
        newborn P92.6
    short stature R62.52
    specified type NEC R62.59
  energy R53.83
  financial resources Z59.6

Lack of *(Continued)*
  food T73.0
  growth R62.52
  heating Z59.1
  housing (permanent) (temporary) Z59.0
    adequate Z59.1
  learning experiences in childhood Z62.898
  leisure time (affecting life-style) Z73.2
  material resources Z59.9
  memory —*see also* Amnesia
    mild, following organic brain damage
        F06.8
  ovulation N97.0
  parental supervision or control of child
        Z62.0
  person able to render necessary care Z74.2
  physical exercise Z72.3
  play experience in childhood Z62.898
  posterior occlusal support M26.57
  relaxation (affecting life-style) Z73.2
  sexual
    desire F52.0
    enjoyment F52.1
  shelter Z59.0
  sleep (adequate) Z72.820
  supervision of child by parent Z62.0
  support, posterior occlusal M26.57
  water T73.1
Lacrimal —*see* condition
Lacrimation, abnormal —*see* Epiphora
Lacrimonasal duct —*see* condition
Lactation, lactating (breast) (puerperal,
    postpartum)
  associated
    cracked nipple O92.13
    retracted nipple O92.03
  defective O92.4
  disorder NEC O92.79
  excessive O92.6
  failed (complete) O92.3
    partial O92.4
  mastitis NEC —*see* Mastitis, obstetric
  mother (care and/or examination) Z39.1
  nonpuerperal N64.3
Lacticemia, excessive E87.2
Lacunar skull Q75.8
Laennec's cirrhosis K74.69
  alcoholic K70.30
    with ascites K70.31
Lafora's disease —*see* Epilepsy, generalized,
    idiopathic
Lag, lid (nervous) —*see* Retraction, lid
Lagophthalmos (eyelid) (nervous) H02.209
  cicatricial H02.219
    left H02.216
        lower H02.215
        upper H02.214
    right H02.213
        lower H02.212
        upper H02.211
  keratoconjunctivitis —*see* Keratoconjunctivitis
  left H02.206
    lower H02.205
    upper H02.204
  mechanical H02.229
    left H02.226
        lower H02.225
        upper H02.224
    right H02.223
        lower H02.222
        upper H02.221
  paralytic H02.239
    left H02.236
        lower H02.235
        upper H02.234
    right H02.233
        lower H02.232
        upper H02.231
  right H02.203
    lower H02.202
    upper H02.201

Laki-Lorand factor deficiency —*see* Defect,
    coagulation, specified type NEC
Lalling F80.0
Lambert-Eaton syndrome —*see* Syndrome,
    Lambert-Eaton
Lambliasis, lambliosis A07.1
Landau-Kleffner syndrome —*see* Epilepsy,
    specified NEC
Landouzy-Déjérine dystrophy or
    facioscapulohumeral atrophy G71.0
Landouzy's disease (icterohemorrhagic
    leptospirosis) A27.0
Landry-Guillain-Barré, syndrome or paralysis
    G61.0
Landry's disease or paralysis G61.0
Lane's
  band Q43.3
  kink —*see* Obstruction, intestine
  syndrome K90.2
Langdon Down's syndrome —*see* Trisomy, 21
Lapsed immunization schedule status Z28.3
Large
  baby (regardless of gestational age) (4000g to
        4499g) P08.1
  ear, congenital Q17.1
  physiological cup Q14.2
  stature R68.89
Large-for-dates NEC (infant) (4000g to 4499g)
    P08.1
  affecting management of pregnancy O36.6-
  exceptionally (4500g or more) P08.0
Larsen-Johansson disease
  orosteochondrosis —*see* Osteochondrosis,
    juvenile, patella
Larsen's syndrome (flattened facies and
    multiple congenital dislocations) Q74.8
Larva migrans
  cutaneous B76.9
    Ancylostoma B76.0
  visceral B83.0
Laryngeal —*see* condition
Laryngismus (stridulus) J38.5
  congenital P28.89
  diphtheritic A36.2
Laryngitis (acute) (edematous) (fibrinous)
        (infective) (infiltrative) (malignant)
        (membranous) (phlegmonous)
        (pneumococcal) (pseudomembranous)
        (septic) (subglottic) (suppurative)
        (ulcerative) J04.0
  with
    influenza, flu, or grippe —*see* Influenza,
        with, laryngitis
    tracheitis (acute) —*see* Laryngotracheitis
  atrophic J37.0
  catarrhal J37.0
  chronic J37.0
    with tracheitis (chronic) J37.1
  diphtheritic A36.2
  due to external agent —*see* Inflammation,
        respiratory, upper, due to
  Hemophilus influenzae J04.0
  H. influenzae J04.0
  hypertrophic J37.0
  influenzal —*see* Influenza, with, respiratory
        manifestations NEC
  obstructive J05.0
  sicca J37.0
  spasmodic J05.0
    acute J04.0
  streptococcal J04.0
  stridulous J05.0
  syphilitic (late) A52.73
    congenital A50.59 *[J99]*
    early A50.03 *[J99]*
  tuberculous A15.5
  Vincent's A69.1
Laryngocele (congenital) (ventricular) Q31.3
Laryngofissure J38.7
  congenital Q31.8
Laryngomalacia (congenital) Q31.5

◀ New   ◀▦ Revised   ~~deleted~~ Deleted

Laryngopharyngitis (acute) J06.0
  chronic J37.0
  due to external agent —*see* Inflammation,
    respiratory, upper, due to
Laryngoplegia J38.00
  bilateral J38.02
  unilateral J38.01
Laryngoptosis J38.7
Laryngospasm J38.5
Laryngostenosis J38.6
Laryngotracheitis (acute) (Infectional)
    (infective) (viral) J04.2
  atrophic J37.1
  catarrhal J37.1
  chronic J37.1
  diphtheritic A36.2
  due to external agent —*see* Inflammation,
    respiratory, upper, due to
  Hemophilus influenzae J04.2
  hypertrophic J37.1
  influenzal —*see* Influenza, with, respiratory
    manifestations NEC
  pachydermic J38.7
  sicca J37.1
  spasmodic J38.5
    acute J05.0
  streptococcal J04.2
  stridulous J38.5
  syphilitic (late) A52.73
    congenital A50.59 [J99]
      early A50.03 [J99]
  tuberculous A15.5
  Vincent's A69.1
Laryngotracheobronchitis —*see* Bronchitis
Larynx, laryngeal —*see* condition
Lassa fever A96.2
Lassitude —*see* Weakness
Late
  talker R62.0
  walker R62.0
Late effect (s) —*see* Sequelae
Latent —*see* condition
Laterocession —*see* Lateroversion
Lateroflexion —*see* Lateroversion
Lateroversion
  cervix —*see* Lateroversion, uterus
  uterus, uterine (cervix) (postinfectional)
    (postpartal, old) N85.4
    congenital Q51.818
    in pregnancy or childbirth O34.59-
Lathyrism —*see* Poisoning, food, noxious, plant
Launois' syndrome (pituitary gigantism) E22.0
Launois-Bensaude adenolipomatosis E88.89
Laurence-Moon (-Bardet)-Biedl syndrome
    Q87.89
Lax, laxity —*see also* Relaxation
  ligament (ous) —*see also* Disorder, ligament
    familial M35.7
    knee —*see* Derangement, knee
  skin (acquired) L57.4
    congenital Q82.8
Laxative habit F55.2
Lazy leukocyte syndrome D70.8
Lead miner's lung J63.6
Leak, leakage
  air NEC J93.82
    postprocedural J95.812
  amniotic fluid —*see* Rupture, membranes,
    premature
  blood (microscopic), fetal, into maternal
    circulation affecting management of
    pregnancy —*see* Pregnancy, complicated
    by
  cerebrospinal fluid G96.0
    from spinal (lumbar) puncture G97.0
  device, implant or graft —*see also*
    Complications, by site and type,
    mechanical
    arterial graft NEC —*see* Complication,
      cardiovascular device, mechanical,
      vascular

Leak, leakage (Continued)
  device, implant or graft (Continued)
    breast (implant) T85.43
    catheter NEC T85.638
      dialysis (renal) T82.43
        intraperitoneal T85.631
      infusion NEC T82.534
        spinal (epidural) (subdural) T85.630
      urinary, indwelling T83.038
        cystostomy T83.030
    gastrointestinal —*see* Complications,
      prosthetic device, mechanical,
      gastrointestinal device
    genital NEC T83.498
      penile prosthesis T83.490
    heart NEC —*see* Complication,
      cardiovascular device, mechanical
    joint prosthesis —*see* Complications, joint
      prosthesis, mechanical, specified
      NEC, by site
    ocular NEC —*see* Complications,
      prosthetic device, mechanical, ocular
      device
    orthopedic NEC —*see* Complication,
      orthopedic, device, mechanical
    persistent air J93.82
    specified NEC T85.638
    urinary NEC —*see also* Complication,
      genitourinary, device, urinary,
      mechanical
      graft T83.23
    vascular NEC —*see* Complication,
      cardiovascular device, mechanical
    ventricular intracranial shunt T85.03
  urine —*see* Incontinence
Leaky heart —*see* Endocarditis
Learning defect (specific) F81.9
Leather bottle stomach C16.9
Leber's
  congenital amaurosis H35.50
  optic atrophy (hereditary) H47.22
Lederer's anemia D59.1
Leeches (external) —*see* Hirudiniasis
Leg —*see* condition
Legg (-Calvé)-Perthes disease, syndrome or
    osteochondrosis M91.1-
Legionellosis A48.1
  nonpneumonic A48.2
Legionnaires'
  disease A48.1
    nonpneumonic A48.2
  pneumonia A48.1
Leigh's disease G31.82
Leiner's disease L21.1
Leiofibromyoma —*see* Leiomyoma
Leiomyoblastoma —*see* Neoplasm, connective
    tissue, benign
Leiomyofibroma —*see also* Neoplasm,
    connective tissue, benign
  uterus (cervix) (corpus) D25.9
Leiomyoma —*see also* Neoplasm, connective
    tissue, benign
  bizarre —*see* Neoplasm, connective tissue,
    benign
  cellular —*see* Neoplasm, connective tissue,
    benign
  epithelioid —*see* Neoplasm, connective
    tissue, benign
  uterus (cervix) (corpus) D25.9
    intramural D25.1
    submucous D25.0
    subserosal D25.2
  vascular —*see* Neoplasm, connective tissue,
    benign
Leiomyoma, leiomyomatosis (intravascular) —
    see Neoplasm, connective tissue, uncertain
    behavior
Leiomyosarcoma —*see also* Neoplasm,
    connective tissue, malignant
  epithelioid —*see* Neoplasm, connective
    tissue, malignant

Leiomyosarcoma (Continued)
  myxoid —*see* Neoplasm, connective tissue,
    malignant
Leishmaniasis B55.9
  American (mucocutaneous) B55.2
    cutaneous B55.1
  Asian Desert B55.1
  Brazilian B55.2
  cutaneous (any type) B55.1
  dermal —*see also* Leishmaniasis, cutaneous
    post-kala-azar B55.0
  eyelid B55.1
  infantile B55.0
  Mediterranean B55.0
  mucocutaneous (American) (New World)
    B55.2
  naso-oral B55.2
  nasopharyngeal B55.2
  old world B55.1
  tegumentaria diffusa B55.1
  visceral B55.0
Leishmanoid, dermal —*see also* Leishmaniasis,
    cutaneous
  post-kala-azar B55.0
Lenegre's disease I44.2
Lengthening, leg —*see* Deformity, limb,
    unequal length
Lennert's lymphoma —*see* Lymphoma,
    Lennert's
Lennox-Gastaut syndrome G40.812
  intractable G40.814
    with status epilepticus G40.813
    without status epilepticus G40.814
  not intractable G40.812
    with status epilepticus G40.811
    without status epilepticus G40.812
Lens —*see* condition
Lenticonus (anterior) (posterior) (congenital)
    Q12.8
Lenticular degeneration, progressive E83.01
Lentiglobus (posterior) (congenital) Q12.8
Lentigo (congenital) L81.4
  maligna —*see also* Melanoma, in situ
    melanoma —*see* Melanoma
Lentivirus, as cause of disease classified
    elsewhere B97.31
Leontiasis
  ossium M85.2
  syphilitic (late) A52.78
    congenital A50.59
Lepothrix A48.8
Lepra —*see* Leprosy
Leprechaunism E34.8
Leprosy A30.-
  with muscle disorder A30.9 [M63.80]
    ankle A30.9 [M63.87-]
    foot A30.9 [M63.87-]
    forearm A30.9 [M63.83-]
    hand A30.9 [M63.84-]
    lower leg A30.9 [M63.86-]
    multiple sites A30.9 [M63.89]
    pelvic region A30.9 [M63.85-]
    shoulder region A30.9 [M63.81-]
    specified site NEC A30.9 [M63.88]
    thigh A30.9 [M63.85-]
    upper arm A30.9 [M63.82-]
  anesthetic A30.9
  BB A30.3
  BL A30.4
  borderline (infiltrated) (neuritic) A30.3
    lepromatous A30.4
    tuberculoid A30.2
  BT A30.2
  dimorphous (infiltrated) (neuritic) A30.3
  I A30.0
  indeterminate (macular) (neuritic) A30.0
  lepromatous (diffuse) (infiltrated) (macular)
    (neuritic) (nodular) A30.5
  LL A30.5
  macular (early) (neuritic) (simple) A30.9
  maculoanesthetic A30.9

Leprosy *(Continued)*
  mixed A30.3
  neural A30.9
  nodular A30.5
  primary neuritic A30.3
  specified type NEC A30.8
  TT A30.1
  tuberculoid (major) (minor) A30.1
Leptocytosis, hereditary D56.9
Leptomeningitis (chronic) (circumscribed) (hemorrhagic) (nonsuppurative) —*see* Meningitis
Leptomeningopathy G96.19
Leptospiral —*see* condition
Leptospirochetal —*see* condition
Leptospirosis A27.9
  canicola A27.89
  due to Leptospira interrogans serovar icterohaemorrhagiae A27.0
  icterohemorrhagica A27.0
  pomona A27.89
  Weil's disease A27.0
Leptus dermatitis B88.0
Leriche's syndrome (aortic bifurcation occlusion) I74.09
Leri's pleonosteosis Q78.8
Leri-Weill syndrome Q77.8
Lermoyez' syndrome —*see* Vertigo, peripheral NEC
Lesch-Nyhan syndrome E79.1
Leser-Trélat disease L82.1
  inflamed L82.0
Lesion (s) (nontraumatic)
  abducens nerve —*see* Strabismus, paralytic, sixth nerve
  alveolar process K08.9
  angiocentric immunoproliferative D47.Z9
  anorectal K62.9
  aortic (valve) I35.9
  auditory nerve —*see* subcategory H93.3
  basal ganglion G25.9
  bile duct —*see* Disease, bile duct
  biomechanical M99.9
    specified type NEC M99.89
      abdomen M99.89
      acromioclavicular M99.87
      cervical region M99.81
      cervicothoracic M99.81
      costochondral M99.88
      costovertebral M99.88
      head region M99.80
      hip M99.85
      lower extremity M99.86
      lumbar region M99.83
      lumbosacral M99.83
      occipitocervical M99.80
      pelvic region M99.85
      pubic M99.85
      rib cage M99.88
      sacral region M99.84
      sacrococcygeal M99.84
      sacroiliac M99.84
      specified NEC M99.89
      sternochondral M99.88
      sternoclavicular M99.87
      thoracic region M99.82
      thoracolumbar M99.82
      upper extremity M99.87
  bladder N32.9
  bone —*see* Disorder, bone
  brachial plexus G54.0
  brain G93.9
    congenital Q04.9
    vascular I67.9
      degenerative I67.9
      hypertensive I67.4
  buccal cavity K13.79
  calcified —*see* Calcification
  canthus —*see* Disorder, eyelid
  carate —*see* Pinta, lesions
  cardia K22.9

Lesion *(Continued)*
  cardiac (*see also* Disease, heart) I51.9
    congenital Q24.9
    valvular —*see* Endocarditis
  cauda equina G83.4
  cecum K63.9
  cerebral —*see* Lesion, brain
  cerebrovascular I67.9
    degenerative I67.9
    hypertensive I67.4
  cervical (nerve) root NEC G54.2
  chiasmal —*see* Disorder, optic, chiasm
  chorda tympani G51.8
  coin, lung R91.1
  colon K63.9
  congenital —*see* Anomaly, by site
  conjunctiva H11.9
  conus medullaris —*see* Injury, conus medullaris
  coronary artery —*see* Ischemia, heart
  cranial nerve G52.9
    eighth —*see* Disorder, ear
    eleventh G52.9
    fifth G50.9
    first G52.0
    fourth —*see* Strabismus, paralytic, fourth nerve
    seventh G51.9
    sixth —*see* Strabismus, paralytic, sixth nerve
    tenth G52.2
    twelfth G52.3
  cystic —*see* Cyst
  degenerative —*see* Degeneration
  duodenum K31.9
  edentulous (alveolar) ridge, associated with trauma, due to traumatic occlusion K06.2
  en coup de sabre L94.1
  eyelid —*see* Disorder, eyelid
  gasserian ganglion G50.8
  gastric K31.9
  gastroduodenal K31.9
  gastrointestinal K63.9
  gingiva, associated with trauma K06.2
  glomerular
    focal and segmental (*see also* N00-N07 with fourth character .1) N05.1
    minimal change (*see also* N00-N07 with fourth character .0) N05.0
  heart (organic) —*see* Disease, heart
  hyperchromic, due to pinta (carate) A67.1
  hyperkeratotic —*see* Hyperkeratosis
  hypothalamic E23.7
  ileocecal K63.9
  ileum K63.9
  iliohypogastric nerve G57.8-
  inflammatory —*see* Inflammation
  intestine K63.9
  intracerebral —*see* Lesion, brain
  intrachiasmal (optic) —*see* Disorder, optic, chiasm
  intracranial, space-occupying R90.0
  joint —*see* Disorder, joint
    sacroiliac (old) M53.3
  keratotic —*see* Keratosis
  kidney —*see* Disease, renal
  laryngeal nerve (recurrent) G52.2
  lip K13.0
  liver K76.9
  lumbosacral
    plexus G54.1
    root (nerve) NEC G54.4
  lung (coin) R91.1
  maxillary sinus J32.0
  mitral I05.9
  Morel-Lavallée —*see* Hematoma, by site
  motor cortex NEC G93.89
  mouth K13.79

Lesion *(Continued)*
  nerve G58.9
    femoral G57.2-
    median G56.1-
      carpal tunnel syndrome —*see* Syndrome, carpal tunnel
    plantar G57.6-
    popliteal (lateral) G57.3-
      medial G57.4-
    radial G56.3-
    sciatic G57.0-
    spinal —*see* Injury, nerve, spinal
    ulnar G56.2-
  nervous system, congenital Q07.9
  nonallopathic —*see* Lesion, biomechanical
  nose (internal) J34.89
  obstructive —*see* Obstruction
  obturator nerve G57.8-
  oral mucosa K13.70
  organ or site NEC —*see* Disease, by site
  osteolytic —*see* Osteolysis
  peptic K27.9
  periodontal, due to traumatic occlusion K05.5
  pharynx J39.2
  pigment, pigmented (skin) L81.9
  pinta —*see* Pinta, lesions
  polypoid —*see* Polyp
  prechiasmal (optic) —*see* Disorder, optic, chiasm
  primary (*see also* Syphilis, primary) A51.0
    carate A67.0
    pinta A67.0
    yaws A66.0
  pulmonary J98.4
    valve I37.9
  pylorus K31.9
  rectosigmoid K63.9
  retina, retinal H35.9
  sacroiliac (joint) (old) M53.3
  salivary gland K11.9
    benign lymphoepithelial K11.8
  saphenous nerve G57.8-
  sciatic nerve G57.0-
  secondary —*see* Syphilis, secondary
  shoulder (region) M75.9-
    specified NEC M75.8-
  sigmoid K63.9
  sinus (accessory) (nasal) J34.89
  skin L98.9
    suppurative L08.0
  SLAP S43.43-
  spinal cord G95.9
    congenital Q06.9
  spleen D73.89
  stomach K31.9
  superior glenoid labrum S43.43-
  syphilitic —*see* Syphilis
  tertiary —*see* Syphilis, tertiary
  thoracic root (nerve) NEC G54.3
  tonsillar fossa J35.9
  tooth, teeth K08.9
    white spot
      chewing surface K02.51
      pit and fissure surface K02.51
      smooth surface K02.61
  traumatic —*see* specific type of injury by site
  tricuspid (valve) I07.9
    nonrheumatic I36.9
  trigeminal nerve G50.9
  ulcerated or ulcerative —*see* Ulcer, skin
  uterus N85.9
  vagus nerve G52.2
  valvular —*see* Endocarditis
  vascular I99.9
    affecting central nervous system I67.9
    following trauma NEC T14.8
    umbilical cord, complicating delivery O69.5
  warty —*see* Verruca

◀ New   ◀▥ Revised   ~~deleted~~ Deleted

Lesion *(Continued)*
  white spot (tooth)
    chewing surface K02.51
    pit and fissure surface K02.51
    smooth surface K02.61
Lethargic —*see* condition
Lethargy R53.83
Letterer-Siwe's disease C96.0
Leukemia, leukemic C95.9-
  acute basophilic C94.8-
  acute bilineal C95.0-
  acute erythroid C94.0-
  acute lymphoblastic C91.0-
  acute megakaryoblastic C94.2-
  acute megakaryocytic C94.2-
  acute mixed lineage C95.0-
  acute monoblastic (monoblastic/monocytic)
      C93.0-
  acute monocytic (monoblastic/monocytic)
      C93.0-
  acute myeloblastic (minimal differentiation)
      (with maturation) C92.0-
  acute myeloid
    with
      11q23-abnormality C92.6-
      dysplasia of remaining hematopoesis
          and/or myelodysplastic disease in
          its history C92.A-
      multilineage dysplasia C92.A-
      variation of MLL-gene C92.6-
    M6 (a)(b) C94.0-
    M7 C94.2-
  acute myelomonocytic C92.5-
  acute promyelocytic C92.4-
  adult T-cell (HTLV-1-associated)
      (acute variant) (chronic variant)
      (lymphomatoid variant) (smouldering
      variant) C91.5-
  aggressive NK-cell C94.8-
  AML (1/ETO) (M0) (M1) (M2) (without a
      FAB classification) C92.0-
  AML M3 C92.4-
  AML M4 (Eo with inv(16) or t(16;16))
      C92.5-
  AML M5 C93.0-
  AML M5a C93.0-
  AML M5b C93.0-
  AML Me with t (15;17) and variants C92.4-
  atypical chronic myeloid, BCR/ABL-negative
      C92.2-
  biphenotypic acute C95.0-
  blast cell C95.0-
  Burkitt-type, mature B-cell C91.A-
  chronic lymphocytic, of B-cell type C91.1-
  chronic monocytic C93.1-
  chronic myelogenous (Philadelphia
      chromosome (Ph1) positive) (t(9;22))
      (q34;q11) (with crisis of blast cells)
      C92.1-
  chronic myeloid, BCR/ABL-positive C92.1-
    atypical, BCR/ABL-negative C92.2-
  chronic myelomonocytic C93.1-
  chronic neutrophilic D47.1
  CMML (-1) (-2) (with eosinophilia) C93.1-
  granulocytic (*see also* Category C92) C92.9-
  hairy-cell C91.4-
  juvenile myelomonocytic C93.3-
  lymphoid C91.9-
    specified NEC C91.Z-
  mast cell C94.3-
  mature B-cell, Burkitt-type C91.A-
  monocytic (subacute) C93.9-
    specified NEC C93.Z-
  myelogenous (*see also* Category C92) C92.9-
  myeloid C92.9-
    specified NEC C92.Z-
  plasma cell C90.1-
  plasmacytic C90.1-
  prolymphocytic
    of B-cell type C91.3-
    of T-cell type C91.6-

Leukemia, leukemic *(Continued)*
  specified NEC C94.8-
  stem cell, of unclear lineage C95.0-
  subacute lymphocytic C91.9-
  T-cell large granular lymphocytic C91.Z-
  unspecified cell type C95.9-
    acute C95.0-
    chronic C95.1-
Leukemoid reaction (*see also* Reaction,
    leukemoid) D72.823-
Leukoaraiosis (hypertensive) I67.81
Leukoariosis —*see* Leukoaraiosis
Leukocoria —*see* Disorder, globe, degenerated
    condition, leucocoria
Leukocytopenia D72.819
Leukocytosis D72.829
  eosinophilic D72.1
Leukoderma, leukodermia NEC L81.5
  syphilitic A51.39
    late A52.79
Leukodystrophy E75.29
Leukoedema, oral epithelium K13.29
Leukoencephalitis G04.81
  acute (subacute) hemorrhagic G36.1
    postimmunization or postvaccinal G04.02
  postinfectious G04.01
  subacute sclerosing A81.1
  van Bogaert's (sclerosing) A81.1
Leukoencephalopathy (*see also*
    Encephalopathy) G93.49
  Binswanger's I67.3
  heroin vapor G92
  metachromatic E75.25
  multifocal (progressive) A81.2
  postimmunization and postvaccinal G04.02
  progressive multifocal A81.2
  reversible, posterior G93.6
  van Bogaert's (sclerosing) A81.1
  vascular, progressive I67.3
Leukoerythroblastosis D75.9
Leukokeratosis —*see also* Leukoplakia
  mouth K13.21
  nicotina palati K13.24
  oral mucosa K13.21
  tongue K13.21
  vocal cord J38.3
Leukokraurosis vulva (e) N90.4
Leukoma (cornea) —*see also* Opacity, cornea
  adherent H17.0-
    interfering with central vision —*see* Opacity,
      cornea, central
Leukomalacia, cerebral, newborn P91.2
  periventricular P91.2
Leukomelanopathy, hereditary D72.0
Leukonychia (punctata) (striata) L60.8
  congenital Q84.4
Leukopathia unguium L60.8
  congenital Q84.4
Leukopenia D72.819
  basophilic D72.818
  chemotherapy (cancer) induced D70.1
  congenital D70.0
  cyclic D70.0
  drug induced NEC D70.2
    due to cytoreductive cancer chemotherapy
      D70.1
  eosinophilic D72.818
  familial D70.0
  infantile genetic D70.0
  malignant D70.9
  periodic D70.0
  transitory neonatal P61.5
Leukopenic —*see* condition
Leukoplakia
  anus K62.89
  bladder (postinfectional) N32.89
  buccal K13.21
  cervix (uteri) N88.0
  esophagus K22.8
  gingiva K13.21
  hairy (oral mucosa) (tongue) K13.3

Leukoplakia *(Continued)*
  kidney (pelvis) N28.89
  larynx J38.7
  lip K13.21
  mouth K13.21
  oral epithelium, including tongue (mucosa)
      K13.21
  palate K13.21
  pelvis (kidney) N28.89
  penis (infectional) N48.0
  rectum K62.89
  syphilitic (late) A52.79
  tongue K13.21
  ureter (postinfectional) N28.89
  urethra (postinfectional) N36.8
  uterus N85.8
  vagina N89.4
  vocal cord J38.3
  vulva N90.4
Leukorrhea N89.8
  due to Trichomonas (vaginalis)
      A59.00
  trichomonal A59.00
Leukosarcoma C85.9
Levocardia (isolated) Q24.1
  with situs inversus Q89.3
Levotransposition Q20.5
Lev's disease or syndrome (acquired complete
    heart block) I44.2
Levulosuria —*see* Fructosuria
Levurid L30.2
Lewy body (ies) (dementia) (disease)
    G31.83
Leyden-Moebius dystrophy G71.0
Leydig cell
  carcinoma
    specified site —*see* Neoplasm, malignant,
        by site
    unspecified site
      female C56.9-
      male C62.9-
  tumor
    benign
      specified site —*see* Neoplasm, benign,
          by site
      unspecified site
        female D27.-
        male D29.2-
    malignant
      specified site —*see* Neoplasm,
          malignant, by site
      unspecified site
        female C56.-
        male C62.9-
    specified site —*see* Neoplasm, uncertain
        behavior, by site
    unspecified site
      female D39.1-
      male D40.1-
Leydig-Sertoli cell tumor
  specified site —*see* Neoplasm, benign,
      by site
  unspecified site
    female D27.-
    male D29.2-
LGSIL (Low grade squamous intraepithelial
    lesion on cytologic smear of)
  anus R85.612
  cervix R87.612
  vagina R87.622
Liar, pathologic F60.2
Libido
  decreased R68.82
Libman-Sacks disease M32.11
Lice (infestation) B85.2
  body (Pediculus corporis) B85.1
  crab B85.3
  head (Pediculus capitis) B85.0
  mixed (classifiable to more than one of the
      titles B85.0-B85.3) B85.4
  pubic (Phthirus pubis) B85.3

Lichen L28.0
  albus L90.0
    penis N48.0
    vulva N90.4
  amyloidosis E85.4 *[L99]*
  atrophicus L90.0
    penis N48.0
    vulva N90.4
  congenital Q82.8
  myxedematosus L98.5
  nitidus L44.1
  pilaris Q82.8
    acquired L85.8
  planopilaris L66.1
  planus (chronicus) L43.9
    annularis L43.8
    bullous L43.1
    follicular L66.1
    hypertrophic L43.0
    moniliformis L44.3
    of Wilson L43.9
    specified NEC L43.8
    subacute (active) L43.3
    tropicus L43.3
  ruber
    acuminatus L44.0
    moniliformis L44.3
    planus L43.9
  sclerosus (et atrophicus) L90.0
    penis N48.0
    vulva N90.4
  scrofulosus (primary) (tuberculous) A18.4
  simplex (chronicus) (circumscriptus) L28.0
  striatus L44.2
  urticatus L28.2
Lichenification L28.0
Lichenoides tuberculosis (primary) A18.4
Lichtheim's disease or syndrome —*see*
      Degeneration, combined
Lien migrans D73.89
Ligament —*see* condition
Light
  for gestational age —*see* Light for dates
  headedness R42
Light-for-dates (infant) P05.00
  with weight of
    499 grams or less P05.01
    500-749 grams P05.02
    750-999 grams P05.03
    1000-1249 grams P05.04
    1250-1499 grams P05.05
    1500-1749 grams P05.06
    1750-1999 grams P05.07
    2000-2499 grams P05.08
  affecting management of pregnancy O36.59-
  and small-for-dates —*see* Small for dates
Lightning (effects) (stroke) (struck by) T75.00
  burn —*see* Burn
  foot E53.8
  shock T75.01
  specified effect NEC T75.09
Lightwood-Albright syndrome N25.89
Lightwood's disease or syndrome (renal
      tubular acidosis) N25.89
Ligneous thyroiditis E06.5
Likoff's syndrome I20.8
Limb —*see* condition
Limbic epilepsy personality syndrome F07.0
Limitation, limited
  activities due to disability Z73.6
  cardiac reserve —*see* Disease, heart
  eye muscle duction, traumatic —*see*
      Strabismus, mechanical
  mandibular range of motion M26.52
Lindau (-von Hippel) disease Q85.8
Line (s)
  Beau's L60.4
  Harris' —*see* Arrest, epiphyseal

Line *(Continued)*
  Hudson's (cornea) —*see* Pigmentation,
      cornea, anterior
  Stähli's (cornea) —*see* Pigmentation, cornea,
      anterior
Linea corneae senilis —*see* Change, cornea,
      senile
Lingua
  geographica K14.1
  nigra (villosa) K14.3
  plicata K14.5
  tylosis K13.29
Lingual —*see* condition
Linguatulosis B88.8
Linitis (gastric) plastica C16.9
Lip —*see* condition
Lipedema —*see* Edema
Lipemia —*see also* Hyperlipidemia
  retina, retinalis E78.3
Lipidosis E75.6
  cerebral (infantile) (juvenile) (late) E75.4
  cerebroretinal E75.4
  cerebroside E75.22
  cholesterol (cerebral) E75.5
  glycolipid E75.21
  hepatosplenomegalic E78.3
  sphingomyelin —*see* Niemann-Pick disease
      or syndrome
  sulfatide E75.29
Lipoadenoma —*see* Neoplasm, benign,
      by site
Lipoblastoma —*see* Lipoma
Lipoblastomatosis —*see* Lipoma
Lipochondrodystrophy E76.01
Lipochrome histiocytosis (familial) D71
Lipodermatosclerosis —*see* Varix, leg, with,
      inflammation
  ulcerated —*see* Varix, leg, with, ulcer, with
      inflammation by site
Lipodystrophia progressiva E88.1
Lipodystrophy (progressive) E88.1
  insulin E88.1
  intestinal K90.81
  mesenteric K65.4
Lipofibroma —*see* Lipoma
Lipofuscinosis, neuronal (with ceroidosis)
      E75.4
Lipogranuloma, sclerosing L92.8
Lipogranulomatosis E78.89
Lipoid —*see also* condition
  histiocytosis D76.3
    essential E75.29
  nephrosis N04.9
  proteinosis of Urbach E78.89
Lipoidemia —*see* Hyperlipidemia
Lipoidosis —*see* Lipidosis
Lipoma D17.9
  fetal D17.9
    fat cell D17.9
  infiltrating D17.9
  intramuscular D17.9
  pleomorphic D17.9
  site classification
    arms (skin) (subcutaneous) D17.2-
    connective tissue D17.30
      intra-abdominal D17.5
      intrathoracic D17.4
      peritoneum D17.79
      retroperitoneum D17.79
      specified site NEC D17.39
      spermatic cord D17.6
    face (skin) (subcutaneous) D17.0
    genitourinary organ NEC D17.72
    head (skin) (subcutaneous) D17.0
    intra-abdominal D17.5
    intrathoracic D17.4
    kidney D17.71
    legs (skin) (subcutaneous) D17.2-
    neck (skin) (subcutaneous) D17.0
    peritoneum D17.79
    retroperitoneum D17.79

Lipoma *(Continued)*
  site classification *(Continued)*
    skin D17.30
      specified site NEC D17.39
    specified site NEC D17.79
    spermatic cord D17.6
    subcutaneous D17.30
      specified site NEC D17.39
    trunk (skin) (subcutaneous) D17.1
    unspecified D17.9
  spindle cell D17.9
Lipomatosis E88.2
  dolorosa (Dercum) E88.2
  fetal —*see* Lipoma
  Launois-Bensaude E88.89
Lipomyoma —*see* Lipoma
Lipomyxoma —*see* Lipoma
Lipomyxosarcoma —*see* Neoplasm, connective
      tissue, malignant
Lipoprotein metabolism disorder E78.9
Lipoproteinemia E78.5
  broad-beta E78.2
  floating-beta E78.2
  hyper-pre-beta E78.1
Liposarcoma —*see also* Neoplasm, connective
      tissue, malignant
  dedifferentiated —*see* Neoplasm, connective
      tissue, malignant
  differentiated type —*see* Neoplasm,
      connective tissue, malignant
  embryonal —*see* Neoplasm, connective tissue,
      malignant
  mixed type —*see* Neoplasm, connective
      tissue, malignant
  myxoid —*see* Neoplasm, connective tissue,
      malignant
  pleomorphic —*see* Neoplasm, connective
      tissue, malignant
  round cell —*see* Neoplasm, connective tissue,
      malignant
  well differentiated type —*see* Neoplasm,
      connective tissue, malignant
Liposynovitis prepatellaris E88.89
Lipping, cervix N86
Lipschütz disease or ulcer N76.6
Lipuria R82.0
  schistosomiasis (bilharziasis) B65.0
Lisping F80.0
Lissauer's paralysis A52.17
Lissencephalia, lissencephaly Q04.3
Listeriosis, listerellosis A32.9
  congenital (disseminated) P37.2
  cutaneous A32.0
  neonatal, newborn (disseminated) P37.2
  oculoglandular A32.81
  specified NEC A32.89
Lithemia E79.0
Lithiasis —*see* Calculus
Lithosis J62.8
Lithuria R82.99
Litigation, anxiety concerning Z65.3
Little leaguer's elbow —*see* Epicondylitis,
      medial
Little's disease G80.9
Littre's
  gland —*see* condition
  hernia —*see* Hernia, abdomen
Littritis —*see* Urethritis
Livedo (annularis) (racemosa) (reticularis) R23.1
Liver —*see* condition
Living alone (problems with) Z60.2
  with handicapped person Z74.2
Lloyd's syndrome —*see* Adenomatosis,
      endocrine
Loa loa, loaiasis, loasis B74.3
Lobar —*see* condition
Lobomycosis B48.0
Lobo's disease B48.0
Lobotomy syndrome F07.0
Lobstein (-Ekman) disease or syndrome Q78.0
Lobster-claw hand Q71.6-

◀ New   ◀▥ Revised   ~~deleted~~ Deleted

Lobulation (congenital) —*see also* Anomaly, by site
  kidney, Q63.1
  liver, abnormal Q44.7
  spleen Q89.09
Lobule, lobular —*see* condition
Local, localized —*see* condition
Locked twins causing obstructed labor O66.1
Locked-in state G83.5
Locking
  joint —*see* Derangement, joint, specified type NEC
    knee —*see* Derangement, knee
Lockjaw —*see* Tetanus
Löffler's
  endocarditis I42.3
  eosinophilia J82
  pneumonia J82
  syndrome (eosinophilic pneumonitis) J82
Loiasis (with conjunctival infestation) (eyelid) B74.3
Lone Star fever A77.0
Long
  labor O63.9
    first stage O63.0
    second stage O63.1
  QT syndrome I45.81
Long-term (current) (prophylactic) drug therapy (use of)
  agents affecting estrogen receptors and estrogen levels NEC Z79.818
  anastrozole (Arimidex) Z79.811
  antibiotics Z79.2
    short-term use - omit code
  anticoagulants Z79.01
  anti-inflammatory, non-steroidal (NSAID) Z79.1
  antiplatelet Z79.02
  antithrombotics Z79.02
  aromatase inhibitors Z79.811
  aspirin Z79.82
  birth control pill or patch Z79.3
  bisphosphonates Z79.83
  contraceptive, oral Z79.3
  drug, specified NEC Z79.899
  estrogen receptor downregulators Z79.818
  Evista Z79.810
  exemestane (Aromasin) Z79.811
  Fareston Z79.810
  fulvestrant (Faslodex) Z79.818
  gonadotropin-releasing hormone (GnRH) agonist Z79.818
  goserelin acetate (Zoladex) Z79.818
  hormone replacement (postmenopausal) Z79.890
  insulin Z79.4
  letrozole (Femara) Z79.811
  leuprolide acetate (leuprorelin) (Lupron) Z79.818
  megestrol acetate (Megace) Z79.818
  methadone for pain management Z79.891
  Nolvadex Z79.810
  non-steroidal anti-inflammatories (NSAID) Z79.1
  opiate analgesic Z79.891
  oral contraceptive Z79.3
  raloxifene (Evista) Z79.810
  selective estrogen receptor modulators (SERMs) Z79.810
  steroids
    inhaled Z79.51
    systemic Z79.52
  tamoxifen (Nolvadex) Z79.810
  toremifene (Fareston) Z79.810
Longitudinal stripes or grooves, nails L60.8
  congenital Q84.6
Loop
  intestine —*see* Volvulus
  vascular on papilla (optic) Q14.2

Loose —*see also* condition
  body
    joint M24.00
      ankle M24.07-
      elbow M24.02-
      hand M24.04-
      hip M24.05-
      knee M23.4-
      shoulder (region) M24.01-
      specified site NEC M24.08
      toe M24.07-
      vertebra M24.08
      wrist M24.03-
    knee M23.4-
    sheath, tendon —*see* Disorder, tendon, specified type NEC
  cartilage —*see* Loose, body, joint
  tooth, teeth K08.8
Loosening
  aseptic
    joint prosthesis —*see* Complications, joint prosthesis, mechanical, loosening, by site
    epiphysis —*see* Osteochondropathy
  mechanical
    joint prosthesis —*see* Complications, joint prosthesis, mechanical, loosening, by site
Looser-Milkman (-Debray) syndrome M83.8
Lop ear (deformity) Q17.3
Lorain (-Levi) short stature syndrome E23.0
Lordosis M40.50
  acquired —*see* Lordosis, specified type NEC
  congenital Q76.429
    lumbar region Q76.426
    lumbosacral region Q76.427
    sacral region Q76.428
    sacrococcygeal region Q76.428
    thoracolumbar region Q76.425
  lumbar region M40.56
  lumbosacral region M40.57
  postsurgical M96.4
  postural —*see* Lordosis, specified type NEC
  rachitic (late effect) (sequelae) E64.3
  sequelae of rickets E64.3
  specified type NEC M40.40
    lumbar region M40.46
    lumbosacral region M40.47
    thoracolumbar region M40.45
  thoracolumbar region M40.55
  tuberculous A18.01
Loss (of)
  appetite (*see* Anorexia) R63.0
    hysterical F50.8
    nonorganic origin F50.8
    psychogenic F50.8
  blood —*see* Hemorrhage
  consciousness, transient R55
    traumatic —*see* Injury, intracranial
  control, sphincter, rectum R15.9
    nonorganic origin F98.1
  elasticity, skin R23.4
  family (member) in childhood Z62.898
  fluid (acute) E86.9
    with
      hypernatremia E87.0
      hyponatremia E87.1
  function of labyrinth —*see* subcategory H83.2
  hair, nonscarring —*see* Alopecia
  hearing —*see also* Deafness
    central NOS H90.5
    neural NOS H90.5
    perceptive NOS H90.5
    sensorineural NOS H90.5
    sensory NOS H90.5
  height R29.890
  limb or member, traumatic, current —*see* Amputation, traumatic
  love relationship in childhood Z62.898

Loss (*Continued*)
  memory —*see also* Amnesia
    mild, following organic brain damage F06.8
  mind —*see* Psychosis
  occlusal vertical dimension of fully erupted teeth M26.37
  organ or part —*see* Absence, by site, acquired
  ossicles, ear (partial) H74.32-
  parent in childhood Z63.4
  pregnancy, recurrent N96
    without current pregnancy N96
    care in current pregnancy O26.2-
  recurrent pregnancy —*see* Loss, pregnancy, recurrent
  self-esteem, in childhood Z62.898
  sense of
    smell —*see* Disturbance, sensation, smell
    taste —*see* Disturbance, sensation, taste
    touch R20.8
  sensory R44.9
    dissociative F44.6
  sexual desire F52.0
  sight (acquired) (complete) (congenital) —*see* Blindness
  substance of
    bone —*see* Disorder, bone, density and structure, specified NEC
    cartilage —*see* Disorder, cartilage, specified type NEC
    auricle (ear) —*see* Disorder, pinna, specified type NEC
    vitreous (humor) H15.89
  tooth, teeth —*see* Absence, teeth, acquired
  vision, visual H54.7
    both eyes H54.3
    one eye H54.60
      left (normal vision on right) H54.62
      right (normal vision on left) H54.61
    specified as blindness —*see* Blindness
    subjective
      sudden H53.13-
      transient H53.12-
  vitreous —*see* Prolapse, vitreous
  voice —*see* Aphonia
  weight (abnormal) (cause unknown) R63.4
Louis-Bar syndrome (ataxia-telangiectasia) G11.3
Louping ill (encephalitis) A84.8
Louse, lousiness —*see* Lice
Low
  achiever, school Z55.3
  back syndrome M54.5
  basal metabolic rate R94.8
  birthweight (2499 grams or less) P07.10
    with weight of
      1000-1249 grams P07.14
      1250-1499 grams P07.15
      1500-1749 grams P07.16
      1750-1999 grams P07.17
      2000-2499 grams P07.18
    extreme (999 grams or less) P07.00
      with weight of
        499 grams or less P07.01
        500-749 grams P07.02
        750-999 grams P07.03
    for gestational age —*see* Light for dates
  blood pressure —*see also* Hypotension
    reading (incidental) (isolated) (nonspecific) R03.1
  cardiac reserve —*see* Disease, heart
  function —*see also* Hypofunction
    kidney N28.9
  hematocrit D64.9
  hemoglobin D64.9
  income Z59.6
  level of literacy Z55.0
  lying
    kidney N28.89
    organ or site, congenital —*see* Malposition, congenital

Low *(Continued)*
output syndrome (cardiac) —*see* Failure, heart
platelets (blood) —*see* Thrombocytopenia
reserve, kidney N28.89
salt syndrome E87.1
self esteem R45.81
set ears Q17.4
vision H54.2
one eye (other eye normal) H54.50
left (normal vision on right) H54.52
other eye blind —*see* Blindness
right (normal vision on left) H54.51
Low-density-lipoprotein-type (LDL) hyperlipoproteinemia E78.0
Lowe's syndrome E72.03
Lown-Ganong-Levine syndrome I45.6
LSD reaction (acute) (without dependence) F16.90
with dependence F16.20
L-shaped kidney Q63.8
Ludwig's angina or disease K12.2
Lues (venerea), luetic —*see* Syphilis
Luetscher's syndrome (dehydration) E86.0
Lumbago, lumbalgia M54.5
with sciatica M54.4-
due to intervertebral disc disorder M51.17
due to displacement, intervertebral disc M51.27
with sciatica M51.17
Lumbar —*see* condition
Lumbarization, vertebra, congenital Q76.49
Lumbermen's itch B88.0
Lump —*see* Mass
Lunacy —*see* Psychosis
Lung —*see* condition
Lupoid (miliary) of Boeck D86.3
Lupus
anticoagulant D68.62
with
hemorrhagic disorder D68.312
hypercoagulable state D68.62
finding without diagnosis R76.0
discoid (local) L93.0
erythematosus (discoid) (local) L93.0
disseminated —*see* Lupus, erythematosus, systemic
eyelid H01.129
left H01.126
lower H01.125
upper H01.124
right H01.123
lower H01.122
upper H01.121
profundus L93.2
specified NEC L93.2
subacute cutaneous L93.1
systemic M32.9
with organ or system involvement M32.10
endocarditis M32.11
lung M32.13
pericarditis M32.12
renal (glomerular) M32.14
tubulo-interstitial M32.15
specified organ or system NEC M32.19
drug-induced M32.0
inhibitor (presence of) D68.62
with
hemorrhagic disorder D68.312
hypercoagulable state D68.62
finding without diagnosis R76.0
specified NEC M32.8
exedens A18.4
hydralazine M32.0
correct substance properly administered — *see* Table of Drugs and Chemicals, by drug, adverse effect
overdose or wrong substance given or taken —*see* Table of Drugs and Chemicals, by drug, poisoning

Lupus *(Continued)*
nephritis (chronic) M32.14
nontuberculous, not disseminated L93.0
panniculitis L93.2
pernio (Besnier) D86.3
systemic —*see* Lupus, erythematosus, systemic
tuberculous A18.4
eyelid A18.4
vulgaris A18.4
eyelid A18.4
Luteinoma D27.-
Lutembacher's disease or syndrome (atrial septal defect with mitral stenosis) Q21.1
Luteoma D27.-
Lutz (-Splendore-de Almeida) disease —*see* Paracoccidioidomycosis
Luxation —*see also* Dislocation
eyeball (nontraumatic) —*see* Luxation, globe
birth injury P15.3
globe, nontraumatic H44.82-
lacrimal gland —*see* Dislocation, lacrimal gland
lens (old) (partial) (spontaneous)
congenital Q12.1
syphilitic A50.39
Lycanthropy F22
Lyell's syndrome L51.2
due to drug L51.2
correct substance properly administered — *see* Table of Drugs and Chemicals, by drug, adverse effect
overdose or wrong substance given or taken —*see* Table of Drugs and Chemicals, by drug, poisoning
Lyme disease A69.20
Lymph
gland or node —*see* condition
scrotum —*see* Infestation, filarial
Lymphadenitis I88.9
with ectopic or molar pregnancy O08.0
acute L04.9
axilla L04.2
face L04.0
head L04.0
hip L04.3
limb
lower L04.3
upper L04.2
neck L04.0
shoulder L04.2
specified site NEC L04.8
trunk L04.1
anthracosis (occupational) J60
any site, except mesenteric I88.9
chronic I88.1
subacute I88.1
breast
gestational —*see* Mastitis, obstetric
puerperal, postpartum (nonpurulent) O91.22
chancroidal (congenital) A57
chronic I88.1
mesenteric I88.0
due to
Brugia (malayi) B74.1
timori B74.2
chlamydial lymphogranuloma A55
diphtheria (toxin) A36.89
lymphogranuloma venereum A55
Wuchereria bancrofti B74.0
following ectopic or molar pregnancy O08.0
gonorrheal A54.89
infective —*see* Lymphadenitis, acute
mesenteric (acute) (chronic) (nonspecific) (subacute) I88.0
due to Salmonella typhi A01.09
tuberculous A18.39
mycobacterial A31.8
purulent —*see* Lymphadenitis, acute
pyogenic —*see* Lymphadenitis, acute

Lymphadenitis *(Continued)*
regional, nonbacterial I88.8
septic —*see* Lymphadenitis, acute
subacute, unspecified site I88.1
suppurative —*see* Lymphadenitis, acute
syphilitic (early) (secondary) A51.49
late A52.79
tuberculous —*see* Tuberculosis, lymph gland
venereal (chlamydial) A55
Lymphadenoid goiter E06.3
Lymphadenopathy (generalized) R59.1
angioimmunoblastic, with dysproteinemia (AILD) C86.5
due to toxoplasmosis (acquired) B58.89
congenital (acute) (subacute) (chronic) P37.1
localized R59.0
syphilitic (early) (secondary) A51.49
Lymphadenosis R59.1
Lymphangiectasis I89.0
conjunctiva H11.89
postinfectional I89.0
scrotum I89.0
Lymphangiectatic elephantiasis, nonfilarial I89.0
Lymphangioendothelioma D18.1
malignant —*see* Neoplasm, connective tissue, malignant
Lymphangioleiomyomatosis J84.81
Lymphangioma D18.1
capillary D18.1
cavernous D18.1
cystic D18.1
malignant —*see* Neoplasm, connective tissue, malignant
Lymphangiomyoma D18.1
Lymphangiomyomatosis J84.81
Lymphangiosarcoma —*see* Neoplasm, connective tissue, malignant
Lymphangitis I89.1
with
abscess - code by site under Abscess
cellulitis - code by site under Cellulitis
ectopic or molar pregnancy O08.0
acute L03.91
abdominal wall L03.321
ankle —*see* Lymphangitis, acute, lower limb
arm —*see* Lymphangitis, acute, upper limb
auricle (ear) —*see* Lymphangitis, acute, ear
axilla L03.12-
back (any part) L03.322
buttock L03.327
cervical (meaning neck) L03.222
cheek (external) L03.212
chest wall L03.323
digit
finger —*see* Lymphangitis, acute, finger
toe —*see* Lymphangitis, acute, toe
ear (external) H60.1-
external auditory canal —*see* Lymphangitis, acute, ear
eyelid —*see* Abscess, eyelid
face NEC L03.212
finger (intrathecal) (periosteal) (subcutaneous) (subcuticular) L03.02-
foot —*see* Lymphangitis, acute, lower limb
gluteal (region) L03.327
groin L03.324
hand —*see* Lymphangitis, acute, upper limb
head NEC L03.891
face (any part, except ear, eye and nose) L03.212
heel —*see* Lymphangitis, acute, lower limb
hip —*see* Lymphangitis, acute, lower limb
jaw (region) L03.212
knee —*see* Lymphangitis, acute, lower limb
leg —*see* Lymphangitis, acute, lower limb
lower limb L03.12-
toe —*see* Lymphangitis, acute, toe

Lymphangitis (Continued)
  acute (Continued)
    navel L03.326
    neck (region) L03.222
    orbit, orbital —see Cellulitis, orbit
    pectoral (region) L03.323
    perineal, perineum L03.325
    scalp (any part) L03.891
    shoulder —see Lymphangitis, acute, upper
      limb
    specified site NEC L03.898
    thigh —see Lymphangitis, acute, lower
      limb
    thumb (intrathecal) (periosteal)
      (subcutaneous) (subcuticular) —see
      Lymphangitis, acute, finger
    toe (intrathecal) (periosteal) (subcutaneous)
      (subcuticular) L03.04-
    trunk L03.329
      abdominal wall L03.321
      back (any part) L03.322
      buttock L03.327
      chest wall L03.323
      groin L03.324
      perineal, perineum L03.325
      umbilicus L03.326
    umbilicus L03.326
    upper limb L03.12-
      axilla —see Lymphangitis, acute, axilla
      finger —see Lymphangitis, acute, finger
      thumb —see Lymphangitis, acute, finger
      wrist —see Lymphangitis, acute, upper
        limb
  breast
    gestational —see Mastitis, obstetric
  chancroidal A57
  chronic (any site) I89.1
  due to
    Brugia (malayi) B74.1
      timori B74.2
    Wuchereria bancrofti B74.0
  following ectopic or molar pregnancy O08.89
  penis
    acute N48.29
    gonococcal (acute) (chronic) A54.09
  puerperal, postpartum, childbirth O86.89
  strumous, tuberculous A18.2
  subacute (any site) I89.1
  tuberculous —see Tuberculosis, lymph gland
Lymphatic (vessel) —see condition
Lymphatism E32.8
Lymphectasia I89.0
Lymphedema (acquired) —see also Elephantiasis
  congenital Q82.0
  hereditary (chronic) (idiopathic) Q82.0
  postmastectomy I97.2
  praecox I89.0
  secondary I89.0
  surgical NEC I97.89
    postmastectomy (syndrome) I97.2
Lymphoblastic —see condition
Lymphoblastoma (diffuse) —see Lymphoma,
  lymphoblastic (diffuse)
  giant follicular —see Lymphoma,
    lymphoblastic (diffuse)
  macrofollicular —see Lymphoma,
    lymphoblastic (diffuse)
Lymphocele I89.8
Lymphocytic
  chorioencephalitis (acute) (serous) A87.2
  choriomeningitis (acute) (serous) A87.2
  meningoencephalitis A87.2

Lymphocytoma, benign cutis L98.8
Lymphocytopenia D72.810
Lymphocytosis (symptomatic)
  D72.820
  infectious (acute) B33.8
Lymphoepithelioma —see Neoplasm,
  malignant, by site
Lymphogranuloma (malignant) —see also
  Lymphoma, Hodgkin
  chlamydial A55
  inguinale A55
  venereum (any site) (chlamydial) (with
    stricture of rectum) A55
Lymphogranulomatosis (malignant) —see also
  Lymphoma, Hodgkin
  benign (Boeck's sarcoid) (Schaumann's)
    D86.1
Lymphohistiocytosis, hemophagocytic
  (familial) D76.1
Lymphoid —see condition
Lymphoma (of) (malignant) C85.90
  adult T-cell (HTLV-1-associated)
    (acute variant) (chronic variant)
    (lymphomatoid variant) (smouldering
    variant) C91.5-
  anaplastic large cell
    ALK-negative C84.7-
    ALK-positive C84.6-
    CD30-positive C84.6-
    primary cutaneous C86.6
  angioimmunoblastic T-cell C86.5
  BALT C88.4
  B-cell C85.1-
  B-precursor C83.5-
  blastic NK-cell C86.4
  bronchial-associated lymphoid tissue
    [BALT-lymphoma] C88.4
  Burkitt (atypical) C83.7-
  Burkitt-like C83.7-
  centrocytic C83.1-
  cutaneous follicle center C82.6-
  cutaneous T-cell C84.A-
  diffuse follicle center C82.5-
  diffuse large cell C83.3-
    anaplastic C83.3-
    B-cell C83.3-
    CD30-positive C83.3-
    centroblastic C83.3-
    immunoblastic C83.3-
    plasmablastic C83.3-
    subtype not specified C83.3-
    T-cell rich C83.3-
  enteropathy-type (associated) (intestinal)
    T-cell C86.2
  extranodal marginal zone B-cell
    lymphoma of mucosa-associated
    lymphoid tissue [MALT-lymphoma]
    C88.4
  extranodal NK/T-cell, nasal type
    C86.0
  follicular C82.9-
    grade
      I C82.0-
      II C82.1-
      III C82.2-
      IIIa C82.3-
      IIIb C82.4-
    specified NEC C82.8-
  hepatosplenic T-cell (alpha-beta)
    (gamma-delta) C86.1
  histiocytic C85.9-
    true C96.A

Lymphoma (Continued)
  Hodgkin C81.9
    classical C81.7-
      lymphocyte-rich C81.4-
      lymphocytic depletion C81.3-
      mixed cellularity C81.2-
      nodular sclerosis C81.1-
      specified NEC C81.7-
    lymphocyte-rich classical C81.4-
    lymphocyte depleted classical C81.3-
    mixed cellularity classical C81.2-
    nodular
      lymphocyte predominant C81.0-
      sclerosis classical C81.1-
  intravascular large B-cell C83.8-
  Lennert's C84.4-
  lymphoblastic (diffuse) C83.5-
  lymphoblastic B-cell C83.5-
  lymphoblastic T-cell C83.5-
  lymphoepithelioid C84.4-
  lymphoplasmacytic C83.0-
    with IgM-production C88.0
  MALT C88.4
  mantle cell C83.1-
  mature T-cell NEC C84.4-
  mature T/NK-cell C84.9-
    specified NEC C84.Z-
  mediastinal (thymic) large B-cell
    C85.2-
  Mediterranean C88.3
  mucosa-associated lymphoid tissue
    [MALT-lymphoma] C88.4
  NK/T cell C84.9-
  nodal marginal zone C83.0-
  non-follicular (diffuse) C83.9-
    specified NEC C83.8-
  non-Hodgkin (see also Lymphoma, by type)
    C85.9-
    specified NEC C85.8-
  non-leukemic variant of B-CLL C83.0-
  peripheral T-cell, not classified C84.4-
  primary cutaneous
    anaplastic large cell C86.6
    CD30-positive large T-cell C86.6
  primary effusion B-cell C83.8-
  SALT C88.4
  skin-associated lymphoid tissue [SALT-
    lymphoma] C88.4
  small cell B-cell C83.0-
  splenic marginal zone C83.0-
  subcutaneous panniculitis-like T-cell
    C86.3
  T-precursor C83.5-
  true histiocytic C96.A
Lymphomatosis —see Lymphoma
Lymphopathia venereum, veneris A55
Lymphopenia D72.810
Lymphoplasmacytic leukemia —see Leukemia,
  chronic lymphocytic, B-cell type
Lymphoproliferation, X-linked disease
  D82.3
Lymphoreticulosis, benign (of inoculation)
  A28.1
Lymphorrhea I89.8
Lymphosarcoma (diffuse) (see also Lymphoma)
  C85.9-
Lymphostasis I89.8
Lypemania —see Melancholia
Lysine and hydroxylysine metabolism
  disorder E72.3
Lyssa —see Rabies

M

Macacus ear Q17.3
Maceration, wet feet, tropical (syndrome) T69.02-
MacLeod's syndrome J43.0
Macrocephalia, macrocephaly Q75.3
Macrocheilia, macrochilia (congenital)Q18.6
Macrocolon (see also Megacolon) Q43.1
Macrocornea Q15.8
    with glaucoma Q15.0
Macrocytic —see condition
Macrocytosis D75.89
Macrodactylia, macrodactylism (fingers) (thumbs) Q74.0
    toes Q74.2
Macrodontia K00.2
Macrogenia M26.05
Macrogenitosomia (adrenal) (male) (praecox) E25.9
    congenital E25.0
Macroglobulinemia (idiopathic) (primary) C88.0
    monoclonal (essential) D47.2
    Waldenström C88.0
Macroglossia (congenital) Q38.2
    acquired K14.8
Macrognathia, macrognathism (congenital) (mandibular) (maxillary) M26.09
Macrogyria (congenital) Q04.8
Macrohydrocephalus —see Hydrocephalus
Macromastia —see Hypertrophy, breast
Macrophthalmos Q11.3
    in congenital glaucoma Q15.0
Macropsia H53.15
Macrosigmoid K59.3
    congenital Q43.2
Macrospondylitis, acromegalic E22.0
Macrostomia (congenital) Q18.4
Macrotia (external ear) (congenital) Q17.1
Macula
    cornea, corneal —see Opacity, cornea
    degeneration (atrophic) (exudative) (senile) —see also Degeneration, macula
    hereditary —see Dystrophy, retina
Maculae ceruleae — B85.1
Maculopathy, toxic —see Degeneration, macula, toxic
Madarosis (eyelid) H02.729
    left H02.726
        lower H02.725
        upper H02.724
    right H02.723
        lower H02.722
        upper H02.721
Madelung's
    deformity (radius) Q74.0
    disease
        radial deformity Q74.0
        symmetrical lipomas, neck E88.89
Madness —see Psychosis
Madura
    foot B47.9
        actinomycotic B47.1
        mycotic B47.0
Maduromycosis B47.0
Maffucci's syndrome Q78.4
Magnesium metabolism disorder —see Disorder, metabolism, magnesium
Main en griffe (acquired) —see also Deformity, limb, clawhand
    congenital Q74.0
Maintenance (encounter for)
    antineoplastic chemotherapy Z51.11
    antineoplastic radiation therapy Z51.0
    methadone F11.20
Majocchi's
    disease L81.7
    granuloma B35.8
Major —see condition
Malabar itch (any site) B35.5

Malabsorption K90.9
    calcium K90.89
    carbohydrate K90.4
    disaccharide E73.9
    fat K90.4
    galactose E74.20
    glucose(-galactose) E74.39
    intestinal K90.9
        specified NEC K90.89
    isomaltose E74.31
    lactose E73.9
    methionine E72.19
    monosaccharide E74.39
    postgastrectomy K91.2
    postsurgical K91.2
    protein K90.4
    starch K90.4
    sucrose E74.39
    syndrome K90.9
        postsurgical K91.2
Malacia, bone (adult) M83.9
    juvenile —see Rickets
Malacoplakia
    bladder N32.89
    pelvis (kidney) N28.89
    ureter N28.89
    urethra N36.8
Malacosteon, juvenile —see Rickets
Maladaptation —see Maladjustment
Maladie de Roger Q21.0
Maladjustment
    conjugal Z63.0
        involving divorce or estrangement Z63.5
    educational Z55.4
    family Z63.9
    marital Z63.0
        involving divorce or estrangement Z63.5
    occupational NEC Z56.89
    simple, adult —see Disorder, adjustment
    situational —see Disorder, adjustment
    social Z60.9
        due to
            acculturation difficulty Z60.3
            discrimination and persecution (perceived) Z60.5
            exclusion and isolation Z60.4
            life-cycle (phase of life) transition Z60.0
            rejection Z60.4
            specified reason NEC Z60.8
Malaise R53.81
Malakoplakia —see Malacoplakia
Malaria, malarial (fever) B54
    with
        blackwater fever B50.8
            hemoglobinuric (bilious) B50.8
            hemoglobinuria B50.8
        accidentally induced (therapeutically) - code by type under Malaria
    algid B50.9
    cerebral B50.0 [G94]
    clinically diagnosed (without parasitological confirmation) B54
    congenital NEC P37.4
        falciparum P37.3
    congestion, congestive B54
    continued (fever) B50.9
    estivo-autumnal B50.9
    falciparum B50.9
        with complications NEC B50.8
            cerebral B50.0 [G94]
        severe B50.8
    hemorrhagic B54
    malariae B52.9
        with
            complications NEC B52.8
            glomerular disorder B52.0
    malignant (tertian) —see Malaria, falciparum
    mixed infections — code to first listed type in B50-B53
    ovale B53.0
    parasitologically confirmed NEC B53.8

Malaria, malarial (Continued)
    pernicious, acute —see Malaria, falciparum
    Plasmodium (P.)
        falciparum NEC —see Malaria, falciparum
        malariae NEC B52.9
            with Plasmodium
                falciparum (and or vivax) —see Malaria, falciparum
                vivax —see also Malaria, vivax
                    and falciparum —see Malaria, falciparum
        ovale B53.0
            with Plasmodium malariae —see also Malaria, malariae
                and vivax —see also Malaria, vivax
                    and falciparum —see Malaria, falciparum
        simian B53.1
            with Plasmodium malariae —see also Malaria, malariae
                and vivax —see also Malaria, vivax
                    and falciparum —see Malaria, falciparum
        vivax NEC B51.9
            with Plasmodium falciparum —see Malaria, falciparum
    quartan —see Malaria, malariae
    quotidian —see Malaria, falciparum
    recurrent B54
    remittent B54
    specified type NEC (parasitologically confirmed) B53.8
    spleen B54
    subtertian (fever) —see Malaria, falciparum
    tertian (benign) —see also Malaria, vivax
        malignant B50.9
    tropical B50.9
    typhoid B54
    vivax B51.9
        with
            complications NEC B51.8
            ruptured spleen B51.0
Malassez's disease (cystic) N50.8
Malassimilation K90.9
Mal de los pintos —see Pinta
Mal de mer T75.3
Maldescent, testis Q53.9
    bilateral Q53.20
        abdominal Q53.21
        perineal Q53.22
    unilateral Q53.10
        abdominal Q53.11
        perineal Q53.12
Maldevelopment —see also Anomaly
    brain Q07.9
    colon Q43.9
    hip Q74.2
        congenital dislocation Q65.2
            bilateral Q65.1
            unilateral Q65.0-
    mastoid process Q75.8
    middle ear Q16.4
        except ossicles Q16.4
        ossicles Q16.3
    ossicles Q16.3
    spine Q76.49
    toe Q74.2
Male type pelvis Q74.2
    with disproportion (fetopelvic) O33.3
        causing obstructed labor O65.3
Malformation (congenital) —see also Anomaly
    adrenal gland Q89.1
    affecting multiple systems with skeletal changes NEC Q87.5
    alimentary tract Q45.9
        specified type NEC Q45.8
        upper Q40.9
            specified type NEC Q40.8
    aorta Q25.9
        atresia Q25.2
        coarctation (preductal) (postductal) Q25.1

◀ New   ◀ Revised   ~~deleted~~ Deleted

Malformation (Continued)
  aorta (Continued)
    patent ductus arteriosus Q25.0
    specified type NEC Q25.4
    stenosis (supravalvular) Q25.3
  aortic valve Q23.9
    specified NEC Q23.8
  arteriovenous, aneurysmatic (congenital)
      Q27.30
    brain Q28.2
    cerebral Q28.2
    peripheral Q27.30
      digestive system Q27.33
      lower limb Q27.32
      other specified site Q27.39
      renal vessel Q27.34
      upper limb Q27.31
    precerebral vessels (nonruptured) Q28.0
  auricle
    ear (congenital) Q17.3
      acquired H61.119
        left H61.112
          with right H61.113
        right H61.111
          with left H61.113
  bile duct Q44.5
  bladder Q64.79
    aplasia Q64.5
    diverticulum Q64.6
    exstrophy —see Exstrophy, bladder
    neck obstruction Q64.31
  bone Q79.9
    face Q75.9
      specified type NEC Q75.8
    skull Q75.9
      specified type NEC Q75.8
  brain (multiple) Q04.9
    arteriovenous Q28.2
    specified type NEC Q04.8
  branchial cleft Q18.2
  breast Q83.9
    specified type NEC Q83.8
  broad ligament Q50.6
  bronchus Q32.4
  bursa Q79.9
  cardiac
    chambers Q20.9
      specified type NEC Q20.8
    septum Q21.9
      specified type NEC Q21.8
  cerebral Q04.9
    vessels Q28.3
  cervix uteri Q51.9
    specified type NEC Q51.828
  Chiari
    Type I G93.5
    Type II Q07.01
  choroid (congenital) Q14.3
    plexus Q07.8
  circulatory system Q28.9
  cochlea Q16.5
  cornea Q13.4
  coronary vessels Q24.5
  corpus callosum (congenital) Q04.0
  diaphragm Q79.1
  digestive system NEC, specified type NEC
      Q45.8
  dura Q07.9
    brain Q04.9
    spinal Q06.9
  ear Q17.9
    causing impairment of hearing Q16.9
    external Q17.9
      accessory auricle Q17.0
      causing impairment of hearing Q16.9
        absence of
          auditory canal Q16.1
          auricle Q16.0
        macrotia Q17.1
        microtia Q17.2
        misplacement Q17.4

Malformation (Continued)
  ear (Continued)
    external (Continued)
      misshapen NEC Q17.3
      prominence Q17.5
      specified type NEC Q17.8
    inner Q16.5
    middle Q16.4
      absence of eustachian tube Q16.2
      ossicles (fusion) Q16.3
    ossicles Q16.3
    specified type NEC Q17.8
  epididymis Q55.4
  esophagus Q39.9
    specified type NEC Q39.8
  eye Q15.9
    lid Q10.3
    specified NEC Q15.8
  fallopian tube Q50.6
  genital organ —see Anomaly, genitalia
  great
    artery Q25.9
      aorta —see Malformation, aorta
      pulmonary artery —see Malformation,
          pulmonary, artery
      specified type NEC Q25.8
    vein Q26.9
      anomalous
        portal venous connection Q26.5
        pulmonary venous connection Q26.4
          partial Q26.3
          total Q26.2
      persistent left superior vena cava Q26.1
      portal vein-hepatic artery fistula Q26.6
      specified type NEC Q26.8
      vena cava stenosis, congenital Q26.0
  gum Q38.6
  hair Q84.2
  heart Q24.9
    specified type NEC Q24.8
  integument Q84.9
    specified type NEC Q84.8
  internal ear Q16.5
  intestine Q43.9
    specified type NEC Q43.8
  iris Q13.2
  joint Q74.9
    ankle Q74.2
    lumbosacral Q76.49
    sacroiliac Q74.2
    specified type NEC Q74.8
  kidney Q63.9
    accessory Q63.0
    giant Q63.3
    horseshoe Q63.1
    hydronephrosis Q62.0
    malposition Q63.2
    specified type NEC Q63.8
  lacrimal apparatus Q10.6
  lingual Q38.3
  lip Q38.0
  liver Q44.7
  lung Q33.9
  meninges or membrane (congenital) Q07.9
    cerebral Q04.8
    spinal (cord) Q06.9
  middle ear Q16.4
    ossicles Q16.3
  mitral valve Q23.9
    specified NEC Q23.8
  Mondini's (congenital) (malformation,
      cochlea) Q16.5
  mouth (congenital) Q38.6
  multiple types NEC Q89.7
  musculoskeletal system Q79.9
  myocardium Q24.8
  nail Q84.6
  nervous system (central) Q07.9
  nose Q30.9
    specified type NEC Q30.8
  optic disc Q14.2

Malformation (Continued)
  orbit Q10.7
  ovary Q50.39
  palate Q38.5
  parathyroid gland Q89.2
  pelvic organs or tissues NEC
    in pregnancy or childbirth O34.8-
      causing obstructed labor O65.5
  penis Q55.69
    aplasia Q55.5
    curvature (lateral) Q55.61
    hypoplasia Q55.62
  pericardium Q24.8
  peripheral vascular system Q27.9
    specified type NEC Q27.8
  pharynx Q38.8
  precerebral vessels Q28.1
  prostate Q55.4
  pulmonary
    arteriovenous Q25.72
    artery Q25.9
      atresia Q25.5
      specified type NEC Q25.79
      stenosis Q25.6
    valve Q22.3
  renal artery Q27.2
  respiratory system Q34.9
  retina Q14.1
  scrotum —see Malformation, testis and
      scrotum
  seminal vesicles Q55.4
  sense organs NEC Q07.9
  skin Q82.9
  specified NEC Q89.8
  spinal
    cord Q06.9
    nerve root Q07.8
  spine Q76.49
    kyphosis —see Kyphosis, congenital
    lordosis —see Lordosis, congenital
  spleen Q89.09
  stomach Q40.3
    specified type NEC Q40.2
  teeth, tooth K00.9
  tendon Q79.9
  testis and scrotum Q55.20
    aplasia Q55.0
    hypoplasia Q55.1
    polyorchism Q55.21
    retractile testis Q55.22
    scrotal transposition Q55.23
    specified NEC Q55.29
  thorax, bony Q76.9
  throat Q38.8
  thyroid gland Q89.2
  tongue (congenital) Q38.3
    hypertrophy Q38.2
    tie Q38.1
  trachea Q32.1
  tricuspid valve Q22.9
    specified type NEC Q22.8
  umbilical cord NEC (complicating delivery)
      O69.89
  umbilicus Q89.9
  ureter Q62.8
    agenesis Q62.4
    duplication Q62.5
    malposition —see Malposition, congenital,
        ureter
    obstructive defect —see Defect, obstructive,
        ureter
    vesico-uretero-renal reflux Q62.7
  urethra Q64.79
    aplasia Q64.5
    duplication Q64.74
    posterior valves Q64.2
    prolapse Q64.71
    stricture Q64.32
  urinary system Q64.9
  uterus Q51.9
    specified type NEC Q51.818

Malformation (Continued)
  vagina Q52.4
  vascular system, peripheral Q27.9
  vas deferens Q55.4
    atresia Q55.3
  venous —see Anomaly, vein (s)
  vulva Q52.70
Malfunction —see also Dysfunction
  cardiac electronic device T82.119
    electrode T82.110
    pulse generator T82.111
    specified type NEC T82.118
  catheter device NEC T85.618
    cystostomy T83.010
    dialysis (renal) (vascular) T82.41
      intraperitoneal T85.611
    infusion NEC T82.514
      spinal (epidural) (subdural) T85.610
    urinary, indwelling T83.018
  colostomy K94.03
    valve K94.03
  cystostomy (stoma) N99.512
    catheter T83.010
  enteric stoma K94.13
  enterostomy K94.13
  esophagostomy K94.33
  gastroenteric K31.89
  gastrostomy K94.23
  ileostomy K94.13
    valve K94.13
  jejunostomy K94.13
  pacemaker —see Malfunction, cardiac
    electronic device
  prosthetic device, internal —see
    Complications, prosthetic device, by
    site, mechanical
  tracheostomy J95.03
  urinary device NEC —see Complication,
    genitourinary, device, urinary,
    mechanical
  valve
    colostomy K94.03
    heart T82.09
    ileostomy K94.13
  vascular graft or shunt NEC —see
    Complication, cardiovascular device,
    mechanical, vascular
  ventricular (communicating shunt) T85.01
Malherbe's tumor —see Neoplasm, skin, benign
Malibu disease L98.8-
Malignancy —see also Neoplasm, malignant,
  by site
  unspecified site (primary) C80.1
Malignant —see condition
Malingerer, malingering Z76.5
Mallet finger (acquired) —see Deformity, finger,
  mallet finger
  congenital Q74.0
  sequelae of rickets E64.3
Malleus A24.0
Mallory's bodies R89.7
Mallory-Weiss syndrome K22.6
Malnutrition E46
  degree
    first E44.1
    mild (protein) E44.1
    moderate (protein) E44.0
    second E44.0
    severe (protein-energy) E43
      intermediate form E42
        with
          kwashiorkor (and marasmus) E42
          marasmus E41
    third E43
  following gastrointestinal surgery K91.2
  intrauterine
    light-for-dates —see Light for dates
    small-for-dates —see Small for dates
  lack of care, or neglect (child) (infant) T76.02
    confirmed T74.02
  malignant E40

Malnutrition (Continued)
  protein E46
    calorie E46
      mild E44.1
      moderate E44.0
      severe E43
        intermediate form E42
          with
            kwashiorkor (and marasmus)
              E42
            marasmus E41
    energy E46
      mild E44.1
      moderate E44.0
      severe E43
        intermediate form E42
          with
            kwashiorkor (and marasmus)
              E42
            marasmus E41
  severe (protein-energy) E43
    with
      kwashiorkor (and marasmus) E42
      marasmus E41
Malocclusion (teeth) M26.4
  Angle's M26.219
    class I M26.211
    class II M26.212
    class III M26.213
  due to
    abnormal swallowing M26.59
    mouth breathing M26.59
    tongue, lip or finger habits M26.59
  temporomandibular (joint) M26.69
Malposition
  cervix —see Malposition, uterus
  congenital
    adrenal (gland) Q89.1
    alimentary tract Q45.8
      lower Q43.8
      upper Q40.8
    aorta Q25.4
    appendix Q43.8
    arterial trunk Q20.0
    artery (peripheral) Q27.8
      coronary Q24.5
      digestive system Q27.8
      lower limb Q27.8
      pulmonary Q25.79
      specified site NEC Q27.8
      upper limb Q27.8
    auditory canal Q17.8
      causing impairment of hearing Q16.9
    auricle (ear) Q17.4
      causing impairment of hearing Q16.9
      cervical Q18.2
    biliary duct or passage Q44.5
    bladder (mucosa) —see Exstrophy, bladder
    brachial plexus Q07.8
    brain tissue Q04.8
    breast Q83.8
    bronchus Q32.4
    cecum Q43.8
    clavicle Q74.0
    colon Q43.8
    digestive organ or tract NEC Q45.8
      lower Q43.8
      upper Q40.8
    ear (auricle) (external) Q17.4
      ossicles Q16.3
    endocrine (gland) NEC Q89.2
    epiglottis Q31.8
    eustachian tube Q17.8
    eye Q15.8
    facial features Q18.8
    fallopian tube Q50.6
    finger (s) Q68.1
      supernumerary Q69.0
    foot Q66.9
    gallbladder Q44.1
    gastrointestinal tract Q45.8

Malposition (Continued)
  congenital (Continued)
    genitalia, genital organ (s) or tract
      female Q52.8
        external Q52.79
        internal NEC Q52.8
      male Q55.8
    glottis Q31.8
    hand Q68.1
    heart Q24.8
      dextrocardia Q24.0
        with complete transposition of viscera
          Q89.3
    hepatic duct Q44.5
    hip (joint) Q65.89
    intestine (large) (small) Q43.8
      with anomalous adhesions, fixation or
        malrotation Q43.3
    joint NEC Q68.8
    kidney Q63.2
    larynx Q31.8
    limb Q68.8
      lower Q68.8
      upper Q68.8
    liver Q44.7
    lung (lobe) Q33.8
    nail (s) Q84.6
    nerve Q07.8
    nervous system NEC Q07.8
    nose, nasal (septum) Q30.8
    organ or site not listed —see Anomaly,
      by site
    ovary Q50.39
    pancreas Q45.3
    parathyroid (gland) Q89.2
    patella Q74.1
    peripheral vascular system Q27.8
    pituitary (gland) Q89.2
    respiratory organ or system NEC
      Q34.8
    rib (cage) Q76.6
      supernumerary in cervical region
        Q76.5
    scapula Q74.0
    shoulder Q74.0
    spinal cord Q06.8
    spleen Q89.09
    sternum NEC Q76.7
    stomach Q40.2
    symphysis pubis Q74.2
    thymus (gland) Q89.2
    thyroid (gland) (tissue) Q89.2
      cartilage Q31.8
    toe (s) Q66.9
      supernumerary Q69.2
    tongue Q38.3
    trachea Q32.1
    ureter Q62.60
      deviation Q62.61
      displacement Q62.62
      ectopia Q62.63
      specified type NEC Q62.69
    uterus Q51.818
    vein (s) (peripheral) Q27.8
      great Q26.8
    vena cava (inferior) (superior) Q26.8
  device, implant or graft (see also
    Complications, by site and type,
    mechanical) T85.628
    arterial graft NEC —see Complication,
      cardiovascular device, mechanical,
      vascular
    breast (implant) T85.42
    catheter NEC T85.628
      cystostomy T83.020
      dialysis (renal) T82.42
        intraperitoneal T85.621
      infusion NEC T82.524
        spinal (epidural) (subdural)
          T85.620
      urinary, indwelling T83.028

◄ New   ◄▥ Revised   ~~deleted~~ Deleted

Malposition *(Continued)*
device, implant or graft *(Continued)*
electronic (electrode) (pulse generator)
(stimulator)
bone T84.320
cardiac T82.129
electrode T82.120
pulse generator T82.121
specified type NEC T82.128
nervous system —*see* Complication,
prosthetic device, mechanical,
electronic nervous system
stimulator
urinary —*see* Complication,
genitourinary, device, urinary,
mechanical
fixation, internal (orthopedic) NEC —*see*
Complication, fixation device,
mechanical
gastrointestinal —*see* Complications,
prosthetic device, mechanical,
gastrointestinal device
genital NEC T83.428
intrauterine contraceptive device T83.32
penile prosthesis T83.420
heart NEC —*see* Complication,
cardiovascular device, mechanical
joint prosthesis —*see* Complication, joint
prosthesis, mechanical
ocular NEC —*see* Complications, prosthetic
device, mechanical, ocular device
orthopedic NEC —*see* Complication,
orthopedic, device, mechanical
specified NEC T85.628
urinary NEC —*see also* Complication,
genitourinary, device, urinary,
mechanical
graft T83.22
vascular NEC —*see* Complication,
cardiovascular device, mechanical
ventricular intracranial shunt T85.02
fetus —*see* Pregnancy, complicated by
(management affected by), presentation,
fetal
gallbladder K82.8
gastrointestinal tract, congenital Q45.8
heart, congenital NEC Q24.8
joint prosthesis —*see* Complications, joint
prosthesis, mechanical, displacement,
by site
stomach K31.89
congenital Q40.2
tooth, teeth, fully erupted M26.30
uterus (acute) (acquired) (adherent)
(asymptomatic) (postinfectional)
(postpartal, old) N85.4
anteflexion or anteversion N85.4
congenital Q51.818
flexion N85.4
lateral —*see* Lateroversion, uterus
inversion N85.5
lateral (flexion) (version) —*see*
Lateroversion, uterus
in pregnancy or childbirth —*see*
subcategory O34.5
retroflexion or retroversion —*see*
Retroversion, uterus
Malposture R29.3
Malrotation
cecum Q43.3
colon Q43.3
intestine Q43.3
kidney Q63.2
Malta fever —*see* Brucellosis
Maltreatment
adult
abandonment
confirmed T74.01
suspected T76.01
confirmed T74.91
history of Z91.419

Maltreatment *(Continued)*
adult *(Continued)*
neglect
confirmed T74.01
suspected T76.01
physical abuse
confirmed T74.11
suspected T76.11
psychological abuse
confirmed T74.31
history of Z91.411
suspected T76.31
sexual abuse
confirmed T74.21
suspected T76.21
suspected T76.91
child
abandonment
confirmed T74.02
suspected T76.02
confirmed T74.92
history of —*see* History, personal (of),
abuse
neglect
confirmed T74.02
history of —*see* History, personal (of),
abuse
suspected T76.02
physical abuse
confirmed T74.12
history of —*see* History, personal (of),
abuse
suspected T76.12
psychological abuse
confirmed T74.32
history of —*see* History, personal (of),
abuse
suspected T76.32
sexual abuse
confirmed T74.22
history of —*see* History, personal (of),
abuse
suspected T76.22
suspected T76.92
personal history of Z91.89
Maltworker's lung J67.4
Malunion, fracture —*see* Fracture, by site
Mammillitis N61
puerperal, postpartum O91.02
Mammitis —*see* Mastitis
Mammogram (examination) Z12.39
routine Z12.31
Mammoplasia N62
Management (of)
bone conduction hearing device (implanted)
Z45.320
cardiac pacemaker NEC Z45.018
cerebrospinal fluid drainage device Z45.41
cochlear device (implanted) Z45.321
contraceptive Z30.9
specified NEC Z30.8
implanted device Z45.9
specified NEC Z45.89
infusion pump Z45.1
procreative Z31.9
male factor infertility in female Z31.81
specified NEC Z31.89
prosthesis (external) (*see also* Fitting)
Z44.9
implanted Z45.9
specified NEC Z45.89
renal dialysis catheter Z49.01
vascular access device Z45.2
Mangled —*see* specified injury by site
Mania (monopolar) —*see also* Disorder, mood,
manic episode
with psychotic symptoms F30.2
without psychotic symptoms F30.10
mild F30.11
moderate F30.12
severe F30.13

Mania *(Continued)*
Bell's F30.8
chronic (recurrent) F31.89
hysterical F44.89
puerperal F30.8
recurrent F31.89
Manic-depressive insanity, psychosis, or
syndrome —*see* Disorder, bipolar
Mannosidosis E77.1
Mansonelliasis, mansonellosis B74.4
Manson's
disease B65.1
schistosomiasis B65.1
Manual —*see* condition
Maple-bark-stripper's lung (disease) J67.6
Maple-syrup-urine disease E71.0
Marable's syndrome (celiac artery
compression) I77.4
Marasmus E41
due to malnutrition E41
intestinal E41
nutritional E41
senile R54
tuberculous NEC —*see* Tuberculosis
Marble
bones Q78.2
skin R23.8
Marburg virus disease A98.3
March
fracture —*see* Fracture, traumatic, stress, by
site
hemoglobinuria D59.6
Marchesani (-Weill) syndrome Q87.0
Marchiafava (-Bignami) syndrome or disease
G37.1
Marchiafava-Micheli syndrome D59.5
Marcus Gunn's syndrome Q07.8
Marfan's syndrome —*see* Syndrome, Marfan's
Marie-Bamberger disease —*see*
Osteoarthropathy, hypertrophic, specified
NEC
Marie-Charcot-Tooth neuropathic muscular
atrophy G60.0
Marie's
cerebellar ataxia (late-onset) G11.2
disease or syndrome (acromegaly) E22.0
Marie-Strümpell arthritis, disease or
spondylitis —*see* Spondylitis, ankylosing
Marion's disease (bladder neck obstruction)
N32.0
Marital conflict Z63.0
Mark
port wine Q82.5
raspberry Q82.5
strawberry Q82.5
stretch L90.6
tattoo L81.8
Marker heterochromatin —*see* Extra, marker
chromosomes
Maroteaux-Lamy syndrome (mild) (severe)
E76.29
Marrow (bone)
arrest D61.9
poor function D75.89
Marseilles fever A77.1
Marsh fever —*see* Malaria
Marshall's (hidrotic) ectodermal dysplasia
Q82.4
Marsh's disease (exophthalmic goiter) E05.00
with storm E05.01
Masculinization (female) with adrenal
hyperplasia E25.9
congenital E25.0
Masculinovoblastoma D27.-
Masochism (sexual) F65.51
Mason's lung J62.8
Mass
abdominal R19.00
epigastric R19.06
generalized R19.07
left lower quadrant R19.04

Mass *(Continued)*
  abdominal *(Continued)*
    left upper quadrant R19.02
    periumbilic R19.05
    right lower quadrant R19.03
    right upper quadrant R19.01
    specified site NEC R19.09
  breast N63
  chest R22.2
  cystic —*see* Cyst
  ear H93.8-
  head R22.0
  intra-abdominal (diffuse) (generalized) —*see*
    Mass, abdominal
  kidney N28.89
  liver R16.0
  localized (skin) R22.9
    chest R22.2
    head R22.0
    limb
      lower R22.4-
      upper R22.3-
    neck R22.1
    trunk R22.2
  lung R91.8
  malignant —*see* Neoplasm, malignant,
    by site
  neck R22.1
  pelvic (diffuse) (generalized) —*see* Mass,
    abdominal
  specified organ NEC —*see* Disease, by site
  splenic R16.1
  substernal thyroid —*see* Goiter
  superficial (localized) R22.9
  umbilical (diffuse) (generalized) R19.09
Massive —*see* condition
Mast cell
  disease, systemic tissue D47.0
  leukemia C94.3-
  sarcoma C96.2
  tumor D47.0
    malignant C96.2
Mastalgia N64.4
Masters-Allen syndrome N83.8
Mastitis (acute) (diffuse) (nonpuerperal)
  (subacute) N61
  chronic (cystic) —*see* Mastopathy, cystic
  cystic (Schimmelbusch's type) —*see*
    Mastopathy, cystic
  fibrocystic —*see* Mastopathy, cystic
  infective N61
    newborn P39.0
  interstitial, gestational or puerperal —*see*
    Mastitis, obstetric
  neonatal (noninfective) P83.4
    infective P39.0
  obstetric (interstitial) (nonpurulent)
    associated with
      lactation O91.23
      pregnancy O91.21-
      puerperium O91.22
    purulent
      associated with
        lactation O91.13
        pregnancy O91.11-
        puerperium O91.12
  periductal —*see* Ectasia, mammary duct
  phlegmonous —*see* Mastopathy, cystic
  plasma cell —*see* Ectasia, mammary duct
Mastocytoma D47.0
  malignant C96.2
Mastocytosis Q82.2
  aggressive systemic C96.2
  indolent systemic D47.0
  malignant C96.2
  systemic, associated with clonal hematopoetic
    non-mast-cell disease (SM-AHNMD)
    D47.0
Mastodynia N64.4
Mastoid —*see* condition
Mastoidalgia —*see* subcategory H92.0

Mastoiditis (coalescent) (hemorrhagic)
  (suppurative) H70.9-
  acute, subacute H70.00-
    complicated NEC H70.09-
    subperiosteal H70.01-
  chronic (necrotic) (recurrent) H70.1-
  in (due to)
    infectious disease NEC B99 [H75.0-]
    parasitic disease NEC B89 [H75.0-]
    tuberculosis A18.03
  petrositis —*see* Petrositis
  postauricular fistula —*see* Fistula,
    postauricular
  specified NEC H70.89-
  tuberculous A18.03
Mastopathy, mastopathia N64.9
  chronica cystica —*see* Mastopathy, cystic
  cystic (chronic) (diffuse) N60.1
    with epithelial proliferation N60.3-
  diffuse cystic —*see* Mastopathy, cystic
  estrogenic, oestrogenica N64.89
  ovarian origin N64.89
Mastoplasia, mastoplastia N62
Masturbation (excessive) F98.8
Maternal care (for) —*see* Pregnancy
  (complicated by) (management
  affected by)
Matheiu's disease (leptospiral jaundice)
  A27.0
Mauclaire's disease or osteochondrosis —
  see Osteochondrosis, juvenile, hand,
  metacarpal
Maxcy's disease A75.2
Maxilla, maxillary —*see* condition
May (-Hegglin) anomaly or syndrome
  D72.0
McArdle (-Schmid)(-Pearson) disease
  (glycogen storage) E74.04
McCune-Albright syndrome Q78.1
McQuarrie's syndrome (idiopathic familial
  hypoglycemia) E16.2
Meadow's syndrome Q86.1
Measles (black) (hemorrhagic) (suppressed)
  B05.9
  with
    complications NEC B05.89
    encephalitis B05.0
    intestinal complications B05.4
    keratitis (keratoconjunctivitis) B05.81
    meningitis B05.1
    otitis media B05.3
    pneumonia B05.2
  French —*see* Rubella
  German —*see* Rubella
  Liberty —*see* Rubella
Meatitis, urethral —*see* Urethritis
Meatus, meatal —*see* condition
Meat-wrappers' asthma J68.9
Meckel-Gruber syndrome Q61.9
Meckel's diverticulitis, diverticulum
  (displaced) (hypertrophic) Q43.0
Meconium
  ileus, newborn P76.0
    in cystic fibrosis E84.11
    meaning meconium plug (without cystic
      fibrosis) P76.0
  obstruction, newborn P76.0
    due to fecaliths P76.0
    in mucoviscidosis E84.11
  peritonitis P78.0
  plug syndrome (newborn) NEC P76.0
Median —*see also* condition
  arcuate ligament syndrome I77.4
  bar (prostate) (vesical orifice) —*see*
    Hyperplasia, prostate
  rhomboid glossitis K14.2
Mediastinal shift R93.8
Mediastinitis (acute) (chronic)
  J98.5
  syphilitic A52.73
  tuberculous A15.8

Mediastinopericarditis —*see also* Pericarditis
  acute I30.9
  adhesive I31.0
  chronic I31.8
    rheumatic I09.2
Mediastinum, mediastinal —*see* condition
Medicine poisoning —*see* Table of Drugs and
  Chemicals, by drug, poisoning
Mediterranean
  fever —*see* Brucellosis
    familial E85.0
    tick A77.1
  kala-azar B55.0
  leishmaniasis B55.0
  tick fever A77.1
Medulla —*see* condition
Medullary cystic kidney Q61.5
Medullated fibers
  optic (nerve) Q14.8
  retina Q14.1
Medulloblastoma
  desmoplastic C71.6
  specified site —*see* Neoplasm, malignant, by
    site
  unspecified site C71.6
Medulloepithelioma —*see also* Neoplasm,
  malignant, by site
  teratoid —*see* Neoplasm, malignant, by site
Medullomyoblastoma
  specified site —*see* Neoplasm, malignant, by
    site
  unspecified site C71.6
Meekeren-Ehlers-Danlos syndrome
  Q79.6
Megacolon (acquired) (functional) (not
  Hirschsprung's disease) (in) K59.3
  Chagas' disease B57.32
  congenital, congenitum (aganglionic)
    Q43.1
  Hirschsprung's (disease) Q43.1
  toxic NEC K59.3
    due to Clostridium difficile A04.7
Megaesophagus (functional) K22.0
  congenital Q39.5
  in (due to) Chagas' disease B57.31
Megalencephaly Q04.5
Megalerythema (epidemic) B08.3
Megaloappendix Q43.8
Megalocephalus, megalocephaly NEC Q75.3
Megalocornea Q15.8
  with glaucoma Q15.0
Megalocytic anemia D53.1
Megalodactylia (fingers) (thumbs) (congenital)
  Q74.0
  toes Q74.2
Megaloduodenum Q43.8
Megaloesophagus (functional) K22.0
  congenital Q39.5
Megalogastria (acquired) K31.89
  congenital Q40.2
Megalophthalmos Q11.3
Megalopsia H53.15
Megalosplenia —*see* Splenomegaly
Megaloureter N28.82
  congenital Q62.2
Megarectum K62.89
Megasigmoid K59.3
  congenital Q43.2
Megaureter N28.82
  congenital Q62.2
Megavitamin-B6 syndrome E67.2
Megrim —*see* Migraine
Meibomian
  cyst, infected —*see* Hordeolum
  gland —*see* condition
  sty, stye —*see* Hordeolum
Meibomitis —*see* Hordeolum
Meige-Milroy disease (chronic hereditary
  edema) Q82.0
Meige's syndrome Q82.0
Melalgia, nutritional E53.8

◀ New   ◀⁞⁞ Revised   ~~deleted~~ Deleted

Melancholia F32.9
  climacteric (single episode) F32.8
    recurrent episode F33.9
  hypochondriac F45.29
  intermittent (single episode) F32.8
    recurrent episode F33.9
  involutional (single episode) F32.8
    recurrent episode F33.9
  menopausal (single episode) F32.8
    recurrent episode F33.9
  puerperal F32.8
  reactive (emotional stress or trauma) F32.3
  recurrent F33.9
  senile F03
  stuporous (single episode) F32.8
    recurrent episode F33.9
Melanemia R79.89
Melanoameloblastoma —see Neoplasm, bone, benign
Melanoblastoma —see Melanoma
Melanocarcinoma —see Melanoma
Melanocytoma, eyeball D31.4-
Melanocytosis, neurocutaneous Q82.8
Melanoderma, melanodermia L81.4
Melanodontia, infantile K03.89
Melanodontoclasia K03.89
Melanoepithelioma —see Melanoma
Melanoma (malignant) C43.9
  acral lentiginous, malignant —see Melanoma, skin, by site
  amelanotic —see Melanoma, skin, by site
  balloon cell —see Melanoma, skin, by site
  benign —see Nevus
  desmoplastic, malignant —see Melanoma, skin, by site
  epithelioid cell —see Melanoma, skin, by site
    with spindle cell, mixed —see Melanoma, skin, by site
  in
    giant pigmented nevus —see Melanoma, skin, by site
    Hutchinson's melanotic freckle —see Melanoma, skin, by site
    junctional nevus —see Melanoma, skin, by site
    precancerous melanosis —see Melanoma, skin, by site
  in situ D03.9
    abdominal wall D03.59
    ala nasi D03.39
    ankle D03.7-
    anus, anal (margin) (skin) D03.51
    arm D03.6-
    auditory canal D03.2-
    auricle (ear) D03.2-
    auricular canal (external) D03.2-
    axilla, axillary fold D03.59
    back D03.59
    breast D03.52
    brow D03.39
    buttock D03.59
    canthus (eye) D03.1-
    cheek (external) D03.39
    chest wall D03.59
    chin D03.39
    choroid D03.8
    conjunctiva D03.8
    ear (external) D03.2-
    external meatus (ear) D03.2-
    eye D03.8
    eyebrow D03.39
    eyelid (lower) (upper) D03.1-
    face D03.30
      specified NEC D03.39
    female genital organ (external) NEC D03.8
    finger D03.6-
    flank D03.59
    foot D03.7-
    forearm D03.6-
    forehead D03.39
    foreskin D03.8

Melanoma (Continued)
  in situ (Continued)
    gluteal region D03.59
    groin D03.59
    hand D03.6-
    heel D03.7-
    helix D03.2-
    hip D03.7-
    interscapular region D03.59
    iris D03.8
    jaw D03.39
    knee D03.7-
    labium (majus) (minus) D03.8
    lacrimal gland D03.8
    leg D03.7-
    lip (lower) (upper) D03.0
    lower limb NEC D03.7-
    male genital organ (external) NEC D03.8
    nail D03.9
      finger D03.6-
      toe D03.7-
    neck D03.4
    nose (external) D03.39
    orbit D03.8
    penis D03.8
    perianal skin D03.51
    perineum D03.51
    pinna D03.2-
    popliteal fossa or space D03.7-
    prepuce D03.8
    pudendum D03.8
    retina D03.8
    retrobulbar D03.8
    scalp D03.4
    scrotum D03.8
    shoulder D03.6-
    specified site NEC D03.8
    submammary fold D03.52
    temple D03.39
    thigh D03.7-
    toe D03.7-
    trunk NEC D03.59
    umbilicus D03.59
    upper limb NEC D03.6-
    vulva D03.8
  juvenile —see Nevus
  malignant, of soft parts except skin —see Neoplasm, connective tissue, malignant
  metastatic
    breast C79.81
    genital organ C79.82
    specified site NEC C79.89
  neurotropic, malignant —see Melanoma, skin, by site
  nodular —see Melanoma, skin, by site
  regressing, malignant —see Melanoma, skin, by site
  skin C43.9
    abdominal wall C43.59
    ala nasi C43.31
    ankle C43.7-
    anus, anal (skin) C43.51
    arm C43.6-
    auditory canal (external) C43.2-
    auricle (ear) C43.2-
    auricular canal (external) C43.2-
    axilla, axillary fold C43.59
    back C43.59
    breast (female) (male) C43.52
    brow C43.39
    buttock C43.59
    canthus (eye) C43.1-
    cheek (external) C43.39
    chest wall C43.59
    chin C43.39
    ear (external) C43.2-
    elbow C43.6-
    external meatus (ear) C43.2-
    eyebrow C43.39

Melanoma (Continued)
  skin (Continued)
    eyelid (lower) (upper) C43.1-
    face C43.30
      specified NEC C43.39
    female genital organ (external) NEC C51.9
    finger C43.6-
    flank C43.59
    foot C43.7-
    forearm C43.6-
    forehead C43.39
    foreskin C60.0
    glabella C43.39
    gluteal region C43.59
    groin C43.59
    hand C43.6-
    heel C43.7-
    helix C43.2-
    hip C43.7-
    interscapular region C43.59
    jaw (external) C43.39
    knee C43.7-
    labium C51.9
      majus C51.0
      minus C51.1
    leg C43.7-
    lip (lower) (upper) C43.0
    lower limb NEC C43.7-
    male genital organ (external) NEC C63.9
    nail
      finger C43.6-
      toe C43.7-
    nasolabial groove C43.39
    nates C43.59
    neck C43.4
    nose (external) C43.31
    overlapping site C43.8
    palpebra C43.1-
    penis C60.9
    perianal skin C43.51
    perineum C43.51
    pinna C43.2-
    popliteal fossa or space C43.7-
    prepuce C60.0
    pudendum C51.9
    scalp C43.4
    scrotum C63.2
    shoulder C43.6-
    skin NEC C43.9
    submammary fold C43.52
    temple C43.39
    thigh C43.7-
    toe C43.7-
    trunk NEC C43.59
    umbilicus C43.59
    upper limb NEC C43.6-
    vulva C51.9
      overlapping sites C51.8
  spindle cell
    with epithelioid, mixed —see Melanoma, skin, by site
    type A C69.4-
    type B C69.4-
  superficial spreading —see Melanoma, skin, by site
Melanosarcoma —see also Melanoma
  epithelioid cell —see Melanoma
Melanosis L81.4
  addisonian E27.1
    tuberculous A18.7
  adrenal E27.1
  colon K63.89
  conjunctiva —see Pigmentation, conjunctiva
    congenital Q13.89
  cornea (presenile) (senile) —see also Pigmentation, cornea
    congenital Q13.4
  eye NEC H57.8
    congenital Q15.8
  lenticularis progressiva Q82.1
  liver K76.89

Melanosis *(Continued)*
  precancerous —*see also* Melanoma, in situ
    malignant melanoma in —*see* Melanoma
  Riehl's L81.4
  sclera H15.89
    congenital Q13.89
  suprarenal E27.1
  tar L81.4
  toxic L81.4
Melanuria R82.99
MELAS syndrome E88.41
Melasma L81.1
  adrenal (gland) E27.1
  suprarenal (gland) E27.1
Melena K92.1
  with ulcer - code by site under Ulcer, with
    hemorrhage K27.4
  due to swallowed maternal blood P78.2
  newborn, neonatal P54.1
    due to swallowed maternal blood P78.2
Meleney's
  gangrene (cutaneous) —*see* Ulcer, skin
  ulcer (chronic undermining) —*see* Ulcer, skin
Melioidosis A24.9
  acute A24.1
  chronic A24.2
  fulminating A24.1
  pneumonia A24.1
  pulmonary (chronic) A24.2
    acute A24.1
    subacute A24.2
  sepsis A24.1
  specified NEC A24.3
  subacute A24.2
Melitensis, febris A23.0
Melkersson (-Rosenthal) syndrome G51.2
Mellitus, diabetes —*see* Diabetes
Melorheostosis (bone) —*see* Disorder, bone,
    density and structure, specified NEC
Meloschisis Q18.4
Melotia Q17.4
Membrana
  capsularis lentis posterior Q13.89
  epipapillaris Q14.2
Membranacea placenta O43.19-
Membranaceous uterus N85.8
Membrane (s), membranous —*see also*
    condition
  cyclitic —*see* Membrane, pupillary
  folds, congenital —*see* Web
  Jackson's Q43.3
  over face of newborn P28.9
  premature rupture —*see* Rupture,
    membranes, premature
  pupillary H21.4-
    persistent Q13.89
  retained (with hemorrhage) (complicating
    delivery) O72.2
    without hemorrhage O73.1
  secondary cataract —*see* Cataract, secondary
  unruptured (causing asphyxia) —*see*
    Asphyxia, newborn
  vitreous —*see* Opacity, vitreous, membranes
    and strands
Membranitis —*see* Chorioamnionitis
Memory disturbance, lack or loss —*see also*
    Amnesia
  mild, following organic brain damage F06.8
Menadione deficiency E56.1
Menarche
  delayed E30.0
  precocious E30.1
Mendacity, pathologic F60.2
Mendelson's syndrome (due to anesthesia)
    J95.4
  in labor and delivery O74.0
  in pregnancy O29.01-
  obstetric O74.0
  postpartum, puerperal O89.01
Ménétrier's disease or syndrome K29.60
  with bleeding K29.61

Ménière's disease, syndrome or vertigo H81.0-
Meninges, meningeal —*see* condition
Meningioma —*see also* Neoplasm, meninges,
    benign
  angioblastic —*see* Neoplasm, meninges,
    benign
  angiomatous —*see* Neoplasm, meninges,
    benign
  endotheliomatous —*see* Neoplasm, meninges,
    benign
  fibroblastic —*see* Neoplasm, meninges,
    benign
  fibrous —*see* Neoplasm, meninges, benign
  hemangioblastic —*see* Neoplasm, meninges,
    benign
  hemangiopericytic —*see* Neoplasm,
    meninges, benign
  malignant —*see* Neoplasm, meninges,
    malignant
  meningiothelial —*see* Neoplasm, meninges,
    benign
  meningotheliomatous —*see* Neoplasm,
    meninges, benign
  mixed —*see* Neoplasm, meninges, benign
  multiple —*see* Neoplasm, meninges,
    uncertain behavior
  papillary —*see* Neoplasm, meninges,
    uncertain behavior
  psammomatous —*see* Neoplasm, meninges,
    benign
  syncytial —*see* Neoplasm, meninges, benign
  transitional —*see* Neoplasm, meninges,
    benign
Meningiomatosis (diffuse) —*see* Neoplasm,
    meninges, uncertain behavior
Meningism —*see* Meningismus
Meningismus (infectional) (pneumococcal)
    R29.1
  due to serum or vaccine R29.1
  influenzal —*see* Influenza, with,
    manifestations NEC
Meningitis (basal) (basic) (brain) (cerebral)
    (cervical) (congestive) (diffuse)
    (hemorrhagic) infantile) (membranous)
    (metastatic) (nonspecific) (pontine)
    (progressive) (simple) (spinal) (subacute)
    (sympathetic) (toxic) G03.9
  abacterial G03.0
  actinomycotic A42.81
  adenoviral A87.1
  arbovirus A87.8
  aseptic (acute) G03.0
  bacterial G00.9
    Escherichia coli (E. coli) G00.8
    Friedländer (bacillus) G00.8
    gram-negative G00.9
    H. influenzae G00.0
    Klebsiella G00.8
    pneumococcal G00.1
    specified organism NEC G00.8
    staphylococcal G00.3
    streptococcal (acute) G00.2
  benign recurrent (Mollaret) G03.2
  candidal B37.5
  caseous (tuberculous) A17.0
  cerebrospinal A39.0
  chronic NEC G03.1
  clear cerebrospinal fluid NEC G03.0
  coxsackievirus A87.0
  cryptococcal B45.1
  diplococcal (gram positive) A39.0
  echovirus A87.0
  enteroviral A87.0
  eosinophilic B83.2
  epidemic NEC A39.0
  Escherichia coli (E. coli) G00.8
  fibrinopurulent G00.9
    specified organism NEC G00.8
  Friedländer (bacillus) G00.8
  gonococcal A54.81
  gram-negative cocci G00.9

Meningitis *(Continued)*
  gram-positive cocci G00.9
  Haemophilus (influenzae) G00.0
  H. influenzae G00.0
  in (due to)
    adenovirus A87.1
    African trypanosomiasis B56.9 *[G02]*
    anthrax A22.8
    bacterial disease NEC A48.8 *[G01]*
    Chagas' disease (chronic) B57.41
    chickenpox B01.0
    coccidioidomycosis B38.4
    Diplococcus pneumoniae G00.1
    enterovirus A87.0
    herpes (simplex) virus B00.3
      zoster B02.1
    infectious mononucleosis B27.92
    leptospirosis A27.81
    Listeria monocytogenes A32.11
    Lyme disease A69.21
    measles B05.1
    mumps (virus) B26.1
    neurosyphilis (late) A52.13
    parasitic disease NEC B89 *[G02]*
    poliovirus A80.9 *[G02]*
    preventive immunization, inoculation or
      vaccination G03.8
    rubella B06.02
    Salmonella infection A02.21
    specified cause NEC G03.8
    typhoid fever A01.01
    varicella B01.0
    viral disease NEC A87.8
    whooping cough A37.90
    zoster B02.1
  infectious G00.9
  influenzal (H. influenzae) G00.0
  Klebsiella G00.8
  leptospiral (aseptic) A27.81
  lymphocytic (acute) (benign) (serous)
    A87.2
  meningococcal A39.0
  Mima polymorpha G00.8
  Mollaret (benign recurrent) G03.2
  monilial B37.5
  mycotic NEC B49 *[G02]*
  Neisseria A39.0
  nonbacterial G03.0
  nonpyogenic NEC G03.0
  ossificans G96.19
  pneumococcal G00.1
  poliovirus A80.9 *[G02]*
  postmeasles B05.1
  purulent G00.9
    specified organism NEC G00.8
  pyogenic G00.9
    specified organism NEC G00.8
  Salmonella (arizonae) (Cholerae-Suis)
    (enteritidis) (typhimurium) A02.21
  septic G00.9
    specified organism NEC G00.8
  serosa circumscripta NEC G03.0
  serous NEC G93.2
  specified organism NEC G00.8
  sporotrichosis B42.81
  staphylococcal G00.3
  sterile G03.0
  streptococcal (acute) G00.2
  suppurative G00.9
    specified organism NEC G00.8
  syphilitic (late) (tertiary) A52.13
    acute A51.41
    congenital A50.41
    secondary A51.41
  Torula histolytica (cryptococcal) B45.1
  traumatic (complication of injury)
    T79.8
  tuberculous A17.0
  typhoid A01.01
  viral NEC A87.9
  Yersinia pestis A20.3

◀ New   ◀▥ Revised   ~~deleted~~ Deleted

Meningocele (spinal) —*see also* Spina bifida
  with hydrocephalus —*see* Spina bifida, by
    site, with hydrocephalus
  acquired (traumatic) G96.19
  cerebral —*see* Encephalocele
Meningocerebritis —*see* Meningoencephalitis
Meningococcemia A39.4
  acute A39.2
  chronic A39.3
Meningococcus, meningococcal (*see also*
    condition) A39.9
  adrenalitis, hemorrhagic A39.1
  carrier (suspected) of Z22.31
  meningitis (cerebrospinal) A39.0
Meningoencephalitis (*see also* Encephalitis)
    G04.90
  acute NEC (*see also* Encephalitis, viral) A86
  bacterial NEC G04.2
  California A83.5
  diphasic A84.1
  eosinophilic B83.2
  epidemic A39.81
  herpesviral, herpetic B00.4
    due to herpesvirus 6 B10.01
    due to herpesvirus 7 B10.09
    specified NEC B10.09
  in (due to)
    blastomycosis NEC B40.81
    diseases classified elsewhere G05.3
    free-living amebae B60.2
    Hemophilus influenzae (H. influenzae)
      G04.2
    herpes B00.4
      due to herpesvirus 6 B10.01
      due to herpesvirus 7 B10.09
      specified NEC B10.09
    H. influenzae G00.0
    Lyme disease A69.22
    mercury —*see* subcategory T56.1
    mumps B26.2
    Naegleria (amebae) (organisms) (fowleri)
      B60.2
    Parastrongylus cantonensis B83.2
    toxoplasmosis (acquired) B58.2
      congenital P37.1
  infectious (acute) (viral) A86
  influenzal (H. influenzae) G04.2
  Listeria monocytogenes A32.12
  lymphocytic (serous) A87.2
  mumps B26.2
  parasitic NEC B89 [G05.3]
  pneumococcal G00.1
  primary amebic B60.2
  specific (syphilitic) A52.14
  specified organism NEC G04.81
  staphylococcal G04.2
  streptococcal G04.2
  syphilitic A52.14
  toxic NEC G92
    due to mercury —*see* subcategory
      T56.1
  tuberculous A17.82
  virus NEC A86
Meningoencephalocele —*see also*
    Encephalocele
  syphilitic A52.19
    congenital A50.49
Meningoencephalomyelitis —*see also*
    Meningoencephalitis
  acute NEC (viral) A86
    disseminated G04.00
      postimmunization or postvaccination
        G04.02
      postinfectious G04.01
  due to
    actinomycosis A42.82
    Torula B45.1
    Toxoplasma or toxoplasmosis (acquired)
      B58.2
      congenital P37.1
  postimmunization or postvaccination G04.02

Meningoencephalomyelopathy G96.9
Meningoencephalopathy G96.9
Meningomyelitis —*see also*
    Meningoencephalitis
  bacterial NEC G04.2
  blastomycotic NEC B40.81
  cryptococcal B45.1
  in diseases classified elsewhere G05.4
  meningococcal A39.81
  syphilitic A52.14
  tuberculous A17.82
Meningomyelocele —*see also* Spina bifida
  syphilitic A52.19
Meningomyeloneuritis —*see*
    Meningoencephalitis
Meningoradiculitis —*see* Meningitis
Meningovascular —*see* condition
Menkes' disease or syndrome E83.09
  meaning maple-syrup-urine disease E71.0
Menometrorrhagia N92.1
Menopause, menopausal (asymptomatic)
    (state) Z78.0
  arthritis (any site) NEC —*see* Arthritis,
    specified form NEC
  bleeding N92.4
  depression (single episode) F32.8
    agitated (single episode) F32.2
      recurrent episode F33.9
    psychotic (single episode) F32.8
      recurrent episode F33.9
    recurrent episode F33.9
    melancholia (single episode) F32.8
      recurrent episode F33.9
  paranoid state F22
  premature E28.319
    asymptomatic E28.319
      postirradiation E89.40
      postsurgical E89.40
    symptomatic E28.310
      postirradiation E89.41
      postsurgical E89.41
  psychosis NEC F28
  symptomatic N95.1
  toxic polyarthritis NEC —*see* Arthritis,
    specified form NEC
Menorrhagia (primary) N92.0
  climacteric N92.4
    menopausal N92.4
  menopausal N92.4
  postclimacteric N95.0
  postmenopausal N95.0
  preclimacteric or premenopausal N92.4
  pubertal (menses retained) N92.2
Menostaxis N92.0
Menses, retention N94.89
Menstrual —*see* Menstruation
Menstruation
  absent —*see* Amenorrhea
  anovulatory N97.0
  cycle, irregular N92.6
  delayed N91.0
  disorder N93.9
    psychogenic F45.8
  during pregnancy O20.8
  excessive (with regular cycle) N92.0
    with irregular cycle N92.1
    at puberty N92.2
  frequent N92.0
  infrequent —*see* Oligomenorrhea
  irregular N92.6
    specified NEC N92.5
  latent N92.5
  membranous N92.5
  painful (*see also* Dysmenorrhea) N94.6
    primary N94.4
    psychogenic F45.8
    secondary N94.5
  passage of clots N92.0
  precocious E30.1
  protracted N92.5
  rare —*see* Oligomenorrhea

Menstruation (*Continued*)
  retained N94.89
  retrograde N92.5
  scanty —*see* Oligomenorrhea
  suppression N94.89
  vicarious (nasal) N94.89
Mental —*see also* condition
  deficiency —*see* Disability, intellectual
  deterioration —*see* Psychosis
  disorder —*see* Disorder, mental
  exhaustion F48.8
  insufficiency (congenital) —*see* Disability,
    intellectual
  observation without need for further medical
    care Z03.89
  retardation —*see* Disability, intellectual
  subnormality —*see* Disability, intellectual
  upset —*see* Disorder, mental
Meralgia paresthetica G57.1-
Mercurial —*see* condition
Mercurialism —*see* subcategory T56.1
MERRF syndrome (myoclonic epilepsy
    associated with ragged-red fiber)
    E88.42
Merkel cell tumor —*see* Carcinoma,
    Merkel cell
Merocele —*see* Hernia, femoral
Meromelia
  lower limb —*see* Defect, reduction, lower
    limb
    intercalary
      femur —*see* Defect, reduction, lower
        limb, specified type NEC
      tibiofibular (complete) (incomplete) —
        see Defect, reduction, lower
        limb
  upper limb —*see* Defect, reduction, upper
    limb
    intercalary, humeral, radioulnar —*see*
      Agenesis, arm, with hand present
Merzbacher-Pelizaeus disease E75.29
Mesaortitis —*see* Aortitis
Mesarteritis —*see* Arteritis
Mesencephalitis —*see* Encephalitis
Mesenchymoma —*see also* Neoplasm,
    connective tissue, uncertain behavior
  benign —*see* Neoplasm, connective tissue,
    benign
  malignant —*see* Neoplasm, connective tissue,
    malignant
Mesenteritis
  retractile K65.4
  sclerosing K65.4
Mesentery, mesenteric —*see* condition
Mesiodens, mesiodentes K00.1
Mesio-occlusion M26.213
Mesocolon —*see* condition
Mesonephroma (malignant) —*see* Neoplasm,
    malignant, by site
  benign —*see* Neoplasm, benign, by site
Mesophlebitis —*see* Phlebitis
Mesostromal dysgenesia Q13.89
Mesothelioma (malignant) C45.9
  benign
    mesentery D19.1
    mesocolon D19.1
    omentum D19.1
    peritoneum D19.1
    pleura D19.0
    specified site NEC D19.7
    unspecified site D19.9
  biphasic C45.9
    benign
      mesentery D19.1
      mesocolon D19.1
      omentum D19.1
      peritoneum D19.1
      pleura D19.0
      specified site NEC D19.7
      unspecified site D19.9
  cystic D48.4

M

◀ New   ◀▦ Revised   ~~deleted~~ Deleted

Migraine *(Continued)*
  basilar —*see* Migraine, with aura
  classical —*see* Migraine, with aura
  common —*see* Migraine, without aura
  complicated G43.109
  equivalents —*see* Migraine, with aura
  familiar —*see* Migraine, hemiplegic
  hemiplegic G43.409
    with refractory migraine G43.419
      with status migrainosus G43.411
      without status migrainosus G43.419
    intractable G43.419
      with status migrainosus G43.411
      without status migrainosus G43.419
    not intractable G43.409
      with status migrainosus G43.401
      without status migrainosus G43.409
    without refractory migraine G43.409
      with status migrainosus G43.401
      without status migrainosus G43.409
  intractable G43.919
    with status migrainosus G43.911
    without status migrainosus G43.919
  menstrual G43.829
    with refractory migraine G43.839
      with status migrainosus G43.831
      without status migrainosus G43.839
    intractable G43.839
      with status migrainosus G43.831
      without status migrainosus G43.839
    not intractable G43.829
      with status migrainosus G43.821
      without status migrainosus G43.829
    without refractory migraine G43.829
      with status migrainosus G43.821
      without status migrainosus G43.829
  menstrually related —*see* Migraine,
    menstrual
  not intractable G43.909
    with status migrainosus G43.901
    without status migrainosus G43.919
  ophthalmoplegic G43.B0
    with refractory migraine G43.B1
    intractable G43.B1
    not intractable G43.B0
      without refractory migraine G43.B0
  persistent aura (with, without) cerebral
    infarction —*see* Migraine, with aura,
    persistent
  preceded or accompanied by transient
    focal neurological phenomena —*see*
    Migraine, with aura
  pre-menstrual —*see* Migraine, menstrual
  pure menstrual —*see* Migraine, menstrual
  retinal —*see* Migraine, with aura
  specified NEC G43.809
    intractable G43.819
      with status migrainosus G43.811
      without status migrainosus G43.819
    not intractable G43.809
      with status migrainosus G43.801
      without status migrainosus G43.809
  sporadic —*see* Migraine, hemiplegic
  transformed —*see* Migraine, without aura,
    chronic
  triggered seizures —*see* Migraine, with
    aura
  without aura G43.009
    with refractory migraine G43.019
      with status migrainosus G43.011
      without status migrainosus G43.019
    chronic G43.709
      with refractory migraine G43.719
        with status migrainosus G43.711
        without status migrainosus G43.719
      intractable
        with status migrainosus G43.711
        without status migrainosus G43.719
      not intractable
        with status migrainosus G43.701
        without status migrainosus G43.709

Migraine *(Continued)*
  without aura *(Continued)*
    chronic *(Continued)*
      without refractory migraine G43.709
        with status migrainosus G43.701
        without status migrainosus
          G43.709
    intractable
      with status migrainosus G43.011
      without status migrainosus G43.019
    not intractable
      with status migrainosus G43.001
      without status migrainosus G43.009
    without mention of refractory migraine
      G43.009
      with status migrainosus G43.001
      without status migrainosus G43.009
    without refractory migraine G43.909
      with status migrainosus G43.901
      without status migrainosus G43.919
Migrant, social Z59.0
Migration, anxiety concerning Z60.3
Migratory, migrating —*see also* condition
  person Z59.0
  testis Q55.29
Mikity-Wilson disease or syndrome P27.0
Mikulicz' disease or syndrome K11.8
Miliaria L74.3
  alba L74.1
  apocrine L75.2
  crystallina L74.1
  profunda L74.2
  rubra L74.0
  tropicalis L74.2
Miliary —*see* condition
Milium L72.0
  colloid L57.8
Milk
  crust L21.0
  excessive secretion O92.6
  poisoning —*see* Poisoning, food, noxious
  retention O92.79
  sickness —*see* Poisoning, food, noxious
  spots I31.0
Milk-alkali disease or syndrome E83.52
Milk-leg (deep vessels) (nonpuerperal) —*see*
  Embolism, vein, lower extremity
  complicating pregnancy O22.3-
  puerperal, postpartum, childbirth O87.1
Milkman's disease or syndrome M83.8
Milky urine —*see* Chyluria
Millard-Gubler (-Foville) paralysis or
  syndrome G46.3
Millar's asthma J38.5
Miller-Fisher syndrome G61.0
Mills' disease —*see* Hemiplegia
Millstone maker's pneumoconiosis J62.8
Milroy's disease (chronic hereditary edema)
  Q82.0
Minamata disease T26.1
Miners' asthma or lung J60
Minkowski-Chauffard syndrome —*see*
  Spherocytosis
Minor —*see* condition
Minor's disease (hematomyelia) G95.19
Minot's disease (hemorrhagic disease),
  newborn P53
Minot-von Willebrand-Jurgens disease or
  syndrome (angiohemophilia) D68.0
Minus (and plus) hand (intrinsic) —*see*
  Deformity, limb, specified type NEC,
  forearm
Miosis (pupil) H57.03
Mirizzi's syndrome (hepatic duct stenosis)
  K83.1
Mirror writing F81.0
Misadventure (of) (prophylactic) (therapeutic)
  (see also Complications) T88.9
  administration of insulin (by accident) —*see*
    subcategory T38.3
  infusion —*see* Complications, infusion

Misadventure *(Continued)*
  local applications (of fomentations, plasters,
    etc.) T88.9
    burn or scald —*see* Burn
    specified NEC T88.8
  medical care (early) (late) T88.9
    adverse effect of drugs or chemicals —*see*
      Table of Drugs and Chemicals
  medical care (early) (late)
    burn or scald —*see* Burn
    specified NEC T88.8
  specified NEC T88.8
  surgical procedure (early) (late) —*see*
    Complications, surgical procedure
  transfusion —*see* Complications, transfusion
  vaccination or other immunological
    procedure —*see* Complications,
    vaccination
Miscarriage O03.9
Misdirection, aqueous H40.83-
Misperception, sleep state F51.02
Misplaced, misplacement
  ear Q17.4
  kidney (acquired) N28.89
    congenital Q63.2
  organ or site, congenital NEC —*see*
    Malposition, congenital
Missed
  abortion O02.1
  delivery O36.4
Missing —*see* Absence
Misuse of drugs F19.99
Mitchell's disease (erythromelalgia) I73.81
Mite (s) (infestation) B88.9
  diarrhea B88.0
  grain (itch) B88.0
  hair follicle (itch) B88.0
  in sputum B88.0
Mitral —*see* condition
Mittelschmerz N94.0
Mixed —*see* condition
MNGIE (Mitochondrial Neurogastrointestinal
  Encephalopathy) syndrome E88.49
Mobile, mobility
  cecum Q43.3
  excessive —*see* Hypermobility
  gallbladder, congenital Q44.1
  kidney N28.89
  organ or site, congenital NEC —*see*
    Malposition, congenital
Mobitz heart block (atrioventricular) I44.1
Moebius, Möbius
  disease (ophthalmoplegic migraine) —*see*
    Migraine, ophthalmoplegic
  syndrome Q87.0
    congenital oculofacial paralysis (with other
      anomalies) Q87.0
    ophthalmoplegic migraine —*see* Migraine,
      ophthalmoplegic
Moeller's glossitis K14.0
Mohr's syndrome (Types I and II) Q87.0
Mola destruens D39.2
Molar pregnancy O02.0
Molarization of premolars K00.2
Molding, head (during birth) - omit code
Mole (pigmented) —*see also* Nevus
  blood O02.0
  Breus' O02.0
  cancerous —*see* Melanoma
  carneous O02.0
  destructive D39.2
  fleshy O02.0
  hydatid, hydatidiform (benign) (complicating
    pregnancy) (delivered) (undelivered)
    O01.9
    classical O01.0
    complete O01.0
    incomplete O01.1
    invasive D39.2
    malignant D39.2
    partial O01.1

◀ New ◀━ Revised ~~deleted~~ Deleted

Mounier-Kuhn syndrome (Continued)
  acquired J98.09
    with bronchiectasis J47.9
      with
        exacerbation (acute) J47.1
        lower respiratory infection J47.0
Mountain
  sickness T70.29
    with polycythemia , acquired (acute) D75.1
  tick fever A93.2
Mouse, joint —see Loose, body, joint
  knee M23.4-
Mouth —see condition
Movable
  coccyx —see subcategory M53.2
  kidney N28.89
    congenital Q63.8
  spleen D73.89
Movements, dystonic R25.8
Moyamoya disease I67.5
MRSA (Methicillin resistant Staphylococcus
    aureus)
  infection A49.02
    as the cause of diseases classified
        elsewhere B95.62
  sepsis A41.02
MSSA (Methicillin susceptible Staphylococcus
    aureus)
  infection A49.01
    as the cause of diseases classified
        elsewhere B95.61
  sepsis A41.01
Mucha-Habermann disease L41.0
Mucinosis (cutaneous) (focal) (papular)
    (reticular erythematous) (skin) L98.5
  oral K13.79
Mucocele
  appendix K38.8
  buccal cavity K13.79
  gallbladder K82.1
  lacrimal sac, chronic H04.43-
  nasal sinus J34.1
  nose J34.1
  salivary gland (any) K11.6
  sinus (accessory) (nasal) J34.1
  turbinate (bone) (middle) (nasal) J34.1
  uterus N85.8
Mucolipidosis
  I E77.1
  II, III E77.0
  IV E75.11
Mucopolysaccharidosis E76.3
  beta-gluduronidase deficiency E76.29
  cardiopathy E76.3 [I52]
  Hunter's syndrome E76.1
  Hurler's syndrome E76.01
  Hurler-Scheie syndrome E76.02
  Maroteaux-Lamy syndrome E76.29
  Morquio syndrome E76.219
    A E76.210
    B E76.211
    classic E76.210
  Sanfilippo syndrome E76.22
  Scheie's syndrome E76.03
  specified NEC E76.29
  type
    I
      Hurler's syndrome E76.01
      Hurler-Scheie syndrome E76.02
      Scheie's syndrome E76.03
    II E76.1
    III E76.22
    IV E76.219
    IVA E76.210
    IVB E76.211
    VI E76.29
    VII E76.29
Mucormycosis B46.5
  cutaneous B46.3
  disseminated B46.4
  gastrointestinal B46.2

Mucormycosis (Continued)
  generalized B46.4
  pulmonary B46.0
  rhinocerebral B46.1
  skin B46.3
  subcutaneous B46.3
Mucositis (ulcerative) K12.30
  due to drugs NEC K12.32
  gastrointestinal K92.81
  mouth (oral) (oropharyngeal) K12.30
    due to antineoplastic therapy K12.31
    due to drugs NEC K12.32
    due to radiation K12.33
    specified NEC K12.39
    viral K12.39
  nasal J34.81
  oral cavity —see Mucositis, mouth
  oral soft tissues —see Mucositis, mouth
  vagina and vulva N76.81
Mucositis necroticans agranulocytica —see
    Agranulocytosis
Mucous —see also condition
  patches (syphilitic) A51.39
    congenital A50.07
Mucoviscidosis E84.9
  with meconium obstruction E84.11
Mucus
  asphyxia or suffocation —see Asphyxia,
      mucus
  in stool R19.5
  plug —see Asphyxia, mucus
Muguet B37.0
Mulberry molars (congenital syphilis) A50.52
Müllerian mixed tumor
  specified site —see Neoplasm, malignant, by
      site
  unspecified site C54.9
Multicystic kidney (development) Q61.4
Multiparity (grand) Z64.1
  affecting management of pregnancy, labor
      and delivery (supervision only)
      O09.4-
  requiring contraceptive management —see
      Contraception
Multipartita placenta O43.19-
Multiple, multiplex —see also condition
  digits (congenital) Q69.9
  endocrine neoplasia —see Neoplasia,
      endocrine, multiple [MEN]
  personality F44.81
Mumps B26.9
  arthritis B26.85
  complication NEC B26.89
  encephalitis B26.2
  hepatitis B26.81
  meningitis (aseptic) B26.1
  meningoencephalitis B26.2
  myocarditis B26.82
  oophoritis B26.89
  orchitis B26.0
  pancreatitis B26.3
  polyneuropathy B26.84
Mumu (see also Infestation, filarial) B74.9 [N51]
Münchhausen's syndrome —see Disorder,
    factitious
Münchmeyer's syndrome —see Myositis,
    ossificans, progressiva
Mural —see condition
Murmur (cardiac) (heart) (organic) R01.1
  abdominal R19.15
  aortic (valve) —see Endocarditis, aortic
  benign R01.0
  diastolic —see Endocarditis
  Flint I35.1
  functional R01.0
  Graham Steell I37.1
  innocent R01.0
  mitral (valve) —see Insufficiency, mitral
  nonorganic R01.0
  presystolic, mitral —see Insufficiency, mitral
  pulmonic (valve) I37.8

Murmur (Continued)
  systolic (valvular) —see Endocarditis
  tricuspid (valve) I07.9
  valvular —see Endocarditis
Murri's disease (intermittent hemoglobinuria)
    D59.6
Muscle, muscular —see also condition
  carnitine (palmityltransferase) deficiency
    E71.314
Musculoneuralgia —see Neuralgia
Mushroom-workers' (pickers') disease or lung
    J67.5
Mushrooming hip —see Derangement, joint,
    specified NEC, hip
Mutation (s)
  factor V Leiden D68.51
  surfactant, of lung J84.83
  prothrombin gene D68.52
Mutism —see also Aphasia
  deaf (acquired) (congenital) NEC H91.3
  elective (adjustment reaction) (childhood)
    F94.0
  hysterical F44.4
  selective (childhood) F94.0
MVD (microvillus inclusion disease) Q43.8
MVID (microvillus inclusion disease) Q43.8
Myalgia M79.1
  epidemic (cervical) B33.0
  traumatic NEC T14.8
Myasthenia G70.9
  congenital G70.2
  cordis —see Failure, heart
  developmental G70.2
  gravis G70.00
    with exacerbation (acute) G70.01
    in crisis G70.01
  neonatal, transient P94.0
  pseudoparalytica G70.00
    with exacerbation (acute) G70.01
    in crisis G70.01
  stomach, psychogenic F45.8
  syndrome
    in
      diabetes mellitus —see E08-E13 with .44
      neoplastic disease (see also Neoplasm)
        D49.9 [G73.3]
      pernicious anemia D51.0 [G73.3]
      thyrotoxicosis E05.90 [G73.3]
        with thyroid storm E05.91 [G73.3]
Myasthenic M62.81
Mycelium infection B49
Mycetismus —see Poisoning, food, noxious,
    mushroom
Mycetoma B47.9
  actinomycotic B47.1
  bone (mycotic) B47.9 [M90.80]
  eumycotic B47.0
  foot B47.9
    actinomycotic B47.1
    mycotic B47.0
  madurae NEC B47.9
    mycotic B47.0
  maduromycotic B47.0
  mycotic B47.0
  nocardial B47.1
Mycobacteriosis —see Mycobacterium
Mycobacterium, mycobacterial (infection)
    A31.9
  anonymous A31.9
  atypical A31.9
    cutaneous A31.1
    pulmonary A31.0
      tuberculous —see Tuberculosis,
          pulmonary
    specified site NEC A31.8
  avium (intracellulare complex) A31.0
  balnei A31.1
  Battey A31.0
  chelonei A31.8
  cutaneous A31.1
  extrapulmonary systemic A31.8

M

Mycobacterium, mycobacterial (Continued)
  fortuitum A31.8
  intracellulare (Battey bacillus) A31.0
  kakaferifu A31.8
  kansasii (yellow bacillus) A31.0
  kasongo A31.8
  leprae (see also Leprosy) A30.9
  luciflavum A31.1
  marinum (M. balnei) A31.1
  nonspecific —see Mycobacterium, atypical
  pulmonary (atypical) A31.0
    tuberculous —see Tuberculosis, pulmonary
  scrofulaceum A31.8
  simiae A31.8
  systemic, extrapulmonary A31.8
  szulgai A31.8
  terrae A31.8
  triviale A31.8
  tuberculosis (human, bovine) —see
    Tuberculosis
  ulcerans A31.1
  xenopi A31.8
Mycoplasma (M.) pneumoniae, as cause of
  disease classified elsewhere B96.0
Mycosis, mycotic B49
  cutaneous NEC B36.9
  ear B36.8
  fungoides (extranodal) (solid organ)
    C84.0-
  mouth B37.0
  nails B35.1
  opportunistic B48.8
  skin NEC B36.9
  specified NEC B48.8
  stomatitis B37.0
  vagina, vaginitis (candidal) B37.3
Mydriasis (pupil) H57.04
Myelatelia Q06.1
Myelinolysis, pontine, central G37.2
Myelitis (acute) (ascending) (childhood)
  (chronic) (descending) (diffuse)
  (disseminated) (idiopathic) (pressure)
  (progressive) (spinal cord) (subacute) (see
  also Encephalitis) G04.91
  herpes simplex B00.82
  herpes zoster B02.24
  in diseases classified elsewhere G05.4
  necrotizing, subacute G37.4
  optic neuritis in G36.0
  postchickenpox B01.12
  postherpetic B02.24
  postimmunization G04.02
  postinfectious NEC G04.89
  postvaccinal G04.02
  specified NEC G04.89
  syphilitic (transverse) A52.14
  toxic G92
  transverse (in demyelinating diseases of
    central nervous system) G37.3
  tuberculous A17.82
  varicella B01.12
Myeloblastic —see condition
Myeloblastoma
  granular cell —see also Neoplasm, connective
    tissue
    malignant —see Neoplasm, connective
      tissue, malignant
    tongue D10.1
Myelocele —see Spina bifida
Myelocystocele —see Spina bifida
Myelocytic —see condition
Myelodysplasia D46.9
  specified NEC D46.Z
  spinal cord (congenital) Q06.1
Myelodysplastic syndrome D46.9
  with
    5q deletion D46.C
    isolated del (5q) chromosomal abnormality
      C46.C
  specified NEC D46.Z
Myeloencephalitis —see Encephalitis

Myelofibrosis D75.81
  with myeloid metaplasia D47.4
  acute C94.4-
  idiopathic (chronic) D47.4
  primary D47.1
  secondary D75.81
    in myeloproliferative disease D47.4
Myelogenous —see condition
Myeloid —see condition
Myelokathexis D70.9
Myeloleukodystrophy E75.29
Myelolipoma —see Lipoma
Myeloma (multiple) C90.0-
  monostotic C90.3
    plasma cell C90.0-
  plasma cell C90.0-
  solitary (see also Plasmacytoma, solitary)
    C90.3-
Myelomalacia G95.89
Myelomatosis C90.0-
Myelomeningitis —see Meningoencephalitis
Myelomeningocele (spinal cord) —see Spina
  bifida
Myelo-osteo-musculodysplasia hereditaria
  Q79.8
Myelopathic
  anemia D64.89
  muscle atrophy —see Atrophy, muscle, spinal
  pain syndrome G89.0
Myelopathy (spinal cord) G95.9
  drug-induced G95.89
  in (due to)
    degeneration or displacement,
      intervertebral disc NEC —see
      Disorder, disc, with, myelopathy
    infection —see Encephalitis
    intervertebral disc disorder —see also
      Disorder, disc, with, myelopathy
    mercury —see subcategory T56.1
    neoplastic disease (see also Neoplasm)
      D49.9 [G99.2]
    pernicious anemia D51.0 [G99.2]
    spondylosis —see Spondylosis, with
      myelopathy NEC
  necrotic (subacute) (vascular) G95.19
  radiation-induced G95.89
  spondylogenic NEC —see Spondylosis, with
    myelopathy NEC
  toxic G95.89
  transverse, acute G37.3
  vascular G95.19
  vitamin B12 E53.8 [G32.0]
Myelophthisis D61.82
Myeloradiculitis G04.91
Myeloradiculodysplasia (spinal) Q06.1
Myelosarcoma C92.3-
Myelosclerosis D75.89
  with myeloid metaplasia D47.4
  disseminated, of nervous system G35
  megakaryocytic D47.4
    with myeloid metaplasia D47.4
Myelosis
  acute C92.0-
  aleukemic C92.9-
  chronic D47.1
  erythremic (acute) C94.0-
  megakaryocytic C94.2-
  nonleukemic D72.828
  subacute C92.9-
Myiasis (cavernous) B87.9
  aural B87.4
  creeping B87.0
  cutaneous B87.0
  dermal B87.0
  ear (external) (middle) B87.4
  eye B87.2
  genitourinary B87.81
  intestinal B87.82
  laryngeal B87.3
  nasopharyngeal B87.3
  ocular B87.2

Myiasis (Continued)
  orbit B87.2
  skin B87.0
  specified site NEC B87.89
  traumatic B87.1
  wound B87.1
Myoadenoma, prostate —see Hyperplasia,
  prostate
Myoblastoma
  granular cell —see also Neoplasm, connective
    tissue, benign
    malignant —see Neoplasm, connective
      tissue, malignant
  tongue D10.1
Myocardial —see condition
Myocardiopathy (congestive) (constrictive)
  (familial) (hypertrophic nonobstructive)
  (idiopathic) (infiltrative) (obstructive)
  (primary) (restrictive) (sporadic) (see also
  Cardiomyopathy) I42.9
  alcoholic I42.6
  cobalt-beer I42.6
  glycogen storage E74.02 [I43]
  hypertrophic obstructive I42.1
  in (due to)
    beriberi E51.12
    cardiac glycogenosis E74.02 [I43]
    Friedreich's ataxia G11.1 [I43]
    myotonia atrophica G71.11 [I43]
    progressive muscular dystrophy G71.0
      [I43]
  obscure (African) I42.8
  secondary I42.9
  thyrotoxic E05.90 [I43]
    with storm E05.91 [I43]
  toxic NEC I42.7
Myocarditis (with arteriosclerosis) (chronic)
  (fibroid) (interstitial) (old) (progressive)
  (senile) I51.4
  with
    rheumatic fever (conditions in I00) I09.0
      active —see Myocarditis, acute,
        rheumatic
      inactive or quiescent (with chorea) I09.0
  active I40.9
    rheumatic I01.2
      with chorea (acute) (rheumatic)
        (Sydenham's) I02.0
  acute or subacute (interstitial) I40.9
    due to
      streptococcus (beta-hemolytic) I01.2
    idiopathic I40.1
    rheumatic I01.2
      with chorea (acute) (rheumatic)
        (Sydenham's) I02.0
    specified NEC I40.8
  aseptic of newborn B33.22
  bacterial (acute) I40.0
  Coxsackie (virus) B33.22
  diphtheritic A36.81
  eosinophilic I40.1
  epidemic of newborn (Coxsackie) B33.22
  Fiedler's (acute) (isolated) I40.1
  giant cell (acute) (subacute) I40.1
  gonococcal A54.83
  granulomatous (idiopathic) (isolated)
    (nonspecific) I40.1
  hypertensive —see Hypertension, heart
  idiopathic (granulomatous) I40.1
  in (due to)
    diphtheria A36.81
    epidemic louse-borne typhus A75.0 [I41]
    Lyme disease A69.29
    sarcoidosis D86.85
    scarlet fever A38.1
    toxoplasmosis (acquired) B58.81
    typhoid A01.02
    typhus NEC A75.9 [I41]
  infective I40.0
  influenzal —see Influenza, with, myocarditis
  isolated (acute) I40.1

◀ New   ◀▬ Revised   ~~deleted~~ Deleted

Myocarditis (Continued)
  meningococcal A39.52
  mumps B26.82
  nonrheumatic, active I40.9
  parenchymatous I40.9
  pneumococcal I40.0
  rheumatic (chronic) (inactive) (with chorea)
      I09.0
    active or acute I01.2
      with chorea (acute) (rheumatic)
          (Sydenham's) I02.0
  rheumatoid —see Rheumatoid, carditis
  septic I40.0
  staphylococcal I40.0
  suppurative I40.0
  syphilitic (chronic) A52.06
  toxic I40.8
    rheumatic —see Myocarditis, acute,
        rheumatic
  tuberculous A18.84
  typhoid A01.02
  valvular —see Endocarditis
  virus, viral I40.0
    of newborn (Coxsackie) B33.22
Myocardium, myocardial —see condition
Myocardosis —see Cardiomyopathy
Myoclonus, myoclonic, myoclonia (familial)
      (essential) (multifocal) (simplex) G25.3
  drug-induced G25.3
  epilepsy (see also Epilepsy, generalized,
      specified NEC) G40.4-
    familial (progressive) G25.3
  epileptica G40.409
    with status epilepticus G40.401
  facial G51.3
  familial progressive G25.3
  Friedreich's G25.3
  jerks G25.3
  massive G25.3
  palatal G25.3
  pharyngeal G25.3
Myocytolysis I51.5
Myodiastasis —see Diastasis, muscle
Myoendocarditis —see Endocarditis
Myoepithelioma —see Neoplasm, benign, by
    site
Myofasciitis (acute) —see Myositis
Myofibroma —see also Neoplasm, connective
      tissue, benign
  uterus (cervix) (corpus) —see Leiomyoma
Myofibromatosis D48.1
  infantile Q89.8
Myofibrosis M62.89
  heart —see Myocarditis
  scapulohumeral —see Lesion, shoulder,
      specified NEC
Myofibrositis M79.7
  scapulohumeral —see Lesion, shoulder,
      specified NEC
Myoglobulinuria, myoglobinuria (primary)
    R82.1
Myokymia, facial G51.4
Myolipoma —see Lipoma
Myoma —see also Neoplasm, connective tissue,
      benign
  malignant —see Neoplasm, connective tissue,
      malignant
  prostate D29.1
  uterus (cervix) (corpus) —see Leiomyoma
Myomalacia M62.89
Myometritis —see Endometritis
Myometrium —see condition
Myonecrosis, clostridial A48.0
Myopathy G72.9
  acute
    necrotizing G72.81
    quadriplegic G72.81
  alcoholic G72.1
  benign congenital G71.2
  central core G71.2
  centronuclear G71.2

Myopathy (Continued)
  congenital (benign) G71.2
  critical illness G72.81
  distal G71.0
  drug-induced G72.0
  endocrine NEC E34.9 [G73.7]
  extraocular muscles H05.82-
  facioscapulohumeral G71.0
  hereditary G71.9
    specified NEC G71.8
  immune NEC G72.49
  in (due to)
    Addison's disease E27.1 [G73.7]
    alcohol G72.1
    amyloidosis E85.0 [G73.7]
    cretinism E00.9 [G73.7]
    Cushing's syndrome E24.9 [G73.7]
    drugs G72.0
    endocrine disease NEC E34.9 [G73.7]
    giant cell arteritis M31.6 [G73.7]
    glycogen storage disease E74.00 [G73.7]
    hyperadrenocorticism E24.9 [G73.7]
    hyperparathyroidism NEC E21.3 [G73.7]
    hypoparathyroidism E20.9 [G73.7]
    hypopituitarism E23.0 [G73.7]
    hypothyroidism E03.9 [G73.7]
    infectious disease NEC B99 [G73.7]
    lipid storage disease E75.6 [G73.7]
    metabolic disease NEC E88.9 [G73.7]
    myxedema E03.9 [G73.7]
    parasitic disease NEC B89 [G73.7]
    polyarteritis nodosa M30.0 [G73.7]
    rheumatoid arthritis —see Rheumatoid,
        myopathy
    sarcoidosis D86.87
    scleroderma M34.82
    sicca syndrome M35.03
    Sjögren's syndrome M35.03
    systemic lupus erythematosus M32.19
    thyrotoxicosis (hyperthyroidism) E05.90
        [G73.7]
      with thyroid storm E05.91 [G73.7]
    toxic agent NEC G72.2
  inflammatory NEC G72.49
  intensive care (ICU) G72.81
  limb-girdle G71.0
  mitochondrial NEC G71.3
  myotubular G71.2
  mytonic, proximal (PROMM) G71.11
  nemaline G71.2
  ocular G71.0
  oculopharyngeal G71.0
  of critical illness G72.81
  primary G71.9
    specified NEC G71.8
  progressive NEC G72.89
  proximal myotonic (PROMM) G71.11
  rod G71.2
  scapulohumeral G71.0
  specified NEC G72.89
  toxic G72.2
Myopericarditis —see also Pericarditis
  chronic rheumatic I09.2
Myopia (axial) (congenital) H52.1-
  degenerative (malignant) H44.2-
  malignant H44.2-
  pernicious H44.2-
  progressive high (degenerative) H44.2-
Myosarcoma —see Neoplasm, connective tissue,
    malignant
Myosis (pupil) H57.03
  stromal (endolymphatic) D39.0
Myositis M60.9
  clostridial A48.0
  due to posture —see Myositis, specified type
    NEC
  epidemic B33.0
  fibrosa or fibrous (chronic), Volkmann's
    T79.6
  foreign body granuloma —see Granuloma,
    foreign body

Myositis (Continued)
  in (due to)
    bilharziasis B65.9 [M63.8-]
    cysticercosis B69.81
    leprosy A30.9 [M63.8-]
    mycosis B49 [M63.8-]
    sarcoidosis D86.87
    schistosomiasis B65.9 [M63.8-]
    syphilis
      late A52.78
      secondary A51.49
    toxoplasmosis (acquired) B58.82
    trichinellosis B75 [M63.8-]
    tuberculosis A18.09
  inclusion body [IBM] G72.41
  infective M60.009
    arm M60.002
      left M60.001
      right M60.000
    leg M60.005
      left M60.004
      right M60.003
    lower limb M60.005
      ankle M60.07-
      foot M60.07-
      lower leg M60.06-
      thigh M60.05-
      toe M60.07-
    multiple sites M60.09
    specified site NEC M60.08
    upper limb M60.002
      finger M60.04-
      forearm M60.03-
      hand M60.04-
      shoulder region M60.01-
      upper arm M60.02-
  interstitial M60.10
    ankle M60.17-
    foot M60.17-
    forearm M60.13-
    hand M60.14-
    lower leg M60.16-
    multiple sites M60.19
    shoulder region M60.11-
    specified site NEC M60.18
    thigh M60.15-
    upper arm M60.12-
  mycotic B49 [M63.8-]
  ossificans or ossifying (circumscripta) —see
      also Ossification, muscle, specified NEC
    in (due to)
      burns M61.30
        ankle M61.37-
        foot M61.37-
        forearm M61.33-
        hand M61.34-
        lower leg M61.36-
        multiple sites M61.39
        pelvic region M61.35-
        shoulder region M61.31-
        specified site NEC M61.38
        thigh M61.35-
        upper arm M61.32-
      quadriplegia or paraplegia M61.20
        ankle M61.27-
        foot M61.27-
        forearm M61.23-
        hand M61.24-
        lower leg M61.26-
        multiple sites M61.29
        pelvic region M61.25-
        shoulder region M61.21-
        specified site NEC M61.28
        thigh M61.25-
        upper arm M61.22-
    progressiva M61.10
      ankle M61.17-
      finger M61.14-
      foot M61.17-
      forearm M61.13-
      hand M61.14-

Myositis (Continued)
  ossificans or ossifying (Continued)
    progressiva (Continued)
      lower leg M61.16-
      multiple sites M61.19
      pelvic region M61.15-
      shoulder region M61.11-
      specified site NEC M61.18
      thigh M61.15-
      toe M61.17-
      upper arm M61.12-
    traumatica M61.00
      ankle M61.07-
      foot M61.07-
      forearm M61.03-
      hand M61.04-
      lower leg M61.06-
      multiple sites M61.09
      pelvic region M61.05-
      shoulder region M61.01-
      specified site NEC M61.08
      thigh M61.05-
      upper arm M61.02-
  purulent —see Myositis, infective
  specified type NEC M60.80
    ankle M60.87-
    foot M60.87-
    forearm M60.83-
    hand M60.84-
    lower leg M60.86-
    multiple sites M60.89
    pelvic region M60.85-

Myositis (Continued)
  specified type NEC (Continued)
    shoulder region M60.81-
    specified site NEC M60.88
    thigh M60.85-
    upper arm M60.82-
  suppurative —see Myositis, infective
  traumatic (old) —see Myositis, specified type
    NEC
Myospasia impulsiva F95.2
Myotonia (acquisita) (intermittens) M62.89
  atrophica G71.11
  chondrodystrophic G71.13
  congenita (acetazolamide responsive)
    (dominant) (recessive) G71.12
  drug-induced G71.14
  dystrophica G71.11
  fluctuans G71.19
  levior G71.12
  permanens G71.19
  symptomatic G71.19
Myotonic pupil —see Anomaly, pupil, function,
  tonic pupil
Myriapodiasis B88.2
Myringitis H73.2-
  with otitis media —see Otitis, media
  acute H73.00-
    bullous H73.01-
    specified NEC H73.09-
  bullous —see Myringitis, acute, bullous
  chronic H73.1-
Mysophobia F40.228

Mytilotoxism —see Poisoning, fish
Myxadenitis labialis K13.0
Myxedema (adult) (idiocy) (infantile) (juvenile)
  (see also Hypothyroidism) E03.9
  circumscribed E05.90
    with storm E05.91
  coma E03.5
  congenital E00.1
  cutis L98.5
  localized (pretibial) E05.90
    with storm E05.91
  papular L98.5
Myxochondrosarcoma —see Neoplasm,
  cartilage, malignant
Myxofibroma —see Neoplasm, connective
  tissue, benign
  odontogenic —see Cyst, calcifying
    odontogenic
Myxofibrosarcoma —see Neoplasm, connective
  tissue, malignant
Myxolipoma D17.9
Myxoliposarcoma —see Neoplasm, connective
  tissue, malignant
Myxoma —see also Neoplasm, connective tissue,
  benign
  nerve sheath —see Neoplasm, nerve,
    benign
  odontogenic —see Cyst, calcifying
    odontogenic
Myxosarcoma —see Neoplasm, connective
  tissue, malignant

M

◀ New   ◀▥ Revised   ~~deleted~~ Deleted

N

Naegeli's
   disease Q82.8
   leukemia, monocytic C93.1-
Naegleriasis (with meningoencephalitis) B60.2
Naffziger's syndrome G54.0
Naga sore —see Ulcer, skin
Nägele's pelvis M95.5
   with disproportion (fetopelvic) O33.0
      causing obstructed labor O65.0
Nail —see also condition
   biting F98.8
   patella syndrome Q87.2
Nanism, nanosomia —see Dwarfism
Nanophyetiasis B66.8
Nanukayami A27.89
Napkin rash L22
Narcolepsy G47.419
   with cataplexy G47.411
   in conditions classified elsewhere G47.429
      with cataplexy G47.421
Narcosis R06.89
Narcotism —see Dependence
NARP (Neuropathy, Ataxia and Retinitis
   pigmentosa) syndrome E88.49
Narrow
   anterior chamber angle H40.03-
   pelvis —see Contraction, pelvis
Narrowing —see also Stenosis
   artery I77.1
      auditory, internal I65.8
      basilar —see Occlusion, artery, basilar
      carotid —see Occlusion, artery, carotid
      cerebellar —see Occlusion, artery, cerebellar
      cerebral —see Occlusion artery, cerebral
      choroidal —see Occlusion, artery, cerebral,
         specified NEC
      communicating posterior —see Occlusion,
         artery, cerebral, specified NEC
      coronary —see also Disease, heart, ischemic,
         atherosclerotic
         congenital Q24.5
         syphilitic A50.54 [I52]
         due to syphilis NEC A52.06
      hypophyseal —see Occlusion, artery,
         cerebral, specified NEC
      pontine —see Occlusion, artery, cerebral,
         specified NEC
      precerebral —see Occlusion, artery,
         precerebral
      vertebral —see Occlusion, artery, vertebral
   auditory canal (external) —see Stenosis,
      external ear canal
   eustachian tube —see Obstruction, eustachian
      tube
   eyelid —see Disorder, eyelid function
   larynx J38.6
   mesenteric artery K55.0
   palate M26.89
   palpebral fissure —see Disorder, eyelid
      function
   ureter N13.5
      with infection N13.6
   urethra —see Stricture, urethra
Narrowness, abnormal, eyelid Q10.3
Nasal —see condition
Nasolachrymal, nasolacrimal —see condition
Nasopharyngeal —see also condition
   pituitary gland Q89.2
   torticollis M43.6
Nasopharyngitis (acute) (infective)
   (streptococcal) (subacute) J00
   chronic (suppurative) (ulcerative) J31.1
Nasopharynx, nasopharyngeal —see condition
Natal tooth, teeth K00.6
Nausea (without vomiting) R11.0
   with vomiting R11.2
   gravidarum —see Hyperemesis, gravidarum
   marina T75.3
   navalis T75.3

Navel —see condition
Neapolitan fever —see Brucellosis
Near drowning T75.1
Nearsightedness —see Myopia
Near-syncope R55
Nebula, cornea —see Opacity, cornea
Necator americanus infestation B76.1
Necatoriasis B76.1
Neck —see condition
Necrobiosis R68.89
   lipoidica NEC L92.1
      with diabetes —see E08-E13 with .620
Necrolysis, toxic epidermal L51.2
   due to drug
      correct substance properly administered —
         see Table of Drugs and Chemicals, by
         drug, adverse effect
      overdose or wrong substance given or
         taken —see Table of Drugs and
         Chemicals, by drug, poisoning
Necrophilia F65.89
Necrosis, necrotic (ischemic) —see also
   Gangrene
   adrenal (capsule) (gland) E27.49
   amputation stump (surgical) (late)
      T87.50
      arm T87.5-
      leg T87.5-
   antrum J32.0
   aorta (hyaline) —see also Aneurysm, aorta
      cystic medial —see Dissection, aorta
   artery I77.5
   bladder (aseptic) (sphincter) N32.89
   bone (see also Osteonecrosis) M87.9
      aseptic or avascular —see Osteonecrosis
         idiopathic M87.00
      ethmoid J32.2
      jaw M27.2
      tuberculous —see Tuberculosis, bone
   brain I67.89
   breast (aseptic) (fat) (segmental) N64.1
   bronchus J98.09
   central nervous system NEC I67.89
   cerebellar I67.89
   cerebral I67.89
   colon K55.0
   cornea H18.40
   cortical (acute) (renal) N17.1
   cystic medial (aorta) —see Dissection, aorta
   dental pulp K04.1
   esophagus K22.8
   ethmoid (bone) J32.2
   eyelid —see Disorder, eyelid, degenerative
   fat, fatty (generalized) —see also Disorder, soft
      tissue, specified type NEC
      abdominal wall K65.4
      breast (aseptic) (segmental) N64.1
      localized —see Degeneration, by site,
         fatty
      mesentery K65.4
      omentum K65.4
      pancreas K86.8
      peritoneum K65.4
      skin (subcutaneous), newborn P83.0
      subcutaneous, due to birth injury P15.6
   gallbladder —see Cholecystitis, acute
   heart —see Infarct, myocardium
   hip, aseptic or avascular —see Osteonecrosis,
      by type, femur
   intestine (acute) (hemorrhagic) (massive)
      K55.0
   jaw M27.2
   kidney (bilateral) N28.0
      acute N17.9
      cortical (acute) (bilateral) N17.1
         with ectopic or molar pregnancy
            O08.4
      medullary (bilateral) (in acute renal
         failure) (papillary) N17.2
      papillary (bilateral) (in acute renal
         failure) N17.2

Necrosis, necrotic (Continued)
   kidney (Continued)
      tubular N17.0
         with ectopic or molar pregnancy O08.4
         complicating
            abortion —see Abortion, by type,
               complicated by, tubular necrosis
            ectopic or molar pregnancy O08.4
            pregnancy —see Pregnancy,
               complicated by, diseases of,
               specified type or system NEC
         following ectopic or molar pregnancy
            O08.4
         traumatic T79.5
   larynx J38.7
   liver (with hepatic failure) (cell) —see Failure,
      hepatic
      hemorrhagic, central K76.2
   lung J85.0
   lymphatic gland —see Lymphadenitis, acute
   mammary gland (fat) (segmental) N64.1
   mastoid (chronic) —see Mastoiditis, chronic
   medullary (acute) (renal) N17.2
   mesentery K55.0
      fat K65.4
   mitral valve —see Insufficiency, mitral
   myocardium, myocardial —see Infarct,
      myocardium
   nose J34.0
   omentum (with mesenteric infarction)
      K55.0
      fat K65.4
   orbit, orbital —see Osteomyelitis, orbit
   ossicles, ear —see Abnormal, ear ossicles
   ovary N70.92
   pancreas (aseptic) (duct) (fat) K86.8
      acute (infective) —see Pancreatitis, acute
      infective —see Pancreatitis, acute
   papillary (acute) (renal) N17.2
   perineum N90.89
   peritoneum (with mesenteric infarction)
      K55.0
      fat K65.4
   pharynx J02.9
      in granulocytopenia —see Neutropenia
      Vincent's A69.1
   phosphorus —see subcategory T54.2
   pituitary (gland) (postpartum) (Sheehan)
      E23.0
   pressure —see Ulcer, pressure, by site
   pulmonary J85.0
   pulp (dental) K04.1
   radiation —see Necrosis, by site
   radium —see Necrosis, by site
   renal —see Necrosis, kidney
   sclera H15.89
   scrotum N50.8
   skin or subcutaneous tissue NEC I96
   spine, spinal (column) —see also
      Osteonecrosis, by type, vertebra
      cord G95.19
   spleen D73.5
   stomach K31.89
   stomatitis (ulcerative) A69.0
   subcutaneous fat, newborn P83.8
   subendocardial (acute) I21.4
      chronic I25.89
   suprarenal (capsule) (gland) E27.49
   testis N50.8
   thymus (gland) E32.8
   tonsil J35.8
   trachea J39.8
   tuberculous NEC —see Tuberculosis
   tubular (acute) (anoxic) (renal) (toxic) N17.0
      postprocedural N99.0
   vagina N89.8
   vertebra —see also Osteonecrosis, by type,
      vertebra
      tuberculous A18.01
   vulva N90.89
   X-ray —see Necrosis, by site

Necrospermia —see Infertility, male
Need (for)
  care provider because (of)
    assistance with personal care Z74.1
    continuous supervision required Z74.3
    impaired mobility Z74.09
    no other household member able to render
      care Z74.2
    specified reason NEC Z74.8
  immunization —see Vaccination
  vaccination —see Vaccination
Neglect
  adult
    confirmed T74.01
    history of Z91.412
    suspected T76.01
  child (childhood)
    confirmed T74.02
    history of Z62.812
    suspected T76.02
  emotional, in childhood Z62.898
  hemispatial R41.4
  left-sided R41.4
  sensory R41.4
  visuospatial R41.4
Neisserian infection NEC —see Gonococcus
Nelaton's syndrome G60.8
Nelson's syndrome E24.1
Nematodiasis (intestinal) B82.0
  Ancylostoma B76.0
Neonatal —see also Newborn
  acne L70.4
  bradycardia P29.12
  screening, abnormal findings on P09
  tachycardia P29.11
  tooth, teeth K00.6
Neonatorum —see condition
Neoplasia
  endocrine, multiple (MEN) E31.20
    type I E31.21
    type IIA E31.22
    type IIB E31.23
  intraepithelial (histologically confirmed)
    anal (AIN) (histologically confirmed)
      K62.82
      grade I K62.82
      grade II K62.82
      severe D01.3
    cervical glandular (histologically
      confirmed) D06.9
    cervix (uteri) (CIN) (histologically
      confirmed) N87.9
      glandular D06.9
      grade I N87.0
      grade II N87.1
      grade III (severe dysplasia) —see also
        Carcinoma, cervix uteri, in situ
        D06.9
    prostate (histologically confirmed) (PIN I)
      (PIN II) N42.3
      grade I N42.3
      grade II N42.3
      severe D07.5
    vagina (histologically confirmed) (VAIN)
      N89.3
      grade I N89.0
      grade II N89.1
      grade III (severe dysplasia) D07.2
    vulva (histologically confirmed) (VIN)
      N90.3
      grade I N90.0
      grade II N90.1
      grade III (severe dysplasia) D07.1
Neoplasm, neoplastic —see also Table of
    Neoplasms
  lipomatous, benign —see Lipoma
Neovascularization
  ciliary body —see Disorder, iris, vascular
  cornea H16.40-
    deep H16.44-
    ghost vessels —see Ghost, vessels

Neovascularization (Continued)
  cornea (Continued)
    localized H16.43-
    pannus —see Pannus
  iris —see Disorder, iris, vascular
  retina H35.05-
Nephralgia N23
Nephritis, nephritic (albuminuric) (azotemic)
    (congenital) (disseminated) (epithelial)
    (familial) (focal) (granulomatous)
    (hemorrhagic) (infantile) (nonsuppurative,
    excretory) (uremic) N05.9
  with
    dense deposit disease N05.6
    diffuse
      crescentic glomerulonephritis N05.7
      endocapillary proliferative
        glomerulonephritis N05.4
      membranous glomerulonephritis
        N05.2
      mesangial proliferative
        glomerulonephritis N05.3
      mesangiocapillary glomerulonephritis
        N05.5
    edema —see Nephrosis
    focal and segmental glomerular lesions
      N05.1
    foot process disease N04.9
    glomerular lesion
      diffuse sclerosing N05.8
      hypocomplementemic —see Nephritis,
        membranoproliferative
      IgA —see Nephropathy, IgA
      lobular, lobulonodular —see Nephritis,
        membranoproliferative
      nodular —see Nephritis,
        membranoproliferative
    lesion of
      glomerulonephritis, proliferative
        N05.8
      renal necrosis N05.9
    minor glomerular abnormality N05.0
    specified morphological changes NEC
      N05.8
  acute N00.9
    with
      dense deposit disease N00.6
      diffuse
        crescentic glomerulonephritis
          N00.7
        endocapillary proliferative
          glomerulonephritis N00.4
        membranous glomerulonephritis
          N00.2
        mesangial proliferative
          glomerulonephritis N00.3
        mesangiocapillary glomerulonephritis
          N00.5
      focal and segmental glomerular lesions
        N00.1
      minor glomerular abnormality N00.0
      specified morphological changes NEC
        N00.8
  amyloid E85.4 [N08]
  antiglomerular basement membrane (anti-
    GBM) antibody NEC
    in Goodpasture's syndrome M31.0
  antitubular basement membrane
    (tubulo-interstitial) NEC N12
    toxic —see Nephropathy, toxic
  arteriolar —see Hypertension, kidney
  arteriosclerotic —see Hypertension,
    kidney
  ascending —see Nephritis, tubulo-interstitial
  atrophic N03.9
  Balkan (endemic) N15.0
  calculous, calculus —see Calculus,
    kidney
  cardiac —see Hypertension, kidney
  cardiovascular —see Hypertension,
    kidney

Nephritis, nephritic (Continued)
  chronic N03.9
    with
      dense deposit disease N03.6
      diffuse
        crescentic glomerulonephritis
          N03.7
        endocapillary proliferative
          glomerulonephritis N03.4
        membranous glomerulonephritis
          N03.2
        mesangial proliferative
          glomerulonephritis N03.3
        mesangiocapillary glomerulonephritis
          N03.5
      focal and segmental glomerular lesions
        N03.1
      minor glomerular abnormality
        N03.0
      specified morphological changes
        NEC N03.8
    arteriosclerotic —see Hypertension,
      kidney
  cirrhotic N26.9
  complicating pregnancy O26.83-
  croupous N00.9
  degenerative —see Nephrosis
  diffuse sclerosing N05.8
  due to
    diabetes mellitus —see E08-E13 with .21
    subacute bacterial endocarditis I33.0
    systemic lupus erythematosus (chronic)
      M32.14
    typhoid fever A01.09
  gonococcal (acute) (chronic) A54.21
  hypocomplementemic —see Nephritis,
    membranoproliferative
  IgA —see Nephropathy, IgA
  immune complex (circulating) NEC N05.8
  infective —see Nephritis, tubulo-interstitial
  interstitial —see Nephritis, tubulo-interstitial
  lead N14.3
  membranoproliferative (diffuse) (type 1 or 3)
    (see also N00-N07 with fourth character
    .5) N05.5
    type 2 (see also N00-N07 with fourth
      character .6) N05.6
  minimal change N05.0
  necrotic, necrotizing NEC (see also
    N00-N07 with fourth character .8)
    N05.8
  nephrotic —see Nephrosis
  nodular —see Nephritis,
    membranoproliferative
  polycystic Q61.3
    adult type Q61.2
    autosomal
      dominant Q61.2
      recessive NEC Q61.19
    childhood type NEC Q61.19
    infantile type NEC Q61.19
  poststreptococcal N05.9
    acute N00.9
    chronic N03.9
  rapidly progressive N01.9
  proliferative NEC (see also N00-N07 with
    fourth character .8) N05.8
  purulent —see Nephritis, tubulo-interstitial
  rapidly progressive N01.9
    with
      dense deposit disease N01.6
      diffuse
        crescentic glomerulonephritis N01.7
        endocapillary proliferative
          glomerulonephritis N01.4
        membranous glomerulonephritis
          N01.2
        mesangial proliferative
          glomerulonephritis N01.3
        mesangiocapillary glomerulonephritis
          N01.5

◀ New   ◀▦ Revised   ~~deleted~~ Deleted

Nephritis, nephritic *(Continued)*
  rapidly progressive *(Continued)*
    with *(Continued)*
      focal and segmental glomerular lesions N01.1
      minor glomerular abnormality N01.0
      specified morphological changes NEC N01.8
  salt losing or wasting NEC N28.89
  saturnine N14.3
  sclerosing, diffuse N05.8
  septic —*see* Nephritis, tubulo-interstitial
  specified pathology NEC *(see also* N00-N07 with fourth character .8) N05.8
  subacute N01.9
  suppurative —*see* Nephritis, tubulo-interstitial
  syphilitic (late) A52.75
    congenital A50.59 *[N08]*
    early (secondary) A51.44
  toxic —*see* Nephropathy, toxic
  tubal, tubular —*see* Nephritis, tubulo-interstitial
  tuberculous A18.11
  tubulo-interstitial (in) N12
    acute (infectious) N10
    chronic (infectious) N11.9
      nonobstructive N11.8
        reflux-associated N11.0
      obstructive N11.1
      specified NEC N11.8
    due to
      brucellosis A23.9 *[N16]*
      cryoglobulinemia D89.1 *[N16]*
      glycogen storage disease E74.00 *[N16]*
      Sjögren's syndrome M35.04
  vascular —*see* Hypertension, kidney
  war N00.9
Nephroblastoma (epithelial) (mesenchymal) C64-
Nephrocalcinosis E83.59 *[N29]*
Nephrocystitis, pustular —*see* Nephritis, tubulo-interstitial
Nephrolithiasis (congenital) (pelvis) (recurrent) —*see also* Calculus, kidney
Nephroma C64-
  mesoblastic D41.0-
Nephronephritis —*see* Nephrosis
Nephronophthisis Q61.5
Nephropathia epidemica A98.5
Nephropathy *(see also* Nephritis) N28.9
  with
    edema —*see* Nephrosis
    glomerular lesion —*see* Glomerulonephritis
  amyloid, hereditary E85.0
  analgesic N14.0
    with medullary necrosis, acute N17.2
  Balkan (endemic) N15.0
  chemical —*see* Nephropathy, toxic
  diabetic —*see* E08-E13 with .21
  drug-induced N14.2
    specified NEC N14.1
  focal and segmental hyalinosis or sclerosis N02.1
  heavy metal-induced N14.3
  hereditary NEC N07.9
    with
      dense deposit disease N07.6
      diffuse
        crescentic glomerulonephritis N07.7
        endocapillary proliferative glomerulonephritis N07.4
        membranous glomerulonephritis N07.2
        mesangial proliferative glomerulonephritis N07.3
        mesangiocapillary glomerulonephritis N07.5

Nephropathy *(Continued)*
  hereditary NEC *(Continued)*
    with *(Continued)*
      focal and segmental glomerular lesions N07.1
      minor glomerular abnormality N07.0
      specified morphological changes NEC N07.8
  hypercalcemic N25.89
  hypertensive —*see* Hypertension, kidney
  hypokalemic (vacuolar) N25.89
  IgA N02.8
    with glomerular lesion N02.9
      focal and segmental hyalinosis or sclerosis N02.1
      membranoproliferative (diffuse) N02.5
      membranous (diffuse) N02.2
      mesangial proliferative (diffuse) N02.3
      mesangiocapillary (diffuse) N02.5
      proliferative NEC N02.8
      specified pathology NEC N02.8
  lead N14.3
  membranoproliferative (diffuse) N02.5
  membranous (diffuse) N02.2
  mesangial (IgA/IgG) —*see* Nephropathy, IgA
    proliferative (diffuse) N02.3
  mesangiocapillary (diffuse) N02.5
  obstructive N13.8
  phenacetin N17.2
  phosphate-losing N25.0
  potassium depletion N25.89
  pregnancy-related O26.83-
  proliferative NEC *(see also* N00-N07 with fourth character .8) N05.8
  protein-losing N25.89
  saturnine N14.3
  sickle-cell D57.- *[N08]*
  toxic NEC N14.4
    due to
      drugs N14.2
        analgesic N14.0
        specified NEC N14.1
      heavy metals N14.3
  vasomotor N17.0
  water-losing N25.89
Nephroptosis N28.83
Nephropyosis —*see* Abscess, kidney
Nephrorrhagia N28.89
Nephrosclerosis (arteriolar) (arteriosclerotic) (chronic) (hyaline) —*see also* Hypertension, kidney
  hyperplastic —*see* Hypertension, kidney
  senile N26.9
Nephrosis, nephrotic (Epstein's) (syndrome) (congenital) N04.9
  with
    foot process disease N04.9
    glomerular lesion N04.1
    hypocomplementemic N04.5
  acute N04.9
  anoxic —*see* Nephrosis, tubular
  chemical —*see* Nephrosis, tubular
  cholemic K76.7
  diabetic —*see* E08-E13 with .21
  Finnish type (congenital) Q89.8
  hemoglobin N10
  hemoglobinuric —*see* Nephrosis, tubular
  in
    amyloidosis E85.4 *[N08]*
    diabetes mellitus —*see* E08-E13 with .21
    epidemic hemorrhagic fever A98.5
    malaria (malariae) B52.0
  ischemic —*see* Nephrosis, tubular
  lipoid N04.9
  lower nephron —*see* Nephrosis, tubular
  malarial (malariae) B52.0
  minimal change N04.0
  myoglobin N10
  necrotizing —*see* Nephrosis, tubular
  osmotic (sucrose) N25.89
  radiation N04.9

Nephrosis, nephrotic *(Continued)*
  syphilitic (late) A52.75
  toxic —*see* Nephrosis, tubular
  tubular (acute) N17.0
    postprocedural N99.0
    radiation N04.9
Nephrosonephritis, hemorrhagic (endemic) A98.5
Nephrostomy
  attention to Z43.6
  status Z93.6
Nerve —*see also* condition
  injury —*see* Injury, nerve, by body site
Nerves R45.0
Nervous *(see also* condition) R45.0
  heart F45.8
  stomach F45.8
  tension R45.0
Nervousness R45.0
Nesidioblastoma
  pancreas D13.7
  specified site NEC —*see* Neoplasm, benign, by site
  unspecified site D13.7
Nettleship's syndrome Q82.2
Neumann's disease or syndrome L10.1
Neuralgia, neuralgic (acute) M79.2
  accessory (nerve) G52.8
  acoustic (nerve) —*see* subcategory H93.3
  auditory (nerve) —*see* subcategory H93.3
  ciliary G44.009
    intractable G44.001
    not intractable G44.009
  cranial
    nerve —*see also* Disorder, nerve, cranial
      fifth or trigeminal —*see* Neuralgia, trigeminal
    postherpetic, postzoster B02.29
  ear —*see* subcategory H92.0
  facialis vera G51.1
  Fothergill's —*see* Neuralgia, trigeminal
  glossopharyngeal (nerve) G52.1
  Horton's G44.099
    intractable G44.091
    not intractable G44.099
  Hunt's B02.21
  hypoglossal (nerve) G52.3
  infraorbital —*see* Neuralgia, trigeminal
  malarial —*see* Malaria
  migrainous G44.009
    intractable G44.001
    not intractable G44.009
  Morton's G57.6-
  nerve, cranial —*see* Disorder, nerve, cranial
  nose G52.0
  occipital M54.81
  olfactory G52.0
  penis N48.9
  perineum R10.2
  postherpetic NEC B02.29
    trigeminal B02.22
  pubic region R10.2
  scrotum R10.2
  Sluder's G44.89
  specified nerve NEC G58.8
  spermatic cord R10.2
  sphenopalatine (ganglion) G90.09
  trifacial —*see* Neuralgia, trigeminal
  trigeminal G50.0
    postherpetic, postzoster B02.22
  vagus (nerve) G52.2
  writer's F48.8
    organic G25.89
Neurapraxia —*see* Injury, nerve
Neurasthenia F48.8
  cardiac F45.8
  gastric F45.8
  heart F45.8

Neurilemmoma —*see also* Neoplasm, nerve, benign
  acoustic (nerve) D33.3
  malignant —*see also* Neoplasm, nerve, malignant
    acoustic (nerve) C72.4
Neurilemmosarcoma —*see* Neoplasm, nerve, malignant
Neurinoma —*see* Neoplasm, nerve, benign
Neurinomatosis —*see* Neoplasm, nerve, uncertain behavior
Neuritis (rheumatoid) M79.2
  abducens (nerve) —*see* Strabismus, paralytic, sixth nerve
  accessory (nerve) G52.8
  acoustic (nerve) (*see also* subcategory) H93.3
    in (due to)
      infectious disease NEC B99 [H94.0-]
      parasitic disease NEC B89 [H94.0-]
    syphilitic A52.15
  alcoholic G62.1
    with psychosis —*see* Psychosis, alcoholic
  amyloid, any site E85.4 [G63]
  auditory (nerve) —*see* subcategory H93.3
  brachial —*see* Radiculopathy
    due to displacement, intervertebral disc —*see* Disorder, disc, cervical, with neuritis
  cranial nerve
    due to Lyme disease A69.22
    eighth or acoustic or auditory —*see* subcategory H93.3
    eleventh or accessory G52.8
    fifth or trigeminal G51.0
    first or olfactory G52.0
    fourth or trochlear —*see* Strabismus, paralytic, fourth nerve
    second or optic —*see* Neuritis, optic
    seventh or facial G51.8
      newborn (birth injury) P11.3
    sixth or abducent —*see* Strabismus, paralytic, sixth nerve
    tenth or vagus G52.2
    third or oculomotor —*see* Strabismus, paralytic, third nerve
    twelfth or hypoglossal G52.3
  Déjérine-Sottas G60.0
  diabetic (mononeuropathy) —*see* E08-E13 with .41
    polyneuropathy —*see* E08-E13 with .42
  due to
    beriberi E51.11
    displacement, prolapse or rupture, intervertebral disc —*see* Disorder, disc, with, radiculopathy
    herniation, nucleus pulposus M51.9 [G55]
  endemic E51.11
  facial G51.8
    newborn (birth injury) P11.3
  general —*see* Polyneuropathy
  geniculate ganglion G51.1
    due to herpes (zoster) B02.21
  gouty M10.00 [G63]
  hypoglossal (nerve) G52.3
  ilioinguinal (nerve) G57.9-
  infectious (multiple) NEC G61.0
  interstitial hypertrophic progressive G60.0
  lumbar M54.16
  lumbosacral M54.17
  multiple —*see also* Polyneuropathy
    endemic E51.11
    infective, acute G61.0
  multiplex endemica E51.11
  nerve root —*see* Radiculopathy
  oculomotor (nerve) —*see* Strabismus, paralytic, third nerve
  olfactory nerve G52.0
  optic (nerve) (hereditary) (sympathetic) H46.9
    with demyelination G36.0
    in myelitis G36.0
    nutritional H46.2

Neuritis (Continued)
  optic (Continued)
    papillitis —*see* Papillitis, optic
    retrobulbar H46.1-
    specified type NEC H46.8
    toxic H46.3
  peripheral (nerve) G62.9
    multiple —*see* Polyneuropathy
    single —*see* Mononeuritis
  pneumogastric (nerve) G52.2
  postherpetic, postzoster B02.29
  progressive hypertrophic interstitial G60.0
  retrobulbar —*see also* Neuritis, optic, retrobulbar
    in (due to)
      late syphilis A52.15
      meningococcal infection A39.82
    meningococcal A39.82
    syphilitic A52.15
  sciatic (nerve) —*see also* Sciatica
    due to displacement of intervertebral disc —*see* Disorder, disc, with, radiculopathy
  serum (*see also* Reaction, serum) T80.69
  shoulder-girdle G54.5
  specified nerve NEC G58.8
  spinal (nerve) root —*see* Radiculopathy
  syphilitic A52.15
  thenar (median) G56.1-
  thoracic M54.14
  toxic NEC G62.2
  trochlear (nerve) —*see* Strabismus, paralytic, fourth nerve
  vagus (nerve) G52.2
Neuroastrocytoma —*see* Neoplasm, uncertain behavior, by site
Neuroavitaminosis E56.9 [G99.8]
Neuroblastoma
  olfactory C30.0
  specified site —*see* Neoplasm, malignant, by site
  unspecified site C74.90
Neurochorioretinitis —*see* Chorioretinitis
Neurocirculatory asthenia F45.8
Neurocysticercosis B69.0
Neurocytoma —*see* Neoplasm, benign, by site
Neurodermatitis (circumscribed) (circumscripta) (local) L28.0
  atopic L20.81
  diffuse (Brocq) L20.81
  disseminated L20.81
Neuroencephalomyelopathy, optic G36.0
Neuroepithelioma —*see also* Neoplasm, malignant, by site
  olfactory C30.0
Neurofibroma —*see also* Neoplasm, nerve, benign
  melanotic —*see* Neoplasm, nerve, benign
  multiple —*see* Neurofibromatosis
  plexiform —*see* Neoplasm, nerve, benign
Neurofibromatosis (multiple) (nonmalignant) Q85.00
  acoustic Q85.02
  malignant —*see* Neoplasm, nerve, malignant
  specified NEC Q85.09
  type 1 (von Recklinghausen) Q85.01
  type 2 Q85.02
Neurofibrosarcoma —*see* Neoplasm, nerve, malignant
Neurogenic —*see also* condition
  bladder (*see also* Dysfunction, bladder, neuromuscular) N31.9
    cauda equina syndrome G83.4
  bowel NEC K59.2
  heart F45.8
Neuroglioma —*see* Neoplasm, uncertain behavior, by site
Neurolabyrinthitis (of Dix and Hallpike) —*see* Neuronitis, vestibular
Neurolathyrism —*see* Poisoning, food, noxious, plant

Neuroleprosy A30.9
Neuroma —*see also* Neoplasm, nerve, benign
  acoustic (nerve) D33.3
  amputation (stump) (traumatic) (surgical complication) (late) T87.3-
    arm T87.3-
    leg T87.3-
  digital (toe) G57.6-
  interdigital (toe) G58.8
    lower limb G57.8-
    upper limb G56.8-
  intermetatarsal G57.8-
  Morton's G57.6-
  nonneoplastic
    arm G56.9-
    leg G57.9-
    lower extremity G57.9-
    upper extremity G56.9-
  optic (nerve) D33.3
  plantar G57.6-
  plexiform —*see* Neoplasm, nerve, benign
  surgical (nonneoplastic)
    arm G56.9-
    leg G57.9-
    lower extremity G57.9-
    upper extremity G56.9-
Neuromyalgia —*see* Neuralgia
Neuromyasthenia (epidemic) (postinfectious) G93.3
Neuromyelitis G36.9
  ascending G61.0
  optica G36.0
Neuromyopathy G70.9
  paraneoplastic D49.9 [G13.0]
Neuromyotonia (Isaacs) G71.19
Neuronevus —*see* Nevus
Neuronitis G58.9
  ascending (acute) G57.2-
  vestibular H81.2-
Neuroparalytic —*see* condition
Neuropathy, neuropathic G62.9
  acute motor G62.81
  alcoholic G62.1
    with psychosis —*see* Psychosis, alcoholic
  arm G56.9-
  autonomic, peripheral —*see* Neuropathy, peripheral, autonomic
  axillary G56.9-
  bladder N31.9
    atonic (motor) (sensory) N31.2
    autonomous N31.2
    flaccid N31.2
    nonreflex N31.2
    reflex N31.1
    uninhibited N31.0
  brachial plexus G54.0
  cervical plexus G54.2
  chronic
    progressive segmentally demyelinating G62.89
    relapsing demyelinating G62.89
  Déjérine-Sottas G60.0
  diabetic —*see* E08-E13 with .40
    mononeuropathy —*see* E08-E13 with .41
    polyneuropathy —*see* E08-E13 with .42
  entrapment G58.9
    iliohypogastric nerve G57.8-
    ilioinguinal nerve G57.8-
    lateral cutaneous nerve of thigh G57.1-
    median nerve G56.0-
    obturator nerve G57.8-
    peroneal nerve G57.3-
    posterior tibial nerve G57.5-
    saphenous nerve G57.8-
    ulnar nerve G56.2-
  facial nerve G51.9
  hereditary G60.9
    motor and sensory (types I-IV) G60.0
    sensory G60.8
    specified NEC G60.8

Neuropathy, neuropathic *(Continued)*
hypertrophic G60.0
  Charcot-Marie-Tooth G60.0
  Déjérine-Sottas G60.0
  interstitial progressive G60.0
  of infancy G60.0
  Refsum G60.1
idiopathic G60.9
  progressive G60.3
  specified NEC G60.8
in association with hereditary ataxia G60.2
intercostal G58.0
ischemic —*see* Disorder, nerve
Jamaica (ginger) G62.2
leg NEC G57.9-
lower extremity G57.9-
lumbar plexus G54.1
median nerve G56.1-
motor and sensory —*see also* Polyneuropathy
  hereditary (types I-IV) G60.0
multiple (acute) (chronic) —*see*
  Polyneuropathy
optic (nerve) —*see also* Neuritis, optic
  ischemic H47.01-
paraneoplastic (sensorial) (Denny Brown)
  D49.9 *[G13.0]*
peripheral (nerve) *(see also* Polyneuropathy)
  G62.9
  autonomic G90.9
    idiopathic G90.09
    in (due to)
      amyloidosis E85.4 *[G99.0]*
      diabetes mellitus —*see* E08-E13 with
        .43
      endocrine disease NEC E34.9 *[G99.0]*
      gout M10.00 *[G99.0]*
      hyperthyroidism E05.90 *[G99.0]*
        with thyroid storm E05.91 *[G99.0]*
      metabolic disease NEC E88.9 *[G99.0]*
  idiopathic G60.9
    progressive G60.3
  in (due to)
    antitetanus serum G62.0
    arsenic G62.2
    drugs NEC G62.0
    lead G62.2
    organophosphate compounds G62.2
    toxic agent NEC G62.2
plantar nerves G57.6-
progressive
  hypertrophic interstitial G60.0
  inflammatory G62.81
radicular NEC —*see* Radiculopathy
sacral plexus G54.1
sciatic G57.0-
serum G61.1
toxic NEC G62.2
trigeminal sensory G50.8
ulnar nerve G56.2-
uremic N18.9 *[G63]*
vitamin B12 E53.8 *[G63]*
  with anemia (pernicious) D51.0 *[G63]*
    due to dietary deficiency D51.3 *[G63]*
Neurophthisis —*see also* Disorder, nerve
peripheral, diabetic —*see* E08-E13 with .42
Neuroretinitis —*see* Chorioretinitis
Neuroretinopathy, hereditary optic H47.22
Neurosarcoma —*see* Neoplasm, nerve,
  malignant
Neurosclerosis —*see* Disorder, nerve
Neurosis, neurotic F48.9
anankastic F42
anxiety (state) F41.1
  panic type F41.0
asthenic F48.8
bladder F45.8
cardiac (reflex) F45.8
cardiovascular F45.8
character F60.9
colon F45.8
compensation F68.1

Neurosis, neurotic *(Continued)*
compulsive, compulsion F42
conversion F44.9
craft F48.8
cutaneous F45.8
depersonalization F48.1
depressive (reaction) (type) F34.1
environmental F48.8
excoriation L98.1
fatigue F48.8
functional —*see* Disorder, somatoform
gastric F45.8
gastrointestinal F45.8
heart F45.8
hypochondriacal F45.21
hysterical F44.9
incoordination F45.8
  larynx F45.8
  vocal cord F45.8
intestine F45.8
larynx (sensory) F45.8
  hysterical F44.4
mixed NEC F48.8
musculoskeletal F45.8
obsessional F42
obsessive-compulsive F42
occupational F48.8
ocular NEC F45.8
organ —*see* Disorder, somatoform
pharynx F45.8
phobic F40.9
posttraumatic (situational) F43.10
  acute F43.11
  chronic F43.12
psychasthenic (type) F48.8
railroad F48.8
rectum F45.8
respiratory F45.8
rumination F45.8
sexual F65.9
situational F48.8
social F40.10
  generalized F40.11
specified type NEC F48.8
state F48.9
  with depersonalization episode F48.1
stomach F45.8
traumatic F43.10
  acute F43.11
  chronic F43.12
vasomotor F45.8
visceral F45.8
war F48.8
Neurospongioblastosis diffusa Q85.1
Neurosyphilis (arrested) (early) (gumma) (late)
  (latent) (recurrent) (relapse) A52.3
with ataxia (cerebellar) (locomotor) (spastic)
  (spinal) A52.19
aneurysm (cerebral) A52.05
arachnoid (adhesive) A52.13
arteritis (any artery) (cerebral) A52.04
asymptomatic A52.2
congenital A50.40
dura (mater) A52.13
general paresis A52.17
hemorrhagic A52.05
juvenile (asymptomatic) (meningeal)
  A50.40
leptomeninges (aseptic) A52.13
meningeal, meninges (adhesive) A52.13
meningitis A52.13
meningovascular (diffuse) A52.13
optic atrophy A52.15
parenchymatous (degenerative) A52.19
paresis, paretic A52.17
  juvenile A50.45
remission in (sustained) A52.3
serological (without symptoms) A52.2
specified nature or site NEC A52.19
tabes, tabetic (dorsalis) A52.11
  juvenile A50.45

Neurosyphilis *(Continued)*
taboparesis A52.17
  juvenile A50.45
thrombosis (cerebral) A52.05
vascular (cerebral) NEC A52.05
Neurothekeoma —*see* Neoplasm, nerve, benign
Neurotic —*see* Neurosis
Neurotoxemia —*see* Toxemia
Neutroclusion M26.211
Neutropenia, neutropenic (chronic) (genetic)
  (idiopathic) (immune) (infantile)
  (malignant) (pernicious) (splenic) D70.9
congenital (primary) D70.0
cyclic D70.4
cytoreductive cancer chemotherapy sequela
  D70.1
drug-induced D70.2
  due to cytoreductive cancer chemotherapy
    D70.1
due to infection D70.3
fever D70.9
neonatal, transitory (isoimmune) (maternal
  transfer) P61.5
periodic D70.4
secondary (cyclic) (periodic) (splenic) D70.4
  drug-induced D70.2
    due to cytoreductive cancer
      chemotherapy D70.1
toxic D70.8
Neutrophilia, hereditary giant D72.0
Nevocarcinoma —*see* Melanoma
Nevus D22.9
achromic —*see* Neoplasm, skin, benign
amelanotic —*see* Neoplasm, skin, benign
angiomatous D18.00
  intra-abdominal D18.03
  intracranial D18.02
  skin D18.01
  specified site NEC D18.09
araneus I78.1
balloon cell —*see* Neoplasm, skin, benign
bathing trunk D48.5
blue —*see* Neoplasm, skin, benign
  cellular —*see* Neoplasm, skin, benign
  giant —*see* Neoplasm, skin, benign
  Jadassohn's —*see* Neoplasm, skin, benign
  malignant —*see* Melanoma
capillary D18.00
  intra-abdominal D18.03
  intracranial D18.02
  skin D18.01
  specified site NEC D18.09
cavernous D18.00
  intra-abdominal D18.03
  intracranial D18.02
  skin D18.01
  specified site NEC D18.09
cellular —*see* Neoplasm, skin, benign
  blue —*see* Neoplasm, skin, benign
choroid D31.3-
comedonicus Q82.5
conjunctiva D31.0-
dermal —*see* Neoplasm, skin, benign
  with epidermal nevus —*see* Neoplasm,
    skin, benign
dysplastic —*see* Neoplasm, skin, benign
eye D31.9-
flammeus Q82.5
hemangiomatous D18.00
  intra-abdominal D18.03
  intracranial D18.02
  skin D18.01
  specified site NEC D18.09
iris D31.4-
lacrimal gland D31.5-
lymphatic D18.1
magnocellular
  specified site —*see* Neoplasm, benign, by
    site
  unspecified site D31.40
malignant —*see* Melanoma

Nevus *(Continued)*
  meaning hemangioma D18.00
    intra-abdominal D18.03
    intracranial D18.02
    skin D18.01
    specified site NEC D18.09
  mouth (mucosa) D10.30
    specified site NEC D10.39
    white sponge Q38.6
  multiplex Q85.1
  non-neoplastic I78.1
  oral mucosa D10.30
    specified site NEC D10.39
    white sponge Q38.6
  orbit D31.6-
  pigmented
    giant *(see also* Neoplasm, skin, uncertain
      behavior) D48.5
      malignant melanoma in —*see* Melanoma
  portwine Q82.5
  retina D31.2-
  retrobulbar D31.6-
  sanguineous Q82.5
  senile I78.1
  skin D22.9
    abdominal wall D22.5
    ala nasi D22.39
    ankle D22.7-
    anus, anal D22.5
    arm D22.6-
    auditory canal (external) D22.2-
    auricle (ear) D22.2-
    auricular canal (external) D22.2-
    axilla, axillary fold D22.5
    back D22.5
    breast D22.5
    brow D22.39
    buttock D22.5
    canthus (eye) D22.1-
    cheek (external) D22.39
    chest wall D22.5
    chin D22.39
    ear (external) D22.2-
    external meatus (ear) D22.2-
    eyebrow D22.39
    eyelid (lower) (upper) D22.1-
    face D22.30
      specified NEC D22.39
    female genital organ (external) NEC
      D28.0
    finger D22.6-
    flank D22.5
    foot D22.7-
    forearm D22.6-
    forehead D22.39
    foreskin D29.0
    genital organ (external) NEC
      female D28.0
      male D29.9
    gluteal region D22.5
    groin D22.5
    hand D22.6-
    heel D22.7-
    helix D22.2-
    hip D22.7-
    interscapular region D22.5
    jaw D22.39
    knee D22.7-
    labium (majus) (minus) D28.0
    leg D22.7-
    lip (lower) (upper) D22.0
    lower limb D22.7-
    male genital organ (external) D29.9
    nail D22.9
      finger D22.6-
      toe D22.7-
    nasolabial groove D22.39
    nates D22.5
    neck D22.4
    nose (external) D22.39
    palpebra D22.1-

Nevus *(Continued)*
  skin *(Continued)*
    penis D29.0
    perianal skin D22.5
    perineum D22.5
    pinna D22.2-
    popliteal fossa or space D22.7-
    prepuce D29.0
    pudendum D28.0
    scalp D22.4
    scrotum D29.4
    shoulder D22.6-
    submammary fold D22.5
    temple D22.39
    thigh D22.7-
    toe D22.7-
    trunk NEC D22.5
    umbilicus D22.5
    upper limb D22.6-
    vulva D28.0
  specified site NEC —*see* Neoplasm, benign,
    by site
  spider I78.1
  stellar I78.1
  strawberry Q82.5
  Sutton's —*see* Neoplasm, skin, benign
  unius lateris Q82.5
  Unna's Q82.5
  vascular Q82.5
  verrucous Q82.5
Newborn (infant) (liveborn) (singleton)
  Z38.2
  abstinence syndrome P96.1
  acne L70.4
  affected by (suspected to be)
    abnormalities of membranes P02.9
      specified NEC P02.8
    abruptio placenta P02.1
    amino-acid metabolic disorder, transitory
      P74.8
    amniocentesis (while in utero) P00.6
    amnionitis P02.7
    apparent life threatening event (ALTE)
      R68.13
    bleeding (into)
      cerebral cortex P52.22
      germinal matrix P52.0
      ventricles P52.1
    breech delivery P03.0
    cardiac arrest P29.81
    cardiomyopathy I42.8
      congenital I42.4
    cerebral ischemia P91.0
    Cesarean delivery P03.4
    chemotherapy agents P04.1
    chorioamnionitis P02.7
    cocaine (crack) P04.41
    complications of labor and delivery
      P03.9
      specified NEC P03.89
    compression of umbilical cord NEC
      P02.5
    contracted pelvis P03.1
    delivery P03.9
      Cesarean P03.4
      forceps P03.2
      vacuum extractor P03.3
    entanglement (knot) in umbilical cord
      P02.5
    environmental chemicals P04.6
    fetal (intrauterine)
      growth retardation P05.9
      malnutrition not light or small for
        gestational age P05.2
    forceps delivery P03.2
    heart rate abnormalities
      bradycardia P29.12
      intrauterine P03.819
        before onset of labor P03.810
        during labor P03.811
      tachycardia P29.11

Newborn *(Continued)*
  affected by *(Continued)*
    hemorrhage (antepartum) P02.1
      cerebellar (nontraumatic) P52.6
      intracerebral (nontraumatic) P52.4
      intracranial (nontraumatic) P52.9
        specified NEC P52.8
      intraventricular (nontraumatic) P52.3
        grade 1 P52.0
        grade 2 P52.1
        grade 3 P52.21
        grade 4 P52.22
      posterior fossa (nontraumatic) P52.6
      subarachnoid (nontraumatic) P52.5
      subependymal P52.0
        with intracerebral extension P52.22
        with intraventricular extension P52.1
          with enlargment of ventricles
            P52.21
        without intraventricular extension
          P52.0
    hypoxic ischemic encephalopathy [HIE]
      P91.60
      mild P91.61
      moderate P91.62
      severe P91.63
    induction of labor P03.89
    intestinal perforation P78.0
    intrauterine (fetal) blood loss P50.9
      due to (from)
        cut end of co-twin cord P50.5
        hemorrhage into
          co-twin P50.3
          maternal circulation P50.4
        placenta P50.2
        ruptured cord blood P50.1
        vasa previa P50.0
      specified NEC P50.8
    intrauterine (fetal) hemorrhage P50.9
    intrauterine (in utero) procedure P96.5
    malpresentation (malposition) NEC P03.1
    maternal (complication of) (use of)
      alcohol P04.3
      analgesia (maternal) P04.0
      anesthesia (maternal) P04.0
      blood loss P02.1
      circulatory disease P00.3
      condition P00.9
        specified NEC P00.89
      delivery P03.9
        Cesarean P03.4
        forceps P03.2
        vacuum extractor P03.3
      diabetes mellitus (pre-existing) P70.1
      disorder P00.9
        specified NEC P00.89
      drugs (addictive) (illegal) NEC P04.49
      ectopic pregnancy P01.4
      gestational diabetes P70.0
      hemorrhage P02.1
      hypertensive disorder P00.0
      incompetent cervix P01.0
      infectious disease P00.2
      injury P00.5
      labor and delivery P03.9
      malpresentation before labor P01.7
      maternal death P01.6
      medical procedure P00.7
      medication P04.1
      multiple pregnancy P01.5
      nutritional disorder P00.4
      oligohydramnios P01.2
      parasitic disease P00.2
      periodontal disease P00.81
      placenta previa P02.0
      polyhydramnios P01.3
      precipitate delivery P03.5
      pregnancy P01.9
        specified P01.8
      premature rupture of membranes P01.1
      renal disease P00.1

Newborn *(Continued)*
  affected by *(Continued)*
    maternal *(Continued)*
      respiratory disease P00.3
      surgical procedure P00.6
      urinary tract disease P00.1
      uterine contraction (abnormal) P03.6
     meconium peritonitis P78.0
     medication (legal) (maternal use) (prescribed) P04.1
     membrane abnormalities P02.9
      specified NEC P02.8
     membranitis P02.7
     methamphetamine (s) P04.49
     mixed metabolic and respiratory acidosis P84
     neonatal abstinence syndrome P96.1
     noxious substances transmitted via placenta or breast milk P04.9
      specified NEC P04.8
     nutritional supplements P04.5
     placenta previa P02.0
     placental
      abnormality (functional) (morphological) P02.20
       specified NEC P02.29
      dysfunction P02.29
      infarction P02.29
      insufficiency P02.29
      separation NEC P02.1
      transfusion syndromes P02.3
     placentitis P02.7
     precipitate delivery P03.5
     prolapsed cord P02.4
     respiratory arrest P28.81
     slow intrauterine growth P05.9
     tobacco P04.2
     twin to twin transplacental transfusion P02.3
     umbilical cord (tightly) around neck P02.5
     umbilical cord condition P02.60
      short cord P02.69
      specified NEC P02.69
     uterine contractions (abnormal) P03.6
     vasa previa P02.69
      from intrauterine blood loss P50.0
  apnea P28.3
   obstructive P28.4
   primary P28.3
   specified P28.4
  born in hospital Z38.00
   by cesarean Z38.01
  born outside hospital Z38.1
  breast buds P96.89
  breast engorgement P83.4
  check-up —*see* Newborn, examination
  convulsion P90
  dehydration P74.1
  examination
   8 to 28 days old Z00.111
   under 8 days old Z00.110
  fever P81.9
   environmentally-induced P81.0
  hyperbilirubinemia P59.9
   of prematurity P59.0
  hypernatremia P74.2
  hyponatremia P74.2
  infection P39.9
   candidal P37.5
   specified NEC P39.8
   urinary tract P39.3
  jaundice P59.8
   due to
    breast milk inhibitor P59.3
    hepatocellular damage P59.20
     specified NEC P59.29
    preterm delivery P59.0
   of prematurity P59.0
   specified NEC P59.8
  late metabolic acidosis P74.0

Newborn *(Continued)*
  mastitis P39.0
   infective P39.0
   noninfective P83.4
  multiple born NEC Z38.8
   born in hospital Z38.68
    by cesarean Z38.69
   born outside hospital Z38.7
  omphalitis P38.9
   with mild hemorrhage P38.1
   without hemorrhage P38.9
  post-term P08.21
  prolonged gestation (over 42 completed weeks) P08.22
  quadruplet Z38.8
   born in hospital Z38.63
    by cesarean Z38.64
   born outside hospital Z38.7
  quintuplet Z38.8
   born in hospital Z38.65
    by cesarean Z38.66
   born outside hospital Z38.7
  seizure P90
  sepsis (congenital) P36.9
   due to
    anaerobes NEC P36.5
    Escherichia coli P36.4
    Staphylococcus P36.30
     aureus P36.2
     specified NEC P36.39
    Streptococcus P36.10
     group B P36.0
     specified NEC P36.19
   specified NEC P36.8
  triplet Z38.8
   born in hospital Z38.61
    by cesarean Z38.62
   born outside hospital Z38.7
  twin Z38.5
   born in hospital Z38.30
    by cesarean Z38.31
   born outside hospital Z38.4
  vomiting P92.09
   bilious P92.01
  weight check Z00.111
Newcastle conjunctivitis or disease B30.8
Nezelof's syndrome (pure alymphocytosis) D81.4
Niacin (amide) deficiency E52
Nicolas (-Durand)-Favre disease A55
Nicotine —*see* Tobacco
Nicotinic acid deficiency E52
Niemann-Pick disease or syndrome E75.249
  specified NEC E75.248
  type
   A E75.240
   B E75.241
   C E75.242
   D E75.243
Night
  blindness —*see* Blindness, night
  sweats R61
  terrors (child) F51.4
Nightmares (REM sleep type) F51.5
Nipple —*see* condition
Nisbet's chancre A57
Nishimoto (-Takeuchi) disease I67.5
Nitritoid crisis or reaction —*see* Crisis, nitritoid
Nitrosohemoglobinemia D74.8
Njovera A65
Nocardiosis, nocardiasis A43.9
  cutaneous A43.1
  lung A43.0
  pneumonia A43.0
  pulmonary A43.0
  specified site NEC A43.8
Nocturia R35.1
  psychogenic F45.8
Nocturnal —*see* condition
Nodal rhythm I49.8

Node (s) —*see also* Nodule
  Bouchard's (with arthropathy) M15.2
  Haygarth's M15.8
  Heberden's (with arthropathy) M15.1
  larynx J38.7
  lymph —*see* condition
  milker's B08.03
  Osler's I33.0
  Schmorl's —*see* Schmorl's disease
  singer's J38.2
  teacher's J38.2
  tuberculous —*see* Tuberculosis, lymph gland
  vocal cord J38.2
Nodule (s), nodular
  actinomycotic —*see* Actinomycosis
  breast NEC N63
  colloid (cystic), thyroid E04.1
  cutaneous —*see* Swelling, localized
  endometrial (stromal) D26.1
  Haygarth's M15.8
  inflammatory —*see* Inflammation
  juxta-articular
   syphilitic A52.77
   yaws A66.7
  larynx J38.7
  lung, solitary (subsegmental branch of the bronchial tree) R91.1
   multiple R91.8
  milker's B08.03
  prostate N40.2
   with lower urinary tract symptoms (LUTS) N40.3
   without lower urinary tract symptoms (LUTS) N40.2
  pulmonary, solitary (subsegmental branch of the bronchial tree) R91.1
  retrocardiac R09.89
  rheumatoid M06.30
   ankle M06.37-
   elbow M06.32-
   foot joint M06.37-
   hand joint M06.34-
   hip M06.35-
   knee M06.36-
   multiple site M06.39
   shoulder M06.31-
   vertebra M06.38
   wrist M06.33-
  scrotum (inflammatory) N49.2
  singer's J38.2
  solitary, lung (subsegmental branch of the bronchial tree) R91.1
   multiple R91.8
  subcutaneous —*see* Swelling, localized
  teacher's J38.2
  thyroid (cold) (gland) (nontoxic) E04.1
   with thyrotoxicosis E05.20
    with thyroid storm E05.21
   toxic or with hyperthyroidism E05.20
    with thyroid storm E05.21
  vocal cord J38.2
Noma (gangrenous) (hospital) (infective) A69.0
  auricle I96
  mouth A69.0
  pudendi N76.89
  vulvae N76.89
Nomad, nomadism Z59.0
Nonautoimmune hemolytic anemia D59.4
  drug-induced D59.2
Nonclosure —*see also* Imperfect, closure
  ductus arteriosus (Botallo's) Q25.0
  foramen
   botalli Q21.1
   ovale Q21.1
Noncompliance Z91.19
  with
   dialysis Z91.15
   dietary regimen Z91.11
   medical treatment

Noncompliance (Continued)
  with (Continued)
    medication regimen NEC Z91.14
      underdosing (see also Table of Drugs and
        Chemicals, categories T36-T50, with
        final character 6) Z91.14
        intentional NEC Z91.128
          due to financial hardship of patient
          Z91.120
        unintentional NEC Z91.138
          due to patient's age related debility
          Z91.130
    renal dialysis Z91.15
Nondescent (congenital) —see also Malposition,
  congenital
  cecum Q43.3
  colon Q43.3
  testicle Q53.9
    bilateral Q53.20
      abdominal Q53.21
      perineal Q53.22
    unilateral Q53.10
      abdominal Q53.11
      perineal Q53.12
Nondevelopment
  brain Q02
    part of Q04.3
  heart Q24.8
  organ or site, congenital NEC —see
    Hypoplasia
Nonengagement
  head NEC O32.4
    in labor, causing obstructed labor O64.8
Nonexanthematous tick fever A93.2
Nonexpansion, lung (newborn) P28.0
Nonfunctioning
  cystic duct (see also Disease, gallbladder)
    K82.8
  gallbladder (see also Disease, gallbladder)
    K82.8
  kidney N28.9
  labyrinth —see subcategory H83.2

Non-Hodgkin lymphoma NEC —see
  Lymphoma, non-Hodgkin
Nonimplantation, ovum N97.2
Noninsufflation, fallopian tube N97.1
Non-ketotic hyperglycinemia E72.51
Nonne-Milroy syndrome Q82.0
Nonovulation N97.0
Nonpatent fallopian tube N97.1
Nonpneumatization, lung NEC P28.0
Nonrotation —see Malrotation
Nonsecretion, urine —see Anuria
Nonunion
  fracture—see Fracture, by site
  organ or site, congenital NEC —see Imperfect,
    closure
  symphysis pubis, congenital Q74.2
Nonvisualization, gallbladder R93.2
Nonvital, nonvitalized tooth K04.99
Non-working side interference
  M26.56
Noonan's syndrome Q87.1
Normocytic anemia (infectional) due to blood
  loss (chronic) D50.0
  acute D62
Norrie's disease (congenital) Q15.8
North American blastomycosis B40.9
Norwegian itch B86
Nose, nasal —see condition
Nosebleed R04.0
Nose-picking F98.8
Nosomania F45.21
Nosophobia F45.22
Nostalgia F43.20
Notch of iris Q13.2
Notching nose, congenital (tip) Q30.2
Nothnagel's
  syndrome —see Strabismus, paralytic, third
    nerve
  vasomotor acroparesthesia I73.89
Novy's relapsing fever A68.9
  louse-borne A68.0
  tick-borne A68.1

Noxious
  foodstuffs, poisoning by —see Poisoning,
    food, noxious, plant
  substances transmitted through placenta or
    breast milk P04.9
Nucleus pulposus —see condition
Numbness R20.0
Nuns' knee —see Bursitis, prepatellar
Nursemaid's elbow S53.03-
Nutcracker esophagus K22.4
Nutmeg liver K76.1
Nutrient element deficiency E61.9
  specified NEC E61.8
Nutrition deficient or insufficient (see also
  Malnutrition) E46
  due to
    insufficient food T73.0
    lack of
      care (child) T76.02
        adult T76.01
      food T73.0
Nutritional stunting E45
Nyctalopia (night blindness) —see Blindness,
  night
Nycturia R35.1
  psychogenic F45.8
Nymphomania F52.8
Nystagmus H55.00
  benign paroxysmal —see Vertigo, benign
    paroxysmal
  central positional H81.4-
  congenital H55.01
  dissociated H55.04
  latent H55.02
  miners' H55.09
  positional
    benign paroxysmal H81.4-
    central H81.4-
  specified form NEC H55.09
  visual deprivation H55.03

O

Obermeyer's relapsing fever (European) A68.0
Obesity E66.9
  with alveolar hyperventilation E66.2
  adrenal E27.8
  complicating
    childbirth O99.214
    pregnancy O99.21-
    puerperium O99.215
  constitutional E66.8
  dietary counseling and surveillance Z71.3
  drug-induced E66.1
  due to
    drug E66.1
    excess calories E66.09
      morbid E66.01
      severe E66.01
  endocrine E66.8
  endogenous E66.8
  familial E66.8
  glandular E66.8
  hypothyroid —see Hypothyroidism
  morbid E66.01
    with alveolar hypoventilation E66.2
    due to excess calories E66.01
  nutritional E66.09
  pituitary E23.6
  severe E66.01
  specified type NEC E66.8
Oblique —see condition
Obliteration
  appendix (lumen) K38.8
  artery I77.1
  bile duct (noncalculous) K83.1
  common duct (noncalculous) K83.1
  cystic duct —see Obstruction, gallbladder
  disease, arteriolar I77.1
  endometrium N85.8
  eye, anterior chamber —see Disorder, globe, hypotony
  fallopian tube N97.1
  lymphatic vessel I89.0
    due to mastectomy I97.2
  organ or site, congenital NEC —see Atresia, by site
  ureter N13.5
    with infection N13.6
  urethra —see Stricture, urethra
  vein I87.8
  vestibule (oral) K08.8
Observation (following) (for) (without need for further medical care) Z04.9
  accident NEC Z04.3
    at work Z04.2
    transport Z04.1
  adverse effect of drug Z03.6
  alleged rape or sexual assault (victim), ruled out
    adult Z04.41
    child Z04.42
  criminal assault Z04.8
  development state
    adolescent Z00.3
    period of rapid growth in childhood Z00.2
    puberty Z00.3
  disease, specified NEC Z03.89
  following work accident Z04.2
  growth and development state —see Observation, development state
  injuries (accidental) NEC —see also Observation, accident
  newborn (for suspected condition, ruled out) —see Newborn, affected by (suspected to be), maternal (complication of) (use of)
  postpartum
    immediately after delivery Z39.0
    routine follow-up Z39.2

Observation (Continued)
  pregnancy (normal) (without complication) Z34.9-
    high risk O09.9-
  suicide attempt, alleged NEC Z03.89
    self-poisoning Z03.6
  suspected, ruled out —see also Suspected condition, ruled out
    abuse, physical
      adult Z04.71
      child Z04.72
    accident at work Z04.2
    adult battering victim Z04.71
    child battering victim Z04.72
    condition NEC Z03.89
      newborn —see Newborn, affected by (suspected to be), maternal (complication of) (use of)
    drug poisoning or adverse effect Z03.6
    exposure (to)
      anthrax Z03.810
      biological agent NEC Z03.818
    inflicted injury NEC Z04.8
    suicide attempt, alleged Z03.89
      self-poisoning Z03.6
    toxic effects from ingested substance (drug) (poison) Z03.6
  toxic effects from ingested substance (drug) (poison) Z03.6
Obsession, obsessional state F42
Obsessive-compulsive neurosis or reaction F42
Obstetric embolism, septic —see Embolism, obstetric, septic
Obstetrical trauma (complicating delivery) O71.9
  with or following ectopic or molar pregnancy O08.6
  specified type NEC O71.89
Obstipation —see Constipation
Obstruction, obstructed, obstructive
  airway J98.8
    with
      allergic alveolitis J67.9
      asthma J45.909
        with
          exacerbation (acute) J45.901
          status asthmaticus J45.902
      bronchiectasis J47.9
        with
          exacerbation (acute) J47.1
          lower respiratory infection J47.0
      bronchitis (chronic) J44.9
      emphysema J43.9
    chronic J44.9
      with
        allergic alveolitis —see Pneumonitis, hypersensitivity
        bronchiectasis J47.9
          with
            exacerbation (acute) J47.1
            lower respiratory infection J47.0
    due to
      foreign body —see Foreign body, by site, causing asphyxia
      inhalation of fumes or vapors J68.9
      laryngospasm J38.5
  ampulla of Vater K83.1
  aortic (heart) (valve) —see Stenosis, aortic
  aortoiliac I74.09
  aqueduct of Sylvius G91.1
    congenital Q03.0
      with spina bifida —see Spina bifida, by site, with hydrocephalus
  Arnold-Chiari —see Arnold-Chiari disease
  artery (see also Embolism, artery) I74.9
    basilar (complete) (partial) —see Occlusion, artery, basilar
    carotid (complete) (partial) —see Occlusion, artery, carotid
    cerebellar —see Occlusion, artery, cerebellar

Obstruction, obstructed, obstructive (Continued)
  artery (Continued)
    cerebral (anterior) (middle) (posterior) — see Occlusion, artery, cerebral
    precerebral —see Occlusion, artery, precerebral
    renal N28.0
    retinal NEC —see Occlusion, artery, retina
    vertebral (complete) (partial) —see Occlusion, artery, vertebral
  band (intestinal) K56.69
  bile duct or passage (common) (hepatic) (noncalculous) K83.1
    with calculus K80.51
    congenital (causing jaundice) Q44.3
  biliary (duct) (tract) K83.1
    gallbladder K82.0
  bladder-neck (acquired) N32.0
    congenital Q64.31
    due to hyperplasia (hypertrophy) of prostate —see Hyperplasia, prostate
  bowel —see Obstruction, intestine
  bronchus J98.09
  canal, ear —see Stenosis, external ear canal
  cardia K22.2
  caval veins (inferior) (superior) I87.1
  cecum —see Obstruction, intestine
  circulatory I99.8
  colon —see Obstruction, intestine
  common duct (noncalculous) K83.1
  coronary (artery) —see Occlusion, coronary
  cystic duct —see also Obstruction, gallbladder
    with calculus K80.21
  device, implant or graft (see also Complications, by site and type, mechanical) T85.698
    arterial graft NEC —see Complication, cardiovascular device, mechanical, vascular
    catheter NEC T85.628
      cystostomy T83.090
      dialysis (renal) T82.49
        intraperitoneal T85.691
      infusion NEC T82.594
        spinal (epidural) (subdural) T85.690
      urinary, indwelling T83.098
    due to infection T85.79
    gastrointestinal —see Complications, prosthetic device, mechanical, gastrointestinal device
    genital NEC T83.498
      intrauterine contraceptive device T83.39
      penile prosthesis T83.490
    heart NEC —see Complication, cardiovascular device, mechanical
    joint prosthesis —see Complications, joint prosthesis, mechanical, specified NEC, by site
    orthopedic NEC —see Complication, orthopedic, device, mechanical
    specified NEC T85.628
    urinary NEC —see also Complication, genitourinary, device, urinary, mechanical
      graft T83.29
    vascular NEC —see Complication, cardiovascular device, mechanical
    ventricular intracranial shunt T85.09
  due to foreign body accidentally left in operative wound T81.529
  duodenum K31.5
  ejaculatory duct N50.8
  esophagus K22.2
  eustachian tube (complete) (partial) H68.10-
    cartilagenous (extrinsic) H68.13-
      intrinsic H68.12-
    osseous H68.11-
  fallopian tube (bilateral) N97.1

Obstruction, obstructed, obstructive
   (Continued)
  fecal K56.41
    with hernia —*see* Hernia, by site, with
      obstruction
  foramen of Monro (congenital) Q03.8
    with spina bifida —*see* Spina bifida,
      by site, with hydrocephalus
  foreign body —*see* Foreign body
  gallbladder K82.0
    with calculus, stones K80.21
    congenital Q44.1
  gastric outlet K31.1
  gastrointestinal —*see* Obstruction, intestine
  hepatic K76.89
    duct (noncalculous) K83.1
  hepatobiliary K83.1
  ileum —*see* Obstruction, intestine
  iliofemoral (artery) I74.5
  intestine K56.60
    with
      adhesions (intestinal) (peritoneal)
        K56.5
    adynamic K56.0
    by gallstone K56.3
    congenital (small) Q41.9
      large Q42.9
        specified part NEC Q42.8
    neurogenic K56.0
      Hirschsprung's disease or megacolon
        Q43.1
    newborn P76.9
      due to
        fecaliths P76.8
        inspissated milk P76.2
        meconium (plug) P76.0
          in mucoviscidosis E84.11
        specified NEC P76.8
    postoperative K91.3
    reflex K56.0
    specified NEC K56.69
    volvulus K56.2
  intracardiac ball valve prosthesis T82.09
  jejunum —*see* Obstruction, intestine
  joint prosthesis —*see* Complications, joint
    prosthesis, mechanical, specified NEC,
    by site
  kidney (calices) N28.89
  labor —*see* Delivery
  lacrimal (passages) (duct)
    by
      dacryolith —*see* Dacryolith
      stenosis —*see* Stenosis, lacrimal
    congenital Q10.5
    neonatal H04.53-
  lacrimonasal duct —*see* Obstruction,
    lacrimal
  lacteal, with steatorrhea K90.2
  laryngitis —*see* Laryngitis
  larynx NEC J38.6
    congenital Q31.8
  lung J98.4
    disease, chronic J44.9
  lymphatic I89.0
  meconium (plug)
    newborn P76.0
      due to fecaliths P76.0
      in mucoviscidosis E84.11
  mitral —*see* Stenosis, mitral
  nasal J34.89
  nasolacrimal duct —*see also* Obstruction,
    lacrimal
    congenital Q10.5
  nasopharynx J39.2
  nose J34.89
  organ or site, congenital NEC —*see* Atresia,
    by site
  pancreatic duct K86.8
  parotid duct or gland K11.8
  pelviureteral junction N13.5
    congenital Q62.39

Obstruction, obstructed, obstructive
   (Continued)
  pharynx J39.2
  portal (circulation) (vein) I81
  prostate —*see also* Hyperplasia, prostate
    valve (urinary) N32.0
  pulmonary valve (heart) I37.0
  pyelonephritis (chronic) N11.1
  pylorus
    adult K31.1
    congenital or infantile Q40.0
  rectosigmoid —*see* Obstruction,
    intestine
  rectum K62.4
  renal N28.89
    outflow N13.8
    pelvis, congenital Q62.39
  respiratory J98.8
    chronic J44.9
  retinal (vessels) H34.9
  salivary duct (any) K11.8
    with calculus K11.5
  sigmoid —*see* Obstruction, intestine
  sinus (accessory) (nasal) J34.89
  Stensen's duct K11.8
  stomach NEC K31.89
    acute K31.0
    congenital Q40.2
    due to pylorospasm K31.3
  submandibular duct K11.8
  submaxillary gland K11.8
    with calculus K11.5
  thoracic duct I89.0
  thrombotic —*see* Thrombosis
  trachea J39.8
  tracheostomy airway J95.03
  tricuspid (valve) —*see* Stenosis,
    tricuspid
  upper respiratory, congenital Q34.8
  ureter (functional) (pelvic junction) NEC
    N13.5
    with
      hydronephrosis N13.1
        with infection N13.6
      pyelonephritis (chronic) N11.1
    congenital Q62.39
    due to calculus —*see* Calculus, ureter
  urethra NEC N36.8
    congenital Q64.39
  urinary (moderate) N13.9
    due to hyperplasia (hypertrophy) of
      prostate —*see* Hyperplasia,
      prostate
    organ or tract (lower) N13.9
    prostatic valve N32.0
    specified NEC N13.8
  uropathy N13.9
  uterus N85.8
  vagina N89.5
  valvular —*see* Endocarditis
  vein, venous I87.1
    caval (inferior) (superior) I87.1
    thrombotic —*see* Thrombosis
  vena cava (inferior) (superior) I87.1
  vesical NEC N32.0
  vesicourethral orifice N32.0
    congenital Q64.31
  vessel NEC I99.8
Obturator —*see* condition
Occlusal wear, teeth K03.0
Occlusio pupillae —*see* Membrane,
  pupillary
Occlusion, occluded
  anus K62.4
    congenital Q42.3
      with fistula Q42.2
  aortoiliac (chronic) I74.09
  aqueduct of Sylvius G91.1
    congenital Q03.0
      with spina bifida —*see* Spina bifida, by
      site, with hydrocephalus

Occlusion, occluded *(Continued)*
  artery (*see also* Embolism, artery) I74.9
    auditory, internal I65.8
    basilar I65.1
      with
        infarction I63.22
          due to
            embolism I63.12
            thrombosis I63.02
    brain or cerebral I66.9
      with infarction (due to) I63.5
        embolism I63.4
        thrombosis I63.3
    carotid I65.2-
      with
        infarction I63.23-
          due to
            embolism I63.13-
            thrombosis I63.03-
    cerebellar (anterior inferior) (posterior
      inferior) (superior) I66.3
      with infarction I63.54-
        due to
          embolism I63.44-
          thrombosis I63.34-
    cerebral I66.9
      with infarction I63.50
        due to
          embolism I63.40
            specified NEC I63.49
          thrombosis I63.30
            specified NEC I63.39
      anterior I66.1-
        with infarction I63.52-
          due to
            embolism I63.42-
            thrombosis I63.32-
      middle I66.0-
        with infarction I63.51-
          due to
            embolism I63.41-
            thrombosis I63.31-
      posterior I66.2-
        with infarction I63.53-
          due to
            embolism I63.43-
            thrombosis I63.33-
      specified NEC I66.8
        with infarction I63.59
          due to
            embolism I63.4
            thrombosis I63.3
    choroidal (anterior) —*see* Occlusion,
      artery, cerebral, specified NEC
    communicating posterior —*see*
      Occlusion, artery, precerebral,
      specified NEC
    complete
      coronary I25.82
      extremities I70.92
    coronary (acute) (thrombotic) (without
      myocardial infarction) I24.0
      with myocardial infarction —*see*
        Infarction, myocardium
      chronic total I25.82
      complete I25.82
      healed or old I25.2
      total (chronic) I25.82
    hypophyseal —*see* Occlusion, artery,
      precerebral, specified NEC
    iliac I74.5
    lower extremities due to stenosis or
      stricture I77.1
    mesenteric (embolic) (thrombotic)
      K55.0
    perforating —*see* Occlusion, artery,
      cerebral, specified NEC
    peripheral I77.9
      thrombotic or embolic I74.4
    pontine —*see* Occlusion, artery, cerebral,
      specified NEC

◀ New   ◀▥ Revised   ~~deleted~~ Deleted

Occlusion, occluded *(Continued)*
  artery *(Continued)*
    precerebral I65.9
      with infarction I63.20
        due to
          embolism I63.10
            specified NEC I63.19
          thrombosis I63.00
            specified NEC I63.09
        specified NEC I63.29
      basilar —*see* Occlusion, artery, basilar
      carotid —*see* Occlusion, artery, carotid
      puerperal O88.23
      specified NEC I65.8
        with infarction I63.29
          due to
            embolism I63.19
            thrombosis I63.00
      vertebral —*see* Occlusion, artery,
          vertebral
    renal N28.0
    retinal
      branch H34.23-
      central H34.1-
      partial H34.21-
      transient H34.0-
    spinal —*see* Occlusion, artery, precerebral,
        vertebral
    total (chronic)
      coronary I25.82
      extremities I70.92
    vertebral I65.0-
      with
        infarction I63.21-
          due to
            embolism I63.11-
            thrombosis I63.01-
  basilar artery —*see* Occlusion, artery, basilar
  bile duct (common) (hepatic) (noncalculous)
      K83.1
  bowel —*see* Obstruction, intestine
  carotid (artery) (common) (internal) —*see*
      Occlusion, artery, carotid
  centric (of teeth) M26.59
    maximum intercuspation discrepancy
        M26.55
  cerebellar (artery) —*see* Occlusion, artery,
      cerebellar
  cerebral (artery) —*see* Occlusion, artery,
      cerebral
  cerebrovascular —*see also* Occlusion, artery,
      cerebral
    with infarction I63.5
  cervical canal —*see* Stricture, cervix
  cervix (uteri) —*see* Stricture, cervix
  choanal Q30.0
  choroidal (artery) —*see* Occlusion, artery,
      precerebral, specified NEC
  colon —*see* Obstruction, intestine
  communicating posterior artery —*see*
      Occlusion, artery, precerebral, specified
      NEC
  coronary (artery) (vein) (thrombotic) —*see
      also* Infarct, myocardium
    chronic total I25.82
    healed or old I25.2
    not resulting in infarction I24.0
    total (chronic) I25.82
  cystic duct —*see* Obstruction, gallbladder
  embolic —*see* Embolism
  fallopian tube N97.1
    congenital Q50.6
  gallbladder —*see also* Obstruction,
      gallbladder
    congenital (causing jaundice) Q44.1
  gingiva, traumatic K06.2
  hymen N89.6
    congenital Q52.3
  hypophyseal (artery) —*see* Occlusion, artery,
      precerebral, specified NEC
  iliac artery I74.5

Occlusion, occluded *(Continued)*
  intestine —*see* Obstruction, intestine
  lacrimal passages —*see* Obstruction, lacrimal
  lung J98.4
  lymph or lymphatic channel I89.0
  mammary duct N64.89
  mesenteric artery (embolic) (thrombotic)
      K55.0
  nose J34.89
    congenital Q30.0
  organ or site, congenital NEC —*see* Atresia,
      by site
  oviduct N97.1
    congenital Q50.6
  peripheral arteries
    due to stricture or stenosis I77.1
    upper extremity I74.2
  pontine (artery) —*see* Occlusion, artery,
      precerebral, specified NEC
  posterior lingual, of mandibular teeth M26.29
  precerebral artery —*see* Occlusion, artery,
      precerebral
  punctum lacrimale —*see* Obstruction,
      lacrimal
  pupil —*see* Membrane, pupillary
  pylorus, adult (*see also* Stricture, pylorus)
      K31.1
  renal artery N28.0
  retina, retinal
    artery —*see* Occlusion, artery, retinal
    vein (central) H34.81-
      engorgement H34.82-
      tributary H34.83-
    vessels H34.9
  spinal artery —*see* Occlusion, artery,
      precerebral, vertebral
  teeth (mandibular) (posterior lingual)
      M26.29
  thoracic duct I89.0
  thrombotic —*see* Thrombosis, artery
  traumatic
    edentulous (alveolar) ridge K06.2
    gingiva K06.2
    periodontal K05.5
  tubal N97.1
  ureter (complete) (partial) N13.5
    congenital Q62.10
  ureteropelvic junction N13.5
    congenital Q62.11
  ureterovesical orifice N13.5
    congenital Q62.12
  urethra —*see* Stricture, urethra
  uterus N85.8
  vagina N89.5
  vascular NEC I99.8
  vein —*see* Thrombosis
    retinal —*see* Occlusion, retinal, vein
  vena cava (inferior) (superior) —*see*
      Embolism, vena cava
  ventricle (brain) NEC G91.1
  vertebral (artery) —*see* Occlusion, artery,
      vertebral
  vessel (blood) I99.8
  vulva N90.5
Occult
  blood in feces (stools) R19.5
Occupational
  problems NEC Z56.89
Ochlophobia —*see* Agoraphobia
Ochronosis (endogenous) E70.29
Ocular muscle —*see* condition
Oculogyric crisis or disturbance H51.8
  psychogenic F45.8
Oculomotor syndrome H51.9
Oculopathy
  syphilitic NEC A52.71
    congenital
      early A50.01
      late A50.30
    early (secondary) A51.43
    late A52.71

Oddi's sphincter spasm K83.4
Odontalgia K08.8
Odontoameloblastoma —*see* Cyst, calcifying
    odontogenic
Odontoclasia K03.89
Odontodysplasia, regional K00.4
Odontogenesis imperfecta K00.5
Odontoma (ameloblastic) (complex)
    (compound) (fibroameloblastic) —*see* Cyst,
    calcifying odontogenic
Odontomyelitis (closed) (open) K04.0
Odontorrhagia K08.8
Odontosarcoma, ameloblastic C41.1
  upper jaw (bone) C41.0
Oestriasis —*see* Myiasis
Oguchi's disease H53.63
Ohara's disease —*see* Tularemia
Oidiomycosis —*see* Candidiasis
Oidium albicans infection —*see* Candidiasis
Old (previous) myocardial infarction
    I25.2
Old age (without mention of debility)
    R54-
  dementia F03
Olfactory —*see* condition
Oligemia —*see* Anemia
Oligoastrocytoma
  specified site —*see* Neoplasm, malignant,
      by site
  unspecified site C71.9
Oligocythemia D64.9
Oligodendroblastoma
  specified site —*see* Neoplasm, malignant
  unspecified site C71.9
Oligodendroglioma
  anaplastic type
    specified site —*see* Neoplasm, malignant,
        by site
    unspecified site C71.9
  specified site —*see* Neoplasm, malignant,
      by site
  unspecified site C71.9
Oligodontia —*see* Anodontia
Oligoencephalon Q02
Oligohidrosis L74.4
Oligohydramnios O41.0-
Oligohydrosis L74.4
Oligomenorrhea N91.5
  primary N91.3
  secondary N91.4
Oligophrenia —*see also* Disability, intellectual
  phenylpyruvic E70.0
Oligospermia N46.11
  due to
    drug therapy N46.121
    efferent duct obstruction N46.123
    infection N46.122
    radiation N46.124
    specified cause NEC N46.129
    systemic disease N46.125
Oligotrichia —*see* Alopecia
Oliguria R34
  with, complicating or following ectopic or
      molar pregnancy O08.4
  postprocedural N99.0
Ollier's disease Q78.4
Omenotocele —*see* Hernia, abdomen, specified
    site NEC
Omentitis —*see* Peritonitis
Omentum, omental —*see* condition
Omphalitis (congenital) (newborn) P38.9
  with mild hemorrhage P38.1
  without hemorrhage P38.9
  not of newborn L08.82
  tetanus A33
Omphalocele Q79.2
Omphalomesenteric duct, persistent
    Q43.0
Omphalorrhagia, newborn P51.9
Omsk hemorrhagic fever A98.1
Onanism (excessive) F98.8

Onchocerciasis, onchocercosis B73.1
  with
    eye disease B73.00
      endophthalmitis B73.01
      eyelid B73.09
      glaucoma B73.02
      specified NEC B73.09
    eye NEC B73.00
    eyelid B73.09
Oncocytoma —see Neoplasm, benign, by site
Oncovirus, as cause of disease classified
    elsewhere B97.32
Ondine's curse —see Apnea, sleep
Oneirophrenia F23
Onychauxis L60.2
  congenital Q84.5
Onychia —see also Cellulitis, digit
  with lymphangitis —see Lymphangitis, acute,
      digit
  candidal B37.2
  dermatophytic B35.1
Onychitis —see also Cellulitis, digit
  with lymphangitis —see Lymphangitis, acute,
      digit
Onychocryptosis L60.0
Onychodystrophy L60.3
  congenital Q84.6
Onychogryphosis, onychogryposis L60.2
Onycholysis L60.1
Onychomadesis L60.8
Onychomalacia L60.3
Onychomycosis (finger) (toe) B35.1
Onycho-osteodysplasia Q79.8
Onychophagia F98.8
Onychophosis L60.8
Onychoptosis L60.8
Onychorrhexis L60.3
  congenital Q84.6
Onychoschizia L60.3
Onyxis (finger) (toe) L60.0
Onyxitis —see also Cellulitis, digit
  with lymphangitis —see Lymphangitis, acute,
      digit
Oophoritis (cystic) (infectional) (interstitial)
    N70.92
  with salpingitis N70.93
  acute N70.02
    with salpingitis N70.03
  chronic N70.12
    with salpingitis N70.13
  complicating abortion —see Abortion, by
      type, complicated by, oophoritis
Oophorocele N83.4
Opacity, opacities
  cornea H17.-
    central H17.1-
    congenital Q13.3
    degenerative —see Degeneration, cornea
    hereditary —see Dystrophy, cornea
    inflammatory —see Keratitis
    minor H17.81-
    peripheral H17.82-
    sequelae of trachoma (healed) B94.0
    specified NEC H17.89
  enamel (teeth) (fluoride) (nonfluoride)
      K00.3
  lens —see Cataract
  snowball —see Deposit, crystalline
  vitreous (humor) NEC H43.39-
    congenital Q14.0
    membranes and strands H43.31-
Opalescent dentin (hereditary) K00.5
Open, opening
  abnormal, organ or site, congenital —see
      Imperfect, closure
  angle with
    borderline
      findings
        high risk H40.02-
        low risk H40.01-
      intraocular pressure H40.00-

Open, opening (Continued)
  angle with (Continued)
    cupping of discs H40.01-
    glaucoma (primary) —see Glaucoma, open
        angle
  bite
    anterior M26.220
    posterior M26.221
  false —see Imperfect, closure
  margin on tooth restoration K08.51
  restoration margins of tooth K08.51
  wound —see Wound, open
Operational fatigue F48.8
Operative —see condition
Operculitis —see Periodontitis
Operculum —see Break, retina
Ophiasis L63.2
Ophthalmia (see also Conjunctivitis) H10.9
  actinic rays —see Photokeratitis
  allergic (acute) —see Conjunctivitis, acute,
      atopic
  blennorrhagic (gonococcal) (neonatorum)
      A54.31
  diphtheritic A36.86
  Egyptian A71.1
  electrica —see Photokeratitis
  gonococcal (neonatorum) A54.31
  metastatic —see Endophthalmitis, purulent
  migraine —see Migraine, ophthalmoplegic
  neonatorum, newborn P39.1
    gonococcal A54.31
  nodosa H16.24-
  purulent —see Conjunctivitis, acute,
      mucopurulent
  spring —see Conjunctivitis, acute, atopic
  sympathetic —see Uveitis, sympathetic
Ophthalmitis —see Ophthalmia
Ophthalmocele (congenital) Q15.8
Ophthalmoneuromyelitis G36.0
Ophthalmoplegia —see also Strabismus,
    paralytic
  anterior internuclear —see Ophthalmoplegia,
      internuclear
  ataxia-areflexia G61.0
  diabetic —see E08-E13 with .39
  exophthalmic E05.00
    with thyroid storm E05.01
  external H49.88-
    progressive H49.4-
      with pigmentary retinopathy —see
          Kearns-Sayre syndrome
    total H49.3-
  internal (complete) (total) H52.51-
  internuclear H51.2-
  migraine —see Migraine, ophthalmoplegic
  Parinaud's H49.88-
  progressive external —see Ophthalmoplegia,
      external, progressive
  supranuclear, progressive G23.1
  total (external) —see Ophthalmoplegia,
      external, total
Opioid (s)
  abuse —see Abuse, drug, opioids
  dependence —see Dependence, drug, opioids
Opisthognathism M26.09
Opisthorchiasis (felineus) (viverrini) B66.0
Opitz' disease D73.2
Opiumism —see Dependence, drug, opioid
Oppenheim's disease G70.2
Oppenheim-Urbach disease (necrobiosis
    lipoidica diabeticorum) —see E08-E13 with
    .620
Optic nerve —see condition
Orbit —see condition
Orchioblastoma C62.9-
Orchitis (gangrenous) (nonspecific) (septic)
    (suppurative) N45.2
  blennorrhagic (gonococcal) (acute) (chronic)
      A54.23
  chlamydial A56.19
  filarial (see also Infestation, filarial) B74.9
    [N51]

Orchitis (Continued)
  gonococcal (acute) (chronic) A54.23
  mumps B26.0
  syphilitic A52.76
  tuberculous A18.15
Orf (virus disease) B08.02
Organic —see also condition
  brain syndrome F09
  heart —see Disease, heart
  mental disorder F09
  psychosis F09
Orgasm
  anejaculatory N53.13
Oriental
  bilharziasis B65.2
  schistosomiasis B65.2
Orifice —see condition
Origin of both great vessels from right
    ventricle Q20.1
Ormond's disease (with ureteral obstruction)
    N13.5
  with infection N13.6
Ornithine metabolism disorder E72.4
Ornithinemia (Type I) (Type II) E72.4
Ornithosis A70
Orotaciduria, oroticaciduria (congenital)
    (hereditary) (pyrimidine deficiency) E79.8
  anemia D53.0
Orthodontics
  adjustment Z46.4
  fitting Z46.4
Orthopnea R06.01
Orthopoxvirus B08.09
  specified NEC B08.09
Os, uterus —see condition
Osgood-Schlatter disease or
    osteochondrosis —see Osteochondrosis,
    juvenile, tibia
Osler (-Weber)-Rendu disease I78.0
Osler's nodes I33.0
Osmidrosis L75.0
Osseous —see condition
Ossification
  artery —see Arteriosclerosis
  auricle (ear) —see Disorder, pinna, specified
      type NEC
  bronchial J98.09
  cardiac —see Degeneration, myocardial
  cartilage (senile) —see Disorder, cartilage,
      specified type NEC
  coronary (artery) —see Disease, heart,
      ischemic, atherosclerotic
  diaphragm J98.6
  ear, middle —see Otosclerosis
  falx cerebri G96.19
  fontanel, premature Q75.0
  heart —see also Degeneration, myocardial
    valve —see Endocarditis
  larynx J38.7
  ligament —see Disorder, tendon, specified
      type NEC
    posterior longitudinal —see
        Spondylopathy, specified NEC
  meninges (cerebral) (spinal) G96.19
  multiple, eccentric centers —see Disorder,
      bone, development or growth
  muscle —see also Calcification, muscle
    due to burns —see Myositis, ossificans, in,
        burns
    paralytic —see Myositis, ossificans, in,
        quadriplegia
    progressive —see Myositis, ossificans,
        progressiva
  specified NEC M61.50
    ankle M61.57-
    foot M61.57-
    forearm M61.53-
    hand M61.54-
    lower leg M61.56-
    multiple sites M61.59
    pelvic region M61.55-

◀ New   ◀◀ Revised   ~~deleted~~ Deleted

Ossification *(Continued)*
  muscle *(Continued)*
    specified NEC *(Continued)*
      shoulder region M61.51-
      specified site NEC M61.58
      thigh M61.55-
      upper arm M61.52-
      traumatic —*see* Myositis, ossificans, traumatica
  myocardium, myocardial —*see* Degeneration, myocardial
  penis N48.89
  periarticular —*see* Disorder, joint, specified type NEC
  pinna —*see* Disorder, pinna, specified type NEC
  rider's bone —*see* Ossification, muscle, specified NEC
  sclera H15.89
  subperiosteal, post-traumatic M89.8X-
  tendon —*see* Disorder, tendon, specified type NEC
  trachea J39.8
  tympanic membrane —*see* Disorder, tympanic membrane, specified NEC
  vitreous (humor) —*see* Deposit, crystalline
Osteitis —*see also* Osteomyelitis
  alveolar M27.3
  condensans M85.30
    ankle M85.37-
    foot M85.37-
    forearm M85.33-
    hand M85.34-
    lower leg M85.36-
    multiple site M85.39
    neck M85.38
    rib M85.38
    shoulder M85.31-
    skull M85.38
    specified site NEC M85.38
    thigh M85.35-
    toe M85.37-
    upper arm M85.32-
    vertebra M85.38
  deformans M88.9
    in (due to)
      malignant neoplasm of bone C41.9 *[M90.60]*
      neoplastic disease (*see also* Neoplasm) D49.9 *[M90.60]*
        carpus D49.9 *[M90.64-]*
        clavicle D49.9 *[M90.61-]*
        femur D49.9 *[M90.65-]*
        fibula D49.9 *[M90.66-]*
        finger D49.9 *[M90.64-]*
        humerus D49.9 *[M90.62-]*
        ilium D49.9 *[M90.65-]*
        ischium D49.9 *[M90.65-]*
        metacarpus D49.9 *[M90.64-]*
        metatarsus D49.9 *[M90.67-]*
        multiple sites D49.9 *[M90.69]*
        neck D49.9 *[M90.68]*
        radius D49.9 *[M90.63-]*
        rib D49.9 *[M90.68]*
        scapula D49.9 *[M90.61-]*
        skull D49.9 *[M90.68]*
        tarsus D49.9 *[M90.67-]*
        tibia D49.9 *[M90.66-]*
        toe D49.9 *[M90.67-]*
        ulna D49.9 *[M90.63-]*
        vertebra D49.9 *[M90.68]*
    skull M88.0
    specified NEC —*see* Paget's disease, bone, by site
    vertebra M88.1
  due to yaws A66.6
  fibrosa NEC —*see* Cyst, bone, by site
    circumscripta —*see* Dysplasia, fibrous, bone NEC

Osteitis *(Continued)*
  fibrosa NEC *(Continued)*
    cystica (generalisata) E21.0
    disseminata Q78.1
    osteoplastica E21.0
  fragilitans Q78.0
  Garr's (sclerosing) —*see* Osteomyelitis, specified type NEC
  jaw (acute) (chronic) (lower) (suppurative) (upper) M27.2
  parathyroid E21.0
  petrous bone (acute) (chronic) —*see* Petrositis
  sclerotic, nonsuppurative —*see* Osteomyelitis, specified type NEC
  tuberculosa A18.09
    cystica D86.89
    multiplex cystoides D86.89
Osteoarthritis M19.90
  ankle M19.07-
  elbow M19.02-
  foot joint M19.07-
  generalized M15.9
    erosive M15.4
    primary M15.0
    specified NEC M15.8
  hand joint M19.04-
    first carpometacarpal joint M18.9-
  hip M16.1-
    bilateral M16.0
    due to hip dysplasia (unilateral) M16.3-
      bilateral M16.2
  interphalangeal
    distal (Heberden) M15.1
    proximal (Bouchard) M15.2
  knee M17.9-
    bilateral M17.0
  post-traumatic NEC M19.92
    ankle M19.17-
    elbow M19.12-
    foot joint M19.17-
    hand joint M19.14-
      first carpometacarpal joint M18.3-
        bilateral M18.2
    hip M16.5-
      bilateral M16.4
    knee M17.3-
      bilateral M17.2
    shoulder M19.11-
    wrist M19.13-
  primary M19.91
    ankle M19.07-
    elbow M19.02-
    foot joint M19.07-
    hand joint M19.04-
      first carpometacarpal joint M18.1-
        bilateral M18.0
    hip M16.1-
      bilateral M16.0
    knee M17.1-
      bilateral M17.0
    shoulder M19.01-
    spine —*see* Spondylosis
    wrist M19.03-
  secondary M19.93
    ankle M19.27-
    elbow M19.22-
    foot joint M19.27-
    hand joint M19.24-
      first carpometacarpal joint M18.5-
        bilateral M18.4
    hip M16.7
      bilateral M16.6
    knee M17.5
      bilateral M17.4
    multiple M15.3
    shoulder M19.21-
    spine —*see* Spondylosis
    wrist M19.23-
  shoulder M19.01-
  spine —*see* Spondylosis
  wrist M19.03-

Osteoarthropathy (hypertrophic) M19.90
  ankle —*see* Osteoarthritis, primary, ankle
  elbow —*see* Osteoarthritis, primary, elbow
  foot joint —*see* Osteoarthritis, primary, foot
  hand joint —*see* Osteoarthritis, primary, hand joint
  knee joint —*see* Osteoarthritis, primary, knee
  multiple site —*see* Osteoarthritis, primary, multiple joint
  pulmonary —*see also* Osteoarthropathy, specified type NEC
    hypertrophic —*see* Osteoarthropathy, hypertrophic, specified type NEC
  secondary —*see* Osteoarthropathy, specified type NEC
  secondary hypertrophic —*see* Osteoarthropathy, specified type NEC
  shoulder —*see* Osteoarthritis, primary, shoulder
  specified joint NEC —*see* Osteoarthritis, primary, specified joint NEC
  specified type NEC M89.40
    carpus M89.44-
    clavicle M89.41-
    femur M89.45-
    fibula M89.46-
    finger M89.44-
    humerus M89.42-
    ilium M89.459
    ischium M89.459
    metacarpus M89.44-
    metatarsus M89.47-
    multiple sites M89.49
    neck M89.48
    radius M89.43-
    rib M89.48
    scapula M89.41-
    skull M89.48
    tarsus M89.47-
    tibia M89.46-
    toe M89.47-
    ulna M89.43-
    vertebra M89.48
  spine —*see* Spondylosis
  wrist —*see* Osteoarthritis, primary, wrist
Osteoarthrosis (degenerative) (hypertrophic) (joint) —*see also* Osteoarthritis
  deformans alkaptonurica E70.29 *[M36.8]*
  erosive M15.4
  generalized M15.9
    primary M15.0
  polyarticular M15.9
  spine —*see* Spondylosis
Osteoblastoma —*see* Neoplasm, bone, benign
  aggressive —*see* Neoplasm, bone, uncertain behavior
Osteochondroarthrosis deformans endemica —*see* Disease, Kaschin-Beck
Osteochondritis —*see also* Osteochondropathy, by site
  Brailsford's —*see* Osteochondrosis, juvenile, radius
  dissecans M93.20
    ankle M93.27-
    elbow M93.22-
    foot M93.27-
    hand M93.24-
    hip M93.25-
    knee M93.26-
    multiple sites M93.29
    shoulder joint M93.21-
    specified site NEC M93.28
    wrist M93.23-
  juvenile M92.9
    patellar —*see* Osteochondrosis, juvenile, patella
  syphilitic (congenital) (early) A50.02 *[M90.80]*
    ankle A50.02 *[M90.87-]*
    elbow A50.02 *[M90.82-]*
    foot A50.02 *[M90.87-]*
    forearm A50.02 *[M90.83-]*

Osteodystrophy Q78.9
  azotemic N25.0
  congenital Q78.9
  parathyroid, secondary E21.1
  renal N25.0
Osteofibroma —*see* Neoplasm, bone, benign
Osteofibrosarcoma —*see* Neoplasm, bone, malignant
Osteogenesis imperfecta Q78.0
Osteogenic —*see* condition
Osteolysis M89.50
  carpus M89.54-
  clavicle M89.51-
  femur M89.55-
  fibula M89.56-
  finger M89.54-
  humerus M89.52-
  ilium M89.559
  ischium M89.559
  joint prosthesis (periprosthetic) —*see* Complications, joint prosthesis, mechanical, periprosthetic, osteolysis, by site
  metacarpus M89.54-
  metatarsus M89.57-
  multiple sites M89.59
  neck M89.58
  periprosthetic —*see* Complications, joint prosthesis, mechanical, periprosthetic, osteolysis, by site
  radius M89.53-
  rib M89.58
  scapula M89.51-
  skull M89.58
  tarsus M89.57-
  tibia M89.56-
  toe M89.57-
  ulna M89.53-
  vertebra M89.58
Osteoma —*see also* Neoplasm, bone, benign
  osteoid —*see also* Neoplasm, bone, benign
    giant —*see* Neoplasm, bone, benign
Osteomalacia M83.9
  adult M83.9
    drug-induced NEC M83.5
    due to
      malabsorption (postsurgical) M83.2
      malnutrition M83.3
    specified NEC M83.8
  aluminium-induced M83.4
  infantile —*see* Rickets
  juvenile —*see* Rickets
  oncogenic E83.89
  pelvis M83.8
  puerperal M83.0
  senile M83.1
  vitamin-D-resistant in adults E83.31 *[M90.8-]*
    carpus E83.31 *[M90.84-]*
    clavicle E83.31 *[M90.81-]*
    femur E83.31 *[M90.85-]*
    fibula E83.31 *[M90.86-]*
    finger E83.31 *[M90.84-]*
    humerus E83.31 *[M90.82-]*
    ilium E83.31 *[M90.859]*
    ischium E83.31 *[M90.859]*
    metacarpus E83.31 *[M90.84-]*
    metatarsus E83.31 *[M90.87-]*
    multiple sites E83.31 *[M90.89]*
    neck E83.31 *[M90.88]*
    radius E83.31 *[M90.83-]*
    rib E83.31 *[M90.88]*
    scapula E83.31 *[M90.819]*
    skull E83.31 *[M90.88]*
    tarsus E83.31 *[M90.879]*
    tibia E83.31 *[M90.869]*
    toe E83.31 *[M90.879]*
    ulna E83.31 *[M90.839]*
    vertebra E83.31 *[M90.88]*

Osteomyelitis (general) (infective) (localized) (neonatal) (purulent) (septic) (staphylococcal) (streptococcal) (suppurative) (with periostitis) M86.9
  acute M86.10
    carpus M86.14-
    clavicle M86.11-
    femur M86.15-
    fibula M86.16-
    finger M86.14-
    hematogenous M86.00
      carpus M86.04-
      clavicle M86.01-
      femur M86.05-
      fibula M86.06-
      finger M86.04-
      humerus M86.02-
      ilium M86.059
      ischium M86.059
      mandible M27.2
      metacarpus M86.04-
      metatarsus M86.07-
      multiple sites M86.09
      neck M86.08
      orbit H05.02-
      petrous bone —*see* Petrositis
      radius M86.03-
      rib M86.08
      scapula M86.01-
      skull M86.08
      tarsus M86.07-
      tibia M86.06-
      toe M86.07-
      ulna M86.03-
      vertebra —*see* Osteomyelitis, vertebra
    humerus M86.12-
    ilium M86.159
    ischium M86.159
    mandible M27.2
    metacarpus M86.14-
    metatarsus M86.17-
    multiple sites M86.19
    neck M86.18
    orbit H05.02-
    petrous bone —*see* Petrositis
    radius M86.13-
    rib M86.18
    scapula M86.11-
    skull M86.18
    tarsus M86.17-
    tibia M86.16-
    toe M86.17-
    ulna M86.13-
    vertebra —*see* Osteomyelitis, vertebra
  chronic (or old) M86.60
    with draining sinus M86.40
      carpus M86.44-
      clavicle M86.41-
      femur M86.45-
      fibula M86.46-
      finger M86.44-
      humerus M86.42-
      ilium M86.459
      ischium M86.459
      mandible M27.2
      metacarpus M86.44-
      metatarsus M86.47-
      multiple sites M86.49
      neck M86.48
      orbit H05.02-
      petrous bone —*see* Petrositis
      radius M86.43-
      rib M86.48
      scapula M86.41-
      skull M86.48
      tarsus M86.47-
      tibia M86.46-
      toe M86.47-
      ulna M86.43-
      vertebra —*see* Osteomyelitis, vertebra
    carpus M86.64-

Osteomyelitis *(Continued)*
  chronic *(Continued)*
    clavicle M86.61-
    femur M86.65-
    fibula M86.66-
    finger M86.64-
    hematogenous NEC M86.50
      carpus M86.54-
      clavicle M86.51-
      femur M86.55-
      fibula M86.56-
      finger M86.54-
      humerus M86.52-
      ilium M86.559
      ischium M86.559
      mandible M27.2
      metacarpus M86.54-
      metatarsus M86.57-
      multifocal M86.30
        carpus M86.34-
        clavicle M86.31-
        femur M86.35-
        fibula M86.36-
        finger M86.34-
        humerus M86.32-
        ilium M86.359
        ischium M86.359
        metacarpus M86.34-
        metatarsus M86.37-
        multiple sites M86.39
        neck M86.38
        radius M86.33-
        rib M86.38
        scapula M86.31-
        skull M86.38
        tarsus M86.37-
        tibia M86.36-
        toe M86.37-
        ulna M86.33-
        vertebra —*see* Osteomyelitis, vertebra
      multiple sites M86.59
      neck M86.58
      orbit H05.02-
      petrous bone —*see* Petrositis
      radius M86.53-
      rib M86.58
      scapula M86.51-
      skull M86.58
      tarsus M86.57-
      tibia M86.56-
      toe M86.57-
      ulna M86.53-
      vertebra —*see* Osteomyelitis, vertebra
    humerus M86.62-
    ilium M86.659
    ischium M86.659
    mandible M27.2
    metacarpus M86.64-
    metatarsus M86.67-
    multifocal —*see* Osteomyelitis, chronic, hematogenous, multifocal
    multiple sites M86.69
    neck M86.68
    orbit H05.02-
    petrous bone —*see* Petrositis
    radius M86.63-
    rib M86.68
    scapula M86.61-
    skull M86.68
    tarsus M86.67-
    tibia M86.66-
    toe M86.67-
    ulna M86.63-
    vertebra —*see* Osteomyelitis, vertebra
  echinococcal B67.2
  Garr's —*see* Osteomyelitis, specified type NEC
  jaw (acute) (chronic) (lower) (neonatal) (suppurative) (upper) M27.2
  nonsuppurating —*see* Osteomyelitis, specified type NEC

Osteomyelitis (Continued)
  orbit H05.02-
  petrous bone —see Petrositis
  Salmonella (arizonae) (cholerae-suis)
      (enteritidis) (typhimurium) A02.24
  sclerosing, nonsuppurative —see
      Osteomyelitis, specified type NEC
  specified type NEC (see also subcategory)
      M86.8X-
    mandible M27.2
    orbit H05.02-
    petrous bone —see Petrositis
    vertebra —see Osteomyelitis, vertebra
  subacute M86.20
    carpus M86.24-
    clavicle M86.21-
    femur M86.25-
    fibula M86.26-
    finger M86.24-
    humerus M86.22-
    mandible M27.2
    metacarpus M86.24-
    metatarsus M86.27-
    multiple sites M86.29
    neck M86.28
    orbit H05.02-
    petrous bone —see Petrositis
    radius M86.23-
    rib M86.28
    scapula M86.21-
    skull M86.28
    tarsus M86.27-
    tibia M86.26-
    toe M86.27-
    ulna M86.23-
    vertebra —see Osteomyelitis, vertebra
  syphilitic A52.77
    congenital (early) A50.02 [M90.80]
  tuberculous —see Tuberculosis, bone
  typhoid A01.05
  vertebra M46.20
    cervical region M46.22
    cervicothoracic region M46.23
    lumbar region M46.26
    lumbosacral region M46.27
    occipito-atlanto-axial region M46.21
    sacrococcygeal region M46.28
    thoracic region M46.24
    thoracolumbar region M46.25
Osteomyelofibrosis D75.89
Osteomyelosclerosis D75.89
Osteonecrosis M87.9
  due to
    drugs —see Osteonecrosis, secondary, due
        to, drugs
    trauma —see Osteonecrosis, secondary, due
        to, trauma
  idiopathic aseptic M87.00
    ankle M87.07-
    carpus M87.03-
    clavicle M87.01-
    femur M87.05-
    fibula M87.06-
    finger M87.04-
    humerus M87.02-
    ilium M87.050
    ischium M87.050
    metacarpus M87.04-
    metatarsus M87.07-
    multiple sites M87.09
    neck M87.08
    pelvis M87.050
    radius M87.03-
    rib M87.08
    scapula M87.01-
    skull M87.08
    tarsus M87.07-
    tibia M87.06-
    toe M87.07-
    ulna M87.03-
    vertebra M87.08

Osteonecrosis (Continued)
  secondary NEC M87.30
    carpus M87.33-
    clavicle M87.31-
    due to
      drugs M87.10
        carpus M87.13-
        clavicle M87.11-
        femur M87.15-
        fibula M87.16-
        finger M87.14-
        humerus M87.12-
        ilium M87.159
        ischium M87.159
        jaw M87.180
        metacarpus M87.14-
        metatarsus M87.17-
        multiple sites M87.19
        neck M87.18
        radius M87.13-
        rib M87.18
        scapula M87.11-
        skull M87.18
        tarsus M87.17-
        tibia M87.16-
        toe M87.17-
        ulna M87.13-
        vertebra M87.18
      hemoglobinopathy NEC D58.2 [M90.50]
        carpus D58.2 [M90.54-]
        clavicle D58.2 [M90.51-]
        femur D58.2 [M90.55-]
        fibula D58.2 [M90.56-]
        finger D58.2 [M90.54-]
        humerus D58.2 [M90.52-]
        ilium D58.2 [M90.55-]
        ischium D58.2 [M90.55-]
        metacarpus D58.2 [M90.54-]
        metatarsus D58.2 [M90.57-]
        multiple sites D58.2 [M90.58]
        neck D58.2 [M90.58]
        radius D58.2 [M90.53-]
        rib D58.2 [M90.58]
        scapula D58.2 [M90.51-]
        skull D58.2 [M90.58]
        tarsus D58.2 [M90.57-]
        tibia D58.2 [M90.56-]
        toe D58.2 [M90.57-]
        ulna D58.2 [M90.53-]
        vertebra D58.2 [M90.58]
      trauma (previous) M87.20
        carpus M87.23-
        clavicle M87.21-
        femur M87.25-
        fibula M87.26-
        finger M87.24-
        humerus M87.22-
        ilium M87.25-
        ischium M87.25-
        metacarpus M87.24-
        metatarsus M87.27-
        multiple sites M87.29
        neck M87.28
        radius M87.23-
        rib M87.28
        scapula M87.21-
        skull M87.28
        tarsus M87.27-
        tibia M87.26-
        toe M87.27-
        ulna M87.23-
        vertebra M87.28
      femur M87.35-
      fibula M87.36-
      finger M87.34-
      humerus M87.32
      ilium M87.350
    in
      caisson disease T70.3 [M90.50]
        carpus T70.3 [M90.54-]
        clavicle T70.3 [M90.51-]

Osteonecrosis (Continued)
  secondary NEC (Continued)
    in (Continued)
      caisson disease (Continued)
        femur T70.3 [M90.55-]
        fibula T70.3 [M90.56-]
        finger T70.3 [M90.54-]
        humerus T70.3 [M90.52-]
        ilium T70.3 [M90.55-]
        ischium T70.3 [M90.55-]
        metacarpus T70.3 [M90.54-]
        metatarsus T70.3 [M90.57-]
        multiple sites T70.3 [M90.59]
        neck T70.3 [M90.58]
        radius T70.3 [M90.53-]
        rib T70.3 [M90.58]
        scapula T70.3 [M90.51-]
        skull T70.3 [M90.58]
        tarsus T70.3 [M90.57-]
        tibia T70.3 [M90.56-]
        toe T70.3 [M90.57-]
        ulna T70.3 [M90.53-]
        vertebra T70.3 [M90.58]
      ischium M87.350
      metacarpus M87.34-
      metatarsus M87.37-
      multiple site M87.39
      neck M87.38
      radius M87.33-
      rib M87.38
      scapula M87.319
      skull M87.38
      tarsus M87.379
      tibia M87.366
      toe M87.379
      ulna M87.33-
      vertebra M87.38
    specified type NEC M87.80
      carpus M87.83-
      clavicle M87.81-
      femur M87.85-
      fibula M87.86-
      finger M87.84-
      humerus M87.82-
      ilium M87.85-
      ischium M87.85-
      metacarpus M87.84-
      metatarsus M87.87-
      multiple sites M87.89
      neck M87.88
      radius M87.83-
      rib M87.88-
      scapula M87.81-
      skull M87.88
      tarsus M87.87-
      tibia M87.86-
      toe M87.87-
      ulna M87.83-
      vertebra M87.88
Osteo-onycho-arthro-dysplasia Q79.8
Osteo-onychodysplasia, hereditary Q79.8
Osteopathia condensans disseminata Q78.8
Osteopathy —see also Osteomyelitis,
    Osteonecrosis, Osteoporosis
  after poliomyelitis M89.60
    carpus M89.64-
    clavicle M89.61-
    femur M89.65-
    fibula M89.66-
    finger M89.64-
    humerus M89.62-
    ilium M89.659
    ischium M89.659
    metacarpus M89.64-
    metatarsus M89.67-
    multiple sites M89.69
    neck M89.68
    radius M89.63-
    rib M89.68
    scapula M89.61-
    skull M89.68

◀ New   ◀▥ Revised   deleted Deleted

Osteopathy (Continued)
  after poliomyelitis (Continued)
    tarsus M89.67-
    tibia M89.66-
    toe M89.67-
    ulna M89.63-
    vertebra M89.68
  in (due to)
    renal osteodystrophy N25.0
    specified diseases classified elsewhere —
      see subcategory M90.8
Osteopenia M85.8-
  borderline M85.8-
Osteoperiostitis —see Osteomyelitis, specified
  type NEC
Osteopetrosis (familial) Q78.2
Osteophyte M25.70
  ankle M25.77-
  elbow M25.72-
  foot joint M25.77-
  hand joint M25.74-
  hip M25.75-
  knee M25.76-
  shoulder M25.71-
  spine M25.78
  vertebrae M25.78
  wrist M25.73-
Osteopoikilosis Q78.8
Osteoporosis (female) (male) M81.0
  with current pathological fracture M80.00
  age-related M81.0
    with current pathologic fracture M80.00
      carpus M80.04-
      clavicle M80.01-
      fibula M80.06-
      finger M80.04-
      humerus M80.02-
      ilium M80.05-
      ischium M80.05-
      metacarpus M80.04-
      metatarsus M80.07-
      pelvis M80.05-
      radius M80.03-
      scapula M80.01-
      tarsus M80.07-
      tibia M80.06-
      toe M80.07-
      ulna M80.03-
      vertebra M80.08
  disuse M81.8
    with current pathological fracture M80.80
      carpus M80.84-
      clavicle M80.81-
      fibula M80.86-
      finger M80.84-
      humerus M80.82-
      ilium M80.85-
      ischium M80.85-
      metacarpus M80.84-
      metatarsus M80.87-
      pelvis M80.85-
      radius M80.83-
      scapula M80.81-
      tarsus M80.87-
      tibia M80.86-
      toe M80.87-
      ulna M80.83-
      vertebra M80.88
  drug-induced —see Osteoporosis, specified
    type NEC
  idiopathic —see Osteoporosis, specified type
    NEC
  involutional —see Osteoporosis, age-related
  Lequesne M81.6
  localized M81.6
  postmenopausal M81.0
    with pathological fracture M80.00
      carpus M80.04-
      clavicle M80.01-
      fibula M80.06-
      finger M80.04-

Osteoporosis (Continued)
  postmenopausal (Continued)
    with pathological fracture (Continued)
      humerus M80.02-
      ilium M80.05-
      ischium M80.05-
      metacarpus M80.04-
      metatarsus M80.07-
      pelvis M80.05-
      radius M80.03-
      scapula M80.01-
      tarsus M80.07-
      tibia M80.06-
      toe M80.07-
      ulna M80.03-
      vertebra M80.08
  postoophorectomy —see Osteoporosis,
    specified type NEC
  postsurgical malabsorption —see
    Osteoporosis, specified type NEC
  post-traumatic —see Osteoporosis, specified
    type NEC
  senile —see Osteoporosis, age-related
  specified type NEC M81.8
    with pathological fracture M80.80
      carpus M80.84-
      clavicle M80.81-
      fibula M80.86-
      finger M80.84-
      humerus M80.82-
      ilium M80.85-
      ischium M80.85-
      metacarpus M80.84-
      metatarsus M80.87-
      pelvis M80.85-
      radius M80.83-
      scapula M80.81-
      tarsus M80.87-
      tibia M80.86-
      toe M80.87-
      ulna M80.83-
      vertebra M80.88
Osteopsathyrosis (idiopathica) Q78.0
Osteoradionecrosis, jaw (acute) (chronic)
  (lower) (suppurative) (upper) M27.2
Osteosarcoma (any form) —see Neoplasm,
  bone, malignant
Osteosclerosis Q78.2
  acquired M85.8-
  congenita Q77.4
  fragilitas (generalisata) Q78.2
  myelofibrosis D75.81
Osteosclerotic anemia D64.89
Osteosis
  cutis L94.2
  renal fibrocystic N25.0
Österreicher-Turner syndrome Q87.2
Ostium
  atrioventriculare commune Q21.2
  primum (arteriosum) (defect) (persistent)
    Q21.2
  secundum (arteriosum) (defect) (patent)
    (persistent) Q21.1
Ostrum-Furst syndrome Q75.8
Otalgia —see subcategory H92.0
Otitis (acute) H66.90
  with effusion —see also Otitis, media,
    nonsuppurative
    purulent —see Otitis, media,
      suppurative
  adhesive —see subcategory H74.1
  chronic —see also Otitis, media, chronic
    with effusion —see also Otitis, media,
      nonsuppurative, chronic
  externa H60.9-
    abscess —see Abscess, ear, external
    acute (noninfective) H60.50-
      actinic H60.51-
      chemical H60.52-
      contact H60.53-
      eczematoid H60.54-

Otitis (Continued)
  externa (Continued)
    acute (Continued)
      infective —see Otitis, externa, infective
      reactive H60.55-
      specified NEC H60.59-
    cellulitis —see Cellulitis, ear
    chronic H60.6-
    diffuse —see Otitis, externa, infective,
      diffuse
    hemorrhagic —see Otitis, externa, infective,
      hemorrhagic
    in (due to)
      aspergillosis B44.89
      candidiasis B37.84
      erysipelas A46 [H62.40]
      herpes (simplex) virus infection B00.1
        zoster B02.8
      impetigo L01.00 [H62.40]
      infectious disease NEC B99 [H62.4-]
      mycosis NEC B36.9 [H62.40]
      parasitic disease NEC B89 [H62.40]
      viral disease NEC B34.9 [H62.40]
      zoster B02.8
    infective NEC H60.39-
      abscess —see Abscess, ear, external
      cellulitis —see Cellulitis, ear
      diffuse H60.31-
      hemorrhagic H60.32-
      swimmer's ear —see Swimmer's, ear
    malignant H60.2-
    mycotic B36.9 [H62.40]
    necrotizing —see Otitis, externa, malignant
    Pseudomonas aeruginosa —see Otitis,
      externa, malignant
    reactive —see Otitis, externa, acute, reactive
    specified NEC —see subcategory H60.8
    tropical B36.8
  insidiosa —see Otosclerosis
  interna —see subcategory H83.0
  media (hemorrhagic) (staphylococcal)
    (streptococcal) H66.9-
    with effusion (nonpurulent) —see Otitis,
      media, nonsuppurative
    acute, subacute H66.90
      allergic —see Otitis, media,
        nonsuppurative, acute, allergic
      exudative —see Otitis, media,
        nonsuppurative, acute
      mucoid —see Otitis, media,
        nonsuppurative, acute
      necrotizing —see also Otitis, media,
        suppurative, acute
        in
          measles B05.3
          scarlet fever A38.0
      nonsuppurative NEC —see Otitis, media,
        nonsuppurative, acute
      purulent —see Otitis, media,
        suppurative, acute
      sanguinous —see Otitis, media,
        nonsuppurative, acute
      secretory —see Otitis, media,
        nonsuppurative, acute, serous
      seromucinous —see Otitis, media,
        nonsuppurative, acute
      serous —see Otitis, media,
        nonsuppurative, acute, serous
      suppurative —see Otitis, media,
        suppurative, acute
    allergic —see Otitis, media, nonsuppurative
    catarrhal —see Otitis, media,
      nonsuppurative
    chronic H66.90
      with effusion (nonpurulent) —see Otitis,
        media, nonsuppurative, chronic
      allergic —see Otitis, media,
        nonsuppurative, chronic, allergic
      benign suppurative —see Otitis,
        media, suppurative, chronic,
        tubotympanic

Otitis (Continued)
  media (Continued)
    chronic (Continued)
      catarrhal —see Otitis, media,
        nonsuppurative, chronic, serous
      exudative —see Otitis, media,
        nonsuppurative, chronic
      mucinous —see Otitis, media,
        nonsuppurative, chronic, mucoid
      mucoid —see Otitis, media,
        nonsuppurative, chronic, mucoid
      nonsuppurative NEC —see Otitis, media,
        nonsuppurative, chronic
      purulent —see Otitis, media,
        suppurative, chronic
      secretory —see Otitis, media,
        nonsuppurative, chronic, mucoid
      seromucinous —see Otitis, media,
        nonsuppurative, chronic
      serous —see Otitis, media,
        nonsuppurative, chronic, serous
      suppurative —see Otitis, media,
        suppurative, chronic
      transudative —see Otitis, media,
        nonsuppurative, chronic, mucoid
    exudative —see Otitis, media,
      nonsuppurative
    in (due to) (with)
      influenza —see Influenza, with, otitis
        media
      measles B05.3
      scarlet fever A38.0
      tuberculosis A18.6
      viral disease NEC B34.- [H67.-]
    mucoid —see Otitis, media,
      nonsuppurative
    nonsuppurative H65.9-
      acute or subacute NEC H65.19-
        allergic H65.11-
          recurrent H65.11-
        recurrent H65.19-
        secretory —see Otitis, media,
          nonsuppurative, serous
        serous H65.0-
          recurrent H65.0-
      chronic H65.49-
        allergic H65.41-
        mucoid H65.3-
        serous H65.2-
    postmeasles B05.3
    purulent —see Otitis, media, suppurative
    secretory —see Otitis, media,
      nonsuppurative
    seromucinous —see Otitis, media,
      nonsuppurative
    serous —see Otitis, media, nonsuppurative
    suppurative H66.4-
      acute H66.00-
        with rupture of ear drum H66.01-
        recurrent H66.00-
          with rupture of ear drum H66.01-
      chronic (see also subcategory) H66.3
        atticoantral H66.2-
        benign —see Otitis, media,
          suppurative, chronic,
          tubotympanic
        tubotympanic H66.1-
    transudative —see Otitis, media,
      nonsuppurative
    tuberculous A18.6

Otocephaly Q18.2
Otolith syndrome —see subcategory H81.8
Otomycosis (diffuse) NEC B36.9 [H62.40]
  in
    aspergillosis B44.89
    candidiasis B37.84
    moniliasis B37.84
Otoporosis —see Otosclerosis
Otorrhagia (nontraumatic) H92.2-
  traumatic - code by Type of injury
Otorrhea H92.1-
  cerebrospinal G96.0
Otosclerosis (general) H80.9-
  cochlear (endosteal) H80.2-
  involving
    otic capsule —see Otosclerosis, cochlear
    oval window
      nonobliterative H80.0-
      obliterative H80.1-
    round window —see Otosclerosis, cochlear
  nonobliterative —see Otosclerosis, involving,
    oval window, nonobliterative
  obliterative —see Otosclerosis, involving, oval
    window, obliterative
  specified NEC H80.8-
Otospongiosis —see Otosclerosis
Otto's disease or pelvis M24.7
Outcome of delivery Z37.9
  multiple births Z37.9
    all liveborn Z37.50
      quadruplets Z37.52
      quintuplets Z37.53
      sextuplets Z37.54
      specified number NEC Z37.59
      triplets Z37.51
    all stillborn Z37.7
    some liveborn Z37.60
      quadruplets Z37.62
      quintuplets Z37.63
      sextuplets Z37.64
      specified number NEC Z37.69
      triplets Z37.61
  single NEC Z37.9
    liveborn Z37.0
    stillborn Z37.1
  twins NEC Z37.9
    both liveborn Z37.2
    both stillborn Z37.4
    one liveborn, one stillborn Z37.3
Outlet —see condition
Ovalocytosis (congenital) (hereditary) —see
  Elliptocytosis
Ovarian —see Condition
Ovariocele N83.4
Ovaritis (cystic) —see Oophoritis
Ovary, ovarian —see also condition
  resistant syndrome E28.39
  vein syndrome N13.8
Overactive —see also Hyperfunction
  adrenal cortex NEC E27.0
  bladder N32.81
  hypothalamus E23.3
  thyroid —see Hyperthyroidism
Overactivity R46.3
  child —see Disorder, attention-deficit
    hyperactivity
Overbite (deep) (excessive) (horizontal)
  (vertical) M26.29
Overbreathing —see Hyperventilation
Overconscientious personality F60.5

Overdevelopment —see Hypertrophy
Overdistension —see Distension
Overdose, overdosage (drug) —see Table
  of Drugs and Chemicals, by drug,
  poisoning
Overeating R63.2
  nonorganic origin F50.8
  psychogenic F50.8
Overexertion (effects) (exhaustion) T73.3
Overexposure (effects) T73.9
  exhaustion T73.2
Overfeeding —see Overeating
  newborn P92.4
Overfill, endodontic M27.52
Overgrowth, bone —see Hypertrophy, bone
Overhanging of dental restorative material
  (unrepairable) K08.52
Overheated (places) (effects) —see Heat
Overjet (excessive horizontal) M26.23
Overlaid, overlying (suffocation) —see Asphyxia,
  traumatic, due to mechanical threat
Overlap, excessive horizontal (teeth) M26.23
Overlapping toe (acquired) —see also
  Deformity, toe, specified NEC
  congenital (fifth toe) Q66.89
Overload
  circulatory, due to transfusion (blood) (blood
    components) (TACO) E87.71
  fluid E87.70
    due to transfusion (blood) (blood
      components) E87.71
    specified NEC E87.79
  iron, due to repeated red blood cell
    transfusions E83.111
  potassium (K) E87.5
  sodium (Na) E87.0
Overnutrition —see Hyperalimentation
Overproduction —see also Hypersecretion
  ACTH E27.0
  catecholamine E27.5
  growth hormone E22.0
Overprotection, child by parent Z62.1
Overriding
  aorta Q25.4
  finger (acquired) —see Deformity, finger
    congenital Q68.1
  toe (acquired) —see also Deformity, toe,
    specified NEC
    congenital Q66.89
Overstrained R53.83
  heart —see Hypertrophy, cardiac
Overuse, muscle NEC M70.8-
Overweight E66.3
Overworked R53.83
Oviduct —see condition
Ovotestis Q56.0
Ovulation (cycle)
  failure or lack of N97.0
  pain N94.0
Ovum —see condition
Owren's disease or syndrome (parahemophilia)
  D68.2
Ox heart —see Hypertrophy, cardiac
Oxalosis E72.53
Oxaluria E72.53
Oxycephaly, oxycephalic Q75.0
  syphilitic, congenital A50.02
Oxyuriasis B80
Oxyuris vermicularis (infestation) B80
Ozena J31.0

◄ New   ◄═ Revised   ~~deleted~~ Deleted

P

Pachyderma, pachydermia L85.9
  larynx (verrucosa) J38.7
Pachydermatocele (congenital) Q82.8
Pachydermoperiostosis —*see also*
    Osteoarthropathy, hypertrophic, specified
    type NEC
  clubbed nail M89.40 *[L62]*
Pachygyria Q04.3
Pachymeningitis (adhesive) (basal) (brain)
    (cervical) (chronic) (circumscribed)
    (external) (fibrous) (hemorrhagic)
    (hypertrophic) (internal) (purulent)
    (spinal) (suppurative) —*see* Meningitis
Pachyonychia (congenital) Q84.5
Pacinian tumor —*see* Neoplasm, skin, benign
Pad, knuckle or Garrod's M72.1
Paget-Schroetter syndrome I82.890
Paget's disease
  with infiltrating duct carcinoma —*see*
    Neoplasm, breast, malignant
  bone M88.9
    carpus M88.84-
    clavicle M88.81-
    femur M88.85-
    fibula M88.86-
    finger M88.84-
    humerus M88.82-
    ilium M88.85-
    in neoplastic disease —*see* Osteitis,
      deformans, in neoplastic disease
    ischium M88.85-
    metacarpus M88.84-
    metatarsus M88.87-
    multiple sites M88.89
    neck M88.88
    radius M88.83-
    rib M88.88
    scapula M88.81-
    skull M88.0
    tarsus M88.87-
    tibia M88.86-
    toe M88.87-
    ulna M88.83-
    vertebra M88.88
  breast (female) C50.01-
    male C50.02-
  extramammary —*see also* Neoplasm, skin,
    malignant
    anus C21.0
      margin C44.590
      skin C44.590
  intraductal carcinoma —*see* Neoplasm,
    breast, malignant
  malignant —*see* Neoplasm, skin, malignant
    breast (female) C50.01-
      male C50.02-
    unspecified site (female) C50.01-
      male C50.02-
  mammary —*see* Paget's disease, breast
  nipple —*see* Paget's disease, breast
  osteitis deformans —*see* Paget's disease, bone
Pain (s) (*see also* Painful) R52
  abdominal R10.9
    colic R10.83
    generalized R10.84
      with acute abdomen R10.0
    lower R10.30
      left quadrant R10.32
      pelvic or perineal R10.2
      periumbilical R10.33
      right quadrant R10.31
    rebound —*see* Tenderness, abdominal,
      rebound
    severe with abdominal rigidity R10.0
    tenderness —*see* Tenderness, abdominal
    upper R10.10
      epigastric R10.13
      left quadrant R10.12
      right quadrant R10.11

Pain *(Continued)*
  acute R52
    due to trauma G89.11
    neoplasm related G89.3
    postprocedural NEC G89.18
    post-thoracotomy G89.12
    specified by site — code to Pain, by site
  adnexa (uteri) R10.2
  anginoid —*see* Pain, precordial
  anus K62.89
  arm —*see* Pain, limb, upper
  axillary (axilla) M79.62-
  back (postural) M54.9
  bladder R39.89
    associated with micturition —*see*
      Micturition, painful
  bone —*see* Disorder, bone, specified type
    NEC
  breast N64.4
  broad ligament R10.2
  cancer associated (acute) (chronic) G89.3
  cecum —*see* Pain, abdominal
  cervicobrachial M53.1
  chest (central) R07.9
    anterior wall R07.89
    atypical R07.89
    ischemic I20.9
    musculoskeletal R07.89
    non-cardiac R07.89
    on breathing R07.1
    pleurodynia R07.81
    precordial R07.2
    wall (anterior) R07.89
  chronic G89.29
    associated with significant psychosocial
      dysfunction G89.4
    due to trauma G89.21
    neoplasm related G89.3
    postoperative NEC G89.28
    postprocedural NEC G89.28
    post-thoracotomy G89.22
    specified NEC G89.29
  coccyx M53.3
  colon —*see* Pain, abdominal
  coronary —*see* Angina
  costochondral R07.1
  diaphragm R07.1
  due to cancer G89.3
  due to device, implant or graft (*see also*
    Complications, by site and type,
    specified NEC) T85.84
    arterial graft NEC T82.848
    breast (implant) T85.84
    catheter NEC T85.84
      dialysis (renal) T82.848
        intraperitoneal T85.84
      infusion NEC T82.848
        spinal (epidural) (subdural) T85.84
      urinary (indwelling) T83.84
    electronic (electrode) (pulse generator)
      (stimulator)
      bone T84.84
      cardiac T82.847
      nervous system (brain) (peripheral
        nerve) (spinal) T85.84
      urinary T83.84
    fixation, internal (orthopedic) NEC
      T84.84
    gastrointestinal (bile duct) (esophagus)
      T85.84
    genital NEC T83.84
    heart NEC T82.847
    infusion NEC T85.84
    joint prosthesis T84.84
    ocular (corneal graft) (orbital implant)
      NEC T85.84
    orthopedic NEC T84.84
    specified NEC T85.84
    urinary NEC T83.84
    vascular NEC T82.848
    ventricular intracranial shunt T85.84

Pain *(Continued)*
  due to malignancy (primary) (secondary)
    G89.3
  ear —*see* subcategory H92.0
  epigastric, epigastrium R10.13
  eye —*see* Pain, ocular
  face, facial R51
    atypical G50.1
  female genital organs NEC N94.89
  finger —*see* Pain, limb, upper
  flank —*see* Pain, abdominal
  foot —*see* Pain, limb, lower
  gallbladder K82.9
  gas (intestinal) R14.1
  gastric —*see* Pain, abdominal
  generalized NOS R52
  genital organ
    female N94.89
    male N50.8
  groin —*see* Pain, abdominal, lower
  hand —*see* Pain, limb, upper
  head —*see* Headache
  heart —*see* Pain, precordial
  infra-orbital —*see* Neuralgia, trigeminal
  intercostal R07.82
  intermenstrual N94.0
  jaw R68.84
  joint M25.50
    ankle M25.57-
    elbow M25.52-
    finger M79.64-
    foot M25.57-
    hand M79.64-
    hip M25.55-
    knee M25.56-
    shoulder M25.51-
    toe M25.57-
    wrist M25.53-
  kidney N23
  laryngeal R07.0
  leg —*see* Pain, limb, lower
  limb M79.609
    lower M79.60-
      foot M79.67-
      lower leg M79.66-
      thigh M79.65-
      toe M79.67-
    upper M79.60-
      axilla M79.62-
      finger M79.64-
      forearm M79.63-
      hand M79.64-
      upper arm M79.62-
  loin M54.5
  low back M54.5
  lumbar region M54.5
  mandibular R68.84
  mastoid —*see* subcategory H92.0
  maxilla R68.84
  menstrual (*see also* Dysmenorrhea) N94.6
  metacarpophalangeal (joint) —*see* Pain, joint,
    hand
  metatarsophalangeal (joint) —*see* Pain, joint,
    foot
  mouth K13.79
  muscle —*see* Myalgia
  musculoskeletal (*see also* Pain, by site) M79.1
  myofascial M79.1
  nasal J34.89
  nasopharynx J39.2
  neck NEC M54.2
  nerve NEC —*see* Neuralgia
  neuromuscular —*see* Neuralgia
  nose J34.89
  ocular H57.1-
  ophthalmic —*see* Pain, ocular
  orbital region —*see* Pain, ocular
  ovary N94.89
  over heart —*see* Pain, precordial
  ovulation N94.0
  pelvic (female) R10.2

Pain *(Continued)*
  penis N48.89
  pericardial —*see* Pain, precordial
  perineal, perineum R10.2
  pharynx J39.2
  pleura, pleural, pleuritic R07.81
  postoperative NOS G89.18
  postprocedural NOS G89.18
  post-thoracotomy G89.12
  precordial (region) R07.2
  premenstrual N94.3
  psychogenic (persistent) (any site) F45.41
  radicular (spinal) —*see* Radiculopathy
  rectum K62.89
  respiration R07.1
  retrosternal R07.2
  rheumatoid, muscular —*see* Myalgia
  rib R07.81
  root (spinal) —*see* Radiculopathy
  round ligament (stretch) R10.2
  sacroiliac M53.3
  sciatic —*see* Sciatica
  scrotum N50.8
  seminal vesicle N50.8
  shoulder M25.51-
  spermatic cord N50.8
  spinal root —*see* Radiculopathy
  spine M54.9
    cervical M54.2
    low back M54.5
      with sciatica M54.4-
    thoracic M54.6
  stomach —*see* Pain, abdominal
  substernal R07.2
  temporomandibular (joint) M26.62
  testis N50.8
  thoracic spine M54.6
    with radicular and visceral pain
      M54.14
  throat R07.0
  tibia —*see* Pain, limb, lower
  toe —*see* Pain, limb, lower
  tongue K14.6
  tooth K08.8
  trigeminal —*see* Neuralgia, trigeminal
  tumor associated G89.3
  ureter N23
  urinary (organ) (system) N23
  uterus NEC N94.89
  vagina R10.2
  vertebrogenic (syndrome) M54.89
  vesical R39.89
    associated with micturition —*see*
      Micturition, painful
  vulva R10.2
Painful —*see also* Pain
  coitus
    female N94.1
    male N53.12
    psychogenic F52.6
  ejaculation (semen) N53.12
    psychogenic F52.6
  erection —*see* Priapism
  feet syndrome E53.8
  joint replacement (hip) (knee) T84.84
  menstruation —*see* Dysmenorrhea
    psychogenic F45.8
  micturition —*see* Micturition, painful
  respiration R07.1
  scar NEC L90.5
  wire sutures T81.89
Painter's colic —*see* subcategory T56.0
Palate —*see* condition
Palatoplegia K13.79
Palatoschisis —*see* Cleft, palate
Palilalia R48.8
Palliative care Z51.5
Pallor R23.1
  optic disc, temporal —*see* Atrophy, optic
Palmar —*see also* condition
  fascia —*see* condition

Palpable
  cecum K63.89
  kidney N28.89
  ovary N83.8
  prostate N42.9
  spleen —*see* Splenomegaly
Palpitations (heart) R00.2
  psychogenic F45.8
Palsy (*see also* Paralysis) G83.9
  atrophic diffuse (progressive) G12.22
  Bell's —*see also* Palsy, facial
    newborn P11.3
  brachial plexus NEC G54.0
    newborn (birth injury) P14.3
  brain —*see* Palsy, cerebral
  bulbar (progressive) (chronic) G12.22
    of childhood (Fazio-Londe) G12.1
    pseudo NEC G12.29
    supranuclear (progressive) G23.1
  cerebral (congenital) G80.9
    ataxic G80.4
    athetoid G80.3
    choreathetoid G80.3
    diplegic G80.8
      spastic G80.1
    dyskinetic G80.3
      athetoid G80.3
      choreathetoid G80.3
      distonic G80.3
    dystonic G80.3
    hemiplegic G80.8
      spastic G80.2
    mixed G80.8
    monoplegic G80.8
      spastic G80.1
    paraplegic G80.8
      spastic G80.1
    quadriplegic G80.8
      spastic G80.0
    spastic G80.1
      diplegic G80.1
      hemiplegic G80.2
      monoplegic G80.1
      quadriplegic G80.0
      specified NEC G80.1
      tetrapelgic G80.0
    specified NEC G80.8
    syphilitic A52.12
      congenital A50.49
    tetraplegic G80.8
      spastic G80.0
  cranial nerve —*see also* Disorder, nerve,
    cranial
    multiple G52.7
      in
        infectious disease B99 *[G53]*
        neoplastic disease (*see also* Neoplasm)
          D49.9 *[G53]*
        parasitic disease B89 *[G53]*
        sarcoidosis D86.82
  creeping G12.22
  diver's T70.3
  Erb's P14.0
  facial G51.0
    newborn (birth injury) P11.3
  glossopharyngeal G52.1
  Klumpke (-Déjérine) P14.1
  lead —*see* subcategory T56.0
  median nerve (tardy) G56.1-
  nerve G58.9
    specified NEC G58.8
  peroneal nerve (acute) (tardy) G57.3-
  progressive supranuclear G23.1
  pseudobulbar NEC G12.29
  radial nerve (acute) G56.3-
  seventh nerve —*see also* Palsy, facial
    newborn P11.3
  shaking —*see* Parkinsonism
  spastic (cerebral) (spinal) G80.1
  ulnar nerve (tardy) G56.2-
  wasting G12.29

Paludism —*see* Malaria
Panangiitis M30.0
Panaris, panaritium —*see also* Cellulitis, digit
  with lymphangitis —*see* Lymphangitis, acute,
    digit
Panarteritis nodosa M30.0
  brain or cerebral I67.7
Pancake heart R93.1
  with cor pulmonale (chronic) I27.81
Pancarditis (acute) (chronic) I51.89
  rheumatic I09.89
    active or acute I01.8
Pancoast's syndrome or tumor C34.1-
Pancolitis, ulcerative (chronic) K51.00
  with
    abscess K51.014
    complication K51.019
    fistula K51.013
    obstruction K51.012
    rectal bleeding K51.011
    specified complication NEC K51.018
Pancreas, pancreatic —*see* condition
Pancreatitis (annular) (apoplectic) (calcareous)
    (edematous) (hemorrhagic) (malignant)
    (recurrent) (subacute) (suppurative) K85.9
  acute K85.9
    alcohol induced K85.2
    biliary K85.1
    drug induced K85.3
    gallstone K85.1
    idiopathic K85.0
    specified NEC K85.8
  chronic (infectious) K86.1
    alcohol-induced K86.0
    recurrent K86.1
    relapsing K86.1
  cystic (chronic) K86.1
  cytomegaloviral B25.2
  fibrous (chronic) K86.1
  gallstone K85.1
  gangrenous K85.8
  interstitial (chronic) K86.1
    acute K85.8
  mumps B26.3
  recurrent (chronic) K86.1
  relapsing, chronic K86.1
  syphilitic A52.74
Pancreatoblastoma —*see* Neoplasm, pancreas,
  malignant
Pancreolithiasis K86.8
Pancytolysis D75.89
Pancytopenia (acquired) D61.818
  with
    malformations D61.09
    myelodysplastic syndrome —*see*
      Syndrome, myelodysplastic
  antineoplastic chemotherapy induced
    D61.810
  congenital D61.09
  drug-induced NEC D61.811
Panencephalitis, subacute, sclerosing
  A81.1
Panhematopenia D61.9
  congenital D61.09
  constitutional D61.09
  splenic, primary D73.1
Panhemocytopenia D61.9
  congenital D61.09
  constitutional D61.09
Panhypogonadism E29.1
Panhypopituitarism E23.0
  prepubertal E23.0
Panic (attack) (state) F41.0
  reaction to exceptional stress (transient)
    F43.0
Panmyelopathy, familial, constitutional
  D61.09
Panmyelophthisis D61.82
  congenital D61.09
Panmyelosis (acute) (with myelofibrosis)
  C94.4-

◀ New ◀◀◀ Revised ~~deleted~~ Deleted

Panner's disease —*see* Osteochondrosis, juvenile, humerus
Panneuritis endemica E51.11
Panniculitis (nodular) (nonsuppurative) M79.3
  back M54.00
    cervical region M54.02
    cervicothoracic region M54.03
    lumbar region M54.06
    lumbosacral region M54.07
    multiple sites M54.09
    occipito-atlanto-axial region M54.01
    sacrococcygeal region M54.08
    thoracic region M54.04
    thoracolumbar region M54.05
  lupus L93.2
  mesenteric K65.4
  neck M54.02
    cervicothoracic region M54.03
    occipito-atlanto-axial region M54.01
  relapsing M35.6
Panniculus adiposus (abdominal) E65
Pannus (allergic) (cornea) (degenerativus) (keratic) H16.42-
  abdominal (symptomatic) E65
  trachomatosus, trachomatous (active) A71.1
Panophthalmitis H44.01-
Pansinusitis (chronic) (hyperplastic) (nonpurulent) (purulent) J32.4
  acute J01.40
    recurrent J01.41
  tuberculous A15.8
Panuveitis (sympathetic) H44.11-
Panvalvular disease I08.9
  specified NEC I08.8
Papanicolaou smear, cervix Z12.4
  as part of routine gynecological examination Z01.419
    with abnormal findings Z01.411
  for suspected neoplasm Z12.4
  nonspecific abnormal finding R87.619
  routine Z01.419
    with abnormal findings Z01.411
Papilledema (choked disc) H47.10
  associated with
    decreased ocular pressure H47.12
    increased intracranial pressure H47.11
    retinal disorder H47.13
  Foster-Kennedy syndrome H47.14-
Papillitis H46.00
  anus K62.89
  chronic lingual K14.4
  necrotizing, kidney N17.2
  optic H46.0-
  rectum K62.89
  renal, necrotizing N17.2
  tongue K14.0
Papilloma —*see also* Neoplasm, benign, by site
  acuminatum (female) (male) (anogenital) A63.0
  benign pinta (primary) A67.0
  bladder (urinary) (transitional cell) D41.4
  choroid plexus (lateral ventricle) (third ventricle) D33.0
    anaplastic C71.5
    fourth ventricle D33.1
    malignant C71.5
  renal pelvis (transitional cell) D41.1-
    benign D30.1-
  Schneiderian
    specified site —*see* Neoplasm, benign, by site
    unspecified site D14.0
  serous surface
    borderline malignancy
      specified site —*see* Neoplasm, uncertain behavior, by site
      unspecified site D39.10
    specified site —*see* Neoplasm, benign, by site
    unspecified site D27.9

Papilloma (*Continued*)
  transitional (cell)
    bladder (urinary) D41.4
    inverted type —*see* Neoplasm, uncertain behavior, by site
    renal pelvis D41.1-
    ureter D41.2-
  ureter (transitional cell) D41.2-
    benign D30.2-
  urothelial —*see* Neoplasm, uncertain behavior, by site
  villous —*see* Neoplasm, uncertain behavior, by site
    adenocarcinoma in —*see* Neoplasm, malignant, by site
    in situ —*see* Neoplasm, in situ
  yaws, plantar or palmar A66.1
Papillomata, multiple, of yaws A66.1
Papillomatosis —*see also* Neoplasm, benign, by site
  confluent and reticulated L83
  cystic, breast —*see* Mastopathy, cystic
  ductal, breast —*see* Mastopathy, cystic
  intraductal (diffuse) —*see* Neoplasm, benign, by site
  subareolar duct D24-
Papillomavirus, as cause of disease classified elsewhere B97.7
Papillon-Léage and Psaume syndrome Q87.0
Papule (s) R23.8
  carate (primary) A67.0
  fibrous, of nose D22.39
  Gottron's L94.4
  pinta (primary) A67.0
Papulosis
  lymphomatoid C86.6
  malignant I77.89
Papyraceous fetus O31.0-
Para-albuminemia E88.09
Paracephalus Q89.7
Parachute mitral valve Q23.2
Paracoccidioidomycosis B41.9
  disseminated B41.7
  generalized B41.7
  mucocutaneous-lymphangitic B41.8
  pulmonary B41.0
  specified NEC B41.8
  visceral B41.8
Paradentosis K05.4
Paraffinoma T88.8
Paraganglioma D44.7
  adrenal D35.0-
    malignant C74.1-
  aortic body D44.7
    malignant C75.5
  carotid body D44.6
    malignant C75.4
  chromaffin —*see also* Neoplasm, benign, by site
    malignant —*see* Neoplasm, malignant, by site
  extra-adrenal D44.7
    malignant C75.5
      specified site —*see* Neoplasm, malignant, by site
      unspecified site C75.5
    specified site —*see* Neoplasm, uncertain behavior, by site
    unspecified site D44.7
  gangliocytic D13.2
    specified site —*see* Neoplasm, benign, by site
    unspecified site D13.2
  glomus jugulare D44.7
    malignant C75.5
  jugular D44.7
  malignant C75.5
    specified site —*see* Neoplasm, malignant, by site
    unspecified site C75.5

Paraganglioma (*Continued*)
  nonchromaffin D44.7
    malignant C75.5
      specified site —*see* Neoplasm, malignant, by site
      unspecified site C75.5
    specified site —*see* Neoplasm, uncertain behavior, by site
    unspecified site D44.7
  parasympathetic D44.7
    specified site —*see* Neoplasm, uncertain behavior, by site
    unspecified site D44.7
  specified site —*see* Neoplasm, uncertain behavior, by site
  sympathetic D44.7
    specified site —*see* Neoplasm, uncertain behavior, by site
    unspecified site D44.7
  unspecified site D44.7
Parageusia R43.2
  psychogenic F45.8
Paragonimiasis B66.4
Paragranuloma, Hodgkin —*see* Lymphoma, Hodgkin, classical, specified NEC
Parahemophilia (*see also* Defect, coagulation) D68.2
Parakeratosis R23.4
  variegata L41.0
Paralysis, paralytic (complete) (incomplete) G83.9
  with
    syphilis A52.17
  abducens, abducent (nerve) —*see* Strabismus, paralytic, sixth nerve
  abductor, lower extremity G57.9-
  accessory nerve G52.8
  accommodation —*see also* Paresis, of accommodation
    hysterical F44.89
  acoustic nerve (except Deafness) —*see* subcategory H93.3
  agitans (*see also* Parkinsonism) G20
    arteriosclerotic G21.4
  alternating (oculomotor) G83.89
  amyotrophic G12.21
  ankle G57.9-
  anus (sphincter) K62.89
  arm —*see* Monoplegia, upper limb
  ascending (spinal), acute G61.0
  association G12.29
  asthenic bulbar G70.00
    with exacerbation (acute) G70.01
    in crisis G70.01
  ataxic (hereditary) G11.9
    general (syphilitic) A52.17
  atrophic G58.9
    infantile, acute —*see* Poliomyelitis, paralytic
    progressive G12.22
    spinal (acute) —*see* Poliomyelitis, paralytic
  axillary G54.0
  Babinski-Nageotte's G83.89
  Bell's G51.0
    newborn P11.3
  Benedikt's G46.3
  birth injury P14.9
    spinal cord P11.5
  bladder (neurogenic) (sphincter) N31.2
  bowel, colon or intestine K56.0
  brachial plexus G54.0
    birth injury P14.3
    newborn (birth injury) P14.3
  brain G83.9
    diplegia G83.0
    triplegia G83.89
  bronchial J98.09
  Brown-Séquard G83.81

Paralysis, paralytic *(Continued)*
  bulbar (chronic) (progressive) G12.22
    infantile —*see* Poliomyelitis, paralytic
    poliomyelitic —*see* Poliomyelitis, paralytic
    pseudo G12.29
  bulbospinal G70.00
    with exacerbation (acute) G70.01
    in crisis G70.01
  cardiac (*see also* Failure, heart) I50.9
  cerebrocerebellar, diplegic G80.1
  cervical
    plexus G54.2
    sympathetic G90.09
  Céstan-Chenais G46.3
  Charcot-Marie-Tooth type G60.0
  Clark's G80.9
  colon K56.0
  compressed air T70.3
  compression
    arm G56.9-
    leg G57.9-
    lower extremity G57.9-
    upper extremity G56.9-
  congenital (cerebral) —*see* Palsy, cerebral
  conjugate movement (gaze) (of eye) H51.0
    cortical (nuclear) (supranuclear) H51.0
  cordis —*see* Failure, heart
  cranial or cerebral nerve G52.9
  creeping G12.22
  crossed leg G83.89
  crutch —*see* Injury, brachial plexus
  deglutition R13.0
    hysterical F44.4
  dementia A52.17
  descending (spinal) NEC G12.29
  diaphragm (flaccid) J98.6
    due to accidental dissection of phrenic
      nerve during procedure —*see*
      Puncture, accidental complicating
      surgery
  digestive organs NEC K59.8
  diplegic —*see* Diplegia
  divergence (nuclear) H51.8
  diver's T70.3
  Duchenne's
    birth injury P14.0
    due to or associated with
      motor neuron disease G12.22
      muscular dystrophy G71.0
    due to intracranial or spinal birth injury —*see*
      Palsy, cerebral
  embolic (current episode) I63.4
  Erb (-Duchenne) (birth) (newborn) P14.0
  Erb's syphilitic spastic spinal A52.17
  esophagus K22.8
  eye muscle (extrinsic) H49.9
    intrinsic —*see also* Paresis, of
      accommodation
  facial (nerve) G51.0
    birth injury P11.3
    congenital P11.3
    following operation NEC —*see* Puncture,
      accidental complicating surgery
    newborn (birth injury) P11.3
  familial (recurrent) (periodic) G72.3
    spastic G11.4
  fauces J39.2
  finger G56.9-
  gait R26.1
  gastric nerve (nondiabetic) G52.2
  gaze, conjugate H51.0
  general (progressive) (syphilitic) A52.17
    juvenile A50.45
  glottis J38.00
    bilateral J38.02
    unilateral J38.01
  gluteal G54.1
  Gubler (-Millard) G46.3
  hand —*see* Monoplegia, upper limb
  heart —*see* Arrest, cardiac
  hemiplegic —*see* Hemiplegia

Paralysis, paralytic *(Continued)*
  hyperkalemic periodic (familial) G72.3
  hypoglossal (nerve) G52.3
  hypokalemic periodic G72.3
  hysterical F44.4
  ileus K56.0
  infantile (*see also* Poliomyelitis, paralytic)
    A80.30
    bulbar —*see* Poliomyelitis, paralytic
    cerebral —*see* Palsy, cerebral
    spastic —*see* Palsy, cerebral, spastic
  infective —*see* Poliomyelitis, paralytic
  inferior nuclear G83.9
  internuclear —*see* Ophthalmoplegia,
    internuclear
  intestine K56.0
  iris H57.09
    due to diphtheria (toxin) A36.89
  ischemic, Volkmann's (complicating trauma)
    T79.6
  Jackson's G83.89
  jake —*see* Poisoning, food, noxious, plant
  Jamaica ginger (jake) G62.2
  juvenile general A50.45
  Klumpke (-Déjérine) (birth) (newborn) P14.1
  labioglossal (laryngeal) (pharyngeal) G12.29
  Landry's G61.0
  laryngeal nerve (recurrent) (superior)
    (unilateral) J38.00
    bilateral J38.02
    unilateral J38.01
  larynx J38.00
    bilateral J38.02
    due to diphtheria (toxin) A36.2
    unilateral J38.01
  lateral G12.21
  lead —*see* subcategory T56.0
  left side —*see* Hemiplegia
  leg G83.1-
    both —*see* Paraplegia
    crossed G83.89
    hysterical F44.4
    psychogenic F44.4
    transient or transitory R29.818
      traumatic NEC —*see* Injury, nerve, leg
  levator palpebrae superioris —*see*
    Blepharoptosis, paralytic
  limb —*see* Monoplegia
  lip K13.0
  Lissauer's A52.17
  lower limb —*see* Monoplegia, lower limb
    both —*see* Paraplegia
  lung J98.4
  median nerve G56.1-
  medullary (tegmental) G83.89
  mesencephalic NEC G83.89
    tegmental G83.89
  middle alternating G83.89
  Millard-Gubler-Foville G46.3
  monoplegic —*see* Monoplegia
  motor G83.9
  muscle, muscular NEC G72.89
    due to nerve lesion G58.9
    eye (extrinsic) H49.9
      intrinsic —*see* Paresis, of accommodation
      oblique —*see* Strabismus, paralytic,
        fourth nerve
    iris sphincter H21.9
    ischemic (Volkmann's) (complicating
      trauma) T79.6
    progressive G12.21
    pseudohypertrophic G71.0
  musculocutaneous nerve G56.9-
  musculospiral G56.9-
  nerve —*see also* Disorder, nerve
    abducent —*see* Strabismus, paralytic, sixth
      nerve
    accessory G52.8
    auditory (except Deafness) —*see*
      subcategory H93.3
    birth injury P14.9

Paralysis, paralytic *(Continued)*
  nerve *(Continued)*
    cranial or cerebral G52.9
    facial G51.0
      birth injury P11.3
      congenital P11.3
      newborn (birth injury) P11.3
    fourth or trochlear —*see* Strabismus,
      paralytic, fourth nerve
    newborn (birth injury) P14.9
    oculomotor —*see* Strabismus, paralytic,
      third nerve
    phrenic (birth injury) P14.2
    radial G56.3-
    seventh or facial G51.0
      newborn (birth injury) P11.3
    sixth or abducent —*see* Strabismus,
      paralytic, sixth nerve
    syphilitic A52.15
    third or oculomotor —*see* Strabismus,
      paralytic, third nerve
    trigeminal G50.9
    trochlear —*see* Strabismus, paralytic,
      fourth nerve
    ulnar G56.2-
  normokalemic periodic G72.3
  ocular H49.9
    alternating G83.89
  oculofacial, congenital (Moebius) Q87.0
  oculomotor (external bilateral) (nerve) —*see*
    Strabismus, paralytic, third nerve
  palate (soft) K13.79
  paratrigeminal G50.9
  periodic (familial) (hyperkalemic)
    (hypokalemic) (myotonic)
    (normokalemic) (potassium sensitive)
    (secondary) G72.3
  peripheral autonomic nervous system —*see*
    Neuropathy, peripheral, autonomic
  peroneal (nerve) G57.3-
  pharynx J39.2
  phrenic nerve G56.8-
  plantar nerve (s) G57.6-
  pneumogastric nerve G52.2
  poliomyelitis (current) —*see* Poliomyelitis,
    paralytic
  popliteal nerve G57.3-
  postepileptic transitory G83.84
  progressive (atrophic) (bulbar) (spinal)
    G12.22
    general A52.17
    infantile acute —*see* Poliomyelitis, paralytic
    supranuclear G23.1
  pseudobulbar G12.29
  pseudohypertrophic (muscle) G71.0
  psychogenic F44.4
  quadriceps G57.9-
  quadriplegic —*see* Tetraplegia
  radial nerve G56.3-
  rectus muscle (eye) H49.9
  recurrent isolated sleep G47.53
  respiratory (muscle) (system) (tract) R06.81
    center NEC G93.89
    congenital P28.89
    newborn P28.89
  right side —*see* Hemiplegia
  saturnine —*see* subcategory T56.0
  sciatic nerve G57.0-
  senile G83.9
  shaking —*see* Parkinsonism
  shoulder G56.9-
  sleep, recurrent isolated G47.53
  spastic G83.9
    cerebral —*see* Palsy, cerebral, spastic
    congenital (cerebral) —*see* Palsy, cerebral,
      spastic
    familial G11.4
    hereditary G11.4
    quadriplegic G80.0
    syphilitic (spinal) A52.17
  sphincter, bladder —*see* Paralysis, bladder

◀ New   ◀▦ Revised   ~~deleted~~ Deleted

Paralysis, paralytic (Continued)
  spinal (cord) G83.9
    accessory nerve G52.8
    acute —see Poliomyelitis, paralytic
    ascending acute G61.0
    atrophic (acute) —see also Poliomyelitis,
      paralytic
      spastic, syphilitic A52.17
    congenital NEC —see Palsy, cerebral
    hereditary G95.89
    infantile —see Poliomyelitis, paralytic
    progressive G12.21
    sequelae NEC G83.89
  sternomastoid G52.8
  stomach K31.84
    diabetic —see Diabetes, by type, with
      gastroparesis
    nerve G52.2
      diabetic —see Diabetes, by type, with
        gastroparesis
  stroke —see Infarct, brain
  subcapsularis G56.8-
  supranuclear (progressive) G23.1
  sympathetic G90.8
    cervical G90.09
    nervous system —see Neuropathy,
      peripheral, autonomic
  syndrome G83.9
    specified NEC G83.89
  syphilitic spastic spinal (Erb's) A52.17
  thigh G57.9-
  throat J39.2
    diphtheritic A36.0
    muscle J39.2
  thrombotic (current episode) I63.3
  thumb G56.9-
  tick —see Toxicity, venom, arthropod,
    specified NEC
  Todd's (postepileptic transitory paralysis)
    G83.84
  toe G57.6-
  tongue K14.8
  transient R29.5
    arm or leg NEC R29.818
    traumatic NEC —see Injury, nerve
  trapezius G52.8
  traumatic, transient NEC —see Injury,
    nerve
  trembling —see Parkinsonism
  triceps brachii G56.9-
  trigeminal nerve G50.9
  trochlear (nerve) —see Strabismus, paralytic,
    fourth nerve
  ulnar nerve G56.2-
  upper limb —see Monoplegia, upper limb
  uremic N18.9 [G99.8]
  uveoparotitic D86.89
  uvula K13.79
    postdiphtheritic A36.0
  vagus nerve G52.2
  vasomotor NEC G90.8
  velum palati K13.79
  vesical —see Paralysis, bladder
  vestibular nerve (except Vertigo) —see
    subcategory H93.3
  vocal cords J38.00
    bilateral J38.02
    unilateral J38.01
  Volkmann's (complicating trauma) T79.6
  wasting Q12.29
  Weber's G46.3
  wrist G56.9-
Paramedial urethrovesical orifice Q64.79
Paramenia N92.6
Parametritis (see also Disease, pelvis,
    inflammatory) N73.2
  acute N73.0
  complicating abortion —see Abortion, by
    type, complicated by, parametritis
Parametrium, parametric —see condition
Paramnesia —see Amnesia

Paramolar K00.1
Paramyloidosis E85.8
Paramyoclonus multiplex G25.3
Paramyotonia (congenita) G71.19
Parangi —see Yaws
Paranoia (querulans) F22
  senile F03
Paranoid
  dementia (senile) F03
    praecox —see Schizophrenia
  personality F60.0
  psychosis (climacteric) (involutional)
    (menopausal) F22
    psychogenic (acute) F23
    senile F03
  reaction (acute) F23
    chronic F22
  schizophrenia F20.0
  state (climacteric) (involutional)
    (menopausal) (simple) F22
    senile F03
  tendencies F60.0
  traits F60.0
  trends F60.0
  type, psychopathic personality F60.0
Paraparesis —see Paraplegia
Paraphasia R47.02
Paraphilia F65.9
Paraphimosis (congenital) N47.2
  chancroidal A57
Paraphrenia, paraphrenic (late) F22
  schizophrenia F20.0
Paraplegia (lower) G82.20
  ataxic —see Degeneration, combined, spinal
    cord
  complete G82.21
  congenital (cerebral) G80.8
    spastic G80.1
  familial spastic G11.4
  functional (hysterical) F44.4
  hereditary, spastic G11.4
  hysterical F44.4
  incomplete G82.22
  Pott's A18.01
  psychogenic F44.4
  spastic
    Erb's spinal, syphilitic A52.17
    hereditary G11.4
    tropical G04.1
  syphilitic (spastic) A52.17
  tropical spastic G04.1
Parapoxvirus B08.60
  specified NEC B08.69
Paraproteinemia D89.2
  benign (familial) D89.2
  monoclonal D47.2
  secondary to malignant disease D47.2
Parapsoriasis L41.9
  en plaques L41.4
  guttata L41.1
  large plaque L41.4
  retiform, retiformis L41.5
  small plaque L41.3
  specified NEC L41.8
  varioliformis (acuta) L41.0
Parasitic —see also condition
  disease NEC B89
  stomatitis B37.0
  sycosis (beard) (scalp) B35.0
  twin Q89.4
Parasitism B89
  intestinal B82.9
  skin B88.9
  specified —see Infestation
Parasitophobia F40.218
Parasomnia G47.50
  due to
    alcohol
      abuse F10.182
      dependence F10.282
      use F10.982

Parasomnia (Continued)
  due to (Continued)
    amphetamines
      abuse F15.182
      dependence F15.282
      use F15.982
    caffeine
      abuse F15.182
      dependence F15.282
      use F15.982
    cocaine
      abuse F14.182
      dependence F14.282
      use F14.982
    drug NEC
      abuse F19.182
      dependence F19.282
      use F19.982
    opioid
      abuse F11.182
      dependence F11.282
      use F11.982
    psychoactive substance NEC
      abuse F19.182
      dependence F19.282
      use F19.982
    sedative, hypnotic, or anxiolytic
      abuse F13.182
      dependence F13.282
      use F13.982
    stimulant NEC
      abuse F15.182
      dependence F15.282
      use F15.982
  in conditions classified elsewhere G47.54
  nonorganic origin F51.8
  organic G47.50
  specified NEC G47.59
Paraspadias Q54.9
Paraspasmus facialis G51.8
Parasuicide (attempt)
  history of (personal) Z91.5
    in family Z81.8
Parathyroid gland —see condition
Parathyroid tetany E20.9
Paratrachoma A74.0
Paratyphilitis —see Appendicitis
Paratyphoid (fever) —see Fever, paratyphoid
Paratyphus —see Fever, paratyphoid
Paraurethral duct Q64.79
  nonorganic origin F51.5
Paraurethritis —see also Urethritis
  gonococcal (acute) (chronic) (with abscess)
    A54.1
Paravaccinia NEC B08.04
Paravaginitis —see Vaginitis
Parencephalitis —see also Encephalitis
  sequelae G09
Parent-child conflict —see Conflict, parent-child
  estrangement NEC Z62.890
Paresis —see also Paralysis
  accommodation —see Paresis, of
    accommodation
  Bernhardt's G57.1-
  bladder (sphincter) —see also Paralysis,
    bladder
    tabetic A52.17
  bowel, colon or intestine K56.0
  extrinsic muscle, eye H49.9
  general (progressive) (syphilitic) A52.17
    juvenile A50.45
  heart —see Failure, heart
  insane (syphilitic) A52.17
  juvenile (general) A50.45
  of accommodation H52.52-
  peripheral progressive (idiopathic) G60.3
  pseudohypertrophic G71.0
  senile G83.9
  syphilitic (general) A52.17
    congenital A50.45
  vesical NEC N31.2

Paresthesia —*see also* Disturbance, sensation
   Bernhardt G57.1-
Paretic —*see* condition
Parinaud's
   conjunctivitis H10.89
   oculoglandular syndrome H10.89
   ophthalmoplegia H49.88
Parkinsonism (idiopathic) (primary) G20
   with neurogenic orthostatic hypotension
      (symptomatic) G90.3
   arteriosclerotic G21.4
   dementia G31.83 *[F02.80]*
      with behavioral disturbance G31.83
         [F02.81]
   due to
      drugs NEC G21.19
         neuroleptic G21.11
   neuroleptic induced G21.11
   postencephalitic G21.3
   secondary G21.9
      due to
         arteriosclerosis G21.4
         drugs NEC G21.19
            neuroleptic G21.11
         encephalitis G21.3
         external agents NEC G21.2
         syphilis A52.19
         specified NEC G21.8
   syphilitic A52.19
   treatment-induced NEC G21.19
   vascular G21.4
Parkinson's disease, syndrome or tremor —*see*
   Parkinsonism
Parodontitis —*see* Periodontitis
Parodontosis K05.4
Paronychia —*see also* Cellulitis, digit
   with lymphangitis —*see* Lymphangitis, acute,
      digit
   candidal (chronic) B37.2
   tuberculous (primary) A18.4
Parorexia (psychogenic) F50.8
Parosmia R43.1
   psychogenic F45.8
Parotid gland —*see* condition
Parotitis, parotiditis (allergic) (nonspecific
   toxic) (purulent) (septic) (suppurative) —
   see also Sialoadenitis
   epidemic —*see* Mumps
   infectious —*see* Mumps
   postoperative K91.89
   surgical K91.89
Parrot fever A70
Parrot's disease (early congenital syphilitic
   pseudoparalysis) A50.02
Parry-Romberg syndrome G51.8
Parry's disease or syndrome E05.00
   with thyroid storm E05.01
Pars planitis —*see* Cyclitis
Parsonage (-Aldren)-Turner syndrome G54.5
Parson's disease (exophthalmic goiter)
   E05.00
   with thyroid storm E05.01
Particolored infant Q82.8
Parturition —*see* Delivery
Parulis K04.7
   with sinus K04.6
Parvovirus, as cause of disease classified
   elsewhere B97.6
Pasini and Pierini's atrophoderma L90.3
Passage
   false, urethra N36.5
   meconium (newborn) during delivery
      P03.82
   of sounds or bougies —*see* Attention to,
      artificial, opening
Passive —*see* condition
   smoking Z77.22
Pasteurella septica A28.0
Pasteurellosis —*see* Infection, Pasteurella
PAT (paroxysmal atrial tachycardia) I47.1
Patau's syndrome —*see* Trisomy, 13

Patches
   mucous (syphilitic) A51.39
      congenital A50.07
   smokers' (mouth) K13.24
Patellar —*see* condition
Patent —*see also* Imperfect, closure
   canal of Nuck Q52.4
   cervix N88.3
   ductus arteriosus or Botallo's Q25.0
   foramen
      botalli Q21.1
      ovale Q21.1
   interauricular septum Q21.1
   interventricular septum Q21.0
   omphalomesenteric duct Q43.0
   os (uteri) —*see* Patent, cervix
   ostium secundum Q21.1
   urachus Q64.4
   vitelline duct Q43.0
Paterson (-Brown)(-Kelly) syndrome or web
   D50.1
Pathologic, pathological —*see also* condition
   asphyxia R09.01
   fire-setting F63.1
   gambling F63.0
   ovum O02.0
   resorption, tooth K03.3
   stealing F63.2
Pathology (of) —*see* Disease
   periradicular, associated with previous
      endodontic treatment NEC M27.59
Pattern, sleep-wake, irregular G47.23
Patulous —*see also* Imperfect, closure
   (congenital)
   alimentary tract Q45.8
      lower Q43.8
      upper Q40.8
   eustachian tube H69.0-
Pause, sinoatrial I49.5
Paxton's disease B36.2
Pearl (s)
   enamel K00.2
   Epstein's K09.8
Pearl-worker's disease —*see* Osteomyelitis,
   specified type NEC
Pectenosis K62.4
Pectoral —*see* condition
Pectus
   carinatum (congenital) Q67.7
      acquired M95.4
      rachitic sequelae (late effect) E64.3
   excavatum (congenital) Q67.6
      acquired M95.4
      rachitic sequelae (late effect) E64.3
   recurvatum (congenital) Q67.6
Pedatrophia E41
Pederosis F65.4
Pediculosis (infestation) B85.2
   capitis (head-louse) (any site) B85.0
   corporis (body-louse) (any site) B85.1
   eyelid B85.0
   mixed (classifiable to more than one of the
      titles B85.0-B85.3) B85.4
   pubis (pubic louse) (any site) B85.3
   vestimenti B85.1
   vulvae B85.3
Pediculus (infestation) —*see* Pediculosis
Pedophilia F65.4
Peg-shaped teeth K00.2
Pelade —*see* Alopecia, areata
Pelger-Huët anomaly or syndrome D72.0
Peliosis (rheumatica) D69.0
   hepatis K76.4
      with toxic liver disease K71.8
Pelizaeus-Merzbacher disease E75.29
Pellagra (alcoholic) (with polyneuropathy) E52
Pellagra-cerebellar-ataxia-renal aminoaciduria
   syndrome E72.02
Pellegrini (-Stieda) disease or syndrome —*see*
   Bursitis, tibial collateral
Pellizzi's syndrome E34.8

Pel's crisis A52.11
Pelvic —*see also* condition
   examination (periodic) (routine) Z01.419
      with abnormal findings Z01.411
   kidney, congenital Q63.2
Pelviolithiasis —*see* Calculus, kidney
Pelviperitonitis —*see also* Peritonitis, pelvic
   gonococcal A54.24
   puerperal O85
Pelvis —*see* condition or type
Pemphigoid L12.9
   benign, mucous membrane L12.1
   bullous L12.0
   cicatricial L12.1
   juvenile L12.2
   ocular L12.1
   specified NEC L12.8
Pemphigus L10.9
   benign familial (chronic) Q82.8
   Brazilian L10.3
   circinatus L13.0
   conjunctiva L12.1
   drug-induced L10.5
   erythematosus L10.4
   foliaceous L10.2
   gangrenous —*see* Gangrene
   neonatorum L01.03
   ocular L12.1
   paraneoplastic L10.81
   specified NEC L10.89
   syphilitic (congenital) A50.06
   vegetans L10.1
   vulgaris L10.0
   wildfire L10.3
Pendred's syndrome E07.1
Pendulous
   abdomen, in pregnancy —*see* Pregnancy,
      complicated by, abnormal, pelvic organs
      or tissues NEC
   breast N64.89
Penetrating wound —*see also* Puncture
   with internal injury —*see* Injury, by site
   eyeball —*see* Puncture, eyeball
   orbit (with or without foreign body) —*see*
      Puncture, orbit
   uterus by instrument with or following
      ectopic or molar pregnancy O08.6
Penicillosis B48.4
Penis —*see* condition
Penitis N48.29
Pentalogy of Fallot Q21.8
Pentasomy X syndrome Q97.1
Pentosuria (essential) E74.8
Percreta placenta O43.23-
Peregrinating patient —*see* Disorder, factitious
Perforation, perforated (nontraumatic) (of)
   accidental during procedure (blood vessel)
      (nerve) (organ) —*see* Complication,
      accidental puncture or laceration
   antrum —*see* Sinusitis, maxillary
   appendix K35.2
   atrial septum, multiple Q21.1
   attic, ear —*see* Perforation, tympanum, attic
   bile duct (common) (hepatic) K83.2
      cystic K82.2
   bladder (urinary)
      with or following ectopic or molar
         pregnancy O08.6
      obstetrical trauma O71.5
      traumatic S37.29
         at delivery O71.5
   bowel K63.1
      with or following ectopic or molar
         pregnancy O08.6
      newborn P78.0
      obstetrical trauma O71.5
      traumatic —*see* Laceration, intestine
   broad ligament N83.8
      with or following ectopic or molar
         pregnancy O08.6
      obstetrical trauma O71.6

◀ New   ◀◀ Revised   ~~deleted~~ Deleted

Perforation, perforated (Continued)
  by
    device, implant or graft (see also
        Complications, by site and type,
        mechanical) T85.628
      arterial graft NEC —see Complication,
          cardiovascular device, mechanical,
          vascular
      breast (implant) T85.49
      catheter NEC T85.698
        cystostomy T83.090
        dialysis (renal) T82.49
          intraperitoneal T85.691
        infusion NEC T82.594
          spinal (epidural) (subdural)
              T85.690
      electronic (electrode) (pulse generator)
          (stimulator)
        bone T84.390
        cardiac T82.199
          electrode T82.190
          pulse generator T82.191
          specified type NEC T82.198
        nervous system —see Complication,
            prosthetic device, mechanical,
            electronic nervous system
            stimulator
        urinary —see Complication,
            genitourinary, device, urinary,
            mechanical
      fixation, internal (orthopedic) NEC —see
          Complication, fixation device,
          mechanical
      gastrointestinal —see Complications,
          prosthetic device, mechanical,
          gastrointestinal device
      genital NEC T83.498
        intrauterine contraceptive device
            T83.39
        penile prosthesis T83.490
      heart NEC —see Complication,
          cardiovascular device,
          mechanical
      joint prosthesis —see Complications,
          joint prosthesis, mechanical,
          specified NEC, by site
      ocular NEC —see Complications,
          prosthetic device, mechanical,
          ocular device
      orthopedic NEC —see Complication,
          orthopedic, device, mechanical
      specified NEC T85.628
      urinary NEC —see also Complication,
          genitourinary, device, urinary,
          mechanical
        graft T83.29
        urinary, indwelling T83.098
      vascular NEC —see Complication,
          cardiovascular device,
          mechanical
      ventricular intracranial shunt
          T85.09
    foreign body left accidentally in
        operative wound T81.539
    instrument (any) during a procedure,
        accidental —see Puncture, accidental
        complicating surgery
  cecum K35.2
  cervix (uteri) N88.8
    with or following ectopic or molar
        pregnancy O08.6
    obstetrical trauma O71.3
  colon K63.1
    newborn P78.0
    obstetrical trauma O71.5
    traumatic —see Laceration, intestine,
        large
  common duct (bile) K83.2
  cornea (due to ulceration) —see Ulcer,
      cornea, perforated
  cystic duct K82.2

Perforation, perforated (Continued)
  diverticulum (intestine) K57.80
    with bleeding K57.81
    large intestine K57.20
      with
        bleeding K57.21
        small intestine K57.40
          with bleeding K57.41
    small intestine K57.00
      with
        bleeding K57.01
        large intestine K57.40
          with bleeding K57.41
  ear drum —see Perforation, tympanum
  esophagus K22.3
  ethmoidal sinus —see Sinusitis, ethmoidal
  frontal sinus —see Sinusitis, frontal
  gallbladder K82.2
  heart valve —see Endocarditis
  ileum K63.1
    newborn P78.0
    obstetrical trauma O71.5
    traumatic —see Laceration, intestine, small
  instrumental, surgical (accidental) (blood
      vessel) (nerve) (organ) —see Puncture,
      accidental complicating surgery
  intestine NEC K63.1
    with ectopic or molar pregnancy O08.6
    newborn P78.0
    obstetrical trauma O71.5
    traumatic —see Laceration, intestine
    ulcerative NEC K63.1
      newborn P78.0
  jejunum, jejunal K63.1
    obstetrical trauma O71.5
    traumatic —see Laceration, intestine, small
    ulcer —see Ulcer, gastrojejunal, with
        perforation
  joint prosthesis —see Complications, joint
      prosthesis, mechanical, specified NEC,
      by site
  mastoid (antrum) (cell) —see Disorder,
      mastoid, specified NEC
  maxillary sinus —see Sinusitis, maxillary
  membrana tympani —see Perforation,
      tympanum
  nasal
    septum J34.89
      congenital Q30.3
      syphilitic A52.73
    sinus J34.89
      congenital Q30.8
      due to sinusitis —see Sinusitis
  palate (see also Cleft, palate) Q35.9
    syphilitic A52.79
  palatine vault (see also Cleft, palate, hard)
      Q35.1
    syphilitic A52.79
    congenital A50.59
  pars flaccida (ear drum) —see Perforation,
      tympanum, attic
  pelvic
    floor S31.030
      with
        ectopic or molar pregnancy O08.6
        penetration into retroperitoneal space
            S31.031
        retained foreign body S31.040
          with penetration into
              retroperitoneal space S31.041
      following ectopic or molar pregnancy
          O08.6
      obstetrical trauma O70.1
    organ S37.99
      adrenal gland S37.818
      bladder —see Perforation, bladder
      fallopian tube S37.599
        bilateral S37.592
        unilateral S37.591
      kidney S37.09-
        obstetrical trauma O71.5

Perforation, perforated (Continued)
  pelvic (Continued)
    organ (Continued)
      ovary S37.499
        bilateral S37.492
        unilateral S37.491
      prostate S37.828
      specified organ NEC S37.898
      ureter —see Perforation, ureter
      urethra —see Perforation, urethra
      uterus —see Perforation, uterus
    perineum —see Laceration, perineum
  pharynx J39.2
  rectum K63.1
    newborn P78.0
    obstetrical trauma O71.5
    traumatic S36.63
  root canal space due to endodontic treatment
      M27.51
  sigmoid K63.1
    newborn P78.0
    obstetrical trauma O71.5
    traumatic S36.533
  sinus (accessory) (chronic) (nasal) J34.89
  sphenoidal sinus —see Sinusitis, sphenoidal
  surgical (accidental) (by instrument) (blood
      vessel) (nerve) (organ) —see Puncture,
      accidental complicating surgery
  traumatic
    external —see Puncture
    eye —see Puncture, eyeball
    internal organ —see Injury, by site
  tympanum, tympanic (membrane) (persistent
      post-traumatic) (postinflammatory)
      H72.9-
    attic H72.1-
      multiple —see Perforation, tympanum,
          multiple
      total —see Perforation, tympanum, total
    central H72.0-
      multiple —see Perforation, tympanum,
          multiple
      total —see Perforation, tympanum, total
    marginal NEC —see subcategory H72.2
    multiple H72.81-
    pars flaccida —see Perforation, tympanum,
        attic
    total H72.82-
    traumatic, current episode S09.2-
  typhoid, gastrointestinal —see Typhoid
  ulcer —see Ulcer, by site, with perforation
  ureter N28.89
    traumatic S37.19
  urethra N36.8
    with ectopic or molar pregnancy O08.6
    following ectopic or molar pregnancy
        O08.6
    obstetrical trauma O71.5
    traumatic S37.39
      at delivery O71.5
  uterus
    with ectopic or molar pregnancy O08.6
    by intrauterine contraceptive device T83.39
    following ectopic or molar pregnancy
        O08.6
    obstetrical trauma O71.1
    traumatic S37.69
      obstetric O71.1
  uvula K13.79
    syphilitic A52.79
  vagina
    obstetrical trauma O71.4
    other trauma - see Puncture, vagina
Periadenitis mucosa necrotica recurrens K12.0
Periappendicitis (acute) —see Appendicitis
Periarteritis nodosa (disseminated) (infectious)
    (necrotizing) M30.0
Periarthritis (joint) —see also Enthesopathy
  Duplay's M75.0-
  gonococcal A54.42
  humeroscapularis —see Capsulitis, adhesive

Periarthritis *(Continued)*
  scapulohumeral —*see* Capsulitis, adhesive
  shoulder —*see* Capsulitis, adhesive
  wrist M77.2-
Periarthrosis (angioneural) —*see*
  Enthesopathy
Pericapsulitis, adhesive (shoulder) —*see*
  Capsulitis, adhesive
Pericarditis (with decompensation) (with
    effusion) I31.9
  with rheumatic fever (conditions in I00)
    active —*see* Pericarditis, rheumatic
    inactive or quiescent I09.2
  acute (hemorrhagic) (nonrheumatic) (Sicca)
    I30.9
    with chorea (acute) (rheumatic)
      (Sydenham's) I02.0
    benign I30.8
    nonspecific I30.0
    rheumatic I01.0
      with chorea (acute) (Sydenham's)
        I02.0
  adhesive or adherent (chronic) (external)
    (internal) I31.0
    acute —*see* Pericarditis, acute
    rheumatic I09.2
  bacterial (acute) (subacute) (with serous or
    seropurulent effusion) I30.1
  calcareous I31.1
  cholesterol (chronic) I31.8
    acute I30.9
  chronic (nonrheumatic) I31.9
    rheumatic I09.2
  constrictive (chronic) I31.1
  coxsackie B33.23
  fibrinocaseous (tuberculous) A18.84
  fibrinopurulent I30.1
  fibrinous I30.8
  fibrous I31.0
  gonococcal A54.83
  idiopathic I30.0
  in systemic lupus erythematosus M32.12
  infective I30.1
  meningococcal A39.53
  neoplastic (chronic) I31.8
    acute I30.9
  obliterans, obliterating I31.0
  plastic I31.0
  pneumococcal I30.1
  postinfarction I24.1
  purulent I30.1
  rheumatic (active) (acute) (with effusion)
    (with pneumonia) I01.0
    with chorea (acute) (rheumatic)
      (Sydenham's) I02.0
    chronic or inactive (with chorea) I09.2
  rheumatoid —*see* Rheumatoid, carditis
  septic I30.1
  serofibrinous I30.8
  staphylococcal I30.1
  streptococcal I30.1
  suppurative I30.1
  syphilitic A52.06
  tuberculous A18.84
  uremic N18.9 *[I32]*
  viral I30.1
Pericardium, pericardial —*see* condition
Pericellulitis —*see* Cellulitis
Pericementitis (chronic) (suppurative) —*see also*
  Periodontitis
  acute K05.20
    generalized K05.22
    localized K05.21
Perichondritis
  auricle —*see* Perichondritis, ear
  bronchus J98.09
  ear (external) H61.00-
    acute H61.01-
    chronic H61.02-
    external auditory canal —*see* Perichondritis,
      ear

Perichondritis *(Continued)*
  larynx J38.7
    syphilitic A52.73
    typhoid A01.09
  nose J34.89
  pinna —*see* Perichondritis, ear
  trachea J39.8
Periclasia K05.4
Pericoronitis —*see* Periodontitis
Pericystitis N30.90
  with hematuria N30.91
Peridiverticulitis (intestine) K57.92
  cecum —*see* Diverticulitis, intestine, large
  colon —*see* Diverticulitis, intestine, large
  duodenum —*see* Diverticulitis, intestine,
    small
  intestine —*see* Diverticulitis, intestine
  jejunum —*see* Diverticulitis, intestine, small
  rectosigmoid —*see* Diverticulitis, intestine,
    large
  rectum —*see* Diverticulitis, intestine, large
  sigmoid —*see* Diverticulitis, intestine, large
Periendocarditis —*see* Endocarditis
Periepididymitis N45.1
Perifolliculitis L01.02
  abscedens, caput, scalp L66.3
  capitis, abscedens (et suffodiens) L66.3
  superficial pustular L01.02
Perihepatitis K65.8
Perilabyrinthitis (acute) —*see* subcategory
  H83.0
Perimeningitis —*see* Meningitis
Perimetritis —*see* Endometritis
Perimetrosalpingitis —*see* Salpingo-oophoritis
Perineocele N81.81
Perinephric, perinephritic —*see* condition
Perinephritis —*see also* Infection, kidney
  purulent —*see* Abscess, kidney
Perineum, perineal —*see* condition
Perineuritis NEC —*see* Neuralgia
Periodic —*see* condition
Periodontitis (chronic) (complex) (compound)
    (local) (simplex) K05.30
  acute K05.20
    generalized K05.22
    localized K05.21
  apical K04.5
    acute (pulpal origin) K04.4
  generalized K05.32
  localized K05.31
Periodontoclasia K05.4
Periodontosis (juvenile) K05.4
Periods —*see also* Menstruation
  heavy N92.0
  irregular N92.6
  shortened intervals (irregular) N92.1
Perionychia —*see also* Cellulitis, digit
  with lymphangitis —*see* Lymphangitis, acute,
    digit
Perioophoritis —*see* Salpingo-oophoritis
Periorchitis N45.2
Periosteum, periosteal —*see* condition
Periostitis (albuminosa) (circumscribed)
    (diffuse) (infective) (monomelic) —*see also*
    Osteomyelitis
  alveolar M27.3
  alveolodental M27.3
  dental M27.3
  gonorrheal A54.43
  jaw (lower) (upper) M27.2
  orbit H05.03-
  syphilitic A52.77
    congenital (early) A50.02 *[M90.80]*
    secondary A51.46
  tuberculous —*see* Tuberculosis, bone
  yaws (hypertrophic) (early) (late) A66.6
    [M90.80]
Periostosis (hyperplastic) —*see also* Disorder,
    bone, specified type NEC
  with osteomyelitis —*see* Osteomyelitis,
    specified type NEC

Peripartum
  cardiomyopathy O90.3
Periphlebitis —*see* Phlebitis
Periproctitis K62.89
Periprostatitis —*see* Prostatitis
Perirectal —*see* condition
Perirenal —*see* condition
Perisalpingitis —*see* Salpingo-oophoritis
Perisplenitis (infectional) D73.89
Peristalsis, visible or reversed R19.2
Peritendinitis —*see* Enthesopathy
Peritoneum, peritoneal —*see* condition
Peritonitis (adhesive) (bacterial) (fibrinous)
    (hemorrhagic) (idiopathic) (localized)
    (perforative) (primary) (with adhesions)
    (with effusion) K65.9
  with or following
    abscess K65.1
    appendicitis K35.2
      with perforation or rupture K35.2
      generalized K35.2
      localized K35.3
    diverticular disease (intestine) K57.80
      with bleeding K57.81
      ectopic or molar pregnancy O08.0
      large intestine K57.20
        with
          bleeding K57.21
          small intestine K57.40
            with bleeding K57.41
      small intestine K57.00
        with
          bleeding K57.01
          large intestine K57.40
            with bleeding K57.41
  acute (generalized) K65.0
  aseptic T81.61
  bile, biliary K65.3
  chemical T81.61
  chlamydial A74.81
  chronic proliferative K65.8
  complicating abortion —*see* Abortion, by
    type, complicated by, pelvic peritonitis
  congenital P78.1
  diaphragmatic K65.0
  diffuse K65.0
  diphtheritic A36.89
  disseminated K65.0
  due to
    bile K65.3
    foreign
      body or object accidentally left during
        a procedure (instrument) (sponge)
        (swab) T81.599
      substance accidentally left during a
        procedure (chemical) (powder)
        (talc) T81.61
    talc T81.61
    urine K65.8
  eosinophilic K65.8
    acute K65.0
  fibrocaseous (tuberculous) A18.31
  fibropurulent K65.0
  following ectopic or molar pregnancy O08.0
  general (ized) K65.0
  gonococcal A54.85
  meconium (newborn) P78.0
  neonatal P78.1
    meconium P78.0
  pancreatic K65.0
  paroxysmal, familial E85.0
    benign E85.0
  pelvic
    female N73.5
      acute N73.3
      chronic N73.4
        with adhesions N73.6
    male K65.0
  periodic, familial E85.0
  proliferative, chronic K65.8
  puerperal, postpartum, childbirth O85

Peritonitis (Continued)
  purulent K65.0
  septic K65.0
  specified NEC K65.8
  spontaneous bacterial K65.2
  subdiaphragmatic K65.0
  subphrenic K65.0
  suppurative K65.0
  syphilitic A52.74
    congenital (early) A50.08 [K67]
  talc T81.61
  tuberculous A18.31
  urine K65.8
Peritonsillar —see condition
Peritonsillitis J36
Perityphlitis K37
Periureteritis N28.89
Periurethral —see condition
Periurethritis (gangrenous) —see Urethritis
Periuterine —see condition
Perivaginitis —see Vaginitis
Perivasculitis, retinal H35.06-
Perivasitis (chronic) N49.1
Perivesiculitis (seminal) —see Vesiculitis
Perlèche NEC K13.0
  due to
    candidiasis B37.83
    moniliasis B37.83
    riboflavin deficiency E53.0
    vitamin B2 (riboflavin) deficiency E53.0
Pernicious —see condition
Pernio, perniosis T69.1
Perpetrator (of abuse) —see Index to External
  Causes of Injury, Perpetrator
Persecution
  delusion F22
  social Z60.5
Perseveration (tonic) R48.8
Persistence, persistent (congenital)
  anal membrane Q42.3
    with fistula Q42.2
  arteria stapedia Q16.3
  atrioventricular canal Q21.2
  branchial cleft Q18.0
  bulbus cordis in left ventricle Q21.8
  canal of Cloquet Q14.0
  capsule (opaque) Q12.8
  cilioretinal artery or vein Q14.8
  cloaca Q43.7
  communication —see Fistula, congenital
  convolutions
    aortic arch Q25.4
    fallopian tube Q50.6
    oviduct Q50.6
    uterine tube Q50.6
  double aortic arch Q25.4
  ductus arteriosus (Botalli) Q25.0
  fetal
    circulation P29.3
    form of cervix (uteri) Q51.828
    hemoglobin, hereditary (HPFH) D56.4
  foramen
    Botalli Q21.1
    ovale Q21.1
  Gartner's duct Q52.4
  hemoglobin, fetal (hereditary) (HPFH)
    D56.4
  hyaloid
    artery (generally incomplete) Q14.0
    system Q14.8
  hymen, in pregnancy or childbirth —see
    Pregnancy, complicated by, abnormal,
    vulva
  lanugo Q84.2
  left
    posterior cardinal vein Q26.8
    root with right arch of aorta Q25.4
    superior vena cava Q26.1
  Meckel's diverticulum Q43.0
    malignant —see Table of Neoplasms, small
      intestine, malignant

Persistence, persistent (Continued)
  mucosal disease (middle ear) —see
    Otitis, media, suppurative, chronic,
    tubotympanic
  nail (s), anomalous Q84.6
  omphalomesenteric duct Q43.0
  organ or site not listed —see Anomaly, by site
  ostium
    atrioventriculare commune Q21.2
    primum Q21.2
    secundum Q21.1
  ovarian rests in fallopian tube Q50.6
  pancreatic tissue in intestinal tract Q43.8
  primary (deciduous)
    teeth K00.6
    vitreous hyperplasia Q14.0
  pupillary membrane Q13.89
  rhesus (Rh)titer —see Complication (s),
    transfusion, incompatibility reaction,
    Rh (factor)
  right aortic arch Q25.4
  sinus
    urogenitalis
      female Q52.8
      male Q55.8
    venosus with imperfect incorporation in
      right auricle Q26.8
  thymus (gland) (hyperplasia) E32.0
  thyroglossal duct Q89.2
  thyrolingual duct Q89.2
  truncus arteriosus or communis Q20.0
  tunica vasculosa lentis Q12.2
  umbilical sinus Q64.4
  urachus Q64.4
  vitelline duct Q43.0
Person (with)
  admitted for clinical research, as a control
    subject (normal comparison)
    (participant) Z00.6
  awaiting admission to adequate facility
    elsewhere Z75.1
  concern (normal) about sick person in family
    Z63.6
  consulting on behalf of another Z71.0
  feigning illness Z76.5
  living (in)
    without
      adequate housing (heating) (space) Z59.1
      housing (permanent) (temporary) Z59.0
      person able to render necessary care
        Z74.2
      shelter Z59.0
    alone Z60.2
    boarding school Z59.3
    residential institution Z59.3
  on waiting list Z75.1
  sick or handicapped in family Z63.6
Personality (disorder) F60.9
  accentuation of traits (type A pattern) Z73.1
  affective F34.0
  aggressive F60.3
  amoral F60.2
  anacastic, anankastic F60.5
  antisocial F60.2
  anxious F60.6
  asocial F60.2
  asthenic F60.7
  avoidant F60.6
  borderline F60.3
  change due to organic condition (enduring)
    F07.0
  compulsive F60.5
  cycloid F34.0
  cyclothymic F34.0
  dependent F60.7
  depressive F34.1
  dissocial F60.2
  dual F44.81
  eccentric F60.89
  emotionally unstable F60.3
  expansive paranoid F60.0

Personality (Continued)
  explosive F60.3
  fanatic F60.0
  haltose type F60.89
  histrionic F60.4
  hyperthymic F34.0
  hypothymic F34.1
  hysterical F60.4
  immature F60.89
  inadequate F60.7
  labile (emotional) F60.3
  mixed (nonspecific) F60.81
  morally defective F60.2
  multiple F44.81
  narcissistic F60.81
  obsessional F60.5
  obsessive (-compulsive) F60.5
  organic F07.0
  overconscientious F60.5
  paranoid F60.0
  passive (-dependent) F60.7
  passive-aggressive F60.89
  pathologic F60.9
  pattern defect or disturbance F60.9
  pseudopsychopathic (organic) F07.0
  pseudoretarded (organic) F07.0
  psychoinfantile F60.4
  psychoneurotic NEC F60.89
  psychopathic F60.2
  querulant F60.0
  sadistic F60.89
  schizoid F60.1
  self-defeating F60.7
  sensitive paranoid F60.0
  sociopathic (amoral) (antisocial) (asocial)
    (dissocial) F60.2
  specified NEC F60.89
  type A Z73.1
  unstable (emotional) F60.3
Perthes' disease —see Legg-Calvé-Perthes
  disease
Pertussis (see also Whooping cough)
  A37.90
Perversion, perverted
  appetite F50.8
    psychogenic F50.8
  function
    pituitary gland E23.2
      posterior lobe E22.2
  sense of smell and taste R43.8
    psychogenic F45.8
  sexual —see Deviation, sexual
Pervious, congenital —see also Imperfect,
  closure
  ductus arteriosus Q25.0
Pes (congenital) —see also Talipes
  acquired —see also Deformity, limb, foot,
    specified NEC
    planus —see Deformity, limb, flat foot
  adductus Q66.89
  cavus Q66.7
  deformity NEC, acquired —see Deformity,
    limb, foot, specified NEC
  planus (acquired) (any degree) —see also
    Deformity, limb, flat foot
    rachitic sequelae (late effect) E64.3
  valgus Q66.6
Pest, pestis —see Plague
Petechia, petechiae R23.3
  newborn P54.5
Petechial typhus A75.9
Peter's anomaly Q13.4
Petit mal seizure —see Epilepsy, generalized,
  specified NEC
Petit's hernia —see Hernia, abdomen, specified
  site NEC
Petrellidosis B48.2
Petrositis H70.20-
  acute H70.21-
  chronic H70.22-
Peutz-Jeghers disease or syndrome Q85.8

Peyronie's disease N48.6
Pfeiffer's disease —see Mononucleosis, infectious
Phagedena (dry) (moist) (sloughing) —see also Gangrene
  geometric L88
  penis N48.29
  tropical —see Ulcer, skin
  vulva N76.6
Phagedenic —see condition
Phakoma H35.89
Phakomatosis (see also specific eponymous syndromes) Q85.9
  Bourneville's Q85.1
  specified NEC Q85.8
Phantom limb syndrome (without pain) G54.7
  with pain G54.6
Pharyngeal pouch syndrome D82.1
Pharyngitis (acute) (catarrhal) (gangrenous) (infective) (malignant) (membranous) (phlegmonous) (pseudomembranous) (simple) (subacute) (suppurative) (ulcerative) (viral) J02.9
  with influenza, flu, or grippe —see Influenza, with, pharyngitis
  aphthous B08.5
  atrophic J31.2
  chlamydial A56.4
  chronic (atrophic) (granular) (hypertrophic) J31.2
  coxsackievirus B08.5
  diphtheritic A36.0
  enteroviral vesicular B08.5
  follicular (chronic) J31.2
  fusospirochetal A69.1
  gonococcal A54.5
  granular (chronic) J31.2
  herpesviral B00.2
  hypertrophic J31.2
  infectional, chronic J31.2
  influenzal —see Influenza, with, respiratory manifestations NEC
  lymphonodular, acute (enteroviral) B08.8
  pneumococcal J02.8
  purulent J02.9
  putrid J02.9
  septic J02.0
  sicca J31.2
  specified organism NEC J02.8
  staphylococcal J02.8
  streptococcal J02.0
  syphilitic, congenital (early) A50.03
  tuberculous A15.8
  vesicular, enteroviral B08.5
  viral NEC J02.8
Pharyngoconjunctivitis, viral B30.2
Pharyngolaryngitis (acute) J06.0
  chronic J37.0
Pharyngoplegia J39.2
Pharyngotonsillitis, herpesviral B00.2
Pharyngotracheitis, chronic J42
Pharynx, pharyngeal —see condition
Phenomenon
  Arthus' —see Arthus' phenomenon
  jaw-winking Q07.8
  lupus erythematosus (LE) cell M32.9
  Raynaud's (secondary) I73.00
    with gangrene I73.01
  vasomotor R55
  vasospastic I73.9
  vasovagal R55
  Wenckebach's I44.1
Phenylketonuria E70.1
  classical E70.0
  maternal E70.1
Pheochromoblastoma
  specified site —see Neoplasm, malignant, by site
  unspecified site C74.10

Pheochromocytoma
  malignant
    specified site —see Neoplasm, malignant, by site
    unspecified site C74.10
  specified site —see Neoplasm, benign, by site
  unspecified site D35.00
Pheohyphomycosis —see Chromomycosis
Pheomycosis —see Chromomycosis
Phimosis (congenital) (due to infection) N47.1
  chancroidal A57
Phlebectasia —see also Varix
  congenital Q27.4
Phlebitis (infective) (pyemic) (septic) (suppurative) I80.9
  antepartum —see Thrombophlebitis, antepartum
  blue —see Phlebitis, leg, deep
  breast, superficial I80.8
  cavernous (venous) sinus —see Phlebitis, intracranial (venous) sinus
  cerebral (venous) sinus —see Phlebitis, intracranial (venous) sinus
  chest wall, superficial I80.8
  cranial (venous) sinus —see Phlebitis, intracranial (venous) sinus
  deep (vessels) —see Phlebitis, leg, deep
  due to implanted device —see Complications, by site and type, specified NEC
  during or resulting from a procedure T81.72
  femoral vein (superficial) I80.1-
  femoropopliteal vein I80.0-
  gestational —see Phlebopathy, gestational
  hepatic veins I80.8
  iliofemoral —see Phlebitis, femoral vein
  intracranial (venous) sinus (any) G08
    nonpyogenic I67.6
  intraspinal venous sinuses and veins G08
    nonpyogenic G95.19
  lateral (venous) sinus —see Phlebitis, intracranial (venous) sinus
  leg I80.3
    antepartum —see Thrombophlebitis, antepartum
    deep (vessels) NEC I80.20-
      iliac I80.21-
      popliteal vein I80.22-
      specified vessel NEC I80.29-
      tibial vein I80.23-
    femoral vein (superficial) I80.1-
    superficial (vessels) I80.0-
  longitudinal sinus —see Phlebitis, intracranial (venous) sinus
  lower limb —see Phlebitis, leg
  migrans, migrating (superficial) I82.1
  pelvic
    with ectopic or molar pregnancy O08.0
    following ectopic or molar pregnancy O08.0
    puerperal, postpartum O87.1
  popliteal vein —see Phlebitis, leg, deep, popliteal
  portal (vein) K75.1
  postoperative T81.72
  pregnancy —see Thrombophlebitis, antepartum
  puerperal, postpartum, childbirth O87.0
    deep O87.1
    pelvic O87.1
    superficial O87.0
  retina —see Vasculitis, retina
  saphenous (accessory) (great) (long) (small) —see Phlebitis, leg, superficial
  sinus (meninges) —see Phlebitis, intracranial (venous) sinus
  specified site NEC I80.8
  syphilitic A52.09
  tibial vein —see Phlebitis, leg, deep, tibial
  ulcerative I80.9
    leg —see Phlebitis, leg
  umbilicus I80.8

Phlebitis (Continued)
  uterus (septic) —see Endometritis
  varicose (leg) (lower limb) —see Varix, leg, with, inflammation
Phlebofibrosis I87.8
Phleboliths I87.8
Phlebopathy
  gestational O22.9-
  puerperal O87.9
Phlebosclerosis I87.8
Phlebothrombosis —see also Thrombosis
  antepartum —see Thrombophlebitis, antepartum
  pregnancy —see Thrombophlebitis, antepartum
  puerperal —see Thrombophlebitis, puerperal
Phlebotomus fever A93.1
Phlegmasia
  alba dolens O87.1
    nonpuerperal —see Phlebitis, femoral vein
  cerulea dolens —see Phlebitis, leg, deep
Phlegmon —see Abscess
Phlegmonous —see condition
Phlyctenulosis (allergic) (keratoconjunctivitis) (nontuberculous) —see also Keratoconjunctivitis
  cornea —see Keratoconjunctivitis
  tuberculous A18.52
Phobia, phobic F40.9
  animal F40.218
    spiders F40.210
  examination F40.298
  reaction F40.9
  simple F40.298
  social F40.10
    generalized F40.11
  specific (isolated) F40.298
    animal F40.218
      spiders F40.210
    blood F40.230
    injection F40.231
    injury F40.233
    men F40.290
    natural environment F40.228
      thunderstorms F40.220
    situational F40.248
      bridges F40.242
      closed in spaces F40.240
      flying F40.243
      heights F40.241
    specified focus NEC F40.298
    transfusion F40.231
    women F40.291
  specified NEC F40.8
    medical care NEC F40.232
  state F40.9
Phocas' disease —see Mastopathy, cystic
Phocomelia Q73.1
  lower limb —see Agenesis, leg, with foot present
  upper limb —see Agenesis, arm, with hand present
Phoria H50.50
Phosphate-losing tubular disorder N25.0
Phosphatemia E83.39
Phosphaturia E83.39
Photodermatitis (sun) L56.8
  chronic L57.8
  due to drug L56.8
  light other than sun L59.8
Photokeratitis H16.13-
Photophobia H53.14-
Photophthalmia —see Photokeratitis
Photopsia H53.19
Photoretinitis —see Retinopathy, solar
Photosensitivity, photosensitization (sun) skin L56.8
  light other than sun L59.8
Phrenitis —see Encephalitis
Phrynoderma (vitamin A deficiency) E50.8

◀ New   ◀║║ Revised   deleted Deleted

Phthiriasis (pubis) B85.3
  with any infestation classifiable to
    B85.0-B85.2 B85.4
Phthirus infestation —*see* Phthiriasis
Phthisis —*see also* Tuberculosis
  bulbi (infectional) —*see* Disorder, globe,
    degenerated condition, atrophy
  eyeball (due to infection) —*see* Disorder,
    globe, degenerated condition, atrophy
Phycomycosis —*see* Zygomycosis
Physalopteriasis B81.8
Physical restraint status Z78.1
Phytobezoar T18.9
  intestine T18.3
  stomach T18.2
Pian —*see* Yaws
Pianoma A66.1
Pica F50.8
  in adults F50.8
  infant or child F98.3
Picking, nose F98.8
Pick-Niemann disease —*see* Niemann-Pick
    disease or syndrome
Pick's
  cerebral atrophy G31.01 [F02.80]
    with behavioral disturbance G31.01
      [F02.81]
  disease or syndrome (brain) G31.01 [F02.80]
    with behavioral disturbance G31.01
      [F02.81]
Pickwickian syndrome E66.2
Piebaldism E70.39
Piedra (beard) (scalp) B36.8
  black B36.3
  white B36.2
Pierre Robin deformity or syndrome Q87.0
Pierson's disease or osteochondrosis M91.0
Pig-bel A05.2
Pigeon
  breast or chest (acquired) M95.4
    congenital Q67.7
    rachitic sequelae (late effect) E64.3
  breeder's disease or lung J67.2
  fancier's disease or lung J67.2
  toe —*see* Deformity, toe, specified NEC
Pigmentation (abnormal) (anomaly) L81.9
  conjunctiva H11.13-
  cornea (anterior) H18.01-
    posterior H18.05-
    stromal H18.06-
  diminished melanin formation NEC L81.6
  iron L81.8
  lids, congenital Q82.8
  limbus corneae —*see* Pigmentation, cornea
  metals L81.8
  optic papilla, congenital Q14.2
  retina, congenital (grouped) (nevoid) Q14.1
  scrotum, congenital Q82.8
  tattoo L81.8
Piles (*see also* Hemorrhoids) K64.9
Pili
  annulati or torti (congenital) Q84.1
  incarnati L73.1
Pill roller hand (intrinsic) —*see* Parkinsonism
Pilomatrixoma —*see* Neoplasm, skin, benign
  malignant —*see* Neoplasm, skin, malignant
Pilonidal —*see* condition
Pimple R23.8
Pinched nerve —*see* Neuropathy, entrapment
Pindborg tumor —*see* Cyst, calcifying
    odontogenic
Pineal body or gland —*see* condition
Pinealoblastoma C75.3
Pinealoma D44.5
  malignant C75.3
Pineoblastoma C75.3
Pineocytoma D44.5
Pinguecula H11.15-
Pingueculitis H10.81-
Pinhole meatus (*see also* Stricture, urethra)
    N35.9

Pink
  disease —*see* subcategory T56.1
  eye —*see* Conjunctivitis, acute, mucopurulent
Pinkus' disease (lichen nitidus) L44.1
Pinpoint
  meatus —*see* Stricture, urethra
  os (uteri) —*see* Stricture, cervix
Pins and needles R20.2
Pinta A67.9
  cardiovascular lesions A67.2
  chancre (primary) A67.0
  erythematous plaques A67.1
  hyperchromic lesions A67.1
  hyperkeratosis A67.1
  lesions A67.9
    cardiovascular A67.2
    hyperchromic A67.1
    intermediate A67.1
    late A67.2
    mixed A67.3
    primary A67.0
    skin (achromic) (cicatricial) (dyschromic)
      A67.2
      hyperchromic A67.1
      mixed (achromic and hyperchromic)
        A67.3
  papule (primary) A67.0
  skin lesions (achromic) (cicatricial)
    (dyschromic) A67.2
    hyperchromic A67.1
    mixed (achromic and hyperchromic) A67.3
  vitiligo A67.2
Pintids A67.1
Pinworm (disease) (infection) (infestation) B80
Piroplasmosis B60.0
Pistol wound —*see* Gunshot wound
Pitcher's elbow —*see* Derangement, joint,
    specified type NEC, elbow
Pithecoid pelvis Q74.2
  with disproportion (fetopelvic) O33.0
    causing obstructed labor O65.0
Pithiatism F48.8
Pitted —*see* Pitting
Pitting —*see also* Edema R60.9
  lip R60.0
  nail L60.8
  teeth K00.4
Pituitary gland —*see* condition
Pituitary-snuff-taker's disease J67.8
Pityriasis (capitis) L21.0
  alba L30.5
  circinata (et maculata) L42
  furfuracea L21.0
  Hebra's L26
  lichenoides L41.0
    chronica L41.1
    et varioliformis (acuta) L41.0
  maculata (et circinata) L30.5
  nigra B36.1
  pilaris, Hebra's L44.0
  rosea L42
  rotunda L44.8
  rubra (Hebra) pilaris L44.0
  simplex L30.5
  specified type NEC L30.5
  streptogenes L30.5
  versicolor (scrotal) B36.0
Placenta, placental —*see* Pregnancy,
  complicated by (care of) (management
  affected by), specified condition
Placentitis O41.14-
Plagiocephaly Q67.3
Plague A20.9
  abortive A20.8
  ambulatory A20.8
  asymptomatic A20.8
  bubonic A20.0
  cellulocutaneous A20.1
  cutaneobubonic A20.1
  lymphatic gland A20.0
  meningitis A20.3

Plague (Continued)
  pharyngeal A20.8
  pneumonic (primary) (secondary) A20.2
  pulmonary, pulmonic A20.2
  septicemic A20.7
  tonsillar A20.8
    septicemic A20.7
Planning, family
  contraception Z30.9
  procreation Z31.69
Plaque (s)
  artery, arterial —*see* Arteriosclerosis
  calcareous —*see* Calcification
  coronary, lipid rich I25.83
  epicardial I31.8
  erythematous, of pinta A67.1
  Hollenhorst's —*see* Occlusion, artery, retina
  lipid rich, coronary I25.83
  pleural (without asbestos) J92.9
    with asbestos J92.0
  tongue K13.29
Plasmacytoma C90.3-
  extramedullary C90.2-
  medullary C90.0-
  solitary C90.3-
Plasmacytopenia D72.818
Plasmacytosis D72.822
Plaster ulcer —*see* Ulcer, pressure, by site
Plateau iris syndrome (post-iridectomy)
    (postprocedural) (without glaucoma)
    H21.82
  with glaucoma H40.22-
Platybasia Q75.8
Platyonychia (congenital) Q84.6
  acquired L60.8
Platypelloid pelvis M95.5
  with disproportion (fetopelvic) O33.0
    causing obstructed labor O65.0
  congenital Q74.2
Platyspondylisis Q76.49
Plaut (-Vincent) disease (*see also* Vincent's)
    A69.1
Plethora R23.2
  newborn P61.1
Pleura, pleural —*see* condition
Pleuralgia R07.81
Pleurisy (acute) (adhesive) (chronic) (costal)
    (diaphragmatic) (double) (dry) (fibrinous)
    (fibrous) (interlobar) (latent) (plastic)
    (primary) (residual) (sicca) (sterile)
    (subacute) (unresolved) R09.1
  with
    adherent pleura J86.0
    effusion J90
      chylous, chyliform J94.0
      tuberculous (non primary) A15.6
        primary (progressive) A15.7
    tuberculosis —*see* Pleurisy, tuberculous
      (non primary)
  encysted —*see* Pleurisy, with effusion
  exudative —*see* Pleurisy, with effusion
  fibrinopurulent, fibropurulent —*see*
    Pyothorax
  hemorrhagic —*see* Hemothorax
  pneumococcal J90
  purulent —*see* Pyothorax
  septic —*see* Pyothorax
  serofibrinous —*see* Pleurisy, with effusion
  seropurulent —*see* Pyothorax
  serous —*see* Pleurisy, with effusion
  staphylococcal J86.9
  streptococcal J90
  suppurative —*see* Pyothorax
  traumatic (post) (current) —*see* Injury,
    intrathoracic, pleura
  tuberculous (with effusion) (non primary)
    A15.6
    primary (progressive) A15.7
Pleuritis sicca —*see* Pleurisy
Pleurobronchopneumonia —*see* Pneumonia,
    broncho

Pleurodynia R07.81
  epidemic B33.0
  viral B33.0
Pleuropericarditis —see also Pericarditis
  acute I30.9
Pleuropneumonia (acute) (bilateral) (double)
    (septic) (see also Pneumonia) J18.8
  chronic —see Fibrosis, lung
Pleuro-pneumonia-like-organism (PPLO),
    as cause of disease classified elsewhere
    B96.0
Pleurorrhea —see Pleurisy, with effusion
Plexitis, brachial G54.0
Plica
  polonica B85.0
  syndrome, knee M67.5
  tonsil J35.8
Plicated tongue K14.5
Plug
  bronchus NEC J98.09
  meconium (newborn) NEC syndrome P76.0
  mucus —see Asphyxia, mucus
Plumbism —see subcategory T56.0
Plummer's disease E05.20
  with thyroid storm E05.21
Plummer-Vinson syndrome D50.1
Pluricarential syndrome of infancy E40
Plus (and minus) hand (intrinsic) —see
    Deformity, limb, specified type NEC,
    forearm
Pneumathemia —see Air, embolism
Pneumatic hammer (drill) syndrome T75.21
Pneumatocele (lung) J98.4
  intracranial G93.89
  tension J44.9
Pneumatosis
  cystoides intestinalis K63.89
  intestinalis K63.89
  peritonei K66.8
Pneumaturia R39.89
Pneumoblastoma —see Neoplasm, lung,
    malignant
Pneumocephalus G93.89
Pneumococcemia A40.3
Pneumococcus, pneumococcal —see condition
Pneumoconiosis (due to) (inhalation of) J64
  with tuberculosis (any type in A15) J65
  aluminum J63.0
  asbestos J61
  bagasse, bagassosis J67.1
  bauxite J63.1
  beryllium J63.2
  coal miners' (simple) J60
  coalworkers' (simple) J60
  collier's J60
  cotton dust J66.0
  diatomite (diatomaceous earth) J62.8
  dust
    inorganic NEC J63.6
    lime J62.8
    marble J62.8
    organic NEC J66.8
  fumes or vapors (from silo) J68.9
  graphite J63.3
  grinder's J62.8
  kaolin J62.8
  mica J62.8
  millstone maker's J62.8
  mineral fibers NEC J61
  miner's J60
  moldy hay J67.0
  potter's J62.8
  rheumatoid —see Rheumatoid, lung
  sandblaster's J62.8
  silica, silicate NEC J62.8
    with carbon J60
  stonemason's J62.8
  talc (dust) J62.0
Pneumocystis carinii pneumonia B59
Pneumocystis jiroveci (pneumonia) B59
Pneumocystosis (with pneumonia) B59

Pneumohemopericardium I31.2
Pneumohemothorax J94.2
  traumatic S27.2
Pneumohydropericardium —see Pericarditis
Pneumohydrothorax —see Hydrothorax
Pneumomediastinum J98.2
  congenital or perinatal P25.2
Pneumomycosis B49 [J99]
Pneumonia (acute) (double) (migratory)
    (purulent) (septic) (unresolved) J18.9
  with
    influenza —see Influenza, with, pneumonia
    lung abscess J85.1
      due to specified organism —see
        Pneumonia, in (due to)
  adenoviral J12.0
  adynamic J18.2
  alba A50.04
  allergic (eosinophilic) J82
  alveolar —see Pneumonia, lobar
  anaerobes J15.8
  anthrax A22.1
  apex, apical —see Pneumonia, lobar
  Ascaris B77.81
  aspiration J69.0
    due to
      aspiration of microorganisms
        bacterial J15.9
        viral J12.9
      food (regurgitated) J69.0
      gastric secretions J69.0
      milk (regurgitated) J69.0
      oils, essences J69.1
      solids, liquids NEC J69.8
      vomitus J69.0
    newborn P24.81
      amniotic fluid (clear) P24.11
      blood P24.21
      food (regurgitated) P24.31
      liquor (amnii) P24.11
      meconium P24.01
      milk P24.31
      mucus P24.11
      specified NEC P24.81
      stomach contents P24.31
    postprocedural J95.4
  atypical NEC J18.9
  bacillus J15.9
    specified NEC J15.8
  bacterial J15.9
    specified NEC J15.8
  Bacteroides (fragilis) (oralis)
    (melaninogenicus) J15.8
  basal, basic, basilar —see Pneumonia, by type
  bronchiolitis obliterans organized (BOOP)
    J84.89
  broncho-, bronchial (confluent) (croupous)
    (diffuse) (disseminated) (hemorrhagic)
    (involving lobes) (lobar) (terminal) J18.0
    allergic (eosinophilic) J82
    aspiration —see Pneumonia, aspiration
    bacterial J15.9
      specified NEC J15.8
    chronic —see Fibrosis, lung
    diplococcal J13
    Eaton's agent J15.7
    Escherichia coli (E. coli) J15.5
    Friedländer's bacillus J15.0
    Hemophilus influenzae J14
    hypostatic J18.2
    inhalation (see also Pneumonia, aspiration
      due to fumes or vapors (chemical) J68.0
      of oils or essences J69.1
    Klebsiella (pneumoniae) J15.0
    lipid, lipoid J69.1
      endogenous J84.89
    Mycoplasma (pneumoniae) J15.7
    pleuro-pneumonia-like-organisms (PPLO)
      J15.7
    pneumococcal J13
    Proteus J15.6

Pneumonia (Continued)
  broncho-, bronchial (Continued)
    Pseudomonas J15.1
    Serratia marcescens J15.6
    specified organism NEC J16.8
    staphylococcal —see Pneumonia,
      staphylococcal
    streptococcal NEC J15.4
      group B J15.3
      pneumoniae J13
    viral, virus —see Pneumonia, viral
  Butyrivibrio (fibriosolvens) J15.8
  Candida B37.1
  caseous —see Tuberculosis, pulmonary
  catarrhal —see Pneumonia, broncho
  chlamydial J16.0
    congenital P23.1
  cholesterol J84.89
  cirrhotic (chronic) —see Fibrosis, lung
  Clostridium (haemolyticum) (novyi) J15.8
  confluent —see Pneumonia, broncho
  congenital (infective) P23.9
    due to
      bacterium NEC P23.6
      Chlamydia P23.1
      Escherichia coli P23.4
      Haemophilus influenzae P23.6
      infective organism NEC P23.8
      Klebsiella pneumoniae P23.6
      Mycoplasma P23.6
      Pseudomonas P23.5
      Staphylococcus P23.2
      Streptococcus (except group B) P23.6
        group B P23.3
      viral agent P23.0
    specified NEC P23.8
  croupous —see Pneumonia, lobar
  cryptogenic organizing J84.116
  cytomegalic inclusion B25.0
  cytomegaloviral B25.0
  deglutition —see Pneumonia, aspiration
  desquamative interstitial J84.117
  diffuse —see Pneumonia, broncho
  diplococcal, diplococcus (broncho-) (lobar)
    J13
  disseminated (focal) —see Pneumonia,
    broncho
  Eaton's agent J15.7
  embolic, embolism —see Embolism,
    pulmonary
  Enterobacter J15.6
  eosinophilic J82
  Escherichia coli (E. coli) J15.5
  Eubacterium J15.8
  fibrinous —see Pneumonia, lobar
  fibroid, fibrous (chronic) —see Fibrosis, lung
  Friedländer's bacillus J15.0
  Fusobacterium (nucleatum) J15.8
  gangrenous J85.0
  giant cell (measles) B05.2
  gonococcal A54.84
  gram-negative bacteria NEC J15.6
    anaerobic J15.8
  Hemophilus influenzae (broncho) (lobar) J14
  human metapneumovirus J12.3
  hypostatic (broncho) (lobar) J18.2
  in (due to)
    actinomycosis A42.0
    adenovirus J12.0
    anthrax A22.1
    ascariasis B77.81
    aspergillosis B44.9
    Bacillus anthracis A22.1
    Bacterium anitratum J15.6
    candidiasis B37.1
    chickenpox B01.2
    Chlamydia J16.0
      neonatal P23.1
    coccidioidomycosis B38.2
      acute B38.0
      chronic B38.1

◀ New ◀◀ Revised ~~deleted~~ Deleted

Pneumonia (Continued)
  in (Continued)
    cytomegalovirus disease B25.0
    Diplococcus (pneumoniae) J13
    Eaton's agent J15.7
    Enterobacter J15.6
    Escherichia coli (E. coli) J15.5
    Friedländer's bacillus J15.0
    fumes and vapors (chemical) (inhalation) J68.0
    gonorrhea A54.84
    Hemophilus influenzae (H. influenzae) J14
    Herellea J15.6
    histoplasmosis B39.2
      acute B39.0
      chronic B39.1
    human metapneumovirus J12.3
    Klebsiella (pneumoniae) J15.0
    measles B05.2
    Mycoplasma (pneumoniae) J15.7
    nocardiosis, nocardiasis A43.0
    ornithosis A70
    parainfluenza virus J12.2
    pleuro-pneumonia-like-organism (PPLO) J15.7
    pneumococcus J13
    pneumocystosis (Pneumocystis carinii) (Pneumocystis jiroveci) B59
    Proteus J15.6
    Pseudomonas NEC J15.1
      pseudomallei A24.1
    psittacosis A70
    Q fever A78
    respiratory syncytial virus J12.1
    rheumatic fever I00 [J17]
    rubella B06.81
    Salmonella (infection) A02.22
      typhi A01.03
    schistosomiasis B65.9 [J17]
    Serratia marcescens J15.6
    specified
      bacterium NEC J15.8
      organism NEC J16.8
    spirochetal NEC A69.8
    Staphylococcus J15.20
      aureus (methicillin susceptible) (MSSA) J15.211
        methicillin resistant (MRSA) J15.212
      specified NEC J15.29
    Streptococcus J15.4
      group B J15.3
      pneumoniae J13
      specified NEC J15.4
    toxoplasmosis B58.3
    tularemia A21.2
    typhoid (fever) A01.03
    varicella B01.2
    virus —see Pneumonia, viral
    whooping cough A37.91
      due to
        Bordetella parapertussis A37.11
        Bordetella pertussis A37.01
        specified NEC A37.81
    Yersinia pestis A20.2
  inhalation of food or vomit —see Pneumonia, aspiration
  interstitial J84.9
    chronic J84.111
    desquamative J84.117
    due to
      collagen vascular disease J84.17
      known underlying cause J84.17
    idiopathic NOS J84.111
    in disease classified elsewhere J84.17
    lymphocytic (due to collagen vascular disease) (in diseases classified elsewhere) J84.17
    lymphoid J84.2

Pneumonia (Continued)
  interstitial (Continued)
    non-specific J84.89
      due to
        collagen vascular disease J84.17
        known underlying cause J84.17
      idiopathic J84.113
      in diseases classified elsewhere J84.17
    plasma cell B59
    pseudomonas J15.1
    usual J84.112
      due to collagen vascular disease J84.17
      idiopathic J84.112
      in diseases classified elsewhere J84.17
  Klebsiella (pneumoniae) J15.0
  lipid, lipoid (exogenous) J69.1
    endogenous J84.89
  lobar (disseminated) (double) (interstitial) J18.1
    bacterial J15.9
      specified NEC J15.8
    chronic —see Fibrosis, lung
    Escherichia coli (E. coli) J15.5
    Friedländer's bacillus J15.0
    Hemophilus influenzae J14
    hypostatic J18.2
    Klebsiella (pneumoniae) J15.0
    pneumococcal J13
    Proteus J15.6
    Pseudomonas J15.1
    specified organism NEC J16.8
    staphylococcal —see Pneumonia, staphylococcal
    streptococcal NEC J15.4
    Streptococcus pneumoniae J13
    viral, virus —see Pneumonia, viral
  lobular —see Pneumonia, broncho
  Löffler's J82
  lymphoid interstitial J84.2
  massive —see Pneumonia, lobar
  meconium P24.01
  MSSA (methicillin susceptible Staphylococcus aureus) J15.211
  multilobar —see Pneumonia, by type
  Mycoplasma (pneumoniae) J15.7
  necrotic J85.0
  neonatal P23.9
    aspiration —see Aspiration, by substance, with pneumonia
  nitrogen dioxide J68.9
  organizing J84.89
    due to
      collagen vascular disease J84.17
      known underlying cause J84.17
    in diseases classified elsewhere J84.17
  orthostatic J18.2
  parainfluenza virus J12.2
  parenchymatous —see Fibrosis, lung
  passive J18.2
  patchy —see Pneumonia, broncho
  Peptococcus J15.8
  Peptostreptococcus J15.8
  plasma cell (of infants) B59
  pleurolobar —see Pneumonia, lobar
  pleuro-pneumonia-like organism (PPLO) J15.7
  pneumococcal (broncho) (lobar) J13
  Pneumocystis (carinii) (jiroveci) B59
  postinfectional NEC B99 [J17]
  postmeasles B05.2
  Proteus J15.6
  Pseudomonas J15.1
  psittacosis A70
  radiation J70.0
  respiratory syncytial virus J12.1
  resulting from a procedure J95.89
  rheumatic I00 [J17]
  Salmonella (arizonae) (cholerae-suis) (enteritidis) (typhimurium) A02.22
    typhi A01.03
    typhoid fever A01.03

Pneumonia (Continued)
  SARS-associated coronavirus J12.81
  segmented, segmental —see Pneumonia, broncho-
  Serratia marcescens J15.6
  specified NEC J18.8
    bacterium NEC J15.8
    organism NEC J16.8
    virus NEC J12.89
  spirochetal NEC A69.8
  staphylococcal (broncho) (lobar) J15.20
    aureus (methicillin susceptible) (MSSA) J15.211
      methicillin resistant (MRSA) J15.212
    specified NEC J15.29
  static, stasis J18.2
  streptococcal NEC (broncho) (lobar) J15.4
    group
      A J15.4
      B J15.3
      specified NEC J15.4
  Streptococcus pneumoniae J13
  syphilitic, congenital (early) A50.04
  traumatic (complication) (early) (secondary) T79.8
  tuberculous (any) —see Tuberculosis, pulmonary
  tularemic A21.2
  varicella B01.2
  Veillonella J15.8
  ventilator associated J95.851
  viral, virus (broncho) (interstitial) (lobar) J12.9
    adenoviral J12.0
    congenital P23.0
    human metapneumovirus J12.3
    parainfluenza J12.2
    respiratory syncytial J12.1
    SARS-associated coronavirus J12.81
    specified NEC J12.89
  white (congenital) A50.04
Pneumonic —see condition
Pneumonitis (acute) (primary) —see also Pneumonia
  air-conditioner J67.7
  allergic (due to) J67.9
    organic dust NEC J67.8
    red cedar dust J67.8
    sequoiosis J67.8
    wood dust J67.8
  aspiration J69.0
    due to
      anesthesia J95.4
        during
          labor and delivery O74.0
          pregnancy O29.01-
          puerperium O89.01
      fumes or gases J68.0
      obstetric O74.0
  chemical (due to gases, fumes or vapors) (inhalation) J68.0
    due to anesthesia J95.4
  cholesterol J84.89
  chronic —see Fibrosis, lung
  congenital rubella P35.0
  crack (cocaine) J68.0
  due to
    beryllium J68.0
    cadmium J68.0
    crack (cocaine) J68.0
    detergent J69.8
    fluorocarbon-polymer J68.0
    food, vomit (aspiration) J69.0
    fumes or vapors J68.0
    gases, fumes or vapors (inhalation) J68.0
    inhalation
      blood J69.8
      essences J69.1
      food (regurgitated), milk, vomit J69.0
      oils, essences J69.1
      saliva J69.0
      solids, liquids NEC J69.8

Pneumonitis *(Continued)*
  due to *(Continued)*
    manganese J68.0
    nitrogen dioxide J68.0
    oils, essences J69.1
    solids, liquids NEC J69.8
    toxoplasmosis (acquired) B58.3
      congenital P37.1
    vanadium J68.0
    ventilator J95.851
  eosinophilic J82
  hypersensitivity J67.9
    air conditioner lung J67.7
    bagassosis J67.1
    bird fancier's lung J67.2
    farmer's lung J67.0
    maltworker's lung J67.4
    maple bark-stripper's lung J67.6
    mushroom worker's lung J67.5
    specified organic dust NEC J67.8
    suberosis J67.3
  interstitial (chronic) J84.89
    acute J84.114
    lymphoid J84.2
    non-specific J84.89
      idiopathic J84.113
  lymphoid, interstitial J84.2
  meconium P24.01
  postanesthetic J95.4
    correct substance properly administered — *see* Table of Drugs and Chemcials, by drug, adverse effect
    in labor and delivery O74.0
    in pregnancy O29.01-
    obstetric O74.0
    overdose or wrong substance given or taken (by accident) —*see* Table of Drugs and Chemicals, by drug, poisoning
    postpartum, puerperal O89.01
  postoperative J95.4
    obstetric O74.0
  radiation J70.0
  rubella, congenital P35.0
  ventilation (air-conditioning) J67.7
  ventilator associated J95.851
  wood-dust J67.8
Pneumonoconiosis —*see* Pneumoconiosis
Pneumoparotid K11.8
Pneumopathy NEC J98.4
  alveolar J84.09
  due to organic dust NEC J66.8
  parietoalveolar J84.09
Pneumopericarditis —*see also* Pericarditis
  acute I30.9
Pneumopericardium —*see also* Pericarditis
  congenital P25.3
  newborn P25.3
  traumatic (post) —*see* Injury, heart
Pneumophagia (psychogenic) F45.8
Pneumopleurisy, pneumopleuritis *(see also* Pneumonia) J18.8
Pneumopyopericardium I30.1
Pneumopyothorax —*see* Pyopneumothorax
  with fistula J86.0
Pneumorrhagia —*see also* Hemorrhage, lung
  tuberculous —*see* Tuberculosis, pulmonary
Pneumothorax NOS J93.9
  acute J93.83
  chronic J93.81
  congenital P25.1
  perinatal period P25.1
  postprocedural J95.811
  specified NEC J93.83
  spontaneous NOS J93.83
    newborn P25.1
    primary J93.11
    secondary J93.12
    tension J93.0
  tense valvular, infectional J93.0
  tension (spontaneous) J93.0

Pneumothorax NOS *(Continued)*
  traumatic S27.0
    with hemothorax S27.2
  tuberculous —*see* Tuberculosis, pulmonary
Podagra *(see also* Gout) M10.9
Podencephalus Q01.9
Poikilocytosis R71.8
Poikiloderma L81.6
  Civatte's L57.3
  congenital Q82.8
  vasculare atrophicans L94.5
Poikilodermatomyositis M33.10
  with
    myopathy M33.12
    respiratory involvement M33.11
    specified organ involvement NEC M33.19
Pointed ear (congenital) Q17.3
Poison ivy, oak, sumac or other plant dermatitis (allergic) (contact) L23.7
Poisoning (acute) —*see also* Table of Drugs and Chemicals
  algae and toxins T65.82-
  Bacillus B (aertrycke) (cholerae (suis)) (paratyphosus) (suipestifer) A02.9
    botulinus A05.1
  bacterial toxins A05.9
  berries, noxious —*see* Poisoning, food, noxious, berries
  botulism A05.1
  ciguatera fish T61.0-
  Clostridium botulinum A05.1
  death-cap (Amanita phalloides) (Amanita verna) —*see* Poisoning, food, noxious, mushrooms
  drug —*see* Table of Drugs and Chemicals, by drug, poisoning
  epidemic, fish (noxious) —*see* Poisoning, seafood
    bacterial A05.9
  fava bean D55.0
  fish (noxious) T61.9-
    bacterial —*see* Intoxication, foodborne, by agent
    ciguatera fish —*see* Poisoning, ciguatera fish
    scombroid fish —*see* Poisoning, scombroid fish
    specified type NEC T61.77-
  food (acute) (diseased) (infected) (noxious) NEC T62.9-
    bacterial —*see* Intoxication, foodborne, by agent
    due to
      Bacillus (aertrycke) (choleraesuis) (paratyphosus) (suipestifer) A02.9
        botulinus A05.1
      Clostridium (perfringens) (Welchii) A05.2
      salmonella (aertrycke) (callinarum) (choleraesuis) (enteritidis) (paratyphi) (suipestifer) A02.9
        with
          gastroenteritis A02.0
          sepsis A02.1
      staphylococcus A05.0
      Vibrio
        parahaemolyticus A05.3
        vulnificus A05.5
    noxious or naturally toxic T62.9-
      berries —*see* subcategory T62.1-
      fish —*see* Poisoning, seafood
      mushrooms —*see* subcategory T62.0X-
      plants NEC —*see* subcategory T62.2X-
      seafood —*see* Poisoning, seafood
      specified NEC —*see* subcategory T62.8X-
    ichthyotoxism —*see* Poisoning, seafood
    kreotoxism, food A05.9
    latex T65.81-
    lead T56.0-
    mushroom —*see* Poisoning, food, noxious, mushroom

Poisoning *(Continued)*
  mussels —*see also* Poisoning, shellfish
    bacterial —*see* Intoxication, foodborne, by agent
  nicotine (tobacco) T65.2-
  noxious foodstuffs —*see* Poisoning, food, noxious
  plants, noxious —*see* Poisoning, food, noxious, plants NEC
  ptomaine —*see* Poisoning, food
  radiation J70.0
  Salmonella (arizonae) (cholerae-suis) (enteritidis) (typhimurium) A02.9
  scombroid fish T61.1-
  seafood (noxious) T61.9-
    bacterial —*see* Intoxication, foodborne, by agent
    fish —*see* Poisoning, fish
    shellfish —*see* Poisoning, shellfish
    specified NEC —*see* subcategory T61.8X-
  shellfish (amnesic) (azaspiracid) (diarrheic) (neurotoxic) (noxious) (paralytic) T61.78-
    bacterial —*see* Intoxication, foodborne, by agent
    ciguatera mollusk —*see* Poisoning, ciguatera fish
  specified substance NEC T65.891
  Staphylococcus, food A05.0
  tobacco (nicotine) T65.2-
  water E87.79
Poker spine —*see* Spondylitis, ankylosing
Poland syndrome Q79.8
Polioencephalitis (acute) (bulbar) A80.9
  inferior G12.22
  influenzal —*see* Influenza, with, encephalopathy
  superior hemorrhagic (acute) (Wernicke's) E51.2
  Wernicke's E51.2
Polioencephalomyelitis (acute) (anterior) A80.9
  with beriberi E51.2
Polioencephalopathy, superior hemorrhagic E51.2
  with
    beriberi E51.11
    pellagra E52
Poliomeningoencephalitis —*see* Meningoencephalitis
Poliomyelitis (acute) (anterior) (epidemic) A80.9
  with paralysis (bulbar) —*see* Poliomyelitis, paralytic
  abortive A80.4
  ascending (progressive) —*see* Poliomyelitis, paralytic
  bulbar (paralytic) —*see* Poliomyelitis, paralytic
  congenital P35.8
  nonepidemic A80.9
  nonparalytic A80.4
  paralytic A80.30
    specified NEC A80.39
    vaccine-associated A80.0
    wild virus
      imported A80.1
      indigenous A80.2
  spinal, acute A80.9
Poliosis (eyebrow) (eyelashes) L67.1
  circumscripta, acquired L67.1
Pollakiuria R35.0
  psychogenic F45.8
Pollinosis J30.1
Pollitzer's disease L73.2
Polyadenitis —*see also* Lymphadenitis
  malignant A20.0
Polyalgia M79.89
Polyangiitis M30.0
  microscopic M31.7
  overlap syndrome M30.8

Polyarteritis
microscopic M31.7
nodosa M30.0
with lung involvement M30.1
juvenile M30.2
related condition NEC M30.8
Polyarthralgia —see Pain, joint
Polyarthritis, polyarthropathy (see also
Arthritis) M13.0
due to or associated with other specified
conditions —see Arthritis
epidemic (Australian) (with exanthema)
B33.1
infective —see Arthritis, pyogenic or pyemic
inflammatory M06.4
juvenile (chronic) (seronegative) M08.3
migratory —see Fever, rheumatic
rheumatic, acute —see Fever, rheumatic
Polyarthrosis M15.9
post-traumatic M15.3
primary M15.0
specified NEC M15.8
Polycarential syndrome of infancy E40
Polychondritis (atrophic) (chronic) —see also
Disorder, cartilage, specified type NEC
relapsing M94.1
Polycoria Q13.2
Polycystic (disease)
degeneration, kidney Q61.3
autosomal dominant (adult type) Q61.2
autosomal recessive (infantile type) NEC
Q61.19
kidney Q61.3
autosomal
dominant Q61.2
recessive NEC Q61.19
autosomal dominant (adult type) Q61.2
autosomal recessive (childhood type) NEC
Q61.19
infantile type NEC Q61.19
liver Q44.6
lung J98.4
congenital Q33.0
ovary, ovaries E28.2
spleen Q89.09
Polycythemia (secondary) D75.1
acquired D75.1
benign (familial) D75.0
due to
donor twin P61.1
erythropoietin D75.1
fall in plasma volume D75.1
high altitude D75.1
maternal-fetal transfusion P61.1
stress D75.1
emotional D75.1
erythropoietin D75.1
familial (benign) D75.0
Gaisböck's (hypertonica) D75.1
high altitude D75.1
hypertonica D75.1
hypoxemic D75.1
neonatorum P61.1
nephrogenous D75.1
relative D75.1
secondary D75.1
spurious D75.1
stress D75.1
vera D45
Polycytosis cryptogenica D75.1
Polydactylism, polydactyly Q69.9
toes Q69.2
Polydipsia R63.1
Polydystrophy, pseudo-Hurler E77.0
Polyembryoma —see Neoplasm, malignant,
by site
Polyglandular
deficiency E31.0
dyscrasia E31.9
dysfunction E31.9
syndrome E31.8

Polyhydramnios O40.-
Polymastia Q83.1
Polymenorrhea N92.0
Polymyalgia M35.3
arteritica, giant cell M31.5
rheumatica M35.3
with giant cell arteritis M31.5
Polymyositis (acute) (chronic) (hemorrhagic)
M33.20
with
myopathy M33.22
respiratory involvement M33.21
skin involvement —see
Dermatopolymyositis
specified organ involvement NEC M33.29
ossificans (generalisata) (progressiva) —see
Myositis, ossificans, progressiva
Polyneuritis, polyneuritic —see also
Polyneuropathy
acute (post-)infective G61.0
alcoholic G62.1
cranialis G52.7
demyelinating, chronic inflammatory (CIDP)
G61.81
diabetic —see Diabetes, polyneuropathy
diphtheritic A36.83
due to lack of vitamin NEC E56.9 [G63]
endemic E51.11
erythredema —see subcategory T56.1
febrile, acute G61.0
hereditary ataxic G60.1
idiopathic, acute G61.0
infective (acute) G61.0
inflammatory, chronic demyelinating (CIDP)
G61.81
nutritional E63.9 [G63]
postinfective (acute) G61.0
specified NEC G62.89
Polyneuropathy (peripheral) G62.9
alcoholic G62.1
amyloid (Portuguese) E85.1 [G63]
arsenical G62.2
critical illness G62.81
demyelinating, chronic inflammatory (CIDP)
G61.81
diabetic —see Diabetes, polyneuropathy
drug-induced G62.0
hereditary G60.9
specified NEC G60.8
idiopathic G60.9
progressive G60.3
in (due to)
alcohol G62.1
sequelae G65.2
amyloidosis, familial (Portuguese) E85.1
[G63]
antitetanus serum G61.1
arsenic G62.2
sequelae G65.2
avitaminosis NEC E56.9 [G63]
beriberi E51.11
collagen vascular disease NEC M35.9 [G63]
deficiency (of)
B (-complex) vitamins E53.9 [G63]
vitamin B6 E53.1 [G63]
diabetes —see Diabetes, polyneuropathy
diphtheria A36.83
drug or medicament G62.0
correct substance properly
administered —see Table of Drugs
and Chemicals, by drug, adverse
effect
overdose or wrong substance given or
taken —see Table of Drugs and
Chemicals, by drug, poisoning
endocrine disease NEC E34.9 [G63]
herpes zoster B02.23
hypoglycemia E16.2 [G63]
infectious
disease NEC B99 [G63]
mononucleosis B27.91

Polyneuropathy (Continued)
in (Continued)
lack of vitamin NEC E56.9 [G63]
lead G62.2
sequelae G65.2
leprosy A30.9 [G63]
Lyme disease A69.22
metabolic disease NEC E88.9 [G63]
microscopic polyangiitis M31.7 [G63]
mumps B26.84
neoplastic disease (see also Neoplasm)
D49.9 [G63]
nutritional deficiency NEC E63.9 [G63]
organophosphate compounds G62.2
sequelae G65.2
parasitic disease NEC B89 [G63]
pellagra E52 [G63]
polyarteritis nodosa M30.0
porphyria E80.20 [G63]
radiation G62.82
rheumatoid arthritis —see Rheumatoid,
polyneuropathy
sarcoidosis D86.89
serum G61.1
syphilis (late) A52.15
congenital A50.43
systemic
connective tissue disorder M35.9
[G63]
lupus erythematosus M32.19
toxic agent NEC G62.2
sequelae G65.2
triorthocresyl phosphate G62.2
sequelae G65.2
tuberculosis A17.89
uremia N18.9 [G63]
vitamin B12 deficiency E53.8 [G63]
with anemia (pernicious) D51.0
[G63]
due to dietary deficiency D51.3
[G63]
zoster B02.23
inflammatory G61.9
chronic demyelinating (CIDP) G61.81
sequelae G65.1
specified NEC G61.89
lead G62.2
sequelae G65.2
nutritional NEC E63.9 [G63]
postherpetic (zoster) B02.23
progressive G60.3
radiation-induced G62.82
sensory (hereditary) (idiopathic) G60.8
specified NEC G62.89
syphilitic (late) A52.15
congenital A50.43
Polyopia H53.8
Polyorchism, polyorchidism Q55.21
Polyosteoarthritis (see also Osteoarthritis,
generalized) M15.9-
post-traumatic M15.3
specified NEC M15.8
Polyostotic fibrous dysplasia Q78.1
Polyotia Q17.0
Polyp, polypus
accessory sinus J33.8
adenocarcinoma in —see Neoplasm,
malignant, by site
adenocarcinoma in situ in —see Neoplasm, in
situ, by site
adenoid tissue J33.0
adenomatous —see also Neoplasm, benign,
by site
adenocarcinoma in —see Neoplasm,
malignant, by site
adenocarcinoma in situ in —see Neoplasm,
in situ, by site
carcinoma in —see Neoplasm, malignant,
by site
carcinoma in situ in —see Neoplasm, in
situ, by site

Polyp, polypus *(Continued)*
  adenomatous *(Continued)*
    multiple —*see* Neoplasm, benign
      adenocarcinoma in —*see* Neoplasm,
        malignant, by site
      adenocarcinoma in situ in —*see*
        Neoplasm, in situ, by site
  antrum J33.8
  anus, anal (canal) K62.0
  Bartholin's gland N84.3
  bladder D41.4
  carcinoma in —*see* Neoplasm, malignant, by
    site
  carcinoma in situ in —*see* Neoplasm, in situ,
    by site
  cecum D12.0
  cervix (uteri) N84.1
    in pregnancy or childbirth —*see* Pregnancy,
      complicated by, abnormal, cervix
    mucous N84.1
    nonneoplastic N84.1
  choanal J33.0
  cholesterol K82.4
  clitoris N84.3
  colon K63.5
    adenomatous D12.6
    ascending D12.2
    cecum D12.0
    descending D12.4
    inflammatory K51.40
      with
        abscess K51.414
        complication K51.419
          specified NEC K51.418
        fistula K51.413
        intestinal obstruction K51.412
        rectal bleeding K51.411
    sigmoid D12.5
    transverse D12.3
  corpus uteri N84.0
  dental K04.0
  duodenum K31.7
  ear (middle) H74.4-
  endometrium N84.0
  ethmoidal (sinus) J33.8
  fallopian tube N84.8
  female genital tract N84.9
    specified NEC N84.8
  frontal (sinus) J33.8
  gallbladder K82.4
  gingiva, gum K06.8
  labia, labium (majus) (minus) N84.3
  larynx (mucous) J38.1
    adenomatous D14.1
  malignant —*see* Neoplasm, malignant, by site
  maxillary (sinus) J33.8
  middle ear —*see* Polyp, ear (middle)
  myometrium N84.0
  nares
    anterior J33.9
    posterior J33.0
  nasal (mucous) J33.9
    cavity J33.0
    septum J33.0
  nasopharyngeal J33.0
  nose (mucous) J33.9
  oviduct N84.8
  pharynx J39.2
  placenta O90.89
  prostate —*see* Enlargement, enlarged,
    prostate
  pudenda, pudendum N84.3
  pulpal (dental) K04.0
  rectum (nonadenomatous) K62.1
    adenomatous —*see* Polyp, adenomatous
  septum (nasal) J33.0
  sinus (accessory) (ethmoidal) (frontal)
    (maxillary) (sphenoidal) J33.8
  sphenoidal (sinus) J33.8
  stomach K31.7
    adenomatous D13.1

Polyp, polypus *(Continued)*
  tube, fallopian N84.8
  turbinate, mucous membrane J33.8
  umbilical, newborn P83.6
  ureter N28.89
  urethra N36.2
  uterus (body) (corpus) (mucous) N84.0
    cervix N84.1
    in pregnancy or childbirth —*see* Pregnancy,
      complicated by, tumor, uterus
  vagina N84.2
  vocal cord (mucous) J38.1
  vulva N84.3
Polyphagia R63.2
Polyploidy Q92.7
Polypoid —*see* condition
Polyposis —*see also* Polyp
  coli (adenomatous) D12.6
    adenocarcinoma in C18.9
    adenocarcinoma in situ in —*see* Neoplasm,
      in situ, by site
    carcinoma in C18.9
  colon (adenomatous) D12.6
  familial D12.6
    adenocarcinoma in situ in —*see* Neoplasm,
      in situ, by site
  intestinal (adenomatous) D12.6
  malignant lymphomatous C83.1
  multiple, adenomatous (*see also* Neoplasm,
    benign) D36.9
Polyradiculitis —*see* Polyneuropathy
Polyradiculoneuropathy (acute) (postinfective)
  (segmentally demyelinating) G61.0
Polyserositis
  due to pericarditis I31.1
  pericardial I31.1
  periodic, familial E85.0
  tuberculous A19.9
    acute A19.1
    chronic A19.8
Polysplenia syndrome Q89.09
Polysyndactyly (*see also* Syndactylism,
  syndactyly) Q70.4
Polytrichia L68.3
Polyunguia Q84.6
Polyuria R35.8
  nocturnal R35.1
  psychogenic F45.8
Pompe's disease (glycogen storage) E74.02
Pompholyx L30.1
Poncet's disease (tuberculous rheumatism)
  A18.09
Pond fracture —*see* Fracture, skull
Ponos B55.0
Pons, pontine —*see* condition
Poor
  aesthetic of existing restoration of tooth
    K08.56
  contractions, labor O62.2
  gingival margin to tooth restoration K08.51
  personal hygiene R46.0
  prenatal care, affecting management of
    pregnancy —*see* Pregnancy, complicated
    by, insufficient, prenatal care
  sucking reflex (newborn) R29.2
  urinary stream R39.12
  vision NEC H54.7
Poradenitis, nostras inguinalis or venerea A55
Porencephaly (congenital) (developmental)
  (true) Q04.6
  acquired G93.0
  nondevelopmental G93.0
  traumatic (post) F07.89
Porocephaliasis B88.8
Porokeratosis Q82.8
Poroma, eccrine —*see* Neoplasm, skin, benign
Porphyria (South African) E80.20
  acquired E80.20
  acute intermittent (hepatic) (Swedish) E80.21
  cutanea tarda (hereditary) (symptomatic)
    E80.1

Porphyria *(Continued)*
  due to drugs E80.20
    correct substance properly administered —
      see Table of Drugs and Chemicals, by
      drug, adverse effect
    overdose or wrong substance given or
      taken —*see* Table of Drugs and
      Chemicals, by drug, poisoning
  erythropoietic (congenital) (hereditary)
    E80.0
  hepatocutaneous type E80.1
  secondary E80.20
  toxic NEC E80.20
  variegata E80.20
Porphyrinuria —*see* Porphyria
Porphyruria —*see* Porphyria
Portal —*see* condition
Port wine nevus, mark, or stain Q82.5
Posadas-Wernicke disease B38.9
Positive
  culture (nonspecific)
    blood R78.81
    bronchial washings R84.5
    cerebrospinal fluid R83.5
    cervix uteri R87.5
    nasal secretions R84.5
    nipple discharge R89.5
    nose R84.5
      staphylococcus (Methicillin susceptible)
        Z22.321
        Methicillin resistant Z22.322
    peritoneal fluid R85.5
    pleural fluid R84.5
    prostatic secretions R86.5
    saliva R85.5
    seminal fluid R86.5
    sputum R84.5
    synovial fluid R89.5
    throat scrapings R84.5
    urine R82.7
    vagina R87.5
    vulva R87.5
    wound secretions R89.5
  PPD (skin test) R76.11
  serology for syphilis A53.0
    with signs or symptoms - code as Syphilis,
      by site and stage
    false R76.8
  skin test, tuberculin (without active
    tuberculosis) R76.11
  test, human immunodeficiency virus (HIV)
    R75
  VDRL A53.0
    with signs or symptoms - code by site and
      stage under Syphilis A53.9
  Wassermann reaction A53.0
Postcardiotomy syndrome I97.0
Postcaval ureter Q62.62
Postcholecystectomy syndrome K91.5
Postclimacteric bleeding N95.0
Postcommissurotomy syndrome I97.0
Postconcussional syndrome F07.81
Postcontusional syndrome F07.81
Postcricoid region —*see* condition
Post-dates (40-42 weeks) (pregnancy) (mother)
  O48.0
  more than 42 weeks gestation O48.1
Postencephalitic syndrome F07.89
Posterior —*see* condition
Posterolateral sclerosis (spinal cord) —*see*
  Degeneration, combined
Postexanthematous —*see* condition
Postfebrile —*see* condition
Postgastrectomy dumping syndrome K91.1
Posthemiplegic chorea —*see* Monoplegia
Posthemorrhagic anemia (chronic) D50.0
  acute D62
  newborn P61.3
Postherpetic neuralgia (zoster) B02.29
  trigeminal B02.22
Posthitis N47.7

◀ New   ◀▥ Revised   ~~deleted~~ Deleted

Postimmunization complication or reaction — *see* Complications, vaccination

Postinfectious —*see* condition

Postlaminectomy syndrome NEC M96.1

Postleukotomy syndrome F07.0

Postmastectomy lymphedema (syndrome) I97.2

Postmaturity, postmature (over 42 weeks)
  maternal (over 42 weeks gestation) O48.1
  newborn P08.22

Postmeasles complication NEC (*see also* condition) B05.89

Postmenopausal
  endometrium (atrophic) N95.8
    suppurative (*see also* Endometritis) N71.9
  osteoporosis —*see* Osteoporosis, postmenopausal

Postnasal drip R09.82
  due to
    allergic rhinitis —*see* Rhinitis, allergic
    common cold J00
    gastroesophageal reflux —*see* Reflux, gastroesophageal
    nasopharyngitis —*see* Nasopharyngitis
    other know condition — code to condition
    sinusitis —*see* Sinusitis

Postnatal —*see* condition

Postoperative (postprocedural) —*see* Complication, postoperative
  pneumothorax, therapeutic Z98.3
  state NEC Z98.89

Postpancreatectomy hyperglycemia E89.1

Postpartum —*see* Puerperal

Postphlebitic syndrome —*see* Syndrome, postthrombotic

Postpolio (myelitic) syndrome G14

Postpoliomyelitic —*see also* condition
  osteopathy —*see* Osteopathy, after poliomyelitis

Postprocedural —*see also* Postoperative
  hypoinsulinemia E89.1

Postschizophrenic depression F32.8

Postsurgery status —*see also* Status (post)
  pneumothorax, therapeutic Z98.3

Post-term (40-42 weeks) (pregnancy) (mother) O48.0
  infant P08.21
  more than 42 weeks gestation (mother) O48.1

Post-traumatic brain syndrome, nonpsychotic F07.81

Post-typhoid abscess A01.09

Postures, hysterical F44.2

Postvaccinal reaction or complication —*see* Complications, vaccination

Postvalvulotomy syndrome I97.0

Potain's
  disease (pulmonary edema) —*see* Edema, lung
  syndrome (gastrectasis with dyspepsia) K31.0

Potter's
  asthma J62.8
  facies Q60.6
  lung J62.8
  syndrome (with renal agenesis) Q60.6

Pott's
  curvature (spinal) A18.01
  disease or paraplegia A18.01
  spinal curvature A18.01
  tumor, puffy —*see* Osteomyelitis, specified type NEC

Pouch
  bronchus Q32.4
  Douglas' —*see* condition
  esophagus, esophageal, congenital Q39.6
    acquired K22.5
  gastric K31.4
  Hartmann's K82.8
  pharynx, pharyngeal (congenital) Q38.7

Pouchitis K91.850

Poultrymen's itch B88.0

Poverty NEC Z59.6
  extreme Z59.5

Poxvirus NEC B08.8

Prader-Willi syndrome Q87.1

Preauricular appendage or tag Q17.0

Prebetalipoproteinemia (acquired) (essential) (familial) (hereditary) (primary) (secondary) E78.1
  with chylomicronemia E78.3

Precipitate labor or delivery O62.3

Preclimacteric bleeding (menorrhagia) N92.4

Precocious
  adrenarche E30.1
  menarche E30.1
  menstruation E30.1
  pubarche E30.1
  puberty E30.1
    central E22.8
  sexual development NEC E30.1
  thelarche E30.8

Precocity, sexual (constitutional) (cryptogenic) (female) (idiopathic) (male) E30.1
  with adrenal hyperplasia E25.9
    congenital E25.0

Precordial pain R07.2

Predeciduous teeth K00.2

Prediabetes, prediabetic R73.09
  complicating
    pregnancy —*see* Pregnancy, complicated by, diseases of, specified type or system NEC
    puerperium O99.89

Predislocation status of hip at birth Q65.6

Pre-eclampsia O14.9-
  with pre-existing hypertension —*see* Hypertension, complicating pregnancy, pre-existing, with, pre-eclampsia
  mild O14.0-
  moderate O14.0-
  severe O14.1-
    with hemolysis, elevated liver enzymes and low platelet count (HELLP) O14.2-

Pre-eruptive color change, teeth, tooth K00.8

Pre-excitation atrioventricular conduction I45.6

Preglaucoma H40.00-

Pregnancy (single) (uterine) —*see also* Delivery and Puerperal

---

Note: The Tabular must be reviewed for assignment of the appropriate character indicating the trimester of the pregnancy

Note: The Tabular must be reviewed for assignment of appropriate seventh character for multiple gestation codes in Chapter 15

---

  abdominal (ectopic) O00.0
    with viable fetus O36.7-
  ampullar O00.1
  biochemical O02.81
  broad ligament O00.8
  cervical O00.8
  chemical O02.81
  complicated NOS O26.9-
  complicated by (care of) (management affected by)
    abnormal, abnormality
      cervix O34.4-
        causing obstructed labor O65.5
      cord (umbilical) O69.9
      findings on antenatal screening of mother O28.9
        biochemical O28.1
        chromosomal O28.5
        cytological O28.2
        genetic O28.5
        hematological O28.0
        radiological O28.4
        specified NEC O28.8
        ultrasonic O28.3
      glucose (tolerance) NEC O99.810

Pregnancy (Continued)
  complicated by (Continued)
    abnormal, abnormality (Continued)
      pelvic organs O34.9-
        specified NEC O34.8-
          causing obstructed labor O65.5
      pelvis (bony) (major) NEC O33.0
      perineum O34.7-
      position
        placenta O44.1-
          without hemorrhage O44.0-
        uterus O34.59-
      uterus O34.59-
        causing obstructed labor O65.5
        congenital O34.0-
      vagina O34.6-
        causing obstructed labor O65.5
      vulva O34.7-
        causing obstructed labor O65.5
    abruptio placentae —*see* Abruptio placentae
    abscess or cellulitis
      bladder O23.1-
      breast O91.11-
      genital organ or tract O23.9-
    abuse
      physical O9A.31-
      psychological O9A.51-
      sexual O9A.41-
    adverse effect anesthesia O29.9-
      aspiration pneumonitis O29.01-
      cardiac arrest O29.11-
      cardiac complication NEC O29.19-
      cardiac failure O29.12-
      central nervous system complication NEC O29.29-
      cerebral anoxia O29.21-
      failed or difficult intubation O29.6-
      inhalation of stomach contents or secretions NOS O29.01-
      local, toxic reaction O29.3X
      Mendelson's syndrome O29.01-
      pressure collapse of lung O29.02-
      pulmonary complications NEC O29.09-
      specified NEC O29.8X
      spinal and epidural type NEC O29.5X
        induced headache O29.4-
    albuminuria O12.1-
    alcohol use O99.31-
    amnionitis O41.12-
    anaphylactoid syndrome of pregnancy O88.01-
    anemia (conditions in D50-D64) (pre-existing) O99.01-
      complicating the puerperium O99.03
    antepartum hemorrhage O46.9-
      with coagulation defect —*see* Hemorrhage, antepartum, with coagulation defect
      specified NEC O46.8X-
    appendicitis O99.61-
    atrophy (yellow) (acute) liver (subacute) O26.61-
    bariatric surgery status O99.84-
    bicornis or bicornuate uterus O34.59-
    biliary tract problems O26.61-
    breech presentation O32.1
    cardiovascular diseases (conditions in I00-I09, I20-I52, I70-I99) O99.41-
    cerebrovascular disorders (conditions in I60-I69) O99.41-
    cervical shortening O26.87-
    cervicitis O23.51-
    chloasma (gravidarum) O26.89-
    cholecystitis O99.61-
    cholestasis (intrahepatic) O26.61-
    chorioamnionitis O41.12-
    circulatory system disorder (conditions in I00-I09, I20-I99, O99.41-)
    compound presentation O32.6
    conjoined twins O30.02-

P

Pregnancy *(Continued)*
  complicated by *(Continued)*
    connective system disorders (conditions in M00-M99) O99.89
    contracted pelvis (general) O33.1
      inlet O33.2
      outlet O33.3
    convulsions (eclamptic) (uremic) *(see also* Eclampsia) O15.9-
    cracked nipple O92.11-
    cystitis O23.1-
    cystocele O34.8-
    death of fetus (near term) O36.4
      early pregnancy O02.1
      of one fetus or more in multiple gestation O31.2-
    deciduitis O41.14-
    decreased fetal movement O36.81-
    dental problems O99.61-
    diabetes (mellitus) O24.91-
      gestational (pregnancy induced) *—see* Diabetes, gestational
      pre-existing O24.31-
        specified NEC O24.81-
        type 1 O24.01-
        type 2 O24.11-
    digestive system disorders (conditions in K00-K93) O99.61-
    diseases of *—see* Pregnancy, complicated by, specified body system disease
      biliary tract O26.61-
      blood NEC (conditions in D65-D77) O99.11-
      liver O26.61-
      specified NEC O99.89
    disorders of *—see* Pregnancy, complicated by, specified body system disorder
    amniotic fluid and membranes O41.9-
      specified NEC O41.8X-
      biliary tract O26.61-
      ear and mastoid process (conditions in H60-H95) O99.89
      eye and adnexa (conditions in H00-H59) O99.89
      liver O26.61-
      skin (conditions in L00-L99) O99.71-
      specified NEC O99.89
    displacement, uterus NEC O34.59-
      causing obstructed labor O65.5
    disproportion (due to) O33.9
      fetal deformities NEC O33.7
      generally contracted pelvis O33.1
      hydrocephalic fetus O33.6
      inlet contraction of pelvis O33.2
      mixed maternal and fetal origin O33.4
      specified NEC O33.8
    double uterus O34.59-
      causing obstructed labor O65.5
    drug use (conditions in F11-F19) O99.32-
    eclampsia, eclamptic (coma) (convulsions) (delirium) (nephritis) (uremia) *(see also* Eclampsia) O15-
    ectopic pregnancy *—see* Pregnancy, ectopic
    edema O12.0-
      with
        gestational hypertension, mild *(see also* Pre-eclampsia) O14.0-
        proteinuria O12.2-
    effusion, amniotic fluid *—see* Pregnancy, complicated by, premature rupture of membranes
    elderly
      multigravida O09.52-
      primigravida O09.51-
    embolism *(see also* Embolism, obstetric, pregnancy) O88.-
    endocrine diseases NEC O99.28-
    endometritis O86.12
    excessive weight gain O26.0-
    exhaustion O26.81-
      during labor and delivery O75.81

Pregnancy *(Continued)*
  complicated by *(Continued)*
    face presentation O32.3
    failed induction of labor O61.9
    failed or difficult intubation for anesthesia O29.6-
      instrumental O61.1
      mechanical O61.1
      medical O61.0
      specified NEC O61.8
      surgical O61.1
    false labor (pains) O47.9
      at or after 37 completed weeks of pregnancy O47.1
      before 37 completed weeks of pregnancy O47.0-
    fatigue O26.81-
      during labor and delivery O75.81
    fatty metamorphosis of liver O26.61-
    female genital mutilation O34.8- *[N90.81-]*
    fetal (maternal care for)
      abnormality or damage O35.9
        acid-base balance O68
        specified type NEC O35.8
      acidemia O68
      acidosis O68
      alkalosis O68
      anemia and thrombocytopenia O36.82-
      anencephaly O35.0
      chromosomal abnormality (conditions in Q90-Q99) O35.1
      conjoined twins O30.02-
      damage from
        amniocentesis O35.7
        biopsy procedures O35.7
        drug addiction O35.5
        hematological investigation O35.7
        intrauterine contraceptive device O35.7
        maternal
          alcohol addiction O35.4
          cytomegalovirus infection O35.3
          disease NEC O35.8
          drug addiction O35.5
          listeriosis O35.8
          rubella O35.3
          toxoplasmosis O35.8
          viral infection O35.3
        medical procedure NEC O35.7
        radiation O35.6
      death (near term) O36.4
        early pregnancy O02.1
      decreased movement O36.81-
      disproportion due to deformity (fetal) O33.7
      excessive growth (large for dates) O36.6-
      growth retardation O36.59-
        light for dates O36.59-
        small for dates O36.59-
      heart rate irregularity (bradycardia) (decelerations) (tachycardia) O76
      hereditary disease O35.2
      hydrocephalus O35.0
      intrauterine death O36.4
      poor growth O36.59-
        light for dates O36.59-
        small for dates O36.59-
      problem O36.9-
        specified NEC O36.89-
      reduction (elective) O31.3-
      selective termination O31.3-
      spina bifida O35.0
      thrombocytopenia O36.82-
    fibroid (tumor) (uterus) O34.1-
    fissure of nipple O92.11-
    gallstones O99.61-
    gastric banding status O99.84-
    gastric bypass status O99.84-
    genital herpes (asymptomatic) (history of) (inactive) O98.51-
    genital tract infection O23.9-

Pregnancy *(Continued)*
  complicated by *(Continued)*
    glomerular diseases (conditions in N00-N07) O26.83-
      with hypertension, pre-existing *—see* Hypertension, complicating, pregnancy, pre-existing, with, renal disease
    gonorrhea O98.21-
    grand multiparity O09.4
    habitual aborter *—see* Pregnancy, complicated by, recurrent pregnancy loss
    HELLP syndrome (hemolysis, elevated liver enzymes and low platelet count) O14.2-
    hemorrhage
      antepartum *—see* Hemorrhage, antepartum
      before 20 completed weeks gestation O20.9
        specified NEC O20.8
      due to premature separation, placenta *(see also* Abruptio placentae) O45.9-
      early O20.9
        specified NEC O20.8
      threatened abortion O20.0
    hemorrhoids O22.4-
    hepatitis (viral) O98.41-
    herniation of uterus O34.59-
    high
      head at term O32.4
      risk *—see* Supervision (of) (for), high-risk
    history of in utero procedure during previous pregnancy O09.82-
    HIV O98.71-
    human immunodeficiency virus (HIV) disease O98.71-
    hydatidiform mole *(see also* Mole, hydatidiform) O01.9-
    hydramnios O40.-
    hydrocephalic fetus (disproportion) O33.6
    hydrops
      amnii O40.-
      fetalis O36.2-
        associated with isoimmunization *(see also* Pregnancy, complicated by, isoimmunization) O36.11-
    hydrorrhea O42.90
    hyperemesis (gravidarum) (mild) *(see also* Hyperemesis, gravidarum) O21.0-
    hypertension *—see* Hypertension, complicating pregnancy
    hypertensive
      heart and renal disease, pre-existing *— see* Hypertension, complicating, pregnancy, pre-existing, with, heart disease, with renal disease
      heart disease, pre-existing *—see* Hypertension, complicating, pregnancy, pre-existing, with, heart disease
      renal disease, pre-existing *—see* Hypertension, complicating, pregnancy, pre-existing, with, renal disease
    hypotension O26.5-
    immune disorders NEC (conditions in D80-D89) O99.11-
    incarceration, uterus O34.51-
    incompetent cervix O34.3-
    inconclusive fetal viability O36.80
    infection (s) O98.91-
      amniotic fluid or sac O41.10-
      bladder O23.1-
      carrier state NEC O99.830
        streptococcus B O99.820
      genital organ or tract O23.9-
        specified NEC O23.59-
      genitourinary tract O23.9-

◀ New   ⬅ Revised   ~~deleted~~ Deleted

Pregnancy (Continued)
  complicated by (Continued)
    infection (Continued)
      gonorrhea O98.21-
      hepatitis (viral) O98.41-
      HIV O98.71-
      human immunodeficiency virus (HIV)
        O98.71-
      kidney O23.0-
      nipple O91.01-
      parasitic disease O98.91-
        specified NEC O98.81-
      protozoal disease O98.61-
      sexually transmitted NEC O98.31-
      specified type NEC O98.81-
      syphilis O98.11-
      tuberculosis O98.01-
      urethra O23.2-
      urinary (tract) O23.4-
        specified NEC O23.3-
      viral disease O98.51-
    injury or poisoning (conditions in S00-T88)
      O9A.21-
      due to abuse
        physical O9A.31-
        psychological O9A.51-
        sexual O9A.41-
    insufficient
      prenatal care O09.3-
      weight gain O26.1-
    insulin resistance O26.89
    intrauterine fetal death (near term) O36.4
      early pregnancy O02.1
      multiple gestation (one fetus or more)
        O31.2-
    isoimmunization O36.11-
      anti-A sensitization O36.11-
      anti-B sensitization O36.19-
      Rh O36.09-
        anti-D antibody O36.01-
      specified NEC O36.19-
    laceration of uterus NEC O71.81
    malformation
      placenta, placental (vessel) O43.10-
        specified NEC O43.19-
      uterus (congenital) O34.0-
    malnutrition (conditions in E40-E46) O25.1-
    maternal hypotension syndrome O26.5-
    mental disorders (conditions in F01-F09,
      F20-F99) O99.34-
      alcohol use O99.31-
      drug use O99.32-
      smoking O99.33-
    mentum presentation O32.3
    metabolic disorders O99.28-
    missed
      abortion O02.1
      delivery O36.4
    multiple gestations O30.9-
      conjoined twins O30.02-
      quadruplet —see Pregnancy, quadruplet
      specified complication NEC O31.8X-
      specified number of multiples NEC —see
        Pregnancy, multiple (gestation),
        specified NEC
      triplet —see Pregnancy, triplet
      twin —see Pregnancy, twin
    musculoskeletal condition (conditions is
      M00-M99) O99.89
    necrosis, liver (conditions in K72) O26.61-
    neoplasm
      benign
        cervix O34.4-
        corpus uteri O34.1-
        uterus O34.1-
      malignant O9A.11-
    nephropathy NEC O26.83-
    nervous system condition (conditions in
      G00-G99) O99.35-
    nutritional diseases NEC O99.28-
    obesity (pre-existing) O99.21-

Pregnancy (Continued)
  complicated by (Continued)
    obesity surgery status O99.84-
    oblique lie or presentation O32.2
    older mother —see Pregnancy, complicated
      by, elderly
    oligohydramnios O41.0-
      with premature rupture of membranes
        (see also Pregnancy, complicated by,
        premature rupture of membranes)
        O42-
    onset (spontaneous) of labor after 37
      completed weeks of gestation but
      before 39 completed weeks gestation,
      with delivery by (planned) cesarean
      section O75.82
    oophoritis O23.52-
    overdose, drug (see also Table of Drugs
      and Chemicals, by drug, poisoning)
      O9A.21-
    oversize fetus O33.5
    papyraceous fetus O31.0-
    pelvic inflammatory disease O99.89
    periodontal disease O99.61-
    peripheral neuritis O26.82-
    peritoneal (pelvic) adhesions O99.89
    phlebitis O22.9-
    phlebopathy O22.9-
    phlebothrombosis (superficial) O22.2-
      deep O22.3-
    placenta accreta O43.21-
    placenta increta O43.22-
    placenta percreta O43.23-
    placenta previa O44.1-
      without hemorrhage O44.0-
    placental disorder O43.9-
      specified NEC O43.89-
    placental dysfunction O43.89-
    placental infarction O43.81-
    placental insufficiency O36.51-
    placental transfusion syndromes
      fetomaternal O43.01-
      fetus to fetus O43.02-
      maternofetal O43.01-
    placentitis O41.14-
    pneumonia O99.51-
    poisoning (see also Table of Drugs and
      Chemicals) O9A.21-
    polyhydramnios O40-
    polymorphic eruption of pregnancy
      O26.86
    poor obstetric history NEC O09.29-
    postmaturity (post-term) (40 to 42 weeks)
      O48.0
      more than 42 completed weeks gestation
        (prolonged) O48.1
    pre-eclampsia O14.9-
      mild O14.0-
      moderate O14.0-
      severe O14.1-
        with hemolysis, elevated liver
          enzymes and low platelet count
          (HELLP) O14.2-
    premature labor —see Pregnancy,
      complicated by, preterm labor
    premature rupture of membranes O42.90
      with onset of labor
        within 24 hours O42.00
          after 37 weeks gestation O42.02
          pre-term (before 37 completed
            weeks of gestation) O42.01-
        after 24 hours O42.10
          after 37 weeks gestation O42.12
          pre-term (before 37 completed
            weeks of gestation) O42.11-
        after 37 weeks gestation O42.92
        full-term O42.92
        pre-term (before 37 completed weeks of
          gestation) O42.91-
    premature separation of placenta - (see also
      Abruptio placentae) O45.9-

Pregnancy (Continued)
  complicated by (Continued)
    presentation, fetal —see Delivery,
      complicated by, malposition
    preterm delivery O60.10
    preterm labor
      with delivery O60.10
        preterm O60.10
        term O60.20
      second trimester
        with preterm delivery
          second trimester O60.12
          third trimester O60.13
        with term delivery O60.22
        without delivery O60.02
      third trimester
        with term delivery O60.23
        with third trimester preterm delivery
          O60.14
        without delivery O60.03
      without delivery O60.00
        second trimester O60.02
        third trimester O60.03
    previous history of —see Pregnancy,
      supervision of, high-risk
    prolapse, uterus O34.52-
    proteinuria (gestational) O12.1-
      with edema O12.2-
    pruritic urticarial papules and plaques of
      pregnancy (PUPPP) O26.86
    pruritus (neurogenic) O26.89-
    psychosis or psychoneurosis (puerperal)
      F53
    ptyalism O26.89-
    PUPPP (pruritic urticarial papules and
      plaques of pregnancy) O26.86
    pyelitis O23.0-
    recurrent pregnancy loss O26.2-
    renal disease or failure NEC O26.83-
      with secondary hypertension,
        pre-existing —see Hypertension,
        complicating, pregnancy,
        pre-existing, secondary
      hypertensive, pre-existing —see
        Hypertension, complicating,
        pregnancy, pre-existing, with, renal
        disease
    respiratory condition (conditions in
      J00-J99) O99.51-
    retained, retention
      dead ovum O02.0
      intrauterine contraceptive device
        O26.3-
    retroversion, uterus O34.53-
    Rh immunization, incompatibility or
      sensitization NEC O36.09-
      anti-D antibody O36.01-
    rupture
      amnion (premature) (see also Pregnancy,
        complicated by, premature rupture
        of membranes) O42-
      membranes (premature) (see also
        Pregnancy, complicated by,
        premature rupture of membranes)
        O42-
      uterus (during labor) O71.1
        before onset of labor O71.0-
    salivation (excessive) O26.89-
    salpingitis O23.52-
    salpingo-oophoritis O23.52-
    sepsis (conditions in A40, A41) O98.81-
    size date discrepancy (uterine) O26.84-
    skin condition (conditions in L00-L99)
      O99.71-
    smoking (tobacco) O99.33-
    social problem O09.7-
    specified condition NEC O26.89-
    spotting O26.85-
    streptococcus B carrier state O99.820
    subluxation of symphysis (pubis) O26.71-
    syphilis (conditions in A50-A53) O98.11-

◀ New   ◀▥ Revised   ~~deleted~~ Deleted

Pregnancy *(Continued)*
 supervision of *(Continued)*
  high-risk *(Continued)*
   due to *(Continued)*
    in utero procedure during previous
      pregnancy O09.82-
    in vitro fertilization O09.81-
    molar pregnancy O09.1-
    multiple previous pregnancies O09.4-
    older mother —*see* Pregnancy,
      supervision of, elderly mother
    poor reproductive or obstetric history
      NEC O09.29-
    pre-term labor O09.21-
    previous
      neonatal death O09.29-
    social problems O09.7-
    specified NEC O09.89-
    very young mother —*see* Pregnancy,
      supervision, young mother
  resulting from in vitro fertilization
    O09.81-
 normal Z34.9-
  first Z34.0-
  specified NEC Z34.8-
 young mother
  multigravida O09.62-
  primigravida O09.61-
 triplet O30.10-
  with
   two or more monoamniotic fetuses
     O30.12-
   two or more monochorionic fetuses
     O30.11-
  two or more monoamniotic fetuses O30.12-
  two or more monochorionic fetuses O30.11-
  unable to determine number of placenta
    and number of amniotic sacs O30.19-
  unspecified number of placenta and
    unspecified number of amniotic sacs
    O30.10-
 tubal (with abortion) (with rupture) O00.1
 twin O30.00-
  conjoined O30.02-
  dichorionic/diamniotic (two placenta, two
    amniotic sacs) O30.04-
  monochorionic/diamniotic (one placenta,
    two amniotic sacs) O30.03-
  monochorionic/monoamniotic (one
    placenta, one amniotic sac) O30.01-
  unable to determine number of placenta
    and number of amniotic sacs O30.09-
  unspecified number of placenta and
    unspecified number of amniotic sacs
    O30.00-
 unwanted Z64.0
 weeks of gestation
  8 weeks Z3A.08
  9 weeks Z3A.09
  10 weeks Z3A.10
  11 weeks Z3A.11
  12 weeks Z3A.12
  13 weeks Z3A.13
  14 weeks Z3A.14
  15 weeks Z3A.15
  16 weeks Z3A.16
  17 weeks Z3A.17
  18 weeks Z3A.18
  19 weeks Z3A.19
  20 weeks Z3A.20
  21 weeks Z3A.21
  22 weeks Z3A.22
  23 weeks Z3A.23
  24 weeks Z3A.24
  25 weeks Z3A.25
  26 weeks Z3A.26
  27 weeks Z3A.27
  28 weeks Z3A.28
  29 weeks Z3A.29
  30 weeks Z3A.30
  31 weeks Z3A.31
  32 weeks Z3A.32

Pregnancy *(Continued)*
 weeks of gestation *(Continued)*
  33 weeks Z3A.33
  34 weeks Z3A.34
  35 weeks Z3A.35
  36 weeks Z3A.36
  37 weeks Z3A.37
  38 weeks Z3A.38
  39 weeks Z3A.39
  40 weeks Z3A.40
  41 weeks Z3A.41
  42 weeks Z3A.42
  greater than 42 weeks Z3A.49
  less than 8 weeks Z3A.01
  not specified Z3A.00
Preiser's disease —*see* Osteonecrosis,
  secondary, due to, trauma, metacarpus
Pre-kwashiorkor —*see* Malnutrition, severe
Preleukemia (syndrome) D46.9
Preluxation, hip, congenital Q65.6
Premature —*see also* condition
 adrenarche E27.0
 aging E34.8
 beats I49.40
  atrial I49.1
  auricular I49.1
  supraventricular I49.1
 birth NEC —*see* Preterm, newborn
 closure, foramen ovale Q21.8
 contraction
  atrial I49.1
  atrioventricular I49.49
  auricular I49.1
  auriculoventricular I49.2
  heart (extrasystole) I49.49
  junctional I49.2
  ventricular I49.3
 delivery (*see also* Pregnancy, complicated by,
   preterm labor) O60.10
 ejaculation F52.4
 infant NEC —*see* Preterm, newborn
  light-for-dates —*see* Light for dates
 labor —*see* Pregnancy, complicated by,
   preterm labor
 lungs P28.0
 menopause E28.319
  asymptomatic E28.319
  symptomatic E28.310
 newborn
  extreme (less than 28 completed weeks) —
    see Immaturity, extreme
  less than 37 completed weeks —*see*
    Preterm, newborn
 puberty E30.1
 rupture membranes or amnion —*see*
   Pregnancy, complicated by, premature
   rupture of membranes
 senility E34.8
 thelarche E30.8
 ventricular systole I49.3
Prematurity NEC (less than 37 completed
  weeks) —*see* Preterm, newborn
 extreme (less than 28 completed weeks) —*see*
   Immaturity, extreme
Premenstrual
 dysphoric disorder (PMDD) N94.3
 tension (syndrome) N94.3
Premolarization, cuspids K00.2
Prenatal
 care, normal pregnancy —*see* Pregnancy,
   normal
 screening of mother Z36
 teeth K00.6
Preparatory care for subsequent treatment
  NEC
 for dialysis Z49.01
  peritoneal Z49.02
Prepartum —*see* condition
Preponderance, left or right ventricular I51.7
Prepuce —*see* condition
PRES (posterior reversible encephalopathy
  syndrome) I67.83

Presbycardia R54
Presbycusis, presbyacusia H91.1-
Presbyesophagus K22.8
Presbyophrenia F03
Presbyopia H52.4
Prescription of contraceptives (initial) Z30.019
 emergency (postcoital) Z30.012
 implantable subdermal Z30.019
 injectable Z30.013
 intrauterine contraceptive device Z30.014
 pills Z30.011
 postcoital (emergency) Z30.012
 repeat Z30.40
  implantable subdermal Z30.49
  injectable Z30.42
  pills Z30.41
  specified type NEC Z30.49
 specified type NEC Z30.018
Presence (of)
 ankle-joint implant (functional) (prosthesis)
   Z96.66-
 aortocoronary (bypass) graft Z95.1
 arterial-venous shunt (dialysis) Z99.2
 artificial
  eye (globe) Z97.0
  heart (fully implantable) (mechanical)
    Z95.812
   valve Z95.2
  larynx Z96.3
  lens (intraocular) Z96.1
  limb (complete) (partial) Z97.1-
   arm Z97.1-
    bilateral Z97.15
   leg Z97.1-
    bilateral Z97.16
 audiological implant (functional) Z96.29
 bladder implant (functional) Z96.0
 bone
  conduction hearing device Z96.29
  implant (functional) NEC Z96.7
  joint (prosthesis) —*see* Presence, joint
    implant
 cardiac
  defibrillator (functional) (with synchronous
    cardiac pacemaker)Z95.810
  implant or graft Z95.9
   specified type NEC Z95.818
  pacemaker Z95.0
 cerebrospinal fluid drainage device Z98.2
 cochlear implant (functional) Z96.21
 contact lens (es) Z97.3
 coronary artery graft or prosthesis Z95.5
 CSF shunt Z98.2
 dental prosthesis device Z97.2
 dentures Z97.2
 device (external) NEC Z97.8
  cardiac NEC Z95.818
  heart assist Z95.811
  implanted (functional) Z96.9
   specified NEC Z96.89
  prosthetic Z97.8
 ear implant Z96.20
  cochlear implant Z96.21
  myringotomy tube Z96.22
  specified type NEC Z96.29
 elbow-joint implant (functional) (prosthesis)
   Z96.62-
 endocrine implant (functional) NEC Z96.49
 eustachian tube stent or device (functional)
   Z96.29
 external hearing-aid or device Z97.4
 finger-joint implant (functional) (prosthetic)
   Z96.69-
 functional implant Z96.9
  specified NEC Z96.89
 graft
  cardiac NEC Z95.818
  vascular NEC Z95.828
 hearing-aid or device (external) Z97.4
  implant (bone) (cochlear) (functional)
    Z96.21
 heart assist device Z95.811

Presence *(Continued)*
  heart valve implant (functional) Z95.2
    prosthetic Z95.2
    specified type NEC Z95.4
    xenogenic Z95.3
  hip-joint implant (functional) (prosthesis) Z96.64-
  implanted device (artificial) (functional) (prosthetic) Z96.9
    automatic cardiac defibrillator (with synchronous cardiac pacemaker) Z95.810
    cardiac pacemaker Z95.0
    cochlear Z96.21
    dental Z96.5
    heart Z95.812
    heart valve Z95.2
      prosthetic Z95.2
      specified NEC Z95.4
      xenogenic Z95.3
    insulin pump Z96.41
    intraocular lens Z96.1
    joint Z96.60
      ankle Z96.66-
      elbow Z96.62-
      finger Z96.69-
      hip Z96.64-
      knee Z96.65-
      shoulder Z96.61-
      specified NEC Z96.698
      wrist Z96.63-
    larynx Z96.3
    myringotomy tube Z96.22
    otological Z96.20
      cochlear Z96.21
      eustachian stent Z96.29
      myringotomy Z96.22
      specified NEC Z96.29
      stapes Z96.29
    skin Z96.81
    skull plate Z96.7
    specified NEC Z96.89
    urogenital Z96.0
  insulin pump (functional) Z96.41
  intestinal bypass or anastomosis Z98.0
  intraocular lens (functional) Z96.1
  intrauterine contraceptive device (IUD) Z97.5
  intravascular implant (functional) (prosthetic) NEC Z95.9
    coronary artery Z95.5
    defibrillator (with synchronous cardiac pacemaker) Z95.810
    peripheral vessel (with angioplasty) Z95.820
  joint implant (prosthetic) (any) Z96.60
    ankle —*see* Presence, ankle joint implant
    elbow —*see* Presence, elbow joint implant
    finger —*see* Presence, finger joint implant
    hip —*see* Presence, hip joint implant
    knee —*see* Presence, knee joint implant
    shoulder —*see* Presence, shoulder joint implant
    specified joint NEC Z96.698
    wrist —*see* Presence, wrist joint implant
  knee-joint implant (functional) (prosthesis) Z96.65-
  laryngeal implant (functional) Z96.3
  mandibular implant (dental) Z96.5
  myringotomy tube (s) Z96.22
  orthopedic-joint implant (prosthetic) (any) — *see* Presence, joint implant
  otological implant (functional) Z96.29
  shoulder-joint implant (functional) (prosthesis) Z96.61-
  skull-plate implant Z96.7
  spectacles Z97.3
  stapes implant (functional) Z96.29
  systemic lupus erythematosus [SLE] inhibitor D68.62
  tendon implant (functional) (graft) Z96.7
  tooth root (s) implant Z96.5

Presence *(Continued)*
  ureteral stent Z96.0
  urethral stent Z96.0
  urogenital implant (functional) Z96.0
  vascular implant or device Z95.9
    access port device Z95.828
    specified type NEC Z95.828
  wrist-joint implant (functional) (prosthesis) Z96.63-
Presenile —*see also* condition
  dementia F03
  premature aging E34.8
Presentation, fetal —*see* Delivery, complicated by, malposition
Prespondylolisthesis (congenital) Q76.2
Pressure
  area, skin —*see* Ulcer, pressure, by site
  brachial plexus G54.0
  brain G93.5
    injury at birth NEC P11.1
  cerebral —*see* Pressure, brain
  chest R07.89
  cone, tentorial G93.5
  hyposystolic —*see also* Hypotension
    incidental reading, without diagnosis of hypotension R03.1
  increased
    intracranial (benign) G93.2
      injury at birth P11.0
    intraocular H40.05-
  lumbosacral plexus G54.1
  mediastinum J98.5
  necrosis (chronic) —*see* Ulcer, pressure, by site
  parental, inappropriate (excessive) Z62.6
  sore (chronic) —*see* Ulcer, pressure, by site
  spinal cord G95.20
  ulcer (chronic) —*see* Ulcer, pressure, by site
  venous, increased I87.8
Pre-syncope R55
Preterm
  delivery (*see also* Pregnancy, complicated by, preterm labor) O60.10
  labor —*see* Pregnancy, complicated by, preterm labor
  newborn (infant) P07.30
    gestational age
      28 completed weeks (28 weeks, 0 days through 28 weeks, 6 days) P07.31
      29 completed weeks (29 weeks, 0 days through 29 weeks, 6 days) P07.32
      30 completed weeks (30 weeks, 0 days through 30 weeks, 6 days) P07.33
      31 completed weeks (31 weeks, 0 days through 31 weeks, 6 days) P07.34
      32 completed weeks (32 weeks, 0 days through 32 weeks, 6 days) P07.35
      33 completed weeks (33 weeks, 0 days through 33 weeks, 6 days) P07.36
      34 completed weeks (34 weeks, 0 days through 34 weeks, 6 days) P07.37
      35 completed weeks (35 weeks, 0 days through 35 weeks, 6 days) P07.38
      36 completed weeks (36 weeks, 0 days through 36 weeks, 6 days) P07.39
Previa
  placenta (low) (marginal) (partial) (total) (with hemorrhage) O44.1-
    without hemorrhage O44.0-
  vasa O69.4
Priapism N48.30
  due to
    disease classified elsewhere N48.32
    drug N48.33
    specified cause NEC N48.39
    trauma N48.31
Prickling sensation (skin) R20.2
Prickly heat L74.0
Primary —*see* condition

Primigravida
  elderly, affecting management of pregnancy, labor and delivery (supervision only) — *see* Pregnancy, complicated by, elderly, primigravida
  older, affecting management of pregnancy, labor and delivery (supervision only) — *see* Pregnancy, complicated by, elderly, primigravida
  very young, affecting management of pregnancy, labor and delivery (supervision only) —*see* Pregnancy, complicated by, young mother, primigravida
Primipara
  elderly, affecting management of pregnancy, labor and delivery (supervision only) — *see* Pregnancy, complicated by, elderly, primigravida
  older, affecting management of pregnancy, labor and delivery (supervision only) — *see* Pregnancy, complicated by, elderly, primigravida
  very young, affecting management of pregnancy, labor and delivery (supervision only) —*see* Pregnancy, complicated by, young mother, primigravida
Primus varus (bilateral) Q66.2
PRIND (Prolonged reversible ischemic neurologic deficit) I63.9
Pringle's disease (tuberous sclerosis)Q85.1
Prinzmetal angina I20.1
Prizefighter ear —*see* Cauliflower ear
Problem (with) (related to)
  academic Z55.8
  acculturation Z60.3
  adjustment (to)
    change of job Z56.1
    life-cycle transition Z60.0
    pension Z60.0
    retirement Z60.0
  adopted child Z62.821
  alcoholism in family Z63.72
  atypical parenting situation Z62.9
  bankruptcy Z59.8
  behavioral (adult) F69
    drug seeking Z72.89
  birth of sibling affecting child Z62.898
  care (of)
    provider dependency Z74.9
      specified NEC Z74.8
    sick or handicapped person in family or household Z63.6
  child
    abuse (affecting the child) —*see* Maltreatment, child
    custody or support proceedings Z65.3
    in care of non-parental family member Z62.21
    in foster care Z62.21
    in welfare custody Z62.21
    living in orphanage or group home Z62.22
  child-rearing Z62.9
    specified NEC Z62.898
  communication (developmental) F80.9
  conflict or discord (with)
    boss Z56.4
    classmates Z55.4
    counselor Z64.4
    employer Z56.4
    family Z63.9
      specified NEC Z63.8
    probation officer Z64.4
    social worker Z64.4
    teachers Z55.4
    workmates Z56.4
  conviction in legal proceedings Z65.0
    with imprisonment Z65.1
  counselor Z64.4
  creditors Z59.8

◄ New ◄|||| Revised ~~deleted~~ Deleted

Problem *(Continued)*
digestive K92.9
drug addict in family Z63.72
ear —*see* Disorder, ear
economic Z59.9
  affecting care Z59.9
  specified NEC Z59.8
education Z55.9
  specified NEC Z55.8
employment Z56.9
  change of job Z56.1
  discord Z56.4
  environment Z56.5
  sexual harassment Z56.81
  specified NEC Z56.89
  stress NEC Z56.6
  stressful schedule Z56.3
  threat of job loss Z56.2
  unemployment Z56.0
enuresis, child F98.0
eye H57.9
failed examinations (school) Z55.2
falling Z91.81
family *(see also* Disruption, family) Z63.9-
  specified NEC Z63.8
feeding (elderly) (infant) R63.3
  newborn P92.9
    breast P92.5
    overfeeding P92.4
    slow P92.2
    specified NEC P92.8
    underfeeding P92.3
  nonorganic F50.8
finance Z59.9
  specified NEC Z59.8
foreclosure on loan Z59.8
foster child Z62.822
frightening experience (s) in childhood
  Z62.898
genital NEC
  female N94.9
  male N50.9
health care Z75.9
  specified NEC Z75.8
hearing —*see* Deafness
homelessness Z59.0
housing Z59.9
  inadequate Z59.1
  isolated Z59.8
  specified NEC Z59.8
identity (of childhood) F93.8
illegitimate pregnancy (unwanted) Z64.0
illiteracy Z55.0
impaired mobility Z74.09
imprisonment or incarceration Z65.1
inadequate teaching affecting education
  Z55.8
inappropriate (excessive) parental pressure
  Z62.6
influencing health status NEC Z78.9
in-law Z63.1
institutionalization, affecting child
  Z62.22
intrafamilial communication Z63.8
jealousy, child F93.8
landlord Z59.2
language (developmental) F80.9
learning (developmental) F81.9
legal Z65.3
  conviction without imprisonment Z65.0
  imprisonment Z65.1
  release from prison Z65.2
life-management Z73.9
  specified NEC Z73.89
life-style Z72.9
  gambling Z72.6
  high-risk sexual behavior (heterosexual)
    Z72.51
    bisexual Z72.53
    homosexual Z72.52
  inappropriate eating habits Z72.4

Problem *(Continued)*
life-style *(Continued)*
  self-damaging behavior NEC Z72.89
  specified NEC Z72.89
  tobacco use Z72.0
literacy Z55.9
  low level Z55.0
  specified NEC Z55.8
living alone Z60.2
lodgers Z59.2
loss of love relationship in childhood Z62.898
marital Z63.0
  involving
    divorce Z63.5
    estrangement Z63.5
    gender identity F66
mastication K08.8
medical
  care, within family Z63.6
  facilities Z75.9
    specified NEC Z75.8
mental F48.9
multiparity Z64.1
negative life events in childhood Z62.9
  altered pattern of family relationships
    Z62.898
  frightening experience Z62.898
  loss of
    love relationship Z62.898
    self-esteem Z62.898
  physical abuse (alleged) —*see*
    Maltreatment, child
  removal from home Z62.29
  specified event NEC Z62.898
neighbor Z59.2
neurological NEC R29.818
new step-parent affecting child Z62.898
none (feared complaint unfounded) Z71.1
occupational NEC Z56.89
parent-child —*see* Conflict, parent-child
personal hygiene Z91.89
personality F69
phase-of-life transition, adjustment Z60.0
presence of sick or disabled person in family
  or household Z63.79
  needing care Z63.6
primary support group (family) Z63.9
  specified NEC Z63.8
probation officer Z64.4
psychiatric F99
psychosexual (development) F66
psychosocial Z65.9
  specified NEC Z65.8
relationship Z63.9
  childhood F93.8
release from prison Z65.2
removal from home affecting child Z62.29
seeking and accepting known hazardous and
  harmful
  behavioral or psychological interventions
    Z65.8
  chemical, nutritional or physical
    interventions Z65.8
sexual function (nonorganic) F52.9
sight H54.7
sleep disorder, child F51.9
smell —*see* Disturbance, sensation, smell
social
  environment Z60.9
    specified NEC Z60.8
  exclusion and rejection Z60.4
  worker Z64.4
speech R47.9
  developmental F80.9
  specified NEC R47.89
swallowing —*see* Dysphagia
taste —*see* Disturbance, sensation, taste
tic, child F95.0
underachievement in school Z55.3
unemployment Z56.0
  threatened Z56.2

Problem *(Continued)*
unwanted pregnancy Z64.0
upbringing Z62.9
  specified NEC Z62.898
urinary N39.9
voice production R47.89
work schedule (stressful) Z56.3
Procedure (surgical)
  for purpose other than remedying health
    state Z41.9
    specified NEC Z41.8
  not done Z53.9
    because of
      administrative reasons Z53.8
      contraindication Z53.09
        smoking Z53.01
      patient's decision Z53.20
        for reasons of belief or group pressure
          Z53.1
        left against medical advice (AMA)
          Z53.21
      specified reason NEC Z53.29
    specified reason NEC Z53.8
Procidentia (uteri) N81.3
Proctalgia K62.89
  fugax K59.4
  spasmodic K59.4
Proctitis K62.89
  amebic (acute) A06.0
  chlamydial A56.3
  gonococcal A54.6
  granulomatous —*see* Enteritis, regional, large
    intestine
  herpetic A60.1
  radiation K62.7
  tuberculous A18.32
  ulcerative (chronic) K51.20
    with
      complication K51.219
        abscess K51.214
        fistula K51.213
        obstruction K51.212
        rectal bleeding K51.211
        specified NEC K51.218
Proctocele
  female (without uterine prolapse) N81.6
    with uterine prolapse N81.2
      complete N81.3
  male K62.3
Proctocolitis, mucosal —*see* Rectosigmoiditis,
  ulcerative
Proctoptosis K62.3
Proctorrhagia K62.5
Proctosigmoiditis K63.89
  ulcerative (chronic) —*see* Rectosigmoiditis,
    ulcerative
Proctospasm K59.4
  psychogenic F45.8
Profichet's disease —*see* Disorder, soft tissue,
  specified type NEC
Progeria E34.8
Prognathism (mandibular) (maxillary)
  M26.19
Progonoma (melanotic) —*see* Neoplasm,
  benign, by site
Progressive —*see* condition
Prolactinoma
  specified site —*see* Neoplasm, benign,
    by site
  unspecified site D35.2
Prolapse, prolapsed
  anus, anal (canal) (sphincter) K62.2
  arm or hand O32.2
    causing obstructed labor O64.4
  bladder (mucosa) (sphincter) (acquired)
    congenital Q79.4
    female —*see* Cystocele
    male N32.89
  breast implant (prosthetic) T85.49
  cecostomy K94.09
  cecum K63.4

Prolapse, prolapsed *(Continued)*
  cervix, cervical (hypertrophied) N81.2
    anterior lip, obstructing labor O65.5
    congenital Q51.828
    postpartal, old N81.2
    stump N81.85
  ciliary body (traumatic) —*see* Laceration,
      eye(ball), with prolapse or loss of
      interocular tissue
  colon (pedunculated) K63.4
  colostomy K94.09
  disc (intervertebral) —*see* Displacement,
      intervertebral disc
  eye implant (orbital) T85.398
    lens (ocular) —*see* Complications,
        intraocular lens
  fallopian tube N83.4
  gastric (mucosa) K31.89
  genital, female N81.9
    specified NEC N81.89
  globe, nontraumatic —*see* Luxation, globe
  ileostomy bud K94.19
  intervertebral disc —*see* Displacement,
      intervertebral disc
  intestine (small) K63.4
  iris (traumatic) —*see* Laceration, eye(ball),
      with prolapse or loss of interocular
      tissue
    nontraumatic H21.89
  kidney N28.83
    congenital Q63.2
  laryngeal muscles or ventricle J38.7
  liver K76.89
  meatus urinarius N36.8
  mitral (valve) I34.1
  ocular lens implant —*see* Complications,
      intraocular lens
  organ or site, congenital NEC —*see*
      Malposition, congenital
  ovary N83.4
  pelvic floor, female N81.89
  perineum, female N81.89
  rectum (mucosa) (sphincter) K62.3
    due to trichuris trichuria B79
  spleen D73.89
  stomach K31.89
  umbilical cord
    complicating delivery O69.0
  urachus, congenital Q64.4
  ureter N28.89
    with obstruction N13.5
      with infection N13.6
  ureterovesical orifice N28.89
  urethra (acquired) (infected) (mucosa)
      N36.8
    congenital Q64.71
  urinary meatus N36.8
    congenital Q64.72
  uterovaginal N81.4
    complete N81.3
    incomplete N81.2
  uterus (with prolapse of vagina) N81.4
    complete N81.3
    congenital Q51.818
    first degree N81.2
    in pregnancy or childbirth —*see*
        Pregnancy, complicated by,
        abnormal, uterus
    incomplete N81.2
    postpartal (old) N81.4
    second degree N81.2
    third degree N81.3
  uveal (traumatic) —*see* Laceration, eye(ball),
      with prolapse or loss of interocular
      tissue
  vagina (anterior) (wall) —*see* Cystocele
    with prolapse of uterus N81.4
      complete N81.3
      incomplete N81.2
      posterior wall N81.6
      posthysterectomy N99.3

Prolapse, prolapsed *(Continued)*
  vitreous (humor) H43.0-
    in wound —*see* Laceration, eye(ball), with
        prolapse or loss of interocular tissue
  womb —*see* Prolapse, uterus
Prolapsus, female N81.9
  specified NEC N81.89
Proliferation (s)
  primary cutaneous CD30-positive large T-cell
      C86.6
Proliferative —*see* condition
Prolonged, prolongation (of)
  bleeding (time) (idiopathic) R79.1
  coagulation (time) R79.1
  gestation (over 42 completed weeks)
    mother O48.1
    newborn P08.22
  interval I44.0
  labor O63.9
    first stage O63.0
    second stage O63.1
  partial thromboplastin time (PTT) R79.1
  pregnancy (more than 42 weeks gestation)
      O48.1
  prothrombin time R79.1
  QT interval I45.81
  uterine contractions in labor O62.4
Prominence, prominent
  with disproportion (fetopelvic) O33.0
    causing obstructed labor O65.0
  auricle (congenital) (ear) Q17.5
  ischial spine or sacral promontory
  nose (congenital) acquired M95.0
Promiscuity —*see* High, risk, sexual behavior
Pronation
  ankle —*see* Deformity, limb, foot, specified
      NEC
  foot —*see also* Deformity, limb, foot, specified
      NEC
    congenital Q74.2
Prophylactic
  administration of
    antibiotics, long-term Z79.2
      short-term use - omit code
    drug (*see also* Long-term (current) drug
        therapy (use of)) Z79.899-
    medication Z79.899
  organ removal (for neoplasia management)
      Z40.00
    breast Z40.01
    ovary Z40.02
    specified site NEC Z40.09
  surgery Z40.9
    for risk factors related to malignant
        neoplasm —*see* Prophylactic, organ
        removal
    specified NEC Z40.8
  vaccination Z23
Propionic acidemia E71.121
Proptosis (ocular) —*see also* Exophthalmos
  thyroid —*see* Hyperthyroidism, with goiter
Prosection, anxiety concerning Z65.3
Prosopagnosia R48.3
Prostadynia N42.81
Prostate, prostatic —*see* condition
Prostatism —*see* Hyperplasia, prostate
Prostatitis (congestive) (suppurative) (with
    cystitis) N41.9
  acute N41.0
  cavitary N41.8
  chronic N41.1
  diverticular N41.8
  due to Trichomonas (vaginalis) A59.02
  fibrous N41.1
  gonococcal (acute) (chronic) A54.22
  granulomatous N41.4
  hypertrophic N41.1
  subacute N41.1
  trichomonal A59.02
  tuberculous A18.14
Prostatocystitis N41.3

Prostatorrhea N42.89
Prostatosis N42.82
Prostration R53.83
  heat —*see also* Heat, exhaustion
    anhydrotic T67.3
    due to
      salt (and water) depletion T67.4
      water depletion T67.3
  nervous F48.8
  senile R54
Protanomaly (anomalous trichromat) H53.54
Protanopia (complete) (incomplete) H53.54
Protection (against) (from) —*see* Prophylactic
Protein
  deficiency NEC —*see* Malnutrition
  malnutrition —*see* Malnutrition
  sickness (*see also* Reaction, serum) T80.69
Proteinemia R77.9
Proteinosis
  alveolar (pulmonary) J84.01
  lipid or lipoid (of Urbach) E78.89
Proteinuria R80.9
  Bence Jones R80.3
  complicating pregnancy —*see* Proteinuria,
      gestational
  gestational O12.1-
    with edema O12.2-
  idiopathic R80.0
  isolated R80.0
    with glomerular lesion N06.9
      dense deposit disease N06.6
      diffuse
        crescentic glomerulonephritis N06.7
        endocapillary proliferative
            glomerulonephritis N06.4
        mesangiocapillary glomerulonephritis
            N06.5
      focal and segmental hyalinosis or
          sclerosis N06.1
      membranous (diffuse) N06.2
      mesangial proliferative (diffuse)
          N06.3
      minimal change N06.0
      specified pathology NEC N06.8
  orthostatic R80.2
    with glomerular lesion —*see* Proteinuria,
        isolated, with glomerular lesion
  persistent R80.1
    with glomerular lesion —*see* Proteinuria,
        isolated, with glomerular lesion
  postural R80.2
    with glomerular lesion —*see* Proteinuria,
        isolated, with glomerular lesion
  pre-eclamptic —*see* Pre-eclampsia
  specified type NEC R80.8
Proteolysis, pathologic D65
Proteus (mirabilis) (morganii), as cause of
    disease classified elsewhere B96.4
Prothrombin gene mutation D68.52
Protoporphyria, erythropoietic E80.0
Protozoal —*see also* condition
  disease B64
    specified NEC B60.8
Protrusion, protrusio
  acetabuli M24.7
  acetabulum (into pelvis) M24.7
  device, implant or graft (*see also*
      Complications, by site and type,
      mechanical) T85.698
    arterial graft NEC —*see* Complication,
        cardiovascular device, mechanical,
        vascular
    breast (implant) T85.49
    catheter NEC T85.698
      cystostomy T83.090
      dialysis (renal) T82.49
        intraperitoneal T85.691
      infusion NEC T82.594
        spinal (epidural) (subdural)
            T85.690
      urinary, indwelling T83.098

◀ New　　◀▥ Revised　　~~deleted~~ Deleted

Protrusion, protrusio (Continued)
  device, implant or graft (Continued)
    electronic (electrode) (pulse generator)
        (stimulator)
      bone T84.390
        nervous system —see Complication,
            prosthetic device, mechanical,
            electronic nervous system
            stimulator
    fixation, internal (orthopedic) NEC —see
        Complication, fixation device,
        mechanical
    gastrointestinal —see Complications,
        prosthetic device, mechanical,
        gastrointestinal device
    genital NEC T83.498
      intrauterine contraceptive device
          T83.39
      penile prosthesis T83.490
    heart NEC —see Complication,
        cardiovascular device, mechanical
    joint prosthesis —see Complications, joint
        prosthesis, mechanical, specified
        NEC, by site
    ocular NEC —see Complications, prosthetic
        device, mechanical, ocular device
    orthopedic NEC —see Complication,
        orthopedic, device, mechanical
    specified NEC T85.628
    urinary NEC —see also Complication,
        genitourinary, device, urinary,
        mechanical
      graft T83.29
    vascular NEC —see Complication,
        cardiovascular device, mechanical
    ventricular intracranial shunt T85.09
  intervertebral disc —see Displacement,
      intervertebral disc
  joint prosthesis —see Complications, joint
      prosthesis, mechanical, specified NEC,
      by site
  nucleus pulposus —see Displacement,
      intervertebral disc
Prune belly (syndrome) Q79.4
Prurigo (ferox) (gravis) (Hebrae) (Hebra's)
    (mitis) (simplex) L28.2
  Besnier's L20.0
  estivalis L56.4
  nodularis L28.1
  psychogenic F45.8
Pruritus, pruritic (essential) L29.9
  ani, anus L29.0
    psychogenic F45.8
  anogenital L29.3
    psychogenic F45.8
  due to onchocerca volvulus B73.1
  gravidarum —see Pregnancy, complicated by,
      specified pregnancy-related condition
      NEC
  hiemalis L29.8
  neurogenic (any site) F45.8
  perianal L29.0
  psychogenic (any site) F45.8
  scroti, scrotum L29.1
    psychogenic F45.8
  senile, senilis L29.8
  specified NEC L29.8
    psychogenic F45.8
  Trichomonas A59.9
  vulva, vulvae L29.2
    psychogenic F45.8
Pseudarthrosis, pseudoarthrosis (bone) —see
    Nonunion, fracture
  clavicle, congenital Q74.0
  joint, following fusion or arthrodesis
      M96.0
Pseudoaneurysm —see Aneurysm
Pseudoangina (pectoris) —see Angina
Pseudoangioma I81
Pseudoarteriosus Q28.8
Pseudoarthrosis —see Pseudarthrosis

Pseudobulbar affect (PBA) F48.2
Pseudochromhidrosis L67.8
Pseudocirrhosis, liver, pericardial I31.1
Pseudocowpox B08.03
Pseudocoxalgia M91.3-
Pseudocroup J38.5
Pseudo-Cushing's syndrome, alcohol-induced
    E24.4
Pseudocyesis F45.8
Pseudocyst
  lung J98.4
  pancreas K86.3
  retina —see Cyst, retina
Pseudoelephantiasis neuroarthritica
    Q82.0
Pseudoexfoliation, capsule (lens) —see
    Cataract, specified NEC
Pseudofolliculitis barbae L73.1
Pseudoglioma H44.89
Pseudohemophilia (Bernuth's) (hereditary)
    (type B) D68.0
  Type A D69.8
  vascular D69.8
Pseudohermaphroditism Q56.3
  adrenal E25.8
  female Q56.2
    with adrenocortical disorder E25.8
    without adrenocortical disorder
        Q56.2
  adrenal, congenital E25.0
  male Q56.1
    with
      adrenocortical disorder E25.8
      androgen resistance E34.51
      cleft scrotum Q56.1
      feminizing testis E34.51
      5-alpha-reductase deficiency E29.1
    without gonadal disorder Q56.1
  adrenal E25.8
Pseudo-Hurler's polydystrophy E77.0
Pseudohydrocephalus G93.2
Pseudohypertrophic muscular dystrophy
    (Erb's) G71.0
Pseudohypertrophy, muscle G71.0
Pseudohypoparathyroidism E20.1
Pseudoinsomnia F51.03
Pseudoleukemia, infantile D64.89
Pseudomembranous —see condition
Pseudomeningocele (cerebral) (infective) (post-
    traumatic) G96.19
  postprocedural (spinal) G97.82
Pseudomenses (newborn) P54.6
Pseudomenstruation (newborn) P54.6
Pseudomonas
  aeruginosa, as cause of disease classified
      elsewhere B96.5
  mallei infection A24.0
    as cause of disease classified elsewhere
        B96.5
  pseudomallei, as cause of disease classified
      elsewhere B96.5
Pseudomyotonia G71.19
Pseudomyxoma peritonei C78.6
Pseudoneuritis, optic (nerve) (disc) (papilla),
    congenital Q14.2
Pseudo-obstruction intestine (acute) (chronic)
    (idiopathic) (intermittent secondary)
    (primary) K59.8
Pseudopapilledema H47.33-
  congenital Q14.2
Pseudoparalysis
  arm or leg R29.818
  atonic, congenital P94.2
Pseudopelade L66.0
Pseudophakia Z96.1
Pseudopolyarthritis, rhizomelic M35.3
Pseudopolycythemia D75.1
Pseudopseudohypoparathyroidism
    E20.1
Pseudopterygium H11.81-
Pseudoptosis (eyelid) —see Blepharochalasis

Pseudopuberty, precocious
  female heterosexual E25.8
  male isosexual E25.8
Pseudorickets (renal) N25.0
Pseudorubella B08.20
Pseudosclerema, newborn P83.8
Pseudosclerosis (brain)
  Jakob's —see Creutzfeldt-Jakob disease or
      syndrome
  of Westphal (Strüümpell) E83.01
  spastic —see Creutzfeldt-Jakob disease or
      syndrome
Pseudotetanus —see Convulsions
Pseudotetany R29.0
  hysterical F44.5
Pseudotruncus arteriosus Q25.4
Pseudotuberculosis A28.2
  enterocolitis A04.8
  pasteurella (infection) A28.0
Pseudotumor
  cerebri G93.2
  orbital H05.11-
Pseudoxanthoma elasticum Q82.8
Psilosis (sprue) (tropical) K90.1
  nontropical K90.0
Psittacosis A70
Psoitis M60.88
Psoriasis L40.9
  arthropathic L40.50
    arthritis mutilans L40.52
    distal interphalangeal L40.51
    juvenile L40.54
    other specified L40.59
    spondylitis L40.53
  buccal K13.29
  flexural L40.8
  guttate L40.4
  mouth K13.29
  nummular L40.0
  plaque L40.0
  psychogenic F54
  pustular (generalized) L40.1
    palmaris et plantaris L40.3
  specified NEC L40.8
  vulgaris L40.0
Psychasthenia F48.8
Psychiatric disorder or problem F99
Psychogenic —see also condition
  factors associated with physical conditions
      F54
Psychological and behavioral factors affecting
    medical condition F59
Psychoneurosis, psychoneurotic —see also
    Neurosis
  anxiety (state) F41.1
  depersonalization F48.1
  hypochondriacal F45.21
  hysteria F44.9
  neurasthenic F48.8
  personality NEC F60.89
Psychopathy, psychopathic
  affectionless F94.2
  autistic F84.5
  constitution, post-traumatic F07.81
  personality —see Disorder, personality
  sexual —see Deviation, sexual
  state F60.2
Psychosexual identity disorder of childhood
    F64.2
Psychosis, psychotic F29
  acute (transient) F23
    hysterical F44.9
  affective —see Disorder, mood
  alcoholic F10.959
    with
      abuse F10.159
      anxiety disorder F10.980
        with
          abuse F10.180
          dependence F10.280
      delirium tremens F10.231

P

Psychosis, psychotic *(Continued)*
 alcoholic *(Continued)*
  with *(Continued)*
   delusions F10.950
    with
     abuse F10.150
     dependence F10.250
   dementia F10.97
    with dependence F10.27
   dependence F10.259
   hallucinosis F10.951
    with
     abuse F10.151
     dependence F10.251
   mood disorder F10.94
    with
     abuse F10.14
     dependence F10.24
   paranoia F10.950
    with
     abuse F10.150
     dependence F10.250
  persisting amnesia F10.96
   with dependence F10.26
  amnestic confabulatory F10.96
   with dependence F10.26
  delirium tremens F10.231
  Korsakoff's, Korsakov's, Korsakow's F10.26
  paranoid type F10.950
   with
    abuse F10.150
    dependence F10.250
 anergastic —*see* Psychosis, organic
 arteriosclerotic (simple type) (uncomplicated) F01.50
  with behavioral disturbance F01.51
 childhood F84.0
  atypical F84.8
 climacteric —*see* Psychosis, involutional
 confusional F29
  acute or subacute F05
  reactive F23
 cycloid F23
 depressive —*see* Disorder, depressive
 disintegrative (childhood) F84.3
 drug-induced —*see* F11-F19 with .x59
  paranoid and hallucinatory states —*see* F11-F19 with .x50 or .x51
 due to or associated with
  addiction, drug —*see* F11-F19 with .X59
  dependence
   alcohol F10.259
   drug —*see* F11-F19 with .x59
  epilepsy F06.8
  Huntington's chorea F06.8
  ischemia, cerebrovascular (generalized) F06.8
  multiple sclerosis F06.8
  physical disease F06.8
  presenile dementia F03
  senile dementia F03
  vascular disease (arteriosclerotic) (cerebral) F01.50
   with behavioral disturbance F01.51
 epileptic F06.8
 episode F23
  due to or associated with physical condition F06.8
 exhaustive F43.0
 hallucinatory, chronic F28
 hypomanic F30.8
 hysterical (acute) F44.9
 induced F24
 infantile F84.0
  atypical F84.8
 infective (acute) (subacute) F05
 involutional F28
  depressive —*see* Disorder, depressive
  melancholic —*see* Disorder, depressive
  paranoid (state) F22

Psychosis, psychotic *(Continued)*
 Korsakoff's, Korsakov's, Korsakow's (nonalcoholic) F04
  alcoholic F10.96
   in dependence F10.26
 induced by other psychoactive substance —*see* categories F11-F19
  with .x5x
 mania, manic (single episode) F30.2
  recurrent type F31.89
 manic-depressive —*see* Disorder, mood
 menopausal —*see* Psychosis, involutional
 mixed schizophrenic and affective F25.8
 multi-infarct (cerebrovascular) F01.50
  with behavioral disturbance F01.51
 nonorganic F29
  specified NEC F28
 organic F09
  due to or associated with
   arteriosclerosis (cerebral) —*see* Psychosis, arteriosclerotic
   cerebrovascular disease, arteriosclerotic —*see* Psychosis, arteriosclerotic
   childbirth —*see* Psychosis, puerperal
   Creutzfeldt-Jakob disease or syndrome —*see* Creutzfeldt-Jakob disease or syndrome
   dependence, alcohol F10.259
   disease
    alcoholic liver F10.259
    brain, arteriosclerotic —*see* Psychosis, arteriosclerotic
    cerebrovascular F01.50
     with behavioral disturbance F01.51
    Creutzfeldt-Jakob —*see* Creutzfeldt-Jakob disease or syndrome
    endocrine or metabolic F06.8
     acute or subacute F05
    liver, alcoholic F10.259
   epilepsy transient (acute) F05
   infection
    brain (intracranial) F06.8
     acute or subacute F05
   intoxication
    alcoholic (acute) F10.259
    drug F19 with .X59 F11-
   ischemia, cerebrovascular (generalized) —*see* Psychosis, arteriosclerotic
   puerperium —*see* Psychosis, puerperal
   trauma, brain (birth) (from electric current) (surgical) F06.8
    acute or subacute F05
  infective F06.8
   acute or subacute F05
  post-traumatic F06.8
   acute or subacute F05
 paranoiac F22
 paranoid (climacteric) (involutional) (menopausal) F22
  psychogenic (acute) F23
  schizophrenic F20.0
  senile F03
 postpartum F53
 presbyophrenic (type) F03
 presenile F03
 psychogenic (paranoid) F23
  depressive F32.3
 puerperal F53
  specified type —*see* Psychosis, by type
 reactive (brief) (transient) (emotional stress) (psychological trauma) F23
  depressive F32.3
   recurrent F33.3
  excitative type F30.8
 schizoaffective F25.9
  depressive type F25.1
  manic type F25.0
 schizophrenia, schizophrenic —*see* Schizophrenia

Psychosis, psychotic *(Continued)*
 schizophrenia-like, in epilepsy F06.2
 schizophreniform F20.81
  affective type F25.9
  brief F23
  confusional type F23
  depressive type F25.1
  manic type F25.0
  mixed type F25.0
 senile NEC F03
  depressed or paranoid type F03
  simple deterioration F03
  specified type — code to condition
 shared F24
 situational (reactive) F23
 symbiotic (childhood) F84.3
 symptomatic F09
Psychosomatic —*see* Disorder, psychosomatic
Psychosyndrome, organic F07.9
Psychotic episode due to or associated with physical condition F06.8
Pterygium (eye) H11.00-
 amyloid H11.01-
 central H11.02-
 colli Q18.3
 double H11.03-
 peripheral
  progressive H11.05-
  stationary H11.04-
 recurrent H11.06-
Ptilosis (eyelid) —*see* Madarosis
Ptomaine (poisoning) —*see* Poisoning, food
Ptosis —*see also* Blepharoptosis
 adiposa (false) —*see* Blepharoptosis
 breast N64.81
 cecum K63.4
 colon K63.4
 congenital (eyelid) Q10.0
  specified site NEC —*see* Anomaly, by site
 eyelid —*see* Blepharoptosis
  congenital Q10.0
 gastric K31.89
 intestine K63.4
 kidney N28.83
 liver K76.89
 renal N28.83
 splanchnic K63.4
 spleen D73.89
 stomach K31.89
 viscera K63.4
PTP D69.51
Ptyalism (periodic) K11.7
 hysterical F45.8
 pregnancy —*see* Pregnancy, complicated by, specified pregnancy-related condition NEC
 psychogenic F45.8
Ptyalolithiasis K11.5
Pubarche, precocious E30.1
Pubertas praecox E30.1
Puberty (development state) Z00.3
 bleeding (excessive) N92.2
 delayed E30.0
 precocious (constitutional) (cryptogenic) (idiopathic) E30.1
  central E22.8
  due to
   ovarian hyperfunction E28.1
    estrogen E28.0
   testicular hyperfunction E29.0
 premature E30.1
  due to
   adrenal cortical hyperfunction E25.8
   pineal tumor E34.8
   pituitary (anterior) hyperfunction E22.8
Puckering, macula —*see* Degeneration, macula, puckering
Pudenda, pudendum —*see* condition
Puente's disease (simple glandular cheilitis) K13.0

Puerperal, puerperium (complicated by, complications)
abnormal glucose (tolerance test) O99.815
abscess
  areola O91.02
    associated with lactation O91.03
  Bartholin's gland O86.19
  breast O91.12
    associated with lactation O91.13
  cervix (uteri) O86.11
  genital organ NEC O86.19
  kidney O86.21
  mammary O91.12
    associated with lactation O91.13
  nipple O91.02
    associated with lactation O91.03
  peritoneum O85
  subareolar O91.12
    associated with lactation O91.13
  urinary tract —*see* Puerperal, infection, urinary
  uterus O86.12
  vagina (wall) O86.13
  vaginorectal O86.13
  vulvovaginal gland O86.13
adnexitis O86.19
afibrinogenemia, or other coagulation defect O72.3
albuminuria (acute) (subacute) —*see* Proteinuria, gestational
alcohol use O99.315
anemia O90.81
  pre-existing (pre-pregnancy) O99.03
anesthetic death O89.8
apoplexy O99.43
bariatric surgery status O99.845
blood disorder NEC O99.13
blood dyscrasia O72.3
cardiomyopathy O90.3
cerebrovascular disorder (conditions in I60-I69) O99.43
cervicitis O86.11
circulatory system disorder O99.43
coagulopathy (any) O72.3
complications O90.9
  specified NEC O90.89
convulsions —*see* Eclampsia
cystitis O86.22
cystopyelitis O86.29
delirium NEC F05
diabetes O24.93
  gestational —*see* Puerperal, gestational diabetes
  pre-existing O24.33
    specified NEC O24.83
    type 1 O24.03
    type 2 O24.13
digestive system disorder O99.63
disease O90.9
  breast NEC O92.29
  cerebrovascular (acute) O99.43
  nonobstetric NEC O99.89
  tubo-ovarian O86.19
  Valsuani's O99.03
disorder O90.9
  biliary tract O26.63
  lactation O92.70
  liver O26.63
  nonobstetric NEC O99.89
disruption
  cesarean wound O90.0
  episiotomy wound O90.1
  perineal laceration wound O90.1
drug use O99.325
eclampsia (with pre-existing hypertension) O15.2
embolism (pulmonary) (blood clot) —*see* Embolism, obstetric, puerperal
endocrine, nutritional or metabolic disease NEC O99.285
endophlebitis —*see* Puerperal, phlebitis

Puerperal, puerperium (*Continued*)
endotrachelitis O86.11
failure
  lactation (complete) O92.3
    partial O92.4
  renal, acute O90.4
fever (of unknown origin) O86.4
  septic O85
fissure, nipple O92.12
  associated with lactation O92.13
fistula
  breast (due to mastitis) O91.12
    associated with lactation O91.13
  nipple O91.02
    associated with lactation O91.03
galactophoritis O91.22
  associated with lactation O91.23
galactorrhea O92.6
gastric banding status O99.845
gastric bypass status O99.845
gastrointestinal disease NEC O99.63
gestational diabetes O24.439
  diet controlled O24.430
  insulin (and diet) controlled O24.434
gonorrhea O98.23
hematoma, subdural O99.43
hemiplegia, cerebral O99.355-
  due to cerebrovascular disorder O99.43
hemorrhage O72.1
  brain O99.43
  bulbar O99.43
  cerebellar O99.43
  cerebral O99.43
  cortical O99.43
  delayed or secondary O72.2
  extradural O99.43
  internal capsule O99.43
  intracranial O99.43
  intrapontine O99.43
  meningeal O99.43
  pontine O99.43
  retained placenta O72.0
  subarachnoid O99.43
  subcortical O99.43
  subdural O99.43
  third stage O72.0
  uterine, delayed O72.2
  ventricular O99.43
hemorrhoids O87.2
hepatorenal syndrome O90.4
hypertension —*see* Hypertension, complicating, puerperium
hypertrophy, breast O92.29
induration breast (fibrous) O92.29
infection O86.4
  cervix O86.11
  generalized O85
  genital tract NEC O86.19
    obstetric surgical wound O86.0
  kidney (bacillus coli) O86.21
  maternal O98.93
    carrier state NEC O99.835
    gonorrhea O98.23
    human immunodeficiency virus (HIV) O98.73
    protozoal O98.63
    sexually transmitted NEC O98.33
    specified NEC O98.83
    streptococcus B carrier state O99.825
    syphilis O98.13
    tuberculosis O98.03
    viral hepatitis O98.43
    viral NEC O98.53
  nipple O91.02
    associated with lactation O91.03
  peritoneum O85
  renal O86.21
  specified NEC O86.89

Puerperal, puerperium (*Continued*)
infection (*Continued*)
  urinary (asymptomatic) (tract) NEC O86.20
    bladder O86.22
    kidney O86.21
    specified site NEC O86.29
    urethra O86.22
  vagina O86.13
  vein —*see* Puerperal, phlebitis
ischemia, cerebral O99.43
lymphangitis O86.89
  breast O91.22
    associated with lactation O91.23
malignancy O9A.13
malnutrition O25.3
mammillitis O91.02
  associated with lactation O91.03
mammitis O91.22
  associated with lactation O91.23
mania F30.8
mastitis O91.22
  associated with lactation O91.23
  purulent O91.12
    associated with lactation O91.13
melancholia —*see* Disorder, depressive
mental disorder NEC O99.345
metroperitonitis O85
metrorrhagia —*see* Hemorrhage, postpartum
metrosalpingitis O86.19
metrovaginitis O86.13
milk leg O87.1
monoplegia, cerebral O99.43
mood disturbance O90.6
necrosis, liver (acute) (subacute) (conditions in subcategory K72.0) O26.63
  with renal failure O90.4
nervous system disorder O99.355
neuritis O90.89
obesity (pre-existing prior to pregnancy) O99.215
obesity surgery status O99.845
occlusion, precerebral artery O99.43
paralysis
  bladder (sphincter) O90.89
  cerebral O99.43
paralytic stroke O99.43
parametritis O85
paravaginitis O86.13
pelviperitonitis O85
perimetritis O86.12
perimetrosalpingitis O86.19
perinephritis O86.21
periphlebitis —*see* Puerperal phlebitis
peritoneal infection O85
peritonitis (pelvic) O85
perivaginitis O86.13
phlebitis O87.0
  deep O87.1
  pelvic O87.1
  superficial O87.0
phlebothrombosis, deep O87.1
phlegmasia alba dolens O87.1
placental polyp O90.89
pneumonia, embolic —*see* Embolism, obstetric, puerperal
pre-eclampsia —*see* Pre-eclampsia
psychosis F53
pyelitis O86.21
pyelocystitis O86.29
pyelonephritis O86.21
pyelonephrosis O86.21
pyemia O85
pyocystitis O86.29
pyohemia O85
pyometra O86.12
pyonephritis O86.21
pyosalpingitis O86.19
pyrexia (of unknown origin) O86.4
renal
  disease NEC O90.89
  failure O90.4

Puerperal, puerperium (Continued)
  respiratory disease NEC O99.53
  retention
    decidua —see Retention, decidua
    placenta O72.0
    secundines —see Retention,
      secundines
  retrated nipple O92.02
  salpingo-ovaritis O86.19
  salpingoperitonitis O85
  secondary perineal tear O90.1
  sepsis O85
  sepsis (pelvic) O85
  septic thrombophlebitis O86.81
  skin disorder NEC O99.73
  specified condition NEC O99.89
  stroke O99.43
  subinvolution (uterus) O90.89
  subluxation of symphysis (pubis)
      O26.73
  suppuration —see Puerperal, abscess
  tetanus A34
  thelitis O91.02
    associated with lactation O91.03
  thrombocytopenia O72.3
  thrombophlebitis (superficial) O87.0
    deep O87.1
    pelvic O87.1
    septic O86.81
  thrombosis (venous) —see Thrombosis,
      puerperal
  thyroiditis O90.5
  toxemia (eclamptic) (pre-eclamptic)
      (with convulsions) O15.2
  trauma, non-obstetric O9A.23
    caused by abuse (physical) (suspected)
        O9A.33
      confirmed O9A.33
      psychological (suspected)
          O9A.53
        confirmed O9A.53
      sexual (suspected) O9A.43
        confirmed O9A.43
  uremia (due to renal failure)
      O90.4
  urethritis O86.22
  vaginitis O86.13
  varicose veins (legs) O87.4
    vulva or perineum O87.8
  venous O87.9
  vulvitis O86.19
  vulvovaginitis O86.13
  white leg O87.1
Puerperium —see Puerperal
Pulmolithiasis J98.4
Pulmonary —see condition
Pulpitis (acute) (anachoretic) (chronic)
    (hyperplastic) (irreversible) (putrescent)
    (reversible) (suppurative) (ulcerative)
    K04.0
Pulpless tooth K04.99
Pulse
  alternating R00.8
  bigeminal R00.8
  fast R00.0
  feeble, rapid due to shock following injury
      T79.4
  rapid R00.0
  weak R09.89
Pulsus alternans or trigeminus R00.8
Punch drunk F07.81
Punctum lacrimale occlusion —see Obstruction,
    lacrimal
Puncture
  abdomen, abdominal
    wall S31.139
      with
        foreign body S31.149
        penetration into peritoneal cavity
            S31.639
          with foreign body S31.649

Puncture (Continued)
  abdomen, abdominal (Continued)
    wall (Continued)
      epigastric region S31.132
        with
          foreign body S31.142
          penetration into peritoneal cavity
              S31.632
            with foreign body S31.642
      left
        lower quadrant S31.134
          with
            foreign body S31.144
            penetration into peritoneal cavity
                S31.634
              with foreign body S31.644
        upper quadrant S31.131
          with
            foreign body S31.141
            penetration into peritoneal cavity
                S31.631
              with foreign body S31.641
      periumbilic region S31.135
        with
          foreign body S31.145
          penetration into peritoneal cavity
              S31.635
            with foreign body S31.645
      right
        lower quadrant S31.133
          with
            foreign body S31.143
            penetration into peritoneal cavity
                S31.633
              with foreign body S31.643
        upper quadrant S31.130
          with
            foreign body S31.140
            penetration into peritoneal cavity
                S31.630
              with foreign body S31.640
    accidental, complicating surgery —see
        Complication, accidental puncture or
        laceration
    alveolar (process) —see Puncture, oral cavity
    ankle S91.039
      with
        foreign body S91.049
      left S91.032
        with
          foreign body S91.042
      right S91.031
        with
          foreign body S91.041
    anus S31.833
      with foreign body S31.834
    arm (upper) S41.139
      with foreign body S41.149
      left S41.132
        with foreign body S41.142
      lower —see Puncture, forearm
      right S41.131
        with foreign body S41.141
    auditory canal (external) (meatus) —see
        Puncture, ear
    auricle, ear —see Puncture, ear
    axilla —see Puncture, arm
    back —see also Puncture, thorax, back
      lower S31.030
        with
          foreign body S31.040
            with penetration into
                retroperitoneal space S31.041
          penetration into retroperitoneal space
              S31.031
    bladder (traumatic) S37.29
      nontraumatic N32.89
    breast S21.039
      with foreign body S21.049
      left S21.032
        with foreign body S21.042

Puncture (Continued)
  breast (Continued)
    right S21.031
      with foreign body S21.041
    buttock S31.803
      with foreign body S31.804
      left S31.823
        with foreign body S31.824
      right S31.813
        with foreign body S31.814
    by
      device, implant or graft —see
          Complications, by site and type,
          mechanical
      foreign body left accidentally in operative
          wound T81.539
      instrument (any) during a procedure,
          accidental —see Puncture, accidental
          complicating surgery
    calf —see Puncture, leg
    canaliculus lacrimalis —see Puncture,
        eyelid
    canthus, eye —see Puncture, eyelid
    cervical esophagus S11.23
      with foreign body S11.24
    cheek (external) S01.439
      with foreign body S01.449
      internal —see Puncture, oral cavity
      left S01.432
        with foreign body S01.442
      right S01.431
        with foreign body S01.441
    chest wall —see Puncture, thorax
    chin —see Puncture, head, specified site NEC
    clitoris —see Puncture, vulva
    costal region —see Puncture, thorax
    digit (s)
      foot —see Puncture, toe
      hand —see Puncture, finger
    ear (canal) (external) S01.339
      with foreign body S01.349
      drum S09.2-
      left S01.332
        with foreign body S01.342
      right S01.331
        with foreign body S01.341
    elbow S51.039
      with
        foreign body S51.049
      left S51.032
        with
          foreign body S51.042
      right S51.031
        with
          foreign body S51.041
    epididymis —see Puncture, testis
    epigastric region —see Puncture, abdomen,
        wall, epigastric
    epiglottis S11.83
      with foreign body S11.84
    esophagus
      cervical S11.23
        with foreign body S11.24
      thoracic S27.818
    eyeball S05.6-
      with foreign body S05.5-
    eyebrow —see Puncture, eyelid
    eyelid S01.13-
      with foreign body S01.14-
      left S01.132
        with foreign body S01.142
      right S01.131
        with foreign body S01.141
    face NEC —see Puncture, head, specified site
        NEC
    finger (s) S61.239
      with
        damage to nail S61.339
          with
            foreign body S61.349
        foreign body S61.249

◀ New   ◀⟨⟨ Revised   ~~deleted~~ Deleted

Puncture (Continued)
  finger (Continued)
    index S61.238
      with
        damage to nail S61.338
          with
            foreign body S61.348
        foreign body S61.248
      left S61.231
        with
          damage to nail S61.331
            with
              foreign body S61.341
          foreign body S61.241
      right S61.230
        with
          damage to nail S61.330
            with
              foreign body S61.340
          foreign body S61.240
    little S61.238
      with
        damage to nail S61.338
          with
            foreign body S61.348
        foreign body S61.248
      left S61.237
        with
          damage to nail S61.337
            with
              foreign body S61.347
          foreign body S61.247
      right S61.236
        with
          damage to nail S61.336
            with
              foreign body S61.346
          foreign body S61.246
    middle S61.238
      with
        damage to nail S61.338
          with
            foreign body S61.348
        foreign body S61.248
      left S61.233
        with
          damage to nail S61.333
            with
              foreign body S61.343
          foreign body S61.243
      right S61.232
        with
          damage to nail S61.332
            with
              foreign body S61.342
          foreign body S61.242
    ring S61.238
      with
        damage to nail S61.338
          with
            foreign body S61.348
        foreign body S61.248
      left S61.235
        with
          damage to nail S61.335
            with
              foreign body S61.345
          foreign body S61.245
      right S61.234
        with
          damage to nail S61.334
            with
              foreign body S61.344
          foreign body S61.244
  flank S31.139
    with foreign body S31.149
  foot (except toe (s) alone) S91.339
    with foreign body S91.349
    left S91.332
      with foreign body S91.342

Puncture (Continued)
  foot (Continued)
    right S91.331
      with foreign body S91.341
    toe —see Puncture, toe
  forearm S51.839
    with
      foreign body S51.849
    elbow only —see Puncture, elbow
    left S51.832
      with
        foreign body S51.842
    right S51.831
      with
        foreign body S51.841
  forehead —see Puncture, head, specified site
    NEC
  genital organs, external
    female S31.532
      with foreign body S31.542
      vagina —see Puncture, vagina
      vulva —see Puncture, vulva
    male S31.531
      with foreign body S31.541
      penis —see Puncture, penis
      scrotum —see Puncture, scrotum
      testis —see Puncture, testis
  groin —see Puncture, abdomen, wall
  gum —see Puncture, oral cavity
  hand S61.439
    with
      foreign body S61.449
    finger —see Puncture, finger
    left S61.432
      with
        foreign body S61.442
    right S61.431
      with
        foreign body S61.441
    thumb —see Puncture, thumb
  head S01.93
    with foreign body S01.94
    cheek —see Puncture, cheek
    ear —see Puncture, ear
    eyelid —see Puncture, eyelid
    lip —see Puncture, oral cavity
    nose —see Puncture, nose
    oral cavity —see Puncture, oral cavity
    scalp S01.03
      with foreign body S01.04
    specified site NEC S01.83
      with foreign body S01.84
    temporomandibular area —see Puncture,
      cheek
  heart S26.99
    with hemopericardium S26.09
    without hemopericardium S26.19
  heel —see Puncture, foot
  hip S71.039
    with foreign body S71.049
    left S71.032
      with foreign body S71.042
    right S71.031
      with foreign body S71.041
  hymen —see Puncture, vagina
  hypochondrium —see Puncture, abdomen,
    wall
  hypogastric region —see Puncture, abdomen,
    wall
  inguinal region —see Puncture, abdomen,
    wall
  instep —see Puncture, foot
  internal organs —see Injury, by site
  interscapular region —see Puncture, thorax,
    back
  intestine
    large
      colon S36.599
        ascending S36.590
        descending S36.592
        sigmoid S36.593

Puncture (Continued)
  intestine (Continued)
    large (Continued)
      colon (Continued)
        specified site NEC S36.598
        transverse S36.591
      rectum S36.69
    small S36.499
      duodenum S36.490
      specified site NEC S36.498
  intra-abdominal organ S36.99
    gallbladder S36.128
    intestine —see Puncture, intestine
    liver S36.118
    pancreas —see Puncture, pancreas
    peritoneum S36.81
    specified site NEC S36.898
    spleen S36.09
    stomach S36.39
  jaw —see Puncture, head, specified site
    NEC
  knee S81.039
    with foreign body S81.049
    left S81.032
      with foreign body S81.042
    right S81.031
      with foreign body S81.041
  labium (majus) (minus) —see Puncture,
    vulva
  lacrimal duct —see Puncture, eyelid
  larynx S11.013
    with foreign body S11.014
  leg (lower) S81.839
    with foreign body S81.849
    foot —see Puncture, foot
    knee —see Puncture, knee
    left S81.832
      with foreign body S81.842
    right S81.831
      with foreign body S81.841
    upper —see Puncture, thigh
  lip S01.531
    with foreign body S01.541
  loin —see Puncture, abdomen, wall
  lower back —see Puncture, back, lower
  lumbar region —see Puncture, back, lower
  malar region —see Puncture, head, specified
    site NEC
  mammary —see Puncture, breast
  mastoid region —see Puncture, head,
    specified site NEC
  mouth —see Puncture, oral cavity
  nail
    finger —see Puncture, finger, with damage
      to nail
    toe —see Puncture, toe, with damage to
      nail
  nasal (septum) (sinus) —see Puncture,
    nose
  nasopharynx —see Puncture, head, specified
    site NEC
  neck S11.93
    with foreign body S11.94
    involving
      cervical esophagus —see Puncture,
        cervical esophagus
      larynx —see Puncture, larynx
      pharynx —see Puncture, pharynx
      thyroid gland —see Puncture, thyroid
        gland
      trachea —see Puncture, trachea
    specified site NEC S11.83
      with foreign body S11.84
  nose (septum) (sinus) S01.23
    with foreign body S01.24
  ocular —see Puncture, eyeball - oral cavity
    S01.532
    with foreign body S01.542
  orbit S05.4-
  palate —see Puncture, oral cavity
  palm —see Puncture, hand

◀ New   ◀◀ Revised   ~~deleted~~ Deleted

Purulent —*see* condition
Pus
  in
    stool R19.5
    urine N39.0
  tube (rupture) —*see* Salpingo-oophoritis
Pustular rash L08.0
Pustule (nonmalignant) L08.9
  malignant A22.0
Pustulosis palmaris et plantaris L40.3
Putnam (-Dana) disease or syndrome —*see*
    Degeneration, combined
Putrescent pulp (dental) K04.1
Pyarthritis, pyarthrosis —*see* Arthritis,
    pyogenic or pyemic
  tuberculous —*see* Tuberculosis, joint
Pyelectasis —*see* Hydronephrosis
Pyelitis (congenital) (uremic) —*see also*
    Pyelonephritis
  with
    calculus —*see* category N20
      with hydronephrosis N13.2
    contracted kidney N11.9
  acute N10
  chronic N11.9
    with calculus —*see* category N20
      with hydronephrosis N13.2
  cystica N28.84
  puerperal (postpartum) O86.21
  tuberculous A18.11
Pyelocystitis —*see* Pyelonephritis
Pyelonephritis —*see also* Nephritis,
    tubulo-interstitial
  with
    calculus —*see* category N20
      with hydronephrosis N13.2
    contracted kidney N11.9
  acute N10
  calculous —*see* category N20
    with hydronephrosis N13.2
  chronic N11.9
    with calculus —*see* category N20
      with hydronephrosis N13.2
    associated with ureteral obstruction or
      stricture N11.1
    nonobstructive N11.8
      with reflux (vesicoureteral) N11.0
    obstructive N11.1
    specified NEC N11.8
  in (due to)
    brucellosis A23.9 *[N16]*
    cryoglobulinemia (mixed) D89.1 *[N16]*
    cystinosis E72.04
    diphtheria A36.84

Pyelonephritis *(Continued)*
  in *(Continued)*
    glycogen storage disease E74.09 *[N16]*
    leukemia NEC C95.9- *[N16]*
    lymphoma NEC C85.90 *[N16]*
    multiple myeloma C90.0- *[N16]*
    obstruction N11.1
    Salmonella infection A02.25
    sarcoidosis D86.84
    sepsis A41.9 *[N16]*
    Sjögren's disease M35.04
    toxoplasmosis B58.83
    transplant rejection T86.91 *[N16]*
    Wilson's disease E83.01 *[N16]*
  nonobstructive N12
    with reflux (vesicoureteral) N11.0
    chronic N11.8
  syphilitic A52.75
Pyelonephrosis (obstructive) N11.1
  chronic N11.9
Pyelophlebitis I80.8
Pyeloureteritis cystica N28.85
Pyemia, pyemic (fever) (infection) (purulent) —
    see also Sepsis
  joint —*see* Arthritis, pyogenic or pyemic
  liver K75.1
  pneumococcal A40.3
  portal K75.1
  postvaccinal T88.0
  puerperal, postpartum, childbirth O85
  specified organism NEC A41.89
  tuberculous —*see* Tuberculosis, miliary
Pygopagus Q89.4
Pyknoepilepsy (idiopathic) —*see* Pyknolepsy
Pyknolepsy G40.A09
  intractable G40.A19
    with status epilepticus G40.A11
    without status epilepticus G40.A19
  not intractable G40.A09
    with status epilepticus G40.A01
    without status epilepticus G40.A09
Pylephlebitis K75.1
Pyle's syndrome Q78.5
Pylethrombophlebitis K75.1
Pylethrombosis K75.1
Pyloritis K29.90
  with bleeding K29.91
Pylorospasm (reflex) NEC K31.3
  congenital or infantile Q40.0
  neurotic F45.8
  newborn Q40.0
  psychogenic F45.8
Pylorus, pyloric —*see* condition

Pyoarthrosis —*see* Arthritis, pyogenic or
    pyemic
Pyocele
  mastoid —*see* Mastoiditis, acute
  sinus (accessory) —*see* Sinusitis
  turbinate (bone) J32.9
  urethra (*see also* Urethritis) N34.0
Pyocolpos —*see* Vaginitis
Pyocystitis N30.80
  with hematuria N30.81
Pyoderma, pyodermia L08.0
  gangrenosum L88
  newborn P39.4
  phagedenic L88
  vegetans L08.81
Pyodermatitis L08.0
  vegetans L08.81
Pyogenic —*see* condition
Pyohydronephrosis N13.6
Pyometra, pyometrium, pyometritis —*see*
    Endometritis
Pyomyositis (tropical) —*see* Myositis, infective
Pyonephritis N12
Pyonephrosis N13.6
  tuberculous A18.11
Pyo-oophoritis —*see* Salpingo-oophoritis
Pyo-ovarium —*see* Salpingo-oophoritis
Pyopericarditis, pyopericardium I30.1
Pyophlebitis —*see* Phlebitis
Pyopneumopericardium I30.1
Pyopneumothorax (infective) J86.9
  with fistula J86.0
  tuberculous NEC A15.6
Pyosalpinx, pyosalpingitis —*see also*
    Salpingo-oophoritis
Pyothorax J86.9
  with fistula J86.0
  tuberculous NEC A15.6
Pyoureter N28.89
  tuberculous A18.11
Pyramidopallidonigral syndrome G20
Pyrexia (of unknown origin) R50.9
  atmospheric T67.0
  during labor NEC O75.2
  heat T67.0
  newborn P81.9
    environmentally-induced P81.0
  persistent R50.9
  puerperal O86.4
Pyroglobulinemia NEC E88.09
Pyromania F63.1
Pyrosis R12
Pyuria (bacterial) N39.0

Q

Q fever A78
  with pneumonia A78
Quadricuspid aortic valve Q23.8
Quadrilateral fever A78
Quadriparesis —*see* Quadriplegia
  meaning muscle weakness M62.81
Quadriplegia G82.50-
  complete
    C1-C4 level G82.51
    C5-C7 level G82.53
  congenital (cerebral) (spinal) G80.8
    spastic G80.0

Quadriplegia (*Continued*)
  embolic (current episode) I63.4
  functional R53.2
  incomplete
    C1-C4 level G82.52
    C5-C7 level G82.54
  thrombotic (current episode) I63.3
  traumatic — code to injury with seventh
    character S
    current episode —*see* Injury, spinal (cord),
      cervical
Quadruplet, pregnancy —*see* Pregnancy,
  quadruplet
Quarrelsomeness F60.3

Queensland fever A77.3
Quervain's disease M65.4
  thyroid E06.1
Queyrat's erythroplasia D07.4
  penis D07.4
  specified site —*see* Neoplasm, skin,
    in situ
  unspecified site D07.4
Quincke's disease or edema T78.3
  hereditary D84.1
Quinsy (gangrenous) J36
Quintan fever A79.0
Quintuplet, pregnancy —*see* Pregnancy,
  quintuplet

R

Rabbit fever —see Tularemia
Rabies A82.9
  contact Z20.3
  exposure to Z20.3
  inoculation reaction —see Complications, vaccination
  sylvatic A82.0
  urban A82.1
Rachischisis —see Spina bifida
Rachitic —see also condition
  deformities of spine (late effect) (sequelae) E64.3
  pelvis (late effect) (sequelae) E64.3
    with disproportion (fetopelvic) O33.0
      causing obstructed labor O65.0
Rachitis, rachitism (acute) (tarda) —see also Rickets
  renalis N25.0
  sequelae E64.3
Radial nerve —see condition
Radiation
  burn —see Burn
  effects NOS T66
  sickness NOS T66
  therapy, encounter for Z51.0
Radiculitis (pressure) (vertebrogenic) —see Radiculopathy
Radiculomyelitis —see also Encephalitis
  toxic, due to
    Clostridium tetani A35
    Corynebacterium diphtheriae A36.82
Radiculopathy M54.10
  cervical region M54.12
  cervicothoracic region M54.13
  due to
    disc disorder
      C3 M50.11
      C4 M50.11
      C5 M50.12
      C6 M50.12
      C7 M50.12
      C8 M50.13
    displacement of intervertebral disc —see Disorder, disc, with, radiculopathy
  leg M54.1-
  lumbar region M54.16
  lumbosacral region M54.17
  occipito-atlanto-axial region M54.11
  postherpetic B02.29
  sacrococcygeal region M54.18
  syphilitic A52.11
  thoracic region (with visceral pain) M54.14
  thoracolumbar region M54.15
Radiodermal burns (acute, chronic, or occupational) —see Burn
Radiodermatitis L58.9
  acute L58.0
  chronic L58.1
Radiotherapy session Z51.0
Rage, meaning rabies —see Rabies
Ragpicker's disease A22.1
Ragsorter's disease A22.1
Raillietiniasis B71.8
Railroad neurosis F48.8
Railway spine F48.8
Raised —see also Elevated
  antibody titer R76.0
Rake teeth, tooth M26.39
Rales R09.89
Ramifying renal pelvis Q63.8
Ramsay-Hunt disease or syndrome (see also Hunt's disease) B02.21
  meaning dyssynergia cerebellaris myoclonica G11.1
Ranula K11.6
  congenital Q38.4

Rape
  adult
    confirmed T74.21
    suspected T76.21
  alleged, observation or examination, ruled out
    adult Z04.41
    child Z04.42
  child
    confirmed T74.22
    suspected T76.22
Rapid
  feeble pulse, due to shock, following injury T79.4
  heart (beat) R00.0
    psychogenic F45.8
  second stage (delivery) O62.3
  time-zone change syndrome —see Disorder, sleep, circadian rhythm, psychogenic
Rarefaction, bone —see Disorder, bone, density and structure, specified NEC
Rash (toxic) R21
  canker A38.9
  diaper L22
  drug (internal use) L27.0
    contact (see also Dermatitis, due to, drugs, external) L25.1
  following immunization T88.1
  food —see Dermatitis, due to, food
  heat L74.0
  napkin (psoriasiform) L22
  nettle —see Urticaria
  pustular L08.0
  rose R21
    epidemic B06.9
  scarlet A38.9
  serum (see also Reaction, serum) T80.69
  wandering tongue K14.1
Rasmussen aneurysm —see Tuberculosis, pulmonary
Rasmussen encephalitis G04.81
Rat-bite fever A25.9
  due to Streptobacillus moniliformis A25.1
  spirochetal (morsus muris) A25.0
Rathke's pouch tumor D44.3
Raymond (-Céstan) syndrome I65.8
Raynaud's disease, phenomenon or syndrome (secondary) I73.00
  with gangrene (symmetric) I73.01
RDS (newborn) (type I) P22.0
  type II P22.1
Reaction —see also Disorder
  adaptation —see Disorder, adjustment
  adjustment (anxiety) (conduct disorder) (depressiveness) (distress) —see Disorder, adjustment
    with
      mutism, elective (child) (adolescent) F94.0
  adverse
    food (any) (ingested) NEC T78.1
      anaphylactic —see Shock, anaphylactic, due to food
  anaphylactoid —see Shock, anaphylactic
  affective —see Disorder, mood
  allergic —see Allergy
  anaphylactic —see Shock, anaphylactic
  anesthesia —see Anesthesia, complication
  antitoxin (prophylactic) (therapeutic) —see Complications, vaccination
  anxiety F41.1
  Arthus —see Arthus' phenomenon
  asthenic F48.8
  combat and operational stress F43.0
  compulsive F42
  conversion F44.9
  crisis, acute F43.0
  deoxyribonuclease (DNA) (DNase) hypersensitivity D69.2
  depressive (single episode) F32.9
    affective (single episode) F31.4
      recurrent episode F33.9
    neurotic F34.1
    psychoneurotic F34.1

Reaction (Continued)
  depressive (Continued)
    psychotic F32.3
    recurrent —see Disorder, depressive, recurrent
  dissociative F44.9
  drug NEC T88.7
    addictive —see Dependence, drug
      transmitted via placenta or breast milk —see Absorption, drug, addictive, through placenta
    allergic —see Allergy, drug
    lichenoid L43.2
    newborn P93.8
      gray baby syndrome P93.0
    overdose or poisoning (by accident) —see Table of Drugs and Chemicals, by drug, poisoning
    photoallergic L56.1
    phototoxic L56.0
    withdrawal —see Dependence, by drug, with, withdrawal
      infant of dependent mother P96.1
      newborn P96.1
    wrong substance given or taken (by accident) —see Table of Drugs and Chemicals, by drug, poisoning
  fear F40.9
    child (abnormal) F93.8
  febrile nonhemolytic transfusion (FNHTR) R50.84
  fluid loss, cerebrospinal G97.1
  foreign
    body NEC —see Granuloma, foreign body
      in operative wound (inadvertently left) —see Foreign body, accidentally left during a procedure
    substance accidentally left during a procedure (chemical) (powder) (talc) T81.60
      aseptic peritonitis T81.61
      body or object (instrument) (sponge) (swab) —see Foreign body, accidentally left during a procedure
      specified reaction NEC T81.69
  grief —see Disorder, adjustment
  Herxheimer's R68.89
  hyperkinetic —see Hyperkinesia
  hypochondriacal F45.20
  hypoglycemic, due to insulin E16.0
    with coma (diabetic) —see Diabetes, coma nondiabetic E15
    therapeutic misadventure —see subcategory T38.3
  hypomanic F30.8
  hysterical F44.9
  immunization —see Complications, vaccination
  incompatibility
    ABO blood group (infusion) (transfusion) —see Complication (s), transfusion, incompatibility reaction, ABO
      delayed serologic T80.39
    minor blood group (Duffy) (E) (K(ell)) (Kidd) (Lewis) (M) (N) (P) (S) T80.89
    Rh (factor) (infusion) (transfusion) —see Complication (s), transfusion, incompatibility reaction, Rh (factor)
  inflammatory —see Infection
  infusion —see Complications, infusion
  inoculation (immune serum) —see Complications, vaccination
  insulin T38.3-
  involutional psychotic —see Disorder, depressive
  leukemoid D72.823
    basophilic D72.823
    lymphocytic D72.823
    monocytic D72.823
    myelocytic D72.823
    neutrophilic D72.823

Reaction *(Continued)*
  LSD (acute)
    due to drug abuse —*see* Abuse, drug,
        hallucinogen
    due to drug dependence —*see* Dependence,
        drug, hallucinogen
  lumbar puncture G97.1
  manic-depressive —*see* Disorder, bipolar
  neurasthenic F48.8
  neurogenic —*see* Neurosis
  neurotic F48.9
  neurotic-depressive F34.1
  nitritoid —*see* Crisis, nitritoid - obsessive-
        compulsive F42
  nonspecific
    to
      cell mediated immunity measurement
          of gamma interferon antigen
          response without active
          tuberculosis R76.12
      QuantiFERON-TB test (QFT) without
          active tuberculosis R76.12
      tuberculin test (*see also* Reaction,
          tuberculin skin test) R76.11
  obsessive-compulsive F42
  organic, acute or subacute —*see* Delirium
  paranoid (acute) F23
    chronic F22
    senile F03
  passive dependency F60.7
  phobic F40.9
  post-traumatic stress, uncomplicated
      Z73.3
  psychogenic F99
  psychoneurotic —*see also* Neurosis
    compulsive F42
    depersonalization F48.1
    depressive F34.1
    hypochondriacal F45.20
    neurasthenic F48.8
    obsessive F42
  psychophysiologic —*see* Disorder,
      somatoform
  psychosomatic —*see* Disorder, somatoform
  psychotic —*see* Psychosis
  scarlet fever toxin —*see* Complications,
      vaccination
  schizophrenic F23
    acute (brief) (undifferentiated) F23
    latent F21
    undifferentiated (acute) (brief) F23
  serological for syphilis —*see* Serology for
      syphilis
  serum T80.69
    anaphylactic (immediate) (*see also* Shock,
        anaphylactic) T80.59
    specified reaction NEC
      due to
        administration of blood and blood
            products T80.61
        immunization T80.62
        serum specified NEC T80.69
        vaccination T80.62
  situational —*see* Disorder, adjustment
  somatization —*see* Disorder, somatoform
  spinal puncture G97.1
  stress (severe) F43.9
    acute (agitation) ("daze") (disorientation)
        (disturbance of consciousness) (flight
        reaction) (fugue) F43.0
    specified NEC F43.8
  surgical procedure —*see* Complications,
      surgical procedure
  tetanus antitoxin —*see* Complications,
      vaccination
  toxic, to local anesthesia T81.89
    in labor and delivery O74.4
    in pregnancy O29.3X-
    postpartum, puerperal O89.3
  toxin-antitoxin —*see* Complications,
      vaccination

Reaction *(Continued)*
  transfusion (blood) (bone marrow)
      (lymphocytes) (allergic) —*see*
      Complications, transfusion
  tuberculin skin test, abnormal R76.11
  vaccination (any) —*see* Complications,
      vaccination
  withdrawing, child or adolescent F93.8
Reactive airway disease —*see* Asthma
Reactive depression —*see* Reaction, depressive
Rearrangement
  chromosomal
    balanced (in) Q95.9
      abnormal individual (autosomal) Q95.2
      non-sex (autosomal) chromosomes
          Q95.2
      sex/non-sex chromosomes Q95.3
      specified NEC Q95.8
Recalcitrant patient —*see* Noncompliance
Recanalization, thrombus —*see* Thrombosis
Recession, receding
  chamber angle (eye) H21.55-
  chin M26.09
  gingival (generalized) (localized)
      (postinfective) (postoperative) K06.0
Recklinghausen's disease Q85.01
  bones E21.0
Reclus' disease (cystic) —*see* Mastopathy, cystic
Recrudescent typhus (fever) A75.1
Recruitment, auditory H93.21-
Rectalgia K62.89
Rectitis K62.89
Rectocele
  female (without uterine prolapse) N81.6
    with uterine prolapse N81.4
      incomplete N81.2
  in pregnancy —*see* Pregnancy, complicated
      by, abnormal, pelvic organs or tissues
      NEC
  male K62.3
Rectosigmoid junction —*see* condition
Rectosigmoiditis K63.89
  ulcerative (chronic) K51.30
    with
      complication K51.319
        abscess K51.314
        fistula K51.313
        obstruction K51.312
        rectal bleeding K51.311
        specified NEC K51.318
Rectourethral —*see* condition
Rectovaginal —*see* condition
Rectovesical —*see* condition
Rectum, rectal —*see* condition
Recurrent —*see* condition
  pregnancy loss —*see* Loss (of), pregnancy,
      recurrent
Red bugs B88.0
Red-cedar lung or pneumonitis J67.8
Red tide (*see also* Table of Drugs and Chemicals)
    T65.82-
Reduced
  mobility Z74.09
  ventilatory or vital capacity R94.2
Redundant, redundancy
  anus (congenital) Q43.8
  clitoris N90.89
  colon (congenital) Q43.8
  foreskin (congenital) N47.8
  intestine (congenital) Q43.8
  labia N90.6
  organ or site, congenital NEC —*see* Accessory
  panniculus (abdominal) E65
  prepuce (congenital) N47.8
  pylorus K31.89
  rectum (congenital) Q43.8
  scrotum N50.8
  sigmoid (congenital) Q43.8
  skin (of face) L57.4
    eyelids —*see* Blepharochalasis
  stomach K31.89

Reduplication —*see* Duplication
Reflex R29.2
  hyperactive gag J39.2
  pupillary, abnormal —*see* Anomaly, pupil,
      function
  vasoconstriction I73.9
  vasovagal R55
Reflux K21.9
  acid K21.9
  esophageal K21.9
    with esophagitis K21.0
    newborn P78.83
  gastroesophageal K21.9
    with esophagitis K21.0
  mitral —*see* Insufficiency, mitral
  ureteral —*see* Reflux, vesicoureteral
  vesicoureteral (with scarring) N13.70
    with
      nephropathy N13.729
        with hydroureter N13.739
          bilateral N13.732
          unilateral N13.731
        without hydroureter N13.729
          bilateral N13.722
          unilateral N13.721
      bilateral N13.722
      unilateral N13.721
      pyelonephritis (chronic) N11.0
    without nephropathy N13.71
    congenital Q62.7
Reforming, artificial openings —*see* Attention
    to, artificial, opening
Refractive error —*see* Disorder, refraction
Refsum's disease or syndrome G60.1
Refusal of
  food, psychogenic F50.8
  treatment (because of) Z53.20
    left against medical advice (AMA) Z53.21
    patient's decision NEC Z53.29
    reasons of belief or group pressure Z53.1
Regional —*see* condition
Regurgitation R11.10
  aortic (valve) —*see* Insufficiency, aortic
  food —*see also* Vomiting
    with reswallowing —*see* Rumination
    newborn P92.1
  gastric contents —*see* Vomiting
  heart —*see* Endocarditis
  mitral (valve) —*see* Insufficiency, mitral
    congenital Q23.3
  myocardial —*see* Endocarditis
  pulmonary (valve) (heart) I37.1
    congenital Q22.2
    syphilitic A52.03
  tricuspid —*see* Insufficiency, tricuspid
  valve, valvular —*see* Endocarditis
    congenital Q24.8
  vesicoureteral —*see* Reflux, vesicoureteral
Reichmann's disease or syndrome K31.89
Reifenstein syndrome E34.52
Reinsertion, contraceptive device Z30.433
Reiter's disease, syndrome, or urethritis
    M02.30
  ankle M02.37-
  elbow M02.32-
  foot joint M02.37-
  hand joint M02.34-
  hip M02.35-
  knee M02.36-
  multiple site M02.39
  shoulder M02.31-
  vertebra M02.38
  wrist M02.33-
Rejection
  food, psychogenic F50.8
  transplant T86.91
    bone T86.830
      marrow T86.01
    cornea T86.840
    heart T86.21
      with lung (s) T86.31

◀ New   ◀ Revised   ~~deleted~~ Deleted

Rejection *(Continued)*
 transplant *(Continued)*
  intestine T86.850
  kidney T86.11
  liver T86.41
  lung (s) T86.810
   with heart T86.31
  organ (immune or nonimmune cause)
   T86.91
  pancreas T86.890
  skin (allograft) (autograft) T86.820
  specified NEC T86.890
  stem cell (peripheral blood) (umbilical
   cord) T86.5
Relapsing fever A68.9
 Carter's (Asiatic) A68.1
 Dutton's (West African) A68.1
 Koch's A68.9
 louse-borne (epidemic) A68.0
 Novy's (American) A68.1
 Obermeyers's (European) A68.0
 Spirillum A68.9
 tick-borne (endemic) A68.1
Relationship
 occlusal
  open anterior M26.220
  open posterior M26.221
Relaxation
 anus (sphincter) K62.89
  psychogenic F45.8
 arch (foot) —*see also* Deformity, limb, flat
  foot
 back ligaments —*see* Instability, joint, spine
 bladder (sphincter) N31.2
 cardioesophageal K21.9
 cervix —*see* Incompetency, cervix
 diaphragm J98.6
 joint (capsule) (ligament) (paralytic) —*see*
  Flail, joint
  congenital NEC Q74.8
 lumbosacral (joint) —*see* subcategory M53.2
 pelvic floor N81.89
 perineum N81.89
 posture R29.3
 rectum (sphincter) K62.89
 sacroiliac (joint) —*see* subcategory M53.2
 scrotum N50.8
 urethra (sphincter) N36.44
 vesical N31.2
Release from prison, anxiety concerning
 Z65.2
Remains
 canal of Cloquet Q14.0
 capsule (opaque) Q14.8
Remittent fever (malarial) B54
Remnant
 canal of Cloquet Q14.0
 capsule (opaque) Q14.8
 cervix, cervical stump (acquired)
  (postoperative) N88.8
 cystic duct, postcholecystectomy K91.5
 fingernail L60.8
  congenital Q84.6
 meniscus, knee —*see* Derangement, knee,
  meniscus, specified NEC
 thyroglossal duct Q89.2
 tonsil J35.8
  infected (chronic) J35.01
 urachus Q64.4
Removal (from) (of)
 artificial
  arm Z44.00-
   complete Z44.01-
   partial Z44.02-
  eye Z44.2-
  leg Z44.10-
   complete Z44.11-
   partial Z44.12-
 breast implant Z45.81
 cardiac pulse generator (battery) (end-of-life)
  Z45.010

Removal *(Continued)*
 catheter (urinary) (indwelling) Z46.6
  from artificial opening —*see* Attention to,
   artificial, opening
  non-vascular Z46.82
  vascular NEC Z45.2
 device Z46.9
  contraceptive Z30.432
  implanted NEC Z45.89
  specified NEC Z46.89
 drains Z48.03
 dressing (nonsurgical) Z48.00
  surgical Z48.01
 external
  fixation device — code to fracture with
   seventh character D
  prosthesis, prosthetic device Z44.9
   breast Z44.3-
   specified NEC Z44.8
 home in childhood (to foster home or
  institution) Z62.29
 ileostomy Z43.2
 insulin pump Z46.81
 myringotomy device (stent) (tube) Z45.82
 nervous system device NEC Z46.2
  brain neuropacemaker Z46.2
  visual substitution device Z46.2
   implanted Z45.31
 non-vascular catheter Z46.82
 organ, prophylactic (for neoplasia
  management) —*see* Prophylactic, organ
  removal
 orthodontic device Z46.4
 staples Z48.02
 stent
  ureteral Z46.6
 suture Z48.02
 urinary device Z46.6
 vascular access device or catheter Z45.2
Ren
 arcuatus Q63.1
 mobile, mobilis N28.89
  congenital Q63.8
 unguliformis Q63.1
Renal —*see* condition
Rendu-Osler-Weber disease or syndrome I78.0
Reninoma D41.0-
Renon-Delille syndrome E23.3
Reovirus, as cause of disease classified
 elsewhere B97.5
Repeated falls NEC R29.6
Replaced chromosome by dicentric ring Q93.2
Replacement by artificial or mechanical device
 or prosthesis of
 bladder Z96.0
 blood vessel NEC Z95.828
 bone NEC Z96.7
 cochlea Z96.21
 coronary artery Z95.5
 eustachian tube Z96.29
 eye globe Z97.0
 heart Z95.812
  valve Z95.2
   prosthetic Z95.2
   specified NEC Z95.4
   xenogenic Z95.3
 intestine Z96.89
 joint Z96.60
  hip —*see* Presence, hip joint implant
  knee —*see* Presence, knee joint implant
  specified site NEC Z96.698
 larynx Z96.3
 lens Z96.1
 limb (s) —*see* Presence, artificial, limb
 mandible NEC (for tooth root implant (s))
  Z96.5
 organ NEC Z96.89
 peripheral vessel NEC Z95.828
 stapes Z96.29
 teeth Z97.2
 tendon Z96.7

Replacement by artificial or mechanical device
 or prosthesis of *(Continued)*
 tissue NEC Z96.89
 tooth root (s) Z96.5
 vessel NEC Z95.828
  coronary (artery) Z95.5
Request for expert evidence Z04.8
Reserve, decreased or low
 cardiac —*see* Disease, heart
 kidney N28.89
Residual —*see also* condition
 ovary syndrome N99.83
 state, schizophrenic F20.5
 urine R39.19
Resistance, resistant (to)
 activated protein C D68.51
 complicating pregnancy O26.89
 insulin E88.81
 organism (s)
  to
   drug
    aminoglycosides Z16.29
    amoxicillin Z16.11
    ampicillin Z16.11
    antibiotic (s) Z16.20
     multiple Z16.24
     specified NEC Z16.29
    antifungal Z16.32
    antimicrobial (single) Z16.30
     multiple Z16.35
     specified NEC Z16.39
    antimycbacterial (single) Z16.341
     multiple Z16.342
    antiparasitic Z16.31
    antiviral Z16.33
    beta lactam antibiotics Z16.10
     specified NEC Z16.19
    cephalosporins Z16.19
    extended beta lactamase (ESBL)
     Z16.12
    fluoroquinolones Z16.23
    macrolides Z16.29
    methicillin —*see* MRSA
    multiple drugs (MDRO)
     antibiotics Z16.24
    penicillins Z16.11
    quinine (and related compounds)
     Z16.31
    quinolones Z16.23
    sulfonamides Z16.29
    tetracyclines Z16.29
    tuberculostatics (single) Z16.341
     multiple Z16.342
    vancomycin Z16.21
     related antibiotics Z16.22
 thyroid hormone E07.89
Resorption
 dental (roots) K03.3
  alveoli M26.79
 teeth (external) (internal) (pathological)
  (roots) K03.3
Respiration
 Cheyne-Stokes R06.3
 decreased due to shock, following injury
  T79.4
 disorder of, psychogenic F45.8
 insufficient, or poor R06.89
  newborn P28.5
 painful R07.1
 sighing, psychogenic F45.8
Respiratory —*see also* condition
 distress syndrome (newborn) (type I)
  P22.0
  type II P22.1
 syncytial virus, as cause of disease classified
  elsewhere B97.4
Respite care Z75.5
Response (drug)
 photoallergic L56.1
 phototoxic L56.0
Restless legs (syndrome) G25.81

Restlessness R45.1
Restoration (of)
    dental
        aesthetically inadequate or displeasing
            K08.56
        defective K08.50
            specified NEC K08.59
        failure of marginal integrity K08.51
        failure of periodontal anatomical intergrity
            K08.54
        organ continuity from previous sterilization
            (tuboplasty) (vasoplasty) Z31.0
            aftercare Z31.42
        tooth (existing)
            contours biologically incompatible with
                oral health K08.54
            open margins K08.51
            overhanging K08.52
            poor aesthetic K08.56
            poor gingival margins K08.51
        unsatisfactory, of tooth K08.50
            specified NEC K08.59
Restorative material (dental)
    allergy to K08.55
    fractured K08.539
        with loss of material K08.531
        without loss of material K08.530
    unrepairable overhanging of K08.52
Restriction of housing space Z59.1
Rests, ovarian, in fallopian tube Q50.6
Restzustand (schizophrenic) F20.5
Retained —see also Retention
    cholelithiasis following cholecystectomy
        K91.86
    foreign body fragments (type of) Z18.9
        acrylics Z18.2
        animal quill (s) or spines Z18.31
        cement Z18.83
        concrete Z18.83
        crystalline Z18.83
        depleted isotope Z18.09
        depleted uranium Z18.01
        diethylhexylphthalates Z18.2
        glass Z18.81
        isocyanate Z18.2
        magnetic metal Z18.11
        metal Z18.10
        nonmagnetic metal Z18.12
        nontherapeutic radioactive Z18.09
        organic NEC Z18.39
        plastic Z18.2
        quill (s) (animal) Z18.31
        radioactive (nontherapeutic) NEC
            Z18.09
        specified NEC Z18.89
        spine (s) (animal) Z18.31
        stone Z18.83
        tooth (teeth) Z18.32
        wood Z18.33
    fragments (type of) Z18.9
        acrylics Z18.2
        animal quill (s) or spines Z18.31
        cement Z18.83
        concrete Z18.83
        crystalline Z18.83
        depleted isotope Z18.09
        depleted uranium Z18.01
        diethylhexylphthalates Z18.2
        glass Z18.81
        isocyanate Z18.2
        magnetic metal Z18.11
        metal Z18.10
        nonmagnectic metal Z18.12
        nontherapeutic radioactive Z18.09
        organic NEC Z18.39
        plastic Z18.2
        quill (s) (animal) Z18.31
        radioactive (nontherapeutic) NEC
            Z18.09
        specified NEC Z18.89
        spine (s) (animal) Z18.31

Retained (Continued)
    fragments (Continued)
        stone Z18.83
        tooth (teeth) Z18.32
        wood Z18.33
    gallstones, following cholecystectomy K91.86
Retardation
    development, developmental, specific —see
        Disorder, developmental
    endochondral bone growth —see Disorder,
        bone, development or growth
    growth R62.50
        due to malnutrition E45
    mental —see Disability, intellectual
    motor function, specific F82
    physical (child) R62.52
        due to malnutrition E45
    reading (specific) F81.0
    spelling (specific) (without reading disorder)
        F81.81
Retching —see Vomiting
Retention —see also Retained
    bladder —see Retention, urine
    carbon dioxide E87.2
    cholelithiasis following cholecystectomy
        K91.86
    cyst —see Cyst
    dead
        fetus (at or near term) (mother) O36.4
            early fetal death O02.1
        ovum O02.0
    decidua (fragments) (following delivery)
        (with hemorrhage) O72.2
        without hemorrhage O73.1
    deciduous tooth K00.6
    dental root K08.3
    fecal —see Constipation
    fetus
        dead O36.4
            early O02.1
    fluid R60.9
    foreign body —see also Foreign body, retained
        current trauma - code as Foreign body, by
            site or type
    gallstones, following cholecystectomy
        K91.86
    gastric K31.89
    intrauterine contraceptive device, in
        pregnancy —see Pregnancy, complicated
        by, retention, intrauterine device
    membranes (complicating delivery) (with
        hemorrhage) O72.2
        with abortion —see Abortion, by type
        without hemorrhage O73.1
    meniscus —see Derangement, meniscus
    menses N94.89
    milk (puerperal, postpartum) O92.79
    nitrogen, extrarenal R39.2
    ovary syndrome N99.83
    placenta (total) (with hemorrhage) O72.0
        without hemorrhage O73.0
        portions or fragments (with hemorrhage)
            O72.2
            without hemorrhage O73.1
    products of conception
        early pregnancy (dead fetus) O02.1
        following
            delivery (with hemorrhage) O72.2
                without hemorrhage O73.1
    secundines (following delivery) (with
        hemorrhage) O72.0
        without hemorrhage O73.0
        complicating puerperium (delayed
            hemorrhage) O72.2
        partial O72.2
            without hemorrhage O73.1
    smegma, clitoris N90.89
    urine R33.9
        drug-induced R33.0
        due to hyperplasia (hypertrophy) of
            prostate —see Hyperplasia, prostate

Retention (Continued)
    urine (Continued)
        organic R33.8
            drug-induced R33.0
        psychogenic F45.8
        specified NEC R33.8
    water (in tissues) —see Edema
Reticular erythematous mucinosis L98.5
Reticulation, dust —see Pneumoconiosis
Reticulocytosis R70.1
Reticuloendotheliosis
    acute infantile C96.0
    leukemic C91.4-
    malignant C96.9
    nonlipid C96.0
Reticulohistiocytoma (giant-cell) D76.3
Reticuloid, actinic L57.1
Reticulosis (skin)
    acute of infancy C96.0
    hemophagocytic, familial D76.1
    histiocytic medullary C96.9
    lipomelanotic I89.8
    malignant (midline) C86.0
    nonlipid C96.0
    polymorphic C86.0
    Sézary —see Sézary disease
Retina, retinal —see also condition
    dark area D49.81
Retinitis —see also Inflammation, chorioretinal
    albuminurica N18.9 [H32]
    diabetic —see Diabetes, retinitis
    disciformis —see Degeneration, macula
    focal —see Inflammation, chorioretinal,
        focal
    gravidarum —see Pregnancy, complicated by,
        specified pregnancy-related condition
        NEC
    juxtapapillaris —see Inflammation,
        chorioretinal, focal, juxtapapillary
    luetic —see Retinitis, syphilitic
    pigmentosa H35.52
    proliferans —see Disorder, globe,
        degenerative, specified type NEC
    proliferating —see Disorder, globe,
        degenerative, specified type NEC
    renal N18.9 [H32]
    syphilitic (early) (secondary) A51.43
        central, recurrent A52.71
        congenital (early) A50.01 [H32]
        late A52.71
    tuberculous A18.53
Retinoblastoma C69.2-
    differentiated C69.2-
    undifferentiated C69.2-
Retinochoroiditis —see also Inflammation,
    chorioretinal
    disseminated —see Inflammation,
        chorioretinal, disseminated
        syphilitic A52.71
    focal —see Inflammation, chorioretinal
    juxtapapillaris —see Inflammation,
        chorioretinal, focal, juxtapapillary
Retinopathy (background) H35.00
    arteriosclerotic I70.8 [H35.0-]
    atherosclerotic I70.8 [H35.0-]
    central serous —see Chorioretinopathy,
        central serous
    Coats H35.02-
    diabetic —see Diabetes, retinopathy
    exudative H35.02-
    hypertensive H35.03-
    in (due to)
        diabetes —see Diabetes, retinopathy
    sickle-cell disorders D57.- [H36]
    of prematurity H35.10-
        stage 0 H35.11-
        stage 1 H35.12-
        stage 2 H35.13-
        stage 3 H35.14-
        stage 4 H35.15-
        stage 5 H35.16-

◀ New   ⬅ Revised   ~~deleted~~ Deleted

Retinopathy *(Continued)*
  pigmentary, congenital —*see* Dystrophy,
    retina
  proliferative NEC H35.2-
    diabetic —*see* Diabetes, retinopathy,
      proliferative
    sickle-cell D57.- *[H36]*
  solar H31.02-
Retinoschisis H33.10-
  congenital Q14.1
  specified type NEC H33.19-
Retortamoniasis A07.8
Retractile testis Q55.22
Retraction
  cervix —*see* Retroversion, uterus
  drum (membrane) —*see* Disorder, tympanic
    membrane, specified NEC
  finger —*see* Deformity, finger
  lid H02.539
    left H02.536
      lower H02.535
      upper H02.534
    right H02.533
      lower H02.532
      upper H02.531
  lung J98.4
  mediastinum J98.5
  nipple N64.53
    associated with
      lactation O92.03
      pregnancy O92.01-
      puerperium O92.02
    congenital Q83.8
  palmar fascia M72.0
  pleura —*see* Pleurisy
  ring, uterus (Bandl's) (pathological) O62.4
  sternum (congenital) Q76.7
    acquired M95.4
  uterus —*see* Retroversion, uterus
  valve (heart) —*see* Endocarditis
Retrobulbar —*see* condition
Retrocecal —*see* condition
Retrocession —*see* Retroversion
Retrodisplacement —*see* Retroversion
Retroflection, retroflexion —*see* Retroversion
Retrognathia, retrognathism (mandibular)
  (maxillary) M26.19
Retrograde menstruation N92.5
Retroperineal —*see* condition
Retroperitoneal —*see* condition
Retroperitonitis K68.9
Retropharyngeal —*see* condition
Retroplacental —*see* condition
Retroposition —*see* Retroversion
Retroprosthetic membrane T85.398
Retrosternal thyroid (congenital) Q89.2
Retroversion, retroverted
  cervix —*see* Retroversion, uterus
  female NEC —*see* Retroversion, uterus
  iris H21.89
  testis (congenital) Q55.29
  uterus (acquired) (acute) (any
    degree) (asymptomatic) (cervix)
    (postinfectional) (postpartal, old)
    N85.4
    congenital Q51.818
    in pregnancy O34.53-
Retrovirus, as cause of disease classified
  elsewhere B97.30
  human
    immunodeficiency, type 2 (HIV 2) B97.35
    T-cell lymphotropic
      type I (HTLV-I) B97.33
      type II (HTLV-II) B97.34
  lentivirus B97.31
  oncovirus B97.32
  specified NEC B97.39
Retrusion, premaxilla (developmental)
  M26.09
Rett's disease or syndrome F84.2
Reverse peristalsis R19.2

Reye's syndrome G93.7
Rh (factor)
  hemolytic disease (newborn) P55.0
  incompatibility, immunization or
    sensitization
    affecting management of pregnancy NEC
      O36.09-
      anti-D antibody O36.01-
    newborn P55.0
    transfusion reaction —*see* Complication (s),
      transfusion, incompatibility reaction,
      Rh (factor)
  negative mother affecting newborn P55.0
  titer elevated —*see* Complication (s),
    transfusion, incompatibility reaction,
    Rh (factor)
  transfusion reaction —*see* Complication (s),
    transfusion, incompatibility reaction,
    Rh (factor)
Rhabdomyolysis (idiopathic) NEC M62.82
  traumatic T79.6
Rhabdomyoma —*see also* Neoplasm, connective
  tissue, benign
  adult —*see* Neoplasm, connective tissue,
    benign
  fetal —*see* Neoplasm, connective tissue, benign
  glycogenic —*see* Neoplasm, connective tissue,
    benign
Rhabdomyosarcoma (any type) —*see*
  Neoplasm, connective tissue, malignant
Rhabdosarcoma —*see* Rhabdomyosarcoma
Rhesus (factor) incompatibility —*see* Rh,
  incompatibility
Rheumatic (acute) (subacute) (chronic)
  adherent pericardium I09.2
  coronary arteritis I01.9
  degeneration, myocardium I09.0
  fever (acute) —*see* Fever, rheumatic
  heart —*see* Disease, heart, rheumatic
  myocardial degeneration —*see* Degeneration,
    myocardium
  myocarditis (chronic) (inactive) (with chorea)
    I09.0
    with chorea (acute) (rheumatic)
      (Sydenham's) I02.0
    active or acute I01.2
  pancarditis, acute I01.8
    with chorea (acute (rheumatic)
      Sydenham's) I02.0
  pericarditis (active) (acute) (with effusion)
    (with pneumonia) I01.0
    with chorea (acute) (rheumatic)
      (Sydenham's) I02.0
    chronic or inactive I09.2
  pneumonia I00 *[J17]*
  torticollis M43.6
  typhoid fever A01.09
Rheumatism (articular) (neuralgic)
  (nonarticular) M79.0
  gout —*see* Arthritis, rheumatoid
  intercostal, meaning Tietze's disease M94.0
  palindromic (any site) M12.30
    ankle M12.37-
    elbow M12.32-
    foot joint M12.37-
    hand joint M12.34-
    hip M12.35-
    knee M12.36-
    multiple site M12.39
    shoulder M12.31-
    specified joint NEC M12.38
    vertebrae M12.38
    wrist M12.33-
  sciatic M54.4-
Rheumatoid —*see also* condition
  arthritis —*see also* Arthritis, rheumatoid
    with involvement of organs NEC M05.60
      ankle M05.67-
      elbow M05.62-
      foot joint M05.67-
      hand joint M05.64-

Rheumatoid *(Continued)*
  arthritis *(Continued)*
    with involvement of organs NEC
      (Continued)
      hip M05.65-
      knee M05.66-
      multiple site M05.69
      shoulder M05.61-
      vertebra —*see* Spondylitis, ankylosing
      wrist M05.63-
    seronegative —*see* Arthritis, rheumatoid,
      seronegative
    seropositive —*see* Arthritis, rheumatoid,
      seropositive
  carditis M05.30
    ankle M05.37-
    elbow M05.32-
    foot joint M05.37-
    hand joint M05.34-
    hip M05.35-
    knee M05.36-
    multiple site M05.39
    shoulder M05.31-
    vertebra —*see* Spondylitis, ankylosing
    wrist M05.33-
  endocarditis —*see* Rheumatoid, carditis
  lung (disease) M05.10
    ankle M05.17-
    elbow M05.12-
    foot joint M05.17-
    hand joint M05.14-
    hip M05.15-
    knee M05.16-
    multiple site M05.19
    shoulder M05.11-
    vertebra —*see* Spondylitis, ankylosing
    wrist M05.13-
  myocarditis —*see* Rheumatoid, carditis
  myopathy M05.40
    ankle M05.47-
    elbow M05.42-
    foot joint M05.47-
    hand joint M05.44-
    hip M05.45-
    knee M05.46-
    multiple site M05.49
    shoulder M05.41-
    vertebra —*see* Spondylitis, ankylosing
    wrist M05.43-
  pericarditis —*see* Rheumatoid, carditis
  polyarthritis —*see* Arthritis, rheumatoid
  polyneuropathy M05.50
    ankle M05.57-
    elbow M05.52-
    foot joint M05.57-
    hand joint M05.54-
    hip M05.55-
    knee M05.56-
    multiple site M05.59
    shoulder M05.51-
    vertebra —*see* Spondylitis, ankylosing
    wrist M05.53-
  vasculitis M05.20
    ankle M05.27-
    elbow M05.22-
    foot joint M05.27-
    hand joint M05.24-
    hip M05.25-
    knee M05.26-
    multiple site M05.29
    shoulder M05.21-
    vertebra —*see* Spondylitis, ankylosing
    wrist M05.23-
Rhinitis (atrophic) (catarrhal) (chronic)
  (croupous) (fibrinous) (granulomatous)
  (hyperplastic) (hypertrophic)
  (membranous) (obstructive) (purulent)
  (suppurative) (ulcerative) J31.0
  with
    sore throat —*see* Nasopharyngitis
  acute J00

Rhinitis (*Continued*)
  allergic J30.9
    with asthma J45.909
      with
        exacerbation (acute) J45.901
        status asthmaticus J45.902
    due to
      food J30.5
      pollen J30.1
    nonseasonal J30.89
    perennial J30.89
    seasonal NEC J30.2
    specified NEC J30.89
  infective J00
  pneumococcal J00
  syphilitic A52.73
    congenital A50.05 [*J99*]
  tuberculous A15.8
  vasomotor J30.0
Rhinoantritis (chronic) —*see* Sinusitis, maxillary
Rhinodacryolith —*see* Dacryolith
Rhinolith (nasal sinus) J34.89
Rhinomegaly J34.89
Rhinopharyngitis (acute) (subacute) —*see also* Nasopharyngitis
  chronic J31.1
  destructive ulcerating A66.5
  mutilans A66.5
Rhinophyma L71.1
Rhinorrhea J34.89
  cerebrospinal (fluid) G96.0
  paroxysmal —*see* Rhinitis, allergic
  spasmodic —*see* Rhinitis, allergic
Rhinosalpingitis —*see* Salpingitis, eustachian
Rhinoscleroma A48.8
Rhinosporidiosis B48.1
Rhinovirus infection NEC B34.8
Rhizomelic chondrodysplasia punctata E71.540
Rhythm
  atrioventricular nodal I49.8
  disorder I49.9
    coronary sinus I49.8
    ectopic I49.8
    nodal I49.8
  escape I49.9
  heart, abnormal I49.9
  idioventricular I44.2
  nodal I49.8
  sleep, inversion G47.2-
    nonorganic origin —*see* Disorder, sleep, circadian rhythm, psychogenic
Rhytidosis facialis L98.8
Rib —*see also* condition
  cervical Q76.5
Riboflavin deficiency E53.0
Rice bodies —*see also* Loose, body, joint
  knee M23.4-
Richter syndrome —*see* Leukemia, chronic lymphocytic, B-cell type
Richter's hernia —*see* Hernia, abdomen, with obstruction
Ricinism —*see* Poisoning, food, noxious, plant
Rickets (active) (acute) (adolescent) (chest wall) (congenital) (current) (infantile) (intestinal) E55.0
  adult —*see* Osteomalacia
  celiac K90.0
  hypophosphatemic with nephrotic-glycosuric dwarfism E72.09
  inactive E64.3
  kidney N25.0
  renal N25.0
  sequelae, any E64.3
  vitamin-D-resistant E83.31 [*M90.80*]
Rickettsial disease A79.9
  specified type NEC A79.89
Rickettsialpox (Rickettsia akari) A79.1

Rickettsiosis A79.9
  due to
    Ehrlichia sennetsu A79.81
    Rickettsia akari (rickettsialpox) A79.1
  specified type NEC A79.89
  tick-borne A77.9
  vesicular A79.1
Rider's bone —*see* Ossification, muscle, specified NEC
Ridge, alveolus —*see also* condition
  flabby K06.8
Ridged ear, congenital Q17.3
Riedel's
  lobe, liver Q44.7
  struma, thyroiditis or disease E06.5
Rieger's anomaly or syndrome Q13.81
Riehl's melanosis L81.4
Rietti-Greppi-Micheli anemia D56.9
Rieux's hernia —*see* Hernia, abdomen, specified site NEC
Riga (-Fede) disease K14.0
Riggs' disease —*see* Periodontitis
Right middle lobe syndrome J98.11
Rigid, rigidity —*see also* condition
  abdominal R19.30
    with severe abdominal pain R10.0
      epigastric R19.36
      generalized R19.37
      left lower quadrant R19.34
      left upper quadrant R19.32
      periumbilic R19.35
      right lower quadrant R19.33
      right upper quadrant R19.31
  articular, multiple, congenital Q68.8
  cervix (uteri) in pregnancy —*see* Pregnancy, complicated by, abnormal, cervix
  hymen (acquired) (congenital) N89.6
  nuchal R29.1
  pelvic floor in pregnancy —*see* Pregnancy, complicated by, abnormal, pelvic organs or tissues NEC
  perineum or vulva in pregnancy —*see* Pregnancy, complicated by, abnormal, vulva
  spine —*see* Dorsopathy, specified NEC
  vagina in pregnancy —*see* Pregnancy, complicated by, abnormal, vagina
Rigors R68.89
  with fever R50.9
Riley-Day syndrome G90.1
RIND (reversible ischemic neurologic deficit) I63.9
Ring (s)
  aorta (vascular) Q25.4
  Bandl's O62.4
  contraction, complicating delivery O62.4
  esophageal, lower (muscular) K22.2
  Fleischer's (cornea) H18.04-
  hymenal, tight (acquired) (congenital) N89.6
  Kayser-Fleischer (cornea) H18.04-
  retraction, uterus, pathological O62.4
  Schatzki's (esophagus) (lower) K22.2
    congenital Q39.3
  Soemmerring's —*see* Cataract, secondary
  vascular (congenital) Q25.8
    aorta Q25.4
Ringed hair (congenital) Q84.1
Ringworm B35.9
  beard B35.0
  black dot B35.0
  body B35.4
  Burmese B35.5
  corporeal B35.4
  foot B35.3
  groin B35.6
  hand B35.2
  honeycomb B35.0
  nails B35.1
  perianal (area) B35.6
  scalp B35.0

Ringworm (*Continued*)
  specified NEC B35.8
  Tokelau B35.5
Rise, venous pressure I87.8
Risk, suicidal
  meaning personal history of attempted suicide Z91.5
  meaning suicidal ideation —*see* Ideation, suicidal
Ritter's disease L00
Rivalry, sibling Z62.891
Rivalta's disease A42.2
River blindness B73.01
Robert's pelvis Q74.2
  with disproportion (fetopelvic) O33.0
    causing obstructed labor O65.0
Robin (-Pierre) syndrome Q87.0
Robinow-Silvermann-Smith syndrome Q87.1
Robinson's (hidrotic) ectodermal dysplasia or syndrome Q82.4
Robles' disease B73.01
Rocky Mountain (spotted) fever A77.0
Roetheln —*see* Rubella
Roger's disease Q21.0
Rokitansky-Aschoff sinuses (gallbladder) K82.8
Rolando's fracture (displaced) S62.22-
  nondisplaced S62.22-
Romano-Ward (prolonged QT interval) syndrome I45.81
Romberg's disease or syndrome G51.8
Roof, mouth —*see* condition
Rosacea L71.9
  acne L71.9
  keratitis L71.8
  specified NEC L71.8
Rosary, rachitic E55.0
Rose
  cold J30.1
  fever J30.1
  rash R21
    epidemic B06.9
Rosenbach's erysipeloid A26.0
Rosenthal's disease or syndrome D68.1
Roseola B09
  infantum B08.20
    due to human herpesvirus 6 B08.21
    due to human herpesvirus 7 B08.22
Ross River disease or fever B33.1
Rossbach's disease K31.89
  psychogenic F45.8
Rostan's asthma (cardiac) —*see* Failure, ventricular, left
Rotation
  anomalous, incomplete or insufficient, intestine Q43.3
  cecum (congenital) Q43.3
  colon (congenital) Q43.3
  spine, incomplete or insufficient —*see* Dorsopathy, deforming, specified NEC
  tooth, teeth, fully erupted M26.35
  vertebra, incomplete or insufficient —*see* Dorsopathy, deforming, specified NEC
Rotes Quérol disease or syndrome —*see* Hyperostosis, ankylosing
Roth (-Bernhardt) disease or syndrome —*see* Meralgia paraesthetica
Rothmund (-Thomson) syndrome Q82.8
Rotor's disease or syndrome E80.6
Round
  back (with wedging of vertebrae) —*see* Kyphosis
    sequelae (late effect) of rickets E64.3
  worms (large) (infestation) NEC B82.0
    Ascariasis (*see also* Ascariasis) B77.9
Roussy-Lévy syndrome G60.0
Rubella (German measles) B06.9
  complication NEC B06.09
    neurological B06.00
  congenital P35.0
  contact Z20.4

New   Revised   ~~deleted~~ Deleted

Rubella *(Continued)*
  exposure to Z20.4
  maternal
    care for (suspected) damage to fetus O35.3
    manifest rubella in infant P35.0
    suspected damage to fetus affecting
        management of pregnancy O35.3
  specified complications NEC B06.89
Rubeola (meaning measles) —*see* Measles
  meaning rubella —*see* Rubella
Rubeosis, iris —*see* Disorder, iris, vascular
Rubinstein-Taybi syndrome Q87.2
Rudimentary (congenital) —*see also* Agenesis
  arm —*see* Defect, reduction, upper limb
  bone Q79.9
  cervix uteri Q51.828
  eye Q11.2
  lobule of ear Q17.3
  patella Q74.1
  respiratory organs in thoracopagus Q89.4
  tracheal bronchus Q32.4
  uterus Q51.818
    in male Q56.1
  vagina Q52.0
Ruled out condition —*see* Observation,
    suspected
Rumination R11.10
  with nausea R11.2
  disorder of infancy F98.21
  neurotic F42
  newborn P92.1
  obsessional F42
  psychogenic F42
Runeberg's disease D51.0
Runny nose R09.89
Rupia (syphilitic) A51.39
  congenital A50.06
  tertiary A52.79
Rupture, ruptured
  abscess (spontaneous) - code by site under
    Abscess
  aneurysm —*see* Aneurysm
  anus (sphincter) —*see* Laceration, anus
  aorta, aortic I71.8
    abdominal I71.3
    arch I71.1
    ascending I71.1
    descending I71.8
      abdominal I71.3
      thoracic I71.1
    syphilitic A52.01
    thoracoabdominal I71.5
    thorax, thoracic I71.1
    transverse I71.1
    traumatic —*see* Injury, aorta, laceration,
        major
    valve or cusp (*see also* Endocarditis, aortic)
        I35.8
  appendix (with peritonitis) K35.2
  arteriovenous fistula, brain I60.8
  artery I77.2
    brain —*see* Hemorrhage, intracranial,
        intracerebral
    coronary —*see* Infarct, myocardium
    heart —*see* Infarct, myocardium
    pulmonary I28.8
    traumatic (complication) —*see* Injury,
        blood vessel
  bile duct (common) (hepatic) K83.2
    cystic K82.2
  bladder (sphincter) (nontraumatic)
    (spontaneous) N32.89
    following ectopic or molar pregnancy
        O08.6
    obstetrical trauma O71.5
    traumatic S37.29
  blood vessel —*see also* Hemorrhage
    brain —*see* Hemorrhage, intracranial,
        intracerebral
    heart —*see* Infarct, myocardium
    traumatic (complication) —*see* Injury,
        blood vessel, laceration, major, by site

bone —*see* Fracture
bowel (nontraumatic) K63.1
brain
  aneurysm (congenital) —*see also*
      Hemorrhage, intracranial,
      subarachnoid
    syphilitic A52.05
  hemorrhagic —*see* Hemorrhage,
      intracranial, intracerebral
capillaries I78.8
cardiac (auricle) (ventricle) (wall) I23.3
  with hemopericardium I23.0
  infectional I40.9
  traumatic —*see* Injury, heart
cartilage (articular) (current) —*see also* Sprain
  knee S83.3-
  semilunar —*see* Tear, meniscus
cecum (with peritonitis) K65.0
  with peritoneal abscess K35.3
  traumatic S36.598
celiac artery, traumatic —*see* Injury, blood
    vessel, celiac artery, laceration, major
cerebral aneurysm (congenital) (*see*
    Hemorrhage, intracranial,
    subarachnoid)
cervix (uteri)
  with ectopic or molar pregnancy O08.6
  following ectopic or molar pregnancy
      O08.6
  obstetrical trauma O71.3
  traumatic S37.69
chordae tendineae NEC I51.1
  concurrent with acute myocardial
      infarction —*see* Infarct, myocardium
  following acute myocardial infarction
      (current complication) I23.4
choroid (direct) (indirect) (traumatic) H31.32-
circle of Willis I60.6
colon (nontraumatic) K63.1
  traumatic —*see* Injury, intestine, large
cornea (traumatic) —*see* Injury, eye, laceration
coronary (artery) (thrombotic) —*see* Infarct,
    myocardium
corpus luteum (infected) (ovary) N83.1
cyst —*see* Cyst
cystic duct K82.2
Descemet's membrane —*see* Change, corneal
    membrane, Descemet's, rupture
  traumatic —*see* Injury, eye, laceration
diaphragm, traumatic —*see* Injury,
    intrathoracic, diaphragm
disc —*see* Rupture, intervertebral disc
diverticulum (intestine) K57.80
  with bleeding K57.81
  bladder N32.3
  large intestine K57.20
    with
      bleeding K57.21
      small intestine K57.40
        with bleeding K57.41
  small intestine K57.00
    with
      bleeding K57.01
      large intestine K57.40
        with bleeding K57.41
duodenal stump K31.89
ear drum (nontraumatic) —*see also*
    Perforation, tympanum
  traumatic S09.2-
    due to blast injury —*see* Injury, blast, ear
esophagus K22.3
eye (without prolapse or loss of intraocular
    tissue) —*see* Injury, eye, laceration
fallopian tube NEC (nonobstetric)
    (nontraumatic) N83.8
  due to pregnancy O00.1
fontanel P13.1
gallbladder K82.2
  traumatic S36.128
gastric —*see also* Rupture, stomach
  vessel K92.2

globe (eye) (traumatic) —*see* Injury, eye,
    laceration
graafian follicle (hematoma) N83.0
heart —*see* Rupture, cardiac
hymen (nontraumatic) (nonintentional)
    N89.8
internal organ, traumatic —*see* Injury, by site
intervertebral disc —*see* Displacement,
    intervertebral disc
  traumatic —*see* Rupture, traumatic,
      intervertebral disc
intestine NEC (nontraumatic) K63.1
  traumatic —*see* Injury, intestine
iris —*see also* Abnormality, pupillary
  traumatic —*see* Injury, eye, laceration
joint capsule, traumatic —*see* Sprain
kidney (traumatic) S37.06-
  birth injury P15.8
  nontraumatic N28.89
lacrimal duct (traumatic) —*see* Injury, eye,
    specified site NEC
lens (cataract) (traumatic) —*see* Cataract,
    traumatic
ligament, traumatic —*see* Rupture, traumatic,
    ligament, by site
liver S36.116
  birth injury P15.0
lymphatic vessel I89.8
marginal sinus (placental) (with
    hemorrhage) —*see* Hemorrhage,
    antepartum, specified cause NEC
membrana tympani (nontraumatic) —*see*
    Perforation, tympanum
membranes (spontaneous)
  artificial
    delayed delivery following O75.5
  delayed delivery following —*see*
      Pregnancy, complicated by,
      premature rupture of membranes
meningeal artery I60.8
meniscus (knee) —*see also* Tear, meniscus
  old —*see* Derangement, meniscus
  site other than knee - code as Sprain
mesenteric artery, traumatic —*see* Injury,
    mesenteric, artery, laceration, major
mesentery (nontraumatic) K66.8
  traumatic —*see* Injury, intra-abdominal,
      specified, site NEC
mitral (valve) I34.8
muscle (traumatic) —*see also* Strain
  diastasis —*see* Diastasis, muscle
  nontraumatic M62.10
    ankle M62.17-
    foot M62.17-
    forearm M62.13-
    hand M62.14-
    lower leg M62.16-
    pelvic region M62.15-
    shoulder region M62.11-
    specified site NEC M62.18
    thigh M62.15-
    upper arm M62.12-
  traumatic —*see* Strain, by site
musculotendinous junction NEC,
    nontraumatic —*see* Rupture, tendon,
    spontaneous
mycotic aneurysm causing cerebral
    hemorrhage —*see* Hemorrhage,
    intracranial, subarachnoid
myocardium, myocardial —*see* Rupture,
    cardiac
  traumatic —*see* Injury, heart
nontraumatic, meaning hernia —*see* Hernia
obstructed —*see* Hernia, by site, obstructed
operation wound —*see* Disruption, wound,
    operation
ovary, ovarian N83.8
  corpus luteum cyst N83.1
  follicle (graafian) N83.0
oviduct (nonobstetric) (nontraumatic) N83.8
  due to pregnancy O00.1

Rupture, ruptured *(Continued)*
  pancreas (nontraumatic) K86.8
    traumatic S36.299
  papillary muscle NEC I51.2
    following acute myocardial infarction
      (current complication) I23.5
  pelvic
    floor, complicating delivery O70.1
    organ NEC, obstetrical trauma O71.5
  perineum (nonobstetric) (nontraumatic)
    N90.89
    complicating delivery —*see* Delivery,
      complicated, by, laceration, anus
      (sphincter)
  postoperative wound —*see* Disruption,
    wound, operation
  prostate (traumatic) S37.828
  pulmonary
    artery I28.8
    valve (heart) I37.8
    vein I28.8
    vessel I28.8
  pus tube —*see* Salpingitis
  pyosalpinx —*see* Salpingitis
  rectum (nontraumatic) K63.1
    traumatic S36.69
  retina, retinal (traumatic) (without
    detachment) —*see also* Break, retina
    with detachment —*see* Detachment, retina,
      with retinal, break
  rotator cuff (nontraumatic) M75.10-
    complete M75.12-
    incomplete M75.11-
  sclera —*see* Injury, eye, laceration
  sigmoid (nontraumatic) K63.1
    traumatic S36.593
  spinal cord —*see also* Injury, spinal cord, by
    region
    due to injury at birth P11.5
    newborn (birth injury) P11.5
  spleen (traumatic) S36.09
    birth injury P15.1
    congenital (birth injury) P15.1
    due to P. vivax malaria B51.0
    nontraumatic D73.5
    spontaneous D73.5
  splenic vein R58
    traumatic —*see* Injury, blood vessel,
      splenic vein
  stomach (nontraumatic) (spontaneous)
    K31.89
    traumatic S36.39
  supraspinatus (complete) (incomplete)
    (nontraumatic) —*see* Tear, rotator
    cuff
  symphysis pubis
    obstetric O71.6
    traumatic S33.4
  synovium (cyst) M66.10
    ankle M66.17-
    elbow M66.12-
    finger M66.14-
    foot M66.17-
    forearm M66.13-
    hand M66.14-
    pelvic region M66.15-
    shoulder region M66.11-
    specified site NEC M66.18
    thigh M66.15-
    toe M66.17-
    upper arm M66.12-
    wrist M66.13-
  tendon (traumatic) —*see* Strain
    nontraumatic (spontaneous) M66.9
      ankle M66.87-
      extensor M66.20
        ankle M66.27-
        foot M66.27-
        forearm M66.23-
        hand M66.24-
        lower leg M66.26-
        multiple sites M66.29

Rupture, ruptured *(Continued)*
  tendon *(Continued)*
    nontraumatic *(Continued)*
      extensor *(Continued)*
        pelvic region M66.25-
        shoulder region M66.21-
        specified site NEC M66.28
        thigh M66.25-
        upper arm M66.22-
      flexor M66.30
        ankle M66.37-
        foot M66.37-
        forearm M66.33-
        hand M66.34-
        lower leg M66.36-
        multiple sites M66.39
        pelvic region M66.35-
        shoulder region M66.31-
        specified site NEC M66.38
        thigh M66.35-
        upper arm M66.32-
      foot M66.87-
      forearm M66.83-
      hand M66.84-
      lower leg M66.86-
      multiple sites M66.89
      pelvic region M66.85-
      shoulder region M66.81-
      specified
        site NEC M66.88
        tendon M66.80
      thigh M66.85-
      upper arm M66.82-
  thoracic duct I89.8
  tonsil J35.8
  traumatic
    aorta —*see* Injury, aorta, laceration, major
    diaphragm —*see* Injury, intrathoracic,
      diaphragm
    external site —*see* Wound, open, by site
    eye —*see* Injury, eye, laceration
    internal organ —*see* Injury, by site
    intervertebral disc
      cervical S13.0
      lumbar S33.0
      thoracic S23.0
    kidney S37.06-
    ligament —*see also* Sprain
      ankle —*see* Sprain, ankle
      carpus —*see* Rupture, traumatic,
        ligament, wrist
      collateral (hand) —*see* Rupture,
        traumatic, ligament, finger,
        collateral
      finger (metacarpophalangeal)
        (interphalangeal) S63.40-
        collateral S63.41-
          index S63.41-
          little S63.41-
          middle S63.41-
          ring S63.41-
        index S63.40-
        little S63.40-
        middle S63.40-
        palmar S63.42-
          index S63.42-
          little S63.42-
          middle S63.42-
          ring S63.42-
        ring S63.40-
        specified site NEC S63.499
          index S63.49-
          little S63.49-
          middle S63.49-
          ring S63.49-
        volar plate S63.43-
          index S63.43-
          little S63.43-
          middle S63.43-
          ring S63.43-
      foot —*see* Sprain, foot
      radial collateral S53.2-

Rupture, ruptured *(Continued)*
  traumatic *(Continued)*
    ligament *(Continued)*
      radiocarpal —*see* Rupture, traumatic,
        ligament, wrist, radiocarpal
      ulnar collateral S53.3-
      ulnocarpal —*see* Rupture, traumatic,
        ligament, wrist, ulnocarpal
      wrist S63.30-
        collateral S63.31-
        radiocarpal S63.32-
        specified site NEC S63.39-
        ulnocarpal (palmar) S63.33-
    liver S36.116
    membrana tympani —*see* Rupture, ear
      drum, traumatic
    muscle or tendon —*see* Strain
    myocardium —*see* Injury, heart
    pancreas S36.299
    rectum S36.69
    sigmoid S36.593
    spleen S36.09
    stomach S36.39
    symphysis pubis S33.4
    tympanum, tympanic (membrane) —*see*
      Rupture, ear drum, traumatic
    ureter S37.19
    uterus S37.69
    vagina —*see* Injury, vagina
    vena cava —*see* Injury, vena cava,
      laceration, major
  tricuspid (heart) (valve) I07.8
  tube, tubal (nonobstetric) (nontraumatic)
    N83.8
    abscess —*see* Salpingitis
    due to pregnancy O00.1
  tympanum, tympanic (membrane)
    (nontraumatic) (*see also* Perforation,
    tympanic membrane) H72.9-
    traumatic —*see* Rupture, ear drum,
      traumatic
  umbilical cord, complicating delivery
    O69.89
  ureter (traumatic) S37.19
    nontraumatic N28.89
  urethra (nontraumatic) N36.8
    with ectopic or molar pregnancy
      O08.6
    following ectopic or molar pregnancy
      O08.6
    obstetrical trauma O71.5
    traumatic S37.39
  uterosacral ligament (nonobstetric)
    (nontraumatic) N83.8
  uterus (traumatic) S37.69
    before labor O71.0-
    during or after labor O71.1
    nonpuerperal, nontraumatic N85.8
    pregnant (during labor) O71.1
      before labor O71.0-
  vagina —*see* Injury, vagina
  valve, valvular (heart) —*see* Endocarditis
  varicose vein —*see* Varix
  varix —*see* Varix
  vena cava R58
    traumatic —*see* Injury, vena cava,
      laceration, major
  vesical (urinary) N32.89
  vessel (blood) R58
    pulmonary I28.8
    traumatic —*see* Injury, blood vessel
  viscus R19.8
  vulva complicating delivery O70.0
Russell-Silver syndrome Q87.1
Russian spring-summer type encephalitis
  A84.0
Rust's disease (tuberculous cervical spondylitis)
  A18.01
Ruvalcaba-Myhre-Smith syndrome
  E71.440
Rytand-Lipsitch syndrome I44.2

◀ New   ◀▥ Revised   ~~deleted~~ Deleted

S

Saber, sabre shin or tibia (syphilitic) A50.56
[M90.8-]
Sac lacrimal —*see* condition
Saccharomyces infection B37.9
Saccharopinuria E72.3
Saccular —*see* condition
Sacculation
  aorta (nonsyphilitic) —*see* Aneurysm,
    aorta
  bladder N32.3
  intralaryngeal (congenital) (ventricular)
    Q31.3
  larynx (congenital) (ventricular) Q31.3
  organ or site, congenital —*see* Distortion
  pregnant uterus —*see* Pregnancy, complicated
    by, abnormal, uterus
  ureter N28.89
  urethra N36.1
  vesical N32.3
Sachs' amaurotic familial idiocy or disease
  E75.02
Sachs-Tay disease E75.02
Sacks-Libman disease M32.11
Sacralgia M53.3
Sacralization Q76.49
Sacrodynia M53.3
Sacroiliac joint —*see* condition
Sacroiliitis NEC M46.1
Sacrum —*see* condition
Saddle
  back —*see* Lordosis
  embolus
    abdominal aorta I74.01
    pulmonary artery I26.92
      with acute cor pulmonale I26.02
  injury — code to condition
  nose M95.0
    due to syphilis A50.57
Sadism (sexual) F65.52
Sadness, postpartal O90.6
Sadomasochism F65.50
Saemisch's ulcer (cornea) —*see* Ulcer, cornea,
  central
Sahib disease B55.0
Sailors' skin L57.8
Saint
  Anthony's fire —*see* Erysipelas
  triad —*see* Hernia, diaphragm
  Vitus' dance —*see* Chorea, Sydenham's
Salaam
  attack (s) —*see* Epilepsy, spasms
  tic R25.8
Salicylism
  abuse F55.8
  overdose or wrong substance given —*see*
    Table of Drugs and Chemicals, by drug,
    poisoning
Salivary duct or gland —*see* condition
Salivation, excessive K11.7
Salmonella —*see* Infection, Salmonella
Salmonellosis A02.0
Salpingitis (catarrhal) (fallopian tube) (nodular)
  (pseudofollicular) (purulent) (septic)
  N70.91
  with oophoritis N70.93
  acute N70.01
    with oophoritis N70.03
  chlamydial A56.11
  chronic N70.11
    with oophoritis N70.13
  complicating abortion —*see* Abortion, by
    type, complicated by, salpingitis
  ear —*see* Salpingitis, eustachian
  eustachian (tube) H68.00-
    acute H68.01-
    chronic H68.02-
  follicularis N70.11
    with oophoritis N70.13
  gonococcal (acute) (chronic) A54.24

Salpingitis (Continued)
  interstitial, chronic N70.11
    with oophoritis N70.13
  isthmica nodosa N70.11
    with oophoritis N70.13
  specific (gonococcal) (acute) (chronic) A54.24
  tuberculous (acute) (chronic) A18.17
  venereal (gonococcal) (acute) (chronic) A54.24
Salpingocele N83.4
Salpingo-oophoritis (catarrhal) (purulent)
  (ruptured) (septic) (suppurative) N70.93
  acute N70.03
    with ectopic or molar pregnancy O08.0
    following ectopic or molar pregnancy
      O08.0
    gonococcal A54.24
  chronic N70.13
  following ectopic or molar pregnancy O08.0
  gonococcal (acute) (chronic) A54.24
  puerperal O86.19
  specific (gonococcal) (acute) (chronic) A54.24
  subacute N70.03
  tuberculous (acute) (chronic) A18.17
  venereal (gonococcal) (acute) (chronic)
    A54.24
Salpingo-ovaritis —*see* Salpingo-oophoritis
Salpingoperitonitis —*see* Salpingo-oophoritis
Salzmann's nodular dystrophy —*see*
  Degeneration, cornea, nodular
Sampson's cyst or tumor N80.1
San Joaquin (Valley) fever B38.0
Sandblaster's asthma, lung or pneumoconiosis
  J62.8
Sander's disease (paranoia) F22
Sandfly fever A93.1
Sandhoff's disease E75.01
Sanfilippo (Type B) (Type C) (Type D)
  syndrome E76.22
Sanger-Brown ataxia G11.2
Sao Paulo fever or typhus A77.0
Saponification, mesenteric K65.8
Sarcocele (benign)
  syphilitic A52.76
    congenital A50.59
Sarcocystosis A07.8
Sarcoepiplocele —*see* Hernia
Sarcoepiplomphalocele Q79.2
Sarcoid —*see also* Sarcoidosis
  arthropathy D86.86
  Boeck's D86.9
  Darier-Roussy D86.3
  iridocyclitis D86.83
  meningitis D86.81
  myocarditis D86.85
  myositis D86.87
  pyelonephritis D86.84
  Spiegler-Fendt L08.89
Sarcoidosis D86.9
  with
    cranial nerve palsies D86.82
    hepatic granuloma D86.89
    polyarthritis D86.86
    tubulo-interstitial nephropathy D86.84
  combined sites NEC D86.89
  lung D86.0
    and lymph nodes D86.2
  lymph nodes D86.1
    and lung D86.2
  meninges D86.81
  skin D86.3
  specified type NEC D86.89
Sarcoma (of) —*see also* Neoplasm, connective
  tissue, malignant
  alveolar soft part —*see* Neoplasm, connective
    tissue, malignant
  ameloblastic C41.1
    upper jaw (bone) C41.0
  botryoid —*see* Neoplasm, connective tissue,
    malignant
  botryoides —*see* Neoplasm, connective tissue,
    malignant

Sarcoma (Continued)
  cerebellar C71.6
    circumscribed (arachnoidal) C71.6
    circumscribed (arachnoidal) cerebellar
      C71.6
  clear cell —*see also* Neoplasm, connective
    tissue, malignant
    kidney C64.-
  dendritic cells (accessory cells) C96.4
  embryonal —*see* Neoplasm, connective tissue,
    malignant
  endometrial (stromal) C54.1
    isthmus C54.0
  epithelioid (cell) —*see* Neoplasm, connective
    tissue, malignant
  Ewing's —*see* Neoplasm, bone, malignant
  follicular dendritic cell C96.4
  germinoblastic (diffuse) —*see* Lymphoma,
    diffuse, large cell
    follicular —*see* Lymphoma, follicular,
      specified NEC
  giant cell (except of bone) —*see also* Neoplasm,
    connective tissue, malignant
    bone —*see* Neoplasm, bone, malignant
  glomoid —*see* Neoplasm, connective tissue,
    malignant
  granulocytic C92.3-
  hemangioendothelial —*see* Neoplasm,
    connective tissue, malignant
  hemorrhagic, multiple —*see* Sarcoma,
    Kaposi's
  histiocytic C96.A
  Hodgkin —*see* Lymphoma, Hodgkin
  immunoblastic (diffuse) —*see* Lymphoma,
    diffuse large cell
  interdigitating dendritic cell C96.4
  Kaposi's
    colon C46.4
    connective tissue C46.1
    gastrointestinal organ C46.4
    lung C46.5-
    lymph node (s) C46.3
    palate (hard) (soft) C46.2
    rectum C46.4
    skin C46.0
    specified site NEC C46.7
    stomach C46.4
    unspecified site C46.9
  Kupffer cell C22.3
  Langerhans cell C96.4
  leptomeningeal —*see* Neoplasm, meninges,
    malignant
  liver NEC C22.4
  lymphangioendothelial —*see* Neoplasm,
    connective tissue, malignant
  lymphoblastic —*see* Lymphoma,
    lymphoblastic (diffuse)
  lymphocytic —*see* Lymphoma, small cell
    B-cell
  mast cell C96.2
  melanotic —*see* Melanoma
  meningeal —*see* Neoplasm, meninges,
    malignant
  meningothelial —*see* Neoplasm, meninges,
    malignant
  mesenchymal —*see also* Neoplasm,
    connective tissue, malignant
    mixed —*see* Neoplasm, connective tissue,
      malignant
  mesothelial —*see* Mesothelioma
  monstrocellular
    specified site —*see* Neoplasm, malignant,
      by site
    unspecified site C71.9
  myeloid C92.3-
  neurogenic —*see* Neoplasm, nerve,
    malignant
  odontogenic C41.1
    upper jaw (bone) C41.0
  osteoblastic —*see* Neoplasm, bone,
    malignant

Sarcoma *(Continued)*
- osteogenic —*see also* Neoplasm, bone, malignant
  - juxtacortical —*see* Neoplasm, bone, malignant
  - periosteal —*see* Neoplasm, bone, malignant
  - periosteal —*see also* Neoplasm, bone, malignant
  - osteogenic —*see* Neoplasm, bone, malignant
- pleomorphic cell —*see* Neoplasm, connective tissue, malignant
- reticulum cell (diffuse) —*see* Lymphoma, diffuse large cell
  - nodular —*see* Lymphoma, follicular
  - pleomorphic cell type —*see* Lymphoma, diffuse large cell
- rhabdoid —*see* Neoplasm, malignant, by site
- round cell —*see* Neoplasm, connective tissue, malignant
- small cell —*see* Neoplasm, connective tissue, malignant
- soft tissue —*see* Neoplasm, connective tissue, malignant
- spindle cell —*see* Neoplasm, connective tissue, malignant
- stromal (endometrial) C54.1
  - isthmus C54.0
- synovial —*see also* Neoplasm, connective tissue, malignant
  - biphasic —*see* Neoplasm, connective tissue, malignant
  - epithelioid cell —*see* Neoplasm, connective tissue, malignant
  - spindle cell —*see* Neoplasm, connective tissue, malignant
Sarcomatosis
- meningeal —*see* Neoplasm, meninges, malignant
- specified site NEC —*see* Neoplasm, connective tissue, malignant
- unspecified site C80.1
Sarcosinemia E72.59
Sarcosporidiosis (intestinal) A07.8
Satiety, early R68.81
Saturnine —*see* condition
Saturnism
- overdose or wrong substance given or taken —*see* Table of Drugs and Chemicals, by drug, poisoning
Satyriasis F52.8
Sauriasis —*see* Ichthyosis
SBE (subacute bacterial endocarditis) I33.0
Scabies (any site) B86
Scabs R23.4
Scaglietti-Dagnini syndrome E22.0
Scald —*see* Burn
Scalenus anticus (anterior) **syndrome** G54.0
Scales R23.4
Scaling, skin R23.4
Scalp —*see* condition
Scapegoating affecting child Z62.3
Scaphocephaly Q75.0
Scapulalgia M89.8X1
Scapulohumeral myopathy G71.0
Scar, scarring (*see also* Cicatrix) L90.5
- adherent L90.5
- atrophic L90.5
- cervix
  - in pregnancy or childbirth —*see* Pregnancy, complicated by, abnormal cervix
- cheloid L91.0
- chorioretinal H31.00-
  - posterior pole macula H31.01-
  - postsurgical H59.81-
  - solar retinopathy H31.02-
  - specified type NEC H31.09-
- choroid —*see* Scar, chorioretinal
- conjunctiva H11.24-

Scar, scarring *(Continued)*
- cornea H17.9
  - xerophthalmic —*see also* Opacity, cornea
    - vitamin A deficiency E50.6
- duodenum, obstructive K31.5
- hypertrophic L91.0
- keloid L91.0
- labia N90.89
- lung (base) J98.4
- macula —*see* Scar, chorioretinal, posterior pole
- muscle M62.89
- myocardium, myocardial I25.2
- painful L90.5
- posterior pole (eye) —*see* Scar, chorioretinal, posterior pole
- retina —*see* Scar, chorioretinal
- trachea J39.8
- uterus N85.8
  - in pregnancy O34.29
- vagina N89.8
  - postoperative N99.2
- vulva N90.89
Scarabiasis B88.2
Scarlatina (anginosa) (maligna) (ulcerosa) A38.9
- myocarditis (acute) A38.1
  - old —*see* Myocarditis
- otitis media A38.0
Scarlet fever (albuminuria) (angina) A38.9
Schamberg's disease (progressive pigmentary dermatosis) L81.7
Schatzki's ring (acquired) (esophagus) (lower) K22.2
- congenital Q39.3
Schaufenster krankheit I20.8
Schaumann's
- benign lymphogranulomatosis D86.1
- disease or syndrome —*see* Sarcoidosis
Scheie's syndrome E76.03
Schenck's disease B42.1
Scheuermann's disease or osteochondrosis —*see* Osteochondrosis, juvenile, spine
Schilder (-Flatau) **disease** G37.0
Schilling-type monocytic leukemia C93.0-
Schimmelbusch's disease, cystic mastitis, or hyperplasia —*see* Mastopathy, cystic
Schistosoma infestation —*see* Infestation, Schistosoma
Schistosomiasis B65.9
- with muscle disorder B65.9 *[M63.80]*
  - ankle B65.9 *[M63.87-]*
  - foot B65.9 *[M63.87-]*
  - forearm B65.9 *[M63.83-]*
  - hand B65.9 *[M63.84-]*
  - lower leg B65.9 *[M63.86-]*
  - multiple sites B65.9 *[M63.89]*
  - pelvic region B65.9 *[M63.85-]*
  - shoulder region B65.9 *[M63.81-]*
  - specified site NEC B65.9 *[M63.88]*
  - thigh B65.9 *[M63.85-]*
  - upper arm B65.9 *[M63.82-]*
- Asiatic B65.2
- bladder B65.0
- chestermani B65.8
- colon B65.1
- cutaneous B65.3
- due to
  - S. haematobium B65.0
  - S. japonicum B65.2
  - S. mansoni B65.1
  - S. mattheii B65.8
- Eastern B65.2
- genitourinary tract B65.0
- intestinal B65.1
- lung NEC B65.9 *[J99]*
  - pneumonia B65.9 *[J17]*
- Manson's (intestinal) B65.1
- oriental B65.2
- pulmonary NEC B65.9 *[J99]*
  - pneumonia B65.9

Schistosomiasis *(Continued)*
- Schistosoma
  - haematobium B65.0
  - japonicum B65.2
  - mansoni B65.1
  - specified type NEC B65.8
  - urinary B65.0
  - vesical B65.0
Schizencephaly Q04.6
Schizoaffective psychosis F25.9
Schizodontia K00.2
Schizoid personality F60.1
Schizophrenia, schizophrenic F20.9
- acute (brief) (undifferentiated) F23
- atypical (form) F20.3
- borderline F21
- catalepsy F20.2
- catatonic (type) (excited) (withdrawn) F20.2
- cenesthopathic, cenesthesiopathic F20.89
- childhood type F84.5
- chronic undifferentiated F20.5
- cyclic F25.0
- disorganized (type) F20.1
- flexibilitas cerea F20.2
- hebephrenic (type) F20.1
- incipient F21
- latent F21
- negative type F20.5
- paranoid (type) F20.0
- paraphrenic F20.0
- post-psychotic depression F32.8
- prepsychotic F21
- prodromal F21
- pseudoneurotic F21
- pseudopsychopathic F21
- reaction F23
- residual (state) (type) F20.5
- restzustand F20.5
- schizoaffective (type) —*see* Psychosis, schizoaffective
- simple (type) F20.89
- simplex F20.89
- specified type NEC F20.89
- stupor F20.2
- syndrome of childhood F84.5
- undifferentiated (type) F20.3
  - chronic F20.5
Schizothymia (persistent) F60.1
Schlatter-Osgood disease or osteochondrosis —*see* Osteochondrosis, juvenile, tibia
Schlatter's tibia —*see* Osteochondrosis, juvenile, tibia
Schmidt's syndrome (polyglandular, autoimmune) E31.0
Schmincke's carcinoma or tumor —*see* Neoplasm, nasopharynx, malignant
Schmitz (-Stutzer) **dysentery** A03.0
Schmorl's disease or nodes
- lumbar region M51.46
- lumbosacral region M51.47
- sacrococcygeal region M53.3
- thoracic region M51.44
- thoracolumbar region M51.45
Schneiderian
- papilloma —*see* Neoplasm, nasopharynx benign
  - specified site —*see* Neoplasm, benign, by site
  - unspecified site D14.0
  - specified site —*see* Neoplasm, malignant, by site
  - unspecified site C30.0
Scholte's syndrome (malignant carcinoid) E34.0
Scholz (-Bielchowsky-Henneberg) **disease or syndrome** E75.25
Schönlein (-Henoch) **disease or purpura** (primary) (rheumatic) D69.0
Schottmuller's disease A01.4
Schroeder's syndrome (endocrine hypertensive) E27.0

◀ New   ◀▥ Revised   ~~deleted~~ Deleted

Schüller-Christian disease or syndrome C96.5
Schultze's type acroparesthesia, simple I73.89
Schultz's disease or syndrome —*see*
    Agranulocytosis
Schwalbe-Ziehen-Oppenheim disease G24.1
Schwannoma —*see also* Neoplasm, nerve,
    benign
    malignant —*see also* Neoplasm, nerve,
        malignant
        with rhabdomyoblastic differentiation —
            see Neoplasm, nerve, malignant
    melanocytic —*see* Neoplasm, nerve, benign
    pigmented —*see* Neoplasm, nerve, benign
Schwannomatosis Q85.03
Schwartz (-Jampel) syndrome G71.13
Schwartz-Bartter syndrome E22.2
Schweniger-Buzzi anetoderma L90.1
Sciatic —*see* condition
Sciatica (infective)
    with lumbago M54.4-
        due to intervertebral disc disorder —*see*
            Disorder, disc, with, radiculopathy
    due to displacement of intervertebral disc
        (with lumbago) —*see* Disorder, disc,
        with, radiculopathy
    wallet M54.3-
Scimitar syndrome Q26.8
Sclera —*see* condition
Sclerectasia H15.84-
Scleredema
    adultorum —*see* Sclerosis, systemic
    Buschke's —*see* Sclerosis, systemic
    newborn P83.0
Sclerema (adiposum) (edematosum)
    (neonatorum) (newborn) P83.0
    adultorum —*see* Sclerosis, systemic
Scleriasis —*see* Scleroderma
Scleritis H15.00-
    with corneal involvement H15.04-
    anterior H15.01-
    brawny H15.02-
    in (due to) zoster B02.34
    posterior H15.03-
    specified type NEC H15.09-
    syphilitic A52.71
    tuberculous (nodular) A18.51
Sclerochoroiditis H31.8
Scleroconjunctivitis —*see* Scleritis
Sclerocystic ovary syndrome E28.2
Sclerodactyly, sclerodactylia L94.3
Scleroderma, sclerodermia (acrosclerotic)
    (diffuse) (generalized) (progressive)
    (pulmonary) (*see also* Sclerosis, systemic)
    M34.9-
    circumscribed L94.0
    linear L94.1
    localized L94.0
    newborn P83.8
    systemic M34.9
Sclerokeratitis H16.8
    tuberculous A18.52
Scleroma nasi A48.8
Scleromalacia (perforans) H15.05-
Scleromyxedema L98.5
Sclérose en plaques G35
Sclerosis, sclerotic
    adrenal (gland) E27.8
    Alzheimer's —*see* Disease, Alzheimer's
    amyotrophic (lateral) G12.21
    aorta, aortic I70.0
        valve —*see* Endocarditis, aortic
    artery, arterial, arteriolar, arteriovascular —
        see Arteriosclerosis
    ascending multiple G35
    brain (generalized) (lobular) G37.9
        artery, arterial I67.2
        diffuse G37.0
        disseminated G35
        insular G35
        Krabbe's E75.23
        miliary G35

Sclerosis, sclerotic (*Continued*)
    brain (*Continued*)
        multiple G35
        presenile (Alzheimer's) —*see* Disease,
            Alzheimer's, early onset
        senile (arteriosclerotic) I67.2
        stem, multiple G35
        tuberous Q85.1
    bulbar, multiple G35
    bundle of His I44.39
    cardiac —*see* Disease, heart, ischemic,
        atherosclerotic
    cardiorenal —*see* Hypertension, cardiorenal
    cardiovascular —*see also* Disease,
        cardiovascular
        renal —*see* Hypertension, cardiorenal
    cerebellar —*see* Sclerosis, brain
    cerebral —*see* Sclerosis, brain
    cerebrospinal (disseminated) (multiple) G35
    cerebrovascular I67.2
    choroid —*see* Degeneration, choroid
    combined (spinal cord) —*see also*
        Degeneration, combined
        multiple G35
    concentric (Balo) G37.5
    cornea —*see* Opacity, cornea
    coronary (artery) I25.10
        with angina pectoris —*see* Arteriosclerosis,
            coronary (artery),
    corpus cavernosum
        female N90.89
        male N48.6
    diffuse (brain) (spinal cord) G37.0
    disseminated G35
    dorsal G35
    dorsolateral (spinal cord) —*see* Degeneration,
        combined
    endometrium N85.5
    extrapyramidal G25.9
    eye, nuclear (senile) —*see* Cataract, senile,
        nuclear
    focal and segmental (glomerular) (*see also*
        N00-N07 with fourth character .1)
        N05.1
    Friedreich's (spinal cord) G11.1
    funicular (spermatic cord) N50.8
    general (vascular) —*see* Arteriosclerosis
    gland (lymphatic) I89.8
    hepatic K74.1
        alcoholic K70.2
    hereditary
        cerebellar G11.9
        spinal (Friedreich's ataxia) G11.1
    hippocampal G93.81
    insular G35
    kidney —*see* Sclerosis, renal
    larynx J38.7
    lateral (amyotrophic) (descending) (primary)
        (spinal) G12.21
    lens, senile nuclear —*see* Cataract, senile,
        nuclear
    liver K74.1
        with fibrosis K74.2
            alcoholic K70.2
        alcoholic K70.2
        cardiac K76.1
    lung —*see* Fibrosis, lung
    mastoid —*see* Mastoiditis, chronic
    mesial temporal G93.81
    mitral I05.8
    Mönckeberg's (medial) —*see* Arteriosclerosis,
        extremities
    multiple (brain stem) (cerebral) (generalized)
        (spinal cord) G35
    myocardium, myocardial —*see* Disease, heart,
        ischemic, atherosclerotic
    nuclear (senile), eye —*see* Cataract, senile,
        nuclear
    ovary N83.8
    pancreas K86.8
    penis N48.6

Sclerosis, sclerotic (*Continued*)
    peripheral arteries —*see* Arteriosclerosis,
        extremities
    plaques G35
    pluriglandular E31.8
    polyglandular E31.8
    posterolateral (spinal cord) —*see*
        Degeneration, combined
    presenile (Alzheimer's) —*see* Disease,
        Alzheimer's, early onset
    primary, lateral G12.29
    progressive, systemic M34.0
    pulmonary —*see* Fibrosis, lung
        artery I27.0
        valve (heart) —*see* Endocarditis,
            pulmonary
    renal N26.9
        with
            cystine storage disease E72.09
            hypertensive heart disease (conditions
                in I11) —*see* Hypertension,
                cardiorenal
            arteriolar (hyaline) (hyperplastic) —*see*
                Hypertension, kidney
    retina (senile) (vascular) H35.00
    senile (vascular) —*see* Arteriosclerosis
    spinal (cord) (progressive) G95.89
        ascending G61.0
        combined —*see also* Degeneration,
            combined
            multiple G35
            syphilitic A52.11
        disseminated G35
        dorsolateral —*see* Degeneration, combined
        hereditary (Friedreich's) (mixed form)
            G11.1
        lateral (amyotrophic) G12.21
        multiple G35
        posterior (syphilitic) A52.11
    stomach K31.89
    subendocardial, congenital I42.4
    systemic M34.9
        with
            lung involvement M34.81
            myopathy M34.82
            polyneuropathy M34.83
        drug-induced M34.2
        due to chemicals NEC M34.2
        progressive M34.0
        specified NEC M34.89
    temporal (mesial) G93.81
    tricuspid (heart) (valve) I07.8
    tuberous (brain) Q85.1
    tympanic membrane —*see* Disorder,
        tympanic membrane, specified NEC
    valve, valvular (heart) —*see* Endocarditis
    vascular —*see* Arteriosclerosis
    vein I87.8
Scoliosis (acquired) (postural) M41.9
    adolescent (idiopathic) —*see* Scoliosis,
        idiopathic, juvenile
    congenital Q67.5
        due to bony malformation Q76.3
        failure of segmentation (hemivertebra)
            Q76.3
        hemivertebra fusion Q76.3
        postural Q67.5
    idiopathic M41.20
        adolescent M41.129
            cervical region M41.122
            cervicothoracic region M41.123
            lumbar region M41.126
            lumbosacral region M41.127
            thoracic region M41.124
            thoracolumbar region M41.125
        cervical region M41.22
        cervicothoracic region M41.23
        infantile M41.00
            cervical region M41.02
            cervicothoracic region M41.03
            lumbar region M41.06

Scoliosis *(Continued)*
  idiopathic *(Continued)*
    infantile *(Continued)*
      lumbosacral region M41.07
      sacrococcygeal region M41.08
      thoracic region M41.04
      thoracolumbar region M41.05
    juvenile M41.119
      cervical region M41.112
      cervicothoracic region M41.113
      lumbar region M41.116
      lumbosacral region M41.117
      thoracic region M41.114
      thoracolumbar region M41.115
    lumbar region M41.26
    lumbosacral region M41.27
    thoracic region M41.24
    thoracolumbar region M41.25
  neuromuscular M41.40
    cervical region M41.42
    cervicothoracic region M41.43
    lumbar region M41.46
    lumbosacral region M41.47
    occipito-atlanto-axial region M41.41
    thoracic region M41.44
    thoracolumbar region M41.45
  paralytic —*see* Scoliosis, neuromuscular
  postradiation therapy M96.5
  rachitic (late effect or sequelae) E64.3
    [M49.80]
    cervical region E64.3 *[M49.82]*
    cervicothoracic region E64.3 *[M49.83]*
    lumbar region E64.3 *[M49.86]*
    lumbosacral region E64.3 *[M49.87]*
    multiple sites E64.3 *[M49.89]*
    occipito-atlanto-axial region E64.3 *[M49.81]*
    sacrococcygeal region E64.3 *[M49.88]*
    thoracic region E64.3 *[M49.84]*
    thoracolumbar region E64.3 *[M49.85]*
  sciatic M54.4-
  secondary (to) NEC M41.50
    cerebral palsy, Friedreich's ataxia,
      poliomyelitis, neuromuscular
      disorders —*see* Scoliosis,
      neuromuscular
    cervical region M41.52
    cervicothoracic region M41.53
    lumbar region M41.56
    lumbosacral region M41.57
    thoracic region M41.54
    thoracolumbar region M41.55
  specified form NEC M41.80
    cervical region M41.82
    cervicothoracic region M41.83
    lumbar region M41.86
    lumbosacral region M41.87
    thoracic region M41.84
    thoracolumbar region M41.85
  thoracogenic M41.30
    thoracic region M41.34
    thoracolumbar region M41.35
  tuberculous A18.01
Scoliotic pelvis
  with disproportion (fetopelvic) O33.0
    causing obstructed labor O65.0
Scorbutus, scorbutic —*see also* Scurvy
  anemia D53.2
Scotoma (arcuate) (Bjerrum) (central) (ring) —
    see also Defect, visual field, localized,
    scotoma
  scintillating H53.19
Scratch —*see* Abrasion
Scratchy throat R09.89
Screening (for) Z13.9
  alcoholism Z13.89
  anemia Z13.0
  anomaly, congenital Z13.89
  antenatal, of mother Z36
  arterial hypertension Z13.6
  arthropod-borne viral disease NEC Z11.59
  bacteriuria, asymptomatic Z13.89

Screening *(Continued)*
  behavioral disorder Z13.89
  brain injury, traumatic Z13.850
  bronchitis, chronic Z13.83
  brucellosis Z11.2
  cardiovascular disorder Z13.6
  cataract Z13.5
  chlamydial diseases Z11.8
  cholera Z11.0
  chromosomal abnormalities (nonprocreative)
    NEC Z13.79
  colonoscopy Z12.11
  congenital
    dislocation of hip Z13.89
    eye disorder Z13.5
    malformation or deformation Z13.89
  contamination NEC Z13.88
  cystic fibrosis Z13.228
  dengue fever Z11.59
  dental disorder Z13.84
  depression Z13.89
  developmental handicap Z13.4
    in early childhood Z13.4
  diabetes mellitus Z13.1
  diphtheria Z11.2
  disability, intellectual Z13.4
  disease or disorder Z13.9
    bacterial NEC Z11.2
      intestinal infectious Z11.0
      respiratory tuberculosis Z11.1
    blood or blood-forming organ Z13.0
    cardiovascular Z13.6
    Chagas' Z11.6
    chlamydial Z11.8
    dental Z13.89
    developmental Z13.4
    digestive tract NEC Z13.818
      lower GI Z13.811
      upper GI Z13.810
    ear Z13.5
    endocrine Z13.29
    eye Z13.5
    genitourinary Z13.89
    heart Z13.6
    human immunodeficiency virus (HIV)
      infection Z11.4
    immunity Z13.0
    infection
      intestinal Z11.0
      specified NEC Z11.6
    infectious Z11.9
    mental Z13.89
    metabolic Z13.228
    neurological Z13.89
    nutritional Z13.21
      metabolic Z13.228
        lipoid disorders Z13.220
    protozoal Z11.6
      intestinal Z11.0
    respiratory Z13.83
    rheumatic Z13.828
    rickettsial Z11.8
    sexually-transmitted NEC Z11.3
      human immunodeficiency virus (HIV)
      Z11.4
    sickle-cell (trait) Z13.0
    skin Z13.89
    specified NEC Z13.89
    spirochetal Z11.8
    thyroid Z13.29
    vascular Z13.6
    venereal Z11.3
    viral NEC Z11.59
      human immunodeficiency virus (HIV)
      Z11.4
      intestinal Z11.0
  elevated titer Z13.89
  emphysema Z13.83
  encephalitis, viral (mosquito- or tick-borne)
    Z11.59
  exposure to contaminants (toxic) Z13.88

Screening *(Continued)*
  fever
    dengue Z11.59
    hemorrhagic Z11.59
    yellow Z11.59
  filariasis Z11.6
  galactosemia Z13.228
  gastrointestinal condition Z13.818
  genetic (nonprocreative)- for procreative
    management —*see* Testing, genetic, for
    procreative management
    disease carrier status (nonprocreative)
      Z13.71
    specified NEC (nonprocreative) Z13.79
  genitourinary condition Z13.89
  glaucoma Z13.5
  gonorrhea Z11.3
  gout Z13.89
  helminthiasis (intestinal) Z11.6
  hematopoietic malignancy Z12.89
  hemoglobinopathies NEC Z13.0
  hemorrhagic fever Z11.59
  Hodgkin disease Z12.89
  human immunodeficiency virus (HIV)
    Z11.4
  human papillomavirus Z11.51
  hypertension Z13.6
  immunity disorders Z13.0
  infection
    mycotic Z11.8
    parasitic Z11.8
  ingestion of radioactive substance Z13.88
  intellectual disability Z13.4
  intestinal
    helminthiasis Z11.6
    infectious disease Z11.0
  leishmaniasis Z11.6
  leprosy Z11.2
  leptospirosis Z11.8
  leukemia Z12.89
  lymphoma Z12.89
  malaria Z11.6
  malnutrition Z13.29
    metabolic Z13.228
    nutritional Z13.21
  measles Z11.59
  mental disorder Z13.89
  metabolic errors, inborn Z13.228
  multiphasic Z13.89
  musculoskeletal disorder Z13.828
    osteoporosis Z13.820
  mycoses Z11.8
  myocardial infarction (acute) Z13.6
  neoplasm (malignant) (of) Z12.9
    bladder Z12.6
    blood Z12.89
    breast Z12.39
      routine mammogram Z12.31
    cervix Z12.4
    colon Z12.11
    genitourinary organs NEC Z12.79
      bladder Z12.6
      cervix Z12.4
      ovary Z12.73
      prostate Z12.5
      testis Z12.71
      vagina Z12.72
    hematopoietic system Z12.89
    intestinal tract Z12.10
      colon Z12.11
      rectum Z12.12
      small intestine Z12.13
    lung Z12.2
    lymph (glands) Z12.89
    nervous system Z12.82
    oral cavity Z12.81
    prostate Z12.5
    rectum Z12.12
    respiratory organs Z12.2
    skin Z12.83
    small intestine Z12.13

◀ New   ◀▥ Revised   ~~deleted~~ Deleted

Screening *(Continued)*
  neoplasm *(Continued)*
    specified site NEC Z12.89
    stomach Z12.0
  nephropathy Z13.89
  nervous system disorders NEC Z13.858
  neurological condition Z13.89
  osteoporosis Z13.820
  parasitic infestation Z11.9
    specified NEC Z11.8
  phenylketonuria Z13.228
  plague Z11.2
  poisoning (chemical) (heavy metal) Z13.88
  poliomyelitis Z11.59
  postnatal, chromosomal abnormalities Z13.89
  prenatal, of mother Z36
  protozoal disease Z11.6
    intestinal Z11.0
  pulmonary tuberculosis Z11.1
  radiation exposure Z13.88
  respiratory condition Z13.83
  respiratory tuberculosis Z11.1
  rheumatoid arthritis Z13.828
  rubella Z11.59
  schistosomiasis Z11.6
  sexually-transmitted disease NEC Z11.3
    human immunodeficiency virus (HIV) Z11.4
  sickle-cell disease or trait Z13.0
  skin condition Z13.89
  sleeping sickness Z11.6
  special Z13.9
    specified NEC Z13.89
  syphilis Z11.3
  tetanus Z11.2
  trachoma Z11.8
  traumatic brain injury Z13.850
  trypanosomiasis Z11.6
  tuberculosis, respiratory Z11.1
  venereal disease Z11.3
  viral encephalitis (mosquito- or tick-borne) Z11.59
  whooping cough Z11.2
  worms, intestinal Z11.6
  yaws Z11.8
  yellow fever Z11.59
Scrofula, scrofulosis (tuberculosis of cervical lymph glands) A18.2
Scrofulide (primary) (tuberculous) A18.4
Scrofuloderma, scrofulodermia (any site) (primary) A18.4
Scrofulosus lichen (primary) (tuberculous) A18.4
Scrofulous —*see* condition
Scrotal tongue K14.5
Scrotum —*see* condition
Scurvy, scorbutic E54
  anemia D53.2
  gum E54
  infantile E54
  rickets E55.0 [M90.80]
Sealpox B08.62
Seasickness T75.3
Seatworm (infection) (infestation) B80
Sebaceous —*see also* condition
  cyst —*see* Cyst, sebaceous
Seborrhea, seborrheic L21.9
  capillitii R23.8
  capitis L21.0
  dermatitis L21.9
    infantile L21.1
  eczema L21.9
    infantile L21.1
  sicca L21.0
Seckel's syndrome Q87.1
Seclusion, pupil —*see* Membrane, pupillary
Second hand tobacco smoke exposure (acute) (chronic) Z77.22
  in the perinatal period P96.81

Secondary
  dentin (in pulp) K04.3
  neoplasm, secondaries —*see* Table of Neoplasms, secondary
Secretion
  antidiuretic hormone, inappropriate E22.2
  catecholamine, by pheochromocytoma E27.5
  hormone
    antidiuretic, inappropriate (syndrome) E22.2
    by
      carcinoid tumor E34.0
      pheochromocytoma E27.5
    ectopic NEC E34.2
  urinary
    excessive R35.8
    suppression R34
Section
  nerve, traumatic —*see* Injury, nerve
Segmentation, incomplete (congenital) —*see also* Fusion
  bone NEC Q78.8
  lumbosacral (joint) (vertebra) Q76.49
Seitelberger's syndrome (infantile neuraxonal dystrophy) G31.89
Seizure (s) (*see also* Convulsions) R56.9
  akinetic —*see* Epilepsy, generalized, specified NEC
  atonic —*see* Epilepsy, generalized, specified NEC
  autonomic (hysterical) F44.5
  convulsive —*see* Convulsions
  cortical (focal) (motor) —*see* Epilepsy, localization-related, symptomatic, with simple partial seizures
  disorder (*see also* Epilepsy) G40.909
  due to stroke —*see* Sequelae (of), disease, cerebrovascular, by type, specified NEC
  epileptic —*see* Epilepsy
  febrile (simple) R56.00
    with status epilepticus G40.901
    complex (atypical) (complicated) R56.01
      with status epilepticus G40.901
  grand mal G40.409
    intractable G40.419
      with status epilepticus G40.411
      without status epilepticus G40.419
    not intractable G40.409
      with status epilepticus G40.401
      without status epilepticus G40.409
  heart —*see* Disease, heart
  hysterical F44.5
  intractable G40.919
    with status epilepticus G40.911
  Jacksonian (focal) (motor type) (sensory type) —*see* Epilepsy, localization-related, symptomatic, with simple partial seizures
  newborn P90
  nonspecific epileptic
    atonic —*see* Epilepsy, generalized, specified NEC
    clonic —*see* Epilepsy, generalized, specified NEC
    myoclonic —*see* Epilepsy, generalized, specified NEC
    tonic —*see* Epilepsy, generalized, specified NEC
    tonic-clonic —*see* Epilepsy, generalized, specified NEC
  partial, developing into secondarily generalized seizures
    complex —*see* Epilepsy, localization-related, symptomatic, with complex partial seizures
    simple —*see* Epilepsy, localization-related, symptomatic, with simple partial seizures

Seizure *(Continued)*
  petit mal G40.409
    intractable G40.419
      with status epilepticus G40.411
      without status epilepticus G40.419
    not intractable G40.409
      with status epilepticus G40.401
      without status epilepticus G40.409
  post traumatic R56.1
  recurrent G40.909
  specified NEC G40.89
  uncinate —*see* Epilepsy, localization-related, symptomatic, with complex partial seizures
Selenium deficiency, dietary E59
Self-damaging behavior (life-style) Z72.89
Self-harm (attempted)
  history (personal) Z91.5
    in family Z81.8
Self-mutilation (attempted)
  history (personal) Z91.5
    in family Z81.8
Self-poisoning
  history (personal) Z91.5
    in family Z81.8
  observation following (alleged) attempt Z03.6
Semicoma R40.1
Seminal vesiculitis N49.0
Seminoma C62.9-
  specified site —*see* Neoplasm, malignant, by site
Senear-Usher disease or syndrome L10.4
Senectus R54
Senescence (without mention of psychosis) R54
Senile, senility (*see also* condition) R41.81
  with
    acute confusional state F05
    mental changes NOS F03
    psychosis NEC —*see* Psychosis, senile
  asthenia R54
  cervix (atrophic) N88.8
  debility R54
  endometrium (atrophic) N85.8
  fallopian tube (atrophic) —*see* Atrophy, fallopian tube
  heart (failure) R54
  ovary (atrophic) —*see* Atrophy, ovary
  premature E34.8
  vagina, vaginitis (atrophic) N95.2
  wart L82.1
Sensation
  burning (skin) R20.8
    tongue K14.6
  loss of R20.8
  prickling (skin) R20.2
  tingling (skin) R20.2
Sense loss
  smell —*see* Disturbance, sensation, smell
  taste —*see* Disturbance, sensation, taste
  touch R20.8
Sensibility disturbance (cortical) (deep) (vibratory) R20.9
Sensitive, sensitivity —*see also* Allergy
  carotid sinus G90.01
  child (excessive) F93.8
  cold, autoimmune D59.1
  dentin K03.89
  latex Z91.040
  methemoglobin D74.8
  tuberculin, without clinical or radiological symptoms R76.11
  visual
    glare H53.71
    impaired contrast H53.72
Sensitiver Beziehungswahn F22
Sensitization, auto-erythrocytic D69.2
Separation
  anxiety, abnormal (of childhood) F93.0
  apophysis, traumatic - code as Fracture, by site
  choroid —*see* Detachment, choroid

Separation (Continued)
epiphysis, epiphyseal
nontraumatic —see also
Osteochondropathy, specified type
NEC
upper femoral —see Slipped, epiphysis,
upper femoral
traumatic - code as Fracture, by site
fracture —see Fracture
infundibulum cardiac from right ventricle by
a partition Q24.3
joint (traumatic) (current) - code by site under
Dislocation
pubic bone, obstetrical trauma O71.6
retina, retinal —see Detachment, retina
symphysis pubis, obstetrical trauma O71.6
tracheal ring, incomplete, congenital Q32.1
Sepsis (generalized) (unspecified organism)
A41.9
with
organ dysfunction (acute) (multiple) R65.20
with septic shock R65.21
actinomycotic A42.7
adrenal hemorrhage syndrome
(meningococcal) A39.1
anaerobic A41.4
Bacillus anthracis A22.7
Brucella (see also Brucellosis) A23.9
candidal B37.7
cryptogenic A41.9
due to device, implant or graft T85.79
arterial graft NEC T82.7
breast (implant) T85.79
catheter NEC T85.79
dialysis (renal) T82.7
intraperitoneal T85.71
infusion NEC T82.7
spinal (epidural) (subdural) T85.79
urinary (indwelling) T83.51
ectopic or molar pregnancy O08.82
electronic (electrode) (pulse generator)
(stimulator)
bone T84.7
cardiac T82.7
nervous system (brain) (peripheral
nerve) (spinal) T85.79
urinary T83.59
fixation, internal (orthopedic) —see
Complication, fixation device,
infection
gastrointestinal (bile duct) (esophagus)
T85.79
genital T83.6
heart NEC T82.7
valve (prosthesis) T82.6
graft T82.7
joint prosthesis —see Complication, joint
prosthesis, infection
ocular (corneal graft) (orbital implant)
T85.79
orthopedic NEC T84.7
fixation device, internal —see
Complication, fixation device,
infection
specified NEC T85.79
vascular T82.7
ventricular intracranial shunt T85.79
during labor O75.3
Enterococcus A41.81
Erysipelothrix (rhusiopathiae) (erysipeloid)
A26.7
Escherichia coli (E. coli) A41.5
extraintestinal yersiniosis A28.2
following
abortion (subsequent episode) O08.0
current episode —see Abortion
ectopic or molar pregnancy O08.82
immunization T88.0
infusion, therapeutic injection or
transfusion NEC T80.29
gangrenous A41.9

Sepsis (Continued)
gonococcal A54.86
Gram-negative (organism) A41.5
anaerobic A41.4
Haemophilus influenzae A41.3
herpesviral B00.7
intra-abdominal K65.1
intraocular —see Endophthalmitis, purulent
Listeria monocytogenes A32.7
localized — code to specific localized
infection
in operation wound T81.4
skin —see Abscess
malleus A24.0
melioidosis A24.1
meningeal —see Meningitis
meningococcal A39.4
acute A39.2
chronic A39.3
MSSA (Methicillin susceptible
Staphylococcus aureus) A41.01
newborn P36.9
due to
anaerobes NEC P36.5
Escherichia coli P36.4
Staphylococcus P36.30
aureus P36.2
specified NEC P36.39
Streptococcus P36.10
group B P36.0
specified NEC P36.19
specified NEC P36.8
Pasteurella multocida A28.0
pelvic, puerperal, postpartum, childbirth O85
pneumococcal A40.3
postprocedural T81.4
puerperal, postpartum, childbirth (pelvic)
O85
Salmonella (arizonae) (cholerae-suis)
(enteritidis) (typhimurium) A02.1
severe R65.20
with septic shock R65.21
Shigella (see also Dysentery, bacillary) A03.9
skin, localized —see Abscess
specified organism NEC A41.89
Staphylococcus, staphylococcal A41.2
aureus (methicillin susceptible) (MSSA)
A41.01
methicillin resistant (MRSA) A41.02
coagulase-negative A41.1
specified NEC A41.1
Streptococcus, streptococcal A40.9
agalactiae A40.1
group
A A40.0
B A40.1
D A41.81
neonatal P36.10
group B P36.0
specified NEC P36.19
pneumoniae A40.3
pyogenes A40.0
specified NEC A40.8
tracheostomy stoma J95.02
tularemic A21.7
umbilical, umbilical cord (newborn) —see
Sepsis, newborn
Yersinia pestis A20.7
Septate —see Septum
Septic —see condition
arm —see Cellulitis, upper limb
with lymphangitis —see Lymphangitis,
acute, upper limb
embolus —see Embolism
finger —see Cellulitis, digit
with lymphangitis —see Lymphangitis,
acute, digit
foot —see Cellulitis, lower limb
with lymphangitis —see Lymphangitis,
acute, lower limb
gallbladder (acute) K81.0

Septic (Continued)
hand —see Cellulitis, upper limb
with lymphangitis —see Lymphangitis,
acute, upper limb
joint —see Arthritis, pyogenic or pyemic
leg —see Cellulitis, lower limb
with lymphangitis —see Lymphangitis,
acute, lower limb
nail —see also Cellulitis, digit
with lymphangitis —see Lymphangitis,
acute, digit
sore —see also Abscess
throat J02.0
streptococcal J02.0
spleen (acute) D73.89
teeth, tooth (pulpal origin) K04.4
throat —see Pharyngitis
thrombus —see Thrombosis
toe —see Cellulitis, digit
with lymphangitis —see Lymphangitis,
acute, digit
tonsils, chronic J35.01
with adenoiditis J35.03
uterus —see Endometritis
Septicemia A41.9
meaning sepsis —see Sepsis
Septum, septate (congenital) —see also
Anomaly, by site
anal Q42.3
with fistula Q42.2
aqueduct of Sylvius Q03.0
with spina bifida —see Spina bifida, by site,
with hydrocephalus
uterus (complete) (partial) Q51.2
vagina Q52.10
in pregnancy —see Pregnancy, complicated
by, abnormal vagina
causing obstructed labor O65.5
longitudinal (with or without obstruction)
Q52.12
transverse Q52.11
Sequelae (of) —see also condition
abscess, intracranial or intraspinal (conditions
in G06) G09
amputation — code to injury with seventh
character S
burn and corrosion — code to injury with
seventh character S
calcium deficiency E64.8
cerebrovascular disease —see Sequelae,
disease, cerebrovascular
childbirth O94
contusion — code to injury with seventh
character S
corrosion —see Sequelae, burn and
corrosion
crushing injury — code to injury with
seventh character S
disease
cerebrovascular I69.90
alteration of sensation I69.998
aphasia I69.920
apraxia I69.990
ataxia I69.993
cognitive deficits I69.91
disturbance of vision I69.998
dysarthria I69.922
dysphagia I69.991
dysphasia I69.921
facial droop I69.992
facial weakness I69.992
fluency disorder I69.923
hemiplegia I69.95-
hemorrhage
intracerebral —see Sequelae,
hemorrhage, intracerebral
intracranial, nontraumatic NEC —
see Sequelae, hemorrhage,
intracranial, nontraumatic
subarachnoid —see Sequelae,
hemorrhage, subarachnoid

◀ New ◀▥ Revised ~~deleted~~ Deleted

Sequelae *(Continued)*
  disease *(Continued)*
    cerebrovascular *(Continued)*
      language deficit I69.928
      monoplegia
        lower limb I69.84-
        upper limb I69.93-
      paralytic syndrome I69.96-
      specified effect NEC I69.998
      specified type NEC I69.80
        alteration of sensation I69.898
        aphasia I69.820
        apraxia I69.890
        ataxia I69.893
        cognitive deficits I69.81
        disturbance of vision I69.898
        dysarthria I69.822
        dysphagia I69.891
        dysphasia I69.821
        facial droop I69.892
        facial weakness I69.892
        fluency disorder I69.823
        hemiplegia I69.85-
        language deficit I69.828
        monoplegia
          lower limb I69.84-
          upper limb I69.83-
        paralytic syndrome I69.86-
        specified effect NEC I69.898
      speech deficit I69.928
        speech deficit I69.828
      stroke NOS —*see* Sequelae, stroke
        NOS
  dislocation — code to injury with seventh
    character S
  encephalitis or encephalomyelitis (conditions
    in G04) G09
    in infectious disease NEC B94.8
    viral B94.1
  external cause — code to injury with seventh
    character S
  foreign body entering natural orifice — code
    to injury with seventh character S
  fracture — code to injury with seventh
    character S
  frostbite — code to injury with seventh
    character S
  Hansen's disease B92
  hemorrhage
    intracerebral I69.10
      alteration of sensation I69.198
      aphasia I69.120
      apraxia I69.190
      ataxia I69.193
      cognitive deficits I69.11
      disturbance of vision I69.198
      dysarthria I69.122
      dysphagia I69.191
      dysphasia I69.121
      facial droop I69.192
      facial weakness I69.192
      fluency disorder I69.123
      hemiplegia I69.15-
      language deficit NEC I69.128
      monoplegia
        lower limb I69.14-
        upper limb I69.13-
      paralytic syndrome I69.16-
      specified effect NEC I69.198
      speech deficit NEC I69.128
    intracranial, nontraumatic NEC I69.20
      alteration of sensation I69.298
      aphasia I69.220
      apraxia I69.290
      ataxia I69.293
      cognitive deficits I69.21
      disturbance of vision I69.298
      dysarthria I69.222
      dysphagia I69.291
      dysphasia I69.221
      facial droop I69.292

Sequelae *(Continued)*
  hemorrhage *(Continued)*
    intracranial, nontraumatic NEC
      (Continued)
      facial weakness I69.292
      fluency disorder I69.223
      hemiplegia I69.25-
      language deficit NEC I69.228
      monoplegia
        lower limb I69.24-
        upper limb I69.23-
      paralytic syndrome I69.26-
      specified effect NEC I69.298
      speech deficit NEC I69.228
    subarachnoid I69.00
      alteration of sensation I69.098
      aphasia I69.020
      apraxia I69.090
      ataxia I69.093
      cognitive deficits I69.01
      disturbance of vision I69.098
      dysarthria I69.022
      dysphagia I69.091
      dysphasia I69.021
      facial droop I69.092
      facial weakness I69.092
      fluency disorder I69.023
      hemiplegia I69.05-
      language deficit NEC I69.028
      monoplegia
        lower limb I69.04-
        upper limb I69.03-
      paralytic syndrome I69.06-
      specified effect NEC I69.098
      speech deficit NEC I69.028
  hepatitis, viral B94.2
  hyperalimentation E68
  infarction
    cerebral I69.30
      alteration of sensation I69.398
      aphasia I69.320
      apraxia I69.390
      ataxia I69.393
      cognitive deficits I69.31
      disturbance of vision I69.398
      dysarthria I69.322
      dysphagia I69.391
      dysphasia I69.321
      facial droop I69.392
      facial weakness I69.392
      fluency disorder I69.323
      hemiplegia I69.35-
      language deficit NEC I69.328
      monoplegia
        lower limb I69.34-
        upper limb I69.33-
      paralytic syndrome I69.36-
      specified effect NEC I69.398
      speech deficit NEC I69.328
  infection, pyogenic, intracranial or intraspinal
    G09
  infectious disease B94.9
    specified NEC B94.8
  injury — code to injury with seventh
    character S
  leprosy B92
  meningitis
    bacterial (conditions in G00) G09
    other or unspecified cause (conditions in
      G03) G09
  muscle (and tendon) injury — code to injury
    with seventh character S
  myelitis —*see* Sequelae, encephalitis
  niacin deficiency E64.8
  nutritional deficiency E64.9
    specified NEC E64.8
  obstetrical condition O94
  parasitic disease B94.9
  phlebitis or thrombophlebitis of intracranial
    or intraspinal venous sinuses and veins
    (conditions in G08) G09

Sequelae *(Continued)*
  poisoning — code to poisoning with seventh
    character S
    nonmedicinal substance —*see* Sequelae,
      toxic effect, nonmedicinal substance
  poliomyelitis (acute) B91
  pregnancy O94
  protein-energy malnutrition E64.0
  puerperium O94
  rickets E64.3
  selenium deficiency E64.8
  sprain and strain — code to injury with
    seventh character S
  stroke NOS I69.30
    alteration in sensation I69.398
    aphasia I69.320
    apraxia I69.390
    ataxia I69.393
    cognitive deficits I69.31
    disturbance of vision I69.398
    dysarthria I69.322
    dysphagia I69.391
    dysphasia I69.321
    facial droop I69.392
    facial weakness I69.392
    hemiplegia I69.35-
    language deficit NEC I69.328
    monoplegia
      lower limb I69.34-
      upper limb I69.33-
    paralytic syndrome I69.36-
    specified effect NEC I69.398
    speech deficit NEC I69.328
  tendon and muscle injury — code to injury
    with seventh character S
  thiamine deficiency E64.8
  trachoma B94.0
  tuberculosis B90.9
    bones and joints B90.2
    central nervous system B90.0
    genitourinary B90.1
    pulmonary (respiratory) B90.9
    specified organs NEC B90.8
  viral
    encephalitis B94.1
    hepatitis B94.2
  vitamin deficiency NEC E64.8
    A E64.1
    B E64.8
    C E64.2
  wound, open — code to injury with seventh
    character S
Sequestration —*see also* Sequestrum
  lung, congenital Q33.2
Sequestrum
  bone —*see* Osteomyelitis, chronic
  dental M27.2
  jaw bone M27.2
  orbit —*see* Osteomyelitis, orbit
  sinus (accessory) (nasal) —*see* Sinusitis
Sequoiosis lung or pneumonitis J67.8
Serology for syphilis
  doubtful
    with signs or symptoms - code by site and
      stage under Syphilis
    follow-up of latent syphilis —*see* Syphilis,
      latent
    negative, with signs or symptoms — code by
      site and stage under Syphilis
  positive A53.0
    with signs or symptoms - code by site and
      stage under Syphilis
  reactivated A53.0
Seroma —*see also* Hematoma
  traumatic, secondary and recurrent
    T79.2
Seropurulent —*see* condition
Serositis, multiple K65.8
  pericardial I31.1
  peritoneal K65.8
Serous —*see* condition

◀ New ◀||| Revised ~~deleted~~ Deleted

Short, shortening, shortness *(Continued)*
common bile duct, congenital Q44.5
cord (umbilical), complicating delivery O69.3
cystic duct, congenital Q44.5
esophagus (congenital) Q39.8
femur (acquired) —*see* Deformity, limb,
    unequal length, femur
    congenital —*see* Defect, reduction, lower
      limb, longitudinal, femur
frenum, frenulum, linguae (congenital) Q38.1
hip (acquired) —*see also* Deformity, limb,
    unequal length
    congenital Q65.89
leg (acquired) —*see also* Deformity, limb,
    unequal length
    congenital Q72.81-
    lower leg —*see also* Deformity, limb,
      unequal length
limbed stature, with immunodeficiency D82.2
lower limb (acquired) —*see also* Deformity,
    limb, unequal length
    congenital Q72.81-
organ or site, congenital NEC —*see* Distortion
palate, congenital Q38.5
radius (acquired) —*see also* Deformity, limb,
    unequal length
    congenital —*see* Defect, reduction, upper
      limb, longitudinal, radius
rib syndrome Q77.2
stature (child) (hereditary) (idiopathic) NEC
    R62.52
    constitutional E34.3
    due to endocrine disorder E34.3
    Laron-type E34.3
tendon —*see also* Contraction, tendon
    with contracture of joint —*see* Contraction,
      joint
    Achilles (acquired) M67.0-
      congenital Q66.89
    congenital Q79.8
thigh (acquired) —*see also* Deformity, limb,
    unequal length, femur
    congenital —*see* Defect, reduction, lower
      limb, longitudinal, femur
tibialis anterior (tendon) —*see* Contraction,
    tendon
umbilical cord
    complicating delivery O69.3
upper limb, congenital —*see* Defect,
    reduction, upper limb, specified type
    NEC
urethra N36.8
uvula, congenital Q38.5
vagina (congenital) Q52.4
Shortsightedness —*see* Myopia
Shoshin (acute fulminating beriberi) E51.11
Shoulder —*see* condition
Shovel-shaped incisors K00.2
Shower, thromboembolic —*see* Embolism
Shunt
arterial-venous (dialysis) Z99.2
arteriovenous, pulmonary (acquired) I28.0
    congenital Q25.72
cerebral ventricle (communicating) in situ
    Z98.2
surgical, prosthetic, with complications —*see*
    Complications, cardiovascular, device
    or implant Shutdown, renal N28.9
Shutdown, renal N28.9
Shy-Drager syndrome G90.3
Sialadenitis, sialadenosis (any gland) (chronic)
    (periodic) (suppurative) —*see* Sialoadenitis
Sialectasia K11.8
Sialidosis E77.1
Sialitis, silitis (any gland) (chronic)
    (suppurative) —*see* Sialoadenitis
Sialoadenitis (any gland) (periodic)
    (suppurative) K11.20
acute K11.21
    recurrent K11.22
chronic K11.23

Sialoadenopathy K11.9
Sialoangitis —*see* Sialoadenitis
Sialodochitis (fibrinosa) —*see* Sialoadenitis
Sialodocholithiasis K11.5
Sialolithiasis K11.5
Sialometaplasia, necrotizing K11.8
Sialorrhea —*see also* Ptyalism
periodic —*see* Sialoadenitis
Sialosis K11.7
Siamese twin Q89.4
Sibling rivalry Z62.891
Sicard's syndrome G52.7
Sicca syndrome M35.00
with
    keratoconjunctivitis M35.01
    lung involvement M35.02
    myopathy M35.03
    renal tubulo-interstitial disorders M35.04
    specified organ involvement NEC M35.09
Sick R69
or handicapped person in family Z63.79
    needing care at home Z63.6
sinus (syndrome) I49.5
Sick-euthyroid syndrome E07.81
Sickle-cell
anemia —*see* Disease, sickle-cell
trait D57.3
Sicklemia —*see also* Disease, sickle-cell
trait D57.3
Sickness
air (travel) T75.3
airplane T75.3
alpine T70.29
altitude T70.20
Andes T70.29
aviator's T70.29
balloon T70.29
car T75.3
compressed air T70.3
decompression T70.3
green D50.8
milk —*see* Poisoning, food, noxious
motion T75.3
mountain T70.29
    acute D75.1
protein (*see also* Reaction, serum) T80.69
radiation T66
roundabout (motion) T75.3
sea T75.3
serum NEC (*see also* Reaction, serum) T80.69
sleeping (African) B56.9
    by Trypanosoma B56.9
      brucei
        gambiense B56.0
        rhodesiense B56.1
    East African B56.1
    Gambian B56.0
    Rhodesian B56.1
    West African B56.0
swing (motion) T75.3
train (railway) (travel) T75.3
travel (any vehicle) T75.3
Sideropenia —*see* Anemia, iron deficiency
Siderosilicosis J62.8
Siderosis (lung) J63.4
eye (globe) —*see* Disorder, globe,
    degenerative, siderosis
Siemens' syndrome (ectodermal dysplasia) Q82.8
Sighing R06.89
psychogenic F45.8
Sigmoid —*see also* condition
flexure —*see* condition
kidney Q63.1
Sigmoiditis (*see also* Enteritis) K52.9
infectious A09
noninfectious K52.9
Silfversköld's syndrome Q78.9
Silicosiderosis J62.8
Silicosis, silicotic (simple) (complicated) J62.8
with tuberculosis J65
Silicotuberculosis J65

Silo-fillers' disease J68.8
bronchitis J68.0
pneumonitis J68.0
pulmonary edema J68.1
Silver's syndrome Q87.1
Simian malaria B53.1
Simmonds' cachexia or disease E23.0
Simons' disease or syndrome (progressive
    lipodystrophy) E88.1
Simple, simplex —*see* condition
Simulation, conscious (of illness) Z76.5
Simultanagnosia (asimultagnosia) R48.3
Sin Nombre virus disease (Hantavirus)
    (cardio)-pulmonary syndrome) B33.4
Sinding-Larsen disease or osteochondrosis —
    see Osteochondrosis, juvenile, patella
Singapore hemorrhagic fever A91
Singer's node or nodule J38.2
Single
atrium Q21.2
coronary artery Q24.5
umbilical artery Q27.0
ventricle Q20.4
Singultus R06.6
epidemicus B33.0
Sinus —*see also* Fistula
abdominal K63.89
arrest I45.5
arrhythmia I49.8
bradycardia R00.1
branchial cleft (internal) (external) Q18.0
coccygeal —*see* Sinus, pilonidal
dental K04.6
dermal (congenital) Q06.8
    with abscess Q06.8
    coccygeal, pilonidal —*see* Sinus,
      coccygeal
infected, skin NEC L08.89
marginal, ruptured or bleeding —*see*
    Hemorrhage, antepartum, specified
    cause NEC
medial, face and neck Q18.8
pause I45.5
pericranii Q01.9
pilonidal (infected) (rectum) L05.92
    with abscess L05.02
preauricular Q18.1
rectovaginal N82.3
Rokitansky-Aschoff (gallbladder) K82.8
sacrococcygeal (dermoid) (infected) —*see*
    Sinus, pilonidal
tachycardia R00.0
    paroxysmal I47.1
tarsi syndrome M25.57-
testis N50.8
tract (postinfective) —*see* Fistula
urachus Q64.4
Sinusitis (accessory) (chronic) (hyperplastic)
    (nasal) (nonpurulent) (purulent) J32.9
acute J01.90
    ethmoidal J01.20
      recurrent J01.21
    frontal J01.10
      recurrent J01.11
    involving more than one sinus, other than
      pansinusitis J01.80
      recurrent J01.81
    maxillary J01.00
      recurrent J01.01
    pansinusitis J01.40
      recurrent J01.41
    recurrent J01.91
    specified NEC J01.80
      recurrent J01.81
    sphenoidal J01.30
      recurrent J01.31
allergic —*see* Rhinitis, allergic
due to high altitude T70.1
ethmoidal J32.2
    acute J01.20
      recurrent J01.21

Sinusitis (Continued)
  frontal J32.1
    acute J01.10
      recurrent J01.11
  influenzal —see Influenza, with, respiratory
    manifestations NEC
  involving more than one sinus but not
    pansinusitis J32.8
    acute J01.80
      recurrent J01.81
  maxillary J32.0
    acute J01.00
      recurrent J01.01
  sphenoidal J32.3
    acute J01.30
      recurrent J01.31
  tuberculous, any sinus A15.8
Sinusitis-bronchiectasis-situs inversus
  (syndrome) (triad) Q89.3
Sipple's syndrome E31.22
Sirenomelia (syndrome) Q87.2
Siriasis T67.0
Sirkari's disease B55.0
Siti A65
Situation, psychiatric F99
Situational
  disturbance (transient) —see Disorder,
    adjustment
    acute F43.0
  maladjustment —see Disorder, adjustment
  reaction —see Disorder, adjustment
    acute F43.0
Situs inversus or transversus (abdominalis)
  (thoracis) Q89.3
Sixth disease B08.20
  due to human herpesvirus 6 B08.21
  due to human herpesvirus 7 B08.22
Sjögren-Larsson syndrome Q87.1
Sjögren's syndrome or disease —see Sicca
  syndrome
Skeletal —see condition
Skene's gland —see condition
Skenitis —see Urethritis
Skerljevo A65
Skevas-Zerfus disease —see Toxicity, venom,
  marine animal, sea anemone
Skin —see also condition
  clammy R23.1
  donor —see Donor, skin
  hidebound M35.9
Slate-dressers' or slate-miners' lung J62.8
Sleep
  apnea —see Apnea, sleep
  deprivation Z72.820
  disorder or disturbance G47.9
    child F51.9
    nonorganic origin F51.9
    specified NEC G47.8
  disturbance G47.9
    nonorganic origin F51.9
  drunkenness F51.9
  rhythm inversion G47.2-
  terrors F51.4
  walking F51.3
    hysterical F44.89
Sleep hygiene
  abuse Z72.821
  inadequate Z72.821
  poor Z72.821
Sleeping sickness —see Sickness, sleeping
Sleeplessness —see Insomnia
  menopausal N95.11
Sleep-wake schedule disorder G47.20
Slim disease (in HIV infection) B20
Slipped, slipping
  epiphysis (traumatic) —see also
    Osteochondropathy, specified type
    NEC
    capital femoral (traumatic)
      acute (on chronic) S79.01-
      current traumatic - code as Fracture, by site

Slipped, slipping (Continued)
  epiphysis (Continued)
    upper femoral (nontraumatic) M93.00-
      acute M93.01-
        on chronic M93.03-
      chronic M93.02-
  intervertebral disc —see Displacement,
    intervertebral disc
  ligature, umbilical P51.8
  patella —see Disorder, patella, derangement
    NEC
  rib M89.8X8
  sacroiliac joint —see subcategory M53.2
  tendon —see Disorder, tendon
  ulnar nerve, nontraumatic —see Lesion,
    nerve, ulnar
  vertebra NEC —see Spondylolisthesis
Slocumb's syndrome E27.0
Sloughing (multiple) (phagedena) (skin) —see
  also Gangrene
  abscess —see Abscess
  appendix K38.8
  fascia —see Disorder, soft tissue, specified
    type NEC
  scrotum N50.8
  tendon —see Disorder, tendon
  transplanted organ —see Rejection, transplant
  ulcer —see Ulcer, skin
Slow
  feeding, newborn P92.2
  flow syndrome, coronary I20.8
  heart(beat) R00.1
Slowing, urinary stream R39.19
Sluder's neuralgia (syndrome) G44.89
Slurred, slurring speech R47.81
Small (ness)
  for gestational age —see Small for dates
  introitus, vagina N89.6
  kidney (unknown cause) N27.9
    bilateral N27.1
    unilateral N27.0
  ovary (congenital) Q50.39
  pelvis
    with disproportion (fetopelvic) O33.1
      causing obstructed labor O65.1
  uterus N85.8
  white kidney N03.9
Small-and-light-for-dates —see Small for
  dates
Small-for-dates (infant) P05.10
  with weight of
    499 grams or less P05.11
    500-749 grams P05.12
    750-999 grams P05.13
    1000-1249 grams P05.14
    1250-1499 grams P05.15
    1500-1749 grams P05.16
    1750-1999 grams P05.17
    2000-2499 grams P05.18
Smallpox B03
Smearing, fecal R15.1
Smith-Lemli-Opitz syndrome E78.72
Smith's fracture S52.54-
Smoker —see Dependence, drug, nicotine
Smoker's
  bronchitis J41.0
  cough J41.0
  palate K13.24
  throat J31.2
  tongue K13.24
Smoking
  passive Z77.22
Smothering spells R06.81
Snaggle teeth, tooth M26.39
Snapping
  finger —see Trigger finger
  hip —see Derangement, joint, specified type
    NEC, hip
    involving the iliotiblial band M76.3-
  knee —see Derangement, knee
    involving the iliotiblial band M76.3-

**Sneddon-Wilkinson disease or syndrome (sub-
  corneal pustular dermatosis)** L13.1
Sneezing (intractable) R06.7
Sniffing
  cocaine
    abuse —see Abuse, drug, cocaine
    dependence —see Dependence, drug,
      cocaine
  gasoline
    abuse —see Abuse, drug, inhalant
    dependence —see Dependence, drug,
      inhalant
  glue (airplane)
    abuse —see Abuse, drug, inhalant
    drug dependence —see Dependence, drug,
      inhalant
Sniffles
  newborn P28.89
Snoring R06.83
Snow blindness —see Photokeratitis
Snuffles (non-syphilitic) R06.5
  newborn P28.89
  syphilitic (infant) A50.05 [J99]
Social
  exclusion Z60.4
    due to discrimination or persecution
      (perceived) Z60.5
  migrant Z59.0
    acculturation difficulty Z60.3
  rejection Z60.4
    due to discrimination or persecution
      Z60.5
  role conflict NEC Z73.5
  skills inadequacy NEC Z73.4
  transplantation Z60.3
Sodoku A25.0
Soemmerring's ring —see Cataract, secondary
Soft —see also condition
  nails L60.3
Softening
  bone —see Osteomalacia
  brain (necrotic) (progressive) G93.89
    congenital Q04.8
    embolic I63.4
    hemorrhagic —see Hemorrhage,
      intracranial, intracerebral
    occlusive I63.5
    thrombotic I63.3
  cartilage M94.2-
    patella M22.4-
  cerebellar —see Softening, brain
  cerebral —see Softening, brain
  cerebrospinal —see Softening, brain
  myocardial, heart —see Degeneration,
    myocardial
  spinal cord G95.89
  stomach K31.89
Soldier's
  heart F45.8
  patches I31.0
Solitary
  cyst, kidney N28.1
  kidney, congenital Q60.0
Solvent abuse —see Abuse, drug, inhalant
  dependence —see Dependence, drug,
    inhalant
Somatization reaction, somatic reaction —see
  Disorder, somatoform
Somnambulism F51.3
  hysterical F44.89
Somnolence R40.0
  nonorganic origin F51.11
Sonne dysentery A03.3
Soor B37.0
Sore
  bed —see Ulcer, pressure, by site
  chiclero B55.1
  Delhi B55.1
  desert —see Ulcer, skin
  eye H57.1-
  Lahore B55.1

◀ New   ◀▥ Revised   ~~deleted~~ Deleted

Sore (Continued)
  mouth K13.79
    canker K12.0
  muscle M79.1
  Naga —see Ulcer, skin
  of skin —see Ulcer, skin - oriental B55.1
  pressure —see Ulcer, pressure, by site
  skin L98.9
  soft A57
  throat (acute) —see also Pharyngitis
    with influenza, flu, or grippe —see
        Influenza, with, respiratory
        manifestations NEC
    chronic J31.2
    coxsackie (virus) B08.5
    diphtheritic A36.0
    herpesviral B00.2
    influenzal —see Influenza, with, respiratory
        manifestations NEC
    septic J02.0
    streptococcal (ulcerative) J02.0
    viral NEC J02.8
      coxsackie B08.5
  tropical —see Ulcer, skin
  veldt —see Ulcer, skin
Soto's syndrome (cerebral gigantism) Q87.3
South African cardiomyopathy syndrome I42.8
Southeast Asian hemorrhagic fever A91
Spacing
  abnormal, tooth, teeth, fully erupted M26.30
  excessive, tooth, fully erupted M26.32
Spade-like hand (congenital) Q68.1
Spading nail L60.8
  congenital Q84.6
Spanish collar N47.1
Sparganosis B70.1
Spasm (s), spastic, spasticity (see also condition)
    R25.2
  accommodation —see Spasm, of
      accommodation
  ampulla of Vater K83.4
  anus, ani (sphincter) (reflex) K59.4
    psychogenic F45.8
  artery I73.9
    cerebral G45.9
  Bell's G51.3
  bladder (sphincter, external or internal)
      N32.89
    psychogenic F45.8
  bronchus, bronchiole J98.01
  cardia K22.0
  cardiac I20.1
  carpopedal —see Tetany
  cerebral (arteries) (vascular) G45.9
  cervix, complicating delivery O62.4
  ciliary body (of accommodation) —see Spasm,
      of accommodation
  colon K58.9
    with diarrhea K58.0
    psychogenic F45.8
  common duct K83.8
  compulsive —see Tic
  conjugate H51.8
  coronary (artery) I20.1
  diaphragm (reflex) R06.6
    epidemic B33.0
    psychogenic F45.8
  duodenum K59.8
  epidemic diaphragmatic (transient) B33.0
  esophagus (diffuse) K22.4
    psychogenic F45.8
  facial G51.3
  fallopian tube N83.8
  gastrointestinal (tract) K31.89
    psychogenic F45.8
  glottis J38.5
    hysterical F44.4
    psychogenic F45.8
      conversion reaction F44.4
    reflex through recurrent laryngeal nerve
        J38.5

Spasm (s), spastic, spasticity (Continued)
  habit —see Tic
  heart I20.1
  hemifacial (clonic) G51.3
  hourglass —see Contraction, hourglass
  hysterical F44.4
  infantile —see Epilepsy, spasms
  inferior oblique, eye H51.8
  intestinal (see also Syndrome, irritable bowel)
      K58.9
    psychogenic F45.8
  larynx, laryngeal J38.5
    hysterical F44.4
    psychogenic F45.8
      conversion reaction F44.4
  levator palpebrae superioris —see Disorder,
      eyelid function
  muscle NEC M62.838
    back M62.830
  nerve, trigeminal G51.0
  nervous F45.8
  nodding F98.4
  occupational F48.8
  oculogyric H51.8
    psychogenic F45.8
  of accommodation H52.53-
  ophthalmic artery —see Occlusion, artery,
      retina
  perineal, female N94.89
  peroneo-extensor —see also Deformity, limb,
      flat foot
  pharynx (reflex) J39.2
    hysterical F45.8
    psychogenic F45.8
  psychogenic F45.8
  pylorus NEC K31.3
    adult hypertrophic K31.89
    congenital or infantile Q40.0
    psychogenic F45.8
  rectum (sphincter) K59.4
    psychogenic F45.8
  retinal (artery) —see Occlusion, artery, retina
  sigmoid (see also Syndrome, irritable bowel)
      K58.9
    psychogenic F45.8
  sphincter of Oddi K83.4
  stomach K31.89
    neurotic F45.8
  throat J39.2
    hysterical F45.8
    psychogenic F45.8
  tic F95.9
    chronic F95.1
    transient of childhood F95.0
  tongue K14.8
  torsion (progressive) G24.1
  trigeminal nerve —see Neuralgia, trigeminal
  ureter N13.5
  urethra (sphincter) N35.9
  uterus N85.8
    complicating labor O62.4
  vagina N94.2
    psychogenic F52.5
  vascular I73.9
  vasomotor I73.9
  vein NEC I87.8
  viscera —see Pain, abdominal
Spasmodic —see condition
Spasmophilia —see Tetany
Spasmus nutans F98.4
Spastic, spasticity —see also Spasm
  child (cerebral) (congenital) (paralysis) G80.1
Speaker's throat R49.8
Specific, specified —see condition
Speech
  defect, disorder, disturbance, impediment
      R47.9
    psychogenic, in childhood and adolescence
        F98.8
    slurring R47.81
    specified NEC R47.89

Spencer's disease A08.19
Spens' syndrome (syncope with heart block)
    I45.9
Sperm counts (fertility testing) Z31.41
  postvasectomy Z30.8
  reversal Z31.42
Spermatic cord —see condition
Spermatocele N43.40
  congenital Q55.4
  multiple N43.42
  single N43.41
Spermatocystitis N49.0
Spermatocytoma C62.9-
  specified site —see Neoplasm, malignant, by
      site
Spermatorrhea N50.8
Sphacelus —see Gangrene
Sphenoidal —see condition
Sphenoiditis (chronic) —see Sinusitis,
    sphenoidal
Sphenopalatine ganglion neuralgia
    G90.09
Sphericity, increased, lens (congenital)
    Q12.4
Spherocytosis (congenital) (familial)
    (hereditary) D58.0
  hemoglobin disease D58.0
  sickle-cell (disease) D57.8-
Spherophakia Q12.4
Sphincter —see condition
Sphincteritis, sphincter of Oddi —see
    Cholangitis
Sphingolipidosis E75.3
  specified NEC E75.29
Sphingomyelinosis E75.3
Spicule tooth K00.2
Spider
  bite —see Toxicity, venom, spider
  fingers —see Syndrome, Marfan's
  nevus I78.1
  toes —see Syndrome, Marfan's
  vascular I78.1
Spiegler-Fendt
  benign lymphocytoma L98.8
  sarcoid L08.89
Spielmeyer-Vogt disease E75.4
Spina bifida (aperta) Q05.9
  with hydrocephalus NEC Q05.4
  cervical Q05.5
    with hydrocephalus Q05.0
  dorsal Q05.6
    with hydrocephalus Q05.1
  lumbar Q05.7
    with hydrocephalus Q05.2
  lumbosacral Q05.7
    with hydrocephalus Q05.2
  occulta Q76.0
  sacral Q05.8
    with hydrocephalus Q05.3
  thoracic Q05.6
    with hydrocephalus Q05.1
  thoracolumbar Q05.6
    with hydrocephalus Q05.1
Spindle, Krukenberg's —see Pigmentation,
    cornea, posterior
Spine, spinal —see condition
Spiradenoma (eccrine) —see Neoplasm, skin,
    benign
Spirillosis A25.0
Spirillum
  minus A25.0
  obermeieri infection A68.0
Spirochetal —see condition
Spirochetosis A69.9
  arthritic, arthritica A69.9
  bronchopulmonary A69.8
  icterohemorrhagic A27.0
  lung A69.8
Spirometrosis B70.1
Spitting blood —see Hemoptysis
Splanchnoptosis K63.4

Spleen, splenic —*see* condition
Splenectasis —*see* Splenomegaly
Splenitis (interstitial) (malignant) (nonspecific)
    D73.89
  malarial (*see also* Malaria) B54 [*D77*]
  tuberculous A18.85
Splenocele D73.89
Splenomegaly, splenomegalia (Bengal)
    (cryptogenic) (idiopathic) (tropical) R16.1
  with hepatomegaly R16.2
  cirrhotic D73.2
  congenital Q89.09
  congestive, chronic D73.2
  Egyptian B65.1
  Gaucher's E75.22
  malarial (*see also* Malaria) B54 [*D77*]
  neutropenic D73.81
  Niemann-Pick —*see* Niemann-Pick disease or
    syndrome
  siderotic D73.2
  syphilitic A52.79
    congenital (early) A50.08 [*D77*]
Splenopathy D73.9
Splenoptosis D73.89
Splenosis D73.89
Splinter —*see* Foreign body, superficial, by site
Split, splitting
  foot Q72.7-
  heart sounds R01.2
  lip, congenital —*see* Cleft, lip
  nails L60.3
  urinary stream R39.13
Spondylarthrosis —*see* Spondylosis
Spondylitis (chronic) —*see also* Spondylopathy,
    inflammatory
  ankylopoietica —*see* Spondylitis, ankylosing
  ankylosing (chronic) M45.9
    with lung involvement M45.9 [*J99*]
    cervical region M45.2
    cervicothoracic region M45.3
    juvenile M08.1
    lumbar region M45.6
    lumbosacral region M45.7
    multiple sites M45.0
    occipito-atlanto-axial region M45.1
    sacrococcygeal region M45.8
    thoracic region M45.4
    thoracolumbar region M45.5
  atrophic (ligamentous) —*see* Spondylitis,
    ankylosing
  deformans (chronic) —*see* Spondylosis
  gonococcal A54.41
  gouty M10.08
  in (due to)
    brucellosis A23.9 [*M49.80*]
      cervical region A23.9 [*M49.82*]
      cervicothoracic region A23.9 [*M49.83*]
      lumbar region A23.9 [*M49.86*]
      lumbosacral region A23.9 [*M49.87*]
      multiple sites A23.9 [*M49.89*]
      occipito-atlanto-axial region A23.9
        [*M49.81*]
      sacrococcygeal region A23.9 [*M49.88*]
      thoracic region A23.9 [*M49.84*]
      thoracolumbar region A23.9 [*M49.85*]
    enterobacteria (*see also* subcategory M49.8)
      A04.9
    tuberculosis A18.01
  infectious NEC —*see* Spondylopathy,
    infective
  juvenile ankylosing (chronic) M08.1
  Kümmell's —*see* Spondylopathy, traumatic
  Marie-Strümpell —*see* Spondylitis,
    ankylosing
  muscularis —*see* Spondylopathy, specified
    NEC
  psoriatic L40.53
  rheumatoid —*see* Spondylitis, ankylosing
  rhizomelica —*see* Spondylitis, ankylosing
  sacroiliac NEC M46.1
  senescent, senile —*see* Spondylosis

Spondylitis (*Continued*)
  traumatic (chronic) or post-traumatic —*see*
    Spondylopathy, traumatic
  tuberculous A18.01
  typhosa A01.05
Spondylolisthesis (acquired) (degenerative)
    M43.10
  with disproportion (fetopelvic) O33.0
    causing obstructed labor O65.0
  cervical region M43.12
  cervicothoracic region M43.13
  congenital Q76.2
  lumbar region M43.16
  lumbosacral region M43.17
  multiple sites M43.19
  occipito-atlanto-axial region M43.11
  sacrococcygeal region M43.18
  thoracic region M43.14
  thoracolumbar region M43.15
  traumatic (old) M43.10
    acute
      fifth cervical (displaced) S12.430
        nondisplaced S12.431
        specified type NEC (displaced)
          S12.450
          nondisplaced S12.451
        type III S12.44
      fourth cervical (displaced) S12.330
        nondisplaced S12.331
        specified type NEC (displaced)
          S12.350
          nondisplaced S12.351
        type III S12.34
      second cervical (displaced) S12.130
        nondisplaced S12.131
        specified type NEC (displaced)
          S12.150
          nondisplaced S12.151
        type III S12.14
      seventh cervical (displaced) S12.630
        nondisplaced S12.631
        specified type NEC (displaced)
          S12.650
          nondisplaced S12.651
        type III S12.64
      sixth cervical (displaced) S12.530
        nondisplaced S12.531
        specified type NEC (displaced)
          S12.550
          nondisplaced S12.551
        type III S12.54
      third cervical (displaced) S12.230
        nondisplaced S12.231
        specified type NEC (displaced)
          S12.250
          nondisplaced S12.251
        type III S12.24
Spondylolysis (acquired) M43.00
  cervical region M43.02
  cervicothoracic region M43.03
  congenital Q76.2
  lumbar region M43.06
  lumbosacral region M43.07
    with disproportion (fetopelvic) O33.0
      causing obstructed labor O65.8
  multiple sites M43.09
  occipito-atlanto-axial region M43.01
  sacrococcygeal region M43.08
  thoracic region M43.04
  thoracolumbar region M43.05
Spondylopathy M48.9
  infective NEC M46.50
    cervical region M46.52
    cervicothoracic region M46.53
    lumbar region M46.56
    lumbosacral region M46.57
    multiple sites M46.59
    occipito-atlanto-axial region M46.51
    sacrococcygeal region M46.58
    thoracic region M46.54
    thoracolumbar region M46.55

Spondylopathy (*Continued*)
  inflammatory M46.90
    cervical region M46.92
    cervicothoracic region M46.93
    lumbar region M46.96
    lumbosacral region M46.97
    multiple sites M46.99
    occipito-atlanto-axial region M46.91
    sacrococcygeal region M46.98
    specified type NEC M46.80
      cervical region M46.82
      cervicothoracic region M46.83
      lumbar region M46.86
      lumbosacral region M46.87
      multiple sites M46.89
      occipito-atlanto-axial region M46.81
      sacrococcygeal region M46.88
      thoracic region M46.84
      thoracolumbar region M46.85
    thoracic region M46.94
    thoracolumbar region M46.95
  neuropathic, in
    syringomyelia and syringobulbia G95.0
    tabes dorsalis A52.11
  specified NEC —*see* subcategory M48.8
  traumatic M48.30
    cervical region M48.32
    cervicothoracic region M48.33
    lumbar region M48.36
    lumbosacral region M48.37
    occipito-atlanto-axial region M48.31
    sacrococcygeal region M48.38
    thoracic region M48.34
    thoracolumbar region M48.35
Spondylosis M47.9
  with
    disproportion (fetopelvic) O33.0
      causing obstructed labor O65.0
    myelopathy NEC M47.10
      cervical region M47.12
      cervicothoracic region M47.13
      lumbar region M47.16
      occipito-atlanto-axial region
        M47.11
      thoracic region M47.14
      thoracolumbar region M47.15
    radiculopathy M47.20
      cervical region M47.22
      cervicothoracic region M47.23
      lumbar region M47.26
      lumbosacral region M47.27
      occipito-atlanto-axial region
        M47.21
      sacrococcygeal region M47.28
      thoracic region M47.24
      thoracolumbar region M47.25
  without myelopathy or radiculopathy
    M47.819
    cervical region M47.812
    cervicothoracic region M47.813
    lumbar region M47.816
    lumbosacral region M47.817
    occipito-atlanto-axial region M47.811
    sacrococcygeal region M47.818
    thoracic region M47.814
    thoracolumbar region M47.815
  specified NEC M47.899
    cervical region M47.892
    cervicothoracic region M47.893
    lumbar region M47.896
    lumbosacral region M47.897
    occipito-atlanto-axial region M47.891
    sacrococcygeal region M47.898
    thoracic region M47.894
    thoracolumbar region M47.895
  traumatic —*see* Spondylopathy, traumatic
Sponge
  inadvertently left in operation wound —*see*
    Foreign body, accidentally left during a
    procedure
  kidney (medullary) Q61.5

◀ New   ◀ Revised   ~~deleted~~ Deleted

Sponge-diver's disease —see Toxicity, venom, marine animal, sea anemone
Spongioblastoma (any type) —see Neoplasm, malignant, by site
   specified site —see Neoplasm, malignant, by site
   unspecified site C71.9
Spongioneuroblastoma —see Neoplasm, malignant, by site
Spontaneous —see also condition
   fracture (cause unknown) —see Fracture, pathological
Spoon nail L60.3
   congenital Q84.6
Sporadic —see condition
Sporothrix schenckii infection —see Sporotrichosis
Sporotrichosis B42.9
   arthritis B42.82
   disseminated B42.7
   generalized B42.7
   lymphocutaneous (fixed) (progressive) B42.1
   pulmonary B42.0
   specified NEC B42.89
Spots, spotting (in) (of)
   Bitot's —see also Pigmentation, conjunctiva
      in the young child E50.1
         vitamin A deficiency E50.1
   café, au lait L81.3
   Cayenne pepper I78.1
   cotton wool, retina —see Occlusion, artery, retina
   de Morgan's (senile angiomas) I78.1
   Fuchs' black (myopic) H44.2-
   intermenstrual (regular) N92.0
      irregular N92.1
   Koplik's B05.9
   liver L81.4
   pregnancy O26.85-
   purpuric R23.3
   ruby I78.1
Spotted fever (see Fever, spotted) N92.3
Sprain (joint) (ligament)
   acromioclavicular joint or ligament S43.5-
   ankle S93.40-
      calcaneofibular ligament S93.41-
      deltoid ligament S93.42-
      internal collateral ligament —see Sprain, ankle, specified ligament NEC
      specified ligament NEC S93.49-
      talofibular ligament —see Sprain, ankle, specified ligament NEC
      tibiofibular ligament S93.43-
   anterior longitudinal, cervical S13.4
   atlas, atlanto-axial, atlanto-occipital S13.4
   breast bone —see Sprain, sternum
   calcaneofibular —see Sprain, ankle
   carpal —see Sprain, wrist
   carpometacarpal —see Sprain, hand, specified site NEC
   cartilage
      costal S23.41
      semilunar (knee) —see Sprain, knee, specified site NEC
         with current tear —see Tear, meniscus
      thyroid region S13.5
      xiphoid —see Sprain, sternum
   cervical, cervicodorsal, cervicothoracic S13.4
   chondrosternal S23.421
   coracoclavicular S43.8-
   coracohumeral S43.41-
   coronary, knee —see Sprain, knee, specified site NEC
   costal cartilage S23.41
   cricoarytenoid articulation or ligament S13.5
   cricothyroid articulation S13.5
   cruciate, knee —see Sprain, knee, cruciate
   deltoid, ankle —see Sprain, ankle
   dorsal (spine) S23.3

Sprain (Continued)
   elbow S53.40-
      radial collateral ligament S53.43-
      radiohumeral S53.41-
      rupture
         radial collateral ligament —see Rupture, traumatic, ligament, radial collateral
         ulnar collateral ligament —see Rupture, traumatic, ligament, ulnar collateral
      specified type NEC S53.49-
      ulnar collateral ligament S53.44-
      ulnohumeral S53.42-
   femur, head —see Sprain, hip
   fibular collateral, knee —see Sprain, knee, collateral
   fibulocalcaneal —see Sprain, ankle
   finger (s) S63.61-
      index S63.61-
      interphalangeal (joint) S63.63-
         index S63.63-
         little S63.63-
         middle S63.63-
         ring S63.63-
      little S63.61-
      metacarpophalangeal (joint) S63.65-
      middle S63.61-
      ring S63.61-
      specified site NEC S63.69-
         index S63.69-
         little S63.69-
         middle S63.69-
         ring S63.69-
   foot S93.60-
      specified ligament NEC S93.69-
      tarsal ligament S93.61-
      tarsometatarsal ligament S93.62-
      toe —see Sprain, toe
   hand S63.9-
      finger —see Sprain, finger
      specified site NEC —see subcategory S63.8
      thumb —see Sprain, thumb
   head S03.9
   hip S73.10-
      iliofemoral ligament S73.11-
      ischiocapsular (ligament) S73.12-
      specified NEC S73.19-
   iliofemoral —see Sprain, hip
   innominate
      acetabulum —see Sprain, hip
      sacral junction S33.6
   internal
      collateral, ankle —see Sprain, ankle
      semilunar cartilage —see Sprain, knee, specified site NEC
   interphalangeal
      finger —see Sprain, finger, interphalangeal (joint)
      toe —see Sprain, toe, interphalangeal joint
   ischiocapsular —see Sprain, hip
   ischiofemoral —see Sprain, hip
   jaw (articular disc) (cartilage) (meniscus) S03.4
      old M26.69
   knee S83.9-
      collateral ligament S83.40-
         lateral (fibular) S83.42-
         medial (tibial) S83.41-
      cruciate ligament S83.50-
         anterior S83.51-
         posterior S83.52-
      lateral (fibular) collateral ligament S83.42-
      medial (tibial) collateral ligament S83.41-
      patellar ligament S76.11-
      specified site NEC S83.8X-
      superior tibiofibular joint (ligament) S83.6-
   lateral collateral, knee —see Sprain, knee, collateral
   lumbar (spine) S33.5
   lumbosacral S33.9

Sprain (Continued)
   mandible (articular disc) S03.4
      old M26.69
   medial collateral, knee —see Sprain, knee, collateral
   meniscus
      jaw S03.4
         old M26.69
      knee —see Sprain, knee, specified site NEC
         with current tear —see Tear, meniscus
            old —see Derangement, knee, meniscus, due to old tear
      mandible S03.4
         old M26.69
   metacarpal (distal) (proximal) —see Sprain, hand, specified site NEC
   metacarpophalangeal —see Sprain, finger, metacarpophalangeal (joint)
   metatarsophalangeal —see Sprain, toe, metatarsophalangeal joint
   midcarpal —see Sprain, hand, specified site NEC
   midtarsal —see Sprain, foot, specified site NEC
   neck S13.9
      anterior longitudinal cervical ligament S13.4
      atlanto-axial joint S13.4
      atlanto-occipital joint S13.4
      cervical spine S13.4
      cricoarytenoid ligament S13.5
      cricothyroid ligament S13.5
      specified site NEC S13.8
      thyroid region (cartilage) S13.5
   nose S03.8
   orbicular, hip —see Sprain, hip
   patella —see Sprain, knee, specified site NEC
   patellar ligament S76.11-
   pelvis NEC S33.8
   phalanx
      finger —see Sprain, finger
      toe —see Sprain, toe
   pubofemoral —see Sprain, hip
   radiocarpal —see Sprain, wrist
   radiohumeral —see Sprain, elbow
   radius, collateral —see Rupture, traumatic, ligament, radial collateral
   rib (cage) S23.41
   rotator cuff (capsule) S43.42-
   sacroiliac (region)
      chronic or old —see subcategory M53.2
      joint S33.6
   scaphoid (hand) —see Sprain, hand, specified site NEC
   scapula (r) —see Sprain, shoulder girdle, specified site NEC
   semilunar cartilage (knee) —see Sprain, knee, specified site NEC
      with current tear —see Tear, meniscus
         old —see Derangement, knee, meniscus, due to old tear
   shoulder joint S43.40-
      acromioclavicular joint (ligament) —see Sprain, acromioclavicular joint
      blade —see Sprain, shoulder, girdle, specified site NEC
      coracoclavicular joint (ligament) —see Sprain, coracoclavicular joint
      coracohumeral ligament —see Sprain, coracohumeral joint
      girdle S43.9-
         specified site NEC S43.8-
      rotator cuff —see Sprain, rotator cuff
      specified site NEC S43.49-
      sternoclavicular joint (ligament) —see Sprain, sternoclavicular joint
   spine
      cervical S13.4
      lumbar S33.5
      thoracic S23.3
   sternoclavicular joint S43.6-

Sprain *(Continued)*
  sternum S23.429
    chondrosternal joint S23.421
    specified site NEC S23.428
    sternoclavicular (joint) (ligament)
      S23.420
  symphysis
    jaw S03.4
      old M26.69
    mandibular S03.4
      old M26.69
  talofibular —*see* Sprain, ankle
  tarsal —*see* Sprain, foot, specified site NEC
  tarsometatarsal —*see* Sprain, foot, specified
    site NEC
  temporomandibular S03.4
    old M26.69
  thorax S23.9
    ribs S23.41
    specified site NEC S23.8
    spine S23.3
    sternum —*see* Sprain, sternum
  thumb S63.60-
    interphalangeal (joint) S63.62-
    metacarpophalangeal (joint) S63.64-
    specified site NEC S63.68-
  thyroid cartilage or region S13.5
  tibia (proximal end) —*see* Sprain, knee,
    specified site NEC
  tibial collateral, knee —*see* Sprain, knee,
    collateral
  tibiofibular
    distal —*see* Sprain, ankle
    superior —*see* Sprain, knee, specified site
      NEC
  toe (s) S93.50-
    great S93.50-
    interphalangeal joint S93.51-
      great S93.51-
      lesser S93.51-
    lesser S93.50-
    metatarsophalangeal joint S93.52-
      great S93.52-
      lesser S93.52-
  ulna, collateral —*see* Rupture, traumatic,
    ligament, ulnar collateral
  ulnohumeral —*see* Sprain, elbow
  wrist S63.50-
    carpal S63.51-
    radiocarpal S63.52-
    specified site NEC S63.59-
  xiphoid cartilage —*see* Sprain, sternum
Sprengel's deformity (congenital) Q74.0
Sprue (tropical) K90.1
  celiac K90.0
  idiopathic K90.0
  meaning thrush B37.0
  nontropical K90.0
Spur, bone —*see also* Enthesopathy
  calcaneal M77.3-
  iliac crest M76.2-
  nose (septum) J34.89
Spurway's syndrome Q78.0
Sputum
  abnormal (amount) (color) (odor) (purulent)
    R09.3
  blood-stained R04.2
  excessive (cause unknown) R09.3
Squamous —*see also* condition
  epithelium in
    cervical canal (congenital) Q51.828
    uterine mucosa (congenital) Q51.818
Squashed nose M95.0
  congenital Q67.4
Squeeze, diver's T70.3
Squint —*see also* Strabismus
  accommodative —*see* Strabismus, convergent
    concomitant
St. Hubert's disease A82.9
Stab —*see also* Laceration
  internal organs —*see* Injury, by site

Stafne's cyst or cavity M27.0
Staggering gait R26.0
  hysterical F44.4
Staghorn calculus —*see* Calculus, kidney
Stähli's line (cornea) (pigment) —*see*
  Pigmentation, cornea, anterior
Stain, staining
  meconium (newborn) P96.83
  port wine Q82.5
  tooth, teeth (hard tissues) (extrinsic) K03.6
    due to
      accretions K03.6
      deposits (betel) (black) (green) (materia
        alba) (orange) (soft) (tobacco) K03.6
      metals (copper) (silver) K03.7
      nicotine K03.6
      pulpal bleeding K03.7
      tobacco K03.6
    intrinsic K00.8
Stammering (*see also* Disorder, fluency) F80.81
Standstill
  auricular I45.5
  cardiac —*see* Arrest, cardiac
  sinoatrial I45.5
  ventricular —*see* Arrest, cardiac
Stannosis J63.5
Stanton's disease —*see* Melioidosis
Staphylitis (acute) (catarrhal) (chronic)
  (gangrenous) (membranous) (suppurative)
  (ulcerative) K12.2
Staphylococcal scalded skin syndrome L00
Staphylococcemia A41.2
Staphylococcus, staphylococcal —*see also*
  condition
  as cause of disease classified elsewhere
    B95.8
    aureus (methicillin susceptible) (MSSA)
      B95.61
      methicillin resistant (MRSA) B95.62
    specified NEC, as cause of disease classified
      elsewhere B95.7
Staphyloma (sclera)
  cornea H18.72-
  equatorial H15.81-
  localized (anterior) H15.82-
  posticum H15.83-
  ring H15.85-
Stargardt's disease —*see* Dystrophy, retina
Starvation (inanition) (due to lack of food)
  T73.0
  edema —*see* Malnutrition, severe
Stasis
  bile (noncalculous) K83.1
  bronchus J98.09
    with infection —*see* Bronchitis
  cardiac —*see* Failure, heart, congestive
  cecum K59.8
  colon K59.8
  dermatitis —*see* Varix, leg, with,
    inflammation
  duodenal K31.5
  eczema —*see* Varix, leg, with, inflammation
  edema —*see* Hypertension, venous (chronic),
    idiopathic
  foot T69.0-
  ileocecal coil K59.8
  ileum K59.8
  intestinal K59.8
  jejunum K59.8
  kidney N19
  liver (cirrhotic) K76.1
  lymphatic I89.8
  pneumonia J18.2
  pulmonary —*see* Edema, lung
  rectal K59.8
  renal N19
    tubular N17.0
  ulcer —*see* Varix, leg, with, ulcer
    without varicose veins I87.2
  urine —*see* Retention, urine
  venous I87.8

State (of)
  affective and paranoid, mixed, organic
    psychotic F06.8
  agitated R45.1
    acute reaction to stress F43.0
  anxiety (neurotic) F41.1
  apprehension F41.1
  burn-out Z73.0
  climacteric, female Z78.0
    symptomatic N95.1
  compulsive F42
    mixed with obsessional thoughts
      F42
  confusional (psychogenic) F44.89
    acute —*see also* Delirium
      with
        arteriosclerotic dementia F01.50
          with behavioral disturbance
            F01.51
        senility or dementia F05
    alcoholic F10.231
    epileptic F05
    reactive (from emotional stress,
      psychological trauma) F44.89
    subacute —*see* Delirium
  convulsive —*see* Convulsions
  crisis F43.0
  depressive F32.9
    neurotic F34.1
  dissociative F44.9
  emotional shock (stress) R45.7
  hypercoagulation —*see* Hypercoagulable
  locked-in G83.5
  menopausal Z78.0
    symptomatic N95.1
  neurotic F48.9
    with depersonalization F48.1
  obsessional F42
  oneiroid (schizophrenia-like) F23
  organic
    hallucinatory (nonalcoholic) F06.0
    paranoid (-hallucinatory) F06.2
  panic F41.0
  paranoid F22
    climacteric F22
    involutional F22
    menopausal F22
    organic F06.2
    senile F03
    simple F22
  persistent vegetative R40.3
  phobic F40.9
  postleukotomy F07.0
  pregnant, incidental Z33.1
  psychogenic, twilight F44.89
  psychopathic (constitutional) F60.2
  psychotic, organic —*see also* Psychosis,
    organic
    mixed paranoid and affective F06.8
    senile or presenile F03
    transient NEC F06.8
      with
        depression F06.31
        hallucinations F06.0
  residual schizophrenic F20.5
  restlessness R45.1
  stress (emotional) R45.7
  tension (mental) F48.9
    specified NEC F48.8
  transient organic psychotic NEC F06.8
    depressive type F06.31
    hallucinatory type F06.30
  twilight
    epileptic F05
    psychogenic F44.89
  vegetative, persistent R40.3
  vital exhaustion Z73.0
  withdrawal —*see* Withdrawal, state
Status (post) —*see also* Presence (of)
  absence, epileptic —*see* Epilepsy, by type,
    with status epilepticus

◀ New   ◀≡ Revised   ~~deleted~~ Deleted

Status *(Continued)*
  administration of tPA (rtPA) in a different
      facility within the last 24 hours prior to
      admission to the current facility
      Z92.82
  adrenalectomy (unilateral) (bilateral) E89.6
  anastomosis Z98.0
  anginosus I20.9
  angioplasty (peripheral) Z98.62
    with implant Z95.820
      coronary artery Z98.61
        with implant Z95.5
  aortocoronary bypass Z95.1
  arthrodesis Z98.1
  artificial opening (of) Z93.9
    gastrointestinal tract Z93.4
    specified NEC Z93.8
    urinary tract Z93.6
    vagina Z93.8
  asthmaticus —*see* Asthma, by type, with
      status asthmaticus
  awaiting organ transplant Z76.82
  bariatric surgery Z98.84
  bed confinement Z74.01
  bleb, filtering (vitreous), after glaucoma
      surgery Z98.83
  breast implant Z98.82
    removal Z98.86
  cataract extraction Z98.4-
  cholecystectomy Z90.49
  clitorectomy N90.811
    with excision of labia minora N90.812
  colectomy (complete) (partial) Z90.49
  colonization —*see* Carrier (suspected) of
  colostomy Z93.3
  convulsivus idiopathicus —*see* Epilepsy, by
      type, with status epilepticus
  coronary artery angioplasty —*see* Status,
      angioplasty, coronary artery
  cystectomy (urinary bladder) Z90.6
  cystostomy Z93.50
    appendico-vesicostomy Z93.52
    cutaneous Z93.51
    specified NEC Z93.59
  delinquent immunization Z28.3
  dental Z98.818
    crown Z98.811
    fillings Z98.811
    restoration Z98.811
    sealant Z98.810
    specified NEC Z98.818
  deployment (current) (military) Z56.82
  dialysis (hemodialysis) (peritoneal) Z99.2
  do not resuscitate (DNR) Z66
  donor —*see* Donor
  embedded fragments —*see* Retained, foreign
      body fragments (type of)
  embedded splinter —*see* Retained, foreign
      body fragments (type of)
  enterostomy Z93.4
  epileptic, epilepticus (*see also* Epilepsy, by
      type, with status epilepticus) G40.901
  estrogen receptor
    negative Z17.1
    positive Z17.0
  female genital cutting —*see* Female genital
      mutilation status
  female genital mutilation —*see* Female genital
      mutilation status
  filtering (vitreous) bleb after glaucoma
      surgery Z98.83
  gastrectomy (complete) (partial) Z90.3
  gastric banding Z98.84
  gastric bypass for obesity Z98.84
  gastrostomy Z93.1
  human immunodeficiency virus (HIV)
      infection, asymptomatic Z21
  hysterectomy (complete) (total) Z90.710
    partial (with remaining cervial stump)
        Z90.711
  ileostomy Z93.2

Status *(Continued)*
  implant
    breast Z98.82
  infibulation N90.813
  intestinal bypass Z98.0
  jejunostomy Z93.4
  lapsed immunization schedule Z28.3
  laryngectomy Z90.02
  lymphaticus E32.8
  marmoratus G80.3
  mastectomy (unilateral) (bilateral) Z90.1-
  military deployment status (current)
      Z56.82
    in theater or in support of military war,
        peacekeeping and humanitarian
        operations Z56.82
  nephrectomy (unilateral) (bilateral) Z90.5
  nephrostomy Z93.6
  obesity surgery Z98.84
  oophorectomy
    bilateral Z90.722
    unilateral Z90.721
  organ replacement
    by artificial or mechanical device or
        prosthesis of
      artery Z95.828
      bladder Z96.0
      blood vessel Z95.828
      breast Z97.8
      eye globe Z97.0
      heart Z95.812
        valve Z95.2
      intestine Z97.8
      joint Z96.60
        hip —*see* Presence, hip joint implant
        knee —*see* Presence, knee joint
            implant
        specified site NEC Z96.698
      kidney Z97.8
      larynx Z96.3
      lens Z96.1
      limbs —*see* Presence, artificial, limb
      liver Z97.8
      lung Z97.8
      pancreas Z97.8
    by organ transplant (heterologous)
        (homologous) —*see* Transplant
  pacemaker
    brain Z96.89
    cardiac Z95.0
    specified NEC Z96.89
  pancreatectomy Z90.410
    complete Z90.410
    partial Z90.411
    total Z90.410
  pneumonectomy (complete) (partial) Z90.2
  pneumothorax, therapeutic Z98.3
  postcommotio cerebri F07.81
  postoperative (postprocedural) NEC
      Z98.89
    breast implant Z98.82
    dental Z98.818
      crown Z98.811
      fillings Z98.811
      restoration Z98.811
      sealant Z98.810
      specified NEC Z98.818
    pneumothorax, therapeutic Z98.3
  postpartum (routine follow-up) Z39.2
    care immediately after delivery Z39.0
  postsurgical (postprocedural) NEC Z98.89
    pneumothorax, therapeutic Z98.3
  pregnancy, incidental Z33.1
  prosthesis coronary angioplasty Z95.5
  pseudophakia Z96.1
  renal dialysis (hemodialysis) (peritoneal)
      Z99.2
  retained foreign body —*see* Retained, foreign
      body fragments (type of)
  reversed jejunal transposition (for bypass)
      Z98.0

Status *(Continued)*
  salpingo-oophorectomy
    bilateral Z90.722
    unilateral Z90.721
  sex reassignment surgery status Z87.890
  shunt
    arteriovenous (for dialysis) Z99.2
    cerebrospinal fluid Z98.2
    ventricular (communicating) (for
        drainage) Z98.2
  splenectomy Z90.81
  thymicolymphaticus E32.8
  thymicus E32.8
  thymolymphaticus E32.8
  thyroidectomy (hypothyroidism) E89.0
  tooth (teeth) extraction (*see also* Absence,
      teeth, acquired) K08.409
  tPA (rtPA) administration in a different
      facility within the last 24 hours prior to
      admission to current facility Z92.82
  tracheostomy Z93.0
  transplant —*see* Transplant
    organ removed Z98.85
  tubal ligation Z98.51
  underimmunization Z28.3
  ureterostomy Z93.6
  urethrostomy Z93.6
  vagina, artificial Z93.8
  vasectomy Z98.52
  wheelchair confinement Z99.3
Stealing
  child problem F91.8
    in company with others Z72.810
  pathological (compulsive) F63.2
Steam burn —*see* Burn
Steatocystoma multiplex L72.2
Steatohepatitis (nonalcoholic) (NASH)
    K75.81
Steatoma L72.3
  eyelid (cystic) —*see* Dermatosis, eyelid
    infected —*see* Hordeolum
Steatorrhea (chronic) K90.4
  with lacteal obstruction K90.2
  idiopathic (adult) (infantile) K90.0
  pancreatic K90.3
  primary K90.0
  tropical K90.1
Steatosis E88.89
  heart —*see* Degeneration, myocardial
  kidney N28.89
  liver NEC K76.0
Steele-Richardson-Olszewski disease or
    syndrome G23.1
Steinbrocker's syndrome G90.8
Steinert's disease G71.11
Stein-Leventhal syndrome E28.2
Stein's syndrome E28.2
STEMI (*see also* - Infarct, myocardium, ST
    elevation) I21.3
Stenocardia I20.8
Stenocephaly Q75.8
Stenosis, stenotic (cicatricial) —*see also* Stricture
  ampulla of Vater K83.1
  anus, anal (canal) (sphincter) K62.4
    and rectum K62.4
    congenital Q42.3
      with fistula Q42.2
  aorta (ascending) (supraventricular)
      (congenital) Q25.3
    arteriosclerotic I70.0
    calcified I70.0
  aortic (valve) I35.0
    with insufficiency I35.2
    congenital Q23.0
    rheumatic I06.0
      with
        incompetency, insufficiency or
            regurgitation I06.2
        with mitral (valve) disease I08.0
          with tricuspid (valve) disease
              I08.3

Stenosis, stenotic *(Continued)*
  aortic *(Continued)*
    rheumatic *(Continued)*
      with *(Continued)*
        mitral (valve) disease I08.0
          with tricuspid (valve) disease
            I08.3
        tricuspid (valve) disease I08.2
          with mitral (valve) disease I08.3
      specified cause NEC I35.0
      syphilitic A52.03
  aqueduct of Sylvius (congenital) Q03.0
    with spina bifida —*see* Spina bifida,
      by site, with hydrocephalus
    acquired G91.1
  artery NEC *(see also* Arteriosclerosis)
    I77.1
    celiac I77.4
    cerebral —*see* Occlusion, artery, cerebral
    extremities —*see* Arteriosclerosis,
      extremities
    precerebral —*see* Occlusion, artery,
      precerebral
    pulmonary (congenital) Q25.6
      acquired I28.8
    renal I70.1
  bile duct (common) (hepatic) K83.1
    congenital Q44.3
  bladder-neck (acquired) N32.0
    congenital Q64.31
  brain G93.89
  bronchus J98.09
    congenital Q32.3
    syphilitic A52.72
  cardia (stomach) K22.2
    congenital Q39.3
  cardiovascular —*see* Disease, cardiovascular
  caudal M48.08
  cervix, cervical (canal) N88.2
    congenital Q51.828
    in pregnancy or childbirth —*see* Pregnancy,
      complicated by, abnormal cervix
  colon —*see also* Obstruction, intestine
    congenital Q42.9
      specified NEC Q42.8
  colostomy K94.03
  common (bile) duct K83.1
    congenital Q44.3
  coronary (artery) —*see* Disease, heart,
    ischemic, atherosclerotic
  cystic duct —*see* Obstruction, gallbladder
  due to presence of device, implant or graft
    (see also Complications, by site and type,
      specified NEC) T85.85
    arterial graft NEC T82.858
    breast (implant) T85.85
    catheter T85.85
      dialysis (renal) T82.858
        intraperitoneal T85.85
      infusion NEC T82.858
        spinal (epidural) (subdural) T85.85
      urinary (indwelling) T83.85
    fixation, internal (orthopedic) NEC
      T84.85
    gastrointestinal (bile duct) (esophagus)
      T85.85
    genital NEC T83.85
    heart NEC T82.857
    joint prosthesis T84.85
    ocular (corneal graft) (orbital implant)
      NEC T85.85
    orthopedic NEC T84.85
    specified NEC T85.85
    urinary NEC T83.85
    vascular NEC T82.858
    ventricular intracranial shunt T85.85
  duodenum K31.5
    congenital Q41.0
  ejaculatory duct NEC N50.8
  endocervical os —*see* Stenosis, cervix
  enterostomy K94.13

Stenosis, stenotic *(Continued)*
  esophagus K22.2
    congenital Q39.3
    syphilitic A52.79
      congenital A50.59 *[K23]*
  eustachian tube —*see* Obstruction, eustachian
    tube
  external ear canal (acquired) H61.30-
    congenital Q16.1
    due to
      inflammation H61.32-
      trauma H61.31-
    postprocedural H95.81-
    specified cause NEC H61.39-
  gallbladder —*see* Obstruction, gallbladder
  glottis J38.6
  heart valve (congenital) Q24.8
    aortic Q23.0
    mitral Q23.2
    pulmonary Q22.1
    tricuspid Q22.4
  hepatic duct K83.1
  hymen N89.6
  hypertrophic subaortic (idiopathic) I42.1
  ileum K56.69
    congenital Q41.2
  infundibulum cardia Q24.3
  intervertebral foramina —*see also* Lesion,
    biomechanical, specified NEC
    connective tissue M99.79
      abdomen M99.79
      cervical region M99.71
      cervicothoracic M99.71
      head region M99.70
      lumbar region M99.73
      lumbosacral M99.73
      occipitocervical M99.70
      sacral region M99.74
      sacrococcygeal M99.74
      sacroiliac M99.74
      specified NEC M99.79
      thoracic region M99.72
      thoracolumbar M99.72
    disc M99.79
      abdomen M99.79
      cervical region M99.71
      cervicothoracic M99.71
      head region M99.70
      lower extremity M99.76
      lumbar region M99.73
      lumbosacral M99.73
      occipitocervical M99.70
      pelvic M99.75
      rib cage M99.78
      sacral region M99.74
      sacrococcygeal M99.74
      sacroiliac M99.74
      specified NEC M99.79
      thoracic region M99.72
      thoracolumbar M99.72
      upper extremity M99.77
    osseous M99.69
      abdomen M99.69
      cervical region M99.61
      cervicothoracic M99.61
      head region M99.60
      lower extremity M99.66
      lumbar region M99.63
      lumbosacral M99.63
      occipitocervical M99.60
      pelvic M99.65
      rib cage M99.68
      sacral region M99.64
      sacrococcygeal M99.64
      sacroiliac M99.64
      specified NEC M99.69
      thoracic region M99.62
      thoracolumbar M99.62
      upper extremity M99.67
    subluxation —*see* Stenosis, intervertebral
      foramina, osseous

Stenosis, stenotic *(Continued)*
  intestine —*see also* Obstruction, intestine
    congenital (small) Q41.9
      large Q42.9
        specified NEC Q42.8
      specified NEC Q41.8
  jejunum K56.69
    congenital Q41.1
  lacrimal (passage)
    canaliculi H04.54-
    congenital Q10.5
    duct H04.55-
    punctum H04.56-
    sac H04.57-
  lacrimonasal duct —*see* Stenosis, lacrimal,
    duct
    congenital Q10.5
  larynx J38.6
    congenital NEC Q31.8
      subglottic Q31.1
    syphilitic A52.73
      congenital A50.59 *[J99]*
  mitral (chronic) (inactive) (valve) I05.0
    with
      aortic valve disease I08.0
      incompetency, insufficiency or
        regurgitation I05.2
    active or acute I01.1
      with rheumatic or Sydenham's chorea
        I02.0
    congenital Q23.2
    specified cause, except rheumatic I34.2
    syphilitic A52.03
  myocardium, myocardial —*see also*
    Degeneration, myocardial
    hypertrophic subaortic (idiopathic) I42.1
  nares (anterior) (posterior) J34.89
    congenital Q30.0
  nasal duct —*see also* Stenosis, lacrimal, duct
    congenital Q10.5
  nasolacrimal duct —*see also* Stenosis, lacrimal,
    duct
    congenital Q10.5
  neural canal —*see also* Lesion, biomechanical,
    specified NEC
    connective tissue M99.49
      abdomen M99.49
      cervical region M99.41
      cervicothoracic M99.41
      head region M99.40
      lower extremity M99.46
      lumbar region M99.43
      lumbosacral M99.43
      occipitocervical M99.40
      pelvic M99.45
      rib cage M99.48
      sacral region M99.44
      sacrococcygeal M99.44
      sacroiliac M99.44
      specified NEC M99.49
      thoracic region M99.42
      thoracolumbar M99.42
      upper extremity M99.47
    intervertebral disc M99.59
      abdomen M99.59
      cervical region M99.51
      cervicothoracic M99.51
      head region M99.50
      lower extremity M99.56
      lumbar region M99.53
      lumbosacral M99.53
      occipitocervical M99.50
      pelvic M99.55
      rib cage M99.58
      sacral region M99.54
      sacrococcygeal M99.54
      sacroiliac M99.54
      specified NEC M99.59
      thoracic region M99.52
      thoracolumbar M99.52
      upper extremity M99.57

Stenosis, stenotic *(Continued)*
  neural canal *(Continued)*
    osseous M99.39
      abdomen M99.39
      cervical region M99.31
      cervicothoracic M99.31
      head region M99.30
      lower extremity M99.36
      lumbar region M99.33
      lumbosacral M99.33
      occipitocervical M99.30
      pelvic M99.35
      rib cage M99.38
      sacral region M99.34
      sacrococcygeal M99.34
      sacroiliac M99.34
      specified NEC M99.39
      thoracic region M99.32
      thoracolumbar M99.32
      upper extremity M99.37
    subluxation M99.29
      cervical region M99.21
      cervicothoracic M99.21
      head region M99.20
      lower extremity M99.26
      lumbar region M99.23
      lumbosacral M99.23
      occipitocervical M99.20
      pelvic M99.25
      rib cage M99.28
      sacral region M99.24
      sacrococcygeal M99.24
      sacroiliac M99.24
      specified NEC M99.29
      thoracic region M99.22
      thoracolumbar M99.22
      upper extremity M99.27
  organ or site, congenital NEC —*see* Atresia, by site
  papilla of Vater K83.1
  pulmonary (artery) (congenital) Q25.6
    with ventricular septal defect, transposition of aorta, and hypertrophy of right ventricle Q21.3
    acquired I28.8
    in tetralogy of Fallot Q21.3
    infundibular Q24.3
    subvalvular Q24.3
    supravalvular Q25.6
    valve I37.0
      with insufficiency I37.2
      congenital Q22.1
      rheumatic I09.89
        with aortic, mitral or tricuspid (valve) disease I08.8
    vein, acquired I28.8
    vessel NEC I28.8
  pulmonic (congenital) Q22.1
    infundibular Q24.3
    subvalvular Q24.3
  pylorus (hypertrophic) (acquired) K31.1
    adult K31.1
    congenital Q40.0
    infantile Q40.0
  rectum (sphincter) —*see* Stricture, rectum
  renal artery I70.1
    congenital Q27.1
  salivary duct (any) K11.8
  sphincter of Oddi K83.1
  spinal M48.00
    cervical region M48.02
    cervicothoracic region M48.03
    lumbar region M48.06
    lumbosacral region M48.07
    occipito-atlanto-axial region M48.01
    sacrococcygeal region M48.08
    thoracic region M48.04
    thoracolumbar region M48.05
  stomach, hourglass K31.2

Stenosis, stenotic *(Continued)*
  subaortic (congenital) Q24.4
    hypertrophic (idiopathic) I42.1
  subglottic J38.6
    congenital Q31.1
    postprocedural J95.5
  trachea J39.8
    congenital Q32.1
    syphilitic A52.73
    tuberculous NEC A15.5
  tracheostomy J95.03
  tricuspid (valve) I07.0
    with
      aortic (valve) disease I08.2
      incompetency, insufficiency or regurgitation I07.2
        with aortic (valve) disease I08.2
          with mitral (valve) disease I08.3
      mitral (valve) disease I08.1
        with aortic (valve) disease I08.3
    congenital Q22.4
    nonrheumatic I36.0
      with insufficiency I36.2
  tubal N97.1
  ureter —*see* Atresia, ureter
  ureteropelvic junction, congenital Q62.11
  ureterovesical orifice, congenital Q62.12
  urethra (valve) —*see also* Stricture, urethra
    congenital Q64.32
  urinary meatus, congenital Q64.33
  vagina N89.5
    congenital Q52.4
    in pregnancy —*see* Pregnancy, complicated by, abnormal vagina
      causing obstructed labor O65.5
  valve (cardiac) (heart) (*see also* Endocarditis) I38
    congenital Q24.8
    aortic Q23.0
    mitral Q23.2
    pulmonary Q22.1
    tricuspid Q22.4
  vena cava (inferior) (superior) I87.1
    congenital Q26.0
  vesicourethral orifice Q64.31
  vulva N90.5
Stent jail T82.897
Stercolith (impaction) K56.41
  appendix K38.1
Stercoraceous, stercoral ulcer K63.3
  anus or rectum K62.6
Stereotypies NEC F98.4
Sterility —*see* Infertility
Sterilization —*see* Encounter (for), sterilization
Sternalgia —*see* Angina
Sternopagus Q89.4
Sternum bifidum Q76.7
Steroid
  effects (adverse) (adrenocortical) (iatrogenic)
    cushingoid E24.2
      correct substance properly administered —*see* Table of Drugs and Chemicals, by drug, adverse effect
      overdose or wrong substance given or taken —*see* Table of Drugs and Chemicals, by drug, poisoning
    diabetes —*see* category E09
      correct substance properly administered —*see* Table of Drugs and Chemicals, by drug, adverse effect
      overdose or wrong substance given or taken —*see* Table of Drugs and Chemicals, by drug, poisoning
    fever R50.2
    insufficiency E27.3
      correct substance properly administered —*see* Table of Drugs and Chemicals, by drug, adverse effect

Steroid *(Continued)*
  effects *(Continued)*
    insufficiency *(Continued)*
      overdose or wrong substance given or taken —*see* Table of Drugs and Chemicals, by drug, poisoning
    responder H40.04-
Stevens-Johnson disease or syndrome L51.1
  toxic epidermal necrolysis overlap L51.3
Stewart-Morel syndrome M85.2
Sticker's disease B08.3
Sticky eye —*see* Conjunctivitis, acute, mucopurulent
Stieda's disease —*see* Bursitis, tibial collateral
Stiff neck —*see* Torticollis
Stiff-man syndrome G25.82
Stiffness, joint NEC M25.60-
  ankle M25.67-
  ankylosis —*see* Ankylosis, joint
  contracture —*see* Contraction, joint
  elbow M25.62-
  foot M25.67-
  hand M25.64-
  hip M25.65-
  knee M25.66-
  shoulder M25.61-
  wrist M25.63-
Stigmata congenital syphilis A50.59
Stillbirth P95
Still-Felty syndrome —*see* Felty's syndrome
Still's disease or syndrome (juvenile) M08.20
  adult-onset M06.1
  ankle M08.27-
  elbow M08.22-
  foot joint M08.27-
  hand joint M08.24-
  hip M08.25-
  knee M08.26-
  multiple site M08.29
  shoulder M08.21-
  vertebra M08.28
  wrist M08.23-
Stimulation, ovary E28.1
Sting (venomous) (with allergic or anaphylactic shock) —*see* Table of Drugs and Chemicals, by animal or substance, poisoning
Stippled epiphyses Q78.8
Stitch
  abscess T81.4
  burst (in operation wound) —*see* Disruption, wound, operation
Stokes-Adams disease or syndrome I45.9
Stokes' disease E05.00
  with thyroid storm E05.01
Stokvis (-Talma) disease D74.8
Stoma malfunction
  colostomy K94.03
  enterostomy K94.13
  gastrostomy K94.23
  ileostomy K94.13
  tracheostomy J95.03
Stomach —*see* condition
Stomatitis (denture) (ulcerative) K12.1
  angular K13.0
    due to dietary or vitamin deficiency E53.0
  aphthous K12.0
  bovine B08.61
  candidal B37.0
  catarrhal K12.1
  diphtheritic A36.89
  due to
    dietary deficiency E53.0
    thrush B37.0
    vitamin deficiency
      B group NEC E53.9
      B2 (riboflavin) E53.0
  epidemic B08.8
  epizootic B08.8
  follicular K12.1
  gangrenous A69.0
  Geotrichum B48.3

Stomatitis *(Continued)*
  herpesviral, herpetic B00.2
  herpetiformis K12.0
  malignant K12.1
  membranous acute K12.1
  monilial B37.0
  mycotic B37.0
  necrotizing ulcerative A69.0
  parasitic B37.0
  septic K12.1
  spirochetal A69.1
  suppurative (acute) K12.2
  ulceromembranous A69.1
  vesicular K12.1
    with exanthem (enteroviral) B08.4
    virus disease A93.8
  Vincent's A69.1
Stomatocytosis D58.8
Stomatomycosis B37.0
Stomatorrhagia K13.79
Stone (s) —*see also* Calculus
  bladder (diverticulum) N21.0
  cystine E72.09
  heart syndrome I50.1
  kidney N20.0
  prostate N42.0
  pulpal (dental) K04.2
  renal N20.0
  salivary gland or duct (any) K11.5
  urethra (impacted) N21.1
  urinary (duct) (impacted) (passage) N20.9
    bladder (diverticulum) N21.0
    lower tract N21.9
    specified NEC N21.8
  xanthine E79.8 [N22]
Stonecutter's lung J62.8
Stonemason's asthma, disease, lung or
  pneumoconiosis J62.8
Stoppage
  heart —*see* Arrest, cardiac
  urine —*see* Retention, urine
Storm, thyroid —*see* Thyrotoxicosis
Strabismus (congenital) (nonparalytic) H50.9
  concomitant H50.40
    convergent —*see* Strabismus, convergent
      concomitant
    divergent —*see* Strabismus, divergent
      concomitant
  convergent concomitant H50.00
    accommodative component H50.43
    alternating H50.05
      with
        A pattern H50.06
        specified nonconcomitances NEC
          H50.08
        V pattern H50.07
    monocular H50.01-
      with
        A pattern H50.02-
        specified nonconcomitances NEC
          H50.04-
        V pattern H50.03-
    intermittent H50.31-
      alternating H50.32
  cyclotropia H50.1-
  divergent concomitant H50.10
    alternating H50.15
      with
        A pattern H50.16
        specified nonconcomitances NEC
          H50.18
        V pattern H50.17
    monocular H50.11-
      with
        A pattern H50.12-
        specified nonconcomitances NEC
          H50.14-
        V pattern H50.13-
    intermittent H50.33-
      alternating H50.34
  Duane's syndrome H50.81-

Strabismus *(Continued)*
  due to adhesions, scars H50.69
  heterophoria H50.50
    alternating H50.55
    cyclophoria H50.54
    esophoria H50.51
    exophoria H50.52
    vertical H50.53
  heterotropia H50.40
    intermittent H50.30
  hypertropia H50.2-
  hypotropia —*see* Hypertropia
  latent H50.50
  mechanical H50.60
    Brown's sheath syndrome H50.61-
    specified type NEC H50.69
  monofixation syndrome H50.42
  paralytic H49.9
    abducens nerve H49.2-
    fourth nerve H49.1-
    Kearns-Sayre syndrome H49.81-
    ophthalmoplegia (external)
      progressive H49.4-
        with pigmentary retinopathy
          H49.81-
      total H49.3-
    sixth nerve H49.2-
    specified type NEC H49.88-
    third nerve H49.0-
    trochlear nerve H49.1-
  specified type NEC H50.89
  vertical H50.2-
Strain
  back S39.012
  cervical S16.1
  eye NEC —*see* Disturbance, vision,
    subjective
  heart —*see* Disease, heart
  low back S39.012
  mental NOS Z73.3
    work-related Z56.6
  muscle (tendon) —*see* Injury, muscle, by site,
    strain
  neck S16.1
  physical NOS Z73.3
    work-related Z56.6
  postural —*see also* Disorder, soft tissue, due
    to use
  psychological NEC Z73.3
  tendon —*see* Injury, muscle, by site, strain
Straining, on urination R39.16
Strand, vitreous —*see* Opacity, vitreous,
  membranes and strands
Strangulation, strangulated —*see also*
  Asphyxia, traumatic
  appendix K38.8
  bladder-neck N32.0
  bowel or colon K56.2
  food or foreign body —*see* Foreign body, by
    site
  hemorrhoids —*see* Hemorrhoids, with
    complication
  hernia —*see also* Hernia, by site, with
    obstruction
    with gangrene —*see* Hernia, by site, with
      gangrene
  intestine (large) (small) K56.2
    with hernia —*see also* Hernia, by site, with
      obstruction
      with gangrene —*see* Hernia, by site, with
        gangrene
  mesentery K56.2
  mucus —*see* Asphyxia, mucus
  omentum K56.2
  organ or site, congenital NEC —*see* Atresia,
    by site
  ovary —*see* Torsion, ovary
  penis N48.89
    foreign body T19.4
  rupture —*see* Hernia, by site, with
    obstruction

Strangulation, strangulated *(Continued)*
  stomach due to hernia —*see also* Hernia, by
    site, with obstruction
    with gangrene —*see* Hernia, by site, with
      gangrene
  vesicourethral orifice N32.0
Strangury R30.0
Straw itch B88.0
Strawberry
  gallbladder K82.4
  mark Q82.5
  tongue (red) (white) K14.3
Streak (s)
  macula, angioid H35.33
  ovarian Q50.32
Strephosymbolia F81.0
  secondary to organic lesion R48.8
Streptobacillary fever A25.1
Streptobacillosis A25.1
Streptobacillus moniliformis A25.1
Streptococcus, streptococcal —*see also*
  condition
  as cause of disease classified elsewhere
    B95.5
  group
    A, as cause of disease classified elsewhere
      B95.0
    B, as cause of disease classified elsewhere
      B95.1
    D, as cause of disease classified elsewhere
      B95.2
  pneumoniae, as cause of disease classified
    elsewhere B95.3
  specified NEC, as cause of disease classified
    elsewhere B95.4
Streptomycosis B47.1
Streptotrichosis A48.8
Stress F43.9
  family —*see* Disruption, family
  fetal P84
    complicating pregnancy O77.9
      due to drug administration O77.1
  mental NEC Z73.3
    work-related Z56.6
  physical NEC Z73.3
    work-related Z56.6
  polycythemia D75.1
  reaction (*see also* Reaction, stress) F43.9
  work schedule Z56.3
Stretching, nerve —*see* Injury, nerve
Striae albicantes, atrophicae or distensae
  (cutis) L90.6
Stricture —*see also* Stenosis
  ampulla of Vater K83.1
  anus (sphincter) K62.4
    congenital Q42.3
      with fistula Q42.2
    infantile Q42.3
      with fistula Q42.2
  aorta (ascending) (congenital) Q25.3
    arteriosclerotic I70.0
    calcified I70.0
    supravalvular, congenital Q25.3
  aortic (valve) —*see* Stenosis, aortic
  aqueduct of Sylvius (congenital) Q03.0
    with spina bifida —*see* Spina bifida, by site,
      with hydrocephalus
    acquired G91.1
  artery I77.1
    basilar —*see* Occlusion, artery, basilar
    carotid —*see* Occlusion, artery, carotid
    celiac I77.4
    congenital (peripheral) Q27.8
      cerebral Q28.3
      coronary Q24.5
      digestive system Q27.8
      lower limb Q27.8
      retinal Q14.1
      specified site NEC Q27.8
      umbilical Q27.0
      upper limb Q27.8

Stricture *(Continued)*
  artery *(Continued)*
    coronary —*see* Disease, heart, ischemic, atherosclerotic
      congenital Q24.5
    precerebral —*see* Occlusion, artery, precerebral
    pulmonary (congenital) Q25.6
      acquired I28.8
    renal I70.1
    vertebral —*see* Occlusion, artery, vertebral
  auditory canal (external) (congenital)
    acquired —*see* Stenosis, external ear canal
  bile duct (common) (hepatic) K83.1
    congenital Q44.3
    postoperative K91.89
  bladder N32.89
    neck N32.0
  bowel —*see* Obstruction, intestine
  brain G93.89
  bronchus J98.09
    congenital Q32.3
    syphilitic A52.72
  cardia (stomach) K22.2
    congenital Q39.3
  cardiac —*see also* Disease, heart
    orifice (stomach) K22.2
  cecum —*see* Obstruction, intestine
  cervix, cervical (canal) N88.2
    congenital Q51.828
    in pregnancy —*see* Pregnancy, complicated by, abnormal cervix
      causing obstructed labor O65.5
  colon —*see also* Obstruction, intestine
    congenital Q42.9
      specified NEC Q42.8
  colostomy K94.03
  common (bile) duct K83.1
  coronary (artery) —*see* Disease, heart, ischemic, atherosclerotic
  cystic duct —*see* Obstruction, gallbladder
  digestive organs NEC, congenital Q45.8
  duodenum K31.5
    congenital Q41.0
  ear canal (external) (congenital) Q16.1
    acquired —*see* Stricture, auditory canal, acquired
  ejaculatory duct N50.8
  enterostomy K94.13
  esophagus K22.2
    congenital Q39.3
    syphilitic A52.79
      congenital A50.59 *[K23]*
  eustachian tube —*see also* Obstruction, eustachian tube
    congenital Q17.8
  fallopian tube N97.1
    gonococcal A54.24
    tuberculous A18.17
  gallbladder —*see* Obstruction, gallbladder
  glottis J38.6
  heart —*see also* Disease, heart
    valve (*see also* Endocarditis) I38
      aortic Q23.0
      mitral Q23.4
      pulmonary Q22.1
      tricuspid Q22.4
  hepatic duct K83.1
  hourglass, of stomach K31.2
  hymen N89.6
  hypopharynx J39.2
  ileum K56.69
    congenital Q41.2
  intestine —*see also* Obstruction, intestine
    congenital (small) Q41.9
      large Q42.9
        specified NEC Q42.8
      specified NEC Q41.8
    ischemic K55.1
  jejunum K56.69
    congenital Q41.1

Stricture *(Continued)*
  lacrimal passages —*see also* Stenosis, lacrimal
    congenital Q10.5
  larynx J38.6
    congenital NEC Q31.8
      subglottic Q31.1
    syphilitic A52.73
      congenital A50.59 *[J99]*
  meatus
    ear (congenital) Q16.1
      acquired —*see* Stricture, auditory canal, acquired
    osseous (ear) (congenital) Q16.1
      acquired —*see* Stricture, auditory canal, acquired
    urinarius —*see also* Stricture, urethra
      congenital Q64.33
  mitral (valve) —*see* Stenosis, mitral
  myocardium, myocardial I51.5
    hypertrophic subaortic (idiopathic) I42.1
  nares (anterior) (posterior) J34.89
    congenital Q30.0
  nasal duct —*see also* Stenosis, lacrimal, duct
    congenital Q10.5
  nasolacrimal duct —*see also* Stenosis, lacrimal, duct
    congenital Q10.5
  nasopharynx J39.2
    syphilitic A52.73
  nose J34.89
    congenital Q30.0
  nostril (anterior) (posterior) J34.89
    congenital Q30.0
    syphilitic A52.73
      congenital A50.59 *[J99]*
  organ or site, congenital NEC —*see* Atresia, by site
  os uteri —*see* Stricture, cervix
  osseous meatus (ear) (congenital) Q16.1
    acquired —*see* Stricture, auditory canal, acquired
  oviduct —*see* Stricture, fallopian tube
  pelviureteric junction (congenital) Q62.11
  penis, by foreign body T19.4
  pharynx J39.2
  prostate N42.89
  pulmonary, pulmonic
    artery (congenital) Q25.6
      acquired I28.8
      noncongenital I28.8
    infundibulum (congenital) Q24.3
    valve I37.0
      congenital Q22.1
    vein, acquired I28.8
    vessel NEC I28.8
  punctum lacrimale —*see also* Stenosis, lacrimal, punctum
    congenital Q10.5
  pylorus (hypertrophic) K31.1
    adult K31.1
    congenital Q40.0
    infantile Q40.0
  rectosigmoid K56.69
  rectum (sphincter) K62.4
    congenital Q42.1
      with fistula Q42.0
    due to
      chlamydial lymphogranuloma A55
      irradiation K91.89
      lymphogranuloma venereum A55
    gonococcal A54.6
    inflammatory (chlamydial) A55
    syphilitic A52.74
    tuberculous A18.32
  renal artery I70.1
    congenital Q27.1
  salivary duct or gland (any) K11.8
  sigmoid (flexure) —*see* Obstruction, intestine
  spermatic cord N50.8

Stricture *(Continued)*
  stoma (following) (of)
    colostomy K94.03
    enterostomy K94.13
    gastrostomy K94.23
    ileostomy K94.13
    tracheostomy J95.03
  stomach K31.89
    congenital Q40.2
    hourglass K31.2
  subaortic Q24.4
    hypertrophic (acquired) (idiopathic) I42.1
  subglottic J38.6
  syphilitic NEC A52.79
  trachea J39.8
    congenital Q32.1
    syphilitic A52.73
    tuberculous NEC A15.5
  tracheostomy J95.03
  tricuspid (valve) —*see* Stenosis, tricuspid
  tunica vaginalis N50.8
  ureter (postoperative) N13.5
    with
      hydronephrosis N13.1
        with infection N13.6
      pyelonephritis (chronic) N11.1
    congenital —*see* Atresia, ureter
    tuberculous A18.11
  ureteropelvic junction (congenital) Q62.11
  ureterovesical orifice N13.5
    with infection N13.6
  urethra (organic) (spasmodic) N35.9
    associated with schistosomiasis B65.0 *[N37]*
    congenital Q64.39
      valvular (posterior) Q64.2
    due to
      infection —*see* Stricture, urethra, postinfective
      trauma —*see* Stricture, urethra, post-traumatic
    gonococcal, gonorrheal A54.01
    infective NEC —*see* Stricture, urethra, postinfective
    late effect (sequelae) of injury —*see* Stricture, urethra, post-traumatic
    postcatheterization —*see* Stricture, urethra, postprocedural
    postinfective NEC
      female N35.12
      male N35.119
        anterior urethra N35.114
        bulbous urethra N35.112
        meatal N35.111
        membranous urethra N35.113
    postobstetric N35.021
    postoperative —*see* Stricture, urethra, postprocedural
    postprocedural
      female N99.12
      male N99.114
        anterior urethra N99.113
        bulbous urethra N99.111
        meatal N99.110
        membranous urethra N99.112
    post-traumatic
      female N35.028
        due to childbirth N35.021
      male N35.014
        anterior urethra N35.013
        bulbous urethra N35.011
        meatal N35.010
        membranous urethra N35.012
    sequela (late effect) of
      childbirth N35.021
      injury —*see* Stricture, urethra, post-traumatic
    specified cause NEC N35.8
    syphilitic A52.76
    traumatic —*see* Stricture, urethra, post-traumatic
    valvular (posterior), congenital Q64.2

Stricture *(Continued)*
    urinary meatus —*see* Stricture, urethra
    uterus, uterine (synechiae) N85.6
        os (external) (internal) —*see* Stricture,
            cervix
    vagina (outlet) —*see* Stenosis, vagina
    valve (cardiac) (heart) —*see also* Endocarditis
        congenital
            aortic Q23.0
            mitral Q23.2
            pulmonary Q22.1
            tricuspid Q22.4
    vas deferens N50.8
        congenital Q55.4
    vein I87.1
    vena cava (inferior) (superior) NEC I87.1
        congenital Q26.0
    vesicourethral orifice N32.0
        congenital Q64.31
    vulva (acquired) N90.5
Stridor R06.1
    congenital (larynx) P28.89
Stridulous —*see* condition
Stroke (apoplectic) (brain) (embolic) (ischemic)
        (paralytic) (thrombotic) I63.9
    epileptic —*see* Epilepsy
    heat T67.0
    in evolution I63.9
    intraoperative
        during cardiac surgery I97.810
        during other surgery I97.811
    lightning —*see* Lightning
    meaning
        cerebral hemorrhage — code to
            Hemorrhage, intracranial
        cerebral infarction — code to Infarction,
            cerebral
    postprocedural
        following cardiac surgery I97.820
        following other surgery I97.821
    unspecified (NOS) I63.9
Stromatosis, endometrial D39.0
Strongyloidiasis, strongyloidosis B78.9
    cutaneous B78.1
    disseminated B78.7
    intestinal B78.0
Strophulus pruriginosus L28.2
Struck by lightning —*see* Lightning
Struma —*see also* Goiter
    Hashimoto E06.3
    lymphomatosa E06.3
    nodosa (simplex) E04.9
        endemic E01.2
            multinodular E01.1
        multinodular E04.2
            iodine-deficiency related E01.1
        toxic or with hyperthyroidism E05.20
            with thyroid storm E05.21
            multinodular E05.20
                with thyroid storm E05.21
            uninodular E05.10
                with thyroid storm E05.11
        toxicosa E05.20
            with thyroid storm E05.21
            multinodular E05.20
                with thyroid storm E05.21
            uninodular E05.10
                with thyroid storm E05.11
        uninodular E04.1
    ovarii D27.-
    Riedel's E06.5
Strumipriva cachexia E03.4
Strümpell-Marie spine —*see* Spondylitis,
        ankylosing
Strümpell-Westphal pseudosclerosis E83.01
Stuart deficiency disease (factor X) D68.2
Stuart-Prower factor deficiency (factor X)
        D68.2
Student's elbow —*see* Bursitis, elbow,
        olecranon
Stump —*see* Amputation

Stunting, nutritional E45
Stupor (catatonic) R40.1
    depressive F32.8
    dissociative F44.2
    manic F30.2
    manic-depressive F31.89
    psychogenic (anergic) F44.2
    reaction to exceptional stress (transient)
        F43.0
Sturge (-Weber) (-Dimitri) (-Kalischer) **disease
    or syndrome** Q85.8
Stuttering F80.81
    adult onset F98.5
    childhood onset F80.81
    following cerebrovascular disease —
        see Disorder, fluency, following
        cerebrovascular disease
    in conditions classified elsewhere R47.82
Sty, stye (external) (internal) (meibomian)
        (zeisian) —*see* Hordeolum
Subacidity, gastric K31.89
    psychogenic F45.8
Subacute —*see* condition
Subarachnoid —*see* condition
Subcortical —*see* condition
Subcostal syndrome, nerve compression —*see*
        Mononeuropathy, upper limb, specified
        site NEC
Subcutaneous, subcuticular —*see* condition
Subdural —*see* condition
Subendocardium —*see* condition
Subependymoma
    specified site —*see* Neoplasm, uncertain
        behavior, by site
    unspecified site D43.2
Suberosis J67.3
Subglossitis —*see* Glossitis
Subhemophilia D66
Subinvolution
    breast (postlactational) (postpuerperal)
        N64.89
    puerperal O90.89
    uterus (chronic) (nonpuerperal) N85.3
        puerperal O90.89
Sublingual —*see* condition
Sublinguitis —*see* Sialoadenitis
Subluxatable hip Q65.6
Subluxation —*see also* Dislocation
    acromioclavicular S43.11-
    ankle S93.0-
    atlantoaxial, recurrent M43.4
        with myelopathy M43.3
    carpometacarpal (joint) NEC S63.05-
        thumb S63.04-
    complex, vertebral —*see* Complex,
        subluxation
    congenital —*see also* Malposition,
        congenital
        hip —*see* Dislocation, hip, congenital,
            partial
        joint (excluding hip)
            lower limb Q68.8
            shoulder Q68.8
            upper limb Q68.8
    elbow (traumatic) S53.10-
        anterior S53.11-
        lateral S53.14-
        medial S53.13-
        posterior S53.12-
        specified type NEC S53.19-
    finger S63.20-
        index S63.20-
        interphalangeal S63.22-
            distal S63.24-
                index S63.24-
                little S63.24-
                middle S63.24-
                ring S63.24-
            index S63.22-
            little S63.22-
            middle S63.22-

Subluxation *(Continued)*
    finger *(Continued)*
        interphalangeal *(Continued)*
            proximal S63.23-
                index S63.23-
                little S63.23-
                middle S63.23-
                ring S63.23-
            ring S63.22-
        little S63.20-
        metacarpophalangeal S63.21-
            index S63.21-
            little S63.21-
            middle S63.21-
            ring S63.21-
        middle S63.20-
        ring S63.20-
    foot S93.30-
        specified site NEC S93.33-
        tarsal joint S93.31-
        tarsometatarsal joint S93.32-
        toe —*see* Subluxation, toe
    hip S73.00-
        anterior S73.03-
            obturator S73.02-
        central S73.04-
        posterior S73.01-
    interphalangeal (joint)
        finger S63.22-
            distal joint S63.24-
                index S63.24-
                little S63.24-
                middle S63.24-
                ring S63.24-
            index S63.22-
            little S63.22-
            middle S63.22-
            proximal joint S63.23-
                index S63.23-
                little S63.23-
                middle S63.23-
                ring S63.23-
            ring S63.22-
        thumb S63.12-
            distal joint S63.14-
            proximal joint S63.13-
        toe S93.13-
            great S93.13-
            lesser S93.13-
    joint prosthesis —*see* Complications, joint
        prosthesis, mechanical, displacement,
        by site
    knee S83.10-
        cap —*see* Subluxation, patella
        patella —*see* Subluxation, patella
        proximal tibia
            anteriorly S83.11-
            laterally S83.14-
            medially S83.13-
            posteriorly S83.12-
        specified type NEC S83.19-
    lens —*see* Dislocation, lens, partial
    ligament, traumatic —*see* Sprain, by site
    metacarpal (bone)
        proximal end S63.06-
    metacarpophalangeal (joint)
        finger S63.21-
            index S63.21-
            little S63.21-
            middle S63.21-
            ring S63.21-
        thumb S63.11-
    metatarsophalangeal joint S93.14-
        great toe S93.14-
        lesser toe S93.14-
    midcarpal (joint) S63.03-
    patella S83.00-
        lateral S83.01-
        recurrent (nontraumatic) —*see* Dislocation,
            patella, recurrent, incomplete
        specified type NEC S83.09-

◀ New   ◀▥ Revised   ~~deleted~~ Deleted

Subluxation (Continued)
  pathological —see Dislocation, pathological
  radial head S53.00-
    anterior S53.01-
    nursemaid's elbow S53.03-
    posterior S53.02-
    specified type NEC S53.09-
  radiocarpal (joint) S63.02-
  radioulnar (joint)
    distal S63.01-
    proximal —see Subluxation, elbow
  shoulder
    congenital Q68.8
    girdle S43.30-
      scapula S43.31-
      specified site NEC S43.39-
    traumatic S43.00-
      anterior S43.01-
      inferior S43.03-
      posterior S43.02-
      specified type NEC S43.08-
  sternoclavicular (joint) S43.20-
    anterior S43.21-
    posterior S43.22-
  symphysis (pubis)
  thumb S63.103
    interphalangeal joint —see Subluxation,
        interphalangeal (joint), thumb
    metacarpophalangeal joint —see
        Subluxation, metacarpophalangeal
        (joint), thumb
  toe (s) S93.10-
    great S93.10-
      interphalangeal joint S93.13-
      metatarsophalangeal joint S93.14-
    interphalangeal joint S93.13-
    lesser S93.10-
      interphalangeal joint S93.13-
      metatarsophalangeal joint S93.14-
    metatarsophalangeal joint S93.149
  ulnohumeral joint —see Subluxation, elbow
  vertebral
    recurrent NEC —see subcategory M43.5
    traumatic
      cervical S13.100
        atlantoaxial joint S13.120
        atlantooccipital joint S13.110
        atloidooccipital joint S13.110
        joint between
          C0 and C1 S13.110
          C1 and C2 S13.120
          C2 and C3 S13.130
          C3 and C4 S13.140
          C4 and C5 S13.150
          C5 and C6 S13.160
          C6 and C7 S13.170
          C7 and T1 S13.180
        occipitoatloid joint S13.110
      lumbar S33.100
        joint between
          L1 and L2 S33.110
          L2 and L3 S33.120
          L3 and L4 S33.130
          L4 and L5 S33.140
      thoracic S23.100
        joint between
          T1 and T2 S23.110
          T2 and T3 S23.120
          T3 and T4 S23.122
          T4 and T5 S23.130
          T5 and T6 S23.132
          T6 and T7 S23.140
          T7 and T8 S23.142
          T8 and T9 S23.150
          T9 and T10 S23.152
          T10 and T11 S23.160
          T11 and T12 S23.162
          T12 and L1 S23.170
  ulna
    distal end S63.07-
    proximal end —see Subluxation, elbow

Subluxation (Continued)
  wrist (carpal bone) S63.00-
    carpometacarpal joint —see Subluxation,
        carpometacarpal (joint)
    distal radioulnar joint —see Subluxation,
        radioulnar (joint), distal
    metacarpal bone, proximal —see
        Subluxation, metacarpal (bone),
        proximal end
    midcarpal —see Subluxation, midcarpal
        (joint)
    radiocarpal joint —see Subluxation,
        radiocarpal (joint)
    recurrent —see Dislocation, recurrent, wrist
    specified site NEC S63.09-
    ulna —see Subluxation, ulna, distal end
Submaxillary —see condition
Submersion (fatal) (nonfatal) T75.1
Submucous —see condition
Subnormal, subnormality
  accommodation (old age) H52.4
  mental —see Disability, intellectual
  temperature (accidental) T68
Subphrenic —see condition
Subscapular nerve —see condition
Subseptus uterus Q51.2
Subsiding appendicitis K36
Substernal thyroid E04.9
  congenital Q89.2
Substitution disorder F44.9
Subtentorial —see condition
Subthyroidism (acquired) —see also
    Hypothyroidism
  congenital E03.1
Succenturiate placenta O43.19-
Sucking thumb, child (excessive) F98.8
Sudamen, sudamina L74.1
Sudanese kala-azar B55.0
Sudden
  hearing loss —see Deafness, sudden
  heart failure —see Failure, heart
Sudeck's atrophy, disease, or syndrome —see
    Algoneurodystrophy
Suffocation —see Asphyxia, traumatic
Sugar
  blood
    high (transient) R73.9
    low (transient) E16.2
  in urine R81
Suicide, suicidal (attempted) T14.91
  by poisoning —see Table of Drugs and
      Chemicals
  history of (personal) Z91.5
    in family Z81.8
  ideation —see Ideation, suicidal
  risk
    meaning personal history of attempted
        suicide Z91.5
    meaning suicidal ideation —see Ideation,
        suicidal
  tendencies
    meaning personal history of attempted
        suicide Z91.5
    meaning suicidal ideation —see Ideation,
        suicidal
  trauma —see nature of injury by site
Suipestifer infection —see Infection, salmonella
Sulfhemoglobinemia, sulphemoglobinemia
    (acquired) (with methemoglobinemia)
    D74.8
Sumatran mite fever A75.3
Summer —see condition
Sunburn L55.9
  first degree L55.0
  second degree L55.1
  third degree L55.2
SUNCT (short lasting unilateral neuralgiform
    headache with conjunctival injection and
    tearing) G44.059
  intractable G44.051
  not intractable G44.059

Sunken acetabulum —see Derangement, joint,
    specified type NEC, hip
Sunstroke T67.0
Superfecundation —see Pregnancy,
    multiple
Superfetation —see Pregnancy, multiple
Superinvolution (uterus) N85.8
Supernumerary (congenital)
  aortic cusps Q23.8
  auditory ossicles Q16.3
  bone Q79.8
  breast Q83.1
  carpal bones Q74.0
  cusps, heart valve NEC Q24.8
    aortic Q23.8
    mitral Q23.2
    pulmonary Q22.3
  digit (s) Q69.9
  ear (lobule) Q17.0
  fallopian tube Q50.6
  finger Q69.0
  hymen Q52.4
  kidney Q63.0
  lacrimonasal duct Q10.6
  lobule (ear) Q17.0
  mitral cusps Q23.2
  muscle Q79.8
  nipple (s) Q83.3
  organ or site not listed —see Accessory
  ossicles, auditory Q16.3
  ovary Q50.31
  oviduct Q50.6
  pulmonary, pulmonic cusps Q22.3
  rib Q76.6
    cervical or first (syndrome) Q76.5
  roots (of teeth) K00.2
  spleen Q89.09
  tarsal bones Q74.2
  teeth K00.1
  testis Q55.29
  thumb Q69.1
  toe Q69.2
  uterus Q51.2
  vagina Q52.1
  vertebra Q76.49
Supervision (of)
  contraceptive —see Prescription,
      contraceptives
  dietary (for) Z71.3
    allergy (food) Z71.3
    colitis Z71.3
    diabetes mellitus Z71.3
    food allergy or intolerance Z71.3
    gastritis Z71.3
    hypercholesterolemia Z71.3
    hypoglycemia Z71.3
    intolerance (food) Z71.3
    obesity Z71.3
    specified NEC Z71.3
  healthy infant or child Z76.2
    foundling Z76.1
  high-risk pregnancy —see Pregnancy,
      complicated by, high, risk
  lactation Z39.1
  pregnancy —see Pregnancy, supervision of
Supplemental teeth K00.1
Suppression
  binocular vision H53.34
  lactation O92.5
  menstruation N94.89
  ovarian secretion E28.39
  renal N28.9
  urine, urinary secretion R34
Suppuration, suppurative —see also condition
  accessory sinus (chronic) —see Sinusitis
  adrenal gland
  antrum (chronic) —see Sinusitis,
      maxillary
  bladder —see Cystitis
  brain G06.0
    sequelae G09

Suppuration, suppurative *(Continued)*
  breast N61
    puerperal, postpartum or gestational —*see*
      Mastitis, obstetric, purulent
  dental periosteum M27.3
  ear (middle) —*see also* Otitis, media
    external NEC —*see* Otitis, externa,
      infective
    internal —*see* subcategory H83.0
  ethmoidal (chronic) (sinus) —*see* Sinusitis,
    ethmoidal
  fallopian tube —*see* Salpingo-oophoritis
  frontal (chronic) (sinus) —*see* Sinusitis,
    frontal
  gallbladder (acute) K81.0
  gum K05.20
    generalized K05.22
    localized K05.21
  intracranial G06.0
  joint —*see* Arthritis, pyogenic or pyemic
  labyrinthine —*see* subcategory H83.0
  lung —*see* Abscess, lung
  mammary gland N61
    puerperal, postpartum O91.12
      associated with lactation O91.13
  maxilla, maxillary M27.2
    sinus (chronic) —*see* Sinusitis, maxillary
  muscle —*see* Myositis, infective
  nasal sinus (chronic) —*see* Sinusitis
  pancreas, acute K85.8
  parotid gland —*see* Sialoadenitis
  pelvis, pelvic
    female —*see* Disease, pelvis, inflammatory
    male K65.0
  pericranial —*see* Osteomyelitis
  salivary duct or gland (any) —*see*
    Sialoadenitis
  sinus (accessory) (chronic) (nasal) —*see*
    Sinusitis
  sphenoidal sinus (chronic) —*see* Sinusitis,
    sphenoidal
  thymus (gland) E32.1
  thyroid (gland) E06.0
  tonsil —*see* Tonsillitis
  uterus —*see* Endometritis
Supraeruption of tooth (teeth) M26.34
Supraglottitis J04.30
  with obstruction J04.31
Suprarenal (gland) —*see* condition
Suprascapular nerve —*see* condition
Suprasellar —*see* condition
Surfer's knots or nodules S89.8-
Surgical
  emphysema T81.82
  procedures, complication or misadventure —
    see Complications, surgical procedures
  shock T81.10
Surveillance (of) (for) —*see also* Observation
  alcohol abuse Z71.41
  contraceptive —*see* Prescription,
    contraceptives
  dietary Z71.3
  drug abuse Z71.51
Susceptibility to disease, genetic Z15.89
  malignant neoplasm Z15.09
    breast Z15.01
    endometrium Z15.04
    ovary Z15.02
    prostate Z15.03
    specified NEC Z15.09
  multiple endocrine neoplasia Z15.81
Suspected condition, ruled out —*see also*
  Observation, suspected
  amniotic cavity and membrane Z03.71
  cervical shortening Z03.75
  fetal anomaly Z03.73
  fetal growth Z03.74
  maternal and fetal conditions NEC Z03.79
  oligohydramnios Z03.71
  placental problem Z03.72
  polyhydramnios Z03.71

Suspended uterus
  in pregnancy or childbirth —*see* Pregnancy,
    complicated by, abnormal uterus
Sutton's nevus D22.9
Suture
  burst (in operation wound) T81.31
    external operation wound T81.31
    internal operation wound T81.32
  inadvertently left in operation wound —*see*
    Foreign body, accidentally left during a
    procedure
  removal Z48.02
Swab inadvertently left in operation wound —
  see Foreign body, accidentally left during
  a procedure
Swallowed, swallowing
  difficulty —*see* Dysphagia
  foreign body —*see* Foreign body, alimentary
    tract
Swan-neck deformity (finger) —*see* Deformity,
  finger, swan-neck
Swearing, compulsive F42
  in Gilles de la Tourette's syndrome F95.2
Sweat, sweats
  fetid L75.0
  night R61
Sweating, excessive R61
Sweeley-Klionsky disease E75.21
Sweet's disease or dermatosis L98.2
Swelling (of) R60.9
  abdomen, abdominal (not referable to any
    particular organ) —*see* Mass,
    abdominal
  ankle —*see* Effusion, joint, ankle
  arm M79.89
    forearm M79.89
  breast N63
  Calabar B74.3
  cervical gland R59.0
  chest, localized R22.2
  ear H93.8-
  extremity (lower) (upper) —*see* Disorder, soft
    tissue, specified type NEC
  finger M79.89
  foot M79.89
  glands R59.9
    generalized R59.1
    localized R59.0
  hand M79.89
  head (localized) R22.0
  inflammatory —*see* Inflammation
  intra-abdominal —*see* Mass, abdominal
  joint —*see* Effusion, joint
  leg M79.89
    lower M79.89
  limb —*see* Disorder, soft tissue, specified type
    NEC
  localized (skin) R22.9
    chest R22.2
    head R22.0
    limb
      lower —*see* Mass, localized, limb,
        lower
      upper —*see* Mass, localized, limb,
        upper
    neck R22.1
    trunk R22.2
  neck (localized) R22.1
  pelvic —*see* Mass, abdominal
  scrotum N50.8
  splenic —*see* Splenomegaly
  testis N50.8
  toe M79.89
  umbilical R19.09
  wandering, due to Gnathostoma
    (spinigerum) B83.1
  white —*see* Tuberculosis, arthritis
Swift (-Feer) disease
  overdose or wrong substance given or
    taken —*see* Table of Drugs and
    Chemicals, by drug, poisoning

Swimmer's
  cramp T75.1
  ear H60.33-
  itch B65.3
Swimming in the head R42
Swollen —*see* Swelling
Swyer syndrome Q99.1
Sycosis L73.8
  barbae (not parasitic) L73.8
  contagiosa (mycotic) B35.0
  lupoides L73.8
  mycotic B35.0
  parasitic B35.0
  vulgaris L73.8
Sydenham's chorea —*see* Chorea, Sydenham's
Sylvatic yellow fever A95.0
Sylvest's disease B33.0
Symblepharon H11.23-
  congenital Q10.3
Symond's syndrome G93.2
Sympathetic —*see* condition
Sympatheticotonia G90.8
Sympathicoblastoma
  specified site —*see* Neoplasm, malignant, by
    site
  unspecified site C74.90
Sympathogonioma —*see* Sympathicoblastoma
Symphalangy (fingers) (toes) Q70.9
Symptoms NEC R68.89
  breast NEC N64.59
  development NEC R63.8
  factitious, self-induced —*see* Disorder,
    factitious
  genital organs, female R10.2
  involving
    abdomen NEC R19.8
    appearance NEC R46.89
    awareness R41.9
      altered mental status R41.82
      amnesia —*see* Amnesia
      borderline intellectual functioning
        R41.83
      coma —*see* Coma
      disorientation R41.0
      neurologic neglect syndrome R41.4
      senile cognitive decline R41.81
      specified symptom NEC R41.89
    behavior NEC R46.89
    cardiovascular system NEC R09.89
    chest NEC R09.89
    circulatory system NEC R09.89
    cognitive functions R41.9
      altered mental status R41.82
      amnesia —*see* Amnesia
      borderline intellectual functioning
        R41.83
      coma —*see* Coma
      disorientation R41.0
      neurologic neglect syndrome R41.4
      senile cognitive decline R41.81
      specified symptom NEC R41.89
    development NEC R62.50
    digestive system NEC R19.8
    emotional state NEC R45.89
      emotional lability R45.86
    food and fluid intake R63.8
    general perceptions and sensations
      R44.9
      specified NEC R44.8
    musculoskeletal system R29.91
      specified NEC R29.898
    nervous system R29.90
      specified NEC R29.818
    pelvis NEC R19.8
    respiratory system NEC R09.89
    skin and integument R23.9
    urinary system R39.9
  menopausal N95.1
  metabolism NEC R63.8
  neurotic F48.8
  of infancy R68.19

◀ New   ◀◀◀ Revised   ~~deleted~~ Deleted

Symptoms NEC *(Continued)*
  pelvis NEC, female R10.2
  skin and integument NEC R23.9
  subcutaneous tissue NEC R23.9
Sympus Q74.2
Syncephalus Q89.4
Synchondrosis
  abnormal (congenital) Q78.8
  ischiopubic M91.0
Synchysis (scintillans) (senile) (vitreous body)
    H43.89
Syncope (near) (pre-) R55
  anginosa I20.8
  bradycardia R00.1
  cardiac R55
  carotid sinus G90.01
  due to spinal (lumbar) puncture G97.1
  heart R55
  heat T67.1
  laryngeal R05
  psychogenic F48.8
  tussive R05
  vasoconstriction R55
  vasodepressor R55
  vasomotor R55
  vasovagal R55
Syndactylism, syndactyly Q70.9
  complex (with synostosis)
    fingers Q70.0-
    toes Q70.2-
  simple (without synostosis)
    fingers Q70.1-
    toes Q70.3-
Syndrome —*see also* Disease
  5q minus NOS D46.C
  48,XXXX Q97.1
  49,XXXXX Q97.1
  abdominal
    acute R10.0
    muscle deficiency Q79.4
  abnormal innervation H02.519
    left H02.516
      lower H02.515
      upper H02.514
    right H02.513
      lower H02.512
      upper H02.511
  abstinence, neonatal P96.1
  acid pulmonary aspiration, obstetric O74.0
  acquired immunodeficiency —*see* Human,
      immunodeficiency virus (HIV)
      disease
  acute abdominal R10.0
  acute respiratory distress (adult) (child) J80
  Adair-Dighton Q78.0
  Adams-Stokes (-Morgagni) I45.9
  adiposogenital E23.6
  adrenal
    hemorrhage (meningococcal) A39.1
    meningococcic A39.1
  adrenocortical —*see* Cushing's, syndrome
  adrenogenital E25.9
    congenital, associated with enzyme
      deficiency E25.0
  afferent loop NEC K91.89
  Alagille's Q44.7
  alcohol withdrawal (without convulsions) —
      see Dependence, alcohol, with,
      withdrawal
  Alder's D72.0
  Aldrich (-Wiskott) D82.0
  alien hand R41.4
  Alport Q87.81
  alveolar hypoventilation E66.2
  alveolocapillary block J84.10
  amnesic, amnestic (confabulatory) (due to) —
      see Disorder, amnesic
  amyostatic (Wilson's disease) E83.01
  androgen insensitivity E34.50
    complete E34.51
    partial E34.52

Syndrome *(Continued)*
  androgen resistance (*see also* Syndrome,
      androgen insensitivity) E34.50
  Angelman Q93.5
  anginal —*see* Angina
  ankyloglossia superior Q38.1
  anterior
    chest wall R07.89
    cord G83.82
    spinal artery G95.19
      compression M47.019
        cervical region M47.012
        cervicothoracic region M47.013
        lumbar region M47.016
        occipito-atlanto-axial region M47.011
        thoracic region M47.014
        thoracolumbar region M47.015
    tibial M76.81-
  antibody deficiency D80.9
    agammaglobulinemic D80.1
      hereditary D80.0
    congenital D80.0
    hypogammaglobulinemic D80.1
      hereditary D80.0
  anticardiolipin (-antibody) D68.61
  antiphospholipid (-antibody) D68.61
  aortic
    arch M31.4
    bifurcation I74.09
  aortomesenteric duodenum occlusion K31.5
  apical ballooning (transient left ventricular)
      I51.81
  arcuate ligament I77.4
  argentaffin, argintaffinoma E34.0
  Arnold-Chiari —*see* Arnold-Chiari disease
  Arrillaga-Ayerza I27.0
  Asherman's N85.6
  aspiration, of newborn —*see* Aspiration, by
      substance, with pneumonia
    meconium P24.01
  ataxia-telangiectasia G11.3
  auriculotemporal G50.8
  autoerythrocyte sensitization (Gardner-
      Diamond) D69.2
  autoimmune lymphoproliferative [ALPS]
      D89.82
  autoimmune polyglandular E31.0
  autosomal —*see* Abnormal, autosomes
  Avellis' G46.8
  Ayerza (-Arrillaga) I27.0
  Babinski-Nageotte G83.89
  Bakwin-Krida Q79.8
  bare lymphocyte D81.6
  Barré-Guillain G61.0
  Barré-Liéou M53.0
  Barrett's —*see* Barrett's, esophagus
  Barsony-Polgar K22.4
  Barsony-Teschendorf K22.4
  Barth E78.71
  Bartter's E26.81
  basal cell nevus Q87.89
  Basedow's E05.00
    with thyroid storm E05.01
  basilar artery G45.0
  Batten-Steinert G71.11
  battered
    baby or child —*see* Maltreatment, child,
      physical abuse
    spouse —*see* Maltreatment, adult, physical
      abuse
  Beals Q87.40
  Beau's I51.5
  Beck's I65.8
  Benedikt's G46.3
  Béquez César (-Steinbrinck-Chédiak-Higashi)
      D70.330
  Bernhardt-Roth —*see* Meralgia paresthetica
  Bernheim's I50.9
  big spleen D73.1
  bilateral polycystic ovarian E28.2
  Bing-Horton's —*see* Horton's headache

Syndrome *(Continued)*
  Birt-Hogg-Dube syndrome Q87.89
  Björck (-Thorsen) E34.0
  black
    lung J60
    widow spider bite —*see* Toxicity, venom,
      spider, black widow
  Blackfan-Diamond D61.01
  blind loop K90.2
    congenital Q43.8
    postsurgical K91.2
  blue sclera Q78.0
  blue toe I75.02-
  Boder-Sedgewick G11.3
  Boerhaave's K22.3
  Borjeson Forssman Lehmann Q89.8
  Bouillaud's I01.9
  Bourneville (-Pringle) Q85.1
  Bouveret (-Hoffman) I47.9
  brachial plexus G54.0
  bradycardia-tachycardia I49.5
  brain (nonpsychotic) F09
    with psychosis, psychotic reaction F09
    acute or subacute —*see* Delirium
    congenital —*see* Disability, intellectual
    organic F09
      post-traumatic (nonpsychotic) F07.81
        psychotic F09
    personality change F07.0
    postcontusional F07.81
    post-traumatic, nonpsychotic F07.81
    psycho-organic F09
    psychotic F06.8
  brain stem stroke G46.3
  Brandt's (acrodermatitis enteropathica) E83.2
  broad ligament laceration N83.8
  Brock's J98.11
  bronze baby P83.8
  Brown-Sequard G83.81
  bubbly lung P27.0
  Buchem's M85.2
  Budd-Chiari I82.0
  bulbar (progressive) G12.22
  Bürger-Grütz E78.3
  Burke's K86.8
  Burnett's (milk-alkali) E83.52
  burning feet E53.9
  Bywaters' T79.5
  Call-Fleming I67.841
  carbohydrate-deficient glycoprotein (CDGS)
      E77.8
  carcinogenic thrombophlebitis I82.1
  carcinoid E34.0
  cardiac asthma I50.1
  cardiacos negros I27.0
  cardiofaciocutaneous Q87.89
  cardiopulmonary-obesity E66.2
  cardiorenal —*see* Hypertension, cardiorenal
  cardiorespiratory distress (idiopathic),
      newborn P22.0
  cardiovascular renal —*see* Hypertension,
      cardiorenal
  carotid
    artery (hemispheric) (internal) G45.1
    body G90.01
    sinus G90.01
  carpal tunnel G56.0-
  Cassidy (-Scholte) E34.0
  cat-cry Q93.4
  cat eye Q92.8
  cauda equina G83.4
  causalgia —*see* Causalgia
  celiac K90.0
    artery compression I77.4
    axis I77.4
  central pain G89.0
  cerebellar
    hereditary G11.9
    stroke G46.4
  cerebellomedullary malformation —*see* Spina
      bifida

Syndrome *(Continued)*
  cerebral
    artery
      anterior G46.1
      middle G46.0
      posterior G46.2
    gigantism E22.0
  cervical (root) M53.1
    disc —*see* Disorder, disc, cervical, with
      neuritis
    fusion Q76.1
    posterior, sympathicus M53.0
    rib Q76.5
    sympathetic paralysis G90.2
  cervicobrachial (diffuse) M53.1
  cervicocranial M53.0
  cervicodorsal outlet G54.2
  cervicothoracic outlet G54.0
  Céstan (-Raymond) I65.8
  Charcot's (angina cruris) (intermittent
    claudication) I73.9
  Charcot-Weiss-Baker G90.09
  CHARGE Q89.8
  Chédiak-Higashi (-Steinbrinck) E70.330
  chest wall R07.1
  Chiari's (hepatic vein thrombosis) I82.0
  Chilaiditi's Q43.3
  child maltreatment —*see* Maltreatment,
    child
  chondrocostal junction M94.0
  chondroectodermal dysplasia Q77.6
  chromosome 4 short arm deletion Q93.3
  chromosome 5 short arm deletion Q93.4
  chronic
    pain G89.4
      personality F68.8
  Clarke-Hadfield K86.8
  Clerambault's automatism G93.89
  Clouston's (hidrotic ectodermal dysplasia)
    Q82.4
  clumsiness, clumsy child F82
  cluster headache G44.009
    intractable G44.001
    not intractable G44.009
  Coffin-Lowry Q89.8
  cold injury (newborn) P80.0
  combined immunity deficiency D81.9
  compartment (deep) (posterior) (traumatic)
    T79.A0
    abdomen T79.A3
    lower extremity (hip, buttock, thigh, leg,
      foot, toes) T79.A2
    nontraumatic
      abdomen M79.A3
      lower extremity (hip, buttock, thigh, leg,
        foot, toes) M79.A2-
      specified site NEC M79.A9
      upper extremity (shoulder, arm, forearm,
        wrist, hand, fingers) M79.A1-
    postprocedural —*see* Syndrome
      compartment, nontraumatic
    specified site NEC T79.A9
    upper extremity (shoulder, arm, forearm,
      wrist, hand, fingers) T79.A1
  complex regional pain —*see* Syndrome, pain,
    complex regional
  compression T79.5
    anterior spinal —*see* Syndrome, anterior,
      spinal artery, compression
    cauda equina G83.4
    celiac artery I77.4
    vertebral artery M47.029
      cervical region M47.022
      occipito-atlanto-axial region M47.021
  concussion F07.81
  congenital
    affecting multiple systems NEC Q87.89
    central alveolar hypoventilation G47.35
    facial diplegia Q87.0
    muscular hypertrophy-cerebral Q87.89
    oculo-auriculovertebral Q87.0

Syndrome *(Continued)*
  congenital *(Continued)*
    oculofacial diplegia (Moebius) Q87.0
    rubella (manifest) P35.0
  congestion-fibrosis (pelvic), female N94.89
  congestive dysmenorrhea N94.6
  Conn's E26.01
  connective tissue M35.9
    overlap NEC M35.1
  conus medullaris G95.81
  cord
    anterior G83.82
    posterior G83.83
  coronary
    acute NEC I24.9
    insufficiency or intermediate I20.0
    slow flow I20.8
  Costen's (complex) M26.69
  costochondral junction M94.0
  costoclavicular G54.0
  costovertebral E22.0
  Cowden Q85.8
  craniovertebral M53.0
  Creutzfeldt-Jakob —*see* Creutzfeldt-Jakob
    disease or syndrome
  cri-du-chat Q93.4
  crib death R99
  cricopharyngeal —*see* Dysphagia
  croup J05.0
  CRPS I —*see* Syndrome, pain, complex
    regional I
  crush T79.5
  cryptophthalmos Q87.0
  cubital tunnel —*see* Lesion, nerve, ulnar
  Curschmann (-Batten) (-Steinert) G71.11
  Cushing's E24.9
    alcohol-induced E24.4
    drug-induced E24.2
    due to
      alcohol
      drugs E24.2
      ectopic ACTH E24.3
      overproduction of pituitary ACTH E24.0
    overdose or wrong substance given or
      taken —*see* Table of Drugs and
      Chemicals, by drug, poisoning
    pituitary-dependent E24.0
    specified type NEC E24.8
  cystic duct stump K91.5
  Dana-Putnam D51.0
  Danbolt (-Cross) (acrodermatitis
    enteropathica) E83.2
  Dandy-Walker Q03.1
    with spina bifida Q07.01
  Danlos' Q79.8
  defibrination —*see also* Fibrinolysis
    with
      antepartum hemorrhage —*see*
        Hemorrhage, antepartum, with
        coagulation defect
      intrapartum hemorrhage —*see*
        Hemorrhage, complicating,
        delivery
      newborn P60
      postpartum O72.3
  Degos' I77.8
  Déjérine-Roussy G89.0
  delayed sleep phase G47.21
  demyelinating G37.9
  dependence —*see* F10-F19 with fourth
    character .2
  depersonalization (-derealization) F48.1
  De Quervain E34.51
  de Toni-Fanconi (-Debré) E72.09
    with cystinosis E72.04
  diabetes mellitus-hypertension-nephrosis —
    see Diabetes, nephrosis
  diabetes mellitus in newborn infant P70.2
  diabetes-nephrosis —*see* Diabetes, nephrosis
  diabetic amyotrophy —*see* Diabetes,
    amyotrophy

Syndrome *(Continued)*
  Diamond-Blackfan D61.01
  Diamond-Gardener D69.2
  DIC (diffuse or disseminated intravascular
    coagulopathy) D65
  di George's D82.1
  Dighton's Q78.0
  disequilibrium E87.8
  Döhle body-panmyelopathic D72.0
  dorsolateral medullary G46.4
  double athetosis G80.3
  Down (*see also* Down syndrome) Q90.9
  Dresbach's (elliptocytosis) D58.1
  Dressler's (postmyocardial infarction)
    I24.1
    postcardiotomy I97.0
  drug withdrawal, infant of dependent mother
    P96.1
  dry eye H04.12-
  due to abnormality
    chromosomal Q99.9
      sex
        female phenotype Q97.9
        male phenotype Q98.9
      specified NEC Q99.8
  dumping (postgastrectomy) K91.1
    nonsurgical K31.89
  Dupré's (meningism) R29.1
  dysmetabolic X E88.81
  dyspraxia, developmental F82
  Eagle-Barrett Q79.4
  Eaton-Lambert —*see* Syndrome,
    Lambert-Eaton
  Ebstein's Q22.5
  ectopic ACTH E24.3
  eczema-thrombocytopenia D82.0
  Eddowes' Q78.0
  effort (psychogenic) F45.8
  Ehlers-Danlos Q79.6
  Eisenmenger's I27.89
  Ekman's Q78.0
  electric feet E53.8
  Ellis-van Creveld Q77.6
  empty nest Z60.0
  endocrine-hypertensive E27.0
  entrapment —*see* Neuropathy,
    entrapment
  eosinophilia-myalgia M35.8
  epileptic —*see also* Epilepsy, by type
    absence G40.A09
      intractable G40.A19
        with status epilepticus G40.A11
        without status epilepticus G40.A19
      not intractable G40.A09
        with status epilepticus G40.A01
        without status epilepticus G40.A09
  Erdheim-Chester (ECD) E88.89
  Erdheim's E22.0
  erythrocyte fragmentation D59.4
  Evans D69.41
  exhaustion F48.8
  extrapyramidal G25.9
    specified NEC G25.89
  eye retraction —*see* Strabismus
  eyelid-malar-mandible Q87.0
  Faber's D50.9
  facial pain, paroxysmal G50.0
  Fallot's Q21.3
  familial eczema-thrombocytopenia
    (Wiskott-Aldrich) D82.0
  Fanconi (-de Toni) (-Debré) E72.09
    with cystinosis E72.04
  Fanconi's (anemia) (congenital pancytopenia)
    D61.09
  fatigue
    chronic R53.82
    psychogenic F48.8
  faulty bowel habit K59.3
  Feil-Klippel (brevicollis) Q76.1
  Felty's —*see* Felty's syndrome
  fertile eunuch E23.0

◀ New   ◀ Revised   ~~deleted~~ Deleted

Syndrome *(Continued)*
  fetal
    alcohol (dysmorphic) Q86.0
    hydantoin Q86.1
  Fiedler's I40.1
  first arch Q87.0
  fish odor E72.8
  Fisher's G61.0
  Fitzhugh-Curtis
    due to
      Chlamydia trachomatis A74.81
      Neisseria gonorrhorea (gonococcal
        peritonitis) A54.85
  Fitz's K85.8
  Flajani (-Basedow) E05.00
    with thyroid storm E05.01
  flatback —*see* Flatback syndrome
  floppy
    baby P94.2
    iris (intraoeprative) (IFIS) H21.81
    mitral valve I34.1
  flush E34.0
  Foix-Alajouanine G95.19
  Fong's Q79.8
  foramen magnum G93.5
  Foster-Kennedy H47.14-
  Foville's (peduncular) G46.3
  fragile X Q99.2
  Franceschetti Q75.4
  Frey's
    auriculotemporal G50.8
    hyperhidrosis L74.52
  Friderichsen-Waterhouse A39.1
  Froin's G95.89
  frontal lobe F07.0
  Fukuhara E88.49
  functional
    bowel K59.9
    prepubertal castrate E29.1
  Gaisböck's D75.1
  ganglion (basal ganglia brain) G25.9
    geniculi G51.1
  Gardner-Diamond D69.2
  gastroesophageal
    junction K22.0
    laceration-hemorrhage K22.6
  gastrojejunal loop obstruction K91.89
  Gee-Herter-Heubner K90.0
  Gelineau's G47.419
    with cataplexy G47.411
  genito-anorectal A55
  Gerstmann-Sträussler-Scheinker (GSS)
    A81.82
  Gianotti-Crosti L44.4
  giant platelet (Bernard-Soulier) D69.1
  Gilles de la Tourette's F95.2
  goiter-deafness E07.1
  Goldberg Q89.8
  Goldberg-Maxwell E34.51
  Good's D83.8
  Gopalan' (burning feet) E53.8
  Gorlin's Q87.89
  Gougerot-Blum L81.7
  Gouley's I31.1
  Gower's R55
  gray or grey (newborn) P93.0
    platelet D69.1
  Gubler-Millard G46.3
  Guillain-Barré (-Strohl) G61.0
  gustatory sweating G50.8
  Hadfield-Clarke K86.8
  hair tourniquet —*see* Constriction, external,
    by site
  Hamman's J98.19
  hand-foot L27.1
  hand-shoulder G90.8
  hantavirus (cardio)-pulmonary (HPS) (HCPS)
    B33.4
  happy puppet Q93.5
  Harada's H30.81-
  Hayem-Faber D50.9

Syndrome *(Continued)*
  headache NEC G44.89
    complicated NEC G44.59
  Heberden's I20.8
  Hedinger's E34.0
  Hegglin's D72.0
  HELLP (hemolysis, elevated liver enzymes
    and low platelet count) O14.2-
  hemolytic-uremic D59.3
  hemophagocytic, infection-associated
    D76.2
  Henoch-Schönlein D69.0
  hepatic flexure K59.8
  hepatopulmonary K76.81
  hepatorenal K76.7
    following delivery O90.4
    postoperative or postprocedural K91.83
    postpartum, puerperal O90.4
  hepatourologic K76.7
  Herter (-Gee) (nontropical sprue) K90.0
  Heubner-Herter K90.0
  Heyd's K76.7
  Hilger's G90.09
  histamine-like (fish poisoning) —*see*
    Poisoning, fish
  histiocytic D76.3
  histiocytosis NEC D76.3
  HIV infection, acute B20
  Hoffmann-Werdnig G12.0
  Hollander-Simons E88.1
  Hoppe-Goldflam G70.00
    with exacerbation (acute) G70.01
    in crisis G70.01
  Horner's G90.2
  hungry bone E83.81
  hunterian glossitis D51.0
  Hutchinson's triad A50.53
  hyperabduction G54.0
  hyperammonemia-hyperornithinemia-
    homocitrullinemia E72.4
  hypereosinophilic (idiopathic) D72.1
  hyperimmunoglobulin E (IgE) D82.4
  hyperkalemic E87.5
  hyperkinetic —*see* Hyperkinesia
  hypermobility M35.7
  hypernatremia E87.0
  hyperosmolarity E87.0
  hyperperfusion G97.82
  hypersplenic D73.1
  hypertransfusion, newborn P61.1
  hyperventilation F45.8
  hyperviscosity (of serum)
    polycythemic D75.1
    sclerothymic D58.8
  hypoglycemic (familial) (neonatal) E16.2
  hypokalemic E87.6
  hyponatremic E87.1
  hypopituitarism E23.0
  hypoplastic left-heart Q23.4
  hypopotassemia E87.6
  hyposmolality E87.1
  hypotension, maternal O26.5-
  hypothenar hammer I73.89
  ICF (intravascular coagulation-fibrinolysis)
    D65
  idiopathic
    cardiorespiratory distress, newborn P22.0
    nephrotic (infantile) N04.9
  iliotibial band M76.3-
  immobility, immobilization (paraplegic)
    M62.3
  immune reconstitution D89.3
  immune reconstitution inflammatory [IRIS]
    D89.3
  immunity deficiency, combined D81.9
  immunodeficiency
    acquired —*see* Human, immunodeficiency
      virus (HIV) disease
    combined D81.9
  impending coronary I20.0
  impingement, shoulder M75.4-

Syndrome *(Continued)*
  inappropriate secretion of antidiuretic
    hormone E22.2
  infant
    gestational diabetes P70.0
    of diabetic mother P70.1
  infantilism (pituitary) E23.0
  inferior vena cava I87.1
  inspissated bile (newborn) P59.1
  institutional (childhood) F94.2
  insufficient sleep F51.12
  intermediate coronary (artery) I20.0
  interspinous ligament —*see* Spondylopathy,
    specified NEC
  intestinal
    carcinoid E34.0
    knot K56.2
  intravascular coagulation-fibrinolysis (ICF)
    D65
  iodine-deficiency, congenital E00.9
    type
      mixed E00.2
      myxedematous E00.1
      neurological E00.0
  IRDS (idiopathic respiratory distress,
    newborn) P22.0
  irritable
    bowel K58.9
      with diarrhea K58.0
      psychogenic F45.8
    heart (psychogenic) F45.8
    weakness F48.8
  ischemic bowel (transient) K55.9
    chronic K55.1
    due to mesenteric artery insufficiency
      K55.1
  IVC (intravascular coagulopathy) D65
  Ivemark's Q89.01
  Jaccoud's —*see* Arthropathy, postrheumatic,
    chronic
  Jackson's G83.89
  Jakob-Creutzfeldt —*see* Creutzfeldt-Jakob
    disease or syndrome
  jaw-winking Q07.8
  Jervell-Lange-Nielsen I45.81
  jet lag G47.25
  Job's D71
  Joseph-Diamond-Blackfan D61.01
  jugular foramen G52.7
  Kabuki Q89.8
  Kanner's (autism) F84.0
  Kartagener's Q89.3
  Kelly's D50.1
  Kimmelsteil-Wilson —*see* Diabetes, specified
    type, with Kimmelsteil-Wilson disease
  Klein (e)-Levine G47.13
  Klippel-Feil (brevicollis) Q76.1
  Köhler-Pellegrini-Steida —*see* Bursitis, tibial
    collateral
  König's K59.8
  Korsakoff (-Wernicke) (nonalcoholic) F04
    alcoholic F10.26
  Kostmann's D70.0
  Krabbe's congenital muscle hypoplasia Q79.8
  labyrinthine —*see* subcategory H83.2
  lacunar NEC G46.7
  Lambert-Eaton G70.80
    in
      neoplastic disease G73.1
      specified disease NEC G70.81
  Landau-Kleffner —*see* Epilepsy, specified
    NEC
  Larsen's Q74.8
  lateral
    cutaneous nerve of thigh G57.1-
    medullary G46.4
  Launois' E22.0
  lazy
    leukocyte D70.8
    posture M62.3
  Lemiere I80.8

S

Syndrome *(Continued)*
  Lennox-Gastaut G40.812
    intractable G40.814
      with status epilepticus G40.813
      without status epilepticus G40.814
    not intractable G40.812
      with status epilepticus G40.811
      without status epilepticus G40.812
  lenticular, progressive E83.01
  Leopold-Levi's E05.90
  Lev's I44.2
  Li-Fraumeni Z15.01
  Lichtheim's D51.0
  Lightwood's N25.89
  Lignac (de Toni) (-Fanconi) (-Debré) E72.09
    with cystinosis E72.04
  Likoff's I20.8
  limbic epilepsy personality F07.0
  liver-kidney K76.7
  lobotomy F07.0
  Loffler's J82
  long arm 18 or 21 deletion Q93.89
  long QT I45.81
  Louis-Barré G11.3
  low
    atmospheric pressure T70.29
    back M54.5
    output (cardiac) I50.9
  lower radicular, newborn (birth injury) P14.8
  Luetscher's (dehydration) E86.0
  Lupus anticoagulant D68.62
  Lutembacher's Q21.1
  macrophage activation D76.1
    due to infection D76.2
  magnesium-deficiency R29.0
  Mal de Debarquement R42
  malabsorption K90.9
    postsurgical K91.2
  malformation, congenital, due to
    alcohol Q86.0
    exogenous cause NEC Q86.8
    hydantoin Q86.1
    warfarin Q86.2
  malignant
    carcinoid E34.0
    neuroleptic G21.0
  Mallory-Weiss K22.6
  mandibulofacial dysostosis Q75.4
  manic-depressive —*see* Disorder, bipolar, affective
  maple-syrup-urine E71.0
  Marable's I77.4
  Marfan's Q87.40
    with
      cardiovascular manifestations Q87.418
        aortic dilation Q87.410
      ocular manifestations Q87.42
      skeletal manifestations Q87.43
  Marie's (acromegaly) E22.0
  maternal hypotension —*see* Syndrome, hypotension, maternal
  May (-Hegglin) D72.0
  McArdle (-Schmidt) (-Pearson) E74.04
  McQuarrie's E16.2
  meconium plug (newborn) P76.0
  median arcuate ligament I77.4
  Meekeren-Ehlers-Danlos Q79.6
  megavitamin-B6 E67.2
  Meige G24.4
  MELAS E88.41
  Mendelson's O74.0
  MERRF (myoclonic epilepsy associated with ragged-red fibers) E88.42
  mesenteric
    artery (superior) K55.1
    vascular insufficiency K55.1
  metabolic E88.81
  metastatic carcinoid E34.0
  micrognathia-glossoptosis Q87.0
  midbrain NEC G93.89
  middle lobe (lung) J98.19

Syndrome *(Continued)*
  middle radicular G54.0
  migraine (*see also* Migraine) G43.909-
  Mikulicz' K11.8
  milk-alkali E83.52
  Millard-Gubler G46.3
  Miller-Dieker Q93.88
  Miller-Fisher G61.0
  Minkowski-Chauffard D58.0
  Mirizzi's K83.1
  MNGIE (Mitochondrial Neurogastrointestinal Encephalopathy) E88.49
  Möbius, ophthalmoplegic migraine —*see* Migraine, ophthalmoplegic
  monofixation H50.42
  Morel-Moore M85.2
  Morel-Morgagni M85.2
  Morgagni (-Morel) (-Stewart) M85.2
  Morgagni-Adams-Stokes I45.9
  Mounier-Kuhn Q32.4
    with bronchiectasis J47.9
      with
        exacerbation (acute) J47.1
        lower respiratory infection J47.0
    acquired J98.09
      with bronchiectasis J47.9
        with
          exacerbation (acute) J47.1
          lower respiratory infection J47.0
  mucocutaneous lymph node (acute febrile) (MCLS) M30.3
  multiple endocrine neoplasia (MEN) —*see* Neoplasia, endocrine, multiple (MEN}
  multiple operations —*see* Disorder, factitious
  myasthenic G70.9
    in
      diabetes mellitus —*see* Diabetes, amyotrophy
      endocrine disease NEC E34.9 *[G73.3]*
      neoplastic disease (*see also* Neoplasm) D49.9 *[G73.3]*
      thyrotoxicosis (hyperthyroidism) E05.90 *[G73.3]*
        with thyroid storm E05.91 *[G73.3]*
  myelodysplastic D46.9
    with
      5q deletion D46.C
      isolated del (5q) chromosomal abnormality D46.C
    lesions, low grade D46.20
    specified NEC D46.Z
  myelopathic pain G89.0
  myeloproliferative (chronic) D47.1
  myofascial pain M79.1
  Naffziger's G54.0
  nail patella Q87.2
  NARP (Neuropathy, Ataxia and Retinitis pigmentosa) E88.49
  neonatal abstinence P96.1
  nephritic —*see also* Nephritis
    with edema —*see* Nephrosis
    acute N00.9
    chronic N03.9
    rapidly progressive N01.9
  nephrotic (congenital) (*see also* Nephrosis) N04.9
    with
      dense deposit disease N04.6
      diffuse
        crescentic glomerulonephritis N04.7
        endocapillary proliferative glomerulonephritis N04.4
        membranous glomerulonephritis N04.2
        mesangial proliferative glomerulonephritis N04.3
        mesangiocapillary glomerulonephritis N04.5
      focal and segmental glomerular lesions N04.1

Syndrome *(Continued)*
  nephrotic *(Continued)*
    with *(Continued)*
      minor glomerular abnormality N04.0
      specified morphological changes NEC N04.8
    diabetic —*see* Diabetes, nephrosis
  neurologic neglect R41.4
  Nezelof's D81.4
  Nonne-Milroy-Meige Q82.0
  Nothnagel's vasomotor acroparesthesia I73.89
  oculomotor H51.9
  ophthalmoplegia-cerebellar ataxia —*see* Strabismus, paralytic, third nerve
  oral-facial-digital Q87.0
  organic
    affective F06.30
    amnesic (not alcohol- or drug-induced) F04
    brain F09
    depressive F06.31
    hallucinosis F06.0
    personality F07.0
  Ormond's N13.5
  oro-facial-digital Q87.0
  os trigonum Q68.8
  Osler-Weber-Rendu I78.0
  osteoporosis-osteomalacia M83.8
  Osterreicher-Turner Q79.8
  otolith —*see* subcategory H81.8
  oto-palatal-digital Q87.0
  outlet (thoracic) G54.0
  ovary
    polycystic E28.2
    resistant E28.39
    sclerocystic E28.2
  Owren's D68.2
  Paget-Schroetter I82.890
  pain —*see also* Pain
    complex regional I G90.50
      lower limb G90.52-
      specified site NEC G90.59
      upper limb G90.51-
    complex regional II —*see* Causalgia
  painful
    bruising D69.2
    feet E53.8
    prostate N42.81
  paralysis agitans —*see* Parkinsonism
  paralytic G83.9
    specified NEC G83.89
  Parinaud's H51.0
  parkinsonian —*see* Parkinsonism
  Parkinson's —*see* Parkinsonism
  paroxysmal facial pain G50.0
  Parry's E05.00
    with thyroid storm E05.01
  Parsonage (-Aldren)-Turner G54.5
  patella clunk M25.86-
  Paterson (-Brown) (-Kelly) D50.1
  pectoral girdle I77.89
  pectoralis minor I77.89
  Pelger-Huet D72.0
  pellagra-cerebellar ataxia-renal aminoaciduria E72.02
  pellagroid E52
  Pellegrini-Stieda —*see* Bursitis, tibial collateral
  pelvic congestion-fibrosis, female N94.89
  penta X Q97.1
  peptic ulcer —*see* Ulcer, peptic
  perabduction I77.89
  periodic headache, in adults and children — *see* Headache, periodic syndromes in adults and children
  periurethral fibrosis N13.5
  phantom limb (without pain) G54.7
    with pain G54.6
  pharyngeal pouch D82.1
  Pick's (heart) (liver) I31.1
  Pickwickian E66.2

◀ New   ⬅ Revised   ~~deleted~~ Deleted

Syndrome *(Continued)*
  PIE (pulmonary infiltration with
      eosinophilia) J82
  pigmentary pallidal degeneration
      (progressive) G23.0
  pineal E34.8
  pituitary E22.0
  placental transfusion —*see* Pregnancy,
      complicated by, placental transfusion
      syndromes
  plantar fascia M72.2
  plateau iris (post-iridectomy)
      (postprocedural) H21.82
  Plummer-Vinson D50.1
  pluricarential of infancy E40
  plurideficiency E40
  pluriglandular (compensatory) E31.8
      autoimmune E31.0
  pneumatic hammer T75.21
  polyangiitis overlap M30.8
  polycarential of infancy E40
  polyglandular E31.8
      autoimmune E31.0
  polysplenia Q89.09
  pontine NEC G93.89
  popliteal
      artery entrapment I77.89
      web Q87.89
  postcardiac injury
      postcardiotomy I97.0
      postmyocardial infarction I24.1
  postcardiotomy I97.0
  post chemoembolization — code to
      associated conditions
  postcholecystectomy K91.5
  postcommissurotomy I97.0
  postconcussional F07.81
  postcontusional F07.81
  postencephalitic F07.89
  posterior
      cervical sympathetic M53.0
      cord G83.83
      fossa compression G93.5
      reversible encephalopathy (PRES) I67.83
  postgastrectomy (dumping) K91.1
  postgastric surgery K91.1
  postinfarction I24.1
  postlaminectomy NEC M96.1
  postleukotomy F07.0
  postmastectomy lymphedema I97.2
  postmyocardial infarction I24.1
  postoperative NEC T81.9
      blind loop K90.2
  postpartum panhypopituitary (Sheehan)
      E23.0
  postpolio (myelitic) G14
  postthrombotic I87.009
      with
          inflammation I87.02-
              with ulcer I87.03-
          specified complication NEC I87.09-
          ulcer I87.01-
              with inflammation I87.03-
      asymptomatic I87.00-
  postvagotomy K91.1
  postvalvulotomy I97.0
  postviral NEC G93.3
      fatigue G93.3
  Potain's K31.0
  potassium intoxication E87.5
  precerebral artery (multiple) (bilateral)
      G45.2
  preinfarction I20.0
  preleukemic D46.9
  premature senility E34.8
  premenstrual dysphoric N94.3
  premenstrual tension N94.3
  Prinzmetal-Massumi R07.1
  prune belly Q79.4
  pseudocarpal tunnel (sublimis) —*see*
      Syndrome, carpal tunnel

Syndrome *(Continued)*
  pseudoparalytica G70.00
      with exacerbation (acute) G70.01
      in crisis G70.01
  pseudo -Turner's Q87.1
  psycho-organic (nonpsychotic severity) F07.9
      acute or subacute F05
      depressive type F06.31
      hallucinatory type F06.0
      nonpsychotic severity F07.0
      specified NEC F07.89
  pulmonary
      arteriosclerosis I27.0
      dysmaturity (Wilson-Mikity) P27.0
      hypoperfusion (idiopathic) P22.0
      renal (hemorrhagic) (Goodpasture's) M31.0
  pure
      motor lacunar G46.5
      sensory lacunar G46.6
  Putnam-Dana D51.0
  pyramidopallidonigral G20
  pyriformis —*see* Lesion, nerve, sciatic
  QT interval prolongation I45.81
  radicular NEC —*see* Radiculopathy
      upper limbs, newborn (birth injury) P14.3
  rapid time-zone change G47.25
  Rasmussen G04.81
  Raymond (-Céstan) I65.8
  Raynaud's I73.00
      with gangrene I73.01
  RDS (respiratory distress syndrome,
      newborn) P22.0
  reactive airways dysfunction J68.3
  Refsum's G60.1
  Reifenstein E34.52
  renal glomerulohyalinosis-diabetic —*see*
      Diabetes, nephrosis
  Rendu-Osler-Weber I78.0
  residual ovary N99.83
  resistant ovary E28.39
  respiratory
      distress
          acute J80
          adult J80
          child J80
          newborn (idiopathic) (type I) P22.0
          type II P22.1
  restless legs G25.81
  retinoblastoma (familial) C69.2
  retroperitoneal fibrosis N13.5
  retroviral seroconversion (acute) Z21
  Reye's G93.7
  Richter —*see* Leukemia, chronic lymphocytic,
      B-cell type
  Ridley's I50.1
  right
      heart, hypoplastic Q22.6
      ventricular obstruction —*see* Failure, heart,
          congestive
  Romano-Ward (prolonged QT interval) I45.81
  rotator cuff, shoulder (*see also* Tear, rotator
      cuff) M75.10-
  Rotes Quérol —*see* Hyperostosis, ankylosing
  Roth —*see* Meralgia paresthetica
  rubella (congenital) P35.0
  Ruvalcaba-Myhre-Smith E71.440
  Rytand-Lipsitch I44.2
  salt
      depletion E87.1
          due to heat NEC T67.8
              causing heat exhaustion or prostration
                  T67.4
      low E87.1
  salt-losing N28.89
  Scaglietti-Dagnini E22.0
  scalenus anticus (anterior) G54.0
  scapulocostal —*see* Mononeuropathy, upper
      limb, specified site NEC
  scapuloperoneal G71.0
  schizophrenic, of childhood NEC F84.5
  Schnitzler D47.2

Syndrome *(Continued)*
  Scholte's E34.0
  Schroeder's E27.0
  Schüller-Christian C96.5
  Schwachman's —*see* Syndrome,
      Shwachman's
  Schwartz (-Jampel) G71.13
  Schwartz-Bartter E22.2
  scimitar Q26.8
  sclerocystic ovary E28.2
  Seitelberger's G31.89
  septicemic adrenal hemorrhage A39.1
  seroconversion, retroviral (acute) Z21
  serous meningitis G93.2
  severe acute respiratory (SARS) J12.81
  shaken infant T74.4
  shock (traumatic) T79.4
      kidney N17.0
          following crush injury T79.5
      toxic A48.3
  shock-lung J80
  Shone's — code to specific anomalies
  short
      bowel K91.2
      rib Q77.2
  shoulder-hand —*see* Algoneurodystrophy
  Shwachman's D70.4
  sicca —*see* Sicca syndrome
  sick
      cell E87.1
      sinus I49.5
  sick-euthyroid E07.81
  sideropenic D50.1
  Siemens' ectodermal dysplasia Q82.4
  Silfversköld's Q78.9
  Simons' E88.1
  sinus tarsi M25.57-
  sinusitis-bronchiectasis-situs inversus
      Q89.3
  Sipple's E31.22
  sirenomelia Q87.2
  Slocumb's E27.0
  slow flow, coronary I20.8
  Sluder's G44.89
  Smith-Magenis Q93.88
  Sneddon-Wilkinson L13.1
  Sotos' E22.0
  South African cardiomyopathy I42.8
  spasmodic
      upward movement, eyes H51.8
      winking F95.8
  Spen's I45.9
  splenic
      agenesis Q89.01
      flexure K59.8
      neutropenia D73.81
  Spurway's Q78.0
  staphylococcal scalded skin L00
  Stein-Leventhal E28.2
  Stein's E28.2
  Stevens-Johnson syndrome L51.1
      toxic epidermal necrolysis overlap L51.3
  Stewart-Morel M85.2
  Stickler Q89.8
  stiff baby Q89.8
  stiff man G25.82
  Still-Felty —*see* Felty's syndrome
  Stokes (-Adams) I45.9
  stone heart I50.1
  straight back, congenital Q76.49
  subclavian steal G45.8
  subcoracoid-pectoralis minor G54.0
  subcostal nerve compression I77.89
  subphrenic interposition Q43.3
  superior
      cerebellar artery I63.8
      mesenteric artery K55.1
      semi-circular canal dehiscence H83.8X-
      vena cava I87.1
  supine hypotensive (maternal) —*see*
      Syndrome, hypotension, maternal

Syndrome *(Continued)*
  suprarenal cortical E27.0
  supraspinatus *(see also* Tear, rotator cuff)
      M75.10-
  Susac G93.49
  swallowed blood P78.2
  sweat retention L74.0
  Swyer Q99.1
  Symond's G93.2
  sympathetic
      cervical paralysis G90.2
      pelvic, female N94.89
  systemic inflammatory response (SIRS), of
      non-infectious origin (without organ
      dysfunction) R65.10
      with acute organ dysfunction R65.11
  tachycardia-bradycardia I49.5
  takotsubo I51.81
  TAR (thrombocytopenia with absent radius)
      Q87.2
  tarsal tunnel G57.5-
  teething K00.7
  tegmental G93.89
  telangiectasic-pigmentation-cataract
      Q82.8
  temporal pyramidal apex *—see* Otitis,
      media, suppurative, acute
  temporomandibular joint-pain-dysfunction
      M26.62
  Terry's H44.2-
  testicular feminization *(see also* Syndrome,
      androgen insensitivity) E34.51
  thalamic pain (hyperesthetic) G89.0
  thoracic outlet (compression) G54.0
  Thorson-Björck E34.0
  thrombocytopenia with absent radius (TAR)
      Q87.2
  thyroid-adrenocortical insufficiency E31.0
  tibial
      anterior M76.81-
      posterior M76.82-
  Tietze's M94.0
  time-zone (rapid) G47.25
  Toni-Fanconi E72.09
      with cystinosis E72.04
  Touraine's Q79.8
  tourniquet *—see* Constriction, external,
      by site
  toxic shock A48.3
  transient left ventricular apical ballooning
      I51.81
  traumatic vasospastic T75.22
  Treacher Collins Q75.4
  triple X, female Q97.0
  trisomy Q92.9
      13 Q91.7
          meiotic nondisjunction Q91.4
          mitotic nondisjunction Q91.5
          mosaicism Q91.5
          translocation Q91.6
      18 Q91.3
          meiotic nondisjunction Q91.0
          mitotic nondisjunction Q91.1
          mosaicism Q91.1
          translocation Q91.2
      20 (q)(p) Q92.8
      21 Q90.9
          meiotic nondisjunction Q90.0
          mitotic nondisjunction Q90.1
          mosaicism Q90.1
          translocation Q90.2
      22 Q92.8
  tropical wet feet T69.0-
  Trousseau's I82.1
  tumor lysis (following antineoplastic
      chemotherapy) (spontaneous) NEC
      E88.3
  Twiddler's (due to)
      automatic implantable defibrillator
          T82.198
      cardiac pacemaker T82.198

Syndrome *(Continued)*
  Unverricht (-Lundborg) *—see* Epilepsy,
      generalized, idiopathic
  upward gaze H51.8
  uremia, chronic *(see also* Disease, kidney,
      chronic) N18.9
  urethral N34.3
  urethro-oculo-articular *—see* Reiter's disease
  urohepatic K76.7
  vago-hypoglossal G52.7
  van Buchem's M85.2
  van der Hoeve's Q78.0
  vascular NEC in cerebrovascular disease
      G46.8
  vasoconstriction, reversible cerebrovascular
      I67.841
  vasomotor I73.9
  vasospastic (traumatic) T75.22
  vasovagal R55
  VATER Q87.2
  velo-cardio-facial Q93.81
  vena cava (inferior) (superior) (obstruction)
      I87.1
  vertebral
      artery G45.0
          compression *—see* Syndrome, anterior,
              spinal artery, compression
      steal G45.0
  vertebro-basilar artery G45.0
  vertebrogenic (pain) M54.89
  vertiginous *—see* Disorder, vestibular
      function
  Vinson-Plummer D50.1
  virus B34.9
  visceral larva migrans B83.0
  visual disorientation H53.8
  vitamin B6 deficiency E53.1
  vitreal corneal H59.01-
  vitreous (touch) H59.01-
  Vogt-Koyanagi H20.82-
  Volkmann's T79.6
  von Schroetter's I82.890
  von Willebrand (-Jürgen) D68.0
  Waldenström-Kjellberg D50.1
  Wallenberg's G46.3
  water retention E87.79
  Waterhouse (-Friderichsen) A39.1
  Weber-Gubler G46.3
  Weber-Leyden G46.3
  Weber's G46.3
  Wegener's M31.30
      with
          kidney involvement M31.31
          lung involvement M31.30
              with kidney involvement M31.31
  Weingarten's (tropical eosinophilia) J82
  Weiss-Baker G90.09
  Werdnig-Hoffman G12.0
  Wermer's E31.21
  Werner's E34.8
  Wernicke-Korsakoff (nonalcoholic) F04
      alcoholic F10.26
  West's *—see* Epilepsy, spasms
  Westphal-Strümpell E83.01
  wet
      feet (maceration) (tropical) T69.0-
      lung, newborn P22.1
  whiplash S13.4
  whistling face Q87.0
  Wilkie's K55.1
  Wilkinson-Sneddon L13.1
  Willebrand (-Jürgens) D68.0
  Wilson's (hepatolenticular degeneration)
      E83.01
  Wiskott-Aldrich D82.0
  withdrawal *—see* Withdrawal, state
      drug
          infant of dependent mother P96.1
          therapeutic use, newborn P96.2
  Woakes' (ethmoiditis) J33.1
  Wright's (hyperabduction) I77.89

Syndrome *(Continued)*
  X I20.9
  XXXX Q97.1
  XXXXX Q97.1
  XXXXY Q98.1
  XXY Q98.0
  yellow nail L60.5
  Zahorsky's B08.5
  Zellweger syndrome E71.510
  Zellweger-like syndrome E71.541
Synechia (anterior) (iris) (posterior) (pupil) —
    see also Adhesions, iris
  intra-uterine (traumatic) N85.6
Synesthesia R20.8
Syngamiasis, syngamosis B83.3
Synodontia K00.2
Synorchidism, synorchism Q55.1
Synostosis (congenital) Q78.8
  astragalo-scaphoid Q74.2
  radioulnar Q74.0
Synovial sarcoma *—see* Neoplasm, connective
    tissue, malignant
Synovioma (malignant) *—see also* Neoplasm,
    connective tissue, malignant
  benign *—see* Neoplasm, connective tissue,
      benign
Synoviosarcoma *—see* Neoplasm, connective
    tissue, malignant
Synovitis *—see also* Tenosynovitis
  crepitant
      hand M70.0-
      wrist M70.03-
  gonococcal A54.49
  gouty *—see* Gout, idiopathic
  in (due to)
      crystals M65.8-
      gonorrhea A54.49
      syphilis (late) A52.78
      use, overuse, pressure *—see* Disorder, soft
          tissue, due to use
  infective NEC *—see* Tenosynovitis, infective
      NEC
  specified NEC *—see* Tenosynovitis, specified
      type NEC
  syphilitic A52.78
      congenital (early) A50.02
  toxic *—see* Synovitis, transient
  transient M67.3-
      ankle M67.37-
      elbow M67.32-
      foot joint M67.37-
      hand joint M67.34-
      hip M67.35-
      knee M67.36-
      multiple site M67.39
      pelvic region M67.35-
      shoulder M67.31-
      specified joint NEC M67.38
      wrist M67.33-
  traumatic, current *—see* Sprain
  tuberculous *—see* Tuberculosis, synovitis
  villonodular (pigmented) M12.2-
      ankle M12.27-
      elbow M12.22-
      foot joint M12.27-
      hand joint M12.24-
      hip M12.25-
      knee M12.26-
      multiple site M12.29
      pelvic region M12.25-
      shoulder M12.21-
      specified joint NEC M12.28
      vertebrae M12.28
      wrist M12.23-
Syphilid A51.39
  congenital A50.06
  newborn A50.06
  tubercular (late) A52.79
Syphilis, syphilitic (acquired) A53.9
  abdomen (late) A52.79
  acoustic nerve A52.15

Syphilis, syphilitic *(Continued)*
adenopathy (secondary) A51.49
adrenal (gland) (with cortical hypofunction) A52.79
age under 2 years NOS —*see also* Syphilis, congenital, early
　acquired A51.9
alopecia (secondary) A51.32
anemia (late) A52.79 *[D63.8]*
aneurysm (aorta) (ruptured) A52.01
　central nervous system A52.05
　congenital A50.54 *[I79.0]*
anus (late) A52.74
　primary A51.1
　secondary A51.39
aorta (arch) (abdominal) (thoracic) A52.02
　aneurysm A52.01
aortic (insufficiency) (regurgitation) (stenosis) A52.03
　aneurysm A52.01
arachnoid (adhesive) (cerebral) (spinal) A52.13
asymptomatic —*see* Syphilis, latent
ataxia (locomotor) A52.11
atrophoderma maculatum A51.39
auricular fibrillation A52.06
bladder (late) A52.76
bone A52.77
　secondary A51.46
brain A52.17
breast (late) A52.79
bronchus (late) A52.72
bubo (primary) A51.0
bulbar palsy A52.19
bursa (late) A52.78
cardiac decompensation A52.06
cardiovascular A52.00
central nervous system (late) (recurrent) (relapse) (tertiary) A52.3
　with
　　ataxia A52.11
　　general paralysis A52.17
　　　juvenile A50.45
　　paresis (general) A52.17
　　　juvenile A50.45
　　tabes (dorsalis) A52.11
　　　juvenile A50.45
　　taboparesis A52.17
　　　juvenile A50.45
　aneurysm A52.05
　congenital A50.40
　juvenile A50.40
　remission in (sustained) A52.3
　serology doubtful, negative, or positive A52.3
　specified nature or site NEC A52.19
　vascular A52.05
cerebral A52.17
　meningovascular A52.13
　nerves (multiple palsies) A52.15
　sclerosis A52.17
　thrombosis A52.05
cerebrospinal (tabetic type) A52.12
cerebrovascular A52.05
cervix (late) A52.76
chancre (multiple) A51.0
　extragenital A51.2
　Rollet's A51.0
Charcot's joint A52.16
chorioretinitis A51.43
　congenital A50.01
　late A52.71
　prenatal A50.01
choroiditis —*see* Syphilitic chorioretinitis
choroidoretinitis —*see* Syphilitic chorioretinitis
ciliary body (secondary) A51.43
　late A52.71
colon (late) A52.74
combined spinal sclerosis A52.11
condyloma (latum) A51.31

Syphilis, syphilitic *(Continued)*
congenital A50.9
　with
　　paresis (general) A50.45
　　tabes (dorsalis) A50.45
　　taboparesis A50.45
　chorioretinitis, choroiditis A50.01 *[H32]*
　early, or less than 2 years after birth NEC A50.2
　　with manifestations —*see* Syphilis, congenital, early, symptomatic
　　latent (without manifestations) A50.1
　　　negative spinal fluid test A50.1
　　　serology positive A50.1
　　symptomatic A50.09
　　　cutaneous A50.06
　　　mucocutaneous A50.07
　　　oculopathy A50.01
　　　osteochondropathy A50.02
　　　pharyngitis A50.03
　　　pneumonia A50.04
　　　rhinitis A50.05
　　　visceral A50.08
　interstitial keratitis A50.31
　juvenile neurosyphilis A50.45
　late, or 2 years or more after birth NEC A50.7
　　chorioretinitis, choroiditis A50.32
　　interstitial keratitis A50.31
　　juvenile neurosyphilis A50.45
　　latent (without manifestations) A50.6
　　　negative spinal fluid test A50.6
　　　serology positive A50.6
　　symptomatic or with manifestations NEC A50.59
　　　arthropathy A50.55
　　　cardiovascular A50.54
　　　Clutton's joints A50.51
　　　Hutchinson's teeth A50.52
　　　Hutchinson's triad A50.53
　　　osteochondropathy A50.56
　　　saddle nose A50.57
conjugal A53.9
　tabes A53.11
conjunctiva (late) A52.71
contact Z20.2
cord bladder A52.19
cornea, late A52.71
coronary (artery) (sclerosis) A52.06
coryza, congenital A50.05
cranial nerve A52.15
　multiple palsies A52.15
cutaneous —*see* Syphilis, skin
dacryocystitis (late) A52.71
degeneration, spinal cord A52.12
dementia paralytica A52.17
　juvenilis A50.45
destruction of bone A52.77
dilatation, aorta A52.01
due to blood transfusion A53.9
dura mater A52.13
ear A52.79
　inner A52.79
　　nerve (eighth) A52.15
　　neurorecurrence A52.15
early A51.9
　cardiovascular A52.00
　central nervous system A52.3
　latent (without manifestations) (less than 2 years after infection) A51.5
　　negative spinal fluid test A51.5
　　serological relapse after treatment A51.5
　　serology positive A51.5
　relapse (treated, untreated) A51.9
　skin A51.39
　symptomatic A51.9
　　extragenital chancre A51.2
　　primary, except extragenital chancre A51.0

Syphilis, syphilitic *(Continued)*
early *(Continued)*
　symptomatic *(Continued)*
　　secondary *(see also* Syphilis, secondary) A51.39
　　relapse (treated, untreated) A51.49
　　ulcer A51.39
eighth nerve (neuritis) A52.15
endemic A65
endocarditis A52.03
　aortic A52.03
　pulmonary A52.03
epididymis (late) A52.76
epiglottis (late) A52.73
epiphysitis (congenital) (early) A50.02
episcleritis (late) A52.71
esophagus A52.79
eustachian tube A52.73
exposure to Z20.2
eye A52.71
eyelid (late) (with gumma) A52.71
fallopian tube (late) A52.76
fracture A52.77
gallbladder (late) A52.74
gastric (polyposis) (late) A52.74
general A53.9
　paralysis A52.17
　　juvenile A50.45
genital (primary) A51.0
glaucoma A52.71
gumma NEC A52.79
　cardiovascular system A52.00
　central nervous system A52.3
　congenital A50.59
heart (block) (decompensation) (disease) (failure) A52.06 *[I52]*
　valve NEC A52.03
hemianesthesia A52.19
hemianopsia A52.71
hemiparesis A52.17
hemiplegia A52.17
hepatic artery A52.09
hepatitis A52.74
hepatomegaly, congenital A50.08
hereditaria tarda —*see* Syphilis, congenital, late
hereditary —*see* Syphilis, congenital
Hutchinson's teeth A50.52
hyalitis A52.71
inactive —*see* Syphilis, latent
infantum —*see* Syphilis, congenital
inherited —*see* Syphilis, congenital
internal ear A52.79
intestine (late) A52.74
iris, iritis (secondary) A51.43
　late A52.71
joint (late) A52.77
keratitis (congenital) (interstitial) (late) A50.31
kidney (late) A52.75
lacrimal passages (late) A52.71
larynx (late) A52.73
late A52.9
　cardiovascular A52.00
　central nervous system A52.3
　kidney A52.75
　latent or 2 years or more after infection (without manifestations) A52.8
　　negative spinal fluid test A52.8
　　serology positive A52.8
　paresis A52.17
　specified site NEC A52.79
　symptomatic or with manifestations A52.79
　tabes A52.11
latent A53.0
　with signs or symptoms - code by site and stage under Syphilis
　central nervous system A52.2
　date of infection unspecified A53.0
　early, or less than 2 years after infection A51.5

Syphilis, syphilitic (Continued)
  latent (Continued)
    follow-up of latent syphilis A53.0
      date of infection unspecified A53.0
      late, or 2 years or more after infection
        A52.8
    late, or 2 years or more after infection
      A52.8
    positive serology (only finding) A53.0
      date of infection unspecified A53.0
      early, or less than 2 years after infection
        A51.5
      late, or 2 years or more after infection
        A52.8
  lens (late) A52.71
  leukoderma A51.39
    late A52.79
  lienitis A52.79
  lip A51.39
    chancre (primary) A51.2
    late A52.79
  Lissauer's paralysis A52.17
  liver A52.74
  locomotor ataxia A52.11
  lung A52.72
  lymph gland (early) (secondary) A51.49
    late A52.79
  lymphadenitis (secondary) A51.49
  macular atrophy of skin A51.39
    striated A52.79
  mediastinum (late) A52.73
  meninges (adhesive) (brain) (spinal cord)
    A52.13
  meningitis A52.13
    acute (secondary) A51.41
    congenital A50.41
  meningoencephalitis A52.14
  meningovascular A52.13
    congenital A50.41
  mesarteritis A52.09
    brain A52.04
  middle ear A52.77
  mitral stenosis A52.03
  monoplegia A52.17
  mouth (secondary) A51.39
    late A52.79
  mucocutaneous (secondary) A51.39
    late A52.79
  mucous
    membrane (secondary) A51.39
      late A52.79
    patches A51.39
      congenital A50.07
  mulberry molars A50.52
  muscle A52.78
  myocardium A52.06
  nasal sinus (late) A52.73
  neonatorum —see Syphilis, congenital
  nephrotic syndrome (secondary)
    A51.44
  nerve palsy (any cranial nerve)
    A52.15
    multiple A52.15
  nervous system, central A52.3
  neuritis A52.15
    acoustic A52.15
  neurorecidive of retina A52.19
  neuroretinitis A52.19
  newborn —see Syphilis, congenital
  nodular superficial (late) A52.79
  nonvenereal A65
  nose (late) A52.73
    saddle back deformity A50.57
  occlusive arterial disease A52.09
  oculopathy A52.71
  ophthalmic (late) A52.71
  optic nerve (atrophy) (neuritis) (papilla)
    A52.15
  orbit (late) A52.71
  organic A53.9
  osseous (late) A52.77

Syphilis, syphilitic (Continued)
  osteochondritis (congenital) (early) A50.02
    [M90.80]
  osteoporosis A52.77
  ovary (late) A52.76
  oviduct (late) A52.76
  palate (late) A52.79
  pancreas (late) A52.74
  paralysis A52.17
    general A52.17
      juvenile A50.45
  paresis (general) A52.17
    juvenile A50.45
  paresthesia A52.19
  Parkinson's disease or syndrome A52.19
  paroxysmal tachycardia A52.06
  pemphigus (congenital) A50.06
  penis (chancre) A51.0
    late A52.76
  pericardium A52.06
  perichondritis, larynx (late) A52.73
  periosteum (late) A52.77
    congenital (early) A50.02 [M90.80]
    early (secondary) A51.46
  peripheral nerve A52.79
  petrous bone (late) A52.77
  pharynx (late) A52.73
    secondary A51.39
  pituitary (gland) A52.79
  pleura (late) A52.73
  pneumonia, white A50.04
  pontine lesion A52.17
  portal vein A52.09
  primary A51.0
    anal A51.1
    and secondary —see Syphilis, secondary
    central nervous system A52.3
    extragenital chancre NEC A51.2
    fingers A51.2
    genital A51.0
    lip A51.2
    specified site NEC A51.2
    tonsils A51.2
  prostate (late) A52.76
  ptosis (eyelid) A52.71
  pulmonary (late) A52.72
    artery A52.09
  pyelonephritis (late) A52.75
  recently acquired, symptomatic A51.9
  rectum (late) A52.74
  respiratory tract (late) A52.73
  retina, late A52.71
  retrobulbar neuritis A52.15
  salpingitis A52.76
  sclera (late) A52.71
  sclerosis
    cerebral A52.17
    coronary A52.06
    multiple A52.11
  scotoma (central) A52.71
  scrotum (late) A52.76
  secondary (and primary) A51.49
    adenopathy A51.49
    anus A51.39
    bone A51.46
    chorioretinitis, choroiditis A51.43
    hepatitis A51.45
    liver A51.45
    lymphadenitis A51.49
    meningitis (acute) A51.41
    mouth A51.39
    mucous membranes A51.39
    periosteum, periostitis A51.46
    pharynx A51.39
    relapse (treated, untreated) A51.49
    skin A51.39
    specified form NEC A51.49
    tonsil A51.39
    ulcer A51.39
    viscera NEC A51.49
    vulva A51.39

Syphilis, syphilitic (Continued)
  seminal vesicle (late) A52.76
  seronegative with signs or symptoms -
    code by site and stage under
    Syphilis
  seropositive
    with signs or symptoms - code
      by site and stage under
      Syphilis
    follow-up of latent syphilis —see Syphilis,
      latent
    only finding —see Syphilis, latent
  seventh nerve (paralysis) A52.15
  sinus, sinusitis (late) A52.73
  skeletal system A52.77
  skin (with ulceration) (early) (secondary)
    A51.39
    late or tertiary A52.79
  small intestine A52.74
  spastic spinal paralysis A52.17
  spermatic cord (late) A52.76
  spinal (cord) A52.12
  spleen A52.79
  splenomegaly A52.79
  spondylitis A52.77
  staphyloma A52.71
  stigmata (congenital) A50.59
  stomach A52.74
  synovium A52.78
  tabes dorsalis (late) A52.11
    juvenile A50.45
  tabetic type A52.11
    juvenile A50.45
  taboparesis A52.17
    juvenile A50.45
  tachycardia A52.06
  tendon (late) A52.78
  tertiary A52.9
    with symptoms NEC A52.79
    cardiovascular A52.00
    central nervous system A52.3
    multiple NEC A52.79
    specified site NEC A52.79
  testis A52.76
  thorax A52.73
  throat A52.73
  thymus (gland) (late) A52.79
  thyroid (late) A52.79
  tongue (late) A52.79
  tonsil (lingual) (late) A52.73
    primary A51.2
    secondary A51.39
  trachea (late) A52.73
  tunica vaginalis (late) A52.76
  ulcer (any site) (early) (secondary)
    A51.39
    late A52.79
    perforating A52.79
      foot A52.11
  urethra (late) A52.76
  urogenital (late) A52.76
  uterus (late) A52.76
  uveal tract (secondary) A51.43
    late A52.71
  uveitis (secondary) A51.43
    late A52.71
  uvula (late) (perforated) A52.79
  vagina A51.0
    late A52.76
  valvulitis NEC A52.03
  vascular A52.00
    brain (cerebral) A52.05
  ventriculi A52.74
  vesicae urinariae (late) A52.76
  viscera (abdominal) (late) A52.74
    secondary A51.49
  vitreous (opacities) (late) A52.71
    hemorrhage A52.71
  vulva A51.0
    late A52.76
    secondary A51.39

◀ New   ◀⫶⫶ Revised   ~~deleted~~ Deleted

Syphiloma A52.79
   cardiovascular system A52.00
   central nervous system A52.3
   circulatory system A52.00
   congenital A50.59
Syphilophobia F45.29
Syringadenoma —*see also* Neoplasm, skin, benign
   papillary —*see* Neoplasm, skin, benign
Syringobulbia G95.0

Syringocystadenoma —*see* Neoplasm, skin, benign
   papillary —*see* Neoplasm, skin, benign
Syringoma —*see also* Neoplasm, skin, benign
   chondroid —*see* Neoplasm, skin, benign
Syringomyelia G95.0
Syringomyelitis —*see* Encephalitis
Syringomyelocele —*see* Spina bifida
Syringopontia G95.0

System, systemic —*see also* condition
   disease, combined —*see* Degeneration, combined
   inflammatory response syndrome (SIRS) of non-infectious origin (without organ dysfunction) R65.10
   with acute organ dysfunction R65.11
lupus erythematosus M32.9
   inhibitor present D68.62

T

Tabacism, tabacosis, tabagism —*see also*
    Poisoning, tobacco
  meaning dependence (without remission)
    F17.200
    with
      disorder F17.299
        remission F17.211
        specified disorder NEC F17.298
        withdrawal F17.203
Tabardillo A75.9
  flea-borne A75.2
  louse-borne A75.0
Tabes, tabetic A52.10
  with
    central nervous system syphilis A52.10
    Charcot's joint A52.16
    cord bladder A52.19
    crisis, viscera (any) A52.19
    paralysis, general A52.17
    paresis (general) A52.17
    perforating ulcer (foot) A52.19
  arthropathy (Charcot) A52.16
  bladder A52.19
  bone A52.11
  cerebrospinal A52.12
  congenital A50.45
  conjugal A52.10
  dorsalis A52.11
    juvenile A50.49
  juvenile A50.49
  latent A52.19
  mesenterica A18.39
  paralysis, insane, general A52.17
  spasmodic A52.17
  syphilis (cerebrospinal) A52.12
Taboparalysis A52.17
Taboparesis (remission) A52.17
  juvenile A50.45
TAC (trigeminal autonomic cephalgia) NEC
    G44.099
  intractable G44.091
  not intractable G44.099
Tache noir S60.22-
Tachyalimentation K91.2
Tachyarrhythmia, tachyrhythmia —*see*
    Tachycardia
Tachycardia R00.0
  atrial (paroxysmal) I47.1
  auricular I47.1
  AV nodal re-entry (re-entrant) I47.1
  junctional (paroxysmal) I47.1
  newborn P29.11
  nodal (paroxysmal) I47.1
  non-paroxysmal AV nodal I45.89
  paroxysmal (sustained) (nonsustained)
    I47.9
    with sinus bradycardia I49.5
    atrial (PAT) I47.1
    atrioventricular (AV) (re-entrant) I47.1
      psychogenic F54
    junctional I47.1
      ectopic I47.1
    nodal I47.1
    psychogenic (atrial) (supraventricular)
      (ventricular) F54
    supraventricular (sustained) I47.1
      psychogenic F54
    ventricular I47.2
      psychogenic F54
  psychogenic F45.8
  sick sinus I49.5
  sinoauricular NOS R00.0
    paroxysmal I47.1
  sinus [sinusal] NOS R00.0
    paroxysmal I47.1
  supraventricular I47.1
  ventricular (paroxysmal) (sustained) I47.2
    psychogenic F54
Tachygastria K31.89

Tachypnea R06.82
  hysterical F45.8
  newborn (idiopathic) (transitory) P22.1
  psychogenic F45.8
  transitory, of newborn P22.1
TACO (transfusion associated circulatory
    overload) E87.71
Taenia (infection) (infestation) B68.9
  diminuta B71.0
  echinococcal infestation B67.90
  mediocanellata B68.1
  nana B71.0
  saginata B68.1
  solium (intestinal form) B68.0
    larval form —*see* Cysticercosis
Taeniasis (intestine) —*see* Taenia
Tag (hypertrophied skin) (infected) L91.8
  adenoid J35.8
  anus K64.4
  hemorrhoidal K64.4
  hymen N89.8
  perineal N90.89
  preauricular Q17.0
  sentinel K64.4
  skin L91.8
    accessory (congenital) Q82.8
    anus K64.4
    congenital Q82.8
    preauricular Q17.0
  tonsil J35.8
  urethra, urethral N36.8
  vulva N90.89
Tahyna fever B33.8
Takahara's disease E80.3
Takayasu's disease or syndrome M31.4
Talcosis (pulmonary) J62.0
Talipes (congenital) Q66.89
  acquired, planus —*see* Deformity, limb, flat
    foot
  asymmetric Q66.89
  calcaneovalgus Q66.4
  calcaneovarus Q66.1
  calcaneus Q66.89
  cavus Q66.7
  equinovalgus Q66.6
  equinovarus Q66.0
  equinus Q66.89
  percavus Q66.7
  planovalgus Q66.6
  planus (acquired) (any degree) —*see also*
    Deformity, limb, flat foot
    congenital Q66.5-
    due to rickets (sequelae) E64.3
  valgus Q66.6
  varus Q66.3
Tall stature, constitutional E34.4
Talma's disease M62.89
Talon noir S90.3-
  hand S60.22-
  heel S90.3-
  toe S90.1-
Tamponade, heart I31.4
Tanapox (virus disease) B08.71
Tangier disease E78.6
Tantrum, child problem F91.8
Tapeworm (infection) (infestation) —*see*
    Infestation, tapeworm
Tapia's syndrome G52.7
TAR (thrombocytopenia with absent radius)
    syndrome Q87.2
Tarral-Besnier disease L44.0
Tarsal tunnel syndrome —*see* Syndrome, tarsal
    tunnel
Tarsalgia —*see* Pain, limb, lower
Tarsitis (eyelid) H01.8
  syphilitic A52.71
  tuberculous A18.4
Tartar (teeth) (dental calculus) K03.6
Tattoo (mark) L81.8
Tauri's disease E74.09
Taurodontism K00.2

Taussig-Bing syndrome Q20.1
Taybi's syndrome Q87.2
Tay-Sachs amaurotic familial idiocy or disease
    E75.02
TBI (traumatic brain injury) —*see* category
    S06
Teacher's node or nodule J38.2
Tear, torn (traumatic) —*see also* Laceration
  with abortion —*see* Abortion
  annular fibrosis M51.35
  anus, anal (sphincter) S31.831
    complicating delivery
      with third degree perineal laceration
        O70.2
        with mucosa O70.3
      without third degree perineal laceration
        O70.4
    nontraumatic (healed) (old) K62.81
  articular cartilage, old —*see* Derangement,
    joint, articular cartilage, by site
  bladder
    with ectopic or molar pregnancy O08.6
    following ectopic or molar pregnancy
      O08.6
    obstetrical O71.5
    traumatic —*see* Injury, bladder
  bowel
    with ectopic or molar pregnancy O08.6
    following ectopic or molar pregnancy
      O08.6
    obstetrical trauma O71.5
  broad ligament
    with ectopic or molar pregnancy O08.6
    following ectopic or molar pregnancy
      O08.6
    obstetrical trauma O71.6
  bucket handle (knee) (meniscus) —*see* Tear,
    meniscus
  capsule, joint —*see* Sprain
  cartilage —*see also* Sprain
    articular, old —*see* Derangement, joint,
      articular cartilage, by site
  cervix
    with ectopic or molar pregnancy O08.6
    following ectopic or molar pregnancy
      O08.6
    obstetrical trauma (current) O71.3
    old N88.1
    traumatic —*see* Injury, uterus
  dural G97.41
    nontraumatic G96.11
  internal organ —*see* Injury, by site
  knee cartilage
    articular (current) S83.3-
    old —*see* Derangement, knee, meniscus,
      due to old tear
  ligament —*see* Sprain
  meniscus (knee) (current injury) S83.209
    bucket-handle S83.20-
    lateral
      bucket-handle S83.25-
      complex S83.27-
      peripheral S83.26-
      specified type NEC S83.28-
    medial
      bucket-handle S83.21-
      complex S83.23-
      peripheral S83.22-
      specified type NEC S83.24-
    old —*see* Derangement, knee, meniscus,
      due to old tear
    site other than knee - code as Sprain
    specified type NEC S83.20-
  muscle —*see* Strain
  pelvic
    floor, complicating delivery O70.1
    organ NEC, obstetrical trauma O71.5
      with ectopic or molar pregnancy O08.6
      following ectopic or molar pregnancy
        O08.6
  perineal, secondary O90.1

◀ New   ◀▥ Revised   ~~deleted~~ Deleted

Tear, torn *(Continued)*
- periurethral tissue, obstetrical trauma O71.82
  - with ectopic or molar pregnancy O08.6
  - following ectopic or molar pregnancy O08.6
- rectovaginal septum —*see* Laceration, vagina
- retina, retinal (without detachment) (horseshoe) —*see also* Break, retina, horseshoe
  - with detachment —*see* Detachment, retina, with retinal, break
- rotator cuff (nontraumatic) M75.10-
  - complete M75.12-
  - incomplete M75.11-
  - traumatic S46.01-
  - capsule S43.42-
- semilunar cartilage, knee —*see* Tear, meniscus
- supraspinatus (complete) (incomplete) (nontraumatic) (*see also* Tear, rotator cuff) M75.10-
- tendon —*see* Strain
- tentorial, at birth P10.4
- umbilical cord
  - complicating delivery O69.89
- urethra
  - with ectopic or molar pregnancy O08.6
  - following ectopic or molar pregnancy O08.6
  - obstetrical trauma O71.5
- uterus —*see* Injury, uterus
- vagina —*see* Laceration, vagina
- vessel, from catheter —*see* Puncture, accidental complicating surgery
- vulva, complicating delivery O70.0

Tear-stone —*see* Dacryolith
Teeth —*see also* condition
- grinding
  - psychogenic F45.8
  - sleep related G47.63
Teething (syndrome) K00.7
Telangiectasia, telangiectasis (verrucous) I78.1
- ataxic (cerebellar) (Louis-Bar) G11.3
- familial I78.0
- hemorrhagic, hereditary (congenital) (senile) I78.0
- hereditary, hemorrhagic (congenital) (senile) I78.0
- juxtafoveal H35.07-
- macular H35.07-
- parafoveal H35.07-
- retinal (idiopathic) (juxtafoveal) (macular) (parafoveal) H35.07-
- spider I78.1
Telephone scatologia F65.89
Telescoped bowel or intestine K56.1
- congenital Q43.8
Temperature
- body, high (of unknown origin) R50.9
- cold, trauma from T69.9
  - newborn P80.0
  - specified effect NEC T69.8
Temple —*see* condition
Temporal —*see* condition
Temporomandibular joint pain-dysfunction syndrome M26.62
Temporosphenoidal —*see* condition
Tendency
- bleeding —*see* Defect, coagulation
- suicide
  - meaning personal history of attempted suicide Z91.5
  - meaning suicidal ideation —*see* Ideation, suicidal
- to fall R29.6
Tenderness, abdominal R10.819
- epigastric R10.816
- generalized R10.817
- left lower quadrant R10.814
- left upper quadrant R10.812
- periumbilic R10.815

Tenderness, abdominal *(Continued)*
- rebound R10.829
  - epigastric R10.826
  - generalized R10.827
  - left lower quadrant R10.824
  - left upper quadrant R10.822
  - periumbilic R10.825
  - right lower quadrant R10.823
  - right upper quadrant R10.821
- right lower quadrant R10.813
- right upper quadrant R10.811
Tendinitis, tendonitis —*see also* Enthesopathy
- Achilles M76.6-
- adhesive —*see* Tenosynovitis, specified type NEC
  - shoulder —*see* Capsulitis, adhesive
- bicipital M75.2-
- calcific M65.2-
  - ankle M65.27-
  - foot M65.27-
  - forearm M65.23-
  - hand M65.24-
  - lower leg M65.26-
  - multiple sites M65.29
  - pelvic region M65.25-
  - shoulder M75.3-
  - specified site NEC M65.28
  - thigh M65.25-
  - upper arm M65.22-
- due to use, overuse, pressure —*see also* Disorder, soft tissue, due to use
  - specified NEC —*see* Disorder, soft tissue, due to use, specified NEC
- gluteal M76.0-
- patellar M76.5-
- peroneal M76.7-
- psoas M76.1-
- tibial (posterior) M76.82-
  - anterior M76.81-
- trochanteric —*see* Bursitis, hip, trochanteric
Tendon —*see* condition
Tendosynovitis —*see* Tenosynovitis
Tenesmus (rectal) R19.8
- vesical R30.1
Tennis elbow —*see* Epicondylitis, lateral
Tenonitis —*see also* Tenosynovitis
- eye (capsule) H05.04-
Tenontosynovitis —*see* Tenosynovitis
Tenontothecitis —*see* Tenosynovitis
Tenophyte —*see* Disorder, synovium, specified type NEC
Tenosynovitis (*see also* Synovitis) M65.9
- adhesive —*see* Tenosynovitis, specified type NEC
  - shoulder —*see* Capsulitis, adhesive
- bicipital (calcifying) —*see* Tendinitis, bicipital
- gonococcal A54.49
- in (due to)
  - crystals M65.8-
  - gonorrhea A54.49
  - syphilis (late) A52.78
  - use, overuse, pressure —*see also* Disorder, soft tissue, due to use
    - specified NEC —*see* Disorder, soft tissue, due to use, specified NEC
- infective NEC M65.1-
  - ankle M65.17-
  - foot M65.17-
  - forearm M65.13-
  - hand M65.14-
  - lower leg M65.16-
  - multiple sites M65.19
  - pelvic region M65.15-
  - shoulder region M65.11-
  - specified site NEC M65.18
  - thigh M65.15-
  - upper arm M65.12-
- radial styloid M65.4
- shoulder region M65.81-
  - adhesive —*see* Capsulitis, adhesive

Tenosynovitis *(Continued)*
- specified type NEC M65.88-
  - ankle M65.87-
  - foot M65.87-
  - forearm M65.83-
  - hand M65.84-
  - lower leg M65.86-
  - multiple sites M65.89
  - pelvic region M65.85-
  - shoulder region M65.81-
  - specified site NEC M65.88
  - thigh M65.85-
  - upper arm M65.82-
- tuberculous —*see* Tuberculosis, tenosynovitis
Tenovaginitis —*see* Tenosynovitis
Tension
- arterial, high —*see also* Hypertension
  - without diagnosis of hypertension R03.0
- headache G44.209
  - intractable G44.201
  - not intractable G44.209
- nervous R45.0
- pneumothorax J93.0
- premenstrual N94.3
- state (mental) F48.9
Tentorium —*see* condition
Teratencephalus Q89.8
Teratism Q89.7
Teratoblastoma (malignant) —*see* Neoplasm, malignant, by site
Teratocarcinoma —*see also* Neoplasm, malignant, by site
- liver C22.7
Teratoma (solid) —*see also* Neoplasm, uncertain behavior, by site
- with embryonal carcinoma, mixed —*see* Neoplasm, malignant, by site
- with malignant transformation —*see* Neoplasm, malignant, by site
- adult (cystic) —*see* Neoplasm, benign, by site
- benign —*see* Neoplasm, benign, by site
- combined with choriocarcinoma —*see* Neoplasm, malignant, by site
- cystic (adult) —*see* Neoplasm, benign, by site
- differentiated —*see* Neoplasm, benign, by site
- embryonal —*see also* Neoplasm, malignant, by site
  - liver C22.7
- immature —*see* Neoplasm, malignant, by site
- liver C22.7
  - adult, benign, cystic, differentiated type or mature D13.4
- malignant —*see also* Neoplasm, malignant, by site
  - anaplastic —*see* Neoplasm, malignant, by site
  - intermediate —*see* Neoplasm, malignant, by site
    - specified site —*see* Neoplasm, malignant, by site
    - unspecified site C62.90
  - undifferentiated —*see* Neoplasm, malignant, by site
- mature —*see* Neoplasm, uncertain behavior, by site
- malignant —*see* Neoplasm, by site, malignant, by site
- ovary D27.-
  - embryonal, immature or malignant C56-
- solid —*see* Neoplasm, uncertain behavior, by site
- testis C62.9-
  - adult, benign, cystic, differentiated type or mature D29.2-
  - scrotal C62.1-
  - undescended C62.0-
Termination
- anomalous —*see also* Malposition, congenital
  - right pulmonary vein Q26.3
- pregnancy, elective Z33.2

Ternidens diminutus infestation B81.8
Ternidensiasis B81.8
Terror (s) night (child) F51.4
Terrorism, victim of Z65.4
Terry's syndrome H44.2-
Tertiary —see condition
Test, tests, testing (for)
  adequacy (for dialysis)
    hemodialysis Z49.31
    peritoneal Z49.32
  blood pressure Z01.30
    abnormal reading —see Blood, pressure
  blood typing Z01.83
    Rh typing Z01.83
  blood-alcohol Z04.8
    positive —see Findings, abnormal, in
      blood
  blood-drug Z04.8
    positive —see Findings, abnormal, in
      blood
  cardiac pulse generator (battery) Z45.010
  fertility Z31.41
  genetic
    disease carrier status for procreative
      management
        female Z31.430
        male Z31.440
    male partner of patient with recurrent
      pregnancy loss Z31.441
    procreative management NEC
        female Z31.438
        male Z31.448
  hearing Z01.10
    with abnormal findings NEC Z01.118
  HIV (human immunodeficiency virus)
    nonconclusive (in infants) R75
    positive Z21
    seropositive Z21
  immunity status Z01.84
  intelligence NEC Z01.89
  laboratory (as part of a general medical
    examination) Z00.00
    with abnormal finding Z00.01
    for medicolegal reason NEC Z04.8
  male partner of patient with recurrent
    pregnancy loss Z31.441
  Mantoux (for tuberculosis) Z11.1
    abnormal result R76.11
  pregnancy, positive first pregnancy —see
    Pregnancy, normal, first
  procreative Z31.49
    fertility Z31.41
  skin, diagnostic
    allergy Z01.82
      special screening examination —see
        Screening, by name of disease
    Mantoux Z11.1
    tuberculin Z11.1
  specified NEC Z01.89
  tuberculin Z11.1
    abnormal result R76.11
  vision Z01.00
    with abnormal findings Z01.01
  Wassermann Z11.3
    positive —see Serology for syphilis,
      positive
Testicle, testicular, testis —see also condition
  feminization syndrome (see also Syndrome,
    androgen insensitivity) E34.51
  migrans Q55.29
Tetanus, tetanic (cephalic) (convulsions) A35
  with
    abortion A34
    ectopic or molar pregnancy O08.0
    following ectopic or molar pregnancy
      O08.0
    inoculation reaction (due to serum) —see
      Complications, vaccination
  neonatorum A33
  obstetrical A34
  puerperal, postpartum, childbirth A34

Tetany (due to) R29.0
  alkalosis E87.3
  associated with rickets E55.0
  convulsions R29.0
    hysterical F44.5
  functional (hysterical) F44.5
  hyperkinetic R29.0
    hysterical F44.5
  hyperpnea R06.4
    hysterical F44.5
    psychogenic F45.8
  hyperventilation (see also Hyperventilation)
    R06.4
    hysterical F44.5
  neonatal (without calcium or magnesium
    deficiency) P71.3
  parathyroid (gland) E20.9
  parathyroprival E89.2
  post- (para)thyroidectomy E89.2
  postoperative E89.2
  pseudotetany R29.0
  psychogenic (conversion reaction) F44.5
Tetralogy of Fallot Q21.3
Tetraplegia (chronic) (see also Quadriplegia)
  G82.50-
Thailand hemorrhagic fever A91
Thalassanemia —see Thalassemia
Thalassemia (anemia) (disease) D56.9
  with other hemoglobinopathy D56.8
  alpha (major) (severe) (triple gene defect)
    D56.0
    minor D56.3
    silent carrier D56.3
    trait D56.3
  beta (severe) D56.1
    homozygous D56.1
    major D56.1
    minor D56.3
    trait D56.3
  delta-beta (homozygous) D56.2
    minor D56.3
    trait D56.3
  dominant D56.8
  hemoglobin
    C D56.8
    E-beta D56.5
  intermedia D56.1
  major D56.1
  minor D56.3
  mixed D56.8
  sickle-cell —see Disease, sickle-cell,
    thalassemia
  specified type NEC D56.8
  trait D56.3
  variants D56.8
Thanatophoric dwarfism or short stature Q77.1
Thaysen-Gee disease (nontropical sprue) K90.0
Thaysen's disease K90.0
Thecoma D27-
  luteinized D27-
  malignant C56-
Thelarche, premature E30.8
Thelaziasis B83.8
Thelitis N61
  puerperal, postpartum or gestational —see
    Infection, nipple
Therapeutic —see condition
Therapy
  drug, long-term (current) (prophylactic)
    agents affecting estrogen receptors and
      estrogen levels NEC Z79.818
    anastrozole (Arimidex) Z79.811
    antibiotics Z79.2
      short-term use - omit code
    anticoagulants Z79.01
    anti-inflammatory Z79.1
    antiplatelet Z79.02
    antithrombotics Z79.02
    aromatase inhibitors Z79.811
    aspirin Z79.82
    birth control pill or patch Z79.3

Therapy (Continued)
  drug, long-term (Continued)
    bisphosphonates Z79.83
    contraceptive, oral Z79.3
    drug, specified NEC Z79.899
    estrogen receptor downregulators
      Z79.818
    Evista Z79.810
    exemestane (Aromasin) Z79.811
    Fareston Z79.810
    fulvestrant (Faslodex) Z79.818
    gonadotropin-releasing hormone (GnRH)
      agonist Z79.818
    goserelin acetate (Zoladex) Z79.818
    hormone replacement (postmenopausal)
      Z79.890
    insulin Z79.4
    letrozole (Femara) Z79.811
    leuprolide acetate (leuprorelin) (Lupron)
      Z79.818
    megestrol acetate (Megace) Z79.818
    methadone
      for pain management Z79.891
      maintenance therapy F11.20
    Nolvadex Z79.810
    opiate analgesic Z79.891
    oral contraceptive Z79.3
    raloxifene (Evista) Z79.810
    selective estrogen receptor modulators
      (SERMs) Z79.810
    short term - omit code
    steroids
      inhaled Z79.51
      systemic Z79.52
    tamoxifen (Nolvadex) Z79.810
    toremifene (Fareston) Z79.810
Thermic —see condition
Thermography (abnormal) (see also Abnormal,
    diagnostic imaging) R93.8
  breast R92.8
Thermoplegia T67.0
Thesaurismosis, glycogen —see Disease,
    glycogen storage
Thiamin deficiency E51.9
  specified NEC E51.8
Thiaminic deficiency with beriberi E51.11
Thibierge-Weissenbach syndrome —see
    Sclerosis, systemic
Thickening
  bone —see Hypertrophy, bone
  breast N64.59
  endometrium R93.8
  epidermal L85.9
    specified NEC L85.8
  hymen N89.6
  larynx J38.7
  nail L60.2
    congenital Q84.5
  periosteal —see Hypertrophy, bone
  pleura J92.9
    with asbestos J92.0
  skin R23.4
  subepiglottic J38.7
  tongue K14.8
  valve, heart —see Endocarditis
Thigh —see condition
Thinning vertebra —see Spondylopathy,
    specified NEC
Thirst, excessive R63.1
  due to deprivation of water T73.1
Thomsen disease G71.12
Thoracic —see also condition
  kidney Q63.2
  outlet syndrome G54.0
Thoracogastroschisis (congenital) Q79.8
Thoracopagus Q89.4
Thorax —see condition
Thorn's syndrome N28.89
Thorson-Björck syndrome E34.0
Threadworm (infection) (infestation)
    B80

Threatened
  abortion O20.0
    with subsequent abortion O03.9
  job loss, anxiety concerning Z56.2
  labor (without delivery) O47.9
    after 37 completed weeks of gestation
      O47.1
    before 37 completed weeks of gestation
      O47.0-
  loss of job, anxiety concerning Z56.2
  miscarriage O20.0
  unemployment, anxiety concerning Z56.2
Three-day fever A93.1
Threshers' lung J67.0
Thrix annulata (congenital) Q84.1
Throat —see condition
Thrombasthenia (Glanzmann) (hemorrhagic)
  (hereditary) D69.1
Thromboangiitis I73.1
  obliterans (general) I73.1
    cerebral I67.89
    vessels
      brain I67.89
      spinal cord I67.89
Thromboarteritis —see Arteritis
Thromboasthenia (Glanzmann) (hemorrhagic)
  (hereditary) D69.1
Thrombocytasthenia (Glanzmann) D69.1
Thrombocythemia (essential) (hemorrhagic)
  (idiopathic) (primary) D47.3
Thrombocytopathy (dystrophic) (granulopenic)
  D69.1
Thrombocytopenia, thrombocytopenic D69.6
  with absent radius (TAR) Q87.2
  congenital D69.42
  dilutional D69.59
  due to
    drugs D69.59
    extracorporeal circulation of blood D69.59
    (massive)blood transfusion D69.59
    platelet alloimmunization D69.59
  essential D69.3
  heparin induced (HIT) D75.82
  hereditary D69.42
  idiopathic D69.3
  neonatal, transitory P61.0
    due to
      exchange transfusion P61.0
      idiopathic maternal thrombocytopenia
        P61.0
      isoimmunization P61.0
  primary NEC D69.49
    idiopathic D69.3
  puerperal, postpartum O72.3
  secondary D69.59
  transient neonatal P61.0
Thrombocytosis, essential D47.3
  primary D47.3
Thromboembolism —see Embolism
Thrombopathy (Bernard-Soulier) D69.1
  constitutional D68.0
  Willebrand-Jurgens D68.0
Thrombopenia —see Thrombocytopenia
Thrombophilia D68.59
  primary NEC D68.59
  secondary NEC D68.69
  specified NEC D68.69
Thrombophlebitis I80.9
  antepartum O22.2-
    deep O22.3-
    superficial O22.2-
  cavernous (venous) sinus G08
    complicating pregnancy O22.5-
    nonpyogenic I67.6
  cerebral (sinus) (vein) G08
    nonpyogenic I67.6
    sequelae G09
  due to implanted device —see Complications,
    by site and type, specified NEC
  during or resulting from a procedure NEC
    T81.72

Thrombophlebitis (Continued)
  femoral vein (superficial) I80.1-
  femoropopliteal vein I80.0-
  hepatic (vein) I80.8
  idiopathic, recurrent I82.1
  iliofemoral I80.1-
  intracranial venous sinus (any) G08
    nonpyogenic I67.6
    sequelae G09
  intraspinal venous sinuses and veins G08
    nonpyogenic G95.19
  lateral (venous) sinus G08
    nonpyogenic I67.6
  leg I80.299
    superficial I80.0-
  longitudinal (venous) sinus G08
    nonpyogenic I67.6
  lower extremity I80.299
  migrans, migrating I82.1
  pelvic
    with ectopic or molar pregnancy O08.0
    following ectopic or molar pregnancy
      O08.0
    puerperal O87.1
  popliteal vein —see Phlebitis, leg, deep,
    popliteal
  portal (vein) K75.1
  postoperative T81.72
  pregnancy —see Thrombophlebitis,
    antepartum
  puerperal, postpartum, childbirth O87.0
    deep O87.1
    pelvic O87.1
    septic O86.81
    superficial O87.0
  saphenous (greater) (lesser) I80.0-
  sinus (intracranial) G08
    nonpyogenic I67.6
  specified site NEC I80.8
  tibial vein I80.23-
Thrombosis, thrombotic (bland) (multiple)
  (progressive) (silent) (vessel) I82.90
  anal K64.5
  antepartum —see Thrombophlebitis,
    antepartum
  aorta, aortic I74.10
    abdominal I74.09
      saddle I74.01
    bifurcation I74.09
    saddle I74.01
    specified site NEC I74.19
    terminal I74.09
    thoracic I74.11
    valve —see Endocarditis, aortic
  apoplexy I63.3
  artery, arteries (postinfectional) I74.9
    auditory, internal —see Occlusion, artery,
      precerebral, specified NEC
    basilar —see Occlusion, artery, basilar
    carotid (common) (internal) —see
      Occlusion, artery, carotid
    cerebellar (anterior inferior) (posterior
      inferior) (superior) —see Occlusion,
      artery, cerebellar
    cerebral —see Occlusion, artery, cerebral
    choroidal (anterior) —see Occlusion, artery,
      cerebral, specified NEC
    communicating, posterior —see Occlusion,
      artery, cerebral, specified NEC
    coronary —see also Infarct, myocardium
      not resulting in infarction I24.0
    hepatic I74.8
    hypophyseal —see Occlusion, artery,
      cerebral, specified NEC
    iliac I74.5
    limb I74.4
      lower I74.3
      upper I74.2
    meningeal, anterior or posterior —see
      Occlusion, artery, cerebral, specified
      NEC

Thrombosis, thrombotic (Continued)
  artery, arteries (Continued)
    mesenteric (with gangrene) K55.0
    ophthalmic —see Occlusion, artery, retina
    pontine —see Occlusion, artery, cerebral,
      specified NEC
    precerebral —see Occlusion, artery,
      precerebral
    pulmonary (iatrogenic) —see Embolism,
      pulmonary
    renal N28.0
    retinal —see Occlusion, artery, retina
    spinal, anterior or posterior G95.11
    traumatic NEC T14.8
    vertebral —see Occlusion, artery, vertebral
  atrium, auricular —see also Infarct,
    myocardium
    following acute myocardial infarction
      (current complication) I23.6
    not resulting in infarction I24.0
  basilar (artery) —see Occlusion, artery,
    basilar
  brain (artery) (stem) —see also Occlusion,
    artery, cerebral
    due to syphilis A52.05
    puerperal O99.43
    sinus —see Thrombosis, intracranial
      venous sinus
  capillary I78.8
  cardiac —see also Infarct, myocardium
    not resulting in infarction I24.0
    valve —see Endocarditis
  carotid (artery) (common) (internal) —see
    Occlusion, artery, carotid
  cavernous (venous) sinus —see Thrombosis,
    intracranial venous sinus
  cerebellar artery (anterior inferior) (posterior
    inferior) (superior) I66.3
  cerebral (artery) —see Occlusion, artery,
    cerebral
  cerebrovenous sinus —see also Thrombosis,
    intracranial venous sinus
    puerperium O87.3
  chronic I82.91
  coronary (artery) (vein) —see also Infarct,
    myocardium
    not resulting in infarction I24.0
  corpus cavernosum N48.89
  cortical I66.9
  deep —see Embolism, vein, lower extremity
  due to device, implant or graft (see also
    Complications, by site and type,
    specified NEC) T85.86
    arterial graft NEC T82.868
    breast (implant) T85.86
    catheter NEC T85.86
      dialysis (renal) T82.868
        intraperitoneal T85.86
      infusion NEC T82.868
        spinal (epidural) (subdural) T85.86
      urinary (indwelling) T83.86
    electronic (electrode) (pulse generator)
      (stimulator)
      bone T84.86
      cardiac T82.867
      nervous system (brain) (peripheral
        nerve) (spinal) T85.86
      urinary T83.86
    fixation, internal (orthopedic) NEC T84.86
    gastrointestinal (bile duct) (esophagus)
      T85.86
    genital NEC T83.86
    heart T82.867
    joint prosthesis T84.86
    ocular (corneal graft) (orbital implant)
      NEC T85.86
    orthopedic NEC T84.86
    specified NEC T85.86
    urinary NEC T83.86
    vascular NEC T82.868
    ventricular intracranial shunt T85.86

Thrombosis, thrombotic *(Continued)*
  during the puerperium —*see* Thrombosis,
      puerperal
  endocardial —*see also* Infarct, myocardium
      not resulting in infarction I24.0
  eye —*see* Occlusion, retina
  genital organ
      female NEC N94.89
          pregnancy —*see* Thrombophlebitis,
              antepartum
      male N50.1
  gestational —*see* Phlebopathy, gestational
  heart (chamber) —*see also* Infarct,
      myocardium
      not resulting in infarction I24.0
  hepatic (vein) I82.0
      artery I74.8
  history (of) Z86.718
  intestine (with gangrene) K55.0
  intracardiac NEC (apical) (atrial) (auricular)
      (ventricular) (old) I51.3
  intracranial (arterial) I66.9
      venous sinus (any) G08
          nonpyogenic origin I67.6
          puerperium O87.3
  intramural —*see also* Infarct, myocardium
      not resulting in infarction I24.0
  intraspinal venous sinuses and veins G08
      nonpyogenic G95.19
  kidney (artery) N28.0
  lateral (venous) sinus —*see* Thrombosis,
      intracranial venous sinus
  leg —*see* Thrombosis, vein, lower
      extremity
      arterial I74.3
  liver (venous) I82.0
      artery I74.8
      portal vein I81
  longitudinal (venous) sinus —*see* Thrombosis,
      intracranial venous sinus
  lower limb —*see* Thrombosis, vein, lower
      extremity
  lung (iatrogenic) (postoperative) —*see*
      Embolism, pulmonary
  meninges (brain) (arterial) I66.8
  mesenteric (artery) (with gangrene) K55.0
      vein (inferior) (superior) I81
  mitral I34.8
  mural —*see also* Infarct, myocardium
      due to syphilis A52.06
      not resulting in infarction I24.0
  omentum (with gangrene) K55.0
  ophthalmic —*see* Occlusion, retina
  pampiniform plexus (male) N50.1
  parietal —*see also* Infarct, myocardium
      not resulting in infarction I24.0
  penis, superficial vein N48.81
  perianal venous K64.5
  peripheral arteries I74.4
      upper I74.2
  personal history (of) Z86.718
  portal I81
      due to syphilis A52.09
  precerebral artery —*see* Occlusion, artery,
      precerebral
  puerperal, postpartum O87.0
      brain (artery) O99.43
          venous (sinus) O87.3
      cardiac O99.43
      cerebral (artery) O99.43
          venous (sinus) O87.3
      superficial O87.0
  pulmonary (artery) (iatrogenic)
      (postoperative) (vein) —*see* Embolism,
      pulmonary
  renal (artery) N28.0
      vein I82.3
  resulting from presence of device, implant or
      graft —*see* Complications, by site and
      type, specified NEC
  retina, retinal —*see* Occlusion, retina

Thrombosis, thrombotic *(Continued)*
  scrotum N50.1
  seminal vesicle N50.1
  sigmoid (venous) sinus —*see* Thrombosis,
      intracranial venous sinus
  sinus, intracranial (any) —*see* Thrombosis,
      intracranial venous sinus
  specified site NEC I82.890
      chronic I82.891
  spermatic cord N50.1
  spinal cord (arterial) G95.11
      due to syphilis A52.09
      pyogenic origin G06.1
  spleen, splenic D73.5
      artery I74.8
  testis N50.1
  traumatic NEC T14.8
  tricuspid I07.8
  tumor —*see* Neoplasm, by site
  tunica vaginalis N50.1
  umbilical cord (vessels), complicating
      delivery O69.5
  vas deferens N50.1
  vein (acute) I82.90
      antecubital I82.61-
          chronic I82.71-
      axillary I82.A1-
          chronic I82.A2-
      basilic I82.61-
          chronic I82.71-
      brachial I82.62-
          chronic I82.72-
      brachiocephalic (innominate) I82.290
          chronic I82.291
      cerebral, nonpyogenic I67.6
      cephalic I82.61-
          chronic I82.71-
      chronic I82.91
      deep (DVT) I82.40-
          calf I82.4Z-
              chronic I82.5Z-
          lower leg I82.4Z-
              chronic I82.5Z-
          thigh I82.4Y-
              chronic I82.5Y-
          upper leg I82.4Y
              chronic I82.5y-
      femoral I82.41-
          chronic I82.51-
      iliac (iliofemoral) I82.42-
          chronic I82.52-
      innominate I82.290
          chronic I82.291
      internal jugular I82.C1-
          chronic I82.C2-
      lower extremity
          deep I82.40-
              chronic I82.50-
              specified NEC I82.49-
                  chronic NEC I82.59-
          distal
              deep I82.4Z-
          proximal
              deep I82.4Y-
                  chronic I82.5Y-
          superficial I82.81-
      perianal K64.5
      popliteal I82.43-
          chronic I82.53-
      radial I82.62-
          chronic I82.72-
      renal I82.3
      saphenous (greater) (lesser) I82.81-
      specified NEC I82.890
          chronic NEC I82.891
      subclavian I82.B1-
          chronic I82.B2-
      thoracic NEC I82.290
          chronic I82.291
      tibial I82.44-
          chronic I82.54-

Thrombosis, thrombotic *(Continued)*
  vein *(Continued)*
      ulnar I82.62-
          chronic I82.72-
      upper extremity I82.60-
          chronic I82.70-
          deep I82.62-
              chronic I82.72-
          superficial I82.61-
              chronic I82.71-
      vena cava
          inferior I82.220
              chronic I82.221
          superior I82.210
              chronic I82.211
      venous, perianal K64.5
      ventricle —*see also* Infarct, myocardium
          following acute myocardial infarction
              (current complication) I23.6
          not resulting in infarction I24.0
Thrombus —*see* Thrombosis
Thrush —*see also* Candidiasis
  newborn P37.5
  oral B37.0
  vaginal B37.3
Thumb —*see also* condition
  sucking (child problem) F98.8
Thymitis E32.8
Thymoma (benign) D15.0
  malignant C37
Thymus, thymic (gland) —*see* condition
Thyrocele —*see* Goiter
Thyroglossal —*see also* condition
  cyst Q89.2
  duct, persistent Q89.2
Thyroid (gland) (body) —*see also* condition
  hormone resistance E07.89
  lingual Q89.2
  nodule (cystic) (nontoxic) (single) E04.1
Thyroiditis E06.9
  acute (nonsuppurative) (pyogenic)
      (suppurative) E06.0
  autoimmune E06.3
  chronic (nonspecific) (sclerosing) E06.5
      with thyrotoxicosis, transient E06.2
      fibrous E06.5
      lymphadenoid E06.3
      lymphocytic E06.3
      lymphoid E06.3
  de Quervain's E06.1
  drug-induced E06.4
  fibrous (chronic) E06.5
  giant-cell (follicular) E06.1
  granulomatous (de Quervain) (subacute)
      E06.1
  Hashimoto's (struma lymphomatosa)
      E06.3
  iatrogenic E06.4
  ligneous E06.5
  lymphocytic (chronic) E06.3
  lymphoid E06.3
  lymphomatous E06.3
  nonsuppurative E06.1
  postpartum, puerperal O90.5
  pseudotuberculous E06.1
  pyogenic E06.0
  radiation E06.4
  Riedel's E06.5
  subacute (granulomatous) E06.1
  suppurative E06.0
  tuberculous A18.81
  viral E06.1
  woody E06.5
Thyrolingual duct, persistent Q89.2
Thyromegaly E01.0
Thyrotoxic
  crisis —*see* Thyrotoxicosis
  heart disease or failure (*see also*
      Thyrotoxicosis) E05.90 *[143]*
      with thyroid storm E05.91 *[143]*
  storm —*see* Thyrotoxicosis

◀ New   ◀◀ Revised   ~~deleted~~ Deleted

Thyrotoxicosis (recurrent) E05.90
  with
    goiter (diffuse) E05.00
      with thyroid storm E05.01
      adenomatous uninodular E05.10
        with thyroid storm E05.11
      multinodular E05.20
        with thyroid storm E05.21
      nodular E05.20
        with thyroid storm E05.21
      uninodular E05.10
        with thyroid storm E05.11
    infiltrative
      dermopathy E05.00
        with thyroid storm E05.01
      ophthalmopathy E05.00
        with thyroid storm E05.01
    single thyroid nodule E05.10
      with thyroid storm E05.11
    thyroid storm E05.91
  due to
    ectopic thyroid nodule or tissue E05.30
      with thyroid storm E05.31
    ingestion of (excessive) thyroid material
      E05.40
      with thyroid storm E05.41
    overproduction of thyroid-stimulating
      hormone E05.80
      with thyroid storm E05.81
    specified cause NEC E05.80
      with thyroid storm E05.81
  factitia E05.40
    with thyroid storm E05.41
  heart E05.90 [I43]
    with thyroid storm E05.91 [I43]
    failure E05.90 [I43]
  neonatal (transient) P72.1
  transient with chronic thyroiditis E06.2
Tibia vara —see Osteochondrosis, juvenile, tibia
Tic (disorder) F95.9
  breathing F95.8
  child problem F95.0
  compulsive F95.1
  de la Tourette F95.2
  degenerative (generalized) (localized) G25.69
    facial G25.69
  disorder
    chronic
      motor F95.1
      vocal F95.1
    combined vocal and multiple motor F95.2
    transient F95.0
  douloureux G50.0
    atypical G50.1
    postherpetic, postzoster B02.22
  drug-induced G25.61
  eyelid F95.8
  habit F95.9
    chronic F95.1
    transient of childhood F95.0
  lid, transient of childhood F95.0
  motor-verbal F95.2
  occupational F48.8
  orbicularis F95.8
    transient of childhood F95.0
  organic origin G25.69
  postchoreic G25.69
  psychogenic, compulsive F95.1
  salaam R25.8
  spasm (motor or vocal) F95.9
    chronic F95.1
    transient of childhood F95.0
  specified NEC F95.8
Tick-borne —see condition
Tietze's disease or syndrome M94.0
Tight, tightness
  anus K62.89
  chest R07.89
  fascia (lata) M62.89
  foreskin (congenital) N47.1
  hymen, hymenal ring N89.6

Tight, tightness (Continued)
  introitus (acquired) (congenital) N89.6
  rectal sphincter K62.89
  tendon —see Short, tendon
  urethral sphincter N35.9
Tilting vertebra —see Dorsopathy, deforming,
    specified NEC
Timidity, child F93.8
Tin-miner's lung J63.5
Tinea (intersecta) (tarsi) B35.9
  amiantacea L44.8
  asbestina B35.0
  barbae B35.0
  beard B35.0
  black dot B35.0
  blanca B36.2
  capitis B35.0
  corporis B35.4
  cruris B35.6
  flava B36.0
  foot B35.3
  furfuracea B36.0
  imbricata (Tokelau) B35.5
  kerion B35.0
  manuum B35.2
  microsporic —see Dermatophytosis
  nigra B36.1
  nodosa —see Piedra
  pedis B35.3
  scalp B35.0
  specified site NEC B35.8
  sycosis B35.0
  tonsurans B35.0
  trichophytic —see Dermatophytosis
  unguium B35.1
  versicolor B36.0
Tingling sensation (skin) R20.2
Tinnitus (audible) (aurium) (subjective) —see
    subcategory H93.1
Tipped tooth (teeth) M26.33
Tipping
  pelvis M95.5
    with disproportion (fetopelvic) O33.0
      causing obstructed labor O65.0
  tooth (teeth), fully erupted M26.33
Tiredness R53.83
Tissue —see condition
Tobacco (nicotine)
  dependence —see Dependence, drug, nicotine
  harmful use Z72.0
  heart —see Tobacco, toxic effect
  maternal use, affecting newborn P04.2
  toxic effect —see Table of Drugs and
      Chemicals, by substance, poisoning
    chewing tobacco —see Table of Drugs
        and Chemicals, by substance,
        poisoning
    cigarettes —see Table of Drugs and
        Chemicals, by substance,
        poisoning
  use Z72.0
    complicating
      childbirth O99.334
      pregnancy O99.33-
      puerperium O99.335
    counseling and surveillance Z71.6
  withdrawal state —see Dependence, drug,
      nicotine
Tocopherol deficiency E56.0
Todd's
  cirrhosis K74.3
  paralysis (postepileptic) (transitory) G83.84
Toe —see condition
Toilet, artificial opening —see Attention to,
    artificial, opening
Tokelau (ringworm) B35.5
Tollwut —see Rabies
Tommaselli's disease R31.9
  correct substance properly administered —see
      Table of Drugs and Chemicals, by drug,
      adverse effect

Tommaselli's disease (Continued)
  overdose or wrong substance given or
      taken —see Table of Drugs and
      Chemicals, by drug, poisoning
Tongue —see also condition
  tie Q38.1
Tonic pupil —see Anomaly, pupil, function,
    tonic pupil
Toni-Fanconi syndrome (cystinosis) E72.09
  with cystinosis E72.04
Tonsil —see condition
Tonsillitis (acute) (catarrhal) (croupous)
    (follicular) (gangrenous) (infective)
    (lacunar) (lingual) (malignant)
    (membranous) (parenchymatous)
    (phlegmonous) (pseudomembranous)
    (purulent) (septic) (subacute)
    (suppurative) (toxic) (ulcerative)
    (vesicular) (viral) J03.90
  chronic J35.01
    with adenoiditis J35.03
  diphtheritic A36.0
  hypertrophic J35.01
    with adenoiditis J35.03
  recurrent J03.91
  specified organism NEC J03.80
    recurrent J03.81
  staphylococcal J03.80
    recurrent J03.81
  streptococcal J03.00
    recurrent J03.01
  tuberculous A15.8
  Vincent's A69.1
Tooth, teeth —see condition
Toothache K08.8
Topagnosis R20.8
Tophi —see Gout, chronic
TORCH infection —see Infection, congenital
  without active infection P00.2
Torn —see Tear
Tornwaldt's cyst or disease J39.2
Torsion
  accessory tube —see Torsion, fallopian tube
  adnexa (female) —see Torsion, fallopian tube
  aorta, acquired I77.1
  appendix epididymis N44.04
  appendix testis N44.03
  bile duct (common) (hepatic) K83.8
    congenital Q44.5
  bowel, colon or intestine K56.2
  cervix —see Malposition, uterus
  cystic duct K82.8
  dystonia —see Dystonia, torsion
  epididymis (appendix) N44.04
  fallopian tube N83.52
    with ovary N83.53
  gallbladder K82.8
    congenital Q44.1
  hydatid of Morgagni
    female N83.52
    male N44.03
  kidney (pedicle) (leading to infarction)
    N28.0
  Meckel's diverticulum (congenital) Q43.0
    malignant —see Table of Neoplasms, small
        intestine, malignant
  mesentery K56.2
  omentum K56.2
  organ or site, congenital NEC —see Anomaly,
      by site
  ovary (pedicle) N83.51
    with fallopian tube N83.53
    congenital Q50.2
  oviduct —see Torsion, fallopian tube
  penis (acquired) N48.82
    congenital Q55.63
  spasm —see Dystonia, torsion
  spermatic cord N44.02
    extravaginal N44.01
    intravaginal N44.02
  spleen D73.5

Torsion *(Continued)*
　testis, testicle N44.00
　　appendix N44.03
　tibia —*see* Deformity, limb, specified type
　　NEC, lower leg
　uterus —*see* Malposition, uterus
Torticollis (intermittent) (spastic) M43.6
　congenital (sternomastoid) Q68.0
　due to birth injury P15.8
　hysterical F44.4
　ocular R29.891
　psychogenic F45.8
　　conversion reaction F44.4
　rheumatic M43.6
　rheumatoid M06.88
　spasmodic G24.3
　traumatic, current S13.4
Tortipelvis G24.1
Tortuous
　artery I77.1
　organ or site, congenital NEC —*see* Distortion
　retinal vessel, congenital Q14.1
　ureter N13.8
　urethra N36.8
　vein —*see* Varix
Torture, victim of Z65.4
Torula, torular (histolytica) (infection) —*see*
　Cryptococcosis
Torulosis —*see* Cryptococcosis
Torus (mandibularis) (palatinus) M27.0
　fracture —*see* Fracture, by site, torus
Touraine's syndrome Q79.8
Tourette's syndrome F95.2
Tourniquet syndrome —*see* Constriction,
　external, by site
Tower skull Q75.0
　with exophthalmos Q87.0
Toxemia R68.89
　bacterial —*see* Sepsis
　burn —*see* Burn
　eclamptic (with pre-existing hypertension) —
　　see Eclampsia
　erysipelatous —*see* Erysipelas
　fatigue R68.89
　food —*see* Poisoning, food
　gastrointestinal K52.1
　intestinal K52.1
　kidney —*see* Uremia
　malarial —*see* Malaria
　myocardial —*see* Myocarditis, toxic
　of pregnancy —*see* Pre-eclampsia
　pre-eclamptic —*see* Pre-eclampsia
　small intestine K52.1
　staphylococcal, due to food A05.0
　stasis R68.89
　uremic —*see* Uremia
　urinary —*see* Uremia
Toxemica cerebropathia psychica
　(nonalcoholic) F04
　alcoholic —*see* Alcohol, amnestic disorder
Toxic (poisoning) —*see also* condition T65.91
　effect —*see* Table of Drugs and Chemicals, by
　　substance, poisoning
　shock syndrome A48.3
　thyroid (gland) —*see* Thyrotoxicosis
Toxicemia —*see* Toxemia
Toxicity —*see* Table of Drugs and Chemicals, by
　substance, poisoning
　fava bean D55.0
　food, noxious —*see* Poisoning, food
　from drug or nonmedicinal substance —*see*
　　Table of Drugs and Chemicals, by
　　drug
Toxicosis —*see also* Toxemia
　capillary, hemorrhagic D69.0
Toxinfection, gastrointestinal K52.1
Toxocariasis B83.0
Toxoplasma, toxoplasmosis (acquired) B58.9
　with
　　hepatitis B58.1
　　meningoencephalitis B58.2
　　ocular involvement B58.00

Toxoplasma, toxoplasmosis *(Continued)*
　with *(Continued)*
　　other organ involvement B58.89
　　pneumonia, pneumonitis B58.3
　congenital (acute) (subacute) (chronic) P37.1
　maternal, manifest toxoplasmosis in infant
　　(acute) (subacute) (chronic) P37.1
tPA (rtPA) administation in a different facility
　within the last 24 hours prior to admission
　to current facility Z92.82
Trabeculation, bladder N32.89
Trachea —*see* condition
Tracheitis (catarrhal) (infantile) (membranous)
　(plastic) (septal) (suppurative) (viral)
　J04.10
　with
　　bronchitis (15 years of age and above) J40
　　　acute or subacute —*see* Bronchitis,
　　　　acute
　　　chronic J42
　　　tuberculous NEC A15.5
　　　under 15 years of age J20.9
　　laryngitis (acute) J04.2
　　　chronic J37.1
　　　tuberculous NEC A15.5
　acute J04.10
　　with obstruction J04.11
　chronic J42
　　with
　　　bronchitis (chronic) J42
　　　laryngitis (chronic) J37.1
　diphtheritic (membranous) A36.89
　due to external agent —*see* Inflammation,
　　respiratory, upper, due to
　syphilitic A52.73
　tuberculous A15.5
Trachelitis (nonvenereal) —*see* Cervicitis
Tracheobronchial —*see* condition
Tracheobronchitis (15 years of age and
　above) —*see also* Bronchitis
　due to
　　Bordetella bronchiseptica A37.80
　　　with pneumonia A37.81
　　Francisella tularensis A21.8
Tracheobronchomegaly Q32.4
　with bronchiectasis J47.9
　　with
　　　exacerbation (acute) J47.1
　　　lower respiratory infection J47.0
　acquired J98.09
　　with bronchiectasis J47.9
　　　with
　　　　exacerbation (acute) J47.1
　　　　lower respiratory infection J47.0
Tracheobronchopneumonitis —*see* Pneumonia,
　broncho-
Tracheocele (external) (internal) J39.8
　congenital Q32.1
Tracheomalacia J39.8
　congenital Q32.0
Tracheopharyngitis (acute) J06.9
　chronic J42
　due to external agent —*see* Inflammation,
　　respiratory, upper, due to
Tracheostenosis J39.8
Tracheostomy
　complication —*see* Complication,
　　tracheostomy
　status Z93.0
　　attention to Z43.0
　　malfunctioning J95.03
Trachoma, trachomatous A71.9
　active (stage) A71.1
　contraction of conjunctiva A71.1
　dubium A71.0
　healed or sequelae B94.0
　initial (stage) A71.0
　pannus A71.1
　Türck's J37.0
Traction, vitreomacular H43.82-
Train sickness T75.3

Trait (s)
　Hb-S D57.3
　hemoglobin
　　abnormal NEC D58.2
　　　with thalassemia D56.3
　　C —*see* Disease, hemoglobin C
　　S (Hb-S) D57.3
　Lepore D56.3
　personality, accentuated Z73.1
　sickle-cell D57.3
　　with elliptocytosis or spherocytosis
　　　D57.3
　type A personality Z73.1
Tramp Z59.0
Trance R41.89
　hysterical F44.89
Transaminasemia R74.0
Transection
　abdomen (partial) S38.3
　aorta (incomplete) —*see also* Injury, aorta
　　complete —*see* Injury, aorta, laceration,
　　　major
　carotid artery (incomplete) —*see also* Injury,
　　blood vessel, carotid, laceration
　　complete —*see* Injury, blood vessel, carotid,
　　　laceration, major
　celiac artery (incomplete) S35.211
　　branch (incomplete) S35.291
　　　complete S35.292
　　complete S35.212
　innominate
　　artery (incomplete) —*see also* Injury, blood
　　　vessel, thoracic, innominate, artery,
　　　laceration
　　　complete —*see* Injury, blood vessel,
　　　　thoracic, innominate, artery,
　　　　laceration, major
　　vein (incomplete) —*see also* Injury, blood
　　　vessel, thoracic, innominate, vein,
　　　laceration
　　　complete —*see* Injury, blood vessel,
　　　　thoracic, innominate, vein,
　　　　laceration, major
　jugular vein (external) (incomplete) —*see*
　　also Injury, blood vessel, jugular vein,
　　laceration
　　complete —*see* Injury, blood vessel, jugular
　　　vein, laceration, major
　　internal (incomplete) —*see also* Injury,
　　　blood vessel, jugular vein, internal,
　　　laceration
　　　complete —*see* Injury, blood vessel,
　　　　jugular vein, internal, laceration,
　　　　major
　mesenteric artery (incomplete) —*see also*
　　Injury, mesenteric, artery, laceration
　　complete —*see* Injury, mesenteric artery,
　　　laceration, major
　pulmonary vessel (incomplete) —*see*
　　also Injury, blood vessel, thoracic,
　　pulmonary, laceration
　　complete —*see* Injury, blood vessel,
　　　thoracic, pulmonary, laceration,
　　　major
　subclavian —*see* Transection, innominate
　vena cava (incomplete) —*see also* Injury, vena
　　cava
　　complete —*see* Injury, vena cava,
　　　laceration, major
　vertebral artery (incomplete) —*see also*
　　Injury, blood vessel, vertebral,
　　laceration
　　complete —*see* Injury, blood vessel,
　　　vertebral, laceration, major
Transfusion
　associated (red blood cell) hemochromatosis
　　E83.111
　blood
　　ABO incompatible —*see* Complication (s),
　　　transfusion, incompatibility reaction,
　　　ABO

Transfusion (Continued)
  blood (Continued)
    minor·blood group (Duffy) (E) (K(ell))
        (Kidd) (Lewis) (M) (N) (P) (S) T80.89
      reaction or complication —see
          Complications, transfusion
    fetomaternal (mother) —see Pregnancy,
        complicated by, placenta, transfusion
        syndrome
    maternofetal (mother) —see Pregnancy,
        complicated by, placenta, transfusion
        syndrome
    placental (syndrome) (mother) —see
        Pregnancy, complicated by, placenta,
        transfusion syndrome
    reaction (adverse) —see Complications,
        transfusion
    related acute lung injury (TRALI) J95.84
    twin-to-twin —see Pregnancy, complicated by,
        placenta, transfusion syndrome, fetus
        to fetus
Transient (meaning homeless) (see also
      condition) Z59.0
Translocation
  balanced autosomal Q95.9
    in normal individual Q95.0
  chromosomes NEC Q99.8
    balanced and insertion in normal
        individual Q95.0
  Down's syndrome Q90.2
  trisomy
    13 Q91.6
    18 Q91.2
    21 Q90.2
Translucency, iris —see Degeneration, iris
Transmission of chemical substances through
      the placenta —see Absorption, chemical,
      through placenta
Transparency, lung, unilateral J43.0
Transplant (ed) (status) Z94.9
  awaiting organ Z76.82
  bone Z94.6
    marrow Z94.81
  candidate Z76.82
  complication —see Complication, transplant
  cornea Z94.7
  heart Z94.1
    and lung (s) Z94.3
    valve Z95.2
      prosthetic Z95.2
      specified NEC Z95.4
      xenogenic Z95.3
  intestine Z94.82
  kidney Z94.0
  liver Z94.4
  lung (s) Z94.2
    and heart Z94.3
  organ (failure) (infection) (rejection)Z94.9
    removal status Z98.85
  pancreas Z94.83
  skin Z94.5
  social Z60.3
  specified organ or tissue NEC Z94.89
  stem cells Z94.84
  tissue Z94.9
Transplants, ovarian, endometrial N80.1
Transposed —see Transposition
Transposition (congenital) —see also
      Malposition, congenital
  abdominal viscera Q89.3
  aorta (dextra) Q20.3
  appendix Q43.8
  colon Q43.8
  corrected Q20.5
  great vessels (complete) (partial) Q20.3
  heart Q24.0
    with complete transposition of viscera
        Q89.3
  intestine (large) (small) Q43.8
  reversed jejunal (for bypass) (status) Z98.0
  scrotum Q55.23

Transposition (Continued)
  stomach Q40.2
    with general transposition of viscera Q89.3
  tooth, teeth, fully erupted M26.30
  vessels, great (complete) (partial) Q20.3
  viscera (abdominal) (thoracic) Q89.3
Transsexualism F64.1
Transvestism, transvestitism (dual-role) F64.1
  fetishistic F65.1
Trapped placenta (with hemorrhage) O72.0
  without hemorrhage O73.0
Trauma, traumatism —see also Injury
  acoustic —see subcategory H83.3
  birth —see Birth, injury
  complicating ectopic or molar pregnancy
      O08.6
  during delivery O71.9
  following ectopic or molar pregnancy O08.6
  obstetric O71.9
    specified NEC O71.89
Traumatic —see also condition
  brain injury —see category S06
Treacher Collins syndrome Q75.4
Treitz's hernia —see Hernia, abdomen, specified
      site NEC
Trematode infestation —see Infestation, fluke
Trematodiasis —see Infestation, fluke
Trembling paralysis —see Parkinsonism
Tremor (s) R25.1
  drug induced G25.1
  essential (benign) G25.0
  familial G25.0
  hereditary G25.0
  hysterical F44.4
  intention G25.2
  medication induced postural G25.1
  mercurial —see subcategory T56.1
  Parkinson's —see Parkinsonism
  psychogenic (conversion reaction) F44.4
  senilis R54
  specified type NEC G25.2
Trench
  fever A79.0
  foot —see Immersion, foot
  mouth A69.1
Treponema pallidum infection —see Syphilis
Treponematosis
  due to
    T. pallidum —see Syphilis
    T. pertenue —see Yaws
Triad
  Hutchinson's (congenital syphilis) A50.53
  Kartagener's Q89.3
  Saint's —see Hernia, diaphragm
Trichiasis (eyelid) H02.059
  with entropion —see Entropion
  left H02.056
    lower H02.055
    upper H02.054
  right H02.053
    lower H02.052
    upper H02.051
Trichinella spiralis (infection) (infestation) B75
Trichinellosis, trichiniasis, trichinelliasis,
      trichinosis B75
  with muscle disorder B75 [M63.80]
    ankle B75 [M63.87-]
    foot B75 [M63.87-]
    forearm B75 [M63.83-]
    hand B75 [M63.84-]
    lower leg B75 [M63.86-]
    multiple sites B75 [M63.89]
    pelvic region B75 [M63.85-]
    shoulder region B75 [M63.81-]
    specified site NEC B75 [M63.88]
    thigh B75 [M63.85-]
    upper arm B75 [M63.82-]

Trichobezoar T18.9
  intestine T18.3
  stomach T18.2
Trichocephaliasis, trichocephalosis B79
Trichocephalus infestation B79
Trichoclasis L67.8
Trichoepithelioma —see also Neoplasm, skin,
      benign
  malignant —see Neoplasm, skin, malignant
Trichofolliculoma —see Neoplasm, skin,
      benign
Tricholemmoma —see Neoplasm, skin,
      benign
Trichomoniasis A59.9
  bladder A59.03
  cervix A59.09
  intestinal A07.8
  prostate A59.02
  seminal vesicles A59.09
  specified site NEC A59.8
  urethra A59.03
  urogenitalis A59.00
  vagina A59.01
  vulva A59.01
Trichomycosis
  axillaris A48.8
  nodosa, nodularis B36.8
Trichonodosis L67.8
Trichophytid, trichophyton infection —see
      Dermatophytosis
Trichophytobezoar T18.9
  intestine T18.3
  stomach T18.2
Trichophytosis —see Dermatophytosis
Trichoptilosis L67.8
Trichorrhexis (nodosa) (invaginata) L67.0
Trichosis axillaris A48.8
Trichosporosis nodosa B36.2
Trichostasis spinulosa (congenital) Q84.1
Trichostrongyliasis, trichostrongylosis (small
      intestine) B81.2
Trichostrongylus infection B81.2
Trichotillomania F63.3
Trichromat, trichromatopsia, anomalous
      (congenital) H53.55
Trichuriasis B79
Trichuris trichiura (infection) (infestation) (any
      site) B79
Tricuspid (valve) —see condition
Trifid —see also Accessory
  kidney (pelvis) Q63.8
  tongue Q38.3
Trigeminal neuralgia —see Neuralgia,
      trigeminal
Trigeminy R00.8
Trigger finger (acquired) M65.30
  congenital Q74.0
  index finger M65.32-
  little finger M65.35-
  middle finger M65.33-
  ring finger M65.34-
  thumb M65.31-
Trigonitis (bladder) (chronic)
      (pseudomembranous) N30.30
  with hematuria N30.31
Trigonocephaly Q75.0
Trilocular heart —see Cor triloculare
Trimethylaminuria E72.52
Tripartite placenta O43.19-
Triphalangeal thumb Q74.0
Triple —see also Accessory
  kidneys Q63.0
  uteri Q51.818
  X, female Q97.0
Triplegia G83.89
  congenital G80.8
Triplet (newborn) —see also Newborn, triplet
  complicating pregnancy —see Pregnancy,
      triplet
Triplication —see Accessory
Triploidy Q92.7

Trismus R25.2
  neonatorum A33
  newborn A33
Trisomy (syndrome) Q92.9
  13 (partial) Q91.7
    meiotic nondisjunction Q91.4
    mitotic nondisjunction Q91.5
    mosaicism Q91.5
    translocation Q91.6
  18 (partial) Q91.3
    meiotic nondisjunction Q91.0
    mitotic nondisjunction Q91.1
    mosaicism Q91.1
    translocation Q91.2
  20 Q92.8
  21 (partial) Q90.9
    meiotic nondisjunction Q90.0
    mitotic nondisjunction Q90.1
    mosaicism Q90.1
    translocation Q90.2
  22 Q92.8
  autosomes Q92.9
  chromosome specified NEC Q92.8
    partial Q92.2
      due to unbalanced translocation Q92.5
    specified NEC Q92.8
    whole (nonsex chromosome)
      meiotic nondisjunction Q92.0
      mitotic nondisjunction Q92.1
      mosaicism Q92.1
  due to
    dicentrics —see Extra, marker
      chromosomes
    extra rings —see Extra, marker
      chromosomes
    isochromosomes —see Extra, marker
      chromosomes
  specified NEC Q92.8
  whole chromosome Q92.9
    meiotic nondisjunction Q92.0
    mitotic nondisjunction Q92.1
    mosaicism Q92.1
    partial Q92.9
    specified NEC Q92.8
Tritanomaly, tritanopia H53.55
Trombiculosis, trombiculiasis, trombidiosis
  B88.0
Trophedema (congenital) (hereditary) Q82.0
Trophoblastic disease (see also Mole,
  hydatidiform) O01.9
Tropholymphedema Q82.0
Trophoneurosis NEC G96.8
  disseminated M34.9
Tropical —see condition
Trouble —see also Disease
  heart —see Disease, heart
  kidney —see Disease, renal
  nervous R45.0
  sinus —see Sinusitis
Trousseau's syndrome (thrombophlebitis
  migrans) I82.1
Truancy, childhood
  from school Z72.810
Truncus
  arteriosus (persistent) Q20.0
  communis Q20.0
Trunk —see condition
Trypanosomiasis
  African B56.9
    by Trypanosoma brucei
      gambiense B56.0
      rhodesiense B56.1
  American —see Chagas' disease
  Brazilian —see Chagas' disease
  by Trypanosoma
    brucei gambiense B56.0
    brucei rhodesiense B56.1
    cruzi —see Chagas' disease
  gambiensis, Gambian B56.0
  rhodesiensis, Rhodesian B56.1
  South American —see Chagas' disease

Trypanosomiasis (Continued)
  where
    African trypanosomiasis is prevalent B56.9
    Chagas' disease is prevalent B57.2
T-shaped incisors K00.2
Tsutsugamushi (disease) (fever) A75.3
Tube, tubal, tubular —see condition
Tubercle —see also Tuberculosis
  brain, solitary A17.81
  Darwin's Q17.8
  Ghon, primary infection A15.7
Tuberculid, tuberculide (indurating,
  subcutaneous) (lichenoid) (miliary)
  (papulonecrotic) (primary) (skin) A18.4
Tuberculoma —see also Tuberculosis
  brain A17.81
  meninges (cerebral) (spinal) A17.1
  spinal cord A17.81
Tuberculosis, tubercular, tuberculous
  (calcification) (calcified) (caseous)
  (chromogenic acid-fast bacilli)
  (degeneration) (fibrocaseous) (fistula)
  (interstitial) (isolated circumscribed
  lesions) (necrosis) (parenchymatous)
  (ulcerative) A15.9
  with pneumoconiosis (any condition in
    J60-J64) J65
  abdomen (lymph gland) A18.39
  abscess (respiratory) A15.9
    bone A18.03
      hip A18.02
      knee A18.02
      sacrum A18.01
      specified site NEC A18.03
      spinal A18.01
      vertebra A18.01
    brain A17.81
    breast A18.89
    Cowper's gland A18.15
    dura (mater) (cerebral) (spinal) A17.81
    epidural (cerebral) (spinal) A17.81
    female pelvis A18.17
    frontal sinus A15.8
    genital organs NEC A18.10
    genitourinary A18.10
    gland (lymphatic) —see Tuberculosis,
      lymph gland
    hip A18.02
    intestine A18.32
    ischiorectal A18.32
    joint NEC A18.02
      hip A18.02
      knee A18.02
      specified NEC A18.02
      vertebral A18.01
    kidney A18.11
    knee A18.02
    latent A76.11
    lumbar (spine) A18.01
    lung —see Tuberculosis, pulmonary
    meninges (cerebral) (spinal) A17.0
    muscle A18.09
    perianal (fistula) A18.32
    perinephritic A18.11
    perirectal A18.32
    rectum A18.32
    retropharyngeal A15.8
    sacrum A18.01
    scrofulous A18.2
    scrotum A18.15
    skin (primary) A18.4
    spinal cord A17.81
    spine or vertebra (column) A18.01
    subdiaphragmatic A18.31
    testis A18.15
    urinary A18.13
    uterus A18.17
  accessory sinus —see Tuberculosis, sinus
  Addison's disease A18.7
  adenitis —see Tuberculosis, lymph gland
  adenoids A15.8

Tuberculosis, tubercular, tuberculous
  (Continued)
  adenopathy —see Tuberculosis, lymph gland
  adherent pericardium A18.84
  adnexa (uteri) A18.17
  adrenal (capsule) (gland) A18.7
  alimentary canal A18.32
  anemia A18.89
  ankle (joint) (bone) A18.02
  anus A18.32
  apex, apical —see Tuberculosis, pulmonary
  appendicitis, appendix A18.32
  arachnoid A17.0
  artery, arteritis A18.89
    cerebral A18.89
  arthritis (chronic) (synovial) A18.02
    spine or vertebra (column) A18.01
  articular —see Tuberculosis, joint
  ascites A18.31
  asthma —see Tuberculosis, pulmonary
  axilla, axillary (gland) A18.2
  bladder A18.12
  bone A18.03
    hip A18.02
    knee A18.02
    limb NEC A18.03
    sacrum A18.01
    spine or vertebral column A18.01
  bowel (miliary) A18.32
  brain A17.81
  breast A18.89
  broad ligament A18.17
  bronchi, bronchial, bronchus A15.5
    ectasia, ectasis (bronchiectasis) —see
      Tuberculosis, pulmonary
    fistula A15.5
      primary (progressive) A15.7
    gland or node A15.4
      primary (progressive) A15.7
    lymph gland or node A15.4
      primary (progressive) A15.7
  bronchiectasis —see Tuberculosis, pulmonary
  bronchitis A15.5
  bronchopleural A15.6
  bronchopneumonia, bronchopneumonic —see
    Tuberculosis, pulmonary
  bronchorrhagia A15.5
  bronchotracheal A15.5
  bronze disease A18.7
  buccal cavity A18.83
  bulbourethral gland A18.15
  bursa A18.09
  cachexia A15.9
  cardiomyopathy A18.84
  caries —see Tuberculosis, bone
  cartilage A18.02
    intervertebral A18.01
  catarrhal —see Tuberculosis, respiratory
  cecum A18.32
  cellulitis (primary) A18.4
  cerebellum A17.81
  cerebral, cerebrum A17.81
  cerebrospinal A17.81
    meninges A17.0
  cervical (lymph gland or node) A18.2
  cervicitis, cervix (uteri) A18.16
  chest —see Tuberculosis, respiratory
  chorioretinitis A18.53
  choroid, choroiditis A18.53
  ciliary body A18.54
  colitis A18.32
  collier's J65
  colliquativa (primary) A18.4
  colon A18.32
  complex, primary A15.7
  congenital P37.0
  conjunctiva A18.59
  connective tissue (systemic) A18.89
  contact Z20.1
  cornea (ulcer) A18.52
  Cowper's gland A18.15

Tuberculosis, tubercular, tuberculous
(Continued)
coxae A18.02
coxalgia A18.02
cul-de-sac of Douglas A18.17
curvature, spine A18.01
cutis (colliquativa) (primary) A18.4
cyst, ovary A18.18
cystitis A18.12
dactylitis A18.03
diarrhea A18.32
diffuse —*see* Tuberculosis, miliary
digestive tract A18.32
disseminated —*see* Tuberculosis, miliary
duodenum A18.32
dura (mater) (cerebral) (spinal) A17.0
   abscess (cerebral) (spinal) A17.81
dysentery A18.32
ear (inner) (middle) A18.6
   bone A18.03
   external (primary) A18.4
   skin (primary) A18.4
elbow A18.02
emphysema —*see* Tuberculosis, pulmonary
empyema A15.6
encephalitis A17.82
endarteritis A18.89
endocarditis A18.84
   aortic A18.84
   mitral A18.84
   pulmonary A18.84
   tricuspid A18.84
endocrine glands NEC A18.82
endometrium A18.17
enteric, enterica, enteritis A18.32
enterocolitis A18.32
epididymis, epididymitis A18.15
epidural abscess (cerebral) (spinal) A17.81
epiglottis A15.5
episcleritis A18.51
erythema (induratum) (nodosum) (primary)
   A18.4
esophagus A18.83
eustachian tube A18.6
exposure (to) Z20.1
exudative —*see* Tuberculosis, pulmonary
eye A18.50
eyelid (primary) (lupus) A18.4
fallopian tube (acute) (chronic) A18.17
fascia A18.09
fauces A15.8
female pelvic inflammatory disease A18.17
finger A18.03
first infection A15.7
gallbladder A18.83
ganglion A18.09
gastritis A18.83
gastrocolic fistula A18.32
gastroenteritis A18.32
gastrointestinal tract A18.32
general, generalized —*see* Tuberculosis,
   miliary
genital organs A18.10
genitourinary A18.10
genu A18.02
glandula suprarenalis A18.7
glandular, general A18.2
glottis A15.5
grinder's J65
gum A18.83
hand A18.03
heart A18.84
hematogenous —*see* Tuberculosis, miliary
hemoptysis —*see* Tuberculosis, pulmonary
hemorrhage NEC —*see* Tuberculosis,
   pulmonary
hemothorax A15.6
hepatitis A18.83
hilar lymph nodes A15.4
   primary (progressive) A15.7
hip (joint) (disease) (bone) A18.02

Tuberculosis, tubercular, tuberculous
(Continued)
hydropneumothorax A15.6
hydrothorax A15.6
hypoadrenalism A18.7
hypopharynx A15.8
ileocecal (hyperplastic) A18.32
ileocolitis A18.32
ileum A18.32
iliac spine (superior) A18.03
immunological findings only A15.7
indurativa (primary) A18.4
infantile A15.7
infection A15.9
   without clinical manifestations A15.7
infraclavicular gland A18.2
inguinal gland A18.2
inguinalis A18.2
intestine (any part) A18.32
iridocyclitis A18.54
iris, iritis A18.54
ischiorectal A18.32
jaw A18.03
jejunum A18.32
joint A18.02
   vertebral A18.01
keratitis (interstitial) A18.52
keratoconjunctivitis A18.52
kidney A18.11
knee (joint) A18.02
kyphosis, kyphoscoliosis A18.01
laryngitis A15.5
larynx A15.5
latent R76.11
leptomeninges, leptomeningitis (cerebral)
   (spinal) A17.0
lichenoides (primary) A18.4
linguae A18.83
lip A18.83
liver A18.83
lordosis A18.01
lung —*see* Tuberculosis, pulmonary
lupus vulgaris A18.4
lymph gland or node (peripheral) A18.2
   abdomen A18.39
   bronchial A15.4
      primary (progressive) A15.7
   cervical A18.2
   hilar A15.4
      primary (progressive) A15.7
   intrathoracic A15.4
      primary (progressive) A15.7
   mediastinal A15.4
      primary (progressive) A15.7
   mesenteric A18.39
   retroperitoneal A18.39
   tracheobronchial A15.4
      primary (progressive) A15.7
lymphadenitis —*see* Tuberculosis, lymph
   gland
lymphangitis —*see* Tuberculosis, lymph
   gland
lymphatic (gland) (vessel) —*see* Tuberculosis,
   lymph gland
mammary gland A18.89
marasmus A15.9
mastoiditis A18.03
mediastinal lymph gland or node
   A15.4
   primary (progressive) A15.7
mediastinitis A15.8
   primary (progressive) A15.7
mediastinum A15.8
   primary (progressive) A15.7
medulla A17.81
melanosis, Addisonian A18.7
meninges, meningitis (basilar) (cerebral)
   (cerebrospinal) (spinal) A17.0
meningoencephalitis A17.82
mesentery, mesenteric (gland or node)
   A18.39

Tuberculosis, tubercular, tuberculous
(Continued)
miliary A19.9
   acute A19.2
      multiple sites A19.1
      single specified site A19.0
   chronic A19.8
   specified NEC A19.8
millstone makers' J65
miner's J65
molder's J65
mouth A18.83
multiple A19.9
   acute A19.1
   chronic A19.8
muscle A18.09
myelitis A17.82
myocardium, myocarditis A18.84
nasal (passage) (sinus) A15.8
nasopharynx A15.8
neck gland A18.2
nephritis A18.11
nerve (mononeuropathy) A17.83
nervous system A17.9
nose (septum) A15.8
ocular A18.50
omentum A18.31
oophoritis (acute) (chronic) A18.17
optic (nerve trunk) (papilla) A18.59
orbit A18.59
orchitis A18.15
organ, specified NEC A18.89
osseous —*see* Tuberculosis, bone
osteitis —*see* Tuberculosis, bone
osteomyelitis —*see* Tuberculosis, bone
otitis media A18.6
ovary, ovaritis (acute) (chronic) A18.17
oviduct (acute) (chronic) A18.17
pachymeningitis A17.0
palate (soft) A18.83
pancreas A18.83
papulonecrotic (a) (primary) A18.4
parathyroid glands A18.82
paronychia (primary) A18.4
parotid gland or region A18.83
pelvis (bony) A18.03
penis A18.15
peribronchitis A15.5
pericardium, pericarditis A18.84
perichondritis, larynx A15.5
periostitis —*see* Tuberculosis, bone
perirectal fistula A18.32
peritoneum NEC A18.31
peritonitis A18.31
pharynx, pharyngitis A15.8
phlyctenulosis (keratoconjunctivitis) A18.52
phthisis NEC —*see* Tuberculosis, pulmonary
pituitary gland A18.82
pleura, pleural, pleurisy, pleuritis (fibrinous)
   (obliterative) (purulent) (simple plastic)
   (with effusion) A15.6
   primary (progressive) A15.7
pneumonia, pneumonic —*see* Tuberculosis,
   pulmonary
pneumothorax (spontaneous) (tense
   valvular) —*see* Tuberculosis, pulmonary
polyneuropathy A17.89
polyserositis A19.9
   acute A19.1
   chronic A19.8
potter's J65
prepuce A18.15
primary (complex) A15.7
proctitis A18.32
prostate, prostatitis A18.14
pulmonalis —*see* Tuberculosis, pulmonary
pulmonary (cavitated) (fibrotic) (infiltrative)
   (nodular) A15.0
   childhood type or first infection A15.7
   primary (complex) A15.7
pyelitis A18.11

Tuberculosis, tubercular, tuberculous
(Continued)
pyelonephritis A18.11
pyemia —*see* Tuberculosis, miliary
pyonephrosis A18.11
pyopneumothorax A15.6
pyothorax A15.6
rectum (fistula) (with abscess) A18.32
reinfection stage —*see* Tuberculosis,
   pulmonary
renal A18.11
renis A18.11
respiratory A15.9
  primary A15.7
  specified site NEC A15.8
retina, retinitis A18.53
retroperitoneal (lymph gland or node)
   A18.39
rheumatism NEC A18.09
rhinitis A15.8
sacroiliac (joint) A18.01
sacrum A18.01
salivary gland A18.83
salpingitis (acute) (chronic) A18.17
sandblaster's J65
sclera A18.51
scoliosis A18.01
scrofulous A18.2
scrotum A18.15
seminal tract or vesicle A18.15
senile A15.9
septic —*see* Tuberculosis, miliary
shoulder (joint) A18.02
  blade A18.03
sigmoid A18.32
sinus (any nasal) A15.8
  bone A18.03
  epididymis A18.15
skeletal NEC A18.03
skin (any site) (primary) A18.4
small intestine A18.32
soft palate A18.83
spermatic cord A18.15
spine, spinal (column) A18.01
  cord A17.81
  medulla A17.81
  membrane A17.0
  meninges A17.0
spleen, splenitis A18.85
spondylitis A18.01
sternoclavicular joint A18.02
stomach A18.83
stonemason's J65
subcutaneous tissue (cellular) (primary)
   A18.4
subcutis (primary) A18.4
subdeltoid bursa A18.83
submaxillary (region) A18.83
supraclavicular gland A18.2
suprarenal (capsule) (gland) A18.7
swelling, joint (*see also* category M01) (*see also*
   Tuberculosis, joint) A18.02
symphysis pubis A18.02
synovitis A18.09
  articular A18.02
  spine or vertebra A18.01
systemic —*see* Tuberculosis, miliary
tarsitis A18.4
tendon (sheath) —*see* Tuberculosis,
   tenosynovitis
tenosynovitis A18.09
  spine or vertebra A18.01
testis A18.15
throat A15.8
thymus gland A18.82
thyroid gland A18.81
tongue A18.83
tonsil, tonsillitis A15.8
trachea, tracheal A15.5
  lymph gland or node A15.4
   primary (progressive) A15.7

Tuberculosis, tubercular, tuberculous
(Continued)
  tracheobronchial A15.5
  lymph gland or node A15.4
   primary (progressive) A15.7
tubal (acute) (chronic) A18.17
tunica vaginalis A18.15
ulcer (skin) (primary) A18.4
  bowel or intestine A18.32
  specified NEC - code under Tuberculosis,
   by site
unspecified site A15.9
ureter A18.11
urethra, urethral (gland) A18.13
urinary organ or tract A18.13
uterus A18.17
uveal tract A18.54
uvula A18.83
vagina A18.18
vas deferens A18.15
verruca, verrucosa (cutis) (primary)
   A18.4
vertebra (column) A18.01
vesiculitis A18.15
vulva A18.18
wrist (joint) A18.02
Tuberculum
Carabelli (*see* Note at) K00.2
occlusal (*see* Note at) K00.2
paramolare K00.2
Tuberosity, enitre maxillary M26.07
Tuberous sclerosis (brain) Q85.1
Tubo-ovarian —*see* condition
Tuboplasty, after previous sterilization
   Z31.0
aftercare Z31.42
Tubotympanitis, catarrhal (chronic) —*see*
  Otitis, media, nonsuppurative, chronic,
  serous
Tularemia A21.9
with
  conjunctivitis A21.1
  pneumonia A21.2
abdominal A21.3
bronchopneumonic A21.2
conjunctivitis A21.1
cryptogenic A21.3
enteric A21.3
gastrointestinal A21.3
generalized A21.7
ingestion A21.3
intestinal A21.3
oculoglandular A21.1
ophthalmic A21.1
pneumonia (any), pneumonic A21.2
pulmonary A21.2
sepsis A21.7
specified NEC A21.8
typhoidal A21.7
ulceroglandular A21.0
Tularensis conjunctivitis A21.1
Tumefaction —*see also* Swelling
liver —*see* Hypertrophy, liver
Tumor —*see also* Neoplasm, unspecified
  behavior, by site
acinar cell —*see* Neoplasm, uncertain
  behavior, by site
acinic cell —*see* Neoplasm, uncertain
  behavior, by site
adenocarcinoid —*see* Neoplasm, malignant,
  by site
adenomatoid —*see also* Neoplasm, benign,
  by site
  odontogenic —*see* Cyst, calcifying
   odontogenic
adnexal (skin) —*see* Neoplasm, skin, benign,
  by site
adrenal
  cortical (benign) D35.0-
   malignant C74.0-
  rest —*see* Neoplasm, benign, by site

Tumor *(Continued)*
alpha-cell
  malignant
   pancreas C25.4
   specified site NEC —*see* Neoplasm,
    malignant, by site
   unspecified site C25.4
  pancreas D13.7
  specified site NEC —*see* Neoplasm, benign,
   by site
  unspecified site D13.7
aneurysmal —*see* Aneurysm
aortic body D44.7
  malignant C75.5
Askin's —*see* Neoplasm, connective tissue,
  malignant
basal cell (*see also* Neoplasm, skin, uncertain
  behavior) D48.5
Bednar —*see* Neoplasm, skin, malignant
benign (unclassified) —*see* Neoplasm, benign,
  by site
beta-cell
  malignant
   pancreas C25.4
   specified site NEC —*see* Neoplasm,
    malignant, by site
   unspecified site C25.4
  pancreas D13.7
  specified site NEC —*see* Neoplasm, benign,
   by site
  unspecified site D13.7
Brenner D27.9
  borderline malignancy D39.1-
  malignant C56-
  proliferating D39.1
bronchial alveolar, intravascular D38.1
Brooke's —*see* Neoplasm, skin, benign
brown fat —*see* Lipoma
Burkitt —*see* Lymphoma, Burkitt
calcifying epithelial odontogenic —*see* Cyst,
  calcifying odontogenic
carcinoid
  benign D3A.00
   appendix D3A.020
   ascending colon D3A.022
   bronchus (lung) D3A.090
   cecum D3A.021
   colon D3A.029
   descending colon D3A.024
   duodenum D3A.010
   foregut NOS D3A.094
   hindgut NOS D3A.096
   ileum D3A.012
   jejunum D3A.011
   kidney D3A.093
   large intestine D3A.029
   lung (bronchus) D3A.090
   midgut NOS D3A.095
   rectum D3A.026
   sigmoid colon D3A.025
   small intestine D3A.019
   specified NEC D3A.098
   stomach D3A.092
   thymus D3A.091
   transverse colon D3A.023
  malignant C7A.00
   appendix C7A.020
   ascending colon C7A.022
   bronchus (lung) C7A.090
   cecum C7A.021
   colon C7A.029
   descending colon C7A.024
   duodenum C7A.010
   foregut NOS C7A.094
   hindgut NOS C7A.096
   ileum C7A.012
   jejunum C7A.011
   kidney C7A.093
   large intestine C7A.029
   lung (bronchus) C7A.090
   midgut NOS C7A.095

◄ New   ◄▮ Revised   ~~deleted~~ Deleted

Tumor *(Continued)*
  carcinoid *(Continued)*
    malignant *(Continued)*
      rectum C7A.026
      sigmoid colon C7A.025
      small intestine C7A.019
      specified NEC C7A.098
      stomach C7A.092
      thymus C7A.091
      transverse colon C7A.023
    mesentary metastasis C7B.04
    secondary C7B.00
      bone C7B.03
      distant lymph nodes C7B.01
      liver C7B.02
      peritoneum C7B.04
      specified NEC C7B.09
  carotid body D44.6
    malignant C75.4
  cells —*see also* Neoplasm, unspecified
      behavior, by site
    benign —*see* Neoplasm, benign, by site
    malignant —*see* Neoplasm, malignant, by
        site
    uncertain whether benign or malignant —
        see Neoplasm, uncertain behavior,
        by site
  cervix, in pregnancy or childbirth —*see*
      Pregnancy, complicated by, tumor,
      cervix
  chondromatous giant cell —*see* Neoplasm,
      bone, benign
  chromaffin —*see also* Neoplasm, benign, by
      site
    malignant —*see* Neoplasm, malignant, by
        site
  Cock's peculiar L72.3
  Codman's —*see* Neoplasm, bone, benign
  dentigerous, mixed —*see* Cyst, calcifying
      odontogenic
  dermoid —*see* Neoplasm, benign, by site
    with malignant transformation C56-
  desmoid (extra-abdominal) —*see also*
      Neoplasm, connective tissue, uncertain
      behavior
    abdominal —*see* Neoplasm, connective
        tissue, uncertain behavior
  embolus —*see* Neoplasm, secondary,
      by site
  embryonal (mixed) —*see also* Neoplasm,
      uncertain behavior, by site
    liver C22.7
  endodermal sinus
    specified site —*see* Neoplasm, malignant,
        by site
    unspecified site
      female C56.-
      male C62.90
  epithelial
    benign —*see* Neoplasm, benign, by site
    malignant —*see* Neoplasm, malignant, by
        site
  Ewing's —*see* Neoplasm, bone, malignant,
      by site
  fatty —*see* Lipoma
  fibroid —*see* Leiomyoma
  G cell
    malignant
      pancreas C25.4
      specified site NEC —*see* Neoplasm,
          malignant, by site
      unspecified site C25.4
    specified site —*see* Neoplasm, uncertain
        behavior, by site
    unspecified site D37.8
  germ cell —*see also* Neoplasm, malignant,
      by site
    mixed —*see* Neoplasm, malignant,
        by site
  ghost cell, odontogenic —*see* Cyst, calcifying
      odontogenic

Tumor *(Continued)*
  giant cell —*see also* Neoplasm, uncertain
      behavior, by site
    bone D48.0
      malignant —*see* Neoplasm, bone,
          malignant
    chondromatous —*see* Neoplasm, bone,
        benign
    malignant —*see* Neoplasm, malignant, by
        site
    soft parts —*see* Neoplasm, connective
        tissue, uncertain behavior
      malignant —*see* Neoplasm, connective
          tissue, malignant
  glomus D18.00
    intra-abdominal D18.03
    intracranial D18.02
    jugulare D44.7
      malignant C75.5
    skin D18.01
    specified site NEC D18.09
  gonadal stromal —*see* Neoplasm, uncertain
      behavior, by site
  granular cell —*see also* Neoplasm, connective
      tissue, benign
    malignant —*see* Neoplasm, connective
        tissue, malignant
  granulosa cell D39.1-
    juvenile D39.1-
    malignant C56-
  granulosa cell-theca cell D39.1-
    malignant C56-
  Grawitz's C64-
  hemorrhoidal —*see* Hemorrhoids
  hilar cell D27-
  hilus cell D27-
  Hurthle cell (benign) D34
    malignant C73
  hydatid —*see* Echinococcus
  hypernephroid —*see also* Neoplasm,
      uncertain behavior, by site
  interstitial cell —*see also* Neoplasm, uncertain
      behavior, by site
    benign —*see* Neoplasm, benign, by site
    malignant —*see* Neoplasm, malignant, by
        site
  intravascular bronchial alveolar D38.1
  islet cell —*see* Neoplasm, benign, by site
    malignant —*see* Neoplasm, malignant, by
        site
      pancreas C25.4
      specified site NEC —*see* Neoplasm,
          malignant, by site
      unspecified site C25.4
    pancreas D13.7
    specified site NEC —*see* Neoplasm, benign,
        by site
    unspecified site D13.7
  juxtaglomerular D41.0-
  Klatskin's C24.0
  Krukenberg's C79.6-
  Leydig cell —*see* Neoplasm, uncertain
      behavior, by site
    benign —*see* Neoplasm, benign, by site
      specified site —*see* Neoplasm, benign,
          by site
      unspecified site
        female D27.9
        male D29.20
    malignant —*see* Neoplasm, malignant, by
        site
      specified site —*see* Neoplasm,
          malignant, by site
      unspecified site
        female C56.9
        male C62.90
    specified site —*see* Neoplasm, uncertain
        behavior, by site
    unspecified site
      female D39.10
      male D40.10

Tumor *(Continued)*
  lipid cell, ovary D27-
  lipoid cell, ovary D27-
  malignant (*see also* Neoplasm, malignant, by
      site) C80.1
    fusiform cell (type) C80.1
    giant cell (type) C80.1
    localized, plasma cell —*see* Plasmacytoma,
        solitary
    mixed NEC C80.1
    small cell (type) C80.1
    spindle cell (type) C80.1
    unclassified C80.1
  mast cell D47.0
    malignant C96.2
  melanotic, neuroectodermal —*see* Neoplasm,
      benign, by site
  Merkel cell —*see* Carcinoma, Merkel cell
  mesenchymal
    malignant —*see* Neoplasm, connective
        tissue, malignant
    mixed —*see* Neoplasm, connective tissue,
        uncertain behavior
  mesodermal, mixed —*see also* Neoplasm,
      malignant, by site
    liver C22.4
  mesonephric —*see also* Neoplasm, uncertain
      behavior, by site
    malignant —*see* Neoplasm, malignant, by
        site
  metastatic
    from specified site —*see* Neoplasm,
        malignant, by site
    of specified site —*see* Neoplasm,
        malignant, by site
    to specified site —*see* Neoplasm, secondary,
        by site
  mixed NEC —*see also* Neoplasm, benign, by
      site
    malignant —*see* Neoplasm, malignant, by
        site
  mucinous of low malignant potential
    specified site —*see* Neoplasm, malignant,
        by site
    unspecified site C56.9
  mucocarcinoid
    specified site —*see* Neoplasm, malignant,
        by site
    unspecified site C18.1
  mucoepidermoid —*see* Neoplasm, uncertain
      behavior, by site
  Müllerian, mixed
    specified site —*see* Neoplasm, malignant,
        by site
    unspecified site C54.9
  myoepithelial —*see* Neoplasm, benign,
      by site
  neuroectodermal (peripheral) —*see*
      Neoplasm, malignant, by site
  primitive
    specified site —*see* Neoplasm,
        malignant, by site
    unspecified site C71.9
  neuroendocrine D3A.8
    malignant poorly differentiated
        C7A.1
    secondary NEC C7B.8
    specified NEC C7A.8
  neurogenic olfactory C30.0
  nonencapsulated sclerosing C73
  odontogenic (adenomatoid) (benign)
      (calcifying epithelial) (keratocystic)
      (squamous) —*see* Cyst, calcifying
      odontogenic
    malignant C41.1
      upper jaw (bone) C41.0
  ovarian stromal D39.1-
  ovary, in pregnancy —*see* Pregnancy,
      complicated by
  pacinian —*see* Neoplasm, skin, benign
  Pancoast's —*see* Pancoast's syndrome

Tumor *(Continued)*
papillary —*see also* Papilloma
  cystic D37.9
  mucinous of low malignant potential C56-
    specified site —*see* Neoplasm,
      malignant, by site
    unspecified site C56.9
  serous of low malignant potential
    specified site —*see* Neoplasm,
      malignant, by site
    unspecified site C56.9
pelvic, in pregnancy or childbirth —*see*
  Pregnancy, complicated by
phantom F45.8
phyllodes D48.6-
  benign D24-
  malignant —*see* Neoplasm, breast,
    malignant
Pindborg —*see* Cyst, calcifying odontogenic
placental site trophoblastic D39.2
plasma cell (malignant) (localized) —*see*
  Plasmacytoma, solitary
polyvesicular vitelline
  specified site —*see* Neoplasm, malignant,
    by site
  unspecified site
    female C56.9
    male C62.90
Pott's puffy —*see* Osteomyelitis, specified
  NEC
Rathke's pouch D44.3
retinal anlage —*see* Neoplasm, benign,
  by site
salivary gland type, mixed —*see* Neoplasm,
  salivary gland, benign
  malignant —*see* Neoplasm, salivary gland,
    malignant
Sampson's N80.1
Schmincke's —*see* Neoplasm, nasopharynx,
  malignant
sclerosing stromal D27-
sebaceous —*see* Cyst, sebaceous
secondary —*see* Neoplasm, secondary,
  by site
  carcinoid C7B.00
    bone C7B.03
    distant lymph nodes C7B.01
    liver C7B.02
    peritoneum C7B.04
    specified NEC C7B.09
  neuroendocrine NEC C7B.8
serous of low malignant potential
  specified site —*see* Neoplasm, malignant,
    by site
  unspecified site C56.9
Sertoli cell —*see* Neoplasm, benign, by site
  with lipid storage
    specified site —*see* Neoplasm, benign,
      by site
    unspecified site
      female D27.9
      male D29.20
  specified site —*see* Neoplasm, benign, by
    site
  unspecified site
    female D27.9
    male D29.20
Sertoli-Leydig cell —*see* Neoplasm, benign,
  by site
  specified site —*see* Neoplasm, benign, by
    site
  unspecified site
    female D27.9
    male D29.20
sex cord(-stromal) —*see* Neoplasm, uncertain
  behavior, by site
  with annular tubules D39.1-
skin appendage —*see* Neoplasm, skin,
  benign
smooth muscle —*see* Neoplasm, connective
  tissue, uncertain behavior

Tumor *(Continued)*
soft tissue
  benign —*see* Neoplasm, connective tissue,
    benign
  malignant —*see* Neoplasm, connective
    tissue, malignant
sternomastoid (congenital) Q68.0
stromal
  endometrial D39.0
  gastric D48.1
    benign D21.4
    malignant C16.9
    uncertain behavior D48.1
  gastrointestinal
    benign D21.4
    malignant C49.4
    uncertain behavior D48.1
  intestine
    benign D21.4
    malignant C49.4
    uncertain behavior D48.1
  ovarian D39.1-
  stomach
    benign D21.4
    malignant C16.9
    uncertain behavior D48.1
sweat gland —*see also* Neoplasm, skin,
  uncertain behavior
  benign —*see* Neoplasm, skin, benign
  malignant —*see* Neoplasm, skin, malignant
syphilitic, brain A52.17
testicular D40.10
testicular stromal D40.1-
theca cell D27.-
theca cell-granulosa cell D39.1-
Triton, malignant —*see* Neoplasm, nerve,
  malignant
trophoblastic, placental site D39.2
turban D23.4
uterus (body), in pregnancy or childbirth —
  see Pregnancy, complicated by, tumor,
  uterus
vagina, in pregnancy or childbirth —*see*
  Pregnancy, complicated by
varicose —*see* Varix
von Recklinghausen's —*see*
  Neurofibromatosis
vulva or perineum, in pregnancy or
  childbirth —*see* Pregnancy, complicated
  by
  causing obstructed labor O65.5
Warthin's —*see* Neoplasm, salivary gland,
  benign
Wilms' C64-
yolk sac —*see* Neoplasm, malignant, by site
  specified site —*see* Neoplasm, malignant,
    by site
  unspecified site
    female C56.9
    male C62.90
Tumor lysis syndrome (following
  antineoplastic chemotherapy)
  (spontaneous) NEC E88.3
Tumorlet —*see* Neoplasm, uncertain behavior,
  by site
Tungiasis B88.1
Tunica vasculosa lentis Q12.2
Turban tumor D23.4
Türck's trachoma J37.0
Turner-Kieser syndrome Q79.8
Turner-like syndrome Q87.1
Turner's
  hypoplasia (tooth) K00.4
  syndrome Q96.9
    specified NEC Q96.8
  tooth K00.4
Turner-Ullrich syndrome Q96.9
Tussis convulsiva —*see* Whooping cough
Twiddler's syndrome (due to)
  automatic implantable defibrillator T82.198
  cardiac pacemaker T82.198

Twilight state
  epileptic F05
  psychogenic F44.89
Twin (newborn) —*see also* Newborn, twin
  conjoined Q89.4
  pregnancy —*see* Pregnancy, twin, conjoined
Twinning, teeth K00.2
Twist, twisted
  bowel, colon or intestine K56.2
  hair (congenital) Q84.1
  mesentery K56.2
  omentum K56.2
  organ or site, congenital NEC —*see* Anomaly,
    by site
  ovarian pedicle —*see* Torsion, ovary
Twitching R25.3
Tylosis (acquired) L84
  buccalis K13.29
  linguae K13.29
  palmaris et plantaris (congenital) (inherited)
    Q82.8
    acquired L85.1
Tympanism R14.0
Tympanites (abdominal) (intestinal) R14.0
Tympanitis —*see* Myringitis
Tympanosclerosis —*see* subcategory H74.0
Tympanum —*see* condition
Tympany
  abdomen R14.0
  chest R09.89
Type A behavior pattern Z73.1
Typhlitis —*see* Appendicitis
Typhoenteritis —*see* Typhoid
Typhoid (abortive) (ambulant) (any site)
  (clinical) (fever) (hemorrhagic) (infection)
  (intermittent) (malignant) (rheumatic)
  (Widal negative) A01.00
  with pneumonia A01.03
  abdominal A01.09
  arthritis A01.04
  carrier (suspected) of Z22.0
  cholecystitis (current) A01.09
  endocarditis A01.02
  heart involvement A01.02
  inoculation reaction —*see* Complications,
    vaccination
  meningitis A01.01
  mesenteric lymph nodes A01.09
  myocarditis A01.02
  osteomyelitis A01.05
  perichondritis, larynx A01.09
  pneumonia A01.03
  specified NEC A01.09
  spine A01.05
  ulcer (perforating) A01.09
Typhomalaria (fever) —*see* Malaria
Typhomania A01.00
Typhoperitonitis A01.09
Typhus (fever) A75.9
  abdominal, abdominalis —*see* Typhoid
  African tick A77.1
  amarillic A95.9
  brain A75.9 *[G94]*
  cerebral A75.9 *[G94]*
  classical A75.0
  due to Rickettsia
    prowazekii A75.0
      recrudescent A75.1
    tsutsugamushi A75.3
    typhi A75.2
  endemic (flea-borne) A75.2
  epidemic (louse-borne) A75.0
  exanthematic NEC A75.0
  exanthematicus SAI A75.0
    brillii SAI A75.1
    mexicanus SAI A75.2
    typhus murinus A75.2
  flea-borne A75.2
  India tick A77.1
  Kenya (tick) A77.1
  louse-borne A75.0

Typhus (Continued)
   Mexican A75.2
   mite-borne A75.3
   murine A75.2
   North Asian tick-borne A77.2
   petechial A75.9
   Queensland tick A77.3
   rat A75.2

Typhus (Continued)
   recrudescent A75.1
   recurrens —see Fever, relapsing
   Sao Paulo A77.0
   scrub (China) (India) (Malaysia) (New
      Guinea) A75.3
   shop (of Malaysia) A75.2
   Siberian tick A77.2

Typhus (Continued)
   tick-borne A77.9
   tropical (mite-borne) A75.3
Tyrosinemia E70.21
   newborn, transitory P74.5
Tyrosinosis E70.21
Tyrosinuria E70.29

U

Uhl's anomaly or disease Q24.8
Ulcer, ulcerated, ulcerating, ulceration, ulcerative
  alveolar process M27.3
  amebic (intestine) A06.1
    skin A06.7
  anastomotic —see Ulcer, gastrojejunal
  anorectal K62.6
  antral —see Ulcer, stomach
  anus (sphincter) (solitary) K62.6
  aorta —see Aneurysm
  aphthous (oral) (recurrent) K12.0
    genital organ (s)
      female N76.6
      male N50.8
  artery I77.2
  atrophic —see Ulcer, skin
    decubitus —see Ulcer, pressure, by site
  back L98.429
    with
      bone necrosis L98.424
      exposed fat layer L98.422
      muscle necrosis L98.423
      skin breakdown only L98.421
  Barrett's (esophagus) K22.10
    with bleeding K22.11
  bile duct (common) (hepatic) K83.8
  bladder (solitary) (sphincter) NEC N32.89
    bilharzial B65.9 [N33]
    in schistosomiasis (bilharzial) B65.9 [N33]
    submucosal —see Cystitis, interstitial
    tuberculous A18.12
  bleeding K27.4
  bone —see Osteomyelitis, specified type NEC
  bowel —see Ulcer, intestine
  breast N61
  bronchus J98.09
  buccal (cavity) (traumatic) K12.1
  Buruli A31.1
  buttock L98.419
    with
      bone necrosis L98.414
      exposed fat layer L98.412
      muscle necrosis L98.413
      skin breakdown only L98.411
  cancerous —see Neoplasm, malignant, by site
  cardia K22.10
    with bleeding K22.11
  cardioesophageal (peptic) K22.10
    with bleeding K22.11
  cecum —see Ulcer, intestine
  cervix (uteri) (decubitus) (trophic) N86
    with cervicitis N72
  chancroidal A57
  chiclero B55.1
  chronic (cause unknown) —see Ulcer, skin
  Cochin-China B55.1
  colon —see Ulcer, intestine
  conjunctiva H10.89
  cornea H16.00-
    with hypopyon H16.03-
      central H16.01-
      dendritic (herpes simplex) B00.52
      marginal H16.04-
      Mooren's H16.05-
      mycotic H16.06-
      perforated H16.07-
      ring H16.02-
      tuberculous (phlyctenular) A18.52
  corpus cavernosum (chronic) N48.5
  crural —see Ulcer, lower limb
  Curling's —see Ulcer, peptic, acute
  Cushing's —see Ulcer, peptic, acute
  cystic duct K82.8
  cystitis (interstitial) —see Cystitis, interstitial
  decubitus —see Ulcer, pressure, by site
  dendritic, cornea (herpes simplex) B00.52
  diabetes, diabetic —see Diabetes, ulcer
  Dieulafoy's K25.0

Ulcer, ulcerated, ulcerating, ulceration, ulcerative (Continued)
  due to
    infection NEC —see Ulcer, skin
    radiation NEC L59.8
    trophic disturbance (any region) —see Ulcer, skin
    X-ray L58.1
  duodenum, duodenal (eroded) (peptic) K26.9
    with
      hemorrhage K26.4
        and perforation K26.6
      perforation K26.5
    acute K26.3
      with
        hemorrhage K26.0
          and perforation K26.2
        perforation K26.1
    chronic K26.7
      with
        hemorrhage K26.4
          and perforation K26.6
        perforation K26.5
  dysenteric A09
  elusive —see Cystitis, interstitial
  endocarditis (acute) (chronic) (subacute) I28.8
  epiglottis J38.7
  esophagus (peptic) K22.10
    with bleeding K22.11
    due to
      aspirin K22.10
        with bleeding K22.11
      gastrointestinal reflux disease K21.0
      ingestion of chemical or medicament K22.10
        with bleeding K22.11
    fungal K22.10
      with bleeding K22.11
    infective K22.10
      with bleeding K22.11
    varicose —see Varix, esophagus
  eyelid (region) H01.8
  fauces J39.2
  Fenwick (-Hunner) (solitary) —see Cystitis, interstitial
  fistulous —see Ulcer, skin
  foot (indolent) (trophic) —see Ulcer, lower limb
  frambesial, initial A66.0
  frenum (tongue) K14.0
  gallbladder or duct K82.8
  gangrenous —see Gangrene
  gastric —see Ulcer, stomach
  gastrocolic —see Ulcer, gastrojejunal
  gastroduodenal —see Ulcer, peptic
  gastroesophageal —see Ulcer, stomach
  gastrointestinal —see Ulcer, gastrojejunal
  gastrojejunal (peptic) K28.9
    with
      hemorrhage K28.4
        and perforation K28.6
      perforation K28.5
    acute K28.3
      with
        hemorrhage K28.0
          and perforation K28.2
        perforation K28.1
    chronic K28.7
      with
        hemorrhage K28.4
          and perforation K28.6
        perforation K28.5
  gastrojejunocolic —see Ulcer, gastrojejunal
  gingiva K06.8
  gingivitis K05.10
    nonplaque induced K05.11
    plaque induced K05.10
  glottis J38.7
  granuloma of pudenda A58
  gum K06.8
  gumma, due to yaws A66.4

Ulcer, ulcerated, ulcerating, ulceration, ulcerative (Continued)
  heel —see Ulcer, lower limb
  hemorrhoid (see also Hemorrhoids, by degree) K64.8
  Hunner's —see Cystitis, interstitial
  hypopharynx J39.2
  hypopyon (chronic) (subacute) —see Ulcer, cornea, with hypopyon
  hypostaticum —see Ulcer, varicose
  ileum —see Ulcer, intestine
  intestine, intestinal K63.3
    with perforation K63.1
    amebic A06.1
    duodenal —see Ulcer, duodenum
    granulocytopenic (with hemorrhage) —see Neutropenia
    marginal —see Ulcer, gastrojejunal
    perforating K63.1
      newborn P78.0
    primary, small intestine K63.3
    rectum K62.6
    stercoraceous, stercoral K63.3
    tuberculous A18.32
    typhoid (fever) —see Typhoid
    varicose I86.8
  jejunum, jejunal —see Ulcer, gastrojejunal
  keratitis —see Ulcer, cornea
  knee —see Ulcer, lower limb
  labium (majus) (minus) N76.6
  laryngitis —see Laryngitis
  larynx (aphthous) (contact) J38.7
    diphtheritic A36.2
  leg —see Ulcer, lower limb
  lip K13.0
  Lipschütz's N76.6
  lower limb (atrophic) (chronic) (neurogenic) (perforating) (pyogenic) (trophic) (tropical) L97.909
    with
      bone necrosis L97.904
      exposed fat layer L97.902
      muscle necrosis L97.903
      skin breakdown only L97.901
    ankle L97.309
      with
        bone necrosis L97.304
        exposed fat layer L97.302
        muscle necrosis L97.303
        skin breakdown only L97.301
      left L97.329
        with
          bone necrosis L97.324
          exposed fat layer L97.322
          muscle necrosis L97.323
          skin breakdown only L97.321
      right L97.319
        with
          bone necrosis L97.314
          exposed fat layer L97.312
          muscle necrosis L97.313
          skin breakdown only L97.311
    calf L97.209
      with
        bone necrosis L97.204
        exposed fat layer L97.202
        muscle necrosis L97.203
        skin breakdown only L97.201
      left L97.229
        with
          bone necrosis L97.224
          exposed fat layer L97.222
          muscle necrosis L97.223
          skin breakdown only L97.221
      right L97.219
        with
          bone necrosis L97.214
          exposed fat layer L97.212
          muscle necrosis L97.213
          skin breakdown only L97.211
    decubitus —see Ulcer, pressure, by site

◀ New   ◀▥ Revised   ~~deleted~~ Deleted

Ulcer, ulcerated, ulcerating, ulceration,
ulcerative (Continued)
  lower limb (Continued)
    foot specified NEC L97.509
      with
        bone necrosis L97.504
        exposed fat layer L97.502
        muscle necrosis L97.503
        skin breakdown only L97.501
      left L97.529
        with
          bone necrosis L97.524
          exposed fat layer L97.522
          muscle necrosis L97.523
          skin breakdown only L97.521
      right L97.519
        with
          bone necrosis L97.514
          exposed fat layer L97.512
          muscle necrosis L97.513
          skin breakdown only L97.511
    heel L97.409
      with
        bone necrosis L97.404
        exposed fat layer L97.402
        muscle necrosis L97.403
        skin breakdown only L97.401
      left L97.429
        with
          bone necrosis L97.424
          exposed fat layer L97.422
          muscle necrosis L97.423
          skin breakdown only L97.421
      right L97.419
        with
          bone necrosis L97.414
          exposed fat layer L97.412
          muscle necrosis L97.413
          skin breakdown only L97.411
    left L97.929
      with
        bone necrosis L97.924
        exposed fat layer L97.922
        muscle necrosis L97.923
        skin breakdown only L97.921
    lower leg NOS L97.909
      with
        bone necrosis L97.904
        exposed fat layer L97.902
        muscle necrosis L97.903
        skin breakdown only L97.901
      left L97.929
        with
          bone necrosis L97.924
          exposed fat layer L97.922
          muscle necrosis L97.923
          skin breakdown only L97.921
      right L97.919
        with
          bone necrosis L97.914
          exposed fat layer L97.912
          muscle necrosis L97.913
          skin breakdown only L97.911
    specified site NEC L97.809
      with
        bone necrosis L97.804
        exposed fat layer L97.802
        muscle necrosis L97.803
        skin breakdown only L97.801
      left L97.829
        with
          bone necrosis L97.824
          exposed fat layer L97.822
          muscle necrosis L97.823
          skin breakdown only L97.821
      right L97.819
        with
          bone necrosis L97.814
          exposed fat layer L97.812
          muscle necrosis L97.813
          skin breakdown only L97.811

Ulcer, ulcerated, ulcerating, ulceration,
ulcerative (Continued)
  lower limb (Continued)
    midfoot L97.409
      with
        bone necrosis L97.404
        exposed fat layer L97.402
        muscle necrosis L97.403
        skin breakdown only L97.401
      left L97.429
        with
          bone necrosis L97.424
          exposed fat layer L97.422
          muscle necrosis L97.423
          skin breakdown only L97.421
      right L97.419
        with
          bone necrosis L97.414
          exposed fat layer L97.412
          muscle necrosis L97.413
          skin breakdown only L97.411
    right L97.919
      with
        bone necrosis L97.914
        exposed fat layer L97.912
        muscle necrosis L97.913
        skin breakdown only L97.911
    thigh L97.109
      with
        bone necrosis L97.104
        exposed fat layer L97.102
        muscle necrosis L97.103
        skin breakdown only L97.101
      left L97.129
        with
          bone necrosis L97.124
          exposed fat layer L97.122
          muscle necrosis L97.123
          skin breakdown only L97.121
      right L97.119
        with
          bone necrosis L97.114
          exposed fat layer L97.112
          muscle necrosis L97.113
          skin breakdown only L97.111
    toe L97.509
      with
        bone necrosis L97.504
        exposed fat layer L97.502
        muscle necrosis L97.503
        skin breakdown only L97.501
      left L97.529
        with
          bone necrosis L97.524
          exposed fat layer L97.522
          muscle necrosis L97.523
          skin breakdown only L97.521
      right L97.519
        with
          bone necrosis L97.514
          exposed fat layer L97.512
          muscle necrosis L97.513
          skin breakdown only L97.511
  leprous A30.1
  syphilitic A52.19
  varicose —see Varix, leg, with, ulcer
  luetic —see Ulcer, syphilitic
  lung J98.4
    tuberculous —see Tuberculosis, pulmonary
  malignant —see Neoplasm, malignant, by site
  marginal NEC —see Ulcer, gastrojejunal
  meatus (urinarius) N34.2
  Meckel's diverticulum Q43.0
    malignant —see Table of Neoplasms, small
      intestine, malignant
  Meleney's (chronic undermining) —see Ulcer,
    skin
  Mooren's (cornea) —see Ulcer, cornea,
    Mooren's
  mycobacterial (skin) A31.1
  nasopharynx J39.2

Ulcer, ulcerated, ulcerating, ulceration,
ulcerative (Continued)
  neck, uterus N86
  neurogenic NEC —see Ulcer, skin
  nose, nasal (passage) (infective) (septum)
    J34.0
    skin —see Ulcer, skin
    spirochetal A69.8
    varicose (bleeding) I86.8
  oral mucosa (traumatic) K12.1
  palate (soft) K12.1
  penis (chronic) N48.5
  peptic (site unspecified) K27.9
    with
      hemorrhage K27.4
        and perforation K27.6
      perforation K27.5
    acute K27.3
      with
        hemorrhage K27.0
          and perforation K27.2
        perforation K27.1
    chronic K27.7
      with
        hemorrhage K27.4
          and perforation K27.6
        perforation K27.5
    esophagus K22.10
      with bleeding K22.11
    newborn P78.82
  perforating K27.5
    skin —see Ulcer, skin
  peritonsillar J35.8
  phagedenic (tropical) —see Ulcer, skin
  pharynx J39.2
  phlebitis —see Phlebitis
  plaster —see Ulcer, pressure, by site
  popliteal space —see Ulcer, lower limb
  postpyloric —see Ulcer, duodenum
  prepuce N47.7
  prepyloric —see Ulcer, stomach
  pressure (pressure area) L89.9-
    ankle L89.5-
    back L89.1-
    buttock L89.3-
    coccyx L89.15-
    contiguous site of back, buttock, hip L89.4-
    elbow L89.0-
    face L89.81-
    head L89.81-
    heel L89.6-
    hip L89.2-
    sacral region (tailbone) L89.15-
    specified site NEC L89.89-
    stage 1 (healing) (pre-ulcer skin changes
        limited to persistent focal edema)
      ankle L89.5-
      back L89.1-
      buttock L89.3-
      coccyx L89.15-
      contiguous site of back, buttock, hip
        L89.4-
      elbow L89.0-
      face L89.81-
      head L89.81-
      heel L89.6-
      hip L89.2-
      sacral region (tailbone) L89.15-
      specified site NEC L89.89-
    stage 2 (healing) (abrasion, blister, partial
        thickness skin loss involving
        epidermis and/or dermis)
      ankle L89.5-
      back L89.1-
      buttock L89.3-
      coccyx L89.15-
      contiguous site of back, buttock, hip
        L89.4-
      elbow L89.0-
      face L89.81-
      head L89.81-

◀ New   ◀⊪ Revised   deleted Deleted

Ulcer, ulcerated, ulcerating, ulceration, ulcerative (Continued)
pressure (Continued)
stage 2 (Continued)
heel L89.6-
hip L89.2-
sacral region (tailbone) L89.15-
specified site NEC L89.89-
stage 3 (healing) (full thickness skin loss involving damage or necrosis of subcutaneous tissue)
ankle L89.5-
back L89.1-
buttock L89.3-
coccyx L89.15-
contiguous site of back, buttock, hip L89.4-
elbow L89.0-
face L89.81-
head L89.81-
heel L89.6-
hip L89.2-
sacral region (tailbone) L89.15-
specified site NEC L89.89-
stage 4 (healing) (necrosis of soft tissues through to underlying muscle, tendon, or bone)
ankle L89.5-
back L89.1-
buttock L89.3-
coccyx L89.15-
contiguous site of back, buttock, hip L89.4-
elbow L89.0-
face L89.81-
head L89.81-
heel L89.6-
hip L89.2-
sacral region (tailbone) L89.15-
specified site NEC L89.89-
unspecified stage
ankle L89.5-
back L89.1-
buttock L89.3-
coccyx L89.15-
contiguous site of back, buttock, hip L89.4-
elbow L89.0-
face L89.81-
head L89.81-
heel L89.6-
hip L89.2-
sacral region (tailbone) L89.15-
specified site NEC L89.89-
unstageable
ankle L89.5-
back L89.1-
buttock L89.3-
coccyx L89.15-
contiguous site of back, buttock, hip L89.4-
elbow L89.0-
face L89.81-
head L89.81-
heel L89.6-
hip L89.2-
sacral region (tailbone) L89.15-
specified site NEC L89.89-
primary of intestine K63.3
with perforation K63.1
prostate N41.9
pyloric —see Ulcer, stomach
rectosigmoid K63.3
with perforation K63.1
rectum (sphincter) (solitary) K62.6
stercoraceous, stercoral K62.6
retina —see Inflammation, chorioretinal
rodent —see also Neoplasm, skin, malignant
sclera —see Scleritis
scrofulous (tuberculous) A18.2

Ulcer, ulcerated, ulcerating, ulceration, ulcerative (Continued)
scrotum N50.8
tuberculous A18.15
varicose I86.1
seminal vesicle N50.8
sigmoid —see Ulcer, intestine
skin (atrophic) (chronic) (neurogenic) (non-healing) (perforating) (pyogenic) (trophic) (tropical) L98.499
with gangrene —see Gangrene
amebic A06.7
back —see Ulcer, back
buttock —see Ulcer, buttock
decubitus —see Ulcer, pressure
lower limb —see Ulcer, lower limb
mycobacterial A31.1
specified site NEC L98.499
with
bone necrosis L98.494
exposed fat layer L98.492
muscle necrosis L98.493
skin breakdown only L98.491
tuberculous (primary) A18.4
varicose —see Ulcer, varicose
sloughing —see Ulcer, skin
solitary, anus or rectum (sphincter) K62.6
sore throat J02.9
streptococcal J02.0
spermatic cord N50.8
spine (tuberculous) A18.01
stasis (venous) —see Varix, leg, with, ulcer
without varicose veins I87.2
stercoraceous, stercoral K63.3
with perforation K63.1
anus or rectum K62.6
stoma, stomal —see Ulcer, gastrojejunal
stomach (eroded) (peptic) (round) K25.9
with
hemorrhage K25.4
and perforation K25.6
perforation K25.5
acute K25.3
with
hemorrhage K25.0
and perforation K25.2
perforation K25.1
chronic K25.7
with
hemorrhage K25.4
and perforation K25.6
perforation K25.5
stomal —see Ulcer, gastrojejunal
stomatitis K12.1
stress —see Ulcer, peptic
strumous (tuberculous) A18.2
submucosal, bladder —see Cystitis, interstitial
syphilitic (any site) (early) (secondary) A51.39
late A52.79
perforating A52.79
foot A52.11
testis N50.8
thigh —see Ulcer, lower limb
throat J39.2
diphtheritic A36.0
toe —see Ulcer, lower limb
tongue (traumatic) K14.0
tonsil J35.8
diphtheritic A36.0
trachea J39.8
trophic —see Ulcer, skin
tropical —see Ulcer, skin
tuberculous —see Tuberculosis, ulcer
tunica vaginalis N50.8
turbinate J34.89
typhoid (perforating) —see Typhoid

Ulcer, ulcerated, ulcerating, ulceration, ulcerative (Continued)
unspecified site —see Ulcer, skin
urethra (meatus) —see Urethritis
uterus N85.8
cervix N86
with cervicitis N72
neck N86
with cervicitis N72
vagina N76.5
in Behçet's disease M35.2 [N77.0]
pessary N89.8
valve, heart I33.0
varicose (lower limb, any part) —see also Varix, leg, with, ulcer
broad ligament I86.2
esophagus —see Varix, esophagus
inflamed or infected —see Varix, leg, with ulcer, with inflammation
nasal septum I86.8
perineum I86.3
scrotum I86.1
specified site NEC I86.8
sublingual I86.0
vulva I86.3
vas deferens N50.8
vulva (acute) (infectional) N76.6
in (due to)
Behçet's disease M35.2 [N77.0]
herpesviral (herpes simplex) infection A60.04
tuberculosis A18.18
vulvobuccal, recurring N76.6
X-ray L58.1
yaws A66.4
Ulcerosa scarlatina A38.8
Ulcus —see also Ulcer
cutis tuberculosum A18.4
duodeni —see Ulcer, duodenum
durum (syphilitic) A51.0
extragenital A51.2
gastrojejunale —see Ulcer, gastrojejunal
hypostaticum —see Ulcer, varicose
molle (cutis) (skin) A57
serpens corneae —see Ulcer, cornea, central
ventriculi —see Ulcer, stomach
Ulegyria Q04.8
Ulerythema
ophryogenes, congenital Q84.2
sycosiforme L73.8
Ullrich(-Bonnevie)(-Turner) syndrome Q87.1
Ullrich-Feichtiger syndrome Q87.0
Ulnar —see condition
Ulorrhagia, ulorrhea K06.8
Umbilicus, umbilical —see condition
Unacceptable
contours of tooth K08.54
morphology of tooth K08.54
Unavailability (of)
bed at medical facility Z75.1
health service-related agencies Z75.4
medical facilities (at) Z75.3
due to
investigation by social service agency Z75.2
lack of services at home Z75.0
remoteness from facility Z75.3
waiting list Z75.1
home Z75.0
outpatient clinic Z75.3
schooling Z55.1
social service agencies Z75.4
Uncinaria americana infestation B76.1
Uncinariasis B76.9
Uncongenial work Z56.5
Unconscious (ness) —see Coma
Underachievement in school Z55.3
Underdevelopment —see also Undeveloped
nose Q30.1
sexual E30.0

◀ New ◀▥ Revised ~~deleted~~ Deleted

Underdosing (*see also* Table of Drugs and
Chemicals, categories T36-T50, with final
character 6) Z91.14
  intentional NEC Z91.128
    due to financial hardship of patient
Z91.120
  unintentional NEC Z91.138
    due to patient's age related debility
Z91.130
Underfeeding, newborn P92.3
Underfill, endodontic M27.53
Underimmunization status Z28.3
Undernourishment —*see* Malnutrition
Undernutrition —*see* Malnutrition
Under observation —*see* Observation
Underweight R63.6
  for gestational age —*see* Light for dates
Underwood's disease P83.0
Undescended —*see also* Malposition, congenital
  cecum Q43.3
  colon Q43.3
  testicle —*see* Cryptorchid
Undeveloped, undevelopment —*see also*
Hypoplasia
  brain (congenital) Q02
  cerebral (congenital) Q02
  heart Q24.8
  lung Q33.6
  testis E29.1
  uterus E30.0
Undiagnosed (disease) R69
Undulant fever —*see* Brucellosis
Unemployment, anxiety concerning Z56.0
  threatened Z56.2
Unequal length (acquired) (limb) —*see also*
Deformity, limb, unequal length
  leg —*see also* Deformity, limb, unequal
length
    congenital Q72.9-
Unextracted dental root K08.3
Unguis incarnatus L60.0
Unhappiness R45.2
Unicornate uterus Q51.4
Unilateral —*see also* condition
  development, breast N64.89
  organ or site, congenital NEC —*see* Agenesis,
by site
Unilocular heart Q20.8
Union, abnormal —*see also* Fusion
  larynx and trachea Q34.8
Universal mesentery Q43.3
Unrepairable overhanging of dental
restorative materials K08.52
Unsatisfactory
  restoration of tooth K08.50
    specified NEC K08.59
  sample of cytologic smear
    anus R85.615
    cervix R87.615
    vagina R87.625
  surroundings Z59.1
  work Z56.5
Unsoundness of mind —*see* Psychosis
Unstable
  back NEC —*see* Instability, joint, spine
  hip (congenital) Q65.6
    acquired —*see* Derangement, joint,
specified type NEC, hip
  joint —*see* Instability, joint
    secondary to removal of joint prosthesis
M96.89
  lie (mother) O32.0
  lumbosacral joint (congenital)
    acquired —*see* subcategory M53.2
  sacroiliac —*see* subcategory M53.2
  spine NEC —*see* Instability, joint, spine
Unsteadiness on feet R26.81
Untruthfulness, child problem F91.8
Unverricht(-Lundborg) disease or epilepsy —
see Epilepsy, generalized, idiopathic
Unwanted pregnancy Z64.0

Upbringing, institutional Z62.22
  away from parents NEC Z62.29
  in care of non-parental family member Z62.21
  in foster care Z62.21
  in orphanage or group home Z62.22
  in welfare custody Z62.21
Upper respiratory —*see* condition
Upset
  gastric K30
  gastrointestinal K30
    psychogenic F45.8
  intestinal (large) (small) K59.9
    psychogenic F45.8
  menstruation N93.9
  mental F48.9
  stomach K30
    psychogenic F45.8
Urachus —*see also* condition
  patent or persistent Q64.4
Urbach-Oppenheim disease (necrobiosis
lipoidica diabeticorum) —*see* E08-E13 with
.620
Urbach's lipoid proteinosis E78.89
Urbach-Wiethe disease E78.89
Urban yellow fever A95.1
Urea
  blood, high —*see* Uremia
  cycle metabolism disorder —*see* Disorder,
urea cycle metabolism
Uremia, uremic N19
  with
    ectopic or molar pregnancy O08.4
    polyneuropathy N18.9 *[G63]*
  chronic (*see also* Disease, kidney, chronic)
N18.9
    due to hypertension —*see* Hypertensive,
kidney
  complicating
    ectopic or molar pregnancy O08.4
  congenital P96.0
  extrarenal R39.2
  following ectopic or molar pregnancy O08.4
  newborn P96.0
  prerenal R39.2
Ureter, ureteral —*see* condition
Ureteralgia N23
Ureterectasis —*see* Hydroureter
Ureteritis N28.89
  cystica N28.86
  due to calculus N20.1
    with calculus, kidney N20.2
      with hydronephrosis N13.2
  gonococcal (acute) (chronic) A54.21
  nonspecific N28.89
Ureterocele N28.89
  congenital (orthotopic) Q62.31
    ectopic Q62.32
Ureterolith, ureterolithiasis —*see* Calculus,
ureter
Ureterostomy
  attention to Z43.6
  status Z93.6
Urethra, urethral —*see* condition
Urethralgia R39.89
Urethritis (anterior) (posterior) N34.2
  calculous N21.1
  candidal B37.41
  chlamydial A56.01
  diplococcal (gonococcal) A54.01
    with abscess (accessory gland)
(periurethral) A54.1
  gonococcal A54.01
    with abscess (accessory gland)
(periurethral) A54.1
  nongonococcal N34.1
    Reiter's —*see* Reiter's disease
  nonspecific N34.1
  nonvenereal N34.1
  postmenopausal N34.2
  puerperal O86.22
  Reiter's —*see* Reiter's disease

Urethritis (*Continued*)
  specified NEC N34.2
  trichomonal or due to Trichomonas
(vaginalis) A59.03
Urethrocele N81.0
  with
    cystocele —*see* Cystocele
    prolapse of uterus —*see* Prolapse, uterus
Urethrolithiasis (with colic or infection) N21.1
Urethrorectal —*see* condition
Urethrorrhagia N36.8
Urethrorrhea R36.9
Urethrostomy
  attention to Z43.6
  status Z93.6
Urethrotrigonitis —*see* Trigonitis
Urethrovaginal —*see* condition
Urgency
  fecal R15.2
  hypertensive —*see* Hypertension
  urinary N39.41
Urhidrosis, uridrosis L74.8
Uric acid in blood (increased) E79.0
Uricacidemia (asymptomatic) E79.0
Uricemia (asymptomatic) E79.0
Uricosuria R82.99
Urinary —*see* condition
Urination
  frequent R35.0
  painful R30.9
Urine
  blood in —*see* Hematuria
  discharge, excessive R35.8
  enuresis, nonorganic origin F98.0
  extravasation R39.0
  frequency R35.0
  incontinence R32
    nonorganic origin F98.0
  intermittent stream R39.19
  pus in N39.0
  retention or stasis R33.9
    organic R33.8
      drug-induced R33.0
    psychogenic F45.8
  secretion
    deficient R34
    excessive R35.8
    frequency R35.0
  stream
    intermittent R39.19
    slowing R39.19
    splitting R39.13
    weak R39.12
Urinemia —*see* Uremia
Urinoma, urethra N36.8
Uroarthritis, infectious (Reiter's) —*see* Reiter's
disease
Urodialysis R34
Urolithiasis —*see* Calculus, urinary
Uronephrosis —*see* Hydronephrosis
Uropathy N39.9
  obstructive N13.9
    specified NEC N13.8
  reflux N13.9
    specified NEC N13.8
  vesicoureteral reflux-associated —*see* Reflux,
vesicoureteral
Urosepsis — code to condition
Urticaria L50.9
  with angioneurotic edema T78.3
    hereditary D84.1
  allergic L50.0
  cholinergic L50.5
  chronic L50.8
  cold, familial L50.2
  contact L50.6
  dermatographic L50.3
  due to
    cold or heat L50.2
    drugs L50.0
    food L50.0

Urticaria (Continued)
  due to (Continued)
    inhalants L50.0
    plants L50.6
    serum (see also Reaction, serum) T80.69
  factitial L50.3
  giant T78.3
    hereditary D84.1
  gigantea T78.3
  idiopathic L50.1
  larynx T78.3
    hereditary D84.1
  neonatorum P83.8
  nonallergic L50.1
  papulosa (Hebra) L28.2
  pigmentosa Q82.2
  recurrent periodic L50.8
  serum (see also Reaction, serum) T80.69
  solar L56.3
  specified type NEC L50.8
  thermal (cold) (heat) L50.2
  vibratory L50.4
  xanthelasmoidea Q82.2
Use (of)
  alcohol F10.99
    with sleep disorder F10.982
    harmful —see Abuse, alcohol
  amphetamines —see Use, stimulant NEC
  caffeine —see Use, stimulant NEC
  cannabis F12.90
    with
      anxiety disorder F12.980
      intoxication F12.929
        with
          delirium F12.921
          perceptual disturbance F12.922
        uncomplicated F12.920
      other specified disorder F12.988
      psychosis F12.959
        delusions F12.950
        hallucinations F12.951
      unspecified disorder F12.99
  cocaine F14.90
    with
      anxiety disorder F14.980
      intoxication F14.929
        with
          delirium F14.921
          perceptual disturbance F14.922
        uncomplicated F14.920
      other specified disorder F14.988
      psychosis F14.959
        delusions F14.950
        hallucinations F14.951
      sexual dysfunction F14.981
      sleep disorder F14.982
      unspecified disorder F14.99
    harmful —see Abuse, drug, cocaine
  drug (s) NEC F19.90
    with sleep disorder F19.982
    harmful —see Abuse, drug, by type
  hallucinogen NEC F16.90
    with
      anxiety disorder F16.980
      intoxication F16.929
        with
          delirium F16.921
        uncomplicated F16.920
      mood disorder F16.94
      other specified disorder F16.988
      perception disorder (flashbacks)
        F16.983

Use (Continued)
  hallucinogen NEC (Continued)
    with (Continued)
      psychosis F16.959
        delusions F16.950
        hallucinations F16.951
      unspecified disorder F16.99
    harmful —see Abuse, drug, hallucinogen
      NEC
  inhalants F18.90
    with
      anxiety disorder F18.980
      intoxication F18.929
        with delirium F18.921
        uncomplicated F18.920
      mood disorder F18.94
      other specified disorder F18.988
      persisting dementia F18.97
      psychosis F18.959
        delusions F18.950
        hallucinations F18.951
      unspecified disorder F18.99
    harmful —see Abuse, drug, inhalant
  methadone F11.20
  nonprescribed drugs F19.90
    harmful —see Abuse, non-psychoactive
      substance
  opioid F11.90
    with
      disorder F11.99
        mood F11.94
        sleep F11.982
        specified type NEC F11.988
      intoxication F11.929
        with
          delirium F11.921
          perceptual disturbance
            F11.922
        uncomplicated F11.920
      withdrawal F11.93
    harmful —see Abuse, drug, opioid
  patent medicines F19.90
    harmful —see Abuse, non-psychoactive
      substance
  psychoactive drug NEC F19.90
    with
      anxiety disorder F19.980
      intoxication F19.929
        with
          delirium F19.921
          perceptual disturbance
            F19.922
        uncomplicated F19.920
      mood disorder F19.94
      other specified disorder F19.988
      persisting
        amnestic disorder F19.96
        dementia F19.97
      psychosis F19.959
        delusions F19.950
        hallucinations F19.951
      sexual dysfunction F19.981
      sleep disorder F19.982
      unspecified disorder F19.99
      withdrawal F19.939
        with
          delirium F19.931
          perceptual disturbance
            F19.932
        uncomplicated F19.930
    harmful —see Abuse, drug NEC,
      psychoactive NEC

Use (Continued)
  sedative, hypnotic, or anxiolytic F13.90
    with
      anxiety disorder F13.980
      intoxication F13.929
        with
          delirium F13.921
        uncomplicated F13.920
      other specified disorder F13.988
      persisting
        amnestic disorder F13.96
        dementia F13.97
      psychosis F13.959
        delusions F13.950
        hallucinations F13.951
      sexual dysfunction F13.981
      sleep disorder F13.982
      unspecified disorder F13.99
    harmful —see Abuse, drug, sedative,
      hypnotic, or anxiolytic
  stimulant NEC F15.90
    with
      anxiety disorder F15.980
      intoxication F15.929
        with
          delirium F15.921
          perceptual disturbance F15.922
        uncomplicated F15.920
      mood disorder F15.94
      other specified disorder F15.988
      psychosis F15.959
        delusions F15.950
        hallucinations F15.951
      sexual dysfunction F15.981
      sleep disorder F15.982
      unspecified disorder F15.99
      withdrawal F15.93
    harmful —see Abuse, drug, stimulant NEC
  tobacco Z72.0
    with dependence —see Dependence, drug,
      nicotine
  volatile solvents (see also Use, inhalant) F18.90
    harmful —see Abuse, drug, inhalant
Usher-Senear disease or syndrome L10.4
Uta B55.1
Uteromegaly N85.2
Uterovaginal —see condition
Uterovesical —see condition
Uveal —see condition
Uveitis (anterior) —see also Iridocyclitis
  acute —see Iridocyclitis, acute
  chronic —see Iridocyclitis, chronic
  due to toxoplasmosis (acquired) B58.09
    congenital P37.1
  granulomatous —see Iridocyclitis, chronic
  heterochromic —see Cyclitis, Fuchs'
    heterochromic
  lens-induced —see Iridocyclitis, lens-induced
  posterior —see Chorioretinitis
  sympathetic H44.13-
  syphilitic (secondary) A51.43
    congenital (early) A50.01
    late A52.71
  tuberculous A18.54
Uveoencephalitis —see Inflammation,
  chorioretinal
Uveokeratitis —see Iridocyclitis
Uveoparotitis D86.89
Uvula —see condition
Uvulitis (acute) (catarrhal) (chronic)
  (membranous) (suppurative) (ulcerative)
  K12.2

V

Vaccination (prophylactic)
  complication or reaction —*see* Complications, vaccination
  delayed Z28.9
  encounter for Z23
  not done —*see* Immunization, not done, because (of)
Vaccinia (generalized) (localized) T88.1
  without vaccination B08.011
  congenital P35.8
Vacuum, in sinus (accessory) (nasal) J34.89
Vagabond, vagabondage Z59.0
Vagabond's disease B85.1
Vagina, vaginal —*see* condition
Vaginalitis (tunica) (testis) N49.1
Vaginismus (reflex) N94.2
  functional F52.5
  nonorganic F52.5
  psychogenic F52.5
  secondary N94.2
Vaginitis (acute) (circumscribed) (diffuse) (emphysematous) (nonvenereal) (ulcerative) N76.0
  with ectopic or molar pregnancy O08.0
  amebic A06.82
  atrophic, postmenopausal N95.2
  bacterial N76.0
  blennorrhagic (gonococcal) A54.02
  candidal B37.3
  chlamydial A56.02
  chronic N76.1
  due to Trichomonas (vaginalis) A59.01
  following ectopic or molar pregnancy O08.0
  gonococcal A54.02
    with abscess (accessory gland) (periurethral) A54.1
  granuloma A58
  in (due to)
    candidiasis B37.3
    herpesviral (herpes simplex) infection A60.04
    pinworm infection B80 [N77.1]
  monilial B37.3
  mycotic (candidal) B37.3
  postmenopausal atrophic N95.2
  puerperal (postpartum) O86.13
  senile (atrophic) N95.2
  subacute or chronic N76.1
  syphilitic (early) A51.0
    late A52.76
  trichomonal A59.01
  tuberculous A18.18
Vaginosis —*see* Vaginitis
Vagotonia G52.2
Vagrancy Z59.0
VAIN —*see* Neoplasia, intraepithelial, vagina
Vallecula —*see* condition
Valley fever B38.0
Valsuani's disease —*see* Anemia, obstetric
Valve, valvular (formation) —*see also* condition
  cerebral ventricle (communicating) in situ Z98.2
  cervix, internal os Q51.828
  congenital NEC —*see* Atresia, by site
  ureter (pelvic junction) (vesical orifice) Q62.39
  urethra (congenital) (posterior) Q64.2
Valvulitis (chronic) —*see* Endocarditis
Valvulopathy —*see* Endocarditis
Van Bogaert's leukoencephalopathy (sclerosing) (subacute) A81.1
Van Bogaert-Scherer-Epstein disease or syndrome E75.5
Van Buchem's syndrome M85.2
Van Creveld-von Gierke disease E74.01
Van der Hoeve (-de Kleyn) syndrome Q78.0
Van der Woude's syndrome Q38.0
Van Neck's disease or osteochondrosis M91.0
Vanishing lung J44.9

Vapor asphyxia or suffocation T59.9
  specified agent —*see* Table of Drugs and Chemicals
Variance, lethal ball, prosthetic heart valve T82.09
Variants, thalassemic D56.8
Variations in hair color L67.1
Varicella B01.9
  with
    complications NEC B01.89
    encephalitis B01.11
    encephalomyelitis B01.11
    meningitis B01.0
    myelitis B01.12
    pneumonia B01.2
  congenital P35.8
Varices —*see* Varix
Varicocele (scrotum) (thrombosed) I86.1
  ovary I86.2
  perineum I86.3
  spermatic cord (ulcerated) I86.1
Varicose
  aneurysm (ruptured) I77.0
  dermatitis —*see* Varix, leg, with, inflammation
  eczema —*see* Varix, leg, with, inflammation
  phlebitis —*see* Varix, with, inflammation
  tumor —*see* Varix
  ulcer (lower limb, any part) —*see also* Varix, leg, with, ulcer
    anus (*see also* Hemorrhoids) K64.8
    esophagus —*see* Varix, esophagus
    inflamed or infected —*see* Varix, leg, with ulcer, with inflammation
    nasal septum I86.8
    perineum I86.3
    scrotum I86.1
    specified site NEC I86.8
  vein —*see* Varix
  vessel —*see* Varix, leg
Varicosis, varicosities, varicosity —*see* Varix
Variola (major) (minor) B03
Varioloid B03
Varix (lower limb) (ruptured) I83.90
  with
    edema I83.899
    inflammation I83.10
      with ulcer (venous) I83.209
    pain I83.819
    specified complication NEC I83.899
    stasis dermatitis I83.10
      with ulcer (venous) I83.209
    swelling I83.899
    ulcer I83.009
      with inflammation I83.209
  aneurysmal I77.0
  asymptomatic I83.9-
  bladder I86.2
  broad ligament I86.2
  complicating
    childbirth (lower extremity) O87.4
      anus or rectum O87.2
      genital (vagina, vulva or perineum) O87.8
    pregnancy (lower extremity) O22.0-
      anus or rectum O22.4-
      genital (vagina, vulva or perineum) O22.1-
    puerperium (lower extremity) O87.4
      anus or rectum O87.2
      genital (vagina, vulva, perineum) O87.8
  congenital (any site) Q27.8
  esophagus (idiopathic) (primary) (ulcerated) I85.00
    bleeding I85.01
    congenital Q27.8
    in (due to)
      alcoholic liver disease I85.10
        bleeding I85.11
      cirrhosis of liver I85.10
        bleeding I85.11

Varix (Continued)
  esophagus (Continued)
    in (Continued)
      portal hypertension I85.10
        bleeding I85.11
      schistosomiasis I85.10
        bleeding I85.11
      toxic liver disease I85.10
        bleeding I85.11
    secondary I85.10
      bleeding I85.11
  gastric I86.4
  inflamed or infected I83.10
    ulcerated I83.209
  labia (majora) I86.3
  leg (asymptomatic) I83.90
    with
      edema I83.899
      inflammation I83.10
        with ulcer —*see* Varix, leg, with, ulcer, with inflammation by site
      pain I83.819
      specified complication NEC I83.899
      swelling I83.899
      ulcer I83.009
        with inflammation I83.209
        ankle I83.003
          with inflammation I83.203
        calf I83.002
          with inflammation I83.202
        foot NEC I83.005
          with inflammation I83.205
        heel I83.004
          with inflammation I83.204
        lower leg NEC I83.008
          with inflammation I83.208
        midfoot I83.004
          with inflammation I83.204
        thigh I83.001
          with inflammation I83.201
  bilateral (asymptomatic) I83.93
    with
      edema I83.893
      pain I83.813
      specified complication NEC I83.893
      swelling I83.893
      ulcer I83.009
        with inflammation I83.209
  left (asymptomatic) I83.92
    with
      edema I83.892
      inflammation I83.12
        with ulcer —*see* Varix, leg, with, ulcer, with inflammation by site
      pain I83.812
      specified complication NEC I83.892
      swelling I83.892
      ulcer I83.029
        with inflammation I83.229
        ankle I83.023
          with inflammation I83.223
        calf I83.022
          with inflammation I83.222
        foot NEC I83.025
          with inflammation I83.225
        heel I83.024
          with inflammation I83.224
        lower leg NEC I83.028
          with inflammation I83.228
        midfoot I83.024
          with inflammation I83.224
        thigh I83.021
          with inflammation I83.221
  right (asymptomatic) I83.91
    with
      edema I83.891
      inflammation I83.11
        with ulcer —*see* Varix, leg, with, ulcer, with inflammation by site

Varix (*Continued*)
 leg (*Continued*)
  right (*Continued*)
   with (*Continued*)
    pain I83.811
    specified complication NEC I83.891
    swelling I83.891
    ulcer I83.019
     with inflammation I83.219
     ankle I83.013
      with inflammation I83.213
     calf I83.012
      with inflammation I83.212
     foot NEC I83.015
      with inflammation I83.215
     heel I83.014
      with inflammation I83.214
     lower leg NEC I83.018
      with inflammation I83.218
     midfoot I83.014
      with inflammation I83.214
     thigh I83.011
      with inflammation I83.211
 nasal septum I86.8
 orbit I86.8
  congenital Q27.8
 ovary I86.2
 papillary I78.1
 pelvis I86.2
 perineum I86.3
 pharynx I86.8
 placenta O43.89-
 renal papilla I86.8
 retina H35.09
 scrotum (ulcerated) I86.1
 sigmoid colon I86.8
 specified site NEC I86.8
 spinal (cord) (vessels) I86.8
 spleen, splenic (vein) (with phlebolith) I86.8
 stomach I86.4
 sublingual I86.0
 ulcerated I83.009
  inflamed or infected I83.209
 uterine ligament I86.2
 vagina I86.8
 vocal cord I86.8
 vulva I86.3
Vas deferens —*see* condition
Vas deferentitis N49.1
Vasa previa O69.4
 hemorrhage from, affecting newborn P50.0
Vascular —*see also* condition
 loop on optic papilla Q14.2
 spasm I73.9
 spider I78.1
Vascularization, cornea —*see* Neovascularization, cornea
Vasculitis I77.6
 allergic D69.0
 cryoglobulinemic D89.1
 disseminated I77.6
 hypocomplementemic M31.8
 kidney I77.89
 livedoid L95.0
 nodular L95.8
 retina H35.06-
 rheumatic —*see* Fever, rheumatic
 rheumatoid —*see* Rheumatoid, vasculitis
 skin (limited to) L95.9
  specified NEC L95.8
Vasculopathy, necrotizing M31.9
 cardiac allograft T86.290
 specified NEC M31.8
Vasitis (nodosa) N49.1
 tuberculous A18.15
Vasodilation I73.9
Vasomotor —*see* condition
Vasoplasty, after previous sterilization Z31.0
 aftercare Z31.42

Vasospasm (vasoconstriction) I73.9
 cerebral (cerebrovascular) (artery) I67.848
  reversible I67.841
 coronary I20.1
 nerve
  arm —*see* Mononeuropathy, upper limb
  brachial plexus G54.0
  cervical plexus G54.2
  leg —*see* Mononeuropathy, lower limb
 peripheral NOS I73.9
 retina (artery) —*see* Occlusion, artery, retina
Vasospastic —*see* condition
Vasovagal attack (paroxysmal) R55
 psychogenic F45.8
VATER syndrome Q87.2
Vater's ampulla —*see* condition
Vegetation, vegetative
 adenoid (nasal fossa) J35.8
 endocarditis (acute) (any valve) (subacute) I33.0
 heart (mycotic) (valve) I33.0
Veil
 Jackson's Q43.3
Vein, venous —*see* condition
Veldt sore —*see* Ulcer, skin
Velpeau's hernia —*see* Hernia, femoral
Venereal
 bubo A55
 disease A64
 granuloma inguinale A58
 lymphogranuloma (Durand-Nicolas-Favre) A55
Venofibrosis I87.8
Venom, venomous —*see* Table of Drugs and Chemicals, by animal or substance, poisoning
Venous —*see* condition
Ventilator lung, newborn P27.8
Ventral —*see* condition
Ventricle, ventricular —*see also* condition
 escape I49.3
 inversion Q20.5
Ventriculitis (cerebral) (*see also* Encephalitis) G04.90
Ventriculostomy status Z98.2
Vernet's syndrome G52.7
Verneuil's disease (syphilitic bursitis) A52.78
Verruca (due to HPV) (filiformis) (simplex) (viral) (vulgaris) B07.9
 acuminata A63.0
 necrogenica (primary) (tuberculosa) A18.4
 plana B07.8
 plantaris B07.0
 seborrheica L82.1
  inflamed L82.0
 senile (seborrheic) L82.1
  inflamed L82.0
 tuberculosa (primary) A18.4
 venereal A63.0
Verrucosities —*see* Verruca
Verruga peruana, peruviana A44.1
Version
 with extraction
 cervix —*see* Malposition, uterus
 uterus (postinfectional) (postpartal, old) —*see* Malposition, uterus
Vertebra, vertebral —*see* condition
Vertical talus (congenital) Q66.80
 left foot Q66.82
 right foot Q66.81
Vertigo R42
 auditory —*see* Vertigo, aural
 aural H81.31-
 benign paroxysmal (positional) H81.1-
 central (origin) H81.4-
 cerebral H81.4-
 Dix and Hallpike (epidemic) —*see* Neuronitis, vestibular
 due to infrasound T75.23

Vertigo (*Continued*)
 epidemic A88.1
  Dix and Hallpike —*see* Neuronitis, vestibular
  Pedersen's —*see* Neuronitis, vestibular
  vestibular neuronitis —*see* Neuronitis, vestibular
 hysterical F44.89
 infrasound T75.23
 labyrinthine —*see* subcategory H81.0
 laryngeal R05
 malignant positional H81.4-
 Ménière's —*see* subcategory H81.40
 menopausal N95.11
 otogenic —*see* Vertigo, aural
 paroxysmal positional, benign —*see* Vertigo, benign paroxysmal
 Pedersen's (epidemic) —*see* Neuronitis, vestibular
 peripheral NEC H81.39-
 positional
  benign paroxysmal —*see* Vertigo, benign paroxysmal
  malignant H81.4-
Very-low-density-lipoprotein-type (VLDL) hyperlipoproteinemia E78.1
Vesania —*see* Psychosis
Vesical —*see* condition
Vesicle
 cutaneous R23.8
 seminal —*see* condition
 skin R23.8
Vesicocolic —*see* condition
Vesicoperineal —*see* condition
Vesicorectal —*see* condition
Vesicourethrorectal —*see* condition
Vesicovaginal —*see* condition
Vesicular —*see* condition
Vesiculitis (seminal) N49.0
 amebic A06.82
 gonorrheal (acute) (chronic) A54.23
 trichomonal A59.09
 tuberculous A18.15
Vestibulitis (ear) (*see also* subcategory) H83.0
 nose (external) J34.89
 vulvar N94.810
Vestibulopathy, acute peripheral (recurrent) — *see* Neuronitis, vestibular
Vestige, vestigial —*see also* Persistence
 branchial Q18.0
 structures in vitreous Q14.0
Vibration
 adverse effects T75.20
  pneumatic hammer syndrome T75.21
  specified effect NEC T75.29
  vasospastic syndrome T75.22
  vertigo from infrasound T75.23
 exposure (occupational) Z57.7
 vertigo T75.23
Vibriosis A28.9
Victim (of)
 crime Z65.4
 disaster Z65.5
 terrorism Z65.4
 torture Z65.4
 war Z65.5
Vidal's disease L28.0
Villaret's syndrome G52.7
Villous —*see* condition
VIN —*see* Neoplasia, intraepithelial, vulva
Vincent's infection (angina) (gingivitis) A69.1
 stomatitis NEC A69.1
Vinson-Plummer syndrome D50.1
Violence, physical R45.6
Viosterol deficiency —*see* Deficiency, calciferol
Vipoma —*see* Neoplasm, malignant, by site
Viremia B34.9
Virilism (adrenal) E25.9
 congenital E25.0

◄ New   ◄ Revised   ~~deleted~~ Deleted

Virilization (female) (suprarenal) E25.9
  congenital E25.0
  isosexual E28.2
Virulent bubo A57
Virus, viral —*see also* condition
  as cause of disease classified elsewhere
    B97.89
  cytomegalovirus B25.9
  human immunodeficiency (HIV) —*see*
    Human, immunodeficiency virus (HIV)
    disease
  infection —*see* Infection, virus
  specified NEC B34.8
  swine influenza (viruses that normally cause
    infections in pigs) (*see also* Influenza,
    due to, identified novel influenza A
    virus) J09.X2
  West Nile (fever) A92.30
    with
      complications NEC A92.39
      cranial nerve disorders A92.32
      encephalitis A92.31
      encephalomyelitis A92.31
      neurologic manifestation NEC A92.32
      optic neuritis A92.32
      polyradiculitis A92.32
Viscera, visceral —*see* condition
Visceroptosis K63.4
Visible peristalsis R19.2
Vision, visual
  binocular, suppression H53.34
  blurred, blurring H53.8
    hysterical F44.6
  defect, defective NEC H54.7
  disorientation (syndrome) H53.8
  disturbance H53.9
    hysterical F44.6
  double H53.2
  examination Z01.00
    with abnormal findings Z01.01
  field, limitation (defect) —*see* Defect, visual
    field
  hallucinations R44.1
  halos H53.19
  loss —*see* Loss, vision
    sudden —*see* Disturbance, vision,
      subjective, loss, sudden
  low (both eyes) —*see* Low, vision
  perception, simultaneous without fusion
    H53.33
Vitality, lack or want of R53.83
  newborn P96.89
Vitamin deficiency —*see* Deficiency, vitamin
Vitelline duct, persistent Q43.0
Vitiligo L80
  eyelid H02.739
    left H02.736
      lower H02.735
      upper H02.734

Vitiligo *(Continued)*
  eyelid *(Continued)*
    right H02.733
      lower H02.732
      upper H02.731
  pinta A67.2
  vulva N90.89
Vitreal corneal syndrome H59.01-
Vitreoretinopathy, proliferative —*see also*
  Retinopathy, proliferative
  with retinal detachment —*see* Detachment,
    retina, traction
Vitreous —*see also* condition
  touch syndrome —*see* Complication,
    postprocedural, following cataract
    surgery
Vocal cord —*see* condition
Vogt-Koyanagi syndrome H20.82-
Vogt's disease or syndrome G80.3
Vogt-Spielmeyer amaurotic idiocy or disease
  E75.4
Voice
  change R49.9
    specified NEC R49.8
  loss —*see* Aphonia
Volhynian fever A79.0
Volkmann's ischemic contracture or paralysis
  (complicating trauma) T79.6
Volvulus (bowel) (colon) (duodenum)
  (intestine) K56.2
  with perforation K56.2
  congenital Q43.8
  fallopian tube —*see* Torsion, fallopian
    tube
  oviduct —*see* Torsion, fallopian tube
  stomach (due to absence of gastrocolic
    ligament) K31.89
Vomiting R11.10
  with nausea R11.2
  without nausea R11.11
  asphyxia —*see* Foreign body, by site, causing
    asphyxia, gastric contents
  bilious (cause unknown) R11.14
    following gastro-intestinal surgery
      K91.0
    in newborn P92.01
  blood —*see* Hematemesis
  causing asphyxia, choking, or suffocation —
    see Foreign body, by site
  cyclical G43.A0
    with refractory migraine G43.A1
    intractable G43.A1
    not intractable G43.A0
    psychogenic F50.8
    without refractory migraine G43.A0
  fecal mater R11.13
  following gastrointestinal surgery
    K91.0
    psychogenic F50.8

Vomiting *(Continued)*
  functional K31.89
  hysterical F50.8
  nervous F50.8
  neurotic F50.8
  newborn NEC P92.09
    bilious P92.01
  periodic R11.10
    psychogenic F50.8
  projectile R11.12
  psychogenic F50.8
  uremic —*see* Uremia
Vomito negro —*see* Fever, yellow
Von Bezold's abscess —*see* Mastoiditis,
  acute
Von Economo-Cruchet disease A85.8
Von Eulenburg's disease G71.19
Von Gierke's disease E74.01
Von Hippel (-Lindau) disease or syndrome
  Q85.8
Von Jaksch's anemia or disease D64.89
Von Recklinghausen
  disease (neurofibromatosis) Q85.01
    bones E21.0
Von Schroetter's syndrome I82.890
Von Willebrand (-Jurgens)(-Minot) disease or
  syndrome D68.0
Von Zumbusch's disease L40.1
Voyeurism F65.3
Vrolik's disease Q78.0
Vulva —*see* condition
Vulvismus N94.2
Vulvitis (acute) (allergic) (atrophic)
  (hypertrophic) (intertriginous) (senile)
  N76.2
  with ectopic or molar pregnancy O08.0
  adhesive, congenital Q52.79
  blennorrhagic (gonococcal) A54.02
  candidal B37.3
  chlamydial A56.02
  due to Haemophilus ducreyi A57
  following ectopic or molar pregnancy
    O08.0
  gonococcal A54.02
    with abscess (accessory gland)
      (periurethral) A54.1
  herpesviral A60.04
  leukoplakic N90.4
  monilial B37.3
  puerperal (postpartum) O86.19
  subacute or chronic N76.3
  syphilitic (early) A51.0
    late A52.76
  trichomonal A59.01
  tuberculous A18.18
Vulvodynia N94.819
  specified NEC N94.818
Vulvorectal —*see* condition
Vulvovaginitis (acute) —*see* Vaginitis

W

Waiting list, person on Z75.1
  for organ transplant Z76.82
  undergoing social agency investigation Z75.2
Waldenström
  hypergammaglobulinemia D89.0
  syndrome or macroglobulinemia C88.0
Waldenström-Kjellberg syndrome D50.1
Walking
  difficulty R26.2
    psychogenic F44.4
  sleep F51.3
    hysterical F44.89
Wall, abdominal —see condition
Wallenberg's disease or syndrome G46.3
Wallgren's disease I87.8
Wandering
  gallbladder, congenital Q44.1
  in diseases classified elsewhere Z91.83
  kidney, congenital Q63.8
  organ or site, congenital NEC —see
    Malposition, congenital, by site
  pacemaker (heart) I49.8
  spleen D73.89
War neurosis F48.8
Wart (due to HPV) (filiform) (infectious) (viral)
    B07.9
  anogenital region (venereal) A63.0
  common B07.8
  external genital organs (venereal) A63.0
  flat B07.8
  Hassall-Henle's (of cornea) H18.49
  Peruvian A44.1
  plantar B07.0
  prosector (tuberculous) A18.4
  seborrheic L82.1
    inflamed L82.0
  senile (seborrheic) L82.1
    inflamed L82.0
  tuberculous A18.4
  venereal A63.0
Warthin's tumor —see Neoplasm, salivary
    gland, benign
Wassilieff's disease A27.0
Wasting
  disease R64
    due to malnutrition E41
  extreme (due to malnutrition) E41
  muscle NEC —see Atrophy, muscle
Water
  clefts (senile cataract) —see Cataract, senile,
    incipient
  deprivation of T73.1
  intoxication E87.79
  itch B76.9
  lack of T73.1
  loading E87.70
  on
    brain —see Hydrocephalus
    chest J94.8
  poisoning E87.79
Waterbrash R12
Waterhouse(-Friderichsen) syndrome or
    disease (meningococcal) A39.1
Water-losing nephritis N25.89
Watermelon stomach K31.819
  with hemorrhage K31.811
  without hemorrhage K31.819
Watsoniasis B66.8
Wax in ear —see Impaction, cerumen
Weak, weakening, weakness (generalized)
    R53.1
  arches (acquired) —see also Deformity, limb,
    flat foot
  bladder (sphincter) R32
  facial R29.810
    following
      cerebrovascular disease I69.992
        cerebral infarction I69.392
        intracerebral hemorrhage I69.192

Weak, weakening, weakness (Continued)
  facial (Continued)
    following (Continued)
      cerebrovascular disease (Continued)
        nontraumatic intracranial hemorrhage
          NEC I69.292
        specified disease NEC I69.892
        stroke I69.392
        subarachnoid hemorrhage I69.092
  foot (double) —see Weak, arches
  heart, cardiac —see Failure, heart
  mind F70
  muscle M62.81
  myocardium —see Failure, heart
  newborn P96.89
  pelvic fundus N81.89
  pubocervical tissue N81.82
  rectovaginal tissue N81.83
  senile R54
  urinary stream R39.12
  valvular —see Endocarditis
Wear, worn (with normal or routine use)
  articular bearing surface of internal joint
    prosthesis —see Complications, joint
    prosthesis, mechanical, wear of articular
    bearing surfaces, by site
  device, implant or graft —see Complications,
    by site, mechanical complication
  tooth, teeth (approximal) (hard tissues)
    (interproximal) (occlusal) K03.0
Weather, weathered
  effects of
    cold T69.9
      specified effect NEC T69.8
    hot —see Heat
  skin L57.8
Weaver's syndrome Q87.3
Web, webbed (congenital)
  duodenal Q43.8
  esophagus Q39.4
  fingers Q70.1
  larynx (glottic) (subglottic) Q31.0
  neck (pterygium colli) Q18.3
  Paterson-Kelly D50.1
  popliteal syndrome Q87.89
  toes Q70.3
Weber-Christian disease M35.6
Weber-Cockayne syndrome (epidermolysis
    bullosa) Q81.8
Weber-Gubler syndrome G46.3
Weber-Leyden syndrome G46.3
Weber-Osler syndrome I78.0
Weber's paralysis or syndrome G46.3
Wedge-shaped or wedging vertebra —see
    Collapse, vertebra NEC
Wegener's granulomatosis or syndrome
    M31.30
  with
    kidney involvement M31.31
    lung involvement M31.30
      with kidney involvement M31.31
Wegner's disease A50.02
Weight
  1000-2499 grams at birth (low) —see Low,
    birthweight
  999 grams or less at birth (extremely low) —
    see Low, birthweight, extreme
  gain (abnormal) (excessive) R63.5
    in pregnancy —see Pregnancy, complicated
      by, excessive weight gain
    low —see Pregnancy, complicated by,
      insufficient, weight gain
  loss (abnormal) (cause unknown) R63.4
Weightlessness (effect of) T75.82
Weil (l)-Marchesani syndrome Q87.1
Weil's disease A27.0
Weingarten's syndrome J82
Weir Mitchell's disease I73.81
Weiss-Baker syndrome G90.09
Wells' disease L98.3
Wen —see Cyst, sebaceous

Wenckebach's block or phenomenon I44.1
Werdnig-Hoffmann syndrome (muscular
    atrophy) G12.0
Werlhof's disease D69.3
Werner-His disease A79.0
Wermer's disease or syndrome E31.21
Werner's disease or syndrome E34.8
Wernicke-Korsakoff's syndrome or psychosis
    (alcoholic) F10.96
  with dependence F10.26
  drug-induced
    due to drug abuse —see Abuse, drug, by
      type, with amnestic disorder
    due to drug dependence —see Dependence,
      drug, by type, with amnestic disorder
  nonalcoholic F04
Wernicke-Posadas disease B38.9
Wernicke's
  developmental aphasia F80.2
  disease or syndrome E51.2
  encephalopathy E51.2
  polioencephalitis, superior E51.2
West African fever B50.8
Westphal-Strümpell syndrome E83.01
West's syndrome —see Epilepsy, spasms
Wet
  feet, tropical (maceration) (syndrome) —see
    Immersion, foot
  lung (syndrome), newborn P22.1
Wharton's duct —see condition
Wheal —see Urticaria
Wheezing R06.2
Whiplash injury S13.4
Whipple's disease (see also subcategory M14.8-)
    K90.81
Whipworm (disease) (infection) (infestation)
    B79
Whistling face Q87.0
White —see also condition
  kidney, small N03.9
  leg, puerperal, postpartum, childbirth O87.1
  mouth B37.0
  patches of mouth K13.29
  spot lesions, teeth
    chewing surface K02.51
    pit and fissure surface K02.51
    smooth surface K02.61
Whitehead L70.0
Whitlow —see also Cellulitis, digit
  with lymphangitis —see Lymphangitis, acute,
    digit
  herpesviral B00.89
Whitmore's disease or fever —see Melioidosis
Whooping cough A37.90
  with pneumonia A37.91
    due to Bordetella
      bronchiseptica A37.81
      parapertussis A37.11
      pertussis A37.01
    specified organism NEC A37.81
  due to
    Bordetella
      bronchiseptica A37.80
        with pneumonia A37.81
      parapertussis A37.10
        with pneumonia A37.11
      pertussis A37.00
        with pneumonia A37.01
    specified NEC A37.80
      with pneumonia A37.81
Wichman's asthma J38.5
Wide cranial sutures, newborn P96.3
Widening aorta —see Ectasia, aorta
  with aneurysm —see Aneurysm, aorta
Wilkie's disease or syndrome K55.1
Wilkinson-Sneddon disease or syndrome
    L13.1
Willebrand (-Jürgens) thrombopathy D68.0
Willige-Hunt disease or syndrome G23.1
Wilms' tumor C64-
Wilson-Mikity syndrome P27.0

◀ New   ◀▥ Revised   ~~deleted~~ Deleted

Wilson's
  disease or syndrome E83.01
  hepatolenticular degeneration E83.01
  lichen ruber L43.9
Window —*see also* Imperfect, closure
  aorticopulmonary Q21.4
Winter —*see* condition
Wiskott-Aldrich syndrome D82.0
Withdrawal state —*see also* Dependence, drug
    by type, with withdrawal
  newborn
    correct therapeutic substance properly
      administered P96.2
    infant of dependent mother P96.1
    therapeutic substance, neonatal P96.2
Witts' anemia D50.8
Witzelsucht F07.0
Woakes' ethmoiditis or syndrome J33.1
Wolff-Hirschorn syndrome Q93.3
Wolff-Parkinson-White syndrome I45.6
Wolhynian fever A79.0
Wolman's disease E75.5
Wood lung or pneumonitis J67.8
Woolly, wooly hair (congenital) (nevus)
  Q84.1
Woolsorter's disease A22.1
Word
  blindness (congenital) (developmental)
    F81.0
  deafness (congenital) (developmental)
    H93.25
Worm (s) (infection) (infestation) —*see also*
    Infestation, helminth
  guinea B72
  in intestine NEC B82.0
Worm-eaten soles A66.3
Worn out —*see* Exhaustion
  cardiac
    defibrillator (with synchronous cardiac
      pacemaker) Z45.02
    pacemaker
      battery Z45.010
      lead Z45.018
  device, implant or graft —*see* Complications,
    by site, mechanical
Worried well Z71.1
Worries R45.82
Wound, open
  abdomen, abdominal
    wall S31.109
      with penetration into peritoneal cavity
        S31.609
      bite —*see* Bite, abdomen, wall
      epigastric region S31.102
        with penetration into peritoneal cavity
          S31.602
        bite —*see* Bite, abdomen, wall,
          epigastric region
        laceration —*see* Laceration, abdomen,
          wall, epigastric region
        puncture —*see* Puncture, abdomen,
          wall, epigastric region
      laceration —*see* Laceration, abdomen,
        wall
      left
        lower quadrant S31.104
          with penetration into peritoneal
            cavity S31.604
          bite —*see* Bite, abdomen, wall, left,
            lower quadrant
          laceration —*see* Laceration,
            abdomen, wall, left, lower
            quadrant
          puncture —*see* Puncture,
            abdomen, wall, left, lower
            quadrant
        upper quadrant S31.101
          with penetration into peritoneal
            cavity S31.601
          bite —*see* Bite, abdomen, wall, left,
            upper quadrant

Wound, open *(Continued)*
  abdomen, abdominal *(Continued)*
    wall *(Continued)*
      left *(Continued)*
        upper quadrant *(Continued)*
          laceration —*see* Laceration,
            abdomen, wall, left, upper
            quadrant
          puncture —*see* Puncture, abdomen,
            wall, left, upper quadrant
      periumbilic region S31.105
        with penetration into peritoneal cavity
          S31.605
        bite —*see* Bite, abdomen, wall,
          periumbilic region
        laceration —*see* Laceration, abdomen,
          wall, periumbilic region
        puncture —*see* Puncture, abdomen,
          wall, periumbilic region
      puncture —*see* Puncture, abdomen, wall
      right
        lower quadrant S31.103
          with penetration into peritoneal
            cavity S31.603
          bite —*see* Bite, abdomen, wall, right,
            lower quadrant
          laceration —*see* Laceration,
            abdomen, wall, right, lower
            quadrant
          puncture —*see* Puncture, abdomen,
            wall, right, lower quadrant
        upper quadrant S31.100
          with penetration into peritoneal
            cavity S31.600
          bite —*see* Bite, abdomen, wall, right,
            upper quadrant
          laceration —*see* Laceration,
            abdomen, wall, right, upper
            quadrant
          puncture —*see* Puncture, abdomen,
            wall, right, upper quadrant
    alveolar (process) —*see* Wound, open, oral
      cavity
    ankle S91.00-
      bite —*see* Bite, ankle
      laceration —*see* Laceration, ankle
      puncture —*see* Puncture, ankle
    antecubital space —*see* Wound, open, elbow
    anterior chamber, eye —*see* Wound, open,
      ocular
    anus S31.839
      bite S31.835
      laceration —*see* Laceration, anus
      puncture —*see* Puncture, anus
    arm (upper) S41.10-
      with amputation —*see* Amputation,
        traumatic, arm
      bite —*see* Bite, arm
      forearm —*see* Wound, open, forearm
      laceration —*see* Laceration, arm
      puncture —*see* Puncture, arm
    auditory canal (external) (meatus) —*see*
      Wound, open, ear
    auricle, ear —*see* Wound, open, ear
    axilla —*see* Wound, open, arm
    back —*see also* Wound, open, thorax, back
      lower S31.000
        with penetration into retroperitoneal
          space S31.001
        bite —*see* Bite, back, lower
        laceration —*see* Laceration, back,
          lower
        puncture —*see* Puncture, back, lower
    bite —*see* Bite
    blood vessel —*see* Injury, blood vessel
    breast S21.00-
      with amputation —*see* Amputation,
        traumatic, breast
      bite —*see* Bite, breast
      laceration —*see* Laceration, breast
      puncture —*see* Puncture, breast

Wound, open *(Continued)*
  buttock S31.809
    bite —*see* Bite, buttock
    laceration —*see* Laceration, buttock
    left S31.829
    puncture —*see* Puncture, buttock
    right S31.819
  calf —*see* Wound, open, leg
  canaliculus lacrimalis —*see* Wound,
    open, eyelid
  canthus, eye —*see* Wound, open,
    eyelid
  cervical esophagus S11.20
    bite S11.25
    laceration —*see* Laceration, esophagus,
      traumatic, cervical
    puncture —*see* Puncture, cervical
      esophagus
  cheek (external) S01.40-
    bite —*see* Bite, cheek
    internal —*see* Wound, open, oral
      cavity
    laceration —*see* Laceration, cheek
    puncture —*see* Puncture, cheek
  chest wall —*see* Wound, open, thorax
  chin —*see* Wound, open, head, specified site
    NEC
  choroid —*see* Wound, open, ocular
  ciliary body (eye) —*see* Wound, open,
    ocular
  clitoris S31.40
    with amputation —*see* Amputation,
      traumatic, clitoris
    bite S31.45
    laceration —*see* Laceration, vulva
    puncture —*see* Puncture, vulva
  conjunctiva —*see* Wound, open, ocular
  cornea —*see* Wound, open, ocular
  costal region —*see* Wound, open, thorax
  Descemet's membrane —*see* Wound, open,
    ocular
  digit (s)
    foot —*see* Wound, open, toe
    hand —*see* Wound, open, finger
  ear (canal) (external) S01.30-
    with amputation —*see* Amputation,
      traumatic, ear
    bite —*see* Bite, ear
    drum S09.2-
    laceration —*see* Laceration, ear
    puncture —*see* Puncture, ear
  elbow S51.00-
    bite —*see* Bite, elbow
    laceration —*see* Laceration, elbow
    puncture —*see* Puncture, elbow
  epididymis —*see* Wound, open, testis
  epigastric region S31.102
    with penetration into peritoneal cavity
      S31.602
    bite —*see* Bite, abdomen, wall, epigastric
      region
    laceration —*see* Laceration, abdomen, wall,
      epigastric region
    puncture —*see* Puncture, abdomen, wall,
      epigastric region
  epiglottis —*see* Wound, open, neck, specified
    site NEC
  esophagus (thoracic) S27.819
    cervical —*see* Wound, open, cervical
      esophagus
    laceration S27.813
    specified type NEC S27.818
  eye —*see* Wound, open, ocular
  eyeball —*see* Wound, open, ocular
  eyebrow —*see* Wound, open, eyelid
  eyelid S01.10-
    bite —*see* Bite, eyelid
    laceration —*see* Laceration, eyelid
    puncture —*see* Puncture, eyelid
  face NEC —*see* Wound, open, head, specified
    site NEC

Wound, open *(Continued)*
finger (s) S61.209
  with
    amputation —*see* Amputation,
      traumatic, finger
    damage to nail S61.309
  bite —*see* Bite, finger
  index S61.208
    with
      damage to nail S61.308
    left S61.201
      with
        damage to nail S61.301
    right S61.200
      with
        damage to nail S61.300
    laceration —*see* Laceration, finger
  little S61.208
    with
      damage to nail S61.308
    left S61.207
      with damage to nail S61.307
    right S61.206
      with damage to nail S61.306
  middle S61.208
    with
      damage to nail S61.308
    left S61.203
      with damage to nail S61.303
    right S61.202
      with damage to nail S61.302
  puncture —*see* Puncture, finger
  ring S61.208
    with
      damage to nail S61.308
    left S61.205
      with damage to nail S61.305
    right S61.204
      with damage to nail S61.304
flank —*see* Wound, open, abdomen, wall
foot (except toe (s) alone) S91.30-
  with amputation —*see* Amputation,
    traumatic, foot
  bite —*see* Bite, foot
  laceration —*see* Laceration, foot
  puncture —*see* Puncture, foot
  toe —*see* Wound, open, toe
forearm S51.80-
  with
    amputation —*see* Amputation,
      traumatic, forearm
  bite —*see* Bite, forearm
  elbow only —*see* Wound, open, elbow
  laceration —*see* Laceration, forearm
  puncture —*see* Puncture, forearm
forehead —*see* Wound, open, head, specified
  site NEC
genital organs, external
  with amputation —*see* Amputation,
    traumatic, genital organs
  bite —*see* Bite, genital organ
  female S31.502
    vagina S31.40
    vulva S31.40
  laceration —*see* Laceration, genital
    organ
  male S31.501
    penis S31.20
    scrotum S31.30
    testes S31.30
  puncture —*see* Puncture, genital organ
globe (eye) —*see* Wound, open, ocular
groin —*see* Wound, open, abdomen, wall
gum —*see* Wound, open, oral cavity
hand S61.40-
  with
    amputation —*see* Amputation,
      traumatic, hand
  bite —*see* Bite, hand
  finger (s) —*see* Wound, open, finger
  laceration —*see* Laceration, hand

Wound, open *(Continued)*
hand *(Continued)*
  puncture —*see* Puncture, hand
  thumb —*see* Wound, open, thumb
head S01.90
  bite —*see* Bite, head
  cheek —*see* Wound, open, cheek
  ear —*see* Wound, open, ear
  eyelid —*see* Wound, open, eyelid
  laceration —*see* Laceration, head
  lip —*see* Wound, open, lip
  nose S01.20
  oral cavity —*see* Wound, open, oral cavity
  puncture —*see* Puncture, head
  scalp —*see* Wound, open, scalp
  specified site NEC S01.80
  temporomandibular area —*see* Wound,
    open, cheek
heel —*see* Wound, open, foot
hip S71.00-
  with amputation —*see* Amputation,
    traumatic, hip
  bite —*see* Bite, hip
  laceration —*see* Laceration, hip
  puncture —*see* Puncture, hip
hymen S31.40
  bite —*see* Bite, vulva
  laceration —*see* Laceration, vagina
  puncture —*see* Puncture, vagina
hypochondrium S31.109
  bite —*see* Bite, hypochondrium
  laceration —*see* Laceration,
    hypochondrium
  puncture —*see* Puncture, hypochondrium
hypogastric region S31.109
  bite —*see* Bite, hypogastric region
  laceration —*see* Laceration, hypogastric
    region
  puncture —*see* Puncture, hypogastric
    region
iliac (region) —*see* Wound, open, inguinal
  region
inguinal region S31.109
  bite —*see* Bite, abdomen, wall, lower
    quadrant
  laceration —*see* Laceration, inguinal region
  puncture —*see* Puncture, inguinal region
instep —*see* Wound, open, foot
interscapular region —*see* Wound, open,
  thorax, back
intraocular —*see* Wound, open, ocular
iris —*see* Wound, open, ocular
jaw —*see* Wound, open, head, specified site
  NEC
knee S81.00-
  bite —*see* Bite, knee
  laceration —*see* Laceration, knee
  puncture —*see* Puncture, knee
labium (majus) (minus) —*see* Wound, open,
  vulva
laceration —*see* Laceration, by site
lacrimal duct —*see* Wound, open, eyelid
larynx S11.019
  bite —*see* Bite, larynx
  laceration —*see* Laceration, larynx
  puncture —*see* Puncture, larynx
left
  lower quadrant S31.104
    with penetration into peritoneal cavity
      S31.604
    bite —*see* Bite, abdomen, wall, left, lower
      quadrant
    laceration —*see* Laceration, abdomen,
      wall, left, lower quadrant
    puncture —*see* Puncture, abdomen, wall,
      left, lower quadrant
  upper quadrant S31.101
    with penetration into peritoneal cavity
      S31.601
    bite —*see* Bite, abdomen, wall, left,
      upper quadrant

Wound, open *(Continued)*
left *(Continued)*
  upper quadrant *(Continued)*
    laceration —*see* Laceration, abdomen,
      wall, left, upper quadrant
    puncture —*see* Puncture, abdomen, wall,
      left, upper quadrant
leg (lower) S81.80-
  with amputation —*see* Amputation,
    traumatic, leg
  ankle —*see* Wound, open, ankle
  bite —*see* Bite, leg
  foot —*see* Wound, open, foot
  knee —*see* Wound, open, knee
  laceration —*see* Laceration, leg
  puncture —*see* Puncture, leg
  toe —*see* Wound, open, toe
  upper —*see* Wound, open, thigh
lip S01.501
  bite —*see* Bite, lip
  laceration —*see* Laceration, lip
  puncture —*see* Puncture, lip
loin S31.109
  bite —*see* Bite, abdomen, wall
  laceration —*see* Laceration, loin
  puncture —*see* Puncture, loin
lower back —*see* Wound, open, back,
  lower
lumbar region —*see* Wound, open, back,
  lower
malar region —*see* Wound, open, head,
  specified site NEC
mammary —*see* Wound, open, breast
mastoid region —*see* Wound, open, head,
  specified site NEC
mouth —*see* Wound, open, oral cavity
nail
  finger —*see* Wound, open, finger, with
    damage to nail
  toe —*see* Wound, open, toe, with damage
    to nail
nape (neck) —*see* Wound, open, neck
nasal (septum) (sinus) —*see* Wound, open,
  nose
nasopharynx —*see* Wound, open, head,
  specified site NEC
neck S11.90
  bite —*see* Bite, neck
  involving
    cervical esophagus S11.20
    larynx —*see* Wound, open, larynx
    pharynx S11.20
    thyroid S11.10
    trachea (cervical) S11.029
      bite —*see* Bite, trachea
      laceration S11.021
        with foreign body S11.022
      puncture S11.023
        with foreign body S11.024
  laceration —*see* Laceration, neck
  puncture —*see* Puncture, neck
  specified site NEC S11.80
  specified type NEC S11.89
nose (septum) (sinus) S01.20
  with amputation —*see* Amputation,
    traumatic, nose
  bite —*see* Bite, nose
  laceration —*see* Laceration, nose
  puncture —*see* Puncture, nose
ocular S05.90
  avulsion (traumatic enucleation) S05.7-
  eyeball S05.6-
    with foreign body S05.5-
  eyelid —*see* Wound, open, eyelid
  laceration and rupture S05.3-
    with prolapse or loss of intraocular
      tissue S05.2-
  orbit (penetrating) (with or without foreign
    body) S05.4-
  periocular area —*see* Wound, open, eyelid
  specified NEC S05.8X-

◀ New   ◀▦ Revised   ~~deleted~~ Deleted

Wound, open *(Continued)*
  oral cavity S01.502
    bite S01.552
    laceration —*see* Laceration, oral cavity
    puncture —*see* Puncture, oral cavity
  orbit —*see* Wound, open, ocular, orbit
  palate —*see* Wound, open, oral cavity
  palm —*see* Wound, open, hand
  pelvis, pelvic —*see also* Wound, open, back,
      lower
    girdle —*see* Wound, open, hip
  penetrating —*see* Puncture, by site
  penis S31.20
    with amputation —*see* Amputation,
        traumatic, penis
    bite S31.25
    laceration —*see* Laceration, penis
    puncture —*see* Puncture, penis
  perineum
    bite —*see* Bite, perineum
    female S31.502
    laceration —*see* Laceration, perineum
    male S31.501
    puncture —*see* Puncture, perineum
  periocular area (with or without lacrimal
        passages) —*see* Wound, open, eyelid
  periumbilic region S31.105
    with penetration into peritoneal cavity
        S31.605
    bite —*see* Bite, abdomen, wall, periumbilic
        region
    laceration —*see* Laceration, abdomen, wall,
        periumbilic region
    puncture —*see* Puncture, abdomen, wall,
        periumbilic region
  phalanges
    finger —*see* Wound, open, finger
    toe —*see* Wound, open, toe
  pharynx S11.20
  pinna —*see* Wound, open, ear
  popliteal space —*see* Wound, open, knee
  prepuce —*see* Wound, open, penis
  pubic region —*see* Wound, open, back,
      lower
  pudendum —*see* Wound, open, genital
      organs, external
  puncture wound —*see* Puncture
  rectovaginal septum —*see* Wound, open,
      vagina
  right
    lower quadrant S31.103
      with penetration into peritoneal cavity
          S31.603
      bite —*see* Bite, abdomen, wall, right,
          lower quadrant
      laceration —*see* Laceration, abdomen,
          wall, right, lower quadrant
      puncture —*see* Puncture, abdomen, wall,
          right, lower quadrant
    upper quadrant S31.100
      with penetration into peritoneal cavity
          S31.600
      bite —*see* Bite, abdomen, wall, right,
          upper quadrant
      laceration —*see* Laceration, abdomen,
          wall, right, upper quadrant
      puncture —*see* Puncture, abdomen, wall,
          right, upper quadrant
  sacral region —*see* Wound, open, back,
      lower
  sacroiliac region —*see* Wound, open, back,
      lower
  salivary gland —*see* Wound, open, oral
      cavity

Wound, open *(Continued)*
  scalp S01.00
    bite S01.05
    laceration —*see* Laceration, scalp
    puncture —*see* Puncture, scalp
  scalpel, newborn (birth injury) P15.8
  scapular region —*see* Wound, open, shoulder
  sclera —*see* Wound, open, ocular
  scrotum S31.30
    with amputation —*see* Amputation,
        traumatic, scrotum
    bite S31.35
    laceration —*see* Laceration, scrotum
    puncture —*see* Puncture, scrotum
  shin —*see* Wound, open, leg
  shoulder S41.00-
    with amputation —*see* Amputation,
        traumatic, arm
    bite —*see* Bite, shoulder
    laceration —*see* Laceration, shoulder
    puncture —*see* Puncture, shoulder
  skin NOS T14.8
  spermatic cord —*see* Wound, open, testis
  sternal region —*see* Wound, open, thorax,
      front wall
  submaxillary region —*see* Wound, open,
      head, specified site NEC
  submental region —*see* Wound, open, head,
      specified site NEC
  subungual
    finger (s) —*see* Wound, open, finger
    toe (s) —*see* Wound, open, toe
  supraclavicular region —*see* Wound, open,
      neck, specified site NEC
  temple, temporal region —*see* Wound, open,
      head, specified site NEC
  temporomandibular area —*see* Wound, open,
      cheek
  testis S31.30
    with amputation —*see* Amputation,
        traumatic, testes
    bite S31.35
    laceration —*see* Laceration, testis
    puncture —*see* Puncture, testis
  thigh S71.10-
    with amputation —*see* Amputation,
        traumatic, hip
    bite —*see* Bite, thigh
    laceration —*see* Laceration, thigh
    puncture —*see* Puncture, thigh
  thorax, thoracic (wall) S21.90
    back S21.20-
      with penetration S21.40
    bite —*see* Bite, thorax
    breast —*see* Wound, open, breast
    front S21.10-
      with penetration S21.30
    laceration —*see* Laceration, thorax
    puncture —*see* Puncture, thorax
  throat —*see* Wound, open, neck
  thumb S61.009
    with
      amputation —*see* Amputation,
          traumatic, thumb
      damage to nail S61.109
    bite —*see* Bite, thumb
    laceration —*see* Laceration, thumb
    left S61.002
      with
        damage to nail S61.102
    puncture —*see* Puncture, thumb
    right S61.001
      with
        damage to nail S61.101

Wound, open *(Continued)*
  thyroid (gland) —*see* Wound, open, neck,
      thyroid
  toe (s) S91.109
    with
      amputation —*see* Amputation,
          traumatic, toe
      damage to nail S91.209
    bite —*see* Bite, toe
    great S91.103
      with
        damage to nail S91.203
      left S91.102
        with
          damage to nail S91.202
      right S91.101
        with
          damage to nail S91.201
    laceration —*see* Laceration, toe
    lesser S91.106
      with
        damage to nail S91.206
      left S91.105
        with
          damage to nail S91.205
      right S91.104
        with
          damage to nail S91.204
    puncture —*see* Puncture, toe
  tongue —*see* Wound, open, oral cavity
  trachea (cervical region) —*see* Wound, open,
      neck, trachea
  tunica vaginalis —*see* Wound, open, testis
  tympanum, tympanic membrane S09.2-
    laceration —*see* Laceration, ear, drum
    puncture —*see* Puncture, tympanum
  umbilical region —*see* Wound, open,
      abdomen, wall, periumbilic region
  uvula —*see* Wound, open, oral cavity
  vagina S31.40
    bite S31.45
    laceration —*see* Laceration, vagina
    puncture —*see* Puncture, vagina
  vitreous (humor) —*see* Wound, open,
      ocular
  vocal cord S11.039
    bite —*see* Bite, vocal cord
    laceration S11.031
      with foreign body S11.032
    puncture S11.033
      with foreign body S11.034
  vulva S31.40
    with amputation —*see* Amputation,
        traumatic, vulva
    bite S31.45
    laceration —*see* Laceration, vulva
    puncture —*see* Puncture, vulva
  wrist S61.50-
    bite —*see* Bite, wrist
    laceration —*see* Laceration, wrist
    puncture —*see* Puncture, wrist
Wound, superficial —*see* Injury *(see also*
    specified injury type)
Wright's syndrome G54.0
Wrist —*see* condition
Wrong drug (by accident) (given in error) —
    see Table of Drugs and Chemicals, by
    drug, poisoning
Wry neck —*see* Torticollis
Wuchereria (bancrofti) infestation B74.0
Wuchereriasis B74.0
Wuchernde Struma Langhans C73

X

Xanthelasma (eyelid) (palpebrarum) H02.60
  left H02.66
    lower H02.65
    upper H02.64
  right H02.63
    lower H02.62
    upper H02.61
Xanthelasmatosis (essential) E78.2
Xanthinuria, hereditary E79.8
Xanthoastrocytoma
  specified site —see Neoplasm, malignant, by
    site
  unspecified site C71.9
Xanthofibroma —see Neoplasm, connective
  tissue, benign
Xanthogranuloma D76.3
Xanthoma (s), xanthomatosis (primary)
    (familial) (hereditary) E75.5
  with
    hyperlipoproteinemia
      Type I E78.3
      Type III E78.2
      Type IV E78.1
      Type V E78.3
  bone (generalisata) C96.5
  cerebrotendinous E75.5
  cutaneotendinous E75.5

Xanthoma (s), xanthomatosis (Continued)
  disseminatum (skin) E78.2
  eruptive E78.2
  hypercholesterinemic E78.0
  hypercholesterolemic E78.0
  hyperlipidemic E78.5
  joint E75.5
  multiple (skin) E78.2
  tendon (sheath) E75.5
  tuberosum E78.2
  tuberous E78.2
  tubo-eruptive E78.2
  verrucous, oral mucosa K13.4
Xanthosis R23.8
Xenophobia F40.10
Xeroderma —see also Ichthyosis
  acquired L85.0
    eyelid H01.149
      left H01.146
        lower H01.145
        upper H01.144
      right H01.143
        lower H01.142
        upper H01.141
  pigmentosum Q82.1
  vitamin A deficiency E50.8
Xerophthalmia (vitamin A deficiency) E50.7
  unrelated to vitamin A deficiency —see
    Keratoconjunctivitis

Xerosis
  conjunctiva H11.14-
    with Bitot's spots —see also Pigmentation,
      conjunctiva
      vitamin A deficiency E50.1
    vitamin A deficiency E50.0
  cornea H18.89-
    with ulceration —see Ulcer, cornea
      vitamin A deficiency E50.3
    vitamin A deficiency E50.2
  cutis L85.3
  skin L85.3
Xerostomia K11.7
Xiphopagus Q89.4
XO syndrome Q96.9
X-ray (of)
  abnormal findings —see Abnormal,
    diagnostic imaging
  breast (mammogram) (routine) Z12.31
  chest
    routine (as part of a general medical
      examination) Z00.00
    with abnormal findings Z00.01
  routine (as part of a general medical
    examination) Z00.00
  with abnormal findings Z00.01
XXXXY syndrome Q98.1
XXY syndrome Q98.0

◀ New   ◀ Revised   deleted Deleted

Y

Yaba pox virus disease B08.72
Yatapoxvirus B08.70
  specified NEC B08.79
Yawning R06.89
  psychogenic F45.8
Yaws A66.9
  bone lesions A66.6
  butter A66.1
  chancre A66.0
  cutaneous, less than five years after infection
    A66.2
  early (cutaneous) (macular) (maculopapular)
    (micropapular) (papular) A66.2
    frambeside A66.2
    skin lesions NEC A66.2
  eyelid A66.2
  ganglion A66.6
  gangosis, gangosa A66.5
  gumma, gummata A66.4
    bone A66.6
  gummatous
    frambeside A66.4
    osteitis A66.6
    periostitis A66.6
  hydrarthrosis (see also subcategory M14.8-)
    A66.6
  hyperkeratosis (early) (late) A66.3

Yaws (Continued)
  initial lesions A66.0
  joint lesions (see also subcategory M14.8-)
    A66.6
  juxta-articular nodules A66.7
  late nodular (ulcerated) A66.4
  latent (without clinical manifestations) (with
    positive serology) A66.8
  mother A66.0
  mucosal A66.7
  multiple papillomata A66.1
  nodular, late (ulcerated) A66.4
  osteitis A66.6
  papilloma, plantar or palmar A66.1
  periostitis (hypertrophic) A66.6
  specified NEC A66.7
  ulcers A66.4
  wet crab A66.1
Yeast infection (see also Candidiasis) B37.9
Yellow
  atrophy (liver) —see Failure, hepatic
  fever —see Fever, yellow
  jack —see Fever, yellow
  jaundice —see Jaundice
  nail syndrome L60.5
Yersiniosis —see also Infection, Yersinia
  extraintestinal A28.2
  intestinal A04.6

Z

Zahorsky's syndrome (herpangina) B08.5
Zellweger's syndrome Q87.89
Zenker's diverticulum (esophagus) K22.5
Ziehen-Oppenheim disease G24.1
Zieve's syndrome K70.0
Zinc
  deficiency, dietary E60
  metabolism disorder E83.2
Zollinger-Ellison syndrome E16.4
Zona —see Herpes, zoster
Zoophobia F40.218
Zoster (herpes) —see Herpes, zoster
Zygomycosis B46.9
  specified NEC B46.8
Zymotic —see condition

ICD-10-CM
Table of Neoplasms

	Malignant Primary	Malignant Secondary	Ca in situ	Benign	Uncertain Behavior	Unspecified Behavior
The list below gives the code numbers for neoplasms by anatomical site. For each site there are six possible code numbers according to whether the neoplasm in question is malignant, benign, in situ, of uncertain behavior, or of unspecified nature. The description of the neoplasm will often indicate which of the six columns is appropriate; e.g., malignant melanoma of skin, benign fibroadenoma of breast, carcinoma in situ of cervix uteri.						
Where such descriptors are not present, the remainder of the Index should be consulted where guidance is given to the appropriate column for each morphological (histological) variety listed; e.g., Mesonephroma — *see Neoplasm, malignant;* Embryoma — *see also Neoplasm, uncertain behavior;* Disease, Bowen's — *see Neoplasm, skin, in situ.* However, the guidance in the Index can be overridden if one of the descriptors mentioned above is present; e.g., malignant adenoma of colon is coded to C18.9 and not to D12.6 as the adjective "malignant" overrides the Index entry "Adenoma — *see also Neoplasm, benign.*"						
Codes listed with a dash -, following the code have a required additional character for laterality. The tablular must be reviewed for the complete code.						
Neoplasm, neoplastic	C80.1	C79.9	D09.9	D36.9	D48.9	D49.9
abdomen, abdominal	C76.2	C79.8-	D09.8	D36.7	D48.7	D49.89
cavity	C76.2	C79.8-	D09.8	D36.7	D48.7	D49.89
organ	C76.2	C79.8-	D09.8	D36.7	D48.7	D49.89
viscera	C76.2	C79.8-	D09.8	D36.7	D48.7	D49.89
wall — *see also Neoplasm, abdomen, wall, skin*	C44.509	C79.2-	D04.5	D23.5	D48.5	D49.2
connective tissue	C49.4	C79.8-	—	D21.4	D48.1	D49.2
skin	C44.509					
basal cell carcinoma	C44.519	—	—	—	—	—
specified type NEC	C44.599	—	—	—	—	—
squamous cell carcinoma	C44.529	—	—	—	—	—
abdominopelvic	C76.8	C79.8-	—	D36.7	D48.7	D49.89
accessory sinus — *see Neoplasm, sinus*						
acoustic nerve	C72.4-	C79.49	—	D33.3	D43.3	D49.7
adenoid (pharynx) (tissue)	C11.1	C79.89	D00.08	D10.6	D37.05	D49.0
adipose tissue — *see also Neoplasm, connective tissue*	C49.4	C79.89	—	D21.9	D48.1	D49.2
adnexa (uterine)	C57.4	C79.89	D07.39	D28.7	D39.8	D49.5
adrenal	C74.9-	C79.7-	D09.3	D35.0-	D44.1-	D49.7
capsule	C74.9-	C79.7-	D09.3	D35.0-	D44.1-	D49.7
cortex	C74.0-	C79.7-	D09.3	D35.0-	D44.1-	D49.7
gland	C74.9-	C79.7-	D09.3	D35.0-	D44.1-	D49.7
medulla	C74.1-	C79.7-	D09.3	D35.0-	D44.1-	D49.7
ala nasi (external) — *see also Neoplasm, skin, nose*	C44.301	C79.2	D04.39	D23.39	D48.5	D49.2
alimentary canal or tract NEC	C26.9	C78.80	D01.9	D13.9	D37.9	D49.0
alveolar	C03.9	C79.89	D00.03	D10.39	D37.09	D49.0
mucosa	C03.9	C79.89	D00.03	D10.39	D37.09	D49.0
lower	C03.1	C79.89	D00.03	D10.39	D37.09	D49.0
upper	C03.0	C79.89	D00.03	D10.39	D37.09	D49.0
ridge or process	C41.1	C79.51	—	D16.5-	D48.0	D49.2
carcinoma	C03.9	C79.8-	—	—	—	—
lower	C03.1	C79.8-	—	—	—	—
upper	C03.0	C79.8-	—	—	—	—

TABLE OF NEOPLASMS

	Malignant Primary	Malignant Secondary	Ca in situ	Benign	Uncertain Behavior	Unspecified Behavior
alveolar *(Continued)*						
ridge or process *(Continued)*						
lower	C41.1	C79.51	—	D16.5-	D48.0	D49.2
mucosa	C03.9	C79.89	D00.03	D10.39	D37.09	D49.0
lower	C03.1	C79.89	D00.03	D10.39	D37.09	D49.0
upper	C03.0	C79.89	D00.03	D10.39	D37.09	D49.0
upper	C41.0	C79.51	—	D16.4-	D48.0	D49.2
sulcus	C06.1	C79.89	D00.02	D10.39	D37.09	D49.0
alveolus	C03.9	C79.89	D00.03	D10.39	D37.09	D49.0
lower	C03.1	C79.89	D00.03	D10.39	D37.09	D49.0
upper	C03.0	C79.89	D00.03	D10.39	D37.09	D49.0
ampulla of Vater	C24.1	C78.89	D01.5	D13.5	D37.6	D49.0
ankle NEC	C76.5-	C79.89	D04.7-	D36.7	D48.7	D49.89
anorectum, anorectal (junction)	C21.8	C78.5	D01.3	D12.9	D37.8	D49.0
antecubital fossa or space	C76.4-	C79.89	D04.6-	D36.7	D48.7	D49.89
antrum (Highmore) (maxillary)	C31.0	C78.39	D02.3	D14.0	D38.5	D49.1
pyloric	C16.3	C78.89	D00.2	D13.1	D37.1	D49.0
tympanicum	C30.1	C78.39	D02.3	D14.0	D38.5	D49.1
anus, anal	C21.0	C78.5	D01.3	D12.9	D37.8	D49.0
canal	C21.1	C78.5	D01.3	D12.9	D37.8	D49.0
cloacogenic zone	C21.2	C78.5	D01.3	D12.9	D37.8	D49.0
margin — *see also Neoplasm, anus, skin*	C44.500	C79.2	D04.5	D23.5	D48.5	D49.2
overlapping lesion with rectosigmoid junction or rectum	C21.8	—	—	—	—	—
skin	C44.500	C79.2	D04.5	D23.5	D48.5	D49.2
basal cell carcinoma	C44.510	—	—	—	—	—
specified type NEC	C44.590	—	—	—	—	—
squamous cell carcinoma	C44.520	—	—	—	—	—
sphincter	C21.1	C78.5	D01.3	D12.9	D37.8	D49.0
aorta (thoracic)	C49.3	C79.89	—	D21.3	D48.1	D49.2
abdominal	C49.4	C79.89	—	D21.4	D48.1	D49.2
aortic body	C75.5	C79.89	—	D35.6	D44.7	D49.7
aponeurosis	C49.9	C79.89	—	D21.9	D48.1	D49.2
palmar	C49.1-	C79.89	—	D21.1-	D48.1	D49.2
plantar	C49.2-	C79.89	—	D21.2-	D48.1	D49.2
appendix	C18.1	C78.5	D01.0	D12.1	D37.3	D49.0
arachnoid	C70.9	C79.49	—	D32.9	D42.9	D49.7
cerebral	C70.0	C79.32	—	D32.0	D42.0	D49.7
spinal	C70.1	C79.49	—	D32.1	D42.1	D49.7
areola	C50.0-	C79.81	D05.-	D24.-	D48.6-	D49.3
arm NEC	C76.4-	C79.89	D04.6-	D36.7	D48.7	D49.89
artery — *see Neoplasm, connective tissue*						

	Malignant Primary	Malignant Secondary	Ca in situ	Benign	Uncertain Behavior	Unspecified Behavior
aryepiglottic fold	C13.1	C79.89	D00.08	D10.7	D37.05	D49.0
hypopharyngeal aspect	C13.1	C79.89	D00.08	D10.7	D37.05	D49.0
laryngeal aspect	C32.1	C78.39	D02.0	D14.1	D38.0	D49.1
marginal zone	C13.1	C79.89	D00.08	D10.7	D37.05	D49.0
arytenoid (cartilage)	C32.3	C78.39	D02.0	D14.1	D38.0	D49.1
fold — see Neoplasm, aryepiglottic						
associated with transplanted organ	C80.2	—	—	—	—	—
atlas	C41.2	C79.51	—	D16.6	D48.0	D49.2
atrium, cardiac	C38.0	C79.89	—	D15.1	D48.7	D49.89
auditory						
canal (external) (skin) A81	C44.20-	C79.2	D04.2-	D23.2-	D48.5	D49.2
internal	C30.1	C78.39	D02.3	D14.0	D38.5	D49.1
nerve	C72.4-	C79.49	—	D33.3	D43.3	D49.7
tube	C30.1	C78.39	D02.3	D14.0	D38.5	D49.1
opening	C11.2	C79.89	D00.08	D10.6	D37.05	D49.0
auricle, ear — see also Neoplasm, skin, ear	C44.20-	C79.2	D04.2-	D23.2-	D48.5	D49.2
auricular canal (external) — see also Neoplasm, skin, ear	C44.20-	C79.2	D04.2-	D23.2-	D48.5	D49.2
internal	C30.1	C78.39	D02.3	D14.0	D38.5	D49.2
autonomic nerve or nervous system NEC (see Neoplasm, nerve, peripheral)						
axilla, axillary	C76.1	C79.89	D09.8	D36.7	D48.7	D49.89
fold — see also Neoplasm, skin, trunk	C44.509	C79.2	D04.5	D23.5	D48.5	D49.2
back NEC	C76.8	C79.89	D04.5	D36.7	D48.7	D49.89
Bartholin's gland	C51.0	C79.82	D07.1	D28.0	D39.8	D49.5
basal ganglia	C71.0	C79.31	—	D33.0	D43.0	D49.6
basis pedunculi	C71.7	C79.31	—	D33.1	D43.1	D49.6
bile or biliary (tract)	C24.9	C78.89	D01.5	D13.5	D37.6	D49.0
canaliculi (biliferi) (intrahepatic)	C22.1	C78.7	D01.5	D13.4	D37.6	D49.0
canals, interlobular	C22.1	C78.89	D01.5	D13.4	D37.6	D49.0
duct or passage (common) (cystic) (extrahepatic)	C24.0	C78.89	D01.5	D13.5	D37.6	D49.0
interlobular	C22.1	C78.89	D01.5	D13.4	D37.6	D49.0
intrahepatic	C22.1	C78.7	D01.5	D13.4	D37.6	D49.0
and extrahepatic	C24.8	C78.89	D01.5	D13.5	D37.6	D49.0
bladder (urinary)	C67.9	C79.11	D09.0	D30.3	D41.4	D49.4
dome	C67.1	C79.11	D09.0	D30.3	D41.4	D49.4
neck	C67.5	C79.11	D09.0	D30.3	D41.4	D49.4
orifice	C67.9	C79.11	D09.0	D30.3	D41.4	D49.4
ureteric	C67.6	C79.11	D09.0	D30.3	D41.4	D49.4
urethral	C67.5	C79.11	D09.0	D30.3	D41.4	D49.4
overlapping lesion	C67.8	—	—	—	—	—
sphincter	C67.8	C79.11	D09.0	D30.3	D41.4	D49.4
trigone	C67.0	C79.11	D09.0	D30.3	D41.4	D49.4
urachus	C67.7	C79.11	D09.0	D30.3	D41.4	D49.4

TABLE OF NEOPLASMS

	Malignant Primary	Malignant Secondary	Ca in situ	Benign	Uncertain Behavior	Unspecified Behavior
bladder (urinary) *(Continued)*						
wall	C67.9	C79.11	D09.0	D30.3	D41.4	D49.4
anterior	C67.3	C79.11	D09.0	D30.3	D41.4	D49.4
lateral	C67.2	C79.11	D09.0	D30.3	D41.4	D49.4
posterior	C67.4	C79.11	D09.0	D30.3	D41.4	D49.4
blood vessel — *see Neoplasm, connective tissue*						
bone (periosteum)	C41.9	C79.51	—	D16.9-	D48.0	D49.2
acetabulum	C41.4	C79.51	—	D16.8-	D48.0	D49.2
ankle	C40.3-	C79.51	—	D16.3-	—	—
arm NEC	C40.0-	C79.51	—	D16.0-	—	—
astragalus	C40.3-	C79.51	—	D16.3-	—	—
atlas	C41.2	C79.51	—	D16.6-	D48.0	D49.2
axis	C41.2	C79.51	—	D16.6-	D48.0	D49.2
back NEC	C41.2	C79.51	—	D16.6-	D48.0	D49.2
calcaneus	C40.3-	C79.51	—	D16.3-	—	—
calvarium	C41.0	C79.51	—	D16.4-	D48.0	D49.2
carpus (any)	C40.1-	C79.51	—	D16.1-	—	—
cartilage NEC	C41.9	C79.51	—	D16.9-	D48.0	D49.2
clavicle	C41.3	C79.51	—	D16.7-	D48.0	D49.2
clivus	C41.0	C79.51	—	D16.4-	D48.0	D49.2
coccygeal vertebra	C41.4	C79.51	—	D16.8-	D48.0	D49.2
coccyx	C41.4	C79.51	—	D16.8-	D48.0	D49.2
costal cartilage	C41.3	C79.51	—	D16.7-	D48.0	D49.2
costovertebral joint	C41.3	C79.51	—	D16.7-	D48.0	D49.2
cranial	C41.0	C79.51	—	D16.4-	D48.0	D49.2
cuboid	C40.3-	C79.51	—	D16.3-	—	—
cuneiform	C41.9	C79.51	—	D16.9-	D48.0	D49.2
elbow	C40.0-	C79.51	—	D16.0-	—	—
ethmoid (labyrinth)	C41.0	C79.51	—	D16.4-	D48.0	D49.2
face	C41.0	C79.51	—	D16.4-	D48.0	D49.2
femur (any part)	C40.2-	C79.51	—	D16.2-	—	—
fibula (any part)	C40.2-	C79.51	—	D16.2-	—	—
finger (any)	C40.1-	C79.51	—	D16.1-	—	—
foot	C40.3-	C79.51	—	D16.3-	—	—
forearm	C40.0-	C79.51	—	D16.0-	—	—
frontal	C41.0	C79.51	—	D16.4-	D48.0	D49.2
hand	C40.1-	C79.51	—	D16.1-	—	—
heel	C40.3-	C79.51	—	D16.3-	—	—
hip	C41.4	C79.51	—	D16.8-	D48.0	D49.2
humerus (any part)	C40.0-	C79.51	—	D16.0-	—	—
hyoid	C41.0	C79.51	—	D16.4-	D48.0	D49.2
ilium	C41.4	C79.51	—	D16.8-	D48.0	D49.2
innominate	C41.4	C79.51	—	D16.8-	D48.0	D49.2

◀ New ◀ Revised ~~deleted~~ Deleted

	Malignant Primary	Malignant Secondary	Ca in situ	Benign	Uncertain Behavior	Unspecified Behavior
bone *(Continued)*						
intervertebral cartilage or disc	C41.2	C79.51	—	D16.6-	D48.0	D49.2
ischium	C41.4	C79.51	—	D16.8-	D48.0	D49.2
jaw (lower)	C41.1	C79.51	—	D16.5-	D48.0	D49.2
knee	C40.2-	C79.51	—	D16.2-	—	—
leg NEC	C40.2-	C79.51	—	D16.2-	—	—
limb NEC	C40.9-	C79.51	—	D16.9-	—	—
lower (long bones)	C40.2-	C79.51	—	D16.2-	—	—
short bones	C40.3-	C79.51	—	D16.3-	—	—
upper (long bones)	C40.0-	C79.51	—	D16.0-	—	—
short bones	C40.1-	C79.51	—	D16.1-	—	—
malar	C41.0	C79.51	—	D16.4-	D48.0	D49.2
mandible	C41.1	C79.51	—	D16.5-	D48.0	D49.2
marrow NEC (any bone)	C96.9	C79.52	—	—	D47.9	D49.89
mastoid	C41.0	C79.51	—	D16.4-	D48.0	D49.2
maxilla, maxillary (superior)	C41.0	C79.51	—	D16.4-	D48.0	D49.2
inferior	C41.1	C79.51	—	D16.5-	D48.0	D49.2
metacarpus (any)	C40.1-	C79.51	—	D16.1-	—	—
metatarsus (any)	C40.3-	C79.51	—	D16.3-	—	—
overlapping sites	C40.8-	—	—	—	—	—
navicular						
ankle	C40.3-	C79.51	—	—	—	—
hand	C40.1-	C79.51	—	—	—	—
nose, nasal	C41.0	C79.51	—	D16.4-	D48.0	D49.2
occipital	C41.0	C79.51	—	D16.4-	D48.0	D49.2
orbit	C41.0	C79.51	—	D16.4-	D48.0	D49.2
parietal	C41.0	C79.51	—	D16.4-	D48.0	D49.2
patella	C40.2-	C79.51	—	—	—	—
pelvic	C41.4	C79.51	—	D16.8	D48.0	D49.2
phalanges						
foot	C40.3-	C79.51	—	—	—	—
hand	C40.1-	C79.51	—	—	—	—
pubic	C41.4	C79.51	—	D16.8	D48.0	D49.2
radius (any part)	C40.0-	C79.51	—	D16.0-	—	—
rib	C41.3	C79.51	—	D16.7	D48.0	D49.2
sacral vertebra	C41.4	C79.51	—	D16.8	D48.0	D49.2
sacrum	C41.4	C79.51	—	D16.8	D48.0	D49.2
scaphoid					—	—
of ankle	C40.3-	C79.51	—	—	—	—
of hand	C40.1-	C79.51	—	—	—	—
scapula (any part)	C40.0-	C79.51	—	D16.0-	—	—
sella turcica	C41.0	C79.51	—	D16.4-	D48.0	D49.2
shoulder	C40.0-	C79.51	—	D16.0-	—	—

◄ New ◄ Revised deleted Deleted

TABLE OF NEOPLASMS

	Malignant Primary	Malignant Secondary	Ca in situ	Benign	Uncertain Behavior	Unspecified Behavior
bone *(Continued)*						
skull	C41.0	C79.51	—	D16.4-	D48.0	D49.2
sphenoid	C41.0	C79.51	—	D16.4-	D48.0	D49.2
spine, spinal (column)	C41.2	C79.51	—	D16.6	D48.0	D49.2
coccyx	C41.4	C79.51	—	D16.8	D48.0	D49.2
sacrum	C41.4	C79.51	—	D16.8	D48.0	D49.2
sternum	C41.3	C79.51	—	D16.7	D48.0	D49.2
tarsus (any)	C40.3-	C79.51	—	—	—	—
temporal	C41.0	C79.51	—	D16.4-	D48.0	D49.2
thumb	C40.1-	C79.51	—	—	—	—
tibia (any part)	C40.2-	C79.51	—	—	—	—
toe (any)	C40.3-	C79.51	—	—	—	—
trapezium	C40.1-	C79.51	—	—	—	—
trapezoid	C40.1-	C79.51	—	—	—	—
turbinate	C41.0	C79.51	—	D16.4-	D48.0	D49.2
ulna (any part)	C40.0-	C79.51	—	D16.0-	—	—
unciform	C40.1-	C79.51	—	—	—	—
vertebra (column)	C41.2	C79.51	—	D16.6	D48.0	D49.2
coccyx	C41.4	C79.51	—	D16.8	D48.0	D49.2
sacrum	C41.4	C79.51	—	D16.8	D48.0	D49.2
vomer	C41.0	C79.51	—	D16.4-	D48.0	D49.2
wrist	C40.1-	C79.51	—	—	—	—
xiphoid process	C41.3	C79.51	—	D16.7	D48.0	D49.2
zygomatic	C41.0	C79.51	—	D16.4-	D48.0	D49.2
book-leaf (mouth)	C06.89	C79.89	D00.00	D10.39	D37.09	D49.0
bowel — *see* Neoplasm, intestine						
brachial plexus	C47.1-	C79.89	—	D36.12	D48.2	D49.2
brain NEC	C71.9	C79.31	—	D33.2	D43.2	D49.6
basal ganglia	C71.0	C79.31	—	D33.0	D43.0	D49.6
cerebellopontine angle	C71.6	C79.31	—	D33.1	D43.1	D49.6
cerebellum NOS	C71.6	C79.31	—	D33.1	D43.1	D49.6
cerebrum	C71.0	C79.31	—	D33.0	D43.0	D49.6
choroid plexus	C71.7	C79.31	—	D33.1	D43.1	D49.6
corpus callosum	C71.8	C79.31	—	D33.2	D43.2	D49.6
corpus striatum	C71.0	C79.31	—	D33.0	D43.0	D49.6
cortex (cerebral)	C71.0	C79.31	—	D33.0	D43.0	D49.6
frontal lobe	C71.1	C79.31	—	D33.0	D43.0	D49.6
globus pallidus	C71.0	C79.31	—	D33.0	D43.0	D49.6
hippocampus	C71.2	C79.31	—	D33.0	D43.0	D49.6
hypothalamus	C71.0	C79.31	—	D33.0	D43.0	D49.6
internal capsule	C71.0	C79.31	—	D33.0	D43.0	D49.6
medulla oblongata	C71.7	C79.31	—	D33.1	D43.1	D49.6
meninges	C70.0	C79.32	—	D32.0	D42.0	D49.7

◀ New   ◀▥ Revised   ~~deleted~~ Deleted

	Malignant Primary	Malignant Secondary	Ca in situ	Benign	Uncertain Behavior	Unspecified Behavior
brain NEC *(Continued)*						
midbrain	C71.7	C79.31	—	D33.1	D43.1	D49.6
occipital lobe	C71.4	C79.31	—	D33.0	D43.0	D49.6
overlapping lesion	C71.8	C79.31	—	—	—	—
parietal lobe	C71.3	C79.31	—	D33.0	D43.0	D49.6
peduncle	C71.7	C79.31	—	D33.1	D43.1	D49.6
pons	C71.7	C79.31	—	D33.1	D43.1	D49.6
stem	C71.7	C79.31	—	D33.1	D43.1	D49.6
tapetum	C71.8	C79.31	—	D33.2	D43.2	D49.6
temporal lobe	C71.2	C79.31	—	D33.0	D43.0	D49.6
thalamus	C71.0	C79.31	—	D33.0	D43.0	D49.6
uncus	C71.2	C79.31	—	D33.0	D43.0	D49.6
ventricle (floor)	C71.5	C79.31	—	D33.0	D43.0	D49.6
fourth	C71.7	C79.31	—	D33.1	D43.1	D49.6
branchial (cleft) (cyst) (vestiges)	C10.4	C79.89	D00.08	D10.5	D37.05	D49.0
breast (connective tissue) (glandular tissue) (soft parts)	C50.9-	C79.81	D05.-	D24.-	D48.6-	D49.3
areola	C50.0-	C79.81	D05.-	D24.-	D48.6-	D49.3
axillary tail	C50.6-	C79.81	D05.-	D24.-	D48.6-	D49.3
central portion	C50.1-	C79.81	D05.-	D24.-	D48.6-	D49.3
inner	C50.8-	C79.81	D05.-	D24.-	D48.6-	D49.3
lower	C50.8-	C79.81	D05.-	D24.-	D48.6-	D49.3
lower-inner quadrant	C50.3-	C79.81	D05.-	D24.-	D48.6-	D49.3
lower-outer quadrant	C50.5-	C79.81	D05.-	D24.-	D48.6-	D49.3
mastectomy site (skin) — *see also Neoplasm, breast, skin*	C44.501	C79.2	—	—	—	—
specified as breast tissue	C50.8-	C79.81	—	—	—	—
midline	C50.8-	C79.81	D05.-	D24.-	D48.6-	D49.3
nipple	C50.0-	C79.81	D05.-	D24.-	D48.6-	D49.3
outer	C50.8-	C79.81	D05.-	D24.-	D48.6-	D49.3
overlapping lesion	C50.8-	—	—	—	—	—
skin	C44.501	C79.2	D04.5	D23.5	D48.5	D49.2
basal cell carcinoma	C44.511	—	—	—	—	—
specified type NEC	C44.591	—	—	—	—	—
squamous cell carcinoma	C44.521	—	—	—	—	—
tail (axillary)	C50.6-	C79.81	D05.-	D24.-	D48.6-	D49.3
upper	C50.8-	C79.81	D05.-	D24.-	D48.6-	D49.3
upper-inner quadrant	C50.2-	C79.81	D05.-	D24.-	D48.6-	D49.3
upper-outer quadrant	C50.4-	C79.81	D05.-	D24.-	D48.6-	D49.3
broad ligament	C57.1	C79.82	D07.39	D28.2	D39.8	D49.5
bronchiogenic, bronchogenic (lung)	C34.9-	C78.0-	D02.2-	D14.3-	D38.1	D49.1
bronchiole	C34.9-	C78.0-	D02.2-	D14.3-	D38.1	D49.1
bronchus	C34.9-	C78.0-	D02.2-	D14.3-	D38.1	D49.1
carina	C34.0-	C78.0-	D02.2-	D14.3-	D38.1	D49.1
lower lobe of lung	C34.3-	C78.0-	D02.2-	D14.3-	D38.1	D49.1

	Malignant Primary	Malignant Secondary	Ca in situ	Benign	Uncertain Behavior	Unspecified Behavior
bronchus (Continued)						
main	C34.0-	C78.0-	D02.2-	D14.3-	D38.1	D49.1
middle lobe of lung	C34.2	C78.0-	D02.21	D14.31	D38.1	D49.1
overlapping lesion	C34.8-	—	—	—	—	—
upper lobe of lung	C34.1-	C78.0-	D02.2-	D14.3-	D38.1	D49.1
brow	C44.309	C79.2	D04.39	D23.39	D48.5	D49.2
basal cell carcinoma	C44.319	—	—	—	—	—
specified type NEC	C44.399	—	—	—	—	—
squamous cell carcinoma	C44.329	—	—	—	—	—
buccal (cavity)	C06.9	C79.89	D00.00	D10.39	D37.09	D49.0
commissure	C06.0	C79.89	D00.02	D10.39	D37.09	D49.0
groove (lower) (upper)	C06.1	C79.89	D00.02	D10.39	D37.09	D49.0
mucosa	C06.0	C79.89	D00.02	D10.39	D37.09	D49.0
sulcus (lower) (upper)	C06.1	C79.89	D00.02	D10.39	D37.09	D49.0
bulbourethral gland	C68.0	C79.19	D09.19	D30.4	D41.3	D49.5
bursa — see Neoplasm, connective tissue						
buttock NEC	C76.3	C79.89	D04.5	D36.7	D48.7	D49.89
calf	C76.5-	C79.89	D04.7-	D36.7	D48.7	D49.89
calvarium	C41.0	C79.51	—	D16.4-	D48.0	D49.2
calyx, renal	C65.-	C79.0-	D09.19	D30.1-	D41.1-	D49.5
canal						
anal	C21.1	C78.5	D01.3	D12.9	D37.8	D49.0
auditory (external) — see also Neoplasm, skin, ear	C44.20-	C79.2	D04.2-	D23.2-	D48.5	D49.2
auricular (external) — see also Neoplasm, skin, ear	C44.20-	C79.2	D04.2-	D23.2-	D48.5	D49.2
canaliculi, biliary (biliferi) (intrahepatic)	C22.1	C78.7	D01.5	D13.4	D37.6	D49.0
canthus (eye) (inner) (outer)	C44.10-	C79.2	D04.1-	D23.1-	D48.5	D49.2
basal cell carcinoma	C44.11-	—	—	—	—	—
specified type NEC	C44.19-	—	—	—	—	—
squamous cell carcinoma	C44.12-	—	—	—	—	—
capillary — see Neoplasm, connective tissue						
caput coli	C18.0	C78.5	D01.0	D12.0	D37.4	D49.0
carcinoid — see Tumor, carcinoid						
cardia (gastric)	C16.0	C78.89	D00.2	D13.1	D37.1	D49.0
cardiac orifice (stomach)	C16.0	C78.89	D00.2	D13.1	D37.1	D49.0
cardio-esophageal junction	C16.0	C78.89	D00.2	D13.1	D37.1	D49.0
cardio-esophagus	C16.0	C78.89	D00.2	D13.1	D37.1	D49.0
carina (bronchus)	C34.0-	C78.0-	D02.2-	D14.3-	D38.1	D49.1
carotid (artery)	C49.0	C79.89	—	D21.0	D48.1	D49.2
body	C75.4	C79.89	—	D35.5	D44.6	D49.7
carpus (any bone)	C40.1-	C79.51	—	D16.1-	—	—
cartilage (articular) (joint) NEC — see also Neoplasm, bone	C41.9	C79.51	—	D16.9-	D48.0	D49.2
arytenoid	C32.3	C78.39	D02.0	D14.1	D38.0	D49.1
auricular	C49.0	C79.89	—	D21.0	D48.1	D49.2

◀ New ◀ Revised deleted Deleted

	Malignant Primary	Malignant Secondary	Ca in situ	Benign	Uncertain Behavior	Unspecified Behavior
cartilage NEC *(Continued)*						
bronchi	C34.0-	C78.39	—	D14.3-	D38.1	D49.1
costal	C41.3	C79.51	—	D16.7	D48.0	D49.2
cricoid	C32.3	C78.39	D02.0	D14.1	D38.0	D49.1
cuneiform	C32.3	C78.39	D02.0	D14.1	D38.0	D49.1
ear (external)	C49.0	C79.89	—	D21.0	D48.1	D49.2
ensiform	C41.3	C79.51	—	D16.7	D48.0	D49.2
epiglottis	C32.1	C78.39	D02.0	D14.1	D38.0	D49.1
anterior surface	C10.1-	C79.89	D00.08	D10.5	D37.05	D49.0
eyelid	C49.0	C79.89	—	D21.0	D48.1	D49.2
intervertebral	C41.2	C79.51	—	D16.6	D48.0	D49.2
larynx, laryngeal	C32.3	C78.39	D02.0	D14.1	D38.0	D49.1
nose, nasal	C30.0	C78.39	D02.3	D14.0	D38.5	D49.1
pinna	C49.0	C79.89	—	D21.0	D48.1	D49.2
rib	C41.3	C79.51	—	D16.7	D48.0	D49.2
semilunar (knee)	C40.2-	C79.51	—	D16.2-	D48.0	D49.2
thyroid	C32.3	C78.39	D02.0	D14.1	D38.0	D49.1
trachea	C33	C78.39	D02.1	D14.2	D38.1	D49.1
cauda equina	C72.1	C79.49	—	D33.4	D43.4	D49.7
cavity						
buccal	C06.9	C79.89	D00.00	D10.30	D37.09	D49.0
nasal	C30.0	C78.39	D02.3	D14.0	D38.5	D49.1
oral	C06.9	C79.89	D00.00	D10.30	D37.09	D49.0
peritoneal	C48.2	C78.6	—	D20.1	D48.4	D49.0
tympanic	C30.1	C78.39	D02.3	D14.0	D38.5	D49.1
cecum	C18.0	C78.5	D01.0	D12.0	D37.4	D49.0
central nervous system	C72.9	C79.40	—	—	—	—
cerebellopontine (angle)	C71.6	C79.31	—	D33.1	D43.1	D49.6
cerebellum, cerebellar	C71.6	C79.31	—	D33.1	D43.1	D49.6
cerebrum, cerebral (cortex) (hemisphere) (white matter)	C71.0	C79.31	—	D33.0	D43.0	D49.6
meninges	C70.0	C79.32	—	D32.0	D42.0	D49.7
peduncle	C71.7	C79.31	—	D33.1	D43.1	D49.6
ventricle	C71.5	C79.31	—	D33.0	D43.0	D49.6
fourth	C71.7	C79.31	—	D33.1	D43.1	D49.6
cervical region	C76.0	C79.89	D09.8	D36.7	D48.7	D49.89
cervix (cervical) (uteri) (uterus)	C53.9	C79.82	D06.9	D26.0	D39.0	D49.5
canal	C53.0	C79.82	D06.0	D26.0	D39.0	D49.5
endocervix (canal) (gland)	C53.0	C79.82	D06.0	D26.0	D39.0	D49.5
exocervix	C53.1	C79.82	D06.1	D26.0	D39.0	D49.5
external os	C53.1	C79.82	D06.1	D26.0	D39.0	D49.5
internal os	C53.0	C79.82	D06.0	D26.0	D39.0	D49.5
nabothian gland	C53.0	C79.82	D06.0	D26.0	D39.0	D49.5
overlapping lesion	C53.8	—	—	—	—	—

	Malignant Primary	Malignant Secondary	Ca in situ	Benign	Uncertain Behavior	Unspecified Behavior
cervix (Continued)						
squamocolumnar junction	C53.8	C79.82	D06.7	D26.0	D39.0	D49.5
stump	C53.8	C79.82	D06.7	D26.0	D39.0	D49.5
cheek	C76.0	C79.89	D09.8	D36.7	D48.7	D49.89
external	C44.309	C79.2	D04.39	D23.39	D48.5	D49.2
basal cell carcinoma	C44.319	—	—	—	—	—
specified type NEC	C44.399	—	—	—	—	—
squamous cell carcinoma	C44.329	—	—	—	—	—
inner aspect	C06.0	C79.89	D00.02	D10.39	D37.09	D49.0
internal	C06.0	C79.89	D00.02	D10.39	D37.09	D49.0
mucosa	C06.0	C79.89	D00.02	D10.39	D37.09	D49.0
chest (wall) NEC	C76.1	C79.89	D09.8	D36.7	D48.7	D49.89
chiasma opticum	C72.3-	C79.49	—	D33.3	D43.3	D49.7
chin	C44.309	C79.2	D04.39	D23.39	D48.5	D49.2
basal cell carcinoma	C44.319	—	—	—	—	—
specified type NEC	C44.399	—	—	—	—	—
squamous cell carcinoma	C44.329	—	—	—	—	—
choana	C11.3	C79.89	D00.08	D10.6	D37.05	D49.0
cholangiole	C22.1	C78.89	D01.5	D13.4	D37.6	D49.0
choledochal duct	C24.0	C78.89	D01.5	D13.5	D37.6	D49.0
choroid	C69.3-	C79.49	D09.2-	D31.3-	D48.7	D49.81
plexus	C71.5	C79.31	—	D33.0	D43.0	D49.6
ciliary body	C69.4-	C79.49	D09.2-	D31.4-	D48.7	D49.89
clavicle	C41.3	C79.51	—	D16.7	D48.0	D49.2
clitoris	C51.2	C79.82	D07.1	D28.0	D39.8	D49.5
clivus	C41.0	C79.51	—	D16.4-	D48.0	D49.2
cloacogenic zone	C21.2	C78.5	D01.3	D12.9	D37.8	D49.0
coccygeal						
body or glomus	C49.5	C79.89	—	D21.5	D48.1	D49.2
vertebra	C41.4	C79.51	—	D16.8	D48.0	D49.2
coccyx	C41.4	C79.51	—	D16.8	D48.0	D49.2
colon — see also Neoplasm, intestine, large	C18.9	C78.5	—	—	—	—
with rectum	C19	C78.5	D01.1	D12.7	D37.5	D49.0
column, spinal — see Neoplasm, spine						
columnella — see also Neoplasm, skin, face	C44.390	C79.2	D04.39	D23.39	D48.5	D49.2
commissure						
labial, lip	C00.6	C79.89	D00.01	D10.39	D37.01	D49.0
laryngeal	C32.0	C78.39	D02.0	D14.1	D38.0	D49.1
common (bile) duct	C24.0	C78.89	D01.5	D13.5	D37.6	D49.0
concha — see also Neoplasm, skin, ear	C44.20-	C79.2	D04.2-	D23.2-	D48.5	D49.2
nose	C30.0	C78.39	D02.3	D14.0	D38.5	D49.1
conjunctiva	C69.0-	C79.49	D09.2-	D31.0-	D48.7	D49.89

◀ New ◀▦ Revised ~~deleted~~ Deleted

	Malignant Primary	Malignant Secondary	Ca in situ	Benign	Uncertain Behavior	Unspecified Behavior
connective tissue NEC	C49.9	C79.89	—	D21.9	D48.1	D49.2

Note: For neoplasms of connective tissue (blood vessel, bursa, fascia, ligament, muscle, peripheral nerves, sympathetic and parasympathetic nerves and ganglia, synovia, tendon, etc.) or of morphological types that indicate connective tissue, code according to the list under "Neoplasm, connective tissue". For sites that do not appear in this list, code to neoplasm of that site; e.g., fibrosarcoma, pancreas (C25.9)

Note: Morphological types that indicate connective tissue appear in their proper place in the alphabetic index with the instruction "*see Neoplasm, connective tissue ....*"

	Malignant Primary	Malignant Secondary	Ca in situ	Benign	Uncertain Behavior	Unspecified Behavior
abdomen	C49.4	C79.89	—	D21.4	D48.1	D49.2
abdominal wall	C49.4	C79.89	—	D21.4	D48.1	D49.2
ankle	C49.2-	C79.89	—	D21.2-	D48.1	D49.2
antecubital fossa or space	C49.1-	C79.89	—	D21.1-	D48.1	D49.2
arm	C49.1-	C79.89	—	D21.1-	D48.1	D49.2
auricle (ear)	C49.0	C79.89	—	D21.0	D48.1	D49.2
axilla	C49.3	C79.89	—	D21.3	D48.1	D49.2
back	C49.6	C79.89	—	D21.6	D48.1	D49.2
breast — *see Neoplasm, breast*						
buttock	C49.5	C79.89	—	D21.5	D48.1	D49.2
calf	C49.2-	C79.89	—	D21.2-	D48.1	D49.2
cervical region	C49.0	C79.89	—	D21.0	D48.1	D49.2
cheek	C49.0	C79.89	—	D21.0	D48.1	D49.2
chest (wall)	C49.3	C79.89	—	D21.3	D48.1	D49.2
chin	C49.0	C79.89	—	D21.0	D48.1	D49.2
diaphragm	C49.3	C79.89	—	D21.3	D48.1	D49.2
ear (external)	C49.0	C79.89	—	D21.0	D48.1	D49.2
elbow	C49.1-	C79.89	—	D21.1-	D48.1	D49.2
extrarectal	C49.5	C79.89	—	D21.5	D48.1	D49.2
extremity	C49.9	C79.89	—	D21.9	D48.1	D49.2
lower	C49.2-	C79.89	—	D21.2-	D48.1	D49.2
upper	C49.1-	C79.89	—	D21.1-	D48.1	D49.2
eyelid	C49.0	C79.89	—	D21.0	D48.1	D49.2
face	C49.0	C79.89	—	D21.0	D48.1	D49.2
finger	C49.1-	C79.89	—	D21.1-	D48.1	D49.2
flank	C49.6	C79.89	—	D21.6	D48.1	D49.2
foot	C49.2-	C79.89	—	D21.2-	D48.1	D49.2
forearm	C49.1-	C79.89	—	D21.1-	D48.1	D49.2
forehead	C49.0	C79.89	—	D21.0	D48.1	D49.2
gastric	C49.4	C79.89	—	D21.4	D48.1	D49.2
gastrointestinal	C49.4	C79.89	—	D21.4	D48.1	D49.2
gluteal region	C49.5	C79.89	—	D21.5	D48.1	D49.2
great vessels NEC	C49.3	C79.89	—	D21.3	D48.1	D49.2
groin	C49.5	C79.89	—	D21.5	D48.1	D49.2
hand	C49.1-	C79.89	—	D21.1-	D48.1	D49.2

TABLE OF NEOPLASMS

TABLE OF NEOPLASMS

	Malignant Primary	Malignant Secondary	Ca in situ	Benign	Uncertain Behavior	Unspecified Behavior
connective tissue NEC *(Continued)*						
head	C49.0	C79.89	—	D21.0	D48.1	D49.2
heel	C49.2-	C79.89	—	D21.2-	D48.1	D49.2
hip	C49.2-	C79.89	—	D21.2-	D48.1	D49.2
hypochondrium	C49.4	C79.89	—	D21.4	D48.1	D49.2
iliopsoas muscle	C49.5	C79.89	—	D21.5	D48.1	D49.2
infraclavicular region	C49.3	C79.89	—	D21.3	D48.1	D49.2
inguinal (canal) (region)	C49.5	C79.89	—	D21.5	D48.1	D49.2
intestinal	C49.4	C79.89	—	D21.4	D48.1	D49.2
intrathoracic	C49.3	C79.89	—	D21.3	D48.1	D49.2
ischiorectal fossa	C49.5	C79.89	—	D21.5	D48.1	D49.2
jaw	C03.9	C79.89	D00.03	D10.39	D48.1	D49.0
knee	C49.2-	C79.89	—	D21.2-	D48.1	D49.2
leg	C49.2-	C79.89	—	D21.2-	D48.1	D49.2
limb NEC	C49.9	C79.89	—	D21.9	D48.1	D49.2
lower	C49.2-	C79.89	—	D21.2-	D48.1	D49.2
upper	C49.1-	C79.89	—	D21.1-	D48.1	D49.2
nates	C49.5	C79.89	—	D21.5	D48.1	D49.2
neck	C49.0	C79.89	—	D21.0	D48.1	D49.2
orbit	C69.6-	C79.49	D09.2-	D31.6-	D48.1	D49.89
overlapping lesion	C49.8	—	—	—	—	—
pararectal	C49.5	C79.89	—	D21.5	D48.1	D49.2
para-urethral	C49.5	C79.89	—	D21.5	D48.1	D49.2
paravaginal	C49.5	C79.89	—	D21.5	D48.1	D49.2
pelvis (floor)	C49.5	C79.89	—	D21.5	D48.1	D49.2
pelvo-abdominal	C49.8	C79.89	—	D21.6	D48.1	D49.2
perineum	C49.5	C79.89	—	D21.5	D48.1	D49.2
perirectal (tissue)	C49.5	C79.89	—	D21.5	D48.1	D49.2
periurethral (tissue)	C49.5	C79.89	—	D21.5	D48.1	D49.2
popliteal fossa or space	C49.2-	C79.89	—	D21.2-	D48.1	D49.2
presacral	C49.5	C79.89	—	D21.5	D48.1	D49.2
psoas muscle	C49.4	C79.89	—	D21.4	D48.1	D49.2
pterygoid fossa	C49.0	C79.89	—	D21.0	D48.1	D49.2
rectovaginal septum or wall	C49.5	C79.89	—	D21.5	D48.1	D49.2
rectovesical	C49.5	C79.89	—	D21.5	D48.1	D49.2
retroperitoneum	C48.0	C78.6	—	D20.0	D48.3	D49.0
sacrococcygeal region	C49.5	C79.89	—	D21.5	D48.1	D49.2
scalp	C49.0	C79.89	—	D21.0	D48.1	D49.2
scapular region	C49.3	C79.89	—	D21.3	D48.1	D49.2
shoulder	C49.1-	C79.89	—	D21.1-	D48.1	D49.2
skin (dermis) NEC—*see also Neoplasm, skin, by site*	C44.90	C79.2	D04.9	D23.9	D48.5	D49.2
stomach	C49.4	C79.89	—	D21.4	D48.1	D49.2
submental	C49.0	C79.89	—	D21.0	D48.1	D49.2

◀ New   ◀▥ Revised   ~~deleted~~ Deleted

	Malignant Primary	Malignant Secondary	Ca in situ	Benign	Uncertain Behavior	Unspecified Behavior
connective tissue NEC *(Continued)*						
supraclavicular region	C49.0	C79.89	—	D21.0	D48.1	D49.2
temple	C49.0	C79.89	—	D21.0	D48.1	D49.2
temporal region	C49.0	C79.89	—	D21.0	D48.1	D49.2
thigh	C49.2-	C79.89	—	D21.2-	D48.1	D49.2
thoracic (duct) (wall)	C49.3	C79.89	—	D21.3	D48.1	D49.2
thorax	C49.3	C79.89	—	D21.3	D48.1	D49.2
thumb	C49.1-	C79.89	—	D21.1-	D48.1	D49.2
toe	C49.2-	C79.89	—	D21.2-	D48.1	D49.2
trunk	C49.6	C79.89	—	D21.6	D48.1	D49.2
umbilicus	C49.4	C79.89	—	D21.4	D48.1	D49.2
vesicorectal	C49.5	C79.89	—	D21.5	D48.1	D49.2
wrist	C49.1-	C79.89	—	D21.1-	D48.1	D49.2
conus medullaris	C72.0	C79.49	—	D33.4	D43.4	D49.7
cord (true) (vocal)	C32.0	C78.39	D02.0	D14.1	D38.0	D49.1
false	C32.1	C78.39	D02.0	D14.1	D38.0	D49.1
spermatic	C63.1-	C79.82	D07.69	D29.8	D40.8	D49.5
spinal (cervical) (lumbar) (thoracic)	C72.0	C79.49	—	D33.4	D43.4	D49.7
cornea (limbus)	C69.1-	C79.49	D09.2-	D31.1-	D48.7	D49.89
corpus						
albicans	C56.-	C79.6-	D07.39	D27.-	D39.1-	D49.5
callosum, brain	C71.0	C79.31	—	D33.2	D43.2	D49.6
cavernosum	C60.2	C79.82	D07.4	D29.0	D40.8	D49.5
gastric	C16.2	C78.89	D00.2	D13.1	D37.1	D49.0
overlapping sites	C54.8	—	—	—	—	—
penis	C60.2	C79.82	D07.4	D29.0	D40.8	D49.5
striatum, cerebrum	C71.0	C79.31	—	D33.0	D43.0	D49.6
uteri	C54.9	C79.82	D07.0	D26.1	D39.0	D49.5
isthmus	C54.0	C79.82	D07.0	D26.1	D39.0	D49.5
cortex						
adrenal	C74.0-	C79.7-	D09.3	D35.0-	D44.1-	D49.7
cerebral	C71.0	C79.31	—	D33.0	D43.0	D49.6
costal cartilage	C41.3	C79.51	—	D16.7	D48.0	D49.2
costovertebral joint	C41.3	C79.51	—	D16.7	D48.0	D49.2
Cowper's gland	C68.0	C79.19	D09.19	D30.4	D41.3	D49.5
cranial (fossa, any)	C71.9	C79.31	—	D33.2	D43.2	D49.6
meninges	C70.0	C79.32	—	D32.0	D42.0	D49.7
nerve	C72.50	C79.49	—	D33.3	D43.3	D49.7
specified NEC	C72.59	C79.49	—	D33.3	D43.3	D49.7
craniobuccal pouch	C75.2	C79.89	D09.3	D35.2	D44.3	D49.7
craniopharyngeal (duct) (pouch)	C75.2	C79.89	D09.3	D35.3	D44.4	D49.7
cricoid	C13.0	C79.89	D00.08	D10.7	D37.05	D49.0
cartilage	C32.3	C78.39	D02.0	D14.1	D38.0	D49.1

TABLE OF NEOPLASMS

	Malignant Primary	Malignant Secondary	Ca in situ	Benign	Uncertain Behavior	Unspecified Behavior
cricopharynx	C13.0	C79.89	D00.08	D10.7	D37.05	D49.0
crypt of Morgagni	C21.8	C78.5	D01.3	D12.9	D37.8	D49.0
crystalline lens	C69.4-	C79.49	D09.2-	D31.4-	D48.7	D49.89
cul-de-sac (Douglas')	C48.1	C78.6	—	D20.1	D48.4	D49.0
cuneiform cartilage	C32.3	C78.39	D02.0	D14.1	D38.0	D49.1
cutaneous — see Neoplasm, skin						
cutis — see Neoplasm, skin						
cystic (bile) duct (common)	C24.0	C78.89	D01.5	D13.5	D37.6	D49.0
dermis — see Neoplasm, skin						
diaphragm	C49.3	C79.89	—	D21.3	D48.1	D49.2
digestive organs, system, tube, or tract NEC	C26.9	C78.89	D01.9	D13.9	D37.9	D49.0
disc, intervertebral	C41.2	C79.51	—	D16.6	D48.0	D49.2
disease, generalized	C80.0	—	—	—	—	—
disseminated	C80.0	—	—	—	—	—
Douglas' cul-de-sac or pouch	C48.1	C78.6	—	D20.1	D48.4	D49.0
duodenojejunal junction	C17.8	C78.4	D01.49	D13.39	D37.2	D49.0
duodenum	C17.0	C78.4	D01.49	D13.2	D37.2	D49.0
dura (cranial) (mater)	C70.9	C79.49	—	D32.9	D42.9	D49.7
cerebral	C70.0	C79.32	—	D32.0	D42.0	D49.7
spinal	C70.1	C79.49	—	D32.1	D42.1	D49.7
ear (external) — see also Neoplasm, skin, ear	C44.20-	C79.2	D04.2-	D23.2-	D48.5	D49.2
auricle or auris — see also Neoplasm, skin, ear	C44.20-	C79.2	D04.2-	D23.2-	D48.5	D49.2
canal, external — see also Neoplasm, skin, ear	C44.20-	C79.2	D04.2-	D23.2-	D48.5	D49.2
cartilage	C49.0	C79.89	—	D21.0	D48.1	D49.2
external meatus — see also Neoplasm, skin, ear	C44.20-	C79.2	D04.2-	D23.2-	D48.5	D49.2
inner	C30.1	C78.39	D02.3	D14.0	D38.5	D49.1
lobule — see also Neoplasm, skin, ear	C44.20-	C79.2	D04.2-	D23.2-	D48.5	D49.2
middle	C30.1	C78.39	D02.3	D14.0	D38.5	D49.1
overlapping lesion with accessory sinuses	C31.8	—	—	—	—	—
skin	C44.20-	C79.2	D04.2-	D23.2-	D48.5	D49.2
basal cell carcinoma	C44.21-	—	—	—	—	—
specified type NEC	C44.29-	—	—	—	—	—
squamous cell carcinoma	C44.22-	—	—	—	—	—
earlobe	C44.20-	C79.2	D04.2-	D23.2-	D48.5	D49.2
basal cell carcinoma	C44.21-	—	—	—	—	—
specified type NEC	C44.29-	—	—	—	—	—
squamous cell carcinoma	C44.22-	—	—	—	—	—
ejaculatory duct	C63.7	C79.82	D07.69	D29.8	D40.8	D49.5
elbow NEC	C76.4-	C79.89	D04.6-	D36.7	D48.7	D49.89
endocardium	C38.0	C79.89	—	D15.1	D48.7	D49.89
endocervix (canal) (gland)	C53.0	C79.82	D06.0	D26.0	D39.0	D49.5
endocrine gland NEC	C75.9	C79.89	D09.3	D35.9	D44.9	D49.7
pluriglandular	C75.8	C79.89	D09.3	D35.7	D44.9	D49.7

◀ New   ◀▥ Revised   ~~deleted~~ Deleted

	Malignant Primary	Malignant Secondary	Ca in situ	Benign	Uncertain Behavior	Unspecified Behavior
endometrium (gland) (stroma)	C54.1	C79.82	D07.0	D26.1	D39.0	D49.5
ensiform cartilage	C41.3	C79.51	—	D16.7	D48.0	D49.2
enteric — see Neoplasm, intestine						
ependyma (brain)	C71.5	C79.31	—	D33.0	D43.0	D49.6
fourth ventricle	C71.7	C79.31	—	D33.1	D43.1	D49.6
epicardium	C38.0	C79.89	—	D15.1	D48.7	D49.89
epididymis	C63.0-	C79.82	D07.69	D29.3-	D40.8	D49.5
epidural	C72.9	C79.49	—	D33.9	D43.9	D49.7
epiglottis	C32.1	C78.39	D02.0	D14.1	D38.0	D49.1
anterior aspect or surface	C10.1	C79.89	D00.08	D10.5	D37.05	D49.0
cartilage	C32.3	C78.39	D02.0	D14.1	D38.0	D49.1
free border (margin)	C10.1	C79.89	D00.08	D10.5	D37.05	D49.0
junctional region	C10.8	C79.89	D00.08	D10.5	D37.05	D49.0
posterior (laryngeal) surface	C32.1	C78.39	D02.0	D14.1	D38.0	D49.1
suprahyoid portion	C32.1	C78.39	D02.0	D14.1	D38.0	D49.1
esophagogastric junction	C16.0	C78.89	D00.2	D13.1	D37.1	D49.0
esophagus	C15.9	C78.89	D00.1	D13.0	D37.8	D49.0
abdominal	C15.5	C78.89	D00.1	D13.0	D37.8	D49.0
cervical	C15.3	C78.89	D00.1	D13.0	D37.8	D49.0
distal (third)	C15.5	C78.89	D00.1	D13.0	D37.8	D49.0
lower (third)	C15.5	C78.89	D00.1	D13.0	D37.8	D49.0
middle (third)	C15.4	C78.89	D00.1	D13.0	D37.8	D49.0
overlapping lesion	C15.8	—	—	—	—	—
proximal (third)	C15.3	C78.89	D00.1	D13.0	D37.8	D49.0
thoracic	C15.4	C78.89	D00.1	D13.0	D37.8	D49.0
upper (third)	C15.3	C78.89	D00.1	D13.0	D37.8	D49.0
ethmoid (sinus)	C31.1	C78.39	D02.3	D14.0	D38.5	D49.1
bone or labyrinth	C41.0	C79.51	—	D16.4-	D48.0	D49.2
eustachian tube	C30.1	C78.39	D02.3	D14.0	D38.5	D49.1
exocervix	C53.1	C79.82	D06.1	D26.0	D39.0	D49.5
external						
meatus (ear) — see also Neoplasm, skin, ear	C44.20-	C79.2	D04.2-	D23.2-	D48.5	D49.2
os, cervix uteri	C53.1	C79.82	D06.1	D26.0	D39.0	D49.5
extradural	C72.9	C79.49	—	D33.9	D43.9	D49.7
extrahepatic (bile) duct	C24.0	C78.89	D01.5	D13.5	D37.6	D49.0
overlapping lesion with gallbladder	C24.8	—	—	—	—	—
extraocular muscle	C69.6-	C79.49	D09.2-	D31.6-	D48.7	D49.89
extrarectal	C76.3	C79.89	D09.8	D36.7	D48.7	D49.89
extremity	C76.8	C79.89	D04.8	D36.7	D48.7	D49.89
lower	C76.5-	C79.89	D04.7-	D36.7	D48.7	D49.89
upper	C76.4-	C79.89	D04.6-	D36.7	D48.7	D49.89
eye NEC	C69.9-	C79.49	D09.2	D31.9	D48.7	D49.89
overlapping sites	C69.8	—	—	—	—	—
eyeball	C69.9-	C79.49	D09.2-	D31.9-	D48.7	D49.89

TABLE OF NEOPLASMS

	Malignant Primary	Malignant Secondary	Ca in situ	Benign	Uncertain Behavior	Unspecified Behavior
eyebrow	C44.309	C79.2	D04.39	D23.39	D48.5	D49.2
basal cell carcinoma	C44.319	—	—	—	—	—
specified type NEC	C44.399	—	—	—	—	—
squamous cell carcinoma	C44.329	—	—	—	—	—
eyelid (lower) (skin) (upper)	C44.10-	—	—	—	—	—
basal cell carcinoma	C44.11-	—	—	—	—	—
cartilage	C49.0	C79.89	—	D21.0	D48.1	D49.2
specified type NEC	C44.19-	—	—	—	—	—
squamous cell carcinoma	C44.12-	—	—	—	—	—
face NEC	C76.0	C79.89	D04.39	D36.7	D48.7	D49.89
fallopian tube (accessory)	C57.0-	C79.82	D07.39	D28.2	D39.8	D49.5
falx (cerebella) (cerebri)	C70.0	C79.32	—	D32.0	D42.0	D49.7
fascia — see also Neoplasm, connective tissue						
palmar	C49.1-	C79.89	—	D21.1-	D48.1	D49.2
plantar	C49.2-	C79.89	—	D21.2-	D48.1	D49.2
fatty tissue — see Neoplasm, connective tissue						
fauces, faucial NEC	C10.9	C79.89	D00.08	D10.5	D37.05	D49.0
pillars	C09.1	C79.89	D00.08	D10.5	D37.05	D49.0
tonsil	C09.9	C79.89	D00.08	D10.4	D37.05	D49.0
femur (any part)	C40.2-	—	—	D16.2-	—	—
fetal membrane	C58	C79.82	D07.0	D26.7	D39.2	D49.5
fibrous tissue — see Neoplasm, connective tissue						
fibula (any part)	C40.2-	C79.51	—	D16.2-	—	—
filum terminale	C72.0	C79.49	—	D33.4	D43.4	D49.7
finger NEC	C76.4-	C79.89	D04.6-	D36.7	D48.7	D49.89
flank NEC	C76.8	C79.89	D04.5	D36.7	D48.7	D49.89
follicle, nabothian	C53.0	C79.82	D06.0	D26.0	D39.0	D49.5
foot NEC	C76.5-	C79.89	D04.7-	D36.7	D48.7	D49.89
forearm NEC	C76.4-	C79.89	D04.6-	D36.7	D48.7	D49.89
forehead (skin)	C44.309	C79.2	D04.39	D23.39	D48.5	D49.2
basal cell carcinoma	C44.319	—	—	—	—	—
specified type NEC	C44.399	—	—	—	—	—
squamous cell carcinoma	C44.329	—	—	—	—	—
foreskin	C60.0	C79.82	D07.4	D29.0	D40.8	D49.5
fornix						
pharyngeal	C11.3	C79.89	D00.08	D10.6	D37.05	D49.0
vagina	C52	C79.82	D07.2	D28.1	D39.8	D49.5
fossa (of)						
anterior (cranial)	C71.9	C79.31	—	D33.2	D43.2	D49.6
cranial	C71.9	C79.31	—	D33.2	D43.2	D49.6
ischiorectal	C76.3	C79.89	D09.8	D36.7	D48.7	D49.89
middle (cranial)	C71.9	C79.31	—	D33.2	D43.2	D49.6
piriform	C12	C79.89	D00.08	D10.7	D37.05	D49.0

◄ New   ◀◀◀ Revised   ~~deleted~~ Deleted

	Malignant Primary	Malignant Secondary	Ca in situ	Benign	Uncertain Behavior	Unspecified Behavior
fossa *(Continued)*						
pituitary	C75.1	C79.89	D09.3	D35.2	D44.3	D49.7
posterior (cranial)	C71.9	C79.31	—	D33.2	D43.2	D49.6
pterygoid	C49.0	C79.89	—	D21.0	D48.1	D49.2
pyriform	C12	C79.89	D00.08	D10.7	D37.05	D49.0
Rosenmuller	C11.2	C79.89	D00.08	D10.6	D37.05	D49.0
tonsillar	C09.0	C79.89	D00.08	D10.5	D37.05	D49.0
fourchette	C51.9	C79.82	D07.1	D28.0	D39.8	D49.5
frenulum						
labii — *see Neoplasm, lip, internal*						
linguae	C02.2	C79.89	D00.07	D10.1	D37.02	D49.0
frontal						
bone	C41.0	C79.51	—	D16.4-	D48.0	D49.2
lobe, brain	C71.1	C79.31	—	D33.0	D43.0	D49.6
pole	C71.1	C79.31	—	D33.0	D43.0	D49.6
sinus	C31.2	C78.39	D02.3	D14.0	D38.5	D49.1
fundus						
stomach	C16.1	C78.89	D00.2	D13.1	D37.1	D49.0
uterus	C54.3	C79.82	D07.0	D26.1	D39.0	D49.5
gall duct (extrahepatic)	C24.0	C78.89	D01.5	D13.5	D37.6	D49.0
intrahepatic	C22.1	C78.7	D01.5	D13.4	D37.6	D49.0
gallbladder	C23	C78.89	D01.5	D13.5	D37.6	D49.0
overlapping lesion with extrahepatic bile ducts	C24.8	—	—	—	—	—
ganglia — *see also Neoplasm, nerve, peripheral*	C47.9	C79.89	—	D36.10	D48.2	D49.2
basal	C71.0	C79.31	—	D33.0	D43.0	D49.6
cranial nerve	C72.50	C79.49	—	D33.3	D43.3	D49.7
Gartner's duct	C52	C79.82	D07.2	D28.1	D39.8	D49.5
gastric — *see Neoplasm, stomach*						
gastrocolic	C26.9	C78.89	D01.9	D13.9	D37.9	D49.0
gastroesophageal junction	C16.0	C78.89	D00.2	D13.1	D37.1	D49.0
gastrointestinal (tract) NEC	C26.9	C78.89	D01.9	D13.9	D37.9	D49.0
generalized	C80.0	—	—	—	—	—
genital organ or tract						
female NEC	C57.9	C79.82	D07.30	D28.9	D39.9	D49.5
overlapping lesion	C57.8	—	—	—	—	—
specified site NEC	C57.7	C79.82	D07.39	D28.7	D39.8	D49.5
male NEC	C63.9	C79.82	D07.60	D29.9	D40.9	D49.5
overlapping lesion	C63.8	—	—	—	—	—
specified site NEC	C63.7	C79.82	D07.69	D29.8	D40.8	D49.5
genitourinary tract						
female	C57.9	C79.82	D07.30	D28.9	D39.9	D49.5
male	C63.9	C79.82	D07.60	D29.9	D40.9	D49.5

TABLE OF NEOPLASMS

	Malignant Primary	Malignant Secondary	Ca in situ	Benign	Uncertain Behavior	Unspecified Behavior
gingiva (alveolar) (marginal)	C03.9	C79.89	D00.03	D10.39	D37.09	D49.0
lower	C03.1	C79.89	D00.03	D10.39	D37.09	D49.0
mandibular	C03.1	C79.89	D00.03	D10.39	D37.09	D49.0
maxillary	C03.0	C79.89	D00.03	D10.39	D37.09	D49.0
upper	C03.0	C79.89	D00.03	D10.39	D37.09	D49.0
gland, glandular (lymphatic) (system) — see also Neoplasm, lymph gland						
endocrine NEC	C75.9	C79.89	D09.3	D35.9	D44.9	D49.7
salivary — see Neoplasm, salivary gland						
glans penis	C60.1	C79.82	D07.4	D29.0	D40.8	D49.5
globus pallidus	C71.0	C79.31	—	D33.0	D43.0	D49.6
glomus						
coccygeal	C49.5	C79.89	—	D21.5	D48.1	D49.2
jugularis	C75.5	C79.89	—	D35.6	D44.7	D49.7
glosso-epiglottic fold(s)	C10.1	C79.89	D00.08	D10.5	D37.05	D49.0
glossopalatine fold	C09.1	C79.89	D00.08	D10.5	D37.05	D49.0
glossopharyngeal sulcus	C09.0	C79.89	D00.08	D10.5	D37.05	D49.0
glottis	C32.0	C78.39	D02.0	D14.1	D38.0	D49.1
gluteal region	C76.3	C79.89	D04.5	D36.7	D48.7	D49.89
great vessels NEC	C49.3	C79.89	—	D21.3	D48.1	D49.2
groin NEC	C76.3	C79.89	D04.5	D36.7	D48.7	D49.89
gum	C03.9	C79.89	D00.03	D10.39	D37.09	D49.0
lower	C03.1	C79.89	D00.03	D10.39	D37.09	D49.0
upper	C03.0	C79.89	D00.03	D10.39	D37.09	D49.0
hand NEC	C76.4-	C79.89	D04.6-	D36.7	D48.7	D49.89
head NEC	C76.0	C79.89	D04.4	D36.7	D48.7	D49.89
heart	C38.0	C79.89	—	D15.1	D48.7	D49.89
heel NEC	C76.5-	C79.89	D04.7-	D36.7	D48.7	D49.89
helix — see also Neoplasm, skin, ear	C44.20-	C79.2	D04.2-	D23.2-	D48.5	D49.2
hematopoietic, hemopoietic tissue NEC	C96.9	—	—	—	—	—
specified NEC	C96.Z	—	—	—	—	—
hemisphere, cerebral	C71.0	C79.31	—	D33.0	D43.0	D49.6
hemorrhoidal zone	C21.1	C78.5	D01.3	D12.9	D37.8	D49.0
hepatic — see also Index to disease, by histology	C22.9	C78.7	D01.5	D13.4	D37.6	D49.0
duct (bile)	C24.0	C78.89	D01.5	D13.5	D37.6	D49.0
flexure (colon)	C18.3	C78.5	D01.0	D12.3	D37.4	D49.0
primary	C22.8	C78.7	D01.5	D13.4	D37.6	D49.0
hepatobiliary	C24.9	C79.89	D01.5	D13.5	D37.6	D49.0
hepatoblastoma	C22.2	C78.7	D01.5	D13.4	D37.6	D49.0
hepatoma	C22.0	C78.7	D01.5	D13.4	D37.6	D49.0
hilus of lung	C34.0-	C78.0-	D02.2-	D14.3-	D38.1	D49.1
hip NEC	C76.5-	C79.89	D04.7-	D36.7	D48.7	D49.89
hippocampus, brain	C71.2	C79.31	—	D33.0	D43.0	D49.6
humerus (any part)	C40.0-	C79.51	—	D16.0-	—	—
hymen	C52	C79.82	D07.2	D28.1	D39.8	D49.5

◀ New   ◀▦ Revised   ~~deleted~~ Deleted

	Malignant Primary	Malignant Secondary	Ca in situ	Benign	Uncertain Behavior	Unspecified Behavior
hypopharynx, hypopharyngeal NEC	C13.9	C79.89	D00.08	D10.7	D37.05	D49.0
overlapping lesion	C13.8	—	—	—	—	—
postcricoid region	C13.0	C79.89	D00.08	D10.7	D37.05	D49.0
posterior wall	C13.2	C79.89	D00.08	D10.7	D37.05	D49.0
pyriform fossa (sinus)	C12	C79.89	D00.08	D10.7	D37.05	D49.0
hypophysis	C75.1	C79.89	D09.3	D35.2	D44.3	D49.7
hypothalamus	C71.0	C79.31	—	D33.0	D43.0	D49.6
ileocecum, ileocecal (coil) (junction) (valve)	C18.0	C78.5	D01.0	D12.0	D37.4	D49.0
ileum	C17.2	C78.4	D01.49	D13.39	D37.2	D49.0
ilium	C41.4	C79.51	—	D16.8	D48.0	D49.2
immunoproliferative NEC	C88.9	—	—	—	—	—
infraclavicular (region)	C76.1	C79.89	D04.5	D36.7	D48.7	D49.89
inguinal (region)	C76.3	C79.89	D04.5	D36.7	D48.7	D49.89
insula	C71.0	C79.31	—	D33.0	D43.0	D49.6
insular tissue (pancreas)	C25.4	C78.89	D01.7	D13.7	D37.8	D49.0
brain	C71.0	C79.31	—	D33.0	D43.0	D49.6
interarytenoid fold	C13.1	C79.89	D00.08	D10.7	D37.05	D49.0
hypopharyngeal aspect	C13.1	C79.89	D00.08	D10.7	D37.05	D49.0
laryngeal aspect	C32.1	C78.39	D02.0	D14.1	D38.0	D49.1
marginal zone	C13.1	C79.89	D00.08	D10.7	D37.05	D49.0
interdental papillae	C03.9	C79.89	D00.03	D10.39	D37.09	D49.0
lower	C03.1	C79.89	D00.03	D10.39	D37.09	D49.0
upper	C03.0	C79.89	D00.03	D10.39	D37.09	D49.0
internal						
capsule	C71.0	C79.31	—	D33.0	D43.0	D49.6
os (cervix)	C53.0	C79.82	D06.0	D26.0	D39.0	D49.5
intervertebral cartilage or disc	C41.2	C79.51	—	D16.6	D48.0	D49.2
intestine, intestinal	C26.0	C78.80	D01.40	D13.9	D37.8	D49.0
large	C18.9	C78.5	D01.0	D12.6	D37.4	D49.0
appendix	C18.1	C78.5	D01.0	D12.1	D37.3	D49.0
caput coli	C18.0	C78.5	D01.0	D12.0	D37.4	D49.0
cecum	C18.0	C78.5	D01.0	D12.0	D37.4	D49.0
colon	C18.9	C78.5	D01.0	D12.6	D37.4	D49.0
and rectum	C19	C78.5	D01.1	D12.7	D37.5	D49.0
ascending	C18.2	C78.5	D01.0	D12.2	D37.4	D49.0
caput	C18.0	C78.5	D01.0	D12.0	D37.4	D49.0
descending	C18.6	C78.5	D01.0	D12.4	D37.4	D49.0
distal	C18.6	C78.5	D01.0	D12.4	D37.4	D49.0
left	C18.6	C78.5	D01.0	D12.4	D37.4	D49.0
overlapping lesion	C18.8	—	—	—	—	—
pelvic	C18.7	C78.5	D01.0	D12.5	D37.4	D49.0
right	C18.2	C78.5	D01.0	D12.2	D37.4	D49.0
sigmoid (flexure)	C18.7	C78.5	D01.0	D12.5	D37.4	D49.0
transverse	C18.4	C78.5	D01.0	D12.3	D37.4	D49.0

TABLE OF NEOPLASMS

	Malignant Primary	Malignant Secondary	Ca in situ	Benign	Uncertain Behavior	Unspecified Behavior
intestine, intestinal *(Continued)*						
large *(Continued)*						
hepatic flexure	C18.3	C78.5	D01.0	D12.3	D37.4	D49.0
ileocecum, ileocecal (coil) (valve)	C18.0	C78.5	D01.0	D12.0	D37.4	D49.0
overlapping lesion	C18.8	—	—	—	—	—
sigmoid flexure (lower) (upper)	C18.7	C78.5	D01.0	D12.5	D37.4	D49.0
splenic flexure	C18.5	C78.5	D01.0	D12.3	D37.4	D49.0
small	C17.9	C78.4	D01.40	D13.30	D37.2	D49.0
duodenum	C17.0	C78.4	D01.49	D13.2	D37.2	D49.0
ileum	C17.2	C78.4	D01.49	D13.39	D37.2	D49.0
jejunum	C17.1	C78.4	D01.49	D13.39	D37.2	D49.0
overlapping lesion	C17.8	—	—	—	—	—
tract NEC	C26.0	C78.89	D01.40	D13.9	D37.8	D49.0
intra-abdominal	C76.2	C79.89	D09.8	D36.7	D48.7	D49.89
intracranial NEC	C71.9	C79.31	—	D33.2	D43.2	D49.6
intrahepatic (bile) duct	C22.1	C78.7	D01.5	D13.4	D37.6	D49.0
intraocular	C69.9-	C79.49	D09.2-	D31.9-	D48.7	D49.89
intraorbital	C69.6-	C79.49	D09.2-	D31.6-	D48.7	D49.89
intrasellar	C75.1	C79.89	D09.3	D35.2	D44.3	D49.7
intrathoracic (cavity) (organs)	C76.1	C79.89	D09.8	D15.9	D48.7	D49.89
specified NEC	C76.1	C79.89	D09.8	D15.7	—	—
iris	C69.4-	C79.49	D09.2-	D31.4-	D48.7	D49.89
ischiorectal (fossa)	C76.3	C79.89	D09.8	D36.7	D48.7	D49.89
ischium	C41.4	C79.51	—	D16.8	D48.0	D49.2
island of Reil	C71.0	C79.31	—	D33.0	D43.0	D49.6
islands or islets of Langerhans	C25.4	C78.89	D01.7	D13.7	D37.8	D49.0
isthmus uteri	C54.0	C79.82	D07.0	D26.1	D39.0	D49.5
jaw	C76.0	C79.89	D09.8	D36.7	D48.7	D49.89
bone	C41.1	C79.51	—	D16.5-	D48.0	D49.2
lower	C41.1	C79.51	—	D16.5-	—	—
upper	C41.0	C79.51	—	D16.4-	—	—
carcinoma (any type) (lower) (upper)	C76.0	C79.89	—	—	—	—
skin — *see also Neoplasm, skin, face*	C44.309	C79.2	D04.39	D23.39	D48.5	D49.2
soft tissues	C03.9	C79.89	D00.03	D10.39	D37.09	D49.0
lower	C03.1	C79.89	D00.03	D10.39	D37.09	D49.0
upper	C03.0	C79.89	D00.03	D10.39	D37.09	D49.0
jejunum	C17.1	C78.4	D01.49	D13.39	D37.2	D49.0
joint NEC — *see also Neoplasm, bone*	C41.9	C79.51	—	D16.9-	D48.0	D49.2
acromioclavicular	C40.0-	C79.51	—	D16.0-	—	—
bursa or synovial membrane — *see Neoplasm, connective tissue*						
costovertebral	C41.3	C79.51	—	D16.7	D48.0	D49.2
sternocostal	C41.3	C79.51	—	D16.7	D48.0	D49.2
temporomandibular	C41.1	C79.51	—	D16.5-	D48.0	D49.2

◄ New   ◄▥ Revised   ~~deleted~~ Deleted

	Malignant Primary	Malignant Secondary	Ca in situ	Benign	Uncertain Behavior	Unspecified Behavior
junction						
anorectal	C21.8	C78.5	D01.3	D12.9	D37.8	D49.0
cardioesophageal	C16.0	C78.89	D00.2	D13.1	D37.1	D49.0
esophagogastric	C16.0	C78.89	D00.2	D13.1	D37.1	D49.0
gastroesophageal	C16.0	C78.89	D00.2	D13.1	D37.1	D49.0
hard and soft palate	C05.9	C79.89	D00.00	D10.39	D37.09	D49.0
ileocecal	C18.0	C78.5	D01.0	D12.0	D37.4	D49.0
pelvirectal	C19	C78.5	D01.1	D12.7	D37.5	D49.0
pelviureteric	C65.-	C79.0-	D09.19	D30.1-	D41.1-	D49.5
rectosigmoid	C19	C78.5	D01.1	D12.7	D37.5	D49.0
squamocolumnar, of cervix	C53.8	C79.82	D06.7	D26.0	D39.0	D49.5
Kaposi's sarcoma — see Kaposi's, sarcoma						
kidney (parenchymal)	C64.-	C79.0-	D09.19	D30.0-	D41.0-	D49.5
calyx	C65.-	C79.0-	D09.19	D30.1-	D41.1-	D49.5
hilus	C65.-	C79.0-	D09.19	D30.1-	D41.1-	D49.5
pelvis	C65.-	C79.0-	D09.19	D30.1-	D41.1-	D49.5
knee NEC	C76.5-	C79.89	D04.7-	D36.7	D48.7	D49.89
labia (skin)	C51.9	C79.82	D07.1	D28.0	D39.8	D49.5
majora	C51.0	C79.82	D07.1	D28.0	D39.8	D49.5
minora	C51.1	C79.82	D07.1	D28.0	D39.8	D49.5
labial — see also Neoplasm, lip	C00.9	C79.89	D00.01	D10.0	D37.01	D49.0
sulcus (lower) (upper)	C06.1	C79.89	D00.02	D10.39	D37.09	D49.0
labium (skin)	C51.9	C79.82	D07.1	D28.0	D39.8	D49.5
majus	C51.0	C79.82	D07.1	D28.0	D39.8	D49.5
minus	C51.1	C79.82	D07.1	D28.0	D39.8	D49.5
lacrimal						
canaliculi	C69.5-	C79.49	D09.2-	D31.5-	D48.7	D49.89
duct (nasal)	C69.5-	C79.49	D09.2-	D31.5-	D48.7	D49.89
gland	C69.5-	C79.49	D09.2-	D31.5-	D48.7	D49.89
punctum	C69.5-	C79.49	D09.2-	D31.5-	D48.7	D49.89
sac	C69.5-	C79.49	D09.2-	D31.5-	D48.7	D49.89
Langerhans, islands or islets	C25.4	C78.89	D01.7	D13.7	D37.8	D49.0
laryngopharynx	C13.9	C79.89	D00.08	D10.7	D37.05	D49.0
larynx, laryngeal NEC	C32.9	C78.39	D02.0	D14.1	D38.0	D49.1
aryepiglottic fold	C32.1	C78.39	D02.0	D14.1	D38.0	D49.1
cartilage (arytenoid) (cricoid) (cuneiform) (thyroid)	C32.3	C78.39	D02.0	D14.1	D38.0	D49.1
commissure (anterior) (posterior)	C32.0	C78.39	D02.0	D14.1	D38.0	D49.1
extrinsic NEC	C32.1	C78.39	D02.0	D14.1	D38.0	D49.1
meaning hypopharynx	C13.9	C79.89	D00.08	D10.7	D37.05	D49.0
interarytenoid fold	C32.1	C78.39	D02.0	D14.1	D38.0	D49.1
intrinsic	C32.0	C78.39	D02.0	D14.1	D38.0	D49.1
overlapping lesion	C32.8	—	—	—	—	—
ventricular band	C32.1	C78.39	D02.0	D14.1	D38.0	D49.1
leg NEC	C76.5-	C79.89	D04.7-	D36.7	D48.7	D49.89

TABLE OF NEOPLASMS

	Malignant Primary	Malignant Secondary	Ca in situ	Benign	Uncertain Behavior	Unspecified Behavior
lens, crystalline	C69.4-	C79.49	D09.2-	D31.4-	D48.7	D49.89
lid (lower) (upper)	C44.10-	C79.2	D04.1-	D23.1-	D48.5	D49.2
basal cell carcinoma	C44.11-	—	—	—	—	—
specified type NEC	C44.19-	—	—	—	—	—
squamous cell carcinoma	C44.12-	—	—	—	—	—
ligament — see also Neoplasm, connective tissue						
broad	C57.1	C79.82	D07.39	D28.2	D39.8	D49.5
Mackenrodt's	C57.7	C79.82	D07.39	D28.7	D39.8	D49.5
non-uterine — see Neoplasm, connective tissue						
round	C57.2	C79.82	—	D28.2	D39.8	D49.5
sacro-uterine	C57.3	C79.82	—	D28.2	D39.8	D49.5
uterine	C57.3	C79.82	—	D28.2	D39.8	D49.5
utero-ovarian	C57.7	C79.82	D07.39	D28.2	D39.8	D49.5
uterosacral	C57.3	C79.82	—	D28.2	D39.8	D49.5
limb	C76.8	C79.89	D04.8	D36.7	D48.7	D49.89
lower	C76.5-	C79.89	D04.7-	D36.7	D48.7	D49.89
upper	C76.4-	C79.89	D04.6-	D36.7	D48.7	D49.89
limbus of cornea	C69.1-	C79.49	D09.2-	D31.1-	D48.7	D49.89
lingual NEC — see also Neoplasm, tongue	C02.9	C79.89	D00.07	D10.1	D37.02	D49.0
lingula, lung	C34.1-	C78.0-	D02.2-	D14.3-	D38.1	D49.1
lip	C00.9	C79.89	D00.01	D10.0	D37.01	D49.0
buccal aspect — see Neoplasm, lip, internal						
commissure	C00.6	C79.89	D00.01	D10.0	D37.01	D49.0
external	C00.2	C79.89	D00.01	D10.0	D37.01	D49.0
lower	C00.1	C79.89	D00.01	D10.0	D37.01	D49.0
upper	C00.0	C79.89	D00.01	D10.0	D37.01	D49.0
frenulum — see Neoplasm, lip, internal						
inner aspect — see Neoplasm, lip, internal						
internal	C00.5	C79.89	D00.01	D10.0	D37.01	D49.0
lower	C00.4	C79.89	D00.01	D10.0	D37.01	D49.0
upper	C00.3	C79.89	D00.01	D10.0	D37.01	D49.0
lipstick area	C00.2	C79.89	D00.01	D10.0	D37.01	D49.0
lower	C00.1	C79.89	D00.01	D10.0	D37.01	D49.0
upper	C00.0	C79.89	D00.01	D10.0	D37.01	D49.0
lower	C00.1	C79.89	D00.01	D10.0	D37.01	D49.0
internal	C00.4	C79.89	D00.01	D10.0	D37.01	D49.0
mucosa — see Neoplasm, lip, internal						
oral aspect — see Neoplasm, lip, internal						
overlapping lesion	C00.8	—	—	—	—	—
with oral cavity or pharynx	C14.8	—	—	—	—	—
skin (commissure) (lower) (upper)	C44.00	C79.2	D04.0	D23.0	D48.5	D49.2
basal cell carcinoma	C44.01	—	—	—	—	—
specified type NEC	C44.09	—	—	—	—	—
squamous cell carcinoma	C44.02	—	—	—	—	—

◀ New   ◀▥ Revised   ~~deleted~~ Deleted

	Malignant Primary	Malignant Secondary	Ca in situ	Benign	Uncertain Behavior	Unspecified Behavior
lip *(Continued)*						
upper	C00.0	C79.89	D00.01	D10.0	D37.01	D49.0
internal	C00.3	C79.89	D00.01	D10.0	D37.01	D49.0
vermilion border	C00.2	C79.89	D00.01	D10.0	D37.01	D49.0
lower	C00.1	C79.89	D00.01	D10.0	D37.01	D49.0
upper	C00.0	C79.89	D00.01	D10.0	D37.01	D49.0
lipomatous — *see Lipoma, by site*						
liver — *see also Index to disease, by histology*	C22.9	C78.7	D01.5	D13.4	D37.6	D49.0
primary	C22.8	C78.7	D01.5	D13.4	D37.6	D49.0
lumbosacral plexus	C47.5	C79.89	—	D36.16	D48.2	D49.2
lung	C34.9-	C78.0-	D02.2-	D14.3-	D38.1	D49.1
azygos lobe	C34.1-	C78.0-	D02.2-	D14.3-	D38.1	D49.1
carina	C34.0-	C78.0-	D02.2-	D14.3-	D38.1	D49.1
hilus	C34.0-	C78.0-	D02.2-	D14.3-	D38.1	D49.1
lingula	C34.1-	C78.0-	D02.2-	D14.3-	D38.1	D49.1
lobe NEC	C34.9-	C78.0-	D02.2-	D14.3-	D38.1	D49.1
lower lobe	C34.3-	C78.0-	D02.2-	D14.3-	D38.1	D49.1
main bronchus	C34.0-	C78.0-	D02.2-	D14.3-	D38.1	D49.1
mesothelioma — *see Mesothelioma*						
middle lobe	C34.2	C78.0-	D02.21	D14.31	D38.1	D49.1
overlapping lesion	C34.8-	—	—	—	—	—
upper lobe	C34.1-	C78.0-	D02.2-	D14.3-	D38.1	D49.1
lymph, lymphatic channel NEC	C49.9	C79.89	—	D21.9	D48.1	D49.2
gland (secondary)	—	C77.9	—	D36.0	D48.7	D49.89
abdominal	—	C77.2	—	D36.0	D48.7	D49.89
aortic	—	C77.2	—	D36.0	D48.7	D49.89
arm	—	C77.3	—	D36.0	D48.7	D49.89
auricular (anterior) (posterior)	—	C77.0	—	D36.0	D48.7	D49.89
axilla, axillary	—	C77.3	—	D36.0	D48.7	D49.89
brachial	—	C77.3	—	D36.0	D48.7	D49.89
bronchial	—	C77.1	—	D36.0	D48.7	D49.89
bronchopulmonary	—	C77.1	—	D36.0	D48.7	D49.89
celiac	—	C77.2	—	D36.0	D48.7	D49.89
cervical	—	C77.0	—	D36.0	D48.7	D49.89
cervicofacial	—	C77.0	—	D36.0	D48.7	D49.89
Cloquet	—	C77.4	—	D36.0	D48.7	D49.89
colic	—	C77.2	—	D36.0	D48.7	D49.89
common duct	—	C77.2	—	D36.0	D48.7	D49.89
cubital	—	C77.3	—	D36.0	D48.7	D49.89
diaphragmatic	—	C77.1	—	D36.0	D48.7	D49.89
epigastric, inferior	—	C77.1	—	D36.0	D48.7	D49.89
epitrochlear	—	C77.3	—	D36.0	D48.7	D49.89
esophageal	—	C77.1	—	D36.0	D48.7	D49.89
face	—	C77.0	—	D36.0	D48.7	D49.89

	Malignant Primary	Malignant Secondary	Ca in situ	Benign	Uncertain Behavior	Unspecified Behavior
lymph, lymphatic channel NEC *(Continued)*						
gland *(Continued)*						
femoral	—	C77.4	—	D36.0	D48.7	D49.89
gastric	—	C77.2	—	D36.0	D48.7	D49.89
groin	—	C77.4	—	D36.0	D48.7	D49.89
head	—	C77.0	—	D36.0	D48.7	D49.89
hepatic	—	C77.2	—	D36.0	D48.7	D49.89
hilar (pulmonary)	—	C77.1	—	D36.0	D48.7	D49.89
splenic	—	C77.2	—	D36.0	D48.7	D49.89
hypogastric	—	C77.5	—	D36.0	D48.7	D49.89
ileocolic	—	C77.2	—	D36.0	D48.7	D49.89
iliac	—	C77.5	—	D36.0	D48.7	D49.89
infraclavicular	—	C77.3	—	D36.0	D48.7	D49.89
inguina, inguinal	—	C77.4	—	D36.0	D48.7	D49.89
innominate	—	C77.1	—	D36.0	D48.7	D49.89
intercostal	—	C77.1	—	D36.0	D48.7	D49.89
intestinal	—	C77.2	—	D36.0	D48.7	D49.89
intrabdominal	—	C77.2	—	D36.0	D48.7	D49.89
intrapelvic	—	C77.5	—	D36.0	D48.7	D49.89
intrathoracic	—	C77.1	—	D36.0	D48.7	D49.89
jugular	—	C77.0	—	D36.0	D48.7	D49.89
leg	—	C77.4	—	D36.0	D48.7	D49.89
limb						
lower	—	C77.4	—	D36.0	D48.7	D49.89
upper	—	C77.3	—	D36.0	D48.7	D49.89
lower limb	—	C77.4	—	D36.0	D48.7	D49.89
lumbar	—	C77.2	—	D36.0	D48.7	D49.89
mandibular	—	C77.0	—	D36.0	D48.7	D49.89
mediastinal	—	C77.1	—	D36.0	D48.7	D49.89
mesenteric (inferior) (superior)	—	C77.2	—	D36.0	D48.7	D49.89
midcolic	—	C77.2	—	D36.0	D48.7	D49.89
multiple sites in categories C77.0 - C77.5	—	C77.8	—	D36.0	D48.7	D49.89
neck	—	C77.0	—	D36.0	D48.7	D49.89
obturator	—	C77.5	—	D36.0	D48.7	D49.89
occipital	—	C77.0	—	D36.0	D48.7	D49.89
pancreatic	—	C77.2	—	D36.0	D48.7	D49.89
para-aortic	—	C77.2	—	D36.0	D48.7	D49.89
paracervical	—	C77.5	—	D36.0	D48.7	D49.89
parametrial	—	C77.5	—	D36.0	D48.7	D49.89
parasternal	—	C77.1	—	D36.0	D48.7	D49.89
parotid	—	C77.0	—	D36.0	D48.7	D49.89
pectoral	—	C77.3	—	D36.0	D48.7	D49.89
pelvic	—	C77.5	—	D36.0	D48.7	D49.89

◀ New   ◀▥ Revised   ~~deleted~~ Deleted

	Malignant Primary	Malignant Secondary	Ca in situ	Benign	Uncertain Behavior	Unspecified Behavior
lymph, lymphatic channel NEC *(Continued)*						
gland *(Continued)*						
peri-aortic	—	C77.2	—	D36.0	D48.7	D49.89
peripancreatic	—	C77.2	—	D36.0	D48.7	D49.89
popliteal	—	C77.4	—	D36.0	D48.7	D49.89
porta hepatis	—	C77.2	—	D36.0	D48.7	D49.89
portal	—	C77.2	—	D36.0	D48.7	D49.89
preauricular	—	C77.0	—	D36.0	D48.7	D49.89
prelaryngeal	—	C77.0	—	D36.0	D48.7	D49.89
presymphysial	—	C77.5	—	D36.0	D48.7	D49.89
pretracheal	—	C77.0	—	D36.0	D48.7	D49.89
primary (any site) NEC	C96.9	—	—	—	—	—
pulmonary (hiler)	—	C77.1	—	D36.0	D48.7	D49.89
pyloric	—	C77.2	—	D36.0	D48.7	D49.89
retroperitoneal	—	C77.2	—	D36.0	D48.7	D49.89
retropharyngeal	—	C77.0	—	D36.0	D48.7	D49.89
Rosenmuller's	—	C77.4	—	D36.0	D48.7	D49.89
sacral	—	C77.5	—	D36.0	D48.7	D49.89
scalene	—	C77.0	—	D36.0	D48.7	D49.89
site NEC	—	C77.9	—	D36.0	D48.7	D49.89
splenic (hilar)	—	C77.2	—	D36.0	D48.7	D49.89
subclavicular	—	C77.3	—	D36.0	D48.7	D49.89
subinguinal	—	C77.4	—	D36.0	D48.7	D49.89
sublingual	—	C77.0	—	D36.0	D48.7	D49.89
submandibular	—	C77.0	—	D36.0	D48.7	D49.89
submaxillary	—	C77.0	—	D36.0	D48.7	D49.89
submental	—	C77.0	—	D36.0	D48.7	D49.89
subscapular	—	C77.3	—	D36.0	D48.7	D49.89
supraclavicular	—	C77.0	—	D36.0	D48.7	D49.89
thoracic	—	C77.1	—	D36.0	D48.7	D49.89
tibial	—	C77.4	—	D36.0	D48.7	D49.89
tracheal	—	C77.1	—	D36.0	D48.7	D49.89
tracheobronchial	—	C77.1	—	D36.0	D48.7	D49.89
upper limb	—	C77.3	—	D36.0	D48.7	D49.89
Virchow's	—	C77.0	—	D36.0	D48.7	D49.89
node — *see also Neoplasm, lymph gland*						
primary NEC	C96.9	—	—	—	—	—
vessel — *see also Neoplasm, connective tissue*	C49.9	C79.89	—	D21.9	D48.1	D49.2
Mackenrodt's ligament	C57.7	C79.82	D07.39	D28.7	D39.8	D49.5
malar	C41.0	C79.51	—	D16.4-	D48.0	D49.2
region — *see Neoplasm, cheek*						
mammary gland — *see Neoplasm, breast*						

	Malignant Primary	Malignant Secondary	Ca in situ	Benign	Uncertain Behavior	Unspecified Behavior
mandible	C41.1	C79.51	—	D16.5-	D48.0	D49.2
alveolar						
mucosa (carcinoma)	C03.1	C79.89	D00.03	D10.39	D37.09	D49.0
ridge or process	C41.1	C79.51	—	D16.5-	D48.0	D49.2
marrow (bone) NEC	C96.9	C79.52	—	—	D47.9	D49.89
mastectomy site (skin) — see also Neoplasm, breast, skin	C44.501	C79.2	—	—	—	—
specified as breast tissue	C50.8-	C79.81	—	—	—	—
mastoid (air cells) (antrum) (cavity)	C30.1	C78.39	D02.3	D14.0	D38.5	D49.1
bone or process	C41.0	C79.51	—	D16.4-	D48.0	D49.2
maxilla, maxillary (superior)	C41.0	C79.51	—	D16.4-	D48.0	D49.2
alveolar						
mucosa	C03.0	C79.89	D00.03	D10.39	D37.09	D49.0
ridge or process (carcinoma)	C41.0	C79.51	—	D16.4-	D48.0	D49.2
antrum	C31.0	C78.39	D02.3	D14.0	D38.5	D49.1
carcinoma	C03.0	C79.51	—	—	—	—
inferior — see Neoplasm, mandible						
sinus	C31.0	C78.39	D02.3	D14.0	D38.5	D49.1
meatus external (ear) — see also Neoplasm, skin, ear	C44.20-	C79.2	D04.2-	D23.2-	D48.5	D49.2
Meckel diverticulum, malignant	C17.3	C78.4	D01.49	D13.39	D37.2	D49.0
mediastinum, mediastinal	C38.3	C78.1	—	D15.2	D38.3	D49.89
anterior	C38.1	C78.1	—	D15.2	D38.3	D49.89
posterior	C38.2	C78.1	—	D15.2	D38.3	D49.89
medulla						
adrenal	C74.1-	C79.7-	D09.3	D35.0-	D44.1-	D49.7
oblongata	C71.7	C79.31	—	D33.1	D43.1	D49.6
meibomian gland	C44.10-	C79.2	D04.1-	D23.1-	D48.5	D49.2
basal cell carcinoma	C44.11-	—	—	—	—	—
specified type NEC	C44.19-	—	—	—	—	—
squamous cell carcinoma	C44.12-	—	—	—	—	—
melanoma — see Melanoma						
meninges	C70.9	C79.49	—	D32.9	D42.9	D49.7
brain	C70.0	C79.32	—	D32.0	D42.0	D49.7
cerebral	C70.0	C79.32	—	D32.0	D42.0	D49.7
crainial	C70.0	C79.32	—	D32.0	D42.0	D49.7
intracranial	C70.0	C79.32	—	D32.0	D42.0	D49.7
spinal (cord)	C70.1	C79.49	—	D32.1	D42.1	D49.7
meniscus, knee joint (lateral) (medial)	C40.2-	C79.51	—	D16.2-	D48.0	D49.2
Merkel cell — see Carcinoma, Merkel cell						
mesentery, mesenteric	C48.1	C78.6	—	D20.1	D48.4	D49.0
mesoappendix	C48.1	C78.6	—	D20.1	D48.4	D49.0
mesocolon	C48.1	C78.6	—	D20.1	D48.4	D49.0
mesopharynx — see Neoplasm, oropharynx						
mesosalpinx	C57.1	C79.82	D07.39	D28.2	D39.8	D49.5

	Malignant Primary	Malignant Secondary	Ca in situ	Benign	Uncertain Behavior	Unspecified Behavior
mesothelial tissue — *see Mesothelioma*						
mesothelioma — *see Mesothelioma*						
mesovarium	C57.1	C79.82	D07.39	D28.2	D39.8	D49.5
metacarpus (any bone)	C40.1-	C79.51	—	D16.1-	—	—
metastatic NEC — *see also Neoplasm, by site, secondary*	—	C79.9	—	—	—	—
metatarsus (any bone)	C40.3-	C79.51	—	D16.3-	—	—
midbrain	C71.7	C79.31	—	D33.1	D43.1	D49.6
milk duct — *see Neoplasm, breast*						
mons						
pubis	C51.9	C79.82	D07.1	D28.0	D39.8	D49.5
veneris	C51.9	C79.82	D07.1	D28.0	D39.8	D49.5
motor tract	C72.9	C79.49	—	D33.9	D43.9	D49.7
brain	C71.9	C79.31	—	D33.2	D43.2	D49.6
cauda equina	C72.1	C79.49	—	D33.4	D43.4	D49.7
spinal	C72.0	C79.49	—	D33.4	D43.4	D49.7
mouth	C06.9	C79.89	D00.00	D10.30	D37.09	D49.0
book-leaf	C06.89	C79.89	—	—	—	—
floor	C04.9	C79.89	D00.06	D10.2	D37.09	D49.0
anterior portion	C04.0	C79.89	D00.06	D10.2	D37.09	D49.0
lateral portion	C04.1	C79.89	D00.06	D10.2	D37.09	D49.0
overlapping lesion	C04.8	—	—	—	—	—
overlapping NEC	C06.80	—	—	—	—	—
roof	C05.9	C79.89	D00.00	D10.39	D37.09	D49.0
specified part NEC	C06.89	C79.89	D00.00	D10.39	D37.09	D49.0
vestibule	C06.1	C79.89	D00.00	D10.39	D37.09	D49.0
mucosa						
alveolar (ridge or process)	C03.9	C79.89	D00.03	D10.39	D37.09	D49.0
lower	C03.1	C79.89	D00.03	D10.39	D37.09	D49.0
upper	C03.0	C79.89	D00.03	D10.39	D37.09	D49.0
buccal	C06.0	C79.89	D00.02	D10.39	D37.09	D49.0
cheek	C06.0	C79.89	D00.02	D10.39	D37.09	D49.0
lip — *see Neoplasm, lip, internal*						
nasal	C30.0	C78.39	D02.3	D14.0	D38.5	D49.1
oral	C06.0	C79.89	D00.02	D10.39	D37.09	D49.0
Mullerian duct						
female	C57.7	C79.82	D07.39	D28.7	D39.8	D49.5
male	C63.7	C79.82	D07.69	D29.8	D40.8	D49.5
muscle — *see also Neoplasm, connective tissue*						
extraocular	C69.6-	C79.49	D09.2-	D31.6-	D48.7	D49.89
myocardium	C38.0	C79.89	—	D15.1	D48.7	D49.89
myometrium	C54.2	C79.82	D07.0	D26.1	D39.0	D49.5
myopericardium	C38.0	C79.89	—	D15.1	D48.7	D49.89
nabothian gland (follicle)	C53.0	C79.82	D06.0	D26.0	D39.0	D49.5

TABLE OF NEOPLASMS

	Malignant Primary	Malignant Secondary	Ca in situ	Benign	Uncertain Behavior	Unspecified Behavior
nail — see also Neoplasm, skin, limb	C44.90	C79.2	D04.9	D23.9	D48.5	D49.2
finger — see also Neoplasm, skin, limb, upper	C44.60-	C79.2	D04.6-	D23.6-	D48.5	D49.2
toe — see also Neoplasm, skin, limb, lower	C44.70-	C79.2	D04.7-	D23.7-	D48.5	D49.2
nares, naris (anterior) (posterior)	C30.0	C78.39	D02.3	D14.0	D38.5	D49.1
nasal — see Neoplasm, nose						
nasolabial groove — see also Neoplasm, skin, face	C44.309	C79.2	D04.39	D23.39	D48.5	D49.2
nasolacrimal duct	C69.5-	C79.49	D09.2-	D31.5-	D48.7	D49.89
nasopharynx, nasopharyngeal	C11.9	C79.89	D00.08	D10.6	D37.05	D49.0
floor	C11.3	C79.89	D00.08	D10.6	D37.05	D49.0
overlapping lesion	C11.8	—	—	—	—	—
roof	C11.0	C79.89	D00.08	D10.6	D37.05	D49.0
wall	C11.9	C79.89	D00.08	D10.6	D37.05	D49.0
anterior	C11.3	C79.89	D00.08	D10.6	D37.05	D49.0
lateral	C11.2	C79.89	D00.08	D10.6	D37.05	D49.0
posterior	C11.1	C79.89	D00.08	D10.6	D37.05	D49.0
superior	C11.0	C79.89	D00.08	D10.6	D37.05	D49.0
nates — see also Neoplasm, skin, trunk	C44.509	C79.2	D04.5	D23.5	D48.5	D49.2
neck NEC	C76.0	C79.89	D09.8	D36.7	D48.7	D49.89
skin	C44.40	—	—	—	—	—
basal cell carcinoma	C44.41	—	—	—	—	—
specified type NEC	C44.49	—	—	—	—	—
squamous cell carcinoma	C44.42	—	—	—	—	—
nerve (ganglion)	C47.9	C79.89	—	D36.10	D48.2	D49.2
abducens	C72.59	C79.49	—	D33.3	D43.3	D49.7
accessory (spinal)	C72.59	C79.49	—	D33.3	D43.3	D49.7
acoustic	C72.4-	C79.49	—	D33.3	D43.3	D49.7
auditory	C72.4-	C79.49	—	D33.3	D43.3	D49.7
autonomic NEC — see also Neoplasm, nerve, peripheral	C47.9	C79.89	—	D36.10	D48.2	D49.2
brachial	C47.1-	C79.89	—	D36.12	D48.2	D49.2
cranial	C72.50	C79.49	—	D33.3	D43.3	D49.7
specified NEC	C72.59	C79.49	—	D33.3	D43.3	D49.7
facial	C72.59	C79.49	—	D33.3	D43.3	D49.7
femoral	C47.2-	C79.89	—	D36.13	D48.2	D49.2
ganglion NEC — see also Neoplasm, nerve, peripheral	C47.9	C79.89	—	D36.10	D48.2	D49.2
glossopharyngeal	C72.59	C79.49	—	D33.3	D43.3	D49.7
hypoglossal	C72.59	C79.49	—	D33.3	D43.3	D49.7
intercostal	C47.3	C79.89	—	D36.14	D48.2	D49.2
lumbar	C47.6	C79.89	—	D36.17	D48.2	D49.2
median	C47.1-	C79.89	—	D36.12	D48.2	D49.2
obturator	C47.2-	C79.89	—	D36.13	D48.2	D49.2
oculomotor	C72.59	C79.49	—	D33.3	D43.3	D49.7
olfactory	C47.2-	C79.49	—	D33.3	D43.3	D49.7
optic	C72.3-	C79.49	—	D33.3	D43.3	D49.7
parasympathetic NEC	C47.9	C79.89	—	D36.10	D48.2	D49.2

◀ New ◀ Revised ~~deleted~~ Deleted

	Malignant Primary	Malignant Secondary	Ca in situ	Benign	Uncertain Behavior	Unspecified Behavior
nerve *(Continued)*						
peripheral NEC	C47.9	C79.89	—	D36.10	D48.2	D49.2
abdomen	C47.4	C79.89	—	D36.15	D48.2	D49.2
abdominal wall	C47.4	C79.89	—	D36.15	D48.2	D49.2
ankle	C47.2-	C79.89	—	D36.13	D48.2	D49.2
antecubital fossa or space	C47.1-	C79.89	—	D36.12	D48.2	D49.2
arm	C47.1-	C79.89	—	D36.12	D48.2	D49.2
auricle (ear)	C47.0	C79.89	—	D36.11	D48.2	D49.2
axilla	C47.3	C79.89	—	D36.12	D48.2	D49.2
back	C47.6	C79.89	—	D36.17	D48.2	D49.2
buttock	C47.5	C79.89	—	D36.16	D48.2	D49.2
calf	C47.2-	C79.89	—	D36.13	D48.2	D49.2
cervical region	C47.0	C79.89	—	D36.11	D48.2	D49.2
cheek	C47.0	C79.89	—	D36.11	D48.2	D49.2
chest (wall)	C47.3	C79.89	—	D36.14	D48.2	D49.2
chin	C47.0	C79.89	—	D36.11	D48.2	D49.2
ear (external)	C47.0	C79.89	—	D36.11	D48.2	D49.2
elbow	C47.1-	C79.89	—	D36.12	D48.2	D49.2
extrarectal	C47.5	C79.89	—	D36.16	D48.2	D49.2
extremity	C47.9	C79.89	—	D36.10	D48.2	D49.2
lower	C47.2-	C79.89	—	D36.13	D48.2	D49.2
upper	C47.1-	C79.89	—	D36.12	D48.2	D49.2
eyelid	C47.0	C79.89	—	D36.11	D48.2	D49.2
face	C47.0	C79.89	—	D36.11	D48.2	D49.2
finger	C47.1-	C79.89	—	D36.12	D48.2	D49.2
flank	C47.6	C79.89	—	D36.17	D48.2	D49.2
foot	C47.2-	C79.89	—	D36.13	D48.2	D49.2
forearm	C47.1-	C79.89	—	D36.12	D48.2	D49.2
forehead	C47.0	C79.89	—	D36.11	D48.2	D49.2
gluteal region	C47.5	C79.89	—	D36.16	D48.2	D49.2
groin	C47.5	C79.89	—	D36.16	D48.2	D49.2
hand	C47.1-	C79.89	—	D36.12	D48.2	D49.2
head	C47.0	C79.89	—	D36.11	D48.2	D49.2
heel	C47.2-	C79.89	—	D36.13	D48.2	D49.2
hip	C47.2-	C79.89	—	D36.13	D48.2	D49.2
infraclavicular region	C47.3	C79.89	—	D36.14	D48.2	D49.2
inguinal (canal) (region)	C47.5	C79.89	—	D36.16	D48.2	D49.2
intrathoracic	C47.3	C79.89	—	D36.14	D48.2	D49.2
ischiorectal fossa	C47.5	C79.89	—	D36.16	D48.2	D49.2
knee	C47.2-	C79.89	—	D36.13	D48.2	D49.2
leg	C47.2-	C79.89	—	D36.13	D48.2	D49.2
limb NEC	C47.9	C79.89	—	D36.10	D48.2	D49.2
lower	C47.2-	C79.89	—	D36.13	D48.2	D49.2
upper	C47.1-	C79.89	—	D36.12	D48.2	D49.2

	Malignant Primary	Malignant Secondary	Ca in situ	Benign	Uncertain Behavior	Unspecified Behavior
nerve *(Continued)*						
peripheral NEC *(Continued)*						
nates	C47.5	C79.89	—	D36.16	D48.2	D49.2
neck	C47.0	C79.89	—	D36.11	D48.2	D49.2
orbit	C69.6-	C79.49	—	D31.6-	D48.7	D49.2
pararectal	C47.5	C79.89	—	D36.16	D48.2	D49.2
paraurethral	C47.5	C79.89	—	D36.16	D48.2	D49.2
paravaginal	C47.5	C79.89	—	D36.16	D48.2	D49.2
pelvis (floor)	C47.5	C79.89	—	D36.16	D48.2	D49.2
pelvoabdominal	C47.8	C79.89	—	D36.17	D48.2	D49.2
perineum	C47.5	C79.89	—	D36.16	D48.2	D49.2
perirectal (tissue)	C47.5	C79.89	—	D36.16	D48.2	D49.2
periurethral (tissue)	C47.5	C79.89	—	D36.16	D48.2	D49.2
popliteal fossa or space	C47.2-	C79.89	—	D36.13	D48.2	D49.2
presacral	C47.5	C79.89	—	D36.16	D48.2	D49.2
pterygoid fossa	C47.0	C79.89	—	D36.11	D48.2	D49.2
rectovaginal septum or wall	C47.5	C79.89	—	D36.16	D48.2	D49.2
rectovesical	C47.5	C79.89	—	D36.16	D48.2	D49.2
sacrococcygeal region	C47.5	C79.89	—	D36.16	D48.2	D49.2
scalp	C47.0	C79.89	—	D36.11	D48.2	D49.2
scapular region	C47.3	C79.89	—	D36.14	D48.2	D49.2
shoulder	C47.1-	C79.89	—	D36.12	D48.2	D49.2
submental	C47.0	C79.89	—	D36.11	D48.2	D49.2
supraclavicular region	C47.0	C79.89	—	D36.11	D48.2	D49.2
temple	C47.0	C79.89	—	D36.11	D48.2	D49.2
temporal region	C47.0	C79.89	—	D36.11	D48.2	D49.2
thigh	C47.2-	C79.89	—	D36.13	D48.2	D49.2
thoracic (duct) (wall)	C47.3	C79.89	—	D36.14	D48.2	D49.2
thorax	C47.3	C79.89	—	D36.14	D48.2	D49.2
thumb	C47.1-	C79.89	—	D36.12	D48.2	D49.2
toe	C47.2-	C79.89	—	D36.13	D48.2	D49.2
trunk	C47.6	C79.89	—	D36.17	D48.2	D49.2
umbilicus	C47.4	C79.89	—	D36.15	D48.2	D49.2
vesicorectal	C47.5	C79.89	—	D36.16	D48.2	D49.2
wrist	C47.1-	C79.89	—	D36.12	D48.2	D49.2
radial	C47.1-	C79.89	—	D36.12	D48.2	D49.2
sacral	C47.5	C79.89	—	D36.16	D48.2	D49.2
sciatic	C47.2-	C79.89	—	D36.13	D48.2	D49.2
spinal NEC	C47.9	C79.89	—	D36.10	D48.2	D49.2
accessory	C72.59	C79.49	—	D33.3	D43.3	D49.7
sympathetic NEC — *see also Neoplasm, nerve, peripheral*	C47.9	C79.89	—	D36.10	D48.2	D49.2
trigeminal	C72.59	C79.49	—	D33.3	D43.3	D49.7
trochlear	C72.59	C79.49	—	D33.3	D43.3	D49.7

◀ New ◀ Revised ~~deleted~~ Deleted

	Malignant Primary	Malignant Secondary	Ca in situ	Benign	Uncertain Behavior	Unspecified Behavior
nerve *(Continued)*						
ulnar	C47.1-	C79.89	—	D36.12	D48.2	D49.2
vagus	C72.59	C79.49	—	D33.3	D43.3	D49.7
nervous system (central)	C72.9	C79.40	—	D33.9	D43.9	D49.7
autonomic — *see Neoplasm, nerve, peripheral*						
parasympathetic — *see Neoplasm, nerve, peripheral*						
specified site NEC	—	C79.49	—	D33.7	D43.8	—
sympathetic — *see Neoplasm, nerve, peripheral*						
nevus — *see Nevus*						
nipple	C50.0-	C79.81	D05.-	D24.-	—	—
nose, nasal	C76.0	C79.89	D09.8	D36.7	D48.7	D49.89
ala (external) (nasi) — *see also Neoplasm, nose, skin*	C44.301	C79.2	D04.39	D23.39	D48.5	D49.2
bone	C41.0	C79.51	—	D16.4-	D48.0	D49.2
cartilage	C30.0	C78.39	D02.3	D14.0	D38.5	D49.1
cavity	C30.0	C78.39	D02.3	D14.0	D38.5	D49.1
choana	C11.3	C79.89	D00.08	D10.6	D37.05	D49.0
external (skin) — *see also Neoplasm, nose, skin*	C44.301	C79.2	D04.39	D23.39	D48.5	D49.2
fossa	C30.0	C78.39	D02.3	D14.0	D38.5	D49.1
internal	C30.0	C78.39	D02.3	D14.0	D38.5	D49.1
mucosa	C30.0	C78.39	D02.3	D14.0	D38.5	D49.1
septum	C30.0	C78.39	D02.3	D14.0	D38.5	D49.1
posterior margin	C11.3	C79.89	D00.08	D10.6	D37.05	D49.0
sinus — *see Neoplasm, sinus*						
skin	C44.301	C79.2	D04.39	D23.39	D48.5	D49.2
basal cell carcinoma	C44.311	—	—	—	—	—
specified type NEC	C44.391	—	—	—	—	—
squamous cell carcinoma	C44.321	—	—	—	—	—
turbinate (mucosa)	C30.0	C78.39	D02.3	D14.0	D38.5	D49.1
bone	C41.0	C79.51	—	D16.4-	D48.0	D49.2
vestibule	C30.0	C78.39	D02.3	D14.0	D38.5	D49.1
nostril	C30.0	C78.39	D02.3	D14.0	D38.5	D49.1
nucleus pulposus	C41.2	C79.51	—	D16.6	D48.0	D49.2
occipital						
bone	C41.0	C79.51	—	D16.4-	D48.0	D49.2
lobe or pole, brain	C71.4	C79.31	—	D33.0	D43.0	D49.6
odontogenic — *see Neoplasm, jaw bone*						
olfactory nerve or bulb	C72.2-	C79.49	—	D33.3	D43.3	D49.7
olive (brain)	C71.7	C79.31	—	D33.1	D43.1	D49.6
omentum	C48.1	C78.6	—	D20.1	D48.4	D49.0
operculum (brain)	C71.0	C79.31	—	D33.0	D43.0	D49.6
optic nerve, chiasm, or tract	C72.3-	C79.49	—	D33.3	D43.3	D49.7
oral (cavity)	C06.9	C79.89	D00.00	D10.30	D37.09	D49.0
ill-defined	C14.8	C79.89	D00.00	D10.30	D37.09	D49.0
mucosa	C06.0	C79.89	D00.02	D10.39	D37.09	D49.0

	Malignant Primary	Malignant Secondary	Ca in situ	Benign	Uncertain Behavior	Unspecified Behavior
orbit	C69.6-	C79.49	D09.2-	D31.6-	D48.7	D49.89
autonomic nerve	C69.6-	C79.49	—	D31.6-	D48.7	D49.2
bone	C41.0	C79.51	—	D16.4-	D48.0	D49.2
eye	C69.6-	C79.49	D09.2-	D31.6-	D48.7	D49.89
peripheral nerves	C69.6-	C79.49	—	D31.6-	D48.7	D49.2
soft parts	C69.6-	C79.49	D09.2-	D31.6-	D48.7	D49.89
organ of Zuckerkandl	C75.5	C79.89	—	D35.6	D44.7	D49.7
oropharynx	C10.9	C79.89	D00.08	D10.5	D37.05	D49.0
branchial cleft (vestige)	C10.4	C79.89	D00.08	D10.5	D37.05	D49.0
junctional region	C10.8	C79.89	D00.08	D10.5	D37.05	D49.0
lateral wall	C10.2	C79.89	D00.08	D10.5	D37.05	D49.0
overlapping lesion	C10.8	—	—	—	—	—
pillars or fauces	C09.1	C79.89	D00.08	D10.5	D37.05	D49.0
posterior wall	C10.3	C79.89	D00.08	D10.5	D37.05	D49.0
vallecula	C10.0	C79.89	D00.08	D10.5	D37.05	D49.0
os						
external	C53.1	C79.82	D06.1	D26.0	D39.0	D49.5
internal	C53.0	C79.82	D06.0	D26.0	D39.0	D49.5
ovary	C56.-	C79.6-	D07.39	D27.-	D39.1-	D49.5
oviduct	C57.0-	C79.82	D07.39	D28.2	D39.8	D49.5
palate	C05.9	C79.89	D00.00	D10.39	D37.09	D49.0
hard	C05.0	C79.89	D00.05	D10.39	D37.09	D49.0
junction of hard and soft palate	C05.9	C79.89	D00.00	D10.39	D37.09	D49.0
overlapping lesions	C05.8	—	—	—	—	—
soft	C05.1	C79.89	D00.04	D10.39	D37.09	D49.0
nasopharyngeal surface	C11.3	C79.89	D00.08	D10.6	D37.05	D49.0
posterior surface	C11.3	C79.89	D00.08	D10.6	D37.05	D49.0
superior surface	C11.3	C79.89	D00.08	D10.6	D37.05	D49.0
palatoglossal arch	C09.1	C79.89	D00.00	D10.5	D37.09	D49.0
palatopharyngeal arch	C09.1	C79.89	D00.00	D10.5	D37.09	D49.0
pallium	C71.0	C79.31	—	D33.0	D43.0	D49.6
palpebra	C44.10-	C79.2	D04.1-	D23.1-	D48.5	D49.2
basal cell carcinoma	C44.11-	—	—	—	—	—
specified type NEC	C44.19-	—	—	—	—	—
squamous cell carcinoma	C44.12-	—	—	—	—	—
pancreas	C25.9	C78.89	D01.7	D13.6	D37.8	D49.0
body	C25.1	C78.89	D01.7	D13.6	D37.8	D49.0
duct (of Santorini) (of Wirsung)	C25.3	C78.89	D01.7	D13.6	D37.8	D49.0
ectopic tissue	C25.7	C78.89	—	D13.6	D37.8	D49.0
head	C25.0	C78.89	D01.7	D13.6	D37.8	D49.0
islet cells	C25.4	C78.89	D01.7	D13.7	D37.8	D49.0
neck	C25.7	C78.89	D01.7	D13.6	D37.8	D49.0
overlapping lesion	C25.8	—	—	—	—	—
tail	C25.2	C78.89	D01.7	D13.6	D37.8	D49.0

◀ New   ◀ Revised   ~~deleted~~ Deleted

	Malignant Primary	Malignant Secondary	Ca in situ	Benign	Uncertain Behavior	Unspecified Behavior
para-aortic body	C75.5	C79.89	—	D35.6	D44.7	D49.7
paraganglion NEC	C75.5	C79.89	—	D35.6	D44.7	D49.7
parametrium	C57.3	C79.82	—	D28.2	D39.8	D49.5
paranephric	C48.0	C78.6	—	D20.0	D48.3	D49.0
pararectal	C76.3	C79.89	—	D36.7	D48.7	D49.89
parasagittal (region)	C76.0	C79.89	D09.8	D36.7	D48.7	D49.89
parasellar	C72.9	C79.49	—	D33.9	D43.8	D49.7
parathyroid (gland)	C75.0	C79.89	D09.3	D35.1	D44.2	D49.7
paraurethral	C76.3	C79.89	—	D36.7	D48.7	D49.89
gland	C68.1	C79.19	D09.19	D30.8	D41.8	D49.5
paravaginal	C76.3	C79.89	—	D36.7	D48.7	D49.89
parenchyma, kidney	C64.-	C79.0-	D09.19	D30.0-	D41.0-	D49.5
parietal						
bone	C41.0	C79.51	—	D16.4-	D48.0	D49.2
lobe, brain	C71.3	C79.31	—	D33.0	D43.0	D49.6
paroophoron	C57.1	C79.82	D07.39	D28.2	D39.8	D49.5
parotid (duct) (gland)	C07	C79.89	D00.00	D11.0	D37.030	D49.0
parovarium	C57.1	C79.82	D07.39	D28.2	D39.8	D49.5
patella	C40.20	C79.51	—	—	—	—
peduncle, cerebral	C71.7	C79.31	—	D33.1	D43.1	D49.6
pelvirectal junction	C19	C78.5	D01.1	D12.7	D37.5	D49.0
pelvis, pelvic	C76.3	C79.89	D09.8	D36.7	D48.7	D49.89
bone	C41.4	C79.51	—	D16.8	D48.0	D49.2
floor	C76.3	C79.89	D09.8	D36.7	D48.7	D49.89
renal	C65.-	C79.0-	D09.19	D30.1-	D41.1-	D49.5
viscera	C76.3	C79.89	D09.8	D36.7	D48.7	D49.89
wall	C76.3	C79.89	D09.8	D36.7	D48.7	D49.89
pelvo-abdominal	C76.8	C79.89	D09.8	D36.7	D48.7	D49.89
penis	C60.9	C79.82	D07.4	D29.0	D40.8	D49.5
body	C60.2	C79.82	D07.4	D29.0	D40.8	D49.5
corpus (cavernosum)	C60.2	C79.82	D07.4	D29.0	D40.8	D49.5
glans	C60.1	C79.82	D07.4	D29.0	D40.8	D49.5
overlapping sites	C60.8	—	—	—	—	—
skin NEC	C60.9	C79.82	D07.4	D29.0	D40.8	D49.5
periadrenal (tissue)	C48.0	C78.6	—	D20.0	D48.3	D49.0
perianal (skin) — see also Neoplasm, anus, skin	C44.500	C79.2	D04.5	D23.5	D48.5	D49.2
pericardium	C38.0	C79.89	—	D15.1	D48.7	D49.89
perinephric	C48.0	C78.6	—	D20.0	D48.3	D49.0
perineum	C76.3	C79.89	D09.8	D36.7	D48.7	D49.89
periodontal tissue NEC	C03.9	C79.89	D00.03	D10.39	D37.09	D49.0
periosteum — see Neoplasm, bone						
peripancreatic	C48.0	C78.6	—	D20.0	D48.3	D49.0
peripheral nerve NEC	C47.9	C79.89	—	D36.10	D48.2	D49.2
perirectal (tissue)	C76.3	C79.89	—	D36.7	D48.7	D49.89

TABLE OF NEOPLASMS

	Malignant Primary	Malignant Secondary	Ca in situ	Benign	Uncertain Behavior	Unspecified Behavior
perirenal (tissue)	C48.0	C78.6	—	D20.0	D48.3	D49.0
peritoneum, peritoneal (cavity)	C48.2	C78.6	—	D20.1	D48.4	D49.0
benign mesothelial tissue — see Mesothelioma, benign						
overlapping lesion	C48.8	—	—	—	—	—
with digestive organs	C26.9	—	—	—	—	—
parietal	C48.1	C78.6	—	D20.1	D48.4	D49.0
pelvic	C48.1	C78.6	—	D20.1	D48.4	D49.0
specified part NEC	C48.1	C78.6	—	D20.1	D48.4	D49.0
peritonsillar (tissue)	C76.0	C79.89	D09.8	D36.7	D48.7	D49.89
periurethral tissue	C76.3	C79.89	—	D36.7	D48.7	D49.89
phalanges						
foot	C40.3-	C79.51	—	D16.3-	—	—
hand	C40.1-	C79.51	—	D16.1-	—	—
pharynx, pharyngeal	C14.0	C79.89	D00.08	D10.9	D37.05	D49.0
bursa	C11.1	C79.89	D00.08	D10.6	D37.05	D49.0
fornix	C11.3	C79.89	D00.08	D10.6	D37.05	D49.0
recess	C11.2	C79.89	D00.08	D10.6	D37.05	D49.0
region	C14.0	C79.89	D00.08	D10.9	D37.05	D49.0
tonsil	C11.1	C79.89	D00.08	D10.6	D37.05	D49.0
wall (lateral) (posterior)	C14.0	C79.89	D00.08	D10.9	D37.05	D49.0
pia mater	C70.9	C79.40	—	D32.9	D42.9	D49.7
cerebral	C70.0	C79.32	—	D32.0	D42.0	D49.7
cranial	C70.0	C79.32	—	D32.0	D42.0	D49.7
spinal	C70.1	C79.49	—	D32.1	D42.1	D49.7
pillars of fauces	C09.1	C79.89	D00.08	D10.5	D37.05	D49.0
pineal (body) (gland)	C75.3	C79.89	D09.3	D35.4	D44.5	D49.7
pinna (ear) NEC — see also Neoplasm, skin, ear	C44.20-	C79.2	D04.2-	D23.2-	D48.5	D49.2
piriform fossa or sinus	C12	C79.89	D00.08	D10.7	D37.05	D49.0
pituitary (body) (fossa) (gland) (lobe)	C75.1	C79.89	D09.3	D35.2	D44.3	D49.7
placenta	C58	C79.82	D07.0	D26.7	D39.2	D49.5
pleura, pleural (cavity)	C38.4	C78.2	—	D19.0	D38.2	D49.1
overlapping lesion with heart or mediastinum	C38.8	—	—	—	—	—
parietal	C38.4	C78.2	—	D19.0	D38.2	D49.1
visceral	C38.4	C78.2	—	D19.0	D38.2	D49.1
plexus						
brachial	C47.1-	C79.89	—	D36.12	D48.2	D49.2
cervical	C47.0	C79.89	—	D36.11	D48.2	D49.2
choroid	C71.5	C79.31	—	D33.0	D43.0	D49.6
lumbosacral	C47.5	C79.89	—	D36.16	D48.2	D49.2
sacral	C47.5	C79.89	—	D36.16	D48.2	D49.2
pluriendocrine	C75.8	C79.89	D09.3	D35.7	D44.9	D49.7
pole						
frontal	C71.1	C79.31	—	D33.0	D43.0	D49.6
occipital	C71.4	C79.31	—	D33.0	D43.0	D49.6

◀ New ◀◀ Revised ~~deleted~~ Deleted

	Malignant Primary	Malignant Secondary	Ca in situ	Benign	Uncertain Behavior	Unspecified Behavior
pons (varolii)	C71.7	C79.31	—	D33.1	D43.1	D49.6
popliteal fossa or space	C76.5-	C79.89	D04.7-	D36.7	D48.7	D49.89
postcricoid (region)	C13.0	C79.89	D00.08	D10.7	D37.05	D49.0
posterior fossa (cranial)	C71.9	C79.31	—	D33.2	D43.2	D49.6
postnasal space	C11.9	C79.89	D00.08	D10.6	D37.05	D49.0
prepuce	C60.0	C79.82	D07.4	D29.0	D40.8	D49.5
prepylorus	C16.4	C78.89	D00.2	D13.1	D37.1	D49.0
presacral (region)	C76.3	C79.89	—	D36.7	D48.7	D49.89
prostate (gland)	C61	C79.82	D07.5	D29.1	D40.0	D49.5
utricle	C68.0	C79.19	D09.19	D30.4	D41.3	D49.5
pterygoid fossa	C49.0	C79.89	—	D21.0	D48.1	D49.2
pubic bone	C41.4	C79.51	—	D16.8	D48.0	D49.2
pudenda, pudendum (femaie)	C51.9	C79.82	D07.1	D28.0	D39.8	D49.5
pulmonary—see also Neoplasm, lung	C34.9-	C78.0-	D02.2-	D14.3-	D38.1	D49.1
putamen	C71.0	C79.31		D33.0	D43.0	D49.6
pyloric						
antrum	C16.3	C78.89	D00.2	D13.1	D37.1	D49.0
canal	C16.4	C78.89	D00.2	D13.1	D37.1	D49.0
pylorus	C16.4	C78.89	D00.2	D13.1	D37.1	D49.0
pyramid (brain)	C71.7	C79.31	—	D33.1	D43.1	D49.6
pyriform fossa or sinus	C12	C79.89	D00.08	D10.7	D37.05	D49.0
radius (any part)	C40.0-	C79.51	—	D16.0-	—	—
Rathke's pouch	C75.1	C79.89	D09.3	D35.2	D44.3	D49.7
rectosigmoid (junction)	C19	C78.5	D01.1	D12.7	D37.5	D49.0
overlapping lesion with anus or rectum	C21.8	—	—	—	—	—
rectouterine pouch	C48.1	C78.6	—	D20.1	D48.4	D49.0
rectovaginal septum or wall	C76.3	C79.89	D09.8	D36.7	D48.7	D49.89
rectovesical septum	C76.3	C79.89	D09.8	D36.7	D48.7	D49.89
rectum (ampulla)	C20	C78.5	D01.2	D12.8	D37.5	D49.0
and colon	C19	C78.5	D01.1	D12.7	D37.5	D49.0
overlapping lesion with anus or rectosigmoid junction	C21.8	—	—	—	—	—
renal	C64.-	C79.0-	D09.19	D30.0-	D41.0-	D49.5
calyx	C65.-	C79.0-	D09.19	D30.1-	D41.1-	D49.5
hilus	C65.-	C79.0-	D09.19	D30.1-	D41.1-	D49.5
parenchyma	C64.-	C79.0-	D09.19	D30.0-	D41.0-	D49.5
pelvis	C65.-	C79.0-	D09.19	D30.1-	D41.1-	D49.5
respiratory						
organs or system NEC	C39.9	C78.30	D02.4	D14.4	D38.6	D49.1
tract NEC	C39.9	C78.30	D02.4	D14.4	D38.5	D49.1
upper	C39.0	C78.30	D02.4	D14.4	D38.5	D49.1
retina	C69.2-	C79.49	D09.2-	D31.2-	D48.7	D49.81
retrobulbar	C69.6-	C79.49	—	D31.6-	D48.7	D49.89
retrocecal	C48.0	C78.6	—	D20.0	D48.3	D49.0
retromolar (area) (triangle) (trigone)	C06.2	C79.89	D00.00	D10.39	D37.09	D49.0

TABLE OF NEOPLASMS

	Malignant Primary	Malignant Secondary	Ca in situ	Benign	Uncertain Behavior	Unspecified Behavior
retro-orbital	C76.0	C79.89	D09.8	D36.7	D48.7	D49.89
retroperitoneal (space) (tissue)	C48.0	C78.6	—	D20.0	D48.3	D49.0
retroperitoneum	C48.0	C78.6	—	D20.0	D48.3	D49.0
retropharyngeal	C14.0	C79.89	D00.08	D10.9	D37.05	D49.0
retrovesical (septum)	C76.3	C79.89	D09.8	D36.7	D48.7	D49.89
rhinencephalon	C71.0	C79.31	—	D33.0	D43.0	D49.6
rib	C41.3	C79.51	—	D16.7	D48.0	D49.2
Rosenmuller's fossa	C11.2	C79.89	D00.08	D10.6	D37.05	D49.0
round ligament	C57.2	C79.82	—	D28.2	D39.8	D49.5
sacrococcyx, sacrococcygeal	C41.4	C79.51	—	D16.8	D48.0	D49.2
region	C76.3	C79.89	D09.8	D36.7	D48.7	D49.89
sacrouterine ligament	C57.3	C79.82	—	D28.2	D39.8	D49.5
sacrum, sacral (vertebra)	C41.4	C79.51	—	D16.8	D48.0	D49.2
salivary gland or duct (major)	C08.9	C79.89	D00.00	D11.9	D37.039	D49.0
minor NEC	C06.9	C79.89	D00.00	D10.39	D37.04	D49.0
overlapping lesion	C08.9	—	—	—	—	—
parotid	C07	C79.89	D00.00	D11.0	D37.030	D49.0
pluriglandular	C08.9	C79.89	D00.00	D11.9	D37.039	D49.0
sublingual	C08.1	C79.89	D00.00	D11.7	D37.031	D49.0
submandibular	C08.0	C79.89	D00.00	D11.7	D37.032	D49.0
submaxillary	C08.0	C79.89	D00.00	D11.7	D37.032	D49.0
salpinx (uterine)	C57.0-	C79.82	D07.39	D28.2	D39.8	D49.5
Santorini's duct	C25.3	C78.89	D01.7	D13.6	D37.8	D49.0
scalp	C44.40	C79.2	D04.4	D23.4	D48.5	D49.2
basal cell carcinoma	C44.41	—	—	—	—	—
specified type NEC	C44.49	—	—	—	—	—
squamous cell carcinoma	C44.42	—	—	—	—	—
scapula (any part)	C40.0-	C79.51	—	D16.0-	—	—
scapular region	C76.1	C79.89	D09.8	D36.7	D48.7	D49.89
scar NEC — see also Neoplasm, skin, by site	C44.90	C79.2	D04.9	D23.9	D48.5	D49.2
sciatic nerve	C47.2-	C79.89	—	D36.13	D48.2	D49.2
sclera	C69.4-	C79.49	D09.2-	D31.4-	D48.7	D49.89
scrotum (skin)	C63.2	C79.82	D07.61	D29.4	D40.8	D49.5
sebaceous gland — see Neoplasm, skin						
sella turcica	C75.1	C79.89	D09.3	D35.2	D44.3	D49.7
bone	C41.0	C79.51	—	D16.4-	D48.0	D49.2
semilunar cartilage (knee)	C40.2-	C79.51	—	D16.2-	D48.0	D49.2
seminal vesicle	C63.7	C79.82	D07.69	D29.8	D40.8	D49.5
septum						
nasal	C30.0	C78.39	D02.3	D14.0	D38.5	D49.1
posterior margin	C11.3	C79.89	D00.08	D10.6	D37.05	D49.0
rectovaginal	C76.3	C79.89	D09.8	D36.7	D48.7	D49.89
rectovesical	C76.3	C79.89	D09.8	D36.7	D48.7	D49.89

◀ New ◀▦ Revised ~~deleted~~ Deleted

	Malignant Primary	Malignant Secondary	Ca in situ	Benign	Uncertain Behavior	Unspecified Behavior
septum *(Continued)*						
urethrovaginal	C57.9	C79.82	D07.30	D28.9	D39.9	D49.5
vesicovaginal	C57.9	C79.82	D07.30	D28.9	D39.9	D49.5
shoulder NEC	C76.4-	C79.89	D04.6-	D36.7	D48.7	D49.89
sigmoid flexure (lower) (upper)	C18.7	C78.5	D01.0	D12.5	D37.4	D49.0
sinus (accessory)	C31.9	C78.39	D02.3	D14.0	D38.5	D49.1
bone (any)	C41.0	C79.51	—	D16.4-	D48.0	D49.2
ethmoidal	C31.1	C78.39	D02.3	D14.0	D38.5	D49.1
frontal	C31.2	C78.39	D02.3	D14.0	D38.5	D49.1
maxillary	C31.0	C78.39	D02.3	D14.0	D38.5	D49.1
nasal, paranasal NEC	C31.9	C78.39	D02.3	D14.0	D38.5	D49.1
overlapping lesion	C31.8	—	—	—	—	—
pyriform	C12	C79.89	D00.08	D10.7	D37.05	D49.0
sphenoid	C31.3	C78.39	D02.3	D14.0	D38.5	D49.1
skeleton, skeletal NEC	C41.9	C79.51	—	D16.9-	D48.0	D49.2
Skene's gland	C68.1	C79.19	D09.19	D30.8	D41.8	D49.5
skin NOS	C44.90	C79.2	D04.9	D23.9	D48.5	D49.2
abdominal wall	C44.509	C79.2	D04.5	D23.5	D48.5	D49.2
basal cell carcinoma	C44.519	—	—	—	—	—
specified type NEC	C44.599	—	—	—	—	—
squamous cell carcinoma	C44.529	—	—	—	—	—
ala nasi — *see also Neoplasm, nose, skin*	C44.301	C79.2	D04.39	D23.39	D48.5	D49.2
ankle — *see also Neoplasm, skin, limb, lower*	C44.70-	C79.2	D04.7-	D23.7-	D48.5	D49.2
antecubital space — *see also Neoplasm, skin, limb, upper*	C44.60-	C79.2	D04.6-	D23.6-	D48.5	D49.2
anus	C44.500	C79.2	D04.5	D23.5	D48.5	D49.2
basal cell carcinoma	C44.510	—	—	—	—	—
specified type NEC	C44.590	—	—	—	—	—
squamous cell carcinoma	C44.520	—	—	—	—	—
arm — *see also Neoplasm, skin, limb, upper*	C44.60-	C79.2	D04.6-	D23.6-	D48.5	D49.2
auditory canal (external) — *see also Neoplasm, skin, ear*	C44.20-	C79.2	D04.2-	D23.2-	D48.5	D49.2
auricle (ear) — *see also Neoplasm, skin, ear*	C44.20-	C79.2	D04.2-	D23.2-	D48.5	D49.2
auricular canal (external) — *see also Neoplasm, skin, ear*	C44.20-	C79.2	D04.2-	D23.2-	D48.5	D49.2
axilla, axillary fold — *see also Neoplasm, skin, trunk*	C44.509	C79.2	D04.5	D23.5	D48.5	D49.2
back — *see also Neoplasm, skin, trunk*	C44.509	C79.2	D04.5	D23.5	D48.5	D49.2
basal cell carcinoma	C44.91					
breast	C44.501	C79.2	D04.5	D23.5	D48.5	D49.2
basal cell carcinoma	C44.511	—	—	—	—	—
specified type NEC	C44.591	—	—	—	—	—
squamous cell carcinoma	C44.521	—	—	—	—	—
brow — *see also Neoplasm, skin, face*	C44.309	C79.2	D04.39	D23.39	D48.5	D49.2
buttock — *see also Neoplasm, skin, trunk*	C44.509	C79.2	D04.5	D23.5	D48.5	D49.2
calf — *see also Neoplasm, skin, limb, lower*	C44.70-	C79.2	D04.7-	D23.7-	D48.5	D49.2

TABLE OF NEOPLASMS

	Malignant Primary	Malignant Secondary	Ca in situ	Benign	Uncertain Behavior	Unspecified Behavior
skin NOS *(Continued)*						
canthus (eye) (inner) (outer)	C44.10-	C79.2	D04.1-	D23.1-	D48.5	D49.2
basal cell carcinoma	C44.11-	—	—	—	—	—
specified type NEC	C44.19-	—	—	—	—	—
squamous cell carcinoma	C44.12-	—	—	—	—	—
cervical region — *see also Neoplasm, skin, neck*	C44.40	C79.2	D04.4	D23.4	D48.5	D49.2
cheek (external) — *see also Neoplasm, skin, face*	C44.309	C79.2	D04.39	D23.39	D48.5	D49.2
chest (wall) — *see also Neoplasm, skin, trunk*	C44.509	C79.2	D04.5	D23.5	D48.5	D49.2
chin — *see also Neoplasm, skin, face*	C44.309	C79.2	D04.39	D23.39	D48.5	D49.2
clavicular area — *see also Neoplasm, skin, trunk*	C44.509	C79.2	D04.5	D23.5	D48.5	D49.2
clitoris	C51.2	C79.82	D07.1	D28.0	D39.8	D49.5
columnella — *see also Neoplasm, skin, face*	C44.309	C79.2	D04.39	D23.39	D48.5	D49.2
concha — *see also Neoplasm, skin, ear*	C44.20-	C79.2	D04.2-	D23.2-	D48.5	D49.2
ear (external)	C44.20-	C79.2	D04.2-	D23.2-	D48.5	D49.2
basal cell carcinoma	C44.21-	—	—	—	—	—
specified type NEC	C44.29-	—	—	—	—	—
squamous cell carcinoma	C44.22-	—	—	—	—	—
elbow — *see also Neoplasm, skin, limb, upper*	C44.60-	C79.2	D04.6-	D23.6-	D48.5	D49.2
eyebrow — *see also Neoplasm, skin, face*	C44.309	C79.2	D04.39	D23.39	D48.5	D49.2
eyelid	C44.10-	C79.2	D04.1-	D23.1-	D48.5	D49.2
basal cell carcinoma	C44.11-	—	—	—	—	—
specified type NEC	C44.19-	—	—	—	—	—
squamous cell carcinoma	C44.12-	—	—	—	—	—
face NOS	C44.300	C79.2	D04.30	D23.30	D48.5	D49.2
basal cell carcinoma	C44.310	—	—	—	—	—
specified type NEC	C44.390	—	—	—	—	—
squamous cell carcinoma	C44.320	—	—	—	—	—
female genital organs (external)	C51.9	C79.82	D07.1	D28.0	D39.8	D49.5
clitoris	C51.2	C79.82	D07.1	D28.0	D39.8	D49.5
labium NEC	C51.9	C79.82	D07.1	D28.0	D39.8	D49.5
majus	C51.0	C79.82	D07.1	D28.0	D39.8	D49.5
minus	C51.1	C79.82	D07.1	D28.0	D39.8	D49.5
pudendum	C51.9	C79.82	D07.1	D28.0	D39.8	D49.5
vulva	C51.9	C79.82	D07.1	D28.0	D39.8	D49.5
finger — *see also Neoplasm, skin, limb, upper*	C44.60-	C79.2	D04.6-	D23.6-	D48.5	D49.2
flank — *see also Neoplasm, skin, trunk*	C44.509	C79.2	D04.5	D23.5	D48.5	D49.2
foot — *see also Neoplasm, skin, limb, lower*	C44.70-	C79.2	D04.7-	D23.7-	D48.5	D49.2
forearm — *see also Neoplasm, skin, limb, upper*	C44.60-	C79.2	D04.6-	D23.6-	D48.5	D49.2
forehead — *see also Neoplasm, skin, face*	C44.309	C79.2	D04.39	D23.39	D48.5	D49.2
glabella — *see also Neoplasm, skin, face*	C44.309	C79.2	D04.39	D23.39	D48.5	D49.2
gluteal region — *see also Neoplasm, skin, trunk*	C44.509	C79.2	D04.5	D23.5	D48.5	D49.2
groin — *see also Neoplasm, skin, trunk*	C44.509	C79.2	D04.5	D23.5	D48.5	D49.2
hand — *see also Neoplasm, skin, limb, upper*	C44.60-	C79.2	D04.6-	D23.6-	D48.5	D49.2

◀ New　◀▥ Revised　~~deleted~~ Deleted

	Malignant Primary	Malignant Secondary	Ca in situ	Benign	Uncertain Behavior	Unspecified Behavior
skin NOS *(Continued)*						
head NEC — *see also Neoplasm, skin, scalp*	C44.40	C79.2	D04.4	D23.4	D48.5	D49.2
heel — *see also Neoplasm, skin, limb, lower*	C44.70-	C79.2	D04.7-	D23.7-	D48.5	D49.2
helix — *see also Neoplasm, skin, ear*	C44.20-	C79.2	D04.2-	D23.2-	D48.5	D49.2
hip — *see also Neoplasm, skin, limb, lower*	C44.70-	C79.2	D04.7-	D23.7-	D48.5	D49.2
infraclavicular region — *see also Neoplasm, skin, trunk*	C44.509	C79.2	D04.5	D23.5	D48.5	D49.2
inguinal region — *see also Neoplasm, skin, trunk*	C44.509	C79.2	D04.5	D23.5	D48.5	D49.2
jaw — *see also Neoplasm, skin, face*	C44.309	C79.2	D04.39	D23.39	D48.5	D49.2
Kaposi's sarcoma — *see Kaposi's, sarcoma, skin*						
knee — *see also Neoplasm, skin, limb, lower*	C44.70-	C79.2	D04.7-	D23.7-	D48.5	D49.2
labia						
majora	C51.0	C79.82	D07.1	D28.0	D39.8	D49.5
minora	C51.1	C79.82	D07.1	D28.0	D39.8	D49.5
leg — *see also Neoplasm, skin, limb, lower*	C44.70-	C79.2	D04.7-	D23.7-	D48.5	D49.2
lid (lower) (upper)	C44.10-	C79.2	D04.1-	D23.1-	D48.5	D49.2
basal cell carcinoma	C44.11-	—	—	—	—	—
specified type NEC	C44.19-	—	—	—	—	—
squamous cell carcinoma	C44.12-	—	—	—	—	—
limb NEC	C44.90	C79.2	D04.9	D23.9	D48.5	D49.2
basal cell carcinoma	C44.91					
lower	C44.70-	C79.2	D04.7-	D23.7-	D48.5	D49.2
basal cell carcinoma	C44.71-	—	—	—	—	—
specified type NEC	C44.79-	—	—	—	—	—
squamous cell carcinoma	C44.72-	—	—	—	—	—
upper	C44.60-	C79.2	D04.6-	D23.6-	D48.5	D49.2
basal cell carcinoma	C44.61-	—	—	—	—	—
specified type NEC	C44.69-	—	—	—	—	—
squamous cell carcinoma	C44.62-	—	—	—	—	—
lip (lower) (upper)	C44.00	C79.2	D04.0	D23.0	D48.5	D49.2
basal cell carcinoma	C44.01	—	—	—	—	—
specified type NEC	C44.09	—	—	—	—	—
squamous cell carcinoma	C44.02	—	—	—	—	—
male genital organs	C63.9	C79.82	D07.60	D29.9	D40.8	D49.5
penis	C60.9	C79.82	D07.4	D29.0	D40.8	D49.5
prepuce	C60.0	C79.82	D07.4	D29.0	D40.8	D49.5
scrotum	C63.2	C79.82	D07.61	D29.4	D40.8	D49.5
mastectomy site (skin) — *see also Neoplasm, skin, breast*	C44.501	C79.2	—	—	—	—
specified as breast tissue	C50.8-	C79.81	—	—	—	—
meatus, acoustic (external) — *see also Neoplasm, skin, ear*	C44.20-	C79.2	D04.2-	D23.2-	D48.5	D49.2
melanotic — *see Melanoma*						
Merkel cell — *see Carcinoma, Merkel cell*						
nates — *see also Neoplasm, skin, trunk*	C44.509	C79.2	D04.5	D23.5	D48.5	D49.2

◀ New   ◀▥ Revised   ~~deleted~~ Deleted

	Malignant Primary	Malignant Secondary	Ca in situ	Benign	Uncertain Behavior	Unspecified Behavior
skin NOS *(Continued)*						
neck	C44.40	C79.2	D04.4	D23.4	D48.5	D49.2
basal cell carcinoma	C44.41	—	—	—	—	—
specified type NEC	C44.49	—	—	—	—	—
squamous cell carcinoma	C44.42	—	—	—	—	—
nevus — *see Nevus, skin*						
nose (external) — *see also Neoplasm, nose, skin*	C44.301	C79.2	D04.39	D23.39	D48.5	D49.2
overlapping lesion	C44.80	—	—	—	—	—
basal cell carcinoma	C44.81	—	—	—	—	—
specified type NEC	C44.89	—	—	—	—	—
squamous cell carcinoma	C44.82	—	—	—	—	—
palm — *see also Neoplasm, skin, limb, upper*	C44.60-	C79.2	D04.6-	D23.6-	D48.5	D49.2
palpebra	C44.10-	C79.2	D04.1-	D23.1-	D48.5	D49.2
basal cell carcinoma	C44.11-	—	—	—	—	—
specified type NEC	C44.19-	—	—	—	—	—
squamous cell carcinoma	C44.12-	—	—	—	—	—
penis NEC	C60.9	C79.82	D07.4	D29.0	D40.8	D49.5
perianal — *see also Neoplasm, skin, anus*	C44.500	C79.2	D04.5	D23.5	D48.5	D49.2
perineum — *see also Neoplasm, skin, anus*	C44.500	C79.2	D04.5	D23.5	D48.5	D49.2
pinna — *see also Neoplasm, skin, ear*	C44.20-	C79.2	D04.2-	D23.2-	D48.5	D49.2
plantar — *see also Neoplasm, skin, limb, lower*	C44.70-	C79.2	D04.7-	D23.7-	D48.5	D49.2
popliteal fossa or space — *see also Neoplasm, skin, limb, lower*	C44.70-	C79.2	D04.7-	D23.7-	D48.5	D49.2
prepuce	C60.0	C79.82	D07.4	D29.0	D40.8	D49.5
pubes — *see also Neoplasm, skin, trunk*	C44.509	C79.2	D04.5	D23.5	D48.5	D49.2
sacrococcygeal region — *see also Neoplasm, skin, trunk*	C44.509	C79.2	D04.5	D23.5	D48.5	D49.2
scalp	C44.40	C79.2	D04.4	D23.4	D48.5	D49.2
basal cell carcinoma	C44.41	—	—	—	—	—
specified type NEC	C44.49	—	—	—	—	—
squamous cell carcinoma	C44.42	—	—	—	—	—
scapular region — *see also Neoplasm, skin, trunk*	C44.509	C79.2	D04.5	D23.5	D48.5	D49.2
scrotum	C63.2	C79.82	D07.61	D29.4	D40.8	D49.5
shoulder — *see also Neoplasm, skin, limb, upper*	C44.60-	C79.2	D04.6-	D23.6-	D48.5	D49.2
sole (foot) — *see also Neoplasm, skin, limb, lower*	C44.70-	C79.2	D04.7-	D23.7-	D48.5	D49.2
specified sites NEC	C44.80	C79.2	D04.8	D23.9	D48.5	D49.2
basal cell carcinoma	C44.81	—	—	—	—	—
specified type NEC	C44.89	—	—	—	—	—
squamous cell carcinoma	C44.82	—	—	—	—	—
specified type NEC	C44.99	—	—	—	—	—
squamous cell carcinoma	C44.92	—	—	—	—	—
submammary fold — *see also Neoplasm, skin, trunk*	C44.509	C79.2	D04.5	D23.5	D48.5	D49.2
supraclavicular region — *see also Neoplasm, skin, neck*	C44.40	C79.2	D04.4	D23.4	D48.5	D49.2
temple — *see also Neoplasm, skin, face*	C44.309	C79.2	D04.39	D23.39	D48.5	D49.2
thigh — *see also Neoplasm, skin, limb, lower*	C44.70-	C79.2	D04.7-	D23.7-	D48.5	D49.2
thoracic wall — *see also Neoplasm, skin, trunk*	C44.509	C79.2	D04.5	D23.5	D48.5	D49.2

◀ New ◀▥▥ Revised ~~deleted~~ Deleted

	Malignant Primary	Malignant Secondary	Ca in situ	Benign	Uncertain Behavior	Unspecified Behavior
skin NOS *(Continued)*						
thumb — *see also Neoplasm, skin, limb, upper*	C44.60-	C79.2	D04.6-	D23.6-	D48.5	D49.2
toe — *see also Neoplasm, skin, limb, lower*	C44.70-	C79.2	D04.7-	D23.7-	D48.5	D49.2
tragus — *see also Neoplasm, skin, ear*	C44.20-	C79.2	D04.2-	D23.2-	D48.5	D49.2
trunk	C44.509	C79.2	D04.5	D23.5	D48.5	D49.2
basal cell carcinoma	C44.519	—	—	—	—	—
specified type NEC	C44.599	—	—	—	—	—
squamous cell carcinoma	C44.529	—	—	—	—	—
umbilicus — *see also Neoplasm, skin, trunk*	C44.509	C79.2	D04.5	D23.5	D48.5	D49.2
vulva	C51.9	C79.82	D07.1	D28.0	D39.8	D49.5
overlapping lesion	C51.8	—	—	—	—	—
wrist — *see also Neoplasm, skin, limb, upper*	C44.60-	C79.2	D04.6-	D23.6-	D48.5	D49.2
skull	C41.0	C79.51	—	D16.4-	D48.0	D49.2
soft parts or tissues — *see Neoplasm, connective tissue*						
specified site NEC	C76.8	C79.89	D09.8	D36.7	D48.7	D49.89
spermatic cord	C63.1-	C79.82	D07.69	D29.8	D40.8	D49.5
sphenoid	C31.3	C78.39	D02.3	D14.0	D38.5	D49.1
bone	C41.0	C79.51	—	D16.4-	D48.0	D49.2
sinus	C31.3	C78.39	D02.3	D14.0	D38.5	D49.1
sphincter						
anal	C21.1	C78.5	D01.3	D12.9	D37.8	D49.0
of Oddi	C24.0	C78.89	D01.5	D13.5	D37.6	D49.0
spine, spinal (column)	C41.2	C79.51	—	D16.6	D48.0	D49.2
bulb	C71.7	C79.31	—	D33.1	D43.1	D49.6
coccyx	C41.4	C79.51	—	D16.8	D48.0	D49.2
cord (cervical) (lumbar) (sacral) (thoracic)	C72.0	C79.49	—	D33.4	D43.4	D49.7
dura mater	C70.1	C79.49	—	D32.1	D42.1	D49.7
lumbosacral	C41.2	C79.51	—	D16.6	D48.0	D49.2
marrow NEC	C96.9	C79.52	—	—	D47.9	D49.89
membrane	C70.1	C79.49	—	D32.1	D42.1	D49.7
meninges	C70.1	C79.49	—	D32.1	D42.1	D49.7
nerve (root)	C47.9	C79.89	—	D36.10	D48.2	D49.2
pia mater	C70.1	C79.49	—	D32.1	D42.1	D49.7
root	C47.9	C79.89	—	D36.10	D48.2	D49.2
sacrum	C41.4	C79.51	—	D16.8	D48.0	D49.2
spleen, splenic NEC	C26.1	C78.89	D01.7	D13.9	D37.8	D49.0
flexure (colon)	C18.5	C78.5	D01.0	D12.3	D37.4	D49.0
stem, brain	C71.7	C79.31	—	D33.1	D43.1	D49.6
Stensen's duct	C07	C79.89	D00.00	D11.0	D37.030	D49.0
sternum	C41.3	C79.51	—	D16.7	D48.0	D49.2
stomach	C16.9	C78.89	D00.2	D13.1	D37.1	D49.0
antrum (pyloric)	C16.3	C78.89	D00.2	D13.1	D37.1	D49.0
body	C16.2	C78.89	D00.2	D13.1	D37.1	D49.0
cardia	C16.0	C78.89	D00.2	D13.1	D37.1	D49.0

	Malignant Primary	Malignant Secondary	Ca in situ	Benign	Uncertain Behavior	Unspecified Behavior
stomach *(Continued)*						
cardiac orifice	C16.0	C78.89	D00.2	D13.1	D37.1	D49.0
corpus	C16.2	C78.89	D00.2	D13.1	D37.1	D49.0
fundus	C16.1	C78.89	D00.2	D13.1	D37.1	D49.0
greater curvature NEC	C16.6	C78.89	D00.2	D13.1	D37.1	D49.0
lesser curvature NEC	C16.5	C78.89	D00.2	D13.1	D37.1	D49.0
overlapping lesion	C16.8	—	—	—	—	—
prepylorus	C16.4	C78.89	D00.2	D13.1	D37.1	D49.0
pylorus	C16.4	C78.89	D00.2	D13.1	D37.1	D49.0
wall NEC	C16.9	C78.89	D00.2	D13.1	D37.1	D49.0
anterior NEC	C16.8	C78.89	D00.2	D13.1	D37.1	D49.0
posterior NEC	C16.8	C78.89	D00.2	D13.1	D37.1	D49.0
stroma, endometrial	C54.1	C79.82	D07.0	D26.1	D39.0	D49.5
stump, cervical	C53.8	C79.82	D06.7	D26.0	D39.0	D49.5
subcutaneous (nodule) (tissue) NEC — *see Neoplasm, connective tissue*						
subdural	C70.9	C79.32	—	D32.9	D42.9	D49.7
subglottis, subglottic	C32.2	C78.39	D02.0	D14.1	D38.0	D49.1
sublingual	C04.9	C79.89	D00.06	D10.2	D37.09	D49.0
gland or duct	C08.1	C79.89	D00.00	D11.7	D37.031	D49.0
submandibular gland	C08.0	C79.89	D00.00	D11.7	D37.032	D49.0
submaxillary gland or duct	C08.0	C79.89	D00.00	D11.7	D37.032	D49.0
submental	C76.0	C79.89	D09.8	D36.7	D48.7	D49.89
subpleural	C34.9-	C78.0-	D02.2-	D14.3-	D38.1	D49.1
substernal	C38.1	C78.1	—	D15.2	D38.3	D49.89
sudoriferous, sudoriparous gland, site unspecified	C44.90	C79.2	D04.9	D23.9	D48.5	D49.2
specified site — *see Neoplasm, skin*						
supraclavicular region	C76.0	C79.89	D09.8	D36.7	D48.7	D49.89
supraglottis	C32.1	C78.39	D02.0	D14.1	D38.0	D49.1
suprarenal	C74.9-	C79.7-	D09.3	D35.0-	D44.1-	D49.7
capsule	C74.9-	C79.7-	D09.3	D35.0-	D44.1-	D49.7
cortex	C74.0-	C79.7-	D09.3	D35.0-	D44.1-	D49.7
gland	C74.9-	C79.7-	D09.3	D35.0-	D44.1-	D49.7
medulla	C74.1-	C79.7-	D09.3	D35.0-	D44.1-	D49.7
suprasellar (region)	C71.9	C79.31	—	D33.2	D43.2	D49.6
supratentorial (brain) NEC	C71.0	C79.31	—	D33.0	D43.0	D49.6
sweat gland (apocrine) (eccrine), site unspecified	C44.90	C79.2	D04.9	D23.9	D48.5	D49.2
specified site — *see Neoplasm, skin*						
sympathetic nerve or nervous system NEC	C47.9	C79.89	—	D36.10	D48.2	D49.2
symphysis pubis	C41.4	C79.51	—	D16.8	D48.0	D49.2
synovial membrane — *see Neoplasm, connective tissue*						
tapetum, brain	C71.8	C79.31	—	D33.2	D43.2	D49.6
tarsus (any bone)	C40.3-	C79.51	—	D16.3-	—	—
temple (skin) — *see also Neoplasm, skin, face*	C44.309	C79.2	D04.39	D23.39	D48.5	D49.2

◀ New   ◀ⁱⁱⁱ Revised   ~~deleted~~ Deleted

	Malignant Primary	Malignant Secondary	Ca in situ	Benign	Uncertain Behavior	Unspecified Behavior
temporal						
bone	C41.0	C79.51	—	D16.4-	D48.0	D49.2
lobe or pole	C71.2	C79.31	—	D33.0	D43.0	D49.6
region	C76.0	C79.89	D09.8	D36.7	D48.7	D49.89
skin — see also Neoplasm, skin, face	C44.309	C79.2	D04.39	D23.39	D48.5	D49.2
tendon (sheath) — see Neoplasm, connective tissue						
tentorium (cerebelli)	C70.0	C79.32	—	D32.0	D42.0	D49.7
testis, testes	C62.9-	C79.82	D07.69	D29.2-	D40.1-	D49.5
descended	C62.1-	C79.82	D07.69	D29.2-	D40.1-	D49.5
ectopic	C62.0-	C79.82	D07.69	D29.2-	D40.1-	D49.5
retained	C62.0-	C79.82	D07.69	D29.2-	D40.1-	D49.5
scrotal	C62.1-	C79.82	D07.69	D29.2-	D40.1-	D49.5
undescended	C62.0-	C79.82	D07.69	D29.2-	D40.1-	D49.5
unspecified whether descended or undescended	C62.9-	C79.82	D07.69	D29.2-	D40.1-	D49.5
thalamus	C71.0	C79.31	—	D33.0	D43.0	D49.6
thigh NEC	C76.5-	C79.89	D04.7-	D36.7	D48.7	D49.89
thorax, thoracic (cavity) (organs NEC)	C76.1	C79.89	D09.8	D36.7	D48.7	D49.89
duct	C49.3	C79.89	—	D21.3	D48.1	D49.2
wall NEC	C76.1	C79.89	D09.8	D36.7	D48.7	D49.89
throat	C14.0	C79.89	D00.08	D10.9	D37.05	D49.0
thumb NEC	C76.4-	C79.89	D04.6-	D36.7	D48.7	D49.89
thymus (gland)	C37	C79.89	D09.3	D15.0	D38.4	D49.89
thyroglossal duct	C73	C79.89	D09.3	D34	D44.0	D49.7
thyroid (gland)	C73	C79.89	D09.3	D34	D44.0	D49.7
cartilage	C32.3	C78.39	D02.0	D14.1	D38.0	D49.1
tibia (any part)	C40.2-	C79.51	—	D16.2-	—	—
toe NEC	C76.5-	C79.89	D04.7-	D36.7	D48.7	D49.89
tongue	C02.9	C79.89	D00.07	D10.1	D37.02	D49.0
anterior (two-thirds) NEC	C02.3	C79.89	D00.07	D10.1	D37.02	D49.0
dorsal surface	C02.0	C79.89	D00.07	D10.1	D37.02	D49.0
ventral surface	C02.2	C79.89	D00.07	D10.1	D37.02	D49.0
base (dorsal surface)	C01	C79.89	D00.07	D10.1	D37.02	D49.0
border (lateral)	C02.1	C79.89	D00.07	D10.1	D37.02	D49.0
dorsal surface NEC	C02.0	C79.89	D00.07	D10.1	D37.02	D49.0
fixed part NEC	C01	C79.89	D00.07	D10.1	D37.02	D49.0
foreamen cecum	C02.0	C79.89	D00.07	D10.1	D37.02	D49.0
frenulum linguae	C02.2	C79.89	D00.07	D10.1	D37.02	D49.0
junctional zone	C02.8	C79.89	D00.07	D10.1	D37.02	D49.0
margin (lateral)	C02.1	C79.89	D00.07	D10.1	D37.02	D49.0
midline NEC	C02.0	C79.89	D00.07	D10.1	D37.02	D49.0
mobile part NEC	C02.3	C79.89	D00.07	D10.1	D37.02	D49.0
overlapping lesion	C02.8	—	—	—	—	—
posterior (third)	C01	C79.89	D00.07	D10.1	D37.02	D49.0

TABLE OF NEOPLASMS

	Malignant Primary	Malignant Secondary	Ca in situ	Benign	Uncertain Behavior	Unspecified Behavior
tongue *(Continued)*						
root	C01	C79.89	D00.07	D10.1	D37.02	D49.0
surface (dorsal)	C02.0	C79.89	D00.07	D10.1	D37.02	D49.0
base	C01	C79.89	D00.07	D10.1	D37.02	D49.0
ventral	C02.2	C79.89	D00.07	D10.1	D37.02	D49.0
tip	C02.1	C79.89	D00.07	D10.1	D37.02	D49.0
tonsil	C02.4	C79.89	D00.07	D10.1	D37.02	D49.0
tonsil	C09.9	C79.89	D00.08	D10.4	D37.05	D49.0
fauces, faucial	C09.9	C79.89	D00.08	D10.4	D37.05	D49.0
lingual	C02.4	C79.89	D00.07	D10.1	D37.02	D49.0
overlapping sites	C09.8	—	—	—	—	—
palatine	C09.9	C79.89	D00.08	D10.4	D37.05	D49.0
pharyngeal	C11.1	C79.89	D00.08	D10.6	D37.05	D49.0
pillar (anterior) (posterior)	C09.1	C79.89	D00.08	D10.5	D37.05	D49.0
tonsillar fossa	C09.0	C79.89	D00.08	D10.5	D37.05	D49.0
tooth socket NEC	C03.9	C79.89	D00.03	D10.39	D37.09	D49.0
trachea (cartilage) (mucosa)	C33	C78.39	D02.1	D14.2	D38.1	D49.1
overlapping lesion with bronchus or lung	C34.8-	—	—	—	—	—
tracheobronchial	C34.8-	C78.39	D02.1	D14.2	D38.1	D49.1
overlapping lesion with lung	C34.8-	—	—	—	—	—
tragus — *see also Neoplasm, skin, ear*	C44.20-	C79.2	D04.2-	D23.2-	D48.5	D49.2
trunk NEC	C76.8	C79.89	D04.5	D36.7	D48.7	D49.89
tubo-ovarian	C57.8	C79.82	D07.39	D28.7	D39.8	D49.5
tunica vaginalis	C63.7	C79.82	D07.69	D29.8	D40.8	D49.5
turbinate (bone)	C41.0	C79.51	—	D16.4-	D48.0	D49.2
nasal	C30.0	C78.39	D02.3	D14.0	D38.5	D49.1
tympanic cavity	C30.1	C78.39	D02.3	D14.0	D38.5	D49.1
ulna (any part)	C40.0-	C79.51	—	D16.0-	—	—
umbilicus, umbilical — *see also Neoplasm, skin, trunk*	C44.509	C79.2	D04.5	D23.5	D48.5	D49.2
uncus, brain	C71.2	C79.31	—	D33.0	D43.0	D49.6
unknown site or unspecified	C80.1	C79.9	D09.9	D36.9	D48.9	D49.9
urachus	C67.7	C79.11	D09.0	D30.3	D41.4	D49.4
ureter, ureteral	C66.-	C79.19	D09.19	D30.2-	D41.2-	D49.5
orifice (bladder)	C67.6	C79.11	D09.0	D30.3	D41.4	D49.4
ureter-bladder (junction)	C67.6	C79.11	D09.0	D30.3	D41.4	D49.4
urethra, urethral (gland)	C68.0	C79.19	D09.19	D30.4	D41.3	D49.5
orifice, internal	C67.5	C79.11	D09.0	D30.3	D41.4	D49.4
urethrovaginal (septum)	C57.9	C79.82	D07.30	D28.9	D39.8	D49.5
urinary organ or system	C68.9	C79.10	D09.10	D30.9	D41.9	D49.5
bladder — *see Neoplasm, bladder*						
overlapping lesion	C68.8	—	—	—	—	—
specified sites NEC	C68.8	C79.19	D09.19	D30.8	D41.8	D49.5

◀ New ◀▥ Revised ~~deleted~~ Deleted

	Malignant Primary	Malignant Secondary	Ca in situ	Benign	Uncertain Behavior	Unspecified Behavior
utero-ovarian	C57.8	C79.82	D07.39	D28.7	D39.8	D49.5
ligament	C57.1	C79.82	D07.39	D28.2	D39.8	D49.5
uterosacral ligament	C57.3	C79.82	—	D28.2	D39.8	D49.5
uterus, uteri, uterine	C55	C79.82	D07.0	D26.9	D39.0	D49.5
adnexa NEC	C57.4	C79.82	D07.39	D28.7	D39.8	D49.5
body	C54.9	C79.82	D07.0	D26.1	D39.0	D49.5
cervix	C53.9	C79.82	D06.9	D26.0	D39.0	D49.5
cornu	C54.9	C79.82	D07.0	D26.1	D39.0	D49.5
corpus	C54.9	C79.82	D07.0	D26.1	D39.0	D49.5
endocervix (canal) (gland)	C53.0	C79.82	D06.0	D26.0	D39.0	D49.5
endometrium	C54.1	C79.82	D07.0	D26.1	D39.0	D49.5
exocervix	C53.1	C79.82	D06.1	D26.0	D39.0	D49.5
external os	C53.1	C79.82	D06.1	D26.0	D39.0	D49.5
fundus	C54.3	C79.82	D07.0	D26.1	D39.0	D49.5
internal os	C53.0	C79.82	D06.0	D26.0	D39.0	D49.5
isthmus	C54.0	C79.82	D07.0	D26.1	D39.0	D49.5
ligament	C57.3	C79.82	—	D28.2	D39.8	D49.5
broad	C57.1	C79.82	D07.39	D28.2	D39.8	D49.5
round	C57.2	C79.82	—	D28.2	D39.8	D49.5
lower segment	C54.0	C79.82	D07.0	D26.1	D39.0	D49.5
myometrium	C54.2	C79.82	D07.0	D26.1	D39.0	D49.5
overlapping sites	C54.8	—	—	—	—	—
squamocolumnar junction	C53.8	C79.82	D06.7	D26.0	D39.0	D49.5
tube	C57.0-	C79.82	D07.39	D28.2	D39.8	D49.5
utricle, prostatic	C68.0	C79.19	D09.19	D30.4	D41.3	D49.5
uveal tract	C69.4-	C79.49	D09.2-	D31.4-	D48.7	D49.89
uvula	C05.2	C79.89	D00.04	D10.39	D37.09	D49.0
vagina, vaginal (fornix) (vault) (wall)	C52	C79.82	D07.2	D28.1	D39.8	D49.5
vaginovesical	C57.9	C79.82	D07.30	D28.9	D39.9	D49.5
septum	C57.9	C79.82	D07.30	D28.9	D39.9	D49.5
vallecula (epiglottis)	C10.0	C79.89	D00.08	D10.5	D37.05	D49.0
vas deferens	C63.1-	C79.82	D07.69	D29.8	D40.8	D49.5
vascular — see Neoplasm, connective tissue						
Vater's ampulla	C24.1	C78.89	D01.5	D13.5	D37.6	D49.0
vein, venous — see Neoplasm, connective tissue						
vena cava (abdominal) (inferior)	C49.4	C79.89	—	D21.4	D48.1	D49.2
superior	C49.3	C79.89	—	D21.3	D48.1	D49.2
ventricle (cerebral) (floor) (lateral) (third)	C71.5	C79.31	—	D33.0	D43.0	D49.6
cardiac (left) (right)	C38.0	C79.89	—	D15.1	D48.7	D49.89
fourth	C71.7	C79.31	—	D33.1	D43.1	D49.6
ventricular band of larynx	C32.1	C78.39	D02.0	D14.1	D38.0	D49.1
ventriculus — see Neoplasm, stomach						

◀ New   ◀═ Revised   ~~deleted~~ Deleted

	Malignant Primary	Malignant Secondary	Ca in situ	Benign	Uncertain Behavior	Unspecified Behavior
vermillion border — see Neoplasm, lip						
vermis, cerebellum	C71.6	C79.31	—	D33.1	D43.1	D49.6
vertebra (column)	C41.2	C79.51	—	D16.6	D48.0	D49.2
coccyx	C41.4	C79.51	—	D16.8-	D48.0	D49.2
marrow NEC	C96.9	C79.52	—	—	D47.9	D49.89
sacrum	C41.4	C79.51	—	D16.8-	D48.0	D49.2
vesical — see Neoplasm, bladder						
vesicle, seminal	C63.7	C79.82	D07.69	D29.8	D40.8	D49.5
vesicocervical tissue	C57.9	C79.82	D07.30	D28.9	D39.9	D49.5
vesicorectal	C76.3	C79.82	D09.8	D36.7	D48.7	D49.89
vesicovaginal	C57.9	C79.82	D07.30	D28.9	D39.9	D49.5
septum	C57.9	C79.82	D07.30	D28.9	D39.8	D49.5
vessel (blood) — see Neoplasm, connective tissue						
vestibular gland, greater	C51.0	C79.82	D07.1	D28.0	D39.8	D49.5
vestibule						
mouth	C06.1	C79.89	D00.00	D10.39	D37.09	D49.0
nose	C30.0	C78.39	D02.3	D14.0	D38.5	D49.1
Virchow's gland	C77.0	C77.0	—	D36.0	D48.7	D49.89
viscera NEC	C76.8	C79.89	D09.8	D36.7	D48.7	D49.89
vocal cords (true)	C32.0	C78.39	D02.0	D14.1	D38.0	D49.1
false	C32.1	C78.39	D02.0	D14.1	D38.0	D49.1
vomer	C41.0	C79.51	—	D16.4-	D48.0	D49.2
vulva	C51.9	C79.82	D07.1	D28.0	D39.8	D49.5
vulvovaginal gland	C51.0	C79.82	D07.1	D28.0	D39.8	D49.5
Waldeyer's ring	C14.2	C79.89	D00.08	D10.9	D37.05	D49.0
Wharton's duct	C08.0	C79.89	D00.00	D11.7	D37.032	D49.0
white matter (central) (cerebral)	C71.0	C79.31	—	D33.0	D43.0	D49.6
windpipe	C33	C78.39	D02.1	D14.2	D38.1	D49.1
Wirsung's duct	C25.3	C78.89	D01.7	D13.6	D37.8	D49.0
wolffian (body) (duct)						
female	C57.7	C79.82	D07.39	D28.7	D39.8	D49.5
male	C63.7	C79.82	D07.69	D29.8	D40.8	D49.5
womb — see Neoplasm, uterus						
wrist NEC	C76.4-	C79.89	D04.6-	D36.7	D48.7	D49.89
xiphoid process	C41.3	C79.51	—	D16.7	D48.0	D49.2
Zuckerkandl organ	C75.5	C79.89	—	D35.6	D44.7	D49.7

◀ New ◀|||| Revised ~~deleted~~ Deleted

ICD-10-CM
Table of Drugs and Chemicals

ICD-10-CM
Table of Drugs and Chemicals

Substance	External Cause (T-Code)					
	Poisoning, Accidental (Unintentional)	Poisoning, Intentional Self-Harm	Poisoning, Assault	Poisoning, Undetermined	Adverse Effect	Underdosing
#						
1-propanol	T51.3X1	T51.3X2	T51.3X3	T51.3X4	—	—
2-propanol	T51.2X1	T51.2X2	T51.2X3	T51.2X4	—	—
2,4-D (dichlorophen-oxyacetic acid)	T60.3X1	T60.3X2	T60.3X3	T60.3X4	—	—
2,4-toluene diisocyanate	T65.0X1	T65.0X2	T65.0X3	T65.0X4	—	—
2,4,5-T (trichloro-phenoxyacetic acid)	T60.1X1	T60.1X2	T60.1X3	T60.1X4	—	—
14-hydroxydihydro-morphinone	T40.2X1	T40.2X2	T40.2X3	T40.2X4	T40.2X5	T40.2X6
A						
ABOB	T37.5X1	T37.5X2	T37.5X3	T37.5X4	T37.5X5	T37.5X6
Abrine	T62.2X1	T62.2X2	T62.2X3	T62.2X4	—	—
Abrus (seed)	T62.2X1	T62.2X2	T62.2X3	T62.2X4	—	—
Absinthe	T51.0X1	T51.0X2	T51.0X3	T51.0X4	—	—
beverage	T51.0X1	T51.0X2	T51.0X3	T51.0X4	—	—
Acaricide	T60.8X1	T60.8X2	T60.8X3	T60.8X4	—	—
Acebutolol	T44.7X1	T44.7X2	T44.7X3	T44.7X4	T44.7X5	T44.7X6
Acecarbromal	T42.6X1	T42.6X2	T42.6X3	T42.6X4	T42.6X5	T42.6X6
Aceclidine	T44.1X1	T44.1X2	T44.1X3	T44.1X4	T44.1X5	T44.1X6
Acedapsone	T37.0X1	T37.0X2	T37.0X3	T37.0X4	T37.0X5	T37.0X6
Acefylline piperazine	T48.6X1	T48.6X2	T48.6X3	T48.6X4	T48.6X5	T48.6X6
Acemorphan	T40.2X1	T40.2X2	T40.2X3	T40.2X4	T40.2X5	T40.2X6
Acenocoumarin	T45.511	T45.512	T45.513	T45.514	T45.515	T45.516
Acenocoumarol	T45.511	T45.512	T45.513	T45.514	T45.515	T45.516
Acepifylline	T48.6X1	T48.6X2	T48.6X3	T48.6X4	T48.6X5	T48.6X6
Acepromazine	T43.3X1	T43.3X2	T43.3X3	T43.3X4	T43.3X5	T43.3X6
Acesulfamethoxypyridazine	T37.0X1	T37.0X2	T37.0X3	T37.0X4	T37.0X5	T37.0X6
Acetal	T52.8X1	T52.8X2	T52.8X3	T52.8X4	—	—
Acetaldehyde (vapor)	T52.8X1	T52.8X2	T52.8X3	T52.8X4	—	—
liquid	T65.891	T65.892	T65.893	T65.894	—	—
P-Acetamidophenol	T39.1X1	T39.1X2	T39.1X3	T39.1X4	T39.1X5	T39.1X6
Acetaminophen	T39.1X1	T39.1X2	T39.1X3	T39.1X4	T39.1X5	T39.1X6
Acetaminosalol	T39.1X1	T39.1X2	T39.1X3	T39.1X4	T39.1X5	T39.1X6
Acetanilide	T39.1X1	T39.1X2	T39.1X3	T39.1X4	T39.1X5	T39.1X6
Acetarsol	T37.3X1	T37.3X2	T37.3X3	T37.3X4	T37.3X5	T37.3X6
Acetazolamide	T50.2X1	T50.2X2	T50.2X3	T50.2X4	T50.2X5	T50.2X6
Acetiamine	T45.2X1	T45.2X2	T45.2X3	T45.2X4	T45.2X5	T45.2X6
Acetic						
acid	T54.2X1	T54.2X2	T54.2X3	T54.2X4	—	—
with sodium acetate (ointment)	T49.3X1	T49.3X2	T49.3X3	T49.3X4	T49.3X5	T49.3X6
ester (solvent) (vapor)	T52.8X1	T52.8X2	T52.8X3	T52.8X4	—	—

◄ New ◄‖‖ Revised ~~deleted~~ Deleted

TABLE OF DRUGS AND CHEMICALS

Substance	Poisoning, Accidental (Unintentional)	Poisoning, Intentional Self-Harm	Poisoning, Assault	Poisoning, Undetermined	Adverse Effect	Underdosing
	External Cause (T-Code)					
Acetic *(Continued)*						
acid *(Continued)*						
irrigating solution	T50.3X1	T50.3X2	T50.3X3	T50.3X4	T50.3X5	T50.3X6
medicinal (lotion)	T49.2X1	T49.2X2	T49.2X3	T49.2X4	T49.2X5	T49.2X6
anhydride	T65.891	T65.892	T65.893	T65.894	—	—
ether (vapor)	T52.8X1	T52.8X2	T52.8X3	T52.8X4	—	—
Acetohexamide	T38.3X1	T38.3X2	T38.3X3	T38.3X4	T38.3X5	T38.3X6
Acetohydroxamic acid	T50.991	T50.992	T50.993	T50.994	T50.995	T50.996
Acetomenaphthone	T45.7X1	T45.7X2	T45.7X3	T45.7X4	T45.7X5	T45.7X6
Acetomorphine	T40.1X1	T40.1X2	T40.1X3	T40.1X4	—	—
Acetone (oils)	T52.4X1	T52.4X2	T52.4X3	T52.4X4	—	—
chlorinated	T52.4X1	T52.4X2	T52.4X3	T52.4X4	—	—
vapor	T52.4X1	T52.4X2	T52.4X3	T52.4X4	—	—
Acetonitrile	T52.8X1	T52.8X2	T52.8X3	T52.8X4	—	—
Acetophenazine	T43.3X1	T43.3X2	T43.3X3	T43.3X4	T43.3X5	T43.3X6
Acetophenetedin	T39.1X1	T39.1X2	T39.1X3	T39.1X4	T39.1X5	T39.1X6
Acetophenone	T52.4X1	T52.4X2	T52.4X3	T52.4X4	—	—
Acetorphine	T40.2X1	T40.2X2	T40.2X3	T40.2X4	—	—
Acetosulfone (sodium)	T37.1X1	T37.1X2	T37.1X3	T37.1X4	T37.1X5	T37.1X6
Acetrizoate (sodium)	T50.8X1	T50.8X2	T50.8X3	T50.8X4	T50.8X5	T50.8X6
Acetylcarbromal	T42.6X1	T42.6X2	T42.6X3	T42.6X4	T42.6X5	T42.6X6
Acetrizoic acid	T50.8X1	T50.8X2	T50.8X3	T50.8X4	T50.8X5	T50.8X6
Acetyl						
bromide	T53.6X1	T53.6X2	T53.6X3	T53.6X4	—	—
chloride	T53.6X1	T53.6X2	T53.6X3	T53.6X4	—	—
Acetylcholine						
chloride	T44.1X1	T44.1X2	T44.1X3	T44.1X4	T44.1X5	T44.1X6
derivative	T44.1X1	T44.1X2	T44.1X3	T44.1X4	T44.1X5	T44.1X6
Acetylcysteine	T48.4X1	T48.4X2	T48.4X3	T48.4X4	T48.4X5	T48.4X6
Acetyldigitoxin	T46.0X1	T46.0X2	T46.0X3	T46.0X4	T46.0X5	T46.0X6
Acetyldigoxin	T46.0X1	T46.0X2	T46.0X3	T46.0X4	T46.0X5	T46.0X6
Acetyldihydrocodeine	T40.2X1	T40.2X2	T40.2X3	T40.2X4	—	—
Acetyldihydrocodeinone	T40.2X1	T40.2X2	T40.2X3	T40.2X4	—	—
Acetylene (gas)	T59.891	T59.892	T59.893	T59.894	—	—
dichloride	T53.6X1	T53.6X2	T53.6X3	T53.6X4	—	—
incomplete combustion of	T58.11	T58.12	T58.13	T58.14	—	—
industrial	T59.891	T59.892	T59.893	T59.894	—	—
tetrachloride	T53.6X1	T53.6X2	T53.6X3	T53.6X4	—	—
vapor	T53.6X1	T53.6X2	T53.6X3	T53.6X4	—	—
Acetylphenylhydrazine	T39.8X1	T39.8X2	T39.8X3	T39.8X4	T39.8X5	T39.8X6

◀ New   ◀≣ Revised   ~~deleted~~ Deleted

Substance	External Cause (T-Code)					
	Poisoning, Accidental (Unintentional)	Poisoning, Intentional Self-Harm	Poisoning, Assault	Poisoning, Undetermined	Adverse Effect	Underdosing
Acetylpheneturide	T42.6X1	T42.6X2	T42.6X3	T42.6X4	T42.6X5	T42.6X6
Acetylsalicylic acid (salts)	T39.011	T39.012	T39.013	T39.014	T39.015	T39.016
enteric coated	T39.011	T39.012	T39.013	T39.014	T39.015	T39.016
Acetylsulfamethoxypyridazine	T37.0X1	T37.0X2	T37.0X3	T37.0X4	T37.0X5	T37.0X6
Achromycin	T36.4X1	T36.4X2	T36.4X3	T36.4X4	T36.4X5	T36.4X6
ophthalmic preparation	T49.5X1	T49.5X2	T49.5X3	T49.5X4	T49.5X5	T49.5X6
topical NEC	T49.0X1	T49.0X2	T49.0X3	T49.0X4	T49.0X5	T49.0X6
Aciclovir	T37.5X1	T37.5X2	T37.5X3	T37.5X4	T37.5X5	T37.5X6
Acid (corrosive) NEC	T54.2X1	T54.2X2	T54.2X3	T54.2X4	—	—
Acidifying agent NEC	T50.901	T50.902	T50.903	T50.904	T50.905	T50.906
Acipimox	T46.6X1	T46.6X2	T46.6X3	T46.6X4	T46.6X5	T46.6X6
Acitretin	T50.991	T50.992	T50.993	T50.994	T50.995	T50.996
Aclarubicin	T45.1X1	T45.1X2	T45.1X3	T45.1X4	T45.1X5	T45.1X6
Aclatonium napadisilate	T48.1X1	T48.1X2	T48.1X3	T48.1X4	T48.1X5	T48.1X6
Aconite (wild)	T46.991	T46.992	T46.993	T46.994	T46.995	T46.996
Aconitine	T46.991	T46.992	T46.993	T46.994	T46.995	T46.996
Aconitum ferox	T46.991	T46.992	T46.993	T46.994	T46.995	T46.996
Acridine	T65.6X1	T65.6X2	T65.6X3	T65.6X4	—	—
vapor	T59.891	T59.892	T59.893	T59.894	—	—
Acriflavine	T37.91	T37.92	T37.93	T37.94	T37.95	T37.96
Acriflavinium chloride	T49.0X1	T49.0X2	T49.0X3	T49.0X4	T49.0X5	T49.0X6
Acrinol	T49.0X1	T49.0X2	T49.0X3	T49.0X4	T49.0X5	T49.0X6
Acrisorcin	T49.0X1	T49.0X2	T49.0X3	T49.0X4	T49.0X5	T49.0X6
Acrivastine	T45.0X1	T45.0X2	T45.0X3	T45.0X4	T45.0X5	T45.0X6
Acrolein (gas)	T59.891	T59.892	T59.893	T59.894	—	—
liquid	T54.1X1	T54.1X2	T54.1X3	T54.1X4	—	—
Acrylamide	T65.891	T65.892	T65.893	T65.894	—	—
Acrylic resin	T49.3X1	T49.3X2	T49.3X3	T49.3X4	T49.3X5	T49.3X6
Acrylonitrile	T65.891	T65.892	T65.893	T65.894	—	—
Actaea spicata	T62.2X1	T62.2X2	T62.2X3	T62.2X4	—	—
berry	T62.1X1	T62.1X2	T62.1X3	T62.1X4	—	—
Acterol	T37.3X1	T37.3X2	T37.3X3	T37.3X4	T37.3X5	T37.3X6
ACTH	T38.811	T38.812	T38.813	T38.814	T38.815	T38.816
Actinomycin C	T45.1X1	T45.1X2	T45.1X3	T45.1X4	T45.1X5	T45.1X6
Actinomycin D	T45.1X1	T45.1X2	T45.1X3	T45.1X4	T45.1X5	T45.1X6
Activated charcoal — see also Charcoal, medicinal	T47.6X1	T47.6X2	T47.6X3	T47.6X4	T47.6X5	T47.6X6
Acyclovir	T37.5X1	T37.5X2	T37.5X3	T37.5X4	T37.5X5	T37.5X6
Adenine	T45.2X1	T45.2X2	T45.2X3	T45.2X4	T45.2X5	T45.2X6
arabinoside	T37.5X1	T37.5X2	T37.5X3	T37.5X4	T37.5X5	T37.5X6
Adenosine (phosphate)	T46.2X1	T46.2X2	T46.2X3	T46.2X4	T46.2X5	T46.2X6

TABLE OF DRUGS AND CHEMICALS

Substance	External Cause (T-Code)					
	Poisoning, Accidental (Unintentional)	Poisoning, Intentional Self-Harm	Poisoning, Assault	Poisoning, Undetermined	Adverse Effect	Underdosing
ADH	T38.891	T38.892	T38.893	T38.894	T38.895	T38.896
Adhesive NEC	T65.891	T65.892	T65.893	T65.894	—	—
Adicillin	T36.0X1	T36.0X2	T36.0X3	T36.0X4	T36.0X5	T36.0X6
Adiphenine	T44.3X1	T44.3X2	T44.3X3	T44.3X4	T44.3X5	T44.3X6
Adipiodone	T50.8X1	T50.8X2	T50.8X3	T50.8X4	T50.8X5	T50.8X6
Adjunct, pharmaceutical	T50.901	T50.902	T50.903	T50.904	T50.905	T50.906
Adrenal (extract, cortex or medulla) (glucocorticoids) (hormones) (mineralocorticoids)	T38.0X1	T38.0X2	T38.0X3	T38.0X4	T38.0X5	T38.0X6
ENT agent	T49.6X1	T49.6X2	T49.6X3	T49.6X4	T49.6X5	T49.6X6
ophthalmic preparation	T49.5X1	T49.5X2	T49.5X3	T49.5X4	T49.5X5	T49.5X6
topical NEC	T49.0X1	T49.0X2	T49.0X3	T49.0X4	T49.0X5	T49.0X6
Adrenaline	T44.5X1	T44.5X2	T44.5X3	T44.5X4	T44.5X5	T44.5X6
Adrenalin — see Adrenaline						
Adrenergic NEC	T44.901	T44.902	T44.903	T44.904	T44.905	T44.906
blocking agent NEC	T44.8X1	T44.8X2	T44.8X3	T44.8X4	T44.8X5	T44.8X6
beta, heart	T44.7X1	T44.7X2	T44.7X3	T44.7X4	T44.7X5	T44.7X6
specified NEC	T44.991	T44.992	T44.993	T44.994	T44.995	T44.996
Adrenochrome						
(mono) semicarbazone	T46.991	T46.992	T46.993	T46.994	T46.995	T46.996
derivative	T46.991	T46.992	T46.993	T46.994	T46.995	T46.996
Adrenocorticotrophic hormone	T38.811	T38.812	T38.813	T38.814	T38.815	T38.816
Adrenocorticotrophin	T38.811	T38.812	T38.813	T38.814	T38.815	T38.816
Adriamycin	T45.1X1	T45.1X2	T45.1X3	T45.1X4	T45.1X5	T45.1X6
Aerosol spray NEC	T65.91	T65.92	T65.93	T65.94	—	—
Aerosporin	T36.8X1	T36.8X2	T36.8X3	T36.8X4	T36.8X5	T36.8X6
ENT agent	T49.6X1	T49.6X2	T49.6X3	T49.6X4	T49.6X5	T49.6X6
ophthalmic preparation	T49.5X1	T49.5X2	T49.5X3	T49.5X4	T49.5X5	T49.5X6
topical NEC	T49.0X1	T49.0X2	T49.0X3	T49.0X4	T49.0X5	T49.0X6
Aethusa cynapium	T62.2X1	T62.2X2	T62.2X3	T62.2X4	—	—
Afghanistan black	T40.7X1	T40.7X2	T40.7X3	T40.7X4	T40.7X5	T40.7X6
Aflatoxin	T64.01	T64.02	T64.03	T64.04	—	—
Afloqualone	T42.8X1	T42.8X2	T42.8X3	T42.8X4	T42.8X5	T42.8X6
African boxwood	T62.2X1	T62.2X2	T62.2X3	T62.2X4	—	—
Agar	T47.4X1	T47.4X2	T47.4X3	T47.4X4	T47.4X5	T47.4X6
Agonist						
predominantly						
alpha-adrenoreceptor	T44.4X1	T44.4X2	T44.4X3	T44.4X4	T44.4X5	T44.4X6
beta-adrenoreceptor	T44.5X1	T44.5X2	T44.5X3	T44.5X4	T44.5X5	T44.5X6
Agricultural agent NEC	T65.91	T65.92	T65.93	T65.94	—	—
Agrypnal	T42.3X1	T42.3X2	T42.3X3	T42.3X4	T42.3X5	T42.3X6

◀ New ◀ Revised ~~deleted~~ Deleted

Substance	External Cause (T-Code)					
	Poisoning, Accidental (Unintentional)	Poisoning, Intentional Self-Harm	Poisoning, Assault	Poisoning, Undetermined	Adverse Effect	Underdosing
AHLG	T50.Z11	T50.Z12	T50.Z13	T50.Z14	T50.Z15	T50.Z16
Air contaminant(s), source/type NOS	T65.91	T65.92	T65.93	T65.94	—	—
Ajmaline	T46.2X1	T46.2X2	T46.2X3	T46.2X4	T46.2X5	T46.2X6
Akritoin	T37.8X1	T37.8X2	T37.8X3	T37.8X4	T37.8X5	T37.8X6
Akee	T62.1X1	T62.1X2	T62.1X3	T62.1X4	—	—
Akrinol	T49.0X1	T49.0X2	T49.0X3	T49.0X4	T49.0X5	T49.0X6
Alacepril	T46.4X1	T46.4X2	T46.4X3	T46.4X4	T46.4X5	T46.4X6
Alantolactone	T37.4X1	T37.4X2	T37.4X3	T37.4X4	T37.4X5	T37.4X6
Albamycin	T36.8X1	T36.8X2	T36.8X3	T36.8X4	T36.8X5	T36.8X6
Albendazole	T37.4X1	T37.4X2	T37.4X3	T37.4X4	T37.4X5	T37.4X6
Albumin						
bovine	T45.8X1	T45.8X2	T45.8X3	T45.8X4	T45.8X5	T45.8X6
human serum	T45.8X1	T45.8X2	T45.8X3	T45.8X4	T45.8X5	T45.8X6
salt-poor	T45.8X1	T45.8X2	T45.8X3	T45.8X4	T45.8X5	T45.8X6
normal human serum	T45.8X1	T45.8X2	T45.8X3	T45.8X4	T45.8X5	T45.8X6
Albuterol	T48.6X1	T48.6X2	T48.6X3	T48.6X4	T48.6X5	T48.6X6
Albutoin	T42.0X1	T42.0X2	T42.0X3	T42.0X4	T42.0X5	T42.0X6
Alclometasone	T49.0X1	T49.0X2	T49.0X3	T49.0X4	T49.0X5	T49.0X6
Alcohol	T51.91	T51.92	T51.93	T51.94	—	—
absolute	T51.0X1	T51.0X2	T51.0X3	T51.0X4	—	—
beverage	T51.0X1	T51.0X2	T51.0X3	T51.0X4	—	—
allyl	T51.8X1	T51.8X2	T51.8X3	T51.8X4	—	—
amyl	T51.3X1	T51.3X2	T51.3X3	T51.3X4	—	—
antifreeze	T51.1X1	T51.1X2	T51.1X3	T51.1X4	—	—
beverage	T51.0X1	T51.0X2	T51.0X3	T51.0X4	—	—
butyl	T51.3X1	T51.3X2	T51.3X3	T51.3X4	—	—
dehydrated	T51.0X1	T51.0X2	T51.0X3	T51.0X4	—	—
beverage	T51.0X1	T51.0X2	T51.0X3	T51.0X4	—	—
denatured	T51.0X1	T51.0X2	T51.0X3	T51.0X4	—	—
deterrent NEC	T50.6X1	T50.6X2	T50.6X3	T50.6X4	T50.6X5	T50.6X6
diagnostic (gastric function)	T50.8X1	T50.8X2	T50.8X3	T50.8X4	T50.8X5	T50.8X6
ethyl	T51.0X1	T51.0X2	T51.0X3	T51.0X4	—	—
beverage	T51.0X1	T51.0X2	T51.0X3	T51.0X4	—	—
grain	T51.0X1	T51.0X2	T51.0X3	T51.0X4	—	—
beverage	T51.0X1	T51.0X2	T51.0X3	T51.0X4	—	—
industrial	T51.0X1	T51.0X2	T51.0X3	T51.0X4	—	—
isopropyl	T51.2X1	T51.2X2	T51.2X3	T51.2X4	—	—
methyl	T51.1X1	T51.1X2	T51.1X3	T51.1X4	—	—
preparation for consumption	T51.0X1	T51.0X2	T51.0X3	T51.0X4	—	—

TABLE OF DRUGS AND CHEMICALS

Substance	External Cause (T-Code)					
	Poisoning, Accidental (Unintentional)	Poisoning, Intentional Self-Harm	Poisoning, Assault	Poisoning, Undetermined	Adverse Effect	Underdosing
Alcohol *(Continued)*						
propyl	T51.3X1	T51.3X2	T51.3X3	T51.3X4	—	—
secondary	T51.2X1	T51.2X2	T51.2X3	T51.2X4	—	—
radiator	T51.1X1	T51.1X2	T51.1X3	T51.1X4	—	—
rubbing	T51.2X1	T51.2X2	T51.2X3	T51.2X4	—	—
specified type NEC	T51.8X1	T51.8X2	T51.8X3	T51.8X4	—	—
surgical	T51.0X1	T51.0X2	T51.0X3	T51.0X4	—	—
vapor (from any type of Alcohol)	T59.891	T59.892	T59.893	T59.894	—	—
wood	T51.1X1	T51.1X2	T51.1X3	T51.1X4	—	—
Alcuronium (chloride)	T48.1X1	T48.1X2	T48.1X3	T48.1X4	T48.1X5	T48.1X6
Aldactone	T50.0X1	T50.0X2	T50.0X3	T50.0X4	T50.0X5	T50.0X6
Aldesulfone sodium	T37.1X1	T37.1X2	T37.1X3	T37.1X4	T37.1X5	T37.1X6
Aldicarb	T60.0X1	T60.0X2	T60.0X3	T60.0X4	—	—
Aldomet	T46.5X1	T46.5X2	T46.5X3	T46.5X4	T46.5X5	T46.5X6
Aldosterone	T50.0X1	T50.0X2	T50.0X3	T50.0X4	T50.0X5	T50.0X6
Aldrin (dust)	T60.1X1	T60.1X2	T60.1X3	T60.1X4	—	—
Aleve — *see Naproxen*						
Alexitol sodium	T47.1X1	T47.1X2	T47.1X3	T47.1X4	T47.1X5	T47.1X6
Alfacalcidol	T45.2X1	T45.2X2	T45.2X3	T45.2X4	T45.2X5	T45.2X6
Alfadolone	T41.1X1	T41.1X2	T41.1X3	T41.1X4	T41.1X5	T41.1X6
Alfaxalone	T41.1X1	T41.1X2	T41.1X3	T41.1X4	T41.1X5	T41.1X6
Alfentanil	T40.4X1	T40.4X2	T40.4X3	T40.4X4	T40.4X5	T40.4X6
Alfuzosin (hydrochloride)	T44.8X1	T44.8X2	T44.8X3	T44.8X4	T44.8X5	T44.8X6
Algae (harmful) (toxin)	T65.821	T65.822	T65.823	T65.824	—	—
Algeldrate	T47.1X1	T47.1X2	T47.1X3	T47.1X4	T47.1X5	T47.1X6
Algin	T47.8X1	T47.8X2	T47.8X3	T47.8X4	T47.8X5	T47.8X6
Alglucerase	T45.3X1	T45.3X2	T45.3X3	T45.3X4	T45.3X5	T45.3X6
Alidase	T45.3X1	T45.3X2	T45.3X3	T45.3X4	T45.3X5	T45.3X6
Alimemazine	T43.3X1	T43.3X2	T43.3X3	T43.3X4	T43.3X5	T43.3X6
Aliphatic thiocyanates	T65.0X1	T65.0X2	T65.0X3	T65.0X4	—	—
Alizapride	T45.0X1	T45.0X2	T45.0X3	T45.0X4	T45.0X5	T45.0X6
Alkali (caustic)	T54.3X1	T54.3X2	T54.3X3	T54.3X4	—	—
Alkalizing agent NEC	T50.901	T50.902	T50.903	T50.904	T50.905	T50.906
Alkaline antiseptic solution (aromatic)	T49.6X1	T49.6X2	T49.6X3	T49.6X4	T49.6X5	T49.6X6
Alkalinizing agents (medicinal)	T50.901	T50.902	T50.903	T50.904	T50.905	T50.906
Alka-seltzer	T39.011	T39.012	T39.013	T39.014	T39.015	T39.016
Alkavervir	T46.5X1	T46.5X2	T46.5X3	T46.5X4	T46.5X5	T46.5X6
Alkonium (bromide)	T49.0X1	T49.0X2	T49.0X3	T49.0X4	T49.0X5	T49.0X6
Alkylating drug NEC	T45.1X1	T45.1X2	T45.1X3	T45.1X4	T45.1X5	T45.1X6
antimyeloproliferative	T45.1X1	T45.1X2	T45.1X3	T45.1X4	T45.1X5	T45.1X6
lymphatic	T45.1X1	T45.1X2	T45.1X3	T45.1X4	T45.1X5	T45.1X6

◀ New ◀⁞⁞⁞ Revised ~~deleted~~ Deleted

Substance	External Cause (T-Code)					
	Poisoning, Accidental (Unintentional)	Poisoning, Intentional Self-Harm	Poisoning, Assault	Poisoning, Undetermined	Adverse Effect	Underdosing
Alkylisocyanate	T65.0X1	T65.0X2	T65.0X3	T65.0X4	—	—
Allantoin	T49.411	T49.412	T49.413	T49.414	T49.415	T49.416
Allegron	T43.0X1	T43.0X2	T43.0X3	T43.0X4	T43.0X5	T43.0X6
Allethrin	T49.0X1	T49.0X2	T49.0X3	T49.0X4	T49.0X5	T49.0X6
Allobarbital	T42.3X1	T42.3X2	T42.3X3	T42.3X4	T42.3X5	T42.3X6
Allopurinol	T50.4X1	T50.4X2	T50.4X3	T50.4X4	T50.4X5	T50.4X6
Allyl						
alcohol	T51.8X1	T51.8X2	T51.8X3	T51.8X4	—	—
disulfide	T46.6X1	T46.6X2	T46.6X3	T46.6X4	T46.6X5	T46.6X6
Allylestrenol	T38.5X1	T38.5X2	T38.5X3	T38.5X4	T38.5X5	T38.5X6
Allylisopropylacetylurea	T42.6X1	T42.6X2	T42.6X3	T42.6X4	T42.6X5	T42.6X6
Allylisopropylmalonylurea	T42.3X1	T42.3X2	T42.3X3	T42.3X4	T42.3X5	T42.3X6
Allylthiourea	T49.3X1	T49.3X2	T49.3X3	T49.3X4	T49.3X5	T49.3X6
Allyltribromide	T42.6X1	T42.6X2	T42.6X3	T42.6X4	T42.6X5	T42.6X6
Allypropymal	T42.3X1	T42.3X2	T42.3X3	T42.3X4	T42.3X5	T42.3X6
Almagate	T47.1X1	T47.1X2	T47.1X3	T47.1X4	T47.1X5	T47.1X6
Almasilate	T47.1X1	T47.1X2	T47.1X3	T47.1X4	T47.1X5	T47.1X6
Almitrine	T50.7X1	T50.7X2	T50.7X3	T50.7X4	T50.7X5	T50.7X6
Aloes	T47.2X1	T47.2X2	T47.2X3	T47.2X4	T47.2X5	T47.2X6
Aloglutamol	T47.1X1	T47.1X2	T47.1X3	T47.1X4	T47.1X5	T47.1X6
Aloin	T47.2X1	T47.2X2	T47.2X3	T47.2X4	T47.2X5	T47.2X6
Aloxidone	T42.2X1	T42.2X2	T42.2X3	T42.2X4	T42.2X5	T42.2X6
Alpha						
acetyldigoxin	T46.0X1	T46.0X2	T46.0X3	T46.0X4	T46.0X5	T46.0X6
adrenergic blocking drug	T44.6X1	T44.6X2	T44.6X3	T44.6X4	T44.6X5	T44.6X6
amylase	T45.3X1	T45.3X2	T45.3X3	T45.3X4	T45.3X5	T45.3X6
tocoferol (acetate)	T45.2X1	T45.2X2	T45.2X3	T45.2X4	T45.2X5	T45.2X6
tocopherol	T45.2X1	T45.2X2	T45.2X3	T45.2X4	T45.2X5	T45.2X6
Alphadolone	T41.1X1	T41.1X2	T41.1X3	T41.1X4	T41.1X5	T41.1X6
Alphaprodine	T40.4X1	T40.4X2	T40.4X3	T40.4X4	T40.4X5	T40.4X6
Alphaxalone	T41.1X1	T41.1X2	T41.1X3	T41.1X4	T41.1X5	T41.1X6
Alprazolam	T42.4X1	T42.4X2	T42.4X3	T42.4X4	T42.4X5	T42.4X6
Alprenolol	T44.7X1	T44.7X2	T44.7X3	T44.7X4	T44.7X5	T44.7X6
Alprostadil	T46.7X1	T46.7X2	T46.7X3	T46.7X4	T46.7X5	T46.7X6
Alsactide	T38.811	T38.812	T38.813	T38.814	T38.815	T38.816
Alseroxylon	T46.5X1	T46.5X2	T46.5X3	T46.5X4	T46.5X5	T46.5X6
Alteplase	T45.611	T45.612	T45.613	T45.614	T45.615	T45.616
Altizide	T50.2X1	T50.2X2	T50.2X3	T50.2X4	T50.2X5	T50.2X6
Altretamine	T45.1X1	T45.1X2	T45.1X3	T45.1X4	T45.1X5	T45.1X6

◀ New   ◀▥ Revised   ~~deleted~~ Deleted

Substance	Poisoning, Accidental (Unintentional)	Poisoning, Intentional Self-Harm	Poisoning, Assault	Poisoning, Undetermined	Adverse Effect	Underdosing
			External Cause (T-Code)			
Alum (medicinal)	T49.4X1	T49.4X2	T49.4X3	T49.4X4	T49.4X5	T49.4X6
nonmedicinal (ammonium) (potassium)	T56.891	T56.892	T56.893	T56.894	—	—
Aluminium, aluminum						
acetate	T49.2X1	T49.2X2	T49.2X3	T49.2X4	T49.2X5	T49.2X6
solution	T49.0X1	T49.0X2	T49.0X3	T49.0X4	T49.0X5	T49.0X6
aspirin	T39.011	T39.012	T39.013	T39.014	T39.015	T39.016
bis (acetylsalicylate)	T39.011	T39.012	T39.013	T39.014	T39.015	T39.016
carbonate (gel, basic)	T47.1X1	T47.1X2	T47.1X3	T47.1X4	T47.1X5	T47.1X6
chlorhydroxide-complex	T47.1X1	T47.1X2	T47.1X3	T47.1X4	T47.1X5	T47.1X6
chloride	T49.2X1	T49.2X2	T49.2X3	T49.2X4	T49.2X5	T49.2X6
clofibrate	T46.6X1	T46.6X2	T46.6X3	T46.6X4	T46.6X5	T46.6X6
diacetate	T49.2X1	T49.2X2	T49.2X3	T49.2X4	T49.2X5	T49.2X6
glycinate	T47.1X1	T47.1X2	T47.1X3	T47.1X4	T47.1X5	T47.1X6
hydroxide (gel)	T47.1X1	T47.1X2	T47.1X3	T47.1X4	T47.1X5	T47.1X6
hydroxide-magnesium carb. gel	T47.1X1	T47.1X2	T47.1X3	T47.1X4	T47.1X5	T47.1X6
magnesium silicate	T47.1X1	T47.1X2	T47.1X3	I47.1X4	I47.1X5	T47.1X6
nicotinate	T46.7X1	T46.7X2	T46.7X3	T46.7X4	T46.7X5	T46.7X6
ointment (surgical) (topical)	T49.3X1	T49.3X2	T49.3X3	T49.3X4	T49.3X5	T49.3X6
phosphate	T47.1X1	T47.1X2	T47.1X3	T47.1X4	T47.1X5	T47.1X6
salicylate	T39.091	T39.092	T39.093	T39.094	T39.095	T39.096
silicate	T47.1X1	T47.1X2	T47.1X3	T47.1X4	T47.1X5	T47.1X6
sodium silicate	T47.1X1	T47.1X2	T47.1X3	T47.1X4	T47.1X5	T47.1X6
subacetate	T49.2X1	T49.2X2	T49.2X3	T49.2X4	T49.2X5	T49.2X6
sulfate	T49.0X1	T49.0X2	T49.0X3	T49.0X4	T49.0X5	T49.0X6
tannate	T47.6X1	T47.6X2	T47.6X3	T47.6X4	T47.6X5	T47.6X6
topical NEC	T49.3X1	T49.3X2	T49.3X3	T49.3X4	T49.3X5	T49.3X6
Alurate	T42.3X1	T42.3X2	T42.3X3	T42.3X4	T42.3X5	T42.3X6
Alverine	T44.3X1	T44.3X2	T44.3X3	T44.3X4	T44.3X5	T44.3X6
Alvodine	T40.2X1	T40.2X2	T40.2X3	T40.2X4	T40.2X5	T40.2X6
Amanita phalloides	T62.0X1	T62.0X2	T62.0X3	T62.0X4	—	—
Amanitine	T62.0X1	T62.0X2	T62.0X3	T62.0X4	—	—
Amantadine	T42.8X1	T42.8X2	T42.8X3	T42.8X4	T42.8X5	T42.8X6
Ambazone	T49.6X1	T49.6X2	T49.6X3	T49.6X4	T49.6X5	T49.6X6
Ambenonium (chloride)	T44.0X1	T44.0X2	T44.0X3	T44.0X4	T44.0X5	T44.0X6
Ambroxol	T48.4X1	T48.4X2	T48.4X3	T48.4X4	T48.4X5	T48.4X6
Ambuphylline	T48.6X1	T48.6X2	T48.6X3	T48.6X4	T48.6X5	T48.6X6
Ambutonium bromide	T44.3X1	T44.3X2	T44.3X3	T44.3X4	T44.3X5	T44.3X6
Amcinonide	T49.0X1	T49.0X2	T49.0X3	T49.0X4	T49.0X5	T49.0X6
Amdinocilline	T36.0X1	T36.0X2	T36.0X3	T36.0X4	T36.0X5	T36.0X6

◀ New   ◀▬ Revised   ~~deleted~~ Deleted

Substance	External Cause (T-Code)					
	Poisoning, Accidental (Unintentional)	Poisoning, Intentional Self-Harm	Poisoning, Assault	Poisoning, Undetermined	Adverse Effect	Underdosing
Ametazole	T50.8X1	T50.8X2	T50.8X3	T50.8X4	T50.8X5	T50.8X6
Amethocaine	T41.3X1	T41.3X2	T41.3X3	T41.3X4	T41.3X5	T41.3X6
regional	T41.3X1	T41.3X2	T41.3X3	T41.3X4	T41.3X5	T41.3X6
spinal	T41.3X1	T41.3X2	T41.3X3	T41.3X4	T41.3X5	T41.3X6
Amethopterin	T45.1X1	T45.1X2	T45.1X3	T45.1X4	T45.1X5	T45.1X6
Amezinium metilsulfate	T44.991	T44.992	T44.993	T44.994	T44.995	T44.996
Amfebutamone	T43.291	T43.292	T43.293	T43.294	T43.295	T43.296
Amfepramone	T50.5X1	T50.5X2	T50.5X3	T50.5X4	T50.5X5	T50.5X6
Amfetamine	T43.621	T43.622	T43.623	T43.624	T43.625	T43.626
Amfetaminil	T43.621	T43.622	T43.623	T43.624	T43.625	T43.626
Amfomycin	T36.8X1	T36.8X2	T36.8X3	T36.8X4	T36.8X5	T36.8X6
Amidefrine mesilate	T48.5X1	T48.5X2	T48.5X3	T48.5X4	T48.5X5	T48.5X6
Amidone	T40.3X1	T40.3X2	T40.3X3	T40.3X4	T40.3X5	T40.3X6
Amidopyrine	T39.2X1	T39.2X2	T39.2X3	T39.2X4	T39.2X5	T39.2X6
Amidotrizoate	T50.8X1	T50.8X2	T50.8X3	T50.8X4	T50.8X5	T50.8X6
Amiflamine	T43.1X1	T43.1X2	T43.1X3	T43.1X4	T43.1X5	T43.1X6
Amikacin	T36.5X1	T36.5X2	T36.5X3	T36.5X4	T36.5X5	T36.5X6
Amikhelline	T46.3X1	T46.3X2	T46.3X3	T46.3X4	T46.3X5	T46.3X6
Amiloride	T50.2X1	T50.2X2	T50.2X3	T50.2X4	T50.2X5	T50.2X6
Aminacrine	T49.0X1	T49.0X2	T49.0X3	T49.0X4	T49.0X5	T49.0X6
Amineptine	T43.011	T43.012	T43.013	T43.014	T43.015	T43.016
Aminitrozole	T37.3X1	T37.3X2	T37.3X3	T37.3X4	T37.3X5	T37.3X6
Aminoacetic acid (derivatives)	T50.3X1	T50.3X2	T50.3X3	T50.3X4	T50.3X5	T50.3X6
Amino acids	T50.3X1	T50.3X2	T50.3X3	T50.3X4	T50.3X5	T50.3X6
Aminoacridine	T49.0X1	T49.0X2	T49.0X3	T49.0X4	T49.0X5	T49.0X6
Aminobenzoic acid (-p)	T49.3X1	T49.3X2	T49.3X3	T49.3X4	T49.3X5	T49.3X6
4-Aminobutyric acid	T43.8X1	T43.8X2	T43.8X3	T43.8X4	T43.8X5	T43.8X6
Aminocaproic acid	T45.621	T45.622	T45.623	T45.624	T45.625	T45.626
Aminofenazone	T39.2X1	T39.2X2	T39.2X3	T39.2X4	T39.2X5	T39.2X6
Aminoethylisothiourium	T45.8X1	T45.8X2	T45.8X3	T45.8X4	T45.8X5	T45.8X6
Aminoglutethimide	T45.1X1	T45.1X2	T45.1X3	T45.1X4	T45.1X5	T45.1X6
Aminohippuric acid	T50.8X1	T50.8X2	T50.8X3	T50.8X4	T50.8X5	T50.8X6
Aminomethylbenzoic acid	T45.691	T45.692	T45.693	T45.694	T45.695	T45.696
Aminometradine	T50.2X1	T50.2X2	T50.2X3	T50.2X4	T50.2X5	T50.2X6
Aminopentamide	T44.3X1	T44.3X2	T44.3X3	T44.3X4	T44.3X5	T44.3X6
Aminophenazone	T39.2X1	T39.2X2	T39.2X3	T39.2X4	T39.2X5	T39.2X6
Aminophenol	T54.0X1	T54.0X2	T54.0X3	T54.0X4	—	—
4-Aminophenol derivatives	T39.1X1	T39.1X2	T39.1X3	T39.1X4	T39.1X5	T39.1X6
Aminophenylpyridone	T43.591	T43.592	T43.593	T43.594	T43.595	T43.596

TABLE OF DRUGS AND CHEMICALS

Substance	External Cause (T-Code)					
	Poisoning, Accidental (Unintentional)	Poisoning, Intentional Self-Harm	Poisoning, Assault	Poisoning, Undetermined	Adverse Effect	Underdosing
Aminophylline	T48.6X1	T48.6X2	T48.6X3	T48.6X4	T48.6X5	T48.6X6
Aminopterin sodium	T45.1X1	T45.1X2	T45.1X3	T45.1X4	T45.1X5	T45.1X6
Aminopyrine	T39.2X1	T39.2X2	T39.2X3	T39.2X4	T39.2X5	T39.2X6
8-Aminoquinoline drugs	T37.2X1	T37.2X2	T37.2X3	T37.2X4	T37.2X5	T37.2X6
Aminorex	T50.5X1	T50.5X2	T50.5X3	T50.5X4	T50.5X5	T50.5X6
Aminosalicylic acid	T37.1X1	T37.1X2	T37.1X3	T37.1X4	T37.1X5	T37.1X6
Aminosalylum	T37.1X1	T37.1X2	T37.1X3	T37.1X4	T37.1X5	T37.1X6
Amiodarone	T46.2X1	T46.2X2	T46.2X3	T46.2X4	T46.2X5	T46.2X6
Amiphenazole	T50.7X1	T50.7X2	T50.7X3	T50.7X4	T50.7X5	T50.7X6
Amiquinsin	T46.5X1	T46.5X2	T46.5X3	T46.5X4	T46.5X5	T46.5X6
Amisometradine	T50.2X1	T50.2X2	T50.2X3	T50.2X4	T50.2X5	T50.2X6
Amisulpride	T43.591	T43.592	T43.593	T43.594	T43.595	T43.596
Amitriptyline	T43.021	T43.022	T43.023	T43.024	T43.025	T43.026
Amitriptylinoxide	T43.021	T43.022	T43.023	T43.024	T43.025	T43.026
Amlexanox	T48.6X1	T48.6X2	T48.6X3	T48.6X4	T48.6X5	T48.6X6
Ammonia (fumes) (gas) (vapor)	T59.891	T59.892	T59.893	T59.894	—	—
aromatic spirit	T48.991	T48.992	T48.993	T48.994	T48.995	T48.996
liquid (household)	T54.3X1	T54.3X2	T54.3X3	T54.3X4	—	—
Ammoniated mercury	T49.0X1	T49.0X2	T49.0X3	T49.0X4	T49.0X5	T49.0X6
Ammonium						
acid tartrate	T49.5X1	T49.5X2	T49.5X3	T49.5X4	T49.5X5	T49.5X6
bromide	T42.6X1	T42.6X2	T42.6X3	T42.6X4	T42.6X5	T42.6X6
carbonate	T54.3X1	T54.3X2	T54.3X3	T54.3X4	—	—
chloride	T50.991	T50.992	T50.993	T50.994	T50.995	T50.996
expectorant	T48.4X1	T48.4X2	T48.4X3	T48.4X4	T48.4X5	T48.4X6
compounds (household) NEC	T54.3X1	T54.3X2	T54.3X3	T54.3X4	—	—
fumes (any usage)	T59.891	T59.892	T59.893	T59.894	—	—
industrial	T54.3X1	T54.3X2	T54.3X3	T54.3X4	—	—
ichthyosulronate	T49.4X1	T49.4X2	T49.4X3	T49.4X4	T49.4X5	T49.4X6
mandelate	T37.91	T37.92	T37.93	T37.94	T37.95	T37.96
sulfamate	T60.3X1	T60.3X2	T60.3X3	T60.3X4	—	—
sulfonate resin	T47.8X1	T47.8X2	T47.8X3	T47.8X4	T47.8X5	T47.8X6
Amobarbital (sodium)	T42.3X1	T42.3X2	T42.3X3	T42.3X4	T42.3X5	T42.3X6
Amodiaquine	T37.2X1	T37.2X2	T37.2X3	T37.2X4	T37.2X5	T37.2X6
Amopyroquin(e)	T37.2X1	T37.2X2	T37.2X3	T37.2X4	T37.2X5	T37.2X6
Amoxapine	T43.011	T43.012	T43.013	T43.014	T43.015	T43.016
Amoxicillin	T36.0X1	T36.0X2	T36.0X3	T36.0X4	T36.0X5	T36.0X6
Amperozide	T43.591	T43.592	T43.593	T43.594	T43.595	T43.596
Amphenidone	T43.591	T43.592	T43.593	T43.594	T43.595	T43.596
Amphetamine NEC	T43.621	T43.622	T43.623	T43.624	T43.625	T43.626

◀ New   ◀ Revised   ~~deleted~~ Deleted

Substance	Poisoning, Accidental (Unintentional)	Poisoning, Intentional Self-Harm	Poisoning, Assault	Poisoning, Undetermined	Adverse Effect	Underdosing
	External Cause (T-Code)					
Amphomycin	T36.8X1	T36.8X2	T36.8X3	T36.8X4	T36.8X5	T36.8X6
Amphotalide	T37.4X1	T37.4X2	T37.4X3	T37.4X4	T37.4X5	T37.4X6
Amphotericin B	T36.7X1	T36.7X2	T36.7X3	T36.7X4	T36.7X5	T36.7X6
topical	T49.0X1	T49.0X2	T49.0X3	T49.0X4	T49.0X5	T49.0X6
Ampicillin	T36.0X1	T36.0X2	T36.0X3	T36.0X4	T36.0X5	T36.0X6
Amprotropine	T44.3X1	T44.3X2	T44.3X3	T44.3X4	T44.3X5	T44.3X6
Amsacrine	T45.1X1	T45.1X2	T45.1X3	T45.1X4	T45.1X5	T45.1X6
Amygdaline	T62.2X1	T62.2X2	T62.2X3	T62.2X4	—	—
Amyl						
acetate	T52.8X1	T52.8X2	T52.8X3	T52.8X4	—	—
vapor	T59.891	T59.892	T59.893	T59.894	—	—
alcohol	T51.3X1	T51.3X2	T51.3X3	T51.3X4	—	—
chloride	T53.6X1	T53.6X2	T53.6X3	T53.6X4	—	—
formate	T52.8X1	T52.8X2	T52.8X3	T52.8X4	—	—
nitrite	T46.3X1	T46.3X2	T46.3X3	T46.3X4	T46.3X5	T46.3X6
propionate	T65.891	T65.892	T65.893	T65.894	—	—
Amylase	T47.5X1	T47.5X2	T47.5X3	T47.5X4	T47.5X5	T47.5X6
Amyleine, regional	T41.3X1	T41.3X2	T41.3X3	T41.3X4	T41.3X5	T41.3X6
Amylene						
dichloride	T53.6X1	T53.6X2	T53.6X3	T53.6X4	—	—
hydrate	T51.3X1	T51.3X2	T51.3X3	T51.3X4	—	—
Amylmetacresol	T49.6X1	T49.6X2	T49.6X3	T49.6X4	T49.6X5	T49.6X6
Amylobarbitone	T42.3X1	T42.3X2	T42.3X3	T42.3X4	T42.3X5	T42.3X6
Amylocaine, regional	T41.3X1	T41.3X2	T41.3X3	T41.3X4	T41.3X5	T41.3X6
infiltration (subcutaneous)	T41.3X1	T41.3X2	T41.3X3	T41.3X4	T41.3X5	T41.3X6
nerve block (peripheral) (plexus)	T41.3X1	T41.3X2	T41.3X3	T41.3X4	T41.3X5	T41.3X6
spinal	T41.3X1	T41.3X2	T41.3X3	T41.3X4	T41.3X5	T41.3X6
topical (surface)	T41.3X1	T41.3X2	T41.3X3	T41.3X4	T41.3X5	T41.3X6
Amylopectin	T47.6X1	T47.6X2	T47.6X3	T47.6X4	T47.6X5	T47.6X6
Amytal (sodium)	T42.3X1	T42.3X2	T42.3X3	T42.3X4	T42.3X5	T42.3X6
Anabolic steroid	T38.7X1	T38.7X2	T38.7X3	T38.7X4	T38.7X5	T38.7X6
Analeptic NEC	T50.7X1	T50.7X2	T50.7X3	T50.7X4	T50.7X5	T50.7X6
Analgesic	T39.91	T39.92	T39.93	T39.94	T39.95	T39.96
anti-inflammatory NEC	T39.91	T39.92	T39.93	T39.94	T39.95	T39.96
propionic acid derivative	T39.311	T39.312	T39.313	T39.314	T39.315	T39.316
antirheumatic NEC	T39.4X1	T39.4X2	T39.4X3	T39.4X4	T39.4X5	T39.4X6
aromatic NEC	T39.1X1	T39.1X2	T39.1X3	T39.1X4	T39.1X5	T39.1X6
narcotic NEC	T40.601	T40.602	T40.603	T40.604	T40.605	T40.606
combination	T40.601	T40.602	T40.603	T40.604	T40.605	T40.606
obstetric	T40.601	T40.602	T40.603	T40.604	T40.605	T40.606

TABLE OF DRUGS AND CHEMICALS

Substance	Poisoning, Accidental (Unintentional)	Poisoning, Intentional Self-Harm	Poisoning, Assault	Poisoning, Undetermined	Adverse Effect	Underdosing
Analgesic *(Continued)*						
non-narcotic NEC	T39.91	T39.92	T39.93	T39.94	T39.95	T39.96
combination	T39.91	T39.92	T39.93	T39.94	T39.95	T39.96
pyrazole	T39.2X1	T39.2X2	T39.2X3	T39.2X4	T39.2X5	T39.2X6
specified NEC	T39.8X1	T39.8X2	T39.8X3	T39.8X4	T39.8X5	T39.8X6
Analgin	T39.2X1	T39.2X2	T39.2X3	T39.2X4	T39.2X5	T39.2X6
Anamirta cocculus	T62.1X1	T62.1X2	T62.1X3	T62.1X4	—	—
Ancillin	T36.0X1	T36.0X2	T36.0X3	T36.0X4	T36.0X5	T36.0X6
Ancrod	T45.691	T45.692	T45.693	T45.694	T45.695	T45.696
Androgen	T38.7X1	T38.7X2	T38.7X3	T38.7X4	T38.7X5	T38.7X6
Androgen-estrogen mixture	T38.7X1	T38.7X2	T38.7X3	T38.7X4	T38.7X5	T38.7X6
Androstalone	T38.7X1	T38.7X2	T38.7X3	T38.7X4	T38.7X5	T38.7X6
Androstanolone	T38.7X1	T38.7X2	T38.7X3	T38.7X4	T38.7X5	T38.7X6
Androsterone	T38.7X1	T38.7X2	T38.7X3	T38.7X4	T38.7X5	T38.7X6
Anemone pulsatilla	T62.2X1	T62.2X2	T62.2X3	T62.2X4	—	—
Anesthesia						
caudal	T41.3X1	T41.3X2	T41.3X3	T41.3X4	T41.3X5	T41.3X6
endotracheal	T41.0X1	T41.0X2	T41.0X3	T41.0X4	T41.0X5	T41.0X6
epidural	T41.3X1	T41.3X2	T41.3X3	T41.3X4	T41.3X5	T41.3X6
inhalation	T41.0X1	T41.0X2	T41.0X3	T41.0X4	T41.0X5	T41.0X6
local	T41.3X1	T41.3X2	T41.3X3	T41.3X4	T41.3X5	T41.3X6
mucosal	T41.3X1	T41.3X2	T41.3X3	T41.3X4	T41.3X5	T41.3X6
muscle relaxation	T48.1X1	T48.1X2	T48.1X3	T48.1X4	T48.1X5	T48.1X6
nerve blocking	T41.3X1	T41.3X2	T41.3X3	T41.3X4	T41.3X5	T41.3X6
plexus blocking	T41.3X1	T41.3X2	T41.3X3	T41.3X4	T41.3X5	T41.3X6
potentiated	T41.201	T41.202	T41.203	T41.204	T41.205	T41.206
rectal	T41.201	T41.202	T41.203	T41.204	T41.205	T41.206
general	T41.201	T41.202	T41.203	T41.204	T41.205	T41.206
local	T41.3X1	T41.3X2	T41.3X3	T41.3X4	T41.3X5	T41.3X6
regional	T41.3X1	T41.3X2	T41.3X3	T41.3X4	T41.3X5	T41.3X6
surface	T41.3X1	T41.3X2	T41.3X3	T41.3X4	T41.3X5	T41.3X6
Anesthetic NEC — *see also Anesthesia*	T41.41	T41.42	T41.43	T41.44	T41.45	T41.46
with muscle relaxant	T41.201	T41.202	T41.203	T41.204	T41.205	T41.206
general	T41.201	T41.202	T41.203	T41.204	T41.205	T41.206
local	T41.3X1	T41.3X2	T41.3X3	T41.3X4	T41.3X5	T41.3X6
gaseous NEC	T41.0X1	T41.0X2	T41.0X3	T41.0X4	T41.0X5	T41.0X6
general NEC	T41.201	T41.202	T41.203	T41.204	T41.205	T41.206
halogenated hydrocarbon derivatives NEC	T41.0X1	T41.0X2	T41.0X3	T41.0X4	T41.0X5	T41.0X6
infiltration NEC	T41.3X1	T41.3X2	T41.3X3	T41.3X4	T41.3X5	T41.3X6
intravenous NEC	T41.1X1	T41.1X2	T41.1X3	T41.1X4	T41.1X5	T41.1X6

◀ New ◀▥ Revised ~~deleted~~ Deleted

Substance	External Cause (T-Code)					
	Poisoning, Accidental (Unintentional)	Poisoning, Intentional Self-Harm	Poisoning, Assault	Poisoning, Undetermined	Adverse Effect	Underdosing
Anesthetic NEC *(Continued)*						
local NEC	T41.3X1	T41.3X2	T41.3X3	T41.3X4	T41.3X5	T41.3X6
rectal	T41.201	T41.202	T41.203	T41.204	T41.205	T41.206
general	T41.201	T41.202	T41.203	T41.204	T41.205	T41.206
local	T41.3X1	T41.3X2	T41.3X3	T41.3X4	T41.3X5	T41.3X6
regional NEC	T41.3X1	T41.3X2	T41.3X3	T41.3X4	T41.3X5	T41.3X6
spinal NEC	T41.3X1	T41.3X2	T41.3X3	T41.3X4	T41.3X5	T41.3X6
thiobarbiturate	T41.1X1	T41.1X2	T41.1X3	T41.1X4	T41.1X5	T41.1X6
topical	T41.3X1	T41.3X2	T41.3X3	T41.3X4	T41.3X5	T41.3X6
Aneurine	T45.2X1	T45.2X2	T45.2X3	T45.2X4	T45.2X5	T45.2X6
Angio-Conray	T50.8X1	T50.8X2	T50.8X3	T50.8X4	T50.8X5	T50.8X6
Angiotensin	T44.5X1	T44.5X2	T44.5X3	T44.5X4	T44.5X5	T44.5X6
Angiotensinamide	T44.991	T44.992	T44.993	T44.994	T44.995	T44.996
Anhydrohydroxy-progesterone	T38.5X1	T38.5X2	T38.5X3	T38.5X4	T38.5X5	T38.5X6
Anhydron	T50.2X1	T50.2X2	T50.2X3	T50.2X4	T50.2X5	T50.2X6
Anileridine	T40.4X1	T40.4X2	T40.4X3	T40.4X4	T40.4X5	T40.4X6
Aniline (dye) (liquid)	T65.3X1	T65.3X2	T65.3X3	T65.3X4	—	—
analgesic	T39.1X1	T39.1X2	T39.1X3	T39.1X4	T39.1X5	T39.1X6
derivatives, therapeutic NEC	T39.1X1	T39.1X2	T39.1X3	T39.1X4	T39.1X5	T39.1X6
vapor	T65.3X1	T65.3X2	T65.3X3	T65.3X4	—	—
Anise oil	T47.5X1	T47.5X2	T47.5X3	T47.5X4	T47.5X5	T47.5X6
Aniscoropine	T44.3X1	T44.3X2	T44.3X3	T44.3X4	T44.3X5	T44.3X6
Anisidine	T65.3X1	T65.3X2	T65.3X3	T65.3X4	—	—
Anisindione	T45.511	T45.512	T45.513	T45.514	T45.515	T45.516
Anisotropine methyl-bromide	T44.3X1	T44.3X2	T44.3X3	T44.3X4	T44.3X5	T44.3X6
Anistreplase	T45.611	T45.612	T45.613	T45.614	T45.615	T45.616
Anorexiant (central)	T50.5X1	T50.5X2	T50.5X3	T50.5X4	T50.5X5	T50.5X6
Anorexic agents	T50.5X1	T50.5X2	T50.5X3	T50.5X4	T50.5X5	T50.5X6
Ansamycin	T36.6X1	T36.6X2	T36.6X3	T36.6X4	T36.6X5	T36.6X6
Ant (bite) (sting)	T63.421	T63.422	T63.423	T63.424	—	—
Antabuse	T50.6X1	T50.6X2	T50.6X3	T50.6X4	T50.6X5	T50.6X6
Ant poison—*see Insecticide*						
Antacid NEC	T47.1X1	T47.1X2	T47.1X3	T47.1X4	T47.1X5	T47.1X6
Antagonist						
Aldosterone	T50.0X1	T50.0X2	T50.0X3	T50.0X4	T50.0X5	T50.0X6
alpha-adrenoreceptor	T44.6X1	T44.6X2	T44.6X3	T44.6X4	T44.6X5	T44.6X6
anticoagulant	T45.7X1	T45.7X2	T45.7X3	T45.7X4	T45.7X5	T45.7X6
beta-adrenoreceptor	T44.7X1	T44.7X2	T44.7X3	T44.7X4	T44.7X5	T44.7X6
extrapyramidal NEC	T44.3X1	T44.3X2	T44.3X3	T44.3X4	T44.3X5	T44.3X6
folic acid	T45.1X1	T45.1X2	T45.1X3	T45.1X4	T45.1X5	T45.1X6

TABLE OF DRUGS AND CHEMICALS

Substance	External Cause (T-Code)					
	Poisoning, Accidental (Unintentional)	Poisoning, Intentional Self-Harm	Poisoning, Assault	Poisoning, Undetermined	Adverse Effect	Underdosing
Antagonist *(Continued)*						
H2 receptor	T47.0X1	T47.0X2	T47.0X3	T47.0X4	T47.0X5	T47.0X6
heavy metal	T45.8X1	T45.8X2	T45.8X3	T45.8X4	T45.8X5	T45.8X6
narcotic analgesic	T50.7X1	T50.7X2	T50.7X3	T50.7X4	T50.7X5	T50.7X6
opiate	T50.7X1	T50.7X2	T50.7X3	T50.7X4	T50.7X5	T50.7X6
pyrimidine	T45.1X1	T45.1X2	T45.1X3	T45.1X4	T45.1X5	T45.1X6
serotonin	T46.5X1	T46.5X2	T46.5X3	T46.5X4	T46.5X5	T46.5X6
Antazolin(e)	T45.0X1	T45.0X2	T45.0X3	T45.0X4	T45.0X5	T45.0X6
Anterior pituitary hormone NEC	T38.811	T38.812	T38.813	T38.814	T38.815	T38.816
Anthelmintic NEC	T37.4X1	T37.4X2	T37.4X3	T37.4X4	T37.4X5	T37.4X6
Anthiolimine	T37.4X1	T37.4X2	T37.4X3	T37.4X4	T37.4X5	T37.4X6
Anthralin	T49.4X1	T49.4X2	T49.4X3	T49.4X4	T49.4X5	T49.4X6
Anthramycin	T45.1X1	T45.1X2	T45.1X3	T45.1X4	T45.1X5	T45.1X6
Antiadrenergic NEC	T44.8X1	T44.8X2	T44.8X3	T44.8X4	T44.8X5	T44.8X6
Antiallergic NEC	T45.0X1	T45.0X2	T45.0X3	T45.0X4	T45.0X5	T45.0X6
Anti-anemic (drug) (preparation)	T45.8X1	T45.8X2	T45.8X3	T45.8X4	T45.8X5	T45.8X6
Antiandrogen NEC	T38.6X1	T38.6X2	T38.6X3	T38.6X4	T38.6X5	T38.6X6
Antianxiety drug NEC	T43.501	T43.502	T43.503	T43.504	T43.505	T43.506
Antiaris toxicaria	T65.891	T65.892	T65.893	T65.894	—	—
Antiarteriosclerotic drug	T46.6X1	T46.6X2	T46.6X3	T46.6X4	T46.6X5	T46.6X6
Antiasthmatic drug NEC	T48.6X1	T48.6X2	T48.6X3	T48.6X4	T48.6X5	T48.6X6
Antibiotic NEC	T36.91	T36.92	T36.93	T36.94	T36.95	T36.96
aminoglycoside	T36.5X1	T36.5X2	T36.5X3	T36.5X4	T36.5X5	T36.5X6
anticancer	T45.1X1	T45.1X2	T45.1X3	T45.1X4	T45.1X5	T45.1X6
antifungal	T36.7X1	T36.7X2	T36.7X3	T36.7X4	T36.7X5	T36.7X6
antimycobacterial	T36.5X1	T36.5X2	T36.5X3	T36.5X4	T36.5X5	T36.5X6
antineoplastic	T45.1X1	T45.1X2	T45.1X3	T45.1X4	T45.1X5	T45.1X6
cephalosporin (group)	T36.1X1	T36.1X2	T36.1X3	T36.1X4	T36.1X5	T36.1X6
chloramphenicol (group)	T36.2X1	T36.2X2	T36.2X3	T36.2X4	T36.2X5	T36.2X6
ENT	T49.6X1	T49.6X2	T49.6X3	T49.6X4	T49.6X5	T49.6X6
eye	T49.5X1	T49.5X2	T49.5X3	T49.5X4	T49.5X5	T49.5X6
fungicidal (local)	T49.0X1	T49.0X2	T49.0X3	T49.0X4	T49.0X5	T49.0X6
intestinal	T36.8X1	T36.8X2	T36.8X3	T36.8X4	T36.8X5	T36.8X6
b-lactam NEC	T36.1X1	T36.1X2	T36.1X3	T36.1X4	T36.1X5	T36.1X6
local	T49.0X1	T49.0X2	T49.0X3	T49.0X4	T49.0X5	T49.0X6
macrolides	T36.3X1	T36.3X2	T36.3X3	T36.3X4	T36.3X5	T36.3X6
polypeptide	T36.8X1	T36.8X2	T36.8X3	T36.8X4	T36.8X5	T36.8X6
specified NEC	T36.8X1	T36.8X2	T36.8X3	T36.8X4	T36.8X5	T36.8X6
tetracycline (group)	T36.4X1	T36.4X2	T36.4X3	T36.4X4	T36.4X5	T36.4X6
throat	T49.6X1	T49.6X2	T49.6X3	T49.6X4	T49.6X5	T49.6X6

◀ New ◀▥ Revised ~~deleted~~ Deleted

Substance	Poisoning, Accidental (Unintentional)	Poisoning, Intentional Self-Harm	Poisoning, Assault	Poisoning, Undetermined	Adverse Effect	Underdosing
	External Cause (T-Code)					
Anticancer agents NEC	T45.1X1	T45.1X2	T45.1X3	T45.1X4	T45.1X5	T45.1X6
Anticholesterolemic drug NEC	T46.6X1	T46.6X2	T46.6X3	T46.6X4	T46.6X5	T46.6X6
Anticholinergic NEC	T44.3X1	T44.3X2	T44.3X3	T44.3X4	T44.3X5	T44.3X6
Anticholinesterase	T44.0X1	T44.0X2	T44.0X3	T44.0X4	T44.0X5	T44.0X6
organophosphorus	T44.0X1	T44.0X2	T44.0X3	T44.0X4	T44.0X5	T44.0X6
insecticide	T60.0X1	T60.0X2	T60.0X3	T60.0X4	—	—
nerve gas	T59.891	T59.892	T59.893	T59.894	—	—
reversible	T44.0X1	T44.0X2	T44.0X3	T44.0X4	T44.0X5	T44.0X6
ophthalmological	T49.5X1	T49.5X2	T49.5X3	T49.5X4	T49.5X5	T49.5X6
Anticoagulant NEC	T45.511	T45.512	T45.513	T45.514	T45.515	T45.516
Antagonist	T45.7X1	T45.7X2	T45.7X3	T45.7X4	T45.7X5	T45.7X6
Anti-common-cold drug NEC	T48.5X1	T48.5X2	T48.5X3	T48.5X4	T48.5X5	T48.5X6
Anticonvulsant	T42.71	T42.72	T42.73	T42.74	T42.75	T42.76
barbiturate	T42.3X1	T42.3X2	T42.3X3	T42.3X4	T42.3X5	T42.3X6
combination (with barbiturate)	T42.3X1	T42.3X2	T42.3X3	T42.3X4	T42.3X5	T42.3X6
hydantoin	T42.0X1	T42.0X2	T42.0X3	T42.0X4	T42.0X5	T42.0X6
hypnotic NEC	T42.6X1	T42.6X2	T42.6X3	T42.6X4	T42.6X5	T42.6X6
oxazolidinedione	T42.2X1	T42.2X2	T42.2X3	T42.2X4	T42.2X5	T42.2X6
pyrimidinedione	T42.6X1	T42.6X2	T42.6X3	T42.6X4	T42.6X5	T42.6X6
specified NEC	T42.6X1	T42.6X2	T42.6X3	T42.6X4	T42.6X5	T42.6X6
succinimide	T42.2X1	T42.2X2	T42.2X3	T42.2X4	T42.2X5	T42.2X6
Anti-D immunoglobulin (human)	T50.Z11	T50.Z12	T50.Z13	T50.Z14	T50.Z15	T50.Z16
Antidepressant NEC	T43.201	T43.202	T43.203	T43.204	T43.205	T43.206
monoamine oxidase inhibitor	T43.1X1	T43.1X2	T43.1X3	T43.1X4	T43.1X5	T43.1X6
selective serotonin norepinephrine reuptake inhibitor	T43.211	T43.212	T43.213	T43.214	T43.215	T43.216
selective serotonin reuptake inhibitor	T43.221	T43.222	T43.223	T43.224	T43.225	T43.226
specified NEC	T43.291	T43.292	T43.293	T43.294	T43.295	T43.296
tetracyclic	T43.021	T43.022	T43.023	T43.024	T43.025	T43.026
triazolopyridine	T43.221	T43.222	T43.223	T43.224	T43.225	T43.226
tricyclic	T43.011	T43.012	T43.013	T43.014	T43.015	T43.016
Antidiabetic NEC	T38.3X1	T38.3X2	T38.3X3	T38.3X4	T38.3X5	T38.3X6
biguanide	T38.3X1	T38.3X2	T38.3X3	T38.3X4	T38.3X5	T38.3X6
and sulfonyl combined	T38.3X1	T38.3X2	T38.3X3	T38.3X4	T38.3X5	T38.3X6
combined	T38.3X1	T38.3X2	T38.3X3	T38.3X4	T38.3X5	T38.3X6
sulfonylurea	T38.3X1	T38.3X2	T38.3X3	T38.3X4	T38.3X5	T38.3X6
Antidiarrheal drug NEC	T47.6X1	T47.6X2	T47.6X3	T47.6X4	T47.6X5	T47.6X6
absorbent	T47.6X1	T47.6X2	T47.6X3	T47.6X4	T47.6X5	T47.6X6
Antidiphtheria serum	T50.Z11	T50.Z12	T50.Z13	T50.Z14	T50.Z15	T50.Z16
Antidiuretic hormone	T38.891	T38.892	T38.893	T38.894	T38.895	T38.896

◀ New ◀▥ Revised ~~deleted~~ Deleted

Substance	Poisoning, Accidental (Unintentional)	Poisoning, Intentional Self-Harm	Poisoning, Assault	Poisoning, Undetermined	Adverse Effect	Underdosing
	External Cause (T-Code)					
Antidote NEC	T50.6X1	T50.6X2	T50.6X3	T50.6X4	T50.6X5	T50.6X6
heavy metal	T45.8X1	T45.8X2	T45.8X3	T45.8X4	T45.8X5	T45.8X6
Antidysrhythmic NEC	T46.2X1	T46.2X2	T46.2X3	T46.2X4	T46.2X5	T46.2X6
Antiemetic drug	T45.0X1	T45.0X2	T45.0X3	T45.0X4	T45.0X5	T45.0X6
Antiepilepsy agent	T42.71	T42.72	T42.73	T42.74	T42.75	T42.76
combination	T42.5X1	T42.5X2	T42.5X3	T42.5X4	T42.5X5	T42.5X6
mixed	T42.5X1	T42.5X2	T42.5X3	T42.5X4	T42.5X5	T42.5X6
specified, NEC	T42.6X1	T42.6X2	T42.6X3	T42.6X4	T42.6X5	T42.6X6
Antiestrogen NEC	T38.6X1	T38.6X2	T38.6X3	T38.6X4	T38.6X5	T38.6X6
Antifertility pill	T38.4X1	T38.4X2	T38.4X3	T38.4X4	T38.4X5	T38.4X6
Antifibrinolytic drug	T45.621	T45.622	T45.623	T45.624	T45.625	T45.626
Antifilarial drug	T37.4X1	T37.4X2	T37.4X3	T37.4X4	T37.4X5	T37.4X6
Antiflatulent	T47.5X1	T47.5X2	T47.5X3	T47.5X4	T47.5X5	T47.5X6
Antifreeze	T65.91	T65.92	T65.93	T65.94	—	—
alcohol	T51.1X1	T51.1X2	T51.1X3	T51.1X4	—	—
ethylene glycol	T51.8X1	T51.8X2	T51.8X3	T51.8X4	—	—
Antifungal						
antibiotic (systemic)	T36.7X1	T36.7X2	T36.7X3	T36.7X4	T36.7X5	T36.7X6
anti-infective NEC	T37.91	T37.92	T37.93	T37.94	T37.95	T37.96
disinfectant, local	T49.0X1	T49.0X2	T49.0X3	T49.0X4	T49.0X5	T49.0X6
nonmedicinal (spray)	T60.3X1	T60.3X2	T60.3X3	T60.3X4	—	—
topical	T49.0X1	T49.0X2	T49.0X3	T49.0X4	T49.0X5	T49.0X6
Anti-gastric-secretion drug NEC	T47.1X1	T47.1X2	T47.1X3	T47.1X4	T47.1X5	T47.1X6
Antigonadotrophin NEC	T38.6X1	T38.6X2	T38.6X3	T38.6X4	T38.6X5	T38.6X6
Antihallucinogen	T43.501	T43.502	T43.503	T43.504	T43.505	T43.506
Antihelmintics	T37.4X1	T37.4X2	T37.4X3	T37.4X4	T37.4X5	T37.4X6
Antihemophilic						
factor	T45.8X1	T45.8X2	T45.8X3	T45.8X4	T45.8X5	T45.8X6
fraction	T45.8X1	T45.8X2	T45.8X3	T45.8X4	T45.8X5	T45.8X6
globulin concentrate	T45.7X1	T45.7X2	T45.7X3	T45.7X4	T45.7X5	T45.7X6
human plasma	T45.8X1	T45.8X2	T45.8X3	T45.8X4	T45.8X5	T45.8X6
plasma, dried	T45.7X1	T45.7X2	T45.7X3	T45.7X4	T45.7X5	T45.7X6
Antihemorrhoidal preparation	T49.2X1	T49.2X2	T49.2X3	T49.2X4	T49.2X5	T49.2X6
Antiheparin drug	T45.7X1	T45.7X2	T45.7X3	T45.7X4	T45.7X5	T45.7X6
Antihistamine	T45.0X1	T45.0X2	T45.0X3	T45.0X4	T45.0X5	T45.0X6
Antihookworm drug	T37.4X1	T37.4X2	T37.4X3	T37.4X4	T37.4X5	T37.4X6
Anti-human lymphocytic globulin	T50.Z11	T50.Z12	T50.Z13	T50.Z14	T50.Z15	T50.Z16
Antihyperlipidemic drug	T46.6X1	T46.6X2	T46.6X3	T46.6X4	T46.6X5	T46.6X6
Antihypertensive drug NEC	T46.5X1	T46.5X2	T46.5X3	T46.5X4	T46.5X5	T46.5X6

◀ New   ◀▥ Revised   d̶e̶l̶e̶t̶e̶d̶ Deleted

Substance	External Cause (T-Code)					
	Poisoning, Accidental (Unintentional)	Poisoning, Intentional Self-Harm	Poisoning, Assault	Poisoning, Undetermined	Adverse Effect	Underdosing
Anti-infective NEC	T37.91	T37.92	T37.93	T37.94	T37.95	T37.96
anthelmintic	T37.4X1	T37.4X2	T37.4X3	T37.4X4	T37.4X5	T37.4X6
antibiotics	T36.91	T36.92	T36.93	T36.94	T36.95	T36.96
specified NEC	T36.8X1	T36.8X2	T36.8X3	T36.8X4	T36.8X5	T36.8X6
antimalarial	T37.2X1	T37.2X2	T37.2X3	T37.2X4	T37.2X5	T37.2X6
antimycobacterial NEC	T37.1X1	T37.1X2	T37.1X3	T37.1X4	T37.1X5	T37.1X6
antibiotics	T36.5X1	T36.5X2	T36.5X3	T36.5X4	T36.5X5	T36.5X6
antiprotozoal NEC	T37.3X1	T37.3X2	T37.3X3	T37.3X4	T37.3X5	T37.3X6
blood	T37.2X1	T37.2X2	T37.2X3	T37.2X4	T37.2X5	T37.2X6
antiviral	T37.5X1	T37.5X2	T37.5X3	T37.5X4	T37.5X5	T37.5X6
arsenical	T37.8X1	T37.8X2	T37.8X3	T37.8X4	T37.8X5	T37.8X6
bismuth, local	T49.0X1	T49.0X2	T49.0X3	T49.0X4	T49.0X5	T49.0X6
ENT	T49.6X1	T49.6X2	T49.6X3	T49.6X4	T49.6X5	T49.6X6
eye NEC	T49.5X1	T49.5X2	T49.5X3	T49.5X4	T49.5X5	T49.5X6
heavy metals NEC	T37.8X1	T37.8X2	T37.8X3	T37.8X4	T37.8X5	T37.8X6
local NEC	T49.0X1	T49.0X2	T49.0X3	T49.0X4	T49.0X5	T49.0X6
specified NEC	T49.0X1	T49.0X2	T49.0X3	T49.0X4	T49.0X5	T49.0X6
mixed	T37.91	T37.92	T37.93	T37.94	T37.95	T37.96
ophthalmic preparation	T49.5X1	T49.5X2	T49.5X3	T49.5X4	T49.5X5	T49.5X6
topical NEC	T49.0X1	T49.0X2	T49.0X3	T49.0X4	T49.0X5	T49.0X6
Anti-inflammatory drug NEC	T49.0X1	T49.0X2	T49.0X3	T49.0X4	T49.0X5	T49.0X6
local	T49.0X1	T49.0X2	T49.0X3	T49.0X4	T49.0X5	T49.0X6
nonsteroidal NEC	T39.391	T39.392	T39.393	T39.394	T39.395	T39.396
propionic acid derivative	T39.311	T39.312	T39.313	T39.314	T39.315	T39.316
specified NEC	T39.391	T39.392	T39.393	T39.394	T39.395	T39.396
Antikaluretic	T50.3X1	T50.3X2	T50.3X3	T50.3X4	T50.3X5	T50.3X6
Antiknock (tetraethyl lead)	T56.0X1	T56.0X2	T56.0X3	T56.0X4	—	—
Antilipemic drug NEC	T46.6X1	T46.6X2	T46.6X3	T46.6X4	T46.6X5	T46.6X6
Antimalarial	T37.2X1	T37.2X2	T37.2X3	T37.2X4	T37.2X5	T37.2X6
prophylactic NEC	T37.2X1	T37.2X2	T37.2X3	T37.2X4	T37.2X5	T37.2X6
pyrimidine derivative	T37.2X1	T37.2X2	T37.2X3	T37.2X4	T37.2X5	T37.2X6
Antimetabolite	T45.1X1	T45.1X2	T45.1X3	T45.1X4	T45.1X5	T45.1X6
Antimitotic agent	T45.1X1	T45.1X2	T45.1X3	T45.1X4	T45.1X5	T45.1X6
Antimony (compounds) (vapor) NEC	T56.891	T56.892	T56.893	T56.894	—	—
anti-infectives	T37.8X1	T37.8X2	T37.8X3	T37.8X4	T37.8X5	T37.8X6
dimercaptosuccinate	T37.3X1	T37.3X2	T37.3X3	T37.3X4	T37.3X5	T37.3X6
hydride	T56.891	T56.892	T56.893	T56.894	—	—
pesticide (vapor)	T60.8X1	T60.8X2	T60.8X3	T60.8X4	—	—
potassium (sodium) tartrate	T37.8X1	T37.8X2	T37.8X3	T37.8X4	T37.8X5	T37.8X6

TABLE OF DRUGS AND CHEMICALS

Substance	External Cause (T-Code)					
	Poisoning, Accidental (Unintentional)	Poisoning, Intentional Self-Harm	Poisoning, Assault	Poisoning, Undetermined	Adverse Effect	Underdosing
Antimony NEC *(Continued)*						
sodium dimercaptosuccinate	T37.3X1	T37.3X2	T37.3X3	T37.3X4	T37.3X5	T37.3X6
tartrated	T37.8X1	T37.8X2	T37.8X3	T37.8X4	T37.8X5	T37.8X6
Antimuscarinic NEC	T44.3X1	T44.3X2	T44.3X3	T44.3X4	T44.3X5	T44.3X6
Antimycobacterial drug NEC	T37.1X1	T37.1X2	T37.1X3	T37.1X4	T37.1X5	T37.1X6
antibiotics	T36.5X1	T36.5X2	T36.5X3	T36.5X4	T36.5X5	T36.5X6
combination	T37.1X1	T37.1X2	T37.1X3	T37.1X4	T37.1X5	T37.1X6
Antinausea drug	T45.0X1	T45.0X2	T45.0X3	T45.0X4	T45.0X5	T45.0X6
Antinematode drug	T37.4X1	T37.4X2	T37.4X3	T37.4X4	T37.4X5	T37.4X6
Antineoplastic NEC	T45.1X1	T45.1X2	T45.1X3	T45.1X4	T45.1X5	T45.1X6
alkaloidal	T45.1X1	T45.1X2	T45.1X3	T45.1X4	T45.1X5	T45.1X6
antibiotics	T45.1X1	T45.1X2	T45.1X3	T45.1X4	T45.1X5	T45.1X6
combination	T45.1X1	T45.1X2	T45.1X3	T45.1X4	T45.1X5	T45.1X6
estrogen	T38.5X1	T38.5X2	T38.5X3	T38.5X4	T38.5X5	T38.5X6
steroid	T38.7X1	T38.7X2	T38.7X3	T38.7X4	T38.7X5	T38.7X6
Antiparasitic drug (systemic)	T37.91	T37.92	T37.93	T37.94	T37.95	T37.96
local	T49.0X1	T49.0X2	T49.0X3	T49.0X4	T49.0X5	T49.0X6
specified NEC	T37.8X1	T37.8X2	T37.8X3	T37.8X4	T37.8X5	T37.8X6
Antiparkinsonism drug NEC	T42.8X1	T42.8X2	T42.8X3	T42.8X4	T42.8X5	T42.8X6
Antiperspirant NEC	T49.2X1	T49.2X2	T49.2X3	T49.2X4	T49.2X5	T49.2X6
Antiphlogistic NEC	T39.4X1	T39.4X2	T39.4X3	T39.4X4	T39.4X5	T39.4X6
Antiplatyhelmintic drug	T37.4X1	T37.4X2	T37.4X3	T37.4X4	T37.4X5	T37.4X6
Antiprotozoal drug NEC	T37.3X1	T37.3X2	T37.3X3	T37.3X4	T37.3X5	T37.3X6
blood	T37.2X1	T37.2X2	T37.2X3	T37.2X4	T37.2X5	T37.2X6
local	T49.0X1	T49.0X2	T49.0X3	T49.0X4	T49.0X5	T49.0X6
Antipruritic drug NEC	T49.1X1	T49.1X2	T49.1X3	T49.1X4	T49.1X5	T49.1X6
Antipsychotic drug	T43.501	T43.502	T43.503	T43.504	T43.505	T43.506
specified NEC	T43.591	T43.592	T43.593	T43.594	T43.595	T43.596
Antipyretic	T39.91	T39.92	T39.93	T39.94	T39.95	T39.96
specified NEC	T39.8X1	T39.8X2	T39.8X3	T39.8X4	T39.8X5	T39.8X6
Antipyrine	T39.2X1	T39.2X2	T39.2X3	T39.2X4	T39.2X5	T39.2X6
Antirabies hyperimmune serum	T50.Z11	T50.Z12	T50.Z13	T50.Z14	T50.Z15	T50.Z16
Antirheumatic NEC	T39.4X1	T39.4X2	T39.4X3	T39.4X4	T39.4X5	T39.4X6
Antirigidity drug NEC	T42.8X1	T42.8X2	T42.8X3	T42.8X4	T42.8X5	T42.8X6
Antischistosomal drug	T37.4X1	T37.4X2	T37.4X3	T37.4X4	T37.4X5	T37.4X6
Antiscorpion sera	T50.Z11	T50.Z12	T50.Z13	T50.Z14	T50.Z15	T50.Z16
Antiseborrheics	T49.4X1	T49.4X2	T49.4X3	T49.4X4	T49.4X5	T49.4X6
Antiseptics (external) (medicinal)	T49.0X1	T49.0X2	T49.0X3	T49.0X4	T49.0X5	T49.0X6
Antistine	T45.0X1	T45.0X2	T45.0X3	T45.0X4	T45.0X5	T45.0X6
Antitapeworm drug	T37.4X1	T37.4X2	T37.4X3	T37.4X4	T37.4X5	T37.4X6

◄ New   ◄▦ Revised   ~~deleted~~ Deleted

Substance	Poisoning, Accidental (Unintentional)	Poisoning, Intentional Self-Harm	Poisoning, Assault	Poisoning, Undetermined	Adverse Effect	Underdosing
	External Cause (T-Code)					
Antitetanus immunoglobulin	T50.Z11	T50.Z12	T50.Z13	T50.Z14	T50.Z15	T50.Z16
Antithyroid drug NEC	T38.2X1	T38.2X2	T38.2X3	T38.2X4	T38.2X5	T38.2X6
Antitoxin	T50.Z11	T50.Z12	T50.Z13	T50.Z14	T50.Z15	T50.Z16
diphtheria	T50.Z11	T50.Z12	T50.Z13	T50.Z14	T50.Z15	T50.Z16
gas gangrene	T50.Z11	T50.Z12	T50.Z13	T50.Z14	T50.Z15	T50.Z16
tetanus	T50.Z11	T50.Z12	T50.Z13	T50.Z14	T50.Z15	T50.Z16
Antitoxin, any	T50.901	T50.902	T50.903	T50.904	T50.905	T50.906
Antitrichomonal drug	T37.3X1	T37.3X2	T37.3X3	T37.3X4	T37.3X5	T37.3X6
Antituberculars	T37.1X1	T37.1X2	T37.1X3	T37.1X4	T37.1X5	T37.1X6
antibiotics	T36.5X1	T36.5X2	T36.5X3	T36.5X4	T36.5X5	T36.5X6
Antitussive NEC	T48.3X1	T48.3X2	T48.3X3	T48.3X4	T48.3X5	T48.3X6
codeine mixture	T40.2X1	T40.2X2	T40.2X3	T40.2X4	T40.2X5	T40.2X6
opiate	T40.2X1	T40.2X2	T40.2X3	T40.2X4	T40.2X5	T40.2X6
Antivaricose drug	T46.8X1	T46.8X2	T46.8X3	T46.8X4	T46.8X5	T46.8X6
Antivenin, antivenom (sera)	T50.Z11	T50.Z12	T50.Z13	T50.Z14	T50.Z15	T50.Z16
crotaline	T50.Z11	T50.Z12	T50.Z13	T50.Z14	T50.Z15	T50.Z16
spider bite	T50.Z11	T50.Z12	T50.Z13	T50.Z14	T50.Z15	T50.Z16
Antivertigo drug	T45.0X1	T45.0X2	T45.0X3	T45.0X4	T45.0X5	T45.0X6
Antiviral drug NEC	T37.5X1	T37.5X2	T37.5X3	T37.5X4	T37.5X5	T37.5X6
eye	T49.5X1	T49.5X2	T49.5X3	T49.5X4	T49.5X5	T49.5X6
Antiwhipworm drug	T37.4X1	T37.4X2	T37.4X3	T37.4X4	T37.4X5	T37.4X6
Ant poisons — see Pesticides						
Antrol — see also by specific chemical substance	T60.91	T60.92	T60.93	T60.94	—	—
fungicide	T60.91	T60.92	T60.93	T60.94	—	—
ANTU (alpha naphthylthiourea)	T60.4X1	T60.4X2	T60.4X3	T60.4X4	—	—
Apalcillin	T36.0X1	T36.0X2	T36.0X3	T36.0X4	T36.0X5	T36.0X6
APC	T48.5X1	T48.5X2	T48.5X3	T48.5X4	T48.5X5	T48.5X6
Aplonidine	T44.4X1	T44.4X2	T44.4X3	T44.4X4	T44.4X5	T44.4X6
Apomorphine	T47.7X1	T47.7X2	T47.7X3	T47.7X4	T47.7X5	T47.7X6
Appetite depressants, central	T50.5X1	T50.5X2	T50.5X3	T50.5X4	T50.5X5	T50.5X6
Apraclonidine (hydrochloride)	T44.4X1	T44.4X2	T44.4X3	T44.4X4	T44.4X5	T44.4X6
Apresoline	T46.5X1	T46.5X2	T46.5X3	T46.5X4	T46.5X5	T46.5X6
Aprindine	T46.2X1	T46.2X2	T46.2X3	T46.2X4	T46.2X5	T46.2X6
Aprobarbital	T42.3X1	T42.3X2	T42.3X3	T42.3X4	T42.3X5	T42.3X6
Apronalide	T42.6X1	T42.6X2	T42.6X3	T42.6X4	T42.6X5	T42.6X6
Aprotinin	T45.621	T45.622	T45.623	T45.624	T45.625	T45.626
Aptocaine	T41.3X1	T41.3X2	T41.3X3	T41.3X4	T41.3X5	T41.3X6
Aqua fortis	T54.2X1	T54.2X2	T54.2X3	T54.2X4	—	—
Ara-A	T37.5X1	T37.5X2	T37.5X3	T37.5X4	T37.5X5	T37.5X6
Ara-C	T45.1X1	T45.1X2	T45.1X3	T45.1X4	T45.1X5	T45.1X6

◀ New   ◀▥ Revised   d̶e̶l̶e̶t̶e̶d̶ Deleted

TABLE OF DRUGS AND CHEMICALS

Substance	Poisoning, Accidental (Unintentional)	Poisoning, Intentional Self-Harm	Poisoning, Assault	Poisoning, Undetermined	Adverse Effect	Underdosing
			External Cause (T-Code)			
Arachis oil	T49.3X1	T49.3X2	T49.3X3	T49.3X4	T49.3X5	T49.3X6
cathartic	T47.4X1	T47.4X2	T47.4X3	T47.4X4	T47.4X5	T47.4X6
Aralen	T37.2X1	T37.2X2	T37.2X3	T37.2X4	T37.2X5	T37.2X6
Arecoline	T44.1X1	T44.1X2	T44.1X3	T44.1X4	T44.1X5	T44.1X6
Arginine	T50.991	T50.992	T50.993	T50.994	T50.995	T50.996
glutamate	T50.991	T50.992	T50.993	T50.994	T50.995	T50.996
Argyrol	T49.0X1	T49.0X2	T49.0X3	T49.0X4	T49.0X5	T49.0X6
ENT agent	T49.6X1	T49.6X2	T49.6X3	T49.6X4	T49.6X5	T49.6X6
ophthalmic preparation	T49.5X1	T49.5X2	T49.5X3	T49.5X4	T49.5X5	T49.5X6
Aristocort	T38.0X1	T38.0X2	T38.0X3	T38.0X4	T38.0X5	T38.0X6
ENT agent	T49.6X1	T49.6X2	T49.6X3	T49.6X4	T49.6X5	T49.6X6
ophthalmic preparation	T49.5X1	T49.5X2	T49.5X3	T49.5X4	T49.5X5	T49.5X6
topical NEC	T49.0X1	T49.0X2	T49.0X3	T49.0X4	T49.0X5	T49.0X6
Aromatics, corrosive	T54.1X1	T54.1X2	T54.1X3	T54.1X4	—	—
disinfectants	T54.1X1	T54.1X2	T54.1X3	T54.1X4	—	—
Arsenate of lead	T57.0X1	T57.0X2	T57.0X3	T57.0X4	—	—
herbicide	T57.0X1	T57.0X2	T57.0X3	T57.0X4	—	—
Arsenic, arsenicals (compounds) (dust) (vapor) NEC	T57.0X1	T57.0X2	T57.0X3	T57.0X4	—	—
anti-infectives	T37.8X1	T37.8X2	T37.8X3	T37.8X4	T37.8X5	T37.8X6
pesticide (dust) (fumes)	T57.0X1	T57.0X2	T57.0X3	T57.0X4	—	—
Arsine (gas)	T57.0X1	T57.0X2	T57.0X3	T57.0X4	—	—
Arsphenamine (silver)	T37.8X1	T37.8X2	T37.8X3	T37.8X4	T37.8X5	T37.8X6
Arsthinol	T37.3X1	T37.3X2	T37.3X3	T37.3X4	T37.3X5	T37.3X6
Artane	T44.3X1	T44.3X2	T44.3X3	T44.3X4	T44.3X5	T44.3X6
Arthropod (venomous) NEC	T63.481	T63.482	T63.483	T63.484	—	—
Articaine	T41.3X1	T41.3X2	T41.3X3	T41.3X4	T41.3X5	T41.3X6
Asbestos	T57.8X1	T57.8X2	T57.8X3	T57.8X4	—	—
Ascaridole	T37.4X1	T37.4X2	T37.4X3	T37.4X4	T37.4X5	T37.4X6
Ascorbic acid	T45.2X1	T45.2X2	T45.2X3	T45.2X4	T45.2X5	T45.2X6
Asiaticoside	T49.0X1	T49.0X2	T49.0X3	T49.0X4	T49.0X5	T49.0X6
Asparaginase	T45.1X1	T45.1X2	T45.1X3	T45.1X4	T45.1X5	T45.1X6
Aspidium (oleoresin)	T37.4X1	T37.4X2	T37.4X3	T37.4X4	T37.4X5	T37.4X6
Aspirin (aluminum) (soluble)	T39.011	T39.012	T39.013	T39.014	T39.015	T39.016
Aspoxicillin	T36.0X1	T36.0X2	T36.0X3	T36.0X4	T36.0X5	T36.0X6
Astemizole	T45.0X1	T45.0X2	T45.0X3	T45.0X4	T45.0X5	T45.0X6
Astringent (local)	T49.2X1	T49.2X2	T49.2X3	T49.2X4	T49.2X5	T49.2X6
specified NEC	T49.2X1	T49.2X2	T49.2X3	T49.2X4	T49.2X5	T49.2X6
Astromicin	T36.5X1	T36.5X2	T36.5X3	T36.5X4	T36.5X5	T36.5X6
Ataractic drug NEC	T43.501	T43.502	T43.503	T43.504	T43.505	T43.506

◀ New   ◀▥ Revised   ~~deleted~~ Deleted

Substance	External Cause (T-Code)					
	Poisoning, Accidental (Unintentional)	Poisoning, Intentional Self-Harm	Poisoning, Assault	Poisoning, Undetermined	Adverse Effect	Underdosing
Atenolol	T44.7X1	T44.7X2	T44.7X3	T44.7X4	T44.7X5	T44.7X6
Atonia drug, intestinal	T47.4X1	T47.4X2	T47.4X3	T47.4X4	T47.4X5	T47.4X6
Atophan	T50.4X1	T50.4X2	T50.4X3	T50.4X4	T50.4X5	T50.4X6
Atracurium besilate	T48.1X1	T48.1X2	T48.1X3	T48.1X4	T48.1X5	T48.1X6
Atropine	T44.3X1	T44.3X2	T44.3X3	T44.3X4	T44.3X5	T44.3X6
derivative	T44.3X1	T44.3X2	T44.3X3	T44.3X4	T44.3X5	T44.3X6
methonitrate	T44.3X1	T44.3X2	T44.3X3	T44.3X4	T44.3X5	T44.3X6
Attapulgite	T47.6X1	T47.6X2	T47.6X3	T47.6X4	T47.6X5	T47.6X6
Attenuvax	T50.991	T50.992	T50.993	T50.994	T50.995	T50.996
Auramine	T65.891	T65.892	T65.893	T65.894	—	—
dye	T65.6X1	T65.6X2	T65.6X3	T65.6X4	—	—
fungicide	T60.3X1	T60.3X2	T60.3X3	T60.3X4	—	—
Auranofin	T39.4X1	T39.4X2	T39.4X3	T39.4X4	T39.4X5	T39.4X6
Aurantiin	T46.991	T46.992	T46.993	T46.994	T46.995	T46.996
Aureomycin	T36.4X1	T36.4X2	T36.4X3	T36.4X4	T36.4X5	T36.4X6
ophthalmic preparation	T49.5X1	T49.5X2	T49.5X3	T49.5X4	T49.5X5	T49.5X6
topical NEC	T49.0X1	T49.0X2	T49.0X3	T49.0X4	T49.0X5	T49.0X6
Aurothioglucose	T39.4X1	T39.4X2	T39.4X3	T39.4X4	T39.4X5	T39.4X6
Aurothioglycanide	T39.4X1	T39.4X2	T39.4X3	T39.4X4	T39.4X5	T39.4X6
Aurothiomalate sodium	T39.4X1	T39.4X2	T39.4X3	T39.4X4	T39.4X5	T39.4X6
Aurotioprol	T39.4X1	T39.4X2	T39.4X3	T39.4X4	T39.4X5	T39.4X6
Automobile fuel	T52.0X1	T52.0X2	T52.0X3	T52.0X4	—	—
Autonomic nervous system agent NEC	T44.901	T44.902	T44.903	T44.904	T44.905	T44.906
Avlosulfon	T37.1X1	T37.1X2	T37.1X3	T37.1X4	T37.1X5	T37.1X6
Avomine	T42.6X1	T42.6X2	T42.6X3	T42.6X4	T42.6X5	T42.6X6
Axerophthol	T45.2X1	T45.2X2	T45.2X3	T45.2X4	T45.2X5	T45.2X6
Azacitidine	T45.1X1	T45.1X2	T45.1X3	T45.1X4	T45.1X5	T45.1X6
Azacyclonol	T43.591	T43.592	T43.593	T43.594	T43.595	T43.596
Azadirachta	T60.2X1	T60.2X2	T60.2X3	T60.2X4	—	—
Azanidazole	T37.3X1	T37.3X2	T37.3X3	T37.3X4	T37.3X5	T37.3X6
Azapetine	T46.7X1	T46.7X2	T46.7X3	T46.7X4	T46.7X5	T46.7X6
Azapropazone	T39.2X1	T39.2X2	T39.2X3	T39.2X4	T39.2X5	T39.2X6
Azaribine	T45.1X1	T45.1X2	T45.1X3	T45.1X4	T45.1X5	T45.1X6
Azaserine	T45.1X1	T45.1X2	T45.1X3	T45.1X4	T45.1X5	T45.1X6
Azatadine	T45.0X1	T45.0X2	T45.0X3	T45.0X4	T45.0X5	T45.0X6
Azatepa	T45.1X1	T45.1X2	T45.1X3	T45.1X4	T45.1X5	T45.1X6
Azathioprine	T45.1X1	T45.1X2	T45.1X3	T45.1X4	T45.1X5	T45.1X6
Azelaic acid	T49.0X1	T49.0X2	T49.0X3	T49.0X4	T49.0X5	T49.0X6
Azelastine	T45.0X1	T45.0X2	T45.0X3	T45.0X4	T45.0X5	T45.0X6

TABLE OF DRUGS AND CHEMICALS

◀ New   ◀▥ Revised   ~~deleted~~ Deleted

Substance	External Cause (T-Code)					
	Poisoning, Accidental (Unintentional)	Poisoning, Intentional Self-Harm	Poisoning, Assault	Poisoning, Undetermined	Adverse Effect	Underdosing
Azidocillin	T36.0X1	T36.0X2	T36.0X3	T36.0X4	T36.0X5	T36.0X6
Azidothymidine	T37.5X1	T37.5X2	T37.5X3	T37.5X4	T37.5X5	T37.5X6
Azinphos (ethyl) (methyl)	T60.0X1	T60.0X2	T60.0X3	T60.0X4	—	—
Aziridine (chelating)	T54.1X1	T54.1X2	T54.1X3	T54.1X4	—	—
Azithromycin	T36.3X1	T36.3X2	T36.3X3	T36.3X4	T36.3X5	T36.3X6
Azlocillin	T36.01	T36.02	T36.03	T36.04	T36.05	T36.06
Azobenzene smoke	T65.3X1	T65.3X2	T65.3X3	T65.3X4	—	—
acaricide	T60.8X1	T60.8X2	T60.8X3	T60.8X4	—	—
Azosulfamide	T37.0X1	T37.0X2	T37.0X3	T37.0X4	T37.0X5	T37.0X6
AZT	T37.5X1	T37.5X2	T37.5X3	T37.5X4	T37.5X5	T37.5X6
Aztreonam	T36.1X1	T36.1X2	T36.1X3	T36.1X4	T36.1X5	T36.1X6
Azulfidine	T37.0X1	T37.0X2	T37.0X3	T37.0X4	T37.0X5	T37.0X6
Azuresin	T50.8X1	T50.8X2	T50.8X3	T50.8X4	T50.8X5	T50.8X6
B						
Bacampicillin	T36.0X1	T36.0X2	T36.0X3	T36.0X4	T36.0X5	T36.0X6
Bacillus						
lactobacillus	T47.8X1	T47.8X2	T47.8X3	T47.8X4	T47.8X5	T47.8X6
subtilis	T47.6X1	T47.6X2	T47.6X3	T47.6X4	T47.6X5	T47.6X6
Bacimycin	T49.0X1	T49.0X2	T49.0X3	T49.0X4	T49.0X5	T49.0X6
ophthalmic preparation	T49.5X1	T49.5X2	T49.5X3	T49.5X4	T49.5X5	T49.5X6
Bacitracin zinc	T49.0X1	T49.0X2	T49.0X3	T49.0X4	T49.0X5	T49.0X6
with neomycin	T49.0X1	T49.0X2	T49.0X3	T49.0X4	T49.0X5	T49.0X6
ENT agent	T49.6X1	T49.6X2	T49.6X3	T49.6X4	T49.6X5	T49.6X6
ophthalmic preparation	T49.5X1	T49.5X2	T49.5X3	T49.5X4	T49.5X5	T49.5X6
topical NEC	T49.0X1	T49.0X2	T49.0X3	T49.0X4	T49.0X5	T49.0X6
Baclofen	T42.8X1	T42.8X2	T42.8X3	T42.8X4	T42.8X5	T42.8X6
Baking soda	T50.991	T50.992	T50.993	T50.994	T50.995	T50.996
BAL	T45.8X1	T45.8X2	T45.8X3	T45.8X4	T45.8X5	T45.8X6
Bambuterol	T48.6X1	T48.6X2	T48.6X3	T48.6X4	T48.6X5	T48.6X6
Bamethan (sulfate)	T46.7X1	T46.7X2	T46.7X3	T46.7X4	T46.7X5	T46.7X6
Bamifylline	T48.6X1	T48.6X2	T48.6X3	T48.6X4	T48.6X5	T48.6X6
Bamipine	T45.0X1	T45.0X2	T45.0X3	T45.0X4	T45.0X5	T45.0X6
Baneberry — see Actaea spicata						
Banewort — see Belladonna						
Barbenyl	T42.3X1	T42.3X2	T42.3X3	T42.3X4	T42.3X5	T42.3X6
Barbexaclone	T42.6X1	T42.6X2	T42.6X3	T42.6X4	T42.6X5	T42.6X6
Barbital	T42.3X1	T42.3X2	T42.3X3	T42.3X4	T42.3X5	T42.3X6
sodium	T42.3X1	T42.3X2	T42.3X3	T42.3X4	T42.3X5	T42.3X6
Barbitone	T42.3X1	T42.3X2	T42.3X3	T42.3X4	T42.3X5	T42.3X6

◄ New   ◀⫶⫶⫶ Revised   ~~deleted~~ Deleted

Substance	External Cause (T-Code)					
	Poisoning, Accidental (Unintentional)	Poisoning, Intentional Self-Harm	Poisoning, Assault	Poisoning, Undetermined	Adverse Effect	Underdosing
Barbiturate NEC	T42.3X1	T42.3X2	T42.3X3	T42.3X4	T42.3X5	T42.3X6
with tranquilizer	T42.3X1	T42.3X2	T42.3X3	T42.3X4	T42.3X5	T42.3X6
anesthetic (intravenous)	T41.1X1	T41.1X2	T41.1X3	T41.1X4	T41.1X5	T41.1X6
Barium (carbonate) (chloride) (sulfite)	T57.8X1	T57.8X2	T57.8X3	T57.8X4	—	—
diagnostic agent	T50.8X1	T50.8X2	T50.8X3	T50.8X4	T50.8X5	T50.8X6
pesticide	T60.4X1	T60.4X2	T60.4X3	T60.4X4	—	—
rodenticide	T60.4X1	T60.4X2	T60.4X3	T60.4X4	—	—
sulfate (medicinal)	T50.8X1	T50.8X2	T50.8X3	T50.8X4	T50.8X5	T50.8X6
Barrier cream	T49.3X1	T49.3X2	T49.3X3	T49.3X4	T49.3X5	T49.3X6
Basic fuchsin	T49.0X1	T49.0X2	T49.0X3	T49.0X4	T49.0X5	T49.0X6
Battery acid or fluid	T54.2X1	T54.2X2	T54.2X3	T54.2X4	—	—
Bay rum	T51.8X1	T51.8X2	T51.8X3	T51.8X4	—	—
BCG (vaccine)	T50.A91	T50.A92	T50.A93	T50.A94	T50.A95	T50.A96
BCNU	T45.1X1	T45.1X2	T45.1X3	T45.1X4	T45.1X5	T45.1X6
Bearsfoot	T62.2X1	T62.2X2	T62.2X3	T62.2X4	—	—
Beclamide	T42.6X1	T42.6X2	T42.6X3	T42.6X4	T42.6X5	T42.6X6
Beclomethasone	T44.5X1	T44.5X2	T44.5X3	T44.5X4	T44.5X5	T44.5X6
Bee (sting) (venom)	T63.441	T63.442	T63.443	T63.444	—	—
Befunolol	T49.5X1	T49.5X2	T49.5X3	T49.5X4	T49.5X5	T49.5X6
Bekanamycin	T36.5X1	T36.5X2	T36.5X3	T36.5X4	T36.5X5	T36.5X6
Belladonna— see also Nightshade						
alkaloids	T44.3X1	T44.3X2	T44.3X3	T44.3X4	T44.3X5	T44.3X6
extract	T44.3X1	T44.3X2	T44.3X3	T44.3X4	T44.3X5	T44.3X6
herb	T44.3X1	T44.3X2	T44.3X3	T44.3X4	T44.3X5	T44.3X6
Bemegride	T50.7X1	T50.7X2	T50.7X3	T50.7X4	T50.7X5	T50.7X6
Benactyzine	T44.3X1	T44.3X2	T44.3X3	T44.3X4	T44.3X5	T44.3X6
Benadryl	T45.0X1	T45.0X2	T45.0X3	T45.0X4	T45.0X5	T45.0X6
Benaprizine	T44.3X1	T44.3X2	T44.3X3	T44.3X4	T44.3X5	T44.3X6
Benazepril	T46.4X1	T46.4X2	T46.4X3	T46.4X4	T46.4X5	T46.4X6
Bencyclane	T46.7X1	T46.7X2	T46.7X3	T46.7X4	T46.7X5	T46.7X6
Bendazol	T46.3X1	T46.3X2	T46.3X3	T46.3X4	T46.3X5	T46.3X6
Bendrofluazide	T50.2X1	T50.2X2	T50.2X3	T50.2X4	T50.2X5	T50.2X6
Bendroflumethiazide	T50.2X1	T50.2X2	T50.2X3	T50.2X4	T50.2X5	T50.2X6
Benemid	T50.4X1	T50.4X2	T50.4X3	T50.4X4	T50.4X5	T50.4X6
Benethamine penicillin	T36.0X1	T36.0X2	T36.0X3	T36.0X4	T36.0X5	T36.0X6
Benisone	T49.0X1	T49.0X2	T49.0X3	T49.0X4	T49.0X5	T49.0X6
Benexate	T47.1X1	T47.1X2	T47.1X3	T47.1X4	T47.1X5	T47.1X6
Benfluorex	T46.6X1	T46.6X2	T46.6X3	T46.6X4	T46.6X5	T46.6X6
Benfotiamine	T45.2X1	T45.2X2	T45.2X3	T45.2X4	T45.2X5	T45.2X6
Benomyl	T60.0X1	T60.0X2	T60.0X3	T60.0X4	—	—

◀ New   ◀▥ Revised   ~~deleted~~ Deleted

Substance	External Cause (T-Code)					
	Poisoning, Accidental (Unintentional)	Poisoning, Intentional Self-Harm	Poisoning, Assault	Poisoning, Undetermined	Adverse Effect	Underdosing
Benoquin	T49.8X1	T49.8X2	T49.8X3	T49.8X4	T49.8X5	T49.8X6
Benoxinate	T41.3X1	T41.3X2	T41.3X3	T41.3X4	T41.3X5	T41.3X6
Benperidol	T43.4X1	T43.4X2	T43.4X3	T43.4X4	T43.4X5	T43.4X6
Benproperine	T48.3X1	T48.3X2	T48.3X3	T48.3X4	T48.3X5	T48.3X6
Benserazide	T42.8X1	T42.8X2	T42.8X3	T42.8X4	T42.8X5	T42.8X6
Bentazepam	T42.4X1	T42.4X2	T42.4X3	T42.4X4	T42.4X5	T42.4X6
Bentiromide	T50.8X1	T50.8X2	T50.8X3	T50.8X4	T50.8X5	T50.8X6
Bentonite	T49.3X1	T49.3X2	T49.3X3	T49.3X4	T49.3X5	T49.3X6
Benzalbutyramide	T46.6X1	T46.6X2	T46.6X3	T46.6X4	T46.6X5	T46.6X6
Benzalkonium (chloride)	T49.0X1	T49.0X2	T49.0X3	T49.0X4	T49.0X5	T49.0X6
ophthalmic preparation	T49.5X1	T49.5X2	T49.5X3	T49.5X4	T49.5X5	T49.5X6
Benzamine	T41.3X1	T41.3X2	T41.3X3	T41.3X4	T41.3X5	T41.3X6
lactate	T49.1X1	T49.1X2	T49.1X3	T49.1X4	T49.1X5	T49.1X6
Benzamidosalicylate (calcium)	T37.1X1	T37.1X2	T37.1X3	T37.1X4	T37.1X5	T37.1X6
Benzamphetamine	T50.5X1	T50.5X2	T50.5X3	T50.5X4	T50.5X5	T50.5X6
Benzapril hydrochloride	T46.5X1	T46.5X2	T46.5X3	T46.5X4	T46.5X5	T46.5X6
Benzathine benzylpenicillin	T36.0X1	T36.0X2	T36.0X3	T36.0X4	T36.0X5	T36.0X6
Benzathine penicillin	T36.0X1	T36.0X2	T36.0X3	T36.0X4	T36.0X5	T36.0X6
Benzatropine	T42.8X1	T42.8X2	T42.8X3	T42.8X4	T42.8X5	T42.8X6
Benzbromarone	T50.4X1	T50.4X2	T50.4X3	T50.4X4	T50.4X5	T50.4X6
Benzcarbimine	T45.1X1	T45.1X2	T45.1X3	T45.1X4	T45.1X5	T45.1X6
Benzedrex	T44.991	T44.992	T44.993	T44.994	T44.995	T44.996
Benzedrine (amphetamine)	T43.621	T43.622	T43.623	T43.624	T43.625	T43.626
Benzenamine	T65.3X1	T65.3X2	T65.3X3	T65.3X4	—	—
Benzene	T52.1X1	T52.1X2	T52.1X3	T52.1X4	—	—
homologues (acetyl) (dimethyl) (methyl) (solvent)	T52.2X1	T52.2X2	T52.2X3	T52.2X4	—	—
Benzethonium (chloride)	T49.0X1	T49.0X2	T49.0X3	T49.0X4	T49.0X5	T49.0X6
Benzfetamine	T50.5X1	T50.5X2	T50.5X3	T50.5X4	T50.5X5	T50.5X6
Benzhexol	T44.3X1	T44.3X2	T44.3X3	T44.3X4	T44.3X5	T44.3X6
Benzhydramine (chloride)	T45.0X1	T45.0X2	T45.0X3	T45.0X4	T45.0X5	T45.0X6
Benzidine	T65.891	T65.892	T65.893	T65.894	—	—
Benzilonium bromide	T44.3X1	T44.3X2	T44.3X3	T44.3X4	T44.3X5	T44.3X6
Benzimidazole	T60.3X1	T60.3X2	T60.3X3	T60.3X4	—	—
Benzin(e) — see Ligroin						
Benziodarone	T46.3X1	T46.3X2	T46.3X3	T46.3X4	T46.3X5	T46.3X6
Benznidazole	T37.3X1	T37.3X2	T37.3X3	T37.3X4	T37.3X5	T37.3X6
Benzocaine	T41.3X1	T41.3X2	T41.3X3	T41.3X4	T41.3X5	T41.3X6
Benzoctamine	T43.0X1	T43.0X2	T43.0X3	T43.0X4	T43.0X5	T43.0X6
Benzodiapin	T42.4X1	T42.4X2	T42.4X3	T42.4X4	T42.4X5	T42.4X6
Benzodiazepine NEC	T42.4X1	T42.4X2	T42.4X3	T42.4X4	T42.4X5	T42.4X6

◀ New   ◀▥ Revised   ~~deleted~~ Deleted

Substance	Poisoning, Accidental (Unintentional)	Poisoning, Intentional Self-Harm	Poisoning, Assault	Poisoning, Undetermined	Adverse Effect	Underdosing
	External Cause (T-Code)					
Benzoic acid	T49.0X1	T49.0X2	T49.0X3	T49.0X4	T49.0X5	T49.0X6
with salicylic acid	T49.0X1	T49.0X2	T49.0X3	T49.0X4	T49.0X5	T49.0X6
Benzoin (tincture)	T48.5X1	T48.5X2	T48.5X3	T48.5X4	T48.5X5	T48.5X6
Benzol (benzene)	T52.1X1	T52.1X2	T52.1X3	T52.1X4	—	—
vapor	T52.0X1	T52.0X2	T52.0X3	T52.0X4	—	—
Benzomorphan	T40.2X1	T40.2X2	T40.2X3	T40.2X4	T40.2X5	T40.2X6
Benzonatate	T48.3X1	T48.3X2	T48.3X3	T48.3X4	T48.3X5	T48.3X6
Benzophenones	T49.3X1	T49.3X2	T49.3X3	T49.3X4	T49.3X5	T49.3X6
Benzopyrone	T46.991	T46.992	T46.993	T46.994	T46.995	T46.996
Benzothiadiazides	T50.2X1	T50.2X2	T50.2X3	T50.2X4	T50.2X5	T50.2X6
Benzoxonium chloride	T49.0X1	T49.0X2	T49.0X3	T49.0X4	T49.0X5	T49.0X6
Benzoyl peroxide	T49.0X1	T49.0X2	T49.0X3	T49.0X4	T49.0X5	T49.0X6
Benzoylpas calcium	T37.1X1	T37.1X2	T37.1X3	T37.1X4	T37.1X5	T37.1X6
Benzperidin	T43.591	T43.592	T43.593	T43.594	T43.595	T43.596
Benzperidol	T43.591	T43.592	T43.593	T43.594	T43.595	T43.596
Benzphetamine	T50.5X1	T50.5X2	T50.5X3	T50.5X4	T50.5X5	T50.5X6
Benzpyrinium bromide	T44.1X1	T44.1X2	T44.1X3	T44.1X4	T44.1X5	T44.1X6
Benzquinamide	T45.0X1	T45.0X2	T45.0X3	T45.0X4	T45.0X5	T45.0X6
Benzthiazide	T50.2X1	T50.2X2	T50.2X3	T50.2X4	T50.2X5	T50.2X6
Benztropine						
anticholinergic	T44.3X1	T44.3X2	T44.3X3	T44.3X4	T44.3X5	T44.3X6
antiparkinson	T42.8X1	T42.8X2	T42.8X3	T42.8X4	T42.8X5	T42.8X6
Benzydamine	T49.0X1	T49.0X2	T49.0X3	T49.0X4	T49.0X5	T49.0X6
Benzyl						
acetate	T52.8X1	T52.8X2	T52.8X3	T52.8X4	—	—
alcohol	T49.0X1	T49.0X2	T49.0X3	T49.0X4	T49.0X5	T49.0X6
benzoate	T49.0X1	T49.0X2	T49.0X3	T49.0X4	T49.0X5	T49.0X6
Benzoic acid	T49.0X1	T49.0X2	T49.0X3	T49.0X4	T49.0X5	T49.0X6
morphine	T40.2X1	T40.2X2	T40.2X3	T40.2X4	—	—
nicotinate	T46.6X1	T46.6X2	T46.6X3	T46.6X4	T46.6X5	T46.6X6
penicillin	T36.0X1	T36.0X2	T36.0X3	T36.0X4	T36.0X5	T36.0X6
Benzylhydrochlorthia-zide	T50.2X1	T50.2X2	T50.2X3	T50.2X4	T50.2X5	T50.2X6
Benzylpenicillin	T36.0X1	T36.0X2	T36.0X3	T36.0X4	T36.0X5	T36.0X6
Benzylthiouracil	T38.2X1	T38.2X2	T38.2X3	T38.2X4	T38.2X5	T38.2X6
Bephenium hydroxy-naphthoate	T37.4X1	T37.4X2	T37.4X3	T37.4X4	T37.4X5	T37.4X6
Bepridil	T46.1X1	T46.1X2	T46.1X3	T46.1X4	T46.1X5	T46.1X6
Bergamot oil	T65.891	T65.892	T65.893	T65.894	—	—
Bergapten	T50.991	T50.992	T50.993	T50.994	T50.995	T50.996
Berries, poisonous	T62.1X1	T62.1X2	T62.1X3	T62.1X4	—	—
Beryllium (compounds)	T56.7X1	T56.7X2	T56.7X3	T56.7X4	—	—

TABLE OF DRUGS AND CHEMICALS

Substance	Poisoning, Accidental (Unintentional)	Poisoning, Intentional Self-Harm	Poisoning, Assault	Poisoning, Undetermined	Adverse Effect	Underdosing
			External Cause (T-Code)			
b-acetyldigoxin	T46.0X1	T46.0X2	T46.0X3	T46.0X4	T46.0X5	T46.0X6
beta adrenergic blocking agent, heart	T44.7X1	T44.7X2	T44.7X3	T44.7X4	T44.7X5	T44.7X6
b-benzalbutyramide	T46.6X1	T46.6X2	T46.6X3	T46.6X4	T46.6X5	T46.6X6
Betacarotene	T45.2X1	T45.2X2	T45.2X3	T45.2X4	T45.2X5	T45.2X6
b-eucaine	T49.1X1	T49.1X2	T49.1X3	T49.1X4	T49.1X5	T49.1X6
Beta-Chlor	T42.6X1	T42.6X2	T42.6X3	T42.6X4	T42.6X5	T42.6X6
b-galactosidase	T47.5X1	T47.5X2	T47.5X3	T47.5X4	T47.5X5	T47.5X6
Betahistine	T46.7X1	T46.7X2	T46.7X3	T46.7X4	T46.7X5	T46.7X6
Betaine	T47.5X1	T47.5X2	T47.5X3	T47.5X4	T47.5X5	T47.5X6
Betamethasone	T49.0X1	T49.0X2	T49.0X3	T49.0X4	T49.0X5	T49.0X6
topical	T49.0X1	T49.0X2	T49.0X3	T49.0X4	T49.0X5	T49.0X6
Betamicin	T36.8X1	T36.8X2	T36.8X3	T36.8X4	T36.8X5	T36.8X6
Betanidine	T46.5X1	T46.5X2	T46.5X3	T46.5X4	T46.5X5	T46.5X6
b-sitosterol(s)	T46.6X1	T46.6X2	T46.6X3	T46.6X4	T46.6X5	T46.6X6
Betaxolol	T44.7X1	T44.7X2	T44.7X3	I44.7X4	T44.7X5	T44.7X6
Betazole	T50.8X1	T50.8X2	T50.8X3	T50.8X4	T50.8X5	T50.8X6
Bethanechol	T44.1X1	T44.1X2	T44.1X3	T44.1X4	T44.1X5	T44.1X6
chloride	T44.1X1	T44.1X2	T44.1X3	T44.1X4	T44.1X5	T44.1X6
Bethanidine	T46.5X1	T46.5X2	T46.5X3	T46.5X4	T46.5X5	T46.5X6
Betoxycaine	T41.3X1	T41.3X2	T41.3X3	T41.3X4	T41.3X5	T41.3X6
Betula oil	T49.3X1	T49.3X2	T49.3X3	T49.3X4	T49.3X5	T49.3X6
Bevantolol	T44.7X1	T44.7X2	T44.7X3	T44.7X4	T44.7X5	T44.7X6
Bevonium metilsulfate	T44.3X1	T44.3X2	T44.3X3	T44.3X4	T44.3X5	T44.3X6
Bezafibrate	T46.6X1	T46.6X2	T46.6X3	T46.6X4	T46.6X5	T46.6X6
Bezitramide	T40.4X1	T40.4X2	T40.4X3	T40.4X4	T40.4X5	T40.4X6
BHA	T50.991	T50.992	T50.993	T50.994	T50.995	T50.996
Bhang	T40.7X1	T40.7X2	T40.7X3	T40.7X4	T40.7X5	T40.7X6
BHC (medicinal)	T49.0X1	T49.0X2	T49.0X3	T49.0X4	T49.0X5	T49.0X6
nonmedicinal (vapor)	T53.6X1	T53.6X2	T53.6X3	T53.6X4	—	—
Bialamicol	T37.3X1	T37.3X2	T37.3X3	T37.3X4	T37.3X5	T37.3X6
Bibenzonium bromide	T48.3X1	T48.3X2	T48.3X3	T48.3X4	T48.3X5	T48.3X6
Bibrocathol	T49.5X1	T49.5X2	T49.5X3	T49.5X4	T49.5X5	T49.5X6
Bichloride of mercury — see Mercury, chloride						
Bichromates (calcium) (potassium) (sodium) (crystals)	T57.8X1	T57.8X2	T57.8X3	T57.8X4	—	—
fumes	T56.2X1	T56.2X2	T56.2X3	T56.2X4	—	—
Biclotymol	T49.6X1	T49.6X2	T49.6X3	T49.6X4	T49.6X5	T49.6X6
Bicucculine	T50.7X1	T50.7X2	T50.7X3	T50.7X4	T50.7X5	T50.7X6
Bifemelane	T43.291	T43.292	T43.293	T43.294	T43.295	T43.296
Biguanide derivatives, oral	T38.3X1	T38.3X2	T38.3X3	T38.3X4	T38.3X5	T38.3X6

◀ New   ◀⁃ Revised   ~~deleted~~ Deleted

Substance	Poisoning, Accidental (Unintentional)	Poisoning, Intentional Self-Harm	Poisoning, Assault	Poisoning, Undetermined	Adverse Effect	Underdosing
			External Cause (T-Code)			
Biligrafin	T50.8X1	T50.8X2	T50.8X3	T50.8X4	T50.8X5	T50.8X6
Bile salts	T47.5X1	T47.5X2	T47.5X3	T47.5X4	T47.5X5	T47.5X6
Bilopaque	T50.8X1	T50.8X2	T50.8X3	T50.8X4	T50.8X5	T50.8X6
Binifibrate	T46.6X1	T46.6X2	T46.6X3	T46.6X4	T46.6X5	T46.6X6
Binitrobenzol	T65.3X1	T65.3X2	T65.3X3	T65.3X4	—	—
Bioflavonoid(s)	T46.991	T46.992	T46.993	T46.994	T46.995	T46.996
Biological substance NEC	T50.901	T50.902	T50.903	T50.904	T50.905	T50.906
Biotin	T45.2X1	T45.2X2	T45.2X3	T45.2X4	T45.2X5	T45.2X6
Biperiden	T44.3X1	T44.3X2	T44.3X3	T44.3X4	T44.3X5	T44.3X6
Bisacodyl	T47.2X1	T47.2X2	T47.2X3	T47.2X4	T47.2X5	T47.2X6
Bisbentiamine	T45.2X1	T45.2X2	T45.2X3	T45.2X4	T45.2X5	T45.2X6
Bisbutiamine	T45.2X1	T45.2X2	T45.2X3	T45.2X4	T45.2X5	T45.2X6
Bisdequalinium (salts) (diacetate)	T49.6X1	T49.6X2	T49.6X3	T49.6X4	T49.6X5	T49.6X6
Bishydroxycoumarin	T45.511	T45.512	T45.513	T45.514	T45.515	T45.516
Bismarsen	T37.8X1	T37.8X2	T37.8X3	T37.8X4	T37.8X5	T37.8X6
Bismuth salts	T47.6X1	T47.6X2	T47.6X3	T47.6X4	T47.6X5	T47.6X6
aluminate	T47.1X1	T47.1X2	T47.1X3	T47.1X4	T47.1X5	T47.1X6
anti-infectives	T37.8X1	T37.8X2	T37.8X3	T37.8X4	T37.8X5	T37.8X6
formic iodide	T49.0X1	T49.0X2	T49.0X3	T49.0X4	T49.0X5	T49.0X6
glycolylarsenate	T49.0X1	T49.0X2	T49.0X3	T49.0X4	T49.0X5	T49.0X6
nonmedicinal (compounds) NEC	T65.91	T65.92	T65.93	T65.94	—	—
subcarbonate	T47.6X1	T47.6X2	T47.6X3	T47.6X4	T47.6X5	T47.6X6
subsalicylate	T37.8X1	T37.8X2	T37.8X3	T37.8X4	T37.8X5	T37.8X6
sulfarsphenamine	T37.8X1	T37.8X2	T37.8X3	T37.8X4	T37.8X5	T37.8X6
Bisoprolol	T44.7X1	T44.7X2	T44.7X3	T44.7X4	T44.7X5	T44.7X6
Bisoxatin	T47.2X1	T47.2X2	T47.2X3	T47.2X4	T47.2X5	T47.2X6
Bisulepin (hydrochloride)	T45.0X1	T45.0X2	T45.0X3	T45.0X4	T45.0X5	T45.0X6
Bithionol	T37.8X1	T37.8X2	T37.8X3	T37.8X4	T37.8X5	T37.8X6
anthelminthic	T37.4X1	T37.4X2	T37.4X3	T37.4X4	T37.4X5	T37.4X6
Bitolterol	T48.6X1	T48.6X2	T48.6X3	T48.6X4	T48.6X5	T48.6X6
Bitoscanate	T37.4X1	T37.4X2	T37.4X3	T37.4X4	T37.4X5	T37.4X6
Bitter almond oil	T62.8X1	T62.8X2	T62.8X3	T62.8X4	—	—
Bittersweet	T62.2X1	T62.2X2	T62.2X3	T62.2X4	—	—
Black						
flag	T60.91	T60.92	T60.93	T60.94	—	—
henbane	T62.2X1	T62.2X2	T62.2X3	T62.2X4	—	—
leaf (40)	T60.91	T60.92	T60.93	T60.94	—	—
widow spider (bite)	T63.311	T63.312	T63.313	T63.314	—	—
antivenin	T50.Z11	T50.Z12	T50.Z13	T50.Z14	T50.Z15	T50.Z16
Blast furnace gas (carbon monoxide from)	T58.8X1	T58.8X2	T58.8X3	T58.8X4	—	—

◀ New   ◀▥ Revised   ~~deleted~~ Deleted

TABLE OF DRUGS AND CHEMICALS

Substance	Poisoning, Accidental (Unintentional)	Poisoning, Intentional Self-Harm	Poisoning, Assault	Poisoning, Undetermined	Adverse Effect	Underdosing
				External Cause (T-Code)		
Bleach	T54.91	T54.92	T54.93	T54.94	—	—
Bleaching agent (medicinal)	T49.4X1	T49.4X2	T49.4X3	T49.4X4	T49.4X5	T49.4X6
Bleomycin	T45.1X1	T45.1X2	T45.1X3	T45.1X4	T45.1X5	T45.1X6
Blockain	T41.3X1	T41.3X2	T41.3X3	T41.3X4	T41.3X5	T41.3X6
infiltration (subcutaneous)	T41.3X1	T41.3X2	T41.3X3	T41.3X4	T41.3X5	T41.3X6
nerve block (peripheral) (plexus)	T41.3X1	T41.3X2	T41.3X3	T41.3X4	T41.3X5	T41.3X6
topical (surface)	T41.3X1	T41.3X2	T41.3X3	T41.3X4	T41.3X5	T41.3X6
Blockers, calcium channel	T46.1X1	T46.1X2	T46.1X3	T46.1X4	T46.1X5	T46.1X6
Blood (derivatives) (natural) (plasma) (whole)	T45.8X1	T45.8X2	T45.8X3	T45.8X4	T45.8X5	T45.8X6
dried	T45.8X1	T45.8X2	T45.8X3	T45.8X4	T45.8X5	T45.8X6
drug affecting NEC	T45.91	T45.92	T45.93	T45.94	T45.95	T45.96
expander NEC	T45.8X1	T45.8X2	T45.8X3	T45.8X4	T45.8X5	T45.8X6
fraction NEC	T45.8X1	T45.8X2	T45.8X3	T45.8X4	T45.8X5	T45.8X6
substitute (macromolecular)	T45.8X1	T45.8X2	T45.8X3	T45.8X4	T45.8X5	T45.8X6
Blue velvet	T40.2X1	T40.2X2	T40.2X3	T40.2X4	—	—
Bone meal	T62.8X1	T62.8X2	T62.8X3	T62.8X4	—	—
Bonine	T45.0X1	T45.0X2	T45.0X3	T45.0X4	T45.0X5	T45.0X6
Bopindolol	T44.7X1	T44.7X2	T44.7X3	T44.7X4	T44.7X5	T44.7X6
Boracic acid	T49.0X1	T49.0X2	T49.0X3	T49.0X4	T49.0X5	T49.0X6
ENT agent	T49.6X1	T49.6X2	T49.6X3	T49.6X4	T49.6X5	T49.6X6
ophthalmic preparation	T49.5X1	T49.5X2	T49.5X3	T49.5X4	T49.5X5	T49.5X6
Borane complex	T57.8X1	T57.8X2	T57.8X3	T57.8X4	—	—
Borate(s)	T57.8X1	T57.8X2	T57.8X3	T57.8X4	—	—
buffer	T50.991	T50.992	T50.993	T50.994	T50.995	T50.996
cleanser	T54.91	T54.92	T54.93	T54.94	—	—
sodium	T57.8X1	T57.8X2	T57.8X3	T57.8X4	—	—
Borax (cleanser)	T54.91	T54.92	T54.93	T54.94	—	—
Bordeaux mixture	T60.3X1	T60.3X2	T60.3X3	T60.3X4	—	—
Boric acid	T49.0X1	T49.0X2	T49.0X3	T49.0X4	T49.0X5	T49.0X6
ENT agent	T49.6X1	T49.6X2	T49.6X3	T49.6X4	T49.6X5	T49.6X6
ophthalmic preparation	T49.5X1	T49.5X2	T49.5X3	T49.5X4	T49.5X5	T49.5X6
Bornaprine	T44.3X1	T44.3X2	T44.3X3	T44.3X4	T44.3X5	T44.3X6
Boron	T57.8X1	T57.8X2	T57.8X3	T57.8X4	—	—
hydride NEC	T57.8X1	T57.8X2	T57.8X3	T57.8X4	—	—
fumes or gas	T57.8X1	T57.8X2	T57.8X3	T57.8X4	—	—
trifluoride	T59.891	T59.892	T59.893	T59.894	—	—
Botox	T48.291	T48.292	T48.293	T48.294	T48.295	T48.296
Botulinus anti-toxin (type A, B)	T50.Z11	T50.Z12	T50.Z13	T50.Z14	T50.Z15	T50.Z16
Brake fluid vapor	T59.891	T59.892	T59.893	T59.894	—	—
Brallobarbital	T42.3X1	T42.3X2	T42.3X3	T42.3X4	T42.3X5	T42.3X6

◀ New   ◀☰ Revised   ~~deleted~~ Deleted

Substance	External Cause (T-Code)					
	Poisoning, Accidental (Unintentional)	Poisoning, Intentional Self-Harm	Poisoning, Assault	Poisoning, Undetermined	Adverse Effect	Underdosing
Bran (wheat)	T47.4X1	T47.4X2	T47.4X3	T47.4X4	T47.4X5	T47.4X6
Brass (fumes)	T56.891	T56.892	T56.893	T56.894	—	—
Brasso	T52.0X1	T52.0X2	T52.0X3	T52.0X4	—	—
Bretylium tosilate	T46.2X1	T46.2X2	T46.2X3	T46.2X4	T46.2X5	T46.2X6
Brevital (sodium)	T41.1X1	T41.1X2	T41.1X3	T41.1X4	T41.1X5	T41.1X6
Brinase	T45.3X1	T45.3X2	T45.3X3	T45.3X4	T45.3X5	T45.3X6
British antilewisite	T45.8X1	T45.8X2	T45.8X3	T45.8X4	T45.8X5	T45.8X6
Brodifacoum	T60.4X1	T60.4X2	T60.4X3	T60.4X4	—	—
Bromal (hydrate)	T42.6X1	T42.6X2	T42.6X3	T42.6X4	T42.6X5	T42.6X6
Bromazepam	T42.4X1	T42.4X2	T42.4X3	T42.4X4	T42.4X5	T42.4X6
Bromazine	T45.0X1	T45.0X2	T45.0X3	T45.0X4	T45.0X5	T45.0X6
Brombenzylcyanide	T59.3X1	T59.3X2	T59.3X3	T59.3X4	—	—
Bromelains	T45.3X1	T45.3X2	T45.3X3	T45.3X4	T45.3X5	T45.3X6
Bromethalin	T60.4X1	T60.4X2	T60.4X3	T60.4X4	—	—
Bromhexine	T48.4X1	T48.4X2	T48.4X3	T48.4X4	T48.4X5	T48.4X6
Bromide salts	T42.6X1	T42.6X2	T42.6X3	T42.6X4	T42.6X5	T42.6X6
Bromindione	T45.511	T45.512	T45.513	T45.514	T45.515	T45.516
Bromine						
compounds (medicinal)	T42.6X1	T42.6X2	T42.6X3	T42.6X4	T42.6X5	T42.6X6
sedative	T42.6X1	T42.6X2	T42.6X3	T42.6X4	T42.6X5	T42.6X6
vapor	T59.891	T59.892	T59.893	T59.894	—	—
Bromisovalum	T42.6X1	T42.6X2	T42.6X3	T42.6X4	T42.6X5	T42.6X6
Bromisoval	T42.6X1	T42.6X2	T42.6X3	T42.6X4	T42.6X5	T42.6X6
Bromobenzylcyanide	T59.3X1	T59.3X2	T59.3X3	T59.3X4	—	—
Bromochlorosalicylani-lide	T49.0X1	T49.0X2	T49.0X3	T49.0X4	T49.0X5	T49.0X6
Bromocriptine	T42.8X1	T42.8X2	T42.8X3	T42.8X4	T42.8X5	T42.8X6
Bromodiphenhydramine	T45.0X1	T45.0X2	T45.0X3	T45.0X4	T45.0X5	T45.0X6
Bromoform	T42.6X1	T42.6X2	T42.6X3	T42.6X4	T42.6X5	T42.6X6
Bromophenol blue reagent	T50.991	T50.992	T50.993	T50.994	T50.995	T50.996
Bromopride	T47.8X1	T47.8X2	T47.8X3	T47.8X4	T47.8X5	T47.8X6
Bromosalicylchloranitide	T49.0X1	T49.0X2	T49.0X3	T49.0X4	T49.0X5	T49.0X6
Bromosalicylhydroxamic acid	T37.1X1	T37.1X2	T37.1X3	T37.1X4	T37.1X5	T37.1X6
Bromo-seltzer	T39.1X1	T39.1X2	T39.1X3	T39.1X4	T39.1X5	T39.1X6
Bromoxynil	T60.3X1	T60.3X2	T60.3X3	T60.3X4	—	—
Bromperidol	T43.4X1	T43.4X2	T43.4X3	T43.4X4	T43.4X5	T43.4X6
Brompheniramine	T45.0X1	T45.0X2	T45.0X3	T45.0X4	T45.0X5	T45.0X6
Bromsulfophthalein	T50.8X1	T50.8X2	T50.8X3	T50.8X4	T50.8X5	T50.8X6
Bromural	T42.6X1	T42.6X2	T42.6X3	T42.6X4	T42.6X5	T42.6X6
Bromvaletone	T42.6X1	T42.6X2	T42.6X3	T42.6X4	T42.6X5	T42.6X6
Bronchodilator NEC	T48.6X1	T48.6X2	T48.6X3	T48.6X4	T48.6X5	T48.6X6

◀ New   ◀▥ Revised   ~~deleted~~ Deleted

Substance	External Cause (T-Code)					
	Poisoning, Accidental (Unintentional)	Poisoning, Intentional Self-Harm	Poisoning, Assault	Poisoning, Undetermined	Adverse Effect	Underdosing
Brotizolam	T42.4X1	T42.4X2	T42.4X3	T42.4X4	T42.4X5	T42.4X6
Brovincamine	T46.7X1	T46.7X2	T46.7X3	T46.7X4	T46.7X5	T46.7X6
Brown spider (bite) (venom)	T63.391	T63.392	T63.393	T63.394	—	—
Brown recluse spider (bite) (venom)	T63.331	T63.332	T63.333	T63.334	—	—
Broxaterol	T48.6X1	T48.6X2	T48.6X3	T48.6X4	T48.6X5	T48.6X6
Broxuridine	T45.1X1	T45.1X2	T45.1X3	T45.1X4	T45.1X5	T45.1X6
Broxyquinoline	T37.8X1	T37.8X2	T37.8X3	T37.8X4	T37.8X5	T37.8X6
Bruceine	T48.291	T48.292	T48.293	T48.294	T48.295	T48.296
Brucia	T62.2X1	T62.2X2	T62.2X3	T62.2X4	—	—
Brucine	T65.1X1	T65.1X2	T65.1X3	T65.1X4	—	—
Brunswick green — see Copper						
Bruten — see Ibuprofen						
Bryonia	T47.2X1	T47.2X2	T47.2X3	T47.2X4	T47.2X5	T47.2X6
Buclizine	T45.0X1	T45.0X2	T45.0X3	T45.0X4	T45.0X5	T45.0X6
Buclosamide	T49.0X1	T49.0X7	T49.0X3	T49.0X4	T49.0X5	T49.0X6
Budesonide	T44.5X1	T44.5X2	T44.5X3	T44.5X4	T44.5X5	T44.5X6
Budralazine	T46.5X1	T46.5X2	T46.5X3	T46.5X4	T46.5X5	T46.5X6
Bufferin	T39.011	T39.012	T39.013	T39.014	T39.015	T39.016
Buflomedil	T46.7X1	T46.7X2	T46.7X3	T46.7X4	T46.7X5	T46.7X6
Buformin	T38.3X1	T38.3X2	T38.3X3	T38.3X4	T38.3X5	T38.3X6
Bufotenine	T40.991	T40.992	T40.993	T40.994	—	—
Bufrolin	T48.6X1	T48.6X2	T48.6X3	T48.6X4	T48.6X5	T48.6X6
Bufylline	T48.6X1	T48.6X2	T48.6X3	T48.6X4	T48.6X5	T48.6X6
Bulk filler	T50.5X1	T50.5X2	T50.5X3	T50.5X4	T50.5X5	T50.5X6
cathartic	T47.4X1	T47.4X2	T47.4X3	T47.4X4	T47.4X5	T47.4X6
Bumetanide	T50.1X1	T50.1X2	T50.1X3	T50.1X4	T50.1X5	T50.1X6
Bunaftine	T46.2X1	T46.2X2	T46.2X3	T46.2X4	T46.2X5	T46.2X6
Bunamiodyl	T50.8X1	T50.8X2	T50.8X3	T50.8X4	T50.8X5	T50.8X6
Bunazosin	T44.6X1	T44.6X2	T44.6X3	T44.6X4	T44.6X5	T44.6X6
Bunitrolol	T44.7X1	T44.7X2	T44.7X3	T44.7X4	T44.7X5	T44.7X6
Buphenine	T46.7X1	T46.7X2	T46.7X3	T46.7X4	T46.7X5	T46.7X6
Bupivacaine	T41.3X1	T41.3X2	T41.3X3	T41.3X4	T41.3X5	T41.3X6
infiltration (subcutaneous)	T41.3X1	T41.3X2	T41.3X3	T41.3X4	T41.3X5	T41.3X6
nerve block (peripheral) (plexus)	T41.3X1	T41.3X2	T41.3X3	T41.3X4	T41.3X5	T41.3X6
spinal	T41.3X1	T41.3X2	T41.3X3	T41.3X4	T41.3X5	T41.3X6
Bupranolol	T44.7X1	T44.7X2	T44.7X3	T44.7X4	T44.7X5	T44.7X6
Buprenorphine	T40.4X1	T40.4X2	T40.4X3	T40.4X4	T40.4X5	T40.4X6
Bupropion	T43.291	T43.292	T43.293	T43.294	T43.295	T43.296
Burimamide	T47.1X1	T47.1X2	T47.1X3	T47.1X4	T47.1X5	T47.1X6
Buserelin	T38.891	T38.892	T38.893	T38.894	T38.895	T38.896

◀ New   ◀⫶⫶ Revised   ~~deleted~~ Deleted

Substance	External Cause (T-Code)					
	Poisoning, Accidental (Unintentional)	Poisoning, Intentional Self-Harm	Poisoning, Assault	Poisoning, Undetermined	Adverse Effect	Underdosing
Buspirone	T43.591	T43.592	T43.593	T43.594	T43.595	T43.596
Busulfan, busulphan	T45.1X1	T45.1X2	T45.1X3	T45.1X4	T45.1X5	T45.1X6
Butabarbital (sodium)	T42.3X1	T42.3X2	T42.3X3	T42.3X4	T42.3X5	T42.3X6
Butabarbitone	T42.3X1	T42.3X2	T42.3X3	T42.3X4	T42.3X5	T42.3X6
Butabarpal	T42.3X1	T42.3X2	T42.3X3	T42.3X4	T42.3X5	T42.3X6
Butacaine	T41.3X1	T41.3X2	T41.3X3	T41.3X4	T41.3X5	T41.3X6
Butalamine	T46.7X1	T46.7X2	T46.7X3	T46.7X4	T46.7X5	T46.7X6
Butalbital	T42.3X1	T42.3X2	T42.3X3	T42.3X4	T42.3X5	T42.3X6
Butallylonal	T42.3X1	T42.3X2	T42.3X3	T42.3X4	T42.3X5	T42.3X6
Butamben	T41.3X1	T41.3X2	T41.3X3	T41.3X4	T41.3X5	T41.3X6
Butamirate	T48.3X1	T48.3X2	T48.3X3	T48.3X4	T48.3X5	T48.3X6
Butane (distributed in mobile container)	T59.891	T59.892	T59.893	T59.894	—	—
distributed through pipes	T59.891	T59.892	T59.893	T59.894	—	—
incomplete combustion	T58.11	T58.12	T58.13	T58.14	—	—
Butanilicaine	T41.3X1	T41.3X2	T41.3X3	T41.3X4	T41.3X5	T41.3X6
Butanol	T51.3X1	T51.3X2	T51.3X3	T51.3X4	—	—
Butanone, 2-butanone	T52.4X1	T52.4X2	T52.4X3	T52.4X4	—	—
Butantrone	T49.4X1	T49.4X2	T49.4X3	T49.4X4	T49.4X5	T49.4X6
Butaperazine	T43.3X1	T43.3X2	T43.3X3	T43.3X4	T43.3X5	T43.3X6
Butazolidin	T39.2X1	T39.2X2	T39.2X3	T39.2X4	T39.2X5	T39.2X6
Butetamate	T48.6X1	T48.6X2	T48.6X3	T48.6X4	T48.6X5	T48.6X6
Butethal	T42.3X1	T42.3X2	T42.3X3	T42.3X4	T42.3X5	T42.3X6
Butethamate	T44.3X1	T44.3X2	T44.3X3	T44.3X4	T44.3X5	T44.3X6
Buthalitone (sodium)	T41.1X1	T41.1X2	T41.1X3	T41.1X4	T41.1X5	T41.1X6
Butisol (sodium)	T42.3X1	T42.3X2	T42.3X3	T42.3X4	T42.3X5	T42.3X6
Butizide	T50.2X1	T50.2X2	T50.2X3	T50.2X4	T50.2X5	T50.2X6
Butobarbital	T42.3X1	T42.3X2	T42.3X3	T42.3X4	T42.3X5	T42.3X6
sodium	T42.3X1	T42.3X2	T42.3X3	T42.3X4	T42.3X5	T42.3X6
Butobarbitone	T42.3X1	T42.3X2	T42.3X3	T42.3X4	T42.3X5	T42.3X6
Butoconazole (nitrate)	T49.0X1	T49.0X2	T49.0X3	T49.0X4	T49.0X5	T49.0X6
Butorphanol	T40.4X1	T40.4X2	T40.4X3	T40.4X4	T40.4X5	T40.4X6
Butriptyline	T43.011	T43.012	T43.013	T43.014	T43.015	T43.016
Butropium bromide	T44.3X1	T44.3X2	T44.3X3	T44.3X4	T44.3X5	T44.3X6
Buttercups	T62.2X1	T62.2X2	T62.2X3	T62.2X4	—	—
Butter of antimony — *see* Antimony						
Butyl						
acetate (secondary)	T52.8X1	T52.8X2	T52.8X3	T52.8X4	—	—
alcohol	T51.3X1	T51.3X2	T51.3X3	T51.3X4	—	—
aminobenzoate	T41.3X1	T41.3X2	T41.3X3	T41.3X4	T41.3X5	T41.3X6
butyrate	T52.8X1	T52.8X2	T52.8X3	T52.8X4	—	—

TABLE OF DRUGS AND CHEMICALS

Substance	Poisoning, Accidental (Unintentional)	Poisoning, Intentional Self-Harm	Poisoning, Assault	Poisoning, Undetermined	Adverse Effect	Underdosing
Butyl *(Continued)*						
carbinol	T51.3X1	T51.3X2	T51.3X3	T51.3X4	—	—
carbitol	T52.3X1	T52.3X2	T52.3X3	T52.3X4	—	—
cellosolve	T52.3X1	T52.3X2	T52.3X3	T52.3X4	—	—
chloral (hydrate)	T42.6X1	T42.6X2	T42.6X3	T42.6X4	T42.6X5	T42.6X6
formate	T52.8X1	T52.8X2	T52.8X3	T52.8X4	—	—
lactate	T52.8X1	T52.8X2	T52.8X3	T52.8X4	—	—
propionate	T52.8X1	T52.8X2	T52.8X3	T52.8X4	—	—
scopolamine bromide	T44.3X1	T44.3X2	T44.3X3	T44.3X4	T44.3X5	T44.3X6
thiobarbital sodium	T41.1X1	T41.1X2	T41.1X3	T41.1X4	T41.1X5	T41.1X6
Butylated hydroxy-anisole	T50.991	T50.992	T50.993	T50.994	T50.995	T50.996
Butylchloral hydrate	T42.6X1	T42.6X2	T42.6X3	T42.6X4	T42.6X5	T42.6X6
Butyltoluene	T52.2X1	T52.2X2	T52.2X3	T52.2X4	—	—
Butyn	T41.3X1	T41.3X2	T41.3X3	T41.3X4	T41.3X5	T41.3X6
Butyrophenone (-based tranquilizers)	T43.4X1	T43.4X2	T43.4X3	T43.4X4	T43.4X5	T43.4X6
C						
Cabergoline	T42.8X1	T42.8X2	T42.8X3	T42.8X4	T42.8X5	T42.8X6
Cacodyl, cacodylic acid	T57.0X1	T57.0X2	T57.0X3	T57.0X4	—	—
Cactinomycin	T45.1X1	T45.1X2	T45.1X3	T45.1X4	T45.1X5	T45.1X6
Cade oil	T49.4X1	T49.4X2	T49.4X3	T49.4X4	T49.4X5	T49.4X6
Cadexomer iodine	T49.0X1	T49.0X2	T49.0X3	T49.0X4	T49.0X5	T49.0X6
Cadmium (chloride) (fumes) (oxide)	T56.3X1	T56.3X2	T56.3X3	T56.3X4	—	—
sulfide (medicinal) NEC	T49.4X1	T49.4X2	T49.4X3	T49.4X4	T49.4X5	T49.4X6
Cadralazine	T46.5X1	T46.5X2	T46.5X3	T46.5X4	T46.5X5	T46.5X6
Caffeine	T43.611	T43.612	T43.613	T43.614	T43.615	T43.616
Calabar bean	T62.2X1	T62.2X2	T62.2X3	T62.2X4	—	—
Caladium seguinum	T62.2X1	T62.2X2	T62.2X3	T62.2X4	—	—
Calamine (lotion)	T49.3X1	T49.3X2	T49.3X3	T49.3X4	T49.3X5	T49.3X6
Calcifediol	T45.2X1	T45.2X2	T45.2X3	T45.2X4	T45.2X5	T45.2X6
Calciferol	T45.2X1	T45.2X2	T45.2X3	T45.2X4	T45.2X5	T45.2X6
Calcitonin	T50.991	T50.992	T50.993	T50.994	T50.995	T50.996
Calcitriol	T45.2X1	T45.2X2	T45.2X3	T45.2X4	T45.2X5	T45.2X6
Calcium	T50.3X1	T50.3X2	T50.3X3	T50.3X4	T50.3X5	T50.3X6
actylsalicylate	T39.011	T39.012	T39.013	T39.014	T39.015	T39.016
benzamidosalicylate	T37.1X1	T37.1X2	T37.1X3	T37.1X4	T37.1X5	T37.1X6
bromide	T42.6X1	T42.6X2	T42.6X3	T42.6X4	T42.6X5	T42.6X6
bromolactobionate	T42.6X1	T42.6X2	T42.6X3	T42.6X4	T42.6X5	T42.6X6
carbaspirin	T39.011	T39.012	T39.013	T39.014	T39.015	T39.016
carbimide	T50.6X1	T50.6X2	T50.6X3	T50.6X4	T50.6X5	T50.6X6

◀ New ◀ Revised ~~deleted~~ Deleted

Substance	Poisoning, Accidental (Unintentional)	Poisoning, Intentional Self-Harm	Poisoning, Assault	Poisoning, Undetermined	Adverse Effect	Underdosing
Calcium *(Continued)*						
carbonate	T47.1X1	T47.1X2	T47.1X3	T47.1X4	T47.1X5	T47.1X6
chloride	T50.991	T50.992	T50.993	T50.994	T50.995	T50.996
anhydrous	T50.991	T50.992	T50.993	T50.994	T50.995	T50.996
cyanide	T57.8X1	T57.8X2	T57.8X3	T57.8X4	—	—
dioctyl sulfosuccinate	T47.4X1	T47.4X2	T47.4X3	T47.4X4	T47.4X5	T47.4X6
disodium edathamil	T45.8X1	T45.8X2	T45.8X3	T45.8X4	T45.8X5	T45.8X6
disodium edetate	T45.8X1	T45.8X2	T45.8X3	T45.8X4	T45.8X5	T45.8X6
dobesilate	T46.991	T46.992	T46.993	T46.994	T46.995	T46.996
EDTA	T45.8X1	T45.8X2	T45.8X3	T45.8X4	T45.8X5	T45.8X6
ferrous citrate	T45.4X1	T45.4X2	T45.4X3	T45.4X4	T45.4X5	T45.4X6
folinate	T45.8X1	T45.8X2	T45.8X3	T45.8X4	T45.8X5	T45.8X6
glubionate	T50.3X1	T50.3X2	T50.3X3	T50.3X4	T50.3X5	T50.3X6
gluconate	T50.3X1	T50.3X2	T50.3X3	T50.3X4	T50.3X5	T50.3X6
gluconogalactogluconate	T50.3X1	T50.3X2	T50.3X3	T50.3X4	T50.3X5	T50.3X6
hydrate, hydroxide	T54.3X1	T54.3X2	T54.3X3	T54.3X4	—	—
hypochlorite	T54.3X1	T54.3X2	T54.3X3	T54.3X4	—	—
iodide	T48.4X1	T48.4X2	T48.4X3	T48.4X4	T48.4X5	T48.4X6
ipodate	T50.8X1	T50.8X2	T50.8X3	T50.8X4	T50.8X5	T50.8X6
lactate	T50.3X1	T50.3X2	T50.3X3	T50.3X4	T50.3X5	T50.3X6
leucovorin	T45.8X1	T45.8X2	T45.8X3	T45.8X4	T45.8X5	T45.8X6
mandelate	T37.91	T37.92	T37.93	T37.94	T37.95	T37.96
oxide	T54.3X1	T54.3X2	T54.3X3	T54.3X4	—	—
pantothenate	T45.2X1	T45.2X2	T45.2X3	T45.2X4	T45.2X5	T45.2X6
phosphate	T50.3X1	T50.3X2	T50.3X3	T50.3X4	T50.3X5	T50.3X6
salicylate	T39.091	T39.092	T39.093	T39.094	T39.095	T39.096
salts	T50.3X1	T50.3X2	T50.3X3	T50.3X4	T50.3X5	T50.3X6
Calculus-dissolving drug	T50.991	T50.992	T50.993	T50.994	T50.995	T50.996
Calomel	T49.0X1	T49.0X2	T49.0X3	T49.0X4	T49.0X5	T49.0X6
Caloric agent	T50.3X1	T50.3X2	T50.3X3	T50.3X4	T50.3X5	T50.3X6
Calusterone	T38.7X1	T38.7X2	T38.7X3	T38.7X4	T38.7X5	T38.7X6
Camazepam	T42.4X1	T42.4X2	T42.4X3	T42.4X4	T42.4X5	T42.4X6
Camomile	T49.0X1	T49.0X2	T49.0X3	T49.0X4	T49.0X5	T49.0X6
Camoquin	T37.2X1	T37.2X2	T37.2X3	T37.2X4	T37.2X5	T37.2X6
Camphor						
insecticide	T60.2X1	T60.2X2	T60.2X3	T60.2X4	—	—
medicinal	T49.8X1	T49.8X2	T49.8X3	T49.8X4	T49.8X5	T49.8X6
Camylofin	T44.3X1	T44.3X2	T44.3X3	T44.3X4	T44.3X5	T44.3X6
Cancer chemotherapy drug regimen	T45.1X1	T45.1X2	T45.1X3	T45.1X4	T45.1X5	T45.1X6
Candeptin	T49.0X1	T49.0X2	T49.0X3	T49.0X4	T49.0X5	T49.0X6

◀ New   ◀▥ Revised   ~~deleted~~ Deleted

TABLE OF DRUGS AND CHEMICALS

Substance	Poisoning, Accidental (Unintentional)	Poisoning, Intentional Self-Harm	Poisoning, Assault	Poisoning, Undetermined	Adverse Effect	Underdosing
					External Cause (T-Code)	
Candicidin	T49.0X1	T49.0X2	T49.0X3	T49.0X4	T49.0X5	T49.0X6
Cannabinol	T40.7X1	T40.7X2	T40.7X3	T40.7X4	T40.7X5	T40.7X6
Cannabis (derivatives)	T40.7X1	T40.7X2	T40.7X3	T40.7X4	T40.7X5	T40.7X6
Canned heat	T51.1X1	T51.1X2	T51.1X3	T51.1X4	—	—
Canrenoic acid	T50.0X1	T50.0X2	T50.0X3	T50.0X4	T50.0X5	T50.0X6
Canrenone	T50.0X1	T50.0X2	T50.0X3	T50.0X4	T50.0X5	T50.0X6
Cantharides, cantharidin, cantharis	T49.8X1	T49.8X2	T49.8X3	T49.8X4	T49.8X5	T49.8X6
Canthaxanthin	T50.991	T50.992	T50.993	T50.994	T50.995	T50.996
Capillary-active drug NEC	T46.901	T46.902	T46.903	T46.904	T46.905	T46.906
Capreomycin	T36.8X1	T36.8X2	T36.8X3	T36.8X4	T36.8X5	T36.8X6
Capsicum	T49.4X1	T49.4X2	T49.4X3	T49.4X4	T49.4X5	T49.4X6
Captafol	T60.3X1	T60.3X2	T60.3X3	T60.3X4	—	—
Captan	T60.3X1	T60.3X2	T60.3X3	T60.3X4	—	—
Captodiame, captodiamine	T43.591	T43.592	T43.593	T43.594	T43.595	T43.596
Captopril	T46.4X1	T46.4X2	T46.4X3	T46.4X4	T46.4X5	T46.4X6
Caramiphen	T44.3X1	T44.3X2	T44.3X3	T44.3X4	T44.3X5	T44.3X6
Carazolol	T44.7X1	T44.7X2	T44.7X3	T44.7X4	T44.7X5	T44.7X6
Carbachol	T44.1X1	T44.1X2	T44.1X3	T44.1X4	T44.1X5	T44.1X6
Carbacrylamine (resin)	T50.3X1	T50.3X2	T50.3X3	T50.3X4	T50.3X5	T50.3X6
Carbamate (insecticide)	T60.0X1	T60.0X2	T60.0X3	T60.0X4	—	—
Carbamate (sedative)	T42.6X1	T42.6X2	T42.6X3	T42.6X4	T42.6X5	T42.6X6
herbicide	T60.0X1	T60.0X2	T60.0X3	T60.0X4	—	—
insecticide	T60.0X1	T60.0X2	T60.0X3	T60.0X4	—	—
Carbamazepine	T42.1X1	T42.1X2	T42.1X3	T42.1X4	T42.1X5	T42.1X6
Carbamide	T47.3X1	T47.3X2	T47.3X3	T47.3X4	T47.3X5	T47.3X6
peroxide	T49.0X1	T49.0X2	T49.0X3	T49.0X4	T49.0X5	T49.0X6
topical	T49.8X1	T49.8X2	T49.8X3	T49.8X4	T49.8X5	T49.8X6
Carbamylcholine chloride	T44.1X1	T44.1X2	T44.1X3	T44.1X4	T44.1X5	T44.1X6
Carbaril	T60.0X1	T60.0X2	T60.0X3	T60.0X4	—	—
Carbarsone	T37.3X1	T37.3X2	T37.3X3	T37.3X4	T37.3X5	T37.3X6
Carbaryl	T60.0X1	T60.0X2	T60.0X3	T60.0X4	—	—
Carbaspirin	T39.011	T39.012	T39.013	T39.014	T39.015	T39.016
Carbazochrome (salicylate) (sodium sulfonate)	T49.4X1	T49.4X2	T49.4X3	T49.4X4	T49.4X5	T49.4X6
Carbenicillin	T36.0X1	T36.0X2	T36.0X3	T36.0X4	T36.0X5	T36.0X6
Carbenoxolone	T47.1X1	T47.1X2	T47.1X3	T47.1X4	T47.1X5	T47.1X6
Carbetapentane	T48.3X1	T48.3X2	T48.3X3	T48.3X4	T48.3X5	T48.3X6
Carbethyl salicylate	T39.091	T39.092	T39.093	T39.094	T39.095	T39.096
Carbidopa (with levodopa)	T42.8X1	T42.8X2	T42.8X3	T42.8X4	T42.8X5	T42.8X6
Carbimazole	T38.2X1	T38.2X2	T38.2X3	T38.2X4	T38.2X5	T38.2X6

◀ New   ⬅ Revised   ~~deleted~~ Deleted

Substance	External Cause (T-Code)					
	Poisoning, Accidental (Unintentional)	Poisoning, Intentional Self-Harm	Poisoning, Assault	Poisoning, Undetermined	Adverse Effect	Underdosing
Carbinol	T51.1X1	T51.1X2	T51.1X3	T51.1X4	—	—
Carbinoxamine	T45.0X1	T45.0X2	T45.0X3	T45.0X4	T45.0X5	T45.0X6
Carbiphene	T39.8X1	T39.8X2	T39.8X3	T39.8X4	T39.8X5	T39.8X6
Carbitol	T52.3X1	T52.3X2	T52.3X3	T52.3X4	—	—
Carbocaine	T41.3X1	T41.3X2	T41.3X3	T41.3X4	T41.3X5	T41.3X6
infiltration (subcutaneous)	T41.3X1	T41.3X2	T41.3X3	T41.3X4	T41.3X5	T41.3X6
nerve block (peripheral) (plexus)	T41.3X1	T41.3X2	T41.3X3	T41.3X4	T41.3X5	T41.3X6
topical (surface)	T41.3X1	T41.3X2	T41.3X3	T41.3X4	T41.3X5	T41.3X6
Carbo medicinalis	T47.6X1	T47.6X2	T47.6X3	T47.6X4	T47.6X5	T47.6X6
Carbomycin	T36.8X1	T36.8X2	T36.8X3	T36.8X4	T36.8X5	T36.8X6
Carbocisteine	T48.4X1	T48.4X2	T48.4X3	T48.4X4	T48.4X5	T48.4X6
Carbocromen	T46.3X1	T46.3X2	T46.3X3	T46.3X4	T46.3X5	T46.3X6
Carbol fuchsin	T49.0X1	T49.0X2	T49.0X3	T49.0X4	T49.0X5	T49.0X6
Carbolic acid—see also Phenol	T54.0X1	T54.0X2	T54.0X3	T54.0X4	—	—
Carbolonium (bromide)	T48.1X1	T48.1X2	T48.1X3	T48.1X4	T48.1X5	T48.1X6
Carbon						
bisulfide (liquid)	T65.4X1	T65.4X2	T65.4X3	T65.4X4	—	—
vapor	T65.4X1	T65.4X2	T65.4X3	T65.4X4		
dioxide (gas)	T59.7X1	T59.7X2	T59.7X3	T59.7X4	—	—
medicinal	T41.5X1	T41.5X2	T41.5X3	T41.5X4	T41.5X5	T41.5X6
nonmedicinal	T59.7X1	T59.7X2	T59.7X3	T59.7X4	—	—
snow	T49.4X1	T49.4X2	T49.4X3	T49.4X4	T49.4X5	T49.4X6
disulfide (liquid)	T65.4X1	T65.4X2	T65.4X3	T65.4X4		
vapor	T65.4X1	T65.4X2	T65.4X3	T65.4X4		
monoxide (from incomplete combustion)	T58.91	T58.92	T58.93	T58.94	—	—
blast furnace gas	T58.8X1	T58.8X2	T58.8X3	T58.8X4	—	—
butane (distributed in mobile container)	T58.11	T58.12	T58.13	T58.14	—	—
distributed through pipes	T58.11	T58.12	T58.13	T58.14	—	—
charcoal fumes	T58.2X1	T58.2X2	T58.2X3	T58.2X4	—	—
coal	T58.2X1	T58.2X2	T58.2X3	T58.2X4		
coke (in domestic stoves, fireplaces)	T58.2X1	T58.2X2	T58.2X3	T58.2X4	—	—
gas (piped)	T58.11	T58.12	T58.13	T58.14	—	—
solid (in domestic stoves, fireplaces)	T58.2X1	T58.2X2	T58.2X3	T58.2X4	—	—
exhaust gas (motor) not in transit	T58.01	T58.02	T58.03	T58.04	—	—
combustion engine, any not in watercraft	T58.01	T58.02	T58.03	T58.04	—	—
farm tractor, not in transit	T58.01	T58.02	T58.03	T58.04	—	—
gas engine	T58.01	T58.02	T58.03	T58.04	—	—
motor pump	T58.01	T58.02	T58.03	T58.04	—	—
motor vehicle, not in transit	T58.01	T58.02	T58.03	T58.04	—	—

TABLE OF DRUGS AND CHEMICALS

Substance	External Cause (T-Code)					
	Poisoning, Accidental (Unintentional)	Poisoning, Intentional Self-Harm	Poisoning, Assault	Poisoning, Undetermined	Adverse Effect	Underdosing
Carbon *(Continued)*						
monoxide *(Continued)*						
fuel (in domestic use)	T58.2X1	T58.2X2	T58.2X3	T58.2X4	—	—
gas (piped)	T58.11	T58.12	T58.13	T58.14	—	—
in mobile container	T58.11	T58.12	T58.13	T58.14	—	—
utility	T58.11	T58.12	T58.13	T58.14	—	—
in mobile container	T58.11	T58.12	T58.13	T58.14	—	—
piped (natural)	T58.11	T58.12	T58.13	T58.14	—	—
illuminating gas	T58.11	T58.12	T58.13	T58.14	—	—
industrial fuels or gases, any	T58.8X1	T58.8X2	T58.8X3	T58.8X4	—	—
kerosene (in domestic stoves, fireplaces)	T58.2X1	T58.2X2	T58.2X3	T58.2X4	—	—
kiln gas or vapor	T58.8X1	T58.8X2	T58.8X3	T58.8X4	—	—
motor exhaust gas, not in transit	T58.01	T58.02	T58.03	T58.04	—	—
piped gas (manufactured) (natural)	T58.11	T58.12	T58.13	T58.14	—	—
producer gas	T58.8X1	T58.8X2	T58.8X3	T58.8X4	—	—
propane (distributed in mobile container)	T58.11	T58.12	T58.13	T58.14	—	—
distributed through pipes	T58.11	T58.12	T58.13	T58.14	—	—
specified source NEC	T58.8X1	T58.8X2	T58.8X3	T58.8X4	—	—
stove gas	T58.11	T58.12	T58.13	T58.14	—	—
piped	T58.11	T58.12	T58.13	T58.14	—	—
utility gas	T58.11	T58.12	T58.13	T58.14	—	—
piped	T58.11	T58.12	T58.13	T58.14	—	—
water gas	T58.11	T58.12	T58.13	T58.14	—	—
wood (in domestic stoves, fireplaces)	T58.2X1	T58.2X2	T58.2X3	T58.2X4	—	—
tetrachloride (vapor) NEC	T53.0X1	T53.0X2	T53.0X3	T53.0X4	—	—
liquid (cleansing agent) NEC	T53.0X1	T53.0X2	T53.0X3	T53.0X4	—	—
solvent	T53.0X1	T53.0X2	T53.0X3	T53.0X4	—	—
Carbonic acid gas	T59.7X1	T59.7X2	T59.7X3	T59.7X4	—	—
anhydrase inhibitor NEC	T50.2X1	T50.2X2	T50.2X3	T50.2X4	T50.2X5	T50.2X6
Carbophenothion	T60.0X1	T60.0X2	T60.0X3	T60.0X4		
Carboplatin	T45.1X1	T45.1X2	T45.1X3	T45.1X4	T45.1X5	T45.1X6
Carboprost	T48.0X1	T48.0X2	T48.0X3	T48.0X4	T48.0X5	T48.0X6
Carboquone	T45.1X1	T45.1X2	T45.1X3	T45.1X4	T45.1X5	T45.1X6
Carbowax	T49.3X1	T49.3X2	T49.3X3	T49.3X4	T49.3X5	T49.3X6
Carboxymethyl-cellulose	T47.4X1	T47.4X2	T47.4X3	T47.4X4	T47.4X5	T47.4X6
S-Carboxymethyl-cysteine	T48.4X1	T48.4X2	T48.4X3	T48.4X4	T48.4X5	T48.4X6
Carbrital	T42.3X1	T42.3X2	T42.3X3	T42.3X4	T42.3X5	T42.3X6
Carbromal	T42.6X1	T42.6X2	T42.6X3	T42.6X4	T42.6X5	T42.6X6
Carbutamide	T38.3X1	T38.3X2	T38.3X3	T38.3X4	T38.3X5	T38.3X6
Carbuterol	T48.6X1	T48.6X2	T48.6X3	T48.6X4	T48.6X5	T48.6X6

◀ New ◀◀ Revised ~~deleted~~ Deleted

Substance	External Cause (T-Code)					
	Poisoning, Accidental (Unintentional)	Poisoning, Intentional Self-Harm	Poisoning, Assault	Poisoning, Undetermined	Adverse Effect	Underdosing
Cardiac						
depressants	T46.2X1	T46.2X2	T46.2X3	T46.2X4	T46.2X5	T46.2X6
rhythm regulator	T46.2X1	T46.2X2	T46.2X3	T46.2X4	T46.2X5	T46.2X6
specified NEC	T46.2X1	T46.2X2	T46.2X3	T46.2X4	T46.2X5	T46.2X6
Cardiografin	T50.8X1	T50.8X2	T50.8X3	T50.8X4	T50.8X5	T50.8X6
Cardio-green	T50.8X1	T50.8X2	T50.8X3	T50.8X4	T50.8X5	T50.8X6
Cardiotonic (glycoside) NEC	T46.0X1	T46.0X2	T46.0X3	T46.0X4	T46.0X5	T46.0X6
Cardiovascular drug NEC	T46.901	T46.902	T46.903	T46.904	T46.905	T46.906
Cardrase	T50.2X1	T50.2X2	T50.2X3	T50.2X4	T50.2X5	T50.2X6
Carfusin	T49.0X1	T49.0X2	T49.0X3	T49.0X4	T49.0X5	T49.0X6
Carfecillin	T36.0X1	T36.0X2	T36.0X3	T36.0X4	T36.0X5	T36.0X6
Carfenazine	T43.3X1	T43.3X2	T43.3X3	T43.3X4	T43.3X5	T43.3X6
Carindacillin	T36.0X1	T36.0X2	T36.0X3	T36.0X4	T36.0X5	T36.0X6
Carisoprodol	T42.8X1	T42.8X2	T42.8X3	T42.8X4	T42.8X5	T42.8X6
Carmellose	T47.4X1	T47.4X2	T47.4X3	T47.4X4	T47.4X5	T47.4X6
Carminative	T47.5X1	T47.5X2	T47.5X3	T47.5X4	T47.5X5	T47.5X6
Carmofur	T45.1X1	T45.1X2	T45.1X3	T45.1X4	T45.1X5	T45.1X6
Carmustine	T45.1X1	T45.1X2	T45.1X3	T45.1X4	T45.1X5	T45.1X6
Carotene	T45.2X1	T45.2X2	T45.2X3	T45.2X4	T45.2X5	T45.2X6
Carphenazine	T43.3X1	T43.3X2	T43.3X3	T43.3X4	T43.3X5	T43.3X6
Carpipramine	T42.4X1	T42.4X2	T42.4X3	T42.4X4	T42.4X5	T42.4X6
Carprofen	T39.311	T39.312	T39.313	T39.314	T39.315	T39.316
Carpronium chloride	T44.3X1	T44.3X2	T44.3X3	T44.3X4	T44.3X5	T44.3X6
Carrageenan	T47.8X1	T47.8X2	T47.8X3	T47.8X4	T47.8X5	T47.8X6
Carteolol	T44.7X1	T44.7X2	T44.7X3	T44.7X4	T44.7X5	T44.7X6
Carter's Little Pills	T47.2X1	T47.2X2	T47.2X3	T47.2X4	T47.2X5	T47.2X6
Cascara (sagrada)	T47.2X1	T47.2X2	T47.2X3	T47.2X4	T47.2X5	T47.2X6
Cassava	T62.2X1	T62.2X2	T62.2X3	T62.2X4	—	—
Castellani's paint	T49.0X1	T49.0X2	T49.0X3	T49.0X4	T49.0X5	T49.0X6
Castor						
bean	T62.2X1	T62.2X2	T62.2X3	T62.2X4	—	—
oil	T47.2X1	T47.2X2	T47.2X3	T47.2X4	T47.2X5	T47.2X6
Catalase	T45.3X1	T45.3X2	T45.3X3	T45.3X4	T45.3X5	T45.3X6
Caterpillar (sting)	T63.431	T63.432	T63.433	T63.434	—	—
Catha (edulis) (tea)	T43.691	T43.692	T43.693	T43.694	—	—
Cathartic NEC	T47.4X1	T47.4X2	T47.4X3	T47.4X4	T47.4X5	T47.4X6
anthacene derivative	T47.2X1	T47.2X2	T47.2X3	T47.2X4	T47.2X5	T47.2X6
bulk	T47.4X1	T47.4X2	T47.4X3	T47.4X4	T47.4X5	T47.4X6
contact	T47.2X1	T47.2X2	T47.2X3	T47.2X4	T47.2X5	T47.2X6
emollient NEC	T47.4X1	T47.4X2	T47.4X3	T47.4X4	T47.4X5	T47.4X6

TABLE OF DRUGS AND CHEMICALS

Substance	External Cause (T-Code)					
	Poisoning, Accidental (Unintentional)	Poisoning, Intentional Self-Harm	Poisoning, Assault	Poisoning, Undetermined	Adverse Effect	Underdosing
Cathartic NEC *(Continued)*						
irritant NEC	T47.2X1	T47.2X2	T47.2X3	T47.2X4	T47.2X5	T47.2X6
mucilage	T47.4X1	T47.4X2	T47.4X3	T47.4X4	T47.4X5	T47.4X6
saline	T47.3X1	T47.3X2	T47.3X3	T47.3X4	T47.3X5	T47.3X6
vegetable	T47.2X1	T47.2X2	T47.2X3	T47.2X4	T47.2X5	T47.2X6
Cathine	T50.5X1	T50.5X2	T50.5X3	T50.5X4	T50.5X5	T50.5X6
Cathomycin	T36.8X1	T36.8X2	T36.8X3	T36.8X4	T36.8X5	T36.8X6
Cation exchange resin	T50.3X1	T50.3X2	T50.3X3	T50.3X4	T50.3X5	T50.3X6
Caustic(s) NEC	T54.91	T54.92	T54.93	T54.94	—	—
alkali	T54.3X1	T54.3X2	T54.3X3	T54.3X4	—	—
hydroxide	T54.3X1	T54.3X2	T54.3X3	T54.3X4	—	—
potash	T54.3X1	T54.3X2	T54.3X3	T54.3X4	—	—
soda	T54.3X1	T54.3X2	T54.3X3	T54.3X4	—	—
specified NEC	T54.91	T54.92	T54.93	T54.94	—	—
Ceepryn	T49.0X1	T49.0X2	T49.0X3	T49.0X4	T49.0X5	T49.0X6
ENT agent	T49.6X1	T49.6X2	T49.6X3	T49.6X4	T49.6X5	T49.6X6
lozenges	T49.6X1	T49.6X2	T49.6X3	T49.6X4	T49.6X5	T49.6X6
Cefacetrile	T36.1X1	T36.1X2	T36.1X3	T36.1X4	T36.1X5	T36.1X6
Cefaclor	T36.1X1	T36.1X2	T36.1X3	T36.1X4	T36.1X5	T36.1X6
Cefadroxil	T36.1X1	T36.1X2	T36.1X3	T36.1X4	T36.1X5	T36.1X6
Cefalexin	T36.1X1	T36.1X2	T36.1X3	T36.1X4	T36.1X5	T36.1X6
Cefaloglycin	T36.1X1	T36.1X2	T36.1X3	T36.1X4	T36.1X5	T36.1X6
Cefaloridine	T36.1X1	T36.1X2	T36.1X3	T36.1X4	T36.1X5	T36.1X6
Cefalosporins	T36.1X1	T36.1X2	T36.1X3	T36.1X4	T36.1X5	T36.1X6
Cefalotin	T36.1X1	T36.1X2	T36.1X3	T36.1X4	T36.1X5	T36.1X6
Cefamandole	T36.1X1	T36.1X2	T36.1X3	T36.1X4	T36.1X5	T36.1X6
Cefamycin antibiotic	T36.1X1	T36.1X2	T36.1X3	T36.1X4	T36.1X5	T36.1X6
Cefapirin	T36.1X1	T36.1X2	T36.1X3	T36.1X4	T36.1X5	T36.1X6
Cefatrizine	T36.1X1	T36.1X2	T36.1X3	T36.1X4	T36.1X5	T36.1X6
Cefazedone	T36.1X1	T36.1X2	T36.1X3	T36.1X4	T36.1X5	T36.1X6
Cefazolin	T36.1X1	T36.1X2	T36.1X3	T36.1X4	T36.1X5	T36.1X6
Cefbuperazone	T36.1X1	T36.1X2	T36.1X3	T36.1X4	T36.1X5	T36.1X6
Cefetamet	T36.1X1	T36.1X2	T36.1X3	T36.1X4	T36.1X5	T36.1X6
Cefixime	T36.1X1	T36.1X2	T36.1X3	T36.1X4	T36.1X5	T36.1X6
Cefmenoxime	T36.1X1	T36.1X2	T36.1X3	T36.1X4	T36.1X5	T36.1X6
Cefmetazole	T36.1X1	T36.1X2	T36.1X3	T36.1X4	T36.1X5	T36.1X6
Cefminox	T36.1X1	T36.1X2	T36.1X3	T36.1X4	T36.1X5	T36.1X6
Cefonicid	T36.1X1	T36.1X2	T36.1X3	T36.1X4	T36.1X5	T36.1X6
Cefoperazone	T36.1X1	T36.1X2	T36.1X3	T36.1X4	T36.1X5	T36.1X6

◀ New   ◀▥ Revised   ~~deleted~~ Deleted

Substance	Poisoning, Accidental (Unintentional)	Poisoning, Intentional Self-Harm	Poisoning, Assault	Poisoning, Undetermined	Adverse Effect	Underdosing
Ceforanide	T36.1X1	T36.1X2	T36.1X3	T36.1X4	T36.1X5	T36.1X6
Cefotaxime	T36.1X1	T36.1X2	T36.1X3	T36.1X4	T36.1X5	T36.1X6
Cefotetan	T36.1X1	T36.1X2	T36.1X3	T36.1X4	T36.1X5	T36.1X6
Cefotiam	T36.1X1	T36.1X2	T36.1X3	T36.1X4	T36.1X5	T36.1X6
Cefoxitin	T36.1X1	T36.1X2	T36.1X3	T36.1X4	T36.1X5	T36.1X6
Cefpimizole	T36.1X1	T36.1X2	T36.1X3	T36.1X4	T36.1X5	T36.1X6
Cefpiramide	T36.1X1	T36.1X2	T36.1X3	T36.1X4	T36.1X5	T36.1X6
Cefradine	T36.1X1	T36.1X2	T36.1X3	T36.1X4	T36.1X5	T36.1X6
Cefroxadine	T36.1X1	T36.1X2	T36.1X3	T36.1X4	T36.1X5	T36.1X6
Cefsulodin	T36.1X1	T36.1X2	T36.1X3	T36.1X4	T36.1X5	T36.1X6
Ceftazidime	T36.1X1	T36.1X2	T36.1X3	T36.1X4	T36.1X5	T36.1X6
Cefteram	T36.1X1	T36.1X2	T36.1X3	T36.1X4	T36.1X5	T36.1X6
Ceftezole	T36.1X1	T36.1X2	T36.1X3	T36.1X4	T36.1X5	T36.1X6
Ceftizoxime	T36.1X1	T36.1X2	T36.1X3	T36.1X4	T36.1X5	T36.1X6
Ceftriaxone	T36.1X1	T36.1X2	T36.1X3	T36.1X4	T36.1X5	T36.1X6
Cefuroxime	T36.1X1	T36.1X2	T36.1X3	T36.1X4	T36.1X5	T36.1X6
Cefuzonam	T36.1X1	T36.1X2	T36.1X3	T36.1X4	T36.1X5	T36.1X6
Celestone	T38.0X1	T38.0X2	T38.0X3	T38.0X4	T38.0X5	T38.0X6
topical	T49.0X1	T49.0X2	T49.0X3	T49.0X4	T49.0X5	T49.0X6
Celiprolol	T44.7X1	T44.7X2	T44.7X3	T44.7X4	T44.7X5	T44.7X6
Cellosolve	T52.91	T52.92	T52.93	T52.94	—	—
Cell stimulants and proliferants	T49.8X1	T49.8X2	T49.8X3	T49.8X4	T49.8X5	T49.8X6
Cellulose						
cathartic	T47.4X1	T47.4X2	T47.4X3	T47.4X4	T47.4X5	T47.4X6
hydroxyethyl	T47.4X1	T47.4X2	T47.4X3	T47.4X4	T47.4X5	T47.4X6
nitrates (topical)	T49.3X1	T49.3X2	T49.3X3	T49.3X4	T49.3X5	T49.3X6
oxidized	T49.4X1	T49.4X2	T49.4X3	T49.4X4	T49.4X5	T49.4X6
Centipede (bite)	T63.411	T63.412	T63.413	T63.414	—	—
Central nervous system						
depressants	T42.71	T42.72	T42.73	T42.74	T42.75	T42.76
anesthetic (general) NEC	T41.201	T41.202	T41.203	T41.204	T41.205	T41.206
gases NEC	T41.0X1	T41.0X2	T41.0X3	T41.0X4	T41.0X5	T41.0X6
intravenous	T41.1X1	T41.1X2	T41.1X3	T41.1X4	T41.1X5	T41.1X6
barbiturates	T42.3X1	T42.3X2	T42.3X3	T42.3X4	T42.3X5	T42.3X6
benzodiazepines	T42.4X1	T42.4X2	T42.4X3	T42.4X4	T42.4X5	T42.4X6
bromides	T42.6X1	T42.6X2	T42.6X3	T42.6X4	T42.6X5	T42.6X6
cannabis sativa	T40.7X1	T40.7X2	T40.7X3	T40.7X4	T40.7X5	T40.7X6
chloral hydrate	T42.6X1	T42.6X2	T42.6X3	T42.6X4	T42.6X5	T42.6X6
ethanol	T51.0X1	T51.0X2	T51.0X3	T51.0X4	—	—

Substance	External Cause (T-Code)					
	Poisoning, Accidental (Unintentional)	Poisoning, Intentional Self-Harm	Poisoning, Assault	Poisoning, Undetermined	Adverse Effect	Underdosing
Central nervous system *(Continued)*						
depressants *(Continued)*						
hallucinogenics	T40.901	T40.902	T40.903	T40.904	T40.905	T40.906
hypnotics	T42.71	T42.72	T42.73	T42.74	T42.75	T42.76
specified NEC	T42.6X1	T42.6X2	T42.6X3	T42.6X4	T42.6X5	T42.6X6
muscle relaxants	T42.8X1	T42.8X2	T42.8X3	T42.8X4	T42.8X5	T42.8X6
paraldehyde	T42.6X1	T42.6X2	T42.6X3	T42.6X4	T42.6X5	T42.6X6
sedatives; sedative-hypnotics	T42.71	T42.72	T42.73	T42.74	T42.75	T42.76
mixed NEC	T42.6X1	T42.6X2	T42.6X3	T42.6X4	T42.6X5	T42.6X6
specified NEC	T42.6X1	T42.6X2	T42.6X3	T42.6X4	T42.6X5	T42.6X6
muscle-tone depressants	T42.8X1	T42.8X2	T42.8X3	T42.8X4	T42.8X5	T42.8X6
stimulants	T43.601	T43.602	T43.603	T43.604	T43.605	T43.606
amphetamines	T43.621	T43.622	T43.623	T43.624	T43.625	T43.626
analeptics	T50.7X1	T50.7X2	T50.7X3	T50.7X4	T50.7X5	T50.7X6
antidepressants	T43.201	T43.202	T43.203	T43.204	T43.205	T43.206
opiate antagonists	T50.7X1	T50.7X2	T50.7X3	T50.7X4	T50.7X5	T50.7X6
specified NEC	T43.691	T43.692	T43.693	T43.694	T43.695	T43.696
Cephalexin	T36.1X1	T36.1X2	T36.1X3	T36.1X4	T36.1X5	T36.1X6
Cephaloglycin	T36.1X1	T36.1X2	T36.1X3	T36.1X4	T36.1X5	T36.1X6
Cephaloridine	T36.1X1	T36.1X2	T36.1X3	T36.1X4	T36.1X5	T36.1X6
Cephalosporins	T36.1X1	T36.1X2	T36.1X3	T36.1X4	T36.1X5	T36.1X6
N (adicillin)	T36.0X1	T36.0X2	T36.0X3	T36.0X4	T36.0X5	T36.0X6
Cephalothin	T36.1X1	T36.1X2	T36.1X3	T36.1X4	T36.1X5	T36.1X6
Cephalotin	T36.1X1	T36.1X2	T36.1X3	T36.1X4	T36.1X5	T36.1X6
Cephradine	T36.1X1	T36.1X2	T36.1X3	T36.1X4	T36.1X5	T36.1X6
Cerbera (odallam)	T62.2X1	T62.2X2	T62.2X3	T62.2X4	—	—
Cerberin	T46.0X1	T46.0X2	T46.0X3	T46.0X4	T46.0X5	T46.0X6
Cerebral stimulants	T43.601	T43.602	T43.603	T43.604	T43.605	T43.606
psychotherapeutic	T43.601	T43.602	T43.603	T43.604	T43.605	T43.606
specified NEC	T43.691	T43.692	T43.693	T43.694	T43.695	T43.696
Cerium oxalate	T45.0X1	T45.0X2	T45.0X3	T45.0X4	T45.0X5	T45.0X6
Cerous oxalate	T45.0X1	T45.0X2	T45.0X3	T45.0X4	T45.0X5	T45.0X6
Ceruletide	T50.8X1	T50.8X2	T50.8X3	T50.8X4	T50.8X5	T50.8X6
Cetalkonium (chloride)	T49.0X1	T49.0X2	T49.0X3	T49.0X4	T49.0X5	T49.0X6
Cethexonium chloride	T49.0X1	T49.0X2	T49.0X3	T49.0X4	T49.0X5	T49.0X6
Cetiedil	T46.7X1	T46.7X2	T46.7X3	T46.7X4	T46.7X5	T46.7X6
Cetirizine	T45.0X1	T45.0X2	T45.0X3	T45.0X4	T45.0X5	T45.0X6
Cetomacrogol	T50.991	T50.992	T50.993	T50.994	T50.995	T50.996
Cetotiamine	T45.2X1	T45.2X2	T45.2X3	T45.2X4	T45.2X5	T45.2X6

◀ New ◀▥ Revised ~~deleted~~ Deleted

Substance	External Cause (T-Code)					
	Poisoning, Accidental (Unintentional)	Poisoning, Intentional Self-Harm	Poisoning, Assault	Poisoning, Undetermined	Adverse Effect	Underdosing
Cetoxime	T45.0X1	T45.0X2	T45.0X3	T45.0X4	T45.0X5	T45.0X6
Cetraxate	T47.1X1	T47.1X2	T47.1X3	T47.1X4	T47.1X5	T47.1X6
Cetrimide	T49.0X1	T49.0X2	T49.0X3	T49.0X4	T49.0X5	T49.0X6
Cetrimonium (bromide)	T49.0X1	T49.0X2	T49.0X3	T49.0X4	T49.0X5	T49.0X6
Cetylpyridinium chloride	T49.0X1	T49.0X2	T49.0X3	T49.0X4	T49.0X5	T49.0X6
ENT agent	T49.6X1	T49.6X2	T49.6X3	T49.6X4	T49.6X5	T49.6X6
lozenges	T49.6X1	T49.6X2	T49.6X3	T49.6X4	T49.6X5	T49.6X6
Cevadillasee Sabadilla						
Cevitamic acid	T45.2X1	T45.2X2	T45.2X3	T45.2X4	T45.2X5	T45.2X6
Chalk, precipitated	T47.1X1	T47.1X2	T47.1X3	T47.1X4	T47.1X5	T47.1X6
Chamomile	T49.0X1	T49.0X2	T49.0X3	T49.0X4	T49.0X5	T49.0X6
Ch'an su	T46.0X1	T46.0X2	T46.0X3	T46.0X4	T46.0X5	T46.0X6
Charcoal	T47.6X1	T47.6X2	T47.6X3	T47.6X4	T47.6X5	T47.6X6
activated — *see also Charcoal, medicinal*	T47.6X1	T47.6X2	T47.6X3	T47.6X4	T47.6X5	T47.6X6
fumes (Carbon monoxide)	T58.2X1	T58.2X2	T58.2X3	T58.2X4	—	—
industrial	T58.8X1	T58.8X2	T58.8X3	T58.8X4	—	—
medicinal (activated)	T47.6X1	T47.6X2	T47.6X3	T47.6X4	T47.6X5	T47.6X6
antidiarrheal	T47.6X1	T47.6X2	T47.6X3	T47.6X4	T47.6X5	T47.6X6
poison control	T47.8X1	T47.8X2	T47.8X3	T47.8X4	T47.8X5	T47.8X6
specified use other than for diarrhea	T47.8X1	T47.8X2	T47.8X3	T47.8X4	T47.8X5	T47.8X6
topical	T49.8X1	T49.8X2	T49.8X3	T49.8X4	T49.8X5	T49.8X6
Chaulmosulfone	T37.1X1	T37.1X2	T37.1X3	T37.1X4	T37.1X5	T37.1X6
Chelating agent NEC	T50.6X1	T50.6X2	T50.6X3	T50.6X4	T50.6X5	T50.6X6
Chelidonium majus	T62.2X1	T62.2X2	T62.2X3	T62.2X4	—	—
Chemical substance NEC	T65.91	T65.92	T65.93	T65.94	—	—
Chenodeoxycholic acid	T47.5X1	T47.5X2	T47.5X3	T47.5X4	T47.5X5	T47.5X6
Chenodiol	T47.5X1	T47.5X2	T47.5X3	T47.5X4	T47.5X5	T47.5X6
Chenopodium	T37.4X1	T37.4X2	T37.4X3	T37.4X4	T37.4X5	T37.4X6
Cherry laurel	T62.2X1	T62.2X2	T62.2X3	T62.2X4	—	—
Chinidin(e)	T46.2X1	T46.2X2	T46.2X3	T46.2X4	T46.2X5	T46.2X6
Chiniofon	T37.8X1	T37.8X2	T37.8X3	T37.8X4	T37.8X5	T37.8X6
Chlophedianol	T48.3X1	T48.3X2	T48.3X3	T48.3X4	T48.3X5	T48.3X6
Chloral	T42.6X1	T42.6X2	T42.6X3	T42.6X4	T42.6X5	T42.6X6
derivative	T42.6X1	T42.6X2	T42.6X3	T42.6X4	T42.6X5	T42.6X6
hydrate	T42.6X1	T42.6X2	T42.6X3	T42.6X4	T42.6X5	T42.6X6
Chloralamide	T42.6X1	T42.6X2	T42.6X3	T42.6X4	T42.6X5	T42.6X6
Chloralodol	T42.6X1	T42.6X2	T42.6X3	T42.6X4	T42.6X5	T42.6X6
Chloralose	T60.4X1	T60.4X2	T60.4X3	T60.4X4	—	—
Chlorambucil	T45.1X1	T45.1X2	T45.1X3	T45.1X4	T45.1X5	T45.1X6

TABLE OF DRUGS AND CHEMICALS

	External Cause (T-Code)					
Substance	Poisoning, Accidental (Unintentional)	Poisoning, Intentional Self-Harm	Poisoning, Assault	Poisoning, Undetermined	Adverse Effect	Underdosing
Chloramine	T57.8X1	T57.8X2	T57.8X3	T57.8X4	—	—
T	T49.0X1	T49.0X2	T49.0X3	T49.0X4	T49.0X5	T49.0X6
topical	T49.0X1	T49.0X2	T49.0X3	T49.0X4	T49.0X5	T49.0X6
Chloramphenicol	T36.2X1	T36.2X2	T36.2X3	T36.2X4	T36.2X5	T36.2X6
ENT agent	T49.6X1	T49.6X2	T49.6X3	T49.6X4	T49.6X5	T49.6X6
ophthalmic preparation	T49.5X1	T49.5X2	T49.5X3	T49.5X4	T49.5X5	T49.5X6
topical NEC	T49.0X1	T49.0X2	T49.0X3	T49.0X4	T49.0X5	T49.0X6
Chlorate (potassium) (sodium) NEC	T60.3X1	T60.3X2	T60.3X3	T60.3X4	—	—
herbicide	T60.3X1	T60.3X2	T60.3X3	T60.3X4	—	—
Chlorazanil	T50.2X1	T50.2X2	T50.2X3	T50.2X4	T50.2X5	T50.2X6
Chlorbenzene, chlorbenzol	T53.7X1	T53.7X2	T53.7X3	T53.7X4	—	—
Chlorbenzoxamine	T44.3X1	T44.3X2	T44.3X3	T44.3X4	T44.3X5	T44.3X6
Chlorbutol	T42.6X1	T42.6X2	T42.6X3	T42.6X4	T42.6X5	T42.6X6
Chlorcyclizine	T45.0X1	T45.0X2	T45.0X3	T45.0X4	T45.0X5	T45.0X6
Chlordan(e) (dust)	T60.1X1	T60.1X2	T60.1X3	T60.1X4	—	—
Chlordantoin	T49.0X1	T49.0X2	T49.0X3	T49.0X4	T49.0X5	T49.0X6
Chlordiazepoxide	T42.4X1	T42.4X2	T42.4X3	T42.4X4	T42.4X5	T42.4X6
Chlordiethyl benzamide	T49.3X1	T49.3X2	T49.3X3	T49.3X4	T49.3X5	T49.3X6
Chloresium	T49.8X1	T49.8X2	T49.8X3	T49.8X4	T49.8X5	T49.8X6
Chlorethiazol	T42.6X1	T42.6X2	T42.6X3	T42.6X4	T42.6X5	T42.6X6
Chlorethyl — see Ethyl chloride						
Chloretone	T42.6X1	T42.6X2	T42.6X3	T42.6X4	T42.6X5	T42.6X6
Chlorex	T53.6X1	T53.6X2	T53.6X3	T53.6X4	—	—
insecticide	T60.1X1	T60.1X2	T60.1X3	T60.1X4	—	—
Chlorfenvinphos	T60.0X1	T60.0X2	T60.0X3	T60.0X4	—	—
Chlorhexadol	T42.6X1	T42.6X2	T42.6X3	T42.6X4	T42.6X5	T42.6X6
Chlorhexamide	T45.1X1	T45.1X2	T45.1X3	T45.1X4	T45.1X5	T45.1X6
Chlorhexidine	T49.0X1	T49.0X2	T49.0X3	T49.0X4	T49.0X5	T49.0X6
Chlorhydroxyquinolin	T49.0X1	T49.0X2	T49.0X3	T49.0X4	T49.0X5	T49.0X6
Chloride of lime (bleach)	T54.3X1	T54.3X2	T54.3X3	T54.3X4	—	—
Chlorimipramine	T43.011	T43.012	T43.013	T43.014	T43.015	T43.016
Chlorinated						
camphene	T53.6X1	T53.6X2	T53.6X3	T53.6X4	—	—
diphenyl	T53.7X1	T53.7X2	T53.7X3	T53.7X4	—	—
hydrocarbons NEC	T53.91	T53.92	T53.93	T53.94	—	—
solvents	T53.91	T53.92	T53.93	T53.94	—	—
lime (bleach)	T54.3X1	T54.3X2	T54.3X3	T54.3X4	—	—
and boric acid solution	T49.0X1	T49.0X2	T49.0X3	T49.0X4	T49.0X5	T49.0X6
naphthalene (insecticide)	T60.1X1	T60.1X2	T60.1X3	T60.1X4	—	—
industrial (non-pesticide)	T53.7X1	T53.7X2	T53.7X3	T53.7X4	—	—

◀ New   ◀▥ Revised   ~~deleted~~ Deleted

Substance	Poisoning, Accidental (Unintentional)	Poisoning, Intentional Self-Harm	Poisoning, Assault	Poisoning, Undetermined	Adverse Effect	Underdosing
			External Cause (T-Code)			
Chlorinated *(Continued)*						
pesticide NEC	T60.8X1	T60.8X2	T60.8X3	T60.8X4	—	—
soda — *see also sodium hypochlorite*						
solution	T49.0X1	T49.0X2	T49.0X3	T49.0X4	T49.0X5	T49.0X6
Chlorine (fumes) (gas)	T59.4X1	T59.4X2	T59.4X3	T59.4X4	—	—
bleach	T54.3X1	T54.3X2	T54.3X3	T54.3X4	—	—
compound gas NEC	T59.4X1	T59.4X2	T59.4X3	T59.4X4	—	—
disinfectant	T59.4X1	T59.4X2	T59.4X3	T59.4X4	—	—
releasing agents NEC	T59.4X1	T59.4X2	T59.4X3	T59.4X4	—	—
Chlorisondamine chloride	T46.991	T46.992	T46.993	T46.994	T46.995	T46.996
Chlormadinone	T38.5X1	T38.5X2	T38.5X3	T38.5X4	T38.5X5	T38.5X6
Chlormephos	T60.0X1	T60.0X2	T60.0X3	T60.0X4	—	—
Chlormerodrin	T50.2X1	T50.2X2	T50.2X3	T50.2X4	T50.2X5	T50.2X6
Chlormethiazole	T42.6X1	T42.6X2	T42.6X3	T42.6X4	T42.6X5	T42.6X6
Chlormethine	T45.1X1	T45.1X2	T45.1X3	T45.1X4	T45.1X5	T45.1X6
Chlormethylenecycline	T36.4X1	T36.4X2	T36.4X3	T36.4X4	T36.4X5	T36.4X6
Chlormezanone	T42.6X1	T42.6X2	T42.6X3	T42.6X4	T42.6X5	T42.6X6
Chloroacetic acid	T60.3X1	T60.3X2	T60.3X3	T60.3X4	—	—
Chloroacetone	T59.3X1	T59.3X2	T59.3X3	T59.3X4	—	—
Chloroacetophenone	T59.3X1	T59.3X2	T59.3X3	T59.3X4	—	—
Chloroaniline	T53.7X1	T53.7X2	T53.7X3	T53.7X4	—	—
Chlorobenzene, chlorobenzol	T53.7X1	T53.7X2	T53.7X3	T53.7X4	—	—
Chlorobromomethane (fire extinguisher)	T53.6X1	T53.6X2	T53.6X3	T53.6X4	—	—
Chlorobutanol	T49.0X1	T49.0X2	T49.0X3	T49.0X4	T49.0X5	T49.0X6
Chlorocresol	T49.0X1	T49.0X2	T49.0X3	T49.0X4	T49.0X5	T49.0X6
Chlorodehydro-methyltestosterone	T38.7X1	T38.7X2	T38.7X3	T38.7X4	T38.7X5	T38.7X6
Chlorodinitrobenzene	T53.7X1	T53.7X2	T53.7X3	T53.7X4	—	—
dust or vapor	T53.7X1	T53.7X2	T53.7X3	T53.7X4	—	—
Chlorodiphenyl	T53.7X1	T53.7X2	T53.7X3	T53.7X4	—	—
Chloroethane — *see Ethyl chloride*						
Chloroethylene	T53.6X1	T53.6X2	T53.6X3	T53.6X4	—	—
Chlorofluorocarbons	T53.5X1	T53.5X2	T53.5X3	T53.5X4	—	—
Chloroform (fumes) (vapor)	T53.1X1	T53.1X2	T53.1X3	T53.1X4	—	—
anesthetic	T41.0X1	T41.0X2	T41.0X3	T41.0X4	T41.0X5	T41.0X6
solvent	T53.1X1	T53.1X2	T53.1X3	T53.1X4	—	—
water, concentrated	T41.0X1	T41.0X2	T41.0X3	T41.0X4	T41.0X5	T41.0X6
Chloroguanide	T37.2X1	T37.2X2	T37.2X3	T37.2X4	T37.2X5	T37.2X6
Chloromycetin	T36.2X1	T36.2X2	T36.2X3	T36.2X4	T36.2X5	T36.2X6
ENT agent	T49.6X1	T49.6X2	T49.6X3	T49.6X4	T49.6X5	T49.6X6
ophthalmic preparation	T49.5X1	T49.5X2	T49.5X3	T49.5X4	T49.5X5	T49.5X6

◀ New　◀▥ Revised　~~deleted~~ Deleted

Substance	External Cause (T-Code)					
	Poisoning, Accidental (Unintentional)	Poisoning, Intentional Self-Harm	Poisoning, Assault	Poisoning, Undetermined	Adverse Effect	Underdosing
Chloromycetin (Continued)						
otic solution	T49.6X1	T49.6X2	T49.6X3	T49.6X4	T49.6X5	T49.6X6
topical NEC	T49.0X1	T49.0X2	T49.0X3	T49.0X4	T49.0X5	T49.0X6
Chloronitrobenzene	T53.7X1	T53.7X2	T53.7X3	T53.7X4	—	—
dust or vapor	T53.7X1	T53.7X2	T53.7X3	T53.7X4	—	—
Chlorophacinone	T60.4X1	T60.4X2	T60.4X3	T60.4X4		
Chlorophenol	T53.7X1	T53.7X2	T53.7X3	T53.7X4	—	—
Chlorophenothane	T60.1X1	T60.1X2	T60.1X3	T60.1X4		
Chlorophyll	T50.991	T50.992	T50.993	T50.994	T50.995	T50.996
Chloropicrin (fumes)	T53.6X1	T53.6X2	T53.6X3	T53.6X4	—	—
fumigant	T60.8X1	T60.8X2	T60.8X3	T60.8X4		
fungicide	T60.3X1	T60.3X2	T60.3X3	T60.3X4	—	—
pesticide	T60.8X1	T60.8X2	T60.8X3	T60.8X4	—	—
Chloroprocaine	T41.3X1	T41.3X2	T41.3X3	T41.3X4	T41.3X5	T41.3X6
infiltration (subcutaneous)	T41.3X1	T41.3X2	T41.3X3	T41.3X4	T41.3X5	T41.3X6
nerve block (peripheral) (plexus)	T41.3X1	T41.3X2	T41.3X3	T41.3X4	T41.3X5	T41.3X6
spinal	T41.3X1	T41.3X2	T41.3X3	T41.3X4	T41.3X5	T41.3X6
Chloroptic	T49.5X1	T49.5X2	T49.5X3	T49.5X4	T49.5X5	T49.5X6
Chloropurine	T45.1X1	T45.1X2	T45.1X3	T45.1X4	T45.1X5	T45.1X6
Chloropyramine	T45.0X1	T45.0X2	T45.0X3	T45.0X4	T45.0X5	T45.0X6
Chloropyrifos	T60.0X1	T60.0X2	T60.0X3	T60.0X4	—	—
Chloropyrilene	T45.0X1	T45.0X2	T45.0X3	T45.0X4	T45.0X5	T45.0X6
Chloroquine	T37.2X1	T37.2X2	T37.2X3	T37.2X4	T37.2X5	T37.2X6
Chlorothalonil	T60.3X1	T60.3X2	T60.3X3	T60.3X4	—	—
Chlorothen	T45.0X1	T45.0X2	T45.0X3	T45.0X4	T45.0X5	T45.0X6
Chlorothiazide	T50.2X1	T50.2X2	T50.2X3	T50.2X4	T50.2X5	T50.2X6
Chlorothymol	T49.4X1	T49.4X2	T49.4X3	T49.4X4	T49.4X5	T49.4X6
Chlorotrianisene	T38.5X1	T38.5X2	T38.5X3	T38.5X4	T38.5X5	T38.5X6
Chlorovinyldichloro-arsine, not in war	T57.0X1	T57.0X2	T57.0X3	T57.0X4	—	—
Chloroxine	T49.4X1	T49.4X2	T49.4X3	T49.4X4	T49.4X5	T49.4X6
Chloroxylenol	T49.0X1	T49.0X2	T49.0X3	T49.0X4	T49.0X5	T49.0X6
Chlorphenamine	T45.0X1	T45.0X2	T45.0X3	T45.0X4	T45.0X5	T45.0X6
Chlorphenesin	T42.8X1	T42.8X2	T42.8X3	T42.8X4	T42.8X5	T42.8X6
topical (antifungal)	T49.0X1	T49.0X2	T49.0X3	T49.0X4	T49.0X5	T49.0X6
Chlorpheniramine	T45.0X1	T45.0X2	T45.0X3	T45.0X4	T45.0X5	T45.0X6
Chlorphenoxamine	T45.0X1	T45.0X2	T45.0X3	T45.0X4	T45.0X5	T45.0X6
Chlorphentermine	T50.5X1	T50.5X2	T50.5X3	T50.5X4	T50.5X5	T50.5X6
Chlorprocaine — see Chloroprocaine						
Chlorproguanil	T37.2X1	T37.2X2	T37.2X3	T37.2X4	T37.2X5	T37.2X6
Chlorpromazine	T43.3X1	T43.3X2	T43.3X3	T43.3X4	T43.3X5	T43.3X6

◄ New   ⇇ Revised   ~~deleted~~ Deleted

Substance	External Cause (T-Code)					
	Poisoning, Accidental (Unintentional)	Poisoning, Intentional Self-Harm	Poisoning, Assault	Poisoning, Undetermined	Adverse Effect	Underdosing
Chlorpropamide	T38.3X1	T38.3X2	T38.3X3	T38.3X4	T38.3X5	T38.3X6
Chlorprothixene	T43.4X1	T43.4X2	T43.4X3	T43.4X4	T43.4X5	T43.4X6
Chlorquinaldol	T49.0X1	T49.0X2	T49.0X3	T49.0X4	T49.0X5	T49.0X6
Chlorquinol	T49.0X1	T49.0X2	T49.0X3	T49.0X4	T49.0X5	T49.0X6
Chlortalidone	T50.2X1	T50.2X2	T50.2X3	T50.2X4	T50.2X5	T50.2X6
Chlortetracycline	T36.4X1	T36.4X2	T36.4X3	T36.4X4	T36.4X5	T36.4X6
Chlorthalidone	T50.2X1	T50.2X2	T50.2X3	T50.2X4	T50.2X5	T50.2X6
Chlorthiophos	T60.0X1	T60.0X2	T60.0X3	T60.0X4	—	—
Chlorotrianisene	T38.5X1	T38.5X2	T38.5X3	T38.5X4	T38.5X5	T38.5X6
Chlor-Trimeton	T45.0X1	T45.0X2	T45.0X3	T45.0X4	T45.0X5	T45.0X6
Chlorthion	T60.0X1	T60.0X2	T60.0X3	T60.0X4	—	—
Chlorzoxazone	T42.8X1	T42.8X2	T42.8X3	T42.8X4	T42.8X5	T42.8X6
Choke damp	T59.7X1	T59.7X2	T59.7X3	T59.7X4	—	—
Cholagogues	T47.5X1	T47.5X2	T47.5X3	T47.5X4	T47.5X5	T47.5X6
Cholebrine	T50.8X1	T50.8X2	T50.8X3	T50.8X4	T50.8X5	T50.8X6
Cholecalciferol	T45.2X1	T45.2X2	T45.2X3	T45.2X4	T45.2X5	T45.2X6
Cholecystokinin	T50.8X1	T50.8X2	T50.8X3	T50.8X4	T50.8X5	T50.8X6
Cholera vaccine	T50.A91	T50.A92	T50.A93	T50.A94	T50.A95	T50.A96
Choleretic	T47.5X1	T47.5X2	T47.5X3	T47.5X4	T47.5X5	T47.5X6
Cholesterol-lowering agents	T46.6X1	T46.6X2	T46.6X3	T46.6X4	T46.6X5	T46.6X6
Cholestyramine (resin)	T46.6X1	T46.6X2	T46.6X3	T46.6X4	T46.6X5	T46.6X6
Cholic acid	T47.5X1	T47.5X2	T47.5X3	T47.5X4	T47.5X5	T47.5X6
Choline	T48.6X1	T48.6X2	T48.6X3	T48.6X4	T48.6X5	T48.6X6
chloride	T50.991	T50.992	T50.993	T50.994	T50.995	T50.996
dihydrogen citrate	T50.991	T50.992	T50.993	T50.994	T50.995	T50.996
salicylate	T39.091	T39.092	T39.093	T39.094	T39.095	T39.096
theophyllinate	T48.6X1	T48.6X2	T48.6X3	T48.6X4	T48.6X5	T48.6X6
Cholinergic (drug) NEC	T44.1X1	T44.1X2	T44.1X3	T44.1X4	T44.1X5	T44.1X6
muscle tone enhancer	T44.1X1	T44.1X2	T44.1X3	T44.1X4	T44.1X5	T44.1X6
organophosphorus	T44.0X1	T44.0X2	T44.0X3	T44.0X4	T44.0X5	T44.0X6
insecticide	T60.0X1	T60.0X2	T60.0X3	T60.0X4	—	—
nerve gas	T59.891	T59.892	T59.893	T59.894	—	—
trimethyl ammonium propanediol	T44.1X1	T44.1X2	T44.1X3	T44.1X4	T44.1X5	T44.1X6
Cholinesterase reactivator	T50.6X1	T50.6X2	T50.6X3	T50.6X4	T50.6X5	T50.6X6
Cholografin	T50.8X1	T50.8X2	T50.8X3	T50.8X4	T50.8X5	T50.8X6
Chorionic gonadotropin	T38.891	T38.892	T38.893	T38.894	T38.895	T38.896
Chromate	T56.2X1	T56.2X2	T56.2X3	T56.2X4	—	—
dust or mist	T56.2X1	T56.2X2	T56.2X3	T56.2X4	—	—
lead — see also lead	T56.0X1	T56.0X2	T56.0X3	T56.0X4	—	—
paint	T56.0X1	T56.0X2	T56.0X3	T56.0X4	—	—

◀ New   ◀▥ Revised   ~~deleted~~ Deleted

Substance	External Cause (T-Code)					
	Poisoning, Accidental (Unintentional)	Poisoning, Intentional Self-Harm	Poisoning, Assault	Poisoning, Undetermined	Adverse Effect	Underdosing
Chromic						
acid	T56.2X1	T56.2X2	T56.2X3	T56.2X4	—	—
dust or mist	T56.2X1	T56.2X2	T56.2X3	T56.2X4	—	—
phosphate 32P	T45.1X1	T45.1X2	T45.1X3	T45.1X4	T45.1X5	T45.1X6
Chromium	T56.2X1	T56.2X2	T56.2X3	T56.2X4	—	—
compounds — see Chromate						
sesquioxide	T50.8X1	T50.8X2	T50.8X3	T50.8X4	T50.8X5	T50.8X6
Chromomycin A3	T45.1X1	T45.1X2	T45.1X3	T45.1X4	T45.1X5	T45.1X6
Chromonar	T46.3X1	T46.3X2	T46.3X3	T46.3X4	T46.3X5	T46.3X6
Chromyl chloride	T56.2X1	T56.2X2	T56.2X3	T56.2X4	—	—
Chrysarobin	T49.4X1	T49.4X2	T49.4X3	T49.4X4	T49.4X5	T49.4X6
Chrysazin	T47.2X1	T47.2X2	T47.2X3	T47.2X4	T47.2X5	T47.2X6
Chymar	T45.3X1	T45.3X2	T45.3X3	T45.3X4	T45.3X5	T45.3X6
ophthalmic preparation	T49.5X1	T49.5X2	T49.5X3	T49.5X4	T49.5X5	T49.5X6
Chymopapain	T45.3X1	T45.3X2	T45.3X3	T45.3X4	T45.3X5	T45.3X6
Chymotrypsin	T45.3X1	T45.3X2	T45.3X3	T45.3X4	T45.3X5	T45.3X6
ophthalmic preparation	T49.5X1	T49.5X2	T49.5X3	T49.5X4	T49.5X5	T49.5X6
Cianidanol	T50.991	T50.992	T50.993	T50.994	T50.995	T50.996
Cianopramine	T43.011	T43.012	T43.013	T43.014	T43.015	T43.016
Cibenzoline	T46.2X1	T46.2X2	T46.2X3	T46.2X4	T46.2X5	T46.2X6
Ciclacillin	T36.0X1	T36.0X2	T36.0X3	T36.0X4	T36.0X5	T36.0X6
Ciclobarbital — see Hexobarbital						
Ciclonicate	T46.7X1	T46.7X2	T46.7X3	T46.7X4	T46.7X5	T46.7X6
Ciclopirox (olamine)	T49.0X1	T49.0X2	T49.0X3	T49.0X4	T49.0X5	T49.0X6
Ciclosporin	T45.1X1	T45.1X2	T45.1X3	T45.1X4	T45.1X5	T45.1X6
Cicuta maculata or virosa	T62.2X1	T62.2X2	T62.2X3	T62.2X4	—	—
Cicutoxin	T62.2X1	T62.2X2	T62.2X3	T62.2X4	—	—
Cigarette lighter fluid	T52.0X1	T52.0X2	T52.0X3	T52.0X4	—	—
Cigarettes (tobacco)	T65.221	T65.222	T65.223	T65.224	—	—
Ciguatoxin	T61.01	T61.02	T61.03	T61.04	—	—
Cilazapril	T46.4X1	T46.4X2	T46.4X3	T46.4X4	T46.4X5	T46.4X6
Cimetidine	T47.0X1	T47.0X2	T47.0X3	T47.0X4	T47.0X5	T47.0X6
Cimetropium bromide	T44.3X1	T44.3X2	T44.3X3	T44.3X4	T44.3X5	T44.3X6
Cinchocaine	T41.3X1	T41.3X2	T41.3X3	T41.3X4	T41.3X5	T41.3X6
topical (surface)	T41.3X1	T41.3X2	T41.3X3	T41.3X4	T41.3X5	T41.3X6
Cinchona	T37.2X1	T37.2X2	T37.2X3	T37.2X4	T37.2X5	T37.2X6
Cinchonine alkaloids	T37.2X1	T37.2X2	T37.2X3	T37.2X4	T37.2X5	T37.2X6
Cinchophen	T50.4X1	T50.4X2	T50.4X3	T50.4X4	T50.4X5	T50.4X6
Cinepazide	T46.7X1	T46.7X2	T46.7X3	T46.7X4	T46.7X5	T46.7X6
Cinnamedrine	T48.5X1	T48.5X2	T48.5X3	T48.5X4	T48.5X5	T48.5X6

◄ New　◄▦ Revised　deleted Deleted

Substance	Poisoning, Accidental (Unintentional)	Poisoning, Intentional Self-Harm	Poisoning, Assault	Poisoning, Undetermined	Adverse Effect	Underdosing
Cinnarizine	T45.0X1	T45.0X2	T45.0X3	T45.0X4	T45.0X5	T45.0X6
Cinoxacin	T37.8X1	T37.8X2	T37.8X3	T37.8X4	T37.8X5	T37.8X6
Ciprofibrate	T46.6X1	T46.6X2	T46.6X3	T46.6X4	T46.6X5	T46.6X6
Ciprofloxacin	T36.8X1	T36.8X2	T36.8X3	T36.8X4	T36.8X5	T36.8X6
Cisapride	T47.8X1	T47.8X2	T47.8X3	T47.8X4	T47.8X5	T47.8X6
Cisplatin	T45.1X1	T45.1X2	T45.1X3	T45.1X4	T45.1X5	T45.1X6
Citalopram	T43.221	T43.222	T43.223	T43.224	T43.225	T43.226
Citanest	T41.3X1	T41.3X2	T41.3X3	T41.3X4	T41.3X5	T41.3X6
infiltration (subcutaneous)	T41.3X1	T41.3X2	T41.3X3	T41.3X4	T41.3X5	T41.3X6
nerve block (peripheral) (plexus)	T41.3X1	T41.3X2	T41.3X3	T41.3X4	T41.3X5	T41.3X6
Citric acid	T47.5X1	T47.5X2	T47.5X3	T47.5X4	T47.5X5	T47.5X6
Citrovorum (factor)	T45.8X1	T45.8X2	T45.8X3	T45.8X4	T45.8X5	T45.8X6
Claviceps purpurea	T62.2X1	T62.2X2	T62.2X3	T62.2X4	—	—
Clavulanic acid	T36.1X1	T36.1X2	T36.1X3	T36.1X4	T36.1X5	T36.1X6
Cleaner, cleansing agent, type not specified	T65.891	T65.892	T65.893	T65.894	—	—
of paint or varnish	T52.91	T52.92	T52.93	T52.94	—	—
specified type NEC	T65.891	T65.892	T65.893	T65.894	—	—
Clebopride	T47.8X1	T47.8X2	T47.8X3	T47.8X4	T47.8X5	T47.8X6
Clefamide	T37.3X1	T37.3X2	T37.3X3	T37.3X4	T37.3X5	T37.3X6
Clemastine	T45.0X1	T45.0X2	T45.0X3	T45.0X4	T45.0X5	T45.0X6
Clematis vitalba	T62.2X1	T62.2X2	T62.2X3	T62.2X4	—	—
Clemizole	T45.0X1	T45.0X2	T45.0X3	T45.0X4	T45.0X5	T45.0X6
penicillin	T36.0X1	T36.0X2	T36.0X3	T36.0X4	T36.0X5	T36.0X6
Clenbuterol	T48.6X1	T48.6X2	T48.6X3	T48.6X4	T48.6X5	T48.6X6
Clidinium bromide	T44.3X1	T44.3X2	T44.3X3	T44.3X4	T44.3X5	T44.3X6
Clindamycin	T36.8X1	T36.8X2	T36.8X3	T36.8X4	T36.8X5	T36.8X6
Clinofibrate	T46.6X1	T46.6X2	T46.6X3	T46.6X4	T46.6X5	T46.6X6
Clioquinol	T37.8X1	T37.8X2	T37.8X3	T37.8X4	T37.8X5	T37.8X6
Cliradon	T40.2X1	T40.2X2	T40.2X3	T40.2X4	—	—
Clobazam	T42.4X1	T42.4X2	T42.4X3	T42.4X4	T42.4X5	T42.4X6
Clobenzorex	T50.5X1	T50.5X2	T50.5X3	T50.5X4	T50.5X5	T50.5X6
Clobetasol	T49.0X1	T49.0X2	T49.0X3	T49.0X4	T49.0X5	T49.0X6
Clobetasone	T49.0X1	T49.0X2	T49.0X3	T49.0X4	T49.0X5	T49.0X6
Clobutinol	T48.3X1	T48.3X2	T48.3X3	T48.3X4	T48.3X5	T48.3X6
Clocapramine	T43.0X1	T43.0X2	T43.0X3	T43.0X4	T43.0X5	T43.0X6
Clocortolone	T38.0X1	T38.0X2	T38.0X3	T38.0X4	T38.0X5	T38.0X6
Clodantoin	T49.0X1	T49.0X2	T49.0X3	T49.0X4	T49.0X5	T49.0X6
Clodronic acid	T50.991	T50.992	T50.993	T50.994	T50.995	T50.996
Clofazimine	T37.1X1	T37.1X2	T37.1X3	T37.1X4	T37.1X5	T37.1X6
Clofedanol	T48.3X1	T48.3X2	T48.3X3	T48.3X4	T48.3X5	T48.3X6

◀ New   ◀◀ Revised   ~~deleted~~ Deleted

Substance	Poisoning, Accidental (Unintentional)	Poisoning, Intentional Self-Harm	Poisoning, Assault	Poisoning, Undetermined	Adverse Effect	Underdosing
			External Cause (T-Code)			
Clofenamide	T50.2X1	T50.2X2	T50.2X3	T50.2X4	T50.2X5	T50.2X6
Clofenotane	T49.0X1	T49.0X2	T49.0X3	T49.0X4	T49.0X5	T49.0X6
Clofezone	T39.2X1	T39.2X2	T39.2X3	T39.2X4	T39.2X5	T39.2X6
Clofibrate	T46.6X1	T46.6X2	T46.6X3	T46.6X4	T46.6X5	T46.6X6
Clofibride	T46.6X1	T46.6X2	T46.6X3	T46.6X4	T46.6X5	T46.6X6
Cloforex	T50.5X1	T50.5X2	T50.5X3	T50.5X4	T50.5X5	T50.5X6
Clomacran	T43.0X1	T43.0X2	T43.0X3	T43.0X4	T43.0X5	T43.0X6
Clomethiazole	T42.6X1	T42.6X2	T42.6X3	T42.6X4	T42.6X5	T42.6X6
Clometocillin	T36.0X1	T36.0X2	T36.0X3	T36.0X4	T36.0X5	T36.0X6
Clomifene	T38.5X1	T38.5X2	T38.5X3	T38.5X4	T38.5X5	T38.5X6
Clomiphene	T38.5X1	T38.5X2	T38.5X3	T38.5X4	T38.5X5	T38.5X6
Clomipramine	T43.011	T43.012	T43.013	T43.014	T43.015	T43.016
Clomocycline	T36.4X1	T36.4X2	T36.4X3	T36.4X4	T36.4X5	T36.4X6
Clonazepam	T42.4X1	T42.4X2	T42.4X3	T42.4X4	T42.4X5	T42.4X6
Clonidine	T46.5X1	T46.5X2	T46.5X3	T46.5X4	T46.5X5	T46.5X6
Clonixin	T39.8X1	T39.8X2	T39.8X3	T39.8X4	T39.8X5	T39.8X6
Clopamide	T50.2X1	T50.2X2	T50.2X3	T50.2X4	T50.2X5	T50.2X6
Clopenthixol	T43.4X1	T43.4X2	T43.4X3	T43.4X4	T43.4X5	T43.4X6
Cloperastine	T48.3X1	T48.3X2	T48.3X3	T48.3X4	T48.3X5	T48.3X6
Clophedianol	T48.3X1	T48.3X2	T48.3X3	T48.3X4	T48.3X5	T48.3X6
Cloponone	T36.2X1	T36.2X2	T36.2X3	T36.2X4	T36.2X5	T36.2X6
Cloprednol	T38.0X1	T38.0X2	T38.0X3	T38.0X4	T38.0X5	T38.0X6
Cloral betaine	T42.6X1	T42.6X2	T42.6X3	T42.6X4	T42.6X5	T42.6X6
Cloramfenicol	T36.2X1	T36.2X2	T36.2X3	T36.2X4	T36.2X5	T36.2X6
Clorazepate (dipotassium)	T42.4X1	T42.4X2	T42.4X3	T42.4X4	T42.4X5	T42.4X6
Clorexolone	T50.2X1	T50.2X2	T50.2X3	T50.2X4	T50.2X5	T50.2X6
Clorox (bleach)	T54.91	T54.92	T54.93	T54.94	—	—
Clorfenamine	T45.0X1	T45.0X2	T45.0X3	T45.0X4	T45.0X5	T45.0X6
Clorgiline	T43.1X1	T43.1X2	T43.1X3	T43.1X4	T43.1X5	T43.1X6
Clorotepine	T44.3X1	T44.3X2	T44.3X3	T44.3X4	T44.3X5	T44.3X6
Clorprenaline	T48.6X1	T48.6X2	T48.6X3	T48.6X4	T48.6X5	T48.6X6
Clortermine	T50.5X1	T50.5X2	T50.5X3	T50.5X4	T50.5X5	T50.5X6
Clotiapine	T43.591	T43.592	T43.593	T43.594	T43.595	T43.596
Clotiazepam	T42.4X1	T42.4X2	T42.4X3	T42.4X4	T42.4X5	T42.4X6
Clotibric acid	T46.6X1	T46.6X2	T46.6X3	T46.6X4	T46.6X5	T46.6X6
Clotrimazole	T49.0X1	T49.0X2	T49.0X3	T49.0X4	T49.0X5	T49.0X6
Cloxacillin	T36.0X1	T36.0X2	T36.0X3	T36.0X4	T36.0X5	T36.0X6
Cloxazolam	T42.4X1	T42.4X2	T42.4X3	T42.4X4	T42.4X5	T42.4X6
Cloxiquine	T49.0X1	T49.0X2	T49.0X3	T49.0X4	T49.0X5	T49.0X6
Clozapine	T42.4X1	T42.4X2	T42.4X3	T42.4X4	T42.4X5	T42.4X6

◀ New   ◀▥ Revised   deleted Deleted

Substance	External Cause (T-Code)					
	Poisoning, Accidental (Unintentional)	Poisoning, Intentional Self-Harm	Poisoning, Assault	Poisoning, Undetermined	Adverse Effect	Underdosing
Coagulant NEC	T45.7X1	T45.7X2	T45.7X3	T45.7X4	T45.7X5	T45.7X6
Coal (carbon monoxide from) — see also Carbon, monoxide, coal	T58.2X1	T58.2X2	T58.2X3	T58.2X4	—	—
oil — see Kerosene						
tar	T49.1X1	T49.1X2	T49.1X3	T49.1X4	T49.1X5	T49.1X6
fumes	T59.891	T59.892	T59.893	T59.894	—	—
medicinal (ointment)	T49.4X1	T49.4X2	T49.4X3	T49.4X4	T49.4X5	T49.4X6
analgesics NEC	T39.2X1	T39.2X2	T39.2X3	T39.2X4	T39.2X5	T39.2X6
naphtha (solvent)	T52.0X1	T52.0X2	T52.0X3	T52.0X4		
Cobalamine	T45.2X1	T45.2X2	T45.2X3	T45.2X4	T45.2X5	T45.2X6
Cobalt (nonmedicinal) (fumes) (industrial)	T56.891	T56.892	T56.893	T56.894		
medicinal (trace) (chloride)	T45.8X1	T45.8X2	T45.8X3	T45.8X4	T45.8X5	T45.8X6
Cobra (venom)	T63.041	T63.042	T63.043	T63.044		
Coca (leaf)	T40.5X1	T40.5X2	T40.5X3	T40.5X4	T40.5X5	T40.5X6
Cocaine	T40.5X1	T40.5X2	T40.5X3	T40.5X4	T40.5X5	T40.5X6
topical anesthetic	T41.3X1	T41.3X2	T41.3X3	T41.3X4	T41.3X5	T41.3X6
Cocarboxylase	T45.3X1	T45.3X2	T45.3X3	T45.3X4	T45.3X5	T45.3X6
Coccidioidin	T50.8X1	T50.8X2	T50.8X3	T50.8X4	T50.8X5	T50.8X6
Cocculus indicus	T62.1X1	T62.1X2	T62.1X3	T62.1X4		
Cochineal	T65.6X1	T65.6X2	T65.6X3	T65.6X4		
medicinal products	T50.991	T50.992	T50.993	T50.994	T50.995	T50.996
Codeine	T40.2X1	T40.2X2	T40.2X3	T40.2X4	T40.2X5	T40.2X6
Cod-liver oil	T45.2X1	T45.2X2	T45.2X3	T45.2X4	T45.2X5	T45.2X6
Coenzyme A	T50.991	T50.992	T50.993	T50.994	T50.995	T50.996
Coffee	T62.8X1	T62.8X2	T62.8X3	T62.8X4	—	—
Cogalactoisomerase	T50.991	T50.992	T50.993	T50.994	T50.995	T50.996
Cogentin	T44.3X1	T44.3X2	T44.3X3	T44.3X4	T44.3X5	T44.3X6
Coke fumes or gas (carbon monoxide)	T58.2X1	T58.2X2	T58.2X3	T58.2X4	—	—
industrial use	T58.8X1	T58.8X2	T58.8X3	T58.8X4	—	—
Colace	T47.4X1	T47.4X2	T47.4X3	T47.4X4	T47.4X5	T47.4X6
Colaspase	T45.1X1	T45.1X2	T45.1X3	T45.1X4	T45.1X5	T45.1X6
Colchicine	T50.4X1	T50.4X2	T50.4X3	T50.4X4	T50.4X5	T50.4X6
Colchicum	T62.2X1	T62.2X2	T62.2X3	T62.2X4	—	—
Cold cream	T49.3X1	T49.3X2	T49.3X3	T49.3X4	T49.3X5	T49.3X6
Colecalciferol	T45.2X1	T45.2X2	T45.2X3	T45.2X4	T45.2X5	T45.2X6
Colestipol	T46.6X1	T46.6X2	T46.6X3	T46.6X4	T46.6X5	T46.6X6
Colestyramine	T46.6X1	T46.6X2	T46.6X3	T46.6X4	T46.6X5	T46.6X6
Colimycin	T36.8X1	T36.8X2	T36.8X3	T36.8X4	T36.8X5	T36.8X6
Colistimethate	T36.8X1	T36.8X2	T36.8X3	T36.8X4	T36.8X5	T36.8X6
Colistin	T36.8X1	T36.8X2	T36.8X3	T36.8X4	T36.8X5	T36.8X6
sulfate (eye preparation)	T49.5X1	T49.5X2	T49.5X3	T49.5X4	T49.5X5	T49.5X6

TABLE OF DRUGS AND CHEMICALS

Substance	External Cause (T-Code)					
	Poisoning, Accidental (Unintentional)	Poisoning, Intentional Self-Harm	Poisoning, Assault	Poisoning, Undetermined	Adverse Effect	Underdosing
Collagen	T50.991	T50.992	T50.993	T50.994	T50.995	T50.996
Collagenase	T49.4X1	T49.4X2	T49.4X3	T49.4X4	T49.4X5	T49.4X6
Collodion	T49.3X1	T49.3X2	T49.3X3	T49.3X4	T49.3X5	T49.3X6
Colocynth	T47.2X1	T47.2X2	T47.2X3	T47.2X4	T47.2X5	T47.2X6
Colophony adhesive	T49.3X1	T49.3X2	T49.3X3	T49.3X4	T49.3X5	T49.3X6
Colorant — see also Dye	T50.991	T50.992	T50.993	T50.994	T50.995	T50.996
Coloring matter — see Dye(s)						
Combustion gas (after combustion) — see Carbon, monoxide						
prior to combustion	T59.891	T59.892	T59.893	T59.894	—	—
Compazine	T43.3X1	T43.3X2	T43.3X3	T43.3X4	T43.3X5	T43.3X6
Compound						
42 (warfarin)	T60.4X1	T60.4X2	T60.4X3	T60.4X4	—	—
269 (endrin)	T60.1X1	T60.1X2	T60.1X3	T60.1X4	—	—
497 (dieldrin)	T60.1X1	T60.1X2	T60.1X3	T60.1X4	—	—
1080 (sodium fluoroacetate)	T60.4X1	T60.4X2	T60.4X3	T60.4X4	—	—
3422 (parathion)	T60.0X1	T60.0X2	T60.0X3	T60.0X4	—	—
3911 (phorate)	T60.0X1	T60.0X2	T60.0X3	T60.0X4	—	—
3956 (toxaphene)	T60.1X1	T60.1X2	T60.1X3	T60.1X4	—	—
4049 (malathion)	T60.0X1	T60.0X2	T60.0X3	T60.0X4	—	—
4069 (malathion)	T60.0X1	T60.0X2	T60.0X3	T60.0X4	—	—
4124 (dicapthon)	T60.0X1	T60.0X2	T60.0X3	T60.0X4	—	—
E (cortisone)	T38.0X1	T38.0X2	T38.0X3	T38.0X4	T38.0X5	T38.0X6
F (hydrocortisone)	T38.0X1	T38.0X2	T38.0X3	T38.0X4	T38.0X5	T38.0X6
Congener, anabolic	T38.7X1	T38.7X2	T38.7X3	T38.7X4	T38.7X5	T38.7X6
Congo red	T50.8X1	T50.8X2	T50.8X3	T50.8X4	T50.8X5	T50.8X6
Coniine, conine	T62.2X1	T62.2X2	T62.2X3	T62.2X4	—	—
Conium (maculatum)	T62.2X1	T62.2X2	T62.2X3	T62.2X4	—	—
Conjugated estrogenic substances	T38.5X1	T38.5X2	T38.5X3	T38.5X4	T38.5X5	T38.5X6
Contac	T48.5X1	T48.5X2	T48.5X3	T48.5X4	T48.5X5	T48.5X6
Contact lens solution	T49.5X1	T49.5X2	T49.5X3	T49.5X4	T49.5X5	T49.5X6
Contraceptive (oral)	T38.4X1	T38.4X2	T38.4X3	T38.4X4	T38.4X5	T38.4X6
vaginal	T49.8X1	T49.8X2	T49.8X3	T49.8X4	T49.8X5	T49.8X6
Contrast medium, radiography	T50.8X1	T50.8X2	T50.8X3	T50.8X4	T50.8X5	T50.8X6
Convallaria glycosides	T46.0X1	T46.0X2	T46.0X3	T46.0X4	T46.0X5	T46.0X6
Convallaria majalis	T62.2X1	T62.2X2	T62.2X3	T62.2X4	—	—
berry	T62.1X1	T62.1X2	T62.1X3	T62.1X4	—	—
Copper (dust) (fumes) (nonmedicinal) NEC	T56.4X1	T56.4X2	T56.4X3	T56.4X4	—	—
arsenate, arsenite	T57.0X1	T57.0X2	T57.0X3	T57.0X4	—	—
insecticide	T60.2X1	T60.2X2	T60.2X3	T60.2X4	—	—

◀ New   ◀ Revised   ~~deleted~~ Deleted

Substance	Poisoning, Accidental (Unintentional)	Poisoning, Intentional Self-Harm	Poisoning, Assault	Poisoning, Undetermined	Adverse Effect	Underdosing
External Cause (T-Code)						
Copper NEC *(Continued)*						
emetic	T47.7X1	T47.7X2	T47.7X3	T47.7X4	T47.7X5	T47.7X6
fungicide	T60.3X1	T60.3X2	T60.3X3	T60.3X4	—	—
gluconate	T49.0X1	T49.0X2	T49.0X3	T49.0X4	T49.0X5	T49.0X6
insecticide	T60.2X1	T60.2X2	T60.2X3	T60.2X4	—	—
medicinal (trace)	T45.8X1	T45.8X2	T45.8X3	T45.8X4	T45.8X5	T45.8X6
oleate	T49.0X1	T49.0X2	T49.0X3	T49.0X4	T49.0X5	T49.0X6
sulfate	T56.4X1	T56.4X2	T56.4X3	T56.4X4	—	—
cupric	T56.4X1	T56.4X2	T56.4X3	T56.4X4	—	—
fungicide	T60.3X1	T60.3X2	T60.3X3	T60.3X4	—	—
medicinal						
ear	T49.6X1	T49.6X2	T49.6X3	T49.6X4	T49.6X5	T49.6X6
emetic	T47.7X1	T47.7X2	T47.7X3	T47.7X4	T47.7X5	T47.7X6
eye	T49.5X1	T49.5X2	T49.5X3	T49.5X4	T49.5X5	T49.5X6
cuprous	T56.4X1	T56.4X2	T56.4X3	T56.4X4	—	—
fungicide	T60.3X1	T60.3X2	T60.3X3	T60.3X4	—	—
medicinal						
ear	T49.6X1	T49.6X2	T49.6X3	T49.6X4	T49.6X5	T49.6X6
emetic	T47.7X1	T47.7X2	T47.7X3	T47.7X4	T47.7X5	T47.7X6
eye	T49.5X1	T49.5X2	T49.5X3	T49.5X4	T49.5X5	T49.5X6
Copperhead snake (bite) (venom)	T63.061	T63.062	T63.063	T63.064	—	—
Coral (sting)	T63.691	T63.692	T63.693	T63.694	—	—
snake (bite) (venom)	T63.021	T63.022	T63.023	T63.024	—	—
Corbadrine	T49.6X1	T49.6X2	T49.6X3	T49.6X4	T49.6X5	T49.6X6
Cordran	T49.0X1	T49.0X2	T49.0X3	T49.0X4	T49.0X5	T49.0X6
Cordite	T65.891	T65.892	T65.893	T65.894	—	—
vapor	T59.891	T59.892	T59.893	T59.894	—	—
Corn cures	T49.4X1	T49.4X2	T49.4X3	T49.4X4	T49.4X5	T49.4X6
Cornhusker's lotion	T49.3X1	T49.3X2	T49.3X3	T49.3X4	T49.3X5	T49.3X6
Corn starch	T49.3X1	T49.3X2	T49.3X3	T49.3X4	T49.3X5	T49.3X6
Coronary vasodilator NEC	T46.3X1	T46.3X2	T46.3X3	T46.3X4	T46.3X5	T46.3X6
Corrosive NEC	T54.91	T54.92	T54.93	T54.94	—	—
acid NEC	T54.2X1	T54.2X2	T54.2X3	T54.2X4	—	—
aromatics	T54.1X1	T54.1X2	T54.1X3	T54.1X4	—	—
disinfectant	T54.1X1	T54.1X2	T54.1X3	T54.1X4	—	—
fumes NEC	T54.91	T54.92	T54.93	T54.94	—	—
specified NEC	T54.91	T54.92	T54.93	T54.94	—	—
sublimate	T56.1X1	T56.1X2	T56.1X3	T56.1X4	—	—
Cortate	T38.0X1	T38.0X2	T38.0X3	T38.0X4	T38.0X5	T38.0X6

◀ New   ◀ Revised   ~~deleted~~ Deleted

TABLE OF DRUGS AND CHEMICALS

Substance	Poisoning, Accidental (Unintentional)	Poisoning, Intentional Self-Harm	Poisoning, Assault	Poisoning, Undetermined	Adverse Effect	Underdosing
			External Cause (T-Code)			
Cort-Dome	T38.0X1	T38.0X2	T38.0X3	T38.0X4	T38.0X5	T38.0X6
ENT agent	T49.6X1	T49.6X2	T49.6X3	T49.6X4	T49.6X5	T49.6X6
ophthalmic preparation	T49.5X1	T49.5X2	T49.5X3	T49.5X4	T49.5X5	T49.5X6
topical NEC	T49.0X1	T49.0X2	T49.0X3	T49.0X4	T49.0X5	T49.0X6
Cortef	T38.0X1	T38.0X2	T38.0X3	T38.0X4	T38.0X5	T38.0X6
ENT agent	T49.6X1	T49.6X2	T49.6X3	T49.6X4	T49.6X5	T49.6X6
ophthalmic preparation	T49.5X1	T49.5X2	T49.5X3	T49.5X4	T49.5X5	T49.5X6
topical NEC	T49.0X1	T49.0X2	T49.0X3	T49.0X4	T49.0X5	T49.0X6
Corticosteroid	T38.0X1	T38.0X2	T38.0X3	T38.0X4	T38.0X5	T38.0X6
ENT agent	T49.6X1	T49.6X2	T49.6X3	T49.6X4	T49.6X5	T49.6X6
mineral	T50.0X1	T50.0X2	T50.0X3	T50.0X4	T50.0X5	T50.0X6
ophthalmic	T49.5X1	T49.5X2	T49.5X3	T49.5X4	T49.5X5	T49.5X6
topical NEC	T49.0X1	T49.0X2	T49.0X3	T49.0X4	T49.0X5	T49.0X6
Corticotropin	T38.811	T38.812	T38.813	T38.814	T38.815	T38.816
Cortisol	T49.0X1	T49.0X2	T49.0X3	T49.0X4	T49.0X5	T49.0X6
ENT agent	T49.6X1	T49.6X2	T49.6X3	T49.6X4	T49.6X5	T49.6X6
ophthalmic preparation	T49.5X1	T49.5X2	T49.5X3	T49.5X4	T49.5X5	T49.5X6
topical NEC	T49.0X1	T49.0X2	T49.0X3	T49.0X4	T49.0X5	T49.0X6
Cortisone (acetate)	T38.0X1	T38.0X2	T38.0X3	T38.0X4	T38.0X5	T38.0X6
ENT agent	T49.6X1	T49.6X2	T49.6X3	T49.6X4	T49.6X5	T49.6X6
ophthalmic preparation	T49.5X1	T49.5X2	T49.5X3	T49.5X4	T49.5X5	T49.5X6
topical NEC	T49.0X1	T49.0X2	T49.0X3	T49.0X4	T49.0X5	T49.0X6
Cortivazol	T38.0X1	T38.0X2	T38.0X3	T38.0X4	T38.0X5	T38.0X6
Cortogen	T38.0X1	T38.0X2	T38.0X3	T38.0X4	T38.0X5	T38.0X6
ENT agent	T49.6X1	T49.6X2	T49.6X3	T49.6X4	T49.6X5	T49.6X6
ophthalmic preparation	T49.5X1	T49.5X2	T49.5X3	T49.5X4	T49.5X5	T49.5X6
Cortone	T38.0X1	T38.0X2	T38.0X3	T38.0X4	T38.0X5	T38.0X6
ENT agent	T49.6X1	T49.6X2	T49.6X3	T49.6X4	T49.6X5	T49.6X6
ophthalmic preparation	T49.5X1	T49.5X2	T49.5X3	T49.5X4	T49.5X5	T49.5X6
Cortril	T38.0X1	T38.0X2	T38.0X3	T38.0X4	T38.0X5	T38.0X6
ENT agent	T49.6X1	T49.6X2	T49.6X3	T49.6X4	T49.6X5	T49.6X6
ophthalmic preparation	T49.5X1	T49.5X2	T49.5X3	T49.5X4	T49.5X5	T49.5X6
topical NEC	T49.0X1	T49.0X2	T49.0X3	T49.0X4	T49.0X5	T49.0X6
Corynebacterium parvum	T45.1X1	T45.1X2	T45.1X3	T45.1X4	T45.1X5	T45.1X6
Cosmetic preparation	T49.8X1	T49.8X2	T49.8X3	T49.8X4	T49.8X5	T49.8X6
Cosmetics	T49.8X1	T49.8X2	T49.8X3	T49.8X4	T49.8X5	T49.8X6
Cosyntropin	T38.811	T38.812	T38.813	T38.814	T38.815	T38.816
Cotarnine	T45.7X1	T45.7X2	T45.7X3	T45.7X4	T45.7X5	T45.7X6
Co-trimoxazole	T36.8X1	T36.8X2	T36.8X3	T36.8X4	T36.8X5	T36.8X6
Cottonseed oil	T49.3X1	T49.3X2	T49.3X3	T49.3X4	T49.3X5	T49.3X6

◀ New   ◀▥ Revised   ~~deleted~~ Deleted

Substance	External Cause (T-Code)					
	Poisoning, Accidental (Unintentional)	Poisoning, Intentional Self-Harm	Poisoning, Assault	Poisoning, Undetermined	Adverse Effect	Underdosing
Cough mixture (syrup)	T48.4X1	T48.4X2	T48.4X3	T48.4X4	T48.4X5	T48.4X6
containing opiates	T40.2X1	T40.2X2	T40.2X3	T40.2X4	T40.2X5	T40.2X6
expectorants	T48.4X1	T48.4X2	T48.4X3	T48.4X4	T48.4X5	T48.4X6
Coumadin	T45.511	T45.512	T45.513	T45.514	T45.515	T45.516
rodenticide	T60.4X1	T60.4X2	T60.4X3	T60.4X4	—	—
Coumaphos	T60.0X1	T60.0X2	T60.0X3	T60.0X4	—	—
Coumarin	T45.511	T45.512	T45.513	T45.514	T45.515	T45.516
Coumetarol	T45.511	T45.512	T45.513	T45.514	T45.515	T45.516
Cowbane	T62.2X1	T62.2X2	T62.2X3	T62.2X4	—	—
Cozyme	T45.2X1	T45.2X2	T45.2X3	T45.2X4	T45.2X5	T45.2X6
Crack	T40.5X1	T40.5X2	T40.5X3	T40.5X4	—	—
Crataegus extract	T46.0X1	T46.0X2	T46.0X3	T46.0X4	T46.0X5	T46.0X6
Creolin	T54.1X1	T54.1X2	T54.1X3	T54.1X4	—	—
disinfectant	T54.1X1	T54.1X2	T54.1X3	T54.1X4	—	—
Creosol (compound)	T49.0X1	T49.0X2	T49.0X3	T49.0X4	T49.0X5	T49.0X6
Creosote (coal tar) (beechwood)	T49.0X1	T49.0X2	T49.0X3	T49.0X4	T49.0X5	T49.0X6
medicinal (expectorant)	T48.4X1	T48.4X2	T48.4X3	T48.4X4	T48.4X5	T48.4X6
syrup	T48.4X1	T48.4X2	T48.4X3	T48.4X4	T48.4X5	T48.4X6
Cresol(s)	T49.0X1	T49.0X2	T49.0X3	T49.0X4	T49.0X5	T49.0X6
and soap solution	T49.0X1	T49.0X2	T49.0X3	T49.0X4	T49.0X5	T49.0X6
Cresyl acetate	T49.0X1	T49.0X2	T49.0X3	T49.0X4	T49.0X5	T49.0X6
Cresylic acid	T49.0X1	T49.0X2	T49.0X3	T49.0X4	T49.0X5	T49.0X6
Crimidine	T60.4X1	T60.4X2	T60.4X3	T60.4X4	—	—
Croconazole	T37.8X1	T37.8X2	T37.8X3	T37.8X4	T37.8X5	T37.8X6
Cromoglicic acid	T48.6X1	T48.6X2	T48.6X3	T48.6X4	T48.6X5	T48.6X6
Cromolyn	T48.6X1	T48.6X2	T48.6X3	T48.6X4	T48.6X5	T48.6X6
Cromonar	T46.3X1	T46.3X2	T46.3X3	T46.3X4	T46.3X5	T46.3X6
Cropropamide	T39.8X1	T39.8X2	T39.8X3	T39.8X4	T39.8X5	T39.8X6
with crotethamide	T50.7X1	T50.7X2	T50.7X3	T50.7X4	T50.7X5	T50.7X6
Crotamiton	T49.0X1	T49.0X2	T49.0X3	T49.0X4	T49.0X5	T49.0X6
Crotethamide	T39.8X1	T39.8X2	T39.8X3	T39.8X4	T39.8X5	T39.8X6
with cropropamide	T50.7X1	T50.7X2	T50.7X3	T50.7X4	T50.7X5	T50.7X6
Croton (oil)	T47.2X1	T47.2X2	T47.2X3	T47.2X4	T47.2X5	T47.2X6
chloral	T42.6X1	T42.6X2	T42.6X3	T42.6X4	T42.6X5	T42.6X6
Crude oil	T52.0X1	T52.0X2	T52.0X3	T52.0X4	—	—
Cryogenine	T39.8X1	T39.8X2	T39.8X3	T39.8X4	T39.8X5	T39.8X6
Cryolite (vapor)	T60.1X1	T60.1X2	T60.1X3	T60.1X4	—	—
insecticide	T60.1X1	T60.1X2	T60.1X3	T60.1X4	—	—
Cryptenamine (tannates)	T46.5X1	T46.5X2	T46.5X3	T46.5X4	T46.5X5	T46.5X6
Crystal violet	T49.0X1	T49.0X2	T49.0X3	T49.0X4	T49.0X5	T49.0X6

◄ New   ◀▥ Revised   ~~deleted~~ Deleted

Substance	Poisoning, Accidental (Unintentional)	Poisoning, Intentional Self-Harm	Poisoning, Assault	Poisoning, Undetermined	Adverse Effect	Underdosing
	External Cause (T-Code)					
Cuckoopint	T62.2X1	T62.2X2	T62.2X3	T62.2X4	—	—
Cumetharol	T45.511	T45.512	T45.513	T45.514	T45.515	T45.516
Cupric						
acetate	T60.3X1	T60.3X2	T60.3X3	T60.3X4	—	—
acetoarsenite	T57.0X1	T57.0X2	T57.0X3	T57.0X4	—	—
arsenate	T57.0X1	T57.0X2	T57.0X3	T57.0X4	—	—
gluconate	T49.0X1	T49.0X2	T49.0X3	T49.0X4	T49.0X5	T49.0X6
oleate	T49.0X1	T49.0X2	T49.0X3	T49.0X4	T49.0X5	T49.0X6
sulfate	T56.4X1	T56.4X2	T56.4X3	T56.4X4	—	—
Cuprous sulfate — see also Copper sulfate	T56.4X1	T56.4X2	T56.4X3	T56.4X4	—	—
Curare, curarine	T48.1X1	T48.1X2	T48.1X3	T48.1X4	T48.1X5	T48.1X6
Cyamemazine	T43.3X1	T43.3X2	T43.3X3	T43.3X4	T43.3X5	T43.3X6
Cyamopsis tetragono-loba	T46.6X1	T46.6X2	T46.6X3	T46.6X4	T46.6X5	T46.6X6
Cyanacetyl hydrazide	T37.1X1	T37.1X2	T37.1X3	T37.1X4	T37.1X5	T37.1X6
Cyanic acid (gas)	T59.891	T59.892	T59.893	T59.894	—	—
Cyanide(s) (compounds) (potassium) (sodium) NEC	T65.0X1	T65.0X2	T65.0X3	T65.0X4	—	—
dust or gas (inhalation) NEC	T57.3X1	T57.3X2	T57.3X3	T57.3X4	—	—
fumigant	T65.0X1	T65.0X2	T65.0X3	T65.0X4	—	—
hydrogen	T57.3X1	T57.3X2	T57.3X3	T57.3X4	—	—
mercuric — see Mercury						
pesticide (dust) (fumes)	T65.0X1	T65.0X2	T65.0X3	T65.0X4	—	—
Cyanoacrylate adhesive	T49.3X1	T49.3X2	T49.3X3	T49.3X4	T49.3X5	T49.3X6
Cyanocobalamin	T45.8X1	T45.8X2	T45.8X3	T45.8X4	T45.8X5	T45.8X6
Cyanogen (chloride) (gas) NEC	T59.891	T59.892	T59.893	T59.894	—	—
Cyclacillin	T36.0X1	T36.0X2	T36.0X3	T36.0X4	T36.0X5	T36.0X6
Cyclaine	T41.3X1	T41.3X2	T41.3X3	T41.3X4	T41.3X5	T41.3X6
Cyclamate	T50.991	T50.992	T50.993	T50.994	T50.995	T50.996
Cyclamen europaeum	T62.2X1	T62.2X2	T62.2X3	T62.2X4	—	—
Cyclandelate	T46.7X1	T46.7X2	T46.7X3	T46.7X4	T46.7X5	T46.7X6
Cyclazocine	T50.7X1	T50.7X2	T50.7X3	T50.7X4	T50.7X5	T50.7X6
Cyclizine	T45.0X1	T45.0X2	T45.0X3	T45.0X4	T45.0X5	T45.0X6
Cyclobarbital	T42.3X1	T42.3X2	T42.3X3	T42.3X4	T42.3X5	T42.3X6
Cyclobarbitone	T42.3X1	T42.3X2	T42.3X3	T42.3X4	T42.3X5	T42.3X6
Cyclobenzaprine	T48.1X1	T48.1X2	T48.1X3	T48.1X4	T48.1X5	T48.1X6
Cyclodrine	T44.3X1	T44.3X2	T44.3X3	T44.3X4	T44.3X5	T44.3X6
Cycloguanil embonate	T37.2X1	T37.2X2	T37.2X3	T37.2X4	T37.2X5	T37.2X6
Cycloheptadiene	T43.291	T43.292	T43.293	T43.294	T43.295	T43.296
Cyclohexane	T52.8X1	T52.8X2	T52.8X3	T52.8X4	—	—
Cyclohexanol	T51.8X1	T51.8X2	T51.8X3	T51.8X4	—	—
Cyclohexanone	T52.4X1	T52.4X2	T52.4X3	T52.4X4	—	—

◀ New ◀▥ Revised ~~deleted~~ Deleted

Substance	Poisoning, Accidental (Unintentional)	Poisoning, Intentional Self-Harm	Poisoning, Assault	Poisoning, Undetermined	Adverse Effect	Underdosing
	External Cause (T-Code)					
Cycloheximide	T60.3X1	T60.3X2	T60.3X3	T60.3X4	—	—
Cyclohexyl acetate	T52.8X1	T52.8X2	T52.8X3	T52.8X4	—	—
Cycloleucin	T45.1X1	T45.1X2	T45.1X3	T45.1X4	T45.1X5	T45.1X6
Cyclomethycaine	T41.3X1	T41.3X2	T41.3X3	T41.3X4	T41.3X5	T41.3X6
Cyclopentamine	T44.4X1	T44.4X2	T44.4X3	T44.4X4	T44.4X5	T44.4X6
Cyclopenthiazide	T50.2X1	T50.2X2	T50.2X3	T50.2X4	T50.2X5	T50.2X6
Cyclopentolate	T44.3X1	T44.3X2	T44.3X3	T44.3X4	T44.3X5	T44.3X6
Cyclophosphamide	T45.1X1	T45.1X2	T45.1X3	T45.1X4	T45.1X5	T45.1X6
Cycloplegic drug	T49.5X1	T49.5X2	T49.5X3	T49.5X4	T49.5X5	T49.5X6
Cyclopropane	T41.291	T41.292	T41.293	T41.294	T41.295	T41.296
Cyclopyrabital	T39.8X1	T39.8X2	T39.8X3	T39.8X4	T39.8X5	T39.8X6
Cycloserine	T37.1X1	T37.1X2	T37.1X3	T37.1X4	T37.1X5	T37.1X6
Cyclosporin	T45.1X1	T45.1X2	T45.1X3	T45.1X4	T45.1X5	T45.1X6
Cyclothiazide	T50.2X1	T50.2X2	T50.2X3	T50.2X4	T50.2X5	T50.2X6
Cycrimine	T44.3X1	T44.3X2	T44.3X3	T44.3X4	T44.3X5	T44.3X6
Cyhalothrin	T60.1X1	T60.1X2	T60.1X3	T60.1X4	—	—
Cymarin	T46.0X1	T46.0X2	T46.0X3	T46.0X4	T46.0X5	T46.0X6
Cypermethrin	T60.1X1	T60.1X2	T60.1X3	T60.1X4	—	—
Cyphenothrin	T60.2X1	T60.2X2	T60.2X3	T60.2X4	—	—
Cyproheptadine	T45.0X1	T45.0X2	T45.0X3	T45.0X4	T45.0X5	T45.0X6
Cyprolidol	T43.291	T43.292	T43.293	T43.294	T43.295	T43.296
Cyproterone	T38.6X1	T38.6X2	T38.6X3	T38.6X4	T38.6X5	T38.6X6
Cysteamine	T50.6X1	T50.6X2	T50.6X3	T50.6X4	T50.6X5	T50.6X6
Cytarabine	T45.1X1	T45.1X2	T45.1X3	T45.1X4	T45.1X5	T45.1X6
Cytisus						
laburnum	T62.2X1	T62.2X2	T62.2X3	T62.2X4	—	—
scoparius	T62.2X1	T62.2X2	T62.2X3	T62.2X4	—	—
Cytochrome C	T47.5X1	T47.5X2	T47.5X3	T47.5X4	T47.5X5	T47.5X6
Cytomel	T38.1X1	T38.1X2	T38.1X3	T38.1X4	T38.1X5	T38.1X6
Cytosine arabinoside	T45.1X1	T45.1X2	T45.1X3	T45.1X4	T45.1X5	T45.1X6
Cytoxan	T45.1X1	T45.1X2	T45.1X3	T45.1X4	T45.1X5	T45.1X6
Cytozyme	T45.7X1	T45.7X2	T45.7X3	T45.7X4	T45.7X5	T45.7X6
2,4-D	T60.3X1	T60.3X2	T60.3X3	T60.3X4	—	—
D						
Dacarbazine	T45.1X1	T45.1X2	T45.1X3	T45.1X4	T45.1X5	T45.1X6
Dactinomycin	T45.1X1	T45.1X2	T45.1X3	T45.1X4	T45.1X5	T45.1X6
DADPS	T37.1X1	T37.1X2	T37.1X3	T37.1X4	T37.1X5	T37.1X6
Dakin's solution	T49.0X1	T49.0X2	T49.0X3	T49.0X4	T49.0X5	T49.0X6
Dalapon (sodium)	T60.3X1	T60.3X2	T60.3X3	T60.3X4	—	—

TABLE OF DRUGS AND CHEMICALS

TABLE OF DRUGS AND CHEMICALS

Substance	Poisoning, Accidental (Unintentional)	Poisoning, Intentional Self-Harm	Poisoning, Assault	Poisoning, Undetermined	Adverse Effect	Underdosing
Dalmane	T42.4X1	T42.4X2	T42.4X3	T42.4X4	T42.4X5	T42.4X6
Danazol	T38.6X1	T38.6X2	T38.6X3	T38.6X4	T38.6X5	T38.6X6
Danilone	T45.511	T45.512	T45.513	T45.514	T45.515	T45.516
Danthron	T47.2X1	T47.2X2	T47.2X3	T47.2X4	T47.2X5	T47.2X6
Dantrolene	T42.8X1	T42.8X2	T42.8X3	T42.8X4	T42.8X5	T42.8X6
Dantron	T47.2X1	T47.2X2	T47.2X3	T47.2X4	T47.2X5	T47.2X6
Daphne (gnidium) (mezereum)	T62.2X1	T62.2X2	T62.2X3	T62.2X4	—	—
berry	T62.1X1	T62.1X2	T62.1X3	T62.1X4	—	—
Dapsone	T37.1X1	T37.1X2	T37.1X3	T37.1X4	T37.1X5	T37.1X6
Daraprim	T37.2X1	T37.2X2	T37.2X3	T37.2X4	T37.2X5	T37.2X6
Darnel	T62.2X1	T62.2X2	T62.2X3	T62.2X4	—	—
Darvon	T39.8X1	T39.8X2	T39.8X3	T39.8X4	T39.8X5	T39.8X6
Daunomycin	T45.1X1	T45.1X2	T45.1X3	T45.1X4	T45.1X5	T45.1X6
Daunorubicin	T45.1X1	T45.1X2	T45.1X3	T45.1X4	T45.1X5	T45.1X6
DBI	T38.3X1	T38.3X2	T38.3X3	T38.3X4	T38.3X5	T38.3X6
D-Con	T60.91	T60.92	T60.93	T60.94	—	—
insecticide	T60.2X1	T60.2X2	T60.2X3	T60.2X4	—	—
rodenticide	T60.4X1	T60.4X2	T60.4X3	T60.4X4	—	—
DDAVP	T38.891	T38.892	T38.893	T38.894	T38.895	T38.896
DDE (bis(chlorophenyl)-dichloroethylene)	T60.2X1	T60.2X2	T60.2X3	T60.2X4	—	—
DDS	T37.1X1	T37.1X2	T37.1X3	T37.1X4	T37.1X5	T37.1X6
DDT (dust)	T60.1X1	T60.1X2	T60.1X3	T60.1X4	—	—
Deadly nightshade — *see also Belladonna*	T62.2X1	T62.2X2	T62.2X3	T62.2X4	—	—
berry	T62.1X1	T62.1X2	T62.1X3	T62.1X4	—	—
Deamino-D-arginine vasopressin	T38.891	T38.892	T38.893	T38.894	T38.895	T38.896
Deanol (aceglumate)	T50.991	T50.992	T50.993	T50.994	T50.995	T50.996
Debrisoquine	T46.5X1	T46.5X2	T46.5X3	T46.5X4	T46.5X5	T46.5X6
Decaborane	T57.8X1	T57.8X2	T57.8X3	T57.8X4	—	—
fumes	T59.891	T59.892	T59.893	T59.894	—	—
Decadron	T38.0X1	T38.0X2	T38.0X3	T38.0X4	T38.0X5	T38.0X6
ENT agent	T49.6X1	T49.6X2	T49.6X3	T49.6X4	T49.6X5	T49.6X6
ophthalmic preparation	T49.5X1	T49.5X2	T49.5X3	T49.5X4	T49.5X5	T49.5X6
topical NEC	T49.0X1	T49.0X2	T49.0X3	T49.0X4	T49.0X5	T49.0X6
Decahydronaphthalene	T52.8X1	T52.8X2	T52.8X3	T52.8X4	—	—
Decalin	T52.8X1	T52.8X2	T52.8X3	T52.8X4	—	—
Decamethonium (bromide)	T48.1X1	T48.1X2	T48.1X3	T48.1X4	T48.1X5	T48.1X6
Decholin	T47.5X1	T47.5X2	T47.5X3	T47.5X4	T47.5X5	T47.5X6
Declomycin	T36.4X1	T36.4X2	T36.4X3	T36.4X4	T36.4X5	T36.4X6
Decongestant, nasal (mucosa)	T48.5X1	T48.5X2	T48.5X3	T48.5X4	T48.5X5	T48.5X6
combination	T48.5X1	T48.5X2	T48.5X3	T48.5X4	T48.5X5	T48.5X6

◀ New   ◀‖‖ Revised   ~~deleted~~ Deleted

Substance	External Cause (T-Code)					
	Poisoning, Accidental (Unintentional)	Poisoning, Intentional Self-Harm	Poisoning, Assault	Poisoning, Undetermined	Adverse Effect	Underdosing
Deet	T60.8X1	T60.8X2	T60.8X3	T60.8X4	—	—
Deferoxamine	T45.8X1	T45.8X2	T45.8X3	T45.8X4	T45.8X5	T45.8X6
Deflazacort	T38.0X1	T38.0X2	T38.0X3	T38.0X4	T38.0X5	T38.0X6
Deglycyrrhizinized extract of licorice	T48.4X1	T48.4X2	T48.4X3	T48.4X4	T48.4X5	T48.4X6
Dehydrocholic acid	T47.5X1	T47.5X2	T47.5X3	T47.5X4	T47.5X5	T47.5X6
Dehydroemetine	T37.3X1	T37.3X2	T37.3X3	T37.3X4	T37.3X5	T37.3X6
Dekalin	T52.8X1	T52.8X2	T52.8X3	T52.8X4	—	—
Delalutin	T38.5X1	T38.5X2	T38.5X3	T38.5X4	T38.5X5	T38.5X6
Delphinium	T62.2X1	T62.2X2	T62.2X3	T62.2X4	—	—
Deltasone	T38.0X1	T38.0X2	T38.0X3	T38.0X4	T38.0X5	T38.0X6
Deltra	T38.0X1	T38.0X2	T38.0X3	T38.0X4	T38.0X5	T38.0X6
Delvinal	T42.3X1	T42.3X2	T42.3X3	T42.3X4	T42.3X5	T42.3X6
Delorazepam	T42.4X1	T42.4X2	T42.4X3	T42.4X4	T42.4X5	T42.4X6
Deltamethrin	T60.1X1	T60.1X2	T60.1X3	T60.1X4	—	—
Demecarium (bromide)	T49.5X1	T49.5X2	T49.5X3	T49.5X4	T49.5X5	T49.5X6
Demeclocycline	T36.4X1	T36.4X2	T36.4X3	T36.4X4	T36.4X5	T36.4X6
Demecolcine	T45.1X1	T45.1X2	T45.1X3	T45.1X4	T45.1X5	T45.1X6
Demegestone	T38.5X1	T38.5X2	T38.5X3	T38.5X4	T38.5X5	T38.5X6
Demelanizing agents	T49.8X1	T49.8X2	T49.8X3	T49.8X4	T49.8X5	T49.8X6
Demephion -O and -S	T60.0X1	T60.0X2	T60.0X3	T60.0X4	—	—
Demerol	T40.2X1	T40.2X2	T40.2X3	T40.2X4	T40.2X5	T40.2X6
Demethylchlortetracycline	T36.4X1	T36.4X2	T36.4X3	T36.4X4	T36.4X5	T36.4X6
Demethyltetracycline	T36.4X1	T36.4X2	T36.4X3	T36.4X4	T36.4X5	T36.4X6
Demeton -O and -S	T60.0X1	T60.0X2	T60.0X3	T60.0X4	—	—
Demulcent (external)	T49.3X1	T49.3X2	T49.3X3	T49.3X4	T49.3X5	T49.3X6
specified NEC	T49.3X1	T49.3X2	T49.3X3	T49.3X4	T49.3X5	T49.3X6
Demulen	T38.4X1	T38.4X2	T38.4X3	T38.4X4	T38.4X5	T38.4X6
Denatured alcohol	T51.0X1	T51.0X2	T51.0X3	T51.0X4	—	—
Dendrid	T49.5X1	T49.5X2	T49.5X3	T49.5X4	T49.5X5	T49.5X6
Dental drug, topical application NEC	T49.7X1	T49.7X2	T49.7X3	T49.7X4	T49.7X5	T49.7X6
Dentifrice	T49.7X1	T49.7X2	T49.7X3	T49.7X4	T49.7X5	T49.7X6
Deodorant spray (feminine hygiene)	T49.8X1	T49.8X2	T49.8X3	T49.8X4	T49.8X5	T49.8X6
Deoxycortone	T50.0X1	T50.0X2	T50.0X3	T50.0X4	T50.0X5	T50.0X6
2-Deoxy-5-fluorouridine	T45.1X1	T45.1X2	T45.1X3	T45.1X4	T45.1X5	T45.1X6
5-Deoxy-5-fluorouridine	T45.1X1	T45.1X2	T45.1X3	T45.1X4	T45.1X5	T45.1X6
Deoxyribonuclease (pancreatic)	T45.3X1	T45.3X2	T45.3X3	T45.3X4	T45.3X5	T45.3X6
Depilatory	T49.4X1	T49.4X2	T49.4X3	T49.4X4	T49.4X5	T49.4X6
Deprenalin	T42.8X1	T42.8X2	T42.8X3	T42.8X4	T42.8X5	T42.8X6
Deprenyl	T42.8X1	T42.8X2	T42.8X3	T42.8X4	T42.8X5	T42.8X6

TABLE OF DRUGS AND CHEMICALS

Substance	Poisoning, Accidental (Unintentional)	Poisoning, Intentional Self-Harm	Poisoning, Assault	Poisoning, Undetermined	Adverse Effect	Underdosing
			External Cause (T-Code)			
Depressant, appetite	T50.5X1	T50.5X2	T50.5X3	T50.5X4	T50.5X5	T50.5X6
Depressant						
appetite, central	T50.5X1	T50.5X2	T50.5X3	T50.5X4	T50.5X5	T50.5X6
cardiac	T46.2X1	T46.2X2	T46.2X3	T46.2X4	T46.2X5	T46.2X6
central nervous system (anesthetic) — *see also Central nervous system, depressants*	T42.71	T42.72	T42.73	T42.74	T42.75	T42.76
general anesthetic	T41.201	T41.202	T41.203	T41.204	T41.205	T41.206
muscle tone	T42.8X1	T42.8X2	T42.8X3	T42.8X4	T42.8X5	T42.8X6
muscle tone, central	T42.8X1	T42.8X2	T42.8X3	T42.8X4	T42.8X5	T42.8X6
psychotherapeutic	T43.501	T43.502	T43.503	T43.504	T43.505	T43.506
Deptropine	T45.0X1	T45.0X2	T45.0X3	T45.0X4	T45.0X5	T45.0X6
Dequalinium (chloride)	T49.0X1	T49.0X2	T49.0X3	T49.0X4	T49.0X5	T49.0X6
Derris root	T60.2X1	T60.2X2	T60.2X3	T60.2X4	—	—
Deserpidine	T43.011	T43.012	T43.013	T43.014	T43.015	T43.016
Desferrioxamine	T45.8X1	T45.8X2	T45.8X3	T45.8X4	T45.8X5	T45.8X6
Desipramine	T43.0X1	T43.0X2	T43.0X3	T43.0X4	T43.0X5	T43.0X6
Deslanoside	T46.0X1	T46.0X2	T46.0X3	T46.0X4	T46.0X5	T46.0X6
Desloughing agent	T49.4X1	T49.4X2	T49.4X3	T49.4X4	T49.4X5	T49.4X6
Desmethylimipramine	T43.011	T43.012	T43.013	T43.014	T43.015	T43.016
Desmopressin	T38.891	T38.892	T38.893	T38.894	T38.895	T38.896
Desocodeine	T40.2X1	T40.2X2	T40.2X3	T40.2X4	T40.2X5	T40.2X6
Desogestrel	T38.5X1	T38.5X2	T38.5X3	T38.5X4	T38.5X5	T38.5X6
Desomorphine	T40.2X1	T40.2X2	T40.2X3	T40.2X4	—	—
Desonide	T49.0X1	T49.0X2	T49.0X3	T49.0X4	T49.0X5	T49.0X6
Desoximetasone	T49.0X1	T49.0X2	T49.0X3	T49.0X4	T49.0X5	T49.0X6
Desoxycorticosteroid	T50.0X1	T50.0X2	T50.0X3	T50.0X4	T50.0X5	T50.0X6
Desoxycortone	T50.0X1	T50.0X2	T50.0X3	T50.0X4	T50.0X5	T50.0X6
Desoxyephedrine	T43.621	T43.622	T43.623	T43.624	T43.625	T43.626
Detaxtran	T46.6X1	T46.6X2	T46.6X3	T46.6X4	T46.6X5	T46.6X6
Detergent	T49.2X1	T49.2X2	T49.2X3	T49.2X4	T49.2X5	T49.2X6
external medication	T49.2X1	T49.2X2	T49.2X3	T49.2X4	T49.2X5	T49.2X6
local	T49.2X1	T49.2X2	T49.2X3	T49.2X4	T49.2X5	T49.2X6
medicinal	T49.2X1	T49.2X2	T49.2X3	T49.2X4	T49.2X5	T49.2X6
nonmedicinal	T55.1X1	T55.1X2	T55.1X3	T55.1X4	—	—
specified NEC	T55.1X1	T55.1X2	T55.1X3	T55.1X4	T55.1X5	T55.1X6
Deterrent, alcohol	T50.6X1	T50.6X2	T50.6X3	T50.6X4	T50.6X5	T50.6X6
Detoxifying agent	T50.6X1	T50.6X2	T50.6X3	T50.6X4	T50.6X5	T50.6X6
Detrothyronine	T38.1X1	T38.1X2	T38.1X3	T38.1X4	T38.1X5	T38.1X6
Dettol (external medication)	T49.0X1	T49.0X2	T49.0X3	T49.0X4	T49.0X5	T49.0X6

◀ New ◀▥ Revised ~~deleted~~ Deleted

Substance	External Cause (T-Code)					
	Poisoning, Accidental (Unintentional)	Poisoning, Intentional Self-Harm	Poisoning, Assault	Poisoning, Undetermined	Adverse Effect	Underdosing
Dexamethasone	T38.0X1	T38.0X2	T38.0X3	T38.0X4	T38.0X5	T38.0X6
ENT agent	T49.6X1	T49.6X2	T49.6X3	T49.6X4	T49.6X5	T49.6X6
ophthalmic preparation	T49.5X1	T49.5X2	T49.5X3	T49.5X4	T49.5X5	T49.5X6
topical NEC	T49.0X1	T49.0X2	T49.0X3	T49.0X4	T49.0X5	T49.0X6
Dexamfetamine	T43.621	T43.622	T43.623	T43.624	T43.625	T43.626
Dexamphetamine	T43.621	T43.622	T43.623	T43.624	T43.625	T43.626
Dexbrompheniramine	T45.0X1	T45.0X2	T45.0X3	T45.0X4	T45.0X5	T45.0X6
Dexchlorpheniramine	T45.0X1	T45.0X2	T45.0X3	T45.0X4	T45.0X5	T45.0X6
Dexedrine	T43.621	T43.622	T43.623	T43.624	T43.625	T43.626
Dexetimide	T44.3X1	T44.3X2	T44.3X3	T44.3X4	T44.3X5	T44.3X6
Dexfenfluramine	T50.5X1	T50.5X2	T50.5X3	T50.5X4	T50.5X5	T50.5X6
Dexpanthenol	T45.2X1	T45.2X2	T45.2X3	T45.2X4	T45.2X5	T45.2X6
Dextran (40) (70) (150)	T45.8X1	T45.8X2	T45.8X3	T45.8X4	T45.8X5	T45.8X6
Dextriferron	T45.4X1	T45.4X2	T45.4X3	T45.4X4	T45.4X5	T45.4X6
Dextroamphetamine	T43.621	T43.622	T43.623	T43.624	T43.625	T43.626
Dextro calcium pantothenate	T45.2X1	T45.2X2	T45.2X3	T45.2X4	T45.2X5	T45.2X6
Dextromethorphan	T48.3X1	T48.3X2	T48.3X3	T48.3X4	T48.3X5	T48.3X6
Dextromoramide	T40.4X1	T40.4X2	T40.4X3	T40.4X4	—	—
topical	T49.8X1	T49.8X2	T49.8X3	T49.8X4	T49.8X5	T49.8X6
Dextro pantothenyl alcohol	T45.2X1	T45.2X2	T45.2X3	T45.2X4	T45.2X5	T45.2X6
Dextropropoxyphene	T40.4X1	T40.4X2	T40.4X3	T40.4X4	T40.4X5	T40.4X6
Dextrorphan	T40.2X1	T40.2X2	T40.2X3	T40.2X4	T40.2X5	T40.2X6
Dextrose	T50.3X1	T50.3X2	T50.3X3	T50.3X4	T50.3X5	T50.3X6
concentrated solution, intravenous	T46.8X1	T46.8X2	T46.8X3	T46.8X4	T46.8X5	T46.8X6
Dextrothyroxin	T38.1X1	T38.1X2	T38.1X3	T38.1X4	T38.1X5	T38.1X6
Dextrothyroxine sodium	T38.1X1	T38.1X2	T38.1X3	T38.1X4	T38.1X5	T38.1X6
DFP	T44.0X1	T44.0X2	T44.0X3	T44.0X4	T44.0X5	T44.0X6
DHE	T37.3X1	T37.3X2	T37.3X3	T37.3X4	T37.3X5	T37.3X6
45	T46.5X1	T46.5X2	T46.5X3	T46.5X4	T46.5X5	T46.5X6
Diabinese	T38.3X1	T38.3X2	T38.3X3	T38.3X4	T38.3X5	T38.3X6
Diacetone alcohol	T52.4X1	T52.4X2	T52.4X3	T52.4X4	—	—
Diacetyl monoxime	T50.991	T50.992	T50.993	T50.994	—	—
Diacetylmorphine	T40.1X1	T40.1X2	T40.1X3	T40.1X4	—	—
Diachylon plaster	T49.4X1	T49.4X2	T49.4X3	T49.4X4	T49.4X5	T49.4X6
Diaethylstilboestrolum	T38.5X1	T38.5X2	T38.5X3	T38.5X4	T38.5X5	T38.5X6
Diagnostic agent NEC	T50.8X1	T50.8X2	T50.8X3	T50.8X4	T50.8X5	T50.8X6
Dial (soap)	T49.2X1	T49.2X2	T49.2X3	T49.2X4	T49.2X5	T49.2X6
sedative	T42.3X1	T42.3X2	T42.3X3	T42.3X4	T42.3X5	T42.3X6
Dialkyl carbonate	T52.91	T52.92	T52.93	T52.94	—	—

TABLE OF DRUGS AND CHEMICALS

Substance	Poisoning, Accidental (Unintentional)	Poisoning, Intentional Self-Harm	Poisoning, Assault	Poisoning, Undetermined	Adverse Effect	Underdosing
Diallylbarbituric acid	T42.3X1	T42.3X2	T42.3X3	T42.3X4	T42.3X5	T42.3X6
Diallymal	T42.3X1	T42.3X2	T42.3X3	T42.3X4	T42.3X5	T42.3X6
Dialysis solution (intraperitoneal)	T50.3X1	T50.3X2	T50.3X3	T50.3X4	T50.3X5	T50.3X6
Diaminodiphenylsulfone	T37.1X1	T37.1X2	T37.1X3	T37.1X4	T37.1X5	T37.1X6
Diamorphine	T40.1X1	T40.1X2	T40.1X3	T40.1X4	—	—
Diamox	T50.2X1	T50.2X2	T50.2X3	T50.2X4	T50.2X5	T50.2X6
Diamthazole	T49.0X1	T49.0X2	T49.0X3	T49.0X4	T49.0X5	T49.0X6
Dianthone	T47.2X1	T47.2X2	T47.2X3	T47.2X4	T47.2X5	T47.2X6
Diaphenylsulfone	T37.0X1	T37.0X2	T37.0X3	T37.0X4	T37.0X5	T37.0X6
Diasone (sodium)	T37.1X1	T37.1X2	T37.1X3	T37.1X4	T37.1X5	T37.1X6
Diastase	T47.5X1	T47.5X2	T47.5X3	T47.5X4	T47.5X5	T47.5X6
Diatrizoate	T50.8X1	T50.8X2	T50.8X3	T50.8X4	T50.8X5	T50.8X6
Diazepam	T42.4X1	T42.4X2	T42.4X3	T42.4X4	T42.4X5	T42.4X6
Diazinon	T60.0X1	T60.0X2	T60.0X3	T60.0X4	—	—
Diazomethane (gas)	T59.891	T59.892	T59.893	T59.894	—	—
Diazoxide	T46.5X1	T46.5X2	T46.5X3	T46.5X4	T46.5X5	T46.5X6
Dibekacin	T36.5X1	T36.5X2	T36.5X3	T36.5X4	T36.5X5	T36.5X6
Dibenamine	T44.6X1	T44.6X2	T44.6X3	T44.6X4	T44.6X5	T44.6X6
Dibenzepin	T43.011	T43.012	T43.013	T43.014	T43.015	T43.016
Dibenzheptropine	T45.0X1	T45.0X2	T45.0X3	T45.0X4	T45.0X5	T45.0X6
Dibenzyline	T44.6X1	T44.6X2	T44.6X3	T44.6X4	T44.6X5	T44.6X6
Diborane (gas)	T59.891	T59.892	T59.893	T59.894	—	—
Dibromochloropropane	T60.8X1	T60.8X2	T60.8X3	T60.8X4	—	—
Dibromodulcitol	T45.1X1	T45.1X2	T45.1X3	T45.1X4	T45.1X5	T45.1X6
Dibromoethane	T53.6X1	T53.6X2	T53.6X3	T53.6X4	—	—
Dibromomannitol	T45.1X1	T45.1X2	T45.1X3	T45.1X4	T45.1X5	T45.1X6
Dibromopropamidine isethionate	T49.0X1	T49.0X2	T49.0X3	T49.0X4	T49.0X5	T49.0X6
Dibrompropamidine	T49.0X1	T49.0X2	T49.0X3	T49.0X4	T49.0X5	T49.0X6
Dibucaine	T41.3X1	T41.3X2	T41.3X3	T41.3X4	T41.3X5	T41.3X6
topical (surface)	T41.3X1	T41.3X2	T41.3X3	T41.3X4	T41.3X5	T41.3X6
Dibunate sodium	T48.3X1	T48.3X2	T48.3X3	T48.3X4	T48.3X5	T48.3X6
Dibutoline sulfate	T44.3X1	T44.3X2	T44.3X3	T44.3X4	T44.3X5	T44.3X6
Dicamba	T60.3X1	T60.3X2	T60.3X3	T60.3X4	—	—
Dicapthon	T60.0X1	T60.0X2	T60.0X3	T60.0X4	—	—
Dichlobenil	T60.3X1	T60.3X2	T60.3X3	T60.3X4	—	—
Dichlone	T60.3X1	T60.3X2	T60.3X3	T60.3X4	—	—
Dichloralphenozone	T42.6X1	T42.6X2	T42.6X3	T42.6X4	T42.6X5	T42.6X6
Dichlorbenzidine	T65.3X1	T65.3X2	T65.3X3	T65.3X4	—	—
Dichlorhydrin	T52.8X1	T52.8X2	T52.8X3	T52.8X4	—	—
Dichlorhydroxyquinoline	T37.8X1	T37.8X2	T37.8X3	T37.8X4	T37.8X5	T37.8X6

◀ New ◀⦙⦙ Revised ~~deleted~~ Deleted

Substance	Poisoning, Accidental (Unintentional)	Poisoning, Intentional Self-Harm	Poisoning, Assault	Poisoning, Undetermined	Adverse Effect	Underdosing
			External Cause (T-Code)			
Dichlorobenzene	T53.7X1	T53.7X2	T53.7X3	T53.7X4	—	—
Dichlorobenzyl alcohol	T49.6X1	T49.6X2	T49.6X3	T49.6X4	T49.6X5	T49.6X6
Dichlorodifluoromethane	T53.5X1	T53.5X2	T53.5X3	T53.5X4	—	—
Dichloroethane	T52.8X1	T52.8X2	T52.8X3	T52.8X4	—	—
Sym-Dichloroethyl ether	T53.6X1	T53.6X2	T53.6X3	T53.6X4	—	—
Dichloroethyl sulfide, not in war	T59.891	T59.892	T59.893	T59.894	—	—
Dichloroethylene	T53.6X1	T53.6X2	T53.6X3	T53.6X4	—	—
Dichloroformoxine, not in war	T59.891	T59.892	T59.893	T59.894	—	—
Dichlorohydrin, alpha-dichlorohydrin	T52.8X1	T52.8X2	T52.8X3	T52.8X4	—	—
Dichloromethane (solvent)	T53.4X1	T53.4X2	T53.4X3	T53.4X4	—	—
vapor	T53.4X1	T53.4X2	T53.4X3	T53.4X4	—	—
Dichloronaphthoquinone	T60.3X1	T60.3X2	T60.3X3	T60.3X4	—	—
Dichlorophen	T37.4X1	T37.4X2	T37.4X3	T37.4X4	T37.4X5	T37.4X6
2,4-Dichlorophenoxy-acetic acid	T60.3X1	T60.3X2	T60.3X3	T60.3X4	—	—
Dichloropropene	T60.3X1	T60.3X2	T60.3X3	T60.3X4	—	—
Dichloropropionic acid	T60.3X1	T60.3X2	T60.3X3	T60.3X4	—	—
Dichlorphenamide	T50.2X1	T50.2X2	T50.2X3	T50.2X4	T50.2X5	T50.2X6
Dichlorvos	T60.0X1	T60.0X2	T60.0X3	T60.0X4	—	—
Diclofenac	T39.391	T39.392	T39.393	T39.394	T39.395	T39.396
Diclofenamide	T50.2X1	T50.2X2	T50.2X3	T50.2X4	T50.2X5	T50.2X6
Diclofensine	T43.291	T43.292	T43.293	T43.294	T43.295	T43.296
Diclonixine	T39.8X1	T39.8X2	T39.8X3	T39.8X4	T39.8X5	T39.8X6
Dicloxacillin	T36.0X1	T36.0X2	T36.0X3	T36.0X4	T36.0X5	T36.0X6
Dicophane	T49.0X1	T49.0X2	T49.0X3	T49.0X4	T49.0X5	T49.0X6
Dicoumarol, dicoumarin, dicumarol	T45.511	T45.512	T45.513	T45.514	T45.515	T45.516
Dicrotophos	T60.0X1	T60.0X2	T60.0X3	T60.0X4	—	—
Dicyanogen (gas)	T65.0X1	T65.0X2	T65.0X3	T65.0X4	—	—
Dicyclomine	T44.3X1	T44.3X2	T44.3X3	T44.3X4	T44.3X5	T44.3X6
Dicycloverine	T44.3X1	T44.3X2	T44.3X3	T44.3X4	T44.3X5	T44.3X6
Dideoxycytidine	T37.5X1	T37.5X2	T37.5X3	T37.5X4	T37.5X5	T37.5X6
Dideoxyinosine	T37.5X1	T37.5X2	T37.5X3	T37.5X4	T37.5X5	T37.5X6
Dieldrin (vapor)	T60.1X1	T60.1X2	T60.1X3	T60.1X4	—	—
Diemal	T42.3X1	T42.3X2	T42.3X3	T42.3X4	T42.3X5	T42.3X6
Dienestrol	T38.5X1	T38.5X2	T38.5X3	T38.5X4	T38.5X5	T38.5X6
Dienoestrol	T38.5X1	T38.5X2	T38.5X3	T38.5X4	T38.5X5	T38.5X6
Dietetic drug NEC	T50.901	T50.902	T50.903	T50.904	T50.905	T50.906
Diethazine	T42.8X1	T42.8X2	T42.8X3	T42.8X4	T42.8X5	T42.8X6
Diethyl						
barbituric acid	T42.3X1	T42.3X2	T42.3X3	T42.3X4	T42.3X5	T42.3X6
carbamazine	T37.4X1	T37.4X2	T37.4X3	T37.4X4	T37.4X5	T37.4X6

Substance	External Cause (T-Code)					
	Poisoning, Accidental (Unintentional)	Poisoning, Intentional Self-Harm	Poisoning, Assault	Poisoning, Undetermined	Adverse Effect	Underdosing
Diethyl *(Continued)*						
carbinol	T51.3X1	T51.3X2	T51.3X3	T51.3X4	—	—
carbonate	T52.8X1	T52.8X2	T52.8X3	T52.8X4	—	—
ether (vapor) — *see also ether*	T41.0X1	T41.0X2	T41.0X3	T41.0X4	T41.0X5	T41.0X6
oxide	T52.8X1	T52.8X2	T52.8X3	T52.8X4	—	—
propion	T50.5X1	T50.5X2	T50.5X3	T50.5X4	T50.5X5	T50.5X6
stilbestrol	T38.5X1	T38.5X2	T38.5X3	T38.5X4	T38.5X5	T38.5X6
toluamide (nonmedicinal)	T60.8X1	T60.8X2	T60.8X3	T60.8X4	—	—
medicinal	T49.3X1	T49.3X2	T49.3X3	T49.3X4	T49.3X5	T49.3X6
Diethylcarbamazine	T37.4X1	T37.4X2	T37.4X3	T37.4X4	T37.4X5	T37.4X6
Diethylene						
dioxide	T52.8X1	T52.8X2	T52.8X3	T52.8X4	—	—
glycol (monoacetate) (monobutyl ether) (monoethyl ether)	T52.3X1	T52.3X2	T52.3X3	T52.3X4	—	—
Diethylhexylphthalate	T65.891	T65.892	T65.893	T65.894	—	—
Diethylpropion	T50.5X1	T50.5X2	T50.5X3	T50.5X4	T50.5X5	T50.5X6
Diethylstilbestrol	T38.5X1	T38.5X2	T38.5X3	T38.5X4	T38.5X5	T38.5X6
Diethylstilboestrol	T38.5X1	T38.5X2	T38.5X3	T38.5X4	T38.5X5	T38.5X6
Diethylsulfone-diethylmethane	T42.6X1	T42.6X2	T42.6X3	T42.6X4	T42.6X5	T42.6X6
Diethyltoluamide	T49.0X1	T49.0X2	T49.0X3	T49.0X4	T49.0X5	T49.0X6
Diethyltryptamine (DET)	T40.991	T40.992	T40.993	T40.994	—	—
Difebarbamate	T42.3X1	T42.3X2	T42.3X3	T42.3X4	T42.3X5	T42.3X6
Difencloxazine	T40.2X1	T40.2X2	T40.2X3	T40.2X4	T40.2X5	T40.2X6
Difenidol	T45.0X1	T45.0X2	T45.0X3	T45.0X4	T45.0X5	T45.0X6
Difenoxin	T47.6X1	T47.6X2	T47.6X3	T47.6X4	T47.6X5	T47.6X6
Difetarsone	T37.3X1	T37.3X2	T37.3X3	T37.3X4	T37.3X5	T37.3X6
Diffusin	T45.3X1	T45.3X2	T45.3X3	T45.3X4	T45.3X5	T45.3X6
Diflorasone	T49.0X1	T49.0X2	T49.0X3	T49.0X4	T49.0X5	T49.0X6
Diflubenzuron	T60.1X1	T60.1X2	T60.1X3	T60.1X4	—	—
Diflos	T44.0X1	T44.0X2	T44.0X3	T44.0X4	T44.0X5	T44.0X6
Diflucortolone	T49.0X1	T49.0X2	T49.0X3	T49.0X4	T49.0X5	T49.0X6
Diflunisal	T39.091	T39.092	T39.093	T39.094	T39.095	T39.096
Difluoromethyldopa	T42.8X1	T42.8X2	T42.8X3	T42.8X4	T42.8X5	T42.8X6
Difluorophate	T44.0X1	T44.0X2	T44.0X3	T44.0X4	T44.0X5	T44.0X6
Digestant NEC	T47.5X1	T47.5X2	T47.5X3	T47.5X4	T47.5X5	T47.5X6
Digitalin(e)	T46.0X1	T46.0X2	T46.0X3	T46.0X4	T46.0X5	T46.0X6
Digitalis (leaf) (glycoside)	T46.0X1	T46.0X2	T46.0X3	T46.0X4	T46.0X5	T46.0X6
lanata	T46.0X1	T46.0X2	T46.0X3	T46.0X4	T46.0X5	T46.0X6
purpurea	T46.0X1	T46.0X2	T46.0X3	T46.0X4	T46.0X5	T46.0X6
Digitoxin	T46.0X1	T46.0X2	T46.0X3	T46.0X4	T46.0X5	T46.0X6

◀ New ◀▥ Revised ~~deleted~~ Deleted

Substance	External Cause (T-Code)					
	Poisoning, Accidental (Unintentional)	Poisoning, Intentional Self-Harm	Poisoning, Assault	Poisoning, Undetermined	Adverse Effect	Underdosing
Digitoxose	T46.0X1	T46.0X2	T46.0X3	T46.0X4	T46.0X5	T46.0X6
Digoxin	T46.0X1	T46.0X2	T46.0X3	T46.0X4	T46.0X5	T46.0X6
Digoxine	T46.0X1	T46.0X2	T46.0X3	T46.0X4	T46.0X5	T46.0X6
Dihydralazine	T46.5X1	T46.5X2	T46.5X3	T46.5X4	T46.5X5	T46.5X6
Dihydrazine	T46.5X1	T46.5X2	T46.5X3	T46.5X4	T46.5X5	T46.5X6
Dihydrocodeinone	T40.2X1	T40.2X2	T40.2X3	T40.2X4	T40.2X5	T40.2X6
Dihydroergocornine	T46.7X1	T46.7X2	T46.7X3	T46.7X4	T46.7X5	T46.7X6
Dihydroergocristine (mesilate)	T46.7X1	T46.7X2	T46.7X3	T46.7X4	T46.7X5	T46.7X6
Dihydroergokryptine	T46.7X1	T46.7X2	T46.7X3	T46.7X4	T46.7X5	T46.7X6
Dihydroergotamine	T46.5X1	T46.5X2	T46.5X3	T46.5X4	T46.5X5	T46.5X6
Dihydroergotoxine	T46.7X1	T46.7X2	T46.7X3	T46.7X4	T46.7X5	T46.7X6
mesilate	T46.7X1	T46.7X2	T46.7X3	T46.7X4	T46.7X5	T46.7X6
Dihydrohydroxycodein-one	T40.2X1	T40.2X2	T40.2X3	T40.2X4	T40.2X5	T40.2X6
Dihydrohydroxymorphinone	T40.2X1	T40.2X2	T40.2X3	T40.2X4	T40.2X5	T40.2X6
Dihydroisocodeine	T40.2X1	T40.2X2	T40.2X3	T40.2X4	T40.2X5	T40.2X6
Dihydromorphine	T40.2X1	T40.2X2	T40.2X3	T40.2X4	—	—
Dihydromorphinone	T40.2X1	T40.2X2	T40.2X3	T40.2X4	T40.2X5	T40.2X6
Dihydrostreptomycin	T36.5X1	T36.5X2	T36.5X3	T36.5X4	T36.5X5	T36.5X6
Dihydrotachysterol	T45.2X1	T45.2X2	T45.2X3	T45.2X4	T45.2X5	T45.2X6
Dihydroxyaluminum aminoacetate	T47.1X1	T47.1X2	T47.1X3	T47.1X4	T47.1X5	T47.1X6
Dihydroxyaluminum sodium carbonate	T47.1X1	T47.1X2	T47.1X3	T47.1X4	T47.1X5	T47.1X6
Dihydroxyanthraquinone	T47.2X1	T47.2X2	T47.2X3	T47.2X4	T47.2X5	T47.2X6
Dihydroxycodeinone	T40.2X1	T40.2X2	T40.2X3	T40.2X4	T40.2X5	T40.2X6
Dihydroxypropyl theophylline	T50.2X1	T50.2X2	T50.2X3	T50.2X4	T50.2X5	T50.2X6
Diiodohydroxyquin	T37.8X1	T37.8X2	T37.8X3	T37.8X4	T37.8X5	T37.8X6
topical	T49.0X1	T49.0X2	T49.0X3	T49.0X4	T49.0X5	T49.0X6
Diiodohydroxyquinoline	T37.8X1	T37.8X2	T37.8X3	T37.8X4	T37.8X5	T37.8X6
Diiodotyrosine	T38.2X1	T38.2X2	T38.2X3	T38.2X4	T38.2X5	T38.2X6
Diisopromine	T44.3X1	T44.3X2	T44.3X3	T44.3X4	T44.3X5	T44.3X6
Diisopropylamine	T46.3X1	T46.3X2	T46.3X3	T46.3X4	T46.3X5	T46.3X6
Diisopropylfluorophosphonate	T44.0X1	T44.0X2	T44.0X3	T44.0X4	T44.0X5	T44.0X6
Dilantin	T42.0X1	T42.0X2	T42.0X3	T42.0X4	T42.0X5	T42.0X6
Dilaudid	T40.2X1	T40.2X2	T40.2X3	T40.2X4	T40.2X5	T40.2X6
Dilazep	T46.3X1	T46.3X2	T46.3X3	T46.3X4	T46.3X5	T46.3X6
Dill	T47.5X1	T47.5X2	T47.5X3	T47.5X4	T47.5X5	T47.5X6
Diloxanide	T37.3X1	T37.3X2	T37.3X3	T37.3X4	T37.3X5	T37.3X6
Diltiazem	T46.1X1	T46.1X2	T46.1X3	T46.1X4	T46.1X5	T46.1X6
Dimazole	T49.0X1	T49.0X2	T49.0X3	T49.0X4	T49.0X5	T49.0X6
Dimefline	T50.7X1	T50.7X2	T50.7X3	T50.7X4	T50.7X5	T50.7X6

◀ New ◀▥ Revised ~~deleted~~ Deleted

	External Cause (T-Code)					
Substance	Poisoning, Accidental (Unintentional)	Poisoning, Intentional Self-Harm	Poisoning, Assault	Poisoning, Undetermined	Adverse Effect	Underdosing
Dimefox	T60.0X1	T60.0X2	T60.0X3	T60.0X4	—	—
Dimemorfan	T48.3X1	T48.3X2	T48.3X3	T48.3X4	T48.3X5	T48.3X6
Dimenhydrinate	T45.0X1	T45.0X2	T45.0X3	T45.0X4	T45.0X5	T45.0X6
Dimercaprol (British anti-lewisite)	T45.8X1	T45.8X2	T45.8X3	T45.8X4	T45.8X5	T45.8X6
Dimercaptopropanol	T45.8X1	T45.8X2	T45.8X3	T45.8X4	T45.8X5	T45.8X6
Dimestrol	T38.5X1	T38.5X2	T38.5X3	T38.5X4	T38.5X5	T38.5X6
Dimetane	T45.0X1	T45.0X2	T45.0X3	T45.0X4	T45.0X5	T45.0X6
Dimethicone	T47.1X1	T47.1X2	T47.1X3	T47.1X4	T47.1X5	T47.1X6
Dimethindene	T45.0X1	T45.0X2	T45.0X3	T45.0X4	T45.0X5	T45.0X6
Dimethisoquin	T49.1X1	T49.1X2	T49.1X3	T49.1X4	T49.1X5	T49.1X6
Dimethisterone	T38.5X1	T38.5X2	T38.5X3	T38.5X4	T38.5X5	T38.5X6
Dimethoate	T60.0X1	T60.0X2	T60.0X3	T60.0X4	—	—
Dimethocaine	T41.3X1	T41.3X2	T41.3X3	T41.3X4	T41.3X5	T41.3X6
Dimethoxanate	T48.3X1	T48.3X2	T48.3X3	T48.3X4	T48.3X5	T48.3X6
Dimethyl						
arsine, arsinic acid	T57.0X1	T57.0X2	T57.0X3	T57.0X4	—	—
carbinol	T51.2X1	T51.2X2	T51.2X3	T51.2X4	—	—
carbonate	T52.8X1	T52.8X2	T52.8X3	T52.8X4	—	—
diguanide	T38.3X1	T38.3X2	T38.3X3	T38.3X4	T38.3X5	T38.3X6
ketone	T52.4X1	T52.4X2	T52.4X3	T52.4X4	—	—
vapor	T52.4X1	T52.4X2	T52.4X3	T52.4X4	—	—
meperidine	T40.2X1	T40.2X2	T40.2X3	T40.2X4	T40.2X5	T40.2X6
parathion	T60.0X1	T60.0X2	T60.0X3	T60.0X4	—	—
phthlate	T49.3X1	T49.3X2	T49.3X3	T49.3X4	T49.3X5	T49.3X6
polysiloxane	T47.8X1	T47.8X2	T47.8X3	T47.8X4	T47.8X5	T47.8X6
sulfate (fumes)	T59.891	T59.892	T59.893	T59.894	—	—
liquid	T65.891	T65.892	T65.893	T65.894	—	—
sulfoxide (nonmedicinal)	T52.8X1	T52.8X2	T52.8X3	T52.8X4	—	—
medicinal	T49.4X1	T49.4X2	T49.4X3	T49.4X4	T49.4X5	T49.4X6
tryptamine	T40.991	T40.992	T40.993	T40.994	—	—
tubocurarine	T48.1X1	T48.1X2	T48.1X3	T48.1X4	T48.1X5	T48.1X6
Dimethylamine sulfate	T49.4X1	T49.4X2	T49.4X3	T49.4X4	T49.4X5	T49.4X6
Dimethylformamide	T52.8X1	T52.8X2	T52.8X3	T52.8X4	—	—
Dimethyltubocurarinium chloride	T48.1X1	T48.1X2	T48.1X3	T48.1X4	T48.1X5	T48.1X6
Dimeticone	T47.1X1	T47.1X2	T47.1X3	T47.1X4	T47.1X5	T47.1X6
Dimetilan	T60.0X1	T60.0X2	T60.0X3	T60.0X4	—	—
Dimetindene	T45.0X1	T45.0X2	T45.0X3	T45.0X4	T45.0X5	T45.0X6
Dimetotiazine	T43.3X1	T43.3X2	T43.3X3	T43.3X4	T43.3X5	T43.3X6

◀ New   ◀ Revised   ~~deleted~~ Deleted

Substance	External Cause (T-Code)					
	Poisoning, Accidental (Unintentional)	Poisoning, Intentional Self-Harm	Poisoning, Assault	Poisoning, Undetermined	Adverse Effect	Underdosing
Dimorpholamine	T50.7X1	T50.7X2	T50.7X3	T50.7X4	T50.7X5	T50.7X6
Dimoxyline	T46.3X1	T46.3X2	T46.3X3	T46.3X4	T46.3X5	T46.3X6
Dinitrobenzene	T65.3X1	T65.3X2	T65.3X3	T65.3X4	—	—
vapor	T59.891	T59.892	T59.893	T59.894	—	—
Dinitrobenzol	T65.3X1	T65.3X2	T65.3X3	T65.3X4	—	—
vapor	T59.891	T59.892	T59.893	T59.894	—	—
Dinitrobutylphenol	T65.3X1	T65.3X2	T65.3X3	T65.3X4	—	—
Dinitro (-ortho-)cresol (pesticide) (spray)	T65.3X1	T65.3X2	T65.3X3	T65.3X4	—	—
Dinitrocyclohexylphenol	T65.3X1	T65.3X2	T65.3X3	T65.3X4	—	—
Dinitrophenol	T65.3X1	T65.3X2	T65.3X3	T65.3X4	—	—
Dinoprost	T48.0X1	T48.0X2	T48.0X3	T48.0X4	T48.0X5	T48.0X6
Dinoprostone	T48.0X1	T48.0X2	T48.0X3	T48.0X4	T48.0X5	T48.0X6
Dinoseb	T60.3X1	T60.3X2	T60.3X3	T60.3X4	—	—
Dioctyl sulfosuccinate (calcium) (sodium)	T47.4X1	T47.4X2	T47.4X3	T47.4X4	T47.4X5	T47.4X6
Diodone	T50.8X1	T50.8X2	T50.8X3	T50.8X4	T50.8X5	T50.8X6
Diodoquin	T37.8X1	T37.8X2	T37.8X3	T37.8X4	T37.8X5	T37.8X6
Dionin	T40.2X1	T40.2X2	T40.2X3	T40.2X4	T40.2X5	T40.2X6
Diosmin	T46.991	T46.992	T46.993	T46.994	T46.995	T46.996
Dioxane	T52.8X1	T52.8X2	T52.8X3	T52.8X4	—	—
Dioxathion	T60.0X1	T60.0X2	T60.0X3	T60.0X4	—	—
Dioxin	T53.7X1	T53.7X2	T53.7X3	T53.7X4	—	—
Dioxopromethazine	T43.3X1	T43.3X2	T43.3X3	T43.3X4	T43.3X5	T43.3X6
Dioxyline	T46.3X1	T46.3X2	T46.3X3	T46.3X4	T46.3X5	T46.3X6
Dipentene	T52.8X1	T52.8X2	T52.8X3	T52.8X4	—	—
Diperodon	T41.3X1	T41.3X2	T41.3X3	T41.3X4	T41.3X5	T41.3X6
Diphacinone	T60.4X1	T60.4X2	T60.4X3	T60.4X4	—	—
Diphemanil	T44.3X1	T44.3X2	T44.3X3	T44.3X4	T44.3X5	T44.3X6
metilsulfate	T44.3X1	T44.3X2	T44.3X3	T44.3X4	T44.3X5	T44.3X6
Diphenadione	T45.511	T45.512	T45.513	T45.514	T45.515	T45.516
rodenticide	T60.4X1	T60.4X2	T60.4X3	T60.4X4	—	—
Diphenhydramine	T45.0X1	T45.0X2	T45.0X3	T45.0X4	T45.0X5	T45.0X6
Diphenidol	T45.0X1	T45.0X2	T45.0X3	T45.0X4	T45.0X5	T45.0X6
Diphenoxylate	T47.6X1	T47.6X2	T47.6X3	T47.6X4	T47.6X5	T47.6X6
Diphenylamine	T65.3X1	T65.3X2	T65.3X3	T65.3X4	—	—
Diphenylbutazone	T39.2X1	T39.2X2	T39.2X3	T39.2X4	T39.2X5	T39.2X6
Diphenylchloroarsine, not in war	T57.0X1	T57.0X2	T57.0X3	T57.0X4	—	—
Diphenylhydantoin	T42.0X1	T42.0X2	T42.0X3	T42.0X4	T42.0X5	T42.0X6
Diphenylmethane dye	T52.1X1	T52.1X2	T52.1X3	T52.1X4		

◀ New ◀▥ Revised ~~deleted~~ Deleted

Substance	Poisoning, Accidental (Unintentional)	Poisoning, Intentional Self-Harm	Poisoning, Assault	Poisoning, Undetermined	Adverse Effect	Underdosing
Diphenylpyraline	T45.0X1	T45.0X2	T45.0X3	T45.0X4	T45.0X5	T45.0X6
Diphtheria						
antitoxin	T50.Z11	T50.Z12	T50.Z13	T50.Z14	T50.Z15	T50.Z16
toxoid	T50.A91	T50.A92	T50.A93	T50.A94	T50.A95	T50.A96
with tetanus toxoid	T50.A21	T50.A22	T50.A23	T50.A24	T50.A25	T50.A26
with pertussis component	T50.A11	T50.A12	T50.A13	T50.A14	T50.A15	T50.A16
vaccine (combination)	T50.A91	T50.A92	T50.A93	T50.A94	T50.A95	T50.A96
combination						
including pertussis	T50.A11	T50.A12	T50.A13	T50.A14	T50.A15	T50.A16
without pertussis	T50.A21	T50.A22	T50.A23	T50.A24	T50.A25	T50.A26
Diphylline	T50.2X1	T50.2X2	T50.2X3	T50.2X4	T50.2X5	T50.2X6
Dipipanone	T40.4X1	T40.4X2	T40.4X3	T40.4X4	—	—
Dipivefrine	T49.5X1	T49.5X2	T49.5X3	T49.5X4	T49.5X5	T49.5X6
Diplovax	T50.B91	T50.B92	T50.B93	T50.B94	T50.B95	T50.B96
Diprophylline	T50.2X1	T50.2X2	T50.2X3	T50.2X4	T50.2X5	T50.2X6
Dipropyline	T48.291	T48.292	T48.293	T48.294	T48.295	T48.296
Dipyridamole	T46.3X1	T46.3X2	T46.3X3	T46.3X4	T46.3X5	T46.3X6
Dipyrone	T39.2X1	T39.2X2	T39.2X3	T39.2X4	T39.2X5	T39.2X6
Diquat (dibromide)	T60.3X1	T60.3X2	T60.3X3	T60.3X4	—	—
Disinfectant	T65.891	T65.892	T65.893	T65.894	—	—
alkaline	T54.3X1	T54.3X2	T54.3X3	T54.3X4	—	—
aromatic	T54.1X1	T54.1X2	T54.1X3	T54.1X4	—	—
intestinal	T37.8X1	T37.8X2	T37.8X3	T37.8X4	T37.8X5	T37.8X6
Disipal	T42.8X1	T42.8X2	T42.8X3	T42.8X4	T42.8X5	T42.8X6
Disodium edetate	T50.6X1	T50.6X2	T50.6X3	T50.6X4	T50.6X5	T50.6X6
Disoprofol	T41.291	T41.292	T41.293	T41.294	T41.295	T41.296
Disopyramide	T46.2X1	T46.2X2	T46.2X3	T46.2X4	T46.2X5	T46.2X6
Distigmine (bromide)	T44.0X1	T44.0X2	T44.0X3	T44.0X4	T44.0X5	T44.0X6
Disulfamide	T50.2X1	T50.2X2	T50.2X3	T50.2X4	T50.2X5	T50.2X6
Disulfanilamide	T37.0X1	T37.0X2	T37.0X3	T37.0X4	T37.0X5	T37.0X6
Disulfiram	T50.6X1	T50.6X2	T50.6X3	T50.6X4	T50.6X5	T50.6X6
Disulfoton	T60.0X1	T60.0X2	T60.0X3	T60.0X4	—	—
Dithiazanine iodide	T37.4X1	T37.4X2	T37.4X3	T37.4X4	T37.4X5	T37.4X6
Dithiocarbamate	T60.0X1	T60.0X2	T60.0X3	T60.0X4	—	—
Dithranol	T49.4X1	T49.4X2	T49.4X3	T49.4X4	T49.4X5	T49.4X6
Diucardin	T50.2X1	T50.2X2	T50.2X3	T50.2X4	T50.2X5	T50.2X6
Diupres	T50.2X1	T50.2X2	T50.2X3	T50.2X4	T50.2X5	T50.2X6
Diuretic NEC	T50.2X1	T50.2X2	T50.2X3	T50.2X4	T50.2X5	T50.2X6
benzothiadiazine	T50.2X1	T50.2X2	T50.2X3	T50.2X4	T50.2X5	T50.2X6
carbonic acid anhydrase inhibitors	T50.2X1	T50.2X2	T50.2X3	T50.2X4	T50.2X5	T50.2X6

◀ New   ◀ Revised   ~~deleted~~ Deleted

	External Cause (T-Code)					
Substance	Poisoning, Accidental (Unintentional)	Poisoning, Intentional Self-Harm	Poisoning, Assault	Poisoning, Undetermined	Adverse Effect	Underdosing
Diuretic NEC *(Continued)*						
furfuryl NEC	T50.2X1	T50.2X2	T50.2X3	T50.2X4	T50.2X5	T50.2X6
loop (high-ceiling)	T50.1X1	T50.1X2	T50.1X3	T50.1X4	T50.1X5	T50.1X6
mercurial NEC	T50.2X1	T50.2X2	T50.2X3	T50.2X4	T50.2X5	T50.2X6
osmotic	T50.2X1	T50.2X2	T50.2X3	T50.2X4	T50.2X5	T50.2X6
purine NEC	T50.2X1	T50.2X2	T50.2X3	T50.2X4	T50.2X5	T50.2X6
saluretic NEC	T50.2X1	T50.2X2	T50.2X3	T50.2X4	T50.2X5	T50.2X6
sulfonamide	T50.2X1	T50.2X2	T50.2X3	T50.2X4	T50.2X5	T50.2X6
thiazide NEC	T50.2X1	T50.2X2	T50.2X3	T50.2X4	T50.2X5	T50.2X6
xanthine	T50.2X1	T50.2X2	T50.2X3	T50.2X4	T50.2X5	T50.2X6
Diurgin	T50.2X1	T50.2X2	T50.2X3	T50.2X4	T50.2X5	T50.2X6
Diuril	T50.2X1	T50.2X2	T50.2X3	T50.2X4	T50.2X5	T50.2X6
Diuron	T60.3X1	T60.3X2	T60.3X3	T60.3X4	—	—
Divalproex	T42.6X1	T42.6X2	T42.6X3	T42.6X4	T42.6X5	T42.6X6
Divinyl ether	T41.0X1	T41.0X2	T41.0X3	T41.0X4	T41.0X5	T41.0X6
Dixanthogen	T49.0X1	T49.0X2	T49.0X3	T49.0X4	T49.0X5	T49.0X6
Dixyrazine	T43.3X1	T43.3X2	T43.3X3	T43.3X4	T43.3X5	T43.3X6
D-lysergic acid diethylamide	T40.8X1	T40.8X2	T40.8X3	T40.8X4	—	—
DMCT	T36.4X1	T36.4X2	T36.4X3	T36.4X4	T36.4X5	T36.4X6
DMSO — *see Dimethyl sulfoxide*						
DNBP	T60.3X1	T60.3X2	T60.3X3	T60.3X4	—	—
DNOC	T65.3X1	T65.3X2	T65.3X3	T65.3X4	—	—
DOCA	T38.0X1	T38.0X2	T38.0X3	T38.0X4	T38.0X5	T38.0X6
Dobutamine	T44.5X1	T44.5X2	T44.5X3	T44.5X4	T44.5X5	T44.5X6
Docusate sodium	T47.4X1	T47.4X2	T47.4X3	T47.4X4	T47.4X5	T47.4X6
Dodicin	T49.0X1	T49.0X2	T49.0X3	T49.0X4	T49.0X5	T49.0X6
Dofamium chloride	T49.0X1	T49.0X2	T49.0X3	T49.0X4	T49.0X5	T49.0X6
Dolophine	T40.3X1	T40.3X2	T40.3X3	T40.3X4	T40.3X5	T40.3X6
Doloxene	T39.8X1	T39.8X2	T39.8X3	T39.8X4	T39.8X5	T39.8X6
Domestic gas (after combustion) — *see Gas, utility*						
prior to combustion	T59.891	T59.892	T59.893	T59.894	—	—
Domiodol	T48.4X1	T48.4X2	T48.4X3	T48.4X4	T48.4X5	T48.4X6
Domiphen (bromide)	T49.0X1	T49.0X2	T49.0X3	T49.0X4	T49.0X5	T49.0X6
Domperidone	T45.0X1	T45.0X2	T45.0X3	T45.0X4	T45.0X5	T45.0X6
Dopa	T42.8X1	T42.8X2	T42.8X3	T42.8X4	T42.8X5	T42.8X6
Dopamine	T44.991	T44.992	T44.993	T44.994	T44.995	T44.996
Doriden	T42.6X1	T42.6X2	T42.6X3	T42.6X4	T42.6X5	T42.6X6
Dormiral	T42.3X1	T42.3X2	T42.3X3	T42.3X4	T42.3X5	T42.3X6
Dormison	T42.6X1	T42.6X2	T42.6X3	T42.6X4	T42.6X5	T42.6X6
Dornase	T48.4X1	T48.4X2	T48.4X3	T48.4X4	T48.4X5	T48.4X6

◀ New　◀IIII Revised　~~deleted~~ Deleted

Substance	Poisoning, Accidental (Unintentional)	Poisoning, Intentional Self-Harm	Poisoning, Assault	Poisoning, Undetermined	Adverse Effect	Underdosing
	External Cause (T-Code)					
Dorsacaine	T41.3X1	T41.3X2	T41.3X3	T41.3X4	T41.3X5	T41.3X6
Dosulepin	T43.011	T43.012	T43.013	T43.014	T43.015	T43.016
Dothiepin	T43.011	T43.012	T43.013	T43.014	T43.015	T43.016
Doxantrazole	T48.6X1	T48.6X2	T48.6X3	T48.6X4	T48.6X5	T48.6X6
Doxapram	T50.7X1	T50.7X2	T50.7X3	T50.7X4	T50.7X5	T50.7X6
Doxazosin	T44.6X1	T44.6X2	T44.6X3	T44.6X4	T44.6X5	T44.6X6
Doxepin	T43.011	T43.012	T43.013	T43.014	T43.015	T43.016
Doxifluridine	T45.1X1	T45.1X2	T45.1X3	T45.1X4	T45.1X5	T45.1X6
Doxorubicin	T45.1X1	T45.1X2	T45.1X3	T45.1X4	T45.1X5	T45.1X6
Doxycycline	T36.4X1	T36.4X2	T36.4X3	T36.4X4	T36.4X5	T36.4X6
Doxylamine	T45.0X1	T45.0X2	T45.0X3	T45.0X4	T45.0X5	T45.0X6
Dramamine	T45.0X1	T45.0X2	T45.0X3	T45.0X4	T45.0X5	T45.0X6
Drano (drain cleaner)	T54.3X1	T54.3X2	T54.3X3	T54.3X4	—	—
Dressing, live pulp	T49.7X1	T49.7X2	T49.7X3	T49.7X4	T49.7X5	T49.7X6
Drocode	T40.2X1	T40.2X2	T40.2X3	T40.2X4	T40.2X5	T40.2X6
Dromoran	T40.2X1	T40.2X2	T40.2X3	T40.2X4	T40.2X5	T40.2X6
Dromostanolone	T38.7X1	T38.7X2	T38.7X3	T38.7X4	T38.7X5	T38.7X6
Dronabinol	T40.7X1	T40.7X2	T40.7X3	T40.7X4	T40.7X5	T40.7X6
Droperidol	T43.591	T43.592	T43.593	T43.594	T43.595	T43.596
Dropropizine	T48.3X1	T48.3X2	T48.3X3	T48.3X4	T48.3X5	T48.3X6
Drostanolone	T38.7X1	T38.7X2	T38.7X3	T38.7X4	T38.7X5	T38.7X6
Drotaverine	T44.3X1	T44.3X2	T44.3X3	T44.3X4	T44.3X5	T44.3X6
Drotrecogin alfa	T45.511	T45.512	T45.513	T45.514	T45.515	T45.516
Drug NEC	T50.901	T50.902	T50.903	T50.904	T50.905	T50.906
specified NEC	T50.991	T50.992	T50.993	T50.994	T50.995	T50.996
DTIC	T45.1X1	T45.1X2	T45.1X3	T45.1X4	T45.1X5	T45.1X6
Duboisine	T44.3X1	T44.3X2	T44.3X3	T44.3X4	T44.3X5	T44.3X6
Dulcolax	T47.2X1	T47.2X2	T47.2X3	T47.2X4	T47.2X5	T47.2X6
Duponol (C) (EP)	T49.2X1	T49.2X2	T49.2X3	T49.2X4	T49.2X5	T49.2X6
Durabolin	T38.7X1	T38.7X2	T38.7X3	T38.7X4	T38.7X5	T38.7X6
Dyclone	T41.3X1	T41.3X2	T41.3X3	T41.3X4	T41.3X5	T41.3X6
Dyclonine	T41.3X1	T41.3X2	T41.3X3	T41.3X4	T41.3X5	T41.3X6
Dydrogesterone	T38.5X1	T38.5X2	T38.5X3	T38.5X4	T38.5X5	T38.5X6
Dye NEC	T65.6X1	T65.6X2	T65.6X3	T65.6X4	—	—
antiseptic	T49.0X1	T49.0X2	T49.0X3	T49.0X4	T49.0X5	T49.0X6
diagnostic agents	T50.8X1	T50.8X2	T50.8X3	T50.8X4	T50.8X5	T50.8X6
pharmaceutical NEC	T50.901	T50.902	T50.903	T50.904	T50.905	T50.906
Dyflos	T44.0X1	T44.0X2	T44.0X3	T44.0X4	T44.0X5	T44.0X6
Dymelor	T38.3X1	T38.3X2	T38.3X3	T38.3X4	T38.3X5	T38.3X6

◀ New ◀▥ Revised deleted Deleted

Substance	External Cause (T-Code)					
	Poisoning, Accidental (Unintentional)	Poisoning, Intentional Self-Harm	Poisoning, Assault	Poisoning, Undetermined	Adverse Effect	Underdosing
Dynamite	T65.3X1	T65.3X2	T65.3X3	T65.3X4	—	—
fumes	T59.891	T59.892	T59.893	T59.894	—	—
Dyphylline	T44.3X1	T44.3X2	T44.3X3	T44.3X4	T44.3X5	T44.3X6
E						
Ear drug NEC	T49.6X1	T49.6X2	T49.6X3	T49.6X4	T49.6X5	T49.6X6
Ear preparations	T49.6X1	T49.6X2	T49.6X3	T49.6X4	T49.6X5	T49.6X6
Econazole	T49.0X1	T49.0X2	T49.0X3	T49.0X4	T49.0X5	T49.0X6
Ecothiopate iodide	T49.5X1	T49.5X2	T49.5X3	T49.5X4	T49.5X5	T49.5X6
Echothiophate, echothiopate, ecothiopate	T49.5X1	T49.5X2	T49.5X3	T49.5X4	T49.5X5	T49.5X6
Ecstasy	T43.621	T43.622	T43.623	T43.624	T43.625	T43.626
Ectylurea	T42.6X1	T42.6X2	T42.6X3	T42.6X4	T42.6X5	T42.6X6
Edathamil disodium	T45.8X1	T45.8X2	T45.8X3	T45.8X4	T45.8X5	T45.8X6
Edecrin	T50.1X1	T50.1X2	T50.1X3	T50.1X4	T50.1X5	T50.1X6
Edetate, disodium (calcium)	T45.8X1	T45.8X2	T45.8X3	T45.8X4	T45.8X5	T45.8X6
Edoxudine	T49.5X1	T49.5X2	T49.5X3	T49.5X4	T49.5X5	T49.5X6
Edrophonium	T44.0X1	T44.0X2	T44.0X3	T44.0X4	T44.0X5	T44.0X6
chloride	T44.0X1	T44.0X2	T44.0X3	T44.0X4	T44.0X5	T44.0X6
EDTA	T50.6X1	T50.6X2	T50.6X3	T50.6X4	T50.6X5	T50.6X6
Eflornithine	T37.2X1	T37.2X2	T37.2X3	T37.2X4	T37.2X5	T37.2X6
Efloxate	T46.3X1	T46.3X2	T46.3X3	T46.3X4	T46.3X5	T46.3X6
Elase	T49.8X1	T49.8X2	T49.8X3	T49.8X4	T49.8X5	T49.8X6
Elastase	T47.5X1	T47.5X2	T47.5X3	T47.5X4	T47.5X5	T47.5X6
Elaterium	T47.2X1	T47.2X2	T47.2X3	T47.2X4	T47.2X5	T47.2X6
Elcatonin	T50.991	T50.992	T50.993	T50.994	T50.995	T50.996
Elder	T62.2X1	T62.2X2	T62.2X3	T62.2X4	—	—
berry (unripe)	T62.1X1	T62.1X2	T62.1X3	T62.1X4	—	—
Electrolyte balance drug	T50.3X1	T50.3X2	T50.3X3	T50.3X4	T50.3X5	T50.3X6
Electrolytes NEC	T50.3X1	T50.3X2	T50.3X3	T50.3X4	T50.3X5	T50.3X6
Electrolytic agent NEC	T50.3X1	T50.3X2	T50.3X3	T50.3X4	T50.3X5	T50.3X6
Elemental diet	T50.901	T50.902	T50.903	T50.904	T50.905	T50.906
Elliptinium acetate	T45.1X1	T45.1X2	T45.1X3	T45.1X4	T45.1X5	T45.1X6
Embramine	T45.0X1	T45.0X2	T45.0X3	T45.0X4	T45.0X5	T45.0X6
Emepronium (salts)	T44.3X1	T44.3X2	T44.3X3	T44.3X4	T44.3X5	T44.3X6
bromide	T44.3X1	T44.3X2	T44.3X3	T44.3X4	T44.3X5	T44.3X6
Emetic NEC	T47.7X1	T47.7X2	T47.7X3	T47.7X4	T47.7X5	T47.7X6
Emetine	T37.3X1	T37.3X2	T37.3X3	T37.3X4	T37.3X5	T37.3X6
Emollient NEC	T49.3X1	T49.3X2	T49.3X3	T49.3X4	T49.3X5	T49.3X6
Emorfazone	T39.8X1	T39.8X2	T39.8X3	T39.8X4	T39.8X5	T39.8X6

Substance	Poisoning, Accidental (Unintentional)	Poisoning, Intentional Self-Harm	Poisoning, Assault	Poisoning, Undetermined	Adverse Effect	Underdosing
Emylcamate	T43.591	T43.592	T43.593	T43.594	T43.595	T43.596
Enalapril	T46.4X1	T46.4X2	T46.4X3	T46.4X4	T46.4X5	T46.4X6
Enalaprilat	T46.4X1	T46.4X2	T46.4X3	T46.4X4	T46.4X5	T46.4X6
Encainide	T46.2X1	T46.2X2	T46.2X3	T46.2X4	T46.2X5	T46.2X6
Endocaine	T41.3X1	T41.3X2	T41.3X3	T41.3X4	T41.3X5	T41.3X6
Endosulfan	T60.2X1	T60.2X2	T60.2X3	T60.2X4	—	—
Endothall	T60.3X1	T60.3X2	T60.3X3	T60.3X4	—	—
Endralazine	T46.5X1	T46.5X2	T46.5X3	T46.5X4	T46.5X5	T46.5X6
Endrin	T60.1X1	T60.1X2	T60.1X3	T60.1X4	—	—
Enflurane	T41.0X1	T41.0X2	T41.0X3	T41.0X4	T41.0X5	T41.0X6
Enhexymal	T42.3X1	T42.3X2	T42.3X3	T42.3X4	T42.3X5	T42.3X6
Enocitabine	T45.1X1	T45.1X2	T45.1X3	T45.1X4	T45.1X5	T45.1X6
Enovid	T38.4X1	T38.4X2	T38.4X3	T38.4X4	T38.4X5	T38.4X6
Enoxacin	T36.8X1	T36.8X2	T36.8X3	T36.8X4	T36.8X5	T36.8X6
Enoxaparin (sodium)	T45.511	T45.512	T45.513	T45.514	T45.515	T45.516
Enpiprazole	T43.591	T43.592	T43.593	T43.594	T43.595	T43.596
Enprofylline	T48.6X1	T48.6X2	T48.6X3	T48.6X4	T48.6X5	T48.6X6
Enprostil	T47.1X1	T47.1X2	T47.1X3	T47.1X4	T47.1X5	T47.1X6
ENT preparations (anti-infectives)	T49.6X1	T49.6X2	T49.6X3	T49.6X4	T49.6X5	T49.6X6
Enviomycin	T36.8X1	T36.8X2	T36.8X3	T36.8X4	T36.8X5	T36.8X6
Enzodase	T45.3X1	T45.3X2	T45.3X3	T45.3X4	T45.3X5	T45.3X6
Enzyme NEC	T45.3X1	T45.3X2	T45.3X3	T45.3X4	T45.3X5	T45.3X6
depolymerizing	T49.8X1	T49.8X2	T49.8X3	T49.8X4	T49.8X5	T49.8X6
fibrolytic	T45.3X1	T45.3X2	T45.3X3	T45.3X4	T45.3X5	T45.3X6
gastric	T47.5X1	T47.5X2	T47.5X3	T47.5X4	T47.5X5	T47.5X6
intestinal	T47.5X1	T47.5X2	T47.5X3	T47.5X4	T47.5X5	T47.5X6
local action	T49.4X1	T49.4X2	T49.4X3	T49.4X4	T49.4X5	T49.4X6
proteolytic	T49.4X1	T49.4X2	T49.4X3	T49.4X4	T49.4X5	T49.4X6
thrombolytic	T45.3X1	T45.3X2	T45.3X3	T45.3X4	T45.3X5	T45.3X6
EPAB	T41.3X1	T41.3X2	T41.3X3	T41.3X4	T41.3X5	T41.3X6
Epanutin	T42.0X1	T42.0X2	T42.0X3	T42.0X4	T42.0X5	T42.0X6
Ephedra	T44.991	T44.992	T44.993	T44.994	T44.995	T44.996
Ephedrine	T44.991	T44.992	T44.993	T44.994	T44.995	T44.996
Epichlorhydrin, epichlorohydrin	T52.8X1	T52.8X2	T52.8X3	T52.8X4	—	—
Epicillin	T36.0X1	T36.0X2	T36.0X3	T36.0X4	T36.0X5	T36.0X6
Epiestriol	T38.5X1	T38.5X2	T38.5X3	T38.5X4	T38.5X5	T38.5X6
Epilim — *see Sodium valproate*						
Epimestrol	T38.5X1	T38.5X2	T38.5X3	T38.5X4	T38.5X5	T38.5X6
Epinephrine	T44.5X1	T44.5X2	T44.5X3	T44.5X4	T44.5X5	T44.5X6

◀ New   ◀▥ Revised   ~~deleted~~ Deleted

Substance	External Cause (T-Code)					
	Poisoning, Accidental (Unintentional)	Poisoning, Intentional Self-Harm	Poisoning, Assault	Poisoning, Undetermined	Adverse Effect	Underdosing
Epirubicin	T45.1X1	T45.1X2	T45.1X3	T45.1X4	T45.1X5	T45.1X6
Epitiostanol	T38.7X1	T38.7X2	T38.7X3	T38.7X4	T38.7X5	T38.7X6
Epitizide	T50.2X1	T50.2X2	T50.2X3	T50.2X4	T50.2X5	T50.2X6
EPN	T60.0X1	T60.0X2	T60.0X3	T60.0X4	—	—
EPO	T45.8X1	T45.8X2	T45.8X3	T45.8X4	T45.8X5	T45.8X6
Epoetin alpha	T45.8X1	T45.8X2	T45.8X3	T45.8X4	T45.8X5	T45.8X6
Epomediol	T50.991	T50.992	T50.993	T50.994	T50.995	T50.996
Epoprostenol	T45.521	T45.522	T45.523	T45.524	T45.525	T45.526
Epoxy resin	T65.891	T65.892	T65.893	T65.894	—	—
Eprazinone	T48.4X1	T48.4X2	T48.4X3	T48.4X4	T48.4X5	T48.4X6
Epsilon amino-caproic acid	T45.621	T45.622	T45.623	T45.624	T45.625	T45.626
Epsom salt	T47.3X1	T47.3X2	T47.3X3	T47.3X4	T47.3X5	T47.3X6
Eptazocine	T40.4X1	T40.4X2	T40.4X3	T40.4X4	T40.4X5	T40.4X6
Equanil	T43.591	T43.592	T43.593	T43.594	T43.595	T43.596
Equisetum	T62.2X1	T62.2X2	T62.2X3	T62.2X4	—	—
diuretic	T50.2X1	T50.2X2	T50.2X3	T50.2X4	T50.2X5	T50.2X6
Ergobasine	T48.0X1	T48.0X2	T48.0X3	T48.0X4	T48.0X5	T48.0X6
Ergocalciferol	T45.2X1	T45.2X2	T45.2X3	T45.2X4	T45.2X5	T45.2X6
Ergoloid mesylates	T46.7X1	T46.7X2	T46.7X3	T46.7X4	T46.7X5	T46.7X6
Ergometrine	T48.0X1	T48.0X2	T48.0X3	T48.0X4	T48.0X5	T48.0X6
Ergonovine	T48.0X1	T48.0X2	T48.0X3	T48.0X4	T48.0X5	T48.0X6
Ergot NEC	T64.81	T64.82	T64.83	T64.84	—	—
derivative	T48.0X1	T48.0X2	T48.0X3	T48.0X4	T48.0X5	T48.0X6
medicinal (alkaloids)	T48.0X1	T48.0X2	T48.0X3	T48.0X4	T48.0X5	T48.0X6
prepared	T48.0X1	T48.0X2	T48.0X3	T48.0X4	T48.0X5	T48.0X6
Ergotamine	T46.5X1	T46.5X2	T46.5X3	T46.5X4	T46.5X5	T46.5X6
Ergotocine	T48.0X1	T48.0X2	T48.0X3	T48.0X4	T48.0X5	T48.0X6
Ergotrate	T48.0X1	T48.0X2	T48.0X3	T48.0X4	T48.0X5	T48.0X6
Eritrityl tetranitrate	T46.3X1	T46.3X2	T46.3X3	T46.3X4	T46.3X5	T46.3X6
Erythrityl tetranitrate	T46.3X1	T46.3X2	T46.3X3	T46.3X4	T46.3X5	T46.3X6
Erythrol tetranitrate	T46.3X1	T46.3X2	T46.3X3	T46.3X4	T46.3X5	T46.3X6
Erythromycin (salts)	T36.3X1	T36.3X2	T36.3X3	T36.3X4	T36.3X5	T36.3X6
ophthalmic preparation	T49.5X1	T49.5X2	T49.5X3	T49.5X4	T49.5X5	T49.5X6
topical NEC	T49.0X1	T49.0X2	T49.0X3	T49.0X4	T49.0X5	T49.0X6
Erythropoietin	T45.8X1	T45.8X2	T45.8X3	T45.8X4	T45.8X5	T45.8X6
human	T45.8X1	T45.8X2	T45.8X3	T45.8X4	T45.8X5	T45.8X6
Escin	T46.991	T46.992	T46.993	T46.994	T46.995	T46.996
Esculin	T45.2X1	T45.2X2	T45.2X3	T45.2X4	T45.2X5	T45.2X6
Esculoside	T45.2X1	T45.2X2	T45.2X3	T45.2X4	T45.2X5	T45.2X6

Substance	External Cause (T-Code)					
	Poisoning, Accidental (Unintentional)	Poisoning, Intentional Self-Harm	Poisoning, Assault	Poisoning, Undetermined	Adverse Effect	Underdosing
ESDT (ether-soluble tar distillate)	T49.1X1	T49.1X2	T49.1X3	T49.1X4	T49.1X5	T49.1X6
Eserine	T49.5X1	T49.5X2	T49.5X3	T49.5X4	T49.5X5	T49.5X6
Esflurbiprofen	T39.311	T39.312	T39.313	T39.314	T39.315	T39.316
Eskabarb	T42.3X1	T42.3X2	T42.3X3	T42.3X4	T42.3X5	T42.3X6
Eskalith	T43.8X1	T43.8X2	T43.8X3	T43.8X4	T43.8X5	T43.8X6
Esmolol	T44.7X1	T44.7X2	T44.7X3	T44.7X4	T44.7X5	T44.7X6
Estanozolol	T38.7X1	T38.7X2	T38.7X3	T38.7X4	T38.7X5	T38.7X6
Estazolam	T42.4X1	T42.4X2	T42.4X3	T42.4X4	T42.4X5	T42.4X6
Estradiol	T38.5X1	T38.5X2	T38.5X3	T38.5X4	T38.5X5	T38.5X6
with testosterone	T38.7X1	T38.7X2	T38.7X3	T38.7X4	T38.7X5	T38.7X6
benzoate	T38.5X1	T38.5X2	T38.5X3	T38.5X4	T38.5X5	T38.5X6
Estramustine	T45.1X1	T45.1X2	T45.1X3	T45.1X4	T45.1X5	T45.1X6
Estriol	T38.5X1	T38.5X2	T38.5X3	T38.5X4	T38.5X5	T38.5X6
Estrogen	T38.5X1	T38.5X2	T38.5X3	T38.5X4	T38.5X5	T38.5X6
with progesterone	T38.5X1	T38.5X2	T38.5X3	T38.5X4	T38.5X5	T38.5X6
conjugated	T38.5X1	T38.5X2	T38.5X3	T38.5X4	T38.5X5	T38.5X6
Estrone	T38.5X1	T38.5X2	T38.5X3	T38.5X4	T38.5X5	T38.5X6
Estropipate	T38.5X1	T38.5X2	T38.5X3	T38.5X4	T38.5X5	T38.5X6
Etacrynate sodium	T50.1X1	T50.1X2	T50.1X3	T50.1X4	T50.1X5	T50.1X6
Etacrynic acid	T50.1X1	T50.1X2	T50.1X3	T50.1X4	T50.1X5	T50.1X6
Etafedrine	T48.6X1	T48.6X2	T48.6X3	T48.6X4	T48.6X5	T48.6X6
Etafenone	T46.3X1	T46.3X2	T46.3X3	T46.3X4	T46.3X5	T46.3X6
Etambutol	T37.1X1	T37.1X2	T37.1X3	T37.1X4	T37.1X5	T37.1X6
Etamiphyllin	T48.6X1	T48.6X2	T48.6X3	T48.6X4	T48.6X5	T48.6X6
Etamivan	T50.7X1	T50.7X2	T50.7X3	T50.7X4	T50.7X5	T50.7X6
Etamsylate	T45.7X1	T45.7X2	T45.7X3	T45.7X4	T45.7X5	T45.7X6
Etebenecid	T50.4X1	T50.4X2	T50.4X3	T50.4X4	T50.4X5	T50.4X6
Ethacridine	T49.0X1	T49.0X2	T49.0X3	T49.0X4	T49.0X5	T49.0X6
Ethacrynic acid	T50.1X1	T50.1X2	T50.1X3	T50.1X4	T50.1X5	T50.1X6
Ethadione	T42.2X1	T42.2X2	T42.2X3	T42.2X4	T42.2X5	T42.2X6
Ethambutol	T37.1X1	T37.1X2	T37.1X3	T37.1X4	T37.1X5	T37.1X6
Ethamide	T50.2X1	T50.2X2	T50.2X3	T50.2X4	T50.2X5	T50.2X6
Ethamivan	T50.7X1	T50.7X2	T50.7X3	T50.7X4	T50.7X5	T50.7X6
Ethamsylate	T45.7X1	T45.7X2	T45.7X3	T45.7X4	T45.7X5	T45.7X6
Ethanol	T51.0X1	T51.0X2	T51.0X3	T51.0X4	—	—
beverage	T51.0X1	T51.0X2	T51.0X3	T51.0X4	—	—
Ethanolamine oleate	T46.8X1	T46.8X2	T46.8X3	T46.8X4	T46.8X5	T46.8X6
Ethaverine	T44.3X1	T44.3X2	T44.3X3	T44.3X4	T44.3X5	T44.3X6
Ethchlorvynol	T42.6X1	T42.6X2	T42.6X3	T42.6X4	T42.6X5	T42.6X6
Ethebenecid	T50.4X1	T50.4X2	T50.4X3	T50.4X4	T50.4X5	T50.4X6

◀ New ◀ Revised deleted Deleted

Substance	Poisoning, Accidental (Unintentional)	Poisoning, Intentional Self-Harm	Poisoning, Assault	Poisoning, Undetermined	Adverse Effect	Underdosing
	External Cause (T-Code)					
Ether (vapor)	T41.0X1	T41.0X2	T41.0X3	T41.0X4	T41.0X5	T41.0X6
anesthetic	T41.0X1	T41.0X2	T41.0X3	T41.0X4	T41.0X5	T41.0X6
divinyl	T41.0X1	T41.0X2	T41.0X3	T41.0X4	T41.0X5	T41.0X6
ethyl (medicinal)	T41.0X1	T41.0X2	T41.0X3	T41.0X4	T41.0X5	T41.0X6
nonmedicinal	T52.8X1	T52.8X2	T52.8X3	T52.8X4	—	—
petroleum — *see Ligroin*						
solvent	T52.8X1	T52.8X2	T52.8X3	T52.8X4	—	—
Ethiazide	T50.2X1	T50.2X2	T50.2X3	T50.2X4	T50.2X5	T50.2X6
Ethidium chloride (vapor)	T59.891	T59.892	T59.893	T59.894	—	—
Ethinamate	T42.6X1	T42.6X2	T42.6X3	T42.6X4	T42.6X5	T42.6X6
Ethinylestradiol, ethinyloestradiol	T38.5X1	T38.5X2	T38.5X3	T38.5X4	T38.5X5	T38.5X6
with						
levonorgestrel	T38.4X1	T38.4X2	T38.4X3	T38.4X4	T38.4X5	T38.4X6
norethisterone	T38.4X1	T38.4X2	T38.4X3	T38.4X4	T38.4X5	T38.4X6
Ethiodized oil (131 I)	T50.8X1	T50.8X2	T50.8X3	T50.8X4	T50.8X5	T50.8X6
Ethion	T60.0X1	T60.0X2	T60.0X3	T60.0X4	—	—
Ethionamide	T37.1X1	T37.1X2	T37.1X3	T37.1X4	T37.1X5	T37.1X6
Ethioniamide	T37.1X1	T37.1X2	T37.1X3	T37.1X4	T37.1X5	T37.1X6
Ethisterone	T38.5X1	T38.5X2	T38.5X3	T38.5X4	T38.5X5	T38.5X6
Ethobral	T42.3X1	T42.3X2	T42.3X3	T42.3X4	T42.3X5	T42.3X6
Ethocaine (infiltration) (topical)	T41.3X1	T41.3X2	T41.3X3	T41.3X4	T41.3X5	T41.3X6
nerve block (peripheral) (plexus)	T41.3X1	T41.3X2	T41.3X3	T41.3X4	T41.3X5	T41.3X6
spinal	T41.3X1	T41.3X2	T41.3X3	T41.3X4	T41.3X5	T41.3X6
Ethoheptazine	T40.4X1	T40.4X2	T40.4X3	T40.4X4	T40.4X5	T40.4X6
Ethopropazine	T44.3X1	T44.3X2	T44.3X3	T44.3X4	T44.3X5	T44.3X6
Ethosuximide	T42.2X1	T42.2X2	T42.2X3	T42.2X4	T42.2X5	T42.2X6
Ethotoin	T42.0X1	T42.0X2	T42.0X3	T42.0X4	T42.0X5	T42.0X6
Ethoxazene	T37.91	T37.92	T37.93	T37.94	T37.95	T37.96
Ethoxazorutoside	T46.991	T46.992	T46.993	T46.994	T46.995	T46.996
2-Ethoxyethanol	T52.3X1	T52.3X2	T52.3X3	T52.3X4	—	—
Ethoxzolamide	T50.2X1	T50.2X2	T50.2X3	T50.2X4	T50.2X5	T50.2X6
Ethyl						
acetate	T52.8X1	T52.8X2	T52.8X3	T52.8X4	—	—
alcohol	T51.0X1	T51.0X2	T51.0X3	T51.0X4	—	—
beverage	T51.0X1	T51.0X2	T51.0X3	T51.0X4	—	—
aldehyde (vapor)	T59.891	T59.892	T59.893	T59.894	—	—
liquid	T52.8X1	T52.8X2	T52.8X3	T52.8X4	—	—
aminobenzoate	T41.3X1	T41.3X2	T41.3X3	T41.3X4	T41.3X5	T41.3X6
aminophenothiazine	T43.3X1	T43.3X2	T43.3X3	T43.3X4	T43.3X5	T43.3X6
benzoate	T52.8X1	T52.8X2	T52.8X3	T52.8X4	—	—

TABLE OF DRUGS AND CHEMICALS

	External Cause (T-Code)					
Substance	Poisoning, Accidental (Unintentional)	Poisoning, Intentional Self-Harm	Poisoning, Assault	Poisoning, Undetermined	Adverse Effect	Underdosing
Ethyl *(Continued)*						
biscoumacetate	T45.511	T45.512	T45.513	T45.514	T45.515	T45.516
bromide (anesthetic)	T41.0X1	T41.0X2	T41.0X3	T41.0X4	T41.0X5	T41.0X6
carbamate	T45.1X1	T45.1X2	T45.1X3	T45.1X4	T45.1X5	T45.1X6
carbinol	T51.3X1	T51.3X2	T51.3X3	T51.3X4	—	—
carbonate	T52.8X1	T52.8X2	T52.8X3	T52.8X4	—	—
chaulmoograte	T37.1X1	T37.1X2	T37.1X3	T37.1X4	T37.1X5	T37.1X6
chloride (anesthetic)	T41.0X1	T41.0X2	T41.0X3	T41.0X4	T41.0X5	T41.0X6
anesthetic (local)	T41.3X1	T41.3X2	T41.3X3	T41.3X4	T41.3X5	T41.3X6
inhaled	T41.0X1	T41.0X2	T41.0X3	T41.0X4	T41.0X5	T41.0X6
local	T49.4X1	T49.4X2	T49.4X3	T49.4X4	T49.4X5	T49.4X6
solvent	T53.6X1	T53.6X2	T53.6X3	T53.6X4	—	—
dibunate	T48.3X1	T48.3X2	T48.3X3	T48.3X4	T48.3X5	T48.3X6
dichloroarsine (vapor)	T57.0X1	T57.0X2	T57.0X3	T57.0X4	—	—
estranol	T38.7X1	T38.7X2	T38.7X3	T38.7X4	T38.7X5	T38.7X6
ether — *see also ether*	T52.8X1	T52.8X2	T52.8X3	T52.8X4	—	—
formate NEC (solvent)	T52.0X1	T52.0X2	T52.0X3	T52.0X4	—	—
fumarate	T49.4X1	T49.4X2	T49.4X3	T49.4X4	T49.4X5	T49.4X6
hydroxyisobutyrate NEC (solvent)	T52.8X1	T52.8X2	T52.8X3	T52.8X4	—	—
iodoacetate	T59.3X1	T59.3X2	T59.3X3	T59.3X4	—	—
lactate NEC (solvent)	T52.8X1	T52.8X2	T52.8X3	T52.8X4	—	—
loflazepate	T42.4X1	T42.4X2	T42.4X3	T42.4X4	T42.4X5	T42.4X6
mercuric chloride	T56.1X1	T56.1X2	T56.1X3	T56.1X4	—	—
methylcarbinol	T51.8X1	T51.8X2	T51.8X3	T51.8X4	—	—
morphine	T40.2X1	T40.2X2	T40.2X3	T40.2X4	T40.2X5	T40.2X6
noradrenaline	T48.6X1	T48.6X2	T48.6X3	T48.6X4	T48.6X5	T48.6X6
oxybutyrate NEC (solvent)	T52.8X1	T52.8X2	T52.8X3	T52.8X4	—	—
Ethylene (gas)	T59.891	T59.892	T59.893	T59.894	—	—
anesthetic (general)	T41.0X1	T41.0X2	T41.0X3	T41.0X4	T41.0X5	T41.0X6
chlorohydrin	T52.8X1	T52.8X2	T52.8X3	T52.8X4	—	—
vapor	T53.6X1	T53.6X2	T53.6X3	T53.6X4	—	—
dichloride	T52.8X1	T52.8X2	T52.8X3	T52.8X4	—	—
vapor	T53.6X1	T53.6X2	T53.6X3	T53.6X4	—	—
dinitrate	T52.3X1	T52.3X2	T52.3X3	T52.3X4	—	—
glycol(s)	T52.8X1	T52.8X2	T52.8X3	T52.8X4	—	—
dinitrate	T52.3X1	T52.3X2	T52.3X3	T52.3X4	—	—
monobutyl ether	T52.3X1	T52.3X2	T52.3X3	T52.3X4	—	—
imine	T54.1X1	T54.1X2	T54.1X3	T54.1X4	—	—
oxide (fumigant) (nonmedicinal)	T59.891	T59.892	T59.893	T59.894	—	—
medicinal	T49.0X1	T49.0X2	T49.0X3	T49.0X4	T49.0X5	T49.0X6

◀ New ◀‖‖ Revised ~~deleted~~ Deleted

Substance	Poisoning, Accidental (Unintentional)	Poisoning, Intentional Self-Harm	Poisoning, Assault	Poisoning, Undetermined	Adverse Effect	Underdosing
			External Cause (T-Code)			
Ethylenediamine theophylline	T48.6X1	T48.6X2	T48.6X3	T48.6X4	T48.6X5	T48.6X6
Ethylenediaminetetra-acetic acid	T50.6X1	T50.6X2	T50.6X3	T50.6X4	T50.6X5	T50.6X6
Ethylenedinitrilotetra-acetate	T50.6X1	T50.6X2	T50.6X3	T50.6X4	T50.6X5	T50.6X6
Ethylestrenol	T38.7X1	T38.7X2	T38.7X3	T38.7X4	T38.7X5	T38.7X6
Ethylhydroxycellulose	T47.4X1	T47.4X2	T47.4X3	T47.4X4	T47.4X5	T47.4X6
Ethylidene						
chloride NEC	T53.6X1	T53.6X2	T53.6X3	T53.6X4	—	—
diacetate	T60.3X1	T60.3X2	T60.3X3	T60.3X4	—	—
dicoumarin	T45.511	T45.512	T45.513	T45.514	T45.515	T45.516
dicoumarol	T45.511	T45.512	T45.513	T45.514	T45.515	T45.516
diethyl ether	T52.0X1	T52.0X2	T52.0X3	T52.0X4	—	—
Ethylmorphine	T40.2X1	T40.2X2	T40.2X3	T40.2X4	T40.2X5	T40.2X6
Ethylnorepinephrine	T48.6X1	T48.6X2	T48.6X3	T48.6X4	T48.6X5	T48.6X6
Ethylparachlorophen-oxyisobutyrate	T46.6X1	T46.6X2	T46.6X3	T46.6X4	T46.6X5	T46.6X6
Ethynodiol	T38.4X1	T38.4X2	T38.4X3	T38.4X4	T38.4X5	T38.4X6
with mestranol diacetate	T38.4X1	T38.4X2	T38.4X3	T38.4X4	T38.4X5	T38.4X6
Etidocaine	T41.3X1	T41.3X2	T41.3X3	T41.3X4	T41.3X5	T41.3X6
infiltration (subcutaneous)	T41.3X1	T41.3X2	T41.3X3	T41.3X4	T41.3X5	T41.3X6
nerve (peripheral) (plexus)	T41.3X1	T41.3X2	T41.3X3	T41.3X4	T41.3X5	T41.3X6
Etidronate	T50.991	T50.992	T50.993	T50.994	T50.995	T50.996
Etidronic acid (disodium salt)	T50.991	T50.992	T50.993	T50.994	T50.995	T50.996
Etifoxine	T42.6X1	T42.6X2	T42.6X3	T42.6X4	T42.6X5	T42.6X6
Etilefrine	T44.4X1	T44.4X2	T44.4X3	T44.4X4	T44.4X5	T44.4X6
Etilfen	T42.3X1	T42.3X2	T42.3X3	T42.3X4	T42.3X5	T42.3X6
Etinodiol	T38.4X1	T38.4X2	T38.4X3	T38.4X4	T38.4X5	T38.4X6
Etiroxate	T46.6X1	T46.6X2	T46.6X3	T46.6X4	T46.6X5	T46.6X6
Etizolam	T42.4X1	T42.4X2	T42.4X3	T42.4X4	T42.4X5	T42.4X6
Etodolac	T39.391	T39.392	T39.393	T39.394	T39.395	T39.396
Etofamide	T37.3X1	T37.3X2	T37.3X3	T37.3X4	T37.3X5	T37.3X6
Etofibrate	T46.6X1	T46.6X2	T46.6X3	T46.6X4	T46.6X5	T46.6X6
Etofylline	T46.7X1	T46.7X2	T46.7X3	T46.7X4	T46.7X5	T46.7X6
clofibrate	T46.6X1	T46.6X2	T46.6X3	T46.6X4	T46.6X5	T46.6X6
Etoglucid	T45.1X1	T45.1X2	T45.1X3	T45.1X4	T45.1X5	T45.1X6
Etomidate	T41.1X1	T41.1X2	T41.1X3	T41.1X4	T41.1X5	T41.1X6
Etomide	T39.8X1	T39.8X2	T39.8X3	T39.8X4	T39.8X5	T39.8X6
Etomidoline	T44.3X1	T44.3X2	T44.3X3	T44.3X4	T44.3X5	T44.3X6
Etoposide	T45.1X1	T45.1X2	T45.1X3	T45.1X4	T45.1X5	T45.1X6
Etorphine	T40.2X1	T40.2X2	T40.2X3	T40.2X4	T40.2X5	T40.2X6
Etoval	T42.3X1	T42.3X2	T42.3X3	T42.3X4	T42.3X5	T42.3X6
Etozolin	T50.1X1	T50.1X2	T50.1X3	T50.1X4	T50.1X5	T50.1X6

◀ New   ◀||| Revised   ~~deleted~~ Deleted

TABLE OF DRUGS AND CHEMICALS

Substance	External Cause (T-Code)					
	Poisoning, Accidental (Unintentional)	Poisoning, Intentional Self-Harm	Poisoning, Assault	Poisoning, Undetermined	Adverse Effect	Underdosing
Etretinate	T50.991	T50.992	T50.993	T50.994	T50.995	T50.996
Etryptamine	T43.691	T43.692	T43.693	T43.694	T43.695	T43.696
Etybenzatropine	T44.3X1	T44.3X2	T44.3X3	T44.3X4	T44.3X5	T44.3X6
Etynodiol	T38.4X1	T38.4X2	T38.4X3	T38.4X4	T38.4X5	T38.4X6
Eucaine	T41.3X1	T41.3X2	T41.3X3	T41.3X4	T41.3X5	T41.3X6
Eucalyptus oil	T49.7X1	T49.7X2	T49.7X3	T49.7X4	T49.7X5	T49.7X6
Eucatropine	T49.5X1	T49.5X2	T49.5X3	T49.5X4	T49.5X5	T49.5X6
Eucodal	T40.2X1	T40.2X2	T40.2X3	T40.2X4	T40.2X5	T40.2X6
Euneryl	T42.3X1	T42.3X2	T42.3X3	T42.3X4	T42.3X5	T42.3X6
Euphthalmine	T44.3X1	T44.3X2	T44.3X3	T44.3X4	T44.3X5	T44.3X6
Eurax	T49.0X1	T49.0X2	T49.0X3	T49.0X4	T49.0X5	T49.0X6
Euresol	T49.4X1	T49.4X2	T49.4X3	T49.4X4	T49.4X5	T49.4X6
Euthroid	T38.1X1	T38.1X2	T38.1X3	T38.1X4	T38.1X5	T38.1X6
Evans blue	T50.8X1	T50.8X2	T50.8X3	T50.8X4	T50.8X5	T50.8X6
Evipal	T42.3X1	T42.3X2	T42.3X3	T42.3X4	T42.3X5	T42.3X6
sodium	T41.1X1	T41.1X2	T41.1X3	T41.1X4	T41.1X5	T41.1X6
Evipan	T42.3X1	T42.3X2	T42.3X3	T42.3X4	T42.3X5	T42.3X6
sodium	T41.1X1	T41.1X2	T41.1X3	T41.1X4	T41.1X5	T41.1X6
Exalamide	T49.0X1	T49.0X2	T49.0X3	T49.0X4	T49.0X5	T49.0X6
Exalgin	T39.1X1	T39.1X2	T39.1X3	T39.1X4	T39.1X5	T39.1X6
Excipients, pharmaceutical	T50.901	T50.902	T50.903	T50.904	T50.905	T50.906
Exhaust gas (engine) (motor vehicle)	T58.01	T58.02	T58.03	T58.04	—	—
Ex-Lax (phenolphthalein)	T47.2X1	T47.2X2	T47.2X3	T47.2X4	T47.2X5	T47.2X6
Expectorant NEC	T48.4X1	T48.4X2	T48.4X3	T48.4X4	T48.4X5	T48.4X6
Extended insulin zinc suspension	T38.3X1	T38.3X2	T38.3X3	T38.3X4	T38.3X5	T38.3X6
External medications (skin) (mucous membrane)	T49.91	T49.92	T49.93	T49.94	T49.95	T49.96
dental agent	T49.7X1	T49.7X2	T49.7X3	T49.7X4	T49.7X5	T49.7X6
ENT agent	T49.6X1	T49.6X2	T49.6X3	T49.6X4	T49.6X5	T49.6X6
ophthalmic preparation	T49.5X1	T49.5X2	T49.5X3	T49.5X4	T49.5X5	T49.5X6
specified NEC	T49.8X1	T49.8X2	T49.8X3	T49.8X4	T49.8X5	T49.8X6
Extrapyramidal antagonist NEC	T44.3X1	T44.3X2	T44.3X3	T44.3X4	T44.3X5	T44.3X6
Eye agents (anti-infective)	T49.5X1	T49.5X2	T49.5X3	T49.5X4	T49.5X5	T49.5X6
Eye drug NEC	T49.5X1	T49.5X2	T49.5X3	T49.5X4	T49.5X5	T49.5X6
F						
FAC (fluorouracil + doxorubicin + cyclophosphamide)	T45.1X1	T45.1X2	T45.1X3	T45.1X4	T45.1X5	T45.1X6
Factor						
I (fibrinogen)	T45.8X1	T45.8X2	T45.8X3	T45.8X4	T45.8X5	T45.8X6
III (thromboplastin)	T45.8X1	T45.8X2	T45.8X3	T45.8X4	T45.8X5	T45.8X6
VIII (antihemophilic Factor) (Concentrate)	T45.8X1	T45.8X2	T45.8X3	T45.8X4	T45.8X5	T45.8X6

◀ New ◀ Revised ~~deleted~~ Deleted

	External Cause (T-Code)					
Substance	Poisoning, Accidental (Unintentional)	Poisoning, Intentional Self-Harm	Poisoning, Assault	Poisoning, Undetermined	Adverse Effect	Underdosing
Factor *(Continued)*						
IX complex	T45.7X1	T45.7X2	T45.7X3	T45.7X4	T45.7X5	T45.7X6
human	T45.8X1	T45.8X2	T45.8X3	T45.8X4	T45.8X5	T45.8X6
Famotidine	T47.0X1	T47.0X2	T47.0X3	T47.0X4	T47.0X5	T47.0X6
Fat suspension, intravenous	T50.991	T50.992	T50.993	T50.994	T50.995	T50.996
Fazadinium bromide	T48.1X1	T48.1X2	T48.1X3	T48.1X4	T48.1X5	T48.1X6
Febarbamate	T42.3X1	T42.3X2	T42.3X3	T42.3X4	T42.3X5	T42.3X6
Fecal softener	T47.4X1	T47.4X2	T47.4X3	T47.4X4	T47.4X5	T47.4X6
Fedrilate	T48.3X1	T48.3X2	T48.3X3	T48.3X4	T48.3X5	T48.3X6
Felodipine	T46.1X1	T46.1X2	T46.1X3	T46.1X4	T46.1X5	T46.1X6
Felypressin	T38.891	T38.892	T38.893	T38.894	T38.895	T38.896
Femoxetine	T43.221	T43.222	T43.223	T43.224	T43.225	T43.226
Fenalcomine	T46.3X1	T46.3X2	T46.3X3	T46.3X4	T46.3X5	T46.3X6
Fenamisal	T37.1X1	T37.1X2	T37.1X3	T37.1X4	T37.1X5	T37.1X6
Fenazone	T39.2X1	T39.2X2	T39.2X3	T39.2X4	T39.2X5	T39.2X6
Fenbendazole	T37.4X1	T37.4X2	T37.4X3	T37.4X4	T37.4X5	T37.4X6
Fenbutrazate	T50.5X1	T50.5X2	T50.5X3	T50.5X4	T50.5X5	T50.5X6
Fencamfamine	T43.691	T43.692	T43.693	T43.694	T43.695	T43.696
Fendiline	T46.1X1	T46.1X2	T46.1X3	T46.1X4	T46.1X5	T46.1X6
Fenetylline	T43.691	T43.692	T43.693	T43.694	T43.695	T43.696
Fenflumizole	T39.391	T39.392	T39.393	T39.394	T39.395	T39.396
Fenfluramine	T50.5X1	T50.5X2	T50.5X3	T50.5X4	T50.5X5	T50.5X6
Fenobarbital	T42.3X1	T42.3X2	T42.3X3	T42.3X4	T42.3X5	T42.3X6
Fenofibrate	T46.6X1	T46.6X2	T46.6X3	T46.6X4	T46.6X5	T46.6X6
Fenoprofen	T39.311	T39.312	T39.313	T39.314	T39.315	T39.316
Fenoterol	T48.6X1	T48.6X2	T48.6X3	T48.6X4	T48.6X5	T48.6X6
Fenoverine	T44.3X1	T44.3X2	T44.3X3	T44.3X4	T44.3X5	T44.3X6
Fenoxazoline	T48.5X1	T48.5X2	T48.5X3	T48.5X4	T48.5X5	T48.5X6
Fenproporex	T50.5X1	T50.5X2	T50.5X3	T50.5X4	T50.5X5	T50.5X6
Fenquizone	T50.2X1	T50.2X2	T50.2X3	T50.2X4	T50.2X5	T50.2X6
Fentanyl	T40.4X1	T40.4X2	T40.4X3	T40.4X4	T40.4X5	T40.4X6
Fentazin	T43.3X1	T43.3X2	T43.3X3	T43.3X4	T43.3X5	T43.3X6
Fenthion	T60.0X1	T60.0X2	T60.0X3	T60.0X4	—	—
Fenticlor	T49.0X1	T49.0X2	T49.0X3	T49.0X4	T49.0X5	T49.0X6
Fenylbutazone	T39.2X1	T39.2X2	T39.2X3	T39.2X4	T39.2X5	T39.2X6
Feprazone	T39.2X1	T39.2X2	T39.2X3	T39.2X4	T39.2X5	T39.2X6
Fer de lance (bite) (venom)	T63.061	T63.062	T63.063	T63.064	—	—
Ferric — *see also Iron*						
chloride	T45.4X1	T45.4X2	T45.4X3	T45.4X4	T45.4X5	T45.4X6
citrate	T45.4X1	T45.4X2	T45.4X3	T45.4X4	T45.4X5	T45.4X6

Substance	Poisoning, Accidental (Unintentional)	Poisoning, Intentional Self-Harm	Poisoning, Assault	Poisoning, Undetermined	Adverse Effect	Underdosing
			External Cause (T-Code)			
Ferric *(Continued)*						
hydroxide						
colloidal	T45.4X1	T45.4X2	T45.4X3	T45.4X4	T45.4X5	T45.4X6
polymaltose	T45.4X1	T45.4X2	T45.4X3	T45.4X4	T45.4X5	T45.4X6
pyrophosphate	T45.4X1	T45.4X2	T45.4X3	T45.4X4	T45.4X5	T45.4X6
Ferritin	T45.4X1	T45.4X2	T45.4X3	T45.4X4	T45.4X5	T45.4X6
Ferrocholinate	T45.4X1	T45.4X2	T45.4X3	T45.4X4	T45.4X5	T45.4X6
Ferrodextrane	T45.4X1	T45.4X2	T45.4X3	T45.4X4	T45.4X5	T45.4X6
Ferropolimaler	T45.4X1	T45.4X2	T45.4X3	T45.4X4	T45.4X5	T45.4X6
Ferrous — *see also Iron*						
phosphate	T45.4X1	T45.4X2	T45.4X3	T45.4X4	T45.4X5	T45.4X6
salt	T45.4X1	T45.4X2	T45.4X3	T45.4X4	T45.4X5	T45.4X6
with folic acid	T45.4X1	T45.4X2	T45.4X3	T45.4X4	T45.4X5	T45.4X6
Ferrous fumerate, gluconate, lactate, salt NEC, sulfate (medicinal)	T45.4X1	T45.4X2	T45.4X3	T45.4X4	T45.4X5	T45.4X6
Ferrovanadium (fumes)	T59.891	T59.892	T59.893	T59.894	—	—
Ferrum — *see Iron*						
Fertilizers NEC	T65.891	T65.892	T65.893	T65.894	—	—
with herbicide mixture	T60.3X1	T60.3X2	T60.3X3	T60.3X4	—	—
Fetoxilate	T47.6X1	T47.6X2	T47.6X3	T47.6X4	T47.6X5	T47.6X6
Fiber, dietary	T47.4X1	T47.4X2	T47.4X3	T47.4X4	T47.4X5	T47.4X6
Fibrinogen (human)	T45.8X1	T45.8X2	T45.8X3	T45.8X4	T45.8X5	T45.8X6
Fibrinolysin (human)	T45.691	T45.692	T45.693	T45.694	T45.695	T45.696
Fibrinolysis						
affecting drug	T45.601	T45.602	T45.603	T45.604	T45.605	T45.606
inhibitor NEC	T45.621	T45.622	T45.623	T45.624	T45.625	T45.626
Fibrinolytic drug	T45.611	T45.612	T45.613	T45.614	T45.615	T45.616
Filix mas	T37.4X1	T37.4X2	T37.4X3	T37.4X4	T37.4X5	T37.4X6
Filtering cream	T49.3X1	T49.3X2	T49.3X3	T49.3X4	T49.3X5	T49.3X6
Fiorinal	T39.011	T39.012	T39.013	T39.014	T39.015	T39.016
Firedamp	T59.891	T59.892	T59.893	T59.894	—	—
Fish, noxious, nonbacterial	T61.91	T61.92	T61.93	T61.94	—	—
ciguatera	T61.01	T61.02	T61.03	T61.04	—	—
scombroid	T61.11	T61.12	T61.13	T61.14	—	—
shell	T61.781	T61.782	T61.783	T61.784	—	—
specified NEC	T61.771	T61.772	T61.773	T61.774	—	—
Flagyl	T37.3X1	T37.3X2	T37.3X3	T37.3X4	T37.3X5	T37.3X6
Flavine adenine dinucleotide	T45.2X1	T45.2X2	T45.2X3	T45.2X4	T45.2X5	T45.2X6
Flavodic acid	T46.991	T46.992	T46.993	T46.994	T46.995	T46.996
Flavoxate	T44.3X1	T44.3X2	T44.3X3	T44.3X4	T44.3X5	T44.3X6

◀ New   ◀ Revised   ~~deleted~~ Deleted

Substance	External Cause (T-Code)					
	Poisoning, Accidental (Unintentional)	Poisoning, Intentional Self-Harm	Poisoning, Assault	Poisoning, Undetermined	Adverse Effect	Underdosing
Flaxedil	T48.1X1	T48.1X2	T48.1X3	T48.1X4	T48.1X5	T48.1X6
Flaxseed (medicinal)	T49.3X1	T49.3X2	T49.3X3	T49.3X4	T49.3X5	T49.3X6
Flecainide	T46.2X1	T46.2X2	T46.2X3	T46.2X4	T46.2X5	T46.2X6
Fleroxacin	T36.8X1	T36.8X2	T36.8X3	T36.8X4	T36.8X5	T36.8X6
Floctafenine	T39.8X1	T39.8X2	T39.8X3	T39.8X4	T39.8X5	T39.8X6
Flomax	T44.6X1	T44.6X2	T44.6X3	T44.6X4	T44.6X5	T44.6X6
Flomoxef	T36.1X1	T36.1X2	T36.1X3	T36.1X4	T36.1X5	T36.1X6
Flopropione	T44.3X1	T44.3X2	T44.3X3	T44.3X4	T44.3X5	T44.3X6
Florantyrone	T47.5X1	T47.5X2	T47.5X3	T47.5X4	T47.5X5	T47.5X6
Floraquin	T37.8X1	T37.8X2	T37.8X3	T37.8X4	T37.8X5	T37.8X6
Florinef	T38.0X1	T38.0X2	T38.0X3	T38.0X4	T38.0X5	T38.0X6
ENT agent	T49.6X1	T49.6X2	T49.6X3	T49.6X4	T49.6X5	T49.6X6
ophthalmic preparation	T49.5X1	T49.5X2	T49.5X3	T49.5X4	T49.5X5	T49.5X6
topical NEC	T49.0X1	T49.0X2	T49.0X3	T49.0X4	T49.0X5	T49.0X6
Flowers of sulfur	T49.4X1	T49.4X2	T49.4X3	T49.4X4	T49.4X5	T49.4X6
Floxuridine	T45.1X1	T45.1X2	T45.1X3	T45.1X4	T45.1X5	T45.1X6
Fluanisone	T43.4X1	T43.4X2	T43.4X3	T43.4X4	T43.4X5	T43.4X6
Flubendazole	T37.4X1	T37.4X2	T37.4X3	T37.4X4	T37.4X5	T37.4X6
Fluclorolone acetonide	T49.0X1	T49.0X2	T49.0X3	T49.0X4	T49.0X5	T49.0X6
Flucloxacillin	T36.0X1	T36.0X2	T36.0X3	T36.0X4	T36.0X5	T36.0X6
Fluconazole	T37.8X1	T37.8X2	T37.8X3	T37.8X4	T37.8X5	T37.8X6
Flucytosine	T37.8X1	T37.8X2	T37.8X3	T37.8X4	T37.8X5	T37.8X6
Fludeoxyglucose (18F)	T50.8X1	T50.8X2	T50.8X3	T50.8X4	T50.8X5	T50.8X6
Fludiazepam	T42.4X1	T42.4X2	T42.4X3	T42.4X4	T42.4X5	T42.4X6
Fludrocortisone	T50.0X1	T50.0X2	T50.0X3	T50.0X4	T50.0X5	T50.0X6
ENT agent	T49.6X1	T49.6X2	T49.6X3	T49.6X4	T49.6X5	T49.6X6
ophthalmic preparation	T49.5X1	T49.5X2	T49.5X3	T49.5X4	T49.5X5	T49.5X6
topical NEC	T49.0X1	T49.0X2	T49.0X3	T49.0X4	T49.0X5	T49.0X6
Fludroxycortide	T49.0X1	T49.0X2	T49.0X3	T49.0X4	T49.0X5	T49.0X6
Flufenamic acid	T39.391	T39.392	T39.393	T39.394	T39.395	T39.396
Fluindione	T45.511	T45.512	T45.513	T45.514	T45.515	T45.516
Flumequine	T37.8X1	T37.8X2	T37.8X3	T37.8X4	T37.8X5	T37.8X6
Flumethasone	T49.0X1	T49.0X2	T49.0X3	T49.0X4	T49.0X5	T49.0X6
Flumethiazide	T50.2X1	T50.2X2	T50.2X3	T50.2X4	T50.2X5	T50.2X6
Flumidin	T37.5X1	T37.5X2	T37.5X3	T37.5X4	T37.5X5	T37.5X6
Flunarizine	T46.7X1	T46.7X2	T46.7X3	T46.7X4	T46.7X5	T46.7X6
Flunidazole	T37.8X1	T37.8X2	T37.8X3	T37.8X4	T37.8X5	T37.8X6
Flunisolide	T48.6X1	T48.6X2	T48.6X3	T48.6X4	T48.6X5	T48.6X6
Flunitrazepam	T42.4X1	T42.4X2	T42.4X3	T42.4X4	T42.4X5	T42.4X6

◀ New ◀ Revised ~~deleted~~ Deleted

Substance	External Cause (T-Code)					
	Poisoning, Accidental (Unintentional)	Poisoning, Intentional Self-Harm	Poisoning, Assault	Poisoning, Undetermined	Adverse Effect	Underdosing
Fluocinolone (acetonide)	T49.0X1	T49.0X2	T49.0X3	T49.0X4	T49.0X5	T49.0X6
Fluocinonide	T49.0X1	T49.0X2	T49.0X3	T49.0X4	T49.0X5	T49.0X6
Fluocortin (butyl)	T49.0X1	T49.0X2	T49.0X3	T49.0X4	T49.0X5	T49.0X6
Fluocortolone	T49.0X1	T49.0X2	T49.0X3	T49.0X4	T49.0X5	T49.0X6
Fluohydrocortisone	T38.0X1	T38.0X2	T38.0X3	T38.0X4	T38.0X5	T38.0X6
ENT agent	T49.6X1	T49.6X2	T49.6X3	T49.6X4	T49.6X5	T49.6X6
ophthalmic preparation	T49.5X1	T49.5X2	T49.5X3	T49.5X4	T49.5X5	T49.5X6
topical NEC	T49.0X1	T49.0X2	T49.0X3	T49.0X4	T49.0X5	T49.0X6
Fluonid	T49.0X1	T49.0X2	T49.0X3	T49.0X4	T49.0X5	T49.0X6
Fluopromazine	T43.3X1	T43.3X2	T43.3X3	T43.3X4	T43.3X5	T43.3X6
Fluoroacetate	T60.8X1	T60.8X2	T60.8X3	T60.8X4	—	—
Fluorescein	T50.8X1	T50.8X2	T50.8X3	T50.8X4	T50.8X5	T50.8X6
Fluorhydrocortisone	T50.0X1	T50.0X2	T50.0X3	T50.0X4	T50.0X5	T50.0X6
Fluoride (nonmedicinal) (pesticide) (sodium) NEC	T60.8X1	T60.8X2	T60.8X3	T60.8X4	—	—
hydrogen — see Hydrofluoric acid						
medicinal NEC	T50.991	T50.992	T50.993	T50.994	T50.995	T50.996
dental use	T49.7X1	T49.7X2	T49.7X3	T49.7X4	T49.7X5	T49.7X6
not pesticide NEC	T54.91	T54.92	T54.93	T54.94	—	—
stannous	T49.7X1	T49.7X2	T49.7X3	T49.7X4	T49.7X5	T49.7X6
Fluorinated corticosteroids	T38.0X1	T38.0X2	T38.0X3	T38.0X4	T38.0X5	T38.0X6
Fluorine (gas)	T59.5X1	T59.5X2	T59.5X3	T59.5X4	—	—
salt — see Fluoride(s)						
Fluoristan	T49.7X1	T49.7X2	T49.7X3	T49.7X4	T49.7X5	T49.7X6
Fluormetholone	T49.0X1	T49.0X2	T49.0X3	T49.0X4	T49.0X5	T49.0X6
Fluoroacetate	T60.8X1	T60.8X2	T60.8X3	T60.8X4	—	—
Fluorocarbon monomer	T53.6X1	T53.6X2	T53.6X3	T53.6X4	—	—
Fluorocytosine	T37.8X1	T37.8X2	T37.8X3	T37.8X4	T37.8X5	T37.8X6
Fluorodeoxyuridine	T45.1X1	T45.1X2	T45.1X3	T45.1X4	T45.1X5	T45.1X6
Fluorometholone	T49.0X1	T49.0X2	T49.0X3	T49.0X4	T49.0X5	T49.0X6
ophthalmic preparation	T49.5X1	T49.5X2	T49.5X3	T49.5X4	T49.5X5	T49.5X6
Fluorophosphate insecticide	T60.0X1	T60.0X2	T60.0X3	T60.0X4	—	—
Fluorosol	T46.3X1	T46.3X2	T46.3X3	T46.3X4	T46.3X5	T46.3X6
Fluorouracil	T45.1X1	T45.1X2	T45.1X3	T45.1X4	T45.1X5	T45.1X6
Fluorphenylalanine	T49.5X1	T49.5X2	T49.5X3	T49.5X4	T49.5X5	T49.5X6
Fluothane	T41.0X1	T41.0X2	T41.0X3	T41.0X4	T41.0X5	T41.0X6
Fluoxetine	T43.221	T43.222	T43.223	T43.224	T43.225	T43.226
Fluoxymesterone	T38.7X1	T38.7X2	T38.7X3	T38.7X4	T38.7X5	T38.7X6
Flupenthixol	T43.4X1	T43.4X2	T43.4X3	T43.4X4	T43.4X5	T43.4X6
Flupentixol	T43.4X1	T43.4X2	T43.4X3	T43.4X4	T43.4X5	T43.4X6
Fluphenazine	T43.3X1	T43.3X2	T43.3X3	T43.3X4	T43.3X5	T43.3X6

◀ New ◀▥ Revised ~~deleted~~ Deleted

Substance	External Cause (T-Code)					
	Poisoning, Accidental (Unintentional)	Poisoning, Intentional Self-Harm	Poisoning, Assault	Poisoning, Undetermined	Adverse Effect	Underdosing
Fluprednidene	T49.0X1	T49.0X2	T49.0X3	T49.0X4	T49.0X5	T49.0X6
Fluprednisolone	T38.0X1	T38.0X2	T38.0X3	T38.0X4	T38.0X5	T38.0X6
Fluradoline	T39.8X1	T39.8X2	T39.8X3	T39.8X4	T39.8X5	T39.8X6
Flurandrenolide	T49.0X1	T49.0X2	T49.0X3	T49.0X4	T49.0X5	T49.0X6
Flurandrenolone	T49.0X1	T49.0X2	T49.0X3	T49.0X4	T49.0X5	T49.0X6
Flurazepam	T42.4X1	T42.4X2	T42.4X3	T42.4X4	T42.4X5	T42.4X6
Flurbiprofen	T39.311	T39.312	T39.313	T39.314	T39.315	T39.316
Flurobate	T49.0X1	T49.0X2	T49.0X3	T49.0X4	T49.0X5	T49.0X6
Flurotyl	T43.291	T43.292	T43.293	T43.294	T43.295	T43.296
Fluroxene	T41.0X1	T41.0X2	T41.0X3	T41.0X4	T41.0X5	T41.0X6
Fluspirilene	T43.591	T43.592	T43.593	T43.594	T43.595	T43.596
Flutamide	T38.6X1	T38.6X2	T38.6X3	T38.6X4	T38.6X5	T38.6X6
Flutazolam	T42.4X1	T42.4X2	T42.4X3	T42.4X4	T42.4X5	T42.4X6
Fluticasone propionate	T49.1X1	T49.1X2	T49.1X3	T49.1X4	T49.1X5	T49.1X6
Flutoprazepam	T42.4X1	T42.4X2	T42.4X3	T42.4X4	T42.4X5	T42.4X6
Flutropium bromide	T48.6X1	T48.6X2	T48.6X3	T48.6X4	T48.6X5	T48.6X6
Fluvoxamine	T43.221	T43.222	T43.223	T43.224	T43.225	T43.226
Folacin	T45.8X1	T45.8X2	T45.8X3	T45.8X4	T45.8X5	T45.8X6
Folic acid	T45.8X1	T45.8X2	T45.8X3	T45.8X4	T45.8X5	T45.8X6
with ferrous salt	T45.2X1	T45.2X2	T45.2X3	T45.2X4	T45.2X5	T45.2X6
antagonist	T45.1X1	T45.1X2	T45.1X3	T45.1X4	T45.1X5	T45.1X6
Folinic acid	T45.8X1	T45.8X2	T45.8X3	T45.8X4	T45.8X5	T45.8X6
Folium stramoniae	T48.6X1	T48.6X2	T48.6X3	T48.6X4	T48.6X5	T48.6X6
Follicle-stimulating hormone, human	T38.811	T38.812	T38.813	T38.814	T38.815	T38.816
Folpet	T60.3X1	T60.3X2	T60.3X3	T60.3X4	—	—
Fominoben	T48.3X1	T48.3X2	T48.3X3	T48.3X4	T48.3X5	T48.3X6
Food, foodstuffs, noxious, nonbacterial, NEC	T62.91	T62.92	T62.93	T62.94	—	—
berries	T62.1X1	T62.1X2	T62.1X3	T62.1X4	—	—
fish—see also Fish	T61.91	T61.92	T61.93	T61.94	—	—
mushrooms	T62.0X1	T62.0X2	T62.0X3	T62.0X4	—	—
plants	T62.2X1	T62.2X2	T62.2X3	T62.2X4	—	—
seafood	T61.91	T61.92	T61.93	T61.94	—	—
specified NEC	T61.8X1	T61.8X2	T61.8X3	T61.8X4	—	—
seeds	T62.2X1	T62.2X2	T62.2X3	T62.2X4	—	—
shellfish	T61.781	T61.782	T61.783	T61.784	—	—
specified NEC	T62.8X1	T62.8X2	T62.8X3	T62.8X4	—	—
Fool's parsley	T62.2X1	T62.2X2	T62.2X3	T62.2X4	—	—
Formaldehyde (solution), gas or vapor	T59.2X1	T59.2X2	T59.2X3	T59.2X4	—	—
fungicide	T60.3X1	T60.3X2	T60.3X3	T60.3X4	—	—

◀ New   ◀▥ Revised   ~~deleted~~ Deleted

TABLE OF DRUGS AND CHEMICALS

	External Cause (T-Code)					
Substance	Poisoning, Accidental (Unintentional)	Poisoning, Intentional Self-Harm	Poisoning, Assault	Poisoning, Undetermined	Adverse Effect	Underdosing
Formalin	T59.2X1	T59.2X2	T59.2X3	T59.2X4	—	—
fungicide	T60.3X1	T60.3X2	T60.3X3	T60.3X4	—	—
vapor	T59.2X1	T59.2X2	T59.2X3	T59.2X4	—	—
Formic acid	T54.2X1	T54.2X2	T54.2X3	T54.2X4		
vapor	T59.891	T59.892	T59.893	T59.894		
Foscarnet sodium	T37.5X1	T37.5X2	T37.5X3	T37.5X4	T37.5X5	T37.5X6
Fosfestrol	T38.5X1	T38.5X2	T38.5X3	T38.5X4	T38.5X5	T38.5X6
Fosfomycin	T36.8X1	T36.8X2	T36.8X3	T36.8X4	T36.8X5	T36.8X6
Fosfonet sodium	T37.5X1	T37.5X2	T37.5X3	T37.5X4	T37.5X5	T37.5X6
Fosinopril	T46.4X1	T46.4X2	T46.4X3	T46.4X4	T46.4X5	T46.4X6
sodium	T46.4X1	T46.4X2	T46.4X3	T46.4X4	T46.4X5	T46.4X6
Fowler's solution	T57.0X1	T57.0X2	T57.0X3	T57.0X4	—	—
Foxglove	T62.2X1	T62.2X2	T62.2X3	T62.2X4	—	—
Framycetin	T36.5X1	T36.5X2	T36.5X3	T36.5X4	T36.5X5	T36.5X6
Frangula	T47.2X1	T47.2X2	T47.2X3	T47.2X4	T47.2X5	T47.2X6
extract	T47.2X1	T47.2X2	T47.2X3	T47.2X4	T47.2X5	T47.2X6
Frei antigen	T50.8X1	T50.8X2	T50.8X3	T50.8X4	T50.8X5	T50.8X6
Freon	T53.5X1	T53.5X2	T53.5X3	T53.5X4	—	—
Fructose	T50.3X1	T50.3X2	T50.3X3	T50.3X4	T50.3X5	T50.3X6
Frusemide	T50.1X1	T50.1X2	T50.1X3	T50.1X4	T50.1X5	T50.1X6
FSH	T38.811	T38.812	T38.813	T38.814	T38.815	T38.816
Ftorafur	T45.1X1	T45.1X2	T45.1X3	T45.1X4	T45.1X5	T45.1X6
Fuel						
automobile	T52.0X1	T52.0X2	T52.0X3	T52.0X4	—	—
exhaust gas, not in transit	T58.01	T58.02	T58.03	T58.04	—	—
vapor NEC	T52.0X1	T52.0X2	T52.0X3	T52.0X4	—	—
gas (domestic use) — see also Carbon, monoxide, fuel, utility	T59.891	T59.892	T59.893	T59.894	—	—
utility	T59.891	T59.892	T59.893	T59.894	—	—
in mobile container	T59.891	T59.892	T59.893	T59.894	—	—
incomplete combustion of — see Carbon, monoxide, fuel, utility						
piped (natural)	T59.891	T59.892	T59.893	T59.894	—	—
industrial, incomplete combustion	T58.8X1	T58.8X2	T58.8X3	T58.8X4	—	—
Fugillin	T36.8X1	T36.8X2	T36.8X3	T36.8X4	T36.8X5	T36.8X6
Fulminate of mercury	T56.1X1	T56.1X2	T56.1X3	T56.1X4	—	—
Fulvicin	T36.7X1	T36.7X2	T36.7X3	T36.7X4	T36.7X5	T36.7X6
Fumadil	T36.8X1	T36.8X2	T36.8X3	T36.8X4	T36.8X5	T36.8X6
Fumagillin	T36.8X1	T36.8X2	T36.8X3	T36.8X4	T36.8X5	T36.8X6
Fumaric acid	T49.4X1	T49.4X2	T49.4X3	T49.4X4	T49.4X5	T49.4X6
Fumes (from)	T59.91	T59.92	T59.93	T59.94	—	—
carbon monoxide — see Carbon, monoxide						
charcoal (domestic use) — see Charcoal, fumes						

◀ New   ◀▥ Revised   ~~deleted~~ Deleted

Substance	External Cause (T-Code)					
	Poisoning, Accidental (Unintentional)	Poisoning, Intentional Self-Harm	Poisoning, Assault	Poisoning, Undetermined	Adverse Effect	Underdosing
Fumes *(Continued)*						
chloroform — *see Chloroform*						
coke (in domestic stoves, fireplaces) — *see Coke, fumes*						
corrosive NEC	T54.91	T54.92	T54.93	T54.94	—	—
ether — *see ether*						
freons	T53.5X1	T53.5X2	T53.5X3	T53.5X4	—	—
hydrocarbons	T59.891	T59.892	T59.893	T59.894	—	—
petroleum (liquefied)	T59.891	T59.892	T59.893	T59.894	—	—
distributed through pipes (pure or mixed with air)	T59.891	T59.892	T59.893	T59.894	—	—
lead — *see lead*						
metal — *see Metals, or the specified metal*						
nitrogen dioxide	T59.0X1	T59.0X2	T59.0X3	T59.0X4	—	—
pesticides — *see Pesticides*						
petroleum (liquefied)	T59.891	T59.892	T59.893	T59.894	—	—
distributed through pipes (pure or mixed with air)	T59.891	T59.892	T59.893	T59.894	—	—
polyester	T59.891	T59.892	T59.893	T59.894	—	—
specified source NEC — *see also substance specified*	T59.891	T59.892	T59.893	T59.894	—	—
sulfur dioxide	T59.1X1	T59.1X2	T59.1X3	T59.1X4	—	—
Fumigant NEC	T60.91	T60.92	T60.93	T60.94		
Fungi, noxious, used as food	T62.0X1	T62.0X2	T62.0X3	T62.0X4	—	—
Fungicide NEC (nonmedicinal)	T60.3X1	T60.3X2	T60.3X3	T60.3X4	—	—
Fungizone	T36.7X1	T36.7X2	T36.7X3	T36.7X4	T36.7X5	T36.7X6
topical	T49.0X1	T49.0X2	T49.0X3	T49.0X4	T49.0X5	T49.0X6
Furacin	T49.0X1	T49.0X2	T49.0X3	T49.0X4	T49.0X5	T49.0X6
Furadantin	T37.91	T37.92	T37.93	T37.94	T37.95	T37.96
Furazolidone	T37.8X1	T37.8X2	T37.8X3	T37.8X4	T37.8X5	T37.8X6
Furazolium chloride	T49.0X1	T49.0X2	T49.0X3	T49.0X4	T49.0X5	T49.0X6
Furfural	T52.8X1	T52.8X2	T52.8X3	T52.8X4	—	—
Furnace (coal burning) (domestic), gas from industrial	T58.2X1	T58.2X2	T58.2X3	T58.2X4	—	—
industrial	T58.8X1	T58.8X2	T58.8X3	T58.8X4	—	—
Furniture polish	T65.891	T65.892	T65.893	T65.894	—	—
Furosemide	T50.1X1	T50.1X2	T50.1X3	T50.1X4	T50.1X5	T50.1X6
Furoxone	T37.91	T37.92	T37.93	T37.94	T37.95	T37.96
Fursultiamine	T45.2X1	T45.2X2	T45.2X3	T45.2X4	T45.2X5	T45.2X6
Fusafungine	T36.8X1	T36.8X2	T36.8X3	T36.8X4	T36.8X5	T36.8X6
Fusel oil (any) (amyl) (butyl) (propyl), vapor	T51.3X1	T51.3X2	T51.3X3	T51.3X4	—	—
Fusidate (ethanolamine) (sodium)	T36.8X1	T36.8X2	T36.8X3	T36.8X4	T36.8X5	T36.8X6
Fusidic acid	T36.8X1	T36.8X2	T36.8X3	T36.8X4	T36.8X5	T36.8X6
Fytic acid, nonasodium	T50.6X1	T50.6X2	T50.6X3	T50.6X4	T50.6X5	T50.6X6

Substance	External Cause (T-Code)					
	Poisoning, Accidental (Unintentional)	Poisoning, Intentional Self-Harm	Poisoning, Assault	Poisoning, Undetermined	Adverse Effect	Underdosing
G						
GABA	T43.8X1	T43.8X2	T43.8X3	T43.8X4	T43.8X5	T43.8X6
Gadopentetic acid	T50.8X1	T50.8X2	T50.8X3	T50.8X4	T50.8X5	T50.8X6
Galactose	T50.3X1	T50.3X2	T50.3X3	T50.3X4	T50.3X5	T50.3X6
b-Galactosidase	T47.5X1	T47.5X2	T47.5X3	T47.5X4	T47.5X5	T47.5X6
Galantamine	T44.0X1	T44.0X2	T44.0X3	T44.0X4	T44.0X5	T44.0X6
Gallamine (triethiodide)	T48.1X1	T48.1X2	T48.1X3	T48.1X4	T48.1X5	T48.1X6
Gallium citrate	T50.991	T50.992	T50.993	T50.994	T50.995	T50.996
Gallopamil	T46.1X1	T46.1X2	T46.1X3	T46.1X4	T46.1X5	T46.1X6
Gamboge	T47.2X1	T47.2X2	T47.2X3	T47.2X4	T47.2X5	T47.2X6
Gamimune	T50.Z11	T50.Z12	T50.Z13	T50.Z14	T50.Z15	T50.Z16
Gamma-aminobutyric acid	T43.8X1	T43.8X2	T43.8X3	T43.8X4	T43.8X5	T43.8X6
Gamma-benzene hexachloride (medicinal)	T49.0X1	T49.0X2	T49.0X3	T49.0X4	T49.0X5	T49.0X6
nonmedicinal, vapor	T53.6X1	T53.6X2	T53.6X3	T53.6X4	—	—
Gamma-BHC (medicinal) — *see also Gamma-benzene hexachloride*	T49.0X1	T49.0X2	T49.0X3	T49.0X4	T49.0X5	T49.0X6
Gamma globulin	T50.Z11	T50.Z12	T50.Z13	T50.Z14	T50.Z15	T50.Z16
Gamulin	T50.Z11	T50.Z12	T50.Z13	T50.Z14	T50.Z15	T50.Z16
Ganciclovir (sodium)	T37.5X1	T37.5X2	T37.5X3	T37.5X4	T37.5X5	T37.5X6
Ganglionic blocking drug NEC	T44.2X1	T44.2X2	T44.2X3	T44.2X4	T44.2X5	T44.2X6
specified NEC	T44.2X1	T44.2X2	T44.2X3	T44.2X4	T44.2X5	T44.2X6
Ganja	T40.7X1	T40.7X2	T40.7X3	T40.7X4	T40.7X5	T40.7X6
Garamycin	T36.5X1	T36.5X2	T36.5X3	T36.5X4	T36.5X5	T36.5X6
ophthalmic preparation	T49.5X1	T49.5X2	T49.5X3	T49.5X4	T49.5X5	T49.5X6
topical NEC	T49.0X1	T49.0X2	T49.0X3	T49.0X4	T49.0X5	T49.0X6
Gardenal	T42.3X1	T42.3X2	T42.3X3	T42.3X4	T42.3X5	T42.3X6
Gardepanyl	T42.3X1	T42.3X2	T42.3X3	T42.3X4	T42.3X5	T42.3X6
Gas	T59.91	T59.92	T59.93	T59.94	—	—
acetylene	T59.891	T59.892	T59.893	T59.894	—	—
incomplete combustion of	T58.11	T58.12	T58.13	T58.14		
air contaminants, source or type not specified	T59.91	T59.92	T59.93	T59.94	—	—
anesthetic	T41.0X1	T41.0X2	T41.0X3	T41.0X4	T41.0X5	T41.0X6
blast furnace	T58.8X1	T58.8X2	T58.8X3	T58.8X4	—	—
butane — *see butane*						
carbon monoxide — *see Carbon, monoxide*						
chlorine	T59.4X1	T59.4X2	T59.4X3	T59.4X4	—	—
coal	T58.2X1	T58.2X2	T58.2X3	T58.2X4	—	—
cyanide	T57.3X1	T57.3X2	T57.3X3	T57.3X4	—	—
dicyanogen	T65.0X1	T65.0X2	T65.0X3	T65.0X4	—	—
domestic — *see Domestic gas*	T57.91	T57.92	T57.93	T57.94	—	—

◀ New   ◀◀ Revised   ~~deleted~~ Deleted

Substance	External Cause (T-Code)					
	Poisoning, Accidental (Unintentional)	Poisoning, Intentional Self-Harm	Poisoning, Assault	Poisoning, Undetermined	Adverse Effect	Underdosing
Gas *(Continued)*						
exhaust	T57.91	T57.92	T57.93	T57.94	—	—
from utility (for cooking, heating, or lighting) (after combustion) — *see Carbon, monoxide, fuel, utility*						
prior to combustion	T59.891	T59.892	T59.893	T59.894	—	—
from wood or coal-burning stove or fireplace	T57.91	T57.92	T57.93	T57.94	—	—
fuel (domestic use) (after combustion) — *see also Carbon, monoxide, fuel*	T57.91	T57.92	T57.93	T57.94	—	—
industrial use	T58.8X1	T58.8X2	T58.8X3	T58.8X4	—	—
prior to combustion	T59.891	T59.892	T59.893	T59.894	—	—
utility	T59.891	T59.892	T59.893	T59.894	—	—
in mobile container	T59.891	T59.892	T59.893	T59.894	—	—
incomplete combustion of — *see Carbon, monoxide, fuel, utility*						
piped (natural)	T59.891	T59.892	T59.893	T59.894	—	—
garage	T58.01	T58.02	T58.03	T58.04	—	—
hydrocarbon NEC	T59.891	T59.892	T59.893	T59.894	—	—
incomplete combustion of — *see Carbon, monoxide, fuel, utility*						
liquefied — *see butane*						
piped	T59.891	T59.892	T59.893	T59.894	—	—
hydrocyanic acid	T65.0X1	T65.0X2	T65.0X3	T65.0X4	—	—
illuminating (after combustion)	T58.11	T58.12	T58.13	T58.14	—	—
prior to combustion	T59.891	T59.892	T59.893	T59.894	—	—
incomplete combustion, any — *see Carbon, monoxide*						
kiln	T58.8X1	T58.8X2	T58.8X3	T58.8X4	—	—
lacrimogenic	T59.3X1	T59.3X2	T59.3X3	T59.3X4	—	—
liquefied petroleum — *see butane*						
marsh	T59.891	T59.892	T59.893	T59.894	—	—
motor exhaust, not in transit	T58.01	T58.02	T58.03	T58.04	—	—
mustard, not in war	T59.891	T59.892	T59.893	T59.894	—	—
natural	T59.891	T59.892	T59.893	T59.894	—	—
nerve, not in war	T59.91	T59.92	T59.93	T59.94	—	—
oil	T52.0X1	T52.0X2	T52.0X3	T52.0X4	—	—
petroleum (liquefied) (distributed in mobile containers)	T59.891	T59.892	T59.893	T59.894	—	—
piped (pure or mixed with air)	T59.891	T59.892	T59.893	T59.894	—	—
piped (manufactured) (natural) NEC	T59.891	T59.892	T59.893	T59.894	—	—
producer	T58.8X1	T58.8X2	T58.8X3	T58.8X4	—	—
propane — *see propane*						
refrigerant (chlorofluoro-carbon)	T53.5X1	T53.5X2	T53.5X3	T53.5X4	—	—
not chlorofluoro-carbon	T59.891	T59.892	T59.893	T59.894	—	—
sewer	T59.91	T59.92	T59.93	T59.94	—	—
specified source NEC	T59.91	T59.92	T59.93	T59.94	—	—

◀ New   ◀▥ Revised   ~~deleted~~ Deleted

	External Cause (T-Code)					
Substance	Poisoning, Accidental (Unintentional)	Poisoning, Intentional Self-Harm	Poisoning, Assault	Poisoning, Undetermined	Adverse Effect	Underdosing
Gas *(Continued)*						
stove (after combustion)	T58.11	T58.12	T58.13	T58.14	—	—
tear	T59.3X1	T59.3X2	T59.3X3	T59.3X4	—	—
therapeutic	T41.5X1	T41.5X2	T41.5X3	T41.5X4	T41.5X5	T41.5X6
utility (for cooking, heating, or lighting) (piped) NEC	T59.891	T59.892	T59.893	T59.894	—	—
in mobile container	T59.891	T59.892	T59.893	T59.894	—	—
incomplete combustion of — *see* Carbon, monoxide, fuel, utility						
piped (natural)	T59.891	T59.892	T59.893	T59.894	—	—
water	T58.11	T58.12	T58.13	T58.14	—	—
incomplete combustion of — *see* Carbon, monoxide, fuel, utility						
Gaseous substance — *see* Gas						
Gasoline	T52.0X1	T52.0X2	T52.0X3	T52.0X4	—	—
vapor	T52.0X1	T52.0X2	T52.0X3	T52.0X4	—	—
Gastric enzymes	T47.5X1	T47.5X2	T47.5X3	T47.5X4	T47.5X5	T47.5X6
Gastrografin	T50.8X1	T50.8X2	T50.8X3	T50.8X4	T50.8X5	T50.8X6
Gastrointestinal drug	T47.91	T47.92	T47.93	T47.94	T47.95	T47.96
biological	T47.8X1	T47.8X2	T47.8X3	T47.8X4	T47.8X5	T47.8X6
specified NEC	T47.8X1	T47.8X2	T47.8X3	T47.8X4	T47.8X5	T47.8X6
Gaultheria procumbens	T62.2X1	T62.2X2	T62.2X3	T62.2X4	—	—
Gelatin (intravenous)	T45.8X1	T45.8X2	T45.8X3	T45.8X4	T45.8X5	T45.8X6
absorbable (sponge)	T45.7X1	T45.7X2	T45.7X3	T45.7X4	T45.7X5	T45.7X6
Gefarnate	T44.3X1	T44.3X2	T44.3X3	T44.3X4	T44.3X5	T44.3X6
Gelfilm	T49.8X1	T49.8X2	T49.8X3	T49.8X4	T49.8X5	T49.8X6
Gelfoam	T45.7X1	T45.7X2	T45.7X3	T45.7X4	T45.7X5	T45.7X6
Gelsemine	T50.991	T50.992	T50.993	T50.994	T50.995	T50.996
Gelsemium (sempervirens)	T62.2X1	T62.2X2	T62.2X3	T62.2X4	—	—
Gemeprost	T48.0X1	T48.0X2	T48.0X3	T48.0X4	T48.0X5	T48.0X6
Gemfibrozil	T46.6X1	T46.6X2	T46.6X3	T46.6X4	T46.6X5	T46.6X6
Gemonil	T42.3X1	T42.3X2	T42.3X3	T42.3X4	T42.3X5	T42.3X6
Gentamicin	T36.5X1	T36.5X2	T36.5X3	T36.5X4	T36.5X5	T36.5X6
ophthalmic preparation	T49.5X1	T49.5X2	T49.5X3	T49.5X4	T49.5X5	T49.5X6
topical NEC	T49.0X1	T49.0X2	T49.0X3	T49.0X4	T49.0X5	T49.0X6
Gentian	T47.5X1	T47.5X2	T47.5X3	T47.5X4	T47.5X5	T47.5X6
violet	T49.0X1	T49.0X2	T49.0X3	T49.0X4	T49.0X5	T49.0X6
Gepefrine	T44.4X1	T44.4X2	T44.4X3	T44.4X4	T44.4X5	T44.4X6
Gestonorone caproate	T38.5X1	T38.5X2	T38.5X3	T38.5X4	T38.5X5	T38.5X6
Gexane	T49.0X1	T49.0X2	T49.0X3	T49.0X4	T49.0X5	T49.0X6
Gila monster (venom)	T63.111	T63.112	T63.113	T63.114	—	—
Ginger	T47.5X1	T47.5X2	T47.5X3	T47.5X4	T47.5X5	T47.5X6
Jamaica — *see* Jamaica, ginger						

◀ New ◀▥ Revised ~~deleted~~ Deleted

Substance	Poisoning, Accidental (Unintentional)	Poisoning, Intentional Self-Harm	Poisoning, Assault	Poisoning, Undetermined	Adverse Effect	Underdosing
	External Cause (T-Code)					
Gitalin	T46.0X1	T46.0X2	T46.0X3	T46.0X4	T46.0X5	T46.0X6
amorphous	T46.0X1	T46.0X2	T46.0X3	T46.0X4	T46.0X5	T46.0X6
Gitaloxin	T46.0X1	T46.0X2	T46.0X3	T46.0X4	T46.0X5	T46.0X6
Gitoxin	T46.0X1	T46.0X2	T46.0X3	T46.0X4	T46.0X5	T46.0X6
Glafenine	T39.8X1	T39.8X2	T39.8X3	T39.8X4	T39.8X5	T39.8X6
Glandular extract (medicinal) NEC	T50.Z91	T50.Z92	T50.Z93	T50.Z94	T50.Z95	T50.Z96
Glaucarubin	T37.3X1	T37.3X2	T37.3X3	T37.3X4	T37.3X5	T37.3X6
Glibenclamide	T38.3X1	T38.3X2	T38.3X3	T38.3X4	T38.3X5	T38.3X6
Glibornuride	T38.3X1	T38.3X2	T38.3X3	T38.3X4	T38.3X5	T38.3X6
Gliclazide	T38.3X1	T38.3X2	T38.3X3	T38.3X4	T38.3X5	T38.3X6
Glimidine	T38.3X1	T38.3X2	T38.3X3	T38.3X4	T38.3X5	T38.3X6
Glipizide	T38.3X1	T38.3X2	T38.3X3	T38.3X4	T38.3X5	T38.3X6
Gliquidone	T38.3X1	T38.3X2	T38.3X3	T38.3X4	T38.3X5	T38.3X6
Glisolamide	T38.3X1	T38.3X2	T38.3X3	T38.3X4	T38.3X5	T38.3X6
Glisoxepide	T38.3X1	T38.3X2	T38.3X3	T38.3X4	T38.3X5	T38.3X6
Globin zinc insulin	T38.3X1	T38.3X2	T38.3X3	T38.3X4	T38.3X5	T38.3X6
Globulin						
antilymphocytic	T50.Z11	T50.Z12	T50.Z13	T50.Z14	T50.Z15	T50.Z16
antirhesus	T50.Z11	T50.Z12	T50.Z13	T50.Z14	T50.Z15	T50.Z16
antivenin	T50.Z11	T50.Z12	T50.Z13	T50.Z14	T50.Z15	T50.Z16
antiviral	T50.Z11	T50.Z12	T50.Z13	T50.Z14	T50.Z15	T50.Z16
Glucagon	T38.3X1	T38.3X2	T38.3X3	T38.3X4	T38.3X5	T38.3X6
Glucocorticoids	T38.0X1	T38.0X2	T38.0X3	T38.0X4	T38.0X5	T38.0X6
Glucocorticosteroid	T38.0X1	T38.0X2	T38.0X3	T38.0X4	T38.0X5	T38.0X6
Gluconic acid	T50.991	T50.992	T50.993	T50.994	T50.995	T50.996
Glucosamine sulfate	T39.4X1	T39.4X2	T39.4X3	T39.4X4	T39.4X5	T39.4X6
Glucose	T50.3X1	T50.3X2	T50.3X3	T50.3X4	T50.3X5	T50.3X6
with sodium chloride	T50.3X1	T50.3X2	T50.3X3	T50.3X4	T50.3X5	T50.3X6
Glucosulfone sodium	T37.1X1	T37.1X2	T37.1X3	T37.1X4	T37.1X5	T37.1X6
Glucurolactone	T47.8X1	T47.8X2	T47.8X3	T47.8X4	T47.8X5	T47.8X6
Glue NEC	T52.8X1	T52.8X2	T52.8X3	T52.8X4	—	—
Glutamic acid	T47.5X1	T47.5X2	T47.5X3	T47.5X4	T47.5X5	T47.5X6
Glutaral (medicinal)	T49.0X1	T49.0X2	T49.0X3	T49.0X4	T49.0X5	T49.0X6
nonmedicinal	T65.891	T65.892	T65.893	T65.894	—	—
Glutaraldehyde (nonmedicinal)	T65.891	T65.892	T65.893	T65.894	—	—
medicinal	T49.0X1	T49.0X2	T49.0X3	T49.0X4	T49.0X5	T49.0X6
Glutathione	T50.6X1	T50.6X2	T50.6X3	T50.6X4	T50.6X5	T50.6X6
Glutethimide	T42.6X1	T42.6X2	T42.6X3	T42.6X4	T42.6X5	T42.6X6
Glyburide	T38.3X1	T38.3X2	T38.3X3	T38.3X4	T38.3X5	T38.3X6

◀ New   ◀⫴ Revised   ~~deleted~~ Deleted

Substance	Poisoning, Accidental (Unintentional)	Poisoning, Intentional Self-Harm	Poisoning, Assault	Poisoning, Undetermined	Adverse Effect	Underdosing
Glycerin	T47.4X1	T47.4X2	T47.4X3	T47.4X4	T47.4X5	T47.4X6
Glycerol	T47.4X1	T47.4X2	T47.4X3	T47.4X4	T47.4X5	T47.4X6
borax	T49.6X1	T49.6X2	T49.6X3	T49.6X4	T49.6X5	T49.6X6
intravenous	T50.3X1	T50.3X2	T50.3X3	T50.3X4	T50.3X5	T50.3X6
iodinated	T48.4X1	T48.4X2	T48.4X3	T48.4X4	T48.4X5	T48.4X6
Glycerophosphate	T50.991	T50.992	T50.993	T50.994	T50.995	T50.996
Glyceryl						
gualacolate	T48.4X1	T48.4X2	T48.4X3	T48.4X4	T48.4X5	T48.4X6
nitrate	T46.3X1	T46.3X2	T46.3X3	T46.3X4	T46.3X5	T46.3X6
triacetate (topical)	T49.0X1	T49.0X2	T49.0X3	T49.0X4	T49.0X5	T49.0X6
trinitrate	T46.3X1	T46.3X2	T46.3X3	T46.3X4	T46.3X5	T46.3X6
Glycine	T50.3X1	T50.3X2	T50.3X3	T50.3X4	T50.3X5	T50.3X6
Glyclopyramide	T38.3X1	T38.3X2	T38.3X3	T38.3X4	T38.3X5	T38.3X6
Glycobiarsol	T37.3X1	T37.3X2	T37.3X3	T37.3X4	T37.3X5	T37.3X6
Glycols (ether)	T52.3X1	T52.3X2	T52.3X3	T52.3X4	—	—
Glyconiazide	T37.1X1	T37.1X2	T37.1X3	T37.1X4	T37.1X5	T37.1X6
Glycopyrrolate	T44.3X1	T44.3X2	T44.3X3	T44.3X4	T44.3X5	T44.3X6
Glycopyrronium	T44.3X1	T44.3X2	T44.3X3	T44.3X4	T44.3X5	T44.3X6
bromide	T44.3X1	T44.3X2	T44.3X3	T44.3X4	T44.3X5	T44.3X6
Glycoside, cardiac (stimulant)	T46.0X1	T46.0X2	T46.0X3	T46.0X4	T46.0X5	T46.0X6
Glycyrclamide	T38.3X1	T38.3X2	T38.3X3	T38.3X4	T38.3X5	T38.3X6
Glycyrrhiza extract	T48.4X1	T48.4X2	T48.4X3	T48.4X4	T48.4X5	T48.4X6
Glycyrrhizic acid	T48.4X1	T48.4X2	T48.4X3	T48.4X4	T48.4X5	T48.4X6
Glycyrrhizinate potassium	T48.4X1	T48.4X2	T48.4X3	T48.4X4	T48.4X5	T48.4X6
Glymidine sodium	T38.3X1	T38.3X2	T38.3X3	T38.3X4	T38.3X5	T38.3X6
Glyphosate	T60.3X1	T60.3X2	T60.3X3	T60.3X4	—	—
Glyphylline	T48.6X1	T48.6X2	T48.6X3	T48.6X4	T48.6X5	T48.6X6
Gold						
colloidal (I98Au)	T45.1X1	T45.1X2	T45.1X3	T45.1X4	T45.1X5	T45.1X6
salts	T39.4X1	T39.4X2	T39.4X3	T39.4X4	T39.4X5	T39.4X6
Golden sulfide of antimony	T56.891	T56.892	T56.893	T56.894	—	—
Goldylocks	T62.2X1	T62.2X2	T62.2X3	T62.2X4	—	—
Gonadal tissue extract	T38.901	T38.902	T38.903	T38.904	T38.905	T38.906
female	T38.5X1	T38.5X2	T38.5X3	T38.5X4	T38.5X5	T38.5X6
male	T38.7X1	T38.7X2	T38.7X3	T38.7X4	T38.7X5	T38.7X6
Gonadorelin	T38.891	T38.892	T38.893	T38.894	T38.895	T38.896
Gonadotropin	T38.891	T38.892	T38.893	T38.894	T38.895	T38.896
chorionic	T38.891	T38.892	T38.893	T38.894	T38.895	T38.896
pituitary	T38.811	T38.812	T38.813	T38.814	T38.815	T38.816
Goserelin	T45.1X1	T45.1X2	T45.1X3	T45.1X4	T45.1X5	T45.1X6

◀ New ◀ Revised ~~deleted~~ Deleted

Substance	External Cause (T-Code)					
	Poisoning, Accidental (Unintentional)	Poisoning, Intentional Self-Harm	Poisoning, Assault	Poisoning, Undetermined	Adverse Effect	Underdosing
Grain alcohol	T51.0X1	T51.0X2	T51.0X3	T51.0X4	—	—
Gramicidin	T49.0X1	T49.0X2	T49.0X3	T49.0X4	T49.0X5	T49.0X6
Granisetron	T45.0X1	T45.0X2	T45.0X3	T45.0X4	T45.0X5	T45.0X6
Gratiola officinalis	T62.2X1	T62.2X2	T62.2X3	T62.2X4	—	—
Grease	T65.891	T65.892	T65.893	T65.894	—	—
Green hellebore	T62.2X1	T62.2X2	T62.2X3	T62.2X4	—	—
Green soap	T49.2X1	T49.2X2	T49.2X3	T49.2X4	T49.2X5	T49.2X6
Grifulvin	T36.7X1	T36.7X2	T36.7X3	T36.7X4	T36.7X5	T36.7X6
Griseofulvin	T36.7X1	T36.7X2	T36.7X3	T36.7X4	T36.7X5	T36.7X6
Growth hormone	T38.811	T38.812	T38.813	T38.814	T38.815	T38.816
Guaiacol derivatives	T48.4X1	T48.4X2	T48.4X3	T48.4X4	T48.4X5	T48.4X6
Guaiac reagent	T50.991	T50.992	T50.993	T50.994	T50.995	T50.996
Guaifenesin	T48.4X1	T48.4X2	T48.4X3	T48.4X4	T48.4X5	T48.4X6
Guaimesal	T48.4X1	T48.4X2	T48.4X3	T48.4X4	T48.4X5	T48.4X6
Guaiphenesin	T48.4X1	T48.4X2	T48.4X3	T48.4X4	T48.4X5	T48.4X6
Guamecycline	T36.4X1	T36.4X2	T36.4X3	T36.4X4	T36.4X5	T36.4X6
Guanabenz	T46.5X1	T46.5X2	T46.5X3	T46.5X4	T46.5X5	T46.5X6
Guanacline	T46.5X1	T46.5X2	T46.5X3	T46.5X4	T46.5X5	T46.5X6
Guanadrel	T46.5X1	T46.5X2	T46.5X3	T46.5X4	T46.5X5	T46.5X6
Guanatol	T37.2X1	T37.2X2	T37.2X3	T37.2X4	T37.2X5	T37.2X6
Guanethidine	T46.5X1	T46.5X2	T46.5X3	T46.5X4	T46.5X5	T46.5X6
Guanfacine	T46.5X1	T46.5X2	T46.5X3	T46.5X4	T46.5X5	T46.5X6
Guano	T65.891	T65.892	T65.893	T65.894	—	—
Guanochlor	T46.5X1	T46.5X2	T46.5X3	T46.5X4	T46.5X5	T46.5X6
Guanoclor	T46.5X1	T46.5X2	T46.5X3	T46.5X4	T46.5X5	T46.5X6
Guanoctine	T46.5X1	T46.5X2	T46.5X3	T46.5X4	T46.5X5	T46.5X6
Guanoxabenz	T46.5X1	T46.5X2	T46.5X3	T46.5X4	T46.5X5	T46.5X6
Guanoxan	T46.5X1	T46.5X2	T46.5X3	T46.5X4	T46.5X5	T46.5X6
Guar gum (medicinal)	T46.6X1	T46.6X2	T46.6X3	T46.6X4	T46.6X5	T46.6X6
H						
Hachimycin	T36.7X1	T36.7X2	T36.7X3	T36.7X4	T36.7X5	T36.7X6
Hair						
dye	T49.4X1	T49.4X2	T49.4X3	T49.4X4	T49.4X5	T49.4X6
preparation NEC	T49.4X1	T49.4X2	T49.4X3	T49.4X4	T49.4X5	T49.4X6
Halazepam	T42.4X1	T42.4X2	T42.4X3	T42.4X4	T42.4X5	T42.4X6
Halcinolone	T49.0X1	T49.0X2	T49.0X3	T49.0X4	T49.0X5	T49.0X6
Halcinonide	T49.0X1	T49.0X2	T49.0X3	T49.0X4	T49.0X5	T49.0X6
Halethazole	T49.0X1	T49.0X2	T49.0X3	T49.0X4	T49.0X5	T49.0X6
Hallucinogen NEC	T40.901	T40.902	T40.903	T40.904	T40.905	T40.906

TABLE OF DRUGS AND CHEMICALS

Substance	External Cause (T-Code)					
	Poisoning, Accidental (Unintentional)	Poisoning, Intentional Self-Harm	Poisoning, Assault	Poisoning, Undetermined	Adverse Effect	Underdosing
Halofantrine	T37.2X1	T37.2X2	T37.2X3	T37.2X4	T37.2X5	T37.2X6
Halofenate	T46.6X1	T46.6X2	T46.6X3	T46.6X4	T46.6X5	T46.6X6
Halometasone	T49.0X1	T49.0X2	T49.0X3	T49.0X4	T49.0X5	T49.0X6
Haloperidol	T43.4X1	T43.4X2	T43.4X3	T43.4X4	T43.4X5	T43.4X6
Haloprogin	T49.0X1	T49.0X2	T49.0X3	T49.0X4	T49.0X5	T49.0X6
Halotex	T49.0X1	T49.0X2	T49.0X3	T49.0X4	T49.0X5	T49.0X6
Halothane	T41.0X1	T41.0X2	T41.0X3	T41.0X4	T41.0X5	T41.0X6
Haloxazolam	T42.4X1	T42.4X2	T42.4X3	T42.4X4	T42.4X5	T42.4X6
Halquinols	T49.0X1	T49.0X2	T49.0X3	T49.0X4	T49.0X5	T49.0X6
Hamamelis	T49.2X1	T49.2X2	T49.2X3	T49.2X4	T49.2X5	T49.2X6
Haptendextran	T45.8X1	T45.8X2	T45.8X3	T45.8X4	T45.8X5	T45.8X6
Harmonyl	T46.5X1	T46.5X2	T46.5X3	T46.5X4	T46.5X5	T46.5X6
Hartmann's solution	T50.3X1	T50.3X2	T50.3X3	T50.3X4	T50.3X5	T50.3X6
Hashish	T40.7X1	T40.7X2	T40.7X3	T40.7X4	T40.7X5	T40.7X6
Hawaiian Woodrose seeds	T40.991	T40.992	T40.993	T40.994	—	—
HCB	T60.3X1	T60.3X2	T60.3X3	T60.3X4	—	—
HCH	T53.6X1	T53.6X2	T53.6X3	T53.6X4	—	—
medicinal	T49.0X1	T49.0X2	T49.0X3	T49.0X4	T49.0X5	T49.0X6
HCN	T57.3X1	T57.3X2	T57.3X3	T57.3X4	—	—
Headache cures, drugs, powders NEC	T50.901	T50.902	T50.903	T50.904	T50.905	T50.906
Heavenly Blue (morning glory)	T40.991	T40.992	T40.993	T40.994	—	—
Heavy metal antidote	T45.8X1	T45.8X2	T45.8X3	T45.8X4	T45.8X5	T45.8X6
Hedaquinium	T49.0X1	T49.0X2	T49.0X3	T49.0X4	T49.0X5	T49.0X6
Hedge hyssop	T62.2X1	T62.2X2	T62.2X3	T62.2X4	—	—
Heet	T49.8X1	T49.8X2	T49.8X3	T49.8X4	T49.8X5	T49.8X6
Helium	T48.991	T48.992	T48.993	T48.994	T48.995	T48.996
Helenin	T37.4X1	T37.4X2	T37.4X3	T37.4X4	T37.4X5	T37.4X6
Hellebore (black) (green) (white)	T62.2X1	T62.2X2	T62.2X3	T62.2X4	—	—
Helium (nonmedicinal) NEC	T59.891	T59.892	T59.893	T59.894	—	—
medicinal	T48.991	T48.992	T48.993	T48.994	T48.995	T48.996
Hematin	T45.8X1	T45.8X2	T45.8X3	T45.8X4	T45.8X5	T45.8X6
Hematinic preparation	T45.8X1	T45.8X2	T45.8X3	T45.8X4	T45.8X5	T45.8X6
Hemlock	T62.2X1	T62.2X2	T62.2X3	T62.2X4	—	—
Hemostatic	T45.621	T45.622	T45.623	T45.624	T45.625	T45.626
drug, systemic	T45.621	T45.622	T45.623	T45.624	T45.625	T45.626
Hemostyptic	T49.4X1	T49.4X2	T49.4X3	T49.4X4	T49.4X5	T49.4X6
Henbane	T62.2X1	T62.2X2	T62.2X3	T62.2X4	—	—
Heparin (sodium)	T45.511	T45.512	T45.513	T45.514	T45.515	T45.516
action reverser	T45.7X1	T45.7X2	T45.7X3	T45.7X4	T45.7X5	T45.7X6
Heparin-fraction	T45.511	T45.512	T45.513	T45.514	T45.515	T45.516

◀ New　◀▥ Revised　~~deleted~~ Deleted

Substance	External Cause (T-Code)					
	Poisoning, Accidental (Unintentional)	Poisoning, Intentional Self-Harm	Poisoning, Assault	Poisoning, Undetermined	Adverse Effect	Underdosing
Heparinoid (systemic)	T45.511	T45.512	T45.513	T45.514	T45.515	T45.516
Hepatic secretion stimulant	T47.8X1	T47.8X2	T47.8X3	T47.8X4	T47.8X5	T47.8X6
Hepatitis B						
immune globulin	T50.Z11	T50.Z12	T50.Z13	T50.Z14	T50.Z15	T50.Z16
vaccine	T50.B91	T50.B92	T50.B93	T50.B94	T50.B95	T50.B96
Hepronicate	T46.7X1	T46.7X2	T46.7X3	T46.7X4	T46.7X5	T46.7X6
Heptabarb	T42.3X1	T42.3X2	T42.3X3	T42.3X4	T42.3X5	T42.3X6
Heptabarbitone	T42.3X1	T42.3X2	T42.3X3	T42.3X4	T42.3X5	T42.3X6
Heptabarbital	T42.3X1	T42.3X2	T42.3X3	T42.3X4	T42.3X5	T42.3X6
Heptachlor	T60.1X1	T60.1X2	T60.1X3	T60.1X4	—	—
Heptalgin	T40.2X1	T40.2X2	T40.2X3	T40.2X4	T40.2X5	T40.2X6
Heptaminol	T46.3X1	T46.3X2	T46.3X3	T46.3X4	T46.3X5	T46.3X6
Herbicide NEC	T60.3X1	T60.3X2	T60.3X3	T60.3X4	—	—
Heroin	T40.1X1	T40.1X2	T40.1X3	T40.1X4	—	—
Herplex	T49.5X1	T49.5X2	T49.5X3	T49.5X4	T49.5X5	T49.5X6
HES	T45.8X1	T45.8X2	T45.8X3	T45.8X4	T45.8X5	T45.8X6
Hesperidin	T46.991	T46.992	T46.993	T46.994	T46.995	T46.996
Hetacillin	T36.0X1	T36.0X2	T36.0X3	T36.0X4	T36.0X5	T36.0X6
Hetastarch	T45.8X1	T45.8X2	T45.8X3	T45.8X4	T45.8X5	T45.8X6
HETP	T60.0X1	T60.0X2	T60.0X3	T60.0X4	—	—
Hexachlorobenzene (vapor)	T60.3X1	T60.3X2	T60.3X3	T60.3X4	—	—
Hexachlorocyclohexane	T53.6X1	T53.6X2	T53.6X3	T53.6X4	—	—
Hexachlorophene	T49.0X1	T49.0X2	T49.0X3	T49.0X4	T49.0X5	T49.0X6
Hexadiline	T46.3X1	T46.3X2	T46.3X3	T46.3X4	T46.3X5	T46.3X6
Hexadimethrine (bromide)	T45.7X1	T45.7X2	T45.7X3	T45.7X4	T45.7X5	T45.7X6
Hexadylamine	T46.3X1	T46.3X2	T46.3X3	T46.3X4	T46.3X5	T46.3X6
Hexaethyl tetraphosphate	T60.0X1	T60.0X2	T60.0X3	T60.0X4	—	—
Hexafluorenium bromide	T48.1X1	T48.1X2	T48.1X3	T48.1X4	T48.1X5	T48.1X6
Hexafluorodiethyl ether	T43.291	T43.292	T43.293	T43.294	T43.295	T43.296
Hexafluronium (bromide)	T48.1X1	T48.1X2	T48.1X3	T48.1X4	T48.1X5	T48.1X6
Hexahydrobenzol	T52.8X1	T52.8X2	T52.8X3	T52.8X4	—	—
Hexahydrocresol(s)	T51.8X1	T51.8X2	T51.8X3	T51.8X4	—	—
arsenide	T57.0X1	T57.0X2	T57.0X3	T57.0X4	—	—
arseniurated	T57.0X1	T57.0X2	T57.0X3	T57.0X4	—	—
cyanide	T57.3X1	T57.3X2	T57.3X3	T57.3X4	—	—
gas	T59.891	T59.892	T59.893	T59.894	—	—
Fluoride (liquid)	T57.8X1	T57.8X2	T57.8X3	T57.8X4	—	—
vapor	T59.891	T59.892	T59.893	T59.894	—	—
phophorated	T60.0X1	T60.0X2	T60.0X3	T60.0X4	—	—
sulfate	T57.8X1	T57.8X2	T57.8X3	T57.8X4	—	—

TABLE OF DRUGS AND CHEMICALS

Substance	Poisoning, Accidental (Unintentional)	Poisoning, Intentional Self-Harm	Poisoning, Assault	Poisoning, Undetermined	Adverse Effect	Underdosing
Hexahydrocresol(s) *(Continued)*						
sulfide (gas)	T59.6X1	T59.6X2	T59.6X3	T59.6X4	—	—
arseniurated	T57.0X1	T57.0X2	T57.0X3	T57.0X4	—	—
sulfurated	T57.8X1	T57.8X2	T57.8X3	T57.8X4	—	—
Hexahydrophenol	T51.8X1	T51.8X2	T51.8X3	T51.8X4	—	—
Hexa-germ	T49.2X1	T49.2X2	T49.2X3	T49.2X4	T49.2X5	T49.2X6
Hexalen	T51.8X1	T51.8X2	T51.8X3	T51.8X4	—	—
Hexamethonium bromide	T44.2X1	T44.2X2	T44.2X3	T44.2X4	T44.2X5	T44.2X6
Hexamethylene	T52.8X1	T52.8X2	T52.8X3	T52.8X4	—	—
Hexamethylmelamine	T45.1X1	T45.1X2	T45.1X3	T45.1X4	T45.1X5	T45.1X6
Hexamidine	T49.0X1	T49.0X2	T49.0X3	T49.0X4	T49.0X5	T49.0X6
Hexamine (mandelate)	T37.8X1	T37.8X2	T37.8X3	T37.8X4	T37.8X5	T37.8X6
Hexanone, 2-hexanone	T52.4X1	T52.4X2	T52.4X3	T52.4X4	—	—
Hexanuorenium	T48.1X1	T48.1X2	T48.1X3	T48.1X4	T48.1X5	T48.1X6
Hexapropymate	T42.6X1	T42.6X2	T42.6X3	T42.6X4	T42.6X5	T42.6X6
Hexasonium iodide	T44.3X1	T44.3X2	T44.3X3	T44.3X4	T44.3X5	T44.3X6
Hexcarbacholine bromide	T48.1X1	T48.1X2	T48.1X3	T48.1X4	T48.1X5	T48.1X6
Hexemal	T42.3X1	T42.3X2	T42.3X3	T42.3X4	T42.3X5	T42.3X6
Hexestrol	T38.5X1	T38.5X2	T38.5X3	T38.5X4	T38.5X5	T38.5X6
Hexethal (sodium)	T42.3X1	T42.3X2	T42.3X3	T42.3X4	T42.3X5	T42.3X6
Hexetidine	T37.8X1	T37.8X2	T37.8X3	T37.8X4	T37.8X5	T37.8X6
Hexobarbital	T42.3X1	T42.3X2	T42.3X3	T42.3X4	T42.3X5	T42.3X6
rectal	T41.291	T41.292	T41.293	T41.294	T41.295	T41.296
sodium	T41.1X1	T41.1X2	T41.1X3	T41.1X4	T41.1X5	T41.1X6
Hexobendine	T46.3X1	T46.3X2	T46.3X3	T46.3X4	T46.3X5	T46.3X6
Hexocyclium	T44.3X1	T44.3X2	T44.3X3	T44.3X4	T44.3X5	T44.3X6
metilsulfate	T44.3X1	T44.3X2	T44.3X3	T44.3X4	T44.3X5	T44.3X6
Hexoestrol	T38.5X1	T38.5X2	T38.5X3	T38.5X4	T38.5X5	T38.5X6
Hexone	T52.4X1	T52.4X2	T52.4X3	T52.4X4	—	—
Hexoprenaline	T48.6X1	T48.6X2	T48.6X3	T48.6X4	T48.6X5	T48.6X6
Hexylcaine	T41.3X1	T41.3X2	T41.3X3	T41.3X4	T41.3X5	T41.3X6
Hexylresorcinol	T52.2X1	T52.2X2	T52.2X3	T52.2X4	—	—
HGH (human growth hormone)	T38.811	T38.812	T38.813	T38.814	T38.815	T38.816
Hinkle's pills	T47.2X1	T47.2X2	T47.2X3	T47.2X4	T47.2X5	T47.2X6
Histalog	T50.8X1	T50.8X2	T50.8X3	T50.8X4	T50.8X5	T50.8X6
Histamine (phosphate)	T50.8X1	T50.8X2	T50.8X3	T50.8X4	T50.8X5	T50.8X6
Histoplasmin	T50.8X1	T50.8X2	T50.8X3	T50.8X4	T50.8X5	T50.8X6
Holly berries	T62.2X1	T62.2X2	T62.2X3	T62.2X4	—	—
Homatropine	T44.3X1	T44.3X2	T44.3X3	T44.3X4	T44.3X5	T44.3X6
methylbromide	T44.3X1	T44.3X2	T44.3X3	T44.3X4	T44.3X5	T44.3X6

◀ New ◀ Revised ~~deleted~~ Deleted

Substance	Poisoning, Accidental (Unintentional)	Poisoning, Intentional Self-Harm	Poisoning, Assault	Poisoning, Undetermined	Adverse Effect	Underdosing
			External Cause (T-Code)			
Homochlorcyclizine	T45.0X1	T45.0X2	T45.0X3	T45.0X4	T45.0X5	T45.0X6
Homosalate	T49.3X1	T49.3X2	T49.3X3	T49.3X4	T49.3X5	T49.3X6
Homo-tet	T50.Z11	T50.Z12	T50.Z13	T50.Z14	T50.Z15	T50.Z16
Hormone	T38.801	T38.802	T38.803	T38.804	T38.805	T38.806
adrenal cortical steroids	T38.0X1	T38.0X2	T38.0X3	T38.0X4	T38.0X5	T38.0X6
androgenic	T38.7X1	T38.7X2	T38.7X3	T38.7X4	T38.7X5	T38.7X6
anterior pituitary NEC	T38.811	T38.812	T38.813	T38.814	T38.815	T38.816
antidiabetic agents	T38.3X1	T38.3X2	T38.3X3	T38.3X4	T38.3X5	T38.3X6
antidiuretic	T38.891	T38.892	T38.893	T38.894	T38.895	T38.896
cancer therapy	T45.1X1	T45.1X2	T45.1X3	T45.1X4	T45.1X5	T45.1X6
follicle stimulating	T38.811	T38.812	T38.813	T38.814	T38.815	T38.816
gonadotropic	T38.891	T38.892	T38.893	T38.894	T38.895	T38.896
pituitary	T38.811	T38.812	T38.813	T38.814	T38.815	T38.816
growth	T38.811	T38.812	T38.813	T38.814	T38.815	T38.816
luteinizing	T38.811	T38.812	T38.813	T38.814	T38.815	T38.816
ovarian	T38.5X1	T38.5X2	T38.5X3	T38.5X4	T38.5X5	T38.5X6
oxytocic	T48.0X1	T48.0X2	T48.0X3	T48.0X4	T48.0X5	T48.0X6
parathyroid (derivatives)	T50.991	T50.992	T50.993	T50.994	T50.995	T50.996
pituitary (posterior) NEC	T38.891	T38.892	T38.893	T38.894	T38.895	T38.896
anterior	T38.811	T38.812	T38.813	T38.814	T38.815	T38.816
specified, NEC	T38.891	T38.892	T38.893	T38.894	T38.895	T38.896
thyroid	T38.1X1	T38.1X2	T38.1X3	T38.1X4	T38.1X5	T38.1X6
Hornet (sting)	T63.451	T63.452	T63.453	T63.454	—	—
Horse anti-human lymphocytic serum	T50.Z11	T50.Z12	T50.Z13	T50.Z14	T50.Z15	T50.Z16
Horticulture agent NEC	T65.91	T65.92	T65.93	T65.94	—	—
with pesticide	T60.91	T60.92	T60.93	T60.94	—	—
Human						
albumin	T45.8X1	T45.8X2	T45.8X3	T45.8X4	T45.8X5	T45.8X6
growth hormone (HGH)	T38.811	T38.812	T38.813	T38.814	T38.815	T38.816
immune serum	T50.Z11	T50.Z12	T50.Z13	T50.Z14	T50.Z15	T50.Z16
Hyaluronidase	T45.3X1	T45.3X2	T45.3X3	T45.3X4	T45.3X5	T45.3X6
Hyazyme	T45.3X1	T45.3X2	T45.3X3	T45.3X4	T45.3X5	T45.3X6
Hycodan	T40.2X1	T40.2X2	T40.2X3	T40.2X4	T40.2X5	T40.2X6
Hydantoin derivative NEC	T42.0X1	T42.0X2	T42.0X3	T42.0X4	T42.0X5	T42.0X6
Hydeltra	T38.0X1	T38.0X2	T38.0X3	T38.0X4	T38.0X5	T38.0X6
Hydergine	T44.6X1	T44.6X2	T44.6X3	T44.6X4	T44.6X5	T44.6X6
Hydrabamine penicillin	T36.0X1	T36.0X2	T36.0X3	T36.0X4	T36.0X5	T36.0X6
Hydralazine	T46.5X1	T46.5X2	T46.5X3	T46.5X4	T46.5X5	T46.5X6
Hydrargaphen	T49.0X1	T49.0X2	T49.0X3	T49.0X4	T49.0X5	T49.0X6

◀ New ◀‖‖ Revised ~~deleted~~ Deleted

TABLE OF DRUGS AND CHEMICALS

Substance	External Cause (T-Code)					
	Poisoning, Accidental (Unintentional)	Poisoning, Intentional Self-Harm	Poisoning, Assault	Poisoning, Undetermined	Adverse Effect	Underdosing
Hydrargyri amino-chloridum	T49.0X1	T49.0X2	T49.0X3	T49.0X4	T49.0X5	T49.0X6
Hydrastine	T48.291	T48.292	T48.293	T48.294	T48.295	T48.296
Hydrazine	T54.1X1	T54.1X2	T54.1X3	T54.1X4	—	—
monoamine oxidase inhibitors	T43.1X1	T43.1X2	T43.1X3	T43.1X4	T43.1X5	T43.1X6
Hydrazoic acid, azides	T54.2X1	T54.2X2	T54.2X3	T54.2X4	—	—
Hydriodic acid	T48.4X1	T48.4X2	T48.4X3	T48.4X4	T48.4X5	T48.4X6
Hydrocarbon gas	T59.891	T59.892	T59.893	T59.894	—	—
incomplete combustion of—see Carbon, monoxide, fuel, utility						
liquefied (mobile container)	T59.891	T59.892	T59.893	T59.894	—	—
piped (natural)	T59.891	T59.892	T59.893	T59.894	—	—
Hydrochloric acid (liquid)	T54.2X1	T54.2X2	T54.2X3	T54.2X4	—	—
medicinal (digestant)	T47.5X1	T47.5X2	T47.5X3	T47.5X4	T47.5X5	T47.5X6
vapor	T59.891	T59.892	T59.893	T59.894	—	—
Hydrochlorothiazide	T50.2X1	T50.2X2	T50.2X3	T50.2X4	T50.2X5	T50.2X6
Hydrocodone	T40.2X1	T40.2X2	T40.2X3	T40.2X4	T40.2X5	T40.2X6
Hydrocortisone (derivatives)	T49.0X1	T49.0X2	T49.0X3	T49.0X4	T49.0X5	T49.0X6
aceponate	T49.0X1	T49.0X2	T49.0X3	T49.0X4	T49.0X5	T49.0X6
ENT agent	T49.6X1	T49.6X2	T49.6X3	T49.6X4	T49.6X5	T49.6X6
ophthalmic preparation	T49.5X1	T49.5X2	T49.5X3	T49.5X4	T49.5X5	T49.5X6
topical NEC	T49.0X1	T49.0X2	T49.0X3	T49.0X4	T49.0X5	T49.0X6
Hydrocortone	T38.0X1	T38.0X2	T38.0X3	T38.0X4	T38.0X5	T38.0X6
ENT agent	T49.6X1	T49.6X2	T49.6X3	T49.6X4	T49.6X5	T49.6X6
ophthalmic preparation	T49.5X1	T49.5X2	T49.5X3	T49.5X4	T49.5X5	T49.5X6
topical NEC	T49.0X1	T49.0X2	T49.0X3	T49.0X4	T49.0X5	T49.0X6
Hydrocyanic acid (liquid)	T57.3X1	T57.3X2	T57.3X3	T57.3X4	—	—
gas	T65.0X1	T65.0X2	T65.0X3	T65.0X4	—	—
Hydroflumethiazide	T50.2X1	T50.2X2	T50.2X3	T50.2X4	T50.2X5	T50.2X6
Hydrofluoric acid (liquid)	T54.2X1	T54.2X2	T54.2X3	T54.2X4	—	—
vapor	T59.891	T59.892	T59.893	T59.894	—	—
Hydrogen	T59.891	T59.892	T59.893	T59.894	—	—
arsenide	T57.0X1	T57.0X2	T57.0X3	T57.0X4	—	—
arseniureted	T57.0X1	T57.0X2	T57.0X3	T57.0X4	—	—
chloride	T57.8X1	T57.8X2	T57.8X3	T57.8X4	—	—
cyanide (salts)	T57.3X1	T57.3X2	T57.3X3	T57.3X4	—	—
gas	T57.3X1	T57.3X2	T57.3X3	T57.3X4	—	—
Fluoride	T59.5X1	T59.5X2	T59.5X3	T59.5X4	—	—
vapor	T59.5X1	T59.5X2	T59.5X3	T59.5X4	—	—
peroxide	T49.0X1	T49.0X2	T49.0X3	T49.0X4	T49.0X5	T49.0X6
phosphureted	T57.1X1	T57.1X2	T57.1X3	T57.1X4	—	—

◀ New   ⬅ Revised   deleted Deleted

Substance	External Cause (T-Code)					
	Poisoning, Accidental (Unintentional)	Poisoning, Intentional Self-Harm	Poisoning, Assault	Poisoning, Undetermined	Adverse Effect	Underdosing
Hydrogen *(Continued)*						
sulfide	T59.6X1	T59.6X2	T59.6X3	T59.6X4	—	—
arseniureted	T57.0X1	T57.0X2	T57.0X3	T57.0X4	—	—
sulfureted	T59.6X1	T59.6X2	T59.6X3	T59.6X4	—	—
Hydromethylpyridine	T46.7X1	T46.7X2	T46.7X3	T46.7X4	T46.7X5	T46.7X6
Hydromorphinol	T40.2X1	T40.2X2	T40.2X3	T40.2X4	—	—
Hydromorphinone	T40.2X1	T40.2X2	T40.2X3	T40.2X4	T40.2X5	T40.2X6
Hydromorphone	T40.2X1	T40.2X2	T40.2X3	T40.2X4	T40.2X5	T40.2X6
Hydromox	T50.2X1	T50.2X2	T50.2X3	T50.2X4	T50.2X5	T50.2X6
Hydrophilic lotion	T49.3X1	T49.3X2	T49.3X3	T49.3X4	T49.3X5	T49.3X6
Hydroquinidine	T46.2X1	T46.2X2	T46.2X3	T46.2X4	T46.2X5	T46.2X6
Hydroquinone	T52.2X1	T52.2X2	T52.2X3	T52.2X4	—	—
vapor	T59.891	T59.892	T59.893	T59.894	—	—
Hydrosulfuric acid (gas)	T59.6X1	T59.6X2	T59.6X3	T59.6X4	—	—
Hydrotalcite	T47.1X1	T47.1X2	T47.1X3	T47.1X4	T47.1X5	T47.1X6
Hydrous wool fat	T49.3X1	T49.3X2	T49.3X3	T49.3X4	T49.3X5	T49.3X6
Hydroxide, caustic	T54.3X1	T54.3X2	T54.3X3	T54.3X4	—	—
Hydroxocobalamin	T45.8X1	T45.8X2	T45.8X3	T45.8X4	T45.8X5	T45.8X6
Hydroxyamphetamine	T49.5X1	T49.5X2	T49.5X3	T49.5X4	T49.5X5	T49.5X6
Hydroxycarbamide	T45.1X1	T45.1X2	T45.1X3	T45.1X4	T45.1X5	T45.1X6
Hydroxychloroquine	T37.8X1	T37.8X2	T37.8X3	T37.8X4	T37.8X5	T37.8X6
Hydroxydihydrocodeinone	T40.2X1	T40.2X2	T40.2X3	T40.2X4	T40.2X5	T40.2X6
Hydroxyestrone	T38.5X1	T38.5X2	T38.5X3	T38.5X4	T38.5X5	T38.5X6
Hydroxyethyl starch	T45.8X1	T45.8X2	T45.8X3	T45.8X4	T45.8X5	T45.8X6
Hydroxymethylpentanone	T52.4X1	T52.4X2	T52.4X3	T52.4X4	—	—
Hydroxyphenamate	T43.591	T43.592	T43.593	T43.594	T43.595	T43.596
Hydroxyphenylbutazone	T39.2X1	T39.2X2	T39.2X3	T39.2X4	T39.2X5	T39.2X6
Hydroxyprogesterone	T38.5X1	T38.5X2	T38.5X3	T38.5X4	T38.5X5	T38.5X6
caproate	T38.5X1	T38.5X2	T38.5X3	T38.5X4	T38.5X5	T38.5X6
Hydroxyquinoline (derivatives) NEC	T37.8X1	T37.8X2	T37.8X3	T37.8X4	T37.8X5	T37.8X6
Hydroxystilbamidine	T37.3X1	T37.3X2	T37.3X3	T37.3X4	T37.3X5	T37.3X6
Hydroxytoluene (nonmedicinal)	T54.0X1	T54.0X2	T54.0X3	T54.0X4	—	—
medicinal	T49.0X1	T49.0X2	T49.0X3	T49.0X4	T49.0X5	T49.0X6
Hydroxyurea	T45.1X1	T45.1X2	T45.1X3	T45.1X4	T45.1X5	T45.1X6
Hydroxyzine	T43.591	T43.592	T43.593	T43.594	T43.595	T43.596
Hyoscine	T44.3X1	T44.3X2	T44.3X3	T44.3X4	T44.3X5	T44.3X6
Hyoscyamine	T44.3X1	T44.3X2	T44.3X3	T44.3X4	T44.3X5	T44.3X6
Hyoscyamus	T44.3X1	T44.3X2	T44.3X3	T44.3X4	T44.3X5	T44.3X6
dry extract	T44.3X1	T44.3X2	T44.3X3	T44.3X4	T44.3X5	T44.3X6

◀ New   ◀▥ Revised   ~~deleted~~ Deleted

TABLE OF DRUGS AND CHEMICALS

Substance	External Cause (T-Code)					
	Poisoning, Accidental (Unintentional)	Poisoning, Intentional Self-Harm	Poisoning, Assault	Poisoning, Undetermined	Adverse Effect	Underdosing
Hypaque	T50.8X1	T50.8X2	T50.8X3	T50.8X4	T50.8X5	T50.8X6
Hypertussis	T50.Z11	T50.Z12	T50.Z13	T50.Z14	T50.Z15	T50.Z16
Hypnotic	T42.71	T42.72	T42.73	T42.74	T42.75	T42.76
anticonvulsant	T42.71	T42.72	T42.73	T42.74	T42.75	T42.76
specified NEC	T42.6X1	T42.6X2	T42.6X3	T42.6X4	T42.6X5	T42.6X6
Hypochlorite	T49.0X1	T49.0X2	T49.0X3	T49.0X4	T49.0X5	T49.0X6
Hypophysis, posterior	T38.891	T38.892	T38.893	T38.894	T38.895	T38.896
Hypotensive NEC	T46.5X1	T46.5X2	T46.5X3	T46.5X4	T46.5X5	T46.5X6
Hypromellose	T49.5X1	T49.5X2	T49.5X3	T49.5X4	T49.5X5	T49.5X6
I						
Ibacitabine	T37.5X1	T37.5X2	T37.5X3	T37.5X4	T37.5X5	T37.5X6
Ibopamine	T44.991	T44.992	T44.993	T44.994	T44.995	T44.996
Ibufenac	T39.311	T39.312	T39.313	T39.314	T39.315	T39.316
Ibuprofen	T39.311	T39.312	T39.313	T39.314	T39.315	T39.316
Ibuproxam	T39.311	T39.312	T39.313	T39.314	T39.315	T39.316
Ibuterol	T48.6X1	T48.6X2	T48.6X3	T48.6X4	T48.6X5	T48.6X6
Ichthammol	T49.0X1	T49.0X2	T49.0X3	T49.0X4	T49.0X5	T49.0X6
Ichthyol	T49.4X1	T49.4X2	T49.4X3	T49.4X4	T49.4X5	T49.4X6
Idarubicin	T45.1X1	T45.1X2	T45.1X3	T45.1X4	T45.1X5	T45.1X6
Idrocilamide	T42.8X1	T42.8X2	T42.8X3	T42.8X4	T42.8X5	T42.8X6
Ifenprodil	T46.7X1	T46.7X2	T46.7X3	T46.7X4	T46.7X5	T46.7X6
Ifosfamide	T45.1X1	T45.1X2	T45.1X3	T45.1X4	T45.1X5	T45.1X6
Iletin	T38.3X1	T38.3X2	T38.3X3	T38.3X4	T38.3X5	T38.3X6
Ilex	T62.2X1	T62.2X2	T62.2X3	T62.2X4	—	—
Illuminating gas (after combustion)	T58.11	T58.12	T58.13	T58.14	—	—
prior to combustion	T59.891	T59.892	T59.893	T59.894	—	—
Ilopan	T45.2X1	T45.2X2	T45.2X3	T45.2X4	T45.2X5	T45.2X6
Iloprost	T46.7X1	T46.7X2	T46.7X3	T46.7X4	T46.7X5	T46.7X6
Ilotycin	T36.3X1	T36.3X2	T36.3X3	T36.3X4	T36.3X5	T36.3X6
ophthalmic preparation	T49.5X1	T49.5X2	T49.5X3	T49.5X4	T49.5X5	T49.5X6
topical NEC	T49.0X1	T49.0X2	T49.0X3	T49.0X4	T49.0X5	T49.0X6
Imidazole-4-carboxamide	T45.1X1	T45.1X2	T45.1X3	T45.1X4	T45.1X5	T45.1X6
Imipenem	T36.0X1	T36.0X2	T36.0X3	T36.0X4	T36.0X5	T36.0X6
Imipramine	T43.011	T43.012	T43.013	T43.014	T43.015	T43.016
Iminostilbene	T42.1X1	T42.1X2	T42.1X3	T42.1X4	T42.1X5	T42.1X6
Immu-G	T50.Z11	T50.Z12	T50.Z13	T50.Z14	T50.Z15	T50.Z16
Immuglobin	T50.Z11	T50.Z12	T50.Z13	T50.Z14	T50.Z15	T50.Z16
Immune						
globulin	T50.Z11	T50.Z12	T50.Z13	T50.Z14	T50.Z15	T50.Z16
serum globulin	T50.Z11	T50.Z12	T50.Z13	T50.Z14	T50.Z15	T50.Z16

◄ New   ◄ Revised   deleted Deleted

Substance	External Cause (T-Code)					
	Poisoning, Accidental (Unintentional)	Poisoning, Intentional Self-Harm	Poisoning, Assault	Poisoning, Undetermined	Adverse Effect	Underdosing
Immunoglobin human (intravenous) (normal)	T50.Z11	T50.Z12	T50.Z13	T50.Z14	T50.Z15	T50.Z16
unmodified	T50.Z11	T50.Z12	T50.Z13	T50.Z14	T50.Z15	T50.Z16
Immunosuppressive drug	T45.1X1	T45.1X2	T45.1X3	T45.1X4	T45.1X5	T45.1X6
Immu-tetanus	T50.Z11	T50.Z12	T50.Z13	T50.Z14	T50.Z15	T50.Z16
Indalpine	T43.221	T43.222	T43.223	T43.224	T43.225	T43.226
Indanazoline	T48.5X1	T48.5X2	T48.5X3	T48.5X4	T48.5X5	T48.5X6
Indandione (derivatives)	T45.511	T45.512	T45.513	T45.514	T45.515	T45.516
Indapamide	T46.5X1	T46.5X2	T46.5X3	T46.5X4	T46.5X5	T46.5X6
Indendione (derivatives)	T45.511	T45.512	T45.513	T45.514	T45.515	T45.516
Indenolol	T44.7X1	T44.7X2	T44.7X3	T44.7X4	T44.7X5	T44.7X6
Inderal	T44.7X1	T44.7X2	T44.7X3	T44.7X4	T44.7X5	T44.7X6
Indian						
hemp	T40.7X1	T40.7X2	T40.7X3	T40.7X4	T40.7X5	T40.7X6
tobacco	T62.2X1	T62.2X2	T62.2X3	T62.2X4	—	—
Indigo carmine	T50.8X1	T50.8X2	T50.8X3	T50.8X4	T50.8X5	T50.8X6
Indobufen	T45.521	T45.522	T45.523	T45.524	T45.525	T45.526
Indocin	T39.2X1	T39.2X2	T39.2X3	T39.2X4	T39.2X5	T39.2X6
Indocyanine green	T50.8X1	T50.8X2	T50.8X3	T50.8X4	T50.8X5	T50.8X6
Indometacin	T39.391	T39.392	T39.393	T39.394	T39.395	T39.396
Indomethacin	T39.391	T39.392	T39.393	T39.394	T39.395	T39.396
farnesil	T39.4X1	T39.4X2	T39.4X3	T39.4X4	T39.4X5	T39.4X6
Indoramin	T44.6X1	T44.6X2	T44.6X3	T44.6X4	T44.6X5	T44.6X6
Industrial						
alcohol	T51.0X1	T51.0X2	T51.0X3	T51.0X4	—	—
fumes	T59.891	T59.892	T59.893	T59.894	—	—
solvents (fumes) (vapors)	T52.91	T52.92	T52.93	T52.94	—	—
Influenza vaccine	T50.B91	T50.B92	T50.B93	T50.B94	T50.B95	T50.B96
Ingested substance NEC	T65.91	T65.92	T65.93	T65.94	—	—
INH	T37.1X1	T37.1X2	T37.1X3	T37.1X4	T37.1X5	T37.1X6
Inhalation, gas (noxious) — see Gas						
Inhibitor						
angiotensin-converting enzyme	T46.4X1	T46.4X2	T46.4X3	T46.4X4	T46.4X5	T46.4X6
carbonic anhydrase	T50.2X1	T50.2X2	T50.2X3	T50.2X4	T50.2X5	T50.2X6
fibrinolysis	T45.621	T45.622	T45.623	T45.624	T45.625	T45.626
monoamine oxidase NEC	T43.1X1	T43.1X2	T43.1X3	T43.1X4	T43.1X5	T43.1X6
hydrazine	T43.1X1	T43.1X2	T43.1X3	T43.1X4	T43.1X5	T43.1X6
postsynaptic	T43.8X1	T43.8X2	T43.8X3	T43.8X4	T43.8X5	T43.8X6
prothrombin synthesis	T45.511	T45.512	T45.513	T45.514	T45.515	T45.516
Ink	T65.891	T65.892	T65.893	T65.894	—	—
Inorganic substance NEC	T57.91	T57.92	T57.93	T57.94	—	—

TABLE OF DRUGS AND CHEMICALS

Substance	External Cause (T-Code)					
	Poisoning, Accidental (Unintentional)	Poisoning, Intentional Self-Harm	Poisoning, Assault	Poisoning, Undetermined	Adverse Effect	Underdosing
Inosine pranobex	T37.5X1	T37.5X2	T37.5X3	T37.5X4	T37.5X5	T37.5X6
Inositol	T50.991	T50.992	T50.993	T50.994	T50.995	T50.996
nicotinate	T46.7X1	T46.7X2	T46.7X3	T46.7X4	T46.7X5	T46.7X6
Inproquone	T45.1X1	T45.1X2	T45.1X3	T45.1X4	T45.1X5	T45.1X6
Insect (sting), venomous	T63.481	T63.482	T63.483	T63.484	—	—
ant	T63.421	T63.422	T63.423	T63.424	—	—
bee	T63.441	T63.442	T63.443	T63.444	—	—
caterpillar	T63.431	T63.432	T63.433	T63.434	—	—
hornet	T63.451	T63.452	T63.453	T63.454	—	—
wasp	T63.461	T63.462	T63.463	T63.464	—	—
Insecticide NEC	T60.91	T60.92	T60.93	T60.94	—	—
carbamate	T60.0X1	T60.0X2	T60.0X3	T60.0X4	—	—
chlorinated	T60.1X1	T60.1X2	T60.1X3	T60.1X4	—	—
mixed	T60.91	T60.92	T60.93	T60.94	—	—
organochlorine	T60.1X1	T60.1X2	T60.1X3	T60.1X4	—	—
organophosphorus	T60.0X1	T60.0X2	T60.0X3	T60.0X4	—	—
Insular tissue extract	T38.3X1	T38.3X2	T38.3X3	T38.3X4	T38.3X5	T38.3X6
Insulin (amorphous) (globin) (isophane) (Lente) (NPH) (Semilente) (Ultralente)	T38.3X1	T38.3X2	T38.3X3	T38.3X4	T38.3X5	T38.3X6
defalan	T38.3X1	T38.3X2	T38.3X3	T38.3X4	T38.3X5	T38.3X6
human	T38.3X1	T38.3X2	T38.3X3	T38.3X4	T38.3X5	T38.3X6
injection, soluble	T38.3X1	T38.3X2	T38.3X3	T38.3X4	T38.3X5	T38.3X6
biphasic	T38.3X1	T38.3X2	T38.3X3	T38.3X4	T38.3X5	T38.3X6
intermediate acting	T38.3X1	T38.3X2	T38.3X3	T38.3X4	T38.3X5	T38.3X6
protamine zinc	T38.3X1	T38.3X2	T38.3X3	T38.3X4	T38.3X5	T38.3X6
slow acting	T38.3X1	T38.3X2	T38.3X3	T38.3X4	T38.3X5	T38.3X6
zinc						
protamine injection	T38.3X1	T38.3X2	T38.3X3	T38.3X4	T38.3X5	T38.3X6
suspension (amorphous) (crystalline)	T38.3X1	T38.3X2	T38.3X3	T38.3X4	T38.3X5	T38.3X6
Interferon (alpha) (beta) (gamma)	T37.5X1	T37.5X2	T37.5X3	T37.5X4	T37.5X5	T37.5X6
Intestinal motility control drug	T47.6X1	T47.6X2	T47.6X3	T47.6X4	T47.6X5	T47.6X6
biological	T47.8X1	T47.8X2	T47.8X3	T47.8X4	T47.8X5	T47.8X6
Intranarcon	T41.1X1	T41.1X2	T41.1X3	T41.1X4	T41.1X5	T41.1X6
Intravenous						
amino acids	T50.991	T50.992	T50.993	T50.994	T50.995	T50.996
fat suspension	T50.991	T50.992	T50.993	T50.994	T50.995	T50.996
Inulin	T50.8X1	T50.8X2	T50.8X3	T50.8X4	T50.8X5	T50.8X6
Invert sugar	T50.3X1	T50.3X2	T50.3X3	T50.3X4	T50.3X5	T50.3X6
Inza — see Naproxen						
Iobenzamic acid	T50.8X1	T50.8X2	T50.8X3	T50.8X4	T50.8X5	T50.8X6
Iocarmic acid	T50.8X1	T50.8X2	T50.8X3	T50.8X4	T50.8X5	T50.8X6

◀ New   ◀▥ Revised   ~~deleted~~ Deleted

Substance	Poisoning, Accidental (Unintentional)	Poisoning, Intentional Self-Harm	Poisoning, Assault	Poisoning, Undetermined	Adverse Effect	Underdosing
			External Cause (T-Code)			
Iocetamic acid	T50.8X1	T50.8X2	T50.8X3	T50.8X4	T50.8X5	T50.8X6
Iodamide	T50.8X1	T50.8X2	T50.8X3	T50.8X4	T50.8X5	T50.8X6
Iodide NEC — see also Iodine	T49.0X1	T49.0X2	T49.0X3	T49.0X4	T49.0X5	T49.0X6
mercury (ointment)	T49.0X1	T49.0X2	T49.0X3	T49.0X4	T49.0X5	T49.0X6
methylate	T49.0X1	T49.0X2	T49.0X3	T49.0X4	T49.0X5	T49.0X6
potassium (expectorant) NEC	T48.4X1	T48.4X2	T48.4X3	T48.4X4	T48.4X5	T48.4X6
Iodinated						
contrast medium	T50.8X1	T50.8X2	T50.8X3	T50.8X4	T50.8X5	T50.8X6
glycerol	T48.4X1	T48.4X2	T48.4X3	T48.4X4	T48.4X5	T48.4X6
human serum albumin (131I)	T50.8X1	T50.8X2	T50.8X3	T50.8X4	T50.8X5	T50.8X6
Iodine (antiseptic, external) (tincture) NEC	T49.0X1	T49.0X2	T49.0X3	T49.0X4	T49.0X5	T49.0X6
125 — see also Radiation sickness, and Exposure to radioactivce isotopes	T50.8X1	T50.8X2	T50.8X3	T50.8X4	T50.8X5	T50.8X6
therapeutic	T50.991	T50.992	T50.993	T50.994	T50.995	T50.996
131 — see also Radiation sickness, and Exposure to radioactivce isotopes	T50.8X1	T50.8X2	T50.8X3	T50.8X4	T50.8X5	T50.8X6
therapeutic	T38.2X1	T38.2X2	T38.2X3	T38.2X4	T38.2X5	T38.2X6
diagnostic	T50.8X1	T50.8X2	T50.8X3	T50.8X4	T50.8X5	T50.8X6
for thyroid conditions (antithyroid)	T38.2X1	T38.2X2	T38.2X3	T38.2X4	T38.2X5	T38.2X6
solution	T49.0X1	T49.0X2	T49.0X3	T49.0X4	T49.0X5	T49.0X6
vapor	T59.891	T59.892	T59.893	T59.894	—	—
Iodipamide	T50.8X1	T50.8X2	T50.8X3	T50.8X4	T50.8X5	T50.8X6
Iodized (poppy seed) oil	T50.8X1	T50.8X2	T50.8X3	T50.8X4	T50.8X5	T50.8X6
Iodobismitol	T37.8X1	T37.8X2	T37.8X3	T37.8X4	T37.8X5	T37.8X6
Iodochlorhydroxyquin	T37.8X1	T37.8X2	T37.8X3	T37.8X4	T37.8X5	T37.8X6
topical	T49.0X1	T49.0X2	T49.0X3	T49.0X4	T49.0X5	T49.0X6
Iodochlorhydroxyquino-line	T37.8X1	T37.8X2	T37.8X3	T37.8X4	T37.8X5	T37.8X6
Iodocholesterol (131I)	T50.8X1	T50.8X2	T50.8X3	T50.8X4	T50.8X5	T50.8X6
Iodoform	T49.0X1	T49.0X2	T49.0X3	T49.0X4	T49.0X5	T49.0X6
Iodohippuric acid	T50.8X1	T50.8X2	T50.8X3	T50.8X4	T50.8X5	T50.8X6
Iodopanoic acid	T50.8X1	T50.8X2	T50.8X3	T50.8X4	T50.8X5	T50.8X6
Iodophthalein (sodium)	T50.8X1	T50.8X2	T50.8X3	T50.8X4	T50.8X5	T50.8X6
Iodopyracet	T50.8X1	T50.8X2	T50.8X3	T50.8X4	T50.8X5	T50.8X6
Iodoquinol	T37.8X1	T37.8X2	T37.8X3	T37.8X4	T37.8X5	T37.8X6
Iodoxamic acid	T50.8X1	T50.8X2	T50.8X3	T50.8X4	T50.8X5	T50.8X6
Iofendylate	T50.8X1	T50.8X2	T50.8X3	T50.8X4	T50.8X5	T50.8X6
Ioglycamic acid	T50.8X1	T50.8X2	T50.8X3	T50.8X4	T50.8X5	T50.8X6
Iohexol	T50.8X1	T50.8X2	T50.8X3	T50.8X4	T50.8X5	T50.8X6
Ion exchange resin						
anion	T47.8X1	T47.8X2	T47.8X3	T47.8X4	T47.8X5	T47.8X6
cation	T50.3X1	T50.3X2	T50.3X3	T50.3X4	T50.3X5	T50.3X6

◀ New   ◀▥ Revised   ~~deleted~~ Deleted

Substance	External Cause (T-Code)					
	Poisoning, Accidental (Unintentional)	Poisoning, Intentional Self-Harm	Poisoning, Assault	Poisoning, Undetermined	Adverse Effect	Underdosing
Ion exchange resin *(Continued)*						
cholestyramine	T46.6X1	T46.6X2	T46.6X3	T46.6X4	T46.6X5	T46.6X6
intestinal	T47.8X1	T47.8X2	T47.8X3	T47.8X4	T47.8X5	T47.8X6
Iopamidol	T50.8X1	T50.8X2	T50.8X3	T50.8X4	T50.8X5	T50.8X6
Iopanoic acid	T50.8X1	T50.8X2	T50.8X3	T50.8X4	T50.8X5	T50.8X6
Iophenoic acid	T50.8X1	T50.8X2	T50.8X3	T50.8X4	T50.8X5	T50.8X6
Iopodate, sodium	T50.8X1	T50.8X2	T50.8X3	T50.8X4	T50.8X5	T50.8X6
Iopodic acid	T50.8X1	T50.8X2	T50.8X3	T50.8X4	T50.8X5	T50.8X6
Iopromide	T50.8X1	T50.8X2	T50.8X3	T50.8X4	T50.8X5	T50.8X6
Iopydol	T50.8X1	T50.8X2	T50.8X3	T50.8X4	T50.8X5	T50.8X6
Iotalamic acid	T50.8X1	T50.8X2	T50.8X3	T50.8X4	T50.8X5	T50.8X6
Iothalamate	T50.8X1	T50.8X2	T50.8X3	T50.8X4	T50.8X5	T50.8X6
Iothiouracil	T38.2X1	T38.2X2	T38.2X3	T38.2X4	T38.2X5	T38.2X6
Iotrol	T50.8X1	T50.8X2	T50.8X3	T50.8X4	T50.8X5	T50.8X6
Iotrolan	T50.8X1	T50.8X2	T50.8X3	T50.8X4	T50.8X5	T50.8X6
Iotroxate	T50.8X1	T50.8X2	T50.8X3	T50.8X4	T50.8X5	T50.8X6
Iotroxic acid	T50.8X1	T50.8X2	T50.8X3	T50.8X4	T50.8X5	T50.8X6
Ioversol	T50.8X1	T50.8X2	T50.8X3	T50.8X4	T50.8X5	T50.8X6
Ioxaglate	T50.8X1	T50.8X2	T50.8X3	T50.8X4	T50.8X5	T50.8X6
Ioxaglic acid	T50.8X1	T50.8X2	T50.8X3	T50.8X4	T50.8X5	T50.8X6
Ioxitalamic acid	T50.8X1	T50.8X2	T50.8X3	T50.8X4	T50.8X5	T50.8X6
Ipecac	T47.7X1	T47.7X2	T47.7X3	T47.7X4	T47.7X5	T47.7X6
Ipecacuanha	T48.4X1	T48.4X2	T48.4X3	T48.4X4	T48.4X5	T48.4X6
Ipodate, calcium	T50.8X1	T50.8X2	T50.8X3	T50.8X4	T50.8X5	T50.8X6
Ipral	T42.3X1	T42.3X2	T42.3X3	T42.3X4	T42.3X5	T42.3X6
Ipratropium (bromide)	T48.6X1	T48.6X2	T48.6X3	T48.6X4	T48.6X5	T48.6X6
Ipriflavone	T46.3X1	T46.3X2	T46.3X3	T46.3X4	T46.3X5	T46.3X6
Iprindole	T43.011	T43.012	T43.013	T43.014	T43.015	T43.016
Iproclozide	T43.1X1	T43.1X2	T43.1X3	T43.1X4	T43.1X5	T43.1X6
Iprofenin	T50.8X1	T50.8X2	T50.8X3	T50.8X4	T50.8X5	T50.8X6
Iproheptine	T49.2X1	T49.2X2	T49.2X3	T49.2X4	T49.2X5	T49.2X6
Iproniazid	T43.1X1	T43.1X2	T43.1X3	T43.1X4	T43.1X5	T43.1X6
Iproplatin	T45.1X1	T45.1X2	T45.1X3	T45.1X4	T45.1X5	T45.1X6
Iproveratril	T46.1X1	T46.1X2	T46.1X3	T46.1X4	T46.1X5	T46.1X6
Iron (compounds) (medicinal) NEC	T45.4X1	T45.4X2	T45.4X3	T45.4X4	T45.4X5	T45.4X6
ammonium	T45.4X1	T45.4X2	T45.4X3	T45.4X4	T45.4X5	T45.4X6
dextran injection	T45.4X1	T45.4X2	T45.4X3	T45.4X4	T45.4X5	T45.4X6
nonmedicinal	T56.891	T56.892	T56.893	T56.894	—	—

◀ New ◀ Revised ~~deleted~~ Deleted

Substance	External Cause (T-Code)					
	Poisoning, Accidental (Unintentional)	Poisoning, Intentional Self-Harm	Poisoning, Assault	Poisoning, Undetermined	Adverse Effect	Underdosing
Iron NEC *(Continued)*						
salts	T45.4X1	T45.4X2	T45.4X3	T45.4X4	T45.4X5	T45.4X6
sorbitex	T45.4X1	T45.4X2	T45.4X3	T45.4X4	T45.4X5	T45.4X6
sorbitol citric acid complex	T45.4X1	T45.4X2	T45.4X3	T45.4X4	T45.4X5	T45.4X6
Irrigating fluid (vaginal)	T49.8X1	T49.8X2	T49.8X3	T49.8X4	T49.8X5	T49.8X6
eye	T49.5X1	T49.5X2	T49.5X3	T49.5X4	T49.5X5	T49.5X6
Isepamicin	T36.5X1	T36.5X2	T36.5X3	T36.5X4	T36.5X5	T36.5X6
Isoaminile (citrate)	T48.3X1	T48.3X2	T48.3X3	T48.3X4	T48.3X5	T48.3X6
Isoamyl nitrite	T46.3X1	T46.3X2	T46.3X3	T46.3X4	T46.3X5	T46.3X6
Isobenzan	T60.1X1	T60.1X2	T60.1X3	T60.1X4	—	—
Isobutyl acetate	T52.8X1	T52.8X2	T52.8X3	T52.8X4	—	—
Isocarboxazid	T43.1X1	T43.1X2	T43.1X3	T43.1X4	T43.1X5	T43.1X6
Isoconazole	T49.0X1	T49.0X2	T49.0X3	T49.0X4	T49.0X5	T49.0X6
Isocyanate	T65.0X1	T65.0X2	T65.0X3	T65.0X4	—	—
Isoephedrine	T44.991	T44.992	T44.993	T44.994	T44.995	T44.996
Isoetarine	T48.6X1	T48.6X2	T48.6X3	T48.6X4	T48.6X5	T48.6X6
Isoethadione	T42.2X1	T42.2X2	T42.2X3	T42.2X4	T42.2X5	T42.2X6
Isoetharine	T44.5X1	T44.5X2	T44.5X3	T44.5X4	T44.5X5	T44.5X6
Isoflurane	T41.0X1	T41.0X2	T41.0X3	T41.0X4	T41.0X5	T41.0X6
Isoflurophate	T44.0X1	T44.0X2	T44.0X3	T44.0X4	T44.0X5	T44.0X6
Isomaltose, ferric complex	T45.4X1	T45.4X2	T45.4X3	T45.4X4	T45.4X5	T45.4X6
Isometheptene	T44.3X1	T44.3X2	T44.3X3	T44.3X4	T44.3X5	T44.3X6
Isoniazid	T37.1X1	T37.1X2	T37.1X3	T37.1X4	T37.1X5	T37.1X6
with						
rifampicin	T36.6X1	T36.6X2	T36.6X3	T36.6X4	T36.6X5	T36.6X6
thioacetazone	T37.1X1	T37.1X2	T37.1X3	T37.1X4	T37.1X5	T37.1X6
Isonicotinic acid hydrazide	T37.1X1	T37.1X2	T37.1X3	T37.1X4	T37.1X5	T37.1X6
Isonipecaine	T40.4X1	T40.4X2	T40.4X3	T40.4X4	T40.4X5	T40.4X6
Isopentaquine	T37.2X1	T37.2X2	T37.2X3	T37.2X4	T37.2X5	T37.2X6
Isophane insulin	T38.3X1	T38.3X2	T38.3X3	T38.3X4	T38.3X5	T38.3X6
Isophorone	T65.891	T65.892	T65.893	T65.894	—	—
Isophosphamide	T45.1X1	T45.1X2	T45.1X3	T45.1X4	T45.1X5	T45.1X6
Isopregnenone	T38.5X1	T38.5X2	T38.5X3	T38.5X4	T38.5X5	T38.5X6
Isoprenaline	T48.6X1	T48.6X2	T48.6X3	T48.6X4	T48.6X5	T48.6X6
Isopromethazine	T43.3X1	T43.3X2	T43.3X3	T43.3X4	T43.3X5	T43.3X6
Isopropamide	T44.3X1	T44.3X2	T44.3X3	T44.3X4	T44.3X5	T44.3X6
iodide	T44.3X1	T44.3X2	T44.3X3	T44.3X4	T44.3X5	T44.3X6
Isopropanol	T51.2X1	T51.2X2	T51.2X3	T51.2X4	—	—

Substance	Poisoning, Accidental (Unintentional)	Poisoning, Intentional Self-Harm	Poisoning, Assault	Poisoning, Undetermined	Adverse Effect	Underdosing
Isopropyl						
acetate	T52.8X1	T52.8X2	T52.8X3	T52.8X4	—	—
alcohol	T51.2X1	T51.2X2	T51.2X3	T51.2X4	—	—
medicinal	T49.4X1	T49.4X2	T49.4X3	T49.4X4	T49.4X5	T49.4X6
ether	T52.8X1	T52.8X2	T52.8X3	T52.8X4	—	—
Isopropylaminophena-zone	T39.2X1	T39.2X2	T39.2X3	T39.2X4	T39.2X5	T39.2X6
Isoproterenol	T48.6X1	T48.6X2	T48.6X3	T48.6X4	T48.6X5	T48.6X6
Isosorbide dinitrate	T46.3X1	T46.3X2	T46.3X3	T46.3X4	T46.3X5	T46.3X6
Isothipendyl	T45.0X1	T45.0X2	T45.0X3	T45.0X4	T45.0X5	T45.0X6
Isotretinoin	T50.991	T50.992	T50.993	T50.994	T50.995	T50.996
Isoxazolyl penicillin	T36.0X1	T36.0X2	T36.0X3	T36.0X4	T36.0X5	T36.0X6
Isoxicam	T39.391	T39.392	T39.393	T39.394	T39.395	T39.396
Isoxsuprine	T46.7X1	T46.7X2	T46.7X3	T46.7X4	T46.7X5	T46.7X6
Ispagula	T47.4X1	T47.4X2	T47.4X3	T47.4X4	T47.4X5	T47.4X6
husk	T47.4X1	T47.4X2	T47.4X3	T47.4X4	T47.4X5	T47.4X6
Isradipine	T46.1X1	T46.1X2	T46.1X3	T46.1X4	T46.1X5	T46.1X6
I-thyroxine sodium	T38.1X1	T38.1X2	T38.1X3	T38.1X4	T38.1X5	T38.1X6
Itraconazole	T37.8X1	T37.8X2	T37.8X3	T37.8X4	T37.8X5	T37.8X6
Itramin tosilate	T46.3X1	T46.3X2	T46.3X3	T46.3X4	T46.3X5	T46.3X6
Ivermectin	T37.4X1	T37.4X2	T37.4X3	T37.4X4	T37.4X5	T37.4X6
Izoniazid	T37.1X1	T37.1X2	T37.1X3	T37.1X4	T37.1X5	T37.1X6
with thioacetazone	T37.1X1	T37.1X2	T37.1X3	T37.1X4	T37.1X5	T37.1X6
J						
Jalap	T47.2X1	T47.2X2	T47.2X3	T47.2X4	T47.2X5	T47.2X6
Jamaica						
dogwood (bark)	T39.8X1	T39.8X2	T39.8X3	T39.8X4	T39.8X5	T39.8X6
ginger	T65.891	T65.892	T65.893	T65.894	—	—
root	T62.2X1	T62.2X2	T62.2X3	T62.2X4	—	—
Jatropha	T62.2X1	T62.2X2	T62.2X3	T62.2X4	—	—
curcas	T62.2X1	T62.2X2	T62.2X3	T62.2X4	—	—
Jectofer	T45.4X1	T45.4X2	T45.4X3	T45.4X4	T45.4X5	T45.4X6
Jellyfish (sting)	T63.621	T63.622	T63.623	T63.624	—	—
Jequirity (bean)	T62.2X1	T62.2X2	T62.2X3	T62.2X4	—	—
Jimson weed (stramonium)	T62.2X1	T62.2X2	T62.2X3	T62.2X4	—	—
seeds	T62.2X1	T62.2X2	T62.2X3	T62.2X4	—	—
Josamycin	T36.3X1	T36.3X2	T36.3X3	T36.3X4	T36.3X5	T36.3X6
Juniper tar	T49.1X1	T49.1X2	T49.1X3	T49.1X4	T49.1X5	T49.1X6

◀ New   ◀||| Revised   ~~deleted~~ Deleted

Substance	Poisoning, Accidental (Unintentional)	Poisoning, Intentional Self-Harm	Poisoning, Assault	Poisoning, Undetermined	Adverse Effect	Underdosing
External Cause (T-Code)						
K						
Kallidinogenase	T46.7X1	T46.7X2	T46.7X3	T46.7X4	T46.7X5	T46.7X6
Kallikrein	T46.7X1	T46.7X2	T46.7X3	T46.7X4	T46.7X5	T46.7X6
Kanamycin	T36.5X1	T36.5X2	T36.5X3	T36.5X4	T36.5X5	T36.5X6
Kantrex	T36.5X1	T36.5X2	T36.5X3	T36.5X4	T36.5X5	T36.5X6
Kaolin	T47.6X1	T47.6X2	T47.6X3	T47.6X4	T47.6X5	T47.6X6
light	T47.6X1	T47.6X2	T47.6X3	T47.6X4	T47.6X5	T47.6X6
Karaya (gum)	T47.4X1	T47.4X2	T47.4X3	T47.4X4	T47.4X5	T47.4X6
Kebuzone	T39.2X1	T39.2X2	T39.2X3	T39.2X4	T39.2X5	T39.2X6
Kelevan	T60.1X1	T60.1X2	T60.1X3	T60.1X4	—	—
Kemithal	T41.1X1	T41.1X2	T41.1X3	T41.1X4	T41.1X5	T41.1X6
Kenacort	T38.0X1	T38.0X2	T38.0X3	T38.0X4	T38.0X5	T38.0X6
Keratolytic drug NEC	T49.4X1	T49.4X2	T49.4X3	T49.4X4	T49.4X5	T49.4X6
anthracene	T49.4X1	T49.4X2	T49.4X3	T49.4X4	T49.4X5	T49.4X6
Keratoplastic NEC	T49.4X1	T49.4X2	T49.4X3	T49.4X4	T49.4X5	T49.4X6
Kerosene, kerosine (fuel) (solvent) NEC	T52.0X1	T52.0X2	T52.0X3	T52.0X4	—	—
insecticide	T52.0X1	T52.0X2	T52.0X3	T52.0X4	—	—
vapor	T52.0X1	T52.0X2	T52.0X3	T52.0X4	—	—
Ketamine	T41.291	T41.292	T41.293	T41.294	T41.295	T41.296
Ketazolam	T42.4X1	T42.4X2	T42.4X3	T42.4X4	T42.4X5	T42.4X6
Ketazon	T39.2X1	T39.2X2	T39.2X3	T39.2X4	T39.2X5	T39.2X6
Ketobemidone	T40.4X1	T40.4X2	T40.4X3	T40.4X4	—	—
Ketoconazole	T49.0X1	T49.0X2	T49.0X3	T49.0X4	T49.0X5	T49.0X6
Ketols	T52.4X1	T52.4X2	T52.4X3	T52.4X4	—	—
Ketone oils	T52.4X1	T52.4X2	T52.4X3	T52.4X4	—	—
Ketoprofen	T39.311	T39.312	T39.313	T39.314	T39.315	T39.316
Ketorolac	T39.8X1	T39.8X2	T39.8X3	T39.8X4	T39.8X5	T39.8X6
Ketotifen	T45.0X1	T45.0X2	T45.0X3	T45.0X4	T45.0X5	T45.0X6
Khat	T43.691	T43.692	T43.693	T43.694	—	—
Khellin	T46.3X1	T46.3X2	T46.3X3	T46.3X4	T46.3X5	T46.3X6
Khelloside	T46.3X1	T46.3X2	T46.3X3	T46.3X4	T46.3X5	T46.3X6
Kiln gas or vapor (carbon monoxide)	T58.8X1	T58.8X2	T58.8X3	T58.8X4	—	—
Kitasamycin	T36.3X1	T36.3X2	T36.3X3	T36.3X4	T36.3X5	T36.3X6
Konsyl	T47.4X1	T47.4X2	T47.4X3	T47.4X4	T47.4X5	T47.4X6
Kosam seed	T62.2X1	T62.2X2	T62.2X3	T62.2X4	—	—
Krait (venom)	T63.091	T63.092	T63.093	T63.094	—	—
Kwell (insecticide)	T60.1X1	T60.1X2	T60.1X3	T60.1X4	—	—
anti-infective (topical)	T49.0X1	T49.0X2	T49.0X3	T49.0X4	T49.0X5	T49.0X6

◀ New ◀‖‖ Revised ~~deleted~~ Deleted

Substance	External Cause (T-Code)					
	Poisoning, Accidental (Unintentional)	Poisoning, Intentional Self-Harm	Poisoning, Assault	Poisoning, Undetermined	Adverse Effect	Underdosing
L						
Labetalol	T44.8X1	T44.8X2	T44.8X3	T44.8X4	T44.8X5	T44.8X6
Laburnum (seeds)	T62.2X1	T62.2X2	T62.2X3	T62.2X4	—	—
leaves	T62.2X1	T62.2X2	T62.2X3	T62.2X4	—	—
Lachesine	T49.5X1	T49.5X2	T49.5X3	T49.5X4	T49.5X5	T49.5X6
Lacidipine	T46.5X1	T46.5X2	T46.5X3	T46.5X4	T46.5X5	T46.5X6
Lacquer	T65.6X1	T65.6X2	T65.6X3	T65.6X4	—	—
Lacrimogenic gas	T59.3X1	T59.3X2	T59.3X3	T59.3X4	—	—
Lactated potassic saline	T50.3X1	T50.3X2	T50.3X3	T50.3X4	T50.3X5	T50.3X6
Lactic acid	T49.8X1	T49.8X2	T49.8X3	T49.8X4	T49.8X5	T49.8X6
Lactobacillus						
acidophilus	T47.6X1	T47.6X2	T47.6X3	T47.6X4	T47.6X5	T47.6X6
compound	T47.6X1	T47.6X2	T47.6X3	T47.6X4	T47.6X5	T47.6X6
bifidus, lyophilized	T47.6X1	T47.6X2	T47.6X3	T47.6X4	T47.6X5	T47.6X6
bulgaricus	T47.6X1	T47.6X2	T47.6X3	T47.6X4	T47.6X5	T47.6X6
sporogenes	T47.6X1	T47.6X2	T47.6X3	T47.6X4	T47.6X5	T47.6X6
Lactoflavin	T45.2X1	T45.2X2	T45.2X3	T45.2X4	T45.2X5	T45.2X6
Lactose (as excipient)	T50.901	T50.902	T50.903	T50.904	T50.905	T50.906
Lactuca (virosa) (extract)	T42.6X1	T42.6X2	T42.6X3	T42.6X4	T42.6X5	T42.6X6
Lactucarium	T42.6X1	T42.6X2	T42.6X3	T42.6X4	T42.6X5	T42.6X6
Lactulose	T47.3X1	T47.3X2	T47.3X3	T47.3X4	T47.3X5	T47.3X6
Laevo — see Levo-						
Lanatosides	T46.0X1	T46.0X2	T46.0X3	T46.0X4	T46.0X5	T46.0X6
Lanolin	T49.3X1	T49.3X2	T49.3X3	T49.3X4	T49.3X5	T49.3X6
Largactil	T43.3X1	T43.3X2	T43.3X3	T43.3X4	T43.3X5	T43.3X6
Larkspur	T62.2X1	T62.2X2	T62.2X3	T62.2X4	—	—
Laroxyl	T43.011	T43.012	T43.013	T43.014	T43.015	T43.016
Lassar's paste	T49.4X1	T49.4X2	T49.4X3	T49.4X4	T49.4X5	T49.4X6
Lasix	T50.1X1	T50.1X2	T50.1X3	T50.1X4	T50.1X5	T50.1X6
Latamoxef	T36.1X1	T36.1X2	T36.1X3	T36.1X4	T36.1X5	T36.1X6
Latex	T65.811	T65.812	T65.813	T65.814	—	—
Lathyrus (seed)	T62.2X1	T62.2X2	T62.2X3	T62.2X4	—	—
Laudanum	T40.0X1	T40.0X2	T40.0X3	T40.0X4	T40.0X5	T40.0X6
Laudexium	T48.1X1	T48.1X2	T48.1X3	T48.1X4	T48.1X5	T48.1X6
Laughing gas	T41.0X1	T41.0X2	T41.0X3	T41.0X4	T41.0X5	T41.0X6
Laurel, black or cherry	T62.2X1	T62.2X2	T62.2X3	T62.2X4	—	—
Laurolinium	T49.0X1	T49.0X2	T49.0X3	T49.0X4	T49.0X5	T49.0X6
Lauryl sulfoacetate	T49.2X1	T49.2X2	T49.2X3	T49.2X4	T49.2X5	T49.2X6

◀ New   ◀▥ Revised   ~~deleted~~ Deleted

	External Cause (T-Code)					
Substance	Poisoning, Accidental (Unintentional)	Poisoning, Intentional Self-Harm	Poisoning, Assault	Poisoning, Undetermined	Adverse Effect	Underdosing
Laxative NEC	T47.4X1	T47.4X2	T47.4X3	T47.4X4	T47.4X5	T47.4X6
osmotic	T47.3X1	T47.3X2	T47.3X3	T47.3X4	T47.3X5	T47.3X6
saline	T47.3X1	T47.3X2	T47.3X3	T47.3X4	T47.3X5	T47.3X6
stimulant	T47.2X1	T47.2X2	T47.2X3	T47.2X4	T47.2X5	T47.2X6
L-dopa	T42.8X1	T42.8X2	T42.8X3	T42.8X4	T42.8X5	T42.8X6
Lead (dust) (fumes) (vapor) NEC	T56.0X1	T56.0X2	T56.0X3	T56.0X4	—	—
acetate	T49.2X1	T49.2X2	T49.2X3	T49.2X4	T49.2X5	T49.2X6
alkyl (fuel additive)	T56.0X1	T56.0X2	T56.0X3	T56.0X4	—	—
anti-infectives	T37.8X1	T37.8X2	T37.8X3	T37.8X4	T37.8X5	T37.8X6
antiknock compound (tetraethyl)	T56.0X1	T56.0X2	T56.0X3	T56.0X4	—	—
arsenate, arsenite (dust) (herbicide) (insecticide) (vapor)	T57.0X1	T57.0X2	T57.0X3	T57.0X4	—	—
carbonate	T56.0X1	T56.0X2	T56.0X3	T56.0X4	—	—
paint	T56.0X1	T56.0X2	T56.0X3	T56.0X4	—	—
chromate	T56.0X1	T56.0X2	T56.0X3	T56.0X4	—	—
paint	T56.0X1	T56.0X2	T56.0X3	T56.0X4	—	—
dioxide	T56.0X1	T56.0X2	T56.0X3	T56.0X4	—	—
inorganic	T56.0X1	T56.0X2	T56.0X3	T56.0X4	—	—
iodide	T56.0X1	T56.0X2	T56.0X3	T56.0X4	—	—
pigment (paint)	T56.0X1	T56.0X2	T56.0X3	T56.0X4	—	—
monoxide (dust)	T56.0X1	T56.0X2	T56.0X3	T56.0X4	—	—
paint	T56.0X1	T56.0X2	T56.0X3	T56.0X4	—	—
organic	T56.0X1	T56.0X2	T56.0X3	T56.0X4	—	—
oxide	T56.0X1	T56.0X2	T56.0X3	T56.0X4	—	—
paint	T56.0X1	T56.0X2	T56.0X3	T56.0X4	—	—
paint	T56.0X1	T56.0X2	T56.0X3	T56.0X4	—	—
salts	T56.0X1	T56.0X2	T56.0X3	T56.0X4	—	—
specified compound NEC	T56.0X1	T56.0X2	T56.0X3	T56.0X4	—	—
tetra-ethyl	T56.0X1	T56.0X2	T56.0X3	T56.0X4	—	—
Lebanese red	T40.7X1	T40.7X2	T40.7X3	T40.7X4	T40.7X5	T40.7X6
Lefetamine	T39.8X1	T39.8X2	T39.8X3	T39.8X4	T39.8X5	T39.8X6
Lenperone	T43.4X1	T43.4X2	T43.4X3	T43.4X4	T43.4X5	T43.4X6
Lente lietin (insulin)	T38.3X1	T38.3X2	T38.3X3	T38.3X4	T38.3X5	T38.3X6
Leptazol	T50.7X1	T50.7X2	T50.7X3	T50.7X4	T50.7X5	T50.7X6
Leptophos	T60.0X1	T60.0X2	T60.0X3	T60.0X4	—	—
Leritine	T40.2X1	T40.2X2	T40.2X3	T40.2X4	T40.2X5	T40.2X6
Letosteine	T48.4X1	T48.4X2	T48.4X3	T48.4X4	T48.4X5	T48.4X6
Letter	T38.1X1	T38.1X2	T38.1X3	T38.1X4	T38.1X5	T38.1X6
Lettuce opium	T42.6X1	T42.6X2	T42.6X3	T42.6X4	T42.6X5	T42.6X6
Leucinocaine	T41.3X1	T41.3X2	T41.3X3	T41.3X4	T41.3X5	T41.3X6

◀ New   ◀ Revised   ~~deleted~~ Deleted

TABLE OF DRUGS AND CHEMICALS

TABLE OF DRUGS AND CHEMICALS

Substance	External Cause (T-Code)					
	Poisoning, Accidental (Unintentional)	Poisoning, Intentional Self-Harm	Poisoning, Assault	Poisoning, Undetermined	Adverse Effect	Underdosing
Leucocianidol	T46.991	T46.992	T46.993	T46.994	T46.995	T46.996
Leucovorin (factor)	T45.8X1	T45.8X2	T45.8X3	T45.8X4	T45.8X5	T45.8X6
Leukeran	T45.1X1	T45.1X2	T45.1X3	T45.1X4	T45.1X5	T45.1X6
Leuprolide	T38.891	T38.892	T38.893	T38.894	T38.895	T38.896
Levalbuterol	T48.6X1	T48.6X2	T48.6X3	T48.6X4	T48.6X5	T48.6X6
Levallorphan	T50.7X1	T50.7X2	T50.7X3	T50.7X4	T50.7X5	T50.7X6
Levamisole	T37.4X1	T37.4X2	T37.4X3	T37.4X4	T37.4X5	T37.4X6
Levanil	T42.6X1	T42.6X2	T42.6X3	T42.6X4	T42.6X5	T42.6X6
Levarterenol	T44.4X1	T44.4X2	T44.4X3	T44.4X4	T44.4X5	T44.4X6
Levdropropizine	T48.3X1	T48.3X2	T48.3X3	T48.3X4	T48.3X5	T48.3X6
Levobunolol	T49.5X1	T49.5X2	T49.5X3	T49.5X4	T49.5X5	T49.5X6
Levocabastine (hydrochloride)	T45.0X1	T45.0X2	T45.0X3	T45.0X4	T45.0X5	T45.0X6
Levocarnitine	T50.991	T50.992	T50.993	T50.994	T50.995	T50.996
Levodopa	T42.8X1	T42.8X2	T42.8X3	T42.8X4	T42.8X5	T42.8X6
with carbidopa	T42.8X1	T42.8X2	T42.8X3	T42.8X4	T42.8X5	T42.8X6
Levo-dromoran	T40.2X1	T40.2X2	T40.2X3	T40.2X4	T40.2X5	T40.2X6
Levoglutamide	T50.991	T50.992	T50.993	T50.994	T50.995	T50.996
Levoid	T38.1X1	T38.1X2	T38.1X3	T38.1X4	T38.1X5	T38.1X6
Levo-iso-methadone	T40.3X1	T40.3X2	T40.3X3	T40.3X4	T40.3X5	T40.3X6
Levomepromazine	T43.3X1	T43.3X2	T43.3X3	T43.3X4	T43.3X5	T43.3X6
Levonordefrin	T49.6X1	T49.6X2	T49.6X3	T49.6X4	T49.6X5	T49.6X6
Levonorgestrel	T38.4X1	T38.4X2	T38.4X3	T38.4X4	T38.4X5	T38.4X6
with ethinylestradiol	T38.5X1	T38.5X2	T38.5X3	T38.5X4	T38.5X5	T38.5X6
Levopromazine	T43.3X1	T43.3X2	T43.3X3	T43.3X4	T43.3X5	T43.3X6
Levoprome	T42.6X1	T42.6X2	T42.6X3	T42.6X4	T42.6X5	T42.6X6
Levopropoxyphene	T40.4X1	T40.4X2	T40.4X3	T40.4X4	T40.4X5	T40.4X6
Levopropylhexedrine	T50.5X1	T50.5X2	T50.5X3	T50.5X4	T50.5X5	T50.5X6
Levoproxyphylline	T48.6X1	T48.6X2	T48.6X3	T48.6X4	T48.6X5	T48.6X6
Levorphanol	T40.4X1	T40.4X2	T40.4X3	T40.4X4	T40.4X5	T40.4X6
Levothyroxine	T38.1X1	T38.1X2	T38.1X3	T38.1X4	T38.1X5	T38.1X6
sodium	T38.1X1	T38.1X2	T38.1X3	T38.1X4	T38.1X5	T38.1X6
Levsin	T44.3X1	T44.3X2	T44.3X3	T44.3X4	T44.3X5	T44.3X6
Levulose	T50.3X1	T50.3X2	T50.3X3	T50.3X4	T50.3X5	T50.3X6
Lewisite (gas), not in war	T57.0X1	T57.0X2	T57.0X3	T57.0X4	—	—
Librium	T42.4X1	T42.4X2	T42.4X3	T42.4X4	T42.4X5	T42.4X6
Lidex	T49.0X1	T49.0X2	T49.0X3	T49.0X4	T49.0X5	T49.0X6
Lidocaine	T41.3X1	T41.3X2	T41.3X3	T41.3X4	T41.3X5	T41.3X6
regional	T41.3X1	T41.3X2	T41.3X3	T41.3X4	T41.3X5	T41.3X6
spinal	T41.3X1	T41.3X2	T41.3X3	T41.3X4	T41.3X5	T41.3X6
Lidofenin	T50.8X1	T50.8X2	T50.8X3	T50.8X4	T50.8X5	T50.8X6

◀ New   ◀▥ Revised   d̶e̶l̶e̶t̶e̶d̶ Deleted

Substance	Poisoning, Accidental (Unintentional)	Poisoning, Intentional Self-Harm	Poisoning, Assault	Poisoning, Undetermined	Adverse Effect	Underdosing
	External Cause (T-Code)					
Lidoflazine	T46.1X1	T46.1X2	T46.1X3	T46.1X4	T46.1X5	T46.1X6
Lighter fluid	T52.0X1	T52.0X2	T52.0X3	T52.0X4	—	—
Lignin hemicellulose	T47.6X1	T47.6X2	T47.6X3	T47.6X4	T47.6X5	T47.6X6
Lignocaine	T41.3X1	T41.3X2	T41.3X3	T41.3X4	T41.3X5	T41.3X6
regional	T41.3X1	T41.3X2	T41.3X3	T41.3X4	T41.3X5	T41.3X6
spinal	T41.3X1	T41.3X2	T41.3X3	T41.3X4	T41.3X5	T41.3X6
Ligroin(e) (solvent)	T52.0X1	T52.0X2	T52.0X3	T52.0X4	—	—
vapor	T59.891	T59.892	T59.893	T59.894	—	—
Ligustrum vulgare	T62.2X1	T62.2X2	T62.2X3	T62.2X4	—	—
Lily of the valley	T62.2X1	T62.2X2	T62.2X3	T62.2X4	—	—
Lime (chloride)	T54.3X1	T54.3X2	T54.3X3	T54.3X4	—	—
Limonene	T52.8X1	T52.8X2	T52.8X3	T52.8X4	—	—
Lincomycin	T36.8X1	T36.8X2	T36.8X3	T36.8X4	T36.8X5	T36.8X6
Lindane (insecticide) (nonmedicinal) (vapor)	T53.6X1	T53.6X2	T53.6X3	T53.6X4	—	—
medicinal	T49.0X1	T49.0X2	T49.0X3	T49.0X4	T49.0X5	T49.0X6
Liniments NEC	T49.91	T49.92	T49.93	T49.94	T49.95	T49.96
Linoleic acid	T46.6X1	T46.6X2	T46.6X3	T46.6X4	T46.6X5	T46.6X6
Linolenic acid	T46.6X1	T46.6X2	T46.6X3	T46.6X4	T46.6X5	T46.6X6
Linseed	T47.4X1	T47.4X2	T47.4X3	T47.4X4	T47.4X5	T47.4X6
Liothyronine	T38.1X1	T38.1X2	T38.1X3	T38.1X4	T38.1X5	T38.1X6
Liotrix	T38.1X1	T38.1X2	T38.1X3	T38.1X4	T38.1X5	T38.1X6
Lipancreatin	T47.5X1	T47.5X2	T47.5X3	T47.5X4	T47.5X5	T47.5X6
Lipo-alprostadil	T46.7X1	T46.7X2	T46.7X3	T46.7X4	T46.7X5	T46.7X6
Lipo-Lutin	T38.5X1	T38.5X2	T38.5X3	T38.5X4	T38.5X5	T38.5X6
Lipotropic drug NEC	T50.901	T50.902	T50.903	T50.904	T50.905	T50.906
Liquefied petroleum gases	T59.891	T59.892	T59.893	T59.894	—	—
piped (pure or mixed with air)	T59.891	T59.892	T59.893	T59.894	—	—
Liquid						
paraffin	T47.4X1	T47.4X2	T47.4X3	T47.4X4	T47.4X5	T47.4X6
petrolatum	T47.4X1	T47.4X2	T47.4X3	T47.4X4	T47.4X5	T47.4X6
topical	T49.3X1	T49.3X2	T49.3X3	T49.3X4	T49.3X5	T49.3X6
specified NEC	T65.891	T65.892	T65.893	T65.894	—	—
substance	T65.91	T65.92	T65.93	T65.94	—	—
Liquor creosolis compositus	T65.891	T65.892	T65.893	T65.894	—	—
Liquorice	T48.4X1	T48.4X2	T48.4X3	T48.4X4	T48.4X5	T48.4X6
extract	T47.8X1	T47.8X2	T47.8X3	T47.8X4	T47.8X5	T47.8X6
Lirugen	T50.991	T50.992	T50.993	T50.994	T50.995	T50.996
Lisinopril	T46.4X1	T46.4X2	T46.4X3	T46.4X4	T46.4X5	T46.4X6
Lisuride	T42.8X1	T42.8X2	T42.8X3	T42.8X4	T42.8X5	T42.8X6
Lithane	T43.8X1	T43.8X2	T43.8X3	T43.8X4	T43.8X5	T43.8X6

TABLE OF DRUGS AND CHEMICALS

Substance	External Cause (T-Code)					
	Poisoning, Accidental (Unintentional)	Poisoning, Intentional Self-Harm	Poisoning, Assault	Poisoning, Undetermined	Adverse Effect	Underdosing
Lithium	T56.891	T56.892	T56.893	T56.894	—	—
gluconate	T43.591	T43.592	T43.593	T43.594	T43.595	T43.596
salts (carbonate)	T43.591	T43.592	T43.593	T43.594	T43.595	T43.596
Lithonate	T43.8X1	T43.8X2	T43.8X3	T43.8X4	T43.8X5	T43.8X6
Liver						
extract	T45.8X1	T45.8X2	T45.8X3	T45.8X4	T45.8X5	T45.8X6
for parenteral use	T45.8X1	T45.8X2	T45.8X3	T45.8X4	T45.8X5	T45.8X6
fraction 1	T45.8X1	T45.8X2	T45.8X3	T45.8X4	T45.8X5	T45.8X6
hydrolysate	T45.8X1	T45.8X2	T45.8X3	T45.8X4	T45.8X5	T45.8X6
Lizard (bite) (venom)	T63.121	T63.122	T63.123	T63.124	—	—
LMD	T45.8X1	T45.8X2	T45.8X3	T45.8X4	T45.8X5	T45.8X6
Lobelia	T62.2X1	T62.2X2	T62.2X3	T62.2X4	—	—
Lobeline	T50.7X1	T50.7X2	T50.7X3	T50.7X4	T50.7X5	T50.7X6
Local action drug NEC	T49.8X1	T49.8X2	T49.8X3	T49.8X4	T49.8X5	T49.8X6
Locorten	T49.0X1	T49.0X2	T49.0X3	T49.0X4	T49.0X5	T49.0X6
Lofepramine	T43.011	T43.012	T43.013	T43.014	T43.015	T43.016
Lolium temulentum	T62.2X1	T62.2X2	T62.2X3	T62.2X4	—	—
Lomotil	T47.6X1	T47.6X2	T47.6X3	T47.6X4	T47.6X5	T47.6X6
Lomustine	T45.1X1	T45.1X2	T45.1X3	T45.1X4	T45.1X5	T45.1X6
Lonidamine	T45.1X1	T45.1X2	T45.1X3	T45.1X4	T45.1X5	T45.1X6
Loperamide	T47.6X1	T47.6X2	T47.6X3	T47.6X4	T47.6X5	T47.6X6
Loprazolam	T42.4X1	T42.4X2	T42.4X3	T42.4X4	T42.4X5	T42.4X6
Lorajmine	T46.2X1	T46.2X2	T46.2X3	T46.2X4	T46.2X5	T46.2X6
Loratidine	T45.0X1	T45.0X2	T45.0X3	T45.0X4	T45.0X5	T45.0X6
Lorazepam	T42.4X1	T42.4X2	T42.4X3	T42.4X4	T42.4X5	T42.4X6
Lorcainide	T46.2X1	T46.2X2	T46.2X3	T46.2X4	T46.2X5	T46.2X6
Lormetazepam	T42.4X1	T42.4X2	T42.4X3	T42.4X4	T42.4X5	T42.4X6
Lotions NEC	T49.91	T49.92	T49.93	T49.94	T49.95	T49.96
Lotusate	T42.3X1	T42.3X2	T42.3X3	T42.3X4	T42.3X5	T42.3X6
Lovastatin	T46.6X1	T46.6X2	T46.6X3	T46.6X4	T46.6X5	T46.6X6
Loxapine	T43.591	T43.592	T43.593	T43.594	T43.595	T43.596
Lowila	T49.2X1	T49.2X2	T49.2X3	T49.2X4	T49.2X5	T49.2X6
Lozenges (throat)	T49.6X1	T49.6X2	T49.6X3	T49.6X4	T49.6X5	T49.6X6
LSD	T40.8X1	T40.8X2	T40.8X3	T40.8X4	—	—
L-Tryptophan — see amino acid						
Lubricant, eye	T49.5X1	T49.5X2	T49.5X3	T49.5X4	T49.5X5	T49.5X6
Lubricating oil NEC	T52.0X1	T52.0X2	T52.0X3	T52.0X4	—	—
Lucanthone	T37.4X1	T37.4X2	T37.4X3	T37.4X4	T37.4X5	T37.4X6
Luminal	T42.3X1	T42.3X2	T42.3X3	T42.3X4	T42.3X5	T42.3X6
Lung irritant (gas) NEC	T59.91	T59.92	T59.93	T59.94	—	—

◀ New ◀ Revised ~~deleted~~ Deleted

Substance	Poisoning, Accidental (Unintentional)	Poisoning, Intentional Self-Harm	Poisoning, Assault	Poisoning, Undetermined	Adverse Effect	Underdosing
	External Cause (T-Code)					
Luteinizing hormone	T38.811	T38.812	T38.813	T38.814	T38.815	T38.816
Lutocylol	T38.5X1	T38.5X2	T38.5X3	T38.5X4	T38.5X5	T38.5X6
Lutromone	T38.5X1	T38.5X2	T38.5X3	T38.5X4	T38.5X5	T38.5X6
Lututrin	T48.291	T48.292	T48.293	T48.294	T48.295	T48.296
Lye (Concentrated)	T54.3X1	T54.3X2	T54.3X3	T54.3X4	—	—
Lygranum (skin test)	T50.8X1	T50.8X2	T50.8X3	T50.8X4	T50.8X5	T50.8X6
Lymecycline	T36.4X1	T36.4X2	T36.4X3	T36.4X4	T36.4X5	T36.4X6
Lymphogranuloma venereum antigen	T50.8X1	T50.8X2	T50.8X3	T50.8X4	T50.8X5	T50.8X6
Lynestrenol	T38.4X1	T38.4X2	T38.4X3	T38.4X4	T38.4X5	T38.4X6
Lypressin	T38.891	T38.892	T38.893	T38.894	T38.895	T38.896
Lyovac Sodium Edecrin	T50.1X1	T50.1X2	T50.1X3	T50.1X4	T50.1X5	T50.1X6
Lysergic acid diethylamide	T40.8X1	T40.8X2	T40.8X3	T40.8X4	—	—
Lysergide	T40.8X1	T40.8X2	T40.8X3	T40.8X4	—	—
Lysine vasopressin	T38.891	T38.892	T38.893	T38.894	T38.895	T38.896
Lysol	T54.1X1	T54.1X2	T54.1X3	T54.1X4	—	—
Lysozyme	T49.0X1	T49.0X2	T49.0X3	T49.0X4	T49.0X5	T49.0X6
Lytta (vitatta)	T49.8X1	T49.8X2	T49.8X3	T49.8X4	T49.8X5	T49.8X6
M						
Mace	T59.3X1	T59.3X2	T59.3X3	T59.3X4	—	—
Macrogol	T50.991	T50.992	T50.993	T50.994	T50.995	T50.996
Macrolide						
anabolic drug	T38.7X1	T38.7X2	T38.7X3	T38.7X4	T38.7X5	T38.7X6
antibiotic	T36.3X1	T36.3X2	T36.3X3	T36.3X4	T36.3X5	T36.3X6
Mafenide	T49.0X1	T49.0X2	T49.0X3	T49.0X4	T49.0X5	T49.0X6
Magaldrate	T47.1X1	T47.1X2	T47.1X3	T47.1X4	T47.1X5	T47.1X6
Magic mushroom	T40.991	T40.992	T40.993	T40.994	—	—
Magnamycin	T36.8X1	T36.8X2	T36.8X3	T36.8X4	T36.8X5	T36.8X6
Magnesia magma	T47.1X1	T47.1X2	T47.1X3	T47.1X4	T47.1X5	T47.1X6
Magnesium NEC	T56.891	T56.892	T56.893	T56.894	—	—
carbonate	T47.1X1	T47.1X2	T47.1X3	T47.1X4	T47.1X5	T47.1X6
citrate	T47.4X1	T47.4X2	T47.4X3	T47.4X4	T47.4X5	T47.4X6
hydroxide	T47.1X1	T47.1X2	T47.1X3	T47.1X4	T47.1X5	T47.1X6
oxide	T47.1X1	T47.1X2	T47.1X3	T47.1X4	T47.1X5	T47.1X6
peroxide	T49.0X1	T49.0X2	T49.0X3	T49.0X4	T49.0X5	T49.0X6
salicylate	T39.091	T39.092	T39.093	T39.094	T39.095	T39.096
silicofluoride	T50.3X1	T50.3X2	T50.3X3	T50.3X4	T50.3X5	T50.3X6
sulfate	T47.4X1	T47.4X2	T47.4X3	T47.4X4	T47.4X5	T47.4X6
thiosulfate	T45.0X1	T45.0X2	T45.0X3	T45.0X4	T45.0X5	T45.0X6
trisilicate	T47.1X1	T47.1X2	T47.1X3	T47.1X4	T47.1X5	T47.1X6

Substance	Poisoning, Accidental (Unintentional)	Poisoning, Intentional Self-Harm	Poisoning, Assault	Poisoning, Undetermined	Adverse Effect	Underdosing
Malathion (medicinal)	T49.0X1	T49.0X2	T49.0X3	T49.0X4	T49.0X5	T49.0X6
insecticide	T60.0X1	T60.0X2	T60.0X3	T60.0X4	—	—
Male fern extract	T37.4X1	T37.4X2	T37.4X3	T37.4X4	T37.4X5	T37.4X6
M-AMSA	T45.1X1	T45.1X2	T45.1X3	T45.1X4	T45.1X5	T45.1X6
Mandelic acid	T37.8X1	T37.8X2	T37.8X3	T37.8X4	T37.8X5	T37.8X6
Manganese (dioxide) (salts)	T57.2X1	T57.2X2	T57.2X3	T57.2X4	—	—
medicinal	T50.991	T50.992	T50.993	T50.994	T50.995	T50.996
Mannitol	T47.3X1	T47.3X2	T47.3X3	T47.3X4	T47.3X5	T47.3X6
hexanitrate	T46.3X1	T46.3X2	T46.3X3	T46.3X4	T46.3X5	T46.3X6
Mannomustine	T45.1X1	T45.1X2	T45.1X3	T45.1X4	T45.1X5	T45.1X6
MAO inhibitors	T43.1X1	T43.1X2	T43.1X3	T43.1X4	T43.1X5	T43.1X6
Mapharsen	T37.8X1	T37.8X2	T37.8X3	T37.8X4	T37.8X5	T37.8X6
Maphenide	T49.0X1	T49.0X2	T49.0X3	T49.0X4	T49.0X5	T49.0X6
Maprotiline	T43.021	T43.022	T43.023	T43.024	T43.025	T43.026
Marcaine	T41.3X1	T41.3X2	T41.3X3	T41.3X4	T41.3X5	T41.3X6
infiltration (subcutaneous)	T41.3X1	T41.3X2	T41.3X3	T41.3X4	T41.3X5	T41.3X6
nerve block (peripheral) (plexus)	T41.3X1	T41.3X2	T41.3X3	T41.3X4	T41.3X5	T41.3X6
Marezine	T45.0X1	T45.0X2	T45.0X3	T45.0X4	T45.0X5	T45.0X6
Marihuana	T40.7X1	T40.7X2	T40.7X3	T40.7X4	T40.7X5	T40.7X6
Marijuana	T40.7X1	T40.7X2	T40.7X3	T40.7X4	T40.7X5	T40.7X6
Marine (sting)	T63.691	T63.692	T63.693	T63.694	—	—
animals (sting)	T63.691	T63.692	T63.693	T63.694	—	—
plants (sting)	T63.711	T63.712	T63.713	T63.714	—	—
Marplan	T43.1X1	T43.1X2	T43.1X3	T43.1X4	T43.1X5	T43.1X6
Marsh gas	T59.891	T59.892	T59.893	T59.894	—	—
Marsilid	T43.1X1	T43.1X2	T43.1X3	T43.1X4	T43.1X5	T43.1X6
Matulane	T45.1X1	T45.1X2	T45.1X3	T45.1X4	T45.1X5	T45.1X6
Mazindol	T50.5X1	T50.5X2	T50.5X3	T50.5X4	T50.5X5	T50.5X6
MCPA	T60.3X1	T60.3X2	T60.3X3	T60.3X4	—	—
MDMA	T43.621	T43.622	T43.623	T43.624	T43.625	T43.626
Meadow saffron	T62.2X1	T62.2X2	T62.2X3	T62.2X4	—	—
Measles virus vaccine (attenuated)	T50.B91	T50.B92	T50.B93	T50.B94	T50.B95	T50.B96
Meat, noxious	T62.8X1	T62.8X2	T62.8X3	T62.8X4		
Meballymal	T42.3X1	T42.3X2	T42.3X3	T42.3X4	T42.3X5	T42.3X6
Mebanazine	T43.1X1	T43.1X2	T43.1X3	T43.1X4	T43.1X5	T43.1X6
Mebaral	T42.3X1	T42.3X2	T42.3X3	T42.3X4	T42.3X5	T42.3X6
Mebendazole	T37.4X1	T37.4X2	T37.4X3	T37.4X4	T37.4X5	T37.4X6
Mebeverine	T44.3X1	T44.3X2	T44.3X3	T44.3X4	T44.3X5	T44.3X6
Mebhydrolin	T45.0X1	T45.0X2	T45.0X3	T45.0X4	T45.0X5	T45.0X6
Mebumal	T42.3X1	T42.3X2	T42.3X3	T42.3X4	T42.3X5	T42.3X6

◀ New   ◀▥ Revised   ~~deleted~~ Deleted

Substance	Poisoning, Accidental (Unintentional)	Poisoning, Intentional Self-Harm	Poisoning, Assault	Poisoning, Undetermined	Adverse Effect	Underdosing
Mebutamate	T43.591	T43.592	T43.593	T43.594	T43.595	T43.596
Mecamylamine	T44.2X1	T44.2X2	T44.2X3	T44.2X4	T44.2X5	T44.2X6
Mechlorethamine	T45.1X1	T45.1X2	T45.1X3	T45.1X4	T45.1X5	T45.1X6
Mecillinam	T36.0X1	T36.0X2	T36.0X3	T36.0X4	T36.0X5	T36.0X6
Meclizine (hydrochloride)	T45.0X1	T45.0X2	T45.0X3	T45.0X4	T45.0X5	T45.0X6
Meclocycline	T36.4X1	T36.4X2	T36.4X3	T36.4X4	T36.4X5	T36.4X6
Meclofenamate	T39.391	T39.392	T39.393	T39.394	T39.395	T39.396
Meclofenamic acid	T39.391	T39.392	T39.393	T39.394	T39.395	T39.396
Meclofenoxate	T43.691	T43.692	T43.693	T43.694	T43.695	T43.696
Meclozine	T45.0X1	T45.0X2	T45.0X3	T45.0X4	T45.0X5	T45.0X6
Mecobalamin	T45.8X1	T45.8X2	T45.8X3	T45.8X4	T45.8X5	T45.8X6
Mecoprop	T60.3X1	T60.3X2	T60.3X3	T60.3X4	—	—
Mecrilate	T49.3X1	T49.3X2	T49.3X3	T49.3X4	T49.3X5	T49.3X6
Mecysteine	T48.4X1	T48.4X2	T48.4X3	T48.4X4	T48.4X5	T48.4X6
Medazepam	T42.4X1	T42.4X2	T42.4X3	T42.4X4	T42.4X5	T42.4X6
Medicament NEC	T50.901	T50.902	T50.903	T50.904	T50.905	T50.906
Medinal	T42.3X1	T42.3X2	T42.3X3	T42.3X4	T42.3X5	T42.3X6
Medomin	T42.3X1	T42.3X2	T42.3X3	T42.3X4	T42.3X5	T42.3X6
Medrogestone	T38.5X1	T38.5X2	T38.5X3	T38.5X4	T38.5X5	T38.5X6
Medroxalol	T44.8X1	T44.8X2	T44.8X3	T44.8X4	T44.8X5	T44.8X6
Medroxyprogesterone acetate (depot)	T38.5X1	T38.5X2	T38.5X3	T38.5X4	T38.5X5	T38.5X6
Medrysone	T49.0X1	T49.0X2	T49.0X3	T49.0X4	T49.0X5	T49.0X6
Mefenamic acid	T39.391	T39.392	T39.393	T39.394	T39.395	T39.396
Mefenorex	T50.5X1	T50.5X2	T50.5X3	T50.5X4	T50.5X5	T50.5X6
Mefloquine	T37.2X1	T37.2X2	T37.2X3	T37.2X4	T37.2X5	T37.2X6
Mefruside	T50.2X1	T50.2X2	T50.2X3	T50.2X4	T50.2X5	T50.2X6
Megahallucinogen	T40.901	T40.902	T40.903	T40.904	T40.905	T40.906
Megestrol	T38.5X1	T38.5X2	T38.5X3	T38.5X4	T38.5X5	T38.5X6
Meglumine						
antimoniate	T37.8X1	T37.8X2	T37.8X3	T37.8X4	T37.8X5	T37.8X6
diatrizoate	T50.8X1	T50.8X2	T50.8X3	T50.8X4	T50.8X5	T50.8X6
iodipamide	T50.8X1	T50.8X2	T50.8X3	T50.8X4	T50.8X5	T50.8X6
iotroxate	T50.8X1	T50.8X2	T50.8X3	T50.8X4	T50.8X5	T50.8X6
MEK (methyl ethyl ketone)	T52.4X1	T52.4X2	T52.4X3	T52.4X4	—	—
Meladrazine	T44.3X1	T44.3X2	T44.3X3	T44.3X4	T44.3X5	T44.3X6
Meladinin	T49.3X1	T49.3X2	T49.3X3	T49.3X4	T49.3X5	T49.3X6
Melaleuca alternifolia oil	T49.0X1	T49.0X2	T49.0X3	T49.0X4	T49.0X5	T49.0X6
Melanizing agents	T49.3X1	T49.3X2	T49.3X3	T49.3X4	T49.3X5	T49.3X6
Melanocyte-stimulating hormone	T38.891	T38.892	T38.893	T38.894	T38.895	T38.896
Melarsonyl potassium	T37.3X1	T37.3X2	T37.3X3	T37.3X4	T37.3X5	T37.3X6

◀ New   ◀ Revised   deleted Deleted

Substance	External Cause (T-Code)					
	Poisoning, Accidental (Unintentional)	Poisoning, Intentional Self-Harm	Poisoning, Assault	Poisoning, Undetermined	Adverse Effect	Underdosing
Melarsoprol	T37.3X1	T37.3X2	T37.3X3	T37.3X4	T37.3X5	T37.3X6
Melia azedarach	T62.2X1	T62.2X2	T62.2X3	T62.2X4	—	—
Melitracen	T43.011	T43.012	T43.013	T43.014	T43.015	T43.016
Mellaril	T43.3X1	T43.3X2	T43.3X3	T43.3X4	T43.3X5	T43.3X6
Meloxine	T49.3X1	T49.3X2	T49.3X3	T49.3X4	T49.3X5	T49.3X6
Melperone	T43.4X1	T43.4X2	T43.4X3	T43.4X4	T43.4X5	T43.4X6
Melphalan	T45.1X1	T45.1X2	T45.1X3	T45.1X4	T45.1X5	T45.1X6
Memantine	T43.8X1	T43.8X2	T43.8X3	T43.8X4	T43.8X5	T43.8X6
Menadiol	T45.7X1	T45.7X2	T45.7X3	T45.7X4	T45.7X5	T45.7X6
sodium sulfate	T45.7X1	T45.7X2	T45.7X3	T45.7X4	T45.7X5	T45.7X6
Menadione	T45.7X1	T45.7X2	T45.7X3	T45.7X4	T45.7X5	T45.7X6
sodium bisulfite	T45.7X1	T45.7X2	T45.7X3	T45.7X4	T45.7X5	T45.7X6
Menaphthone	T45.7X1	T45.7X2	T45.7X3	T45.7X4	T45.7X5	T45.7X6
Menaquinone	T45.7X1	T45.7X2	T45.7X3	T45.7X4	T45.7X5	T45.7X6
Menatetrenone	T45.7X1	T45.7X2	T45.7X3	T45.7X4	T45.7X5	T45.7X6
Meningococcal vaccine	T50.A91	T50.A92	T50.A93	T50.A94	T50.A95	T50.A96
Menningovax (-AC) (-C)	T50.A91	T50.A92	T50.A93	T50.A94	T50.A95	T50.A96
Menotropins	T38.811	T38.812	T38.813	T38.814	T38.815	T38.816
Menthol	T48.5X1	T48.5X2	T48.5X3	T48.5X4	T48.5X5	T48.5X6
Mepacrine	T37.2X1	T37.2X2	T37.2X3	T37.2X4	T37.2X5	T37.2X6
Meparfynol	T42.6X1	T42.6X2	T42.6X3	T42.6X4	T42.6X5	T42.6X6
Mepartricin	T36.7X1	T36.7X2	T36.7X3	T36.7X4	T36.7X5	T36.7X6
Mepazine	T43.3X1	T43.3X2	T43.3X3	T43.3X4	T43.3X5	T43.3X6
Mepenzolate	T44.3X1	T44.3X2	T44.3X3	T44.3X4	T44.3X5	T44.3X6
bromide	T44.3X1	T44.3X2	T44.3X3	T44.3X4	T44.3X5	T44.3X6
Meperidine	T40.4X1	T40.4X2	T40.4X3	T40.4X4	T40.4X5	T40.4X6
Mephebarbital	T42.3X1	T42.3X2	T42.3X3	T42.3X4	T42.3X5	T42.3X6
Mephenamin(e)	T42.8X1	T42.8X2	T42.8X3	T42.8X4	T42.8X5	T42.8X6
Mephenesin	T42.8X1	T42.8X2	T42.8X3	T42.8X4	T42.8X5	T42.8X6
Mephenhydramine	T45.0X1	T45.0X2	T45.0X3	T45.0X4	T45.0X5	T45.0X6
Mephenoxalone	T42.8X1	T42.8X2	T42.8X3	T42.8X4	T42.8X5	T42.8X6
Mephentermine	T44.991	T44.992	T44.993	T44.994	T44.995	T44.996
Mephenytoin	T42.0X1	T42.0X2	T42.0X3	T42.0X4	T42.0X5	T42.0X6
with phenobarbital	T42.3X1	T42.3X2	T42.3X3	T42.3X4	T42.3X5	T42.3X6
Mephobarbital	T42.3X1	T42.3X2	T42.3X3	T42.3X4	T42.3X5	T42.3X6
Mephosfolan	T60.0X1	T60.0X2	T60.0X3	T60.0X4	—	—
Mepindolol	T44.7X1	T44.7X2	T44.7X3	T44.7X4	T44.7X5	T44.7X6
Mepiperphenidol	T44.3X1	T44.3X2	T44.3X3	T44.3X4	T44.3X5	T44.3X6
Mepitiostane	T38.7X1	T38.7X2	T38.7X3	T38.7X4	T38.7X5	T38.7X6

◀ New   ◀▥ Revised   ~~deleted~~ Deleted

Substance	Poisoning, Accidental (Unintentional)	Poisoning, Intentional Self-Harm	Poisoning, Assault	Poisoning, Undetermined	Adverse Effect	Underdosing
			External Cause (T-Code)			
Mepivacaine	T41.3X1	T41.3X2	T41.3X3	T41.3X4	T41.3X5	T41.3X6
epidural	T41.3X1	T41.3X2	T41.3X3	T41.3X4	T41.3X5	T41.3X6
Meprednisone	T38.0X1	T38.0X2	T38.0X3	T38.0X4	T38.0X5	T38.0X6
Meprobam	T43.591	T43.592	T43.593	T43.594	T43.595	T43.596
Meprobamate	T43.591	T43.592	T43.593	T43.594	T43.595	T43.596
Meproscillarin	T46.0X1	T46.0X2	T46.0X3	T46.0X4	T46.0X5	T46.0X6
Meprylcaine	T41.3X1	T41.3X2	T41.3X3	T41.3X4	T41.3X5	T41.3X6
Meptazinol	T39.8X1	T39.8X2	T39.8X3	T39.8X4	T39.8X5	T39.8X6
Mepyramine	T45.0X1	T45.0X2	T45.0X3	T45.0X4	T45.0X5	T45.0X6
Mequitazine	T43.3X1	T43.3X2	T43.3X3	T43.3X4	T43.3X5	T43.3X6
Meralluride	T50.2X1	T50.2X2	T50.2X3	T50.2X4	T50.2X5	T50.2X6
Merbaphen	T50.2X1	T50.2X2	T50.2X3	T50.2X4	T50.2X5	T50.2X6
Merbromin	T49.0X1	T49.0X2	T49.0X3	T49.0X4	T49.0X5	T49.0X6
Mercaptobenzothiazole salts	T49.0X1	T49.0X2	T49.0X3	T49.0X4	T49.0X5	T49.0X6
Mercaptomerin	T50.2X1	T50.2X2	T50.2X3	T50.2X4	T50.2X5	T50.2X6
Mercaptopurine	T45.1X1	T45.1X2	T45.1X3	T45.1X4	T45.1X5	T45.1X6
Mercumatilin	T50.2X1	T50.2X2	T50.2X3	T50.2X4	T50.2X5	T50.2X6
Mercuramide	T50.2X1	T50.2X2	T50.2X3	T50.2X4	T50.2X5	T50.2X6
Mercurochrome	T49.0X1	T49.0X2	T49.0X3	T49.0X4	T49.0X5	T49.0X6
Mercurophylline	T50.2X1	T50.2X2	T50.2X3	T50.2X4	T50.2X5	T50.2X6
Mercury, mercurial, mercuric, mercurous (compounds) (cyanide) (fumes) (nonmedicinal) (vapor) NEC	T56.1X1	T56.1X2	T56.1X3	T56.1X4	—	—
ammoniated	T49.0X1	T49.0X2	T49.0X3	T49.0X4	T49.0X5	T49.0X6
anti-infective						
local	T49.0X1	T49.0X2	T49.0X3	T49.0X4	T49.0X5	T49.0X6
systemic	T37.8X1	T37.8X2	T37.8X3	T37.8X4	T37.8X5	T37.8X6
topical	T49.0X1	T49.0X2	T49.0X3	T49.0X4	T49.0X5	T49.0X6
chloride (ammoniated)	T49.0X1	T49.0X2	T49.0X3	T49.0X4	T49.0X5	T49.0X6
fungicide	T56.1X1	T56.1X2	T56.1X3	T56.1X4	—	—
diuretic NEC	T50.2X1	T50.2X2	T50.2X3	T50.2X4	T50.2X5	T50.2X6
fungicide	T56.1X1	T56.1X2	T56.1X3	T56.1X4	—	—
organic (fungicide)	T56.1X1	T56.1X2	T56.1X3	T56.1X4	—	—
oxide, yellow	T49.0X1	T49.0X2	T49.0X3	T49.0X4	T49.0X5	T49.0X6
Mersalyl	T50.2X1	T50.2X2	T50.2X3	T50.2X4	T50.2X5	T50.2X6
Merthiolate	T49.0X1	T49.0X2	T49.0X3	T49.0X4	T49.0X5	T49.0X6
ophthalmic preparation	T49.5X1	T49.5X2	T49.5X3	T49.5X4	T49.5X5	T49.5X6
Meruvax	T50.B91	T50.B92	T50.B93	T50.B94	T50.B95	T50.B96
Mesalazine	T47.8X1	T47.8X2	T47.8X3	T47.8X4	T47.8X5	T47.8X6
Mescal buttons	T40.991	T40.992	T40.993	T40.994	—	—

◀ New ◀▥▥ Revised ~~deleted~~ Deleted

TABLE OF DRUGS AND CHEMICALS

Substance	External Cause (T-Code)					
	Poisoning, Accidental (Unintentional)	Poisoning, Intentional Self-Harm	Poisoning, Assault	Poisoning, Undetermined	Adverse Effect	Underdosing
Mescaline	T40.991	T40.992	T40.993	T40.994	—	—
Mesna	T48.4X1	T48.4X2	T48.4X3	T48.4X4	T48.4X5	T48.4X6
Mesoglycan	T46.6X1	T46.6X2	T46.6X3	T46.6X4	T46.6X5	T46.6X6
Mesoridazine	T43.3X1	T43.3X2	T43.3X3	T43.3X4	T43.3X5	T43.3X6
Mestanolone	T38.7X1	T38.7X2	T38.7X3	T38.7X4	T38.7X5	T38.7X6
Mesterolone	T38.7X1	T38.7X2	T38.7X3	T38.7X4	T38.7X5	T38.7X6
Mestranol	T38.5X1	T38.5X2	T38.5X3	T38.5X4	T38.5X5	T38.5X6
Mesulergine	T42.8X1	T42.8X2	T42.8X3	T42.8X4	T42.8X5	T42.8X6
Mesulfen	T49.0X1	T49.0X2	T49.0X3	T49.0X4	T49.0X5	T49.0X6
Mesuximide	T42.2X1	T42.2X2	T42.2X3	T42.2X4	T42.2X5	T42.2X6
Metabutethamine	T41.3X1	T41.3X2	T41.3X3	T41.3X4	T41.3X5	T41.3X6
Metactesylacetate	T49.0X1	T49.0X2	T49.0X3	T49.0X4	T49.0X5	T49.0X6
Metacycline	T36.4X1	T36.4X2	T36.4X3	T36.4X4	T36.4X5	T36.4X6
Metaldehyde (snail killer) NEC	T60.8X1	T60.8X2	T60.8X3	T60.8X4	—	—
Metals (heavy) (nonmedicinal)	T56.91	T56.92	T56.93	T56.94	—	—
dust, fumes, or vapor NEC	T56.91	T56.92	T56.93	T56.94	—	—
light NEC	T56.91	T56.92	T56.93	T56.94	—	—
dust, fumes, or vapor NEC	T56.91	T56.92	T56.93	T56.94	—	—
specified NEC	T56.891	T56.892	T56.893	T56.894	—	—
thallium	T56.811	T56.812	T56.813	T56.814	—	—
Metamfetamine	T43.621	T43.622	T43.623	T43.624	T43.625	T43.626
Metamizole sodium	T39.2X1	T39.2X2	T39.2X3	T39.2X4	T39.2X5	T39.2X6
Metampicillin	T36.0X1	T36.0X2	T36.0X3	T36.0X4	T36.0X5	T36.0X6
Metamucil	T47.4X1	T47.4X2	T47.4X3	T47.4X4	T47.4X5	T47.4X6
Metaphen	T49.0X1	T49.0X2	T49.0X3	T49.0X4	T49.0X5	T49.0X6
Metandienone	T38.7X1	T38.7X2	T38.7X3	T38.7X4	T38.7X5	T38.7X6
Metandrostenolone	T38.7X1	T38.7X2	T38.7X3	T38.7X4	T38.7X5	T38.7X6
Metaphos	T60.0X1	T60.0X2	T60.0X3	T60.0X4	—	—
Metapramine	T43.011	T43.012	T43.013	T43.014	T43.015	T43.016
Metaproterenol	T48.291	T48.292	T48.293	T48.294	T48.295	T48.296
Metaraminol	T44.4X1	T44.4X2	T44.4X3	T44.4X4	T44.4X5	T44.4X6
Metaxalone	T42.8X1	T42.8X2	T42.8X3	T42.8X4	T42.8X5	T42.8X6
Metenolone	T38.7X1	T38.7X2	T38.7X3	T38.7X4	T38.7X5	T38.7X6
Metergoline	T42.8X1	T42.8X2	T42.8X3	T42.8X4	T42.8X5	T42.8X6
Metescufylline	T46.991	T46.992	T46.993	T46.994	T46.995	T46.996
Metetoin	T42.0X1	T42.0X2	T42.0X3	T42.0X4	T42.0X5	T42.0X6
Metformin	T38.3X1	T38.3X2	T38.3X3	T38.3X4	T38.3X5	T38.3X6
Methacholine	T44.1X1	T44.1X2	T44.1X3	T44.1X4	T44.1X5	T44.1X6
Methacycline	T36.4X1	T36.4X2	T36.4X3	T36.4X4	T36.4X5	T36.4X6
Methadone	T40.3X1	T40.3X2	T40.3X3	T40.3X4	T40.3X5	T40.3X6

◀ New ◀️ Revised ~~deleted~~ Deleted

Substance	Poisoning, Accidental (Unintentional)	Poisoning, Intentional Self-Harm	Poisoning, Assault	Poisoning, Undetermined	Adverse Effect	Underdosing
	External Cause (T-Code)					
Methallenestril	T38.5X1	T38.5X2	T38.5X3	T38.5X4	T38.5X5	T38.5X6
Methallenoestril	T38.5X1	T38.5X2	T38.5X3	T38.5X4	T38.5X5	T38.5X6
Methamphetamine	T43.621	T43.622	T43.623	T43.624	T43.625	T43.626
Methampyrone	T39.2X1	T39.2X2	T39.2X3	T39.2X4	T39.2X5	T39.2X6
Methandienone	T38.7X1	T38.7X2	T38.7X3	T38.7X4	T38.7X5	T38.7X6
Methandriol	T38.7X1	T38.7X2	T38.7X3	T38.7X4	T38.7X5	T38.7X6
Methandrostenolone	T38.7X1	T38.7X2	T38.7X3	T38.7X4	T38.7X5	T38.7X6
Methane	T59.891	T59.892	T59.893	T59.894	—	—
Methanethiol	T59.891	T59.892	T59.893	T59.894	—	—
Methaniazide	T37.1X1	T37.1X2	T37.1X3	T37.1X4	T37.1X5	T37.1X6
Methanol (vapor)	T51.1X1	T51.1X2	T51.1X3	T51.1X4	—	—
Methantheline	T44.3X1	T44.3X2	T44.3X3	T44.3X4	T44.3X5	T44.3X6
Methanthelinium bromide	T44.3X1	T44.3X2	T44.3X3	T44.3X4	T44.3X5	T44.3X6
Methaphenilene	T45.0X1	T45.0X2	T45.0X3	T45.0X4	T45.0X5	T45.0X6
Methapyrilene	T45.0X1	T45.0X2	T45.0X3	T45.0X4	T45.0X5	T45.0X6
Methaqualone (compound)	T42.6X1	T42.6X2	T42.6X3	T42.6X4	T42.6X5	T42.6X6
Metharbital	T42.3X1	T42.3X2	T42.3X3	T42.3X4	T42.3X5	T42.3X6
Methazolamide	T50.2X1	T50.2X2	T50.2X3	T50.2X4	T50.2X5	T50.2X6
Methdilazine	T43.3X1	T43.3X2	T43.3X3	T43.3X4	T43.3X5	T43.3X6
Methedrine	T43.621	T43.622	T43.623	T43.624	T43.625	T43.626
Methenamine (mandelate)	T37.8X1	T37.8X2	T37.8X3	T37.8X4	T37.8X5	T37.8X6
Methenolone	T38.7X1	T38.7X2	T38.7X3	T38.7X4	T38.7X5	T38.7X6
Methergine	T48.0X1	T48.0X2	T48.0X3	T48.0X4	T48.0X5	T48.0X6
Methetoin	T42.0X1	T42.0X2	T42.0X3	T42.0X4	T42.0X5	T42.0X6
Methiacil	T38.2X1	T38.2X2	T38.2X3	T38.2X4	T38.2X5	T38.2X6
Methicillin	T36.0X1	T36.0X2	T36.0X3	T36.0X4	T36.0X5	T36.0X6
Methimazole	T38.2X1	T38.2X2	T38.2X3	T38.2X4	T38.2X5	T38.2X6
Methiodal sodium	T50.8X1	T50.8X2	T50.8X3	T50.8X4	T50.8X5	T50.8X6
Methionine	T50.991	T50.992	T50.993	T50.994	T50.995	T50.996
Methisazone	T37.5X1	T37.5X2	T37.5X3	T37.5X4	T37.5X5	T37.5X6
Methisoprinol	T37.5X1	T37.5X2	T37.5X3	T37.5X4	T37.5X5	T37.5X6
Methitural	T42.3X1	T42.3X2	T42.3X3	T42.3X4	T42.3X5	T42.3X6
Methixene	T44.3X1	T44.3X2	T44.3X3	T44.3X4	T44.3X5	T44.3X6
Methobarbital, methobarbitone	T42.3X1	T42.3X2	T42.3X3	T42.3X4	T42.3X5	T42.3X6
Methocarbamol	T42.8X1	T42.8X2	T42.8X3	T42.8X4	T42.8X5	T42.8X6
skeletal muscle relaxant	T48.1X1	T48.1X2	T48.1X3	T48.1X4	T48.1X5	T48.1X6
Methohexital	T41.1X1	T41.1X2	T41.1X3	T41.1X4	T41.1X5	T41.1X6
Methohexitone	T41.1X1	T41.1X2	T41.1X3	T41.1X4	T41.1X5	T41.1X6
Methoin	T42.0X1	T42.0X2	T42.0X3	T42.0X4	T42.0X5	T42.0X6
Methopholine	T39.8X1	T39.8X2	T39.8X3	T39.8X4	T39.8X5	T39.8X6

TABLE OF DRUGS AND CHEMICALS

◀ New　◀▥ Revised　~~deleted~~ Deleted

	External Cause (T-Code)					
Substance	Poisoning, Accidental (Unintentional)	Poisoning, Intentional Self-Harm	Poisoning, Assault	Poisoning, Undetermined	Adverse Effect	Underdosing
Methopromazine	T43.3X1	T43.3X2	T43.3X3	T43.3X4	T43.3X5	T43.3X6
Methorate	T48.3X1	T48.3X2	T48.3X3	T48.3X4	T48.3X5	T48.3X6
Methoserpidine	T46.5X1	T46.5X2	T46.5X3	T46.5X4	T46.5X5	T46.5X6
Methotrexate	T45.1X1	T45.1X2	T45.1X3	T45.1X4	T45.1X5	T45.1X6
Methotrimeprazine	T43.3X1	T43.3X2	T43.3X3	T43.3X4	T43.3X5	T43.3X6
Methoxa-Dome	T49.3X1	T49.3X2	T49.3X3	T49.3X4	T49.3X5	T49.3X6
Methoxamine	T44.4X1	T44.4X2	T44.4X3	T44.4X4	T44.4X5	T44.4X6
Methoxsalen	T50.991	T50.992	T50.993	T50.994	T50.995	T50.996
Methoxyaniline	T65.3X1	T65.3X2	T65.3X3	T65.3X4	—	—
Methoxybenzyl penicillin	T36.0X1	T36.0X2	T36.0X3	T36.0X4	T36.0X5	T36.0X6
Methoxychlor	T53.7X1	T53.7X2	T53.7X3	T53.7X4	—	—
Methoxy-DDT	T53.7X1	T53.7X2	T53.7X3	T53.7X4	—	—
2-Methoxyethanol	T52.3X1	T52.3X2	T52.3X3	T52.3X4	—	—
Methoxyflurane	T41.0X1	T41.0X2	T41.0X3	T41.0X4	T41.0X5	T41.0X6
Methoxyphenamine	T48.6X1	T48.6X2	T48.6X3	T48.6X4	T48.6X5	T48.6X6
Methoxypromazine	T43.3X1	T43.3X2	T43.3X3	T43.3X4	T43.3X5	T43.3X6
5-Methoxypsoralen (5-MOP)	T50.991	T50.992	T50.993	T50.994	T50.995	T50.996
8-Methoxypsoralen (8-MOP)	T50.991	T50.992	T50.993	T50.994	T50.995	T50.996
Methscopolamine bromide	T44.3X1	T44.3X2	T44.3X3	T44.3X4	T44.3X5	T44.3X6
Methsuximide	T42.2X1	T42.2X2	T42.2X3	T42.2X4	T42.2X5	T42.2X6
Methyclothiazide	T50.2X1	T50.2X2	T50.2X3	T50.2X4	T50.2X5	T50.2X6
Methyl						
acetate	T52.4X1	T52.4X2	T52.4X3	T52.4X4	—	—
acetone	T52.4X1	T52.4X2	T52.4X3	T52.4X4	—	—
acrylate	T65.891	T65.892	T65.893	T65.894	—	—
alcohol	T51.1X1	T51.1X2	T51.1X3	T51.1X4	—	—
aminophenol	T65.3X1	T65.3X2	T65.3X3	T65.3X4	—	—
amphetamine	T43.621	T43.622	T43.623	T43.624	T43.625	T43.626
androstanolone	T38.7X1	T38.7X2	T38.7X3	T38.7X4	T38.7X5	T38.7X6
atropine	T44.3X1	T44.3X2	T44.3X3	T44.3X4	T44.3X5	T44.3X6
benzene	T52.2X1	T52.2X2	T52.2X3	T52.2X4	—	—
benzoate	T52.8X1	T52.8X2	T52.8X3	T52.8X4	—	—
benzol	T52.2X1	T52.2X2	T52.2X3	T52.2X4	—	—
bromide (gas)	T59.891	T59.892	T59.893	T59.894	—	—
fumigant	T60.8X1	T60.8X2	T60.8X3	T60.8X4	—	—
butanol	T51.3X1	T51.3X2	T51.3X3	T51.3X4	—	—
carbinol	T51.1X1	T51.1X2	T51.1X3	T51.1X4	—	—
carbonate	T52.8X1	T52.8X2	T52.8X3	T52.8X4	—	—
CCNU	T45.1X1	T45.1X2	T45.1X3	T45.1X4	T45.1X5	T45.1X6
cellosolve	T52.91	T52.92	T52.93	T52.94	—	—

◀ New ◀▥ Revised ~~deleted~~ Deleted

Substance	Poisoning, Accidental (Unintentional)	Poisoning, Intentional Self-Harm	Poisoning, Assault	Poisoning, Undetermined	Adverse Effect	Underdosing
			External Cause (T-Code)			
Methyl *(Continued)*						
cellulose	T47.4X1	T47.4X2	T47.4X3	T47.4X4	T47.4X5	T47.4X6
chloride (gas)	T59.891	T59.892	T59.893	T59.894	—	—
chloroformate	T59.3X1	T59.3X2	T59.3X3	T59.3X4	—	—
cyclohexane	T52.8X1	T52.8X2	T52.8X3	T52.8X4	—	—
cyclohexanol	T51.8X1	T51.8X2	T51.8X3	T51.8X4	—	—
cyclohexanone	T52.8X1	T52.8X2	T52.8X3	T52.8X4	—	—
cyclohexyl acetate	T52.8X1	T52.8X2	T52.8X3	T52.8X4	—	—
demeton	T60.0X1	T60.0X2	T60.0X3	T60.0X4	—	—
dihydromorphinone	T40.2X1	T40.2X2	T40.2X3	T40.2X4	T40.2X5	T40.2X6
ergometrine	T48.0X1	T48.0X2	T48.0X3	T48.0X4	T48.0X5	T48.0X6
ergonovine	T48.0X1	T48.0X2	T48.0X3	T48.0X4	T48.0X5	T48.0X6
ethyl ketone	T52.4X1	T52.4X2	T52.4X3	T52.4X4	—	—
glucamine antimonate	T37.8X1	T37.8X2	T37.8X3	T37.8X4	T37.8X5	T37.8X6
hydrazine	T65.891	T65.892	T65.893	T65.894	—	—
iodide	T65.891	T65.892	T65.893	T65.894	—	—
isobutyl ketone	T52.4X1	T52.4X2	T52.4X3	T52.4X4	—	—
isothiocyanate	T60.3X1	T60.3X2	T60.3X3	T60.3X4	—	—
mercaptan	T59.891	T59.892	T59.893	T59.894	—	—
morphine NEC	T40.2X1	T40.2X2	T40.2X3	T40.2X4	T40.2X5	T40.2X6
nicotinate	T49.4X1	T49.4X2	T49.4X3	T49.4X4	T49.4X5	T49.4X6
paraben	T49.0X1	T49.0X2	T49.0X3	T49.0X4	T49.0X5	T49.0X6
parafynol	T42.6X1	T42.6X2	T42.6X3	T42.6X4	T42.6X5	T42.6X6
parathion	T60.0X1	T60.0X2	T60.0X3	T60.0X4	—	—
peridol	T43.4X1	T43.4X2	T43.4X3	T43.4X4	T43.4X5	T43.4X6
phenidate	T43.631	T43.632	T43.633	T43.634	T43.635	T43.636
prednisolone	T38.0X1	T38.0X2	T38.0X3	T38.0X4	T38.0X5	T38.0X6
ENT agent	T49.6X1	T49.6X2	T49.6X3	T49.6X4	T49.6X5	T49.6X6
ophthalmic preparation	T49.5X1	T49.5X2	T49.5X3	T49.5X4	T49.5X5	T49.5X6
topical NEC	T49.0X1	T49.0X2	T49.0X3	T49.0X4	T49.0X5	T49.0X6
propylcarbinol	T51.3X1	T51.3X2	T51.3X3	T51.3X4	—	—
rosaniline NEC	T49.0X1	T49.0X2	T49.0X3	T49.0X4	T49.0X5	T49.0X6
salicylate	T49.2X1	T49.2X2	T49.2X3	T49.2X4	T49.2X5	T49.2X6
sulfate (fumes)	T59.891	T59.892	T59.893	T59.894	—	—
liquid	T52.8X1	T52.8X2	T52.8X3	T52.8X4	—	—
sulfonal	T42.6X1	T42.6X2	T42.6X3	T42.6X4	T42.6X5	T42.6X6
testosterone	T38.7X1	T38.7X2	T38.7X3	T38.7X4	T38.7X5	T38.7X6
thiouracil	T38.2X1	T38.2X2	T38.2X3	T38.2X4	T38.2X5	T38.2X6
Methylamphetamine	T43.621	T43.622	T43.623	T43.624	T43.625	T43.626
Methylated spirit	T51.1X1	T51.1X2	T51.1X3	T51.1X4	—	—

◀ New   ◀|||| Revised   ~~deleted~~ Deleted

Substance	Poisoning, Accidental (Unintentional)	Poisoning, Intentional Self-Harm	Poisoning, Assault	Poisoning, Undetermined	Adverse Effect	Underdosing
	External Cause (T-Code)					
Methylatropine nitrate	T44.3X1	T44.3X2	T44.3X3	T44.3X4	T44.3X5	T44.3X6
Methylbenactyzium bromide	T44.3X1	T44.3X2	T44.3X3	T44.3X4	T44.3X5	T44.3X6
Methylbenzethonium chloride	T49.0X1	T49.0X2	T49.0X3	T49.0X4	T49.0X5	T49.0X6
Methylcellulose	T47.4X1	T47.4X2	T47.4X3	T47.4X4	T47.4X5	T47.4X6
laxative	T47.4X1	T47.4X2	T47.4X3	T47.4X4	T47.4X5	T47.4X6
Methylchlorophenoxy-acetic acid	T60.3X1	T60.3X2	T60.3X3	T60.3X4	—	—
Methyldopa	T46.5X1	T46.5X2	T46.5X3	T46.5X4	T46.5X5	T46.5X6
Methyldopate	T46.5X1	T46.5X2	T46.5X3	T46.5X4	T46.5X5	T46.5X6
Methylene						
blue	T50.6X1	T50.6X2	T50.6X3	T50.6X4	T50.6X5	T50.6X6
chloride or dichloride (solvent) NEC	T53.4X1	T53.4X2	T53.4X3	T53.4X4	—	—
Methylenedioxyamphet-amine	T43.621	T43.622	T43.623	T43.624	T43.625	T43.626
Methylenedioxymethamphetamine	T43.621	T43.622	T43.623	T43.624	T43.625	T43.626
Methylergometrine	T48.0X1	T48.0X2	T48.0X3	T48.0X4	T48.0X5	T48.0X6
Methylergonovine	T48.0X1	T48.0X2	T48.0X3	T48.0X4	T48.0X5	T48.0X6
Methylestrenolone	T38.5X1	T38.5X2	T38.5X3	T38.5X4	T38.5X5	T38.5X6
Methylethyl cellulose	T50.991	T50.992	T50.993	T50.994	T50.995	T50.996
Methylhexabital	T42.3X1	T42.3X2	T42.3X3	T42.3X4	T42.3X5	T42.3X6
Methylmorphine	T40.2X1	T40.2X2	T40.2X3	T40.2X4	T40.2X5	T40.2X6
Methylparaben (ophthalmic)	T49.5X1	T49.5X2	T49.5X3	T49.5X4	T49.5X5	T49.5X6
Methylparafynol	T42.6X1	T42.6X2	T42.6X3	T42.6X4	T42.6X5	T42.6X6
Methylpentynol, methylpenthynol	T42.6X1	T42.6X2	T42.6X3	T42.6X4	T42.6X5	T42 6X6
Methylphenidate	T43.631	T43.632	T43.633	T43.634	T43.635	T43.636
Methylphenobarbital	T42.3X1	T42.3X2	T42.3X3	T42.3X4	T42.3X5	T42.3X6
Methylpolysiloxane	T47.1X1	T47.1X2	T47.1X3	T47.1X4	T47.1X5	T47.1X6
Methylprednisolone — see Methyl, prednisolone						
Methylrosaniline	T49.0X1	T49.0X2	T49.0X3	T49.0X4	T49.0X5	T49.0X6
Methylrosanilinium chloride	T49.0X1	T49.0X2	T49.0X3	T49.0X4	T49.0X5	T49.0X6
Methyltestosterone	T38.7X1	T38.7X2	T38.7X3	T38.7X4	T38.7X5	T38.7X6
Methylthionine chloride	T50.6X1	T50.6X2	T50.6X3	T50.6X4	T50.6X5	T50.6X6
Methylthioninium chloride	T50.6X1	T50.6X2	T50.6X3	T50.6X4	T50.6X5	T50.6X6
Methylthiouracil	T38.2X1	T38.2X2	T38.2X3	T38.2X4	T38.2X5	T38.2X6
Methyprylon	T42.6X1	T42.6X2	T42.6X3	T42.6X4	T42.6X5	T42.6X6
Methysergide	T46.5X1	T46.5X2	T46.5X3	T46.5X4	T46.5X5	T46.5X6
Metiamide	T47.1X1	T47.1X2	T47.1X3	T47.1X4	T47.1X5	T47.1X6
Meticillin	T36.0X1	T36.0X2	T36.0X3	T36.0X4	T36.0X5	T36.0X6
Meticrane	T50.2X1	T50.2X2	T50.2X3	T50.2X4	T50.2X5	T50.2X6
Metildigoxin	T46.0X1	T46.0X2	T46.0X3	T46.0X4	T46.0X5	T46.0X6
Metipranolol	T49.5X1	T49.5X2	T49.5X3	T49.5X4	T49.5X5	T49.5X6

◀ New   ◀▥ Revised   ~~deleted~~ Deleted

	External Cause (T-Code)					
Substance	Poisoning, Accidental (Unintentional)	Poisoning, Intentional Self-Harm	Poisoning, Assault	Poisoning, Undetermined	Adverse Effect	Underdosing
Metirosine	T46.5X1	T46.5X2	T46.5X3	T46.5X4	T46.5X5	T46.5X6
Metisazone	T37.5X1	T37.5X2	T37.5X3	T37.5X4	T37.5X5	T37.5X6
Metixene	T44.3X1	T44.3X2	T44.3X3	T44.3X4	T44.3X5	T44.3X6
Metizoline	T48.5X1	T48.5X2	T48.5X3	T48.5X4	T48.5X5	T48.5X6
Metoclopramide	T45.0X1	T45.0X2	T45.0X3	T45.0X4	T45.0X5	T45.0X6
Metofenazate	T43.3X1	T43.3X2	T43.3X3	T43.3X4	T43.3X5	T43.3X6
Metofoline	T39.8X1	T39.8X2	T39.8X3	T39.8X4	T39.8X5	T39.8X6
Metolazone	T50.2X1	T50.2X2	T50.2X3	T50.2X4	T50.2X5	T50.2X6
Metopon	T40.2X1	T40.2X2	T40.2X3	T40.2X4	T40.2X5	T40.2X6
Metoprine	T45.1X1	T45.1X2	T45.1X3	T45.1X4	T45.1X5	T45.1X6
Metoprolol	T44.7X1	T44.7X2	T44.7X3	T44.7X4	T44.7X5	T44.7X6
Metrifonate	T60.0X1	T60.0X2	T60.0X3	T60.0X4	—	—
Metrizamide	T50.8X1	T50.8X2	T50.8X3	T50.8X4	T50.8X5	T50.8X6
Metrizoic acid	T50.8X1	T50.8X2	T50.8X3	T50.8X4	T50.8X5	T50.8X6
Metronidazole	T37.8X1	T37.8X2	T37.8X3	T37.8X4	T37.8X5	T37.8X6
Metycaine	T41.3X1	T41.3X2	T41.3X3	T41.3X4	T41.3X5	T41.3X6
infiltration (subcutaneous)	T41.3X1	T41.3X2	T41.3X3	T41.3X4	T41.3X5	T41.3X6
nerve block (peripheral) (plexus)	T41.3X1	T41.3X2	T41.3X3	T41.3X4	T41.3X5	T41.3X6
topical (surface)	T41.3X1	T41.3X2	T41.3X3	T41.3X4	T41.3X5	T41.3X6
Metyrapone	T50.8X1	T50.8X2	T50.8X3	T50.8X4	T50.8X5	T50.8X6
Mevinphos	T60.0X1	T60.0X2	T60.0X3	T60.0X4	—	—
Mexazolam	T42.4X1	T42.4X2	T42.4X3	T42.4X4	T42.4X5	T42.4X6
Mexenone	T49.3X1	T49.3X2	T49.3X3	T49.3X4	T49.3X5	T49.3X6
Mexiletine	T46.2X1	T46.2X2	T46.2X3	T46.2X4	T46.2X5	T46.2X6
Mezereon	T62.2X1	T62.2X2	T62.2X3	T62.2X4	—	—
berries	T62.1X1	T62.1X2	T62.1X3	T62.1X4	—	—
Mezlocillin	T36.0X1	T36.0X2	T36.0X3	T36.0X4	T36.0X5	T36.0X6
Mianserin	T43.021	T43.022	T43.023	T43.024	T43.025	T43.026
Micatin	T49.0X1	T49.0X2	T49.0X3	T49.0X4	T49.0X5	T49.0X6
Miconazole	T49.0X1	T49.0X2	T49.0X3	T49.0X4	T49.0X5	T49.0X6
Micronomicin	T36.5X1	T36.5X2	T36.5X3	T36.5X4	T36.5X5	T36.5X6
Midazolam	T42.4X1	T42.4X2	T42.4X3	T42.4X4	T42.4X5	T42.4X6
Midecamycin	T36.3X1	T36.3X2	T36.3X3	T36.3X4	T36.3X5	T36.3X6
Mifepristone	T38.6X1	T38.6X2	T38.6X3	T38.6X4	T38.6X5	T38.6X6
Milk of magnesia	T47.1X1	T47.1X2	T47.1X3	T47.1X4	T47.1X5	T47.1X6
Millipede (tropical) (venomous)	T63.411	T63.412	T63.413	T63.414	—	—
Miltown	T43.591	T43.592	T43.593	T43.594	T43.595	T43.596
Milverine	T44.3X1	T44.3X2	T44.3X3	T44.3X4	T44.3X5	T44.3X6
Minaprine	T43.291	T43.292	T43.293	T43.294	T43.295	T43.296

Substance	External Cause (T-Code)					
	Poisoning, Accidental (Unintentional)	Poisoning, Intentional Self-Harm	Poisoning, Assault	Poisoning, Undetermined	Adverse Effect	Underdosing
Minaxolone	T41.291	T41.292	T41.293	T41.294	T41.295	T41.296
Mineral						
acids	T54.2X1	T54.2X2	T54.2X3	T54.2X4	—	—
oil (laxative) (medicinal)	T47.4X1	T47.4X2	T47.4X3	T47.4X4	T47.4X5	T47.4X6
emulsion	T47.2X1	T47.2X2	T47.2X3	T47.2X4	T47.2X5	T47.2X6
nonmedicinal	T52.0X1	T52.0X2	T52.0X3	T52.0X4	—	—
topical	T49.3X1	T49.3X2	T49.3X3	T49.3X4	T49.3X5	T49.3X6
salt NEC	T50.3X1	T50.3X2	T50.3X3	T50.3X4	T50.3X5	T50.3X6
spirits	T52.0X1	T52.0X2	T52.0X3	T52.0X4	—	—
Mineralocorticosteroid	T50.0X1	T50.0X2	T50.0X3	T50.0X4	T50.0X5	T50.0X6
Minocycline	T36.4X1	T36.4X2	T36.4X3	T36.4X4	T36.4X5	T36.4X6
Minoxidil	T46.7X1	T46.7X2	T46.7X3	T46.7X4	T46.7X5	T46.7X6
Miokamycin	T36.3X1	T36.3X2	T36.3X3	T36.3X4	T36.3X5	T36.3X6
Miotic drug	T49.5X1	T49.5X2	T49.5X3	T49.5X4	T49.5X5	T49.5X6
Mipafox	T60.0X1	T60.0X2	T60.0X3	T60.0X4	—	—
Mirex	T60.1X1	T60.1X2	T60.1X3	T60.1X4	—	—
Mirtazapine	T43.021	T43.022	T43.023	T43.024	T43.025	T43.026
Misonidazole	T37.3X1	T37.3X2	T37.3X3	T37.3X4	T37.3X5	T37.3X6
Misoprostol	T47.1X1	T47.1X2	T47.1X3	T47.1X4	T47.1X5	T47.1X6
Mithramycin	T45.1X1	T45.1X2	T45.1X3	T45.1X4	T45.1X5	T45.1X6
Mitobronitol	T45.1X1	T45.1X2	T45.1X3	T45.1X4	T45.1X5	T45.1X6
Mitoguazone	T45.1X1	T45.1X2	T45.1X3	T45.1X4	T45.1X5	T45.1X6
Mitolactol	T45.1X1	T45.1X2	T45.1X3	T45.1X4	T45.1X5	T45.1X6
Mitomycin	T45.1X1	T45.1X2	T45.1X3	T45.1X4	T45.1X5	T45.1X6
Mitopodozide	T45.1X1	T45.1X2	T45.1X3	T45.1X4	T45.1X5	T45.1X6
Mitotane	T45.1X1	T45.1X2	T45.1X3	T45.1X4	T45.1X5	T45.1X6
Mitoxantrone	T45.1X1	T45.1X2	T45.1X3	T45.1X4	T45.1X5	T45.1X6
Mivacurium chloride	T48.1X1	T48.1X2	T48.1X3	T48.1X4	T48.1X5	T48.1X6
Miyari bacteria	T47.6X1	T47.6X2	T47.6X3	T47.6X4	T47.6X5	T47.6X6
Moclobemide	T43.1X1	T43.1X2	T43.1X3	T43.1X4	T43.1X5	T43.1X6
Moderil	T46.5X1	T46.5X2	T46.5X3	T46.5X4	T46.5X5	T46.5X6
Mofebutazone	T39.2X1	T39.2X2	T39.2X3	T39.2X4	T39.2X5	T39.2X6
Mogadon — see Nitrazepam						
Molindone	T43.591	T43.592	T43.593	T43.594	T43.595	T43.596
Molsidomine	T46.3X1	T46.3X2	T46.3X3	T46.3X4	T46.3X5	T46.3X6
Mometasone	T49.0X1	T49.0X2	T49.0X3	T49.0X4	T49.0X5	T49.0X6
Monistat	T49.0X1	T49.0X2	T49.0X3	T49.0X4	T49.0X5	T49.0X6
Monkshood	T62.2X1	T62.2X2	T62.2X3	T62.2X4	—	—
Monoamine oxidase inhibitor NEC	T43.1X1	T43.1X2	T43.1X3	T43.1X4	T43.1X5	T43.1X6
hydrazine	T43.1X1	T43.1X2	T43.1X3	T43.1X4	T43.1X5	T43.1X6

◀ New ◀▥ Revised ~~deleted~~ Deleted

Substance	External Cause (T-Code)					
	Poisoning, Accidental (Unintentional)	Poisoning, Intentional Self-Harm	Poisoning, Assault	Poisoning, Undetermined	Adverse Effect	Underdosing
Monobenzone	T49.4X1	T49.4X2	T49.4X3	T49.4X4	T49.4X5	T49.4X6
Monochloroacetic acid	T60.3X1	T60.3X2	T60.3X3	T60.3X4	—	—
Monochlorobenzene	T53.7X1	T53.7X2	T53.7X3	T53.7X4	—	—
Monoethanolamine	T46.8X1	T46.8X2	T46.8X3	T46.8X4	T46.8X5	T46.8X6
oleate	T46.8X1	T46.8X2	T46.8X3	T46.8X4	T46.8X5	T46.8X6
Monooctanoin	T50.991	T50.992	T50.993	T50.994	T50.995	T50.996
Monophenylbutazone	T39.2X1	T39.2X2	T39.2X3	T39.2X4	T39.2X5	T39.2X6
Monosodium glutamate	T65.891	T65.892	T65.893	T65.894	—	—
Monosulfiram	T49.0X1	T49.0X2	T49.0X3	T49.0X4	T49.0X5	T49.0X6
Monoxide, carbon—see Carbon, monoxide	T57.91	T57.92	T57.93	T57.94	—	—
Monoxidine hydrochloride	T46.1X1	T46.1X2	T46.1X3	T46.1X4	T46.1X5	T46.1X6
Monuron	T60.3X1	T60.3X2	T60.3X3	T60.3X4		
Moperone	T43.4X1	T43.4X2	T43.4X3	T43.4X4	T43.4X5	T43.4X6
Mopidamol	T45.1X1	T45.1X2	T45.1X3	T45.1X4	T45.1X5	T45.1X6
MOPP (mechlorethamine + vincristine + prednisone + procarbazine)	T45.1X1	T45.1X2	T45.1X3	T45.1X4	T45.1X5	T45.1X6
Morfin	T40.2X1	T40.2X2	T40.2X3	T40.2X4	T40.2X5	T40.2X6
Morinamide	T37.1X1	T37.1X2	T37.1X3	T37.1X4	T37.1X5	T37.1X6
Morning glory seeds	T40.991	T40.992	T40.993	T40.994	—	—
Moroxydine	T37.5X1	T37.5X2	T37.5X3	T37.5X4	T37.5X5	T37.5X6
Morphazinamide	T37.1X1	T37.1X2	T37.1X3	T37.1X4	T37.1X5	T37.1X6
Morphine	T40.2X1	T40.2X2	T40.2X3	T40.2X4	T40.2X5	T40.2X6
antagonist	T50.7X1	T50.7X2	T50.7X3	T50.7X4	T50.7X5	T50.7X6
Morpholinylethylmorphine	T40.2X1	T40.2X2	T40.2X3	T40.2X4	—	—
Morsuximide	T42.2X1	T42.2X2	T42.2X3	T42.2X4	T42.2X5	T42.2X6
Mosapramine	T43.591	T43.592	T43.593	T43.594	T43.595	T43.596
Moth balls—see also Pesticides	T60.2X1	T60.2X2	T60.2X3	T60.2X4	—	—
naphthalene	T60.2X1	T60.2X2	T60.2X3	T60.2X4	—	—
paradichlorobenzene	T60.1X1	T60.1X2	T60.1X3	T60.1X4	—	—
Motor exhaust gas	T58.01	T58.02	T58.03	T58.04	—	—
Mouthwash (antiseptic) (zinc chloride)	T49.6X1	T49.6X2	T49.6X3	T49.6X4	T49.6X5	T49.6X6
Moxastine	T45.0X1	T45.0X2	T45.0X3	T45.0X4	T45.0X5	T45.0X6
Moxaverine	T44.3X1	T44.3X2	T44.3X3	T44.3X4	T44.3X5	T44.3X6
Moxifensine	T43.291	T43.292	T43.293	T43.294	T43.295	T43.296
Moxisylyte	T46.7X1	T46.7X2	T46.7X3	T46.7X4	T46.7X5	T46.7X6
Mucilage, plant	T47.4X1	T47.4X2	T47.4X3	T47.4X4	T47.4X5	T47.4X6
Mucolytic drug	T48.4X1	T48.4X2	T48.4X3	T48.4X4	T48.4X5	T48.4X6
Mucomyst	T48.4X1	T48.4X2	T48.4X3	T48.4X4	T48.4X5	T48.4X6
Mucous membrane agents (external)	T49.91	T49.92	T49.93	T49.94	T49.95	T49.96
specified NEC	T49.8X1	T49.8X2	T49.8X3	T49.8X4	T49.8X5	T49.8X6

◀ New ◀◀ Revised ~~deleted~~ Deleted

TABLE OF DRUGS AND CHEMICALS

Substance	Poisoning, Accidental (Unintentional)	Poisoning, Intentional Self-Harm	Poisoning, Assault	Poisoning, Undetermined	Adverse Effect	Underdosing
	External Cause (T-Code)					
Mumps						
immune globulin (human)	T50.Z11	T50.Z12	T50.Z13	T50.Z14	T50.Z15	T50.Z16
skin test antigen	T50.8X1	T50.8X2	T50.8X3	T50.8X4	T50.8X5	T50.8X6
vaccine	T50.B91	T50.B92	T50.B93	T50.B94	T50.B95	T50.B96
Mumpsvax	T50.B91	T50.B92	T50.B93	T50.B94	T50.B95	T50.B96
Mupirocin	T49.0X1	T49.0X2	T49.0X3	T49.0X4	T49.0X5	T49.0X6
Muriatic acid — *see Hydrochloric acid*						
Muromonab-CD3	T45.1X1	T45.1X2	T45.1X3	T45.1X4	T45.1X5	T45.1X6
Muscle relaxant — *see Relaxant, muscle*						
Muscle-action drug NEC	T48.201	T48.202	T48.203	T48.204	T48.205	T48.206
Muscle affecting agents NEC	T48.201	T48.202	T48.203	T48.204	T48.205	T48.206
oxytocic	T48.0X1	T48.0X2	T48.0X3	T48.0X4	T48.0X5	T48.0X6
relaxants	T48.201	T48.202	T48.203	T48.204	T48.205	T48.206
central nervous system	T42.8X1	T42.8X2	T42.8X3	T42.8X4	T42.8X5	T42.8X6
skeletal	T48.1X1	T48.1X2	T48.1X3	T48.1X4	T48.1X5	T48.1X6
smooth	T44.3X1	T44.3X2	T44.3X3	T44.3X4	T44.3X5	T44.3X6
Muscle-tone depressant, central NEC	T42.8X1	T42.8X2	T42.8X3	T42.8X4	T42.8X5	T42.8X6
specified NEC	T42.8X1	T42.8X2	T42.8X3	T42.8X4	T42.8X5	T42.8X6
Mushroom, noxious	T62.0X1	T62.0X2	T62.0X3	T62.0X4	—	—
Mussel, noxious	T61.781	T61.782	T61.783	T61.784	—	—
Mustard (emetic)	T47.7X1	T47.7X2	T47.7X3	T47.7X4	T47.7X5	T47.7X6
black	T47.7X1	T47.7X2	T47.7X3	T47.7X4	T47.7X5	T47.7X6
gas, not in war	T59.91	T59.92	T59.93	T59.94	—	—
nitrogen	T45.1X1	T45.1X2	T45.1X3	T45.1X4	T45.1X5	T45.1X6
Mustine	T45.1X1	T45.1X2	T45.1X3	T45.1X4	T45.1X5	T45.1X6
M-vac	T45.1X1	T45.1X2	T45.1X3	T45.1X4	T45.1X5	T45.1X6
Mycifradin	T36.5X1	T36.5X2	T36.5X3	T36.5X4	T36.5X5	T36.5X6
topical	T49.0X1	T49.0X2	T49.0X3	T49.0X4	T49.0X5	T49.0X6
Mycitracin	T36.8X1	T36.8X2	T36.8X3	T36.8X4	T36.8X5	T36.8X6
ophthalmic preparation	T49.5X1	T49.5X2	T49.5X3	T49.5X4	T49.5X5	T49.5X6
Mycostatin	T36.7X1	T36.7X2	T36.7X3	T36.7X4	T36.7X5	T36.7X6
topical	T49.0X1	T49.0X2	T49.0X3	T49.0X4	T49.0X5	T49.0X6
Mycotoxins	T64.81	T64.82	T64.83	T64.84	—	—
aflatoxin	T64.01	T64.02	T64.03	T64.04	—	—
specified NEC	T64.81	T64.82	T64.83	T64.84	—	—
Mydriacyl	T44.3X1	T44.3X2	T44.3X3	T44.3X4	T44.3X5	T44.3X6
Mydriatic drug	T49.5X1	T49.5X2	T49.5X3	T49.5X4	T49.5X5	T49.5X6
Myelobromal	T45.1X1	T45.1X2	T45.1X3	T45.1X4	T45.1X5	T45.1X6
Myleran	T45.1X1	T45.1X2	T45.1X3	T45.1X4	T45.1X5	T45.1X6
Myochrysin(e)	T39.2X1	T39.2X2	T39.2X3	T39.2X4	T39.2X5	T39.2X6

◀ New   ◀▥ Revised   ~~deleted~~ Deleted

Substance	Poisoning, Accidental (Unintentional)	Poisoning, Intentional Self-Harm	Poisoning, Assault	Poisoning, Undetermined	Adverse Effect	Underdosing
	External Cause (T-Code)					
Myoneural blocking agents	T48.1X1	T48.1X2	T48.1X3	T48.1X4	T48.1X5	T48.1X6
Myralact	T49.0X1	T49.0X2	T49.0X3	T49.0X4	T49.0X5	T49.0X6
Myristica fragrans	T62.2X1	T62.2X2	T62.2X3	T62.2X4	—	—
Myristicin	T65.891	T65.892	T65.893	T65.894	—	—
Mysoline	T42.3X1	T42.3X2	T42.3X3	T42.3X4	T42.3X5	T42.3X6
N						
Nabilone	T40.7X1	T40.7X2	T40.7X3	T40.7X4	T40.7X5	T40.7X6
Nabumetone	T39.391	T39.392	T39.393	T39.394	T39.395	T39.396
Nadolol	T44.7X1	T44.7X2	T44.7X3	T44.7X4	T44.7X5	T44.7X6
Nafcillin	T36.0X1	T36.0X2	T36.0X3	T36.0X4	T36.0X5	T36.0X6
Nafoxidine	T38.6X1	T38.6X2	T38.6X3	T38.6X4	T38.6X5	T38.6X6
Naftazone	T46.991	T46.992	T46.993	T46.994	T46.995	T46.996
Naftidrofuryl (oxalate)	T46.7X1	T46.7X2	T46.7X3	T46.7X4	T46.7X5	T46.7X6
Naftifine	T49.0X1	T49.0X2	T49.0X3	T49.0X4	T49.0X5	T49.0X6
Nail polish remover	T52.91	T52.92	T52.93	T52.94	—	—
Nalbuphine	T40.4X1	T40.4X2	T40.4X3	T40.4X4	T40.4X5	T40.4X6
Naled	T60.0X1	T60.0X2	T60.0X3	T60.0X4	—	—
Nalidixic acid	T37.8X1	T37.8X2	T37.8X3	T37.8X4	T37.8X5	T37.8X6
Nalorphine	T50.7X1	T50.7X2	T50.7X3	T50.7X4	T50.7X5	T50.7X6
Naloxone	T50.7X1	T50.7X2	T50.7X3	T50.7X4	T50.7X5	T50.7X6
Naltrexone	T50.7X1	T50.7X2	T50.7X3	T50.7X4	T50.7X5	T50.7X6
Namenda	T43.8X1	T43.8X2	T43.8X3	T43.8X4	T43.8X5	T43.8X6
Nandrolone	T38.7X1	T38.7X2	T38.7X3	T38.7X4	T38.7X5	T38.7X6
Naphazoline	T48.5X1	T48.5X2	T48.5X3	T48.5X4	T48.5X5	T48.5X6
Naphtha (painters') (petroleum)	T52.0X1	T52.0X2	T52.0X3	T52.0X4	—	—
solvent	T52.0X1	T52.0X2	T52.0X3	T52.0X4	—	—
vapor	T52.0X1	T52.0X2	T52.0X3	T52.0X4	—	—
Naphthalene (non-chlorinated)	T60.2X1	T60.2X2	T60.2X3	T60.2X4	—	—
chlorinated	T60.1X1	T60.1X2	T60.1X3	T60.1X4	—	—
vapor	T60.1X1	T60.1X2	T60.1X3	T60.1X4	—	—
insecticide or moth repellent	T60.2X1	T60.2X2	T60.2X3	T60.2X4	—	—
chlorinated	T60.1X1	T60.1X2	T60.1X3	T60.1X4	—	—
vapor	T60.2X1	T60.2X2	T60.2X3	T60.2X4	—	—
chlorinated	T60.1X1	T60.1X2	T60.1X3	T60.1X4	—	—
Naphthol	T65.891	T65.892	T65.893	T65.894	—	—
Naphthylamine	T65.891	T65.892	T65.893	T65.894	—	—
Naphthylthiourea (ANTU)	T60.4X1	T60.4X2	T60.4X3	T60.4X4	—	—
Naprosyn — see Naproxen						
Naproxen	T39.311	T39.312	T39.313	T39.314	T39.315	T39.316

Substance	External Cause (T-Code)					
	Poisoning, Accidental (Unintentional)	Poisoning, Intentional Self-Harm	Poisoning, Assault	Poisoning, Undetermined	Adverse Effect	Underdosing
Narcotic (drug)	T40.601	T40.602	T40.603	T40.604	T40.605	T40.606
analgesic NEC	T40.601	T40.602	T40.603	T40.604	T40.605	T40.606
antagonist	T50.7X1	T50.7X2	T50.7X3	T50.7X4	T50.7X5	T50.7X6
specified NEC	T40.691	T40.692	T40.693	T40.694	T40.695	T40.696
synthetic	T40.4X1	T40.4X2	T40.4X3	T40.4X4	T40.4X5	T40.4X6
Narcotine	T48.3X1	T48.3X2	T48.3X3	T48.3X4	T48.3X5	T48.3X6
Nardil	T43.1X1	T43.1X2	T43.1X3	T43.1X4	T43.1X5	T43.1X6
Nasal drug NEC	T49.6X1	T49.6X2	T49.6X3	T49.6X4	T49.6X5	T49.6X6
Natamycin	T49.0X1	T49.0X2	T49.0X3	T49.0X4	T49.0X5	T49.0X6
Natrium cyanide — *see* Cyanide(s)						
Natural gas	T59.891	T59.892	T59.893	T59.894	—	—
incomplete combustion	T57.91	T57.92	T57.93	T57.94	—	—
Natural						
blood (product)	T45.8X1	T45.8X2	T45.8X3	T45.8X4	T45.8X5	T45.8X6
gas (piped)	T59.891	T59.892	T59.893	T59.894	—	—
incomplete combustion	T58.11	T58.12	T58.13	T58.14	—	—
Nealbarbital	T42.3X1	T42.3X2	T42.3X3	T42.3X4	T42.3X5	T42.3X6
Nectadon	T48.3X1	T48.3X2	T48.3X3	T48.3X4	T48.3X5	T48.3X6
Nedocromil	T48.6X1	T48.6X2	T48.6X3	T48.6X4	T48.6X5	T48.6X6
Nefopam	T39.8X1	T39.8X2	T39.8X3	T39.8X4	T39.8X5	T39.8X6
Nematocyst (sting)	T63.691	T63.692	T63.693	T63.694	—	—
Nembutal	T42.3X1	T42.3X2	T42.3X3	T42.3X4	T42.3X5	T42.3X6
Nemonapride	T43.591	T43.592	T43.593	T43.594	T43.595	T43.596
Neoarsphenamine	T37.8X1	T37.8X2	T37.8X3	T37.8X4	T37.8X5	T37.8X6
Neocinchophen	T50.4X1	T50.4X2	T50.4X3	T50.4X4	T50.4X5	T50.4X6
Neomycin (derivatives)	T36.5X1	T36.5X2	T36.5X3	T36.5X4	T36.5X5	T36.5X6
with						
bacitracin	T49.0X1	T49.0X2	T49.0X3	T49.0X4	T49.0X5	T49.0X6
neostigmine	T44.0X1	T44.0X2	T44.0X3	T44.0X4	T44.0X5	T44.0X6
ENT agent	T49.6X1	T49.6X2	T49.6X3	T49.6X4	T49.6X5	T49.6X6
ophthalmic preparation	T49.5X1	T49.5X2	T49.5X3	T49.5X4	T49.5X5	T49.5X6
topical NEC	T49.0X1	T49.0X2	T49.0X3	T49.0X4	T49.0X5	T49.0X6
Neonal	T42.3X1	T42.3X2	T42.3X3	T42.3X4	T42.3X5	T42.3X6
Neoprontosil	T37.0X1	T37.0X2	T37.0X3	T37.0X4	T37.0X5	T37.0X6
Neosalvarsan	T37.8X1	T37.8X2	T37.8X3	T37.8X4	T37.8X5	T37.8X6
Neosilversalvarsan	T37.8X1	T37.8X2	T37.8X3	T37.8X4	T37.8X5	T37.8X6
Neosporin	T36.8X1	T36.8X2	T36.8X3	T36.8X4	T36.8X5	T36.8X6
ENT agent	T49.6X1	T49.6X2	T49.6X3	T49.6X4	T49.6X5	T49.6X6
opthalmic preparation	T49.5X1	T49.5X2	T49.5X3	T49.5X4	T49.5X5	T49.5X6
topical NEC	T49.0X1	T49.0X2	T49.0X3	T49.0X4	T49.0X5	T49.0X6

◀ New ◀▥ Revised ~~deleted~~ Deleted

Substance	External Cause (T-Code)					
	Poisoning, Accidental (Unintentional)	Poisoning, Intentional Self-Harm	Poisoning, Assault	Poisoning, Undetermined	Adverse Effect	Underdosing
Neostigmine bromide	T44.0X1	T44.0X2	T44.0X3	T44.0X4	T44.0X5	T44.0X6
Neraval	T42.3X1	T42.3X2	T42.3X3	T42.3X4	T42.3X5	T42.3X6
Neravan	T42.3X1	T42.3X2	T42.3X3	T42.3X4	T42.3X5	T42.3X6
Nerium oleander	T62.2X1	T62.2X2	T62.2X3	T62.2X4	—	—
Nerve gas, not in war	T59.91	T59.92	T59.93	T59.94	—	—
Nesacaine	T41.3X1	T41.3X2	T41.3X3	T41.3X4	T41.3X5	T41.3X6
infiltration (subcutaneous)	T41.3X1	T41.3X2	T41.3X3	T41.3X4	T41.3X5	T41.3X6
nerve block (peripheral) (plexus)	T41.3X1	T41.3X2	T41.3X3	T41.3X4	T41.3X5	T41.3X6
Netilmicin	T36.5X1	T36.5X2	T36.5X3	T36.5X4	T36.5X5	T36.5X6
Neurobarb	T42.3X1	T42.3X2	T42.3X3	T42.3X4	T42.3X5	T42.3X6
Neuroleptic drug NEC	T43.501	T43.502	T43.503	T43.504	T43.505	T43.506
Neuromuscular blocking drug	T48.1X1	T48.1X2	T48.1X3	T48.1X4	T48.1X5	T48.1X6
Neutral insulin injection	T38.3X1	T38.3X2	T38.3X3	T38.3X4	T38.3X5	T38.3X6
Neutral spirits	T51.0X1	T51.0X2	T51.0X3	T51.0X4	—	—
beverage	T51.0X1	T51.0X2	T51.0X3	T51.0X4	—	—
Niacin	T46.7X1	T46.7X2	T46.7X3	T46.7X4	T46.7X5	T46.7X6
Niacinamide	T45.2X1	T45.2X2	T45.2X3	T45.2X4	T45.2X5	T45.2X6
Nialamide	T43.1X1	T43.1X2	T43.1X3	T43.1X4	T43.1X5	T43.1X6
Niaprazine	T42.6X1	T42.6X2	T42.6X3	T42.6X4	T42.6X5	T42.6X6
Nicametate	T46.7X1	T46.7X2	T46.7X3	T46.7X4	T46.7X5	T46.7X6
Nicardipine	T46.1X1	T46.1X2	T46.1X3	T46.1X4	T46.1X5	T46.1X6
Nicergoline	T46.7X1	T46.7X2	T46.7X3	T46.7X4	T46.7X5	T46.7X6
Nickel (carbonyl) (tetra-carbonyl) (fumes) (vapor)	T56.891	T56.892	T56.893	T56.894	—	—
Nickelocene	T56.891	T56.892	T56.893	T56.894	—	—
Niclosamide	T37.4X1	T37.4X2	T37.4X3	T37.4X4	T37.4X5	T37.4X6
Nicofuranose	T46.7X1	T46.7X2	T46.7X3	T46.7X4	T46.7X5	T46.7X6
Nicomorphine	T40.2X1	T40.2X2	T40.2X3	T40.2X4	—	—
Nicorandil	T46.3X1	T46.3X2	T46.3X3	T46.3X4	T46.3X5	T46.3X6
Nicotiana (plant)	T62.2X1	T62.2X2	T62.2X3	T62.2X4	—	—
Nicotinamide	T45.2X1	T45.2X2	T45.2X3	T45.2X4	T45.2X5	T45.2X6
Nicotine (insecticide) (spray) (sulfate) NEC	T60.2X1	T60.2X2	T60.2X3	T60.2X4	—	—
from tobacco	T65.291	T65.292	T65.293	T65.294	—	—
cigarettes	T65.221	T65.222	T65.223	T65.224	—	—
not insecticide	T65.291	T65.292	T65.293	T65.294	—	—
Nicotinic acid	T46.7X1	T46.7X2	T46.7X3	T46.7X4	T46.7X5	T46.7X6
Nicotinyl alcohol	T46.7X1	T46.7X2	T46.7X3	T46.7X4	T46.7X5	T46.7X6
Nicoumalone	T45.511	T45.512	T45.513	T45.514	T45.515	T45.516
Nifedipine	T46.1X1	T46.1X2	T46.1X3	T46.1X4	T46.1X5	T46.1X6
Nifenazone	T39.2X1	T39.2X2	T39.2X3	T39.2X4	T39.2X5	T39.2X6
Nifuraldezone	T37.91	T37.92	T37.93	T37.94	T37.95	T37.96

◀ New   ◀▥▥ Revised   ~~deleted~~ Deleted

Substance	Poisoning, Accidental (Unintentional)	Poisoning, Intentional Self-Harm	Poisoning, Assault	Poisoning, Undetermined	Adverse Effect	Underdosing
			External Cause (T-Code)			
Nifuratel	T37.8X1	T37.8X2	T37.8X3	T37.8X4	T37.8X5	T37.8X6
Nifurtimox	T37.3X1	T37.3X2	T37.3X3	T37.3X4	T37.3X5	T37.3X6
Nifurtoinol	T37.8X1	T37.8X2	T37.8X3	T37.8X4	T37.8X5	T37.8X6
Nightshade, deadly (solanum) — see also Belladonna	T62.2X1	T62.2X2	T62.2X3	T62.2X4	—	—
berry	T62.1X1	T62.1X2	T62.1X3	T62.1X4	—	—
Nikethamide	T50.7X1	T50.7X2	T50.7X3	T50.7X4	T50.7X5	T50.7X6
Nilstat	T36.7X1	T36.7X2	T36.7X3	T36.7X4	T36.7X5	T36.7X6
topical	T49.0X1	T49.0X2	T49.0X3	T49.0X4	T49.0X5	T49.0X6
Nilutamide	T38.6X1	T38.6X2	T38.6X3	T38.6X4	T38.6X5	T38.6X6
Nimesulide	T39.391	T39.392	T39.393	T39.394	T39.395	T39.396
Nimetazepam	T42.4X1	T42.4X2	T42.4X3	T42.4X4	T42.4X5	T42.4X6
Nimodipine	T46.1X1	T46.1X2	T46.1X3	T46.1X4	T46.1X5	T46.1X6
Nimorazole	T37.3X1	T37.3X2	T37.3X3	T37.3X4	T37.3X5	T37.3X6
Nimustine	T45.1X1	T45.1X2	T45.1X3	T45.1X4	T45.1X5	T45.1X6
Niridazole	T37.4X1	T37.4X2	T37.4X3	T37.4X4	T37.4X5	T37.4X6
Nisentil	T40.2X1	T40.2X2	T40.2X3	T40.2X4	T40.2X5	T40.2X6
Nisoldipine	T46.1X1	T46.1X2	T46.1X3	T46.1X4	T46.1X5	T46.1X6
Nitramine	T65.3X1	T65.3X2	T65.3X3	T65.3X4	—	—
Nitrate, organic	T46.3X1	T46.3X2	T46.3X3	T46.3X4	T46.3X5	T46.3X6
Nitrazepam	T42.4X1	T42.4X2	T42.4X3	T42.4X4	T42.4X5	T42.4X6
Nitrefazole	T50.6X1	T50.6X2	T50.6X3	T50.6X4	T50.6X5	T50.6X6
Nitrendipine	T46.1X1	T46.1X2	T46.1X3	T46.1X4	T46.1X5	T46.1X6
Nitric						
acid (liquid)	T54.2X1	T54.2X2	T54.2X3	T54.2X4	—	—
vapor	T59.891	T59.892	T59.893	T59.894	—	—
oxide (gas)	T59.0X1	T59.0X2	T59.0X3	T59.0X4	—	—
Nitrimidazine	T37.3X1	T37.3X2	T37.3X3	T37.3X4	T37.3X5	T37.3X6
Nitrite, amyl (medicinal) (vapor)	T46.3X1	T46.3X2	T46.3X3	T46.3X4	T46.3X5	T46.3X6
Nitroaniline	T65.3X1	T65.3X2	T65.3X3	T65.3X4	—	—
vapor	T59.891	T59.892	T59.893	T59.894	—	—
Nitrobenzene, nitrobenzol	T65.3X1	T65.3X2	T65.3X3	T65.3X4	—	—
vapor	T65.3X1	T65.3X2	T65.3X3	T65.3X4	—	—
Nitrocellulose	T65.891	T65.892	T65.893	T65.894	—	—
lacquer	T65.891	T65.892	T65.893	T65.894	—	—
Nitrodiphenyl	T65.3X1	T65.3X2	T65.3X3	T65.3X4	—	—
Nitrofural	T49.0X1	T49.0X2	T49.0X3	T49.0X4	T49.0X5	T49.0X6
Nitrofurantoin	T37.8X1	T37.8X2	T37.8X3	T37.8X4	T37.8X5	T37.8X6
Nitrofurazone	T49.0X1	T49.0X2	T49.0X3	T49.0X4	T49.0X5	T49.0X6
Nitrogen	T59.0X1	T59.0X2	T59.0X3	T59.0X4	—	—
mustard	T45.1X1	T45.1X2	T45.1X3	T45.1X4	T45.1X5	T45.1X6

◀ New   ◀▥ Revised   d̶e̶l̶e̶t̶e̶d̶ Deleted

Substance	External Cause (T-Code)					
	Poisoning, Accidental (Unintentional)	Poisoning, Intentional Self-Harm	Poisoning, Assault	Poisoning, Undetermined	Adverse Effect	Underdosing
Nitroglycerin, nitro-glycerol (medicinal)	T46.3X1	T46.3X2	T46.3X3	T46.3X4	T46.3X5	T46.3X6
nonmedicinal	T65.5X1	T65.5X2	T65.5X3	T65.5X4	—	—
fumes	T65.5X1	T65.5X2	T65.5X3	T65.5X4	—	—
Nitroglycol	T52.3X1	T52.3X2	T52.3X3	T52.3X4	—	—
Nitrohydrochloric acid	T54.2X1	T54.2X2	T54.2X3	T54.2X4	—	—
Nitromersol	T49.0X1	T49.0X2	T49.0X3	T49.0X4	T49.0X5	T49.0X6
Nitronaphthalene	T65.891	T65.892	T65.893	T65.894	—	—
Nitrophenol	T54.0X1	T54.0X2	T54.0X3	T54.0X4	—	—
Nitropropane	T52.8X1	T52.8X2	T52.8X3	T52.8X4	—	—
Nitroprusside	T46.5X1	T46.5X2	T46.5X3	T46.5X4	T46.5X5	T46.5X6
Nitrosodimethylamine	T65.3X1	T65.3X2	T65.3X3	T65.3X4	—	—
Nitrothiazol	T37.4X1	T37.4X2	T37.4X3	T37.4X4	T37.4X5	T37.4X6
Nitrotoluene, nitrotoluol	T65.3X1	T65.3X2	T65.3X3	T65.3X4	—	—
vapor	T65.3X1	T65.3X2	T65.3X3	T65.3X4	—	—
Nitrous						
acid (liquid)	T54.2X1	T54.2X2	T54.2X3	T54.2X4	—	—
fumes	T59.891	T59.892	T59.893	T59.894	—	—
ether spirit	T46.3X1	T46.3X2	T46.3X3	T46.3X4	T46.3X5	T46.3X6
oxide	T41.0X1	T41.0X2	T41.0X3	T41.0X4	T41.0X5	T41.0X6
Nitroxoline	T37.8X1	T37.8X2	T37.8X3	T37.8X4	T37.8X5	T37.8X6
Nitrozone	T49.0X1	T49.0X2	T49.0X3	T49.0X4	T49.0X5	T49.0X6
Nizatidine	T47.0X1	T47.0X2	T47.0X3	T47.0X4	T47.0X5	T47.0X6
Nizofenone	T43.8X1	T43.8X2	T43.8X3	T43.8X4	T43.8X5	T43.8X6
Noctec	T42.6X1	T42.6X2	T42.6X3	T42.6X4	T42.6X5	T42.6X6
Noludar	T42.6X1	T42.6X2	T42.6X3	T42.6X4	T42.6X5	T42.6X6
Noptil	T42.3X1	T42.3X2	T42.3X3	T42.3X4	T42.3X5	T42.3X6
Nomegestrol	T38.5X1	T38.5X2	T38.5X3	T38.5X4	T38.5X5	T38.5X6
Nomifensine	T43.291	T43.292	T43.293	T43.294	T43.295	T43.296
Nonoxinol	T49.8X1	T49.8X2	T49.8X3	T49.8X4	T49.8X5	T49.8X6
Nonylphenoxy (polyethoxy-ethanol)	T49.8X1	T49.8X2	T49.8X3	T49.8X4	T49.8X5	T49.8X6
Noptil	T42.3X1	T42.3X2	T42.3X3	T42.3X4	T42.3X5	T42.3X6
Noradrenaline	T44.4X1	T44.4X2	T44.4X3	T44.4X4	T44.4X5	T44.4X6
Noramidopyrine	T39.2X1	T39.2X2	T39.2X3	T39.2X4	T39.2X5	T39.2X6
methanesulfonate sodium	T39.2X1	T39.2X2	T39.2X3	T39.2X4	T39.2X5	T39.2X6
Norbormide	T60.4X1	T60.4X2	T60.4X3	T60.4X4	—	—
Nordazepam	T42.4X1	T42.4X2	T42.4X3	T42.4X4	T42.4X5	T42.4X6
Norepinephrine	T44.4X1	T44.4X2	T44.4X3	T44.4X4	T44.4X5	T44.4X6
Norethandrolone	T38.7X1	T38.7X2	T38.7X3	T38.7X4	T38.7X5	T38.7X6
Norethindrone	T38.4X1	T38.4X2	T38.4X3	T38.4X4	T38.4X5	T38.4X6

◀ New   ◀||| Revised   ~~deleted~~ Deleted

TABLE OF DRUGS AND CHEMICALS

Substance	External Cause (T-Code)					
	Poisoning, Accidental (Unintentional)	Poisoning, Intentional Self-Harm	Poisoning, Assault	Poisoning, Undetermined	Adverse Effect	Underdosing
Norethisterone (acetate) (enantate)	T38.4X1	T38.4X2	T38.4X3	T38.4X4	T38.4X5	T38.4X6
with ethinylestradiol	T38.5X1	T38.5X2	T38.5X3	T38.5X4	T38.5X5	T38.5X6
Noretynodrel	T38.5X1	T38.5X2	T38.5X3	T38.5X4	T38.5X5	T38.5X6
Norfenefrine	T44.4X1	T44.4X2	T44.4X3	T44.4X4	T44.4X5	T44.4X6
Norfloxacin	T36.8X1	T36.8X2	T36.8X3	T36.8X4	T36.8X5	T36.8X6
Norgestrel	T38.4X1	T38.4X2	T38.4X3	T38.4X4	T38.4X5	T38.4X6
Norgestrienone	T38.4X1	T38.4X2	T38.4X3	T38.4X4	T38.4X5	T38.4X6
Norlestrin	T38.4X1	T38.4X2	T38.4X3	T38.4X4	T38.4X5	T38.4X6
Norlutin	T38.4X1	T38.4X2	T38.4X3	T38.4X4	T38.4X5	T38.4X6
Normal serum albumin (human), salt-poor	T45.8X1	T45.8X2	T45.8X3	T45.8X4	T45.8X5	T45.8X6
Normethandrone	T38.5X1	T38.5X2	T38.5X3	T38.5X4	T38.5X5	T38.5X6
Normison—see Benzodiazepines						
Normorphine	T40.2X1	T40.2X2	T40.2X3	T40.2X4	—	—
Norpseudoephedrine	T50.5X1	T50.5X2	T50.5X3	T50.5X4	T50.5X5	T50.5X6
Nortestosterone (furanpropionate)	T38.7X1	T38.7X2	T38.7X3	T38.7X4	T38.7X5	T38.7X6
Nortriptyline	T43.011	T43.012	T43.013	T43.014	T43.015	T43.016
Noscapine	T48.3X1	T48.3X2	T48.3X3	T48.3X4	T48.3X5	T48.3X6
Nose preparations	T49.6X1	T49.6X2	T49.6X3	T49.6X4	T49.6X5	T49.6X6
Novobiocin	T36.5X1	T36.5X2	T36.5X3	T36.5X4	T36.5X5	T36.5X6
Novocain (infiltration) (topical)	T41.3X1	T41.3X2	T41.3X3	T41.3X4	T41.3X5	T41.3X6
nerve block (peripheral) (plexus)	T41.3X1	T41.3X2	T41.3X3	T41.3X4	I41.3X5	T41.3X6
spinal	T41.3X1	T41.3X2	T41.3X3	T41.3X4	T41.3X5	T41.3X6
Noxious foodstuff	T62.91	T62.92	T62.93	T62.94	—	—
specified NEC	T62.8X1	T62.8X2	T62.8X3	T62.8X4	—	—
Noxiptiline	T43.011	T43.012	T43.013	T43.014	T43.015	T43.016
Noxytiolin	T49.0X1	T49.0X2	T49.0X3	T49.0X4	T49.0X5	T49.0X6
NPH lletin (insulin)	T38.3X1	T38.3X2	T38.3X3	T38.3X4	T38.3X5	T38.3X6
Numorphan	T40.2X1	T40.2X2	T40.2X3	T40.2X4	T40.2X5	T40.2X6
Nunol	T42.3X1	T42.3X2	T42.3X3	T42.3X4	T42.3X5	T42.3X6
Nupercaine (spinal anesthetic)	T41.3X1	T41.3X2	T41.3X3	T41.3X4	T41.3X5	T41.3X6
topical (surface)	T41.3X1	T41.3X2	T41.3X3	T41.3X4	T41.3X5	T41.3X6
Nutmeg oil (liniment)	T49.3X1	T49.3X2	T49.3X3	T49.3X4	T49.3X5	T49.3X6
Nutritional supplement	T50.901	T50.902	T50.903	T50.904	T50.905	T50.906
Nux vomica	T65.1X1	T65.1X2	T65.1X3	T65.1X4	—	—
Nydrazid	T37.1X1	T37.1X2	T37.1X3	T37.1X4	T37.1X5	T37.1X6
Nylidrin	T46.7X1	T46.7X2	T46.7X3	T46.7X4	T46.7X5	T46.7X6
Nystatin	T36.7X1	T36.7X2	T36.7X3	T36.7X4	T36.7X5	T36.7X6
topical	T49.0X1	T49.0X2	T49.0X3	T49.0X4	T49.0X5	T49.0X6
Nytol	T45.0X1	T45.0X2	T45.0X3	T45.0X4	T45.0X5	T45.0X6

◀ New   ◀▥ Revised   ~~deleted~~ Deleted

Substance	External Cause (T-Code)					
	Poisoning, Accidental (Unintentional)	Poisoning, Intentional Self-Harm	Poisoning, Assault	Poisoning, Undetermined	Adverse Effect	Underdosing
O						
Obidoxime chloride	T50.6X1	T50.6X2	T50.6X3	T50.6X4	T50.6X5	T50.6X6
Octafonium (chloride)	T49.3X1	T49.3X2	T49.3X3	T49.3X4	T49.3X5	T49.3X6
Octamethyl pyrophos-phoramide	T60.0X1	T60.0X2	T60.0X3	T60.0X4	—	—
Octanoin	T50.991	T50.992	T50.993	T50.994	T50.995	T50.996
Octatropine methyl-bromide	T44.3X1	T44.3X2	T44.3X3	T44.3X4	T44.3X5	T44.3X6
Octotiamine	T45.2X1	T45.2X2	T45.2X3	T45.2X4	T45.2X5	T45.2X6
Octoxinol (9)	T49.8X1	T49.8X2	T49.8X3	T49.8X4	T49.8X5	T49.8X6
Octreotide	T38.991	T38.992	T38.993	T38.994	T38.995	T38.996
Octyl nitrite	T46.3X1	T46.3X2	T46.3X3	T46.3X4	T46.3X5	T46.3X6
Oestradiol	T38.5X1	T38.5X2	T38.5X3	T38.5X4	T38.5X5	T38.5X6
Oestriol	T38.5X1	T38.5X2	T38.5X3	T38.5X4	T38.5X5	T38.5X6
Oestrogen	T38.5X1	T38.5X2	T38.5X3	T38.5X4	T38.5X5	T38.5X6
Oestrone	T38.5X1	T38.5X2	T38.5X3	T38.5X4	T38.5X5	T38.5X6
Ofloxacin	T36.8X1	T36.8X2	T36.8X3	T36.8X4	T36.8X5	T36.8X6
Oil (of)	T65.891	T65.892	T65.893	T65.894	—	—
bitter almond	T62.8X1	T62.8X2	T62.8X3	T62.8X4	—	—
cloves	T49.7X1	T49.7X2	T49.7X3	T49.7X4	T49.7X5	T49.7X6
colors	T65.6X1	T65.6X2	T65.6X3	T65.6X4	—	—
fumes	T59.891	T59.892	T59.893	T59.894	—	—
lubricating	T52.0X1	T52.0X2	T52.0X3	T52.0X4	—	—
Niobe	T52.8X1	T52.8X2	T52.8X3	T52.8X4	—	—
vitriol (liquid)	T54.2X1	T54.2X2	T54.2X3	T54.2X4	—	—
fumes	T54.2X1	T54.2X2	T54.2X3	T54.2X4	—	—
wintergreen (bitter) NEC	T49.3X1	T49.3X2	T49.3X3	T49.3X4	T49.3X5	T49.3X6
Oily preparation (for skin)	T49.3X1	T49.3X2	T49.3X3	T49.3X4	T49.3X5	T49.3X6
Ointment NEC	T49.3X1	T49.3X2	T49.3X3	T49.3X4	T49.3X5	T49.3X6
Olanzapine	T43.591	T43.592	T43.593	T43.594	T43.595	T43.596
Oleander	T62.2X1	T62.2X2	T62.2X3	T62.2X4	—	—
Oleandomycin	T36.3X1	T36.3X2	T36.3X3	T36.3X4	T36.3X5	T36.3X6
Oleandrin	T46.0X1	T46.0X2	T46.0X3	T46.0X4	T46.0X5	T46.0X6
Oleic acid	T46.6X1	T46.6X2	T46.6X3	T46.6X4	T46.6X5	T46.6X6
Oleovitamin A	T45.2X1	T45.2X2	T45.2X3	T45.2X4	T45.2X5	T45.2X6
Oleum ricini	T47.2X1	T47.2X2	T47.2X3	T47.2X4	T47.2X5	T47.2X6
Olive oil (medicinal) NEC	T47.4X1	T47.4X2	T47.4X3	T47.4X4	T47.4X5	T47.4X6
Olivomycin	T45.1X1	T45.1X2	T45.1X3	T45.1X4	T45.1X5	T45.1X6
Olsalazine	T47.8X1	T47.8X2	T47.8X3	T47.8X4	T47.8X5	T47.8X6
Omeprazole	T47.1X1	T47.1X2	T47.1X3	T47.1X4	T47.1X5	T47.1X6

◀ New   ◀ Revised   ~~deleted~~ Deleted

Substance	Poisoning, Accidental (Unintentional)	Poisoning, Intentional Self-Harm	Poisoning, Assault	Poisoning, Undetermined	Adverse Effect	Underdosing
	External Cause (T-Code)					
OMPA	T60.0X1	T60.0X2	T60.0X3	T60.0X4	—	—
Ondansetron	T45.0X1	T45.0X2	T45.0X3	T45.0X4	T45.0X5	T45.0X6
Oncovin	T45.1X1	T45.1X2	T45.1X3	T45.1X4	T45.1X5	T45.1X6
Ophthaine	T41.3X1	T41.3X2	T41.3X3	T41.3X4	T41.3X5	T41.3X6
Ophthetic	T41.3X1	T41.3X2	T41.3X3	T41.3X4	T41.3X5	T41.3X6
Opiate NEC	T40.601	T40.602	T40.603	T40.604	T40.605	T40.606
antagonists	T50.7X1	T50.7X2	T50.7X3	T50.7X4	T50.7X5	T50.7X6
Opioid NEC	T40.2X1	T40.2X2	T40.2X3	T40.2X4	T40.2X5	T40.2X6
Opipramol	T43.011	T43.012	T43.013	T43.014	T43.015	T43.016
Opium alkaloids (total)	T40.0X1	T40.0X2	T40.0X3	T40.0X4	T40.0X5	T40.0X6
standardized powdered	T40.0X1	T40.0X2	T40.0X3	T40.0X4	T40.0X5	T40.0X6
tincture (camphorated)	T40.0X1	T40.0X2	T40.0X3	T40.0X4	T40.0X5	T40.0X6
Oracon	T38.4X1	T38.4X2	T38.4X3	T38.4X4	T38.4X5	T38.4X6
Oragrafin	T50.8X1	T50.8X2	T50.8X3	T50.8X4	T50.8X5	T50.8X6
Oral contraceptives	T38.4X1	T38.4X2	T38.4X3	T38.4X4	T38.4X5	T38.4X6
Oral rehydration salts	T50.3X1	T50.3X2	T50.3X3	T50.3X4	T50.3X5	T50.3X6
Orazamide	T50.991	T50.992	T50.993	T50.994	T50.995	T50.996
Orciprenaline	T48.291	T48.292	T48.293	T48.294	T48.295	T48.296
Organidin	T48.4X1	T48.4X2	T48.4X3	T48.4X4	T48.4X5	T48.4X6
Organonitrate NEC	T46.3X1	T46.3X2	T46.3X3	T46.3X4	T46.3X5	T46.3X6
Organophosphates	T60.0X1	T60.0X2	T60.0X3	T60.0X4	—	—
Orimune	T50.B91	T50.B92	T50.B93	T50.B94	T50.B95	T50.B96
Orinase	T38.3X1	T38.3X2	T38.3X3	T38.3X4	T38.3X5	T38.3X6
Ormeloxifene	T38.6X1	T38.6X2	T38.6X3	T38.6X4	T38.6X5	T38.6X6
Ornidazole	T37.3X1	T37.3X2	T37.3X3	T37.3X4	T37.3X5	T37.3X6
Ornithine aspartate	T50.991	T50.992	T50.993	T50.994	T50.995	T50.996
Ornoprostil	T47.1X1	T47.1X2	T47.1X3	T47.1X4	T47.1X5	T47.1X6
Orphenadrine (hydrochloride)	T42.8X1	T42.8X2	T42.8X3	T42.8X4	T42.8X5	T42.8X6
Ortal (sodium)	T42.3X1	T42.3X2	T42.3X3	T42.3X4	T42.3X5	T42.3X6
Orthoboric acid	T49.0X1	T49.0X2	T49.0X3	T49.0X4	T49.0X5	T49.0X6
ENT agent	T49.6X1	T49.6X2	T49.6X3	T49.6X4	T49.6X5	T49.6X6
ophthalmic preparation	T49.5X1	T49.5X2	T49.5X3	T49.5X4	T49.5X5	T49.5X6
Orthocaine	T41.3X1	T41.3X2	T41.3X3	T41.3X4	T41.3X5	T41.3X6
Orthodichlorobenzene	T53.7X1	T53.7X2	T53.7X3	T53.7X4	—	—
Ortho-Novum	T38.4X1	T38.4X2	T38.4X3	T38.4X4	T38.4X5	T38.4X6
Orthotolidine (reagent)	T54.2X1	T54.2X2	T54.2X3	T54.2X4	—	—
Osmic acid (liquid)	T54.2X1	T54.2X2	T54.2X3	T54.2X4	—	—
fumes	T54.2X1	T54.2X2	T54.2X3	T54.2X4	—	—
Osmotic diuretics	T50.2X1	T50.2X2	T50.2X3	T50.2X4	T50.2X5	T50.2X6
Otilonium bromide	T44.3X1	T44.3X2	T44.3X3	T44.3X4	T44.3X5	T44.3X6

◄ New   ◄ Revised   ~~deleted~~ Deleted

Substance	Poisoning, Accidental (Unintentional)	Poisoning, Intentional Self-Harm	Poisoning, Assault	Poisoning, Undetermined	Adverse Effect	Underdosing
Otorhinolaryngological drug NEC	T49.6X1	T49.6X2	T49.6X3	T49.6X4	T49.6X5	T49.6X6
Ouabain(e)	T46.0X1	T46.0X2	T46.0X3	T46.0X4	T46.0X5	T46.0X6
Ovarian						
hormone	T38.5X1	T38.5X2	T38.5X3	T38.5X4	T38.5X5	T38.5X6
stimulant	T38.5X1	T38.5X2	T38.5X3	T38.5X4	T38.5X5	T38.5X6
Ovral	T38.4X1	T38.4X2	T38.4X3	T38.4X4	T38.4X5	T38.4X6
Ovulen	T38.4X1	T38.4X2	T38.4X3	T38.4X4	T38.4X5	T38.4X6
Oxacillin	T36.0X1	T36.0X2	T36.0X3	T36.0X4	T36.0X5	T36.0X6
Oxalic acid	T54.2X1	T54.2X2	T54.2X3	T54.2X4	—	—
ammonium salt	T50.991	T50.992	T50.993	T50.994	T50.995	T50.996
Oxamniquine	T37.4X1	T37.4X2	T37.4X3	T37.4X4	T37.4X5	T37.4X6
Oxanamide	T43.591	T43.592	T43.593	T43.594	T43.595	T43.596
Oxandrolone	T38.7X1	T38.7X2	T38.7X3	T38.7X4	T38.7X5	T38.7X6
Oxantel	T37.4X1	T37.4X2	T37.4X3	T37.4X4	T37.4X5	T37.4X6
Oxapium iodide	T44.3X1	T44.3X2	T44.3X3	T44.3X4	T44.3X5	T44.3X6
Oxaprotiline	T43.021	T43.022	T43.023	T43.024	T43.025	T43.026
Oxaprozin	T39.311	T39.312	T39.313	T39.314	T39.315	T39.316
Oxatomide	T45.0X1	T45.0X2	T45.0X3	T45.0X4	T45.0X5	T45.0X6
Oxazepam	T42.4X1	T42.4X2	T42.4X3	T42.4X4	T42.4X5	T42.4X6
Oxazimedrine	T50.5X1	T50.5X2	T50.5X3	T50.5X4	T50.5X5	T50.5X6
Oxazolam	T42.4X1	T42.4X2	T42.4X3	T42.4X4	T42.4X5	T42.4X6
Oxazolidine derivatives	T42.2X1	T42.2X2	T42.2X3	T42.2X4	T42.2X5	T42.2X6
Oxazolidinedione (derivative)	T42.2X1	T42.2X2	T42.2X3	T42.2X4	T42.2X5	T42.2X6
Ox bile extract	T47.5X1	T47.5X2	T47.5X3	T47.5X4	T47.5X5	T47.5X6
Oxcarbazepine	T42.1X1	T42.1X2	T42.1X3	T42.1X4	T42.1X5	T42.1X6
Oxedrine	T44.4X1	T44.4X2	T44.4X3	T44.4X4	T44.4X5	T44.4X6
Oxeladin (citrate)	T48.3X1	T48.3X2	T48.3X3	T48.3X4	T48.3X5	T48.3X6
Oxendolone	T38.5X1	T38.5X2	T38.5X3	T38.5X4	T38.5X5	T38.5X6
Oxetacaine	T41.3X1	T41.3X2	T41.3X3	T41.3X4	T41.3X5	T41.3X6
Oxethazine	T41.3X1	T41.3X2	T41.3X3	T41.3X4	T41.3X5	T41.3X6
Oxetorone	T39.8X1	T39.8X2	T39.8X3	T39.8X4	T39.8X5	T39.8X6
Oxiconazole	T49.0X1	T49.0X2	T49.0X3	T49.0X4	T49.0X5	T49.0X6
Oxidizing agent NEC	T54.91	T54.92	T54.93	T54.94	—	—
Oxipurinol	T50.4X1	T50.4X2	T50.4X3	T50.4X4	T50.4X5	T50.4X6
Oxitriptan	T43.291	T43.292	T43.293	T43.294	T43.295	T43.296
Oxitropium bromide	T48.6X1	T48.6X2	T48.6X3	T48.6X4	T48.6X5	T48.6X6
Oxodipine	T46.1X1	T46.1X2	T46.1X3	T46.1X4	T46.1X5	T46.1X6
Oxolamine	T48.3X1	T48.3X2	T48.3X3	T48.3X4	T48.3X5	T48.3X6
Oxolinic acid	T37.8X1	T37.8X2	T37.8X3	T37.8X4	T37.8X5	T37.8X6
Oxomemazine	T43.3X1	T43.3X2	T43.3X3	T43.3X4	T43.3X5	T43.3X6

Substance	External Cause (T-Code)					
	Poisoning, Accidental (Unintentional)	Poisoning, Intentional Self-Harm	Poisoning, Assault	Poisoning, Undetermined	Adverse Effect	Underdosing
Oxophenarsine	T37.3X1	T37.3X2	T37.3X3	T37.3X4	T37.3X5	T37.3X6
Oxprenolol	T44.7X1	T44.7X2	T44.7X3	T44.7X4	T44.7X5	T44.7X6
Oxsoralen	T49.3X1	T49.3X2	T49.3X3	T49.3X4	T49.3X5	T49.3X6
Oxtriphylline	T48.6X1	T48.6X2	T48.6X3	T48.6X4	T48.6X5	T48.6X6
Oxybate sodium	T41.291	T41.292	T41.293	T41.294	T41.295	T41.296
Oxybuprocaine	T41.3X1	T41.3X2	T41.3X3	T41.3X4	T41.3X5	T41.3X6
Oxybutynin	T44.3X1	T44.3X2	T44.3X3	T44.3X4	T44.3X5	T44.3X6
Oxychlorosene	T49.0X1	T49.0X2	T49.0X3	T49.0X4	T49.0X5	T49.0X6
Oxycodone	T40.2X1	T40.2X2	T40.2X3	T40.2X4	T40.2X5	T40.2X6
Oxyfedrine	T46.3X1	T46.3X2	T46.3X3	T46.3X4	T46.3X5	T46.3X6
Oxygen	T41.5X1	T41.5X2	T41.5X3	T41.5X4	T41.5X5	T41.5X6
Oxylone	T49.0X1	T49.0X2	T49.0X3	T49.0X4	T49.0X5	T49.0X6
ophthalmic preparation	T49.5X1	T49.5X2	T49.5X3	T49.5X4	T49.5X5	T49.5X6
Oxymesterone	T38.7X1	T38.7X2	T38.7X3	T38.7X4	T38.7X5	T38.7X6
Oxymetazoline	T48.5X1	T48.5X2	T48.5X3	T48.5X4	T48.5X5	T48.5X6
Oxymetholone	T38.7X1	T38.7X2	T38.7X3	T38.7X4	T38.7X5	T38.7X6
Oxymorphone	T40.2X1	T40.2X2	T40.2X3	T40.2X4	T40.2X5	T40.2X6
Oxypertine	T43.591	T43.592	T43.593	T43.594	T43.595	T43.596
Oxyphenbutazone	T39.2X1	T39.2X2	T39.2X3	T39.2X4	T39.2X5	T39.2X6
Oxyphencyclimine	T44.3X1	T44.3X2	T44.3X3	T44.3X4	T44.3X5	T44.3X6
Oxyphenisatine	T47.2X1	T47.2X2	T47.2X3	T47.2X4	T47.2X5	T47.2X6
Oxyphenonium bromide	T44.3X1	T44.3X2	T44.3X3	T44.3X4	T44.3X5	T44.3X6
Oxypolygelatin	T45.8X1	T45.8X2	T45.8X3	T45.8X4	T45.8X5	T45.8X6
Oxyquinoline (derivatives)	T37.8X1	T37.8X2	T37.8X3	T37.8X4	T37.8X5	T37.8X6
Oxytetracycline	T36.4X1	T36.4X2	T36.4X3	T36.4X4	T36.4X5	T36.4X6
Oxytocic drug NEC	T48.0X1	T48.0X2	T48.0X3	T48.0X4	T48.0X5	T48.0X6
Oxytocin (synthetic)	T48.0X1	T48.0X2	T48.0X3	T48.0X4	T48.0X5	T48.0X6
Ozone	T59.891	T59.892	T59.893	T59.894	—	—
P						
PABA	T49.3X1	T49.3X2	T49.3X3	T49.3X4	T49.3X5	T49.3X6
Packed red cells	T45.8X1	T45.8X2	T45.8X3	T45.8X4	T45.8X5	T45.8X6
Padimate	T49.3X1	T49.3X2	T49.3X3	T49.3X4	T49.3X5	T49.3X6
Paint NEC	T65.6X1	T65.6X2	T65.6X3	T65.6X4	—	—
cleaner	T52.91	T52.92	T52.93	T52.94	—	—
fumes NEC	T59.891	T59.892	T59.893	T59.894	—	—
lead (fumes)	T56.0X1	T56.0X2	T56.0X3	T56.0X4	—	—
solvent NEC	T52.8X1	T52.8X2	T52.8X4	T52.8X4	—	—
stripper	T52.8X1	T52.8X2	T52.8X3	T52.8X4	—	—
Palfium	T40.2X1	T40.2X2	T40.2X3	T40.2X4	—	—

◀ New   ◀⫴ Revised   ~~deleted~~ Deleted

Substance	Poisoning, Accidental (Unintentional)	Poisoning, Intentional Self-Harm	Poisoning, Assault	Poisoning, Undetermined	Adverse Effect	Underdosing
	External Cause (T-Code)					
Palm kernel oil	T50.991	T50.992	T50.993	T50.994	T50.995	T50.996
Paludrine	T37.2X1	T37.2X2	T37.2X3	T37.2X4	T37.2X5	T37.2X6
PAM (pralidoxime)	T50.6X1	T50.6X2	T50.6X3	T50.6X4	T50.6X5	T50.6X6
Pamaquine (naphthoute)	T37.2X1	T37.2X2	T37.2X3	T37.2X4	T37.2X5	T37.2X6
Panadol	T39.1X1	T39.1X2	T39.1X3	T39.1X4	T39.1X5	T39.1X6
Pancreatic						
digestive secretion stimulant	T47.8X1	T47.8X2	T47.8X3	T47.8X4	T47.8X5	T47.8X6
dornase	T45.3X1	T45.3X2	T45.3X3	T45.3X4	T45.3X5	T45.3X6
Pancreatin	T47.5X1	T47.5X2	T47.5X3	T47.5X4	T47.5X5	T47.5X6
Pancrelipase	T47.5X1	T47.5X2	T47.5X3	T47.5X4	T47.5X5	T47.5X6
Pancuronium (bromide)	T48.1X1	T48.1X2	T48.1X3	T48.1X4	T48.1X5	T48.1X6
Pangamic acid	T45.2X1	T45.2X2	T45.2X3	T45.2X4	T45.2X5	T45.2X6
Panthenol	T45.2X1	T45.2X2	T45.2X3	T45.2X4	T45.2X5	T45.2X6
topical	T49.8X1	T49.8X2	T49.8X3	T49.8X4	T49.8X5	T49.8X6
Pantopon	T40.0X1	T40.0X2	T40.0X3	T40.0X4	T40.0X5	T40.0X6
Pantothenic acid	T45.2X1	T45.2X2	T45.2X3	T45.2X4	T45.2X5	T45.2X6
Panwarfin	T45.511	T45.512	T45.513	T45.514	T45.515	T45.516
Papain	T47.5X1	T47.5X2	T47.5X3	T47.5X4	T47.5X5	T47.5X6
digestant	T47.5X1	T47.5X2	T47.5X3	T47.5X4	T47.5X5	T47.5X6
Papaveretum	T40.0X1	T40.0X2	T40.0X3	T40.0X4	T40.0X5	T40.0X6
Papaverine	T44.3X1	T44.3X2	T44.3X3	T44.3X4	T44.3X5	T44.3X6
Para-acetamidophenol	T39.1X1	T39.1X2	T39.1X3	T39.1X4	T39.1X5	T39.1X6
Para-aminobenzoic acid	T49.3X1	T49.3X2	T49.3X3	T49.3X4	T49.3X5	T49.3X6
Para-aminophenol derivatives	T39.1X1	T39.1X2	T39.1X3	T39.1X4	T39.1X5	T39.1X6
Para-aminosalicylic acid	T37.1X1	T37.1X2	T37.1X3	T37.1X4	T37.1X5	T37.1X6
Paracetaldehyde	T42.6X1	T42.6X2	T42.6X3	T42.6X4	T42.6X5	T42.6X6
Paracetamol	T39.1X1	T39.1X2	T39.1X3	T39.1X4	T39.1X5	T39.1X6
Parachlorophenol (camphorated)	T49.0X1	T49.0X2	T49.0X3	T49.0X4	T49.0X5	T49.0X6
Paracodin	T40.2X1	T40.2X2	T40.2X3	T40.2X4	T40.2X5	T40.2X6
Paradione	T42.2X1	T42.2X2	T42.2X3	T42.2X4	T42.2X5	T42.2X6
Paraffin(s) (wax)	T52.0X1	T52.0X2	T52.0X3	T52.0X4	—	—
liquid (medicinal)	T47.4X1	T47.4X2	T47.4X3	T47.4X4	T47.4X5	T47.4X6
nonmedicinal	T52.0X1	T52.0X2	T52.0X3	T52.0X4	—	—
Paraformaldehyde	T60.3X1	T60.3X2	T60.3X3	T60.3X4	—	—
Paraldehyde	T42.6X1	T42.6X2	T42.6X3	T42.6X4	T42.6X5	T42.6X6
Paramethadione	T42.2X1	T42.2X2	T42.2X3	T42.2X4	T42.2X5	T42.2X6
Paramethasone	T38.0X1	T38.0X2	T38.0X3	T38.0X4	T38.0X5	T38.0X6
acetate	T49.0X1	T49.0X2	T49.0X3	T49.0X4	T49.0X5	T49.0X6
Paraoxon	T60.0X1	T60.0X2	T60.0X3	T60.0X4	—	—
Paraquat	T60.3X1	T60.3X2	T60.3X3	T60.3X4	—	—

◀ New   ◀ Revised   ~~deleted~~ Deleted

Substance	Poisoning, Accidental (Unintentional)	Poisoning, Intentional Self-Harm	Poisoning, Assault	Poisoning, Undetermined	Adverse Effect	Underdosing
Parasympatholytic NEC	T44.3X1	T44.3X2	T44.3X3	T44.3X4	T44.3X5	T44.3X6
Parasympathomimetic drug NEC	T44.1X1	T44.1X2	T44.1X3	T44.1X4	T44.1X5	T44.1X6
Parathion	T60.0X1	T60.0X2	T60.0X3	T60.0X4	—	—
Parathormone	T50.991	T50.992	T50.993	T50.994	T50.995	T50.996
Parathyroid extract	T50.991	T50.992	T50.993	T50.994	T50.995	T50.996
Paratyphoid vaccine	T50.A91	T50.A92	T50.A93	T50.A94	T50.A95	T50.A96
Paredrine	T44.4X1	T44.4X2	T44.4X3	T44.4X4	T44.4X5	T44.4X6
Paregoric	T40.0X1	T40.0X2	T40.0X3	T40.0X4	T40.0X5	T40.0X6
Pargyline	T46.5X1	T46.5X2	T46.5X3	T46.5X4	T46.5X5	T46.5X6
Paris green	T57.0X1	T57.0X2	T57.0X3	T57.0X4	—	—
insecticide	T57.0X1	T57.0X2	T57.0X3	T57.0X4	—	—
Parnate	T43.1X1	T43.1X2	T43.1X3	T43.1X4	T43.1X5	T43.1X6
Paromomycin	T36.5X1	T36.5X2	T36.5X3	T36.5X4	T36.5X5	T36.5X6
Paroxypropione	T45.1X1	T45.1X2	T45.1X3	T45.1X4	T45.1X5	T45.1X6
Parzone	T40.2X1	T40.2X2	T40.2X3	T40.2X4	T40.2X5	T40.2X6
PAS	T37.1X1	T37.1X2	T37.1X3	T37.1X4	T37.1X5	T37.1X6
Pasiniazid	T37.1X1	T37.1X2	T37.1X3	T37.1X4	T37.1X5	T37.1X6
PBB (polybrominated biphenyls)	T65.891	T65.892	T65.893	T65.894	—	—
PCB	T65.891	T65.892	T65.893	T65.894	—	—
PCP						
meaning pentachlorophenol	T60.1X1	T60.1X2	T60.1X3	T60.1X4	—	—
fungicide	T60.3X1	T60.3X2	T60.3X3	T60.3X4	—	—
herbicide	T60.3X1	T60.3X2	T60.3X3	T60.3X4	—	—
insecticide	T60.1X1	T60.1X2	T60.1X3	T60.1X4	—	—
meaning phencyclidine	T40.991	T40.992	T40.993	T40.994	—	—
Peach kernel oil (emulsion)	T47.4X1	T47.4X2	T47.4X3	T47.4X4	T47.4X5	T47.4X6
Peanut oil (emulsion) NEC	T47.4X1	T47.4X2	T47.4X3	T47.4X4	T47.4X5	T47.4X6
topical	T49.3X1	T49.3X2	T49.3X3	T49.3X4	T49.3X5	T49.3X6
Pearly Gates (morning glory seeds)	T40.991	T40.992	T40.993	T40.994	—	—
Pecazine	T43.3X1	T43.3X2	T43.3X3	T43.3X4	T43.3X5	T43.3X6
Pectin	T47.6X1	T47.6X2	T47.6X3	T47.6X4	T47.6X5	T47.6X6
Pefloxacin	T37.8X1	T37.8X2	T37.8X3	T37.8X4	T37.8X5	T37.8X6
Pegademase, bovine	T50.Z91	T50.Z92	T50.Z93	T50.Z94	T50.Z95	T50.Z96
Pelletierine tannate	T37.4X1	T37.4X2	T37.4X3	T37.4X4	T37.4X5	T37.4X6
Pemirolast (potassium)	T48.6X1	T48.6X2	T48.6X3	T48.6X4	T48.6X5	T48.6X6
Pemoline	T50.7X1	T50.7X2	T50.7X3	T50.7X4	T50.7X5	T50.7X6
Pempidine	T44.2X1	T44.2X2	T44.2X3	T44.2X4	T44.2X5	T44.2X6
Penamecillin	T36.0X1	T36.0X2	T36.0X3	T36.0X4	T36.0X5	T36.0X6
Penbutolol	T44.7X1	T44.7X2	T44.7X3	T44.7X4	T44.7X5	T44.7X6
Penethamate	T36.0X1	T36.0X2	T36.0X3	T36.0X4	T36.0X5	T36.0X6

◀ New ◀▦ Revised ~~deleted~~ Deleted

	External Cause (T-Code)					
Substance	**Poisoning, Accidental (Unintentional)**	**Poisoning, Intentional Self-Harm**	**Poisoning, Assault**	**Poisoning, Undetermined**	**Adverse Effect**	**Underdosing**
Penfluridol	T43.591	T43.592	T43.593	T43.594	T43.595	T43.596
Penflutizide	T50.2X1	T50.2X2	T50.2X3	T50.2X4	T50.2X5	T50.2X6
Pengitoxin	T46.0X1	T46.0X2	T46.0X3	T46.0X4	T46.0X5	T46.0X6
Penicillamine	T50.6X1	T50.6X2	T50.6X3	T50.6X4	T50.6X5	T50.6X6
Penicillin (any)	T36.0X1	T36.0X2	T36.0X3	T36.0X4	T36.0X5	T36.0X6
Penicillinase	T45.3X1	T45.3X2	T45.3X3	T45.3X4	T45.3X5	T45.3X6
Penicilloyl polylysine	T50.8X1	T50.8X2	T50.8X3	T50.8X4	T50.8X5	T50.8X6
Penimepicycline	T36.4X1	T36.4X2	T36.4X3	T36.4X4	T36.4X5	T36.4X6
Pentachloroethane	T53.6X1	T53.6X2	T53.6X3	T53.6X4	—	—
Pentachloronaphthalene	T53.7X1	T53.7X2	T53.7X3	T53.7X4	—	—
Pentachlorophenol (pesticide)	T60.1X1	T60.1X2	T60.1X3	T60.1X4	—	—
fungicide	T60.3X1	T60.3X2	T60.3X3	T60.3X4	—	—
herbicide	T60.3X1	T60.3X2	T60.3X3	T60.3X4	—	—
insecticide	T60.1X1	T60.1X2	T60.1X3	T60.1X4	—	—
Pentaerythritol tetranitrate	T46.3X1	T46.3X2	T46.3X3	T46.3X4	T46.3X5	T46.3X6
Pentaerythritol	T46.3X1	T46.3X2	T46.3X3	T46.3X4	T46.3X5	T46.3X6
chloral	T42.6X1	T42.6X2	T42.6X3	T42.6X4	T42.6X5	T42.6X6
tetranitrate NEC	T46.3X1	T46.3X2	T46.3X3	T46.3X4	T46.3X5	T46.3X6
Pentagastrin	T50.8X1	T50.8X2	T50.8X3	T50.8X4	T50.8X5	T50.8X6
Pentalin	T53.6X1	T53.6X2	T53.6X3	T53.6X4	—	—
Pentamethonium bromide	T44.2X1	T44.2X2	T44.2X3	T44.2X4	T44.2X5	T44.2X6
Pentamidine	T37.3X1	T37.3X2	T37.3X3	T37.3X4	T37.3X5	T37.3X6
Pentanol	T51.3X1	T51.3X2	T51.3X3	T51.3X4	—	—
Pentapyrrolinium (bitartrate)	T44.2X1	T44.2X2	T44.2X3	T44.2X4	T44.2X5	T44.2X6
Pentaquine	T37.2X1	T37.2X2	T37.2X3	T37.2X4	T37.2X5	T37.2X6
Pentazocine	T40.4X1	T40.4X2	T40.4X3	T40.4X4	T40.4X5	T40.4X6
Pentetrazole	T50.7X1	T50.7X2	T50.7X3	T50.7X4	T50.7X5	T50.7X6
Penthienate bromide	T44.3X1	T44.3X2	T44.3X3	T44.3X4	T44.3X5	T44.3X6
Pentifylline	T46.7X1	T46.7X2	T46.7X3	T46.7X4	T46.7X5	T46.7X6
Pentobarbital	T42.3X1	T42.3X2	T42.3X3	T42.3X4	T42.3X5	T42.3X6
sodium	T42.3X1	T42.3X2	T42.3X3	T42.3X4	T42.3X5	T42.3X6
Pentobarbitone	T42.3X1	T42.3X2	T42.3X3	T42.3X4	T42.3X5	T42.3X6
Pentolonium tartrate	T44.2X1	T44.2X2	T44.2X3	T44.2X4	T44.2X5	T44.2X6
Pentosan polysulfate (sodium)	T39.8X1	T39.8X2	T39.8X3	T39.8X4	T39.8X5	T39.8X6
Pentostatin	T45.1X1	T45.1X2	T45.1X3	T45.1X4	T45.1X5	T45.1X6
Pentothal	T41.1X1	T41.1X2	T41.1X3	T41.1X4	T41.1X5	T41.1X6
Pentoxifylline	T46.7X1	T46.7X2	T46.7X3	T46.7X4	T46.7X5	T46.7X6
Pentoxyverine	T48.3X1	T48.3X2	T48.3X3	T48.3X4	T48.3X5	T48.3X6
Pentrinat	T46.3X1	T46.3X2	T46.3X3	T46.3X4	T46.3X5	T46.3X6
Pentylenetetrazole	T50.7X1	T50.7X2	T50.7X3	T50.7X4	T50.7X5	T50.7X6

TABLE OF DRUGS AND CHEMICALS

◀ New   ◀▦ Revised   ~~deleted~~ Deleted

Substance	External Cause (T-Code)					
	Poisoning, Accidental (Unintentional)	Poisoning, Intentional Self-Harm	Poisoning, Assault	Poisoning, Undetermined	Adverse Effect	Underdosing
Pentylsalicylamide	T37.1X1	T37.1X2	T37.1X3	T37.1X4	T37.1X5	T37.1X6
Pentymal	T42.3X1	T42.3X2	T42.3X3	T42.3X4	T42.3X5	T42.3X6
Peplomycin	T45.1X1	T45.1X2	T45.1X3	T45.1X4	T45.1X5	T45.1X6
Peppermint (oil)	T47.5X1	T47.5X2	T47.5X3	T47.5X4	T47.5X5	T47.5X6
Pepsin	T47.5X1	T47.5X2	T47.5X3	T47.5X4	T47.5X5	T47.5X6
digestant	T47.5X1	T47.5X2	T47.5X3	T47.5X4	T47.5X5	T47.5X6
Pepstatin	T47.1X1	T47.1X2	T47.1X3	T47.1X4	T47.1X5	T47.1X6
Peptavlon	T50.8X1	T50.8X2	T50.8X3	T50.8X4	T50.8X5	T50.8X6
Perazine	T43.3X1	T43.3X2	T43.3X3	T43.3X4	T43.3X5	T43.3X6
Percaine (spinal)	T41.3X1	T41.3X2	T41.3X3	T41.3X4	T41.3X5	T41.3X6
topical (surface)	T41.3X1	T41.3X2	T41.3X3	T41.3X4	T41.3X5	T41.3X6
Perchloroethylene	T53.3X1	T53.3X2	T53.3X3	T53.3X4	—	—
medicinal	T37.4X1	T37.4X2	T37.4X3	T37.4X4	T37.4X5	T37.4X6
vapor	T53.3X1	T53.3X2	T53.3X3	T53.3X4	—	—
Percodan	T40.2X1	T40.2X2	T40.2X3	T40.2X4	T40.2X5	T40.2X6
Percogesic — see also acetaminophen	T45.0X1	T45.0X2	T45.0X3	T45.0X4	T45.0X5	T45.0X6
Percorten	T38.0X1	T38.0X2	T38.0X3	T38.0X4	T38.0X5	T38.0X6
Pergolide	T42.8X1	T42.8X2	T42.8X3	T42.8X4	T42.8X5	T42.8X6
Pergonal	T38.811	T38.812	T38.813	T38.814	T38.815	T38.816
Perhexilene	T46.3X1	T46.3X2	T46.3X3	T46.3X4	T46.3X5	T46.3X6
Perhexiline (maleate)	T46.3X1	T46.3X2	T46.3X3	T46.3X4	T46.3X5	T46.3X6
Periactin	T45.0X1	T45.0X2	T45.0X3	T45.0X4	T45.0X5	T45.0X6
Periciazine	T43.3X1	T43.3X2	T43.3X3	T43.3X4	T43.3X5	T43.3X6
Periclor	T42.6X1	T42.6X2	T42.6X3	T42.6X4	T42.6X5	T42.6X6
Perindopril	T46.4X1	T46.4X2	T46.4X3	T46.4X4	T46.4X5	T46.4X6
Perisoxal	T39.8X1	T39.8X2	T39.8X3	T39.8X4	T39.8X5	T39.8X6
Peritrate	T46.3X1	T46.3X2	T46.3X3	T46.3X4	T46.3X5	T46.3X6
Peritoneal dialysis solution	T50.3X1	T50.3X2	T50.3X3	T50.3X4	T50.3X5	T50.3X6
Perlapine	T42.4X1	T42.4X2	T42.4X3	T42.4X4	T42.4X5	T42.4X6
Permanganate	T65.891	T65.892	T65.893	T65.894	—	—
Permethrin	T60.1X1	T60.1X2	T60.1X3	T60.1X4	—	—
Pernocton	T42.3X1	T42.3X2	T42.3X3	T42.3X4	T42.3X5	T42.3X6
Pernoston	T42.3X1	T42.3X2	T42.3X3	T42.3X4	T42.3X5	T42.3X6
Peronine	T40.2X1	T40.2X2	T40.2X3	T40.2X4	—	—
Perphenazine	T43.3X1	T43.3X2	T43.3X3	T43.3X4	T43.3X5	T43.3X6
Pertofrane	T43.011	T43.012	T43.013	T43.014	T43.015	T43.016
Pertussis						
immune serum (human)	T50.Z11	T50.Z12	T50.Z13	T50.Z14	T50.Z15	T50.Z16
vaccine (with diphtheria toxoid) (with tetanus toxoid)	T50.A11	T50.A12	T50.A13	T50.A14	T50.A15	T50.A16
Peruvian balsam	T49.0X1	T49.0X2	T49.0X3	T49.0X4	T49.0X5	T49.0X6

◀ New   ◀‖‖ Revised   ~~deleted~~ Deleted

Substance	Poisoning, Accidental (Unintentional)	Poisoning, Intentional Self-Harm	Poisoning, Assault	Poisoning, Undetermined	Adverse Effect	Underdosing
Peruvoside	T46.0X1	T46.0X2	T46.0X3	T46.0X4	T46.0X5	T46.0X6
Pesticide (dust) (fumes) (vapor) NEC	T60.91	T60.92	T60.93	T60.94	—	—
arsenic	T57.0X1	T57.0X2	T57.0X3	T57.0X4	—	—
chlorinated	T60.1X1	T60.1X2	T60.1X3	T60.1X4	—	—
cyanide	T65.0X1	T65.0X2	T65.0X3	T65.0X4	—	—
kerosene	T52.0X1	T52.0X2	T52.0X3	T52.0X4	—	—
mixture (of compounds)	T60.91	T60.92	T60.93	T60.94	—	—
naphthalene	T60.2X1	T60.2X2	T60.2X3	T60.2X4	—	—
organochlorine (compounds)	T60.1X1	T60.1X2	T60.1X3	T60.1X4	—	—
petroleum (distillate) (products) NEC	T60.8X1	T60.8X2	T60.8X3	T60.8X4	—	—
specified ingredient NEC	T60.8X1	T60.8X2	T60.8X3	T60.8X4	—	—
strychnine	T65.1X1	T65.1X2	T65.1X3	T65.1X4	—	—
thallium	T60.4X1	T60.4X2	T60.4X3	T60.4X4	—	—
Pethidine	T40.4X1	T40.4X2	T40.4X3	T40.4X4	T40.4X5	T40.4X6
Petrichloral	T42.6X1	T42.6X2	T42.6X3	T42.6X4	T42.6X5	T42.6X6
Petrol	T52.0X1	T52.0X2	T52.0X3	T52.0X4	—	—
vapor	T52.0X1	T52.0X2	T52.0X3	T52.0X4	—	—
Petrolatum	T49.3X1	T49.3X2	T49.3X3	T49.3X4	T49.3X5	T49.3X6
hydrophilic	T49.3X1	T49.3X2	T49.3X3	T49.3X4	T49.3X5	T49.3X6
liquid	T47.4X1	T47.4X2	T47.4X3	T47.4X4	T47.4X5	T47.4X6
topical	T49.3X1	T49.3X2	T49.3X3	T49.3X4	T49.3X5	T49.3X6
nonmedicinal	T52.0X1	T52.0X2	T52.0X3	T52.0X4	—	—
red veterinary	T49.3X1	T49.3X2	T49.3X3	T49.3X4	T49.3X5	T49.3X6
white	T49.3X1	T49.3X2	T49.3X3	T49.3X4	T49.3X5	T49.3X6
Petroleum (products) NEC	T52.0X1	T52.0X2	T52.0X3	T52.0X4	—	—
benzine(s) — *see* Ligroin						
ether — *see* Ligroin						
jelly — *see* Petrolatum						
naphtha — *see* Ligroin						
pesticide	T60.8X1	T60.8X2	T60.8X3	T60.8X4	—	—
solids	T52.0X1	T52.0X2	T52.0X3	T52.0X4	—	—
solvents	T52.0X1	T52.0X2	T52.0X3	T52.0X4	—	—
vapor	T52.0X1	T52.0X2	T52.0X3	T52.0X4	—	—
Peyote	T40.991	T40.992	T40.993	T40.994	—	—
Phanodorm, phanodorn	T42.3X1	T42.3X2	T42.3X3	T42.3X4	T42.3X5	T42.3X6
Phanquinone	T37.3X1	T37.3X2	T37.3X3	T37.3X4	T37.3X5	T37.3X6
Phanquone	T37.3X1	T37.3X2	T37.3X3	T37.3X4	T37.3X5	T37.3X6
Pharmaceutical						
adjunct NEC	T50.901	T50.902	T50.903	T50.904	T50.905	T50.906
excipient NEC	T50.901	T50.902	T50.903	T50.904	T50.905	T50.906

Substance	External Cause (T-Code)					
	Poisoning, Accidental (Unintentional)	Poisoning, Intentional Self-Harm	Poisoning, Assault	Poisoning, Undetermined	Adverse Effect	Underdosing
Pharmaceutical *(Continued)*						
sweetener	T50.901	T50.902	T50.903	T50.904	T50.905	T50.906
viscous agent	T50.901	T50.902	T50.903	T50.904	T50.905	T50.906
Phemitone	T42.3X1	T42.3X2	T42.3X3	T42.3X4	T42.3X5	T42.3X6
Phenacaine	T41.3X1	T41.3X2	T41.3X3	T41.3X4	T41.3X5	T41.3X6
Phenacemide	T42.6X1	T42.6X2	T42.6X3	T42.6X4	T42.6X5	T42.6X6
Phenacetin	T39.1X1	T39.1X2	T39.1X3	T39.1X4	T39.1X5	T39.1X6
Phenadoxone	T40.2X1	T40.2X2	T40.2X3	T40.2X4	—	—
Phenaglycodol	T43.591	T43.592	T43.593	T43.594	T43.595	T43.596
Phenantoin	T42.0X1	T42.0X2	T42.0X3	T42.0X4	T42.0X5	T42.0X6
Phenaphthazine reagent	T50.991	T50.992	T50.993	T50.994	T50.995	T50.996
Phenazocine	T40.4X1	T40.4X2	T40.4X3	T40.4X4	T40.4X5	T40.4X6
Phenazone	T39.2X1	T39.2X2	T39.2X3	T39.2X4	T39.2X5	T39.2X6
Phenazopyridine	T39.8X1	T39.8X2	T39.8X3	T39.8X4	T39.8X5	T39.8X6
Phenbenicillin	T36.0X1	T36.0X2	T36.0X3	T36.0X4	T36.0X5	T36.0X6
Phenbutrazate	T50.5X1	T50.5X2	T50.5X3	T50.5X4	T50.5X5	T50.5X6
Phencyclidine	T40.991	T40.992	T40.993	T40.994	T40.995	T40.996
Phendimetrazine	T50.5X1	T50.5X2	T50.5X3	T50.5X4	T50.5X5	T50.5X6
Phenelzine	T43.1X1	T43.1X2	T43.1X3	T43.1X4	T43.1X5	T43.1X6
Phenemal	T42.3X1	T42.3X2	T42.3X3	T42.3X4	T42.3X5	T42.3X6
Phenergan	T42.6X1	T42.6X2	T42.6X3	T42.6X4	T42.6X5	T42.6X6
Pheneticillin	T36.0X1	T36.0X2	T36.0X3	T36.0X4	T36.0X5	T36.0X6
Pheneturide	T42.6X1	T42.6X2	T42.6X3	T42.6X4	T42.6X5	T42.6X6
Phenformin	T38.3X1	T38.3X2	T38.3X3	T38.3X4	T38.3X5	T38.3X6
Phenglutarimide	T44.3X1	T44.3X2	T44.3X3	T44.3X4	T44.3X5	T44.3X6
Phenicarbazide	T39.8X1	T39.8X2	T39.8X3	T39.8X4	T39.8X5	T39.8X6
Phenindamine	T45.0X1	T45.0X2	T45.0X3	T45.0X4	T45.0X5	T45.0X6
Phenindione	T45.511	T45.512	T45.513	T45.514	T45.515	T45.516
Pheniprazine	T43.1X1	T43.1X2	T43.1X3	T43.1X4	T43.1X5	T43.1X6
Pheniramine	T45.0X1	T45.0X2	T45.0X3	T45.0X4	T45.0X5	T45.0X6
Phenisatin	T47.2X1	T47.2X2	T47.2X3	T47.2X4	T47.2X5	T47.2X6
Phenmetrazine	T50.5X1	T50.5X2	T50.5X3	T50.5X4	T50.5X5	T50.5X6
Phenobal	T42.3X1	T42.3X2	T42.3X3	T42.3X4	T42.3X5	T42.3X6
Phenobarbital	T42.3X1	T42.3X2	T42.3X3	T42.3X4	T42.3X5	T42.3X6
with						
mephenytoin	T42.3X1	T42.3X2	T42.3X3	T42.3X4	T42.3X5	T42.3X6
phenytoin	T42.3X1	T42.3X2	T42.3X3	T42.3X4	T42.3X5	T42.3X6
sodium	T42.3X1	T42.3X2	T42.3X3	T42.3X4	T42.3X5	T42.3X6
Phenobarbitone	T42.3X1	T42.3X2	T42.3X3	T42.3X4	T42.3X5	T42.3X6

◀ New ◀░ Revised ~~deleted~~ Deleted

Substance	External Cause (T-Code)					
	Poisoning, Accidental (Unintentional)	Poisoning, Intentional Self-Harm	Poisoning, Assault	Poisoning, Undetermined	Adverse Effect	Underdosing
Phenobutiodil	T50.8X1	T50.8X2	T50.8X3	T50.8X4	T50.8X5	T50.8X6
Phenoctide	T49.0X1	T49.0X2	T49.0X3	T49.0X4	T49.0X5	T49.0X6
Phenol	T49.0X1	T49.0X2	T49.0X3	T49.0X4	T49.0X5	T49.0X6
disinfectant	T54.0X1	T54.0X2	T54.0X3	T54.0X4	—	—
in oil injection	T46.8X1	T46.8X2	T46.8X3	T46.8X4	T46.8X5	T46.8X6
medicinal	T49.1X1	T49.1X2	T49.1X3	T49.1X4	T49.1X5	T49.1X6
nonmedicinal NEC	T54.0X1	T54.0X2	T54.0X3	T54.0X4	—	—
pesticide	T60.8X1	T60.8X2	T60.8X3	T60.8X4	—	—
red	T50.8X1	T50.8X2	T50.8X3	T50.8X4	T50.8X5	T50.8X6
Phenolic preparation	T49.1X1	T49.1X2	T49.1X3	T49.1X4	T49.1X5	T49.1X6
Phenolphthalein	T47.2X1	T47.2X2	T47.2X3	T47.2X4	T47.2X5	T47.2X6
Phenolsulfonphthalein	T50.8X1	T50.8X2	T50.8X3	T50.8X4	T50.8X5	T50.8X6
Phenomorphan	T40.2X1	T40.2X2	T40.2X3	T40.2X4	—	—
Phenonyl	T42.3X1	T42.3X2	T42.3X3	T42.3X4	T42.3X5	T42.3X6
Phenoperidine	T40.4X1	T40.4X2	T40.4X3	T40.4X4	—	—
Phenopyrazone	T46.991	T46.992	T46.993	T46.994	T46.995	T46.996
Phenoquin	T50.4X1	T50.4X2	T50.4X3	T50.4X4	T50.4X5	T50.4X6
Phenothiazine (psychotropic) NEC	T43.3X1	T43.3X2	T43.3X3	T43.3X4	T43.3X5	T43.3X6
insecticide	T60.2X1	T60.2X2	T60.2X3	T60.2X4	—	—
Phenothrin	T49.0X1	T49.0X2	T49.0X3	T49.0X4	T49.0X5	T49.0X6
Phenoxybenzamine	T46.7X1	T46.7X2	T46.7X3	T46.7X4	T46.7X5	T46.7X6
Phenoxyethanol	T49.0X1	T49.0X2	T49.0X3	T49.0X4	T49.0X5	T49.0X6
Phenoxymethyl penicillin	T36.0X1	T36.0X2	T36.0X3	T36.0X4	T36.0X5	T36.0X6
Phenprobamate	T42.8X1	T42.8X2	T42.8X3	T42.8X4	T42.8X5	T42.8X6
Phenprocoumon	T45.511	T45.512	T45.513	T45.514	T45.515	T45.516
Phensuximide	T42.2X1	T42.2X2	T42.2X3	T42.2X4	T42.2X5	T42.2X6
Phentermine	T50.5X1	T50.5X2	T50.5X3	T50.5X4	T50.5X5	T50.5X6
Phenthicillin	T36.0X1	T36.0X2	T36.0X3	T36.0X4	T36.0X5	T36.0X6
Phentolamine	T46.7X1	T46.7X2	T46.7X3	T46.7X4	T46.7X5	T46.7X6
Phenyl						
butazone	T39.2X1	T39.2X2	T39.2X3	T39.2X4	T39.2X5	T39.2X6
enediamine	T65.3X1	T65.3X2	T65.3X3	T65.3X4	—	—
hydrazine	T65.3X1	T65.3X2	T65.3X3	T65.3X4	—	—
antineoplastic	T45.1X1	T45.1X2	T45.1X3	T45.1X4	T45.1X5	T45.1X6
mercuric compounds — see Mercury						
salicylate	T49.3X1	T49.3X2	T49.3X3	T49.3X4	T49.3X5	T49.3X6
Phenylalanine mustard	T45.1X1	T45.1X2	T45.1X3	T45.1X4	T45.1X5	T45.1X6
Phenylbutazone	T39.2X1	T39.2X2	T39.2X3	T39.2X4	T39.2X5	T39.2X6
Phenylenediamine	T65.3X1	T65.3X2	T65.3X3	T65.3X4	—	—

◀ New   ◀▥ Revised   ~~deleted~~ Deleted

TABLE OF DRUGS AND CHEMICALS

Substance	External Cause (T-Code)					
	Poisoning, Accidental (Unintentional)	Poisoning, Intentional Self-Harm	Poisoning, Assault	Poisoning, Undetermined	Adverse Effect	Underdosing
Phenylephrine	T44.4X1	T44.4X2	T44.4X3	T44.4X4	T44.4X5	T44.4X6
Phenylethylbiguanide	T38.3X1	T38.3X2	T38.3X3	T38.3X4	T38.3X5	T38.3X6
Phenylmercuric						
acetate	T49.0X1	T49.0X2	T49.0X3	T49.0X4	T49.0X5	T49.0X6
borate	T49.0X1	T49.0X2	T49.0X3	T49.0X4	T49.0X5	T49.0X6
nitrate	T49.0X1	T49.0X2	T49.0X3	T49.0X4	T49.0X5	T49.0X6
Phenylmethylbarbitone	T42.3X1	T42.3X2	T42.3X3	T42.3X4	T42.3X5	T42.3X6
Phenylpropanol	T47.5X1	T47.5X2	T47.5X3	T47.5X4	T47.5X5	T47.5X6
Phenylpropanolamine	T44.991	T44.992	T44.993	T44.994	T44.995	T44.996
Phenylsulfthion	T60.0X1	T60.0X2	T60.0X3	T60.0X4	—	—
Phenyltoloxamine	T45.0X1	T45.0X2	T45.0X3	T45.0X4	T45.0X5	T45.0X6
Phenyramidol, phenyramidon	T39.8X1	T39.8X2	T39.8X3	T39.8X4	T39.8X5	T39.8X6
Phenytoin	T42.0X1	T42.0X2	T42.0X3	T42.0X4	T42.0X5	T42.0X6
with Phenobarbital	T42.3X1	T42.3X2	T42.3X3	T42.3X4	T42.3X5	T42.3X6
pHisoHex	T49.2X1	T49.2X2	T49.2X3	T49.2X4	T49.2X5	T49.2X6
Pholcodine	T48.3X1	T48.3X2	T48.3X3	T48.3X4	T48.3X5	T48.3X6
Pholedrine	T46.991	T46.992	T46.993	T46.994	T46.995	T46.996
Phorate	T60.0X1	T60.0X2	T60.0X3	T60.0X4	—	—
Phosdrin	T60.0X1	T60.0X2	T60.0X3	T60.0X4	—	—
Phosfolan	T60.0X1	T60.0X2	T60.0X3	T60.0X4	—	—
Phosgene (gas)	T59.891	T59.892	T59.893	T59.894	—	—
Phosphamidon	T60.0X1	T60.0X2	T60.0X3	T60.0X4	—	—
Phosphate	T65.891	T65.892	T65.893	T65.894	—	—
laxative	T47.4X1	T47.4X2	T47.4X3	T47.4X4	T47.4X5	T47.4X6
organic	T60.0X1	T60.0X2	T60.0X3	T60.0X4	—	—
solvent	T52.91	T52.92	T52.93	T52.94	—	—
tricresyl	T65.891	T65.892	T65.893	T65.894	—	—
Phosphine	T57.1X1	T57.1X2	T57.1X3	T57.1X4	—	—
fumigant	T57.1X1	T57.1X2	T57.1X3	T57.1X4	—	—
Phospholine	T49.5X1	T49.5X2	T49.5X3	T49.5X4	T49.5X5	T49.5X6
Phosphoric acid	T54.2X1	T54.2X2	T54.2X3	T54.2X4	—	—
Phosphorus (compound) NEC	T57.1X1	T57.1X2	T57.1X3	T57.1X4	—	—
pesticide	T60.0X1	T60.0X2	T60.0X3	T60.0X4	—	—
Phthalates	T65.891	T65.892	T65.893	T65.894	—	—
Phthalic anhydride	T65.891	T65.892	T65.893	T65.894	—	—
Phthalimidoglutarimide	T42.6X1	T42.6X2	T42.6X3	T42.6X4	T42.6X5	T42.6X6
Phthalylsulfathiazole	T37.0X1	T37.0X2	T37.0X3	T37.0X4	T37.0X5	T37.0X6
Phylloquinone	T45.7X1	T45.7X2	T45.7X3	T45.7X4	T45.7X5	T45.7X6
Physeptone	T40.3X1	T40.3X2	T40.3X3	T40.3X4	T40.3X5	T40.3X6

◀ New   ◀💧 Revised   ~~deleted~~ Deleted

Substance	Poisoning, Accidental (Unintentional)	Poisoning, Intentional Self-Harm	Poisoning, Assault	Poisoning, Undetermined	Adverse Effect	Underdosing
			External Cause (T-Code)			
Physostigma venenosum	T62.2X1	T62.2X2	T62.2X3	T62.2X4	—	—
Physostigmine	T49.5X1	T49.5X2	T49.5X3	T49.5X4	T49.5X5	T49.5X6
Phytolacca decandra	T62.2X1	T62.2X2	T62.2X3	T62.2X4	—	—
berries	T62.1X1	T62.1X2	T62.1X3	T62.1X4	—	—
Phytomenadione	T45.7X1	T45.7X2	T45.7X3	T45.7X4	T45.7X5	T45.7X6
Phytonadione	T45.7X1	T45.7X2	T45.7X3	T45.7X4	T45.7X5	T45.7X6
Picoperine	T48.3X1	T48.3X2	T48.3X3	T48.3X4	T48.3X5	T48.3X6
Picosulfate (sodium)	T47.2X1	T47.2X2	T47.2X3	T47.2X4	T47.2X5	T47.2X6
Picric (acid)	T54.2X1	T54.2X2	T54.2X3	T54.2X4	—	—
Picrotoxin	T50.7X1	T50.7X2	T50.7X3	T50.7X4	T50.7X5	T50.7X6
Piketoprofen	T49.0X1	T49.0X2	T49.0X3	T49.0X4	T49.0X5	T49.0X6
Pilocarpine	T44.1X1	T44.1X2	T44.1X3	T44.1X4	T44.1X5	T44.1X6
Pilocarpus (jaborandi) extract	T44.1X1	T44.1X2	T44.1X3	T44.1X4	T44.1X5	T44.1X6
Pilsicainide (hydrochloride)	T46.2X1	T46.2X2	T46.2X3	T46.2X4	T46.2X5	T46.2X6
Pimaricin	T36.7X1	T36.7X2	T36.7X3	T36.7X4	T36.7X5	T36.7X6
Pimeclone	T50.7X1	T50.7X2	T50.7X3	T50.7X4	T50.7X5	T50.7X6
Pimelic ketone	T52.8X1	T52.8X2	T52.8X3	T52.8X4	—	—
Pimethixene	T45.0X1	T45.0X2	T45.0X3	T45.0X4	T45.0X5	T45.0X6
Piminodine	T40.2X1	T40.2X2	T40.2X3	T40.2X4	T40.2X5	T40.2X6
Pimozide	T43.591	T43.592	T43.593	T43.594	T43.595	T43.596
Pinacidil	T46.5X1	T46.5X2	T46.5X3	T46.5X4	T46.5X5	T46.5X6
Pinaverium bromide	T44.3X1	T44.3X2	T44.3X3	T44.3X4	T44.3X5	T44.3X6
Pinazepam	T42.4X1	T42.4X2	T42.4X3	T42.4X4	T42.4X5	T42.4X6
Pindolol	T44.7X1	T44.7X2	T44.7X3	T44.7X4	T44.7X5	T44.7X6
Pindone	T60.4X1	T60.4X2	T60.4X3	T60.4X4	—	—
Pine oil (disinfectant)	T65.891	T65.892	T65.893	T65.894	—	—
Pinkroot	T37.4X1	T37.4X2	T37.4X3	T37.4X4	T37.4X5	T37.4X6
Pipadone	T40.2X1	T40.2X2	T40.2X3	T40.2X4	—	—
Pipamazine	T45.0X1	T45.0X2	T45.0X3	T45.0X4	T45.0X5	T45.0X6
Pipamperone	T43.4X1	T43.4X2	T43.4X3	T43.4X4	T43.4X5	T43.4X6
Pipazetate	T48.3X1	T48.3X2	T48.3X3	T48.3X4	T48.3X5	T48.3X6
Pipemidic acid	T37.8X1	T37.8X2	T37.8X3	T37.8X4	T37.8X5	T37.8X6
Pipenzolate bromide	T44.3X1	T44.3X2	T44.3X3	T44.3X4	T44.3X5	T44.3X6
Piperacetazine	T43.3X1	T43.3X2	T43.3X3	T43.3X4	T43.3X5	T43.3X6
Piperacillin	T36.0X1	T36.0X2	T36.0X3	T36.0X4	T36.0X5	T36.0X6
Piperazine	T37.4X1	T37.4X2	T37.4X3	T37.4X4	T37.4X5	T37.4X6
estrone sulfate	T38.5X1	T38.5X2	T38.5X3	T38.5X4	T38.5X5	T38.5X6
Piper cubeba	T62.2X1	T62.2X2	T62.2X3	T62.2X4	—	—
Piperidione	T48.3X1	T48.3X2	T48.3X3	T48.3X4	—	—

◀ New ◀‖‖ Revised ~~deleted~~ Deleted

Substance	External Cause (T-Code)					
	Poisoning, Accidental (Unintentional)	Poisoning, Intentional Self-Harm	Poisoning, Assault	Poisoning, Undetermined	Adverse Effect	Underdosing
Piperidolate	T44.3X1	T44.3X2	T44.3X3	T44.3X4	T44.3X5	T44.3X6
Piperocaine	T41.3X1	T41.3X2	T41.3X3	T41.3X4	T41.3X5	T41.3X6
infiltration (subcutaneous)	T41.3X1	T41.3X2	T41.3X3	T41.3X4	T41.3X5	T41.3X6
nerve block (peripheral) (plexus)	T41.3X1	T41.3X2	T41.3X3	T41.3X4	T41.3X5	T41.3X6
topical (surface)	T41.3X1	T41.3X2	T41.3X3	T41.3X4	T41.3X5	T41.3X6
Piperonyl butoxide	T60.8X1	T60.8X2	T60.8X3	T60.8X4	—	—
Pipethanate	T44.3X1	T44.3X2	T44.3X3	T44.3X4	T44.3X5	T44.3X6
Pipobroman	T45.1X1	T45.1X2	T45.1X3	T45.1X4	T45.1X5	T45.1X6
Pipofezine	T43.0X1	T43.0X2	T43.0X3	T43.0X4	T43.0X5	T43.0X6
Pipotiazine	T43.3X1	T43.3X2	T43.3X3	T43.3X4	T43.3X5	T43.3X6
Pipoxizine	T45.0X1	T45.0X2	T45.0X3	T45.0X4	T45.0X5	T45.0X6
Pipradrol	T43.691	T43.692	T43.693	T43.694	T43.695	T43.696
Piprinhydrinate	T45.0X1	T45.0X2	T45.0X3	T45.0X4	T45.0X5	T45.0X6
Pirarubicin	T45.1X1	T45.1X2	T45.1X3	T45.1X4	T45.1X5	T45.1X6
Pirazinamide	T37.1X1	T37.1X2	T37.1X3	T37.1X4	T37.1X5	T37.1X6
Pirbuterol	T48.6X1	T48.6X2	T48.6X3	T48.6X4	T48.6X5	T48.6X6
Pirenzepine	T47.1X1	T47.1X2	T47.1X3	T47.1X4	T47.1X5	T47.1X6
Piretanide	T50.1X1	T50.1X2	T50.1X3	T50.1X4	T50.1X5	T50.1X6
Piribedil	T42.8X1	T42.8X2	T42.8X3	T42.8X4	T42.8X5	T42.8X6
Piridoxilate	T46.3X1	T46.3X2	T46.3X3	T46.3X4	T46.3X5	T46.3X6
Piritramide	T40.4X1	T40.4X2	T40.4X3	T40.4X4	—	—
Pirlindole	T43.0X1	T43.0X2	T43.0X3	T43.0X4	T43.0X5	T43.0X6
Piromidic acid	T37.8X1	T37.8X2	T37.8X3	T37.8X4	T37.8X5	T37.8X6
Piroxicam	T39.391	T39.392	T39.393	T39.394	T39.395	T39.396
beta-cyclodextrin complex	T39.8X1	T39.8X2	T39.8X3	T39.8X4	T39.8X5	T39.8X6
Pirozadil	T46.6X1	T46.6X2	T46.6X3	T46.6X4	T46.6X5	T46.6X6
Piscidia (bark) (erythrina)	T39.8X1	T39.8X2	T39.8X3	T39.8X4	T39.8X5	T39.8X6
Pitch	T65.891	T65.892	T65.893	T65.894	—	—
Pitkin's solution	T41.3X1	T41.3X2	T41.3X3	T41.3X4	T41.3X5	T41.3X6
Pitocin	T48.0X1	T48.0X2	T48.0X3	T48.0X4	T48.0X5	T48.0X6
Pitressin (tannate)	T38.891	T38.892	T38.893	T38.894	T38.895	T38.896
Pituitary extracts (posterior)	T38.891	T38.892	T38.893	T38.894	T38.895	T38.896
anterior	T38.811	T38.812	T38.813	T38.814	T38.815	T38.816
Pituitrin	T38.891	T38.892	T38.893	T38.894	T38.895	T38.896
Pivampicillin	T36.0X1	T36.0X2	T36.0X3	T36.0X4	T36.0X5	T36.0X6
Pivmecillinam	T36.0X1	T36.0X2	T36.0X3	T36.0X4	T36.0X5	T36.0X6
Placental hormone	T38.891	T38.892	T38.893	T38.894	T38.895	T38.896
Placidyl	T42.6X1	T42.6X2	T42.6X3	T42.6X4	T42.6X5	T42.6X6
Plague vaccine	T50.A91	T50.A92	T50.A93	T50.A94	T50.A95	T50.A96

◀ New   ◀▥ Revised   ~~deleted~~ Deleted

Substance	Poisoning, Accidental (Unintentional)	Poisoning, Intentional Self-Harm	Poisoning, Assault	Poisoning, Undetermined	Adverse Effect	Underdosing
External Cause (T-Code)						
Plant						
food or fertilizer NEC	T65.891	T65.892	T65.893	T65.894	—	—
containing herbicide	T60.3X1	T60.3X2	T60.3X3	T60.3X4	—	—
noxious, used as food	T62.2X1	T62.2X2	T62.2X3	T62.2X4	—	—
berries	T62.1X1	T62.1X2	T62.1X3	T62.1X4	—	—
seeds	T62.2X1	T62.2X2	T62.2X3	T62.2X4	—	—
specified type NEC	T62.2X1	T62.2X2	T62.2X3	T62.2X4	—	—
Plasma	T45.8X1	T45.8X2	T45.8X3	T45.8X4	T45.8X5	T45.8X6
expander NEC	T45.8X1	T45.8X2	T45.8X3	T45.8X4	T45.8X5	T45.8X6
protein fraction (human)	T45.8X1	T45.8X2	T45.8X3	T45.8X4	T45.8X5	T45.8X6
Plasmanate	T45.8X1	T45.8X2	T45.8X3	T45.8X4	T45.8X5	T45.8X6
Plasminogen (tissue) activator	T45.611	T45.612	T45.613	T45.614	T45.615	T45.616
Plaster dressing	T49.3X1	T49.3X2	T49.3X3	T49.3X4	T49.3X5	T49.3X6
Plastic dressing	T49.3X1	T49.3X2	T49.3X3	T49.3X4	T49.3X5	T49.3X6
Plegicil	T43.3X1	T43.3X2	T43.3X3	T43.3X4	T43.3X5	T43.3X6
Plicamycin	T45.1X1	T45.1X2	T45.1X3	T45.1X4	T45.1X5	T45.1X6
Podophyllotoxin	T49.8X1	T49.8X2	T49.8X3	T49.8X4	T49.8X5	T49.8X6
Podophyllum (resin)	T49.4X1	T49.4X2	T49.4X3	T49.4X4	T49.4X5	T49.4X6
Poison NEC	T65.91	T65.92	T65.93	T65.94	—	—
Poisonous berries	T62.1X1	T62.1X2	T62.1X3	T62.1X4	—	—
Pokeweed (any part)	T62.2X1	T62.2X2	T62.2X3	T62.2X4	—	—
Poldine metilsulfate	T44.3X1	T44.3X2	T44.3X3	T44.3X4	T44.3X5	T44.3X6
Polidexide (sulfate)	T46.6X1	T46.6X2	T46.6X3	T46.6X4	T46.6X5	T46.6X6
Polidocanol	T46.8X1	T46.8X2	T46.8X3	T46.8X4	T46.8X5	T46.8X6
Poliomyelitis vaccine	T50.B91	T50.B92	T50.B93	T50.B94	T50.B95	T50.B96
Polish (car) (floor) (furniture) (metal) (porcelain) (silver)	T65.891	T65.892	T65.893	T65.894	—	—
abrasive	T65.891	T65.892	T65.893	T65.894	—	—
porcelain	T65.891	T65.892	T65.893	T65.894	—	—
Poloxalkol	T47.4X1	T47.4X2	T47.4X3	T47.4X4	T47.4X5	T47.4X6
Poloxamer	T47.4X1	T47.4X2	T47.4X3	T47.4X4	T47.4X5	T47.4X6
Polyaminostyrene resins	T50.3X1	T50.3X2	T50.3X3	T50.3X4	T50.3X5	T50.3X6
Polycarbophil	T47.4X1	T47.4X2	T47.4X3	T47.4X4	T47.4X5	T47.4X6
Polychlorinated biphenyl	T65.891	T65.892	T65.893	T65.894	—	—
Polycycline	T36.4X1	T36.4X2	T36.4X3	T36.4X4	T36.4X5	T36.4X6
Polyester fumes	T59.891	T59.892	T59.893	T59.894	—	—
Polyester resin hardener	T52.91	T52.92	T52.93	T52.94	—	—
fumes	T59.891	T59.892	T59.893	T59.894	—	—
Polyestradiol phosphate	T38.5X1	T38.5X2	T38.5X3	T38.5X4	T38.5X5	T38.5X6
Polyethanolamine alkyl sulfate	T49.2X1	T49.2X2	T49.2X3	T49.2X4	T49.2X5	T49.2X6

◀ New   ◀▥ Revised   ~~deleted~~ Deleted

Substance	Poisoning, Accidental (Unintentional)	Poisoning, Intentional Self-Harm	Poisoning, Assault	Poisoning, Undetermined	Adverse Effect	Underdosing
			External Cause (T-Code)			
Polyethylene adhesive	T49.3X1	T49.3X2	T49.3X3	T49.3X4	T49.3X5	T49.3X6
Polyferose	T45.4X1	T45.4X2	T45.4X3	T45.4X4	T45.4X5	T45.4X6
Polygeline	T45.8X1	T45.8X2	T45.8X3	T45.8X4	T45.8X5	T45.8X6
Polymyxin	T36.8X1	T36.8X2	T36.8X3	T36.8X4	T36.8X5	T36.8X6
B	T36.8X1	T36.8X2	T36.8X3	T36.8X4	T36.8X5	T36.8X6
ENT agent	T49.6X1	T49.6X2	T49.6X3	T49.6X4	T49.6X5	T49.6X6
ophthalmic preparation	T49.5X1	T49.5X2	T49.5X3	T49.5X4	T49.5X5	T49.5X6
topical NEC	T49.0X1	T49.0X2	T49.0X3	T49.0X4	T49.0X5	T49.0X6
E sulfate (eye preparation)	T49.5X1	T49.5X2	T49.5X3	T49.5X4	T49.5X5	T49.5X6
Polynoxylin	T49.0X1	T49.0X2	T49.0X3	T49.0X4	T49.0X5	T49.0X6
Polyoestradiol phosphate	T38.5X1	T38.5X2	T38.5X3	T38.5X4	T38.5X5	T38.5X6
Polyoxymethyleneurea	T49.0X1	T49.0X2	T49.0X3	T49.0X4	T49.0X5	T49.0X6
Polysilane	T47.8X1	T47.8X2	T47.8X3	T47.8X4	T47.8X5	T47.8X6
Polytetrafluoroethylene (inhaled)	T59.891	T59.892	T59.893	T59.894	—	—
Polythiazide	T50.2X1	T50.2X2	T50.2X3	T50.2X4	T50.2X5	T50.2X6
Polyvidone	T45.8X1	T45.8X2	T45.8X3	T45.8X4	T45.8X5	T45.8X6
Polyvinylpyrrolidone	T45.8X1	T45.8X2	T45.8X3	T45.8X4	T45.8X5	T45.8X6
Pontocaine (hydrochloride) (infiltration) (topical)	T41.3X1	T41.3X2	T41.3X3	T41.3X4	T41.3X5	T41.3X6
nerve block (peripheral) (plexus)	T41.3X1	T41.3X2	T41.3X3	T41.3X4	T41.3X5	T41.3X6
spinal	T41.3X1	T41.3X2	T41.3X3	T41.3X4	T41.3X5	T41.3X6
Porfiromycin	T45.1X1	T45.1X2	T45.1X3	T45.1X4	T45.1X5	T45.1X6
Posterior pituitary hormone NEC	T38.891	T38.892	T38.893	T38.894	T38.895	T38.896
Pot	T40.7X1	T40.7X2	T40.7X3	T40.7X4	T40.7X5	T40.7X6
Potash (caustic)	T54.3X1	T54.3X2	T54.3X3	T54.3X4	—	—
Potassic saline injection (lactated)	T50.3X1	T50.3X2	T50.3X3	T50.3X4	T50.3X5	T50.3X6
Potassium (salts) NEC	T50.3X1	T50.3X2	T50.3X3	T50.3X4	T50.3X5	T50.3X6
aminobenzoate	T45.8X1	T45.8X2	T45.8X3	T45.8X4	T45.8X5	T45.8X6
aminosalicylate	T37.1X1	T37.1X2	T37.1X3	T37.1X4	T37.1X5	T37.1X6
antimony 'tartrate'	T37.8X1	T37.8X2	T37.8X3	T37.8X4	T37.8X5	T37.8X6
arsenite (solution)	T57.0X1	T57.0X2	T57.0X3	T57.0X4	—	—
bichromate	T56.2X1	T56.2X2	T56.2X3	T56.2X4	—	—
bisulfate	T47.3X1	T47.3X2	T47.3X3	T47.3X4	T47.3X5	T47.3X6
bromide	T42.6X1	T42.6X2	T42.6X3	T42.6X4	T42.6X5	T42.6X6
canrenoate	T50.0X1	T50.0X2	T50.0X3	T50.0X4	T50.0X5	T50.0X6
carbonate	T54.3X1	T54.3X2	T54.3X3	T54.3X4	—	—
chlorate NEC	T65.891	T65.892	T65.893	T65.894	—	—
chloride	T50.3X1	T50.3X2	T50.3X3	T50.3X4	T50.3X5	T50.3X6
citrate	T50.991	T50.992	T50.993	T50.994	T50.995	T50.996
cyanide	T65.0X1	T65.0X2	T65.0X3	T65.0X4		

◀ New ◀▥ Revised ~~deleted~~ Deleted

Substance	Poisoning, Accidental (Unintentional)	Poisoning, Intentional Self-Harm	Poisoning, Assault	Poisoning, Undetermined	Adverse Effect	Underdosing
Potassium NEC *(Continued)*						
ferric hexacyanoferrate (medicinal)	T50.6X1	T50.6X2	T50.6X3	T50.6X4	T50.6X5	T50.6X6
nonmedicinal	T65.891	T65.892	T65.893	T65.894	—	—
Fluoride	T57.8X1	T57.8X2	T57.8X3	T57.8X4	—	—
glucaldrate	T47.1X1	T47.1X2	T47.1X3	T47.1X4	T47.1X5	T47.1X6
hydroxide	T54.3X1	T54.3X2	T54.3X3	T54.3X4	—	—
iodate	T49.0X1	T49.0X2	T49.0X3	T49.0X4	T49.0X5	T49.0X6
iodide	T48.4X1	T48.4X2	T48.4X3	T48.4X4	T48.4X5	T48.4X6
nitrate	T57.8X1	T57.8X2	T57.8X3	T57.8X4	—	—
oxalate	T65.891	T65.892	T65.893	T65.894	—	—
perchlorate (nonmedicinal) NEC	T65.891	T65.892	T65.893	T65.894	—	—
antithyroid	T38.2X1	T38.2X2	T38.2X3	T38.2X4	T38.2X5	T38.2X6
medicinal	T38.2X1	T38.2X2	T38.2X3	T38.2X4	T38.2X5	T38.2X6
Permanganate (nonmedicinal)	T65.891	T65.892	T65.893	T65.894	—	—
medicinal	T49.0X1	T49.0X2	T49.0X3	T49.0X4	T49.0X5	T49.0X6
sulfate	T47.2X1	T47.2X2	T47.2X3	T47.2X4	T47.2X5	T47.2X6
Potassium-removing resin	T50.3X1	T50.3X2	T50.3X3	T50.3X4	T50.3X5	T50.3X6
Potassium-retaining drug	T50.3X1	T50.3X2	T50.3X3	T50.3X4	T50.3X5	T50.3X6
Povidone	T45.8X1	T45.8X2	T45.8X3	T45.8X4	T45.8X5	T45.8X6
iodine	T49.0X1	T49.0X2	T49.0X3	T49.0X4	T49.0X5	T49.0X6
Practolol	T44.7X1	T44.7X2	T44.7X3	T44.7X4	T44.7X5	T44.7X6
Prajmalium bitartrate	T46.2X1	T46.2X2	T46.2X3	T46.2X4	T46.2X5	T46.2X6
Pralidoxime (iodide)	T50.6X1	T50.6X2	T50.6X3	T50.6X4	T50.6X5	T50.6X6
chloride	T50.6X1	T50.6X2	T50.6X3	T50.6X4	T50.6X5	T50.6X6
Pramiverine	T44.3X1	T44.3X2	T44.3X3	T44.3X4	T44.3X5	T44.3X6
Pramocaine	T49.1X1	T49.1X2	T49.1X3	T49.1X4	T49.1X5	T49.1X6
Pramoxine	T49.1X1	T49.1X2	T49.1X3	T49.1X4	T49.1X5	T49.1X6
Prasterone	T38.7X1	T38.7X2	T38.7X3	T38.7X4	T38.7X5	T38.7X6
Pravastatin	T46.6X1	T46.6X2	T46.6X3	T46.6X4	T46.6X5	T46.6X6
Prazepam	T42.4X1	T42.4X2	T42.4X3	T42.4X4	T42.4X5	T42.4X6
Praziquantel	T37.4X1	T37.4X2	T37.4X3	T37.4X4	T37.4X5	T37.4X6
Prazitone	T43.291	T43.292	T43.293	T43.294	T43.295	T43.296
Prazosin	T44.6X1	T44.6X2	T44.6X3	T44.6X4	T44.6X5	T44.6X6
Prednicarbate	T49.0X1	T49.0X2	T49.0X3	T49.0X4	T49.0X5	T49.0X6
Prednimustine	T45.1X1	T45.1X2	T45.1X3	T45.1X4	T45.1X5	T45.1X6
Prednisolone	T38.0X1	T38.0X2	T38.0X3	T38.0X4	T38.0X5	T38.0X6
ENT agent	T49.6X1	T49.6X2	T49.6X3	T49.6X4	T49.6X5	T49.6X6
ophthalmic preparation	T49.5X1	T49.5X2	T49.5X3	T49.5X4	T49.5X5	T49.5X6
steaglate	T49.0X1	T49.0X2	T49.0X3	T49.0X4	T49.0X5	T49.0X6
topical NEC	T49.0X1	T49.0X2	T49.0X3	T49.0X4	T49.0X5	T49.0X6

Substance	External Cause (T-Code)					
	Poisoning, Accidental (Unintentional)	Poisoning, Intentional Self-Harm	Poisoning, Assault	Poisoning, Undetermined	Adverse Effect	Underdosing
Prednisone	T38.0X1	T38.0X2	T38.0X3	T38.0X4	T38.0X5	T38.0X6
Prednylidene	T38.0X1	T38.0X2	T38.0X3	T38.0X4	T38.0X5	T38.0X6
Pregnandiol	T38.5X1	T38.5X2	T38.5X3	T38.5X4	T38.5X5	T38.5X6
Pregneninolone	T38.5X1	T38.5X2	T38.5X3	T38.5X4	T38.5X5	T38.5X6
Preludin	T43.691	T43.692	T43.693	T43.694	T43.695	T43.696
Premarin	T38.5X1	T38.5X2	T38.5X3	T38.5X4	T38.5X5	T38.5X6
Premedication anesthetic	T41.201	T41.202	T41.203	T41.204	T41.205	T41.206
Prenalterol	T44.5X1	T44.5X2	T44.5X3	T44.5X4	T44.5X5	T44.5X6
Prenoxdiazine	T48.3X1	T48.3X2	T48.3X3	T48.3X4	T48.3X5	T48.3X6
Prenylamine	T46.3X1	T46.3X2	T46.3X3	T46.3X4	T46.3X5	T46.3X6
Preparation, local	T49.4X1	T49.4X2	T49.4X3	T49.4X4	T49.4X5	T49.4X6
Preparation H	T49.8X1	T49.8X2	T49.8X3	T49.8X4	T49.8X5	T49.8X6
Preservative (nonmedicinal)	T65.891	T65.892	T65.893	T65.894	—	—
medicinal	T50.901	T50.902	T50.903	T50.904	T50.905	T50.906
wood	T60.91	T60.92	T60.93	T60.94	—	—
Prethcamide	T50.7X1	T50.7X2	T50.7X3	T50.7X4	T50.7X5	T50.7X6
Pride of China	T62.2X1	T62.2X2	T62.2X3	T62.2X4	—	—
Pridinol	T44.3X1	T44.3X2	T44.3X3	T44.3X4	T44.3X5	T44.3X6
Prifinium bromide	T44.3X1	T44.3X2	T44.3X3	T44.3X4	T44.3X5	T44.3X6
Prilocaine	T41.3X1	T41.3X2	T41.3X3	T41.3X4	T41.3X5	T41.3X6
infiltration (subcutaneous)	T41.3X1	T41.3X2	T41.3X3	T41.3X4	T41.3X5	T41.3X6
nerve block (peripheral) (plexus)	T41.3X1	T41.3X2	T41.3X3	T41.3X4	T41.3X5	T41.3X6
regional	T41.3X1	T41.3X2	T41.3X3	T41.3X4	T41.3X5	T41.3X6
Primaquine	T37.2X1	T37.2X2	T37.2X3	T37.2X4	T37.2X5	T37.2X6
Primidone	T42.6X1	T42.6X2	T42.6X3	T42.6X4	T42.6X5	T42.6X6
Primula (veris)	T62.2X1	T62.2X2	T62.2X3	T62.2X4	—	—
Prinadol	T40.2X1	T40.2X2	T40.2X3	T40.2X4	T40.2X5	T40.2X6
Priscol, Priscoline	T44.6X1	T44.6X2	T44.6X3	T44.6X4	T44.6X5	T44.6X6
Pristinamycin	T36.3X1	T36.3X2	T36.3X3	T36.3X4	T36.3X5	T36.3X6
Privet	T62.2X1	T62.2X2	T62.2X3	T62.2X4	—	—
berries	T62.1X1	T62.1X2	T62.1X3	T62.1X4	—	—
Privine	T44.4X1	T44.4X2	T44.4X3	T44.4X4	T44.4X5	T44.4X6
Pro-Banthine	T44.3X1	T44.3X2	T44.3X3	T44.3X4	T44.3X5	T44.3X6
Probarbital	T42.3X1	T42.3X2	T42.3X3	T42.3X4	T42.3X5	T42.3X6
Probenecid	T50.4X1	T50.4X2	T50.4X3	T50.4X4	T50.4X5	T50.4X6
Probucol	T46.6X1	T46.6X2	T46.6X3	T46.6X4	T46.6X5	T46.6X6
Procainamide	T46.2X1	T46.2X2	T46.2X3	T46.2X4	T46.2X5	T46.2X6
Procaine	T41.3X1	T41.3X2	T41.3X3	T41.3X4	T41.3X5	T41.3X6
benzylpenicillin	T36.0X1	T36.0X2	T36.0X3	T36.0X4	T36.0X5	T36.0X6
nerve block (periphreal) (plexus)	T41.3X1	T41.3X2	T41.3X3	T41.3X4	T41.3X5	T41.3X6

◀ New   ◀▥ Revised   deleted Deleted

	External Cause (T-Code)					
Substance	Poisoning, Accidental (Unintentional)	Poisoning, Intentional Self-Harm	Poisoning, Assault	Poisoning, Undetermined	Adverse Effect	Underdosing
Procaine *(Continued)*						
penicillin G	T36.0X1	T36.0X2	T36.0X3	T36.0X4	T36.0X5	T36.0X6
regional	T41.3X1	T41.3X2	T41.3X3	T41.3X4	T41.3X5	T41.3X6
spinal	T41.3X1	T41.3X2	T41.3X3	T41.3X4	T41.3X5	T41.3X6
Procalmidol	T43.591	T43.592	T43.593	T43.594	T43.595	T43.596
Procarbazine	T45.1X1	T45.1X2	T45.1X3	T45.1X4	T45.1X5	T45.1X6
Procaterol	T44.5X1	T44.5X2	T44.5X3	T44.5X4	T44.5X5	T44.5X6
Prochlorperazine	T43.3X1	T43.3X2	T43.3X3	T43.3X4	T43.3X5	T43.3X6
Procyclidine	T44.3X1	T44.3X2	T44.3X3	T44.3X4	T44.3X5	T44.3X6
Producer gas	T58.8X1	T58.8X2	T58.8X3	T58.8X4	—	—
Profadol	T40.4X1	T40.4X2	T40.4X3	T40.4X4	T40.4X5	T40.4X6
Profenamine	T44.3X1	T44.3X2	T44.3X3	T44.3X4	T44.3X5	T44.3X6
Profenil	T44.3X1	T44.3X2	T44.3X3	T44.3X4	T44.3X5	T44.3X6
Proflavine	T49.0X1	T49.0X2	T49.0X3	T49.0X4	T49.0X5	T49.0X6
Progabide	T42.6X1	T42.6X2	T42.6X3	T42.6X4	T42.6X5	T42.6X6
Progestin	T38.5X1	T38.5X2	T38.5X3	T38.5X4	T38.5X5	T38.5X6
oral contraceptive	T38.4X1	T38.4X2	T38.4X3	T38.4X4	T38.4X5	T38.4X6
Progesterone	T38.5X1	T38.5X2	T38.5X3	T38.5X4	T38.5X5	T38.5X6
Progestogen NEC	T38.5X1	T38.5X2	T38.5X3	T38.5X4	T38.5X5	T38.5X6
Progestone	T38.5X1	T38.5X2	T38.5X3	T38.5X4	T38.5X5	T38.5X6
Proglumide	T47.1X1	T47.1X2	T47.1X3	T47.1X4	T47.1X5	T47.1X6
Proguanil	T37.2X1	T37.2X2	T37.2X3	T37.2X4	T37.2X5	T37.2X6
Prolactin	T38.811	T38.812	T38.813	T38.814	T38.815	T38.816
Prolintane	T43.691	T43.692	T43.693	T43.694	T43.695	T43.696
Proloid	T38.1X1	T38.1X2	T38.1X3	T38.1X4	T38.1X5	T38.1X6
Proluton	T38.5X1	T38.5X2	T38.5X3	T38.5X4	T38.5X5	T38.5X6
Promacetin	T37.1X1	T37.1X2	T37.1X3	T37.1X4	T37.1X5	T37.1X6
Promazine	T43.3X1	T43.3X2	T43.3X3	T43.3X4	T43.3X5	T43.3X6
Promedol	T40.2X1	T40.2X2	T40.2X3	T40.2X4	—	—
Promegestone	T38.5X1	T38.5X2	T38.5X3	T38.5X4	T38.5X5	T38.5X6
Promethazine (teoclate)	T43.3X1	T43.3X2	T43.3X3	T43.3X4	T43.3X5	T43.3X6
Promin	T37.1X1	T37.1X2	T37.1X3	T37.1X4	T37.1X5	T37.1X6
Pronase	T45.3X1	T45.3X2	T45.3X3	T45.3X4	T45.3X5	T45.3X6
Pronestyl (hydrochloride)	T46.2X1	T46.2X2	T46.2X3	T46.2X4	T46.2X5	T46.2X6
Pronetalol	T44.7X1	T44.7X2	T44.7X3	T44.7X4	T44.7X5	T44.7X6
Prontosil	T37.0X1	T37.0X2	T37.0X3	T37.0X4	T37.0X5	T37.0X6
Propachlor	T60.3X1	T60.3X2	T60.3X3	T60.3X4	—	—
Propafenone	T46.2X1	T46.2X2	T46.2X3	T46.2X4	T46.2X5	T46.2X6
Propallylonal	T42.3X1	T42.3X2	T42.3X3	T42.3X4	T42.3X5	T42.3X6
Propamidine	T49.0X1	T49.0X2	T49.0X3	T49.0X4	T49.0X5	T49.0X6

TABLE OF DRUGS AND CHEMICALS

TABLE OF DRUGS AND CHEMICALS

Substance	External Cause (T-Code)					
	Poisoning, Accidental (Unintentional)	Poisoning, Intentional Self-Harm	Poisoning, Assault	Poisoning, Undetermined	Adverse Effect	Underdosing
Propane (distributed in mobile container)	T59.891	T59.892	T59.893	T59.894	—	—
distributed through pipes	T59.891	T59.892	T59.893	T59.894	—	—
incomplete combustion	T57.11	T57.12	T57.13	T57.14	—	—
Propanidid	T41.291	T41.292	T41.293	T41.294	T41.295	T41.296
Propanil	T60.3X1	T60.3X2	T60.3X3	T60.3X4	—	—
1-Propanol	T51.3X1	T51.3X2	T51.3X3	T51.3X4	—	—
2-Propanol	T51.2X1	T51.2X2	T51.2X3	T51.2X4	—	—
Propantheline	T44.3X1	T44.3X2	T44.3X3	T44.3X4	T44.3X5	T44.3X6
bromide	T44.3X1	T44.3X2	T44.3X3	T44.3X4	T44.3X5	T44.3X6
Proparacaine	T41.3X1	T41.3X2	T41.3X3	T41.3X4	T41.3X5	T41.3X6
Propatylnitrate	T46.3X1	T46.3X2	T46.3X3	T46.3X4	T46.3X5	T46.3X6
Propicillin	T36.0X1	T36.0X2	T36.0X3	T36.0X4	T36.0X5	T36.0X6
Propiolactone	T49.0X1	T49.0X2	T49.0X3	T49.0X4	T49.0X5	T49.0X6
Propiomazine	T45.0X1	T45.0X2	T45.0X3	T45.0X4	T45.0X5	T45.0X6
Propionaidehyde (medicinal)	T42.6X1	T42.6X2	T42.6X3	T42.6X4	T42.6X5	T42.6X6
Propionate (calcium) (sodium)	T49.0X1	T49.0X2	T49.0X3	T49.0X4	T49.0X5	T49.0X6
Propion gel	T49.0X1	T49.0X2	T49.0X3	T49.0X4	T49.0X5	T49.0X6
Propitocaine	T41.3X1	T41.3X2	T41.3X3	T41.3X4	T41.3X5	T41.3X6
infiltration (subcutaneous)	T41.3X1	T41.3X2	T41.3X3	T41.3X4	T41.3X5	T41.3X6
nerve block (peripheral) (plexus)	T41.3X1	T41.3X2	T41.3X3	T41.3X4	T41.3X5	T41.3X6
Propofol	T41.291	T41.292	T41.293	T41.294	T41.295	T41.296
Propoxur	T60.0X1	T60.0X2	T60.0X3	T60.0X4	—	—
Propoxycaine	T41.3X1	T41.3X2	T41.3X3	T41.3X4	T41.3X5	T41.3X6
infiltration (subcutaneous)	T41.3X1	T41.3X2	T41.3X3	T41.3X4	T41.3X5	T41.3X6
nerve block (peripheral) (plexus)	T41.3X1	T41.3X2	T41.3X3	T41.3X4	T41.3X5	T41.3X6
topical (surface)	T41.3X1	T41.3X2	T41.3X3	T41.3X4	T41.3X5	T41.3X6
Propoxyphene	T40.4X1	T40.4X2	T40.4X3	T40.4X4	T40.4X5	T40.4X6
Propranolol	T44.7X1	T44.7X2	T44.7X3	T44.7X4	T44.7X5	T44.7X6
Propyl						
alcohol	T51.3X1	T51.3X2	T51.3X3	T51.3X4	—	—
carbinol	T51.3X1	T51.3X2	T51.3X3	T51.3X4	—	—
hexadrine	T44.4X1	T44.4X2	T44.4X3	T44.4X4	T44.4X5	T44.4X6
iodone	T50.8X1	T50.8X2	T50.8X3	T50.8X4	T50.8X5	T50.8X6
thiouracil	T38.2X1	T38.2X2	T38.2X3	T38.2X4	T38.2X5	T38.2X6
Propylaminophenothiazine	T43.3X1	T43.3X2	T43.3X3	T43.3X4	T43.3X5	T43.3X6
Propylene	T59.891	T59.892	T59.893	T59.894	—	—
Propylhexedrine	T48.5X1	T48.5X2	T48.5X3	T48.5X4	T48.5X5	T48.5X6
Propyliodone	T50.8X1	T50.8X2	T50.8X3	T50.8X4	T50.8X5	T50.8X6
Propylthiouracil	T38.2X1	T38.2X2	T38.2X3	T38.2X4	T38.2X5	T38.2X6
Propylparaben (ophthalmic)	T49.5X1	T49.5X2	T49.5X3	T49.5X4	T49.5X5	T49.5X6

◀ New ◀▥ Revised ~~deleted~~ Deleted

Substance	External Cause (T-Code)					
	Poisoning, Accidental (Unintentional)	Poisoning, Intentional Self-Harm	Poisoning, Assault	Poisoning, Undetermined	Adverse Effect	Underdosing
Propyphenazone	T39.2X1	T39.2X2	T39.2X3	T39.2X4	T39.2X5	T39.2X6
Proquazone	T39.391	T39.392	T39.393	T39.394	T39.395	T39.396
Proscillaridin	T46.0X1	T46.0X2	T46.0X3	T46.0X4	T46.0X5	T46.0X6
Prostacyclin	T45.521	T45.522	T45.523	T45.524	T45.525	T45.526
Prostaglandin (I2)	T45.521	T45.522	T45.523	T45.524	T45.525	T45.526
E1	T46.7X1	T46.7X2	T46.7X3	T46.7X4	T46.7X5	T46.7X6
E2	T48.0X1	T48.0X2	T48.0X3	T48.0X4	T48.0X5	T48.0X6
F2 alpha	T48.0X1	T48.0X2	T48.0X3	T48.0X4	T48.0X5	T48.0X6
Prostigmin	T44.0X1	T44.0X2	T44.0X3	T44.0X4	T44.0X5	T44.0X6
Prosultiamine	T45.2X1	T45.2X2	T45.2X3	T45.2X4	T45.2X5	T45.2X6
Protamine sulfate	T45.7X1	T45.7X2	T45.7X3	T45.7X4	T45.7X5	T45.7X6
zinc insulin	T38.3X1	T38.3X2	T38.3X3	T38.3X4	T38.3X5	T38.3X6
Protease	T47.5X1	T47.5X2	T47.5X3	T47.5X4	T47.5X5	T47.5X6
Protectant, skin NEC	T49.3X1	T49.3X2	T49.3X3	T49.3X4	T49.3X5	T49.3X6
Protein hydrolysate	T50.991	T50.992	T50.993	T50.994	T50.995	T50.996
Prothiaden — see Dothiepin hydrochloride						
Prothionamide	T37.1X1	T37.1X2	T37.1X3	T37.1X4	T37.1X5	T37.1X6
Prothipendyl	T43.591	T43.592	T43.593	T43.594	T43.595	T43.596
Prothoate	T60.0X1	T60.0X2	T60.0X3	T60.0X4	—	—
Prothrombin						
activator	T45.7X1	T45.7X2	T45.7X3	T45.7X4	T45.7X5	T45.7X6
synthesis inhibitor	T45.511	T45.512	T45.513	T45.514	T45.515	T45.516
Protionamide	T37.1X1	T37.1X2	T37.1X3	T37.1X4	T37.1X5	T37.1X6
Protirelin	T38.891	T38.892	T38.893	T38.894	T38.895	T38.896
Protokylol	T48.6X1	T48.6X2	T48.6X3	T48.6X4	T48.6X5	T48.6X6
Protopam	T50.6X1	T50.6X2	T50.6X3	T50.6X4	T50.6X5	T50.6X6
Protoveratrine(s) (A) (B)	T46.5X1	T46.5X2	T46.5X3	T46.5X4	T46.5X5	T46.5X6
Protriptyline	T43.011	T43.012	T43.013	T43.014	T43.015	T43.016
Provera	T38.5X1	T38.5X2	T38.5X3	T38.5X4	T38.5X5	T38.5X6
Provitamin A	T45.2X1	T45.2X2	T45.2X3	T45.2X4	T45.2X5	T45.2X6
Proxibarbal	T42.3X1	T42.3X2	T42.3X3	T42.3X4	T42.3X5	T42.3X6
Proxymetacaine	T41.3X1	T41.3X2	T41.3X3	T41.3X4	T41.3X5	T41.3X6
Proxyphylline	T48.6X1	T48.6X2	T48.6X3	T48.6X4	T48.6X5	T48.6X6
Prozac — see Fluoxetine hydrochloride						
Prunus						
laurocerasus	T62.2X1	T62.2X2	T62.2X3	T62.2X4	—	—
virginiana	T62.2X1	T62.2X2	T62.2X3	T62.2X4	—	—
Prussian blue						
commercial	T65.891	T65.892	T65.893	T65.894	—	—
therapeutic	T50.6X1	T50.6X2	T50.6X3	T50.6X4	T50.6X5	T50.6X6

◀ New ◀ Revised ~~deleted~~ Deleted

Substance	External Cause (T-Code)					
	Poisoning, Accidental (Unintentional)	Poisoning, Intentional Self-Harm	Poisoning, Assault	Poisoning, Undetermined	Adverse Effect	Underdosing
Prussic acid	T65.0X1	T65.0X2	T65.0X3	T65.0X4	—	—
vapor	T57.3X1	T57.3X2	T57.3X3	T57.3X4	—	—
Pseudoephedrine	T44.991	T44.992	T44.993	T44.994	T44.995	T44.996
Psilocin	T40.991	T40.992	T40.993	T40.994	—	—
Psilocybin	T40.991	T40.992	T40.993	T40.994	—	—
Psilocybine	T40.991	T40.992	T40.993	T40.994	—	—
Psoralene (nonmedicinal)	T65.891	T65.892	T65.893	T65.894	—	—
Psoralens (medicinal)	T50.991	T50.992	T50.993	T50.994	T50.995	T50.996
PSP (phenolsulfonphthalein)	T50.8X1	T50.8X2	T50.8X3	T50.8X4	T50.8X5	T50.8X6
Psychodysleptic drug NEC	T40.901	T40.902	T40.903	T40.904	T40.905	T40.906
Psychostimulant	T43.601	T43.602	T43.603	T43.604	T43.605	T43.606
amphetamine	T43.621	T43.622	T43.623	T43.624	T43.625	T43.626
caffeine	T43.611	T43.612	T43.613	T43.614	T43.615	T43.616
methylphenidate	T43.631	T43.632	T43.633	T43.634	T43.635	T43.636
specified NEC	T43.691	T43.692	T43.693	T43.694	T43.695	T43.696
Psychotherapeutic drug NEC	T43.91	T43.92	T43.93	T43.94	T43.95	T43.96
antidepressants — see also Antidepressant	T43.201	T43.202	T43.203	T43.204	T43.205	T43.206
specified NEC	T43.8X1	T43.8X2	T43.8X3	T43.8X4	T43.8X5	T43.8X6
tranquilizers NEC	T43.501	T43.502	T43.503	T43.504	T43.505	T43.506
Psychotomimetic agents	T40.901	T40.902	T40.903	T40.904	T40.905	T40.906
Psychotropic drug NEC	T43.91	T43.92	T43.93	T43.94	T43.95	T43.96
specified NEC	T43.8X1	T43.8X2	T43.8X3	T43.8X4	T43.8X5	T43.8X6
Psyllium hydrophilic mucilloid	T47.4X1	T47.4X2	T47.4X3	T47.4X4	T47.4X5	T47.4X6
Pteroylglutamic acid	T45.8X1	T45.8X2	T45.8X3	T45.8X4	T45.8X5	T45.8X6
Pteroyltriglutamate	T45.1X1	T45.1X2	T45.1X3	T45.1X4	T45.1X5	T45.1X6
PTFE — see Polytetrafluoroethylene						
Pulp						
devitalizing paste	T49.7X1	T49.7X2	T49.7X3	T49.7X4	T49.7X5	T49.7X6
dressing	T49.7X1	T49.7X2	T49.7X3	T49.7X4	T49.7X5	T49.7X6
Pulsatilla	T62.2X1	T62.2X2	T62.2X3	T62.2X4	—	—
Pumpkin seed extract	T37.4X1	T37.4X2	T37.4X3	T37.4X4	T37.4X5	T37.4X6
Purex (bleach)	T54.91	T54.92	T54.93	T54.94	—	—
Purgative NEC — see also Cathartic	T47.4X1	T47.4X2	T47.4X3	T47.4X4	T47.4X5	T47.4X6
Purine analogue (antineoplastic)	T45.1X1	T45.1X2	T45.1X3	T45.1X4	T45.1X5	T45.1X6
Purine diuretics	T50.2X1	T50.2X2	T50.2X3	T50.2X4	T50.2X5	T50.2X6
Purinethol	T45.1X1	T45.1X2	T45.1X3	T45.1X4	T45.1X5	T45.1X6
PVP	T45.8X1	T45.8X2	T45.8X3	T45.8X4	T45.8X5	T45.8X6
Pyrabital	T39.8X1	T39.8X2	T39.8X3	T39.8X4	T39.8X5	T39.8X6
Pyramidon	T39.2X1	T39.2X2	T39.2X3	T39.2X4	T39.2X5	T39.2X6
Pyrantel	T37.4X1	T37.4X2	T37.4X3	T37.4X4	T37.4X5	T37.4X6

◀ New ◀▥ Revised ~~deleted~~ Deleted

Substance	Poisoning, Accidental (Unintentional)	Poisoning, Intentional Self-Harm	Poisoning, Assault	Poisoning, Undetermined	Adverse Effect	Underdosing
	External Cause (T-Code)					
Pyrathiazine	T45.0X1	T45.0X2	T45.0X3	T45.0X4	T45.0X5	T45.0X6
Pyrazinamide	T37.1X1	T37.1X2	T37.1X3	T37.1X4	T37.1X5	T37.1X6
Pyrazinoic acid (amide)	T37.1X1	T37.1X2	T37.1X3	T37.1X4	T37.1X5	T37.1X6
Pyrazole (derivatives)	T39.2X1	T39.2X2	T39.2X3	T39.2X4	T39.2X5	T39.2X6
Pyrazolone analgesic NEC	T39.2X1	T39.2X2	T39.2X3	T39.2X4	T39.2X5	T39.2X6
Pyrethrin, pyrethrum (nonmedicinal)	T60.2X1	T60.2X2	T60.2X3	T60.2X4	—	—
Pyrethrum extract	T49.0X1	T49.0X2	T49.0X3	T49.0X4	T49.0X5	T49.0X6
Pyribenzamine	T45.0X1	T45.0X2	T45.0X3	T45.0X4	T45.0X5	T45.0X6
Pyridine	T52.8X1	T52.8X2	T52.8X3	T52.8X4	—	—
aldoxime methiodide	T50.6X1	T50.6X2	T50.6X3	T50.6X4	T50.6X5	T50.6X6
aldoxime methyl chloride	T50.6X1	T50.6X2	T50.6X3	T50.6X4	T50.6X5	T50.6X6
vapor	T59.891	T59.892	T59.893	T59.894	—	—
Pyridium	T39.8X1	T39.8X2	T39.8X3	T39.8X4	T39.8X5	T39.8X6
Pyridostigmine bromide	T44.0X1	T44.0X2	T44.0X3	T44.0X4	T44.0X5	T44.0X6
Pyridoxal phosphate	T45.2X1	T45.2X2	T45.2X3	T45.2X4	T45.2X5	T45.2X6
Pyridoxine	T45.2X1	T45.2X2	T45.2X3	T45.2X4	T45.2X5	T45.2X6
Pyrilamine	T45.0X1	T45.0X2	T45.0X3	T45.0X4	T45.0X5	T45.0X6
Pyrimethamine	T37.2X1	T37.2X2	T37.2X3	T37.2X4	T37.2X5	T37.2X6
with sulfadoxine	T37.2X1	T37.2X2	T37.2X3	T37.2X4	T37.2X5	T37.2X6
Pyrimidine antagonist	T45.1X1	T45.1X2	T45.1X3	T45.1X4	T45.1X5	T45.1X6
Pyriminil	T60.4X1	T60.4X2	T60.4X3	T60.4X4	—	—
Pyrithione zinc	T49.4X1	T49.4X2	T49.4X3	T49.4X4	T49.4X5	T49.4X6
Pyrithyldione	T42.6X1	T42.6X2	T42.6X3	T42.6X4	T42.6X5	T42.6X6
Pyrogallic acid	T49.0X1	T49.0X2	T49.0X3	T49.0X4	T49.0X5	T49.0X6
Pyrogallol	T49.0X1	T49.0X2	T49.0X3	T49.0X4	T49.0X5	T49.0X6
Pyroxylin	T49.3X1	T49.3X2	T49.3X3	T49.3X4	T49.3X5	T49.3X6
Pyrrobutamine	T45.0X1	T45.0X2	T45.0X3	T45.0X4	T45.0X5	T45.0X6
Pyrrolizidine alkaloids	T62.8X1	T62.8X2	T62.8X3	T62.8X4	—	—
Pyrvinium chloride	T37.4X1	T37.4X2	T37.4X3	T37.4X4	T37.4X5	T37.4X6
PZI	T38.3X1	T38.3X2	T38.3X3	T38.3X4	T38.3X5	T38.3X6
Q						
Quaalude	T42.6X1	T42.6X2	T42.6X3	T42.6X4	T42.6X5	T42.6X6
Quarternary ammonium						
anti-infective	T49.0X1	T49.0X2	T49.0X3	T49.0X4	T49.0X5	T49.0X6
ganglion blocking	T44.2X1	T44.2X2	T44.2X3	T44.2X4	T44.2X5	T44.2X6
parasympatholytic	T44.3X1	T44.3X2	T44.3X3	T44.3X4	T44.3X5	T44.3X6
Quazepam	T42.4X1	T42.4X2	T42.4X3	T42.4X4	T42.4X5	T42.4X6
Quicklime	T54.3X1	T54.3X2	T54.3X3	T54.3X4	—	—
Quillaja extract	T48.4X1	T48.4X2	T48.4X3	T48.4X4	T48.4X5	T48.4X6

Substance	External Cause (T-Code)					
	Poisoning, Accidental (Unintentional)	Poisoning, Intentional Self-Harm	Poisoning, Assault	Poisoning, Undetermined	Adverse Effect	Underdosing
Quinacrine	T37.2X1	T37.2X2	T37.2X3	T37.2X4	T37.2X5	T37.2X6
Quinaglute	T46.2X1	T46.2X2	T46.2X3	T46.2X4	T46.2X5	T46.2X6
Quinalbarbital	T42.3X1	T42.3X2	T42.3X3	T42.3X4	T42.3X5	T42.3X6
Quinalbarbitone sodium	T42.3X1	T42.3X2	T42.3X3	T42.3X4	T42.3X5	T42.3X6
Quinalphos	T60.0X1	T60.0X2	T60.0X3	T60.0X4	—	—
Quinapril	T46.4X1	T46.4X2	T46.4X3	T46.4X4	T46.4X5	T46.4X6
Quinestradiol	T38.5X1	T38.5X2	T38.5X3	T38.5X4	T38.5X5	T38.5X6
Quinestradol	T38.5X1	T38.5X2	T38.5X3	T38.5X4	T38.5X5	T38.5X6
Quinestrol	T38.5X1	T38.5X2	T38.5X3	T38.5X4	T38.5X5	T38.5X6
Quinethazone	T50.2X1	T50.2X2	T50.2X3	T50.2X4	T50.2X5	T50.2X6
Quingestanol	T38.4X1	T38.4X2	T38.4X3	T38.4X4	T38.4X5	T38.4X6
Quinidine	T46.2X1	T46.2X2	T46.2X3	T46.2X4	T46.2X5	T46.2X6
Quinine	T37.2X1	T37.2X2	T37.2X3	T37.2X4	T37.2X5	T37.2X6
Quiniobine	T37.8X1	T37.8X2	T37.8X3	T37.8X4	T37.8X5	T37.8X6
Quinisocaine	T49.1X1	T49.1X2	T49.1X3	T49.1X4	T49.1X5	T49.1X6
Quinocide	T37.2X1	T37.2X2	T37.2X3	T37.2X4	T37.2X5	T37.2X6
Quinoline (derivatives) NEC	T37.8X1	T37.8X2	T37.8X3	T37.8X4	T37.8X5	T37.8X6
Quinupramine	T43.011	T43.012	T43.013	T43.014	T43.015	T43.016
Quotane	T41.3X1	T41.3X2	T41.3X3	T41.3X4	T41.3X5	T41.3X6
R						
Rabies						
immune globulin (human)	T50.Z11	T50.Z12	T50.Z13	T50.Z14	T50.Z15	T50.Z16
vaccine	T50.B91	T50.B92	T50.B93	T50.B94	T50.B95	T50.B96
Racemoramide	T40.2X1	T40.2X2	T40.2X3	T40.2X4	—	—
Racemorphan	T40.2X1	T40.2X2	T40.2X3	T40.2X4	T40.2X5	T40.2X6
Racepinefrin	T44.5X1	T44.5X2	T44.5X3	T44.5X4	T44.5X5	T44.5X6
Raclopride	T43.591	T43.592	T43.593	T43.594	T43.595	T43.596
Radiator alcohol	T51.1X1	T51.1X2	T51.1X3	T51.1X4	—	—
Radioactive drug NEC	T50.8X1	T50.8X2	T50.8X3	T50.8X4	T50.8X5	T50.8X6
Radio-opaque (drugs) (materials)	T50.8X1	T50.8X2	T50.8X3	T50.8X4	T50.8X5	T50.8X6
Ramifenazone	T39.2X1	T39.2X2	T39.2X3	T39.2X4	T39.2X5	T39.2X6
Ramipril	T46.4X1	T46.4X2	T46.4X3	T46.4X4	T46.4X5	T46.4X6
Ranitidine	T47.0X1	T47.0X2	T47.0X3	T47.0X4	T47.0X5	T47.0X6
Ranunculus	T62.2X1	T62.2X2	T62.2X3	T62.2X4	—	—
Rat poison NEC	T60.4X1	T60.4X2	T60.4X3	T60.4X4	—	—
Rattlesnake (venom)	T63.011	T63.012	T63.013	T63.014	—	—
Raubasine	T46.7X1	T46.7X2	T46.7X3	T46.7X4	T46.7X5	T46.7X6
Raudixin	T46.5X1	T46.5X2	T46.5X3	T46.5X4	T46.5X5	T46.5X6
Rautensin	T46.5X1	T46.5X2	T46.5X3	T46.5X4	T46.5X5	T46.5X6

◀ New   ◀ Revised   ~~deleted~~ Deleted

Substance	External Cause (T-Code)					
	Poisoning, Accidental (Unintentional)	Poisoning, Intentional Self-Harm	Poisoning, Assault	Poisoning, Undetermined	Adverse Effect	Underdosing
Rautina	T46.5X1	T46.5X2	T46.5X3	T46.5X4	T46.5X5	T46.5X6
Rautotal	T46.5X1	T46.5X2	T46.5X3	T46.5X4	T46.5X5	T46.5X6
Rauwiloid	T46.5X1	T46.5X2	T46.5X3	T46.5X4	T46.5X5	T46.5X6
Rauwoldin	T46.5X1	T46.5X2	T46.5X3	T46.5X4	T46.5X5	T46.5X6
Rauwolfia (alkaloids)	T46.5X1	T46.5X2	T46.5X3	T46.5X4	T46.5X5	T46.5X6
Razoxane	T45.1X1	T45.1X2	T45.1X3	T45.1X4	T45.1X5	T45.1X6
Realgar	T57.0X1	T57.0X2	T57.0X3	T57.0X4	—	—
Recombinant (R) — *see specific protein*						
Red blood cells, packed	T45.8X1	T45.8X2	T45.8X3	T45.8X4	T45.8X5	T45.8X6
Red squill (scilliroside)	T60.4X1	T60.4X2	T60.4X3	T60.4X4	—	—
Reducing agent, industrial NEC	T65.891	T65.892	T65.893	T65.894	—	—
Refrigerant gas (chlorofluoro-carbon)	T53.5X1	T53.5X2	T53.5X3	T53.5X4	—	—
not chlorofluoro-carbon	T59.891	T59.892	T59.893	T59.894	—	—
Regroton	T50.2X1	T50.2X2	T50.2X3	T50.2X4	T50.2X5	T50.2X6
Rehydration salts (oral)	T50.3X1	T50.3X2	T50.3X3	T50.3X4	T50.3X5	T50.3X6
Rela	T42.8X1	T42.8X2	T42.8X3	T42.8X4	T42.8X5	T42.8X6
Relaxant, muscle						
anesthetic	T48.1X1	T48.1X2	T48.1X3	T48.1X4	T48.1X5	T48.1X6
central nervous system	T42.8X1	T42.8X2	T42.8X3	T42.8X4	T42.8X5	T42.8X6
skeletal NEC	T48.1X1	T48.1X2	T48.1X3	T48.1X4	T48.1X5	T48.1X6
smooth NEC	T44.3X1	T44.3X2	T44.3X3	T44.3X4	T44.3X5	T44.3X6
Remoxipride	T43.591	T43.592	T43.593	T43.594	T43.595	T43.596
Renese	T50.2X1	T50.2X2	T50.2X3	T50.2X4	T50.2X5	T50.2X6
Renografin	T50.8X1	T50.8X2	T50.8X3	T50.8X4	T50.8X5	T50.8X6
Replacement solution	T50.3X1	T50.3X2	T50.3X3	T50.3X4	T50.3X5	T50.3X6
Reproterol	T48.6X1	T48.6X2	T48.6X3	T48.6X4	T48.6X5	T48.6X6
Rescinnamine	T46.5X1	T46.5X2	T46.5X3	T46.5X4	T46.5X5	T46.5X6
Reserpin(e)	T46.5X1	T46.5X2	T46.5X3	T46.5X4	T46.5X5	T46.5X6
Resorcin, resorcinol (nonmedicinal)	T65.891	T65.892	T65.893	T65.894	—	—
medicinal	T49.4X1	T49.4X2	T49.4X3	T49.4X4	T49.4X5	T49.4X6
Respaire	T48.4X1	T48.4X2	T48.4X3	T48.4X4	T48.4X5	T48.4X6
Respiratory drug NEC	T48.901	T48.902	T48.903	T48.904	T48.905	T48.906
antiasthmatic NEC	T48.6X1	T48.6X2	T48.6X3	T48.6X4	T48.6X5	T48.6X6
anti-common-cold NEC	T48.5X1	T48.5X2	T48.5X3	T48.5X4	T48.5X5	T48.5X6
expectorant NEC	T48.4X1	T48.4X2	T48.4X3	T48.4X4	T48.4X5	T48.4X6
stimulant	T48.901	T48.902	T48.903	T48.904	T48.905	T48.906
Retinoic acid	T49.0X1	T49.0X2	T49.0X3	T49.0X4	T49.0X5	T49.0X6
Retinol	T45.2X1	T45.2X2	T45.2X3	T45.2X4	T45.2X5	T45.2X6
Rh (D) immune globulin (human)	T50.Z11	T50.Z12	T50.Z13	T50.Z14	T50.Z15	T50.Z16
Rhodine	T39.011	T39.012	T39.013	T39.014	T39.015	T39.016

◀ New   ◀|||| Revised   ~~deleted~~ Deleted

TABLE OF DRUGS AND CHEMICALS

Substance	External Cause (T-Code)					
	Poisoning, Accidental (Unintentional)	Poisoning, Intentional Self-Harm	Poisoning, Assault	Poisoning, Undetermined	Adverse Effect	Underdosing
RhoGAM	T50.Z11	T50.Z12	T50.Z13	T50.Z14	T50.Z15	T50.Z16
Rhubarb						
dry extract	T47.2X1	T47.2X2	T47.2X3	T47.2X4	T47.2X5	T47.2X6
tincture, compound	T47.2X1	T47.2X2	T47.2X3	T47.2X4	T47.2X5	T47.2X6
Ribavirin	T37.5X1	T37.5X2	T37.5X3	T37.5X4	T37.5X5	T37.5X6
Riboflavin	T45.2X1	T45.2X2	T45.2X3	T45.2X4	T45.2X5	T45.2X6
Ribostamycin	T36.5X1	T36.5X2	T36.5X3	T36.5X4	T36.5X5	T36.5X6
Ricin	T62.2X1	T62.2X2	T62.2X3	T62.2X4	—	—
Ricinus communis	T62.2X1	T62.2X2	T62.2X3	T62.2X4	—	—
Rickettsial vaccine NEC	T50.A91	T50.A92	T50.A93	T50.A94	T50.A95	T50.A96
Rifabutin	T36.6X1	T36.6X2	T36.6X3	T36.6X4	T36.6X5	T36.6X6
Rifamide	T36.6X1	T36.6X2	T36.6X3	T36.6X4	T36.6X5	T36.6X6
Rifampicin	T36.6X1	T36.6X2	T36.6X3	T36.6X4	T36.6X5	T36.6X6
with isoniazid	T37.1X1	T37.1X2	T37.1X3	T37.1X4	T37.1X5	T37.1X6
Rifampin	T36.6X1	T36.6X2	T36.6X3	T36.6X4	T36.6X5	T36.6X6
Rifamycin	T36.6X1	T36.6X2	T36.6X3	T36.6X4	T36.6X5	T36.6X6
Rifaximin	T36.6X1	T36.6X2	T36.6X3	T36.6X4	T36.6X5	T36.6X6
Rimantadine	T37.5X1	T37.5X2	T37.5X3	T37.5X4	T37.5X5	T37.5X6
Rimazolium metilsulfate	T39.8X1	T39.8X2	T39.8X3	T39.8X4	T39.8X5	T39.8X6
Rimifon	T37.1X1	T37.1X2	T37.1X3	T37.1X4	T37.1X5	T37.1X6
Rimiterol	T48.6X1	T48.6X2	T48.6X3	T48.6X4	T48.6X5	T48.6X6
Ringer (lactate) solution	T50.3X1	T50.3X2	T50.3X3	T50.3X4	T50.3X5	T50.3X6
Ristocetin	T36.8X1	T36.8X2	T36.8X3	T36.8X4	T36.8X5	T36.8X6
Ritalin	T43.631	T43.632	T43.633	T43.634	T43.635	T43.636
Ritodrine	T44.5X1	T44.5X2	T44.5X3	T44.5X4	T44.5X5	T44.5X6
Roach killer — see Insecticide						
Rociverine	T44.3X1	T44.3X2	T44.3X3	T44.3X4	T44.3X5	T44.3X6
Rocky Mountain spotted fever vaccine	T50.A91	T50.A92	T50.A93	T50.A94	T50.A95	T50.A96
Rodenticide NEC	T60.4X1	T60.4X2	T60.4X3	T60.4X4	—	—
Rohypnol	T42.4X1	T42.4X2	T42.4X3	T42.4X4	T42.4X5	T42.4X6
Rokitamycin	T36.3X1	T36.3X2	T36.3X3	T36.3X4	T36.3X5	T36.3X6
Rolaids	T47.1X1	T47.1X2	T47.1X3	T47.1X4	T47.1X5	T47.1X6
Rolitetracycline	T36.4X1	T36.4X2	T36.4X3	T36.4X4	T36.4X5	T36.4X6
Romilar	T48.3X1	T48.3X2	T48.3X3	T48.3X4	T48.3X5	T48.3X6
Ronifibrate	T46.6X1	T46.6X2	T46.6X3	T46.6X4	T46.6X5	T46.6X6
Rosaprostol	T47.1X1	T47.1X2	T47.1X3	T47.1X4	T47.1X5	T47.1X6
Rose bengal sodium (131I)	T50.8X1	T50.8X2	T50.8X3	T50.8X4	T50.8X5	T50.8X6
Rose water ointment	T49.3X1	T49.3X2	T49.3X3	T49.3X4	T49.3X5	T49.3X6
Rosoxacin	T37.8X1	T37.8X2	T37.8X3	T37.8X4	T37.8X5	T37.8X6
Rotenone	T60.2X1	T60.2X2	T60.2X3	T60.2X4	—	—

◀ New   ◀◀◀ Revised   deleted Deleted

Substance	Poisoning, Accidental (Unintentional)	Poisoning, Intentional Self-Harm	Poisoning, Assault	Poisoning, Undetermined	Adverse Effect	Underdosing
Rotoxamine	T45.0X1	T45.0X2	T45.0X3	T45.0X4	T45.0X5	T45.0X6
Rough-on-rats	T60.4X1	T60.4X2	T60.4X3	T60.4X4	—	—
Roxatidine	T47.0X1	T47.0X2	T47.0X3	T47.0X4	T47.0X5	T47.0X6
Roxithromycin	T36.3X1	T36.3X2	T36.3X3	T36.3X4	T36.3X5	T36.3X6
Rt-PA	T45.611	T45.612	T45.613	T45.614	T45.615	T45.616
Rubbing alcohol	T51.2X1	T51.2X2	T51.2X3	T51.2X4	—	—
Rubefacient	T49.4X1	T49.4X2	T49.4X3	T49.4X4	T49.4X5	T49.4X6
Rubella vaccine	T50.B91	T50.B92	T50.B93	T50.B94	T50.B95	T50.B96
Rubelogen	T50.B91	T50.B92	T50.B93	T50.B94	T50.B95	T50.B96
Rubeovax	T50.991	T50.992	T50.993	T50.994	T50.995	T50.996
Rubidium chloride Rb82	T50.8X1	T50.8X2	T50.8X3	T50.8X4	T50.8X5	T50.8X6
Rubidomycin	T45.1X1	T45.1X2	T45.1X3	T45.1X4	T45.1X5	T45.1X6
Rue	T62.2X1	T62.2X2	T62.2X3	T62.2X4	—	—
Rufocromomycin	T45.1X1	T45.1X2	T45.1X3	T45.1X4	T45.1X5	T45.1X6
Russel's viper venin	T45.7X1	T45.7X2	T45.7X3	T45.7X4	T45.7X5	T45.7X6
Ruta (graveolens)	T62.2X1	T62.2X2	T62.2X3	T62.2X4	—	—
Rutinum	T46.991	T46.992	T46.993	T46.994	T46.995	T46.996
Rutoside	T46.991	T46.992	T46.993	T46.994	T46.995	T46.996
S						
Sabadilla (plant)	T62.2X1	T62.2X2	T62.2X3	T62.2X4	—	—
pesticide	T60.2X1	T60.2X2	T60.2X3	T60.2X4	—	—
Saccharated iron oxide	T45.8X1	T45.8X2	T45.8X3	T45.8X4	T45.8X5	T45.8X6
Saccharin	T50.901	T50.902	T50.903	T50.904	T50.905	T50.906
Saccharomyces boulardii	T47.6X1	T47.6X2	T47.6X3	T47.6X4	T47.6X5	T47.6X6
Safflower oil	T46.6X1	T46.6X2	T46.6X3	T46.6X4	T46.6X5	T46.6X6
Safrazine	T43.1X1	T43.1X2	T43.1X3	T43.1X4	T43.1X5	T43.1X6
Salazosulfapyridine	T37.0X1	T37.0X2	T37.0X3	T37.0X4	T37.0X5	T37.0X6
Salbutamol	T48.6X1	T48.6X2	T48.6X3	T48.6X4	T48.6X5	T48.6X6
Salicylamide	T39.091	T39.092	T39.093	T39.094	T39.095	T39.096
Salicylate NEC	T39.091	T39.092	T39.093	T39.094	T39.095	T39.096
methyl	T49.3X1	T49.3X2	T49.3X3	T49.3X4	T49.3X5	T49.3X6
theobromine calcium	T50.2X1	T50.2X2	T50.2X3	T50.2X4	T50.2X5	T50.2X6
Salicylazosulfapyridine	T37.0X1	T37.0X2	T37.0X3	T37.0X4	T37.0X5	T37.0X6
Salicylhydroxamic acid	T49.0X1	T49.0X2	T49.0X3	T49.0X4	T49.0X5	T49.0X6
Salicylic acid	T49.4X1	T49.4X2	T49.4X3	T49.4X4	T49.4X5	T49.4X6
with benzoic acid	T49.4X1	T49.4X2	T49.4X3	T49.4X4	T49.4X5	T49.4X6
congeners	T39.091	T39.092	T39.093	T39.094	T39.095	T39.096
derivative	T39.091	T39.092	T39.093	T39.094	T39.095	T39.096
salts	T39.091	T39.092	T39.093	T39.094	T39.095	T39.096

◀ New ◀▥ Revised ~~deleted~~ Deleted

Substance	External Cause (T-Code)					
	Poisoning, Accidental (Unintentional)	Poisoning, Intentional Self-Harm	Poisoning, Assault	Poisoning, Undetermined	Adverse Effect	Underdosing
Salinazid	T37.1X1	T37.1X2	T37.1X3	T37.1X4	T37.1X5	T37.1X6
Salmeterol	T48.6X1	T48.6X2	T48.6X3	T48.6X4	T48.6X5	T48.6X6
Salol	T49.3X1	T49.3X2	T49.3X3	T49.3X4	T49.3X5	T49.3X6
Salsalate	T39.091	T39.092	T39.093	T39.094	T39.095	T39.096
Salt substitute	T50.901	T50.902	T50.903	T50.904	T50.905	T50.906
Salt-replacing drug	T50.901	T50.902	T50.903	T50.904	T50.905	T50.906
Salt-retaining mineralocorticoid	T50.0X1	T50.0X2	T50.0X3	T50.0X4	T50.0X5	T50.0X6
Saluretic NEC	T50.2X1	T50.2X2	T50.2X3	T50.2X4	T50.2X5	T50.2X6
Saluron	T50.2X1	T50.2X2	T50.2X3	T50.2X4	T50.2X5	T50.2X6
Salvarsan 606 (neosilver) (silver)	T37.8X1	T37.8X2	T37.8X3	T37.8X4	T37.8X5	T37.8X6
Sambucus canadensis	T62.2X1	T62.2X2	T62.2X3	T62.2X4	—	—
berry	T62.1X1	T62.1X2	T62.1X3	T62.1X4	—	—
Sandril	T46.5X1	T46.5X2	T46.5X3	T46.5X4	T46.5X5	T46.5X6
Sanguinaria canadensis	T62.2X1	T62.2X2	T62.2X3	T62.2X4	—	—
Saniflush (cleaner)	T54.2X1	T54.2X2	T54.2X3	T54.2X4	—	—
Santonin	T37.4X1	T37.4X2	T37.4X3	T37.4X4	T37.4X5	T37.4X6
Santyl	T49.8X1	T49.8X2	T49.8X3	T49.8X4	T49.8X5	T49.8X6
Saralasin	T46.5X1	T46.5X2	T46.5X3	T46.5X4	T46.5X5	T46.5X6
Sarcolysin	T45.1X1	T45.1X2	T45.1X3	T45.1X4	T45.1X5	T45.1X6
Sarkomycin	T45.1X1	T45.1X2	T45.1X3	T45.1X4	T45.1X5	T45.1X6
Saroten	T43.011	T43.012	T43.013	T43.014	T43.015	T43.016
Saturnine — see Lead						
Savin (oil)	T49.4X1	T49.4X2	T49.4X3	T49.4X4	T49.4X5	T49.4X6
Scammony	T47.2X1	T47.2X2	T47.2X3	T47.2X4	T47.2X5	T47.2X6
Scarlet red	T49.8X1	T49.8X2	T49.8X3	T49.8X4	T49.8X5	T49.8X6
Scheele's green	T57.0X1	T57.0X2	T57.0X3	T57.0X4	—	—
insecticide	T57.0X1	T57.0X2	T57.0X3	T57.0X4	—	—
Schizontozide (blood) (tissue)	T37.2X1	T37.2X2	T37.2X3	T37.2X4	T37.2X5	T37.2X6
Schradan	T60.0X1	T60.0X2	T60.0X3	T60.0X4	—	—
Schweinfurth green	T57.0X1	T57.0X2	T57.0X3	T57.0X4	—	—
insecticide	T57.0X1	T57.0X2	T57.0X3	T57.0X4	—	—
Scilla, rat poison	T60.4X1	T60.4X2	T60.4X3	T60.4X4	—	—
Scillaren	T60.4X1	T60.4X2	T60.4X3	T60.4X4	—	—
Sclerosing agent	T46.8X1	T46.8X2	T46.8X3	T46.8X4	T46.8X5	T46.8X6
Scombrotoxin	T61.11	T61.12	T61.13	T61.14	—	—
Scopolamine	T44.3X1	T44.3X2	T44.3X3	T44.3X4	T44.3X5	T44.3X6
Scopolia extract	T44.3X1	T44.3X2	T44.3X3	T44.3X4	T44.3X5	T44.3X6
Scouring powder	T65.891	T65.892	T65.893	T65.894	—	—

◀ New   ◀▥ Revised   ~~deleted~~ Deleted

Substance	Poisoning, Accidental (Unintentional)	Poisoning, Intentional Self-Harm	Poisoning, Assault	Poisoning, Undetermined	Adverse Effect	Underdosing
Sea						
anemone (sting)	T63.631	T63.632	T63.633	T63.634	—	—
cucumber (sting)	T63.691	T63.692	T63.693	T63.694	—	—
snake (bite) (venom)	T63.091	T63.092	T63.093	T63.094	—	—
urchin spine (puncture)	T63.691	T63.692	T63.693	T63.694	—	—
Seafood	T61.91	T61.92	T61.93	T61.94	—	—
specified NEC	T61.8X1	T61.8X2	T61.8X3	T61.8X4	—	—
Secbutabarbital	T42.3X1	T42.3X2	T42.3X3	T42.3X4	T42.3X5	T42.3X6
Secbutabarbitone	T42.3X1	T42.3X2	T42.3X3	T42.3X4	T42.3X5	T42.3X6
Secnidazole	T37.3X1	T37.3X2	T37.3X3	T37.3X4	T37.3X5	T37.3X6
Secobarbital	T42.3X1	T42.3X2	T42.3X3	T42.3X4	T42.3X5	T42.3X6
Seconal	T42.3X1	T42.3X2	T42.3X3	T42.3X4	T42.3X5	T42.3X6
Secretin	T50.8X1	T50.8X2	T50.8X3	T50.8X4	T50.8X5	T50.8X6
Sedative NEC	T42.71	T42.72	T42.73	T42.74	T42.75	T42.76
mixed NEC	T42.6X1	T42.6X2	T42.6X3	T42.6X4	T42.6X5	T42.6X6
Sedormid	T42.6X1	T42.6X2	T42.6X3	T42.6X4	T42.6X5	T42.6X6
Seed disinfectant or dressing	T60.8X1	T60.8X2	T60.8X3	T60.8X4	—	—
Seeds (poisonous)	T62.2X1	T62.2X2	T62.2X3	T62.2X4	—	—
Selegiline	T42.8X1	T42.8X2	T42.8X3	T42.8X4	T42.8X5	T42.8X6
Selenium NEC	T56.891	T56.892	T56.893	T56.894	—	—
disulfide or sulfide	T49.4X1	T49.4X2	T49.4X3	T49.4X4	T49.4X5	T49.4X6
fumes	T59.891	T59.892	T59.893	T59.894	—	—
sulfide	T49.4X1	T49.4X2	T49.4X3	T49.4X4	T49.4X5	T49.4X6
Selenomethionine (75Se)	T50.8X1	T50.8X2	T50.8X3	T50.8X4	T50.8X5	T50.8X6
Selsun	T49.4X1	T49.4X2	T49.4X3	T49.4X4	T49.4X5	T49.4X6
Semustine	T45.1X1	T45.1X2	T45.1X3	T45.1X4	T45.1X5	T45.1X6
Senega syrup	T48.4X1	T48.4X2	T48.4X3	T48.4X4	T48.4X5	T48.4X6
Senna	T47.2X1	T47.2X2	T47.2X3	T47.2X4	T47.2X5	T47.2X6
Sennoside A+B	T47.2X1	T47.2X2	T47.2X3	T47.2X4	T47.2X5	T47.2X6
Septisol	T49.2X1	T49.2X2	T49.2X3	T49.2X4	T49.2X5	T49.2X6
Seractide	T38.811	T38.812	T38.813	T38.814	T38.815	T38.816
Serax	T42.4X1	T42.4X2	T42.4X3	T42.4X4	T42.4X5	T42.4X6
Serenesil	T42.6X1	T42.6X2	T42.6X3	T42.6X4	T42.6X5	T42.6X6
Serenium (hydrochloride)	T37.91	T37.92	T37.93	T37.94	T37.95	T37.96
Serepax — see Oxazepam						
Sermorelin	T38.891	T38.892	T38.893	T38.894	T38.895	T38.896
Sernyl	T41.1X1	T41.1X2	T41.1X3	T41.1X4	T41.1X5	T41.1X6
Serotonin	T50.991	T50.992	T50.993	T50.994	T50.995	T50.996

TABLE OF DRUGS AND CHEMICALS

TABLE OF DRUGS AND CHEMICALS

Substance	External Cause (T-Code)					
	Poisoning, Accidental (Unintentional)	Poisoning, Intentional Self-Harm	Poisoning, Assault	Poisoning, Undetermined	Adverse Effect	Underdosing
Serpasil	T46.5X1	T46.5X2	T46.5X3	T46.5X4	T46.5X5	T46.5X6
Serrapeptase	T45.3X1	T45.3X2	T45.3X3	T45.3X4	T45.3X5	T45.3X6
Serum						
antibotulinus	T50.Z11	T50.Z12	T50.Z13	T50.Z14	T50.Z15	T50.Z16
anticytotoxic	T50.Z11	T50.Z12	T50.Z13	T50.Z14	T50.Z15	T50.Z16
antidiphtheria	T50.Z11	T50.Z12	T50.Z13	T50.Z14	T50.Z15	T50.Z16
antimeningococcus	T50.Z11	T50.Z12	T50.Z13	T50.Z14	T50.Z15	T50.Z16
anti-Rh	T50.Z11	T50.Z12	T50.Z13	T50.Z14	T50.Z15	T50.Z16
anti-snake-bite	T50.Z11	T50.Z12	T50.Z13	T50.Z14	T50.Z15	T50.Z16
antitetanic	T50.Z11	T50.Z12	T50.Z13	T50.Z14	T50.Z15	T50.Z16
antitoxic	T50.Z11	T50.Z12	T50.Z13	T50.Z14	T50.Z15	T50.Z16
complement (inhibitor)	T45.8X1	T45.8X2	T45.8X3	T45.8X4	T45.8X5	T45.8X6
convalescent	T50.Z11	T50.Z12	T50.Z13	T50.Z14	T50.Z15	T50.Z16
hemolytic complement	T45.8X1	T45.8X2	T45.8X3	T45.8X4	T45.8X5	T45.8X6
immune (human)	T50.Z11	T50.Z12	T50.Z13	T50.Z14	T50.Z15	T50.Z16
protective NEC	T50.Z11	T50.Z12	T50.Z13	T50.Z14	T50.Z15	T50.Z16
Setastine	T45.0X1	T45.0X2	T45.0X3	T45.0X4	T45.0X5	T45.0X6
Setoperone	T43.591	T43.592	T43.593	T43.594	T43.595	T43.596
Sewer gas	T59.91	T59.92	T59.93	T59.94	—	—
Shampoo	T55.0X1	T55.0X2	T55.0X3	T55.0X4	—	—
Shellfish, noxious, nonbacterial	T61.781	T61.782	T61.783	T61.784	—	—
Sildenafil	T46.7X1	T46.7X2	T46.7X3	T46.7X4	T46.7X5	T46.7X6
Silibinin	T50.991	T50.992	T50.993	T50.994	T50.995	T50.996
Silicone NEC	T65.891	T65.892	T65.893	T65.894	—	—
medicinal	T49.3X1	T49.3X2	T49.3X3	T49.3X4	T49.3X5	T49.3X6
Silvadene	T49.0X1	T49.0X2	T49.0X3	T49.0X4	T49.0X5	T49.0X6
Silver	T49.0X1	T49.0X2	T49.0X3	T49.0X4	T49.0X5	T49.0X6
anti-infectives	T49.0X1	T49.0X2	T49.0X3	T49.0X4	T49.0X5	T49.0X6
arsphenamine	T37.8X1	T37.8X2	T37.8X3	T37.8X4	T37.8X5	T37.8X6
colloidal	T49.0X1	T49.0X2	T49.0X3	T49.0X4	T49.0X5	T49.0X6
nitrate	T49.0X1	T49.0X2	T49.0X3	T49.0X4	T49.0X5	T49.0X6
ophthalmic preparation	T49.5X1	T49.5X2	T49.5X3	T49.5X4	T49.5X5	T49.5X6
toughened (keratolytic)	T49.4X1	T49.4X2	T49.4X3	T49.4X4	T49.4X5	T49.4X6
nonmedicinal (dust)	T56.891	T56.892	T56.893	T56.894	—	—
protein	T49.5X1	T49.5X2	T49.5X3	T49.5X4	T49.5X5	T49.5X6
salvarsan	T37.8X1	T37.8X2	T37.8X3	T37.8X4	T37.8X5	T37.8X6
sulfadiazine	T49.4X1	T49.4X2	T49.4X3	T49.4X4	T49.4X5	T49.4X6
Silymarin	T50.991	T50.992	T50.993	T50.994	T50.995	T50.996
Simaldrate	T47.1X1	T47.1X2	T47.1X3	T47.1X4	T47.1X5	T47.1X6
Simazine	T60.3X1	T60.3X2	T60.3X3	T60.3X4	—	—

◄ New   ◄‖‖ Revised   ~~deleted~~ Deleted

Substance	External Cause (T-Code)					
	Poisoning, Accidental (Unintentional)	Poisoning, Intentional Self-Harm	Poisoning, Assault	Poisoning, Undetermined	Adverse Effect	Underdosing
Simethicone	T47.1X1	T47.1X2	T47.1X3	T47.1X4	T47.1X5	T47.1X6
Simfibrate	T46.6X1	T46.6X2	T46.6X3	T46.6X4	T46.6X5	T46.6X6
Simvastatin	T46.6X1	T46.6X2	T46.6X3	T46.6X4	T46.6X5	T46.6X6
Sincalide	T50.8X1	T50.8X2	T50.8X3	T50.8X4	T50.8X5	T50.8X6
Sinequan	T43.011	T43.012	T43.013	T43.014	T43.015	T43.016
Singoserp	T46.5X1	T46.5X2	T46.5X3	T46.5X4	T46.5X5	T46.5X6
Sintrom	T45.511	T45.512	T45.513	T45.514	T45.515	T45.516
Sisomicin	T36.5X1	T36.5X2	T36.5X3	T36.5X4	T36.5X5	T36.5X6
Sitosterols	T46.6X1	T46.6X2	T46.6X3	T46.6X4	T46.6X5	T46.6X6
Skeletal muscle relaxants	T48.1X1	T48.1X2	T48.1X3	T48.1X4	T48.1X5	T48.1X6
Skin						
agents (external)	T49.91	T49.92	T49.93	T49.94	T49.95	T49.96
specified NEC	T49.8X1	T49.8X2	T49.8X3	T49.8X4	T49.8X5	T49.8X6
test antigen	T50.8X1	T50.8X2	T50.8X3	T50.8X4	T50.8X5	T50.8X6
Sleep-eze	T45.0X1	T45.0X2	T45.0X3	T45.0X4	T45.0X5	T45.0X6
Sleeping draught, pill	T42.71	T42.72	T42.73	T42.74	T42.75	T42.76
Smallpox vaccine	T50.B11	T50.B12	T50.B13	T50.B14	T50.B15	T50.B16
Smelter fumes NEC	T56.91	T56.92	T56.93	T56.94	—	—
Smog	T59.1X1	T59.1X2	T59.1X3	T59.1X4	—	—
Smoke NEC	T59.811	T59.812	T59.813	T59.814	—	—
Smooth muscle relaxant	T44.3X1	T44.3X2	T44.3X3	T44.3X4	T44.3X5	T44.3X6
Snail killer NEC	T60.8X1	T60.8X2	T60.8X3	T60.8X4	—	—
Snake venom or bite	T63.001	T63.002	T63.003	T63.004	—	—
hemocoagulase	T45.7X1	T45.7X2	T45.7X3	T45.7X4	T45.7X5	T45.7X6
Snuff	T65.211	T65.212	T65.213	T65.214	—	—
Soap (powder) (product)	T55.0X1	T55.0X2	T55.0X3	T55.0X4	—	—
enema	T47.4X1	T47.4X2	T47.4X3	T47.4X4	T47.4X5	T47.4X6
medicinal, soft	T49.2X1	T49.2X2	T49.2X3	T49.2X4	T49.2X5	T49.2X6
superfatted	T49.2X1	T49.2X2	T49.2X3	T49.2X4	T49.2X5	T49.2X6
Sobrerol	T48.4X1	T48.4X2	T48.4X3	T48.4X4	T48.4X5	T48.4X6
Soda (caustic)	T54.3X1	T54.3X2	T54.3X3	T54.3X4	—	—
bicarb	T47.1X1	T47.1X2	T47.1X3	T47.1X4	T47.1X5	T47.1X6
chlorinated — *see Sodium, hypochlorite*						
Sodium						
acetosulfone	T37.1X1	T37.1X2	T37.1X3	T37.1X4	T37.1X5	T37.1X6
acetrizoate	T50.8X1	T50.8X2	T50.8X3	T50.8X4	T50.8X5	T50.8X6
acid phosphate	T50.3X1	T50.3X2	T50.3X3	T50.3X4	T50.3X5	T50.3X6
alginate	T47.8X1	T47.8X2	T47.8X3	T47.8X4	T47.8X5	T47.8X6
amidotrizoate	T50.8X1	T50.8X2	T50.8X3	T50.8X4	T50.8X5	T50.8X6
aminopterin	T45.1X1	T45.1X2	T45.1X3	T45.1X4	T45.1X5	T45.1X6

	External Cause (T-Code)					
Substance	Poisoning, Accidental (Unintentional)	Poisoning, Intentional Self-Harm	Poisoning, Assault	Poisoning, Undetermined	Adverse Effect	Underdosing
Sodium *(Continued)*						
amylosulfate	T47.8X1	T47.8X2	T47.8X3	T47.8X4	T47.8X5	T47.8X6
amytal	T42.3X1	T42.3X2	T42.3X3	T42.3X4	T42.3X5	T42.3X6
antimony gluconate	T37.3X1	T37.3X2	T37.3X3	T37.3X4	T37.3X5	T37.3X6
arsenate	T57.0X1	T57.0X2	T57.0X3	T57.0X4	—	—
aurothiomalate	T39.4X1	T39.4X2	T39.4X3	T39.4X4	T39.4X5	T39.4X6
aurothiosulfate	T39.4X1	T39.4X2	T39.4X3	T39.4X4	T39.4X5	T39.4X6
barbiturate	T42.3X1	T42.3X2	T42.3X3	T42.3X4	T42.3X5	T42.3X6
basic phosphate	T47.4X1	T47.4X2	T47.4X3	T47.4X4	T47.4X5	T47.4X6
bicarbonate	T47.1X1	T47.1X2	T47.1X3	T47.1X4	T47.1X5	T47.1X6
bichromate	T57.8X1	T57.8X2	T57.8X3	T57.8X4	—	—
biphosphate	T50.3X1	T50.3X2	T50.3X3	T50.3X4	T50.3X5	T50.3X6
bisulfate	T65.891	T65.892	T65.893	T65.894	—	—
borate						
cleanser	T57.8X1	T57.8X2	T57.8X3	T57.8X4	—	—
eye	T49.5X1	T49.5X2	T49.5X3	T49.5X4	T49.5X5	T49.5X6
therapeutic	T49.8X1	T49.8X2	T49.8X3	T49.8X4	T49.8X5	T49.8X6
bromide	T42.6X1	T42.6X2	T42.6X3	T42.6X4	T42.6X5	T42.6X6
cacodylate (nonmedicinal) NEC	T50.8X1	T50.8X2	T50.8X3	T50.8X4	T50.8X5	T50.8X6
anti-infective	T37.8X1	T37.8X2	T37.8X3	T37.8X4	T37.8X5	T37.8X6
herbicide	T60.3X1	T60.3X2	T60.3X3	T60.3X4	—	—
calcium edetate	T45.8X1	T45.8X2	T45.8X3	T45.8X4	T45.8X5	T45.8X6
carbonate NEC	T54.3X1	T54.3X2	T54.3X3	T54.3X4	—	—
chlorate NEC	T65.891	T65.892	T65.893	T65.894	—	—
herbicide	T54.91	T54.92	T54.93	T54.94	—	—
chloride	T50.3X1	T50.3X2	T50.3X3	T50.3X4	T50.3X5	T50.3X6
with glucose	T50.3X1	T50.3X2	T50.3X3	T50.3X4	T50.3X5	T50.3X6
chromate	T65.891	T65.892	T65.893	T65.894	—	—
citrate	T50.991	T50.992	T50.993	T50.994	T50.995	T50.996
cromoglicate	T48.6X1	T48.6X2	T48.6X3	T48.6X4	T48.6X5	T48.6X6
cyanide	T65.0X1	T65.0X2	T65.0X3	T65.0X4	—	—
cyclamate	T50.3X1	T50.3X2	T50.3X3	T50.3X4	T50.3X5	T50.3X6
dehydrocholate	T45.8X1	T45.8X2	T45.8X3	T45.8X4	T45.8X5	T45.8X6
diatrizoate	T50.8X1	T50.8X2	T50.8X3	T50.8X4	T50.8X5	T50.8X6
dibunate	T48.4X1	T48.4X2	T48.4X3	T48.4X4	T48.4X5	T48.4X6
dioctyl sulfosuccinate	T47.4X1	T47.4X2	T47.4X3	T47.4X4	T47.4X5	T47.4X6
dipantoyl ferrate	T45.8X1	T45.8X2	T45.8X3	T45.8X4	T45.8X5	T45.8X6
edetate	T45.8X1	T45.8X2	T45.8X3	T45.8X4	T45.8X5	T45.8X6
ethacrynate	T50.1X1	T50.1X2	T50.1X3	T50.1X4	T50.1X5	T50.1X6
feredetate	T45.8X1	T45.8X2	T45.8X3	T45.8X4	T45.8X5	T45.8X6

◄ New   ◄▥ Revised   ~~deleted~~ Deleted

Substance	External Cause (T-Code)					
	Poisoning, Accidental (Unintentional)	Poisoning, Intentional Self-Harm	Poisoning, Assault	Poisoning, Undetermined	Adverse Effect	Underdosing
Sodium *(Continued)*						
Fluoride — *see Fluoride*						
fluoroacetate (dust) (pesticide)	T60.4X1	T60.4X2	T60.4X3	T60.4X4	—	—
free salt	T50.3X1	T50.3X2	T50.3X3	T50.3X4	T50.3X5	T50.3X6
fusidate	T36.8X1	T36.8X2	T36.8X3	T36.8X4	T36.8X5	T36.8X6
glucaldrate	T47.1X1	T47.1X2	T47.1X3	T47.1X4	T47.1X5	T47.1X6
glucosulfone	T37.1X1	T37.1X2	T37.1X3	T37.1X4	T37.1X5	T37.1X6
glutamate	T45.8X1	T45.8X2	T45.8X3	T45.8X4	T45.8X5	T45.8X6
hydrogen carbonate	T50.3X1	T50.3X2	T50.3X3	T50.3X4	T50.3X5	T50.3X6
hydroxide	T54.3X1	T54.3X2	T54.3X3	T54.3X4	—	—
hypochlorite (bleach) NEC	T54.3X1	T54.3X2	T54.3X3	T54.3X4	—	—
disinfectant	T54.3X1	T54.3X2	T54.3X3	T54.3X4	—	—
medicinal (anti-infective) (external)	T49.0X1	T49.0X2	T49.0X3	T49.0X4	T49.0X5	T49.0X6
vapor	T54.3X1	T54.3X2	T54.3X3	T54.3X4	—	—
hyposulfite	T49.0X1	T49.0X2	T49.0X3	T49.0X4	T49.0X5	T49.0X6
indigotin disulfonate	T50.8X1	T50.8X2	T50.8X3	T50.8X4	T50.8X5	T50.8X6
iodide	T50.991	T50.992	T50.993	T50.994	T50.995	T50.996
I-131	T50.8X1	T50.8X2	T50.8X3	T50.8X4	T50.8X5	T50.8X6
therapeutic	T38.2X1	T38.2X2	T38.2X3	T38.2X4	T38.2X5	T38.2X6
iodohippurate (131I)	T50.8X1	T50.8X2	T50.8X3	T50.8X4	T50.8X5	T50.8X6
iopodate	T50.8X1	T50.8X2	T50.8X3	T50.8X4	T50.8X5	T50.8X6
iothalamate	T50.8X1	T50.8X2	T50.8X3	T50.8X4	T50.8X5	T50.8X6
iron edetate	T45.4X1	T45.4X2	T45.4X3	T45.4X4	T45.4X5	T45.4X6
lactate (compound solution)	T45.8X1	T45.8X2	T45.8X3	T45.8X4	T45.8X5	T45.8X6
lauryl (sulfate)	T49.2X1	T49.2X2	T49.2X3	T49.2X4	T49.2X5	T49.2X6
(L)-triiodothyronine	T38.1X1	T38.1X2	T38.1X3	T38.1X4	T38.1X5	T38.1X6
magnesium citrate	T50.991	T50.992	T50.993	T50.994	T50.995	T50.996
mersalate	T50.2X1	T50.2X2	T50.2X3	T50.2X4	T50.2X5	T50.2X6
metasilicate	T65.891	T65.892	T65.893	T65.894	—	—
metrizoate	T50.8X1	T50.8X2	T50.8X3	T50.8X4	T50.8X5	T50.8X6
monofluoroacetate (pesticide)	T60.1X1	T60.1X2	T60.1X3	T60.1X4	—	—
morrhuate	T46.8X1	T46.8X2	T46.8X3	T46.8X4	T46.8X5	T46.8X6
nafcillin	T36.0X1	T36.0X2	T36.0X3	T36.0X4	T36.0X5	T36.0X6
nitrate (oxidizing agent)	T65.891	T65.892	T65.893	T65.894	—	—
nitrite	T50.6X1	T50.6X2	T50.6X3	T50.6X4	T50.6X5	T50.6X6
nitroferricyanide	T46.5X1	T46.5X2	T46.5X3	T46.5X4	T46.5X5	T46.5X6
nitroprusside	T46.5X1	T46.5X2	T46.5X3	T46.5X4	T46.5X5	T46.5X6
oxalate	T65.891	T65.892	T65.893	T65.894	—	—
oxide/peroxide	T65.891	T65.892	T65.893	T65.894	—	—
oxybate	T41.291	T41.292	T41.293	T41.294	T41.295	T41.296

Substance	Poisoning, Accidental (Unintentional)	Poisoning, Intentional Self-Harm	Poisoning, Assault	Poisoning, Undetermined	Adverse Effect	Underdosing
	External Cause (T-Code)					
Sodium *(Continued)*						
para-aminohippurate	T50.8X1	T50.8X2	T50.8X3	T50.8X4	T50.8X5	T50.8X6
perborate (nonmedicinal) NEC	T65.891	T65.892	T65.893	T65.894	—	—
medicinal	T49.0X1	T49.0X2	T49.0X3	T49.0X4	T49.0X5	T49.0X6
soap	T55.0X1	T55.0X2	T55.0X3	T55.0X4	—	—
percarbonate — *see Sodium, perborate*						
pertechnetate Tc99m	T50.8X1	T50.8X2	T50.8X3	T50.8X4	T50.8X5	T50.8X6
phosphate						
cellulose	T45.8X1	T45.8X2	T45.8X3	T45.8X4	T45.8X5	T45.8X6
dibasic	T47.2X1	T47.2X2	T47.2X3	T47.2X4	T47.2X5	T47.2X6
monobasic	T47.2X1	T47.2X2	T47.2X3	T47.2X4	T47.2X5	T47.2X6
phytate	T50.6X1	T50.6X2	T50.6X3	T50.6X4	T50.6X5	T50.6X6
picosulfate	T47.2X1	T47.2X2	T47.2X3	T47.2X4	T47.2X5	T47.2X6
polyhydroxyaluminium monocarbonate	T47.1X1	T47.1X2	T47.1X3	T47.1X4	T47.1X5	T47.1X6
polystyrene sulfonate	T50.3X1	T50.3X2	T50.3X3	T50.3X4	T50.3X5	T50.3X6
propionate	T49.0X1	T49.0X2	T49.0X3	T49.0X4	T49.0X5	T49.0X6
propyl hydroxybenzoate	T50.991	T50.992	T50.993	T50.994	T50.995	T50.996
psylliate	T46.8X1	T46.8X2	T46.8X3	T46.8X4	T46.8X5	T46.8X6
removing resins	T50.3X1	T50.3X2	T50.3X3	T50.3X4	T50.3X5	T50.3X6
salicylate	T39.091	T39.092	T39.093	T39.094	T39.095	T39.096
salt NEC	T50.3X1	T50.3X2	T50.3X3	T50.3X4	T50.3X5	T50.3X6
selenate	T60.2X1	T60.2X2	T60.2X3	T60.2X4	—	—
stibogluconate	T37.3X1	T37.3X2	T37.3X3	T37.3X4	T37.3X5	T37.3X6
sulfate	T47.4X1	T47.4X2	T47.4X3	T47.4X4	T47.4X5	T47.4X6
sulfoxone	T37.1X1	T37.1X2	T37.1X3	T37.1X4	T37.1X5	T37.1X6
tetradecyl sulfate	T46.8X1	T46.8X2	T46.8X3	T46.8X4	T46.8X5	T46.8X6
thiopental	T41.1X1	T41.1X2	T41.1X3	T41.1X4	T41.1X5	T41.1X6
thiosalicylate	T39.091	T39.092	T39.093	T39.094	T39.095	T39.096
thiosulfate	T50.6X1	T50.6X2	T50.6X3	T50.6X4	T50.6X5	T50.6X6
tolbutamide	T38.3X1	T38.3X2	T38.3X3	T38.3X4	T38.3X5	T38.3X6
l-triiodothyronine	T38.1X1	T38.1X2	T38.1X3	T38.1X4	T38.1X5	T38.1X6
tyropanoate	T50.8X1	T50.8X2	T50.8X3	T50.8X4	T50.8X5	T50.8X6
valproate	T42.6X1	T42.6X2	T42.6X3	T42.6X4	T42.6X5	T42.6X6
versenate	T50.6X1	T50.6X2	T50.6X3	T50.6X4	T50.6X5	T50.6X6
Sodium-free salt	T50.901	T50.902	T50.903	T50.904	T50.905	T50.906
Sodium-removing resin	T50.3X1	T50.3X2	T50.3X3	T50.3X4	T50.3X5	T50.3X6
Soft soap	T55.0X1	T55.0X2	T55.0X3	T55.0X4	—	—
Solanine	T62.2X1	T62.2X2	T62.2X3	T62.2X4	—	—
berries	T62.1X1	T62.1X2	T62.1X3	T62.1X4	—	—

◀ New ◀╍ Revised ~~deleted~~ Deleted

Substance	External Cause (T-Code)					
	Poisoning, Accidental (Unintentional)	Poisoning, Intentional Self-Harm	Poisoning, Assault	Poisoning, Undetermined	Adverse Effect	Underdosing
Solanum dulcamara	T62.2X1	T62.2X2	T62.2X3	T62.2X4	—	—
berries	T62.1X1	T62.1X2	T62.1X3	T62.1X4	—	—
Solapsone	T37.1X1	T37.1X2	T37.1X3	T37.1X4	T37.1X5	T37.1X6
Solar lotion	T49.3X1	T49.3X2	T49.3X3	T49.3X4	T49.3X5	T49.3X6
Solasulfone	T37.1X1	T37.1X2	T37.1X3	T37.1X4	T37.1X5	T37.1X6
Soldering fluid	T65.891	T65.892	T65.893	T65.894	—	—
Solid substance	T65.91	T65.92	T65.93	T65.94	—	—
specified NEC	T65.891	T65.892	T65.893	T65.894	—	—
Solvent, industrial NEC	T52.91	T52.92	T52.93	T52.94	—	—
naphtha	T52.0X1	T52.0X2	T52.0X3	T52.0X4	—	—
petroleum	T52.0X1	T52.0X2	T52.0X3	T52.0X4	—	—
specified NEC	T52.8X1	T52.8X2	T52.8X3	T52.8X4	—	—
Soma	T42.8X1	T42.8X2	T42.8X3	T42.8X4	T42.8X5	T42.8X6
Somatorelin	T38.891	T38.892	T38.893	T38.894	T38.895	T38.896
Somatostatin	T38.991	T38.992	T38.993	T38.994	T38.995	T38.996
Somatotropin	T38.811	T38.812	T38.813	T38.814	T38.815	T38.816
Somatrem	T38.811	T38.812	T38.813	T38.814	T38.815	T38.816
Somatropin	T38.811	T38.812	T38.813	T38.814	T38.815	T38.816
Sominex	T45.0X1	T45.0X2	T45.0X3	T45.0X4	T45.0X5	T45.0X6
Somnos	T42.6X1	T42.6X2	T42.6X3	T42.6X4	T42.6X5	T42.6X6
Somonal	T42.3X1	T42.3X2	T42.3X3	T42.3X4	T42.3X5	T42.3X6
Soneryl	T42.3X1	T42.3X2	T42.3X3	T42.3X4	T42.3X5	T42.3X6
Soothing syrup	T50.901	T50.902	T50.903	T50.904	T50.905	T50.906
Sopor	T42.6X1	T42.6X2	T42.6X3	T42.6X4	T42.6X5	T42.6X6
Soporific	T42.71	T42.72	T42.73	T42.74	T42.75	T42.76
Soporific drug	T42.71	T42.72	T42.73	T42.74	T42.75	T42.76
specified type NEC	T42.6X1	T42.6X2	T42.6X3	T42.6X4	T42.6X5	T42.6X6
Sorbide nitrate	T46.3X1	T46.3X2	T46.3X3	T46.3X4	T46.3X5	T46.3X6
Sorbitol	T47.4X1	T47.4X2	T47.4X3	T47.4X4	T47.4X5	T47.4X6
Sotalol	T44.7X1	T44.7X2	T44.7X3	T44.7X4	T44.7X5	T44.7X6
Sotradecol	T46.8X1	T46.8X2	T46.8X3	T46.8X4	T46.8X5	T46.8X6
Soysterol	T46.6X1	T46.6X2	T46.6X3	T46.6X4	T46.6X5	T46.6X6
Spacoline	T44.3X1	T44.3X2	T44.3X3	T44.3X4	T44.3X5	T44.3X6
Spanish fly	T49.8X1	T49.8X2	T49.8X3	T49.8X4	T49.8X5	T49.8X6
Sparine	T43.3X1	T43.3X2	T43.3X3	T43.3X4	T43.3X5	T43.3X6
Sparteine	T48.0X1	T48.0X2	T48.0X3	T48.0X4	T48.0X5	T48.0X6
Spasmolytic						
anticholinergics	T44.3X1	T44.3X2	T44.3X3	T44.3X4	T44.3X5	T44.3X6
autonomic	T44.3X1	T44.3X2	T44.3X3	T44.3X4	T44.3X5	T44.3X6

Substance	Poisoning, Accidental (Unintentional)	Poisoning, Intentional Self-Harm	Poisoning, Assault	Poisoning, Undetermined	Adverse Effect	Underdosing
External Cause (T-Code)						
Spasmolytic *(Continued)*						
bronchial NEC	T48.6X1	T48.6X2	T48.6X3	T48.6X4	T48.6X5	T48.6X6
quaternary ammonium	T44.3X1	T44.3X2	T44.3X3	T44.3X4	T44.3X5	T44.3X6
skeletal muscle NEC	T48.1X1	T48.1X2	T48.1X3	T48.1X4	T48.1X5	T48.1X6
Spectinomycin	T36.5X1	T36.5X2	T36.5X3	T36.5X4	T36.5X5	T36.5X6
Speed	T43.621	T43.622	T43.623	T43.624	T43.625	T43.626
Spermicide	T49.8X1	T49.8X2	T49.8X3	T49.8X4	T49.8X5	T49.8X6
Spider (bite) (venom)	T63.391	T63.392	T63.393	T63.394	—	—
antivenin	T50.Z11	T50.Z12	T50.Z13	T50.Z14	T50.Z15	T50.Z16
Spigelia (root)	T37.4X1	T37.4X2	T37.4X3	T37.4X4	T37.4X5	T37.4X6
Spindle inactivator	T50.4X1	T50.4X2	T50.4X3	T50.4X4	T50.4X5	T50.4X6
Spiperone	T43.4X1	T43.4X2	T43.4X3	T43.4X4	T43.4X5	T43.4X6
Spiramycin	T36.3X1	T36.3X2	T36.3X3	T36.3X4	T36.3X5	T36.3X6
Spirapril	T46.4X1	T46.4X2	T46.4X3	T46.4X4	T46.4X5	T46.4X6
Spirilene	T43.591	T43.592	T43.593	T43.594	T43.595	T43.596
Spirit(s) (neutral) NEC	T51.0X1	T51.0X2	T51.0X3	T51.0X4	—	—
beverage	T51.0X1	T51.0X2	T51.0X3	T51.0X4	—	—
industrial	T51.0X1	T51.0X2	T51.0X3	T51.0X4	—	—
mineral	T52.0X1	T52.0X2	T52.0X3	T52.0X4	—	—
of salt — *see Hydrochloric acid*						
surgical	T51.0X1	T51.0X2	T51.0X3	T51.0X4	—	—
Spironolactone	T50.0X1	T50.0X2	T50.0X3	T50.0X4	T50.0X5	T50.0X6
Spiroperidol	T43.4X1	T43.4X2	T43.4X3	T43.4X4	T43.4X5	T43.4X6
Sponge, absorbable (gelatin)	T45.7X1	T45.7X2	T45.7X3	T45.7X4	T45.7X5	T45.7X6
Sporostacin	T49.0X1	T49.0X2	T49.0X3	T49.0X4	T49.0X5	T49.0X6
Spray (aerosol)	T65.91	T65.92	T65.93	T65.94	—	—
cosmetic	T65.891	T65.892	T65.893	T65.894	—	—
medicinal NEC	T50.901	T50.902	T50.903	T50.904	T50.905	T50.906
pesticides — *see Pesticides*						
specified content — *see specific substance*						
Spurge flax	T62.2X1	T62.2X2	T62.2X3	T62.2X4	—	—
Spurges	T62.2X1	T62.2X2	T62.2X3	T62.2X4	—	—
Sputum viscosity-lowering drug	T48.4X1	T48.4X2	T48.4X3	T48.4X4	T48.4X5	T48.4X6
Squill	T46.0X1	T46.0X2	T46.0X3	T46.0X4	T46.0X5	T46.0X6
rat poison	T60.4X1	T60.4X2	T60.4X3	T60.4X4	—	—
Squirting cucumber (cathartic)	T47.2X1	T47.2X2	T47.2X3	T47.2X4	T47.2X5	T47.2X6
Stains	T65.6X1	T65.6X2	T65.6X3	T65.6X4	—	—
Stannous fluoride	T49.7X1	T49.7X2	T49.7X3	T49.7X4	T49.7X5	T49.7X6
Stanolone	T38.7X1	T38.7X2	T38.7X3	T38.7X4	T38.7X5	T38.7X6
Stanozolol	T38.7X1	T38.7X2	T38.7X3	T38.7X4	T38.7X5	T38.7X6

◀ New   ◀▦ Revised   ~~deleted~~ Deleted

Substance	Poisoning, Accidental (Unintentional)	Poisoning, Intentional Self-Harm	Poisoning, Assault	Poisoning, Undetermined	Adverse Effect	Underdosing
Staphisagria or stavesacre (pediculicide)	T49.0X1	T49.0X2	T49.0X3	T49.0X4	T49.0X5	T49.0X6
Starch	T50.901	T50.902	T50.903	T50.904	T50.905	T50.906
Stelazine	T43.3X1	T43.3X2	T43.3X3	T43.3X4	T43.3X5	T43.3X6
Stemetil	T43.3X1	T43.3X2	T43.3X3	T43.3X4	T43.3X5	T43.3X6
Stepronin	T48.4X1	T48.4X2	T48.4X3	T48.4X4	T48.4X5	T48.4X6
Sterculia	T47.4X1	T47.4X2	T47.4X3	T47.4X4	T47.4X5	T47.4X6
Sternutator gas	T59.891	T59.892	T59.893	T59.894	—	—
Steroid	T38.0X1	T38.0X2	T38.0X3	T38.0X4	T38.0X5	T38.0X6
anabolic	T38.7X1	T38.7X2	T38.7X3	T38.7X4	T38.7X5	T38.7X6
androgenic	T38.7X1	T38.7X2	T38.7X3	T38.7X4	T38.7X5	T38.7X6
antineoplastic, hormone	T38.7X1	T38.7X2	T38.7X3	T38.7X4	T38.7X5	T38.7X6
estrogen	T38.5X1	T38.5X2	T38.5X3	T38.5X4	T38.5X5	T38.5X6
ENT agent	T49.6X1	T49.6X2	T49.6X3	T49.6X4	T49.6X5	T49.6X6
ophthalmic preparation	T49.5X1	T49.5X2	T49.5X3	T49.5X4	T49.5X5	T49.5X6
topical NEC	T49.0X1	T49.0X2	T49.0X3	T49.0X4	T49.0X5	T49.0X6
Stibine	T56.891	T56.892	T56.893	T56.894	—	—
Stibogluconate	T37.3X1	T37.3X2	T37.3X3	T37.3X4	T37.3X5	T37.3X6
Stibophen	T37.4X1	T37.4X2	T37.4X3	T37.4X4	T37.4X5	T37.4X6
Stilbamidine (isetionate)	T37.3X1	T37.3X2	T37.3X3	T37.3X4	T37.3X5	T37.3X6
Stilbestrol	T38.5X1	T38.5X2	T38.5X3	T38.5X4	T38.5X5	T38.5X6
Stilboestrol	T38.5X1	T38.5X2	T38.5X3	T38.5X4	T38.5X5	T38.5X6
Stimulant						
central nervous system — see also Psychostimulant	T43.601	T43.602	T43.603	T43.604	T43.605	T43.606
analeptics	T50.7X1	T50.7X2	T50.7X3	T50.7X4	T50.7X5	T50.7X6
opiate antagonist	T50.7X1	T50.7X2	T50.7X3	T50.7X4	T50.7X5	T50.7X6
psychotherapeutic NEC — see also Psychotherapeutic drug	T43.601	T43.602	T43.603	T43.604	T43.605	T43.606
specified NEC	T43.691	T43.692	T43.693	T43.694	T43.695	T43.696
respiratory	T48.901	T48.902	T48.903	T48.904	T48.905	T48.906
Stone-dissolving drug	T50.901	T50.902	T50.903	T50.904	T50.905	T50.906
Storage battery (cells) (acid)	T54.2X1	T54.2X2	T54.2X3	T54.2X4	—	—
Stovaine	T41.3X1	T41.3X2	T41.3X3	T41.3X4	T41.3X5	T41.3X6
infiltration (subcutaneous)	T41.3X1	T41.3X2	T41.3X3	T41.3X4	T41.3X5	T41.3X6
nerve block (peripheral) (plexus)	T41.3X1	T41.3X2	T41.3X3	T41.3X4	T41.3X5	T41.3X6
spinal	T41.3X1	T41.3X2	T41.3X3	T41.3X4	T41.3X5	T41.3X6
topical (surface)	T41.3X1	T41.3X2	T41.3X3	T41.3X4	T41.3X5	T41.3X6
Stovarsal	T37.8X1	T37.8X2	T37.8X3	T37.8X4	T37.8X5	T37.8X6
Stove gas — see Gas, stove	T57.91	T57.92	T57.93	T57.94	—	—
Stoxil	T49.5X1	T49.5X2	T49.5X3	T49.5X4	T49.5X5	T49.5X6
Stramonium	T48.6X1	T48.6X2	T48.6X3	T48.6X4	T48.6X5	T48.6X6
natural state	T62.2X1	T62.2X2	T62.2X3	T62.2X4	—	—

TABLE OF DRUGS AND CHEMICALS

Substance	Poisoning, Accidental (Unintentional)	Poisoning, Intentional Self-Harm	Poisoning, Assault	Poisoning, Undetermined	Adverse Effect	Underdosing
	External Cause (T-Code)					
Streptodornase	T45.3X1	T45.3X2	T45.3X3	T45.3X4	T45.3X5	T45.3X6
Streptoduocin	T36.5X1	T36.5X2	T36.5X3	T36.5X4	T36.5X5	T36.5X6
Streptokinase	T45.611	T45.612	T45.613	T45.614	T45.615	T45.616
Streptomycin (derivative)	T36.5X1	T36.5X2	T36.5X3	T36.5X4	T36.5X5	T36.5X6
Streptonivicin	T36.5X1	T36.5X2	T36.5X3	T36.5X4	T36.5X5	T36.5X6
Streptovarycin	T36.5X1	T36.5X2	T36.5X3	T36.5X4	T36.5X5	T36.5X6
Streptozocin	T45.1X1	T45.1X2	T45.1X3	T45.1X4	T45.1X5	T45.1X6
Streptozotocin	T45.1X1	T45.1X2	T45.1X3	T45.1X4	T45.1X5	T45.1X6
Stripper (paint) (solvent)	T52.8X1	T52.8X2	T52.8X3	T52.8X4	—	—
Strobane	T60.1X1	T60.1X2	T60.1X3	T60.1X4	—	—
Strofantina	T46.0X1	T46.0X2	T46.0X3	T46.0X4	T46.0X5	T46.0X6
Strophanthin (g) (k)	T46.0X1	T46.0X2	T46.0X3	T46.0X4	T46.0X5	T46.0X6
Strophanthus	T46.0X1	T46.0X2	T46.0X3	T46.0X4	T46.0X5	T46.0X6
Strophantin	T46.0X1	T46.0X2	T46.0X3	T46.0X4	T46.0X5	T46.0X6
Strophantin-g	T46.0X1	T46.0X2	T46.0X3	T46.0X4	T46.0X5	T46.0X6
Strychnine (nonmedicinal) (pesticide) (salts)	T65.1X1	T65.1X2	T65.1X3	T65.1X4	—	—
medicinal	T48.291	T48.292	T48.293	T48.294	T48.295	T48.296
Strychnos (ignatii) — see Strychnine						
Styramate	T42.8X1	T42.8X2	T42.8X3	T42.8X4	T42.8X5	T42.8X6
Styrene	T65.891	T65.892	T65.893	T65.894	—	—
Succinimide, antiepileptic or anticonvulsant	T42.2X1	T42.2X2	T42.2X3	T42.2X4	T42.2X5	T42.2X6
mercuric — see Mercury						
Succinylcholine	T48.1X1	T48.1X2	T48.1X3	T48.1X4	T48.1X5	T48.1X6
Succinylsulfathiazole	T37.0X1	T37.0X2	T37.0X3	T37.0X4	T37.0X5	T37.0X6
Sucralfate	T47.1X1	T47.1X2	T47.1X3	T47.1X4	T47.1X5	T47.1X6
Sucrose	T50.3X1	T50.3X2	T50.3X3	T50.3X4	T50.3X5	T50.3X6
Sufentanil	T40.4X1	T40.4X2	T40.4X3	T40.4X4	T40.4X5	T40.4X6
Sulbactam	T36.0X1	T36.0X2	T36.0X3	T36.0X4	T36.0X5	T36.0X6
Sulbenicillin	T36.0X1	T36.0X2	T36.0X3	T36.0X4	T36.0X5	T36.0X6
Sulbentine	T49.0X1	T49.0X2	T49.0X3	T49.0X4	T49.0X5	T49.0X6
Sulfacetamide	T49.0X1	T49.0X2	T49.0X3	T49.0X4	T49.0X5	T49.0X6
ophthalmic preparation	T49.5X1	T49.5X2	T49.5X3	T49.5X4	T49.5X5	T49.5X6
Sulfachlorpyridazine	T37.0X1	T37.0X2	T37.0X3	T37.0X4	T37.0X5	T37.0X6
Sulfacitine	T37.0X1	T37.0X2	T37.0X3	T37.0X4	T37.0X5	T37.0X6
Sulfadiasulfone sodium	T37.0X1	T37.0X2	T37.0X3	T37.0X4	T37.0X5	T37.0X6
Sulfadiazine	T37.0X1	T37.0X2	T37.0X3	T37.0X4	T37.0X5	T37.0X6
silver (topical)	T49.0X1	T49.0X2	T49.0X3	T49.0X4	T49.0X5	T49.0X6
Sulfadimethoxine	T37.0X1	T37.0X2	T37.0X3	T37.0X4	T37.0X5	T37.0X6
Sulfadimidine	T37.0X1	T37.0X2	T37.0X3	T37.0X4	T37.0X5	T37.0X6

◀ New   ◀░ Revised   ~~deleted~~ Deleted

Substance	Poisoning, Accidental (Unintentional)	Poisoning, Intentional Self-Harm	Poisoning, Assault	Poisoning, Undetermined	Adverse Effect	Underdosing
	External Cause (T-Code)					
Sulfadoxine	T37.0X1	T37.0X2	T37.0X3	T37.0X4	T37.0X5	T37.0X6
with pyrimethamine	T37.2X1	T37.2X2	T37.2X3	T37.2X4	T37.2X5	T37.2X6
Sulfaethidole	T37.0X1	T37.0X2	T37.0X3	T37.0X4	T37.0X5	T37.0X6
Sulfafurazole	T37.0X1	T37.0X2	T37.0X3	T37.0X4	T37.0X5	T37.0X6
Sulfaguanidine	T37.0X1	T37.0X2	T37.0X3	T37.0X4	T37.0X5	T37.0X6
Sulfalene	T37.0X1	T37.0X2	T37.0X3	T37.0X4	T37.0X5	T37.0X6
Sulfaloxate	T37.0X1	T37.0X2	T37.0X3	T37.0X4	T37.0X5	T37.0X6
Sulfaloxic acid	T37.0X1	T37.0X2	T37.0X3	T37.0X4	T37.0X5	T37.0X6
Sulfamazone	T39.2X1	T39.2X2	T39.2X3	T39.2X4	T39.2X5	T39.2X6
Sulfamerazine	T37.0X1	T37.0X2	T37.0X3	T37.0X4	T37.0X5	T37.0X6
Sulfameter	T37.0X1	T37.0X2	T37.0X3	T37.0X4	T37.0X5	T37.0X6
Sulfamethazine	T37.0X1	T37.0X2	T37.0X3	T37.0X4	T37.0X5	T37.0X6
Sulfamethizole	T37.0X1	T37.0X2	T37.0X3	T37.0X4	T37.0X5	T37.0X6
Sulfamethoxazole	T37.0X1	T37.0X2	T37.0X3	T37.0X4	T37.0X5	T37.0X6
with trimethoprim	T36.8X1	T36.8X2	T36.8X3	T36.8X4	T36.8X5	T36.8X6
Sulfamethoxydiazine	T37.0X1	T37.0X2	T37.0X3	T37.0X4	T37.0X5	T37.0X6
Sulfamethoxypyridazine	T37.0X1	T37.0X2	T37.0X3	T37.0X4	T37.0X5	T37.0X6
Sulfamethylthiazole	T37.0X1	T37.0X2	T37.0X3	T37.0X4	T37.0X5	T37.0X6
Sulfametoxydiazine	T37.0X1	T37.0X2	T37.0X3	T37.0X4	T37.0X5	T37.0X6
Sulfamidopyrine	T39.2X1	T39.2X2	T39.2X3	T39.2X4	T39.2X5	T39.2X6
Sulfamonomethoxine	T37.0X1	T37.0X2	T37.0X3	T37.0X4	T37.0X5	T37.0X6
Sulfamoxole	T37.0X1	T37.0X2	T37.0X3	T37.0X4	T37.0X5	T37.0X6
Sulfamylon	T49.0X1	T49.0X2	T49.0X3	T49.0X4	T49.0X5	T49.0X6
Sulfan blue (diagnostic dye)	T50.8X1	T50.8X2	T50.8X3	T50.8X4	T50.8X5	T50.8X6
Sulfanilamide	T37.0X1	T37.0X2	T37.0X3	T37.0X4	T37.0X5	T37.0X6
Sulfanilylguanidine	T37.0X1	T37.0X2	T37.0X3	T37.0X4	T37.0X5	T37.0X6
Sulfaperin	T37.0X1	T37.0X2	T37.0X3	T37.0X4	T37.0X5	T37.0X6
Sulfaphenazole	T37.0X1	T37.0X2	T37.0X3	T37.0X4	T37.0X5	T37.0X6
Sulfaphenylthiazole	T37.0X1	T37.0X2	T37.0X3	T37.0X4	T37.0X5	T37.0X6
Sulfaproxyline	T37.0X1	T37.0X2	T37.0X3	T37.0X4	T37.0X5	T37.0X6
Sulfapyridine	T37.0X1	T37.0X2	T37.0X3	T37.0X4	T37.0X5	T37.0X6
Sulfapyrimidine	T37.0X1	T37.0X2	T37.0X3	T37.0X4	T37.0X5	T37.0X6
Sulfarsphenamine	T37.8X1	T37.8X2	T37.8X3	T37.8X4	T37.8X5	T37.8X6
Sulfasalazine	T37.0X1	T37.0X2	T37.0X3	T37.0X4	T37.0X5	T37.0X6
Sulfasuxidine	T37.0X1	T37.0X2	T37.0X3	T37.0X4	T37.0X5	T37.0X6
Sulfasymazine	T37.0X1	T37.0X2	T37.0X3	T37.0X4	T37.0X5	T37.0X6
Sulfated amylopectin	T47.8X1	T47.8X2	T47.8X3	T47.8X4	T47.8X5	T47.8X6
Sulfathiazole	T37.0X1	T37.0X2	T37.0X3	T37.0X4	T37.0X5	T37.0X6
Sulfatostearate	T49.2X1	T49.2X2	T49.2X3	T49.2X4	T49.2X5	T49.2X6

◀ New ◀▥ Revised ~~deleted~~ Deleted

Substance	External Cause (T-Code)					
	Poisoning, Accidental (Unintentional)	Poisoning, Intentional Self-Harm	Poisoning, Assault	Poisoning, Undetermined	Adverse Effect	Underdosing
Sulfinpyrazone	T50.4X1	T50.4X2	T50.4X3	T50.4X4	T50.4X5	T50.4X6
Sulfiram	T49.0X1	T49.0X2	T49.0X3	T49.0X4	T49.0X5	T49.0X6
Sulfisomidine	T37.0X1	T37.0X2	T37.0X3	T37.0X4	T37.0X5	T37.0X6
Sulfisoxazole	T37.0X1	T37.0X2	T37.0X3	T37.0X4	T37.0X5	T37.0X6
ophthalmic preparation	T49.5X1	T49.5X2	T49.5X3	T49.5X4	T49.5X5	T49.5X6
Sulfobromophthalein (sodium)	T50.8X1	T50.8X2	T50.8X3	T50.8X4	T50.8X5	T50.8X6
Sulfobromphthalein	T50.8X1	T50.8X2	T50.8X3	T50.8X4	T50.8X5	T50.8X6
Sulfogaiacol	T48.4X1	T48.4X2	T48.4X3	T48.4X4	T48.4X5	T48.4X6
Sulfomyxin	T36.8X1	T36.8X2	T36.8X3	T36.8X4	T36.8X5	T36.8X6
Sulfonal	T42.6X1	T42.6X2	T42.6X3	T42.6X4	T42.6X5	T42.6X6
Sulfonamide NEC	T37.0X1	T37.0X2	T37.0X3	T37.0X4	T37.0X5	T37.0X6
eye	T49.5X1	T49.5X2	T49.5X3	T49.5X4	T49.5X5	T49.5X6
Sulfonazide	T37.1X1	T37.1X2	T37.1X3	T37.1X4	T37.1X5	T37.1X6
Sulfones	T37.1X1	T37.1X2	T37.1X3	T37.1X4	T37.1X5	T37.1X6
Sulfonethylmethane	T42.6X1	T42.6X2	T42.6X3	T42.6X4	T42.6X5	T42.6X6
Sulfonmethane	T42.6X1	T42.6X2	T42.6X3	T42.6X4	T42.6X5	T42.6X6
Sulfonphthal, sulfonphthol	T50.8X1	T50.8X2	T50.8X3	T50.8X4	T50.8X5	T50.8X6
Sulfonylurea derivatives, oral	T38.3X1	T38.3X2	T38.3X3	T38.3X4	T38.3X5	T38.3X6
Sulforidazine	T43.3X1	T43.3X2	T43.3X3	T43.3X4	T43.3X5	T43.3X6
Sulfoxone	T37.1X1	T37.1X2	T37.1X3	T37.1X4	T37.1X5	T37.1X6
Sulfur, sulfurated, sulfuric, sulfurous, sulfuryl (compounds NEC) (medicinal)	T49.4X1	T49.4X2	T49.4X3	T49.4X4	T49.4X5	T49.4X6
acid	T54.2X1	T54.2X2	T54.2X3	T54.2X4	—	—
dioxide (gas)	T59.1X1	T59.1X2	T59.1X3	T59.1X4	—	—
ether — see Ether(s)						
hydrogen	T59.6X1	T59.6X2	T59.6X3	T59.6X4	—	—
medicinal (keratolytic) (ointment) NEC	T49.4X1	T49.4X2	T49.4X3	T49.4X4	T49.4X5	T49.4X6
ointment	T49.0X1	T49.0X2	T49.0X3	T49.0X4	T49.0X5	T49.0X6
pesticide (vapor)	T60.91	T60.92	T60.93	T60.94	—	—
vapor NEC	T59.891	T59.892	T59.893	T59.894	—	—
Sulfuric acid	T54.2X1	T54.2X2	T54.2X3	T54.2X4	—	—
Sulglicotide	T47.1X1	T47.1X2	T47.1X3	T47.1X4	T47.1X5	T47.1X6
Sulindac	T39.391	T39.392	T39.393	T39.394	T39.395	T39.396
Sulisatin	T47.2X1	T47.2X2	T47.2X3	T47.2X4	T47.2X5	T47.2X6
Sulisobenzone	T49.3X1	T49.3X2	T49.3X3	T49.3X4	T49.3X5	T49.3X6
Sulkowitch's reagent	T50.8X1	T50.8X2	T50.8X3	T50.8X4	T50.8X5	T50.8X6
Sulmetozine	T44.3X1	T44.3X2	T44.3X3	T44.3X4	T44.3X5	T44.3X6
Suloctidil	T46.7X1	T46.7X2	T46.7X3	T46.7X4	T46.7X5	T46.7X6
Sulph — see also Sulf-						
Sulphadiazine	T37.0X1	T37.0X2	T37.0X3	T37.0X4	T37.0X5	T37.0X6
Sulphadimethoxine	T37.0X1	T37.0X2	T37.0X3	T37.0X4	T37.0X5	T37.0X6

◀ New ◀▥ Revised ~~deleted~~ Deleted

Substance	Poisoning, Accidental (Unintentional)	Poisoning, Intentional Self-Harm	Poisoning, Assault	Poisoning, Undetermined	Adverse Effect	Underdosing
Sulphadimidine	T37.0X1	T37.0X2	T37.0X3	T37.0X4	T37.0X5	T37.0X6
Sulphadione	T37.1X1	T37.1X2	T37.1X3	T37.1X4	T37.1X5	T37.1X6
Sulphafurazole	T37.0X1	T37.0X2	T37.0X3	T37.0X4	T37.0X5	T37.0X6
Sulphamethizole	T37.0X1	T37.0X2	T37.0X3	T37.0X4	T37.0X5	T37.0X6
Sulphamethoxazole	T37.0X1	T37.0X2	T37.0X3	T37.0X4	T37.0X5	T37.0X6
Sulphan blue	T50.8X1	T50.8X2	T50.8X3	T50.8X4	T50.8X5	T50.8X6
Sulphaphenazole	T37.0X1	T37.0X2	T37.0X3	T37.0X4	T37.0X5	T37.0X6
Sulphapyridine	T37.0X1	T37.0X2	T37.0X3	T37.0X4	T37.0X5	T37.0X6
Sulphasalazine	T37.0X1	T37.0X2	T37.0X3	T37.0X4	T37.0X5	T37.0X6
Sulphinpyrazone	T50.4X1	T50.4X2	T50.4X3	T50.4X4	T50.4X5	T50.4X6
Sulpiride	T43.591	T43.592	T43.593	T43.594	T43.595	T43.596
Sulprostone	T48.0X1	T48.0X2	T48.0X3	T48.0X4	T48.0X5	T48.0X6
Sulpyrine	T39.2X1	T39.2X2	T39.2X3	T39.2X4	T39.2X5	T39.2X6
Sultamicillin	T36.0X1	T36.0X2	T36.0X3	T36.0X4	T36.0X5	T36.0X6
Sulthiame	T42.6X1	T42.6X2	T42.6X3	T42.6X4	T42.6X5	T42.6X6
Sultiame	T42.6X1	T42.6X2	T42.6X3	T42.6X4	T42.6X5	T42.6X6
Sultopride	T43.591	T43.592	T43.593	T43.594	T43.595	T43.596
Sumatriptan	T39.8X1	T39.8X2	T39.8X3	T39.8X4	T39.8X5	T39.8X6
Sunflower seed oil	T46.6X1	T46.6X2	T46.6X3	T46.6X4	T46.6X5	T46.6X6
Superinone	T48.4X1	T48.4X2	T48.4X3	T48.4X4	T48.4X5	T48.4X6
Suprofen	T39.311	T39.312	T39.313	T39.314	T39.315	T39.316
Suramin (sodium)	T37.4X1	T37.4X2	T37.4X3	T37.4X4	T37.4X5	T37.4X6
Surfacaine	T41.3X1	T41.3X2	T41.3X3	T41.3X4	T41.3X5	T41.3X6
Surital	T41.1X1	T41.1X2	T41.1X3	T41.1X4	T41.1X5	T41.1X6
Sutilains	T45.3X1	T45.3X2	T45.3X3	T45.3X4	T45.3X5	T45.3X6
Suxamethonium (chloride)	T48.1X1	T48.1X2	T48.1X3	T48.1X4	T48.1X5	T48.1X6
Suxethonium (chloride)	T48.1X1	T48.1X2	T48.1X3	T48.1X4	T48.1X5	T48.1X6
Suxibuzone	T39.2X1	T39.2X2	T39.2X3	T39.2X4	T39.2X5	T39.2X6
Sweet oil (birch)	T49.3X1	T49.3X2	T49.3X3	T49.3X4	T49.3X5	T49.3X6
Sweet niter spirit	T46.3X1	T46.3X2	T46.3X3	T46.3X4	T46.3X5	T46.3X6
Sweetener	T50.901	T50.902	T50.903	T50.904	T50.905	T50.906
Sym-dichloroethyl ether	T53.6X1	T53.6X2	T53.6X3	T53.6X4	—	—
Sympatholytic NEC	T44.8X1	T44.8X2	T44.8X3	T44.8X4	T44.8X5	T44.8X6
haloalkylamine	T44.8X1	T44.8X2	T44.8X3	T44.8X4	T44.8X5	T44.8X6
Sympathomimetic NEC	T44.901	T44.902	T44.903	T44.904	T44.905	T44.906
anti-common-cold	T48.5X1	T48.5X2	T48.5X3	T48.5X4	T48.5X5	T48.5X6
bronchodilator	T48.6X1	T48.6X2	T48.6X3	T48.6X4	T48.6X5	T48.6X6
specified NEC	T44.991	T44.992	T44.993	T44.994	T44.995	T44.996
Synagis	T50.B91	T50.B92	T50.B93	T50.B94	T50.B95	T50.B96
Synalar	T49.0X1	T49.0X2	T49.0X3	T49.0X4	T49.0X5	T49.0X6

TABLE OF DRUGS AND CHEMICALS

◀ New   ◀═ Revised   ~~deleted~~ Deleted

Substance	Poisoning, Accidental (Unintentional)	Poisoning, Intentional Self-Harm	Poisoning, Assault	Poisoning, Undetermined	Adverse Effect	Underdosing
			External Cause (T-Code)			
Synthroid	T38.1X1	T38.1X2	T38.1X3	T38.1X4	T38.1X5	T38.1X6
Syntocinon	T48.0X1	T48.0X2	T48.0X3	T48.0X4	T48.0X5	T48.0X6
Syrosingopine	T46.5X1	T46.5X2	T46.5X3	T46.5X4	T46.5X5	T46.5X6
Systemic drug	T45.91	T45.92	T45.93	T45.94	T45.95	T45.96
specified NEC	T45.8X1	T45.8X2	T45.8X3	T45.8X4	T45.8X5	T45.8X6
2,4,5-T	T60.3X1	T60.3X2	T60.3X3	T60.3X4	—	—
T						
Tablets — *see also specified substance*	T50.901	T50.902	T50.903	T50.904	T50.905	T50.906
Tace	T38.5X1	T38.5X2	T38.5X3	T38.5X4	T38.5X5	T38.5X6
Tacrine	T44.0X1	T44.0X2	T44.0X3	T44.0X4	T44.0X5	T44.0X6
Tadalafil	T46.7X1	T46.7X2	T46.7X3	T46.7X4	T46.7X5	T46.7X6
Talampicillin	T36.0X1	T36.0X2	T36.0X3	T36.0X4	T36.0X5	T36.0X6
Talbutal	T42.3X1	T42.3X2	T42.3X3	T42.3X4	T42.3X5	T42.3X6
Talc powder	T49.3X1	T49.3X2	T49.3X3	T49.3X4	T49.3X5	T49.3X6
Talcum	T49.3X1	T49.3X2	T49.3X3	T49.3X4	T49.3X5	T49.3X6
Taleranol	T38.6X1	T38.6X2	T38.6X3	T38.6X4	T38.6X5	T38.6X6
Tamoxifen	T38.6X1	T38.6X2	T38.6X3	T38.6X4	T38.6X5	T38.6X6
Tamsulosin	T44.6X1	T44.6X2	T44.6X3	T44.6X4	T44.6X5	T44.6X6
Tandearil, tanderil	T39.2X1	T39.2X2	T39.2X3	T39.2X4	T39.2X5	T39.2X6
Tannic acid	T49.2X1	T49.2X2	T49.2X3	T49.2X4	T49.2X5	T49.2X6
medicinal (astringent)	T49.2X1	T49.2X2	T49.2X3	T49.2X4	T49.2X5	T49.2X6
Tannin — *see Tannic acid*						
Tansy	T62.2X1	T62.2X2	T62.2X3	T62.2X4	—	—
TAO	T36.3X1	T36.3X2	T36.3X3	T36.3X4	T36.3X5	T36.3X6
Tapazole	T38.2X1	T38.2X2	T38.2X3	T38.2X4	T38.2X5	T38.2X6
Tar NEC	T52.0X1	T52.0X2	T52.0X3	T52.0X4	—	—
camphor	T60.1X1	T60.1X2	T60.1X3	T60.1X4	—	—
distillate	T49.1X1	T49.1X2	T49.1X3	T49.1X4	T49.1X5	T49.1X6
fumes	T59.891	T59.892	T59.893	T59.894	—	—
medicinal	T49.1X1	T49.1X2	T49.1X3	T49.1X4	T49.1X5	T49.1X6
ointment	T49.1X1	T49.1X2	T49.1X3	T49.1X4	T49.1X5	T49.1X6
Taractan	T43.591	T43.592	T43.593	T43.594	T43.595	T43.596
Tarantula (venomous)	T63.321	T63.322	T63.323	T63.324	—	—
Tartar emetic	T37.8X1	T37.8X2	T37.8X3	T37.8X4	T37.8X5	T37.8X6
Tartaric acid	T65.891	T65.892	T65.893	T65.894	—	—
Tartrated antimony (anti-infective)	T37.8X1	T37.8X2	T37.8X3	T37.8X4	T37.8X5	T37.8X6
Tartrate, laxative	T47.4X1	T47.4X2	T47.4X3	T47.4X4	T47.4X5	T47.4X6
Tauromustine	T45.1X1	T45.1X2	T45.1X3	T45.1X4	T45.1X5	T45.1X6
TCA — *see Trichloroacetic acid*						

◀ New ◀▦ Revised ~~deleted~~ Deleted

Substance	Poisoning, Accidental (Unintentional)	Poisoning, Intentional Self-Harm	Poisoning, Assault	Poisoning, Undetermined	Adverse Effect	Underdosing
	External Cause (T-Code)					
TCDD	T53.7X1	T53.7X2	T53.7X3	T53.7X4	—	—
TDI (vapor)	T65.0X1	T65.0X2	T65.0X3	T65.0X4	—	—
Tear						
gas	T59.3X1	T59.3X2	T59.3X3	T59.3X4	—	—
solution	T49.5X1	T49.5X2	T49.5X3	T49.5X4	T49.5X5	T49.5X6
Teclothiazide	T50.2X1	T50.2X2	T50.2X3	T50.2X4	T50.2X5	T50.2X6
Teclozan	T37.3X1	T37.3X2	T37.3X3	T37.3X4	T37.3X5	T37.3X6
Tegafur	T45.1X1	T45.1X2	T45.1X3	T45.1X4	T45.1X5	T45.1X6
Tegretol	T42.1X1	T42.1X2	T42.1X3	T42.1X4	T42.1X5	T42.1X6
Teicoplanin	T36.8X1	T36.8X2	T36.8X3	T36.8X4	T36.8X5	T36.8X6
Telepaque	T50.8X1	T50.8X2	T50.8X3	T50.8X4	T50.8X5	T50.8X6
Tellurium	T56.891	T56.892	T56.893	T56.894	—	—
fumes	T56.891	T56.892	T56.893	T56.894	—	—
TEM	T45.1X1	T45.1X2	T45.1X3	T45.1X4	T45.1X5	T45.1X6
Temazepam	T42.4X1	T42.4X2	T42.4X3	T42.4X4	T42.4X5	T42.4X6
Temocillin	T36.0X1	T36.0X2	T36.0X3	T36.0X4	T36.0X5	T36.0X6
Tenamfetamine	T43.621	T43.622	T43.623	T43.624	T43.625	T43.626
Teniposide	T45.1X1	T45.1X2	T45.1X3	T45.1X4	T45.1X5	T45.1X6
Tenitramine	T46.3X1	T46.3X2	T46.3X3	T46.3X4	T46.3X5	T46.3X6
Tenoglicin	T48.4X1	T48.4X2	T48.4X3	T48.4X4	T48.4X5	T48.4X6
Tenonitrozole	T37.3X1	T37.3X2	T37.3X3	T37.3X4	T37.3X5	T37.3X6
Tenoxicam	T39.391	T39.392	T39.393	T39.394	T39.395	T39.396
TEPA	T45.1X1	T45.1X2	T45.1X3	T45.1X4	T45.1X5	T45.1X6
TEPP	T60.0X1	T60.0X2	T60.0X3	T60.0X4	—	—
Teprotide	T46.5X1	T46.5X2	T46.5X3	T46.5X4	T46.5X5	T46.5X6
Terazosin	T44.6X1	T44.6X2	T44.6X3	T44.6X4	T44.6X5	T44.6X6
Terbufos	T60.0X1	T60.0X2	T60.0X3	T60.0X4	—	—
Terbutaline	T48.6X1	T48.6X2	T48.6X3	T48.6X4	T48.6X5	T48.6X6
Terconazole	T49.0X1	T49.0X2	T49.0X3	T49.0X4	T49.0X5	T49.0X6
Terfenadine	T45.0X1	T45.0X2	T45.0X3	T45.0X4	T45.0X5	T45.0X6
Teriparatide (acetate)	T50.991	T50.992	T50.993	T50.994	T50.995	T50.996
Terizidone	T37.1X1	T37.1X2	T37.1X3	T37.1X4	T37.1X5	T37.1X6
Terlipressin	T38.891	T38.892	T38.893	T38.894	T38.895	T38.896
Terodiline	T46.3X1	T46.3X2	T46.3X3	T46.3X4	T46.3X5	T46.3X6
Teroxalene	T37.4X1	T37.4X2	T37.4X3	T37.4X4	T37.4X5	T37.4X6
Terpin(cis) hydrate	T48.4X1	T48.4X2	T48.4X3	T48.4X4	T48.4X5	T48.4X6
Terramycin	T36.4X1	T36.4X2	T36.4X3	T36.4X4	T36.4X5	T36.4X6
Tertatolol	T44.7X1	T44.7X2	T44.7X3	T44.7X4	T44.7X5	T44.7X6
Tessalon	T48.3X1	T48.3X2	T48.3X3	T48.3X4	T48.3X5	T48.3X6
Testolactone	T38.7X1	T38.7X2	T38.7X3	T38.7X4	T38.7X5	T38.7X6

Substance	External Cause (T-Code)					
	Poisoning, Accidental (Unintentional)	Poisoning, Intentional Self-Harm	Poisoning, Assault	Poisoning, Undetermined	Adverse Effect	Underdosing
Testosterone	T38.7X1	T38.7X2	T38.7X3	T38.7X4	T38.7X5	T38.7X6
Tetanus toxoid or vaccine	T50.A91	T50.A92	T50.A93	T50.A94	T50.A95	T50.A96
antitoxin	T50.Z11	T50.Z12	T50.Z13	T50.Z14	T50.Z15	T50.Z16
immune globulin (human)	T50.Z11	T50.Z12	T50.Z13	T50.Z14	T50.Z15	T50.Z16
toxoid	T50.A91	T50.A92	T50.A93	T50.A94	T50.A95	T50.A96
with diphtheria toxoid	T50.A21	T50.A22	T50.A23	T50.A24	T50.A25	T50.A26
with pertussis	T50.A11	T50.A12	T50.A13	T50.A14	T50.A15	T50.A16
Tetrabenazine	T43.591	T43.592	T43.593	T43.594	T43.595	T43.596
Tetracaine	T41.3X1	T41.3X2	T41.3X3	T41.3X4	T41.3X5	T41.3X6
nerve block (peripheral) (plexus)	T41.3X1	T41.3X2	T41.3X3	T41.3X4	T41.3X5	T41.3X6
regional	T41.3X1	T41.3X2	T41.3X3	T41.3X4	T41.3X5	T41.3X6
spinal	T41.3X1	T41.3X2	T41.3X3	T41.3X4	T41.3X5	T41.3X6
Tetrachlorethylene — see Tetrachloroethylene						
Tetrachlormethiazide	T50.2X1	T50.2X2	T50.2X3	T50.2X4	T50.2X5	T50.2X6
2,3,7,8-Tetrachlorodibenzo-p-dioxin	T53.7X1	T53.7X2	T53.7X3	T53.7X4	—	—
Tetrachloroethane	T53.6X1	T53.6X2	T53.6X3	T53.6X4	—	—
vapor	T53.6X1	T53.6X2	T53.6X3	T53.6X4	—	—
paint or varnish	T53.6X1	T53.6X2	T53.6X3	T53.6X4	—	—
Tetrachloroethylene (liquid)	T53.3X1	T53.3X2	T53.3X3	T53.3X4		
medicinal	T37.4X1	T37.4X2	T37.4X3	T37.4X4	T37.4X5	T37.4X6
vapor	T53.3X1	T53.3X2	T53.3X3	T53.3X4	—	—
Tetrachloromethane — see Carbon tetrachloride						
Tetracosactide	T38.811	T38.812	T38.813	T38.814	T38.815	T38.816
Tetracosactrin	T38.811	T38.812	T38.813	T38.814	T38.815	T38.816
Tetracycline	T36.4X1	T36.4X2	T36.4X3	T36.4X4	T36.4X5	T36.4X6
ophthalmic preparation	T49.5X1	T49.5X2	T49.5X3	T49.5X4	T49.5X5	T49.5X6
topical NEC	T49.0X1	T49.0X2	T49.0X3	T49.0X4	T49.0X5	T49.0X6
Tetradifon	T60.8X1	T60.8X2	T60.8X3	T60.8X4	—	—
Tetradotoxin	T61.771	T61.772	T61.773	T61.774	—	—
Tetraethyl						
lead	T56.0X1	T56.0X2	T56.0X3	T56.0X4	—	—
pyrophosphate	T60.0X1	T60.0X2	T60.0X3	T60.0X4	—	—
Tetraethylammonium chloride	T44.2X1	T44.2X2	T44.2X3	T44.2X4	T44.2X5	T44.2X6
Tetraethylthiuram disulfide	T50.6X1	T50.6X2	T50.6X3	T50.6X4	T50.6X5	T50.6X6
Tetrahydroaminoacridine	T44.0X1	T44.0X2	T44.0X3	T44.0X4	T44.0X5	T44.0X6
Tetrahydrocannabinol	T40.7X1	T40.7X2	T40.7X3	T40.7X4	T40.7X5	T40.7X6
Tetrahydrofuran	T52.8X1	T52.8X2	T52.8X3	T52.8X4	—	—
Tetrahydronaphthalene	T52.8X1	T52.8X2	T52.8X3	T52.8X4	—	—
Tetrahydrozoline	T49.5X1	T49.5X2	T49.5X3	T49.5X4	T49.5X5	T49.5X6
Tetralin	T52.8X1	T52.8X2	T52.8X3	T52.8X4	—	—

◀ New   ◀▥ Revised   ~~deleted~~ Deleted

Substance	Poisoning, Accidental (Unintentional)	Poisoning, Intentional Self-Harm	Poisoning, Assault	Poisoning, Undetermined	Adverse Effect	Underdosing
	External Cause (T-Code)					
Tetramethrin	T60.2X1	T60.2X2	T60.2X3	T60.2X4	—	—
Tetramethylthiuram (disulfide) NEC	T60.3X1	T60.3X2	T60.3X3	T60.3X4	—	—
medicinal	T49.0X1	T49.0X2	T49.0X3	T49.0X4	T49.0X5	T49.0X6
Tetramisole	T37.4X1	T37.4X2	T37.4X3	T37.4X4	T37.4X5	T37.4X6
Tetranicotinoyl fructose	T46.7X1	T46.7X2	T46.7X3	T46.7X4	T46.7X5	T46.7X6
Tetronal	T42.6X1	T42.6X2	T42.6X3	T42.6X4	T42.6X5	T42.6X6
Tetrazepam	T42.4X1	T42.4X2	T42.4X3	T42.4X4	T42.4X5	T42.4X6
Tetryl	T65.3X1	T65.3X2	T65.3X3	T65.3X4	—	—
Tetrylammonium chloride	T44.2X1	T44.2X2	T44.2X3	T44.2X4	T44.2X5	T44.2X6
Tetryzoline	T49.5X1	T49.5X2	T49.5X3	T49.5X4	T49.5X5	T49.5X6
Thalidomide	T45.1X1	T45.1X2	T45.1X3	T45.1X4	T45.1X5	T45.1X6
Thallium (compounds) (dust) NEC	T56.811	T56.812	T56.813	T56.814	—	—
pesticide	T60.4X1	T60.4X2	T60.4X3	T60.4X4	—	—
THC	T40.7X1	T40.7X2	T40.7X3	T40.7X4	T40.7X5	T40.7X6
Thebacon	T48.3X1	T48.3X2	T48.3X3	T48.3X4	T48.3X5	T48.3X6
Thebaine	T40.2X1	T40.2X2	T40.2X3	T40.2X4	T40.2X5	T40.2X6
Thenoic acid	T49.6X1	T49.6X2	T49.6X3	T49.6X4	T49.6X5	T49.6X6
Thenyldiamine	T45.0X1	T45.0X2	T45.0X3	T45.0X4	T45.0X5	T45.0X6
Theobromine (calcium salicylate)	T48.6X1	T48.6X2	T48.6X3	T48.6X4	T48.6X5	T48.6X6
sodium salicylate	T48.6X1	T48.6X2	T48.6X3	T48.6X4	T48.6X5	T48.6X6
Theophyllamine	T48.6X1	T48.6X2	T48.6X3	T48.6X4	T48.6X5	T48.6X6
Theophylline	T48.6X1	T48.6X2	T48.6X3	T48.6X4	T48.6X5	T48.6X6
aminobenzoic acid	T48.6X1	T48.6X2	T48.6X3	T48.6X4	T48.6X5	T48.6X6
ethylenediamine	T48.6X1	T48.6X2	T48.6X3	T48.6X4	T48.6X5	T48.6X6
piperazine p-amino-benzoate	T48.6X1	T48.6X2	T48.6X3	T48.6X4	T48.6X5	T48.6X6
Thiabendazole	T37.4X1	T37.4X2	T37.4X3	T37.4X4	T37.4X5	T37.4X6
Thialbarbital	T41.1X1	T41.1X2	T41.1X3	T41.1X4	T41.1X5	T41.1X6
Thiamazole	T38.2X1	T38.2X2	T38.2X3	T38.2X4	T38.2X5	T38.2X6
Thiambutosine	T37.1X1	T37.1X2	T37.1X3	T37.1X4	T37.1X5	T37.1X6
Thiamine	T45.2X1	T45.2X2	T45.2X3	T45.2X4	T45.2X5	T45.2X6
Thiamphenicol	T36.2X1	T36.2X2	T36.2X3	T36.2X4	T36.2X5	T36.2X6
Thiamylal	T41.1X1	T41.1X2	T41.1X3	T41.1X4	T41.1X5	T41.1X6
sodium	T41.1X1	T41.1X2	T41.1X3	T41.1X4	T41.1X5	T41.1X6
Thiazesim	T43.291	T43.292	T43.293	T43.294	T43.295	T43.296
Thiazides (diuretics)	T50.2X1	T50.2X2	T50.2X3	T50.2X4	T50.2X5	T50.2X6
Thiazinamium metilsulfate	T43.3X1	T43.3X2	T43.3X3	T43.3X4	T43.3X5	T43.3X6
Thiethylperazine	T43.3X1	T43.3X2	T43.3X3	T43.3X4	T43.3X5	T43.3X6
Thimerosal	T49.0X1	T49.0X2	T49.0X3	T49.0X4	T49.0X5	T49.0X6
ophthalmic preparation	T49.5X1	T49.5X2	T49.5X3	T49.5X4	T49.5X5	T49.5X6

◀ New   ◀▥ Revised   ~~deleted~~ Deleted

Substance	External Cause (T-Code)					
	Poisoning, Accidental (Unintentional)	Poisoning, Intentional Self-Harm	Poisoning, Assault	Poisoning, Undetermined	Adverse Effect	Underdosing
Thioacetazone	T37.1X1	T37.1X2	T37.1X3	T37.1X4	T37.1X5	T37.1X6
with isoniazid	T37.1X1	T37.1X2	T37.1X3	T37.1X4	T37.1X5	T37.1X6
Thiobarbital sodium	T41.1X1	T41.1X2	T41.1X3	T41.1X4	T41.1X5	T41.1X6
Thiobarbiturate anesthetic	T41.1X1	T41.1X2	T41.1X3	T41.1X4	T41.1X5	T41.1X6
Thiobismol	T37.8X1	T37.8X2	T37.8X3	T37.8X4	T37.8X5	T37.8X6
Thiobutabarbital sodium	T41.1X1	T41.1X2	T41.1X3	T41.1X4	T41.1X5	T41.1X6
Thiocarbamate (insecticide)	T60.0X1	T60.0X2	T60.0X3	T60.0X4	—	—
Thiocarbamide	T38.2X1	T38.2X2	T38.2X3	T38.2X4	T38.2X5	T38.2X6
Thiocarbarsone	T37.8X1	T37.8X2	T37.8X3	T37.8X4	T37.8X5	T37.8X6
Thiocarlide	T37.1X1	T37.1X2	T37.1X3	T37.1X4	T37.1X5	T37.1X6
Thioctamide	T50.991	T50.992	T50.993	T50.994	T50.995	T50.996
Thioctic acid	T50.991	T50.992	T50.993	T50.994	T50.995	T50.996
Thiofos	T60.0X1	T60.0X2	T60.0X3	T60.0X4	—	—
Thioglycolate	T49.4X1	T49.4X2	T49.4X3	T49.4X4	T49.4X5	T49.4X6
Thioglycolic acid	T65.891	T65.892	T65.893	T65.894	—	—
Thioguanine	T45.1X1	T45.1X2	T45.1X3	T45.1X4	T45.1X5	T45.1X6
Thiomercaptomerin	T50.2X1	T50.2X2	T50.2X3	T50.2X4	T50.2X5	T50.2X6
Thiomerin	T50.2X1	T50.2X2	T50.2X3	T50.2X4	T50.2X5	T50.2X6
Thiomersal	T49.0X1	T49.0X2	T49.0X3	T49.0X4	T49.0X5	T49.0X6
Thionazin	T60.0X1	T60.0X2	T60.0X3	T60.0X4	—	—
Thiopental (sodium)	T41.1X1	T41.1X2	T41.1X3	T41.1X4	T41.1X5	T41.1X6
Thiopentone (sodium)	T41.1X1	T41.1X2	T41.1X3	T41.1X4	T41.1X5	T41.1X6
Thiopropazate	T43.3X1	T43.3X2	T43.3X3	T43.3X4	T43.3X5	T43.3X6
Thioproperazine	T43.3X1	T43.3X2	T43.3X3	T43.3X4	T43.3X5	T43.3X6
Thioridazine	T43.3X1	T43.3X2	T43.3X3	T43.3X4	T43.3X5	T43.3X6
Thiosinamine	T49.3X1	T49.3X2	T49.3X3	T49.3X4	T49.3X5	T49.3X6
Thiotepa	T45.1X1	T45.1X2	T45.1X3	T45.1X4	T45.1X5	T45.1X6
Thiothixene	T43.4X1	T43.4X2	T43.4X3	T43.4X4	T43.4X5	T43.4X6
Thiouracil (benzyl) (methyl) (propyl)	T38.2X1	T38.2X2	T38.2X3	T38.2X4	T38.2X5	T38.2X6
Thiourea	T38.2X1	T38.2X2	T38.2X3	T38.2X4	T38.2X5	T38.2X6
Thiphenamil	T44.3X1	T44.3X2	T44.3X3	T44.3X4	T44.3X5	T44.3X6
Thiram	T60.3X1	T60.3X2	T60.3X3	T60.3X4	—	—
medicinal	T49.2X1	T49.2X2	T49.2X3	T49.2X4	T49.2X5	T49.2X6
Thonzylamine (systemic)	T45.0X1	T45.0X2	T45.0X3	T45.0X4	T45.0X5	T45.0X6
mucosal decongestant	T48.5X1	T48.5X2	T48.5X3	T48.5X4	T48.5X5	T48.5X6
Thorazine	T43.3X1	T43.3X2	T43.3X3	T43.3X4	T43.3X5	T43.3X6
Thorium dioxide suspension	T50.8X1	T50.8X2	T50.8X3	T50.8X4	T50.8X5	T50.8X6
Thornapple	T62.2X1	T62.2X2	T62.2X3	T62.2X4	—	—
Throat drug NEC	T49.6X1	T49.6X2	T49.6X3	T49.6X4	T49.6X5	T49.6X6
Thrombin	T45.7X1	T45.7X2	T45.7X3	T45.7X4	T45.7X5	T45.7X6

◀ New   ⬅ Revised   ~~deleted~~ Deleted

Substance	Poisoning, Accidental (Unintentional)	Poisoning, Intentional Self-Harm	Poisoning, Assault	Poisoning, Undetermined	Adverse Effect	Underdosing
	External Cause (T-Code)					
Thrombolysin	T45.611	T45.612	T45.613	T45.614	T45.615	T45.616
Thromboplastin	T45.7X1	T45.7X2	T45.7X3	T45.7X4	T45.7X5	T45.7X6
Thurfyl nicotinate	T46.7X1	T46.7X2	T46.7X3	T46.7X4	T46.7X5	T46.7X6
Thymol	T49.0X1	T49.0X2	T49.0X3	T49.0X4	T49.0X5	T49.0X6
Thymopentin	T37.5X1	T37.5X2	T37.5X3	T37.5X4	T37.5X5	T37.5X6
Thymoxamine	T46.7X1	T46.7X2	T46.7X3	T46.7X4	T46.7X5	T46.7X6
Thymus extract	T38.891	T38.892	T38.893	T38.894	T38.895	T38.896
Thyreotrophic hormone	T38.811	T38.812	T38.813	T38.814	T38.815	T38.816
Thyroglobulin	T38.1X1	T38.1X2	T38.1X3	T38.1X4	T38.1X5	T38.1X6
Thyroid (hormone)	T38.1X1	T38.1X2	T38.1X3	T38.1X4	T38.1X5	T38.1X6
Thyrolar	T38.1X1	T38.1X2	T38.1X3	T38.1X4	T38.1X5	T38.1X6
Thyrotrophin	T38.811	T38.812	T38.813	T38.814	T38.815	T38.816
Thyrotropic hormone	T38.811	T38.812	T38.813	T38.814	T38.815	T38.816
Thyroxine	T38.1X1	T38.1X2	T38.1X3	T38.1X4	T38.1X5	T38.1X6
Tiabendazole	T37.4X1	T37.4X2	T37.4X3	T37.4X4	T37.4X5	T37.4X6
Tiamizide	T50.2X1	T50.2X2	T50.2X3	T50.2X4	T50.2X5	T50.2X6
Tianeptine	T43.291	T43.292	T43.293	T43.294	T43.295	T43.296
Tiapamil	T46.1X1	T46.1X2	T46.1X3	T46.1X4	T46.1X5	T46.1X6
Tiapride	T43.591	T43.592	T43.593	T43.594	T43.595	T43.596
Tiaprofenic acid	T39.311	T39.312	T39.313	T39.314	T39.315	T39.316
Tiaramide	T39.8X1	T39.8X2	T39.8X3	T39.8X4	T39.8X5	T39.8X6
Ticarcillin	T36.0X1	T36.0X2	T36.0X3	T36.0X4	T36.0X5	T36.0X6
Ticlatone	T49.0X1	T49.0X2	T49.0X3	T49.0X4	T49.0X5	T49.0X6
Ticlopidine	T45.521	T45.522	T45.523	T45.524	T45.525	T45.526
Ticrynafen	T50.1X1	T50.1X2	T50.1X3	T50.1X4	T50.1X5	T50.1X6
Tidiacic	T50.991	T50.992	T50.993	T50.994	T50.995	T50.996
Tiemonium	T44.3X1	T44.3X2	T44.3X3	T44.3X4	T44.3X5	T44.3X6
iodide	T44.3X1	T44.3X2	T44.3X3	T44.3X4	T44.3X5	T44.3X6
Tienilic acid	T50.1X1	T50.1X2	T50.1X3	T50.1X4	T50.1X5	T50.1X6
Tifenamil	T44.3X1	T44.3X2	T44.3X3	T44.3X4	T44.3X5	T44.3X6
Tigan	T45.0X1	T45.0X2	T45.0X3	T45.0X4	T45.0X5	T45.0X6
Tigloidine	T44.3X1	T44.3X2	T44.3X3	T44.3X4	T44.3X5	T44.3X6
Tilactase	T47.5X1	T47.5X2	T47.5X3	T47.5X4	T47.5X5	T47.5X6
Tiletamine	T41.291	T41.292	T41.293	T41.294	T41.295	T41.296
Tilidine	T40.4X1	T40.4X2	T40.4X3	T40.4X4	—	—
Timepidium bromide	T44.3X1	T44.3X2	T44.3X3	T44.3X4	T44.3X5	T44.3X6
Timiperone	T43.4X1	T43.4X2	T43.4X3	T43.4X4	T43.4X5	T43.4X6
Timolol	T44.7X1	T44.7X2	T44.7X3	T44.7X4	T44.7X5	T44.7X6
Tin (chloride) (dust) (oxide) NEC	T56.6X1	T56.6X2	T56.6X3	T56.6X4	—	—
anti-infectives	T37.8X1	T37.8X2	T37.8X3	T37.8X4	T37.8X5	T37.8X6

TABLE OF DRUGS AND CHEMICALS

Substance	External Cause (T-Code)					
	Poisoning, Accidental (Unintentional)	Poisoning, Intentional Self-Harm	Poisoning, Assault	Poisoning, Undetermined	Adverse Effect	Underdosing
Tincture, iodine — *see Iodine*						
Tindal	T43.3X1	T43.3X2	T43.3X3	T43.3X4	T43.3X5	T43.3X6
Tinidazole	T37.3X1	T37.3X2	T37.3X3	T37.3X4	T37.3X5	T37.3X6
Tinoridine	T39.8X1	T39.8X2	T39.8X3	T39.8X4	T39.8X5	T39.8X6
Tiocarlide	T37.1X1	T37.1X2	T37.1X3	T37.1X4	T37.1X5	T37.1X6
Tioclomarol	T45.511	T45.512	T45.513	T45.514	T45.515	T45.516
Tioconazole	T49.0X1	T49.0X2	T49.0X3	T49.0X4	T49.0X5	T49.0X6
Tioguanine	T45.1X1	T45.1X2	T45.1X3	T45.1X4	T45.1X5	T45.1X6
Tiopronin	T50.991	T50.992	T50.993	T50.994	T50.995	T50.996
Tiotixene	T43.4X1	T43.4X2	T43.4X3	T43.4X4	T43.4X5	T43.4X6
Tioxolone	T49.4X1	T49.4X2	T49.4X3	T49.4X4	T49.4X5	T49.4X6
Tipepidine	T48.3X1	T48.3X2	T48.3X3	T48.3X4	T48.3X5	T48.3X6
Tiquizium bromide	T44.3X1	T44.3X2	T44.3X3	T44.3X4	T44.3X5	T44.3X6
Tiratricol	T38.1X1	T38.1X2	T38.1X3	T38.1X4	T38.1X5	T38.1X6
Tisopurine	T50.4X1	T50.4X2	T50.4X3	T50.4X4	T50.4X5	T50.4X6
Titanium (compounds) (vapor)	T56.891	T56.892	T56.893	T56.894	—	—
dioxide	T49.3X1	T49.3X2	T49.3X3	T49.3X4	T49.3X5	T49.3X6
ointment	T49.3X1	T49.3X2	T49.3X3	T49.3X4	T49.3X5	T49.3X6
oxide	T49.3X1	T49.3X2	T49.3X3	T49.3X4	T49.3X5	T49.3X6
tetrachloride	T56.891	T56.892	T56.893	T56.894	—	—
Titanocene	T56.891	T56.892	T56.893	T56.894	—	—
Titroid	T38.1X1	T38.1X2	T38.1X3	T38.1X4	T38.1X5	T38.1X6
Tizanidine	T42.8X1	T42.8X2	T42.8X3	T42.8X4	T42.8X5	T42.8X6
TMTD	T60.3X1	T60.3X2	T60.3X3	T60.3X4	—	—
TNT (fumes)	T65.3X1	T65.3X2	T65.3X3	T65.3X4	—	—
Toadstool	T62.0X1	T62.0X2	T62.0X3	T62.0X4	—	—
Tobacco NEC	T65.291	T65.292	T65.293	T65.294	—	—
cigarettes	T65.221	T65.222	T65.223	T65.224	—	—
Indian	T62.2X1	T62.2X2	T62.2X3	T62.2X4	—	—
smoke, second-hand	T65.221	T65.222	T65.223	T65.224	—	—
Tobramycin	T36.5X1	T36.5X2	T36.5X3	T36.5X4	T36.5X5	T36.5X6
Tocainide	T46.2X1	T46.2X2	T46.2X3	T46.2X4	T46.2X5	T46.2X6
Tocoferol	T45.2X1	T45.2X2	T45.2X3	T45.2X4	T45.2X5	T45.2X6
Tocopherol	T45.2X1	T45.2X2	T45.2X3	T45.2X4	T45.2X5	T45.2X6
acetate	T45.2X1	T45.2X2	T45.2X3	T45.2X4	T45.2X5	T45.2X6
Tocosamine	T48.0X1	T48.0X2	T48.0X3	T48.0X4	T48.0X5	T48.0X6
Todralazine	T46.5X1	T46.5X2	T46.5X3	T46.5X4	T46.5X5	T46.5X6
Tofisopam	T42.4X1	T42.4X2	T42.4X3	T42.4X4	T42.4X5	T42.4X6
Tofranil	T43.011	T43.012	T43.013	T43.014	T43.015	T43.016
Toilet deodorizer	T65.891	T65.892	T65.893	T65.894	—	—

◀ New ◀⫼ Revised ~~deleted~~ Deleted

Substance	Poisoning, Accidental (Unintentional)	Poisoning, Intentional Self-Harm	Poisoning, Assault	Poisoning, Undetermined	Adverse Effect	Underdosing
Tolamolol	T44.7X1	T44.7X2	T44.7X3	T44.7X4	T44.7X5	T44.7X6
Tolazamide	T38.3X1	T38.3X2	T38.3X3	T38.3X4	T38.3X5	T38.3X6
Tolazoline	T46.7X1	T46.7X2	T46.7X3	T46.7X4	T46.7X5	T46.7X6
Tolbutamide (sodium)	T38.3X1	T38.3X2	T38.3X3	T38.3X4	T38.3X5	T38.3X6
Tolciclate	T49.0X1	T49.0X2	T49.0X3	T49.0X4	T49.0X5	T49.0X6
Tolmetin	T39.391	T39.392	T39.393	T39.394	T39.395	T39.396
Tolnaftate	T49.0X1	T49.0X2	T49.0X3	T49.0X4	T49.0X5	T49.0X6
Tolonidine	T46.5X1	T46.5X2	T46.5X3	T46.5X4	T46.5X5	T46.5X6
Toloxatone	T42.6X1	T42.6X2	T42.6X3	T42.6X4	T42.6X5	T42.6X6
Tolperisone	T44.3X1	T44.3X2	T44.3X3	T44.3X4	T44.3X5	T44.3X6
Tolserol	T42.8X1	T42.8X2	T42.8X3	T42.8X4	T42.8X5	T42.8X6
Toluene (liquid)	T52.2X1	T52.2X2	T52.2X3	T52.2X4	—	—
diisocyanate	T65.0X1	T65.0X2	T65.0X3	T65.0X4	—	—
Toluidine	T65.891	T65.892	T65.893	T65.894	—	—
vapor	T59.891	T59.892	T59.893	T59.894	—	—
Toluol (liquid)	T52.2X1	T52.2X2	T52.2X3	T52.2X4	—	—
vapor	T52.2X1	T52.2X2	T52.2X3	T52.2X4	—	—
Toluylenediamine	T65.3X1	T65.3X2	T65.3X3	T65.3X4	—	—
Tolylene-2,4-diisocyanate	T65.0X1	T65.0X2	T65.0X3	T65.0X4	—	—
Tonic NEC	T50.901	T50.902	T50.903	T50.904	T50.905	T50.906
Topical action drug NEC	T49.91	T49.92	T49.93	T49.94	T49.95	T49.96
ear, nose or throat	T49.6X1	T49.6X2	T49.6X3	T49.6X4	T49.6X5	T49.6X6
eye	T49.5X1	T49.5X2	T49.5X3	T49.5X4	T49.5X5	T49.5X6
skin	T49.91	T49.92	T49.93	T49.94	T49.95	T49.96
specified NEC	T49.8X1	T49.8X2	T49.8X4	T49.8X4	T49.8X5	T49.8X6
Toquizine	T44.3X1	T44.3X2	T44.3X3	T44.3X4	T44.3X5	T44.3X6
Toremifene	T38.6X1	T38.6X2	T38.6X3	T38.6X4	T38.6X5	T38.6X6
Tosylchloramide sodium	T49.8X1	T49.8X2	T49.8X3	T49.8X4	T49.8X5	T49.8X6
Toxaphene (dust) (spray)	T60.1X1	T60.1X2	T60.1X3	T60.1X4	—	—
Toxin, diphtheria (Schick Test)	T50.8X1	T50.8X2	T50.8X3	T50.8X4	T50.8X5	T50.8X6
Toxoid						
combined	T50.A21	T50.A22	T50.A23	T50.A24	T50.A25	T50.A26
diphtheria	T50.A91	T50.A92	T50.A93	T50.A94	T50.A95	T50.A96
tetanus	T50.A91	T50.A92	T50.A93	T50.A94	T50.A95	T50.A96
Trace element NEC	T45.8X1	T45.8X2	T45.8X3	T45.8X4	T45.8X5	T45.8X6
Tractor fuel NEC	T52.0X1	T52.0X2	T52.0X3	T52.0X4	—	—
Tragacanth	T50.991	T50.992	T50.993	T50.994	T50.995	T50.996
Tramadol	T40.4X1	T40.4X2	T40.4X3	T40.4X4	T40.4X5	T40.4X6
Tramazoline	T48.5X1	T48.5X2	T48.5X3	T48.5X4	T48.5X5	T48.5X6
Tranexamic acid	T45.621	T45.622	T45.623	T45.624	T45.625	T45.626

◀ New   ◀▥ Revised   ~~deleted~~ Deleted

Substance	External Cause (T-Code)					
	Poisoning, Accidental (Unintentional)	Poisoning, Intentional Self-Harm	Poisoning, Assault	Poisoning, Undetermined	Adverse Effect	Underdosing
Tranilast	T45.0X1	T45.0X2	T45.0X3	T45.0X4	T45.0X5	T45.0X6
Tranquilizer NEC	T43.501	T43.502	T43.503	T43.504	T43.505	T43.506
with hypnotic or sedative	T42.6X1	T42.6X2	T42.6X3	T42.6X4	T42.6X5	T42.6X6
benzodiazepine NEC	T42.4X1	T42.4X2	T42.4X3	T42.4X4	T42.4X5	T42.4X6
butyrophenone NEC	T43.4X1	T43.4X2	T43.4X3	T43.4X4	T43.4X5	T43.4X6
carbamate	T43.591	T43.592	T43.593	T43.594	T43.595	T43.596
dimethylamine	T43.3X1	T43.3X2	T43.3X3	T43.3X4	T43.3X5	T43.3X6
ethylamine	T43.3X1	T43.3X2	T43.3X3	T43.3X4	T43.3X5	T43.3X6
hydroxyzine	T43.591	T43.592	T43.593	T43.594	T43.595	T43.596
major NEC	T43.501	T43.502	T43.503	T43.504	T43.505	T43.506
penothiazine NEC	T43.3X1	T43.3X2	T43.3X3	T43.3X4	T43.3X5	T43.3X6
phenothiazine-based	T43.3X1	T43.3X2	T43.3X3	T43.3X4	T43.3X5	T43.3X6
piperazine NEC	T43.3X1	T43.3X2	T43.3X3	T43.3X4	T43.3X5	T43.3X6
piperidine	T43.3X1	T43.3X2	T43.3X3	T43.3X4	T43.3X5	T43.3X6
propylamine	T43.3X1	T43.3X2	T43.3X3	T43.3X4	T43.3X5	T43.3X6
specified NEC	T43.591	T43.592	T43.593	T43.594	T43.595	T43.596
thioxanthene NEC	T43.591	T43.592	T43.593	T43.594	T43.595	T43.596
Tranxene	T42.4X1	T42.4X2	T42.4X3	T42.4X4	T42.4X5	T42.4X6
Tranylcypromine	T43.1X1	T43.1X2	T43.1X3	T43.1X4	T43.1X5	T43.1X6
Trapidil	T46.3X1	T46.3X2	T46.3X3	T46.3X4	T46.3X5	T46.3X6
Trasentine	T44.3X1	T44.3X2	T44.3X3	T44.3X4	T44.3X5	T44.3X6
Travert	T50.3X1	T50.3X2	T50.3X3	T50.3X4	T50.3X5	T50.3X6
Trazodone	T43.211	T43.212	T43.213	T43.214	T43.215	T43.216
Trecator	T37.1X1	T37.1X2	T37.1X3	T37.1X4	T37.1X5	T37.1X6
Treosulfan	T45.1X1	T45.1X2	T45.1X3	T45.1X4	T45.1X5	T45.1X6
Tretamine	T45.1X1	T45.1X2	T45.1X3	T45.1X4	T45.1X5	T45.1X6
Tretinoin	T49.0X1	T49.0X2	T49.0X3	T49.0X4	T49.0X5	T49.0X6
Tretoquinol	T48.6X1	T48.6X2	T48.6X3	T48.6X4	T48.6X5	T48.6X6
Triacetin	T49.0X1	T49.0X2	T49.0X3	T49.0X4	T49.0X5	T49.0X6
Triacetoxyanthracene	T49.4X1	T49.4X2	T49.4X3	T49.4X4	T49.4X5	T49.4X6
Triacetyloleandomycin	T36.3X1	T36.3X2	T36.3X3	T36.3X4	T36.3X5	T36.3X6
Triamcinolone	T49.0X1	T49.0X2	T49.0X3	T49.0X4	T49.0X5	T49.0X6
ENT agent	T49.6X1	T49.6X2	T49.6X3	T49.6X4	T49.6X5	T49.6X6
hexacetonide	T49.0X1	T49.0X2	T49.0X3	T49.0X4	T49.0X5	T49.0X6
ophthalmic preparation	T49.5X1	T49.5X2	T49.5X3	T49.5X4	T49.5X5	T49.5X6
topical NEC	T49.0X1	T49.0X2	T49.0X3	T49.0X4	T49.0X5	T49.0X6
Triampyzine	T44.3X1	T44.3X2	T44.3X3	T44.3X4	T44.3X5	T44.3X6
Triamterene	T50.2X1	T50.2X2	T50.2X3	T50.2X4	T50.2X5	T50.2X6
Triazine (herbicide)	T60.3X1	T60.3X2	T60.3X3	T60.3X4	—	—
Triaziquone	T45.1X1	T45.1X2	T45.1X3	T45.1X4	T45.1X5	T45.1X6

◄ New   ◄▥ Revised   ~~deleted~~ Deleted

Substance	Poisoning, Accidental (Unintentional)	Poisoning, Intentional Self-Harm	Poisoning, Assault	Poisoning, Undetermined	Adverse Effect	Underdosing
	External Cause (T-Code)					
Triazolam	T42.4X1	T42.4X2	T42.4X3	T42.4X4	T42.4X5	T42.4X6
Triazole (herbicide)	T60.3X1	T60.3X2	T60.3X3	T60.3X4	—	—
Tribenoside	T46.991	T46.992	T46.993	T46.994	T46.995	T46.996
Tribromacetaldehyde	T42.6X1	T42.6X2	T42.6X3	T42.6X4	T42.6X5	T42.6X6
Tribromoethanol, rectal	T41.291	T41.292	T41.293	T41.294	T41.295	T41.296
Tribromomethane	T42.6X1	T42.6X2	T42.6X3	T42.6X4	T42.6X5	T42.6X6
Trichlorethane	T53.2X1	T53.2X2	T53.2X3	T53.2X4	—	—
Trichlorethylene	T53.2X1	T53.2X2	T53.2X3	T53.2X4	—	—
Trichlorfon	T60.0X1	T60.0X2	T60.0X3	T60.0X4	—	—
Trichlormethiazide	T50.2X1	T50.2X2	T50.2X3	T50.2X4	T50.2X5	T50.2X6
Trichlormethine	T45.1X1	T45.1X2	T45.1X3	T45.1X4	T45.1X5	T45.1X6
Trichloroacetic acid, Trichloracetic acid	T54.2X1	T54.2X2	T54.2X3	T54.2X4	—	—
medicinal	T49.4X1	T49.4X2	T49.4X3	T49.4X4	T49.4X5	T49.4X6
Trichloroethane	T53.2X1	T53.2X2	T53.2X3	T53.2X4	—	—
Trichloroethanol	T42.6X1	T42.6X2	T42.6X3	T42.6X4	T42.6X5	T42.6X6
Trichloroethylene (liquid) (vapor)	T53.2X1	T53.2X2	T53.2X3	T53.2X4	—	—
anesthetic (gas)	T41.0X1	T41.0X2	T41.0X3	T41.0X4	T41.0X5	T41.0X6
vapor NEC	T53.2X1	T53.2X2	T53.2X3	T53.2X4	—	—
Trichloroethyl phosphate	T42.6X1	T42.6X2	T42.6X3	T42.6X4	T42.6X5	T42.6X6
Trichlorofluoromethane NEC	T53.5X1	T53.5X2	T53.5X3	T53.5X4	—	—
Trichloronate	T60.0X1	T60.0X2	T60.0X3	T60.0X4	—	—
2,4,5-Trichlorophen-oxyacetic acid	T60.3X1	T60.3X2	T60.3X3	T60.3X4	—	—
Trichloropropane	T53.6X1	T53.6X2	T53.6X3	T53.6X4	—	—
Trichlorotriethylamine	T45.1X1	T45.1X2	T45.1X3	T45.1X4	T45.1X5	T45.1X6
Trichomonacides NEC	T37.3X1	T37.3X2	T37.3X3	T37.3X4	T37.3X5	T37.3X6
Trichomycin	T36.7X1	T36.7X2	T36.7X3	T36.7X4	T36.7X5	T36.7X6
Triclobisonium chloride	T49.0X1	T49.0X2	T49.0X3	T49.0X4	T49.0X5	T49.0X6
Triclocarban	T49.0X1	T49.0X2	T49.0X3	T49.0X4	T49.0X5	T49.0X6
Triclofos	T42.6X1	T42.6X2	T42.6X3	T42.6X4	T42.6X5	T42.6X6
Triclosan	T49.0X1	T49.0X2	T49.0X3	T49.0X4	T49.0X5	T49.0X6
Tricresyl phosphate	T65.891	T65.892	T65.893	T65.894	—	—
solvent	T52.91	T52.92	T52.93	T52.94	—	—
Tricyclamol chloride	T44.3X1	T44.3X2	T44.3X3	T44.3X4	T44.3X5	T44.3X6
Tridesilon	T49.0X1	T49.0X2	T49.0X3	T49.0X4	T49.0X5	T49.0X6
Tridihexethyl iodide	T44.3X1	T44.3X2	T44.3X3	T44.3X4	T44.3X5	T44.3X6
Tridione	T42.2X1	T42.2X2	T42.2X3	T42.2X4	T42.2X5	T42.2X6
Trientine	T45.8X1	T45.8X2	T45.8X3	T45.8X4	T45.8X5	T45.8X6
Triethanolamine NEC	T54.3X1	T54.3X2	T54.3X3	T54.3X4	—	—
detergent	T54.3X1	T54.3X2	T54.3X3	T54.3X4	—	—
trinitrate (biphosphate)	T46.3X1	T46.3X2	T46.3X3	T46.3X4	T46.3X5	T46.3X6

◀ New   ◀▦ Revised   ~~deleted~~ Deleted

Substance	External Cause (T-Code)					
	Poisoning, Accidental (Unintentional)	Poisoning, Intentional Self-Harm	Poisoning, Assault	Poisoning, Undetermined	Adverse Effect	Underdosing
Triethanomelamine	T45.1X1	T45.1X2	T45.1X3	T45.1X4	T45.1X5	T45.1X6
Triethylenemelamine	T45.1X1	T45.1X2	T45.1X3	T45.1X4	T45.1X5	T45.1X6
Triethylenephosphoramide	T45.1X1	T45.1X2	T45.1X3	T45.1X4	T45.1X5	T45.1X6
Triethylenethiophosphoramide	T45.1X1	T45.1X2	T45.1X3	T45.1X4	T45.1X5	T45.1X6
Trifluoperazine	T43.3X1	T43.3X2	T43.3X3	T43.3X4	T43.3X5	T43.3X6
Trifluoroethyl vinyl ether	T41.0X1	T41.0X2	T41.0X3	T41.0X4	T41.0X5	T41.0X6
Trifluperidol	T43.4X1	T43.4X2	T43.4X3	T43.4X4	T43.4X5	T43.4X6
Triflupromazine	T43.3X1	T43.3X2	T43.3X3	T43.3X4	T43.3X5	T43.3X6
Trifluridine	T37.5X1	T37.5X2	T37.5X3	T37.5X4	T37.5X5	T37.5X6
Triflusal	T45.521	T45.522	T45.523	T45.524	T45.525	T45.526
Trihexyphenidyl	T44.3X1	T44.3X2	T44.3X3	T44.3X4	T44.3X5	T44.3X6
Triiodothyronine	T38.1X1	T38.1X2	T38.1X3	T38.1X4	T38.1X5	T38.1X6
Trilene	T41.0X1	T41.0X2	T41.0X3	T41.0X4	T41.0X5	T41.0X6
Trilostane	T38.991	T38.992	T38.993	T38.994	T38.995	T38.996
Trimebutine	T44.3X1	T44.3X2	T44.3X3	T44.3X4	T44.3X5	T44.3X6
Trimecaine	T41.3X1	T41.3X2	T41.3X3	T41.3X4	T41.3X5	T41.3X6
Trimeprazine (tartrate)	T44.3X1	T44.3X2	T44.3X3	T44.3X4	T44.3X5	T44.3X6
Trimetaphan camsilate	T44.2X1	T44.2X2	T44.2X3	T44.2X4	T44.2X5	T44.2X6
Trimetazidine	T46.7X1	T46.7X2	T46.7X3	T46.7X4	T46.7X5	T46.7X6
Trimethadione	T42.2X1	T42.2X2	T42.2X3	T42.2X4	T42.2X5	T42.2X6
Trimethaphan	T44.2X1	T44.2X2	T44.2X3	T44.2X4	T44.2X5	T44.2X6
Trimethidinium	T44.2X1	T44.2X2	T44.2X3	T44.2X4	T44.2X5	T44.2X6
Trimethobenzamide	T45.0X1	T45.0X2	T45.0X3	T45.0X4	T45.0X5	T45.0X6
Trimethoprim	T37.8X1	T37.8X2	T37.8X3	T37.8X4	T37.8X5	T37.8X6
with sulfamethoxazole	T36.8X1	T36.8X2	T36.8X3	T36.8X4	T36.8X5	T36.8X6
Trimethylcarbinol	T51.3X1	T51.3X2	T51.3X3	T51.3X4	—	—
Trimethylpsoralen	T49.3X1	T49.3X2	T49.3X3	T49.3X4	T49.3X5	T49.3X6
Trimeton	T45.0X1	T45.0X2	T45.0X3	T45.0X4	T45.0X5	T45.0X6
Trimetrexate	T45.1X1	T45.1X2	T45.1X3	T45.1X4	T45.1X5	T45.1X6
Trimipramine	T43.011	T43.012	T43.013	T43.014	T43.015	T43.016
Trimustine	T45.1X1	T45.1X2	T45.1X3	T45.1X4	T45.1X5	T45.1X6
Trinitrine	T46.3X1	T46.3X2	T46.3X3	T46.3X4	T46.3X5	T46.3X6
Trinitrobenzol	T65.3X1	T65.3X2	T65.3X3	T65.3X4	—	—
Trinitrophenol	T65.3X1	T65.3X2	T65.3X3	T65.3X4	—	—
Trinitrotoluene (fumes)	T65.3X1	T65.3X2	T65.3X3	T65.3X4	—	—
Trional	T42.6X1	T42.6X2	T42.6X3	T42.6X4	T42.6X5	T42.6X6
Triorthocresyl phosphate	T65.891	T65.892	T65.893	T65.894		
Trioxide of arsenic	T57.0X1	T57.0X2	T57.0X3	T57.0X4	—	—
Trioxysalen	T49.4X1	T49.4X2	T49.4X3	T49.4X4	T49.4X5	T49.4X6
Tripamide	T50.2X1	T50.2X2	T50.2X3	T50.2X4	T50.2X5	T50.2X6

◀ New ◀▥ Revised ~~deleted~~ Deleted

Substance	External Cause (T-Code)					
	Poisoning, Accidental (Unintentional)	Poisoning, Intentional Self-Harm	Poisoning, Assault	Poisoning, Undetermined	Adverse Effect	Underdosing
Triparanol	T46.6X1	T46.6X2	T46.6X3	T46.6X4	T46.6X5	T46.6X6
Tripelennamine	T45.0X1	T45.0X2	T45.0X3	T45.0X4	T45.0X5	T45.0X6
Triperiden	T44.3X1	T44.3X2	T44.3X3	T44.3X4	T44.3X5	T44.3X6
Triperidol	T43.4X1	T43.4X2	T43.4X3	T43.4X4	T43.4X5	T43.4X6
Triphenylphosphate	T65.891	T65.892	T65.893	T65.894	—	—
Triple						
bromides	T42.6X1	T42.6X2	T42.6X3	T42.6X4	T42.6X5	T42.6X6
carbonate	T47.1X1	T47.1X2	T47.1X3	T47.1X4	T47.1X5	T47.1X6
vaccine						
DPT	T50.A11	T50.A12	T50.A13	T50.A14	T50.A15	T50.A16
including pertussis	T50.A11	T50.A12	T50.A13	T50.A14	T50.A15	T50.A16
MMR	T50.B91	T50.B92	—	—	—	—
Triprolidine	T45.0X1	T45.0X2	T45.0X3	T45.0X4	T45.0X5	T45.0X6
Trisodium hydrogen edetate	T50.6X1	T50.6X2	T50.6X4	T50.6X4	T50.6X5	T50.6X6
Trisoralen	T49.3X1	T49.3X2	T49.3X3	T49.3X4	T49.3X5	T49.3X6
Trisulfapyrimidines	T37.0X1	T37.0X2	T37.0X3	T37.0X4	T37.0X5	T37.0X6
Trithiozine	T44.3X1	T44.3X2	T44.3X3	T44.3X4	T44.3X5	T44.3X6
Tritiozine	T44.3X1	T44.3X2	T44.3X3	T44.3X4	T44.3X5	T44.3X6
Tritoqualine	T45.0X1	T45.0X2	T45.0X3	T45.0X4	T45.0X5	T45.0X6
Trofosfamide	T45.1X1	T45.1X2	T45.1X3	T45.1X4	T45.1X5	T45.1X6
Troleandomycin	T36.3X1	T36.3X2	T36.3X3	T36.3X4	T36.3X5	T36.3X6
Trolnitrate (phosphate)	T46.3X1	T46.3X2	T46.3X3	T46.3X4	T46.3X5	T46.3X6
Tromantadine	T37.5X1	T37.5X2	T37.5X3	T37.5X4	T37.5X5	T37.5X6
Trometamol	T50.2X1	T50.2X2	T50.2X3	T50.2X4	T50.2X5	T50.2X6
Tromethamine	T50.2X1	T50.2X2	T50.2X3	T50.2X4	T50.2X5	T50.2X6
Tronothane	T41.3X1	T41.3X2	T41.3X3	T41.3X4	T41.3X5	T41.3X6
Tropacine	T44.3X1	T44.3X2	T44.3X3	T44.3X4	T44.3X5	T44.3X6
Tropatepine	T44.3X1	T44.3X2	T44.3X3	T44.3X4	T44.3X5	T44.3X6
Tropicamide	T44.3X1	T44.3X2	T44.3X3	T44.3X4	T44.3X5	T44.3X6
Trospium chloride	T44.3X1	T44.3X2	T44.3X3	T44.3X4	T44.3X5	T44.3X6
Troxerutin	T46.991	T46.992	T46.993	T46.994	T46.995	T46.996
Troxidone	T42.2X1	T42.2X2	T42.2X3	T42.2X4	T42.2X5	T42.2X6
Tryparsamide	T37.3X1	T37.3X2	T37.3X3	T37.3X4	T37.3X5	T37.3X6
Trypsin	T45.3X1	T45.3X2	T45.3X3	T45.3X4	T45.3X5	T45.3X6
Tryptizol	T43.011	T43.012	T43.013	T43.014	T43.015	T43.016
TSH	T38.811	T38.812	T38.813	T38.814	T38.815	T38.816
Tuaminoheptane	T48.5X1	T48.5X2	T48.5X3	T48.5X4	T48.5X5	T48.5X6
Tuberculin, purified protein derivative (PPD)	T50.8X1	T50.8X2	T50.8X3	T50.8X4	T50.8X5	T50.8X6
Tubocurare	T48.1X1	T48.1X2	T48.1X3	T48.1X4	T48.1X5	T48.1X6
Tubocurarine (chloride)	T48.1X1	T48.1X2	T48.1X3	T48.1X4	T48.1X5	T48.1X6

TABLE OF DRUGS AND CHEMICALS

Substance	Poisoning, Accidental (Unintentional)	Poisoning, Intentional Self-Harm	Poisoning, Assault	Poisoning, Undetermined	Adverse Effect	Underdosing
Tulobuterol	T48.6X1	T48.6X2	T48.6X3	T48.6X4	T48.6X5	T48.6X6
Turpentine (spirits of)	T52.8X1	T52.8X2	T52.8X3	T52.8X4	—	—
vapor	T52.8X1	T52.8X2	T52.8X3	T52.8X4	—	—
Tybamate	T43.591	T43.592	T43.593	T43.594	T43.595	T43.596
Tyloxapol	T48.4X1	T48.4X2	T48.4X3	T48.4X4	T48.4X5	T48.4X6
Tymazoline	T48.5X1	T48.5X2	T48.5X3	T48.5X4	T48.5X5	T48.5X6
Typhoid-paratyphoid vaccine	T50.A91	T50.A92	T50.A93	T50.A94	T50.A95	T50.A96
Typhus vaccine	T50.A91	T50.A92	T50.A93	T50.A94	T50.A95	T50.A96
Tyropanoate	T50.8X1	T50.8X2	T50.8X3	T50.8X4	T50.8X5	T50.8X6
Tyrothricin	T49.6X1	T49.6X2	T49.6X3	T49.6X4	T49.6X5	T49.6X6
ENT agent	T49.6X1	T49.6X2	T49.6X3	T49.6X4	T49.6X5	T49.6X6
ophthalmic preparation	T49.5X1	T49.5X2	T49.5X3	T49.5X4	T49.5X5	T49.5X6
U						
Ufenamate	T39.391	T39.392	T39.393	T39.394	T39.395	T39.396
Ultraviolet light protectant	T49.3X1	T49.3X2	T49.3X3	T49.3X4	T49.3X5	T49.3X6
Undecenoic acid	T49.0X1	T49.0X2	T49.0X3	T49.0X4	T49.0X5	T49.0X6
Undecoylium	T49.0X1	T49.0X2	T49.0X3	T49.0X4	T49.0X5	T49.0X6
Undecylenic acid (derivatives)	T49.0X1	T49.0X2	T49.0X3	T49.0X4	T49.0X5	T49.0X6
Unna's boot	T49.3X1	T49.3X2	T49.3X3	T49.3X4	T49.3X5	T49.3X6
Unsaturated fatty acid	T46.6X1	T46.6X2	T46.6X3	T46.6X4	T46.6X5	T46.6X6
Uracil mustard	T45.1X1	T45.1X2	T45.1X3	T45.1X4	T45.1X5	T45.1X6
Uramustine	T45.1X1	T45.1X2	T45.1X3	T45.1X4	T45.1X5	T45.1X6
Urapidil	T46.5X1	T46.5X2	T46.5X3	T46.5X4	T46.5X5	T46.5X6
Urari	T48.1X1	T48.1X2	T48.1X3	T48.1X4	T48.1X5	T48.1X6
Urate oxidase	T50.4X1	T50.4X2	T50.4X3	T50.4X4	T50.4X5	T50.4X6
Urea	T47.3X1	T47.3X2	T47.3X3	T47.3X4	T47.3X5	T47.3X6
peroxide	T49.0X1	T49.0X2	T49.0X3	T49.0X4	T49.0X5	T49.0X6
stibamine	T37.4X1	T37.4X2	T37.4X3	T37.4X4	T37.4X5	T37.4X6
topical	T49.8X1	T49.8X2	T49.8X3	T49.8X4	T49.8X5	T49.8X6
Urethane	T45.1X1	T45.1X2	T45.1X3	T45.1X4	T45.1X5	T45.1X6
Urginea (maritima) (scilla) — *see Squill*						
Uric acid metabolism drug NEC	T50.4X1	T50.4X2	T50.4X3	T50.4X4	T50.4X5	T50.4X6
Uricosuric agent	T50.4X1	T50.4X2	T50.4X3	T50.4X4	T50.4X5	T50.4X6
Urinary anti-infective	T37.8X1	T37.8X2	T37.8X3	T37.8X4	T37.8X5	T37.8X6
Urofollitropin	T38.811	T38.812	T38.813	T38.814	T38.815	T38.816
Urokinase	T45.611	T45.612	T45.613	T45.614	T45.615	T45.616
Urokon	T50.8X1	T50.8X2	T50.8X3	T50.8X4	T50.8X5	T50.8X6
Ursodeoxycholic acid	T50.991	T50.992	T50.993	T50.994	T50.995	T50.996
Ursodiol	T50.991	T50.992	T50.993	T50.994	T50.995	T50.996

◀ New ◀ Revised ~~deleted~~ Deleted

Substance	External Cause (T-Code)					
	Poisoning, Accidental (Unintentional)	Poisoning, Intentional Self-Harm	Poisoning, Assault	Poisoning, Undetermined	Adverse Effect	Underdosing
Urtica	T62.2X1	T62.2X2	T62.2X3	T62.2X4	—	—
Utility gas—*see Gas, utility*						
V						
Vaccine NEC	T50.Z91	T50.Z92	T50.Z93	T50.Z94	T50.Z95	T50.Z96
antineoplastic	T50.Z91	T50.Z92	T50.Z93	T50.Z94	T50.Z95	T50.Z96
bacterial NEC	T50.A91	T50.A92	T50.A93	T50.A94	T50.A95	T50.A96
with						
other bacterial component	T50.A91	T50.A92	T50.A93	T50.A94	T50.A95	T50.A96
pertussis component	T50.A91	T50.A92	T50.A93	T50.A94	T50.A95	T50.A96
viral-rickettsial component	T50.A91	T50.A92	T50.A93	T50.A94	T50.A95	T50.A96
mixed NEC	T50.A91	T50.A92	T50.A93	T50.A94	T50.A95	T50.A96
BCG	T50.A91	T50.A92	T50.A93	T50.A94	T50.A95	T50.A96
cholera	T50.A91	T50.A92	T50.A93	T50.A94	T50.A95	T50.A96
diphtheria	T50.A91	T50.A92	T50.A93	T50.A94	T50.A95	T50.A96
with tetanus	T50.A21	T50.A22	T50.A23	T50.A24	T50.A25	T50.A26
and pertussis	T50.A11	T50.A12	T50.A13	T50.A14	T50.A15	T50.A16
influenza	T50.B91	T50.B92	T50.B93	T50.B94	T50.B95	T50.B96
measles	T50.B91	T50.B92	T50.B93	T50.B94	T50.B95	T50.B96
with mumps and rubella	T50.B91	T50.B92	T50.B93	T50.B94	T50.B95	T50.B96
meningococcal	T50.A91	T50.A92	T50.A93	T50.A94	T50.A95	T50.A96
mumps	T50.B91	T50.B92	T50.B93	T50.B94	T50.B95	T50.B96
paratyphoid	T50.A91	T50.A92	T50.A93	T50.A94	T50.A95	T50.A96
pertussis	T50.A11	T50.A12	T50.A13	T50.A14	T50.A15	T50.A16
with diphtheria	T50.A11	T50.A12	T50.A13	T50.A14	T50.A15	T50.A16
and tetanus	T50.A11	T50.A12	T50.A13	T50.A14	T50.A15	T50.A16
plague	T50.A91	T50.A92	T50.A93	T50.A94	T50.A95	T50.A96
poliomyelitis	T50.B91	T50.B92	T50.B93	T50.B94	T50.B95	T50.B96
poliovirus	T50.B91	T50.B92	T50.B93	T50.B94	T50.B95	T50.B96
rabies	T50.B91	T50.B92	T50.B93	T50.B94	T50.B95	T50.B96
respiratory syncytial virus	T50.B91	T50.B92	T50.B93	T50.B94	T50.B95	T50.B96
rickettsial NEC	T50.A91	T50.A92	T50.A93	T50.A94	T50.A95	T50.A96
with						
bacterial component	T50.A21	T50.A22	T50.A23	T50.A24	T50.A25	T50.A26
Rocky Mountain spotted fever	T50.A91	T50.A92	T50.A93	T50.A94	T50.A95	T50.A96
rubella	T50.B91	T50.B92	T50.B93	T50.B94	T50.B95	T50.B96
sabin oral	T50.B91	T50.B92	T50.B93	T50.B94	T50.B95	T50.B96
smallpox	T50.B11	T50.B12	T50.B13	T50.B14	T50.B15	T50.B16
TAB	T50.A91	T50.A92	T50.A93	T50.A94	T50.A95	T50.A96
tetanus	T50.A91	T50.A92	T50.A93	T50.A94	T50.A95	T50.A96

◀ New ◀▥ Revised ~~deleted~~ Deleted

TABLE OF DRUGS AND CHEMICALS

Substance	External Cause (T-Code)					
	Poisoning, Accidental (Unintentional)	Poisoning, Intentional Self-Harm	Poisoning, Assault	Poisoning, Undetermined	Adverse Effect	Underdosing
Vaccine NEC *(Continued)*						
typhoid	T50.A91	T50.A92	T50.A93	T50.A94	T50.A95	T50.A96
typhus	T50.A91	T50.A92	T50.A93	T50.A94	T50.A95	T50.A96
viral NEC	T50.B91	T50.B92	T50.B93	T50.B94	T50.B95	T50.B96
yellow fever	T50.B91	T50.B92	T50.B93	T50.B94	T50.B95	T50.B96
Vaccinia immune globulin	T50.Z11	T50.Z12	T50.Z13	T50.Z14	T50.Z15	T50.Z16
Vaginal contraceptives	T49.8X1	T49.8X2	T49.8X3	T49.8X4	T49.8X5	T49.8X6
Valerian						
root	T42.6X1	T42.6X2	T42.6X3	T42.6X4	T42.6X5	T42.6X6
tincture	T42.6X1	T42.6X2	T42.6X3	T42.6X4	T42.6X5	T42.6X6
Valethamate bromide	T44.3X1	T44.3X2	T44.3X3	T44.3X4	T44.3X5	T44.3X6
Valisone	T49.0X1	T49.0X2	T49.0X3	T49.0X4	T49.0X5	T49.0X6
Valium	T42.4X1	T42.4X2	T42.4X3	T42.4X4	T42.4X5	T42.4X6
Valmid	T42.6X1	T42.6X2	T42.6X3	T42.6X4	T42.6X5	T42.6X6
Valnoctamide	T42.6X1	T42.6X2	T42.6X3	T42.6X4	T42.6X5	T42.6X6
Valproate (sodium)	T42.6X1	T42.6X2	T42.6X3	T42.6X4	T42.6X5	T42.6X6
Valproic acid	T42.6X1	T42.6X2	T42.6X3	T42.6X4	T42.6X5	T42.6X6
Valpromide	T42.6X1	T42.6X2	T42.6X3	T42.6X4	T42.6X5	T42.6X6
Vanadium	T56.891	T56.892	T56.893	T56.894	—	—
Vancomycin	T36.8X1	T36.8X2	T36.8X3	T36.8X4	T36.8X5	T36.8X6
Vapor — *see also Gas*	T59.91	T59.92	T59.93	T59.94	—	—
kiln (carbon monoxide)	T58.8X1	T58.8X2	T58.8X3	T58.8X4	—	—
lead — *see lead*						
specified source NEC	T59.891	T59.892	T59.893	T59.894	—	—
Vardenafil	T46.7X1	T46.7X2	T46.7X3	T46.7X4	T46.7X5	T46.7X6
Varicose reduction drug	T46.8X1	T46.8X2	T46.8X3	T46.8X4	T46.8X5	T46.8X6
Varnish	T65.4X1	T65.4X2	T65.4X3	T65.4X4	—	—
cleaner	T52.91	T52.92	T52.93	T52.94	—	—
Vaseline	T49.3X1	T49.3X2	T49.3X3	T49.3X4	T49.3X5	T49.3X6
Vasodilan	T46.7X1	T46.7X2	T46.7X3	T46.7X4	T46.7X5	T46.7X6
Vasodilator						
coronary NEC	T46.3X1	T46.3X2	T46.3X3	T46.3X4	T46.3X5	T46.3X6
peripheral NEC	T46.7X1	T46.7X2	T46.7X3	T46.7X4	T46.7X5	T46.7X6
Vasopressin	T38.891	T38.892	T38.893	T38.894	T38.895	T38.896
Vasopressor drugs	T38.891	T38.892	T38.893	T38.894	T38.895	T38.896
Vecuronium bromide	T48.1X1	T48.1X2	T48.1X3	T48.1X4	T48.1X5	T48.1X6
Vegetable extract, astringent	T49.2X1	T49.2X2	T49.2X3	T49.2X4	T49.2X5	T49.2X6
Venlafaxine	T43.211	T43.212	T43.213	T43.214	T43.215	T43.216

◀ New   ◀▨ Revised   ~~deleted~~ Deleted

Substance	External Cause (T-Code)					
	Poisoning, Accidental (Unintentional)	Poisoning, Intentional Self-Harm	Poisoning, Assault	Poisoning, Undetermined	Adverse Effect	Underdosing
Venom, venomous (bite) (sting)	T63.91	T63.92	T63.93	T63.94	—	—
amphibian NEC	T63.831	T63.832	T63.833	T63.834	—	—
animal NEC	T63.891	T63.892	T63.893	T63.894	—	—
ant	T63.421	T63.422	T63.423	T63.424	—	—
arthropod NEC	T63.481	T63.482	T63.483	T63.484	—	—
bee	T63.441	T63.442	T63.443	T63.444	—	—
centipede	T63.411	T63.412	T63.413	T63.414	—	—
fish	T63.591	T63.592	T63.593	T63.594	—	—
frog	T63.811	T63.812	T63.813	T63.814	—	—
hornet	T63.451	T63.452	T63.453	T63.454	—	—
insect NEC	T63.481	T63.482	T63.483	T63.484	—	—
lizard	T63.121	T63.122	T63.123	T63.124	—	—
marine						
animals	T63.691	T63.692	T63.693	T63.694	—	—
bluebottle	T63.611	T63.612	T63.613	T63.614	—	—
jellyfish NEC	T63.621	T63.622	T63.623	T63.624	—	—
Portugese Man-o-war	T63.611	T63.612	T63.613	T63.614	—	—
sea anemone	T63.631	T63.632	T63.633	T63.634	—	—
specified NEC	T63.691	T63.692	T63.693	T63.694	—	—
fish	T63.591	T63.592	T63.593	T63.594	—	—
plants	T63.711	T63.712	T63.713	T63.714	—	—
sting ray	T63.511	T63.512	T63.513	T63.514	—	—
millipede (tropical)	T63.411	T63.412	T63.413	T63.414	—	—
plant NEC	T63.791	T63.792	T63.793	T63.794	—	—
marine	T63.711	T63.712	T63.713	T63.714	—	—
reptile	T63.191	T63.192	T63.193	T63.194	—	—
gila monster	T63.111	T63.112	T63.113	T63.114	—	—
lizard NEC	T63.121	T63.122	T63.123	T63.124	—	—
scorpion	T63.2X1	T63.2X2	T63.2X3	T63.2X4	—	—
snake	T63.001	T63.002	T63.003	T63.004	—	—
African NEC	T63.081	T63.082	T63.083	T63.084	—	—
American (North) (South) NEC	T63.061	T63.062	T63.063	T63.064	—	—
Asian	T63.081	T63.082	T63.083	T63.084	—	—
Australian	T63.071	T63.072	T63.073	T63.074	—	—
cobra	T63.041	T63.042	T63.043	T63.044	—	—
coral snake	T63.021	T63.022	T63.023	T63.024	—	—
rattlesnake	T63.011	T63.012	T63.013	T63.014	—	—
specified NEC	T63.091	T63.092	T63.093	T63.094	—	—
taipan	T63.031	T63.032	T63.033	T63.034	—	—

◀ New ◀ Revised deleted Deleted

TABLE OF DRUGS AND CHEMICALS

Substance	Poisoning, Accidental (Unintentional)	Poisoning, Intentional Self-Harm	Poisoning, Assault	Poisoning, Undetermined	Adverse Effect	Underdosing
Venom, venomous *(Continued)*						
specified NEC	T63.891	T63.892	T63.893	T63.894	—	—
spider	T63.301	T63.302	T63.303	T63.304	—	—
black widow	T63.311	T63.312	T63.313	T63.314	—	—
brown recluse	T63.331	T63.332	T63.333	T63.334	—	—
specified NEC	T63.391	T63.392	T63.393	T63.394	—	—
tarantula	T63.321	T63.322	T63.323	T63.324	—	—
sting ray	T63.511	T63.512	T63.513	T63.514	—	—
toad	T63.821	T63.822	T63.823	T63.824	—	—
wasp	T63.461	T63.462	T63.463	T63.464	—	—
Venous sclerosing drug NEC	T46.8X1	T46.8X2	T46.8X3	T46.8X4	T46.8X5	T46.8X6
Ventolin — *see Albuterol*						
Verapamil	T46.1X1	T46.1X2	T46.1X3	T46.1X4	T46.1X5	T46.1X6
Veramon	T42.3X1	T42.3X2	T42.3X3	T42.3X4	T42.3X5	T42.3X6
Veratrine	T46.5X1	T46.5X2	T46.5X3	T46.5X4	T46.5X5	T46.5X6
Veratrum						
album	T62.2X1	T62.2X2	T62.2X3	T62.2X4	—	—
alkaloids	T46.5X1	T46.5X2	T46.5X3	T46.5X4	T46.5X5	T46.5X6
viride	T62.2X1	T62.2X2	T62.2X3	T62.2X4	—	—
Verdigris	T60.3X1	T60.3X2	T60.3X3	T60.3X4	—	—
Veronal	T42.3X1	T42.3X2	T42.3X3	T42.3X4	T42.3X5	T42.3X6
Veroxil	T37.4X1	T37.4X2	T37.4X3	T37.4X4	T37.4X5	T37.4X6
Versenate	T50.6X1	T50.6X2	T50.6X3	T50.6X4	T50.6X5	T50.6X6
Versidyne	T39.8X1	T39.8X2	T39.8X3	T39.8X4	T39.8X5	T39.8X6
Vetrabutine	T48.0X1	T48.0X2	T48.0X3	T48.0X4	T48.0X5	T48.0X6
Vidarabine	T37.5X1	T37.5X2	T37.5X3	T37.5X4	T37.5X5	T37.5X6
Vienna						
green	T57.0X1	T57.0X2	T57.0X3	T57.0X4	—	—
insecticide	T60.2X1	T60.2X2	T60.2X3	T60.2X4	—	—
red	T57.0X1	T57.0X2	T57.0X3	T57.0X4	—	—
pharmaceutical dye	T50.991	T50.992	T50.993	T50.994	T50.995	T50.996
Vigabatrin	T42.6X1	T42.6X2	T42.6X3	T42.6X4	T42.6X5	T42.6X6
Viloxazine	T43.291	T43.292	T43.293	T43.294	T43.295	T43.296
Viminol	T39.8X1	T39.8X2	T39.8X3	T39.8X4	T39.8X5	T39.8X6
Vinbarbital, vinbarbitone	T42.3X1	T42.3X2	T42.3X3	T42.3X4	T42.3X5	T42.3X6
Vinblastine	T45.1X1	T45.1X2	T45.1X3	T45.1X4	T45.1X5	T45.1X6
Vinburnine	T46.7X1	T46.7X2	T46.7X3	T46.7X4	T46.7X5	T46.7X6
Vincamine	T45.1X1	T45.1X2	T45.1X3	T45.1X4	T45.1X5	T45.1X6
Vincristine	T45.1X1	T45.1X2	T45.1X3	T45.1X4	T45.1X5	T45.1X6
Vindesine	T45.1X1	T45.1X2	T45.1X3	T45.1X4	T45.1X5	T45.1X6

◀ New ◀꜡ Revised ~~deleted~~ Deleted

Substance	Poisoning, Accidental (Unintentional)	Poisoning, Intentional Self-Harm	Poisoning, Assault	Poisoning, Undetermined	Adverse Effect	Underdosing
	External Cause (T-Code)					
Vinesthene, vinethene	T41.0X1	T41.0X2	T41.0X3	T41.0X4	T41.0X5	T41.0X6
Vinorelbine tartrate	T45.1X1	T45.1X2	T45.1X3	T45.1X4	T45.1X5	T45.1X6
Vinpocetine	T46.7X1	T46.7X2	T46.7X3	T46.7X4	T46.7X5	T46.7X6
Vinyl						
acetate	T65.891	T65.892	T65.893	T65.894	—	—
bital	T42.3X1	T42.3X2	T42.3X3	T42.3X4	T42.3X5	T42.3X6
bromide	T65.891	T65.892	T65.893	T65.894	—	—
chloride	T59.891	T59.892	T59.893	T59.894	—	—
ether	T41.0X1	T41.0X2	T41.0X3	T41.0X4	T41.0X5	T41.0X6
Vinylbital	T42.3X1	T42.3X2	T42.3X3	T42.3X4	T42.3X5	T42.3X6
Vinylidene chloride	T65.891	T65.892	T65.893	T65.894	—	—
Vioform	T37.8X1	T37.8X2	T37.8X3	T37.8X4	T37.8X5	T37.8X6
topical	T49.0X1	T49.0X2	T49.0X3	T49.0X4	T49.0X5	T49.0X6
Viomycin	T36.8X1	T36.8X2	T36.8X3	T36.8X4	T36.8X5	T36.8X6
Viosterol	T45.2X1	T45.2X2	T45.2X3	T45.2X4	T45.2X5	T45.2X6
Viper (venom)	T63.091	T63.092	T63.093	T63.094	—	—
Viprynium	T37.4X1	T37.4X2	T37.4X3	T37.4X4	T37.4X5	T37.4X6
Viquidil	T46.7X1	T46.7X2	T46.7X3	T46.7X4	T46.7X5	T46.7X6
Viral vaccine NEC	T50.B91	T50.B92	T50.B93	T50.B94	T50.B95	T50.B96
Virginiamycin	T36.8X1	T36.8X2	T36.8X3	T36.8X4	T36.8X5	T36.8X6
Virugon	T37.5X1	T37.5X2	T37.5X3	T37.5X4	T37.5X5	T37.5X6
Viscous agent	T50.901	T50.902	T50.903	T50.904	T50.905	T50.906
Visine	T49.5X1	T49.5X2	T49.5X3	T49.5X4	T49.5X5	T49.5X6
Visnadine	T46.3X1	T46.3X2	T46.3X3	T46.3X4	T46.3X5	T46.3X6
Vitamin NEC	T45.2X1	T45.2X2	T45.2X3	T45.2X4	T45.2X5	T45.2X6
A	T45.2X1	T45.2X2	T45.2X3	T45.2X4	T45.2X5	T45.2X6
B NEC	T45.2X1	T45.2X2	T45.2X3	T45.2X4	T45.2X5	T45.2X6
nicotinic acid	T46.7X1	T46.7X2	T46.7X3	T46.7X4	T46.7X5	T46.7X6
B1	T45.2X1	T45.2X2	T45.2X3	T45.2X4	T45.2X5	T45.2X6
B2	T45.2X1	T45.2X2	T45.2X3	T45.2X4	T45.2X5	T45.2X6
B6	T45.2X1	T45.2X2	T45.2X3	T45.2X4	T45.2X5	T45.2X6
B12	T45.2X1	T45.2X2	T45.2X3	T45.2X4	T45.2X5	T45.2X6
B15	T45.2X1	T45.2X2	T45.2X3	T45.2X4	T45.2X5	T45.2X6
C	T45.2X1	T45.2X2	T45.2X3	T45.2X4	T45.2X5	T45.2X6
D	T45.2X1	T45.2X2	T45.2X3	T45.2X4	T45.2X5	T45.2X6
D2	T45.2X1	T45.2X2	T45.2X3	T45.2X4	T45.2X5	T45.2X6
D3	T45.2X1	T45.2X2	T45.2X3	T45.2X4	T45.2X5	T45.2X6
E	T45.2X1	T45.2X2	T45.2X3	T45.2X4	T45.2X5	T45.2X6
E acetate	T45.2X1	T45.2X2	T45.2X3	T45.2X4	T45.2X5	T45.2X6
hematopoietic	T45.8X1	T45.8X2	T45.8X3	T45.8X4	T45.8X5	T45.8X6

Substance	External Cause (T-Code)					
	Poisoning, Accidental (Unintentional)	Poisoning, Intentional Self-Harm	Poisoning, Assault	Poisoning, Undetermined	Adverse Effect	Underdosing
Vitamin NEC *(Continued)*						
K NEC	T45.7X1	T45.7X2	T45.7X3	T45.7X4	T45.7X5	T45.7X6
K1	T45.7X1	T45.7X2	T45.7X3	T45.7X4	T45.7X5	T45.7X6
K2	T45.7X1	T45.7X2	T45.7X3	T45.7X4	T45.7X5	T45.7X6
PP	T45.2X1	T45.2X2	T45.2X3	T45.2X4	T45.2X5	T45.2X6
ulceroprotectant	T47.1X1	T47.1X2	T47.1X3	T47.1X4	T47.1X5	T47.1X6
Vleminckx's solution	T49.4X1	T49.4X2	T49.4X3	T49.4X4	T49.4X5	T49.4X6
Voltaren — *see Diclofenac sodium*						
W						
Warfarin	T45.511	T45.512	T45.513	T45.514	T45.515	T45.516
rodenticide	T60.4X1	T60.4X2	T60.4X3	T60.4X4	—	—
sodium	T60.4X1	T60.4X2	T60.4X3	T60.4X4	—	—
Wasp (sting)	T63.461	T63.462	T63.463	T63.464	—	—
Water						
balance drug	T50.3X1	T50.3X2	T50.3X3	T50.3X4	T50.3X5	T50.3X6
distilled	T50.3X1	T50.3X2	T50.3X3	T50.3X4	T50.3X5	T50.3X6
gas — *see Gas, water*						
incomplete combustion of — *see Carbon, monoxide, fuel, utility*						
hemlock	T62.2X1	T62.2X2	T62.2X3	T62.2X4	—	—
moccasin (venom)	T63.061	T63.062	T63.063	T63.064	—	—
purified	T50.3X1	T50.3X2	T50.3X3	T50.3X4	T50.3X5	T50.3X6
Wax (paraffin) (petroleum)	T52.0X1	T52.0X2	T52.0X3	T52.0X4	—	—
automobile	T65.891	T65.892	T65.893	T65.894	—	—
floor	T52.0X1	T52.0X2	T52.0X3	T52.0X4	—	—
Weed killers NEC	T60.3X1	T60.3X2	T60.3X3	T60.3X4	—	—
Welldorm	T42.6X1	T42.6X2	T42.6X3	T42.6X4	T42.6X5	T42.6X6
White						
arsenic	T57.0X1	T57.0X2	T57.0X3	T57.0X4	—	—
hellebore	T62.2X1	T62.2X2	T62.2X3	T62.2X4	—	—
lotion (keratolytic)	T49.4X1	T49.4X2	T49.4X3	T49.4X4	T49.4X5	T49.4X6
spirit	T52.0X1	T52.0X2	T52.0X3	T52.0X4	—	—
Whitewash	T65.891	T65.892	T65.893	T65.894	—	—
Whole blood (human)	T45.8X1	T45.8X2	T45.8X3	T45.8X4	T45.8X5	T45.8X6
Wild						
black cherry	T62.2X1	T62.2X2	T62.2X3	T62.2X4	—	—
poisonous plants NEC	T62.2X1	T62.2X2	T62.2X3	T62.2X4	—	—
Window cleaning fluid	T65.891	T65.892	T65.893	T65.894	—	—
Wintergreen (oil)	T49.3X1	T49.3X2	T49.3X3	T49.3X4	T49.3X5	T49.3X6

◀ New   ◀▥ Revised   ~~deleted~~ Deleted

Substance	External Cause (T-Code)					
	Poisoning, Accidental (Unintentional)	Poisoning, Intentional Self-Harm	Poisoning, Assault	Poisoning, Undetermined	Adverse Effect	Underdosing
Wisterine	T62.2X1	T62.2X2	T62.2X3	T62.2X4	—	—
Witch hazel	T49.2X1	T49.2X2	T49.2X3	T49.2X4	T49.2X5	T49.2X6
Wood alcohol or spirit	T51.1X1	T51.1X2	T51.1X3	T51.1X4	—	—
Wool fat (hydrous)	T49.3X1	T49.3X2	T49.3X3	T49.3X4	T49.3X5	T49.3X6
Woorali	T48.1X1	T48.1X2	T48.1X3	T48.1X4	T48.1X5	T48.1X6
Wormseed, American	T37.4X1	T37.4X2	T37.4X3	T37.4X4	T37.4X5	T37.4X6
X						
Xamoterol	T44.5X1	T44.5X2	T44.5X3	T44.5X4	T44.5X5	T44.5X6
Xanthine diuretics	T50.2X1	T50.2X2	T50.2X3	T50.2X4	T50.2X5	T50.2X6
Xanthinol nicotinate	T46.7X1	T46.7X2	T46.7X3	T46.7X4	T46.7X5	T46.7X6
Xanthotoxin	T49.3X1	T49.3X2	T49.3X3	T49.3X4	T49.3X5	T49.3X6
Xantinol nicotinate	T46.7X1	T46.7X2	T46.7X3	T46.7X4	T46.7X5	T46.7X6
Xantocillin	T36.0X1	T36.0X2	T36.0X3	T36.0X4	T36.0X5	T36.0X6
Xenon (127Xe) (133Xe)	T50.8X1	T50.8X2	T50.8X3	T50.8X4	T50.8X5	T50.8X6
Xenysalate	T49.4X1	T49.4X2	T49.4X3	T49.4X4	T49.4X5	T49.4X6
Xibornol	T37.8X1	T37.8X2	T37.8X3	T37.8X4	T37.8X5	T37.8X6
Xigris	T45.511	T45.512	T45.513	T45.514	T45.515	T45.516
Xipamide	T50.2X1	T50.2X2	T50.2X3	T50.2X4	T50.2X5	T50.2X6
Xylene (vapor)	T52.2X1	T52.2X2	T52.2X3	T52.2X4	—	—
Xylocaine (infiltration) (topical)	T41.3X1	T41.3X2	T41.3X3	T41.3X4	T41.3X5	T41.3X6
nerve block (peripheral) (plexus)	T41.3X1	T41.3X2	T41.3X3	T41.3X4	T41.3X5	T41.3X6
spinal	T41.3X1	T41.3X2	T41.3X3	T41.3X4	T41.3X5	T41.3X6
Xylol (vapor)	T52.2X1	T52.2X2	T52.2X3	T52.2X4	—	—
Xylometazoline	T48.5X1	T48.5X2	T48.5X3	T48.5X4	T48.5X5	T48.5X6
Y						
Yeast	T45.2X1	T45.2X2	T45.2X3	T45.2X4	T45.2X5	T45.2X6
dried	T45.2X1	T45.2X2	T45.2X3	T45.2X4	T45.2X5	T45.2X6
Yellow						
fever vaccine	T50.B91	T50.B92	T50.B93	T50.B94	T50.B95	T50.B96
jasmine	T62.2X1	T62.2X2	T62.2X3	T62.2X4	—	—
phenolphthalein	T47.2X1	T47.2X2	T47.2X3	T47.2X4	T47.2X5	T47.2X6
Yew	T62.2X1	T62.2X2	T62.2X3	T62.2X4	—	—
Yohimbic acid	T40.991	T40.992	T40.993	T40.994	T40.995	T40.996
Z						
Zactane	T39.8X1	T39.8X2	T39.8X3	T39.8X4	T39.8X5	T39.8X6
Zalcitabine	T37.5X1	T37.5X2	T37.5X3	T37.5X4	T37.5X5	T37.5X6
Zaroxolyn	T50.2X1	T50.2X2	T50.2X3	T50.2X4	T50.2X5	T50.2X6

TABLE OF DRUGS AND CHEMICALS

◀ New ◀════ Revised deleted Deleted

Substance	Poisoning, Accidental (Unintentional)	Poisoning, Intentional Self-Harm	Poisoning, Assault	Poisoning, Undetermined	Adverse Effect	Underdosing
Zephiran (topical)	T49.0X1	T49.0X2	T49.0X3	T49.0X4	T49.0X5	T49.0X6
ophthalmic preparation	T49.5X1	T49.5X2	T49.5X3	T49.5X4	T49.5X5	T49.5X6
Zeranol	T38.7X1	T38.7X2	T38.7X3	T38.7X4	T38.7X5	T38.7X6
Zerone	T51.1X1	T51.1X2	T51.1X3	T51.1X4	—	—
Zidovudine	T37.5X1	T37.5X2	T37.5X3	T37.5X4	T37.5X5	T37.5X6
Zimeldine	T43.221	T43.222	T43.223	T43.224	T43.225	T43.226
Zinc (compounds) (fumes) (vapor) NEC	T56.5X1	T56.5X2	T56.5X3	T56.5X4	—	—
anti-infectives	T49.0X1	T49.0X2	T49.0X3	T49.0X4	T49.0X5	T49.0X6
antivaricose	T46.8X1	T46.8X2	T46.8X3	T46.8X4	T46.8X5	T46.8X6
bacitracin	T49.0X1	T49.0X2	T49.0X3	T49.0X4	T49.0X5	T49.0X6
chloride (mouthwash)	T49.6X1	T49.6X2	T49.6X3	T49.6X4	T49.6X5	T49.6X6
chromate	T56.5X1	T56.5X2	T56.5X3	T56.5X4	—	—
gelatin	T49.3X1	T49.3X2	T49.3X3	T49.3X4	T49.3X5	T49.3X6
oxide	T49.3X1	T49.3X2	T49.3X3	T49.3X4	T49.3X5	T49.3X6
plaster	T49.3X1	T49.3X2	T49.3X3	T49.3X4	T49.3X5	T49.3X6
peroxide	T49.0X1	T49.0X2	T49.0X3	T49.0X4	T49.0X5	T49.0X6
pesticides	T56.5X1	T56.5X2	T56.5X3	T56.5X4	—	—
phosphide	T60.4X1	T60.4X2	T60.4X3	T60.4X4	—	—
pyrithionate	T49.4X1	T49.4X2	T49.4X3	T49.4X4	T49.4X5	T49.4X6
stearate	T49.3X1	T49.3X2	T49.3X3	T49.3X4	T49.3X5	T49.3X6
sulfate	T49.5X1	T49.5X2	T49.5X3	T49.5X4	T49.5X5	T49.5X6
ENT agent	T49.6X1	T49.6X2	T49.6X3	T49.6X4	T49.6X5	T49.6X6
ophthalmic solution	T49.5X1	T49.5X2	T49.5X3	T49.5X4	T49.5X5	T49.5X6
topical NEC	T49.0X1	T49.0X2	T49.0X3	T49.0X4	T49.0X5	T49.0X6
undecylenate	T49.0X1	T49.0X2	T49.0X3	T49.0X4	T49.0X5	T49.0X6
Zineb	T60.0X1	T60.0X2	T60.0X3	T60.0X4	—	—
Zinostatin	T45.1X1	T45.1X2	T45.1X3	T45.1X4	T45.1X5	T45.1X6
Zipeprol	T48.3X1	T48.3X2	T48.3X3	T48.3X4	T48.3X5	T48.3X6
Zofenopril	T46.4X1	T46.4X2	T46.4X3	T46.4X4	T46.4X5	T46.4X6
Zolpidem	T42.6X1	T42.6X2	T42.6X3	T42.6X4	T42.6X5	T42.6X6
Zomepirac	T39.391	T39.392	T39.393	T39.394	T39.395	T39.396
Zopiclone	T42.6X1	T42.6X2	T42.6X3	T42.6X4	T42.6X5	T42.6X6
Zorubicin	T45.1X1	T45.1X2	T45.1X3	T45.1X4	T45.1X5	T45.1X6
Zotepine	T43.591	T43.592	T43.593	T43.594	T43.595	T43.596
Zovant	T45.511	T45.512	T45.513	T45.514	T45.515	T45.516
Zoxazolamine	T42.8X1	T42.8X2	T42.8X3	T42.8X4	T42.8X5	T42.8X6
Zuclopenthixol	T43.4X1	T43.4X2	T43.4X3	T43.4X4	T43.4X5	T43.4X6
Zygadenus (venenosus)	T62.2X1	T62.2X2	T62.2X3	T62.2X4	—	—
Zyprexa	T43.591	T43.592	T43.593	T43.594	T43.595	T43.596

◀ New ◀ Revised deleted Deleted

External Cause
of Injuries Index

A

Abandonment (causing exposure to weather conditions) (with intent to injure or kill) NEC X58
Abuse (adult) (child) (mental) (physical) (sexual) X58
Accident (to) X58
  aircraft (in transit) (powered) —*see also* Accident, transport, aircraft
    due to, caused by cataclysm —*see* Forces of nature, by type
  animal-drawn vehicle —*see* Accident, transport, animal-drawn vehicle occupant
  animal-rider —*see* Accident, transport, animal-rider
  automobile —*see* Accident, transport, car occupant
  bare foot water skiier V94.4
  boat, boating —*see also* Accident, watercraft
    striking swimmer
      powered V94.11
      unpowered V94.12
  bus —*see* Accident, transport, bus occupant
  cable car, not on rails V98.0
    on rails —*see* Accident, transport, streetcar occupant
  car —*see* Accident, transport, car occupant
  caused by, due to
    animal NEC W64
    chain hoist W24.0
    cold (excessive) —*see* Exposure, cold
    corrosive liquid, substance —*see* Table of Drugs and Chemicals
    cutting or piercing instrument —*see* Contact, with, by type of instrument
    drive belt W24.0
    electric
      current —*see* Exposure, electric current
      motor (*see also* Contact, with, by type of machine) W31.3
        current (of) W86.8
    environmental factor NEC X58
    explosive material —*see* Explosion
    fire, flames —*see* Exposure, fire
    firearm missile —*see* Discharge, firearm by type
    heat (excessive) —*see* Heat
    hot —*see* Contact, with, hot
    ignition —*see* Ignition
    lifting device W24.0
    lightning —*see* subcategory T75.0
      causing fire —*see* Exposure, fire
    machine, machinery —*see* Contact, with, by type of machine
    natural factor NEC X58
    pulley (block) W24.0
    radiation —*see* Radiation
    steam X13.1
      inhalation X13.0
      pipe X16
    thunderbolt —*see* subcategory T75.0
      causing fire —*see* Exposure, fire
    transmission device W24.1
  coach —*see* Accident, transport, bus occupant
  coal car —*see* Accident, transport, industrial vehicle occupant
  diving —*see also* Fall, into, water
    with
      drowning or submersion —*see* Drowning
  forklift —*see* Accident, transport, industrial vehicle occupant
  heavy transport vehicle NOS —*see* Accident, transport, truck occupant
  ice yacht V98.2

Accident *(Continued)*
  in
    medical, surgical procedure
      as, or due to misadventure —*see* Misadventure
      causing an abnormal reaction or later complication without mention of misadventure (*see also* Complication of or following, by type of procedure) Y84.9
  land yacht V98.1
  late effect of —*see* W00-X58 with 7th character S
  logging car —*see* Accident, transport, industrial vehicle occupant
  machine, machinery —*see also* Contact, with, by type of machine
  on board watercraft V93.69
    explosion —*see* Explosion, in, watercraft
    fire —*see* Burn, on board watercraft
    powered craft V93.63
      ferry boat V93.61
      fishing boat V93.62
      jetskis V93.63
      liner V93.61
      merchant ship V93.60
      passenger ship V93.61
      sailboat V93.64
  mine tram —*see* Accident, transport, industrial vehicle occupant
  mobility scooter (motorized) —*see* Accident, transport, pedestrian, conveyance, specified type NEC
  motor scooter —*see* Accident, transport, motorcyclist
  motor vehicle NOS (traffic) (*see also* Accident, transport) V89.2
    nontraffic V89.0
    three-wheeled NOS —*see* Accident, transport, three-wheeled motor vehicle occupant
  motorcycle NOS —*see* Accident, transport, motorcyclist
  nonmotor vehicle NOS (nontraffic) (*see also* Accident, transport) V89.1
    traffic NOS V89.3
  nontraffic (victim's mode of transport NOS) V88.9
    collision (between) V88.7
      bus and truck V88.5
      car and:
        bus V88.3
        pickup V88.2
        three-wheeled motor vehicle V88.0
        train V88.6
        truck V88.4
        two-wheeled motor vehicle V88.0
        van V88.2
      specified vehicle NEC and:
        three-wheeled motor vehicle V88.1
        two-wheeled motor vehicle V88.1
    known mode of transport —*see* Accident, transport, by type of vehicle
    noncollision V88.8
  on board watercraft V93.89
    powered craft V93.83
      ferry boat V93.81
      fishing boat V93.82
      jetskis V93.83
      liner V93.81
      merchant ship V93.80
      passenger ship V93.81
    unpowered craft V93.88
      canoe V93.85
      inflatable V93.86
      in tow
        recreational V94.31
        specified NEC V94.32
      kayak V93.85

Accident *(Continued)*
  on board watercraft *(Continued)*
    unpowered craft *(Continued)*
      sailboat V93.84
      surf-board V93.88
      water skis V93.87
      windsurfer V93.88
  parachutist V97.29
    entangled in object V97.21
    injured on landing V97.22
  pedal cycle —*see* Accident, transport, pedal cyclist
  pedestrian (on foot)
    with
      another pedestrian W51
        with fall W03
          due to ice or snow W00.0
      on pedestrian conveyance NEC V00.09
      roller skater (in-line) V00.01
      skate boarder V00.02
      transport vehicle —*see* Accident, transport
    on pedestrian conveyance —*see* Accident, transport, pedestrian, conveyance
  pick-up truck or van —*see* Accident, transport, pickup truck occupant
  quarry truck —*see* Accident, transport, industrial vehicle occupant
  railway vehicle (any) (in motion) —*see* Accident, transport, railway vehicle occupant
    due to cataclysm —*see* Forces of nature, by type
  scooter (non-motorized) —*see* Accident, transport, pedestrian, conveyance, scooter
  sequelae of —*see* W00-X58 with 7th character S
  skateboard —*see* Accident, transport, pedestrian, conveyance, skateboard
  ski (ing) —*see* Accident, transport, pedestrian, conveyance
  lift V98.3
  specified cause NEC X58
  streetcar —*see* Accident, transport, streetcar occupant
  traffic (victim's mode of transport NOS) V87.9
    collision (between) V87.7
      bus and truck V87.5
      car and:
        bus V87.3
        pickup V87.2
        three-wheeled motor vehicle V87.0
        train V87.6
        truck V87.4
        two-wheeled motor vehicle V87.0
        van V87.2
      specified vehicle NEC and:
        three-wheeled motor vehicle V87.1
        two-wheeled motor vehicle V87.1
    known mode of transport —*see* Accident, transport, by type of vehicle
    noncollision V87.8
  transport (involving injury to) V99
    18 wheeler —*see* Accident, transport, truck occupant
    agricultural vehicle occupant (nontraffic) V84.9
      driver V84.5
      hanger-on V84.7
      passenger V84.6
      traffic V84.3
        driver V84.0
        hanger-on V84.2
        passenger V84.1
      while boarding or alighting V84.4

◀ New   ◀▥ Revised   ~~deleted~~ Deleted

Accident (Continued)
 transport (Continued)
  aircraft NEC V97.89
   military NEC V97.818
    with civilian aircraft V97.810
    civilian injured by V97.811
   occupant injured (in)
    nonpowered craft accident
      V96.9
     balloon V96.00
      collision V96.03
      crash V96.01
      explosion V96.05
      fire V96.04
      forced landing V96.02
      specified type NEC V96.09
     glider V96.20
      collision V96.23
      crash V96.21
      explosion V96.25
      fire V96.24
      forced landing V96.22
      specified type NEC V96.29
     hang glider V96.10
      collision V96.13
      crash V96.11
      explosion V96.15
      fire V96.14
      forced landing V96.12
      specified type NEC V96.19
     specified craft NEC V96.8
    powered craft accident V95.9
     fixed wing NEC
      commercial V95.30
       collision V95.33
       crash V95.31
       explosion V95.35
       fire V95.34
       forced landing V95.32
       specified type NEC
         V95.39
      private V95.20
       collision V95.23
       crash V95.21
       explosion V95.25
       fire V95.24
       forced landing V95.22
       specified type NEC
         V95.29
     glider V95.10
      collision V95.13
      crash V95.11
      explosion V95.15
      fire V95.14
      forced landing V95.12
      specified type NEC V95.19
     helicopter V95.00
      collision V95.03
      crash V95.01
      explosion V95.05
      fire V95.04
      forced landing V95.02
      specified type NEC V95.09
     spacecraft V95.40
      collision V95.43
      crash V95.41
      explosion V95.45
      fire V95.44
      forced landing V95.42
      specified type NEC V95.49
     specified craft NEC V95.8
     ultralight V95.10
      collision V95.13
      crash V95.11
      explosion V95.15
      fire V95.14
      forced landing V95.12
      specified type NEC V95.19
    specified accident NEC V97.0
    while boarding or alighting
      V97.1

Accident (Continued)
 transport (Continued)
  aircraft NEC (Continued)
   person (injured by)
    falling from, in or on aircraft V97.0
    machinery on aircraft V97.89
    on ground with aircraft involvement
      V97.39
    rotating propeller V97.32
    struck by object falling from aircraft
      V97.31
    sucked into aircraft jet V97.33
    while boarding or alighting aircraft
      V97.1
  airport (battery-powered) passenger
    vehicle —see Accident, transport,
    industrial vehicle occupant
  all-terrain vehicle occupant (nontraffic)
    V86.99
   driver V86.59
   dune buggy —see Accident, transport,
    dune buggy occupant
   hanger-on V86.79
   passenger V86.69
   snowmobile —see Accident, transport,
    snowmobile occupant
   traffic V86.39
    driver V86.09
    hanger-on V86.29
    passenger V86.19
   while boarding or alighting V86.49
  ambulance occupant (traffic) V86.31
   driver V86.01
   hanger-on V86.21
   nontraffic V86.91
    driver V86.51
    hanger-on V86.71
    passenger V86.61
   passenger V86.11
   while boarding or alighting V86.41
  animal-drawn vehicle occupant (in)
    V80.929
   collision (with)
    animal V80.12
     being ridden V80.711
    animal-drawn vehicle V80.721
    bus V80.42
    car V80.42
    fixed or stationary object V80.82
    military vehicle V80.920
    nonmotor vehicle V80.791
    pedal cycle V80.22
    pedestrian V80.12
    pickup V80.42
    railway train or vehicle V80.62
    specified motor vehicle NEC V80.52
    streetcar V80.731
    truck V80.42
    two-or three-wheeled motor vehicle
      V80.32
    van V80.42
   noncollision V80.02
   specified circumstance NEC V80. 928
  animal-rider V80.919
   collision (with)
    animal V80.11
     being ridden V80.710
    animal-drawn vehicle V80.720
    bus V80.41
    car V80.41
    fixed or stationary object V80.81
    military vehicle V80.910
    nonmotor vehicle V80.790
    pedal cycle V80.21
    pedestrian V80.11
    pickup V80.41
    railway train or vehicle V80.61
    specified motor vehicle NEC
      V80.51
    streetcar V80.730
    truck V80.41

Accident (Continued)
 transport (Continued)
  animal-rider (Continued)
   collision (Continued)
    two- or three-wheeled motor vehicle
      V80.31
    van V80.41
   noncollision V80.018
    specified as horse rider V80.010
   specified circumstance NEC V80.918
  armored car —see Accident, transport,
    truck occupant
  battery-powered truck (baggage) (mail) —
    see Accident, transport, industrial
    vehicle occupant
  bus occupant V79.9
   collision (with)
    animal (traffic) V70.9
     being ridden (traffic) V76.9
      nontraffic V76.3
       while boarding or alighting V76.4
     nontraffic V70.3
      while boarding or alighting V70.4
    animal-drawn vehicle (traffic) V76.9
     nontraffic V76.3
      while boarding or alighting V76.4
    bus (traffic) V74.9
     nontraffic V74.3
      while boarding or alighting V74.4
    car (traffic) V73.9
     nontraffic V73.3
      while boarding or alighting V73.4
    motor vehicle NOS (traffic) V79.60
     nontraffic V79.20
    specified type NEC (traffic) V79.69
     nontraffic V79.29
    pedal cycle (traffic) V71.9
     nontraffic V71.3
      while boarding or alighting V71.4
    pickup truck (traffic) V73.9
     nontraffic V73.3
      while boarding or alighting V73.4
    railway vehicle (traffic) V75.9
     nontraffic V75.3
      while boarding or alighting V75.4
    specified vehicle NEC (traffic) V76.9
     nontraffic V76.3
      while boarding or alighting V76.4
    stationary object (traffic) V77.9
     nontraffic V77.3
      while boarding or alighting V77.4
    streetcar (traffic) V76.9
     nontraffic V76.3
      while boarding or alighting V76.4
    three wheeled motor vehicle (traffic)
      V72.9
     nontraffic V72.3
      while boarding or alighting V72.4
    truck (traffic) V74.9
     nontraffic V74.3
      while boarding or alighting V74.4
    two wheeled motor vehicle (traffic)
      V72.9
     nontraffic V72.3
      while boarding or alighting V72.4
    van (traffic) V73.9
     nontraffic V73.3
      while boarding or alighting V73.4
   driver
    collision (with)
     animal (traffic) V70.5
      being ridden (traffic) V76.5
       nontraffic V76.0
     nontraffic V70.0
     animal-drawn vehicle (traffic)
       V76.5
      nontraffic V76.0
     bus (traffic) V74.5
      nontraffic V74.0
     car (traffic) V73.5
      nontraffic V73.0

A

Accident *(Continued)*
  transport *(Continued)*
    bus occupant *(Continued)*
      driver *(Continued)*
        collision *(Continued)*
          motor vehicle NOS (traffic) V79.40
            nontraffic V79.00
            specified type NEC (traffic)
              V79.49
            nontraffic V79.09
          pedal cycle (traffic) V71.5
            nontraffic V71.0
          pickup truck (traffic) V73.5
            nontraffic V73.0
          railway vehicle (traffic) V75.5
            nontraffic V75.0
          specified vehicle NEC (traffic)
            V76.5
            nontraffic V76.0
          stationary object (traffic) V77.5
            nontraffic V77.0
          streetcar (traffic) V76.5
            nontraffic V76.0
          three wheeled motor vehicle
            (traffic) V72.5
            nontraffic V72.0
          truck (traffic) V74.5
            nontraffic V74.0
          two wheeled motor vehicle (traffic)
            V72.5
            nontraffic V72.0
          van (traffic) V73.5
            nontraffic V73.0
        noncollision accident (traffic) V78.5
          nontraffic V78.0
      hanger-on
        collision (with)
          animal (traffic) V70.7
            being ridden (traffic) V76.7
              nontraffic V76.2
            nontraffic V70.2
          animal-drawn vehicle (traffic) V76.7
            nontraffic V76.2
          bus (traffic) V74.7
            nontraffic V74.2
          car (traffic) V73.7
            nontraffic V73.2
          pedal cycle (traffic) V71.7
            nontraffic V71.2
          pickup truck (traffic) V73.7
            nontraffic V73.2
          railway vehicle (traffic) V75.7
            nontraffic V75.2
          specified vehicle NEC (traffic) V76.7
            nontraffic V76.2
          stationary object (traffic) V77.7
            nontraffic V77.2
          streetcar (traffic) V76.7
            nontraffic V76.2
          three wheeled motor vehicle
            (traffic) V72.7
            nontraffic V72.2
          truck (traffic) V74.7
            nontraffic V74.2
          two wheeled motor vehicle (traffic)
            V72.7
            nontraffic V72.2
          van (traffic) V73.7
            nontraffic V73.2
        noncollision accident (traffic) V78.7
          nontraffic V78.2
        noncollision accident (traffic) V78.9
          nontraffic V78.3
          while boarding or alighting V78.4
        nontraffic V79.3
      passenger
        collision (with)
          animal (traffic) V70.6
            being ridden (traffic) V76.6
              nontraffic V76.1
            nontraffic V70.1

Accident *(Continued)*
  transport *(Continued)*
    bus occupant *(Continued)*
      passenger *(Continued)*
        collision *(Continued)*
          animal-drawn vehicle (traffic) V76.6
            nontraffic V76.1
          bus (traffic) V74.6
            nontraffic V74.1
          car (traffic) V73.6
            nontraffic V73.1
          motor vehicle NOS (traffic) V79.50
            nontraffic V79.10
            specified type NEC (traffic)
              V79.59
            nontraffic V79.19
          pedal cycle (traffic) V71.6
            nontraffic V71.1
          pickup truck (traffic) V73.6
            nontraffic V73.1
          railway vehicle (traffic) V75.6
            nontraffic V75.1
          specified vehicle NEC (traffic) V76.6
            nontraffic V76.1
          stationary object (traffic) V77.6
            nontraffic V77.1
          streetcar (traffic) V76.6
            nontraffic V76.1
          three wheeled motor vehicle
            (traffic) V72.6
            nontraffic V72.1
          truck (traffic) V74.6
            nontraffic V74.1
          two wheeled motor vehicle (traffic)
            V72.6
            nontraffic V72.1
          van (traffic) V73.6
            nontraffic V73.1
        noncollision accident (traffic) V78.6
          nontraffic V78.1
      specified type NEC V79.88
      military vehicle V79.81
    cable car, not on rails V98.0
      on rails —*see* Accident, transport,
        streetcar occupant
    car occupant V49.9
      ambulance occupant —*see* Accident,
        transport, ambulance occupant
      collision (with)
        animal (traffic) V40.9
          being ridden (traffic) V46.9
            nontraffic V46.3
            while boarding or alighting
              V46.4
          nontraffic V40.3
          while boarding or alighting V40.4
        animal-drawn vehicle (traffic) V46.9
          nontraffic V46.3
          while boarding or alighting V46.4
        bus (traffic) V44.9
          nontraffic V44.3
          while boarding or alighting V44.4
        car (traffic) V43.92
          nontraffic V43.32
          while boarding or alighting V43.42
        motor vehicle NOS (traffic) V49.60
          nontraffic V49.20
          specified type NEC (traffic) V49.69
            nontraffic V49.29
        pedal cycle (traffic) V41.9
          nontraffic V41.3
          while boarding or alighting V41.4
        pickup truck (traffic) V43.93
          nontraffic V43.33
          while boarding or alighting V43.43
        railway vehicle (traffic) V45.9
          nontraffic V45.3
          while boarding or alighting V45.4
        specified vehicle NEC (traffic) V46.9
          nontraffic V46.3
          while boarding or alighting V46.4

Accident *(Continued)*
  transport *(Continued)*
    car occupant *(Continued)*
      collision *(Continued)*
        sport utility vehicle (traffic) V43.91
          nontraffic V43.31
          while boarding or alighting V43.41
        stationary object (traffic) V47.92
          nontraffic V47.32
          while boarding or alighting V47.4
        streetcar (traffic) V46.9
          nontraffic V46.3
          while boarding or alighting V46.4
        three wheeled motor vehicle (traffic)
          V42.9
          nontraffic V42.3
          while boarding or alighting V42.4
        truck (traffic) V44.9
          nontraffic V44.3
          while boarding or alighting V44.4
        two wheeled motor vehicle (traffic)
          V42.9
          nontraffic V42.3
          while boarding or alighting V42.4
        van (traffic) V43.94
          nontraffic V43.34
          while boarding or alighting V43.44
      driver
        collision (with)
          animal (traffic) V40.5
            being ridden (traffic) V46.5
              nontraffic V46.0
            nontraffic V40.0
          animal-drawn vehicle (traffic) V46.5
            nontraffic V46.0
          bus (traffic) V44.5
            nontraffic V44.0
          car (traffic) V43.52
            nontraffic V43.02
          motor vehicle NOS (traffic) V49.40
            nontraffic V49.00
            specified type NEC (traffic)
              V49.49
            nontraffic V49.09
          pedal cycle (traffic) V41.5
            nontraffic V41.0
          pickup truck (traffic) V43.53
            nontraffic V43.03
          railway vehicle (traffic) V45.5
            nontraffic V45.0
          specified vehicle NEC (traffic) V46.5
            nontraffic V46.0
          sport utility vehicle (traffic) V43.51
            nontraffic V43.01
          stationary object (traffic) V47.52
            nontraffic V47.02
          streetcar (traffic) V46.5
            nontraffic V46.0
          three wheeled motor vehicle
            (traffic) V42.5
            nontraffic V42.0
          truck (traffic) V44.5
            nontraffic V44.0
          two wheeled motor vehicle (traffic)
            V42.5
            nontraffic V42.0
          van (traffic) V43.54
            nontraffic V43.04
        noncollision accident (traffic) V48.5
          nontraffic V48.0
      hanger-on
        collision (with)
          animal (traffic) V40.7
            being ridden (traffic) V46.7
              nontraffic V46.2
            nontraffic V40.2
          animal-drawn vehicle (traffic)
            V46.7
            nontraffic V46.2
          bus (traffic) V44.7
            nontraffic V44.2

Accident *(Continued)*
transport *(Continued)*
car occupant *(Continued)*
hanger-on *(Continued)*
collision *(Continued)*
car (traffic) V43.72
nontraffic V43.22
pedal cycle (traffic) V41.7
nontraffic V41.2
pickup truck (traffic) V43.73
nontraffic V43.23
railway vehicle (traffic) V45.7
nontraffic V45.2
specified vehicle NEC (traffic) V46.7
nontraffic V46.2
sport utility vehicle (traffic) V43.71
nontraffic V43.21
stationary object (traffic) V47.7
nontraffic V47.2
streetcar (traffic) V46.7
nontraffic V46.2
three wheeled motor vehicle
(traffic) V42.7
nontraffic V42.2
truck (traffic) V44.7
nontraffic V44.2
two wheeled motor vehicle (traffic)
V42.7
nontraffic V42.2
van (traffic) V43.74
nontraffic V43.24
noncollision accident (traffic) V48.7
nontraffic V48.2
noncollision accident (traffic) V48.9
nontraffic V48.3
while boarding or alighting V48.4
nontraffic V49.3
passenger
collision (with)
animal (traffic) V40.6
being ridden (traffic) V46.6
nontraffic V46.1
nontraffic V40.1
animal-drawn vehicle (traffic) V46.6
nontraffic V46.1
bus (traffic) V44.6
nontraffic V44.1
car (traffic) V43.62
nontraffic V43.12
motor vehicle NOS (traffic) V49.50
nontraffic V49.10
specified type NEC (traffic) V49.59
nontraffic V49.19
pedal cycle (traffic) V41.6
nontraffic V41.1
pickup truck (traffic) V43.63
nontraffic V43.13
railway vehicle (traffic) V45.6
nontraffic V45.1
specified vehicle NEC (traffic) V46.6
nontraffic V46.1
sport utility vehicle (traffic) V43.61
nontraffic V43.11
stationary object (traffic) V47.62
nontraffic V47.12
streetcar (traffic) V46.6
nontraffic V46.1
three wheeled motor vehicle
(traffic) V42.6
nontraffic V42.1
truck (traffic) V44.6
nontraffic V44.1
two wheeled motor vehicle (traffic)
V42.6
nontraffic V42.1
van (traffic) V43.64
nontraffic V43.14
noncollision accident (traffic) V48.6
nontraffic V48.1
specified type NEC V49.88
military vehicle V49.81

Accident *(Continued)*
transport *(Continued)*
coal car —*see* Accident, transport,
industrial vehicle occupant
construction vehicle occupant (nontraffic)
V85.9
driver V85.5
hanger-on V85.7
passenger V85.6
traffic V85.3
driver V85.0
hanger-on V85.2
passenger V85.1
while boarding or alighting V85.4
dirt bike rider —*see* Accident, transport,
all-terrain vehicle occupant
due to cataclysm —*see* Forces of nature,
by type
dune buggy occupant (nontraffic) V86.93
driver V86.53
hanger-on V86.73
passenger V86.63
traffic V86.33
driver V86.03
hanger-on V86.23
passenger V86.13
while boarding or alighting V86.43
forklift —*see* Accident, transport, industrial
vehicle occupant
go cart —*see* Accident, transport, all-terrain
vehicle occupant
golf cart —*see* Accident, transport, all-
terrain vehicle occupant
heavy transport vehicle occupant —*see*
Accident, transport, truck occupant
ice yacht V98.2
industrial vehicle occupant (nontraffic)
V83.9
driver V83.5
hanger-on V83.7
passenger V83.6
traffic V83.3
driver V83.0
hanger-on V83.2
passenger V83.1
while boarding or alighting V83.4
interurban electric car —*see* Accident,
transport, streetcar
land yacht V98.1
logging car —*see* Accident, transport,
industrial vehicle occupant
military vehicle occupant (traffic) V86.34
driver V86.04
hanger-on V86.24
nontraffic V86.94
driver V86.54
hanger-on V86.74
passenger V86.64
passenger V86.14
while boarding or alighting V86.44
mine tram —*see* Accident, transport,
industrial vehicle occupant
motor vehicle NEC occupant (traffic) V86.39
driver V86.09
hanger-on V86.29
nontraffic V86.99
driver V86.59
hanger-on V86.79
passenger V86.69
passenger V86.19
while boarding or alighting V86.49
motorcoach —*see* Accident, transport, bus
occupant
motorcyclist V29.9
collision (with)
animal (traffic) V20.9
being ridden (traffic) V26.9
nontraffic V26.2
while boarding or alighting V26.3
nontraffic V20.2
while boarding or alighting V20.3

Accident *(Continued)*
transport *(Continued)*
motorcyclist *(Continued)*
collision *(Continued)*
animal-drawn vehicle (traffic) V26.9
nontraffic V26.2
while boarding or alighting V26.3
bus (traffic) V24.9
nontraffic V24.2
while boarding or alighting V24.3
car (traffic) V23.9
nontraffic V23.2
while boarding or alighting V23.3
motor vehicle NOS (traffic) V29.60
nontraffic V29.20
specified type NEC (traffic) V29.69
nontraffic V29.29
pedal cycle (traffic) V21.9
nontraffic V21.2
while boarding or alighting V21.3
pickup truck (traffic) V23.9
nontraffic V23.2
while boarding or alighting V23.3
railway vehicle (traffic) V25.9
nontraffic V25.2
while boarding or alighting V25.3
specified vehicle NEC (traffic) V26.9
nontraffic V26.2
while boarding or alighting V26.3
stationary object (traffic) V27.9
nontraffic V27.2
while boarding or alighting V27.3
streetcar (traffic) V26.9
nontraffic V26.2
while boarding or alighting V26.3
three wheeled motor vehicle (traffic)
V22.9
nontraffic V22.2
while boarding or alighting V22.3
truck (traffic) V24.9
nontraffic V24.2
while boarding or alighting V24.3
two wheeled motor vehicle (traffic)
V22.9
nontraffic V22.2
while boarding or alighting V22.3
van (traffic) V23.9
nontraffic V23.2
while boarding or alighting V23.3
driver
collision (with)
animal (traffic) V20.4
being ridden (traffic) V26.4
nontraffic V26.0
nontraffic V20.0
animal-drawn vehicle (traffic) V26.4
nontraffic V26.0
bus (traffic) V24.4
nontraffic V24.0
car (traffic) V23.4
nontraffic V23.0
motor vehicle NOS (traffic) V29.40
nontraffic V29.00
specified type NEC (traffic)
V29.49
nontraffic V29.09
pedal cycle (traffic) V21.4
nontraffic V21.0
pickup truck (traffic) V23.4
nontraffic V23.0
railway vehicle (traffic) V25.4
nontraffic V25.0
specified vehicle NEC (traffic) V26.4
nontraffic V26.0
stationary object (traffic) V27.4
nontraffic V27.0
streetcar (traffic) V26.4
nontraffic V26.0
three wheeled motor vehicle
(traffic) V22.4
nontraffic V22.0

Accident *(Continued)*
 transport *(Continued)*
  motorcyclist *(Continued)*
   driver *(Continued)*
    collision *(Continued)*
     truck (traffic) V24.4
      nontraffic V24.0
     two wheeled motor vehicle (traffic) V22.4
      nontraffic V22.0
     van (traffic) V23.4
      nontraffic V23.0
    noncollision accident (traffic) V28.4
     nontraffic V28.0
   noncollision accident (traffic) V28.9
    nontraffic V28.2
    while boarding or alighting V28.3
   nontraffic V29.3
   passenger
    collision (with)
     animal (traffic) V20.5
      being ridden (traffic) V26.5
       nontraffic V26.1
      nontraffic V20.1
     animal-drawn vehicle (traffic) V26.5
      nontraffic V26.1
     bus (traffic) V24.5
      nontraffic V24.1
     car (traffic) V23.5
      nontraffic V23.1
     motor vehicle NOS (traffic) V29.50
      nontraffic V29.10
      specified type NEC (traffic) V29.59
       nontraffic V29.19
     pedal cycle (traffic) V21.5
      nontraffic V21.1
     pickup truck (traffic) V23.5
      nontraffic V23.1
     railway vehicle (traffic) V25.5
      nontraffic V25.1
     specified vehicle NEC (traffic) V26.5
      nontraffic V26.1
     stationary object (traffic) V27.5
      nontraffic V27.1
     streetcar (traffic) V26.5
      nontraffic V26.1
     three wheeled motor vehicle (traffic) V22.5
      nontraffic V22.1
     truck (traffic) V24.5
      nontraffic V24.1
     two wheeled motor vehicle (traffic) V22.5
      nontraffic V22.1
     van (traffic) V23.5
      nontraffic V23.1
    noncollision accident (traffic) V28.5
     nontraffic V28.1
   specified type NEC V29.88
   military vehicle V29.81
  occupant (of)
   aircraft (powered) V95.9
    fixed wing
     commercial —*see* Accident, transport, aircraft, occupant, powered, fixed wing, commercial
     private —*see* Accident, transport, aircraft, occupant, powered, fixed wing, private
    nonpowered V96.9
    specified NEC V95.8
   airport battery-powered vehicle —*see* Accident, transport, industrial vehicle occupant
   all-terrain vehicle (ATV) —*see* Accident, transport, all-terrain vehicle occupant

Accident *(Continued)*
 transport *(Continued)*
  occupant *(Continued)*
   animal-drawn vehicle —*see* Accident, transport, animal-drawn vehicle occupant
   automobile —*see* Accident, transport, car occupant
   balloon V96.00
   battery-powered vehicle —*see* Accident, transport, industrial vehicle occupant
   bicycle —*see* Accident, transport, pedal cyclist
    motorized —*see* Accident, transport, motorcycle rider
   boat NEC —*see* Accident, watercraft
   bulldozer —*see* Accident, transport, construction vehicle occupant
   bus —*see* Accident, transport, bus occupant
   cable car (on rails) —*see also* Accident, transport, streetcar occupant
    not on rails V98.0
   car —*see also* Accident, transport, car occupant
    cable (on rails) —*see also* Accident, transport, streetcar occupant
     not on rails V98.0
   coach —*see* Accident, transport, bus occupant
   coal-car —*see* Accident, transport, industrial vehicle occupant
   digger —*see* Accident, transport, construction vehicle occupant
   dump truck —*see* Accident, transport, construction vehicle occupant
   earth-leveler —*see* Accident, transport, construction vehicle occupant
   farm machinery (self-propelled) —*see* Accident, transport, agricultural vehicle occupant
   forklift —*see* Accident, transport, industrial vehicle occupant
   glider (unpowered) V96.20
    hang V96.10
    powered (microlight) (ultralight) —*see* Accident, transport, aircraft, occupant, powered, glider
   glider (unpowered) NEC V96.20
   hang-glider V96.10
   harvester —*see* Accident, transport, agricultural vehicle occupant
   heavy (transport) vehicle —*see* Accident, transport, truck occupant
   helicopter —*see* Accident, transport, aircraft, occupant, helicopter
   ice-yacht V98.2
   kite (carrying person) V96.8
   land-yacht V98.1
   logging car —*see* Accident, transport, industrial vehicle occupant
   mechanical shovel —*see* Accident, transport, construction vehicle occupant
   microlight —*see* Accident, transport, aircraft, occupant, powered, glider
   minibus —*see* Accident, transport, car occupant
   minivan —*see* Accident, transport, car occupant
   moped —*see* Accident, transport, motorcycle
   motor scooter —*see* Accident, transport, motorcycle
   motorcycle (with sidecar) —*see* Accident, transport, motorcycle
   pedal cycle —*see also* Accident, transport, pedal cyclist
   pick-up (truck) —*see* Accident, transport, pickup truck occupant

Accident *(Continued)*
 transport *(Continued)*
  occupant *(Continued)*
   railway (train) (vehicle) (subterranean) (elevated) —*see* Accident, transport, railway vehicle occupant
   rickshaw —*see* Accident, transport, pedal cycle
    pedal driven —*see* Accident, transport, pedal cyclist
   road-roller —*see* Accident, transport, construction vehicle occupant
   ship NOS V94.9
   ski-lift (chair) (gondola) V98.3
   snowmobile —*see* Accident, transport, snowmobile occupant
   spacecraft, spaceship —*see* Accident, transport, aircraft, occupant, spacecraft
   sport utility vehicle —*see* Accident, transport, car occupant
   streetcar (interurban) (operating on public street or highway) —*see* Accident, transport, streetcar occupant
   SUV —*see* Accident, transport, car occupant
   téléférique V98.0
   three-wheeled vehicle (motorized) —*see also* Accident, transport, three-wheeled motor vehicle occupant
    nonmotorized —*see* Accident, transport, pedal cycle
   tractor (farm) (and trailer) —*see* Accident, transport, agricultural vehicle occupant
   train —*see* Accident, transport, railway vehicle occupant
   tram —*see* Accident, transport, streetcar occupant
    in mine or quarry —*see* Accident, transport, industrial vehicle occupant
   tricycle —*see* Accident, transport, pedal cycle
    motorized —*see* Accident, transport, three-wheeled motor vehicle
   trolley —*see* Accident, transport, streetcar occupant
    in mine or quarry —*see* Accident, transport, industrial vehicle occupant
   tub, in mine or quarry —*see* Accident, transport, industrial vehicle occupant
   ultralight —*see* Accident, transport, aircraft, occupant, powered, glider
   van —*see* Accident, transport, van occupant
   vehicle NEC V89.9
    heavy transport —*see* Accident, transport, truck occupant
    motor (traffic) NEC V89.2
     nontraffic NEC V89.0
   watercraft NOS V94.9
    causing drowning —*see* Drowning, resulting from accident to boat
  parachutist V97.29
   after accident to aircraft —*see* Accident, transport, aircraft
   entangled in object V97.21
   injured on landing V97.22
  pedal cyclist V19.9
   collision (with)
    animal (traffic) V10.9
     being ridden (traffic) V16.9
      nontraffic V16.2
      while boarding or alighting V16.3
     nontraffic V10.2
     while boarding or alighting V10.3

◀ New   ◀▥ Revised   ~~deleted~~ Deleted

Accident *(Continued)*
  transport *(Continued)*
    pedal cyclist *(Continued)*
      collision *(Continued)*
        animal-drawn vehicle (traffic) V16.9
          nontraffic V16.2
          while boarding or alighting V16.3
        bus (traffic) V14.9
          nontraffic V14.2
          while boarding or alighting V14.3
        car (traffic) V13.9
          nontraffic V13.2
          while boarding or alighting V13.3
        motor vehicle NOS (traffic) V19.60
          nontraffic V19.20
          specified type NEC (traffic) V19.69
            nontraffic V19.29
        pedal cycle (traffic) V11.9
          nontraffic V11.2
          while boarding or alighting V11.3
        pickup truck (traffic) V13.9
          nontraffic V13.2
          while boarding or alighting V13.3
        railway vehicle (traffic) V15.9
          nontraffic V15.2
          while boarding or alighting V15.3
        specified vehicle NEC (traffic) V16.9
          nontraffic V16.2
          while boarding or alighting V16.3
        stationary object (traffic) V17.9
          nontraffic V17.2
          while boarding or alighting V17.3
        streetcar (traffic) V16.9
          nontraffic V16.2
          while boarding or alighting V16.3
        three wheeled motor vehicle (traffic)
          V12.9
          nontraffic V12.2
          while boarding or alighting V12.3
        truck (traffic) V14.9
          nontraffic V14.2
          while boarding or alighting V14.3
        two wheeled motor vehicle (traffic)
          V12.9
          nontraffic V12.2
          while boarding or alighting V12.3
        van (traffic) V13.9
          nontraffic V13.2
          while boarding or alighting V13.3
      driver
        collision (with)
          animal (traffic) V10.4
            being ridden (traffic) V16.4
              nontraffic V16.0
            nontraffic V10.0
          animal-drawn vehicle (traffic) V16.4
            nontraffic V16.0
          bus (traffic) V14.4
            nontraffic V14.0
          car (traffic) V13.4
            nontraffic V13.0
          motor vehicle NOS (traffic) V19.40
            nontraffic V19.00
            specified type NEC (traffic)
              V19.49
              nontraffic V19.09
          pedal cycle (traffic) V11.4
            nontraffic V11.0
          pickup truck (traffic) V13.4
            nontraffic V13.0
          railway vehicle (traffic) V15.4
            nontraffic V15.0
          specified vehicle NEC (traffic) V16.4
            nontraffic V16.0
          stationary object (traffic) V17.4
            nontraffic V17.0
          streetcar (traffic) V16.4
            nontraffic V16.0
          three wheeled motor vehicle
            (traffic) V12.4
            nontraffic V12.0

Accident *(Continued)*
  transport *(Continued)*
    pedal cyclist *(Continued)*
      driver *(Continued)*
        collision *(Continued)*
          truck (traffic) V14.4
            nontraffic V14.0
          two wheeled motor vehicle (traffic)
            V12.4
            nontraffic V12.0
          van (traffic) V13.4
            nontraffic V13.0
        noncollision accident (traffic) V18.4
          nontraffic V18.0
        noncollision accident (traffic) V18.9
          nontraffic V18.2
          while boarding or alighting V18.3
        nontraffic V19.3
      passenger
        collision (with)
          animal (traffic) V10.5
            being ridden (traffic) V16.5
              nontraffic V16.1
            nontraffic V10.1
          animal-drawn vehicle (traffic) V16.5
            nontraffic V16.1
          bus (traffic) V14.5
            nontraffic V14.1
          car (traffic) V13.5
            nontraffic V13.1
          motor vehicle NOS (traffic) V19.50
            nontraffic V19.10
            specified type NEC (traffic)
              V19.59
              nontraffic V19.19
          pedal cycle (traffic) V11.5
            nontraffic V11.1
          pickup truck (traffic) V13.5
            nontraffic V13.1
          railway vehicle (traffic) V15.5
            nontraffic V15.1
          specified vehicle NEC (traffic) V16.5
            nontraffic V16.1
          stationary object (traffic) V17.5
            nontraffic V17.1
          streetcar (traffic) V16.5
            nontraffic V16.1
          three wheeled motor vehicle
            (traffic) V12.5
            nontraffic V12.1
          truck (traffic) V14.5
            nontraffic V14.1
          two wheeled motor vehicle (traffic)
            V12.5
            nontraffic V12.1
          van (traffic) V13.5
            nontraffic V13.1
        noncollision accident (traffic) V18.5
          nontraffic V18.1
        specified type NEC V19.88
        military vehicle V19.81
    pedestrian
      conveyance (occupant) V09.9
        babystroller V00.828
          collision (with) V09.9
            animal being ridden or animal
              drawn vehicle V06.99
              nontraffic V06.09
              traffic V06.19
            bus or heavy transport V04.99
              nontraffic V04.09
              traffic V04.19
            car V03.99
              nontraffic V03.09
              traffic V03.19
            pedal cycle V01.99
              nontraffic V01.09
              traffic V01.19
            pick-up truck or van V03.99
              nontraffic V03.09
              traffic V03.19

Accident *(Continued)*
  transport *(Continued)*
    pedestrian *(Continued)*
      conveyance *(Continued)*
        babystroller *(Continued)*
          collision *(Continued)*
            railway (train) (vehicle) V05.99
              nontraffic V05.09
              traffic V05.19
            stationary object V00.822
            streetcar V06.99
              nontraffic V06.09
              traffic V06.19
            two- or three-wheeled motor
              vehicle V02.99
              nontraffic V02.09
              traffic V02.19
            vehicle V09.9
              animal-drawn V06.99
                nontraffic V06.09
                traffic V06.19
              motor
                nontraffic V09.00
                traffic V09.20
        fall V00.821
        nontraffic V09.1
          involving motor vehicle NEC
            V09.00
        traffic V09.3
          involving motor vehicle NEC
            V09.20
        flat-bottomed NEC V00.388
          collision (with) V09.9
            animal being ridden or animal
              drawn vehicle V06.99
              nontraffic V06.09
              traffic V06.19
            bus or heavy transport V04.99
              nontraffic V04.09
              traffic V04.19
            car V03.99
              nontraffic V03.09
              traffic V03.19
            pedal cycle V01.99
              nontraffic V01.09
              traffic V01.19
            pick-up truck or van V03.99
              nontraffic V03.09
              traffic V03.19
            railway (train) (vehicle) V05.99
              nontraffic V05.09
              traffic V05.19
            stationary object V00.382
            streetcar V06.99
              nontraffic V06.09
              traffic V06.19
            two-or three-wheeled motor
              vehicle V02.99
              nontraffic V02.09
              traffic V02.19
            vehicle V09.9
              animal-drawn V06.99
                nontraffic V06.09
                traffic V06.19
              motor
                nontraffic V09.00
                traffic V09.20
        fall V00.381
        nontraffic V09.1
          involving motor vehicle NEC
            V09.00
        snow
          board —*see* Accident, transport,
            pedestrian, conveyance,
            snow board
          ski —*see* Accident, transport,
            pedestrian, conveyance, skis
            (snow)
        traffic V09.3
          involving motor vehicle NEC
            V09.20

Accident *(Continued)*
 transport *(Continued)*
  pedestrian *(Continued)*
   conveyance *(Continued)*
    gliding type NEC V00.288
     collision (with) V09.9
      animal being ridden or animal
       drawn vehicle V06.99
       nontraffic V06.09
       traffic V06.19
      bus or heavy transport
       V04.99
       nontraffic V04.09
       traffic V04.19
      car V03.99
       nontraffic V03.09
       traffic V03.19
      pedal cycle V01.99
       nontraffic V01.09
       traffic V01.19
      pick-up truck or van V03.99
       nontraffic V03.09
       traffic V03.19
      railway (train) (vehicle) V05.99
       nontraffic V05.09
       traffic V05.19
      stationary object V00.282
      streetcar V06.99
       nontraffic V06.09
       traffic V06.19
      two- or three-wheeled motor
       vehicle V02.99
       nontraffic V02.09
       traffic V02.19
      vehicle V09.9
       animal-drawn V06.99
        nontraffic V06.09
        traffic V06.19
       motor
        nontraffic V09.00
        traffic V09.20
     fall V00.281
    heelies —*see* Accident, transport,
      pedestrian, conveyance,
      heelies
    ice skate —*see* Accident, transport,
      pedestrian, conveyance, ice
      skate
    nontraffic V09.1
     involving motor vehicle NEC
       V09.00
    sled —*see* Accident, transport,
      pedestrian, conveyance, sled
    traffic V09.3
     involving motor vehicle NEC
       V09.20
    wheelies —*see* Accident,
      transport, pedestrian,
      conveyance, heelies
   heelies V00.158
    colliding with stationary object
      V00.152
    fall V00.151
   ice skates V00.218
    collision (with) V09.9
     animal being ridden or animal
      drawn vehicle V06.99
      nontraffic V06.09
      traffic V06.19
     bus or heavy transport V04.99
      nontraffic V04.09
      traffic V04.19
     car V03.99
      nontraffic V03.09
      traffic V03.19
     pedal cycle V01.99
      nontraffic V01.09
      traffic V01.19
     pick-up truck or van V03.99
      nontraffic V03.09
      traffic V03.19

Accident *(Continued)*
 transport *(Continued)*
  pedestrian *(Continued)*
   conveyance *(Continued)*
    ice skates *(Continued)*
     collision *(Continued)*
      railway (train) (vehicle)
       V05.99
       nontraffic V05.09
       traffic V05.19
      stationary object V00.212
      streetcar V06.99
       nontraffic V06.09
       traffic V06.19
      two- or three-wheeled motor
       vehicle V02.99
       nontraffic V02.09
       traffic V02.19
      vehicle V09.9
       animal-drawn V06.99
        nontraffic V06.09
        traffic V06.19
       motor
        nontraffic V09.00
        traffic V09.20
     fall V00.211
     nontraffic V09.1
      involving motor vehicle NEC
        V09.00
     traffic V09.3
      involving motor vehicle NEC
        V09.20
    motorized mobility scooter
      V00.838
     collision with stationary object
       V00.832
     fall from V00.831
    nontraffic V09.1
     involving motor vehicle
       V09.00
      military V09.01
      specified type NEC V09.09
    roller skates (non in-line) V00.128
     collision (with) V09.9
      animal being ridden or animal
       drawn vehicle V06.91
       nontraffic V06.01
       traffic V06.11
      bus or heavy transport
       V04.91
       nontraffic V04.01
       traffic V04.11
      car V03.91
       nontraffic V03.01
       traffic V03.11
      pedal cycle V01.91
       nontraffic V01.01
       traffic V01.11
      pick-up truck or van V03.91
       nontraffic V03.01
       traffic V03.11
      railway (train) (vehicle)
       V05.91
       nontraffic V05.01
       traffic V05.11
      stationary object V00.122
      streetcar V06.91
       nontraffic V06.01
       traffic V06.11
      two- or three-wheeled motor
       vehicle V02.91
       nontraffic V02.01
       traffic V02.11
      vehicle V09.9
       animal-drawn V06.91
        nontraffic V06.01
        traffic V06.11
       motor
        nontraffic V09.00
        traffic V09.20
     fall V00.121

Accident *(Continued)*
 transport *(Continued)*
  pedestrian *(Continued)*
   conveyance *(Continued)*
    roller skates *(Continued)*
     in-line V00.118
      collision —*see also* Accident,
       transport, pedestrian,
       conveyance occupant, roller
       skates, collision
       with stationary object
        V00.112
      fall V00.111
      nontraffic V09.1
       involving motor vehicle NEC
        V09.00
      traffic V09.3
       involving motor vehicle NEC
        V09.20
     rolling shoes V00.158
      colliding with stationary object
        V00.152
      fall V00.151
     rolling type NEC V00.188
      collision (with) V09.9
       animal being ridden or animal
        drawn vehicle V06.99
        nontraffic V06.09
        traffic V06.19
       bus or heavy transport V04.99
        nontraffic V04.09
        traffic V04.19
       car V03.99
        nontraffic V03.09
        traffic V03.19
       pedal cycle V01.99
        nontraffic V01.09
        traffic V01.19
       pick-up truck or van V03.99
        nontraffic V03.09
        traffic V03.19
       railway (train) (vehicle)
        V05.99
        nontraffic V05.09
        traffic V05.19
       stationary object V00.182
       streetcar V06.99
        nontraffic V06.09
        traffic V06.19
       two- or three-wheeled motor
        vehicle V02.99
        nontraffic V02.09
        traffic V02.19
       vehicle V09.9
        animal-drawn V06.99
         nontraffic V06.09
         traffic V06.19
        motor
         nontraffic V09.00
         traffic V09.20
      fall V00.181
     in-line roller skate —*see* Accident,
       transport, pedestrian,
       conveyance, roller skate,
       in-line
     nontraffic V09.1
      involving motor vehicle NEC
        V09.00
     roller skate —*see* Accident,
       transport, pedestrian,
       conveyance, roller skate
     scooter (non-motorized) —
       see Accident, transport,
       pedestrian, conveyance,
       scooter
     skateboard —*see* Accident,
       transport, pedestrian,
       conveyance, skateboard
     traffic V09.3
      involving motor vehicle NEC
        V09.20

◀ New ◀▥▥ Revised ~~deleted~~ Deleted

Accident (Continued)
  transport (Continued)
    pedestrian (Continued)
      conveyance (Continued)
        scooter (non-motorized) V00.148
          collision (with) V09.9
            animal being ridden or animal
              drawn vehicle V06.99
              nontraffic V06.09
              traffic V06.19
            bus or heavy transport
              V04.99
              nontraffic V04.09
              traffic V04.19
            car V03.99
              nontraffic V03.09
              traffic V03.19
            pedal cycle V01.99
              nontraffic V01.09
              traffic V01.19
            pick-up truck or van V03.99
              nontraffic V03.09
              traffic V03.19
            railway (train) (vehicle)
              V05.99
              nontraffic V05.09
              traffic V05.19
            stationary object V00.142
            streetcar V06.99
              nontraffic V06.09
              traffic V06.19
            two- or three-wheeled motor
              vehicle V02.99
              nontraffic V02.09
              traffic V02.19
            vehicle V09.9
              animal-drawn V06.99
                nontraffic V06.09
                traffic V06.19
              motor
                nontraffic V09.00
                traffic V09.20
        fall V00.141
        nontraffic V09.1
          involving motor vehicle NEC
            V09.00
        traffic V09.3
          involving motor vehicle NEC
            V09.20
        skate board V00.138
          collision (with) V09.9
            animal being ridden or
              animal drawn vehicle
              V06.92
              nontraffic V06.02
              traffic V06.12
            bus or heavy transport
              V04.92
              nontraffic V04.02
              traffic V04.12
            car V03.92
              nontraffic V03.02
              traffic V03.12
            pedal cycle V01.92
              nontraffic V01.02
              traffic V01.12
            pick-up truck or van V03.92
              nontraffic V03.02
              traffic V03.12
            railway (train) (vehicle)
              V05.92
              nontraffic V05.02
              traffic V05.12
            stationary object V00.132
            streetcar V06.92
              nontraffic V06.02
              traffic V06.12
            two- or three-wheeled motor
              vehicle V02.92
              nontraffic V02.02
              traffic V02.12

Accident (Continued)
  transport (Continued)
    pedestrian (Continued)
      conveyance (Continued)
        skate board (Continued)
          collision (Continued)
            vehicle V09.9
              animal-drawn V06.92
                nontraffic V06.02
                traffic V06.12
              motor
                nontraffic V09.00
                traffic V09.20
          fall V00.131
          nontraffic V09.1
            involving motor vehicle NEC
              V09.00
          traffic V09.3
            involving motor vehicle NEC
              V09.20
        skis (snow) V00.328
          collision (with) V09.9
            animal being ridden or animal
              drawn vehicle V06.99
              nontraffic V06.09
              traffic V06.19
            bus or heavy transport V04.99
              nontraffic V04.09
              traffic V04.19
            car V03.99
              nontraffic V03.09
              traffic V03.19
            pedal cycle V01.99
              nontraffic V01.09
              traffic V01.19
            pick-up truck or van V03.99
              nontraffic V03.09
              traffic V03.19
            railway (train) (vehicle) V05.99
              nontraffic V05.09
              traffic V05.19
            stationary object V00.322
            streetcar V06.99
              nontraffic V06.09
              traffic V06.19
            two- or three-wheeled motor
              vehicle V02.99
              nontraffic V02.09
              traffic V02.19
            vehicle V09.9
              animal-drawn V06.99
                nontraffic V06.09
                traffic V06.19
              motor
                nontraffic V09.00
                traffic V09.20
          fall V00.321
          nontraffic V09.1
            involving motor vehicle NEC
              V09.00
          traffic V09.3
            involving motor vehicle NEC
              V09.20
        sled V00.228
          collision (with) V09.9
            animal being ridden or animal
              drawn vehicle V06.99
              nontraffic V06.09
              traffic V06.19
            bus or heavy transport V04.99
              nontraffic V04.09
              traffic V04.19
            car V03.99
              nontraffic V03.09
              traffic V03.19
            pedal cycle V01.99
              nontraffic V01.09
              traffic V01.19
            pick-up truck or van V03.99
              nontraffic V03.09
              traffic V03.19

Accident (Continued)
  transport (Continued)
    pedestrian (Continued)
      conveyance (Continued)
        sled (Continued)
          collision (Continued)
            railway (train) (vehicle)
              V05.99
              nontraffic V05.09
              traffic V05.19
            stationary object V00.222
            streetcar V06.99
              nontraffic V06.09
              traffic V06.19
            two- or three-wheeled motor
              vehicle V02.99
              nontraffic V02.09
              traffic V02.19
            vehicle V09.9
              animal-drawn V06.99
                nontraffic V06.09
                traffic V06.19
              motor
                nontraffic V09.00
                traffic V09.20
          fall V00.221
          nontraffic V09.1
            involving motor vehicle NEC
              V09.00
          traffic V09.3
            involving motor vehicle NEC
              V09.20
        snow board V00.318
          collision (with) V09.9
            animal being ridden or animal
              drawn vehicle V06.99
              nontraffic V06.09
              traffic V06.19
            bus or heavy transport V04.99
              nontraffic V04.09
              traffic V04.19
            car V03.99
              nontraffic V03.09
              traffic V03.19
            pedal cycle V01.99
              nontraffic V01.09
              traffic V01.19
            pick-up truck or van V03.99
              nontraffic V03.09
              traffic V03.19
            railway (train) (vehicle) V05.99
              nontraffic V05.09
              traffic V05.19
            stationary object V00.312
            streetcar V06.99
              nontraffic V06.09
              traffic V06.19
            two- or three-wheeled motor
              vehicle V02.99
              nontraffic V02.09
              traffic V02.19
            vehicle V09.9
              animal-drawn V06.99
                nontraffic V06.09
                traffic V06.19
              motor
                nontraffic V09.00
                traffic V09.20
          fall V00.311
          nontraffic V09.1
            involving motor vehicle NEC
              V09.00
          traffic V09.3
            involving motor vehicle NEC
              V09.20
        specified type NEC V00.898
          collision (with) V09.9
            animal being ridden or animal
              drawn vehicle V06.99
              nontraffic V06.09
              traffic V06.19

A

Accident *(Continued)*
transport *(Continued)*
pedestrian *(Continued)*
conveyance *(Continued)*
specified type NEC *(Continued)*
collision *(Continued)*
bus or heavy transport V04.99
nontraffic V04.09
traffic V04.19
car V03.99
nontraffic V03.09
traffic V03.19
pedal cycle V01.99
nontraffic V01.09
traffic V01.19
pick-up truck or van V03.99
nontraffic V03.09
traffic V03.19
railway (train) (vehicle) V05.99
nontraffic V05.09
traffic V05.19
stationary object V00.892
streetcar V06.99
nontraffic V06.09
traffic V06.19
two- or three-wheeled motor vehicle V02.99
nontraffic V02.09
traffic V02.19
vehicle V09.9
animal-drawn V06.99
nontraffic V06.09
traffic V06.19
motor
nontraffic V09.00
traffic V09.20
fall V00.891
nontraffic V09.1
involving motor vehicle NEC V09.00
traffic V09.3
involving motor vehicle NEC V09.20
traffic V09.3
involving motor vehicle V09.20
military V09.21
specified type NEC V09.29
wheelchair (powered) V00.818
collision (with) V09.9
animal being ridden or animal drawn vehicle V06.99
nontraffic V06.09
traffic V06.19
bus or heavy transport V04.99
nontraffic V04.09
traffic V04.19
car V03.99
nontraffic V03.09
traffic V03.19
pedal cycle V01.99
nontraffic V01.09
traffic V01.19
pick-up truck or van V03.99
nontraffic V03.09
traffic V03.19
railway (train) (vehicle) V05.99
nontraffic V05.09
traffic V05.19
stationary object V00.812
streetcar V06.99
nontraffic V06.09
traffic V06.19
two- or three-wheeled motor vehicle V02.99
nontraffic V02.09
traffic V02.19

Accident *(Continued)*
transport *(Continued)*
pedestrian *(Continued)*
conveyance *(Continued)*
wheelchair *(Continued)*
collision *(Continued)*
vehicle V09.9
animal-drawn V06.99
nontraffic V06.09
traffic V06.19
motor
nontraffic V09.00
traffic V09.20
fall V00.811
nontraffic V09.1
involving motor vehicle NEC V09.00
traffic V09.3
involving motor vehicle NEC V09.20
wheeled shoe V00.158
colliding with stationary object V00.152
fall V00.151
on foot —*see also* Accident, pedestrian
collision (with)
animal being ridden or animal drawn vehicle V06.90
nontraffic V06.00
traffic V06.10
bus or heavy transport V04.90
nontraffic V04.00
traffic V04.10
car V03.90
nontraffic V03.00
traffic V03.10
pedal cycle V01.90
nontraffic V01.00
traffic V01.10
pick-up truck or van V03.90
nontraffic V03.00
traffic V03.10
railway (train) (vehicle) V05.90
nontraffic V05.00
traffic V05.10
streetcar V06.90
nontraffic V06.00
traffic V06.10
two- or three-wheeled motor vehicle V02.90
nontraffic V02.00
traffic V02.10
vehicle V09.9
animal-drawn V06.90
nontraffic V06.00
traffic V06.10
motor
nontraffic V09.00
traffic V09.20
nontraffic V09.1
involving motor vehicle V09.00
military V09.01
specified type NEC V09.09
traffic V09.3
involving motor vehicle V09.20
military V09.21
specified type NEC V09.29
person NEC (unknown way or transportation) V99
collision (between)
bus (with)
heavy transport vehicle (traffic) V87.5
nontraffic V88.5
car (with)
nontraffic V88.5
bus (traffic) V87.3
nontraffic V88.3
heavy transport vehicle (traffic) V87.4
nontraffic V88.4

Accident *(Continued)*
transport *(Continued)*
person NEC *(Continued)*
collision *(Continued)*
car *(Continued)*
pick-up truck or van (traffic) V87.2
nontraffic V88.2
train or railway vehicle (traffic) V87.6
nontraffic V88.6
two- or three-wheeled motor vehicle (traffic) V87.0
nontraffic V88.0
motor vehicle (traffic) NEC V87.7
nontraffic V88.7
two- or three-wheeled vehicle (with) (traffic)
motor vehicle NEC V87.1
nontraffic V88.1
nonmotor vehicle (collision) (noncollision) (traffic) V87.9
nontraffic V88.9
pickup truck occupant V59.9
collision (with)
animal (traffic) V50.9
being ridden (traffic) V56.9
nontraffic V56.3
while boarding or alighting V56.4
nontraffic V50.3
while boarding or alighting V50.4
animal-drawn vehicle (traffic) V56.9
nontraffic V56.3
while boarding or alighting V56.4
bus (traffic) V54.9
nontraffic V54.3
while boarding or alighting V54.4
car (traffic) V53.9
nontraffic V53.3
while boarding or alighting V53.4
motor vehicle NOS (traffic) V59.60
nontraffic V59.20
specified type NEC (traffic) V59.69
nontraffic V59.29
pedal cycle (traffic) V51.9
nontraffic V51.3
while boarding or alighting V51.4
pickup truck (traffic) V53.9
nontraffic V53.3
while boarding or alighting V53.4
railway vehicle (traffic) V55.9
nontraffic V55.3
while boarding or alighting V55.4
specified vehicle NEC (traffic) V56.9
nontraffic V56.3
while boarding or alighting V56.4
stationary object (traffic) V57.9
nontraffic V57.3
while boarding or alighting V57.4
streetcar (traffic) V56.9
nontraffic V56.3
while boarding or alighting V56.4
three wheeled motor vehicle (traffic) V52.9
nontraffic V52.3
while boarding or alighting V52.4
truck (traffic) V54.9
nontraffic V54.3
while boarding or alighting V54.4
two wheeled motor vehicle (traffic) V52.9
nontraffic V52.3
while boarding or alighting V52.4
van (traffic) V53.9
nontraffic V53.3
while boarding or alighting V53.4
driver
collision (with)
animal (traffic) V50.5
being ridden (traffic) V56.5
nontraffic V56.0
nontraffic V50.0

◄ New ◄▥ Revised ~~deleted~~ Deleted

A

◀ New ◀▥▥ Revised ~~deleted~~ Deleted

Accident *(Continued)*
　transport *(Continued)*
　　three-wheeled motor vehicle occupant
　　　(Continued)
　　　collision *(Continued)*
　　　　specified vehicle NEC (traffic) V36.9
　　　　　nontraffic V36.3
　　　　　while boarding or alighting V36.4
　　　　stationary object (traffic) V37.9
　　　　　nontraffic V37.3
　　　　　while boarding or alighting V37.4
　　　　streetcar (traffic) V36.9
　　　　　nontraffic V36.3
　　　　　while boarding or alighting V36.4
　　　　three wheeled motor vehicle (traffic)
　　　　　V32.9
　　　　　nontraffic V32.3
　　　　　while boarding or alighting V32.4
　　　　truck (traffic) V34.9
　　　　　nontraffic V34.3
　　　　　while boarding or alighting V34.4
　　　　two wheeled motor vehicle (traffic)
　　　　　V32.9
　　　　　nontraffic V32.3
　　　　　while boarding or alighting V32.4
　　　　van (traffic) V33.9
　　　　　nontraffic V33.3
　　　　　while boarding or alighting V33.4
　　　driver
　　　　collision (with)
　　　　　animal (traffic) V30.5
　　　　　　being ridden (traffic) V36.5
　　　　　　　nontraffic V36.0
　　　　　　nontraffic V30.0
　　　　　animal-drawn vehicle (traffic) V36.5
　　　　　　nontraffic V36.0
　　　　　bus (traffic) V34.5
　　　　　　nontraffic V34.0
　　　　　car (traffic) V33.5
　　　　　　nontraffic V33.0
　　　　　motor vehicle NOS (traffic) V39.40
　　　　　　nontraffic V39.00
　　　　　　specified type NEC (traffic)
　　　　　　　V39.49
　　　　　　　　nontraffic V39.09
　　　　　pedal cycle (traffic) V31.5
　　　　　　nontraffic V31.0
　　　　　pickup truck (traffic) V33.5
　　　　　　nontraffic V33.0
　　　　　railway vehicle (traffic) V35.5
　　　　　　nontraffic V35.0
　　　　　specified vehicle NEC (traffic) V36.5
　　　　　　nontraffic V36.0
　　　　　stationary object (traffic) V37.5
　　　　　　nontraffic V37.0
　　　　　streetcar (traffic) V36.5
　　　　　　nontraffic V36.0
　　　　　three wheeled motor vehicle
　　　　　　(traffic) V32.5
　　　　　　nontraffic V32.0
　　　　　truck (traffic) V34.5
　　　　　　nontraffic V34.0
　　　　　two wheeled motor vehicle (traffic)
　　　　　　V32.5
　　　　　　nontraffic V32.0
　　　　　van (traffic) V33.5
　　　　　　nontraffic V33.0
　　　　noncollision accident (traffic) V38.5
　　　　　nontraffic V38.0
　　　hanger-on
　　　　collision (with)
　　　　　animal (traffic) V30.7
　　　　　　being ridden (traffic) V36.7
　　　　　　　nontraffic V36.2
　　　　　　nontraffic V30.2
　　　　　animal-drawn vehicle (traffic) V36.7
　　　　　　nontraffic V36.2
　　　　　bus (traffic) V34.7
　　　　　　nontraffic V34.2
　　　　　car (traffic) V33.7
　　　　　　nontraffic V33.2

Accident *(Continued)*
　transport *(Continued)*
　　three-wheeled motor vehicle occupant
　　　(Continued)
　　　hanger-on *(Continued)*
　　　　collision *(Continued)*
　　　　　pedal cycle (traffic) V31.7
　　　　　　nontraffic V31.2
　　　　　pickup truck (traffic) V33.7
　　　　　　nontraffic V33.2
　　　　　railway vehicle (traffic) V35.7
　　　　　　nontraffic V35.2
　　　　　specified vehicle NEC (traffic) V36.7
　　　　　　nontraffic V36.2
　　　　　stationary object (traffic) V37.7
　　　　　　nontraffic V37.2
　　　　　streetcar (traffic) V36.7
　　　　　　nontraffic V36.2
　　　　　three wheeled motor vehicle
　　　　　　(traffic) V32.7
　　　　　　nontraffic V32.2
　　　　　truck (traffic) V34.7
　　　　　　nontraffic V34.2
　　　　　two wheeled motor vehicle (traffic)
　　　　　　V32.7
　　　　　　nontraffic V32.2
　　　　　van (traffic) V33.7
　　　　　　nontraffic V33.2
　　　　noncollision accident (traffic) V38.7
　　　　　nontraffic V38.2
　　　noncollision accident (traffic) V38.9
　　　　nontraffic V38.3
　　　　while boarding or alighting V38.4
　　　nontraffic V39.3
　　　passenger
　　　　collision (with)
　　　　　animal (traffic) V30.6
　　　　　　being ridden (traffic) V36.6
　　　　　　　nontraffic V36.1
　　　　　　nontraffic V30.1
　　　　　animal-drawn vehicle (traffic) V36.6
　　　　　　nontraffic V36.1
　　　　　bus (traffic) V34.6
　　　　　　nontraffic V34.1
　　　　　car (traffic) V33.6
　　　　　　nontraffic V33.1
　　　　　motor vehicle NOS (traffic) V39.50
　　　　　　nontraffic V39.10
　　　　　　specified type NEC (traffic)
　　　　　　　V39.59
　　　　　　　　nontraffic V39.19
　　　　　pedal cycle (traffic) V31.6
　　　　　　nontraffic V31.1
　　　　　pickup truck (traffic) V33.6
　　　　　　nontraffic V33.1
　　　　　railway vehicle (traffic) V35.6
　　　　　　nontraffic V35.1
　　　　　specified vehicle NEC (traffic)
　　　　　　V36.6
　　　　　　nontraffic V36.1
　　　　　stationary object (traffic) V37.6
　　　　　　nontraffic V37.1
　　　　　streetcar (traffic) V36.6
　　　　　　nontraffic V36.1
　　　　　three wheeled motor vehicle
　　　　　　(traffic) V32.6
　　　　　　nontraffic V32.1
　　　　　truck (traffic) V34.6
　　　　　　nontraffic V34.1
　　　　　two wheeled motor vehicle (traffic)
　　　　　　V32.6
　　　　　　nontraffic V32.1
　　　　　van (traffic) V33.6
　　　　　　nontraffic V33.1
　　　　noncollision accident (traffic) V38.6
　　　　　nontraffic V38.1
　　　specified type NEC V39.89
　　　　military vehicle V39.81
　　　tractor (farm) (and trailer) —*see* Accident,
　　　　transport, agricultural vehicle
　　　　occupant

Accident *(Continued)*
　transport *(Continued)*
　　tram —*see* Accident, transport, streetcar
　　　in mine or quarry —*see* Accident,
　　　　transport, industrial vehicle
　　　　occupant
　　trolley —*see* Accident, transport, streetcar
　　　in mine or quarry —*see* Accident,
　　　　transport, industrial vehicle
　　　　occupant
　　truck (heavy) occupant V69.9
　　　collision (with)
　　　　animal (traffic) V60.9
　　　　　being ridden (traffic) V66.9
　　　　　　nontraffic V66.3
　　　　　　while boarding or alighting V66.4
　　　　　nontraffic V60.3
　　　　　while boarding or alighting V60.4
　　　　animal-drawn vehicle (traffic) V66.9
　　　　　nontraffic V66.3
　　　　　while boarding or alighting V66.4
　　　　bus (traffic) V64.9
　　　　　nontraffic V64.3
　　　　　while boarding or alighting V64.4
　　　　car (traffic) V63.9
　　　　　nontraffic V63.3
　　　　　while boarding or alighting V63.4
　　　　motor vehicle NOS (traffic) V69.60
　　　　　nontraffic V69.20
　　　　　specified type NEC (traffic) V69.69
　　　　　　nontraffic V69.29
　　　　pedal cycle (traffic) V61.9
　　　　　nontraffic V61.3
　　　　　while boarding or alighting V61.4
　　　　pickup truck (traffic) V63.9
　　　　　nontraffic V63.3
　　　　　while boarding or alighting V63.4
　　　　railway vehicle (traffic) V65.9
　　　　　nontraffic V65.3
　　　　　while boarding or alighting V65.4
　　　　specified vehicle NEC (traffic) V66.9
　　　　　nontraffic V66.3
　　　　　while boarding or alighting V66.4
　　　　stationary object (traffic) V67.9
　　　　　nontraffic V67.3
　　　　　while boarding or alighting V67.4
　　　　streetcar (traffic) V66.9
　　　　　nontraffic V66.3
　　　　　while boarding or alighting V66.4
　　　　three wheeled motor vehicle (traffic)
　　　　　V62.9
　　　　　nontraffic V62.3
　　　　　while boarding or alighting V62.4
　　　　truck (traffic) V64.9
　　　　　nontraffic V64.3
　　　　　while boarding or alighting V64.4
　　　　two wheeled motor vehicle (traffic)
　　　　　V62.9
　　　　　nontraffic V62.3
　　　　　while boarding or alighting V62.4
　　　　van (traffic) V63.9
　　　　　nontraffic V63.3
　　　　　while boarding or alighting V63.4
　　　driver
　　　　collision (with)
　　　　　animal (traffic) V60.5
　　　　　　being ridden (traffic) V66.5
　　　　　　　nontraffic V66.0
　　　　　　nontraffic V60.0
　　　　　animal-drawn vehicle (traffic)
　　　　　　V66.5
　　　　　　nontraffic V66.0
　　　　　bus (traffic) V64.5
　　　　　　nontraffic V64.0
　　　　　car (traffic) V63.5
　　　　　　nontraffic V63.0
　　　　　motor vehicle NOS (traffic) V69.40
　　　　　　nontraffic V69.00
　　　　　　specified type NEC (traffic)
　　　　　　　V69.49
　　　　　　　　nontraffic V69.09

◀ New　◀||| Revised　~~deleted~~ Deleted

Accident (Continued)
  transport (Continued)
    truck occupant (Continued)
      driver (Continued)
        collision (Continued)
          pedal cycle (traffic) V61.5
            nontraffic V61.0
          pickup truck (traffic) V63.5
            nontraffic V63.0
          railway vehicle (traffic) V65.5
            nontraffic V65.0
          specified vehicle NEC (traffic) V66.5
            nontraffic V66.0
          stationary object (traffic) V67.5
            nontraffic V67.0
          streetcar (traffic) V66.5
            nontraffic V66.0
          three wheeled motor vehicle
              (traffic) V62.5
            nontraffic V62.0
          truck (traffic) V64.5
            nontraffic V64.0
          two wheeled motor vehicle (traffic)
              V62.5
            nontraffic V62.0
          van (traffic) V63.5
            nontraffic V63.0
        noncollision accident (traffic) V68.5
          nontraffic V68.0
      dump —see Accident, transport,
          construction vehicle occupant
      hanger-on
        collision (with)
          animal (traffic) V60.7
            being ridden (traffic) V66.7
              nontraffic V66.2
            nontraffic V60.2
          animal-drawn vehicle (traffic) V66.7
            nontraffic V66.2
          bus (traffic) V64.7
            nontraffic V64.2
          car (traffic) V63.7
            nontraffic V63.2
          pedal cycle (traffic) V61.7
            nontraffic V61.2
          pickup truck (traffic) V63.7
            nontraffic V63.2
          railway vehicle (traffic) V65.7
            nontraffic V65.2
          specified vehicle NEC (traffic) V66.7
            nontraffic V66.2
          stationary object (traffic) V67.7
            nontraffic V67.2
          streetcar (traffic) V66.7
            nontraffic V66.2
          three wheeled motor vehicle
              (traffic) V62.7
            nontraffic V62.2
          truck (traffic) V64.7
            nontraffic V64.2
          two wheeled motor vehicle (traffic)
              V62.7
            nontraffic V62.2
          van (traffic) V63.7
            nontraffic V63.2
        noncollision accident (traffic) V68.7
          nontraffic V68.2
      noncollision accident (traffic) V68.9
        nontraffic V68.3
        while boarding or alighting V68.4
      nontraffic V69.3
      passenger
        collision (with)
          animal (traffic) V60.6
            being ridden (traffic) V66.6
              nontraffic V66.1
            nontraffic V60.1
          animal-drawn vehicle (traffic) V66.6
            nontraffic V66.1
          bus (traffic) V64.6
            nontraffic V64.1

Accident (Continued)
  transport (Continued)
    truck occupant (Continued)
      passenger (Continued)
        collision (Continued)
          car (traffic) V63.6
            nontraffic V63.1
          motor vehicle NOS (traffic) V69.50
            nontraffic V69.10
            specified type NEC (traffic)
                V69.59
              nontraffic V69.19
          pedal cycle (traffic) V61.6
            nontraffic V61.1
          pickup truck (traffic) V63.6
            nontraffic V63.1
          railway vehicle (traffic) V65.6
            nontraffic V65.1
          specified vehicle NEC (traffic)
              V66.6
            nontraffic V66.1
          stationary object (traffic) V67.6
            nontraffic V67.1
          streetcar (traffic) V66.6
            nontraffic V66.1
          three wheeled motor vehicle
              (traffic) V62.6
            nontraffic V62.1
          truck (traffic) V64.6
            nontraffic V64.1
          two wheeled motor vehicle (traffic)
              V62.6
            nontraffic V62.1
          van (traffic) V63.6
            nontraffic V63.1
        noncollision accident (traffic) V68.6
          nontraffic V68.1
      pickup —see Accident, transport, pickup
          truck occupant
      specified type NEC V69.88
      military vehicle V69.81
    van occupant V59.9
      collision (with)
        animal (traffic) V50.9
          being ridden (traffic) V56.9
            nontraffic V56.3
            while boarding or alighting
                V56.4
          nontraffic V50.3
          while boarding or alighting V50.4
        animal-drawn vehicle (traffic) V56.9
          nontraffic V56.3
          while boarding or alighting V56.4
        bus (traffic) V54.9
          nontraffic V54.3
          while boarding or alighting V54.4
        car (traffic) V53.9
          nontraffic V53.3
          while boarding or alighting V53.4
        motor vehicle NOS (traffic) V59.60
          nontraffic V59.20
          specified type NEC (traffic) V59.69
            nontraffic V59.29
        pedal cycle (traffic) V51.9
          nontraffic V51.3
          while boarding or alighting V51.4
        pickup truck (traffic) V53.9
          nontraffic V53.3
          while boarding or alighting V53.4
        railway vehicle (traffic) V55.9
          nontraffic V55.3
          while boarding or alighting V55.4
        specified vehicle NEC (traffic) V56.9
          nontraffic V56.3
          while boarding or alighting V56.4
        stationary object (traffic) V57.9
          nontraffic V57.3
          while boarding or alighting V57.4
        streetcar (traffic) V56.9
          nontraffic V56.3
          while boarding or alighting V56.4

Accident (Continued)
  transport (Continued)
    van occupant (Continued)
      collision (Continued)
        three wheeled motor vehicle (traffic)
            V52.9
          nontraffic V52.3
          while boarding or alighting V52.4
        truck (traffic) V54.9
          nontraffic V54.3
          while boarding or alighting V54.4
        two wheeled motor vehicle (traffic)
            V52.9
          nontraffic V52.3
          while boarding or alighting V52.4
        van (traffic) V53.9
          nontraffic V53.3
          while boarding or alighting V53.4
      driver
        collision (with)
          animal (traffic) V50.5
            being ridden (traffic) V56.5
              nontraffic V56.0
            nontraffic V50.0
          animal-drawn vehicle (traffic) V56.5
            nontraffic V56.0
          bus (traffic) V54.5
            nontraffic V54.0
          car (traffic) V53.5
            nontraffic V53.0
          motor vehicle NOS (traffic) V59.40
            nontraffic V59.00
            specified type NEC (traffic)
                V59.49
              nontraffic V59.09
          pedal cycle (traffic) V51.5
            nontraffic V51.0
          pickup truck (traffic) V53.5
            nontraffic V53.0
          railway vehicle (traffic) V55.5
            nontraffic V55.0
          specified vehicle NEC (traffic) V56.5
            nontraffic V56.0
          stationary object (traffic) V57.5
            nontraffic V57.0
          streetcar (traffic) V56.5
            nontraffic V56.0
          three wheeled motor vehicle
              (traffic) V52.5
            nontraffic V52.0
          truck (traffic) V54.5
            nontraffic V54.0
          two wheeled motor vehicle (traffic)
              V52.5
            nontraffic V52.0
          van (traffic) V53.5
            nontraffic V53.0
        noncollision accident (traffic) V58.5
          nontraffic V58.0
      hanger-on
        collision (with)
          animal (traffic) V50.7
            being ridden (traffic) V56.7
              nontraffic V56.2
            nontraffic V50.2
          animal-drawn vehicle (traffic) V56.7
            nontraffic V56.2
          bus (traffic) V54.7
            nontraffic V54.2
          car (traffic) V53.7
            nontraffic V53.2
          pedal cycle (traffic) V51.7
            nontraffic V51.2
          pickup truck (traffic) V53.7
            nontraffic V53.2
          railway vehicle (traffic) V55.7
            nontraffic V55.2
          specified vehicle NEC (traffic) V56.7
            nontraffic V56.2
          stationary object (traffic) V57.7
            nontraffic V57.2

Accident *(Continued)*
  transport *(Continued)*
    van occupant *(Continued)*
      hanger-on *(Continued)*
        collision *(Continued)*
          streetcar (traffic) V56.7
            nontraffic V56.2
          three wheeled motor vehicle
            (traffic) V52.7
            nontraffic V52.2
          truck (traffic) V54.7
            nontraffic V54.2
          two wheeled motor vehicle (traffic)
            V52.7
            nontraffic V52.2
          van (traffic) V53.7
            nontraffic V53.2
        noncollision accident (traffic) V58.7
          nontraffic V58.2
      noncollision accident (traffic) V58.9
        nontraffic V58.3
        while boarding or alighting V58.4
      nontraffic V59.3
      passenger
        collision (with)
          animal (traffic) V50.6
            being ridden (traffic) V56.6
              nontraffic V56.1
            nontraffic V50.1
          animal-drawn vehicle (traffic) V56.6
            nontraffic V56.1
          bus (traffic) V54.6
            nontraffic V54.1
          car (traffic) V53.6
            nontraffic V53.1
          motor vehicle NOS (traffic) V59.50
            nontraffic V59.10
            specified type NEC (traffic) V59.59
              nontraffic V59.19
          pedal cycle (traffic) V51.6
            nontraffic V51.1
          pickup truck (traffic) V53.6
            nontraffic V53.1
          railway vehicle (traffic) V55.6
            nontraffic V55.1
          specified vehicle NEC (traffic) V56.6
            nontraffic V56.1
          stationary object (traffic) V57.6
            nontraffic V57.1
          streetcar (traffic) V56.6
            nontraffic V56.1
          three wheeled motor vehicle
            (traffic) V52.6
            nontraffic V52.1
          truck (traffic) V54.6
            nontraffic V54.1
          two wheeled motor vehicle (traffic)
            V52.6
            nontraffic V52.1
          van (traffic) V53.6
            nontraffic V53.1
        noncollision accident (traffic) V58.6
          nontraffic V58.1
      specified type NEC V59.88
        military vehicle V59.81
    watercraft occupant —*see* Accident,
      watercraft
    vehicle NEC V89.9
      animal-drawn NEC —*see* Accident,
        transport, animal-drawn vehicle
        occupant
      special
        agricultural —*see* Accident, transport,
          agricultural vehicle occupant
        construction —*see* Accident, transport,
          construction vehicle occupant
        industrial —*see* Accident, transport,
          industrial vehicle occupant
        three-wheeled NEC (motorized) —*see*
          Accident, transport, three-wheeled
          motor vehicle occupant

Accident *(Continued)*
  watercraft V94.9
    causing
      drowning —*see* Drowning, due to,
        accident to, watercraft
      injury NEC V91.89
        crushed between craft and object
          V91.19
          powered craft V91.13
            ferry boat V91.11
            fishing boat V91.12
            jetskis V91.13
            liner V91.11
            merchant ship V91.10
            passenger ship V91.11
          unpowered craft V91.18
            canoe V91.15
            inflatable V91.16
            kayak V91.15
            sailboat V91.14
            surf-board V91.18
            windsurfer V91.18
        fall on board V91.29
          powered craft V91.23
            ferry boat V91.21
            fishing boat V91.22
            jetskis V91.23
            liner V91.21
            merchant ship V91.20
            passenger ship V91.21
          unpowered craft
            canoe V91.25
            inflatable V91.26
            kayak V91.25
            sailboat V91.24
        fire on board causing burn V91.09
          powered craft V91.03
            ferry boat V91.01
            fishing boat V91.02
            jetskis V91.03
            liner V91.01
            merchant ship V91.00
            passenger ship V91.01
          unpowered craft V91.08
            canoe V91.05
            inflatable V91.06
            kayak V91.05
            sailboat V91.04
            surf-board V91.08
            water skis V91.07
            windsurfer V91.08
        hit by falling object V91.39
          powered craft V91.33
            ferry boat V91.31
            fishing boat V91.32
            jetskis V91.33
            liner V91.31
            merchant ship V91.30
            passenger ship V91.31
          unpowered craft V91.38
            canoe V91.35
            inflatable V91.36
            kayak V91.35
            sailboat V91.34
            surf-board V91.38
            water skis V91.37
            windsurfer V91.38
        specified type NEC V91.89
          powered craft V91.83
            ferry boat V91.81
            fishing boat V91.82
            jetskis V91.83
            liner V91.81
            merchant ship V91.80
            passenger ship V91.81
          unpowered craft V91.88
            canoe V91.85
            inflatable V91.86
            kayak V91.85
            sailboat V91.84
            surf-board V91.88

Accident *(Continued)*
  watercraft *(Continued)*
    causing *(Continued)*
      injury NEC *(Continued)*
        specified type NEC *(Continued)*
          unpowered craft *(Continued)*
            water skis V91.87
            windsurfer V91.88
      due to, caused by cataclysm —*see* Forces of
        nature, by type
      military NEC V94.818
        with civilian watercraft V94.810
        civilian in water injured by V94.811
      nonpowered, struck by
        nonpowered vessel V94.22
        powered vessel V94.21
      specified type NEC V94.89
      striking swimmer
        powered V94.11
        unpowered V94.12
  Acid throwing (assault) Y08.89
  Activity (involving) (of victim at time of event)
    Y93.9
    aerobic and step exercise (class) Y93.A3
    alpine skiing Y93.23
    animal care NEC Y93.K9
    arts and handcrafts NEC Y93.D9
    athletics NEC Y93.79
    athletics played as a team or group NEC
      Y93.69
    athletics played individually NEC Y93.59
    baking Y93.G3
    ballet Y93.41
    barbells Y93.B3
    BASE (Building, Antenna, Span, Earth)
      jumping Y93.33
    baseball Y93.64
    basketball Y93.67
    bathing (personal) Y93.E1
    beach volleyball Y93.68
    bike riding Y93.55
    boogie boarding Y93.18
    bowling Y93.54
    boxing Y93.71
    brass instrument playing Y93.J4
    building construction Y93.H3
    bungee jumping Y93.34
    calisthenics Y93.A2
    canoeing (in calm and turbulent water)
      Y93.16
    capture the flag Y93.6A
    cardiorespiratory exercise NEC Y93.A9
    caregiving (providing) NEC Y93.F9
      bathing Y93.F1
      lifting Y93.F2
    cellular
      communication device Y93.C2
      telephone Y93.C2
    challenge course Y93.A5
    cheerleading Y93.45
    circuit training Y93.A4
    cleaning
      floor Y93.E5
    climbing NEC Y93.39
      mountain Y93.31
      rock Y93.31
      wall Y93.31
    clothing care and maintenance NEC
      Y93.E9
    combatives Y93.75
    computer
      keyboarding Y93.C1
      technology NEC Y93.C9
    confidence course Y93.A5
    construction (building) Y93.H3
    cooking and baking Y93.G3
    cool down exercises Y93.A2
    cricket Y93.69
    crocheting Y93.D1
    cross country skiing Y93.24
    dancing (all types) Y93.41

◀ New   ◀▥ Revised   ~~deleted~~ Deleted

Aerosinusitis —*see* Air, pressure
After-effect, late —*see* Sequelae
Air
  blast in war operations —*see* War operations,
    air blast
  pressure
    change, rapid
      during
        ascent W94.29
          while (in) (surfacing from)
            aircraft W94.23
            deep water diving W94.21
            underground W94.22
        descent W94.39
          in
            aircraft W94.31
            water W94.32
    high, prolonged W94.0
    low, prolonged W94.12
      due to residence or long visit at high
        altitude W94.11
Alpine sickness W94.11
Altitude sickness W94.11
Anaphylactic shock, anaphylaxis —*see* Table of
  Drugs and Chemicals
Andes disease W94.11
Arachnidism, arachnoidism X58
Arson (with intent to injure or kill) X97
Asphyxia, asphyxiation
  by
    food (bone) (seed) —*see* categories T17
      and T18
    gas —*see also* Table of Drugs and Chemicals
      legal
        execution —*see* Legal, intervention,
          gas
        intervention —*see* Legal, intervention,
          gas
  from
    fire —*see also* Exposure, fire
      in war operations —*see* War operations,
        fire
    ignition —*see* Ignition
    vomitus T17.81
  in war operations —*see* War operations,
    restriction of airway
Aspiration
  food (any type) (into respiratory tract) (with
    asphyxia, obstruction respiratory tract,
    suffocation) —*see* categories T17 and T18
  foreign body —*see* Foreign body, aspiration
  vomitus (with asphyxia, obstruction
    respiratory tract, suffocation) T17.81
Assassination (attempt) —*see* Assault
Assault (homicidal) (by) (in) Y09
  arson X97
  bite (of human being) Y04.1
  bodily force Y04.8
    bite Y04.1
    bumping into Y04.2
    sexual —*see* subcategories T74.0, T76.0
    unarmed fight Y04.0

Assault *(Continued)*
  bomb X96.9
    antipersonnel X96.0
    fertilizer X96.3
    gasoline X96.1
    letter X96.2
    petrol X96.1
    pipe X96.3
    specified NEC X96.8
  brawl (hand) (fists) (foot) (unarmed) Y04.0
  burning, burns (by fire) NEC X97
    acid Y08.89
    caustic, corrosive substance Y08.89
    chemical from swallowing caustic,
      corrosive substance —*see* Table of
      Drugs and Chemicals
    cigarette (s) X97
    hot object X98.9
      fluid NEC X98.2
      household appliance X98.3
      specified NEC X98.8
      steam X98.0
      tap water X98.1
      vapors X98.0
    scalding —*see* Assault, burning
    steam X98.0
    vitriol Y08.89
  caustic, corrosive substance (gas) Y08.89
  crashing of
    aircraft Y08.81
    motor vehicle Y03.8
      pushed in front of Y02.0
      run over Y03.0
      specified NEC Y03.8
  cutting or piercing instrument X99.9
    dagger X99.2
    glass X99.0
    knife X99.1
    specified NEC X99.8
    sword X99.2
  dagger X99.2
  drowning (in) X92.9
    bathtub X92.0
    natural water X92.3
    specified NEC X92.8
    swimming pool X92.1
      following fall X92.2
  dynamite X96.8
  explosive (s) (material) X96.9
  fight (hand) (fists) (foot) (unarmed) Y04.0
    with weapon —*see* Assault, by type of
      weapon
  fire X97
  firearm X95.9
    airgun X95.01
    handgun X93
    hunting rifle X94.1
    larger X94.9
      specified NEC X94.8
    machine gun X94.2
    shotgun X94.0
    specified NEC X95.8

Assault *(Continued)*
  from high place Y01
  gunshot (wound) NEC —*see* Assault, firearm,
    by type
  incendiary device X97
  injury Y09
    to child due to criminal abortion attempt
      NEC Y08.89
  knife X99.1
  late effect of —*see* X92-Y08 with 7th character
    S
  placing before moving object NEC Y02.8
    motor vehicle Y02.0
  poisoning —*see* categories T36-T65 with 7th
    character S
  puncture, any part of body —*see* Assault,
    cutting or piercing instrument
  pushing
    before moving object NEC Y02.8
      motor vehicle Y02.0
      subway train Y02.1
      train Y02.1
  rape T74.2-
  scalding —*see* Assault, burning
  sequelae of —*see* X92-Y08 with 7th character
    S
  sexual (by bodily force) T74.2-
  shooting —*see* Assault, firearm
  specified means NEC Y08.89
  stab, any part of body —*see* Assault, cutting
    or piercing instrument
  steam X98.0
  striking against
    other person Y04.2
    sports equipment Y08.09
      baseball bat Y08.02
      hockey stick Y08.01
  struck by
    sports equipment Y08.09
      baseball bat Y08.02
      hockey stick Y08.01
  submersion —*see* Assault, drowning
  violence Y09
  weapon Y09
    blunt Y00
    cutting or piercing —*see* Assault, cutting or
      piercing instrument
    firearm —*see* Assault, firearm
  wound Y09
    cutting —*see* Assault, cutting or piercing
      instrument
    gunshot —*see* Assault, firearm
    knife X99.1
    piercing —*see* Assault, cutting or piercing
      instrument
    puncture —*see* Assault, cutting or piercing
      instrument
    stab —*see* Assault, cutting or piercing
      instrument
Attack by mammals NEC W55.89
Avalanche —*see* Landslide
Aviator's disease —*see* Air, pressure

◀ New   ◀▦ Revised   ~~deleted~~ Deleted

B

Barotitis, barodontalgia, barosinusitis, barotrauma (otitic) (sinus) —*see* Air, pressure
Battered (baby) (child) (person) (syndrome) X58
Bayonet wound W26.1
  in
    legal intervention —*see* Legal, intervention, sharp object, bayonet
    war operations —*see* War operations, combat
  stated as undetermined whether accidental or intentional Y28.8
  suicide (attempt) X78.2
Bean in nose —*see* categories T17 and T18
Bed set on fire NEC —*see* Exposure, fire, uncontrolled, building, bed
Beheading (by guillotine)
  homicide X99.9
  legal execution —*see* Legal, intervention
Bending, injury in —*see* category Y93
Bends —*see* Air, pressure, change
Bite, bitten by
  alligator W58.01
  arthropod (nonvenomous) NEC W57
  bull W55.21
  cat W55.01
  cow W55.21
  crocodile W58.11
  dog W54.0
  goat W55.31
  hoof stock NEC W55.31
  horse W55.11
  human being (accidentally) W50.3
    with intent to injure or kill Y04.1
    as, or caused by, a crowd or human stampede (with fall) W52
    assault Y04.1
    homicide (attempt) Y04.1
    in
      fight Y04.1
  insect (nonvenomous) W57
  lizard (nonvenomous) W59.01
  mammal NEC W55.81
    marine W56.31
  marine animal (nonvenomous) W56.81
  millipede W57
  moray eel W56.51
  mouse W53.01
  person (s) (accidentally) W50.3
    with intent to injure or kill Y04.1
    as, or caused by, a crowd or human stampede (with fall) W52
    assault Y04.1
    homicide (attempt) Y04.1
    in
      fight Y04.1
  pig W55.41
  raccoon W55.51
  rat W53.11
  reptile W59.81
    lizard W59.01
    snake W59.11
    turtle W59.21
      terrestrial W59.81
  rodent W53.81
    mouse W53.01
    rat W53.11
    specified NEC W53.81
    squirrel W53.21
  shark W56.41
  sheep W55.31
  snake (nonvenomous) W59.11
  spider (nonvenomous) W57
  squirrel W53.21
Blast (air) in war operations —*see* War operations, blast
Blizzard X37.2

Blood alcohol level Y90.9
  20-39mg/100ml Y90.1
  40-59mg/100ml Y90.2
  60-79mg/100ml Y90.3
  80-99mg/100ml Y90.4
  100-119mg/100ml Y90.5
  120-199mg/100ml Y90.6
  200-239mg/100ml Y90.7
  less than 20mg/100ml Y90.0
  presence in blood, level not specified Y90.9
Blow X58
  by law-enforcing agent, police (on duty) —*see* Legal, intervention, manhandling
    blunt object —*see* Legal, intervention, blunt object
Blowing up —*see* Explosion
Brawl (hand) (fists) (foot) Y04.0
Breakage (accidental) (part of)
  ladder (causing fall) W11
  scaffolding (causing fall) W12
Broken
  glass, contact with —*see* Contact, with, glass
  power line (causing electric shock) W85
Bumping against, into (accidentally)
  object NEC W22.8
    with fall —*see* Fall, due to, bumping against, object
    caused by crowd or human stampede (with fall) W52
    sports equipment W21.9
  person (s) W51
    with fall W03
      due to ice or snow W00.0
    assault Y04.2
    caused by, a crowd or human stampede (with fall) W52
    homicide (attempt) Y04.2
  sports equipment W21.9
Burn, burned, burning (accidental) (by) (from) (on)
  acid NEC —*see* Table of Drugs and Chemicals
  bed linen —*see* Exposure, fire, uncontrolled, in building, bed
  blowtorch X08.8
    with ignition of clothing NEC X06.2
    nightwear X05
  bonfire, campfire (controlled) —*see also* Exposure, fire, controlled, not in building
    uncontrolled —*see* Exposure, fire, uncontrolled, not in building
  candle X08.8
    with ignition of clothing NEC X06.2
    nightwear X05
  caustic liquid, substance (external) (internal) NEC —*see* Table of Drugs and Chemicals
  chemical (external) (internal) —*see also* Table of Drugs and Chemicals
    in war operations —*see* War operations, fire
  cigar (s) or cigarette (s) X08.8
    with ignition of clothing NEC X06.2
    nightwear X05
  clothes, clothing NEC (from controlled fire) X06.2
    with conflagration —*see* Exposure, fire, uncontrolled, building
    not in building or structure —*see* Exposure, fire, uncontrolled, not in building
  cooker (hot) X15.8
    stated as undetermined whether accidental or intentional Y27.3
    suicide (attempt) X77.3
  electric blanket X16
  engine (hot) X17
  fire, flames —*see* Exposure, fire
  flare, Very pistol —*see* Discharge, firearm NEC

Burn, burned, burning (Continued)
  heat
    from appliance (electrical) (household) X15.8
      cooker X15.8
      hotplate X15.2
      kettle X15.8
      light bulb X15.8
      saucepan X15.3
      skillet X15.3
      stated as undetermined whether accidental or intentional Y27.3
      stove X15.0
      suicide (attempt) X77.3
      toaster X15.1
    in local application or packing during medical or surgical procedure Y63.5
  heating
    appliance, radiator or pipe X16
  homicide (attempt) —*see* Assault, burning
  hot
    air X14.1
    cooker X15.8
    drink X10.0
    engine X17
    fat X10.2
    fluid NEC X12
    food X10.1
    gases X14.1
    heating appliance X16
    household appliance NEC X15.8
    kettle X15.8
    liquid NEC X12
    machinery X17
    metal (molten) (liquid) NEC X18
    object (not producing fire or flames) NEC X19
    oil (cooking) X10.2
    pipe (s) X16
    radiator X16
    saucepan (glass) (metal) X15.3
    stove (kitchen) X15.0
    substance NEC X19
      caustic or corrosive NEC —*see* Table of Drugs and Chemicals
    toaster X15.1
    tool X17
    vapor X13.1
    water (tap) —*see* Contact, with, hot, tap water
  hotplate X15.2
    suicide (attempt) X77.3
  ignition —*see* Ignition
  in war operations —*see* War operations, fire
  inflicted by other person X97
    by hot objects, hot vapor, and steam —*see* Assault, burning, hot object
  internal, from swallowed caustic, corrosive liquid, substance —*see* Table of Drugs and Chemicals
  iron (hot) X15.8
    stated as undetermined whether accidental or intentional Y27.3
    suicide (attempt) X77.3
  kettle (hot) X15.8
    stated as undetermined whether accidental or intentional Y27.3
    suicide (attempt) X77.3
  lamp (flame) X08.8
    with ignition of clothing NEC X06.2
    nightwear X05
  lighter (cigar) (cigarette) X08.8
    with ignition of clothing NEC X06.2
    nightwear X05
  lightning —*see* subcategory T75.0
    causing fire —*see* Exposure, fire
  liquid (boiling) (hot) NEC X12
    stated as undetermined whether accidental or intentional Y27.2
    suicide (attempt) X77.2

Burn, burned, burning *(Continued)*
  local application of externally applied
      substance in medical or surgical care
      Y63.5
  machinery (hot) X17
  matches X08.8
    with ignition of clothing NEC X06.2
      nightwear X05
  mattress —*see* Exposure, fire, uncontrolled,
    building, bed
  medicament, externally applied Y63.5
  metal (hot) (liquid) (molten) NEC X18
  nightwear (nightclothes, nightdress, gown,
    pajamas, robe) X05
  object (hot) NEC X19
  on board watercraft
    due to
      accident to watercraft V91.09
        powered craft V91.03
          ferry boat V91.01
          fishing boat V91.02
          jetskis V91.03
          liner V91.01
          merchant ship V91.00
          passenger ship V91.01
        unpowered craft V91.08
          canoe V91.05
          inflatable V91.06
          kayak V91.05
          sailboat V91.04
          surf-board V91.08
          water skis V91.07
          windsurfer V91.08
      fire on board V93.09
        ferry boat V93.01
        fishing boat V93.02
        jetskis V93.03
        liner V93.01
        merchant ship V93.00
        passenger ship V93.01
        powered craft NEC V93.03
        sailboat V93.04

Burn, burned, burning *(Continued)*
  on board watercraft *(Continued)*
    due to *(Continued)*
      specified heat source NEC on board
        V93.19
        ferry boat V93.11
        fishing boat V93.12
        jetskis V93.13
        liner V93.11
        merchant ship V93.10
        passenger ship V93.11
        powered craft NEC V93.13
        sailboat V93.14
  pipe (hot) X16
    smoking X08.8
      with ignition of clothing NEC X06.2
        nightwear X05
  powder —*see* Powder burn
  radiator (hot) X16
  saucepan (hot) (glass) (metal) X15.3
    stated as undetermined whether
      accidental or intentional
      Y27.3
    suicide (attempt) X77.3
  self-inflicted X76
    stated as undetermined whether
      accidental or intentional
      Y26
  stated as undetermined whether
    accidental or intentional Y27.0
  steam X13.1
    pipe X16
      stated as undetermined whether
        accidental or intentional
        Y27.8
    stated as undetermined whether
      accidental or intentional Y27.0
    suicide (attempt) X77.0
  stove (hot) (kitchen) X15.0
    stated as undetermined whether
      accidental or intentional Y27.3
    suicide (attempt) X77.3

Burn, burned, burning *(Continued)*
  substance (hot) NEC X19
    boiling X12
      stated as undetermined whether
        accidental or intentional Y27.2
      suicide (attempt) X77.2
    molten (metal) X18
  suicide (attempt) NEC X76
    hot
      household appliance X77.3
      object X77.9
  stated as undetermined whether accidental or
    intentional Y27.0
  therapeutic misadventure
    heat in local application or packing during
      medical or surgical procedure Y63.5
    overdose of radiation Y63.2
  toaster (hot) X15.1
    stated as undetermined whether accidental
      or intentional Y27.3
    suicide (attempt) X77.3
  tool (hot) X17
  torch, welding X08.8
    with ignition of clothing NEC X06.2
      nightwear X05
  trash fire (controlled) —*see* Exposure, fire,
    controlled, not in building
    uncontrolled —*see* Exposure, fire,
      uncontrolled, not in building
  vapor (hot) X13.1
    stated as undetermined whether accidental
      or intentional Y27.0
    suicide (attempt) X77.0
  Very pistol —*see* Discharge, firearm NEC
Butted by animal W55.82
  bull W55.22
  cow W55.22
  goat W55.32
  horse W55.12
  pig W55.42
  sheep W55.32

◄ New   ◄▭ Revised   ~~deleted~~ Deleted

C

Caisson disease —*see* Air, pressure, change
Campfire (exposure to) (controlled) —*see also* Exposure, fire, controlled, not in building
  uncontrolled —*see* Exposure, fire, uncontrolled, not in building
Capital punishment (any means) —*see* Legal, intervention
Car sickness T75.3
Casualty (not due to war) NEC X58
  war —*see* War operations
Cat
  bite W55.01
  scratch W55.03
Cataclysm, cataclysmic (any injury) NEC —*see* Forces of nature
Catching fire —*see* Exposure, fire
Caught
  between
    folding object W23.0
    objects (moving) (stationary and moving) W23.0
      and machinery —*see* Contact, with, by type of machine
      stationary W23.1
    sliding door and door frame W23.0
  by, in
    machinery (moving parts of) —*see* Contact, with, by type of machine
    washing-machine wringer W23.0
  under packing crate (due to losing grip) W23.1
Cave-in caused by cataclysmic earth surface movement or eruption —*see* Landslide
Change (s) in air pressure —*see* Air, pressure, change
Choked, choking (on) (any object except food or vomitus)
  food (bone) (seed) —*see* categories T17 and T18
  vomitus T17.81-
Civil insurrection —*see* War operations
Cloudburst (any injury) X37.8
Cold, exposure to (accidental) (excessive) (extreme) (natural) (place) NEC —*see* Exposure, cold
Collapse
  building W20.1
    burning (uncontrolled fire) X00.2
  dam or man-made structure (causing earth movement) X36.0
  machinery —*see* Contact, with, by type of machine
  structure W20.1
    burning (uncontrolled fire) X00.2
Collision (accidental) NEC (*see also* Accident, transport) V89.9
  pedestrian W51
    with fall W03
      due to ice or snow W00.0
      involving pedestrian conveyance —*see* Accident, transport, pedestrian, conveyance
    and
      crowd or human stampede (with fall) W52
      object W22.8
        with fall —*see* Fall, due to, bumping against, object
    person (s) —*see* Collision, pedestrian
  transport vehicle NEC V89.9
    and
      avalanche, fallen or not moving —*see* Accident, transport
        falling or moving —*see* Landslide
      landslide, fallen or not moving —*see* Accident, transport
        falling or moving —*see* Landslide

Collision NEC (*Continued*)
  transport vehicle NEC (*Continued*)
    due to cataclysm —*see* Forces of nature, by type
    intentional, purposeful suicide (attempt) —*see* Suicide, collision
Combustion, spontaneous —*see* Ignition
Complication (delayed) of or following (medical or surgical procedure) Y84.9
  with misadventure —*see* Misadventure
  amputation of limb (s) Y83.5
  anastomosis (arteriovenous) (blood vessel) (gastrojejunal) (tendon) (natural or artificial material) Y83.2
  aspiration (of fluid) Y84.4
    tissue Y84.8
  biopsy Y84.8
  blood
    sampling Y84.7
    transfusion
      procedure Y84.8
  bypass Y83.2
  catheterization (urinary) Y84.6
    cardiac Y84.0
  colostomy Y83.3
  cystostomy Y83.3
  dialysis (kidney) Y84.1
  drug —*see* Table of Drugs and Chemicals
  due to misadventure —*see* Misadventure
  duodenostomy Y83.3
  electroshock therapy Y84.3
  external stoma, creation of Y83.3
  formation of external stoma Y83.3
  gastrostomy Y83.3
  graft Y83.2
  hypothermia (medically-induced) Y84.8
  implant, implantation (of)
    artificial
      internal device (cardiac pacemaker) (electrodes in brain) (heart valve prosthesis) (orthopedic) Y83.1
      material or tissue (for anastomosis or bypass) Y83.2
        with creation of external stoma Y83.3
      natural tissues (for anastomosis or bypass) Y83.2
        with creation of external stoma Y83.3
  infusion
    procedure Y84.8
  injection —*see* Table of Drugs and Chemicals
    procedure Y84.8
  insertion of gastric or duodenal sound Y84.5
  insulin-shock therapy Y84.3
  paracentesis (abdominal) (thoracic) (aspirative) Y84.4
  procedures other than surgical operation —*see* Complication of or following, by type of procedure
  radiological procedure or therapy Y84.2
  removal of organ (partial) (total) NEC Y83.6
  sampling
    blood Y84.7
    fluid NEC Y84.4
    tissue Y84.8
  shock therapy Y84.3
  surgical operation NEC (*see also* Complication of or following, by type of operation) Y83.9
    reconstructive NEC Y83.4
      with
        anastomosis, bypass or graft Y83.2
        formation of external stoma Y83.3
    specified NEC Y83.8
  transfusion —*see also* Table of Drugs and Chemicals
    procedure Y84.8
  transplant, transplantation (heart) (kidney) (liver) (whole organ, any) Y83.0
    partial organ Y83.4
  ureterostomy Y83.3

Complication of or following (*Continued*)
  vaccination —*see also* Table of Drugs and Chemicals
    procedure Y84.8
Compression
  divers' squeeze —*see* Air, pressure, change
  trachea by
    food (lodged in esophagus) —*see* categories T17 and T18
    vomitus (lodged in esophagus) T17.81-
Conflagration —*see* Exposure, fire, uncontrolled
Constriction (external)
  hair W49.01
  jewelry W49.04
  ring W49.04
  rubber band W49.03
  specified item NEC W49.09
  string W49.02
  thread W49.02
Contact (accidental)
  with
    abrasive wheel (metalworking) W31.1
    alligator W58.09
      bite W58.01
      crushing W58.03
      strike W58.02
    amphibian W62.9
      frog W62.0
      toad W62.1
    animal (nonvenomous) NEC W64
      marine W56.89
        bite W56.81
        dolphin —*see* Contact, with, dolphin
        fish NEC —*see* Contact, with, fish
        mammal —*see* Contact, with, mammal, marine
        orca —*see* Contact, with, orca
        sea lion —*see* Contact, with, sea lion
        shark —*see* Contact, with, shark
        strike W56.82
    animate mechanical force NEC W64
    arrow W21.89
      not thrown, projected or falling W45.8
    arthropods (nonvenomous) W57
    axe W27.0
    band-saw (industrial) W31.2
    bayonet —*see* Bayonet wound
    bee (s) X58
    bench-saw (industrial) W31.2
    bird W61.99
      bite W61.91
      chicken —*see* Contact, with, chicken
      duck —*see* Contact, with, duck
      goose —*see* Contact, with, goose
      macaw —*see* Contact, with, macaw
      parrot —*see* Contact, with, parrot
      psittacine —*see* Contact, with, psittacine
      strike W61.92
      turkey —*see* Contact, with, turkey
    blender W29.0
    boiling water X12
      stated as undetermined whether accidental or intentional Y27.2
      suicide (attempt) X77.2
    bore, earth-drilling or mining (land) (seabed) W31.0
    buffalo —*see* Contact, with, hoof stock NEC
    bull W55.29
      bite W55.21
      gored W55.22
      strike W55.22
    bumper cars W31.81
    camel —*see* Contact, with, hoof stock NEC
    can
      lid W45.2
      opener W27.4
        powered W29.0
    cat W55.09
      bite W55.01
      scratch W55.03
    caterpillar (venomous) X58

Contact *(Continued)*
  with *(Continued)*
    centipede (venomous) X58
    chain
      hoist W24.0
        agricultural operations W30.89
      saw W29.3
    chicken W61.39
      peck W61.33
      strike W61.32
    chisel W27.0
    circular saw W31.2
    cobra X58
    combine (harvester) W30.0
    conveyer belt W24.1
    cooker (hot) X15.8
      stated as undetermined whether
        accidental or intentional Y27.3
      suicide (attempt) X77.3
    coral X58
    cotton gin W31.82
    cow W55.29
      bite W55.21
      strike W55.22
    crane W24.0
      agricultural operations W30.89
    crocodile W58.19
      bite W58.11
      crushing W58.13
      strike W58.12
    dagger W26.1
      stated as undetermined whether
        accidental or intentional Y28.2
      suicide (attempt) X78.2
    dairy equipment W31.82
    dart W21.89
      not thrown, projected or falling W45.8
    deer —*see* Contact, with, hoof stock
      NEC
    derrick W24.0
      agricultural operations W30.89
      hay W30.2
    dog W54.8
      bite W54.0
      strike W54.1
    dolphin W56.09
      bite W56.01
      strike W56.02
    donkey —*see* Contact, with, hoof stock
      NEC
    drill (powered) W29.8
      earth (land) (seabed) W31.0
      nonpowered W27.8
    drive belt W24.0
      agricultural operations W30.89
    dry ice —*see* Exposure, cold, man-made
    dryer (clothes) (powered) (spin) W29.2
    duck W61.69
      bite W61.61
      strike W61.62
    earth(-)
      drilling machine (industrial) W31.0
      scraping machine in stationary use
        W31.83
    edge of stiff paper W45.1
    electric
      beater W29.0
      blanket X16
      fan W29.2
        commercial W31.82
      knife W29.1
      mixer W29.0
    elevator (building) W24.0
      agricultural operations W30.89
      grain W30.3
    engine (s), hot NEC X17
    excavating machine W31.0
    farm machine W30.9
    feces —*see* Contact, with, by type of
      animal
    fer de lance X58

Contact *(Continued)*
  with *(Continued)*
    fish W56.59
      bite W56.51
      shark —*see* Contact, with, shark
      strike W56.52
    flying horses W31.81
    forging (metalworking) machine
      W31.1
    fork W27.4
    forklift (truck) W24.0
      agricultural operations W30.89
    frog W62.0
    garden
      cultivator (powered) W29.3
        riding W30.89
      fork W27.1
    gas turbine W31.3
    Gila monster X58
    giraffe —*see* Contact, with, hoof stock
      NEC
    glass (sharp) (broken) W25
      with subsequent fall W18.02
      assault X99.0
      due to fall —*see* Fall, by type
      stated as undetermined whether
        accidental or intentional Y28. 0
      suicide (attempt) X78.0
    goat W55.39
      bite W55.31
      strike W55.32
    goose W61.59
      bite W61.51
      strike W61.52
    hand
      saw W27.0
      tool (not powered) NEC W27.8
        powered W29.8
    harvester W30.0
    hay-derrick W30.2
    heat NEC X19
      from appliance (electrical)
        (household) —*see* Contact, with,
        hot, household appliance
      heating appliance X16
    heating
      appliance (hot) X16
      pad (electric) X16
    hedge-trimmer (powered) W29.3
    hoe W27.1
    hoist (chain) (shaft) NEC W24.0
      agricultural W30.89
    hoof stock NEC W55.39
      bite W55.31
      strike W55.32
    hornet (s) X58
    horse W55.19
      bite W55.11
      strike W55.12
    hot
      air X14.1
        inhalation X14.0
      cooker X15.8
      drinks X10.0
      engine X17
      fats X10.2
      fluids NEC X12
        assault X98.2
        suicide (attempt) X77.2
        undetermined whether accidental or
          intentional Y27.2
      food X10.1
      gases X14.1
        inhalation X14.0
      heating appliance X16
      household appliance X15.8
        assault X98.3
        cooker X15.8
        hotplate X15.2
        kettle X15.8
        light bulb X15.8

Contact *(Continued)*
  with *(Continued)*
    hot *(Continued)*
      household appliance *(Continued)*
        object NEC X19
          assault X98.8
          stated as undetermined whether
            accidental or intentional Y27.9
          suicide (attempt) X77.8
        saucepan X15.3
        skillet X15.3
        stated as undetermined whether
          accidental or intentional Y27.3
        stove X15.0
          suicide (attempt) X77.3
        toaster X15.1
      kettle X15.8
      light bulb X15.8
      liquid NEC (*see also* Burn) X12
        drinks X10.0
        stated as undetermined whether
          accidental or intentional Y27.2
        suicide (attempt) X77.2
        tap water X11.8
          stated as undetermined whether
            accidental or intentional Y27.1
          suicide (attempt) X77.1
      machinery X17
      metal (molten) (liquid) NEC X18
      object (not producing fire or flames)
        NEC X19
      oil (cooking) X10.2
      pipe X16
      plate X15.2
      radiator X16
      saucepan (glass) (metal) X15.3
      skillet X15.3
      stove (kitchen) X15.0
      substance NEC X19
      tap-water X11.8
        assault X98.1
        heated on stove X12
          stated as undetermined whether
            accidental or intentional Y27.2
          suicide (attempt) X77.2
        in bathtub X11.0
        running X11.1
        stated as undetermined whether
          accidental or intentional Y27.1
        suicide (attempt) X77.1
      toaster X15.1
      tool X17
      vapors X13.1
        inhalation X13.0
      water (tap) X11.8
        boiling X12
          stated as undetermined whether
            accidental or intentional Y27.2
          suicide (attempt) X77.2
        heated on stove X12
          stated as undetermined whether
            accidental or intentional Y27.2
          suicide (attempt) X77.2
        in bathtub X11.0
        running X11.1
        stated as undetermined whether
          accidental or intentional Y27.1
        suicide (attempt) X77.1
    hotplate X15.2
    ice-pick W27.4
    insect (nonvenomous) NEC W57
    kettle (hot) X15.8
    knife W26.0
      assault X99.1
      electric W29.1
      stated as undetermined whether
        accidental or intentional Y28.1
      suicide (attempt) X78.1
    lathe (metalworking) W31.1
      turnings W45.8
      woodworking W31.2

Contact *(Continued)*
  with *(Continued)*
    lawnmower (powered) (ridden) W28
      causing electrocution W86.8
        suicide (attempt) X83.1
      unpowered W27.1
    lift, lifting (devices) W24.0
      agricultural operations W30.89
      shaft W24.0
    liquefied gas —*see* Exposure, cold,
      man-made
    liquid air, hydrogen, nitrogen —*see*
      Exposure, cold, man-made
    lizard (nonvenomous) W59.09
      bite W59.01
      strike W59.02
    llama —*see* Contact, with, hoof stock NEC
    macaw W61.19
      bite W61.11
      strike W61.12
    machine, machinery W31.9
      abrasive wheel W31.1
      agricultural including animal-powered
        W30.9
        combine harvester W30.0
        grain storage elevator W30.3
        hay derrick W30.2
        power take-off device W30.1
        reaper W30.0
        specified NEC W30.89
        thresher W30.0
        transport vehicle, stationary W30.81
      band saw W31.2
      bench saw W31.2
      circular saw W31.2
      commercial NEC W31.82
      drilling, metal (industrial) W31.1
      earth-drilling W31.0
      earthmoving or scraping W31.89
      excavating W31.89
      forging machine W31.1
      gas turbine W31.3
      hot X17
      internal combustion engine W31.3
      land drill W31.0
      lathe W31.1
      lifting (devices) W24.0
      metal drill W31.1
      metalworking (industrial) W31.1
      milling, metal W31.1
      mining W31.0
      molding W31.2
      overhead plane W31.2
      power press, metal W31.1
      prime mover W31.3
      printing W31.89
      radial saw W31.2
      recreational W31.81
      roller-coaster W31.81
      rolling mill, metal W31.1
      sander W31.2
      seabed drill W31.0
      shaft
        hoist W31.0
        lift W31.0
      specified NEC W31.89
      spinning W31.89
      steam engine W31.3
      transmission W24.1
      undercutter W31.0
      water driven turbine W31.3
      weaving W31.89
      woodworking or forming (industrial)
        W31.2
    mammal (feces) (urine) W55.89
      bull —*see* Contact, with, bull
      cat —*see* Contact, with, cat
      cow —*see* Contact, with, cow
      goat —*see* Contact, with, goat
      hoof stock —*see* Contact, with, hoof
        stock

Contact *(Continued)*
  with *(Continued)*
    mammal *(Continued)*
      horse —*see* Contact, with, horse
      marine W56.39
        dolphin —*see* Contact, with, dolphin
        orca —*see* Contact, with, orca
        sea lion —*see* Contact, with, sea lion
        specified NEC W56.39
          bite W56.31
          strike W56.32
      pig —*see* Contact, with, pig
      raccoon —*see* Contact, with, raccoon
      rodent —*see* Contact, with, rodent
      sheep —*see* Contact, with, sheep
      specified NEC W55.89
        bite W55.81
        strike W55.82
    marine
      animal W56.89
        bite W56.81
        dolphin —*see* Contact, with, dolphin
        fish NEC —*see* Contact, with, fish
        mammal —*see* Contact, with,
          mammal, marine
        orca —*see* Contact, with, orca
        sea lion —*see* Contact, with, sea lion
        shark —*see* Contact, with, shark
        strike W56.82
    meat
      grinder (domestic) W29.0
        industrial W31.82
        nonpowered W27.4
      slicer (domestic) W29.0
        industrial W31.82
    merry go round W31.81
    metal, (hot) (liquid) (molten) NEC X18
    millipede W57
    nail W45.0
      gun W29.4
    needle (sewing) W27.3
      hypodermic W46.0
        contaminated W46.1
    object (blunt) NEC
      hot NEC X19
      legal intervention —*see* Legal,
        intervention, blunt object
      sharp NEC W45.8
        inflicted by other person NEC W45.8
          stated as
            intentional homicide (attempt) —
              see Assault, cutting or
              piercing instrument
        legal intervention —*see* Legal,
          intervention, sharp object
        self-inflicted X78.9
    orca W56.29
      bite W56.21
      strike W56.22
    overhead plane W31.2
    paper (as sharp object) W45.1
    paper-cutter W27.5
    parrot W61.09
      bite W61.01
      strike W61.02
    pig W55.49
      bite W55.41
      strike W55.42
    pipe, hot X16
    pitchfork W27.1
    plane (metal) (wood) W27.0
      overhead W31.2
    plant thorns, spines, sharp leaves or other
      mechanisms W60
    powered
      garden cultivator W29.3
      household appliance, implement, or
        machine W29.8
      saw (industrial) W31.2
        hand W29.8
    printing machine W31.89

Contact *(Continued)*
  with *(Continued)*
    psittacine bird W61.29
      bite W61.21
      macaw —*see* Contact, with, macaw
      parrot —*see* Contact, with, parrot
      strike W61.22
    pulley (block) (transmission) W24.0
      agricultural operations W30.89
    raccoon W55.59
      bite W55.51
      strike W55.52
    radial-saw (industrial) W31.2
    radiator (hot) X16
    rake W27.1
    rattlesnake X58
    reaper W30.0
    reptile W59.89
      lizard —*see* Contact, with, lizard
      snake —*see* Contact, with, snake
      specified NEC W59.89
        bite W59.81
        crushing W59.83
        strike W59.82
      turtle —*see* Contact, with, turtle
    rivet gun (powered) W29.4
    road scraper —*see* Accident, transport,
      construction vehicle
    rodent (feces) (urine) W53.89
      bite W53.81
      mouse W53.09
        bite W53.01
      rat W53.19
        bite W53.11
      specified NEC W53.89
        bite W53.81
      squirrel W53.29
        bite W53.21
    roller coaster W31.81
    rope NEC W24.0
      agricultural operations W30.89
    saliva —*see* Contact, with, by type of
      animal
    sander W29.8
      industrial W31.2
    saucepan (hot) (glass) (metal) X15.3
    saw W27.0
      band (industrial) W31.2
      bench (industrial) W31.2
      chain W29.3
      hand W27.0
    sawing machine, metal W31.1
    scissors W27.2
    scorpion X58
    screwdriver W27.0
      powered W29.8
    sea
      anemone, cucumber or urchin (spine)
        X58
      lion W56.19
        bite W56.11
        strike W56.12
    serpent —*see* Contact, with, snake, by type
    sewing-machine (electric) (powered)
      W29.2
      not powered W27.8
    shaft (hoist) (lift) (transmission) NEC
      W24.0
      agricultural W30.89
    shark W56.49
      bite W56.41
      strike W56.42
    shears (hand) W27.2
      powered (industrial) W31.1
        domestic W29.2
    sheep W55.39
      bite W55.31
      strike W55.32
    shovel W27.8
      steam —*see* Accident, transport,
        construction vehicle

Contact *(Continued)*
  with *(Continued)*
    snake (nonvenomous) W59.19
      bite W59.11
      crushing W59.13
      strike W59.12
    spade W27.1
    spider (venomous) X58
    spin-drier W29.2
    spinning machine W31.89
    splinter W45.8
    sports equipment W21.9
    staple gun (powered) W29.8
    steam X13.1
      engine W31.3
      inhalation X13.0
      pipe X16
      shovel W31.89
    stove (hot) (kitchen) X15.0
    substance, hot NEC X19
      molten (metal) X18
    sword W26.1
      assault X99.2
      stated as undetermined whether
        accidental or intentional
        Y28.2
      suicide (attempt) X78.2
    tarantula X58
    thresher W30.0
    tin can lid W45.2
    toad W62.1
    toaster (hot) X15.1
    tool W27.8
      hand (not powered) W27.8
        auger W27.0
        axe W27.0
        can opener W27.4
        chisel W27.0
        fork W27.4
        garden W27.1
        handsaw W27.0
        hoe W27.1
        ice-pick W27.4
        kitchen utensil W27.4
        manual
          lawn mower W27.1
          sewing machine W27.8
        meat grinder W27.4
        needle (sewing) W27.3
          hypodermic W46.0
            contaminated W46.1
        paper cutter W27.5
        pitchfork W27.1
        rake W27.1
        scissors W27.2
        screwdriver W27.0
        specified NEC W27.8
        workbench W27.0
      hot X17
      powered W29.8
        blender W29.0
          commercial W31.82
        can opener W29.0
          commercial W31.82
        chainsaw W29.3
        clothes dryer W29.2
          commercial W31.82
        dishwasher W29.2
          commercial W31.82
        edger W29.3
        electric fan W29.2
          commercial W31.82
        electric knife W29.1
        food processor W29.0
          commercial W31.82
        garbage disposal W29.0
          commercial W31.82

Contact *(Continued)*
  with *(Continued)*
    tool *(Continued)*
      powered *(Continued)*
        garden tool W29.3
        hedge trimmer W29.3
        ice maker W29.0
          commercial W31.82
        kitchen appliance W29.0
          commercial W31.82
        lawn mower W28
        meat grinder W29.0
          commercial W31.82
        mixer W29.0
          commercial W31.82
        rototiller W29.3
        sewing machine W29.2
          commercial W31.82
        washing machine W29.2
          commercial W31.82
    transmission device (belt, cable, chain,
      gear, pinion, shaft) W24.1
      agricultural operations W30.89
    turbine (gas) (water-driven) W31.3
    turkey W61.49
      peck W61.43
      strike W61.42
    turtle (nonvenomous) W59.29
      bite W59.21
      strike W59.22
      terrestrial W59.89
        bite W59.81
        crushing W59.83
        strike W59.82
    under-cutter W31.0
    urine —*see* Contact, with, by type of
      animal
    vehicle
      agricultural use (transport) —*see*
        Accident, transport, agricultural
        vehicle
        not on public highway W30.81
      industrial use (transport) —*see*
        Accident, transport, industrial
        vehicle
        not on public highway W31.83
      off-road use (transport) —*see* Accident,
        transport, all-terrain or off-road
        vehicle
        not on public highway W31.83
      special construction use (transport) —*see*
        Accident, transport, construction
        vehicle
        not on public highway W31.83
    venomous
      animal X58
      arthropods X58
      lizard X58
      marine animal NEC X58
      marine plant NEC X58
      millipedes (tropical) X58
      plant (s) X58
      snake X58
      spider X58
    viper X58
    washing-machine (powered) W29.2
    wasp X58
    weaving-machine W31.89
    winch W24.0
      agricultural operations W30.89
    wire NEC W24.0
      agricultural operations W30.89
    wood slivers W45.8
    yellow jacket X58
    zebra —*see* Contact, with, hoof stock
      NEC
Coup de soleil X32

Crash
  aircraft (in transit) (powered) V95.9
    balloon V96.01
    fixed wing NEC (private) V95.21
      commercial V95.31
    glider V96.21
      hang V96.11
      powered V95.11
    helicopter V95.01
    in war operations —*see* War operations,
      destruction of aircraft
    microlight V95.11
    nonpowered V96.9
      specified NEC V96.8
    powered NEC V95.8
    stated as
      homicide (attempt) Y08.81
      suicide (attempt) X83.0
    ultralight V95.11
  spacecraft V95.41
  transport vehicle NEC (*see also* Accident,
    transport) V89.9
    homicide (attempt) Y03.8
    motor NEC (traffic) V89.2
      homicide (attempt) Y03.8
      suicide (attempt) —*see* Suicide, collision
Cruelty (mental) (physical) (sexual) X58
Crushed (accidentally) X58
  between objects (moving) (stationary and
    moving) W23.0
    stationary W23.1
  by
    alligator W58.03
    avalanche NEC —*see* Landslide
    cave-in W20.0
      caused by cataclysmic earth surface
        movement —*see* Landslide
    crocodile W58.13
    crowd or human stampede W52
    falling
      aircraft V97.39
        in war operations —*see* War
          operations, destruction of aircraft
      earth, material W20.0
        caused by cataclysmic earth surface
          movement —*see* Landslide
      object NEC W20.8
    landslide NEC —*see* Landslide
    lizard (nonvenomous) W59.09
    machinery —*see* Contact, with, by type of
      machine
    reptile NEC W59.89
    snake (nonvenomous) W59.13
  in
    machinery —*see* Contact, with, by type of
      machine
Cut, cutting (any part of body) (accidental) —
    see also Contact, with, by object or machine
  during medical or surgical treatment as
    misadventure —*see* Index to Diseases
    and Injuries, Complications
  homicide (attempt) —*see* Assault, cutting or
    piercing instrument
  inflicted by other person —*see* Assault,
    cutting or piercing instrument
  legal
    execution —*see* Legal, intervention
    intervention —*see* Legal, intervention,
      sharp object
  machine NEC (*see also* Contact, with, by type
    of machine) W31.9
  self-inflicted —*see* Suicide, cutting or piercing
    instrument
  suicide (attempt) —*see* Suicide, cutting or
    piercing instrument
Cyclone (any injury) X37.1

D

Decapitation (accidental circumstances)
NEC X58
homicide X99.9
legal execution —see Legal, intervention
Dehydration from lack of water X58
Deprivation X58
Derailment (accidental)
railway (rolling stock) (train) (vehicle)
(without antecedent collision) V81.7
with antecedent collision —see Accident,
transport, railway vehicle occupant
streetcar (without antecedent collision)
V82.7
with antecedent collision —see Accident,
transport, streetcar occupant
Descent
parachute (voluntary) (without accident to
aircraft) V97.29
due to accident to aircraft —see Accident,
transport, aircraft
Desertion X58
Destitution X58
Disability, late effect or sequela of injury —see
Sequelae
Discharge (accidental)
airgun W34.010
assault X95.01
homicide (attempt) X95.01
stated as undetermined whether accidental
or intentional Y24.0
suicide (attempt) X74.01
BB gun —see Discharge, airgun
firearm (accidental) W34.00
assault X95.9
handgun (pistol) (revolver) W32.0
assault X93
homicide (attempt) X93
legal intervention —see Legal,
intervention, firearm, handgun
stated as undetermined whether
accidental or intentional Y22
suicide (attempt) X72
homicide (attempt) X95.9
hunting rifle W33.02
assault X94.1
homicide (attempt) X94.1
legal intervention
injuring
bystander Y35.032
law enforcement personnel
Y35.031
suspect Y35.033
stated as undetermined whether
accidental or intentional Y23.1
suicide (attempt) X73.1
larger W33.00
assault X94.9
homicide (attempt) X94.9
hunting rifle —see Discharge, firearm,
hunting rifle
legal intervention —see Legal,
intervention, firearm by type of
firearm
machine gun —see Discharge, firearm,
machine gun
shotgun —see Discharge, firearm,
shotgun
specified NEC W33.09
assault X94.8
homicide (attempt) X94.8
legal intervention
injuring
bystander Y35.092
law enforcement personnel
Y35.091
suspect Y35.093
stated as undetermined whether
accidental or intentional Y23.8
suicide (attempt) X73.8

Discharge (Continued)
firearm (Continued)
larger (Continued)
stated as undetermined whether
accidental or intentional Y23.9
suicide (attempt) X73.9
legal intervention
injuring
bystander Y35.002
law enforcement personnel Y35.001
suspect Y35.03
using rubber bullet
injuring
bystander Y35.042
law enforcement personnel
Y35.041
suspect Y35.043
machine gun W33.03
assault X94.2
homicide (attempt) X94.2
legal intervention —see Legal,
intervention, firearm, machine gun
stated as undetermined whether
accidental or intentional Y23.3
suicide (attempt) X73.2
pellet gun —see Discharge, airgun
shotgun W33.01
assault X94.0
homicide (attempt) X94.0
legal intervention —see Legal,
intervention, firearm, specified NEC
stated as undetermined whether
accidental or intentional Y23.0
suicide (attempt) X73.0
specified NEC W34.09
assault X95.8
homicide (attempt) X95.8
legal intervention —see Legal,
intervention, firearm, specified NEC
stated as undetermined whether
accidental or intentional Y24.8
suicide (attempt) X74.8
stated as undetermined whether accidental
or intentional Y24.9
suicide (attempt) X74.9
Very pistol W34.09
assault X95.8
homicide (attempt) X95.8
stated as undetermined whether
accidental or intentional Y24.8
suicide (attempt) X74.8
firework (s) W39
stated as undetermined whether accidental
or intentional Y25
gas-operated gun NEC W34.018
airgun —see Discharge, airgun
assault X95.09
homicide (attempt) X95.09
paintball gun —see Discharge, paintball
gun
stated as undetermined whether accidental
or intentional Y24.8
suicide (attempt) X74.09
gun NEC —see also Discharge, firearm NEC
air —see Discharge, airgun
BB —see Discharge, airgun
for single hand use —see Discharge,
firearm, handgun
hand —see Discharge, firearm, handgun
machine —see Discharge, firearm, machine
gun
other specified —see Discharge, firearm
NEC
paintball —see Discharge, paintball gun
pellet —see Discharge, airgun
handgun —see Discharge, firearm, handgun
machine gun —see Discharge, firearm,
machine gun
paintball gun W34.011
assault X95.02
homicide (attempt) X95.02

Discharge (Continued)
paintball gun (Continued)
stated as undetermined whether accidental
or intentional Y24.8
suicide (attempt) X74.02
pistol —see Discharge, firearm, handgun
flare —see Discharge, firearm, Very pistol
pellet —see Discharge, airgun
Very —see Discharge, firearm, Very pistol
revolver —see Discharge, firearm, handgun
rifle (hunting) —see Discharge, firearm,
hunting rifle
shotgun —see Discharge, firearm, shotgun
spring-operated gun NEC W34.018
assault X95.09
homicide (attempt) X95.09
stated as undetermined whether accidental
or intentional Y24.8
suicide (attempt) X74.09
Disease
Andes W94.11
aviator's —see Air, pressure
range W94.11
Diver's disease, palsy, paralysis, squeeze —see
Air, pressure
Diving (into water) —see Accident, diving
Dog bite W54.0
Dragged by transport vehicle NEC (see also
Accident, transport) V09.9
Drinking poison (accidental) —see Table of
Drugs and Chemicals
Dropped (accidentally) while being carried or
supported by other person W04
Drowning (accidental) W74
assault X92.9
due to
accident (to)
machinery —see Contact, with, by type
of machine
watercraft V90.89
burning V90.29
powered V90.23
fishing boat V90.22
jetskis V90.23
merchant ship V90.20
passenger ship V90.21
unpowered V90.28
canoe V90.25
inflatable V90.26
kayak V90.25
sailboat V90.24
water skis V90.27
crushed V90.39
powered V90.33
fishing boat V90.32
jetskis V90.33
merchant ship V90.30
passenger ship V90.31
unpowered V90.38
canoe V90.35
inflatable V90.36
kayak V90.35
sailboat V90.34
water skis V90.37
overturning V90.09
powered V90.03
fishing boat V90.02
jetskis V90.03
merchant ship V90.00
passenger ship V90.01
unpowered V90.08
canoe V90.05
inflatable V90.06
kayak V90.05
sailboat V90.04
sinking V90.19
powered V90.13
fishing boat V90.12
jetskis V90.13
merchant ship V90.10
passenger ship V90.11

Drowning *(Continued)*
  due to *(Continued)*
    accident *(Continued)*
      watercraft *(Continued)*
        sinking *(Continued)*
          unpowered V90.18
            canoe V90.15
            inflatable V90.16
            kayak V90.15
            sailboat V90.14
          specified type NEC V90.89
          powered V90.83
            fishing boat V90.82
            jetskis V90.83
            merchant ship V90.80
            passenger ship V90.81
          unpowered V90.88
            canoe V90.85
            inflatable V90.86
            kayak V90.85
            sailboat V90.84
            water skis V90.87
    avalanche —*see* Landslide
    cataclysmic
      earth surface movement NEC —*see*
        Forces of nature, earth movement
      storm —*see* Forces of nature, cataclysmic
        storm
    cloudburst X37.8
    cyclone X37.1
    fall overboard (from) V92.09
      powered craft V92.03
        ferry boat V92.01
        fishing boat V92.02
        jetskis V92.03
        liner V92.01
        merchant ship V92.00
        passenger ship V92.01
      resulting from
        accident to watercraft —*see* Drowning,
          due to, accident to, watercraft
        being washed overboard (from)
          V92.29
          powered craft V92.23
            ferry boat V92.21
            fishing boat V92.22
            jetskis V92.23
            liner V92.21
            merchant ship V92.20
            passenger ship V92.21
          unpowered craft V92.28
            canoe V92.25
            inflatable V92.26
            kayak V92.25
            sailboat V92.24
            surf-board V92.28
            water skis V92.27
            windsurfer V92.28
        motion of watercraft V92.19
          powered craft V92.13
            ferry boat V92.11
            fishing boat V92.12
            jetskis V92.13
            liner V92.11
            merchant ship V92.10
            passenger ship V92.11
          unpowered craft
            canoe V92.15
            inflatable V92.16
            kayak V92.15
            sailboat V92.14
      unpowered craft V92.08
        canoe V92.05
        inflatable V92.06
        kayak V92.05

Drowning *(Continued)*
  due to *(Continued)*
    fall overboard *(Continued)*
      unpowered craft *(Continued)*
        sailboat V92.04
        surf-board V92.08
        water skis V92.07
        windsurfer V92.08
    hurricane X37.0
    jumping into water from watercraft
      (involved in accident) —*see also*
      Drowning, due to, accident to,
      watercraft
    without accident to or on watercraft
      W16.711
    tidal wave NEC —*see* Forces of nature,
      tidal wave
    torrential rain X37.8
  following
    fall
      into
        bathtub W16.211
        bucket W16.221
        fountain —*see* Drowning, following,
          fall, into, water, specified NEC
        quarry —*see* Drowning, following,
          fall, into, water, specified NEC
        reservoir —*see* Drowning, following,
          fall, into, water, specified NEC
        swimming-pool W16.011
          stated as undetermined whether
            accidental or intentional
            Y21.3
          striking
            bottom W16.021
            wall W16.031
          suicide (attempt) X71.2
        water NOS W16.41
          natural (lake) (open sea) (river)
            (stream) (pond) W16.111
            striking
              bottom W16.121
              side W16.131
          specified NEC W16.311
            striking
              bottom W16.321
              wall W16.331
      overboard NEC —*see* Drowning, due to,
        fall overboard
    jump or dive
      from boat W16.711
        striking bottom W16.721
      into
        fountain —*see* Drowning, following,
          jump or dive, into, water,
          specified NEC
        quarry —*see* Drowning, following,
          jump or dive, into, water,
          specified NEC
        reservoir —*see* Drowning, following,
          jump or dive, into, water,
          specified NEC
        swimming-pool W16.511
          striking
            bottom W16.521
            wall W16.531
          suicide (attempt) X71.2
        water NOS W16.91
          natural (lake) (open sea) (river)
            (stream) (pond) W16.611
          specified NEC W16.811
            striking
              bottom W16.821
              wall W16.831
          striking bottom W16.621

Drowning *(Continued)*
  homicide (attempt) X92.9
  in
    bathtub (accidental) W65
      assault X92.04
      following fall W16.211
        stated as undetermined whether
          accidental or intentional
          Y21.1
      stated as undetermined whether
        accidental or intentional Y21.0
      suicide (attempt) X71.0
    lake —*see* Drowning, in, natural water
    natural water (lake) (open sea) (river)
      (stream) (pond) W69
      assault X92.3
      following
        dive or jump W16.611
          striking bottom W16.621
        fall W16.111
          striking
            bottom W16.121
            side W16.131
      stated as undetermined whether
        accidental or intentional Y21.4
      suicide (attempt) X71.3
    quarry —*see* Drowning, in, specified place
      NEC
    quenching tank —*see* Drowning, in,
      specified place NEC
    reservoir —*see* Drowning, in, specified
      place NEC
    river —*see* Drowning, in, natural water
    sea —*see* Drowning, in, natural water
    specified place NEC W73
      assault X92.8
      following
        dive or jump W16.811
          striking
            bottom W16.821
            wall W16.831
        fall W16.311
          striking
            bottom W16.321
            wall W16.331
      stated as undetermined whether
        accidental or intentional Y21.8
      suicide (attempt) X71.8
    stream —*see* Drowning, in, natural water
    swimming-pool W67
      assault X92.1
        following fall X92.2
      following
        dive or jump W16.511
          striking
            bottom W16.521
            wall W16.531
        fall W16.011
          striking
            bottom W16.021
            wall W16.031
      stated as undetermined whether
        accidental or intentional Y21.2
        following fall Y21.3
      suicide (attempt) X71.1
        following fall X71.2
    war operations —*see* War operations,
      restriction of airway
  resulting from accident to watercraft —*see*
    Drowning, due to, accident, watercraft
  self-inflicted X71.9
  stated as undetermined whether accidental or
    intentional Y21.9
  suicide (attempt) X71.9

◀ New   ◀▦ Revised   ~~deleted~~ Deleted

E

Earth (surface) movement NEC —see Forces of nature, earth movement
Earth falling (on) W20.0
  caused by cataclysmic earth surface movement or eruption —see Landslide
Earthquake (any injury) X34
Effect (s) (adverse) of
  air pressure (any) —see Air, pressure
  cold, excessive (exposure to) —see Exposure, cold
  heat (excessive) —see Heat
  hot place (weather) —see Heat
  insolation X30
  late —see Sequelae
  motion —see Motion
  nuclear explosion or weapon in war operations —see War operations, nuclear weapon
  radiation —see Radiation
  travel —see Travel
Electric shock (accidental) (by) (in) —see Exposure, electric current
Electrocution (accidental) —see Exposure, electric current
Endotracheal tube wrongly placed during anesthetic procedure Y65.3
Entanglement
  in
    bed linen, causing suffocation —see category T71
    wheel of pedal cycle V19.88
Entry of foreign body or material —see Foreign body
Environmental pollution related condition —see Z57
Execution, legal (any method) —see Legal, intervention
Exhaustion
  cold —see Exposure, cold
  due to excessive exertion —see category Y93
  heat —see Heat
Explosion (accidental) (of) (with secondary fire) W40.9
  acetylene W40.1
  aerosol can W36.1
  air tank (compressed) (in machinery) W36.2
  aircraft (in transit) (powered) NEC V95.9
    balloon V96.05
    fixed wing NEC (private) V95.25
      commercial V95.35
    glider V96.25
      hang V96.15
      powered V95.15
    helicopter V95.05
    in war operations —see War operations, destruction of aircraft
    microlight V95.15
    nonpowered V96.9
      specified NEC V96.8
    powered NEC V95.8
    stated as
      homicide (attempt) Y03.8
      suicide (attempt) X83.0
    ultralight V95.15
  anesthetic gas in operating room W40.1
  antipersonnel bomb W40.8
    assault X96.0
    homicide (attempt) X96.0
    suicide (attempt) X75
  assault X96.9
  bicycle tire W37.0
  blasting (cap) (materials) W40.0
  boiler (machinery), not on transport vehicle W35
    on watercraft —see Explosion, in, watercraft
  butane W40.1
  caused by other person X96.9
  coal gas W40.1

Explosion (Continued)
  detonator W40.0
  dump (munitions) W40.8
  dynamite W40.0
    in
      assault X96.8
      homicide (attempt) X96.8
      legal intervention
        injuring
          bystander Y35.112
          law enforcement personnel Y35.111
          suspect Y35.113
      suicide (attempt) X75
  explosive (material) W40.9
    gas W40.1
    in blasting operation W40.0
    specified NEC W40.8
      in
        assault X96.8
        homicide (attempt) X96.8
        legal intervention
          injuring
            bystander Y35.192
            law enforcement personnel Y35.191
            suspect Y35.193
        suicide (attempt) X75
  factory (munitions) W40.8
  fertilizer bomb W40.8
    assault X96.3
    homicide (attempt) X96.3
    suicide (attempt) X75
  fire-damp W40.1
  firearm (parts) NEC W34.19
    airgun W34.110
    BB gun W34.110
    gas, air or spring-operated gun NEC W34.118
    handgun W32.1
    hunting rifle W33.12
    larger firearm W33.10
      specified NEC W33.19
    machine gun W33.13
    paintball gun W34.111
    pellet gun W34.110
    shotgun W33.11
    Very pistol [flare] W34.19
  fireworks W39
  gas (coal) (explosive) W40.1
    cylinder W36.9
      aerosol can W36.1
      air tank W36.2
      pressurized W36.3
      specified NEC W36.8
  gasoline (fumes) (tank) not in moving motor vehicle W40.1
    bomb W40.8
      assault X96.1
      homicide (attempt) X96.1
      suicide (attempt) X75
    in motor vehicle —see Accident, transport, by type of vehicle
  grain store W40.8
  grenade W40.8
    in
      assault X96.8
      homicide (attempt) X96.8
      legal intervention
        injuring
          bystander Y35.192
          law enforcement personnel Y35.191
          suspect Y35.193
      suicide (attempt) X75
  handgun (parts) —see Explosion, firearm, handgun (parts)
  homicide (attempt) X96.9
    antipersonnel bomb —see Explosion, antipersonnel bomb
    fertilizer bomb —see Explosion, fertilizer bomb

Explosion (Continued)
  homicide (Continued)
    gasoline bomb —see Explosion, gasoline bomb
    letter bomb —see Explosion, letter bomb
    pipe bomb —see Explosion, pipe bomb
    specified NEC X96.8
  hose, pressurized W37.8
  hot water heater, tank (in machinery) W35
    on watercraft —see Explosion, in, watercraft
  in, on
    dump W40.8
    factory W40.8
    mine (of explosive gases) NEC W40.1
    watercraft V93.59
      powered craft V93.53
        ferry boat V93.51
        fishing boat V93.52
        jetskis V93.53
        liner V93.51
        merchant ship V93.50
        passenger ship V93.51
        sailboat V93.54
  letter bomb W40.8
    assault X96.2
    homicide (attempt) X96.2
    suicide (attempt) X75
  machinery —see also Contact, with, by type of machine
    on board watercraft —see Explosion, in, watercraft
    pressure vessel —see Explosion, by type of vessel
  methane W40.1
  mine W40.1
  missile NEC W40.8
  mortar bomb W40.8
    in
      assault X96.8
      homicide (attempt) X96.8
      legal intervention
        injuring
          bystander Y35.192
          law enforcement personnel Y35.191
          suspect Y35.193
      suicide (attempt) X75
  munitions (dump) (factory) W40.8
  pipe, pressurized W37.8
    bomb W40.8
      assault X96.4
      homicide (attempt) X96.4
      suicide (attempt) X75
  pressure, pressurized
    cooker W38
    gas tank (in machinery) W36.3
    hose W37.8
    pipe W37.8
    specified device NEC W38
    tire W37.8
      bicycle W37.0
    vessel (in machinery) W38
  propane W40.1
  self-inflicted X75
  shell (artillery) NEC W40.8
    during war operations —see War operations, explosion
    in
      legal intervention
        injuring
          bystander Y35.122
          law enforcement personnel Y35.121
          suspect Y35.123
    war —see War operations, explosion
  spacecraft V95.45
  stated as undetermined whether accidental or intentional Y25
  steam or water lines (in machinery) W37.8
  stove W40.9
  suicide (attempt) X75

Explosion (*Continued*)
- tire, pressurized W37.8
  - bicycle W37.0
- undetermined whether accidental or intentional Y25
- vehicle tire NEC W37.8
  - bicycle W37.0
- war operations —*see* War operations, explosion

Exposure (*to*) X58
- air pressure change —*see* Air, pressure
- cold (accidental) (excessive) (extreme) (natural) (place) X31
  - assault Y08.89
  - due to
    - man-made conditions W93.8
      - dry ice (contact) W93.01
        - inhalation W93.02
      - liquid air (contact) (hydrogen) (nitrogen) W93.11
        - inhalation W93.12
      - refrigeration unit (deep freeze) W93.2
    - suicide (attempt) X83.2
    - weather (conditions) X31
  - homicide (attempt) Y08.89
  - self-inflicted X83.2
- due to abandonment or neglect X58
- electric current W86.8
  - appliance (faulty) W86.8
    - domestic W86.0
  - caused by other person Y08.89
  - conductor (faulty) W86.1
  - control apparatus (faulty) W86.1
  - electric power generating plant, distribution station W86.1
  - electroshock gun —*see* Exposure, electric current, taser
  - high-voltage cable W85
  - homicide (attempt) Y08.89
  - legal execution —*see* Legal, intervention, specified means NEC
  - lightning —*see* subcategory T75.0
  - live rail W86.8
  - misadventure in medical or surgical procedure in electroshock therapy Y63.4
  - motor (electric) (faulty) W86.8
    - domestic W86.0
  - self-inflicted X83.1
  - specified NEC W86.8
    - domestic W86.0
  - stun gun —*see* Exposure, electric current, taser
  - suicide (attempt) X83.1
  - taser W86.8
    - assault Y08.89
    - legal intervention —*see* category Y35
    - self-harm (intentional) X83.8
    - undetermined intent Y33
  - third rail W86.8
  - transformer (faulty) W86.1
  - transmission lines W85
- environmental tobacco smoke X58
- excessive
  - cold —*see* Exposure, cold
  - heat (natural) NEC X30
  - man-made W92
- factor (s) NOS X58
  - environmental NEC X58
    - man-made NEC W99
    - natural NEC —*see* Forces of nature
  - specified NEC X58
- fire, flames (accidental) X08.8
  - assault X97
  - campfire —*see* Exposure, fire, controlled, not in building
  - controlled (in)
    - with ignition (of) clothing (*see also* Ignition, clothes) X06.2
      - nightwear X05

Exposure (*Continued*)
- fire, flames (*Continued*)
  - controlled (*Continued*)
    - bonfire —*see* Exposure, fire, controlled, not in building
    - brazier (in building or structure) —*see also* Exposure, fire, controlled, building
      - not in building or structure —*see* Exposure, fire, controlled, not in building
    - building or structure X02.0
      - with
        - fall from building X02.3
        - from building X02.5
        - injury due to building collapse X02.2
        - smoke inhalation X02.1
      - hit by object from building X02.4
      - specified mode of injury NEC X02.8
    - fireplace, furnace or stove —*see* Exposure, fire, controlled, building
    - not in building or structure X03.0
      - with
        - fall X03.3
        - smoke inhalation X03.1
      - hit by object X03.4
      - specified mode of injury NEC X03.8
    - trash —*see* Exposure, fire, controlled, not in building
  - fireplace —*see* Exposure, fire, controlled, building
  - fittings or furniture (in building or structure) (uncontrolled) —*see* Exposure, fire, uncontrolled, building
  - forest (uncontrolled) —*see* Exposure, fire, uncontrolled, not in building
  - grass (uncontrolled) —*see* Exposure, fire, uncontrolled, not in building
  - hay (uncontrolled) —*see* Exposure, fire, uncontrolled, not in building
  - homicide (attempt) X97
  - ignition of highly flammable material X04
  - in, of, on, starting in
    - machinery —*see* Contact, with, by type of machine
    - motor vehicle (in motion) (*see also* Accident, transport, occupant by type of vehicle) V87.8
      - with collision —*see* Collision
    - railway rolling stock, train, vehicle V81.81
      - with collision —*see* Accident, transport, railway vehicle occupant
    - street car (in motion) V82.8
      - with collision —*see* Accident, transport, streetcar occupant
    - transport vehicle NEC —*see also* Accident, transport
      - with collision —*see* Collision
    - war operations —*see also* War operations, fire
      - from nuclear explosion —*see* War operations, nuclear weapons
    - watercraft (in transit) (not in transit) V91.09
      - localized —*see* Burn, on board watercraft, due to, fire on board
      - powered craft V91.03
        - ferry boat V91.01
        - fishing boat V91.02
        - jet skis V91.03
        - liner V91.01
        - merchant ship V91.00
        - passenger ship V91.01
      - unpowered craft V91.08
        - canoe V91.05
        - inflatable V91.06
        - kayak V91.05
        - sailboat V91.04

Exposure (*Continued*)
- fire, flames (*Continued*)
  - in, of, on, starting in (*Continued*)
    - watercraft (*Continued*)
      - unpowered craft (*Continued*)
        - surf-board V91.08
        - waterskis V91.07
        - windsurfer V91.08
  - lumber (uncontrolled) —*see* Exposure, fire, uncontrolled, not in building
  - mine (uncontrolled) —*see* Exposure, fire, uncontrolled, not in building
  - prairie (uncontrolled) —*see* Exposure, fire, uncontrolled, not in building
  - resulting from
    - explosion —*see* Explosion
    - lightning X08.8
  - self-inflicted X76
  - specified NEC X08.8
  - started by other person X97
  - stated as undetermined whether accidental or intentional Y26
  - stove —*see* Exposure, fire, controlled, building
  - suicide (attempt) X76
  - tunnel (uncontrolled) —*see* Exposure, fire, uncontrolled, not in building
  - uncontrolled
    - in building or structure X00.0
      - with
        - fall from building X00.3
        - injury due to building collapse X00.2
        - jump from building X00.5
        - smoke inhalation X00.1
      - bed X08.00
        - due to
          - cigarette X08.01
          - specified material NEC X08.09
      - furniture NEC X08.20
        - due to
          - cigarette X08.21
          - specified material NEC X08.29
      - hit by object from building X00.4
      - sofa X08.10
        - due to
          - cigarette X08.11
          - specified material NEC X08.19
      - specified mode of injury NEC X00.8
    - not in building or structure (any) X01.0
      - with
        - fall X01.3
        - smoke inhalation X01.1
      - hit by object X01.4
      - specified mode of injury NEC X01.8
  - undetermined whether accidental or intentional Y26
- forces of nature NEC —*see* Forces of nature
- G-forces (abnormal) W49.9
- gravitational forces (abnormal) W49.9
- heat (natural) NEC —*see* Heat
- high-pressure jet (hydraulic) (pneumatic) W49.9
- hydraulic jet W49.9
- inanimate mechanical force W49.9
- jet, high-pressure (hydraulic) (pneumatic) W49.9
- lightning —*see* subcategory T75.0
  - causing fire —*see* Exposure, fire
- mechanical forces NEC W49.9
  - animate NEC W64
  - inanimate NEC W49.9
- noise W42.9
  - supersonic W42.0
- noxious substance —*see* Table of Drugs and Chemical
- pneumatic jet W49.9

Exposure *(Continued)*
    prolonged in deep-freeze unit or refrigerator
        W93.2
    radiation —*see* Radiation
    smoke —*see also* Exposure, fire
        tobacco, second hand Z77.22
    specified factors NEC X58
    sunlight X32
        man-made (sun lamp) W89.8
            tanning bed W89.1
    supersonic waves W42.0
    transmission line (s), electric W85
    vibration W49.9

Exposure *(Continued)*
    waves
        infrasound W49.9
        sound W42.9
        supersonic W42.0
    weather NEC —*see* Forces of nature
External cause status Y99.9
    child assisting in compensated work for
        family Y99.8
    civilian activity done for financial or other
        compensation Y99.0
    civilian activity done for income or pay
        Y99.0

External cause status *(Continued)*
    family member assisting in compensated
        work for other family member Y99.8
    hobby not done for income Y99.8
    leisure activity Y99.8
    military activity Y99.1
    off-duty activity of military personnel Y99.8
    recreation or sport not for income or while a
        student Y99.8
    specified NEC Y99.8
    student activity Y99.8
    volunteer activity Y99.2

F

Factors, supplemental
  alcohol
    blood level
      less than 20mg/100ml Y90.0
      presence in blood, level not specified
        Y90.9
      20-39mg/100ml Y90.1
      40-59mg/100ml Y90.2
      60-79mg/100ml Y90.3
      80-99mg/100ml Y90.4
      100-119mg/100ml Y90.5
      120-199mg/100ml Y90.6
      200-239mg/100ml Y90.7
      240mg/100ml or more Y90.8
      presence in blood, but level not specified
        Y90.9
  environmental-pollution-related condition —
    see Z57
  nosocomial condition Y95
  work-related condition Y99.0
Failure
  in suture or ligature during surgical
    procedure Y65.2
  mechanical, of instrument or apparatus
    (any) (during any medical or surgical
    procedure) Y65.8
  sterile precautions (during medical and
    surgical care) —*see* Misadventure,
    failure, sterile precautions, by type of
    procedure
  to
    introduce tube or instrument Y65.4
      endotracheal tube during anesthesia Y65.3
    make curve (transport vehicle) NEC —*see*
      Accident, transport
    remove tube or instrument Y65.4
Fall, falling (accidental) W19
  building W20.1
    burning (uncontrolled fire) X00.3
  down
    embankment W17.81
    escalator W10.0
    hill W17.81
    ladder W11
    ramp W10.2
    stairs, steps W10.9
  due to
    bumping against
      object W18.00
        sharp glass W18.02
        specified NEC W18.09
        sports equipment W18.01
      person W03
        due to ice or snow W00.0
        on pedestrian conveyance —*see*
          Accident, transport, pedestrian,
          conveyance
    collision with another person W03
      due to ice or snow W00.0
      involving pedestrian conveyance —*see*
        Accident, transport, pedestrian,
        conveyance
    grocery cart tipping over W17.82
    ice or snow W00.9
      from one level to another W00.2
      on stairs or steps W00.1
      involving pedestrian conveyance —*see*
        Accident, transport, pedestrian,
        conveyance
      on same level W00.0
    slipping (on moving sidewalk) W01.0
      with subsequent striking against object
        W01.10
        furniture W01.190
        sharp object W01.119
          glass W01.110
          power tool or machine W01.111
          specified NEC W01.118
        specified NEC W01.198

Fall, falling (Continued)
  due to (Continued)
    striking against
      object W18.00
        sharp glass W18.02
        specified NEC W18.09
        sports equipment W18.01
      person W03
        due to ice or snow W00.0
        on pedestrian conveyance —*see*
          Accident, transport, pedestrian,
          conveyance
    earth (with asphyxia or suffocation (by
      pressure)) —*see* Earth, falling
  from, off, out of
    aircraft NEC (with accident to aircraft
      NEC) V97.0
      while boarding or alighting V97.1
    balcony W13.0
    bed W06
    boat, ship, watercraft NEC (with
      drowning or submersion) —
      see Drowning, due to, fall
      overboard
      with hitting bottom or object V94.0
    bridge W13.1
    building W13.9
      burning (uncontrolled fire) X00.3
    cavity W17.2
    chair W07
    cherry picker W17.89
    cliff W15
    dock W17.4
    embankment W17.81
    escalator W10.0
    flagpole W13.8
    furniture NEC W08
    grocery cart W17.82
    haystack W17.89
    high place NEC W17.89
      stated as undetermined whether
        accidental or intentional Y30
    hole W17.2
    incline W10.2
    ladder W11
    lifting device W17.89
    machine, machinery —*see also* Contact,
      with, by type of machine
      not in operation W17.89
    manhole W17.1
    mobile elevated work platform [MEWP]
      W17.89
    motorized mobility scooter W05.2
    one level to another NEC W17.89
      intentional, purposeful, suicide
        (attempt) X80
      stated as undetermined whether
        accidental or intentional Y30
    pit W17.2
    playground equipment W09.8
      jungle gym W09.2
      slide W09.0
      swing W09.1
    quarry W17.89
    railing W13.9
    ramp W10.2
    roof W13.2
    scaffolding W12
    scooter (nonmotorized) W05.1
      motorized mobility W05.2
    sky lift W17.89
    stairs, steps W10.9
      curb W10.1
      due to ice or snow W00.1
      escalator W10.0
      incline W10.2
      ramp W10.2
      sidewalk curb W10.1
      specified NEC W10.8
    stepladder W11
    storm drain W17.1

Fall, falling (Continued)
  from, off, out of (Continued)
    streetcar NEC V82.6
      with antecedent collision —*see*
        Accident, transport, streetcar
        occupant
      while boarding or alighting V82.4
    structure NEC W13.8
      burning (uncontrolled fire) X00.3
    table W08
    toilet W18.11
      with subsequent striking against object
        W18.12
    train NEC V81.6
      during derailment (without antecedent
        collision) V81.7
      with antecedent collision —*see*
        Accident, transport, railway
        vehicle occupant
      while boarding or alighting V81.4
    transport vehicle after collision —*see*
      Accident, transport, by type of
      vehicle, collision
    tree W14
    vehicle (in motion) NEC (*see also* Accident,
      transport) V89.9
      motor NEC (*see also* Accident, transport,
        occupant, by type of vehicle)
        V87.8
      stationary W17.89
        while boarding or alighting —*see*
          Accident, transport, by type
          of vehicle, while boarding or
          alighting
    viaduct W13.8
    wall W13.8
    watercraft —*see also* Drowning, due to, fall
      overboard
      with hitting bottom or object V94.0
    well W17.0
    wheelchair, non-moving W05.0
      powered —*see* Accident, transport,
        pedestrian, conveyance occupant,
        specified type NEC
    window W13.4
  in, on
    aircraft NEC V97.0
      with accident to aircraft V97.0
      while boarding or alighting
        V97.1
    bathtub (empty) W18.2
      filled W16.212
        causing drowning W16.211
    escalator W10.0
    incline W10.2
    ladder W11
    machine, machinery —*see* Contact, with,
      by type of machine
    object, edged, pointed or sharp (with
      cut) —*see* Fall, by type
    playground equipment W09.8
      jungle gym W09.2
      slide W09.0
      swing W09.1
    ramp W10.2
    scaffolding W12
    shower W18.2
      causing drowning W16.211
    staircase, stairs, steps W10.9
      curb W10.1
      due to ice or snow W00.1
      escalator W10.0
      incline W10.2
      specified NEC W10.8
    streetcar (without antecedent collision)
      V82.5
      with antecedent collision —*see*
        Accident, transport, streetcar
        occupant
      while boarding or alighting
        V82.4

◀ New   ◀|||| Revised   ~~deleted~~ Deleted

Fall, falling (*Continued*)
  in, on (*Continued*)
    train (without antecedent collision) V81.5
      with antecedent collision —*see* Accident,
        transport, railway vehicle occupant
      during derailment (without antecedent
        collision) V81.7
        with antecedent collision —*see*
          Accident, transport, railway
          vehicle occupant
      while boarding or alighting V81.4
    transport vehicle after collision —*see*
      Accident, transport, by type of
      vehicle, collision
    watercraft V93.39
      due to
        accident to craft V91.29
          powered craft V91.23
            ferry boat V91.21
            fishing boat V91.22
            jetskis V91.23
            liner V91.21
            merchant ship V91.20
            passenger ship V91.21
          unpowered craft
            canoe V91.25
            inflatable V91.26
            kayak V91.25
            sailboat V91.24
        powered craft V93.33
          ferry boat V93.31
          fishing boat V93.32
          jetskis V93.33
          liner V93.31
          merchant ship V93.30
          passenger ship V93.31
        unpowered craft V93.38
          canoe V93.35
          inflatable V93.36
          kayak V93.35
          sailboat V93.34
          surf-board V93.38
          windsurfer V93.38
  into
    cavity W17.2
    dock W17.4
    fire —*see* Exposure, fire, by type
    haystack W17.89
    hole W17.2
    lake —*see* Fall, into, water
    manhole W17.1
    moving part of machinery —*see* Contact,
      with, by type of machine
    ocean —*see* Fall, into, water
    opening in surface NEC W17.89
    pit W17.2
    pond —*see* Fall, into, water
    quarry W17.89
    river —*see* Fall, into, water
    shaft W17.89
    storm drain W17.1
    stream —*see* Fall, into, water
    swimming pool —*see also* Fall, into, water,
      in, swimming pool
      empty W17.3
    tank W17.89
    water W16.42
      causing drowning W16.41
      from watercraft —*see* Drowning, due to,
        fall overboard
      hitting diving board W21.4
      in
        bathtub W16.212
          causing drowning W16.211
        bucket W16.222
          causing drowning W16.221
        natural body of water W16.112
          causing drowning W16.111
          striking
            bottom W16.122
              causing drowning W16.121

Fall, falling (*Continued*)
  into (*Continued*)
    water (*Continued*)
      in (*Continued*)
        natural body of water (*Continued*)
          striking (*Continued*)
            side W16.132
              causing drowning W16.131
        specified water NEC W16.312
          causing drowning W16.311
          striking
            bottom W16.322
              causing drowning W16.321
            wall W16.332
              causing drowning W16.331
        swimming pool W16.012
          causing drowning W16.011
          striking
            bottom W16.022
              causing drowning W16.021
            wall W16.032
              causing drowning W16.031
        utility bucket W16.222
          causing drowning W16.221
    well W17.0
  involving
    bed W06
    chair W07
    furniture NEC W08
    glass —*see* Fall, by type
    playground equipment W09.8
      jungle gym W09.2
      slide W09.0
      swing W09.1
    roller blades —*see* Accident, transport,
      pedestrian, conveyance
    skateboard (s) —*see* Accident, transport,
      pedestrian, conveyance
    skates (ice) (in line) (roller) —*see*
      Accident, transport, pedestrian,
      conveyance
    skis —*see* Accident, transport, pedestrian,
      conveyance
    table W08
    wheelchair, non-moving W05.0
      powered —*see* Accident, transport,
        pedestrian, conveyance, specified
        type NEC
  object —*see* Struck by, object, falling
  off
    toilet W18.11
      with subsequent striking against object
        W18.12
  on same level W18.30
    due to
      specified NEC W18.39
      stepping on an object W18.31
  out of
    bed W06
    building NEC W13.8
    chair W07
    furniture NEC W08
    wheelchair, non-moving W05.0
      powered —*see* Accident, transport,
        pedestrian, conveyance, specified
        type NEC
    window W13.4
  over
    animal W01.0
    cliff W15
    embankment W17.81
    small object W01.0
  rock W20.8
  same level W18.30
    from
      being crushed, pushed, or stepped on
        by a crowd or human stampede
        W52
      collision, pushing, shoving, by or with
        other person W03
      slipping, stumbling, tripping W01.0

Fall, falling (*Continued*)
  same level (*Continued*)
    involving ice or snow W00.0
      involving skates (ice) (roller),
        skateboard, skis —*see* Accident,
        transport, pedestrian, conveyance
  snowslide (avalanche) —*see* Landslide
  stone W20.8
  structure W20.1
    burning (uncontrolled fire) X00.3
  through
    bridge W13.1
    floor W13.3
    roof W13.2
    wall W13.8
    window W13.4
  timber W20.8
  tree (caused by lightning) W20.8
  while being carried or supported by other
    person (s) W04
Fallen on by
  animal (not being ridden) NEC W55.89
Felo-de-se —*see* Suicide
Fight (hand) (fists) (foot) —*see* Assault, fight
Fire (accidental) —*see* Exposure, fire
Firearm discharge —*see* Discharge, firearm
**Fireball effects from nuclear explosion in war
  operations** —*see* War operations, nuclear
  weapons
Fireworks (explosion) W39
Flash burns from explosion —*see* Explosion
Flood (any injury) (caused by) X38
  collapse of man-made structure causing earth
    movement X36.0
  tidal wave —*see* Forces of nature, tidal wave
Food (any type) in
  air passages (with asphyxia, obstruction, or
    suffocation) —*see* categories T17 and T18
  alimentary tract causing asphyxia (due to
    compression of trachea) —*see* categories
    T17 and T18
Forces of nature X39.8
  avalanche X36.1
    causing transport accident —*see* Accident,
      transport, by type of vehicle
  blizzard X37.2
  cataclysmic storm X37.9
    with flood X38
    blizzard X37.2
    cloudburst X37.8
    cyclone X37.1
    dust storm X37.3
    hurricane X37.0
    specified storm NEC X37.8
    storm surge X37.0
    tornado X37.1
    twister X37.1
    typhoon X37.0
  cloudburst X37.8
  cold (natural) X31
  cyclone X37.1
  dam collapse causing earth movement X36.0
  dust storm X37.3
  earth movement X36.1
    caused by dam or structure collapse X36.0
    earthquake X34
  earthquake X34
  flood (caused by) X38
    dam collapse X36.0
    tidal wave —*see* Forces of nature, tidal
      wave
  heat (natural) X30
  hurricane X37.0
  landslide X36.1
    causing transport accident —*see* Accident,
      transport, by type of vehicle
  lightning —*see* subcategory T75.0
    causing fire —*see* Exposure, fire
  mudslide X36.1
    causing transport accident —*see* Accident,
      transport, by type of vehicle

Forces of nature (*Continued*)
  radiation (natural) X39.08
    radon X39.01
  radon X39.01
  specified force NEC X39.8
  storm surge X37.0
  structure collapse causing
     earth movement
     X36.0
  sunlight X32
  tidal wave X37.41
    due to
      earthquake X37.41
      landslide X37.43
      storm X37.42
      volcanic eruption X37.41
  tornado X37.1

Forces of nature (*Continued*)
  tsunami X37.41
  twister X37.1
  typhoon X37.0
  volcanic eruption X35
Foreign body
  aspiration - *see* Index to Diseases and
    Injuries. Foreign body, respiratory
    tract
  entering through skin
    W45.8
    can lid W45.2
    nail W45.0
    paper W45.1
    specified NEC 45.8
    splinter W45.8

Forest fire (exposure to) —*see* Exposure, fire,
  uncontrolled, not in building
Found injured X58
  from exposure (to) —*see* Exposure
  on
    highway, road(way), street V89.9
    railway right of way V81.9
Fracture (circumstances unknown or
  unspecified) X58
  due to specified cause NEC X58
Freezing —*see* Exposure, cold
Frostbite X31
  due to man-made conditions —*see* Exposure,
    cold, man-made
Frozen —*see* Exposure, cold

G

Gored by bull W55.22
Gunshot wound W34.00

H

Hailstones, injured by X39.8
Hanged herself or himself —*see* Hanging,
  self-inflicted
Hanging (accidental) (*see also* category T71)
  legal execution —*see* Legal, intervention,
    specified means NEC
Heat (effects of) (excessive) X30
  due to
    man-made conditions W92
      on board watercraft V93.29
        fishing boat V93.22
        merchant ship V93.20
        passenger ship V93.21
        sailboat V93.24
        specified powered craft NEC V93.23
    weather (conditions) X30

Heat (*Continued*)
  from
    electric heating apparatus causing
      burning X16
    nuclear explosion in war operations —
      see War operations, nuclear
      weapons
    inappropriate in local application or
      packing in medical or surgical
      procedure Y63.5
Hemorrhage
  delayed following medical or surgical
    treatment without mention of
    misadventure —*see* Index to Diseases
    and Injuries, Complication(s)
  during medical or surgical treatment as
    misadventure —*see* Index to Diseases
    and Injuries, Complication(s)

High
  altitude (effects) —*see* Air, pressure, low
  level of radioactivity, effects —*see* Radiation
  pressure (effects) —*see* Air, pressure, high
  temperature, effects —*see* Heat
Hit, hitting (accidental) by —*see* Struck by
Hitting against —*see* Striking against
Homicide (attempt) (justifiable) —*see* Assault
Hot
  place, effects —*see also* Heat
  weather, effects X30
House fire (uncontrolled) —*see* Exposure, fire,
  uncontrolled, building
Humidity, causing problem X39.8
Hunger X58
Hurricane (any injury) X37.0
Hypobarism, hypobaropathy —*see* Air,
  pressure, low

F, G, & H

I

Ictus
  caloris —*see also* Heat
  solaris X30
Ignition (accidental) (*see also* Exposure, fire)
    X08.8
  anesthetic gas in operating room W40.1
  apparel X06.2
    from highly flammable material X04
    nightwear X05
  bed linen (sheets) (spreads) (pillows)
      (mattress) —*see* Exposure, fire,
      uncontrolled, building, bed
  benzine X04
  clothes, clothing NEC (from controlled fire)
      X06.2
    from
      highly flammable material X04
  ether X04
    in operating room W40.1
  explosive material —*see* Explosion
  gasoline X04
  jewelry (plastic) (any) X06.0
  kerosene X04
  material
    explosive —*see* Explosion
    highly flammable with secondary
        explosion X04
  nightwear X05
  paraffin X04
  petrol X04
Immersion (accidental) —*see also* Drowning
  hand or foot due to cold (excessive) X31
Implantation of quills of porcupine
    W55.89
Inanition (from) (hunger) X58
  thirst X58.8
Inappropriate operation performed
  correct operation on wrong side or body
      part (wrong side) (wrong site)
      Y65.53
  operation intended for another patient done
      on wrong patient Y65.52
  wrong operation performed on correct
      patient Y65.51
Inattention after, at birth (homicidal intent)
    (infanticidal intent) X58
Incident, adverse
  device
    anesthesiology Y70.8
      accessory Y70.2
      diagnostic Y70.0
      miscellaneous Y70.8
      monitoring Y70.0
      prosthetic Y70.2
      rehabilitative Y70.1
      surgical Y70.3
      therapeutic Y70.1
    cardiovascular Y71.8
      accessory Y71.2
      diagnostic Y71.0
      miscellaneous Y71.8
      monitoring Y71.0
      prosthetic Y71.2
      rehabilitative Y71.1
      surgical Y71.3
      therapeutic Y71.1
    gastroenterology Y73.8
      accessory Y73.2
      diagnostic Y73.0
      miscellaneous Y73.8
      monitoring Y73.0
      prosthetic Y73.2
      rehabilitative Y73.1
      surgical Y73.3
      therapeutic Y73.1
    general
      hospital Y74.8
        accessory Y74.2
        diagnostic Y74.0

Incident, adverse *(Continued)*
  device *(Continued)*
    general *(Continued)*
      hospital *(Continued)*
        miscellaneous Y74.8
        monitoring Y74.0
        prosthetic Y74.2
        rehabilitative Y74.1
        surgical Y74.3
        therapeutic Y74.1
      surgical Y81.8
        accessory Y81.2
        diagnostic Y81.0
        miscellaneous Y81.8
        monitoring Y81.0
        prosthetic Y81.2
        rehabilitative Y81.1
        surgical Y81.3
        therapeutic Y81.1
    gynecological Y76.8
      accessory Y76.2
      diagnostic Y76.0
      miscellaneous Y76.8
      monitoring Y76.0
      prosthetic Y76.2
      rehabilitative Y76.1
      surgical Y76.3
      therapeutic Y76.1
    medical Y82.9
      specified type NEC Y82.8
    neurological Y75.8
      accessory Y75.2
      diagnostic Y75.0
      miscellaneous Y75.8
      monitoring Y75.0
      prosthetic Y75.2
      rehabilitative Y75.1
      surgical Y75.3
      therapeutic Y75.1
    obstetrical Y76.8
      accessory Y76.2
      diagnostic Y76.0
      miscellaneous Y76.8
      monitoring Y76.0
      prosthetic Y76.2
      rehabilitative Y76.1
      surgical Y76.3
      therapeutic Y76.1
    ophthalmic Y77.8
      accessory Y77.2
      diagnostic Y77.0
      miscellaneous Y77.8
      monitoring Y77.0
      prosthetic Y77.2
      rehabilitative Y77.1
      surgical Y77.3
      therapeutic Y77.1
    orthopedic Y79.8
      accessory Y79.2
      diagnostic Y79.0
      miscellaneous Y79.8
      monitoring Y79.0
      prosthetic Y79.2
      rehabilitative Y79.1
      surgical Y79.3
      therapeutic Y79.1
    otorhinolaryngological Y72.8
      accessory Y72.2
      diagnostic Y72.0
      miscellaneous Y72.8
      monitoring Y72.0
      prosthetic Y72.2
      rehabilitative Y72.1
      surgical Y72.3
      therapeutic Y72.1
    personal use Y74.8
      accessory Y74.2
      diagnostic Y74.0
      miscellaneous Y74.8
      monitoring Y74.0
      prosthetic Y74.2

Incident, adverse *(Continued)*
  device *(Continued)*
    personal use *(Continued)*
      rehabilitative Y74.1
      surgical Y74.3
      therapeutic Y74.1
    physical medicine Y80.8
      accessory Y80.2
      diagnostic Y80.0
      miscellaneous Y80.8
      monitoring Y80.0
      prosthetic Y80.2
      rehabilitative Y80.1
      surgical Y80.3
      therapeutic Y80.1
    plastic surgical Y81.8
      accessory Y81.2
      diagnostic Y81.0
      miscellaneous Y81.8
      monitoring Y81.0
      prosthetic Y81.2
      rehabilitative Y81.1
      surgical Y81.3
      therapeutic Y81.1
    radiological Y78.8
      accessory Y78.2
      diagnostic Y78.0
      miscellaneous Y78.8
      monitoring Y78.0
      prosthetic Y78.2
      rehabilitative Y78.1
      surgical Y78.3
      therapeutic Y78.1
    urology Y73.8
      accessory Y73.2
      diagnostic Y73.0
      miscellaneous Y73.8
      monitoring Y73.0
      prosthetic Y73.2
      rehabilitative Y73.1
      surgical Y73.3
      therapeutic Y73.1
Incineration (accidental) —*see* Exposure, fire
Infanticide —*see* Assault
Infrasound waves (causing injury) W49.9
Ingestion
  foreign body (causing injury) (with
      obstruction) —*see* Foreign body,
      alimentary canal
  poisonous
    plant (s) X58
    substance NEC —*see* Table of Drugs and
        Chemicals
Inhalation
  excessively cold substance, man-made —*see*
      Exposure, cold, man-made
  food (any type) (into respiratory tract) (with
      asphyxia, obstruction respiratory tract,
      suffocation) —*see* categories T17 and T18
  foreign body —*see* Foreign body, aspiration
  gastric contents (with asphyxia, obstruction
      respiratory passage, suffocation) T17.81-
  hot air or gases X14.0
  liquid air, hydrogen, nitrogen W93.12
    suicide (attempt) X83.2
  steam X13.0
    assault X98.0
    stated as undetermined whether accidental
        or intentional Y27.0
    suicide (attempt) X77.0
  toxic gas —*see* Table of Drugs and
      Chemicals
  vomitus (with asphyxia, obstruction
      respiratory passage, suffocation)T17.81-
Injury, injured (accidental(ly)) NOS X58
  by, caused by, from
    assault —*see* Assault
    law-enforcing agent, police, in course
        of legal intervention —*see* Legal
        intervention
    suicide (attempt) X83.8

Injury, injured NOS (*Continued*)
  due to, in
    civil insurrection —*see* War
      operations
    fight (*see also* Assault, fight)
      Y04.0
    war operations —*see* War
      operations
  homicide (*see also* Assault) Y09
  inflicted (by)
    in course of arrest (attempted), suppression
      of disturbance, maintenance of order,
      by law-enforcing agents —*see* Legal
      intervention

Injury, injured NOS (*Continued*)
  inflicted (*Continued*)
    other person
      stated as
        accidental X58
        intentional, homicide (attempt) —*see*
          Assault
        undetermined whether accidental or
          intentional Y33
    purposely (inflicted) by other person (s) —*see*
      Assault
    self-inflicted X83.8
      stated as accidental X58
    specified cause NEC X58

Injury, injured NOS (*Continued*)
  undetermined whether accidental or
    intentional Y33
Insolation, effects X30
Insufficient nourishment X58
Interruption of respiration (by)
  food (lodged in esophagus) —*see* categories
    T17 and T18
  vomitus (lodged in esophagus) T17.81-
Intervention, legal —*see* Legal intervention
Intoxication
  drug —*see* Table of Drugs and Chemicals
  poison —*see* Table of Drugs and
    Chemicals

J

Jammed (accidentally)
  between objects (moving) (stationary and
    moving) W23.0
    stationary W23.1
Jumped, jumping
  before moving object NEC X81.8
    motor vehicle X81.0
    subway train X81.1
    train X81.1
    undetermined whether accidental or
      intentional Y31
  from
    boat (into water) voluntarily,
      without accident (to or on boat)
      W16.712
      with
        accident to or on boat —*see* Accident,
          watercraft
        drowning or submersion W16.711
          suicide (attempt) X71.3

Jumped, jumping (*Continued*)
  from (*Continued*)
    boat voluntarily, without accident
      (*Continued*)
        striking bottom W16.722
        causing drowning W16.721
    building (*see also* Jumped, from,
      high place) W13.9
      burning (uncontrolled fire)
        X00.5
    high place NEC W17.89
      suicide (attempt) X80
      undetermined whether accidental or
        intentional Y30
    structure (*see also* Jumped, from, high
      place) W13.9
      burning (uncontrolled fire)
        X00.5
  into water W16.92
    causing drowning W16.91
    from, off watercraft —*see* Jumped, from,
      boat

Jumped, jumping (*Continued*)
  into water (*Continued*)
    in
      natural body W16.612
        causing drowning W16.611
        striking bottom W16.622
          causing drowning W16.621
      specified place NEC W16.812
        causing drowning W16.811
        striking
          bottom W16.822
            causing drowning W16.821
          wall W16.832
            causing drowning W16.831
      swimming pool W16.512
        causing drowning W16.511
        striking
          bottom W16.522
            causing drowning W16.521
          wall W16.532
            causing drowning W16.531
  suicide (attempt) X71.3

K

Kicked by
  animal NEC W55.82
  person (s) (accidentally) W50.1
    with intent to injure or kill Y04.0
    as, or caused by, a crowd or human
      stampede (with fall) W52
    assault Y04.0
    homicide (attempt) Y04.0
    in
      fight Y04.0
      legal intervention
        injuring
          bystander Y35.812
          law enforcement personnel Y35.811
          suspect Y35.813

Kicking against
  object W22.8
    sports equipment W21.9
    stationary W22.09
      sports equipment W21.89
  person —*see* Striking against, person
  sports equipment W21.9
Killed, killing (accidentally) NOS (*see also*
  Injury) X58
  in
    action —*see* War operations
    brawl, fight (hand) (fists) (foot) Y04.0
      by weapon —*see also* Assault
        cutting, piercing —*see* Assault, cutting
          or piercing instrument
        firearm —*see* Discharge, firearm, by
          type, homicide

Killed, killing NOS (*Continued*)
  self
    stated as
      accident NOS X58
      suicide —*see* Suicide
      undetermined whether accidental or
        intentional Y33
Knocked down (accidentally) (by) NOS X58
  animal (not being ridden) NEC —*see also*
    Struck by, by type of animal
  crowd or human stampede W52
  person W51
    in brawl, fight Y04.0
  transport vehicle NEC (*see also* Accident,
    transport) V09.9

◀ New   ◀▦ Revised   ~~deleted~~ Deleted

L

Laceration NEC —*see* Injury
Lack of
  care (helpless person) (infant) (newborn) X58
  food except as result of abandonment or
    neglect X58
    due to abandonment or neglect X58
  water except as result of transport accident X58
    due to transport accident —*see* Accident,
      transport, by type
    helpless person, infant, newborn X58
Landslide (falling on transport vehicle) X36.1
  caused by collapse of man-made structure
    X36.0
Late effect —*see* Sequelae
Legal
  execution (any method) —*see* Legal,
    intervention
  intervention (by)
    baton —*see* Legal, intervention, blunt
      object, baton
    bayonet —*see* Legal, intervention, sharp
      object, bayonet
    blow —*see* Legal, intervention,
      manhandling
    blunt object
      baton
        injuring
          bystander Y35.312
          law enforcement personnel Y35.311
          suspect Y35.313
      injuring
        bystander Y35.302
        law enforcement personnel Y35.301
        suspect Y35.303
      specified NEC
        injuring
          bystander Y35.392
          law enforcement personnel Y35.391
          suspect Y35.393
      stave
        injuring
          bystander Y35.392
          law enforcement personnel Y35.391
          suspect Y35.393
    bomb —*see* Legal, intervention, explosive
    cutting or piercing instrument —*see* Legal,
      intervention, sharp object
    dynamite —*see* Legal, intervention,
      explosive, dynamite
    explosive (s)
      dynamite
        injuring
          bystander Y35.112
          law enforcement personnel Y35.111
          suspect Y35.113
      grenade
        injuring
          bystander Y35.192
          law enforcement personnel Y35.191
          suspect Y35.193
      injuring
        bystander Y35.102
        law enforcement personnel Y35.101
        suspect Y35.103

Legal *(Continued)*
  intervention *(Continued)*
    explosive *(Continued)*
      mortar bomb
        injuring
          bystander Y35.192
          law enforcement personnel
            Y35.191
          suspect Y35.193
      shell
        injuring
          bystander Y35.122
          law enforcement personnel Y35.121
          suspect Y35.123
      specified NEC
        injuring
          bystander Y35.192
          law enforcement personnel Y35.191
          suspect Y35.193
    firearm (s) (discharge)
      handgun
        injuring
          bystander Y35.022
          law enforcement personnel Y35.021
          suspect Y35.023
      injuring
        bystander Y35.002
        law cnforcement personnel Y35.001
        suspect Y35.003
      machine gun
        injuring
          bystander Y35.012
          law enforcement personnel Y35.011
          suspect Y35.013
      rifle pellet
        injuring
          bystander Y35.032
          law enforcement personnel Y35.031
          suspect Y35.033
      rubber bullet
        injuring
          bystander Y35.042
          law cnforcement personnel Y35.041
          suspect Y35.043
      shotgun —*see* Legal, intervention,
        firearm, specified NEC
      specified NEC
        injuring
          bystander Y35.092
          law enforcement personnel Y35.091
          suspect Y35.093
    gas (asphyxiation) (poisoning)
      injuring
        bystander Y35.202
        law enforcement personnel Y35.201
        suspect Y35.203
      specified NEC
        injuring
          bystander Y35.292
          law enforcement personnel Y35.291
          suspect Y35.293
      tear gas
        injuring
          bystander Y35.212
          law enforcement personnel Y35.211
          suspect Y35.213

Legal *(Continued)*
  intervention *(Continued)*
    grenade —*see* Legal, intervention,
      explosive, grenade
    injuring
      bystander Y35.92
      law enforcement personnel Y35.91
      suspect Y35.93
    late effect (of) (*see* with 7th character S)
      Y35
    manhandling
      injuring
        bystander Y35.812
        law enforcement personnel Y35.811
        suspect Y35.813
    sequelae (of) (*see* with 7th character S)
      Y35
    sharp objects
      bayonet
        injuring
          bystander Y35.412
          law enforcement personnel
            Y35.411
          suspect Y35.413
      injuring
        bystander Y35.402
        law enforcement personnel Y35.401
        suspect Y35.403
      specified NEC
        injuring
          bystander Y35.492
          law enforcement personnel
            Y35.491
          suspect Y35.493
    specified means NEC
      injuring
        bystander Y35.892
        law enforcement personnel Y35.891
        suspect Y35.893
    stabbing —*see* Legal, intervention, sharp
      object
    stave —*see* Legal, intervention, blunt
      object, stave
    tear gas —*see* Legal, intervention, gas, tear
      gas
    truncheon —*see* Legal, intervention, blunt
      object, stave
Lightning (shock) (stroke) (struck by) —*see*
  subcategory T75.0
  causing fire —*see* Exposure, fire
Loss of control (transport vehicle) NEC —*see*
  Accident, transport
Lost at sea NOS —*see* Drowning, due to, fall
  overboard
Low
  pressure (effects) —*see* Air, pressure, low
  temperature (effects) —*see* Exposure, cold
Lying before train, vehicle or other moving
  object X81.8
  subway train X81.1
  train X81.1
  undetermined whether accidental or
    intentional Y31
Lynching —*see* Assault

M

Malfunction (mechanism or component) (of)
  firearm
    airgun W34.10
    BB gun W34.110
    gas, air or spring-operated gun NEC
      W34.118
    handgun W32.1
    hunting rifle W33.12
    larger firearm W33.10
      specified NEC W33.19
    machine gun W33.13
    paintball gun W34.111
    pellet gun W34.110
    shotgun W33.11
    specified NEC W34.19
    Very pistol [flare] W34.19
  handgun —*see* Malfunction, firearm,
    handgun
Maltreatment —*see* Perpetrator
Mangled (accidentally) NOS X58
Manhandling (in brawl, fight) Y04.0
  legal intervention —*see* Legal, intervention,
    manhandling
Manslaughter (nonaccidental) —*see* Assault
Mauled by animal NEC W55.89
Medical procedure, complication of
  (delayed or as an abnormal reaction
    without mention of misadventure) —*see*
    Complication of or following, by specified
    type of procedure
  due to or as a result of misadventure —*see*
    Misadventure
Melting (due to fire) —*see also* Exposure, fire
  apparel NEC X06.3
  clothes, clothing NEC X06.3
    nightwear X05
  fittings or furniture (burning building)
    (uncontrolled fire) X00.8
  nightwear X05
  plastic jewelry X06.1
Mental cruelty X58
Military operations (injuries to military and
  civilians occuring during peacetime on
  military property and during routine
  military exercises and operations) (by)
  (from) (involving) Y37.90-
  air blast Y37.20-
  aircraft
    destruction —*see* Military operations,
      destruction of aircraft
  airway restriction —*see* Military operations,
    restriction of airways
  asphyxiation —*see* Military operations,
    restriction of airways
  biological weapons Y37.6X-
  blast Y37.20-
  blast fragments Y37.20-
  blast wave Y37.20-
  blast wind Y37.20-
  bomb Y37.20-
    dirty Y37.50-
    gasoline Y37.31-
    incendiary Y37.31-
    petrol Y37.31-
  bullet Y37.43-
    incendiary Y37.32-
    rubber Y37.41-
  chemical weapons Y37.7X-
  combat
    hand to hand (unarmed) combat
      Y37.44-
    using blunt or piercing object Y37.45-
  conflagration —*see* Military operations, fire
  conventional warfare NEC Y37.49-
  depth-charge Y37.01-
  destruction of aircraft Y37.10-
    due to
      air to air missile Y37.11-
      collision with other aircraft Y37.12-

Military operations (*Continued*)
  destruction of aircraft (*Continued*)
    due to (*Continued*)
      detonation (accidental) of onboard
        munitions and explosives Y37.14-
      enemy fire or explosives Y37.11-
      explosive placed on aircraft Y37.11-
      onboard fire Y37.13-
      rocket propelled grenade [RPG] Y37.11-
      small arms fire Y37.11-
      surface to air missile Y37.11-
    specified NEC Y37.19-
  detonation (accidental) of
    onboard marine weapons Y37.05-
    own munitions or munitions launch device
      Y37.24-
  dirty bomb Y37.50-
  explosion (of) Y37.20-
    aerial bomb Y37.21-
    bomb NOS (*see also* Military operations,
      bomb (s)) Y37.20-
    fragments Y37.20-
    grenade Y37.29-
    guided missile Y37.22-
    improvised explosive device [IED] (person-
      borne) (roadside) (vehicle-borne)
      Y37.23-
    land mine Y37.29-
    marine mine (at sea) (in harbor) Y37.02-
    marine weapon Y37.00-
      specified NEC Y37.09-
    own munitions or munitions launch device
      (accidental) Y37.24-
    sea-based artillery shell Y37.03-
    specified NEC Y37.29-
    torpedo Y37.04-
  fire Y37.30-
    specified NEC Y37.39-
  firearms
    discharge Y37.43-
    pellets Y37.42-
  flamethrower Y37.33-
  fragments (from) (of)
    improvised explosive device [IED] (person-
      borne) (roadside) (vehicle-borne)
      Y37.26-
    munitions Y37.25-
    specified NEC Y37.29-
    weapons Y37.27-
  friendly fire Y37.92-
  hand to hand (unarmed) combat Y37.44-
  hot substances —*see* Military operations, fire
  incendiary bullet Y37.32-
  nuclear weapon (effects of) Y37.50-
    acute radiation exposure Y37.54-
    blast pressure Y37.51-
    direct blast Y37.51-
    direct heat Y37.53-
    fallout exposure Y37.54-
    fireball Y37.53-
    indirect blast (struck or crushed by blast
      debris) (being thrown by blast)
      Y37.52-
    ionizing radiation (immediate exposure)
      Y37.54-
    nuclear radiation Y37.54-
    radiation
      ionizing (immediate exposure) Y37.54-
      nuclear Y37.54-
      thermal Y37.53-
    secondary effects Y37.54-
    specified NEC Y37.59-
    thermal radiation Y37.53-
  restriction of air (airway)
    intentional Y37.46-
    unintentional Y37.47-
  rubber bullets Y37.41-
  shrapnel NOS Y37.29-
  suffocation —*see* Military operations,
    restriction of airways
  unconventional warfare NEC Y37.7X-

Military operations (*Continued*)
  underwater blast NOS Y37.00-
  warfare
    conventional NEC Y37.49-
    unconventional NEC Y37.7X-
  weapon of mass destruction [WMD] Y37.91-
  weapons
    biological weapons Y37.6X-
    chemical Y37.7X-
    nuclear (effects of) Y37.50-
      acute radiation exposure Y37.54-
      blast pressure Y37.51-
      direct blast Y37.51-
      direct heat Y37.53-
      fallout exposure Y37.54-
      fireball Y37.53-
      indirect blast (struck or crushed by blast
        debris) (being thrown by blast)
        Y37.52-
      radiation
        ionizing (immediate exposure) Y37.54-
        nuclear Y37.54-
        thermal Y37.53-
      secondary effects Y37.54-
      specified NEC Y37.59-
    of mass destruction [WMD] Y37.91-
Misadventure (s) to patient (s) during surgical
  or medical care Y69
  contaminated medical or biological substance
    (blood, drug, fluid) Y64.9
    administered (by) NEC Y64.9
      immunization Y64.1
      infusion Y64.0
      injection Y64.1
      specified means NEC Y64.8
      transfusion Y64.0
      vaccination Y64.1
  excessive amount of blood or other fluid
    during transfusion or infusion Y63.0
  failure
    in dosage Y63.9
      electroshock therapy Y63.4
      inappropriate temperature (too hot or
        too cold) in local application and
        packing Y63.5
      infusion
        excessive amount of fluid Y63.0
        incorrect dilution of fluid Y63.1
      insulin-shock therapy Y63.4
      nonadministration of necessary drug or
        biological substance Y63.6
      overdose —*see* Table of Drugs and
        Chemicals
      radiation, in therapy Y63.2
    radiation
      overdose Y63.2
    specified procedure NEC Y63.8
    transfusion
      excessive amount of blood Y63.0
    mechanical, of instrument or apparatus
      (any) (during any procedure) Y65.8
    sterile precautions (during procedure)
      Y62.9
      aspiration of fluid or tissue (by puncture
        or catheterization, except heart)
        Y62.6
      biopsy (except needle aspiration) Y62.8
        needle (aspirating) Y62.6
      blood sampling Y62.6
      catheterization Y62.6
        heart Y62.5
      dialysis (kidney) Y62.2
      endoscopic examination Y62.4
      enema Y62.8
      immunization Y62.3
      infusion Y62.1
      injection Y62.3
      needle biopsy Y62.6
      paracentesis (abdominal) (thoracic)
        Y62.6
      perfusion Y62.2

◀ New   ◀◀ Revised   ~~deleted~~ Deleted

Misadventure (s) to patient (s) during surgical or medical care *(Continued)*
failure *(Continued)*
sterile precautions *(Continued)*
puncture (lumbar) Y62.6
removal of catheter or packing Y62.8
specified procedure NEC Y62.8
surgical operation Y62.0
transfusion Y62.1
vaccination Y62.3
suture or ligature during surgical procedure Y65.2
to introduce or to remove tube or instrument —*see* Failure, to
hemorrhage —*see* Index to Diseases and Injuries, Complication(s)
inadvertent exposure of patient to radiation Y63.3
inappropriate
operation performed —*see* Inappropriate operation performed
temperature (too hot or too cold) in local application or packing Y63.5
infusion *(see also* Misadventure, by type, infusion) Y69
excessive amount of fluid Y63.0
incorrect dilution of fluid Y63.1
wrong fluid Y65.1
mismatched blood in transfusion Y65.0
nonadministration of necessary drug or biological substance Y63.6
overdose —*see* Table of Drugs and Chemicals
radiation (in therapy) Y63.2
perforation —*see* Index to Diseases and Injuries, Complication(s)
performance of inappropriate operation —*see* Inappropriate operation performed
puncture —*see* Index to Diseases and Injuries, Complication(s)
specified type NEC Y65.8
failure
suture or ligature during surgical operation Y65.2
to introduce or to remove tube or instrument —*see* Failure, to
infusion of wrong fluid Y65.1
specified type NEC *(Continued)*
performance of inappropriate operation —*see* Inappropriate operation performed
transfusion of mismatched blood Y65.0
wrong
fluid in infusion Y65.1
placement of endotracheal tube during anesthetic procedure Y65.3
transfusion —*see* Misadventure, by type, transfusion
excessive amount of blood Y63.0
mismatched blood Y65.0
wrong
drug given in error —*see* Table of Drugs and Chemicals
fluid in infusion Y65.1
placement of endotracheal tube during anesthetic procedure Y65.3
Mismatched blood in transfusion Y65.0
Motion sickness T75.3
Mountain sickness W94.11
Mudslide (of cataclysmic nature) —*see* Landslide
Murder (attempt) —*see* Assault

N

Nail, contact with W45.0
gun W29.4
Neglect (criminal) (homicidal intent) X58
Noise (causing injury) (pollution) W42.9
supersonic W42.0

Nonadministration (of)
drug or biological substance (necessary) Y63.6
surgical and medical care Y66
Nosocomial condition Y95

O

Object
falling
from, in, on, hitting
machinery —*see* Contact, with, by type of machine
set in motion by
accidental explosion or rupture of pressure vessel W38
firearm —*see* Discharge, firearm, by type
machine (ry) —*see* Contact, with, by type of machine

Overdose (drug) —*see* Table of Drugs and Chemicals
radiation Y63.2
Overexertion —*see* category Y93
Overexposure (accidental) (to)
cold *(see also* Exposure, cold) X31
due to man-made conditions —*see* Exposure, cold, man-made
heat *(see also* Heat) X30
radiation —*see* Radiation
radioactivity W88.0
sun (sunburn) X32
weather NEC —*see* Forces of nature
wind NEC —*see* Forces of nature

Overheated —*see* Heat
Overturning (accidental)
machinery —*see* Contact, with, by type of machine
transport vehicle NEC *(see also* Accident, transport) V89.9
watercraft (causing drowning, submersion) —*see also* Drowning, due to, accident to, watercraft, overturning
causing injury except drowning or submersion —*see* Accident, watercraft, causing, injury NEC

P

Parachute descent (voluntary) (without accident to aircraft) V97.29
  due to accident to aircraft —*see* Accident, transport, aircraft
Pecked by bird W61.99
Perforation during medical or surgical treatment as misadventure —*see* Index to Diseases and Injuries, Complication(s)
Perpetrator, perpetration, of assault, maltreatment and neglect (by) Y07.9
  boyfriend Y07.03
  brother Y07.410
    stepbrother Y07.435
  coach Y07.53
  cousin
    female Y07.491
    male Y07.490
  daycare provider Y07.519
    at-home
      adult care Y07.512
      childcare Y07.510
    care center
      adult care Y07.513
      childcare Y07.511
  family member NEC Y07.499
  father Y07.11
    adoptive Y07.13
    foster Y07.420
    stepfather Y07.430
  foster father Y07.420
  foster mother Y07.421
  girl friend Y07.04
  healthcare provider Y07.529
    mental health Y07.521
    specified NEC Y07.528
  husband Y07.01
  instructor Y07.53
  mother Y07.12
    adoptive Y07.14
    foster Y07.421
    stepmother Y07.433
  nonfamily member Y07.50
    specified NEC Y07.59
  nurse Y07.528
  occupational therapist Y07.528
  partner of parent
    female Y07.434
    male Y07.432
  physical therapist Y07.528
  sister Y07.411
  speech therapist Y07.528
  stepbrother Y07.435
  stepfather Y07.430
  stepmother Y07.433
  stepsister Y07.436
  teacher Y07.53
  wife Y07.02
Piercing —*see* Contact, with, by type of object or machine
Pinched
  between objects (moving) (stationary and moving) W23.0
    stationary W23.1
Pinned under machine (ry) —*see* Contact, with, by type of machine
Place of occurrence Y92.9
  abandoned house Y92.89
  airplane Y92.813
  airport Y92.520
  ambulatory health services establishment NEC Y92.538
  ambulatory surgery center Y92.530
  amusement park Y92.831
  apartment (co-op) —*see* Place of occurrence, residence, apartment
  assembly hall Y92.29
  bank Y92.510
  barn Y92.71
  baseball field Y92.320

Place of occurrence (*Continued*)
  basketball court Y92.310
  beach Y92.832
  boarding house —*see* Place of occurrence, residence, boarding house
  boat Y92.814
  bowling alley Y92.39
  bridge Y92.89
  building under construction Y92.61
  bus Y92.811
    station Y92.521
  cafe Y92.511
  campsite Y92.833
  campus —*see* Place of occurrence, school
  canal Y92.89
  car Y92.810
  casino Y92.59
  children's home —*see* Place of occurrence, residence, institutional, orphanage
  church Y92.22
  cinema Y92.26
  clubhouse Y92.29
  coal pit Y92.64
  college (community) Y92.214
  condominium —*see* Place of occurrence, residence, apartment
  construction area —*see* Place of occurrence, industrial and construction area
  convalescent home —*see* Place of occurrence, residence, institutional, nursing home
  court-house Y92.240
  cricket ground Y92.328
  cultural building Y92.258
    art gallery Y92.250
    museum Y92.251
    music hall Y92.252
    opera house Y92.253
    specified NEC Y92.258
    theater Y92.254
  dancehall Y92.252
  day nursery Y92.210
  dentist office Y92.531
  derelict house Y92.89
  desert Y92.820
  dock NOS Y92.89
  dockyard Y92.62
  doctor's office Y92.531
  dormitory —*see* Place of occurrence, residence, institutional, school dormitory
  dry dock Y92.62
  factory (building) (premises) Y92.63
  farm (land under cultivation) (outbuildings) Y92.79
    barn Y92.71
    chicken coop Y92.72
    field Y92.73
    hen house Y92.72
    house —*see* Place of occurrence, residence, house
    orchard Y92.74
    specified NEC Y92.79
  football field Y92.321
  forest Y92.821
  freeway Y92.411
  gallery Y92.250
  garage (commercial) Y92.59
    boarding house Y92.044
    military base Y92.135
    mobile home Y92.025
    nursing home Y92.124
    orphanage Y92.114
    private house Y92.015
    reform school Y92.155
  gas station Y92.524
  gasworks Y92.69
  golf course Y92.39
  gravel pit Y92.64
  grocery Y92.512
  gymnasium Y92.39
  handball court Y92.318
  harbor Y92.89

Place of occurrence (*Continued*)
  harness racing course Y92.39
  healthcare provider office Y92.531
  highway (interstate) Y92.411
  hill Y92.828
  hockey rink Y92.330
  home —*see* Place of occurrence, residence
  hospice —*see* Place of occurrence, residence, institutional, nursing home
  hospital Y92.239
    cafeteria Y92.233
    corridor Y92.232
    operating room Y92.234
    patient
      bathroom Y92.231
      room Y92.230
    specified NEC Y92.238
  hotel Y92.59
  house —*see also* Place of occurrence, residence
    abandoned Y92.89
    under construction Y92.61
  industrial and construction area (yard) Y92.69
    building under construction Y92.61
    dock Y92.62
    dry dock Y92.62
    factory Y92.63
    gasworks Y92.69
    mine Y92.64
    oil rig Y92.65
    pit Y92.64
    power station Y92.69
    shipyard Y92.62
    specified NEC Y92.69
    tunnel under construction Y92.69
    workshop Y92.69
  kindergarten Y92.211
  lacrosse field Y92.328
  lake Y92.828
  library Y92.241
  mall Y92.59
  market Y92.512
  marsh Y92.828
  military
    base —*see* Place of occurrence, residence, institutional, military base
    training ground Y92.84
  mine Y92.64
  mosque Y92.22
  motel Y92.59
  motorway (interstate) Y92.411
  mountain Y92.828
  movie-house Y92.26
  museum Y92.251
  music-hall Y92.252
  not applicable Y92.9
  nuclear power station Y92.69
  nursing home —*see* Place of occurrence, residence, institutional, nursing home
  office building Y92.59
  offshore installation Y92.65
  oil rig Y92.65
  old people's home —*see* Place of occurrence, residence, institutional, specified NEC
  opera-house Y92.253
  orphanage —*see* Place of occurrence, residence, institutional, orphanage
  outpatient surgery center Y92.530
  park (public) Y92.830
    amusement Y92.831
  parking garage Y92.89
    lot Y92.481
  pavement Y92.480
  physician office Y92.531
  polo field Y92.328
  pond Y92.828
  post office Y92.242
  power station Y92.69
  prairie Y92.828
  prison —*see* Place of occurrence, residence, institutional, prison

◀ New   ◀■ Revised   ~~deleted~~ Deleted

Place of occurrence *(Continued)*
public
  administration building Y92.248
    city hall Y92.243
    courthouse Y92.240
    library Y92.241
    post office Y92.242
    specified NEC Y92.248
  building NEC Y92.29
  hall Y92.29
  place NOS Y92.89
race course Y92.39
radio station Y92.59
railway line (bridge) Y92.85
ranch (outbuildings) —*see* Place of
  occurrence, farm
recreation area Y92.838
  amusement park Y92.831
  beach Y92.832
  campsite Y92.833
  park (public) Y92.830
  seashore Y92.832
  specified NEC Y92.838
reform school —*see* Place of occurrence,
  residence, institutional, reform school
religious institution Y92.22
residence (non-institutional) (private) Y92.009
  apartment Y92.039
    bathroom Y92.031
    bedroom Y92.032
    kitchen Y92.030
    specified NEC Y92.038
  bathroom Y92.002
  bedroom Y92.003
  boarding house Y92.049
    bathroom Y92.041
    bedroom Y92.042
    driveway Y92.043
    garage Y92.044
    garden Y92.046
    kitchen Y92.040
    specified NEC Y92.048
    swimming pool Y92.045
    yard Y92.046
  dining room Y92.001
  garden Y92.007
  home Y92.009
  house, single family Y92.019
    bathroom Y92.012
    bedroom Y92.013
    dining room Y92.011
    driveway Y92.014
    garage Y92.015
    garden Y92.017
    kitchen Y92.010
    specified NEC Y92.018
    swimming pool Y92.016
    yard Y92.017
  institutional Y92.10
    children's home —*see* Place of
      occurrence, residence, institutional,
      orphanage
    hospice —*see* Place of occurrence,
      residence, institutional, nursing
      home
    military base Y92.139
      barracks Y92.133
      garage Y92.135
      garden Y92.137
      kitchen Y92.130
      mess hall Y92.131
      specified NEC Y92.138
      swimming pool Y92.136
      yard Y92.137
    nursing home Y92.129
      bathroom Y92.121
      bedroom Y92.122
      driveway Y92.123
      garage Y92.124
      garden Y92.126
      kitchen Y92.120

Place of occurrence *(Continued)*
residence *(Continued)*
  institutional *(Continued)*
    nursing home *(Continued)*
      specified NEC Y92.128
      swimming pool Y92.125
      yard Y92.126
    orphanage Y92.119
      bathroom Y92.111
      bedroom Y92.112
      driveway Y92.113
      garage Y92.114
      garden Y92.116
      kitchen Y92.110
      specified NEC Y92.118
      swimming pool Y92.115
      yard Y92.116
    prison Y92.149
      bathroom Y92.142
      cell Y92.143
      courtyard Y92.147
      dining room Y92.141
      kitchen Y92.140
      specified NEC Y92.148
      swimming pool Y92.146
    reform school Y92.159
      bathroom Y92.152
      bedroom Y92.153
      dining room Y92.151
      driveway Y92.154
      garage Y92.155
      garden Y92.157
      kitchen Y92.150
      specified NEC Y92.158
      swimming pool Y92.156
      yard Y92.157
    school dormitory Y92.169
      bathroom Y92.162
      bedroom Y92.163
      dining room Y92.161
      kitchen Y92.160
      specified NEC Y92.168
    specified NEC Y92.199
      bathroom Y92.192
      bedroom Y92.193
      dining room Y92.191
      driveway Y92.194
      garage Y92.195
      garden Y92.197
      kitchen Y92.190
      specified NEC Y92.198
      swimming pool Y92.196
      yard Y92.197
  kitchen Y92.000
  mobile home Y92.029
    bathroom Y92.022
    bedroom Y92.023
    dining room Y92.021
    driveway Y92.024
    garage Y92.025
    garden Y92.027
    kitchen Y92.020
    specified NEC Y92.028
    swimming pool Y92.026
    yard Y92.027
  specified place in residence NEC Y92.008
  specified residence type NEC Y92.099
    bathroom Y92.091
    bedroom Y92.092
    driveway Y92.093
    garage Y92.094
    garden Y92.096
    kitchen Y92.090
    specified NEC Y92.098
    swimming pool Y92.095
    yard Y92.096
restaurant Y92.511
riding school Y92.39
river Y92.828
road Y92.488
rodeo ring Y92.39

Place of occurrence *(Continued)*
rugby field Y92.328
same day surgery center Y92.530
sand pit Y92.64
school (private) (public) (state) Y92.219
  college Y92.214
  daycare center Y92.210
  elementary school Y92.211
  high school Y92.213
  kindergarten Y92.211
  middle school Y92.212
  specified NEC Y92.218
  trace school Y92.215
  university Y92.214
  vocational school Y92.215
sea (shore) Y92.832
senior citizen center Y92.29
service area
  airport Y92.520
  bus station Y92.521
  gas station Y92.524
  highway rest stop Y92.523
  railway station Y92.522
shipyard Y92.62
shop(commercial) Y92.513
sidewalk Y92.480
silo Y92.79
skating rink (roller) Y92.331
  ice Y92.330
slaughter house Y92.86
soccer field Y92.322
specified place NEC Y92.89
sports area Y92.39
  athletic
    court Y92.318
      basketball Y92.310
      specified NEC Y92.318
      squash Y92.311
      tennis Y92.312
    field Y92.328
      baseball Y92.320
      cricket ground Y92.328
      football Y92.321
      hockey Y92.328
      soccer Y92.322
      specified NEC Y92.328
  golf course Y92.39
  gymnasium Y92.39
  riding school Y92.39
  skating rink (roller) Y92.331
    ice Y92.330
  stadium Y92.39
  swimming pool Y92.34
squash court Y92.311
stadium Y92.39
steeplechasing course Y92.39
store Y92.512
stream Y92.828
street and highway Y92.410
  bike path Y92.482
  freeway Y92.411
  highway ramp Y92.415
  interstate highway Y92.411
  local residential or business street
    Y92.414
  motorway Y92.411
  parking lot Y92.481
  parkway Y92.412
  sidewalk Y92.480
  specified NEC Y92.488
  state road Y92.413
subway car Y92.816
supermarket Y92.512
swamp Y92.828
swimming pool (public) Y92.34
  private (at) Y92.095
    boarding house Y92.045
    military base Y92.136
    mobile home Y92.026
    nursing home Y92.125
    orphanage Y92.115

P

Place of occurrence *(Continued)*
 swimming pool *(Continued)*
  private *(Continued)*
   prison Y92.146
   reform school Y92.156
   single family residence
    Y92.016
 synagogue Y92.22
 television station Y92.59
 tennis court Y92.312
 theater Y92.254
 trade area Y92.59
  bank Y92.510
  cafe Y92.511
  casino Y92.59
  garage Y92.59
  hotel Y92.59
  market Y92.512
  office building Y92.59
  radio station Y92.59
  restaurant Y92.511
  shop Y92.513
  shopping mall Y92.59
  store Y92.512
  supermarket Y92.512
  television station Y92.59
  warehouse Y92.59
 trailer park, residential —*see* Place of
  occurrence, residence, mobile
  home
 trailer site NOS Y92.89
 train Y92.815
  station Y92.522
 truck Y92.812
 tunnel under construction Y92. 69
 university Y92.214
 urgent (health) care center Y92.532
 vehicle (transport) Y92.818
  airplane Y92.813
  boat Y92.814
  bus Y92.811
  car Y92.810
  specified NEC Y92.818
  subway car Y92.816
  train Y92.815
  truck Y92.812
 warehouse Y92.59
 water reservoir Y92.89
 wilderness area Y92.828
  desert Y92.820
  forest Y92.821
  marsh Y92.828
  mountain Y92.828
  prairie Y92.828
  specified NEC Y92.828
  swamp Y92.828
 workshop Y92.69
 yard, private Y92.096
  boarding house Y92.046
  mobile home Y92.027
  single family house Y92.017

Place of occurrence *(Continued)*
 youth center Y92.29
 zoo (zoological garden) Y92.834
Plumbism —*see* Table of Drugs and Chemicals,
  lead
Poisoning (accidental) (by) —*see also* Table of
  Drugs and Chemicals
 by plant, thorns, spines, sharp leaves or other
  mechanisms NEC X58
 carbon monoxide
  generated by
   motor vehicle —*see* Accident, transport
   watercraft (in transit) (not in transit)
    V93.89
    ferry boat V93.81
    fishing boat V93.82
    jet skis V93.83
    liner V93.81
    merchant ship V93.80
    passenger ship V93.81
    powered craft NEC V93.83
 caused by injection of poisons into skin by
   plant thorns, spines, sharp leaves X58
  marine or sea plants (venomous) X58
 exhaust gas
  generated by
   motor vehicle —*see* Accident, transport
   watercraft (in transit) (not in transit)
    V93.89
    ferry boat V93.81
    fishing boat V93.82
    jet skis V93.83
    liner V93.81
    merchant ship V93.80
    passenger ship V93.81
    powered craft NEC V93.83
 fumes or smoke due to
  explosion (*see also* Explosion) W40.9
  fire —*see* Exposure, fire
  ignition —*see* Ignition
 gas
  in legal intervention —*see* Legal,
   intervention, gas
  legal execution —*see* Legal, intervention,
   gas
 in war operations —*see* War operations
 legal
  execution —*see* Legal, intervention, gas
  intervention
   by gas —*see* Legal, intervention, gas
   other specified means —*see* Legal,
    intervention, specified means
    NEC
Powder burn (by) (from)
 airgun W34.110
 BB gun W34.110
 firearm NEC W34.19
 gas, air or spring-operated gun NEC
  W34.118
 handgun W32.1
 hunting rifle W33.12

Powder burn *(Continued)*
 larger firearm W33.10
  specified NEC W33.19
 machine gun W33.13
 paintball gun W34.111
 pellet gun W34.110
 shotgun W33.11
 Very pistol [flare] W34.19
Premature cessation (of) surgical and medical
  care Y66
Privation (food) (water) X58
Procedure (operation)
 correct, on wrong side or body part (wrong
  side) (wrong site) Y65.53
 intended for another patient done on wrong
  patient Y65.52
 performed on patient not scheduled for
  surgery Y65.52
 performed on wrong patient Y65.52
 wrong, performed on correct patient Y65.51
Prolonged
 sitting in transport vehicle —*see* Travel, by
  type of vehicle
 stay in
  high altitude as cause of anoxia,
   barodontalgia, barotitis or hypoxia
   W94.11
  weightless environment X52
Pulling, excessive —*see* category Y93
Puncture, puncturing —*see also* Contact, with,
  by type of object or machine
 by
  plant thorns, spines, sharp leaves or other
   mechanisms NEC W60
 during medical or surgical treatment as
  misadventure —*see* Index to Diseases
  and Injuries, Complication(s)
Pushed, pushing (accidental) (injury in)
  (overexertion) —*see also* category Y93
 by other person (s) (accidental) W51
  with fall W03
   due to ice or snow W00.0
  as, or caused by, a crowd or human
   stampede (with fall) W52
 before moving object NEC Y02.8
  motor vehicle Y02.0
  subway train Y02.1
  train Y02.1
 from
  high place NEC
   in accidental circumstances W17.89
   stated as
    intentional, homicide (attempt) Y01
    undetermined whether accidental
     or intentional Y30
  transport vehicle NEC (*see also* Accident,
   transport) V89.9
   stated as
    intentional, homicide (attempt)
     Y08.89

R

Radiation (exposure to)
  arc lamps W89.0
  atomic power plant (malfunction) NEC
    W88.1
  complication of or abnormal reaction to
    medical radiotherapy Y84.2
  electromagnetic, ionizing W88.0
  gamma rays W88.1
  in
    war operations (from or following
      nuclear explosion) —see also War
      operations
    inadvertent exposure of patient (receiving
      test or therapy) Y63.3
  infrared (heaters and lamps) W90.1
    excessive heat from W92
  ionized, ionizing (particles, artificially
    accelerated)
    radioisotopes W88.1
    specified NEC W88.8
    x-rays W88.0
  isotopes, radioactive —see Radiation,
    radioactive isotopes
  laser (s) W90.2
    in war operations —see War operations
    misadventure in medical care Y63.2
  light sources (man-made visible and
    ultraviolet) W89.9
    natural X32
    specified NEC W89.8
    tanning bed W89.1
    welding light W89.0
  man-made visible light W89.9
    specified NEC W89.8
    tanning bed W89.1
    welding light W89.0
  microwave W90.8
  misadventure in medical or surgical
    procedure Y63.2

Radiation (Continued)
  natural NEC X39.08
    radon X39.01
  overdose (in medical or surgical procedure)
    Y63.2
  radar W90.0
  radioactive isotopes (any) W88.1
    atomic power plant malfunction W88.1
    misadventure in medical or surgical
      treatment Y63.2
  radiofrequency W90.0
  radium NEC W88.1
  sun X32
  ultraviolet (light) (man-made) W89.9
    natural X32
    specified NEC W89.8
    tanning bed W89.1
    welding light W89.0
  welding arc, torch, or light W89.0
    excessive heat from W92
  x-rays (hard) (soft) W88.0
Range disease W94.11
Rape (attempted) T74.2-
Rat bite W53.11
Reaction, abnormal to medical procedure (see
    also Complication of or following, by type
    of procedure) Y84.9
  with misadventure —see Misadventure
  biologicals —see Table of Drugs and
    Chemicals
  drugs —see Table of Drugs and
    Chemicals
  vaccine —see Table of Drugs and
    Chemicals
Recoil
  airgun W34.110
  BB gun W34.110
  firearm NEC W34.19
  gas, air or spring-operated gun NEC
    W34.118

Recoil (Continued)
  handgun W32.1
  hunting rifle W33.12
  larger firearm W33.10
    specified NEC W33.19
  machine gun W33.13
  paintball gun W34.111
  pellet W34.110
  shotgun W33.11
  Very pistol [flare] W34.19
Reduction in
  atmospheric pressure —see Air, pressure,
    change
Rock falling on or hitting (accidentally)
    (person) W20.8
  in cave-in W20.0
Run over (accidentally) (by)
  animal (not being ridden) NEC W55.89
  machinery —see Contact, with, by specified
    type of machine
  transport vehicle NEC (see also Accident,
    transport) V09.9
    intentional homicide (attempt) Y03.0
    motor NEC V09.20
      intentional homicide (attempt)
        Y03.0
Running
  before moving object X81.8
    motor vehicle X81.0
Running off, away
  animal (being ridden) (see also Accident,
    transport) V80.918
    not being ridden W55.89
  animal-drawn vehicle NEC (see also Accident,
    transport) V80.928
  highway, road(way), street
    transport vehicle NEC (see also Accident,
      transport) V89.9
Rupture pressurized devices —see Explosion,
    by type of device

S

Saturnism —*see* Table of Drugs and Chemicals, lead
Scald, scalding (accidental) (by) (from) (in) X19
  air (hot) X14.1
  gases (hot) X14.1
  homicide (attempt) —*see* Assault, burning, hot object
  inflicted by other person
    stated as intentional, homicide (attempt) —*see* Assault, burning, hot object
  liquid (boiling) (hot) NEC X12
    stated as undetermined whether accidental or intentional Y27.2
    suicide (attempt) X77.2
  local application of externally applied substance in medical or surgical care Y63.5
  metal (molten) (liquid) (hot) NEC X18
  self-inflicted X77.9
  stated as undetermined whether accidental or intentional Y27.8
  steam X13.1
    assault X98.0
    stated as undetermined whether accidental or intentional Y27.0
    suicide (attempt) X77.0
  suicide (attempt) X77.9
  vapor (hot) X13.1
    assault X98.0
    stated as undetermined whether accidental or intentional Y27.0
    suicide (attempt) X77.0
Scratched by
  cat W55.03
  person (s) (accidentally) W50.4
    with intent to injure or kill Y04.0
    as, or caused by, a crowd or human stampede (with fall) W52
    assault Y04.0
    homicide (attempt) Y04.0
    in
      fight Y04.0
      legal intervention
        injuring
          bystander Y35.892
          law enforcement personnel Y35.891
          suspect Y35.893
Seasickness T75.3
Self-harm NEC —*see also* External cause by type, undetermined whether accidental or intentional
  intentional —*see* Suicide
  poisoning NEC —*see* Table of drugs and biologicals, accident
Self-inflicted (injury) NEC —*see also* External cause by type, undetermined whether accidental or intentional
  intentional —*see* Suicide
  poisoning NEC —*see* Table of drugs and biologicals, accident
Sequelae (of)
  accident NEC —*see* W00-X58 with 7th character S
  assault (homicidal) (any means) —*see* X92-Y08 with 7th character S
  homicide, attempt (any means) —*see* X92-Y08 with 7th character S
  injury undetermined whether accidentally or purposely inflicted —*see* Y21-Y33 with 7th character S
  intentional self-harm (classifiable to X71-X83) —*see* X71-X83 with 7th character S
  legal intervention (*see* with 7th character S Y35)
  motor vehicle accident —*see* V00-V99 with 7th character S
  suicide, attempt (any means) —*see* X71-X83 with 7th character S

Sequelae (*Continued*)
  transport accident —*see* V00-V99 with 7th character S
  war operations —*see* War operations
Shock
  electric —*see* Exposure, electric current
  from electric appliance (any) (faulty) W86.8
    domestic W86.0
    suicide (attempt) X83.1
Shooting, shot (accidental (ly)) —*see also* Discharge, firearm, by type
  herself or himself —*see* Discharge, firearm by type, self-inflicted
  homicide (attempt) —*see* Discharge, firearm by type, homicide
  in war operations —*see* War operations
  inflicted by other person —*see* Discharge, firearm by type, homicide
    accidental —*see* Discharge, firearm, by type of firearm
  legal
    execution —*see* Legal, intervention, firearm
    intervention —*see* Legal, intervention, firearm
  self-inflicted —*see* Discharge, firearm by type, suicide
    accidental —*see* Discharge, firearm, by type of firearm
  suicide (attempt) —*see* Discharge, firearm by type, suicide
Shoving (accidentally) by other person —*see* Pushed, by other person
Sickness
  alpine W94.11
  motion —*see* Motion
  mountain W94.11
Sinking (accidental)
  watercraft (causing drowning, submersion) —*see also* Drowning, due to, accident to, watercraft, sinking
    causing injury except drowning or submersion —*see* Accident, watercraft, causing, injury NEC
Siriasis X32
Slashed wrists —*see* Cut, self-inflicted
Slipping (accidental) (on same level) (with fall) W01.0
  without fall W18.40
    due to
      specified NEC W18.49
      stepping from one level to another W18.43
      stepping into hole or opening W18.42
      stepping on object W18.41
  on
    ice W00.0
      with skates —*see* Accident, transport, pedestrian, conveyance
    mud W01.0
    oil W01.0
    snow W00.0
      with skis —*see* Accident, transport, pedestrian, conveyance
    surface (slippery) (wet) NEC W01.0
Sliver, wood, contact with W45.8
Smoldering (due to fire) —*see* Exposure, fire
Sodomy (attempted) by force T74.2-
Sound waves (causing injury) W42.9
  supersonic W42.0
Splinter, contact with W45.8
Stab, stabbing —*see* Cut
Starvation X58
Status of external cause Y99.9
  child assisting in compensated work for family Y99.8
  civilian activity done for financial or other compensation Y99.0
  civilian activity done for income or pay Y99.0
  family member assisting in compensated work for other family member Y99.8
  hobby not done for income Y99.8

Status of external cause (*Continued*)
  leisure activity Y99.8
  military activity Y99.1
  off-duty activity of military personnel Y99.8
  recreation or sport not for income or while a student Y99.8
  specified NEC Y99.8
  student activity Y99.8
  volunteer activity Y99.2
Stepped on
  by
    animal (not being ridden) NEC W55.89
    crowd or human stampede W52
    person W50.0
Stepping on
  object W22.8
    with fall W18.31
    sports equipment W21.9
    stationary W22.09
      sports equipment W21.89
  person W51
    by crowd or human stampede W52
    sports equipment W21.9
Sting
  arthropod, nonvenomous W57
  insect, nonvenomous W57
Storm (cataclysmic) —*see* Forces of nature, cataclysmic storm
Straining, excessive —*see* category Y93
Strangling —*see* Strangulation
Strangulation (accidental) —*see* category T71
Strenuous movements —*see* category Y93
Striking against
  airbag (automobile) W22.10
    driver side W22.11
    front passenger side W22.12
    specified NEC W22.19
  bottom when
    diving or jumping into water (in) W16.822
      causing drowning W16.821
      from boat W16.722
        causing drowning W16.721
      natural body W16.622
        causing drowning W16.821
      swimming pool W16.522
        causing drowning W16.521
    falling into water (in) W16.322
      causing drowning W16.321
      fountain —*see* Striking against, bottom when, falling into water, specified NEC
      natural body W16.122
        causing drowning W16.121
      reservoir —*see* Striking against, bottom when, falling into water, specified NEC
      specified NEC W16.322
        causing drowning W16.321
      swimming pool W16.022
        causing drowning W16.021
  diving board (swimming-pool) W21.4
  object W22.8
    with
      drowning or submersion —*see* Drowning
      fall —*see* Fall, due to, bumping against, object
    caused by crowd or human stampede (with fall) W52
    furniture W22.03
    lamppost W22.02
    sports equipment W21.9
    stationary W22.09
      sports equipment W21.89
    wall W22.01
  person (s) W51
    with fall W03
      due to ice or snow W00.0
    as, or caused by, a crowd or human stampede (with fall) W52

◀ New   ⬅ Revised   ~~deleted~~ Deleted

Struck by *(Continued)*
  sports equipment *(Continued)*
    bat or racquet
      baseball bat W21.11
        assault Y08.02
      golf club W21.13
        assault Y08.09
      specified NEC W21.19
      tennis racquet W21.12
        assault Y08.09
    cleats (shoe) W21.31
    foot wear NEC W21.39
    football helmet W21.81
    hockey (ice)
      field
        puck W21.221
        stick W21.211
      puck W21.220
      stick W21.210
        assault Y08.01
    skate blades W21.32
    specified NEC W21.89
      assault Y08.09
  thunderbolt —*see* subcategory
    T75.0
  causing fire —*see* Exposure, fire
  transport vehicle NEC *(see also* Accident,
    transport) V09.9
    intentional, homicide (attempt) Y03.0
    motor NEC *(see also* Accident, transport)
      V09.20
      homicide Y03.0
  vehicle (transport) NEC —*see* Accident,
    transport, by type of vehicle
    stationary (falling from jack,
      hydraulic lift, ramp)
      W20.8
Stumbling
  without fall W18.40
    due to
      specified NEC W18.49
      stepping from one level to another
        W18.43
      stepping into hole or opening
        W18.42
      stepping on object W18.41
  over
    animal NEC W01.0
      with fall W18.09
    carpet, rug or (small) object
      W22.8
      with fall W18.09
    person W51
      with fall W03
        due to ice or snow W00.0
Submersion (accidental) —*see* Drowning

Suffocation (accidental) (by external means) (by
    pressure) (mechanical) —*see also* category
    T71
  due to, by
    avalanche —*see* Landslide
    explosion —*see* Explosion
    fire —*see* Exposure, fire
    food, any type (aspiration) (ingestion)
      (inhalation) —*see* categories T17 and
      T18
    ignition —*see* Ignition
    landslide —*see* Landslide
    machine (ry) —*see* Contact, with, by type
      of machine
    vomitus (aspiration) (inhalation)
      T17.81-
  in
    burning building X00.8
Suicide, suicidal (attempted) (by) X83.8
  blunt object X79
  burning, burns X76
    hot object X77.9
      fluid NEC X77.2
      household appliance X77.3
      specified NEC X77.8
      steam X77.0
      tap water X77.1
      vapors X77.0
    caustic substance —*see* Table of Drugs and
      Chemicals
  cold, extreme X83.2
  collision of motor vehicle with
    motor vehicle X82.0
    specified NEC X82.8
    train X82.1
    tree X82.2
  crashing of aircraft X83.0
  cut (any part of body) X78.9
  cutting or piercing instrument X78.9
    dagger X78.2
    glass X78.0
    knife X78.1
    specified NEC X78.8
    sword X78.2
  drowning (in) X71.9
    bathtub X71.0
    natural water X71.3
    specified NEC X71.8
    swimming pool X71.1
      following fall X71.2
  electrocution X83.1
  explosive (s) (material) X75
  fire, flames X76
  firearm X74.9
    airgun X74.01
    handgun X72

Suicide, suicidal *(Continued)*
  firearm *(Continued)*
    hunting rifle X73.1
    larger X73.9
      specified NEC X73.8
    machine gun X73.2
    shotgun X73.0
    specified NEC X74.8
  hanging X83.8
  hot object —*see* Suicide, burning, hot object
  jumping
    before moving object X81.8
      motor vehicle X81.0
      subway train X81.1
      train X81.1
    from high place X80
  late effect of attempt —*see* X71-X83 with 7th
    character S
  lying before moving object, train, vehicle X81.8
  poisoning —*see* Table of Drugs and
    Chemicals
  puncture (any part of body) —*see* Suicide,
    cutting or piercing instrument
  scald —*see* Suicide, burning, hot object
  sequelae of attempt —*see* X71-X83 with 7th
    character S
  sharp object (any) —*see* Suicide, cutting or
    piercing instrument
  shooting —*see* Suicide, firearm
  specified means NEC X83.8
  stab (any part of body) —*see* Suicide, cutting
    or piercing instrument
  steam, hot vapors X77.0
  strangulation X83.8
  submersion —*see* Suicide, drowning
  suffocation X83.8
  wound NEC X83.8
Sunstroke X32
Supersonic waves (causing injury) W42.0
Surgical procedure, complication of (delayed
    or as an abnormal reaction without
    mention of misadventure) —*see also*
    Complication of or following, by type of
    procedure
  due to or as a result of misadventure —*see*
    Misadventure
Swallowed, swallowing
  foreign body —*see* Foreign body, alimentary
    canal
  poison —*see* Table of Drugs and Chemicals
  substance
    caustic or corrosive —*see* Table of Drugs
      and Chemicals
    poisonous —*see* Table of Drugs and
      Chemicals

T

Tackle in sport W03
Terrorism (involving) Y38.80
  biological weapons Y38.6X-
  chemical weapons Y38.7X-
  conflagration Y38.3X-
  drowning and submersion Y38.89-
  explosion Y38.2X-
    destruction of aircraft Y38.1X-
    marine weapons Y38.0X-
  fire Y38.3X-
  firearms Y38.4X-
  hot substances Y38.5X-
  lasers Y38.89-
  nuclear weapons Y38.5X-
  piercing or stabbing instruments
    Y38.89-
  secondary effects Y38.9X-
  specified method NEC Y38.89-
  suicide bomber Y38.81-
Thirst X58
Threat to breathing
  aspiration —see Aspiration
  due to cave-in, falling earth or substance
    NEC —see category T71
Thrown (accidentally)
  against part (any) of or object in transport
    vehicle (in motion) NEC (see also
    Accident, transport)

Thrown (Continued)
  from
    high place, homicide (attempt) Y01
    machinery —see Contact, with, by type of
      machine
    transport vehicle NEC (see also Accident,
      transport) V89.9
  off —see Thrown, from
Thunderbolt —see subcategory T75.0
  causing fire —see Exposure, fire
Tidal wave (any injury) NEC —see Forces of
  nature, tidal wave
Took
  overdose (drug) —see Table of Drugs and
    Chemicals
  poison —see Table of Drugs and
    Chemicals
Tornado (any injury) X37.1
Torrential rain (any injury) X37.8
Torture X58
Trampled by animal NEC W55.89
Trapped (accidentally)
  between objects (moving) (stationary and
    moving) —see Caught
  by part (any) of
    motorcycle V29.88
    pedal cycle V19.88
    transport vehicle NEC (see also Accident,
      transport) V89.9
Travel (effects) (sickness) T75.3

Tree falling on or hitting (accidentally)
  (person) W20.8
Tripping
  without fall W18.40
    due to
      specified NEC W18.49
      stepping from one level to another
        W18.43
      stepping into hole or opening
        W18.42
      stepping on object W18.41
  over
    animal W01.0
      with fall W01.0
    carpet, rug or (small) object W22.8
      with fall W18.09
    person W51
      with fall W03
        due to ice or snow W00.0
Twisted by person (s) (accidentally) W50.2
  with intent to injure or kill Y04.0
  as, or caused by, a crowd or human stampede
    (with fall) W52
  assault Y04.0
  homicide (attempt) Y04.0
  in
    fight Y04.0
    legal intervention —see Legal, intervention,
      manhandling
Twisting, excessive —see category Y93

U

Underdosing of necessary drugs, medicaments
  or biological substances Y63.6
Undetermined intent (contact) (exposure)
  automobile collision Y32
  blunt object Y29
  drowning (submersion) (in) Y21.9
    bathtub Y21.0
      after fall Y21.1
    natural water (lake) (ocean) (pond) (river)
      (stream) Y21.4
    specified place NEC Y21.8
    swimming pool Y21.2
      after fall Y21.3
  explosive material Y25
  fall, jump or push from high place Y30
  falling, lying or running before moving object
    Y31
  fire Y26

Undetermined intent (Continued)
  firearm discharge Y24.9
    airgun (BB) (pellet) Y24.0
    handgun (pistol) (revolver) Y22
    hunting rifle Y23.1
    larger Y23.9
      hunting rifle Y23.1
      machine gun Y23.3
      military Y23.2
      shotgun Y23.0
      specified type NEC Y23.8
    machine gun Y23.3
    military Y23.2
    shotgun Y23.0
    specified type NEC Y24.8
    Very pistol Y24.8
  hot object Y27.9
    fluid NEC Y27.2
    household appliance Y27.3
    specified object NEC Y27.8

Undetermined intent (Continued)
  hot object (Continued)
    steam Y27.0
    tap water Y27.1
    vapor Y27.0
  jump, fall or push from high place Y30
  lying, falling or running before moving object
    Y31
  motor vehicle crash Y32
  push, fall or jump from high place Y30
  running, falling or lying before moving object
    Y31
  sharp object Y28.9
    dagger Y28.2
    glass Y28.0
    knife Y28.1
    specified object NEC Y28.8
    sword Y28.2
  smoke Y26
  specified event NEC Y33

V

Vibration (causing injury) W49.9
Victim (of)
  avalanche —see Landslide
  earth movements NEC —see Forces of nature,
    earth movement
  earthquake X34

Victim (Continued)
  flood —see Flood
  landslide —see Landslide
  lightning —see subcategory T75.0
    causing fire —see Exposure, fire
  storm (cataclysmic) NEC —see Forces of
    nature, cataclysmic storm
  volcanic eruption X35

Volcanic eruption (any injury) X35
Vomitus, gastric contents in air passages
  (with asphyxia, obstruction or
  suffocation) T17.81-

T, U, & V

W

Walked into stationary object (any) W22.09
  furniture W22.03
  lamppost W22.02
  wall W22.01
War operations (injuries to military personnel
    and civilians during war, civil insurrection
    and peacekeeping missions) (by) (from)
    (involving) Y36.90-
  after cessation of hostilities Y36.89-
    explosion (of)
      bomb placed during war operations
        Y36.82-
      mine placed during war operations
        Y36.81-
      specified NEC Y36.88-
  air blast Y36.20-
  aircraft
    destruction —*see* War operations,
      destruction of aircraft
  airway restriction —*see* War operations,
    restriction of airways
  asphyxiation —*see* War operations, restriction
    of airways
  biological weapons Y36.6X-
  blast Y36.20-
  blast fragments Y36.20-
  blast wave Y36.20-
  blast wind Y36.20-
  bomb Y36.20-
    dirty Y36.50-
    gasoline Y36.31-
    incendiary Y36.31-
    petrol Y36.31-
  bullet Y36.43-
    incendiary Y36.32-
    rubber Y36.41-
  chemical weapons Y36.7X-
  combat
    hand to hand (unarmed) combat Y36.44-
    using blunt or piercing object Y36.45-
  conflagration —*see* War operations, fire
  conventional warfare NEC Y36.49-
  depth-charge Y36.01-
  destruction of aircraft Y36.10-
    due to
      air to air missile Y36.11-
      collision with other aircraft Y36.12-
      detonation (accidental) of onboard
        munitions and explosives Y36.14-
      enemy fire or explosives Y36.11-
      explosive placed on aircraft Y36.11-
      onboard fire Y36.13-
      rocket propelled grenade [RPG] Y36.11-
      small arms fire Y36.11-
      surface to air missile Y36.11-
    specified NEC Y36.19-
  detonation (accidental) of
    onboard marine weapons Y36.05-
    own munitions or munitions launch device
      Y36.24-

War operations (*Continued*)
  dirty bomb Y36.50-
  explosion (of) Y36.20-
    aerial bomb Y36.21-
    after cessation of hostilities
      bomb placed during war operations
        Y36.82-
      mine placed during war operations
        Y36.81-
    bomb NOS (*see also* War operations,
      bomb (s)) Y36.20-
    fragments Y36.20-
    grenade Y36.29-
    guided missile Y36.22-
    improvised explosive device [IED]
      (person-borne) (roadside)
      (vehicle-borne) Y36.23-
    land mine Y36.29-
    marine mine (at sea) (in harbor)
      Y36.02-
    marine weapon Y36.00-
      specified NEC Y36.09-
    own munitions or munitions launch
      device (accidental) Y36.24-
    sea-based artillery shell Y36.03-
    specified NEC Y36.29-
    torpedo Y36.04-
  fire Y36.30-
    specified NEC Y36.39-
  firearms
    discharge Y36.43-
    pellets Y36.42-
  flamethrower Y36.33-
  fragments (from) (of)
    improvised explosive device [IED]
      (person-borne) (roadside)
      (vehicle-borne) Y36.26-
    munitions Y36.25-
    specified NEC Y36.29-
    weapons Y36.27-
  friendly fire Y36.92
  hand to hand (unarmed) combat
    Y36.44-
  hot substances —*see* War operations,
    fire
  incendiary bullet Y36.32-
  nuclear weapon (effects of) Y36.50-
    acute radiation exposure Y36.54-
    blast pressure Y36.51-
    direct blast Y36.51-
    direct heat Y36.53-
    fallout exposure Y36.54-
    fireball Y36.53-
    indirect blast (struck or crushed by blast
      debris) (being thrown by blast)
      Y36.52-
    ionizing radiation (immediate exposure)
      Y36.54-
    nuclear radiation Y36.54-
    radiation
      ionizing (immediate exposure)
        Y36.54-

War operations (*Continued*)
  nuclear weapon (*Continued*)
    radiation (*Continued*)
      nuclear Y36.54-
      thermal Y36.53-
    secondary effects Y36.54-
    specified NEC Y36.59-
    thermal radiation Y36.53-
  restriction of air (airway)
    intentional Y36.46-
    unintentional Y36.47-
  rubber bullets Y36.41-
  shrapnel NOS Y36.29-
  suffocation —*see* War operations, restriction
    of airways
  unconventional warfare NEC Y36.7X-
  underwater blast NOS Y36.00-
  warfare
    conventional NEC Y36.49-
    unconventional NEC Y36.7X-
  weapon of mass destruction [WMD] Y36.91
  weapons
    biological weapons Y36.6X-
    chemical Y36.7X-
    nuclear (effects of) Y36.50-
      acute radiation exposure Y36.54-
      blast pressure Y36.51-
      direct blast Y36.51-
      direct heat Y36.53-
      fallout exposure Y36.54-
      fireball Y36.53-
      indirect blast (struck or crushed by blast
        debris) (being thrown by blast)
        Y36.52-
      radiation
        ionizing (immediate exposure) Y36.54-
        nuclear Y36.54-
        thermal Y36.53-
      secondary effects Y36.54-
      specified NEC Y36.59-
    of mass destruction [WMD] Y36.91-
Washed
  away by flood —*see* Flood
  off road by storm (transport vehicle) —*see*
    Forces of nature, cataclysmic storm
Weather exposure NEC —*see* Forces of nature
Weightlessness (causing injury) (effects of) (in
    spacecraft, real or simulated) X52
Work related condition Y99.0
Wound (accidental) NEC (*see also* Injury) X58
  battle (*see also* War operations) Y36.90
  gunshot —*see* Discharge, firearm by type
Wreck transport vehicle NEC (*see also* Accident,
    transport) V89.9
Wrong
  device implanted into correct surgical site
    Y65.51
  fluid in infusion Y65.1
  patient, procedure performed on Y65.52
  procedure (operation) on correct patient
    Y65.51

◀ New   ◀▥ Revised   ~~deleted~~ Deleted

PART III

ICD-10-CM Tabular List of Diseases and Injuries

CHAPTER 1

CERTAIN INFECTIOUS AND PARASITIC DISEASES (A00-B99)

Includes   diseases generally recognized as communicable or transmissible

Use additional code to identify resistance to antimicrobial drugs (Z16.-)

Excludes1   certain localized infections - see body system-related chapters

Excludes2   carrier or suspected carrier of infectious disease (Z22.-)

infectious and parasitic diseases complicating pregnancy, childbirth and the puerperium (O98.-)

infectious and parasitic diseases specific to the perinatal period (P35-P39)

influenza and other acute respiratory infections (J00-J22)

This chapter contains the following blocks:

A00-A09	Intestinal infectious diseases
A15-A19	Tuberculosis
A20-A28	Certain zoonotic bacterial diseases
A30-A49	Other bacterial diseases
A50-A64	Infections with a predominantly sexual mode of transmission
A65-A69	Other spirochetal diseases
A70-A74	Other diseases caused by chlamydiae
A75-A79	Rickettsioses
A80-A89	Viral and prion infections of the central nervous system
A90-A99	Arthropod-borne viral fevers and viral hemorrhagic fevers
B00-B09	Viral infections characterized by skin and mucous membrane lesions
B10	Other human herpesviruses
B15-B19	Viral hepatitis
B20	Human immunodeficiency virus [HIV] disease
B25-B34	Other viral diseases
B35-B49	Mycoses
B50-B64	Protozoal diseases
B65-B83	Helminthiases
B85-B89	Pediculosis, acariasis and other infestations
B90-B94	Sequelae of infectious and parasitic diseases
B95-B97	Bacterial and viral infectious agents
B99	Other infectious diseases

INTESTINAL INFECTIOUS DISEASES (A00-A09)

● **A00**   **Cholera**

A serious, often deadly, infectious disease of the small intestine

    A00.0   **Cholera due to Vibrio cholerae 01, biovar cholerae**
        Classical cholera

    A00.1   **Cholera due to Vibrio cholerae 01, biovar eltor**
        Cholera eltor

    A00.9   **Cholera, unspecified**

● **A01**   **Typhoid and paratyphoid fevers**

Caused by Salmonella typhi and Salmonella paratyphi A, B, and C bacteria

  ● **A01.0**   **Typhoid fever**
        Infection due to Salmonella typhi

      A01.00   **Typhoid fever, unspecified**

      A01.01   **Typhoid meningitis**

      A01.02   **Typhoid fever with heart involvement**
           Typhoid endocarditis
           Typhoid myocarditis

      A01.03   **Typhoid pneumonia**

      A01.04   **Typhoid arthritis**

      A01.05   **Typhoid osteomyelitis**

      A01.09   **Typhoid fever with other complications**

    A01.1   **Paratyphoid fever A**

    A01.2   **Paratyphoid fever B**

Item 1–1   **Salmonella** is a bacterium that lives in the intestines of fowl and mammals and can spread to humans through improper food preparation and cooking. Salmonellosis is an infection with the bacterium. Symptoms include diarrhea, fever, and abdominal cramps 12 to 72 hours after infection. The illness usually lasts 4 to 7 days, and most persons recover without treatment. The diarrhea may be so severe that the patient needs to be hospitalized. Patients with immunocompromised systems in chronic, ill health are more likely to have the infection invade their bloodstream with life-threatening results. For example, patients with sickle cell disease are more prone to salmonella osteomyelitis than others.

    A01.3   **Paratyphoid fever C**

    A01.4   **Paratyphoid fever, unspecified**
        Infection due to Salmonella paratyphi NOS

● **A02**   **Other salmonella infections**

    Includes   infection or foodborne intoxication due to any Salmonella species other than S. typhi and S. paratyphi

    A02.0   **Salmonella enteritis**
        Salmonellosis

    A02.1   **Salmonella sepsis**

  ● **A02.2**   **Localized salmonella infections**

      A02.20   **Localized salmonella infection, unspecified**
         Specified in the documentation as localized, but unspecified as to type

      A02.21   **Salmonella meningitis**
         Specified as localized in the meninges

      A02.22   **Salmonella pneumonia**
         Specified as localized in the lungs

      A02.23   **Salmonella arthritis**
         Specified as localized in the joints

      A02.24   **Salmonella osteomyelitis**
         Specified as localized in bone

      A02.25   **Salmonella pyelonephritis**
        Salmonella tubulo-interstitial nephropathy

      A02.29   **Salmonella with other localized infection**
         Specified as localized (because it is still under localized heading) but does not assign into any of the above codes

    A02.8   **Other specified salmonella infections**
      Any specified salmonella infection which does NOT assign into any of the above codes (not specified as localized)

    A02.9   **Salmonella infection, unspecified**
      Unspecified in the documentation as to specific type of salmonella

● **A03**   **Shigellosis**
    An infectious disease caused by bacteria (Shigella)

    A03.0   **Shigellosis due to Shigella dysenteriae**
        Group A shigellosis [Shiga-Kruse dysentery]

    A03.1   **Shigellosis due to Shigella flexneri**
        Group B shigellosis

    A03.2   **Shigellosis due to Shigella boydii**
        Group C shigellosis

    A03.3   **Shigellosis due to Shigella sonnei**
        Group D shigellosis

    A03.8   **Other shigellosis**

    A03.9   **Shigellosis, unspecified**
        Bacillary dysentery NOS

● **A04**   **Other bacterial intestinal infections**

    Excludes1   bacterial foodborne intoxications, NEC (A05.-)
           tuberculous enteritis (A18.32)

    A04.0   **Enteropathogenic Escherichia coli infection**
      Pertaining to or producing intestinal disease

    A04.1   **Enterotoxigenic Escherichia coli infection**
      Producing or containing intestinal toxin

    A04.2   **Enteroinvasive Escherichia coli infection**
      Capable of penetrating and spreading through intestinal mucosal epithelium

    A04.3   **Enterohemorrhagic Escherichia coli infection**
      Causing bloody diarrhea, resulting from microorganisms

◀ New   ◀|||| Revised   ~~deleted~~ Deleted   **OGCR** Official Guidelines   X Assign placeholder X   ● Use Additional Character(s)

Excludes 1	Excludes 2	Includes	Use additional	Code first	Code also	Unspecified

CHAPTER 1 (A00-B99)

Figure 1-1   Electron micrograph of escherichia coli (E. coli) expressing P fimbriae. (From Mandell, Bennett, & Dolin: Principles and Practice of Infectious Diseases, ed 7, Churchill Livingstone, An Imprint of Elsevier, 2009)

Item 1-2   *Escherichia coli [E. coli]* is a gram-negative bacterium found in the intestinal tracts of humans and animals and is usually nonpathogenic. Pathogenic strains can cause diarrhea or pyogenic (pus-producing) infections. Can be a threat to food safety.

A04.4   **Other intestinal Escherichia coli infections**
Escherichia coli enteritis NOS

A04.5   **Campylobacter enteritis**
Spiral shaped bacterium

A04.6   **Enteritis due to Yersinia enterocolitica**
> **Excludes1**   extraintestinal yersiniosis (A28.2)

Transmitted by infected food /water and person-to-person contact, affecting intestinal tract

A04.7   **Enterocolitis due to Clostridium difficile**
Foodborne intoxication by Clostridium difficile
Pseudomembraneous colitis
Marked by fibrinous deposit (false membrane) with enmeshed necrotic cells

A04.8   **Other specified bacterial intestinal infections**

A04.9   **Bacterial intestinal infection, unspecified**
Bacterial enteritis NOS

● **A05**   **Other bacterial foodborne intoxications, not elsewhere classified**
> **Excludes1**   Clostridium difficile foodborne intoxication and infection (A04.7)
> Escherichia coli infection (A04.0-A04.4)
> listeriosis (A32.-)
> salmonella foodborne intoxication and infection (A02.-)
> toxic effect of noxious foodstuffs (T61-T62)

A05.0   **Foodborne staphylococcal intoxication**

A05.1   **Botulism food poisoning**
Botulism NOS
Classical foodborne intoxication due to Clostridium botulinum
> **Excludes1**   infant botulism (A48.51)
> wound botulism (A48.52)

A05.2   **Foodborne Clostridium perfringens [Clostridium welchii] intoxication**
Type A causes gas gangrene and necrotizing colitis; major cause of food poisoning in humans
Enteritis necroticans
Pig-bel

A05.3   **Foodborne Vibrio parahaemolyticus intoxication**
Organism that survives only in high salt environment (halophilic), major cause of gastroenteritis due to consumption of raw or improperly cooked fish/seafood

A05.4   **Foodborne Bacillus cereus intoxication**
Spore-forming species commonly found in soil, causes food poisoning from formation of intestinal toxins in contaminated foods

A05.5   **Foodborne Vibrio vulnificus intoxication**
Species that survives in high salt environment (halophilic) with infection by eating raw seafood causes septicemia and cellulitis

A05.8   **Other specified bacterial foodborne intoxications**

A05.9   **Bacterial foodborne intoxication, unspecified**

● **A06**   **Amebiasis**
An intestinal illness caused by the microscopic parasite Entamoeba histolytica
> **Includes**   infection due to Entamoeba histolytica
> **Excludes1**   other protozoal intestinal diseases (A07.-)
> **Excludes2**   acanthamebiasis (B60.1-)
> Naegleriasis (B60.2)

A06.0   **Acute amebic dysentery**
Acute amebiasis
Intestinal amebiasis NOS

A06.1   **Chronic intestinal amebiasis**

A06.2   **Amebic nondysenteric colitis**
Pertaining to single cell microorganism

A06.3   **Ameboma of intestine**
Tumorlike mass produced by localized inflammation often in intestine
Ameboma NOS

A06.4   **Amebic liver abscess**
Hepatic amebiasis

A06.5   **Amebic lung abscess**
Amebic abscess of lung (and liver)

A06.6   **Amebic brain abscess**
Amebic abscess of brain (and liver) (and lung)

A06.7   **Cutaneous amebiasis**

● **A06.8**   **Amebic infection of other sites**

    A06.81   **Amebic cystitis**

    A06.82   **Other amebic genitourinary infections**
Amebic balanitis
Amebic vesiculitis
Amebic vulvovaginitis

    A06.89   **Other amebic infections**
Amebic appendicitis
Amebic splenic abscess

A06.9   **Amebiasis, unspecified**

● **A07**   **Other protozoal intestinal diseases**

A07.0   **Balantidiasis**
Balantidial dysentery
Infection by protozoa that may cause diarrhea and dysentery, with ulceration of colonic mucous membranes

A07.1   **Giardiasis [lambliasis]**
Common infection in small intestine spread by contaminated food, water, or direct person-to-person contact

A07.2   **Cryptosporidiosis**
Human infection with protozoa usually seen as self-limited diarrhea in those who work with cattle

A07.3   **Isosporiasis**
Human intestinal disease caused by protozoa
Infection due to Isospora belli and Isospora hominis
Intestinal coccidiosis
Isosporosis

A07.4   **Cyclosporiasis**
Infection by protozoa with most common species infecting humans being C cayetanensis

A07.8   **Other specified protozoal intestinal diseases**
Intestinal microsporidiosis
Intestinal trichomoniasis
Sarcocystosis
Sarcosporidiosis

A07.9   **Protozoal intestinal disease, unspecified**
Flagellate diarrhea
Protozoal colitis
Protozoal diarrhea
Protozoal dysentery

CHAPTER 1 (A00-B99)

◀ New   ◀▦ Revised   ~~deleted~~ Deleted   **OGCR** Official Guidelines   X Assign placeholder X   ● Use Additional Character(s)

| Excludes 1 | Excludes 2 | Includes | Use additional | Code first | Code also | Unspecified |

CHAPTER 1 (A00-B99)

● **A08   Viral and other specified intestinal infections**

> **Excludes1**   influenza with involvement of gastrointestinal
> tract (J09.X3, J10.2, J11.2)

A08.0   Rotaviral enteritis

● **A08.1   Acute gastroenteropathy due to Norwalk agent and
other small round viruses**

> **A08.11   Acute gastroenteropathy due to Norwalk agent**
> Acute gastroenteropathy due to Norovirus
> Acute gastroenteropathy due to Norwalk-like
> agent

> **A08.19   Acute gastroenteropathy due to other small
> round viruses**
> Acute gastroenteropathy due to small round
> virus [SRV] NOS

A08.2   Adenoviral enteritis

● **A08.3   Other viral enteritis**

> **A08.31   Calicivirus enteritis**

> **A08.32   Astrovirus enteritis**

> **A08.39   Other viral enteritis**
> Coxsackie virus enteritis
> Echovirus enteritis
> Enterovirus enteritis NEC
> Torovirus enteritis

A08.4   Viral intestinal infection, unspecified
Viral enteritis NOS
Viral gastroenteritis NOS
Viral gastroenteropathy NOS

A08.8   Other specified intestinal infections

A09   Infectious gastroenteritis and colitis, unspecified
Infectious colitis NOS
Infectious enteritis NOS
Infectious gastroenteritis NOS

> **Excludes1**   colitis NOS (K52.9)
> diarrhea NOS (R19.7)
> enteritis NOS (K52.9)
> gastroenteritis NOS (K52.9)
> noninfective gastroenteritis and colitis,
> unspecified (K52.9)

TUBERCULOSIS (A15-A19)

> **Includes**   infections due to Mycobacterium tuberculosis
> and Mycobacterium bovis

> **Excludes1**   congenital tuberculosis (P37.0)
> nonspecific reaction to test for tuberculosis
> without active tuberculosis (R76.1-)
> pneumoconiosis associated with tuberculosis, any
> type in A15 (J65)
> positive PPD (R76.11)
> positive tuberculin skin test without active
> tuberculosis (R76.11)
> sequelae of tuberculosis (B90.-)
> silicotuberculosis (J65)

● **A15   Respiratory tuberculosis**

A15.0   Tuberculosis of lung
Tuberculous bronchiectasis
Chronic dilatation of bronchi
Tuberculous fibrosis of lung
Tuberculous pneumonia
Tuberculous pneumothorax

A15.4   Tuberculosis of intrathoracic lymph nodes
Tuberculosis of hilar lymph nodes
Tuberculosis of mediastinal lymph nodes
Tuberculosis of tracheobronchial lymph nodes

> **Excludes1**   tuberculosis specified as primary (A15.7)

A15.5   Tuberculosis of larynx, trachea and bronchus
Tuberculosis of bronchus
Tuberculosis of glottis
Tuberculosis of larynx
Tuberculosis of trachea

Figure 1-2   Far advanced bilateral pulmonary tuberculosis before and
after 8 months of treatment with streptomycin, PAS, and isoniazid. (From
Hinshaw HC, Garland LH: Diseases of the Chest, ed 4, Philadelphia, WB
Saunders, 1980)

Item 1–3   Tuberculosis is a common and deadly infectious disease
caused by the *Mycobacterium tuberculosis* organism. The first tuberculosis
infection is called the **primary infection** and most commonly attacks the
lungs but can affect the central nervous system, lymphatic system, circulatory
system, genitourinary system, bones, joints, and even the skin. A **Ghon** lesion
is the **initial lesion.** A **secondary lesion** occurs when the tubercle bacilli
are carried to other areas.

Item 1–4   Although it primarily affects the lungs, the bacteria
Mycobacterium tuberculosis can travel from the pulmonary circulation to
virtually any organ in the body, much as a cancer metastasizes to a secondary
site. If the immune system becomes compromised by age or disease, what
would otherwise be a self-limiting primary tuberculosis in the lungs will develop
in other organs. These are known as extrapulmonary sites.

A15.6   Tuberculous pleurisy
Tuberculosis of pleura
Tuberculous empyema

> **Excludes1**   primary respiratory tuberculosis (A15.7)

A15.7   Primary respiratory tuberculosis

A15.8   Other respiratory tuberculosis
Mediastinal tuberculosis
Nasopharyngeal tuberculosis
Tuberculosis of nose
Tuberculosis of sinus [any nasal]

A15.9   Respiratory tuberculosis unspecified

● **A17   Tuberculosis of nervous system**

A17.0   Tuberculous meningitis
Tuberculosis of meninges (cerebral) (spinal)
Tuberculous leptomeningitis

> **Excludes1**   tuberculous meningoencephalitis
> (A17.82)

A17.1   Meningeal tuberculoma
Tuberculoma of meninges (cerebral) (spinal)

> **Excludes2**   tuberculoma of brain and spinal cord
> (A17.81)

● **A17.8   Other tuberculosis of nervous system**

> **A17.81   Tuberculoma of brain and spinal cord**
> Tuberculous abscess of brain and spinal cord

> **A17.82   Tuberculous meningoencephalitis**
> *Inflammation of brain and meninges; AKA
> cerebromeningitis and encephalomeningitis*
> Tuberculous myelitis

> **A17.83   Tuberculous neuritis**
> Tuberculous mononeuropathy

> **A17.89   Other tuberculosis of nervous system**
> Tuberculous polyneuropathy

A17.9   Tuberculosis of nervous system, unspecified

◀ New   ◀||| Revised   ~~deleted~~ Deleted   OGCR Official Guidelines   X Assign placeholder X   ● Use Additional Character(s)

Excludes 1   Excludes 2   Includes   Use additional   Code first   Code also   Unspecified

● **A18   Tuberculosis of other organs**
   ● **A18.0   Tuberculosis of bones and joints**
      A18.01   Tuberculosis of spine
         Pott's disease or curvature of spine
         Tuberculous arthritis
         Tuberculous osteomyelitis of spine
         Tuberculous spondylitis
      A18.02   Tuberculous arthritis of other joints
         Tuberculosis of hip (joint)
         Tuberculosis of knee (joint)
      A18.03   Tuberculosis of other bones
         Tuberculous mastoiditis
         Tuberculous osteomyelitis
      A18.09   Other musculoskeletal tuberculosis
         Tuberculous myositis
         Tuberculous synovitis
         Tuberculous tenosynovitis
   ● **A18.1   Tuberculosis of genitourinary system**
      A18.10   Tuberculosis of genitourinary system, unspecified
      A18.11   Tuberculosis of kidney and ureter
      A18.12   Tuberculosis of bladder
      A18.13   Tuberculosis of other urinary organs
         Tuberculous urethritis
      A18.14   Tuberculosis of prostate
      A18.15   Tuberculosis of other male genital organs
      A18.16   Tuberculosis of cervix
      A18.17   Tuberculous female pelvic inflammatory disease
         Tuberculous endometritis
         Tuberculous oophoritis and salpingitis
         Oophoritis = inflammation of ovary
         Salpingitis = inflammation of fallopian tube
      A18.18   Tuberculosis of other female genital organs
         Tuberculous ulceration of vulva
   A18.2   Tuberculous peripheral lymphadenopathy
      Tuberculous adenitis
      | Excludes2 | tuberculosis of bronchial and mediastinal lymph nodes (A15.4)
         tuberculosis of mesenteric and retroperitoneal lymph nodes (A18.39)
         tuberculous tracheobronchial adenopathy (A15.4)
   ● **A18.3   Tuberculosis of intestines, peritoneum and mesenteric glands**
      A18.31   Tuberculous peritonitis
         Tuberculous ascites
      A18.32   Tuberculous enteritis
         Tuberculosis of anus and rectum
         Tuberculosis of intestine (large) (small)
      A18.39   Retroperitoneal tuberculosis
         Tuberculosis of mesenteric glands
         Tuberculosis of retroperitoneal (lymph glands)
   A18.4   Tuberculosis of skin and subcutaneous tissue
      Erythema induratum, tuberculous
      Lupus excedens
      Lupus vulgaris NOS
      Lupus vulgaris of eyelid
         Cutaneous tuberculosis characterized by reddish brown plaque on skin surrounded by papules and nodules
      Scrofuloderma
         Type of cutaneous tuberculosis, with direct extension of tuberculosis into skin from underlying structures; AKA tuberculosis colliquativa
      Tuberculosis of external ear
      | Excludes2 | lupus erythematosus (L93.-)
         lupus NOS (M32.9)
         systemic (M32.-)

● **A18.5   Tuberculosis of eye**
   | Excludes2 | lupus vulgaris of eyelid (A18.4)
   A18.50   Tuberculosis of eye, unspecified
   A18.51   Tuberculous episcleritis
      Inflammation of episclera and adjacent tissues
   A18.52   Tuberculous keratitis
      Tuberculous interstitial keratitis
      Tuberculous keratoconjunctivitis (interstitial) (phlyctenular)
      Inflammation of cornea and conjunctiva
   A18.53   Tuberculous chorioretinitis
      Inflammation of choroid and retina; retinochoroiditis
   A18.54   Tuberculous iridocyclitis
      Inflammation of iris and ciliary body
   A18.59   Other tuberculosis of eye
      Tuberculous conjunctivitis
A18.6   Tuberculosis of (inner) (middle) ear
   Tuberculous otitis media
   | Excludes2 | tuberculosis of external ear (A18.4)
      tuberculous mastoiditis (A18.03)
A18.7   Tuberculosis of adrenal glands
   Tuberculous Addison's disease
● **A18.8   Tuberculosis of other specified organs**
   A18.81   Tuberculosis of thyroid gland
   A18.82   Tuberculosis of other endocrine glands
      Tuberculosis of pituitary gland
      Tuberculosis of thymus gland
   A18.83   Tuberculosis of digestive tract organs, not elsewhere classified
      | Excludes1 | tuberculosis of intestine (A18.32)
   A18.84   Tuberculosis of heart
      Tuberculous cardiomyopathy
      Tuberculous endocarditis
      Tuberculous myocarditis
      Tuberculous pericarditis
   A18.85   Tuberculosis of spleen
   A18.89   Tuberculosis of other sites
      Tuberculosis of muscle
      Tuberculous cerebral arteritis

● **A19   Miliary tuberculosis**
   | Includes | disseminated tuberculosis
      generalized tuberculosis
      tuberculous polyserositis
   A19.0   Acute miliary tuberculosis of a single specified site
   A19.1   Acute miliary tuberculosis of multiple sites
   A19.2   Acute miliary tuberculosis, unspecified
   A19.8   Other miliary tuberculosis
   A19.9   Miliary tuberculosis, unspecified

Item 1–5   Miliary tuberculosis can be a life-threatening condition. If a tuberculous lesion enters a blood vessel, immense dissemination of tuberculous organisms can occur if the immune system is weak. High-risk populations—children under 4 years of age, the elderly, or the immunocompromised—are particularly prone to this type of infection. The lesions will have a millet seedlike appearance on chest x-ray. Bronchial washings and biopsy may aid in diagnosis.

CHAPTER 1 (A00-B99)

CERTAIN ZOONOTIC BACTERIAL DISEASES (A20-A28)

● **A20   Plague**
Infectious disease caused by a Yersinia pestis bacterium, transmitted by a rodent flea bite or handling of infected animal

   Includes   infection due to Yersinia pestis

   A20.0   Bubonic plague

   A20.1   Cellulocutaneous plague
   Skin and subcutaneous tissue plague

   A20.2   Pneumonic plague

   A20.3   Plague meningitis

   A20.7   Septicemic plague

   A20.8   Other forms of plague
   Abortive plague
   Asymptomatic plague
   Pestis minor
   Systemic bacterial disease

   A20.9   Plague, unspecified

● **A21   Tularemia**
Caused by Francisella tularensis bacterium found in rodents, rabbits, and hares and transmitted to humans by contact with infected animal tissues or by ticks, biting flies, or mosquitoes

   Includes   deer-fly fever
   infection due to Francisella tularensis
   rabbit fever

   A21.0   Ulceroglandular tularemia
   Most common form of tularemia in humans is painful, swollen, erythematous papule at point of inoculation that ruptures to form shallow ulcer

   A21.1   Oculoglandular tularemia
   Primary site of entry is conjunctival sac, results in granulomatous corneal lesions
   Ophthalmic tularemia

   A21.2   Pulmonary tularemia

   A21.3   Gastrointestinal tularemia
   Abdominal tularemia

   A21.7   Generalized tularemia

   A21.8   Other forms of tularemia

   A21.9   Tularemia, unspecified

● **A22   Anthrax**
An acute infectious disease caused by the spore-forming Bacillus anthracis; occurs in humans exposed to infected animals or tissue from infected animals

   Includes   infection due to Bacillus anthracis

   A22.0   Cutaneous anthrax
   Malignant carbuncle
   Malignant pustule

   A22.1   Pulmonary anthrax
   Inhalation anthrax
   Ragpicker's disease
   Woolsorter's disease

   A22.2   Gastrointestinal anthrax

   A22.7   Anthrax sepsis
   Infectious bacterial disease

   A22.8   Other forms of anthrax
   Anthrax meningitis

   A22.9   Anthrax, unspecified

Item 1-6   Brucellosis: An infectious disease caused by the bacterium Brucella. Humans are infected by contact with contaminated animals or animal products. In humans brucellosis symptoms that are similar to the flu include fever, sweats, headaches, back pains, and physical weakness. Severe infections of the central nervous system or lining of the heart may occur. Brucellosis can also cause chronic symptoms that include recurrent fevers, joint pain, and fatigue.

● **A23   Brucellosis**

   Includes   Malta fever
   Mediterranean fever
   undulant fever

   A23.0   Brucellosis due to Brucella melitensis
   Resulting in flu-like symptoms that may lead to chronic symptoms that include recurrent fevers, joint pain, and fatigue

   A23.1   Brucellosis due to Brucella abortus
   Most common cause of brucellosis in humans; AKA Bang bacillus

   A23.2   Brucellosis due to Brucella suis
   Species found primarily in pigs, rabbits, and reindeer

   A23.3   Brucellosis due to Brucella canis
   Species that causes respiratory tract infection in humans

   A23.8   Other brucellosis

   A23.9   Brucellosis, unspecified

● **A24   Glanders and melioidosis**
Infection, usually of rodents, which spreads to other animals and humans, caused by Burkholderia pseudomallei through break in skin contaminated with infested soil or water

   A24.0   Glanders
   Infection due to Pseudomonas mallei
   Malleus

   A24.1   Acute and fulminating melioidosis
   Melioidosis pneumonia
   Melioidosis sepsis

   A24.2   Subacute and chronic melioidosis

   A24.3   Other melioidosis

   A24.9   Melioidosis, unspecified
   Infection due to Pseudomonas pseudomallei NOS
   Whitmore's disease

● **A25   Rat-bite fevers**
RBF, infectious disease caused by Streptobacillus moniliformis or Spirillum minus.

   A25.0   Spirillosis
   Any disease condition caused by spirilla
   Sodoku

   A25.1   Streptobacillosis
   Acute, febrile human illness caused by bacteria transmitted by rats in most cases, passed from rodent to human via rodent's urine or mucous secretions; AKA rat fever
   Epidemic arthritic erythema
   Haverhill fever
   Streptobacillary rat-bite fever

   A25.9   Rat-bite fever, unspecified

● **A26   Erysipeloid**
Infection with Erysipelothrix rhusiopathiae, occurring often as occupational disease resulting from handling infected fish, shellfish, meat, or poultry

   A26.0   Cutaneous erysipeloid
   Erythema migrans

   A26.7   Erysipelothrix sepsis

   A26.8   Other forms of erysipeloid

   A26.9   Erysipeloid, unspecified

● **A27**   **Leptospirosis**
Occurs most commonly in the tropics

     A27.0   **Leptospirosis icterohemorrhagica**
         Leptospiral or spirochetal jaundice (hemorrhagic)
         Weil's disease

     ● **A27.8**   **Other forms of leptospirosis**
         A27.81   **Aseptic meningitis in leptospirosis**
         A27.89   **Other forms of leptospirosis**

     A27.9   **Leptospirosis, unspecified**

● **A28**   **Other zoonotic bacterial diseases, not elsewhere classified**

     A28.0   **Pasteurellosis**
         Infection of humans or other animals by species of
           Pasteurella

     A28.1   **Cat-scratch disease**
         Cat-scratch fever

     A28.2   **Extraintestinal yersiniosis**
         Infection from Yersinia enterocolitica; AKA enteric
           yersiniosis, intestinal yersiniosis, Yersinia enteritis

         | **Excludes1** | enteritis due to Yersinia enterocolitica
               (A04.6)
               plague (A20.-)

     A28.8   **Other specified zoonotic bacterial diseases, not elsewhere classified**

     A28.9   **Zoonotic bacterial disease, unspecified**

OTHER BACTERIAL DISEASES (A30-A49)

● **A30**   **Leprosy [Hansen's disease]**
Chronic infectious disease attacking the skin, peripheral nerves, and
mucous membranes

     | **Includes** | infection due to Mycobacterium leprae
     | **Excludes1** | sequelae of leprosy (B92)

     A30.0   **Indeterminate leprosy**
         I leprosy

     A30.1   **Tuberculoid leprosy**
         TT leprosy

     A30.2   **Borderline tuberculoid leprosy**
         BT leprosy

     A30.3   **Borderline leprosy**
         BB leprosy

     A30.4   **Borderline lepromatous leprosy**
         BL leprosy

     A30.5   **Lepromatous leprosy**
         LL leprosy

     A30.8   **Other forms of leprosy**

     A30.9   **Leprosy, unspecified**

● **A31**   **Infection due to other mycobacteria**

     | **Excludes2** | leprosy (A30.-)
               tuberculosis (A15-A19)

     A31.0   **Pulmonary mycobacterial infection**
         Infection due to Mycobacterium avium
         Infection due to Mycobacterium intracellulare [Battey
           bacillus]
         Infection due to Mycobacterium kansasii

     A31.1   **Cutaneous mycobacterial infection**
         Buruli ulcer
         Infection due to Mycobacterium marinum
         Infection due to Mycobacterium ulcerans

     A31.2   **Disseminated mycobacterium avium-intracellulare complex (DMAC)**
         MAC sepsis

     A31.8   **Other mycobacterial infections**

     A31.9   **Mycobacterial infection, unspecified**
         Atypical mycobacterial infection NOS
         Mycobacteriosis NOS

● **A32**   **Listeriosis**
Infection caused by Listeria monocytogenes

     | **Includes** | listerial foodborne infection
     | **Excludes1** | neonatal (disseminated) listeriosis (P37.2)

     A32.0   **Cutaneous listeriosis**

     ● **A32.1**   **Listerial meningitis and meningoencephalitis**
         A32.11   **Listerial meningitis**
         A32.12   **Listerial meningoencephalitis**

     A32.7   **Listerial sepsis**

     ● **A32.8**   **Other forms of listeriosis**
         A32.81   **Oculoglandular listeriosis**
           Primary infection site is conjunctival sac, which if
             untreated may result in perforation of cornea
             and optic atrophy

         A32.82   **Listerial endocarditis**
           Exudative and proliferative inflammatory condition
             of endocardium caused by listeria bacteria

         A32.89   **Other forms of listeriosis**
           Listerial cerebral arteritis

     A32.9   **Listeriosis, unspecified**

   A33   **Tetanus neonatorum**
Neonate = newborn

   A34   **Obstetrical tetanus**

   A35   **Other tetanus**
     Tetanus NOS

     | **Excludes1** | tetanus neonatorum (A33)
               obstetrical tetanus (A34)

● **A36**   **Diphtheria**

     A36.0   **Pharyngeal diphtheria**
         Diphtheritic membranous angina
         Tonsillar diphtheria

     A36.1   **Nasopharyngeal diphtheria**

     A36.2   **Laryngeal diphtheria**
         Diphtheritic laryngotracheitis

     A36.3   **Cutaneous diphtheria**
         | **Excludes2** | erythrasma (L08.1)

     ● **A36.8**   **Other diphtheria**
         A36.81   **Diphtheritic cardiomyopathy**
           Diphtheritic myocarditis
         A36.82   **Diphtheritic radiculomyelitis**
         A36.83   **Diphtheritic polyneuritis**
         A36.84   **Diphtheritic tubulo-interstitial nephropathy**
         A36.85   **Diphtheritic cystitis**
         A36.86   **Diphtheritic conjunctivitis**
         A36.89   **Other diphtheritic complications**
           Diphtheritic peritonitis

     A36.9   **Diphtheria, unspecified**

Item 1-7 Diptheria: A highly contagious bacterial disease that results in the formation of an adherent membrane in the throat that may lead to suffocation. In its most poisonous form, it attacks the heart and lungs. It is spread by direct physical contact or breathing the aerosolized secretions of infected individuals. The exact location is specified in the codes.

CHAPTER 1 (A00-B99)

◀ New   ◀ Revised   ~~deleted~~ Deleted   **OGCR** Official Guidelines   X Assign placeholder X   ● Use Additional Character(s)

| Excludes 1 | | Excludes 2 | | Includes | | Use additional | | Code first | | Code also | | Unspecified |

● **A37** **Whooping cough**
    Pertussis is a highly contagious disease caused by the bacterium
    Bordetella pertussis and results in a whooping sounding cough.

  ● **A37.0** **Whooping cough due to Bordetella pertussis**
    A37.00 Whooping cough due to Bordetella pertussis without pneumonia
    A37.01 Whooping cough due to Bordetella pertussis with pneumonia

  ● **A37.1** **Whooping cough due to Bordetella parapertussis**
    A37.10 Whooping cough due to Bordetella parapertussis without pneumonia
    A37.11 Whooping cough due to Bordetella parapertussis with pneumonia

  ● **A37.8** **Whooping cough due to other Bordetella species**
    A37.80 Whooping cough due to other Bordetella species without pneumonia
    A37.81 Whooping cough due to other Bordetella species with pneumonia

  ● **A37.9** **Whooping cough, unspecified species**
    A37.90 Whooping cough, unspecified species without pneumonia
    A37.91 Whooping cough, unspecified species with pneumonia

● **A38** **Scarlet fever**
    Most commonly caused by the bacteria Streptococcus pneumoniae and
    Neisseria meningitides

    Includes scarlatina
    Excludes2 streptococcal sore throat (J02.0)

  A38.0 **Scarlet fever with otitis media**
  A38.1 **Scarlet fever with myocarditis**
  A38.8 **Scarlet fever with other complications**
  A38.9 **Scarlet fever, uncomplicated**
    Scarlet fever, NOS

● **A39** **Meningococcal infection**
    Most commonly caused by the bacteria Streptococcus pneumoniae and
    Neisseria meningitides

  A39.0 **Meningococcal meningitis**
  A39.1 **Waterhouse-Friderichsen syndrome**
    Fulminating complication of meningococcemia
    Meningococcal hemorrhagic adrenalitis
    Meningococcic adrenal syndrome

  A39.2 **Acute meningococcemia**
  A39.3 **Chronic meningococcemia**
  A39.4 **Meningococcemia, unspecified**

  ● **A39.5** **Meningococcal heart disease**
    A39.50 Meningococcal carditis, unspecified
    A39.51 Meningococcal endocarditis
    A39.52 Meningococcal myocarditis
    A39.53 Meningococcal pericarditis

  ● **A39.8** **Other meningococcal infections**
    A39.81 Meningococcal encephalitis
    A39.82 Meningococcal retrobulbar neuritis
      Optic neuritis in portion of optic nerve posterior to
      eyeball; AKA postocular optic neuritis
    A39.83 Meningococcal arthritis
    A39.84 Postmeningococcal arthritis
    A39.89 Other meningococcal infections
      Meningococcal conjunctivitis

  A39.9 **Meningococcal infection, unspecified**
    Meningococcal disease NOS

● **A40** **Streptococcal sepsis**
    Code first
    postprocedural streptococcal sepsis (T81.4)
    streptococcal sepsis during labor (O75.3)
    streptococcal sepsis following abortion or ectopic or molar pregnancy (O03-O07, O08.0)
    streptococcal sepsis following immunization (T88.0)
    streptococcal sepsis following infusion, transfusion or therapeutic injection (T80.2-)
    Excludes1 neonatal (P36.0-P36.1)
      puerperal sepsis (O85)
      sepsis due to Streptococcus, group D (A41.81)

  A40.0 **Sepsis due to streptococcus, group A**
  A40.1 **Sepsis due to streptococcus, group B**
  A40.3 **Sepsis due to Streptococcus pneumoniae**
    Pneumococcal sepsis
  A40.8 **Other streptococcal sepsis**
  A40.9 **Streptococcal sepsis, unspecified**

● **A41** **Other sepsis**
    Code first
    postprocedural sepsis (T81.4)
    sepsis during labor (O75.3)
    sepsis following abortion, ectopic or molar pregnancy (O03-O07, O08.0)
    sepsis following immunization (T88.0)
    sepsis following infusion, transfusion or therapeutic injection (T80.2-)
    Excludes1 bacteremia NOS (R78.81)
      neonatal (P36.-)
      puerperal sepsis (O85)
      sepsis NOS (A41.9)
      streptococcal sepsis (A40.-)
    Excludes2 sepsis (due to) (in) actinomycotic (A42.7)
      sepsis (due to) (in) anthrax (A22.7)
      sepsis (due to) (in) candidal (B37.7)
      sepsis (due to) (in) Erysipelothrix (A26.7)
      sepsis (due to) (in) extraintestinal yersiniosis (A28.2)
      sepsis (due to) (in) gonococcal (A54.86)
      sepsis (due to) (in) herpesviral (B00.7)
      sepsis (due to) (in) listerial (A32.7)
      sepsis (due to) (in) melioidosis (A24.1)
      sepsis (due to) (in) meningococcal (A39.2-A39.4)
      sepsis (due to) (in) plague (A20.7)
      sepsis (due to) (in) tularemia (A21.7)
      toxic shock syndrome (A48.3)

  ● **A41.0** **Sepsis due to Staphylococcus aureus**
    A41.01 Sepsis due to Methicillin susceptible Staphylococcus aureus
      MSSA sepsis
      Staphylococcus aureus sepsis NOS
    A41.02 Sepsis due to Methicillin resistant Staphylococcus aureus

  A41.1 **Sepsis due to other specified staphylococcus**
    Coagulase negative staphylococcus sepsis
  A41.2 **Sepsis due to unspecified staphylococcus**
  A41.3 **Sepsis due to Hemophilus influenzae**
  A41.4 **Sepsis due to anaerobes**
    Excludes1 gas gangrene (A48.0)

  ● **A41.5** **Sepsis due to other Gram-negative organisms**
    A41.50 Gram-negative sepsis, unspecified
      Gram-negative sepsis NOS
    A41.51 Sepsis due to Escherichia coli [E. coli]
    A41.52 Sepsis due to Pseudomonas
      Pseudomonas aeruginosa
    A41.53 Sepsis due to Serratia
    A41.59 Other Gram-negative sepsis

◀ New   ◀▥ Revised   ~~deleted~~ Deleted   **OGCR** Official Guidelines   X Assign placeholder X   ● Use Additional Character(s)

Excludes 1   Excludes 2   Includes   Use additional   Code first   Code also   Unspecified

Item 1–8   Gas gangrene is a necrotizing subcutaneous infection that will cause tissue death. Patients with poor circulation (e.g., diabetes, peripheral nephropathy) will have low oxygen content in their tissues (hypoxia), which allows the Clostridium bacteria to flourish. Gas gangrene often occurs at the site of a surgical wound or trauma. Onset is sudden and dramatic. Treatment can include debridement, amputation, and/or hyperbaric oxygen treatments.

● **A41.8   Other specified sepsis**
     A41.81   Sepsis due to Enterococcus
     A41.89   Other specified sepsis
   A41.9   Sepsis, unspecified organism
       Septicemia NOS

● **A42   Actinomycosis**
     Excludes1   actinomycetoma (B47.1)
   A42.0   Pulmonary actinomycosis
   A42.1   Abdominal actinomycosis
   A42.2   Cervicofacial actinomycosis
   A42.7   Actinomycotic sepsis
● **A42.8   Other forms of actinomycosis**
     A42.81   Actinomycotic meningitis
     A42.82   Actinomycotic encephalitis
     A42.89   Other forms of actinomycosis
   A42.9   Actinomycosis, unspecified

● **A43   Nocardiosis**
   A43.0   Pulmonary nocardiosis
   A43.1   Cutaneous nocardiosis
   A43.8   Other forms of nocardiosis
   A43.9   Nocardiosis, unspecified

● **A44   Bartonellosis**
   A44.0   Systemic bartonellosis
       Oroya fever
   A44.1   Cutaneous and mucocutaneous bartonellosis
       Verruga peruana
   A44.8   Other forms of bartonellosis
   A44.9   Bartonellosis, unspecified

   A46   Erysipelas
     Excludes1   postpartum or puerperal erysipelas (O86.89)

● **A48   Other bacterial diseases, not elsewhere classified**
     Excludes1   actinomycetoma (B47.1)
   A48.0   Gas gangrene
       Clostridial cellulitis
       Clostridial myonecrosis
   A48.1   Legionnaires' disease
   A48.2   Nonpneumonic Legionnaires' disease [Pontiac fever]
   A48.3   Toxic shock syndrome
       Use additional code to identify the organism (B95, B96)
     Excludes1   endotoxic shock NOS (R57.8)
                sepsis NOS (A41.9)
   A48.4   Brazilian purpuric fever
       Systemic Hemophilus aegyptius infection
● **A48.5   Other specified botulism**
       Non-foodborne intoxication due to toxins of
          Clostridium botulinum [C. botulinum]
     Excludes1   food poisoning due to toxins of
                Clostridium botulinum (A05.1)
     A48.51   Infant botulism
     A48.52   Wound botulism
         Non-foodborne botulism NOS
         Use additional code for associated wound
   A48.8   Other specified bacterial diseases

● **A49   Bacterial infection of unspecified site**
     Excludes1   bacterial agents as the cause of diseases classified
                elsewhere (B95-B96)
             chlamydial infection NOS (A74.9)
             meningococcal infection NOS (A39.9)
             rickettsial infection NOS (A79.9)
             spirochetal infection NOS (A69.9)
● **A49.0   Staphylococcal infection, unspecified site**
     A49.01   Methicillin susceptible Staphylococcus aureus infection, unspecified site
         Methicillin susceptible Staphylococcus aureus (MSSA) infection
         Staphylococcus aureus infection NOS
     A49.02   Methicillin resistant Staphylococcus aureus infection, unspecified site
         Methicillin resistant Staphylococcus aureus (MRSA) infection
   A49.1   Streptococcal infection, unspecified site
   A49.2   Hemophilus influenzae infection, unspecified site
       Any of seven bacterium of genus Haemophilus
   A49.3   Mycoplasma infection, unspecified site
       Bacterium of class Mollicutes, unusual group of bacteria distinguished by absence of cell wall
   A49.8   Other bacterial infections of unspecified site
   A49.9   Bacterial infection, unspecified
     Excludes1   bacteremia NOS (R78.81)

INFECTIONS WITH A PREDOMINANTLY SEXUAL MODE OF TRANSMISSION (A50-A64)

     Excludes1   human immunodeficiency virus [HIV] disease (B20)
                nonspecific and nongonococcal urethritis (N34.1)
                Reiter's disease (M02.3-)

● **A50   Congenital syphilis**
● **A50.0   Early congenital syphilis, symptomatic**
       Any congenital syphilitic condition specified as early or manifest less than two years after birth
     A50.01   Early congenital syphilitic oculopathy
     A50.02   Early congenital syphilitic osteochondropathy
     A50.03   Early congenital syphilitic pharyngitis
         Early congenital syphilitic laryngitis
     A50.04   Early congenital syphilitic pneumonia
     A50.05   Early congenital syphilitic rhinitis
     A50.06   Early cutaneous congenital syphilis
     A50.07   Early mucocutaneous congenital syphilis
     A50.08   Early visceral congenital syphilis
     A50.09   Other early congenital syphilis, symptomatic
   A50.1   Early congenital syphilis, latent
       Congenital syphilis without clinical manifestations, with positive serological reaction and negative spinal fluid test, less than two years after birth
   A50.2   Early congenital syphilis, unspecified
       Congenital syphilis NOS less than two years after birth
● **A50.3   Late congenital syphilitic oculopathy**
     Excludes1   Hutchinson's triad (A50.53)
     A50.30   Late congenital syphilitic oculopathy, unspecified
     A50.31   Late congenital syphilitic interstitial keratitis
     A50.32   Late congenital syphilitic chorioretinitis
     A50.39   Other late congenital syphilitic oculopathy

CHAPTER 1 (A00-B99)

Figure 1-3 Chancre of primary syphilis. (From Mandell, Bennett, & Dolin: Principles and Practice of Infectious Diseases, ed 7, Churchill Livingstone, An Imprint of Elsevier, 2009)

Item 1–9 Syphilis, also known as lues, is the most serious of the venereal diseases caused by *Treponema pallidum.* The **primary** stage is characterized by an ulceration known as **chancre,** which usually appears on the genitals but can also develop on the anus, lips, tonsils, breasts, or fingers. Syphilis is easy to cure in its early stages. A single intramuscular injection of penicillin will usually cure a person who has had syphilis for less than a year.

The **secondary** stage is characterized by a rash that can affect any area of the body. **Latent** syphilis is divided into **early,** which is diagnosed within two years of infection, and **late,** which is diagnosed two years or more after infection. Additional doses of penicillin or another antibiotic are needed to treat someone who has had syphilis for longer than a year. For those allergic to penicillin, there are other antibiotic treatments. **Congenital** syphilis is also labeled **early** or **late** based on the time of diagnosis.

- **A50.4 Late congenital neurosyphilis [juvenile neurosyphilis]**
  Use additional code to identify any associated mental disorder
  Excludes1   Hutchinson's triad (A50.53)
  - **A50.40 Late congenital neurosyphilis, unspecified**
    Juvenile neurosyphilis NOS
  - **A50.41 Late congenital syphilitic meningitis**
  - **A50.42 Late congenital syphilitic encephalitis**
  - **A50.43 Late congenital syphilitic polyneuropathy**
  - **A50.44 Late congenital syphilitic optic nerve atrophy**
  - **A50.45 Juvenile general paresis**
    Dementia paralytica juvenilis
    Juvenile tabetoparetic neurosyphilis
  - **A50.49 Other late congenital neurosyphilis**
    Juvenile tabes dorsalis
- **A50.5 Other late congenital syphilis, symptomatic**
  Any congenital syphilitic condition specified as late or manifest two years or more after birth
  - **A50.51 Clutton's joints**
  - **A50.52 Hutchinson's teeth**
  - **A50.53 Hutchinson's triad**
  - **A50.54 Late congenital cardiovascular syphilis**
  - **A50.55 Late congenital syphilitic arthropathy**
  - **A50.56 Late congenital syphilitic osteochondropathy**
  - **A50.57 Syphilitic saddle nose**
  - **A50.59 Other late congenital syphilis, symptomatic**
- **A50.6 Late congenital syphilis, latent**
  Congenital syphilis without clinical manifestations, with positive serological reaction and negative spinal fluid test, two years or more after birth.
- **A50.7 Late congenital syphilis, unspecified**
  Congenital syphilis NOS two years or more after birth.
- **A50.9 Congenital syphilis, unspecified**
- **A51 Early syphilis**
  - **A51.0 Primary genital syphilis**
    Syphilitic chancre NOS
  - **A51.1 Primary anal syphilis**
  - **A51.2 Primary syphilis of other sites**
  - **A51.3 Secondary syphilis of skin and mucous membranes**
    - **A51.31 Condyloma latum**
    - **A51.32 Syphilitic alopecia**
    - **A51.39 Other secondary syphilis of skin**
      Syphilitic leukoderma
      Syphilitic mucous patch
      Excludes1   late syphilitic leukoderma (A52.79)

- **A51.4 Other secondary syphilis**
  - **A51.41 Secondary syphilitic meningitis**
  - **A51.42 Secondary syphilitic female pelvic disease**
  - **A51.43 Secondary syphilitic oculopathy**
    Secondary syphilitic chorioretinitis
    Secondary syphilitic iridocyclitis, iritis
    Secondary syphilitic uveitis
  - **A51.44 Secondary syphilitic nephritis**
  - **A51.45 Secondary syphilitic hepatitis**
  - **A51.46 Secondary syphilitic osteopathy**
  - **A51.49 Other secondary syphilitic conditions**
    Secondary syphilitic lymphadenopathy
    Secondary syphilitic myositis
- **A51.5 Early syphilis, latent**
  Syphilis (acquired) without clinical manifestations, with positive serological reaction and negative spinal fluid test, less than two years after infection.
- **A51.9 Early syphilis, unspecified**
- **A52 Late syphilis**
  - **A52.0 Cardiovascular and cerebrovascular syphilis**
    - **A52.00 Cardiovascular syphilis, unspecified**
    - **A52.01 Syphilitic aneurysm of aorta**
    - **A52.02 Syphilitic aortitis**
    - **A52.03 Syphilitic endocarditis**
      Syphilitic aortic valve incompetence or stenosis
      Syphilitic mitral valve stenosis
      Syphilitic pulmonary valve regurgitation
    - **A52.04 Syphilitic cerebral arteritis**
    - **A52.05 Other cerebrovascular syphilis**
      Syphilitic cerebral aneurysm (ruptured) (non-ruptured)
      Syphilitic cerebral thrombosis
    - **A52.06 Other syphilitic heart involvement**
      Syphilitic coronary artery disease
      Syphilitic myocarditis
      Syphilitic pericarditis
    - **A52.09 Other cardiovascular syphilis**
  - **A52.1 Symptomatic neurosyphilis**
    - **A52.10 Symptomatic neurosyphilis, unspecified**
    - **A52.11 Tabes dorsalis**
      Cognitive decline with progressive degeneration of posterior columns, roots, and ganglia of spinal cord, occur 15-20 years after initial infection of syphilis; AKA Duchenne disease
      Locomotor ataxia (progressive)
      Tabetic neurosyphilis
    - **A52.12 Other cerebrospinal syphilis**
    - **A52.13 Late syphilitic meningitis**
    - **A52.14 Late syphilitic encephalitis**
    - **A52.15 Late syphilitic neuropathy**
      Late syphilitic acoustic neuritis
      Late syphilitic optic (nerve) atrophy
      Late syphilitic polyneuropathy
      Late syphilitic retrobulbar neuritis
    - **A52.16 Charcôt's arthropathy (tabetic)**
      Progressive musculoskeletal condition characterized by joint dislocation, fractures, and deformities, results in progressive destruction of bone and soft tissue of weight-bearing joints
    - **A52.17 General paresis**
      Chronic meningoencephalitis results in loss of cortical function, or progressive dementia and generalized paralysis, occurring 10-20 years after initial infection of syphilis; AKA Bayle disease, dementia paralytica, paralytic dementiaparetic neurosyphilis, syphilitic meningoencephalitis
      Dementia paralytica
    - **A52.19 Other symptomatic neurosyphilis**
      Syphilitic parkinsonism

◀ New   ◀▥ Revised   ~~deleted~~ Deleted   OGCR Official Guidelines   X Assign placeholder X   ● Use Additional Character(s)

| Excludes 1 | Excludes 2 | Includes | Use additional | Code first | Code also | Unspecified |

A52.2 **Asymptomatic neurosyphilis**

A52.3 **Neurosyphilis, unspecified**
  Gumma (syphilitic)
  Destructive lesions of syphilis
  Syphilis (late)
  Syphiloma

● A52.7 **Other symptomatic late syphilis**

    A52.71 **Late syphilitic oculopathy**
  Late syphilitic chorioretinitis
  Late syphilitic episcleritis

    A52.72 **Syphilis of lung and bronchus**

    A52.73 **Symptomatic late syphilis of other respiratory organs**

    A52.74 **Syphilis of liver and other viscera**
  Late syphilitic peritonitis

    A52.75 **Syphilis of kidney and ureter**
  Syphilitic glomerular disease

    A52.76 **Other genitourinary symptomatic late syphilis**
  Late syphilitic female pelvic inflammatory disease

    A52.77 **Syphilis of bone and joint**

    A52.78 **Syphilis of other musculoskeletal tissue**
  Late syphilitic bursitis
  Syphilis [stage unspecified] of bursa
  Syphilis [stage unspecified] of muscle
  Syphilis [stage unspecified] of synovium
  Syphilis [stage unspecified] of tendon

    A52.79 **Other symptomatic late syphilis**
  Late syphilitic leukoderma
  Syphilis of adrenal gland
  Syphilis of pituitary gland
  Syphilis of thyroid gland
  Syphilitic splenomegaly
  Excludes1 syphilitic leukoderma (secondary) (A51.39)

A52.8 **Late syphilis, latent**
  Syphilis (acquired) without clinical manifestations, with positive serological reaction and negative spinal fluid test, two years or more after infection

A52.9 **Late syphilis, unspecified**

● A53 **Other and unspecified syphilis**

  A53.0 **Latent syphilis, unspecified as early or late**
  Latent syphilis NOS
  Positive serological reaction for syphilis

  A53.9 **Syphilis, unspecified**
  Infection due to Treponema pallidum NOS
  Syphilis (acquired) NOS
  Excludes1 syphilis NOS under two years of age (A50.2)

● A54 **Gonococcal infection**

  ● A54.0 **Gonococcal infection of lower genitourinary tract without periurethral or accessory gland abscess**
  Excludes1 gonococcal infection with genitourinary gland abscess (A54.1)
  gonococcal infection with periurethral abscess (A54.1)

    A54.00 **Gonococcal infection of lower genitourinary tract, unspecified**

    A54.01 **Gonococcal cystitis and urethritis, unspecified**

    A54.02 **Gonococcal vulvovaginitis, unspecified**

    A54.03 **Gonococcal cervicitis, unspecified**

    A54.09 **Other gonococcal infection of lower genitourinary tract**

  A54.1 **Gonococcal infection of lower genitourinary tract with periurethral and accessory gland abscess**
  Gonococcal Bartholin's gland abscess

Item 1-10 An STD (sexually transmitted disease) caused by **Neisseria gonorrhoeae** that flourishes in the warm, moist areas of the reproductive tract. Untreated gonorrhea spreads to other parts of the body, causing inflammation of the testes or prostate or pelvic inflammatory disease (PID).

● A54.2 **Gonococcal pelviperitonitis and other gonococcal genitourinary infection**

    A54.21 **Gonococcal infection of kidney and ureter**

    A54.22 **Gonococcal prostatitis**

    A54.23 **Gonococcal infection of other male genital organs**
  Gonococcal epididymitis
  Gonococcal orchitis

    A54.24 **Gonococcal female pelvic inflammatory disease**
  Gonococcal pelviperitonitis
  Excludes1 gonococcal peritonitis (A54.85)

    A54.29 **Other gonococcal genitourinary infections**

● A54.3 **Gonococcal infection of eye**

    A54.30 **Gonococcal infection of eye, unspecified**

    A54.31 **Gonococcal conjunctivitis**
  Form of bacterial conjunctivitis contracted by newborns during delivery; AKA neonatal conjunctivitis
  Ophthalmia neonatorum due to gonococcus

    A54.32 **Gonococcal iridocyclitis**
  Inflammation of iris and of ciliary body due to gonococcal infection

    A54.33 **Gonococcal keratitis**
  Inflammation of cornea due to gonococcal infection; AKA keratoconjunctivitis, keratopathy

    A54.39 **Other gonococcal eye infection**
  Gonococcal endophthalmia

● A54.4 **Gonococcal infection of musculoskeletal system**

    A54.40 **Gonococcal infection of musculoskeletal system, unspecified**

    A54.41 **Gonococcal spondylopathy**
  Disorder of vertebrae due to gonococcal infection; AKA rachiopathy

    A54.42 **Gonococcal arthritis**
  Excludes2 gonococcal infection of spine (A54.41)

    A54.43 **Gonococcal osteomyelitis**
  Excludes2 gonococcal infection of spine (A54.41)

    A54.49 **Gonococcal infection of other musculoskeletal tissue**
  Gonococcal bursitis
  Gonococcal myositis
  Gonococcal synovitis
  Gonococcal tenosynovitis

  A54.5 **Gonococcal pharyngitis**

  A54.6 **Gonococcal infection of anus and rectum**

● A54.8 **Other gonococcal infections**

    A54.81 **Gonococcal meningitis**

    A54.82 **Gonococcal brain abscess**

    A54.83 **Gonococcal heart infection**
  Gonococcal endocarditis
  Gonococcal myocarditis
  Gonococcal pericarditis

    A54.84 **Gonococcal pneumonia**

    A54.85 **Gonococcal peritonitis**
  Excludes1 gonococcal pelviperitonitis (A54.24)

    A54.86 **Gonococcal sepsis**

    A54.89 **Other gonococcal infections**
  Gonococcal keratoderma
  Gonococcal lymphadenitis

  A54.9 **Gonococcal infection, unspecified**

◀ New   ◀◀ Revised   ~~deleted~~ Deleted   **OGCR** Official Guidelines   X Assign placeholder X   ● Use Additional Character(s)

| Excludes 1 | Excludes 2 | Includes | Use additional | Code first | Code also | Unspecified |

A55   Chlamydial lymphogranuloma (venereum)
      Climatic or tropical bubo
      Durand-Nicolas-Favre disease
      Esthiomene
      Lymphogranuloma inguinale

● **A56   Other sexually transmitted chlamydial diseases**
     Includes   sexually transmitted diseases due to Chlamydia trachomatis
     Excludes1   neonatal chlamydial conjunctivitis (P39.1)
                   neonatal chlamydial pneumonia (P23.1)
     Excludes2   chlamydial lymphogranuloma (A55)
                   conditions classified to A74.-

  ● **A56.0   Chlamydial infection of lower genitourinary tract**
       A56.00   Chlamydial infection of lower genitourinary tract, unspecified
       A56.01   Chlamydial cystitis and urethritis
       A56.02   Chlamydial vulvovaginitis
       A56.09   Other chlamydial infection of lower genitourinary tract
                   Chlamydial cervicitis

  ● **A56.1   Chlamydial infection of pelviperitoneum and other genitourinary organs**
       A56.11   Chlamydial female pelvic inflammatory disease
       A56.19   Other chlamydial genitourinary infection
                   Chlamydial epididymitis
                   Chlamydial orchitis

     A56.2   Chlamydial infection of genitourinary tract, unspecified
     A56.3   Chlamydial infection of anus and rectum
     A56.4   Chlamydial infection of pharynx
     A56.8   Sexually transmitted chlamydial infection of other sites

A57   Chancroid
      Ulcus molle
      Sexually transmitted infection caused by bacteria, Haemophilus ducreyi

A58   Granuloma inguinale
      Chronic, progressive, ulcerative granulomatous disease
      Donovanosis

● **A59   Trichomoniasis**
     Excludes2   intestinal trichomoniasis (A07.8)
      A common STD caused by a parasite, Trichomonas vaginalis

  ● **A59.0   Urogenital trichomoniasis**
       A59.00   Urogenital trichomoniasis, unspecified
                   Fluor (vaginalis) due to Trichomonas
                   Leukorrhea (vaginalis) due to Trichomonas
       A59.01   Trichomonal vulvovaginitis
       A59.02   Trichomonal prostatitis
       A59.03   Trichomonal cystitis and urethritis
       A59.09   Other urogenital trichomoniasis
                   Common sexually transmitted disease (STD) caused by single-celled protozoan parasite; AKA trich
                   Trichomonas cervicitis

     A59.8   Trichomoniasis of other sites
     A59.9   Trichomoniasis, unspecified

● **A60   Anogenital herpesviral [herpes simplex] infections**
  ● **A60.0   Herpesviral infection of genitalia and urogenital tract**
       A60.00   Herpesviral infection of urogenital system, unspecified
       A60.01   Herpesviral infection of penis
       A60.02   Herpesviral infection of other male genital organs
       A60.03   Herpesviral cervicitis
       A60.04   Herpesviral vulvovaginitis
                   Herpesviral [herpes simplex] ulceration
                   Herpesviral [herpes simplex] vaginitis
                   Herpesviral [herpes simplex] vulvitis
       A60.09   Herpesviral infection of other urogenital tract

     A60.1   Herpesviral infection of perianal skin and rectum
     A60.9   Anogenital herpesviral infection, unspecified

● **A63   Other predominantly sexually transmitted diseases, not elsewhere classified**
     Excludes2   molluscum contagiosum (B08.1)
                   papilloma of cervix (D26.0)

     A63.0   Anogenital (venereal) warts
                   Anogenital warts due to (human) papillomavirus [HPV]
                   Condyloma acuminatum
     A63.8   Other specified predominantly sexually transmitted diseases

     A64   Unspecified sexually transmitted disease

OTHER SPIROCHETAL DISEASES (A65-A69)

     Excludes2   leptospirosis (A27.-)
                   syphilis (A50-A53)

A65   Nonvenereal syphilis
      Bejel
      Endemic syphilis
      Njovera

● **A66   Yaws**
      Endemic, infectious, tropical disease caused by spirochete, spread by direct contact; AKA frambesia, framboesia, frambesia tropica
     Includes   bouba
                   frambesia (tropica)
                   pian

     A66.0   Initial lesions of yaws
                   Chancre of yaws
                   Frambesia, initial or primary
                   Initial frambesial ulcer
                   Mother yaw

     A66.1   Multiple papillomata and wet crab yaws
                   Frambesioma
                   Pianoma
                   Plantar or palmar papilloma of yaws

     A66.2   Other early skin lesions of yaws
                   Cutaneous yaws, less than five years after infection
                   Early yaws (cutaneous)(macular)(maculopapular)(micropapular)(papular)
                   Frambeside of early yaws

     A66.3   Hyperkeratosis of yaws
                   Hypertrophy of stratum corneum of skin in which there are small, hard, verrucous scales
                   Ghoul hand
                   Hyperkeratosis, palmar or plantar (early) (late) due to yaws
                   Worm-eaten soles

CHAPTER 1 (A00-B99)

A66.4   Gummata and ulcers of yaws
Small, rubbery granuloma with necrotic center and inflamed characteristic of advanced stage of syphilis; AKA syphiloma
Gummatous frambeside
Nodular late yaws (ulcerated)

A66.5   Gangosa
Manifestation of yaws that develops in the soft palate and spreads eroding bone, cartilage, and soft tissue
Rhinopharyngitis mutilans

A66.6   Bone and joint lesions of yaws
Yaws ganglion
Yaws goundou
Yaws gumma, bone
Yaws gummatous osteitis or periostitis
Yaws hydrarthrosis
Yaws osteitis
Yaws periostitis (hypertrophic)

A66.7   Other manifestations of yaws
Juxta-articular nodules of yaws
Mucosal yaws

A66.8   Latent yaws
Yaws without clinical manifestations, with positive serology

A66.9   Yaws, unspecified

● **A67   Pinta [carate]**
Group of nonvenereal diseases caused by Treponema species

A67.0   Primary lesions of pinta
Chancre (primary) of pinta
Papule (primary) of pinta

A67.1   Intermediate lesions of pinta
Erythematous plaques of pinta
Hyperchromic lesions of pinta
Hyperkeratosis of pinta
Pintids

A67.2   Late lesions of pinta
Achromic skin lesions of pinta
Cicatricial skin lesions of pinta
Dyschromic skin lesions of pinta

A67.3   Mixed lesions of pinta
Achromic with hyperchromic skin lesions of pinta [carate]

A67.9   Pinta, unspecified

● **A68   Relapsing fevers**
Includes   recurrent fever
Excludes2   Lyme disease (A69.2-)

A68.0   Louse-borne relapsing fever
Relapsing fever due to Borrelia recurrentis

A68.1   Tick-borne relapsing fever
Relapsing fever due to any Borrelia species other than Borrelia recurrentis

A68.9   Relapsing fever, unspecified

● **A69   Other spirochetal infections**

A69.0   Necrotizing ulcerative stomatitis
Cancrum oris
Fusospirochetal gangrene
Noma
Stomatitis gangrenosa

A69.1   Other Vincent's infections
Fusospirochetal pharyngitis
Necrotizing ulcerative (acute) gingivitis
Necrotizing ulcerative (acute) gingivostomatitis
Spirochetal stomatitis
Trench mouth
Vincent's angina
Vincent's gingivitis

Item 1-11 Cancrum oris, also known as **noma** or **gangrenous stomatitis,** begins as an ulcer of the gingiva and results in a progressive gangrenous process.

● **A69.2   Lyme disease**
Erythema chronicum migrans due to Borrelia burgdorferi

A69.20   Lyme disease, unspecified

A69.21   Meningitis due to Lyme disease

A69.22   Other neurologic disorders in Lyme disease
Cranial neuritis
Meningoencephalitis
Polyneuropathy

A69.23   Arthritis due to Lyme disease

A69.29   Other conditions associated with Lyme disease
Myopericarditis due to Lyme disease

A69.8   Other specified spirochetal infections

A69.9   Spirochetal infection, unspecified

OTHER DISEASES CAUSED BY CHLAMYDIAE (A70-A74)

Excludes1   sexually transmitted chlamydial diseases (A55-A56)

A70   Chlamydia psittaci infections
Ornithosis
Parrot fever
Psittacosis

● **A71   Trachoma**
Excludes1   sequelae of trachoma (B94.0)

A71.0   Initial stage of trachoma
Trachoma dubium

A71.1   Active stage of trachoma
Granular conjunctivitis (trachomatous)
Trachomatous follicular conjunctivitis
Trachomatous pannus

A71.9   Trachoma, unspecified

● **A74   Other diseases caused by chlamydiae**
Excludes1   neonatal chlamydial conjunctivitis (P39.1)
neonatal chlamydial pneumonia (P23.1)
Reiter's disease (M02.3-)
sexually transmitted chlamydial diseases (A55-A56)
Excludes2   chlamydial pneumonia (J16.0)

A74.0   Chlamydial conjunctivitis
Paratrachoma

● **A74.8   Other chlamydial diseases**

A74.81   Chlamydial peritonitis

A74.89   Other chlamydial diseases

A74.9   Chlamydial infection, unspecified
Chlamydiosis NOS

RICKETTSIOSES (A75-A79)

● **A75   Typhus fever**
Excludes1   rickettsiosis due to Ehrlichia sennetsu (A79.81)

A75.0   Epidemic louse-borne typhus fever due to Rickettsia prowazekii
Organisms transmitted between humans via louse
Classical typhus (fever)
Epidemic (louse-borne) typhus

A75.1   Recrudescent typhus [Brill's disease]
Brill-Zinsser disease

A75.2   Typhus fever due to Rickettsia typhi
Murine (flea-borne) typhus

A75.3   Typhus fever due to Rickettsia tsutsugamushi
Scrub (mite-borne) typhus
Tsutsugamushi fever

A75.9   Typhus fever, unspecified
Typhus (fever) NOS

CHAPTER 1 (A00-B99)

Item 1–12   Rickettsioses are diseases spread from ticks, lice, fleas, or mites to humans.

    Typhus is spread to humans chiefly by the fleas of rats.

    Endemic identifies a disease as being present in low numbers of humans at all times, whereas **epidemic** identifies a disease as being present in high numbers of humans at a specific time. Morbidity (death) is higher in epidemic diseases.

    Brill's disease, also known as **Brill-Zinsser disease,** is spread from human to human by body lice and also from the lice of flying squirrels. **Scrub typhus** is spread in the same ways as Brill's disease.

    Malaria is spread to humans by mosquitoes.

● **A77   Spotted fever [tick-borne rickettsioses]**

    A77.0   Spotted fever due to Rickettsia rickettsii
        Rocky Mountain spotted fever
        Sao Paulo fever

    A77.1   Spotted fever due to Rickettsia conorii
        African tick typhus
        Boutonneuse fever
        India tick typhus
        Kenya tick typhus
        Marseilles fever
        Mediterranean tick fever

    A77.2   Spotted fever due to Rickettsia siberica
        North Asian tick fever
        Siberian tick typhus

    A77.3   Spotted fever due to Rickettsia australis
        Queensland tick typhus

●   **A77.4   Ehrlichiosis**
        Type of tick-borne fever caused by bacteria infection
        [Excludes1]   Rickettsiosis due to Ehrlichia sennetsu (A79.81)

        A77.40   Ehrlichiosis, unspecified
        A77.41   Ehrlichiosis chafeensis [E. chafeensis]
        A77.49   Other ehrlichiosis

    A77.8   Other spotted fevers

    A77.9   Spotted fever, unspecified
        Tick-borne typhus NOS

  A78   Q fever
        Infection due to Coxiella burnetii
        Nine Mile fever
        Quadrilateral fever

● **A79   Other rickettsioses**

    A79.0   Trench fever
        Quintan fever
        Wolhynian fever

    A79.1   Rickettsialpox due to Rickettsia akari
        Kew Garden fever
        Vesicular rickettsiosis

●   **A79.8   Other specified rickettsioses**
        A79.81   Rickettsiosis due to Ehrlichia sennetsu
        A79.89   Other specified rickettsioses

    A79.9   Rickettsiosis, unspecified
        Rickettsial infection NOS

VIRAL AND PRION INFECTIONS OF THE CENTRAL NERVOUS SYSTEM (A80-A89)

    [Excludes1]   postpolio syndrome (G14)
                sequelae of poliomyelitis (B91)
                sequelae of viral encephalitis (B94.1)

● **A80   Acute poliomyelitis**

    A80.0   Acute paralytic poliomyelitis, vaccine-associated
    A80.1   Acute paralytic poliomyelitis, wild virus, imported
    A80.2   Acute paralytic poliomyelitis, wild virus, indigenous
●   **A80.3   Acute paralytic poliomyelitis, other and unspecified**
        A80.30   Acute paralytic poliomyelitis, unspecified
        A80.39   Other acute paralytic poliomyelitis
    A80.4   Acute nonparalytic poliomyelitis
    A80.9   Acute poliomyelitis, unspecified

Item 1-13   Acute Poliomyelitis: Also called infantile paralysis and is caused by the poliovirus, which enters the body orally and infects the intestinal wall and then enters the blood stream and central nervous system, causing muscle weakness and paralysis. This disease has been nearly eradicated with the polio vaccine.

● **A81   Atypical virus infections of central nervous system**
    [Includes]   diseases of the central nervous system caused by prions

    [Use additional] code to identify:
    dementia with behavioral disturbance (F02.81)
    dementia without behavioral disturbance (F02.80)

●   **A81.0   Creutzfeldt-Jakob disease**
        A81.00   Creutzfeldt-Jakob disease, unspecified
            Jakob-Creutzfeldt disease, unspecified

        A81.01   Variant Creutzfeldt-Jakob disease
            vCJD

        A81.09   Other Creutzfeldt-Jakob disease
            CJD
            Familial Creutzfeldt-Jakob disease
            Iatrogenic Creutzfeldt-Jakob disease
            Sporadic Creutzfeldt-Jakob disease
            Subacute spongiform encephalopathy (with dementia)

    A81.1   Subacute sclerosing panencephalitis
        Type of viral encephalitis that causes parenchymatous lesions in gray and white matter of brain
        Dawson's inclusion body encephalitis
        Van Bogaert's sclerosing leukoencephalopathy

    A81.2   Progressive multifocal leukoencephalopathy
        Group of diseases affecting white matter of brain
        Multifocal leukoencephalopathy NOS

●   **A81.8   Other atypical virus infections of central nervous system**
        A81.81   Kuru
        A81.82   Gerstmann-Sträussler-Scheinker syndrome
            GSS syndrome
        A81.83   Fatal familial insomnia
            FFI
        A81.89   Other atypical virus infections of central nervous system

    A81.9   Atypical virus infection of central nervous system, unspecified
        Prion diseases of the central nervous system NOS

● **A82   Rabies**
    Viral disease affecting the central nervous system and transmitted from infected mammals to man.
    A82.0   Sylvatic rabies
    A82.1   Urban rabies
    A82.9   Rabies, unspecified

● **A83   Mosquito-borne viral encephalitis**
    Inflammation of the brain caused most commonly by Herpes Simplex virus.
    [Includes]   mosquito-borne viral meningoencephalitis
    [Excludes2]   Venezuelan equine encephalitis (A92.2)
                West Nile fever (A92.3-)
                West Nile virus (A92.3-)

    A83.0   Japanese encephalitis
    A83.1   Western equine encephalitis
    A83.2   Eastern equine encephalitis
    A83.3   St. Louis encephalitis
    A83.4   Australian encephalitis
        Kunjin virus disease
    A83.5   California encephalitis
        California meningoencephalitis
        La Crosse encephalitis

Item 1-14   **Encephalitis** is an inflammation of the brain most often caused by a virus but may also be caused by a bacteria and most commonly transmitted by a mosquito. **Myelitis** is an inflammation of the spinal cord that may disrupt CNS function. Untreated myelitis may rapidly lead to permanent damage to the spinal cord. **Encephalomyelitis** is a general term for an inflammation of the brain and spinal cord.

A83.6   Rocio virus disease
     Mosquito-borne virus

A83.8   Other mosquito-borne viral encephalitis

A83.9   Mosquito-borne viral encephalitis, unspecified

● **A84   Tick-borne viral encephalitis**
> **Includes**   tick-borne viral meningoencephalitis

A84.0   Far Eastern tick-borne encephalitis [Russian spring-summer encephalitis]

A84.1   Central European tick-borne encephalitis

A84.8   Other tick-borne viral encephalitis
     Louping ill
     Powassan virus disease

A84.9   Tick-borne viral encephalitis, unspecified

● **A85   Other viral encephalitis, not elsewhere classified**
> **Includes**   specified viral encephalomyelitis NEC
>   specified viral meningoencephalitis NEC
>
> **Excludes1**   benign myalgic encephalomyelitis (G93.3)
>   encephalitis due to cytomegalovirus (B25.8)
>   encephalitis due to herpesvirus NEC (B10.0-)
>   encephalitis due to herpesvirus [herpes simplex] (B00.4)
>   encephalitis due to measles virus (B05.0)
>   encephalitis due to mumps virus (B26.2)
>   encephalitis due to poliomyelitis virus (A80.-)
>   encephalitis due to zoster (B02.0)
>   lymphocytic choriomeningitis (A87.2)

A85.0   Enteroviral encephalitis
     Enteroviral encephalomyelitis

A85.1   Adenoviral encephalitis
     Adenoviral meningoencephalitis

A85.2   Arthropod-borne viral encephalitis, unspecified
> **Excludes1**   West nile virus with encephalitis (A92.31)

A85.8   Other specified viral encephalitis
     Encephalitis lethargica
     Von Economo-Cruchet disease

A86   Unspecified viral encephalitis
     Viral encephalomyelitis NOS
     Viral meningoencephalitis NOS

● **A87   Viral meningitis**
> **Excludes1**   meningitis due to herpesvirus [herpes simplex] (B00.3)
>   meningitis due to measles virus (B05.1)
>   meningitis due to mumps virus (B26.1)
>   meningitis due to poliomyelitis virus (A80.-)
>   meningitis due to zoster (B02.1)

A87.0   Enteroviral meningitis
     Group of common viruses responsible for the majority of viral meningitis
     Coxsackievirus meningitis
     Echovirus meningitis

A87.1   Adenoviral meningitis

A87.2   Lymphocytic choriomeningitis
     Lymphocytic meningoencephalitis

A87.8   Other viral meningitis

A87.9   Viral meningitis, unspecified

● **A88   Other viral infections of central nervous system, not elsewhere classified**
> **Excludes1**   viral encephalitis NOS (A86)
>   viral meningitis NOS (A87.9)

A88.0   Enteroviral exanthematous fever [Boston exanthem]
     Infectious skin eruption

A88.1   Epidemic vertigo

A88.8   Other specified viral infections of central nervous system

A89   Unspecified viral infection of central nervous system

ARTHROPOD-BORNE VIRAL FEVERS AND VIRAL HEMORRHAGIC FEVERS (A90-A99)

A90   Dengue fever [classical dengue]
     Acute, self-limited disease, characterized by fever, prostration, severe muscle pains, headache, rash, lymphadenopathy, and leukopenia, caused by dengue virus; AKA breakbone, dandy
> **Excludes1**   dengue hemorrhagic fever (A91)

A91   Dengue hemorrhagic fever
     Serious follow-up to regular dengue, with symptoms of hemorrhage

● **A92   Other mosquito-borne viral fevers**
> **Excludes1**   Ross River disease (B33.1)

A92.0   Chikungunya virus disease
     Transmitted by mosquitoes
     Chikungunya (hemorrhagic) fever

A92.1   O'nyong-nyong fever
     Acute, nonfatal febrile disease transmitted by mosquitoes, which clinically resembles dengue and chikungunya

A92.2   Venezuelan equine fever
     Venezuelan equine encephalitis
     Venezuelan equine encephalomyelitis virus disease

● **A92.3   West Nile virus infection**
     West Nile fever

   A92.30   West Nile virus infection, unspecified
       West Nile fever NOS
       West Nile fever without complications
       West Nile virus NOS

   A92.31   West Nile virus infection with encephalitis
       West Nile encephalitis
       West Nile encephalomyelitis

   A92.32   West Nile virus infection with other neurologic manifestation
       Use additional code to specify the neurologic manifestation

   A92.39   West Nile virus infection with other complications
       Use additional code to specify the other conditions

A92.4   Rift Valley fever

A92.8   Other specified mosquito-borne viral fevers

A92.9   Mosquito-borne viral fever, unspecified

● **A93   Other arthropod-borne viral fevers, not elsewhere classified**

A93.0   Oropouche virus disease
     Tropical viral infection
     Oropouche fever

A93.1   Sandfly fever
     Pappataci fever
     Phlebotomus fever

A93.2   Colorado tick fever

A93.8   Other specified arthropod-borne viral fevers
     Piry virus disease
     Vesicular stomatitis virus disease [Indiana fever]

A94   Unspecified arthropod-borne viral fever
     Arboviral fever NOS
     Arbovirus infection NOS

CHAPTER 1 (A00-B99)

● **A95** **Yellow fever**
Acute infectious disease transmitted by mosquitoes
    A95.0 **Sylvatic yellow fever**
        Jungle yellow fever
    A95.1 **Urban yellow fever**
    A95.9 **Yellow fever, unspecified**

● **A96** **Arenaviral hemorrhagic fever**
Virus that causes various hemorrhagic fevers
    A96.0 **Junin hemorrhagic fever**
        Argentinian hemorrhagic fever
    A96.1 **Machupo hemorrhagic fever**
        Transmitted by contact with infected rodents
        Bolivian hemorrhagic fever
    A96.2 **Lassa fever**
        Acute type of hemorrhagic fever caused by contact with
        disease carrying mouse or person
    A96.8 **Other arenaviral hemorrhagic fevers**
    A96.9 **Arenaviral hemorrhagic fever, unspecified**

● **A98** **Other viral hemorrhagic fevers, not elsewhere classified**
    Excludes1 chikungunya hemorrhagic fever (A92.0)
                dengue hemorrhagic fever (A91)
    A98.0 **Crimean-Congo hemorrhagic fever**
        Virus transmitted by ticks and contact with blood, secretions,
        or fluids from infected humans or animals
        Central Asian hemorrhagic fever
    A98.1 **Omsk hemorrhagic fever**
        Transmitted to humans by bites of infected ticks or contact
        with infected muskrats
    A98.2 **Kyasanur Forest disease**
        Transmitted via infected monkeys, voles, ticks
    A98.3 **Marburg virus disease**
        Rare, acute, often fatal type of hemorrhagic fever
    A98.4 **Ebola virus disease**
    A98.5 **Hemorrhagic fever with renal syndrome**
        Epidemic hemorrhagic fever
        Korean hemorrhagic fever
        Russian hemorrhagic fever
        Hantaan virus disease
        Hantavirus disease with renal manifestations
        Nephropathia epidemica
        Songo fever
        Excludes1 hantavirus (cardio)-pulmonary syndrome
                    (B33.4)
    A98.8 **Other specified viral hemorrhagic fevers**

● **A99** **Unspecified viral hemorrhagic fever**

Figure 1-4 Primary herpes simplex in and around the mouth. The infection is usually acquired from siblings or parents and is readily transmitted to other direct contacts. (From Forbes, Jackson: Colour Atlas and Text of Clinical Medicine, International Edition, Mosby, 2002)

Item 1-15 Herpes is a viral disease for which there is no cure. There are two types of the herpes simplex virus: **Type I** causes **cold sores** or **fever blisters**, and **Type II** causes **genital herpes.** The virus can be spread from a sore on the lips to the genitals or from the genitals to the lips.

VIRAL INFECTIONS CHARACTERIZED BY SKIN AND MUCOUS MEMBRANE LESIONS (B00-B09)

● **B00 Herpesviral [herpes simplex] infections**

Excludes1	congenital herpesviral infections (P35.2)
Excludes2	anogenital herpesviral infection (A60.-)
	gammaherpesviral mononucleosis (B27.0-)
	herpangina (B08.5)

B00.0 Eczema herpeticum
  Cutaneous eruption caused by herpes simplex virus (HSV) type 1, HSV-2, coxsackievirus A16, or vaccinia virus
  Kaposi's varicelliform eruption

B00.1 Herpesviral vesicular dermatitis
  Vesicle formation; characteristics include formation of blisters and scabs on feet and legs
  Herpes simplex facialis
  Herpes simplex labialis
  Herpes simplex otitis externa
  Vesicular dermatitis of ear
  Vesicular dermatitis of lip

B00.2 Herpesviral gingivostomatitis and pharyngotonsillitis
  Inflammation involving both gingivae and oral mucosa
  Herpesviral pharyngitis
    Inflammation of pharynx and tonsils; AKA tonsillopharyngitis

B00.3 Herpesviral meningitis

B00.4 Herpesviral encephalitis
  Herpesviral meningoencephalitis
  Simian B disease

| Excludes1 | herpesviral encephalitis due to herpesvirus 6 and 7 (B10.01, B10.09) |
| | non-simplex herpesviral encephalitis (B10.0-) |

● **B00.5 Herpesviral ocular disease**
  B00.50 Herpesviral ocular disease, unspecified
  B00.51 Herpesviral iridocyclitis
    Herpesviral iritis
    Herpesviral uveitis, anterior
  B00.52 Herpesviral keratitis
    Herpesviral keratoconjunctivitis
  B00.53 Herpesviral conjunctivitis
  B00.59 Other herpesviral disease of eye
    Herpesviral dermatitis of eyelid

B00.7 Disseminated herpesviral disease
  Herpesviral sepsis

● **B00.8 Other forms of herpesviral infections**
  B00.81 Herpesviral hepatitis
  B00.82 Herpes simplex myelitis
  B00.89 Other herpesviral infection
    Herpesviral whitlow

B00.9 Herpesviral infection, unspecified
  Herpes simplex infection NOS

Item 1-16 Zoster: Also known as **shingles** and is caused by the same virus as chickenpox. After exposure, the virus lies dormant in nerve tissue and is activated by factors including aging, stress, suppression of the immune system, and certain medication. It begins as a unilateral rash that leads to blisters and sores on the skin. It may involve the nerve pathways of the eye, forehead, nose, and eyelids and may be very painful with long term systemic effects.

● **B01 Varicella [chickenpox]**
  Very contagious disease caused by the varicella zoster virus that results in an itchy outbreak of skin blisters (varicella). The same virus causes shingles (zoster).

  B01.0 Varicella meningitis
  ● **B01.1 Varicella encephalitis, myelitis and encephalomyelitis**
    Postchickenpox encephalitis, myelitis and encephalomyelitis
    B01.11 Varicella encephalitis and encephalomyelitis
      Postchickenpox encephalitis and encephalomyelitis
    B01.12 Varicella myelitis
      Postchickenpox myelitis
  B01.2 Varicella pneumonia
  ● **B01.8 Varicella with other complications**
    B01.81 Varicella keratitis
    B01.89 Other varicella complications
  B01.9 Varicella without complication
    Varicella NOS

● **B02 Zoster [herpes zoster]**

| Includes | shingles |
| | zona |

  B02.0 Zoster encephalitis
    Zoster meningoencephalitis
  B02.1 Zoster meningitis
  ● **B02.2 Zoster with other nervous system involvement**
    B02.21 Postherpetic geniculate ganglionitis
    B02.22 Postherpetic trigeminal neuralgia
    B02.23 Postherpetic polyneuropathy
    B02.24 Postherpetic myelitis
      Herpes zoster myelitis
    B02.29 Other postherpetic nervous system involvement
      Postherpetic radiculopathy
  ● **B02.3 Zoster ocular disease**
    B02.30 Zoster ocular disease, unspecified
    B02.31 Zoster conjunctivitis
    B02.32 Zoster iridocyclitis
    B02.33 Zoster keratitis
      Herpes zoster keratoconjunctivitis
    B02.34 Zoster scleritis
    B02.39 Other herpes zoster eye disease
      Zoster blepharitis
  B02.7 Disseminated zoster
  B02.8 Zoster with other complications
    Herpes zoster otitis externa
  B02.9 Zoster without complications
    Zoster NOS

Figure 1-5 Photograph of eyelids with marginal blepharitis. (From Mandell, Bennett, & Dolin: Principles and Practice of Infectious Diseases, ed 7, Churchill Livingstone, An Imprint of Elsevier, 2009)

Item 1-17 Blepharitis is a common condition in which the eyelid is swollen and yellow scaling and conjunctivitis develop. Usually the hair on the scalp and brow is involved.

◀ New   ◀◀◀ Revised   ~~deleted~~ Deleted   OGCR Official Guidelines   X Assign placeholder X   ● Use Additional Character(s)
Excludes 1   Excludes 2   Includes   Use additional   Code first   Code also   Unspecified
723

CHAPTER 1 (A00-B99)

B03 **Smallpox**
> **Note:** In 1980 the 33rd World Health Assembly declared that smallpox had been eradicated. The classification is maintained for surveillance purposes.

B04 **Monkeypox**
> *Disease occurring in captive monkeys and other mammals that may be transmitted to humans, clinically similar to smallpox*

● B05 **Measles**
> **Includes**   morbilli
> **Excludes1**   subacute sclerosing panencephalitis (A81.1)

B05.0 **Measles complicated by encephalitis**
   Postmeasles encephalitis

B05.1 **Measles complicated by meningitis**
   Postmeasles meningitis

B05.2 **Measles complicated by pneumonia**
   Postmeasles pneumonia

B05.3 **Measles complicated by otitis media**
   Postmeasles otitis media

B05.4 **Measles with intestinal complications**

● B05.8 **Measles with other complications**

   B05.81 **Measles keratitis and keratoconjunctivitis**

   B05.89 **Other measles complications**

B05.9 **Measles without complication**
   Measles NOS

● B06 **Rubella [German measles]**
> **Excludes1**   congenital rubella (P35.0)

● B06.0 **Rubella with neurological complications**

   B06.00 **Rubella with neurological complication, unspecified**

   B06.01 **Rubella encephalitis**
      Rubella meningoencephalitis

   B06.02 **Rubella meningitis**

   B06.09 **Other neurological complications of rubella**

● B06.8 **Rubella with other complications**

   B06.81 **Rubella pneumonia**

   B06.82 **Rubella arthritis**

   B06.89 **Other rubella complications**

B06.9 **Rubella without complication**
   Rubella NOS

● B07 **Viral warts**
> **Includes**   verruca simplex
>   verruca vulgaris
>   viral warts due to human papillomavirus
> **Excludes2**   anogenital (venereal) warts (A63.0)
>   papilloma of bladder (D41.4)
>   papilloma of cervix (D26.0)
>   papilloma larynx (D14.1)

B07.0 **Plantar wart**
   Verruca plantaris

B07.8 **Other viral warts**
   Common wart
   Flat wart
   Verruca plana

B07.9 **Viral wart, unspecified**

● B08 **Other viral infections characterized by skin and mucous membrane lesions, not elsewhere classified**
> **Excludes1**   vesicular stomatitis virus disease (A93.8)

● B08.0 **Other orthopoxvirus infections**
> **Excludes2**   monkeypox (B04)

   ● B08.01 **Cowpox and vaccinia not from vaccine**

      B08.010 **Cowpox**

      B08.011 **Vaccinia not from vaccine**
> **Excludes1**   vaccinia (from vaccination) (generalized) (T88.1)

   B08.02 **Orf virus disease**
      Contagious pustular dermatitis
      Ecthyma contagiosum

   B08.03 **Pseudocowpox [milker's node]**

   B08.04 **Paravaccinia, unspecified**

   B08.09 **Other orthopoxvirus infections**
      Orthopoxvirus infection NOS

B08.1 **Molluscum contagiosum**
   Various skin diseases characterized by soft, rounded, cutaneous lesions

● B08.2 **Exanthema subitum [sixth disease] Roseola infantum**
   Acute, short-lived high fever in infants and young children followed by a rash mainly on the trunk, caused by human herpesvirus 6

   B08.20 **Exanthema subitum [sixth disease], unspecified Roseola infantum, unspecified**

   B08.21 **Exanthema subitum [sixth disease] due to human herpesvirus 6 Roseola infantum due to human herpesvirus 6**
      Virus results in sudden rash; infection results in lifelong persistence

   B08.22 **Exanthema subitum [sixth disease] due to human herpesvirus 7 Roseola infantum due to human herpesvirus 7**

B08.3 **Erythema infectiosum [fifth disease]**
   Moderately contagious, epidemic disease in children caused by B19 virus; onset of rash that begins as redness of cheeks, later there is rash on trunk and limbs; when this fades, there may be central clearing that leaves lacelike pattern

B08.4 **Enteroviral vesicular stomatitis with exanthem**
   Hand, foot and mouth disease
   Check your documentation—this code is HAND, foot, and mouth disease. Code B08.8 is foot and mouth disease.

B08.5 **Enteroviral vesicular pharyngitis**
   Herpangina

● B08.6 **Parapoxvirus infections**

   B08.60 **Parapoxvirus infection, unspecified**

   B08.61 **Bovine stomatitis**

   B08.62 **Sealpox**

   B08.69 **Other parapoxvirus infections**

● B08.7 **Yatapoxvirus infections**

   B08.70 **Yatapoxvirus infection, unspecified**

   B08.71 **Tanapox virus disease**

   B08.72 **Yaba pox virus disease**
      Yaba monkey tumor disease

   B08.79 **Other yatapoxvirus infections**

B08.8 **Other specified viral infections characterized by skin and mucous membrane lesions**
   Enteroviral lymphonodular pharyngitis
   Foot-and-mouth disease
   Check your documentation. Code B08.4 is for HAND, foot, and mouth disease.
   Poxvirus NEC

B09 **Unspecified viral infection characterized by skin and mucous membrane lesions**
   Viral enanthema NOS
   Viral exanthema NOS

◀ New   ◀▥ Revised   ~~deleted~~ Deleted   OGCR Official Guidelines   X Assign placeholder X   ● Use Additional Character(s)

Excludes 1   Excludes 2   Includes   Use additional   Code first   Code also   Unspecified

OTHER HUMAN HERPESVIRUSES (B10)

● **B10   Other human herpesviruses**

Excludes2   cytomegalovirus (B25.9)
Epstein-Barr virus (B27.0-)
herpes NOS (B00.9)
herpes simplex (B00.-)
herpes zoster (B02.-)
human herpesvirus NOS (B00.-)
human herpesvirus 1 and 2 (B00.-)
human herpesvirus 3 (B01.-, B02.-)
human herpesvirus 4 (B27.0-)
human herpesvirus 5 (B25.-)
varicella (B01.-)
zoster (B02.-)

● **B10.0   Other human herpesvirus encephalitis**

Excludes2   herpes encephalitis NOS (B00.4)
herpes simplex encephalitis (B00.4)
human herpesvirus encephalitis (B00.4)
simian B herpes virus encephalitis (B00.4)

B10.01   Human herpesvirus 6 encephalitis
Sudden rash or roseola

B10.09   Other human herpesvirus encephalitis
Human herpesvirus 7 encephalitis
Virus closely related to human herpesvirus 6, but not known to cause any disease

● **B10.8   Other human herpesvirus infection**

B10.81   Human herpesvirus 6 infection
Causative agent of exanthema subitum that results in sudden rash

B10.82   Human herpesvirus 7 infection
Closely related to human herpesvirus 6, but not known cause any disease

B10.89   Other human herpesvirus infection
Human herpesvirus 8 infection
May be the cause of Kaposi sarcoma, a malignant tumor
Kaposi's sarcoma-associated herpesvirus infection

VIRAL HEPATITIS (B15-B19)

Excludes1   sequelae of viral hepatitis (B94.2)
Excludes2   cytomegaloviral hepatitis (B25.1)
herpesviral [herpes simplex] hepatitis (B00.81)

● **B15   Acute hepatitis A**

B15.0   Hepatitis A with hepatic coma

B15.9   Hepatitis A without hepatic coma
Hepatitis A (acute) (viral) NOS

● **B16   Acute hepatitis B**

B16.0   Acute hepatitis B with delta-agent with hepatic coma

B16.1   Acute hepatitis B with delta-agent without hepatic coma

B16.2   Acute hepatitis B without delta-agent with hepatic coma

B16.9   Acute hepatitis B without delta-agent and without hepatic coma
Hepatitis B (acute) (viral) NOS

● **B17   Other acute viral hepatitis**

B17.0   Acute delta-(super) infection of hepatitis B carrier

● **B17.1   Acute hepatitis C**

B17.10   Acute hepatitis C without hepatic coma
Acute hepatitis C NOS

B17.11   Acute hepatitis C with hepatic coma

B17.2   Acute hepatitis E

B17.8   Other specified acute viral hepatitis
Hepatitis non-A non-B (acute) (viral) NEC

B17.9   Acute viral hepatitis, unspecified
Acute hepatitis NOS

Figure 1-6   Hepatitis B viral infection. **A.** Liver parenchyma showing hepatocytes with diffuse granular cytoplasm, so-called ground glass hepatocytes (H&E). **B.** Immunoperoxidase stains from the same case, showing cytoplasmic inclusions of viral particles. (From Kumar: Robbins and Cotran: Pathologic Basis of Disease, ed 8, Saunders, An Imprint of Elsevier, 2009)

Item 1–18   Hepatitis A (HAV) was formerly called epidemic, infectious, short-incubation, or acute catarrhal jaundice hepatitis. The primary transmission mode is the oral–fecal route. **Hepatitis B (HBV)** was formerly called long-incubation period, serum, or homologous serum hepatitis. Transmission modes are through blood from infected persons and from body fluids of infected mother to neonate. **Hepatitis C (HCV),** caused by the hepatitis C virus, is primarily transfusion associated. **Hepatitis D (HDV),** also called delta hepatitis, is caused by the hepatitis D virus in patients formerly or currently infected with hepatitis B. **Hepatitis E (HEV)** is also called enterically transmitted non-A, non-B hepatitis. The primary transmission mode is the oral–fecal route, usually through contaminated water.

● **B18   Chronic viral hepatitis**

B18.0   Chronic viral hepatitis B with delta-agent

B18.1   Chronic viral hepatitis B without delta-agent
Chronic (viral) hepatitis B

B18.2   Chronic viral hepatitis C

B18.8   Other chronic viral hepatitis

B18.9   Chronic viral hepatitis, unspecified

● **B19   Unspecified viral hepatitis**

B19.0   Unspecified viral hepatitis with hepatic coma

● **B19.1   Unspecified viral hepatitis B**

B19.10   Unspecified viral hepatitis B without hepatic coma
Unspecified viral hepatitis B NOS

B19.11   Unspecified viral hepatitis B with hepatic coma

● **B19.2   Unspecified viral hepatitis C**

B19.20   Unspecified viral hepatitis C without hepatic coma
Viral hepatitis C NOS

B19.21   Unspecified viral hepatitis C with hepatic coma

B19.9   Unspecified viral hepatitis without hepatic coma
Viral hepatitis NOS

OGCR Section I. C.1.a

Certain Infectious and Parasitic Diseases (A00-B99)

a. Human Immunodeficiency Virus (HIV) Infections

1) Code only confirmed cases

Code only confirmed cases of HIV infection illness. This is an exception to the hospital inpatient guideline Section II, H.

In this context, "confirmation" does not require documentation of positive serology or culture for HIV; the provider's diagnostic statement that the patient is HIV positive, or has an HIV-related illness is sufficient.

Figure 1-7 Kaposi's sarcoma. There are large confluent hyperpigmented patch-stage lesions with lymphedema. (From Cohen & Powderly: Infectious Diseases, ed 3, Mosby, An Imprint of Elsevier, 2010)

Item 1-19 AIDS (acquired immune deficiency syndrome) is caused by **HIV** (human immunodeficiency virus). HIV affects certain white blood cells (T-4 lymphocytes) and destroys the ability of the cells to fight infections, making patients susceptible to a host of infectious diseases (e.g., **Pneumocystis carinii pneumonia (PCP)**, **Kaposi's sarcoma,** and **lymphoma**). **AIDS-related complex (ARC)** is an early stage of AIDS in which tests for HIV are positive but the symptoms are mild.

HUMAN IMMUNODEFICIENCY VIRUS [HIV] DISEASE (B20)

B20　Human immunodeficiency virus [HIV] disease

> **Includes**　acquired immune deficiency syndrome [AIDS]
> AIDS-related complex [ARC]
> HIV infection, symptomatic

> *Code first* Human immunodeficiency virus [HIV] disease complicating pregnancy, childbirth and the puerperium, if applicable (O98.7-)

> **Use additional** code(s) to identify all manifestations of HIV infection

> **Excludes1**　asymptomatic human immunodeficiency virus [HIV] infection status (Z21)
> exposure to HIV virus (Z20.6)
> inconclusive serologic evidence of HIV (R75)

OTHER VIRAL DISEASES (B25-B34)

● B25　Cytomegaloviral disease
　　AKA: HCMV or Human Herpesvirus 5 (HHV-5)

> **Excludes1**　congenital cytomegalovirus infection (P35.1)
> cytomegaloviral mononucleosis (B27.1-)

　B25.0　Cytomegaloviral pneumonitis

　B25.1　Cytomegaloviral hepatitis

　B25.2　Cytomegaloviral pancreatitis

　B25.8　Other cytomegaloviral diseases
　　　　Cytomegaloviral encephalitis

　B25.9　Cytomegaloviral disease, unspecified

● B26　Mumps

> **Includes**　epidemic parotitis
> infectious parotitis

　　Acute, contagious, viral disease

　B26.0　Mumps orchitis

　B26.1　Mumps meningitis

　B26.2　Mumps encephalitis

　B26.3　Mumps pancreatitis

● B26.8　Mumps with other complications

　　B26.81　Mumps hepatitis

　　B26.82　Mumps myocarditis

　　B26.83　Mumps nephritis

　　B26.84　Mumps polyneuropathy

　　B26.85　Mumps arthritis

　　B26.89　Other mumps complications

　B26.9　Mumps without complication
　　　　Mumps NOS
　　　　Mumps parotitis NOS

● B27　Infectious mononucleosis

> **Includes**　glandular fever
> monocytic angina
> Pfeiffer's disease

● B27.0　Gammaherpesviral mononucleosis
　　AKA: Pfeiffer's disease, infective mononucleosis
　　Mononucleosis due to Epstein-Barr virus

　　B27.00　Gammaherpesviral mononucleosis without complication
　　　　　Infective mononucleosis

　　B27.01　Gammaherpesviral mononucleosis with polyneuropathy

　　B27.02　Gammaherpesviral mononucleosis with meningitis

　　B27.09　Gammaherpesviral mononucleosis with other complications
　　　　　Hepatomegaly in gammaherpesviral mononucleosis

● B27.1　Cytomegaloviral mononucleosis
　　Infectious disease resembling infectious mononucleosis

　　B27.10　Cytomegaloviral mononucleosis without complications

　　B27.11　Cytomegaloviral mononucleosis with polyneuropathy

　　B27.12　Cytomegaloviral mononucleosis with meningitis

　　B27.19　Cytomegaloviral mononucleosis with other complication
　　　　　Hepatomegaly in cytomegaloviral mononucleosis

● B27.8　Other infectious mononucleosis

　　B27.80　Other infectious mononucleosis without complication

　　B27.81　Other infectious mononucleosis with polyneuropathy

　　B27.82　Other infectious mononucleosis with meningitis

　　B27.89　Other infectious mononucleosis with other complication
　　　　　Hepatomegaly in other infectious mononucleosis

● B27.9　Infectious mononucleosis, unspecified

　　B27.90　Infectious mononucleosis, unspecified without complication

　　B27.91　Infectious mononucleosis, unspecified with polyneuropathy

　　B27.92　Infectious mononucleosis, unspecified with meningitis

　　B27.99　Infectious mononucleosis, unspecified with other complication
　　　　　Hepatomegaly in unspecified infectious mononucleosis

● B30　Viral conjunctivitis

> **Excludes1**　herpesviral [herpes simplex] ocular disease (B00.5)
> ocular zoster (B02.3)

　B30.0　Keratoconjunctivitis due to adenovirus
　　　　Epidemic keratoconjunctivitis
　　　　Shipyard eye

　B30.1　Conjunctivitis due to adenovirus
　　　　Acute adenoviral follicular conjunctivitis
　　　　Swimming-pool conjunctivitis

◀ New　⬷ Revised　~~deleted~~ Deleted　OGCR Official Guidelines　X Assign placeholder X　● Use Additional Character(s)

Excludes 1　Excludes 2　Includes　Use additional　Code first　Code also　Unspecified

B30.2 **Viral pharyngoconjunctivitis**

B30.3 **Acute epidemic hemorrhagic conjunctivitis (enteroviral)**
Conjunctivitis due to coxsackievirus 24
Conjunctivitis due to enterovirus 70
Hemorrhagic conjunctivitis (acute)(epidemic)

B30.8 **Other viral conjunctivitis**
Newcastle conjunctivitis

B30.9 **Viral conjunctivitis, unspecified**

● B33 **Other viral diseases, not elsewhere classified**

B33.0 **Epidemic myalgia**
*Acute infectious disease, caused by group A coxsackie viruses
or other enteroviruses with symptoms that include
sudden pain in chest or upper abdomen with fever*
Bornholm disease

B33.1 **Ross River disease**
Epidemic polyarthritis and exanthema
Ross River fever

● B33.2 **Viral carditis**
Coxsackie (virus) carditis

B33.20 **Viral carditis, unspecified**

B33.21 **Viral endocarditis**

B33.22 **Viral myocarditis**

B33.23 **Viral pericarditis**

B33.24 **Viral cardiomyopathy**

B33.3 **Retrovirus infections, not elsewhere classified**
Retrovirus infection NOS

B33.4 **Hantavirus (cardio)-pulmonary syndrome [HPS] [HCPS]**
Hantavirus disease with pulmonary manifestations
Sin nombre virus disease

Use additional code to identify any associated acute
kidney failure (N17.9)

| Excludes1 | hantavirus disease with renal
manifestations (A98.5)
hemorrhagic fever with renal
manifestations (A98.5) |

B33.8 **Other specified viral diseases**

| Excludes1 | anogenital human papillomavirus
infection (A63.0)
viral warts due to human papillomavirus
infection (B07) |

● B34 **Viral infection of unspecified site**

| Excludes1 | anogenital human papillomavirus infection
(A63.0)
cytomegaloviral disease NOS (B25.9)
herpesvirus [herpes simplex] infection NOS
(B00.9)
retrovirus infection NOS (B33.3)
viral agents as the cause of diseases classified
elsewhere (B97.-)
viral warts due to human papillomavirus
infection (B07) |

B34.0 **Adenovirus infection, unspecified**

B34.1 **Enterovirus infection, unspecified**
Intestinal tract infection
Coxsackievirus infection NOS
Echovirus infection NOS

B34.2 **Coronavirus infection, unspecified**

| Excludes1 | pneumonia due to SARS-associated
coronavirus (J12.81) |

B34.3 **Parvovirus infection, unspecified**

B34.4 **Papovavirus infection, unspecified**

B34.8 **Other viral infections of unspecified site**

B34.9 **Viral infection, unspecified**
Viremia NOS

MYCOSES (B35-B49)

| Excludes2 | hypersensitivity pneumonitis due to organic dust
(J67.-)
mycosis fungoides (C84.0-) |

● B35 **Dermatophytosis**
AKA tinea or ringworm

| **Includes** | favus
infections due to species of Epidermophyton,
Micro-sporum and Trichophyton
tinea, any type except those in B36.- |

B35.0 **Tinea barbae and tinea capitis**
Beard ringworm
Kerion
Scalp ringworm
Sycosis, mycotic

B35.1 **Tinea unguium**
*White patches or pits on surface or edges of nails, followed by
infection under nail plate*
Dermatophytic onychia
Dermatophytosis of nail
Onychomycosis
Ringworm of nails

B35.2 **Tinea manuum**
Tinea of hands
Dermatophytosis of hand
Hand ringworm

B35.3 **Tinea pedis**
Tinea affecting feet
Athlete's foot
Dermatophytosis of foot
Foot ringworm

B35.4 **Tinea corporis**
Infecting skin areas other than hands
Ringworm of the body

B35.5 **Tinea imbricata**
*Chronic tropical tinea corporis; AKA Oriental ringworm,
tinea inguinalis, tinea cruris*
Tokelau

B35.6 **Tinea cruris**
*In groin or perineal area, spreading to adjacent regions; AKA
jock itch, eczema marginatum, ringworm of groin, or t
inguinalis*
Dhobi itch
Groin ringworm
Jock itch

B35.8 **Other dermatophytoses**
Disseminated dermatophytosis
Granulomatous dermatophytosis

B35.9 **Dermatophytosis, unspecified**
Ringworm NOS

● B36 **Other superficial mycoses**

B36.0 **Pityriasis versicolor**
*Common, chronic, symptomless disorder that includes
macular patches of various sizes and shapes; AKA liver
spots*
Tinea flava
Tinea versicolor

B36.1 **Tinea nigra**
*Minor fungal infection, with dark lesions, usually on skin of
hands*
Keratomycosis nigricans palmaris
Microsporosis nigra
Pityriasis nigra

B36.2 **White piedra**
*White to light brown nodules on hair of beard, axilla, or
groin; AKA trichosporosis*
Tinea blanca

B36.3 **Black piedra**
*Characterized by small black or brown nodules on shafts of
scalp hair*

B36.8 **Other specified superficial mycoses**

B36.9 **Superficial mycosis, unspecified**

◄ New ◄|||| Revised ~~deleted~~ Deleted OGCR Official Guidelines X Assign placeholder X ● Use Additional Character(s)

| Excludes 1 | Excludes 2 | Includes | Use additional | Code first | Code also | Unspecified |

Figure 1-8   Oral candidiasis (thrush). *(Courtesy of Stephen Raffanti, MD, MPH.)* (From Mandell, Bennett, & Dolin: Principles and Practice of Infectious Diseases, ed 7, Churchill Livingstone, An Imprint of Elsevier, 2009)

Item 1-20 Candidiasis, also called oidiomycosis or moniliasis, is a fungal infection. It most often appears on moist cutaneous areas of the body but can also be responsible for a variety of systemic infections such as endocarditis, meningitis, arthritis, and myositis. Antifungal medications cure most yeast infections.

● **B37 Candidiasis**

> **Includes**   candidosis
> moniliasis

> **Excludes1**   neonatal candidiasis (P37.5)

B37.0 Candidal stomatitis
Oral thrush

B37.1 Pulmonary candidiasis
Candidal bronchitis
Candidal pneumonia

B37.2 Candidiasis of skin and nail
Candidal onychia
Candidal paronychia

> **Excludes2**   diaper dermatitis (L22)

B37.3 Candidiasis of vulva and vagina
Candidal vulvovaginitis
Monilial vulvovaginitis
Vaginal thrush

● **B37.4 Candidiasis of other urogenital sites**

     B37.41 Candidal cystitis and urethritis

     B37.42 Candidal balanitis
        Male condition only

     B37.49 Other urogenital candidiasis
        Candidal pyelonephritis

B37.5 Candidal meningitis

B37.6 Candidal endocarditis

B37.7 Candidal sepsis
Disseminated candidiasis systemic candidiasis

● **B37.8 Candidiasis of other sites**

     B37.81 Candidal esophagitis

     B37.82 Candidal enteritis
        Candidal proctitis

     B37.83 Candidal cheilitis
        Inflammation affecting lip

     B37.84 Candidal otitis externa
        Inflammation of external auditory canal

     B37.89 Other sites of candidiasis
        Infection manifested by invasive candidiasis
        Candidal osteomyelitis

B37.9 Candidiasis, unspecified
Thrush NOS

● **B38 Coccidioidomycosis**
Fungal disease; AKA coccidioidosis, coccidioidal granuloma, Posadas, or Posadas-Wernicke disease

B38.0 Acute pulmonary coccidioidomycosis

B38.1 Chronic pulmonary coccidioidomycosis

B38.2 Pulmonary coccidioidomycosis, unspecified

B38.3 Cutaneous coccidioidomycosis

B38.4 Coccidioidomycosis meningitis

B38.7 Disseminated coccidioidomycosis
Generalized coccidioidomycosis

● **B38.8 Other forms of coccidioidomycosis**

     B38.81 Prostatic coccidioidomycosis

     B38.89 Other forms of coccidioidomycosis

B38.9 Coccidioidomycosis, unspecified

Item 1-21   Bird and bat droppings that fall into the soil give rise to a fungus that can spread airborne spores. When inhaled into the lungs, these spores divide and multiply into lesions. Histoplasmosis capsulatum takes three forms: primary (lodged in the lungs only), chronic (resembles TB), and disseminated (infection has moved to other organs). This is an opportunistic infection in immunosuppressed patients.

● **B39 Histoplasmosis**
Infection resulting from inhalation or ingestion of spores; AKA Darling disease

> **Code first** associated AIDS (B20)

> **Use additional** code for any associated manifestations, such as:
> endocarditis (I39)
> meningitis (G02)
> pericarditis (I32)
> retinitits (H32)

B39.0 Acute pulmonary histoplasmosis capsulati

B39.1 Chronic pulmonary histoplasmosis capsulati

B39.2 Pulmonary histoplasmosis capsulati, unspecified

B39.3 Disseminated histoplasmosis capsulati
Generalized histoplasmosis capsulati

B39.4 Histoplasmosis capsulati, unspecified
American histoplasmosis

B39.5 Histoplasmosis duboisii
African histoplasmosis

B39.9 Histoplasmosis, unspecified

● **B40 Blastomycosis**
Rare and potentially fatal infection caused by inhaling fungus found in moist soil in temperate climates.

> **Excludes1**   Brazilian blastomycosis (B41.-)
> keloidal blastomycosis (B48.0)

B40.0 Acute pulmonary blastomycosis

B40.1 Chronic pulmonary blastomycosis

B40.2 Pulmonary blastomycosis, unspecified

B40.3 Cutaneous blastomycosis

B40.7 Disseminated blastomycosis
Generalized blastomycosis

● **B40.8 Other forms of blastomycosis**

     B40.81 Blastomycotic meningoencephalitis
        Meningomyelitis due to blastomycosis

     B40.89 Other forms of blastomycosis

B40.9 Blastomycosis, unspecified

● **B41 Paracoccidioidomycosis**
Fungal infection usually chronic that begins in lungs, spreads to mucocutaneous areas which may extend to skin, tonsils, gastrointestinal lymphatics, liver, and spleen; AKA Almeida or Lutz-Splendore-Almeida disease, Brazilian or South American blastomycosis, or paracoccidioidal granuloma

> **Includes**   Brazilian blastomycosis
> Lutz' disease

B41.0 Pulmonary paracoccidioidomycosis

B41.7 Disseminated paracoccidioidomycosis
Generalized paracoccidioidomycosis

B41.8 Other forms of paracoccidioidomycosis

B41.9 Paracoccidioidomycosis, unspecified

● **B42 Sporotrichosis**
Chronic fungal infection with nodular lesions

B42.0 Pulmonary sporotrichosis

B42.1 Lymphocutaneous sporotrichosis

B42.7 Disseminated sporotrichosis
Generalized sporotrichosis

● **B42.8 Other forms of sporotrichosis**

     B42.81 Cerebral sporotrichosis
        Meningitis due to sporotrichosis

     B42.82 Sporotrichosis arthritis

     B42.89 Other forms of sporotrichosis

B42.9 Sporotrichosis, unspecified

● **B43**   **Chromomycosis and pheomycotic abscess**
Chronic fungal infection of skin, initiated at site of puncture affecting lower limb or foot (mossy foot)

     B43.0   **Cutaneous chromomycosis**
              Dermatitis verrucosa

     B43.1   **Pheomycotic brain abscess**
              Cerebral chromomycosis

     B43.2   **Subcutaneous pheomycotic abscess and cyst**

     B43.8   **Other forms of chromomycosis**

     B43.9   **Chromomycosis, unspecified**

● **B44**   **Aspergillosis**
Infection marked by inflammatory lesions in skin, ear, orbit, nasal sinuses, lungs, and occasionally bones and meninges

     Includes   aspergilloma

     B44.0   **Invasive pulmonary aspergillosis**

     B44.1   **Other pulmonary aspergillosis**

     B44.2   **Tonsillar aspergillosis**

     B44.7   **Disseminated aspergillosis**
              Generalized aspergillosis

   ● **B44.8**   **Other forms of aspergillosis**

         B44.81   **Allergic bronchopulmonary aspergillosis**

         B44.89   **Other forms of aspergillosis**

     B44.9   **Aspergillosis, unspecified**

● **B45**   **Cryptococcosis**
Infection in the immunocompromised and fatal if left untreated; AKA torulosis, Buschke, or Busse-Buschke disease

     B45.0   **Pulmonary cryptococcosis**

     B45.1   **Cerebral cryptococcosis**
              Cryptococcal meningitis
              Cryptococcosis meningocerebralis

     B45.2   **Cutaneous cryptococcosis**

     B45.3   **Osseous cryptococcosis**

     B45.7   **Disseminated cryptococcosis**
              Generalized cryptococcosis

     B45.8   **Other forms of cryptococcosis**

     B45.9   **Cryptococcosis, unspecified**

● **B46**   **Zygomycosis**
Fungal infections including subcutaneous lesions and infection of sinuses, brain, or lungs

     B46.0   **Pulmonary mucormycosis**
              Fungal infection affecting lung

     B46.1   **Rhinocerebral mucormycosis**

     B46.2   **Gastrointestinal mucormycosis**

     B46.3   **Cutaneous mucormycosis**
              Subcutaneous mucormycosis

     B46.4   **Disseminated mucormycosis**
              Generalized mucormycosis

     B46.5   **Mucormycosis, unspecified**

     B46.8   **Other zygomycoses**
              Entomophthoromycosis

     B46.9   **Zygomycosis, unspecified**
              Phycomycosis NOS

● **B47**   **Mycetoma**
Slow progressive, destructive fungal infection of cutaneous and subcutaneous tissues, fascia, and bone, primarily seen in foot (Madura foot) or leg

     B47.0   **Eumycetoma**
              Madura foot, mycotic Maduromycosis

     B47.1   **Actinomycetoma**

     B47.9   **Mycetoma, unspecified**
              Madura foot NOS

● **B48**   **Other mycoses, not elsewhere classified**

     B48.0   **Lobomycosis**
              Infection with symptoms of red, smooth, hard cutaneous nodules resembling keloids
              Keloidal blastomycosis
              Lobo's disease

     B48.1   **Rhinosporidiosis**
              Chronic, localized granulomatous fungal infection, affecting mucocutaneous tissues, usually of nose characterized by polyps, papillomas, and wartlike lesions

     B48.2   **Allescheriasis**
              Fungal infection
              Infection due to Pseudallescheria boydii

         Excludes1   eumycetoma (B47.0)

     B48.3   **Geotrichosis**
              Fungal infection usually of bronchi, lungs, mouth, or intestinal tract
              Geotrichum stomatitis

     B48.4   **Penicillosis**
              Fungal infection

     B48.8   **Other specified mycoses**
              Adiaspiromycosis
              Infection of tissue and organs by Alternaria
              Infection of tissue and organs by Drechslera
              Infection of tissue and organs by Fusarium
              Infection of tissue and organs by saprophytic fungi NEC

B49   **Unspecified mycosis**
     Fungemia NOS

PROTOZOAL DISEASES (B50-B64)

     Excludes1   amebiasis (A06.-)
                     other protozoal intestinal diseases (A07.-)

● **B50**   **Plasmodium falciparum malaria**
Severe form of malaria that can be fatal

     Includes   mixed infections of Plasmodium falciparum with any other Plasmodium species

     B50.0   **Plasmodium falciparum malaria with cerebral complications**
              Cerebral malaria NOS

     B50.8   **Other severe and complicated Plasmodium falciparum malaria**
              Severe or complicated Plasmodium falciparum malaria NOS

     B50.9   **Plasmodium falciparum malaria, unspecified**

● **B51**   **Plasmodium vivax malaria**

     Includes   mixed infections of Plasmodium vivax with other Plasmodium species, except Plasmodium falciparum

     Excludes1   plasmodium vivax with Plasmodium falciparum (B50.-)

     B51.0   **Plasmodium vivax malaria with rupture of spleen**

     B51.8   **Plasmodium vivax malaria with other complications**

     B51.9   **Plasmodium vivax malaria without complication**
              Plasmodium vivax malaria NOS

● **B52**   **Plasmodium malariae malaria**
Causes fever that recurs at approximately three-day intervals (quartan fever), longer than two-day (tertian) intervals of other malarial parasites

     Includes   mixed infections of Plasmodium malariae with other Plasmodium species, except Plasmodium falciparum and Plasmodium vivax

     Excludes1   plasmodium falciparum (B50.-)
                     plasmodium vivax (B51.-)

     B52.0   **Plasmodium malariae malaria with nephropathy**

     B52.8   **Plasmodium malariae malaria with other complications**

     B52.9   **Plasmodium malariae malaria without complication**
              Plasmodium malariae malaria NOS

CHAPTER 1 (A00-B99)

◀ New   ◀◀ Revised   ~~deleted~~ Deleted   **OGCR** Official Guidelines   X Assign placeholder X   ● Use Additional Character(s)

Excludes 1   Excludes 2   Includes   Use additional   Code first   Code also   Unspecified

● B53   Other specified malaria

B53.0   Plasmodium ovale malaria
Least diagnosed type of malaria spread by female mosquitoes of rare species

Excludes1   plasmodium ovale with Plasmodium falciparum (B50.-)
plasmodium ovale with Plasmodium malariae (B52.-)
plasmodium ovale with Plasmodium vivax (B51.-)

B53.1   Malaria due to simian plasmodia
Malaria-like disease (parasite infection)

Excludes1   malaria due to simian plasmodia with Plasmodium falciparum (B50.-)
malaria due to simian plasmodia with Plasmodium malariae (B52.-)
malaria due to simian plasmodia with Plasmodium ovale (B53.0)
malaria due to simian plasmodia with Plasmodium vivax (B51.-)

B53.8   Other malaria, not elsewhere classified

B54   Unspecified malaria

● B55   Leishmaniasis
Protozoal infection

B55.0   Visceral leishmaniasis
Kala-azar
Post-kala-azar dermal leishmaniasis

B55.1   Cutaneous leishmaniasis

B55.2   Mucocutaneous leishmaniasis

B55.9   Leishmaniasis, unspecified

● B56   African trypanosomiasis
Human African trypanosomiasis (HAT) is transmitted by fly bites

B56.0   Gambiense trypanosomiasis
Infection due to Trypanosoma brucei gambiense
West African sleeping sickness

B56.1   Rhodesiense trypanosomiasis
East African sleeping sickness
Infection due to Trypanosoma brucei rhodesiense

B56.9   African trypanosomiasis, unspecified
Sleeping sickness NOS

● B57   Chagas' disease
Tropical parasitic disease

Includes   American trypanosomiasis
infection due to Trypanosoma cruzi

B57.0   Acute Chagas' disease with heart involvement
Acute Chagas' disease with myocarditis

B57.1   Acute Chagas' disease without heart involvement
Acute Chagas' disease NOS

B57.2   Chagas' disease (chronic) with heart involvement
American trypanosomiasis NOS
Chagas' disease (chronic) NOS
Chagas' disease (chronic) with myocarditis
Trypanosomiasis NOS

● B57.3   Chagas' disease (chronic) with digestive system involvement

B57.30   Chagas' disease with digestive system involvement, unspecified

B57.31   Megaesophagus in Chagas' disease

B57.32   Megacolon in Chagas' disease

B57.39   Other digestive system involvement in Chagas' disease

● B57.4   Chagas' disease (chronic) with nervous system involvement

B57.40   Chagas' disease with nervous system involvement, unspecified

B57.41   Meningitis in Chagas' disease

B57.42   Meningoencephalitis in Chagas' disease

B57.49   Other nervous system involvement in Chagas' disease

B57.5   Chagas' disease (chronic) with other organ involvement

Item 1–22   Toxoplasmosis is caused by the protozoa **Toxoplasma gondii,** of which the house cat can be a host. Human infection occurs when contact is made with materials containing the pathogen, such as feces, contaminated soil, or ingestion of infected lamb, goat, or pork. Of the infected, very few have symptoms because a healthy person's immune system keeps the parasite from causing illness. When the immune system is compromised, symptoms may occur. Clinical symptoms include flu-like symptoms, but the disease progresses to include the eyes and the brain in babies.

● B58   Toxoplasmosis
Infection by protozoon transmitted in cysts in feces of cats

Includes   infection due to Toxoplasma gondii
Excludes1   congenital toxoplasmosis (P37.1)

● B58.0   Toxoplasma oculopathy

B58.00   Toxoplasma oculopathy, unspecified

B58.01   Toxoplasma chorioretinitis

B58.09   Other toxoplasma oculopathy
Toxoplasma uveitis

B58.1   Toxoplasma hepatitis

B58.2   Toxoplasma meningoencephalitis

B58.3   Pulmonary toxoplasmosis

● B58.8   Toxoplasmosis with other organ involvement

B58.81   Toxoplasma myocarditis

B58.82   Toxoplasma myositis

B58.83   Toxoplasma tubulo-interstitial nephropathy
Toxoplasma pyelonephritis

B58.89   Toxoplasmosis with other organ involvement

B58.9   Toxoplasmosis, unspecified

B59   Pneumocystosis
Caused by fungus
Pneumonia due to Pneumocystis carinii
Pneumonia due to Pneumocystis jiroveci

● B60   Other protozoal diseases, not elsewhere classified

Excludes1   cryptosporidiosis (A07.2)
intestinal microsporidiosis (A07.8)
isosporiasis (A07.3)

B60.0   Babesiosis
Tickborne disease caused by microscopic organisms
Piroplasmosis

● B60.1   Acanthamebiasis

B60.10   Acanthamebiasis, unspecified

B60.11   Meningoencephalitis due to Acanthamoeba (culbertsoni)

B60.12   Conjunctivitis due to Acanthamoeba

B60.13   Keratoconjunctivitis due to Acanthamoeba

B60.19   Other acanthamebic disease

B60.2   Naegleriasis
Infection with microscopic organisms
Primary amebic meningoencephalitis

B60.8   Other specified protozoal diseases
Microsporidiosis

B64   Unspecified protozoal disease

HELMINTHIASES (B65-B83)

Diseases or infestations caused by parasitic worms

● B65   Schistosomiasis [bilharziasis]
Infection with flukes (flat parasitic worms)

Includes   snail fever

B65.0   Schistosomiasis due to Schistosoma haematobium [urinary schistosomiasis]

B65.1   Schistosomiasis due to Schistosoma mansoni [intestinal schistosomiasis]

B65.2   Schistosomiasis due to Schistosoma japonicum
Asiatic schistosomiasis

B65.3   Cercarial dermatitis
Swimmer's itch

B65.8 Other schistosomiasis
    Infection due to Schistosoma intercalatum
    Infection due to Schistosoma mattheei
    Infection due to Schistosoma mekongi

B65.9 Schistosomiasis, unspecified

● **B66 Other fluke infections**
    Trematode (parasitic worms)

B66.0 Opisthorchiasis
    Infection due to cat liver fluke
    Infection due to Opisthorchis (felineus)(viverrini)

B66.1 Clonorchiasis
    Chinese liver fluke disease
    Infection due to Clonorchis sinensis
    Oriental liver fluke disease

B66.2 Dicroceliasis
    Liver fluke
    Infection due to Dicrocoelium dendriticum
    Lancet fluke infection

B66.3 Fascioliasis
    Infection due to Fasciola gigantica
    Infection due to Fasciola hepatica
    Infection due to Fasciola indica
    Sheep liver fluke disease

B66.4 Paragonimiasis
    Infection due to Paragonimus species
    Lung fluke disease
    Pulmonary distomiasis

B66.5 Fasciolopsiasis
    Largest intestinal fluke in humans
    Infection due to Fasciolopsis buski
    Intestinal distomiasis

B66.8 Other specified fluke infections
    Echinostomiasis
    Heterophyiasis
    Metagonimiasis
    Nanophyetiasis
    Watsoniasis

B66.9 Fluke infection, unspecified

● **B67 Echinococcosis**
    Larval forms of tapeworms usually of liver or lungs
    Includes hydatidosis

B67.0 Echinococcus granulosus infection of liver

B67.1 Echinococcus granulosus infection of lung

B67.2 Echinococcus granulosus infection of bone

● **B67.3 Echinococcus granulosus infection, other and multiple sites**

    B67.31 Echinococcus granulosus infection, thyroid gland

    B67.32 Echinococcus granulosus infection, multiple sites

    B67.39 Echinococcus granulosus infection, other sites

B67.4 Echinococcus granulosus infection, unspecified
    Dog tapeworm (infection)

B67.5 Echinococcus multilocularis infection of liver

● **B67.6 Echinococcus multilocularis infection, other and multiple sites**

    B67.61 Echinococcus multilocularis infection, multiple sites

    B67.69 Echinococcus multilocularis infection, other sites

B67.7 Echinococcus multilocularis infection, unspecified

B67.8 Echinococcosis, unspecified, of liver

● **B67.9 Echinococcosis, other and unspecified**

    B67.90 Echinococcosis, unspecified
      Echinococcosis NOS

    B67.99 Other echinococcosis

Item 1-23 Echinococcosis: Also known as hydatid disease; is caused by Echinococcus granulosus, E. multilocularis, and E. vogeli tapeworms; and is contracted from infected food. Found in southern South America, the Mediterranean, the Middle East, central Asia, and Africa and uncommon in the United States but has been reported in California, New Mexico, Arizona and Utah. The disease is treated with medication over a long course as it is resistive.

● **B68 Taeniasis**
    Intestinal tapeworm (cestode) infection from raw or undercooked meat of infected animal
    Excludes1 cysticercosis (B69.-)

B68.0 Taenia solium taeniasis
    Pork tapeworm (infection)

B68.1 Taenia saginata taeniasis
    Beef tapeworm (infection)
    Infection due to adult tapeworm Taenia saginata

B68.9 Taeniasis, unspecified

● **B69 Cysticercosis**
    Systemic illness caused by the larvae of pork tapeworm
    Includes cysticerciasis infection due to larval form of Taenia solium

B69.0 Cysticercosis of central nervous system

B69.1 Cysticercosis of eye

● **B69.8 Cysticercosis of other sites**

    B69.81 Myositis in cysticercosis

    B69.89 Cysticercosis of other sites

B69.9 Cysticercosis, unspecified

● **B70 Diphyllobothriasis and sparganosis**
    Infection with tapeworms seen most often from inadequately cooked fish

B70.0 Diphyllobothriasis
    Diphyllobothrium (adult) (latum) (pacificum) infection
    Fish tapeworm (infection)
    Excludes2 larval diphyllobothriasis (B70.1)

B70.1 Sparganosis
    Infection with migrating tapeworm larvae, which invade subcutaneous tissues, causing inflammation and fibrosis that resembles cellulitis
    Infection due to Sparganum (mansoni) (proliferum)
    Infection due to Spirometra larva
    Larval diphyllobothriasis
    Spirometrosis

● **B71 Other cestode infections**

B71.0 Hymenolepiasis
    Intestinal infestation with tapeworms
    Dwarf tapeworm infection
    Rat tapeworm (infection)

B71.1 Dipylidiasis
    Infection with tapeworm common to dogs and cats and seen in children having close contact with infected pets

B71.8 Other specified cestode infections
    Infection by the larval stage of a tapeworm, usually through fruit or vegetables
    Coenurosis

B71.9 Cestode infection, unspecified
    Tapeworm (infection) NOS

B72 Dracunculiasis
    Infection with roundworms
    Includes guinea worm infection
                infection due to Dracunculus medinensis

● **B73 Onchocerciasis**
    Infection with parasitic worm
    Includes onchocerca volvulus infection
                onchocercosis
                river blindness

● **B73.0 Onchocerciasis with eye disease**

    B73.00 Onchocerciasis with eye involvement, unspecified

    B73.01 Onchocerciasis with endophthalmitis

    B73.02 Onchocerciasis with glaucoma

    B73.09 Onchocerciasis with other eye involvement
      Infestation of eyelid due to onchocerciasis

B73.1 Onchocerciasis without eye disease

◀ New   ◀▏▏▏ Revised   ~~deleted~~ Deleted   **OGCR** Official Guidelines   X Assign placeholder X   ● Use Additional Character(s)

Excludes 1   Excludes 2   Includes   Use additional   Code first   Code also   Unspecified

CHAPTER 1 (A00-B99)

● **B74** **Filariasis**
Infestation with slender threadlike worms
> **Excludes2**   onchocerciasis (B73)
>   tropical (pulmonary) eosinophilia NOS (J82)

     B74.0 **Filariasis due to Wuchereria bancrofti**
         Bancroftian elephantiasis
         Bancroftian filariasis

     B74.1 **Filariasis due to Brugia malayi**

     B74.2 **Filariasis due to Brugia timori**

     B74.3 **Loiasis**
         Infection with round worms growing in subcutaneous
            connective tissue
         Calabar swelling
         Eyeworm disease of Africa
         Loa loa infection

     B74.4 **Mansonelliasis**
         Infection with filarial parasite
         Infection due to Mansonella ozzardi
         Infection due to Mansonella perstans
         Infection due to Mansonella streptocerca

     B74.8 **Other filariases**
         Dirofilariasis

     B74.9 **Filariasis, unspecified**

B75 **Trichinellosis**
Infestation with parasitic roundworms ingested in undercooked
*   contaminated meat*
> **Includes**   infection due to Trichinella species trichiniasis

● **B76** **Hookworm diseases**
Occurs in hot, humid parts of world where larvae are soil borne, enter
*   digestive tract through skin of feet/legs or in contaminated food/*
*   water; AKA ground itch*
> **Includes**   uncinariasis

     B76.0 **Ancylostomiasis**
         Infection due to Ancylostoma species

     B76.1 **Necatoriasis**
         Infection due to Necator americanus

     B76.8 **Other hookworm diseases**

     B76.9 **Hookworm disease, unspecified**
         Cutaneous larva migrans NOS

● **B77** **Ascariasis**
Infection by roundworm in small intestine
> **Includes**   ascaridiasis
>   roundworm infection

     B77.0 **Ascariasis with intestinal complications**

    ● **B77.8** **Ascariasis with other complications**
         B77.81   **Ascariasis pneumonia**
         B77.89   **Ascariasis with other complications**

     B77.9 **Ascariasis, unspecified**

● **B78** **Strongyloidiasis**
Infection with adult female roundworms
> **Excludes1**   trichostrongyliasis (B81.2)

     B78.0 **Intestinal strongyloidiasis**

     B78.1 **Cutaneous strongyloidiasis**

     B78.7 **Disseminated strongyloidiasis**

     B78.9 **Strongyloidiasis, unspecified**

B79 **Trichuriasis**
Intestinal infection with roundworms
> **Includes**   trichocephaliasis
>   whipworm (disease)(infection)

B80 **Enterobiasis**
Intestinal infection with pinworms
> **Includes**   oxyuriasis
>   pinworm infection
>   threadworm infection

● **B81** **Other intestinal helminthiases, not elsewhere classified**
Diseases or infestations caused by parasitic worms
> **Excludes1**   angiostrongyliasis due to Parastrongylus
>   cantonensis (B83.2)

     B81.0 **Anisakiasis**
         Roundworm infection via contaminated undercooked infected
            fish or marine mammals
         Infection due to Anisakis larva

     B81.1 **Intestinal capillariasis**
         Infestation with of parasites (nematodes)
         Capillariasis NOS
         Infection due to Capillaria philippinensis
>   **Excludes2**   hepatic capillariasis (B83.8)

     B81.2 **Trichostrongyliasis**

     B81.3 **Intestinal angiostrongyliasis**
         Angiostrongyliasis due to Parastrongylus costaricensis

     B81.4 **Mixed intestinal helminthiases**
         Infection due to intestinal helminths classified to more
            than one of the categories B65.0-B81.3 and B81.8
         Mixed helminthiasis NOS

     B81.8 **Other specified intestinal helminthiases**
         Infection due to Oesophagostomum species
            [esophagostomiasis]
         Infection due to Ternidens diminutus [ternidensiasis]

● **B82** **Unspecified intestinal parasitism**

     B82.0 **Intestinal helminthiasis, unspecified**
         Infected with worms

     B82.9 **Intestinal parasitism, unspecified**

● **B83** **Other helminthiases**
Caused by parasitic worms
> **Excludes1**   capillariasis NOS (B81.1)
> **Excludes2**   intestinal capillariasis (B81.1)

     B83.0 **Visceral larva migrans**
         Prolonged migration of nematode larvae
         Toxocariasis

     B83.1 **Gnathostomiasis**
         Infection with nematode occurring from ingested undercooked
            fish contaminated with larvae; larvae migrate to
            subcutaneous tissue or deeper tissues, results are
            abscesses
         Wandering swelling

     B83.2 **Angiostrongyliasis due to Parastrongylus cantonensis**
         Nematode infection caused by eating contaminated raw
            snails, slugs, or paratenic hosts such as prawns or
            crabs; larval worms migrate to central nervous system
            resulting in eosinophilic meningitis
         Eosinophilic meningoencephalitis due to
            Parastrongylus cantonensis
>   **Excludes2**   intestinal angiostrongyliasis (B81.3)

     B83.3 **Syngamiasis**
         Infestation with gapeworm from turkey, pheasant, guinea fowl,
            goose, and wild birds
         Syngamosis

     B83.4 **Internal hirudiniasis**
         Infestation by leeches
>   **Excludes2**   external hirudiniasis (B88.3)

     B83.8 **Other specified helminthiases**
         Parasitic worm infestation
         Acanthocephaliasis
         Gongylonemiasis
         Hepatic capillariasis
         Metastrongyliasis
         Thelaziasis

     B83.9 **Helminthiasis, unspecified**
         Worms NOS
>   **Excludes1**   intestinal helminthiasis NOS (B82.0)

PEDICULOSIS, ACARIASIS AND OTHER INFESTATIONS (B85-B89)

Infestation of lice

- **B85 Pediculosis and phthiriasis**

  B85.0 Pediculosis due to Pediculus humanus capitis
  Head-louse infestation

  B85.1 Pediculosis due to Pediculus humanus corporis
  Body-louse infestation

  B85.2 Pediculosis, unspecified

  B85.3 Phthiriasis
  Crab or pubic lice
  Infestation by crab-louse
  Infestation by Phthirus pubis

  B85.4 Mixed pediculosis and phthiriasis
  Infestation classifiable to more than one of the categories B85.0-B85.3

B86 Scabies
  Sarcoptic itch
  Contagious dermatitis caused by mites

- **B87 Myiasis**
  Infestation by fly maggots

  Includes   infestation by larva of flies

  B87.0 Cutaneous myiasis
  Creeping myiasis

  B87.1 Wound myiasis
  Traumatic myiasis

  B87.2 Ocular myiasis

  B87.3 Nasopharyngeal myiasis
  Laryngeal myiasis

  B87.4 Aural myiasis

  - **B87.8 Myiasis of other sites**

    B87.81 Genitourinary myiasis

    B87.82 Intestinal myiasis

    B87.89 Myiasis of other sites

  B87.9 Myiasis, unspecified

- **B88 Other infestations**

  B88.0 Other acariasis
  Acarine dermatitis
  Dermatitis due to Demodex species
  Dermatitis due to Dermanyssus gallinae
  Dermatitis due to Liponyssoides sanguineus
  Trombiculosis
  Excludes2   scabies (B86)

  B88.1 Tungiasis [sandflea infestation]
  Inflammatory skin disease caused by infestation of fleas

  B88.2 Other arthropod infestations
  Scarabiasis

  B88.3 External hirudiniasis
  Leech infestation NOS
  Excludes2   internal hirudiniasis (B83.4)

  B88.8 Other specified infestations
  Infection of topical fresh water fish parasite
  Ichthyoparasitism due to Vandellia cirrhosa
  Linguatulosis
  Porocephaliasis

  B88.9 Infestation, unspecified
  Infestation (skin) NOS
  Infestation by mites NOS
  Skin parasites NOS

B89 Unspecified parasitic disease

SEQUELAE OF INFECTIOUS AND PARASITIC DISEASES (B90-B94)

Note: Categories B90-B94 are to be used to indicate conditions in categories A00-B89 as the cause of sequelae, which are themselves classified elsewhere. The 'sequelae' include conditions specified as such; they also include residuals of diseases classifiable to the above categories if there is evidence that the disease itself is no longer present. Codes from these categories are not to be used for chronic infections. Code chronic current infections to active infectious disease as appropriate.

Code first condition resulting from (sequela) the infectious or parasitic disease

- **B90 Sequelae of tuberculosis**
  Condition resulting from tuberculosis

  B90.0 Sequelae of central nervous system tuberculosis

  B90.1 Sequelae of genitourinary tuberculosis

  B90.2 Sequelae of tuberculosis of bones and joints

  B90.8 Sequelae of tuberculosis of other organs
  Excludes2   sequelae of respiratory tuberculosis (B90.9)

  B90.9 Sequelae of respiratory and unspecified tuberculosis
  Sequelae of tuberculosis NOS

B91 Sequelae of poliomyelitis
  Excludes1   postpolio syndrome (G14)

B92 Sequelae of leprosy

- **B94 Sequelae of other and unspecified infectious and parasitic diseases**

  B94.0 Sequelae of trachoma

  B94.1 Sequelae of viral encephalitis

  B94.2 Sequelae of viral hepatitis

  B94.8 Sequelae of other specified infectious and parasitic diseases

  B94.9 Sequelae of unspecified infectious and parasitic disease

  OGCR   Section I.C.1.b

  Certain infectious and parasitic diseases
  Infectious agents as the cause of diseases classified to other chapters
  Certain infections are classified in chapters other than Chapter 1 and no organism is identified as part of the infection code. In these instances, it is necessary to use an additional code from Chapter 1 to identify the organism. A code from category B95, Streptococcus, Staphylococcus, and Enterococcus as the cause of diseases classified to other chapters, B96, Other bacterial agents as the cause of diseases classified to other chapters, or B97, Viral agents as the cause of diseases classified to other chapters, is to be used as an additional code to identify the organism. An instructional note will be found at the infection code advising that an additional organism code is required.

BACTERIAL AND VIRAL INFECTIOUS AGENTS (B95-B97)

Note: These categories are provided for use as supplementary or additional codes to identify the infectious agent(s) in diseases classified elsewhere.

Code the disease first, then the bacterium. Do not report codes from B95-B97 for sepsis.

- **B95 Streptococcus, Staphylococcus, and Enterococcus as the cause of diseases classified elsewhere**

  B95.0 Streptococcus, group A, as the cause of diseases classified elsewhere

  B95.1 Streptococcus, group B, as the cause of diseases classified elsewhere

  B95.2 Enterococcus as the cause of diseases classified elsewhere

  B95.3 Streptococcus pneumoniae as the cause of diseases classified elsewhere

  B95.4 Other streptococcus as the cause of diseases classified elsewhere

---

◀ New   ◀ Revised   ~~deleted~~ Deleted   OGCR Official Guidelines   X Assign placeholder X   ● Use Additional Character(s)

Excludes 1   Excludes 2   Includes   Use additional   Code first   Code also   Unspecified

CHAPTER 1 (A00-B99)

B95.5   Unspecified streptococcus as the cause of diseases classified elsewhere

● **B95.6**   Staphylococcus aureus as the cause of diseases classified elsewhere

    B95.61   Methicillin susceptible Staphylococcus aureus infection as the cause of diseases classified elsewhere
        Methicillin susceptible Staphylococcus aureus (MSSA) infection as the cause of diseases classified elsewhere
        Staphylococcus aureus infection NOS as the cause of diseases classified elsewhere

    B95.62   Methicillin resistant Staphylococcus aureus infection as the cause of diseases classified elsewhere
        Methicillin resistant staphylococcus aureus (MRSA) infection as the cause of diseases classified elsewhere

B95.7   Other staphylococcus as the cause of diseases classified elsewhere

B95.8   Unspecified staphylococcus as the cause of diseases classified elsewhere

● **B96**   Other bacterial agents as the cause of diseases classified elsewhere

B96.0   Mycoplasma pneumoniae [M. pneumoniae] as the cause of diseases classified elsewhere
    Pleuro-pneumonia-like-organism [PPLO]

B96.1   Klebsiella pneumoniae [K. pneumoniae] as the cause of diseases classified elsewhere

● **B96.2**   Escherichia coli [E. coli] as the cause of diseases classified elsewhere

    B96.20   Unspecified Escherichia coli [E. coli] as the cause of diseases classified elsewhere
        Escherichia coli [E. coli] NOS

    B96.21   Shiga toxin-producing Escherichia coli [E. coli] (STEC) O157 as the cause of diseases classified elsewhere
        E. coli O157:H- (nonmotile) with confirmation of Shiga toxin
        E. coli O157 with confirmation of Shiga toxin when H antigen is unknown, or is not H7
        O157:H7 Escherichia coli [E.coli] with or without confirmation of Shiga toxin-production
        Shiga toxin-producing Escherichia coli [E.coli] O157:H7 with or without confirmation of Shiga toxin-production
        STEC O157:H7 with or without confirmation of Shiga toxin-production

    B96.22   Other specified Shiga toxin-producing Escherichia coli [E. coli] (STEC) as the cause of diseases classified elsewhere
        Non-O157 Shiga toxin-producing Escherichia coli [E.coli]
        Non-O157 Shiga toxin-producing Escherichia coli [E.coli] with known O group

    B96.23   Unspecified Shiga toxin-producing Escherichia coli [E. coli] (STEC) as the cause of diseases classified elsewhere
        Shiga toxin-producing Escherichia coli [E. coli] with unspecified O group
        STEC NOS

    B96.29   Other Escherichia coli [E. coli] as the cause of diseases classified elsewhere
        Non-Shiga toxin-producing E. coli

B96.3   Hemophilus influenzae [H. influenzae] as the cause of diseases classified elsewhere

B96.4   Proteus (mirabilis) (morganii) as the cause of diseases classified elsewhere

B96.5   Pseudomonas (aeruginosa) (mallei) (pseudomallei) as the cause of diseases classified elsewhere

B96.6   Bacteroides fragilis [B. fragilis] as the cause of diseases classified elsewhere

B96.7   Clostridium perfringens [C. perfringens] as the cause of diseases classified elsewhere

● **B96.8**   Other specified bacterial agents as the cause of diseases classified elsewhere

    B96.81   Helicobacter pylori [H. pylori] as the cause of diseases classified elsewhere

    B96.82   Vibrio vulnificus as the cause of diseases classified elsewhere

    B96.89   Other specified bacterial agents as the cause of diseases classified elsewhere

● **B97**   Viral agents as the cause of diseases classified elsewhere

B97.0   Adenovirus as the cause of diseases classified elsewhere

● **B97.1**   Enterovirus as the cause of diseases classified elsewhere

    B97.10   Unspecified enterovirus as the cause of diseases classified elsewhere

    B97.11   Coxsackievirus as the cause of diseases classified elsewhere

    B97.12   Echovirus as the cause of diseases classified elsewhere

    B97.19   Other enterovirus as the cause of diseases classified elsewhere

● **B97.2**   Coronavirus as the cause of diseases classified elsewhere

    B97.21   SARS-associated coronavirus as the cause of diseases classified elsewhere
        Excludes1   pneumonia due to SARS-associated coronavirus (J12.81)

    B97.29   Other coronavirus as the cause of diseases classified elsewhere

● **B97.3**   Retrovirus as the cause of diseases classified elsewhere
    Excludes1   human immunodeficiency virus [HIV] disease (B20)

    B97.30   Unspecified retrovirus as the cause of diseases classified elsewhere

    B97.31   Lentivirus as the cause of diseases classified elsewhere

    B97.32   Oncovirus as the cause of diseases classified elsewhere

    B97.33   Human T-cell lymphotrophic virus, type I [HTLV-I] as the cause of diseases classified elsewhere

    B97.34   Human T-cell lymphotrophic virus, type II [HTLV-II] as the cause of diseases classified elsewhere

    B97.35   Human immunodeficiency virus, type 2 [HIV 2] as the cause of diseases classified elsewhere

    B97.39   Other retrovirus as the cause of diseases classified elsewhere

B97.4   Respiratory syncytial virus as the cause of diseases classified elsewhere

B97.5   Reovirus as the cause of diseases classified elsewhere

B97.6   Parvovirus as the cause of diseases classified elsewhere

B97.7   Papillomavirus as the cause of diseases classified elsewhere

Item 1–24 Retrovirus develops by copying its RNA, genetic materials, into the DNA, which then produces new virus particles. It is from the Retroviridae virus family. **Human T-cell lymphotropic virus, Type I (HTLV-I)** is also called human T-cell leukemia virus, Type I, and is a retrovirus thought to cause T-cell leukemia/lymphoma. **Human T-cell lymphotropic virus, Type II (HTLV-II),** is also called human T-cell leukemia virus, Type II, and is a retrovirus associated with hematologic disorders.

  HIV-2 is one of the serotypes of HIV and is usually confined to West Africa, whereas HIV-1 is found worldwide.

◀ New   ◀ Revised   ~~deleted~~ Deleted   OGCR Official Guidelines   X Assign placeholder X   ● Use Additional Character(s)

Excludes 1   Excludes 2   Includes   Use additional   Code first   Code also   Unspecified

● **B97.8** **Other viral agents as the cause of diseases classified elsewhere**

    B97.81 **Human metapneumovirus as the cause of diseases classified elsewhere**

    B97.89 **Other viral agents as the cause of diseases classified elsewhere**

<u>**OTHER INFECTIOUS DISEASES (B99)**</u>

● **B99** **Other and unspecified infectious diseases**

    B99.8 **Other infectious disease**

    B99.9 Unspecified infectious disease

CHAPTER 1 (A00–B99)

Item 2–1 Neoplasm: Neo = new, plasm = growth, development, formation. This new growth (mass, tumor) can be malignant or benign, which is confirmed by the pathology report. Do not assign a code to a neoplasm until you review the pathology report. Certain CPT codes will specify benign or malignant lesion, so be certain the diagnosis code supports the procedure code.

OGCR Section I.C.2

General Guidelines

Chapter 2 of the ICD-10-CM contains the codes for the most benign and all malignant neoplasms. Certain benign neoplasms, such as prostatic adenomas, may be found in the specific body system chapters. To properly code a neoplasm, it is necessary to determine from the record if the neoplasm is benign, in-situ, malignant, or, of uncertain histologic behavior. If malignant, any secondary (metastatic) sites should also be determined.

CHAPTER 2

NEOPLASMS (C00-D49)

This chapter contains the following blocks:

C00-C14	Malignant neoplasms of lip, oral cavity and pharynx
C15-C26	Malignant neoplasms of digestive organs
C30-C39	Malignant neoplasms of respiratory and intrathoracic organs
C40-C41	Malignant neoplasms of bone and articular cartilage
C43-C44	Melanoma and other malignant neoplasms of skin
C45-C49	Malignant neoplasms of mesothelial and soft tissue
C50	Malignant neoplasms of breast
C51-C58	Malignant neoplasms of female genital organs
C60-C63	Malignant neoplasms of male genital organs
C64-C68	Malignant neoplasms of urinary tract
C69-C72	Malignant neoplasms of eye, brain and other parts of central nervous system
C73-C75	Malignant neoplasms of thyroid and other endocrine glands
C7A	Malignant neuroendocrine tumors
C7B	Secondary neuroendocrine tumors
C76-C80	Malignant neoplasms of ill-defined, other secondary and unspecified sites
C81-C96	Malignant neoplasms of lymphoid, hematopoietic and related tissue
D00-D09	In situ neoplasms
D10-D36	Benign neoplasms, except benign neuroendocrine tumors
D3A	Benign neuroendocrine tumors
D37-D48	Neoplasms of uncertain behavior, polycythemia vera and myelodysplastic syndromes
D49	Neoplasms of unspecified behavior

Notes: Functional activity

All neoplasms are classified in this chapter, whether they are functionally active or not. An additional code from Chapter 4 may be used, to identify functional activity associated with any neoplasm.

Morphology [Histology]

Chapter 2 classifies neoplasms primarily by site (topography), with broad groupings for behavior, malignant, in situ, benign, etc. The Table of Neoplasms should be used to identify the correct topography code. In a few cases, such as for malignant melanoma and certain neuroendocrine tumors, the morphology (histologic type) is included in the category and codes.

Primary malignant neoplasms overlapping site boundaries

A primary malignant neoplasm that overlaps two or more contiguous (next to each other) sites should be classified to the subcategory/code .8 ('overlapping lesion'), unless the combination is specifically indexed elsewhere. For multiple neoplasms of the same site that are not contiguous, such as tumors in different quadrants of the same breast, codes for each site should be assigned.

Malignant neoplasm of ectopic tissue

Malignant neoplasms of ectopic tissue are to be coded to the site mentioned, e.g., ectopic pancreatic malignant neoplasms are coded to pancreas, unspecified (C25.9).

MALIGNANT NEOPLASMS (C00-C96)

MALIGNANT NEOPLASMS, STATED OR PRESUMED TO BE PRIMARY (OF SPECIFIED SITES), AND CERTAIN SPECIFIED HISTOLOGIES, EXCEPT NEUROENDOCRINE, AND OF LYMPHOID, HEMATOPOIETIC AND RELATED TISSUE (C00-C75)

MALIGNANT NEOPLASMS OF LIP, ORAL CAVITY AND PHARYNX (C00-C14)

● C00   **Malignant neoplasm of lip**
Use additional code to identify:
   alcohol abuse and dependence (F10.-)
   history of tobacco use (Z87.891)
   tobacco dependence (F17.-)
   tobacco use (Z72.0)

Excludes1	malignant melanoma of lip (C43.0)
	Merkel cell carcinoma of lip (C4A.0)
	other and unspecified malignant neoplasm of skin of lip (C44.0-)

C00.0   **Malignant neoplasm of external upper lip**
   Malignant neoplasm of lipstick area of upper lip
   Malignant neoplasm of upper lip NOS
   Malignant neoplasm of vermilion border of upper lip

C00.1   **Malignant neoplasm of external lower lip**
   Malignant neoplasm of lower lip NOS
   Malignant neoplasm of lipstick area of lower lip
   Malignant neoplasm of vermilion border of lower lip

C00.2   **Malignant neoplasm of external lip, unspecified**
   Malignant neoplasm of vermilion border of lip NOS

C00.3   **Malignant neoplasm of upper lip, inner aspect**
   Malignant neoplasm of buccal aspect of upper lip
   Malignant neoplasm of frenulum of upper lip
   Malignant neoplasm of mucosa of upper lip
   Malignant neoplasm of oral aspect of upper lip

C00.4   **Malignant neoplasm of lower lip, inner aspect**
   Malignant neoplasm of buccal aspect of lower lip
   Malignant neoplasm of frenulum of lower lip
   Malignant neoplasm of mucosa of lower lip
   Malignant neoplasm of oral aspect of lower lip

C00.5   **Malignant neoplasm of lip, unspecified, inner aspect**
   Malignant neoplasm of buccal aspect of lip, unspecified
   Malignant neoplasm of frenulum of lip, unspecified
   Malignant neoplasm of mucosa of lip, unspecified
   Malignant neoplasm of oral aspect of lip, unspecified

C00.6   **Malignant neoplasm of commissure of lip, unspecified**
   Commissure: Site of union of corresponding parts

C00.8   **Malignant neoplasm of overlapping sites of lip**

C00.9   **Malignant neoplasm of lip, unspecified**

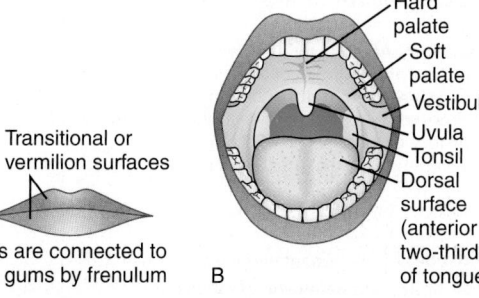

Figure 2-1 Anatomical structures of the mouth and lips. **A.** Transitional or vermilion borders. Lips are connected to the gums by frenulum. **B.** Dorsal surface. **C.** Ventral surface.

C01   Malignant neoplasm of base of tongue
Malignant neoplasm of dorsal surface of base of tongue
Malignant neoplasm of fixed part of tongue NOS
Malignant neoplasm of posterior third of tongue
Use additional code to identify:
alcohol abuse and dependence (F10.-)
history of tobacco use (Z87.891)
tobacco dependence (F17.-)
tobacco use (Z72.0)

●**C02   Malignant neoplasm of other and unspecified parts of tongue**
Use additional code to identify:
alcohol abuse and dependence (F10.-)
history of tobacco use (Z87.891)
tobacco dependence (F17.-)
tobacco use (Z72.0)

C02.0   **Malignant neoplasm of dorsal surface of tongue**
Malignant neoplasm of anterior two-thirds of tongue, dorsal surface
Excludes2   malignant neoplasm of dorsal surface of base of tongue (C01)

C02.1   **Malignant neoplasm of border of tongue**
Malignant neoplasm of tip of tongue

C02.2   **Malignant neoplasm of ventral surface of tongue**
Malignant neoplasm of anterior two-thirds of tongue, ventral surface
Malignant neoplasm of frenulum linguae

C02.3   **Malignant neoplasm of anterior two-thirds of tongue, part unspecified**
Malignant neoplasm of middle third of tongue NOS
Malignant neoplasm of mobile part of tongue NOS

C02.4   **Malignant neoplasm of lingual tonsil**
Lingual tonsil: Aggregation of lymph follicles at root of tongue
Excludes2   malignant neoplasm of tonsil NOS (C09.9)

C02.8   **Malignant neoplasm of overlapping sites of tongue**
Malignant neoplasm of two or more contiguous sites of tongue

C02.9   **Malignant neoplasm of tongue, unspecified**

●C03   **Malignant neoplasm of gum**
Includes   malignant neoplasm of alveolar (ridge) mucosa
malignant neoplasm of gingiva
Use additional code to identify:
alcohol abuse and dependence (F10.-)
history of tobacco use (Z87.891)
tobacco dependence (F17.-)
tobacco use (Z72.0)
Excludes2   malignant odontogenic neoplasms (C41.0-C41.1)

C03.0   **Malignant neoplasm of upper gum**
C03.1   **Malignant neoplasm of lower gum**
C03.9   **Malignant neoplasm of gum, unspecified**

●C04   **Malignant neoplasm of floor of mouth**
Use additional code to identify:
alcohol abuse and dependence (F10.-)
history of tobacco use (Z87.891)
tobacco dependence (F17.-)
tobacco use (Z72.0)

C04.0   **Malignant neoplasm of anterior floor of mouth**
Malignant neoplasm of anterior to the premolar-canine junction

C04.1   **Malignant neoplasm of lateral floor of mouth**
C04.8   **Malignant neoplasm of overlapping sites of floor of mouth**
C04.9   **Malignant neoplasm of floor of mouth, unspecified**

●C05   **Malignant neoplasm of palate**
Use additional code to identify:
alcohol abuse and dependence (F10.-)
history of tobacco use (Z87.891)
tobacco dependence (F17.-)
tobacco use (Z72.0)
Excludes1   Kaposi's sarcoma of palate (C46.2)

C05.0   **Malignant neoplasm of hard palate**
C05.1   **Malignant neoplasm of soft palate**
Excludes2   malignant neoplasm of nasopharyngeal surface of soft palate (C11.3)

C05.2   **Malignant neoplasm of uvula**
C05.8   **Malignant neoplasm of overlapping sites of palate**
C05.9   **Malignant neoplasm of palate, unspecified**
Malignant neoplasm of roof of mouth

●C06   **Malignant neoplasm of other and unspecified parts of mouth**
Use additional code to identify:
alcohol abuse and dependence (F10.-)
history of tobacco use (Z87.891)
tobacco dependence (F17.-)
tobacco use (Z72.0)

C06.0   **Malignant neoplasm of cheek mucosa**
Malignant neoplasm of buccal mucosa NOS
Malignant neoplasm of internal cheek

C06.1   **Malignant neoplasm of vestibule of mouth**
Malignant neoplasm of buccal sulcus (upper) (lower)
Malignant neoplasm of labial sulcus (upper) (lower)

C06.2   **Malignant neoplasm of retromolar area**
●C06.8   **Malignant neoplasm of overlapping sites of other and unspecified parts of mouth**
C06.80   **Malignant neoplasm of overlapping sites of unspecified parts of mouth**
C06.89   **Malignant neoplasm of overlapping sites of other parts of mouth 'book leaf' neoplasm [ventral surface of tongue and floor of mouth]**

C06.9   **Malignant neoplasm of mouth, unspecified**
Malignant neoplasm of minor salivary gland, unspecified site
Malignant neoplasm of oral cavity NOS

◀ New   ◀▥ Revised   ~~deleted~~ Deleted   OGCR Official Guidelines   X Assign placeholder X   ● Use Additional Character(s)
Excludes 1   Excludes 2   Includes   Use additional   Code first   Code also   Unspecified

CHAPTER 2 (C00-D49)   737

CHAPTER 2 (C00–D49)

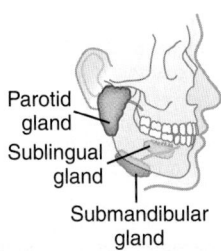

Parotid gland
Sublingual gland
Submandibular gland

Figure 2-2 Major salivary glands.

C07   Malignant neoplasm of parotid gland
    Use additional code to identify:
      alcohol abuse and dependence (F10.-)
      exposure to environmental tobacco smoke (Z77.22)
      exposure to tobacco smoke in the perinatal period (P96.81)
      history of tobacco use (Z87.891)
      occupational exposure to environmental tobacco smoke
        (Z57.31)
      tobacco dependence (F17.-)
      tobacco use (Z72.0)

C08   Malignant neoplasm of other and unspecified major salivary glands
    Includes   malignant neoplasm of salivary ducts
    Use additional code to identify:
      alcohol abuse and dependence (F10.-)
      exposure to environmental tobacco smoke (Z77.22)
      exposure to tobacco smoke in the perinatal period (P96.81)
      history of tobacco use (Z87.891)
      occupational exposure to environmental tobacco smoke
        (Z57.31)
      tobacco dependence (F17.-)
      tobacco use (Z72.0)
    Excludes1   malignant neoplasms of specified minor salivary glands which are classified according to their anatomical location
    Excludes2   malignant neoplasms of minor salivary glands NOS (C06.9)
                  malignant neoplasm of parotid gland (C07)

C08.0   Malignant neoplasm of submandibular gland
      Malignant neoplasm of submaxillary gland

C08.1   Malignant neoplasm of sublingual gland

C08.9   Malignant neoplasm of major salivary gland, unspecified
      Malignant neoplasm of salivary gland (major) NOS

(See Plate 61 on page NAP-25.)

C09   Malignant neoplasm of tonsil
    Use additional code to identify:
      alcohol abuse and dependence (F10.-)
      exposure to environmental tobacco smoke (Z77.22)
      exposure to tobacco smoke in the perinatal period (P96.81)
      history of tobacco use (Z87.891)
      occupational exposure to environmental tobacco smoke
        (Z57.31)
      tobacco dependence (F17.-)
      tobacco use (Z72.0)
    Excludes2   malignant neoplasm of lingual tonsil (C02.4)
                  malignant neoplasm of pharyngeal tonsil (C11.1)

C09.0   Malignant neoplasm of tonsillar fossa
      Surface of palatine (two masses of lymphatic tissue on sides of throat) tonsils

C09.1   Malignant neoplasm of tonsillar pillar (anterior) (posterior)
      Extension from palatine (two masses of lymphatic tissue on sides of throat) tonsils

C09.8   Malignant neoplasm of overlapping sites of tonsil

C09.9   Malignant neoplasm of tonsil, unspecified
      Malignant neoplasm of tonsil NOS
      Malignant neoplasm of faucial tonsils
      Malignant neoplasm of palatine tonsils

C10   Malignant neoplasm of oropharynx
    Area of throat at back of mouth
    Use additional code to identify:
      alcohol abuse and dependence (F10.-)
      exposure to environmental tobacco smoke (Z77.22)
      exposure to tobacco smoke in the perinatal period (P96.81)
      history of tobacco use (Z87.891)
      occupational exposure to environmental tobacco smoke
        (Z57.31)
      tobacco dependence (F17.-)
      tobacco use (Z72.0)
    Excludes2   malignant neoplasm of tonsil (C09.-)

C10.0   Malignant neoplasm of vallecula
      Vallecula, depression or furrow

C10.1   Malignant neoplasm of anterior surface of epiglottis
      Malignant neoplasm of epiglottis, free border [margin]
      Malignant neoplasm of glossoepiglottic fold(s)
    Excludes2   malignant neoplasm of epiglottis (suprahyoid portion) NOS (C32.1)

C10.2   Malignant neoplasm of lateral wall of oropharynx

C10.3   Malignant neoplasm of posterior wall of oropharynx

C10.4   Malignant neoplasm of branchial cleft
      Congenital slitlike openings formed between branchial arches pharyngeal groove
      Malignant neoplasm of branchial cyst [site of neoplasm]

C10.8   Malignant neoplasm of overlapping sites of oropharynx
      Malignant neoplasm of junctional region of oropharynx

C10.9   Malignant neoplasm of oropharynx, unspecified

C11   Malignant neoplasm of nasopharynx
    Use additional code to identify:
      exposure to environmental tobacco smoke (Z77.22)
      exposure to tobacco smoke in the perinatal period (P96.81)
      history of tobacco use (Z87.891)
      occupational exposure to environmental tobacco smoke
        (Z57.31)
      tobacco dependence (F17.-)
      tobacco use (Z72.0)

C11.0   Malignant neoplasm of superior wall of nasopharynx
      Part of pharynx that lies above soft palate
      Malignant neoplasm of roof of nasopharynx

C11.1   Malignant neoplasm of posterior wall of nasopharynx
      Malignant neoplasm of adenoid
      Malignant neoplasm of pharyngeal tonsil

C11.2   Malignant neoplasm of lateral wall of nasopharynx
      Malignant neoplasm of fossa of Rosenmüller
      Malignant neoplasm of opening of auditory tube
      Malignant neoplasm of pharyngeal recess

C11.3   Malignant neoplasm of anterior wall of nasopharynx
      Malignant neoplasm of floor of nasopharynx
      Malignant neoplasm of nasopharyngeal (anterior) (posterior) surface of soft palate
      Malignant neoplasm of posterior margin of nasal choana
      Malignant neoplasm of posterior margin of nasal septum

C11.8   Malignant neoplasm of overlapping sites of nasopharynx

C11.9   Malignant neoplasm of nasopharynx, unspecified
      Malignant neoplasm of nasopharyngeal wall NOS

C12   Malignant neoplasm of pyriform sinus
    Malignant neoplasm of pyriform fossa
    Use additional code to identify:
      exposure to environmental tobacco smoke (Z77.22)
      exposure to tobacco smoke in the perinatal period (P96.81)
      history of tobacco use (Z87.891)
      occupational exposure to environmental tobacco smoke
        (Z57.31)
      tobacco dependence (F17.-)
      tobacco use (Z72.0)

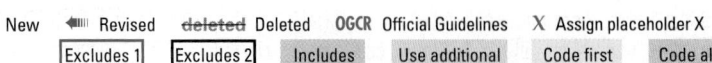

◀ New   ◀▥ Revised   ~~deleted~~ Deleted   **OGCR** Official Guidelines   X Assign placeholder X   ● Use Additional Character(s)

Excludes 1   Excludes 2   Includes   Use additional   Code first   Code also   Unspecified

● C13 **Malignant neoplasm of hypopharynx**

   Use additional code to identify:
   exposure to environmental tobacco smoke (Z77.22)
   exposure to tobacco smoke in the perinatal period (P96.81)
   history of tobacco use (Z87.891)
   occupational exposure to environmental tobacco smoke (Z57.31)
   tobacco dependence (F17.-)
   tobacco use (Z72.0)

   Excludes2 malignant neoplasm of pyriform sinus (C12)

   C13.0 **Malignant neoplasm of postcricoid region**
          Behind the cricoid cartilage of neck

   C13.1 **Malignant neoplasm of aryepiglottic fold, hypopharyngeal aspect**
          Arytenoepiglottic fold, triangular opening between side of epiglottis and apex of arytenoid cartilage
          Malignant neoplasm of aryepiglottic fold, marginal zone
          Malignant neoplasm of aryepiglottic fold NOS
          Malignant neoplasm of interarytenoid fold, marginal zone
          Malignant neoplasm of interarytenoid fold NOS

          Excludes2 malignant neoplasm of aryepiglottic fold or interarytenoid fold, laryngeal aspect (C32.1)

   C13.2 **Malignant neoplasm of posterior wall of hypopharynx**

   C13.8 **Malignant neoplasm of overlapping sites of hypopharynx**

   C13.9 **Malignant neoplasm of hypopharynx, unspecified**
          Malignant neoplasm of hypopharyngeal wall NOS

● C14 **Malignant neoplasm of other and ill-defined sites in the lip, oral cavity and pharynx**

   Use additional code to identify:
   alcohol abuse and dependence (F10.-)
   exposure to environmental tobacco smoke (Z77.22)
   exposure to tobacco smoke in the perinatal period (P96.81)
   history of tobacco use (Z87.891)
   occupational exposure to environmental tobacco smoke (Z57.31)
   tobacco dependence (F17.-)
   tobacco use (Z72.0)

   Excludes1 malignant neoplasm of oral cavity NOS (C06.9)

   C14.0 **Malignant neoplasm of pharynx, unspecified**

   C14.2 **Malignant neoplasm of Waldeyer's ring**

   C14.8 **Malignant neoplasm of overlapping sites of lip, oral cavity and pharynx**
          Primary malignant neoplasm of two or more contiguous sites of lip, oral cavity and pharynx

          Excludes1 'book leaf' neoplasm [ventral surface of tongue and floor of mouth] (C06.89)

MALIGNANT NEOPLASM OF DIGESTIVE ORGANS (C15-C26)

   Excludes1 Kaposi's sarcoma of gastrointestinal sites (C46.4)

● C15 **Malignant neoplasms of esophagus**

   Use additional code to identify:
   alcohol abuse and dependence (F10.-)

   C15.3 **Malignant neoplasm of upper third of esophagus**

   C15.4 **Malignant neoplasm of middle third of esophagus**

   C15.5 **Malignant neoplasm of lower third of esophagus**

          Excludes1 malignant neoplasm of cardio-esophageal junction (C16.0)

   C15.8 **Malignant neoplasm of overlapping sites of esophagus**

   C15.9 **Malignant neoplasm of esophagus, unspecified**

Figure 2-3 The esophagus is the muscular tube that connects the pharynx and the stomach. The 10 inch (25 cm) long esophagus is divided into three parts: **cervical, thoracic,** and **abdominal.**

● C16 **Malignant neoplasm of stomach**

   Use additional code to identify:
   alcohol abuse and dependence (F10.-)

   Excludes2 malignant carcinoid tumor of the stomach (C7A.092)

   C16.0 **Malignant neoplasm of cardia**
          Malignant neoplasm of cardiac orifice
          Malignant neoplasm of cardio-esophageal junction
          Malignant neoplasm of esophagus and stomach
          Malignant neoplasm of gastro-esophageal junction

   C16.1 **Malignant neoplasm of fundus of stomach**

   C16.2 **Malignant neoplasm of body of stomach**

   C16.3 **Malignant neoplasm of pyloric antrum**
          Malignant neoplasm of gastric antrum

   C16.4 **Malignant neoplasm of pylorus**
          Malignant neoplasm of prepylorus
          Malignant neoplasm of pyloric canal

   C16.5 **Malignant neoplasm of lesser curvature of stomach, unspecified**
          Malignant neoplasm of lesser curvature of stomach, not classifiable to C16.1-C16.4

   C16.6 **Malignant neoplasm of greater curvature of stomach, unspecified**
          Malignant neoplasm of greater curvature of stomach, not classifiable to C16.0-C16.4

   C16.8 **Malignant neoplasm of overlapping sites of stomach**

   C16.9 **Malignant neoplasm of stomach, unspecified**
          Gastric cancer NOS

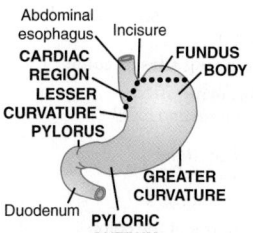

Figure 2-4 Parts of the stomach.

Item 2-2 The esophagus opens into the stomach through the **cardiac orifice,** also called the **cardioesophageal junction.** The **cardia** is adjacent to the cardiac orifice. The stomach widens into the **greater** and **lesser curvatures.** The **pyloric antrum** precedes the **pylorus,** which opens to the duodenum.

CHAPTER 2 (C00-D49)

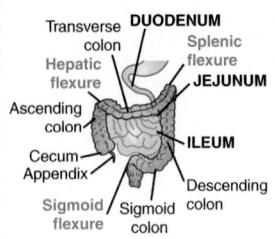

Figure 2-5 Small intestine and colon.

CHAPTER 2 (C00-D49)

● **C17 Malignant neoplasm of small intestine**
　Excludes1 malignant carcinoid tumor of the small intestine (C7A.01)

C17.0 Malignant neoplasm of duodenum
　First or proximal portion of small intestine, extending from pylorus to jejunum

C17.1 Malignant neoplasm of jejunum
　Second section of small intestine, extending from duodenum to ileum

C17.2 Malignant neoplasm of ileum
　Distal and longest portion of small intestine, extending from jejunum to cecum
　Excludes1 malignant neoplasm of ileocecal valve (C18.0)

C17.3 Meckel's diverticulum, malignant
　Appendage of ileum
　Excludes1 Meckel's diverticulum, congenital (Q43.0)

C17.8 Malignant neoplasm of overlapping sites of small intestine

C17.9 Malignant neoplasm of small intestine, unspecified

● **C18 Malignant neoplasm of colon**
　Excludes1 malignant carcinoid tumors of the colon (C7A.02)

C18.0 Malignant neoplasm of cecum
　First section of large intestine
　Malignant neoplasm of ileocecal valve

C18.1 Malignant neoplasm of appendix
　Blind ended tube connected to the cecum; AKA vermiform appendix

C18.2 Malignant neoplasm of ascending colon
　Ascending colon is between cecum and right colic flexure

C18.3 Malignant neoplasm of hepatic flexure
　A flexure is a bending in a structure or organ. Note the three flexures illustrated in Figure 2–5.

C18.4 Malignant neoplasm of transverse colon
　Portion of colon that runs transversely across upper part of abdomen, between right and left colic flexures

C18.5 Malignant neoplasm of splenic flexure
　Bend at junction of transverse and descending colon

C18.6 Malignant neoplasm of descending colon
　Portion between left colic flexure and sigmoid colon at pelvic brim; AKA iliac colon

C18.7 Malignant neoplasm of sigmoid colon
　S-shaped part of colon extending from pelvic brim to third segment of sacrum
　Malignant neoplasm of sigmoid (flexure)
　Excludes1 malignant neoplasm of rectosigmoid junction (C19)

C18.8 Malignant neoplasm of overlapping sites of colon

C18.9 Malignant neoplasm of colon, unspecified
　Malignant neoplasm of large intestine NOS

C19 Malignant neoplasm of rectosigmoid junction
　Malignant neoplasm of colon with rectum
　Malignant neoplasm of rectosigmoid (colon)
　Excludes1 malignant carcinoid tumors of the colon (C7A.02-)

C20 Malignant neoplasm of rectum
　Malignant neoplasm of rectal ampulla
　Excludes1 malignant carcinoid tumor of the rectum (C7A.026)

● **C21 Malignant neoplasm of anus and anal canal**
　Excludes2 malignant carcinoid tumors of the colon (C7A.02-)
　malignant melanoma of anal margin (C43.51)
　malignant melanoma of anal skin (C43.51)
　malignant melanoma of perianal skin (C43.51)
　other and unspecified malignant neoplasm of anal margin (C44.500, C44.510, C44.520, C44.590)
　other and unspecified malignant neoplasm of anal skin (C44.500, C44.510, C44.520, C44.590)
　other and unspecified malignant neoplasm of perianal skin (C44.500, C44.510, C44.520, C44.590)

C21.0 Malignant neoplasm of anus, unspecified

C21.1 Malignant neoplasm of anal canal
　Terminal part of large intestine
　Malignant neoplasm of anal sphincter

C21.2 Malignant neoplasm of cloacogenic zone

C21.8 Malignant neoplasm of overlapping sites of rectum, anus and anal canal
　Malignant neoplasm of anorectal junction
　Malignant neoplasm of anorectum
　Primary malignant neoplasm of two or more contiguous sites of rectum, anus and anal canal

● **C22 Malignant neoplasm of liver and intrahepatic bile ducts**
　Intrahepatic: Within liver
　Use additional code to identify:
　alcohol abuse and dependence (F10.-)
　hepatitis B (B16.-, B18.0-B18.1) hepatitis C (B17.1-, B18.2)
　Excludes1 malignant neoplasm of biliary tract NOS (C24.9)
　secondary malignant neoplasm of liver and intrahepatic bile duct (C78.7)

C22.0 Liver cell carcinoma
　Hepatocellular carcinoma
　Hepatoma

C22.1 Intrahepatic bile duct carcinoma
　Cholangiocarcinoma
　Adenocarcinoma (cancer that originates in glandular tissue) arising from epithelium of intrahepatic bile ducts
　Excludes1 malignant neoplasm of hepatic duct (C24.0)

C22.2 Hepatoblastoma
　Malignant intrahepatic tumor

C22.3 Angiosarcoma of liver
　Kupffer cell sarcoma

C22.4 Other sarcomas of liver

C22.7 Other specified carcinomas of liver

C22.8 Malignant neoplasm of liver, primary, unspecified as to type

C22.9 Malignant neoplasm of liver, not specified as primary or secondary

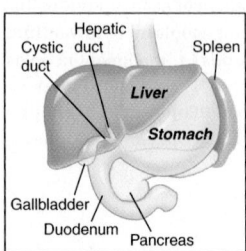

Figure 2-6 Diagram of liver, gallbladder, hepatic duct, pancreas, and spleen. (From Thibodeau and Patton: Anatomy and Physiology, ed 7, Mosby, 2010)

◀ New　◀▥ Revised　~~deleted~~ Deleted　**OGCR** Official Guidelines　X Assign placeholder X　● Use Additional Character(s)
Excludes 1　Excludes 2　Includes　Use additional　Code first　Code also　Unspecified

740

C23   **Malignant neoplasm of gallbladder**

●C24   **Malignant neoplasm of other and unspecified parts of biliary tract**

> **Excludes1**   malignant neoplasm of intrahepatic bile duct (C22.1)

C24.0   **Malignant neoplasm of extrahepatic bile duct**
Extrahepatic = outside the liver
Malignant neoplasm of biliary duct or passage NOS
Malignant neoplasm of common bile duct
Malignant neoplasm of cystic duct
Malignant neoplasm of hepatic duct

C24.1   **Malignant neoplasm of ampulla of Vater**
Union of pancreatic duct and common bile duct

C24.8   **Malignant neoplasm of overlapping sites of biliary tract**
Malignant neoplasm involving both intrahepatic and extrahepatic bile ducts
Primary malignant neoplasm of two or more contiguous sites of biliary tract

C24.9   **Malignant neoplasm of biliary tract, unspecified**

●C25   **Malignant neoplasm of pancreas**
Check documentation for specific site.
Use additional code to identify:
alcohol abuse and dependence (F10.-)

C25.0   **Malignant neoplasm of head of pancreas**

C25.1   **Malignant neoplasm of body of pancreas**

C25.2   **Malignant neoplasm of tail of pancreas**

C25.3   **Malignant neoplasm of pancreatic duct**

C25.4   **Malignant neoplasm of endocrine pancreas**
Malignant neoplasm of islets of Langerhans
That part of the pancreas that acts as endocrine gland and consists of islets of Langerhans
Use additional code to identify any functional activity.

C25.7   **Malignant neoplasm of other parts of pancreas**
Malignant neoplasm of neck of pancreas

C25.8   **Malignant neoplasm of overlapping sites of pancreas**

C25.9   **Malignant neoplasm of pancreas, unspecified**

●C26   **Malignant neoplasm of other and ill-defined digestive organs**

> **Excludes1**   malignant neoplasm of peritoneum and retroperitoneum (C48.-)

C26.0   **Malignant neoplasm of intestinal tract, part unspecified**
Malignant neoplasm of intestine NOS

C26.1   **Malignant neoplasm of spleen**

> **Excludes1**   Hodgkin lymphoma (C81.-)
> non-Hodgkin lymphoma (C82-C85)

C26.9   **Malignant neoplasm of ill-defined sites within the digestive system**
Malignant neoplasm of alimentary canal or tract NOS
Malignant neoplasm of gastrointestinal tract NOS

> **Excludes1**   malignant neoplasm of abdominal NOS (C76.2)
> malignant neoplasm of intra-abdominal NOS (C76.2)

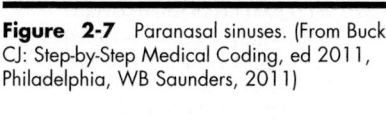

Figure 2-7 Paranasal sinuses. (From Buck CJ: Step-by-Step Medical Coding, ed 2011, Philadelphia, WB Saunders, 2011)

MALIGNANT NEOPLASMS OF RESPIRATORY AND INTRATHORACIC ORGANS (C30-C39)

> **Includes**   malignant neoplasm of middle ear
> **Excludes1**   mesothelioma (C45.-)

●C30   **Malignant neoplasm of nasal cavity and middle ear**

C30.0   **Malignant neoplasm of nasal cavity**
Malignant neoplasm of cartilage of nose
Malignant neoplasm of nasal concha
Malignant neoplasm of internal nose
Malignant neoplasm of septum of nose
Malignant neoplasm of vestibule of nose
Anterior part of nasal cavity

> **Excludes1**   malignant neoplasm of nasal bone (C41.0)
> malignant neoplasm of nose NOS (C76.0)
> malignant neoplasm of olfactory bulb (C72.2-)
> malignant neoplasm of posterior margin of nasal septum and choana (C11.3)
> malignant melanoma of skin of nose (C43.31)
> malignant neoplasm of turbinates (C41.0)
> other and unspecified malignant neoplasm of skin of nose C44.301, C44.311, C44.321, C44.391)

C30.1   **Malignant neoplasm of middle ear**
Malignant neoplasm of antrum tympanicum
Boney cavity or chamber
Malignant neoplasm of auditory tube
Malignant neoplasm of eustachian tube
Malignant neoplasm of inner ear
Malignant neoplasm of mastoid air cells
Malignant neoplasm of tympanic cavity

> **Excludes1**   malignant neoplasm of auricular canal (external) (C43.2-, C44.2-)
> malignant neoplasm of bone of ear (meatus) (C41.0)
> malignant neoplasm of cartilage of ear (C49.0)
> malignant melanoma of skin of (external) ear (C43.2-)
> other and unspecified malignant neoplasm of skin of (external) ear (C44.2-)

●C31   **Malignant neoplasm of accessory sinuses**
Paired sinuses in bones of face

C31.0   **Malignant neoplasm of maxillary sinus**
Malignant neoplasm of antrum (Highmore) (maxillary)

C31.1   **Malignant neoplasm of ethmoidal sinus**

C31.2   **Malignant neoplasm of frontal sinus**

C31.3   **Malignant neoplasm of sphenoid sinus**

C31.8   **Malignant neoplasm of overlapping sites of accessory sinuses**

C31.9   **Malignant neoplasm of accessory sinus, unspecified**

CHAPTER 2 (C00-D49)

Item 2-3 Islets of Langerhans (endocrine producing cells comprising 1% to 2% of the pancreatic mass) make and secrete hormones that regulate the body's production of insulin, glucagon, and stomach acid. Breakdown of the insulin-producing cells can cause diabetes mellitus. Islet cell tumors can be benign or malignant and include glucagonomas, insulinomas, gastrinomas, and neuroendocrine tumor. The neoplasm table must be consulted for the correct neoplasm code.

◀ New   ⬅ Revised   ~~deleted~~ Deleted   **OGCR** Official Guidelines   X Assign placeholder X   ● Use Additional Character(s)

Excludes 1   Excludes 2   Includes   Use additional   Code first   Code also   Unspecified

● **C32   Malignant neoplasm of larynx**
   Use additional code to identify:
      alcohol abuse and dependence (F10.-)
      exposure to environmental tobacco smoke (Z77.22)
      exposure to tobacco smoke in the perinatal period (P96.81)
      history of tobacco use (Z87.891)
      occupational exposure to environmental tobacco smoke
         (Z57.31)
      tobacco dependence (F17.-)
      tobacco use (Z72.0)

   C32.0   Malignant neoplasm of glottis
      Vocal apparatus of larynx, consisting of true vocal cords
         (plicae vocales) and opening between them (rima
         glottidis)
      Malignant neoplasm of intrinsic larynx
      Malignant neoplasm of laryngeal commissure (anterior)
         (posterior)
      Malignant neoplasm of vocal cord (true) NOS
         True *vocal cords ("lower vocal folds") produce vocalization*
            when air from the lungs passes between them. Check
            your documentation. Code C32.1 is for malignant
            neoplasm of the **false** *vocal cords.*

   C32.1   Malignant neoplasm of supraglottis
      Area of pharynx above glottis
      Malignant neoplasm of aryepiglottic fold or
         interarytenoid fold, laryngeal aspect
      Malignant neoplasm of epiglottis (suprahyoid portion)
         NOS
      Malignant neoplasm of extrinsic larynx
      Malignant neoplasm of false vocal cord
         False *vocal cords ("upper vocal folds") are not involved in*
            vocalization. Check your documentation. Code C32.0 is
            for true vocal cords.
      Malignant neoplasm of posterior (laryngeal) surface of
         epiglottis
      Malignant neoplasm of ventricular bands
      | Excludes2 | malignant neoplasm of anterior surface of
               epiglottis (C10.1)
            malignant neoplasm of aryepiglottic
               fold or interarytenoid fold,
               hypopharyngeal aspect (C13.1)
            malignant neoplasm of aryepiglottic fold
               or interarytenoid fold, marginal zone
               (C13.1)
            malignant neoplasm of aryepiglottic fold
               or interarytenoid fold NOS (C13.1)

   C32.2   Malignant neoplasm of subglottis
      Lowest part of larynx from just below vocal cords down to top
         of trachea

   C32.3   Malignant neoplasm of laryngeal cartilage
      Cartilages of larynx, including cricoid, thyroid, and
         epiglottic, and two each of arytenoid, corniculate, and
         cuneiform

   C32.8   Malignant neoplasm of overlapping sites of larynx

   C32.9   Malignant neoplasm of larynx, unspecified

C33   Malignant neoplasm of trachea
   Use additional code to identify:
      exposure to environmental tobacco smoke (Z77.22)
      exposure to tobacco smoke in the perinatal period (P96.81)
      history of tobacco use (Z87.891)
      occupational exposure to environmental tobacco smoke
         (Z57.31)
      tobacco dependence (F17.-)
      tobacco use (Z72.0)

● **C34   Malignant neoplasm of bronchus and lung**
   Use additional code to identify:
      exposure to environmental tobacco smoke (Z77.22)
      exposure to tobacco smoke in the perinatal period (P96.81)
      history of tobacco use (Z87.891)
      occupational exposure to environmental tobacco smoke
         (Z57.31)
      tobacco dependence (F17.-)
      tobacco use (Z72.0)
   | Excludes1 | Kaposi's sarcoma of lung (C46.5-)
            malignant carcinoid tumor of the bronchus and
               lung (C7A.090)

   ● **C34.0   Malignant neoplasm of main bronchus**
      Malignant neoplasm of carina
         Ridgelike structure
      Malignant neoplasm of hilus (of lung)
         Anatomic depression or pit

      **C34.00   Malignant neoplasm of unspecified main
                  bronchus**
      C34.01   Malignant neoplasm of right main bronchus
      C34.02   Malignant neoplasm of left main bronchus

   ● **C34.1   Malignant neoplasm of upper lobe, bronchus or lung**
      **C34.10   Malignant neoplasm of unspecified bronchus
                  or lung**
      **C34.11   Malignant neoplasm of upper lobe, right
                  bronchus or lung**
      **C34.12   Malignant neoplasm of upper lobe, left
                  bronchus or lung**

   C34.2   Malignant neoplasm of middle lobe, bronchus or lung

   ● **C34.3   Malignant neoplasm of lower lobe, bronchus or lung**
      **C34.30   Malignant neoplasm of lower lobe, unspecified
                  bronchus or lung**
      **C34.31   Malignant neoplasm of lower lobe, right
                  bronchus or lung**
      **C34.32   Malignant neoplasm of lower lobe, left
                  bronchus or lung**

   ● **C34.8   Malignant neoplasm of overlapping sites of bronchus
               and lung**
      **C34.80   Malignant neoplasm of overlapping sites
                  of unspecified bronchus and lung**
      **C34.81   Malignant neoplasm of overlapping sites of
                  right bronchus and lung**
      **C34.82   Malignant neoplasm of overlapping sites of left
                  bronchus and lung**

   ● **C34.9   Malignant neoplasm of unspecified part of bronchus or
               lung**
      **C34.90   Malignant neoplasm of unspecified part of
                  unspecified bronchus or lung**
         Lung cancer NOS
      **C34.91   Malignant neoplasm of unspecified part of
                  right bronchus or lung**
      **C34.92   Malignant neoplasm of unspecified part of left
                  bronchus or lung**

C37   Malignant neoplasm of thymus
   | Excludes1 | malignant carcinoid tumor of the thymus
            (C7A.091)

◀ New   ◀▥ Revised   ~~deleted~~ Deleted   **OGCR** Official Guidelines   X Assign placeholder X   ● Use Additional Character(s)
| Excludes 1 | | Excludes 2 | Includes   Use additional   Code first   Code also   Unspecified

● **C38**   **Malignant neoplasm of heart, mediastinum and pleura**
> **Excludes1**   mesothelioma (C45.-)

     C38.0   **Malignant neoplasm of heart**
           Malignant neoplasm of pericardium
> **Excludes1**   malignant neoplasm of great vessels (C49.3)

     C38.1   **Malignant neoplasm of anterior mediastinum**
     C38.2   **Malignant neoplasm of posterior mediastinum**
     C38.3   **Malignant neoplasm of mediastinum, part unspecified**
     C38.4   **Malignant neoplasm of pleura**
     C38.8   **Malignant neoplasm of overlapping sites of heart, mediastinum and pleura**
           Pleura are comprised of serous membrane that lines the thoracic cavity (parietal) and covers the lungs (visceral).

● **C39**   **Malignant neoplasm of other and ill-defined sites in the respiratory system and intrathoracic organs**
       Intrathoracic: within thorax/chest
> Use additional code to identify:
       exposure to environmental tobacco smoke (Z77.22)
       exposure to tobacco smoke in the perinatal period (P96.81)
       history of tobacco use (Z87.891)
       occupational exposure to environmental tobacco smoke (Z57.31)
       tobacco dependence (F17.-)
       tobacco use (Z72.0)
> **Excludes1**   intrathoracic malignant neoplasm NOS (C76.1)
                 thoracic malignant neoplasm NOS (C76.1)

     C39.0   **Malignant neoplasm of upper respiratory tract, part unspecified**
     C39.9   **Malignant neoplasm of lower respiratory tract, part unspecified**
           Malignant neoplasm of respiratory tract NOS

MALIGNANT NEOPLASMS OF BONE AND ARTICULAR CARTILAGE (C40-C41)

> **Includes**   malignant neoplasm of cartilage (articular) (joint)
          malignant neoplasm of periosteum
> **Excludes1**   malignant neoplasm of bone marrow NOS (C96.9)
          malignant neoplasm of synovia (C49.-)

● **C40**   **Malignant neoplasm of bone and articular cartilage of limbs**
> Use additional code to identify major osseous defect, if applicable (M89.7-)

   ● **C40.0**   **Malignant neoplasm of scapula and long bones of upper limb**
       C40.00   **Malignant neoplasm of scapula and long bones of unspecified upper limb**
       C40.01   **Malignant neoplasm of scapula and long bones of right upper limb**
       C40.02   **Malignant neoplasm of scapula and long bones of left upper limb**

   ● **C40.1**   **Malignant neoplasm of short bones of upper limb**
       C40.10   **Malignant neoplasm of short bones of unspecified upper limb**
       C40.11   **Malignant neoplasm of short bones of right upper limb**
       C40.12   **Malignant neoplasm of short bones of left upper limb**

   ● **C40.2**   **Malignant neoplasm of long bones of lower limb**
       C40.20   **Malignant neoplasm of long bones of unspecified lower limb**
       C40.21   **Malignant neoplasm of long bones of right lower limb**
       C40.22   **Malignant neoplasm of long bones of left lower limb**

Figure 2-8   Diagram of skeleton of trunk and limbs with bones labeled. (From Thibodeau and Patton: Anatomy and Physiology, ed 7, Mosby, 2010)

   ● **C40.3**   **Malignant neoplasm of short bones of lower limb**
       C40.30   **Malignant neoplasm of short bones of unspecified lower limb**
       C40.31   **Malignant neoplasm of short bones of right lower limb**
       C40.32   **Malignant neoplasm of short bones of left lower limb**

   ● **C40.8**   **Malignant neoplasm of overlapping sites of bone and articular cartilage of limb**
       C40.80   **Malignant neoplasm of overlapping sites of bone and articular cartilage of unspecified limb**
       C40.81   **Malignant neoplasm of overlapping sites of bone and articular cartilage of right limb**
       C40.82   **Malignant neoplasm of overlapping sites of bone and articular cartilage of left limb**

   ● **C40.9**   **Malignant neoplasm of unspecified bones and articular cartilage of limb**
       C40.90   **Malignant neoplasm of unspecified bones and articular cartilage of unspecified limb**
       C40.91   **Malignant neoplasm of unspecified bones and articular cartilage of right limb**
       C40.92   **Malignant neoplasm of unspecified bones and articular cartilage of left limb**

● **C41**   **Malignant neoplasm of bone and articular cartilage of other and unspecified sites**
> **Excludes1**   malignant neoplasm of bones of limbs (C40.-)
          malignant neoplasm of cartilage of ear (C49.0)
          malignant neoplasm of cartilage of eyelid (C49.0)
          malignant neoplasm of cartilage of larynx (C32.3)
          malignant neoplasm of cartilage of limbs (C40.-)
          malignant neoplasm of cartilage of nose (C30.0)

     C41.0   **Malignant neoplasm of bones of skull and face**
          Malignant neoplasm of maxilla (superior)
          Malignant neoplasm of orbital bone
> **Excludes2**   carcinoma, any type except intraosseous or odontogenic of:
          maxillary sinus (C31.0)
          upper jaw (C03.0)
          malignant neoplasm of jaw bone (lower) (C41.1)

CHAPTER 2 (C00-D49)

◀ New   ⬅ Revised   ~~deleted~~ Deleted   **OGCR** Official Guidelines   X Assign placeholder X   ● Use Additional Character(s)

| Excludes 1 | Excludes 2 | Includes | Use additional | Code first | Code also | Unspecified |

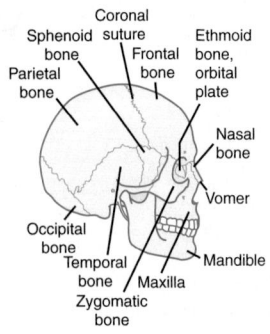

Figure 2-9   Bones of the skull.

Figure 2-10   Malignant melanoma of skin. (From Goldman: Cecil Textbook of Medicine, ed 22, Saunders, 2004)

Item 2–4   **Malignant melanoma** is a serious form of skin cancer that affects the melanocytes (pigment-forming cells) and is caused by ultraviolet (UV) rays from the sun that damage skin. It is most commonly seen in the 40- to 60-year-olds with fair skin, blue or green eyes, and red or blond hair who sunburn easily.

Melanoma can spread very rapidly and is the most deadly form of skin cancer. It is less common than other types of skin cancer. The rate of melanoma is increasing and currently is the leading cause of death from skin disease.

C41.1 Malignant neoplasm of mandible
Malignant neoplasm of inferior maxilla
Malignant neoplasm of lower jaw bone
> **Excludes2**   carcinoma, any type except intraosseous or odontogenic of:
> jaw NOS (C03.9)
> lower (C03.1)
> malignant neoplasm of upper jaw bone (C41.0)

C41.2 Malignant neoplasm of vertebral column
> **Excludes1**   malignant neoplasm of sacrum and coccyx (C41.4)

C41.3 Malignant neoplasm of ribs, sternum and clavicle

C41.4 Malignant neoplasm of pelvic bones, sacrum and coccyx

C41.9 Malignant neoplasm of bone and articular cartilage, unspecified

MELANOMA AND OTHER MALIGNANT NEOPLASMS OF SKIN (C43-C44)

● **C43 Malignant melanoma of skin**
> **Excludes1**   melanoma in situ (D03.-)
> **Excludes2**   malignant melanoma of skin of genital organs (C51-C52, C60.-, C63.-)
> Merkel cell carcinoma (C4A.-)
> sites other than skin-code to malignant neoplasm of the site

C43.0 Malignant melanoma of lip
> **Excludes1**   malignant neoplasm of vermilion border of lip (C00.0-C00.2)

● **C43.1 Malignant melanoma of eyelid, including canthus**
Canthus: Either corner of eye where upper and lower eyelids meet

    C43.10 Malignant melanoma of unspecified eyelid, including canthus

    C43.11 Malignant melanoma of right eyelid, including canthus

    C43.12 Malignant melanoma of left eyelid, including canthus

● **C43.2 Malignant melanoma of ear and external auricular canal**

    C43.20 Malignant melanoma of unspecified ear and external auricular canal

    C43.21 Malignant melanoma of right ear and external auricular canal

    C43.22 Malignant melanoma of left ear and external auricular canal

● **C43.3 Malignant melanoma of other and unspecified parts of face**

    C43.30 Malignant melanoma of unspecified part of face

    C43.31 Malignant melanoma of nose

    C43.39 Malignant melanoma of other parts of face

C43.4 Malignant melanoma of scalp and neck

● **C43.5 Malignant melanoma of trunk**
> **Excludes2**   malignant neoplasm of anus NOS (C21.0)
> malignant neoplasm of scrotum (C63.2)

    C43.51 Malignant melanoma of anal skin
    Malignant melanoma of anal margin
    Malignant melanoma of perianal skin

    C43.52 Malignant melanoma of skin of breast

    C43.59 Malignant melanoma of other part of trunk

● **C43.6 Malignant melanoma of upper limb, including shoulder**

    C43.60 Malignant melanoma of upper limb, including shoulder, unspecified side

    C43.61 Malignant melanoma of right upper limb, including shoulder

    C43.62 Malignant melanoma of left upper limb, including shoulder

● **C43.7 Malignant melanoma of lower limb, including hip**

    C43.70 Malignant melanoma of unspecified lower limb, including hip

    C43.71 Malignant melanoma of right lower limb, including hip

    C43.72 Malignant melanoma of left lower limb, including hip

C43.8 Malignant melanoma of overlapping sites of skin

C43.9 Malignant melanoma of skin, unspecified
Malignant melanoma of unspecified site of skin
Melanoma (malignant) NOS

C4A Merkel cell carcinoma

C4A.0 Merkel cell carcinoma of lip
> **Excludes1**   malignant neoplasm of vermilion border of lip (C00.0-C00.2)

● **C4A.1 Merkel cell carcinoma of eyelid, including canthus**

    C4A.10 Merkel cell carcinoma of unspecified eyelid, including canthus

    C4A.11 Merkel cell carcinoma of right eyelid, including canthus

    C4A.12 Merkel cell carcinoma of left eyelid, including canthus

● **C4A.2 Merkel cell carcinoma of ear and external auricular canal**

    C4A.20 Merkel cell carcinoma of unspecified ear and external auricular canal

    C4A.21 Merkel cell carcinoma of right ear and external auricular canal

    C4A.22 Merkel cell carcinoma of left ear and external auricular canal

CHAPTER 2 (C00-D49)

◀ New   ◀≡ Revised   ~~deleted~~ Deleted   OGCR Official Guidelines   X Assign placeholder X   ● Use Additional Character(s)

Excludes 1   Excludes 2   Includes   Use additional   Code first   Code also   Unspecified

● C4A.3   Merkel cell carcinoma of other and unspecified parts of face
     C4A.30   Merkel cell carcinoma of unspecified part of face
     C4A.31   Merkel cell carcinoma of nose
     C4A.39   Merkel cell carcinoma of other parts of face
   C4A.4   Merkel cell carcinoma of scalp and neck
● C4A.5   Merkel cell carcinoma of trunk

> **Excludes2**   malignant neoplasm of anus NOS (C21.0)
>   malignant neoplasm of scrotum (C63.2)

     C4A.51   Merkel cell carcinoma of anal skin
          Merkel cell carcinoma of anal margin
          Merkel cell carcinoma of perianal skin
     C4A.52   Merkel cell carcinoma of skin of breast
     C4A.59   Merkel cell carcinoma of other part of trunk
● C4A.6   Merkel cell carcinoma of upper limb, including shoulder
     C4A.60   Merkel cell carcinoma of unspecified upper limb, including shoulder
     C4A.61   Merkel cell carcinoma of right upper limb, including shoulder
     C4A.62   Merkel cell carcinoma of left upper limb, including shoulder
● C4A.7   Merkel cell carcinoma of lower limb, including hip
     C4A.70   Merkel cell carcinoma of unspecified lower limb, including hip
     C4A.71   Merkel cell carcinoma of right lower limb, including hip
     C4A.72   Merkel cell carcinoma of left lower limb, including hip
   C4A.8   Merkel cell carcinoma of overlapping sites
   C4A.9   Merkel cell carcinoma, unspecified
          Merkel cell carcinoma of unspecified site
          Merkel cell carcinoma NOS

● C44   Other and unspecified malignant neoplasm of skin

> **Includes**   malignant neoplasm of sebaceous glands
>   malignant neoplasm of sweat glands

> **Excludes1**   Kaposi's sarcoma of skin (C46.0)
>   malignant melanoma of skin (C43.-)
>   malignant neoplasm of skin of genital organs (C51-C52, C60.-, C63.2)
>   Merkel cell carcinoma (C4A.-)

● C44.0   Other and unspecified malignant neoplasm of skin of lip

> **Excludes1**   malignant neoplasm of lip (C00.-)

     C44.00   Unspecified malignant neoplasm of skin of lip
     C44.01   Basal cell carcinoma of skin of lip
     C44.02   Squamous cell carcinoma of skin of lip
     C44.09   Other specified malignant neoplasm of skin of lip
● C44.1   Other and unspecified malignant neoplasm of skin of eyelid, including canthus

> **Excludes1**   connective tissue of eyelid (C49.0)

   ● C44.10   Unspecified malignant neoplasm of skin of eyelid, including canthus
       C44.101   Unspecified malignant neoplasm of skin of unspecified eyelid, including canthus
       C44.102   Unspecified malignant neoplasm of skin of right eyelid, including canthus
       C44.109   Unspecified malignant neoplasm of skin of left eyelid, including canthus

● C44.11   Basal cell carcinoma of skin of eyelid, including canthus
       C44.111   Basal cell carcinoma of skin of unspecified eyelid, including canthus
       C44.112   Basal cell carcinoma of skin of right eyelid, including canthus
       C44.119   Basal cell carcinoma of skin of left eyelid, including canthus
● C44.12   Squamous cell carcinoma of skin of eyelid, including canthus
       C44.121   Squamous cell carcinoma of skin of unspecified eyelid, including canthus
       C44.122   Squamous cell carcinoma of skin of right eyelid, including canthus
       C44.129   Squamous cell carcinoma of skin of left eyelid, including canthus
● C44.19   Other specified malignant neoplasm of skin of eyelid, including canthus
       C44.191   Other specified malignant neoplasm of skin of unspecified eyelid, including canthus
       C44.192   Other specified malignant neoplasm of skin of right eyelid, including canthus
       C44.199   Other specified malignant neoplasm of skin of left eyelid, including canthus
● C44.2   Other and unspecified malignant neoplasm of skin of ear and external auricular canal

> **Excludes1**   connective tissue of ear (C49.0)

   ● C44.20   Unspecified malignant neoplasm of skin of ear and external auricular canal
       C44.201   Unspecified malignant neoplasm of skin of unspecified ear and external auricular canal
       C44.202   Unspecified malignant neoplasm of skin of right ear and external auricular canal
       C44.209   Unspecified malignant neoplasm of skin of left ear and external auricular canal
   ● C44.21   Basal cell carcinoma of skin of ear and external auricular canal
       C44.211   Basal cell carcinoma of skin of unspecified ear and external auricular canal
       C44.212   Basal cell carcinoma of skin of right ear and external auricular canal
       C44.219   Basal cell carcinoma of skin of left ear and external auricular canal
   ● C44.22   Squamous cell carcinoma of skin of ear and external auricular canal
       C44.221   Squamous cell carcinoma of skin of unspecified ear and external auricular canal
       C44.222   Squamous cell carcinoma of skin of right ear and external auricular canal
       C44.229   Squamous cell carcinoma of skin of left ear and external auricular canal

CHAPTER 2 (C00-D49)

● **C44.29** Other specified malignant neoplasm of skin of ear and external auricular canal

  C44.291 Other specified malignant neoplasm of skin of unspecified ear and external auricular canal

  C44.292 Other specified malignant neoplasm of skin of right ear and external auricular canal

  C44.299 Other specified malignant neoplasm of skin of left ear and external auricular canal

● **C44.3** Other and unspecified malignant neoplasm of skin of other and unspecified parts of face

  ● **C44.30** Unspecified malignant neoplasm of skin of other and unspecified parts of face

    C44.300 Unspecified malignant neoplasm of skin of unspecified part of face

    C44.301 Unspecified malignant neoplasm of skin of nose

    C44.309 Unspecified malignant neoplasm of skin of other parts of face

  ● **C44.31** Basal cell carcinoma of skin of other and unspecified parts of face

    C44.310 Basal cell carcinoma of skin of unspecified parts of face

    C44.311 Basal cell carcinoma of skin of nose

    C44.319 Basal cell carcinoma of skin of other parts of face

  ● **C44.32** Squamous cell carcinoma of skin of other and unspecified parts of face

    C44.320 Squamous cell carcinoma of skin of unspecified parts of face

    C44.321 Squamous cell carcinoma of skin of nose

    C44.329 Squamous cell carcinoma of skin of other parts of face

  ● **C44.39** Other specified malignant neoplasm of skin of other and unspecified parts of face

    C44.390 Other specified malignant neoplasm of skin of unspecified parts of face

    C44.391 Other specified malignant neoplasm of skin of nose

    C44.399 Other specified malignant neoplasm of skin of other parts of face

● **C44.4** Other and unspecified malignant neoplasm of skin of scalp and neck

  C44.40 Unspecified malignant neoplasm of skin of scalp and neck

  C44.41 Basal cell carcinoma of skin of scalp and neck

  C44.42 Squamous cell carcinoma of skin of scalp and neck

  C44.49 Other specified malignant neoplasm of skin of scalp and neck

● **C44.5** Other and unspecified malignant neoplasm of skin of trunk

  Excludes1 anus NOS (C21.0)
                 scrotum (C63.2)

  ● **C44.50** Unspecified malignant neoplasm of skin of trunk

    C44.500 Unspecified malignant neoplasm of anal skin
      Unspecified malignant neoplasm of anal margin
      Unspecified malignant neoplasm of perianal skin

    C44.501 Unspecified malignant neoplasm of skin of breast

    C44.509 Unspecified malignant neoplasm of skin of other part of trunk

● **C44.51** Basal cell carcinoma of skin of trunk

  C44.510 Basal cell carcinoma of anal skin
    Basal cell carcinoma of anal margin
    Basal cell carcinoma of perianal skin

  C44.511 Basal cell carcinoma of skin of breast

  C44.519 Basal cell carcinoma of skin of other part of trunk

● **C44.52** Squamous cell carcinoma of skin of trunk

  C44.520 Squamous cell carcinoma of anal skin
    Squamous cell carcinoma of anal margin
    Squamous cell carcinoma of perianal skin

  C44.521 Squamous cell carcinoma of skin of breast

  C44.529 Squamous cell carcinoma of skin of other part of trunk

● **C44.59** Other specified malignant neoplasm of skin of trunk

  C44.590 Other specified malignant neoplasm of anal skin
    Other specified malignant neoplasm of anal margin
    Other specified malignant neoplasm of perianal skin

  C44.591 Other specified malignant neoplasm of skin of breast

  C44.599 Other specified malignant neoplasm of skin of other part of trunk

● **C44.6** Other and unspecified malignant neoplasm of skin of upper limb, including shoulder

  ● **C44.60** Unspecified malignant neoplasm of skin of upper limb, including shoulder

    C44.601 Unspecified malignant neoplasm of skin of unspecified upper limb, including shoulder

    C44.602 Unspecified malignant neoplasm of skin of right upper limb, including shoulder

    C44.609 Unspecified malignant neoplasm of skin of left upper limb, including shoulder

  ● **C44.61** Basal cell carcinoma of skin of upper limb, including shoulder

    C44.611 Basal cell carcinoma of skin of unspecified upper limb, including shoulder

    C44.612 Basal cell carcinoma of skin of right upper limb, including shoulder

    C44.619 Basal cell carcinoma of skin of left upper limb, including shoulder

  ● **C44.62** Squamous cell carcinoma of skin of upper limb, including shoulder

    C44.621 Squamous cell carcinoma of skin of unspecified upper limb, including shoulder

    C44.622 Squamous cell carcinoma of skin of right upper limb, including shoulder

    C44.629 Squamous cell carcinoma of skin of left upper limb, including shoulder

● C44.69   Other specified malignant neoplasm of skin of upper limb, including shoulder

C44.691   Other specified malignant neoplasm of skin of unspecified upper limb, including shoulder

C44.692   Other specified malignant neoplasm of skin of right upper limb, including shoulder

C44.699   Other specified malignant neoplasm of skin of left upper limb, including shoulder

● C44.7   Other and unspecified malignant neoplasm of skin of lower limb, including hip

● C44.70   Unspecified malignant neoplasm of skin of lower limb, including hip

C44.701   Unspecified malignant neoplasm of skin of unspecified lower limb, including hip

C44.702   Unspecified malignant neoplasm of skin of right lower limb, including hip

C44.709   Unspecified malignant neoplasm of skin of left lower limb, including hip

● C44.71   Basal cell carcinoma of skin of lower limb, including hip

C44.711   Basal cell carcinoma of skin of unspecified lower limb, including hip

C44.712   Basal cell carcinoma of skin of right lower limb, including hip

C44.719   Basal cell carcinoma of skin of left lower limb, including hip

● C44.72   Squamous cell carcinoma of skin of lower limb, including hip

C44.721   Squamous cell carcinoma of skin of unspecified lower limb, including hip

C44.722   Squamous cell carcinoma of skin of right lower limb, including hip

C44.729   Squamous cell carcinoma of skin of left lower limb, including hip

● C44.79   Other specified malignant neoplasm of skin of lower limb, including hip

C44.791   Other specified malignant neoplasm of skin of unspecified lower limb, including hip

C44.792   Other specified malignant neoplasm of skin of right lower limb, including hip

C44.799   Other specified malignant neoplasm of skin of left lower limb, including hip

● C44.8   Other and unspecified malignant neoplasm of overlapping sites of skin

C44.80   Unspecified malignant neoplasm of overlapping sites of skin

C44.81   Basal cell carcinoma of overlapping sites of skin

C44.82   Squamous cell carcinoma of overlapping sites of skin

C44.89   Other specified malignant neoplasm of overlapping sites of skin

● C44.9   Other and unspecified malignant neoplasm of skin, unspecified

C44.90   Unspecified malignant neoplasm of skin, unspecified
Malignant neoplasm of unspecified site of skin

C44.91   Basal cell carcinoma of skin, unspecified

C44.92   Squamous cell carcinoma of skin, unspecified

C44.99   Other specified malignant neoplasm of skin, unspecified

MALIGNANT NEOPLASMS OF MESOTHELIAL AND SOFT TISSUE (C45-C49)

● C45   Mesothelioma
Malignant cells develop in protective lining that covers internal organs (mesothelium) caused by exposure to asbestos

C45.0   Mesothelioma of pleura
Excludes 1   other malignant neoplasm of pleura (C38.4)

C45.1   Mesothelioma of peritoneum
Mesothelioma of cul-de-sac
Mesothelioma of mesentery
Mesothelioma of mesocolon
Mesothelioma of omentum
Mesothelioma of peritoneum (parietal) (pelvic)
Excludes 1   other malignant neoplasm of soft tissue of peritoneum (C48.-)

C45.2   Mesothelioma of pericardium
Excludes 1   other malignant neoplasm of pericardium (C38.0)

C45.7   Mesothelioma of other sites

C45.9   Mesothelioma, unspecified

● C46   Kaposi's sarcoma
Code first any human immunodeficiency virus [HIV] disease (B20)

C46.0   Kaposi's sarcoma of skin

C46.1   Kaposi's sarcoma of soft tissue
Kaposi's sarcoma of blood vessel
Kaposi's sarcoma of connective tissue
Kaposi's sarcoma of fascia
Kaposi's sarcoma of ligament
Kaposi's sarcoma of lymphatic(s) NEC
Kaposi's sarcoma of muscle
Excludes 2   Kaposi's sarcoma of lymph glands and nodes (C46.3)

C46.2   Kaposi's sarcoma of palate

C46.3   Kaposi's sarcoma of lymph nodes

C46.4   Kaposi's sarcoma of gastrointestinal sites

● C46.5   Kaposi's sarcoma of lung

C46.50   Kaposi's sarcoma of unspecified lung

C46.51   Kaposi's sarcoma of right lung

C46.52   Kaposi's sarcoma of left lung

C46.7   Kaposi's sarcoma of other sites

C46.9   Kaposi's sarcoma, unspecified
Kaposi's sarcoma of unspecified site

Figure 2-11   Kaposi's sarcoma. There are large confluent hyperpigmented patch-stage lesions with lymphedema. (From Cohen & Powderly: Infectious Diseases, ed 3, Mosby, An Imprint of Elsevier, 2010)

Item 2-5   Kaposi's sarcoma is a cancer that causes patches of abnormal tissue to grow under the skin; in the lining of the mouth, nose, and throat; or in other organs, often beginning and spreading to other organs. Patients who have had organ transplants or patients with AIDS are at high risk for this malignancy.

CHAPTER 2 (C00-D49)

◄ New   ◀▦ Revised   ~~deleted~~ Deleted   **OGCR** Official Guidelines   X Assign placeholder X   ● Use Additional Character(s)

| Excludes 1 | Excludes 2 | Includes | Use additional | Code first | Code also | Unspecified |

● **C47 Malignant neoplasm of peripheral nerves and autonomic nervous system**

> **Includes**   malignant neoplasm of sympathetic and parasympathetic nerves and ganglia
>
> **Excludes1**   Kaposi's sarcoma of soft tissue (C46.1)

   C47.0 Malignant neoplasm of peripheral nerves of head, face and neck

> **Excludes1**   malignant neoplasm of peripheral nerves of orbit (C69.6-)

● **C47.1 Malignant neoplasm of peripheral nerves of upper limb, including shoulder**

     C47.10 Malignant neoplasm of peripheral nerves of unspecified upper limb, including shoulder

     C47.11 Malignant neoplasm of peripheral nerves of right upper limb, including shoulder

     C47.12 Malignant neoplasm of peripheral nerves of left upper limb, including shoulder

● **C47.2 Malignant neoplasm of peripheral nerves of lower limb, including hip**

     C47.20 Malignant neoplasm of peripheral nerves of unspecified lower limb, including hip

     C47.21 Malignant neoplasm of peripheral nerves of right lower limb, including hip

     C47.22 Malignant neoplasm of peripheral nerves of left lower limb, including hip

   C47.3 Malignant neoplasm of peripheral nerves of thorax

   C47.4 Malignant neoplasm of peripheral nerves of abdomen

   C47.5 Malignant neoplasm of peripheral nerves of pelvis

   C47.6 Malignant neoplasm of peripheral nerves of trunk, unspecified

> Malignant neoplasm of peripheral nerves of unspecified part of trunk

   C47.8 Malignant neoplasm of overlapping sites of peripheral nerves and autonomic nervous system

   C47.9 Malignant neoplasm of peripheral nerves and autonomic nervous system, unspecified

> Malignant neoplasm of unspecified site of peripheral nerves and autonomic nervous system

● **C48 Malignant neoplasm of retroperitoneum and peritoneum**

> **Excludes1**   Kaposi's sarcoma of connective tissue (C46.1)
> mesothelioma (C45.-)

   C48.0 Malignant neoplasm of retroperitoneum

> *Behind/outside of peritoneum*

   C48.1 Malignant neoplasm of specified parts of peritoneum

> *Serous membrane lining abdominopelvic walls and covering viscera*
>
> Malignant neoplasm of cul-de-sac
> Malignant neoplasm of mesentery
> Malignant neoplasm of mesocolon
> Malignant neoplasm of omentum
> Malignant neoplasm of parietal peritoneum
> Malignant neoplasm of pelvic peritoneum

   C48.2 Malignant neoplasm of peritoneum, unspecified

   C48.8 Malignant neoplasm of overlapping sites of retroperitoneum and peritoneum

● **C49 Malignant neoplasm of other connective and soft tissue**

> **Includes**   malignant neoplasm of blood vessel
> malignant neoplasm of bursa
> malignant neoplasm of cartilage
> malignant neoplasm of fascia
> malignant neoplasm of fat
> malignant neoplasm of ligament, except uterine
> malignant neoplasm of lymphatic vessel
> malignant neoplasm of muscle
> malignant neoplasm of synovia
> malignant neoplasm of tendon (sheath)
>
> **Excludes1**   malignant neoplasm of cartilage (of):
> articular (C40-C41)
> larynx (C32.3)
> nose (C30.0)
> malignant neoplasm of connective tissue of breast (C50.-)
>
> **Excludes2**   Kaposi's sarcoma of soft tissue (C46.1)
> malignant neoplasm of heart (C38.0)
> malignant neoplasm of peripheral nerves and autonomic nervous system (C47.-)
> malignant neoplasm of peritoneum (C48.2)
> malignant neoplasm of retroperitoneum (C48.0)
> malignant neoplasm of uterine ligament (C57.3)
> mesothelioma (C45.-)

   C49.0 Malignant neoplasm of connective and soft tissue of head, face and neck

> Malignant neoplasm of connective tissue of ear
> Malignant neoplasm of connective tissue of eyelid
>
> **Excludes1**   connective tissue of orbit (C69.6-)

● **C49.1 Malignant neoplasm of connective and soft tissue of upper limb, including shoulder**

     C49.10 Malignant neoplasm of connective and soft tissue of unspecified upper limb, including shoulder

     C49.11 Malignant neoplasm of connective and soft tissue of right upper limb, including shoulder

     C49.12 Malignant neoplasm of connective and soft tissue of left upper limb, including shoulder

● **C49.2 Malignant neoplasm of connective and soft tissue of lower limb, including hip**

     C49.20 Malignant neoplasm of connective and soft tissue of unspecified lower limb, including hip

     C49.21 Malignant neoplasm of connective and soft tissue of right lower limb, including hip

     C49.22 Malignant neoplasm of connective and soft tissue of left lower limb, including hip

   C49.3 Malignant neoplasm of connective and soft tissue of thorax

> Malignant neoplasm of axilla
> Malignant neoplasm of diaphragm
> Malignant neoplasm of great vessels
>
> **Excludes1**   malignant neoplasm of breast (C50.-)
> malignant neoplasm of heart (C38.0)
> malignant neoplasm of mediastinum (C38.1-C38.3)
> malignant neoplasm of thymus (C37)

   C49.4 Malignant neoplasm of connective and soft tissue of abdomen

> Malignant neoplasm of abdominal wall
> Malignant neoplasm of hypochondrium

   C49.5 Malignant neoplasm of connective and soft tissue of pelvis

> Malignant neoplasm of buttock
> Malignant neoplasm of groin
> Malignant neoplasm of perineum

C49.6   **Malignant neoplasm of connective and soft tissue of trunk, unspecified**

     Malignant neoplasm of back NOS

C49.8   **Malignant neoplasm of overlapping sites of connective and soft tissue**

     Primary malignant neoplasm of two or more contiguous sites of connective and soft tissue

C49.9   **Malignant neoplasm of connective and soft tissue, unspecified**

MALIGNANT NEOPLASMS OF BREAST (C50)

● C50   **Malignant neoplasm of breast**

   Includes   connective tissue of breast
         Paget's disease of breast
         Paget's disease of nipple
         Intraductal carcinoma of breast characterized by eczema-like inflammatory skin changes

   Use additional code to identify estrogen receptor status (Z17.0, Z17.1)

   Excludes1   skin of breast (C44.501, C44.511, C44.521, C44.591)

● C50.0   **Malignant neoplasm of nipple and areola**

   ● C50.01   **Malignant neoplasm of nipple and areola, female**

     C50.011   **Malignant neoplasm of nipple and areola, right female breast**

     C50.012   **Malignant neoplasm of nipple and areola, left female breast**

     C50.019   **Malignant neoplasm of nipple and areola, unspecified female breast**

   ● C50.02   **Malignant neoplasm of nipple and areola, male**

     C50.021   **Malignant neoplasm of nipple and areola, right male breast**

     C50.022   **Malignant neoplasm of nipple and areola, left male breast**

     C50.029   **Malignant neoplasm of nipple and areola, unspecified male breast**

● C50.1   **Malignant neoplasm of central portion of breast**

   ● C50.11   **Malignant neoplasm of central portion of breast, female**

     C50.111   **Malignant neoplasm of central portion of right female breast**

     C50.112   **Malignant neoplasm of central portion of left female breast**

     C50.119   **Malignant neoplasm of central portion of unspecified female breast**

   ● C50.12   **Malignant neoplasm of central portion of breast, male**

     C50.121   **Malignant neoplasm of central portion of right male breast**

     C50.122   **Malignant neoplasm of central portion of left male breast**

     C50.129   **Malignant neoplasm of central portion of unspecified male breast**

● C50.2   **Malignant neoplasm of upper-inner quadrant of breast**

   ● C50.21   **Malignant neoplasm of upper-inner quadrant of breast, female**

     C50.211   **Malignant neoplasm of upper-inner quadrant of right female breast**

     C50.212   **Malignant neoplasm of upper-inner quadrant of left female breast**

     C50.219   **Malignant neoplasm of upper-inner quadrant of unspecified female breast**

Figure 2-12   Female breast quadrants and axillary tail.

   ● C50.22   **Malignant neoplasm of upper-inner quadrant of breast, male**

     C50.221   **Malignant neoplasm of upper-inner quadrant of right male breast**

     C50.222   **Malignant neoplasm of upper-inner quadrant of left male breast**

     C50.229   **Malignant neoplasm of upper-inner quadrant of unspecified male breast**

● C50.3   **Malignant neoplasm of lower-inner quadrant of breast**

   ● C50.31   **Malignant neoplasm of lower-inner quadrant of breast, female**

     C50.311   **Malignant neoplasm of lower-inner quadrant of right female breast**

     C50.312   **Malignant neoplasm of lower-inner quadrant of left female breast**

     C50.319   **Malignant neoplasm of lower-inner quadrant of unspecified female breast**

   ● C50.32   **Malignant neoplasm of lower-inner quadrant of breast, male**

     C50.321   **Malignant neoplasm of lower-inner quadrant of right male breast**

     C50.322   **Malignant neoplasm of lower-inner quadrant of left male breast**

     C50.329   **Malignant neoplasm of lower-inner quadrant of unspecified male breast**

● C50.4   **Malignant neoplasm of upper-outer quadrant of breast**

   ● C50.41   **Malignant neoplasm of upper-outer quadrant of breast, female**

     C50.411   **Malignant neoplasm of upper-outer quadrant of right female breast**

     C50.412   **Malignant neoplasm of upper-outer quadrant of left female breast**

     C50.419   **Malignant neoplasm of upper-outer quadrant of unspecified female breast**

   ● C50.42   **Malignant neoplasm of upper-outer quadrant of breast, male**

     C50.421   **Malignant neoplasm of upper-outer quadrant of right male breast**

     C50.422   **Malignant neoplasm of upper-outer quadrant of left male breast**

     C50.429   **Malignant neoplasm of upper-outer quadrant of unspecified male breast**

● C50.5   **Malignant neoplasm of lower-outer quadrant of breast**

   ● C50.51   **Malignant neoplasm of lower-outer quadrant of breast, female**

     C50.511   **Malignant neoplasm of lower-outer quadrant of right female breast**

     C50.512   **Malignant neoplasm of lower-outer quadrant of left female breast**

     C50.519   **Malignant neoplasm of lower-outer quadrant of unspecified female breast**

● C50.52   **Malignant neoplasm of lower-outer quadrant of breast, male**

     C50.521   **Malignant neoplasm of lower-outer quadrant of right male breast**

     C50.522   **Malignant neoplasm of lower-outer quadrant of left male breast**

     C50.529   **Malignant neoplasm of lower-outer quadrant of unspecified male breast**

● C50.6   **Malignant neoplasm of axillary tail of breast**

 ● C50.61   **Malignant neoplasm of axillary tail of breast, female**

     C50.611   **Malignant neoplasm of axillary tail of right female breast**

     C50.612   **Malignant neoplasm of axillary tail of left female breast**

     C50.619   **Malignant neoplasm of axillary tail of unspecified female breast**

 ● C50.62   **Malignant neoplasm of axillary tail of breast, male**

     C50.621   **Malignant neoplasm of axillary tail of right male breast**

     C50.622   **Malignant neoplasm of axillary tail of left male breast**

     C50.629   **Malignant neoplasm of axillary tail of unspecified male breast**

● C50.8   **Malignant neoplasm of overlapping sites of breast**

 ● C50.81   **Malignant neoplasm of overlapping sites of breast, female**

     C50.811   **Malignant neoplasm of overlapping sites of right female breast**

     C50.812   **Malignant neoplasm of overlapping sites of left female breast**

     C50.819   **Malignant neoplasm of overlapping sites of unspecified female breast**

 ● C50.82   **Malignant neoplasm of overlapping sites of breast, male**

     C50.821   **Malignant neoplasm of overlapping sites of right male breast**

     C50.822   **Malignant neoplasm of overlapping sites of left male breast**

     C50.829   **Malignant neoplasm of overlapping sites of unspecified male breast**

● C50.9   **Malignant neoplasm of breast of unspecified site**

 ● C50.91   **Malignant neoplasm of breast of unspecified site, female**

     C50.911   **Malignant neoplasm of unspecified site of right female breast**

     C50.912   **Malignant neoplasm of unspecified site of left female breast**

     C50.919   **Malignant neoplasm of unspecified site of unspecified female breast**

 ● C50.92   **Malignant neoplasm of breast of unspecified site, male**

     C50.921   **Malignant neoplasm of unspecified site of right male breast**

     C50.922   **Malignant neoplasm of unspecified site of left male breast**

     C50.929   **Malignant neoplasm of unspecified site of unspecified male breast**

Figure 2-13   Cervix uteri.

MALIGNANT NEOPLASMS OF FEMALE GENITAL ORGANS (C51-C58)

Includes   malignant neoplasm of skin of female genital organs

● C51   **Malignant neoplasm of vulva**

   Excludes1   carcinoma in situ of vulva (D07.1)

   C51.0   **Malignant neoplasm of labium majus**
      Outer folds of skin external female genitalia
      Malignant neoplasm of Bartholin's [greater vestibular] gland

   C51.1   **Malignant neoplasm of labium minus**
      Two inner folds surrounding vulva in female genitalia

   C51.2   **Malignant neoplasm of clitoris**

   C51.8   **Malignant neoplasm of overlapping sites of vulva**

   C51.9   **Malignant neoplasm of vulva, unspecified**
      Malignant neoplasm of external female genitalia NOS
      Malignant neoplasm of pudendum

 C52   **Malignant neoplasm of vagina**

   Excludes1   carcinoma in situ of vagina (D07.2)

● C53   **Malignant neoplasm of cervix uteri**

   Excludes1   carcinoma in situ of cervix uteri (D06.-)

   C53.0   **Malignant neoplasm of endocervix**
      Inside the cervix

   C53.1   **Malignant neoplasm of exocervix**
      Outside the cervix

   C53.8   **Malignant neoplasm of overlapping sites of cervix uteri**

   C53.9   **Malignant neoplasm of cervix uteri, unspecified**

● C54   **Malignant neoplasm of corpus uteri**

   C54.0   **Malignant neoplasm of isthmus uteri**
      Constricted part of uterus between cervix and body
      Malignant neoplasm of lower uterine segment

   C54.1   **Malignant neoplasm of endometrium**
      Lining of uterus

   C54.2   **Malignant neoplasm of myometrium**
      Middle layer of uterine wall consisting of smooth muscle supporting stromal and vascular tissue

   C54.3   **Malignant neoplasm of fundus uteri**
      Top rounded portion of uterus

   C54.8   **Malignant neoplasm of overlapping sites of corpus uteri**
      Main body of uterus

   C54.9   **Malignant neoplasm of corpus uteri, unspecified**

 C55   **Malignant neoplasm of uterus, part unspecified**

● C56   **Malignant neoplasm of ovary**

   Use additional code to identify any functional activity

   C56.1   **Malignant neoplasm of right ovary**

   C56.2   **Malignant neoplasm of left ovary**

   C56.9   **Malignant neoplasm of unspecified ovary**

● **C57**   **Malignant neoplasm of other and unspecified female genital organs**
   ● **C57.0**   **Malignant neoplasm of fallopian tube**
     Malignant neoplasm of oviduct
     Malignant neoplasm of uterine tube
     C57.00   **Malignant neoplasm of unspecified fallopian tube**
     C57.01   **Malignant neoplasm of right fallopian tube**
     C57.02   **Malignant neoplasm of left fallopian tube**
   ● **C57.1**   **Malignant neoplasm of broad ligament**
     C57.10   **Malignant neoplasm of unspecified broad ligament**
     C57.11   **Malignant neoplasm of right broad ligament**
     C57.12   **Malignant neoplasm of left broad ligament**
   ● **C57.2**   **Malignant neoplasm of round ligament**
     C57.20   **Malignant neoplasm of unspecified round ligament**
     C57.21   **Malignant neoplasm of right round ligament**
     C57.22   **Malignant neoplasm of left round ligament**
   C57.3   **Malignant neoplasm of parametrium**
     Malignant neoplasm of uterine ligament NOS
   C57.4   **Malignant neoplasm of uterine adnexa, unspecified**
   C57.7   **Malignant neoplasm of other specified female genital organs**
     Malignant neoplasm of wolffian body or duct
   C57.8   **Malignant neoplasm of overlapping sites of female genital organs**
     Primary malignant neoplasm of two or more contiguous sites of the female genital organs whose point of origin cannot be determined
     Primary tubo-ovarian malignant neoplasm whose point of origin cannot be determined
     Primary utero-ovarian malignant neoplasm whose point of origin cannot be determined
   C57.9   **Malignant neoplasm of female genital organ, unspecified**
     Malignant neoplasm of female genitourinary tract NOS

  C58   **Malignant neoplasm of placenta**
   Includes   choriocarcinoma NOS
         chorionepithelioma NOS
   Excludes1   chorioadenoma (destruens) (D39.2)
         hydatidiform mole NOS (O01.9)
         invasive hydatidiform mole (D39.2)
         male choriocarcinoma NOS (C62.9-)
         malignant hydatidiform mole (D39.2)

MALIGNANT NEOPLASMS OF MALE GENITAL ORGANS (C60-C63)

   Includes   malignant neoplasm of skin of male genital organs

● **C60**   **Malignant neoplasm of penis**
   C60.0   **Malignant neoplasm of prepuce**
     Malignant neoplasm of foreskin
   C60.1   **Malignant neoplasm of glans penis**
   C60.2   **Malignant neoplasm of body of penis**
     Malignant neoplasm of corpus cavernosum
   C60.8   **Malignant neoplasm of overlapping sites of penis**
   C60.9   **Malignant neoplasm of penis, unspecified**
     Malignant neoplasm of skin of penis NOS

  C61   **Malignant neoplasm of prostate**
   Excludes1   malignant neoplasm of seminal vesicle (C63.7)

Figure 2-14   Penis and other male genital organs.

● **C62**   **Malignant neoplasm of testis**
   Use additional code to identify any functional activity.
   ● **C62.0**   **Malignant neoplasm of undescended testis**
     Malignant neoplasm of ectopic testis
     Malignant neoplasm of retained testis
     C62.00   **Malignant neoplasm of unspecified undescended testis**
     C62.01   **Malignant neoplasm of undescended right testis**
     C62.02   **Malignant neoplasm of undescended left testis**
   ● **C62.1**   **Malignant neoplasm of descended testis**
     Malignant neoplasm of scrotal testis
     C62.10   **Malignant neoplasm of unspecified descended testis, unspecified side**
     C62.11   **Malignant neoplasm of descended right testis**
     C62.12   **Malignant neoplasm of descended left testis**
   ● **C62.9**   **Malignant neoplasm of testis, unspecified whether descended or undescended**
     C62.90   **Malignant neoplasm of unspecified testis, unspecified whether descended or undescended**
       Malignant neoplasm of testis NOS
     C62.91   **Malignant neoplasm of right testis, unspecified whether descended or undescended**
     C62.92   **Malignant neoplasm of left testis, unspecified whether descended or undescended**

● **C63**   **Malignant neoplasm of other and unspecified male genital organs**
   ● **C63.0**   **Malignant neoplasm of epididymis**
     C63.00   **Malignant neoplasm of unspecified epididymis**
     C63.01   **Malignant neoplasm of right epididymis**
     C63.02   **Malignant neoplasm of left epididymis**
   ● **C63.1**   **Malignant neoplasm of spermatic cord**
     C63.10   **Malignant neoplasm of unspecified spermatic cord**
     C63.11   **Malignant neoplasm of right spermatic cord**
     C63.12   **Malignant neoplasm of left spermatic cord**
   C63.2   **Malignant neoplasm of scrotum**
     Malignant neoplasm of skin of scrotum
   C63.7   **Malignant neoplasm of other specified male genital organs**
     Malignant neoplasm of seminal vesicle
     Malignant neoplasm of tunica vaginalis
   C63.8   **Malignant neoplasm of overlapping sites of male genital organs**
     Primary malignant neoplasm of two or more contiguous sites of male genital organs whose point of origin cannot be determined
   C63.9   **Malignant neoplasm of male genital organ, unspecified**
     Malignant neoplasm of male genitourinary tract NOS

CHAPTER 2 (C00-D49)

MALIGNANT NEOPLASMS OF URINARY TRACT (C64-C68)

● **C64** **Malignant neoplasm of kidney, except renal pelvis**

> **Excludes1**   malignant carcinoid tumor of the kidney (C7A.093)
> malignant neoplasm of renal calyces (C65.-)
> malignant neoplasm of renal pelvis (C65.-)

    C64.1   **Malignant neoplasm of right kidney, except renal pelvis**

    C64.2   **Malignant neoplasm of left kidney, except renal pelvis**

    C64.9   **Malignant neoplasm of unspecified kidney, except renal pelvis**

● **C65** **Malignant neoplasm of renal pelvis**

> **Includes**   malignant neoplasm of pelviureteric junction
> malignant neoplasm of renal calyces

    C65.1   **Malignant neoplasm of right renal pelvis**

    C65.2   **Malignant neoplasm of left renal pelvis**

    C65.9   **Malignant neoplasm of unspecified renal pelvis**

● **C66** **Malignant neoplasm of ureter**

> **Excludes1**   malignant neoplasm of ureteric orifice of bladder (C67.6)

    C66.1   **Malignant neoplasm of right ureter**

    C66.2   **Malignant neoplasm of left ureter**

    C66.9   **Malignant neoplasm of unspecified ureter**

● **C67** **Malignant neoplasm of bladder**

    C67.0   **Malignant neoplasm of trigone of bladder**
Triangular area formed by three openings in the floor of urinary bladder

    C67.1   **Malignant neoplasm of dome of bladder**
Vaulted roof

    C67.2   **Malignant neoplasm of lateral wall of bladder**
Side walls

    C67.3   **Malignant neoplasm of anterior wall of bladder**
Front wall

    C67.4   **Malignant neoplasm of posterior wall of bladder**
Back wall

    C67.5   **Malignant neoplasm of bladder neck**
Joining of bladder and urethra
Malignant neoplasm of internal urethral orifice

    C67.6   **Malignant neoplasm of ureteric orifice**
Opening from bladder to ureters

    C67.7   **Malignant neoplasm of urachus**
Embryonic canal that connects the urinary bladder with the structure that forms the umbilical cord (allantois)

    C67.8   **Malignant neoplasm of overlapping sites of bladder**

    C67.9   **Malignant neoplasm of bladder, unspecified**

● **C68** **Malignant neoplasm of other and unspecified urinary organs**

> **Excludes1**   malignant neoplasm of female genitourinary tract NOS (C57.9)
> malignant neoplasm of male genitourinary tract NOS (C63.9)

    C68.0   **Malignant neoplasm of urethra**

> **Excludes1**   malignant neoplasm of urethral orifice of bladder (C67.5)

    C68.1   **Malignant neoplasm of paraurethral glands**
Group of glands of female urethra drained by paraurethral ducts; AKA Skene glands, female prostate

    C68.8   **Malignant neoplasm of overlapping sites of urinary organs**
Primary malignant neoplasm of two or more contiguous sites of urinary organs whose point of origin cannot be determined

    C68.9   **Malignant neoplasm of urinary organ, unspecified**
Malignant neoplasm of urinary system NOS

MALIGNANT NEOPLASMS OF EYE, BRAIN AND OTHER PARTS OF CENTRAL NERVOUS SYSTEM (C69-C72)

● **C69** **Malignant neoplasm of eye and adnexa**

> **Excludes1**   malignant neoplasm of connective tissue of eyelid (C49.0)
> malignant neoplasm of eyelid (skin) (C43.1-, C44.1-)
> malignant neoplasm of optic nerve (C72.3-)

● **C69.0**   **Malignant neoplasm of conjunctiva**

    C69.00   **Malignant neoplasm of unspecified conjunctiva**

    C69.01   **Malignant neoplasm of right conjunctiva**

    C69.02   **Malignant neoplasm of left conjunctiva**

● **C69.1**   **Malignant neoplasm of cornea**

    C69.10   **Malignant neoplasm of unspecified cornea**

    C69.11   **Malignant neoplasm of right cornea**

    C69.12   **Malignant neoplasm of left cornea**

● **C69.2**   **Malignant neoplasm of retina**

> **Excludes1**   dark area on retina (D49.81)
> neoplasm of unspecified behavior of retina and choroid (D49.81)
> retinal freckle (D49.81)

    C69.20   **Malignant neoplasm of unspecified retina**

    C69.21   **Malignant neoplasm of right retina**

    C69.22   **Malignant neoplasm of left retina**

● **C69.3**   **Malignant neoplasm of choroid**

    C69.30   **Malignant neoplasm of unspecified choroid**

    C69.31   **Malignant neoplasm of right choroid**

    C69.32   **Malignant neoplasm of left choroid**

● **C69.4**   **Malignant neoplasm of ciliary body**

    C69.40   **Malignant neoplasm of unspecified ciliary body**

    C69.41   **Malignant neoplasm of right ciliary body**

    C69.42   **Malignant neoplasm of left ciliary body**

● **C69.5**   **Malignant neoplasm of lacrimal gland and duct**
Malignant neoplasm of lacrimal sac
Malignant neoplasm of nasolacrimal duct

    C69.50   **Malignant neoplasm of unspecified lacrimal gland and duct**

    C69.51   **Malignant neoplasm of right lacrimal gland and duct**

    C69.52   **Malignant neoplasm of left lacrimal gland and duct**

● **C69.6**   **Malignant neoplasm of orbit**
Malignant neoplasm of connective tissue of orbit
Malignant neoplasm of extraocular muscle
Malignant neoplasm of peripheral nerves of orbit
Malignant neoplasm of retrobulbar tissue
Malignant neoplasm of retro-ocular tissue

> **Excludes1**   malignant neoplasm of orbital bone (C41.0)

    C69.60   **Malignant neoplasm of unspecified orbit**

    C69.61   **Malignant neoplasm of right orbit**

    C69.62   **Malignant neoplasm of left orbit**

● **C69.8**   **Malignant neoplasm of overlapping sites of eye and adnexa**

    C69.80   **Malignant neoplasm of overlapping sites of unspecified eye and adnexa**

    C69.81   **Malignant neoplasm of overlapping sites of right eye and adnexa**

    C69.82   **Malignant neoplasm of overlapping sites of left eye and adnexa**

● **C69.9**   **Malignant neoplasm of unspecified site of eye**
Malignant neoplasm of eyeball

    C69.90   **Malignant neoplasm of unspecified site of unspecified eye**

    C69.91   **Malignant neoplasm of unspecified site of right eye**

    C69.92   **Malignant neoplasm of unspecified site of left eye**

Figure 2-15 The brain.

● C70 Malignant neoplasm of meninges
    C70.0 Malignant neoplasm of cerebral meninges
    C70.1 Malignant neoplasm of spinal meninges
    C70.9 Malignant neoplasm of meninges, unspecified

● C71 Malignant neoplasm of brain
    Excludes1   malignant neoplasm of cranial nerves
                    (C72.2-C72.5)
                    retrobulbar malignant neoplasm (C69.6-)
    C71.0 Malignant neoplasm of cerebrum, except lobes and
          ventricles
          Malignant neoplasm of supratentorial NOS
    C71.1 Malignant neoplasm of frontal lobe
    C71.2 Malignant neoplasm of temporal lobe
    C71.3 Malignant neoplasm of parietal lobe
    C71.4 Malignant neoplasm of occipital lobe
    C71.5 Malignant neoplasm of cerebral ventricle
          Excludes1   malignant neoplasm of fourth cerebral
                        ventricle (C71.7)
    C71.6 Malignant neoplasm of cerebellum
    C71.7 Malignant neoplasm of brain stem
          Malignant neoplasm of fourth cerebral ventricle
          Infratentorial malignant neoplasm NOS
    C71.8 Malignant neoplasm of overlapping sites of brain
    C71.9 Malignant neoplasm of brain, unspecified

● C72 Malignant neoplasm of spinal cord, cranial nerves and other
    parts of central nervous system
    Excludes1   malignant neoplasm of meninges (C70.-)
                    malignant neoplasm of peripheral nerves and
                      autonomic nervous system (C47.-)
    C72.0 Malignant neoplasm of spinal cord
    C72.1 Malignant neoplasm of cauda equina
          Lower end of spinal column
    ● C72.2 Malignant neoplasm of olfactory nerve
          Malignant neoplasm of olfactory bulb
          C72.20 Malignant neoplasm of unspecified olfactory
                  nerve
          C72.21 Malignant neoplasm of right olfactory nerve
          C72.22 Malignant neoplasm of left olfactory nerve
    ● C72.3 Malignant neoplasm of optic nerve
          C72.30 Malignant neoplasm of unspecified optic nerve
          C72.31 Malignant neoplasm of right optic nerve
          C72.32 Malignant neoplasm of left optic nerve
    ● C72.4 Malignant neoplasm of acoustic nerve
          C72.40 Malignant neoplasm of unspecified acoustic
                  nerve
          C72.41 Malignant neoplasm of right acoustic nerve
          C72.42 Malignant neoplasm of left acoustic nerve

● C72.5 Malignant neoplasm of other and unspecified cranial
    nerves
    C72.50 Malignant neoplasm of unspecified cranial
          nerve
          Malignant neoplasm of cranial nerve NOS
    C72.59 Malignant neoplasm of other cranial nerves
    C72.9 Malignant neoplasm of central nervous
    system, unspecified
          Malignant neoplasm of unspecified site of central
              nervous system
          Malignant neoplasm of nervous system NOS

MALIGNANT NEOPLASMS OF THYROID AND OTHER ENDOCRINE GLANDS (C73-C75)

C73 Malignant neoplasm of thyroid gland
    Use additional code to identify any functional activity

● C74 Malignant neoplasm of adrenal gland
    ● C74.0 Malignant neoplasm of cortex of adrenal gland
          C74.00 Malignant neoplasm of cortex of unspecified
                  adrenal gland
          C74.01 Malignant neoplasm of cortex of right adrenal
                  gland
          C74.02 Malignant neoplasm of cortex of left adrenal
                  gland
    ● C74.1 Malignant neoplasm of medulla of adrenal gland
          Pair of glands situated on top of or above each kidney
          ("suprarenal")
          C74.10 Malignant neoplasm of medulla of unspecified
                  adrenal gland
          C74.11 Malignant neoplasm of medulla of right
                  adrenal gland
          C74.12 Malignant neoplasm of medulla of left adrenal
                  gland
    ● C74.9 Malignant neoplasm of unspecified part of adrenal
          gland
          C74.90 Malignant neoplasm of unspecified part of
                  unspecified adrenal gland
          C74.91 Malignant neoplasm of unspecified part of right
                  adrenal gland
          C74.92 Malignant neoplasm of unspecified part of left
                  adrenal gland

● C75 Malignant neoplasm of other endocrine glands and related
    structures
    Excludes1   malignant carcinoid tumors (C7A.0-)
                    malignant neoplasm of adrenal gland (C74.-)
                    malignant neoplasm of endocrine pancreas
                      (C25.4)
                    malignant neoplasm of islets of Langerhans
                      (C25.4)
                    malignant neoplasm of ovary (C56.-)
                    malignant neoplasm of testis (C62.-)
                    malignant neoplasm of thymus (C37)
                    malignant neoplasm of thyroid gland (C73)
                    malignant neuroendocrine tumors (C7A.-)
    C75.0 Malignant neoplasm of parathyroid gland
    C75.1 Malignant neoplasm of pituitary gland
    C75.2 Malignant neoplasm of craniopharyngeal duct
    C75.3 Malignant neoplasm of pineal gland
    C75.4 Malignant neoplasm of carotid body
    C75.5 Malignant neoplasm of aortic body and other
          paraganglia
    C75.8 Malignant neoplasm with pluriglandular
          involvement, unspecified
    C75.9 Malignant neoplasm of endocrine gland, unspecified

CHAPTER 2 (C00-D49)

◀ New   ◀||||| Revised   ~~deleted~~ Deleted   OGCR Official Guidelines   X Assign placeholder X   ● Use Additional Character(s)
Excludes 1   Excludes 2   Includes   Use additional   Code first   Code also   Unspecified

MALIGNANT NEUROENDOCRINE TUMORS (C7A)

● **C7A** **Malignant neuroendocrine tumors**

Code also any associated multiple endocrine neoplasia [MEN] syndromes (E31.2-)

Use additional code to identify any associated endocrine syndrome, such as:

carcinoid syndrome (E34.0)

Excludes2 malignant pancreatic islet cell tumors (C25.4)
Merkel cell carcinoma (C4A.-)

● **C7A.0** **Malignant carcinoid tumors**

C7A.00 **Malignant carcinoid tumor of unspecified site**

● C7A.01 **Malignant carcinoid tumors of the small intestine**

C7A.010 **Malignant carcinoid tumor of the duodenum**

C7A.011 **Malignant carcinoid tumor of the jejunum**

C7A.012 **Malignant carcinoid tumor of the ileum**

C7A.019 **Malignant carcinoid tumor of the small intestine, unspecified portion**

● C7A.02 **Malignant carcinoid tumors of the appendix, large intestine, and rectum**

C7A.020 **Malignant carcinoid tumor of the appendix**

C7A.021 **Malignant carcinoid tumor of the cecum**

C7A.022 **Malignant carcinoid tumor of the ascending colon**

C7A.023 **Malignant carcinoid tumor of the transverse colon**

C7A.024 **Malignant carcinoid tumor of the descending colon**

C7A.025 **Malignant carcinoid tumor of the sigmoid colon**

C7A.026 **Malignant carcinoid tumor of the rectum**

C7A.029 **Malignant carcinoid tumor of the large intestine, unspecified portion**
Malignant carcinoid tumor of the colon NOS

● C7A.09 **Malignant carcinoid tumors of other sites**

C7A.090 **Malignant carcinoid tumor of the bronchus and lung**

C7A.091 **Malignant carcinoid tumor of the thymus**

C7A.092 **Malignant carcinoid tumor of the stomach**

C7A.093 **Malignant carcinoid tumor of the kidney**

C7A.094 **Malignant carcinoid tumor of the foregut NOS**

C7A.095 **Malignant carcinoid tumor of the midgut NOS**

C7A.096 **Malignant carcinoid tumor of the hindgut NOS**

C7A.098 **Malignant carcinoid tumors of other sites**

C7A.1 **Malignant poorly differentiated neuroendocrine tumors**
Malignant poorly differentiated neuroendocrine tumor NOS
Malignant poorly differentiated neuroendocrine carcinoma, any site
High grade neuroendocrine carcinoma, any site

C7A.8 **Other malignant neuroendocrine tumors**
Secondary neuroendocrine tumors (C7B)

● **C7B** **Secondary neuroendocrine tumors**

Use additional code to identify any functional activity

● **C7B.0** **Secondary carcinoid tumors**

C7B.00 **Secondary carcinoid tumors, unspecified site**

C7B.01 **Secondary carcinoid tumors of distant lymph nodes**

C7B.02 **Secondary carcinoid tumors of liver**

C7B.03 **Secondary carcinoid tumors of bone**

C7B.04 **Secondary carcinoid tumors of peritoneum**
Mesentary metastasis of carcinoid tumor

C7B.09 **Secondary carcinoid tumors of other sites**

C7B.1 **Secondary Merkel cell carcinoma**
Merkel cell carcinoma nodal presentation
Merkel cell carcinoma visceral metastatic presentation

C7B.8 **Other secondary neuroendocrine tumors**

MALIGNANT NEOPLASMS OF ILL-DEFINED, OTHER SECONDARY AND UNSPECIFIED SITES (C76-C80)

● **C76** **Malignant neoplasm of other and ill-defined sites**

Excludes1 malignant neoplasm of female genitourinary tract NOS (C57.9)
malignant neoplasm of male genitourinary tract NOS (C63.9)
malignant neoplasm of lymphoid, hematopoietic and related tissue (C81-C96)
malignant neoplasm of skin (C44.-)
malignant neoplasm of unspecified site NOS (C80.1)

C76.0 **Malignant neoplasm of head, face and neck**
Malignant neoplasm of cheek NOS
Malignant neoplasm of nose NOS

C76.1 **Malignant neoplasm of thorax**
Intrathoracic malignant neoplasm NOS
Malignant neoplasm of axilla NOS
Thoracic malignant neoplasm NOS

C76.2 **Malignant neoplasm of abdomen**

C76.3 **Malignant neoplasm of pelvis**
Malignant neoplasm of groin NOS
Malignant neoplasm of sites overlapping systems within the pelvis
Rectovaginal (septum) malignant neoplasm
Between rectum and vagina
Rectovesical (septum) malignant neoplasm
Between rectum and urinary bladder; AKA vesicorectal

● **C76.4** **Malignant neoplasm of upper limb**

C76.40 **Malignant neoplasm of unspecified upper limb**

C76.41 **Malignant neoplasm of right upper limb**

C76.42 **Malignant neoplasm of left upper limb**

● **C76.5** **Malignant neoplasm of lower limb**

C76.50 **Malignant neoplasm of unspecified lower limb**

C76.51 **Malignant neoplasm of right lower limb**

C76.52 **Malignant neoplasm of left lower limb**

C76.8 **Malignant neoplasm of other specified ill-defined sites**
Malignant neoplasm of overlapping ill-defined sites

● **C77** **Secondary and unspecified malignant neoplasm of lymph nodes**

Excludes1 malignant neoplasm of lymph nodes, specified as primary (C81-C86, C88, C96.-)
mesentary metastasis of carcinoid tumor (C7B.04)
secondary carcinoid tumors of distant lymph nodes (C7B.01)

C77.0 **Secondary and unspecified malignant neoplasm of lymph nodes of head, face and neck**
Secondary and unspecified malignant neoplasm of supraclavicular lymph nodes

C77.1 **Secondary and unspecified malignant neoplasm of intrathoracic lymph nodes**

C77.2 Secondary and unspecified malignant neoplasm of intra-abdominal lymph nodes

C77.3 Secondary and unspecified malignant neoplasm of axilla and upper limb lymph nodes

     Secondary and unspecified malignant neoplasm of pectoral lymph nodes

C77.4 Secondary and unspecified malignant neoplasm of inguinal and lower limb lymph nodes

C77.5 Secondary and unspecified malignant neoplasm of intrapelvic lymph nodes

C77.8 Secondary and unspecified malignant neoplasm of lymph nodes of multiple regions

C77.9 Secondary and unspecified malignant neoplasm of lymph node, unspecified

● C78 Secondary malignant neoplasm of respiratory and digestive organs

    Excludes1 lymph node metastases (C77.0)
             secondary carcinoid tumors of liver (C7B.02)
             secondary carcinoid tumors of peritoneum (C7B.04)

● C78.0 Secondary malignant neoplasm of lung

    C78.00 Secondary malignant neoplasm of unspecified lung

    C78.01 Secondary malignant neoplasm of right lung

    C78.02 Secondary malignant neoplasm of left lung

C78.1 Secondary malignant neoplasm of mediastinum
    Thoracic cavity between pleural cavities

C78.2 Secondary malignant neoplasm of pleura
    Serous membrane covering lungs and lining thoracic cavity

● C78.3 Secondary malignant neoplasm of other and unspecified respiratory organs

    C78.30 Secondary malignant neoplasm of unspecified respiratory organ

    C78.39 Secondary malignant neoplasm of other respiratory organs

C78.4 Secondary malignant neoplasm of small intestine

C78.5 Secondary malignant neoplasm of large intestine and rectum

C78.6 Secondary malignant neoplasm of retroperitoneum and peritoneum

C78.7 Secondary malignant neoplasm of liver and intrahepatic bile duct

● C78.8 Secondary malignant neoplasm of other and unspecified digestive organs

    C78.80 Secondary malignant neoplasm of unspecified digestive organ

    C78.89 Secondary malignant neoplasm of other digestive organs

● C79 Secondary malignant neoplasm of other and unspecified sites

    Excludes1 lymph node metastases (C77.0)
             secondary carcinoid tumors (C7B.-)
             secondary neuroendocrine tumors (C7B.-)

● C79.0 Secondary malignant neoplasm of kidney and renal pelvis

    C79.00 Secondary malignant neoplasm of unspecified kidney and renal pelvis

    C79.01 Secondary malignant neoplasm of right kidney and renal pelvis

    C79.02 Secondary malignant neoplasm of left kidney and renal pelvis

Item 2-6 The adrenal glands are a pair of glands situated on top of or above each kidney ("suprarenal") and chiefly responsible for regulating the stress response through the synthesis of corticosteroids and catecholamines, including cortisol and adrenaline.

● C79.1 Secondary malignant neoplasm of bladder and other and unspecified urinary organs

    C79.10 Secondary malignant neoplasm of unspecified urinary organs

    C79.11 Secondary malignant neoplasm of bladder

    C79.19 Secondary malignant neoplasm of other urinary organs

C79.2 Secondary malignant neoplasm of skin

    Excludes1 secondary Merkel cell carcinoma (C7B.1)

● C79.3 Secondary malignant neoplasm of brain and cerebral meninges

    C79.31 Secondary malignant neoplasm of brain

    C79.32 Secondary malignant neoplasm of cerebral meninges

● C79.4 Secondary malignant neoplasm of other and unspecified parts of nervous system

    C79.40 Secondary malignant neoplasm of unspecified part of nervous system

    C79.49 Secondary malignant neoplasm of other parts of nervous system

● C79.5 Secondary malignant neoplasm of bone and bone marrow

    Excludes1 secondary carcinoid tumors of bone (C7B.03)

    C79.51 Secondary malignant neoplasm of bone

    C79.52 Secondary malignant neoplasm of bone marrow

● C79.6 Secondary malignant neoplasm of ovary

    C79.60 Secondary malignant neoplasm of unspecified ovary

    C79.61 Secondary malignant neoplasm of right ovary

    C79.62 Secondary malignant neoplasm of left ovary

● C79.7 Secondary malignant neoplasm of adrenal gland

    C79.70 Secondary malignant neoplasm of unspecified adrenal gland

    C79.71 Secondary malignant neoplasm of right adrenal gland

    C79.72 Secondary malignant neoplasm of left adrenal gland

● C79.8 Secondary malignant neoplasm of other specified sites

    C79.81 Secondary malignant neoplasm of breast

    C79.82 Secondary malignant neoplasm of genital organs

    C79.89 Secondary malignant neoplasm of other specified sites

C79.9 Secondary malignant neoplasm of unspecified site
    Metastatic cancer NOS
    Metastatic disease NOS

    Excludes1 carcinomatosis NOS (C80.0)
             generalized cancer NOS (C80.0)
             malignant (primary) neoplasm of unspecified site (C80.1)

CHAPTER 2 (C00-D49)

OGCR Section I.C.2.j and k

Disseminated malignant neoplasm, unspecified

j. Code C80.0, Disseminated malignant neoplasm, unspecified, is for use only in those cases where the patient has advanced metastatic disease and no known primary or secondary sites are specified. It should not be used in place of assigning codes for the primary site and all known secondary sites.

Malignant neoplasm without specification of site

k. Code C80.1, Malignant (primary) neoplasm, unspecified, equates to Cancer, unspecified. This code should only be used when no determination can be made as to the primary site of a malignancy. This code should rarely be used in the inpatient setting.

● C80   Malignant neoplasm without specification of site
    Excludes1   malignant carcinoid tumor of unspecified site
                    (C7A.00)
                 malignant neoplasm of specified multiple sites-
                    code to each site

    C80.0   Disseminated malignant neoplasm, unspecified
             Carcinomatosis NOS
             Generalized cancer, unspecified site (primary)
                (secondary)
             Generalized malignancy, unspecified site (primary)
                (secondary)

    C80.1   Malignant (primary) neoplasm, unspecified
             Cancer NOS
             Cancer unspecified site (primary)
             Carcinoma unspecified site (primary)
             Malignancy unspecified site (primary)
             Excludes1   secondary malignant neoplasm of
                            unspecified site (C79.9)

    C80.2   Malignant neoplasm associated with transplanted organ
             Code first complication of transplanted organ (T86.-)
             Use additional code to identify the specific malignancy

    (See Plate 315 on page NAP-1.)

    ### MALIGNANT NEOPLASMS OF LYMPHOID, HEMATOPOIETIC AND RELATED TISSUE (C81-C96)

    Excludes2   Kaposi's sarcoma of lymph nodes (C46.3)
                 secondary and unspecified neoplasm of lymph
                    nodes (C77.-)
                 secondary neoplasm of bone marrow (C79.52)
                 secondary neoplasm of spleen (C78.89)

● C81   Hodgkin lymphoma
         Form of malignant lymphoma with four types, nodular sclerosis,
            mixed cellularity, lymphocyte depleted, and lymphocyte
            predominant
         Excludes1   personal history of Hodgkin lymphoma (Z85.71)

    ● C81.0   Nodular lymphocyte predominant Hodgkin lymphoma
               Least aggressive, least common, typically no symptoms
               Lymphocytic-histiocytic predominance Hodgkin's
                  disease
        C81.00   Nodular lymphocyte predominant Hodgkin
                  lymphoma, unspecified site
        C81.01   Nodular lymphocyte predominant Hodgkin
                  lymphoma, lymph nodes of head, face, and
                  neck
        C81.02   Nodular lymphocyte predominant Hodgkin
                  lymphoma, intrathoracic lymph nodes
        C81.03   Nodular lymphocyte predominant Hodgkin
                  lymphoma, intra-abdominal lymph nodes
        C81.04   Nodular lymphocyte predominant Hodgkin
                  lymphoma, lymph nodes of axilla and upper
                  limb

        C81.05   Nodular lymphocyte predominant Hodgkin
                  lymphoma, lymph nodes of inguinal region and
                  lower limb
        C81.06   Nodular lymphocyte predominant Hodgkin
                  lymphoma, intrapelvic lymph nodes
        C81.07   Nodular lymphocyte predominant Hodgkin
                  lymphoma, spleen
        C81.08   Nodular lymphocyte predominant Hodgkin
                  lymphoma, lymph nodes of multiple sites
        C81.09   Nodular lymphocyte predominant Hodgkin
                  lymphoma, extranodal and solid organ sites

    ● C81.1   Nodular sclerosis classical Hodgkin lymphoma
               Moderately aggressive; most common in young adults
        C81.10   Nodular sclerosis classical Hodgkin
                  lymphoma, unspecified site
        C81.11   Nodular sclerosis classical Hodgkin lymphoma,
                  lymph nodes of head, face, and neck
        C81.12   Nodular sclerosis classical Hodgkin lymphoma,
                  intrathoracic lymph nodes
        C81.13   Nodular sclerosis classical Hodgkin lymphoma,
                  intra-abdominal lymph nodes
        C81.14   Nodular sclerosis classical Hodgkin lymphoma,
                  lymph nodes of axilla and upper limb
        C81.15   Nodular sclerosis classical Hodgkin lymphoma,
                  lymph nodes of inguinal region and lower limb
        C81.16   Nodular sclerosis classical Hodgkin lymphoma,
                  intrapelvic lymph nodes
        C81.17   Nodular sclerosis classical Hodgkin lymphoma,
                  spleen
        C81.18   Nodular sclerosis classical Hodgkin lymphoma,
                  lymph nodes of multiple sites
        C81.19   Nodular sclerosis classical Hodgkin lymphoma,
                  extranodal and solid organ sites

    ● C81.2   Mixed cellularity classical Hodgkin lymphoma
               A type of Hodgkin's that is moderately aggressive with mixed
                  cell types
        C81.20   Mixed cellularity classical Hodgkin
                  lymphoma, unspecified site
        C81.21   Mixed cellularity classical Hodgkin lymphoma,
                  lymph nodes of head, face, and neck
        C81.22   Mixed cellularity classical Hodgkin lymphoma,
                  intrathoracic lymph nodes
        C81.23   Mixed cellularity classical Hodgkin lymphoma,
                  intra-abdominal lymph nodes
        C81.24   Mixed cellularity classical Hodgkin lymphoma,
                  lymph nodes of axilla and upper limb
        C81.25   Mixed cellularity classical Hodgkin lymphoma,
                  lymph nodes of inguinal region and lower limb
        C81.26   Mixed cellularity classical Hodgkin lymphoma,
                  intrapelvic lymph nodes
        C81.27   Mixed cellularity classical Hodgkin lymphoma,
                  spleen
        C81.28   Mixed cellularity classical Hodgkin lymphoma,
                  lymph nodes of multiple sites
        C81.29   Mixed cellularity classical Hodgkin lymphoma,
                  extranodal and solid organ sites

    ● C81.3   Lymphocyte depleted classical Hodgkin lymphoma
               Most aggressive type with poor prognosis
        C81.30   Lymphocyte depleted classical Hodgkin
                  lymphoma, unspecified site
        C81.31   Lymphocyte depleted classical Hodgkin
                  lymphoma, lymph nodes of head, face, and
                  neck
        C81.32   Lymphocyte depleted classical Hodgkin
                  lymphoma, intrathoracic lymph nodes

◀ New   ◀▥ Revised   ~~deleted~~ Deleted   OGCR Official Guidelines   X Assign placeholder X   ● Use Additional Character(s)

Excludes 1   Excludes 2   Includes   Use additional   Code first   Code also   Unspecified

C81.33   Lymphocyte depleted classical Hodgkin lymphoma, intra-abdominal lymph nodes

C81.34   Lymphocyte depleted classical Hodgkin lymphoma, lymph nodes of axilla and upper limb

C81.35   Lymphocyte depleted classical Hodgkin lymphoma, lymph nodes of inguinal region and lower limb

C81.36   Lymphocyte depleted classical Hodgkin lymphoma, intrapelvic lymph nodes

C81.37   Lymphocyte depleted classical Hodgkin lymphoma, spleen

C81.38   Lymphocyte depleted classical Hodgkin lymphoma, lymph nodes of multiple sites

C81.39   Lymphocyte depleted classical Hodgkin lymphoma, extranodal and solid organ sites

● **C81.4   Lymphocyte-rich classical Hodgkin lymphoma**

     Excludes1   nodular lymphocyte predominant Hodgkin lymphoma (C81.0-)

C81.40   Lymphocyte-rich classical Hodgkin lymphoma, unspecified site

C81.41   Lymphocyte-rich classical Hodgkin lymphoma, lymph nodes of head, face, and neck

C81.42   Lymphocyte-rich classical Hodgkin lymphoma, intrathoracic lymph nodes

C81.43   Lymphocyte-rich classical Hodgkin lymphoma, intra-abdominal lymph nodes

C81.44   Lymphocyte-rich classical Hodgkin lymphoma, lymph nodes of axilla and upper limb

C81.45   Lymphocyte-rich classical Hodgkin lymphoma, lymph nodes of inguinal region and lower limb

C81.46   Lymphocyte-rich classical Hodgkin lymphoma, intrapelvic lymph nodes

C81.47   Lymphocyte-rich classical Hodgkin lymphoma, spleen

C81.48   Lymphocyte-rich classical Hodgkin lymphoma, lymph nodes of multiple sites

C81.49   Lymphocyte-rich classical Hodgkin lymphoma, extranodal and solid organ sites

● **C81.7   Other classical Hodgkin lymphoma**

     Classical Hodgkin lymphoma NOS

C81.70   Other classical Hodgkin lymphoma, unspecified site

C81.71   Other classical Hodgkin lymphoma, lymph nodes of head, face, and neck

C81.72   Other classical Hodgkin lymphoma, intrathoracic lymph nodes

C81.73   Other classical Hodgkin lymphoma, intra-abdominal lymph nodes

C81.74   Other classical Hodgkin lymphoma, lymph nodes of axilla and upper limb

C81.75   Other classical Hodgkin lymphoma, lymph nodes of inguinal region and lower limb

C81.76   Other classical Hodgkin lymphoma, intrapelvic lymph nodes

C81.77   Other classical Hodgkin lymphoma, spleen

C81.78   Other classical Hodgkin lymphoma, lymph nodes of multiple sites

C81.79   Other classical Hodgkin lymphoma, extranodal and solid organ sites

● **C81.9   Hodgkin lymphoma, unspecified**

C81.90   Hodgkin lymphoma, unspecified, unspecified site

C81.91   Hodgkin lymphoma, unspecified, lymph nodes of head, face, and neck

C81.92   Hodgkin lymphoma, unspecified, intrathoracic lymph nodes

C81.93   Hodgkin lymphoma, unspecified, intra-abdominal lymph nodes

C81.94   Hodgkin lymphoma, unspecified, lymph nodes of axilla and upper limb

C81.95   Hodgkin lymphoma, unspecified, lymph nodes of inguinal region and lower limb

C81.96   Hodgkin lymphoma, unspecified, intrapelvic lymph nodes

C81.97   Hodgkin lymphoma, unspecified, spleen

C81.98   Hodgkin lymphoma, unspecified, lymph nodes of multiple sites

C81.99   Hodgkin lymphoma, unspecified, extranodal and solid organ sites

● **C82   Follicular lymphoma**

     Group of malignant lymphomas

     Includes   follicular lymphoma with or without diffuse areas

     Excludes1   mature T/NK-cell lymphomas (C84.-) personal history of non-Hodgkin lymphoma (Z85.72)

● **C82.0   Follicular lymphoma grade I**

C82.00   Follicular lymphoma grade I, unspecified site

C82.01   Follicular lymphoma grade I, lymph nodes of head, face, and neck

C82.02   Follicular lymphoma grade I, intrathoracic lymph nodes

C82.03   Follicular lymphoma grade I, intra-abdominal lymph nodes

C82.04   Follicular lymphoma grade I, lymph nodes of axilla and upper limb

C82.05   Follicular lymphoma grade I, lymph nodes of inguinal region and lower limb

C82.06   Follicular lymphoma grade I, intrapelvic lymph nodes

C82.07   Follicular lymphoma grade I, spleen

C82.08   Follicular lymphoma grade I, lymph nodes of multiple sites

C82.09   Follicular lymphoma grade I, extranodal and solid organ sites

● **C82.1   Follicular lymphoma grade II**

C82.10   Follicular lymphoma grade II, unspecified site

C82.11   Follicular lymphoma grade II, lymph nodes of head, face, and neck

C82.12   Follicular lymphoma grade II, intrathoracic lymph nodes

C82.13   Follicular lymphoma grade II, intra-abdominal lymph nodes

C82.14   Follicular lymphoma grade II, lymph nodes of axilla and upper limb

C82.15   Follicular lymphoma grade II, lymph nodes of inguinal region and lower limb

C82.16   Follicular lymphoma grade II, intrapelvic lymph nodes

C82.17   Follicular lymphoma grade II, spleen

C82.18   Follicular lymphoma grade II, lymph nodes of multiple sites

C82.19   Follicular lymphoma grade II, extranodal and solid organ sites

● **C82.2   Follicular lymphoma grade III, unspecified**

C82.20   Follicular lymphoma grade III, unspecified, unspecified site

C82.21   Follicular lymphoma grade III, unspecified, lymph nodes of head, face, and neck

C82.22   Follicular lymphoma grade III, unspecified, intrathoracic lymph nodes

C82.23   Follicular lymphoma grade III, unspecified, intra-abdominal lymph nodes

CHAPTER 2 (C00-D49)

C82.24   Follicular lymphoma grade III, unspecified, lymph nodes of axilla and upper limb

C82.25   Follicular lymphoma grade III, unspecified, lymph nodes of inguinal region and lower limb

C82.26   Follicular lymphoma grade III, unspecified, intrapelvic lymph nodes

C82.27   Follicular lymphoma grade III, unspecified, spleen

C82.28   Follicular lymphoma grade III, unspecified, lymph nodes of multiple sites

C82.29   Follicular lymphoma grade III, unspecified, extranodal and solid organ sites

● C82.3   Follicular lymphoma grade IIIa

C82.30   Follicular lymphoma grade IIIa, unspecified site

C82.31   Follicular lymphoma grade IIIa, lymph nodes of head, face, and neck

C82.32   Follicular lymphoma grade IIIa, intrathoracic lymph nodes

C82.33   Follicular lymphoma grade IIIa, intra-abdominal lymph nodes

C82.34   Follicular lymphoma grade IIIa, lymph nodes of axilla and upper limb

C82.35   Follicular lymphoma grade IIIa, lymph nodes of inguinal region and lower limb

C82.36   Follicular lymphoma grade IIIa, intrapelvic lymph nodes

C82.37   Follicular lymphoma grade IIIa, spleen

C82.38   Follicular lymphoma grade IIIa, lymph nodes of multiple sites

C82.39   Follicular lymphoma grade IIIa, extranodal and solid organ sites

● C82.4   Follicular lymphoma grade IIIb

C82.40   Follicular lymphoma grade IIIb, unspecified site

C82.41   Follicular lymphoma grade IIIb, lymph nodes of head, face, and neck

C82.42   Follicular lymphoma grade IIIb, intrathoracic lymph nodes

C82.43   Follicular lymphoma grade IIIb, intra-abdominal lymph nodes

C82.44   Follicular lymphoma grade IIIb, lymph nodes of axilla and upper limb

C82.45   Follicular lymphoma grade IIIb, lymph nodes of inguinal region and lower limb

C82.46   Follicular lymphoma grade IIIb, intrapelvic lymph nodes

C82.47   Follicular lymphoma grade IIIb, spleen

C82.48   Follicular lymphoma grade IIIb, lymph nodes of multiple sites

C82.49   Follicular lymphoma grade IIIb, extranodal and solid organ sites

● C82.5   Diffuse follicle center lymphoma

C82.50   Diffuse follicle center lymphoma, unspecified site

C82.51   Diffuse follicle center lymphoma, lymph nodes of head, face, and neck

C82.52   Diffuse follicle center lymphoma, intrathoracic lymph nodes

C82.53   Diffuse follicle center lymphoma, intra-abdominal lymph nodes

C82.54   Diffuse follicle center lymphoma, lymph nodes of axilla and upper limb

C82.55   Diffuse follicle center lymphoma, lymph nodes of inguinal region and lower limb

C82.56   Diffuse follicle center lymphoma, intrapelvic lymph nodes

C82.57   Diffuse follicle center lymphoma, spleen

C82.58   Diffuse follicle center lymphoma, lymph nodes of multiple sites

C82.59   Diffuse follicle center lymphoma, extranodal and solid organ sites

● C82.6   Cutaneous follicle center lymphoma

C82.60   Cutaneous follicle center lymphoma, unspecified site

C82.61   Cutaneous follicle center lymphoma, lymph nodes of head, face, and neck

C82.62   Cutaneous follicle center lymphoma, intrathoracic lymph nodes

C82.63   Cutaneous follicle center lymphoma, intra-abdominal lymph nodes

C82.64   Cutaneous follicle center lymphoma, lymph nodes of axilla and upper limb

C82.65   Cutaneous follicle center lymphoma, lymph nodes of inguinal region and lower limb

C82.66   Cutaneous follicle center lymphoma, intrapelvic lymph nodes

C82.67   Cutaneous follicle center lymphoma, spleen

C82.68   Cutaneous follicle center lymphoma, lymph nodes of multiple sites

C82.69   Cutaneous follicle center lymphoma, extranodal and solid organ sites

● C82.8   Other types of follicular lymphoma

C82.80   Other types of follicular lymphoma, unspecified site

C82.81   Other types of follicular lymphoma, lymph nodes of head, face, and neck

C82.82   Other types of follicular lymphoma, intrathoracic lymph nodes

C82.83   Other types of follicular lymphoma, intra-abdominal lymph nodes

C82.84   Other types of follicular lymphoma, lymph nodes of axilla and upper limb

C82.85   Other types of follicular lymphoma, lymph nodes of inguinal region and lower limb

C82.86   Other types of follicular lymphoma, intrapelvic lymph nodes

C82.87   Other types of follicular lymphoma, spleen

C82.88   Other types of follicular lymphoma, lymph nodes of multiple sites

C82.89   Other types of follicular lymphoma, extranodal and solid organ sites

● C82.9   Follicular lymphoma, unspecified

C82.90   Follicular lymphoma, unspecified, unspecified site

C82.91   Follicular lymphoma, unspecified, lymph nodes of head, face, and neck

C82.92   Follicular lymphoma, unspecified, intrathoracic lymph nodes

C82.93   Follicular lymphoma, unspecified, intra-abdominal lymph nodes

C82.94   Follicular lymphoma, unspecified, lymph nodes of axilla and upper limb

C82.95   Follicular lymphoma, unspecified, lymph nodes of inguinal region and lower limb

C82.96   Follicular lymphoma, unspecified, intrapelvic lymph nodes

C82.97   Follicular lymphoma, unspecified, spleen

C82.98   Follicular lymphoma, unspecified, lymph nodes of multiple sites

C82.99   Follicular lymphoma, unspecified, extranodal and solid organ sites

● **C83**   **Non-follicular lymphoma**

> **Excludes1**   personal history of non-Hodgkin lymphoma (Z85.72)

● **C83.0**   **Small cell B-cell lymphoma**
> Lymphoplasmacytic lymphoma
> Nodal marginal zone lymphoma
> Non-leukemic variant of B-CLL
> Splenic marginal zone lymphoma
>
> > **Excludes1**   chronic lymphocytic leukemia (C91.1)
> >   mature T/NK-cell lymphomas (C84.-)
> >   Waldenström macroglobulinemia (C88.0)

   C83.00   Small cell B-cell lymphoma, unspecified site

   C83.01   Small cell B-cell lymphoma, lymph nodes of head, face, and neck

   C83.02   Small cell B-cell lymphoma, intrathoracic lymph nodes

   C83.03   Small cell B-cell lymphoma, intra-abdominal lymph nodes

   C83.04   Small cell B-cell lymphoma, lymph nodes of axilla and upper limb

   C83.05   Small cell B-cell lymphoma, lymph nodes of inguinal region and lower limb

   C83.06   Small cell B-cell lymphoma, intrapelvic lymph nodes

   C83.07   Small cell B-cell lymphoma, spleen

   C83.08   Small cell B-cell lymphoma, lymph nodes of multiple sites

   C83.09   Small cell B-cell lymphoma, extranodal and solid organ sites

● **C83.1**   **Mantle cell lymphoma**
> Centrocytic lymphoma
> Malignant lymphomatous polyposis

   C83.10   Mantle cell lymphoma, unspecified site

   C83.11   Mantle cell lymphoma, lymph nodes of head, face, and neck

   C83.12   Mantle cell lymphoma, intrathoracic lymph nodes

   C83.13   Mantle cell lymphoma, intra-abdominal lymph nodes

   C83.14   Mantle cell lymphoma, lymph nodes of axilla and upper limb

   C83.15   Mantle cell lymphoma, lymph nodes of inguinal region and lower limb

   C83.16   Mantle cell lymphoma, intrapelvic lymph nodes

   C83.17   Mantle cell lymphoma, spleen

   C83.18   Mantle cell lymphoma, lymph nodes of multiple sites

   C83.19   Mantle cell lymphoma, extranodal and solid organ sites

● **C83.3**   **Diffuse large B-cell lymphoma**
> Anaplastic diffuse large B-cell lymphoma
> CD30-positive diffuse large B-cell lymphoma
> Centroblastic diffuse large B-cell lymphoma
> Diffuse large B-cell lymphoma, subtype not specified
> Immunoblastic diffuse large B-cell lymphoma
> Plasmablastic diffuse large B-cell lymphoma
> Diffuse large B-cell lymphoma, subtype not specified
> T-cell rich diffuse large B-cell lymphoma
>
> > **Excludes1**   mediastinal (thymic) large B-cell lymphoma (C85.2-)
> >   mature T/NK-cell lymphomas (C84.-)

   C83.30   Diffuse large B-cell lymphoma, unspecified site

   C83.31   Diffuse large B-cell lymphoma, lymph nodes of head, face, and neck

   C83.32   Diffuse large B-cell lymphoma, intrathoracic lymph nodes

   C83.33   Diffuse large B-cell lymphoma, intra-abdominal lymph nodes

   C83.34   Diffuse large B-cell lymphoma, lymph nodes of axilla and upper limb

   C83.35   Diffuse large B-cell lymphoma, lymph nodes of inguinal region and lower limb

   C83.36   Diffuse large B-cell lymphoma, intrapelvic lymph nodes

   C83.37   Diffuse large B-cell lymphoma, spleen

   C83.38   Diffuse large B-cell lymphoma, lymph nodes of multiple sites

   C83.39   Diffuse large B-cell lymphoma, extranodal and solid organ sites

● **C83.5**   **Lymphoblastic (diffuse) lymphoma**
> *Highly malignant type of non-Hodgkin lymphoma with diffuse infiltration*
> B-precursor lymphoma
> Lymphoblastic B-cell lymphoma
> Lymphoblastic lymphoma NOS
> Lymphoblastic T-cell lymphoma
> T-precursor lymphoma

   C83.50   Lymphoblastic (diffuse) lymphoma, unspecified site

   C83.51   Lymphoblastic (diffuse) lymphoma, lymph nodes of head, face, and neck

   C83.52   Lymphoblastic (diffuse) lymphoma, intrathoracic lymph nodes

   C83.53   Lymphoblastic (diffuse) lymphoma, intra-abdominal lymph nodes

   C83.54   Lymphoblastic (diffuse) lymphoma, lymph nodes of axilla and upper limb

   C83.55   Lymphoblastic (diffuse) lymphoma, lymph nodes of inguinal region and lower limb

   C83.56   Lymphoblastic (diffuse) lymphoma, intrapelvic lymph nodes

   C83.57   Lymphoblastic (diffuse) lymphoma, spleen

   C83.58   Lymphoblastic (diffuse) lymphoma, lymph nodes of multiple sites

   C83.59   Lymphoblastic (diffuse) lymphoma, extranodal and solid organ sites

● **C83.7**   **Burkitt lymphoma**
> *Form of small cell lymphoma*
> Atypical Burkitt lymphoma
> Burkitt-like lymphoma
>
> > **Excludes1**   mature B-cell leukemia Burkitt type (C91.A-)

   C83.70   Burkitt lymphoma, unspecified site

   C83.71   Burkitt lymphoma, lymph nodes of head, face, and neck

   C83.72   Burkitt lymphoma, intrathoracic lymph nodes

   C83.73   Burkitt lymphoma, intra-abdominal lymph nodes

   C83.74   Burkitt lymphoma, lymph nodes of axilla and upper limb

   C83.75   Burkitt lymphoma, lymph nodes of inguinal region and lower limb

   C83.76   Burkitt lymphoma, intrapelvic lymph nodes

   C83.77   Burkitt lymphoma, spleen

   C83.78   Burkitt lymphoma, lymph nodes of multiple sites

   C83.79   Burkitt lymphoma, extranodal and solid organ sites

● **C83.8** **Other non-follicular lymphoma**
Intravascular large B-cell lymphoma
Lymphoid granulomatosis
Primary effusion B-cell lymphoma

> **Excludes1**   mediastinal (thymic) large B-cell
> lymphoma (C85.2-)
> T-cell rich B-cell lymphoma (C83.3-)

C83.80 Other non-follicular lymphoma, unspecified site

C83.81 Other non-follicular lymphoma, lymph nodes of head, face, and neck

C83.82 Other non-follicular lymphoma, intrathoracic lymph nodes

C83.83 Other non-follicular lymphoma, intra-abdominal lymph nodes

C83.84 Other non-follicular lymphoma, lymph nodes of axilla and upper limb

C83.85 Other non-follicular lymphoma, lymph nodes of inguinal region and lower limb

C83.86 Other non-follicular lymphoma, intrapelvic lymph nodes

C83.87 Other non-follicular lymphoma, spleen

C83.88 Other non-follicular lymphoma, lymph nodes of multiple sites

C83.89 Other non-follicular lymphoma, extranodal and solid organ sites

● **C83.9** **Non-follicular (diffuse) lymphoma, unspecified**

C83.90 Non-follicular (diffuse) lymphoma, unspecified, unspecified site

C83.91 Non-follicular (diffuse) lymphoma, unspecified, lymph nodes of head, face, and neck

C83.92 Non-follicular (diffuse) lymphoma, unspecified, intrathoracic lymph nodes

C83.93 Non-follicular (diffuse) lymphoma, unspecified, intra-abdominal lymph nodes

C83.94 Non-follicular (diffuse) lymphoma, unspecified, lymph nodes of axilla and upper limb

C83.95 Non-follicular (diffuse) lymphoma, unspecified, lymph nodes of inguinal region and lower limb

C83.96 Non-follicular (diffuse) lymphoma, unspecified, intrapelvic lymph nodes

C83.97 Non-follicular (diffuse) lymphoma, unspecified, spleen

C83.98 Non-follicular (diffuse) lymphoma, unspecified, lymph nodes of multiple sites

C83.99 Non-follicular (diffuse) lymphoma, unspecified, extranodal and solid organ sites

● **C84** **Mature T/NK-cell lymphomas**

> **Excludes1**   personal history of non-Hodgkin lymphoma
> (Z85.72)

● **C84.0** **Mycosis fungoides**
*Chronic or rapidly progressive form of cutaneous T-cell
lymphoma; AKA granuloma fungoides*

> **Excludes1**   peripheral T-cell lymphoma, not classified
> (C84.4-)

C84.00 Mycosis fungoides, unspecified site

C84.01 Mycosis fungoides, lymph nodes of head, face, and neck

C84.02 Mycosis fungoides, intrathoracic lymph nodes

C84.03 Mycosis fungoides, intra-abdominal lymph nodes

C84.04 Mycosis fungoides, lymph nodes of axilla and upper limb

C84.05 Mycosis fungoides, lymph nodes of inguinal region and lower limb

C84.06 Mycosis fungoides, intrapelvic lymph nodes

C84.07 Mycosis fungoides, spleen

C84.08 Mycosis fungoides, lymph nodes of multiple sites

C84.09 Mycosis fungoides, extranodal and solid organ sites

● **C84.1** **Sézary disease**
Type of cutaneous lymphoma affecting T-cells

C84.10 Sézary disease, unspecified site

C84.11 Sézary disease, lymph nodes of head, face, and neck

C84.12 Sézary disease, intrathoracic lymph nodes

C84.13 Sézary disease, intra-abdominal lymph nodes

C84.14 Sézary disease, lymph nodes of axilla and upper limb

C84.15 Sézary disease, lymph nodes of inguinal region and lower limb

C84.16 Sézary disease, intrapelvic lymph nodes

C84.17 Sézary disease, spleen

C84.18 Sézary disease, lymph nodes of multiple sites

C84.19 Sézary disease, extranodal and solid organ sites

● **C84.4** **Peripheral T-cell lymphoma, not classified**
*Diverse group of blood carcinomas originating from T-cells,
requiring aggressive chemotherapy*
Lennert's lymphoma
Lymphoepithelioid lymphoma
Mature T-cell lymphoma, not elsewhere classified

C84.40 Peripheral T-cell lymphoma, not classified, unspecified site

C84.41 Peripheral T-cell lymphoma, not classified, lymph nodes of head, face, and neck

C84.42 Peripheral T-cell lymphoma, not classified, intrathoracic lymph nodes

C84.43 Peripheral T-cell lymphoma, not classified, intra-abdominal lymph nodes

C84.44 Peripheral T-cell lymphoma, not classified, lymph nodes of axilla and upper limb

C84.45 Peripheral T-cell lymphoma, not classified, lymph nodes of inguinal region and lower limb

C84.46 Peripheral T-cell lymphoma, not classified, intrapelvic lymph nodes

C84.47 Peripheral T-cell lymphoma, not classified, spleen

C84.48 Peripheral T-cell lymphoma, not classified, lymph nodes of multiple sites

C84.49 Peripheral T-cell lymphoma, not classified, extranodal and solid organ sites

● **C84.6** **Anaplastic large cell lymphoma, ALK-positive**
Anaplastic large cell lymphoma, CD30-positive

C84.60 Anaplastic large cell lymphoma, ALK-positive, unspecified site

C84.61 Anaplastic large cell lymphoma, ALK-positive, lymph nodes of head, face, and neck

C84.62 Anaplastic large cell lymphoma, ALK-positive, intrathoracic lymph nodes

C84.63 Anaplastic large cell lymphoma, ALK-positive, intra-abdominal lymph nodes

Item 2-7 Lymphosarcoma, also known as malignant lymphoma, is a cancer of the lymph system exhibiting abnormal cells encompassing an entire lymph node creating a diffuse pattern without any definite organization. Diffuse pattern lymphoma has a more unfavorable survival outlook than those with a follicular or nodular pattern. Reticulosarcoma is the most common aggressive form of non-Hodgkin's lymphoma.

C84.64   Anaplastic large cell lymphoma, ALK-positive, lymph nodes of axilla and upper limb

C84.65   Anaplastic large cell lymphoma, ALK-positive, lymph nodes of inguinal region and lower limb

C84.66   Anaplastic large cell lymphoma, ALK-positive, intrapelvic lymph nodes

C84.67   Anaplastic large cell lymphoma, ALK-positive, spleen

C84.68   Anaplastic large cell lymphoma, ALK-positive, lymph nodes of multiple sites

C84.69   Anaplastic large cell lymphoma, ALK-positive, extranodal and solid organ sites

● C84.7   Anaplastic large cell lymphoma, ALK-negative
> Excludes1   primary cutaneous CD30-positive T-cell proliferations (C86.6-)

C84.70   Anaplastic large cell lymphoma, ALK-negative, unspecified site

C84.71   Anaplastic large cell lymphoma, ALK-negative, lymph nodes of head, face, and neck

C84.72   Anaplastic large cell lymphoma, ALK-negative, intrathoracic lymph nodes

C84.73   Anaplastic large cell lymphoma, ALK-negative, intra-abdominal lymph nodes

C84.74   Anaplastic large cell lymphoma, ALK-negative, lymph nodes of axilla and upper limb

C84.75   Anaplastic large cell lymphoma, ALK-negative, lymph nodes of inguinal region and lower limb

C84.76   Anaplastic large cell lymphoma, ALK-negative, intrapelvic lymph nodes

C84.77   Anaplastic large cell lymphoma, ALK-negative, spleen

C84.78   Anaplastic large cell lymphoma, ALK-negative, lymph nodes of multiple sites

C84.79   Anaplastic large cell lymphoma, ALK-negative, extranodal and solid organ sites

● C84.A   Cutaneous T-cell lymphoma, unspecified

C84.A0   Cutaneous T-cell lymphoma, unspecified, unspecified site

C84.A1   Cutaneous T-cell lymphoma, unspecified lymph nodes of head, face, and neck

C84.A2   Cutaneous T-cell lymphoma, unspecified, intrathoracic lymph nodes

C84.A3   Cutaneous T-cell lymphoma, unspecified, intra-abdominal lymph nodes

C84.A4   Cutaneous T-cell lymphoma, unspecified, lymph nodes of axilla and upper limb

C84.A5   Cutaneous T-cell lymphoma, unspecified, lymph nodes of inguinal region and lower limb

C84.A6   Cutaneous T-cell lymphoma, unspecified, intrapelvic lymph nodes

C84.A7   Cutaneous T-cell lymphoma, unspecified, spleen

C84.A8   Cutaneous T-cell lymphoma, unspecified, lymph nodes of multiple sites

C84.A9   Cutaneous T-cell lymphoma, unspecified, extranodal and solid organ sites

● C84.Z   Other mature T/NK-cell lymphomas
> **Note:** If T-cell lineage or involvement is mentioned in conjunction with a specific lymphoma, code to the more specific description.
> Excludes1   angioimmunoblastic T-cell lymphoma (C86.5)
> blastic NK-cell lymphoma (C86.4)
> enteropathy-type T-cell lymphoma (C86.2)
> extranodal NK-cell lymphoma, nasal type (C86.0)
> hepatosplenic T-cell lymphoma (C86.1)
> primary cutaneous CD30-positive T-cell proliferations (C86.6)
> subcutaneous panniculitis-like T-cell lymphoma (C86.3)
> T-cell leukemia (C91.1-)

C84.Z0   Other mature T/NK-cell lymphomas, unspecified site

C84.Z1   Other mature T/NK-cell lymphomas, lymph nodes of head, face, and neck

C84.Z2   Other mature T/NK-cell lymphomas, intrathoracic lymph nodes

C84.Z3   Other mature T/NK-cell lymphomas, intra-abdominal lymph nodes

C84.Z4   Other mature T/NK-cell lymphomas, lymph nodes of axilla and upper limb

C84.Z5   Other mature T/NK-cell lymphomas, lymph nodes of inguinal region and lower limb

C84.Z6   Other mature T/NK-cell lymphomas, intrapelvic lymph nodes

C84.Z7   Other mature T/NK-cell lymphomas, spleen

C84.Z8   Other mature T/NK-cell lymphomas, lymph nodes of multiple sites

C84.Z9   Other mature T/NK-cell lymphomas, extranodal and solid organ sites

● C84.9   Mature T/NK-cell lymphomas, unspecified
NK/T cell lymphoma NOS
> Excludes1   mature T-cell lymphoma, not elsewhere classified (C84.4-)

C84.90   Mature T/NK-cell lymphomas, unspecified, unspecified site

C84.91   Mature T/NK-cell lymphomas, unspecified, lymph nodes of head, face, and neck

C84.92   Mature T/NK-cell lymphomas, unspecified, intrathoracic lymph nodes

C84.93   Mature T/NK-cell lymphomas, unspecified, intra-abdominal lymph nodes

C84.94   Mature T/NK-cell lymphomas, unspecified, lymph nodes of axilla and upper limb

C84.95   Mature T/NK-cell lymphomas, unspecified, lymph nodes of inguinal region and lower limb

C84.96   Mature T/NK-cell lymphomas, unspecified, intrapelvic lymph nodes

C84.97   Mature T/NK-cell lymphomas, unspecified, spleen

C84.98   Mature T/NK-cell lymphomas, unspecified, lymph nodes of multiple sites

C84.99   Mature T/NK-cell lymphomas, unspecified, extranodal and solid organ sites

CHAPTER 2 (C00-D49)

CHAPTER 2 (C00-D49)

● **C85 Other specified and unspecified types of non-Hodgkin lymphoma**
> Excludes1   other specified types of T/NK-cell lymphoma (C86.-)
> personal history of non-Hodgkin lymphoma (Z85.72)

● **C85.1 Unspecified B-cell lymphoma**
> **Note:** If B-cell lineage or involvement is mentioned in conjunction with a specific lymphoma, code to the more specific description.

- C85.10 Unspecified B-cell lymphoma, unspecified site
- C85.11 Unspecified B-cell lymphoma, lymph nodes of head, face, and neck
- C85.12 Unspecified B-cell lymphoma, intrathoracic lymph nodes
- C85.13 Unspecified B-cell lymphoma, intra-abdominal lymph nodes
- C85.14 Unspecified B-cell lymphoma, lymph nodes of axilla and upper limb
- C85.15 Unspecified B-cell lymphoma, lymph nodes of inguinal region and lower limb
- C85.16 Unspecified B-cell lymphoma, intrapelvic lymph nodes
- C85.17 Unspecified B-cell lymphoma, spleen
- C85.18 Unspecified B-cell lymphoma, lymph nodes of multiple sites
- C85.19 Unspecified B-cell lymphoma, extranodal and solid organ sites

● **C85.2 Mediastinal (thymic) large B-cell lymphoma**
- C85.20 Mediastinal (thymic) large B-cell lymphoma, unspecified site
- C85.21 Mediastinal (thymic) large B-cell lymphoma, lymph nodes of head, face, and neck
- C85.22 Mediastinal (thymic) large B-cell lymphoma, intrathoracic lymph nodes
- C85.23 Mediastinal (thymic) large B-cell lymphoma, intra-abdominal lymph nodes
- C85.24 Mediastinal (thymic) large B-cell lymphoma, lymph nodes of axilla and upper limb
- C85.25 Mediastinal (thymic) large B-cell lymphoma, lymph nodes of inguinal region and lower limb
- C85.26 Mediastinal (thymic) large B-cell lymphoma, intrapelvic lymph nodes
- C85.27 Mediastinal (thymic) large B-cell lymphoma, spleen
- C85.28 Mediastinal (thymic) large B-cell lymphoma, lymph nodes of multiple sites
- C85.29 Mediastinal (thymic) large B-cell lymphoma, extranodal and solid organ sites

● **C85.8 Other specified types of non-Hodgkin lymphoma**
- C85.80 Other specified types of non-Hodgkin lymphoma, unspecified site
- C85.81 Other specified types of non-Hodgkin lymphoma, lymph nodes of head, face, and neck
- C85.82 Other specified types of non-Hodgkin lymphoma, intrathoracic lymph nodes
- C85.83 Other specified types of non-Hodgkin lymphoma, intra-abdominal lymph nodes
- C85.84 Other specified types of non-Hodgkin lymphoma, lymph nodes of axilla and upper limb
- C85.85 Other specified types of non-Hodgkin lymphoma, lymph nodes of inguinal region and lower limb
- C85.86 Other specified types of non-Hodgkin lymphoma, intrapelvic lymph nodes

- C85.87 Other specified types of non-Hodgkin lymphoma, spleen
- C85.88 Other specified types of non-Hodgkin lymphoma, lymph nodes of multiple sites
- C85.89 Other specified types of non-Hodgkin lymphoma, extranodal and solid organ sites

● **C85.9 Non-Hodgkin lymphoma, unspecified**
> Lymphoma NOS
> Malignant lymphoma NOS
> Non-Hodgkin lymphoma NOS

- C85.90 Non-Hodgkin lymphoma, unspecified, unspecified site
- C85.91 Non-Hodgkin lymphoma, unspecified, lymph nodes of head, face, and neck
- C85.92 Non-Hodgkin lymphoma, unspecified, intrathoracic lymph nodes
- C85.93 Non-Hodgkin lymphoma, unspecified, intra-abdominal lymph nodes
- C85.94 Non-Hodgkin lymphoma, unspecified, lymph nodes of axilla and upper limb
- C85.95 Non-Hodgkin lymphoma, unspecified, lymph nodes of inguinal region and lower limb
- C85.96 Non-Hodgkin lymphoma, unspecified, intrapelvic lymph nodes
- C85.97 Non-Hodgkin lymphoma, unspecified, spleen
- C85.98 Non-Hodgkin lymphoma, unspecified, lymph nodes of multiple sites
- C85.99 Non-Hodgkin lymphoma, unspecified, extranodal and solid organ sites

● **C86 Other specified types of T/NK-cell lymphoma**
> Excludes1   anaplastic large cell lymphoma, ALK negative (C84.7-)
> anaplastic large cell lymphoma, ALK positive (C84.6-)
> mature T/NK-cell lymphomas (C84.-)
> other specified types of non-Hodgkin lymphoma (C85.8-)

- C86.0 Extranodal NK/T-cell lymphoma, nasal type
- C86.1 Hepatosplenic T-cell lymphoma
  > Alpha-beta and gamma delta types
- C86.2 Enteropathy-type (intestinal) T-cell lymphoma
  > Enteropathy associated T-cell lymphoma
- C86.3 Subcutaneous panniculitis-like T-cell lymphoma
- C86.4 Blastic NK-cell lymphoma
- C86.5 Angioimmunoblastic T-cell lymphoma
  > Angioimmunoblastic lymphadenopathy with dysproteinemia (AILD)
- C86.6 Primary cutaneous CD30-positive T-cell proliferations
  > Lymphomatoid papulosis
  > Primary cutaneous anaplastic large cell lymphoma
  > Primary cutaneous CD30-positive large T-cell lymphoma

● **C88 Malignant immunoproliferative diseases and certain other B-cell lymphomas**
> *Diseases involving immune system*
> Excludes1   B-cell lymphoma, unspecified (C85.1-)
> personal history of other malignant neoplasms of lymphoid, hematopoietic and related tissues (Z85.79)

- C88.0 Waldenström's macroglobulinemia
  > Lymphoplasmacytic lymphoma with IgM-production
  > Macroglobulinemia (idiopathic) (primary)
  > Excludes1   small cell B-cell lymphoma (C83.0)
- C88.2 Heavy chain disease
  > Franklin disease
  > Gamma heavy chain disease
  > Mu heavy chain disease

C88.3 Immunoproliferative small intestinal disease
    Alpha heavy chain disease
    Mediterranean lymphoma

C88.4 Extranodal marginal zone B-cell lymphoma of mucosa-associated lymphoid tissue [MALT-lymphoma]
    Lymphoma of skin-associated lymphoid tissue [SALT-lymphoma]
    Lymphoma of bronchial-associated lymphoid tissue [BALT-lymphoma]

    | Excludes1 | high malignant (diffuse large B-cell) lymphoma (C83.3-)

C88.8 Other malignant immunoproliferative diseases

C88.9 Malignant immunoproliferative disease, unspecified
    Immunoproliferative disease NOS

● **C90 Multiple myeloma and malignant plasma cell neoplasms**

    | Excludes1 | personal history of other malignant neoplasms of lymphoid, hematopoietic and related tissues (Z85.79)

● **C90.0 Multiple myeloma**
    Kahler's disease
    Medullary plasmacytoma
    Myelomatosis
    Plasma cell myeloma

    | Excludes1 | solitary myeloma (C90.3-)
                    solitary plasmacytoma (C90.3-)

    C90.00 Multiple myeloma not having achieved remission
        Multiple myeloma with failed remission
        Multiple myeloma NOS

    C90.01 Multiple myeloma in remission

    C90.02 Multiple myeloma in relapse

● **C90.1 Plasma cell leukemia**
    Rare type of acute leukemia
    Plasmacytic leukemia

    C90.10 Plasma cell leukemia not having achieved remission
        Plasma cell leukemia with failed remission
        Plasma cell leukemia NOS

    C90.11 Plasma cell leukemia in remission

    C90.12 Plasma cell leukemia in relapse

● **C90.2 Extramedullary plasmacytoma**
    Malignant monoclonal plasma cell tumor growing in soft tissue; AKA plasma cell dyscrasias

    C90.20 Extramedullary plasmacytoma not having achieved remission
        Extramedullary plasmacytoma with failed remission
        Extramedullary plasmacytoma NOS

    C90.21 Extramedullary plasmacytoma in remission

    C90.22 Extramedullary plasmacytoma in relapse

● **C90.3 Solitary plasmacytoma**
    Localized malignant plasma cell tumor NOS
    Plasmacytoma NOS
    Solitary myeloma

    C90.30 Solitary plasmacytoma not having achieved remission
        Solitary plasmacytoma with failed remission
        Solitary plasmacytoma NOS

    C90.31 Solitary plasmacytoma in remission

    C90.32 Solitary plasmacytoma in relapse

Item 2-9 Leukemia is a cancer (acute or chronic) of the blood-forming tissues of the bone marrow. Blood cells all start out as stem cells. They mature and become red cells, white cells, or platelets. There are three main types of leukocytes (white cells that fight infection): monocytes, lymphocytes, and granulocytes. **Acute monocytic leukemia** (AML) affects monocytes. **Acute lymphoid leukemia** (ALL) affects lymphocytes, and **acute myeloid leukemia** (AML) affects cells that typically develop into white blood cells (not lymphocytes), though it may develop in other blood cells.

● **C91 Lymphoid leukemia**
    Type of leukemia affecting circulating cells of lymphoid origin

    | Excludes1 | personal history of leukemia (Z85.6)

● **C91.0 Acute lymphoblastic leukemia [ALL]**
    Note: Code C91.0 should only be used for T-cell and B-cell precursor leukemia

    C91.00 Acute lymphoblastic leukemia not having achieved remission
        Acute lymphoblastic leukemia with failed remission
        Acute lymphoblastic leukemia NOS

    C91.01 Acute lymphoblastic leukemia, in remission

    C91.02 Acute lymphoblastic leukemia, in relapse

● **C91.1 Chronic lymphocytic leukemia of B-cell type**
    Lymphoplasmacytic leukemia
    Richter syndrome

    | Excludes1 | lymphoplasmacytic lymphoma (C83.0-)

    C91.10 Chronic lymphocytic leukemia of B-cell type not having achieved remission
        Chronic lymphocytic leukemia of B-cell type with failed remission
        Chronic lymphocytic leukemia of B-cell type NOS

    C91.11 Chronic lymphocytic leukemia of B-cell type in remission

    C91.12 Chronic lymphocytic leukemia of B-cell type in relapse

● **C91.3 Prolymphocytic leukemia of B-cell type**
    Chronic leukemia with symptoms of large number of circulating lymphocytes

    C91.30 Prolymphocytic leukemia of B-cell type not having achieved remission
        Prolymphocytic leukemia of B-cell type with failed remission
        Prolymphocytic leukemia of B-cell type NOS

    C91.31 Prolymphocytic leukemia of B-cell type, in remission

    C91.32 Prolymphocytic leukemia of B-cell type, in relapse

● **C91.4 Hairy cell leukemia**
    Chronic leukemia with splenomegaly and excessive number of abnormal large mononuclear cells covered by hairlike villi
    Leukemic reticuloendotheliosis

    C91.40 Hairy cell leukemia not having achieved remission
        Hairy cell leukemia with failed remission
        Hairy cell leukemia NOS

    C91.41 Hairy cell leukemia, in remission

    C91.42 Hairy cell leukemia, in relapse

CHAPTER 2 (C00-D49)

Item 2-8 Multiple myeloma is a cancer of a plasma cell (a type of white blood cell) and is an incurable but treatable disease. Immunoproliferative neoplasm is a term for diseases (mostly cancers) in which the immune system cells proliferate.

◀ New   ⬅ Revised   ~~deleted~~ Deleted   **OGCR** Official Guidelines   X Assign placeholder X   ● Use Additional Character(s)

| Excludes 1 | | Excludes 2 | Includes Use additional   Code first Code also Unspecified

CHAPTER 2 (C00-D49)

● **C91.5**   **Adult T-cell lymphoma/leukemia (HTLV-1-associated)**
Acute variant of adult T-cell lymphoma/leukemia (HTLV-1-associated)
Chronic variant of adult T-cell lymphoma/leukemia (HTLV-1-associated)
Lymphomatoid variant of adult T-cell lymphoma/leukemia (HTLV-1-associated)
Smouldering variant of adult T-cell lymphoma/leukemia (HTLV-1-associated)

     C91.50   **Adult T-cell lymphoma/leukemia (HTLV-1-associated) not having achieved remission**
Adult T-cell lymphoma/leukemia (HTLV-1-associated) with failed remission
Adult T-cell lymphoma/leukemia (HTLV-1-associated) NOS

     C91.51   **Adult T-cell lymphoma/leukemia (HTLV-1-associated), in remission**

     C91.52   **Adult T-cell lymphoma/leukemia (HTLV-1-associated), in relapse**

● **C91.6**   **Prolymphocytic leukemia of T-cell type**

     C91.60   **Prolymphocytic leukemia of T-cell type not having achieved remission**
Prolymphocytic leukemia of T-cell type with failed remission
Prolymphocytic leukemia of T-cell type NOS

     C91.61   **Prolymphocytic leukemia of T-cell type, in remission**

     C91.62   **Prolymphocytic leukemia of T-cell type, in relapse**

● **C91.A**   **Mature B-cell leukemia Burkitt-type**

     Excludes1   Burkitt lymphoma (C83.7-)

     C91.A0   **Mature B-cell leukemia Burkitt-type not having achieved remission**
Mature B-cell leukemia Burkitt-type with failed remission
Mature B-cell leukemia Burkitt-type NOS

     C91.A1   **Mature B-cell leukemia Burkitt-type, in remission**

     C91.A2   **Mature B-cell leukemia Burkitt-type, in relapse**

● **C91.Z**   **Other lymphoid leukemia**
T-cell large granular lymphocytic leukemia (associated with rheumatoid arthritis)

     C91.Z0   **Other lymphoid leukemia not having achieved remission**
Other lymphoid leukemia with failed remission
Other lymphoid leukemia NOS

     C91.Z1   **Other lymphoid leukemia, in remission**

     C91.Z2   **Other lymphoid leukemia, in relapse**

● **C91.9**   **Lymphoid leukemia, unspecified**

     C91.90   **Lymphoid leukemia, unspecified not having achieved remission**
Lymphoid leukemia with failed remission
Lymphoid leukemia NOS

     C91.91   **Lymphoid leukemia, unspecified, in remission**

     C91.92   **Lymphoid leukemia, unspecified, in relapse**

● **C92**   **Myeloid leukemia**

     Includes   granulocytic leukemia
myelogenous leukemia

     Excludes1   personal history of leukemia (Z85.6)

● **C92.0**   **Acute myeloblastic leukemia**
Acute myeloblastic leukemia, minimal differentiation
Acute myeloblastic leukemia (with maturation)
Acute myeloblastic leukemia 1/ETO
Acute myeloblastic leukemia M0
Acute myeloblastic leukemia M1
Acute myeloblastic leukemia M2
Acute myeloblastic leukemia with t(8;21)
Acute myeloblastic leukemia (without a FAB classification) NOS
Refractory anemia with excess blasts in transformation [RAEB T]

     Excludes1   acute exacerbation of chronic myeloid leukemia (C92.10)
refractory anemia with excess of blasts not in transformation (D46.2-)

     C92.00   **Acute myeloblastic leukemia, not having achieved remission**
Acute myeloblastic leukemia with failed remission
Acute myeloblastic leukemia NOS

     C92.01   **Acute myeloblastic leukemia, in remission**

     C92.02   **Acute myeloblastic leukemia, in relapse**

● **C92.1**   **Chronic myeloid leukemia, BCR/ABL-positive**
Chronic myelogenous leukemia, Philadelphia chromosome (Ph1) positive
Chronic myelogenous leukemia, t(9;22) (q34;q11)
Chronic myelogenous leukemia with crisis of blast cells

     Excludes1   atypical chronic myeloid leukemia BCR/ABL-negative (C92.2-)
chronic myelomonocytic leukemia (C93.1-)
chronic myeloproliferative disease (D47.1)

     C92.10   **Chronic myeloid leukemia, BCR/ABL-positive, not having achieved remission**
Chronic myeloid leukemia, BCR/ABL-positive with failed remission
Chronic myeloid leukemia, BCR/ABL-positive NOS

     C92.11   **Chronic myeloid leukemia, BCR/ABL-positive, in remission**

     C92.12   **Chronic myeloid leukemia, BCR/ABL-positive, in relapse**

● **C92.2**   **Atypical chronic myeloid leukemia, BCR/ABL-negative**

     C92.20   **Atypical chronic myeloid leukemia, BCR/ABL-negative, not having achieved remission**
Atypical chronic myeloid leukemia, BCR/ABL-negative with failed remission
Atypical chronic myeloid leukemia, BCR/ABL-negative NOS

     C92.21   **Atypical chronic myeloid leukemia, BCR/ABL-negative, in remission**

     C92.22   **Atypical chronic myeloid leukemia, BCR/ABL-negative, in relapse**

● **C92.3**   **Myeloid sarcoma**
A malignant tumor of immature myeloid cells
Chloroma
Granulocytic sarcoma

     C92.30   **Myeloid sarcoma, not having achieved remission**
Myeloid sarcoma with failed remission
Myeloid sarcoma NOS

     C92.31   **Myeloid sarcoma, in remission**

     C92.32   **Myeloid sarcoma, in relapse**

● **C92.4** **Acute promyelocytic leukemia**
　　　　AML M3
　　　　AML Me with t(15;17) and variants

　　C92.40 **Acute promyelocytic leukemia, not having achieved remission**
　　　　　　Acute promyelocytic leukemia with failed remission
　　　　　　Acute promyelocytic leukemia NOS

　　C92.41 **Acute promyelocytic leukemia, in remission**

　　C92.42 **Acute promyelocytic leukemia, in relapse**

● **C92.5** **Acute myelomonocytic leukemia**
　　　　AML M4
　　　　AML M4 Eo with inv(16) or t(16;16)

　　C92.50 **Acute myelomonocytic leukemia, not having achieved remission**
　　　　　　Acute myelomonocytic leukemia with failed remission
　　　　　　Acute myelomonocytic leukemia NOS

　　C92.51 **Acute myelomonocytic leukemia, in remission**

　　C92.52 **Acute myelomonocytic leukemia, in relapse**

● **C92.6** **Acute myeloid leukemia with 11q23-abnormality**
　　　　Acute myeloid leukemia with variation of MLL-gene

　　C92.60 **Acute myeloid leukemia with 11q23-abnormality not having achieved remission**
　　　　　　Acute myeloid leukemia with 11q23-abnormality with failed remission
　　　　　　Acute myeloid leukemia with 11q23-abnormality NOS

　　C92.61 **Acute myeloid leukemia with 11q23-abnormality in remission**

　　C92.62 **Acute myeloid leukemia with 11q23-abnormality in relapse**

● **C92.A** **Acute myeloid leukemia with multilineage dysplasia**
　　　　Acute myeloid leukemia with dysplasia of remaining hematopoesis and/or myelodysplastic disease in its history

　　C92.A0 **Acute myeloid leukemia with multilineage dysplasia, not having achieved remission**
　　　　　　Acute myeloid leukemia with multilineage dysplasia with failed remission
　　　　　　Acute myeloid leukemia with multilineage dysplasia NOS

　　C92.A1 **Acute myeloid leukemia with multilineage dysplasia, in remission**

　　C92.A2 **Acute myeloid leukemia with multilineage dysplasia, in relapse**

● **C92.Z** **Other myeloid leukemia**

　　C92.Z0 **Other myeloid leukemia not having achieved remission**
　　　　　　Myeloid leukemia NEC with failed remission
　　　　　　Myeloid leukemia NEC

　　C92.Z1 **Other myeloid leukemia, in remission**

　　C92.Z2 **Other myeloid leukemia, in relapse**

● **C92.9** **Myeloid leukemia, unspecified**

　　C92.90 **Myeloid leukemia, unspecified, not having achieved remission**
　　　　　　Myeloid leukemia, unspecified with failed remission
　　　　　　Myeloid leukemia, unspecified NOS

　　C92.91 **Myeloid leukemia, unspecified in remission**

　　C92.92 **Myeloid leukemia, unspecified in relapse**

● **C93** **Monocytic leukemia**
　　　Includes monocytoid leukemia
　　　Excludes1 personal history of leukemia (Z85.6)

● **C93.0** **Acute monoblastic/monocytic leukemia**
　　　　AML M5
　　　　AML M5a
　　　　AML M5b

　　C93.00 **Acute monoblastic/monocytic leukemia, not having achieved remission**
　　　　　　Acute monoblastic/monocytic leukemia with failed remission
　　　　　　Acute monoblastic/monocytic leukemia NOS

　　C93.01 **Acute monoblastic/monocytic leukemia, in remission**

　　C93.02 **Acute monoblastic/monocytic leukemia, in relapse**

● **C93.1** **Chronic myelomonocytic leukemia**
　　　　Chronic monocytic leukemia
　　　　CMML-1
　　　　CMML-2
　　　　CMML with eosinophilia

　　C93.10 **Chronic myelomonocytic leukemia not having achieved remission**
　　　　　　Chronic myelomonocytic leukemia with failed remission
　　　　　　Chronic myelomonocytic leukemia NOS

　　C93.11 **Chronic myelomonocytic leukemia, in remission**

　　C93.12 **Chronic myelomonocytic leukemia, in relapse**

● **C93.3** **Juvenile myelomonocytic leukemia**

　　C93.30 **Juvenile myelomonocytic leukemia, not having achieved remission**
　　　　　　Juvenile myelomonocytic leukemia with failed remission
　　　　　　Juvenile myelomonocytic leukemia NOS

　　C93.31 **Juvenile myelomonocytic leukemia, in remission**

　　C93.32 **Juvenile myelomonocytic leukemia, in relapse**

● **C93.Z** **Other monocytic leukemia**

　　C93.Z0 **Other monocytic leukemia, not having achieved remission**
　　　　　　Other monocytic leukemia NOS

　　C93.Z1 **Other monocytic leukemia, in remission**

　　C93.Z2 **Other monocytic leukemia, in relapse**

● **C93.9** **Monocytic leukemia, unspecified**

　　C93.90 **Monocytic leukemia, unspecified, not having achieved remission**
　　　　　　Monocytic leukemia, unspecified with failed remission
　　　　　　Monocytic leukemia, unspecified NOS

　　C93.91 **Monocytic leukemia, unspecified in remission**

　　C93.92 **Monocytic leukemia, unspecified in relapse**

● **C94** **Other leukemias of specified cell type**
　　　Excludes1 leukemic reticuloendotheliosis (C91.4-)
　　　　　　myelodysplastic syndromes (D46.-)
　　　　　　personal history of leukemia (Z85.6)
　　　　　　plasma cell leukemia (C90.1-)

● **C94.0** **Acute erythroid leukemia**
　　　　Acute myeloid leukemia M6(a)(b)
　　　　Erythroleukemia

　　C94.00 **Acute erythroid leukemia, not having achieved remission**
　　　　　　Acute erythroid leukemia with failed remission
　　　　　　Acute erythroid leukemia NOS

　　C94.01 **Acute erythroid leukemia, in remission**

　　C94.02 **Acute erythroid leukemia, in relapse**

CHAPTER 2 (C00-D49)

◀ New　　⬅ Revised　　~~deleted~~ Deleted　　**OGCR** Official Guidelines　　X Assign placeholder X　　● Use Additional Character(s)

Excludes 1　　Excludes 2　　Includes　　Use additional　　Code first　　Code also　　Unspecified

● **C94.2**   **Acute megakaryoblastic leukemia**
Acute myeloid leukemia M7
Acute megakaryocytic leukemia

     C94.20   **Acute megakaryoblastic leukemia not having achieved remission**
Acute megakaryoblastic leukemia with failed remission
Acute megakaryoblastic leukemia NOS

     C94.21   **Acute megakaryoblastic leukemia, in remission**

     C94.22   **Acute megakaryoblastic leukemia, in relapse**

● **C94.3**   **Mast cell leukemia**

     C94.30   **Mast cell leukemia not having achieved remission**
Mast cell leukemia with failed remission
Mast cell leukemia NOS

     C94.31   **Mast cell leukemia, in remission**

     C94.32   **Mast cell leukemia, in relapse**

● **C94.4**   **Acute panmyelosis with myelofibrosis**
Acute myelofibrosis

> **Excludes1**   myelofibrosis NOS (D75.81)
> secondary myelofibrosis NOS (D75.81)

     C94.40   **Acute panmyelosis with myelofibrosis not having achieved remission**
Acute myelofibrosis NOS
Acute panmyelosis with myelofibrosis with failed remission
Acute panmyelosis NOS

     C94.41   **Acute panmyelosis with myelofibrosis, in remission**

     C94.42   **Acute panmyelosis with myelofibrosis, in relapse**

     C94.6   **Myelodysplastic disease, not classified**
Myeloproliferative disease, not classified

● **C94.8**   **Other specified leukemias**
Aggressive NK-cell leukemia
Acute basophilic leukemia

     C94.80   **Other specified leukemias not having achieved remission**
Other specified leukemia with failed remission
Other specified leukemias NOS

     C94.81   **Other specified leukemias, in remission**

     C94.82   **Other specified leukemias, in relapse**

● **C95**   **Leukemia of unspecified cell type**

> **Excludes1**   personal history of leukemia (Z85.6)

● **C95.0**   **Acute leukemia of unspecified cell type**
Acute bilineal leukemia
Acute mixed lineage leukemia
Biphenotypic acute leukemia
Stem cell leukemia of unclear lineage

> **Excludes1**   acute exacerbation of unspecified chronic leukemia (C95.10)

     C95.00   **Acute leukemia of unspecified cell type not having achieved remission**
Acute leukemia of unspecified cell type with failed remission
Acute leukemia NOS

     C95.01   **Acute leukemia of unspecified cell type, in remission**

     C95.02   **Acute leukemia of unspecified cell type, in relapse**

● **C95.1**   **Chronic leukemia of unspecified cell type**

     C95.10   **Chronic leukemia of unspecified cell type not having achieved remission**
Chronic leukemia of unspecified cell type with failed remission
Chronic leukemia NOS

     C95.11   **Chronic leukemia of unspecified cell type, in remission**

     C95.12   **Chronic leukemia of unspecified cell type, in relapse**

● **C95.9**   **Leukemia, unspecified**

     C95.90   **Leukemia, unspecified not having achieved remission**
Leukemia, unspecified with failed remission
Leukemia NOS

     C95.91   **Leukemia, unspecified, in remission**

     C95.92   **Leukemia, unspecified, in relapse**

● **C96**   **Other and unspecified malignant neoplasms of lymphoid, hematopoietic and related tissue**

> **Excludes1**   personal history of other malignant neoplasms of lymphoid, hematopoietic and related tissues (Z85.79)

     C96.0   **Multifocal and multisystemic (disseminated) Langerhans-cell histiocytosis**
Histiocytosis X, multisystemic
Letterer-Siwe disease

> **Excludes1**   adult pulmonary Langerhans cell histiocytosis (J84.82)
> multifocal and unisystemic Langerhans-cell histiocytosis (C96.5)
> unifocal Langerhans-cell histiocytosis (C96.6)

     C96.2   **Malignant mast cell tumor**
Aggressive systemic mastocytosis
Mast cell sarcoma

> **Excludes1**   indolent mastocytosis (D47.0)
> mast cell leukemia (C94.30)
> mastocytosis (congenital) (cutaneous) (Q82.2)

     C96.4   **Sarcoma of dendritic cells (accessory cells)**
Follicular dendritic cell sarcoma
Interdigitating dendritic cell sarcoma
Langerhans cell sarcoma

     C96.5   **Multifocal and unisystemic Langerhans-cell histiocytosis**
Hand-Schüller-Christian disease
Histiocytosis X, multifocal

> **Excludes1**   multifocal and multisystemic (disseminated) Langerhans-cell histiocytosis (C96.0)
> unifocal Langerhans-cell histiocytosis (C96.6)

     C96.6   **Unifocal Langerhans-cell histiocytosis**
Eosinophilic granuloma
Histiocytosis X, unifocal
Histiocytosis X NOS
Langerhans-cell histiocytosis NOS

> **Excludes1**   multifocal and multisysemic (disseminated) Langerhans-cell histiocytosis (C96.0)
> multifocal and unisystemic Langerhans-cell histiocytosis (C96.5)

     C96.A   **Histiocytic sarcoma**
Malignant histiocytosis

     C96.Z   **Other specified malignant neoplasms of lymphoid, hematopoietic and related tissue**

     C96.9   **Malignant neoplasm of lymphoid, hematopoietic and related tissue, unspecified**

In situ is carcinoma involving cells in localized tissues that has not spread to nearby tissues

IN SITU NEOPLASMS (D00-D09)

Includes   Bowen's disease
erythroplasia
grade III intraepithelial neoplasia
Queyrat's erythroplasia

● **D00   Carcinoma in situ of oral cavity, esophagus and stomach**
Excludes1   melanoma in situ (D03.-)
● **D00.0   Carcinoma in situ of lip, oral cavity and pharynx**
Use additional code to identify:
exposure to environmental tobacco smoke (Z77.22)
exposure to tobacco smoke in the perinatal period (P96.81)
history of tobacco use (Z87.891)
occupational exposure to environmental tobacco smoke (Z57.31)
tobacco dependence (F17.-)
tobacco use (Z72.0)
Excludes1   carcinoma in situ of aryepiglottic fold or interarytenoid fold, laryngeal aspect (D02.0)
carcinoma in situ of epiglottis NOS (D02.0)
carcinoma in situ of epiglottis suprahyoid portion (D02.0)
carcinoma in situ of skin of lip (D03.0, D04.0)

D00.00   Carcinoma in situ of oral cavity, unspecified site
D00.01   Carcinoma in situ of labial mucosa and vermilion border
D00.02   Carcinoma in situ of buccal mucosa
D00.03   Carcinoma in situ of gingiva and edentulous alveolar ridge
D00.04   Carcinoma in situ of soft palate
D00.05   Carcinoma in situ of hard palate
D00.06   Carcinoma in situ of floor of mouth
D00.07   Carcinoma in situ of tongue
D00.08   Carcinoma in situ of pharynx
Carcinoma in situ of aryepiglottic fold NOS
Carcinoma in situ of hypopharyngeal aspect of aryepiglottic fold
Carcinoma in situ of marginal zone of aryepiglottic fold

D00.1   Carcinoma in situ of esophagus
D00.2   Carcinoma in situ of stomach

● **D01   Carcinoma in situ of other and unspecified digestive organs**
Excludes1   melanoma in situ (D03.-)
D01.0   Carcinoma in situ of colon
Excludes1   carcinoma in situ of rectosigmoid junction (D01.1)
D01.1   Carcinoma in situ of rectosigmoid junction
D01.2   Carcinoma in situ of rectum
D01.3   Carcinoma in situ of anus and anal canal
Excludes1   carcinoma in situ of anal margin (D04.5)
carcinoma in situ of anal skin (D04.5)
carcinoma in situ of perianal skin (D04.5)
● **D01.4   Carcinoma in situ of other and unspecified parts of intestine**
Excludes1   carcinoma in situ of ampulla of Vater (D01.5)
D01.40   Carcinoma in situ of unspecified part of intestine
D01.49   Carcinoma in situ of other parts of intestine
D01.5   Carcinoma in situ of liver, gallbladder and bile ducts
Carcinoma in situ of ampulla of Vater
D01.7   Carcinoma in situ of other specified digestive organs
Carcinoma in situ of pancreas
D01.9   Carcinoma in situ of digestive organ, unspecified

● **D02   Carcinoma in situ of middle ear and respiratory system**
Use additional code to identify:
exposure to environmental tobacco smoke (Z77.22)
exposure to tobacco smoke in the perinatal period (P96.81)
history of tobacco use (Z87.891)
occupational exposure to environmental tobacco smoke (Z57.31)
tobacco dependence (F17.-)
tobacco use (Z72.0)
Excludes1   melanoma in situ (D03.-)
D02.0   Carcinoma in situ of larynx
Carcinoma in situ of aryepiglottic fold or interarytenoid fold, laryngeal aspect
Carcinoma in situ of epiglottis (suprahyoid portion)
Excludes1   carcinoma in situ of aryepiglottic fold or interarytenoid fold NOS (D00.08)
carcinoma in situ of hypopharyngeal aspect (D00.08)
carcinoma in situ of marginal zone (D00.08)
D02.1   Carcinoma in situ of trachea
● **D02.2   Carcinoma in situ of bronchus and lung**
D02.20   Carcinoma in situ of unspecified bronchus and lung
D02.21   Carcinoma in situ of right bronchus and lung
D02.22   Carcinoma in situ of left bronchus and lung
D02.3   Carcinoma in situ of other parts of respiratory system
Carcinoma in situ of accessory sinuses
Carcinoma in situ of middle ear
Carcinoma in situ of nasal cavities
Excludes1   carcinoma in situ of ear (external) (skin) (D04.2-)
carcinoma in situ of nose NOS (D09.8)
carcinoma in situ of skin of nose (D04.3)
D02.4   Carcinoma in situ of respiratory system, unspecified

● **D03   Melanoma in situ**
D03.0   Melanoma in situ of lip
● **D03.1   Melanoma in situ of eyelid, including canthus**
D03.10   Melanoma in situ of unspecified eyelid, including canthus
D03.11   Melanoma in situ of right eyelid, including canthus
D03.12   Melanoma in situ of left eyelid, including canthus
● **D03.2   Melanoma in situ of ear and external auricular canal**
D03.20   Melanoma in situ of unspecified ear and external auricular canal
D03.21   Melanoma in situ of right ear and external auricular canal
D03.22   Melanoma in situ of left ear and external auricular canal
● **D03.3   Melanoma in situ of other and unspecified parts of face**
D03.30   Melanoma in situ of unspecified part of face
D03.39   Melanoma in situ of other parts of face
D03.4   Melanoma in situ of scalp and neck
● **D03.5   Melanoma in situ of trunk**
D03.51   Melanoma in situ of anal skin
Melanoma in situ of anal margin
Melanoma in situ of perianal skin
D03.52   Melanoma in situ of breast (skin) (soft tissue)
D03.59   Melanoma in situ of other part of trunk
● **D03.6   Melanoma in situ of upper limb, including shoulder**
D03.60   Melanoma in situ of unspecified upper limb, including shoulder
D03.61   Melanoma in situ of right upper limb, including shoulder
D03.62   Melanoma in situ of left upper limb, including shoulder

◀ New   ◀▥ Revised   ~~deleted~~ Deleted   OGCR Official Guidelines   X Assign placeholder X   ● Use Additional Character(s)
Excludes 1   Excludes 2   Includes   Use additional   Code first   Code also   Unspecified
767

CHAPTER 2 (C00-D49)

● **D03.7**   **Melanoma in situ of lower limb, including hip**

     D03.70   Melanoma in situ of unspecified lower limb, including hip

     D03.71   Melanoma in situ of right lower limb, including hip

     D03.72   Melanoma in situ of left lower limb, including hip

   D03.8   **Melanoma in situ of other sites**

     Melanoma in situ of scrotum

     Excludes1   carcinoma in situ of scrotum (D07.61)

   D03.9   **Melanoma in situ, unspecified**

● **D04**   **Carcinoma in situ of skin**

     Excludes1   erythroplasia of Queyrat (penis) NOS (D07.4)

                melanoma in situ (D03.-)

   D04.0   **Carcinoma in situ of skin of lip**

     Excludes1   carcinoma in situ of vermilion border of lip (D00.01)

● **D04.1**   **Carcinoma in situ of skin of eyelid, including canthus**

     D04.10   Carcinoma in situ of skin of unspecified eyelid, including canthus

     D04.11   Carcinoma in situ of skin of right eyelid, including canthus

     D04.12   Carcinoma in situ of skin of left eyelid, including canthus

● **D04.2**   **Carcinoma in situ of skin of ear and external auricular canal**

     D04.20   Carcinoma in situ of skin of unspecified ear and external auricular canal

     D04.21   Carcinoma in situ of skin of right ear and external auricular canal

     D04.22   Carcinoma in situ of skin of left ear and external auricular canal

● **D04.3**   **Carcinoma in situ of skin of other and unspecified parts of face**

     D04.30   Carcinoma in situ of skin of unspecified part of face

     D04.39   Carcinoma in situ of skin of other parts of face

   D04.4   **Carcinoma in situ of skin of scalp and neck**

   D04.5   **Carcinoma in situ of skin of trunk**

     Carcinoma in situ of anal margin

     Carcinoma in situ of anal skin

     Carcinoma in situ of perianal skin

     Carcinoma in situ of skin of breast

     Excludes1   carcinoma in situ of anus NOS (D01.3)

                carcinoma in situ of scrotum (D07.61)

                carcinoma in situ of skin of genital organs (D07.-)

● **D04.6**   **Carcinoma in situ of skin of upper limb, including shoulder**

     D04.60   Carcinoma in situ of skin of unspecified upper limb, including shoulder

     D04.61   Carcinoma in situ of skin of right upper limb, including shoulder

     D04.62   Carcinoma in situ of skin of left upper limb, including shoulder

● **D04.7**   **Carcinoma in situ of skin of lower limb, including hip**

     D04.70   Carcinoma in situ of skin of unspecified lower limb, including hip

     D04.71   Carcinoma in situ of skin of right lower limb, including hip

     D04.72   Carcinoma in situ of skin of left lower limb, including hip

   D04.8   **Carcinoma in situ of skin of other sites**

   D04.9   **Carcinoma in situ of skin, unspecified**

● **D05**   **Carcinoma in situ of breast**

     Excludes1   carcinoma in situ of skin of breast (D04.5)

                melanoma in situ of breast (skin) (D03.5)

                Paget's disease of breast or nipple (C50.-)

● **D05.0**   **Lobular carcinoma in situ of breast**

     D05.00   Lobular carcinoma in situ of unspecified breast

     D05.01   Lobular carcinoma in situ of right breast

     D05.02   Lobular carcinoma in situ of left breast

● **D05.1**   **Intraductal carcinoma in situ of breast**

     D05.10   Intraductal carcinoma in situ of unspecified breast

     D05.11   Intraductal carcinoma in situ of right breast

     D05.12   Intraductal carcinoma in situ of left breast

● **D05.8**   **Other specified type of carcinoma in situ of breast**

     D05.80   Other specified type of carcinoma in situ of unspecified breast

     D05.81   Other specified type of carcinoma in situ of right breast

     D05.82   Other specified type of carcinoma in situ of left breast

● **D05.9**   **Unspecified type of carcinoma in situ of breast**

     D05.90   Unspecified type of carcinoma in situ of unspecified breast

     D05.91   Unspecified type of carcinoma in situ of right breast

     D05.92   Unspecified type of carcinoma in situ of left breast

● **D06**   **Carcinoma in situ of cervix uteri**

     Includes   cervical adenocarcinoma in situ

               cervical intraepithelial glandular neoplasia

               cervical intraepithelial neoplasia III [CIN III]

               severe dysplasia of cervix uteri

     Excludes1   cervical intraepithelial neoplasia II [CIN II] (N87.1)

               cytologic evidence of malignancy of cervix without histologic confirmation (R87.614)

               high grade squamous intraepithelial lesion (HGSIL) of cervix (R87.613)

               melanoma in situ of cervix (D03.5)

               moderate cervical dysplasia (N87.1)

   D06.0   **Carcinoma in situ of endocervix**

   D06.1   **Carcinoma in situ of exocervix**

   D06.7   **Carcinoma in situ of other parts of cervix**

   D06.9   **Carcinoma in situ of cervix, unspecified**

● **D07**   **Carcinoma in situ of other and unspecified genital organs**

     Excludes1   melanoma in situ of trunk (D03.5)

   D07.0   **Carcinoma in situ of endometrium**

   D07.1   **Carcinoma in situ of vulva**

     Severe dysplasia of vulva

     Vulvar intraepithelial neoplasia III [VIN III]

     Excludes1   moderate dysplasia of vulva (N90.1)

               vulvar intraepithelial neoplasia II [VIN II] (N90.1)

   D07.2   **Carcinoma in situ of vagina**

     Severe dysplasia of vagina

     Vaginal intraepithelial neoplasia III [VIN III]

     Excludes1   moderate dysplasia of vagina (N89.1)

               vaginal intraepithelial neoplasia II [VIN II] (N89.1)

● **D07.3**   **Carcinoma in situ of other and unspecified female genital organs**

     D07.30   Carcinoma in situ of unspecified female genital organs

     D07.39   Carcinoma in situ of other female genital organs

◀ New   ◀▥ Revised   ~~deleted~~ Deleted   **OGCR** Official Guidelines   X Assign placeholder X   ● Use Additional Character(s)

Excludes 1   Excludes 2   Includes   Use additional   Code first   Code also   Unspecified

D07.4 **Carcinoma in situ of penis**
Erythroplasia of Queyrat NOS

D07.5 **Carcinoma in situ of prostate**
Prostatic intraepithelial neoplasia III (PIN III)
Severe dysplasia of prostate
Excludes1 dysplasia (mild) (moderate) of prostate
(N42.3)

● D07.6 **Carcinoma in situ of other and unspecified male genital organs**

D07.60 **Carcinoma in situ of unspecified male genital organs**

D07.61 **Carcinoma in situ of scrotum**

D07.69 **Carcinoma in situ of other male genital organs**

● D09 **Carcinoma in situ of other and unspecified sites**
Excludes1 melanoma in situ (D03.-)

D09.0 **Carcinoma in situ of bladder**

● D09.1 **Carcinoma in situ of other and unspecified urinary organs**

D09.10 **Carcinoma in situ of unspecified urinary organ**

D09.19 **Carcinoma in situ of other urinary organs**

● D09.2 **Carcinoma in situ of eye**
Excludes1 carcinoma in situ of skin of eyelid
(D04.1-)

D09.20 **Carcinoma in situ of unspecified eye**

D09.21 **Carcinoma in situ of right eye**

D09.22 **Carcinoma in situ of left eye**

D09.3 **Carcinoma in situ of thyroid and other endocrine glands**
Excludes1 carcinoma in situ of endocrine pancreas
(D01.7)
carcinoma in situ of ovary (D07.39)
carcinoma in situ of testis (D07.69)

D09.8 **Carcinoma in situ of other specified sites**

D09.9 **Carcinoma in situ, unspecified**

BENIGN NEOPLASMS, EXCEPT BENIGN NEUROENDOCRINE TUMORS (D10-D36)

● D10 **Benign neoplasm of mouth and pharynx**

D10.0 **Benign neoplasm of lip**
Benign neoplasm of lip (frenulum) (inner aspect)
(mucosa) (vermilion border)
Excludes1 benign neoplasm of skin of lip (D22.0,
D23.0)

D10.1 **Benign neoplasm of tongue**
Benign neoplasm of lingual tonsil

D10.2 **Benign neoplasm of floor of mouth**

● D10.3 **Other and unspecified parts of mouth**

D10.30 **Benign neoplasm of unspecified part of mouth**

D10.39 **Benign neoplasm of other parts of mouth**
Benign neoplasm of minor salivary gland NOS
Excludes1 benign odontogenic neoplasms
(D16.4-D16.5)
benign neoplasm of mucosa of
lip (D10.0)
benign neoplasm of
nasopharyngeal surface of
soft palate (D10.6)

D10.4 **Benign neoplasm of tonsil**
Benign neoplasm of tonsil (faucial) (palatine)
Excludes1 benign neoplasm of lingual tonsil
(D10.1)
benign neoplasm of pharyngeal tonsil
(D10.6)
benign neoplasm of tonsillar fossa (D10.5)
benign neoplasm of tonsillar pillars
(D10.5)

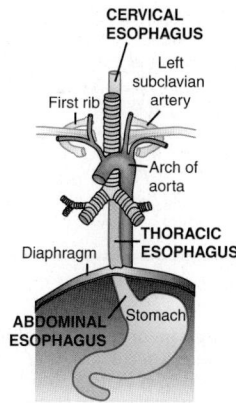

Figure 2-16 The esophagus is the muscular tube that connects the pharynx and the stomach. The 10 inch (25 cm) long esophagus is divided into three parts: **cervical, thoracic,** and **abdominal.**

D10.5 **Benign neoplasm of other parts of oropharynx**
Division of pharynx lying between soft palate and upper edge of epiglottis
Benign neoplasm of epiglottis, anterior aspect
Benign neoplasm of tonsillar fossa
Benign neoplasm of tonsillar pillars
Benign neoplasm of vallecula
Excludes1 benign neoplasm of epiglottis NOS
(D14.1)
benign neoplasm of epiglottis,
suprahyoid portion (D14.1)

D10.6 **Benign neoplasm of nasopharynx**
Segment of pharynx that lies above soft palate
Benign neoplasm of pharyngeal tonsil
Benign neoplasm of posterior margin of septum and choanae

D10.7 **Benign neoplasm of hypopharynx**
Segment of pharynx that lies below upper edge of epiglottis and opens into larynx and esophagus

D10.9 **Benign neoplasm of pharynx, unspecified**

● D11 **Benign neoplasm of major salivary glands**
Excludes1 benign neoplasms of specified minor salivary
glands which are classified according to their
anatomical location
benign neoplasms of minor salivary glands NOS
(D10.39)

D11.0 **Benign neoplasm of parotid gland**

D11.7 **Benign neoplasm of other major salivary glands**
Benign neoplasm of sublingual salivary gland
Benign neoplasm of submandibular salivary gland

D11.9 **Benign neoplasm of major salivary gland, unspecified**

● D12 **Benign neoplasm of colon, rectum, anus and anal canal**
Excludes1 benign carcinoid tumors of the large intestine,
and rectum (D3A.02-)

D12.0 **Benign neoplasm of cecum**
Benign neoplasm of ileocecal valve

D12.1 **Benign neoplasm of appendix**
Excludes1 benign carcinoid tumor of the appendix
(D3A.020)

D12.2 **Benign neoplasm of ascending colon**

D12.3 **Benign neoplasm of transverse colon**
Benign neoplasm of hepatic flexure
Benign neoplasm of splenic flexure
Flexure is a bending in a structure or organ. Note the three flexures illustrated in Figure 2–17. Hepatic = liver, sigmoid = colon, splenic = spleen.

D12.4 **Benign neoplasm of descending colon**

D12.5 **Benign neoplasm of sigmoid colon**

CHAPTER 2 (C00-D49)

◀ New   ⇇ Revised   ~~deleted~~ Deleted   **OGCR** Official Guidelines   X Assign placeholder X   ● Use Additional Character(s)

Excludes 1 | Excludes 2 | Includes | Use additional | Code first | Code also | Unspecified

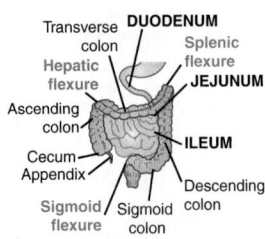

Figure 2-17   Small intestine and colon.

D12.6   **Benign neoplasm of colon, unspecified**
     Adenomatosis of colon
     Benign neoplasm of large intestine NOS
     Polyposis (hereditary) of colon
     Excludes1   inflammatory polyp of colon (K51.4-)
                 polyp of colon NOS (K63.5)

D12.7   **Benign neoplasm of rectosigmoid junction**
     Angle where sigmoid colon becomes rectum

D12.8   **Benign neoplasm of rectum**
     Excludes1   benign carcinoid tumor of the rectum
                 (D3A.026)

D12.9   **Benign neoplasm of anus and anal canal**
     Benign neoplasm of anus NOS
     Excludes1   benign neoplasm of anal margin (D22.5,
                 D23.5)
                 benign neoplasm of anal skin (D22.5,
                 D23.5)
                 benign neoplasm of perianal skin (D22.5,
                 D23.5)

● **D13**   **Benign neoplasm of other and ill-defined parts of digestive system**
     Excludes1   benign stromal tumors of digestive system
                 (D21.4)

D13.0   **Benign neoplasm of esophagus**

D13.1   **Benign neoplasm of stomach**
     Excludes1   benign carcinoid tumor of the stomach
                 (D3A.092)

D13.2   **Benign neoplasm of duodenum**
     Excludes1   benign carcinoid tumor of the duodenum
                 (D3A.010)

● **D13.3**   **Benign neoplasm of other and unspecified parts of small intestine**
     Excludes1   benign carcinoid tumors of the small
                 intestine (D3A.01-)
                 benign neoplasm of ileocecal valve
                 (D12.0)

     D13.30   **Benign neoplasm of unspecified part of small intestine**

     D13.39   **Benign neoplasm of other parts of small intestine**

D13.4   **Benign neoplasm of liver**
     Benign neoplasm of intrahepatic bile ducts

D13.5   **Benign neoplasm of extrahepatic bile ducts**
     Extensions of common hepatic bile duct (tube that collects bile from liver)

D13.6   **Benign neoplasm of pancreas**
     Excludes1   benign neoplasm of endocrine pancreas
                 (D13.7)

D13.7   **Benign neoplasm of endocrine pancreas**
     Pancreatic islets: Cells scattered throughout pancreas
     Islet cell tumor
     Benign neoplasm of islets of Langerhans
     Use additional code to identify any functional activity.

D13.9   **Benign neoplasm of ill-defined sites within the digestive system**
     Benign neoplasm of digestive system NOS
     Benign neoplasm of intestine NOS
     Benign neoplasm of spleen

● **D14**   **Benign neoplasm of middle ear and respiratory system**

D14.0   **Benign neoplasm of middle ear, nasal cavity and accessory sinuses**
     Benign neoplasm of cartilage of nose
     Excludes1   benign neoplasm of auricular canal
                 (external) (D22.2-, D23.2-)
                 benign neoplasm of bone of ear (D16.4)
                 benign neoplasm of bone of nose (D16.4)
                 benign neoplasm of cartilage of ear
                 (D21.0)
                 benign neoplasm of ear (external) (skin)
                 (D22.2-, D23.2-)
                 benign neoplasm of nose NOS (D36.7)
                 benign neoplasm of skin of nose (D22.39,
                 D23.39)
                 benign neoplasm of olfactory bulb (D33.3)
                 benign neoplasm of posterior margin of
                 septum and choanae (D10.6)
                 polyp of accessory sinus (J33.8)
                 polyp of ear (middle) (H74.4)
                 polyp of nasal (cavity) (J33.-)

D14.1   **Benign neoplasm of larynx**
     Adenomatous polyp of larynx
     Benign neoplasm of epiglottis (suprahyoid portion)
     Horseshoe shaped bone in anterior midline of neck between chin and thyroid cartilage
     Excludes1   benign neoplasm of epiglottis, anterior
                 aspect (D10.5)
                 polyp (nonadenomatous) of vocal cord or
                 larynx (J38.1)

D14.2   **Benign neoplasm of trachea**

● **D14.3**   **Benign neoplasm of bronchus and lung**
     Excludes1   benign carcinoid tumor of the bronchus
                 and lung (D3A.090)

     D14.30   **Benign neoplasm of unspecified bronchus and lung**

     D14.31   **Benign neoplasm of right bronchus and lung**

     D14.32   **Benign neoplasm of left bronchus and lung**

D14.4   **Benign neoplasm of respiratory system, unspecified**

● **D15**   **Benign neoplasm of other and unspecified intrathoracic organs**
     Excludes1   benign neoplasm of mesothelial tissue (D19.-)

D15.0   **Benign neoplasm of thymus**
     Excludes1   benign carcinoid tumor of the thymus
                 (D3A.091)

D15.1   **Benign neoplasm of heart**
     Excludes1   benign neoplasm of great vessels (D21.3)

D15.2   **Benign neoplasm of mediastinum**

D15.7   **Benign neoplasm of other specified intrathoracic organs**

D15.9   **Benign neoplasm of intrathoracic organ, unspecified**

● **D16**   **Benign neoplasm of bone and articular cartilage**
     Excludes1   benign neoplasm of connective tissue of ear
                 (D21.0)
                 benign neoplasm of connective tissue of eyelid
                 (D21.0)
                 benign neoplasm of connective tissue of larynx
                 (D14.1)
                 benign neoplasm of connective tissue of nose
                 (D14.0)
                 benign neoplasm of synovia (D21.-)

● **D16.0**   **Benign neoplasm of scapula and long bones of upper limb**

     D16.00   **Benign neoplasm of scapula and long bones of unspecified upper limb**

     D16.01   **Benign neoplasm of scapula and long bones of right upper limb**

     D16.02   **Benign neoplasm of scapula and long bones of left upper limb**

● **D16.1** **Benign neoplasm of short bones of upper limb**
    D16.10   Benign neoplasm of short bones of unspecified upper limb
    D16.11   Benign neoplasm of short bones of right upper limb
    D16.12   Benign neoplasm of short bones of left upper limb

● **D16.2** **Benign neoplasm of long bones of lower limb**
    D16.20   Benign neoplasm of long bones of unspecified lower limb
    D16.21   Benign neoplasm of long bones of right lower limb
    D16.22   Benign neoplasm of long bones of left lower limb

● **D16.3** **Benign neoplasm of short bones of lower limb**
    D16.30   Benign neoplasm of short bones of unspecified lower limb
    D16.31   Benign neoplasm of short bones of right lower limb
    D16.32   Benign neoplasm of short bones of left lower limb

D16.4 **Benign neoplasm of bones of skull and face**
    Benign neoplasm of maxilla (superior)
    Benign neoplasm of orbital bone
      Cavity or socket of skull in which eye and its appendages are located
    Keratocyst of maxilla
    Keratocystic odontogenic tumor of maxilla
    | Excludes1 | benign neoplasm of lower jaw bone (D16.5) |

D16.5 **Benign neoplasm of lower jaw bone**
    Keratocyst of mandible
    Keratocystic odontogenic tumor of mandible

D16.6 **Benign neoplasm of vertebral column**
    | Excludes1 | benign neoplasm of sacrum and coccyx (D16.8) |

D16.7 **Benign neoplasm of ribs, sternum and clavicle**

D16.8 **Benign neoplasm of pelvic bones, sacrum and coccyx**

D16.9 **Benign neoplasm of bone and articular cartilage, unspecified**

● **D17** **Benign lipomatous neoplasm**
    Slow growing benign tumors (rubbery masses) of mature fat cells enclosed in a thin fibrous capsule

D17.0 **Benign lipomatous neoplasm of skin and subcutaneous tissue of head, face and neck**

D17.1 **Benign lipomatous neoplasm of skin and subcutaneous tissue of trunk**

● **D17.2** **Benign lipomatous neoplasm of skin and subcutaneous tissue of limb**
    D17.20   Benign lipomatous neoplasm of skin and subcutaneous tissue of unspecified limb
    D17.21   Benign lipomatous neoplasm of skin and subcutaneous tissue of right arm
    D17.22   Benign lipomatous neoplasm of skin and subcutaneous tissue of left arm
    D17.23   Benign lipomatous neoplasm of skin and subcutaneous tissue of right leg
    D17.24   Benign lipomatous neoplasm of skin and subcutaneous tissue of left leg

● **D17.3** **Benign lipomatous neoplasm of skin and subcutaneous tissue of other and unspecified sites**
    D17.30   Benign lipomatous neoplasm of skin and subcutaneous tissue of unspecified sites
    D17.39   Benign lipomatous neoplasm of skin and subcutaneous tissue of other sites

D17.4 **Benign lipomatous neoplasm of intrathoracic organs**

Figure 2-18 Hemangioma of skin and subcutaneous tissue. (From Yanoff: Ophthalmology, ed 3, Mosby, Inc., 2008)

Item 2–10 **Hemangiomas** are abnormally dense collections of dilated capillaries that occur on the skin or in internal organs. Hemangiomas are both deep and superficial and undergo a rapid growth phase when the size increases rapidly, followed by a rest phase, in which the tumor changes very little, followed by an involutional phase in which the tumor begins to and can disappear altogether. **Lymphangiomas** or cystic hygroma are benign collections of overgrown lymph vessels and, although rare, may occur anywhere but most commonly on the head and neck of children and infants. Visceral organs, lungs, and gastrointestinal tract may also be involved.

D17.5 **Benign lipomatous neoplasm of intra-abdominal organs**
    | Excludes1 | benign lipomatous neoplasm of peritoneum and retroperitoneum (D17.79) |

D17.6 **Benign lipomatous neoplasm of spermatic cord**

● **D17.7** **Benign lipomatous neoplasm of other sites**
    D17.71   Benign lipomatous neoplasm of kidney
    D17.72   Benign lipomatous neoplasm of other genitourinary organ
    D17.79   Benign lipomatous neoplasm of other sites
        Benign lipomatous neoplasm of peritoneum
        Benign lipomatous neoplasm of retroperitoneum

D17.9 **Benign lipomatous neoplasm, unspecified**
    Lipoma NOS

● **D18** **Hemangioma and lymphangioma, any site**
    | Excludes1 | benign neoplasm of glomus jugulare (D35.6) |
    | | blue or pigmented nevus (D22.-) |
    | | nevus NOS (D22.-) |
    | | vascular nevus (Q82.5) |

● **D18.0** **Hemangioma**
    Common type of vascular malformation
    Angioma NOS
    Cavernous nevus
    D18.00   Hemangioma unspecified site
    D18.01   Hemangioma of skin and subcutaneous tissue
    D18.02   Hemangioma of intracranial structures
    D18.03   Hemangioma of intra-abdominal structures
    D18.09   Hemangioma of other sites

D18.1 **Lymphangioma, any site**

● **D19** **Benign neoplasm of mesothelial tissue**
    Mesothelial tissue is the membrane lining several body cavities

D19.0 **Benign neoplasm of mesothelial tissue of pleura**

D19.1 **Benign neoplasm of mesothelial tissue of peritoneum**

D19.7 **Benign neoplasm of mesothelial tissue of other sites**

D19.9 **Benign neoplasm of mesothelial tissue, unspecified**
    Benign mesothelioma NOS

● **D20** **Benign neoplasm of soft tissue of retroperitoneum and peritoneum**
    | Excludes1 | benign lipomatous neoplasm of peritoneum and retroperitoneum (D17.79) |
    | | benign neoplasm of mesothelial tissue (D19.-) |

D20.0 **Benign neoplasm of soft tissue of retroperitoneum**

D20.1 **Benign neoplasm of soft tissue of peritoneum**

CHAPTER 2 (C00-D49)

◀ New   ◀◀◀ Revised   ~~deleted~~ Deleted   **OGCR** Official Guidelines   X Assign placeholder X   ● Use Additional Character(s)

| Excludes 1 | Excludes 2 | Includes | Use additional | Code first | Code also | Unspecified |

● **D21   Other benign neoplasms of connective and other soft tissue**

Includes   benign neoplasm of blood vessel
benign neoplasm of bursa
benign neoplasm of cartilage
benign neoplasm of fascia
benign neoplasm of fat
benign neoplasm of ligament, except uterine
benign neoplasm of lymphatic channel
benign neoplasm of muscle
benign neoplasm of synovia
benign neoplasm of tendon (sheath)
benign stromal tumors

Excludes1   benign neoplasm of articular cartilage (D16.-)
benign neoplasm of cartilage of larynx (D14.1)
benign neoplasm of cartilage of nose (D14.0)
benign neoplasm of connective tissue of breast (D24.-)
benign neoplasm of peripheral nerves and autonomic nervous system (D36.1-)
benign neoplasm of peritoneum (D20.1)
benign neoplasm of retroperitoneum (D20.0)
benign neoplasm of uterine ligament, any (D28.2)
benign neoplasm of vascular tissue (D18.-)
hemangioma (D18.0-)
lipomatous neoplasm (D17.-)
lymphangioma (D18.1)
uterine leiomyoma (D25.-)

D21.0   Benign neoplasm of connective and other soft tissue of head, face and neck
Benign neoplasm of connective tissue of ear
Benign neoplasm of connective tissue of eyelid

> **Excludes1**   benign neoplasm of connective tissue of orbit (D31.6-)

● **D21.1   Benign neoplasm of connective and other soft tissue of upper limb, including shoulder**

D21.10   Benign neoplasm of connective and other soft tissue of unspecified upper limb, including shoulder

D21.11   Benign neoplasm of connective and other soft tissue of right upper limb, including shoulder

D21.12   Benign neoplasm of connective and other soft tissue of left upper limb, including shoulder

● **D21.2   Benign neoplasm of connective and other soft tissue of lower limb, including hip**

D21.20   Benign neoplasm of connective and other soft tissue of unspecified lower limb, including hip

D21.21   Benign neoplasm of connective and other soft tissue of right lower limb, including hip

D21.22   Benign neoplasm of connective and other soft tissue of left lower limb, including hip

D21.3   Benign neoplasm of connective and other soft tissue of thorax
Benign neoplasm of axilla
Benign neoplasm of diaphragm
Benign neoplasm of great vessels

> **Excludes1**   benign neoplasm of heart (D15.1)
> benign neoplasm of mediastinum (D15.2)
> benign neoplasm of thymus (D15.0)

D21.4   Benign neoplasm of connective and other soft tissue of abdomen Benign stromal tumors of abdomen

D21.5   Benign neoplasm of connective and other soft tissue of pelvis

> **Excludes1**   benign neoplasm of any uterine ligament (D28.2)
> uterine leiomyoma (D25.-)

D21.6   Benign neoplasm of connective and other soft tissue of trunk, unspecified
Benign neoplasm of back NOS

D21.9   Benign neoplasm of connective and other soft tissue, unspecified

● **D22   Melanocytic nevi**

Includes   atypical nevus
blue hairy pigmented nevus
nevus NOS

D22.0   Melanocytic nevi of lip
Skin lesions composed of nests of nevus cells with macules/ papules

● **D22.1   Melanocytic nevi of eyelid, including canthus**

D22.10   Melanocytic nevi of unspecified eyelid, including canthus

D22.11   Melanocytic nevi of right eyelid, including canthus

D22.12   Melanocytic nevi of left eyelid, including canthus

● **D22.2   Melanocytic nevi of ear and external auricular canal**

D22.20   Melanocytic nevi of unspecified ear and external auricular canal

D22.21   Melanocytic nevi of right ear and external auricular canal

D22.22   Melanocytic nevi of left ear and external auricular canal

● **D22.3   Melanocytic nevi of other and unspecified parts of face**

D22.30   Melanocytic nevi of unspecified part of face

D22.39   Melanocytic nevi of other parts of face

D22.4   Melanocytic nevi of scalp and neck

D22.5   Melanocytic nevi of trunk
Melanocytic nevi of anal margin
Melanocytic nevi of anal skin
Melanocytic nevi of perianal skin
Melanocytic nevi of skin of breast

● **D22.6   Melanocytic nevi of upper limb, including shoulder**

D22.60   Melanocytic nevi of unspecified upper limb, including shoulder

D22.61   Melanocytic nevi of right upper limb, including shoulder

D22.62   Melanocytic nevi of left upper limb, including shoulder

● **D22.7   Melanocytic nevi of lower limb, including hip**

D22.70   Melanocytic nevi of unspecified lower limb, including hip

D22.71   Melanocytic nevi of right lower limb, including hip

D22.72   Melanocytic nevi of left lower limb, including hip

D22.9   Melanocytic nevi, unspecified

● **D23   Other benign neoplasms of skin**

Includes   benign neoplasm of hair follicles
benign neoplasm of sebaceous glands
benign neoplasm of sweat glands

Excludes1   benign lipomatous neoplasms of skin (D17.0-D17.3)
melanocytic nevi (D22.-)

D23.0   Other benign neoplasm of skin of lip

> **Excludes1**   benign neoplasm of vermilion border of lip (D10.0)

● **D23.1   Other benign neoplasm of skin of eyelid, including canthus**

D23.10   Other benign neoplasm of skin unspecified of eyelid, including canthus

D23.11   Other benign neoplasm of skin of right eyelid, including canthus

D23.12   Other benign neoplasm of skin of left eyelid, including canthus

● **D23.2** **Other benign neoplasm of skin of ear and external auricular canal**

     D23.20 Other benign neoplasm of skin of `unspecified` ear and external auricular canal

     D23.21 Other benign neoplasm of skin of right ear and external auricular canal

     D23.22 Other benign neoplasm of skin of left ear and external auricular canal

● **D23.3** **Other benign neoplasm of skin of other and unspecified parts of face**

     D23.30 Other benign neoplasm of skin of `unspecified` part of face

     D23.39 Other benign neoplasm of skin of other parts of face

  D23.4 **Other benign neoplasm of skin of scalp and neck**

  D23.5 **Other benign neoplasm of skin of trunk**
      Other benign neoplasm of anal margin
      Other benign neoplasm of anal skin
      Other benign neoplasm of perianal skin
      Other benign neoplasm of skin of breast

     | Excludes1 | benign neoplasm of anus NOS (D12.9) |

● **D23.6** **Other benign neoplasm of skin of upper limb, including shoulder**

     D23.60 Other benign neoplasm of skin of `unspecified` upper limb, including shoulder

     D23.61 Other benign neoplasm of skin of right upper limb, including shoulder

     D23.62 Other benign neoplasm of skin of left upper limb, including shoulder

● **D23.7** **Other benign neoplasm of skin of lower limb, including hip**

     D23.70 Other benign neoplasm of skin of `unspecified` lower limb, including hip

     D23.71 Other benign neoplasm of skin of right lower limb, including hip

     D23.72 Other benign neoplasm of skin of left lower limb, including hip

  D23.9 **Other benign neoplasm of skin, `unspecified`**

● **D24** **Benign neoplasm of breast**

     `Includes`   benign neoplasm of connective tissue of breast
               benign neoplasm of soft parts of breast
               fibroadenoma of breast

     | Excludes2 | adenofibrosis of breast (N60.2) |
               benign cyst of breast (N60.-)
               benign mammary dysplasia (N60.-)
               benign neoplasm of skin of breast (D22.5, D23.5)
               fibrocystic disease of breast (N60.-)

  D24.1 **Benign neoplasm of right breast**

  D24.2 **Benign neoplasm of left breast**

  D24.9 **Benign neoplasm of `unspecified` breast**

● **D25** **Leiomyoma of uterus**
     Benign tumors or nodules of the uterine wall

     `Includes`   uterine fibroid
               uterine fibromyoma
               uterine myoma

  D25.0 **Submucous leiomyoma of uterus**

  D25.1 **Intramural leiomyoma of uterus**
      Interstitial leiomyoma of uterus

  D25.2 **Subserosal leiomyoma of uterus**
      Subperitoneal leiomyoma of uterus

  D25.9 **Leiomyoma of uterus, `unspecified`**

● **D26** **Other benign neoplasms of uterus**

  D26.0 **Other benign neoplasm of cervix uteri**

  D26.1 **Other benign neoplasm of corpus uteri**

  D26.7 **Other benign neoplasm of other parts of uterus**

  D26.9 **Other benign neoplasm of uterus, `unspecified`**

Item 2–11   Teratoma: terat = monster, oma = mass, tumor. Alternate terms: dermoid cyst of the ovary, ovarian teratoma. Teratomas are neoplasms and arise from germ cells (ovaries in female and testes in male) and can be benign or malignant. Teratomas have been known to contain hair, nails, and teeth, giving them a bizarre ("monster") appearance.

● **D27** **Benign neoplasm of ovary**
     `Use additional` code to identify any functional activity.

     | Excludes2 | corpus albicans cyst (N83.2) |
                corpus luteum cyst (N83.1)
                endometrial cyst (N80.1)
                follicular (atretic) cyst (N83.0)
                graafian follicle cyst (N83.0)
                ovarian cyst NEC (N83.2)
                ovarian retention cyst (N83.2)

  D27.0 **Benign neoplasm of right ovary**

  D27.1 **Benign neoplasm of left ovary**

  D27.9 **Benign neoplasm of `unspecified` ovary**

● **D28** **Benign neoplasm of other and unspecified female genital organs**

     `Includes`   adenomatous polyp
               benign neoplasm of skin of female genital organs
               benign teratoma

     | Excludes1 | epoophoron cyst (Q50.5) |
                fimbrial cyst (Q50.4)
                Gartner's duct cyst (Q52.4)
                parovarian cyst (Q50.5)

  D28.0 **Benign neoplasm of vulva**

  D28.1 **Benign neoplasm of vagina**

  D28.2 **Benign neoplasm of uterine tubes and ligaments**
      Benign neoplasm of fallopian tube
      Benign neoplasm of uterine ligament (broad) (round)

  D28.7 **Benign neoplasm of other specified female genital organs**

  D28.9 **Benign neoplasm of female genital organ, `unspecified`**

● **D29** **Benign neoplasm of male genital organs**
     `Includes`   benign neoplasm of skin of male genital organs

  D29.0 **Benign neoplasm of penis**

  D29.1 **Benign neoplasm of prostate**
     | Excludes1 | enlarged prostate (N40.-) |

● **D29.2** **Benign neoplasm of testis**
     `Use additional` code to identify any functional activity.

     D29.20 Benign neoplasm of `unspecified` testis

     D29.21 Benign neoplasm of right testis

     D29.22 Benign neoplasm of left testis

● **D29.3** **Benign neoplasm of epididymis**

     D29.30 Benign neoplasm of `unspecified` epididymis

     D29.31 Benign neoplasm of right epididymis

     D29.32 Benign neoplasm of left epididymis

  D29.4 **Benign neoplasm of scrotum**
      Benign neoplasm of skin of scrotum

  D29.8 **Benign neoplasm of other specified male genital organs**
      Benign neoplasm of seminal vesicle
      Benign neoplasm of spermatic cord
      Benign neoplasm of tunica vaginalis

  D29.9 **Benign neoplasm of male genital organ, `unspecified`**

● **D30** **Benign neoplasm of urinary organs**

● **D30.0** **Benign neoplasm of kidney**

     | Excludes1 | benign carcinoid tumor of the kidney (D3A.093) |
                benign neoplasm of renal calyces (D30.1-)
                benign neoplasm of renal pelvis (D30.1-)

     D30.00 Benign neoplasm of `unspecified` kidney

     D30.01 Benign neoplasm of right kidney

     D30.02 Benign neoplasm of left kidney

● D30.1   Benign neoplasm of renal pelvis
   D30.10   Benign neoplasm of unspecified renal pelvis
   D30.11   Benign neoplasm of right renal pelvis
   D30.12   Benign neoplasm of left renal pelvis
● D30.2   Benign neoplasm of ureter
   Excludes1   benign neoplasm of ureteric orifice of
               bladder (D30.3)
   D30.20   Benign neoplasm of unspecified ureter
   D30.21   Benign neoplasm of right ureter
   D30.22   Benign neoplasm of left ureter
D30.3   Benign neoplasm of bladder
        Benign neoplasm of ureteric orifice of bladder
        Benign neoplasm of urethral orifice of bladder
D30.4   Benign neoplasm of urethra
        Excludes1   benign neoplasm of urethral orifice of
                    bladder (D30.3)
D30.8   Benign neoplasm of other specified urinary organs
        Benign neoplasm of paraurethral glands
D30.9   Benign neoplasm of urinary organ, unspecified
        Benign neoplasm of urinary system NOS

● D31   Benign neoplasm of eye and adnexa
        Excludes1   benign neoplasm of connective tissue of eyelid
                    (D21.0)
                    benign neoplasm of optic nerve (D33.3)
                    benign neoplasm of skin of eyelid (D22.1-, D23.1-)
   ● D31.0   Benign neoplasm of conjunctiva
      D31.00   Benign neoplasm of unspecified conjunctiva
      D31.01   Benign neoplasm of right conjunctiva
      D31.02   Benign neoplasm of left conjunctiva
   ● D31.1   Benign neoplasm of cornea
      D31.10   Benign neoplasm of unspecified cornea
      D31.11   Benign neoplasm of right cornea
      D31.12   Benign neoplasm of left cornea
   ● D31.2   Benign neoplasm of retina
        Excludes1   dark area on retina (D49.81)
                    hemangioma of retina (D49.81)
                    neoplasm of unspecified behavior of
                        retina and choroid (D49.81)
                    retinal freckle (D49.81)
      D31.20   Benign neoplasm of unspecified retina
      D31.21   Benign neoplasm of right retina
      D31.22   Benign neoplasm of left retina
   ● D31.3   Benign neoplasm of choroid
      D31.30   Benign neoplasm of unspecified choroid
      D31.31   Benign neoplasm of right choroid
      D31.32   Benign neoplasm of left choroid
   ● D31.4   Benign neoplasm of ciliary body
      D31.40   Benign neoplasm of unspecified ciliary body
      D31.41   Benign neoplasm of right ciliary body
      D31.42   Benign neoplasm of left ciliary body
   ● D31.5   Benign neoplasm of lacrimal gland and duct
        Benign neoplasm of lacrimal sac
        Benign neoplasm of nasolacrimal duct
      D31.50   Benign neoplasm of unspecified lacrimal gland
               and duct
      D31.51   Benign neoplasm of right lacrimal gland and
               duct
      D31.52   Benign neoplasm of left lacrimal gland and
               duct

● D31.6   Benign neoplasm of unspecified site of orbit
        Benign neoplasm of connective tissue of orbit
        Benign neoplasm of extraocular muscle
        Benign neoplasm of peripheral nerves of orbit
        Benign neoplasm of retrobulbar tissue
        Benign neoplasm of retro-ocular tissue
        Excludes1   benign neoplasm of orbital bone (D16.4)
   D31.60   Benign neoplasm of unspecified site of
            unspecified orbit
   D31.61   Benign neoplasm of unspecified site of right
            orbit
   D31.62   Benign neoplasm of unspecified site of left
            orbit
● D31.9   Benign neoplasm of unspecified part of eye
        Benign neoplasm of eyeball
   D31.90   Benign neoplasm of unspecified part of
            unspecified eye
   D31.91   Benign neoplasm of unspecified part of right
            eye
   D31.92   Benign neoplasm of unspecified part of left eye

● D32   Benign neoplasm of meninges
   D32.0   Benign neoplasm of cerebral meninges
   D32.1   Benign neoplasm of spinal meninges
   D32.9   Benign neoplasm of meninges, unspecified
           Meningioma NOS

● D33   Benign neoplasm of brain and other parts of central nervous
        system
        Excludes1   angioma (D18.0-)
                    benign neoplasm of meninges (D32.-)
                    benign neoplasm of peripheral nerves and
                        autonomic nervous system (D36.1-)
                    hemangioma (D18.0-)
                    neurofibromatosis (Q85.0-)
                    retro-ocular benign neoplasm (D31.6-)
   D33.0   Benign neoplasm of brain, supratentorial
        Benign neoplasm of cerebral ventricle
        Benign neoplasm of cerebrum
        Benign neoplasm of frontal lobe
        Benign neoplasm of occipital lobe
        Benign neoplasm of parietal lobe
        Benign neoplasm of temporal lobe
        Excludes1   benign neoplasm of fourth ventricle
                    (D33.1)
   D33.1   Benign neoplasm of brain, infratentorial
        Benign neoplasm of brain stem
        Benign neoplasm of cerebellum
        Benign neoplasm of fourth ventricle
   D33.2   Benign neoplasm of brain, unspecified
   D33.3   Benign neoplasm of cranial nerves
        Benign neoplasm of olfactory bulb
   D33.4   Benign neoplasm of spinal cord
   D33.7   Benign neoplasm of other specified parts of central
           nervous system
   D33.9   Benign neoplasm of central nervous system, unspecified
        Benign neoplasm of nervous system (central) NOS

D34   Benign neoplasm of thyroid gland
      Use additional code to identify any functional activity.

CHAPTER 2 (C00-D49)

● **D35** **Benign neoplasm of other and unspecified endocrine glands**
  Use additional code to identify any functional activity.
  > **Excludes1**   benign neoplasm of endocrine pancreas (D13.7)
  >   benign neoplasm of ovary (D27.-)
  >   benign neoplasm of testis (D29.2.-)
  >   benign neoplasm of thymus (D15.0)

  ● **D35.0** **Benign neoplasm of adrenal gland**
    D35.00   Benign neoplasm of unspecified adrenal gland
    D35.01   Benign neoplasm of right adrenal gland
    D35.02   Benign neoplasm of left adrenal gland
  D35.1   Benign neoplasm of parathyroid gland
  D35.2   Benign neoplasm of pituitary gland
  D35.3   Benign neoplasm of craniopharyngeal duct
  D35.4   Benign neoplasm of pineal gland
  D35.5   Benign neoplasm of carotid body
  D35.6   Benign neoplasm of aortic body and other paraganglia
    Benign tumor of glomus jugulare
  D35.7   Benign neoplasm of other specified endocrine glands
  D35.9   Benign neoplasm of endocrine gland, unspecified
    Benign neoplasm of unspecified endocrine gland

● **D36** **Benign neoplasm of other and unspecified sites**
  D36.0   Benign neoplasm of lymph nodes
    > **Excludes1**   lymphangioma (D18.1)
  ● **D36.1** **Benign neoplasm of peripheral nerves and autonomic nervous system**
    > **Excludes1**   benign neoplasm of peripheral nerves of orbit (D31.6-)
    >   neurofibromatosis (Q85.0-)

    D36.10   Benign neoplasm of peripheral nerves and autonomic nervous system, unspecified
    D36.11   Benign neoplasm of peripheral nerves and autonomic nervous system of face, head, and neck
    D36.12   Benign neoplasm of peripheral nerves and autonomic nervous system, upper limb, including shoulder
    D36.13   Benign neoplasm of peripheral nerves and autonomic nervous system of lower limb, including hip
    D36.14   Benign neoplasm of peripheral nerves and autonomic nervous system of thorax
    D36.15   Benign neoplasm of peripheral nerves and autonomic nervous system of abdomen
    D36.16   Benign neoplasm of peripheral nerves and autonomic nervous system of pelvis
    D36.17   Benign neoplasm of peripheral nerves and autonomic nervous system of trunk, unspecified
  D36.7   Benign neoplasm of other specified sites
    Benign neoplasm of nose NOS
  D36.9   Benign neoplasm, unspecified site

BENIGN NEUROENDOCRINE TUMORS (D3A)

● **D3A** **Benign neuroendocrine tumors**
  Code also any associated multiple endocrine neoplasia [MEN] syndromes (E31.2-)
  Use additional code to identify any associated endocrine syndrome, such as:
    carcinoid syndrome (E34.0)
  > **Excludes2**   benign pancreatic islet cell tumors (D13.7)
  ● **D3A.0** **Benign carcinoid tumors**
    D3A.00   Benign carcinoid tumor of unspecified site
      Carcinoid tumor NOS
    ● **D3A.01** **Benign carcinoid tumors of the small intestine**
      D3A.010   Benign carcinoid tumor of the duodenum
      D3A.011   Benign carcinoid tumor of the jejunum

      D3A.012   Benign carcinoid tumor of the ileum
      D3A.019   Benign carcinoid tumor of the small intestine, unspecified portion
    ● **D3A.02** **Benign carcinoid tumors of the appendix, large intestine, and rectum**
      D3A.020   Benign carcinoid tumor of the appendix
      D3A.021   Benign carcinoid tumor of the cecum
      D3A.022   Benign carcinoid tumor of the ascending colon
      D3A.023   Benign carcinoid tumor of the transverse colon
      D3A.024   Benign carcinoid tumor of the descending colon
      D3A.025   Benign carcinoid tumor of the sigmoid colon
      D3A.026   Benign carcinoid tumor of the rectum
      D3A.029   Benign carcinoid tumor of the large intestine, unspecified portion
        Benign carcinoid tumor of the colon NOS
    ● **D3A.09** **Benign carcinoid tumors of other sites**
      D3A.090   Benign carcinoid tumor of the bronchus and lung
      D3A.091   Benign carcinoid tumor of the thymus
      D3A.092   Benign carcinoid tumor of the stomach
      D3A.093   Benign carcinoid tumor of the kidney
      D3A.094   Benign carcinoid tumor of the foregut NOS
      D3A.095   Benign carcinoid tumor of the midgut NOS
      D3A.096   Benign carcinoid tumor of the hindgut NOS
      D3A.098   Benign carcinoid tumors of other sites
  D3A.8   Other benign neuroendocrine tumors
    Neuroendocrine tumor NOS

NEOPLASMS OF UNCERTAIN BEHAVIOR, POLYCYTHEMIA VERA AND MYELODYSPLASTIC SYNDROMES (D37-D48)

Note: Categories D37-D44, and D48 classify by site neoplasms of uncertain behavior, i.e., histologic confirmation whether the neoplasm is malignant or benign cannot be made.
> **Excludes1**   neoplasms of unspecified behavior (D49.-)

● **D37** **Neoplasm of uncertain behavior of oral cavity and digestive organs**
  > **Excludes1**   stromal tumors of uncertain behavior of digestive system (D48.1)
  ● **D37.0** **Neoplasm of uncertain behavior of lip, oral cavity and pharynx**
    > **Excludes1**   neoplasm of uncertain behavior of aryepiglottic fold or interarytenoid fold, laryngeal aspect (D38.0)
    >   neoplasm of uncertain behavior of epiglottis NOS (D38.0)
    >   neoplasm of uncertain behavior of skin of lip (D48.5)
    >   neoplasm of uncertain behavior of suprahyoid portion of epiglottis (D38.0)

    D37.01   Neoplasm of uncertain behavior of lip
      Neoplasm of uncertain behavior of vermilion border of lip
    D37.02   Neoplasm of uncertain behavior of tongue

◀ New   ⬅⦙⦙ Revised   ~~deleted~~ Deleted   **OGCR** Official Guidelines   **X** Assign placeholder X   ● Use Additional Character(s)

Excludes 1   Excludes 2   Includes   Use additional   Code first   Code also   Unspecified

775

Figure 2-19 Major salivary glands.

Parotid gland
Sublingual gland
Submandibular gland

● **D37.03** **Neoplasm of uncertain behavior of the major salivary glands**
    D37.030 **Neoplasm of uncertain behavior of the parotid salivary glands**
    D37.031 **Neoplasm of uncertain behavior of the sublingual salivary glands**
    D37.032 **Neoplasm of uncertain behavior of the submandibular salivary glands**
    D37.039 **Neoplasm of uncertain behavior of the major salivary glands, unspecified**
D37.04 **Neoplasm of uncertain behavior of the minor salivary glands**
    Neoplasm of uncertain behavior of submucosal salivary glands of lip
    Neoplasm of uncertain behavior of submucosal salivary glands of cheek
    Neoplasm of uncertain behavior of submucosal salivary glands of hard palate
    Neoplasm of uncertain behavior of submucosal salivary glands of soft palate
D37.05 **Neoplasm of uncertain behavior of pharynx**
    Neoplasm of uncertain behavior of aryepiglottic fold of pharynx NOS
    Neoplasm of uncertain behavior of hypopharyngeal aspect of aryepiglottic fold of pharynx
    Neoplasm of uncertain behavior of marginal zone of aryepiglottic fold of pharynx
D37.09 **Neoplasm of uncertain behavior of other specified sites of the oral cavity**
D37.1 **Neoplasm of uncertain behavior of stomach**
D37.2 **Neoplasm of uncertain behavior of small intestine**
D37.3 **Neoplasm of uncertain behavior of appendix**
D37.4 **Neoplasm of uncertain behavior of colon**
D37.5 **Neoplasm of uncertain behavior of rectum**
    Neoplasm of uncertain behavior of rectosigmoid junction
    Rectosigmoid junction: Angle where sigmoid colon becomes rectum
D37.6 **Neoplasm of uncertain behavior of liver, gallbladder and bile ducts**
    Neoplasm of uncertain behavior of ampulla of Vater
    Ampulla of Vater: Enlarged segment of ducts from liver and pancreas at entry point to small intestine
D37.8 **Neoplasm of uncertain behavior of other specified digestive organs**
    Neoplasm of uncertain behavior of anal canal
    Neoplasm of uncertain behavior of anal sphincter
    Neoplasm of uncertain behavior of anus NOS
    Neoplasm of uncertain behavior of esophagus
    Neoplasm of uncertain behavior of intestine NOS
    Neoplasm of uncertain behavior of pancreas
    Excludes1 neoplasm of uncertain behavior of anal margin (D48.5)
        neoplasm of uncertain behavior of anal skin (D48.5)
        neoplasm of uncertain behavior of perianal skin (D48.5)
D37.9 **Neoplasm of uncertain behavior of digestive organ, unspecified**

● **D38** **Neoplasm of uncertain behavior of middle ear and respiratory and intrathoracic organs**
    Excludes1 neoplasm of uncertain behavior of heart (D48.7)
D38.0 **Neoplasm of uncertain behavior of larynx**
    Neoplasm of uncertain behavior of aryepiglottic fold or interarytenoid fold, laryngeal aspect
    Neoplasm of uncertain behavior of epiglottis (suprahyoid portion)
    Excludes1 neoplasm of uncertain behavior of aryepiglottic fold or interarytenoid fold NOS (D37.05)
        neoplasm of uncertain behavior of hypopharyngeal aspect of aryepiglottic fold (D37.05)
        neoplasm of uncertain behavior of marginal zone of aryepiglottic fold (D37.05)
D38.1 **Neoplasm of uncertain behavior of trachea, bronchus and lung**
D38.2 **Neoplasm of uncertain behavior of pleura**
D38.3 **Neoplasm of uncertain behavior of mediastinum**
D38.4 **Neoplasm of uncertain behavior of thymus**
D38.5 **Neoplasm of uncertain behavior of other respiratory organs**
    Neoplasm of uncertain behavior of accessory sinuses
    Neoplasm of uncertain behavior of cartilage of nose
    Neoplasm of uncertain behavior of middle ear
    Neoplasm of uncertain behavior of nasal cavities
    Excludes1 neoplasm of uncertain behavior of ear (external) (skin) (D48.5)
        neoplasm of uncertain behavior of nose NOS (D48.7)
        neoplasm of uncertain behavior of skin of nose (D48.5)
D38.6 **Neoplasm of uncertain behavior of respiratory organ, unspecified**

● **D39** **Neoplasm of uncertain behavior of female genital organs**
D39.0 **Neoplasm of uncertain behavior of uterus**
● **D39.1** **Neoplasm of uncertain behavior of ovary**
    Use additional code to identify any functional activity.
    D39.10 **Neoplasm of uncertain behavior of unspecified ovary**
    D39.11 **Neoplasm of uncertain behavior of right ovary**
    D39.12 **Neoplasm of uncertain behavior of left ovary**
D39.2 **Neoplasm of uncertain behavior of placenta**
    Chorioadenoma destruens
    Invasive hydatidiform mole
    Malignant hydatidiform mole
    Excludes1 hydatidiform mole NOS (O01.9)
D39.8 **Neoplasm of uncertain behavior of other specified female genital organs**
    Neoplasm of uncertain behavior of skin of female genital organs
D39.9 **Neoplasm of uncertain behavior of female genital organ, unspecified**

● **D40** **Neoplasm of uncertain behavior of male genital organs**
D40.0 **Neoplasm of uncertain behavior of prostate**
● **D40.1** **Neoplasm of uncertain behavior of testis**
    D40.10 **Neoplasm of uncertain behavior of unspecified testis**
    D40.11 **Neoplasm of uncertain behavior of right testis**
    D40.12 **Neoplasm of uncertain behavior of left testis**
D40.8 **Neoplasm of uncertain behavior of other specified male genital organs**
    Neoplasm of uncertain behavior of skin of male genital organs
D40.9 **Neoplasm of uncertain behavior of male genital organ, unspecified**

● **D41   Neoplasm of uncertain behavior of urinary organs**
   ● **D41.0   Neoplasm of uncertain behavior of kidney**

> **Excludes1**   neoplasm of uncertain behavior of renal pelvis (D41.1-)

     D41.00   Neoplasm of uncertain behavior of unspecified kidney

     D41.01   Neoplasm of uncertain behavior of right kidney

     D41.02   Neoplasm of uncertain behavior of left kidney

   ● **D41.1   Neoplasm of uncertain behavior of renal pelvis**

     D41.10   Neoplasm of uncertain behavior of unspecified renal pelvis

     D41.11   Neoplasm of uncertain behavior of right renal pelvis

     D41.12   Neoplasm of uncertain behavior of left renal pelvis

   ● **D41.2   Neoplasm of uncertain behavior of ureter**

     D41.20   Neoplasm of uncertain behavior of unspecified ureter

     D41.21   Neoplasm of uncertain behavior of right ureter

     D41.22   Neoplasm of uncertain behavior of left ureter

   D41.3   Neoplasm of uncertain behavior of urethra

   D41.4   Neoplasm of uncertain behavior of bladder

   D41.8   Neoplasm of uncertain behavior of other specified urinary organs

   D41.9   Neoplasm of uncertain behavior of unspecified urinary organ

● **D42   Neoplasm of uncertain behavior of meninges**

   D42.0   Neoplasm of uncertain behavior of cerebral meninges

   D42.1   Neoplasm of uncertain behavior of spinal meninges

   D42.9   Neoplasm of uncertain behavior of meninges, unspecified

● **D43   Neoplasm of uncertain behavior of brain and central nervous system**

> **Excludes1**   neoplasm of uncertain behavior of peripheral nerves and autonomic nervous system (D48.2)

   D43.0   Neoplasm of uncertain behavior of brain, supratentorial
     Superior to tentorium of cerebellum
     Neoplasm of uncertain behavior of cerebral ventricle
     Neoplasm of uncertain behavior of cerebrum
     Neoplasm of uncertain behavior of frontal lobe
     Neoplasm of uncertain behavior of occipital lobe
     Neoplasm of uncertain behavior of parietal lobe
     Neoplasm of uncertain behavior of temporal lobe

> **Excludes1**   neoplasm of uncertain behavior of fourth ventricle (D43.1)

   D43.1   Neoplasm of uncertain behavior of brain, infratentorial
     Beneath the tentorium of cerebellum
     Neoplasm of uncertain behavior of brain stem
     Neoplasm of uncertain behavior of cerebellum
     Neoplasm of uncertain behavior of fourth ventricle

   D43.2   Neoplasm of uncertain behavior of brain, unspecified

   D43.3   Neoplasm of uncertain behavior of cranial nerves

   D43.4   Neoplasm of uncertain behavior of spinal cord

   D43.8   Neoplasm of uncertain behavior of other specified parts of central nervous system

   D43.9   Neoplasm of uncertain behavior of central nervous system, unspecified
     Neoplasm of uncertain behavior of nervous system (central) NOS

● **D44   Neoplasm of uncertain behavior of endocrine glands**

> **Excludes1**   multiple endocrine adenomatosis (E31.2-)
> multiple endocrine neoplasia (E31.2-)
> neoplasm of uncertain behavior of endocrine pancreas (D37.8)
> neoplasm of uncertain behavior of ovary (D39.1-)
> neoplasm of uncertain behavior of testis (D40.1-)
> neoplasm of uncertain behavior of thymus (D38.4)

   D44.0   Neoplasm of uncertain behavior of thyroid gland

   ● **D44.1   Neoplasm of uncertain behavior of adrenal gland**
     Use additional code to identify any functional activity.

     D44.10   Neoplasm of uncertain behavior of unspecified adrenal gland

     D44.11   Neoplasm of uncertain behavior of right adrenal gland

     D44.12   Neoplasm of uncertain behavior of left adrenal gland

   D44.2   Neoplasm of uncertain behavior of parathyroid gland

   D44.3   Neoplasm of uncertain behavior of pituitary gland
     Use additional code to identify any functional activity.

   D44.4   Neoplasm of uncertain behavior of craniopharyngeal duct

   D44.5   Neoplasm of uncertain behavior of pineal gland

   D44.6   Neoplasm of uncertain behavior of carotid body

   D44.7   Neoplasm of uncertain behavior of aortic body and other paraganglia

   D44.9   Neoplasm of uncertain behavior of unspecified endocrine gland

● **D45   Polycythemia vera**

> **Excludes1**   familial polycythemia (D75.0)
> secondary polycythemia (D75.1)

Primary polycythemia. Secondary polycythemia is D75.1. Check your documentation. Polycythemia is caused by too many red blood cells, which increase the thickness of blood (viscosity). This can cause engorgement of the spleen (splenomegaly) with extra RBCs and potential clot formation.

● **D46   Myelodysplastic syndromes**
   Use additional code for adverse effect, if applicable, to identify drug (T36-T50 with fifth or sixth character 5)

> **Excludes2**   drug-induced aplastic anemia (D61.1)

   D46.0   Refractory anemia without ring sideroblasts, so stated
     Refractory anemia without sideroblasts, without excess of blasts

   D46.1   Refractory anemia with ring sideroblasts RARS

   ● **D46.2   Refractory anemia with excess of blasts**
     Form of myelodysplasia with increased immature white blood cells (blasts) in bone marrow

     D46.20   Refractory anemia with excess of blasts, unspecified RAEB NOS

     D46.21   Refractory anemia with excess of blasts 1 RAEB 1
       Bone marrow disease which results in insufficient RBCs (anemia) in which level of blasts is less than 10%

     D46.22   Refractory anemia with excess of blasts 2 RAEB 2
       Bone marrow disease manifested by insufficient numbers of RBCs (anemia) with level of blasts 10-20%

D46.A   **Refractory cytopenia with multilineage dysplasia**

D46.B   **Refractory cytopenia with multilineage dysplasia and ring sideroblasts**
    RCMD RS

D46.C   **Myelodysplastic syndrome with isolated del(5q) chromosomal abnormality**
    Myelodysplastic syndrome with 5q deletion
    5q minus syndrome NOS

D46.4   **Refractory anemia, unspecified**

D46.Z   **Other myelodysplastic syndromes**
> **Excludes1**   chronic myelomonocytic leukemia (C93.1-)

D46.9   **Myelodysplastic syndrome, unspecified**
    Myelodysplasia NOS

● **D47   Other neoplasms of uncertain behavior of lymphoid, hematopoietic and related tissue**

D47.0   **Histiocytic and mast cell tumors of uncertain behavior**
    Indolent systemic mastocytosis
    Mast cell tumor NOS
    Mastocytoma NOS
> **Excludes1**   malignant mast cell tumor (C96.2)
>   mastocytosis (congenital) (cutaneous) (Q82.2)

D47.1   **Chronic myeloproliferative disease**
    Chronic neutrophilic leukemia
    Myeloproliferative disease, unspecified
> **Excludes1**   atypical chronic myeloid leukemia BCR/ABL-negative (C92.2-)
>   chronic myeloid leukemia BCR/ABL-positive (C92.1-)
>   myelofibrosis NOS (D75.81)
>   myelophthisic anemia (D61.82)
>   myelophthisis (D61.82)
>   secondary myelofibrosis NOS (D75.81)

D47.2   **Monoclonal gammopathy**
    Monoclonal gammopathy of undetermined significance [MGUS]

D47.3   **Essential (hemorrhagic) thrombocythemia**
    Essential thrombocytosis
    Idiopathic hemorrhagic thrombocythemia

D47.4   **Osteomyelofibrosis**
    Chronic idiopathic myelofibrosis
    Myelofibrosis (idiopathic) (with myeloid metaplasia)
    Myelosclerosis (megakaryocytic) with myeloid metaplasia
    Secondary myelofibrosis in myeloproliferative disease
> **Excludes1**   acute myelofibrosis (C94.4-)

● D47.Z   **Other specified neoplasms of uncertain behavior of lymphoid, hematopoietic and related tissue**

D47.Z1   **Post-transplant lymphoproliferative disorder (PTLD)**
> *Code first complications of transplanted organs and tissue (T86.-)*

D47.Z9   **Other specified neoplasms of uncertain behavior of lymphoid, hematopoietic and related tissue**
    Histiocytic tumors of uncertain behavior

D47.9   **Neoplasm of uncertain behavior of lymphoid, hematopoietic and related tissue, unspecified**
    Lymphoproliferative disease NOS

● D48   **Neoplasm of uncertain behavior of other and unspecified sites**
> **Excludes1**   neurofibromatosis (nonmalignant) (Q85.0-)

D48.0   **Neoplasm of uncertain behavior of bone and articular cartilage**
> **Excludes1**   neoplasm of uncertain behavior of cartilage of ear (D48.1)
>   neoplasm of uncertain behavior of cartilage of larynx (D38.0)
>   neoplasm of uncertain behavior of cartilage of nose (D38.5)
>   neoplasm of uncertain behavior of connective tissue of eyelid (D48.1)
>   neoplasm of uncertain behavior of synovia (D48.1)

D48.1   **Neoplasm of uncertain behavior of connective and other soft tissue**
    Neoplasm of uncertain behavior of connective tissue of ear
    Neoplasm of uncertain behavior of connective tissue of eyelid
    Stromal tumors of uncertain behavior of digestive system
> **Excludes1**   neoplasm of uncertain behavior of articular cartilage (D48.0)
>   neoplasm of uncertain behavior of cartilage of larynx (D38.0)
>   neoplasm of uncertain behavior of cartilage of nose (D38.5)
>   neoplasm of uncertain behavior of connective tissue of breast (D48.6-)

D48.2   **Neoplasm of uncertain behavior of peripheral nerves and autonomic nervous system**
> **Excludes1**   neoplasm of uncertain behavior of peripheral nerves of orbit (D48.7)

D48.3   **Neoplasm of uncertain behavior of retroperitoneum**

D48.4   **Neoplasm of uncertain behavior of peritoneum**

D48.5   **Neoplasm of uncertain behavior of skin**
    Neoplasm of uncertain behavior of anal margin
    Neoplasm of uncertain behavior of anal skin
    Neoplasm of uncertain behavior of perianal skin
    Neoplasm of uncertain behavior of skin of breast
> **Excludes1**   neoplasm of uncertain behavior of anus NOS (D37.8)
>   neoplasm of uncertain behavior of skin of genital organs (D39.8, D40.8)
>   neoplasm of uncertain behavior of vermilion border of lip (D37.0)

● D48.6   **Neoplasm of uncertain behavior of breast**
    Neoplasm of uncertain behavior of connective tissue of breast
    Cystosarcoma phyllodes
> **Excludes1**   neoplasm of uncertain behavior of skin of breast (D48.5)

D48.60   **Neoplasm of uncertain behavior of unspecified breast**

D48.61   **Neoplasm of uncertain behavior of right breast**

D48.62   **Neoplasm of uncertain behavior of left breast**

D48.7   **Neoplasm of uncertain behavior of other specified sites**
    Neoplasm of uncertain behavior of eye
    Neoplasm of uncertain behavior of heart
    Neoplasm of uncertain behavior of peripheral nerves of orbit
> **Excludes1**   neoplasm of uncertain behavior of connective tissue (D48.1)
>   neoplasm of uncertain behavior of skin of eyelid (D48.5)

D48.9   **Neoplasm of uncertain behavior, unspecified**

● **D49   Neoplasms of unspecified behavior**

> **Note:** Category D49 classifies by site neoplasms of unspecified morphology and behavior. The term 'mass,' unless otherwise stated, is not to be regarded as a neoplastic growth.

> **Includes**   'growth' NOS
> neoplasm NOS
> new growth NOS
> tumor NOS

> **Excludes 1**   neoplasms of uncertain behavior (D37-D44, D48)

D49.0   Neoplasm of unspecified behavior of digestive system

> **Excludes 1**   neoplasm of unspecified behavior of margin of anus (D49.2)
> neoplasm of unspecified behavior of perianal skin (D49.2)
> neoplasm of unspecified behavior of skin of anus (D49.2)

D49.1   Neoplasm of unspecified behavior of respiratory system

D49.2   Neoplasm of unspecified behavior of bone, soft tissue, and skin

> **Excludes 1**   neoplasm of unspecified behavior of anal canal (D49.0)
> neoplasm of unspecified behavior of anus NOS (D49.0)
> neoplasm of unspecified behavior of bone marrow (D49.89)
> neoplasm of unspecified behavior of cartilage of larynx (D49.1)
> neoplasm of unspecified behavior of cartilage of nose (D49.1)
> neoplasm of unspecified behavior of connective tissue of breast (D49.3)
> neoplasm of unspecified behavior of skin of genital organs (D49.5)
> neoplasm of unspecified behavior of vermilion border of lip (D49.0)

D49.3   Neoplasm of unspecified behavior of breast

> **Excludes 1**   neoplasm of unspecified behavior of skin of breast (D49.2)

D49.4   Neoplasm of unspecified behavior of bladder

D49.5   Neoplasm of unspecified behavior of other genitourinary organs

D49.6   Neoplasm of unspecified behavior of brain

> **Excludes 1**   neoplasm of unspecified behavior of cerebral meninges (D49.7)
> neoplasm of unspecified behavior of cranial nerves (D49.7)

D49.7   Neoplasm of unspecified behavior of endocrine glands and other parts of nervous system

> **Excludes 1**   neoplasm of unspecified behavior of peripheral, sympathetic, and parasympathetic nerves and ganglia (D49.2)

● **D49.8   Neoplasm of unspecified behavior of other specified sites**

> **Excludes 1**   neoplasm of unspecified behavior of eyelid (skin) (D49.2)
> neoplasm of unspecified behavior of eyelid cartilage (D49.2)
> neoplasm of unspecified behavior of great vessels (D49.2)
> neoplasm of unspecified behavior of optic nerve (D49.7)

D49.81 Neoplasm of unspecified behavior of retina and choroid
> Dark area on retina
> Retinal freckle

D49.89   Neoplasm of unspecified behavior of other specified sites

D49.9   Neoplasm of unspecified behavior of unspecified site

CHAPTER 3

DISEASES OF THE BLOOD AND BLOOD-FORMING ORGANS AND CERTAIN DISORDERS INVOLVING THE IMMUNE MECHANISM (D50-D89)

Excludes2   autoimmune disease (systemic) NOS (M35.9)
certain conditions originating in the perinatal period (P00-P96)
complications of pregnancy, childbirth and the puerperium (O00-O9A)
congenital malformations, deformations and chromosomal abnormalities (Q00-Q99)
endocrine, nutritional and metabolic diseases (E00-E88)
human immunodeficiency virus [HIV] disease (B20)
injury, poisoning and certain other consequences of external causes (S00-T88)
neoplasms (C00-D49)
symptoms, signs and abnormal clinical and laboratory findings, not elsewhere classified (R00-R94)

This chapter contains the following blocks:

D50-D53	Nutritional anemias
D55-D59	Hemolytic anemias
D60-D64	Aplastic and other anemias and other bone marrow failure syndromes
D65-D69	Coagulation defects, purpura and other hemorrhagic conditions
D70-D77	Other disorders of blood and blood-forming organs
D78	Intraoperative and postprocedural complications of the spleen
D80-D89	Certain disorders involving the immune mechanism

NUTRITIONAL ANEMIAS (D50-D53)

● **D50   Iron deficiency anemia**
A disease characterized by a decrease in the number of red cells (hemoglobin) in the blood.

Includes   asiderotic anemia
hypochromic anemia

D50.0   Iron deficiency anemia secondary to blood loss (chronic)
Posthemorrhagic anemia (chronic)
Excludes1   acute posthemorrhagic anemia (D62)
congenital anemia from fetal blood loss (P61.3)

D50.1   Sideropenic dysphagia
Web-like growth of membranes in throat that makes swallowing difficult
Kelly-Paterson syndrome
Plummer-Vinson syndrome

D50.8   Other iron deficiency anemias
Iron deficiency anemia due to inadequate dietary iron intake

D50.9   Iron deficiency anemia, unspecified

● **D51   Vitamin B12 deficiency anemia**
Excludes1   vitamin B12 deficiency (E53.8)

D51.0   Vitamin B12 deficiency anemia due to intrinsic factor deficiency
Addison anemia
Biermer anemia
Pernicious (congenital) anemia
Congenital intrinsic factor deficiency

D51.1   Vitamin B12 deficiency anemia due to selective vitamin B12 malabsorption with proteinuria
Imerslund (Gräsbeck) syndrome
Megaloblastic hereditary anemia

D51.2   Transcobalamin II deficiency

D51.3   Other dietary vitamin B12 deficiency anemia
Vegan anemia

D51.8   Other vitamin B12 deficiency anemias

D51.9   Vitamin B12 deficiency anemia, unspecified

● **D52   Folate deficiency anemia**
Excludes1   folate deficiency without anemia (E53.8)

D52.0   Dietary folate deficiency anemia
Nutritional megaloblastic anemia

D52.1   Drug-induced folate deficiency anemia
Use additional code for adverse effect, if applicable, to identify drug (T36-T50 with fifth or sixth character 5)

D52.8   Other folate deficiency anemias

D52.9   Folate deficiency anemia, unspecified
Folic acid deficiency anemia NOS

● **D53   Other nutritional anemias**
Includes   megaloblastic anemia unresponsive to vitamin B12 or folate therapy

D53.0   Protein deficiency anemia
Amino-acid deficiency anemia
Orotaciduric anemia
Excludes1   Lesch-Nyhan syndrome (E79.1)

D53.1   Other megaloblastic anemias, not elsewhere classified
Megaloblastic anemia NOS
Excludes1   Di Guglielmo's disease (C94.0)

D53.2   Scorbutic anemia
Anemia resulting from deficiency of ascorbic acid (vitamin C)
Excludes1   scurvy (E54)

D53.8   Other specified nutritional anemias
Anemia associated with deficiency of copper
Anemia associated with deficiency of molybdenum
Anemia associated with deficiency of zinc
Excludes1   nutritional deficiencies without anemia, such as:
copper deficiency NOS (E61.0)
molybdenum deficiency NOS (E61.5)
zinc deficiency NOS (E60)

D53.9   Nutritional anemia, unspecified
Simple chronic anemia
Excludes1   anemia NOS (D64.9)

HEMOLYTIC ANEMIAS (D55-D59)

● **D55   Anemia due to enzyme disorders**
Excludes1   drug-induced enzyme deficiency anemia (D59.2)

D55.0   Anemia due to glucose-6-phosphate dehydrogenase [G6PD] deficiency
Favism
G6PD deficiency anemia

D55.1   Anemia due to other disorders of glutathione metabolism
Anemia (due to) enzyme deficiencies, except G6PD, related to the hexose monophosphate [HMP] shunt pathway
Anemia (due to) hemolytic nonspherocytic (hereditary), type I

D55.2   Anemia due to disorders of glycolytic enzymes
Hemolytic nonspherocytic (hereditary) anemia, type II
Hexokinase deficiency anemia
Pyruvate kinase [PK] deficiency anemia
Triose-phosphate isomerase deficiency anemia
Excludes1   disorders of glycolysis not associated with anemia (E74.8)

D55.3   Anemia due to disorders of nucleotide metabolism

D55.8   Other anemias due to enzyme disorders

D55.9   Anemia due to enzyme disorder, unspecified

● **D56   Thalassemia**
Hereditary disorders characterized by low production of hemoglobin or excessive destruction of red blood cells
> **Excludes1**   sickle-cell thalassemia (D57.4-)

D56.0   Alpha thalassemia
Alpha thalassemia major
Hemoglobin H Constant Spring
Hemoglobin H disease
Hydrops fetalis due to alpha thalassemia
Severe alpha thalassemia
Triple gene defect alpha thalassemia
> Use additional code, if applicable, for hydrops fetalis due to alpha thalassemia (P56.99)
> **Excludes1**   alpha thalassemia trait or minor (D56.3)
> asymptomatic alpha thalassemia (D56.3)
> hydrops fetalis due to isoimmunization (P56.0)
> hydrops fetalis not due to immune hemolysis (P83.2)

D56.1   Beta thalassemia
Beta thalassemia major
Cooley's anemia
Homozygous beta thalassemia
Severe beta thalassemia
Thalassemia intermedia
Thalassemia major
> **Excludes1**   beta thalassemia minor (D56.3)
> beta thalassemia trait (D56.3)
> delta-beta thalassemia (D56.2)
> hemoglobin E-beta thalassemia (D56.5)
> sickle-cell beta thalassemia (D57.4-)

D56.2   Delta-beta thalassemia
Homozygous delta-beta thalassemia
> **Excludes1**   delta-beta thalassemia minor (D56.3)
> delta-beta thalassemia trait (D56.3)

D56.3   Thalassemia minor
Genetic disorders that have in common defective production of hemoglobin
Alpha thalassemia minor
Alpha thalassemia silent carrier
Alpha thalassemia trait
Beta thalassemia minor
Beta thalassemia trait
Delta-beta thalassemia minor
Delta-beta thalassemia trait
Thalassemia trait NOS
> **Excludes1**   alpha thalassemia (D56.0)
> beta thalassemia (D56.1)
> delta-beta thalassemia (D56.2)
> hemoglobin E-beta thalassemia (D56.5)
> sickle-cell trait (D57.3)

D56.4   Hereditary persistence of fetal hemoglobin [HPFH]
Persistent production of hemoglobin

D56.5   Hemoglobin E-beta thalassemia
> **Excludes1**   beta thalassemia (D56.1)
> beta thalassemia minor (D56.3)
> beta thalassemia trait (D56.3)
> delta-beta thalassemia (D56.2)
> delta-beta thalassemia trait (D56.3)
> hemoglobin E disease (D58.2)
> other hemoglobinopathies (D58.2)
> sickle-cell beta thalassemia (D57.4-)

D56.8   Other thalassemias
Dominant thalassemia
Hemoglobin C thalassemia
Mixed thalassemia
Thalassemia with other hemoglobinopathy
> **Excludes1**   hemoglobin C disease (D58.2)
> hemoglobin E disease (D58.2)
> other hemoglobinopathies (D58.2)
> sickle cell anemia (D57.-)
> sickle-cell thalassemia (D57.4)

D56.9   Thalassemia, unspecified
Mediterranean anemia (with other hemoglobinopathy)

● **D57   Sickle-cell disorders**
Inherited disease in which red blood cells, normally disc-shaped, become crescent shaped.
> Use additional code for any associated fever (R50.81)
> **Excludes1**   other hemoglobinopathies (D58.-)

● **D57.0   Hb-SS disease with crisis**
Sickle-cell disease NOS with crisis
Hb-SS disease with vasoocclusive pain

    D57.00   Hb-SS disease with crisis, unspecified
    D57.01   Hb-SS disease with acute chest syndrome
    D57.02   Hb-SS disease with splenic sequestration

D57.1   Sickle-cell disease without crisis Hb-SS disease without crisis
Sickle-cell anemia NOS
Sickle-cell disease NOS
Sickle-cell disorder NOS

● **D57.2   Sickle-cell/Hb-C disease**
Hb-SC disease
Hb-S/Hb-C disease

    D57.20   Sickle-cell/Hb-C disease without crisis
    ● **D57.21   Sickle-cell/Hb-C disease with crisis**

       D57.211   Sickle-cell/Hb-C disease with acute chest syndrome
       D57.212   Sickle-cell/Hb-C disease with splenic sequestration
       D57.219   Sickle-cell/Hb-C disease with crisis, unspecified
          Sickle-cell/Hb-C disease with crisis NOS

D57.3   Sickle-cell trait
Hb-S trait
Heterozygous hemoglobin S

● **D57.4   Sickle-cell thalassemia**
Sickle-cell beta thalassemia
Thalassemia Hb-S disease

    D57.40   Sickle-cell thalassemia without crisis
       Microdrepanocytosis
       Sickle-cell thalassemia NOS

    ● **D57.41   Sickle-cell thalassemia with crisis**
Sickle-cell "crisis" is precipitated when abnormally crescent-shaped red blood cells form clots and interrupt blood flow to major organs, causing severe pain and organ damage.
       Sickle-cell thalassemia with vasoocclusive pain
       D57.411   Sickle-cell thalassemia with acute chest syndrome
       D57.412   Sickle-cell thalassemia with splenic sequestration
       D57.419   Sickle-cell thalassemia with crisis, unspecified
          Sickle-cell thalassemia with crisis NOS

● **D57.8   Other sickle-cell disorders**
Hb-SD disease
Hb-SE disease

    D57.80   Other sickle-cell disorders without crisis
    ● **D57.81   Other sickle-cell disorders with crisis**
       D57.811   Other sickle-cell disorders with acute chest syndrome
       D57.812   Other sickle-cell disorders with splenic sequestration
       D57.819   Other sickle-cell disorders with crisis, unspecified
          Other sickle-cell disorders with crisis NOS

CHAPTER 3 (D50–D89)

◀ New   ◀▥ Revised   ~~deleted~~ Deleted   **OGCR** Official Guidelines   X Assign placeholder X   ● Use Additional Character(s)

| Excludes 1 | Excludes 2 | Includes | Use additional | Code first | Code also | Unspecified |

- **D58**   **Other hereditary hemolytic anemias**
  Genetic condition in which bone marrow is unable to compensate for premature destruction of red blood cells
  > **Excludes1**   hemolytic anemia of the newborn (P55.-)

  D58.0   **Hereditary spherocytosis**
  Presence of spherocytes (spherically shaped red blood cells)
  Acholuric (familial) jaundice
  Congenital (spherocytic) hemolytic icterus
  Minkowski-Chauffard syndrome

  D58.1   **Hereditary elliptocytosis**
  Presence of large numbers of elliptocytes in blood
  Elliptocytosis (congenital)
  Ovalocytosis (congenital) (hereditary)

  D58.2   **Other hemoglobinopathies**
  Abnormal hemoglobin NOS
  Congenital Heinz body anemia
  Hb-C disease
  Hb-D disease
  Hb-E disease
  Hemoglobinopathy NOS
  Unstable hemoglobin hemolytic disease
  > **Excludes1**   familial polycythemia (D75.0)
  > Hb-M disease (D74.0)
  > hemoglobin E-beta thalassemia (D56.5)
  > hereditary persistence of fetal hemoglobin [HPFH] (D56.4)
  > high-altitude polycythemia (D75.1)
  > methemoglobinemia (D74.-)
  > other hemoglobinopathies with thalassemia (D56.8)

  D58.8   **Other specified hereditary hemolytic anemias**
  Stomatocytosis

  D58.9   **Hereditary hemolytic anemia, unspecified**

- **D59**   **Acquired hemolytic anemia**

  D59.0   **Drug-induced autoimmune hemolytic anemia**
  Use additional code for adverse effect, if applicable, to identify drug (T36-T50 with fifth or sixth character 5)

  D59.1   **Other autoimmune hemolytic anemias**
  Autoimmune hemolytic disease (cold type) (warm type)
  Chronic cold hemagglutinin disease
  Cold agglutinin disease
  Cold agglutinin hemoglobinuria
  Cold type (secondary) (symptomatic) hemolytic anemia
  Warm type (secondary) (symptomatic) hemolytic anemia
  > **Excludes1**   Evans syndrome (D69.41)
  > hemolytic disease of newborn (P55.-)
  > paroxysmal cold hemoglobinuria (D59.6)

  D59.2   **Drug-induced nonautoimmune hemolytic anemia**
  Drug-induced enzyme deficiency anemia
  Use additional code for adverse effect, if applicable, to identify drug (T36-T50 with fifth or sixth character 5)

  D59.3   **Hemolytic-uremic syndrome**
  Use additional code to identify associated:
  E. coli infection (B96.2-)
  Pneumococcal pneumonia (J13)
  Shigella dysenteriae (A03.9)

  D59.4   **Other nonautoimmune hemolytic anemias**
  Mechanical hemolytic anemia
  Microangiopathic hemolytic anemia
  Toxic hemolytic anemia

  D59.5   **Paroxysmal nocturnal hemoglobinuria [Marchiafava-Micheli]**
  > **Excludes1**   hemoglobinuria NOS (R82.3)

  D59.6   **Hemoglobinuria due to hemolysis from other external causes**
  Hemoglobinuria from exertion
  March hemoglobinuria
  Paroxysmal cold hemoglobinuria
  Use additional code (Chapter 20) to identify external cause
  > **Excludes1**   hemoglobinuria NOS (R82.3)

  D59.8   **Other acquired hemolytic anemias**

  D59.9   **Acquired hemolytic anemia, unspecified**
  Idiopathic hemolytic anemia, chronic

APLASTIC AND OTHER ANEMIAS AND OTHER BONE MARROW FAILURE SYNDROMES (D60-D64)

- **D60**   **Acquired pure red cell aplasia [erythroblastopenia]**
  Deficiency of erythroblasts
  > **Includes**   red cell aplasia (acquired) (adult) (with thymoma)
  > **Excludes1**   congenital red cell aplasia (D61.01)

  D60.0   **Chronic acquired pure red cell aplasia**
  Lack of development of blood cell

  D60.1   **Transient acquired pure red cell aplasia**

  D60.8   **Other acquired pure red cell aplasias**

  D60.9   **Acquired pure red cell aplasia, unspecified**

- **D61**   **Other aplastic anemias and other bone marrow failure syndromes**
  > **Excludes1**   neutropenia (D70.-)

  - **D61.0**   **Constitutional aplastic anemia**
    Condition where bone marrow is unable to produce blood cells

    D61.01   **Constitutional (pure) red blood cell aplasia**
    Blackfan-Diamond syndrome
    Congenital (pure) red cell aplasia
    Familial hypoplastic anemia
    Primary (pure) red cell aplasia
    Red cell (pure) aplasia of infants
    > **Excludes1**   acquired red cell aplasia (D60.9)

    D61.09   **Other constitutional aplastic anemia**
    Fanconi's anemia
    Pancytopenia with malformations

  D61.1   **Drug-induced aplastic anemia**
  Use additional code for adverse effect, if applicable, to identify drug (T36-T50 with fifth or sixth character 5)

  D61.2   **Aplastic anemia due to other external agents**
  Code first , if applicable, toxic effects of substances chiefly nonmedicinal as to source (T51-T65)

  D61.3   **Idiopathic aplastic anemia**

● **D61.8 Other specified aplastic anemias and other bone marrow failure syndromes**
  ● **D61.81 Pancytopenia**
    Marked deficiency of all the blood elements: Red blood cells (erythrocytes), white blood cells (leukocytes), and platelets (thrombocytes). Check laboratory results.
    Excludes1   pancytopenia (due to) (with) aplastic anemia (D61.9)
       pancytopenia (due to) (with) bone marrow infiltration (D61.82)
       pancytopenia (due to) (with) congenital (pure) red cell aplasia (D61.01)
       pancytopenia (due to) (with) hairy cell leukemia (C91.4-)
       pancytopenia (due to) (with) human immunodeficiency virus disease (B20.-)
       pancytopenia (due to) (with) leukoerythroblastic anemia (D61.82)
       pancytopenia (due to) (with) myelodysplastic syndromes (D46.-)
       pancytopenia (due to) (with) myeloproliferative disease (D47.1)

    D61.810 Antineoplastic chemotherapy induced pancytopenia
      Excludes2   aplastic anemia due to antineoplastic chemotherapy (D61.1)
    D61.811 Other drug-induced pancytopenia
      Excludes2   aplastic anemia due to drugs (D61.1)
    D61.818 Other pancytopenia
  D61.82 Myelophthisis
    Leukoerythroblastic anemia
    Myelophthisic anemia
    Panmyelophthisis
    Code also the underlying disorder, such as:
    malignant neoplasm of breast (C50.-)
    tuberculosis (A15.-)
    Excludes1   idiopathic myelofibrosis (D47.1)
       myelofibrosis NOS (D75.81)
       myelofibrosis with myeloid metaplasia (D47.4)
       primary myelofibrosis (D47.1)
       secondary myelofibrosis (D75.81)
  D61.89 Other specified aplastic anemias and other bone marrow failure syndromes
 D61.9 Aplastic anemia, unspecified
  Hypoplastic anemia NOS
  Medullary hypoplasia

D62 Acute posthemorrhagic anemia
  Excludes1   anemia due to chronic blood loss (D50.0)
     blood loss anemia NOS (D50.0)
     congenital anemia from fetal blood loss (P61.3)

● **D63 Anemia in chronic diseases classified elsewhere**
  D63.0 Anemia in neoplastic disease
    Code first neoplasm (C00-D49)
    Excludes1   anemia due to antineoplastic chemotherapy (D64.81)
       aplastic anemia due to antineoplastic chemotherapy (D61.1)
    OGCR Section I.C.2.e.2.
    2) Anemia associated with chemotherapy, immunotherapy and radiation therapy
    When the admission/encounter is for management of an anemia associated with an adverse effect of the administration of chemotherapy or immunotherapy and the only treatment is for the anemia, the anemia code is sequenced first followed by the appropriate codes for the neoplasm and the adverse effect (T45.1X5, Adverse effect of antineoplastic and immunosuppressive drugs).

  D63.1 Anemia in chronic kidney disease
    Erythropoietin resistant anemia (EPO resistant anemia)
    Code first underlying chronic kidney disease (CKD) (N18.-)
  D63.8 Anemia in other chronic diseases classified elsewhere
    Code first underlying disease, such as:
    diphyllobothriasis (B70.0)
    hookworm disease (B76.0-B76.9)
    hypothyroidism (E00.0-E03.9)
    malaria (B50.0-B54)
    symptomatic late syphilis (A52.79)
    tuberculosis (A18.89)

● **D64 Other anemias**
  Excludes1   refractory anemia (D46.-)
     refractory anemia with excess blasts in transformation [RAEB T] (C92.0-)
  D64.0 Hereditary sideroblastic anemia
    Abnormal production RBCs (erythrocytes)
    Sex-linked hypochromic sideroblastic anemia
  D64.1 Secondary sideroblastic anemia due to disease
    Code first underlying disease
  D64.2 Secondary sideroblastic anemia due to drugs and toxins
    Code first poisoning due to drug or toxin, if applicable (T36-T65 with fifth or sixth character 1-4 or 6)
    Use additional code for adverse effect, if applicable, to identify drug (T36-T50 with fifth or sixth character 5)
  D64.3 Other sideroblastic anemias
    Sideroblastic anemia NOS
    Pyridoxine-responsive sideroblastic anemia NEC
  D64.4 Congenital dyserythropoietic anemia
    Any of several rare hereditary anemias, mostly types of macrocytic anemia
    Dyshematopoietic anemia (congenital)
    Excludes1   Blackfan-Diamond syndrome (D61.01)
       Di Guglielmo's disease (C94.0)
● **D64.8 Other specified anemias**
  D64.81 Anemia due to antineoplastic chemotherapy
    Antineoplastic chemotherapy induced anemia
    Excludes1   anemia in neoplastic disease (D63.0)
       aplastic anemia due to antineoplastic chemotherapy (D61.1)
  D64.89 Other specified anemias
    Infantile pseudoleukemia
 D64.9 Anemia, unspecified

◀ New   ◀ Revised   deleted Deleted   OGCR Official Guidelines   X Assign placeholder X   ● Use Additional Character(s)
Excludes 1   Excludes 2   Includes   Use additional   Code first   Code also   Unspecified
783

COAGULATION DEFECTS, PURPURA AND OTHER HEMORRHAGIC CONDITIONS (D65-D69)

D65   **Disseminated intravascular coagulation [defibrination syndrome]**
Blood clots form and consume all coagulation proteins and platelets and disrupt normal coagulation, resulting in abnormal bleeding
Afibrinogenemia, acquired
Consumption coagulopathy
Diffuse or disseminated intravascular coagulation [DIC]
Fibrinolytic hemorrhage, acquired
Fibrinolytic purpura
Purpura fulminans

> **Excludes1**   disseminated intravascular coagulation (complicating):
>   abortion or ectopic or molar pregnancy (O00-O07, O08.1)
>   in newborn (P60)
>   pregnancy, childbirth and the puerperium (O45.0, O46.0, O67.0, O72.3)

D66   **Hereditary factor VIII deficiency**
Inherited coagulation disorder carried by females but most often affecting males
Classical hemophilia
Deficiency factor VIII (with functional defect)
Hemophilia NOS
Hemophilia A

> **Excludes1**   factor VIII deficiency with vascular defect (D68.0)

D67   **Hereditary factor IX deficiency**
Christmas disease
Factor IX deficiency (with functional defect)
Hemophilia B
Plasma thromboplastin component [PTC] deficiency

● **D68**   **Other coagulation defects**

> **Excludes1**   abnormal coagulation profile (R79.1)
>   coagulation defects complicating abortion or ectopic or molar pregnancy (O00-O07, O08.1)
>   coagulation defects complicating pregnancy, childbirth and the puerperium (O45.0, O46.0, O67.0, O72.3)

   D68.0   **Von Willebrand's disease**
Congenital bleeding disorder
Angiohemophilia
Factor VIII deficiency with vascular defect
Vascular hemophilia

> **Excludes1**   capillary fragility (hereditary) (D69.8)
>   factor VIII deficiency NOS (D66)
>   factor VIII deficiency with functional defect (D66)

   D68.1   **Hereditary factor XI deficiency**
Deficiency of blood coagulation resulting in systemic blood-clotting defect
Hemophilia C
Plasma thromboplastin antecedent [PTA] deficiency
Rosenthal's disease

   D68.2   **Hereditary deficiency of other clotting factors**
Blood clotting disorders caused by hereditary deficiencies of one or more clotting factors
AC globulin deficiency
Congenital afibrinogenemia
Deficiency of factor I [fibrinogen]
Deficiency of factor II [prothrombin]
Deficiency of factor V [labile]
Deficiency of factor VII [stable]
Deficiency of factor X [Stuart-Prower]
Deficiency of factor XII [Hageman]
Deficiency of factor XIII [fibrin stabilizing]
Dysfibrinogenemia (congenital)
Hypoproconvertinemia
Owren's disease
Proaccelerin deficiency

● **D68.3**   **Hemorrhagic disorder due to circulating anticoagulants**
Blood clotting disorders caused by anticoagulants (warfarin and heparin)

●   **D68.31**   **Hemorrhagic disorder due to intrinsic circulating anticoagulants, antibodies, or inhibitors**

     D68.311   **Acquired hemophilia**
Autoimmune hemophilia
Autoimmune inhibitors to clotting factors
Secondary hemophilia

     D68.312   **Antiphospholipid antibody with hemorrhagic disorder**
Lupus anticoagulant (LAC) with hemorrhagic disorder
Systemic lupus erythematosus [SLE] inhibitor with hemorrhagic disorder

> **Excludes1**   antiphospholipid antibody, finding without diagnosis (R76.0)
>   antiphospholipid antibody syndrome (D68.61)
>   antiphospholipid antibody with hypercoagulable state (D68.61)
>   lupus anticoagulant (LAC) finding without diagnosis (R76.0)
>   lupus anticoagulant (LAC) with hypercoagulable state (D68.62)
>   systemic lupus erythematosus [SLE] inhibitor finding without diagnosis (R76.0)
>   systemic lupus erythematosus [SLE] inhibitor with hypercoagulable state (D68.62)

     D68.318   **Other hemorrhagic disorder due to intrinsic circulating anticoagulants, antibodies, or inhibitors**
Antithromboplastinemia
Antithromboplastinogenemia
Hemorrhagic disorder due to intrinsic increase in antithrombin
Hemorrhagic disorder due to intrinsic increase in anti-VIIIa
Hemorrhagic disorder due to intrinsic increase in anti-IXa
Hemorrhagic disorder due to intrinsic increase in anti-XIa

   D68.32   **Hemorrhagic disorder due to extrinsic circulating anticoagulants**
Drug-induced hemorrhagic disorder
Hemorrhagic disorder due to increase in anti-IIa
Hemorrhagic disorder due to increase in anti-Xa
Hyperheparinemia

> Use additional code for adverse effect, if applicable, to identify drug (T45.515, T45.525)

◀ New   ◀▥ Revised   ~~deleted~~ Deleted   **OGCR** Official Guidelines   X Assign placeholder X   ● Use Additional Character(s)

Excludes 1   Excludes 2   Includes   Use additional   Code first   Code also   Unspecified

D68.4 Acquired coagulation factor deficiency
Deficiency of coagulation factor due to liver disease
Deficiency of coagulation factor due to vitamin K deficiency
Excludes1   vitamin K deficiency of newborn (P53)

● **D68.5 Primary thrombophilia**
AKA idiopathic thrombocytopenia, may be acquired or congenital and is a common cause of coagulation disorders.
Primary hypercoagulable states
Excludes1   antiphospholipid syndrome (D68.61)
lupus anticoagulant (D68.62)
secondary activated protein C resistance (D68.69)
secondary antiphospholipid antibody syndrome (D68.69)
secondary lupus anticoagulant with hypercoagulable state (D68.69)
secondary systemic lupus erythematosus [SLE] inhibitor with hypercoagulable state (D68.69)
systemic lupus erythematosus [SLE] inhibitor finding without diagnosis (R76.0)
systemic lupus erythematosus [SLE] inhibitor with hemorrhagic disorder (D68.312)
thrombotic thrombocytopenic purpura (M31.1)

D68.51 Activated protein C resistance
Factor V Leiden mutation

D68.52 Prothrombin gene mutation

D68.59 Other primary thrombophilia
Antithrombin III deficiency
Hypercoagulable state NOS
Primary hypercoagulable state NEC
Primary thrombophilia NEC
Protein C deficiency
Protein S deficiency
Thrombophilia NOS

● **D68.6 Other thrombophilia**
Other hypercoagulable states
Excludes1   diffuse or disseminated intravascular coagulation [DIC] (D65)
heparin induced thrombocytopenia (HIT) (D75.82)
hyperhomocysteinemia (E72.11)

D68.61 Antiphospholipid syndrome
Anticardiolipin syndrome
Antiphospholipid antibody syndrome
Excludes1   anti-phospholipid antibody, finding without diagnosis (R76.0)
anti-phospholipid antibody with hemorrhagic disorder (D68.312)
lupus anticoagulant syndrome (D68.62)

D68.62 Lupus anticoagulant syndrome
Lupus anticoagulant
Presence of systemic lupus erythematosus [SLE] inhibitor
Excludes1   anticardiolipin syndrome (D68.61)
antiphospholipid syndrome (D68.61)
lupus anticoagulant (LAC) finding without diagnosis (R79.0)
lupus anticoagulant (LAC) with hemorrhagic disorder (D68.312)

D68.69 Other thrombophilia
Hypercoagulable states NEC
Secondary hypercoagulable state NOS

D68.8 Other specified coagulation defects
Excludes1   hemorrhagic disease of newborn (P53)

D68.9 Coagulation defect, unspecified

● **D69 Purpura and other hemorrhagic conditions**
Group of conditions characterized by small hemorrhages in skin, mucous membranes, or serosal surfaces
Excludes1   benign hypergammaglobulinemic purpura (D89.0)
cryoglobulinemic purpura (D89.1)
essential (hemorrhagic) thrombocythemia (D47.3)
hemorrhagic thrombocythemia (D47.3)
purpura fulminans (D65)
thrombotic thrombocytopenic purpura (M31.1)
Waldenström hypergammaglobulinemic purpura (D89.0)

D69.0 Allergic purpura
Allergic vasculitis
Nonthrombocytopenic hemorrhagic purpura
Nonthrombocytopenic idiopathic purpura
Purpura anaphylactoid
Purpura Henoch(-Schönlein)
Purpura rheumatica
Vascular purpura
Excludes1   thrombocytopenic hemorrhagic purpura (D69.3)

D69.1 Qualitative platelet defects
Bernard-Soulier [giant platelet] syndrome
Glanzmann's disease
Grey platelet syndrome
Thromboasthenia (hemorrhagic) (hereditary)
Thrombocytopathy
Excludes1   von Willebrand's disease (D68.0)

D69.2 Other nonthrombocytopenic purpura
Purpura NOS
Purpura simplex
Senile purpura

D69.3 Immune thrombocytopenic purpura
Hemorrhagic (thrombocytopenic) purpura
Idiopathic thrombocytopenic purpura
Tidal platelet dysgenesis

● **D69.4 Other primary thrombocytopenia**
Excludes1   transient neonatal thrombocytopenia (P61.0)
Wiskott-Aldrich syndrome (D82.0)

D69.41 Evans syndrome
Acquired hemolytic anemia and thrombocytopenia

D69.42 Congenital and hereditary thrombocytopenia purpura
Congenital thrombocytopenia
Hereditary thrombocytopenia
Code first congential or hereditary disorder, such as:
thrombocytopenia with absent radius (TAR syndrome) (Q87.2)

D69.49 Other primary thrombocytopenia
Megakaryocytic hypoplasia
Primary thrombocytopenia NOS

● **D69.5 Secondary thrombocytopenia**
Acquired reduction of number of platelets required for blood clotting
Excludes1   heparin induced thrombocytopenia (HIT) (D75.82)
transient thrombocytopenia of newborn (P61.0)

D69.51 Posttransfusion purpura
Posttransfusion purpura from whole blood (fresh) or blood products PTP

D69.59 Other secondary thrombocytopenia

D69.6 Thrombocytopenia, unspecified

D69.8 Other specified hemorrhagic conditions
Capillary fragility (hereditary)
Vascular pseudohemophilia

D69.9 Hemorrhagic condition, unspecified

◀ New   ◀▥ Revised   ~~deleted~~ Deleted   **OGCR** Official Guidelines   X Assign placeholder X   ● Use Additional Character(s)

Excludes 1   Excludes 2   Includes   Use additional   Code first   Code also   Unspecified

CHAPTER 3 (D50-D89)

OTHER DISORDERS OF BLOOD AND BLOOD-FORMING ORGANS (D70-D77)

- **D70   Neutropenia**
  Decrease in number of neutrophils (type of white blood cell)
  > **Includes**   agranulocytosis
  > decreased absolute neurophile count (ANC)

  Use additional code for any associated:
  fever (R50.81)
  mucositis (J34.81, K12.3-, K92.81, N76.81)
  > **Excludes1**   neutropenic splenomegaly (D73.81)
  > transient neonatal neutropenia (P61.5)

  - **D70.0   Congenital agranulocytosis**
    Reduced numbers of neutrophils (type of white blood cell)
    Congenital neutropenia
    Infantile genetic agranulocytosis
    Kostmann's disease
  - **D70.1   Agranulocytosis secondary to cancer chemotherapy**
    Decreased numbers of granulocytes (type of white blood cell)
    Code also *underlying neoplasm*
    Use additional code for adverse effect, if applicable, to identify drug (T45.1X5)
  - **D70.2   Other drug-induced agranulocytosis**
    Use additional code for adverse effect, if applicable, to identify drug (T36-T50 with fifth or sixth character 5)
  - **D70.3   Neutropenia due to infection**
  - **D70.4   Cyclic neutropenia**
    Chronic neutropenia (low number of type of white blood cell)
    Cyclic hematopoiesis
    Periodic neutropenia
  - **D70.8   Other neutropenia**
  - **D70.9   Neutropenia, unspecified**

- **D71   Functional disorders of polymorphonuclear neutrophils**
  Polymorphonuclear: varying shapes of nucleus; AKA PMNs
  Cell membrane receptor complex [CR3] defect
  Chronic (childhood) granulomatous disease
  Congenital dysphagocytosis
  Progressive septic granulomatosis

- **D72   Other disorders of white blood cells**
  > **Excludes1**   basophilia (D72.824)
  > immunity disorders (D80-D89)
  > neutropenia (D70)
  > preleukemia (syndrome) (D46.9)

  - **D72.0   Genetic anomalies of leukocytes**
    Alder (granulation) (granulocyte) anomaly
    Alder syndrome
    Hereditary leukocytic hypersegmentation
    Hereditary leukocytic hyposegmentation
    Hereditary leukomelanopathy
    May-Hegglin (granulation) (granulocyte) anomaly
    May-Hegglin syndrome
    Pelger-Huët (granulation) (granulocyte) anomaly
    Pelger-Huët syndrome
    > **Excludes1**   Chédiak (-Steinbrinck)-Higashi syndrome (E70.330)
  - **D72.1   Eosinophilia**
    Formation and accumulation of high number of white cells in blood/tissue
    Allergic eosinophilia
    Hereditary eosinophilia
    > **Excludes1**   Löffler's syndrome (J82)
    > pulmonary eosinophilia (J82)

- **D72.8   Other specified disorders of white blood cells**
  > **Excludes1**   leukemia (C91-C95)
  - **D72.81   Decreased white blood cell count**
    > **Excludes1**   neutropenia (D70.-)
    - **D72.810   Lymphocytopenia**
      Decreased lymphocytes
      Reduction in number of lympho cytes in blood
    - **D72.818   Other decreased white blood cell count**
      Basophilic leukopenia
      Eosinophilic leukopenia
      Monocytopenia
      Other decreased leukocytes
      Plasmacytopenia
    - **D72.819   Decreased white blood cell count, unspecified**
      Decreased leukocytes, unspecified
      Leukocytopenia, unspecified
      Leukopenia
      > **Excludes1**   malignant leukopenia (D70.9)
  - **D72.82   Elevated white blood cell count**
    > **Excludes1**   eosinophilia (D72.1)
    - **D72.820   Lymphocytosis (symptomatic)**
      Elevated lymphocytes
      Excess of normal lymphocytes
    - **D72.821   Monocytosis (symptomatic)**
      > **Excludes1**   infectious mononucleosis (B27.-)
    - **D72.822   Plasmacytosis**
      Presence of excess plasma cells
    - **D72.823   Leukemoid reaction**
      Basophilic leukemoid reaction
      Leukemoid reaction NOS
      Lymphocytic leukemoid reaction
      Monocytic leukemoid reaction
      Myelocytic leukemoid reaction
      Neutrophilic leukemoid reaction
    - **D72.824   Basophilia**
      Increase of basophils in blood
    - **D72.825   Bandemia**
      Bandemia without diagnosis of specific infection
      Excess number of band cells (immature white blood cells) released by bone marrow
      > **Excludes1**   confirmed infection -code to infection
      > leukemia (C91.-, C92.-, C93.-, C94.-, C95.-)
    - **D72.828   Other elevated white blood cell count**
    - **D72.829   Elevated white blood cell count, unspecified**
      Elevated leukocytes, unspecified
      Leukocytosis, unspecified
  - **D72.89   Other specified disorders of white blood cells**
    Abnormality of white blood cells NEC
- **D72.9   Disorder of white blood cells, unspecified**
  Abnormal leukocyte differential NOS

◀ New   ◀▦ Revised   ~~deleted~~ Deleted   OGCR Official Guidelines   X Assign placeholder X   ● Use Additional Character(s)

Excludes 1   Excludes 2   Includes   Use additional   Code first   Code also   Unspecified

CHAPTER 3 (D50-D89)

● **D73 Diseases of spleen**

    D73.0 Hyposplenism
        Diminished functioning of spleen
        Atrophy of spleen
        | **Excludes1** | asplenia (congenital) (Q89.01) |
                     postsurgical absence of spleen (Z90.81)

    D73.1 Hypersplenism
        Accelerated function of spleen
        | **Excludes1** | neutropenic splenomegaly (D73.81) |
                     primary splenic neutropenia (D73.81)
                     splenitis, splenomegaly in late syphilis (A52.79)
                     splenitis, splenomegaly in tuberculosis (A18.85)
                     splenomegaly NOS (R16.1)
                     splenomegaly congenital (Q89.0)

    D73.2 Chronic congestive splenomegaly
        Enlargement of spleen

    D73.3 Abscess of spleen

    D73.4 Cyst of spleen

    D73.5 Infarction of spleen
        Splenic rupture, nontraumatic
        Torsion of spleen
        | **Excludes1** | rupture of spleen due to Plasmodium vivax malaria (B51.0) |
                     traumatic rupture of spleen (S36.03-)

● **D73.8 Other diseases of spleen**

    D73.81 Neutropenic splenomegaly
        Werner-Schultz disease
        Enlarged spleen responding to inadequate number of neutrophils

    D73.89 Other diseases of spleen
        Fibrosis of spleen NOS
        Perisplenitis
        Splenitis NOS

    D73.9 Disease of spleen, unspecified

● **D74 Methemoglobinemia**
    Excessive methemoglobin (form of hemoglobin)

    D74.0 Congenital methemoglobinemia
        Congenital NADH-methemoglobin reductase deficiency
        Hemoglobin-M [Hb-M] disease
        Methemoglobinemia, hereditary

    D74.8 Other methemoglobinemias
        Acquired methemoglobinemia (with sulfhemoglobinemia)
        Toxic methemoglobinemia

    D74.9 Methemoglobinemia, unspecified

● **D75 Other and unspecified diseases of blood and blood-forming organs**
    | **Excludes2** | acute lymphadenitis (L04.-) |
                chronic lymphadenitis (I88.1)
                enlarged lymph nodes (R59.-)
                hypergammaglobulinemia NOS (D89.2)
                lymphadenitis NOS (I88.9)
                mesenteric lymphadenitis (acute) (chronic) (I88.0)

    D75.0 Familial erythrocytosis
        Genetic mutation of gene that results in increased circulating RBCs
        Benign polycythemia
        Familial polycythemia
        | **Excludes1** | hereditary ovalocytosis (D58.1) |

    D75.1 Secondary polycythemia
        Increase in total red cell mass
        Acquired polycythemia
        Emotional polycythemia
        Erythrocytosis NOS
        Hypoxemic polycythemia
        Nephrogenous polycythemia
        Polycythemia due to erythropoietin
        Polycythemia due to fall in plasma volume
        Polycythemia due to high altitude
        Polycythemia due to stress
        Polycythemia NOS
        Relative polycythemia
        | **Excludes1** | polycythemia neonatorum (P61.1) |
                     polycythemia vera (D45)

● **D75.8 Other specified diseases of blood and blood-forming organs**

    D75.81 Myelofibrosis
        Replacing bone marrow by fibrous tissue
        Myelofibrosis NOS
        Secondary myelofibrosis NOS
        Code first the underlying disorder, such as:
            malignant neoplasm of breast (C50.-)
        Use additional code, if applicable, for associated therapy-related myelodysplastic syndrome (D46.-)
        Use additional code for adverse effect, if applicable, to identify drug (T45.1X5)
        | **Excludes1** | acute myelofibrosis (C94.4-) |
                     idiopathic myelofibrosis (D47.1)
                     leukoerythroblastic anemia (D61.82)
                     myelofibrosis with myeloid metaplasia (D47.4)
                     myelophthisic anemia (D61.82)
                     myelophthisis (D61.82)
                     primary myelofibrosis (D47.1)

    D75.82 Heparin induced thrombocytopenia (HIT)

    D75.89 Other specified diseases of blood and blood-forming organs

    D75.9 Disease of blood and blood-forming organs, unspecified

● **D76 Other specified diseases with participation of lymphoreticular and reticulohistiocytic tissue**
    | **Excludes1** | (Abt-) Letterer-Siwe disease (C96.0) |
                eosinophilic granuloma (C96.6)
                Hand-Schüller-Christian disease (C96.5)
                histiocytic sarcoma (C96.A)
                histiocytosis X, multifocal (C96.5)
                histiocytosis X, unifocal (C96.6)
                malignant histiocytosis (C96.A)
                Langerhans-cell histiocytosis, multifocal (C96.5)
                Langerhans-cell histiocytosis NOS (C96.6)
                Langerhans-cell histiocytosis, unifocal (C96.6)
    | **Excludes1** | leukemic reticuloendotheliosis or reticulosis (C91.4-) |
                lipomelanotic reticuloendotheliosis or reticulosis (I89.8)

    D76.1 Hemophagocytic lymphohistiocytosis
        Familial hemophagocytic reticulosis
        Histiocytoses of mononuclear phagocytes

    D76.2 Hemophagocytic syndrome, infection-associated
        Use additional code to identify infectious agent or disease.

    D76.3 Other histiocytosis syndromes
        Reticulohistiocytoma (giant-cell)
        Sinus histiocytosis with massive lymphadenopathy
        Xanthogranuloma

CHAPTER 3 (D50-D89)

D77   Other disorders of blood and blood-forming organs in diseases classified elsewhere

Code first underlying disease, such as:
amyloidosis (E85.-)
congenital early syphilis (A50.0)
echinococcosis (B67.0-B67.9)
malaria (B50.0-B54)
schistosomiasis [bilharziasis] (B65.0-B65.9)
vitamin C deficiency (E54)

> **Excludes1**   rupture of spleen due to Plasmodium vivax malaria (B51.0)
> splenitis, splenomegaly in late syphilis (A52.79)
> splenitis, splenomegaly in tuberculosis (A18.85)

INTRAOPERATIVE AND POSTPROCEDURAL COMPLICATIONS OF THE SPLEEN (D78)

● **D78   Intraoperative and postprocedural complications of the spleen**

  ● **D78.0   Intraoperative hemorrhage and hematoma of the spleen complicating a procedure**

> **Excludes1**   intraoperative hemorrhage and hematoma of the spleen due to accidental puncture or laceration during a procedure (D78.1-)

    D78.01   Intraoperative hemorrhage and hematoma of the spleen complicating a procedure on the spleen

    D78.02   Intraoperative hemorrhage and hematoma of the spleen complicating other procedure

  ● **D78.1   Accidental puncture and laceration of the spleen during a procedure**

    D78.11   Accidental puncture and laceration of the spleen during a procedure on the spleen

    D78.12   Accidental puncture and laceration of the spleen during other procedure

  ● **D78.2   Postprocedural hemorrhage and hematoma of the spleen following a procedure**

    D78.21   Postprocedural hemorrhage and hematoma of the spleen following a procedure on the spleen

    D78.22   Postprocedural hemorrhage and hematoma of the spleen following other procedure

  ● **D78.8   Other intraoperative and postprocedural complications of the spleen**

Use additional code, if applicable, to further specify disorder

    D78.81   Other intraoperative complications of the spleen

    D78.89   Other postprocedural complications of the spleen

---

CERTAIN DISORDERS INVOLVING THE IMMUNE MECHANISM (D80-D89)

Includes   defects in the complement system
immunodeficiency disorders, except human immunodeficiency virus [HIV] disease
sarcoidosis

> **Excludes1**   autoimmune disease (systemic) NOS (M35.9)
> functional disorders of polymorphonuclear neutrophils (D71)
> human immunodeficiency virus [HIV] disease (B20)

● **D80   Immunodeficiency with predominantly antibody defects**

  D80.0   Hereditary hypogammaglobulinemia
Autosomal recessive agammaglobulinemia (Swiss type)
X-linked agammaglobulinemia [Bruton] (with growth hormone deficiency)

  D80.1   Nonfamilial hypogammaglobulinemia
Abnormally low levels of all classes of immunoglobulins
Agammaglobulinemia with immunoglobulin-bearing B-lymphocytes
Common variable agammaglobulinemia [CVAgamma]
Hypogammaglobulinemia NOS

D80.2   Selective deficiency of immunoglobulin A [IgA]

D80.3   Selective deficiency of immunoglobulin G [IgG] subclasses

D80.4   Selective deficiency of immunoglobulin M [IgM]

D80.5   Immunodeficiency with increased immunoglobulin M [IgM]

D80.6   Antibody deficiency with near-normal immunoglobulins or with hyperimmunoglobulinemia
Abnormally high levels of immunoglobulins in serum

D80.7   Transient hypogammaglobulinemia of infancy

D80.8   Other immunodeficiencies with predominantly antibody defects
Kappa light chain deficiency

D80.9   Immunodeficiency with predominantly antibody defects, unspecified

● **D81   Combined immunodeficiencies**

> **Excludes1**   autosomal recessive agammaglobulinemia (Swiss type) (D80.0)

D81.0   Severe combined immunodeficiency [SCID] with reticular dysgenesis

D81.1   Severe combined immunodeficiency [SCID] with low T- and B-cell numbers

D81.2   Severe combined immunodeficiency [SCID] with low or normal B-cell numbers

D81.3   Adenosine deaminase [ADA] deficiency

D81.4   Nezelof's syndrome

D81.5   Purine nucleoside phosphorylase [PNP] deficiency

D81.6   Major histocompatibility complex class I deficiency
Bare lymphocyte syndrome

D81.7   Major histocompatibility complex class II deficiency

● **D81.8   Other combined immunodeficiencies**

  ● **D81.81   Biotin-dependent carboxylase deficiency**
Multiple carboxylase deficiency

> **Excludes1**   biotin-dependent carboxylase deficiency due to dietary deficiency of biotin (E53.8)

    D81.810   Biotinidase deficiency

    D81.818   Other biotin-dependent carboxylase deficiency
Holocarboxylase synthetase deficiency
Other multiple carboxylase deficiency

    D81.819   Biotin-dependent carboxylase deficiency, unspecified
Multiple carboxylase deficiency, unspecified

  D81.89   Other combined immunodeficiencies

D81.9   Combined immunodeficiency, unspecified
Severe combined immunodeficiency disorder [SCID] NOS

● **D82   Immunodeficiency associated with other major defects**

> **Excludes1**   ataxia telangiectasia [Louis-Bar] (G11.3)

D82.0   Wiskott-Aldrich syndrome
X-linked immunodeficiency
Immunodeficiency with thrombocytopenia and eczema

D82.1   Di George's syndrome
Congenital disorder with defective development of third and fourth pharyngeal pouches
Pharyngeal pouch syndrome
Thymic alymphoplasia
Thymic aplasia or hypoplasia with immunodeficiency

D82.2   Immunodeficiency with short-limbed stature

D82.3   Immunodeficiency following hereditary defective response to Epstein-Barr virus
X-linked lymphoproliferative disease

D82.4   **Hyperimmunoglobulin E [IgE] syndrome**
Suspected genetic defect that produces high levels of antibody immunoglobulin (IgE) that causes skin and lung infections and eczema

D82.8   **Immunodeficiency associated with other specified major defects**

D82.9   **Immunodeficiency associated with major defect, unspecified**

● D83   **Common variable immunodeficiency**

D83.0   **Common variable immunodeficiency with predominant abnormalities of B-cell numbers and function**

D83.1   **Common variable immunodeficiency with predominant immunoregulatory T-cell disorders**

D83.2   **Common variable immunodeficiency with autoantibodies to B- or T-cells**

D83.8   **Other common variable immunodeficiencies**

D83.9   **Common variable immunodeficiency, unspecified**

● D84   **Other immunodeficiencies**

D84.0   **Lymphocyte function antigen-1 [LFA-1] defect**

D84.1   **Defects in the complement system**
C1 esterase inhibitor [C1-INH] deficiency

D84.8   **Other specified immunodeficiencies**

D84.9   **Immunodeficiency, unspecified**

● D86   **Sarcoidosis**

D86.0   **Sarcoidosis of lung**

D86.1   **Sarcoidosis of lymph nodes**

D86.2   **Sarcoidosis of lung with sarcoidosis of lymph nodes**

D86.3   **Sarcoidosis of skin**

● D86.8   **Sarcoidosis of other sites**

D86.81   **Sarcoid meningitis**

D86.82   **Multiple cranial nerve palsies in sarcoidosis**

D86.83   **Sarcoid iridocyclitis**
Rare large tumor with irregular surface of iris

D86.84   **Sarcoid pyelonephritis**
Systemic disease of unknown etiology characterized by chronic granulomatous inflammation with tissue destruction of pelvis kidney
Tubulo-interstitial nephropathy in sarcoidosis

D86.85   **Sarcoid myocarditis**

D86.86   **Sarcoid arthropathy**
Polyarthritis in sarcoidosis

D86.87   **Sarcoid myositis**
Granumloma of muscle

D86.89   **Sarcoidosis of other sites**
Hepatic granuloma
Uveoparotid fever [Heerfordt]

D86.9   **Sarcoidosis, unspecified**

Item 3-1 Sarcoidosis: A symptom of an inflammation producing tiny lumps of cells (granulomas) in various organs, most commonly the lungs and lymph nodes, that affect organ function. Cause is unknown occurring primarily in 20- to 40-year-olds, African-American, especially women, and those of Asian, German, Irish, Scandinavian, and Puerto Rican heritage.

● D89   **Other disorders involving the immune mechanism, not elsewhere classified**

   Excludes1   hyperglobulinemia NOS (R77.1)
       monoclonal gammopathy (of undetermined significance) (D47.2)

   Excludes2   transplant failure and rejection (T86.-)

D89.0   **Polyclonal hypergammaglobulinemia**
Benign hypergammaglobulinemic purpura
Polyclonal gammopathy NOS

D89.1   **Cryoglobulinemia**
Cryoglobulin (proteins) in blood that precipitate temperatures below 98.6° F; usually symptomatic of underlying disease
Cryoglobulinemic purpura
Cryoglobulinemic vasculitis
Essential cryoglobulinemia
Idiopathic cryoglobulinemia
Mixed cryoglobulinemia
Primary cryoglobulinemia
Secondary cryoglobulinemia

D89.2   **Hypergammaglobulinemia, unspecified**

D89.3   **Immune reconstitution syndrome**
Immune reconstitution inflammatory syndrome [IRIS]

   Use additional code for adverse effect, if applicable, to identify drug (T36-T50 with fifth or sixth character 5)

● D89.8   **Other specified disorders involving the immune mechanism, not elsewhere classified**

● D89.81   **Graft-versus-host disease**
Code first underlying cause, such as:
complications of transplanted organs and tissue (T86.-)
complications of blood transfusion (T80.89)

   Use additional code to identify associated manifestations, such as:
desquamative dermatitis (L30.8)
diarrhea (R19.7)
elevated bilirubin (R17)
hair loss (L65.9)

D89.810   **Acute graft-versus-host disease**

D89.811   **Chronic graft-versus-host disease**

D89.812   **Acute on chronic graft-versus-host disease**

D89.813   **Graft-versus-host disease, unspecified**

D89.82   **Autoimmune lymphoproliferative syndrome [ALPS]**

D89.89   **Other specified disorders involving the immune mechanism, not elsewhere classified**

   Excludes1   human immunodeficiency virus disease (B20)

D89.9   **Disorder involving the immune mechanism, unspecified**
Immune disease NOS

CHAPTER 3 (D50-D89)

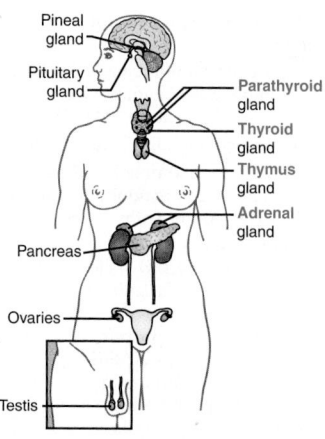

Figure 4-1 The endocrine system. (From Buck CJ: Step-by-Step Medical Coding, ed 2011, Philadelphia, WB Saunders, 2011)

CHAPTER 4

ENDOCRINE, NUTRITIONAL AND METABOLIC DISEASES (E00-E89)

All neoplasms, whether functionally active or not, are classified in Chapter 2. Appropriate codes in this chapter (i.e., E05.8, E07.0, E16-E31, E34.-) may be used as additional codes to indicate either functional activity by neoplasms and ectopic endocrine tissue or hyperfunction and hypofunction of endocrine glands associated with neoplasms and other conditions classified elsewhere.

Excludes1 transitory endocrine and metabolic disorders specific to newborn (P70-P74)

This chapter contains the following blocks:

E00-E07	Disorders of thyroid gland
E08-E13	Diabetes mellitus
E15-E16	Other disorders of glucose regulation and pancreatic internal secretion
E20-E35	Disorders of other endocrine glands
E36	Intraoperative complications of endocrine system
E40-E46	Malnutrition
E50-E64	Other nutritional deficiencies
E65-E68	Overweight, obesity and other hyperalimentation
E70-E88	Metabolic disorders
E89	Postprocedural endocrine and metabolic complications and disorders, not elsewhere classified

DISORDERS OF THYROID GLAND (E00-E07)

● **E00 Congenital iodine-deficiency syndrome**
Use additional code (F70-F79) to identify associated intellectual disabilities.
Excludes1 subclinical iodine-deficiency hypothyroidism (E02)

E00.0 Congenital iodine-deficiency syndrome, neurological type
Endemic cretinism, neurological type

E00.1 Congenital iodine-deficiency syndrome, myxedematous type
Dry, waxy type of swelling (nonpitting edema) with abnormal deposits of mucin in skin (mucinosis) and other tissues
Endemic hypothyroid cretinism
Endemic cretinism, myxedematous type

E00.2 Congenital iodine-deficiency syndrome, mixed type
Endemic cretinism, mixed type

E00.9 Congenital iodine-deficiency syndrome, unspecified
Congenital iodine-deficiency hypothyroidism NOS
Endemic cretinism NOS

Figure 4-2 Goiter is an enlargement of the thyroid gland.

Item 4-1 Simple goiter indicates no nodules are present. The most common type of goiter is a **diffuse colloidal**, also called a **nontoxic** or **endemic** goiter.

● **E01 Iodine-deficiency related thyroid disorders and allied conditions**
Excludes1 congenital iodine-deficiency syndrome (E00.-)
subclinical iodine-deficiency hypothyroidism (E02)

E01.0 Iodine-deficiency related diffuse (endemic) goiter
Thyroid gland is enlarged

E01.1 Iodine-deficiency related multinodular (endemic) goiter
Iodine-deficiency related nodular goiter

E01.2 Iodine-deficiency related (endemic) goiter, unspecified
Endemic goiter NOS

E01.8 Other iodine-deficiency related thyroid disorders and allied conditions
Acquired iodine-deficiency hypothyroidism NOS

E02 Subclinical iodine-deficiency hypothyroidism

● **E03 Other hypothyroidism**
Excludes1 iodine-deficiency related hypothyroidism (E00-E02)
postprocedural hypothyroidism (E89.0)

E03.0 Congenital hypothyroidism with diffuse goiter
Congenital parenchymatous goiter (nontoxic)
Congenital goiter (nontoxic) NOS
Excludes1 transitory congenital goiter with normal function (P72.0)

E03.1 Congenital hypothyroidism without goiter
Aplasia of thyroid (with myxedema)
Congenital atrophy of thyroid
Congenital hypothyroidism NOS

E03.2 Hypothyroidism due to medicaments and other exogenous substances
Code first poisoning due to drug or toxin, if applicable (T36-T65 with fifth or sixth character 1-4 or 6)
Use additional code for adverse effect, if applicable, to identify drug (T36-T50 with fifth or sixth character 5)

E03.3 Postinfectious hypothyroidism

E03.4 Atrophy of thyroid (acquired)
Excludes1 congenital atrophy of thyroid (E03.1)

E03.5 Myxedema coma
Often fatal complication of long-term hypothyroidism

E03.8 Other specified hypothyroidism

E03.9 Hypothyroidism, unspecified
Myxedema NOS

Item 4-2 Hypothyroidism is a condition in which there are insufficient levels of thyroxine. **Cretinism** is congenital hypothyroidism, which can result in mental and physical retardation.

Figure 4-3 Typical appearance of patients with moderately severe primary hypothyroidism or myxedema. (From Larsen: Williams Textbook of Endocrinology, ed 10, Saunders, An Imprint of Elsevier, 2003)

◀ New   ◀▥ Revised   ~~deleted~~ Deleted   **OGCR** Official Guidelines   X Assign placeholder X   ● Use Additional Character(s)

Excludes 1   Excludes 2   Includes   Use additional   Code first   Code also   Unspecified

● **E04** **Other nontoxic goiter**
> **Excludes1** congenital goiter (NOS) (diffuse)
> (parenchymatous) (E03.0)
> iodine-deficiency related goiter (E00-E02)

E04.0 **Nontoxic diffuse goiter**
Thyroid gland is enlarged
Diffuse (colloid) nontoxic goiter
Simple nontoxic goiter

E04.1 **Nontoxic single thyroid nodule**
Colloid nodule (cystic) (thyroid)
Nontoxic uninodular goiter
Thyroid (cystic) nodule NOS

E04.2 **Nontoxic multinodular goiter**
Enlarged thyroid gland with multiple nodules
Cystic goiter NOS
Multinodular (cystic) goiter NOS

E04.8 **Other specified nontoxic goiter**

E04.9 **Nontoxic goiter, unspecified**
Goiter NOS
Nodular goiter (nontoxic) NOS

● **E05** **Thyrotoxicosis [hyperthyroidism]**
Enlarged thyroid gland with multiple nodules
> **Excludes1** chronic thyroiditis with transient thyrotoxicosis
> (E06.2)
> neonatal thyrotoxicosis (P72.1)

● **E05.0** **Thyrotoxicosis with diffuse goiter**
Exophthalmic or toxic goiter NOS
Graves' disease
Toxic diffuse goiter

E05.00 **Thyrotoxicosis with diffuse goiter without thyrotoxic crisis or storm**

E05.01 **Thyrotoxicosis with diffuse goiter with thyrotoxic crisis or storm**

● **E05.1** **Thyrotoxicosis with toxic single thyroid nodule**
Thyrotoxicosis with toxic uninodular goiter

E05.10 **Thyrotoxicosis with toxic single thyroid nodule without thyrotoxic crisis or storm**

E05.11 **Thyrotoxicosis with toxic single thyroid nodule with thyrotoxic crisis or storm**

● **E05.2** **Thyrotoxicosis with toxic multinodular goiter**
Toxic nodular goiter NOS

E05.20 **Thyrotoxicosis with toxic multinodular goiter without thyrotoxic crisis or storm**

E05.21 **Thyrotoxicosis with toxic multinodular goiter with thyrotoxic crisis or storm**

● **E05.3** **Thyrotoxicosis from ectopic thyroid tissue**

E05.30 **Thyrotoxicosis from ectopic thyroid tissue without thyrotoxic crisis or storm**

E05.31 **Thyrotoxicosis from ectopic thyroid tissue with thyrotoxic crisis or storm**

● **E05.4** **Thyrotoxicosis factitia**

E05.40 **Thyrotoxicosis factitia without thyrotoxic crisis or storm**

E05.41 **Thyrotoxicosis factitia with thyrotoxic crisis or storm**

E05.8 **Other thyrotoxicosis**
Overproduction of thyroid-stimulating hormone

E05.80 **Other thyrotoxicosis without thyrotoxic crisis or storm**

E05.81 **Other thyrotoxicosis with thyrotoxic crisis or storm**

● **E05.9** **Thyrotoxicosis, unspecified**
Hyperthyroidism NOS

E05.90 **Thyrotoxicosis, unspecified without thyrotoxic crisis or storm**

E05.91 **Thyrotoxicosis, unspecified with thyrotoxic crisis or storm**

● **E06** **Thyroiditis**
An inflammation of the thyroid gland which results in an inability to convert iodine into thyroid hormone
> **Excludes1** postpartum thyroiditis (O90.5)

E06.0 **Acute thyroiditis**
Abscess of thyroid
Pyogenic thyroiditis
Suppurative thyroiditis
> **Use additional** code (B95-B97) to identify infectious agent.

E06.1 **Subacute thyroiditis**
Inflammation of thyroid gland following viral upper respiratory infection
de Quervain thyroiditis
Giant-cell thyroiditis
Granulomatous thyroiditis
Nonsuppurative thyroiditis
Viral thyroiditis
> **Excludes1** autoimmune thyroiditis (E06.3)

E06.2 **Chronic thyroiditis with transient thyrotoxicosis**
Chronic inflammation of thyroid gland with intermittent overproduction of thyroid hormone
> **Excludes1** autoimmune thyroiditis (E06.3)

E06.3 **Autoimmune thyroiditis**
Hashimoto's thyroiditis
Hashitoxicosis (transient)
Lymphadenoid goiter
Lymphocytic thyroiditis
Struma lymphomatosa

E06.4 **Drug-induced thyroiditis**
> **Use additional** code for adverse effect, if applicable, to identify drug (T36-T50 with fifth or sixth character 5)

E06.5 **Other chronic thyroiditis**
Chronic fibrous thyroiditis
Chronic thyroiditis NOS
Ligneous thyroiditis
Riedel thyroiditis

E06.9 **Thyroiditis, unspecified**

● **E07** **Other disorders of thyroid**

E07.0 **Hypersecretion of calcitonin**
C-cell hyperplasia of thyroid
Hypersecretion of thyrocalcitonin

E07.1 **Dyshormogenetic goiter**
Group of several types of goiter resulting from enzyme defects in hormone synthesis
Familial dyshormogenetic goiter
Pendred's syndrome
> **Excludes1** transitory congenital goiter with normal function (P72.0)

● **E07.8** **Other specified disorders of thyroid**

E07.81 **Sick-euthyroid syndrome**
Euthyroid sick-syndrome

E07.89 **Other specified disorders of thyroid**
Abnormality of thyroid-binding globulin
Hemorrhage of thyroid
Infarction of thyroid

E07.9 **Disorder of thyroid, unspecified**

Figure 4-4 Graves' disease. In Graves' disease, exophthalmos often looks more pronounced than it actually is because of the extreme lid retraction that may occur. This patient, for instance, had minimal proptosis of the left eye but marked lid retraction. (Courtesy Dr. HG Scheie. From Yanoff M, Fine BS: Ocular Pathology, ed 6, St. Louis, Mosby, 2008)

Item 4–3 Thyrotoxicosis is a condition caused by excessive amounts of the thyroid hormone thyroxine production or hyperthyroidism. **Graves' disease is associated with hyperthyroidism** (known as **Basedow's disease** in Europe).

◄ New   ◄ Revised   ~~deleted~~ Deleted   **OGCR** Official Guidelines   X Assign placeholder X   ● Use Additional Character(s)

[Excludes 1] [Excludes 2]   Includes   Use additional   Code first   Code also   Unspecified

OGCR Section I.C.4.a

4.1 Diabetes mellitus

The diabetes mellitus codes are combination codes that include the type of diabetes mellitus, body system affected, and the complications affecting that body system. As many codes within a particular category as are necessary to describe all of the complications of the disease may be used. They should be sequenced based on the reason for a particular visit. Assign as many codes from categories E08–E13 as needed to identify all of the associated conditions that the patient has.

DIABETES MELLITUS (E08-E13)

A metabolic disease that results in persistent hyperglycemia.

● **E08**   **Diabetes mellitus due to underlying condition**

Code first the underlying condition, such as:
congenital rubella (P35.0)
Cushing's syndrome (E24.-)
cystic fibrosis (E84.-)
malignant neoplasm (C00-C96)
malnutrition (E40-E46)
pancreatitis and other diseases of the pancreas (K85-K86.-)

Use additional code to identify any insulin use (Z79.4)

Excludes1   drug or chemical induced diabetes mellitus (E09.-)
gestational diabetes (O24.4-)
neonatal diabetes mellitus (P70.2)
postpancreatectomy diabetes mellitus (E13.-)
postprocedural diabetes mellitus (E13.-)
secondary diabetes mellitus NEC (E13.-)
type 1 diabetes mellitus (E10.-)
type 2 diabetes mellitus (E11.-)

● **E08.0**   **Diabetes mellitus due to underlying condition with hyperosmolarity**

    E08.00   **Diabetes mellitus due to underlying condition with hyperosmolarity without nonketotic hyperglycemic-hyperosmolar coma (NKHHC)**

    E08.01   **Diabetes mellitus due to underlying condition with hyperosmolarity with coma**

● **E08.1**   **Diabetes mellitus due to underlying condition with ketoacidosis**

    E08.10   **Diabetes mellitus due to underlying condition with ketoacidosis without coma**

    E08.11   **Diabetes mellitus due to underlying condition with ketoacidosis with coma**

● **E08.2**   **Diabetes mellitus due to underlying condition with kidney complications**

    E08.21   **Diabetes mellitus due to underlying condition with diabetic nephropathy**
Diabetes mellitus due to underlying condition with intercapillary glomerulosclerosis
Diabetes mellitus due to underlying condition with intracapillary glomerulonephrosis
Diabetes mellitus due to underlying condition with Kimmelstiel-Wilson disease

    E08.22   **Diabetes mellitus due to underlying condition with diabetic chronic kidney disease**
Use additional code to identify stage of chronic kidney disease (N18.1-N18.6)

    E08.29   **Diabetes mellitus due to underlying condition with other diabetic kidney complication**
Renal tubular degeneration in diabetes mellitus due to underlying condition

● **E08.3**   **Diabetes mellitus due to underlying condition with ophthalmic complications**

Changes in blood vessels of retina in which blood vessels swell and leak fluid into retinal surface.

    ● **E08.31**   **Diabetes mellitus due to underlying condition with unspecified diabetic retinopathy**

       E08.311   **Diabetes mellitus due to underlying condition with unspecified diabetic retinopathy with macular edema**

       E08.319   **Diabetes mellitus due to underlying condition with unspecified diabetic retinopathy without macular edema**

    ● **E08.32**   **Diabetes mellitus due to underlying condition with mild nonproliferative diabetic retinopathy**
Diabetes mellitus due to underlying condition with nonproliferative diabetic retinopathy NOS

       E08.321   **Diabetes mellitus due to underlying condition with mild nonproliferative diabetic retinopathy with macular edema**

       E08.329   **Diabetes mellitus due to underlying condition with mild nonproliferative diabetic retinopathy without macular edema**

    ● **E08.33**   **Diabetes mellitus due to underlying condition with moderate nonproliferative diabetic retinopathy**

       E08.331   **Diabetes mellitus due to underlying condition with moderate nonproliferative diabetic retinopathy with macular edema**

       E08.339   **Diabetes mellitus due to underlying condition with moderate nonproliferative diabetic retinopathy without macular edema**

    ● **E08.34**   **Diabetes mellitus due to underlying condition with severe nonproliferative diabetic retinopathy**

       E08.341   **Diabetes mellitus due to underlying condition with severe nonproliferative diabetic retinopathy with macular edema**

       E08.349   **Diabetes mellitus due to underlying condition with severe nonproliferative diabetic retinopathy without macular edema**

    ● **E08.35**   **Diabetes mellitus due to underlying condition with proliferative diabetic retinopathy**

       E08.351   **Diabetes mellitus due to underlying condition with proliferative diabetic retinopathy with macular edema**

       E08.359   **Diabetes mellitus due to underlying condition with proliferative diabetic retinopathy without macular edema**

    E08.36   **Diabetes mellitus due to underlying condition with diabetic cataract**

    E08.39   **Diabetes mellitus due to underlying condition with other diabetic ophthalmic complication**
Use additional code to identify manifestation, such as:
diabetic glaucoma (H40-H42)

● **E08.4**   **Diabetes mellitus due to underlying condition with neurological complications**

     E08.40   Diabetes mellitus due to underlying condition with diabetic neuropathy, unspecified

     E08.41   Diabetes mellitus due to underlying condition with diabetic mononeuropathy

     E08.42   Diabetes mellitus due to underlying condition with diabetic polyneuropathy
         Diabetes mellitus due to underlying condition with diabetic neuralgia

     E08.43   Diabetes mellitus due to underlying condition with diabetic autonomic (poly)neuropathy
         Diabetes mellitus due to underlying condition with diabetic gastroparesis

     E08.44   Diabetes mellitus due to underlying condition with diabetic amyotrophy

     E08.49   Diabetes mellitus due to underlying condition with other diabetic neurological complication

● **E08.5**   **Diabetes mellitus due to underlying condition with circulatory complications**

     E08.51   Diabetes mellitus due to underlying condition with diabetic peripheral angiopathy without gangrene

     E08.52   Diabetes mellitus due to underlying condition with diabetic peripheral angiopathy with gangrene
         Diabetes mellitus due to underlying condition with diabetic gangrene

     E08.59   Diabetes mellitus due to underlying condition with other circulatory complications

● **E08.6**   **Diabetes mellitus due to underlying condition with other specified complications**

     ● **E08.61**   Diabetes mellitus due to underlying condition with diabetic arthropathy

         E08.610   Diabetes mellitus due to underlying condition with diabetic neuropathic arthropathy
            Diabetes mellitus due to underlying condition with Charcôt's joints

         E08.618   Diabetes mellitus due to underlying condition with other diabetic arthropathy

     ● **E08.62**   Diabetes mellitus due to underlying condition with skin complications

         E08.620   Diabetes mellitus due to underlying condition with diabetic dermatitis
            Diabetes mellitus due to underlying condition with diabetic necrobiosis lipoidica

         E08.621   Diabetes mellitus due to underlying condition with foot ulcer
            Use additional code to identify site of ulcer (L97.4-, L97.5-)

         E08.622   Diabetes mellitus due to underlying condition with other skin ulcer
            Use additional code to identify site of ulcer (L97.1-L97.9, L98.41-L98.49)

         E08.628   Diabetes mellitus due to underlying condition with other skin complications

     ● **E08.63**   Diabetes mellitus due to underlying condition with oral complications

         E08.630   Diabetes mellitus due to underlying condition with periodontal disease

         E08.638   Diabetes mellitus due to underlying condition with other oral complications

● **E08.64**   Diabetes mellitus due to underlying condition with hypoglycemia

     E08.641   Diabetes mellitus due to underlying condition with hypoglycemia with coma

     E08.649   Diabetes mellitus due to underlying condition with hypoglycemia without coma

     E08.65   Diabetes mellitus due to underlying condition with hyperglycemia

     E08.69   Diabetes mellitus due to underlying condition with other specified complication
         Use additional code to identify complication

E08.8   Diabetes mellitus due to underlying condition with unspecified complications

E08.9   Diabetes mellitus due to underlying condition without complications

● **E09**   **Drug or chemical induced diabetes mellitus**

Code first poisoning due to drug or toxin, if applicable (T36-T65 with fifth or sixth character 1-4 or 6)

Use additional code for adverse effect, if applicable, to identify drug (T36-T50 with fifth or sixth character 5)

Use additional code to identify any insulin use (Z79.4)

Excludes1	diabetes mellitus due to underlying condition (E08.-)
	gestational diabetes (O24.4-)
	neonatal diabetes mellitus (P70.2)
	postpancreatectomy diabetes mellitus (E13.-)
	postprocedural diabetes mellitus (E13.-)
	secondary diabetes mellitus NEC (E13.-)
	type 1 diabetes mellitus (E10.-)
	type 2 diabetes mellitus (E11.-)

● **E09.0**   **Drug or chemical induced diabetes mellitus with hyperosmolarity**

     E09.00   Drug or chemical induced diabetes mellitus with hyperosmolarity without nonketotic hyperglycemic-hyperosmolar coma (NKHHC)

     E09.01   Drug or chemical induced diabetes mellitus with hyperosmolarity with coma

● **E09.1**   **Drug or chemical induced diabetes mellitus with ketoacidosis**

     E09.10   Drug or chemical induced diabetes mellitus with ketoacidosis without coma

     E09.11   Drug or chemical induced diabetes mellitus with ketoacidosis with coma

● **E09.2**   **Drug or chemical induced diabetes mellitus with kidney complications**

     E09.21   Drug or chemical induced diabetes mellitus with diabetic nephropathy
         Drug or chemical induced diabetes mellitus with intercapillary glomerulosclerosis
         Drug or chemical induced diabetes mellitus with intracapillary glomerulonephrosis
         Drug or chemical induced diabetes mellitus with Kimmelstiel-Wilson disease

     E09.22   Drug or chemical induced diabetes mellitus with diabetic chronic kidney disease
         Use additional code to identify stage of chronic kidney disease (N18.1-N18.6)

     E09.29   Drug or chemical induced diabetes mellitus with other diabetic kidney complication
         Drug or chemical induced diabetes mellitus with renal tubular degeneration

CHAPTER 4 (E00-E90)

● **E09.3 Drug or chemical induced diabetes mellitus with ophthalmic complications**

  ● **E09.31 Drug or chemical induced diabetes mellitus with unspecified diabetic retinopathy**

    E09.311 Drug or chemical induced diabetes mellitus with unspecified diabetic retinopathy with macular edema

    E09.319 Drug or chemical induced diabetes mellitus with unspecified diabetic retinopathy without macular edema

  ● **E09.32 Drug or chemical induced diabetes mellitus with mild nonproliferative diabetic retinopathy**

    Drug or chemical induced diabetes mellitus with nonproliferative diabetic retinopathy NOS

    E09.321 Drug or chemical induced diabetes mellitus with mild nonproliferative diabetic retinopathy with macular edema

    E09.329 Drug or chemical induced diabetes mellitus with mild nonproliferative diabetic retinopathy without macular edema

  ● **E09.33 Drug or chemical induced diabetes mellitus with moderate nonproliferative diabetic retinopathy**

    E09.331 Drug or chemical induced diabetes mellitus with moderate nonproliferative diabetic retinopathy with macular edema

    E09.339 Drug or chemical induced diabetes mellitus with moderate nonproliferative diabetic retinopathy without macular edema

  ● **E09.34 Drug or chemical induced diabetes mellitus with severe nonproliferative diabetic retinopathy**

    E09.341 Drug or chemical induced diabetes mellitus with severe nonproliferative diabetic retinopathy with macular edema

    E09.349 Drug or chemical induced diabetes mellitus with severe nonproliferative diabetic retinopathy without macular edema

  ● **E09.35 Drug or chemical induced diabetes mellitus with proliferative diabetic retinopathy**

    E09.351 Drug or chemical induced diabetes mellitus with proliferative diabetic retinopathy with macular edema

    E09.359 Drug or chemical induced diabetes mellitus with proliferative diabetic retinopathy without macular edema

  E09.36 Drug or chemical induced diabetes mellitus with diabetic cataract

  E09.39 Drug or chemical induced diabetes mellitus with other diabetic ophthalmic complication

    Use additional code to identify manifestation, such as:
      diabetic glaucoma (H40-H42)

● **E09.4 Drug or chemical induced diabetes mellitus with neurological complications**

  E09.40 Drug or chemical induced diabetes mellitus with neurological complications with diabetic neuropathy, unspecified

  E09.41 Drug or chemical induced diabetes mellitus with neurological complications with diabetic mononeuropathy

E09.42 Drug or chemical induced diabetes mellitus with neurological complications with diabetic polyneuropathy

  Drug or chemical induced diabetes mellitus with diabetic neuralgia

E09.43 Drug or chemical induced diabetes mellitus with neurological complications with diabetic autonomic (poly)neuropathy

  Drug or chemical induced diabetes mellitus with diabetic gastroparesis

E09.44 Drug or chemical induced diabetes mellitus with neurological complications with diabetic amyotrophy

E09.49 Drug or chemical induced diabetes mellitus with neurological complications with other diabetic neurological complication

● **E09.5 Drug or chemical induced diabetes mellitus with circulatory complications**

  E09.51 Drug or chemical induced diabetes mellitus with diabetic peripheral angiopathy without gangrene

  E09.52 Drug or chemical induced diabetes mellitus with diabetic peripheral angiopathy with gangrene

    Drug or chemical induced diabetes mellitus with diabetic gangrene

  E09.59 Drug or chemical induced diabetes mellitus with other circulatory complications

● **E09.6 Drug or chemical induced diabetes mellitus with other specified complications**

  ● **E09.61 Drug or chemical induced diabetes mellitus with diabetic arthropathy**

    E09.610 Drug or chemical induced diabetes mellitus with diabetic neuropathic arthropathy

      Drug or chemical induced diabetes mellitus with Charcôt's joints

      Progressive degeneration of weight bearing joint

    E09.618 Drug or chemical induced diabetes mellitus with other diabetic arthropathy

  ● **E09.62 Drug or chemical induced diabetes mellitus with skin complications**

    E09.620 Drug or chemical induced diabetes mellitus with diabetic dermatitis

      Drug or chemical induced diabetes mellitus with diabetic necrobiosis lipoidica

      Necrotizing skin condition

    E09.621 Drug or chemical induced diabetes mellitus with foot ulcer

      Use additional code to identify site of ulcer (L97.4-, L97.5-)

    E09.622 Drug or chemical induced diabetes mellitus with other skin ulcer

      Use additional code to identify site of ulcer (L97.1-L97.9, L98.41-L98.49)

    E09.628 Drug or chemical induced diabetes mellitus with other skin complications

  ● **E09.63 Drug or chemical induced diabetes mellitus with oral complications**

    E09.630 Drug or chemical induced diabetes mellitus with periodontal disease

    E09.638 Drug or chemical induced diabetes mellitus with other oral complications

● E09.64 **Drug or chemical induced diabetes mellitus with hypoglycemia**

    E09.641 **Drug or chemical induced diabetes mellitus with hypoglycemia with coma**

    E09.649 **Drug or chemical induced diabetes mellitus with hypoglycemia without coma**

  E09.65 **Drug or chemical induced diabetes mellitus with hyperglycemia**

  E09.69 **Drug or chemical induced diabetes mellitus with other specified complication**

    Use additional code to identify complication

 E09.8 **Drug or chemical induced diabetes mellitus with unspecified complications**

 E09.9 **Drug or chemical induced diabetes mellitus without complications**

● E10 **Type 1 diabetes mellitus**

Includes brittle diabetes (mellitus)
diabetes (mellitus) due to autoimmune process
diabetes (mellitus) due to immune mediated pancreatic islet beta-cell destruction
idiopathic diabetes (mellitus)
juvenile onset diabetes (mellitus)
ketosis-prone diabetes (mellitus)

Excludes1 diabetes mellitus due to underlying condition (E08.-)
drug or chemical induced diabetes mellitus (E09.-)
gestational diabetes (O24.4-)
hyperglycemia NOS (R73.9)
neonatal diabetes mellitus (P70.2)
postpancreatectomy diabetes mellitus (E13.-)
postprocedural diabetes mellitus (E13.-)
secondary diabetes mellitus NEC (E13.-)
type 2 diabetes mellitus (E11.-)

● E10.1 **Type 1 diabetes mellitus with ketoacidosis**
Acidosis accompanied by accumulation of ketone bodies (ketosis) in body tissues and fluids

  E10.10 **Type 1 diabetes mellitus with ketoacidosis without coma**

  E10.11 **Type 1 diabetes mellitus with ketoacidosis with coma**

● E10.2 **Type 1 diabetes mellitus with kidney complications**

  E10.21 **Type 1 diabetes mellitus with diabetic nephropathy**
Type 1 diabetes mellitus with intercapillary glomerulosclerosis
Type 1 diabetes mellitus with intracapillary glomerulonephrosis
Type 1 diabetes mellitus with Kimmelstiel-Wilson disease

  E10.22 **Type 1 diabetes mellitus with diabetic chronic kidney disease**
Use additional code to identify stage of chronic kidney disease (N18.1-N18.6)

  E10.29 **Type 1 diabetes mellitus with other diabetic kidney complication**
Type 1 diabetes mellitus with renal tubular degeneration

● E10.3 **Type 1 diabetes mellitus with ophthalmic complications**

 ● E10.31 **Type 1 diabetes mellitus with unspecified diabetic retinopathy**

    E10.311 **Type 1 diabetes mellitus with unspecified diabetic retinopathy with macular edema**

    E10.319 **Type 1 diabetes mellitus with unspecified diabetic retinopathy without macular edema**

● E10.32 **Type 1 diabetes mellitus with mild nonproliferative diabetic retinopathy**
Type 1 diabetes mellitus with nonproliferative diabetic retinopathy NOS

  E10.321 **Type 1 diabetes mellitus with mild nonproliferative diabetic retinopathy with macular edema**

  E10.329 **Type 1 diabetes mellitus with mild nonproliferative diabetic retinopathy without macular edema**

● E10.33 **Type 1 diabetes mellitus with moderate nonproliferative diabetic retinopathy**

  E10.331 **Type 1 diabetes mellitus with moderate nonproliferative diabetic retinopathy with macular edema**

  E10.339 **Type 1 diabetes mellitus with moderate nonproliferative diabetic retinopathy without macular edema**

● E10.34 **Type 1 diabetes mellitus with severe nonproliferative diabetic retinopathy**

  E10.341 **Type 1 diabetes mellitus with severe nonproliferative diabetic retinopathy with macular edema**

  E10.349 **Type 1 diabetes mellitus with severe nonproliferative diabetic retinopathy without macular edema**

● E10.35 **Type 1 diabetes mellitus with proliferative diabetic retinopathy**

  E10.351 **Type 1 diabetes mellitus with proliferative diabetic retinopathy with macular edema**

  E10.359 **Type 1 diabetes mellitus with proliferative diabetic retinopathy without macular edema**

  E10.36 **Type 1 diabetes mellitus with diabetic cataract**

  E10.39 **Type 1 diabetes mellitus with other diabetic ophthalmic complication**
Use additional code to identify manifestation, such as:
diabetic glaucoma (H40-H42)

● E10.4 **Type 1 diabetes mellitus with neurological complications**

  E10.40 **Type 1 diabetes mellitus with diabetic neuropathy, unspecified**

  E10.41 **Type 1 diabetes mellitus with diabetic mononeuropathy**

  E10.42 **Type 1 diabetes mellitus with diabetic polyneuropathy**
Type 1 diabetes mellitus with diabetic neuralgia

  E10.43 **Type 1 diabetes mellitus with diabetic autonomic (poly)neuropathy**
Type 1 diabetes mellitus with diabetic gastroparesis

  E10.44 **Type 1 diabetes mellitus with diabetic amyotrophy**

  E10.49 **Type 1 diabetes mellitus with other diabetic neurological complication**

● E10.5 **Type 1 diabetes mellitus with circulatory complications**

  E10.51 **Type 1 diabetes mellitus with diabetic peripheral angiopathy without gangrene**

  E10.52 **Type 1 diabetes mellitus with diabetic peripheral angiopathy with gangrene**
Type 1 diabetes mellitus with diabetic gangrene

  E10.59 **Type 1 diabetes mellitus with other circulatory complications**

● E10.6   **Type 1 diabetes mellitus with other specified complications**
- ● E10.61   **Type 1 diabetes mellitus with diabetic arthropathy**
  - E10.610   **Type 1 diabetes mellitus with diabetic neuropathic arthropathy**
    Type 1 diabetes mellitus with Charcôt's joints
  - E10.618   **Type 1 diabetes mellitus with other diabetic arthropathy**
- ● E10.62   **Type 1 diabetes mellitus with skin complications**
  - E10.620   **Type 1 diabetes mellitus with diabetic dermatitis**
    Type 1 diabetes mellitus with diabetic necrobiosis lipoidica
  - E10.621   **Type 1 diabetes mellitus with foot ulcer**
    Use additional code to identify site of ulcer (L97.4-, L97.5-)
  - E10.622   **Type 1 diabetes mellitus with other skin ulcer**
    Use additional code to identify site of ulcer (L97.1-L97.9, L98.41-L98.49)
  - E10.628   **Type 1 diabetes mellitus with other skin complications**
- ● E10.63   **Type 1 diabetes mellitus with oral complications**
  - E10.630   **Type 1 diabetes mellitus with periodontal disease**
  - E10.638   **Type 1 diabetes mellitus with other oral complications**
- ● E10.64   **Type 1 diabetes mellitus with hypoglycemia**
  - E10.641   **Type 1 diabetes mellitus with hypoglycemia with coma**
  - E10.649   **Type 1 diabetes mellitus with hypoglycemia without coma**
- E10.65   **Type 1 diabetes mellitus with hyperglycemia**
- E10.69   **Type 1 diabetes mellitus with other specified complication**
  Use additional code to identify complication
  Use this code with E10.65 to report hyperosmolarity in a Type 1 patient

E10.8   **Type 1 diabetes mellitus with unspecified complications**

E10.9   **Type 1 diabetes mellitus without complications**

● E11   **Type 2 diabetes mellitus**
> **Includes**   diabetes (mellitus) due to insulin secretory defect
> diabetes NOS
> insulin resistant diabetes (mellitus)

Use additional code to identify any insulin use (Z79.4)

> **Excludes1**   diabetes mellitus due to underlying condition (E08.-)
> drug or chemical induced diabetes mellitus (E09.-)
> gestational diabetes (O24.4-)
> neonatal diabetes mellitus (P70.2)
> postpancreatectomy diabetes mellitus (E13.-)
> postprocedural diabetes mellitus (E13.-)
> secondary diabetes mellitus NEC (E13.-)
> type 1 diabetes mellitus (E10.-)

- ● E11.0   **Type 2 diabetes mellitus with hyperosmolarity**
  - E11.00   **Type 2 diabetes mellitus with hyperosmolarity without nonketotic hyperglycemic-hyperosmolar coma (NKHHC)**
  - E11.01   **Type 2 diabetes mellitus with hyperosmolarity with coma**

- ● E11.2   **Type 2 diabetes mellitus with kidney complications**
  - E11.21   **Type 2 diabetes mellitus with diabetic nephropathy**
    Type 2 diabetes mellitus with intercapillary glomerulosclerosis
    Type 2 diabetes mellitus with intracapillary glomerulonephrosis
    Type 2 diabetes mellitus with Kimmelstiel-Wilson disease
  - E11.22   **Type 2 diabetes mellitus with diabetic chronic kidney disease**
    Use additional code to identify stage of chronic kidney disease (N18.1-N18.6)
  - E11.29   **Type 2 diabetes mellitus with other diabetic kidney complication**
    Type 2 diabetes mellitus with renal tubular degeneration
- ● E11.3   **Type 2 diabetes mellitus with ophthalmic complications**
  - ● E11.31   **Type 2 diabetes mellitus with unspecified diabetic retinopathy**
    - E11.311   **Type 2 diabetes mellitus with unspecified diabetic retinopathy with macular edema**
    - E11.319   **Type 2 diabetes mellitus with unspecified diabetic retinopathy without macular edema**
  - ● E11.32   **Type 2 diabetes mellitus with mild nonproliferative diabetic retinopathy**
    Type 2 diabetes mellitus with nonproliferative diabetic retinopathy NOS
    - E11.321   **Type 2 diabetes mellitus with mild nonproliferative diabetic retinopathy with macular edema**
    - E11.329   **Type 2 diabetes mellitus with mild nonproliferative diabetic retinopathy without macular edema**
  - ● E11.33   **Type 2 diabetes mellitus with moderate nonproliferative diabetic retinopathy**
    - E11.331   **Type 2 diabetes mellitus with moderate nonproliferative diabetic retinopathy with macular edema**
    - E11.339   **Type 2 diabetes mellitus with moderate nonproliferative diabetic retinopathy without macular edema**
  - ● E11.34   **Type 2 diabetes mellitus with severe nonproliferative diabetic retinopathy**
    - E11.341   **Type 2 diabetes mellitus with severe nonproliferative diabetic retinopathy with macular edema**
    - E11.349   **Type 2 diabetes mellitus with severe nonproliferative diabetic retinopathy without macular edema**
  - ● E11.35   **Type 2 diabetes mellitus with proliferative diabetic retinopathy**
    - E11.351   **Type 2 diabetes mellitus with proliferative diabetic retinopathy with macular edema**
    - E11.359   **Type 2 diabetes mellitus with proliferative diabetic retinopathy without macular edema**
  - E11.36   **Type 2 diabetes mellitus with diabetic cataract**
  - E11.39   **Type 2 diabetes mellitus with other diabetic ophthalmic complication**
    Use additional code to identify manifestation, such as:
    diabetic glaucoma (H40-H42)

◀ New   ◀· Revised   ~~deleted~~ Deleted   **OGCR** Official Guidelines   X Assign placeholder X   ● Use Additional Character(s)

Excludes 1   Excludes 2   Includes   Use additional   Code first   Code also   Unspecified

CHAPTER 4 (E00-E90)

● **E11.4**   **Type 2 diabetes mellitus with neurological complications**

   E11.40   **Type 2 diabetes mellitus with diabetic neuropathy, unspecified**

   E11.41   **Type 2 diabetes mellitus with diabetic mononeuropathy**

   E11.42   **Type 2 diabetes mellitus with diabetic polyneuropathy**
       Type 2 diabetes mellitus with diabetic neuralgia

   E11.43   **Type 2 diabetes mellitus with diabetic autonomic (poly)neuropathy**
       Type 2 diabetes mellitus with diabetic gastroparesis

   E11.44   **Type 2 diabetes mellitus with diabetic amyotrophy**

   E11.49   **Type 2 diabetes mellitus with other diabetic neurological complication**

● **E11.5**   **Type 2 diabetes mellitus with circulatory complications**

   E11.51   **Type 2 diabetes mellitus with diabetic peripheral angiopathy without gangrene**

   E11.52   **Type 2 diabetes mellitus with diabetic peripheral angiopathy with gangrene**
       Type 2 diabetes mellitus with diabetic gangrene

   E11.59   **Type 2 diabetes mellitus with other circulatory complications**

● **E11.6**   **Type 2 diabetes mellitus with other specified complications**

  ● **E11.61**   **Type 2 diabetes mellitus with diabetic arthropathy**

     E11.610   **Type 2 diabetes mellitus with diabetic neuropathic arthropathy**
        Type 2 diabetes mellitus with Charcôt's joints

     E11.618   **Type 2 diabetes mellitus with other diabetic arthropathy**

  ● **E11.62**   **Type 2 diabetes mellitus with skin complications**

     E11.620   **Type 2 diabetes mellitus with diabetic dermatitis**
        Type 2 diabetes mellitus with diabetic necrobiosis lipoidica

     E11.621   **Type 2 diabetes mellitus with foot ulcer**
        Use additional code to identify site of ulcer (L97.4-, L97.5-)

     E11.622   **Type 2 diabetes mellitus with other skin ulcer**
        Use additional code to identify site of ulcer (L97.1-L97.9, L98.41-L98.49)

     E11.628   **Type 2 diabetes mellitus with other skin complications**

  ● **E11.63**   **Type 2 diabetes mellitus with oral complications**

     E11.630   **Type 2 diabetes mellitus with periodontal disease**

     E11.638   **Type 2 diabetes mellitus with other oral complications**

  ● **E11.64**   **Type 2 diabetes mellitus with hypoglycemia**

     E11.641   **Type 2 diabetes mellitus with hypoglycemia with coma**

     E11.649   **Type 2 diabetes mellitus with hypoglycemia without coma**

   E11.65   **Type 2 diabetes mellitus with hyperglycemia**

   E11.69   **Type 2 diabetes mellitus with other specified complication**
       Use additional code to identify complication
       Use this code with E11.65 to report DKA in a Type 2 patient

   E11.8   **Type 2 diabetes mellitus with unspecified complications**

   E11.9   **Type 2 diabetes mellitus without complications**

● **E13**   **Other specified diabetes mellitus**

   Includes diabetes mellitus due to genetic defects of beta-cell function
       diabetes mellitus due to genetic defects in insulin action
       postpancreatectomy diabetes mellitus
       postprocedural diabetes mellitus
       secondary diabetes mellitus NEC

   Use additional code to identify any insulin use (Z79.4)

   Excludes1 diabetes (mellitus) due to autoimmune process (E10.-)
       diabetes (mellitus) due to immune mediated pancreatic islet beta-cell destruction (E10.-)
       diabetes mellitus due to underlying condition (E08.-)
       drug or chemical induced diabetes mellitus (E09.-)
       gestational diabetes (O24.4-)
       neonatal diabetes mellitus (P70.2)
       type 2 diabetes mellitus (E11.-)

  ● **E13.0**   **Other specified diabetes mellitus with hyperosmolarity**

     E13.00   **Other specified diabetes mellitus with hyperosmolarity without nonketotic hyperglycemic-hyperosmolar coma (NKHHC)**

     E13.01   **Other specified diabetes mellitus with hyperosmolarity with coma**

  ● **E13.1**   **Other specified diabetes mellitus with ketoacidosis**

     E13.10   **Other specified diabetes mellitus with ketoacidosis without coma**

     E13.11   **Other specified diabetes mellitus with ketoacidosis with coma**

  ● **E13.2**   **Other specified diabetes mellitus with kidney complications**

     E13.21   **Other specified diabetes mellitus with diabetic nephropathy**
        Other specified diabetes mellitus with intercapillary glomerulosclerosis
        Other specified diabetes mellitus with intracapillary glomerulonephrosis
        Other specified diabetes mellitus with Kimmelstiel-Wilson disease

     E13.22   **Other specified diabetes mellitus with diabetic chronic kidney disease**
        Use additional code to identify stage of chronic kidney disease (N18.1-N18.6)

     E13.29   **Other specified diabetes mellitus with other diabetic kidney complication**
        Other specified diabetes mellitus with renal tubular degeneration

  ● **E13.3**   **Other specified diabetes mellitus with ophthalmic complications**

   ● **E13.31**   **Other specified diabetes mellitus with unspecified diabetic retinopathy**

       E13.311   **Other specified diabetes mellitus with unspecified diabetic retinopathy with macular edema**

       E13.319   **Other specified diabetes mellitus with unspecified diabetic retinopathy without macular edema**

   ● **E13.32**   **Other specified diabetes mellitus with mild nonproliferative diabetic retinopathy**
       Other specified diabetes mellitus with nonproliferative diabetic retinopathy NOS

       E13.321   **Other specified diabetes mellitus with mild nonproliferative diabetic retinopathy with macular edema**

       E13.329   **Other specified diabetes mellitus with mild nonproliferative diabetic retinopathy without macular edema**

◀ New   ◀ Revised   ~~deleted~~ Deleted   OGCR Official Guidelines   X Assign placeholder X   ● Use Additional Character(s)

| Excludes 1 | Excludes 2 | Includes | Use additional | Code first | Code also | Unspecified |

● E13.33   Other specified diabetes mellitus with
           moderate nonproliferative diabetic retinopathy
    E13.331   Other specified diabetes mellitus with
              moderate nonproliferative diabetic
              retinopathy with macular edema
    E13.339   Other specified diabetes mellitus with
              moderate nonproliferative diabetic
              retinopathy without macular edema
● E13.34   Other specified diabetes mellitus with severe
           nonproliferative diabetic retinopathy
    E13.341   Other specified diabetes mellitus
              with severe nonproliferative diabetic
              retinopathy with macular edema
    E13.349   Other specified diabetes mellitus
              with severe nonproliferative diabetic
              retinopathy without macular edema
● E13.35   Other specified diabetes mellitus with
           proliferative diabetic retinopathy
    E13.351   Other specified diabetes mellitus with
              proliferative diabetic retinopathy
              with macular edema
    E13.359   Other specified diabetes mellitus with
              proliferative diabetic retinopathy
              without macular edema
  E13.36   Other specified diabetes mellitus with diabetic
           cataract
  E13.39   Other specified diabetes mellitus with other
           diabetic ophthalmic complication
           Use additional code to identify manifestation,
              such as:
              diabetic glaucoma (H40-H42)
● E13.4   Other specified diabetes mellitus with neurological
          complications
  E13.40   Other specified diabetes mellitus with diabetic
           neuropathy, unspecified
  E13.41   Other specified diabetes mellitus with diabetic
           mononeuropathy
  E13.42   Other specified diabetes mellitus with diabetic
           polyneuropathy
           Other specified diabetes mellitus with diabetic
              neuralgia
  E13.43   Other specified diabetes mellitus with diabetic
           autonomic (poly)neuropathy
           Other specified diabetes mellitus with diabetic
              gastroparesis
  E13.44   Other specified diabetes mellitus with diabetic
           amyotrophy
  E13.49   Other specified diabetes mellitus with other
           diabetic neurological complication
● E13.5   Other specified diabetes mellitus with circulatory
          complications
  E13.51   Other specified diabetes mellitus with diabetic
           peripheral angiopathy without gangrene
  E13.52   Other specified diabetes mellitus with diabetic
           peripheral angiopathy with gangrene
           Other specified diabetes mellitus with diabetic
              gangrene
  E13.59   Other specified diabetes mellitus with other
           circulatory complications
● E13.6   Other specified diabetes mellitus with other specified
          complications
● E13.61   Other specified diabetes mellitus with diabetic
           arthropathy
    E13.610   Other specified diabetes mellitus with
              diabetic neuropathic arthropathy
              Other specified diabetes mellitus
                 with Charcôt's joints
    E13.618   Other specified diabetes mellitus with
              other diabetic arthropathy

● E13.62   Other specified diabetes mellitus with skin
           complications
    E13.620   Other specified diabetes mellitus with
              diabetic dermatitis
              Other specified diabetes mellitus with
                 diabetic necrobiosis lipoidica
    E13.621   Other specified diabetes mellitus with
              foot ulcer
              Use additional code to identify site
                 of ulcer (L97.4-, L97.5-)
    E13.622   Other specified diabetes mellitus with
              other skin ulcer
              Use additional code to identify
                 site of ulcer (L97.1-L97.9,
                 L98.41-L98.49)
    E13.628   Other specified diabetes mellitus with
              other skin complications
● E13.63   Other specified diabetes mellitus with oral
           complications
    E13.630   Other specified diabetes mellitus with
              periodontal disease
    E13.638   Other specified diabetes mellitus with
              other oral complications
● E13.64   Other specified diabetes mellitus with
           hypoglycemia
    E13.641   Other specified diabetes mellitus with
              hypoglycemia with coma
    E13.649   Other specified diabetes mellitus with
              hypoglycemia without coma
  E13.65   Other specified diabetes mellitus with
           hyperglycemia
  E13.69   Other specified diabetes mellitus with other
           specified complication
           Use additional code to identify complication
  E13.8   Other specified diabetes mellitus with unspecified
          complications
  E13.9   Other specified diabetes mellitus without complications

OTHER DISORDERS OF GLUCOSE REGULATION AND PANCREATIC INTERNAL SECRETION (E15-E16)

E15   Nondiabetic hypoglycemic coma
      Includes   drug-induced insulin coma in nondiabetic
                   hyperinsulinism with hypoglycemic coma
                   hypoglycemic coma NOS

● E16   Other disorders of pancreatic internal secretion
  E16.0   Drug-induced hypoglycemia without coma
          Use additional code for adverse effect, if applicable,
             to identify drug (T36-T50 with fifth or sixth
             character 5)
  E16.1   Other hypoglycemia
          Functional hyperinsulinism
          Functional nonhyperinsulinemic hypoglycemia
          Hyperinsulinism NOS
          Hyperplasia of pancreatic islet beta cells NOS
          Excludes1   hypoglycemia in infant of diabetic mother
                        (P70.1)
                        neonatal hypoglycemia (P70.4)
  E16.2   Hypoglycemia, unspecified
  E16.3   Increased secretion of glucagon
          Hyperplasia of pancreatic endocrine cells with glucagon
             excess
  E16.4   Increased secretion of gastrin
          Hypergastrinemia
          Hyperplasia of pancreatic endocrine cells with gastrin
             excess
          Zollinger-Ellison syndrome

◀ New   ◀━ Revised   ~~deleted~~ Deleted   OGCR Official Guidelines   X Assign placeholder X   ● Use Additional Character(s)

Excludes 1   Excludes 2   Includes   Use additional   Code first   Code also   Unspecified

CHAPTER 4 (E00-E90)

E16.8   **Other specified disorders of pancreatic internal secretion**
Increased secretion from endocrine pancreas of growth hormone-releasing hormone
Increased secretion from endocrine pancreas of pancreatic polypeptide
Increased secretion from endocrine pancreas of somatostatin
Increased secretion from endocrine pancreas of vasoactive-intestinal polypeptide

E16.9   **Disorder of pancreatic internal secretion, unspecified**
Islet-cell hyperplasia NOS
Pancreatic endocrine cell hyperplasia NOS

DISORDERS OF OTHER ENDOCRINE GLANDS (E20-E35)

Excludes1   galactorrhea (N64.3)
gynecomastia (N62)

● E20   **Hypoparathyroidism**
Greatly reduced function of parathyroid glands; AKA parathyroid insufficiency

Excludes1   Di George's syndrome (D82.1)
postprocedural hypoparathyroidism (E89.2)
tetany NOS (R29.0)
transitory neonatal hypoparathyroidism (P71.4)

E20.0   **Idiopathic hypoparathyroidism**
Rare condition, unknown cause; short dwarf-like with round face

E20.1   **Pseudohypoparathyroidism**
Hereditary condition resembling hypoparathyroidism, but caused by inability to respond to parathyroid hormone

E20.8   **Other hypoparathyroidism**

E20.9   **Hypoparathyroidism, unspecified**
Parathyroid tetany

● E21   **Hyperparathyroidism and other disorders of parathyroid gland**
Excludes1   adult osteomalacia (M83.-)
ectopic hyperparathyroidism (E34.2)
familial hypocalciuric hypercalcemia (E83.52)
hungry bone syndrome (E83.81)
infantile and juvenile osteomalacia (E55.0)

E21.0   **Primary hyperparathyroidism**
Hyperplasia of parathyroid
Osteitis fibrosa cystica generalisata [von Recklinghausen's disease of bone]

E21.1   **Secondary hyperparathyroidism, not elsewhere classified**
Excludes1   secondary hyperparathyroidism of renal origin (N25.81)

E21.2   **Other hyperparathyroidism**
Tertiary hyperparathyroidism
Excludes1   familial hypocalciuric hypercalcemia (E83.52)

E21.3   **Hyperparathyroidism, unspecified**
E21.4   **Other specified disorders of parathyroid gland**
E21.5   **Disorder of parathyroid gland, unspecified**

● E22   **Hyperfunction of pituitary gland**
Excludes1   Cushing's syndrome (E24.-)
Nelson's syndrome (E24.1)
overproduction of ACTH not associated with Cushing's disease (E27.0)
overproduction of pituitary ACTH (E24.0)
overproduction of thyroid-stimulating hormone (E05.8-)

E22.0   **Acromegaly and pituitary gigantism**
Chronic disease caused by hypersecretion of growth hormone
Overproduction of growth hormone
Excludes1   constitutional gigantism (E34.4)
constitutional tall stature (E34.4)
increased secretion from endocrine pancreas of growth hormone-releasing hormone (E16.8)

E22.1   **Hyperprolactinemia**
Increased levels of prolactin
Use additional code for adverse effect, if applicable, to identify drug (T36-T50 with fifth or sixth character 5)

E22.2   **Syndrome of inappropriate secretion of antidiuretic hormone**

E22.8   **Other hyperfunction of pituitary gland**
Central precocious puberty

E22.9   **Hyperfunction of pituitary gland, unspecified**

● E23   **Hypofunction and other disorders of the pituitary gland**
Includes   the listed conditions whether the disorder is in the pituitary or the hypothalamus
Excludes1   postprocedural hypopituitarism (E89.3)

E23.0   **Hypopituitarism**
Fertile eunuch syndrome
Hypogonadotropic hypogonadism
Idiopathic growth hormone deficiency
Isolated deficiency of gonadotropin
Isolated deficiency of growth hormone
Isolated deficiency of pituitary hormone
Kallmann's syndrome
Lorain-Levi short stature
Necrosis of pituitary gland (postpartum)
Panhypopituitarism
Pituitary cachexia
Pituitary insufficiency NOS
Pituitary short stature
Sheehan's syndrome
Simmonds' disease

E23.1   **Drug-induced hypopituitarism**
Use additional code for adverse effect, if applicable, to identify drug (T36-T50 with fifth or sixth character 5)

E23.2   **Diabetes insipidus**
Excludes1   nephrogenic diabetes insipidus (N25.1)

Item 4–4   **Hyperparathyroidism** is an overactive parathyroid gland that secretes excessive parathormone, causing increased levels of circulating calcium. This results in a loss of calcium in the bone (osteoporosis).

Hypoparathyroidism is an underactive parathyroid gland that results in decreased levels of circulating calcium. The primary manifestation is **tetany,** a continuous muscle spasm.

Figure 4-5   **Tetany** caused by hypoparathyroidism.

Item 4–5   **Hyperadrenalism** is overactivity of the adrenal cortex, which secretes corticosteroid hormones. Excessive glucocorticoid hormone results in hyperglycemia (**Cushing's syndrome**), and excessive aldosterone results in **Conn's syndrome. Adrenogenital syndrome** is the result of excessive secretion of androgens, male hormones, which stimulates premature sexual development. **Hypoadrenalism, Addison's disease,** is a condition in which the adrenal glands atrophy.

Figure 4-6   Centripetal and generalized obesity and dorsal kyphosis in a 30-year-old woman with Cushing's disease. (From Larsen: Williams Textbook of Endocrinology, ed 10, Saunders, An Imprint of Elsevier, 2003)

◀ New   ◀||| Revised   ~~deleted~~ Deleted   OGCR Official Guidelines   X Assign placeholder X   ● Use Additional Character(s)

Excludes 1   Excludes 2   Includes   Use additional   Code first   Code also   Unspecified

CHAPTER 4 (E00-E90)

E23.3   **Hypothalamic dysfunction, not elsewhere classified**
> **Excludes1**   Prader-Willi syndrome (Q87.1)
>   Russell-Silver syndrome (Q87.1)

E23.6   **Other disorders of pituitary gland**
> Abscess of pituitary
> Adiposogenital dystrophy

E23.7   **Disorder of pituitary gland, unspecified**

● **E24**   **Cushing's syndrome**
> **Excludes1**   congenital adrenal hyperplasia (E25.0)

E24.0   **Pituitary-dependent Cushing's disease**
> Overproduction of pituitary ACTH
> Pituitary-dependent hypercorticalism

E24.1   **Nelson's syndrome**

E24.2   **Drug-induced Cushing's syndrome**
> Use additional code for adverse effect, if applicable, to identify drug (T36-T50 with fifth or sixth character 5)

E24.3   **Ectopic ACTH syndrome**

E24.4   **Alcohol-induced pseudo-Cushing's syndrome**

E24.8   **Other Cushing's syndrome**

E24.9   **Cushing's syndrome, unspecified**

● **E25**   **Adrenogenital disorders**
> *Disorder of production of steroid hormone in adrenal gland*
> **Includes**   adrenogenital syndromes, virilizing or feminizing, whether acquired or due to adrenal hyperplasia consequent on inborn enzyme defects in hormone synthesis
>   female adrenal pseudohermaphroditism
>   female heterosexual precocious pseudopuberty
>   male isosexual precocious pseudopuberty
>   male macrogenitosomia praecox
>   male sexual precocity with adrenal hyperplasia
>   male virilization (female)
> **Excludes1**   indeterminate sex and pseudohermaphroditism (Q56)
>   chromosomal abnormalities (Q90-Q99)

E25.0   **Congenital adrenogenital disorders associated with enzyme deficiency**
> Congenital adrenal hyperplasia
> 21-Hydroxylase deficiency
> Salt-losing congenital adrenal hyperplasia

E25.8   **Other adrenogenital disorders**
> Idiopathic adrenogenital disorder
> Use additional code for adverse effect, if applicable, to identify drug (T36-T50 with fifth or sixth character 5)

E25.9   **Adrenogenital disorder, unspecified**
> Adrenogenital syndrome NOS

● **E26**   **Hyperaldosteronism**
> *Abnormality of electrolyte metabolism caused by excessive secretion of aldosterone*

● **E26.0**   **Primary hyperaldosteronism**

     E26.01   **Conn's syndrome**
> Code also adrenal adenoma (D35.0-)

     E26.02   **Glucocorticoid-remediable aldosteronism**
> Familial aldosteronism type I

     E26.09   **Other primary hyperaldosteronism**
> Primary aldosteronism due to adrenal hyperplasia (bilateral)

E26.1   **Secondary hyperaldosteronism**

● **E26.8**   **Other hyperaldosteronism**

     E26.81   **Bartter's syndrome**

     E26.89   **Other hyperaldosteronism**

E26.9   **Hyperaldosteronism, unspecified**
> Aldosteronism NOS
> Hyperaldosteronism NOS

● **E27**   **Other disorders of adrenal gland**

E27.0   **Other adrenocortical overactivity**
> Overproduction of ACTH, not associated with Cushing's disease
> Premature adrenarche
> **Excludes1**   Cushing's syndrome (E24.-)

E27.1   **Primary adrenocortical insufficiency**
> Addison's disease
> Autoimmune adrenalitis
> **Excludes1**   Addison only phenotype adrenoleukodystrophy (E71.528)
>   amyloidosis (E85.-)
>   tuberculous Addison's disease (A18.7)
>   Waterhouse-Friderichsen syndrome (A39.1)

E27.2   **Addisonian crisis**
> *Acute onset of adrenocortical insufficiency*
> Adrenal crisis
> Adrenocortical crisis

E27.3   **Drug-induced adrenocortical insufficiency**
> Use additional code for adverse effect, if applicable, to identify drug (T36-T50 with fifth or sixth character 5)

● **E27.4**   **Other and unspecified adrenocortical insufficiency**
> **Excludes1**   adrenoleukodystrophy [Addison-Schilder] (E71.528)
>   Waterhouse-Friderichsen syndrome (A39.1)

     E27.40   **Unspecified adrenocortical insufficiency**
> Adrenocortical insufficiency NOS
> Hypoaldosteronism

     E27.49   **Other adrenocortical insufficiency**
> Adrenal hemorrhage
> Adrenal infarction

E27.5   **Adrenomedullary hyperfunction**
> Adrenomedullary hyperplasia
> Catecholamine hypersecretion

E27.8   **Other specified disorders of adrenal gland**
> Abnormality of cortisol-binding globulin

E27.9   **Disorder of adrenal gland, unspecified**

● **E28**   **Ovarian dysfunction**
> **Excludes1**   isolated gonadotropin deficiency (E23.0)
>   postprocedural ovarian failure (E89.4-)

E28.0   **Estrogen excess**
> Use additional code for adverse effect, if applicable, to identify drug (T36-T50 with fifth or sixth character 5)

E28.1   **Androgen excess**
> Hypersecretion of ovarian androgens
> Use additional code for adverse effect, if applicable, to identify drug (T36-T50 with fifth or sixth character 5)

E28.2   **Polycystic ovarian syndrome**
> Sclerocystic ovary syndrome
> Stein-Leventhal syndrome

● **E28.3**   **Primary ovarian failure**
> **Excludes1**   pure gonadal dysgenesis (Q99.1)
>   Turner's syndrome (Q96.-)

     ● **E28.31**   **Premature menopause**

         E28.310   **Symptomatic premature menopause**
> Symptoms such as flushing, sleeplessness, headache, lack of concentration, associated with premature menopause

         E28.319   **Asymptomatic premature menopause**
> Premature menopause NOS

     E28.39   **Other primary ovarian failure**
> Decreased estrogen
> Resistant ovary syndrome

◄ New   ◄═ Revised   ~~deleted~~ Deleted   **OGCR** Official Guidelines   X Assign placeholder X   ● Use Additional Character(s)

| Excludes 1 | Excludes 2 | Includes | Use additional | Code first | Code also | Unspecified |

E28.8   **Other ovarian dysfunction**
Ovarian hyperfunction NOS
> **Excludes1**   postprocedural ovarian failure (E89.4-)

E28.9   **Ovarian dysfunction, unspecified**

● **E29**   **Testicular dysfunction**
> **Excludes1**   androgen insensitivity syndrome (E34.5-)
> azoospermia or oligospermia NOS (N46.0-N46.1)
> isolated gonadotropin deficiency (E23.0)
> Klinefelter's syndrome (Q98.0-Q98.2, Q98.4)

E29.0   **Testicular hyperfunction**
Hypersecretion of testicular hormones

E29.1   **Testicular hypofunction**
Defective biosynthesis of testicular androgen NOS
5-delta-Reductase deficiency (with male pseudohermaphroditism)
Testicular hypogonadism NOS
> Use additional code for adverse effect, if applicable, to identify drug (T36-T50 with fifth or sixth character 5)
>
> **Excludes1**   postprocedural testicular hypofunction (E89.5)

E29.8   **Other testicular dysfunction**

E29.9   **Testicular dysfunction, unspecified**

● **E30**   **Disorders of puberty, not elsewhere classified**

E30.0   **Delayed puberty**
Constitutional delay of puberty
Delayed sexual development

E30.1   **Precocious puberty**
Sexual maturation at earlier age than normal, or before age 8 in girls and 9 in boys, usually hormonal; AKA sexual precocity or pubertas praecox
Precocious menstruation
> **Excludes1**   Albright (-McCune) (-Sternberg) syndrome (Q78.1)
> central precocious puberty (E22.8)
> congenital adrenal hyperplasia (E25.0)
> female heterosexual precocious pseudopuberty (E25.-)
> male isosexual precocious pseudopuberty (E25.-)

E30.8   **Other disorders of puberty**
Premature thelarche

E30.9   **Disorder of puberty, unspecified**

● **E31**   **Polyglandular dysfunction**
> **Excludes1**   ataxia telangiectasia [Louis-Bar] (G11.3)
> dystrophia myotonica [Steinert] (G71.11)
> pseudohypoparathyroidism (E20.1)

E31.0   **Autoimmune polyglandular failure**
Schmidt's syndrome

E31.1   **Polyglandular hyperfunction**
> **Excludes1**   multiple endocrine adenomatosis (E31.2-)
> multiple endocrine neoplasia (E31.2-)

● **E31.2**   **Multiple endocrine neoplasia [MEN] syndromes**
Adenomatous hyperplasia and malignant tumors in endocrine glands
Multiple endocrine adenomatosis
> Code also any associated malignancies and other conditions associated with the syndromes

E31.20   **Multiple endocrine neoplasia [MEN] syndrome, unspecified**
Multiple endocrine adenomatosis NOS
Multiple endocrine neoplasia [MEN] syndrome NOS

E31.21   **Multiple endocrine neoplasia [MEN] type I**
Wermer's syndrome

E31.22   **Multiple endocrine neoplasia [MEN] type IIA**
Sipple's syndrome

E31.23   **Multiple endocrine neoplasia [MEN] type IIB**

E31.8   **Other polyglandular dysfunction**

E31.9   **Polyglandular dysfunction, unspecified**

● **E32**   **Diseases of thymus**
> **Excludes1**   aplasia or hypoplasia of thymus with immunodeficiency (D82.1)
> myasthenia gravis (G70.0)

E32.0   **Persistent hyperplasia of thymus**
Hypertrophy of thymus

E32.1   **Abscess of thymus**

E32.8   **Other diseases of thymus**
> **Excludes1**   aplasia or hypoplasia with immunodeficiency (D82.1)
> thymoma (D15.0)

E32.9   **Disease of thymus, unspecified**

● **E34**   **Other endocrine disorders**
> **Excludes1**   pseudohypoparathyroidism (E20.1)

E34.0   **Carcinoid syndrome**
> **Note:** May be used as an additional code to identify functional activity associated with a carcinoid tumor.

E34.1   **Other hypersecretion of intestinal hormones**

E34.2   **Ectopic hormone secretion, not elsewhere classified**
> **Excludes1**   ectopic ACTH syndrome (E24.3)

E34.3   **Short stature due to endocrine disorder**
Constitutional short stature
Laron-type short stature
> **Excludes1**   achondroplastic short stature (Q77.4)
> hypochondroplastic short stature (Q77.4)
> nutritional short stature (E45)
> pituitary short stature (E23.0)
> progeria (E34.8)
> renal short stature (N25.0)
> Russell-Silver syndrome (Q87.1)
> short-limbed stature with immunodeficiency (D82.2)
> short stature in specific dysmorphic syndromes - code to syndrome - see Alphabetical Index
> short stature NOS (R62.52)

E34.4   **Constitutional tall stature**
Constitutional gigantism

● **E34.5**   **Androgen insensitivity syndrome**

E34.50   **Androgen insensitivity syndrome, unspecified**
Androgen insensitivity NOS

E34.51   **Complete androgen insensitivity syndrome**
Complete androgen insensitivity
de Quervain syndrome
Goldberg-Maxwell syndrome

E34.52   **Partial androgen insensitivity syndrome**
Partial androgen insensitivity
Reifenstein syndrome

E34.8   **Other specified endocrine disorders**
Pineal gland dysfunction
Progeria
> **Excludes2**   pseudohypoparathyroidism (E20.1)

E34.9   **Endocrine disorder, unspecified**
Endocrine disturbance NOS
Hormone disturbance NOS

E35   **Disorders of endocrine glands in diseases classified elsewhere**
> *Code first underlying disease, such as:*
> late congenital syphilis of thymus gland [Dubois disease] (A50.5)
>
> Use additional code, if applicable, to identify:
> sequelae of tuberculosis of other organs (B90.8)
>
> **Excludes1**   Echinococcus granulosus infection of thyroid gland (B67.3)
> meningococcal hemorrhagic adrenalitis (A39.1)
> syphilis of endocrine gland (A52.79)
> tuberculosis of adrenal gland, except calcification (A18.7)
> tuberculosis of endocrine gland NEC (A18.82)
> tuberculosis of thyroid gland (A18.81)
> Waterhouse-Friderichsen syndrome (A39.1)

INTRAOPERATIVE COMPLICATIONS OF ENDOCRINE SYSTEM (E36)

● **E36   Intraoperative complications of endocrine system**

    Excludes2   postprocedural endocrine and metabolic complications and disorders, not elsewhere classified (E89.-)

● **E36.0   Intraoperative hemorrhage and hematoma of an endocrine system organ or structure complicating a procedure**

     Excludes1   intraoperative hemorrhage and hematoma of an endocrine system organ or structure due to accidental puncture or laceration during a procedure (E36.1-)

    E36.01   Intraoperative hemorrhage and hematoma of an endocrine system organ or structure complicating an endocrine system procedure

    E36.02   Intraoperative hemorrhage and hematoma of an endocrine system organ or structure complicating other procedure

● **E36.1   Accidental puncture and laceration of an endocrine system organ or structure during a procedure**

    E36.11   Accidental puncture and laceration of an endocrine system organ or structure during an endocrine system procedure

    E36.12   Accidental puncture and laceration of an endocrine system organ or structure during other procedure

    E36.8   Other intraoperative complications of endocrine system

      Use additional code, if applicable, to further specify disorder

MALNUTRITION (E40-E46)

    Excludes1   intestinal malabsorption (K90.-)
                  sequelae of protein-calorie malnutrition (E64.0)

    Excludes2   nutritional anemias (D50-D53)
                  starvation (T73.0)

E40   Kwashiorkor

Malnutrition produced by severe protein deficiency
Severe malnutrition with nutritional edema with dyspigmentation of skin and hair

    Excludes1   marasmic kwashiorkor (E42)

E41   Nutritional marasmus

Severe malnutrition with marasmus

    Excludes1   marasmic kwashiorkor (E42)

E42   Marasmic kwashiorkor

Severe protein malnutrition
Intermediate form severe protein-calorie malnutrition
Severe protein-calorie malnutrition with signs of both kwashiorkor and marasmus

E43   Unspecified severe protein-calorie malnutrition

Starvation edema

● **E44   Protein-calorie malnutrition of moderate and mild degree**

    E44.0   Moderate protein-calorie malnutrition

    E44.1   Mild protein-calorie malnutrition

E45   Retarded development following protein-calorie malnutrition

Nutritional short stature
Nutritional stunting
Physical retardation due to malnutrition

E46   Unspecified protein-calorie malnutrition

Malnutrition NOS
Protein-calorie imbalance NOS

    Excludes1   nutritional deficiency NOS (E63.9)

Item 4–6   Bitot's spots are the result of a buildup of keratin debris found on the superficial surface the conjunctiva; oval, triangular, or irregular in shape; and a sign of vitamin A deficiency and associated with night blindness. The disease may progress to **keratomalacia,** which can result in eventual prolapse of the iris and loss of the lens.

Figure 4-7   Bitot's spot on the conjunctiva.

OTHER NUTRITIONAL DEFICIENCIES (E50-E64)

    Excludes2   nutritional anemias (D50-D53)

● **E50   Vitamin A deficiency**

    Excludes1   sequelae of vitamin A deficiency (E64.1)

    E50.0   Vitamin A deficiency with conjunctival xerosis

    E50.1   Vitamin A deficiency with Bitot's spot and conjunctival xerosis

      Bitot's spot in the young child

    E50.2   Vitamin A deficiency with corneal xerosis

    E50.3   Vitamin A deficiency with corneal ulceration and xerosis

    E50.4   Vitamin A deficiency with keratomalacia

      Eye disorder that results in dry cornea caused by vitamin A deficiency

    E50.5   Vitamin A deficiency with night blindness

    E50.6   Vitamin A deficiency with xerophthalmic scars of cornea

      Abnormal dryness and thickening of conjunctiva and cornea due to vitamin A deficiency

    E50.7   Other ocular manifestations of vitamin A deficiency

      Xerophthalmia NOS

    E50.8   Other manifestations of vitamin A deficiency

      Follicular keratosis
      Xeroderma

    E50.9   Vitamin A deficiency, unspecified

      Hypovitaminosis A NOS

● **E51   Thiamine deficiency**

    Excludes1   sequelae of thiamine deficiency (E64.8)

● **E51.1   Beriberi**

    E51.11   Dry beriberi

      Thiamine deficiency with nervous system manifestation most often caused by excessive alcohol consumption
      Beriberi NOS
      Beriberi with polyneuropathy

    E51.12   Wet beriberi

      Thiamine deficiency with cardiovascular manifestation most often caused by excessive alcohol consumption
      Beriberi with cardiovascular manifestations
      Cardiovascular beriberi
      Shoshin disease

    E51.2   Wernicke's encephalopathy

      Acute disease of brain due to thiamine deficiency most often associated with excessive alcohol consumption

    E51.8   Other manifestations of thiamine deficiency

    E51.9   Thiamine deficiency, unspecified

Figure 4-8 The sharply demarcated, characteristic scaling dermatitis of pellagra. (From Kumar: Robbins and Cotran: Pathologic Basis of Disease, ed 8, Saunders, An Imprint of Elsevier, 2009)

Item 4–7 **Pellagra** is associated with a deficiency of niacin and its precursor, **tryptophan.** Characteristics of the condition include diarrhea, dermatitis on exposed skin surfaces, dementia, and death. It is prevalent in developing countries where nutrition is inadequate. **Beriberi** is associated with thiamine deficiency.

E52 Niacin deficiency [pellagra]
    Niacin (-tryptophan) deficiency
    Nicotinamide deficiency
    Pellagra (alcoholic)
    Excludes1 sequelae of niacin deficiency (E64.8)

● **E53 Deficiency of other B group vitamins**
    Excludes1 sequelae of vitamin B deficiency (E64.8)
    E53.0 Riboflavin deficiency
        Ariboflavinosis
        Vitamin B2 deficiency
    E53.1 Pyridoxine deficiency
        Vitamin B6 deficiency
        Excludes1 pyridoxine-responsive sideroblastic anemia (D64.3)
    E53.8 Deficiency of other specified B group vitamins
        Biotin deficiency
        Cyanocobalamin deficiency
        Folate deficiency
        Folic acid deficiency
        Pantothenic acid deficiency
        Vitamin B12 deficiency
        Excludes1 folate deficiency anemia (D52.-)
                   vitamin B12 deficiency anemia (D51.-)
    E53.9 Vitamin B deficiency, unspecified

E54 Ascorbic acid deficiency
    Deficiency of vitamin C
    Scurvy
    Excludes1 scorbutic anemia (D53.2)
              sequelae of vitamin C deficiency (E64.2)

● **E55 Vitamin D deficiency**
    Excludes1 adult osteomalacia (M83.-)
              osteoporosis (M80.-)
              sequelae of rickets (E64.3)
    E55.0 Rickets, active
        Infantile osteomalacia
        Juvenile osteomalacia
        Softening of bone
        Excludes1 celiac rickets (K90.0)
                 Crohn's rickets (K50.-)
                 hereditary vitamin D-dependent rickets (E83.32)
                 inactive rickets (E64.3)
                 renal rickets (N25.0)
                 sequelae of rickets (E64.3)
                 vitamin D-resistant rickets (E83.31)
    E55.9 Vitamin D deficiency, unspecified
        Avitaminosis D

● **E56 Other vitamin deficiencies**
    Excludes1 sequelae of other vitamin deficiencies (E64.8)
    E56.0 Deficiency of vitamin E
    E56.1 Deficiency of vitamin K
        Excludes1 deficiency of coagulation factor due to vitamin K deficiency (D68.4)
                 vitamin K deficiency of newborn (P53)
    E56.8 Deficiency of other vitamins
    E56.9 Vitamin deficiency, unspecified

E58 Dietary calcium deficiency
    Excludes1 disorders of calcium metabolism (E83.5-)
              sequelae of calcium deficiency (E64.8)

E59 Dietary selenium deficiency
    Keshan disease
    Excludes1 sequelae of selenium deficiency (E64.8)

E60 Dietary zinc deficiency

● **E61 Deficiency of other nutrient elements**
    Use additional code for adverse effect, if applicable, to identify drug (T36-T50 with fifth or sixth character 5)
    Excludes1 disorders of mineral metabolism (E83.-)
              iodine deficiency related thyroid disorders (E00-E02)
              sequelae of malnutrition and other nutritional deficiencies (E64.-)
    E61.0 Copper deficiency
    E61.1 Iron deficiency
        Excludes1 iron deficiency anemia (D50.-)
    E61.2 Magnesium deficiency
    E61.3 Manganese deficiency
    E61.4 Chromium deficiency
    E61.5 Molybdenum deficiency
    E61.6 Vanadium deficiency
    E61.7 Deficiency of multiple nutrient elements
    E61.8 Deficiency of other specified nutrient elements
    E61.9 Deficiency of nutrient element, unspecified

● **E63 Other nutritional deficiencies**
    Excludes1 dehydration (E86.0)
              failure to thrive, adult (R62.7)
              failure to thrive, child (R62.51)
              feeding problems in newborn (P92.-)
              sequelae of malnutrition and other nutritional deficiencies (E64.-)
    E63.0 Essential fatty acid [EFA] deficiency
    E63.1 Imbalance of constituents of food intake
    E63.8 Other specified nutritional deficiencies
    E63.9 Nutritional deficiency, unspecified

● **E64 Sequelae of malnutrition and other nutritional deficiencies**
    Pathological condition resulting from disease, injury, or other trauma
    Note: This category is to be used to indicate conditions in categories E43, E44, E46, E50-E63 as the cause of sequelae, which are themselves classified elsewhere. The 'sequelae' include conditions specified as such; they also include the late effects of diseases classifiable to the above categories if the disease itself is no longer present
    Code first condition resulting from (sequela) of malnutrition and other nutritional deficiencies
    E64.0 Sequelae of protein-calorie malnutrition
        Excludes2 retarded development following protein-calorie malnutrition (E45)
    E64.1 Sequelae of vitamin A deficiency
    E64.2 Sequelae of vitamin C deficiency
    E64.3 Sequelae of rickets
    E64.8 Sequelae of other nutritional deficiencies
    E64.9 Sequelae of unspecified nutritional deficiency

◄ New   ◄|||| Revised   ~~deleted~~ Deleted   **OGCR** Official Guidelines   X Assign placeholder X   ● Use Additional Character(s)

Excludes 1   Excludes 2   Includes   Use additional   Code first   Code also   Unspecified   **803**

CHAPTER 4 (E00-E90)

OVERWEIGHT, OBESITY AND OTHER HYPERALIMENTATION (E65-E68)

E65   Localized adiposity
     Fat pad

● **E66   Overweight and obesity**
     Code first obesity complicating pregnancy, childbirth and the puerperium, if applicable (O99.21-)
     Use additional code to identify body mass index (BMI), if known (Z68.-)

     | Excludes1 | adiposogenital dystrophy (E23.6) |
     lipomatosis NOS (E88.2)
     lipomatosis dolorosa [Dercum] (E88.2)
     Prader-Willi syndrome (Q87.1)

  ● **E66.0   Obesity due to excess calories**
       E66.01   Morbid (severe) obesity due to excess calories
           Excludes1   morbid (severe) obesity with alveolar hypoventilation (E66.2)

       E66.09   Other obesity due to excess calories

  E66.1   Drug-induced obesity
     Use additional code for adverse effect, if applicable, to identify drug (T36-T50 with fifth or sixth character 5)

  E66.2   Morbid (severe) obesity with alveolar hypoventilation
     Uncommon condition of unknown cause leading to inadequate ventilation in lungs, even though lungs and airways are normal
     Pickwickian syndrome

  E66.3   Overweight

  E66.8   Other obesity

  E66.9   Obesity, unspecified
     Obesity NOS

● **E67   Other hyperalimentation**
     Ingestion of more than optimal amount of nutrients

     | Excludes1 | hyperalimentation NOS (R63.2) |
     sequelae of hyperalimentation (E68)

  E67.0   Hypervitaminosis A

  E67.1   Hypercarotinemia

  E67.2   Megavitamin-B6 syndrome

  E67.3   Hypervitaminosis D

  E67.8   Other specified hyperalimentation

E68   Sequelae of hyperalimentation
     Code first condition resulting from (sequela) of hyperalimentation

METABOLIC DISORDERS (E70-E88)

     | Excludes1 | androgen insensitivity syndrome (E34.5-) |
     congenital adrenal hyperplasia (E25.0)
     Ehlers-Danlos syndrome (Q79.6)
     hemolytic anemias attributable to enzyme disorders (D55.-)
     Marfan's syndrome (Q87.4)
     5-alpha-reductase deficiency (E29.1)

● **E70   Disorders of aromatic amino-acid metabolism**
  E70.0   Classical phenylketonuria
     Inherited disorder that increases to harmful levels amino acid phenylalanine

  E70.1   Other hyperphenylalaninemias
  ● **E70.2   Disorders of tyrosine metabolism**
       Excludes1   transitory tyrosinemia of newborn (P74.5)

     E70.20   Disorder of tyrosine metabolism, unspecified
       Tyrosine: Nonessential amino acid occurring in most proteins

     E70.21   Tyrosinemia
       Congenital amino acid metabolism
       Hypertyrosinemia

     E70.29   Other disorders of tyrosine metabolism
       Alkaptonuria
       Ochronosis

● **E70.3   Albinism**
     Congenital condition of reduced or absent pigment in eyes, skin, and hair

     E70.30   Albinism, unspecified
  ● **E70.31   Ocular albinism**
       E70.310   X-linked ocular albinism
       E70.311   Autosomal recessive ocular albinism
       E70.318   Other ocular albinism
       E70.319   Ocular albinism, unspecified

  ● **E70.32   Oculocutaneous albinism**
       Partial or total lack of melanin pigment in eyes

       | Excludes1 | Chediak-Higashi syndrome (E70.330) |
       Hermansky-Pudlak syndrome (E70.331)

       E70.320   Tyrosinase negative oculocutaneous albinism
         Albinism I
         Oculocutaneous albinism ty-neg

       E70.321   Tyrosinase positive oculocutaneous albinism
         Albinism II
         Oculocutaneous albinism ty-pos

       E70.328   Other oculocutaneous albinism
         Cross syndrome

       E70.329   Oculocutaneous albinism, unspecified

  ● **E70.33   Albinism with hematologic abnormality**
       E70.330   Chediak-Higashi syndrome
       E70.331   Hermansky-Pudlak syndrome
       E70.338   Other albinism with hematologic abnormality
       E70.339   Albinism with hematologic abnormality, unspecified

     E70.39   Other specified albinism
       Piebaldism

● **E70.4   Disorders of histidine metabolism**
     E70.40   Disorders of histidine metabolism, unspecified
     E70.41   Histidinemia
     E70.49   Other disorders of histidine metabolism

  E70.5   Disorders of tryptophan metabolism

  E70.8   Other disorders of aromatic amino-acid metabolism

  E70.9   Disorder of aromatic amino-acid metabolism, unspecified

● **E71   Disorders of branched-chain amino-acid metabolism and fatty-acid metabolism**
  E71.0   Maple-syrup-urine disease
     Due to defect in amino acid catabolism, causing severe ketoacidosis with smell of maple syrup in urine and on body

● **E71.1   Other disorders of branched-chain amino-acid metabolism**
  ● **E71.11   Branched-chain organic acidurias**
       E71.110   Isovaleric acidemia
       E71.111   3-methylglutaconic aciduria
       E71.118   Other branched-chain organic acidurias

  ● **E71.12   Disorders of propionate metabolism**
       E71.120   Methylmalonic acidemia
       E71.121   Propionic acidemia
       E71.128   Other disorders of propionate metabolism

     E71.19   Other disorders of branched-chain amino-acid metabolism
       Hyperleucine-isoleucinemia
       Hypervalinemia

◀ New   ◀▥ Revised   ~~deleted~~ Deleted   **OGCR** Official Guidelines   X Assign placeholder X   ● Use Additional Character(s)

| Excludes 1 | | Excludes 2 | | Includes | | Use additional | | Code first | | Code also | | Unspecified |

E71.2   Disorder of branched-chain amino-acid metabolism, unspecified

● E71.3   Disorders of fatty-acid metabolism

   Excludes1   peroxisomal disorders (E71.5)
                   Refsum's disease (G60.1)
                   Schilder's disease (G37.0)

   Excludes2   carnitine deficiency due to inborn error of metabolism (E71.42)

   E71.30   Disorder of fatty-acid metabolism, unspecified

● E71.31   Disorders of fatty-acid oxidation

   E71.310   Long chain/very long chain acyl CoA dehydrogenase deficiency
             LCAD
             VLCAD

   E71.311   Medium chain acyl CoA dehydrogenase deficiency
             MCAD

   E71.312   Short chain acyl CoA dehydrogenase deficiency
             SCAD

   E71.313   Glutaric aciduria type II
             Glutaric aciduria type II A
             Glutaric aciduria type II B
             Glutaric aciduria type II C

             Excludes1   glutaric aciduria (type 1) NOS (E72.3)

   E71.314   Muscle carnitine palmitoyltransferase deficiency

   E71.318   Other disorders of fatty-acid oxidation

   E71.32   Disorders of ketone metabolism

   E71.39   Other disorders of fatty-acid metabolism

● E71.4   Disorders of carnitine metabolism

   Excludes1   muscle carnitine palmitoyltransferase deficiency (E71.314)

   E71.40   Disorder of carnitine metabolism, unspecified

   E71.41   Primary carnitine deficiency

   E71.42   Carnitine deficiency due to inborn errors of metabolism

             Code also associated inborn error or metabolism

   E71.43   Iatrogenic carnitine deficiency
             Iatrogenic: Outcomes from activity of physicians
             Carnitine deficiency due to hemodialysis
             Carnitine deficiency due to Valproic acid therapy

● E71.44   Other secondary carnitine deficiency

   E71.440   Ruvalcaba-Myhre-Smith syndrome

   E71.448   Other secondary carnitine deficiency

● E71.5   Peroxisomal disorders
          Class of conditions which lead to disorders of lipid metabolism

   Excludes1   Schilder's disease (G37.0)

   E71.50   Peroxisomal disorder, unspecified

● E71.51   Disorders of peroxisome biogenesis
           Group 1 peroxisomal disorders

           Excludes1   Refsum's disease (G60.1)

   E71.510   Zellweger syndrome

   E71.511   Neonatal adrenoleukodystrophy

             Excludes1   X-linked adrenoleuko-dystrophy (E71.42-)

   E71.518   Other disorders of peroxisome biogenesis

● E71.52   X-linked adrenoleukodystrophy

   E71.520   Childhood cerebral X-linked adrenoleukodystrophy

   E71.521   Adolescent X-linked adrenoleukodystrophy

   E71.522   Adrenomyeloneuropathy

   E71.528   Other X-linked adrenoleukodystrophy
             Addison only phenotype adrenoleukodystrophy
             Addison-Schilder adrenoleukodystrophy

   E71.529   X-linked adrenoleukodystrophy, unspecified type

   E71.53   Other group 2 peroxisomal disorders

● E71.54   Other peroxisomal disorders

   E71.540   Rhizomelic chondrodysplasia punctata
             Rare, severe, inherited disorder with limb shortening, bone and cartilage abnormalities, abnormal facial appearance, severe mental retardation, psychomotor retardation, and cataracts

             Excludes1   chondrodysplasia punctata NOS (Q77.3)

   E71.541   Zellweger-like syndrome

   E71.542   Other group 3 peroxisomal disorders

   E71.548   Other peroxisomal disorders

● E72   Other disorders of amino-acid metabolism

   Excludes1   disorders of:
                   aromatic amino-acid metabolism (E70.-)
                   branched-chain amino-acid metabolism (E71.0-E71.2)
                   fatty-acid metabolism (E71.3)
                   purine and pyrimidine metabolism (E79.-)
                   gout (M1A.-, M10.-)

● E72.0   Disorders of amino-acid transport

   Excludes1   disorders of tryptophan metabolism (E70.5)

   E72.00   Disorders of amino-acid transport, unspecified

   E72.01   Cystinuria
            Hereditary aminoaciduria due to impairment of renal transport with predominant symptom of urinary cystine calculi

   E72.02   Hartnup's disease
            Inborn error of metabolism

   E72.03   Lowe's syndrome
            X-linked disorder with rickets, hydrophthalmia, congenital glaucoma, cataracts, mental retardation, and renal tubule dysfunction

            Use additional code for associated glaucoma (H42)

   E72.04   Cystinosis
            Genetic disease with excessive depostits of amino acid cystine in cells
            Fanconi (-de Toni) (-Debré) syndrome with cystinosis

            Excludes1   Fanconi (-de Toni) (-Debré) syndrome without cystinosis (E72.09)

   E72.09   Other disorders of amino-acid transport
            Fanconi (-de Toni) (-Debré) syndrome, unspecified

CHAPTER 4 (E00-E90)

● **E72.1** **Disorders of sulfur-bearing amino-acid metabolism**
  Excludes1　cystinosis (E72.04)
  　　　　　cystinuria (E72.01)
  　　　　　transcobalamin II deficiency (D51.2)

  E72.10 **Disorders of sulfur-bearing amino-acid metabolism, unspecified**

  E72.11 **Homocystinuria**
  　　　　Cystathionine synthase deficiency

  E72.12 **Methylenetetrahydrofolate reductase deficiency**

  E72.19 **Other disorders of sulfur-bearing amino-acid metabolism**
  　　　　Cystathioninuria
  　　　　Methioninemia
  　　　　Sulfite oxidase deficiency

● **E72.2** **Disorders of urea cycle metabolism**
  Excludes1　disorders of ornithine metabolism (E72.4)

  E72.20 **Disorder of urea cycle metabolism, unspecified**
  　　　　Hyperammonemia
  　　　　Elevated levels of ammonia

  　　　　Excludes1　hyperammonemia-
  　　　　　　　　　hyperornithinemia-
  　　　　　　　　　homocitrullinemia
  　　　　　　　　　syndrome E72.4
  　　　　　　　　transient hyperammonemia of
  　　　　　　　　　newborn (P74.6)

  E72.21 **Argininemia**
  　　　　Disorder in which deficiency of enzyme arginase
  　　　　causes build up of arginine and ammonia in
  　　　　blood

  E72.22 **Arginosuccinic aciduria**
  　　　　Gene disorder of urea cycle resulting accumulation
  　　　　of ammonia

  E72.23 **Citrullinemia**
  　　　　Urea cycle disorder that causes ammonia and other
  　　　　toxic substances to accumulate in blood

  E72.29 **Other disorders of urea cycle metabolism**

E72.3 **Disorders of lysine and hydroxylysine metabolism**
  Glutaric aciduria NOS
  Glutaric aciduria (type I)
  Hydroxylysinemia
  Hyperlysinemia

  Excludes1　glutaric aciduria type II (E71.313)
  　　　　　Refsum's disease (G60.1)
  　　　　　Zellweger syndrome (E71.510)

E72.4 **Disorders of ornithine metabolism**
  Hyperammonemia-Hyperornithinemia-
  　Homocitrullinemia syndrome
  Ornithinemia (types I, II)
  Ornithine transcarbamylase deficiency

  Excludes1　hereditary choroidal dystrophy (H31.2-)

● **E72.5** **Disorders of glycine metabolism**

  E72.50 **Disorder of glycine metabolism, unspecified**

  E72.51 **Non-ketotic hyperglycinemia**

  E72.52 **Trimethylaminuria**

  E72.53 **Hyperoxaluria**
  　　　　Oxalosis
  　　　　Oxaluria

  E72.59 **Other disorders of glycine metabolism**
  　　　　D-glycericacidemia
  　　　　Hyperhydroxyprolinemia
  　　　　Hyperprolinemia (types I, II)
  　　　　Sarcosinemia

E72.8 **Other specified disorders of amino-acid metabolism**
  Disorders of beta-amino-acid metabolism
  Disorders of gamma-glutamyl cycle

E72.9 **Disorder of amino-acid metabolism, unspecified**

● **E73** **Lactose intolerance**
  Intolerance for lactose, due to inherited deficiency of lactase activity in
  intestinal mucosa

  E73.0 **Congenital lactase deficiency**

  E73.1 **Secondary lactase deficiency**

  E73.8 **Other lactose intolerance**

  E73.9 **Lactose intolerance, unspecified**

● **E74** **Other disorders of carbohydrate metabolism**
  Excludes1　diabetes mellitus (E08-E13)
  　　　　　hypoglycemia NOS (E16.2)
  　　　　　increased secretion of glucagon (E16.3)
  　　　　　mucopolysaccharidosis (E76.0-E76.3)

● **E74.0** **Glycogen storage disease**

  E74.00 **Glycogen storage disease, unspecified**

  E74.01 **von Gierke's disease**
  　　　　Type I glycogen storage disease

  E74.02 **Pompe disease**
  　　　　Cardiac glycogenosis
  　　　　Type II glycogen storage disease

  E74.03 **Cori disease**
  　　　　Forbes' disease
  　　　　Type III glycogen storage disease

  E74.04 **McArdle disease**
  　　　　Type V glycogen storage disease

  E74.09 **Other glycogen storage disease**
  　　　　Andersen disease
  　　　　Hers disease
  　　　　Tauri disease
  　　　　Glycogen storage disease, types 0, IV, VI-XI
  　　　　Liver phosphorylase deficiency
  　　　　Muscle phosphofructokinase deficiency

● **E74.1** **Disorders of fructose metabolism**
  　　　　Excludes1　muscle phosphofructokinase deficiency
  　　　　　　　　　(E74.09)

  E74.10 **Disorder of fructose metabolism, unspecified**

  E74.11 **Essential fructosuria**
  　　　　Fructokinase deficiency

  E74.12 **Hereditary fructose intolerance**
  　　　　Fructosemia

  E74.19 **Other disorders of fructose metabolism**
  　　　　Fructose-1, 6-diphosphatase deficiency

● **E74.2** **Disorders of galactose metabolism**

  E74.20 **Disorders of galactose metabolism, unspecified**

  E74.21 **Galactosemia**
  　　　　Genetic disorders resulting from defective simple
  　　　　sugar (galactose) metabolism

  E74.29 **Other disorders of galactose metabolism**
  　　　　Galactokinase deficiency

● **E74.3** **Other disorders of intestinal carbohydrate absorption**
  　　　　Excludes2　lactose intolerance (E73.-)

  E74.31 **Sucrase-isomaltase deficiency**
  　　　　Deficiency in metabolism in intestinal mucosa
  　　　　results in malabsorption of sucrose and starch

  E74.39 **Other disorders of intestinal carbohydrate absorption**
  　　　　Disorder of intestinal carbohydrate absorption
  　　　　　NOS
  　　　　Glucose-galactose malabsorption
  　　　　Sucrase deficiency

E74.4 **Disorders of pyruvate metabolism and gluconeogenesis**
  Deficiency of phosphoenolpyruvate carboxykinase
  Deficiency of pyruvate carboxylase
  Deficiency of pyruvate dehydrogenase

  Excludes1　disorders of pyruvate metabolism and
  　　　　　gluconeogenesis with anemia (D55.-)
  　　　　　Leigh's syndrome (G31.82)

E74.8 **Other specified disorders of carbohydrate metabolism**
  Essential pentosuria
  Renal glycosuria

E74.9 **Disorder of carbohydrate metabolism, unspecified**

◀ New　◀▥ Revised　~~deleted~~ Deleted　**OGCR** Official Guidelines　X Assign placeholder X　● Use Additional Character(s)

Excludes 1　Excludes 2　Includes　Use additional　Code first　Code also　Unspecified

Item 4–8 Leukodystrophy is characterized by degeneration and/or failure of the myelin formation of the central nervous system and sometimes of the peripheral nervous system. The disease is inherited and progressive.

● **E75   Disorders of sphingolipid metabolism and other lipid storage disorders**

  Excludes1   mucolipidosis, types I-III (E77.0-E77.1)
  Refsum's disease (G60.1)

● **E75.0   GM2 gangliosidosis**
  Rare metabolic disorder that causes destruction of nerve cells of brain and spinal cord

  E75.00   GM2 gangliosidosis, unspecified

  E75.01   Sandhoff disease

  E75.02   Tay-Sachs disease

  E75.09   Other GM2 gangliosidosis
  Adult GM2 gangliosidosis
  Juvenile GM2 gangliosidosis

● **E75.1   Other and unspecified gangliosidosis**

  E75.10   Unspecified gangliosidosis
  Gangliosidosis NOS

  E75.11   Mucolipidosis IV
  Disorder with symptoms of psychomotor retardation and severe visual impairment

  E75.19   Other gangliosidosis
  GM1 gangliosidosis
  GM3 gangliosidosis

● **E75.2   Other sphingolipidosis**
  Lysosomal (a particle in a cytoplasm cell that contains digestive enzymes) storage diseases with symptoms of abnormal storage of amino acids

  Excludes1   adrenoleukodystrophy [Addison-Schilder] (E71.528)

  E75.21   Fabry (-Anderson) disease

  E75.22   Gaucher disease

  E75.23   Krabbe disease

● **E75.24   Niemann-Pick disease**

  E75.240   Niemann-Pick disease type A

  E75.241   Niemann-Pick disease type B

  E75.242   Niemann-Pick disease type C

  E75.243   Niemann-Pick disease type D

  E75.248   Other Niemann-Pick disease

  E75.249   Niemann-Pick disease, unspecified

  E75.25   Metachromatic leukodystrophy

  E75.29   Other sphingolipidosis
  Farber's syndrome
  Sulfatase deficiency
  Sulfatide lipidosis

  E75.3   Sphingolipidosis, unspecified

  E75.4   Neuronal ceroid lipofuscinosis
  Batten disease
  Bielschowsky-Jansky disease
  Kufs disease
  Spielmeyer-Vogt disease

  E75.5   Other lipid storage disorders
  Cerebrotendinous cholesterosis [van Bogaert-Scherer-Epstein]
  Wolman's disease

  E75.6   Lipid storage disorder, unspecified

● **E76   Disorders of glycosaminoglycan metabolism**

● **E76.0   Mucopolysaccharidosis, type I**
  Inborn metabolic disorder of enzymes that break down carbohydrates

  E76.01   Hurler's syndrome

  E76.02   Hurler-Scheie syndrome

  E76.03   Scheie's syndrome

  E76.1   Mucopolysaccharidosis, type II
  Inborn metabolic disorder of enzymes that break down carbohydrates occurs in 2-4 year old males
  Hunter's syndrome

● **E76.2   Other mucopolysaccharidoses**

● **E76.21   Morquio mucopolysaccharidoses**

  E76.210   Morquio A mucopolysaccharidoses
  Classic Morquio syndrome
  Morquio syndrome A
  Mucopolysaccharidosis, type IVA

  E76.211   Morquio B mucopolysaccharidoses
  Morquio-like
    mucopolysaccharidoses
  Morquio-like syndrome
  Morquio syndrome B
  Mucopolysaccharidosis, type IVB

  E76.219   Morquio mucopolysaccharidoses, unspecified
  Morquio syndrome
  Mucopolysaccharidosis, type IV

  E76.22   Sanfilippo mucopolysaccharidoses
  Mucopolysaccharidosis, type III (A) (B) (C) (D)
  Sanfilippo A syndrome
  Sanfilippo B syndrome
  Sanfilippo C syndrome
  Sanfilippo D syndrome

  E76.29   Other mucopolysaccharidoses
  beta-Glucuronidase deficiency
  Maroteaux-Lamy (mild) (severe) syndrome
  Mucopolysaccharidosis, types VI, VII

  E76.3   Mucopolysaccharidosis, unspecified

  E76.8   Other disorders of glucosaminoglycan metabolism

  E76.9   Glucosaminoglycan metabolism disorder, unspecified

● **E77   Disorders of glycoprotein metabolism**

  E77.0   Defects in post-translational modification of lysosomal enzymes
  Mucolipidosis II [I-cell disease]
  Mucolipidosis III [pseudo-Hurler polydystrophy]

  E77.1   Defects in glycoprotein degradation
  Aspartylglucosaminuria
  Fucosidosis
  Mannosidosis
  Sialidosis [mucolipidosis I]

  E77.8   Other disorders of glycoprotein metabolism

  E77.9   Disorder of glycoprotein metabolism, unspecified

● **E78   Disorders of lipoprotein metabolism and other lipidemias**

  Excludes1   sphingolipidosis (E75.0-E75.3)

  E78.0   Pure hypercholesterolemia
  Familial hypercholesterolemia
  Fredrickson's hyperlipoproteinemia, type IIa
  Hyperbetalipoproteinemia
  Hyperlipidemia, Group A
  Low-density-lipoprotein-type [LDL] hyperlipoproteinemia

  E78.1   Pure hyperglyceridemia
  Elevated fasting triglycerides
  Endogenous hyperglyceridemia
  Fredrickson's hyperlipoproteinemia, type IV
  Hyperlipidemia, group B
  Hyperprebetalipoproteinemia
  Very-low-density-lipoprotein-type [VLDL] hyperlipoproteinemia

  E78.2   Mixed hyperlipidemia
  Broad- or floating-betalipoproteinemia
  Combined hyperlipidemia NOS
  Elevated cholesterol with elevated triglycerides NEC
  Fredrickson's hyperlipoproteinemia, type IIb or III
  Hyperbetalipoproteinemia with prebetalipoproteinemia
  Hypercholesteremia with endogenous hyperglyceridemia
  Hyperlipidemia, group C
  Tubo-eruptive xanthoma
  Xanthoma tuberosum

  Excludes1   cerebrotendinous cholesterosis [van Bogaert-Scherer-Epstein] (E75.5)
  familial combined hyperlipidemia (E78.4)

CHAPTER 4 (E00-E90)

E78.3 **Hyperchylomicronemia**
    Chylomicron retention disease
    Fredrickson's hyperlipoproteinemia, type I or V
    Hyperlipidemia, group D
    Mixed hyperglyceridemia

E78.4 **Other hyperlipidemia**
    Familial combined hyperlipidemia

E78.5 **Hyperlipidemia, unspecified**

E78.6 **Lipoprotein deficiency**
    Abetalipoproteinemia
    Depressed HDL cholesterol
    High-density lipoprotein deficiency
    Hypoalphalipoproteinemia
    Hypobetalipoproteinemia (familial)
    Lecithin cholesterol acyltransferase deficiency
    Tangier disease

● **E78.7** **Disorders of bile acid and cholesterol metabolism**
    Excludes1   Niemann-Pick disease type C (E75.242)

    E78.70 **Disorder of bile acid and cholesterol metabolism, unspecified**

    E78.71 **Barth syndrome**

    E78.72 **Smith-Lemli-Opitz syndrome**

    E78.79 **Other disorders of bile acid and cholesterol metabolism**

● **E78.8** **Other disorders of lipoprotein metabolism**
    E78.81 **Lipoid dermatoarthritis**

    E78.89 **Other lipoprotein metabolism disorders**

E78.9 **Disorder of lipoprotein metabolism, unspecified**

● **E79** **Disorders of purine and pyrimidine metabolism**
Purines, along with pyrimidines, signal RNA and DNA production
    Excludes1   Ataxia-telangiectasia (Q87.1)
               Bloom's syndrome (Q82.8)
               Cockayne's syndrome (Q87.1)
               calculus of kidney (N20.0)
               combined immunodeficiency disorders (D81.-)
               Fanconi's anemia (D61.09)
               gout (M1A.-, M10.-)
               orotaciduric anemia (D53.0)
               progeria (E34.8)
               Werner's syndrome (E34.8)
               xeroderma pigmentosum (Q82.1)

E79.0 **Hyperuricemia without signs of inflammatory arthritis and tophaceous disease**
    Asymptomatic hyperuricemia

E79.1 **Lesch-Nyhan syndrome**
    HGPRT deficiency

E79.2 **Myoadenylate deaminase deficiency**

E79.8 **Other disorders of purine and pyrimidine metabolism**
    Hereditary xanthinuria

E79.9 **Disorder of purine and pyrimidine metabolism, unspecified**

● **E80** **Disorders of porphyrin and bilirubin metabolism**
Group of chemical compounds in RBC's that combine with iron to form heme
    Includes   defects of catalase and peroxidase

E80.0 **Hereditary erythropoietic porphyria**
    Congenital erythropoietic porphyria
    Erythropoietic protoporphyria

E80.1 **Porphyria cutanea tarda**

● **E80.2** **Other and unspecified porphyria**
    E80.20 **Unspecified porphyria**
        Porphyria NOS

    E80.21 **Acute intermittent (hepatic) porphyria**

    E80.29 **Other porphyria**
        Hereditary coproporphyria

E80.3 **Defects of catalase and peroxidase**
    Acatalasia [Takahara]

E80.4 **Gilbert syndrome**

E80.5 **Crigler-Najjar syndrome**

E80.6 **Other disorders of bilirubin metabolism**
    Dubin-Johnson syndrome
    Rotor's syndrome

E80.7 **Disorder of bilirubin metabolism, unspecified**

● **E83** **Disorders of mineral metabolism**
    Excludes1   dietary mineral deficiency (E58-E61)
               parathyroid disorders (E20-E21)
               vitamin D deficiency (E55.-)

● **E83.0** **Disorders of copper metabolism**
    E83.00 **Disorder of copper metabolism, unspecified**

    E83.01 **Wilson's disease**
        Code also associated Kayser Fleischer ring (H18.04-)

    E83.09 **Other disorders of copper metabolism**
        Menkes' (kinky hair) (steely hair) disease

● **E83.1** **Disorders of iron metabolism**
    Excludes1   iron deficiency anemia (D50.-)
               sideroblastic anemia (D64.0-D64.3)

    E83.10 **Disorder of iron metabolism, unspecified**

    ● **E83.11** **Hemochromatosis**
        E83.110 **Hereditary hemochromatosis**
            Bronzed diabetes
            Pigmentary cirrhosis (of liver)
            Primary (hereditary) hemochromatosis

        E83.111 **Hemochromatosis due to repeated red blood cell transfusions**
            Iron overload due to repeated red blood cell transfusions
            Transfusion (red blood cell) associated hemochromatosis

        E83.118 **Other hemochromatosis**

        E83.119 **Hemochromatosis, unspecified**

    E83.19 **Other disorders of iron metabolism**
        Use additional code, if applicable, for idiopathic pulmonary hemosiderosis (J84.03)

E83.2 **Disorders of zinc metabolism**
    Acrodermatitis enteropathica

● **E83.3** **Disorders of phosphorus metabolism and phosphatases**
    Excludes1   adult osteomalacia (M83.-)
               osteoporosis (M80.-)

    E83.30 **Disorder of phosphorus metabolism, unspecified**

    E83.31 **Familial hypophosphatemia**
        Vitamin D-resistant osteomalacia
        Vitamin D-resistant rickets
        Excludes1   vitamin D-deficiency rickets (E55.0)

    E83.32 **Hereditary vitamin D-dependent rickets (type 1) (type 2)**
        25-hydroxyvitamin D 1-alpha-hydroxylase deficiency
        Pseudovitamin D deficiency
        Vitamin D receptor defect

    E83.39 **Other disorders of phosphorus metabolism**
        Acid phosphatase deficiency
        Hypophosphatasia

● **E83.4** **Disorders of magnesium metabolism**
    E83.40 **Disorders of magnesium metabolism, unspecified**

    E83.41 **Hypermagnesemia**

    E83.42 **Hypomagnesemia**

    E83.49 **Other disorders of magnesium metabolism**

CHAPTER 4 (E00-E90)

● **E83.5**   **Disorders of calcium metabolism**

    Excludes 1   chondrocalcinosis (M11.1-M11.2)
                   hungry bone syndrome (E83.81)
                   hyperparathyroidism (E21.0-E21.3)

    E83.50   Unspecified disorder of calcium metabolism

    E83.51   Hypocalcemia

    E83.52   Hypercalcemia
            Familial hypocalciuric hypercalcemia

    E83.59   Other disorders of calcium metabolism
            Idiopathic hypercalciuria

● **E83.8**   **Other disorders of mineral metabolism**

    E83.81   Hungry bone syndrome

    E83.89   Other disorders of mineral metabolism

   E83.9   **Disorder of mineral metabolism, unspecified**

● **E84**   **Cystic fibrosis**

    Includes   mucoviscidosis

   E84.0   **Cystic fibrosis with pulmonary manifestations**

        Use additional code to identify any infectious organism
            present, such as:
            Pseudomonas (B96.5)

● **E84.1**   **Cystic fibrosis with intestinal manifestations**

    E84.11   Meconium ileus in cystic fibrosis

       Excludes 1   meconium ileus not due to cystic
                      fibrosis (P76.0)

    E84.19   Cystic fibrosis with other intestinal
          manifestations
           Distal intestinal obstruction syndrome

   E84.8   **Cystic fibrosis with other manifestations**

   E84.9   **Cystic fibrosis, unspecified**

● **E85**   **Amyloidosis**

    A disorder resulting from the abnormal deposition of a particular
    protein (amyloid) into tissues of the body.

    Excludes 1   Alzheimer's disease (G30.0-)

   E85.0   **Non-neuropathic heredofamilial amyloidosis**
        Familial Mediterranean fever
        Hereditary amyloid nephropathy

   E85.1   **Neuropathic heredofamilial amyloidosis**
        Amyloid polyneuropathy (Portuguese)

   E85.2   **Heredofamilial amyloidosis, unspecified**

   E85.3   **Secondary systemic amyloidosis**
        Hemodialysis-associated amyloidosis

   E85.4   **Organ-limited amyloidosis**
        Localized amyloidosis

   E85.8   **Other amyloidosis**

   E85.9   **Amyloidosis, unspecified**

● **E86**   **Volume depletion**

    Excludes 1   dehydration of newborn (P74.1)
                 hypovolemic shock NOS (R57.1)
                 postprocedural hypovolemic shock (T81.19)
                 traumatic hypovolemic shock (T79.4)

   E86.0   **Dehydration**
        Excessive loss of body water

   E86.1   **Hypovolemia**
        Diminished volume of circulating blood
        Depletion of volume of plasma

   E86.9   **Volume depletion, unspecified**

Item 4–9 Circulating fluid volume is regulated by the amount of water and sodium ingested, excreted by the kidneys into the urine, and lost through the gastrointestinal tract, lungs, and skin. To maintain blood volume within a normal range, the kidneys regulate the amount of water and sodium lost into the urine. Too much (**fluid overload**) or too little fluid volume (**volume depletion**) will affect blood pressure. Severe cases of vomiting, diarrhea, bleeding, and burns (fluid loss through exposed burn surface area) can contribute to fluid loss. Internal body environment must maintain a precise balance (homeostasis) between too much fluid and too little fluid. This complex balancing mechanism is critical to good health.

● **E87**   **Other disorders of fluid, electrolyte and acid-base balance**

    Excludes 1   diabetes insipidus (E23.2)
                 electrolyte imbalance associated with
                    hyperemesis gravidarum (O21.1)
                 electrolyte imbalance following ectopic or molar
                    pregnancy (O08.5)
                 familial periodic paralysis (G72.3)

   E87.0   **Hyperosmolality and hypernatremia**
        Sodium [Na] excess
        Sodium [Na] overload

   E87.1   **Hypo-osmolality and hyponatremia**
        Sodium [Na] deficiency

      Excludes 1   syndrome of inappropriate secretion of
                     antidiuretic hormone (E22.2)

   E87.2   **Acidosis**
        Acidosis NOS
        Lactic acidosis
        Metabolic acidosis
        Respiratory acidosis

      Excludes 1   diabetic acidosis - see categories E08-E10,
                     E13 with ketoacidosis

   E87.3   **Alkalosis**
        Alkalosis NOS
        Metabolic alkalosis
        Respiratory alkalosis

   E87.4   **Mixed disorder of acid-base balance**

   E87.5   **Hyperkalemia**
        Potassium [K] excess
        Potassium [K] overload

   E87.6   **Hypokalemia**
        Potassium [K] deficiency

● **E87.7**   **Fluid overload**

    Excludes 1   edema NOS (R60.9)
                 fluid retention (R60.9)

    E87.70   Fluid overload, unspecified

    E87.71   Transfusion associated circulatory overload
           Fluid overload due to transfusion (blood)
           (blood components) TACO

    E87.79   Other fluid overload

   E87.8   **Other disorders of electrolyte and fluid balance, not**
        elsewhere classified
        Electrolyte imbalance NOS
        Hyperchloremia
        Hypochloremia

● **E88**   **Other and unspecified metabolic disorders**

    Use additional codes for associated conditions

    Excludes 1   histiocytosis X (chronic) (C96.6)

● **E88.0**   **Disorders of plasma-protein metabolism, not elsewhere**
        classified

      Excludes 1   disorder of lipoprotein metabolism (E78.-)
                   monoclonal gammopathy (of
                     undetermined significance) (D47.2)
                   polyclonal hypergammaglobulinemia
                     (D89.0)
                   Waldenström macroglobulinemia (C88.0)

    E88.01   Alpha-1-antitrypsin deficiency AAT deficiency

    E88.09   Other disorders of plasma-protein metabolism,
          not elsewhere classified
          Bisalbuminemia

   E88.1   **Lipodystrophy, not elsewhere classified**
        Defective fat metabolism resulting in absence of subcutaneous
        fat
        Lipodystrophy NOS

      Excludes 1   Whipple's disease (K90.81)

   E88.2   **Lipomatosis, not elsewhere classified**
        Abnormal tumorlike accumulations of fat in tissue
        Lipomatosis NOS
        Lipomatosis (Check) dolorosa [Dercum]

CHAPTER 4 (E00-E90)

E88.3   Tumor lysis syndrome
　　　Tumor lysis syndrome (spontaneous)
　　　Tumor lysis syndrome following antineoplastic drug
　　　　　chemotherapy
　　　Use additional code for adverse effect, if applicable, to
　　　　　identify drug (T45.1X5)

● **E88.4   Mitochondrial metabolism disorders**
　　　Congenital disorder of metabolism
　　　Excludes1 | disorders of pyruvate metabolism (E74.4)
　　　　　Kearns-Sayre syndrome (H49.81)
　　　　　Leber's disease (H47.22)
　　　　　Leigh's encephalopathy (G31.82)
　　　　　Mitochondrial myopathy, NEC (G71.3)
　　　　　Reye's syndrome (G93.7)

　　**E88.40   Mitochondrial metabolism disorder,
　　　　　　unspecified**

　　E88.41   MELAS syndrome
　　　　　Mitochondrial myopathy, encephalopathy,
　　　　　　　lactic acidosis and stroke-like episodes

　　E88.42   MERRF syndrome
　　　　　Myoclonic epilepsy associated with ragged-red
　　　　　　　fibers
　　　　　Code also myoclonic epilepsy (G40.3-)

　　E88.49   Other mitochondrial metabolism disorders

● **E88.8   Other specified metabolic disorders**
　　E88.81   Metabolic syndrome
　　　　　Dysmetabolic syndrome X
　　　　　Use additional codes for associated
　　　　　　　manifestations, such as:
　　　　　obesity (E66.-)

　　E88.89   Other specified metabolic disorders
　　　　　Launois-Bensaude adenolipomatosis
　　　　　Excludes1 | adult pulmonary Langerhans cell
　　　　　　　histiocytosis (J84.82)

E88.9   Metabolic disorder, unspecified

**POSTPROCEDURAL ENDOCRINE AND METABOLIC COMPLICATIONS
AND DISORDERS, NOT ELSEWHERE CLASSIFIED (E89)**

● **E89   Postprocedural endocrine and metabolic complications and
　　disorders, not elsewhere classified**
　　Excludes2 | intraoperative complications of endocrine system
　　　　　organ or structure (E36.0-, E36.1-, E36.8)

E89.0   Postprocedural hypothyroidism
　　　Postirradiation hypothyroidism
　　　Postsurgical hypothyroidism

E89.1   Postprocedural hypoinsulinemia
　　　Postpancreatectomy hyperglycemia
　　　Postsurgical hypoinsulinemia
　　　Use additional code, if applicable, to identify:
　　　　acquired absence of pancreas (Z90.41-)
　　　　diabetes mellitus (postpancreatectomy)
　　　　　(postprocedural) (E13.-)
　　　　insulin use (Z79.4)
　　　Excludes1 | transient postprocedural hyperglycemia
　　　　　　(R73.9)
　　　　　transient postprocedural hypoglycemia
　　　　　　(E16.2)

E89.2   Postprocedural hypoparathyroidism
　　　Parathyroprival tetany

E89.3   Postprocedural hypopituitarism
　　　Postirradiation hypopituitarism

● **E89.4   Postprocedural ovarian failure**
　　E89.40   Asymptomatic postprocedural ovarian failure
　　　　　Postprocedural ovarian failure NOS

　　E89.41   Symptomatic postprocedural ovarian failure
　　　　　Symptoms such as flushing, sleeplessness,
　　　　　　headache, lack of concentration,
　　　　　　associated with postprocedural
　　　　　　menopause

E89.5   Postprocedural testicular hypofunction

**E89.6   Postprocedural adrenocortical (-medullary)
　　hypofunction**

● **E89.8   Other postprocedural endocrine and metabolic
　　complications and disorders**
　　● **E89.81   Postprocedural hemorrhage and hematoma
　　　　of an endocrine system organ or structure
　　　　following a procedure**
　　　　**E89.810   Postprocedural hemorrhage and
　　　　　　hematoma of an endocrine system
　　　　　　organ or structure following an
　　　　　　endocrine system procedure**

　　　　**E89.811   Postprocedural hemorrhage and
　　　　　　hematoma of an endocrine system
　　　　　　organ or structure following other
　　　　　　procedure**

　　**E89.89   Other postprocedural endocrine and metabolic
　　　　complications and disorders**
　　　　Use additional code, if applicable, to further
　　　　　specify disorder

CHAPTER 5

MENTAL, BEHAVIORAL AND NEURODEVELOPMENTAL DISORDERS (F01-F99)

| **Includes** | disorders of psychological development |
| **Excludes2** | symptoms, signs and abnormal clinical laboratory findings, not elsewhere classified (R00-R99) |

This chapter contains the following blocks:

F01-F09	Mental disorders due to known physiological conditions
F10-F19	Mental and behavioral disorders due to psychoactive substance use
F20-F29	Schizophrenia, schizotypal, delusional, and other non-mood psychotic disorders
F30-F39	Mood [affective] disorders
F40-F48	Anxiety, dissociative, stress-related, somatoform and other nonpsychotic mental disorders
F50-F59	Behavioral syndromes associated with physiological disturbances and physical factors
F60-F69	Disorders of adult personality and behavior
F70-F79	Intellectual disabilities
F80-F89	Pervasive and specific developmental disorders
F90-F98	Behavioral and emotional disorders with onset usually occurring in childhood and adolescence
F99	Unspecified mental disorder

MENTAL DISORDERS DUE TO KNOWN PHYSIOLOGICAL CONDITIONS (F01-F09)

This block comprises a range of mental disorders grouped together on the basis of their having in common a demonstrable etiology in cerebral disease, brain injury, or other insult leading to cerebral dysfunction. The dysfunction may be primary, as in diseases, injuries, and insults that affect the brain directly and selectively; or secondary, as in systemic diseases and disorders that attack the brain only as one of the multiple organs or systems of the body that are involved.

● **F01**   **Vascular dementia**

Vascular dementia as a result of infarction of the brain due to vascular disease, including hypertensive cerebrovascular disease.

| **Includes** | arteriosclerotic dementia |

Code first the underlying physiological condition or sequelae of cerebrovascular disease.

● **F01.5**   **Vascular dementia**

F01.50   **Vascular dementia without behavioral disturbance**

F01.51   **Vascular dementia with behavioral disturbance**
Vascular dementia with aggressive behavior
Vascular dementia with combative behavior
Vascular dementia with violent behavior

Use additional code, if applicable, to identify wandering in vascular dementia (Z91.83)

● **F02**   **Dementia in other diseases classified elsewhere**

Code first the underlying physiological condition, such as:
Alzheimer's (G30.-)
cerebral lipidosis (E75.4)
Creutzfeldt-Jakob disease (A81.0-)
dementia with Lewy bodies (G31.83)
epilepsy and recurrent seizures (G40.-)
frontotemporal dementia (G31.09)
hepatolenticular degeneration (E83.0)
human immunodeficiency virus [HIV] disease (B20)
hypercalcemia (E83.52)
hypothyroidism, acquired (E00-E03.-)
intoxications (T36-T65)
Jakob-Creutzfeldt disease (A81.0-)
multiple sclerosis (G35)
neurosyphilis (A52.17)
niacin deficiency [pellagra] (E52)
Parkinson's disease (G20)
Pick's disease (G31.01)
polyarteritis nodosa (M30.0)
systemic lupus erythematosus (M32.-)
trypanosomiasis (B56.-, B57.-)
vitamin B deficiency (E53.8)

Excludes1	dementia with Parkinsonism (G31.83)
Excludes2	dementia in alcohol and psychoactive substance disorders (F10-F19, with .17, .27, .97)
	vascular dementia (F01.5-)

● **F02.8**   **Dementia in other diseases classified elsewhere**

F02.80   **Dementia in other diseases classified elsewhere without behavioral disturbance**
Dementia in other diseases classified elsewhere NOS

F02.81   **Dementia in other diseases classified elsewhere with behavioral disturbance**
Dementia in other diseases classified elsewhere with aggressive behavior
Dementia in other diseases classified elsewhere with combative behavior
Dementia in other diseases classified elsewhere with violent behavior

Use additional code, if applicable, to identify wandering in dementia in conditions classified elsewhere (Z91.83)

● **F03**   **Unspecified dementia**
Presenile dementia NOS
Presenile psychosis NOS
Primary degenerative dementia NOS
Senile dementia NOS
Senile dementia depressed or paranoid type
Senile psychosis NOS

Excludes1	senility NOS (R41.81)
Excludes2	mild memory disturbance due to known physiological condition (F06.8)
	senile dementia with delirium or acute confusional state (F05)

● **F03.9**   **Unspecified dementia**

F03.90   **Unspecified dementia without behavioral disturbance**
Dementia NOS

F03.91   **Unspecified dementia with behavioral disturbance**
Unspecified dementia with aggressive behavior
Unspecified dementia with combative behavior
Unspecified dementia with violent behavior

Use additional code, if applicable, to identify wandering in unspecified dementia (Z91.83)

Item 5-1 Psychosis was a term formerly applied to any mental disorder but is now restricted to disturbances of a great magnitude in which there is a personality disintegration and loss of contact with reality.

F04   Amnestic disorder due to known physiological condition
    Korsakov's psychosis or syndrome, nonalcoholic
    Code first the underlying physiological condition
    Excludes1   amnesia NOS (R41.3)
                    anterograde amnesia (R41.1)
                    dissociative amnesia (F44.0)
                    retrograde amnesia (R41.2)
    Excludes2   alcohol-induced or unspecified Korsakov's
                    syndrome (F10.26, F10.96)
                    Korsakov's syndrome induced by other
                    psychoactive substances (F13.26, F13.96,
                    F19.16, F19.26, F19.96)

F05   Delirium due to known physiological condition
    Acute or subacute brain syndrome
    Acute or subacute confusional state (nonalcoholic)
    Acute or subacute infective psychosis
    Acute or subacute organic reaction
    Acute or subacute psycho-organic syndrome
    Delirium of mixed etiology
    Delirium superimposed on dementia
    Sundowning
    Code first the underlying physiological condition
    Excludes1   delirium NOS (R41.0)
    Excludes2   delirium tremens alcohol-induced or unspecified
                    (F10.231, F10.921)

● **F06   Other mental disorders due to known physiological condition**
    Includes   mental disorders due to endocrine disorder
                    mental disorders due to exogenous hormone
                    mental disorders due to exogenous toxic
                    substance
                    mental disorders due to primary cerebral disease
                    mental disorders due to somatic illness
                    mental disorders due to systemic disease
                    affecting the brain
    Code first the underlying physiological condition
    Excludes1   unspecified dementia (F03)
    Excludes2   delirium due to known physiological condition
                    (F05)
                    dementia as classified in F01-F02
                    other mental disorders associated with alcohol
                    and other psychoactive substances (F10-F19)

    F06.0   Psychotic disorder with hallucinations due to known physiological condition
        Organic hallucinatory state (nonalcoholic)
        Excludes2   hallucinations and perceptual disturbance
                        induced by alcohol and other
                        psychoactive substances (F10-F19
                        with .151, .251, .951)
                        schizophrenia (F20.-)

    F06.1   Catatonic disorder due to known physiological condition
        Excludes1   catatonic stupor (R40.1)
                        stupor NOS (R40.1)
        Excludes2   catatonic schizophrenia (F20.2)
                        dissociative stupor (F44.2)

    F06.2   Psychotic disorder with delusions due to known physiological condition
        Paranoid and paranoid-hallucinatory organic states
        Schizophrenia-like psychosis in epilepsy
        Excludes2   alcohol and drug-induced psychotic
                        disorder (F10-F19 with .150, .250,
                        .950)
                        brief psychotic disorder (F23)
                        delusional disorder (F22)
                        schizophrenia (F20.-)

● **F06.3   Mood disorder due to known physiological condition**
        Excludes2   mood disorders due to alcohol and other
                        psychoactive
                        substances (F10-F19 with .14, .24, .94)
                        mood disorders, not due to known
                        physiological condition or
                        unspecified (F30-F39)

    F06.30   Mood disorder due to known physiological condition, unspecified

    F06.31   Mood disorder due to known physiological condition with depressive features

    F06.32   Mood disorder due to known physiological condition with major depressive-like episode

    F06.33   Mood disorder due to known physiological condition with manic features

    F06.34   Mood disorder due to known physiological condition with mixed features

    F06.4   Anxiety disorder due to known physiological condition
        Excludes2   anxiety disorders due to alcohol and
                        other psychoactive substances
                        (F10-F19 with .180, .280, .980)
                        anxiety disorders, not due to known
                        physiological condition or
                        unspecified (F40.-, F41.-)

    F06.8   Other specified mental disorders due to known physiological condition
        Epileptic psychosis NOS
        Organic dissociative disorder
        Organic emotionally labile [asthenic] disorder

● **F07   Personality and behavioral disorders due to known physiological condition**
    Code first the underlying physiological condition

    F07.0   Personality change due to known physiological condition
        Frontal lobe syndrome
        Limbic epilepsy personality syndrome
        Lobotomy syndrome
        Organic personality disorder
        Organic pseudopsychopathic personality
        Organic pseudoretarded personality
        Postleucotomy syndrome
        Code first underlying physiological condition
        Excludes1   mild cognitive impairment (G31.84)
                        postconcussional syndrome (F07.81)
                        postencephalitic syndrome (F07.89)
                        signs and symptoms involving emotional
                        state (R45.-)
        Excludes2   specific personality disorder (F60.-)

● **F07.8   Other personality and behavioral disorders due to known physiological condition**

    F07.81   Postconcussional syndrome
        Postcontusional syndrome (encephalopathy)
        Post-traumatic brain syndrome, nonpsychotic
        Use additional code to identify associated
        post-traumatic headache, if applicable
        (G44.3-)
        Excludes1   current concussion (brain)
                        (S06.0-)
                        postencephalitic syndrome
                        (F07.89)

    F07.89   Other personality and behavioral disorders due to known physiological condition
        Postencephalitic syndrome
        Damage to temporal brain lobes with memory loss and abnormal behavior
        Right hemispheric organic affective disorder

    F07.9   Unspecified personality and behavioral disorder due to known physiological condition
        Organic psychosyndrome
        Due to exposure to organic solvents

◄ New   ◄░ Revised   ~~deleted~~ Deleted   **OGCR** Official Guidelines   X Assign placeholder X   ● Use Additional Character(s)
    Excludes 1   Excludes 2   Includes   Use additional   Code first   Code also   Unspecified

F09　Unspecified mental disorder due to known physiological
　　　condition
　　　　　Mental disorder NOS due to known physiological condition
　　　　　Organic brain syndrome NOS
　　　　　Organic mental disorder NOS
　　　　　Organic psychosis NOS
　　　　　Symptomatic psychosis NOS
　　　　　Code first the underlying physiological condition
　　　　　Excludes1　psychosis NOS (F29)

MENTAL AND BEHAVIORAL DISORDERS DUE TO PSYCHOACTIVE SUBSTANCE USE (F10-F19)

● F10　Alcohol related disorders
　　　　　Use additional code for blood alcohol level, if applicable (Y90.-)

● F10.1　Alcohol abuse
　　　　　Excludes1　alcohol dependence (F10.2-)
　　　　　　　　　　　　　　alcohol use, unspecified (F10.9-)
　　　F10.10　Alcohol abuse, uncomplicated
　● F10.12　Alcohol abuse with intoxication
　　　　　F10.120　Alcohol abuse with intoxication,
　　　　　　　　　　uncomplicated
　　　　　F10.121　Alcohol abuse with intoxication,
　　　　　　　　　　delirium
　　　　　F10.129　Alcohol abuse with
　　　　　　　　　　intoxication, unspecified
　　　F10.14　Alcohol abuse with alcohol-induced mood
　　　　　　　　disorder
　● F10.15　Alcohol abuse with alcohol-induced psychotic
　　　　　　　disorder
　　　　　F10.150　Alcohol abuse with alcohol-induced
　　　　　　　　　　psychotic disorder with delusions
　　　　　F10.151　Alcohol abuse with alcohol-
　　　　　　　　　　induced psychotic disorder with
　　　　　　　　　　hallucinations
　　　　　F10.159　Alcohol abuse with alcohol-induced
　　　　　　　　　　psychotic disorder, unspecified
　● F10.18　Alcohol abuse with other alcohol-induced
　　　　　　　disorders
　　　　　F10.180　Alcohol abuse with alcohol-induced
　　　　　　　　　　anxiety disorder
　　　　　F10.181　Alcohol abuse with alcohol-induced
　　　　　　　　　　sexual dysfunction
　　　　　F10.182　Alcohol abuse with alcohol-induced
　　　　　　　　　　sleep disorder
　　　　　F10.188　Alcohol abuse with other alcohol-
　　　　　　　　　　induced disorder
　　　F10.19　Alcohol abuse with unspecified alcohol-
　　　　　　　　induced disorder

● F10.2　Alcohol dependence
　　　　　Excludes1　alcohol abuse (F10.1-)
　　　　　　　　　　　　　　alcohol use, unspecified (F10.9-)
　　　　　Excludes2　toxic effect of alcohol (T51.0-)
　　　F10.20　Alcohol dependence, uncomplicated
　　　F10.21　Alcohol dependence, in remission
　● F10.22　Alcohol dependence with intoxication
　　　　　　Acute drunkenness (in alcoholism)
　　　　　　Excludes1　alcohol dependence with
　　　　　　　　　　　　　withdrawal (F10.23-)
　　　　　F10.220　Alcohol dependence with
　　　　　　　　　　intoxication, uncomplicated
　　　　　F10.221　Alcohol dependence with intoxication
　　　　　　　　　　delirium
　　　　　F10.229　Alcohol dependence with
　　　　　　　　　　intoxication, unspecified

● F10.23　Alcohol dependence with withdrawal
　　　　　Excludes1　alcohol dependence with intoxication
　　　　　　　　　　　　　(F10.22-)
　　　　　F10.230　Alcohol dependence with
　　　　　　　　　　withdrawal, uncomplicated
　　　　　F10.231　Alcohol dependence with withdrawal
　　　　　　　　　　delirium
　　　　　F10.232　Alcohol dependence with withdrawal
　　　　　　　　　　with perceptual disturbance
　　　　　F10.239　Alcohol dependence with
　　　　　　　　　　withdrawal, unspecified
　　　F10.24　Alcohol dependence with alcohol-induced
　　　　　　　　mood disorder
　● F10.25　Alcohol dependence with alcohol-induced
　　　　　　　psychotic disorder
　　　　　F10.250　Alcohol dependence with alcohol-
　　　　　　　　　　induced psychotic disorder with
　　　　　　　　　　delusions
　　　　　F10.251　Alcohol dependence with alcohol-
　　　　　　　　　　induced psychotic disorder with
　　　　　　　　　　hallucinations
　　　　　F10.259　Alcohol dependence with
　　　　　　　　　　alcohol-induced psychotic
　　　　　　　　　　disorder, unspecified
　　　F10.26　Alcohol dependence with alcohol-induced
　　　　　　　　persisting amnestic disorder
　　　F10.27　Alcohol dependence with alcohol-induced
　　　　　　　　persisting dementia
　● F10.28　Alcohol dependence with other alcohol-
　　　　　　　induced disorders
　　　　　F10.280　Alcohol dependence with alcohol-
　　　　　　　　　　induced anxiety disorder
　　　　　F10.281　Alcohol dependence with alcohol-
　　　　　　　　　　induced sexual dysfunction
　　　　　F10.282　Alcohol dependence with alcohol-
　　　　　　　　　　induced sleep disorder
　　　　　F10.288　Alcohol dependence with other
　　　　　　　　　　alcohol-induced disorder
　　　F10.29　Alcohol dependence with unspecified alcohol-
　　　　　　　　induced disorder

● F10.9　Alcohol use, unspecified
　　　　　Excludes1　alcohol abuse (F10.1-)
　　　　　　　　　　　　　　alcohol dependence (F10.2-)
　● F10.92　Alcohol use, unspecified with intoxication
　　　　　F10.920　Alcohol use, unspecified with
　　　　　　　　　　intoxication, uncomplicated
　　　　　F10.921　Alcohol use, unspecified with
　　　　　　　　　　intoxication delirium
　　　　　F10.929　Alcohol use, unspecified with
　　　　　　　　　　intoxication, unspecified
　　　F10.94　Alcohol use, unspecified with alcohol-induced
　　　　　　　　mood disorder
　● F10.95　Alcohol use, unspecified with alcohol-induced
　　　　　　　psychotic disorder
　　　　　F10.950　Alcohol use, unspecified with
　　　　　　　　　　alcohol-induced psychotic disorder
　　　　　　　　　　with delusions
　　　　　F10.951　Alcohol use, unspecified with
　　　　　　　　　　alcohol-induced psychotic disorder
　　　　　　　　　　with hallucinations
　　　　　F10.959　Alcohol use, unspecified with
　　　　　　　　　　alcohol-induced psychotic disorder,
　　　　　　　　　　unspecified
　　　F10.96　Alcohol use, unspecified with alcohol-induced
　　　　　　　　persisting amnestic disorder
　　　F10.97　Alcohol use, unspecified with alcohol-induced
　　　　　　　　persisting dementia

CHAPTER 5 (F01-F99)

CHAPTER 5 (F01-F99)

● F10.98   Alcohol use, unspecified with other alcohol-induced disorders

F10.980   Alcohol use, unspecified with alcohol-induced anxiety disorder

F10.981   Alcohol use, unspecified with alcohol-induced sexual dysfunction

F10.982   Alcohol use, unspecified with alcohol-induced sleep disorder

F10.988   Alcohol use, unspecified with other alcohol-induced disorder

F10.99   Alcohol use, unspecified with unspecified alcohol-induced disorder

● F11   Opioid related disorders

● F11.1   Opioid abuse

Excludes1   opioid dependence (F11.2-)
             opioid use, unspecified (F11.9-)

F11.10   Opioid abuse, uncomplicated

● F11.12   Opioid abuse with intoxication

F11.120   Opioid abuse with intoxication, uncomplicated

F11.121   Opioid abuse with intoxication delirium

F11.122   Opioid abuse with intoxication with perceptual disturbance

F11.129   Opioid abuse with intoxication, unspecified

F11.14   Opioid abuse with opioid-induced mood disorder

● F11.15   Opioid abuse with opioid-induced psychotic disorder

F11.150   Opioid abuse with opioid-induced psychotic disorder with delusions

F11.151   Opioid abuse with opioid-induced psychotic disorder with hallucinations

F11.159   Opioid abuse with opioid-induced psychotic disorder, unspecified

● F11.18   Opioid abuse with other opioid-induced disorder

F11.181   Opioid abuse with opioid-induced sexual dysfunction

F11.182   Opioid abuse with opioid-induced sleep disorder

F11.188   Opioid abuse with other opioid-induced disorder

F11.19   Opioid abuse with unspecified opioid-induced disorder

● F11.2   Opioid dependence

Excludes1   opioid abuse (F11.1-)
             opioid use, unspecified (F11.9-)

Excludes2   opioid poisoning (T40.0--T40.2-)

F11.20   Opioid dependence, uncomplicated

F11.21   Opioid dependence, in remission

● F11.22   Opioid dependence with intoxication

Excludes1   opioid dependence with withdrawal (F11.23)

F11.220   Opioid dependence with intoxication, uncomplicated

F11.221   Opioid dependence with intoxication delirium

F11.222   Opioid dependence with intoxication with perceptual disturbance

F11.229   Opioid dependence with intoxication, unspecified

F11.23   Opioid dependence with withdrawal

Excludes1   opioid dependence with intoxication (F11.22-)

F11.24   Opioid dependence with opioid-induced mood disorder

● F11.25   Opioid dependence with opioid-induced psychotic disorder

F11.250   Opioid dependence with opioid-induced psychotic disorder with delusions

F11.251   Opioid dependence with opioid-induced psychotic disorder with hallucinations

F11.259   Opioid dependence with opioid-induced psychotic disorder, unspecified

● F11.28   Opioid dependence with other opioid-induced disorder

F11.281   Opioid dependence with opioid-induced sexual dysfunction

F11.282   Opioid dependence with opioid-induced sleep disorder

F11.288   Opioid dependence with other opioid-induced disorder

F11.29   Opioid dependence with unspecified opioid-induced disorder

● F11.9   Opioid use, unspecified

Excludes1   opioid abuse (F11.1-)
             opioid dependence (F11.2-)

F11.90   Opioid use, unspecified, uncomplicated

● F11.92   Opioid use, unspecified with intoxication

Excludes1   opioid use, unspecified with withdrawal (F11.93)

F11.920   Opioid use, unspecified with intoxication, uncomplicated

F11.921   Opioid use, unspecified with intoxication delirium

F11.922   Opioid use, unspecified with intoxication with perceptual disturbance

F11.929   Opioid use, unspecified with intoxication, unspecified

F11.93   Opioid use, unspecified with withdrawal

Excludes1   opioid use, unspecified with intoxication (F11.92-)

F11.94   Opioid use, unspecified with opioid-induced mood disorder

● F11.95   Opioid use, unspecified with opioid-induced psychotic disorder

F11.950   Opioid use, unspecified with opioid-induced psychotic disorder with delusions

F11.951   Opioid use, unspecified with opioid-induced psychotic disorder with hallucinations

F11.959   Opioid use, unspecified with opioid-induced psychotic disorder, unspecified

● F11.98   Opioid use, unspecified with other specified opioid-induced disorder

F11.981   Opioid use, unspecified with opioid-induced sexual dysfunction

F11.982   Opioid use, unspecified with opioid-induced sleep disorder

F11.988   Opioid use, unspecified with other opioid-induced disorder

F11.99   Opioid use, unspecified with unspecified opioid-induced disorder

● **F12**   **Cannabis related disorders**
    Includes   marijuana
● **F12.1**   **Cannabis abuse**
    Excludes1   cannabis dependence (F12.2-)
                 cannabis use, unspecified (F12.9-)
     F12.10   Cannabis abuse, uncomplicated
●   F12.12   Cannabis abuse with intoxication
         F12.120   Cannabis abuse with intoxication, uncomplicated
         F12.121   Cannabis abuse with intoxication delirium
         F12.122   Cannabis abuse with intoxication with perceptual disturbance
         F12.129   Cannabis abuse with intoxication, unspecified
●   F12.15   Cannabis abuse with psychotic disorder
         F12.150   Cannabis abuse with psychotic disorder with delusions
         F12.151   Cannabis abuse with psychotic disorder with hallucinations
         F12.159   Cannabis abuse with psychotic disorder, unspecified
●   F12.18   Cannabis abuse with other cannabis-induced disorder
         F12.180   Cannabis abuse with cannabis-induced anxiety disorder
         F12.188   Cannabis abuse with other cannabis-induced disorder
     F12.19   Cannabis abuse with unspecified cannabis-induced disorder
● **F12.2**   **Cannabis dependence**
    Excludes1   cannabis abuse (F12.1-)
                 cannabis use, unspecified (F12.9-)
    Excludes2   cannabis poisoning (T40.7-)
     F12.20   Cannabis dependence, uncomplicated
     F12.21   Cannabis dependence, in remission
●   F12.22   Cannabis dependence with intoxication
         F12.220   Cannabis dependence with intoxication, uncomplicated
         F12.221   Cannabis dependence with intoxication delirium
         F12.222   Cannabis dependence with intoxication with perceptual disturbance
         F12.229   Cannabis dependence with intoxication, unspecified
●   F12.25   Cannabis dependence with psychotic disorder
         F12.250   Cannabis dependence with psychotic disorder with delusions
         F12.251   Cannabis dependence with psychotic disorder with hallucinations
         F12.259   Cannabis dependence with psychotic disorder, unspecified
●   F12.28   Cannabis dependence with other cannabis-induced disorder
         F12.280   Cannabis dependence with cannabis-induced anxiety disorder
         F12.288   Cannabis dependence with other cannabis-induced disorder
     F12.29   Cannabis dependence with unspecified cannabis-induced disorder

● **F12.9**   **Cannabis use, unspecified**
    Excludes1   cannabis abuse (F12.1-)
                 cannabis dependence (F12.2-)
     F12.90   Cannabis use, unspecified, uncomplicated
●   F12.92   Cannabis use, unspecified with intoxication
         F12.920   Cannabis use, unspecified with intoxication, uncomplicated
         F12.921   Cannabis use, unspecified with intoxication delirium
         F12.922   Cannabis use, unspecified with intoxication with perceptual disturbance
         F12.929   Cannabis use, unspecified with intoxication, unspecified
●   F12.95   Cannabis use, unspecified with psychotic disorder
         F12.950   Cannabis use, unspecified with psychotic disorder with delusions
         F12.951   Cannabis use, unspecified with psychotic disorder with hallucinations
         F12.959   Cannabis use, unspecified with psychotic disorder, unspecified
●   F12.98   Cannabis use, unspecified with other cannabis-induced disorder
         F12.980   Cannabis use, unspecified with anxiety disorder
         F12.988   Cannabis use, unspecified with other cannabis-induced disorder
     F12.99   Cannabis use, unspecified with unspecified cannabis-induced disorder

● **F13**   **Sedative, hypnotic, or anxiolytic related disorders**
● **F13.1**   **Sedative, hypnotic or anxiolytic-related abuse**
    Excludes1   sedative, hypnotic or anxiolytic-related dependence (F13.2-)
                 sedative, hypnotic, or anxiolytic use, unspecified (F13.9-)
     F13.10   Sedative, hypnotic or anxiolytic abuse, uncomplicated
●   F13.12   Sedative, hypnotic or anxiolytic abuse with intoxication
         F13.120   Sedative, hypnotic or anxiolytic abuse with intoxication, uncomplicated
         F13.121   Sedative, hypnotic or anxiolytic abuse with intoxication delirium
         F13.129   Sedative, hypnotic or anxiolytic abuse with intoxication, unspecified
     F13.14   Sedative, hypnotic or anxiolytic abuse with sedative, hypnotic or anxiolytic-induced mood disorder
●   F13.15   Sedative, hypnotic or anxiolytic abuse with sedative, hypnotic or anxiolyticinduced psychotic disorder
         F13.150   Sedative, hypnotic or anxiolytic abuse with sedative, hypnotic or anxiolytic-induced psychotic disorder with delusions
         F13.151   Sedative, hypnotic or anxiolytic abuse with sedative, hypnotic or anxiolytic-induced psychotic disorder with hallucinations
         F13.159   Sedative, hypnotic or anxiolytic abuse with sedative, hypnotic or anxiolytic-induced psychotic disorder, unspecified

CHAPTER 5 (F01-F99)

CHAPTER 5 (F01-F99)

● **F13.18**   Sedative, hypnotic or anxiolytic abuse with other sedative, hypnotic or anxiolytic-induced disorders

     F13.180   Sedative, hypnotic or anxiolytic abuse with sedative, hypnotic or anxiolytic-induced anxiety disorder

     F13.181   Sedative, hypnotic or anxiolytic abuse with sedative, hypnotic or anxiolytic-induced sexual dysfunction

     F13.182   Sedative, hypnotic or anxiolytic abuse with sedative, hypnotic or anxiolytic-induced sleep disorder

     F13.188   Sedative, hypnotic or anxiolytic abuse with other sedative, hypnotic or anxiolytic-induced disorder

F13.19   Sedative, hypnotic or anxiolytic abuse with unspecified sedative, hypnotic or anxiolytic-induced disorder

● **F13.2**   Sedative, hypnotic or anxiolytic-related dependence

> **Excludes1**   sedative, hypnotic or anxiolytic-related abuse (F13.1-)
> sedative, hypnotic, or anxiolytic use, unspecified (F13.9-)

> **Excludes2**   sedative, hypnotic, or anxiolytic poisoning (T42.-)

F13.20   Sedative, hypnotic or anxiolytic dependence, uncomplicated

F13.21   Sedative, hypnotic or anxiolytic dependence, in remission

● **F13.22**   Sedative, hypnotic or anxiolytic dependence with intoxication

> **Excludes1**   sedative, hypnotic or anxiolytic dependence with withdrawal (F13.23-)

     F13.220   Sedative, hypnotic or anxiolytic dependence with intoxication, uncomplicated

     F13.221   Sedative, hypnotic or anxiolytic dependence with intoxication delirium

     F13.229   Sedative, hypnotic or anxiolytic dependence with intoxication, unspecified

● **F13.23**   Sedative, hypnotic or anxiolytic dependence with withdrawal

> **Excludes1**   sedative, hypnotic or anxiolytic dependence with intoxication (F13.22-)

     F13.230   Sedative, hypnotic or anxiolytic dependence with withdrawal, uncomplicated

     F13.231   Sedative, hypnotic or anxiolytic dependence with withdrawal delirium

     F13.232   Sedative, hypnotic or anxiolytic dependence with withdrawal with perceptual disturbance

     F13.239   Sedative, hypnotic or anxiolytic dependence with withdrawal, unspecified

F13.24   Sedative, hypnotic or anxiolytic dependence with sedative, hypnotic or anxiolytic-induced mood disorder

● **F13.25**   Sedative, hypnotic or anxiolytic dependence with sedative, hypnotic or anxiolytic-induced psychotic disorder

     F13.250   Sedative, hypnotic or anxiolytic dependence with sedative, hypnotic or anxiolytic-induced psychotic disorder with delusions

     F13.251   Sedative, hypnotic or anxiolytic dependence with sedative, hypnotic or anxiolytic-induced psychotic disorder with hallucinations

     F13.259   Sedative, hypnotic or anxiolytic dependence with sedative, hypnotic or anxiolytic-induced psychotic disorder, unspecified

F13.26   Sedative, hypnotic or anxiolytic dependence with sedative, hypnotic or anxiolytic-induced persisting amnestic disorder

F13.27   Sedative, hypnotic or anxiolytic dependence with sedative, hypnotic or anxiolytic-induced persisting dementia

● **F13.28**   Sedative, hypnotic or anxiolytic dependence with other sedative, hypnotic or anxiolytic-induced disorders

     F13.280   Sedative, hypnotic or anxiolytic dependence with sedative, hypnotic or anxiolytic-induced anxiety disorder

     F13.281   Sedative, hypnotic or anxiolytic dependence with sedative, hypnotic or anxiolytic-induced sexual dysfunction

     F13.282   Sedative, hypnotic or anxiolytic dependence with sedative, hypnotic or anxiolytic-induced sleep disorder

     F13.288   Sedative, hypnotic or anxiolytic dependence with other sedative, hypnotic or anxiolytic-induced disorder

F13.29   Sedative, hypnotic or anxiolytic dependence with unspecified sedative, hypnotic or anxiolytic-induced disorder

● **F13.9**   Sedative, hypnotic or anxiolytic-related use, unspecified

> **Excludes1**   sedative, hypnotic or anxiolytic-related abuse (F13.1-)
> sedative, hypnotic or anxiolytic-related dependence (F13.2-)

F13.90   Sedative, hypnotic, or anxiolytic use, unspecified, uncomplicated

● **F13.92**   Sedative, hypnotic or anxiolytic use, unspecified with intoxication

> **Excludes1**   sedative, hypnotic or anxiolytic use, unspecified with withdrawal (F13.93-)

     F13.920   Sedative, hypnotic or anxiolytic use, unspecified with intoxication, uncomplicated

     F13.921   Sedative, hypnotic or anxiolytic use, unspecified with intoxication delirium

     F13.929   Sedative, hypnotic or anxiolytic use, unspecified with intoxication, unspecified

◄ New   ⬤⫶⫶⫶ Revised   ~~deleted~~ Deleted   **OGCR** Official Guidelines   X Assign placeholder X   ● Use Additional Character(s)

Excludes 1   Excludes 2   Includes   Use additional   Code first   Code also   Unspecified

816

● F13.93   Sedative, hypnotic or anxiolytic use,
           unspecified with withdrawal
           Excludes1   sedative, hypnotic or anxiolytic
                           use, unspecified with
                           intoxication (F13.92-)
   F13.930   Sedative, hypnotic or anxiolytic
             use, unspecified with withdrawal,
             uncomplicated
   F13.931   Sedative, hypnotic or anxiolytic
             use, unspecified with withdrawal
             delirium
   F13.932   Sedative, hypnotic or anxiolytic
             use, unspecified with withdrawal
             with perceptual disturbances
   F13.939   Sedative, hypnotic or anxiolytic
             use, unspecified with withdrawal,
             unspecified
   F13.94   Sedative, hypnotic or anxiolytic
            use, unspecified with sedative, hypnotic or
            anxiolytic-induced mood disorder
● F13.95   Sedative, hypnotic or anxiolytic use,
           unspecified with sedative, hypnotic
           or anxiolytic-induced psychotic disorder
   F13.950   Sedative, hypnotic or anxiolytic
             use, unspecified with sedative,
             hypnotic or anxiolytic-induced
             psychotic disorder with delusions
   F13.951   Sedative, hypnotic or anxiolytic
             use, unspecified with sedative,
             hypnotic or anxiolytic-induced
             psychotic disorder with
             hallucinations
   F13.959   Sedative, hypnotic or anxiolytic
             use, unspecified with sedative,
             hypnotic or anxiolytic-induced
             psychotic disorder, unspecified
   F13.96   Sedative, hypnotic or anxiolytic
            use, unspecified with sedative, hypnotic or
            anxiolytic-induced persisting amnestic disorder
   F13.97   Sedative, hypnotic or anxiolytic
            use, unspecified with sedative, hypnotic or
            anxiolytic-induced persisting dementia
● F13.98   Sedative, hypnotic or anxiolytic use,
           unspecified with other sedative, hypnotic or
           anxiolytic-induced disorders
   F13.980   Sedative, hypnotic or anxiolytic
             use, unspecified with sedative,
             hypnotic or anxiolytic-induced
             anxiety disorder
   F13.981   Sedative, hypnotic or anxiolytic
             use, unspecified with sedative,
             hypnotic or anxiolytic-induced sexual
             dysfunction
   F13.982   Sedative, hypnotic or anxiolytic
             use, unspecified with sedative,
             hypnotic or anxiolytic-induced sleep
             disorder
   F13.988   Sedative, hypnotic or anxiolytic
             use, unspecified with other sedative,
             hypnotic or anxiolytic-induced
             disorder
   F13.99   Sedative, hypnotic or anxiolytic
            use, unspecified with unspecified sedative,
            hypnotic or anxiolytic-induced disorder

● F14   Cocaine related disorders
        Excludes2   other stimulant-related disorders (F15.-)
● F14.1   Cocaine abuse
          Excludes1   cocaine dependence (F14.2-)
                          cocaine use, unspecified (F14.9-)
   F14.10   Cocaine abuse, uncomplicated
● F14.12   Cocaine abuse with intoxication
   F14.120   Cocaine abuse with intoxication,
             uncomplicated
   F14.121   Cocaine abuse with intoxication with
             delirium
   F14.122   Cocaine abuse with intoxication with
             perceptual disturbance
   F14.129   Cocaine abuse with
             intoxication, unspecified
   F14.14   Cocaine abuse with cocaine-induced mood
            disorder
● F14.15   Cocaine abuse with cocaine-induced psychotic
           disorder
   F14.150   Cocaine abuse with cocaine-induced
             psychotic disorder with delusions
   F14.151   Cocaine abuse with cocaine-
             induced psychotic disorder with
             hallucinations
   F14.159   Cocaine abuse with cocaine-induced
             psychotic disorder, unspecified
● F14.18   Cocaine abuse with other cocaine-induced
           disorder
   F14.180   Cocaine abuse with cocaine-induced
             anxiety disorder
   F14.181   Cocaine abuse with cocaine-induced
             sexual dysfunction
   F14.182   Cocaine abuse with cocaine-induced
             sleep disorder
   F14.188   Cocaine abuse with other cocaine-
             induced disorder
   F14.19   Cocaine abuse with unspecified cocaine-
            induced disorder
● F14.2   Cocaine dependence
          Excludes1   cocaine abuse (F14.1-)
                          cocaine use, unspecified (F14.9-)
          Excludes2   cocaine poisoning (T40.5-)
   F14.20   Cocaine dependence, uncomplicated
   F14.21   Cocaine dependence, in remission
● F14.22   Cocaine dependence with intoxication
          Excludes1   cocaine dependence with
                          withdrawal (F14.23)
   F14.220   Cocaine dependence with
             intoxication, uncomplicated
   F14.221   Cocaine dependence with intoxication
             delirium
   F14.222   Cocaine dependence with intoxication
             with perceptual disturbance
   F14.229   Cocaine dependence with
             intoxication, unspecified
   F14.23   Cocaine dependence with withdrawal
          Excludes1   cocaine dependence with
                          intoxication (F14.22-)
   F14.24   Cocaine dependence with cocaine-induced
            mood disorder

◀ New   ◀▥ Revised   ~~deleted~~ Deleted   **OGCR** Official Guidelines   X Assign placeholder X   ● Use Additional Character(s)

| Excludes 1 | Excludes 2 | Includes | Use additional | Code first | Code also | Unspecified |

CHAPTER 5 (F01-F99)

● F14.25   Cocaine dependence with cocaine-induced psychotic disorder

     F14.250   Cocaine dependence with cocaine-induced psychotic disorder with delusions

     F14.251   Cocaine dependence with cocaine-induced psychotic disorder with hallucinations

     F14.259   Cocaine dependence with cocaine-induced psychotic disorder, unspecified

● F14.28   Cocaine dependence with other cocaine-induced disorder

     F14.280   Cocaine dependence with cocaine-induced anxiety disorder

     F14.281   Cocaine dependence with cocaine-induced sexual dysfunction

     F14.282   Cocaine dependence with cocaine-induced sleep disorder

     F14.288   Cocaine dependence with other cocaine-induced disorder

     F14.29   Cocaine dependence with unspecified cocaine-induced disorder

● F14.9   Cocaine use, unspecified

     Excludes1   cocaine abuse (F14.1-)
                   cocaine dependence (F14.2-)

     F14.90   Cocaine use, unspecified, uncomplicated

● F14.92   Cocaine use, unspecified with intoxication

     F14.920   Cocaine use, unspecified with intoxication, uncomplicated

     F14.921   Cocaine use, unspecified with intoxication delirium

     F14.922   Cocaine use, unspecified with intoxication with perceptual disturbance

     F14.929   Cocaine use, unspecified with intoxication, unspecified

     F14.94   Cocaine use, unspecified with cocaine-induced mood disorder

● F14.95   Cocaine use, unspecified with cocaine-induced psychotic disorder

     F14.950   Cocaine use, unspecified with cocaine-induced psychotic disorder with delusions

     F14.951   Cocaine use, unspecified with cocaine-induced psychotic disorder with hallucinations

     F14.959   Cocaine use, unspecified with cocaine-induced psychotic disorder, unspecified

● F14.98   Cocaine use, unspecified with other specified cocaine-induced disorder

     F14.980   Cocaine use, unspecified with cocaine-induced anxiety disorder

     F14.981   Cocaine use, unspecified with cocaine-induced sexual dysfunction

     F14.982   Cocaine use, unspecified with cocaine-induced sleep disorder

     F14.988   Cocaine use, unspecified with other cocaine-induced disorder

     F14.99   Cocaine use, unspecified with unspecified cocaine-induced disorder

● F15   Other stimulant related disorders

     Includes   amphetamine-related disorders
                 caffeine

     Excludes2   cocaine-related disorders (F14.-)

● F15.1   Other stimulant abuse

     Excludes1   other stimulant dependence (F15.2-)
                   other stimulant use, unspecified (F15.9-)

     F15.10   Other stimulant abuse, uncomplicated

● F15.12   Other stimulant abuse with intoxication

     F15.120   Other stimulant abuse with intoxication, uncomplicated

     F15.121   Other stimulant abuse with intoxication delirium

     F15.122   Other stimulant abuse with intoxication with perceptual disturbance

     F15.129   Other stimulant abuse with intoxication, unspecified

     F15.14   Other stimulant abuse with stimulant-induced mood disorder

● F15.15   Other stimulant abuse with stimulant-induced psychotic disorder

     F15.150   Other stimulant abuse with stimulant-induced psychotic disorder with delusions

     F15.151   Other stimulant abuse with stimulant-induced psychotic disorder with hallucinations

     F15.159   Other stimulant abuse with stimulant-induced psychotic disorder, unspecified

● F15.18   Other stimulant abuse with other stimulant-induced disorder

     F15.180   Other stimulant abuse with stimulant-induced anxiety disorder

     F15.181   Other stimulant abuse with stimulant-induced sexual dysfunction

     F15.182   Other stimulant abuse with stimulant-induced sleep disorder

     F15.188   Other stimulant abuse with other stimulant-induced disorder

     F15.19   Other stimulant abuse with unspecified stimulant-induced disorder

● F15.2   Other stimulant dependence

     Excludes1   other stimulant abuse (F15.1-)
                   other stimulant use, unspecified (F15.9-)

     F15.20   Other stimulant dependence, uncomplicated

     F15.21   Other stimulant dependence, in remission

● F15.22   Other stimulant dependence with intoxication

     Excludes1   other stimulant dependence with withdrawal (F15.23)

     F15.220   Other stimulant dependence with intoxication, uncomplicated

     F15.221   Other stimulant dependence with intoxication delirium

     F15.222   Other stimulant dependence with intoxication with perceptual disturbance

     F15.229   Other stimulant dependence with intoxication, unspecified

     F15.23   Other stimulant dependence with withdrawal

     Excludes1   other stimulant dependence with intoxication (F15.22-)

F15.24　　Other stimulant dependence with stimulant-induced mood disorder

● F15.25　　Other stimulant dependence with stimulant-induced psychotic disorder

　　　　F15.250　　Other stimulant dependence with stimulant-induced psychotic disorder with delusions

　　　　F15.251　　Other stimulant dependence with stimulant-induced psychotic disorder with hallucinations

　　　　F15.259　　Other stimulant dependence with stimulant-induced psychotic disorder, unspecified

● F15.28　　Other stimulant dependence with other stimulant-induced disorder

　　　　F15.280　　Other stimulant dependence with stimulant-induced anxiety disorder

　　　　F15.281　　Other stimulant dependence with stimulant-induced sexual dysfunction

　　　　F15.282　　Other stimulant dependence with stimulant-induced sleep disorder

　　　　F15.288　　Other stimulant dependence with other stimulant-induced disorder

F15.29　　Other stimulant dependence with unspecified stimulant-induced disorder

● F15.9　　Other stimulant use, unspecified

　　　Excludes1　　other stimulant abuse (F15.1-)
　　　　　　　　　other stimulant dependence (F15.2-)

F15.90　　Other stimulant use, unspecified, uncomplicated

● F15.92　　Other stimulant use, unspecified with intoxication

　　　Excludes1　　other stimulant use, unspecified with withdrawal (F15.93)

　　　　F15.920　　Other stimulant use, unspecified with intoxication, uncomplicated

　　　　F15.921　　Other stimulant use, unspecified with intoxication delirium

　　　　F15.922　　Other stimulant use, unspecified with intoxication with perceptual disturbance

　　　　F15.929　　Other stimulant use, unspecified with intoxication, unspecified

F15.93　　Other stimulant use, unspecified with withdrawal

　　　Excludes1　　other stimulant use, unspecified with intoxication (F15.92-)

F15.94　　Other stimulant use, unspecified with stimulant-induced mood disorder

● F15.95　　Other stimulant use, unspecified with stimulant-induced psychotic disorder

　　　　F15.950　　Other stimulant use, unspecified with stimulant-induced psychotic disorder with delusions

　　　　F15.951　　Other stimulant use, unspecified with stimulant-induced psychotic disorder with hallucinations

　　　　F15.959　　Other stimulant use, unspecified with stimulant-induced psychotic disorder, unspecified

● F15.98　　Other stimulant use, unspecified with other stimulant-induced disorder

　　　　F15.980　　Other stimulant use, unspecified with stimulant-induced anxiety disorder

　　　　F15.981　　Other stimulant use, unspecified with stimulant-induced sexual dysfunction

　　　　F15.982　　Other stimulant use, unspecified with stimulant-induced sleep disorder

　　　　F15.988　　Other stimulant use, unspecified with other stimulant-induced disorder

F15.99　　Other stimulant use, unspecified with unspecified stimulant-induced disorder

● F16　　Hallucinogen related disorders

　　　Includes　　ecstasy
　　　　　　　　　PCP
　　　　　　　　　phencyclidine

● F16.1　　Hallucinogen abuse

　　　Excludes1　　hallucinogen dependence (F16.2-)
　　　　　　　　　hallucinogen use, unspecified (F16.9-)

F16.10　　Hallucinogen abuse, uncomplicated

● F16.12　　Hallucinogen abuse with intoxication

　　　　F16.120　　Hallucinogen abuse with intoxication, uncomplicated

　　　　F16.121　　Hallucinogen abuse with intoxication with delirium

　　　　F16.122　　Hallucinogen abuse with intoxication with perceptual disturbance

　　　　F16.129　　Hallucinogen abuse with intoxication, unspecified

F16.14　　Hallucinogen abuse with hallucinogen-induced mood disorder

● F16.15　　Hallucinogen abuse with hallucinogen-induced psychotic disorder

　　　　F16.150　　Hallucinogen abuse with hallucinogen-induced psychotic disorder with delusions

　　　　F16.151　　Hallucinogen abuse with hallucinogen-induced psychotic disorder with hallucinations

　　　　F16.159　　Hallucinogen abuse with hallucinogen-induced psychotic disorder, unspecified

● F16.18　　Hallucinogen abuse with other hallucinogen-induced disorder

　　　　F16.180　　Hallucinogen abuse with hallucinogen-induced anxiety disorder

　　　　F16.183　　Hallucinogen abuse with hallucinogen persisting perception disorder (flashbacks)

　　　　F16.188　　Hallucinogen abuse with other hallucinogen-induced disorder

F16.19　　Hallucinogen abuse with unspecified hallucinogen-induced disorder

● F16.2　　Hallucinogen dependence

　　　Excludes1　　hallucinogen abuse (F16.1-)
　　　　　　　　　hallucinogen use, unspecified (F16.9-)

F16.20　　Hallucinogen dependence, uncomplicated

F16.21　　Hallucinogen dependence, in remission

● F16.22　　Hallucinogen dependence with intoxication

　　　　F16.220　　Hallucinogen dependence with intoxication, uncomplicated

　　　　F16.221　　Hallucinogen dependence with intoxication with delirium

　　　　F16.229　　Hallucinogen dependence with intoxication, unspecified

F16.24　　Hallucinogen dependence with hallucinogen-induced mood disorder

● F16.25　　Hallucinogen dependence with hallucinogen-induced psychotic disorder

　　　　F16.250　　Hallucinogen dependence with hallucinogen-induced psychotic disorder with delusions

　　　　F16.251　　Hallucinogen dependence with hallucinogen-induced psychotic disorder with hallucinations

　　　　F16.259　　Hallucinogen dependence with hallucinogen-induced psychotic disorder, unspecified

◀ New　　◀||||| Revised　　deleted Deleted　　OGCR Official Guidelines　　X Assign placeholder X　　● Use Additional Character(s)

Excludes 1　　Excludes 2　　Includes　　Use additional　　Code first　　Code also　　Unspecified

● **F16.28** Hallucinogen dependence with other hallucinogen-induced disorder

     F16.280 Hallucinogen dependence with hallucinogen-induced anxiety disorder

     F16.283 Hallucinogen dependence with hallucinogen persisting perception disorder (flashbacks)

     F16.288 Hallucinogen dependence with other hallucinogen-induced disorder

   F16.29 Hallucinogen dependence with unspecified hallucinogen-induced disorder

● **F16.9** Hallucinogen use, unspecified

     Excludes1   hallucinogen abuse (F16.1-)
               hallucinogen dependence (F16.2-)

   F16.90 Hallucinogen use, unspecified, uncomplicated

● F16.92 Hallucinogen use, unspecified with intoxication

     F16.920 Hallucinogen use, unspecified with intoxication, uncomplicated

     F16.921 Hallucinogen use, unspecified with intoxication with delirium

     F16.929 Hallucinogen use, unspecified with intoxication, unspecified

   F16.94 Hallucinogen use, unspecified with hallucinogen-induced mood disorder

● F16.95 Hallucinogen use, unspecified with hallucinogen-induced psychotic disorder

     F16.950 Hallucinogen use, unspecified with hallucinogen-induced psychotic disorder with delusions

     F16.951 Hallucinogen use, unspecified with hallucinogen-induced psychotic disorder with hallucinations

     F16.959 Hallucinogen use, unspecified with hallucinogen-induced psychotic disorder, unspecified

● F16.98 Hallucinogen use, unspecified with other specified hallucinogen-induced disorder

     F16.980 Hallucinogen use, unspecified with hallucinogen-induced anxiety disorder

     F16.983 Hallucinogen use, unspecified with hallucinogen persisting perception disorder (flashbacks)

     F16.988 Hallucinogen use, unspecified with other hallucinogen-induced disorder

   F16.99 Hallucinogen use, unspecified with unspecified hallucinogen-induced disorder

● **F17** Nicotine dependence

     Excludes1   history of tobacco dependence (Z87.891)
               tobacco use NOS (Z72.0)

     Excludes2   tobacco use (smoking) during pregnancy, childbirth and the puerperium (O99.33-)
               toxic effect of nicotine (T65.2-)

● **F17.2** Nicotine dependence

   ● F17.20 Nicotine dependence, unspecified

     F17.200 Nicotine dependence, unspecified, uncomplicated

     F17.201 Nicotine dependence, unspecified, in remission

     F17.203 Nicotine dependence unspecified, with withdrawal

     F17.208 Nicotine dependence, unspecified, with other nicotine-induced disorders

     F17.209 Nicotine dependence, unspecified, with unspecified nicotine-induced disorders

● F17.21 Nicotine dependence, cigarettes

     F17.210 Nicotine dependence, cigarettes, uncomplicated

     F17.211 Nicotine dependence, cigarettes, in remission

     F17.213 Nicotine dependence, cigarettes, with withdrawal

     F17.218 Nicotine dependence, cigarettes, with other nicotine-induced disorders

     F17.219 Nicotine dependence, cigarettes, with unspecified nicotine-induced disorders

● F17.22 Nicotine dependence, chewing tobacco

     F17.220 Nicotine dependence, chewing tobacco, uncomplicated

     F17.221 Nicotine dependence, chewing tobacco, in remission

     F17.223 Nicotine dependence, chewing tobacco, with withdrawal

     F17.228 Nicotine dependence, chewing tobacco, with other nicotine-induced disorders

     F17.229 Nicotine dependence, chewing tobacco, with unspecified nicotine-induced disorders

● F17.29 Nicotine dependence, other tobacco product

     F17.290 Nicotine dependence, other tobacco product, uncomplicated

     F17.291 Nicotine dependence, other tobacco product, in remission

     F17.293 Nicotine dependence, other tobacco product, with withdrawal

     F17.298 Nicotine dependence, other tobacco product, with other nicotine-induced disorders

     F17.299 Nicotine dependence, other tobacco product, with unspecified nicotine-induced disorders

● **F18** Inhalant related disorders

     Includes   volatile solvents

   ● **F18.1** Inhalant abuse

     Excludes1   inhalant dependence (F18.2-)
               inhalant use, unspecified (F18.9-)

   F18.10 Inhalant abuse, uncomplicated

   ● F18.12 Inhalant abuse with intoxication

     F18.120 Inhalant abuse with intoxication, uncomplicated

     F18.121 Inhalant abuse with intoxication delirium

     F18.129 Inhalant abuse with intoxication, unspecified

   F18.14 Inhalant abuse with inhalant-induced mood disorder

   ● F18.15 Inhalant abuse with inhalant-induced psychotic disorder

     F18.150 Inhalant abuse with inhalant-induced psychotic disorder with delusions

     F18.151 Inhalant abuse with inhalant-induced psychotic disorder with hallucinations

     F18.159 Inhalant abuse with inhalant-induced psychotic disorder, unspecified

   F18.17 Inhalant abuse with inhalant-induced dementia

● F18.18   Inhalant abuse with other inhalant-induced disorders

     F18.180   Inhalant abuse with inhalant-induced anxiety disorder

     F18.188   Inhalant abuse with other inhalant-induced disorder

   F18.19   Inhalant abuse with unspecified inhalant-induced disorder

● F18.2   Inhalant dependence

     Excludes1   inhalant abuse (F18.1-)
                   inhalant use, unspecified (F18.9-)

   F18.20   Inhalant dependence, uncomplicated

   F18.21   Inhalant dependence, in remission

● F18.22   Inhalant dependence with intoxication

     F18.220   Inhalant dependence with intoxication, uncomplicated

     F18.221   Inhalant dependence with intoxication delirium

     F18.229   Inhalant dependence with intoxication, unspecified

   F18.24   Inhalant dependence with inhalant-induced mood disorder

● F18.25   Inhalant dependence with inhalant-induced psychotic disorder

     F18.250   Inhalant dependence with inhalant-induced psychotic disorder with delusions

     F18.251   Inhalant dependence with inhalant-induced psychotic disorder with hallucinations

     F18.259   Inhalant dependence with inhalant-induced psychotic disorder, unspecified

   F18.27   Inhalant dependence with inhalant-induced dementia

● F18.28   Inhalant dependence with other inhalant-induced disorders

     F18.280   Inhalant dependence with inhalant-induced anxiety disorder

     F18.288   Inhalant dependence with other inhalant-induced disorder

   F18.29   Inhalant dependence with unspecified inhalant-induced disorder

● F18.9   Inhalant use, unspecified

     Excludes1   inhalant abuse (F18.1-)
                   inhalant dependence (F18.2-)

   F18.90   Inhalant use, unspecified, uncomplicated

● F18.92   Inhalant use, unspecified with intoxication

     F18.920   Inhalant use, unspecified with intoxication, uncomplicated

     F18.921   Inhalant use, unspecified with intoxication with delirium

     F18.929   Inhalant use, unspecified with intoxication, unspecified

   F18.94   Inhalant use, unspecified with inhalant-induced mood disorder

● F18.95   Inhalant use, unspecified with inhalant-induced psychotic disorder

     F18.950   Inhalant use, unspecified with inhalant-induced psychotic disorder with delusions

     F18.951   Inhalant use, unspecified with inhalant-induced psychotic disorder with hallucinations

     F18.959   Inhalant use, unspecified with inhalant-induced psychotic disorder, unspecified

● F18.97   Inhalant use, unspecified with inhalant-induced persisting dementia

● F18.98   Inhalant use, unspecified with other inhalant-induced disorders

     F18.980   Inhalant use, unspecified with inhalant-induced anxiety disorder

     F18.988   Inhalant use, unspecified with other inhalant-induced disorder

   F18.99   Inhalant use, unspecified with unspecified inhalant-induced disorder

● F19   Other psychoactive substance related disorders

     Includes   polysubstance drug use (indiscriminate drug use)

● F19.1   Other psychoactive substance abuse

     Excludes1   other psychoactive substance dependence (F19.2-)
                   other psychoactive substance use, unspecified (F19.9-)

   F19.10   Other psychoactive substance abuse, uncomplicated

● F19.12   Other psychoactive substance abuse with intoxication

     F19.120   Other psychoactive substance abuse with intoxication, uncomplicated

     F19.121   Other psychoactive substance abuse with intoxication delirium

     F19.122   Other psychoactive substance abuse with intoxication with perceptual disturbances

     F19.129   Other psychoactive substance abuse with intoxication, unspecified

   F19.14   Other psychoactive substance abuse with psychoactive substance-induced mood disorder

● F19.15   Other psychoactive substance abuse with psychoactive substance-induced psychotic disorder

     F19.150   Other psychoactive substance abuse with psychoactive substance-induced psychotic disorder with delusions

     F19.151   Other psychoactive substance abuse with psychoactive substance-induced psychotic disorder with hallucinations

     F19.159   Other psychoactive substance abuse with psychoactive substance-induced psychotic disorder, unspecified

   F19.16   Other psychoactive substance abuse with psychoactive substance-induced persisting amnestic disorder

   F19.17   Other psychoactive substance abuse with psychoactive substance-induced persisting dementia

● F19.18   Other psychoactive substance abuse with other psychoactive substance-induced disorders

     F19.180   Other psychoactive substance abuse with psychoactive substance-induced anxiety disorder

     F19.181   Other psychoactive substance abuse with psychoactive substance-induced sexual dysfunction

     F19.182   Other psychoactive substance abuse with psychoactive substance-induced sleep disorder

     F19.188   Other psychoactive substance abuse with other psychoactive substance-induced disorder

   F19.19   Other psychoactive substance abuse with unspecified psychoactive substance-induced disorder

● **F19.2   Other psychoactive substance dependence**

> **Excludes1**   other psychoactive substance abuse (F19.1-)
>
> other psychoactive substance use, unspecified (F19.9-)

F19.20   Other psychoactive substance dependence, uncomplicated

F19.21   Other psychoactive substance dependence, in remission

● F19.22   Other psychoactive substance dependence with intoxication

> **Excludes1**   other psychoactive substance dependence with withdrawal (F19.23-)

    F19.220   Other psychoactive substance dependence with intoxication, uncomplicated

    F19.221   Other psychoactive substance dependence with intoxication delirium

    F19.222   Other psychoactive substance dependence with intoxication with perceptual disturbance

    F19.229   Other psychoactive substance dependence with intoxication, unspecified

● F19.23   Other psychoactive substance dependence with withdrawal

> **Excludes1**   other psychoactive substance dependence with intoxication (F19.22-)

    F19.230   Other psychoactive substance dependence with withdrawal, uncomplicated

    F19.231   Other psychoactive substance dependence with withdrawal delirium

    F19.232   Other psychoactive substance dependence with withdrawal with perceptual disturbance

    F19.239   Other psychoactive substance dependence with withdrawal, unspecified

F19.24   Other psychoactive substance dependence with psychoactive substance-induced mood disorder

● F19.25   Other psychoactive substance dependence with psychoactive substance-induced psychotic disorder

    F19.250   Other psychoactive substance dependence with psychoactive substance-induced psychotic disorder with delusions

    F19.251   Other psychoactive substance dependence with psychoactive substance-induced psychotic disorder with hallucinations

    F19.259   Other psychoactive substance dependence with psychoactive substance-induced psychotic disorder, unspecified

F19.26   Other psychoactive substance dependence with psychoactive substance-induced persisting amnestic disorder

F19.27   Other psychoactive substance dependence with psychoactive substance-induced persisting dementia

● F19.28   Other psychoactive substance dependence with other psychoactive substance-induced disorders

    F19.280   Other psychoactive substance dependence with psychoactive substance-induced anxiety disorder

    F19.281   Other psychoactive substance dependence with psychoactive substance-induced sexual dysfunction

    F19.282   Other psychoactive substance dependence with psychoactive substance-induced sleep disorder

    F19.288   Other psychoactive substance dependence with other psychoactive substance-induced disorder

F19.29   Other psychoactive substance dependence with unspecified psychoactive substance-induced disorder

● **F19.9   Other psychoactive substance use, unspecified**

> **Excludes1**   other psychoactive substance abuse (F19.1-)
>
> other psychoactive substance dependence (F19.2-)

F19.90   Other psychoactive substance use, unspecified, uncomplicated

● F19.92   Other psychoactive substance use, unspecified with intoxication

> **Excludes1**   other psychoactive substance use, unspecified with withdrawal (F19.93)

    F19.920   Other psychoactive substance use, unspecified with intoxication, uncomplicated

    F19.921   Other psychoactive substance use, unspecified with intoxication with delirium

    F19.922   Other psychoactive substance use, unspecified with intoxication with perceptual disturbance

    F19.929   Other psychoactive substance use, unspecified with intoxication, unspecified

● F19.93   Other psychoactive substance use, unspecified with withdrawal

> **Excludes1**   other psychoactive substance use, unspecified with intoxication (F19.92-)

    F19.930   Other psychoactive substance use, unspecified with withdrawal, uncomplicated

    F19.931   Other psychoactive substance use, unspecified with withdrawal delirium

    F19.932   Other psychoactive substance use, unspecified with withdrawal with perceptual disturbance

    F19.939   Other psychoactive substance use, unspecified with withdrawal, unspecified

F19.94   Other psychoactive substance use, unspecified with psychoactive substance-induced mood disorder

● F19.95   Other psychoactive substance use, unspecified with psychoactive substance-induced psychotic disorder

    F19.950   Other psychoactive substance use, unspecified with psychoactive substance-induced psychotic disorder with delusions

    F19.951   Other psychoactive substance use, unspecified with psychoactive substance-induced psychotic disorder with hallucinations

    F19.959   Other psychoactive substance use, unspecified with psychoactive substance-induced psychotic disorder, unspecified

---

◀ New   ◀▥ Revised   ~~deleted~~ Deleted   **OGCR** Official Guidelines   X Assign placeholder X   ● Use Additional Character(s)

Excludes 1   Excludes 2   Includes   Use additional   Code first   Code also   Unspecified

F19.96   Other psychoactive substance use, unspecified with psychoactive substance-induced persisting amnestic disorder

F19.97   Other psychoactive substance use, unspecified with psychoactive substance-induced persisting dementia

● F19.98   Other psychoactive substance use, unspecified with other psychoactive substance-induced disorders

     F19.980   Other psychoactive substance use, unspecified with psychoactive substance-induced anxiety disorder

     F19.981   Other psychoactive substance use, unspecified with psychoactive substance-induced sexual dysfunction

     F19.982   Other psychoactive substance use, unspecified with psychoactive substance-induced sleep disorder

     F19.988   Other psychoactive substance use, unspecified with other psychoactive substance-induced disorder

F19.99   Other psychoactive substance use, unspecified with unspecified psychoactive substance-induced disorder

SCHIZOPHRENIA, SCHIZOTYPAL, DELUSIONAL, AND OTHER NON-MOOD PSYCHOTIC DISORDERS (F20-F29)

● **F20 Schizophrenia**
Personality disorders characterized by multiple mental and behavioral irregularities (may exhibit disorganized thinking, delusions, and auditory hallucinations).

Excludes1   brief psychotic disorder (F23)
cyclic schizophrenia (F25.0)
mood [affective] disorders with psychotic symptoms (F30.2, F31.2, F31.5, F31.64, F32.3, F33.3)
schizoaffective disorder (F25.-)
schizophrenic reaction NOS (F23)

Excludes2   schizophrenic reaction in:
alcoholism (F10.15-, F10.25-, F10.95-)
brain disease (F06.2)
epilepsy (F06.2)
psychoactive drug use (F11-F19 with .15, .25, .95)
schizotypal disorder (F21)

F20.0 Paranoid schizophrenia
Paraphrenic schizophrenia

Excludes1   involutional paranoid state (F22)
paranoia (F22)

F20.1 Disorganized schizophrenia
Hebephrenic schizophrenia
Hebephrenia

F20.2 Catatonic schizophrenia
Schizophrenic catalepsy
Schizophrenic catatonia
Schizophrenic flexibilitas cerea

Excludes1   catatonic stupor (R40.1)

F20.3 Undifferentiated schizophrenia
Atypical schizophrenia

Excludes1   acute schizophrenia-like psychotic disorder (F23)

Excludes2   post-schizophrenic depression (F32.8)

F20.5 Residual schizophrenia
Restzustand (schizophrenic)
Schizophrenic residual state

● **F20.8 Other schizophrenia**

F20.81 Schizophreniform disorder
Schizophreniform psychosis NOS

F20.89 Other schizophrenia
Cenesthopathic schizophrenia
Simple schizophrenia

F20.9 Schizophrenia, unspecified

F21 Schizotypal disorder
Personality disorder characterized by need for social isolation, odd behavior and thinking, and often unconventional beliefs
Borderline schizophrenia
Latent schizophrenia
Latent schizophrenic reaction
Prepsychotic schizophrenia
Prodromal schizophrenia
Pseudoneurotic schizophrenia
Pseudopsychopathic schizophrenia
Schizotypal personality disorder

Excludes2   Asperger's syndrome (F84.5)
schizoid personality disorder (F60.1)

F22 Delusional disorders
Delusional dysmorphophobia
Involutional paranoid state
Paranoia
Paranoia querulans
Paranoid psychosis
Paranoid state
Paraphrenia (late)
Sensitiver Beziehungswahn

Excludes1   mood [affective] disorders with psychotic symptoms (F30.2, F31.2, F31.5, F31.64, F32.3, F33.3)
paranoid schizophrenia (F20.0)

Excludes2   paranoid personality disorder (F60.0)
paranoid psychosis, psychogenic (F23)
paranoid reaction (F23)

F23 Brief psychotic disorder
Paranoid reaction
Psychogenic paranoid psychosis

Excludes2   mood [affective] disorders with psychotic symptoms (F30.2, F31.2, F31.5, F31.64, F32.3, F33.3)

F24 Shared psychotic disorder
Folie à deux
Induced paranoid disorder
Induced psychotic disorder

● **F25 Schizoaffective disorders**
Mental disorder exhibiting major depressive episode, manic episode, or mixed episode occurs with symptoms of schizophrenia, and mood disorder

Excludes1   mood [affective] disorders with psychotic symptoms (F30.2, F31.2, F31.5, F31.64, F32.3, F33.3)
schizophrenia (F20.-)

F25.0 Schizoaffective disorder, bipolar type
Cyclic schizophrenia
Schizoaffective disorder, manic type
Schizoaffective disorder, mixed type
Schizoaffective psychosis, bipolar type
Schizophreniform psychosis, manic type

F25.1 Schizoaffective disorder, depressive type
Schizoaffective psychosis, depressive type
Schizophreniform psychosis, depressive type

F25.8 Other schizoaffective disorders

F25.9 Schizoaffective disorder, unspecified
Schizoaffective psychosis NOS

F28 Other psychotic disorder not due to a substance or known physiological condition
Chronic hallucinatory psychosis

F29 Unspecified psychosis not due to a substance or known physiological condition
Psychosis NOS

Excludes1   mental disorder NOS (F99)
unspecified mental disorder due to known physiological condition (F09)

◀ New   ◀▥ Revised   ~~deleted~~ Deleted   **OGCR** Official Guidelines   X Assign placeholder X   ● Use Additional Character(s)

Excludes 1   Excludes 2   Includes   Use additional   Code first   Code also   Unspecified

MOOD [AFFECTIVE] DISORDERS (F30-F39)

● **F30   Manic episode**
   Elevated, expansive, or irritable mood

   Includes   bipolar disorder, single manic episode
                    mixed affective episode

   Excludes1   bipolar disorder (F31.-)
                    major depressive disorder, single episode (F32.-)
                    major depressive disorder, recurrent (F33.-)

   ● **F30.1   Manic episode without psychotic symptoms**

      F30.10   Manic episode without psychotic symptoms, unspecified

      F30.11   Manic episode without psychotic symptoms, mild

      F30.12   Manic episode without psychotic symptoms, moderate

      F30.13   Manic episode, severe, without psychotic symptoms

   F30.2   Manic episode, severe with psychotic symptoms
      Manic stupor
      Mania with mood-congruent psychotic symptoms
      Mania with mood-incongruent psychotic symptoms

   F30.3   Manic episode in partial remission

   F30.4   Manic episode in full remission

   F30.8   Other manic episodes
      Abnormality of mood resembling mania but less intense
      Hypomania

   F30.9   Manic episode, unspecified
      Mania NOS

● **F31   Bipolar disorder**
   Mood disorders with history of manic, mixed, or hypomanic episodes

   Includes   manic-depressive illness
                    manic-depressive psychosis
                    manic-depressive reaction

   Excludes1   bipolar disorder, single manic episode (F30.-)
                    major depressive disorder, single episode (F32.-)
                    major depressive disorder, recurrent (F33.-)

   Excludes2   cyclothymia (F34.0)

   F31.0   Bipolar disorder, current episode hypomanic

   ● **F31.1   Bipolar disorder, current episode manic without psychotic features**

      F31.10   Bipolar disorder, current episode manic without psychotic features, unspecified

      F31.11   Bipolar disorder, current episode manic without psychotic features, mild

      F31.12   Bipolar disorder, current episode manic without psychotic features, moderate

      F31.13   Bipolar disorder, current episode manic without psychotic features, severe

   F31.2   Bipolar disorder, current episode manic severe with psychotic features
      Bipolar disorder, current episode manic with mood-congruent psychotic symptoms
      Bipolar disorder, current episode manic with mood-incongruent psychotic symptoms

   ● **F31.3   Bipolar disorder, current episode depressed, mild or moderate severity**

      F31.30   Bipolar disorder, current episode depressed, mild or moderate severity, unspecified

      F31.31   Bipolar disorder, current episode depressed, mild

      F31.32   Bipolar disorder, current episode depressed, moderate

   F31.4   Bipolar disorder, current episode depressed, severe, without psychotic features

   F31.5   Bipolar disorder, current episode depressed, severe, with psychotic features
      Bipolar disorder, current episode depressed with mood-incongruent psychotic symptoms
      Bipolar disorder, current episode depressed with mood-congruent psychotic symptoms

● **F31.6   Bipolar disorder, current episode mixed**

   F31.60   Bipolar disorder, current episode mixed, unspecified

   F31.61   Bipolar disorder, current episode mixed, mild

   F31.62   Bipolar disorder, current episode mixed, moderate

   F31.63   Bipolar disorder, current episode mixed, severe, without psychotic features

   F31.64   Bipolar disorder, current episode mixed, severe, with psychotic features
      Bipolar disorder, current episode mixed with mood-congruent psychotic symptoms
      Bipolar disorder, current episode mixed with mood-incongruent psychotic symptoms

● **F31.7   Bipolar disorder, currently in remission**

   F31.70   Bipolar disorder, currently in remission, most recent episode unspecified

   F31.71   Bipolar disorder, in partial remission, most recent episode hypomanic

   F31.72   Bipolar disorder, in full remission, most recent episode hypomanic

   F31.73   Bipolar disorder, in partial remission, most recent episode manic

   F31.74   Bipolar disorder, in full remission, most recent episode manic

   F31.75   Bipolar disorder, in partial remission, most recent episode depressed

   F31.76   Bipolar disorder, in full remission, most recent episode depressed

   F31.77   Bipolar disorder, in partial remission, most recent episode mixed

   F31.78   Bipolar disorder, in full remission, most recent episode mixed

● **F31.8   Other bipolar disorders**

   F31.81   Bipolar II disorder

   F31.89   Other bipolar disorder
      Recurrent manic episodes NOS

   F31.9   Bipolar disorder, unspecified

● **F32   Major depressive disorder, single episode**

   Includes   single episode of agitated depression
                    single episode of depressive reaction
                    single episode of major depression
                    single episode of psychogenic depression
                    single episode of reactive depression
                    single episode of vital depression

   Excludes1   bipolar disorder (F31.-)
                    manic episode (F30.-)
                    recurrent depressive disorder (F33.-)

   Excludes2   adjustment disorder (F43.2)

   F32.0   Major depressive disorder, single episode, mild

   F32.1   Major depressive disorder, single episode, moderate

   F32.2   Major depressive disorder, single episode, severe without psychotic features

   F32.3   Major depressive disorder, single episode, severe with psychotic features
      Single episode of major depression with mood-congruent psychotic symptoms
      Single episode of major depression with mood-incongruent psychotic symptoms
      Single episode of major depression with psychotic symptoms
      Single episode of psychogenic depressive psychosis
      Single episode of psychotic depression
      Single episode of reactive depressive psychosis

   F32.4   Major depressive disorder, single episode, in partial remission

   F32.5   Major depressive disorder, single episode, in full remission

F32.8   **Other depressive episodes**
     Atypical depression
     Post-schizophrenic depression
     Single episode of 'masked' depression NOS

F32.9   **Major depressive disorder, single episode, unspecified**
     Depression NOS
     Depressive disorder NOS
     Major depression NOS

● **F33**   **Major depressive disorder, recurrent**

     Includes   recurrent episodes of depressive reaction
                   recurrent episodes of endogenous depression
                    recurrent episodes of major depression
                    recurrent episodes of psychogenic depression
                    recurrent episodes of reactive depression
                    recurrent episodes of seasonal depressive
                        disorder
                    recurrent episodes of vital depression

     Excludes1   bipolar disorder (F31.-)
                         manic episode (F30.-)

F33.0   **Major depressive disorder, recurrent, mild**

F33.1   **Major depressive disorder, recurrent, moderate**

F33.2   **Major depressive disorder, recurrent severe without psychotic features**

F33.3   **Major depressive disorder, recurrent, severe with psychotic symptoms**
     Endogenous depression with psychotic symptoms
     Recurrent severe episodes of major depression with mood-congruent psychotic symptoms
     Recurrent severe episodes of major depression with mood-incongruent psychotic symptoms
     Recurrent severe episodes of major depression with psychotic symptoms
     Recurrent severe episodes of psychogenic depressive psychosis
     Recurrent severe episodes of psychotic depression
     Recurrent severe episodes of reactive depressive psychosis

● **F33.4**   **Major depressive disorder, recurrent, in remission**

     F33.40   **Major depressive disorder, recurrent, in remission, unspecified**

     F33.41   **Major depressive disorder, recurrent, in partial remission**

     F33.42   **Major depressive disorder, recurrent, in full remission**

F33.8   **Other recurrent depressive disorders**
     Recurrent brief depressive episodes

F33.9   **Major depressive disorder, recurrent, unspecified**
     Monopolar depression NOS

● **F34**   **Persistent mood [affective] disorders**

F34.0   **Cyclothymic disorder**
     Affective personality disorder
     Cycloid personality
     Cyclothymia
     Cyclothymic personality

F34.1   **Dysthymic disorder**
     Depressive neurosis
     Depressive personality disorder
     Dysthymia
     Neurotic depression
     Persistent anxiety depression

     Excludes2   anxiety depression (mild or not persistent) (F41.8)

F34.8   **Other persistent mood [affective] disorders**

F34.9   **Persistent mood [affective] disorder, unspecified**

F39   **Unspecified mood [affective] disorder**
     Affective psychosis NOS

ANXIETY, DISSOCIATIVE, STRESS-RELATED, SOMATOFORM AND OTHER NONPSYCHOTIC MENTAL DISORDERS (F40-F48)

● **F40**   **Phobic anxiety disorders**
     Irrational fear with avoidance of the feared subject, activity, or situation even though the individual knows that the reaction is excessive.

● **F40.0**   **Agoraphobia**
     Intense, irrational fear of open spaces

     F40.00   **Agoraphobia, unspecified**

     F40.01   **Agoraphobia with panic disorder**
         Panic disorder with agoraphobia

         Excludes1   panic disorder without agoraphobia (F41.0)

     F40.02   **Agoraphobia without panic disorder**

● **F40.1**   **Social phobias**
     Anthropophobia
     Social anxiety disorder of childhood
     Social neurosis

     F40.10   **Social phobia, unspecified**

     F40.11   **Social phobia, generalized**

● **F40.2**   **Specific (isolated) phobias**

     Excludes2   dysmorphophobia (nondelusional) (F45.22)
                        nosophobia (F45.22)

●   **F40.21**   **Animal type phobia**

     F40.210   **Arachnophobia**
                 Fear of spiders

     F40.218   **Other animal type phobia**

●   **F40.22**   **Natural environment type phobia**

     F40.220   **Fear of thunderstorms**

     F40.228   **Other natural environment type phobia**

●   **F40.23**   **Blood, injection, injury type phobia**

     F40.230   **Fear of blood**

     F40.231   **Fear of injections and transfusions**

     F40.232   **Fear of other medical care**

     F40.233   **Fear of injury**

●   **F40.24**   **Situational type phobia**

     F40.240   **Claustrophobia**
                 Fear of closed spaces

     F40.241   **Acrophobia**
                 Fear of heights

     F40.242   **Fear of bridges**

     F40.243   **Fear of flying**

     F40.248   **Other situational type phobia**

●   **F40.29**   **Other specified phobia**

     F40.290   **Androphobia**
                 Fear of men

     F40.291   **Gynephobia**
                 Fear of women

     F40.298   **Other specified phobia**

F40.8   **Other phobic anxiety disorders**
     Phobic anxiety disorder of childhood

F40.9   **Phobic anxiety disorder, unspecified**
     Phobia NOS
     Phobic state NOS

● **F41**   **Other anxiety disorders**

     Excludes2   anxiety in:
                    acute stress reaction (F43.0)
                    transient adjustment reaction (F43.2)
                    neurasthenia (F48.8)
                    psychophysiologic disorders (F45.-)
                    separation anxiety (F93.0)

     F41.0   **Panic disorder [episodic paroxysmal anxiety] without agoraphobia**
         Panic attack
         Panic state

         Excludes1   panic disorder with agoraphobia (F40.01)

◀ New   ◀▥ Revised   ̶d̶e̶l̶e̶t̶e̶d̶ Deleted   **OGCR** Official Guidelines   X Assign placeholder X   ● Use Additional Character(s)

| Excludes 1 | Excludes 2 | Includes | Use additional | Code first | Code also | Unspecified |

825

CHAPTER 5 (F01-F99)

F41.1 **Generalized anxiety disorder**
Anxiety neurosis
Anxiety reaction
Anxiety state
Overanxious disorder
Excludes2   neurasthenia (F48.8)

F41.3 **Other mixed anxiety disorders**

F41.8 **Other specified anxiety disorders**
Anxiety depression (mild or not persistent)
Anxiety hysteria
Mixed anxiety and depressive disorder

F41.9 **Anxiety disorder, unspecified**
Anxiety NOS

● **F42** **Obsessive-compulsive disorder**
Anxiety disorder with recurrent obsessions or compulsions
Anancastic neurosis
Obsessive-compulsive neurosis
Excludes2   obsessive-compulsive personality (disorder)
(F60.5)
obsessive-compulsive symptoms occurring in
depression (F32-F33)
obsessive-compulsive symptoms occurring in
schizophrenia (F20.-)

● **F43** **Reaction to severe stress and adjustment disorders**

F43.0 **Acute stress reaction**
Acute crisis reaction
Acute reaction to stress
Combat and operational stress reaction
Combat fatigue
Crisis state
Psychic shock

● **F43.1** **Post-traumatic stress disorder (PTSD)**
Traumatic neurosis

F43.10 **Post-traumatic stress disorder, unspecified**

F43.11 **Post-traumatic stress disorder, acute**

F43.12 **Post-traumatic stress disorder, chronic**

● **F43.2** **Adjustment disorders**
Culture shock
Grief reaction
Hospitalism in children
Excludes2   separation anxiety disorder of childhood
(F93.0)

F43.20 **Adjustment disorder, unspecified**

F43.21 **Adjustment disorder with depressed mood**

F43.22 **Adjustment disorder with anxiety**

F43.23 **Adjustment disorder with mixed anxiety and
depressed mood**

F43.24 **Adjustment disorder with disturbance of
conduct**

F43.25 **Adjustment disorder with mixed disturbance of
emotions and conduct**

F43.29 **Adjustment disorder with other symptoms**

F43.8 **Other reactions to severe stress**

F43.9 **Reaction to severe stress, unspecified**

● **F44** **Dissociative and conversion disorders**
Includes   conversion hysteria
conversion reaction
hysteria
hysterical psychosis
Excludes2   malingering [conscious simulation] (Z76.5)

F44.0 **Dissociative amnesia**
Sudden loss of memory for personal information
Excludes1   amnesia NOS (R41.3)
anterograde amnesia (R41.1)
retrograde amnesia (R41.2)
Excludes2   alcohol-or other psychoactive substance-
induced amnestic disorder (F10, F13,
F19 with .26, .96)
amnestic disorder due to known
physiological condition (F04)
postictal amnesia in epilepsy (G40.-)

F44.1 **Dissociative fugue**
*Characterized by episode of sudden, unexpected travel with
amnesia for past and partial to total confusion about
identity or assumption of new identity*
Excludes2   postictal fugue in epilepsy (G40.-)

F44.2 **Dissociative stupor**
*Profound diminution or absence of voluntary movement and
responsiveness to external stimuli*
Excludes1   catatonic stupor (R40.1)
stupor NOS (R40.1)
Excludes2   catatonic disorder due to known
physiological condition (F06.1)
depressive stupor (F32, F33)
manic stupor (F30, F31)

F44.4 **Conversion disorder with motor symptom or deficit**
Dissociative motor disorders
Psychogenic aphonia
Psychogenic dysphonia

F44.5 **Conversion disorder with seizures or convulsions**
Dissociative convulsions

F44.6 **Conversion disorder with sensory symptom or deficit**
Dissociative anesthesia and sensory loss
Psychogenic deafness

F44.7 **Conversion disorder with mixed symptom presentation**

● **F44.8** **Other dissociative and conversion disorders**

F44.81 **Dissociative identity disorder**
Multiple personality disorder

F44.89 **Other dissociative and conversion disorders**
Ganser's syndrome
Psychogenic confusion
Psychogenic twilight state
Trance and possession disorders

F44.9 **Dissociative and conversion disorder, unspecified**
Dissociative disorder NOS

OGCR Section I.C.5.a

Pain disorders related to psychological factors

Assign code F45.41, for pain that is exclusively psychological. Code
F45.41, Pain disorder exclusively related to psychological factors,
should be used following the appropriate code from category
G89, Pain, not elsewhere classified, if there is documentation of a
psychological component for a patient with acute or chronic pain.
See Section I.C.6. Pain

● **F45** **Somatoform disorders**
*Mental disorders characterized by symptoms suggesting general
medical condition*
Excludes2   dissociative and conversion disorders (F44.-)
factitious disorders (F68.1-)
hair-plucking (F63.3)
lalling (F80.0)
lisping (F80.0)
malingering [conscious simulation] (Z76.5)
nail-biting (F98.8)
psychological or behavioral factors associated
with disorders or diseases classified
elsewhere (F54)
sexual dysfunction, not due to a substance or
known physiological condition (F52.-)
thumb-sucking (F98.8)
tic disorders (in childhood and adolescence) (F95.-)
Tourette's syndrome (F95.2)
trichotillomania (F63.3)

F45.0 **Somatization disorder**
Briquet's disorder
Multiple psychosomatic disorder

F45.1 **Undifferentiated somatoform disorder**
Undifferentiated psychosomatic disorder

◀ New   ◀||||| Revised   ~~deleted~~ Deleted   OGCR Official Guidelines   X Assign placeholder X   ● Use Additional Character(s)

Excludes 1   Excludes 2   Includes   Use additional   Code first   Code also   Unspecified

● **F45.2**   **Hypochondriacal disorders**
     Persistent, unrealistic preoccupation with possibility of
     having serious disease
     Excludes2   delusional dysmorphophobia (F22)
                      fixed delusions about bodily functions or
                        shape (F22)

   F45.20   **Hypochondriacal disorder, unspecified**

   F45.21   **Hypochondriasis**
          Hypochondriacal neurosis

   F45.22   **Body dysmorphic disorder**
          Dysmorphophobia (nondelusional)
          Nosophobia

   F45.29   **Other hypochondriacal disorders**

● **F45.4**   **Pain disorders related to psychological factors**
     Excludes1   pain NOS (R52)

   F45.41   **Pain disorder exclusively related to**
              psychological factors
          Somatoform pain disorder (persistent)

   F45.42   **Pain disorder with related psychological factors**
          Code also associated acute or chronic pain
          (G89.-)

● **F45.8**   **Other somatoform disorders**
     Psychogenic dysmenorrhea
     Psychogenic dysphagia, including 'globus hystericus'
     Psychogenic pruritus
     Psychogenic torticollis
     Somatoform autonomic dysfunction
     Teeth grinding
     Excludes1   sleep related teeth grinding (G47.63)

● **F45.9**   **Somatoform disorder, unspecified**
     Psychosomatic disorder NOS

● **F48**   **Other nonpsychotic mental disorders**

   F48.1   **Depersonalization-derealization syndrome**

   F48.2   **Pseudobulbar affect**
          Involuntary emotional expression disorder
          Code first underlying cause, if known, such as:
            amyotrophic lateral sclerosis (G12.21)
            multiple sclerosis (G35)
            sequelae of cerebrovascular disease (I69.-)
            sequelae of traumatic intracranial injury (S06.-)

   F48.8   **Other specified nonpsychotic mental disorders**
          Dhat syndrome
          Neurasthenia
          Occupational neurosis, including writer's cramp
          Psychasthenia
          Psychasthenic neurosis
          Psychogenic syncope

   F48.9   **Nonpsychotic mental disorder, unspecified**
          Neurosis NOS

**BEHAVIORAL SYNDROMES ASSOCIATED WITH PHYSIOLOGICAL
DISTURBANCES AND PHYSICAL FACTORS (F50-F59)**

● **F50**   **Eating disorders**
     Excludes1   anorexia NOS (R63.0)
                  feeding difficulties (R63.3)
                  polyphagia (R63.2)
     Excludes2   feeding disorder in infancy or childhood (F98.2-)

● **F50.0**   **Anorexia nervosa**
     Excludes1   loss of appetite (R63.0)
                  psychogenic loss of appetite (F50.8)

   F50.00   **Anorexia nervosa, unspecified**

   F50.01   **Anorexia nervosa, restricting type**

   F50.02   **Anorexia nervosa, binge eating/purging type**
          Excludes1   bulimia nervosa (F50.2)

   F50.2   **Bulimia nervosa**
          Bulimia NOS
          Hyperorexia nervosa
          Excludes1   anorexia nervosa, binge eating/purging
                     type (F50.02)

   F50.8   **Other eating disorders**
          Pica in adults
          Psychogenic loss of appetite
          Excludes2   pica of infancy and childhood (F98.3)

   F50.9   **Eating disorder, unspecified**
          Atypical anorexia nervosa
          Atypical bulimia nervosa

● **F51**   **Sleep disorders not due to a substance or known physiological
condition**
     Excludes2   organic sleep disorders (G47.-)

● **F51.0**   **Insomnia not due to a substance or known physiological
condition**
     Excludes2   alcohol related insomnia (F10.182,
                  F10.282, F10.982)
                drug-related insomnia (F11.182, F11.282,
                  F11.982, F13.182, F13.282, F13.982,
                  F14.182, F14.282, F14.982, F15.182,
                  F15.282, F15.982, F19.182, F19.282,
                  F19.982)
                insomnia NOS (G47.0-)
                insomnia due to known physiological
                  condition (G47.0-)
                organic insomnia (G47.0-)
                sleep deprivation (Z72.820)

   F51.01   **Primary insomnia**
          Idiopathic insomnia

   F51.02   **Adjustment insomnia**

   F51.03   **Paradoxical insomnia**

   F51.04   **Psychophysiologic insomnia**

   F51.05   **Insomnia due to other mental disorder**
          Code also associated mental disorder

   F51.09   **Other insomnia not due to a substance or
known physiological condition**

● **F51.1**   **Hypersomnia not due to a substance or known
physiological condition**
     Hypersomnia: Excessive sleeping/sleepiness
     Excludes2   alcohol related hypersomnia (F10.182,
                  F10.282, F10.982)
                drug-related hypersomnia (F11.182,
                  F11.282, F11.982, F13.182, F13.282,
                  F13.982, F14.182, F14.282, F14.982,
                  F15.182, F15.282, F15.982, F19.182,
                  F19.282, F19.982)
                hypersomnia NOS (G47.10)
                hypersomnia due to known physiological
                  condition (G47.10)
                idiopathic hypersomnia (G47.11, G47.12)
                narcolepsy (G47.4-)

   F51.11   **Primary hypersomnia**

   F51.12   **Insufficient sleep syndrome**
          Excludes1   sleep deprivation (Z72.820)

   F51.13   **Hypersomnia due to other mental disorder**
          Code also associated mental disorder

   F51.19   **Other hypersomnia not due to a substance or
known physiological condition**

   F51.3   **Sleepwalking [somnambulism]**

   F51.4   **Sleep terrors [night terrors]**

   F51.5   **Nightmare disorder**
          Dream anxiety disorder

   F51.8   **Other sleep disorders not due to a substance or known
physiological condition**

   F51.9   **Sleep disorder not due to a substance or known
physiological condition, unspecified**
          Emotional sleep disorder NOS

CHAPTER 5 (F01-F99)

● **F52   Sexual dysfunction not due to a substance or known physiological condition**
> [Excludes2] Dhat syndrome (F48.8)

   F52.0   **Hypoactive sexual desire disorder**
> Anhedonia (sexual)
> *Total loss of feeling of sexual pleasure*
> Lack or loss of sexual desire
> [Excludes1] decreased libido (R68.82)

   F52.1   **Sexual aversion disorder**
> Sexual aversion and lack of sexual enjoyment

● F52.2   **Sexual arousal disorders**
> Failure of genital response

      F52.21   **Male erectile disorder**
> Psychogenic impotence
> [Excludes1] impotence of organic origin (N52.-)
> impotence NOS (N52.-)

      F52.22   **Female sexual arousal disorder**
> Frigidity

● F52.3   **Orgasmic disorder**
> Inhibited orgasm
> Psychogenic anorgasmy

      F52.31   **Female orgasmic disorder**

      F52.32   **Male orgasmic disorder**

   F52.4   **Premature ejaculation**

   F52.5   **Vaginismus not due to a substance or known physiological condition**
> Psychogenic vaginismus
> [Excludes2] vaginismus (due to a known physiological condition) (N94.2)

   F52.6   **Dyspareunia not due to a substance or known physiological condition**
> *Dyspareunia: Difficult or painful sexual intercourse*
> Psychogenic dyspareunia
> [Excludes2] dyspareunia (due to a known physiological condition) (N94.1)

   F52.8   **Other sexual dysfunction not due to a substance or known physiological condition**
> Excessive sexual drive
> Nymphomania
> Satyriasis

   F52.9   **Unspecified sexual dysfunction not due to a substance or known physiological condition**
> Sexual dysfunction NOS

F53   Puerperal psychosis
> Postpartum depression
> *Acute mental illness with sudden onset following childbirth with symptoms of affective psychosis, disorientation, and confusion are prevalent*
> [Excludes1] mood disorders with psychotic features (F30.2, F31.2, F31.5, F31.64, F32.3, F33.3)
> postpartum dysphoria (O90.6)
> psychosis in schizophrenia, schizotypal, delusional, and other psychotic disorders (F20-F29)

F54   Psychological and behavioral factors associated with disorders or diseases classified elsewhere
> Psychological factors affecting physical conditions
> *Code first the associated physical disorder, such as:*
> asthma (J45.-)
> dermatitis (L23-L25)
> gastric ulcer (K25.-)
> mucous colitis (K58.-)
> ulcerative colitis (K51.-)
> urticaria (L50.-)
> [Excludes2] tension-type headache (G44.2)

● **F55   Abuse of non-psychoactive substances**
> [Excludes2] abuse of psychoactive substances (F10-F19)

   F55.0   **Abuse of antacids**

   F55.1   **Abuse of herbal or folk remedies**

   F55.2   **Abuse of laxatives**

   F55.3   **Abuse of steroids or hormones**

   F55.4   **Abuse of vitamins**

   F55.8   **Abuse of other non-psychoactive substances**

  F59   **Unspecified behavioral syndromes associated with physiological disturbances and physical factors**
> Psychogenic physiological dysfunction NOS

DISORDERS OF ADULT PERSONALITY AND BEHAVIOR (F60-F69)

● **F60   Specific personality disorders**
> *Long-term patterns of thoughts and behaviors causing serious problems with relationships and work.*

   F60.0   **Paranoid personality disorder**
> *Hostile, devious, and combative response to disappointments*
> Expansive paranoid personality (disorder)
> Fanatic personality (disorder)
> Querulant personality (disorder)
> Paranoid personality (disorder)
> Sensitive paranoid personality (disorder)
> [Excludes2] paranoia (F22)
> paranoia querulans (F22)
> paranoid psychosis (F22)
> paranoid schizophrenia (F20.0)
> paranoid state (F22)

   F60.1   **Schizoid personality disorder**
> *Detachment from social relationships with minimal emotional experiences and expressions*
> [Excludes2] Asperger's syndrome (F84.5)
> delusional disorder (F22)
> schizoid disorder of childhood (F84.5)
> schizophrenia (F20.-)
> schizotypal disorder (F21)

   F60.2   **Antisocial personality disorder**
> *Continuous and chronic antisocial behavior*
> Amoral personality (disorder)
> Asocial personality (disorder)
> Dissocial personality disorder
> Psychopathic personality (disorder)
> Sociopathic personality (disorder)
> [Excludes1] conduct disorders (F91.-)
> [Excludes2] borderline personality disorder (F60.3)

   F60.3   **Borderline personality disorder**
> *Instability of mood, self-image or sense of self, and interpersonal relationships*
> Aggressive personality (disorder)
> Emotionally unstable personality disorder
> Explosive personality (disorder)
> [Excludes2] antisocial personality disorder (F60.2)

   F60.4   **Histrionic personality disorder**
> *Personality disorder with excessive emotional and attention-seeking behavior*
> Hysterical personality (disorder)
> Psychoinfantile personality (disorder)

   F60.5   **Obsessive-compulsive personality disorder**
> Anankastic personality (disorder)
> Compulsive personality (disorder)
> Obsessional personality (disorder)
> [Excludes2] obsessive-compulsive disorder (F42)

   F60.6   **Avoidant personality disorder**
> Anxious personality disorder

   F60.7   **Dependent personality disorder**
> Asthenic personality (disorder)
> Inadequate personality (disorder)
> Passive personality (disorder)

● **F60.8 Other specific personality disorders**
  F60.81 Narcissistic personality disorder
   Vanity, conceit, egotism or indifference to plight of others

  F60.89 Other specific personality disorders
   Eccentric personality disorder
   'Haltlose' type personality disorder
   Immature personality disorder
   Passive-aggressive personality disorder
   Psychoneurotic personality disorder
   Self-defeating personality disorder

F60.9 Personality disorder, unspecified
  Character disorder NOS
  Character neurosis NOS
  Pathological personality NOS

● **F63 Impulse disorders**
  Excludes2 habitual excessive use of alcohol or psychoactive substances (F10-F19)
      impulse disorders involving sexual behavior (F65.-)

F63.0 Pathological gambling
  Compulsive gambling
  Excludes1 gambling and betting NOS (Z72.6)
  Excludes2 excessive gambling by manic patients (F30, F31)
      gambling in antisocial personality disorder (F60.2)

F63.1 Pyromania
  Pathological fire-setting
  Excludes2 fire-setting (by) (in):
      adult with antisocial personality disorder (F60.2)
      alcohol or psychoactive substance intoxication (F10-F19)
      conduct disorders (F91.-)
      mental disorders due to known physiological condition (F01-F09)
      schizophrenia (F20.-)

F63.2 Kleptomania
  Pathological stealing
  Excludes1 shoplifting as the reason for observation for suspected mental disorder (Z03.8)
  Excludes2 depressive disorder with stealing (F31-F33)
      stealing due to underlying mental condition-code to mental condition
      stealing in mental disorders due to known physiological condition (F01-F09)

F63.3 Trichotillomania
  Hair plucking
  Excludes2 other stereotyped movement disorder (F98.4)

● **F63.8 Other impulse disorders**
  F63.81 Intermittent explosive disorder
  F63.89 Other impulse disorders

F63.9 Impulse disorder, unspecified
  Impulse control disorder NOS

● **F64 Gender identity disorders**
  F64.1 Gender identity disorder in adolescence and adulthood
   Dual role transvestism
   Transsexualism
   Use additional code to identify sex reassignment status (Z87.890)
  Excludes1 gender identity disorder in childhood (F64.2)
  Excludes2 fetishistic transvestism (F65.1)

F64.2 Gender identity disorder of childhood
  Excludes1 gender identity disorder in adolescence and adulthood (F64.1)
  Excludes2 sexual maturation disorder (F66)

F64.8 Other gender identity disorders

F64.9 Gender identity disorder, unspecified
  Gender-role disorder NOS

● **F65 Paraphilias**
  F65.0 Fetishism
   Intense sexual urges and arousing fantasies using inanimate objects

  F65.1 Transvestic fetishism
   Intense sexual urges, arousal, or orgasm associated with fantasized/actual cross-dressing
   Fetishistic transvestism

  F65.2 Exhibitionism

  F65.3 Voyeurism
   Sexual urges or arousal involving real or fantasized observation of unsuspecting people who are naked, disrobing, or engaging in sexual activity

  F65.4 Pedophilia

● **F65.5 Sadomasochism**
  F65.50 Sadomasochism, unspecified
  F65.51 Sexual masochism
  F65.52 Sexual sadism

● **F65.8 Other paraphilias**
  F65.81 Frotteurism
   Sexual arousal or orgasm is achieved by rubbing up against another person (or fantasies of), in crowded place with unsuspecting victim

  F65.89 Other paraphilias
   Necrophilia

F65.9 Paraphilia, unspecified
  Sexual deviation NOS

F66 Other sexual disorders
  Sexual maturation disorder
  Sexual relationship disorder

● **F68 Other disorders of adult personality and behavior**
● **F68.1 Factitious disorder**
  Compensation neurosis
  Elaboration of physical symptoms for psychological reasons
  Hospital hopper syndrome
  Münchhausen's syndrome
  Peregrinating patient
  Excludes2 factitial dermatitis (L98.1)
      person feigning illness (with obvious motivation) (Z76.5)

  F68.10 Factitious disorder, unspecified
  F68.11 Factitious disorder with predominantly psychological signs and symptoms
  F68.12 Factitious disorder with predominantly physical signs and symptoms
  F68.13 Factitious disorder with combined psychological and physical signs and symptoms

F68.8 Other specified disorders of adult personality and behavior

F69 Unspecified disorder of adult personality and behavior

INTELLECTUAL DISABILITIES (F70-F79)

Code first any associated physical or developmental disorders
  Excludes1 borderline intellectual functioning, IQ above 70 to 84 (R41.83)

F70 Mild intellectual disabilities
  IQ level 50-55 to approximately 70
  Mild mental subnormality

◀ New ⬅ Revised ~~deleted~~ Deleted **OGCR** Official Guidelines X Assign placeholder X ● Use Additional Character(s)

Excludes 1 Excludes 2 Includes Use additional Code first Code also Unspecified

829

CHAPTER 5 (F01-F99)

F71   Moderate intellectual disabilities
   IQ level 35-40 to 50-55
   Moderate mental subnormality

F72   Severe intellectual disabilities
   IQ 20-25 to 35-40
   Severe mental subnormality

F73   Profound intellectual disabilities
   IQ level below 20-25
   Profound mental subnormality

F78   Other intellectual disabilities

F79   Unspecified intellectual disabilities
   Mental deficiency NOS
   Mental subnormality NOS

PERVASIVE AND SPECIFIC DEVELOPMENTAL DISORDERS (F80-F89)

● **F80   Specific developmental disorders of speech and language**
   F80.0   Phonological disorder
      Communication disorder of unknown cause, characterized by failure to use age-appropriate sounds
      Dyslalia
      Functional speech articulation disorder
      Lalling
      Lisping
      Phonological developmental disorder
      Speech articulation developmental disorder

      Excludes1   speech articulation impairment due to aphasia NOS (R47.01)
                     speech articulation impairment due to apraxia (R48.2)

      Excludes2   speech articulation impairment due to hearing loss (F80.4)
                     speech articulation impairment due to intellectual disabilities (F70-F79)
                     speech articulation impairment with expressive language developmental disorder (F80.1)
                     speech articulation impairment with mixed receptive expressive language developmental disorder (F80.2)

   F80.1   Expressive language disorder
      Developmental dysphasia or aphasia, expressive type

      Excludes1   mixed receptive-expressive language disorder (F80.2)
                     dysphasia and aphasia NOS (R47.-)

      Excludes2   acquired aphasia with epilepsy [Landau-Kleffner] (G40.80-)
                     intellectual disabilities (F70-F79)
                     pervasive developmental disorders (F84.-)
                     selective mutism (F94.0)

   F80.2   Mixed receptive-expressive language disorder
      Developmental dysphasia or aphasia, receptive type
      Developmental Wernicke's aphasia

      Excludes1   central auditory processing disorder (H93.25)
                     dysphasia or aphasia NOS (R47.-)
                     expressive language disorder (F80.1)
                     expressive type dysphasia or aphasia (F80.1)
                     word deafness (H93.25)

      Excludes2   acquired aphasia with epilepsy [Landau-Kleffner] (G40.80-)
                     intellectual disabilities (F70-F79)
                     pervasive developmental disorders (F84.-)
                     selective mutism (F94.0)

   F80.4   Speech and language development delay due to hearing loss

      Code also type of hearing loss (H90.-, H91.-)

● **F80.8   Other developmental disorders of speech or language**
   F80.81   Childhood onset fluency disorder
      Cluttering NOS
      Stuttering NOS

      Excludes1   adult onset fluency disorder (F98.5)
                     fluency disorder in conditions classified elsewhere (R47.82)
                     fluency disorder (stuttering) following cerebrovascular disease (I69. with final characters -23)

   F80.89   Other developmental disorders of speech and language

   F80.9   Developmental disorder of speech and language, unspecified
      Communication disorder NOS
      Language disorder NOS

● **F81   Specific developmental disorders of scholastic skills**
   F81.0   Specific reading disorder
      'Backward reading'
      Developmental dyslexia
      Specific reading retardation

      Excludes1   alexia NOS (R48.0)
                     dyslexia NOS (R48.0)

   F81.2   Mathematics disorder
      Developmental acalculia
      Developmental arithmetical disorder
      Developmental Gerstmann's syndrome

      Excludes1   acalculia NOS (R48.8)

      Excludes2   arithmetical difficulties associated with a reading disorder (F81.0)
                     arithmetical difficulties associated with a spelling disorder (F81.81)
                     arithmetical difficulties due to inadequate teaching (Z55.8)

● **F81.8   Other developmental disorders of scholastic skills**
   F81.81   Disorder of written expression
      Specific spelling disorder

   F81.89   Other developmental disorders of scholastic skills

   F81.9   Developmental disorder of scholastic skills, unspecified
      Knowledge acquisition disability NOS
      Learning disability NOS
      Learning disorder NOS

F82   Specific developmental disorder of motor function
   Clumsy child syndrome
   Developmental coordination disorder
   Developmental dyspraxia

   Excludes1   abnormalities of gait and mobility (R26.-)
                  lack of coordination (R27.-)

   Excludes2   lack of coordination secondary to intellectual disabilities (F70-F79)

◀ New   ◀▥ Revised   deleted Deleted   OGCR Official Guidelines   X Assign placeholder X   ● Use Additional Character(s)
Excludes 1   Excludes 2   Includes   Use additional   Code first   Code also   Unspecified

● **F84** **Pervasive developmental disorders**
Use additional code to identify any associated medical condition and intellectual disabilities.

     F84.0   **Autistic disorder**
          Infantile autism
          Infantile psychosis
          Kanner's syndrome
          | **Excludes1** | Asperger's syndrome (F84.5)

     F84.2   **Rett's syndrome**
          Neurodevelopmental disorder
          | **Excludes1** | Asperger's syndrome (F84.5)
                            Autistic disorder (F84.0)
                            other childhood disintegrative disorder (F84.3)

     F84.3   **Other childhood disintegrative disorder**
          Dementia infantilis
          At least two years of normal development followed by significant loss of language abilities, social skills, bowel/bladder control, motor skills
          Disintegrative psychosis
          Heller's syndrome
          At least two years of normal development followed by significant loss of language abilities, social skills, bowel/bladder control, motor skills
          Symbiotic psychosis
          Abnormal relationship to mothering figure, characterized by intense separation anxiety, severe regression, giving up of useful speech, and autism
          Use additional code to identify any associated neurological condition.
          | **Excludes1** | Asperger's syndrome (F84.5)
                            Autistic disorder (F84.0)
                            Rett's syndrome (F84.2)

     F84.5   **Asperger's syndrome**
          Developmental disorder
          Asperger's disorder
          Autistic psychopathy
          Schizoid disorder of childhood

     F84.8   **Other pervasive developmental disorders**
          Overactive disorder associated with intellectual disabilities and stereotyped movements

     F84.9   **Pervasive developmental disorder, unspecified**
          Atypical autism

F88   **Other disorders of psychological development**
          Developmental agnosia

F89   **Unspecified disorder of psychological development**
          Developmental disorder NOS

BEHAVIORAL AND EMOTIONAL DISORDERS WITH ONSET USUALLY OCCURRING IN CHILDHOOD AND ADOLESCENCE (F90-F98)

Note: Codes within categories F90-F98 may be used regardless of the age of a patient. These disorders generally have onset within the childhood or adolescent years, but may continue throughout life or not be diagnosed until adulthood.

● **F90** **Attention-deficit hyperactivity disorders**
     Attention deficit disorder with hyperactivity=ADHD
     | **Includes** | attention deficit disorder with hyperactivity
                    attention deficit syndrome with hyperactivity
     | **Excludes2** | anxiety disorders (F40.-, F41.-)
                    mood [affective] disorders (F30-F39)
                    pervasive developmental disorders (F84.-)
                    schizophrenia (F20.-)

     F90.0   **Attention-deficit hyperactivity disorder, predominantly inattentive type**

     F90.1   **Attention-deficit hyperactivity disorder, predominantly hyperactive type**

     F90.2   **Attention-deficit hyperactivity disorder, combined type**

     F90.8   **Attention-deficit hyperactivity disorder, other type**

     F90.9   **Attention-deficit hyperactivity disorder, unspecified type**
          Attention-deficit hyperactivity disorder of childhood or adolescence NOS
          Attention-deficit hyperactivity disorder NOS

● **F91** **Conduct disorders**
     Childhood/adolescence disruptive behavior disorder
     | **Excludes1** | antisocial behavior (Z72.81-)
                    antisocial personality disorder (F60.2)
     | **Excludes2** | conduct problems associated with attention-deficit hyperactivity disorder (F90.-)
                    mood [affective] disorders (F30-F39)
                    pervasive developmental disorders (F84.-)
                    schizophrenia (F20.-)

     F91.0   **Conduct disorder confined to family context**

     F91.1   **Conduct disorder, childhood-onset type**
          Unsocialized conduct disorder
          Conduct disorder, solitary aggressive type
          Unsocialized aggressive disorder

     F91.2   **Conduct disorder, adolescent-onset type**
          Socialized conduct disorder
          Conduct disorder, group type

     F91.3   **Oppositional defiant disorder**

     F91.8   **Other conduct disorders**

     F91.9   **Conduct disorder, unspecified**
          Behavioral disorder NOS
          Conduct disorder NOS
          Disruptive behavior disorder NOS

● **F93** **Emotional disorders with onset specific to childhood**
     F93.0   **Separation anxiety disorder of childhood**
          | **Excludes2** | mood [affective] disorders (F30-F39)
                        nonpsychotic mental disorders (F40-F48)
                        phobic anxiety disorder of childhood (F40.8)
                        social phobia (F40.1)

     F93.8   **Other childhood emotional disorders**
          Identity disorder
          | **Excludes2** | gender identity disorder of childhood (F64.2)

     F93.9   **Childhood emotional disorder, unspecified**

● **F94** **Disorders of social functioning with onset specific to childhood and adolescence**
     F94.0   **Selective mutism**
          Elective mutism
          | **Excludes2** | pervasive developmental disorders (F84.-)
                        schizophrenia (F20.-)
                        specific developmental disorders of speech and language (F80.-)
                        transient mutism as part of separation anxiety in young children (F93.0)

     F94.1   **Reactive attachment disorder of childhood**
          Use additional code to identify any associated failure to thrive or growth retardation
          | **Excludes1** | disinhibited attachment disorder of childhood (F94.2)
                        normal variation in pattern of selective attachment
          | **Excludes2** | Asperger's syndrome (F84.5)
                        maltreatment syndromes (T74.-)
                        sexual or physical abuse in childhood, resulting in psychosocial problems (Z62.81-)

     F94.2   **Disinhibited attachment disorder of childhood**
          Affectionless psychopathy
          Institutional syndrome
          | **Excludes1** | reactive attachment disorder of childhood (F94.1)
          | **Excludes2** | Asperger's syndrome (F84.5)
                        attention-deficit hyperactivity disorders (F90.-)
                        hospitalism in children (F43.2-)

     F94.8   **Other childhood disorders of social functioning**

     F94.9   **Childhood disorder of social functioning, unspecified**

◀ New   ⬅ Revised   ~~deleted~~ Deleted   OGCR Official Guidelines   X Assign placeholder X   ● Use Additional Character(s)

| Excludes 1 | | Excludes 2 | Includes   Use additional   Code first   Code also   Unspecified

Item 5–2 Enuresis: Bed wetting by children at night. Causes can be either psychological or medical (diabetes, urinary tract infections, or abnormalities). **Encopresis:** Overflow incontinence of bowels sometimes resulting from chronic constipation or fecal impaction. Check the documentation for additional diagnoses.

● **F95   Tic disorder**
> *Involuntary twitch*

     F95.0   Transient tic disorder

     F95.1   Chronic motor or vocal tic disorder

     F95.2   Tourette's disorder
> Combined vocal and multiple motor tic disorder [de la Tourette]
> Tourette's syndrome

     F95.8   Other tic disorders

     F95.9   Tic disorder, unspecified
> Tic NOS

● **F98   Other behavioral and emotional disorders with onset usually occurring in childhood and adolescence**

     Excludes2   breath-holding spells (R06.89)
> gender identity disorder of childhood (F64.2)
> Kleine-Levin syndrome (G47.13)
> obsessive-compulsive disorder (F42)
> sleep disorders not due to a substance or known physiological condition (F51.-)

     F98.0   Enuresis not due to a substance or known physiological condition
> *Enuresis: Urinary incontinence*
> Enuresis (primary) (secondary) of nonorganic origin
> Functional enuresis
> Psychogenic enuresis
> Urinary incontinence of nonorganic origin

         Excludes1   enuresis NOS (R32)

     F98.1   Encopresis not due to a substance or known physiological condition
> *Encopresis: Fecal incontinence*
> Functional encopresis
> Incontinence of feces of nonorganic origin
> Psychogenic encopresis

         Use additional code to identify the cause of any coexisting constipation.

         Excludes1   encopresis NOS (R15.-)

●   **F98.2   Other feeding disorders of infancy and childhood**

         Excludes1   feeding difficulties (R63.3)

         Excludes2   anorexia nervosa and other eating disorders (F50.-)
> feeding problems of newborn (P92.-)
> pica of infancy or childhood (F98.3)

     F98.21   Rumination disorder of infancy

     F98.29   Other feeding disorders of infancy and early childhood

     F98.3   Pica of infancy and childhood
> *Craving and eating substances such as paint, clay, or dirt to replace a nutritional deficit in the body.*

     F98.4   Stereotyped movement disorders
> Stereotype/habit disorder

         Excludes1   abnormal involuntary movements (R25.-)

         Excludes2   compulsions in obsessive-compulsive disorder (F42)
> hair plucking (F63.3)
> movement disorders of organic origin (G20-G25)
> nail-biting (F98.8)
> nose-picking (F98.8)
> stereotypies that are part of a broader psychiatric condition (F01-F95)
> thumb-sucking (F98.8)
> tic disorders (F95.-)
> trichotillomania (F63.3)

     F98.5   Adult onset fluency disorder

         Excludes1   childhood onset fluency disorder (F80.81)
> dysphasia (R47.02)
> fluency disorder in conditions classified elsewhere (R47.82)
> fluency disorder (stuttering) following cerebrovascular disease (I69. with final characters -23)
> tic disorders (F95.-)

     F98.8   Other specified behavioral and emotional disorders with onset usually occurring in childhood and adolescence
> Excessive masturbation
> Nail-biting
> Nose-picking
> Thumb-sucking

     F98.9   Unspecified behavioral and emotional disorders with onset usually occurring in childhood and adolescence

UNSPECIFIED MENTAL DISORDER (F99)

F99   Mental disorder, not otherwise specified
> Mental illness NOS

     Excludes1   unspecified mental disorder due to known physiological condition (F09)

◀ New   ◀▪▪▪ Revised   ~~deleted~~ Deleted   **OGCR** Official Guidelines   X Assign placeholder X   ● Use Additional Character(s)

Excludes 1   Excludes 2   Includes   Use additional   Code first   Code also   Unspecified

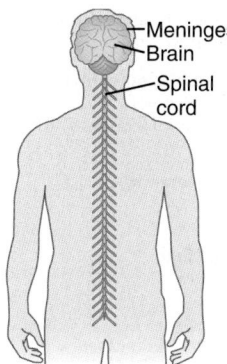
Meninges
Brain
Spinal cord

Figure 6-1   The brain and spinal cord make up the central nervous system.

Item 6–1   The two major classifications of the nervous system are the peripheral nervous system and the central nervous system (CNS). The central nervous system is comprised of the brain and the spinal cord. The peripheral nervous system is comprised of the parasympathetic and sympathetic systems. **Encephalitis** is the swelling of the brain. **Meningitis** is swelling of the covering of the brain, the meninges. Types and causes of brain infections are:

Type	Cause
purulent	bacterial
aseptic/abacterial	viral
chronic meningitis	mycobacterial and fungal

CHAPTER 6

DISEASES OF THE NERVOUS SYSTEM (G00-G99)

Excludes2   certain conditions originating in the perinatal period (P04-P96)
certain infectious and parasitic diseases (A00-B99)
complications of pregnancy, childbirth and the puerperium (O00-O9A)
congenital malformations, deformations, and chromosomal abnormalities (Q00-Q99)
endocrine, nutritional and metabolic diseases (E00-E88)
injury, poisoning and certain other consequences of external causes (S00-T88)
neoplasms (C00-D49)
symptoms, signs and abnormal clinical and laboratory findings, not elsewhere classified (R00-R94)

This chapter contains the following blocks:

G00-G09	Inflammatory diseases of the central nervous system
G10-G14	Systemic atrophies primarily affecting the central nervous system
G20-G26	Extrapyramidal and movement disorders
G30-G32	Other degenerative diseases of the nervous system
G35-G37	Demyelinating diseases of the central nervous system
G40-G47	Episodic and paroxysmal disorders
G50-G59	Nerve, nerve root and plexus disorders
G60-G65	Polyneuropathies and other disorders of the peripheral nervous system
G70-G73	Diseases of myoneural junction and muscle
G80-G83	Cerebral palsy and other paralytic syndromes
G89-G99	Other disorders of the nervous system

INFLAMMATORY DISEASES OF THE CENTRAL NERVOUS SYSTEM (G00-G09)

● **G00**   **Bacterial meningitis, not elsewhere classified**
An infection of the cerebrospinal fluid surrounding the spinal cord and brain.

Includes   bacterial arachnoiditis
bacterial leptomeningitis
bacterial meningitis
bacterial pachymeningitis

Excludes1   bacterial:
meningoencephalitis (G04.2)
meningomyelitis (G04.2)

G00.0   **Hemophilus meningitis**
Meningitis due to Hemophilus influenzae

G00.1   **Pneumococcal meningitis**

G00.2   **Streptococcal meningitis**
Use additional code to further identify organism (B95.0-B95.5)

G00.3   **Staphylococcal meningitis**
Use additional code to further identify organism (B95.61-B95.8)

G00.8   **Other bacterial meningitis**
Meningitis due to Escherichia coli
Meningitis due to Friedländer bacillus
Meningitis due to Klebsiella
Use additional code to further identify organism (B96.-)

G00.9   **Bacterial meningitis, unspecified**
Meningitis due to gram-negative bacteria, unspecified
Purulent meningitis NOS
Pyogenic meningitis NOS
Suppurative meningitis NOS

G01   **Meningitis in bacterial diseases classified elsewhere**
Code first underlying disease
Excludes1   meningitis (in):
gonococcal (A54.81)
leptospirosis (A27.81)
listeriosis (A32.11)
Lyme disease (A69.21)
meningococcal (A39.0)
neurosyphilis (A52.13)
tuberculosis (A17.0)
meningoencephalitis and meningomyelitis in bacterial diseases classified elsewhere (G05)

G02   **Meningitis in other infectious and parasitic diseases classified elsewhere**
Code first underlying disease, such as:
African trypanosomiasis (B56.-)
poliovirus infection (A80.-)
Excludes1   candidal meningitis (B37.5)
coccidioidomycosis meningitis (B38.4)
cryptococcal meningitis (B45.1)
herpesviral [herpes simplex] meningitis (B00.3)
infectious mononucleosis complicated by meningitis (B27.- with fourth character 2)
measles complicated by meningitis (B05.1)
meningoencephalitis and meningomyelitis in other infectious and parasitic diseases classified elsewhere (G05)
mumps meningitis (B26.1)
rubella meningitis (B06.02)
varicella [chickenpox] meningitis (B01.0)
zoster meningitis (B02.1)

● **G03**   **Meningitis due to other and unspecified causes**

> **Includes**   arachnoiditis NOS
> leptomeningitis NOS
> meningitis NOS
> pachymeningitis NOS

> **Excludes1**   meningoencephalitis (G04.-)
> meningomyelitis (G04.-)

G03.0   **Nonpyogenic meningitis**
> Aseptic meningitis
> Nonbacterial meningitis

G03.1   **Chronic meningitis**

G03.2   **Benign recurrent meningitis [Mollaret]**

G03.8   **Meningitis due to other specified causes**

G03.9   **Meningitis, unspecified**
> Arachnoiditis (spinal) NOS

● **G04**   **Encephalitis, myelitis and encephalomyelitis**

> **Includes**   acute ascending myelitis
> meningoencephalitis
> meningomyelitis

> **Excludes1**   encephalopathy NOS (G93.40)
> other noninfectious acute disseminated
> encephalomyelitis (noninfectious ADEM)
> (G04.81)

> **Excludes2**   acute transverse myelitis (G37.3-)
> alcoholic encephalopathy (G31.2)
> benign myalgic encephalomyelitis (G93.3)
> multiple sclerosis (G35)
> subacute necrotizing myelitis (G37.4)
> toxic encephalitis (G92)
> toxic encephalopathy (G92)

● **G04.0**   **Acute disseminated encephalitis and encephalomyelitis (ADEM)**

> **Excludes1**   acute necrotizing hemorrhagic
> encephalopathy (G04.3-)

G04.00   **Acute disseminated encephalitis and encephalomyelitis, unspecified**

G04.01   **Postinfectious acute disseminated encephalitis and encephalomyelitis (postinfectious ADEM)**

> **Excludes1**   post chickenpox encephalitis
> (B01.1)
> post measles encephalitis (B05.0)
> post measles myelitis (B05.1)

G04.02   **Postimmunization acute disseminated encephalitis, myelitis and encephalomyelitis**
> Encephalitis, post immunization
> Encephalomyelitis, post immunization
> Use additional code to identify the vaccine
> (T50.A-, T50.B-, T50.Z-)

G04.1   **Tropical spastic paraplegia**

G04.2   **Bacterial meningoencephalitis and meningomyelitis, not elsewhere classified**

● **G04.3**   **Acute necrotizing hemorrhagic encephalopathy**
> *Sudden and severe CNS disease with pathology of hemorrhages and necrosis of white matter*

> **Excludes1**   acute disseminated encephalitis and
> encephalomyelitis (G04.0-)

G04.30   **Acute necrotizing hemorrhagic encephalopathy, unspecified**

G04.31   **Postinfectious acute necrotizing hemorrhagic encephalopathy**

G04.32   **Postimmunization acute necrotizing hemorrhagic encephalopathy**
> Use additional code to identify vaccine
> (T50.A-, T50.B-, T50.Z-)

G04.39   **Other acute necrotizing hemorrhagic encephalopathy**
> Code also underlying etiology, if applicable

● **G04.8**   **Other encephalitis, myelitis and encephalomyelitis**
> Code also any associated seizure (G40.-, R56.9)

G04.81   **Other encephalitis and encephalomyelitis**
> Noninfectious acute disseminated
> encephalomyelitis (noninfectious ADEM)

G04.89   **Other myelitis**

● **G04.9**   **Encephalitis, myelitis and encephalomyelitis, unspecified**

G04.90   **Encephalitis and encephalomyelitis, unspecified**
> Ventriculitis (cerebral) NOS

G04.91   **Myelitis, unspecified**

● **G05**   **Encephalitis, myelitis and encephalomyelitis in diseases classified elsewhere**

> *Code first underlying disease, such as:*
> human immunodeficiency virus [HIV] disease (B20)
> poliovirus (A80.-)
> suppurative otitis media (H66.01-H66.4)
> trichinellosis (B75)

> **Excludes1**   adenoviral encephalitis, myelitis and
> encephalomyelitis (A85.1)
> congenital toxoplasmosis encephalitis, myelitis
> and encephalomyelitis (P37.1)
> cytomegaloviral encephalitis, myelitis and
> encephalomyelitis (B25.8)
> encephalitis, myelitis and encephalomyelitis (in)
> measles (B05.0)
> encephalitis, myelitis and encephalomyelitis (in)
> systemic lupus erythematosus (M32.19)
> enteroviral encephalitis, myelitis and
> encephalomyelitis (A85.0)
> herpesviral [herpes simplex] encephalitis,
> myelitis and encephalomyelitis (B00.4)
> listerial encephalitis, myelitis and
> éncephalomyelitis (A32.12)
> meningococcal encephalitis, myelitis and
> encephalomyelitis (A39.81)
> mumps encephalitis, myelitis and
> encephalomyelitis (B26.2)
> postchickenpox encephalitis, myelitis and
> encephalomyelitis (B01.1-)
> rubella encephalitis, myelitis and
> encephalomyelitis (B06.01)
> toxoplasmosis encephalitis, myelitis and
> encephalomyelitis (B58.2)
> zoster encephalitis, myelitis and
> encephalomyelitis (B02.0)

G05.3   **Encephalitis and encephalomyelitis in diseases classified elsewhere**
> Meningoencephalitis in diseases classified elsewhere

G05.4   **Myelitis in diseases classified elsewhere**
> Meningomyelitis in diseases classified elsewhere

● **G06**   **Intracranial and intraspinal abscess and granuloma**
> *An accumulation of pus in either the brain or spinal cord*
> Use additional code (B95-B97) to identify infectious agent.

G06.0   **Intracranial abscess and granuloma**
> Brain [any part] abscess (embolic)
> Cerebellar abscess (embolic)
> Cerebral abscess (embolic)
> Intracranial epidural abscess or granuloma
> Intracranial extradural abscess or granuloma
> Intracranial subdural abscess or granuloma
> Otogenic abscess (embolic)

> **Excludes1**   tuberculous intracranial abscess and
> granuloma (A17.81)

G06.1   **Intraspinal abscess and granuloma**
> Abscess (embolic) of spinal cord [any part]
> Intraspinal epidural abscess or granuloma
> Intraspinal extradural abscess or granuloma
> Intraspinal subdural abscess or granuloma

> **Excludes1**   tuberculous intraspinal abscess and
> granuloma (A17.81)

G06.2   **Extradural and subdural abscess, unspecified**

◀ New   ◀▬ Revised   ~~deleted~~ Deleted   OGCR Official Guidelines   X Assign placeholder X   ● Use Additional Character(s)

Excludes 1   Excludes 2   Includes   Use additional   Code first   Code also   Unspecified

G07　Intracranial and intraspinal abscess and granuloma in diseases classified elsewhere

Code first underlying disease, such as:
　　schistosomiasis granuloma of brain (B65.-)

Excludes1　abscess of brain:
　　　　amebic (A06.6)
　　　　chromomycotic (B43.1)
　　　　gonococcal (A54.82)
　　　　tuberculous (A17.81)
　　　　tuberculoma of meninges (A17.1)

G08　Intracranial and intraspinal phlebitis and thrombophlebitis

Septic embolism of intracranial or intraspinal venous sinuses and veins

Septic endophlebitis of intracranial or intraspinal venous sinuses and veins

Septic phlebitis of intracranial or intraspinal venous sinuses and veins

Septic thrombophlebitis of intracranial or intraspinal venous sinuses and veins

Septic thrombosis of intracranial or intraspinal venous sinuses and veins

Excludes1　intracranial phlebitis and thrombophlebitis complicating:
　　　abortion, ectopic or molar pregnancy (O00-O07, O08.7)
　　　pregnancy, childbirth and the puerperium (O22.5, O87.3)
　　　nonpyogenic intracranial phlebitis and thrombophlebitis (I67.6)

Excludes2　intracranial phlebitis and thrombophlebitis complicating nonpyogenic intraspinal phlebitis and thrombophlebitis (G95.1)

G09　Sequelae of inflammatory diseases of central nervous system

Note: Category G09 is to be used to indicate conditions whose primary classification is to G00-G08 as the cause of sequelae, themselves classifiable elsewhere. The 'sequelae' include conditions specified as residuals.

Code first condition resulting from (sequela) of inflammatory diseases of central nervous system

SYSTEMIC ATROPHIES PRIMARILY AFFECTING THE CENTRAL NERVOUS SYSTEM (G10-G14)

G10　Huntington's disease

Genetic disease with degeneration of cells of the nervous system, including brain

Huntington's chorea
Huntington's dementia

● **G11　Hereditary ataxia**

Genetic neurological disorder affecting coordination

Excludes2　cerebral palsy (G80.-)
　　　hereditary and idiopathic neuropathy (G60.-)
　　　metabolic disorders (E70-E88)

G11.0　Congenital nonprogressive ataxia

G11.1　Early-onset cerebellar ataxia
　　Early-onset cerebellar ataxia with essential tremor
　　Early-onset cerebellar ataxia with myoclonus [Hunt's ataxia]
　　Early-onset cerebellar ataxia with retained tendon reflexes
　　Friedreich's ataxia (autosomal recessive)
　　X-linked recessive spinocerebellar ataxia

G11.2　Late-onset cerebellar ataxia

G11.3　Cerebellar ataxia with defective DNA repair
　　Ataxia telangiectasia [Louis-Bar]
　　　Excludes2　Cockayne's syndrome (Q87.1)
　　　　other disorders of purine and pyrimidine metabolism (E79.-)
　　　　xeroderma pigmentosum (Q82.1)

G11.4　Hereditary spastic paraplegia

G11.8　Other hereditary ataxias

G11.9　Hereditary ataxia, unspecified
　　Hereditary cerebellar ataxia NOS
　　Hereditary cerebellar degeneration
　　Hereditary cerebellar disease
　　Hereditary cerebellar syndrome

● **G12　Spinal muscular atrophy and related syndromes**

G12.0　Infantile spinal muscular atrophy, type I [Werdnig-Hoffman]

G12.1　Other inherited spinal muscular atrophy
　　Adult form spinal muscular atrophy
　　Childhood form, type II spinal muscular atrophy
　　Distal spinal muscular atrophy
　　Juvenile form, type III spinal muscular atrophy [Kugelberg-Welander]
　　Progressive bulbar palsy of childhood [Fazio-Londe]
　　Scapuloperoneal form spinal muscular atrophy

● **G12.2　Motor neuron disease**
　　Progressive disease of motor neurons that carry impulses to muscles to move

G12.20　Motor neuron disease, unspecified

G12.21　Amyotrophic lateral sclerosis
　　Lou Gehrig's disease (ALS)
　　Progressive spinal muscle atrophy

G12.22　Progressive bulbar palsy

G12.29　Other motor neuron disease
　　Familial motor neuron disease
　　Primary lateral sclerosis

G12.8　Other spinal muscular atrophies and related syndromes

G12.9　Spinal muscular atrophy, unspecified

● **G13　Systemic atrophies primarily affecting central nervous system in diseases classified elsewhere**

G13.0　Paraneoplastic neuromyopathy and neuropathy
　　Carcinomatous neuromyopathy
　　Sensorial paraneoplastic neuropathy [Denny Brown]
　　Code first underlying neoplasm (C00-D49)

G13.1　Other systemic atrophy primarily affecting central nervous system in neoplastic disease
　　Paraneoplastic limbic encephalopathy
　　Code first underlying neoplasm (C00-D49)

G13.2　Systemic atrophy primarily affecting the central nervous system in myxedema
　　Code first underlying disease, such as:
　　　hypothyroidism (E03.-)
　　　myxedematous congenital iodine deficiency (E00.1)

G13.8　Systemic atrophy primarily affecting central nervous system in other diseases classified elsewhere
　　Code first underlying disease

G14　Postpolio syndrome

Includes　Postpolio myelitic syndrome
Excludes1　sequelae of poliomyelitis (B91)

EXTRAPYRAMIDAL AND MOVEMENT DISORDERS (G20-G26)

G20　Parkinson's disease

Progressive disease of the nervous system that affects muscle coordination

Hemiparkinsonism
Idiopathic Parkinsonism or Parkinson's disease
Paralysis agitans
Parkinsonism or Parkinson's disease NOS
Primary Parkinsonism or Parkinson's disease
Excludes1　dementia with Parkinsonism (G31.83)

Item 6-2 Huntington's chorea is an inherited degenerative disorder of the central nervous system and is characterized by ceaseless, jerky movements and progressive cognitive and behavioral deterioration.

◀ New　　◀▦ Revised　　~~deleted~~ Deleted　　**OGCR** Official Guidelines　　X Assign placeholder X　　● Use Additional Character(s)

| Excludes 1 | Excludes 2 | Includes | Use additional | Code first | Code also | Unspecified |

● **G21   Secondary parkinsonism**
> *Symptoms of Parkinson's caused by medicines, illness, or other nervous system disorder*

> | Excludes1 | dementia with Parkinsonism (G31.83) |
> | --- | --- |
> | | Huntington's disease (G10) |
> | | Shy-Drager syndrome (G90.3) |
> | | syphilitic Parkinsonism (A52.19) |

G21.0   Malignant neuroleptic syndrome
> Use additional code for adverse effect, if applicable, to identify drug (T43.3X5, T43.4X5, T43.505, T43.595)

> | Excludes1 | neuroleptic induced parkinsonism (G21.11) |
> | --- | --- |

● **G21.1   Other drug-induced secondary parkinsonism**

G21.11   Neuroleptic induced parkinsonism
> Use additional code for adverse effect, if applicable, to identify drug (T43.3X5, T43.4X5, T43.505, T43.595)

> | Excludes1 | malignant neuroleptic syndrome (G21.0) |
> | --- | --- |

G21.19   Other drug induced secondary parkinsonism
> Use additional code for adverse effect, if applicable, to identify drug (T36-T50 with fifth or sixth character 5)

G21.2   Secondary parkinsonism due to other external agents
> *Code first (T51-T65) to identify external agent*

G21.3   Postencephalitic parkinsonism

G21.4   Vascular parkinsonism

G21.8   Other secondary parkinsonism

G21.9   Secondary parkinsonism, unspecified

● **G23   Other degenerative diseases of basal ganglia**

> | Excludes2 | multi-system degeneration of the autonomic nervous system (G90.3) |
> | --- | --- |

G23.0   Hallervorden-Spatz disease
> Pigmentary pallidal degeneration

G23.1   Progressive supranuclear ophthalmoplegia [Steele-Richardson-Olszewski]
> Progressive supranuclear palsy

G23.2   Striatonigral degeneration

G23.8   Other specified degenerative diseases of basal ganglia
> Calcification of basal ganglia

G23.9   Degenerative disease of basal ganglia, unspecified

● **G24   Dystonia**
> *Involuntary movements*

> | Includes | dyskinesia |
> | --- | --- |

> | Excludes2 | athetoid cerebral palsy (G80.3) |
> | --- | --- |

● **G24.0   Drug induced dystonia**
> Use additional code for adverse effect, if applicable, to identify drug (T36-T50 with fifth or sixth character 5)

G24.01   Drug induced subacute dyskinesia
> Drug induced blepharospasm
> Drug induced orofacial dyskinesia
> Neuroleptic induced tardive dyskinesia
> Tardive dyskinesia

G24.02   Drug induced acute dystonia
> Acute dystonic reaction to drugs
> Neuroleptic induced acute dystonia

G24.09   Other drug induced dystonia

G24.1   Genetic torsion dystonia
> Dystonia deformans progressiva
> Dystonia musculorum deformans
> Familial torsion dystonia
> Idiopathic familial dystonia
> Idiopathic (torsion) dystonia NOS
> (Schwalbe-) Ziehen-Oppenheim disease

G24.2   Idiopathic nonfamilial dystonia

G24.3   Spasmodic torticollis
> *Head tilts toward one side and chin is elevated and turned toward opposite side (wry neck)*

> | Excludes1 | congenital torticollis (Q68.0) |
> | --- | --- |
> | | hysterical torticollis (F44.4) |
> | | ocular torticollis (R29.891) |
> | | psychogenic torticollis (F45.8) |
> | | torticollis NOS (M43.6) |
> | | traumatic recurrent torticollis (S13.4) |

G24.4   Idiopathic orofacial dystonia
> Orofacial dyskinesia

> | Excludes1 | drug induced orofacial dyskinesia (G24.01) |
> | --- | --- |

G24.5   Blepharospasm
> *Tonic spasm of orbicularis oculi muscle, producing closure of eyelids*

> | Excludes1 | drug induced blepharospasm (G24.01) |
> | --- | --- |

G24.8   Other dystonia
> Acquired torsion dystonia NOS

G24.9   Dystonia, unspecified
> Dyskinesia NOS

● **G25   Other extrapyramidal and movement disorders**
> *Extrapyramidal: Other than pyramidal tracts*

> | Excludes2 | sleep related movement disorders (G47.6-) |
> | --- | --- |

G25.0   Essential tremor
> Familial tremor

> | Excludes1 | tremor NOS (R25.1) |
> | --- | --- |

G25.1   Drug-induced tremor
> Use additional code for adverse effect, if applicable, to identify drug (T36-T50 with fifth or sixth character 5)

G25.2   Other specified forms of tremor
> Intention tremor

G25.3   Myoclonus
> *Shocklike contractions muscle(s)*
> Drug-induced myoclonus
> Palatal myoclonus
> Use additional code for adverse effect, if applicable, to identify drug (T36-T50 with fifth or sixth character 5)

> | Excludes1 | facial myokymia (G51.4) |
> | --- | --- |
> | | myoclonic epilepsy (G40.-) |

G25.4   Drug-induced chorea
> Use additional code for adverse effect, if applicable, to identify drug (T36-T50 with fifth or sixth character 5)

G25.5   Other chorea
> *Continual, involuntary, jerky, movements*
> Chorea NOS

> | Excludes1 | chorea NOS with heart involvement (I02.0) |
> | --- | --- |
> | | Huntington's chorea (G10) |
> | | rheumatic chorea (I02.-) |
> | | Sydenham's chorea (I02.-) |

● **G25.6   Drug induced tics and other tics of organic origin**

G25.61   Drug induced tics
> Use additional code for adverse effect, if applicable, to identify drug (T36-T50 with fifth or sixth character 5)

G25.69   Other tics of organic origin

> | Excludes1 | habit spasm (F95.9) |
> | --- | --- |
> | | tic NOS (F95.9) |
> | | Tourette's syndrome (F95.2) |

● **G25.7   Other and unspecified drug induced movement disorders**
> Use additional code for adverse effect, if applicable, to identify drug (T36-T50 with fifth or sixth character 5)

G25.70   Drug induced movement disorder, unspecified

G25.71   Drug induced akathisia
> Drug induced acathisia
> Neuroleptic induced acute akathisia

G25.79   Other drug induced movement disorders

◀ New   ◀▦ Revised   ~~deleted~~ Deleted   **OGCR** Official Guidelines   X Assign placeholder X   ● Use Additional Character(s)

Excludes 1	Excludes 2	Includes	Use additional	Code first	Code also	Unspecified

CHAPTER 6 (G00-G99)

● **G25.8   Other specified extrapyramidal and movement disorders**
     G25.81   Restless legs syndrome
     G25.82   Stiff-man syndrome
     G25.83   Benign shuddering attacks
     G25.89   Other specified extrapyramidal and movement disorders
   G25.9   Extrapyramidal and movement disorder, unspecified

G26   Extrapyramidal and movement disorders in diseases classified elsewhere
     Code first underlying disease

OTHER DEGENERATIVE DISEASES OF THE NERVOUS SYSTEM (G30-G32)

● **G30   Alzheimer's disease**
   Progressive central neurodegenerative disorder
     Includes   Alzheimer's dementia senile and presenile forms
   Use additional code to identify:
     delirium, if applicable (F05)
     dementia with behavioral disturbance (F02.81)
     dementia without behavioral disturbance (F02.80)
     Excludes 1   senile degeneration of brain NEC (G31.1)
         senile dementia NOS (F03)
         senility NOS (R41.81)
   G30.0   Alzheimer's disease with early onset
   G30.1   Alzheimer's disease with late onset
   G30.8   Other Alzheimer's disease
   G30.9   Alzheimer's disease, unspecified

● **G31   Other degenerative diseases of nervous system, not elsewhere classified**
   Use additional code to identify:
     dementia with behavioral disturbance (F02.81)
     dementia without behavioral disturbance (F02.80)
     Excludes 2   Reye's syndrome (G93.7)
   ● **G31.0   Frontotemporal dementia**
     G31.01   Pick's disease
         Primary progressive aphasia
         Progressive isolated aphasia
     G31.09   Other frontotemporal dementia
         Frontal dementia
   G31.1   Senile degeneration of brain, not elsewhere classified
     Excludes 1   Alzheimer's disease (G30.-)
         senility NOS (R41.81)
   G31.2   Degeneration of nervous system due to alcohol
     Alcoholic cerebellar ataxia
     Alcoholic cerebellar degeneration
     Alcoholic cerebral degeneration
     Alcoholic encephalopathy
     Dysfunction of the autonomic nervous system due to alcohol
     Code also associated alcoholism (F10.-)
   ● **G31.8   Other specified degenerative diseases of nervous system**
     G31.81   Alpers' disease
         Rare neuronal degeneration of cerebral cortex disease of young children
         Grey-matter degeneration
     G31.82   Leigh's disease
         Rare neurometabolic disorder that affects central nervous system
         Subacute necrotizing encephalopathy
     G31.83   Dementia with Lewy bodies
         Closely allied to Parkinson's Disease
         Dementia with Parkinsonism
         Lewy body dementia
         Lewy body disease

     G31.84   Mild cognitive impairment, so stated
         Excludes 1   age related cognitive decline (R41.81)
             altered mental status (R41.82)
             cerebral degeneration (G31.9)
             change in mental status (R41.82)
             cognitive deficits following (sequelae of) cerebral hemorrhage or infarction (I69.01, I69.11, I69.21, I69.31, I69.81, I69.91)
             cognitive impairment due to intracranial or head injury (S06.-)
             dementia (F01.-, F02.-, F03)
             mild memory disturbance (F06.8)
             neurologic neglect syndrome (R41.4)
             personality change, nonpsychotic (F68.8)
     G31.85   Corticobasal degeneration
     G31.89   Other specified degenerative diseases of nervous system
   G31.9   Degenerative disease of nervous system, unspecified

● **G32   Other degenerative disorders of nervous system in diseases classified elsewhere**
   G32.0   Subacute combined degeneration of spinal cord in diseases classified elsewhere
     Dana-Putnam syndrome
     Sclerosis of spinal cord (combined) (dorsolateral) (posterolateral)
     Code first underlying disease, such as:
       anemia (D51.9)
       dietary (D51.3)
       pernicious (D51.0)
       vitamin B12 deficiency (E53.8)
     Excludes 1   syphilitic combined degeneration of spinal cord (A52.11)
   ● **G32.8   Other specified degenerative disorders of nervous system in diseases classified elsewhere**
     Code first underlying disease, such as:
       amyloidosis cerebral degeneration (E85.-)
       cerebral degeneration (due to) hypothyroidism (E00.0-E03.9)
       cerebral degeneration (due to) neoplasm (C00-D49)
       cerebral degeneration (due to) vitamin B deficiency, except thiamine (E52-E53.-)
     Excludes 1   superior hemorrhagic polioencephalitis [Wernicke's encephalopathy] (E51.2)
     G32.81   Cerebellar ataxia in diseases classified elsewhere
         Code first underlying disease, such as:
           celiac disease (with gluten ataxia) (K90.0)
           cerebellar ataxia (in) neoplastic disease (paraneoplastic cerebellar degeneration) (C00-D49)
           non-celiac gluten ataxia (M35.9)
         Excludes 1   systemic atrophy primarily affecting the central nervous system in alcoholic cerebellar ataxia (G31.2)
             systemic atrophy primarily affecting the central nervous system in myxedema (G13.2)
     G32.89   Other specified degenerative disorders of nervous system in diseases classified elsewhere
         Degenerative encephalopathy in diseases classified elsewhere

CHAPTER 6 (G00-G99)

Item 6–3   Multiple sclerosis (MS) is a nervous system disease affecting the brain and spinal cord by damaging the myelin sheath surrounding and protecting nerve cells. The damage slows down/blocks messages between the brain and body. Symptoms are: visual disturbances, muscle weakness, coordination and balance issues, numbness, prickling, thinking and memory problems. The cause is unknown, though it is thought that it may be an autoimmune disease. It affects women more than men, between 20 and 40 years of age. MS can be mild, but it may cause the loss of ability to write, walk, and speak. There is no cure, but medication may slow or control symptoms.

DEMYELINATING DISEASES OF THE CENTRAL NERVOUS SYSTEM (G35-G37)

G35   **Multiple sclerosis**
   Destruction of central nervous system; four types: relapsing remitting, secondary progressive, primary progressive, and progressive relapsing
   Disseminated multiple sclerosis
   Generalized multiple sclerosis
   Multiple sclerosis NOS
   Multiple sclerosis of brain stem
   Multiple sclerosis of cord

● G36   **Other acute disseminated demyelination**
   Excludes1   postinfectious encephalitis and encephalomyelitis NOS (G04.01)

   G36.0   **Neuromyelitis optica [Devic]**
      Inflammatory disorder in which immune system attacks optic nerves and spinal cord producing inflammation of optic nerve (optic neuritis) and spinal cord (myelitis)
      Demyelination in optic neuritis
      Excludes1   optic neuritis NOS (H46)

   G36.1   **Acute and subacute hemorrhagic leukoencephalitis [Hurst]**

   G36.8   **Other specified acute disseminated demyelination**

   G36.9   **Acute disseminated demyelination, unspecified**

● G37   **Other demyelinating diseases of central nervous system**
   Destruction of central nervous system

   G37.0   **Diffuse sclerosis of central nervous system**
      Periaxial encephalitis
      Schilder's disease
      Excludes1   X linked adrenoleukodystrophy (E71.52-)

   G37.1   **Central demyelination of corpus callosum**

   G37.2   **Central pontine myelinolysis**

   G37.3   **Acute transverse myelitis in demyelinating disease of central nervous system**
      Acute transverse myelitis NOS
      Acute transverse myelopathy
      Excludes1   multiple sclerosis (G35)
                     neuromyelitis optica [Devic] (G36.0)

   G37.4   **Subacute necrotizing myelitis of central nervous system**

   G37.5   **Concentric sclerosis [Baló] of central nervous system**

   G37.8   **Other specified demyelinating diseases of central nervous system**

   G37.9   **Demyelinating disease of central nervous system, unspecified**

EPISODIC AND PAROXYSMAL DISORDERS (G40-G47)

● G40   **Epilepsy and recurrent seizures**
   Note: The following terms are to be considered equivalent to intractable: pharmacoresistant (pharmacologically resistant), treatment resistant, refractory (medically) and poorly controlled
   Excludes1   conversion disorder with seizures (F44.5)
                  convulsions NOS (R56.9)
                  hippocampal sclerosis (G93.81)
                  mesial temporal sclerosis (G93.81)
                  post traumatic seizures (R56.1)
                  seizure (convulsive) NOS (R56.9)
                  seizure of newborn (P90)
                  temporal sclerosis (G93.81)
                  Todd's paralysis (G83.8)

● G40.0   **Localization-related (focal) (partial) idiopathic epilepsy and epileptic syndromes with seizures of localized onset**
      Benign childhood epilepsy with centrotemporal EEG spikes
      Childhood epilepsy with occipital EEG paroxysms
      Excludes1   adult onset localization-related epilepsy (G40.1-, G40.2-)

   ● G40.00   **Localization-related (focal) (partial) idiopathic epilepsy and epileptic syndromes with seizures of localized onset, not intractable**
         Localization-related (focal) (partial) idiopathic epilepsy and epileptic syndromes with seizures of localized onset without intractability

      G40.001   **Localization-related (focal) (partial) idiopathic epilepsy and epileptic syndromes with seizures of localized onset, not intractable, with status epilepticus**

      G40.009   **Localization-related (focal) (partial) idiopathic epilepsy and epileptic syndromes with seizures of localized onset, not intractable, without status epilepticus**
            Localization-related (focal) (partial) idiopathic epilepsy and epileptic syndromes with seizures of localized onset NOS

   ● G40.01   **Localization-related (focal) (partial) idiopathic epilepsy and epileptic syndromes with seizures of localized onset, intractable**

      G40.011   **Localization-related (focal) (partial) idiopathic epilepsy and epileptic syndromes with seizures of localized onset, intractable, with status epilepticus**

      G40.019   **Localization-related (focal) (partial) idiopathic epilepsy and epileptic syndromes with seizures of localized onset, intractable, without status epilepticus**

◀ New   ◀▥ Revised   d̶e̶l̶e̶t̶e̶d̶ Deleted   **OGCR** Official Guidelines   X Assign placeholder X   ● Use Additional Character(s)
Excludes 1   Excludes 2   Includes   Use additional   Code first   Code also   Unspecified

● **G40.1**   **Localization-related (focal) (partial) symptomatic epilepsy and epileptic syndromes with simple partial seizures**

     Attacks without alteration of consciousness

     Epilepsia partialis continua [Kozhevnikof]

     Simple partial seizures developing into secondarily generalized seizures

   ● **G40.10**   **Localization-related (focal) (partial) symptomatic epilepsy and epileptic syndromes with simple partial seizures, not intractable**

      Localization-related (focal) (partial) symptomatic epilepsy and epileptic syndromes with simple partial seizures without intractability

     G40.101   **Localization-related (focal) (partial) symptomatic epilepsy and epileptic syndromes with simple partial seizures, not intractable, with status epilepticus**

     G40.109   **Localization-related (focal) (partial) symptomatic epilepsy and epileptic syndromes with simple partial seizures, not intractable, without status epilepticus**

        Localization-related (focal) (partial) symptomatic epilepsy and epileptic syndromes with simple partial seizures NOS

   ● **G40.11**   **Localization-related (focal) (partial) symptomatic epilepsy and epileptic syndromes with simple partial seizures, intractable**

     G40.111   **Localization-related (focal) (partial) symptomatic epilepsy and epileptic syndromes with simple partial seizures, intractable, with status epilepticus**

     G40.119   **Localization-related (focal) (partial) symptomatic epilepsy and epileptic syndromes with simple partial seizures, intractable, without status epilepticus**

● **G40.2**   **Localization-related (focal) (partial) symptomatic epilepsy and epileptic syndromes with complex partial seizures**

     Attacks with alteration of consciousness, often with automatisms

     Complex partial seizures developing into secondarily generalized seizures

   ● **G40.20**   **Localization-related (focal) (partial) symptomatic epilepsy and epileptic syndromes with complex partial seizures, not intractable**

      Localization-related (focal) (partial) symptomatic epilepsy and epileptic syndromes with complex partial seizures without intractability

     G40.201   **Localization-related (focal) (partial) symptomatic epilepsy and epileptic syndromes with complex partial seizures, not intractable, with status epilepticus**

     G40.209   **Localization-related (focal) (partial) symptomatic epilepsy and epileptic syndromes with complex partial seizures, not intractable, without status epilepticus**

        Localization-related (focal) (partial) symptomatic epilepsy and epileptic syndromes with complex partial seizures NOS

● **G40.21**   **Localization-related (focal) (partial) symptomatic epilepsy and epileptic syndromes with complex partial seizures, intractable**

     G40.211   **Localization-related (focal) (partial) symptomatic epilepsy and epileptic syndromes with complex partial seizures, intractable, with status epilepticus**

     G40.219   **Localization-related (focal) (partial) symptomatic epilepsy and epileptic syndromes with complex partial seizures, intractable, without status epilepticus**

● **G40.3**   **Generalized idiopathic epilepsy and epileptic syndromes**

     Code also MERRF syndrome, if applicable (E88.42)

   ● **G40.30**   **Generalized idiopathic epilepsy and epileptic syndromes, not intractable**

      Generalized idiopathic epilepsy and epileptic syndromes without intractability

     G40.301   **Generalized idiopathic epilepsy and epileptic syndromes, not intractable, with status epilepticus**

     G40.309   **Generalized idiopathic epilepsy and epileptic syndromes, not intractable, without status epilepticus**

        Generalized idiopathic epilepsy and epileptic syndromes NOS

   ● **G40.31**   **Generalized idiopathic epilepsy and epileptic syndromes, intractable**

     G40.311   **Generalized idiopathic epilepsy and epileptic syndromes, intractable, with status epilepticus**

     G40.319   **Generalized idiopathic epilepsy and epileptic syndromes, intractable, without status epilepticus**

● **G40.A**   **Absence epileptic syndrome**

     Childhood absence epilepsy [pyknolepsy]

     Juvenile absence epilepsy

     Absence epileptic syndrome, NOS

   ● **G40.A0**   **Absence epileptic syndrome, not intractable**

     G40.A01   **Absence epileptic syndrome, not intractable, with status epilepticus**

     G40.A09   **Absence epileptic syndrome, not intractable, without status epilepticus**

   ● **G40.A1**   **Absence epileptic syndrome, intractable**

     G40.A11   **Absence epileptic syndrome, intractable, with status epilepticus**

     G40.A19   **Absence epileptic syndrome, intractable, without status epilepticus**

● **G40.B**   **Juvenile myoclonic epilepsy [impulsive petit mal]**

   ● **G40.B0**   **Juvenile myoclonic epilepsy, not intractable**

     G40.B01   **Juvenile myoclonic epilepsy, not intractable, with status epilepticus**

     G40.B09   **Juvenile myoclonic epilepsy, not intractable, without status epilepticus**

   ● **G40.B1**   **Juvenile myoclonic epilepsy, intractable**

     G40.B11   **Juvenile myoclonic epilepsy, intractable, with status epilepticus**

     G40.B19   **Juvenile myoclonic epilepsy, intractable, without status epilepticus**

CHAPTER 6 (G00-G99)

● **G40.4 Other generalized epilepsy and epileptic syndromes**
Epilepsy with grand mal seizures on awakening
Epilepsy with myoclonic absences
Epilepsy with myoclonic-astatic seizures
Grand mal seizure NOS
Nonspecific atonic epileptic seizures
Nonspecific clonic epileptic seizures
Nonspecific myoclonic epileptic seizures
Nonspecific tonic epileptic seizures
Nonspecific tonic-clonic epileptic seizures
Symptomatic early myoclonic encephalopathy

  ● **G40.40 Other generalized epilepsy and epileptic syndromes, not intractable**
Other generalized epilepsy and epileptic syndromes without intractability
Other generalized epilepsy and epileptic syndromes NOS

    G40.401 Other generalized epilepsy and epileptic syndromes, not intractable, with status epilepticus

    G40.409 Other generalized epilepsy and epileptic syndromes, not intractable, without status epilepticus

  ● **G40.41 Other generalized epilepsy and epileptic syndromes, intractable**

    G40.411 Other generalized epilepsy and epileptic syndromes, intractable, with status epilepticus

    G40.419 Other generalized epilepsy and epileptic syndromes, intractable, without status epilepticus

● **G40.5 Epileptic seizures related to external causes**
Epileptic seizures related to alcohol
Epileptic seizures related to drugs
Epileptic seizures related to hormonal changes
Epileptic seizures related to sleep deprivation
Epileptic seizures related to stress
Code also, if applicable, associated epilepsy and recurrent seizures (G40.-)
Use additional code for adverse effect, if applicable, to identify drug (T36-T50 with fifth or sixth character 5)

  ● **G40.50 Epileptic seizures related to external causes, not intractable**

    G40.501 Epileptic seizures related to external causes, not intractable, with status epilepticus

    G40.509 Epileptic seizures related to external causes, not intractable, without status epilepticus
Epileptic seizures related to external causes, NOS

● **G40.8 Other epilepsy and recurrent seizures**
Epilepsies and epileptic syndromes undetermined as to whether they are focal or generalized
Landau-Kleffner syndrome

  ● **G40.80 Other epilepsy**

    G40.801 Other epilepsy, not intractable, with status epilepticus
Other epilepsy without intractability with status epilepticus

    G40.802 Other epilepsy, not intractable, without status epilepticus
Other epilepsy NOS
Other epilepsy without intractability without status epilepticus

    G40.803 Other epilepsy, intractable, with status epilepticus

    G40.804 Other epilepsy, intractable, without status epilepticus

  ● **G40.81 Lennox-Gastaut syndrome**

    G40.811 Lennox-Gastaut syndrome, not intractable, with status epilepticus

    G40.812 Lennox-Gastaut syndrome, not intractable, without status epilepticus

    G40.813 Lennox-Gastaut syndrome, intractable, with status epilepticus

    G40.814 Lennox-Gastaut syndrome, intractable, without status epilepticus

  ● **G40.82 Epileptic spasms**
Infantile spasms
Salaam attacks
West's syndrome

    G40.821 Epileptic spasms, not intractable, with status epilepticus

    G40.822 Epileptic spasms, not intractable, without status epilepticus

    G40.823 Epileptic spasms, intractable, with status epilepticus

    G40.824 Epileptic spasms, intractable, without status epilepticus

  G40.89 Other seizures
Excludes1   post traumatic seizures (R56.1)
recurrent seizures NOS (G40.909)
seizure NOS (R56.9)

● **G40.9 Epilepsy, unspecified**

  ● **G40.90 Epilepsy, unspecified, not intractable**
Epilepsy, unspecified, without intractability

    G40.901 Epilepsy, unspecified, not intractable, with status epilepticus

    G40.909 Epilepsy, unspecified, not intractable, without status epilepticus
Epilepsy NOS
Epileptic convulsions NOS
Epileptic fits NOS
Epileptic seizures NOS
Recurrent seizures NOS
Seizure disorder NOS

  ● **G40.91 Epilepsy, unspecified, intractable**
Intractable seizure disorder NOS

    G40.911 Epilepsy, unspecified, intractable, with status epilepticus

    G40.919 Epilepsy, unspecified, intractable, without status epilepticus

● **G43 Migraine**
Note: The following terms are to be considered equivalent to intractable: pharmacoresistant (pharmacologically resistant), treatment resistant, refractory (medically) and poorly controlled
Use additional code for adverse effect, if applicable, to identify drug (T36-T50 with fifth or sixth character 5)
Excludes1   headache NOS (R51)
lower half migraine (G44.00)
Excludes2   headache syndromes (G44.-)

● **G43.0 Migraine without aura**
Neurological disorder, generally recurring headaches without early symptom (aura)
Common migraine
Excludes1   chronic migraine without aura (G43.7-)

  ● **G43.00 Migraine without aura, not intractable**
Neurological disorder, generally recurring headaches without early symptom (aura); resistant to cure, relief, or control
Migraine without aura without mention of refractory migraine

    G43.001 Migraine without aura, not intractable, with status migrainosus

    G43.009 Migraine without aura, not intractable, without status migrainosus
Migraine without aura NOS

◄ New   ◄▥ Revised   ~~deleted~~ Deleted   **OGCR** Official Guidelines   X Assign placeholder X   ● Use Additional Character(s)

Excludes 1   Excludes 2   Includes   Use additional   Code first   Code also   Unspecified

Item 6–4 Migraine headache is described as an intense pulsing or throbbing pain in one area of the head. It can be accompanied by extreme sensitivity to light (photophobic) and sound and is three times more common in women than in men. Symptoms include nausea and vomiting. Research indicates migraine headaches are caused by inherited abnormalities in genes that control the activities of certain cell populations in the brain.

● **G43.01** **Migraine without aura, intractable**
Intractable migraine: Not easily cured or managed; relentless pain from a migraine
Migraine without aura with refractory migraine

     G43.011 **Migraine without aura, intractable, with status migrainosus**

     G43.019 **Migraine without aura, intractable, without status migrainosus**

● **G43.1** **Migraine with aura**
Basilar migraine
Classical migraine
Migraine equivalents
Migraine preceded or accompanied by transient focal neurological phenomena
Migraine triggered seizures
Migraine with acute-onset aura
Migraine with aura without headache (migraine equivalents)
Migraine with prolonged aura
Migraine with typical aura
Retinal migraine
Code also any associated seizure (G40.-, R56.9)
Excludes1   persistent migraine aura (G43.5-, G43.6-)

● **G43.10** **Migraine with aura, not intractable**
Migraine with aura without mention of refractory migraine

     G43.101 **Migraine with aura, not intractable, with status migrainosus**

     G43.109 **Migraine with aura, not intractable, without status migrainosus**
Migraine with aura NOS

● **G43.11** **Migraine with aura, intractable**
Migraine with aura with refractory migraine

     G43.111 **Migraine with aura, intractable, with status migrainosus**

     G43.119 **Migraine with aura, intractable, without status migrainosus**

● **G43.4** **Hemiplegic migraine**
Inherited migraine disorder causing temporary paralysis of one side of body followed by severe headache and nausea
Familial migraine
Sporadic migraine

● **G43.40** **Hemiplegic migraine, not intractable**
Hemiplegic migraine without refractory migraine

     G43.401 **Hemiplegic migraine, not intractable, with status migrainosus**

     G43.409 **Hemiplegic migraine, not intractable, without status migrainosus**
Hemiplegic migraine NOS

● **G43.41** **Hemiplegic migraine, intractable**
Hemiplegic migraine with refractory migraine

     G43.411 **Hemiplegic migraine, intractable, with status migrainosus**

     G43.419 **Hemiplegic migraine, intractable, without status migrainosus**

● **G43.5** **Persistent migraine aura without cerebral infarction**

● **G43.50** **Persistent migraine aura without cerebral infarction, not intractable**
Persistent migraine aura without cerebral infarction, without refractory migraine

     G43.501 **Persistent migraine aura without cerebral infarction, not intractable, with status migrainosus**

     G43.509 **Persistent migraine aura without cerebral infarction, not intractable, without status migrainosus**
Persistent migraine aura NOS

● **G43.51** **Persistent migraine aura without cerebral infarction, intractable**
Persistent migraine aura without cerebral infarction, with refractory migraine

     G43.511 **Persistent migraine aura without cerebral infarction, intractable, with status migrainosus**

     G43.519 **Persistent migraine aura without cerebral infarction, intractable, without status migrainosus**

● **G43.6** **Persistent migraine aura with cerebral infarction**
Visual, motor, or psychic disturbances, paresthesias, and related neurologic abnormalities accompanying migraine
Code also the type of cerebral infarction (I63.-)

● **G43.60** **Persistent migraine aura with cerebral infarction, not intractable**
Persistent migraine aura with cerebral infarction, without refractory migraine

     G43.601 **Persistent migraine aura with cerebral infarction, not intractable, with status migrainosus**

     G43.609 **Persistent migraine aura with cerebral infarction, not intractable, without status migrainosus**

● **G43.61** **Persistent migraine aura with cerebral infarction, intractable**
Persistent migraine aura with cerebral infarction, with refractory migraine

     G43.611 **Persistent migraine aura with cerebral infarction, intractable, with status migrainosus**

     G43.619 **Persistent migraine aura with cerebral infarction, intractable, without status migrainosus**

● **G43.7** **Chronic migraine without aura**
Transformed migraine
Excludes1   migraine without aura (G43.0-)

● **G43.70** **Chronic migraine without aura, not intractable**
Chronic migraine without aura, without refractory migraine

     G43.701 **Chronic migraine without aura, not intractable, with status migrainosus**

     G43.709 **Chronic migraine without aura, not intractable, without status migrainosus**
Chronic migraine without aura NOS

● **G43.71** **Chronic migraine without aura, intractable**
Chronic migraine without aura, with refractory migraine

     G43.711 **Chronic migraine without aura, intractable, with status migrainosus**

     G43.719 **Chronic migraine without aura, intractable, without status migrainosus**

CHAPTER 6 (G00-G99)

● **G43.A   Cyclical vomiting**
    G43.A0   Cyclical vomiting, not intractable
       Cyclical vomiting, without refractory migraine
    G43.A1   Cyclical vomiting, intractable
       Cyclical vomiting, with refractory migraine

● **G43.B   Ophthalmoplegic migraine**
    G43.B0   Ophthalmoplegic migraine, not intractable
       Ophthalmoplegic migraine, without refractory migraine
    G43.B1   Ophthalmoplegic migraine, intractable
       Ophthalmoplegic migraine, with refractory migraine

● **G43.C   Periodic headache syndromes in child or adult**
    G43.C0   Periodic headache syndromes in child or adult, not intractable
       Periodic headache syndromes in child or adult, without refractory migraine
    G43.C1   Periodic headache syndromes in child or adult, intractable
       Periodic headache syndromes in child or adult, with refractory migraine

● **G43.D   Abdominal migraine**
    G43.D0   Abdominal migraine, not intractable
       Abdominal migraine, without refractory migraine
    G43.D1   Abdominal migraine, intractable
       Abdominal migraine, with refractory migraine

● **G43.8   Other migraine**
   ● **G43.80   Other migraine, not intractable**
       Other migraine, without refractory migraine
    G43.801   Other migraine, not intractable, with status migrainosus
    G43.809   Other migraine, not intractable, without status migrainosus
   ● **G43.81   Other migraine, intractable**
       Other migraine, with refractory migraine
    G43.811   Other migraine, intractable, with status migrainosus
    G43.819   Other migraine, intractable, without status migrainosus
   ● **G43.82   Menstrual migraine, not intractable**
       Menstrual headache, not intractable
       Menstrual migraine, without refractory migraine
       Menstrually related migraine, not intractable
       Pre-menstrual headache, not intractable
       Pre-menstrual migraine, not intractable
       Pure menstrual migraine, not intractable
       `Code also` associated premenstrual tension syndrome (N94.3)
    G43.821   Menstrual migraine, not intractable, with status migrainosus
    G43.829   Menstrual migraine, not intractable, without status migrainosus
       Menstrual migraine NOS
   ● **G43.83   Menstrual migraine, intractable**
       Menstrual headache, intractable
       Menstrual migraine, with refractory migraine
       Menstrually related migraine, intractable
       Pre-menstrual headache, intractable
       Pre-menstrual migraine, intractable
       Pure menstrual migraine, intractable
       `Code also` associated premenstrual tension syndrome (N94.3)
    G43.831   Menstrual migraine, intractable, with status migrainosus
    G43.839   Menstrual migraine, intractable, without status migrainosus

● **G43.9   Migraine, unspecified**
   ● **G43.90   Migraine, unspecified, not intractable**
       Migraine, unspecified, without refractory migraine
    G43.901   Migraine, unspecified, not intractable, with status migrainosus
       Status migrainosus NOS
    G43.909   Migraine, unspecified, not intractable, without status migrainosus
       Migraine NOS
   ● **G43.91   Migraine, unspecified, intractable**
       Migraine, unspecified, with refractory migraine
    G43.911   Migraine, unspecified, intractable, with status migrainosus
    G43.919   Migraine, unspecified, intractable, without status migrainosus

● **G44   Other headache syndromes**
   Excludes1   headache NOS (R51)
   Excludes2   atypical facial pain (G50.1)
       headache due to lumbar puncture (G97.1)
       migraines (G43.-)
       trigeminal neuralgia (G50.0)
 ● **G44.0   Cluster headaches and other trigeminal autonomic cephalgias (TAC)**
   ● **G44.00   Cluster headache syndrome, unspecified**
       Ciliary neuralgia
       Cluster headache NOS
       Histamine cephalgia
       Lower half migraine
       Migrainous neuralgia
    G44.001   Cluster headache syndrome, unspecified, intractable
    G44.009   Cluster headache syndrome, unspecified, not intractable
       Cluster headache syndrome NOS
   ● **G44.01   Episodic cluster headache**
    G44.011   Episodic cluster headache, intractable
    G44.019   Episodic cluster headache, not intractable
       Episodic cluster headache NOS
   ● **G44.02   Chronic cluster headache**
    G44.021   Chronic cluster headache, intractable
    G44.029   Chronic cluster headache, not intractable
       Chronic cluster headache NOS
   ● **G44.03   Episodic paroxysmal hemicrania**
       Paroxysmal hemicrania NOS
    G44.031   Episodic paroxysmal hemicrania, intractable
    G44.039   Episodic paroxysmal hemicrania, not intractable
       Episodic paroxysmal hemicrania NOS
   ● **G44.04   Chronic paroxysmal hemicrania**
       Unilateral headache
    G44.041   Chronic paroxysmal hemicrania, intractable
    G44.049   Chronic paroxysmal hemicrania, not intractable
       Chronic paroxysmal hemicrania NOS

- **G44.05** Short lasting unilateral neuralgiform headache with conjunctival injection and tearing (SUNCT)
    - **G44.051** Short lasting unilateral neuralgiform headache with conjunctival injection and tearing (SUNCT), intractable
    - **G44.059** Short lasting unilateral neuralgiform headache with conjunctival injection and tearing (SUNCT), not intractable
        Short lasting unilateral neuralgiform headache with conjunctival injection and tearing (SUNCT) NOS
- **G44.09** Other trigeminal autonomic cephalgias (TAC)
    Cluster headaches
    - **G44.091** Other trigeminal autonomic cephalgias (TAC), intractable
    - **G44.099** Other trigeminal autonomic cephalgias (TAC), not intractable

G44.1 Vascular headache, not elsewhere classified
    Excludes2 cluster headache (G44.0)
    complicated headache syndromes (G44.5-)
    drug-induced headache (G44.4-)
    migraine (G43.-)
    other specified headache syndromes (G44.8-)
    post-traumatic headache (G44.3-)
    tension-type headache (G44.2-)

- **G44.2** Tension-type headache
    - **G44.20** Tension-type headache, unspecified
        - **G44.201** Tension-type headache, unspecified, intractable
        - **G44.209** Tension-type headache, unspecified, not intractable
            Tension headache NOS
    - **G44.21** Episodic tension-type headache
        - **G44.211** Episodic tension-type headache, intractable
        - **G44.219** Episodic tension-type headache, not intractable
            Episodic tension-type headache NOS
    - **G44.22** Chronic tension-type headache
        - **G44.221** Chronic tension-type headache, intractable
        - **G44.229** Chronic tension-type headache, not intractable
            Chronic tension-type headache NOS
- **G44.3** Post-traumatic headache
    - **G44.30** Post-traumatic headache, unspecified
        - **G44.301** Post-traumatic headache, unspecified, intractable
        - **G44.309** Post-traumatic headache, unspecified, not intractable
            Post-traumatic headache NOS
    - **G44.31** Acute post-traumatic headache
        - **G44.311** Acute post-traumatic headache, intractable
        - **G44.319** Acute post-traumatic headache, not intractable
            Acute post-traumatic headache NOS
    - **G44.32** Chronic post-traumatic headache
        - **G44.321** Chronic post-traumatic headache, intractable
        - **G44.329** Chronic post-traumatic headache, not intractable
            Chronic post-traumatic headache NOS

- **G44.4** Drug-induced headache, not elsewhere classified
    Medication overuse headache
    Use additional code for adverse effect, if applicable, to identify drug (T36-T50 with fifth or sixth character 5)
    - **G44.40** Drug-induced headache, not elsewhere classified, not intractable
    - **G44.41** Drug-induced headache, not elsewhere classified, intractable
- **G44.5** Complicated headache syndromes
    - **G44.51** Hemicrania continua
        Persistent unilateral headache
    - **G44.52** New daily persistent headache (NDPH)
    - **G44.53** Primary thunderclap headache
    - **G44.59** Other complicated headache syndrome
- **G44.8** Other specified headache syndromes
    - **G44.81** Hypnic headache
        Benign primary headaches
    - **G44.82** Headache associated with sexual activity
        Orgasmic headache
        Preorgasmic headache
    - **G44.83** Primary cough headache
    - **G44.84** Primary exertional headache
    - **G44.85** Primary stabbing headache
    - **G44.89** Other headache syndrome

- **G45** Transient cerebral ischemic attacks and related syndromes
    Excludes1 neonatal cerebral ischemia (P91.0)
    transient retinal artery occlusion (H34.0-)
    - **G45.0** Vertebro-basilar artery syndrome
    - **G45.1** Carotid artery syndrome (hemispheric)
    - **G45.2** Multiple and bilateral precerebral artery syndromes
    - **G45.3** Amaurosis fugax
        Transient visual loss in one eye
    - **G45.4** Transient global amnesia
        Episode of short-term memory loss, nonrecurrent, lasting few hours
        Excludes1 amnesia NOS (R41.3)
    - **G45.8** Other transient cerebral ischemic attacks and related syndromes
    - **G45.9** Transient cerebral ischemic attack, unspecified
        Spasm of cerebral artery
        TIA
        Transient cerebral ischemia NOS

- **G46** Vascular syndromes of brain in cerebrovascular diseases
    Code first underlying cerebrovascular disease (I60-I69)
    - **G46.0** Middle cerebral artery syndrome
    - **G46.1** Anterior cerebral artery syndrome
    - **G46.2** Posterior cerebral artery syndrome
    - **G46.3** Brain stem stroke syndrome
        Benedikt syndrome
        Claude syndrome
        Foville syndrome
        Millard-Gubler syndrome
        Wallenberg syndrome
        Weber syndrome
    - **G46.4** Cerebellar stroke syndrome
    - **G46.5** Pure motor lacunar syndrome
        Occlusion of single deep penetrating artery
    - **G46.6** Pure sensory lacunar syndrome
    - **G46.7** Other lacunar syndromes
    - **G46.8** Other vascular syndromes of brain in cerebrovascular diseases

CHAPTER 6 (G00-G99)

● **G47   Sleep disorders**
> **Excludes2**   nightmares (F51.5)
> nonorganic sleep disorders (F51.-)
> sleep terrors (F51.4)
> sleepwalking (F51.3)

● **G47.0   Insomnia**
> **Excludes2**   alcohol related insomnia (F10.182,
> F10.282, F10.982)
> drug-related insomnia (F11.182, F11.282,
> F11.982, F13.182, F13.282, F13.982,
> F14.182, F14.282, F14.982, F15.182,
> F15.282, F15.982, F19.182, F19.282,
> F19.982)
> idiopathic insomnia (F51.01)
> insomnia due to a mental disorder (F51.05)
> insomnia not due to a substance or known
> physiological condition (F51.0-)
> nonorganic insomnia (F51.0-)
> primary insomnia (F51.01)
> sleep apnea (G47.3-)

G47.00   Insomnia, unspecified
> Insomnia NOS

G47.01   Insomnia due to medical condition
> Code also associated medical condition

G47.09   Other insomnia

● **G47.1   Hypersomnia**
> **Excludes2**   alcohol-related hypersomnia (F10.182,
> F10.282, F10.982)
> drug-related hypersomnia (F11.182,
> F11.282, F11.982, F13.182, F13.282,
> F13.982, F14.182, F14.282, F14.982,
> F15.182, F15.282, F15.982, F19.182,
> F19.282, F19.982)
> hypersomnia due to a mental disorder
> (F51.13)
> hypersomnia not due to a substance
> or known physiological condition
> (F51.1-)
> primary hypersomnia (F51.11)
> sleep apnea (G47.3-)

G47.10   Hypersomnia, unspecified
> Hypersomnia NOS

G47.11   Idiopathic hypersomnia with long sleep time
> Idiopathic hypersomnia NOS

G47.12   Idiopathic hypersomnia without long sleep time

G47.13   Recurrent hypersomnia
> Kleine-Levin syndrome
> Menstrual related hypersomnia

G47.14   Hypersomnia due to medical condition
> Code also associated medical condition

G47.19   Other hypersomnia

● **G47.2   Circadian rhythm sleep disorders**
> Disorders of the sleep wake schedule
> Inversion of nyctohemeral rhythm
> Inversion of sleep rhythm

G47.20   Circadian rhythm sleep disorder, unspecified type
> Sleep wake schedule disorder NOS

G47.21   Circadian rhythm sleep disorder, delayed sleep phase type
> Delayed sleep phase syndrome

G47.22   Circadian rhythm sleep disorder, advanced sleep phase type

G47.23   Circadian rhythm sleep disorder, irregular sleep wake type
> Irregular sleep-wake pattern

G47.24   Circadian rhythm sleep disorder, free running type

G47.25   Circadian rhythm sleep disorder, jet lag type

G47.26   Circadian rhythm sleep disorder, shift work type

G47.27   Circadian rhythm sleep disorder in conditions classified elsewhere
> Code first underlying condition

G47.29   Other circadian rhythm sleep disorder

● **G47.3   Sleep apnea**
> *Characterized by episodes in which breathing stops during sleep*
> Code also any associated underlying condition
> **Excludes1**   apnea NOS (R06.81)
> Cheyne-Stokes breathing (R06.3)
> pickwickian syndrome (E66.2)
> sleep apnea of newborn (P28.3)

G47.30   Sleep apnea, unspecified
> Sleep apnea NOS

G47.31   Primary central sleep apnea

G47.32   High altitude periodic breathing

G47.33   Obstructive sleep apnea (adult) (pediatric)
> **Excludes1**   obstructive sleep apnea of
> newborn (P28.3)

G47.34   Idiopathic sleep related nonobstructive alveolar hypoventilation
> Sleep related hypoxia

G47.35   Congenital central alveolar hypoventilation syndrome

G47.36   Sleep related hypoventilation in conditions classified elsewhere
> Sleep related hypoxemia in conditions
> classified elsewhere
> Code first underlying condition

G47.37   Central sleep apnea in conditions classified elsewhere
> Code first underlying condition

G47.39   Other sleep apnea

● **G47.4   Narcolepsy and cataplexy**
> *Cataplexy is a disorder evidenced by seizures including
> minor slacking of the facial muscles to complete
> collapse and often affects people who have **narcolepsy**,
> a disorder in which there is great difficulty remaining
> awake during the daytime.*

● **G47.41   Narcolepsy**

G47.411   Narcolepsy with cataplexy

G47.419   Narcolepsy without cataplexy
> Narcolepsy NOS

● **G47.42   Narcolepsy in conditions classified elsewhere**
> Code first underlying condition

**G47.421   Narcolepsy in conditions classified
> elsewhere with cataplexy**

**G47.429   Narcolepsy in conditions classified
> elsewhere without cataplexy**

● **G47.5   Parasomnia**
> **Excludes1**   alcohol induced parasomnia (F10.182,
> F10.282, F10.982)
> drug induced parasomnia (F11.182,
> F11.282, F11.982, F13.182, F13.282,
> F13.982, F14.182, F14.282, F14.982,
> F15.182, F15.282, F15.982, F19.182,
> F19.282, F19.982)
> parasomnia not due to a substance or
> known physiological condition (F51.8)

G47.50   Parasomnia, unspecified
> Parasomnia NOS

G47.51   Confusional arousals

G47.52   REM sleep behavior disorder

G47.53   Recurrent isolated sleep paralysis

G47.54   Parasomnia in conditions classified elsewhere
> Code first underlying condition

G47.59   Other parasomnia

◀ New   ◀▥ Revised   ~~deleted~~ Deleted   **OGCR** Official Guidelines   X Assign placeholder X   ● Use Additional Character(s)

| Excludes 1 | Excludes 2 | Includes | Use additional | Code first | Code also | Unspecified |

Item 6–5   Trigeminal neuralgia, tic douloureux, is a pain syndrome diagnosed from the patient's history alone. The condition is characterized by pain and a brief facial spasm or tic. Pain is unilateral and follows the sensory distribution of cranial nerve V, typically radiating to the maxillary (V2) or mandibular (V3) area.

- **G47.6   Sleep related movement disorders**
  - **Excludes2**   restless legs syndrome (G25.81)
  - **G47.61   Periodic limb movement disorder**
    - Periodic limb movement disorder
  - **G47.62   Sleep related leg cramps**
  - **G47.63   Sleep related bruxism**
    - **Excludes1**   psychogenic bruxism (F45.8)
  - **G47.69   Other sleep related movement disorders**
- **G47.8   Other sleep disorders**
- **G47.9   Sleep disorder, unspecified**
  - Sleep disorder NOS

(See Plate 118 on page NAP-6.)

NERVE, NERVE ROOT AND PLEXUS DISORDERS (G50-G59)

- **Excludes1**   current traumatic nerve, nerve root and plexus disorders - see Injury, nerve by body region
  - neuralgia NOS (M79.2)
  - neuritis NOS (M79.2)
  - peripheral neuritis in pregnancy (O26.82-)
  - radiculitis NOS (M54.1-)

- **G50   Disorders of trigeminal nerve**
  - **Includes**   disorders of 5th cranial nerve
  - **G50.0   Trigeminal neuralgia**
    - Syndrome of paroxysmal facial pain
    - Tic douloureux
  - **G50.1   Atypical facial pain**
  - **G50.8   Other disorders of trigeminal nerve**
  - **G50.9   Disorder of trigeminal nerve, unspecified**

- **G51   Facial nerve disorders**
  - **Includes**   disorders of 7th cranial nerve
  - **G51.0   Bell's palsy**
    - Facial palsy
  - **G51.1   Geniculate ganglionitis**
    - *Rare disorder with symptoms of severe pain deep in ear, spreading to ear canal, outer ear, mastoid or eye regions*
    - **Excludes1**   postherpetic geniculate ganglionitis (B02.21)
  - **G51.2   Melkersson's syndrome**
    - Melkersson-Rosenthal syndrome
  - **G51.3   Clonic hemifacial spasm**
  - **G51.4   Facial myokymia**
    - *Involuntary facial muscle movement*
  - **G51.8   Other disorders of facial nerve**
  - **G51.9   Disorder of facial nerve, unspecified**

- **G52   Disorders of other cranial nerves**
  - **Excludes2**   disorders of acoustic [8th] nerve (H93.3)
    - disorders of optic [2nd] nerve (H46, H47.0)
    - paralytic strabismus due to nerve palsy (H49.0-H49.2)
  - **G52.0   Disorders of olfactory nerve**
    - Disorders of 1st cranial nerve
  - **G52.1   Disorders of glossopharyngeal nerve**
    - Disorder of 9th cranial nerve
    - Glossopharyngeal neuralgia
  - **G52.2   Disorders of vagus nerve**
    - Disorders of pneumogastric [10th] nerve

- **G52.3   Disorders of hypoglossal nerve**
  - Disorders of 12th cranial nerve
- **G52.7   Disorders of multiple cranial nerves**
  - Polyneuritis cranialis
- **G52.8   Disorders of other specified cranial nerves**
- **G52.9   Cranial nerve disorder, unspecified**

- **G53   Cranial nerve disorders in diseases classified elsewhere**
  - *Code first underlying disease, such as:*
    - neoplasm (C00-D49)
  - **Excludes1**   multiple cranial nerve palsy in sarcoidosis (D86.82)
    - multiple cranial nerve palsy in syphilis (A52.15)
    - postherpetic geniculate ganglionitis (B02.21)
    - postherpetic trigeminal neuralgia (B02.22)

- **G54   Nerve root and plexus disorders**
  - *Raiculopathy (nerve root disorder) caused by pressure on nerve root, most common cause is herniation of intervertebral disk. Plexus disorders (plexopathies) are due to compression or injury.*
  - **Excludes1**   current traumatic nerve root and plexus disorders - see nerve injury by body region
    - intervertebral disc disorders (M50-M51)
    - neuralgia or neuritis NOS (M79.2)
    - neuritis or radiculitis brachial NOS (M54.13)
    - neuritis or radiculitis lumbar NOS (M54.16)
    - neuritis or radiculitis lumbosacral NOS (M54.17)
    - neuritis or radiculitis thoracic NOS (M54.14)
    - radiculitis NOS (M54.10)
    - radiculopathy NOS (M54.10)
    - spondylosis (M47.-)
  - **G54.0   Brachial plexus disorders**
    - Thoracic outlet syndrome
  - **G54.1   Lumbosacral plexus disorders**
  - **G54.2   Cervical root disorders, not elsewhere classified**
  - **G54.3   Thoracic root disorders, not elsewhere classified**
  - **G54.4   Lumbosacral root disorders, not elsewhere classified**
  - **G54.5   Neuralgic amyotrophy**
    - Parsonage-Aldren-Turner syndrome
    - Shoulder-girdle neuritis
    - **Excludes1**   neuralgic amyotrophy in diabetes mellitus (E08-E13 with .44)
  - **G54.6   Phantom limb syndrome with pain**
    - *Sensations (cramping, itching) in a limb that no longer exists.*
  - **G54.7   Phantom limb syndrome without pain**
    - Phantom limb syndrome NOS
  - **G54.8   Other nerve root and plexus disorders**
  - **G54.9   Nerve root and plexus disorder, unspecified**

- **G55   Nerve root and plexus compressions in diseases classified elsewhere**
  - *Code first underlying disease, such as:*
    - neoplasm (C00-D49)
  - **Excludes1**   nerve root compression (due to) (in) ankylosing spondylitis (M45.-)
    - nerve root compression (due to) (in)dorsopathies (M53.-, M54.-)
    - nerve root compression (due to) (in)intervertebral disc disorders (M50.1.-, M51.1.-)
    - nerve root compression (due to) (in) spondylopathies (M46.-, M48.-)

Item 6–6   The most common facial nerve disorder is **Bell's Palsy,** which occurs suddenly and results in facial drooping unilaterally. This disorder is the result of a reaction to a virus that causes the facial nerve in the ear to swell resulting in pressure in the bony canal.

◀ New   ⇐ Revised   ~~deleted~~ Deleted   **OGCR** Official Guidelines   X Assign placeholder X   ● Use Additional Character(s)

Excludes 1   Excludes 2   Includes   Use additional   Code first   Code also   Unspecified

(See Plates 472 and 473 on pages NAP-8 and NAP-9.)

- **G56　Mononeuropathies of upper limb**
  > **Excludes1**　current traumatic nerve disorder - see nerve injury by body region

  - **G56.0　Carpal tunnel syndrome**
    - **G56.00**　Carpal tunnel syndrome, unspecified upper limb
    - **G56.01**　Carpal tunnel syndrome, right upper limb
    - **G56.02**　Carpal tunnel syndrome, left upper limb
  - **G56.1　Other lesions of median nerve**
    - **G56.10**　Other lesions of median nerve, unspecified side
    - **G56.11**　Other lesions of median nerve, right upper limb
    - **G56.12**　Other lesions of median nerve, left upper limb
  - **G56.2　Lesion of ulnar nerve**
    Tardy ulnar nerve palsy
    - **G56.20**　Lesion of ulnar nerve, unspecified upper limb
    - **G56.21**　Lesion of ulnar nerve, right upper limb
    - **G56.22**　Lesion of ulnar nerve, left upper limb
  - **G56.3　Lesion of radial nerve**
    - **G56.30**　Lesion of radial nerve, unspecified upper limb
    - **G56.31**　Lesion of radial nerve, right upper limb
    - **G56.32**　Lesion of radial nerve, left upper limb
  - **G56.4　Causalgia of upper limb**
    Intense burning pain and sensitivity to slight touch
    Complex regional pain syndrome II of upper limb
    > **Excludes1**　complex regional pain syndrome I of lower limb (G90.52-)
    > complex regional pain syndrome I of upper limb (G90.51-)
    > complex regional pain syndrome II of lower limb (G57.7-)
    > reflex sympathetic dystrophy of lower limb (G90.52-)
    > reflex sympathetic dystrophy (G90.51-)
    - **G56.40**　Causalgia of unspecified upper limb
    - **G56.41**　Causalgia of right upper limb
    - **G56.42**　Causalgia of left upper limb
  - **G56.8　Other specified mononeuropathies of upper limb**
    Disease of a single nerve
    Interdigital neuroma of upper limb
    - **G56.80**　Other specified mononeuropathies of unspecified upper limb
    - **G56.81**　Other specified mononeuropathies of right upper limb
    - **G56.82**　Other specified mononeuropathies of left upper limb
  - **G56.9　Unspecified mononeuropathy of upper limb**
    Disease of a single nerve
    - **G56.90**　Unspecified mononeuropathy of unspecified upper limb
    - **G56.91**　Unspecified mononeuropathy of right upper limb
    - **G56.92**　Unspecified mononeuropathy of left upper limb

- **G57　Mononeuropathies of lower limb**
  > **Excludes1**　current traumatic nerve disorder - see nerve injury by body region

(See Plates 544 and 545 on pages NAP-10 and NAP-11.)

- **G57.0　Lesion of sciatic nerve**
  > **Excludes1**　sciatica NOS (M54.3-)
  > **Excludes2**　sciatica attributed to intervertebral disc disorder (M51.1.-)
  - **G57.00**　Lesion of sciatic nerve, unspecified lower limb
  - **G57.01**　Lesion of sciatic nerve, right lower limb
  - **G57.02**　Lesion of sciatic nerve, left lower limb
- **G57.1　Meralgia paresthetica**
  Numbness or pain in outer thigh caused by injury to nerve
  Lateral cutaneous nerve of thigh syndrome
  - **G57.10**　Meralgia paresthetica, unspecified lower limb
  - **G57.11**　Meralgia paresthetica, right lower limb
  - **G57.12**　Meralgia paresthetica, left lower limb
- **G57.2　Lesion of femoral nerve**
  - **G57.20**　Lesion of femoral nerve, unspecified lower limb
  - **G57.21**　Lesion of femoral nerve, right lower limb
  - **G57.22**　Lesion of femoral nerve, left lower limb
- **G57.3　Lesion of lateral popliteal nerve**
  Peroneal nerve palsy
  - **G57.30**　Lesion of lateral popliteal nerve, unspecified lower limb
  - **G57.31**　Lesion of lateral popliteal nerve, right lower limb
  - **G57.32**　Lesion of lateral popliteal nerve, left lower limb
- **G57.4　Lesion of medial popliteal nerve**
  - **G57.40**　Lesion of medial popliteal nerve, unspecified lower limb
  - **G57.41**　Lesion of medial popliteal nerve, right lower limb
  - **G57.42**　Lesion of medial popliteal nerve, left lower limb
- **G57.5　Tarsal tunnel syndrome**
  - **G57.50**　Tarsal tunnel syndrome, unspecified lower limb
  - **G57.51**　Tarsal tunnel syndrome, right lower limb
  - **G57.52**　Tarsal tunnel syndrome, left lower limb
- **G57.6　Lesion of plantar nerve**
  Morton's metatarsalgia
  - **G57.60**　Lesion of plantar nerve, unspecified lower limb
  - **G57.61**　Lesion of plantar nerve, right lower limb
  - **G57.62**　Lesion of plantar nerve, left lower limb
- **G57.7　Causalgia of lower limb**
  Complex regional pain syndrome II of lower limb
  > **Excludes1**　complex regional pain syndrome I of lower limb (G90.52-)
  > complex regional pain syndrome I of upper limb (G90.51-)
  > complex regional pain syndrome II of upper limb (G56.4-)
  > reflex sympathetic dystrophy of lower limb (G90.52-)
  > reflex sympathetic dystrophy of upper limb (G90.51-)
  - **G57.70**　Causalgia of unspecified lower limb
  - **G57.71**　Causalgia of right lower limb
  - **G57.72**　Causalgia of left lower limb
- **G57.8　Other specified mononeuropathies of lower limb**
  Interdigital neuroma of lower limb
  - **G57.80**　Other specified mononeuropathies of unspecified lower limb
  - **G57.81**　Other specified mononeuropathies of right lower limb
  - **G57.82**　Other specified mononeuropathies of left lower limb

---

◀ New　◀▥ Revised　d̶e̶l̶e̶t̶e̶d̶ Deleted　**OGCR** Official Guidelines　X Assign placeholder X　● Use Additional Character(s)

846

Excludes 1　Excludes 2　Includes　Use additional　Code first　Code also　Unspecified

● **G57.9**   Unspecified mononeuropathy of lower limb
    G57.90   Unspecified mononeuropathy of unspecified lower limb
    G57.91   Unspecified mononeuropathy of right lower limb
    G57.92   Unspecified mononeuropathy of left lower limb

● **G58**   **Other mononeuropathies**
    G58.0   Intercostal neuropathy
    G58.7   Mononeuritis multiplex
    G58.8   Other specified mononeuropathies
    G58.9   Mononeuropathy, unspecified

G59   **Mononeuropathy in diseases classified elsewhere**
    Code first underlying disease
    Excludes1   diabetic mononeuropathy (E08-E13 with .41)
               syphilitic nerve paralysis (A52.19)
               syphilitic neuritis (A52.15)
               tuberculous mononeuropathy (A17.83)

POLYNEUROPATHIES AND OTHER DISORDERS OF THE PERIPHERAL NERVOUS SYSTEM (G60-G65)

    Excludes1   neuralgia NOS (M79.2)
               neuritis NOS (M79.2)
               peripheral neuritis in pregnancy (O26.82-)
               radiculitis NOS (M54.10)

● **G60**   **Hereditary and idiopathic neuropathy**
    G60.0   **Hereditary motor and sensory neuropathy**
         Charcot-Marie-Tooth disease
         Déjerine-Sottas disease
         Hereditary motor and sensory neuropathy, types I-IV
         Hypertrophic neuropathy of infancy
         Peroneal muscular atrophy (axonal type) (hypertrophic type)
         Roussy-Lévy syndrome
    G60.1   **Refsum's disease**
         Genetic disorder affecting fatty acid metabolism
         Infantile Refsum disease
    G60.2   Neuropathy in association with hereditary ataxia
    G60.3   Idiopathic progressive neuropathy
    G60.8   Other hereditary and idiopathic neuropathies
         Dominantly inherited sensory neuropathy
         Morvan's disease
         Nelaton's syndrome
         Recessively inherited sensory neuropathy
    G60.9   Hereditary and idiopathic neuropathy, unspecified

Item 6-7   The **peripheral nervous system** consists of 31 pairs of spinal nerves, 12 pairs of cranial nerves, and the autonomic nerves, which are divided into the parasympathetic and sympathetic nerves. The cranial nerves are: olfactory (I), optic (II), oculomotor (III), trochlear (IV), trigeminal (V), abducens (VI), facial (VII), vestibulocochlear (VIII), glossopharyngeal (IX), vagus (X), accessory (XI), and hypoglossal (XII).

● **G61**   **Inflammatory polyneuropathy**
    G61.0   **Guillain-Barré syndrome**
         Autoimmune disease affecting peripheral nervous system
         Acute (post-)infective polyneuritis
         Miller Fisher Syndrome
    G61.1   **Serum neuropathy**
         Use additional code for adverse effect, if applicable, to identify serum (T50.-)
   ● **G61.8**   **Other inflammatory polyneuropathies**
        G61.81   Chronic inflammatory demyelinating polyneuritis
        G61.89   Other inflammatory polyneuropathies
    G61.9   Inflammatory polyneuropathy, unspecified

● **G62**   **Other and unspecified polyneuropathies**
    G62.0   **Drug-induced polyneuropathy**
         Use additional code for adverse effect, if applicable, to identify drug (T36-T50 with fifth or sixth character 5)
    G62.1   **Alcoholic polyneuropathy**
         Malfunction of many peripheral nerves throughout the body
    G62.2   **Polyneuropathy due to other toxic agents**
         Code first (T51-T65) *to identify toxic agent*
   ● **G62.8**   **Other specified polyneuropathies**
        G62.81   Critical illness polyneuropathy
            Acute motor neuropathy
        G62.82   Radiation-induced polyneuropathy
            Use additional external cause code (W88-W90, X39.0-) to identify cause
        G62.89   Other specified polyneuropathies
    G62.9   **Polyneuropathy, unspecified**
         Neuropathy NOS

CHAPTER 6 (G00-G99)

Figure 6-2   **A.** Parasympathetic nervous system. **B.** Sympathetic nervous system. (From Buck CJ: Step-by-Step Medical Coding, Philadelphia, WB Saunders, 1998)

◀ New   ⬅ Revised   ~~deleted~~ Deleted   **OGCR** Official Guidelines   X Assign placeholder X   ● Use Additional Character(s)

| Excludes 1 | Excludes 2 | Includes | Use additional | Code first | Code also | Unspecified |

G63   **Polyneuropathy in diseases classified elsewhere**

Code first underlying disease, such as:
     amyloidosis (E85.-)
     endocrine disease, except diabetes (E00-E07, E15-E16,
         E20-E34)
     metabolic diseases (E70-E88)
     neoplasm (C00-D49)
     nutritional deficiency (E40-E64)

> **Excludes1**   polyneuropathy (in):
>   diabetes mellitus (E08-E13 with .42)
>   diphtheria (A36.83)
>   infectious mononucleosis (B27.0-B27.9 with 1)
>   Lyme disease (A69.22)
>   mumps (B26.84)
>   postherpetic (B02.23)
>   rheumatoid arthritis (M05.33)
>   scleroderma (M34.83)
>   systemic lupus erythematosus (M32.19)

G64   **Other disorders of peripheral nervous system**
     Disorder of peripheral nervous system NOS

● G65   **Sequelae of inflammatory and toxic polyneuropathies**

Code first condition resulting from (sequela) of inflammatory and
toxic polyneuropathies

G65.0   **Sequelae of Guillain-Barré syndrome**

G65.1   **Sequelae of other inflammatory polyneuropathy**

G65.2   **Sequelae of toxic polyneuropathy**

DISEASES OF MYONEURAL JUNCTION AND MUSCLE (G70-G73)

● G70   **Myasthenia gravis and other myoneural disorders**

> **Excludes1**   botulism (A05.1, A48.51-A48.52)
>   transient neonatal myasthenia gravis (P94.0)

● G70.0   **Myasthenia gravis**
     Acquired and results in fatigable muscle weakness
     exacerbated by activity and improved with rest.

G70.00   **Myasthenia gravis without (acute) exacerbation**
     Myasthenia gravis NOS

G70.01   **Myasthenia gravis with (acute) exacerbation**
     Myasthenia gravis in crisis

G70.1   **Toxic myoneural disorders**
     Dysfunction at junction of muscle and motor nerve
         (myoneural junction)

     Code first (T51-T65) to identify toxic agent

G70.2   **Congenital and developmental myasthenia**

● G70.8   **Other specified myoneural disorders**

G70.80   **Lambert-Eaton syndrome, unspecified**
     Lambert-Eaton syndrome NOS

G70.81   **Lambert-Eaton syndrome in disease classified**
     elsewhere

     Code first underlying disease

> **Excludes1**   Lambert-Eaton syndrome in
>   neoplastic disease (G73.1)

G70.89   **Other specified myoneural disorders**

G70.9   **Myoneural disorder, unspecified**

● G71   **Primary disorders of muscles**

> **Excludes2**   arthrogryposis multiplex congenita (Q74.3)
>   metabolic disorders (E70-E88)
>   myositis (M60.-)

G71.0   **Muscular dystrophy**
     Autosomal recessive, childhood type, muscular
         dystrophy resembling Duchenne or Becker
         muscular dystrophy
     Benign [Becker] muscular dystrophy
     Benign scapuloperoneal muscular dystrophy with early
         contractures [Emery-Dreifuss]
     Congenital muscular dystrophy NOS
     Congenital muscular dystrophy with specific
         morphological abnormalities of the muscle fiber
     Distal muscular dystrophy
     Facioscapulohumeral muscular dystrophy
     Limb-girdle muscular dystrophy
     Ocular muscular dystrophy
     Oculopharyngeal muscular dystrophy
     Scapuloperoneal muscular dystrophy
     Severe [Duchenne] muscular dystrophy

● G71.1   **Myotonic disorders**
     Inherited disorder that affects muscles tone

G71.11   **Myotonic muscular dystrophy**
     Dystrophia myotonica [Steinert]
     Myotonia atrophica
     Myotonic dystrophy
     Proximal myotonic myopathy (PROMM)
     Steinert disease

G71.12   **Myotonia congenita**
     Acetazolamide responsive myotonia congenita
     Dominant myotonia congenita [Thomsen
         disease]
     Myotonia levior
     Recessive myotonia congenita [Becker disease]

G71.13   **Myotonic chondrodystrophy**
     Chondrodystrophic myotonia
     Congenital myotonic chondrodystrophy
     Schwartz-Jampel disease

G71.14   **Drug induced myotonia**

     Use additional code for adverse effect, if
         applicable, to identify drug (T36-T50 with
         fifth or sixth character 5)

G71.19   **Other specified myotonic disorders**
     Myotonia fluctuans
     Myotonia permanens
     Neuromyotonia [Isaacs]
     Paramyotonia congenita (of von Eulenburg)
     Pseudomyotonia
     Symptomatic myotonia

G71.2   **Congenital myopathies**
     Central core disease
     Fiber-type disproportion
     Minicore disease
     Multicore disease
     Myotubular (centronuclear) myopathy
     Nemaline myopathy

> **Excludes1**   arthrogryposis multiplex congenita
>   (Q74.3)

G71.3   **Mitochondrial myopathy, not elsewhere classified**
     Myopathies associated with increased number of enlarged,
         often abnormal, mitochondria in muscle fibers

> **Excludes1**   Kearns-Sayre syndrome (H49.81)
>   Leber's disease (H47.21)
>   Leigh's encephalopathy (G31.82)
>   mitochondrial metabolism disorders
>   (E88.4.-)
>   Reye's syndrome (G93.7)

G71.8   **Other primary disorders of muscles**

G71.9   **Primary disorder of muscle, unspecified**
     Hereditary myopathy NOS

Item 6–8   Muscular dystrophies (MD) are a group of rare inherited muscle diseases. Voluntary muscles become progressively weaker. In the late stages of MD, fat and connective tissue replace muscle fibers. In some types of muscular dystrophy, heart muscles, other involuntary muscles, and other organs are affected. **Myopathies** is a general term for neuromuscular diseases in which the muscle fibers dysfunction for any one of many reasons, resulting in muscular weakness.

◀ New   ◀▥ Revised   ~~deleted~~ Deleted   OGCR Official Guidelines   X Assign placeholder X   ● Use Additional Character(s)

Excludes 1   Excludes 2   Includes   Use additional   Code first   Code also   Unspecified

● **G72   Other and unspecified myopathies**

> **Excludes1**   arthrogryposis multiplex congenita (Q74.3)
> dermatopolymyositis (M33.-)
> ischemic infarction of muscle (M62.2-)
> myositis (M60.-)
> polymyositis (M33.2.-)

G72.0   Drug-induced myopathy

> Use additional code for adverse effect, if applicable, to identify drug (T36-T50 with fifth or sixth character 5)

G72.1   Alcoholic myopathy

> Use additional code to identify alcoholism (F10.-)

G72.2   Myopathy due to other toxic agents

> *Code first (T51-T65) to identify toxic agent*

G72.3   Periodic paralysis

> Familial periodic paralysis
> Hyperkalemic periodic paralysis (familial)
> Hypokalemic periodic paralysis (familial)
> Myotonic periodic paralysis (familial)
> Normokalemic paralysis (familial)
> Potassium sensitive periodic paralysis
>
> > **Excludes1**   paramyotonia congenita (of von Eulenburg) (G71.19)

● **G72.4   Inflammatory and immune myopathies, not elsewhere classified**

> **G72.41   Inclusion body myositis [IBM]**
>
> **G72.49   Other inflammatory and immune myopathies, not elsewhere classified**
> > Inflammatory myopathy NOS

● **G72.8   Other specified myopathies**

> **G72.81   Critical illness myopathy**
> > Acute necrotizing myopathy
> > Acute quadriplegic myopathy
> > Intensive care (ICU) myopathy
> > Myopathy of critical illness
>
> **G72.89   Other specified myopathies**

G72.9   Myopathy, unspecified

● **G73   Disorders of myoneural junction and muscle in diseases classified elsewhere**

> **G73.1   Lambert-Eaton syndrome in neoplastic disease**
> > *Rare autoimmune disorder affecting calcium channels of nerve-muscle (neuromuscular) junction*
> >
> > *Code first underlying neoplasm (C00-D49)*
> >
> > > **Excludes1**   Lambert-Eaton syndrome not associated with neoplasm (G70.80-G70.81)
>
> **G73.3   Myasthenic syndromes in other diseases classified elsewhere**
> > *Code first underlying disease, such as:*
> > neoplasm (C00-D49)
> > thyrotoxicosis (E05.-)
>
> **G73.7   Myopathy in diseases classified elsewhere**
> > *Code first underlying disease, such as:*
> > hyperparathyroidism (E21.0, E21.3)
> > hypoparathyroidism (E20.-)
> > glycogen storage disease (E74.0)
> > lipid storage disorders (E75.-)
> >
> > > **Excludes1**   myopathy in:
> > > rheumatoid arthritis (M05.32)
> > > sarcoidosis (D86.87)
> > > scleroderma (M34.82)
> > > sicca syndrome [Sjögren] (M35.03)
> > > systemic lupus erythematosus (M32.19)

Item 6–9   **Hemiplegia** is complete paralysis of one side of the body—arm, leg, and trunk. **Hemiparesis** is a generalized weakness or incomplete paralysis of one side of the body. If most activities (eating, writing) are performed with the right hand, the right is the dominant side, and the left is the nondominant side. **Quadriplegia,** also called tetraplegia, is the complete paralysis of all four limbs. **Quadriparesis** is the incomplete paralysis of all four limbs. Nerve damage in C1–C4 is associated with lower limb paralysis, and C5–C7 damage is associated with upper limb paralysis. **Diplegia** is the paralysis of the upper limbs. **Monoplegia** is the complete paralysis of one limb.

CEREBRAL PALSY AND OTHER PARALYTIC SYNDROMES (G80-G83)

● **G80   Cerebral palsy**

> **Excludes1**   hereditary spastic paraplegia (G11.4)

G80.0   Spastic quadriplegic cerebral palsy
> Congenital spastic paralysis (cerebral)

G80.1   Spastic diplegic cerebral palsy
> Spastic cerebral palsy NOS

G80.2   Spastic hemiplegic cerebral palsy

G80.3   Athetoid cerebral palsy
> *Result of damage to cerebellum or basal ganglia responsible for processing neuromuscular signals*
> Double athetosis (syndrome)
> Dyskinetic cerebral palsy
> Dystonic cerebral palsy
> Vogt disease

G80.4   Ataxic cerebral palsy
> *Poor muscle tone and coordination*

G80.8   Other cerebral palsy
> Mixed cerebral palsy syndromes

G80.9   Cerebral palsy, unspecified
> Cerebral palsy NOS

OGCR   Section I.C.6.a.

> Dominant/nondominant side
>
> Codes from category G81, Hemiplegia and hemiparesis, and subcategories, G83.1, Monoplegia of lower limb, G83.2, Monoplegia of upper limb, and G83.3, Monoplegia, unspecified, identify whether the dominant and nondominant side is affected. Should the affected side be documented, but not specified as dominant or nondominant, and the classification system does not indicate a default, code selection is as follows:
>
> - For ambidextrous patients, the default should be dominant.
> - If the left side is affected, the default is non-dominant.
> - If the right side is affected, the default is dominant.

● **G81   Hemiplegia and hemiparesis**

> **Note:**   This category is to be used only when hemiplegia (complete)(incomplete) is reported without further specification, or is stated to be old or longstanding but of unspecified cause. The category is also for use in multiple coding to identify these types of hemiplegia resulting from any cause.
>
> > **Excludes1**   congenital cerebral palsy (G80.-)
> > hemiplegia and hemiparesis due to sequela of cerebrovascular disease (I69.05-, I69.15-, I69.25-, I69.35-, I69.85-, I69.95-)

● **G81.0   Flaccid hemiplegia**

> *Paralysis of half of body with loss of tone of muscles of paralyzed part and absence of tendon reflexes*

G81.00   Flaccid hemiplegia affecting unspecified side

G81.01   Flaccid hemiplegia affecting right dominant side

G81.02   Flaccid hemiplegia affecting left dominant side

G81.03   Flaccid hemiplegia affecting right nondominant side

G81.04   Flaccid hemiplegia affecting left nondominant side

- **G81.1 Spastic hemiplegia**
  Paralysis of half of body with spasticity of muscles of paralyzed part and increased tendon reflexes
  - G81.10 Spastic hemiplegia affecting unspecified side
  - G81.11 Spastic hemiplegia affecting right dominant side
  - G81.12 Spastic hemiplegia affecting left dominant side
  - G81.13 Spastic hemiplegia affecting right nondominant side
  - G81.14 Spastic hemiplegia affecting left nondominant side
- **G81.9 Hemiplegia, unspecified**
  - G81.90 Hemiplegia, unspecified affecting unspecified side
  - G81.91 Hemiplegia, unspecified affecting right dominant side
  - G81.92 Hemiplegia, unspecified affecting left dominant side
  - G81.93 Hemiplegia, unspecified affecting right nondominant side
  - G81.94 Hemiplegia, unspecified affecting left nondominant side

- **G82 Paraplegia (paraparesis) and quadriplegia (quadriparesis)**
  Note: This category is to be used only when the listed conditions are reported without further specification, or are stated to be old or longstanding but of unspecified cause. The category is also for use in multiple coding to identify these conditions resulting from any cause.
  | Excludes1 | congenital cerebral palsy (G80.-) |
  functional quadriplegia (R53.2)
  hysterical paralysis (F44.4)
  - **G82.2 Paraplegia**
    Paralysis of both lower limbs NOS
    Paraparesis (lower) NOS
    Paraplegia (lower) NOS
    - G82.20 Paraplegia, unspecified
    - G82.21 Paraplegia, complete
    - G82.22 Paraplegia, incomplete
  - **G82.5 Quadriplegia**
    Paralysis of all limbs; AKA tetraplegia
    - G82.50 Quadriplegia, unspecified
    - G82.51 Quadriplegia, C1-C4 complete
    - G82.52 Quadriplegia, C1-C4 incomplete
    - G82.53 Quadriplegia, C5-C7 complete
    - G82.54 Quadriplegia, C5-C7 incomplete
- **G83 Other paralytic syndromes**
  Note: This category is to be used only when the listed conditions are reported without further specification, or are stated to be old or longstanding but of unspecified cause. The category is also for use in multiple coding to identify these conditions resulting from any cause.
  | Includes | paralysis (complete) (incomplete), except as in G80-G82 |
  - **G83.0 Diplegia of upper limbs**
    Paralysis affecting limbs on both sides; AKA bilateral paralysis
    Diplegia (upper)
    Paralysis of both upper limbs

- **G83.1 Monoplegia of lower limb**
  Paralysis of limb on one side
  Paralysis of lower limb
  | Excludes1 | monoplegia of lower limbs due to sequela of cerebrovascular disease (I69.04-, I69.14-, I69.24-, I69.34-, I69.84-, I69.94-) |
  - G83.10 Monoplegia of lower limb affecting unspecified side
  - G83.11 Monoplegia of lower limb affecting right dominant side
  - G83.12 Monoplegia of lower limb affecting left dominant side
  - G83.13 Monoplegia of lower limb affecting right nondominant side
  - G83.14 Monoplegia of lower limb affecting left nondominant side
- **G83.2 Monoplegia of upper limb**
  Paralysis of upper limb
  | Excludes1 | monoplegia of upper limbs due to sequela of cerebrovascular disease (I69.03-, I69.13-, I69.23-, I69.33-, I69.83-, I69.93-) |
  - G83.20 Monoplegia of upper limb affecting unspecified side
  - G83.21 Monoplegia of upper limb affecting right dominant side
  - G83.22 Monoplegia of upper limb affecting left dominant side
  - G83.23 Monoplegia of upper limb affecting right nondominant side
  - G83.24 Monoplegia of upper limb affecting left nondominant side
- **G83.3 Monoplegia, unspecified**
  - G83.30 Monoplegia, unspecified affecting unspecified side
  - G83.31 Monoplegia, unspecified affecting right dominant side
  - G83.32 Monoplegia, unspecified affecting left dominant side
  - G83.33 Monoplegia, unspecified affecting right nondominant side
  - G83.34 Monoplegia, unspecified affecting left nondominant side
  - **G83.4 Cauda equina syndrome**
    Aching pain due to compression of spinal nerve roots
    Neurogenic bladder due to cauda equina syndrome
    | Excludes1 | cord bladder NOS (G95.89) |
    neurogenic bladder NOS (N31.9)
  - **G83.5 Locked-in state**
- **G83.8 Other specified paralytic syndromes**
    | Excludes1 | paralytic syndromes due to current spinal cord injury-code to spinal cord injury (S14, S24, S34) |
  - G83.81 Brown-Séquard syndrome
  - G83.82 Anterior cord syndrome
  - G83.83 Posterior cord syndrome
  - G83.84 Todd's paralysis (postepileptic)
  - G83.89 Other specified paralytic syndromes
- **G83.9 Paralytic syndrome, unspecified**

OTHER DISORDERS OF THE NERVOUS SYSTEM (G89-G99)

● **G89   Pain, not elsewhere classified**

Code also related psychological factors associated with pain (F45.42)

Excludes1   generalized pain NOS (R52)
pain disorders exclusively related to psychological factors (F45.41)
pain NOS (R52)

Excludes2   atypical face pain (G50.1)
headache syndromes (G44.-)
localized pain, unspecified type - code to pain by site, such as:
    abdomen pain (R10.-)
    back pain (M54.9)
    breast pain (N64.4)
    chest pain (R07.1-R07.9)
    ear pain (H92.0-)
    eye pain (H57.1)
    headache (R51)
    joint pain (M25.5-)
    limb pain (M79.6-)
    lumbar region pain (M54.5)
    painful urination (R30.9)
    pelvic and perineal pain (R10.2)
    shoulder pain (M25.51-)
    spine pain (M54.-)
    throat pain (R07.0)
    tongue pain (K14.6)
    tooth pain (K08.8)
renal colic (N23)
migraines (G43.-)
myalgia (M79.1)
pain from prosthetic devices, implants, and grafts (T82.84, T83.84, T84.84, T85.84)
phantom limb syndrome with pain (G54.6)
vulvar vestibulitis (N94.810)
vulvodynia (N94.81-)

G89.0   Central pain syndrome
Neurological condition causing intractable pain resulting from damage to CNS
Déjérine-Roussy syndrome
Myelopathic pain syndrome
Thalamic pain syndrome (hyperesthetic)

● **G89.1   Acute pain, not elsewhere classified**

G89.11   Acute pain due to trauma

G89.12   Acute post-thoracotomy pain
Post-thoracotomy pain NOS

G89.18   Other acute postprocedural pain
Postoperative pain NOS
Postprocedural pain NOS

● **G89.2   Chronic pain, not elsewhere classified**

Excludes1   causalgia, lower limb (G57.7-)
causalgia, upper limb (G56.4-)
central pain syndrome (G89.0)
chronic pain syndrome (G89.4)
complex regional pain syndrome II, lower limb (G57.7-)
complex regional pain syndrome II, upper limb (G56.4-)
neoplasm related chronic pain (G89.3)
reflex sympathetic dystrophy (G90.5-)

G89.21   Chronic pain due to trauma

G89.22   Chronic post-thoracotomy pain

G89.28   Other chronic postprocedural pain
Other chronic postoperative pain

G89.29   Other chronic pain

G89.3   Neoplasm related pain (acute) (chronic)
Cancer associated pain
Pain due to malignancy (primary) (secondary)
Tumor associated pain

G89.4   Chronic pain syndrome
Chronic pain associated with significant psychosocial dysfunction

● **G90   Disorders of autonomic nervous system**

Excludes1   dysfunction of the autonomic nervous system due to alcohol (G31.2)

● **G90.0   Idiopathic peripheral autonomic neuropathy**

G90.01   Carotid sinus syncope
Carotid sinus syndrome

G90.09   Other idiopathic peripheral autonomic neuropathy
Idiopathic peripheral autonomic neuropathy NOS

G90.1   Familial dysautonomia [Riley-Day]
Inherited disorder that affects nerve function

G90.2   Horner's syndrome
Due to damage of the sympathetic nervous system
Bernard(-Horner) syndrome
Cervical sympathetic dystrophy or paralysis

G90.3   Multi-system degeneration of the autonomic nervous system
Neurogenic orthostatic hypotension [Shy-Drager]
Excludes1   orthostatic hypotension NOS (I95.1)

G90.4   Autonomic dysreflexia
Syndrome resulting from lesions of spinal cord
Use additional code to identify the cause, such as:
    fecal impaction (K56.41)
    pressure ulcer (pressure area) (L89.-)
    urinary tract infection (N39.0)

● **G90.5   Complex regional pain syndrome I (CRPS I)**
Reflex sympathetic dystrophy
Excludes1   causalgia of lower limb (G57.7-)
causalgia of upper limb (G56.4-)
complex regional pain syndrome II of lower limb (G57.7-)
complex regional pain syndrome II of upper limb (G56.4-)

G90.50   Complex regional pain syndrome I, unspecified

● **G90.51   Complex regional pain syndrome I of upper limb**

G90.511   Complex regional pain syndrome I of right upper limb

G90.512   Complex regional pain syndrome I of left upper limb

G90.513   Complex regional pain syndrome I of upper limb, bilateral

G90.519   Complex regional pain syndrome I of unspecified upper limb

● **G90.52   Complex regional pain syndrome I of lower limb**

G90.521   Complex regional pain syndrome I of right lower limb

G90.522   Complex regional pain syndrome I of left lower limb

G90.523   Complex regional pain syndrome I of lower limb, bilateral

G90.529   Complex regional pain syndrome I of unspecified lower limb

G90.59   Complex regional pain syndrome I of other specified site

G90.8   Other disorders of autonomic nervous system

G90.9   Disorder of the autonomic nervous system, unspecified

● **G91   Hydrocephalus**
Dilatation of cerebral ventricles, accompanied by accumulation of cerebrospinal fluid
Includes   acquired hydrocephalus
Excludes1   Arnold-Chiari syndrome with hydrocephalus (Q07.-)
congenital hydrocephalus (Q03.-)
spina bifida with hydrocephalus (Q05.-)

G91.0   Communicating hydrocephalus
Secondary normal pressure hydrocephalus

G91.1   Obstructive hydrocephalus

CHAPTER 6 (G00-G99)

◀ New   ◀━ Revised   ~~deleted~~ Deleted   **OGCR** Official Guidelines   X Assign placeholder X   ● Use Additional Character(s)

| Excludes 1 | Excludes 2 | Includes | Use additional | Code first | Code also | Unspecified |

G91.2   (Idiopathic) normal pressure hydrocephalus
Normal pressure hydrocephalus NOS

G91.3   Post-traumatic hydrocephalus, unspecified

G91.4   Hydrocephalus in diseases classified elsewhere
Code first underlying condition, such as:
congenital syphilis (A50.4-)
neoplasm (C00-D49)
> **Excludes1**   hydrocephalus due to congenital toxoplasmosis (P37.1)

G91.8   Other hydrocephalus

G91.9   Hydrocephalus, unspecified

G92   Toxic encephalopathy
Disorder or disease of brain caused by chemicals
Toxic encephalitis
Toxic metabolic encephalopathy
Code first (T51-T65) to identify toxic agent

● **G93   Other disorders of brain**

G93.0   Cerebral cysts
Arachnoid cyst
Porencephalic cyst, acquired
> **Excludes1**   acquired periventricular cysts of newborn (P91.1)
> congenital cerebral cysts (Q04.6)

G93.1   Anoxic brain damage, not elsewhere classified
Permanent brain damage by lack of oxygen perfusion through brain tissues.
> **Excludes1**   cerebral anoxia due to anesthesia during labor and delivery (O74.3)
> cerebral anoxia due to anesthesia during the puerperium (O89.2)
> neonatal anoxia (P84)

G93.2   Benign intracranial hypertension
> **Excludes1**   hypertensive encephalopathy (I67.4)

G93.3   Postviral fatigue syndrome
Benign myalgic encephalomyelitis
> **Excludes1**   chronic fatigue syndrome NOS (R53.82)

● **G93.4   Other and unspecified encephalopathy**
> **Excludes1**   alcoholic encephalopathy (G31.2)
> encephalopathy in diseases classified elsewhere (G94)
> hypertensive encephalopathy (I67.4)
> toxic (metabolic) encephalopathy (G92)

G93.40   Encephalopathy, unspecified

G93.41   Metabolic encephalopathy
Septic encephalopathy

G93.49   Other encephalopathy
Encephalopathy NEC

G93.5   Compression of brain
Arnold-Chiari type 1 compression of brain
Compression of brain (stem)
Herniation of brain (stem)
> **Excludes1**   diffuse traumatic compression of brain (S06.2-)
> focal traumatic compression of brain (S06.3-)

G93.6   Cerebral edema
> **Excludes1**   cerebral edema due to birth injury (P11.0)
> traumatic cerebral edema (S06.1-)

G93.7   Reye's syndrome
Life-threatening neurological condition, usually follows viral illness
Code first (T39.0-), if salicylates-induced

● **G93.8   Other specified disorders of brain**

G93.81   Temporal sclerosis
Hippocampal sclerosis
Mesial temporal sclerosis

G93.82   Brain death

G93.89   Other specified disorders of brain
Postradiation encephalopathy

G93.9   Disorder of brain, unspecified

G94   Other disorders of brain in diseases classified elsewhere
Code first underlying disease
> **Excludes1**   encephalopathy in congenital syphilis (A50.49)
> encephalopathy in influenza (J09.X9, J10.81, J11.81)
> encephalopathy in syphilis (A52.19)
> hydrocephalus in diseases classified elsewhere (G91.4)

● **G95   Other and unspecified diseases of spinal cord**
> **Excludes2**   myelitis (G04.-)

G95.0   Syringomyelia and syringobulbia

● **G95.1   Vascular myelopathies**
> **Excludes2**   intraspinal phlebitis and thrombophlebitis, except non-pyogenic (G08)

G95.11   Acute infarction of spinal cord (embolic) (nonembolic)
Anoxia of spinal cord
Arterial thrombosis of spinal cord

G95.19   Other vascular myelopathies
Edema of spinal cord
Hematomyelia
Nonpyogenic intraspinal phlebitis and thrombophlebitis
Subacute necrotic myelopathy

● **G95.2   Other and unspecified cord compression**

G95.20   Unspecified cord compression

G95.29   Other cord compression

● **G95.8   Other specified diseases of spinal cord**
> **Excludes1**   neurogenic bladder NOS (N31.9)
> neurogenic bladder due to cauda equina syndrome (G83.4)
> neuromuscular dysfunction of bladder without spinal cord lesion (N31.-)

G95.81   Conus medullaris syndrome
Damage to gray matter and/or nerve roots in lower end of spinal cord

G95.89   Other specified diseases of spinal cord
Cord bladder NOS
Drug-induced myelopathy
Radiation-induced myelopathy
> **Excludes1**   myelopathy NOS (G95.9)

G95.9   Disease of spinal cord, unspecified
Myelopathy NOS

● **G96   Other disorders of central nervous system**

G96.0   Cerebrospinal fluid leak
> **Excludes1**   cerebrospinal fluid leak from spinal puncture (G97.0)

● **G96.1   Disorders of meninges, not elsewhere classified**

G96.11   Dural tear
> **Excludes1**   accidental puncture or laceration of dura during a procedure (G97.41)

G96.12   Meningeal adhesions (cerebral) (spinal)

G96.19   Other disorders of meninges, not elsewhere classified

G96.8   Other specified disorders of central nervous system

G96.9   Disorder of central nervous system, unspecified

● **G97   Intraoperative and postprocedural complications and disorders of nervous system, not elsewhere classified**
> **Excludes2**   intraoperative and postprocedural cerebrovascular infarction (I97.81-, I97.82-)

G97.0   Cerebrospinal fluid leak from spinal puncture

G97.1   Other reaction to spinal and lumbar puncture
Headache due to lumbar puncture

G97.2   Intracranial hypotension following ventricular shunting

---

◀ New   ◀||| Revised   ~~deleted~~ Deleted   **OGCR** Official Guidelines   X Assign placeholder X   ● Use Additional Character(s)

Excludes 1   Excludes 2   Includes   Use additional   Code first   Code also   Unspecified

● **G97.3** **Intraoperative hemorrhage and hematoma of a nervous system organ or structure complicating a procedure**

> **Excludes1**   intraoperative hemorrhage and hematoma of a nervous system organ or structure due to accidental puncture and laceration during a procedure (G97.4-)

     G97.31 **Intraoperative hemorrhage and hematoma of a nervous system organ or structure complicating a nervous system procedure**

     G97.32 **Intraoperative hemorrhage and hematoma of a nervous system organ or structure complicating other procedure**

● **G97.4** **Accidental puncture and laceration of a nervous system organ or structure during a procedure**

     G97.41 **Accidental puncture or laceration of dura during a procedure**
         Incidental (inadvertent) durotomy

     G97.48 **Accidental puncture and laceration of other nervous system organ or structure during a nervous system procedure**

     G97.49 **Accidental puncture and laceration of other nervous system organ or structure during other procedure**

● **G97.5** **Postprocedural hemorrhage and hematoma of a nervous system organ or structure following a procedure**

     G97.51 **Postprocedural hemorrhage and hematoma of a nervous system organ or structure following a nervous system procedure**

     G97.52 **Postprocedural hemorrhage and hematoma of a nervous system organ or structure following other procedure**

● **G97.8** **Other intraoperative and postprocedural complications and disorders of nervous system**

> Use additional code to further specify disorder

     G97.81 **Other intraoperative complications of nervous system**

     G97.82 **Other postprocedural complications and disorders of nervous system**

● **G98** **Other disorders of nervous system not elsewhere classified**

> **Includes**   nervous system disorder NOS

     G98.0 **Neurogenic arthritis, not elsewhere classified**
         Nonsyphilitic neurogenic arthropathy NEC
         Nonsyphilitic neurogenic spondylopathy NEC

> **Excludes1**   spondylopathy (in):
>   syringomyelia and syringobulbia (G95.0)
>   tabes dorsalis (A52.11)

     G98.8 **Other disorders of nervous system**
         Nervous system disorder NOS

● **G99** **Other disorders of nervous system in diseases classified elsewhere**

     G99.0 **Autonomic neuropathy in diseases classified elsewhere**

> *Code first underlying disease, such as:*
>   amyloidosis (E85.-)
>   gout (M1A.-, M10.-)
>   hyperthyroidism (E05.-)

> **Excludes1**   diabetic autonomic neuropathy (E08-E13 with .43)

     G99.2 **Myelopathy in diseases classified elsewhere**

> *Code first underlying disease, such as:*
>   neoplasm (C00-D49)

> **Excludes1**   myelopathy in:
>   intervertebral disease (M50.0-, M51.0-)
>   spondylosis (M47.0-, M47.1-)

     G99.8 **Other specified disorders of nervous system in diseases classified elsewhere**

> *Code first underlying disorder, such as:*
>   amyloidosis (E85.-)
>   avitaminosis (E56.9)

> **Excludes1**   nervous system involvement in:
>   cysticercosis (B69.0)
>   rubella (B06.0-)
>   syphilis (A52.1-)

CHAPTER 6 (G00-G99)

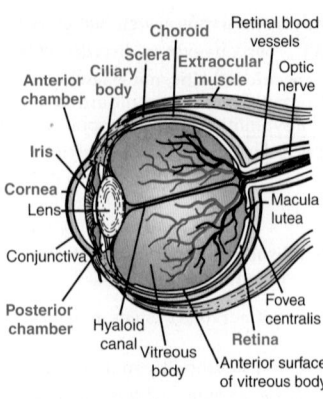

Figure 7–1 Eye and ocular adnexa. (From Buck CJ: Step-by-Step Medical Coding, ed 2011, Philadelphia, WB Saunders, 2011)

(See Plate 87 on page NAP-15.)

CHAPTER 7

DISEASES OF THE EYE AND ADNEXA (H00-H59)

Note: Use an external cause code following the code for the eye condition, if applicable, to identify the cause of the eye condition

> **Excludes2** certain conditions originating in the perinatal period (P04-P96)
> certain infectious and parasitic diseases (A00-B99)
> complications of pregnancy, childbirth and the puerperium (O00-O9A)
> congenital malformations, deformations, and chromosomal abnormalities (Q00-Q99)
> diabetes mellitus related eye conditions (E09.3-, E10.3-, E11.3-, E13.3-)
> endocrine, nutritional and metabolic diseases (E00-E88)
> injury (trauma) of eye and orbit (S05.-)
> injury, poisoning and certain other consequences of external causes (S00-T88)
> neoplasms (C00-D49)
> symptoms, signs and abnormal clinical and laboratory findings, not elsewhere classified (R00-R94)
> syphilis related eye disorders (A50.01, A50.3-, A51.43, A52.71)

This chapter contains the following blocks:

H00-H05	Disorders of eyelid, lacrimal system and orbit
H10-H11	Disorders of conjunctiva
H15-H22	Disorders of sclera, cornea, iris and ciliary body
H25-H28	Disorders of lens
H30-H36	Disorders of choroid and retina
H40-H42	Glaucoma
H43-H44	Disorders of vitreous body and globe
H46-H47	Disorders of optic nerve and visual pathways
H49-H52	Disorders of ocular muscles, binocular movement, accommodation and refraction
H53-H54	Visual disturbances and blindness
H55-H57	Other disorders of eye and adnexa
H59	Intraoperative and postprocedural complications and disorders of eye and adnexa, not elsewhere classified

DISORDERS OF EYELID, LACRIMAL SYSTEM AND ORBIT (H00-H05)

> **Excludes2** open wound of eyelid (S01.1-)
> superficial injury of eyelid (S00.1-, S00.2-)

● **H00   Hordeolum and chalazion**
Hordeolum: inflammatory staphylococcal infection of sebaceous glands of eyelids; AKA stye. Chalazion: eyelid mass

● **H00.0   Hordeolum (externum) (internum) of eyelid**
Bacterial infection (staphylococcus) of the sebaceous gland of the eyelid (stye)

● **H00.01   Hordeolum externum**
Hordeolum NOS
Stye

     H00.011   Hordeolum externum right upper eyelid

     H00.012   Hordeolum externum right lower eyelid

     H00.013   Hordeolum externum right eye, unspecified eyelid

     H00.014   Hordeolum externum left upper eyelid

     H00.015   Hordeolum externum left lower eyelid

     H00.016   Hordeolum externum left eye, unspecified eyelid

     H00.019   Hordeolum externum unspecified eye, unspecified eyelid

● **H00.02   Hordeolum internum**
Infection of meibomian gland

     H00.021   Hordeolum internum right upper eyelid

     H00.022   Hordeolum internum right lower eyelid

     H00.023   Hordeolum internum right eye, unspecified eyelid

     H00.024   Hordeolum internum left upper eyelid

     H00.025   Hordeolum internum left lower eyelid

     H00.026   Hordeolum internum left eye, unspecified eyelid

     H00.029   Hordeolum internum unspecified eye, unspecified eyelid

● **H00.03   Abscess of eyelid**
Furuncle of eyelid

     H00.031   Abscess of right upper eyelid

     H00.032   Abscess of right lower eyelid

     H00.033   Abscess of eyelid right eye, unspecified eyelid

     H00.034   Abscess of left upper eyelid

     H00.035   Abscess of left lower eyelid

     H00.036   Abscess of eyelid left eye, unspecified eyelid

     H00.039   Abscess of eyelid unspecified eye, unspecified eyelid

● **H00.1   Chalazion**
Often caused by accumulation of meibomian gland secretions resulting from a blockage of duct.
Meibomian (gland) cyst

> **Excludes2** infected meibomian gland (H00.02-)

     H00.11   Chalazion right upper eyelid

     H00.12   Chalazion right lower eyelid

     H00.13   Chalazion right eye, unspecified eyelid

     H00.14   Chalazion left upper eyelid

     H00.15   Chalazion left lower eyelid

     H00.16   Chalazion left eye, unspecified eyelid

     H00.19   Chalazion unspecified eye, unspecified eyelid

◀ New   ◀|||| Revised   ~~deleted~~ Deleted   **OGCR** Official Guidelines   X Assign placeholder X   ● Use Additional Character(s)

Excludes 1   Excludes 2   Includes   Use additional   Code first   Code also   Unspecified

● H01   Other inflammation of eyelid
  ● H01.0   Blepharitis
     Inflammation of eyelids
     Excludes1   blepharoconjunctivitis (H10.5-)
    ● H01.00   Unspecified blepharitis
       H01.001   Unspecified blepharitis right upper eyelid
       H01.002   Unspecified blepharitis right lower eyelid
       H01.003   Unspecified blepharitis right eye, unspecified eyelid
       H01.004   Unspecified blepharitis left upper eyelid
       H01.005   Unspecified blepharitis left lower eyelid
       H01.006   Unspecified blepharitis left eye, unspecified eyelid
       H01.009   Unspecified blepharitis unspecified eye, unspecified eyelid
    ● H01.01   Ulcerative blepharitis
       H01.011   Ulcerative blepharitis right upper eyelid
       H01.012   Ulcerative blepharitis right lower eyelid
       H01.013   Ulcerative blepharitis right eye, unspecified eyelid
       H01.014   Ulcerative blepharitis left upper eyelid
       H01.015   Ulcerative blepharitis left lower eyelid
       H01.016   Ulcerative blepharitis left eye, unspecified eyelid
       H01.019   Ulcerative blepharitis unspecified eye, unspecified eyelid
    ● H01.02   Squamous blepharitis
       H01.021   Squamous blepharitis right upper eyelid
       H01.022   Squamous blepharitis right lower eyelid
       H01.023   Squamous blepharitis right eye, unspecified eyelid
       H01.024   Squamous blepharitis left upper eyelid
       H01.025   Squamous blepharitis left lower eyelid
       H01.026   Squamous blepharitis left eye, unspecified eyelid
       H01.029   Squamous blepharitis unspecified eye, unspecified eyelid
  ● H01.1   Noninfectious dermatoses of eyelid
    ● H01.11   Allergic dermatitis of eyelid
       Contact dermatitis of eyelid
       H01.111   Allergic dermatitis of right upper eyelid
       H01.112   Allergic dermatitis of right lower eyelid
       H01.113   Allergic dermatitis of right eye, unspecified eyelid
       H01.114   Allergic dermatitis of left upper eyelid
       H01.115   Allergic dermatitis of left lower eyelid
       H01.116   Allergic dermatitis of left eye, unspecified eyelid
       H01.119   Allergic dermatitis of unspecified eye, unspecified eyelid

● H01.12   Discoid lupus erythematosus of eyelid
     H01.121   Discoid lupus erythematosus of right upper eyelid
     H01.122   Discoid lupus erythematosus of right lower eyelid
     H01.123   Discoid lupus erythematosus of right eye, unspecified eyelid
     H01.124   Discoid lupus erythematosus of left upper eyelid
     H01.125   Discoid lupus erythematosus of left lower eyelid
     H01.126   Discoid lupus erythematosus of left eye, unspecified eyelid
     H01.129   Discoid lupus erythematosus of unspecified eye, unspecified eyelid
● H01.13   Eczematous dermatitis of eyelid
     H01.131   Eczematous dermatitis of right upper eyelid
     H01.132   Eczematous dermatitis of right lower eyelid
     H01.133   Eczematous dermatitis of right eye, unspecified eyelid
     H01.134   Eczematous dermatitis of left upper eyelid
     H01.135   Eczematous dermatitis of left lower eyelid
     H01.136   Eczematous dermatitis of left eye, unspecified eyelid
     H01.139   Eczematous dermatitis of unspecified eye, unspecified eyelid
● H01.14   Xeroderma of eyelid
     Abnormally dry
     H01.141   Xeroderma of right upper eyelid
     H01.142   Xeroderma of right lower eyelid
     H01.143   Xeroderma of right eye, unspecified eyelid
     H01.144   Xeroderma of left upper eyelid
     H01.145   Xeroderma of left lower eyelid
     H01.146   Xeroderma of left eye, unspecified eyelid
     H01.149   Xeroderma of unspecified eye, unspecified eyelid
   H01.8   Other specified inflammations of eyelid
   H01.9   Unspecified inflammation of eyelid
     Inflammation of eyelid NOS

● H02   Other disorders of eyelid
     Turning inward (inversion) of eyelid margin and ingrowing eyelashes
     Excludes1   congenital malformations of eyelid (Q10.0-Q10.3)
  ● H02.0   Entropion and trichiasis of eyelid
    ● H02.00   Unspecified entropion of eyelid
       H02.001   Unspecified entropion of right upper eyelid
       H02.002   Unspecified entropion of right lower eyelid
       H02.003   Unspecified entropion of right eye, unspecified eyelid
       H02.004   Unspecified entropion of left upper eyelid

Figure 7-2   Right lower eyelid entropion. Note the inward rotation of the tarsal plate about the horizontal axis and the resultant contact between the mucocutaneous junction and ocular surface. (From Yanoff: Ophthalmology, ed 3, Mosby, Inc., 2008)

CHAPTER 7 (H00-H59)

H02.005   Unspecified entropion of left lower eyelid

H02.006   Unspecified entropion of left eye, unspecified eyelid

H02.009   Unspecified entropion of unspecified eye, unspecified eyelid

● H02.01   Cicatricial entropion of eyelid
Scar

H02.011   Cicatricial entropion of right upper eyelid

H02.012   Cicatricial entropion of right lower eyelid

H02.013   Cicatricial entropion of right eye, unspecified eyelid

H02.014   Cicatricial entropion of left upper eyelid

H02.015   Cicatricial entropion of left lower eyelid

H02.016   Cicatricial entropion of left eye, unspecified eyelid

H02.019   Cicatricial entropion of unspecified eye, unspecified eyelid

● H02.02   Mechanical entropion of eyelid
Turning inward (inversion) of eyelid margin due to lack of support

H02.021   Mechanical entropion of right upper eyelid

H02.022   Mechanical entropion of right lower eyelid

H02.023   Mechanical entropion of right eye, unspecified eyelid

H02.024   Mechanical entropion of left upper eyelid

H02.025   Mechanical entropion of left lower eyelid

H02.026   Mechanical entropion of left eye, unspecified eyelid

H02.029   Mechanical entropion of unspecified eye, unspecified eyelid

● H02.03   Senile entropion of eyelid
Turning inward (inversion) of eyelid margin due to aging

H02.031   Senile entropion of right upper eyelid

H02.032   Senile entropion of right lower eyelid

H02.033   Senile entropion of right eye, unspecified eyelid

H02.034   Senile entropion of left upper eyelid

H02.035   Senile entropion of left lower eyelid

H02.036   Senile entropion of left eye, unspecified eyelid

H02.039   Senile entropion of unspecified eye, unspecified eyelid

● H02.04   Spastic entropion of eyelid
Turning inward (inversion) of eyelid margin caused by spasm of muscle

H02.041   Spastic entropion of right upper eyelid

H02.042   Spastic entropion of right lower eyelid

H02.043   Spastic entropion of right eye, unspecified eyelid

H02.044   Spastic entropion of left upper eyelid

H02.045   Spastic entropion of left lower eyelid

H02.046   Spastic entropion of left eye, unspecified eyelid

H02.049   Spastic entropion of unspecified eye, unspecified eyelid

● H02.05   Trichiasis without entropian
Ingrowing hairs of eyelashes

H02.051   Trichiasis without entropian right upper eyelid

H02.052   Trichiasis without entropian right lower eyelid

H02.053   Trichiasis without entropian right eye, unspecified eyelid

H02.054   Trichiasis without entropian left upper eyelid

H02.055   Trichiasis without entropian left lower eyelid

H02.056   Trichiasis without entropian left eye, unspecified eyelid

H02.059   Trichiasis without entropian unspecified eye, unspecified eyelid

● H02.1   Ectropion of eyelid
Eversion (pulling away) of eyelid

● H02.10   Unspecified ectropion of eyelid

H02.101   Unspecified ectropion of right upper eyelid

H02.102   Unspecified ectropion of right lower eyelid

H02.103   Unspecified ectropion of right eye, unspecified eyelid

H02.104   Unspecified ectropion of left upper eyelid

H02.105   Unspecified ectropion of left lower eyelid

H02.106   Unspecified ectropion of left eye, unspecified eyelid

H02.109   Unspecified ectropion of unspecified eye, unspecified eyelid

● H02.11   Cicatricial ectropion of eyelid
Pulling of eyelid down and away from eye due to scar or tightening

H02.111   Cicatricial ectropion of right upper eyelid

H02.112   Cicatricial ectropion of right lower eyelid

H02.113   Cicatricial ectropion of right eye, unspecified eyelid

H02.114   Cicatricial ectropion of left upper eyelid

H02.115   Cicatricial ectropion of left lower eyelid

H02.116   Cicatricial ectropion of left eye, unspecified eyelid

H02.119   Cicatricial ectropion of unspecified eye, unspecified eyelid

● H02.12   Mechanical ectropion of eyelid
Eversion (pulling away) of eyelid due to lack of support

H02.121   Mechanical ectropion of right upper eyelid

H02.122   Mechanical ectropion of right lower eyelid

H02.123   Mechanical ectropion of right eye, unspecified eyelid

H02.124   Mechanical ectropion of left upper eyelid

H02.125   Mechanical ectropion of left lower eyelid

H02.126   Mechanical ectropion of left eye, unspecified eyelid

H02.129   Mechanical ectropion of unspecified eye, unspecified eyelid

● H02.13   Senile ectropion of eyelid
           Eversion (pulling away) of eyelid due to age
    H02.131   Senile ectropion of right upper eyelid
    H02.132   Senile ectropion of right lower eyelid
    H02.133   Senile ectropion of right eye,
              unspecified eyelid
    H02.134   Senile ectropion of left upper eyelid
    H02.135   Senile ectropion of left lower eyelid
    H02.136   Senile ectropion of left eye,
              unspecified eyelid
    H02.139   Senile ectropion of unspecified eye,
              unspecified eyelid

● H02.14   Spastic ectropion of eyelid
           *Eversion (pulling away) of eyelid due to tonic
           muscle spasm*
    H02.141   Spastic ectropion of right upper
              eyelid
    H02.142   Spastic ectropion of right lower
              eyelid
    H02.143   Spastic ectropion of right eye,
              unspecified eyelid
    H02.144   Spastic ectropion of left upper eyelid
    H02.145   Spastic ectropion of left lower eyelid
    H02.146   Spastic ectropion of left eye,
              unspecified eyelid
    H02.149   Spastic ectropion of unspecified eye,
              unspecified eyelid

● H02.2   Lagophthalmos
          Condition in which eye cannot completely close
  ● H02.20   Unspecified lagophthalmos
    H02.201   Unspecified lagophthalmos right
              upper eyelid
    H02.202   Unspecified lagophthalmos right
              lower eyelid
    H02.203   Unspecified lagophthalmos right eye,
              unspecified eyelid
    H02.204   Unspecified lagophthalmos left upper
              eyelid
    H02.205   Unspecified lagophthalmos left lower
              eyelid
    H02.206   Unspecified lagophthalmos left eye,
              unspecified eyelid
    H02.209   Unspecified lagophthalmos
              unspecified eye, unspecified eyelid

  ● H02.21   Cicatricial lagophthalmos
             *Upper or lower eyelid does not close due to scar or
             tightening*
    H02.211   Cicatricial lagophthalmos right upper
              eyelid
    H02.212   Cicatricial lagophthalmos right lower
              eyelid
    H02.213   Cicatricial lagophthalmos right eye,
              unspecified eyelid
    H02.214   Cicatricial lagophthalmos left upper
              eyelid
    H02.215   Cicatricial lagophthalmos left lower
              eyelid
    H02.216   Cicatricial lagophthalmos left eye,
              unspecified eyelid
    H02.219   Cicatricial lagophthalmos unspecified
              eye, unspecified eyelid

● H02.22   Mechanical lagophthalmos
           Inability to close lids due to structural disorder
    H02.221   Mechanical lagophthalmos right
              upper eyelid
    H02.222   Mechanical lagophthalmos right
              lower eyelid
    H02.223   Mechanical lagophthalmos right eye,
              unspecified eyelid
    H02.224   Mechanical lagophthalmos left upper
              eyelid
    H02.225   Mechanical lagophthalmos left lower
              eyelid
    H02.226   Mechanical lagophthalmos left eye,
              unspecified eyelid
    H02.229   Mechanical lagophthalmos
              unspecified eye, unspecified eyelid

● H02.23   Paralytic lagophthalmos
           Eyelids do not close due to paralysis
    H02.231   Paralytic lagophthalmos right upper
              eyelid
    H02.232   Paralytic lagophthalmos right lower
              eyelid
    H02.233   Paralytic lagophthalmos right eye,
              unspecified eyelid
    H02.234   Paralytic lagophthalmos left upper
              eyelid
    H02.235   Paralytic lagophthalmos left lower
              eyelid
    H02.236   Paralytic lagophthalmos left eye,
              unspecified eyelid
    H02.239   Paralytic lagophthalmos unspecified
              eye, unspecified eyelid

(See Plate 81, middle, on page NAP-17.)

● H02.3   Blepharochalasis
          *Relaxation of skin of eyelid, due to atrophy of intercellular
          tissue*
          Pseudoptosis
    H02.30   Blepharochalasis unspecified eye, unspecified
             eyelid
    H02.31   Blepharochalasis right upper eyelid
    H02.32   Blepharochalasis right lower eyelid
    H02.33   Blepharochalasis right eye, unspecified eyelid
    H02.34   Blepharochalasis left upper eyelid
    H02.35   Blepharochalasis left lower eyelid
    H02.36   Blepharochalasis left eye, unspecified eyelid

● H02.4   Ptosis of eyelid
          Falling forward, drooping, sagging of eyelid
  ● H02.40   Unspecified ptosis of eyelid
    H02.401   Unspecified ptosis of right eyelid
    H02.402   Unspecified ptosis of left eyelid
    H02.403   Unspecified ptosis of bilateral eyelids
    H02.409   Unspecified ptosis of unspecified
              eyelid

  ● H02.41   Mechanical ptosis of eyelid
    H02.411   Mechanical ptosis of right eyelid
    H02.412   Mechanical ptosis of left eyelid
    H02.413   Mechanical ptosis of bilateral eyelids
    H02.419   Mechanical ptosis of unspecified
              eyelid

Figure 7-3   Ptosis of eyelid. (From Yanoff:
Ophthalmology, ed 3, Mosby, Inc., 2008)

Item 7-1   Ptosis of eyelid is drooping of the upper eyelid over the pupil when
the eyes are fully opened resulting from nerve or muscle damage, which may
require surgical correction.

◀ New   ◀▥ Revised   ~~deleted~~ Deleted   OGCR Official Guidelines   X Assign placeholder X   ● Use Additional Character(s)

| Excludes 1 | Excludes 2 | Includes | Use additional | Code first | Code also | Unspecified |

● **H02.42**   **Myogenic ptosis of eyelid**
     H02.421   **Myogenic ptosis of right eyelid**
     H02.422   **Myogenic ptosis of left eyelid**
     H02.423   **Myogenic ptosis of bilateral eyelids**
     H02.429   **Myogenic ptosis of unspecified eyelid**

● **H02.43**   **Paralytic ptosis of eyelid**
     Neurogenic ptosis of eyelid
     H02.431   **Paralytic ptosis of right eyelid**
     H02.432   **Paralytic ptosis of left eyelid**
     H02.433   **Paralytic ptosis of bilateral eyelids**
     H02.439   **Paralytic ptosis unspecified eyelid**

● **H02.5**   **Other disorders affecting eyelid function**
     Excludes2   blepharospasm (G24.5)
                organic tic (G25.69)
                psychogenic tic (F95.-)

● **H02.51**   **Abnormal innervation syndrome**
     H02.511   **Abnormal innervation syndrome right upper eyelid**
     H02.512   **Abnormal innervation syndrome right lower eyelid**
     H02.513   **Abnormal innervation syndrome right eye, unspecified eyelid**
     H02.514   **Abnormal innervation syndrome left upper eyelid**
     H02.515   **Abnormal innervation syndrome left lower eyelid**
     H02.516   **Abnormal innervation syndrome left eye, unspecified eyelid**
     H02.519   **Abnormal innervation syndrome unspecified eye, unspecified eyelid**

● **H02.52**   **Blepharophimosis**
     Drooping of eyelid with reduced lid size
     Ankyloblepharon
     H02.521   **Blepharophimosis right upper eyelid**
     H02.522   **Blepharophimosis right lower eyelid**
     H02.523   **Blepharophimosis right eye, unspecified eyelid**
     H02.524   **Blepharophimosis left upper eyelid**
     H02.525   **Blepharophimosis left lower eyelid**
     H02.526   **Blepharophimosis left eye, unspecified eyelid**
     H02.529   **Blepharophimosis unspecified eye, unspecified lid**

● **H02.53**   **Eyelid retraction**
     Eyelid lag
     H02.531   **Eyelid retraction right upper eyelid**
     H02.532   **Eyelid retraction right lower eyelid**
     H02.533   **Eyelid retraction right eye, unspecified eyelid**
     H02.534   **Eyelid retraction left upper eyelid**
     H02.535   **Eyelid retraction left lower eyelid**
     H02.536   **Eyelid retraction left eye, unspecified eyelid**
     H02.539   **Eyelid retraction unspecified eye, unspecified lid**

   H02.59   **Other disorders affecting eyelid function**
     Deficient blink reflex
     Sensory disorders

● **H02.6**   **Xanthelasma of eyelid**
     Yellow-to-orange patches or pimples clustered together on eyelid
     H02.60   **Xanthelasma of unspecified eye, unspecified eyelid**
     H02.61   **Xanthelasma of right upper eyelid**
     H02.62   **Xanthelasma of right lower eyelid**
     H02.63   **Xanthelasma of right eye, unspecified eyelid**
     H02.64   **Xanthelasma of left upper eyelid**
     H02.65   **Xanthelasma of left lower eyelid**
     H02.66   **Xanthelasma of left eye, unspecified eyelid**

● **H02.7**   **Other and unspecified degenerative disorders of eyelid and periocular area**
     H02.70   **Unspecified degenerative disorders of eyelid and periocular area**

● **H02.71**   **Chloasma of eyelid and periocular area**
     Dyspigmentation of eyelid
     Hyperpigmentation of eyelid
     H02.711   **Chloasma of right upper eyelid and periocular area**
     H02.712   **Chloasma of right lower eyelid and periocular area**
     H02.713   **Chloasma of right eye, unspecified eyelid and periocular area**
     H02.714   **Chloasma of left upper eyelid and periocular area**
     H02.715   **Chloasma of left lower eyelid and periocular area**
     H02.716   **Chloasma of left eye, unspecified eyelid and periocular area**
     H02.719   **Chloasma of unspecified eye, unspecified eyelid and periocular area**

● **H02.72**   **Madarosis of eyelid and periocular area**
     Loss of eyelashes and/or eyebrows
     Hypotrichosis of eyelid
     H02.721   **Madarosis of right upper eyelid and periocular area**
     H02.722   **Madarosis of right lower eyelid and periocular area**
     H02.723   **Madarosis of right eye, unspecified eyelid and periocular area**
     H02.724   **Madarosis of left upper eyelid and periocular area**
     H02.725   **Madarosis of left lower eyelid and periocular area**
     H02.726   **Madarosis of left eye, unspecified eyelid and periocular area**
     H02.729   **Madarosis of unspecified eye, unspecified eyelid and periocular area**

● **H02.73**   **Vitiligo of eyelid and periocular area**
     Skin pigmentation disease characterized by white patches
     Hypopigmentation of eyelid
     H02.731   **Vitiligo of right upper eyelid and periocular area**
     H02.732   **Vitiligo of right lower eyelid and periocular area**
     H02.733   **Vitiligo of right eye, unspecified eyelid and periocular area**
     H02.734   **Vitiligo of left upper eyelid and periocular area**
     H02.735   **Vitiligo of left lower eyelid and periocular area**
     H02.736   **Vitiligo of left eye, unspecified eyelid and periocular area**
     H02.739   **Vitiligo of unspecified eye, unspecified eyelid and periocular area**

● **H02.79**   **Other degenerative disorders of eyelid and periocular area**

● **H02.8   Other specified disorders of eyelid**
● **H02.81   Retained foreign body in eyelid**

> Use additional code to identify the type of retained foreign body (Z18.-)

> **Excludes1**   laceration of eyelid with foreign body (S01.12-)
> retained intraocular foreign body (H44.6-, H44.7-)
> superficial foreign body of eyelid and periocular area (S00.25-)

H02.811   Retained foreign body in right upper eyelid

H02.812   Retained foreign body in right lower eyelid

H02.813   Retained foreign body in right eye, unspecified eyelid

H02.814   Retained foreign body in left upper eyelid

H02.815   Retained foreign body in left lower eyelid

H02.816   Retained foreign body in left eye, unspecified eyelid

H02.819   Retained foreign body in unspecified eye, unspecified eyelid

● **H02.82   Cysts of eyelid**
Sebaceous cyst of eyelid

H02.821   Cysts of right upper eyelid

H02.822   Cysts of right lower eyelid

H02.823   Cysts of right eye, unspecified eyelid

H02.824   Cysts of left upper eyelid

H02.825   Cysts of left lower eyelid

H02.826   Cysts of left eye, unspecified eyelid

H02.829   Cysts of unspecified eye, unspecified eyelid

● **H02.83   Dermatochalasis of eyelid**
Skin is inelastic and hangs loosely in folds

H02.831   Dermatochalasis of right upper eyelid

H02.832   Dermatochalasis of right lower eyelid

H02.833   Dermatochalasis of right eye, unspecified eyelid

H02.834   Dermatochalasis of left upper eyelid

H02.835   Dermatochalasis of left lower eyelid

H02.836   Dermatochalasis of left eye, unspecified eyelid

H02.839   Dermatochalasis of unspecified eye, unspecified eyelid

● **H02.84   Edema of eyelid**
Hyperemia of eyelid

H02.841   Edema of right upper eyelid

H02.842   Edema of right lower eyelid

H02.843   Edema of right eye, unspecified eyelid

H02.844   Edema of left upper eyelid

H02.845   Edema of left lower eyelid

H02.846   Edema of left eye, unspecified eyelid

H02.849   Edema of unspecified eye, unspecified eyelid

● **H02.85   Elephantiasis of eyelid**
Massive secondary lymphedema with hypertrophy of skin and subcutaneous tissues (pachyderma)

H02.851   Elephantiasis of right upper eyelid

H02.852   Elephantiasis of right lower eyelid

H02.853   Elephantiasis of right eye, unspecified eyelid

H02.854   Elephantiasis of left upper eyelid

H02.855   Elephantiasis of left lower eyelid

H02.856   Elephantiasis of left eye, unspecified eyelid

H02.859   Elephantiasis of unspecified eye, unspecified eyelid

● **H02.86   Hypertrichosis of eyelid**
Excessive growth of hair

H02.861   Hypertrichosis of right upper eyelid

H02.862   Hypertrichosis of right lower eyelid

H02.863   Hypertrichosis of right eye, unspecified eyelid

H02.864   Hypertrichosis of left upper eyelid

H02.865   Hypertrichosis of left lower eyelid

H02.866   Hypertrichosis of left eye, unspecified eyelid

H02.869   Hypertrichosis of unspecified eye, unspecified eyelid

● **H02.87   Vascular anomalies of eyelid**

H02.871   Vascular anomalies of right upper eyelid

H02.872   Vascular anomalies of right lower eyelid

H02.873   Vascular anomalies of right eye, unspecified eyelid

H02.874   Vascular anomalies of left upper eyelid

H02.875   Vascular anomalies of left lower eyelid

H02.876   Vascular anomalies of left eye, unspecified eyelid

H02.879   Vascular anomalies of unspecified eye, unspecified eyelid

H02.89   Other specified disorders of eyelid
Hemorrhage of eyelid

H02.9   Unspecified disorder of eyelid
Disorder of eyelid NOS

● **H04   Disorders of lacrimal system**

> **Excludes1**   congenital malformations of lacrimal system (Q10.4-Q10.6)

● **H04.0   Dacryoadenitis**
Inflammation of lacrimal gland

● **H04.00   Unspecified dacryoadenitis**

H04.001   Unspecified dacryoadenitis, right lacrimal gland

H04.002   Unspecified dacryoadenitis, left lacrimal gland

H04.003   Unspecified dacryoadenitis, bilateral lacrimal glands

H04.009   Unspecified dacryoadenitis, unspecified lacrimal gland

● **H04.01   Acute dacryoadenitis**

H04.011   Acute dacryoadenitis, right lacrimal gland

H04.012   Acute dacryoadenitis, left lacrimal gland

H04.013   Acute dacryoadenitis, bilateral lacrimal glands

H04.019   Acute dacryoadenitis, unspecified lacrimal gland

Figure 7-4   Lacrimal apparatus. (From Buck CJ: Step-by-Step Medical Coding, Philadelphia, WB Saunders, 2006, p 302)

(See Plate 82 on page NAP-19.)

◀ New   ◀═ Revised   ~~deleted~~ Deleted   **OGCR** Official Guidelines   X Assign placeholder X   ● Use Additional Character(s)

| Excludes 1 | Excludes 2 | Includes | Use additional | Code first | Code also | Unspecified |

● **H04.02**   **Chronic dacryoadenitis**

     H04.021   **Chronic dacryoadenitis, right lacrimal gland**

     H04.022   **Chronic dacryoadenitis, left lacrimal gland**

     H04.023   **Chronic dacryoadenitis, bilateral lacrimal gland**

     H04.029   **Chronic dacryoadenitis, unspecified lacrimal gland**

● **H04.03**   **Chronic enlargement of lacrimal gland**

     H04.031   **Chronic enlargement of right lacrimal gland**

     H04.032   **Chronic enlargement of left lacrimal gland**

     H04.033   **Chronic enlargement of bilateral lacrimal glands**

     H04.039   **Chronic enlargement of unspecified lacrimal gland**

● **H04.1**   **Other disorders of lacrimal gland**

  ● **H04.11**   **Dacryops**

     Watery eye or distention of lacrimal duct due to fluid

     H04.111   **Dacryops of right lacrimal gland**

     H04.112   **Dacryops of left lacrimal gland**

     H04.113   **Dacryops of bilateral lacrimal glands**

     H04.119   **Dacryops of unspecified lacrimal gland**

  ● **H04.12**   **Dry eye syndrome**

     Tear film insufficiency, NOS

     H04.121   **Dry eye syndrome of right lacrimal gland**

     H04.122   **Dry eye syndrome of left lacrimal gland**

     H04.123   **Dry eye syndrome of bilateral lacrimal glands**

     H04.129   **Dry eye syndrome of unspecified lacrimal gland**

  ● **H04.13**   **Lacrimal cyst**

     Lacrimal cystic degeneration

     H04.131   **Lacrimal cyst right lacrimal gland**

     H04.132   **Lacrimal cyst left lacrimal gland**

     H04.133   **Lacrimal cyst bilateral lacrimal glands**

     H04.139   **Lacrimal cyst unspecified lacrimal gland**

  ● **H04.14**   **Primary lacrimal gland atrophy**

     H04.141   **Primary lacrimal gland atrophy, right lacrimal gland**

     H04.142   **Primary lacrimal gland atrophy, left lacrimal gland**

     H04.143   **Primary lacrimal gland atrophy, bilateral lacrimal glands**

     H04.149   **Primary lacrimal gland atrophy, unspecified lacrimal gland**

  ● **H04.15**   **Secondary lacrimal gland atrophy**

     H04.151   **Secondary lacrimal gland atrophy, right lacrimal gland**

     H04.152   **Secondary lacrimal gland atrophy, left lacrimal gland**

     H04.153   **Secondary lacrimal gland atrophy, bilateral lacrimal glands**

     H04.159   **Secondary lacrimal gland atrophy, unspecified lacrimal gland**

  ● **H04.16**   **Lacrimal gland dislocation**

     H04.161   **Lacrimal gland dislocation, right lacrimal gland**

     H04.162   **Lacrimal gland dislocation, left lacrimal gland**

     H04.163   **Lacrimal gland dislocation, bilateral lacrimal glands**

     H04.169   **Lacrimal gland dislocation, unspecified lacrimal gland**

   H04.19   **Other specified disorders of lacrimal gland**

● **H04.2**   **Epiphora**

     Overflow of tears due to stricture of lacrimal passages; AKA lacrimation

  ● **H04.20**   **Unspecified epiphora**

     H04.201   **Unspecified epiphora, right lacrimal gland**

     H04.202   **Unspecified epiphora, left lacrimal gland**

     H04.203   **Unspecified epiphora, bilateral lacrimal glands**

     H04.209   **Unspecified epiphora, unspecified lacrimal gland**

  ● **H04.21**   **Epiphora due to excess lacrimation**

     H04.211   **Epiphora due to excess lacrimation, right lacrimal gland**

     H04.212   **Epiphora due to excess lacrimation, left lacrimal gland**

     H04.213   **Epiphora due to excess lacrimation, bilateral lacrimal glands**

     H04.219   **Epiphora due to excess lacrimation, unspecified lacrimal gland**

  ● **H04.22**   **Epiphora due to insufficient drainage**

     H04.221   **Epiphora due to insufficient drainage, right lacrimal gland**

     H04.222   **Epiphora due to insufficient drainage, left lacrimal gland**

     H04.223   **Epiphora due to insufficient drainage, bilateral lacrimal glands**

     H04.229   **Epiphora due to insufficient drainage, unspecified lacrimal gland**

● **H04.3**   **Acute and unspecified inflammation of lacrimal passages**

     Excludes1   neonatal dacryocystitis (P39.1)

  ● **H04.30**   **Unspecified dacryocystitis**

     H04.301   **Unspecified dacryocystitis of right lacrimal passage**

     H04.302   **Unspecified dacryocystitis of left lacrimal passage**

     H04.303   **Unspecified dacryocystitis of bilateral lacrimal passages**

     H04.309   **Unspecified dacryocystitis of unspecified lacrimal passage**

  ● **H04.31**   **Phlegmonous dacryocystitis**

     Cellulitis of lacrimal sac

     H04.311   **Phlegmonous dacryocystitis of right lacrimal passage**

     H04.312   **Phlegmonous dacryocystitis of left lacrimal passage**

     H04.313   **Phlegmonous dacryocystitis of bilateral lacrimal passages**

     H04.319   **Phlegmonous dacryocystitis of unspecified lacrimal passage**

  ● **H04.32**   **Acute dacryocystitis**

     Acute dacryopericystitis

     H04.321   **Acute dacryocystitis of right lacrimal passage**

     H04.322   **Acute dacryocystitis of left lacrimal passage**

     H04.323   **Acute dacryocystitis of bilateral lacrimal passages**

     H04.329   **Acute dacryocystitis of unspecified lacrimal passage**

● **H04.33   Acute lacrimal canaliculitis**
  H04.331   Acute lacrimal canaliculitis of right lacrimal passage
  H04.332   Acute lacrimal canaliculitis of left lacrimal passage
  H04.333   Acute lacrimal canaliculitis of bilateral lacrimal passages
  H04.339   Acute lacrimal canaliculitis of unspecified lacrimal passage
● **H04.4   Chronic inflammation of lacrimal passages**
  ● **H04.41   Chronic dacryocystitis**
    Inflammation of lacrimal sac
    H04.411   Chronic dacryocystitis of right lacrimal passage
    H04.412   Chronic dacryocystitis of left lacrimal passage
    H04.413   Chronic dacryocystitis of bilateral lacrimal passages
    H04.419   Chronic dacryocystitis of unspecified lacrimal passage
  ● **H04.42   Chronic lacrimal canaliculitis**
    Inflammation of lacrimal ducts
    H04.421   Chronic lacrimal canaliculitis of right lacrimal passage
    H04.422   Chronic lacrimal canaliculitis of left lacrimal passage
    H04.423   Chronic lacrimal canaliculitis of bilateral lacrimal passages
    H04.429   Chronic lacrimal canaliculitis of unspecified lacrimal passage
  ● **H04.43   Chronic lacrimal mucocele**
    Accumulation of mucous secretion
    H04.431   Chronic lacrimal mucocele of right lacrimal passage
    H04.432   Chronic lacrimal mucocele of left lacrimal passage
    H04.433   Chronic lacrimal mucocele of bilateral lacrimal passages
    H04.439   Chronic lacrimal mucocele of unspecified lacrimal passage
● **H04.5   Stenosis and insufficiency of lacrimal passages**
  ● **H04.51   Dacryolith**
    Concretion in lacrimal sac/duct; AKA lacrimal calculus
    H04.511   Dacryolith of right lacrimal passage
    H04.512   Dacryolith of left lacrimal passage
    H04.513   Dacryolith of bilateral lacrimal passages
    H04.519   Dacryolith of unspecified lacrimal passage
  ● **H04.52   Eversion of lacrimal punctum**
    Turning out of lacrimal drainage opening
    H04.521   Eversion of right lacrimal punctum
    H04.522   Eversion of left lacrimal punctum
    H04.523   Eversion of bilateral lacrimal punctum
    H04.529   Eversion of unspecified lacrimal punctum
  ● **H04.53   Neonatal obstruction of nasolacrimal duct**
    Excludes1   congenital stenosis and stricture of lacrimal duct (Q10.5)
    H04.531   Neonatal obstruction of right nasolacrimal duct
    H04.532   Neonatal obstruction of left nasolacrimal duct
    H04.533   Neonatal obstruction of bilateral nasolacrimal duct
    H04.539   Neonatal obstruction of unspecified nasolacrimal duct

● **H04.54   Stenosis of lacrimal canaliculi**
  H04.541   Stenosis of right lacrimal canaliculi
  H04.542   Stenosis of left lacrimal canaliculi
  H04.543   Stenosis of bilateral lacrimal canaliculi
  H04.549   Stenosis of unspecified lacrimal canaliculi
● **H04.55   Acquired stenosis of nasolacrimal duct**
  H04.551   Acquired stenosis of right nasolacrimal duct
  H04.552   Acquired stenosis of left nasolacrimal duct
  H04.553   Acquired stenosis of bilateral nasolacrimal duct
  H04.559   Acquired stenosis of unspecified nasolacrimal duct
● **H04.56   Stenosis of lacrimal punctum**
  H04.561   Stenosis of right lacrimal punctum
  H04.562   Stenosis of left lacrimal punctum
  H04.563   Stenosis of bilateral lacrimal punctum
  H04.569   Stenosis of unspecified lacrimal punctum
● **H04.57   Stenosis of lacrimal sac**
  H04.571   Stenosis of right lacrimal sac
  H04.572   Stenosis of left lacrimal sac
  H04.573   Stenosis of bilateral lacrimal sac
  H04.579   Stenosis of unspecified lacrimal sac
● **H04.6   Other changes of lacrimal passages**
  ● **H04.61   Lacrimal fistula**
    H04.611   Lacrimal fistula right lacrimal passage
    H04.612   Lacrimal fistula left lacrimal passage
    H04.613   Lacrimal fistula bilateral lacrimal passages
    H04.619   Lacrimal fistula unspecified lacrimal passage
  H04.69   Other changes of lacrimal passages
● **H04.8   Other disorders of lacrimal system**
  ● **H04.81   Granuloma of lacrimal passages**
    Inflammatory response due to infectious or noninfectious agents
    H04.811   Granuloma of right lacrimal passage
    H04.812   Granuloma of left lacrimal passage
    H04.813   Granuloma of bilateral lacrimal passages
    H04.819   Granuloma of unspecified lacrimal passage
  H04.89   Other disorders of lacrimal system
  H04.9   Disorder of lacrimal system, unspecified
● **H05   Disorders of orbit**
  Excludes1   congenital malformation of orbit (Q10.7)
  ● **H05.0   Acute inflammation of orbit**
    H05.00   Unspecified acute inflammation of orbit
    ● **H05.01   Cellulitis of orbit**
      Infection of soft tissue of orbit
      Abscess of orbit
      H05.011   Cellulitis of right orbit
      H05.012   Cellulitis of left orbit
      H05.013   Cellulitis of bilateral orbits
      H05.019   Cellulitis of unspecified orbit
    ● **H05.02   Osteomyelitis of orbit**
      Infection of boney orbit of eye
      H05.021   Osteomyelitis of right orbit
      H05.022   Osteomyelitis of left orbit
      H05.023   Osteomyelitis of bilateral orbits
      H05.029   Osteomyelitis of unspecified orbit

CHAPTER 7 (H00-H59)

◀ New   ◀▥ Revised   d̶e̶l̶e̶t̶e̶d̶ Deleted   OGCR Official Guidelines   X Assign placeholder X   ● Use Additional Character(s)
Excludes 1 | Excludes 2 | Includes | Use additional | Code first | Code also | Unspecified
861

CHAPTER 7 (H00-H59)

● **H05.03   Periostitis of orbit**
     Inflammation of periosteum (membrane covering bone surface)
    H05.031   Periostitis of right orbit
    H05.032   Periostitis of left orbit
    H05.033   Periostitis of bilateral orbits
    H05.039   Periostitis of unspecified orbit

● **H05.04   Tenonitis of orbit**
     Inflammation of tenon capsule (space enclosing fascia of Tenon between eyeball and fat of orbit)
    H05.041   Tenonitis of right orbit
    H05.042   Tenonitis of left orbit
    H05.043   Tenonitis of bilateral orbits
    H05.049   Tenonitis of unspecified orbit

● **H05.1   Chronic inflammatory disorders of orbit**
    H05.10   Unspecified chronic inflammatory disorders of orbit

● **H05.11   Granuloma of orbit**
     Pseudotumor (inflammatory) of orbit
    H05.111   Granuloma of right orbit
    H05.112   Granuloma of left orbit
    H05.113   Granuloma of bilateral orbits
    H05.119   Granuloma of unspecified orbit

● **H05.12   Orbital myositis**
     Inflammation of extraocular muscles of orbit
    H05.121   Orbital myositis, right orbit
    H05.122   Orbital myositis, left orbit
    H05.123   Orbital myositis, bilateral
    H05.129   Orbital myositis, unspecified orbit

● **H05.2   Exophthalmic conditions**
     Bulging eyes
    H05.20   Unspecified exophthalmos

● **H05.21   Displacement (lateral) of globe**
    H05.211   Displacement (lateral) of globe, right eye
    H05.212   Displacement (lateral) of globe, left eye
    H05.213   Displacement (lateral) of globe, bilateral
    H05.219   Displacement (lateral) of globe, unspecified eye

● **H05.22   Edema of orbit**
     Orbital congestion
    H05.221   Edema of right orbit
    H05.222   Edema of left orbit
    H05.223   Edema of bilateral orbit
    H05.229   Edema of unspecified orbit

● **H05.23   Hemorrhage of orbit**
    H05.231   Hemorrhage of right orbit
    H05.232   Hemorrhage of left orbit
    H05.233   Hemorrhage of bilateral orbit
    H05.239   Hemorrhage of unspecified orbit

● **H05.24   Constant exophthalmos**
     Constant bulging eyes, often symptom of Graves disease
    H05.241   Constant exophthalmos, right eye
    H05.242   Constant exophthalmos, left eye
    H05.243   Constant exophthalmos, bilateral
    H05.249   Constant exophthalmos, unspecified eye

● **H05.25   Intermittent exophthalmos**
     Intermittent bulging eye occurring with bending forward or sharp turning of head
    H05.251   Intermittent exophthalmos, right eye
    H05.252   Intermittent exophthalmos, left eye
    H05.253   Intermittent exophthalmos, bilateral
    H05.259   Intermittent exophthalmos, unspecified eye

● **H05.26   Pulsating exophthalmos**
     Bulging eyes with pulsation and bruit, often due to aneurysm pushing eye forward
    H05.261   Pulsating exophthalmos, right eye
    H05.262   Pulsating exophthalmos, left eye
    H05.263   Pulsating exophthalmos, bilateral
    H05.269   Pulsating exophthalmos, unspecified eye

● **H05.3   Deformity of orbit**
    Excludes1   congenital deformity of orbit (Q10.7)
             hypertelorism (Q75.2)
    H05.30   Unspecified deformity of orbit

● **H05.31   Atrophy of orbit**
    H05.311   Atrophy of right orbit
    H05.312   Atrophy of left orbit
    H05.313   Atrophy of bilateral orbit
    H05.319   Atrophy of unspecified orbit

● **H05.32   Deformity of orbit due to bone disease**
    Code also associated bone disease
    H05.321   Deformity of right orbit due to bone disease
    H05.322   Deformity of left orbit due to bone disease
    H05.323   Deformity of bilateral orbits due to bone disease
    H05.329   Deformity of unspecified orbit due to bone disease

● **H05.33   Deformity of orbit due to trauma or surgery**
    H05.331   Deformity of right orbit due to trauma or surgery
    H05.332   Deformity of left orbit due to trauma or surgery
    H05.333   Deformity of bilateral orbits due to trauma or surgery
    H05.339   Deformity of unspecified orbit due to trauma or surgery

● **H05.34   Enlargement of orbit**
    H05.341   Enlargement of right orbit
    H05.342   Enlargement of left orbit
    H05.343   Enlargement of bilateral orbits
    H05.349   Enlargement of unspecified orbit

● **H05.35   Exostosis of orbit**
    H05.351   Exostosis of right orbit
    H05.352   Exostosis of left orbit
    H05.353   Exostosis of bilateral orbits
    H05.359   Exostosis of unspecified orbit

● **H05.4   Enophthalmos**
     Recessed eyeball into orbit

● **H05.40   Unspecified enophthalmos**
    H05.401   Unspecified enophthalmos, right eye
    H05.402   Unspecified enophthalmos, left eye
    H05.403   Unspecified enophthalmos, bilateral
    H05.409   Unspecified enophthalmos, unspecified eye

◀ New   ◀▥ Revised   ~~deleted~~ Deleted   **OGCR** Official Guidelines   X Assign placeholder X   ● Use Additional Character(s)

Excludes 1   Excludes 2   Includes   Use additional   Code first   Code also   Unspecified

● H05.41   Enophthalmos due to atrophy of orbital tissue
    H05.411   Enophthalmos due to atrophy of orbital tissue, right eye
    H05.412   Enophthalmos due to atrophy of orbital tissue, left eye
    H05.413   Enophthalmos due to atrophy of orbital tissue, bilateral
    H05.419   Enophthalmos due to atrophy of orbital tissue, unspecified eye

● H05.42   Enophthalmos due to trauma or surgery
    H05.421   Enophthalmos due to trauma or surgery, right eye
    H05.422   Enophthalmos due to trauma or surgery, left eye
    H05.423   Enophthalmos due to trauma or surgery, bilateral
    H05.429   Enophthalmos due to trauma or surgery, unspecified eye

● H05.5   Retained (old) foreign body following penetrating wound of orbit
    Retrobulbar foreign body
    Use additional code to identify the type of retained foreign body (Z18.-)
    Excludes1   current penetrating wound of orbit (S05.4-)
    Excludes2   retained foreign body of eyelid (H02.81-) retained intraocular foreign body (H44.6-, H44.7-)
    H05.50   Retained (old) foreign body following penetrating wound of unspecified orbit
    H05.51   Retained (old) foreign body following penetrating wound of right orbit
    H05.52   Retained (old) foreign body following penetrating wound of left orbit
    H05.53   Retained (old) foreign body following penetrating wound of bilateral orbits

● H05.8   Other disorders of orbit
   ● H05.81   Cyst of orbit
    Encephalocele of orbit
    H05.811   Cyst of right orbit
    H05.812   Cyst of left orbit
    H05.813   Cyst of bilateral orbits
    H05.819   Cyst of unspecified orbit
   ● H05.82   Myopathy of extraocular muscles
    Weakness of muscles of eye
    H05.821   Myopathy of extraocular muscles, right orbit
    H05.822   Myopathy of extraocular muscles, left orbit
    H05.823   Myopathy of extraocular muscles, bilateral
    H05.829   Myopathy of extraocular muscles, unspecified orbit
   H05.89   Other disorders of orbit
● H05.9   Unspecified disorder of orbit

DISORDERS OF CONJUNCTIVA (H10-H11)

(See Plate 81, upper, on page NAP-17.)

● H10   Conjunctivitis
    Inflammation of membrane of the inside of the eyelid or on surface of eye (conjunctiva)
    Excludes1   keratoconjunctivitis (H16.2-)

● H10.0   Mucopurulent conjunctivitis
   ● H10.01   Acute follicular conjunctivitis
    H10.011   Acute follicular conjunctivitis, right eye
    H10.012   Acute follicular conjunctivitis, left eye
    H10.013   Acute follicular conjunctivitis, bilateral
    H10.019   Acute follicular conjunctivitis, unspecified eye
   ● H10.02   Other mucopurulent conjunctivitis
    H10.021   Other mucopurulent conjunctivitis, right eye
    H10.022   Other mucopurulent conjunctivitis, left eye
    H10.023   Other mucopurulent conjunctivitis, bilateral
    H10.029   Other mucopurulent conjunctivitis, unspecified eye

● H10.1   Acute atopic conjunctivitis
    Acute papillary conjunctivitis
    H10.10   Acute atopic conjunctivitis, unspecified eye
    H10.11   Acute atopic conjunctivitis, right eye
    H10.12   Acute atopic conjunctivitis, left eye
    H10.13   Acute atopic conjunctivitis, bilateral

● H10.2   Other acute conjunctivitis
   ● H10.21   Acute toxic conjunctivitis
    Acute chemical conjunctivitis
    Code first (T51-T65) to identify chemical and intent
    Excludes1   burn and corrosion of eye and adnexa (T26.-)
    H10.211   Acute toxic conjunctivitis, right eye
    H10.212   Acute toxic conjunctivitis, left eye
    H10.213   Acute toxic conjunctivitis, bilateral
    H10.219   Acute toxic conjunctivitis, unspecified eye
   ● H10.22   Pseudomembranous conjunctivitis
    H10.221   Pseudomembranous conjunctivitis, right eye
    H10.222   Pseudomembranous conjunctivitis, left eye
    H10.223   Pseudomembranous conjunctivitis, bilateral
    H10.229   Pseudomembranous conjunctivitis, unspecified eye
   ● H10.23   Serous conjunctivitis, except viral
    Excludes1   viral conjunctivitis (B30.-)
    H10.231   Serous conjunctivitis, except viral, right eye
    H10.232   Serous conjunctivitis, except viral, left eye
    H10.233   Serous conjunctivitis, except viral, bilateral
    H10.239   Serous conjunctivitis, except viral, unspecified eye

CHAPTER 7 (H00-H59)

- H10.3　Unspecified acute conjunctivitis
  - **Excludes1**　ophthalmia neonatorum NOS (P39.1)
  - H10.30　Unspecified acute conjunctivitis, unspecified eye
  - H10.31　Unspecified acute conjunctivitis, right eye
  - H10.32　Unspecified acute conjunctivitis, left eye
  - H10.33　Unspecified acute conjunctivitis, bilateral
- H10.4　Chronic conjunctivitis
  - H10.40　Unspecified chronic conjunctivitis
    - H10.401　Unspecified chronic conjunctivitis, right eye
    - H10.402　Unspecified chronic conjunctivitis, left eye
    - H10.403　Unspecified chronic conjunctivitis, bilateral
    - H10.409　Unspecified chronic conjunctivitis, unspecified eye
  - H10.41　Chronic giant papillary conjunctivitis
    - *Inflammation of membrane of the inside of the eyelid or on surface of eye often associated with contact lens wear*
    - H10.411　Chronic giant papillary conjunctivitis, right eye
    - H10.412　Chronic giant papillary conjunctivitis, left eye
    - H10.413　Chronic giant papillary conjunctivitis, bilateral
    - H10.419　Chronic giant papillary conjunctivitis, unspecified eye
  - H10.42　Simple chronic conjunctivitis
    - H10.421　Simple chronic conjunctivitis, right eye
    - H10.422　Simple chronic conjunctivitis, left eye
    - H10.423　Simple chronic conjunctivitis, bilateral
    - H10.429　Simple chronic conjunctivitis, unspecified eye
  - H10.43　Chronic follicular conjunctivitis
    - *Inflammation of membrane of the inside of the eyelid or on surface of eye due to topical medications or infection*
    - H10.431　Chronic follicular conjunctivitis, right eye
    - H10.432　Chronic follicular conjunctivitis, left eye
    - H10.433　Chronic follicular conjunctivitis, bilateral
    - H10.439　Chronic follicular conjunctivitis, unspecified eye
  - H10.44　Vernal conjunctivitis
    - *Affecting children, especially boys in which there are flattened papules with thick, gelatinous exudate on conjunctivae on inside of upper lid*
    - **Excludes1**　vernal keratoconjunctivitis with limbar and corneal involvement (H16.26-)
  - H10.45　Other chronic allergic conjunctivitis
- H10.5　Blepharoconjunctivitis
  - *Inflammation of eyelids and conjunctiva*
  - H10.50　Unspecified blepharoconjunctivitis
    - H10.501　Unspecified blepharoconjunctivitis, right eye
    - H10.502　Unspecified blepharoconjunctivitis, left eye
    - H10.503　Unspecified blepharoconjunctivitis, bilateral
    - H10.509　Unspecified blepharoconjunctivitis, unspecified eye

- H10.51　Ligneous conjunctivitis
  - H10.511　Ligneous conjunctivitis, right eye
  - H10.512　Ligneous conjunctivitis, left eye
  - H10.513　Ligneous conjunctivitis, bilateral
  - H10.519　Ligneous conjunctivitis, unspecified eye
- H10.52　Angular blepharoconjunctivitis
  - H10.521　Angular blepharoconjunctivitis, right eye
  - H10.522　Angular blepharoconjunctivitis, left eye
  - H10.523　Angular blepharoconjunctivitis, bilateral
  - H10.529　Angular blepharoconjunctivitis, unspecified eye
- H10.53　Contact blepharoconjunctivitis
  - H10.531　Contact blepharoconjunctivitis, right eye
  - H10.532　Contact blepharoconjunctivitis, left eye
  - H10.533　Contact blepharoconjunctivitis, bilateral
  - H10.539　Contact blepharoconjunctivitis, unspecified eye
- H10.8　Other conjunctivitis
  - H10.81　Pingueculitis
    - *Inflammation of a yellow, raised thickening on the white of the eye associated with chronic dry eyes*
    - **Excludes1**　pinguecula (H11.15-)
    - H10.811　Pingueculitis, right eye
    - H10.812　Pingueculitis, left eye
    - H10.813　Pingueculitis, bilateral
    - H10.819　Pingueculitis, unspecified eye
  - H10.89　Other conjunctivitis
- H10.9　Unspecified conjunctivitis

- H11　Other disorders of conjunctiva
  - **Excludes1**　keratoconjunctivitis (H16.2-)
  - H11.0　Pterygium of eye
    - **Excludes1**　pseudopterygium (H11.81-)
    - H11.00　Unspecified pterygium of eye
      - H11.001　Unspecified pterygium of right eye
      - H11.002　Unspecified pterygium of left eye
      - H11.003　Unspecified pterygium of eye, bilateral
      - H11.009　Unspecified pterygium of unspecified eye
    - H11.01　Amyloid pterygium
      - H11.011　Amyloid pterygium of right eye
      - H11.012　Amyloid pterygium of left eye
      - H11.013　Amyloid pterygium of eye, bilateral
      - H11.019　Amyloid pterygium of unspecified eye

Figure 7-5　Double pterygium. Note both nasal and temporal pterygia in a 57-year-old farmer. (From Yanoff: Ophthalmology, ed 3, Mosby, Inc., 2008)

Item 7–2　Pterygium is Greek for batlike. The condition is characterized by a membrane that extends from the limbus to the center of the cornea and resembles a wing.

● H11.02   Central pterygium of eye
    H11.021   Central pterygium of right eye
    H11.022   Central pterygium of left eye
    H11.023   Central pterygium of eye, bilateral
    H11.029   Central pterygium of unspecified eye

● H11.03   Double pterygium of eye
    H11.031   Double pterygium of right eye
    H11.032   Double pterygium of left eye
    H11.033   Double pterygium of eye, bilateral
    H11.039   Double pterygium of unspecified eye

● H11.04   Peripheral pterygium of eye, stationary
    H11.041   Peripheral pterygium, stationary, right eye
    H11.042   Peripheral pterygium, stationary, left eye
    H11.043   Peripheral pterygium, stationary, bilateral
    H11.049   Peripheral pterygium, stationary, unspecified eye

● H11.05   Peripheral pterygium of eye, progressive
    H11.051   Peripheral pterygium, progressive, right eye
    H11.052   Peripheral pterygium, progressive, left eye
    H11.053   Peripheral pterygium, progressive, bilateral
    H11.059   Peripheral pterygium, progressive, unspecified eye

● H11.06   Recurrent pterygium of eye
    H11.061   Recurrent pterygium of right eye
    H11.062   Recurrent pterygium of left eye
    H11.063   Recurrent pterygium of eye, bilateral
    H11.069   Recurrent pterygium of unspecified eye

● H11.1   Conjunctival degenerations and deposits
    Excludes2   pseudopterygium (H11.81)
    H11.10   Unspecified conjunctival degenerations

● H11.11   Conjunctival deposits
    H11.111   Conjunctival deposits, right eye
    H11.112   Conjunctival deposits, left eye
    H11.113   Conjunctival deposits, bilateral
    H11.119   Conjunctival deposits, unspecified eye

● H11.12   Conjunctival concretions
    White to yellow nodules within or beneath conjunctiva
    H11.121   Conjunctival concretions, right eye
    H11.122   Conjunctival concretions, left eye
    H11.123   Conjunctival concretions, bilateral
    H11.129   Conjunctival concretions, unspecified eye

● H11.13   Conjunctival pigmentations
    Conjunctival argyrosis [argyria]
    H11.131   Conjunctival pigmentations, right eye
    H11.132   Conjunctival pigmentations, left eye
    H11.133   Conjunctival pigmentations, bilateral
    H11.139   Conjunctival pigmentations, unspecified eye

● H11.14   Conjunctival xerosis, unspecified
    Excludes1   xerosis of conjunctiva due to vitamin A deficiency (E50.0, E50.1)
    H11.141   Conjunctival xerosis, unspecified, right eye
    H11.142   Conjunctival xerosis, unspecified, left eye
    H11.143   Conjunctival xerosis, unspecified, bilateral
    H11.149   Conjunctival xerosis, unspecified, unspecified eye

● H11.15   Pinguecula
    Yellowish spot near sclerocorneal junction, usually on nasal side; associated with aging
    Excludes1   pingueculitis (H10.81-)
    H11.151   Pinguecula, right eye
    H11.152   Pinguecula, left eye
    H11.153   Pinguecula, bilateral
    H11.159   Pinguecula, unspecified eye

● H11.2   Conjunctival scars
  ● H11.21   Conjunctival adhesions and strands (localized)
    H11.211   Conjunctival adhesions and strands (localized), right eye
    H11.212   Conjunctival adhesions and strands (localized), left eye
    H11.213   Conjunctival adhesions and strands (localized), bilateral
    H11.219   Conjunctival adhesions and strands (localized), unspecified eye

  ● H11.22   Conjunctival granuloma
    H11.221   Conjunctival granuloma, right eye
    H11.222   Conjunctival granuloma, left eye
    H11.223   Conjunctival granuloma, bilateral
    H11.229   Conjunctival granuloma, unspecified

  ● H11.23   Symblepharon
    Adhesion between tarsal conjunctiva and bulbar conjunctiva
    H11.231   Symblepharon, right eye
    H11.232   Symblepharon, left eye
    H11.233   Symblepharon, bilateral
    H11.239   Symblepharon, unspecified eye

  ● H11.24   Scarring of conjunctiva
    H11.241   Scarring of conjunctiva, right eye
    H11.242   Scarring of conjunctiva, left eye
    H11.243   Scarring of conjunctiva, bilateral
    H11.249   Scarring of conjunctiva, unspecified eye

● H11.3   Conjunctival hemorrhage
    Subconjunctival hemorrhage
    H11.30   Conjunctival hemorrhage, unspecified eye
    H11.31   Conjunctival hemorrhage, right eye
    H11.32   Conjunctival hemorrhage, left eye
    H11.33   Conjunctival hemorrhage, bilateral

● H11.4   Other conjunctival vascular disorders and cysts
  ● H11.41   Vascular abnormalities of conjunctiva
    Conjunctival aneurysm
    H11.411   Vascular abnormalities of conjunctiva, right eye
    H11.412   Vascular abnormalities of conjunctiva, left eye
    H11.413   Vascular abnormalities of conjunctiva, bilateral
    H11.419   Vascular abnormalities of conjunctiva, unspecified eye

CHAPTER 7 (H00-H59)

● **H11.42 Conjunctival edema**
  H11.421 Conjunctival edema, right eye
  H11.422 Conjunctival edema, left eye
  H11.423 Conjunctival edema, bilateral
  H11.429 Conjunctival edema, unspecified eye
● **H11.43 Conjunctival hyperemia**
  H11.431 Conjunctival hyperemia, right eye
  H11.432 Conjunctival hyperemia, left eye
  H11.433 Conjunctival hyperemia, bilateral
  H11.439 Conjunctival hyperemia, unspecified eye
● **H11.44 Conjunctival cysts**
  H11.441 Conjunctival cysts, right eye
  H11.442 Conjunctival cysts, left eye
  H11.443 Conjunctival cysts, bilateral
  H11.449 Conjunctival cysts, unspecified eye
● **H11.8 Other specified disorders of conjunctiva**
  ● **H11.81 Pseudopterygium of conjunctiva**
    Conjunctival scar attached to cornea
    H11.811 Pseudopterygium of conjunctiva, right eye
    H11.812 Pseudopterygium of conjunctiva, left eye
    H11.813 Pseudopterygium of conjunctiva, bilateral
    H11.819 Pseudopterygium of conjunctiva, unspecified eye
  ● **H11.82 Conjunctivochalasis**
    Conjunctiva bulges over eyelid margin or covers lower punctum
    H11.821 Conjunctivochalasis, right eye
    H11.822 Conjunctivochalasis, left eye
    H11.823 Conjunctivochalasis, bilateral
    H11.829 Conjunctivochalasis, unspecified eye
  H11.89 Other specified disorders of conjunctiva
● H11.9 Unspecified disorder of conjunctiva

DISORDERS OF SCLERA, CORNEA, IRIS AND CILIARY BODY (H15-H22)

● **H15 Disorders of sclera**
  ● **H15.0 Scleritis**
    Inflammation of the white (sclera and episclera) of the eye.
    ● **H15.00 Unspecified scleritis**
      H15.001 Unspecified scleritis, right eye
      H15.002 Unspecified scleritis, left eye
      H15.003 Unspecified scleritis, bilateral
      H15.009 Unspecified scleritis, unspecified eye
    ● **H15.01 Anterior scleritis**
      H15.011 Anterior scleritis, right eye
      H15.012 Anterior scleritis, left eye
      H15.013 Anterior scleritis, bilateral
      H15.019 Anterior scleritis, unspecified eye
    ● **H15.02 Brawny scleritis**
      Swelling around the cornea that is gelantinous in appearance
      H15.021 Brawny scleritis, right eye
      H15.022 Brawny scleritis, left eye
      H15.023 Brawny scleritis, bilateral
      H15.029 Brawny scleritis, unspecified eye
    ● **H15.03 Posterior scleritis**
      Sclerotenonitis
      H15.031 Posterior scleritis, right eye
      H15.032 Posterior scleritis, left eye
      H15.033 Posterior scleritis, bilateral
      H15.039 Posterior scleritis, unspecified eye

● **H15.04 Scleritis with corneal involvement**
  H15.041 Scleritis with corneal involvement, right eye
  H15.042 Scleritis with corneal involvement, left eye
  H15.043 Scleritis with corneal involvement, bilateral
  H15.049 Scleritis with corneal involvement, unspecified eye
● **H15.05 Scleromalacia perforans**
  Necrotic without inflammation; usually associated with rheumatoid arthritis
  H15.051 Scleromalacia perforans, right eye
  H15.052 Scleromalacia perforans, left eye
  H15.053 Scleromalacia perforans, bilateral
  H15.059 Scleromalacia perforans, unspecified eye
● **H15.09 Other scleritis**
  Scleral abscess
  H15.091 Other scleritis, right eye
  H15.092 Other scleritis, left eye
  H15.093 Other scleritis, bilateral
  H15.099 Other scleritis, unspecified eye
● **H15.1 Episcleritis**
  Inflammation of the white (sclera and episclera) of the eye.
  ● **H15.10 Unspecified episcleritis**
    H15.101 Unspecified episcleritis, right eye
    H15.102 Unspecified episcleritis, left eye
    H15.103 Unspecified episcleritis, bilateral
    H15.109 Unspecified episcleritis, unspecified eye
  ● **H15.11 Episcleritis periodica fugax**
    Transient, recurrent inflammation of portion of episclera (connective tissue on the surface of the sclera)
    H15.111 Episcleritis periodica fugax, right eye
    H15.112 Episcleritis periodica fugax, left eye
    H15.113 Episcleritis periodica fugax, bilateral
    H15.119 Episcleritis periodica fugax, unspecified eye
  ● **H15.12 Nodular episcleritis**
    Characterized by tender, localized, moveable nodule within inflamed area
    H15.121 Nodular episcleritis, right eye
    H15.122 Nodular episcleritis, left eye
    H15.123 Nodular episcleritis, bilateral
    H15.129 Nodular episcleritis, unspecified eye
● **H15.8 Other disorders of sclera**
  Excludes2 blue sclera (Q13.5)
             degenerative myopia (H44.2-)
  ● **H15.81 Equatorial staphyloma**
    H15.811 Equatorial staphyloma, right eye
    H15.812 Equatorial staphyloma, left eye
    H15.813 Equatorial staphyloma, bilateral
    H15.819 Equatorial staphyloma, unspecified eye
  ● **H15.82 Localized anterior staphyloma**
    H15.821 Localized anterior staphyloma, right eye
    H15.822 Localized anterior staphyloma, left eye
    H15.823 Localized anterior staphyloma, bilateral
    H15.829 Localized anterior staphyloma, unspecified eye

● H15.83   Staphyloma posticum
    H15.831   Staphyloma posticum, right eye
    H15.832   Staphyloma posticum, left eye
    H15.833   Staphyloma posticum, bilateral
    H15.839   Staphyloma posticum, unspecified eye
● H15.84   Scleral ectasia
    H15.841   Scleral ectasia, right eye
    H15.842   Scleral ectasia, left eye
    H15.843   Scleral ectasia, bilateral
    H15.849   Scleral ectasia, unspecified eye
● H15.85   Ring staphyloma
    H15.851   Ring staphyloma, right eye
    H15.852   Ring staphyloma, left eye
    H15.853   Ring staphyloma, bilateral
    H15.859   Ring staphyloma, unspecified eye
H15.89   Other disorders of sclera
H15.9   Unspecified disorder of sclera

● H16   Keratitis
● H16.0   Corneal ulcer
   ● H16.00   Unspecified corneal ulcer
    H16.001   Unspecified corneal ulcer, right eye
    H16.002   Unspecified corneal ulcer, left eye
    H16.003   Unspecified corneal ulcer, bilateral
    H16.009   Unspecified corneal ulcer, unspecified eye
   ● H16.01   Central corneal ulcer
    H16.011   Central corneal ulcer, right eye
    H16.012   Central corneal ulcer, left eye
    H16.013   Central corneal ulcer, bilateral
    H16.019   Central corneal ulcer, unspecified eye
   ● H16.02   Ring corneal ulcer
    H16.021   Ring corneal ulcer, right eye
    H16.022   Ring corneal ulcer, left eye
    H16.023   Ring corneal ulcer, bilateral
    H16.029   Ring corneal ulcer, unspecified eye
   ● H16.03   Corneal ulcer with hypopyon
    H16.031   Corneal ulcer with hypopyon, right eye
    H16.032   Corneal ulcer with hypopyon, left eye
    H16.033   Corneal ulcer with hypopyon, bilateral
    H16.039   Corneal ulcer with hypopyon, unspecified eye

Marginal   Ring   Central   Rosacea   Mooren's
(catarrhal) ulcer   ulcer   corneal ulcer   ulcer   (rodent) ulcer

Figure 7-6   Corneal ulcers: marginal, ring, central corneal, rosacea, and Mooren's.

Item 7–3   An infected ulcer is usually called a **serpiginous** or **hypopyon** ulcer which is a pus sac in the anterior chamber of the eye. **Marginal** ulcers are usually asymptomatic, not primary, and are often superficial and simple. More severe marginal ulcers spread to form a ring ulcer. **Ring** ulcers can extend around the entire corneal periphery. **Central corneal** ulcers develop when there is an abrasion to the epithelium and an infection develops in the eroded area. The **pyocyaneal** ulcer is the most serious corneal infection, which, if left untreated, can lead to loss of the eye.

● H16.04   Marginal corneal ulcer
    H16.041   Marginal corneal ulcer, right eye
    H16.042   Marginal corneal ulcer, left eye
    H16.043   Marginal corneal ulcer, bilateral
    H16.049   Marginal corneal ulcer, unspecified eye
● H16.05   Mooren's corneal ulcer
    H16.051   Mooren's corneal ulcer, right eye
    H16.052   Mooren's corneal ulcer, left eye
    H16.053   Mooren's corneal ulcer, bilateral
    H16.059   Mooren's corneal ulcer, unspecified eye
● H16.06   Mycotic corneal ulcer
    H16.061   Mycotic corneal ulcer, right eye
    H16.062   Mycotic corneal ulcer, left eye
    H16.063   Mycotic corneal ulcer, bilateral
    H16.069   Mycotic corneal ulcer, unspecified eye
● H16.07   Perforated corneal ulcer
    H16.071   Perforated corneal ulcer, right eye
    H16.072   Perforated corneal ulcer, left eye
    H16.073   Perforated corneal ulcer, bilateral
    H16.079   Perforated corneal ulcer, unspecified eye
● H16.1   Other and unspecified superficial keratitis without conjunctivitis
   ● H16.10   Unspecified superficial keratitis
    H16.101   Unspecified superficial keratitis, right eye
    H16.102   Unspecified superficial keratitis, left eye
    H16.103   Unspecified superficial keratitis, bilateral
    H16.109   Unspecified superficial keratitis, unspecified eye
   ● H16.11   Macular keratitis
      Areolar keratitis
      Nummular keratitis
      Stellate keratitis
      Striate keratitis
    H16.111   Macular keratitis, right eye
    H16.112   Macular keratitis, left eye
    H16.113   Macular keratitis, bilateral
    H16.119   Macular keratitis, unspecified eye
   ● H16.12   Filamentary keratitis
    H16.121   Filamentary keratitis, right eye
    H16.122   Filamentary keratitis, left eye
    H16.123   Filamentary keratitis, bilateral
    H16.129   Filamentary keratitis, unspecified eye
   ● H16.13   Photokeratitis
      Snow blindness
      Welders' keratitis
    H16.131   Photokeratitis, right eye
    H16.132   Photokeratitis, left eye
    H16.133   Photokeratitis, bilateral
    H16.139   Photokeratitis, unspecified eye
   ● H16.14   Punctate keratitis
    H16.141   Punctate keratitis, right eye
    H16.142   Punctate keratitis, left eye
    H16.143   Punctate keratitis, bilateral
    H16.149   Punctate keratitis, unspecified eye

◀ New   ◀▥ Revised   ~~deleted~~ Deleted   **OGCR** Official Guidelines   X Assign placeholder X   ● Use Additional Character(s)

Excludes 1   Excludes 2   Includes   Use additional   Code first   Code also   Unspecified

CHAPTER 7 (H00-H59)

● **H16.2   Keratoconjunctivitis**
  ● **H16.20   Unspecified keratoconjunctivitis**
      Superficial keratitis with conjunctivitis NOS
      H16.201   Unspecified keratoconjunctivitis, right eye
      H16.202   Unspecified keratoconjunctivitis, left eye
      H16.203   Unspecified keratoconjunctivitis, bilateral
      H16.209   Unspecified keratoconjunctivitis, unspecified eye

  ● **H16.21   Exposure keratoconjunctivitis**
      H16.211   Exposure keratoconjunctivitis, right eye
      H16.212   Exposure keratoconjunctivitis, left eye
      H16.213   Exposure keratoconjunctivitis, bilateral
      H16.219   Exposure keratoconjunctivitis, unspecified eye

  ● **H16.22   Keratoconjunctivitis sicca, not specified as Sjögren's**
      | Excludes1 | Sjogren's syndrome (M35.01)
      H16.221   Keratoconjunctivitis sicca, not specified as Sjögren's, right eye
      H16.222   Keratoconjunctivitis sicca, not specified as Sjögren's, left eye
      H16.223   Keratoconjunctivitis sicca, not specified as Sjögren's, bilateral
      H16.229   Keratoconjunctivitis sicca, not specified as Sjögren's, unspecified eye

  ● **H16.23   Neurotrophic keratoconjunctivitis**
      H16.231   Neurotrophic keratoconjunctivitis, right eye
      H16.232   Neurotrophic keratoconjunctivitis, left eye
      H16.233   Neurotrophic keratoconjunctivitis, bilateral
      H16.239   Neurotrophic keratoconjunctivitis, unspecified eye

  ● **H16.24   Ophthalmia nodosa**
      H16.241   Ophthalmia nodosa, right eye
      H16.242   Ophthalmia nodosa, left eye
      H16.243   Ophthalmia nodosa, bilateral
      H16.249   Ophthalmia nodosa, unspecified eye

  ● **H16.25   Phlyctenular keratoconjunctivitis**
      H16.251   Phlyctenular keratoconjunctivitis, right eye
      H16.252   Phlyctenular keratoconjunctivitis, left eye
      H16.253   Phlyctenular keratoconjunctivitis, bilateral
      H16.259   Phlyctenular keratoconjunctivitis, unspecified eye

  ● **H16.26   Vernal keratoconjunctivitis, with limbar and corneal involvement**
      | Excludes1 | vernal conjunctivitis without limbar and corneal involvement (H10.44)
      H16.261   Vernal keratoconjunctivitis, with limbar and corneal involvement, right eye
      H16.262   Vernal keratoconjunctivitis, with limbar and corneal involvement, left eye

      H16.263   Vernal keratoconjunctivitis, with limbar and corneal involvement, bilateral
      H16.269   Vernal keratoconjunctivitis, with limbar and corneal involvement, unspecified eye

  ● **H16.29   Other keratoconjunctivitis**
      H16.291   Other keratoconjunctivitis, right eye
      H16.292   Other keratoconjunctivitis, left eye
      H16.293   Other keratoconjunctivitis, bilateral
      H16.299   Other keratoconjunctivitis, unspecified eye

● **H16.3   Interstitial and deep keratitis**
  ● **H16.30   Unspecified interstitial keratitis**
      H16.301   Unspecified interstitial keratitis, right eye
      H16.302   Unspecified interstitial keratitis, left eye
      H16.303   Unspecified interstitial keratitis, bilateral
      H16.309   Unspecified interstitial keratitis, unspecified eye

  ● **H16.31   Corneal abscess**
      H16.311   Corneal abscess, right eye
      H16.312   Corneal abscess, left eye
      H16.313   Corneal abscess, bilateral
      H16.319   Corneal abscess, unspecified eye

  ● **H16.32   Diffuse interstitial keratitis**
      Cogan's syndrome
      H16.321   Diffuse interstitial keratitis, right eye
      H16.322   Diffuse interstitial keratitis, left eye
      H16.323   Diffuse interstitial keratitis, bilateral
      H16.329   Diffuse interstitial keratitis, unspecified eye

  ● **H16.33   Sclerosing keratitis**
      H16.331   Sclerosing keratitis, right eye
      H16.332   Sclerosing keratitis, left eye
      H16.333   Sclerosing keratitis, bilateral
      H16.339   Sclerosing keratitis, unspecified eye

  ● **H16.39   Other interstitial and deep keratitis**
      H16.391   Other interstitial and deep keratitis, right eye
      H16.392   Other interstitial and deep keratitis, left eye
      H16.393   Other interstitial and deep keratitis, bilateral
      H16.399   Other interstitial and deep keratitis, unspecified eye

● **H16.4   Corneal neovascularization**
  ● **H16.40   Unspecified corneal neovascularization**
      H16.401   Unspecified corneal neovascularization, right eye
      H16.402   Unspecified corneal neovascularization, left eye
      H16.403   Unspecified corneal neovascularization, bilateral
      H16.409   Unspecified corneal neovascularization, unspecified eye

  ● **H16.41   Ghost vessels (corneal)**
      H16.411   Ghost vessels (corneal), right eye
      H16.412   Ghost vessels (corneal), left eye
      H16.413   Ghost vessels (corneal), bilateral
      H16.419   Ghost vessels (corneal), unspecified eye

◀ New   ◀▥ Revised   ~~deleted~~ Deleted   **OGCR** Official Guidelines   X Assign placeholder X   ● Use Additional Character(s)

| Excludes 1 | | Excludes 2 | Includes   Use additional   Code first   Code also   Unspecified

● **H16.42 Pannus (corneal)**
    H16.421 Pannus (corneal), right eye
    H16.422 Pannus (corneal), left eye
    H16.423 Pannus (corneal), bilateral
    H16.429 Pannus (corneal), unspecified eye
● **H16.43 Localized vascularization of cornea**
    H16.431 Localized vascularization of cornea, right eye
    H16.432 Localized vascularization of cornea, left eye
    H16.433 Localized vascularization of cornea, bilateral
    H16.439 Localized vascularization of cornea, unspecified eye
● **H16.44 Deep vascularization of cornea**
    H16.441 Deep vascularization of cornea, right eye
    H16.442 Deep vascularization of cornea, left eye
    H16.443 Deep vascularization of cornea, bilateral
    H16.449 Deep vascularization of cornea, unspecified eye

  H16.8 Other keratitis
  H16.9 Unspecified keratitis

● **H17 Corneal scars and opacities**
  ● **H17.0 Adherent leukoma**
    H17.00 Adherent leukoma, unspecified eye
    H17.01 Adherent leukoma, right eye
    H17.02 Adherent leukoma, left eye
    H17.03 Adherent leukoma, bilateral
  ● **H17.1 Central corneal opacity**
    H17.10 Central corneal opacity, unspecified eye
    H17.11 Central corneal opacity, right eye
    H17.12 Central corneal opacity, left eye
    H17.13 Central corneal opacity, bilateral
  ● **H17.8 Other corneal scars and opacities**
    ● **H17.81 Minor opacity of cornea**
       Corneal nebula
      H17.811 Minor opacity of cornea, right eye
      H17.812 Minor opacity of cornea, left eye
      H17.813 Minor opacity of cornea, bilateral
      H17.819 Minor opacity of cornea, unspecified eye
    ● **H17.82 Peripheral opacity of cornea**
      H17.821 Peripheral opacity of cornea, right eye
      H17.822 Peripheral opacity of cornea, left eye
      H17.823 Peripheral opacity of cornea, bilateral
      H17.829 Peripheral opacity of cornea, unspecified eye
    H17.89 Other corneal scars and opacities
  H17.9 Unspecified corneal scar and opacity

● **H18 Other disorders of cornea**
  ● **H18.0 Corneal pigmentations and deposits**
    ● **H18.00 Unspecified corneal deposit**
      H18.001 Unspecified corneal deposit, right eye
      H18.002 Unspecified corneal deposit, left eye
      H18.003 Unspecified corneal deposit, bilateral
      H18.009 Unspecified corneal deposit, unspecified eye
    ● **H18.01 Anterior corneal pigmentations**
      Staehli's line
      H18.011 Anterior corneal pigmentations, right eye
      H18.012 Anterior corneal pigmentations, left eye

      H18.013 Anterior corneal pigmentations, bilateral
      H18.019 Anterior corneal pigmentations, unspecified eye
    ● **H18.02 Argentous corneal deposits**
      H18.021 Argentous corneal deposits, right eye
      H18.022 Argentous corneal deposits, left eye
      H18.023 Argentous corneal deposits, bilateral
      H18.029 Argentous corneal deposits, unspecified eye
    ● **H18.03 Corneal deposits in metabolic disorders**
      Code also associated metabolic disorder
      H18.031 Corneal deposits in metabolic disorders, right eye
      H18.032 Corneal deposits in metabolic disorders, left eye
      H18.033 Corneal deposits in metabolic disorders, bilateral
      H18.039 Corneal deposits in metabolic disorders, unspecified eye
    ● **H18.04 Kayser-Fleischer ring**
      Code also associated Wilson's disease (E83.01)
      H18.041 Kayser-Fleischer ring, right eye
      H18.042 Kayser-Fleischer ring, left eye
      H18.043 Kayser-Fleischer ring, bilateral
      H18.049 Kayser-Fleischer ring, unspecified eye
    ● **H18.05 Posterior corneal pigmentations**
      Krukenberg's spindle
      H18.051 Posterior corneal pigmentations, right eye
      H18.052 Posterior corneal pigmentations, left eye
      H18.053 Posterior corneal pigmentations, bilateral
      H18.059 Posterior corneal pigmentations, unspecified eye
    ● **H18.06 Stromal corneal pigmentations**
      Hematocornea
      H18.061 Stromal corneal pigmentations, right eye
      H18.062 Stromal corneal pigmentations, left eye
      H18.063 Stromal corneal pigmentations, bilateral
      H18.069 Stromal corneal pigmentations, unspecified eye
  ● **H18.1 Bullous keratopathy**
    H18.10 Bullous keratopathy, unspecified eye
    H18.11 Bullous keratopathy, right eye
    H18.12 Bullous keratopathy, left eye
    H18.13 Bullous keratopathy, bilateral
  ● **H18.2 Other and unspecified corneal edema**
    H18.20 Unspecified corneal edema
    ● **H18.21 Corneal edema secondary to contact lens**
      Excludes2 other corneal disorders due to contact lens (H18.82-)
      H18.211 Corneal edema secondary to contact lens, right eye
      H18.212 Corneal edema secondary to contact lens, left eye
      H18.213 Corneal edema secondary to contact lens, bilateral
      H18.219 Corneal edema secondary to contact lens, unspecified eye

CHAPTER 7 (H00-H59)

CHAPTER 7 (H00-H59)

● H18.22   Idiopathic corneal edema
    H18.221   Idiopathic corneal edema, right eye
    H18.222   Idiopathic corneal edema, left eye
    H18.223   Idiopathic corneal edema, bilateral
    H18.229   Idiopathic corneal edema, unspecified eye
● H18.23   Secondary corneal edema
    H18.231   Secondary corneal edema, right eye
    H18.232   Secondary corneal edema, left eye
    H18.233   Secondary corneal edema, bilateral
    H18.239   Secondary corneal edema, unspecified eye
● H18.3   Changes of corneal membranes
    H18.30   Unspecified corneal membrane change
● H18.31   Folds and rupture in Bowman's membrane
    H18.311   Folds and rupture in Bowman's membrane, right eye
    H18.312   Folds and rupture in Bowman's membrane, left eye
    H18.313   Folds and rupture in Bowman's membrane, bilateral
    H18.319   Folds and rupture in Bowman's membrane, unspecified eye
● H18.32   Folds in Descemet's membrane
    H18.321   Folds in Descemet's membrane, right eye
    H18.322   Folds in Descemet's membrane, left eye
    H18.323   Folds in Descemet's membrane, bilateral
    H18.329   Folds in Descemet's membrane, unspecified eye
● H18.33   Rupture in Descemet's membrane
    H18.331   Rupture in Descemet's membrane, right eye
    H18.332   Rupture in Descemet's membrane, left eye
    H18.333   Rupture in Descemet's membrane, bilateral
    H18.339   Rupture in Descemet's membrane, unspecified eye
● H18.4   Corneal degeneration
    Excludes1   Mooren's ulcer (H16.0-)
       recurrent erosion of cornea (H18.83-)
    H18.40   Unspecified corneal degeneration
● H18.41   Arcus senilis
     Senile corneal changes
    H18.411   Arcus senilis, right eye
    H18.412   Arcus senilis, left eye
    H18.413   Arcus senilis, bilateral
    H18.419   Arcus senilis, unspecified eye
● H18.42   Band keratopathy
    H18.421   Band keratopathy, right eye
    H18.422   Band keratopathy, left eye
    H18.423   Band keratopathy, bilateral
    H18.429   Band keratopathy, unspecified eye
    H18.43   Other calcerous corneal degeneration
● H18.44   Keratomalacia
    Excludes1   keratomalacia due to vitamin A deficiency (E50.4)
    H18.441   Keratomalacia, right eye
    H18.442   Keratomalacia, left eye
    H18.443   Keratomalacia, bilateral
    H18.449   Keratomalacia, unspecified eye

● H18.45   Nodular corneal degeneration
    H18.451   Nodular corneal degeneration, right eye
    H18.452   Nodular corneal degeneration, left eye
    H18.453   Nodular corneal degeneration, bilateral
    H18.459   Nodular corneal degeneration, unspecified eye
● H18.46   Peripheral corneal degeneration
    H18.461   Peripheral corneal degeneration, right eye
    H18.462   Peripheral corneal degeneration, left eye
    H18.463   Peripheral corneal degeneration, bilateral
    H18.469   Peripheral corneal degeneration, unspecified eye
    H18.49   Other corneal degeneration
● H18.5   Hereditary corneal dystrophies
    H18.50   Unspecified hereditary corneal dystrophies
    H18.51   Endothelial corneal dystrophy
     Fuchs' dystrophy
    H18.52   Epithelial (juvenile) corneal dystrophy
    H18.53   Granular corneal dystrophy
    H18.54   Lattice corneal dystrophy
    H18.55   Macular corneal dystrophy
    H18.59   Other hereditary corneal dystrophies
● H18.6   Keratoconus
● H18.60   Keratoconus, unspecified
    H18.601   Keratoconus, unspecified, right eye
    H18.602   Keratoconus, unspecified, left eye
    H18.603   Keratoconus, unspecified, bilateral
    H18.609   Keratoconus, unspecified, unspecified eye
● H18.61   Keratoconus, stable
    H18.611   Keratoconus, stable, right eye
    H18.612   Keratoconus, stable, left eye
    H18.613   Keratoconus, stable, bilateral
    H18.619   Keratoconus, stable, unspecified eye
● H18.62   Keratoconus, unstable
     Acute hydrops
    H18.621   Keratoconus, unstable, right eye
    H18.622   Keratoconus, unstable, left eye
    H18.623   Keratoconus, unstable, bilateral
    H18.629   Keratoconus, unstable, unspecified eye

Figure 7-7 Lateral view of the displacement of the cone apex in keratoconus. (From Yanoff: Ophthalmology, ed 3, Mosby, Inc., 2008)

Item 7-4 Keratoconus results in corneal degeneration that begins in childhood, gradually changes the cornea from a round to cone shape, decreasing visual acuity. Treatment includes contact lenses. In severe cases the need for corneal transplant may be the treatment of choice; however, newer technologies may use high frequency radio energy to shrink the edges of the cornea, pulling the central area back to a more normal shape. It can help delay or avoid the need for a corneal transplantation.

◄ New   ◄▥ Revised   ~~deleted~~ Deleted   **OGCR** Official Guidelines   X Assign placeholder X   ● Use Additional Character(s)

Excludes 1   Excludes 2   Includes   Use additional   Code first   Code also   Unspecified

● **H18.7   Other and unspecified corneal deformities**

       Excludes1   congenital malformations of cornea (Q13.3-Q13.4)

     H18.70   Unspecified corneal deformity

● H18.71   Corneal ectasia

       H18.711   Corneal ectasia, right eye

       H18.712   Corneal ectasia, left eye

       H18.713   Corneal ectasia, bilateral

       H18.719   Corneal ectasia, unspecified eye

● H18.72   Corneal staphyloma

       H18.721   Corneal staphyloma, right eye

       H18.722   Corneal staphyloma, left eye

       H18.723   Corneal staphyloma, bilateral

       H18.729   Corneal staphyloma, unspecified eye

● H18.73   Descemetocele

       H18.731   Descemetocele, right eye

       H18.732   Descemetocele, left eye

       H18.733   Descemetocele, bilateral

       H18.739   Descemetocele, unspecified eye

● H18.79   Other corneal deformities

       H18.791   Other corneal deformities, right eye

       H18.792   Other corneal deformities, left eye

       H18.793   Other corneal deformities, bilateral

       H18.799   Other corneal deformities, unspecified eye

● **H18.8   Other specified disorders of cornea**

● H18.81   Anesthesia and hypoesthesia of cornea

       H18.811   Anesthesia and hypoesthesia of cornea, right eye

       H18.812   Anesthesia and hypoesthesia of cornea, left eye

       H18.813   Anesthesia and hypoesthesia of cornea, bilateral

       H18.819   Anesthesia and hypoesthesia of cornea, unspecified eye

● H18.82   Corneal disorder due to contact lens

       Excludes2   corneal edema due to contact lens (H18.21-)

       H18.821   Corneal disorder due to contact lens, right eye

       H18.822   Corneal disorder due to contact lens, left eye

       H18.823   Corneal disorder due to contact lens, bilateral

       H18.829   Corneal disorder due to contact lens, unspecified eye

● H18.83   Recurrent erosion of cornea

       H18.831   Recurrent erosion of cornea, right eye

       H18.832   Recurrent erosion of cornea, left eye

       H18.833   Recurrent erosion of cornea, bilateral

       H18.839   Recurrent erosion of cornea, unspecified eye

● H18.89   Other specified disorders of cornea

       H18.891   Other specified disorders of cornea, right eye

       H18.892   Other specified disorders of cornea, left eye

       H18.893   Other specified disorders of cornea, bilateral

       H18.899   Other specified disorders of cornea, unspecified eye

H18.9   Unspecified disorder of cornea

● **H20   Iridocyclitis**

● **H20.0   Acute and subacute iridocyclitis**

     Acute anterior uveitis

     Acute cyclitis

     Acute iritis

     Subacute anterior uveitis

     Subacute cyclitis

     Subacute iritis

      Excludes1   iridocyclitis, iritis, uveitis (due to) (in) diabetes mellitus (E08-E13 with .39)

              iridocyclitis, iritis, uveitis (due to) (in) diphtheria (A36.89)

              iridocyclitis, iritis, uveitis (due to) (in) gonococcal (A54.32)

              iridocyclitis, iritis, uveitis (due to) (in) herpes (simplex) (B00.51)

              iridocyclitis, iritis, uveitis (due to) (in) herpes zoster (B02.32)

              iridocyclitis, iritis, uveitis (due to) (in) late congenital syphilis (A50.39)

              iridocyclitis, iritis, uveitis (due to) (in) late syphilis (A52.71)

              iridocyclitis, iritis, uveitis (due to) (in) sarcoidosis (D86.83)

              iridocyclitis, iritis, uveitis (due to) (in) syphilis (A51.43)

              iridocyclitis, iritis, uveitis (due to) (in) toxoplasmosis (B58.09)

              iridocyclitis, iritis, uveitis (due to) (in) tuberculosis (A18.54)

     H20.00   Unspecified acute and subacute iridocyclitis

● H20.01   Primary iridocyclitis

       H20.011   Primary iridocyclitis, right eye

       H20.012   Primary iridocyclitis, left eye

       H20.013   Primary iridocyclitis, bilateral

       H20.019   Primary iridocyclitis, unspecified eye

● H20.02   Recurrent acute iridocyclitis

       H20.021   Recurrent acute iridocyclitis, right eye

       H20.022   Recurrent acute iridocyclitis, left eye

       H20.023   Recurrent acute iridocyclitis, bilateral

       H20.029   Recurrent acute iridocyclitis, unspecified eye

● H20.03   Secondary infectious iridocyclitis

       H20.031   Secondary infectious iridocyclitis, right eye

       H20.032   Secondary infectious iridocyclitis, left eye

       H20.033   Secondary infectious iridocyclitis, bilateral

       H20.039   Secondary infectious iridocyclitis, unspecified eye

● H20.04   Secondary noninfectious iridocyclitis

       H20.041   Secondary noninfectious iridocyclitis, right eye

       H20.042   Secondary noninfectious iridocyclitis, left eye

       H20.043   Secondary noninfectious iridocyclitis, bilateral

       H20.049   Secondary noninfectious iridocyclitis, unspecified eye

● H20.05   Hypopyon

       H20.051   Hypopyon, right eye

       H20.052   Hypopyon, left eye

       H20.053   Hypopyon, bilateral

       H20.059   Hypopyon, unspecified eye

CHAPTER 7 (H00-H59)

● **H20.1   Chronic iridocyclitis**
> Use additional code for any associated cataract (H26.21-)
> | **Excludes2** | posterior cyclitis (H30.2-) |
> H20.10   Chronic iridocyclitis, unspecified eye
> H20.11   Chronic iridocyclitis, right eye
> H20.12   Chronic iridocyclitis, left eye
> H20.13   Chronic iridocyclitis, bilateral

● **H20.2   Lens-induced iridocyclitis**
> H20.20   Lens-induced iridocyclitis, unspecified eye
> H20.21   Lens-induced iridocyclitis, right eye
> H20.22   Lens-induced iridocyclitis, left eye
> H20.23   Lens-induced iridocyclitis, bilateral

● **H20.8   Other iridocyclitis**
> | **Excludes2** | glaucomatocyclitis crises (H40.4-) |
> | | posterior cyclitis (H30.2-) |
> | | sympathetic uveitis (H44.13-) |
>
> ● **H20.81   Fuchs' heterochromic cyclitis**
> > H20.811   Fuchs' heterochromic cyclitis, right eye
> > H20.812   Fuchs' heterochromic cyclitis, left eye
> > H20.813   Fuchs' heterochromic cyclitis, bilateral
> > H20.819   Fuchs' heterochromic cyclitis, unspecified eye
>
> ● **H20.82   Vogt-Koyanagi syndrome**
> > H20.821   Vogt-Koyanagi syndrome, right eye
> > H20.822   Vogt-Koyanagi syndrome, left eye
> > H20.823   Vogt-Koyanagi syndrome, bilateral
> > H20.829   Vogt-Koyanagi syndrome, unspecified eye

H20.9   Unspecified iridocyclitis
> Uveitis NOS

● **H21   Other disorders of iris and ciliary body**
> | **Excludes2** | sympathetic uveitis (H44.1-) |
>
> ● **H21.0   Hyphema**
> > | **Excludes1** | traumatic hyphema (S05.1-) |
> > H21.00   Hyphema, unspecified eye
> > H21.01   Hyphema, right eye
> > H21.02   Hyphema, left eye
> > H21.03   Hyphema, bilateral
>
> ● **H21.1   Other vascular disorders of iris and ciliary body**
> > Neovascularization of iris or ciliary body
> > Rubeosis iridis
> > Rubeosis of iris
> >
> > ● **H21.1X   Other vascular disorders of iris and ciliary body**
> > > H21.1X1   Other vascular disorders of iris and ciliary body, right eye
> > > H21.1X2   Other vascular disorders of iris and ciliary body, left eye
> > > H21.1X3   Other vascular disorders of iris and ciliary body, bilateral
> > > H21.1X9   Other vascular disorders of iris and ciliary body, unspecified eye
>
> ● **H21.2   Degeneration of iris and ciliary body**
> > ● **H21.21   Degeneration of chamber angle**
> > > H21.211   Degeneration of chamber angle, right eye
> > > H21.212   Degeneration of chamber angle, left eye
> > > H21.213   Degeneration of chamber angle, bilateral
> > > H21.219   Degeneration of chamber angle, unspecified eye

● **H21.22   Degeneration of ciliary body**
> H21.221   Degeneration of ciliary body, right eye
> H21.222   Degeneration of ciliary body, left eye
> H21.223   Degeneration of ciliary body, bilateral
> H21.229   Degeneration of ciliary body, unspecified eye

● **H21.23   Degeneration of iris (pigmentary)**
> Translucency of iris
> H21.231   Degeneration of iris (pigmentary), right eye
> H21.232   Degeneration of iris (pigmentary), left eye
> H21.233   Degeneration of iris (pigmentary), bilateral
> H21.239   Degeneration of iris (pigmentary), unspecified eye

● **H21.24   Degeneration of pupillary margin**
> H21.241   Degeneration of pupillary margin, right eye
> H21.242   Degeneration of pupillary margin, left eye
> H21.243   Degeneration of pupillary margin, bilateral
> H21.249   Degeneration of pupillary margin, unspecified eye

● **H21.25   Iridoschisis**
> H21.251   Iridoschisis, right eye
> H21.252   Iridoschisis, left eye
> H21.253   Iridoschisis, bilateral
> H21.259   Iridoschisis, unspecified eye

● **H21.26   Iris atrophy (essential) (progressive)**
> H21.261   Iris atrophy (essential) (progressive), right eye
> H21.262   Iris atrophy (essential) (progressive), left eye
> H21.263   Iris atrophy (essential) (progressive), bilateral
> H21.269   Iris atrophy (essential) (progressive), unspecified eye

● **H21.27   Miotic pupillary cyst**
> H21.271   Miotic pupillary cyst, right eye
> H21.272   Miotic pupillary cyst, left eye
> H21.273   Miotic pupillary cyst, bilateral
> H21.279   Miotic pupillary cyst, unspecified eye

H21.29   Other iris atrophy

● **H21.3   Cyst of iris, ciliary body and anterior chamber**
> | **Excludes2** | miotic pupillary cyst (H21.27-) |
>
> ● **H21.30   Idiopathic cysts of iris, ciliary body or anterior chamber**
> > Cyst of iris, ciliary body or anterior chamber NOS
> > H21.301   Idiopathic cysts of iris, ciliary body or anterior chamber, right eye
> > H21.302   Idiopathic cysts of iris, ciliary body or anterior chamber, left eye
> > H21.303   Idiopathic cysts of iris, ciliary body or anterior chamber, bilateral
> > H21.309   Idiopathic cysts of iris, ciliary body or anterior chamber, unspecified eye
>
> ● **H21.31   Exudative cysts of iris or anterior chamber**
> > H21.311   Exudative cysts of iris or anterior chamber, right eye
> > H21.312   Exudative cysts of iris or anterior chamber, left eye
> > H21.313   Exudative cysts of iris or anterior chamber, bilateral
> > H21.319   Exudative cysts of iris or anterior chamber, unspecified eye

CHAPTER 7 (H00-H59)

◀ New   ◀▥ Revised   ~~deleted~~ Deleted   OGCR Official Guidelines   X Assign placeholder X   ● Use Additional Character(s)

 Excludes 1   Excludes 2   Includes   Use additional   Code first   Code also   Unspecified

● H21.32　Implantation cysts of iris, ciliary body or anterior chamber
　　　H21.321　Implantation cysts of iris, ciliary body or anterior chamber, right eye
　　　H21.322　Implantation cysts of iris, ciliary body or anterior chamber, left eye
　　　H21.323　Implantation cysts of iris, ciliary body or anterior chamber, bilateral
　　　H21.329　Implantation cysts of iris, ciliary body or anterior chamber, unspecified eye
● H21.33　Parasitic cyst of iris, ciliary body or anterior chamber
　　　H21.331　Parasitic cyst of iris, ciliary body or anterior chamber, right eye
　　　H21.332　Parasitic cyst of iris, ciliary body or anterior chamber, left eye
　　　H21.333　Parasitic cyst of iris, ciliary body or anterior chamber, bilateral
　　　H21.339　Parasitic cyst of iris, ciliary body or anterior chamber, unspecified eye
● H21.34　Primary cyst of pars plana
　　　H21.341　Primary cyst of pars plana, right eye
　　　H21.342　Primary cyst of pars plana, left eye
　　　H21.343　Primary cyst of pars plana, bilateral
　　　H21.349　Primary cyst of pars plana, unspecified eye
● H21.35　Exudative cyst of pars plana
　　　H21.351　Exudative cyst of pars plana, right eye
　　　H21.352　Exudative cyst of pars plana, left eye
　　　H21.353　Exudative cyst of pars plana, bilateral
　　　H21.359　Exudative cyst of pars plana, unspecified eye
● H21.4　Pupillary membranes
　　　Iris bombé
　　　Pupillary occlusion
　　　Pupillary seclusion
　　　Excludes1　congenital pupillary membranes (Q13.8)
　　　H21.40　Pupillary membranes, unspecified eye
　　　H21.41　Pupillary membranes, right eye
　　　H21.42　Pupillary membranes, left eye
　　　H21.43　Pupillary membranes, bilateral
● H21.5　Other and unspecified adhesions and disruptions of iris and ciliary body
　　　Excludes1　corectopia (Q13.2)
　● H21.50　Unspecified adhesions of iris
　　　　Synechia (iris) NOS
　　　H21.501　Unspecified adhesions of iris, right eye
　　　H21.502　Unspecified adhesions of iris, left eye
　　　H21.503　Unspecified adhesions of iris, bilateral
　　　H21.509　Unspecified adhesions of iris and ciliary body, unspecified eye
　● H21.51　Anterior synechiae (iris)
　　　H21.511　Anterior synechiae (iris), right eye
　　　H21.512　Anterior synechiae (iris), left eye
　　　H21.513　Anterior synechiae (iris), bilateral
　　　H21.519　Anterior synechiae (iris), unspecified eye
　● H21.52　Goniosynechiae
　　　H21.521　Goniosynechiae, right eye
　　　H21.522　Goniosynechiae, left eye
　　　H21.523　Goniosynechiae, bilateral
　　　H21.529　Goniosynechiae, unspecified eye
　● H21.53　Iridodialysis
　　　H21.531　Iridodialysis, right eye
　　　H21.532　Iridodialysis, left eye

　　　H21.533　Iridodialysis, bilateral
　　　H21.539　Iridodialysis, unspecified eye
● H21.54　Posterior synechiae (iris)
　　　H21.541　Posterior synechiae (iris), right eye
　　　H21.542　Posterior synechiae (iris), left eye
　　　H21.543　Posterior synechiae (iris), bilateral
　　　H21.549　Posterior synechiae (iris), unspecified eye
● H21.55　Recession of chamber angle
　　　H21.551　Recession of chamber angle, right eye
　　　H21.552　Recession of chamber angle, left eye
　　　H21.553　Recession of chamber angle, bilateral
　　　H21.559　Recession of chamber angle, unspecified eye
● H21.56　Pupillary abnormalities
　　　Deformed pupil
　　　Ectopic pupil
　　　Rupture of sphincter, pupil
　　　Excludes1　congenital deformity of pupil (Q13.2-)
　　　H21.561　Pupillary abnormality, right eye
　　　H21.562　Pupillary abnormality, left eye
　　　H21.563　Pupillary abnormality, bilateral
　　　H21.569　Pupillary abnormality, unspecified eye
● H21.8　Other specified disorders of iris and ciliary body
　　　H21.81　Floppy iris syndrome
　　　　Intraoperative floppy iris syndrome (IFIS)
　　　　Use additional code for adverse effect, if applicable, to identify drug (T36-T50 with fifth or sixth character 5)
　　　H21.82　Plateau iris syndrome (post-iridectomy) (postprocedural)
　　　H21.89　Other specified disorders of iris and ciliary body
　H21.9　Unspecified disorder of iris and ciliary body

H22　Disorders of iris and ciliary body in diseases classified elsewhere
　　　Code first underlying disease, such as:
　　　gout (M1A.-, M10.-)
　　　leprosy (A30.-)
　　　parasitic disease (B89)

DISORDERS OF LENS (H25-H28)

● H25　Age-related cataract
　　　Senile cataract
　　　Excludes2　capsular glaucoma with pseudoexfoliation of lens (H40.1-)
　● H25.0　Age-related incipient cataract
　● H25.01　Cortical age-related cataract
　　　H25.011　Cortical age-related cataract, right eye
　　　H25.012　Cortical age-related cataract, left eye
　　　H25.013　Cortical age-related cataract, bilateral
　　　H25.019　Cortical age-related cataract, unspecified eye
　● H25.03　Anterior subcapsular polar age-related cataract
　　　H25.031　Anterior subcapsular polar age-related cataract, right eye
　　　H25.032　Anterior subcapsular polar age-related cataract, left eye
　　　H25.033　Anterior subcapsular polar age-related cataract, bilateral
　　　H25.039　Anterior subcapsular polar age-related cataract, unspecified eye

CHAPTER 7 (H00-H59)

Figure 7-8   Age-related cataract.
Nuclear sclerosis and cortical lens opacities
are present. (From Yanoff: Ophthalmology,
ed 3, Mosby, Inc., 2008)

Item 7–5 **Senile** cataracts are linked to the aging process. The most
common area for the formation of a cataract is the cortical area of the lens.
Polar cataracts can be either anterior or posterior. **Anterior polar
cataracts** are more common and are small, white, capsular cataracts located
on the anterior portion of the lens. **Total cataracts,** also called **complete** or
mature, cause an opacity of all fibers of the lens. **Hypermature** describes
a mature cataract with a swollen, milky cortex that covers the entire lens.
Immature, also called **incipient,** cataracts have a clear cortex and are only
slightly opaque. Treatment for all cataracts is the removal of the lens.

● H25.04   Posterior subcapsular polar age-related cataract
    H25.041   Posterior subcapsular polar age-
          related cataract, right eye
    H25.042   Posterior subcapsular polar age-
          related cataract, left eye
    H25.043   Posterior subcapsular polar age-
          related cataract, bilateral
    H25.049   Posterior subcapsular polar age-
          related cataract, unspecified eye
● H25.09   Other age-related incipient cataract
    Coronary age-related cataract
    Punctate age-related cataract
    Water clefts
    H25.091   Other age-related incipient cataract,
          right eye
    H25.092   Other age-related incipient cataract,
          left eye
    H25.093   Other age-related incipient cataract,
          bilateral
    H25.099   Other age-related incipient cataract,
          unspecified eye
● H25.1   Age-related nuclear cataract
    Cataracta brunescens
    Nuclear sclerosis cataract
    H25.10   Age-related nuclear cataract, unspecified eye
    H25.11   Age-related nuclear cataract, right eye
    H25.12   Age-related nuclear cataract, left eye
    H25.13   Age-related nuclear cataract, bilateral
● H25.2   Age-related cataract, morgagnian type
    Age-related hypermature cataract
    H25.20   Age-related cataract, morgagnian type,
         unspecified eye
    H25.21   Age-related cataract, morgagnian type, right
         eye
    H25.22   Age-related cataract, morgagnian type, left eye
    H25.23   Age-related cataract, morgagnian type,
         bilateral
● H25.8   Other age-related cataract
  ● H25.81   Combined forms of age-related cataract
      H25.811   Combined forms of age-related
            cataract, right eye
      H25.812   Combined forms of age-related
            cataract, left eye
      H25.813   Combined forms of age-related
            cataract, bilateral
      H25.819   Combined forms of age-related
            cataract, unspecified eye
    H25.89   Other age-related cataract
● H25.9   Unspecified age-related cataract

● H26   Other cataract
    Excludes1   congenital cataract (Q12.0)
● H26.0   Infantile and juvenile cataract
  ● H26.00   Unspecified infantile and juvenile cataract
      H26.001   Unspecified infantile and juvenile
            cataract, right eye
      H26.002   Unspecified infantile and juvenile
            cataract, left eye
      H26.003   Unspecified infantile and juvenile
            cataract, bilateral
      H26.009   Unspecified infantile and juvenile
            cataract, unspecified eye
  ● H26.01   Infantile and juvenile cortical, lamellar,
      or zonular cataract
      H26.011   Infantile and juvenile cortical,
            lamellar, or zonular cataract, right
            eye
      H26.012   Infantile and juvenile cortical,
            lamellar, or zonular cataract, left eye
      H26.013   Infantile and juvenile cortical,
            lamellar, or zonular cataract,
            bilateral
      H26.019   Infantile and juvenile cortical,
            lamellar, or zonular cataract,
            unspecified eye
  ● H26.03   Infantile and juvenile nuclear cataract
      H26.031   Infantile and juvenile nuclear
            cataract, right eye
      H26.032   Infantile and juvenile nuclear
            cataract, left eye
      H26.033   Infantile and juvenile nuclear
            cataract, bilateral
      H26.039   Infantile and juvenile nuclear
            cataract, unspecified eye
  ● H26.04   Anterior subcapsular polar infantile and
      juvenile cataract
      H26.041   Anterior subcapsular polar infantile
            and juvenile cataract, right eye
      H26.042   Anterior subcapsular polar infantile
            and juvenile cataract, left eye
      H26.043   Anterior subcapsular polar infantile
            and juvenile cataract, bilateral
      H26.049   Anterior subcapsular polar infantile
            and juvenile cataract, unspecified
            eye
  ● H26.05   Posterior subcapsular polar infantile and
      juvenile cataract
      H26.051   Posterior subcapsular polar infantile
            and juvenile cataract, right eye
      H26.052   Posterior subcapsular polar infantile
            and juvenile cataract, left eye
      H26.053   Posterior subcapsular polar infantile
            and juvenile cataract, bilateral
      H26.059   Posterior subcapsular polar infantile
            and juvenile cataract, unspecified
            eye
  ● H26.06   Combined forms of infantile and juvenile
      cataract
      H26.061   Combined forms of infantile and
            juvenile cataract, right eye
      H26.062   Combined forms of infantile and
            juvenile cataract, left eye
      H26.063   Combined forms of infantile and
            juvenile cataract bilateral
      H26.069   Combined forms of infantile and
            juvenile cataract, unspecified eye
    H26.09   Other infantile and juvenile cataract

◀ New   ◀▥ Revised   deleted Deleted   OGCR Official Guidelines   X Assign placeholder X   ● Use Additional Character(s)
Excludes 1   Excludes 2   Includes   Use additional   Code first   Code also   Unspecified

CHAPTER 7 (H00-H59)

● **H26.1**   **Traumatic cataract**
> Use additional code (Chapter 20) to identify external cause

   ● **H26.10**   Unspecified traumatic cataract

     H26.101   Unspecified traumatic cataract, right eye

     H26.102   Unspecified traumatic cataract, left eye

     H26.103   Unspecified traumatic cataract, bilateral

     H26.109   Unspecified traumatic cataract, unspecified eye

   ● **H26.11**   Localized traumatic opacities

     H26.111   Localized traumatic opacities, right eye

     H26.112   Localized traumatic opacities, left eye

     H26.113   Localized traumatic opacities, bilateral

     H26.119   Localized traumatic opacities, unspecified eye

   ● **H26.12**   Partially resolved traumatic cataract

     H26.121   Partially resolved traumatic cataract, right eye

     H26.122   Partially resolved traumatic cataract, left eye

     H26.123   Partially resolved traumatic cataract, bilateral

     H26.129   Partially resolved traumatic cataract, unspecified eye

   ● **H26.13**   Total traumatic cataract

     H26.131   Total traumatic cataract, right eye

     H26.132   Total traumatic cataract, left eye

     H26.133   Total traumatic cataract, bilateral

     H26.139   Total traumatic cataract, unspecified eye

● **H26.2**   **Complicated cataract**

     H26.20   Unspecified complicated cataract
> Cataracta complicata NOS

   ● **H26.21**   Cataract with neovascularization
> Code also associated condition, such as: chronic iridocyclitis (H20.1-)

     H26.211   Cataract with neovascularization, right eye

     H26.212   Cataract with neovascularization, left eye

     H26.213   Cataract with neovascularization, bilateral

     H26.219   Cataract with neovascularization, unspecified eye

   ● **H26.22**   Cataract secondary to ocular disorders (degenerative) (inflammatory)
> Code also associated ocular disorder

     H26.221   Cataract secondary to ocular disorders (degenerative) (inflammatory), right eye

     H26.222   Cataract secondary to ocular disorders (degenerative) (inflammatory), left eye

     H26.223   Cataract secondary to ocular disorders (degenerative) (inflammatory), bilateral

     H26.229   Cataract secondary to ocular disorders (degenerative) (inflammatory), unspecified eye

   ● **H26.23**   Glaucomatous flecks (subcapsular)
> *Code first underlying glaucoma (H40-H42)*

     H26.231   Glaucomatous flecks (subcapsular), right eye

     H26.232   Glaucomatous flecks (subcapsular), left eye

     H26.233   Glaucomatous flecks (subcapsular), bilateral

     H26.239   Glaucomatous flecks (subcapsular), unspecified eye

● **H26.3**   **Drug-induced cataract**
> Toxic cataract
>
> Use additional code for adverse effect, if applicable, to identify drug (T36-T50 with fifth or sixth character 5)

     H26.30   Drug-induced cataract, unspecified eye

     H26.31   Drug-induced cataract, right eye

     H26.32   Drug-induced cataract, left eye

     H26.33   Drug-induced cataract, bilateral

● **H26.4**   **Secondary cataract**

     H26.40   Unspecified secondary cataract

   ● **H26.41**   Soemmering's ring

     H26.411   Soemmering's ring, right eye

     H26.412   Soemmering's ring, left eye

     H26.413   Soemmering's ring, bilateral

     H26.419   Soemmering's ring, unspecified eye

   ● **H26.49**   Other secondary cataract

     H26.491   Other secondary cataract, right eye

     H26.492   Other secondary cataract, left eye

     H26.493   Other secondary cataract, bilateral

     H26.499   Other secondary cataract, unspecified eye

   H26.8   Other specified cataract

   H26.9   Unspecified cataract

● **H27**   **Other disorders of lens**
> **Excludes1**   congenital lens malformations (Q12.-)
> mechanical complications of intraocular lens implant (T85.2)
> pseudophakia (Z96.1)

   ● **H27.0**   Aphakia
> Acquired absence of lens
> Acquired aphakia
> Aphakia due to trauma
>
> **Excludes1**   cataract extraction status (Z98.4-)
> congenital absence of lens (Q12.3)
> congenital aphakia (Q12.3)

     H27.00   Aphakia, unspecified eye

     H27.01   Aphakia, right eye

     H27.02   Aphakia, left eye

     H27.03   Aphakia, bilateral

   ● **H27.1**   Dislocation of lens

     H27.10   Unspecified dislocation of lens

   ● **H27.11**   Subluxation of lens

     H27.111   Subluxation of lens, right eye

     H27.112   Subluxation of lens, left eye

     H27.113   Subluxation of lens, bilateral

     H27.119   Subluxation of lens, unspecified eye

   ● **H27.12**   Anterior dislocation of lens

     H27.121   Anterior dislocation of lens, right eye

     H27.122   Anterior dislocation of lens, left eye

     H27.123   Anterior dislocation of lens, bilateral

     H27.129   Anterior dislocation of lens, unspecified eye

   ● **H27.13**   Posterior dislocation of lens

     H27.131   Posterior dislocation of lens, right eye

     H27.132   Posterior dislocation of lens, left eye

     H27.133   Posterior dislocation of lens, bilateral

     H27.139   Posterior dislocation of lens, unspecified eye

   H27.8   Other specified disorders of lens

   H27.9   Unspecified disorder of lens

CHAPTER 7 (H00-H59)

H28 Cataract in diseases classified elsewhere

Code first underlying disease, such as:
  hypoparathyroidism (E20.-)
  myotonia (G71.1-)
  myxedema (E03.-)
  protein-calorie malnutrition (E40-E46)

| Excludes1 | cataract in diabetes mellitus (E08.36, E09.36, E10.36, E11.36, E13.36) |

DISORDERS OF CHOROID AND RETINA (H30-H36)

(See Plate 90 on page NAP-16.)

● **H30 Chorioretinal inflammation**

  ● **H30.0 Focal chorioretinal inflammation**
    Focal chorioretinitis
    Focal choroiditis
    Focal retinitis
    Focal retinochoroiditis

    ● **H30.00 Unspecified focal chorioretinal inflammation**
      Focal chorioretinitis NOS
      Focal choroiditis NOS
      Focal retinitis NOS
      Focal retinochoroiditis NOS

      H30.001 Unspecified focal chorioretinal inflammation, right eye

      H30.002 Unspecified focal chorioretinal inflammation, left eye

      H30.003 Unspecified focal chorioretinal inflammation, bilateral

      H30.009 Unspecified focal chorioretinal inflammation, unspecified eye

    ● **H30.01 Focal chorioretinal inflammation, juxtapapillary**

      H30.011 Focal chorioretinal inflammation, juxtapapillary, right eye

      H30.012 Focal chorioretinal inflammation, juxtapapillary, left eye

      H30.013 Focal chorioretinal inflammation, juxtapapillary, bilateral

      H30.019 Focal chorioretinal inflammation, juxtapapillary, unspecified eye

    ● **H30.02 Focal chorioretinal inflammation of posterior pole**

      H30.021 Focal chorioretinal inflammation of posterior pole, right eye

      H30.022 Focal chorioretinal inflammation of posterior pole, left eye

      H30.023 Focal chorioretinal inflammation of posterior pole, bilateral

      H30.029 Focal chorioretinal inflammation of posterior pole, unspecified eye

    ● **H30.03 Focal chorioretinal inflammation, peripheral**

      H30.031 Focal chorioretinal inflammation, peripheral, right eye

      H30.032 Focal chorioretinal inflammation, peripheral, left eye

      H30.033 Focal chorioretinal inflammation, peripheral, bilateral

      H30.039 Focal chorioretinal inflammation, peripheral, unspecified eye

    ● **H30.04 Focal chorioretinal inflammation, macular or paramacular**

      H30.041 Focal chorioretinal inflammation, macular or paramacular, right eye

      H30.042 Focal chorioretinal inflammation, macular or paramacular, left eye

      H30.043 Focal chorioretinal inflammation, macular or paramacular, bilateral

      H30.049 Focal chorioretinal inflammation, macular or paramacular, unspecified eye

---

● **H30.1 Disseminated chorioretinal inflammation**
  Disseminated chorioretinitis
  Disseminated choroiditis
  Disseminated retinitis
  Disseminated retinochoroiditis

| Excludes2 | exudative retinopathy (H35.02-) |

  ● **H30.10 Unspecified disseminated chorioretinal inflammation**
    Disseminated chorioretinitis NOS
    Disseminated choroiditis NOS
    Disseminated retinitis NOS
    Disseminated retinochoroiditis NOS

      H30.101 Unspecified disseminated chorioretinal inflammation, right eye

      H30.102 Unspecified disseminated chorioretinal inflammation, left eye

      H30.103 Unspecified disseminated chorioretinal inflammation, bilateral

      H30.109 Unspecified disseminated chorioretinal inflammation, unspecified eye

  ● **H30.11 Disseminated chorioretinal inflammation of posterior pole**

      H30.111 Disseminated chorioretinal inflammation of posterior pole, right eye

      H30.112 Disseminated chorioretinal inflammation of posterior pole, left eye

      H30.113 Disseminated chorioretinal inflammation of posterior pole, bilateral

      H30.119 Disseminated chorioretinal inflammation of posterior pole, unspecified eye

  ● **H30.12 Disseminated chorioretinal inflammation, peripheral**

      H30.121 Disseminated chorioretinal inflammation, peripheral right eye

      H30.122 Disseminated chorioretinal inflammation, peripheral, left eye

      H30.123 Disseminated chorioretinal inflammation, peripheral, bilateral

      H30.129 Disseminated chorioretinal inflammation, peripheral, unspecified eye

  ● **H30.13 Disseminated chorioretinal inflammation, generalized**

      H30.131 Disseminated chorioretinal inflammation, generalized, right eye

      H30.132 Disseminated chorioretinal inflammation, generalized, left eye

      H30.133 Disseminated chorioretinal inflammation, generalized, bilateral

      H30.139 Disseminated chorioretinal inflammation, generalized, unspecified eye

  ● **H30.14 Acute posterior multifocal placoid pigment epitheliopathy**

      H30.141 Acute posterior multifocal placoid pigment epitheliopathy, right eye

      H30.142 Acute posterior multifocal placoid pigment epitheliopathy, left eye

      H30.143 Acute posterior multifocal placoid pigment epitheliopathy, bilateral

      H30.149 Acute posterior multifocal placoid pigment epitheliopathy, unspecified eye

---

● **H30.2 Posterior cyclitis**
   Pars planitis
   H30.20   Posterior cyclitis, unspecified eye
   H30.21   Posterior cyclitis, right eye
   H30.22   Posterior cyclitis, left eye
   H30.23   Posterior cyclitis, bilateral
● **H30.8 Other chorioretinal inflammations**
   ● **H30.81   Harada's disease**
         H30.811   Harada's disease, right eye
         H30.812   Harada's disease, left eye
         H30.813   Harada's disease, bilateral
         H30.819   Harada's disease, unspecified eye
   ● **H30.89   Other chorioretinal inflammations**
         H30.891   Other chorioretinal inflammations, right eye
         H30.892   Other chorioretinal inflammations, left eye
         H30.893   Other chorioretinal inflammations, bilateral
         H30.899   Other chorioretinal inflammations, unspecified eye
● **H30.9 Unspecified chorioretinal inflammation**
   Chorioretinitis NOS
   Choroiditis NOS
   Neuroretinitis NOS
   Retinitis NOS
   Retinochoroiditis NOS
   H30.90   Unspecified chorioretinal inflammation, unspecified eye
   H30.91   Unspecified chorioretinal inflammation, right eye
   H30.92   Unspecified chorioretinal inflammation, left eye
   H30.93   Unspecified chorioretinal inflammation, bilateral

● **H31 Other disorders of choroid**
   ● **H31.0 Chorioretinal scars**
         Excludes2   postsurgical chorioretinal scars (H59.81-)
      ● **H31.00   Unspecified chorioretinal scars**
            H31.001   Unspecified chorioretinal scars, right eye
            H31.002   Unspecified chorioretinal scars, left eye
            H31.003   Unspecified chorioretinal scars, bilateral
            H31.009   Unspecified chorioretinal scars, unspecified eye
      ● **H31.01   Macula scars of posterior pole (postinflammatory) (post-traumatic)**
            Excludes1   postprocedural chorioretinal scar (H59.81-)
            H31.011   Macula scars of posterior pole (postinflammatory) (post-traumatic), right eye
            H31.012   Macula scars of posterior pole (postinflammatory) (post-traumatic), left eye
            H31.013   Macula scars of posterior pole (postinflammatory) (post-traumatic), bilateral
            H31.019   Macula scars of posterior pole (postinflammatory) (post-traumatic), unspecified eye

● **H31.02   Solar retinopathy**
      H31.021   Solar retinopathy, right eye
      H31.022   Solar retinopathy, left eye
      H31.023   Solar retinopathy, bilateral
      H31.029   Solar retinopathy, unspecified eye
● **H31.09   Other chorioretinal scars**
      H31.091   Other chorioretinal scars, right eye
      H31.092   Other chorioretinal scars, left eye
      H31.093   Other chorioretinal scars, bilateral
      H31.099   Other chorioretinal scars, unspecified eye
● **H31.1 Choroidal degeneration**
      Excludes2   angioid streaks of macula (H35.33)
   ● **H31.10   Unspecified choroidal degeneration**
         Choroidal sclerosis NOS
         H31.101   Choroidal degeneration, unspecified, right eye
         H31.102   Choroidal degeneration, unspecified, left eye
         H31.103   Choroidal degeneration, unspecified, bilateral
         H31.109   Choroidal degeneration, unspecified, unspecified eye
   ● **H31.11   Age-related choroidal atrophy**
         H31.111   Age-related choroidal atrophy, right eye
         H31.112   Age-related choroidal atrophy, left eye
         H31.113   Age-related choroidal atrophy, bilateral
         H31.119   Age-related choroidal atrophy, unspecified eye
   ● **H31.12   Diffuse secondary atrophy of choroid**
         H31.121   Diffuse secondary atrophy of choroid, right eye
         H31.122   Diffuse secondary atrophy of choroid, left eye
         H31.123   Diffuse secondary atrophy of choroid, bilateral
         H31.129   Diffuse secondary atrophy of choroid, unspecified eye
● **H31.2 Hereditary choroidal dystrophy**
      Excludes2   hyperornithinemia (E72.4)
                  ornithinemia (E72.4)
      H31.20   Hereditary choroidal dystrophy, unspecified
      H31.21   Choroideremia
      H31.22   Choroidal dystrophy (central areolar) (generalized) (peripapillary)
      H31.23   Gyrate atrophy, choroid
      H31.29   Other hereditary choroidal dystrophy
● **H31.3 Choroidal hemorrhage and rupture**
   ● **H31.30   Unspecified choroidal hemorrhage**
         H31.301   Unspecified choroidal hemorrhage, right eye
         H31.302   Unspecified choroidal hemorrhage, left eye
         H31.303   Unspecified choroidal hemorrhage, bilateral
         H31.309   Unspecified choroidal hemorrhage, unspecified eye

---

◀ New   ◀▥ Revised   ~~deleted~~ Deleted   OGCR Official Guidelines   X Assign placeholder X   ● Use Additional Character(s)

Excludes 1   Excludes 2   Includes   Use additional   Code first   Code also   Unspecified

● **H31.31**   **Expulsive choroidal hemorrhage**
     H31.311   Expulsive choroidal hemorrhage, right eye
     H31.312   Expulsive choroidal hemorrhage, left eye
     H31.313   Expulsive choroidal hemorrhage, bilateral
     H31.319   Expulsive choroidal hemorrhage, unspecified eye

● **H31.32**   **Choroidal rupture**
     H31.321   Choroidal rupture, right eye
     H31.322   Choroidal rupture, left eye
     H31.323   Choroidal rupture, bilateral
     H31.329   Choroidal rupture, unspecified eye

● **H31.4**   **Choroidal detachment**
   ● **H31.40**   **Unspecified choroidal detachment**
     H31.401   Unspecified choroidal detachment, right eye
     H31.402   Unspecified choroidal detachment, left eye
     H31.403   Unspecified choroidal detachment, bilateral
     H31.409   Unspecified choroidal detachment, unspecified eye
   ● **H31.41**   **Hemorrhagic choroidal detachment**
     H31.411   Hemorrhagic choroidal detachment, right eye
     H31.412   Hemorrhagic choroidal detachment, left eye
     H31.413   Hemorrhagic choroidal detachment, bilateral
     H31.419   Hemorrhagic choroidal detachment, unspecified eye
   ● **H31.42**   **Serous choroidal detachment**
     H31.421   Serous choroidal detachment, right eye
     H31.422   Serous choroidal detachment, left eye
     H31.423   Serous choroidal detachment, bilateral
     H31.429   Serous choroidal detachment, unspecified eye

   H31.8   **Other specified disorders of choroid**
   H31.9   **Unspecified disorder of choroid**

H32   **Chorioretinal disorders in diseases classified elsewhere**
     Code first underlying disease, such as:
     congenital toxoplasmosis (P37.1)
     histoplasmosis (B39.-)
     leprosy (A30.-)
     Excludes1   chorioretinitis (in):
                 toxoplasmosis (acquired) (B58.01)
                  tuberculosis (A18.53)

● **H33**   **Retinal detachments and breaks**
     Excludes1   detachment of retinal pigment epithelium (H35.72-, H35.73-)
   ● **H33.0**   **Retinal detachment with retinal break**
     Rhegmatogenous retinal detachment
     Excludes1   serous retinal detachment (without retinal break) (H33.2-)
   ● **H33.00**   **Unspecified retinal detachment with retinal break**
     H33.001   Unspecified retinal detachment with retinal break, right eye
     H33.002   Unspecified retinal detachment with retinal break, left eye

NON-RHEGMATOGENOUS RETINAL DETACHMENT

- Vitreous
- Retina
- Protein-rich fluid in sub-retinal space
- Retinal pigment epithelium

VITREOUS DETACHMENT

- Vitreous
- Posterior hyaloid
- Internal limiting membrane

RHEGMATOGENOUS RETINAL DETACHMENT

- Blood
- Vitreous
- Posterior hyaloid
- Retina
- Retinal tear
- Liquified vitreous
- Retinal pigment epithelium

Figure 7-9   Retinal detachment. (From Kumar: Robbins and Cotran: Pathologic Basis of Disease, ed 7, Saunders, 2005)

Item 7-6   Retinal detachments and defects are conditions of the eye in which the retina separates from the underlying tissue. Initial detachment may be localized, requiring rapid treatment (medical emergency) to avoid the entire retina from detaching which leads to vision loss and blindness.

     H33.003   Unspecified retinal detachment with retinal break, bilateral
     H33.009   Unspecified retinal detachment with retinal break, unspecified eye
   ● **H33.01**   **Retinal detachment with single break**
     H33.011   Retinal detachment with single break, right eye
     H33.012   Retinal detachment with single break, left eye
     H33.013   Retinal detachment with single break, bilateral
     H33.019   Retinal detachment with single break, unspecified eye
   ● **H33.02**   **Retinal detachment with multiple breaks**
     H33.021   Retinal detachment with multiple breaks, right eye
     H33.022   Retinal detachment with multiple breaks, left eye
     H33.023   Retinal detachment with multiple breaks, bilateral
     H33.029   Retinal detachment with multiple breaks, unspecified eye
   ● **H33.03**   **Retinal detachment with giant retinal tear**
     H33.031   Retinal detachment with giant retinal tear, right eye
     H33.032   Retinal detachment with giant retinal tear, left eye
     H33.033   Retinal detachment with giant retinal tear, bilateral
     H33.039   Retinal detachment with giant retinal tear, unspecified eye

◄ New   ◄▦ Revised   ~~deleted~~ Deleted   **OGCR** Official Guidelines   X Assign placeholder X   ● Use Additional Character(s)

| Excludes 1 | Excludes 2 | Includes | Use additional | Code first | Code also | Unspecified |

- **H33.04 Retinal detachment with retinal dialysis**
  - H33.041 Retinal detachment with retinal dialysis, right eye
  - H33.042 Retinal detachment with retinal dialysis, left eye
  - H33.043 Retinal detachment with retinal dialysis, bilateral
  - H33.049 Retinal detachment with retinal dialysis, unspecified eye
- **H33.05 Total retinal detachment**
  - H33.051 Total retinal detachment, right eye
  - H33.052 Total retinal detachment, left eye
  - H33.053 Total retinal detachment, bilateral
  - H33.059 Total retinal detachment, unspecified eye
- **H33.1 Retinoschisis and retinal cysts**

  Excludes1   congenital retinoschisis (Q14.1)
  microcystoid degeneration of retina (H35.42-)

  - **H33.10 Unspecified retinoschisis**
    - H33.101 Unspecified retinoschisis, right eye
    - H33.102 Unspecified retinoschisis, left eye
    - H33.103 Unspecified retinoschisis, bilateral
    - H33.109 Unspecified retinoschisis, unspecified eye
  - **H33.11 Cyst of ora serrata**
    - H33.111 Cyst of ora serrata, right eye
    - H33.112 Cyst of ora serrata, left eye
    - H33.113 Cyst of ora serrata, bilateral
    - H33.119 Cyst of ora serrata, unspecified eye
  - **H33.12 Parasitic cyst of retina**
    - H33.121 Parasitic cyst of retina, right eye
    - H33.122 Parasitic cyst of retina, left eye
    - H33.123 Parasitic cyst of retina, bilateral
    - H33.129 Parasitic cyst of retina, unspecified eye
  - **H33.19 Other retinoschisis and retinal cysts**
    Pseudocyst of retina
    - H33.191 Other retinoschisis and retinal cysts, right eye
    - H33.192 Other retinoschisis and retinal cysts, left eye
    - H33.193 Other retinoschisis and retinal cysts, bilateral
    - H33.199 Other retinoschisis and retinal cysts, unspecified eye
- **H33.2 Serous retinal detachment**
  Retinal detachment NOS
  Retinal detachment without retinal break

  Excludes1   central serous chorioretinopathy (H35.71-)

  H33.20 Serous retinal detachment, unspecified eye
  H33.21 Serous retinal detachment, right eye
  H33.22 Serous retinal detachment, left eye
  H33.23 Serous retinal detachment, bilateral
- **H33.3 Retinal breaks without detachment**

  Excludes1   chorioretinal scars after surgery for detachment (H59.81-)
  peripheral retinal degeneration without break (H35.4-)

- **H33.30 Unspecified retinal break**
  - H33.301 Unspecified retinal break, right eye
  - H33.302 Unspecified retinal break, left eye
  - H33.303 Unspecified retinal break, bilateral
  - H33.309 Unspecified retinal break, unspecified eye
- **H33.31 Horseshoe tear of retina without detachment**
  Operculum of retina without detachment
  - H33.311 Horseshoe tear of retina without detachment, right eye
  - H33.312 Horseshoe tear of retina without detachment, left eye
  - H33.313 Horseshoe tear of retina without detachment, bilateral
  - H33.319 Horseshoe tear of retina without detachment, unspecified eye
- **H33.32 Round hole of retina without detachment**
  - H33.321 Round hole, right eye
  - H33.322 Round hole, left eye
  - H33.323 Round hole, bilateral
  - H33.329 Round hole, unspecified eye
- **H33.33 Multiple defects of retina without detachment**
  - H33.331 Multiple defects of retina without detachment, right eye
  - H33.332 Multiple defects of retina without detachment, left eye
  - H33.333 Multiple defects of retina without detachment, bilateral
  - H33.339 Multiple defects of retina without detachment, unspecified eye
- **H33.4 Traction detachment of retina**
  Proliferative vitreo-retinopathy with retinal detachment
  - H33.40 Traction detachment of retina, unspecified eye
  - H33.41 Traction detachment of retina, right eye
  - H33.42 Traction detachment of retina, left eye
  - H33.43 Traction detachment of retina, bilateral
  H33.8 Other retinal detachments
- **H34 Retinal vascular occlusions**
  Blockage in vessel of the retina

  Excludes1   amaurosis fugax (G45.3)

  - **H34.0 Transient retinal artery occlusion**
    - H34.00 Transient retinal artery occlusion, unspecified eye
    - H34.01 Transient retinal artery occlusion, right eye
    - H34.02 Transient retinal artery occlusion, left eye
    - H34.03 Transient retinal artery occlusion, bilateral
  - **H34.1 Central retinal artery occlusion**
    - H34.10 Central retinal artery occlusion, unspecified eye
    - H34.11 Central retinal artery occlusion, right eye
    - H34.12 Central retinal artery occlusion, left eye
    - H34.13 Central retinal artery occlusion, bilateral
  - **H34.2 Other retinal artery occlusions**
    - **H34.21 Partial retinal artery occlusion**
      Hollenhorst's plaque
      Retinal microembolism
      - H34.211 Partial retinal artery occlusion, right eye
      - H34.212 Partial retinal artery occlusion, left eye
      - H34.213 Partial retinal artery occlusion, bilateral
      - H34.219 Partial retinal artery occlusion, unspecified eye

CHAPTER 7 (H00-H59)

- ●H34.23   Retinal artery branch occlusion
  - H34.231   Retinal artery branch occlusion, right eye
  - H34.232   Retinal artery branch occlusion, left eye
  - H34.233   Retinal artery branch occlusion, bilateral
  - H34.239   Retinal artery branch occlusion, unspecified eye
- ●H34.8   Other retinal vascular occlusions
  - ●H34.81   Central retinal vein occlusion
    - H34.811   Central retinal vein occlusion, right eye
    - H34.812   Central retinal vein occlusion, left eye
    - H34.813   Central retinal vein occlusion, bilateral
    - H34.819   Central retinal vein occlusion, unspecified eye
  - ●H34.82   Venous engorgement
    - Incipient retinal vein occlusion
    - Partial retinal vein occlusion
    - H34.821   Venous engorgement, right eye
    - H34.822   Venous engorgement, left eye
    - H34.823   Venous engorgement, bilateral
    - H34.829   Venous engorgement, unspecified eye
  - ●H34.83   Tributary (branch) retinal vein occlusion
    - H34.831   Tributary (branch) retinal vein occlusion, right eye
    - H34.832   Tributary (branch) retinal vein occlusion, left eye
    - H34.833   Tributary (branch) retinal vein occlusion, bilateral
    - H34.839   Tributary (branch) retinal vein occlusion, unspecified eye
  - H34.9   Unspecified retinal vascular occlusion
- ●H35   Other retinal disorders
  - Excludes2   diabetic retinal disorders (E08.311-E08.359, E09.311-E09.359, E10.311-E10.359, E11.311-E11.359, E13.311-E13.359)
  - ●H35.0   Background retinopathy and retinal vascular changes
    - Code also any associated hypertension (I10.-)
    - H35.00   Unspecified background retinopathy
    - ●H35.01   Changes in retinal vascular appearance
      - Retinal vascular sheathing
      - H35.011   Changes in retinal vascular appearance, right eye
      - H35.012   Changes in retinal vascular appearance, left eye
      - H35.013   Changes in retinal vascular appearance, bilateral
      - H35.019   Changes in retinal vascular appearance, unspecified eye
    - OGCR Section I. C.9.a.5.

      Hypertensive Retinopathy

      Subcategory H35.0, Background retinopathy and retinal vascular changes, should be used with a code from category I10–I15, Hypertensive disease to include the systemic hypertension. The sequencing is based on the reason for the encounter.

- ●H35.02   Exudative retinopathy
  - Coats retinopathy
  - H35.021   Exudative retinopathy, right eye
  - H35.022   Exudative retinopathy, left eye
  - H35.023   Exudative retinopathy, bilateral
  - H35.029   Exudative retinopathy, unspecified eye
- ●H35.03   Hypertensive retinopathy
  - H35.031   Hypertensive retinopathy, right eye
  - H35.032   Hypertensive retinopathy, left eye
  - H35.033   Hypertensive retinopathy, bilateral
  - H35.039   Hypertensive retinopathy, unspecified eye
- ●H35.04   Retinal micro-aneurysms, unspecified
  - H35.041   Retinal micro-aneurysms, unspecified, right eye
  - H35.042   Retinal micro-aneurysms, unspecified, left eye
  - H35.043   Retinal micro-aneurysms, unspecified, bilateral
  - H35.049   Retinal micro-aneurysms, unspecified, unspecified eye
- ●H35.05   Retinal neovascularization, unspecified
  - H35.051   Retinal neovascularization, unspecified, right eye
  - H35.052   Retinal neovascularization, unspecified, left eye
  - H35.053   Retinal neovascularization, unspecified, bilateral
  - H35.059   Retinal neovascularization, unspecified, unspecified eye
- ●H35.06   Retinal vasculitis
  - Eales disease
  - Retinal perivasculitis
  - H35.061   Retinal vasculitis, right eye
  - H35.062   Retinal vasculitis, left eye
  - H35.063   Retinal vasculitis, bilateral
  - H35.069   Retinal vasculitis, unspecified eye
- ●H35.07   Retinal telangiectasis
  - H35.071   Retinal telangiectasis, right eye
  - H35.072   Retinal telangiectasis, left eye
  - H35.073   Retinal telangiectasis, bilateral
  - H35.079   Retinal telangiectasis, unspecified eye
  - H35.09   Other intraretinal microvascular abnormalities
    - Retinal varices
- H35.1   Retinopathy of prematurity
  - ●H35.10   Retinopathy of prematurity, unspecified
    - Retinopathy of prematurity NOS
    - H35.101   Retinopathy of prematurity, unspecified, right eye
    - H35.102   Retinopathy of prematurity, unspecified, left eye
    - H35.103   Retinopathy of prematurity, unspecified, bilateral
    - H35.109   Retinopathy of prematurity, unspecified, unspecified eye
  - ●H35.11   Retinopathy of prematurity, stage 0
    - H35.111   Retinopathy of prematurity, stage 0, right eye
    - H35.112   Retinopathy of prematurity, stage 0, left eye
    - H35.113   Retinopathy of prematurity, stage 0, bilateral
    - H35.119   Retinopathy of prematurity, stage 0, unspecified eye

● H35.12   Retinopathy of prematurity, stage 1
    H35.121   Retinopathy of prematurity, stage 1, right eye
    H35.122   Retinopathy of prematurity, stage 1, left eye
    H35.123   Retinopathy of prematurity, stage 1, bilateral
    H35.129   Retinopathy of prematurity, stage 1, unspecified eye

● H35.13   Retinopathy of prematurity, stage 2
    H35.131   Retinopathy of prematurity, stage 2, right eye
    H35.132   Retinopathy of prematurity, stage 2, left eye
    H35.133   Retinopathy of prematurity, stage 2, bilateral
    H35.139   Retinopathy of prematurity, stage 2, unspecified eye

● H35.14   Retinopathy of prematurity, stage 3
    H35.141   Retinopathy of prematurity, stage 3, right eye
    H35.142   Retinopathy of prematurity, stage 3, left eye
    H35.143   Retinopathy of prematurity, stage 3, bilateral
    H35.149   Retinopathy of prematurity, stage 3, unspecified eye

● H35.15   Retinopathy of prematurity, stage 4
    H35.151   Retinopathy of prematurity, stage 4, right eye
    H35.152   Retinopathy of prematurity, stage 4, left eye
    H35.153   Retinopathy of prematurity, stage 4, bilateral
    H35.159   Retinopathy of prematurity, stage 4, unspecified eye

● H35.16   Retinopathy of prematurity, stage 5
    H35.161   Retinopathy of prematurity, stage 5, right eye
    H35.162   Retinopathy of prematurity, stage 5, left eye
    H35.163   Retinopathy of prematurity, stage 5, bilateral
    H35.169   Retinopathy of prematurity, stage 5, unspecified eye

● H35.17   Retrolental fibroplasia
    H35.171   Retrolental fibroplasia, right eye
    H35.172   Retrolental fibroplasia, left eye
    H35.173   Retrolental fibroplasia, bilateral
    H35.179   Retrolental fibroplasia, unspecified eye

● H35.2   Other non-diabetic proliferative retinopathy
    Proliferative vitreo-retinopathy
    Excludes1   proliferative vitreo-retinopathy with retinal detachment (H33.4-)
    H35.20   Other non-diabetic proliferative retinopathy, unspecified eye
    H35.21   Other non-diabetic proliferative retinopathy, right eye
    H35.22   Other non-diabetic proliferative retinopathy, left eye
    H35.23   Other non-diabetic proliferative retinopathy, bilateral

Item 7–7   Macular degeneration is typically age-related, chronic, and is evidenced by deterioration of the macula (the part of the retina that provides for central field vision), resulting in blurred vision or a blind spot in the center of visual field while not affecting peripheral vision.

● H35.3   Degeneration of macula and posterior pole
    H35.30   Unspecified macular degeneration
        Age-related macular degeneration
    H35.31   Nonexudative age-related macular degeneration
        Atrophic age-related macular degeneration
    H35.32   Exudative age-related macular degeneration
    H35.33   Angioid streaks of macula
● H35.34   Macular cyst, hole, or pseudohole
    H35.341   Macular cyst, hole, or pseudohole, right eye
    H35.342   Macular cyst, hole, or pseudohole, left eye
    H35.343   Macular cyst, hole, or pseudohole, bilateral
    H35.349   Macular cyst, hole, or pseudohole, unspecified eye
● H35.35   Cystoid macular degeneration
    Excludes1   cystoid macular edema following cataract surgery (H59.03-)
    H35.351   Cystoid macular degeneration, right eye
    H35.352   Cystoid macular degeneration, left eye
    H35.353   Cystoid macular degeneration, bilateral
    H35.359   Cystoid macular degeneration, unspecified eye
● H35.36   Drusen (degenerative) of macula
    H35.361   Drusen (degenerative) of macula, right eye
    H35.362   Drusen (degenerative) of macula, left eye
    H35.363   Drusen (degenerative) of macula, bilateral
    H35.369   Drusen (degenerative) of macula, unspecified eye
● H35.37   Puckering of macula
    H35.371   Puckering of macula, right eye
    H35.372   Puckering of macula, left eye
    H35.373   Puckering of macula, bilateral
    H35.379   Puckering of macula, unspecified eye
● H35.38   Toxic maculopathy
    Code first poisoning due to drug or toxin, if applicable (T36-T65 with fifth or sixth character 1-4 or 6)
    Use additional code for adverse effect, if applicable, to identify drug (T36-T50 with fifth or sixth character 5)
    H35.381   Toxic maculopathy, right eye
    H35.382   Toxic maculopathy, left eye
    H35.383   Toxic maculopathy, bilateral
    H35.389   Toxic maculopathy, unspecified eye

CHAPTER 7 (H00-H59)

◀ New   ◀|||| Revised   ~~deleted~~ Deleted   OGCR Official Guidelines   X Assign placeholder X   ● Use Additional Character(s)
Excludes 1   Excludes 2   Includes   Use additional   Code first   Code also   Unspecified

CHAPTER 7 (H00-H59)

● **H35.4**   **Peripheral retinal degeneration**
> **Excludes1**   hereditary retinal degeneration
> (dystrophy) (H35.5-)
> peripheral retinal degeneration with
> retinal break (H33.3-)

     H35.40   Unspecified peripheral retinal degeneration

● **H35.41**   **Lattice degeneration of retina**
> Palisade degeneration of retina

     H35.411   **Lattice degeneration of retina, right eye**

     H35.412   **Lattice degeneration of retina, left eye**

     H35.413   **Lattice degeneration of retina, bilateral**

     H35.419   **Lattice degeneration of retina, unspecified eye**

● **H35.42**   **Microcystoid degeneration of retina**

     H35.421   **Microcystoid degeneration of retina, right eye**

     H35.422   **Microcystoid degeneration of retina, left eye**

     H35.423   **Microcystoid degeneration of retina, bilateral**

     H35.429   **Microcystoid degeneration of retina, unspecified eye**

● **H35.43**   **Paving stone degeneration of retina**

     H35.431   **Paving stone degeneration of retina, right eye**

     H35.432   **Paving stone degeneration of retina, left eye**

     H35.433   **Paving stone degeneration of retina, bilateral**

     H35.439   **Paving stone degeneration of retina, unspecified eye**

● **H35.44**   **Age-related reticular degeneration of retina**

     H35.441   **Age-related reticular degeneration of retina, right eye**

     H35.442   **Age-related reticular degeneration of retina, left eye**

     H35.443   **Age-related reticular degeneration of retina, bilateral**

     H35.449   **Age-related reticular degeneration of retina, unspecified eye**

● **H35.45**   **Secondary pigmentary degeneration**

     H35.451   **Secondary pigmentary degeneration, right eye**

     H35.452   **Secondary pigmentary degeneration, left eye**

     H35.453   **Secondary pigmentary degeneration, bilateral**

     H35.459   **Secondary pigmentary degeneration, unspecified eye**

● **H35.46**   **Secondary vitreoretinal degeneration**

     H35.461   **Secondary vitreoretinal degeneration, right eye**

     H35.462   **Secondary vitreoretinal degeneration, left eye**

     H35.463   **Secondary vitreoretinal degeneration, bilateral**

     H35.469   **Secondary vitreoretinal degeneration, unspecified eye**

● **H35.5**   **Hereditary retinal dystrophy**
> **Excludes1**   dystrophies primarily involving Bruch's
> membrane (H31.1-)

     H35.50   Unspecified hereditary retinal dystrophy

     H35.51   **Vitreoretinal dystrophy**

     H35.52   **Pigmentary retinal dystrophy**
> Albipunctate retinal dystrophy
> Retinitis pigmentosa
> Tapetoretinal dystrophy

     H35.53   **Other dystrophies primarily involving the sensory retina**
> Stargardt's disease

     H35.54   **Dystrophies primarily involving the retinal pigment epithelium**
> Vitelliform retinal dystrophy

● **H35.6**   **Retinal hemorrhage**

     H35.60   **Retinal hemorrhage, unspecified eye**

     H35.61   **Retinal hemorrhage, right eye**

     H35.62   **Retinal hemorrhage, left eye**

     H35.63   **Retinal hemorrhage, bilateral**

● **H35.7**   **Separation of retinal layers**
> **Excludes1**   retinal detachment (serous) (H33.2-)
> rhegmatogenous retinal detachment
> (H33.0-)

     H35.70   Unspecified separation of retinal layers

● **H35.71**   **Central serous chorioretinopathy**

     H35.711   **Central serous chorioretinopathy, right eye**

     H35.712   **Central serous chorioretinopathy, left eye**

     H35.713   **Central serous chorioretinopathy, bilateral**

     H35.719   **Central serous chorioretinopathy, unspecified eye**

● **H35.72**   **Serous detachment of retinal pigment epithelium**

     H35.721   **Serous detachment of retinal pigment epithelium, right eye**

     H35.722   **Serous detachment of retinal pigment epithelium, left eye**

     H35.723   **Serous detachment of retinal pigment epithelium, bilateral**

     H35.729   **Serous detachment of retinal pigment epithelium, unspecified eye**

● **H35.73**   **Hemorrhagic detachment of retinal pigment epithelium**

     H35.731   **Hemorrhagic detachment of retinal pigment epithelium, right eye**

     H35.732   **Hemorrhagic detachment of retinal pigment epithelium, left eye**

     H35.733   **Hemorrhagic detachment of retinal pigment epithelium, bilateral**

     H35.739   **Hemorrhagic detachment of retinal pigment epithelium, unspecified eye**

● **H35.8**   **Other specified retinal disorders**
> **Excludes2**   retinal hemorrhage (H35.6-)

     H35.81   **Retinal edema**
> Retinal cotton wool spots

     H35.82   **Retinal ischemia**

     H35.89   **Other specified retinal disorders**

H35.9   Unspecified retinal disorder

H36   **Retinal disorders in diseases classified elsewhere**
> *Code first underlying disease, such as:*
> lipid storage disorders (E75.-)
> sickle-cell disorders (D57.-)
> **Excludes1**   arteriosclerotic retinopathy (H35.0-)
> diabetic retinopathy (E08.3-, E09.3-, E10.3-, E11.3-,
> E13.3-)

◀ New   ◀▦ Revised   ~~deleted~~ Deleted   OGCR Official Guidelines   X Assign placeholder X   ● Use Additional Character(s)

Excludes 1   Excludes 2   Includes   Use additional   Code first   Code also   Unspecified

GLAUCOMA (H40-H42)

● **H40 Glaucoma**

Intraocular pressure (IOP) that is too high results from too much aqueous humor and because of excess production or inadequate drainage, optic nerve damage and vision loss may occur.

Excludes1 absolute glaucoma (H44.51-)
congenital glaucoma (Q15.0)
traumatic glaucoma due to birth injury (P15.3)

● **H40.0 Glaucoma suspect**

● **H40.00 Preglaucoma, unspecified**

H40.001 Preglaucoma, unspecified, right eye

H40.002 Preglaucoma, unspecified, left eye

H40.003 Preglaucoma, unspecified, bilateral

H40.009 Preglaucoma, unspecified, unspecified eye

● **H40.01 Open angle with borderline findings, low risk**
Open angle, low risk

H40.011 Open angle with borderline findings, low risk, right eye

H40.012 Open angle with borderline findings, low risk, left eye

H40.013 Open angle with borderline findings, low risk, bilateral

H40.019 Open angle with borderline findings, low risk, unspecified eye

● **H40.02 Open angle with borderline findings, high risk**
Open angle, high risk

H40.021 Open angle with borderline findings, high risk, right eye

H40.022 Open angle with borderline findings, high risk, left eye

H40.023 Open angle with borderline findings, high risk, bilateral

H40.029 Open angle with borderline findings, high risk, unspecified eye

● **H40.03 Anatomical narrow angle**
Primary angle closure suspect

H40.031 Anatomical narrow angle, right eye

H40.032 Anatomical narrow angle, left eye

H40.033 Anatomical narrow angle, bilateral

H40.039 Anatomical narrow angle, unspecified eye

● **H40.04 Steroid responder**

H40.041 Steroid responder, right eye

H40.042 Steroid responder, left eye

H40.043 Steroid responder, bilateral

H40.049 Steroid responder, unspecified eye

● **H40.05 Ocular hypertension**

H40.051 Ocular hypertension, right eye

H40.052 Ocular hypertension, left eye

H40.053 Ocular hypertension, bilateral

H40.059 Ocular hypertension, unspecified eye

● **H40.06 Primary angle closure without glaucoma damage**

H40.061 Primary angle closure without glaucoma damage, right eye

H40.062 Primary angle closure without glaucoma damage, left eye

H40.063 Primary angle closure without glaucoma damage, bilateral

H40.069 Primary angle closure without glaucoma damage, unspecified eye

● **H40.1 Open-angle glaucoma**

X● **H40.10 Unspecified open-angle glaucoma**

One of the following 7th characters is to be assigned to code H40.10 to designate the stage of glaucoma

0	stage unspecified
1	mild stage
2	moderate stage
3	severe stage
4	indeterminate stage

X● **H40.11 Primary open-angle glaucoma**
Chronic simple glaucoma

One of the following 7th characters is to be assigned to code H40.11 to designate the stage of glaucoma

0	stage unspecified
1	mild stage
2	moderate stage
3	severe stage
4	indeterminate stage

● **H40.12 Low-tension glaucoma**

One of the following 7th characters is to be assigned to each code in subcategory H40.12 to designate the stage of glaucoma

0	stage unspecified
1	mild stage
2	moderate stage
3	severe stage
4	indeterminate stage

● H40.121 Low-tension glaucoma, right eye

● H40.122 Low-tension glaucoma, left eye

● H40.123 Low-tension glaucoma, bilateral

● H40.129 Low-tension glaucoma, unspecified eye

● **H40.13 Pigmentary glaucoma**

One of the following 7th characters is to be assigned to each code in subcategory H40.13 to designate the stage of glaucoma

0	stage unspecified
1	mild stage
2	moderate stage
3	severe stage
4	indeterminate stage

● H40.131 Pigmentary glaucoma, right eye

● H40.132 Pigmentary glaucoma, left eye

● H40.133 Pigmentary glaucoma, bilateral

● H40.139 Pigmentary glaucoma, unspecified eye

● **H40.14 Capsular glaucoma with pseudoexfoliation of lens**

One of the following 7th characters is to be assigned to each code in subcategory H40.14 to designate the stage of glaucoma

0	stage unspecified
1	mild stage
2	moderate stage
3	severe stage
4	indeterminate stage

● H40.141 Capsular glaucoma with pseudoexfoliation of lens, right eye

● H40.142 Capsular glaucoma with pseudoexfoliation of lens, left eye

CHAPTER 7 (H00-H59)

● H40.143   Capsular glaucoma with pseudoexfoliation of lens, bilateral

● H40.149   Capsular glaucoma with pseudoexfoliation of lens, unspecified eye

● H40.15   Residual stage of open-angle glaucoma

H40.151   Residual stage of open-angle glaucoma, right eye

H40.152   Residual stage of open-angle glaucoma, left eye

H40.153   Residual stage of open-angle glaucoma, bilateral

H40.159   Residual stage of open-angle glaucoma, unspecified eye

● H40.2   Primary angle-closure glaucoma

Excludes1   aqueous misdirection (H40.83-)
malignant glaucoma (H40.83-)

● H40.20   Unspecified primary angle-closure glaucoma

One of the following 7th characters is to be assigned to code H40.20 to designate the stage of glaucoma

0	stage unspecified
1	mild stage
2	moderate stage
3	severe stage
4	indeterminate stage

● H40.21   Acute angle-closure glaucoma

Acute angle-closure glaucoma attack
Acute angle-closure glaucoma crisis

H40.211   Acute angle-closure glaucoma, right eye

H40.212   Acute angle-closure glaucoma, left eye

H40.213   Acute angle-closure glaucoma, bilateral

H40.219   Acute angle-closure glaucoma, unspecified eye

● H40.22   Chronic angle-closure glaucoma

Chronic primary angle closure glaucoma

One of the following 7th characters is to be assigned to each code in subcategory H40.22 to designate the stage of glaucoma

0	stage unspecified
1	mild stage
2	moderate stage
3	severe stage
4	indeterminate stage

● H40.221   Chronic angle-closure glaucoma, right eye

● H40.222   Chronic angle-closure glaucoma, left eye

● H40.223   Chronic angle-closure glaucoma, bilateral

● H40.229   Chronic angle-closure glaucoma, unspecified eye

● H40.23   Intermittent angle-closure glaucoma

H40.231   Intermittent angle-closure glaucoma, right eye

H40.232   Intermittent angle-closure glaucoma, left eye

H40.233   Intermittent angle-closure glaucoma, bilateral

H40.239   Intermittent angle-closure glaucoma, unspecified eye

● H40.24   Residual stage of angle-closure glaucoma

H40.241   Residual stage of angle-closure glaucoma, right eye

H40.242   Residual stage of angle-closure glaucoma, left eye

H40.243   Residual stage of angle-closure glaucoma, bilateral

H40.249   Residual stage of angle-closure glaucoma, unspecified eye

● H40.3   Glaucoma secondary to eye trauma

Code also underlying condition

One of the following 7th characters is to be assigned to each code in subcategory H40.3 to designate the stage of glaucoma

0	stage unspecified
1	mild stage
2	moderate stage
3	severe stage
4	indeterminate stage

X ● H40.30   Glaucoma secondary to eye trauma, unspecified eye

X ● H40.31   Glaucoma secondary to eye trauma, right eye

X ● H40.32   Glaucoma secondary to eye trauma, left eye

X ● H40.33   Glaucoma secondary to eye trauma, bilateral

● H40.4   Glaucoma secondary to eye inflammation

Code also underlying condition

One of the following 7th characters is to be assigned to each code in subcategory H40.4 to designate the stage of glaucoma

0	stage unspecified
1	mild stage
2	moderate stage
3	severe stage
4	indeterminate stage

X ● H40.40   Glaucoma secondary to eye inflammation, unspecified eye

X ● H40.41   Glaucoma secondary to eye inflammation, right eye

X ● H40.42   Glaucoma secondary to eye inflammation, left eye

X ● H40.43   Glaucoma secondary to eye inflammation, bilateral

● H40.5   Glaucoma secondary to other eye disorders

Code also underlying eye disorder

One of the following 7th characters is to be assigned to each code in subcategory H40.5 to designate the stage of glaucoma

0	stage unspecified
1	mild stage
2	moderate stage
3	severe stage
4	indeterminate stage

X ● H40.50   Glaucoma secondary to other eye disorders, unspecified eye

X ● H40.51   Glaucoma secondary to other eye disorders, right eye

X ● H40.52   Glaucoma secondary to other eye disorders, left eye

X ● H40.53   Glaucoma secondary to other eye disorders, bilateral

● **H40.6   Glaucoma secondary to drugs**

> Use additional code for adverse effect, if applicable, to identify drug (T36-T50 with fifth or sixth character 5)

> One of the following 7th characters is to be assigned to each code in subcategory H40.6 to designate the stage of glaucoma

0	stage unspecified
1	mild stage
2	moderate stage
3	severe stage
4	indeterminate stage

X ● **H40.60**   Glaucoma secondary to drugs, unspecified eye
X ● **H40.61**   Glaucoma secondary to drugs, right eye
X ● **H40.62**   Glaucoma secondary to drugs, left eye
X ● **H40.63**   Glaucoma secondary to drugs, bilateral

● **H40.8   Other glaucoma**

    ● **H40.81**   Glaucoma with increased episcleral venous pressure

       H40.811   Glaucoma with increased episcleral venous pressure, right eye
       H40.812   Glaucoma with increased episcleral venous pressure, left eye
       H40.813   Glaucoma with increased episcleral venous pressure, bilateral
       H40.819   Glaucoma with increased episcleral venous pressure, unspecified eye

    ● **H40.82**   Hypersecretion glaucoma

       H40.821   Hypersecretion glaucoma, right eye
       H40.822   Hypersecretion glaucoma, left eye
       H40.823   Hypersecretion glaucoma, bilateral
       H40.829   Hypersecretion glaucoma, unspecified eye

    ● **H40.83**   Aqueous misdirection

> Malignant glaucoma

       H40.831   Aqueous misdirection, right eye
       H40.832   Aqueous misdirection, left eye
       H40.833   Aqueous misdirection, bilateral
       H40.839   Aqueous misdirection, unspecified eye

       H40.89   Other specified glaucoma

    H40.9   Unspecified glaucoma

H42   Glaucoma in diseases classified elsewhere

> *Code first underlying condition, such as:*
> amyloidosis (E85.-)
> aniridia (Q13.1)
> Lowe's syndrome (E72.03)
> Reiger's anomaly (Q13.81)
> specified metabolic disorder (E70-E88)

> **Excludes1**   glaucoma (in):
>   diabetes mellitus (E08.39, E09.39, E10.39, E11.39, E13.39)
>   onchocerciasis (B73.02)
>   syphilis (A52.71)
>   tuberculous (A18.59)

DISORDERS OF VITREOUS BODY AND GLOBE (H43-H44)

● **H43   Disorders of vitreous body**

    ● **H43.0**   Vitreous prolapse

> **Excludes1**   vitreous syndrome following cataract surgery (H59.0-)
> traumatic vitreous prolapse (S05.2-)

       H43.00   Vitreous prolapse, unspecified eye
       H43.01   Vitreous prolapse, right eye
       H43.02   Vitreous prolapse, left eye
       H43.03   Vitreous prolapse, bilateral

    ● **H43.1**   Vitreous hemorrhage

       H43.10   Vitreous hemorrhage, unspecified eye
       H43.11   Vitreous hemorrhage, right eye
       H43.12   Vitreous hemorrhage, left eye
       H43.13   Vitreous hemorrhage, bilateral

    ● **H43.2**   Crystalline deposits in vitreous body

       H43.20   Crystalline deposits in vitreous body, unspecified eye
       H43.21   Crystalline deposits in vitreous body, right eye
       H43.22   Crystalline deposits in vitreous body, left eye
       H43.23   Crystalline deposits in vitreous body, bilateral

● **H43.3   Other vitreous opacities**

    ● **H43.31**   Vitreous membranes and strands

       H43.311   Vitreous membranes and strands, right eye
       H43.312   Vitreous membranes and strands, left eye
       H43.313   Vitreous membranes and strands, bilateral
       H43.319   Vitreous membranes and strands, unspecified eye

    ● **H43.39**   Other vitreous opacities

> Vitreous floaters
> *Small clumps of cells that float in the vitreous of the eye, appearing as black specks or dots in the field of vision and common in the aging eye.*

       H43.391   Other vitreous opacities, right eye
       H43.392   Other vitreous opacities, left eye
       H43.393   Other vitreous opacities, bilateral
       H43.399   Other vitreous opacities, unspecified eye

● **H43.8   Other disorders of vitreous body**

> **Excludes1**   proliferative vitreo-retinopathy with retinal detachment (H33.4)

> **Excludes2**   vitreous abscess (H44.02-)

    ● **H43.81**   Vitreous degeneration

> Vitreous detachment

       H43.811   Vitreous degeneration, right eye
       H43.812   Vitreous degeneration, left eye
       H43.813   Vitreous degeneration, bilateral
       H43.819   Vitreous degeneration, unspecified eye

    ● **H43.82**   Vitreomacular adhesion

> Vitreomacular traction

       H43.821   Vitreomacular adhesion, right eye
       H43.822   Vitreomacular adhesion, left eye
       H43.823   Vitreomacular adhesion, bilateral
       H43.829   Vitreomacular adhesion, unspecified eye

       H43.89   Other disorders of vitreous body

    H43.9   Unspecified disorder of vitreous body

● **H44   Disorders of globe**

> **Includes**   disorders affecting multiple structures of eye

● **H44.0   Purulent endophthalmitis**

> Use additional code to identify organism
> **Excludes1**   bleb associated endophthalmitis (H59.4-)

    ● **H44.00**   Unspecified purulent endophthalmitis

       H44.001   Unspecified purulent endophthalmitis, right eye
       H44.002   Unspecified purulent endophthalmitis, left eye
       H44.003   Unspecified purulent endophthalmitis, bilateral
       H44.009   Unspecified purulent endophthalmitis, unspecified eye

CHAPTER 7 (H00-H59)

- **● H44.01   Panophthalmitis (acute)**
  - H44.011   Panophthalmitis (acute), right eye
  - H44.012   Panophthalmitis (acute), left eye
  - H44.013   Panophthalmitis (acute), bilateral
  - H44.019   Panophthalmitis (acute), unspecified eye
- **● H44.02   Vitreous abscess (chronic)**
  - H44.021   Vitreous abscess (chronic), right eye
  - H44.022   Vitreous abscess (chronic), left eye
  - H44.023   Vitreous abscess (chronic), bilateral
  - H44.029   Vitreous abscess (chronic), unspecified eye
- **● H44.1   Other endophthalmitis**
  - **Excludes1**   bleb associated endophthalmitis (H59.4-)
  - **Excludes2**   ophthalmia nodosa (H16.2-)
  - **● H44.11   Panuveitis**
    - H44.111   Panuveitis, right eye
    - H44.112   Panuveitis, left eye
    - H44.113   Panuveitis, bilateral
    - H44.119   Panuveitis, unspecified eye
  - **● H44.12   Parasitic endophthalmitis, unspecified**
    - H44.121   Parasitic endophthalmitis, unspecified, right eye
    - H44.122   Parasitic endophthalmitis, unspecified, left eye
    - H44.123   Parasitic endophthalmitis, unspecified, bilateral
    - H44.129   Parasitic endophthalmitis, unspecified, unspecified eye
  - **● H44.13   Sympathetic uveitis**
    - H44.131   Sympathetic uveitis, right eye
    - H44.132   Sympathetic uveitis, left eye
    - H44.133   Sympathetic uveitis, bilateral
    - H44.139   Sympathetic uveitis, unspecified eye
  - H44.19   Other endophthalmitis
- **● H44.2   Degenerative myopia**
  - Malignant myopia
  - H44.20   Degenerative myopia, unspecified eye
  - H44.21   Degenerative myopia, right eye
  - H44.22   Degenerative myopia, left eye
  - H44.23   Degenerative myopia, bilateral
- **● H44.3   Other and unspecified degenerative disorders of globe**
  - H44.30   Unspecified degenerative disorder of globe
  - **● H44.31   Chalcosis**
    - H44.311   Chalcosis, right eye
    - H44.312   Chalcosis, left eye
    - H44.313   Chalcosis, bilateral
    - H44.319   Chalcosis, unspecified eye
  - **● H44.32   Siderosis of eye**
    - H44.321   Siderosis of eye, right eye
    - H44.322   Siderosis of eye, left eye
    - H44.323   Siderosis of eye, bilateral
    - H44.329   Siderosis of eye, unspecified eye
  - **● H44.39   Other degenerative disorders of globe**
    - H44.391   Other degenerative disorders of globe, right eye
    - H44.392   Other degenerative disorders of globe, left eye
    - H44.393   Other degenerative disorders of globe, bilateral
    - H44.399   Other degenerative disorders of globe, unspecified eye

- **● H44.4   Hypotony of eye**
  - H44.40   Unspecified hypotony of eye
  - **● H44.41   Flat anterior chamber hypotony of eye**
    - H44.411   Flat anterior chamber hypotony of right eye
    - H44.412   Flat anterior chamber hypotony of left eye
    - H44.413   Flat anterior chamber hypotony of eye, bilateral
    - H44.419   Flat anterior chamber hypotony of unspecified eye
  - **● H44.42   Hypotony of eye due to ocular fistula**
    - H44.421   Hypotony of right eye due to ocular fistula
    - H44.422   Hypotony of left eye due to ocular fistula
    - H44.423   Hypotony of eye due to ocular fistula, bilateral
    - H44.429   Hypotony of unspecified eye due to ocular fistula
  - **● H44.43   Hypotony of eye due to other ocular disorders**
    - H44.431   Hypotony of eye due to other ocular disorders, right eye
    - H44.432   Hypotony of eye due to other ocular disorders, left eye
    - H44.433   Hypotony of eye due to other ocular disorders, bilateral
    - H44.439   Hypotony of eye due to other ocular disorders, unspecified eye
  - **● H44.44   Primary hypotony of eye**
    - H44.441   Primary hypotony of right eye
    - H44.442   Primary hypotony of left eye
    - H44.443   Primary hypotony of eye, bilateral
    - H44.449   Primary hypotony of unspecified eye
- **● H44.5   Degenerated conditions of globe**
  - H44.50   Unspecified degenerated conditions of globe
  - **● H44.51   Absolute glaucoma**
    - H44.511   Absolute glaucoma, right eye
    - H44.512   Absolute glaucoma, left eye
    - H44.513   Absolute glaucoma, bilateral
    - H44.519   Absolute glaucoma, unspecified eye
  - **● H44.52   Atrophy of globe**
    - Phthisis bulbi
    - H44.521   Atrophy of globe, right eye
    - H44.522   Atrophy of globe, left eye
    - H44.523   Atrophy of globe, bilateral
    - H44.529   Atrophy of globe, unspecified eye
  - **● H44.53   Leucocoria**
    - H44.531   Leucocoria, right eye
    - H44.532   Leucocoria, left eye
    - H44.533   Leucocoria, bilateral
    - H44.539   Leucocoria, unspecified eye
- **● H44.6   Retained (old) intraocular foreign body, magnetic**
  - Use additional code to identify magnetic foreign body (Z18.11)
  - **Excludes1**   current intraocular foreign body (S05.-)
  - **Excludes2**   retained foreign body in eyelid (H02.81-)
    - retained (old) foreign body following penetrating wound of orbit (H05.5-)
    - retained (old) intraocular foreign body, nonmagnetic (H44.7-)
  - **● H44.60   Unspecified retained (old) intraocular foreign body, magnetic**
    - H44.601   Unspecified retained (old) intraocular foreign body, magnetic, right eye
    - H44.602   Unspecified retained (old) intraocular foreign body, magnetic, left eye

---

H44.603 Unspecified retained (old) intraocular foreign body, magnetic, bilateral

H44.609 Unspecified retained (old) intraocular foreign body, magnetic, unspecified eye

● H44.61 Retained (old) magnetic foreign body in anterior chamber

H44.611 Retained (old) magnetic foreign body in anterior chamber, right eye

H44.612 Retained (old) magnetic foreign body in anterior chamber, left eye

H44.613 Retained (old) magnetic foreign body in anterior chamber, bilateral

H44.619 Retained (old) magnetic foreign body in anterior chamber, unspecified eye

● H44.62 Retained (old) magnetic foreign body in iris or ciliary body

H44.621 Retained (old) magnetic foreign body in iris or ciliary body, right eye

H44.622 Retained (old) magnetic foreign body in iris or ciliary body, left eye

H44.623 Retained (old) magnetic foreign body in iris or ciliary body, bilateral

H44.629 Retained (old) magnetic foreign body in iris or ciliary body, unspecified eye

● H44.63 Retained (old) magnetic foreign body in lens

H44.631 Retained (old) magnetic foreign body in lens, right eye

H44.632 Retained (old) magnetic foreign body in lens, left eye

H44.633 Retained (old) magnetic foreign body in lens, bilateral

H44.639 Retained (old) magnetic foreign body in lens, unspecified eye

● H44.64 Retained (old) magnetic foreign body in posterior wall of globe

H44.641 Retained (old) magnetic foreign body in posterior wall of globe, right eye

H44.642 Retained (old) magnetic foreign body in posterior wall of globe, left eye

H44.643 Retained (old) magnetic foreign body in posterior wall of globe, bilateral

H44.649 Retained (old) magnetic foreign body in posterior wall of globe, unspecified eye

● H44.65 Retained (old) magnetic foreign body in vitreous body

H44.651 Retained (old) magnetic foreign body in vitreous body, right eye

H44.652 Retained (old) magnetic foreign body in vitreous body, left eye

H44.653 Retained (old) magnetic foreign body in vitreous body, bilateral

H44.659 Retained (old) magnetic foreign body in vitreous body, unspecified eye

● H44.69 Retained (old) intraocular foreign body, magnetic, in other or multiple sites

H44.691 Retained (old) intraocular foreign body, magnetic, in other or multiple sites, right eye

H44.692 Retained (old) intraocular foreign body, magnetic, in other or multiple sites, left eye

H44.693 Retained (old) intraocular foreign body, magnetic, in other or multiple sites, bilateral

H44.699 Retained (old) intraocular foreign body, magnetic, in other or multiple sites, unspecified eye

● H44.7 Retained (old) intraocular foreign body, nonmagnetic

Use additional code to identify nonmagnetic foreign body (Z18.01-Z18.10, Z18.12, Z18.2-Z18.9)

Excludes1 current intraocular foreign body (S05.-)

Excludes2 retained foreign body in eyelid (H02.81-)
retained (old) foreign body following penetrating wound of orbit (H05.5-)
retained (old) intraocular foreign body, magnetic (H44.6-)

● H44.70 Unspecified retained (old) intraocular foreign body, nonmagnetic

H44.701 Unspecified retained (old) intraocular foreign body, nonmagnetic, right eye

H44.702 Unspecified retained (old) intraocular foreign body, nonmagnetic, left eye

H44.703 Unspecified retained (old) intraocular foreign body, nonmagnetic, bilateral

H44.709 Unspecified retained (old) intraocular foreign body, nonmagnetic, unspecified eye

Retained (old) intraocular foreign body NOS

● H44.71 Retained (nonmagnetic) (old) foreign body in anterior chamber

H44.711 Retained (nonmagnetic) (old) foreign body in anterior chamber, right eye

H44.712 Retained (nonmagnetic) (old) foreign body in anterior chamber, left eye

H44.713 Retained (nonmagnetic) (old) foreign body in anterior chamber, bilateral

H44.719 Retained (nonmagnetic) (old) foreign body in anterior chamber, unspecified eye

● H44.72 Retained (nonmagnetic) (old) foreign body in iris or ciliary body

H44.721 Retained (nonmagnetic) (old) foreign body in iris or ciliary body, right eye

H44.722 Retained (nonmagnetic) (old) foreign body in iris or ciliary body, left eye

H44.723 Retained (nonmagnetic) (old) foreign body in iris or ciliary body, bilateral

H44.729 Retained (nonmagnetic) (old) foreign body in iris or ciliary body, unspecified eye

● H44.73 Retained (nonmagnetic) (old) foreign body in lens

H44.731 Retained (nonmagnetic) (old) foreign body in lens, right eye

H44.732 Retained (nonmagnetic) (old) foreign body in lens, left eye

H44.733 Retained (nonmagnetic) (old) foreign body in lens, bilateral

H44.739 Retained (nonmagnetic) (old) foreign body in lens, unspecified eye

● H44.74 Retained (nonmagnetic) (old) foreign body in posterior wall of globe

H44.741 Retained (nonmagnetic) (old) foreign body in posterior wall of globe, right eye

H44.742 Retained (nonmagnetic) (old) foreign body in posterior wall of globe, left eye

H44.743 Retained (nonmagnetic) (old) foreign body in posterior wall of globe, bilateral

H44.749 Retained (nonmagnetic) (old) foreign body in posterior wall of globe, unspecified eye

CHAPTER 7 (H00-H59)

● H44.75　Retained (nonmagnetic) (old) foreign body in vitreous body
　　H44.751　Retained (nonmagnetic) (old) foreign body in vitreous body, right eye
　　H44.752　Retained (nonmagnetic) (old) foreign body in vitreous body, left eye
　　H44.753　Retained (nonmagnetic) (old) foreign body in vitreous body, bilateral
　　H44.759　Retained (nonmagnetic) (old) foreign body in vitreous body, unspecified eye

● H44.79　Retained (old) intraocular foreign body, nonmagnetic, in other or multiple sites
　　H44.791　Retained (old) intraocular foreign body, nonmagnetic, in other or multiple sites, right eye
　　H44.792　Retained (old) intraocular foreign body, nonmagnetic, in other or multiple sites, left eye
　　H44.793　Retained (old) intraocular foreign body, nonmagnetic, in other or multiple sites, bilateral
　　H44.799　Retained (old) intraocular foreign body, nonmagnetic, in other or multiple sites, unspecified eye

● H44.8　Other disorders of globe
　● H44.81　Hemophthalmos
　　　H44.811　Hemophthalmos, right eye
　　　H44.812　Hemophthalmos, left eye
　　　H44.813　Hemophthalmos, bilateral
　　　H44.819　Hemophthalmos, unspecified eye
　● H44.82　Luxation of globe
　　　H44.821　Luxation of globe, right eye
　　　H44.822　Luxation of globe, left eye
　　　H44.823　Luxation of globe, bilateral
　　　H44.829　Luxation of globe, unspecified eye
　　H44.89　Other disorders of globe
　H44.9　Unspecified disorder of globe

(See Plate 86 on page NAP-7.)

DISORDERS OF OPTIC NERVE AND VISUAL PATHWAYS (H46–H47)

● H46　Optic neuritis
　Excludes2　ischemic optic neuropathy (H47.01-)
　　　　　　　neuromyelitis optica [Devic] (G36.0)

● H46.0　Optic papillitis
　　H46.00　Optic papillitis, unspecified eye
　　H46.01　Optic papillitis, right eye
　　H46.02　Optic papillitis, left eye
　　H46.03　Optic papillitis, bilateral
● H46.1　Retrobulbar neuritis
　　Retrobulbar neuritis NOS
　　Excludes1　syphilitic retrobulbar neuritis (A52.15)
　　H46.10　Retrobulbar neuritis, unspecified eye
　　H46.11　Retrobulbar neuritis, right eye
　　H46.12　Retrobulbar neuritis, left eye
　　H46.13　Retrobulbar neuritis, bilateral
　H46.2　Nutritional optic neuropathy
　H46.3　Toxic optic neuropathy
　　　Code first (T51-T65) to identify cause
　H46.8　Other optic neuritis
　H46.9　Unspecified optic neuritis

● H47　Other disorders of optic [2nd] nerve and visual pathways
　● H47.0　Disorders of optic nerve, not elsewhere classified
　　● H47.01　Ischemic optic neuropathy
　　　　H47.011　Ischemic optic neuropathy, right eye
　　　　H47.012　Ischemic optic neuropathy, left eye
　　　　H47.013　Ischemic optic neuropathy, bilateral
　　　　H47.019　Ischemic optic neuropathy, unspecified eye
　　● H47.02　Hemorrhage in optic nerve sheath
　　　　H47.021　Hemorrhage in optic nerve sheath, right eye
　　　　H47.022　Hemorrhage in optic nerve sheath, left eye
　　　　H47.023　Hemorrhage in optic nerve sheath, bilateral
　　　　H47.029　Hemorrhage in optic nerve sheath, unspecified eye
　　● H47.03　Optic nerve hypoplasia
　　　　H47.031　Optic nerve hypoplasia, right eye
　　　　H47.032　Optic nerve hypoplasia, left eye
　　　　H47.033　Optic nerve hypoplasia, bilateral
　　　　H47.039　Optic nerve hypoplasia, unspecified eye
　　● H47.09　Other disorders of optic nerve, not elsewhere classified
　　　　Compression of optic nerve
　　　　H47.091　Other disorders of optic nerve, not elsewhere classified, right eye
　　　　H47.092　Other disorders of optic nerve, not elsewhere classified, left eye
　　　　H47.093　Other disorders of optic nerve, not elsewhere classified, bilateral
　　　　H47.099　Other disorders of optic nerve, not elsewhere classified, unspecified eye
　● H47.1　Papilledema
　　H47.10　Unspecified papilledema
　　H47.11　Papilledema associated with increased intracranial pressure

Figure 7-10　Papilledema. (From Behrma: Nelson Textbook of Pediatrics, ed 17, Saunders, 2004)

Item 7-8　Papilledema is swelling of the optic disc caused by increased intracranial pressure. It is most often bilateral and occurs quickly (hours) or over weeks of time. It is a common symptom of a brain tumor. The term should not be used to describe optic disc swelling with underlying infectious, infiltrative, or inflammatory etiologies.

H47.12   Papilledema associated with decreased ocular pressure
H47.13   Papilledema associated with retinal disorder
● H47.14   Foster-Kennedy syndrome
    H47.141   Foster-Kennedy syndrome, right eye
    H47.142   Foster-Kennedy syndrome, left eye
    H47.143   Foster-Kennedy syndrome, bilateral
    H47.149   Foster-Kennedy syndrome, unspecified eye

● H47.2   Optic atrophy
    H47.20   Unspecified optic atrophy
  ● H47.21   Primary optic atrophy
    H47.211   Primary optic atrophy, right eye
    H47.212   Primary optic atrophy, left eye
    H47.213   Primary optic atrophy, bilateral
    H47.219   Primary optic atrophy, unspecified eye
  H47.22   Hereditary optic atrophy
    Leber's optic atrophy
  ● H47.23   Glaucomatous optic atrophy
    H47.231   Glaucomatous optic atrophy, right eye
    H47.232   Glaucomatous optic atrophy, left eye
    H47.233   Glaucomatous optic atrophy, bilateral
    H47.239   Glaucomatous optic atrophy, unspecified eye
  ● H47.29   Other optic atrophy
    Temporal pallor of optic disc
    H47.291   Other optic atrophy, right eye
    H47.292   Other optic atrophy, left eye
    H47.293   Other optic atrophy, bilateral
    H47.299   Other optic atrophy, unspecified eye

● H47.3   Other disorders of optic disc
  ● H47.31   Coloboma of optic disc
    H47.311   Coloboma of optic disc, right eye
    H47.312   Coloboma of optic disc, left eye
    H47.313   Coloboma of optic disc, bilateral
    H47.319   Coloboma of optic disc, unspecified eye
  ● H47.32   Drusen of optic disc
    H47.321   Drusen of optic disc, right eye
    H47.322   Drusen of optic disc, left eye
    H47.323   Drusen of optic disc, bilateral
    H47.329   Drusen of optic disc, unspecified eye
  ● H47.33   Pseudopapilledema of optic disc
    H47.331   Pseudopapilledema of optic disc, right eye
    H47.332   Pseudopapilledema of optic disc, left eye
    H47.333   Pseudopapilledema of optic disc, bilateral
    H47.339   Pseudopapilledema of optic disc, unspecified eye
  ● H47.39   Other disorders of optic disc
    H47.391   Other disorders of optic disc, right eye
    H47.392   Other disorders of optic disc, left eye
    H47.393   Other disorders of optic disc, bilateral
    H47.399   Other disorders of optic disc, unspecified eye

● H47.4   Disorders of optic chiasm
    Code also underlying condition
  H47.41   Disorders of optic chiasm in (due to) inflammatory disorders
  H47.42   Disorders of optic chiasm in (due to) neoplasm
  H47.43   Disorders of optic chiasm in (due to) vascular disorders
  H47.49   Disorders of optic chiasm in (due to) other disorders

● H47.5   Disorders of other visual pathways
    Disorders of optic tracts, geniculate nuclei and optic radiations
    Code also underlying condition
  ● H47.51   Disorders of visual pathways in (due to) inflammatory disorders
    H47.511   Disorders of visual pathways in (due to) inflammatory disorders, right side
    H47.512   Disorders of visual pathways in (due to) inflammatory disorders, left side
    H47.519   Disorders of visual pathways in (due to) inflammatory disorders, unspecified side
  ● H47.52   Disorders of visual pathways in (due to) neoplasm
    H47.521   Disorders of visual pathways in (due to) neoplasm, right side
    H47.522   Disorders of visual pathways in (due to) neoplasm, left side
    H47.529   Disorders of visual pathways in (due to) neoplasm, unspecified side
  ● H47.53   Disorders of visual pathways in (due to) vascular disorders
    H47.531   Disorders of visual pathways in (due to) vascular disorders, right side
    H47.532   Disorders of visual pathways in (due to) vascular disorders, left side
    H47.539   Disorders of visual pathways in (due to) vascular disorders, unspecified side

● H47.6   Disorders of visual cortex
    Code also underlying condition
    Excludes1   injury to visual cortex S04.04
  ● H47.61   Cortical blindness
    H47.611   Cortical blindness, right side of brain
    H47.612   Cortical blindness, left side of brain
    H47.619   Cortical blindness, unspecified side of brain
  ● H47.62   Disorders of visual cortex in (due to) inflammatory disorders
    H47.621   Disorders of visual cortex in (due to) inflammatory disorders, right side of brain
    H47.622   Disorders of visual cortex in (due to) inflammatory disorders, left side of brain
    H47.629   Disorders of visual cortex in (due to) inflammatory disorders, unspecified side of brain
  ● H47.63   Disorders of visual cortex in (due to) neoplasm
    H47.631   Disorders of visual cortex in (due to) neoplasm, right side of brain
    H47.632   Disorders of visual cortex in (due to) neoplasm, left side of brain
    H47.639   Disorders of visual cortex in (due to) neoplasm, unspecified side of brain

CHAPTER 7 (H00-H59)

● **H47.64**   **Disorders of visual cortex in (due to) vascular disorders**
    H47.641   **Disorders of visual cortex in (due to) vascular disorders, right side of brain**
    H47.642   **Disorders of visual cortex in (due to) vascular disorders, left side of brain**
    H47.649   **Disorders of visual cortex in (due to) vascular disorders, unspecified side of brain**

H47.9   **Unspecified disorder of visual pathways**

DISORDERS OF OCULAR MUSCLES, BINOCULAR MOVEMENT, ACCOMMODATION AND REFRACTION (H49-H52)

| Excludes2 | nystagmus and other irregular eye movements (H55) |

● **H49   Paralytic strabismus**

| Excludes2 | internal ophthalmoplegia (H52.51-)
internuclear ophthalmoplegia (H51.2-)
progressive supranuclear ophthalmoplegia (G23.1) |

  ● **H49.0**   **Third [oculomotor] nerve palsy**
    H49.00   **Third [oculomotor] nerve palsy, unspecified eye**
    H49.01   **Third [oculomotor] nerve palsy, right eye**
    H49.02   **Third [oculomotor] nerve palsy, left eye**
    H49.03   **Third [oculomotor] nerve palsy, bilateral**

  ● **H49.1**   **Fourth [trochlear] nerve palsy**
    H49.10   **Fourth [trochlear] nerve palsy, unspecified eye**
    H49.11   **Fourth [trochlear] nerve palsy, right eye**
    H49.12   **Fourth [trochlear] nerve palsy, left eye**
    H49.13   **Fourth [trochlear] nerve palsy, bilateral**

  ● **H49.2**   **Sixth [abducent] nerve palsy**
    H49.20   **Sixth [abducent] nerve palsy, unspecified eye**
    H49.21   **Sixth [abducent] nerve palsy, right eye**
    H49.22   **Sixth [abducent] nerve palsy, left eye**
    H49.23   **Sixth [abducent] nerve palsy, bilateral**

  ● **H49.3**   **Total (external) ophthalmoplegia**
    H49.30   **Total (external) ophthalmoplegia, unspecified eye**
    H49.31   **Total (external) ophthalmoplegia, right eye**
    H49.32   **Total (external) ophthalmoplegia, left eye**
    H49.33   **Total (external) ophthalmoplegia, bilateral**

  ● **H49.4**   **Progressive external ophthalmoplegia**

| Excludes1 | Kearns-Sayre syndrome (H49.81-) |

    H49.40   **Progressive external ophthalmoplegia, unspecified eye**
    H49.41   **Progressive external ophthalmoplegia, right eye**
    H49.42   **Progressive external ophthalmoplegia, left eye**
    H49.43   **Progressive external ophthalmoplegia, bilateral**

● **H49.8**   **Other paralytic strabismus**
  ● **H49.81**   **Kearns-Sayre syndrome**
     Progressive external ophthalmoplegia with pigmentary retinopathy
     Use additional code for other manifestation, such as:
      heart block (I45.9)
    H49.811   **Kearns-Sayre syndrome, right eye**
    H49.812   **Kearns-Sayre syndrome, left eye**
    H49.813   **Kearns-Sayre syndrome, bilateral**
    H49.819   **Kearns-Sayre syndrome, unspecified eye**

  ● **H49.88**   **Other paralytic strabismus**
     External ophthalmoplegia NOS
    H49.881   **Other paralytic strabismus, right eye**
    H49.882   **Other paralytic strabismus, left eye**
    H49.883   **Other paralytic strabismus, bilateral**
    H49.889   **Other paralytic strabismus, unspecified eye**

H49.9   **Unspecified paralytic strabismus**

● **H50   Other strabismus**
  ● **H50.0**   **Esotropia**
     Convergent concomitant strabismus

| Excludes1 | intermittent esotropia (H50.31-, H50.32) |

    H50.00   **Unspecified esotropia**
  ● **H50.01**   **Monocular esotropia**
    H50.011   **Monocular esotropia, right eye**
    H50.012   **Monocular esotropia, left eye**
  ● **H50.02**   **Monocular esotropia with A pattern**
    H50.021   **Monocular esotropia with A pattern, right eye**
    H50.022   **Monocular esotropia with A pattern, left eye**
  ● **H50.03**   **Monocular esotropia with V pattern**
    H50.031   **Monocular esotropia with V pattern, right eye**
    H50.032   **Monocular esotropia with V pattern, left eye**
  ● **H50.04**   **Monocular esotropia with other noncomitancies**
    H50.041   **Monocular esotropia with other noncomitancies, right eye**
    H50.042   **Monocular esotropia with other noncomitancies, left eye**
    H50.05   **Alternating esotropia**
    H50.06   **Alternating esotropia with A pattern**
    H50.07   **Alternating esotropia with V pattern**
    H50.08   **Alternating esotropia with other noncomitancies**

  ● **H50.1**   **Exotropia**
     Misalignment in which one eye deviates outward (away from nose) while the other fixates normally
     Divergent concomitant strabismus

| Excludes1 | intermittent exotropia (H50.33-, H50.34) |

    H50.10   **Unspecified exotropia**
  ● **H50.11**   **Monocular exotropia**
    H50.111   **Monocular exotropia, right eye**
    H50.112   **Monocular exotropia, left eye**
  ● **H50.12**   **Monocular exotropia with A pattern**
    H50.121   **Monocular exotropia with A pattern, right eye**
    H50.122   **Monocular exotropia with A pattern, left eye**
  ● **H50.13**   **Monocular exotropia with V pattern**
    H50.131   **Monocular exotropia with V pattern, right eye**
    H50.132   **Monocular exotropia with V pattern, left eye**

Item 7–9   Strabismus or esotropia (crossed eyes) is a condition of the extraocular eye muscles, resulting in an inability of the eyes to focus and also affects depth perception.

Figure 7-11   **A.** Image of strabismus. **B.** Exotropia. (**A** from Yanoff: Ophthalmology, ed 3, Mosby, Inc., 2008. **B** from Rakel: Textbook of Family Practice, ed 7, Saunders, 2007)

◀ New   ◀� Revised   ~~deleted~~ Deleted   OGCR Official Guidelines   X Assign placeholder X   ● Use Additional Character(s)

| Excludes 1 | Excludes 2 | Includes | Use additional | Code first | Code also | Unspecified |

- ● H50.14 Monocular exotropia with other noncomitancies
  - H50.141 Monocular exotropia with other noncomitancies, right eye
  - H50.142 Monocular exotropia with other noncomitancies, left eye
  - H50.15 Alternating exotropia
  - H50.16 Alternating exotropia with A pattern
  - H50.17 Alternating exotropia with V pattern
  - H50.18 Alternating exotropia with other noncomitancies
- ● H50.2 Vertical strabismus
  - Hypertropia
  - H50.21 Vertical strabismus, right eye
  - H50.22 Vertical strabismus, left eye
- ● H50.3 Intermittent heterotropia
  - *Displacement of an organ or part of an organ from its normal position*
  - H50.30 Unspecified intermittent heterotropia
  - ● H50.31 Intermittent monocular esotropia
    - H50.311 Intermittent monocular esotropia, right eye
    - H50.312 Intermittent monocular esotropia, left eye
  - H50.32 Intermittent alternating esotropia
  - ● H50.33 Intermittent monocular exotropia
    - H50.331 Intermittent monocular exotropia, right eye
    - H50.332 Intermittent monocular exotropia, left eye
  - H50.34 Intermittent alternating exotropia
- ● H50.4 Other and unspecified heterotropia
  - H50.40 Unspecified heterotropia
  - ● H50.41 Cyclotropia
    - H50.411 Cyclotropia, right eye
    - H50.412 Cyclotropia, left eye
  - H50.42 Monofixation syndrome
  - H50.43 Accommodative component in esotropia
- ● H50.5 Heterophoria
  - *One or both eyes wander away from the position where both eyes are looking together in the same direction*
  - H50.50 Unspecified heterophoria
  - H50.51 Esophoria
    - *Eye deviates inward (toward the nose)*
  - H50.52 Exophoria
    - *Eye deviates outward (toward the ear)*
  - H50.53 Vertical heterophoria
  - H50.54 Cyclophoria
  - H50.55 Alternating heterophoria
- ● H50.6 Mechanical strabismus
  - H50.60 Mechanical strabismus, unspecified
  - ● H50.61 Brown's sheath syndrome
    - H50.611 Brown's sheath syndrome, right eye
    - H50.612 Brown's sheath syndrome, left eye
  - H50.69 Other mechanical strabismus
    - Strabismus due to adhesions
    - Traumatic limitation of duction of eye muscle
- ● H50.8 Other specified strabismus
  - ● H50.81 Duane's syndrome
    - H50.811 Duane's syndrome, right eye
    - H50.812 Duane's syndrome, left eye
  - H50.89 Other specified strabismus
- ● H50.9 Unspecified strabismus

- ● H51 Other disorders of binocular movement
  - H51.0 Palsy (spasm) of conjugate gaze
  - ● H51.1 Convergence insufficiency and excess
    - H51.11 Convergence insufficiency
    - H51.12 Convergence excess
  - ● H51.2 Internuclear ophthalmoplegia
    - H51.20 Internuclear ophthalmoplegia, unspecified eye
    - H51.21 Internuclear ophthalmoplegia, right eye
    - H51.22 Internuclear ophthalmoplegia, left eye
    - H51.23 Internuclear ophthalmoplegia, bilateral
  - H51.8 Other specified disorders of binocular movement
  - H51.9 Unspecified disorder of binocular movement
- ● H52 Disorders of refraction and accommodation
  - ● H52.0 Hypermetropia
    - H52.00 Hypermetropia, unspecified eye
    - H52.01 Hypermetropia, right eye
    - H52.02 Hypermetropia, left eye
    - H52.03 Hypermetropia, bilateral
  - ● H52.1 Myopia
    - **Excludes1** degenerative myopia (H44.2-)
    - H52.10 Myopia, unspecified eye
    - H52.11 Myopia, right eye
    - H52.12 Myopia, left eye
    - H52.13 Myopia, bilateral
  - ● H52.2 Astigmatism
    - ● H52.20 Unspecified astigmatism
      - H52.201 Unspecified astigmatism, right eye
      - H52.202 Unspecified astigmatism, left eye
      - H52.203 Unspecified astigmatism, bilateral
      - H52.209 Unspecified astigmatism, unspecified eye
    - ● H52.21 Irregular astigmatism
      - H52.211 Irregular astigmatism, right eye
      - H52.212 Irregular astigmatism, left eye
      - H52.213 Irregular astigmatism, bilateral
      - H52.219 Irregular astigmatism, unspecified eye
    - ● H52.22 Regular astigmatism
      - H52.221 Regular astigmatism, right eye
      - H52.222 Regular astigmatism, left eye
      - H52.223 Regular astigmatism, bilateral
      - H52.229 Regular astigmatism, unspecified eye
  - ● H52.3 Anisometropia and aniseikonia
    - H52.31 Anisometropia
    - H52.32 Aniseikonia
  - H52.4 Presbyopia
  - ● H52.5 Disorders of accommodation
    - ● H52.51 Internal ophthalmoplegia (complete) (total)
      - H52.511 Internal ophthalmoplegia (complete) (total), right eye
      - H52.512 Internal ophthalmoplegia (complete) (total), left eye
      - H52.513 Internal ophthalmoplegia (complete) (total), bilateral
      - H52.519 Internal ophthalmoplegia (complete) (total), unspecified eye

Item 7–10 Disorders of refraction: **Hypermetropia,** or farsightedness, means focus at a distance is adequate but not on close objects. **Myopia** is near-sightedness or short-sightedness and means the focus on nearby objects is clear but distant objects appear blurred. **Astigmatism** is warping of the curvature of the cornea so light rays entering do not meet a single focal point, resulting in a distorted image. **Anisometropia** is unequal refractive power in which one eye may be myopic (near-sighted) and the other hyperopic (farsighted). **Presbyopia** is the loss of focus on near objects, which occurs with age because the lens loses elasticity.

CHAPTER 7 (H00-H59)

● **H52.52**   **Paresis of accommodation**
     H52.521   Paresis of accommodation, right eye
     H52.522   Paresis of accommodation, left eye
     H52.523   Paresis of accommodation, bilateral
     H52.529   Paresis of accommodation, unspecified eye

● **H52.53**   **Spasm of accommodation**
     H52.531   Spasm of accommodation, right eye
     H52.532   Spasm of accommodation, left eye
     H52.533   Spasm of accommodation, bilateral
     H52.539   Spasm of accommodation, unspecified eye

H52.6   **Other disorders of refraction**

H52.7   **Unspecified disorder of refraction**

VISUAL DISTURBANCES AND BLINDNESS (H53-H54)

● **H53**   **Visual disturbances**

   ● **H53.0**   **Amblyopia ex anopsia**
     Excludes1   amblyopia due to vitamin A deficiency (E50.5)

     ● **H53.00**   **Unspecified amblyopia**
       H53.001   Unspecified amblyopia, right eye
       H53.002   Unspecified amblyopia, left eye
       H53.003   Unspecified amblyopia, bilateral
       H53.009   Unspecified amblyopia, unspecified eye

     ● **H53.01**   **Deprivation amblyopia**
       H53.011   Deprivation amblyopia, right eye
       H53.012   Deprivation amblyopia, left eye
       H53.013   Deprivation amblyopia, bilateral
       H53.019   Deprivation amblyopia, unspecified eye

     ● **H53.02**   **Refractive amblyopia**
       H53.021   Refractive amblyopia, right eye
       H53.022   Refractive amblyopia, left eye
       H53.023   Refractive amblyopia, bilateral
       H53.029   Refractive amblyopia, unspecified eye

     ● **H53.03**   **Strabismic amblyopia**
       Excludes1   strabismus (H50.-)
       H53.031   Strabismic amblyopia, right eye
       H53.032   Strabismic amblyopia, left eye
       H53.033   Strabismic amblyopia, bilateral
       H53.039   Strabismic amblyopia, unspecified eye

   ● **H53.1**   **Subjective visual disturbances**
     Excludes1   subjective visual disturbances due to vitamin A deficiency (E50.5)
                 visual hallucinations (R44.1)

     H53.10   Unspecified subjective visual disturbances

     H53.11   **Day blindness**
       Hemeralopia

     ● **H53.12**   **Transient visual loss**
       Scintillating scotoma
       Excludes1   amaurosis fugax (G45.3-)
                  transient retinal artery occlusion (H34.0-)
       H53.121   Transient visual loss, right eye
       H53.122   Transient visual loss, left eye
       H53.123   Transient visual loss, bilateral
       H53.129   Transient visual loss, unspecified eye

     ● **H53.13**   **Sudden visual loss**
       H53.131   Sudden visual loss, right eye
       H53.132   Sudden visual loss, left eye
       H53.133   Sudden visual loss, bilateral
       H53.139   Sudden visual loss, unspecified eye

     ● **H53.14**   **Visual discomfort**
       Asthenopia
       Photophobia
       H53.141   Visual discomfort, right eye
       H53.142   Visual discomfort, left eye
       H53.143   Visual discomfort, bilateral
       H53.149   Visual discomfort, unspecified

     H53.15   **Visual distortions of shape and size**
       Metamorphopsia

     H53.16   **Psychophysical visual disturbances**

     H53.19   **Other subjective visual disturbances**
       Visual halos

   H53.2   **Diplopia**
     Double vision

   ● **H53.3**   **Other and unspecified disorders of binocular vision**
     H53.30   Unspecified disorder of binocular vision
     H53.31   **Abnormal retinal correspondence**
     H53.32   **Fusion with defective stereopsis**
     H53.33   **Simultaneous visual perception without fusion**
     H53.34   **Suppression of binocular vision**

   ● **H53.4**   **Visual field defects**
     H53.40   Unspecified visual field defects

     ● **H53.41**   **Scotoma involving central area**
       Central scotoma
       H53.411   Scotoma involving central area, right eye
       H53.412   Scotoma involving central area, left eye
       H53.413   Scotoma involving central area, bilateral
       H53.419   Scotoma involving central area, unspecified eye

     ● **H53.42**   **Scotoma of blind spot area**
       Enlarged blind spot
       H53.421   Scotoma of blind spot area, right eye
       H53.422   Scotoma of blind spot area, left eye
       H53.423   Scotoma of blind spot area, bilateral
       H53.429   Scotoma of blind spot area, unspecified eye

     ● **H53.43**   **Sector or arcuate defects**
       Arcuate scotoma
       Bjerrum scotoma
       H53.431   Sector or arcuate defects, right eye
       H53.432   Sector or arcuate defects, left eye
       H53.433   Sector or arcuate defects, bilateral
       H53.439   Sector or arcuate defects, unspecified eye

     ● **H53.45**   **Other localized visual field defect**
       Peripheral visual field defect
       Ring scotoma NOS
       Scotoma NOS
       H53.451   Other localized visual field defect, right eye
       H53.452   Other localized visual field defect, left eye
       H53.453   Other localized visual field defect, bilateral
       H53.459   Other localized visual field defect, unspecified eye

● **H53.46   Homonymous bilateral field defects**
       Homonymous hemianopia
       Homonymous hemianopsia
       Quadrant anopia
       Quadrant anopsia

     H53.461   Homonymous bilateral field defects, right side

     H53.462   Homonymous bilateral field defects, left side

     H53.469   Homonymous bilateral field defects, unspecified side
          Homonymous bilateral field defects NOS

     H53.47   Heteronymous bilateral field defects
       Heteronymous hemianop(s)ia

● **H53.48   Generalized contraction of visual field**

     H53.481   Generalized contraction of visual field, right eye

     H53.482   Generalized contraction of visual field, left eye

     H53.483   Generalized contraction of visual field, bilateral

     H53.489   Generalized contraction of visual field, unspecified eye

● **H53.5   Color vision deficiencies**
       Color blindness

     Excludes2   day blindness (H53.11)

     H53.50   Unspecified color vision deficiencies
       Color blindness NOS

     H53.51   Achromatopsia

     H53.52   Acquired color vision deficiency

     H53.53   Deuteranomaly
       Deuteranopia

     H53.54   Protanomaly
       Protanopia

     H53.55   Tritanomaly
       Tritanopia

     H53.59   Other color vision deficiencies

● **H53.6   Night blindness**

     Excludes1   night blindness due to vitamin A deficiency (E50.5)

     H53.60   Unspecified night blindness

     H53.61   Abnormal dark adaptation curve

     H53.62   Acquired night blindness

     H53.63   Congenital night blindness

     H53.69   Other night blindness

● **H53.7   Vision sensitivity deficiencies**

     H53.71   Glare sensitivity

     H53.72   Impaired contrast sensitivity

   H53.8   Other visual disturbances

   H53.9   Unspecified visual disturbance

● **H54   Blindness and low vision**
     Note: For definition of visual impairment categories see table below.

     Code first any associated underlying cause of the blindness

     Excludes1   amaurosis fugax (G45.3)

   H54.0   Blindness, both eyes
       Visual impairment categories 3, 4, 5 in both eyes.

● **H54.1   Blindness, one eye, low vision other eye**
       Visual impairment categories 3, 4, 5 in one eye, with categories 1 or 2 in the other eye.

     H54.10   Blindness, one eye, low vision other eye, unspecified eyes

     H54.11   Blindness, right eye, low vision left eye

     H54.12   Blindness, left eye, low vision right eye

   H54.2   Low vision, both eyes
       Visual impairment categories 1 or 2 in both eyes.

   H54.3   Unqualified visual loss, both eyes
       Visual impairment category 9 in both eyes.

● **H54.4   Blindness, one eye**
       Visual impairment categories 3, 4, 5 in one eye [normal vision in other eye]

     H54.40   Blindness, one eye, unspecified eye

     H54.41   Blindness, right eye, normal vision left eye

     H54.42   Blindness, left eye, normal vision right eye

● **H54.5   Low vision, one eye**
       Visual impairment categories 1 or 2 in one eye [normal vision in other eye].

     H54.50   Low vision, one eye, unspecified eye

     H54.51   Low vision, right eye, normal vision left eye

     H54.52   Low vision, left eye, normal vision right eye

● **H54.6   Unqualified visual loss, one eye**
       Visual impairment category 9 in one eye [normal vision in other eye].

     H54.60   Unqualified visual loss, one eye, unspecified

     H54.61   Unqualified visual loss, right eye, normal vision left eye

     H54.62   Unqualified visual loss, left eye, normal vision right eye

   H54.7   Unspecified visual loss
       Visual impairment category 9 NOS

   H54.8   Legal blindness, as defined in USA
       Blindness NOS according to USA definition

     Excludes1   legal blindness with specification of impairment level (H54.0-H54.7)

     Note: The table below gives a classification of severity of visual impairment recommended by a WHO Study Group on the Prevention of Blindness, Geneva, 6-10 November 1972.

     The term 'low vision' in category H54 comprises categories 1 and 2 of the table, the term 'blindness' categories 3, 4 and 5, and the term 'unqualified visual loss' category 9.

     If the extent of the visual field is taken into account, patients with a field no greater than 10 but greater than 5 around central fixation should be placed in category 3 and patients with a field no greater than 5 around central fixation should be placed in category 4, even if the central acuity is not impaired.

Category of visual impairment	Visual acuity with best possible correction	
	Maximum less than:	**Minimum equal to or better than:**
	6/18	6/60
3/10 (0.3)	1/10 (0.1)	
20/70	20/200	
	6/60	3/60
1/10 (0.1)	1/20 (0.05)	
20/200	20/400	
	3/60	1/60 (finger counting at one meter)
1/20 (0.05)	1/50 (0.02)	
20/400	5/300 (20/1200)	
	1/60 (finger counting at one meter)	Light perception
1/50 (0.02)		
5/300		
	No light perception	
	Undetermined or unspecified	

CHAPTER 7 (H00-H59)

CHAPTER 7 (H00-H59)

OTHER DISORDERS OF EYE AND ADNEXA (H55-H57)

● **H55 Nystagmus and other irregular eye movements**

● **H55.0 Nystagmus**

Rapid, involuntary movements of the eyes in the horizontal or vertical direction.

H55.00 Unspecified nystagmus

H55.01 Congenital nystagmus

H55.02 Latent nystagmus

H55.03 Visual deprivation nystagmus

H55.04 Dissociated nystagmus

H55.09 Other forms of nystagmus

● **H55.8 Other irregular eye movements**

H55.81 Saccadic eye movements

H55.89 Other irregular eye movements

● **H57 Other disorders of eye and adnexa**

● **H57.0 Anomalies of pupillary function**

H57.00 Unspecified anomaly of pupillary function

H57.01 Argyll Robertson pupil, atypical

> Excludes1   syphilitic Argyll Robertson pupil (A52.19)

H57.02 Anisocoria

H57.03 Miosis

H57.04 Mydriasis

● H57.05 Tonic pupil

H57.051 Tonic pupil, right eye

H57.052 Tonic pupil, left eye

H57.053 Tonic pupil, bilateral

H57.059 Tonic pupil, unspecified eye

H57.09 Other anomalies of pupillary function

● **H57.1 Ocular pain**

H57.10 Ocular pain, unspecified eye

H57.11 Ocular pain, right eye

H57.12 Ocular pain, left eye

H57.13 Ocular pain, bilateral

H57.8 Other specified disorders of eye and adnexa

H57.9 Unspecified disorder of eye and adnexa

INTRAOPERATIVE AND POSTPROCEDURAL COMPLICATIONS AND DISORDERS OF EYE AND ADNEXA, NOT ELSEWHERE CLASSIFIED (H59)

● **H59 Intraoperative and postprocedural complications and disorders of eye and adnexa, not elsewhere classified**

> Excludes1   mechanical complication of intraocular lens (T85.2)
> mechanical complication of other ocular prosthetic devices, implants and grafts (T85.3)
> pseudophakia (Z96.1)
> secondary cataracts (H26.4-)

● **H59.0 Disorders of the eye following cataract surgery**

● H59.01 Keratopathy (bullous aphakic) following cataract surgery

Vitreal corneal syndrome
Vitreous (touch) syndrome

H59.011 Keratopathy (bullous aphakic) following cataract surgery, right eye

H59.012 Keratopathy (bullous aphakic) following cataract surgery, left eye

H59.013 Keratopathy (bullous aphakic) following cataract surgery, bilateral

H59.019 Keratopathy (bullous aphakic) following cataract surgery, unspecified eye

● H59.02 Cataract (lens) fragments in eye following cataract surgery

H59.021 Cataract (lens) fragments in eye following cataract surgery, right eye

H59.022 Cataract (lens) fragments in eye following cataract surgery, left eye

H59.023 Cataract (lens) fragments in eye following cataract surgery, bilateral

H59.029 Cataract (lens) fragments in eye following cataract surgery, unspecified eye

● H59.03 Cystoid macular edema following cataract surgery

H59.031 Cystoid macular edema following cataract surgery, right eye

H59.032 Cystoid macular edema following cataract surgery, left eye

H59.033 Cystoid macular edema following cataract surgery, bilateral

H59.039 Cystoid macular edema following cataract surgery, unspecified eye

● H59.09 Other disorders of the eye following cataract surgery

H59.091 Other disorders of the right eye following cataract surgery

H59.092 Other disorders of the left eye following cataract surgery

H59.093 Other disorders of the eye following cataract surgery, bilateral

H59.099 Other disorders of unspecified eye following cataract surgery

● **H59.1 Intraoperative hemorrhage and hematoma of eye and adnexa complicating a procedure**

> Excludes1   intraoperative hemorrhage and hematoma of eye and adnexa due to accidental puncture or laceration during a procedure (H59.2-)

● H59.11 Intraoperative hemorrhage and hematoma of eye and adnexa complicating an ophthalmic procedure

H59.111 Intraoperative hemorrhage and hematoma of right eye and adnexa complicating an ophthalmic procedure

H59.112 Intraoperative hemorrhage and hematoma of left eye and adnexa complicating an ophthalmic procedure

H59.113 Intraoperative hemorrhage and hematoma of eye and adnexa complicating an ophthalmic procedure, bilateral

H59.119 Intraoperative hemorrhage and hematoma of unspecified eye and adnexa complicating an ophthalmic procedure

● H59.12 Intraoperative hemorrhage and hematoma of eye and adnexa complicating other procedure

H59.121 Intraoperative hemorrhage and hematoma of right eye and adnexa complicating other procedure

H59.122 Intraoperative hemorrhage and hematoma of left eye and adnexa complicating other procedure

H59.123 Intraoperative hemorrhage and hematoma of eye and adnexa complicating other procedure, bilateral

H59.129 Intraoperative hemorrhage and hematoma of unspecified eye and adnexa complicating other procedure

◀ New   ◀‖‖ Revised   ~~deleted~~ Deleted   OGCR Official Guidelines   X Assign placeholder X   ● Use Additional Character(s)

Excludes 1   Excludes 2   Includes   Use additional   Code first   Code also   Unspecified

● H59.2   Accidental puncture and laceration of eye and adnexa during a procedure

  ● H59.21   Accidental puncture and laceration of eye and adnexa during an ophthalmic procedure

    H59.211   Accidental puncture and laceration of right eye and adnexa during an ophthalmic procedure

    H59.212   Accidental puncture and laceration of left eye and adnexa during an ophthalmic procedure

    H59.213   Accidental puncture and laceration of eye and adnexa during an ophthalmic procedure, bilateral

    H59.219   Accidental puncture and laceration of unspecified eye and adnexa during an ophthalmic procedure

  ● H59.22   Accidental puncture and laceration of eye and adnexa during other procedure

    H59.221   Accidental puncture and laceration of right eye and adnexa during other procedure

    H59.222   Accidental puncture and laceration of left eye and adnexa during other procedure

    H59.223   Accidental puncture and laceration of eye and adnexa during other procedure, bilateral

    H59.229   Accidental puncture and laceration of unspecified eye and adnexa during other procedure

● H59.3   Postprocedural hemorrhage and hematoma of eye and adnexa following a procedure

  ● H59.31   Postprocedural hemorrhage and hematoma of eye and adnexa following an ophthalmic procedure

    H59.311   Postprocedural hemorrhage and hematoma of right eye and avdnexa following an ophthalmic procedure

    H59.312   Postprocedural hemorrhage and hematoma of left eye and adnexa following an ophthalmic procedure

    H59.313   Postprocedural hemorrhage and hematoma of eye and adnexa following an ophthalmic procedure, bilateral

    H59.319   Postprocedural hemorrhage and hematoma of unspecified eye and adnexa following an ophthalmic procedure

● H59.32   Postprocedural hemorrhage and hematoma of eye and adnexa following other procedure

    H59.321   Postprocedural hemorrhage and hematoma of right eye and adnexa following other procedure

    H59.322   Postprocedural hemorrhage and hematoma of left eye and adnexa following other procedure

    H59.323   Postprocedural hemorrhage and hematoma of eye and adnexa following other procedure, bilateral

    H59.329   Postprocedural hemorrhage and hematoma of unspecified eye and adnexa following other procedure

● H59.4   Inflammation (infection) of postprocedural bleb
Postprocedural blebitis

  Excludes1   filtering (vitreous) bleb after glaucoma surgery status (Z98.83)

  H59.40   Inflammation (infection) of postprocedural bleb, unspecified

  H59.41   Inflammation (infection) of postprocedural bleb, stage 1

  H59.42   Inflammation (infection) of postprocedural bleb, stage 2

  H59.43   Inflammation (infection) of postprocedural bleb, stage 3
Bleb endophthalmitis

● H59.8   Other intraoperative and postprocedural complications and disorders of eye and adnexa, not elsewhere classified

  ● H59.81   Chorioretinal scars after surgery for detachment

    H59.811   Chorioretinal scars after surgery for detachment, right eye

    H59.812   Chorioretinal scars after surgery for detachment, left eye

    H59.813   Chorioretinal scars after surgery for detachment, bilateral

    H59.819   Chorioretinal scars after surgery for detachment, unspecified eye

  H59.88   Other intraoperative complications of eye and adnexa, not elsewhere classified

  H59.89   Other postprocedural complications and disorders of eye and adnexa, not elsewhere classified

CHAPTER 7 (H00–H59)

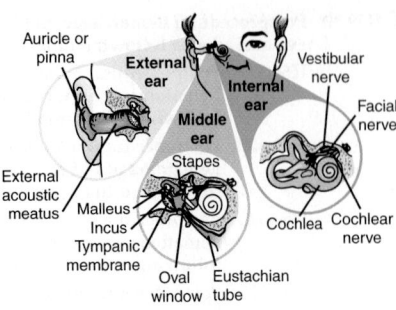

Figure 8-1   Auditory system. (From Buck CJ: Step-by-Step Medical Coding, ed 2010, Philadelphia, WB Saunders, 2010)

(See Plate 92 on page NAP-20.)

CHAPTER 8

DISEASES OF THE EAR AND MASTOID PROCESS (H60-H95)

Note: Use an external cause code following the code for the ear condition, if applicable, to identify the cause of the ear condition

Excludes2	certain conditions originating in the perinatal period (P04-P96)
	certain infectious and parasitic diseases (A00-B99)
	complications of pregnancy, childbirth and the puerperium (O00-O9A)
	congenital malformations, deformations and chromosomal abnormalities (Q00-Q99)
	endocrine, nutritional and metabolic diseases (E00-E88)
	injury, poisoning and certain other consequences of external causes (S00-T88)
	neoplasms (C00-D49)
	symptoms, signs and abnormal clinical and laboratory findings, not elsewhere classified (R00-R94)

This chapter contains the following blocks:

H60-H62	Diseases of external ear
H65-H75	Diseases of middle ear and mastoid
H80-H83	Diseases of inner ear
H90-H94	Other disorders of ear
H95	Intraoperative and postprocedural complications and disorders of ear and mastoid process, not elsewhere classified

DISEASES OF EXTERNAL EAR (H60-H62)

● **H60**   **Otitis externa**

● **H60.0**   **Abscess of external ear**
  Boil of external ear
  Carbuncle of auricle or external auditory canal
  Furuncle of external ear

  H60.00   Abscess of external ear, unspecified ear
  H60.01   Abscess of right external ear
  H60.02   Abscess of left external ear
  H60.03   Abscess of external ear, bilateral

● **H60.1**   **Cellulitis of external ear**
  Cellulitis of auricle
  Cellulitis of external auditory canal

  H60.10   Cellulitis of external ear, unspecified ear
  H60.11   Cellulitis of right external ear
  H60.12   Cellulitis of left external ear
  H60.13   Cellulitis of external ear, bilateral

● **H60.2**   **Malignant otitis externa**
  H60.20   Malignant otitis externa, unspecified ear
  H60.21   Malignant otitis externa, right ear
  H60.22   Malignant otitis externa, left ear
  H60.23   Malignant otitis externa, bilateral

● **H60.3**   **Other infective otitis externa**
  ● **H60.31**   **Diffuse otitis externa**
    H60.311   Diffuse otitis externa, right ear
    H60.312   Diffuse otitis externa, left ear
    H60.313   Diffuse otitis externa, bilateral
    H60.319   Diffuse otitis externa, unspecified ear
  ● **H60.32**   **Hemorrhagic otitis externa**
    H60.321   Hemorrhagic otitis externa, right ear
    H60.322   Hemorrhagic otitis externa, left ear
    H60.323   Hemorrhagic otitis externa, bilateral
    H60.329   Hemorrhagic otitis externa, unspecified ear
  ● **H60.33**   **Swimmer's ear**
    H60.331   Swimmer's ear, right ear
    H60.332   Swimmer's ear, left ear
    H60.333   Swimmer's ear, bilateral
    H60.339   Swimmer's ear, unspecified ear
  ● **H60.39**   **Other infective otitis externa**
    H60.391   Other infective otitis externa, right ear
    H60.392   Other infective otitis externa, left ear
    H60.393   Other infective otitis externa, bilateral
    H60.399   Other infective otitis externa, unspecified ear

● **H60.4**   **Cholesteatoma of external ear**
  Keratosis obturans of external ear (canal)

Excludes2	cholesteatoma of middle ear (H71.-)
	recurrent cholesteatoma of postmastoidectomy cavity (H95.0-)

  H60.40   Cholesteatoma of external ear, unspecified ear
  H60.41   Cholesteatoma of right external ear
  H60.42   Cholesteatoma of left external ear
  H60.43   Cholesteatoma of external ear, bilateral

● **H60.5**   **Acute noninfective otitis externa**
  ● **H60.50**   **Unspecified acute noninfective otitis externa**
    Acute otitis externa NOS
    H60.501   Unspecified acute noninfective otitis externa, right ear
    H60.502   Unspecified acute noninfective otitis externa, left ear
    H60.503   Unspecified acute noninfective otitis externa, bilateral
    H60.509   Unspecified acute noninfective otitis externa, unspecified ear
  ● **H60.51**   **Acute actinic otitis externa**
    H60.511   Acute actinic otitis externa, right ear
    H60.512   Acute actinic otitis externa, left ear
    H60.513   Acute actinic otitis externa, bilateral
    H60.519   Acute actinic otitis externa, unspecified ear
  ● **H60.52**   **Acute chemical otitis externa**
    H60.521   Acute chemical otitis externa, right ear
    H60.522   Acute chemical otitis externa, left ear
    H60.523   Acute chemical otitis externa, bilateral
    H60.529   Acute chemical otitis externa, unspecified ear
  ● **H60.53**   **Acute contact otitis externa**
    H60.531   Acute contact otitis externa, right ear
    H60.532   Acute contact otitis externa, left ear
    H60.533   Acute contact otitis externa, bilateral
    H60.539   Acute contact otitis externa, unspecified ear

● H60.54   Acute eczematoid otitis externa

     H60.541   Acute eczematoid otitis externa, right ear

     H60.542   Acute eczematoid otitis externa, left ear

     H60.543   Acute eczematoid otitis externa, bilateral

     H60.549   Acute eczematoid otitis externa, unspecified ear

● H60.55   Acute reactive otitis externa

     H60.551   Acute reactive otitis externa, right ear

     H60.552   Acute reactive otitis externa, left ear

     H60.553   Acute reactive otitis externa, bilateral

     H60.559   Acute reactive otitis externa, unspecified ear

● H60.59   Other noninfective acute otitis externa

     H60.591   Other noninfective acute otitis externa, right ear

     H60.592   Other noninfective acute otitis externa, left ear

     H60.593   Other noninfective acute otitis externa, bilateral

     H60.599   Other noninfective acute otitis externa, unspecified ear

● H60.6   Unspecified chronic otitis externa

     H60.60   Unspecified chronic otitis externa, unspecified ear

     H60.61   Unspecified chronic otitis externa, right ear

     H60.62   Unspecified chronic otitis externa, left ear

     H60.63   Unspecified chronic otitis externa, bilateral

● H60.8   Other otitis externa

   ● H60.8X   Other otitis externa

     H60.8X1   Other otitis externa, right ear

     H60.8X2   Other otitis externa, left ear

     H60.8X3   Other otitis externa, bilateral

     H60.8X9   Other otitis externa, unspecified ear

● H60.9   Unspecified otitis externa

     H60.90   Unspecified otitis externa, unspecified ear

     H60.91   Unspecified otitis externa, right ear

     H60.92   Unspecified otitis externa, left ear

     H60.93   Unspecified otitis externa, bilateral

● H61   Other disorders of external ear

   ● H61.0   Chondritis and perichondritis of external ear

     Chondrodermatitis nodularis chronica helicis

     Perichondritis of auricle

     Perichondritis of pinna

     ● H61.00   Unspecified perichondritis of external ear

     H61.001   Unspecified perichondritis of right external ear

     H61.002   Unspecified perichondritis of left external ear

     H61.003   Unspecified perichondritis of external ear, bilateral

     H61.009   Unspecified perichondritis of external ear, unspecified ear

     ● H61.01   Acute perichondritis of external ear

     H61.011   Acute perichondritis of right external ear

     H61.012   Acute perichondritis of left external ear

     H61.013   Acute perichondritis of external ear, bilateral

     H61.019   Acute perichondritis of external ear, unspecified ear

● H61.02   Chronic perichondritis of external ear

     H61.021   Chronic perichondritis of right external ear

     H61.022   Chronic perichondritis of left external ear

     H61.023   Chronic perichondritis of external ear, bilateral

     H61.029   Chronic perichondritis of external ear, unspecified ear

● H61.03   Chondritis of external ear

     Chondritis of auricle

     Chondritis of pinna

     H61.031   Chondritis of right external ear

     H61.032   Chondritis of left external ear

     H61.033   Chondritis of external ear, bilateral

     H61.039   Chondritis of external ear, unspecified ear

● H61.1   Noninfective disorders of pinna

     Excludes2   cauliflower ear (M95.1-)

                  gouty tophi of ear (M1A.-)

   ● H61.10   Unspecified noninfective disorders of pinna

     Disorder of pinna NOS

     H61.101   Unspecified noninfective disorders of pinna, right ear

     H61.102   Unspecified noninfective disorders of pinna, left ear

     H61.103   Unspecified noninfective disorders of pinna, bilateral

     H61.109   Unspecified noninfective disorders of pinna, unspecified ear

   ● H61.11   Acquired deformity of pinna

     Acquired deformity of auricle

     Excludes2   cauliflower ear (M95.1-)

     H61.111   Acquired deformity of pinna, right ear

     H61.112   Acquired deformity of pinna, left ear

     H61.113   Acquired deformity of pinna, bilateral

     H61.119   Acquired deformity of pinna, unspecified ear

   ● H61.12   Hematoma of pinna

     Hematoma of auricle

     H61.121   Hematoma of pinna, right ear

     H61.122   Hematoma of pinna, left ear

     H61.123   Hematoma of pinna, bilateral

     H61.129   Hematoma of pinna, unspecified ear

   ● H61.19   Other noninfective disorders of pinna

     H61.191   Noninfective disorders of pinna, right ear

     H61.192   Noninfective disorders of pinna, left ear

     H61.193   Noninfective disorders of pinna, bilateral

     H61.199   Noninfective disorders of pinna, unspecified ear

● H61.2   Impacted cerumen

     Wax in ear

     H61.20   Impacted cerumen, unspecified ear

     H61.21   Impacted cerumen, right ear

     H61.22   Impacted cerumen, left ear

     H61.23   Impacted cerumen, bilateral

CHAPTER 8 (H60-H95)

● **H61.3 Acquired stenosis of external ear canal**
Collapse of external ear canal
> **Excludes1**   postprocedural stenosis of external ear canal (H95.81-)

● **H61.30 Acquired stenosis of external ear canal, unspecified**
     H61.301 Acquired stenosis of right external ear canal, unspecified
     H61.302 Acquired stenosis of left external ear canal, unspecified
     H61.303 Acquired stenosis of external ear canal, unspecified, bilateral
     H61.309 Acquired stenosis of external ear canal, unspecified, unspecified ear

● **H61.31 Acquired stenosis of external ear canal secondary to trauma**
     H61.311 Acquired stenosis of right external ear canal secondary to trauma
     H61.312 Acquired stenosis of left external ear canal secondary to trauma
     H61.313 Acquired stenosis of external ear canal secondary to trauma, bilateral
     H61.319 Acquired stenosis of external ear canal secondary to trauma, unspecified ear

● **H61.32 Acquired stenosis of external ear canal secondary to inflammation and infection**
     H61.321 Acquired stenosis of right external ear canal secondary to inflammation and infection
     H61.322 Acquired stenosis of left external ear canal secondary to inflammation and infection
     H61.323 Acquired stenosis of external ear canal secondary to inflammation and infection, bilateral
     H61.329 Acquired stenosis of external ear canal secondary to inflammation and infection, unspecified ear

● **H61.39 Other acquired stenosis of external ear canal**
     H61.391 Other acquired stenosis of right external ear canal
     H61.392 Other acquired stenosis of left external ear canal
     H61.393 Other acquired stenosis of external ear canal, bilateral
     H61.399 Other acquired stenosis of external ear canal, unspecified ear

● **H61.8 Other specified disorders of external ear**
● **H61.81 Exostosis of external canal**
     H61.811 Exostosis of right external canal
     H61.812 Exostosis of left external canal
     H61.813 Exostosis of external canal, bilateral
     H61.819 Exostosis of external canal, unspecified ear

● **H61.89 Other specified disorders of external ear**
     H61.891 Other specified disorders of right external ear
     H61.892 Other specified disorders of left external ear
     H61.893 Other specified disorders of external ear, bilateral
     H61.899 Other specified disorders of external ear, unspecified ear

● **H61.9 Disorder of external ear, unspecified**
     H61.90 Disorder of external ear, unspecified, unspecified ear
     H61.91 Disorder of right external ear, unspecified
     H61.92 Disorder of left external ear, unspecified
     H61.93 Disorder of external ear, unspecified, bilateral

● **H62 Disorders of external ear in diseases classified elsewhere**
● **H62.4 Otitis externa in other diseases classified elsewhere**
Code first underlying disease, such as:
   erysipelas (A46)
   impetigo (L01.0)
> **Excludes1**   otitis externa (in):
>   candidiasis (B37.84)
>   herpes viral [herpes simplex] (B00.1)
>   herpes zoster (B02.8)

     H62.40 Otitis externa in other diseases classified elsewhere, unspecified ear
     H62.41 Otitis externa in other diseases classified elsewhere, right ear
     H62.42 Otitis externa in other diseases classified elsewhere, left ear
     H62.43 Otitis externa in other diseases classified elsewhere, bilateral

● **H62.8 Other disorders of external ear in diseases classified elsewhere**
Code first underlying disease, such as:
   gout (M1A.-, M10.-)
● **H62.8X Other disorders of external ear in diseases classified elsewhere**
     H62.8X1 Other disorders of right external ear in diseases classified elsewhere
     H62.8X2 Other disorders of left external ear in diseases classified elsewhere
     H62.8X3 Other disorders of external ear in diseases classified elsewhere, bilateral
     H62.8X9 Other disorders of external ear in diseases classified elsewhere, unspecified ear

---

DISEASES OF MIDDLE EAR AND MASTOID (H65-H75)

(See Plate 94 on page NAP-21.)

● **H65 Nonsuppurative otitis media**
Bacterial or viral infection or inflammation of the middle ear; may result in fluid accumulation with pain and temporary hearing loss.
> **Includes**   nonsuppurative otitis media with myringitis

Use additional code for any associated perforated tympanic membrane (H72.-)
Use additional code to identify:
   exposure to environmental tobacco smoke (Z77.22)
   exposure to tobacco smoke in the perinatal period (P96.81)
   history of tobacco use (Z87.891)
   occupational exposure to environmental tobacco smoke (Z57.31)
   tobacco dependence (F17.-)
   tobacco use (Z72.0)

● **H65.0 Acute serous otitis media**
Acute and subacute secretory otitis
     H65.00 Acute serous otitis media, unspecified ear
     H65.01 Acute serous otitis media, right ear
     H65.02 Acute serous otitis media, left ear
     H65.03 Acute serous otitis media, bilateral
     H65.04 Acute serous otitis media, recurrent, right ear
     H65.05 Acute serous otitis media, recurrent, left ear
     H65.06 Acute serous otitis media, recurrent, bilateral
     H65.07 Acute serous otitis media, recurrent, unspecified ear

● **H65.1 Other acute nonsuppurative otitis media**
> **Excludes1**   otitic barotrauma (T70.0)
>   otitis media (acute) NOS (H66.9)

● **H65.11 Acute and subacute allergic otitis media (mucoid) (sanguinous) (serous)**
     H65.111 Acute and subacute allergic otitis media (mucoid) (sanguinous) (serous), right ear

            H65.112   Acute and subacute allergic otitis media (mucoid) (sanguinous) (serous), left ear

            H65.113   Acute and subacute allergic otitis media (mucoid) (sanguinous) (serous), bilateral

            H65.114   Acute and subacute allergic otitis media (mucoid) (sanguinous) (serous), recurrent, right ear

            H65.115   Acute and subacute allergic otitis media (mucoid) (sanguinous) (serous), recurrent, left ear

            H65.116   Acute and subacute allergic otitis media (mucoid) (sanguinous) (serous), recurrent, bilateral

            H65.117   Acute and subacute allergic otitis media (mucoid) (sanguinous) (serous), recurrent, unspecified ear

            H65.119   Acute and subacute allergic otitis media (mucoid) (sanguinous) (serous), unspecified ear

● **H65.19**   Other acute nonsuppurative otitis media
      Acute and subacute mucoid otitis media
      Acute and subacute nonsuppurative otitis media NOS
      Acute and subacute sanguinous otitis media
      Acute and subacute seromucinous otitis media

            H65.191   Other acute nonsuppurative otitis media, right ear

            H65.192   Other acute nonsuppurative otitis media, left ear

            H65.193   Other acute nonsuppurative otitis media, bilateral

            H65.194   Other acute nonsuppurative otitis media, recurrent, right ear

            H65.195   Other acute nonsuppurative otitis media, recurrent, left ear

            H65.196   Other acute nonsuppurative otitis media, recurrent, bilateral

            H65.197   Other acute nonsuppurative otitis media recurrent, unspecified ear

            H65.199   Other acute nonsuppurative otitis media, unspecified ear

● **H65.2**   Chronic serous otitis media
      Chronic tubotympanal catarrh

     H65.20   Chronic serous otitis media, unspecified ear

     H65.21   Chronic serous otitis media, right ear

     H65.22   Chronic serous otitis media, left ear

     H65.23   Chronic serous otitis media, bilateral

● **H65.3**   Chronic mucoid otitis media
      Chronic mucinous otitis media
      Chronic secretory otitis media
      Chronic transudative otitis media
      Glue ear

      Excludes1   adhesive middle ear disease (H74.1)

     H65.30   Chronic mucoid otitis media, unspecified ear

     H65.31   Chronic mucoid otitis media, right ear

     H65.32   Chronic mucoid otitis media, left ear

     H65.33   Chronic mucoid otitis media, bilateral

● **H65.4**   Other chronic nonsuppurative otitis media

   ● **H65.41**   Chronic allergic otitis media

            H65.411   Chronic allergic otitis media, right ear

            H65.412   Chronic allergic otitis media, left ear

            H65.413   Chronic allergic otitis media, bilateral

            H65.419   Chronic allergic otitis media, unspecified ear

● **H65.49**   Other chronic nonsuppurative otitis media
      Chronic exudative otitis media
      Chronic nonsuppurative otitis media NOS
      Chronic otitis media with effusion (nonpurulent)
      Chronic seromucinous otitis media

            H65.491   Other chronic nonsuppurative otitis media, right ear

            H65.492   Other chronic nonsuppurative otitis media, left ear

            H65.493   Other chronic nonsuppurative otitis media, bilateral

            H65.499   Other chronic nonsuppurative otitis media, unspecified ear

● **H65.9**   Unspecified nonsuppurative otitis media
      Allergic otitis media NOS
      Catarrhal otitis media NOS
      Exudative otitis media NOS
      Mucoid otitis media NOS
      Otitis media with effusion (nonpurulent) NOS
      Secretory otitis media NOS
      Seromucinous otitis media NOS
      Serous otitis media NOS
      Transudative otitis media NOS

     H65.90   Unspecified nonsuppurative otitis media, unspecified ear

     H65.91   Unspecified nonsuppurative otitis media, right ear

     H65.92   Unspecified nonsuppurative otitis media, left ear

     H65.93   Unspecified nonsuppurative otitis media, bilateral

● **H66**   Suppurative and unspecified otitis media
     Suppurative: Discharging pus

     Includes   suppurative and unspecified otitis media with myringitis

   Use additional code to identify:
     exposure to environmental tobacco smoke (Z77.22)
     exposure to tobacco smoke in the perinatal period (P96.81)
     history of tobacco use (Z87.891)
     occupational exposure to environmental tobacco smoke (Z57.31)
     tobacco dependence (F17.-)
     tobacco use (Z72.0)

   ● **H66.0**   Acute suppurative otitis media

     ● **H66.00**   Acute suppurative otitis media without spontaneous rupture of ear drum

            H66.001   Acute suppurative otitis media without spontaneous rupture of ear drum, right ear

            H66.002   Acute suppurative otitis media without spontaneous rupture of ear drum, left ear

            H66.003   Acute suppurative otitis media without spontaneous rupture of ear drum, bilateral

            H66.004   Acute suppurative otitis media without spontaneous rupture of ear drum, recurrent, right ear

            H66.005   Acute suppurative otitis media without spontaneous rupture of ear drum, recurrent, left ear

            H66.006   Acute suppurative otitis media without spontaneous rupture of ear drum, recurrent, bilateral

            H66.007   Acute suppurative otitis media without spontaneous rupture of ear drum, recurrent, unspecified ear

            H66.009   Acute suppurative otitis media without spontaneous rupture of ear drum, unspecified ear

● H66.01   Acute suppurative otitis media with spontaneous rupture of ear drum

    H66.011   Acute suppurative otitis media with spontaneous rupture of ear drum, right ear

    H66.012   Acute suppurative otitis media with spontaneous rupture of ear drum, left ear

    H66.013   Acute suppurative otitis media with spontaneous rupture of ear drum, bilateral

    H66.014   Acute suppurative otitis media with spontaneous rupture of ear drum, recurrent, right ear

    H66.015   Acute suppurative otitis media with spontaneous rupture of ear drum, recurrent, left ear

    H66.016   Acute suppurative otitis media with spontaneous rupture of ear drum, recurrent, bilateral

    H66.017   Acute suppurative otitis media with spontaneous rupture of ear drum, recurrent, unspecified ear

    H66.019   Acute suppurative otitis media with spontaneous rupture of ear drum, unspecified ear

● H66.1   Chronic tubotympanic suppurative otitis media

    Benign chronic suppurative otitis media
    Chronic tubotympanic disease

    Use additional code for any associated perforated tympanic membrane (H72.-)

    H66.10   Chronic tubotympanic suppurative otitis media, unspecified

    H66.11   Chronic tubotympanic suppurative otitis media, right ear

    H66.12   Chronic tubotympanic suppurative otitis media, left ear

    H66.13   Chronic tubotympanic suppurative otitis media, bilateral

● H66.2   Chronic atticoantral suppurative otitis media

    Chronic atticoantral disease

    Use additional code for any associated perforated tympanic membrane (H72.-)

    H66.20   Chronic atticoantral suppurative otitis media, unspecified ear

    H66.21   Chronic atticoantral suppurative otitis media, right ear

    H66.22   Chronic atticoantral suppurative otitis media, left ear

    H66.23   Chronic atticoantral suppurative otitis media, bilateral

● H66.3   Other chronic suppurative otitis media

    Chronic suppurative otitis media NOS

    Use additional code for any associated perforated tympanic membrane (H72.-)

    Excludes1   tuberculous otitis media (A18.6)

● H66.3X   Other chronic suppurative otitis media

    H66.3X1   Other chronic suppurative otitis media, right ear

    H66.3X2   Other chronic suppurative otitis media, left ear

    H66.3X3   Other chronic suppurative otitis media, bilateral

    H66.3X9   Other chronic suppurative otitis media, unspecified ear

● H66.4   Suppurative otitis media, unspecified

    Purulent otitis media NOS

    Use additional code for any associated perforated tympanic membrane (H72.-)

    H66.40   Suppurative otitis media, unspecified, unspecified ear

    H66.41   Suppurative otitis media, unspecified, right ear

    H66.42   Suppurative otitis media, unspecified, left ear

    H66.43   Suppurative otitis media, unspecified, bilateral

● H66.9   Otitis media, unspecified

    Otitis media NOS
    Acute otitis media NOS
    Chronic otitis media NOS

    Use additional code for any associated perforated tympanic membrane (H72.-)

    H66.90   Otitis media, unspecified, unspecified ear

    H66.91   Otitis media, unspecified, right ear

    H66.92   Otitis media, unspecified, left ear

    H66.93   Otitis media, unspecified, bilateral

● H67   Otitis media in diseases classified elsewhere

    Code first underlying disease, such as:
    viral disease NEC (B00-B34)

    Use additional code for any associated perforated tympanic membrane (H72.-)

    Excludes1   otitis media in:
        influenza (J09.X9, J10.83, J11.83)
        measles (B05.3)
        scarlet fever (A38.0)
        tuberculosis (A18.6)

    H67.1   Otitis media in diseases classified elsewhere, right ear

    H67.2   Otitis media in diseases classified elsewhere, left ear

    H67.3   Otitis media in diseases classified elsewhere, bilateral

    H67.9   Otitis media in diseases classified elsewhere, unspecified ear

● H68   Eustachian salpingitis and obstruction

   ● H68.0   Eustachian salpingitis

     ● H68.00   Unspecified Eustachian salpingitis

      H68.001   Unspecified Eustachian salpingitis, right ear

      H68.002   Unspecified Eustachian salpingitis, left ear

      H68.003   Unspecified Eustachian salpingitis, bilateral

      H68.009   Unspecified Eustachian salpingitis, unspecified ear

     ● H68.01   Acute Eustachian salpingitis

      H68.011   Acute Eustachian salpingitis, right ear

      H68.012   Acute Eustachian salpingitis, left ear

      H68.013   Acute Eustachian salpingitis, bilateral

      H68.019   Acute Eustachian salpingitis, unspecified ear

     ● H68.02   Chronic Eustachian salpingitis

      H68.021   Chronic Eustachian salpingitis, right ear

      H68.022   Chronic Eustachian salpingitis, left ear

      H68.023   Chronic Eustachian salpingitis, bilateral

      H68.029   Chronic Eustachian salpingitis, unspecified ear

- **H68.1 Obstruction of Eustachian tube**
  Stenosis of Eustachian tube
  Stricture of Eustachian tube
  - **H68.10 Unspecified obstruction of Eustachian tube**
    - H68.101 Unspecified obstruction of Eustachian tube, right ear
    - H68.102 Unspecified obstruction of Eustachian tube, left ear
    - H68.103 Unspecified obstruction of Eustachian tube, bilateral
    - H68.109 Unspecified obstruction of Eustachian tube, unspecified ear
  - **H68.11 Osseous obstruction of Eustachian tube**
    - H68.111 Osseous obstruction of Eustachian tube, right ear
    - H68.112 Osseous obstruction of Eustachian tube, left ear
    - H68.113 Osseous obstruction of Eustachian tube, bilateral
    - H68.119 Osseous obstruction of Eustachian tube, unspecified ear
  - **H68.12 Intrinsic cartilagenous obstruction of Eustachian tube**
    - H68.121 Intrinsic cartilagenous obstruction of Eustachian tube, right ear
    - H68.122 Intrinsic cartilagenous obstruction of Eustachian tube, left ear
    - H68.123 Intrinsic cartilagenous obstruction of Eustachian tube, bilateral
    - H68.129 Intrinsic cartilagenous obstruction of Eustachian tube, unspecified ear
  - **H68.13 Extrinsic cartilagenous obstruction of Eustachian tube**
    Compression of Eustachian tube
    - H68.131 Extrinsic cartilagenous obstruction of Eustachian tube, right ear
    - H68.132 Extrinsic cartilagenous obstruction of Eustachian tube, left ear
    - H68.133 Extrinsic cartilagenous obstruction of Eustachian tube, bilateral
    - H68.139 Extrinsic cartilagenous obstruction of Eustachian tube, unspecified ear
- **H69 Other and unspecified disorders of Eustachian tube**
  - **H69.0 Patulous Eustachian tube**
    - H69.00 Patulous Eustachian tube, unspecified ear
    - H69.01 Patulous Eustachian tube, right ear
    - H69.02 Patulous Eustachian tube, left ear
    - H69.03 Patulous Eustachian tube, bilateral
  - **H69.8 Other specified disorders of Eustachian tube**
    - H69.80 Other specified disorders of Eustachian tube, unspecified ear
    - H69.81 Other specified disorders of Eustachian tube, right ear
    - H69.82 Other specified disorders of Eustachian tube, left ear
    - H69.83 Other specified disorders of Eustachian tube, bilateral
  - **H69.9 Unspecified Eustachian tube disorder**
    - H69.90 Unspecified Eustachian tube disorder, unspecified ear
    - H69.91 Unspecified Eustachian tube disorder, right ear
    - H69.92 Unspecified Eustachian tube disorder, left ear
    - H69.93 Unspecified Eustachian tube disorder, bilateral

- **H70 Mastoiditis and related conditions**
  - **H70.0 Acute mastoiditis**
    Abscess of mastoid
    Empyema of mastoid
    - **H70.00 Acute mastoiditis without complications**
      - H70.001 Acute mastoiditis without complications, right ear
      - H70.002 Acute mastoiditis without complications, left ear
      - H70.003 Acute mastoiditis without complications, bilateral
      - H70.009 Acute mastoiditis without complications, unspecified ear
    - **H70.01 Subperiosteal abscess of mastoid**
      - H70.011 Subperiosteal abscess of mastoid, right ear
      - H70.012 Subperiosteal abscess of mastoid, left ear
      - H70.013 Subperiosteal abscess of mastoid, bilateral
      - H70.019 Subperiosteal abscess of mastoid, unspecified ear
    - **H70.09 Acute mastoiditis with other complications**
      - H70.091 Acute mastoiditis with other complications, right ear
      - H70.092 Acute mastoiditis with other complications, left ear
      - H70.093 Acute mastoiditis with other complications, bilateral
      - H70.099 Acute mastoiditis with other complications, unspecified ear
  - **H70.1 Chronic mastoiditis**
    Caries of mastoid
    Fistula of mastoid
    Excludes1 tuberculous mastoiditis (A18.03)
    - H70.10 Chronic mastoiditis, unspecified ear
    - H70.11 Chronic mastoiditis, right ear
    - H70.12 Chronic mastoiditis, left ear
    - H70.13 Chronic mastoiditis, bilateral
  - **H70.2 Petrositis**
    Inflammation of petrous bone
    - **H70.20 Unspecified petrositis**
      - H70.201 Unspecified petrositis, right ear
      - H70.202 Unspecified petrositis, left ear
      - H70.203 Unspecified petrositis, bilateral
      - H70.209 Unspecified petrositis, unspecified ear
    - **H70.21 Acute petrositis**
      - H70.211 Acute petrositis, right ear
      - H70.212 Acute petrositis, left ear
      - H70.213 Acute petrositis, bilateral
      - H70.219 Acute petrositis, unspecified ear
    - **H70.22 Chronic petrositis**
      - H70.221 Chronic petrositis, right ear
      - H70.222 Chronic petrositis, left ear
      - H70.223 Chronic petrositis, bilateral
      - H70.229 Chronic petrositis, unspecified ear
  - **H70.8 Other mastoiditis and related conditions**
    Excludes1 preauricular sinus and cyst (Q18.1)
    sinus, fistula, and cyst of branchial cleft (Q18.0)
    - **H70.81 Postauricular fistula**
      - H70.811 Postauricular fistula, right ear
      - H70.812 Postauricular fistula, left ear
      - H70.813 Postauricular fistula, bilateral
      - H70.819 Postauricular fistula, unspecified ear

◀ New   Revised   ~~deleted~~ Deleted   OGCR Official Guidelines   X Assign placeholder X   ● Use Additional Character(s)
Excludes 1   Excludes 2   Includes   Use additional   Code first   Code also   Unspecified

CHAPTER 8 (H60-H95)

901

Item 8–1 Mastoiditis is an infection of the portion of the temporal bone of the skull that is behind the ear (mastoid process) caused by an untreated otitis media, leading to an infection of the surrounding structures which may include the brain.

● H70.89 Other mastoiditis and related conditions
  H70.891 Other mastoiditis and related conditions, right ear
  H70.892 Other mastoiditis and related conditions, left ear
  H70.893 Other mastoiditis and related conditions, bilateral
  H70.899 Other mastoiditis and related conditions, unspecified ear
● H70.9 Unspecified mastoiditis
  H70.90 Unspecified mastoiditis, unspecified ear
  H70.91 Unspecified mastoiditis, right ear
  H70.92 Unspecified mastoiditis, left ear
  H70.93 Unspecified mastoiditis, bilateral

● H71 Cholesteatoma of middle ear
  Excludes2 cholesteatoma of external ear (H60.4-)
  recurrent cholesteatoma of postmastoidectomy cavity (H95.0-)
● H71.0 Cholesteatoma of attic
  H71.00 Cholesteatoma of attic, unspecified ear
  H71.01 Cholesteatoma of attic, right ear
  H71.02 Cholesteatoma of attic, left ear
  H71.03 Cholesteatoma of attic, bilateral
● H71.1 Cholesteatoma of tympanum
  H71.10 Cholesteatoma of tympanum, unspecified ear
  H71.11 Cholesteatoma of tympanum, right ear
  H71.12 Cholesteatoma of tympanum, left ear
  H71.13 Cholesteatoma of tympanum, bilateral
● H71.2 Cholesteatoma of mastoid
  H71.20 Cholesteatoma of mastoid, unspecified ear
  H71.21 Cholesteatoma of mastoid, right ear
  H71.22 Cholesteatoma of mastoid, left ear
  H71.23 Cholesteatoma of mastoid, bilateral
● H71.3 Diffuse cholesteatosis
  H71.30 Diffuse cholesteatosis, unspecified ear
  H71.31 Diffuse cholesteatosis, right ear
  H71.32 Diffuse cholesteatosis, left ear
  H71.33 Diffuse cholesteatosis, bilateral
● H71.9 Unspecified cholesteatoma
  H71.90 Unspecified cholesteatoma, unspecified ear
  H71.91 Unspecified cholesteatoma, right ear
  H71.92 Unspecified cholesteatoma, left ear
  H71.93 Unspecified cholesteatoma, bilateral

(See Plate 93 on page NAP-21.)

● H72 Perforation of tympanic membrane
  Hole or rupture in ear drum
  Includes persistent post-traumatic perforation of ear drum
  postinflammatory perforation of ear drum
  Code first any associated otitis media (H65.-, H66.1-, H66.2-, H66.3-, H66.4-, H66.9-, H67.-)
  Excludes1 acute suppurative otitis media with rupture of the tympanic membrane (H66.01-)
  traumatic rupture of ear drum (S09.2-)
● H72.0 Central perforation of tympanic membrane
  H72.00 Central perforation of tympanic membrane, unspecified ear
  H72.01 Central perforation of tympanic membrane, right ear

H72.02 Central perforation of tympanic membrane, left ear
H72.03 Central perforation of tympanic membrane, bilateral
● H72.1 Attic perforation of tympanic membrane
  Perforation of pars flaccida
  H72.10 Attic perforation of tympanic membrane, unspecified ear
  H72.11 Attic perforation of tympanic membrane, right ear
  H72.12 Attic perforation of tympanic membrane, left ear
  H72.13 Attic perforation of tympanic membrane, bilateral
● H72.2 Other marginal perforations of tympanic membrane
● H72.2X Other marginal perforations of tympanic membrane
  H72.2X1 Other marginal perforations of tympanic membrane, right ear
  H72.2X2 Other marginal perforations of tympanic membrane, left ear
  H72.2X3 Other marginal perforations of tympanic membrane, bilateral
  H72.2X9 Other marginal perforations of tympanic membrane, unspecified ear
● H72.8 Other perforations of tympanic membrane
● H72.81 Multiple perforations of tympanic membrane
  H72.811 Multiple perforations of tympanic membrane, right ear
  H72.812 Multiple perforations of tympanic membrane, left ear
  H72.813 Multiple perforations of tympanic membrane, bilateral
  H72.819 Multiple perforations of tympanic membrane, unspecified ear
● H72.82 Total perforations of tympanic membrane
  H72.821 Total perforations of tympanic membrane, right ear
  H72.822 Total perforations of tympanic membrane, left ear
  H72.823 Total perforations of tympanic membrane, bilateral
  H72.829 Total perforations of tympanic membrane, unspecified ear
● H72.9 Unspecified perforation of tympanic membrane
  H72.90 Unspecified perforation of tympanic membrane, unspecified ear
  H72.91 Unspecified perforation of tympanic membrane, right ear
  H72.92 Unspecified perforation of tympanic membrane, left ear
  H72.93 Unspecified perforation of tympanic membrane, bilateral

● H73 Other disorders of tympanic membrane
● H73.0 Acute myringitis
  Excludes1 acute myringitis with otitis media (H65, H66)
● H73.00 Unspecified acute myringitis
  Acute tympanitis NOS
  H73.001 Acute myringitis, right ear
  H73.002 Acute myringitis, left ear
  H73.003 Acute myringitis, bilateral
  H73.009 Acute myringitis, unspecified ear
● H73.01 Bullous myringitis
  H73.011 Bullous myringitis, right ear
  H73.012 Bullous myringitis, left ear
  H73.013 Bullous myringitis, bilateral
  H73.019 Bullous myringitis, unspecified ear

● **H73.09**   Other acute myringitis
     H73.091   Other acute myringitis, right ear
     H73.092   Other acute myringitis, left ear
     H73.093   Other acute myringitis, bilateral
     H73.099   Other acute myringitis, unspecified ear

● **H73.1**   Chronic myringitis
     Chronic tympanitis
     Excludes1   chronic myringitis with otitis media (H65, H66)
     H73.10   Chronic myringitis, unspecified ear
     H73.11   Chronic myringitis, right ear
     H73.12   Chronic myringitis, left ear
     H73.13   Chronic myringitis, bilateral

● **H73.2**   Unspecified myringitis
     H73.20   Unspecified myringitis, unspecified ear
     H73.21   Unspecified myringitis, right ear
     H73.22   Unspecified myringitis, left ear
     H73.23   Unspecified myringitis, bilateral

● **H73.8**   Other specified disorders of tympanic membrane
   ● **H73.81**   Atrophic flaccid tympanic membrane
     H73.811   Atrophic flaccid tympanic membrane, right ear
     H73.812   Atrophic flaccid tympanic membrane, left ear
     H73.813   Atrophic flaccid tympanic membrane, bilateral
     H73.819   Atrophic flaccid tympanic membrane, unspecified ear
   ● **H73.82**   Atrophic nonflaccid tympanic membrane
     H73.821   Atrophic nonflaccid tympanic membrane, right ear
     H73.822   Atrophic nonflaccid tympanic membrane, left ear
     H73.823   Atrophic nonflaccid tympanic membrane, bilateral
     H73.829   Atrophic nonflaccid tympanic membrane, unspecified ear
   ● **H73.89**   Other specified disorders of tympanic membrane
     H73.891   Other specified disorders of tympanic membrane, right ear
     H73.892   Other specified disorders of tympanic membrane, left ear
     H73.893   Other specified disorders of tympanic membrane, bilateral
     H73.899   Other specified disorders of tympanic membrane, unspecified ear

● **H73.9**   Unspecified disorder of tympanic membrane
     H73.90   Unspecified disorder of tympanic membrane, unspecified ear
     H73.91   Unspecified disorder of tympanic membrane, right ear
     H73.92   Unspecified disorder of tympanic membrane, left ear
     H73.93   Unspecified disorder of tympanic membrane, bilateral

● **H74**   Other disorders of middle ear mastoid
     Excludes2   mastoiditis (H70.-)
   ● **H74.0**   Tympanosclerosis
     H74.01   Tympanosclerosis, right ear
     H74.02   Tympanosclerosis, left ear
     H74.03   Tympanosclerosis, bilateral
     H74.09   Tympanosclerosis, unspecified ear

● **H74.1**   Adhesive middle ear disease
     Adhesive otitis
     Excludes1   glue ear (H65.3-)
     H74.11   Adhesive right middle ear disease
     H74.12   Adhesive left middle ear disease
     H74.13   Adhesive middle ear disease, bilateral
     H74.19   Adhesive middle ear disease, unspecified ear

● **H74.2**   Discontinuity and dislocation of ear ossicles
     H74.20   Discontinuity and dislocation of ear ossicles, unspecified ear
     H74.21   Discontinuity and dislocation of right ear ossicles
     H74.22   Discontinuity and dislocation of left ear ossicles
     H74.23   Discontinuity and dislocation of ear ossicles, bilateral

● **H74.3**   Other acquired abnormalities of ear ossicles
   ● **H74.31**   Ankylosis of ear ossicles
     H74.311   Ankylosis of ear ossicles, right ear
     H74.312   Ankylosis of ear ossicles, left ear
     H74.313   Ankylosis of ear ossicles, bilateral
     H74.319   Ankylosis of ear ossicles, unspecified ear
   ● **H74.32**   Partial loss of ear ossicles
     H74.321   Partial loss of ear ossicles, right ear
     H74.322   Partial loss of ear ossicles, left ear
     H74.323   Partial loss of ear ossicles, bilateral
     H74.329   Partial loss of ear ossicles, unspecified ear
   ● **H74.39**   Other acquired abnormalities of ear ossicles
     H74.391   Other acquired abnormalities of right ear ossicles
     H74.392   Other acquired abnormalities of left ear ossicles
     H74.393   Other acquired abnormalities of ear ossicles, bilateral
     H74.399   Other acquired abnormalities of ear ossicles, unspecified ear

● **H74.4**   Polyp of middle ear
     H74.40   Polyp of middle ear, unspecified ear
     H74.41   Polyp of right middle ear
     H74.42   Polyp of left middle ear
     H74.43   Polyp of middle ear, bilateral

● **H74.8**   Other specified disorders of middle ear and mastoid
   ● **H74.8X**   Other specified disorders of middle ear and mastoid
     H74.8X1   Other specified disorders of right middle ear and mastoid
     H74.8X2   Other specified disorders of left middle ear and mastoid
     H74.8X3   Other specified disorders of middle ear and mastoid, bilateral
     H74.8X9   Other specified disorders of middle ear and mastoid, unspecified ear

● **H74.9**   Unspecified disorder of middle ear and mastoid
     H74.90   Unspecified disorder of middle ear and mastoid, unspecified ear
     H74.91   Unspecified disorder of right middle ear and mastoid
     H74.92   Unspecified disorder of left middle ear and mastoid
     H74.93   Unspecified disorder of middle ear and mastoid, bilateral

CHAPTER 8 (H60-H95)

◀ New   ◀⁞⁞⁞ Revised   ~~deleted~~ Deleted   **OGCR** Official Guidelines   X Assign placeholder X   ● Use Additional Character(s)

Excludes 1   Excludes 2   Includes   Use additional   Code first   Code also   Unspecified

903

● **H75　Other disorders of middle ear and mastoid in diseases classified elsewhere**

　Code first underlying disease

　● **H75.0　Mastoiditis in infectious and parasitic diseases classified elsewhere**

　　| Excludes1 | mastoiditis (in):
　　　　　　　　　syphilis (A52.77)
　　　　　　　　　tuberculosis (A18.03) |

　　H75.00　Mastoiditis in infectious and parasitic diseases classified elsewhere, unspecified ear

　　H75.01　Mastoiditis in infectious and parasitic diseases classified elsewhere, right ear

　　H75.02　Mastoiditis in infectious and parasitic diseases classified elsewhere, left ear

　　H75.03　Mastoiditis in infectious and parasitic diseases classified elsewhere, bilateral

　● **H75.8　Other specified disorders of middle ear and mastoid in diseases classified elsewhere**

　　H75.80　Other specified disorders of middle ear and mastoid in diseases classified elsewhere, unspecified ear

　　H75.81　Other specified disorders of right middle ear and mastoid in diseases classified elsewhere

　　H75.82　Other specified disorders of left middle ear and mastoid in diseases classified elsewhere

　　H75.83　Other specified disorders of middle ear and mastoid in diseases classified elsewhere, bilateral

---

DISEASES OF INNER EAR (H80-H83)

(See Plate 95 on page NAP-21.)

● **H80　Otosclerosis**

　Inherited middle ear spongelike bone growth causing hearing loss

　| Includes | Otospongiosis |

　● **H80.0　Otosclerosis involving oval window, nonobliterative**

　　H80.00　Otosclerosis involving oval window, nonobliterative, unspecified ear

　　H80.01　Otosclerosis involving oval window, nonobliterative, right ear

　　H80.02　Otosclerosis involving oval window, nonobliterative, left ear

　　H80.03　Otosclerosis involving oval window, nonobliterative, bilateral

　● **H80.1　Otosclerosis involving oval window, obliterative**

　　H80.10　Otosclerosis involving oval window, obliterative, unspecified ear

　　H80.11　Otosclerosis involving oval window, obliterative, right ear

　　H80.12　Otosclerosis involving oval window, obliterative, left ear

　　H80.13　Otosclerosis involving oval window, obliterative, bilateral

　● **H80.2　Cochlear otosclerosis**

　　Otosclerosis involving otic capsule
　　Otosclerosis involving round window

　　H80.20　Cochlear otosclerosis, unspecified ear

　　H80.21　Cochlear otosclerosis, right ear

　　H80.22　Cochlear otosclerosis, left ear

　　H80.23　Cochlear otosclerosis, bilateral

　● **H80.8　Other otosclerosis**

　　H80.80　Other otosclerosis, unspecified ear

　　H80.81　Other otosclerosis, right ear

　　H80.82　Other otosclerosis, left ear

　　H80.83　Other otosclerosis, bilateral

● **H80.9　Unspecified otosclerosis**

　　H80.90　Unspecified otosclerosis, unspecified ear

　　H80.91　Unspecified otosclerosis, right ear

　　H80.92　Unspecified otosclerosis, left ear

　　H80.93　Unspecified otosclerosis, bilateral

● **H81　Disorders of vestibular function**

　| Excludes1 | epidemic vertigo (A88.1)
　　　　　　　　vertigo NOS (R42) |

　● **H81.0　Ménière's disease**

　　Vestibular disorder that produces recurring symptoms including severe and intermittent hearing loss including the feeling of ear pressure or pain.

　　Labyrinthine hydrops
　　Ménière's syndrome or vertigo

　　H81.01　Ménière's disease, right ear

　　H81.02　Ménière's disease, left ear

　　H81.03　Ménière's disease, bilateral

　　H81.09　Ménière's disease, unspecified ear

　● **H81.1　Benign paroxysmal vertigo**

　　H81.10　Benign paroxysmal vertigo, unspecified ear

　　H81.11　Benign paroxysmal vertigo, right ear

　　H81.12　Benign paroxysmal vertigo, left ear

　　H81.13　Benign paroxysmal vertigo, bilateral

　● **H81.2　Vestibular neuronitis**

　　H81.20　Vestibular neuronitis, unspecified ear

　　H81.21　Vestibular neuronitis, right ear

　　H81.22　Vestibular neuronitis, left ear

　　H81.23　Vestibular neuronitis, bilateral

　● **H81.3　Other peripheral vertigo**

　　● **H81.31　Aural vertigo**

　　　H81.311　Aural vertigo, right ear

　　　H81.312　Aural vertigo, left ear

　　　H81.313　Aural vertigo, bilateral

　　　H81.319　Aural vertigo, unspecified ear

　　● **H81.39　Other peripheral vertigo**

　　　Lermoyez' syndrome
　　　Otogenic vertigo
　　　Peripheral vertigo NOS

　　　H81.391　Other peripheral vertigo, right ear

　　　H81.392　Other peripheral vertigo, left ear

　　　H81.393　Other peripheral vertigo, bilateral

　　　H81.399　Other peripheral vertigo, unspecified ear

　● **H81.4　Vertigo of central origin**

　　Central positional nystagmus

　　H81.41　Vertigo of central origin, right ear

　　H81.42　Vertigo of central origin, left ear

　　H81.43　Vertigo of central origin, bilateral

　　H81.49　Vertigo of central origin, unspecified ear

　● **H81.8　Other disorders of vestibular function**

　　● **H81.8X　Other disorders of vestibular function**

　　　H81.8X1　Other disorders of vestibular function, right ear

　　　H81.8X2　Other disorders of vestibular function, left ear

　　　H81.8X3　Other disorders of vestibular function, bilateral

　　　H81.8X9　Other disorders of vestibular function, unspecified ear

---

● H81.9 **Unspecified disorder of vestibular function**
Vertiginous syndrome NOS

H81.90 **Unspecified** disorder of vestibular function, unspecified ear

H81.91 **Unspecified** disorder of vestibular function, right ear

H81.92 **Unspecified** disorder of vestibular function, left ear

H81.93 **Unspecified** disorder of vestibular function, bilateral

● H82 **Vertiginous syndromes in diseases classified elsewhere**
Code first underlying disease
Excludes1 epidemic vertigo (A88.1)

H82.1 **Vertiginous syndromes in diseases classified elsewhere, right ear**

H82.2 **Vertiginous syndromes in diseases classified elsewhere, left ear**

H82.3 **Vertiginous syndromes in diseases classified elsewhere, bilateral**

H82.9 **Vertiginous syndromes in diseases classified elsewhere, unspecified ear**

● H83 **Other diseases of inner ear**

● H83.0 **Labyrinthitis**
Balance disorder that follows URI or head injury.

H83.01 **Labyrinthitis, right ear**

H83.02 **Labyrinthitis, left ear**

H83.03 **Labyrinthitis, bilateral**

H83.09 **Labyrinthitis, unspecified ear**

● H83.1 **Labyrinthine fistula**

H83.11 **Labyrinthine fistula, right ear**

H83.12 **Labyrinthine fistula, left ear**

H83.13 **Labyrinthine fistula, bilateral**

H83.19 **Labyrinthine fistula, unspecified ear**

● H83.2 **Labyrinthine dysfunction**
Labyrinthine hypersensitivity
Labyrinthine hypofunction
Labyrinthine loss of function

● H83.2X **Labyrinthine dysfunction**

H83.2X1 **Labyrinthine dysfunction, right ear**

H83.2X2 **Labyrinthine dysfunction, left ear**

H83.2X3 **Labyrinthine dysfunction, bilateral**

H83.2X9 **Labyrinthine dysfunction, unspecified ear**

● H83.3 **Noise effects on inner ear**
Acoustic trauma of inner ear
Noise-induced hearing loss of inner ear

● H83.3X **Noise effects on inner ear**

H83.3X1 **Noise effects on right inner ear**

H83.3X2 **Noise effects on left inner ear**

H83.3X3 **Noise effects on inner ear, bilateral**

H83.3X9 **Noise effects on inner ear, unspecified ear**

● H83.8 **Other specified diseases of inner ear**

● H83.8X **Other specified diseases of inner ear**

H83.8X1 **Other specified diseases of right inner ear**

H83.8X2 **Other specified diseases of left inner ear**

H83.8X3 **Other specified diseases of inner ear, bilateral**

H83.8X9 **Other specified diseases of inner ear, unspecified ear**

● H83.9 **Unspecified disease of inner ear**

H83.90 **Unspecified disease of inner ear, unspecified ear**

H83.91 **Unspecified disease of right inner ear**

H83.92 **Unspecified disease of left inner ear**

H83.93 **Unspecified disease of inner ear, bilateral**

OTHER DISORDERS OF EAR (H90-H94)

● H90 **Conductive and sensorineural hearing loss**
Excludes1 deaf nonspeaking NEC (H91.3)
deafness NOS (H91.9-)
hearing loss NOS (H91.9-)
noise-induced hearing loss (H83.3-)
ototoxic hearing loss (H91.0-)
sudden (idiopathic) hearing loss (H91.2-)

H90.0 **Conductive hearing loss, bilateral**

● H90.1 **Conductive hearing loss, unilateral with unrestricted hearing on the contralateral side**

H90.11 **Conductive hearing loss, unilateral, right ear, with unrestricted hearing on the contralateral side**

H90.12 **Conductive hearing loss, unilateral, left ear, with unrestricted hearing on the contralateral side**

H90.2 **Conductive hearing loss, unspecified**
Conductive deafness NOS

H90.3 **Sensorineural hearing loss, bilateral**

● H90.4 **Sensorineural hearing loss, unilateral with unrestricted hearing on the contralateral side**

H90.41 **Sensorineural hearing loss, unilateral, right ear, with unrestricted hearing on the contralateral side**

H90.42 **Sensorineural hearing loss, unilateral, left ear, with unrestricted hearing on the contralateral side**

H90.5 **Unspecified sensorineural hearing loss**
Central hearing loss NOS
Congenital deafness NOS
Neural hearing loss NOS
Perceptive hearing loss NOS
Sensorineural deafness NOS
Sensory hearing loss NOS
Excludes1 abnormal auditory perception (H93.2-)
psychogenic deafness (F44.6)

H90.6 **Mixed conductive and sensorineural hearing loss, bilateral**

● H90.7 **Mixed conductive and sensorineural hearing loss, unilateral with unrestricted hearing on the contralateral side**

H90.71 **Mixed conductive and sensorineural hearing loss, unilateral, right ear, with unrestricted hearing on the contralateral side**

H90.72 **Mixed conductive and sensorineural hearing loss, unilateral, left ear, with unrestricted hearing on the contralateral side**

H90.8 **Mixed conductive and sensorineural hearing loss, unspecified**

● H91 **Other and unspecified hearing loss**
Excludes1 abnormal auditory perception (H93.2-)
hearing loss as classified in H90.-
impacted cerumen (H61.2-)
noise-induced hearing loss (H83.3-)
psychogenic deafness (F44.6)
transient ischemic deafness (H93.01-)

● H91.0 **Ototoxic hearing loss**
Code first poisoning due to drug or toxin, if applicable (T36-T65 with fifth or sixth character 1-4 or 6)
Use additional code for adverse effect, if applicable, to identify drug (T36-T50 with fifth or sixth character 5)

H91.01 **Ototoxic hearing loss, right ear**

H91.02 **Ototoxic hearing loss, left ear**

H91.03 **Ototoxic hearing loss, bilateral**

H91.09 **Ototoxic hearing loss, unspecified ear**

CHAPTER 8 (H60-H95)

◀ New   ◀‖‖ Revised   ~~deleted~~ Deleted   **OGCR** Official Guidelines   X Assign placeholder X   ● Use Additional Character(s)

| Excludes 1 | Excludes 2 | Includes | Use additional | Code first | Code also | Unspecified |

CHAPTER 8 (H60-H95)

● **H91.1 Presbycusis**
Presbyacusia

    H91.10   Presbycusis, unspecified ear
    H91.11   Presbycusis, right ear
    H91.12   Presbycusis, left ear
    H91.13   Presbycusis, bilateral

● **H91.2 Sudden idiopathic hearing loss**
Sudden hearing loss NOS

    H91.20   Sudden idiopathic hearing loss, unspecified ear
    H91.21   Sudden idiopathic hearing loss, right ear
    H91.22   Sudden idiopathic hearing loss, left ear
    H91.23   Sudden idiopathic hearing loss, bilateral

  H91.3 Deaf nonspeaking, not elsewhere classified

● **H91.8 Other specified hearing loss**
  ● **H91.8X   Other specified hearing loss**
      H91.8X1   Other specified hearing loss, right ear
      H91.8X2   Other specified hearing loss, left ear
      H91.8X3   Other specified hearing loss, bilateral
      H91.8X9   Other specified hearing loss, unspecified ear

● **H91.9 Unspecified hearing loss**
Deafness NOS
High frequency deafness
Low frequency deafness

    H91.90   Unspecified hearing loss, unspecified ear
    H91.91   Unspecified hearing loss, right ear
    H91.92   Unspecified hearing loss, left ear
    H91.93   Unspecified hearing loss, bilateral

● **H92   Otalgia and effusion of ear**
  ● **H92.0 Otalgia**
    H92.01   Otalgia, right ear
    H92.02   Otalgia, left ear
    H92.03   Otalgia, bilateral
    H92.09   Otalgia, unspecified ear

  ● **H92.1 Otorrhea**
    Excludes1   leakage of cerebrospinal fluid through ear (G96.0)
    H92.10   Otorrhea, unspecified ear
    H92.11   Otorrhea, right ear
    H92.12   Otorrhea, left ear
    H92.13   Otorrhea, bilateral

  ● **H92.2 Otorrhagia**
    Excludes1   traumatic otorrhagia - code to injury
    H92.20   Otorrhagia, unspecified ear
    H92.21   Otorrhagia, right ear
    H92.22   Otorrhagia, left ear
    H92.23   Otorrhagia, bilateral

● **H93   Other disorders of ear, not elsewhere classified**
  ● **H93.0 Degenerative and vascular disorders of ear**
    Excludes1   presbycusis (H91.1)
    ● **H93.01   Transient ischemic deafness**
      H93.011   Transient ischemic deafness, right ear
      H93.012   Transient ischemic deafness, left ear
      H93.013   Transient ischemic deafness, bilateral
      H93.019   Transient ischemic deafness, unspecified ear

    ● **H93.09   Unspecified degenerative and vascular disorders of ear**
      H93.091   Unspecified degenerative and vascular disorders of right ear
      H93.092   Unspecified degenerative and vascular disorders of left ear
      H93.093   Unspecified degenerative and vascular disorders of ear, bilateral
      H93.099   Unspecified degenerative and vascular disorders of unspecified ear

● **H93.1 Tinnitus**
Perception of sound (ringing, buzzing, humming, whistling tunes, or singing)

    H93.11   Tinnitus, right ear
    H93.12   Tinnitus, left ear
    H93.13   Tinnitus, bilateral
    H93.19   Tinnitus, unspecified ear

● **H93.2 Other abnormal auditory perceptions**
    Excludes2   auditory hallucinations (R44.0)

  ● **H93.21   Auditory recruitment**
    H93.211   Auditory recruitment, right ear
    H93.212   Auditory recruitment, left ear
    H93.213   Auditory recruitment, bilateral
    H93.219   Auditory recruitment, unspecified ear

  ● **H93.22   Diplacusis**
    H93.221   Diplacusis, right ear
    H93.222   Diplacusis, left ear
    H93.223   Diplacusis, bilateral
    H93.229   Diplacusis, unspecified ear

  ● **H93.23   Hyperacusis**
    H93.231   Hyperacusis, right ear
    H93.232   Hyperacusis, left ear
    H93.233   Hyperacusis, bilateral
    H93.239   Hyperacusis, unspecified ear

  ● **H93.24   Temporary auditory threshold shift**
    H93.241   Temporary auditory threshold shift, right ear
    H93.242   Temporary auditory threshold shift, left ear
    H93.243   Temporary auditory threshold shift, bilateral
    H93.249   Temporary auditory threshold shift, unspecified ear

    H93.25   Central auditory processing disorder
      Congenital auditory imperception
      Word deafness
      Excludes1   mixed receptive-expressive language disorder (F80.2)

  ● **H93.29   Other abnormal auditory perceptions**
    H93.291   Other abnormal auditory perceptions, right ear
    H93.292   Other abnormal auditory perceptions, left ear
    H93.293   Other abnormal auditory perceptions, bilateral
    H93.299   Other abnormal auditory perceptions, unspecified ear

● **H93.3 Disorders of acoustic nerve**
Disorder of 8th cranial nerve
    Excludes1   acoustic neuroma (D33.3)
                  syphilitic acoustic neuritis (A52.15)

  ● **H93.3X   Disorders of acoustic nerve**
    H93.3X1   Disorders of right acoustic nerve
    H93.3X2   Disorders of left acoustic nerve
    H93.3X3   Disorders of bilateral acoustic nerves
    H93.3X9   Disorders of unspecified acoustic nerve

● **H93.8 Other specified disorders of ear**
  ● **H93.8X   Other specified disorders of ear**
    H93.8X1   Other specified disorders of right ear
    H93.8X2   Other specified disorders of left ear
    H93.8X3   Other specified disorders of ear, bilateral
    H93.8X9   Other specified disorders of ear, unspecified ear

◀ New   ◀▦ Revised   ~~deleted~~ Deleted   OGCR Official Guidelines   X Assign placeholder X   ● Use Additional Character(s)

Excludes 1   Excludes 2   Includes   Use additional   Code first   Code also   Unspecified

● **H93.9**   **Unspecified disorder of ear**
     H93.90   Unspecified disorder of ear, unspecified ear
     H93.91   Unspecified disorder of right ear
     H93.92   Unspecified disorder of left ear
     H93.93   Unspecified disorder of ear, bilateral

● **H94**   **Other disorders of ear in diseases classified elsewhere**
   ● **H94.0**   **Acoustic neuritis in infectious and parasitic diseases classified elsewhere**

> *Code first underlying disease, such as:*
> parasitic disease (B65-B89)

> **Excludes1**   acoustic neuritis (in):
> herpes zoster (B02.29)
> syphilis (A52.15)

     H94.00   Acoustic neuritis in infectious and parasitic diseases classified elsewhere, unspecified ear
     H94.01   Acoustic neuritis in infectious and parasitic diseases classified elsewhere, right ear
     H94.02   Acoustic neuritis in infectious and parasitic diseases classified elsewhere, left ear
     H94.03   Acoustic neuritis in infectious and parasitic diseases classified elsewhere, bilateral

   ● **H94.8**   **Other specified disorders of ear in diseases classified elsewhere**

> *Code first underlying disease, such as:*
> congenital syphilis (A50.0)

> **Excludes1**   aural myiasis (B87.4)
> syphilitic labyrinthitis (A52.79)

     H94.80   Other specified disorders of ear in diseases classified elsewhere, unspecified ear
     H94.81   Other specified disorders of right ear in diseases classified elsewhere
     H94.82   Other specified disorders of left ear in diseases classified elsewhere
     H94.83   Other specified disorders of ear in diseases classified elsewhere, bilateral

● **H95**   **Intraoperative and postprocedural complications and disorders of ear and mastoid process, not elsewhere classified**
   ● **H95.0**   **Recurrent cholesteatoma of postmastoidectomy cavity**
     H95.00   Recurrent cholesteatoma of postmastoidectomy cavity, unspecified ear
     H95.01   Recurrent cholesteatoma of postmastoidectomy cavity, right ear
     H95.02   Recurrent cholesteatoma of postmastoidectomy cavity, left ear
     H95.03   Recurrent cholesteatoma of postmastoidectomy cavity, bilateral ears

   ● **H95.1**   **Other disorders of ear and mastoid process following mastoidectomy**
     ● **H95.11**   **Chronic inflammation of postmastoidectomy cavity**
       H95.111   Chronic inflammation of postmastoidectomy cavity, right ear
       H95.112   Chronic inflammation of postmastoidectomy cavity, left ear
       H95.113   Chronic inflammation of postmastoidectomy cavity, bilateral ears
       H95.119   Chronic inflammation of postmastoidectomy cavity, unspecified ear
     ● **H95.12**   **Granulation of postmastoidectomy cavity**
       H95.121   Granulation of postmastoidectomy cavity, right ear
       H95.122   Granulation of postmastoidectomy cavity, left ear
       H95.123   Granulation of postmastoidectomy cavity, bilateral ears
       H95.129   Granulation of postmastoidectomy cavity, unspecified ear

   ● **H95.13**   **Mucosal cyst of postmastoidectomy cavity**
       H95.131   Mucosal cyst of postmastoidectomy cavity, right ear
       H95.132   Mucosal cyst of postmastoidectomy cavity, left ear
       H95.133   Mucosal cyst of postmastoidectomy cavity, bilateral ears
       H95.139   Mucosal cyst of postmastoidectomy cavity, unspecified ear
   ● **H95.19**   **Other disorders following mastoidectomy**
       H95.191   Other disorders following mastoidectomy, right ear
       H95.192   Other disorders following mastoidectomy, left ear
       H95.193   Other disorders following mastoidectomy, bilateral ears
       H95.199   Other disorders following mastoidectomy, unspecified ear

   ● **H95.2**   **Intraoperative hemorrhage and hematoma of ear and mastoid process complicating a procedure**

> **Excludes1**   intraoperative hemorrhage and hematoma of ear and mastoid process due to accidental puncture or laceration during a procedure (H95.3-)

     H95.21   Intraoperative hemorrhage and hematoma of ear and mastoid process complicating a procedure on the ear and mastoid process
     H95.22   Intraoperative hemorrhage and hematoma of ear and mastoid process complicating other procedure

   ● **H95.3**   **Accidental puncture and laceration of ear and mastoid process during a procedure**
     H95.31   Accidental puncture and laceration of the ear and mastoid process during a procedure on the ear and mastoid process
     H95.32   Accidental puncture and laceration of the ear and mastoid process during other procedure

   ● **H95.4**   **Postprocedural hemorrhage and hematoma of ear and mastoid process following a procedure**
     H95.41   Postprocedural hemorrhage and hematoma of ear and mastoid process following a procedure on the ear and mastoid process
     H95.42   Postprocedural hemorrhage and hematoma of ear and mastoid process following other procedure

   ● **H95.8**   **Other intraoperative and postprocedural complications and disorders of the ear and mastoid process, not elsewhere classified**

> **Excludes2**   postprocedural complications and disorders following mastoidectomy (H95.0-, H95.1-)

     ● **H95.81**   **Postprocedural stenosis of external ear canal**
       H95.811   Postprocedural stenosis of right external ear canal
       H95.812   Postprocedural stenosis of left external ear canal
       H95.813   Postprocedural stenosis of external ear canal, bilateral
       H95.819   Postprocedural stenosis of unspecified external ear canal
     H95.88   Other intraoperative complications and disorders of the ear and mastoid process, not elsewhere classified

> *Use additional code, if applicable, to further specify disorder*

     H95.89   Other postprocedural complications and disorders of the ear and mastoid process, not elsewhere classified

> *Use additional code, if applicable, to further specify disorder*

CHAPTER 8 (H60-H95)

◀ New   ◀|||| Revised   ~~deleted~~ Deleted   **OGCR** Official Guidelines   X Assign placeholder X   ● Use Additional Character(s)

| Excludes 1 | Excludes 2 | Includes | Use additional | Code first | Code also | Unspecified |

Pulmonary valve

Aortic valve

RA

Mitral valve

Tricuspid valve

RV

LV

Figure 9-1 Cardiovascular valves.

Item 9–1 Rheumatic fever is the inflammation of the valve(s) of the heart, usually the mitral or aortic, which leads to valve damage. Rheumatic heart inflammations are usually **pericarditis** (sac surrounding heart), **endocarditis** (heart cavity), or **myocarditis** (heart muscle).

CHAPTER 9   DISEASES OF THE CIRCULATORY SYSTEM (I00-I99)

Excludes2   certain conditions originating in the perinatal period (P04-P96)
certain infectious and parasitic diseases (A00-B99)
complications of pregnancy, childbirth and the puerperium (O00-O9A)
congenital malformations, deformations, and chromosomal abnormalities (Q00-Q99)
endocrine, nutritional and metabolic diseases (E00-E88)
injury, poisoning and certain other consequences of external causes (S00-T88)
neoplasms (C00-D49)
symptoms, signs and abnormal clinical and laboratory findings, not elsewhere classified (R00-R94)
systemic connective tissue disorders (M30-M36)
transient cerebral ischemic attacks and related syndromes (G45.-)

This chapter contains the following blocks:

I00-I02	Acute rheumatic fever
I05-I09	Chronic rheumatic heart diseases
I10-I15	Hypertensive diseases
I20-I25	Ischemic heart diseases
I26-I28	Pulmonary heart disease and diseases of pulmonary circulation
I30-I52	Other forms of heart disease
I60-I69	Cerebrovascular diseases
I70-I79	Diseases of arteries, arterioles and capillaries
I80-I89	Diseases of veins, lymphatic vessels and lymph nodes, not elsewhere classified
I95-I99	Other and unspecified disorders of the circulatory system

ACUTE RHEUMATIC FEVER (I00-I02)

I00   Rheumatic fever without heart involvement
Includes   arthritis, rheumatic, acute or subacute
Excludes1   rheumatic fever with heart involvement (I01.0-I01.9)

● **I01   Rheumatic fever with heart involvement**
Excludes1   chronic diseases of rheumatic origin (I05-I09) unless rheumatic fever is also present or there is evidence of reactivation or activity of the rheumatic process.

I01.0   Acute rheumatic pericarditis
Any condition in I00 with pericarditis
Rheumatic pericarditis (acute)
Excludes1   acute pericarditis not specified as rheumatic (I30.-)

I01.1   Acute rheumatic endocarditis
Any condition in I00 with endocarditis or valvulitis
Acute rheumatic valvulitis

I01.2   Acute rheumatic myocarditis
Any condition in I00 with myocarditis

Item 9–2 Rheumatic chorea, also called Sydenham's, juvenile, minor, simple, or St. Vitus' dance, is a major symptom of rheumatic fever and is characterized by ceaseless, involuntary, jerky, purposeless movements.

I01.8   Other acute rheumatic heart disease
Any condition in I00 with other or multiple types of heart involvement
Acute rheumatic pancarditis

I01.9   Acute rheumatic heart disease, unspecified
Any condition in I00 with unspecified type of heart involvement
Rheumatic carditis, acute
Rheumatic heart disease, active or acute

● **I02   Rheumatic chorea**
Includes   Sydenham's chorea
Excludes1   chorea NOS (G25.5)
Huntington's chorea (G10)

I02.0   Rheumatic chorea with heart involvement
Chorea NOS with heart involvement
Rheumatic chorea with heart involvement of any type classifiable under I01.-

I02.9   Rheumatic chorea without heart involvement
Rheumatic chorea NOS

CHRONIC RHEUMATIC HEART DISEASES (I05-I09)

● **I05   Rheumatic mitral valve diseases**
Includes   conditions classifiable to both I05.0 and I05.2-I05.9, whether specified as rheumatic or not
Excludes1   mitral valve disease specified as nonrheumatic (I34.-)
mitral valve disease with aortic and/or tricuspid valve involvement (I08.-)

I05.0   Rheumatic mitral stenosis
Mitral (valve) obstruction (rheumatic)

I05.1   Rheumatic mitral insufficiency
Rheumatic mitral incompetence
Rheumatic mitral regurgitation
Excludes1   mitral insufficiency not specified as rheumatic (I34.0)

I05.2   Rheumatic mitral stenosis with insufficiency
Rheumatic mitral stenosis with incompetence or regurgitation

I05.8   Other rheumatic mitral valve diseases
Rheumatic mitral (valve) failure

I05.9   Rheumatic mitral valve disease, unspecified
Rheumatic mitral (valve) disorder (chronic) NOS

● **I06   Rheumatic aortic valve diseases**
Excludes1   aortic valve disease not specified as rheumatic (I35.-)
aortic valve disease with mitral and/or tricuspid valve involvement (I08.-)

I06.0   Rheumatic aortic stenosis
Rheumatic aortic (valve) obstruction

I06.1   Rheumatic aortic insufficiency
Rheumatic aortic incompetence
Rheumatic aortic regurgitation

(See Plate 244 on page NAP-30.)

Item 9–3 Mitral stenosis is the narrowing of the mitral valve separating the left atrium from the left ventricle. **Mitral insufficiency** is the improper closure of the mitral valve which may lead to enlargement (hypertrophy) of the left atrium.

Item 9–4 Aortic stenosis is the narrowing of the aortic valve located between the left ventricle and the aorta. **Aortic insufficiency** is the improper closure of the aortic valve which may lead to enlargement (hypertrophy) of the left ventricle.

◀ New   ◀▥ Revised   ~~deleted~~ Deleted   OGCR Official Guidelines   X Assign placeholder X   ● Use Additional Character(s)

Excludes 1   Excludes 2   Includes   Use additional   Code first   Code also   Unspecified

I06.2   **Rheumatic aortic stenosis with insufficiency**
Rheumatic aortic stenosis with incompetence or
regurgitation

I06.8   **Other rheumatic aortic valve diseases**

I06.9   **Rheumatic aortic valve disease, unspecified**
Rheumatic aortic (valve) disease NOS

● **I07**   **Rheumatic tricuspid valve diseases**

    Includes   rheumatic tricuspid valve diseases specified as
rheumatic or unspecified

    Excludes1   tricuspid valve disease specified as nonrheumatic
(I36.-)
tricuspid valve disease with aortic and/or mitral
valve involvement (I08.-)

I07.0   **Rheumatic tricuspid stenosis**
Tricuspid (valve) stenosis (rheumatic)

I07.1   **Rheumatic tricuspid insufficiency**
Tricuspid (valve) insufficiency (rheumatic)

I07.2   **Rheumatic tricuspid stenosis and insufficiency**

I07.8   **Other rheumatic tricuspid valve diseases**

I07.9   **Rheumatic tricuspid valve disease, unspecified**
Rheumatic tricuspid valve disorder NOS

● **I08**   **Multiple valve diseases**

    Includes   multiple valve diseases specified as rheumatic or
unspecified

    Excludes1   endocarditis, valve unspecified (I38)
multiple valve disease specified a nonrheumatic
(I34.-, I35.-, I36.-, I37.-, I38.-, Q22.-, Q23.-,
Q24.8-)
rheumatic valve disease NOS (I09.1)

I08.0   **Rheumatic disorders of both mitral and aortic valves**
Involvement of both mitral and aortic valves specified
as rheumatic or unspecified

I08.1   **Rheumatic disorders of both mitral and tricuspid valves**

I08.2   **Rheumatic disorders of both aortic and tricuspid valves**

I08.3   **Combined rheumatic disorders of mitral, aortic and
tricuspid valves**

I08.8   **Other rheumatic multiple valve diseases**

I08.9   **Rheumatic multiple valve disease, unspecified**

● **I09**   **Other rheumatic heart diseases**

I09.0   **Rheumatic myocarditis**

    Excludes1   myocarditis not specified as rheumatic
(I51.4)

I09.1   **Rheumatic diseases of endocardium, valve unspecified**
Rheumatic endocarditis (chronic)
Rheumatic valvulitis (chronic)

    Excludes1   endocarditis, valve unspecified (I38)

I09.2   **Chronic rheumatic pericarditis**
Adherent pericardium, rheumatic
Chronic rheumatic mediastinopericarditis
Chronic rheumatic myopericarditis

    Excludes1   chronic pericarditis not specified as
rheumatic (I31.-)

● **I09.8**   **Other specified rheumatic heart diseases**

   I09.81   **Rheumatic heart failure**

     Use additional code to identify type of heart
failure (I50.-)

   I09.89   **Other specified rheumatic heart diseases**
Rheumatic disease of pulmonary valve

I09.9   **Rheumatic heart disease, unspecified**
Rheumatic carditis

    Excludes1   rheumatoid carditis (M05.31)

Item 9–5 Hypertension is caused by high arterial blood pressure in the arteries. **Essential, primary,** or **idiopathic** hypertension occurs without identifiable organic cause. **Secondary** hypertension is that which has an organic cause. **Malignant** hypertension is severely elevated blood pressure. **Benign** hypertension is mildly elevated blood pressure.

HYPERTENSIVE DISEASES (I10-I15)

Use additional code to identify:
exposure to environmental tobacco smoke (Z77.22)
history of tobacco use (Z87.891)
occupational exposure to environmental tobacco
smoke (Z57.31)
tobacco dependence (F17.-)
tobacco use (Z72.0)

    Excludes1   hypertensive disease complicating pregnancy,
childbirth and the puerperium (O10-O11,
O13-O16)
neonatal hypertension (P29.2)
primary pulmonary hypertension (I27.0)

I10   **Essential (primary) hypertension**

    Includes   high blood pressure
hypertension (arterial) (benign) (essential)
(malignant) (primary) (systemic)

    Excludes1   hypertensive disease complicating pregnancy,
childbirth and the puerperium (O10-O11,
O13-O16)

    Excludes2   essential (primary) hypertension involving
vessels of brain (I60-I69)
essential (primary) hypertension involving
vessels of eye (H35.0-)

● **I11**   **Hypertensive heart disease**

    Includes   any condition in I51.4-I51.9 due to hypertension

   I11.0   **Hypertensive heart disease with heart failure**
Hypertensive heart failure

     Use additional code to identify type of heart failure
(I50.-)

   I11.9   **Hypertensive heart disease without heart failure**
Hypertensive heart disease NOS

OGCR Section I.C.9.a.2

Hypertensive Chronic Kidney Disease

Assign codes from category I12, Hypertensive chronic kidney disease, when both hypertension and a condition classifiable to category N18, Chronic kidney disease (CKD), are present. Unlike hypertension with heart disease, ICD-10-CM presumes a cause-and-effect relationship and classifies chronic kidney disease with hypertension as hypertensive chronic kidney disease.

The appropriate code from category N18 should be used as a secondary code with a code from category I12 to identify the stage of chronic kidney disease.

See Section I.C.14. Chronic kidney disease.

If a patient has hypertensive chronic kidney disease and acute renal failure, an additional code for the acute renal failure is required.

● **I12**   **Hypertensive chronic kidney disease**

    Includes   any condition in N18 and N26 - due to
hypertension
arteriosclerosis of kidney
arteriosclerotic nephritis (chronic) (interstitial)
hypertensive nephropathy
nephrosclerosis

    Excludes1   hypertension due to kidney disease (I15.0, I15.1)
renovascular hypertension (I15.0)
secondary hypertension (I15.-)

    Excludes2   acute kidney failure (N17.-)

   I12.0   **Hypertensive chronic kidney disease with stage 5
chronic kidney disease or end stage renal disease**

     Use additional code to identify the stage of chronic
kidney disease (N18.5, N18.6)

◄ New   ⬅ Revised   ~~deleted~~ Deleted   **OGCR** Official Guidelines   X Assign placeholder X   ● Use Additional Character(s)

Excludes 1   Excludes 2   Includes   Use additional   Code first   Code also   Unspecified

I12.9   **Hypertensive chronic kidney disease with stage 1 through stage 4 chronic kidney disease, or unspecified chronic kidney disease**
     Hypertensive chronic kidney disease NOS
     Hypertensive renal disease NOS
     Use additional code to identify the stage of chronic kidney disease (N18.1-N18.4, N18.9)

OGCR Section I.c.9.a.6

Hypertensive Heart and Chronic Kidney Disease

Assign codes from combination category I13, Hypertensive heart and chronic kidney disease, when both hypertensive kidney disease and hypertensive heart disease are stated in the diagnosis. Assume a relationship between the hypertension and the chronic kidney disease, whether or not the condition is so designated. If heart failure is present, assign an additional code from category I50 to identify the type of heart failure.

The appropriate code from category N18, Chronic kidney disease, should be used as a secondary code with a code from category I13 to identify the stage of chronic kidney disease.

See Section I.C.14. Chronic kidney disease.

The codes in category I13, Hypertensive heart and chronic kidney disease, are combination codes that include hypertension, heart disease and chronic kidney disease. The Includes note at I13 specifies that the conditions included at I11 and I12 are included together in I13. If a patient has hypertension, heart disease and chronic kidney disease then a code from I13 should be used, not individual codes for hypertension, heart disease and chronic kidney disease, or codes from I11 or I12.

For patients with both acute renal failure and chronic kidney disease an additional code for acute renal failure is required.

● **I13**   **Hypertensive heart and chronic kidney disease**
     Includes   any condition in I11.- with any condition in I12.-
          cardiorenal disease
          cardiovascular renal disease

   I13.0   **Hypertensive heart and chronic kidney disease with heart failure and stage 1 through stage 4 chronic kidney disease, or unspecified chronic kidney disease**
       Use additional code to identify type of heart failure (I50.-)
       Use additional code to identify stage of chronic kidney disease (N18.1-N18.4, N18.9)

●   **I13.1**   **Hypertensive heart and chronic kidney disease without heart failure**
       I13.10   **Hypertensive heart and chronic kidney disease without heart failure, with stage 1 through stage 4 chronic kidney disease, or unspecified chronic kidney disease**
          Hypertensive heart disease and hypertensive chronic kidney disease NOS
          Use additional code to identify the stage of chronic kidney disease (N18.1-N18.4, N18.9)
       I13.11   **Hypertensive heart and chronic kidney disease without heart failure, with stage 5 chronic kidney disease, or end stage renal disease**
          Use additional code to identify the stage of chronic kidney disease (N18.5, N18.6)

   I13.2   **Hypertensive heart and chronic kidney disease with heart failure and with stage 5 chronic kidney disease, or end stage renal disease**
       Use additional code to identify type of heart failure (I50.-)
       Use additional code to identify the stage of chronic kidney disease (N18.5, N18.6)

OGCR Section I.9.a.6

Hypertension, Secondary

Secondary hypertension is due to an underlying condition. Two codes are required: one to identify the underlying etiology and one from category I15 to identify the hypertension. Sequencing of codes is determined by the reason for admission/encounter.

● **I15**   **Secondary hypertension**
     Code also underlying condition
     Excludes1   postprocedural hypertension (I97.3)
     Excludes2   secondary hypertension involving vessels of brain (I60-I69)
          secondary hypertension involving vessels of eye (H35.0-)

   I15.0   **Renovascular hypertension**
   I15.1   **Hypertension secondary to other renal disorders**
   I15.2   **Hypertension secondary to endocrine disorders**
   I15.8   **Other secondary hypertension**
   I15.9   **Secondary hypertension, unspecified**

ISCHEMIC HEART DISEASES (I20-I25)

Use additional code to identify presence of hypertension (I10-I15)

● **I20**   **Angina pectoris**
     Chest pain/discomfort due to lack of oxygen to the heart muscle. Principal symptom of myocardial infarction.
     Use additional code to identify:
       exposure to environmental tobacco smoke (Z77.22)
       history of tobacco use (Z87.891)
       occupational exposure to environmental tobacco smoke (Z57.31)
       tobacco dependence (F17.-)
       tobacco use (Z72.0)
     Excludes1   angina pectoris with atherosclerotic heart disease of native coronary arteries (I25.1-)
          atherosclerosis of coronary artery bypass graft(s) and coronary artery of transplanted heart with angina pectoris (I25.7-)
          postinfarction angina (I23.7)

   I20.0   **Unstable angina**
       Accelerated angina
       Crescendo angina
       De novo effort angina
       Intermediate coronary syndrome
       Preinfarction syndrome
       Worsening effort angina

   I20.1   **Angina pectoris with documented spasm**
       Angiospastic angina
       Prinzmetal angina
       Spasm-induced angina
       Variant angina

   I20.8   **Other forms of angina pectoris**
       Angina equivalent
       Angina of effort
       Coronary slow flow syndrome
       Stenocardia
       Use additional code(s) for symptoms associated with angina equivalent

   I20.9   **Angina pectoris, unspecified**
       Angina NOS
       Anginal syndrome
       Cardiac angina
       Ischemic chest pain

OGCR See Section I.c.9.e.3

Acute myocardial infarction, unspecified
Code I21.3, ST elevation (STEMI) myocardial infarction of unspecified site, is the default for unspecified acute myocardial infarction. If only STEMI or transmural MI without the site is documented, assign I21.3.

I21   **ST elevation (STEMI) and non-ST elevation (NSTEMI) myocardial infarction**

     Includes   cardiac infarction
                  coronary (artery) embolism
                  coronary (artery) occlusion
                  coronary (artery) rupture
                  coronary (artery) thrombosis
                  infarction of heart, myocardium, or ventricle
                  myocardial infarction specified as acute or with a stated duration of 4 weeks (28 days) or less from onset

     Use additional code, if applicable, to identify:
         exposure to environmental tobacco smoke (Z77.22)
         history of tobacco use (Z87.891)
         occupational exposure to environmental tobacco smoke (Z57.31)
         status post administration of tPA (rtPA) in a different facility within the last 24 hours prior to admission to current facility (Z92.82)
         tobacco dependence (F17.-)
         tobacco use (Z72.0)

     Excludes2   old myocardial infarction (I25.2)
                   postmyocardial infarction syndrome (I24.1)
                   subsequent myocardial infarction (I22.-)

● **I21.0**   **ST elevation (STEMI) myocardial infarction of anterior wall**

     I21.01   **ST elevation (STEMI) myocardial infarction involving left main coronary artery**

     I21.02   **ST elevation (STEMI) myocardial infarction involving left anterior descending coronary artery**
            ST elevation (STEMI) myocardial infarction involving diagonal coronary artery

     I21.09   **ST elevation (STEMI) myocardial infarction involving other coronary artery of anterior wall**
            Acute transmural myocardial infarction of anterior wall
            Anteroapical transmural (Q wave) infarction (acute)
            Anterolateral transmural (Q wave) infarction (acute)
            Anteroseptal transmural (Q wave) infarction (acute)
            Transmural (Q wave) infarction (acute) (of) anterior (wall) NOS

● **I21.1**   **ST elevation (STEMI) myocardial infarction of inferior wall**

     I21.11   **ST elevation (STEMI) myocardial infarction involving right coronary artery**
            Inferoposterior transmural (Q wave) infarction (acute)

     I21.19   **ST elevation (STEMI) myocardial infarction involving other coronary artery of inferior wall**
            Acute transmural myocardial infarction of inferior wall
            Inferolateral transmural (Q wave) infarction (acute)
            Transmural (Q wave) infarction (acute) (of) diaphragmatic wall
            Transmural (Q wave) infarction (acute) (of) inferior (wall) NOS

         Excludes2   ST elevation (STEMI) myocardial infarction involving left circumflex coronary artery (I21.21)

● **I21.2**   **ST elevation (STEMI) myocardial infarction of other sites**

     I21.21   **ST elevation (STEMI) myocardial infarction involving left circumflex coronary artery**
            ST elevation (STEMI) myocardial infarction involving oblique marginal coronary artery

     I21.29   **ST elevation (STEMI) myocardial infarction involving other sites**
            Acute transmural myocardial infarction of other sites
            Apical-lateral transmural (Q wave) infarction (acute)
            Basal-lateral transmural (Q wave) infarction (acute)
            High lateral transmural (Q wave) infarction (acute)
            Lateral (wall) NOS transmural (Q wave) infarction (acute)
            Posterior (true) transmural (Q wave) infarction (acute)
            Posterobasal transmural (Q wave) infarction (acute)
            Posterolateral transmural (Q wave) infarction (acute)
            Posteroseptal transmural (Q wave) infarction (acute)
            Septal transmural (Q wave) infarction (acute) NOS

   I21.3   **ST elevation (STEMI) myocardial infarction of unspecified site**
         Acute transmural myocardial infarction of unspecified site
         Myocardial infarction (acute) NOS
         Transmural (Q wave) myocardial infarction NOS

   I21.4   **Non-ST elevation (NSTEMI) myocardial infarction**
         Acute subendocardial myocardial infarction
         Non-Q wave myocardial infarction NOS
         Nontransmural myocardial infarction NOS

CHAPTER 9 (I00-I99)

● **I22**   **Subsequent ST elevation (STEMI) and non-ST elevation (NSTEMI) myocardial infarction**

> **Includes**   acute myocardial infarction occurring within four weeks (28 days) of a previous acute myocardial infarction, regardless of site
> cardiac infarction
> coronary (artery) embolism
> coronary (artery) occlusion
> coronary (artery) rupture
> coronary (artery) thrombosis
> infarction of heart, myocardium, or ventricle
> recurrent myocardial infarction
> reinfarction of myocardium
> rupture of heart, myocardium, or ventricle

> **Use additional** code, if applicable, to identify:
> exposure to environmental tobacco smoke (Z77.22)
> history of tobacco use (Z87.891)
> occupational exposure to environmental tobacco smoke (Z57.31)
> status post administration of tPA (rtPA) in a different facility within the last 24 hours prior to admission to current facility (Z92.82)
> tobacco dependence (F17.-)
> tobacco use (Z72.0)

I22.0   **Subsequent ST elevation (STEMI) myocardial infarction of anterior wall**
> Subsequent acute transmural myocardial infarction of anterior wall
> Subsequent transmural (Q wave) infarction (acute)(of) anterior (wall) NOS
> Subsequent anteroapical transmural (Q wave) infarction (acute)
> Subsequent anterolateral transmural (Q wave) infarction (acute)
> Subsequent anteroseptal transmural (Q wave) infarction (acute)

I22.1   **Subsequent ST elevation (STEMI) myocardial infarction of inferior wall**
> Subsequent acute transmural myocardial infarction of inferior wall
> Subsequent transmural (Q wave) infarction (acute)(of) diaphragmatic wall
> Subsequent transmural (Q wave) infarction (acute)(of) inferior (wall) NOS
> Subsequent inferolateral transmural (Q wave) infarction (acute)
> Subsequent inferoposterior transmural (Q wave) infarction (acute)

I22.2   **Subsequent non-ST elevation (NSTEMI) myocardial infarction**
> Subsequent acute subendocardial myocardial infarction
> Subsequent non-Q wave myocardial infarction NOS
> Subsequent nontransmural myocardial infarction NOS

I22.8   **Subsequent ST elevation (STEMI) myocardial infarction of other sites**
> Subsequent acute transmural myocardial infarction of other sites
> Subsequent apical-lateral transmural (Q wave) myocardial infarction (acute)
> Subsequent basal-lateral transmural (Q wave) myocardial infarction (acute)
> Subsequent high lateral transmural (Q wave) myocardial infarction (acute)
> Subsequent transmural (Q wave) myocardial infarction (acute)(of) lateral (wall) NOS
> Subsequent posterior (true) transmural (Q wave) myocardial infarction (acute)
> Subsequent posterobasal transmural (Q wave) myocardial infarction (acute)
> Subsequent posterolateral transmural (Q wave) myocardial infarction (acute)
> Subsequent posteroseptal transmural (Q wave) myocardial infarction (acute)
> Subsequent septal NOS transmural (Q wave) myocardial infarction (acute)

I22.9   **Subsequent ST elevation (STEMI) myocardial infarction of unspecified site**
> Subsequent acute myocardial infarction of unspecified site
> Subsequent myocardial infarction (acute) NOS

● **I23**   **Certain current complications following ST elevation (STEMI) and non-ST elevation (NSTEMI) myocardial infarction (within the 28 day period)**

I23.0   **Hemopericardium as current complication following acute myocardial infarction**
> **Excludes1**   hemopericardium not specified as current complication following acute myocardial infarction (I31.2)

I23.1   **Atrial septal defect as current complication following acute myocardial infarction**
> **Excludes1**   acquired atrial septal defect not specified as current complication following acute myocardial infarction (I51.0)

I23.2   **Ventricular septal defect as current complication following acute myocardial infarction**
> **Excludes1**   acquired ventricular septal defect not specified as current complication following acute myocardial infarction (I51.0)

I23.3   **Rupture of cardiac wall without hemopericardium as current complication following acute myocardial infarction**

I23.4   **Rupture of chordae tendineae as current complication following acute myocardial infarction**
> **Excludes1**   rupture of chordae tendineae not specified as current complication following acute myocardial infarction (I51.1)

I23.5   **Rupture of papillary muscle as current complication following acute myocardial infarction**
> **Excludes1**   rupture of papillary muscle not specified as current complication following acute myocardial infarction (I51.2)

I23.6   **Thrombosis of atrium, auricular appendage, and ventricle as current complications following acute myocardial infarction**
> **Excludes1**   thrombosis of atrium, auricular appendage, and ventricle not specified as current complication following acute myocardial infarction (I51.3)

I23.7   **Postinfarction angina**

I23.8   **Other current complications following acute myocardial infarction**

● **I24**   **Other acute ischemic heart diseases**
> **Excludes1**   angina pectoris (I20.-)
> transient myocardial ischemia in newborn (P29.4)

I24.0   **Acute coronary thrombosis not resulting in myocardial infarction**
> Acute coronary (artery) (vein) embolism not resulting in myocardial infarction
> Acute coronary (artery) (vein) occlusion not resulting in myocardial infarction
> Acute coronary (artery) (vein) thromboembolism not resulting in myocardial infarction
> **Excludes1**   atherosclerotic heart disease (I25.1-)

I24.1   **Dressler's syndrome**
> Postmyocardial infarction syndrome
> **Excludes1**   postinfarction angina (I23.7)

I24.8   **Other forms of acute ischemic heart disease**

I24.9   **Acute ischemic heart disease, unspecified**
> **Excludes1**   ischemic heart disease (chronic) NOS (I25.9)

Item 9–6 Classification is based on the location of the atherosclerosis. **"Of native coronary artery"** indicates the atherosclerosis is within an original heart artery. **"Of autologous vein bypass graft"** indicates that the atherosclerosis is within a vein graft that was taken from within the patient. **"Of nonautologous biological bypass graft"** indicates the atherosclerosis is within a vessel grafted from other than the patient. **"Of artery bypass graft"** indicates the atherosclerosis is within an artery that was grafted from within the patient.

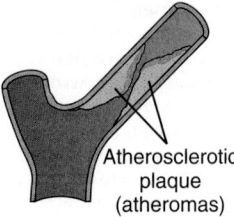

Figure 9-2 Atherosclerotic plaque.

Atherosclerotic plaque (atheromas)

● **I25 Chronic ischemic heart disease**

Use additional code to identify:
chronic total occlusion of coronary artery (I25.82)
exposure to environmental tobacco smoke (Z77.22)
history of tobacco use (Z87.891)
occupational exposure to environmental tobacco smoke (Z57.31)
tobacco dependence (F17.-)
tobacco use (Z72.0)

OGCR See Section I.9.b.

Atherosclerotic Coronary Artery Disease and Angina

ICD-10-CM has combination codes for atherosclerotic heart disease with angina pectoris. The subcategories for these codes are I25.11, Atherosclerotic heart disease of native coronary artery with angina pectoris and I25.7, Atherosclerosis of coronary artery bypass graft(s) and coronary artery of transplanted heart with angina pectoris.

When using one of these combination codes it is not necessary to use an additional code for angina pectoris. A causal relationship can be assumed in a patient with both atherosclerosis and angina pectoris, unless the documentation indicates the angina is due to something other than the atherosclerosis.

If a patient with coronary artery disease is admitted due to an acute myocardial infarction (AMI), the AMI should be sequenced before the coronary artery disease.

See Section I.C.9. Acute myocardial infarction (AMI)

(See Plates 218 and 219 on pages NAP-26 and NAP-27.)

● **I25.1 Atherosclerotic heart disease of native coronary artery**
Disease in which fatty deposits form on the walls of arteries
Atherosclerotic cardiovascular disease
Coronary (artery) atheroma
Coronary (artery) atherosclerosis
Coronary (artery) disease
Coronary (artery) sclerosis

Use additional code, if applicable, to identify:
coronary atherosclerosis due to calcified coronary lesion (I25.84)
coronary atherosclerosis due to lipid rich plaque (I25.83)

Excludes2 atheroembolism (I75.-)
atherosclerosis of coronary artery bypass graft(s) and transplanted heart (I25.7-)

I25.10 Atherosclerotic heart disease of native coronary artery without angina pectoris
Atherosclerotic heart disease NOS

● **I25.11 Atherosclerotic heart disease of native coronary artery with angina pectoris**

I25.110 Atherosclerotic heart disease of native coronary artery with unstable angina pectoris

Excludes1 unstable angina without atherosclerotic heart disease (I20.0)

I25.111 Atherosclerotic heart disease of native coronary artery with angina pectoris with documented spasm

Excludes1 angina pectoris with documented spasm without atherosclerotic heart disease (I20.1)

I25.118 Atherosclerotic heart disease of native coronary artery with other forms of angina pectoris

Excludes1 other forms of angina pectoris without atherosclerotic heart disease (I20.8)

I25.119 Atherosclerotic heart disease of native coronary artery with unspecified angina pectoris
Atherosclerotic heart disease with angina NOS
Atherosclerotic heart disease with ischemic chest pain

Excludes1 unspecified angina pectoris without atherosclerotic heart disease (I20.9)

I25.2 Old myocardial infarction
Healed myocardial infarction
Past myocardial infarction diagnosed by ECG or other investigation, but currently presenting no symptoms

I25.3 Aneurysm of heart
Mural aneurysm
Ventricular aneurysm

● **I25.4 Coronary artery aneurysm and dissection**

I25.41 Coronary artery aneurysm
Coronary arteriovenous fistula, acquired

Excludes1 congenital coronary (artery) aneurysm (Q24.5)

I25.42 Coronary artery dissection

I25.5 Ischemic cardiomyopathy
Excludes2 coronary atherosclerosis (I25.1-, I25.7-)

I25.6 Silent myocardial ischemia

● **I25.7 Atherosclerosis of coronary artery bypass graft(s) and coronary artery of transplanted heart with angina pectoris**

Use additional code, if applicable, to identify:
coronary atherosclerosis due to calcified coronary lesion (I25.84)
coronary atherosclerosis due to lipid rich plaque (I25.83)

Excludes1 atherosclerosis of bypass graft(s) of transplanted heart without angina pectoris (I25.812)
atherosclerosis of coronary artery bypass graft(s) without angina pectoris (I25.810)
atherosclerosis of native coronary artery of transplanted heart without angina pectoris (I25.811)
embolism or thrombus of coronary artery bypass graft(s) (T82.8-)

CHAPTER 9 (I00-I99)

● **I25.70** **Atherosclerosis of coronary artery bypass graft(s), unspecified, with angina pectoris**

     I25.700 **Atherosclerosis of coronary artery bypass graft(s), unspecified, with unstable angina pectoris**

         Excludes 1   unstable angina pectoris without atherosclerosis of coronary artery bypass graft (I20.0)

     I25.701 **Atherosclerosis of coronary artery bypass graft(s), unspecified, with angina pectoris with documented spasm**

         Excludes 1   angina pectoris with documented spasm without atherosclerosis of coronary artery bypass graft (I20.1)

     I25.708 **Atherosclerosis of coronary artery bypass graft(s), unspecified, with other forms of angina pectoris**

         Excludes 1   other forms of angina pectoris without atherosclerosis of coronary artery bypass graft (I20.8)

     I25.709 **Atherosclerosis of coronary artery bypass graft(s), unspecified, with unspecified angina pectoris**

         Excludes 1   unspecified angina pectoris without atherosclerosis of coronary artery bypass graft (I20.9)

● **I25.71** **Atherosclerosis of autologous vein coronary artery bypass graft(s) with angina pectoris**

     I25.710 **Atherosclerosis of autologous vein coronary artery bypass graft(s) with unstable angina pectoris**

         Excludes 1   unstable angina without atherosclerosis of autologous vein coronary artery bypass graft(s) (I20.0)

     I25.711 **Atherosclerosis of autologous vein coronary artery bypass graft(s) with angina pectoris with documented spasm**

         Excludes 1   angina pectoris with documented spasm without atherosclerosis of autologous vein coronary artery bypass graft(s) (I20.1)

     I25.718 **Atherosclerosis of autologous vein coronary artery bypass graft(s) with other forms of angina pectoris**

         Excludes 1   other forms of angina pectoris without atherosclerosis of autologous vein coronary artery bypass graft(s) (I20.8)

     I25.719 **Atherosclerosis of autologous vein coronary artery bypass graft(s) with unspecified angina pectoris**

         Excludes 1   unspecified angina pectoris without atherosclerosis of autologous vein coronary artery bypass graft(s) (I20.9)

● **I25.72** **Atherosclerosis of autologous artery coronary artery bypass graft(s) with angina pectoris**

Atherosclerosis of internal mammary artery graft with angina pectoris

     I25.720 **Atherosclerosis of autologous artery coronary artery bypass graft(s) with unstable angina pectoris**

         Excludes 1   unstable angina without atherosclerosis of autologous artery coronary artery bypass graft(s) (I20.0)

     I25.721 **Atherosclerosis of autologous artery coronary artery bypass graft(s) with angina pectoris with documented spasm**

         Excludes 1   angina pectoris with documented spasm without atherosclerosis of autologous artery coronary artery bypass graft(s) (I20.1)

     I25.728 **Atherosclerosis of autologous artery coronary artery bypass graft(s) with other forms of angina pectoris**

         Excludes 1   other forms of angina pectoris without atherosclerosis of autologous artery coronary artery bypass graft(s) (I20.8)

     I25.729 **Atherosclerosis of autologous artery coronary artery bypass graft(s) with unspecified angina pectoris**

         Excludes 1   unspecified angina pectoris without atherosclerosis of autologous artery coronary artery bypass graft(s) (I20.9)

◀ New   ◀▭ Revised   ~~deleted~~ Deleted   OGCR Official Guidelines   X Assign placeholder X   ● Use Additional Character(s)

Excludes 1   Excludes 2   Includes   Use additional   Code first   Code also   Unspecified

● **I25.73**   **Atherosclerosis of nonautologous biological coronary artery bypass graft(s) with angina pectoris**

     I25.730   **Atherosclerosis of nonautologous biological coronary artery bypass graft(s) with unstable angina pectoris**

         | Excludes1 | unstable angina without atherosclerosis of nonautologous biological coronary artery bypass graft(s) (I20.0)

     I25.731   **Atherosclerosis of nonautologous biological coronary artery bypass graft(s) with angina pectoris with documented spasm**

         | Excludes1 | angina pectoris with documented spasm without atherosclerosis of nonautologous biological coronary artery bypass graft(s) (I20.1)

     I25.738   **Atherosclerosis of nonautologous biological coronary artery bypass graft(s) with other forms of angina pectoris**

         | Excludes1 | other forms of angina pectoris without atherosclerosis of nonautologous biological coronary artery bypass graft(s) (I20.8)

     I25.739   **Atherosclerosis of nonautologous biological coronary artery bypass graft(s) with unspecified angina pectoris**

         | Excludes1 | unspecified angina pectoris without atherosclerosis of nonautologous biological coronary artery bypass graft(s) (I20.9)

● **I25.75**   **Atherosclerosis of native coronary artery of transplanted heart with angina pectoris**

     | Excludes1 | atherosclerosis of native coronary artery of transplanted heart without angina pectoris (I25.811)

     I25.750   **Atherosclerosis of native coronary artery of transplanted heart with unstable angina**

     I25.751   **Atherosclerosis of native coronary artery of transplanted heart with angina pectoris with documented spasm**

     I25.758   **Atherosclerosis of native coronary artery of transplanted heart with other forms of angina pectoris**

     I25.759   **Atherosclerosis of native coronary artery of transplanted heart with unspecified angina pectoris**

● **I25.76**   **Atherosclerosis of bypass graft of coronary artery of transplanted heart with angina pectoris**

     | Excludes1 | atherosclerosis of bypass graft of coronary artery of transplanted heart without angina pectoris (I25.812)

     I25.760   **Atherosclerosis of bypass graft of coronary artery of transplanted heart with unstable angina**

     I25.761   **Atherosclerosis of bypass graft of coronary artery of transplanted heart with angina pectoris with documented spasm**

     I25.768   **Atherosclerosis of bypass graft of coronary artery of transplanted heart with other forms of angina pectoris**

     I25.769   **Atherosclerosis of bypass graft of coronary artery of transplanted heart with unspecified angina pectoris**

● **I25.79**   **Atherosclerosis of other coronary artery bypass graft(s) with angina pectoris**

     I25.790   **Atherosclerosis of other coronary artery bypass graft(s) with unstable angina pectoris**

         | Excludes1 | unstable angina without atherosclerosis of other coronary artery bypass graft(s) (I20.0)

     I25.791   **Atherosclerosis of other coronary artery bypass graft(s) with angina pectoris with documented spasm**

         | Excludes1 | angina pectoris with documented spasm without atherosclerosis of other coronary artery bypass graft(s) (I20.1)

     I25.798   **Atherosclerosis of other coronary artery bypass graft(s) with other forms of angina pectoris**

         | Excludes1 | other forms of angina pectoris without atherosclerosis of other coronary artery bypass graft(s) (I20.8)

     I25.799   **Atherosclerosis of other coronary artery bypass graft(s) with unspecified angina pectoris**

         | Excludes1 | unspecified angina pectoris without atherosclerosis of other coronary artery bypass graft(s) (I20.9)

CHAPTER 9 (I00–I99)

● **I25.8   Other forms of chronic ischemic heart disease**
   ● **I25.81   Atherosclerosis of other coronary vessels without angina pectoris**
        Use additional code, if applicable, to identify: coronary atherosclerosis due to calcified coronary lesion (I25.84) coronary atherosclerosis due to lipid rich plaque (I25.83)

        | Excludes1 | atherosclerotic heart disease of native coronary artery without angina pectoris (I25.10) |

        I25.810   Atherosclerosis of coronary artery bypass graft(s) without angina pectoris
            Atherosclerosis of coronary artery bypass graft NOS

            | Excludes1 | atherosclerosis of coronary bypass graft(s) with angina pectoris (I25.70- -I25.73-, I25.79-) |

        I25.811   Atherosclerosis of native coronary artery of transplanted heart without angina pectoris
            Atherosclerosis of native coronary artery of transplanted heart NOS

            | Excludes1 | atherosclerosis of native coronary artery of transplanted heart with angina pectoris (I25.75-) |

        I25.812   Atherosclerosis of bypass graft of coronary artery of transplanted heart without angina pectoris
            Atherosclerosis of bypass graft of transplanted heart NOS

            | Excludes1 | atherosclerosis of bypass graft of transplanted heart with angina pectoris (I25.76) |

   I25.82   Chronic total occlusion of coronary artery
        Complete occlusion of coronary artery
        Total occlusion of coronary artery
        Code first coronary atherosclerosis (I25.1-, I25.7-, I25.81-)

        | Excludes1 | acute coronary occlusion with myocardial infarction (I21.-, I22.-) acute coronary occlusion without myocardial infarction (I24.0) |

   I25.83   Coronary atherosclerosis due to lipid rich plaque
        Code first coronary atherosclerosis (I25.1-, I25.7-, I25.81-)

  ● **I25.84   Coronary atherosclerosis due to calcified coronary lesion**
        Coronary atherosclerosis due to severely calcified coronary lesion
        Code first coronary atherosclerosis (I25.1-, I25.7-, I25.81-)

   I25.89   Other forms of chronic ischemic heart disease

I25.9   Chronic ischemic heart disease, unspecified
    Ischemic heart disease (chronic) NOS

Item 9–7   Pulmonary heart disease or **cor pulmonale** is right ventricle hypertrophy or RVH as a result of a respiratory disorder increasing back flow pressure to the right ventricle. Left untreated, cor pulmonale leads to right-heart failure and death.

PULMONARY HEART DISEASE AND DISEASES OF PULMONARY CIRCULATION (I26-I28)

● **I26   Pulmonary embolism**

   | Includes | pulmonary (acute)(artery)(vein) infarction pulmonary (acute)(artery)(vein) thromboembolism pulmonary (acute)(artery)(vein) thrombosis |

   | Excludes2 | chronic pulmonary embolism (I27.82) personal history of pulmonary embolism (Z86.711) pulmonary embolism due to trauma (T79.0, T79.1) pulmonary embolism due to complications of surgical and medical care (T80.0, T81.7-, T82.8-) pulmonary embolism complicating abortion, ectopic or molar pregnancy (O00-O07, O08.2) pulmonary embolism complicating pregnancy, childbirth and the puerperium (O88.-) septic (non-pulmonary) arterial embolism (I76) |

 ● **I26.0   Pulmonary embolism with acute cor pulmonale**
   I26.01   Septic pulmonary embolism with acute cor pulmonale
        Code first underlying infection

   I26.02   Saddle embolus of pulmonary artery with acute cor pulmonale

   I26.09   Other pulmonary embolism with acute cor pulmonale
        Acute cor pulmonale NOS

 ● **I26.9   Pulmonary embolism without acute cor pulmonale**
   I26.90   Septic pulmonary embolism without acute cor pulmonale
        Code first underlying infection

   I26.92   Saddle embolus of pulmonary artery without acute cor pulmonale

   I26.99   Other pulmonary embolism without acute cor pulmonale
        Acute pulmonary embolism NOS
        Pulmonary embolism NOS

● **I27   Other pulmonary heart diseases**
   I27.0   Primary pulmonary hypertension
      | Excludes1 | pulmonary hypertension NOS (I27.2) secondary pulmonary hypertension (I27.2) |

   I27.1   Kyphoscoliotic heart disease

   I27.2   Other secondary pulmonary hypertension
        Pulmonary hypertension NOS
        Code also associated underlying condition

 ● **I27.8   Other specified pulmonary heart diseases**
   I27.81   Cor pulmonale (chronic)
        Cor pulmonale NOS
        | Excludes1 | acute cor pulmonale (I26.0-) |

   I27.82   Chronic pulmonary embolism
        Use additional code, if applicable, for associated long-term (current) use of anticoagulants (Z79.01)
        | Excludes1 | personal history of pulmonary embolism (Z86.711) |

   I27.89   Other specified pulmonary heart diseases
        Eisenmenger's complex
        Eisenmenger's syndrome
        | Excludes1 | Eisenmenger's defect (Q21.8) |

   I27.9   Pulmonary heart disease, unspecified
        Chronic cardiopulmonary disease

● **I28   Other diseases of pulmonary vessels**
    I28.0   Arteriovenous fistula of pulmonary vessels
        Excludes1   congenital arteriovenous fistula (Q25.72)
    I28.1   Aneurysm of pulmonary artery
        Excludes1   congenital aneurysm (Q25.79)
                congenital arteriovenous aneurysm
                    (Q25.72)
    I28.8   Other diseases of pulmonary vessels
        Pulmonary arteritis
        Pulmonary endarteritis
        Rupture of pulmonary vessels
        Stenosis of pulmonary vessels
        Stricture of pulmonary vessels
    I28.9   Disease of pulmonary vessels, unspecified

OTHER FORMS OF HEART DISEASE (I30-I52)

● **I30   Acute pericarditis**
    Inflammation of pericardium (sac surrounding the heart) caused by
    an infection.
      Includes   acute mediastinopericarditis
                acute myopericarditis
                acute pericardial effusion
                acute pleuropericarditis
                acute pneumopericarditis
      Excludes1   Dressler's syndrome (I24.1)
              rheumatic pericarditis (acute) (I01.0)
    I30.0   Acute nonspecific idiopathic pericarditis
    I30.1   Infective pericarditis
        Pneumococcal pericarditis
        Pneumopyopericardium
        Purulent pericarditis
        Pyopericarditis
        Pyopericardium
        Pyopneumopericardium
        Staphylococcal pericarditis
        Streptococcal pericarditis
        Suppurative pericarditis
        Viral pericarditis
        Use additional code (B95-B97) to identify infectious
           agent
    I30.8   Other forms of acute pericarditis
    I30.9   Acute pericarditis, unspecified

● **I31   Other diseases of pericardium**
      Excludes1   diseases of pericardium specified as rheumatic
              (I09.2)
              postcardiotomy syndrome (I97.0)
              traumatic injury to pericardium (S26.-)
    I31.0   Chronic adhesive pericarditis
        Accretio cordis
        Adherent pericardium
        Adhesive mediastinopericarditis
    I31.1   Chronic constrictive pericarditis
        Concretio cordis
        Pericardial calcification
    I31.2   Hemopericardium, not elsewhere classified
        Excludes1   hemopericardium as current complication
                following acute myocardial
                infarction (I23.0)
    I31.3   Pericardial effusion (noninflammatory)
        Chylopericardium
        Excludes1   acute pericardial effusion (I30.9)
    I31.4   Cardiac tamponade
        Code first underlying cause
    I31.8   Other specified diseases of pericardium
        Epicardial plaques
        Focal pericardial adhesions
    I31.9   Disease of pericardium, unspecified
        Pericarditis (chronic) NOS

I32   Pericarditis in diseases classified elsewhere
    Code first underlying disease
      Excludes1   pericarditis (in):
              coxsackie (virus) (B33.23)
              gonococcal (A54.83)
              meningococcal (A39.53)
              rheumatoid (arthritis) (M05.31)
              syphilitic (A52.06)
              systemic lupus erythematosus (M32.12)
              tuberculosis (A18.84)

● **I33   Acute and subacute endocarditis**
    Inflammation/infection of lining of heart, affecting heart valves
    including replacement valves and is usually caused by a
    bacterial infection
      Excludes1   acute rheumatic endocarditis (I01.1)
              endocarditis NOS (I38)
    I33.0   Acute and subacute infective endocarditis
        Bacterial endocarditis (acute) (subacute)
        Infective endocarditis (acute) (subacute) NOS
        Endocarditis lenta (acute) (subacute)
        Malignant endocarditis (acute) (subacute)
        Purulent endocarditis (acute) (subacute)
        Septic endocarditis (acute) (subacute)
        Ulcerative endocarditis (acute) (subacute)
        Vegetative endocarditis (acute) (subacute)
        Use additional code (B95-B97) to identify infectious
           agent
    I33.9   Acute and subacute endocarditis, unspecified
        Acute endocarditis NOS
        Acute myoendocarditis NOS
        Acute periendocarditis NOS
        Subacute endocarditis NOS
        Subacute myoendocarditis NOS
        Subacute periendocarditis NOS

● **I34   Nonrheumatic mitral valve disorders**
      Excludes1   mitral valve disease (I05.9)
              mitral valve failure (I05.8)
              mitral valve stenosis (I05.0)
              mitral valve disorder of unspecified cause with
                diseases of aortic and/or tricuspid valve(s)
                (I08.-)
              mitral valve disorder of unspecified cause with
                mitral stenosis or obstruction (I05.0)
              mitral valve disorder specified as congenital
                (Q23.2, Q23.3)
              mitral valve disorder specified as rheumatic
                (I05.-)
    I34.0   Nonrheumatic mitral (valve) insufficiency
        Nonrheumatic mitral (valve) incompetence NOS
        Nonrheumatic mitral (valve) regurgitation NOS
    I34.1   Nonrheumatic mitral (valve) prolapse
        Floppy nonrheumatic mitral valve syndrome
        Excludes1   Marfan's syndrome (Q87.4-)
    I34.2   Nonrheumatic mitral (valve) stenosis
    I34.8   Other nonrheumatic mitral valve disorders
    I34.9   Nonrheumatic mitral valve disorder, unspecified

● **I35   Nonrheumatic aortic valve disorders**
      Excludes1   aortic valve disorder of unspecified cause but
              with diseases of mitral and/or tricuspid
              valve(s) (I08.-)
              aortic valve disorder specified as congenital
                (Q23.0, Q23.1)
              aortic valve disorder specified as rheumatic (I06.-)
              hypertrophic subaortic stenosis (I42.1)
    I35.0   Nonrheumatic aortic (valve) stenosis
    I35.1   Nonrheumatic aortic (valve) insufficiency
        Nonrheumatic aortic (valve) incompetence NOS
        Nonrheumatic aortic (valve) regurgitation NOS
    I35.2   Nonrheumatic aortic (valve) stenosis with insufficiency
    I35.8   Other nonrheumatic aortic valve disorders
    I35.9   Nonrheumatic aortic valve disorder, unspecified

CHAPTER 9 (I00-I99)

◀ New   ◀▦ Revised   ~~deleted~~ Deleted   OGCR Official Guidelines   X Assign placeholder X   ● Use Additional Character(s)

| Excludes 1 | Excludes 2 | Includes | Use additional | Code first | Code also | Unspecified |

CHAPTER 9 (I00-I99)

● **I36**   **Nonrheumatic tricuspid valve disorders**

     Excludes1   tricuspid valve disorders of unspecified cause (I07.-)

                 tricuspid valve disorders specified as congenital (Q22.4, Q22.8, Q22.9)

                 tricuspid valve disorders specified as rheumatic (I07.-)

                 tricuspid valve disorders with aortic and/or mitral valve involvement (I08.-)

   I36.0   **Nonrheumatic tricuspid (valve) stenosis**

   I36.1   **Nonrheumatic tricuspid (valve) insufficiency**
       Nonrheumatic tricuspid (valve) incompetence
       Nonrheumatic tricuspid (valve) regurgitation

   I36.2   **Nonrheumatic tricuspid (valve) stenosis with insufficiency**

   I36.8   **Other nonrheumatic tricuspid valve disorders**

   I36.9   **Nonrheumatic tricuspid valve disorder, unspecified**

● **I37**   **Nonrheumatic pulmonary valve disorders**

     Excludes1   pulmonary valve disorder specified as congenital (Q22.1, Q22.2, Q22.3)

                 pulmonary valve disorder specified as rheumatic (I09.89)

   I37.0   **Nonrheumatic pulmonary valve stenosis**

   I37.1   **Nonrheumatic pulmonary valve insufficiency**
       Nonrheumatic pulmonary valve incompetence
       Nonrheumatic pulmonary valve regurgitation

   I37.2   **Nonrheumatic pulmonary valve stenosis with insufficiency**

   I37.8   **Other nonrheumatic pulmonary valve disorders**

   I37.9   **Nonrheumatic pulmonary valve disorder, unspecified**

   I38   **Endocarditis, valve unspecified**

     Includes   endocarditis (chronic) NOS
                 valvular incompetence NOS
                 valvular insufficiency NOS
                 valvular regurgitation NOS
                 valvular stenosis NOS
                 valvulitis (chronic) NOS

     Excludes1   congenital insufficiency of cardiac valve NOS (Q24.8)

                 congenital stenosis of cardiac valve NOS (Q24.8)
                 endocardial fibroelastosis (I42.4)
                 endocarditis specified as rheumatic (I09.1)

   I39   **Endocarditis and heart valve disorders in diseases classified elsewhere**

     Code first underlying disease, such as:
       Q fever (A78)

     Excludes1   endocardial involvement in:
                 candidiasis (B37.6)
                 gonococcal infection (A54.83)
                 Libman-Sacks disease (M32.11)
                 listerosis (A32.82)
                 meningococcal infection (A39.51)
                 rheumatoid arthritis (M05.31)
                 syphilis (A52.03)
                 tuberculosis (A18.84)
                 typhoid fever (A01.02)

● **I40**   **Acute myocarditis**

     Inflammation of heart muscle due to infection (viral/bacterial).

     Includes   subacute myocarditis

     Excludes1   acute rheumatic myocarditis (I01.2)

   I40.0   **Infective myocarditis**
       Septic myocarditis
       Use additional code (B95-B97) to identify infectious agent

   I40.1   **Isolated myocarditis**
       Fiedler's myocarditis
       Giant cell myocarditis
       Idiopathic myocarditis

   I40.8   **Other acute myocarditis**

   I40.9   **Acute myocarditis, unspecified**

   I41   **Myocarditis in diseases classified elsewhere**

     Code first underlying disease, such as:
       typhus (A75.0-A75.9)

     Excludes1   myocarditis (in):
                 Chagas' disease (chronic) (B57.2)
                 acute (B57.0)
                 coxsackie (virus) infection (B33.22)
                 diphtheritic (A36.81)
                 gonococcal (A54.83)
                 influenzal (J09.X9, J10.82, J11.82)
                 meningococcal (A39.52)
                 mumps (B26.82)
                 rheumatoid arthritis (M05.31)
                 sarcoid (D86.85)
                 syphilis (A52.06)
                 toxoplasmosis (B58.81)
                 tuberculous (A18.84)

● **I42**   **Cardiomyopathy**

     Disease of the heart muscle resulting in an abnormally enlarged, weakened, thickened, and/or stiffened muscles

     Includes   myocardiopathy

     Code first pre-existing cardiomyopathy complicating pregnancy and puerperium (O99.4)

     Excludes1   ischemic cardiomyopathy (I25.5)
                 peripartum cardiomyopathy (O90.3)

     Excludes2   ventricular hypertrophy (I51.7)

   I42.0   **Dilated cardiomyopathy**
       Congestive cardiomyopathy

   I42.1   **Obstructive hypertrophic cardiomyopathy**
       Hypertrophic subaortic stenosis (idiopathic)

   I42.2   **Other hypertrophic cardiomyopathy**
       Nonobstructive hypertrophic cardiomyopathy

   I42.3   **Endomyocardial (eosinophilic) disease**
       Endomyocardial (tropical) fibrosis
       Löffler's endocarditis

   I42.4   **Endocardial fibroelastosis**
       Congenital cardiomyopathy
       Elastomyofibrosis

   I42.5   **Other restrictive cardiomyopathy**
       Constrictive cardiomyopathy NOS

   I42.6   **Alcoholic cardiomyopathy**
       Code also presence of alcoholism (F10.-)

   I42.7   **Cardiomyopathy due to drug and external agent**
       Code first poisoning due to drug or toxin, if applicable (T36-T65 with fifth or sixth character 1-4 or 6)
       Use additional code for adverse effect, if applicable, to identify drug (T36-T50 with fifth or sixth character 5)

   I42.8   **Other cardiomyopathies**

   I42.9   **Cardiomyopathy, unspecified**
       Cardiomyopathy (primary) (secondary) NOS

   I43   **Cardiomyopathy in diseases classified elsewhere**

     Code first underlying disease, such as:
       amyloidosis (E85.-)
       glycogen storage disease (E74.0)
       gout (M10.0-)
       thyrotoxicosis (E05.0-E05.9-)

     Excludes1   cardiomyopathy (in):
                 coxsackie (virus) (B33.24)
                 diphtheria (A36.81)
                 sarcoidosis (D86.85)
                 tuberculosis (A18.84)

● **I44**   **Atrioventricular and left bundle-branch block**
Conduction problem resulting in arrhythmias/dysrhythmias due to a lack of electrical impulses being transmitted normally through the heart.

   I44.0   **Atrioventricular block, first degree**

   I44.1   **Atrioventricular block, second degree**
      Atrioventricular block, type I and II
      Möbitz block, type I and II
      Second degree block, type I and II
      Wenckebach's block

   I44.2   **Atrioventricular block, complete**
      Complete heart block NOS
      Third degree block

●   **I44.3**   **Other and unspecified atrioventricular block**
      Atrioventricular block NOS

     I44.30   **Unspecified atrioventricular block**

     I44.39   **Other atrioventricular block**

   I44.4   **Left anterior fascicular block**

   I44.5   **Left posterior fascicular block**

●   **I44.6**   **Other and unspecified fascicular block**

     I44.60   **Unspecified fascicular block**
        Left bundle-branch hemiblock NOS

     I44.69   **Other fascicular block**

   I44.7   **Left bundle-branch block, unspecified**

● **I45**   **Other conduction disorders**

   I45.0   **Right fascicular block**

●   **I45.1**   **Other and unspecified right bundle-branch block**

     I45.10   **Unspecified right bundle-branch block**
        Right bundle-branch block NOS

     I45.19   **Other right bundle-branch block**

   I45.2   **Bifascicular block**

   I45.3   **Trifascicular block**

   I45.4   **Nonspecific intraventricular block**
      Bundle-branch block NOS

   I45.5   **Other specified heart block**
      Sinoatrial block
      Sinoauricular block

     | Excludes1 | heart block NOS (I45.9)

   I45.6   **Pre-excitation syndrome**
      Accelerated atrioventricular conduction
      Accessory atrioventricular conduction
      Anomalous atrioventricular excitation
      Lown-Ganong-Levine syndrome
      Pre-excitation atrioventricular conduction
      Wolff-Parkinson-White syndrome

●   **I45.8**   **Other specified conduction disorders**

     I45.81   **Long QT syndrome**

     I45.89   **Other specified conduction disorders**
        Atrioventricular [AV] dissociation
        Interference dissociation
        Isorhythmic dissociation
        Nonparoxysmal AV nodal tachycardia

   I45.9   **Conduction disorder, unspecified**
      Heart block NOS
      Stokes-Adams syndrome

● **I46**   **Cardiac arrest**

   | Excludes1 | cardiogenic shock (R57.0)

   I46.2   **Cardiac arrest due to underlying cardiac condition**
      Code first underlying cardiac condition

   I46.8   **Cardiac arrest due to other underlying condition**
      Code first underlying condition

   I46.9   **Cardiac arrest, cause unspecified**

● **I47**   **Paroxysmal tachycardia**
Code first tachycardia complicating:
      abortion or ectopic or molar pregnancy (O00-O07, O08.8)
      obstetric surgery and procedures (O75.4)

   | Excludes1 | tachycardia NOS (R00.0)
         sinoauricular tachycardia NOS (R00.0)
         sinus [sinusal] tachycardia NOS (R00.0)

   I47.0   **Re-entry ventricular arrhythmia**

   I47.1   **Supraventricular tachycardia**
      Atrial (paroxysmal) tachycardia
      Atrioventricular [AV] (paroxysmal) tachycardia
      Atrioventricular re-entrant (nodal) tachycardia [AVNRT] [AVRT]
      Junctional (paroxysmal) tachycardia
      Nodal (paroxysmal) tachycardia

   I47.2   **Ventricular tachycardia**

   I47.9   **Paroxysmal tachycardia, unspecified**
      Bouveret (-Hoffman) syndrome

● **I48**   **Atrial fibrillation and flutter**
Most common abnormal heart rhythm (arrhythmia) presenting as irregular, rapid beating (tachycardia) of the heart's upper chamber.

   I48.0   **Paroxysmal atrial fibrillation**

   I48.1   **Persistent atrial fibrillation**
      Rapid contractions of the upper heart chamber

   I48.2   **Chronic atrial fibrillation**
      Permanent atrial fibrillation

   I48.3   **Typical atrial flutter**
      Type I atrial flutter

   I48.4   **Atypical atrial flutter**
      Type II atrial flutter

●   **I48.9**   **Unspecified atrial fibrillation and atrial flutter**

     I48.91   **Unspecified atrial fibrillation**

     I48.92   **Unspecified atrial flutter**

● **I49**   **Other cardiac arrhythmias**
Code first cardiac arrhythmia complicating:
      abortion or ectopic or molar pregnancy (O00-O07, O08.8)
      obstetric surgery and procedures (O75.4)

   | Excludes1 | bradycardia NOS (R00.1)
         neonatal dysrhythmia (P29.1-)
         sinoatrial bradycardia (R00.1)
         sinus bradycardia (R00.1)
         vagal bradycardia (R00.1)

●   **I49.0**   **Ventricular fibrillation and flutter**

     I49.01   **Ventricular fibrillation**

     I49.02   **Ventricular flutter**

   I49.1   **Atrial premature depolarization**
      Atrial premature beats

   I49.2   **Junctional premature depolarization**

   I49.3   **Ventricular premature depolarization**

●   **I49.4**   **Other and unspecified premature depolarization**

     I49.40   **Unspecified premature depolarization**
        Premature beats NOS

     I49.49   **Other premature depolarization**
        Ectopic beats
        Extrasystoles
        Extrasystolic arrhythmias
        Premature contractions

   I49.5   **Sick sinus syndrome**
      Tachycardia-bradycardia syndrome

   I49.8   **Other specified cardiac arrhythmias**
      Coronary sinus rhythm disorder
      Ectopic rhythm disorder
      Nodal rhythm disorder

   I49.9   **Cardiac arrhythmia, unspecified**
      Arrhythmia (cardiac) NOS

CHAPTER 9 (I00-I99)

◀ New   ⬅ Revised   ~~deleted~~ Deleted   **OGCR** Official Guidelines   X Assign placeholder X   ● Use Additional Character(s)

| Excludes 1 | | Excludes 2 | Includes   Use additional   Code first   Code also   Unspecified

CHAPTER 9 (I00-I99)

Item 9–8 Congestive heart failure (CHF) is a condition in which the left ventricle of the heart cannot pump enough blood to the body. The blood flow from the heart slows or returns to the heart from the venous system back flow resulting in congestion (fluid accumulation) particularly in the abdomen. Most commonly, fluid collects in the lungs and results in shortness of breath, especially when in a reclining position.

● **I50**   **Heart failure**

Code first heart failure complicating abortion or ectopic or molar pregnancy (O00-O07, O08.8)
heart failure due to hypertension (I11.0)
heart failure due to hypertension with chronic kidney disease (I13.-)
heart failure following surgery (I97.13-)
obstetric surgery and procedures (O75.4)
rheumatic heart failure (I09.81)

   Excludes1   cardiac arrest (I46.-)
              neonatal cardiac failure (P29.0)

   I50.1   **Left ventricular failure**
       Cardiac asthma
       Edema of lung with heart disease NOS
       Edema of lung with heart failure
       Left heart failure
       Pulmonary edema with heart disease NOS
       Pulmonary edema with heart failure

       Excludes1   edema of lung without heart disease or heart failure (J81.-)
                   pulmonary edema without heart disease or failure (J81.-)

● **I50.2**   **Systolic (congestive) heart failure**

       Excludes1   combined systolic (congestive) and diastolic (congestive) heart failure (I50.4-)

       I50.20   **Unspecified systolic (congestive) heart failure**

       I50.21   **Acute systolic (congestive) heart failure**
             Presenting a short and relatively severe episode

       I50.22   **Chronic systolic (congestive) heart failure**
             Long-lasting, presenting over time

       I50.23   **Acute on chronic systolic (congestive) heart failure**
             Combination code. What was a chronic condition now has an acute exacerbation (to make more severe).

● **I50.3**   **Diastolic (congestive) heart failure**

       Excludes1   combined systolic (congestive) and diastolic (congestive) heart failure (I50.4-)

       I50.30   **Unspecified diastolic (congestive) heart failure**

       I50.31   **Acute diastolic (congestive) heart failure**

       I50.32   **Chronic diastolic (congestive) heart failure**

       I50.33   **Acute on chronic diastolic (congestive) heart failure**

● **I50.4**   **Combined systolic (congestive) and diastolic (congestive) heart failure**

       I50.40   **Unspecified combined systolic (congestive) and diastolic (congestive) heart failure**

       I50.41   **Acute combined systolic (congestive) and diastolic (congestive) heart failure**

       I50.42   **Chronic combined systolic (congestive) and diastolic (congestive) heart failure**

       I50.43   **Acute on chronic combined systolic (congestive) and diastolic (congestive) heart failure**

   I50.9   **Heart failure, unspecified**
       Biventricular (heart) failure NOS
       Cardiac, heart or myocardial failure NOS
       Congestive heart disease
       Congestive heart failure NOS
       Right ventricular failure (secondary to left heart failure)

       Excludes1   fluid overload (E87.70)

● **I51**   **Complications and ill-defined descriptions of heart disease**

   Excludes1   any condition in I51.4-I51.9 due to hypertension (I11.-)
              any condition in I51.4-I51.9 due to hypertension and chronic kidney disease (I13.-)
              heart disease specified as rheumatic (I00-I09)

   I51.0   **Cardiac septal defect, acquired**
       Acquired septal atrial defect (old)
       Acquired septal auricular defect (old)
       Acquired septal ventricular defect (old)

       Excludes1   cardiac septal defect as current complication following acute myocardial infarction (I23.1, I23.2)

   I51.1   **Rupture of chordae tendineae, not elsewhere classified**

       Excludes1   rupture of chordae tendineae as current complication following acute myocardial infarction (I23.4)

   I51.2   **Rupture of papillary muscle, not elsewhere classified**

       Excludes1   rupture of papillary muscle as current complication following acute myocardial infarction (I23.5)

   I51.3   **Intracardiac thrombosis, not elsewhere classified**
       Apical thrombosis (old)
       Atrial thrombosis (old)
       Auricular thrombosis (old)
       Mural thrombosis (old)
       Ventricular thrombosis (old)

       Excludes1   intracardiac thrombosis as current complication following acute myocardial infarction (I23.6)

   I51.4   **Myocarditis, unspecified**
       Chronic (interstitial) myocarditis
       Myocardial fibrosis
       Myocarditis NOS

       Excludes1   acute or subacute myocarditis (I40.-)

   I51.5   **Myocardial degeneration**
       Fatty degeneration of heart or myocardium
       Myocardial disease
       Senile degeneration of heart or myocardium

   I51.7   **Cardiomegaly**
       Cardiac dilatation
       Cardiac hypertrophy
       Ventricular dilatation

● **I51.8**   **Other ill-defined heart diseases**

       I51.81   **Takotsubo syndrome**
             Reversible left ventricular dysfunction following sudden emotional stress
             Stress induced cardiomyopathy
             Takotsubo cardiomyopathy
             Transient left ventricular apical ballooning syndrome

       I51.89   **Other ill-defined heart diseases**
             Carditis (acute)(chronic)
             Pancarditis (acute)(chronic)

   I51.9   **Heart disease, unspecified**

I52   **Other heart disorders in diseases classified elsewhere**

     Code first underlying disease, such as:
       congenital syphilis (A50.5)
       mucopolysaccharidosis (E76.3)
       schistosomiasis (B65.0-B65.9)

   Excludes1   heart disease (in):
              gonococcal infection (A54.83)
              meningococcal infection (A39.50)
              rheumatoid arthritis (M05.31)
              syphilis (A52.06)

◀ New   ◀◀ Revised   ~~deleted~~ Deleted   **OGCR** Official Guidelines   X Assign placeholder X   ● Use Additional Character(s)

     Excludes 1   Excludes 2   Includes   Use additional   Code first   Code also   Unspecified

CEREBROVASCULAR DISEASES (I60-I69)

Use additional code to identify presence of:
　　alcohol abuse and dependence (F10.-)
　　exposure to environmental tobacco smoke (Z77.22)
　　history of tobacco use (Z87.891)
　　hypertension (I10-I15)
　　occupational exposure to environmental tobacco smoke
　　　　(Z57.31)
　　tobacco dependence (F17.-)
　　tobacco use (Z72.0)

　　Excludes1　transient cerebral ischemic attacks and related
　　　　　　　syndromes (G45.-)
　　　　　　　traumatic intracranial hemorrhage (S06.-)

● I60　Nontraumatic subarachnoid hemorrhage
　　　　Includes　ruptured cerebral aneurysm
　　　　Excludes1　sequelae of subarachnoid hemorrhage (I69.0-)
　　　　　　　　　syphilitic ruptured cerebral aneurysm (A52.05)

● I60.0　Nontraumatic subarachnoid hemorrhage from carotid
　　　　　siphon and bifurcation
　　　　I60.00　Nontraumatic subarachnoid hemorrhage from
　　　　　　　　unspecified carotid siphon and bifurcation
　　　　I60.01　Nontraumatic subarachnoid hemorrhage from
　　　　　　　　right carotid siphon and bifurcation
　　　　I60.02　Nontraumatic subarachnoid hemorrhage from
　　　　　　　　left carotid siphon and bifurcation

● I60.1　Nontraumatic subarachnoid hemorrhage from middle
　　　　　cerebral artery
　　　　I60.10　Nontraumatic subarachnoid hemorrhage from
　　　　　　　　unspecified middle cerebral artery
　　　　I60.11　Nontraumatic subarachnoid hemorrhage from
　　　　　　　　right middle cerebral artery
　　　　I60.12　Nontraumatic subarachnoid hemorrhage from
　　　　　　　　left middle cerebral artery

● I60.2　Nontraumatic subarachnoid hemorrhage from anterior
　　　　　communicating artery
　　　　I60.20　Nontraumatic subarachnoid hemorrhage from
　　　　　　　　unspecified anterior communicating artery
　　　　I60.21　Nontraumatic subarachnoid hemorrhage from
　　　　　　　　right anterior communicating artery
　　　　I60.22　Nontraumatic subarachnoid hemorrhage from
　　　　　　　　left anterior communicating artery

● I60.3　Nontraumatic subarachnoid hemorrhage from posterior
　　　　　communicating artery
　　　　I60.30　Nontraumatic subarachnoid hemorrhage from
　　　　　　　　unspecified posterior communicating artery
　　　　I60.31　Nontraumatic subarachnoid hemorrhage from
　　　　　　　　right posterior communicating artery
　　　　I60.32　Nontraumatic subarachnoid hemorrhage from
　　　　　　　　left posterior communicating artery

　I60.4　Nontraumatic subarachnoid hemorrhage from basilar
　　　　　artery

● I60.5　Nontraumatic subarachnoid hemorrhage from vertebral
　　　　　artery
　　　　I60.50　Nontraumatic subarachnoid hemorrhage from
　　　　　　　　unspecified vertebral artery
　　　　I60.51　Nontraumatic subarachnoid hemorrhage from
　　　　　　　　right vertebral artery
　　　　I60.52　Nontraumatic subarachnoid hemorrhage from
　　　　　　　　left vertebral artery

　I60.6　Nontraumatic subarachnoid hemorrhage from other
　　　　　intracranial arteries

　I60.7　Nontraumatic subarachnoid hemorrhage from
　　　　　unspecified intracranial artery
　　　　　Ruptured (congenital) berry aneurysm
　　　　　Ruptured (congenital) cerebral aneurysm
　　　　　Subarachnoid hemorrhage (nontraumatic) from cerebral
　　　　　　　artery NOS
　　　　　Subarachnoid hemorrhage (nontraumatic) from
　　　　　　　communicating artery NOS
　　　　　Excludes1　berry aneurysm, nonruptured (I67.1)

　I60.8　Other nontraumatic subarachnoid hemorrhage
　　　　　Meningeal hemorrhage
　　　　　Rupture of cerebral arteriovenous malformation

　I60.9　Nontraumatic subarachnoid hemorrhage, unspecified

● I61　Nontraumatic intracerebral hemorrhage
　　　　Excludes1　sequelae of intracerebral hemorrhage (I69.1-)

　　I61.0　Nontraumatic intracerebral hemorrhage in hemisphere,
　　　　　subcortical
　　　　　Deep intracerebral hemorrhage (nontraumatic)

　　I61.1　Nontraumatic intracerebral hemorrhage in hemisphere,
　　　　　cortical
　　　　　Cerebral lobe hemorrhage (nontraumatic)
　　　　　Superficial intracerebral hemorrhage (nontraumatic)

　　I61.2　Nontraumatic intracerebral hemorrhage in hemisphere,
　　　　　unspecified

　　I61.3　Nontraumatic intracerebral hemorrhage in brain stem

　　I61.4　Nontraumatic intracerebral hemorrhage in cerebellum

　　I61.5　Nontraumatic intracerebral hemorrhage, intraventricular

　　I61.6　Nontraumatic intracerebral hemorrhage, multiple
　　　　　localized

　　I61.8　Other nontraumatic intracerebral hemorrhage

　　I61.9　Nontraumatic intracerebral hemorrhage, unspecified

● I62　Other and unspecified nontraumatic intracranial hemorrhage
　　　　Excludes1　sequelae of intracranial hemorrhage (I69.2)

● I62.0　Nontraumatic subdural hemorrhage
　　　　I62.00　Nontraumatic subdural hemorrhage,
　　　　　　　　unspecified
　　　　I62.01　Nontraumatic acute subdural hemorrhage
　　　　I62.02　Nontraumatic subacute subdural hemorrhage
　　　　I62.03　Nontraumatic chronic subdural hemorrhage

　I62.1　Nontraumatic extradural hemorrhage
　　　　　Nontraumatic epidural hemorrhage

　I62.9　Nontraumatic intracranial hemorrhage, unspecified

(See Plate 141 on page NAP-28.)

● I63　Cerebral infarction
　　　　Includes　occlusion and stenosis of cerebral and precerebral
　　　　　　　　　arteries, resulting in cerebral infarction
　　　　Use additional code, if applicable, to identify status post
　　　　　administration of tPA (rtPA) in a different facility within
　　　　　the last 24 hours prior to admission to current facility
　　　　　(Z92.82)
　　　　Excludes1　sequelae of cerebral infarction (I69.3-)

● I63.0　Cerebral infarction due to thrombosis of precerebral
　　　　　arteries
　　　　I63.00　Cerebral infarction due to thrombosis of
　　　　　　　　unspecified precerebral artery
　　● I63.01　Cerebral infarction due to thrombosis of
　　　　　　　　vertebral artery
　　　　　　　　I63.011　Cerebral infarction due to thrombosis
　　　　　　　　　　　　　of right vertebral artery
　　　　　　　　I63.012　Cerebral infarction due to thrombosis
　　　　　　　　　　　　　of left vertebral artery
　　　　　　　　I63.019　Cerebral infarction due to thrombosis
　　　　　　　　　　　　　of unspecified vertebral artery
　　　　I63.02　Cerebral infarction due to thrombosis of basilar
　　　　　　　　artery
　　● I63.03　Cerebral infarction due to thrombosis of carotid
　　　　　　　　artery
　　　　　　　　I63.031　Cerebral infarction due to thrombosis
　　　　　　　　　　　　　of right carotid artery
　　　　　　　　I63.032　Cerebral infarction due to thrombosis
　　　　　　　　　　　　　of left carotid artery
　　　　　　　　I63.039　Cerebral infarction due to thrombosis
　　　　　　　　　　　　　of unspecified carotid artery
　　　　I63.09　Cerebral infarction due to thrombosis of other
　　　　　　　　precerebral artery

◀ New　　◀▥ Revised　　d̶e̶l̶e̶t̶e̶d̶ Deleted　　OGCR Official Guidelines　　X Assign placeholder X　　● Use Additional Character(s)

| Excludes 1 | Excludes 2 | Includes | Use additional | Code first | Code also | Unspecified |

● **I63.1**   **Cerebral infarction due to embolism of precerebral arteries**

     I63.10   Cerebral infarction due to embolism of unspecified precerebral artery

     ● I63.11   Cerebral infarction due to embolism of vertebral artery

         I63.111   Cerebral infarction due to embolism of right vertebral artery

         I63.112   Cerebral infarction due to embolism of left vertebral artery

         I63.119   Cerebral infarction due to embolism of unspecified vertebral artery

     I63.12   Cerebral infarction due to embolism of basilar artery

     ● I63.13   Cerebral infarction due to embolism of carotid artery

         I63.131   Cerebral infarction due to embolism of right carotid artery

         I63.132   Cerebral infarction due to embolism of left carotid artery

         I63.139   Cerebral infarction due to embolism of unspecified carotid artery

     I63.19   Cerebral infarction due to embolism of other precerebral artery

● **I63.2**   **Cerebral infarction due to unspecified occlusion or stenosis of precerebral arteries**

     I63.20   Cerebral infarction due to unspecified occlusion or stenosis of unspecified precerebral arteries

     ● I63.21   Cerebral infarction due to unspecified occlusion or stenosis of vertebral arteries

         I63.211   Cerebral infarction due to unspecified occlusion or stenosis of right vertebral arteries

         I63.212   Cerebral infarction due to unspecified occlusion or stenosis of left vertebral arteries

         I63.219   Cerebral infarction due to unspecified occlusion or stenosis of unspecified vertebral arteries

     I63.22   Cerebral infarction due to unspecified occlusion or stenosis of basilar arteries

     ● I63.23   Cerebral infarction due to unspecified occlusion or stenosis of carotid arteries

         I63.231   Cerebral infarction due to unspecified occlusion or stenosis of right carotid arteries

         I63.232   Cerebral infarction due to unspecified occlusion or stenosis of left carotid arteries

         I63.239   Cerebral infarction due to unspecified occlusion or stenosis of unspecified carotid arteries

     I63.29   Cerebral infarction due to unspecified occlusion or stenosis of other precerebral arteries

● **I63.3**   **Cerebral infarction due to thrombosis of cerebral arteries**

     I63.30   Cerebral infarction due to thrombosis of unspecified cerebral artery

     ● I63.31   Cerebral infarction due to thrombosis of middle cerebral artery

         I63.311   Cerebral infarction due to thrombosis of right middle cerebral artery

         I63.312   Cerebral infarction due to thrombosis of left middle cerebral artery

         I63.319   Cerebral infarction due to thrombosis of unspecified middle cerebral artery

     ● I63.32   Cerebral infarction due to thrombosis of anterior cerebral artery

         I63.321   Cerebral infarction due to thrombosis of right anterior cerebral artery

         I63.322   Cerebral infarction due to thrombosis of left anterior cerebral artery

         I63.329   Cerebral infarction due to thrombosis of unspecified anterior cerebral artery

     ● I63.33   Cerebral infarction due to thrombosis of posterior cerebral artery

         I63.331   Cerebral infarction due to thrombosis of right posterior cerebral artery

         I63.332   Cerebral infarction due to thrombosis of left posterior cerebral artery

         I63.339   Cerebral infarction due to thrombosis of unspecified posterior cerebral artery

     ● I63.34   Cerebral infarction due to thrombosis of cerebellar artery

         I63.341   Cerebral infarction due to thrombosis of right cerebellar artery

         I63.342   Cerebral infarction due to thrombosis of left cerebellar artery

         I63.349   Cerebral infarction due to thrombosis of unspecified cerebellar artery

     I63.39   Cerebral infarction due to thrombosis of other cerebral artery

● **I63.4**   **Cerebral infarction due to embolism of cerebral arteries**

     I63.40   Cerebral infarction due to embolism of unspecified cerebral artery

     ● I63.41   Cerebral infarction due to embolism of middle cerebral artery

         I63.411   Cerebral infarction due to embolism of right middle cerebral artery

         I63.412   Cerebral infarction due to embolism of left middle cerebral artery

         I63.419   Cerebral infarction due to embolism of unspecified middle cerebral artery

     ● I63.42   Cerebral infarction due to embolism of anterior cerebral artery

         I63.421   Cerebral infarction due to embolism of right anterior cerebral artery

         I63.422   Cerebral infarction due to embolism of left anterior cerebral artery

         I63.429   Cerebral infarction due to embolism of unspecified anterior cerebral artery

     ● I63.43   Cerebral infarction due to embolism of posterior cerebral artery

         I63.431   Cerebral infarction due to embolism of right posterior cerebral artery

         I63.432   Cerebral infarction due to embolism of left posterior cerebral artery

         I63.439   Cerebral infarction due to embolism of unspecified posterior cerebral artery

     ● I63.44   Cerebral infarction due to embolism of cerebellar artery

         I63.441   Cerebral infarction due to embolism of right cerebellar artery

         I63.442   Cerebral infarction due to embolism of left cerebellar artery

         I63.449   Cerebral infarction due to embolism of unspecified cerebellar artery

     I63.49   Cerebral infarction due to embolism of other cerebral artery

● I63.5   Cerebral infarction due to unspecified occlusion or stenosis of cerebral arteries

    I63.50   Cerebral infarction due to unspecified occlusion or stenosis of unspecified cerebral artery

   ● I63.51   Cerebral infarction due to unspecified occlusion or stenosis of middle cerebral artery

      I63.511   Cerebral infarction due to unspecified occlusion or stenosis of right middle cerebral artery

      I63.512   Cerebral infarction due to unspecified occlusion or stenosis of left middle cerebral artery

      I63.519   Cerebral infarction due to unspecified occlusion or stenosis of unspecified middle cerebral artery

   ● I63.52   Cerebral infarction due to unspecified occlusion or stenosis of anterior cerebral artery

      I63.521   Cerebral infarction due to unspecified occlusion or stenosis of right anterior cerebral artery

      I63.522   Cerebral infarction due to unspecified occlusion or stenosis of left anterior cerebral artery

      I63.529   Cerebral infarction due to unspecified occlusion or stenosis of unspecified anterior cerebral artery

   ● I63.53   Cerebral infarction due to unspecified occlusion or stenosis of posterior cerebral artery

      I63.531   Cerebral infarction due to unspecified occlusion or stenosis of right posterior cerebral artery

      I63.532   Cerebral infarction due to unspecified occlusion or stenosis of left posterior cerebral artery

      I63.539   Cerebral infarction due to unspecified occlusion or stenosis of unspecified posterior cerebral artery

   ● I63.54   Cerebral infarction due to unspecified occlusion or stenosis of cerebellar artery

      I63.541   Cerebral infarction due to unspecified occlusion or stenosis of right cerebellar artery

      I63.542   Cerebral infarction due to unspecified occlusion or stenosis of left cerebellar artery

      I63.549   Cerebral infarction due to unspecified occlusion or stenosis of unspecified cerebellar artery

    I63.59   Cerebral infarction due to unspecified occlusion or stenosis of other cerebral artery

I63.6   Cerebral infarction due to cerebral venous thrombosis, nonpyogenic

I63.8   Other cerebral infarction

I63.9   Cerebral infarction, unspecified
    Stroke NOS

● I65   Occlusion and stenosis of precerebral arteries, not resulting in cerebral infarction

   Includes   embolism of precerebral artery
            narrowing of precerebral artery
            obstruction (complete) (partial) of precerebral artery
            thrombosis of precerebral artery

   Excludes1   insufficiency, NOS, of precerebral artery (G45.-)
            insufficiency of precerebral arteries causing cerebral infarction (I63.0-I63.2)

  ● I65.0   Occlusion and stenosis of vertebral artery

    I65.01   Occlusion and stenosis of right vertebral artery

    I65.02   Occlusion and stenosis of left vertebral artery

    I65.03   Occlusion and stenosis of bilateral vertebral arteries

    I65.09   Occlusion and stenosis of unspecified vertebral artery

  I65.1   Occlusion and stenosis of basilar artery

  ● I65.2   Occlusion and stenosis of carotid artery

    I65.21   Occlusion and stenosis of right carotid artery

    I65.22   Occlusion and stenosis of left carotid artery

    I65.23   Occlusion and stenosis of bilateral carotid arteries

    I65.29   Occlusion and stenosis of unspecified carotid artery

  I65.8   Occlusion and stenosis of other precerebral arteries

  I65.9   Occlusion and stenosis of unspecified precerebral artery
    Occlusion and stenosis of precerebral artery NOS

● I66   Occlusion and stenosis of cerebral arteries, not resulting in cerebral infarction

   Includes   embolism of cerebral artery
            narrowing of cerebral artery
            obstruction (complete) (partial) of cerebral artery
            thrombosis of cerebral artery

   Excludes1   occlusion and stenosis of cerebral artery causing cerebral infarction (I63.3-I63.5)

  ● I66.0   Occlusion and stenosis of middle cerebral artery

    I66.01   Occlusion and stenosis of right middle cerebral artery

    I66.02   Occlusion and stenosis of left middle cerebral artery

    I66.03   Occlusion and stenosis of bilateral middle cerebral arteries

    I66.09   Occlusion and stenosis of unspecified middle cerebral artery

  ● I66.1   Occlusion and stenosis of anterior cerebral artery

    I66.11   Occlusion and stenosis of right anterior cerebral artery

    I66.12   Occlusion and stenosis of left anterior cerebral artery

    I66.13   Occlusion and stenosis of bilateral anterior cerebral arteries

    I66.19   Occlusion and stenosis of unspecified anterior cerebral artery

  ● I66.2   Occlusion and stenosis of posterior cerebral artery

    I66.21   Occlusion and stenosis of right posterior cerebral artery

    I66.22   Occlusion and stenosis of left posterior cerebral artery

    I66.23   Occlusion and stenosis of bilateral posterior cerebral arteries

    I66.29   Occlusion and stenosis of unspecified posterior cerebral artery

  I66.3   Occlusion and stenosis of cerebellar arteries

  I66.8   Occlusion and stenosis of other cerebral arteries
    Occlusion and stenosis of perforating arteries

  I66.9   Occlusion and stenosis of unspecified cerebral artery

CHAPTER 9 (I00-I99)

● **I67**   **Other cerebrovascular diseases**
> Excludes1   sequelae of the listed conditions (I69.8)

    I67.0   **Dissection of cerebral arteries, nonruptured**
> > Excludes1   ruptured cerebral arteries (I60.7)

    I67.1   **Cerebral aneurysm, nonruptured**
        Cerebral aneurysm NOS
        Cerebral arteriovenous fistula, acquired
        Internal carotid artery aneurysm, intracranial portion
        Internal carotid artery aneurysm, NOS
> > Excludes1   congenital cerebral aneurysm,
> >   nonruptured (Q28.-)
> >   ruptured cerebral aneurysm (I60.7)

    I67.2   **Cerebral atherosclerosis**
        Atheroma of cerebral and precerebral arteries

    I67.3   **Progressive vascular leukoencephalopathy**
        Binswanger's disease

    I67.4   **Hypertensive encephalopathy**

    I67.5   **Moyamoya disease**

    I67.6   **Nonpyogenic thrombosis of intracranial venous system**
        Nonpyogenic thrombosis of cerebral vein
        Nonpyogenic thrombosis of intracranial venous sinus
> > Excludes1   nonpyogenic thrombosis of intracranial
> >   venous system causing infarction
> >   (I63.6)

    I67.7   **Cerebral arteritis, not elsewhere classified**
        Granulomatous angiitis of the nervous system
> > Excludes1   allergic granulomatous angiitis (M30.1)

●   **I67.8**   **Other specified cerebrovascular diseases**

      I67.81   **Acute cerebrovascular insufficiency**
           Acute cerebrovascular insufficiency
              unspecified as to location or reversibility

      I67.82   **Cerebral ischemia**
           Chronic cerebral ischemia

      I67.83   **Posterior reversible encephalopathy syndrome**
           PRES

●   **I67.84**   **Cerebral vasospasm and vasoconstriction**

        I67.841   **Reversible cerebrovascular**
              vasoconstriction syndrome
               Call-Fleming syndrome
               Code first underlying condition, if
                 applicable, such as eclampsia
                 (O15.00-O15.9)

        I67.848   **Other cerebrovascular vasospasm and**
              vasoconstriction

      I67.89   **Other cerebrovascular disease**

    I67.9   **Cerebrovascular disease, unspecified**

● **I68**   **Cerebrovascular disorders in diseases classified elsewhere**

    I68.0   **Cerebral amyloid angiopathy**
        Code first underlying amyloidosis (E85.-)

    I68.2   **Cerebral arteritis in other diseases classified elsewhere**
        Code first underlying disease
> > Excludes1   cerebral arteritis (in):
> >   listerosis (A32.89)
> >   systemic lupus erythematosus (M32.19)
> >   syphilis (A52.04)
> >   tuberculosis (A18.89)

    I68.8   **Other cerebrovascular disorders in diseases classified elsewhere**
        Code first underlying disease
> > Excludes1   syphilitic cerebral aneurysm (A52.05)

OGCR Section I.c.9.d.

Sequelae of Cerebrovascular Disease

1) Category I69, Sequelae of Cerebrovascular disease

Category I69 is used to indicate conditions classifiable to categories I60-I67 as the causes of sequela (neurologic deficits), themselves classified elsewhere. These "late effects" include neurologic deficits that persist after initial onset of conditions classifiable to categories I60-I67. The neurologic deficits caused by cerebrovascular disease may be present from the onset of may arise at any time after the onset of the condition classifiable to categories I60-I67.

Codes from category I69, Sequelae of cerebrovascular disease, that specify hemiplegia, hemiparesis and monoplegia identify whether the dominant or nondominant side is affected. Should the affected side be documented, but not specified as dominant or nondominant, and the classification system does not indicate a default, code selection is as follows:

For ambidextrous patients, the default should be dominant.

If the left side is affected, the default is non-dominant.

If the right side is affected, the default is dominant.

2) Codes from category I69 with codes from I60-I67

Codes from category I69 may be assigned on a health care record with codes from I60-I67, if the patient has a current cerebrovascular disease and deficits from an old cerebrovascular disease.

● **I69**   **Sequelae of cerebrovascular disease**
      Note: Category I69 is to be used to indicate conditions in I60-I67 as the cause of sequelae. The 'sequelae' include conditions specified as such or as residuals which may occur at any time after the onset of the causal condition.
> > Excludes1   personal history of cerebral infarction without
> >   residual deficit (Z86.73)
> >   personal history of prolonged reversible ischemic
> >   neurologic deficit (PRIND) (Z86.73)
> >   personal history of reversible ischemic
> >   neurologcial deficit (RIND) (Z86.73)
> >   sequelae of traumatic intracranial injury (S06.-)
> >   transient ischemic attack (TIA) (G45.9)

●   **I69.0**   **Sequelae of nontraumatic subarachnoid hemorrhage**

      I69.00   **Unspecified sequelae of nontraumatic subarachnoid hemorrhage**

      I69.01   **Cognitive deficits following nontraumatic subarachnoid hemorrhage**

●   **I69.02**   **Speech and language deficits following nontraumatic subarachnoid hemorrhage**

        I69.020   **Aphasia following nontraumatic subarachnoid hemorrhage**

        I69.021   **Dysphasia following nontraumatic subarachnoid hemorrhage**

        I69.022   **Dysarthria following nontraumatic subarachnoid hemorrhage**

        I69.023   **Fluency disorder following nontraumatic subarachnoid hemorrhage**
              Stuttering following nontraumatic subarachnoid hemorrhage

        I69.028   **Other speech and language deficits following nontraumatic subarachnoid hemorrhage**

● **I69.03**   **Monoplegia of upper limb following nontraumatic subarachnoid hemorrhage**

     I69.031   **Monoplegia of upper limb following nontraumatic subarachnoid hemorrhage affecting right dominant side**

     I69.032   **Monoplegia of upper limb following nontraumatic subarachnoid hemorrhage affecting left dominant side**

     I69.033   **Monoplegia of upper limb following nontraumatic subarachnoid hemorrhage affecting right non-dominant side**

     I69.034   **Monoplegia of upper limb following nontraumatic subarachnoid hemorrhage affecting left non-dominant side**

     I69.039   **Monoplegia of upper limb following nontraumatic subarachnoid hemorrhage affecting unspecified side**

● **I69.04**   **Monoplegia of lower limb following nontraumatic subarachnoid hemorrhage**

     I69.041   **Monoplegia of lower limb following nontraumatic subarachnoid hemorrhage affecting right dominant side**

     I69.042   **Monoplegia of lower limb following nontraumatic subarachnoid hemorrhage affecting left dominant side**

     I69.043   **Monoplegia of lower limb following nontraumatic subarachnoid hemorrhage affecting right non-dominant side**

     I69.044   **Monoplegia of lower limb following nontraumatic subarachnoid hemorrhage affecting left non-dominant side**

     I69.049   **Monoplegia of lower limb following nontraumatic subarachnoid hemorrhage affecting unspecified side**

● **I69.05**   **Hemiplegia and hemiparesis following nontraumatic subarachnoid hemorrhage**

     I69.051   **Hemiplegia and hemiparesis following nontraumatic subarachnoid hemorrhage affecting right dominant side**

     I69.052   **Hemiplegia and hemiparesis following nontraumatic subarachnoid hemorrhage affecting left dominant side**

     I69.053   **Hemiplegia and hemiparesis following nontraumatic subarachnoid hemorrhage affecting right non-dominant side**

     I69.054   **Hemiplegia and hemiparesis following nontraumatic subarachnoid hemorrhage affecting left non-dominant side**

     I69.059   **Hemiplegia and hemiparesis following nontraumatic subarachnoid hemorrhage affecting unspecified side**

● **I69.06**   **Other paralytic syndrome following nontraumatic subarachnoid hemorrhage**

     Use additional code to identify type of paralytic syndrome, such as:
     locked-in state (G83.5)
     quadriplegia (G82.5-)

     Excludes1   hemiplegia/hemiparesis following nontraumatic subarachnoid hemorrhage (I69.05-)
                 monoplegia of lower limb following nontraumatic subarachnoid hemorrhage (I69.04-)
                 monoplegia of upper limb following nontraumatic subarachnoid hemorrhage (I69.03-)

     I69.061   **Other paralytic syndrome following nontraumatic subarachnoid hemorrhage affecting right dominant side**

     I69.062   **Other paralytic syndrome following nontraumatic subarachnoid hemorrhage affecting left dominant side**

     I69.063   **Other paralytic syndrome following nontraumatic subarachnoid hemorrhage affecting right non-dominant side**

     I69.064   **Other paralytic syndrome following nontraumatic subarachnoid hemorrhage affecting left non-dominant side**

     I69.065   **Other paralytic syndrome following nontraumatic subarachnoid hemorrhage, bilateral**

     I69.069   **Other paralytic syndrome following nontraumatic subarachnoid hemorrhage affecting unspecified side**

● **I69.09**   **Other sequelae of nontraumatic subarachnoid hemorrhage**

     I69.090   **Apraxia following nontraumatic subarachnoid hemorrhage**

     I69.091   **Dysphagia following nontraumatic subarachnoid hemorrhage**

         Use additional code to identify the type of dysphagia, if known (R13.1-)

     I69.092   **Facial weakness following nontraumatic subarachnoid hemorrhage**

         Facial droop following nontraumatic subarachnoid hemorrhage

     I69.093   **Ataxia following nontraumatic subarachnoid hemorrhage**

     I69.098   **Other sequelae following nontraumatic subarachnoid hemorrhage**

         Alterations of sensation following nontraumatic subarachnoid hemorrhage
         Disturbance of vision following nontraumatic subarachnoid hemorrhage

         Use additional code to identify the sequelae

CHAPTER 9 (I00-I99)

● I69.1   Sequelae of nontraumatic intracerebral hemorrhage

  I69.10   Unspecified sequelae of nontraumatic
           intracerebral hemorrhage

  I69.11   Cognitive deficits following nontraumatic
           intracerebral hemorrhage

● I69.12   Speech and language deficits following
           nontraumatic intracerebral hemorrhage

    I69.120   Aphasia following nontraumatic
              intracerebral hemorrhage

    I69.121   Dysphasia following nontraumatic
              intracerebral hemorrhage

    I69.122   Dysarthria following nontraumatic
              intracerebral hemorrhage

    I69.123   Fluency disorder following
              nontraumatic intracerebral
              hemorrhage
                Stuttering following nontraumatic
                  subarachnoid hemorrhage

    I69.128   Other speech and language deficits
              following nontraumatic intracerebral
              hemorrhage

● I69.13   Monoplegia of upper limb following
           nontraumatic intracerebral hemorrhage

    I69.131   Monoplegia of upper limb following
              nontraumatic intracerebral
              hemorrhage affecting right dominant
              side

    I69.132   Monoplegia of upper limb following
              nontraumatic intracerebral
              hemorrhage affecting left dominant
              side

    I69.133   Monoplegia of upper limb following
              nontraumatic intracerebral
              hemorrhage affecting right non-
              dominant side

    I69.134   Monoplegia of upper limb following
              nontraumatic intracerebral
              hemorrhage affecting left non-
              dominant side

    I69.139   Monoplegia of upper limb following
              nontraumatic intracerebral
              hemorrhage affecting unspecified side

● I69.14   Monoplegia of lower limb following
           nontraumatic intracerebral hemorrhage

    I69.141   Monoplegia of lower limb following
              nontraumatic intracerebral
              hemorrhage affecting right dominant
              side

    I69.142   Monoplegia of lower limb following
              nontraumatic intracerebral
              hemorrhage affecting left dominant
              side

    I69.143   Monoplegia of lower limb following
              nontraumatic intracerebral
              hemorrhage affecting right non-
              dominant side

    I69.144   Monoplegia of lower limb following
              nontraumatic intracerebral
              hemorrhage affecting left non-
              dominant side

    I69.149   Monoplegia of lower limb following
              nontraumatic intracerebral
              hemorrhage affecting unspecified side

● I69.15   Hemiplegia and hemiparesis following
           nontraumatic intracerebral hemorrhage

    I69.151   Hemiplegia and hemiparesis
              following nontraumatic intracerebral
              hemorrhage affecting right dominant
              side

    I69.152   Hemiplegia and hemiparesis
              following nontraumatic intracerebral
              hemorrhage affecting left dominant
              side

    I69.153   Hemiplegia and hemiparesis
              following nontraumatic intracerebral
              hemorrhage affecting right non-
              dominant side

    I69.154   Hemiplegia and hemiparesis
              following nontraumatic intracerebral
              hemorrhage affecting left non-
              dominant side

    I69.159   Hemiplegia and hemiparesis
              following nontraumatic intracerebral
              hemorrhage affecting unspecified side

● I69.16   Other paralytic syndrome following
           nontraumatic intracerebral hemorrhage

           Use additional code to identify type of
             paralytic syndrome, such as:
             locked-in state (G83.5)
             quadriplegia (G82.5-)

           Excludes1   hemiplegia/hemiparesis
                         following nontraumatic
                         intracerebral hemorrhage
                         (I69.15-)
                       monoplegia of lower limb
                         following nontraumatic
                         intracerebral hemorrhage
                         (I69.14-)
                       monoplegia of upper limb
                         following nontraumatic
                         intracerebral hemorrhage
                         (I69.13-)

    I69.161   Other paralytic syndrome following
              nontraumatic intracerebral
              hemorrhage affecting right dominant
              side

    I69.162   Other paralytic syndrome following
              nontraumatic intracerebral
              hemorrhage affecting left dominant
              side

    I69.163   Other paralytic syndrome following
              nontraumatic intracerebral
              hemorrhage affecting right non-
              dominant side

    I69.164   Other paralytic syndrome following
              nontraumatic intracerebral
              hemorrhage affecting left non-
              dominant side

    I69.165   Other paralytic syndrome following
              nontraumatic intracerebral
              hemorrhage, bilateral

    I69.169   Other paralytic syndrome following
              nontraumatic intracerebral
              hemorrhage affecting unspecified side

⬤ **I69.19** **Other sequelae of nontraumatic intracerebral hemorrhage**
  I69.190 **Apraxia following nontraumatic intracerebral hemorrhage**
  I69.191 **Dysphagia following nontraumatic intracerebral hemorrhage**
    Use additional code to identify the type of dysphagia, if known (R13.1-)
  I69.192 **Facial weakness following nontraumatic intracerebral hemorrhage**
    Facial droop following nontraumatic intracerebral hemorrhage
  I69.193 **Ataxia following nontraumatic intracerebral hemorrhage**
  I69.198 **Other sequelae of nontraumatic intracerebral hemorrhage**
    Alteration of sensations following nontraumatic intracerebral hemorrhage
    Disturbance of vision following nontraumatic intracerebral hemorrhage
    Use additional code to identify the sequelae

⬤ **I69.2** **Sequelae of other nontraumatic intracranial hemorrhage**
  I69.20 **Unspecified sequelae of other nontraumatic intracranial hemorrhage**
  I69.21 **Cognitive deficits following other nontraumatic intracranial hemorrhage**
  ⬤ **I69.22** **Speech and language deficits following other nontraumatic intracranial hemorrhage**
    I69.220 **Aphasia following other nontraumatic intracranial hemorrhage**
    I69.221 **Dysphasia following other nontraumatic intracranial hemorrhage**
    I69.222 **Dysarthria following other nontraumatic intracranial hemorrhage**
    I69.223 **Fluency disorder following other nontraumatic intracranial hemorrhage**
      Stuttering following nontraumatic subarachnoid hemorrhage
    I69.228 **Other speech and language deficits following other nontraumatic intracranial hemorrhage**
  ⬤ **I69.23** **Monoplegia of upper limb following other nontraumatic intracranial hemorrhage**
    I69.231 **Monoplegia of upper limb following other nontraumatic intracranial hemorrhage affecting right dominant side**
    I69.232 **Monoplegia of upper limb following other nontraumatic intracranial hemorrhage affecting left dominant side**
    I69.233 **Monoplegia of upper limb following other nontraumatic intracranial hemorrhage affecting right non-dominant side**
    I69.234 **Monoplegia of upper limb following other nontraumatic intracranial hemorrhage affecting left non-dominant side**
    I69.239 **Monoplegia of upper limb following other nontraumatic intracranial hemorrhage affecting unspecified side**

⬤ **I69.24** **Monoplegia of lower limb following other nontraumatic intracranial hemorrhage**
  I69.241 **Monoplegia of lower limb following other nontraumatic intracranial hemorrhage affecting right dominant side**
  I69.242 **Monoplegia of lower limb following other nontraumatic intracranial hemorrhage affecting left dominant side**
  I69.243 **Monoplegia of lower limb following other nontraumatic intracranial hemorrhage affecting right non-dominant side**
  I69.244 **Monoplegia of lower limb following other nontraumatic intracranial hemorrhage affecting left non-dominant side**
  I69.249 **Monoplegia of lower limb following other nontraumatic intracranial hemorrhage affecting unspecified side**
⬤ **I69.25** **Hemiplegia and hemiparesis following other nontraumatic intracranial hemorrhage**
  I69.251 **Hemiplegia and hemiparesis following other nontraumatic intracranial hemorrhage affecting right dominant side**
  I69.252 **Hemiplegia and hemiparesis following other nontraumatic intracranial hemorrhage affecting left dominant side**
  I69.253 **Hemiplegia and hemiparesis following other nontraumatic intracranial hemorrhage affecting right non-dominant side**
  I69.254 **Hemiplegia and hemiparesis following other nontraumatic intracranial hemorrhage affecting left non-dominant side**
  I69.259 **Hemiplegia and hemiparesis following other nontraumatic intracranial hemorrhage affecting unspecified side**
⬤ **I69.26** **Other paralytic syndrome following other nontraumatic intracranial hemorrhage**
    Use additional code to identify type of paralytic syndrome, such as:
    locked-in state (G83.5)
    quadriplegia (G82.5-)
    Excludes1 hemiplegia/hemiparesis following other nontraumatic intracranial hemorrhage (I69.25-)
    monoplegia of lower limb following other nontraumatic intracranial hemorrhage (I69.24-)
    monoplegia of upper limb following other nontraumatic intracranial hemorrhage (I69.23-)
  I69.261 **Other paralytic syndrome following other nontraumatic intracranial hemorrhage affecting right dominant side**
  I69.262 **Other paralytic syndrome following other nontraumatic intracranial hemorrhage affecting left dominant side**

CHAPTER 9 (I00-I99)

◀ New   ◀▥ Revised   ~~deleted~~ Deleted   OGCR Official Guidelines   X Assign placeholder X   ⬤ Use Additional Character(s)
Excludes 1   Excludes 2   Includes   Use additional   Code first   Code also   Unspecified

927

I69.263   Other paralytic syndrome following other nontraumatic intracranial hemorrhage affecting right non-dominant side

I69.264   Other paralytic syndrome following other nontraumatic intracranial hemorrhage affecting left non-dominant side

I69.265   Other paralytic syndrome following other nontraumatic intracranial hemorrhage, bilateral

I69.269   Other paralytic syndrome following other nontraumatic intracranial hemorrhage affecting unspecified side

● I69.29   Other sequelae of other nontraumatic intracranial hemorrhage

     I69.290   Apraxia following other nontraumatic intracranial hemorrhage

     I69.291   Dysphagia following other nontraumatic intracranial hemorrhage

         Use additional code to identify the type of dysphagia, if known (R13.1-)

     I69.292   Facial weakness following other nontraumatic intracranial hemorrhage

         Facial droop following other nontraumatic intracranial hemorrhage

     I69.293   Ataxia following other nontraumatic intracranial hemorrhage

     I69.298   Other sequelae of other nontraumatic intracranial hemorrhage

         Alteration of sensation following other nontraumatic intracranial hemorrhage

         Disturbance of vision following other nontraumatic intracranial hemorrhage

         Use additional code to identify the sequelae

● I69.3   Sequelae of cerebral infarction

     Sequelae of stroke NOS

   I69.30   Unspecified sequelae of cerebral infarction

   I69.31   Cognitive deficits following cerebral infarction

● I69.32   Speech and language deficits following cerebral infarction

     I69.320   Aphasia following cerebral infarction

     I69.321   Dysphasia following cerebral infarction

     I69.322   Dysarthria following cerebral infarction

     I69.323   Fluency disorder following cerebral infarction

         Stuttering following nontraumatic subarachnoid hemorrhage

     I69.328   Other speech and language deficits following cerebral infarction

● I69.33   Monoplegia of upper limb following cerebral infarction

     I69.331   Monoplegia of upper limb following cerebral infarction affecting right dominant side

     I69.332   Monoplegia of upper limb following cerebral infarction affecting left dominant side

I69.333   Monoplegia of upper limb following cerebral infarction affecting right non-dominant side

I69.334   Monoplegia of upper limb following cerebral infarction affecting left non-dominant side

I69.339   Monoplegia of upper limb following cerebral infarction affecting unspecified side

● I69.34   Monoplegia of lower limb following cerebral infarction

     I69.341   Monoplegia of lower limb following cerebral infarction affecting right dominant side

     I69.342   Monoplegia of lower limb following cerebral infarction affecting left dominant side

     I69.343   Monoplegia of lower limb following cerebral infarction affecting right non-dominant side

     I69.344   Monoplegia of lower limb following cerebral infarction affecting left non-dominant side

     I69.349   Monoplegia of lower limb following cerebral infarction affecting unspecified side

● I69.35   Hemiplegia and hemiparesis following cerebral infarction

     I69.351   Hemiplegia and hemiparesis following cerebral infarction affecting right dominant side

     I69.352   Hemiplegia and hemiparesis following cerebral infarction affecting left dominant side

     I69.353   Hemiplegia and hemiparesis following cerebral infarction affecting right non-dominant side

     I69.354   Hemiplegia and hemiparesis following cerebral infarction affecting left non-dominant side

     I69.359   Hemiplegia and hemiparesis following cerebral infarction affecting unspecified side

● I69.36   Other paralytic syndrome following cerebral infarction

     Use additional code to identify type of paralytic syndrome, such as:
     locked-in state (G83.5)
     quadriplegia (G82.5-)

     Excludes1   hemiplegia/hemiparesis following cerebral infarction (I69.35-)
         monoplegia of lower limb following cerebral infarction (I69.34-)
         monoplegia of upper limb following cerebral infarction (I69.33-)

     I69.361   Other paralytic syndrome following cerebral infarction affecting right dominant side

     I69.362   Other paralytic syndrome following cerebral infarction affecting left dominant side

     I69.363   Other paralytic syndrome following cerebral infarction affecting right non-dominant side

◀ New   ◀▥▥ Revised   deleted Deleted   OGCR Official Guidelines   X Assign placeholder X   ● Use Additional Character(s)

Excludes 1   Excludes 2   Includes   Use additional   Code first   Code also   Unspecified

I69.364　　Other paralytic syndrome following cerebral infarction affecting left non-dominant side

I69.365　　Other paralytic syndrome following cerebral infarction, bilateral

I69.369　　Other paralytic syndrome following cerebral infarction affecting unspecified side

● I69.39　Other sequelae of cerebral infarction

I69.390　　Apraxia following cerebral infarction

I69.391　　Dysphagia following cerebral infarction

> Use additional code to identify the type of dysphagia, if known (R13.1-)

I69.392　　Facial weakness following cerebral infarction

> Facial droop following cerebral infarction

I69.393　　Ataxia following cerebral infarction

I69.398　　Other sequelae of cerebral infarction

> Alteration of sensation following cerebral infarction
> Disturbance of vision following cerebral infarction
> Use additional code to identify the sequelae

● I69.8　Sequelae of other cerebrovascular diseases

> **Excludes1**　sequelae of traumatic intracranial injury (S06.-)

I69.80　　Unspecified sequelae of other cerebrovascular disease

I69.81　　Cognitive deficits following other cerebrovascular disease

● I69.82　Speech and language deficits following other cerebrovascular disease

I69.820　　Aphasia following other cerebrovascular disease

I69.821　　Dysphasia following other cerebrovascular disease

I69.822　　Dysarthria following other cerebrovascular disease

I69.823　　Fluency disorder following other cerebrovascular disease

> Stuttering following nontraumatic subarachnoid hemorrhage

I69.828　　Other speech and language deficits following other cerebrovascular disease

● I69.83　Monoplegia of upper limb following other cerebrovascular disease

I69.831　　Monoplegia of upper limb following other cerebrovascular disease affecting right dominant side

I69.832　　Monoplegia of upper limb following other cerebrovascular disease affecting left dominant side

I69.833　　Monoplegia of upper limb following other cerebrovascular disease affecting right non-dominant side

I69.834　　Monoplegia of upper limb following other cerebrovascular disease affecting left non-dominant side

I69.839　　Monoplegia of upper limb following other cerebrovascular disease affecting unspecified side

● I69.84　Monoplegia of lower limb following other cerebrovascular disease

I69.841　　Monoplegia of lower limb following other cerebrovascular disease affecting right dominant side

I69.842　　Monoplegia of lower limb following other cerebrovascular disease affecting left dominant side

I69.843　　Monoplegia of lower limb following other cerebrovascular disease affecting right non-dominant side

I69.844　　Monoplegia of lower limb following other cerebrovascular disease affecting left non-dominant side

I69.849　　Monoplegia of lower limb following other cerebrovascular disease affecting unspecified side

● I69.85　Hemiplegia and hemiparesis following other cerebrovascular disease

I69.851　　Hemiplegia and hemiparesis following other cerebrovascular disease affecting right dominant side

I69.852　　Hemiplegia and hemiparesis following other cerebrovascular disease affecting left dominant side

I69.853　　Hemiplegia and hemiparesis following other cerebrovascular disease affecting right non-dominant side

I69.854　　Hemiplegia and hemiparesis following other cerebrovascular disease affecting left non-dominant side

I69.859　　Hemiplegia and hemiparesis following other cerebrovascular disease affecting unspecified side

● I69.86　Other paralytic syndrome following other cerebrovascular disease

> Use additional code to identify type of paralytic syndrome, such as:
> locked-in state (G83.5)
> quadriplegia (G82.5-)

> **Excludes1**　hemiplegia/hemiparesis following other cerebrovascular disease (I69.85-)
> monoplegia of lower limb following other cerebrovascular disease (I69.84-)
> monoplegia of upper limb following other cerebrovascular disease (I69.83-)

I69.861　　Other paralytic syndrome following other cerebrovascular disease affecting right dominant side

I69.862　　Other paralytic syndrome following other cerebrovascular disease affecting left dominant side

I69.863　　Other paralytic syndrome following other cerebrovascular disease affecting right non-dominant side

I69.864　　Other paralytic syndrome following other cerebrovascular disease affecting left non-dominant side

I69.865　　Other paralytic syndrome following other cerebrovascular disease, bilateral

I69.869　　Other paralytic syndrome following other cerebrovascular disease affecting unspecified side

CHAPTER 9 (I00-I99)

● **I69.89**   **Other sequelae of other cerebrovascular disease**

     I69.890   **Apraxia following other cerebrovascular disease**

     I69.891   **Dysphagia following other cerebrovascular disease**

         Use additional code to identify the type of dysphagia, if known (R13.1-)

     I69.892   **Facial weakness following other cerebrovascular disease**

         Facial droop following other cerebrovascular disease

     I69.893   **Ataxia following other cerebrovascular disease**

     I69.898   **Other sequelae of other cerebrovascular disease**

         Alteration of sensation following other cerebrovascular disease

         Disturbance of vision following other cerebrovascular disease

         Use additional code to identify the sequelae

● **I69.9**   **Sequelae of unspecified cerebrovascular diseases**

   Excludes1   sequelae of stroke (I69.3)   sequelae of traumatic intracranial injury (S06.-)

   I69.90   **Unspecified sequelae of unspecified cerebrovascular disease**

   I69.91   **Cognitive deficits following unspecified cerebrovascular disease**

● **I69.92**   **Speech and language deficits following unspecified cerebrovascular disease**

     I69.920   **Aphasia following unspecified cerebrovascular disease**

     I69.921   **Dysphasia following unspecified cerebrovascular disease**

     I69.922   **Dysarthria following unspecified cerebrovascular disease**

     I69.923   **Fluency disorder following unspecified cerebrovascular disease**

         Stuttering following nontraumatic subarachnoid hemorrhage

     I69.928   **Other speech and language deficits following unspecified cerebrovascular disease**

● **I69.93**   **Monoplegia of upper limb following unspecified cerebrovascular disease**

     I69.931   **Monoplegia of upper limb following unspecified cerebrovascular disease affecting right dominant side**

     I69.932   **Monoplegia of upper limb following unspecified cerebrovascular disease affecting left dominant side**

     I69.933   **Monoplegia of upper limb following unspecified cerebrovascular disease affecting right non-dominant side**

     I69.934   **Monoplegia of upper limb following unspecified cerebrovascular disease affecting left non-dominant side**

     I69.939   **Monoplegia of upper limb following unspecified cerebrovascular disease affecting unspecified side**

● **I69.94**   **Monoplegia of lower limb following unspecified cerebrovascular disease**

     I69.941   **Monoplegia of lower limb following unspecified cerebrovascular disease affecting right dominant side**

     I69.942   **Monoplegia of lower limb following unspecified cerebrovascular disease affecting left dominant side**

     I69.943   **Monoplegia of lower limb following unspecified cerebrovascular disease affecting right non-dominant side**

     I69.944   **Monoplegia of lower limb following unspecified cerebrovascular disease affecting left non-dominant side**

     I69.949   **Monoplegia of lower limb following unspecified cerebrovascular disease affecting unspecified side**

● **I69.95**   **Hemiplegia and hemiparesis following unspecified cerebrovascular disease**

     I69.951   **Hemiplegia and hemiparesis following unspecified cerebrovascular disease affecting right dominant side**

     I69.952   **Hemiplegia and hemiparesis following unspecified cerebrovascular disease affecting left dominant side**

     I69.953   **Hemiplegia and hemiparesis following unspecified cerebrovascular disease affecting right non-dominant side**

     I69.954   **Hemiplegia and hemiparesis following unspecified cerebrovascular disease affecting left non-dominant side**

     I69.959   **Hemiplegia and hemiparesis following unspecified cerebrovascular disease affecting unspecified side**

● **I69.96**   **Other paralytic syndrome following unspecified cerebrovascular disease**

   Use additional code to identify type of paralytic syndrome, such as:
   locked-in state (G83.5)
   quadriplegia (G82.5-)

   Excludes1   hemiplegia/hemiparesis following unspecified cerebrovascular disease (I69.95-)
     monoplegia of lower limb following unspecified cerebrovascular disease (I69.94-)
     monoplegia of upper limb following unspecified cerebrovascular disease (I69.93-)

     I69.961   **Other paralytic syndrome following unspecified cerebrovascular disease affecting right dominant side**

     I69.962   **Other paralytic syndrome following unspecified cerebrovascular disease affecting left dominant side**

     I69.963   **Other paralytic syndrome following unspecified cerebrovascular disease affecting right non-dominant side**

     I69.964   **Other paralytic syndrome following unspecified cerebrovascular disease affecting left non-dominant side**

     I69.965   **Other paralytic syndrome following unspecified cerebrovascular disease, bilateral**

     I69.969   **Other paralytic syndrome following unspecified cerebrovascular disease affecting unspecified side**

● I69.99   **Other sequelae of unspecified cerebrovascular disease**

    I69.990   **Apraxia following unspecified cerebrovascular disease**

    I69.991   **Dysphagia following unspecified cerebrovascular disease**
        Use additional code to identify the type of dysphagia, if known (R13.1-)

    I69.992   **Facial weakness following unspecified cerebrovascular disease**
        Facial droop following unspecified cerebrovascular disease

    I69.993   **Ataxia following unspecified cerebrovascular disease**

    I69.998   **Other sequelae following unspecified cerebrovascular disease**
        Alteration in sensation following unspecified cerebrovascular disease
        Disturbance of vision following unspecified cerebrovascular disease
        Use additional code to identify the sequelae

DISEASES OF ARTERIES, ARTERIOLES AND CAPILLARIES (I70-I79)

● **I70**   **Atherosclerosis**

    Includes   arteriolosclerosis
        arterial degeneration
        arteriosclerosis
        arteriosclerotic vascular disease
        arteriovascular degeneration
        atheroma
        endarteritis deformans or obliterans
        senile arteritis
        senile endarteritis
        vascular degeneration

    Use additional code to identify:
        exposure to environmental tobacco smoke (Z77.22)
        history of tobacco use (Z87.891)
        occupational exposure to environmental tobacco smoke (Z57.31)
        tobacco dependence (F17.-)
        tobacco use (Z72.0)

    Excludes2   arteriosclerotic cardiovascular disease (I25.1-)
        arteriosclerotic heart disease (I25.1-)
        atheroembolism (I75.-)
        cerebral atherosclerosis (I67.2)
        coronary atherosclerosis (I25.1-)
        mesenteric atherosclerosis (K55.1)
        precerebral atherosclerosis (I67.2)
        primary pulmonary atherosclerosis (I27.0)

  I70.0   **Atherosclerosis of aorta**

  I70.1   **Atherosclerosis of renal artery**
    Goldblatt's kidney
    Excludes2   atherosclerosis of renal arterioles (I12.-)

(See Plates 500, 501, and 502 on pages NAP-12 – NAP-14.)

● I70.2   **Atherosclerosis of native arteries of the extremities**
    Mönckeberg's (medial) sclerosis
    Use additional code, if applicable, to identify chronic total occlusion of artery of extremity (I70.92)
    Excludes2   atherosclerosis of bypass graft of extremities (I70.30-I70.79)

● I70.20   **Unspecified atherosclerosis of native arteries of extremities**

    I70.201   **Unspecified atherosclerosis of native arteries of extremities, right leg**

    I70.202   **Unspecified atherosclerosis of native arteries of extremities, left leg**

    I70.203   **Unspecified atherosclerosis of native arteries of extremities, bilateral legs**

    I70.208   **Unspecified atherosclerosis of native arteries of extremities, other extremity**

    I70.209   **Unspecified atherosclerosis of native arteries of extremities, unspecified extremity**

● I70.21   **Atherosclerosis of native arteries of extremities with intermittent claudication**

    I70.211   **Atherosclerosis of native arteries of extremities with intermittent claudication, right leg**

    I70.212   **Atherosclerosis of native arteries of extremities with intermittent claudication, left leg**

    I70.213   **Atherosclerosis of native arteries of extremities with intermittent claudication, bilateral legs**

    I70.218   **Atherosclerosis of native arteries of extremities with intermittent claudication, other extremity**

    I70.219   **Atherosclerosis of native arteries of extremities with intermittent claudication, unspecified extremity**

● I70.22   **Atherosclerosis of native arteries of extremities with rest pain**
    Includes   any condition classifiable to I70.21-

    I70.221   **Atherosclerosis of native arteries of extremities with rest pain, right leg**

    I70.222   **Atherosclerosis of native arteries of extremities with rest pain, left leg**

    I70.223   **Atherosclerosis of native arteries of extremities with rest pain, bilateral legs**

    I70.228   **Atherosclerosis of native arteries of extremities with rest pain, other extremity**

    I70.229   **Atherosclerosis of native arteries of extremities with rest pain, unspecified extremity**

● I70.23   **Atherosclerosis of native arteries of right leg with ulceration**
    Includes   any condition classifiable to I70.211 and I70.221
    Use additional code to identify severity of ulcer (L97.-)

    I70.231   **Atherosclerosis of native arteries of right leg with ulceration of thigh**

    I70.232   **Atherosclerosis of native arteries of right leg with ulceration of calf**

    I70.233   **Atherosclerosis of native arteries of right leg with ulceration of ankle**

    I70.234   **Atherosclerosis of native arteries of right leg with ulceration of heel and midfoot**
        Atherosclerosis of native arteries of right leg with ulceration of plantar surface of midfoot

    I70.235   **Atherosclerosis of native arteries of right leg with ulceration of other part of foot**
        Atherosclerosis of native arteries of right leg extremities with ulceration of toe

    I70.238   **Atherosclerosis of native arteries of right leg with ulceration of other part of lower right leg**

    I70.239   **Atherosclerosis of native arteries of right leg with ulceration of unspecified site**

◀ New   ◀|||| Revised   ~~deleted~~ Deleted   **OGCR** Official Guidelines   **X** Assign placeholder X   ● Use Additional Character(s)

| Excludes 1 | Excludes 2 | Includes | Use additional | Code first | Code also | Unspecified |

● **I70.24** **Atherosclerosis of native arteries of left leg with ulceration**

> **Includes**   any condition classifiable to I70.212 and I70.222

> Use additional code to identify severity of ulcer (L97.-)

I70.241 Atherosclerosis of native arteries of left leg with ulceration of thigh

I70.242 Atherosclerosis of native arteries of left leg with ulceration of calf

I70.243 Atherosclerosis of native arteries of left leg with ulceration of ankle

I70.244 Atherosclerosis of native arteries of left leg with ulceration of heel and midfoot
> Atherosclerosis of native arteries of left leg with ulceration of plantar surface of midfoot

I70.245 Atherosclerosis of native arteries of left leg with ulceration of other part of foot
> Atherosclerosis of native arteries of left leg extremities with ulceration of toe

I70.248 Atherosclerosis of native arteries of left leg with ulceration of other part of lower left leg

I70.249 Atherosclerosis of native arteries of left leg with ulceration of unspecified site

I70.25 **Atherosclerosis of native arteries of other extremities with ulceration**

> **Includes**   any condition classifiable to I70.218 and I70.228

> Use additional code to identify the severity of the ulcer (L98.49-)

● **I70.26** **Atherosclerosis of native arteries of extremities with gangrene**

> **Includes**   any condition classifiable to I70.21-, I70.22-, I70.23-, I70.24-, and I70.25-

> Use additional code to identify the severity of any ulcer (L97.-, L98.49-), if applicable

I70.261 Atherosclerosis of native arteries of extremities with gangrene, right leg

I70.262 Atherosclerosis of native arteries of extremities with gangrene, left leg

I70.263 Atherosclerosis of native arteries of extremities with gangrene, bilateral legs

I70.268 Atherosclerosis of native arteries of extremities with gangrene, other extremity

I70.269 Atherosclerosis of native arteries of extremities with gangrene, unspecified extremity

● **I70.29** **Other atherosclerosis of native arteries of extremities**

I70.291 Other atherosclerosis of native arteries of extremities, right leg

I70.292 Other atherosclerosis of native arteries of extremities, left leg

I70.293 Other atherosclerosis of native arteries of extremities, bilateral legs

I70.298 Other atherosclerosis of native arteries of extremities, other extremity

I70.299 Other atherosclerosis of native arteries of extremities, unspecified extremity

● **I70.3** **Atherosclerosis of unspecified type of bypass graft(s) of the extremities**

> Use additional code, if applicable, to identify chronic total occlusion of artery of extremity (I70.92)

> **Excludes1**   embolism or thrombus of bypass graft(s) of extremities (T82.8-)

● **I70.30** **Unspecified atherosclerosis of unspecified type of bypass graft(s) of the extremities**

70.301 Unspecified atherosclerosis of unspecified type of bypass graft(s) of the extremities, right leg

I70.302 Unspecified atherosclerosis of unspecified type of bypass graft(s) of the extremities, left leg

I70.303 Unspecified atherosclerosis of unspecified type of bypass graft(s) of the extremities, bilateral legs

I70.308 Unspecified atherosclerosis of unspecified type of bypass graft(s) of the extremities, other extremity

I70.309 Unspecified atherosclerosis of unspecified type of bypass graft(s) of the extremities, unspecified extremity

● **I70.31** **Atherosclerosis of unspecified type of bypass graft(s) of the extremities with intermittent claudication**

I70.311 Atherosclerosis of unspecified type of bypass graft(s) of the extremities with intermittent claudication, right leg

I70.312 Atherosclerosis of unspecified type of bypass graft(s) of the extremities with intermittent claudication, left leg

I70.313 Atherosclerosis of unspecified type of bypass graft(s) of the extremities with intermittent claudication, bilateral legs

I70.318 Atherosclerosis of unspecified type of bypass graft(s) of the extremities with intermittent claudication, other extremity

I70.319 Atherosclerosis of unspecified type of bypass graft(s) of the extremities with intermittent claudication, unspecified extremity

● **I70.32** **Atherosclerosis of unspecified type of bypass graft(s) of the extremities with rest pain**

> **Includes**   any condition classifiable to I70.31-

I70.321 Atherosclerosis of unspecified type of bypass graft(s) of the extremities with rest pain, right leg

I70.322 Atherosclerosis of unspecified type of bypass graft(s) of the extremities with rest pain, left leg

I70.323 Atherosclerosis of unspecified type of bypass graft(s) of the extremities with rest pain, bilateral legs

I70.328 Atherosclerosis of unspecified type of bypass graft(s) of the extremities with rest pain, other extremity

I70.329 Atherosclerosis of unspecified type of bypass graft(s) of the extremities with rest pain, unspecified extremity

● **I70.33** **Atherosclerosis of unspecified type of bypass graft(s) of the right leg with ulceration**

> **Includes** any condition classifiable to I70.311 and I70.321

Use additional code to identify severity of ulcer (L97.-)

I70.331 **Atherosclerosis of unspecified type of bypass graft(s) of the right leg with ulceration of thigh**

I70.332 **Atherosclerosis of unspecified type of bypass graft(s) of the right leg with ulceration of calf**

I70.333 **Atherosclerosis of unspecified type of bypass graft(s) of the right leg with ulceration of ankle**

I70.334 **Atherosclerosis of unspecified type of bypass graft(s) of the right leg with ulceration of heel and midfoot**
> Atherosclerosis of unspecified type of bypass graft(s) of right leg with ulceration of plantar surface of midfoot

I70.335 **Atherosclerosis of unspecified type of bypass graft(s) of the right leg with ulceration of other part of foot**
> Atherosclerosis of unspecified type of bypass graft(s) of the right leg with ulceration of toe

I70.338 **Atherosclerosis of unspecified type of bypass graft(s) of the right leg with ulceration of other part of lower leg**

I70.339 **Atherosclerosis of unspecified type of bypass graft(s) of the right leg with ulceration of unspecified site**

● **I70.34** **Atherosclerosis of unspecified type of bypass graft(s) of the left leg with ulceration**

> **Includes** any condition classifiable to I70.312 and I70.322

Use additional code to identify severity of ulcer (L97.-)

I70.341 **Atherosclerosis of unspecified type of bypass graft(s) of the left leg with ulceration of thigh**

I70.342 **Atherosclerosis of unspecified type of bypass graft(s) of the left leg with ulceration of calf**

I70.343 **Atherosclerosis of unspecified type of bypass graft(s) of the left leg with ulceration of ankle**

I70.344 **Atherosclerosis of unspecified type of bypass graft(s) of the left leg with ulceration of heel and midfoot**
> Atherosclerosis of unspecified type of bypass graft(s) of left leg with ulceration of plantar surface of midfoot

I70.345 **Atherosclerosis of unspecified type of bypass graft(s) of the left leg with ulceration of other part of foot**
> Atherosclerosis of unspecified type of bypass graft(s) of the left leg with ulceration of toe

I70.348 **Atherosclerosis of unspecified type of bypass graft(s) of the left leg with ulceration of other part of lower leg**

I70.349 **Atherosclerosis of unspecified type of bypass graft(s) of the left leg with ulceration of unspecified site**

I70.35 **Atherosclerosis of unspecified type of bypass graft(s) of other extremity with ulceration**

> **Includes** any condition classifiable to I70.318 and I70.328

Use additional code to identify severity of ulcer (L98.49-)

● **I70.36** **Atherosclerosis of unspecified type of bypass graft(s) of the extremities with gangrene**

> **Includes** any condition classifiable to I70.31-, I70.32-, I70.33-, I70.34-, I70.35

Use additional code to identify the severity of any ulcer (L97.-, L98.49-), if applicable

I70.361 **Atherosclerosis of unspecified type of bypass graft(s) of the extremities with gangrene, right leg**

I70.362 **Atherosclerosis of unspecified type of bypass graft(s) of the extremities with gangrene, left leg**

I70.363 **Atherosclerosis of unspecified type of bypass graft(s) of the extremities with gangrene, bilateral legs**

I70.368 **Atherosclerosis of unspecified type of bypass graft(s) of the extremities with gangrene, other extremity**

I70.369 **Atherosclerosis of unspecified type of bypass graft(s) of the extremities with gangrene, unspecified extremity**

● **I70.39** **Other atherosclerosis of unspecified type of bypass graft(s) of the extremities**

I70.391 **Other atherosclerosis of unspecified type of bypass graft(s) of the extremities, right leg**

I70.392 **Other atherosclerosis of unspecified type of bypass graft(s) of the extremities, left leg**

I70.393 **Other atherosclerosis of unspecified type of bypass graft(s) of the extremities, bilateral legs**

I70.398 **Other atherosclerosis of unspecified type of bypass graft(s) of the extremities, other extremity**

I70.399 **Other atherosclerosis of unspecified type of bypass graft(s) of the extremities, unspecified extremity**

● **I70.4** **Atherosclerosis of autologous vein bypass graft(s) of the extremities**

Use additional code, if applicable, to identify chronic total occlusion of artery of extremity (I70.92)

● **I70.40** **Unspecified atherosclerosis of autologous vein bypass graft(s) of the extremities**

I70.401 **Unspecified atherosclerosis of autologous vein bypass graft(s) of the extremities, right leg**

I70.402 **Unspecified atherosclerosis of autologous vein bypass graft(s) of the extremities, left leg**

I70.403 **Unspecified atherosclerosis of autologous vein bypass graft(s) of the extremities, bilateral legs**

I70.408 **Unspecified atherosclerosis of autologous vein bypass graft(s) of the extremities, other extremity**

I70.409 **Unspecified atherosclerosis of autologous vein bypass graft(s) of the extremities, unspecified extremity**

CHAPTER 9 (I00-I99)

◀ New   ◀▥ Revised   ~~deleted~~ Deleted   OGCR Official Guidelines   X Assign placeholder X   ● Use Additional Character(s)

| Excludes 1 | Excludes 2 | Includes | Use additional | Code first | Code also | Unspecified |

● **I70.41**   **Atherosclerosis of autologous vein bypass graft(s) of the extremities with intermittent claudication**

    I70.411   Atherosclerosis of autologous vein bypass graft(s) of the extremities with intermittent claudication, right leg

    I70.412   Atherosclerosis of autologous vein bypass graft(s) of the extremities with intermittent claudication, left leg

    I70.413   Atherosclerosis of autologous vein bypass graft(s) of the extremities with intermittent claudication, bilateral legs

    I70.418   Atherosclerosis of autologous vein bypass graft(s) of the extremities with intermittent claudication, other extremity

    I70.419   Atherosclerosis of autologous vein bypass graft(s) of the extremities with intermittent claudication, unspecified extremity

● **I70.42**   **Atherosclerosis of autologous vein bypass graft(s) of the extremities with rest pain**

    Includes   any condition classifiable to I70.41-

    I70.421   Atherosclerosis of autologous vein bypass graft(s) of the extremities with rest pain, right leg

    I70.422   Atherosclerosis of autologous vein bypass graft(s) of the extremities with rest pain, left leg

    I70.423   Atherosclerosis of autologous vein bypass graft(s) of the extremities with rest pain, bilateral legs

    I70.428   Atherosclerosis of autologous vein bypass graft(s) of the extremities with rest pain, other extremity

    I70.429   Atherosclerosis of autologous vein bypass graft(s) of the extremities with rest pain, unspecified extremity

● **I70.43**   **Atherosclerosis of autologous vein bypass graft(s) of the right leg with ulceration**

    Includes   any condition classifiable to I70.411 and I70.421

    Use additional code to identify severity of ulcer (L97.-)

    I70.431   Atherosclerosis of autologous vein bypass graft(s) of the right leg with ulceration of thigh

    I70.432   Atherosclerosis of autologous vein bypass graft(s) of the right leg with ulceration of calf

    I70.433   Atherosclerosis of autologous vein bypass graft(s) of the right leg with ulceration of ankle

    I70.434   Atherosclerosis of autologous vein bypass graft(s) of the right leg with ulceration of heel and midfoot
       Atherosclerosis of autologous vein bypass graft(s) of right leg with ulceration of plantar surface of midfoot

    I70.435   Atherosclerosis of autologous vein bypass graft(s) of the right leg with ulceration of other part of foot
       Atherosclerosis of autologous vein bypass graft(s) of right leg with ulceration of toe

    I70.438   Atherosclerosis of autologous vein bypass graft(s) of the right leg with ulceration of other part of lower leg

    I70.439   Atherosclerosis of autologous vein bypass graft(s) of the right leg with ulceration of unspecified site

● **I70.44**   **Atherosclerosis of autologous vein bypass graft(s) of the left leg with ulceration**

    Includes   any condition classifiable to I70.412 and I70.422

    Use additional code to identify severity of ulcer (L97.-)

    I70.441   Atherosclerosis of autologous vein bypass graft(s) of the left leg with ulceration of thigh

    I70.442   Atherosclerosis of autologous vein bypass graft(s) of the left leg with ulceration of calf

    I70.443   Atherosclerosis of autologous vein bypass graft(s) of the left leg with ulceration of ankle

    I70.444   Atherosclerosis of autologous vein bypass graft(s) of the left leg with ulceration of heel and midfoot
       Atherosclerosis of autologous vein bypass graft(s) of left leg with ulceration of plantar surface of midfoot

    I70.445   Atherosclerosis of autologous vein bypass graft(s) of the left leg with ulceration of other part of foot
       Atherosclerosis of autologous vein bypass graft(s) of left leg with ulceration of toe

    I70.448   Atherosclerosis of autologous vein bypass graft(s) of the left leg with ulceration of other part of lower leg

    I70.449   Atherosclerosis of autologous vein bypass graft(s) of the left leg with ulceration of unspecified site

I70.45   **Atherosclerosis of autologous vein bypass graft(s) of other extremity with ulceration**

    Includes   any condition classifiable to I70.418, I70.428, and I70.438

    Use additional code to identify severity of ulcer (L98.49-)

● **I70.46**   **Atherosclerosis of autologous vein bypass graft(s) of the extremities with gangrene**

    Includes   any condition classifiable to I70.41-, I70.42-, and I70.43-, I70.44-, I70.45

    Use additional code to identify the severity of any ulcer (L97.-, L98.49-), if applicable

    I70.461   Atherosclerosis of autologous vein bypass graft(s) of the extremities with gangrene, right leg

    I70.462   Atherosclerosis of autologous vein bypass graft(s) of the extremities with gangrene, left leg

    I70.463   Atherosclerosis of autologous vein bypass graft(s) of the extremities with gangrene, bilateral legs

    I70.468   Atherosclerosis of autologous vein bypass graft(s) of the extremities with gangrene, other extremity

    I70.469   Atherosclerosis of autologous vein bypass graft(s) of the extremities with gangrene, unspecified extremity

● **I70.49**   **Other atherosclerosis of autologous vein bypass graft(s) of the extremities**

    I70.491   Other atherosclerosis of autologous vein bypass graft(s) of the extremities, right leg

    I70.492   Other atherosclerosis of autologous vein bypass graft(s) of the extremities, left leg

    I70.493   Other atherosclerosis of autologous vein bypass graft(s) of the extremities, bilateral legs

    I70.498   Other atherosclerosis of autologous vein bypass graft(s) of the extremities, other extremity

    I70.499   Other atherosclerosis of autologous vein bypass graft(s) of the extremities, **unspecified** extremity

● **I70.5**   **Atherosclerosis of nonautologous biological bypass graft(s) of the extremities**

    Use additional code, if applicable, to identify chronic total occlusion of artery of extremity (I70.92)

   ● **I70.50**   **Unspecified atherosclerosis of nonautologous biological bypass graft(s) of the extremities**

    I70.501   **Unspecified** atherosclerosis of nonautologous biological bypass graft(s) of the extremities, right leg

    I70.502   **Unspecified** atherosclerosis of nonautologous biological bypass graft(s) of the extremities, left leg

    I70.503   **Unspecified** atherosclerosis of nonautologous biological bypass graft(s) of the extremities, bilateral legs

    I70.508   **Unspecified** atherosclerosis of nonautologous biological bypass graft(s) of the extremities, other extremity

    I70.509   **Unspecified** atherosclerosis of nonautologous biological bypass graft(s) of the extremities, unspecified extremity

   ● **I70.51**   **Atherosclerosis of nonautologous biological bypass graft(s) of the extremities intermittent claudication**

    I70.511   Atherosclerosis of nonautologous biological bypass graft(s) of the extremities with intermittent claudication, right leg

    I70.512   Atherosclerosis of nonautologous biological bypass graft(s) of the extremities with intermittent claudication, left leg

    I70.513   Atherosclerosis of nonautologous biological bypass graft(s) of the extremities with intermittent claudication, bilateral legs

    I70.518   Atherosclerosis of nonautologous biological bypass graft(s) of the extremities with intermittent claudication, other extremity

    I70.519   Atherosclerosis of nonautologous biological bypass graft(s) of the extremities with intermittent claudication, **unspecified** extremity

● **I70.52**   **Atherosclerosis of nonautologous biological bypass graft(s) of the extremities with rest pain**

    Includes   any condition classifiable to I70.51-

    I70.521   Atherosclerosis of nonautologous biological bypass graft(s) of the extremities with rest pain, right leg

    I70.522   Atherosclerosis of nonautologous biological bypass graft(s) of the extremities with rest pain, left leg

    I70.523   Atherosclerosis of nonautologous biological bypass graft(s) of the extremities with rest pain, bilateral legs

    I70.528   Atherosclerosis of nonautologous biological bypass graft(s) of the extremities with rest pain, other extremity

    I70.529   Atherosclerosis of nonautologous biological bypass graft(s) of the extremities with rest pain, **unspecified** extremity

● **I70.53**   **Atherosclerosis of nonautologous biological bypass graft(s) of the right leg with ulceration**

    Includes   any condition classifiable to I70.511 and I70.521

    Use additional code to identify severity of ulcer (L97.-)

    I70.531   Atherosclerosis of nonautologous biological bypass graft(s) of the right leg with ulceration of thigh

    I70.532   Atherosclerosis of nonautologous biological bypass graft(s) of the right leg with ulceration of calf

    I70.533   Atherosclerosis of nonautologous biological bypass graft(s) of the right leg with ulceration of ankle

    I70.534   Atherosclerosis of nonautologous biological bypass graft(s) of the right leg with ulceration of heel and midfoot

      Atherosclerosis of nonautologous biological bypass graft(s) of right leg with ulceration of plantar surface of midfoot

    I70.535   Atherosclerosis of nonautologous biological bypass graft(s) of the right leg with ulceration of other part of foot

      Atherosclerosis of nonautologous biological bypass graft(s) of the right leg with ulceration of toe

    I70.538   Atherosclerosis of nonautologous biological bypass graft(s) of the right leg with ulceration of other part of lower leg

    I70.539   Atherosclerosis of nonautologous biological bypass graft(s) of the right leg with ulceration of **unspecified** site

CHAPTER 9 (I00–I99)

● **I70.54** **Atherosclerosis of nonautologous biological bypass graft(s) of the left leg with ulceration**

> **Includes**   any condition classifiable to I70.512 and I70.522

> Use additional code to identify severity of ulcer (L97.-)

  I70.541 **Atherosclerosis of nonautologous biological bypass graft(s) of the left leg with ulceration of thigh**

  I70.542 **Atherosclerosis of nonautologous biological bypass graft(s) of the left leg with ulceration of calf**

  I70.543 **Atherosclerosis of nonautologous biological bypass graft(s) of the left leg with ulceration of ankle**

  I70.544 **Atherosclerosis of nonautologous biological bypass graft(s) of the left leg with ulceration of heel and midfoot**

> Atherosclerosis of nonautologous biological bypass graft(s) of left leg with ulceration of plantar surface of midfoot

  I70.545 **Atherosclerosis of nonautologous biological bypass graft(s) of the left leg with ulceration of other part of foot**

> Atherosclerosis of nonautologous biological bypass graft(s) of the left leg with ulceration of toe

  I70.548 **Atherosclerosis of nonautologous biological bypass graft(s) of the left leg with ulceration of other part of lower leg**

  I70.549 **Atherosclerosis of nonautologous biological bypass graft(s) of the left leg with ulceration of unspecified site**

I70.55 **Atherosclerosis of nonautologous biological bypass graft(s) of other extremity with ulceration**

> **Includes**   any condition classifiable to I70.518, I70.528, and I70.538

> Use additional code to identify severity of ulcer (L98.49)

● **I70.56** **Atherosclerosis of nonautologous biological bypass graft(s) of the extremities with gangrene**

> **Includes**   any condition classifiable to I70.51-, I70.52-, and I70.53-, I70.54, I70.55

> Use additional code to identify the severity of any ulcer (L97.-, L98.49-), if applicable

  I70.561 **Atherosclerosis of nonautologous biological bypass graft(s) of the extremities with gangrene, right leg**

  I70.562 **Atherosclerosis of nonautologous biological bypass graft(s) of the extremities with gangrene, left leg**

  I70.563 **Atherosclerosis of nonautologous biological bypass graft(s) of the extremities with gangrene, bilateral legs**

  I70.568 **Atherosclerosis of nonautologous biological bypass graft(s) of the extremities with gangrene, other extremity**

  I70.569 **Atherosclerosis of nonautologous biological bypass graft(s) of the extremities with gangrene, unspecified extremity**

● **I70.59** **Other atherosclerosis of nonautologous biological bypass graft(s) of the extremities**

  I70.591 **Other atherosclerosis of nonautologous biological bypass graft(s) of the extremities, right leg**

  I70.592 **Other atherosclerosis of nonautologous biological bypass graft(s) of the extremities, left leg**

  I70.593 **Other atherosclerosis of nonautologous biological bypass graft(s) of the extremities, bilateral legs**

  I70.598 **Other atherosclerosis of nonautologous biological bypass graft(s) of the extremities, other extremity**

  I70.599 **Other atherosclerosis of nonautologous biological bypass graft(s) of the extremities, unspecified extremity**

● **I70.6** **Atherosclerosis of nonbiological bypass graft(s) of the extremities**

> Use additional code, if applicable, to identify chronic total occlusion of artery of extremity (I70.92)

● **I70.60** **Unspecified atherosclerosis of nonbiological bypass graft(s) of the extremities**

  I70.601 **Unspecified atherosclerosis of nonbiological bypass graft(s) of the extremities, right leg**

  I70.602 **Unspecified atherosclerosis of nonbiological bypass graft(s) of the extremities, left leg**

  I70.603 **Unspecified atherosclerosis of nonbiological bypass graft(s) of the extremities, bilateral legs**

  I70.608 **Unspecified atherosclerosis of nonbiological bypass graft(s) of the extremities, other extremity**

  I70.609 **Unspecified atherosclerosis of nonbiological bypass graft(s) of the extremities, unspecified extremity**

● **I70.61** **Atherosclerosis of nonbiological bypass graft(s) of the extremities with intermittent claudication**

  I70.611 **Atherosclerosis of nonbiological bypass graft(s) of the extremities with intermittent claudication, right leg**

  I70.612 **Atherosclerosis of nonbiological bypass graft(s) of the extremities with intermittent claudication, left leg**

  I70.613 **Atherosclerosis of nonbiological bypass graft(s) of the extremities with intermittent claudication, bilateral legs**

  I70.618 **Atherosclerosis of nonbiological bypass graft(s) of the extremities with intermittent claudication, other extremity**

  I70.619 **Atherosclerosis of nonbiological bypass graft(s) of the extremities with intermittent claudication, unspecified extremity**

● **I70.62**   Atherosclerosis of nonbiological bypass graft(s) of the extremities with rest pain
> **Includes**   any condition classifiable to I70.61-

    I70.621   Atherosclerosis of nonbiological bypass graft(s) of the extremities with rest pain, right leg

    I70.622   Atherosclerosis of nonbiological bypass graft(s) of the extremities with rest pain, left leg

    I70.623   Atherosclerosis of nonbiological bypass graft(s) of the extremities with rest pain, bilateral legs

    I70.628   Atherosclerosis of nonbiological bypass graft(s) of the extremities with rest pain, other extremity

    I70.629   Atherosclerosis of nonbiological bypass graft(s) of the extremities with rest pain, unspecified extremity

● **I70.63**   Atherosclerosis of nonbiological bypass graft(s) of the right leg with ulceration
> **Includes**   any condition classifiable to I70.611 and I70.621

> Use additional code to identify severity of ulcer (L97.-)

    I70.631   Atherosclerosis of nonbiological bypass graft(s) of the right leg with ulceration of thigh

    I70.632   Atherosclerosis of nonbiological bypass graft(s) of the right leg with ulceration of calf

    I70.633   Atherosclerosis of nonbiological bypass graft(s) of the right leg with ulceration of ankle

    I70.634   Atherosclerosis of nonbiological bypass graft(s) of the right leg with ulceration of heel and midfoot
> Atherosclerosis of nonbiological bypass graft(s) of right leg with ulceration of plantar surface of midfoot

    I70.635   Atherosclerosis of nonbiological bypass graft(s) of the right leg with ulceration of other part of foot
> Atherosclerosis of nonbiological bypass graft(s) of the right leg with ulceration of toe

    I70.638   Atherosclerosis of nonbiological bypass graft(s) of the right leg with ulceration of other part of lower leg

    I70.639   Atherosclerosis of nonbiological bypass graft(s) of the right leg with ulceration of unspecified site

● **I70.64**   Atherosclerosis of nonbiological bypass graft(s) of the left leg with ulceration
> **Includes**   any condition classifiable to I70.612 and I70.622

> Use additional code to identify severity of ulcer (L97.-)

    I70.641   Atherosclerosis of nonbiological bypass graft(s) of the left leg with ulceration of thigh

    I70.642   Atherosclerosis of nonbiological bypass graft(s) of the left leg with ulceration of calf

    I70.643   Atherosclerosis of nonbiological bypass graft(s) of the left leg with ulceration of ankle

    I70.644   Atherosclerosis of nonbiological bypass graft(s) of the left leg with ulceration of heel and midfoot
> Atherosclerosis of nonbiological bypass graft(s) of left leg with ulceration of plantar surface of midfoot

    I70.645   Atherosclerosis of nonbiological bypass graft(s) of the left leg with ulceration of other part of foot
> Atherosclerosis of nonbiological bypass graft(s) of the left leg with ulceration of toe

    I70.648   Atherosclerosis of nonbiological bypass graft(s) of the left leg with ulceration of other part of lower leg

    I70.649   Atherosclerosis of nonbiological bypass graft(s) of the left leg with ulceration of unspecified site

  I70.65   Atherosclerosis of nonbiological bypass graft(s) of other extremity with ulceration
> **Includes**   any condition classifiable to I70.618 and I70.628

> Use additional code to identify severity of ulcer (L98.49-)

● **I70.66**   Atherosclerosis of nonbiological bypass graft(s) of the extremities with gangrene
> **Includes**   any condition classifiable to I70.61-, I70.62-, I70.63-, I70.64-, I70.65

> Use additional code to identify the severity of any ulcer (L97.-, L98.49-), if applicable

    I70.661   Atherosclerosis of nonbiological bypass graft(s) of the extremities with gangrene, right leg

    I70.662   Atherosclerosis of nonbiological bypass graft(s) of the extremities with gangrene, left leg

    I70.663   Atherosclerosis of nonbiological bypass graft(s) of the extremities with gangrene, bilateral legs

    I70.668   Atherosclerosis of nonbiological bypass graft(s) of the extremities with gangrene, other extremity

    I70.669   Atherosclerosis of nonbiological bypass graft(s) of the extremities with gangrene, unspecified extremity

● **I70.69**   Other atherosclerosis of nonbiological bypass graft(s) of the extremities

    I70.691   Other atherosclerosis of nonbiological bypass graft(s) of the extremities, right leg

    I70.692   Other atherosclerosis of nonbiological bypass graft(s) of the extremities, left leg

    I70.693   Other atherosclerosis of nonbiological bypass graft(s) of the extremities, bilateral legs

    I70.698   Other atherosclerosis of nonbiological bypass graft(s) of the extremities, other extremity

    I70.699   Other atherosclerosis of nonbiological bypass graft(s) of the extremities, unspecified extremity

CHAPTER 9 (I00-I99)

CHAPTER 9 (I00-I99)

● **I70.7**   **Atherosclerosis of other type of bypass graft(s) of the extremities**

Use additional code, if applicable, to identify chronic total occlusion of artery of extremity (I70.92)

● **I70.70**   **Unspecified atherosclerosis of other type of bypass graft(s) of the extremities**

I70.701   Unspecified atherosclerosis of other type of bypass graft(s) of the extremities, right leg

I70.702   Unspecified atherosclerosis of other type of bypass graft(s) of the extremities, left leg

I70.703   Unspecified atherosclerosis of other type of bypass graft(s) of the extremities, bilateral legs

I70.708   Unspecified atherosclerosis of other type of bypass graft(s) of the extremities, other extremity

I70.709   Unspecified atherosclerosis of other type of bypass graft(s) of the extremities, unspecified extremity

● **I70.71**   **Atherosclerosis of other type of bypass graft(s) of the extremities with intermittent claudication**

I70.711   Atherosclerosis of other type of bypass graft(s) of the extremities with intermittent claudication, right leg

I70.712   Atherosclerosis of other type of bypass graft(s) of the extremities with intermittent claudication, left leg

I70.713   Atherosclerosis of other type of bypass graft(s) of the extremities with intermittent claudication, bilateral legs

I70.718   Atherosclerosis of other type of bypass graft(s) of the extremities with intermittent claudication, other extremity

I70.719   Atherosclerosis of other type of bypass graft(s) of the extremities with intermittent claudication, unspecified extremity

● **I70.72**   **Atherosclerosis of other type of bypass graft(s) of the extremities with rest pain**

Includes   any condition classifiable to I70.71-

I70.721   Atherosclerosis of other type of bypass graft(s) of the extremities with rest pain, right leg

I70.722   Atherosclerosis of other type of bypass graft(s) of the extremities with rest pain, left leg

I70.723   Atherosclerosis of other type of bypass graft(s) of the extremities with rest pain, bilateral legs

I70.728   Atherosclerosis of other type of bypass graft(s) of the extremities with rest pain, other extremity

I70.729   Atherosclerosis of other type of bypass graft(s) of the extremities with rest pain, unspecified extremity

● **I70.73**   **Atherosclerosis of other type of bypass graft(s) of the right leg with ulceration**

Includes   any condition classifiable to I70.711 and I70.721

Use additional code to identify severity of ulcer (L97.-)

I70.731   Atherosclerosis of other type of bypass graft(s) of the right leg with ulceration of thigh

I70.732   Atherosclerosis of other type of bypass graft(s) of the right leg with ulceration of calf

I70.733   Atherosclerosis of other type of bypass graft(s) of the right leg with ulceration of ankle

I70.734   Atherosclerosis of other type of bypass graft(s) of the right leg with ulceration of heel and midfoot

Atherosclerosis of other type of bypass graft(s) of right leg with ulceration of plantar surface of midfoot

I70.735   Atherosclerosis of other type of bypass graft(s) of the right leg with ulceration of other part of foot

Atherosclerosis of other type of bypass graft(s) of right leg with ulceration of toe

I70.738   Atherosclerosis of other type of bypass graft(s) of the right leg with ulceration of other part of lower leg

I70.739   Atherosclerosis of other type of bypass graft(s) of the right leg with ulceration of unspecified site

● **I70.74**   **Atherosclerosis of other type of bypass graft(s) of the left leg with ulceration**

Includes   any condition classifiable to I70.712 and I70.722

Use additional code to identify severity of ulcer (L97.-)

I70.741   Atherosclerosis of other type of bypass graft(s) of the left leg with ulceration of thigh

I70.742   Atherosclerosis of other type of bypass graft(s) of the left leg with ulceration of calf

I70.743   Atherosclerosis of other type of bypass graft(s) of the left leg with ulceration of ankle

I70.744   Atherosclerosis of other type of bypass graft(s) of the left leg with ulceration of heel and midfoot

Atherosclerosis of other type of bypass graft(s) of left leg with ulceration of plantar surface of midfoot

I70.745   Atherosclerosis of other type of bypass graft(s) of the left leg with ulceration of other part of foot

Atherosclerosis of other type of bypass graft(s) of left leg with ulceration of toe

I70.748   Atherosclerosis of other type of bypass graft(s) of the left leg with ulceration of other part of lower leg

I70.749   Atherosclerosis of other type of bypass graft(s) of the left leg with ulceration of unspecified site

I70.75   Atherosclerosis of other type of bypass graft(s) of other extremity with ulceration

Includes   any condition classifiable to I70.718 and I70.728

Use additional code to identify severity of ulcer (L98.49)

● **I70.76**   **Atherosclerosis of other type of bypass graft(s) of the extremities with gangrene**

Includes   any condition classifiable to I70.71-, I70.72-, I70.73-, I70.74-, I70.75

Use additional code to identify the severity of any ulcer (L97.-, L98.49-), if applicable

I70.761   Atherosclerosis of other type of bypass graft(s) of the extremities with gangrene, right leg

◄ New   ◄▮▮▮ Revised   ~~deleted~~ Deleted   **OGCR** Official Guidelines   X Assign placeholder X   ● Use Additional Character(s)

Excludes 1   Excludes 2   Includes   Use additional   Code first   Code also   Unspecified

I70.762 Atherosclerosis of other type of bypass graft(s) of the extremities with gangrene, left leg

I70.763 Atherosclerosis of other type of bypass graft(s) of the extremities with gangrene, bilateral legs

I70.768 Atherosclerosis of other type of bypass graft(s) of the extremities with gangrene, other extremity

I70.769 Atherosclerosis of other type of bypass graft(s) of the extremities with gangrene, unspecified extremity

● I70.79 Other atherosclerosis of other type of bypass graft(s) of the extremities

I70.791 Other atherosclerosis of other type of bypass graft(s) of the extremities, right leg

I70.792 Other atherosclerosis of other type of bypass graft(s) of the extremities, left leg

I70.793 Other atherosclerosis of other type of bypass graft(s) of the extremities, bilateral legs

I70.798 Other atherosclerosis of other type of bypass graft(s) of the extremities, other extremity

I70.799 Other atherosclerosis of other type of bypass graft(s) of the extremities, unspecified extremity

I70.8 Atherosclerosis of other arteries

● I70.9 Other and unspecified atherosclerosis

I70.90 Unspecified atherosclerosis

I70.91 Generalized atherosclerosis

I70.92 Chronic total occlusion of artery of the extremities
Complete occlusion of artery of the extremities
Total occlusion of artery of the extremities
Code first atherosclerosis of arteries of the extremities (I70.2-, I70.3-, I70.4-, I70.5-, I70.6-, I70.7-)

● I71 Aortic aneurysm and dissection
Excludes1 aortic ectasia (I77.81-)
syphilitic aortic aneurysm (A52.01)
traumatic aortic aneurysm (S25.09, S35.09)

● I71.0 Dissection of aorta
I71.00 Dissection of unspecified site of aorta
I71.01 Dissection of thoracic aorta
I71.02 Dissection of abdominal aorta
I71.03 Dissection of thoracoabdominal aorta

I71.1 Thoracic aortic aneurysm, ruptured
I71.2 Thoracic aortic aneurysm, without rupture
I71.3 Abdominal aortic aneurysm, ruptured
I71.4 Abdominal aortic aneurysm, without rupture
I71.5 Thoracoabdominal aortic aneurysm, ruptured
I71.6 Thoracoabdominal aortic aneurysm, without rupture
I71.8 Aortic aneurysm of unspecified site, ruptured
Rupture of aorta NOS
I71.9 Aortic aneurysm of unspecified site, without rupture
Aneurysm of aorta
Dilatation of aorta
Hyaline necrosis of aorta

● I72 Other aneurysm
Includes aneurysm (cirsoid) (false) (ruptured)
Excludes2 acquired aneurysm (I77.0)
aneurysm (of) aorta (I71.-)
aneurysm (of) arteriovenous NOS (Q27.3-)
carotid artery dissection (I77.71)
cerebral (nonruptured) aneurysm (I67.1)
coronary aneurysm (I25.4)
coronary artery dissection (I25.42)
dissection of artery NEC (I77.79)
heart aneurysm (I25.3)
iliac artery dissection (I77.72)
pulmonary artery aneurysm (I28.1)
renal artery dissection (I77.73)
retinal aneurysm (H35.0)
ruptured cerebral aneurysm (I60.7)
varicose aneurysm (I77.0)
vertebral artery dissection (I77.74)

I72.0 Aneurysm of carotid artery
Aneurysm of common carotid artery
Aneurysm of external carotid artery
Aneurysm of internal carotid artery, extracranial portion
Excludes1 aneurysm of internal carotid artery, intracranial portion (I67.1)
aneurysm of internal carotid artery NOS (I67.1)

I72.1 Aneurysm of artery of upper extremity
I72.2 Aneurysm of renal artery
I72.3 Aneurysm of iliac artery
I72.4 Aneurysm of artery of lower extremity
I72.8 Aneurysm of other specified arteries
I72.9 Aneurysm of unspecified site

● I73 Other peripheral vascular diseases
Excludes2 chilblains (T69.1)
frostbite (T33-T34)
immersion hand or foot (T69.0-)
spasm of cerebral artery (G45.9)

● I73.0 Raynaud's syndrome
Diminishing oxygen supply to fingers, toes, nose, and ears when exposed to temperature changes or stress
Raynaud's disease
Raynaud's phenomenon (secondary)
I73.00 Raynaud's syndrome without gangrene
I73.01 Raynaud's syndrome with gangrene

I73.1 Thromboangiitis obliterans [Buerger's disease]
Inflammatory occlusive disease resulting in poor circulation to the legs, feet, and sometimes the hands due to progressive inflammatory narrowing and eventually obliteration of the small arteries

● I73.8 Other specified peripheral vascular diseases
Excludes1 diabetic (peripheral) angiopathy (E08-E13 with .51-.52)
I73.81 Erythromelalgia
I73.89 Other specified peripheral vascular diseases
Acrocyanosis
Erythrocyanosis
Simple acroparesthesia [Schultze's type]
Vasomotor acroparesthesia [Nothnagel's type]

I73.9 Peripheral vascular disease, unspecified
Intermittent claudication
Peripheral angiopathy NOS
Spasm of artery
Excludes1 atherosclerosis of the extremities (I70.2--I70.7-)

Item 9–9 An **embolus** is a mass of undissolved matter present in the blood that is transported by the blood current. A **thrombus** is a blood clot that occludes or shuts off a vessel. When a thrombus is dislodged, it becomes an embolus.

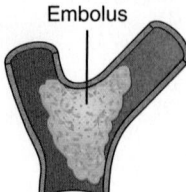

Embolus

Figure 9-3 An arterial embolus.

● **I74**   **Arterial embolism and thrombosis**

     Includes   embolic infarction
                   embolic occlusion
                   thrombotic infarction
                   thrombotic occlusion

Code first embolism and thrombosis complicating abortion or ectopic or molar pregnancy (O00-O07, O08.2)
     embolism and thrombosis complicating pregnancy, childbirth and the puerperium (O88.-)

     Excludes2   atheroembolism (I75.-)
                   basilar embolism and thrombosis (I63.0-I63.2, I65.1)
                   carotid embolism and thrombosis (I63.0-I63.2, I65.2)
                   cerebral embolism and thrombosis (I63.3-I63.5, I66.-)
                   coronary embolism and thrombosis (I21-I25)
                   mesenteric embolism and thrombosis (K55.0)
                   ophthalmic embolism and thrombosis (H34.-)
                   precerebral embolism and thrombosis NOS (I63.0-I63.2, I65.9)
                   pulmonary embolism and thrombosis (I26.-)
                   renal embolism and thrombosis (N28.0)
                   retinal embolism and thrombosis (H34.-)
                   septic embolism and thrombosis (I76)
                   vertebral embolism and thrombosis (I63.0-I63.2, I65.0)

● **I74.0**   **Embolism and thrombosis of abdominal aorta**

     I74.01   **Saddle embolus of abdominal aorta**

     I74.09   **Other arterial embolism and thrombosis of abdominal aorta**
             Aortic bifurcation syndrome
             Aortoiliac obstruction
             Leriche's syndrome

● **I74.1**   **Embolism and thrombosis of other and unspecified parts of aorta**

     I74.10   **Embolism and thrombosis of unspecified parts of aorta**

     I74.11   **Embolism and thrombosis of thoracic aorta**

     I74.19   **Embolism and thrombosis of other parts of aorta**

     I74.2   **Embolism and thrombosis of arteries of the upper extremities**

     I74.3   **Embolism and thrombosis of arteries of the lower extremities**

     I74.4   **Embolism and thrombosis of arteries of extremities, unspecified**
             Peripheral arterial embolism NOS

     I74.5   **Embolism and thrombosis of iliac artery**

     I74.8   **Embolism and thrombosis of other arteries**

     I74.9   **Embolism and thrombosis of unspecified artery**

● **I75**   **Atheroembolism**

     Includes   atherothrombotic microembolism
                   cholesterol embolism

● **I75.0**   **Atheroembolism of extremities**

  ● **I75.01**   **Atheroembolism of upper extremity**

     I75.011   **Atheroembolism of right upper extremity**

     I75.012   **Atheroembolism of left upper extremity**

     I75.013   **Atheroembolism of bilateral upper extremities**

     I75.019   **Atheroembolism of unspecified upper extremity**

  ● **I75.02**   **Atheroembolism of lower extremity**

     I75.021   **Atheroembolism of right lower extremity**

     I75.022   **Atheroembolism of left lower extremity**

     I75.023   **Atheroembolism of bilateral lower extremities**

     I75.029   **Atheroembolism of unspecified lower extremity**

● **I75.8**   **Atheroembolism of other sites**

     I75.81   **Atheroembolism of kidney**
             Use additional code for any associated acute kidney failure and chronic kidney disease (N17.-, N18.-)

     I75.89   **Atheroembolism of other site**

I76   **Septic arterial embolism**

     Code first underlying infection, such as:
        infective endocarditis (I33.0)
        lung abscess (J85.-)

     Use additional code to identify the site of the embolism (I74.-)

     Excludes2   septic pulmonary embolism (I26.01, I26.90)

● **I77**   **Other disorders of arteries and arterioles**

     Excludes2   collagen (vascular) diseases (M30-M36)
                   hypersensitivity angiitis (M31.0)
                   pulmonary artery (I28.-)

     I77.0   **Arteriovenous fistula, acquired**
             Aneurysmal varix
             Arteriovenous aneurysm, acquired

       Excludes1   arteriovenous aneurysm NOS (Q27.3-)
                   presence of arteriovenous shunt (fistula) for dialysis (Z99.2)
                   traumatic - see injury of blood vessel by body region

       Excludes2   cerebral (I67.1)
                   coronary (I25.4)

     I77.1   **Stricture of artery**
             Narrowing of artery

     I77.2   **Rupture of artery**
             Erosion of artery
             Fistula of artery
             Ulcer of artery

       Excludes1   traumatic rupture of artery - see injury of blood vessel by body region

     I77.3   **Arterial fibromuscular dysplasia**
             Fibromuscular hyperplasia (of) carotid artery
             Fibromuscular hyperplasia (of) renal artery

     I77.4   **Celiac artery compression syndrome**

     I77.5   **Necrosis of artery**

I77.6   **Arteritis, unspecified**
      Aortitis NOS
      Endarteritis NOS
      Excludes1   arteritis or endarteritis:
               aortic arch (M31.4)
               cerebral NEC (I67.7)
               coronary (I25.89)
               deformans (I70.-)
               giant cell (M31.5., M31.6)
               obliterans (I70.-)
               senile (I70.-)

I77.7   **Other arterial dissection**
      Excludes2   dissection of aorta (I71.0-)
               dissection of coronary artery (I25.42)
   I77.71   **Dissection of carotid artery**
   I77.72   **Dissection of iliac artery**
   I77.73   **Dissection of renal artery**
   I77.74   **Dissection of vertebral artery**
   I77.79   **Dissection of other artery**

I77.8   **Other specified disorders of arteries and arterioles**
   I77.81   **Aortic ectasia**
        Ectasis aorta
        Excludes1   aortic aneurysm and dissection
                 (I71.0-)
      I77.810   **Thoracic aortic ectasia**
      I77.811   **Abdominal aortic ectasia**
      I77.812   **Thoracoabdominal aortic ectasia**
      I77.819   **Aortic ectasia, unspecified site**
   I77.89   **Other specified disorders of arteries and arterioles**

I77.9   **Disorder of arteries and arterioles, unspecified**

I78   **Diseases of capillaries**
   I78.0   **Hereditary hemorrhagic telangiectasia**
        Rendu-Osler-Weber disease
   I78.1   **Nevus, non-neoplastic**
        Araneus nevus   Spider nevus
        Senile nevus   Stellar nevus
        Excludes1   nevus NOS (D22.-)
                vascular NOS (Q82.5)
        Excludes2   blue nevus (D22.-)
                flammeus nevus (Q82.5)
                hairy nevus (D22.-)
                melanocytic nevus (D22.-)
                pigmented nevus (D22.-)
                portwine nevus (Q82.5)
                sanguineous nevus (Q82.5)
                strawberry nevus (Q82.5)
                verrucous nevus (Q82.5)
   I78.8   **Other diseases of capillaries**
   I78.9   **Disease of capillaries, unspecified**

I79   **Disorders of arteries, arterioles and capillaries in diseases classified elsewhere**
   I79.0   **Aneurysm of aorta in diseases classified elsewhere**
        Code first underlying disease
        Excludes1   syphilitic aneurysm (A52.01)
   I79.1   **Aortitis in diseases classified elsewhere**
        Code first underlying disease
        Excludes1   syphilitic aortitis (A52.02)
   I79.8   **Other disorders of arteries, arterioles and capillaries in diseases classified elsewhere**
        Code first underlying disease, such as:
          amyloidosis (E85.-)
        Excludes1   diabetic (peripheral) angiopathy
                 (E08-E13 with .51-.52)
                syphilitic endarteritis (A52.09)
                tuberculous endarteritis (A18.89)

DISEASES OF VEINS, LYMPHATIC VESSELS AND LYMPH NODES, NOT ELSEWHERE CLASSIFIED (I80-I89)

I80   **Phlebitis and thrombophlebitis**
      Inflammation of a vein with infiltration of walls (phlebitis).
      Includes   endophlebitis
                inflammation, vein
                periphlebitis
                suppurative phlebitis
      Code first phlebitis and thrombophlebitis complicating
         abortion, ectopic or molar pregnancy (O00-O07, O08.7)
         phlebitis and thrombophlebitis complicating pregnancy,
         childbirth and the puerperium (O22.-, O87.-)
      Excludes1   venous embolism and thrombosis of lower
                 extremities (I82.4-, I82.5-, I82.81-)

   I80.0   **Phlebitis and thrombophlebitis of superficial vessels of lower extremities**
        Phlebitis and thrombophlebitis of femoropopliteal vein
      I80.00   **Phlebitis and thrombophlebitis of superficial vessels of unspecified lower extremity**
      I80.01   **Phlebitis and thrombophlebitis of superficial vessels of right lower extremity**
      I80.02   **Phlebitis and thrombophlebitis of superficial vessels of left lower extremity**
      I80.03   **Phlebitis and thrombophlebitis of superficial vessels of lower extremities, bilateral**

   I80.1   **Phlebitis and thrombophlebitis of femoral vein**
      I80.10   **Phlebitis and thrombophlebitis of unspecified femoral vein**
      I80.11   **Phlebitis and thrombophlebitis of right femoral vein**
      I80.12   **Phlebitis and thrombophlebitis of left femoral vein**
      I80.13   **Phlebitis and thrombophlebitis of femoral vein, bilateral**

   I80.2   **Phlebitis and thrombophlebitis of other and unspecified deep vessels of lower extremities**
      I80.20   **Phlebitis and thrombophlebitis of unspecified deep vessels of lower extremities**
        I80.201   **Phlebitis and thrombophlebitis of unspecified deep vessels of right lower extremity**
        I80.202   **Phlebitis and thrombophlebitis of unspecified deep vessels of left lower extremity**
        I80.203   **Phlebitis and thrombophlebitis of unspecified deep vessels of lower extremities, bilateral**
        I80.209   **Phlebitis and thrombophlebitis of unspecified deep vessels of unspecified lower extremity**
      I80.21   **Phlebitis and thrombophlebitis of iliac vein**
        I80.211   **Phlebitis and thrombophlebitis of right iliac vein**
        I80.212   **Phlebitis and thrombophlebitis of left iliac vein**
        I80.213   **Phlebitis and thrombophlebitis of iliac vein, bilateral**
        I80.219   **Phlebitis and thrombophlebitis of unspecified iliac vein**
      I80.22   **Phlebitis and thrombophlebitis of popliteal vein**
        I80.221   **Phlebitis and thrombophlebitis of right popliteal vein**
        I80.222   **Phlebitis and thrombophlebitis of left popliteal vein**
        I80.223   **Phlebitis and thrombophlebitis of popliteal vein, bilateral**
        I80.229   **Phlebitis and thrombophlebitis of unspecified popliteal vein**

◀ New   ⬅ Revised   ~~deleted~~ Deleted   **OGCR** Official Guidelines   X Assign placeholder X   ● Use Additional Character(s)

Excludes 1	Excludes 2	Includes	Use additional	Code first	Code also	Unspecified

CHAPTER 9 (I00-I99)

● I80.23   Phlebitis and thrombophlebitis of tibial vein

    I80.231   Phlebitis and thrombophlebitis of right tibial vein

    I80.232   Phlebitis and thrombophlebitis of left tibial vein

    I80.233   Phlebitis and thrombophlebitis of tibial vein, bilateral

    I80.239   Phlebitis and thrombophlebitis of unspecified tibial vein

● I80.29   Phlebitis and thrombophlebitis of other deep vessels of lower extremities

    I80.291   Phlebitis and thrombophlebitis of other deep vessels of right lower extremity

    I80.292   Phlebitis and thrombophlebitis of other deep vessels of left lower extremity

    I80.293   Phlebitis and thrombophlebitis of other deep vessels of lower extremity, bilateral

    I80.299   Phlebitis and thrombophlebitis of other deep vessels of unspecified lower extremity

I80.3   Phlebitis and thrombophlebitis of lower extremities, unspecified

I80.8   Phlebitis and thrombophlebitis of other sites

I80.9   Phlebitis and thrombophlebitis of unspecified site

I81   **Portal vein thrombosis**
    Portal (vein) obstruction

> **Excludes2**   hepatic vein thrombosis (I82.0)
>   phlebitis of portal vein (K75.1)

● I82   **Other venous embolism and thrombosis**

    Code first venous embolism and thrombosis complicating:
      abortion, ectopic or molar pregnancy (O00-O07, O08.7)
      pregnancy, childbirth and the puerperium (O22.-, O87.-)

> **Excludes2**   venous embolism and thrombosis (of):
>   cerebral (I63.6, I67.6)
>   coronary (I21-I25)
>   intracranial and intraspinal, septic or NOS (G08)
>   intracranial, nonpyogenic (I67.6)
>   intraspinal, nonpyogenic (G95.1)
>   mesenteric (K55.0)
>   portal (I81)
>   pulmonary (I26.-)

I82.0   **Budd-Chiari syndrome**
    Hepatic vein thrombosis

I82.1   **Thrombophlebitis migrans**
    "White leg" is the other term to describe a migrating thrombus.

● I82.2   **Embolism and thrombosis of vena cava and other thoracic veins**

  ● I82.21   Embolism and thrombosis of superior vena cava

    I82.210   Acute embolism and thrombosis of superior vena cava
                Embolism and thrombosis of superior vena cava NOS

    I82.211   Chronic embolism and thrombosis of superior vena cava

  ● I82.22   Embolism and thrombosis of inferior vena cava

    I82.220   Acute embolism and thrombosis of inferior vena cava
                Embolism and thrombosis of inferior vena cava NOS

    I82.221   Chronic embolism and thrombosis of inferior vena cava

● I82.29   Embolism and thrombosis of other thoracic veins
    Embolism and thrombosis of brachiocephalic (innominate) vein

    I82.290   Acute embolism and thrombosis of other thoracic veins

    I82.291   Chronic embolism and thrombosis of other thoracic veins

I82.3   Embolism and thrombosis of renal vein

● I82.4   Acute embolism and thrombosis of deep veins of lower extremity

  I82.40   Acute embolism and thrombosis of unspecified deep veins of lower extremity
    Deep vein thrombosis NOS
    DVT NOS

> **Excludes1**   acute embolism and thrombosis of unspecified deep veins of distal lower extremity (I82.4Z-)
>   acute embolism and thrombosis of unspecified deep veins of proximal lower extremity (I82.4Y-)

    I82.401   Acute embolism and thrombosis of unspecified deep veins of right lower extremity

    I82.402   Acute embolism and thrombosis of unspecified deep veins of left lower extremity

    I82.403   Acute embolism and thrombosis of unspecified deep veins of lower extremity, bilateral

    I82.409   Acute embolism and thrombosis of unspecified deep veins of unspecified lower extremity

● I82.41   Acute embolism and thrombosis of femoral vein

    I82.411   Acute embolism and thrombosis of right femoral vein

    I82.412   Acute embolism and thrombosis of left femoral vein

    I82.413   Acute embolism and thrombosis of femoral vein, bilateral

    I82.419   Acute embolism and thrombosis of unspecified femoral vein

● I82.42   Acute embolism and thrombosis of iliac vein

    I82.421   Acute embolism and thrombosis of right iliac vein

    I82.422   Acute embolism and thrombosis of left iliac vein

    I82.423   Acute embolism and thrombosis of iliac vein, bilateral

    I82.429   Acute embolism and thrombosis of unspecified iliac vein

● I82.43   Acute embolism and thrombosis of popliteal vein

    I82.431   Acute embolism and thrombosis of right popliteal vein

    I82.432   Acute embolism and thrombosis of left popliteal vein

    I82.433   Acute embolism and thrombosis of popliteal vein, bilateral

    I82.439   Acute embolism and thrombosis of unspecified popliteal vein

● **I82.44**   Acute embolism and thrombosis of tibial vein

    I82.441   Acute embolism and thrombosis of right tibial vein

    I82.442   Acute embolism and thrombosis of left tibial vein

    I82.443   Acute embolism and thrombosis of tibial vein, bilateral

    I82.449   Acute embolism and thrombosis of unspecified tibial vein

● **I82.49**   Acute embolism and thrombosis of other specified deep vein of lower extremity

    I82.491   Acute embolism and thrombosis of other specified deep vein of right lower extremity

    I82.492   Acute embolism and thrombosis of other specified deep vein of left lower extremity

    I82.493   Acute embolism and thrombosis of other specified deep vein of lower extremity, bilateral

    I82.499   Acute embolism and thrombosis of other specified deep vein of unspecified lower extremity

● **I82.4Y**   Acute embolism and thrombosis of unspecified deep veins of proximal lower extremity

    Acute embolism and thrombosis of deep vein of thigh NOS

    Acute embolism and thrombosis of deep vein of upper leg NOS

    I82.4Y1   Acute embolism and thrombosis of unspecified deep veins of right proximal lower extremity

    I82.4Y2   Acute embolism and thrombosis of unspecified deep veins of left proximal lower extremity

    I82.4Y3   Acute embolism and thrombosis of unspecified deep veins of proximal lower extremity, bilateral

    I82.4Y9   Acute embolism and thrombosis of unspecified deep veins of unspecified proximal lower extremity

● **I82.4Z**   Acute embolism and thrombosis of unspecified deep veins of distal lower extremity

    Acute embolism and thrombosis of deep vein of calf NOS

    Acute embolism and thrombosis of deep vein of lower leg NOS

    I82.4Z1   Acute embolism and thrombosis of unspecified deep veins of right distal lower extremity

    I82.4Z2   Acute embolism and thrombosis of unspecified deep veins of left distal lower extremity

    I82.4Z3   Acute embolism and thrombosis of unspecified deep veins of distal lower extremity, bilateral

    I82.4Z9   Acute embolism and thrombosis of unspecified deep veins of unspecified distal lower extremity

● **I82.5**   Chronic embolism and thrombosis of deep veins of lower extremity

    Use additional code, if applicable, for associated long-term (current) use of anticoagulants (Z79.01)

    Excludes1   personal history of venous embolism and thrombosis (Z86.718)

● **I82.50**   Chronic embolism and thrombosis of unspecified deep veins of lower extremity

    Excludes1   chronic embolism and thrombosis of unspecified deep veins of distal lower extremity (I82.5Z-)

         chronic embolism and thrombosis of unspecified deep veins of proximal lower extremity (I82.5Y-)

    I82.501   Chronic embolism and thrombosis of unspecified deep veins of right lower extremity

    I82.502   Chronic embolism and thrombosis of unspecified deep veins of left lower extremity

    I82.503   Chronic embolism and thrombosis of unspecified deep veins of lower extremity, bilateral

    I82.509   Chronic embolism and thrombosis of unspecified deep veins of unspecified lower extremity

● **I82.51**   Chronic embolism and thrombosis of femoral vein

    I82.511   Chronic embolism and thrombosis of right femoral vein

    I82.512   Chronic embolism and thrombosis of left femoral vein

    I82.513   Chronic embolism and thrombosis of femoral vein, bilateral

    I82.519   Chronic embolism and thrombosis of unspecified femoral vein

● **I82.52**   Chronic embolism and thrombosis of iliac vein

    I82.521   Chronic embolism and thrombosis of right iliac vein

    I82.522   Chronic embolism and thrombosis of left iliac vein

    I82.523   Chronic embolism and thrombosis of iliac vein, bilateral

    I82.529   Chronic embolism and thrombosis of unspecified iliac vein

● **I82.53**   Chronic embolism and thrombosis of popliteal vein

    I82.531   Chronic embolism and thrombosis of right popliteal vein

    I82.532   Chronic embolism and thrombosis of left popliteal vein

    I82.533   Chronic embolism and thrombosis of popliteal vein, bilateral

    I82.539   Chronic embolism and thrombosis of unspecified popliteal vein

● **I82.54**   Chronic embolism and thrombosis of tibial vein

    I82.541   Chronic embolism and thrombosis of right tibial vein

    I82.542   Chronic embolism and thrombosis of left tibial vein

    I82.543   Chronic embolism and thrombosis of tibial vein, bilateral

    I82.549   Chronic embolism and thrombosis of unspecified tibial vein

CHAPTER 9 (I00-I99)

Item 9–10 Varicose/Varicosities (varix = singular, varices = plural): Enlarged, engorged, tortuous, twisted vascular vessels (veins, arteries, lymphatics). As such, the condition can present in various parts of the body, although the most familiar locations are the lower extremities. A common complication of varices is thrombophlebitis. Varicosities of the anus and rectum are called hemorrhoids.

Figure 9-4 Varicose veins of the legs. (From Goldman: Cecil Medicine, ed 23, Saunders, 2008)

● **I82.59 Chronic embolism and thrombosis of other specified deep vein of lower extremity**
- I82.591 Chronic embolism and thrombosis of other specified deep vein of right lower extremity
- I82.592 Chronic embolism and thrombosis of other specified deep vein of left lower extremity
- I82.593 Chronic embolism and thrombosis of other specified deep vein of lower extremity, bilateral
- I82.599 Chronic embolism and thrombosis of other specified deep vein of unspecified lower extremity

● **I82.5Y Chronic embolism and thrombosis of unspecified deep veins of proximal lower extremity**
Chronic embolism and thrombosis of deep veins of thigh NOS
Chronic embolism and thrombosis of deep veins of upper leg NOS
- I82.5Y1 Chronic embolism and thrombosis of unspecified deep veins of right proximal lower extremity
- I82.5Y2 Chronic embolism and thrombosis of unspecified deep veins of left proximal lower extremity
- I82.5Y3 Chronic embolism and thrombosis of unspecified deep veins of proximal lower extremity, bilateral
- I82.5Y9 Chronic embolism and thrombosis of unspecified deep veins of unspecified proximal lower extremity

● **I82.5Z Chronic embolism and thrombosis of unspecified deep veins of distal lower extremity**
Chronic embolism and thrombosis of deep veins of calf NOS
Chronic embolism and thrombosis of deep veins of lower leg NOS
- I82.5Z1 Chronic embolism and thrombosis of unspecified deep veins of right distal lower extremity
- I82.5Z2 Chronic embolism and thrombosis of unspecified deep veins of left distal lower extremity
- I82.5Z3 Chronic embolism and thrombosis of unspecified deep veins of distal lower extremity, bilateral
- I82.5Z9 Chronic embolism and thrombosis of unspecified deep veins of unspecified distal lower extremity

● **I82.6 Acute embolism and thrombosis of veins of upper extremity**
● **I82.60 Acute embolism and thrombosis of unspecified veins of upper extremity**
- I82.601 Acute embolism and thrombosis of unspecified veins of right upper extremity
- I82.602 Acute embolism and thrombosis of unspecified veins of left upper extremity
- I82.603 Acute embolism and thrombosis of unspecified veins of upper extremity, bilateral
- I82.609 Acute embolism and thrombosis of unspecified veins of unspecified upper extremity

● **I82.61 Acute embolism and thrombosis of superficial veins of upper extremity**
Acute embolism and thrombosis of antecubital vein
Acute embolism and thrombosis of basilic vein
Acute embolism and thrombosis of cephalic vein
- I82.611 Acute embolism and thrombosis of superficial veins of right upper extremity
- I82.612 Acute embolism and thrombosis of superficial veins of left upper extremity
- I82.613 Acute embolism and thrombosis of superficial veins of upper extremity, bilateral
- I82.619 Acute embolism and thrombosis of superficial veins of unspecified upper extremity

● **I82.62 Acute embolism and thrombosis of deep veins of upper extremity**
Acute embolism and thrombosis of brachial vein
Acute embolism and thrombosis of radial vein
Acute embolism and thrombosis of ulnar vein
- I82.621 Acute embolism and thrombosis of deep veins of right upper extremity
- I82.622 Acute embolism and thrombosis of deep veins of left upper extremity
- I82.623 Acute embolism and thrombosis of deep veins of upper extremity, bilateral
- I82.629 Acute embolism and thrombosis of deep veins of unspecified upper extremity

● **I82.7 Chronic embolism and thrombosis of veins of upper extremity**
Use additional code, if applicable, for associated long-term (current) use of anticoagulants (Z79.01)
Excludes1 personal history of venous embolism and thrombosis (Z86.718)

● **I82.70 Chronic embolism and thrombosis of unspecified veins of upper extremity**
- I82.701 Chronic embolism and thrombosis of unspecified veins of right upper extremity
- I82.702 Chronic embolism and thrombosis of unspecified veins of left upper extremity
- I82.703 Chronic embolism and thrombosis of unspecified veins of upper extremity, bilateral
- I82.709 Chronic embolism and thrombosis of unspecified veins of unspecified upper extremity

◄ New ⬅ Revised deleted Deleted OGCR Official Guidelines X Assign placeholder X ● Use Additional Character(s)
944
Excludes 1 Excludes 2 Includes Use additional Code first Code also Unspecified

● **I82.71 Chronic embolism and thrombosis of superficial veins of upper extremity**
Chronic embolism and thrombosis of antecubital vein
Chronic embolism and thrombosis of basilic vein
Chronic embolism and thrombosis of cephalic vein

　I82.711 Chronic embolism and thrombosis of superficial veins of right upper extremity

　I82.712 Chronic embolism and thrombosis of superficial veins of left upper extremity

　I82.713 Chronic embolism and thrombosis of superficial veins of upper extremity, bilateral

　I82.719 Chronic embolism and thrombosis of superficial veins of unspecified upper extremity

● **I82.72 Chronic embolism and thrombosis of deep veins of upper extremity**
Chronic embolism and thrombosis of brachial vein
Chronic embolism and thrombosis of radial vein
Chronic embolism and thrombosis of ulnar vein

　I82.721 Chronic embolism and thrombosis of deep veins of right upper extremity

　I82.722 Chronic embolism and thrombosis of deep veins of left upper extremity

　I82.723 Chronic embolism and thrombosis of deep veins of upper extremity, bilateral

　I82.729 Chronic embolism and thrombosis of deep veins of unspecified upper extremity

● **I82.A Embolism and thrombosis of axillary vein**

● **I82.A1 Acute embolism and thrombosis of axillary vein**

　I82.A11 Acute embolism and thrombosis of right axillary vein

　I82.A12 Acute embolism and thrombosis of left axillary vein

　I82.A13 Acute embolism and thrombosis of axillary vein, bilateral

　I82.A19 Acute embolism and thrombosis of unspecified axillary vein

● **I82.A2 Chronic embolism and thrombosis of axillary vein**

　I82.A21 Chronic embolism and thrombosis of right axillary vein

　I82.A22 Chronic embolism and thrombosis of left axillary vein

　I82.A23 Chronic embolism and thrombosis of axillary vein, bilateral

　I82.A29 Chronic embolism and thrombosis of unspecified axillary vein

● **I82.B Embolism and thrombosis of subclavian vein**

● **I82.B1 Acute embolism and thrombosis of subclavian vein**

　I82.B11 Acute embolism and thrombosis of right subclavian vein

　I82.B12 Acute embolism and thrombosis of left subclavian vein

　I82.B13 Acute embolism and thrombosis of subclavian vein, bilateral

　I82.B19 Acute embolism and thrombosis of unspecified subclavian vein

● **I82.B2 Chronic embolism and thrombosis of subclavian vein**

　I82.B21 Chronic embolism and thrombosis of right subclavian vein

　I82.B22 Chronic embolism and thrombosis of left subclavian vein

　I82.B23 Chronic embolism and thrombosis of subclavian vein, bilateral

　I82.B29 Chronic embolism and thrombosis of unspecified subclavian vein

● **I82.C Embolism and thrombosis of internal jugular vein**

● **I82.C1 Acute embolism and thrombosis of internal jugular vein**

　I82.C11 Acute embolism and thrombosis of right internal jugular vein

　I82.C12 Acute embolism and thrombosis of left internal jugular vein

　I82.C13 Acute embolism and thrombosis of internal jugular vein, bilateral

　I82.C19 Acute embolism and thrombosis of unspecified internal jugular vein

● **I82.C2 Chronic embolism and thrombosis of internal jugular vein**

　I82.C21 Chronic embolism and thrombosis of right internal jugular vein

　I82.C22 Chronic embolism and thrombosis of left internal jugular vein

　I82.C23 Chronic embolism and thrombosis of internal jugular vein, bilateral

　I82.C29 Chronic embolism and thrombosis of unspecified internal jugular vein

● **I82.8 Embolism and thrombosis of other specified veins**
Use additional code, if applicable, for associated long-term (current) use of anticoagulants (Z79.01)

● **I82.81 Embolism and thrombosis of superficial veins of lower extremities**
Embolism and thrombosis of saphenous vein (greater) (lesser)

　I82.811 Embolism and thrombosis of superficial veins of right lower extremities

　I82.812 Embolism and thrombosis of superficial veins of left lower extremities

　I82.813 Embolism and thrombosis of superficial veins of lower extremities, bilateral

　I82.819 Embolism and thrombosis of superficial veins of unspecified lower extremities

● **I82.89 Embolism and thrombosis of other specified veins**

　I82.890 Acute embolism and thrombosis of other specified veins

　I82.891 Chronic embolism and thrombosis of other specified veins

● **I82.9 Embolism and thrombosis of unspecified vein**

　I82.90 Acute embolism and thrombosis of unspecified vein
Embolism of vein NOS
Thrombosis (vein) NOS

　I82.91 Chronic embolism and thrombosis of unspecified vein

CHAPTER 9 (I00-I99)

◀ New　◀▥ Revised　~~deleted~~ Deleted　OGCR Official Guidelines　X Assign placeholder X　● Use Additional Character(s)

Excludes 1　Excludes 2　Includes　Use additional　Code first　Code also　Unspecified

● **I83** **Varicose veins of lower extremities**
    Excludes1 varicose veins complicating pregnancy (O22.0-)
                varicose veins complicating the puerperium
                (O87.4)

  ● **I83.0** **Varicose veins of lower extremities with ulcer**
      Use additional code to identify severity of ulcer (L97.-)

    ● **I83.00** **Varicose veins of unspecified lower extremity with ulcer**

      I83.001 **Varicose veins of unspecified lower extremity with ulcer of thigh**

      I83.002 **Varicose veins of unspecified lower extremity with ulcer of calf**

      I83.003 **Varicose veins of unspecified lower extremity with ulcer of ankle**

      I83.004 **Varicose veins of unspecified lower extremity with ulcer of heel and midfoot**
          Varicose veins of unspecified lower extremity with ulcer of plantar surface of midfoot

      I83.005 **Varicose veins of unspecified lower extremity with ulcer other part of foot**
          Varicose veins of unspecified lower extremity with ulcer of toe

      I83.008 **Varicose veins of unspecified lower extremity with ulcer other part of lower leg**

      I83.009 **Varicose veins of unspecified lower extremity with ulcer of unspecified site**

    ● **I83.01** **Varicose veins of right lower extremity with ulcer**

      I83.011 **Varicose veins of right lower extremity with ulcer of thigh**

      I83.012 **Varicose veins of right lower extremity with ulcer of calf**

      I83.013 **Varicose veins of right lower extremity with ulcer of ankle**

      I83.014 **Varicose veins of right lower extremity with ulcer of heel and midfoot**
          Varicose veins of right lower extremity with ulcer of plantar surface of midfoot

      I83.015 **Varicose veins of right lower extremity with ulcer other part of foot**
          Varicose veins of right lower extremity with ulcer of toe

      I83.018 **Varicose veins of right lower extremity with ulcer other part of lower leg**

      I83.019 **Varicose veins of right lower extremity with ulcer of unspecified site**

    ● **I83.02** **Varicose veins of left lower extremity with ulcer**

      I83.021 **Varicose veins of left lower extremity with ulcer of thigh**

      I83.022 **Varicose veins of left lower extremity with ulcer of calf**

      I83.023 **Varicose veins of left lower extremity with ulcer of ankle**

      I83.024 **Varicose veins of left lower extremity with ulcer of heel and midfoot**
          Varicose veins of left lower extremity with ulcer of plantar surface of midfoot

      I83.025 **Varicose veins of left lower extremity with ulcer other part of foot**
          Varicose veins of left lower extremity with ulcer of toe

      I83.028 **Varicose veins of left lower extremity with ulcer other part of lower leg**

      I83.029 **Varicose veins of left lower extremity with ulcer of unspecified site**

  ● **I83.1** **Varicose veins of lower extremities with inflammation**
      Stasis dermatitis

    I83.10 **Varicose veins of unspecified lower extremity with inflammation**

    I83.11 **Varicose veins of right lower extremity with inflammation**

    I83.12 **Varicose veins of left lower extremity with inflammation**

  ● **I83.2** **Varicose veins of lower extremities with both ulcer and inflammation**
      Use additional code to identify severity of ulcer (L97.-)

    ● **I83.20** **Varicose veins of unspecified lower extremity with both ulcer and inflammation**

      I83.201 **Varicose veins of unspecified lower extremity with both ulcer of thigh and inflammation**

      I83.202 **Varicose veins of unspecified lower extremity with both ulcer of calf and inflammation**

      I83.203 **Varicose veins of unspecified lower extremity with both ulcer of ankle and inflammation**

      I83.204 **Varicose veins of unspecified lower extremity with both ulcer of heel and midfoot and inflammation**
          Varicose veins of unspecified lower extremity with both ulcer of plantar surface of midfoot and inflammation

      I83.205 **Varicose veins of unspecified lower extremity with both ulcer other part of foot and inflammation**
          Varicose veins of unspecified lower extremity with both ulcer of toe and inflammation

      I83.208 **Varicose veins of unspecified lower extremity with both ulcer of other part of lower extremity and inflammation**

      I83.209 **Varicose veins of unspecified lower extremity with both ulcer of unspecified site and inflammation**

    ● **I83.21** **Varicose veins of right lower extremity with both ulcer and inflammation**

      I83.211 **Varicose veins of right lower extremity with both ulcer of thigh and inflammation**

      I83.212 **Varicose veins of right lower extremity with both ulcer of calf and inflammation**

      I83.213 **Varicose veins of right lower extremity with both ulcer of ankle and inflammation**

      I83.214 **Varicose veins of right lower extremity with both ulcer of heel and midfoot and inflammation**
          Varicose veins of right lower extremity with both ulcer of plantar surface of midfoot and inflammation

◀ New   ⬅ Revised   ~~deleted~~ Deleted   OGCR Official Guidelines   X Assign placeholder X   ● Use Additional Character(s)

Excludes 1   Excludes 2   Includes   Use additional   Code first   Code also   Unspecified

I83.215   **Varicose veins of right lower extremity with both ulcer other part of foot and inflammation**
Varicose veins of right lower extremity with both ulcer of toe and inflammation

I83.218   **Varicose veins of right lower extremity with both ulcer of other part of lower extremity and inflammation**

I83.219   **Varicose veins of right lower extremity with both ulcer of unspecified site and inflammation**

● I83.22   **Varicose veins of left lower extremity with both ulcer and inflammation**

I83.221   **Varicose veins of left lower extremity with both ulcer of thigh and inflammation**

I83.222   **Varicose veins of left lower extremity with both ulcer of calf and inflammation**

I83.223   **Varicose veins of left lower extremity with both ulcer of ankle and inflammation**

I83.224   **Varicose veins of left lower extremity with both ulcer of heel and midfoot and inflammation**
Varicose veins of left lower extremity with both ulcer of plantar surface of midfoot and inflammation

I83.225   **Varicose veins of left lower extremity with both ulcer other part of foot and inflammation**
Varicose veins of left lower extremity with both ulcer of toe and inflammation

I83.228   **Varicose veins of left lower extremity with both ulcer of other part of lower extremity and inflammation**

I83.229   **Varicose veins of left lower extremity with both ulcer of unspecified site and inflammation**

● I83.8   **Varicose veins of lower extremities with other complications**

● I83.81   **Varicose veins of lower extremities with pain**

I83.811   **Varicose veins of right lower extremities with pain**

I83.812   **Varicose veins of left lower extremities with pain**

I83.813   **Varicose veins of bilateral lower extremities with pain**

I83.819   **Varicose veins of unspecified lower extremities with pain**

● I83.89   **Varicose veins of lower extremities with other complications**
Varicose veins of lower extremities with edema
Varicose veins of lower extremities with swelling

I83.891   **Varicose veins of right lower extremities with other complications**

I83.892   **Varicose veins of left lower extremities with other complications**

I83.893   **Varicose veins of bilateral lower extremities with other complications**

I83.899   **Varicose veins of unspecified lower extremities with other complications**

● I83.9   **Asymptomatic varicose veins of lower extremities**
Phlebectasia of lower extremities
Varicose veins of lower extremities
Varix of lower extremities

I83.90   **Asymptomatic varicose veins of unspecified lower extremity**
Varicose veins NOS

I83.91   **Asymptomatic varicose veins of right lower extremity**

I83.92   **Asymptomatic varicose veins of left lower extremity**

I83.93   **Asymptomatic varicose veins of bilateral lower extremities**

● I85   **Esophageal varices**
Use additional code to identify:
alcohol abuse and dependence (F10.-)

● I85.0   **Esophageal varices**
Idiopathic esophageal varices
Primary esophageal varices

I85.00   **Esophageal varices without bleeding**
Esophageal varices NOS

I85.01   **Esophageal varices with bleeding**

● I85.1   **Secondary esophageal varices**
Esophageal varices secondary to alcoholic liver disease
Esophageal varices secondary to cirrhosis of liver
Esophageal varices secondary to schistosomiasis
Esophageal varices secondary to toxic liver disease
Code first underlying disease

I85.10   **Secondary esophageal varices without bleeding**

I85.11   **Secondary esophageal varices with bleeding**

● I86   **Varicose veins of other sites**
> Excludes1 | varicose veins of unspecified site (I83.9-)
> Excludes2 | retinal varices (H35.0-)

I86.0   **Sublingual varices**

I86.1   **Scrotal varices**
Varicocele

I86.2   **Pelvic varices**

I86.3   **Vulval varices**
> Excludes1 | vulval varices complicating childbirth and the puerperium (O87.8)
> vulval varices complicating pregnancy (O22.1-)

I86.4   **Gastric varices**

I86.8   **Varicose veins of other specified sites**
Varicose ulcer of nasal septum

● I87   **Other disorders of veins**

● I87.0   **Postthrombotic syndrome**
Chronic venous hypertension due to deep vein thrombosis
Postphlebitic syndrome
> Excludes1 | chronic venous hypertension without deep vein thrombosis (I87.3-)

● I87.00   **Postthrombotic syndrome without complications**
Asymptomatic Postthrombotic syndrome

I87.001   **Postthrombotic syndrome without complications of right lower extremity**

I87.002   **Postthrombotic syndrome without complications of left lower extremity**

I87.003   **Postthrombotic syndrome without complications of bilateral lower extremity**

I87.009   **Postthrombotic syndrome without complications of unspecified extremity**
Postthrombotic syndrome NOS

● **I87.01** **Postthrombotic syndrome with ulcer**

     Use additional code to specify site and severity of ulcer (L97.-)

   I87.011 **Postthrombotic syndrome with ulcer of right lower extremity**

   I87.012 **Postthrombotic syndrome with ulcer of left lower extremity**

   I87.013 **Postthrombotic syndrome with ulcer of bilateral lower extremity**

   I87.019 **Postthrombotic syndrome with ulcer of unspecified lower extremity**

● **I87.02** **Postthrombotic syndrome with inflammation**

   I87.021 **Postthrombotic syndrome with inflammation of right lower extremity**

   I87.022 **Postthrombotic syndrome with inflammation of left lower extremity**

   I87.023 **Postthrombotic syndrome with inflammation of bilateral lower extremity**

   I87.029 **Postthrombotic syndrome with inflammation of unspecified lower extremity**

● **I87.03** **Postthrombotic syndrome with ulcer and inflammation**

     Use additional code to specify site and severity of ulcer (L97.-)

   I87.031 **Postthrombotic syndrome with ulcer and inflammation of right lower extremity**

   I87.032 **Postthrombotic syndrome with ulcer and inflammation of left lower extremity**

   I87.033 **Postthrombotic syndrome with ulcer and inflammation of bilateral lower extremity**

   I87.039 **Postthrombotic syndrome with ulcer and inflammation of unspecified lower extremity**

● **I87.09** **Postthrombotic syndrome with other complications**

   I87.091 **Postthrombotic syndrome with other complications of right lower extremity**

   I87.092 **Postthrombotic syndrome with other complications of left lower extremity**

   I87.093 **Postthrombotic syndrome with other complications of bilateral lower extremity**

   I87.099 **Postthrombotic syndrome with other complications of unspecified lower extremity**

I87.1 **Compression of vein**

     Stricture of vein

     Vena cava syndrome (inferior) (superior)

     Excludes2   compression of pulmonary vein (I28.8)

I87.2 **Venous insufficiency (chronic) (peripheral)**

● **I87.3** **Chronic venous hypertension (idiopathic)**

     Stasis edema

     Excludes1   chronic venous hypertension due to deep vein thrombosis (I87.0-)

                varicose veins of lower extremities (I83.-)

● **I87.30** **Chronic venous hypertension (idiopathic) without complications**

     Asymptomatic chronic venous hypertension (idiopathic)

   I87.301 **Chronic venous hypertension (idiopathic) without complications of right lower extremity**

   I87.302 **Chronic venous hypertension (idiopathic) without complications of left lower extremity**

   I87.303 **Chronic venous hypertension (idiopathic) without complications of bilateral lower extremity**

   I87.309 **Chronic venous hypertension (idiopathic) without complications of unspecified lower extremity**

     Chronic venous hypertension NOS

● **I87.31** **Chronic venous hypertension (idiopathic) with ulcer**

     Use additional code to specify site and severity of ulcer (L97.-)

   I87.311 **Chronic venous hypertension (idiopathic) with ulcer of right lower extremity**

   I87.312 **Chronic venous hypertension (idiopathic) with ulcer of left lower extremity**

   I87.313 **Chronic venous hypertension (idiopathic) with ulcer of bilateral lower extremity**

   I87.319 **Chronic venous hypertension (idiopathic) with ulcer of unspecified lower extremity**

● **I87.32** **Chronic venous hypertension (idiopathic) with inflammation**

   I87.321 **Chronic venous hypertension (idiopathic) with inflammation of right lower extremity**

   I87.322 **Chronic venous hypertension (idiopathic) with inflammation of left lower extremity**

   I87.323 **Chronic venous hypertension (idiopathic) with inflammation of bilateral lower extremity**

   I87.329 **Chronic venous hypertension (idiopathic) with inflammation of unspecified lower extremity**

● **I87.33** **Chronic venous hypertension (idiopathic) with ulcer and inflammation**

     Use additional code to specify site and severity of ulcer (L97.-)

   I87.331 **Chronic venous hypertension (idiopathic) with ulcer and inflammation of right lower extremity**

   I87.332 **Chronic venous hypertension (idiopathic) with ulcer and inflammation of left lower extremity**

   I87.333 **Chronic venous hypertension (idiopathic) with ulcer and inflammation of bilateral lower extremity**

   I87.339 **Chronic venous hypertension (idiopathic) with ulcer and inflammation of unspecified lower extremity**

● **I87.39** **Chronic venous hypertension (idiopathic) with other complications**

   I87.391 **Chronic venous hypertension (idiopathic) with other complications of right lower extremity**

   I87.392 **Chronic venous hypertension (idiopathic) with other complications of left lower extremity**

   I87.393 **Chronic venous hypertension (idiopathic) with other complications of bilateral lower extremity**

   I87.399 **Chronic venous hypertension (idiopathic) with other complications of unspecified lower extremity**

I87.8 **Other specified disorders of veins**

     Phlebosclerosis

     Venofibrosis

I87.9 **Disorder of vein, unspecified**

◄ New   ◄▦ Revised   ~~deleted~~ Deleted   OGCR Official Guidelines   X Assign placeholder X   ● Use Additional Character(s)

Excludes 1   Excludes 2   Includes   Use additional   Code first   Code also   Unspecified

● **I88**   **Nonspecific lymphadenitis**

> **Excludes1**   acute lymphadenitis, except mesenteric (L04.-)
> enlarged lymph nodes NOS (R59.-)
> human immunodeficiency virus [HIV] disease
>   resulting in generalized lymphadenopathy
>   (B20)

I88.0   **Nonspecific mesenteric lymphadenitis**
     Mesenteric lymphadenitis (acute)(chronic)

I88.1   **Chronic lymphadenitis, except mesenteric**
     Adenitis
     Lymphadenitis

I88.8   **Other nonspecific lymphadenitis**

I88.9   **Nonspecific lymphadenitis, unspecified**
     Lymphadenitis NOS

● **I89**   **Other noninfective disorders of lymphatic vessels and lymph nodes**

> **Excludes1**   chylocele, tunica vaginalis (nonfilarial) NOS
>   (N50.8)
> enlarged lymph nodes NOS (R59.-)
> filarial chylocele (B74.-)
> hereditary lymphedema (Q82.0)

I89.0   **Lymphedema, not elsewhere classified**
     Elephantiasis (nonfilarial) NOS
     Lymphangiectasis
     Obliteration, lymphatic vessel
     Praecox lymphedema
     Secondary lymphedema

> **Excludes1**   postmastectomy lymphedema (I97.2)

I89.1   **Lymphangitis**
     Chronic lymphangitis
     Lymphangitis NOS
     Subacute lymphangitis

> **Excludes1**   acute lymphangitis (L03.-)

I89.8   **Other specified noninfective disorders of lymphatic vessels and lymph nodes**
     Chylocele (nonfilarial)
     Chylous ascites
     Chylous cyst
     Lipomelanotic reticulosis
     Lymph node or vessel fistula
     Lymph node or vessel infarction
     Lymph node or vessel rupture

I89.9   **Noninfective disorder of lymphatic vessels and lymph nodes, unspecified**
     Disease of lymphatic vessels NOS

OTHER AND UNSPECIFIED DISORDERS OF THE CIRCULATORY SYSTEM (I95-I99)

● **I95**   **Hypotension**
     Subnormal arterial blood pressure

> **Excludes1**   cardiovascular collapse (R57.9)
> maternal hypotension syndrome (O26.5-)
> nonspecific low blood pressure reading NOS
>   (R03.1)

I95.0   **Idiopathic hypotension**

I95.1   **Orthostatic hypotension**
     Hypotension, postural
     *Moving from a sitting or reclining position to a standing
     position precipitates a sudden drop in blood pressure
     (hypotension).*

> **Excludes1**   neurogenic orthostatic hypotension [Shy-
>   Drager] (G90.3)
> orthostatic hypotension due to drugs
>   (I95.2)

I95.2   **Hypotension due to drugs**
     Orthostatic hypotension due to drugs
     Use additional code for adverse effect, if applicable,
       to identify drug (T36-T50 with fifth or sixth
       character 5)

I95.3   **Hypotension of hemodialysis**
     Intra-dialytic hypotension

● **I95.8**   **Other hypotension**

     I95.81   **Postprocedural hypotension**

     I95.89   **Other hypotension**
       Chronic hypotension

I95.9   **Hypotension, unspecified**

● **I96**   **Gangrene, not elsewhere classified**
     Gangrenous cellulitis

> **Excludes1**   gangrene in atherosclerosis of native arteries of
>   the extremities (I70.26)
> gangrene of certain specified sites - *see*
>   Alphabetical Index
> gangrene in diabetes mellitus (E08-E13)
> gangrene in hernia (K40.1, K40.4, K41.1, K41.4,
>   K42.1, K43.1-, K44.1, K45.1, K46.1)
> gangrene in other peripheral vascular diseases
>   (I73.-)
> gas gangrene (A48.0)
> pyoderma gangrenosum (L88)

● **I97**   **Intraoperative and postprocedural complications and disorders of circulatory system, not elsewhere classified**

> **Excludes2**   postprocedural shock (T81.1-)

I97.0   **Postcardiotomy syndrome**

● **I97.1**   **Other postprocedural cardiac functional disturbances**

> **Excludes2**   acute pulmonary insufficiency following
>   thoracic surgery (J95.1)
> intraoperative cardiac functional
>   disturbances (I97.7-)

   ● **I97.11**   **Postprocedural cardiac insufficiency**

     I97.110   **Postprocedural cardiac insufficiency following cardiac surgery**

     I97.111   **Postprocedural cardiac insufficiency following other surgery**

   ● **I97.12**   **Postprocedural cardiac arrest**

     I97.120   **Postprocedural cardiac arrest following cardiac surgery**

     I97.121   **Postprocedural cardiac arrest following other surgery**

   ● **I97.13**   **Postprocedural heart failure**
     Use additional code to identify the heart
       failure (I50.-)

     I97.130   **Postprocedural heart failure following cardiac surgery**

     I97.131   **Postprocedural heart failure following other surgery**

   ● **I97.19**   **Other postprocedural cardiac functional disturbances**
     Use additional code, if applicable, to further
       specify disorder

     I97.190   **Other postprocedural cardiac functional disturbances following cardiac surgery**

     I97.191   **Other postprocedural cardiac functional disturbances following other surgery**

I97.2   **Postmastectomy lymphedema syndrome**
     Elephantiasis due to mastectomy
     Obliteration of lymphatic vessels

I97.3   **Postprocedural hypertension**

◄ New   ◄ Revised   ~~deleted~~ Deleted   **OGCR** Official Guidelines   X Assign placeholder X   ● Use Additional Character(s)

Excludes 1   Excludes 2   Includes   Use additional   Code first   Code also   Unspecified

● **I97.4** **Intraoperative hemorrhage and hematoma of a circulatory system organ or structure complicating a procedure**

> **Excludes1**   intraoperative hemorrhage and hematoma of a circulatory system organ or structure due to accidental puncture and laceration during a procedure (I97.5-)

> **Excludes2**   intraoperative cerebrovascular hemorrhage complicating a procedure (G97.3-)

● **I97.41** **Intraoperative hemorrhage and hematoma of a circulatory system organ or structure complicating a circulatory system procedure**

     I97.410   **Intraoperative hemorrhage and hematoma of a circulatory system organ or structure complicating a cardiac catheterization**

     I97.411   **Intraoperative hemorrhage and hematoma of a circulatory system organ or structure complicating a cardiac bypass**

     I97.418   **Intraoperative hemorrhage and hematoma of a circulatory system organ or structure complicating other circulatory system procedure**

     I97.42   **Intraoperative hemorrhage and hematoma of a circulatory system organ or structure complicating other procedure**

● **I97.5** **Accidental puncture and laceration of a circulatory system organ or structure during a procedure**

> **Excludes2**   accidental puncture and laceration of brain during a procedure (G97.4-)

     I97.51   **Accidental puncture and laceration of a circulatory system organ or structure during a circulatory system procedure**

     I97.52   **Accidental puncture and laceration of a circulatory system organ or structure during other procedure**

● **I97.6** **Postprocedural hemorrhage and hematoma of a circulatory system organ or structure following a procedure**

> **Excludes2**   postprocedural cerebrovascular hemorrhage complicating a procedure (G97.5-)

● **I97.61** **Postprocedural hemorrhage and hematoma of a circulatory system organ or structure following a circulatory system procedure**

     I97.610   **Postprocedural hemorrhage and hematoma of a circulatory system organ or structure following a cardiac catheterization**

     I97.611   **Postprocedural hemorrhage and hematoma of a circulatory system organ or structure following cardiac bypass**

     I97.618   **Postprocedural hemorrhage and hematoma of a circulatory system organ or structure following other circulatory system procedure**

     I97.62   **Postprocedural hemorrhage and hematoma of a circulatory system organ or structure following other procedure**

● **I97.7** **Intraoperative cardiac functional disturbances**

> **Excludes2**   acute pulmonary insufficiency following thoracic surgery (J95.1)
> postprocedural cardiac functional disturbances (I97.1-)

● **I97.71** **Intraoperative cardiac arrest**

     I97.710   **Intraoperative cardiac arrest during cardiac surgery**

     I97.711   **Intraoperative cardiac arrest during other surgery**

● **I97.79** **Other intraoperative cardiac functional disturbances**

> Use additional code, if applicable, to further specify disorder

     I97.790   **Other intraoperative cardiac functional disturbances during cardiac surgery**

     I97.791   **Other intraoperative cardiac functional disturbances during other surgery**

● **I97.8** **Other intraoperative and postprocedural complications and disorders of the circulatory system, not elsewhere classified**

> Use additional code, if applicable, to further specify disorder

● **I97.81** **Intraoperative cerebrovascular infarction**

     I97.810   **Intraoperative cerebrovascular infarction during cardiac surgery**

     I97.811   **Intraoperative cerebrovascular infarction during other surgery**

● **I97.82** **Postprocedural cerebrovascular infarction**

     I97.820   **Postprocedural cerebrovascular infarction during cardiac surgery**

     I97.821   **Postprocedural cerebrovascular infarction during other surgery**

     I97.88   **Other intraoperative complications of the circulatory system, not elsewhere classified**

     I97.89   **Other postprocedural complications and disorders of the circulatory system, not elsewhere classified**

● **I99** **Other and unspecified disorders of circulatory system**

     I99.8   **Other disorder of circulatory system**

     I99.9   **Unspecified disorder of circulatory system**

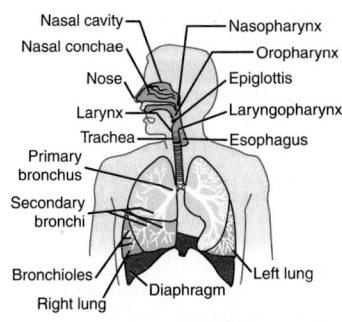

Figure 10–1 Respiratory system. (From Buck CJ: Step-by-Step Medical Coding, ed 2011, Philadelphia, WB Saunders, 2011)

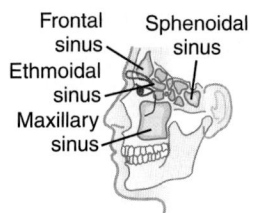

Figure 10-2 Paranasal sinuses. (From Buck CJ: Step-by-Step Medical Coding, ed 2011, Philadelphia, WB Saunders, 2011)

Item 10–1 Pharyngitis is painful inflammation of the pharynx (sore throat). Ninety percent of the infections are caused by a virus with the remaining being bacterial and rarely a fungus (candidiasis). Other irritants such as pollutants, chemicals, or smoke may cause similar symptoms.

OGCR See Section I.C., Chapter 10

Chronic Obstructive Pulmonary Disease (COPD) and Asthma

CHAPTER 10

DISEASES OF THE RESPIRATORY SYSTEM (J00-J99)

Note: When a respiratory condition is described as occurring in more than one site and is not specifically indexed, it should be classified to the lower anatomic site (e.g., tracheobronchitis to bronchitis in J40).

Use additional code, where applicable, to identify:
exposure to environmental tobacco smoke (Z77.22)
exposure to tobacco smoke in the perinatal period (P96.81)
history of tobacco use (Z87.891)
occupational exposure to environmental tobacco smoke (Z57.31)
tobacco dependence (F17.-)
tobacco use (Z72.0)

Excludes2 certain conditions originating in the perinatal period (P04-P96)
certain infectious and parasitic diseases (A00-B99)
complications of pregnancy, childbirth and the puerperium (O00-O99A)
congenital malformations, deformations and chromosomal abnormalities (Q00-Q99)
endocrine, nutritional and metabolic diseases (E00-E88)
injury, poisoning and certain other consequences of external causes (S00-T88)
neoplasms (C00-D49)
smoke inhalation (T59.81-)
symptoms, signs and abnormal clinical and laboratory findings, not elsewhere classified (R00-R94)

This chapter contains the following blocks:

J00-J06	Acute upper respiratory infections
J09-J18	Influenza and pneumonia
J20-J22	Other acute lower respiratory infections
J30-J39	Other diseases of upper respiratory tract
J40-J47	Chronic lower respiratory diseases
J60-J70	Lung diseases due to external agents
J80-J84	Other respiratory diseases principally affecting the interstitium
J85-J86	Suppurative and necrotic conditions of the lower respiratory tract
J90-J94	Other diseases of the pleura
J95	Intraoperative and postprocedural complications and disorders of respiratory system, not elsewhere classified
J96-J99	Other diseases of the respiratory system

ACUTE UPPER RESPIRATORY INFECTIONS (J00-J06)

Excludes1 chronic obstructive pulmonary disease with acute lower respiratory infection (J44.0)
influenza virus with other respiratory manifestations (J09.X2, J10.1, J11.1)

J00   Acute nasopharyngitis [common cold]
Acute rhinitis
Coryza (acute)
Infective nasopharyngitis NOS
Infective rhinitis
Nasal catarrh, acute
Nasopharyngitis NOS

Excludes1 acute pharyngitis (J02.-)
acute sore throat NOS (J02.9)
pharyngitis NOS (J02.9)
rhinitis NOS (J31.0)
sore throat NOS (J02.9)

Excludes2 allergic rhinitis (J30.1-J30.9)
chronic pharyngitis (J31.2)
chronic rhinitis (J31.0)
chronic sore throat (J31.2)
nasopharyngitis, chronic (J31.1)
vasomotor rhinitis (J30.0)

(See Plate 49 on page NAP-24.)

● **J01   Acute sinusitis**
Includes acute abscess of sinus
acute empyema of sinus
acute infection of sinus
acute inflammation of sinus
acute suppuration of sinus

Use additional code (B95-B97) to identify infectious agent.
Excludes1 sinusitis NOS (J32.9)
Excludes2 chronic sinusitis (J32.0-J32.8)

● **J01.0   Acute maxillary sinusitis**
Acute antritis
  J01.00   Acute maxillary sinusitis, unspecified
  J01.01   Acute recurrent maxillary sinusitis
● **J01.1   Acute frontal sinusitis**
  J01.10   Acute frontal sinusitis, unspecified
  J01.11   Acute recurrent frontal sinusitis
● **J01.2   Acute ethmoidal sinusitis**
  J01.20   Acute ethmoidal sinusitis, unspecified
  J01.21   Acute recurrent ethmoidal sinusitis
● **J01.3   Acute sphenoidal sinusitis**
  J01.30   Acute sphenoidal sinusitis, unspecified
  J01.31   Acute recurrent sphenoidal sinusitis
● **J01.4   Acute pansinusitis**
  J01.40   Acute pansinusitis, unspecified
  J01.41   Acute recurrent pansinusitis

CHAPTER 10 (J00-J99)

● **J01.8**   **Other acute sinusitis**
    J01.80   **Other acute sinusitis**
        Acute sinusitis involving more than one sinus but not pansinusitis
    J01.81   **Other acute recurrent sinusitis**
        Acute recurrent sinusitis involving more than one sinus but not pansinusitis

● **J01.9**   **Acute sinusitis, unspecified**
    J01.90   **Acute sinusitis, unspecified**
    J01.91   **Acute recurrent sinusitis, unspecified**

● **J02**   **Acute pharyngitis**
    Includes   acute sore throat
    Excludes1   acute laryngopharyngitis (J06.0)
        peritonsillar abscess (J36)
        pharyngeal abscess (J39.1)
        retropharyngeal abscess (J39.0)
    Excludes2   chronic pharyngitis (J31.2)
    J02.0   **Streptococcal pharyngitis**
        Septic pharyngitis
        Streptococcal sore throat
        Excludes2   scarlet fever (A38.-)
    J02.8   **Acute pharyngitis due to other specified organisms**
        Use additional code (B95-B97) to identify infectious agent
        Excludes1   pharyngitis due to coxsackie virus (B08.5)
            pharyngitis due to gonococcus (A54.5)
            acute pharyngitis due to herpes [simplex] virus (B00.2)
            acute pharyngitis due to infectious mononucleosis (B27.-)
            enteroviral vesicular pharyngitis (B08.5)
    J02.9   **Acute pharyngitis, unspecified**
        Gangrenous pharyngitis (acute)
        Infective pharyngitis (acute) NOS
        Pharyngitis (acute) NOS
        Sore throat (acute) NOS
        Suppurative pharyngitis (acute)
        Ulcerative pharyngitis (acute)

● **J03**   **Acute tonsillitis**
    Inflammation of pharyngeal tonsils caused by virus or bacteria
    Excludes1   acute sore throat (J02.-)
        hypertrophy of tonsils (J35.1)
        peritonsillar abscess (J36)
        sore throat NOS (J02.9)
        streptococcal sore throat (J02.0)
    Excludes2   chronic tonsillitis (J35.0)
● **J03.0**   **Streptococcal tonsillitis**
    J03.00   **Acute streptococcal tonsillitis, unspecified**
    J03.01   **Acute recurrent streptococcal tonsillitis**
● **J03.8**   **Acute tonsillitis due to other specified organisms**
    Use additional code (B95-B97) to identify infectious agent.
    Excludes1   diphtheritic tonsillitis (A36.0)
        herpesviral pharyngotonsillitis (B00.2)
        streptococcal tonsillitis (J03.0)
        tuberculous tonsillitis (A15.8)
        Vincent's tonsillitis (A69.1)
    J03.80   **Acute tonsillitis due to other specified organisms**
    J03.81   **Acute recurrent tonsillitis due to other specified organisms**
● **J03.9**   **Acute tonsillitis, unspecified**
    Follicular tonsillitis (acute)
    Gangrenous tonsillitis (acute)
    Infective tonsillitis (acute)
    Tonsillitis (acute) NOS
    Ulcerative tonsillitis (acute)
    J03.90   **Acute tonsillitis, unspecified**
    J03.91   **Acute recurrent tonsillitis, unspecified**

Item 10–2   **Laryngitis** is an inflammation of the larynx (voice box) resulting in hoarse voice or the complete loss of the voice. **Tracheitis** is an inflammation of the trachea (often following a URI) commonly caused by *staphylococcus aureus* resulting in inspiratory stridor (crowing sound on inspiration) and a croup like cough.

● **J04**   **Acute laryngitis and tracheitis**
    Use additional code (B95-B97) to identify infectious agent.
    Excludes1   acute obstructive laryngitis [croup] and epiglottitis (J05.-)
    Excludes2   laryngismus (stridulus) (J38.5)
    J04.0   **Acute laryngitis**
        Edematous laryngitis (acute)
        Laryngitis (acute) NOS
        Subglottic laryngitis (acute)
        Suppurative laryngitis (acute)
        Ulcerative laryngitis (acute)
        Excludes1   acute obstructive laryngitis (J05.0)
        Excludes2   chronic laryngitis (J37.0)
● **J04.1**   **Acute tracheitis**
    Acute viral tracheitis
    Catarrhal tracheitis (acute)
    Tracheitis (acute) NOS
    Excludes2   chronic tracheitis (J42)
    J04.10   **Acute tracheitis without obstruction**
    J04.11   **Acute tracheitis with obstruction**
    J04.2   **Acute laryngotracheitis**
        Laryngotracheitis NOS
        Tracheitis (acute) with laryngitis (acute)
        Excludes1   acute obstructive laryngotracheitis (J05.0)
        Excludes2   chronic laryngotracheitis (J37.1)
● **J04.3**   **Supraglottitis, unspecified**
    J04.30   **Supraglottitis, unspecified, without obstruction**
    J04.31   **Supraglottitis, unspecified, with obstruction**

● **J05**   **Acute obstructive laryngitis [croup] and epiglottitis**
    Use additional code (B95-B97) to identify infectious agent.
    J05.0   **Acute obstructive laryngitis [croup]**
        Obstructive laryngitis (acute) NOS
        Obstructive laryngotracheitis NOS
    J05.1   **Acute epiglottitis**
        Excludes2   epiglottitis, chronic (J37.0)
    J05.10   **Acute epiglottitis without obstruction**
        Epiglottitis NOS
    J05.11   **Acute epiglottitis with obstruction**

● **J06**   **Acute upper respiratory infections of multiple and unspecified sites**
    Excludes1   acute respiratory infection NOS (J22)
        streptococcal pharyngitis (J02.0)
    J06.0   **Acute laryngopharyngitis**
    J06.9   **Acute upper respiratory infection, unspecified**
        Upper respiratory disease, acute
        Upper respiratory infection NOS

◀ New   ◀▥ Revised   ~~deleted~~ Deleted   OGCR Official Guidelines   X Assign placeholder X   ● Use Additional Character(s)

Excludes 1   Excludes 2   Includes   Use additional   Code first   Code also   Unspecified

INFLUENZA AND PNEUMONIA (J09-J18)

Excludes2 allergic or eosinophilic pneumonia (J82)
aspiration pneumonia NOS (J69.0)
meconium pneumonia (P24.01)
neonatal aspiration pneumonia (P24.-)
pneumonia due to solids and liquids (J69.-)
congenital pneumonia (P23.9)
lipid pneumonia (J69.1)
rheumatic pneumonia (I00)
ventilator associated pneumonia (J95.851)

● **J09** **Influenza due to certain identified influenza viruses**

Excludes1 influenza due to other influenza viruses (J10.-)
influenza due to unidentified influenza virus (J11.-)
seasonal influenza due to other identified influenza virus (J10.-)
seasonal influenza due to unidentified influenza virus (J11.-)

● **J09.X** **Influenza due to identified novel influenza A virus**
Avian influenza
Bird influenza
Influenza A/H5N1
Influenza of other animal origin, not bird or swine
Swine influenza virus (viruses that normally cause infections in pigs)

J09.X1 **Influenza due to identified novel influenza A virus with pneumonia**

Code also , if applicable, associated:
lung abscess (J85.1)
other specified type of pneumonia

J09.X2 **Influenza due to identified novel influenza A virus with other respiratory manifestations**
Influenza due to identified novel influenza A virus NOS
Influenza due to identified novel influenza A virus with laryngitis
Influenza due to identified novel influenza A virus with pharyngitis
Influenza due to identified novel influenza A virus with upper respiratory symptoms

Use additional code, if applicable, for associated:
pleural effusion (J91.8)
sinusitis (J01.-)

J09.X3 **Influenza due to identified novel influenza A virus with gastrointestinal manifestations**
Influenza due to identified novel influenza A virus gastroenteritis

Excludes1 'intestinal flu' [viral gastroenteritis] (A08.-)

J09.X9 **Influenza due to identified novel influenza A virus with other manifestations**
Influenza due to identified novel influenza A virus with encephalopathy
Influenza due to identified novel influenza A virus with myocarditis
Influenza due to identified novel influenza A virus with otitis media

Use additional code to identify manifestation

● **J10** **Influenza due to other identified influenza virus**

Excludes1 influenza due to avian influenza virus (J09.X-)
influenza due to swine flu (J09.X-)
influenza due to unidentified influenza virus (J11.-)

● **J10.0** **Influenza due to other identified influenza virus with pneumonia**

Code also associated lung abscess, if applicable (J85.1)

J10.00 **Influenza due to other identified influenza virus with unspecified type of pneumonia**

J10.01 **Influenza due to other identified influenza virus with the same other identified influenza virus pneumonia**

J10.08 **Influenza due to other identified influenza virus with other specified pneumonia**

Code also other specified type of pneumonia

J10.1 **Influenza due to other identified influenza virus with other respiratory manifestations**
Influenza due to other identified influenza virus NOS
Influenza due to other identified influenza virus with laryngitis
Influenza due to other identified influenza virus with pharyngitis
Influenza due to other identified influenza virus with upper respiratory symptoms

Use additional code for associated pleural effusion, if applicable (J91.8)

Use additional code for associated sinusitis, if applicable (J01.-)

J10.2 **Influenza due to other identified influenza virus with gastrointestinal manifestations**
Influenza due to other identified influenza virus gastroenteritis

Excludes1 'intestinal flu' [viral gastroenteritis] (A08.-)

● **J10.8** **Influenza due to other identified influenza virus with other manifestations**

J10.81 **Influenza due to other identified influenza virus with encephalopathy**

J10.82 **Influenza due to other identified influenza virus with myocarditis**

J10.83 **Influenza due to other identified influenza virus with otitis media**

Use additional code for any associated perforated tympanic membrane (H72.-)

J10.89 **Influenza due to other identified influenza virus with other manifestations**

Use additional codes to identify the manifestations

● **J11** **Influenza due to unidentified influenza virus**

● **J11.0** **Influenza due to unidentified influenza virus with pneumonia**

Code also associated lung abscess, if applicable (J85.1)

J11.00 **Influenza due to unidentified influenza virus with unspecified type of pneumonia**
Influenza with pneumonia NOS

J11.08 **Influenza due to unidentified influenza virus with specified pneumonia**

Code also other specified type of pneumonia

CHAPTER 10 (J00-J99)

J11.1   **Influenza due to unidentified influenza virus with other respiratory manifestations**
Influenza NOS
Influenzal laryngitis NOS
Influenzal pharyngitis NOS
Influenza with upper respiratory symptoms NOS
> Use additional code for associated pleural effusion, if applicable (J91.8)
> Use additional code for associated sinusitis, if applicable (J01.-)

J11.2   **Influenza due to unidentified influenza virus with gastrointestinal manifestations**
Influenza gastroenteritis NOS
> **Excludes1**   'intestinal flu' [viral gastroenteritis] (A08.-)

● **J11.8**   **Influenza due to unidentified influenza virus with other manifestations**

     J11.81   **Influenza due to unidentified influenza virus with encephalopathy**
         Influenzal encephalopathy NOS

     J11.82   **Influenza due to unidentified influenza virus with myocarditis**
         Influenzal myocarditis NOS

     J11.83   **Influenza due to unidentified influenza virus with otitis media**
         Influenzal otitis media NOS
         > Use additional code for any associated perforated tympanic membrane (H72.-)

     J11.89   **Influenza due to unidentified influenza virus with other manifestations**
         > Use additional codes to identify the manifestations

● **J12**   **Viral pneumonia, not elsewhere classified**
> **Includes**   bronchopneumonia due to viruses other than influenza viruses
> *Code first associated influenza, if applicable (J09.X1, J10.0-, J11.0-)*
> Code also associated abscess, if applicable (J85.1)
> **Excludes1**   aspiration pneumonia due to anesthesia during labor and delivery (O74.0)
> aspiration pneumonia due to anesthesia during pregnancy (O29)
> aspiration pneumonia due to anesthesia during puerperium (O89.0)
> aspiration pneumonia due to solids and liquids (J69.-)
> aspiration pneumonia NOS (J69.0)
> congenital pneumonia (P23.0)
> congenital rubella pneumonitis (P35.0)
> interstitial pneumonia NOS (J84.9)
> lipid pneumonia (J69.1)
> neonatal aspiration pneumonia (P24.-)

J12.0   **Adenoviral pneumonia**

J12.1   **Respiratory syncytial virus pneumonia**

J12.2   **Parainfluenza virus pneumonia**

J12.3   **Human metapneumovirus pneumonia**

● **J12.8**   **Other viral pneumonia**

     J12.81   **Pneumonia due to SARS-associated coronavirus**
         Severe acute respiratory syndrome NOS

     J12.89   **Other viral pneumonia**

J12.9   **Viral pneumonia, unspecified**

Item 10–3   Pneumonia is an infection of the lungs, caused by a variety of microorganisms, including viruses, most commonly the Streptococcus pneumoniae (pneumococcus) bacteria, fungi, and parasites. Pneumonia occurs when the immune system is weakened, often by a URI or influenza.

J13   **Pneumonia due to Streptococcus pneumoniae**
Bronchopneumonia due to S. pneumoniae
> *Code first associated influenza, if applicable (J09.X1, J10.0-, J11.0-)*
> Code also associated abscess, if applicable (J85.1)
> **Excludes1**   congenital pneumonia due to S. pneumoniae (P23.6)
> lobar pneumonia, unspecified organism (J18.1)
> pneumonia due to other streptococci (J15.3-J15.4)

J14   **Pneumonia due to Hemophilus influenzae**
Bronchopneumonia due to H. influenzae
> *Code first associated influenza, if applicable (J09.X1, J10.0-, J11.0-)*
> Code also associated abscess, if applicable (J85.1)
> **Excludes1**   congenital pneumonia due to H. influenzae (P23.6)

● **J15**   **Bacterial pneumonia, not elsewhere classified**
> **Includes**   bronchopneumonia due to bacteria other than S. pneumoniae and H. influenzae
> *Code first associated influenza, if applicable (J09.X1, J10.0-, J11.0-)*
> Code also associated abscess, if applicable (J85.1)
> **Excludes1**   chlamydial pneumonia (J16.0)
> congenital pneumonia (P23.-)
> Legionnaires' disease (A48.1)
> spirochetal pneumonia (A69.8)

J15.0   **Pneumonia due to Klebsiella pneumoniae**

J15.1   **Pneumonia due to Pseudomonas**

● **J15.2**   **Pneumonia due to staphylococcus**

     J15.20   **Pneumonia due to staphylococcus, unspecified**

     ● **J15.21**   **Pneumonia due to staphylococcus aureus**

         J15.211   **Pneumonia due to Methicillin susceptible Staphylococcus aureus**
             MSSA pneumonia
             Pneumonia due to Staphylococcus aureus NOS

         J15.212   **Pneumonia due to Methicillin resistant Staphylococcus aureus**

     J15.29   **Pneumonia due to other staphylococcus**

J15.3   **Pneumonia due to streptococcus, group B**

J15.4   **Pneumonia due to other streptococci**
> **Excludes1**   pneumonia due to streptococcus, group B (J15.3)
> pneumonia due to Streptococcus pneumoniae (J13)

J15.5   **Pneumonia due to Escherichia coli**

J15.6   **Pneumonia due to other aerobic Gram-negative bacteria**
Pneumonia due to Serratia marcescens

J15.7   **Pneumonia due to Mycoplasma pneumoniae**

J15.8   **Pneumonia due to other specified bacteria**

J15.9   **Unspecified bacterial pneumonia**
Pneumonia due to gram-positive bacteria

● **J16**   **Pneumonia due to other infectious organisms, not elsewhere classified**
> *Code first associated influenza, if applicable (J09.X1, J10.0-, J11.0-)*
> Code also associated abscess, if applicable (J85.1)
> **Excludes1**   congenital pneumonia (P23.-)
> ornithosis (A70)
> pneumocystosis (B59)
> pneumonia NOS (J18.9)

J16.0   **Chlamydial pneumonia**

J16.8   **Pneumonia due to other specified infectious organisms**

J17   Pneumonia in diseases classified elsewhere

Code first underlying disease, such as:
     Q fever (A78)
     rheumatic fever (I00)
     schistosomiasis (B65.0-B65.9)

   Excludes1   candidial pneumonia (B37.1)
              chlamydial pneumonia (J16.0)
              gonorrheal pneumonia (A54.84)
              histoplasmosis pneumonia (B39.0-B39.2)
              measles pneumonia (B05.2)
              nocardiosis pneumonia (A43.0)
              pneumocystosis (B59)
              pneumonia due to Pneumocystis carinii (B59)
              pneumonia due to Pneumocystis jiroveci (B59)
              pneumonia in actinomycosis (A42.0)
              pneumonia in anthrax (A22.1)
              pneumonia in ascariasis (B77.81)
              pneumonia in aspergillosis (B44.0-B44.1)
              pneumonia in coccidioidomycosis (B38.0-B38.2)
              pneumonia in cytomegalovirus disease (B25.0)
              pneumonia in toxoplasmosis (B58.3)
              rubella pneumonia (B06.81)
              salmonella pneumonia (A02.22)
              spirochetal infection NEC with pneumonia (A69.8)
              tularemia pneumonia (A21.2)
              typhoid fever with pneumonia (A01.03)
              varicella pneumonia (B01.2)
              whooping cough with pneumonia (A37 with fifth-character 1)

● J18   Pneumonia, unspecified organism

Code first associated influenza, if applicable (J09.X1, J10.0-, J11.0-)

   Excludes1   abscess of lung with pneumonia (J85.1)
              aspiration pneumonia due to anesthesia during labor and delivery (O74.0)
              aspiration pneumonia due to anesthesia during pregnancy (O29)
              aspiration pneumonia due to anesthesia during puerperium (O89.0)
              aspiration pneumonia due to solids and liquids (J69.-)
              aspiration pneumonia NOS (J69.0)
              congenital pneumonia (P23.0)
              drug-induced interstitial lung disorder (J70.2-J70.4)
              interstitial pneumonia NOS (J84.9)
              lipid pneumonia (J69.1)
              neonatal aspiration pneumonia (P24.-)
              pneumonitis due to external agents (J67-J70)
              pneumonitis due to fumes and vapors (J68.0)
              usual interstitial pneumonia (J84.17)

J18.0   Bronchopneumonia, unspecified organism

   Excludes1   hypostatic bronchopneumonia (J18.2)
              lipid pneumonia (J69.1)

   Excludes2   acute bronchiolitis (J21.-)
              chronic bronchiolitis (J44.9)

J18.1   Lobar pneumonia, unspecified organism

J18.2   Hypostatic pneumonia, unspecified organism
       Hypostatic bronchopneumonia
       Passive pneumonia

J18.8   Other pneumonia, unspecified organism

J18.9   Pneumonia, unspecified organism

OTHER ACUTE LOWER RESPIRATORY INFECTIONS (J20-J22)

   Excludes2   chronic obstructive pulmonary disease with acute lower respiratory infection (J44.0)

● J20   Acute bronchitis

Inflammation/irritation of the bronchial tubes lasting 2-3 weeks, most commonly caused by a virus.

   Includes   acute and subacute bronchitis (with) bronchospasm
              acute and subacute bronchitis (with) tracheitis
              acute and subacute bronchitis (with) tracheobronchitis, acute
              acute and subacute fibrinous bronchitis
              acute and subacute membranous bronchitis
              acute and subacute purulent bronchitis
              acute and subacute septic bronchitis

   Excludes1   bronchitis NOS (J40)
              tracheobronchitis NOS (J40)

   Excludes2   acute bronchitis with bronchiectasis (J47.0)
              acute bronchitis with chronic obstructive asthma (J44.0)
              acute bronchitis with chronic obstructive pulmonary disease (J44.0)
              allergic bronchitis NOS (J45.909-)
              bronchitis due to chemicals, fumes and vapors (J68.0)
              chronic bronchitis NOS (J42)
              chronic mucopurulent bronchitis (J41.1)
              chronic obstructive bronchitis (J44.-)
              chronic obstructive tracheobronchitis (J44.-)
              chronic simple bronchitis (J41.0)
              chronic tracheobronchitis (J42)

J20.0   Acute bronchitis due to Mycoplasma pneumoniae

J20.1   Acute bronchitis due to Hemophilus influenzae

J20.2   Acute bronchitis due to streptococcus

J20.3   Acute bronchitis due to coxsackievirus

J20.4   Acute bronchitis due to parainfluenza virus

J20.5   Acute bronchitis due to respiratory syncytial virus

J20.6   Acute bronchitis due to rhinovirus

J20.7   Acute bronchitis due to echovirus

J20.8   Acute bronchitis due to other specified organisms

J20.9   Acute bronchitis, unspecified

● J21   Acute bronchiolitis

Bronchiolitis obliterans with organizing pneumonia (BOOP) inflammation of bronchioles and surrounding tissue in lung.

   Includes   acute bronchiolitis with bronchospasm
   Excludes2   respiratory bronchiolitis interstitial lung disease (J84.115)

J21.0   Acute bronchiolitis due to respiratory syncytial virus

J21.1   Acute bronchiolitis due to human metapneumovirus

J21.8   Acute bronchiolitis due to other specified organisms

J21.9   Acute bronchiolitis, unspecified
       Bronchiolitis (acute)

   Excludes1   chronic bronchiolitis (J44.-)

J22   Unspecified acute lower respiratory infection
       Acute (lower) respiratory (tract) infection NOS

   Excludes1   upper respiratory infection (acute) (J06.9)

CHAPTER 10 (J00-J99)

OTHER DISEASES OF UPPER RESPIRATORY TRACT (J30–J39)

● **J30   Vasomotor and allergic rhinitis**

    Includes   spasmodic rhinorrhea

    Excludes1   allergic rhinitis with asthma (bronchial) (J45.909)
                 rhinitis NOS (J31.0)

  J30.0   Vasomotor rhinitis

  J30.1   Allergic rhinitis due to pollen
        Allergy NOS due to pollen
        Hay fever
        Pollinosis

  J30.2   Other seasonal allergic rhinitis

  J30.5   Allergic rhinitis due to food

  ● **J30.8   Other allergic rhinitis**

      J30.81   Allergic rhinitis due to animal (cat) (dog) hair and dander

      J30.89   Other allergic rhinitis
            Perennial allergic rhinitis

  J30.9   Allergic rhinitis, unspecified

● **J31   Chronic rhinitis, nasopharyngitis and pharyngitis**

  Use additional code to identify:
    exposure to environmental tobacco smoke (Z77.22)
    exposure to tobacco smoke in the perinatal period (P96.81)
    history of tobacco use (Z87.891)
    occupational exposure to environmental tobacco smoke (Z57.31)
    tobacco dependence (F17.-)
    tobacco use (Z72.0)

  J31.0   Chronic rhinitis
      Atrophic rhinitis (chronic)
      Granulomatous rhinitis (chronic)
      Hypertrophic rhinitis (chronic)
      Obstructive rhinitis (chronic)
      Ozena
      Purulent rhinitis (chronic)
      Rhinitis (chronic) NOS
      Ulcerative rhinitis (chronic)

      Excludes1   allergic rhinitis (J30.1–J30.9)
                 vasomotor rhinitis (J30.0)

  J31.1   Chronic nasopharyngitis
      Excludes2   acute nasopharyngitis (J00)

  J31.2   Chronic pharyngitis
      Chronic sore throat
      Atrophic pharyngitis (chronic)
      Granular pharyngitis (chronic)
      Hypertrophic pharyngitis (chronic)
      Excludes2   acute pharyngitis (J02.9)

● **J32   Chronic sinusitis**

    Includes   sinus abscess
               sinus empyema
               sinus infection
               sinus suppuration

  Use additional code to identify:
    exposure to environmental tobacco smoke (Z77.22)
    exposure to tobacco smoke in the perinatal period (P96.81)
    history of tobacco use (Z87.891)
    infectious agent (B95-B97)
    occupational exposure to environmental tobacco smoke (Z57.31)
    tobacco dependence (F17.-)
    tobacco use (Z72.0)

    Excludes2   acute sinusitis (J01.-)

  J32.0   Chronic maxillary sinusitis
      Antritis (chronic)
      Maxillary sinusitis NOS

  J32.1   Chronic frontal sinusitis
      Frontal sinusitis NOS

Item 10–4   Nasal polyps are an abnormal growth of tissue (tumor) projecting from a mucous membrane and attached to the surface by a narrow elongated stalk (pedunculated). Nasal polyps usually originate in the ethmoid sinus but also may occur in the maxillary sinus. Symptoms are nasal block, sinusitis, anosmia, and secondary infections.

  J32.2   Chronic ethmoidal sinusitis
      Ethmoidal sinusitis NOS
      Excludes1   Woakes' ethmoiditis (J33.1)

  J32.3   Chronic sphenoidal sinusitis
      Sphenoidal sinusitis NOS

  J32.4   Chronic pansinusitis
      Pansinusitis NOS

  J32.8   Other chronic sinusitis
      Sinusitis (chronic) involving more than one sinus but not pansinusitis

  J32.9   Chronic sinusitis, unspecified
      Sinusitis (chronic) NOS

● **J33   Nasal polyp**

  Use additional code to identify:
    exposure to environmental tobacco smoke (Z77.22)
    exposure to tobacco smoke in the perinatal period (P96.81)
    history of tobacco use (Z87.891)
    occupational exposure to environmental tobacco smoke (Z57.31)
    tobacco dependence (F17.-)
    tobacco use (Z72.0)

    Excludes1   adenomatous polyps (D14.0)

  J33.0   Polyp of nasal cavity
      Choanal polyp
      Nasopharyngeal polyp

  J33.1   Polypoid sinus degeneration
      Woakes' syndrome or ethmoiditis

  J33.8   Other polyp of sinus
      Accessory polyp of sinus
      Ethmoidal polyp of sinus
      Maxillary polyp of sinus
      Sphenoidal polyp of sinus

  J33.9   Nasal polyp, unspecified

● **J34   Other and unspecified disorders of nose and nasal sinuses**
    Excludes2   varicose ulcer of nasal septum (I86.8)

  J34.0   Abscess, furuncle and carbuncle of nose
      Cellulitis of nose
      Necrosis of nose
      Ulceration of nose

  J34.1   Cyst and mucocele of nose and nasal sinus

  J34.2   Deviated nasal septum
      Deflection or deviation of septum (nasal) (acquired)
      Excludes1   congenital deviated nasal septum (Q67.4)

  J34.3   Hypertrophy of nasal turbinates

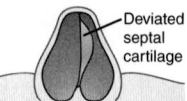
Deviated septal cartilage

Figure 10-3   Deviated nasal septum.

Item 10–5   A **deviated nasal septum** is the displacement of the septal cartilage that separates the nares. This displacement causes obstructed air flow through the nasal passages. A child can be born with this displacement (congenital), or the condition may be acquired through trauma, such as a sports injury. Symptoms include nasal block, sinusitis, and related secondary infections. Septoplasty is surgical repair of this condition.

◄ New   ◄▥ Revised   ~~deleted~~ Deleted   OGCR Official Guidelines   X Assign placeholder X   ● Use Additional Character(s)

Excludes 1   Excludes 2   Includes   Use additional   Code first   Code also   Unspecified

● **J34.8   Other specified disorders of nose and nasal sinuses**

    J34.81   Nasal mucositis (ulcerative)

      Code also type of associated therapy, such as:
       antineoplastic and immunosuppressive
        drugs (T45.1X-)
       radiological procedure and radiotherapy
        (Y84.2)

       Excludes2   gastrointestinal mucositis
           (ulcerative) (K92.81)
           mucositis (ulcerative) of vagina
            and vulva (N76.81)
           oral mucositis (ulcerative)
            (K12.3-)

    J34.89   Other specified disorders of nose and nasal sinuses
      Perforation of nasal septum NOS
      Rhinolith

   J34.9   Unspecified disorder of nose and nasal sinuses

● **J35   Chronic diseases of tonsils and adenoids**

   Use additional code to identify:
   exposure to environmental tobacco smoke (Z77.22)
   exposure to tobacco smoke in the perinatal period (P96.81)
   history of tobacco use (Z87.891)
   occupational exposure to environmental tobacco smoke
    (Z57.31)
   tobacco dependence (F17.-)
   tobacco use (Z72.0)

● **J35.0   Chronic tonsillitis and adenoiditis**

     Excludes2   acute tonsillitis (J03.-)

   J35.01   Chronic tonsillitis

   J35.02   Chronic adenoiditis

   J35.03   Chronic tonsillitis and adenoiditis

  J35.1   Hypertrophy of tonsils
    Enlargement of tonsils

     Excludes1   hypertrophy of tonsils with tonsillitis
         (J35.0-)

  J35.2   Hypertrophy of adenoids
    Enlargement of adenoids

     Excludes1   hypertrophy of adenoids with adenoiditis
         (J35.0-)

  J35.3   Hypertrophy of tonsils with hypertrophy of adenoids

     Excludes1   hypertrophy of tonsils and adenoids with
         tonsillitis and adenoiditis (J35.03)

  J35.8   Other chronic diseases of tonsils and adenoids
    Adenoid vegetations
    Amygdalolith
    Calculus, tonsil
    Cicatrix of tonsil (and adenoid)
    Tonsillar tag
    Ulcer of tonsil

  J35.9   Chronic disease of tonsils and adenoids, unspecified
    Disease (chronic) of tonsils and adenoids NOS

J36   Peritonsillar abscess

    Includes   abscess of tonsil
        peritonsillar cellulitis
        quinsy

   Use additional code (B95-B97) to identify infectious agent.

    Excludes1   acute tonsillitis (J03.-)
        chronic tonsillitis (J35.0)
        retropharyngeal abscess (J39.0)
        tonsillitis NOS (J03.9-)

● **J37   Chronic laryngitis and laryngotracheitis**

   Use additional code to identify:
   exposure to environmental tobacco smoke (Z77.22)
   exposure to tobacco smoke in the perinatal period (P96.81)
   history of tobacco use (Z87.891)
   infectious agent (B95-B97)
   occupational exposure to environmental tobacco smoke
    (Z57.31)
   tobacco dependence (F17.-)
   tobacco use (Z72.0)

  J37.0   Chronic laryngitis
    Catarrhal laryngitis
    Hypertrophic laryngitis
    Sicca laryngitis

     Excludes2   acute laryngitis (J04.0)
         obstructive (acute) laryngitis (J05.0)

  J37.1   Chronic laryngotracheitis
    Laryngitis, chronic, with tracheitis (chronic)
    Tracheitis, chronic, with laryngitis

     Excludes1   chronic tracheitis (J42)
     Excludes2   acute laryngotracheitis (J04.2)
         acute tracheitis (J04.1)

● **J38   Diseases of vocal cords and larynx, not elsewhere classified**

   Use additional code to identify:
   exposure to environmental tobacco smoke (Z77.22)
   exposure to tobacco smoke in the perinatal period (P96.81)
   history of tobacco use (Z87.891)
   occupational exposure to environmental tobacco smoke
    (Z57.31)
   tobacco dependence (F17.-)
   tobacco use (Z72.0)

    Excludes1   congenital laryngeal stridor (P28.89)
        obstructive laryngitis (acute) (J05.0)
        postprocedural subglottic stenosis (J95.5)
        stridor (R06.1)
        ulcerative laryngitis (J04.0)

● **J38.0   Paralysis of vocal cords and larynx**
    Laryngoplegia
    Paralysis of glottis

   J38.00   Paralysis of vocal cords and larynx, unspecified

   J38.01   Paralysis of vocal cords and larynx, unilateral

   J38.02   Paralysis of vocal cords and larynx, bilateral

  J38.1   Polyp of vocal cord and larynx

     Excludes1   adenomatous polyps (D14.1)

  J38.2   Nodules of vocal cords
    Chorditis (fibrinous)(nodosa)(tuberosa)
    Singer's nodes
    Teacher's nodes

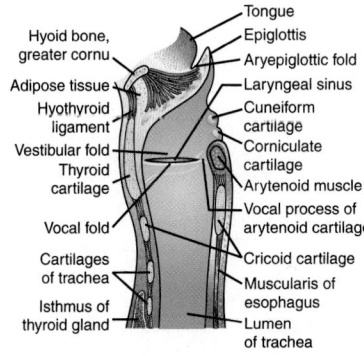

Figure 10-4   Coronal section of the larynx.

Item 10–6 The **larynx** extends from the tongue to the trachea and is divided into an upper and lower portion separated by folds. The framework of the larynx is cartilage composed of the single cricoid, thyroid, and epiglottic cartilages, and the paired arytenoid, cuneiform, and corniculate cartilages.

CHAPTER 10 (J00-J99)

J38.3 **Other diseases of vocal cords**
    Abscess of vocal cords
    Cellulitis of vocal cords
    Granuloma of vocal cords
    Leukokeratosis of vocal cords
    Leukoplakia of vocal cords

J38.4 **Edema of larynx**
    Edema (of) glottis
    Subglottic edema
    Supraglottic edema

> **Excludes1**   acute obstructive laryngitis [croup] (J05.0)
>   edematous laryngitis (J04.0)

J38.5 **Laryngeal spasm**
    Laryngismus (stridulus)

J38.6 **Stenosis of larynx**

J38.7 **Other diseases of larynx**
    Abscess of larynx
    Cellulitis of larynx
    Disease of larynx NOS
    Necrosis of larynx
    Pachyderma of larynx
    Perichondritis of larynx
    Ulcer of larynx

● **J39** **Other diseases of upper respiratory tract**

> **Excludes1**   acute respiratory infection NOS (J22)
>   acute upper respiratory infection (J06.9)
>   upper respiratory inflammation due to chemicals, gases, fumes or vapors (J68.2)

J39.0 **Retropharyngeal and parapharyngeal abscess**
    Peripharyngeal abscess

> **Excludes1**   peritonsillar abscess (J36)

J39.1 **Other abscess of pharynx**
    Cellulitis of pharynx
    Nasopharyngeal abscess

J39.2 **Other diseases of pharynx**
    Cyst of pharynx
    Edema of pharynx

> **Excludes2**   chronic pharyngitis (J31.2)
>   ulcerative pharyngitis (J02.9)

J39.3 **Upper respiratory tract hypersensitivity reaction, site unspecified**

> **Excludes1**   hypersensitivity reaction of upper respiratory tract, such as:
>   extrinsic allergic alveolitis (J67.9)
>   pneumoconiosis (J60-J67.9)

J39.8 **Other specified diseases of upper respiratory tract**

J39.9 **Disease of upper respiratory tract, unspecified**

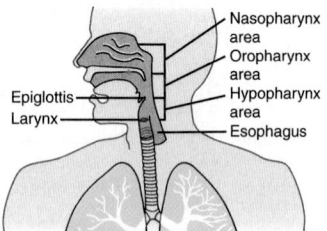

Figure 10-5   The pharynx.

Item 10-7   The **pharynx** is the passage for both food and air between the mouth and the esophagus and is divided into three areas: nasopharynx, oropharynx, and hypopharynx. The hypopharynx branches into the esophagus and the voice box.

Item 10-8   **Chronic bronchitis** is usually defined as being present in any patient who has persistent cough with sputum production for at least three months in at least two consecutive years. **Simple chronic bronchitis** is marked by a productive cough but no pathological airflow obstruction. **Chronic obstructive pulmonary disease (COPD)** is a group of conditions— bronchitis, emphysema, asthma, bronchiectasis, allergic alveolitis—marked by dyspnea. **Catarrhal** bronchitis is an acute form of bronchitis marked by profuse mucus and pus production (**mucopurulent** discharge). **Croupous** bronchitis, also known as pseudomembranous, fibrinous, plastic, exudative, or membranous, is marked by a violent cough and dyspnea.

CHRONIC LOWER RESPIRATORY DISEASES (J40-J47)

> **Excludes1**   bronchitis due to chemicals, gases, fumes and vapors (J68.0)
>
> **Excludes2**   cystic fibrosis (E84.-)

J40 **Bronchitis, not specified as acute or chronic**
    Bronchitis NOS
    Catarrhal bronchitis
    Bronchitis with tracheitis NOS
    Tracheobronchitis NOS

Use additional code to identify:
    exposure to environmental tobacco smoke (Z77.22)
    exposure to tobacco smoke in the perinatal period (P96.81)
    history of tobacco use (Z87.891)
    occupational exposure to environmental tobacco smoke (Z57.31)
    tobacco dependence (F17.-)
    tobacco use (Z72.0)

> **Excludes1**   acute bronchitis (J20.-)
>   allergic bronchitis NOS (J45.909-)
>   asthmatic bronchitis NOS (J45.9-)
>   bronchitis due to chemicals, gases, fumes and vapors (J68.0)

● **J41** **Simple and mucopurulent chronic bronchitis**

Use additional code to identify:
    exposure to environmental tobacco smoke (Z77.22)
    exposure to tobacco smoke in the perinatal period (P96.81)
    history of tobacco use (Z87.891)
    occupational exposure to environmental tobacco smoke (Z57.31)
    tobacco dependence (F17.-)
    tobacco use (Z72.0)

> **Excludes1**   chronic bronchitis NOS (J42)
>   chronic obstructive bronchitis (J44.-)

J41.0 **Simple chronic bronchitis**

J41.1 **Mucopurulent chronic bronchitis**

J41.8 **Mixed simple and mucopurulent chronic bronchitis**

J42 **Unspecified chronic bronchitis**
    Chronic bronchitis NOS
    Chronic tracheitis
    Chronic tracheobronchitis

Use additional code to identify:
    exposure to environmental tobacco smoke (Z77.22)
    exposure to tobacco smoke in the perinatal period (P96.81)
    history of tobacco use (Z87.891)
    occupational exposure to environmental tobacco smoke (Z57.31)
    tobacco dependence (F17.-)
    tobacco use (Z72.0)

> **Excludes1**   chronic asthmatic bronchitis (J44.-)
>   chronic bronchitis with airways obstruction (J44.-)
>   chronic emphysematous bronchitis (J44.-)
>   chronic obstructive pulmonary disease NOS (J44.9)
>   simple and mucopurulent chronic bronchitis (J41.-)

◀ New   ◀▬ Revised   ~~deleted~~ Deleted   **OGCR** Official Guidelines   X Assign placeholder X   ● Use Additional Character(s)

Excludes 1   Excludes 2   Includes   Use additional   Code first   Code also   Unspecified

● **J43   Emphysema**

> Use additional code to identify:
>> exposure to environmental tobacco smoke (Z77.22)
>> history of tobacco use (Z87.891)
>> occupational exposure to environmental tobacco smoke (Z57.31)
>> tobacco dependence (F17.-)
>> tobacco use (Z72.0)

> **Excludes1**   compensatory emphysema (J98.3)
>> emphysema due to inhalation of chemicals, gases, fumes or vapors (J68.4)
>> emphysema with chronic (obstructive) bronchitis (J44.-)
>> emphysematous (obstructive) bronchitis (J44.-)
>> interstitial emphysema (J98.2)
>> mediastinal emphysema (J98.2)
>> neonatal interstitial emphysema (P25.0)
>> surgical (subcutaneous) emphysema (T81.82)
>> traumatic subcutaneous emphysema (T79.7)

J43.0   Unilateral pulmonary emphysema [MacLeod's syndrome]
> Swyer-James syndrome
> Unilateral emphysema
> Unilateral hyperlucent lung
> Unilateral pulmonary artery functional hypoplasia
> Unilateral transparency of lung

J43.1   Panlobular emphysema
> Panacinar emphysema

J43.2   Centrilobular emphysema

J43.8   Other emphysema

J43.9   Emphysema, unspecified
> Bullous emphysema (lung)(pulmonary)
> Emphysema (lung)(pulmonary) NOS
> Emphysematous bleb
> Vesicular emphysema (lung)(pulmonary)

● **J44   Other chronic obstructive pulmonary disease**

> **Includes**   asthma with chronic obstructive pulmonary disease
>> chronic asthmatic (obstructive) bronchitis
>> chronic bronchitis with airways obstruction
>> chronic bronchitis with emphysema
>> chronic emphysematous bronchitis
>> chronic obstructive asthma
>> chronic obstructive bronchitis
>> chronic obstructive tracheobronchitis

> Code also type of asthma, if applicable (J45.-)

> Use additional code to identify:
>> exposure to environmental tobacco smoke (Z77.22)
>> history of tobacco use (Z87.891)
>> occupational exposure to environmental tobacco smoke (Z57.31)
>> tobacco dependence (F17.-)
>> tobacco use (Z72.0)

> **Excludes1**   bronchiectasis (J47.-)
>> chronic bronchitis NOS (J42)
>> chronic simple and mucopurulent bronchitis (J41.-)
>> chronic tracheitis (J42)
>> chronic tracheobronchitis (J42)
>> emphysema without chronic bronchitis (J43.-)
>> lung diseases due to external agents (J60-J70)

J44.0   Chronic obstructive pulmonary disease with acute lower respiratory infection
> Use additional code to identify the infection

J44.1   Chronic obstructive pulmonary disease with (acute) exacerbation
> Decompensated COPD
> Decompensated COPD with (acute) exacerbation

>> **Excludes2**   chronic obstructive pulmonary disease [COPD] with acute bronchitis (J44.0)

J44.9   Chronic obstructive pulmonary disease, unspecified
> Chronic obstructive airway disease NOS
> Chronic obstructive lung disease NOS

Item 10–9   **Asthma** is a bronchial condition marked by airway obstruction, hyper-responsiveness, and inflammation. **Extrinsic** asthma, also known as allergic asthma, is characterized by the same symptoms that occur with exposure to allergens and is divided into the following types: **atopic, occupational, and allergic bronchopulmonary aspergillosis. Intrinsic** asthma occurs in patients who have no history of allergy or sensitivities to allergens and is divided into the following types: **nonreaginic and pharmacologic. Status asthmaticus** is the most severe form of asthma attack and can last for days or weeks.

● **J45   Asthma**
> Allergic (predominantly) asthma
> Allergic bronchitis NOS
> Allergic rhinitis with asthma
> Atopic asthma
> Extrinsic allergic asthma
> Hay fever with asthma
> Idiosyncratic asthma
> Intrinsic nonallergic asthma
> Nonallergic asthma

> Use additional code to identify:
>> exposure to environmental tobacco smoke (Z77.22)
>> exposure to tobacco smoke in the perinatal period (P96.81)
>> history of tobacco use (Z87.891)
>> occupational exposure to environmental tobacco smoke (Z57.31)
>> tobacco dependence (F17.-)
>> tobacco use (Z72.0)

> **Excludes1**   detergent asthma (J69.8)
>> eosinophilic asthma (J82)
>> lung diseases due to external agents (J60-J70)
>> miner's asthma (J60)
>> wheezing NOS (R06.2)
>> wood asthma (J67.8)

> **Excludes2**   asthma with chronic obstructive pulmonary disease (J44.9)
>> chronic asthmatic (obstructive) bronchitis (J44.9)
>> chronic obstructive asthma (J44.9)

● **J45.2   Mild intermittent asthma**

J45.20   Mild intermittent asthma, uncomplicated
> Mild intermittent asthma NOS

J45.21   Mild intermittent asthma with (acute) exacerbation

J45.22   Mild intermittent asthma with status asthmaticus

● **J45.3   Mild persistent asthma**

J45.30   Mild persistent asthma, uncomplicated
> Mild persistent asthma NOS

J45.31   Mild persistent asthma with (acute) exacerbation

J45.32   Mild persistent asthma with status asthmaticus

● **J45.4   Moderate persistent asthma**

J45.40   Moderate persistent asthma, uncomplicated
> Moderate persistent asthma NOS

J45.41   Moderate persistent asthma with (acute) exacerbation

J45.42   Moderate persistent asthma with status asthmaticus

● **J45.5   Severe persistent asthma**

J45.50   Severe persistent asthma, uncomplicated
> Severe persistent asthma NOS

J45.51   Severe persistent asthma with (acute) exacerbation

J45.52   Severe persistent asthma with status asthmaticus

● **J45.9   Other and unspecified asthma**
   ● **J45.90   Unspecified asthma**
      Asthmatic bronchitis NOS
      Childhood asthma NOS
      Late onset asthma
      J45.901   Unspecified asthma with (acute) exacerbation
      J45.902   Unspecified asthma with status asthmaticus
      J45.909   Unspecified asthma, uncomplicated
         Asthma NOS
   ● **J45.99   Other asthma**
      J45.990   Exercise induced bronchospasm
      J45.991   Cough variant asthma
      J45.998   Other asthma

● **J47   Bronchiectasis**
   Includes   bronchiolectasis
   Use additional code to identify:
      exposure to environmental tobacco smoke (Z77.22)
      exposure to tobacco smoke in the perinatal period (P96.81)
      history of tobacco use (Z87.891)
      occupational exposure to environmental tobacco smoke (Z57.31)
      tobacco dependence (F17.-)
      tobacco use (Z72.0)
   Excludes1   congenital bronchiectasis (Q33.4)
      tuberculous bronchiectasis (current disease) (A15.0)
   J47.0   Bronchiectasis with acute lower respiratory infection
      Bronchiectasis with acute bronchitis
   J47.1   Bronchiectasis with (acute) exacerbation
   J47.9   Bronchiectasis, uncomplicated
      Bronchiectasis NOS

LUNG DISEASES DUE TO EXTERNAL AGENTS (J60-J70)

   Excludes2   asthma (J45.-)
      malignant neoplasm of bronchus and lung (C34.-)

J60   Coalworker's pneumoconiosis
   Anthracosilicosis
   Anthracosis
   Black lung disease
   Coalworker's lung
   Excludes1   coalworker pneumoconiosis with tuberculosis, any type in A15 (J65)

J61   Pneumoconiosis due to asbestos and other mineral fibers
   Asbestosis
   Excludes1   pleural plaque with asbestosis (J92.0)
      pneumoconiosis with tuberculosis, any type in A15 (J65)

● **J62   Pneumoconiosis due to dust containing silica**
   Includes   silicotic fibrosis (massive) of lung
   Excludes1   pneumoconiosis with tuberculosis, any type in A15 (J65)
   J62.0   Pneumoconiosis due to talc dust
   J62.8   Pneumoconiosis due to other dust containing silica
      Silicosis NOS

Figure 10-6 Progressive massive fibrosis superimposed on coal workers' pneumoconiosis. The large, blackened scars are located principally in the upper lobe. (From Cotran R, Kumar V, Collins T: Robbins Pathologic Basis of Disease, ed 8, Philadelphia, WB Saunders, 2009. Courtesy of Dr. Warner Laquer, Dr. Jerome Kleinerman, and the National Institute of Occupational Safety and Health, Morgantown, WV)

Item 10–10   Pneumoconiosis refers to a lung condition resulting from exposure to inorganic or organic airborne particles, such as coal dust or moldy hay, as well as chemical fumes and vapors, such as insecticides. In this condition, the lungs retain the airborne particles.

● **J63   Pneumoconiosis due to other inorganic dusts**
   Excludes1   pneumoconiosis with tuberculosis, any type in A15 (J65)
   J63.0   Aluminosis (of lung)
   J63.1   Bauxite fibrosis (of lung)
   J63.2   Berylliosis
   J63.3   Graphite fibrosis (of lung)
   J63.4   Siderosis
   J63.5   Stannosis
   J63.6   Pneumoconiosis due to other specified inorganic dusts

J64   Unspecified pneumoconiosis
   Excludes1   pneumonoconiosis with tuberculosis, any type in A15 (J65)

J65   Pneumoconiosis associated with tuberculosis
   Any condition in J60-J64 with tuberculosis, any type in A15
   Silicotuberculosis

● **J66   Airway disease due to specific organic dust**
   Excludes2   allergic alveolitis (J67.-)
      asbestosis (J61)
      bagassosis (J67.1)
      farmer's lung (J67.0)
      hypersensitivity pneumonitis due to organic dust (J67.-)
      reactive airways dysfunction syndrome (J68.3)
   J66.0   Byssinosis
      Airway disease due to cotton dust
   J66.1   Flax-dressers' disease
   J66.2   Cannabinosis
   J66.8   Airway disease due to other specific organic dusts

● **J67   Hypersensitivity pneumonitis due to organic dust**
   Includes   allergic alveolitis and pneumonitis due to inhaled organic dust and particles of fungal, actinomycetic or other origin
   Excludes1   pneumonitis due to inhalation of chemicals, gases, fumes or vapors (J68.0)
   J67.0   Farmer's lung
      Harvester's lung
      Haymaker's lung
      Moldy hay disease
   J67.1   Bagassosis
      Bagasse disease
      Bagasse pneumonitis
   J67.2   Bird fancier's lung
      Budgerigar fancier's disease or lung
      Pigeon fancier's disease or lung
   J67.3   Suberosis
      Corkhandler's disease or lung
      Corkworker's disease or lung
   J67.4   Maltworker's lung
      Alveolitis due to Aspergillus clavatus
   J67.5   Mushroom-worker's lung
   J67.6   Maple-bark-stripper's lung
      Alveolitis due to Cryptostroma corticale
      Cryptostromosis
   J67.7   Air conditioner and humidifier lung
      Allergic alveolitis due to fungal, thermophilic actinomycetes and other organisms growing in ventilation [air conditioning] systems

J67.8   **Hypersensitivity pneumonitis due to other organic dusts**
    Cheese-washer's lung
    Coffee-worker's lung
    Fish-meal worker's lung
    Furrier's lung
    Sequoiosis

J67.9   **Hypersensitivity pneumonitis due to unspecified organic dust**
    Allergic alveolitis (extrinsic) NOS
    Hypersensitivity pneumonitis NOS

● **J68**   **Respiratory conditions due to inhalation of chemicals, gases, fumes and vapors**
    Code first (T51-T65) to identify cause
    Use additional code to identify associated respiratory conditions, such as:
    acute respiratory failure (J96.0-)

J68.0   **Bronchitis and pneumonitis due to chemicals, gases, fumes and vapors**
    Chemical bronchitis (acute)

J68.1   **Pulmonary edema due to chemicals, gases, fumes and vapors**
    Chemical pulmonary edema (acute) (chronic)
    Excludes1   pulmonary edema (acute) (chronic) NOS (J81.-)

J68.2   **Upper respiratory inflammation due to chemicals, gases, fumes and vapors, not elsewhere classified**

J68.3   **Other acute and subacute respiratory conditions due to chemicals, gases, fumes and vapors**
    Reactive airways dysfunction syndrome

J68.4   **Chronic respiratory conditions due to chemicals, gases, fumes and vapors**
    Emphysema (diffuse) (chronic) due to inhalation of chemicals, gases, fumes and vapors
    Obliterative bronchiolitis (chronic) (subacute) due to inhalation of chemicals, gases, fumes and vapors
    Pulmonary fibrosis (chronic) due to inhalation of chemicals, gases, fumes and vapors
    Excludes1   chronic pulmonary edema due to chemicals, gases, fumes and vapors (J68.1)

J68.8   **Other respiratory conditions due to chemicals, fumes and vapors**

J68.9   **Unspecified respiratory condition due to chemicals, gases, fumes and vapors**

● **J69**   **Pneumonitis due to solids and liquids**
    Excludes1   neonatal aspiration syndromes (P24.-)
    postprocedural pneumonitis (J95.4)

J69.0   **Pneumonitis due to inhalation of food and vomit**
    Aspiration pneumonia NOS
    Aspiration pneumonia (due to) food (regurgitated)
    Aspiration pneumonia (due to) gastric secretions
    Aspiration pneumonia (due to) milk
    Aspiration pneumonia (due to) vomit
    Code also any associated foreign body in respiratory tract (T17.-)
    Excludes1   chemical pneumonitis due to anesthesia (J95.4)
    obstetric aspiration pneumonitis (O74.0)

J69.1   **Pneumonitis due to inhalation of oils and essences**
    Exogenous lipoid pneumonia
    Lipid pneumonia NOS
    Code first (T51-T65) to identify substance
    Excludes1   endogenous lipoid pneumonia (J84.89)

J69.8   **Pneumonitis due to inhalation of other solids and liquids**
    Pneumonitis due to aspiration of blood
    Pneumonitis due to aspiration of detergent
    Code first (T51-T65) to identify substance

● **J70**   **Respiratory conditions due to other external agents**

J70.0   **Acute pulmonary manifestations due to radiation**
    Radiation pneumonitis
    Use additional code (W88-W90, X39.0-) to identify the external cause

J70.1   **Chronic and other pulmonary manifestations due to radiation**
    Fibrosis of lung following radiation
    Use additional code (W88-W90, X39.0-) to identify the external cause

J70.2   **Acute drug-induced interstitial lung disorders**
    Use additional code for adverse effect, if applicable, to identify drug (T36-T50 with fifth or sixth character 5)
    Excludes1   interstitial pneumonia NOS (J84.9)
    lymphoid interstitial pneumonia (J84.2)

J70.3   **Chronic drug-induced interstitial lung disorders**
    Use additional code for adverse effect, if applicable, to identify drug (T36-T50 with fifth or sixth character 5)
    Excludes1   interstitial pneumonia NOS (J84.9)
    lymphoid interstitial pneumonia (J84.2)

J70.4   **Drug-induced interstitial lung disorders, unspecified**
    Use additional code for adverse effect, if applicable, to identify drug (T36-T50 with fifth or sixth character 5)
    Excludes1   interstitial pneumonia NOS (J84.9)
    lymphoid interstitial pneumonia (J84.2)

J70.5   **Respiratory conditions due to smoke inhalation**
    Smoke inhalation NOS
    Excludes1   smoke inhalation due to chemicals, gases, fumes and vapors (J68.9)

J70.8   **Respiratory conditions due to other specified external agents**
    Code first (T51-T65) to identify the external agent

J70.9   **Respiratory conditions due to unspecified external agent**
    Code first (T51-T65) to identify the external agent

OTHER RESPIRATORY DISEASES PRINCIPALLY AFFECTING THE INTERSTITIUM (J80-J84)

J80   **Acute respiratory distress syndrome**
    Acute respiratory distress syndrome in adult or child
    Adult hyaline membrane disease
    Excludes1   respiratory distress syndrome in newborn (perinatal) (P22.0)

● **J81**   **Pulmonary edema**
    Use additional code to identify:
    exposure to environmental tobacco smoke (Z77.22)
    history of tobacco use (Z87.891)
    occupational exposure to environmental tobacco smoke (Z57.31)
    tobacco dependence (F17.-)
    tobacco use (Z72.0)
    Excludes1   chemical (acute) pulmonary edema (J68.1)
    hypostatic pneumonia (J18.2)
    passive pneumonia (J18.2)
    pulmonary edema due to external agents (J60-J70)
    pulmonary edema with heart disease NOS (I50.1)
    pulmonary edema with heart failure (I50.1)

J81.0   **Acute pulmonary edema**
    Acute edema of lung

J81.1   **Chronic pulmonary edema**
    Pulmonary congestion (chronic) (passive)
    Pulmonary edema NOS

CHAPTER 10 (J00-J99)

J82   Pulmonary eosinophilia, not elsewhere classified
Allergic pneumonia
Eosinophilic asthma
Eosinophilic pneumonia
Löffler's pneumonia
Tropical (pulmonary) eosinophilia NOS
Excludes1   pulmonary eosinophilia due to aspergillosis
(B44.-)
pulmonary eosinophilia due to drugs (J70.2-J70.4)
pulmonary eosinophilia due to specified parasitic
infection (B50-B83)
pulmonary eosinophilia due to systemic
connective tissue disorders (M30-M36)
pulmonary infiltrate NOS (R91.8)

● **J84   Other interstitial pulmonary diseases**
Excludes1   drug-induced interstitial lung disorders
(J70.2-J70.4)
interstitial emphysema (J98.2)
lung diseases due to external agents (J60-J70)

● **J84.0   Alveolar and parieto-alveolar conditions**

J84.01   Alveolar proteinosis

J84.02   Pulmonary alveolar microlithiasis

J84.03   Idiopathic pulmonary hemosiderosis
Essential brown induration of lung
Code first underlying disease, such as:
disorders of iron metabolism (E83.1-)
Excludes1   acute idiopathic pulmonary
hemorrhage in infants
[AIPHI] (R04.81)

J84.09   Other alveolar and parieto-alveolar conditions

● **J84.1   Other interstitial pulmonary diseases with fibrosis**
Excludes1   pulmonary fibrosis (chronic) due to
inhalation of chemicals, gases, fumes
or vapors (J68.4)
pulmonary fibrosis (chronic) following
radiation (J70.1)

J84.10   Pulmonary fibrosis, unspecified
Capillary fibrosis of lung
Cirrhosis of lung (chronic) NOS
Fibrosis of lung (atrophic) (chronic) (confluent)
(massive) (perialveolar) (peribronchial)
NOS
Induration of lung (chronic) NOS
Postinflammatory pulmonary fibrosis

● **J84.11   Idiopathic interstitial pneumonia**
Excludes1   lymphoid interstitial pneumonia
(J84.2)
pneumocystis pneumonia (B59)

**J84.111   Idiopathic interstitial pneumonia, not
otherwise specified**

J84.112   Idiopathic pulmonary fibrosis
Cryptogenic fibrosing alveolitis
Idiopathic fibrosing alveolitis

**J84.113   Idiopathic non-specific interstitial
pneumonitis**
Excludes1   non-specific interstitial
pneumonia NOS,
or due to known
underlying cause
(J84.89)

J84.114   Acute interstitial pneumonitis
Hamman-Rich syndrome
Excludes1   pneumocystis
pneumonia (B59)

**J84.115   Respiratory bronchiolitis interstitial
lung disease**

J84.116   Cryptogenic organizing pneumonia
Excludes1   organizing pneumonia
NOS, or due
to known
underlying cause
(J84.89)

J84.117   Desquamative interstitial pneumonia

**J84.17   Other interstitial pulmonary diseases with
fibrosis in diseases classified elsewhere**
Interstitial pneumonia (nonspecific) (usual)
due to collagen vascular disease
Interstitial pneumonia (nonspecific) (usual) in
diseases classified elsewhere
Organizing pneumonia due to collagen
vascular disease
Organizing pneumonia in diseases classified
elsewhere
Code first underlying disease, such as:
progressive systemic sclerosis (M34.0)
rheumatoid arthritis (M05.00-M06.9)
systemic lupus erythematosis (M32.0-M32.9)

J84.2   Lymphoid interstitial pneumonia
Lymphoid interstitial pneumonitis

● **J84.8   Other specified interstitial pulmonary diseases**
Excludes1   exogenous lipoid pneumonia (J69.1)
unspecified lipoid pneumonia (J69.1)

J84.81   Lymphangioleiomyomatosis
Lymphangiomyomatosis

J84.82   Adult pulmonary Langerhans cell histiocytosis
Adult PLCH

J84.83   Surfactant mutations of the lung

● **J84.84   Other interstitial lung diseases of childhood**

**J84.841   Neuroendocrine cell hyperplasia of
infancy**

J84.842   Pulmonary interstitial glycogenosis

**J84.843   Alveolar capillary dysplasia with vein
misalignment**

**J84.848   Other interstitial lung diseases of
childhood**

J84.89   Other specified interstitial pulmonary diseases
Endogenous lipoid pneumonia
Interstitial pneumonitis
Non-specific interstitial pneumonitis NOS
Organizing pneumonia due to known
underlying cause
Organizing pneumonia NOS
Code first, if applicable:
poisoning due to drug or toxin (T51-T65
with fifth or sixth character to indicate
intent), for toxic pneumonopathy
underlying cause of pneumonopathy, if
known
Use additional code, for adverse effect, to
identify drug (T36-T50 with fifth or sixth
character 5), if drug-induced
Excludes1   cryptogenic organizing
pneumonia (J84.116)
idiopathic non-specific
interstitial pneumonitis
(J84.113)
lipoid pneumonia, exogenous or
unspecified (J69.1)
lymphoid interstitial pneumonia
(J84.2)

J84.9   Interstitial pulmonary disease, unspecified
Interstitial pneumonia NOS

Figure 10-7 Bullous emphysema with large
subpleural bullae *(upper left)*. (From Kumar:
Robbins and Cotran: Pathologic Basis of Disease,
ed 8, Saunders, An Imprint of Elsevier, 2009)

◄ New   ◄▯▯▯ Revised   d̶e̶l̶e̶t̶e̶d̶ Deleted   OGCR Official Guidelines   X Assign placeholder X   ● Use Additional Character(s)

Excludes 1   Excludes 2   Includes   Use additional   Code first   Code also   Unspecified

Item 10–11 Empyema is a condition in which pus accumulates in a body cavity. Empyema **with fistula** occurs when the pus passes from one cavity to another organ or structure.

SUPPURATIVE AND NECROTIC CONDITIONS OF THE LOWER RESPIRATORY TRACT (J85-J86)

● J85   **Abscess of lung and mediastinum**
   Use additional code (B95-B97) to identify infectious agent.

   J85.0   **Gangrene and necrosis of lung**
   J85.1   **Abscess of lung with pneumonia**
       Code also the type of pneumonia
   J85.2   **Abscess of lung without pneumonia**
       Abscess of lung NOS
   J85.3   **Abscess of mediastinum**

● J86   **Pyothorax**
   Use additional code (B95-B97) to identify infectious agent.
   Excludes1   abscess of lung (J85.-)
       pyothorax due to tuberculosis (A15.6)

   J86.0   **Pyothorax with fistula**
       Bronchocutaneous fistula
       Bronchopleural fistula
       Hepatopleural fistula
       Mediastinal fistula
       Pleural fistula
       Thoracic fistula
       Any condition classifiable to J86.9 with fistula

   J86.9   **Pyothorax without fistula**
       Abscess of pleura
       Abscess of thorax
       Empyema (chest) (lung) (pleura)
       Fibrinopurulent pleurisy
       Purulent pleurisy
       Pyopneumothorax
       Septic pleurisy
       Seropurulent pleurisy
       Suppurative pleurisy

OTHER DISEASES OF THE PLEURA (J90-J94)

J90   **Pleural effusion, not elsewhere classified**
       Encysted pleurisy
       Pleural effusion NOS
       Pleurisy with effusion (exudative) (serous)
   Excludes1   chylous (pleural) effusion (J94.0)
       malignant pleural effusion (J91.0))
       pleurisy NOS (R09.1)
       tuberculous pleural effusion (A15.6)

● J91   **Pleural effusion in conditions classified elsewhere**
   Excludes2   pleural effusion in heart failure (I50.-)
       pleural effusion in systemic lupus erythematosus (M32.13)

   J91.0   **Malignant pleural effusion**
       Code first underlying neoplasm

   J91.8   **Pleural effusion in other conditions classified elsewhere**
       Code first underlying disease, such as:
       filariasis (B74.0-B74.9)
       influenza (J09.X2, J10.1, J11.1)

● J92   **Pleural plaque**
   Includes   pleural thickening
   J92.0   **Pleural plaque with presence of asbestos**
   J92.9   **Pleural plaque without asbestos**
       Pleural plaque NOS

● J93   **Pneumothorax and air leak**
   Collapsed lung
   Excludes1   congenital or perinatal pneumothorax (P25.1)
       postprocedural air leak (J95.812)
       postprocedural pneumothorax (J95.811)
       traumatic pneumothorax (S27.0)
       tuberculous (current disease) pneumothorax (A15.-)
       pyopneumothorax (J86.-)

   J93.0   **Spontaneous tension pneumothorax**
       Tension pneumothorax (most serious type) occurs when air (positive pressure) collects in the pleural space

   ● J93.1   **Other spontaneous pneumothorax**
       J93.11   **Primary spontaneous pneumothorax**
       J93.12   **Secondary spontaneous pneumothorax**
           Code first underlying condition, such as:
           catamenial pneumothorax due to endometriosis (N80.8)
           cystic fibrosis (E84.-)
           eosinophilic pneumonia (J82)
           lymphangioleiomyomatosis (J84.81)
           malignant neoplasm of bronchus and lung (C34.-)
           Marfan's syndrome (Q87.4)
           pneumonia due to Pneumocystis carinii (B59)
           secondary malignant neoplasm of lung (C78.0-)
           spontaneous rupture of the esophagus (K22.3)

   ● J93.8   **Other pneumothorax and air leak**
       J93.81   **Chronic pneumothorax**
       J93.82   **Other air leak**
           Persistent air leak
       J93.83   **Other pneumothorax**
           Acute pneumothorax
           Spontaneous pneumothorax NOS

   J93.9   **Pneumothorax, unspecified**
       Pneumothorax NOS

● J94   **Other pleural conditions**
   Excludes1   pleurisy NOS (R09.1)
       traumatic hemopneumothorax (S27.2)
       traumatic hemothorax (S27.1)
       tuberculous pleural conditions (current disease) (A15.-)

   J94.0   **Chylous effusion**
       Chyliform effusion
   J94.1   **Fibrothorax**
   J94.2   **Hemothorax**
       Hemopneumothorax
   J94.8   **Other specified pleural conditions**
       Hydropneumothorax
       Hydrothorax
   J94.9   **Pleural condition, unspecified**

CHAPTER 10 (J00-J99)

INTRAOPERATIVE AND POSTPROCEDURAL COMPLICATIONS AND DISORDERS OF RESPIRATORY SYSTEM, NOT ELSEWHERE CLASSIFIED (J95)

● **J95** **Intraoperative and postprocedural complications and disorders of respiratory system, not elsewhere classified**

> **Excludes2** aspiration pneumonia (J69.-)
> emphysema (subcutaneous) resulting from a procedure (T81.82)
> hypostatic pneumonia (J18.2)
> pulmonary manifestations due to radiation (J70.0- J70.1)

● **J95.0** **Tracheostomy complications**

J95.00 Unspecified tracheostomy complication

J95.01 Hemorrhage from tracheostomy stoma

J95.02 Infection of tracheostomy stoma

> Use additional code to identify type of infection, such as:
> cellulitis of neck (L03.8)
> sepsis (A40, A41.-)

J95.03 Malfunction of tracheostomy stoma
> Mechanical complication of tracheostomy stoma
> Obstruction of tracheostomy airway
> Tracheal stenosis due to tracheostomy

J95.04 Tracheo-esophageal fistula following tracheostomy

J95.09 Other tracheostomy complication

J95.1 **Acute pulmonary insufficiency following thoracic surgery**

> **Excludes2** functional disturbances following cardiac surgery (I97.0, I97.1-)

J95.2 **Acute pulmonary insufficiency following nonthoracic surgery**

> **Excludes2** functional disturbances following cardiac surgery (I97.0, I97.1-)

J95.3 **Chronic pulmonary insufficiency following surgery**

> **Excludes2** functional disturbances following cardiac surgery (I97.0, I97.1-)

J95.4 **Chemical pneumonitis due to anesthesia**
> Mendelson's syndrome
> Postprocedural aspiration pneumonia
> Use additional code for adverse effect, if applicable, to identify drug (T41.- with fifth or sixth character 5)

> **Excludes1** aspiration pneumonitis due to anesthesia complicating labor and delivery (O74.0)
> aspiration pneumonitis due to anesthesia complicating pregnancy (O29)
> aspiration pneumonitis due to anesthesia complicating the puerperium (O89.01)

J95.5 **Postprocedural subglottic stenosis**

● **J95.6** **Intraoperative hemorrhage and hematoma of a respiratory system organ or structure complicating a procedure**

> **Excludes1** intraoperative hemorrhage and hematoma of a respiratory system organ or structure due to accidental puncture and laceration during procedure (J95.7-)

J95.61 Intraoperative hemorrhage and hematoma of a respiratory system organ or structure complicating a respiratory system procedure

J95.62 Intraoperative hemorrhage and hematoma of a respiratory system organ or structure complicating other procedure

● **J95.7** **Accidental puncture and laceration of a respiratory system organ or structure during a procedure**

> **Excludes2** postprocedural pneumothorax (J95.811)

J95.71 Accidental puncture and laceration of a respiratory system organ or structure during a respiratory system procedure

J95.72 Accidental puncture and laceration of a respiratory system organ or structure during other procedure

● **J95.8** **Other intraoperative and postprocedural complications and disorders of respiratory system, not elsewhere classified**

● **J95.81** Postprocedural pneumothorax and air leak

J95.811 Postprocedural pneumothorax

J95.812 Postprocedural air leak

● **J95.82** Postprocedural respiratory failure

> **Excludes1** Respiratory failure in other conditions (J96.-)

J95.821 Acute postprocedural respiratory failure
> Postprocedural respiratory failure NOS

J95.822 Acute and chronic postprocedural respiratory failure

● **J95.83** Postprocedural hemorrhage and hematoma of a respiratory system organ or structure following a procedure

J95.830 Postprocedural hemorrhage and hematoma of a respiratory system organ or structure following a respiratory system procedure

J95.831 Postprocedural hemorrhage and hematoma of a respiratory system organ or structure following other procedure

J95.84 Transfusion-related acute lung injury (TRALI)

● **J95.85** Complication of respirator [ventilator]

J95.850 Mechanical complication of respirator

> **Excludes1** encounter for respirator [ventilator] dependence during power failure (Z99.12)

J95.851 Ventilator associated pneumonia
> Ventilator associated pneumonitis
> Use additional code to identify the organism, if known (B95.-, B96.-, B97.-)

> **Excludes1** ventilator lung in newborn (P27.8)

J95.859 Other complication of respirator [ventilator]

J95.88 Other intraoperative complications of respiratory system, not elsewhere classified

J95.89 Other postprocedural complications and disorders of respiratory system, not elsewhere classified
> Use additional code to identify disorder, such as:
> aspiration pneumonia (J69.-)
> bacterial or viral pneumonia (J12-J18)

> **Excludes2** acute pulmonary insufficiency following thoracic surgery (J95.1)
> postprocedural subglottic stenosis (J95.5)

OTHER DISEASES OF THE RESPIRATORY SYSTEM (J96-J99)

● **J96   Respiratory failure, not elsewhere classified**

$\quad$ **Excludes1**$\quad$ acute respiratory distress syndrome (J80)
$\qquad$ cardiorespiratory failure (R09.2)
$\qquad$ newborn respiratory distress syndrome (P22.0)
$\qquad$ postprocedural respiratory failure (J95.82-)
$\qquad$ respiratory arrest (R09.2)
$\qquad$ respiratory arrest of newborn (P28.81)
$\qquad$ respiratory failure of newborn (P28.5)

● **J96.0$\quad$Acute respiratory failure**

$\quad$ **J96.00$\quad$Acute respiratory failure, unspecified whether with hypoxia or hypercapnia**

$\quad$ **J96.01$\quad$Acute respiratory failure with hypoxia**

$\quad$ **J96.02$\quad$Acute respiratory failure with hypercapnia**

● **J96.1$\quad$Chronic respiratory failure**

$\quad$ **J96.10$\quad$Chronic respiratory failure, unspecified whether with hypoxia or hypercapnia**

$\quad$ **J96.11$\quad$Chronic respiratory failure with hypoxia**

$\quad$ **J96.12$\quad$Chronic respiratory failure with hypercapnia**

● **J96.2$\quad$Acute and chronic respiratory failure**
$\qquad$ Acute on chronic respiratory failure

$\quad$ **J96.20$\quad$Acute and chronic respiratory failure, unspecified whether with hypoxia or hypercapnia**

$\quad$ **J96.21$\quad$Acute and chronic respiratory failure with hypoxia**

$\quad$ **J96.22$\quad$Acute and chronic respiratory failure with hypercapnia**

● **J96.9$\quad$Respiratory failure, unspecified**

$\quad$ **J96.90$\quad$Respiratory failure, unspecified, unspecified whether with hypoxia or hypercapnia**

$\quad$ **J96.91$\quad$Respiratory failure, unspecified with hypoxia**

$\quad$ **J96.92$\quad$Respiratory failure, unspecified with hypercapnia**

● **J98   Other respiratory disorders**
$\quad$ Use additional code to identify:
$\qquad$ exposure to environmental tobacco smoke (Z77.22)
$\qquad$ exposure to tobacco smoke in the perinatal period (P96.81)
$\qquad$ history of tobacco use (Z87.891)
$\qquad$ occupational exposure to environmental tobacco smoke (Z57.31)
$\qquad$ tobacco dependence (F17.-)
$\qquad$ tobacco use (Z72.0)

$\quad$ **Excludes1**$\quad$ newborn apnea (P28.4)
$\qquad$ newborn sleep apnea (P28.3)

$\quad$ **Excludes2**$\quad$ apnea NOS (R06.81)
$\qquad$ sleep apnea (G47.3-)

● **J98.0$\quad$Diseases of bronchus, not elsewhere classified**

$\quad$ **J98.01$\quad$Acute bronchospasm**

$\qquad$ **Excludes1**$\quad$ acute bronchiolitis with bronchospasm (J21.-)
$\qquad\qquad$ acute bronchitis with bronchospasm (J20.-)
$\qquad\qquad$ asthma (J45.-)
$\qquad\qquad$ exercise induced bronchospasm (J45.990)

$\quad$ **J98.09$\quad$Other diseases of bronchus, not elsewhere classified**
$\qquad$ Broncholithiasis
$\qquad$ Calcification of bronchus
$\qquad$ Stenosis of bronchus
$\qquad$ Tracheobronchial collapse
$\qquad$ Tracheobronchial dyskinesia
$\qquad$ Ulcer of bronchus

● **J98.1$\quad$Pulmonary collapse**

$\quad$ **Excludes1**$\quad$ therapeutic collapse of lung status (Z98.3)

$\quad$ **J98.11$\quad$Atelectasis**

$\qquad$ **Excludes1**$\quad$ newborn atelectasis
$\qquad\qquad$ tuberculous atelectasis (current disease) (A15)

$\quad$ **J98.19$\quad$Other pulmonary collapse**

J98.2$\quad$Interstitial emphysema
$\quad$ Mediastinal emphysema

$\quad$ **Excludes1**$\quad$ emphysema NOS (J43.9)
$\qquad$ emphysema in newborn (P25.0)
$\qquad$ surgical emphysema (subcutaneous) (T81.82)
$\qquad$ traumatic subcutaneous emphysema (T79.7)

J98.3$\quad$Compensatory emphysema

J98.4$\quad$Other disorders of lung
$\quad$ Calcification of lung
$\quad$ Cystic lung disease (acquired)
$\quad$ Lung disease NOS
$\quad$ Pulmolithiasis

$\quad$ **Excludes1**$\quad$ acute interstitial pneumonitis (J84.114)
$\qquad$ pulmonary insufficiency following surgery (J95.1-J95.2)

J98.5$\quad$Diseases of mediastinum, not elsewhere classified
$\quad$ Fibrosis of mediastinum
$\quad$ Hernia of mediastinum
$\quad$ Retraction of mediastinum
$\quad$ Mediastinitis

$\quad$ **Excludes2**$\quad$ abscess of mediastinum (J85.3)

J98.6$\quad$Disorders of diaphragm
$\quad$ Diaphragmatitis
$\quad$ Paralysis of diaphragm
$\quad$ Relaxation of diaphragm

$\quad$ **Excludes1**$\quad$ congenital malformation of diaphragm NEC (Q79.1)
$\qquad$ congenital diaphragmatic hernia (Q79.0)

$\quad$ **Excludes2**$\quad$ diaphragmatic hernia (K44.-)

J98.8$\quad$Other specified respiratory disorders

J98.9$\quad$Respiratory disorder, unspecified
$\quad$ Respiratory disease (chronic) NOS

J99   Respiratory disorders in diseases classified elsewhere
$\quad$ *Code first underlying disease, such as:*
$\qquad$ amyloidosis (E85.-)
$\qquad$ ankylosing spondylitis (M45)
$\qquad$ congenital syphilis (A50.5)
$\qquad$ cryoglobulinemia (D89.1)
$\qquad$ early congenital syphilis (A50.0)
$\qquad$ schistosomiasis (B65.0-B65.9)

$\quad$ **Excludes1**$\quad$ respiratory disorders in:
$\qquad$ amebiasis (A06.5)
$\qquad$ blastomycosis (B40.0-B40.2)
$\qquad$ candidiasis (B37.1)
$\qquad$ coccidioidomycosis (B38.0-B38.2)
$\qquad$ cystic fibrosis with pulmonary manifestations (E84.0)
$\qquad$ dermatomyositis (M33.01, M33.11)
$\qquad$ histoplasmosis (B39.0-B39.2)
$\qquad$ late syphilis (A52.72, A52.73)
$\qquad$ polymyositis (M33.21)
$\qquad$ sicca syndrome (M35.02)
$\qquad$ systemic lupus erythematosus (M32.13)
$\qquad$ systemic sclerosis (M34.81)
$\qquad$ Wegener's granulomatosis (M31.30-M31.31)

CHAPTER 10 (J00-J99)

◀ New $\quad$ ◀⫶⫶ Revised $\quad$ ~~deleted~~ Deleted $\quad$ **OGCR** Official Guidelines $\quad$ X Assign placeholder X $\quad$ ● Use Additional Character(s)

Excludes 1 $\quad$ Excludes 2 $\quad$ Includes $\quad$ Use additional $\quad$ Code first $\quad$ Code also $\quad$ Unspecified

965

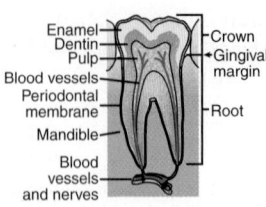

Figure 11-1 Anatomy of a tooth.

Item 11-1 Anodontia is the congenital absence of teeth. **Hypodontia** is partial anodontia. **Oligodontia** is the congenital absence of some teeth, whereas **supernumerary** is having more teeth than the normal number. **Mesiodens** are small extra teeth that often appear in pairs, although single small teeth are not uncommon.

CHAPTER 11

DISEASES OF THE DIGESTIVE SYSTEM (K00-K95)

Excludes2 certain conditions originating in the perinatal period (P04-P96)
certain infectious and parasitic diseases (A00-B99)
complications of pregnancy, childbirth and the puerperium (O00-O9A)
congenital malformations, deformations and chromosomal abnormalities (Q00-Q99)
endocrine, nutritional and metabolic diseases (E00-E88)
injury, poisoning and certain other consequences of external causes (S00-T88)
neoplasms (C00-D49)
symptoms, signs and abnormal clinical and laboratory findings, not elsewhere classified (R00-R94)

This chapter contains the following blocks:

K00-K14	Diseases of oral cavity and salivary glands
K20-K31	Diseases of esophagus, stomach and duodenum
K35-K38	Diseases of appendix
K40-K46	Hernia
K50-K52	Noninfective enteritis and colitis
K55-K64	Other diseases of intestines
K65-K68	Diseases of peritoneum and retroperitoneum
K70-K77	Diseases of liver
K80-K87	Disorders of gallbladder, biliary tract and pancreas
K90-K95	Other diseases of the digestive system

DISEASES OF ORAL CAVITY AND SALIVARY GLANDS (K00-K14)

● **K00 Disorders of tooth development and eruption**
Excludes2 embedded and impacted teeth (K01.-)
K00.0 Anodontia
Hypodontia
Oligodontia
Excludes1 acquired absence of teeth (K08.1-)
K00.1 Supernumerary teeth
Distomolar
Fourth molar
Mesiodens
Paramolar
Supplementary teeth
Excludes2 supernumerary roots (K00.2)

K00.2 Abnormalities of size and form of teeth
Concrescence of teeth
Fusion of teeth
Gemination of teeth
Dens evaginatus
Dens in dente
Dens invaginatus
Enamel pearls
Macrodontia
Microdontia
Peg-shaped [conical] teeth
Supernumerary roots
Taurodontism
Tuberculum paramolare
Excludes1 abnormalities of teeth due to congenital syphilis (A50.5)
tuberculum Carabelli, which is regarded as a normal variation and should not be coded
K00.3 Mottled teeth
Dental fluorosis
Mottling of enamel
Nonfluoride enamel opacities
Excludes2 deposits [accretions] on teeth (K03.6)
K00.4 Disturbances in tooth formation
Aplasia and hypoplasia of cementum
Dilaceration of tooth
Enamel hypoplasia (neonatal) (postnatal) (prenatal)
Regional odontodysplasia
Turner's tooth
Excludes1 Hutchinson's teeth and mulberry molars in congenital syphilis (A50.5)
Excludes2 mottled teeth (K00.3)
K00.5 Hereditary disturbances in tooth structure, not elsewhere classified
Amelogenesis imperfecta
Dentinogenesis imperfecta
Odontogenesis imperfecta
Dentinal dysplasia
Shell teeth
K00.6 Disturbances in tooth eruption
Dentia praecox
Natal tooth
Neonatal tooth
Premature eruption of tooth
Premature shedding of primary [deciduous] tooth
Prenatal teeth
Retained [persistent] primary tooth
Excludes2 embedded and impacted teeth (K01.-)
K00.7 Teething syndrome
K00.8 Other disorders of tooth development
Color changes during tooth formation
Intrinsic staining of teeth NOS
Excludes2 posteruptive color changes (K03.7)
K00.9 Disorder of tooth development, unspecified
Disorder of odontogenesis NOS

● **K01 Embedded and impacted teeth**
Excludes1 abnormal position of fully erupted teeth (M26.3-)
K01.0 Embedded teeth
K01.1 Impacted teeth

◀ New ◀ Revised deleted Deleted OGCR Official Guidelines X Assign placeholder X ● Use Additional Character(s)
Excludes 1 Excludes 2 Includes Use additional Code first Code also Unspecified
966

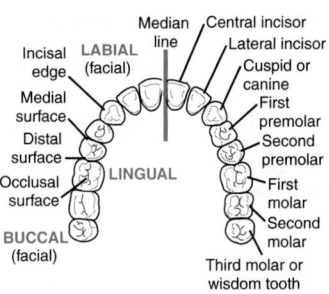

Figure 11-2 The permanent teeth within the dental arch.

Item 11-2 Each dental arch (jaw) normally contains 16 teeth. Tooth decay or **dental caries** is a disease of the enamel, dentin, and cementum of the tooth and can result in a cavity.

● **K02   Dental caries**
> **Includes**   dental cavities
>   tooth decay

> **K02.3   Arrested dental caries**
> > Arrested coronal and root caries

● **K02.5   Dental caries on pit and fissure surface**
> > Dental caries on chewing surface of tooth

> > **K02.51   Dental caries on pit and fissure surface limited to enamel**
> > > White spot lesions [initial caries] on pit and fissure surface of tooth

> > **K02.52   Dental caries on pit and fissure surface penetrating into dentin**

> > **K02.53   Dental caries on pit and fissure surface penetrating into pulp**

● **K02.6   Dental caries on smooth surface**

> > **K02.61   Dental caries on smooth surface limited to enamel**
> > > White spot lesions [initial caries] on smooth surface of tooth

> > **K02.62   Dental caries on smooth surface penetrating into dentin**

> > **K02.63   Dental caries on smooth surface penetrating into pulp**

> **K02.7   Dental root caries**

> **K02.9   Dental caries, unspecified**

● **K03   Other diseases of hard tissues of teeth**
> **Excludes2**   bruxism (F45.8)
>   dental caries (K02.-)
>   teeth-grinding NOS (F45.8)

> **K03.0   Excessive attrition of teeth**
> > Approximal wear of teeth
> > Occlusal wear of teeth

> **K03.1   Abrasion of teeth**
> > Dentifrice abrasion of teeth
> > Habitual abrasion of teeth
> > Occupational abrasion of teeth
> > Ritual abrasion of teeth
> > Traditional abrasion of teeth
> > Wedge defect NOS

> **K03.2   Erosion of teeth**
> > Erosion of teeth due to diet
> > Erosion of teeth due to drugs and medicaments
> > Erosion of teeth due to persistent vomiting
> > Erosion of teeth NOS
> > Idiopathic erosion of teeth
> > Occupational erosion of teeth

> **K03.3   Pathological resorption of teeth**
> > Internal granuloma of pulp
> > Resorption of teeth (external)

> **K03.4   Hypercementosis**
> > Cementation hyperplasia

> **K03.5   Ankylosis of teeth**

> **K03.6   Deposits [accretions] on teeth**
> > Betel deposits [accretions] on teeth
> > Black deposits [accretions] on teeth
> > Extrinsic staining of teeth NOS
> > Green deposits [accretions] on teeth
> > Materia alba deposits [accretions] on teeth
> > Orange deposits [accretions] on teeth
> > Staining of teeth NOS
> > Subgingival dental calculus
> > Supragingival dental calculus
> > Tobacco deposits [accretions] on teeth

> **K03.7   Posteruptive color changes of dental hard tissues**
> > **Excludes2**   deposits [accretions] on teeth (K03.6)

● **K03.8   Other specified diseases of hard tissues of teeth**
> > **K03.81   Cracked tooth**
> > > **Excludes1**   asymptomatic craze lines in enamel - omit code
> > > > broken or fractured tooth due to trauma (S02.5)

> > **K03.89   Other specified diseases of hard tissues of teeth**

> **K03.9   Disease of hard tissues of teeth, unspecified**

K04   Diseases of pulp and periapical tissues
> **K04.0   Pulpitis**
> > Acute pulpitis
> > Chronic (hyperplastic) (ulcerative) pulpitis
> > Irreversible pulpitis
> > Reversible pulpitis

> **K04.1   Necrosis of pulp**
> > Pulpal gangrene

> **K04.2   Pulp degeneration**
> > Denticles
> > Pulpal calcifications
> > Pulpal stones

> **K04.3   Abnormal hard tissue formation in pulp**
> > Secondary or irregular dentine

> **K04.4   Acute apical periodontitis of pulpal origin**
> > Acute apical periodontitis NOS
> > **Excludes1**   acute periodontitis (K05.2-)

> **K04.5   Chronic apical periodontitis**
> > Apical or periapical granuloma
> > Apical periodontitis NOS
> > **Excludes1**   chronic periodontitis (K05.3-)

> **K04.6   Periapical abscess with sinus**
> > Dental abscess with sinus
> > Dentoalveolar abscess with sinus

> **K04.7   Periapical abscess without sinus**
> > Dental abscess without sinus
> > Dentoalveolar abscess without sinus
> > Periapical abscess without sinus

> **K04.8   Radicular cyst**
> > Apical (periodontal) cyst
> > Periapical cyst
> > Residual radicular cyst
> > **Excludes2**   lateral periodontal cyst (K09.0)

● **K04.9   Other and unspecified diseases of pulp and periapical tissues**
> > **K04.90   Unspecified diseases of pulp and periapical tissues**
> > **K04.99   Other diseases of pulp and periapical tissues**

◄ New   ⫷▏ Revised   ~~deleted~~ Deleted   OGCR Official Guidelines   X Assign placeholder X   ● Use Additional Character(s)

Excludes 1   Excludes 2   Includes   Use additional   Code first   Code also   Unspecified

CHAPTER 11 (K00-K95)

Item 11-3 **Acute gingivitis,** also known as orilitis or ulitis, is the short-term, severe inflammation of the gums (gingiva) caused by bacteria. **Chronic gingivitis** is persistent inflammation of the gums. When the gingivitis moves into the periodontium it is called periodontitis, also known as paradentitis.

● **K05 Gingivitis and periodontal diseases**

Use additional code to identify:
  alcohol abuse and dependence (F10.-)
  exposure to environmental tobacco smoke (Z77.22)
  exposure to tobacco smoke in the perinatal period (P96.81)
  history of tobacco use (Z87.891)
  occupational exposure to environmental tobacco smoke
    (Z57.31)
  tobacco dependence (F17.-)
  tobacco use (Z72.0)

● **K05.0 Acute gingivitis**

  | Excludes1 | acute necrotizing ulcerative gingivitis
    (A69.1)
    herpesviral [herpes simplex]
      gingivostomatitis (B00.2)

  K05.00 Acute gingivitis, plaque induced
    Acute gingivitis NOS

  K05.01 Acute gingivitis, non-plaque induced

● **K05.1 Chronic gingivitis**

  Desquamative gingivitis (chronic)
  Gingivitis (chronic) NOS
  Hyperplastic gingivitis (chronic)
  Simple marginal gingivitis (chronic)
  Ulcerative gingivitis (chronic)

  K05.10 Chronic gingivitis, plaque induced
    Chronic gingivitis NOS
    Gingivitis NOS

  K05.11 Chronic gingivitis, non-plaque induced

● **K05.2 Aggressive periodontitis**
  Acute pericoronitis

  | Excludes1 | acute apical periodontitis (K04.4)
    periapical abscess (K04.7)
    periapical abscess with sinus (K04.6)

  K05.20 Aggressive periodontitis, unspecified

  K05.21 Aggressive periodontitis, localized
    Periodontal abscess

  K05.22 Aggressive periodontitis, generalized

● **K05.3 Chronic periodontitis**
  Chronic pericoronitis
  Complex periodontitis
  Periodontitis NOS
  Simplex periodontitis

  | Excludes1 | chronic apical periodontitis (K04.5)

  K05.30 Chronic periodontitis, unspecified

  K05.31 Chronic periodontitis, localized

  K05.32 Chronic periodontitis, generalized

  K05.4 Periodontosis
    Juvenile periodontosis

  K05.5 Other periodontal diseases

  | Excludes2 | leukoplakia of gingiva (K13.21)

  K05.6 Periodontal disease, unspecified

● **K06 Other disorders of gingiva and edentulous alveolar ridge**

  | Excludes2 | acute gingivitis (K05.0)
    atrophy of edentulous alveolar ridge (K08.2)
    chronic gingivitis (K05.1)
    gingivitis NOS (K05.1)

  K06.0 Gingival recession
    Gingival recession (generalized) (localized)
      (postinfective) (postprocedural)

  K06.1 Gingival enlargement
    Gingival fibromatosis

  K06.2 Gingival and edentulous alveolar ridge lesions associated with trauma
    Irritative hyperplasia of edentulous ridge [denture
      hyperplasia]

    Use additional code (Chapter 20) to identify external
      cause or denture status (Z97.2)

  K06.8 Other specified disorders of gingiva and edentulous alveolar ridge
    Fibrous epulis
    Flabby alveolar ridge
    Giant cell epulis
    Peripheral giant cell granuloma of gingiva
    Pyogenic granuloma of gingiva

    | Excludes2 | gingival cyst (K09.0)

  K06.9 Disorder of gingiva and edentulous alveolar ridge, unspecified

● **K08 Other disorders of teeth and supporting structures**

  | Excludes2 | dentofacial anomalies [including malocclusion]
    (M26.-)
    disorders of jaw (M27.-)

  K08.0 Exfoliation of teeth due to systemic causes
    Code also underlying systemic condition

● **K08.1 Complete loss of teeth**
  Acquired loss of teeth, complete

  | Excludes1 | congenital absence of teeth (K00.0)
    exfoliation of teeth due to systemic causes
      (K08.0)
    partial loss of teeth (K08.4-)

  ● **K08.10 Complete loss of teeth, unspecified cause**

    K08.101 Complete loss of teeth, unspecified cause, class I

    K08.102 Complete loss of teeth, unspecified cause, class II

    K08.103 Complete loss of teeth, unspecified cause, class III

    K08.104 Complete loss of teeth, unspecified cause, class IV

    K08.109 Complete loss of teeth, unspecified cause, unspecified class
      Edentulism NOS

  ● **K08.11 Complete loss of teeth due to trauma**

    K08.111 Complete loss of teeth due to trauma, class I

    K08.112 Complete loss of teeth due to trauma, class II

    K08.113 Complete loss of teeth due to trauma, class III

    K08.114 Complete loss of teeth due to trauma, class IV

    K08.119 Complete loss of teeth due to trauma, unspecified class

  ● **K08.12 Complete loss of teeth due to periodontal diseases**

    K08.121 Complete loss of teeth due to periodontal diseases, class I

    K08.122 Complete loss of teeth due to periodontal diseases, class II

    K08.123 Complete loss of teeth due to periodontal diseases, class III

    K08.124 Complete loss of teeth due to periodontal diseases, class IV

    K08.129 Complete loss of teeth due to periodontal diseases, unspecified class

- **K08.13   Complete loss of teeth due to caries**
  - K08.131   Complete loss of teeth due to caries, class I
  - K08.132   Complete loss of teeth due to caries, class II
  - K08.133   Complete loss of teeth due to caries, class III
  - K08.134   Complete loss of teeth due to caries, class IV
  - K08.139   Complete loss of teeth due to caries, unspecified class
- **K08.19   Complete loss of teeth due to other specified cause**
  - K08.191   Complete loss of teeth due to other specified cause, class I
  - K08.192   Complete loss of teeth due to other specified cause, class II
  - K08.193   Complete loss of teeth due to other specified cause, class III
  - K08.194   Complete loss of teeth due to other specified cause, class IV
  - K08.199   Complete loss of teeth due to other specified cause, unspecified class
- **K08.2   Atrophy of edentulous alveolar ridge**
  - K08.20   Unspecified atrophy of edentulous alveolar ridge
    - Atrophy of the mandible NOS
    - Atrophy of the maxilla NOS
  - K08.21   **Minimal atrophy of the mandible**
    - Minimal atrophy of the edentulous mandible
  - K08.22   **Moderate atrophy of the mandible**
    - Moderate atrophy of the edentulous mandible
  - K08.23   **Severe atrophy of the mandible**
    - Severe atrophy of the edentulous mandible
  - K08.24   **Minimal atrophy of maxilla**
    - Minimal atrophy of the edentulous maxilla
  - K08.25   **Moderate atrophy of the maxilla**
    - Moderate atrophy of the edentulous maxilla
  - K08.26   **Severe atrophy of the maxilla**
    - Severe atrophy of the edentulous maxilla
- **K08.3   Retained dental root**
- **K08.4   Partial loss of teeth**
  - Acquired loss of teeth, partial
  - | Excludes1 | complete loss of teeth (K08.1-)
    - congenital absence of teeth (K00.0)
  - | Excludes2 | exfoliation of teeth due to systemic causes (K08.0)
  - **K08.40   Partial loss of teeth, unspecified cause**
    - K08.401   Partial loss of teeth, unspecified cause, class I
    - K08.402   Partial loss of teeth, unspecified cause, class II
    - K08.403   Partial loss of teeth, unspecified cause, class III
    - K08.404   Partial loss of teeth, unspecified cause, class IV
    - K08.409   Partial loss of teeth, unspecified cause, unspecified class
      - Tooth extraction status NOS

- **K08.41   Partial loss of teeth due to trauma**
  - K08.411   Partial loss of teeth due to trauma, class I
  - K08.412   Partial loss of teeth due to trauma, class II
  - K08.413   Partial loss of teeth due to trauma, class III
  - K08.414   Partial loss of teeth due to trauma, class IV
  - K08.419   Partial loss of teeth due to trauma, unspecified class
- **K08.42   Partial loss of teeth due to periodontal diseases**
  - K08.421   Partial loss of teeth due to periodontal diseases, class I
  - K08.422   Partial loss of teeth due to periodontal diseases, class II
  - K08.423   Partial loss of teeth due to periodontal diseases, class III
  - K08.424   Partial loss of teeth due to periodontal diseases, class IV
  - K08.429   Partial loss of teeth due to periodontal diseases, unspecified class
- **K08.43   Partial loss of teeth due to caries**
  - K08.431   Partial loss of teeth due to caries, class I
  - K08.432   Partial loss of teeth due to caries, class II
  - K08.433   Partial loss of teeth due to caries, class III
  - K08.434   Partial loss of teeth due to caries, class IV
  - K08.439   Partial loss of teeth due to caries, unspecified class
- **K08.49   Partial loss of teeth due to other specified cause**
  - K08.491   Partial loss of teeth due to other specified cause, class I
  - K08.492   Partial loss of teeth due to other specified cause, class II
  - K08.493   Partial loss of teeth due to other specified cause, class III
  - K08.494   Partial loss of teeth due to other specified cause, class IV
  - K08.499   Partial loss of teeth due to other specified cause, unspecified class
- **K08.5   Unsatisfactory restoration of tooth**
  - Defective bridge, crown, filling
  - Defective dental restoration
  - | Excludes1 | dental restoration status (Z98.811)
  - | Excludes2 | endosseous dental implant failure (M27.6-)
    - unsatisfactory endodontic treatment (M27.5-)
  - **K08.50   Unsatisfactory restoration of tooth, unspecified**
    - Defective dental restoration NOS
  - **K08.51   Open restoration margins of tooth**
    - Dental restoration failure of marginal integrity
    - Open margin on tooth restoration
    - Poor gingival margin to tooth restoration
  - **K08.52   Unrepairable overhanging of dental restorative materials**
    - Overhanging of tooth restoration

CHAPTER 11 (K00-K95)

● **K08.53** **Fractured dental restorative material**
> **Excludes1** cracked tooth (K03.81)
>   traumatic fracture of tooth
>   (S02.5)

> **K08.530** **Fractured dental restorative material without loss of material**
> **K08.531** **Fractured dental restorative material with loss of material**
> **K08.539** **Fractured dental restorative material, unspecified**

K08.54 **Contour of existing restoration of tooth biologically incompatible with oral health**
> Dental restoration failure of periodontal anatomical integrity
> Unacceptable contours of existing restoration of tooth
> Unacceptable morphology of existing restoration of tooth

K08.55 **Allergy to existing dental restorative material**
> Use additional code to identify the specific type of allergy

K08.56 **Poor aesthetic of existing restoration of tooth**
> Dental restoration aesthetically inadequate or displeasing

K08.59 **Other unsatisfactory restoration of tooth**
> Other defective dental restoration

K08.8 **Other specified disorders of teeth and supporting structures**
> Enlargement of alveolar ridge NOS
> Irregular alveolar process
> Toothache NOS

K08.9 **Disorder of teeth and supporting structures, unspecified**

● **K09** **Cysts of oral region, not elsewhere classified**
> **Includes** lesions showing histological features both of aneurysmal cyst and of another fibro-osseous lesion
> **Excludes2** cysts of jaw (M27.0-, M27.4-)
>   radicular cyst (K04.8)

K09.0 **Developmental odontogenic cysts**
> Dentigerous cyst
> Eruption cyst
> Follicular cyst
> Gingival cyst
> Lateral periodontal cyst
> Primordial cyst
> **Excludes2** keratocysts (D16.4, D16.5)
>   odontogenic keratocystic tumors (D16.4, D16.5)

K09.1 **Developmental (nonodontogenic) cysts of oral region**
> Cyst (of) incisive canal
> Cyst (of) palatine of papilla
> Globulomaxillary cyst
> Median palatal cyst
> Nasoalveolar cyst
> Nasolabial cyst
> Nasopalatine duct cyst

K09.8 **Other cysts of oral region, not elsewhere classified**
> Dermoid cyst
> Epidermoid cyst
> Lymphoepithelial cyst
> Epstein's pearl

K09.9 **Cyst of oral region, unspecified**

Item 11–4 Atrophy is wasting away of a tissue or organ, whereas **hypertrophy** is overdevelopment or enlargement of a tissue or organ. **Sialoadenitis** is salivary gland inflammation. **Parotitis** is the inflammation of the parotid gland. In the epidemic form, parotitis is also known as mumps. **Sialolithiasis** is the formation of calculus within a salivary gland. **Mucocele** is a polyp composed of mucus.

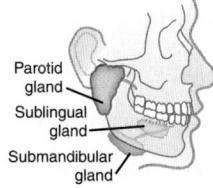

Figure 11-3 Major salivary glands.

Parotid gland
Sublingual gland
Submandibular gland

(See Plate 61 on page NAP-25.)

● **K11** **Diseases of salivary glands**
> Use additional code to identify:
>   alcohol abuse and dependence (F10.-)
>   exposure to environmental tobacco smoke (Z77.22)
>   exposure to tobacco smoke in the perinatal period (P96.81)
>   history of tobacco use (Z87.891)
>   occupational exposure to environmental tobacco smoke (Z57.31)
>   tobacco dependence (F17.-)
>   tobacco use (Z72.0)

K11.0 **Atrophy of salivary gland**
K11.1 **Hypertrophy of salivary gland**
● **K11.2** **Sialoadenitis**
> Parotitis
> **Excludes1** epidemic parotitis (B26.-)
>   mumps (B26.-)
>   uveoparotid fever [Heerfordt] (D86.89)

> **K11.20** **Sialoadenitis, unspecified**
> **K11.21** **Acute sialoadenitis**
>> **Excludes1** acute recurrent sialoadenitis (K11.22)
> **K11.22** **Acute recurrent sialoadenitis**
> **K11.23** **Chronic sialoadenitis**

K11.3 **Abscess of salivary gland**
K11.4 **Fistula of salivary gland**
> **Excludes1** congenital fistula of salivary gland (Q38.4)

K11.5 **Sialolithiasis**
> Calculus of salivary gland or duct
> Stone of salivary gland or duct

K11.6 **Mucocele of salivary gland**
> Mucous extravasation cyst of salivary gland
> Mucous retention cyst of salivary gland
> Ranula

K11.7 **Disturbances of salivary secretion**
> Hypoptyalism
> Ptyalism
> Xerostomia
> **Excludes2** dry mouth NOS (R68.2)

K11.8 **Other diseases of salivary glands**
> Benign lymphoepithelial lesion of salivary gland
> Mikulicz' disease
> Necrotizing sialometaplasia
> Sialectasia
> Stenosis of salivary duct
> Stricture of salivary duct
> **Excludes1** sicca syndrome [Sjögren] (M35.0-)

K11.9 **Disease of salivary gland, unspecified**
> Sialoadenopathy NOS

CHAPTER 11 (K00-K95)

Item 11–5 **Stomatitis** is the inflammation of the oral mucosa. **Mucositis** is the inflammation of the mucous membranes lining the digestive tract from the mouth to the anus. It is a common side effect of chemotherapy and of radiotherapy that involves any part of the digestive tract.

● **K12   Stomatitis and related lesions**
   Use additional code to identify:
     alcohol abuse and dependence (F10.-)
     exposure to environmental tobacco smoke (Z77.22)
     exposure to tobacco smoke in the perinatal period (P96.81)
     history of tobacco use (Z87.891)
     occupational exposure to environmental tobacco smoke (Z57.31)
     tobacco dependence (F17.-)
     tobacco use (Z72.0)
   Excludes1   cancrum oris (A69.0)
       cheilitis (K13.0)
       gangrenous stomatitis (A69.0)
       herpesviral [herpes simplex] gingivostomatitis (B00.2)
       noma (A69.0)

K12.0   Recurrent oral aphthae
   Aphthous stomatitis (major) (minor)
   Bednar's aphthae
   Periadenitis mucosa necrotica recurrens
   Recurrent aphthous ulcer
   Stomatitis herpetiformis

K12.1   Other forms of stomatitis
   Stomatitis NOS
   Denture stomatitis
   Ulcerative stomatitis
   Vesicular stomatitis
   Excludes1   acute necrotizing ulcerative stomatitis (A69.1)
       Vincent's stomatitis (A69.1)

K12.2   Cellulitis and abscess of mouth
   Cellulitis of mouth (floor)
   Submandibular abscess
   Excludes2   abscess of salivary gland (K11.3)
       abscess of tongue (K14.0)
       periapical abscess (K04.6-K04.7)
       periodontal abscess (K05.21)
       peritonsillar abscess (J36)

● **K12.3   Oral mucositis (ulcerative)**
   Mucositis (oral) (oropharyneal)
   Excludes2   gastrointestinal mucositis (ulcerative) (K92.81)
       mucositis (ulcerative) of vagina and vulva (N76.81)
       nasal mucositis (ulcerative) (J34.81)

   K12.30   Oral mucositis (ulcerative), unspecified
   K12.31   Oral mucositis (ulcerative) due to antineoplastic therapy
     Use additional code for adverse effect, if applicable, to identify antineoplastic and immunosuppressive drugs (T45.1X5)
     Use additional code for other antineoplastic therapy, such as:
       radiological procedure and radiotherapy (Y84.2)
   K12.32   Oral mucositis (ulcerative) due to other drugs
     Use additional code for adverse effect, if applicable, to identify drug (T36-T50 with fifth or sixth character 5)
   K12.33   Oral mucositis (ulcerative) due to radiation
     Use additional external cause code (W88-W90, X39.0-) to identify cause
   K12.39   Other oral mucositis (ulcerative)
     Viral oral mucositis (ulcerative)

● **K13   Other diseases of lip and oral mucosa**
   Includes   epithelial disturbances of tongue
   Use additional code to identify:
     alcohol abuse and dependence (F10.-)
     exposure to environmental tobacco smoke (Z77.22)
     exposure to tobacco smoke in the perinatal period (P96.81)
     history of tobacco use (Z87.891)
     occupational exposure to environmental tobacco smoke (Z57.31)
     tobacco dependence (F17.-)
     tobacco use (Z72.0)
   Excludes2   certain disorders of gingiva and edentulous alveolar ridge (K05-K06)
       cysts of oral region (K09.-)
       diseases of tongue (K14.-)
       stomatitis and related lesions (K12.-)

K13.0   Diseases of lips
   Abscess of lips   Exfoliative cheilitis
   Angular cheilitis   Fistula of lips
   Cellulitis of lips   Glandular cheilitis
   Cheilitis NOS   Hypertrophy of lips
   Cheilodynia   Perlèche NEC
   Cheilosis
   Excludes1   ariboflavinosis (E53.0)
       cheilitis due to radiation-related disorders (L55-L59)
       congenital fistula of lips (Q38.0)
       congenital hypertrophy of lips (Q18.6)
       Perlèche due to candidiasis (B37.83)
       Perlèche due to riboflavin deficiency (E53.0)

K13.1   Cheek and lip biting
● **K13.2   Leukoplakia and other disturbances of oral epithelium, including tongue**
   Excludes1   carcinoma in situ of oral epithelium (D00.0-)
       hairy leukoplakia (K13.3)

   K13.21   Leukoplakia of oral mucosa, including tongue
     Considered precancerous and evidenced by thickened white patches of epithelium on mucous membranes
     Leukokeratosis of oral mucosa
     Leukoplakia of gingiva, lips, tongue
     Excludes1   hairy leukoplakia (K13.3)
       leukokeratosis nicotina palati (K13.24)

   K13.22   Minimal keratinized residual ridge mucosa
     Minimal keratinization of alveolar ridge mucosa
   K13.23   Excessive keratinized residual ridge mucosa
     Excessive keratinization of alveolar ridge mucosa
   K13.24   Leukokeratosis nicotina palati
     Smoker's palate
   K13.29   Other disturbances of oral epithelium, including tongue
     Erythroplakia of mouth or tongue
     Focal epithelial hyperplasia of mouth or tongue
     Leukoedema of mouth or tongue
     Other oral epithelium disturbances

K13.3   Hairy leukoplakia

Figure 11-4   Oral leukoplakia and associated squamous carcinoma. (From Feldman: Sleisenger & Fordtran's Gastrointestinal and Liver Disease, ed 8, Saunders, An Imprint of Elsevier, 2006)

◀ New   ◀▦ Revised   ~~deleted~~ Deleted   **OGCR** Official Guidelines   X Assign placeholder X   ● Use Additional Character(s)
Excludes 1   Excludes 2   Includes   Use additional   Code first   Code also   Unspecified

K13.4   **Granuloma and granuloma-like lesions of oral mucosa**
       Eosinophilic granuloma
       Granuloma pyogenicum
       Verrucous xanthoma

K13.5   **Oral submucous fibrosis**
       Submucous fibrosis of tongue

K13.6   **Irritative hyperplasia of oral mucosa**
     Excludes2   irritative hyperplasia of edentulous ridge
                   [denture hyperplasia] (K06.2)

● **K13.7**   **Other and unspecified lesions of oral mucosa**

(See Plate 58 on page NAP-23.)

     K13.70   **Unspecified lesions of oral mucosa**

     K13.79   **Other lesions of oral mucosa**
            Focal oral mucinosis

● **K14**   **Diseases of tongue**
     Use additional code to identify:
       alcohol abuse and dependence (F10.-)
       exposure to environmental tobacco smoke (Z77.22)
       history of tobacco use (Z87.891)
       occupational exposure to environmental tobacco smoke
             (Z57.31)
       tobacco dependence (F17.-)
       tobacco use (Z72.0)
     Excludes2   erythroplakia (K13.29)
                   focal epithelial hyperplasia (K13.29)
                   leukedema of tongue (K13.29)
                   leukoplakia of tongue (K13.21)
                   hairy leukoplakia (K13.3)
                   macroglossia (congenital) (Q38.2)
                   submucous fibrosis of tongue (K13.5)

K14.0   **Glossitis**
       Abscess of tongue
       Ulceration (traumatic) of tongue
     Excludes1   atrophic glossitis (K14.4)

K14.1   **Geographic tongue**
       Benign migratory glossitis
       Glossitis areata exfoliativa

K14.2   **Median rhomboid glossitis**

K14.3   **Hypertrophy of tongue papillae**
       Black hairy tongue
       Coated tongue
       Hypertrophy of foliate papillae
       Lingua villosa nigra

K14.4   **Atrophy of tongue papillae**
       Atrophic glossitis

K14.5   **Plicated tongue**
       Fissured tongue   Scrotal tongue
       Furrowed tongue
     Excludes1   fissured tongue, congenital (Q38.3)

K14.6   **Glossodynia**
       Glossopyrosis   Painful tongue

K14.8   **Other diseases of tongue**
       Atrophy of tongue   Glossocele
       Crenated tongue   Glossoptosis
       Enlargement of tongue   Hypertrophy of tongue

K14.9   **Disease of tongue, unspecified**
       Glossopathy NOS

DISEASES OF ESOPHAGUS, STOMACH AND DUODENUM (K20-K31)
     Excludes2   hiatus hernia (K44.-)

● **K20**   **Esophagitis**
     Use additional code to identify:
       alcohol abuse and dependence (F10.-)
     Excludes1   erosion of esophagus (K22.1-)
                esophagitis with gastro-esophageal reflux disease
                   (K21.0)
                reflux esophagitis (K21.0)
                ulcerative esophagitis (K22.1-)
     Excludes2   eosinophilic gastritis or gastroenteritis (K52.81)

K20.0   **Eosinophilic esophagitis**

K20.8   **Other esophagitis**
       Abscess of esophagus

K20.9   **Esophagitis, unspecified**
       Esophagitis NOS

● **K21**   **Gastro-esophageal reflux disease**
     Excludes1   newborn esophageal reflux (P78.83)

K21.0   **Gastro-esophageal reflux disease with esophagitis**
       Reflux esophagitis

K21.9   **Gastro-esophageal reflux disease without esophagitis**
       Esophageal reflux NOS

● **K22**   **Other diseases of esophagus**
     Excludes2   esophageal varices (I85.-)

K22.0   **Achalasia of cardia**
       Achalasia NOS
       Cardiospasm
     Excludes1   congenital cardiospasm (Q39.5)

● **K22.1**   **Ulcer of esophagus**
       Barrett's ulcer
       Erosion of esophagus
       Fungal ulcer of esophagus
       Peptic ulcer of esophagus
       Ulcer of esophagus due to ingestion of chemicals
       Ulcer of esophagus due to ingestion of drugs and
             medicaments
       Ulcerative esophagitis
       Code first poisoning due to drug or toxin, if applicable
            (T36-T65 with fifth or sixth character 1-4 or 6)
       Use additional code for adverse effect, if applicable,
            to identify drug (T36-T50 with fifth or sixth
            character 5)
     Excludes1   Barrett's esophagus (K22.87-)

K22.10   **Ulcer of esophagus without bleeding**
       Ulcer of esophagus NOS

K22.11   **Ulcer of esophagus with bleeding**
     Excludes2   bleeding esophageal varices
                   (I85.01, I85.11)

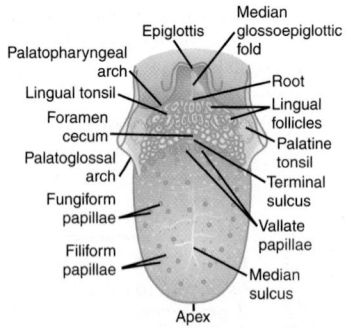

Epiglottis
Median glossoepiglottic fold
Palatopharyngeal arch
Lingual tonsil
Foramen cecum
Palatoglossal arch
Fungiform papillae
Filiform papillae
Root
Lingual follicles
Palatine tonsil
Terminal sulcus
Vallate papillae
Median sulcus
Apex

Figure 11-5   Structure of the tongue.

Item 11–6 Esophageal reflux is the return flow of the contents of the stomach to the esophagus and is referred to as GERD and/or "heartburn." **Gastroesophageal reflux** is the return flow of the contents of the stomach and duodenum to the esophagus. **Esophageal leukoplakia** are white areas on the mucous membrane of the esophagus for which no specific cause can be identified.

◄ New   ◄ Revised   ~~deleted~~ Deleted   OGCR Official Guidelines   X Assign placeholder X   ● Use Additional Character(s)

Excludes 1   Excludes 2   Includes   Use additional   Code first   Code also   Unspecified

CHAPTER 11 (K00-K95)

Figure 11-6 The esophagus is the muscular tube that connects the pharynx and the stomach. The 10 inch (25 cm) long esophagus is divided into three parts: **cervical, thoracic,** and **abdominal.**

Figure 11-7 A. Ulcer. **B.** Perforated ulcer. **C.** Laparoscopic view of a perforated duodenal ulcer *(arrow)* with fibrinous exudate on the adjacent peritoneum. (**C** from Feldman: Sleisenger & Fordtran's Gastrointestinal and Liver Disease, ed 8, Saunders, An Imprint of Elsevier, 2006)

Item 11–8 Gastric ulcers are lesions of the stomach that result in the death of the tissue and a defect of the surface. **Perforated ulcers** are those in which the lesion penetrates the gastric wall, leaving a hole. **Peptic ulcers** are lesions of the stomach or the duodenum. **Peptic** refers to the gastric juice, pepsin.

● **K25   Gastric ulcer**

     Includes   erosion (acute) of stomach
                   pylorus ulcer (peptic)
                   stomach ulcer (peptic)

     Use additional code to identify:
       alcohol abuse and dependence (F10.-)

     Excludes1   acute gastritis (K29.0-)
                  peptic ulcer NOS (K27.-)

     K25.0   Acute gastric ulcer with hemorrhage
     K25.1   Acute gastric ulcer with perforation
     K25.2   Acute gastric ulcer with both hemorrhage and perforation
     K25.3   Acute gastric ulcer without hemorrhage or perforation
     K25.4   Chronic or unspecified gastric ulcer with hemorrhage
     K25.5   Chronic or unspecified gastric ulcer with perforation
     K25.6   Chronic or unspecified gastric ulcer with both hemorrhage and perforation
     K25.7   Chronic gastric ulcer without hemorrhage or perforation
     K25.9   Gastric ulcer, unspecified as acute or chronic, without hemorrhage or perforation

● **K26   Duodenal ulcer**

     Includes   erosion (acute) of duodenum
                   duodenum ulcer (peptic)
                   postpyloric ulcer (peptic)

     Use additional code to identify:
       alcohol abuse and dependence (F10.-)

     Excludes1   peptic ulcer NOS (K27.-)

     K26.0   Acute duodenal ulcer with hemorrhage
     K26.1   Acute duodenal ulcer with perforation
     K26.2   Acute duodenal ulcer with both hemorrhage and perforation
     K26.3   Acute duodenal ulcer without hemorrhage or perforation
     K26.4   Chronic or unspecified duodenal ulcer with hemorrhage
     K26.5   Chronic or unspecified duodenal ulcer with perforation
     K26.6   Chronic or unspecified duodenal ulcer with both hemorrhage and perforation
     K26.7   Chronic duodenal ulcer without hemorrhage or perforation
     K26.9   Duodenal ulcer, unspecified as acute or chronic, without hemorrhage or perforation

K22.2   Esophageal obstruction
     Compression of esophagus
     Constriction of esophagus
     Stenosis of esophagus
     Stricture of esophagus
     Excludes1   congenital stenosis or stricture of esophagus (Q39.3)

K22.3   Perforation of esophagus
     Rupture of esophagus
     Excludes1   traumatic perforation of (thoracic) esophagus (S27.8-)

K22.4   Dyskinesia of esophagus
     Difficulty in moving
     Corkscrew esophagus
     Diffuse esophageal spasm
     Spasm of esophagus
     Excludes1   cardiospasm (K22.0)

K22.5   Diverticulum of esophagus, acquired
     Esophageal pouch, acquired
     Excludes1   diverticulum of esophagus (congenital) (Q39.6)

K22.6   Gastro-esophageal laceration-hemorrhage syndrome
     Mallory-Weiss syndrome

● **K22.7   Barrett's esophagus**
     Barrett's disease
     Barrett's syndrome
     Excludes1   Barrett's ulcer (K22.1)
                  malignant neoplasm of esophagus (C15.-)

     K22.70   Barrett's esophagus without dysplasia
          Barrett's esophagus NOS

     ● **K22.71   Barrett's esophagus with dysplasia**
          K22.710   Barrett's esophagus with low grade dysplasia
          K22.711   Barrett's esophagus with high grade dysplasia
          K22.719   Barrett's esophagus with dysplasia, unspecified

K22.8   Other specified diseases of esophagus
     Hemorrhage of esophagus NOS
     Excludes2   esophageal varices (I85.-)
                  Paterson-Kelly syndrome (D50.1)

K22.9   Disease of esophagus, unspecified

K23   Disorders of esophagus in diseases classified elsewhere
     Code first underlying disease, such as:
     congenital syphilis (A50.5)
     Excludes1   late syphilis (A52.79)
                  megaesophagus due to Chagas' disease (B57.31)
                  tuberculosis (A18.83)

Item 11-7 Achalasia is a condition in which the smooth muscle fibers of the esophagus do not relax. Most frequently, this condition occurs at the esophagogastric sphincter. **Cardiospasm,** also known as **megaesophagus,** is achalasia of the thoracic esophagus.

CHAPTER 11 (K00-K95)

 New   ◀▥▥ Revised   ~~deleted~~ Deleted   **OGCR** Official Guidelines   X Assign placeholder X   ● Use Additional Character(s)

| Excludes 1 | Excludes 2 | Includes | Use additional | Code first | Code also | Unspecified |

● **K27   Peptic ulcer, site unspecified**

> **Includes**   gastroduodenal ulcer NOS
>   peptic ulcer NOS
>
> Use additional code to identify:
>   alcohol abuse and dependence (F10.-)
>
> **Excludes1**   peptic ulcer of newborn (P78.82)

K27.0   Acute peptic ulcer, site unspecified, with hemorrhage

K27.1   Acute peptic ulcer, site unspecified, with perforation

K27.2   Acute peptic ulcer, site unspecified, with both hemorrhage and perforation

K27.3   Acute peptic ulcer, site unspecified, without hemorrhage or perforation

K27.4   Chronic or unspecified peptic ulcer, site unspecified, with hemorrhage

K27.5   Chronic or unspecified peptic ulcer, site unspecified, with perforation

K27.6   Chronic or unspecified peptic ulcer, site unspecified, with both hemorrhage and perforation

K27.7   Chronic peptic ulcer, site unspecified, without hemorrhage or perforation

K27.9   Peptic ulcer, site unspecified, unspecified as acute or chronic, without hemorrhage or perforation

● **K28   Gastrojejunal ulcer**

> **Includes**   anastomotic ulcer (peptic) or erosion
>   gastrocolic ulcer (peptic) or erosion
>   gastrointestinal ulcer (peptic) or erosion
>   gastrojejunal ulcer (peptic) or erosion
>   jejunal ulcer (peptic) or erosion
>   marginal ulcer (peptic) or erosion
>   stomal ulcer (peptic) or erosion
>
> Use additional code to identify:
>   alcohol abuse and dependence (F10.-)
>
> **Excludes1**   primary ulcer of small intestine (K63.3)

K28.0   Acute gastrojejunal ulcer with hemorrhage

K28.1   Acute gastrojejunal ulcer with perforation

K28.2   Acute gastrojejunal ulcer with both hemorrhage and perforation

K28.3   Acute gastrojejunal ulcer without hemorrhage or perforation

K28.4   Chronic or unspecified gastrojejunal ulcer with hemorrhage

K28.5   Chronic or unspecified gastrojejunal ulcer with perforation

K28.6   Chronic or unspecified gastrojejunal ulcer with both hemorrhage and perforation

K28.7   Chronic gastrojejunal ulcer without hemorrhage or perforation

K28.9   Gastrojejunal ulcer, unspecified as acute or chronic, without hemorrhage or perforation

● **K29   Gastritis and duodenitis**

> **Excludes1**   eosinophilic gastritis or gastroenteritis (K52.81)
>   Zollinger-Ellison syndrome (E16.4)

● K29.0   Acute gastritis

> Use additional code to identify:
>   alcohol abuse and dependence (F10.-)
>
> **Excludes1**   erosion (acute) of stomach (K25.-)

K29.00   Acute gastritis without bleeding

K29.01   Acute gastritis with bleeding

● K29.2   Alcoholic gastritis

> Use additional code to identify:
>   alcohol abuse and dependence (F10.-)

K29.20   Alcoholic gastritis without bleeding

K29.21   Alcoholic gastritis with bleeding

Item 11-9   Gastritis is a severe inflammation of the stomach. **Atrophic gastritis** is a chronic inflammation of the stomach that results in destruction of the cells of the mucosa of the stomach. Duodenitis is an inflammation of the duodenum, the first section of the small intestine.

● K29.3   Chronic superficial gastritis

K29.30   Chronic superficial gastritis without bleeding

K29.31   Chronic superficial gastritis with bleeding

● K29.4   Chronic atrophic gastritis
          Gastric atrophy

K29.40   Chronic atrophic gastritis without bleeding

K29.41   Chronic atrophic gastritis with bleeding

● K29.5   Unspecified chronic gastritis
          Chronic antral gastritis
          Chronic fundal gastritis

K29.50   Unspecified chronic gastritis without bleeding

K29.51   Unspecified chronic gastritis with bleeding

● K29.6   Other gastritis
          Giant hypertrophic gastritis
          Granulomatous gastritis
          Ménétrier's disease

K29.60   Other gastritis without bleeding

K29.61   Other gastritis with bleeding

● K29.7   Gastritis, unspecified

K29.70   Gastritis, unspecified, without bleeding

K29.71   Gastritis, unspecified, with bleeding

● K29.8   Duodenitis

K29.80   Duodenitis without bleeding

K29.81   Duodenitis with bleeding

● K29.9   Gastroduodenitis, unspecified

K29.90   Gastroduodenitis, unspecified, without bleeding

K29.91   Gastroduodenitis, unspecified, with bleeding

K30   **Functional dyspepsia**
          Indigestion

> **Excludes1**   dyspepsia NOS (R10.13)
>   heartburn (R12)
>   nervous dyspepsia (F45.8)
>   neurotic dyspepsia (F45.8)
>   psychogenic dyspepsia (F45.8)

● K31   **Other diseases of stomach and duodenum**
          Includes   functional disorders of stomach

> **Excludes2**   diabetic gastroparesis (E08.43, E09.43, E10.43, E11.43, E13.43)
>   diverticulum of duodenum (K57.00-K57.13)

K31.0   Acute dilatation of stomach
          Acute distention of stomach

K31.1   Adult hypertrophic pyloric stenosis
          Pyloric stenosis NOS

> **Excludes1**   congenital or infantile pyloric stenosis (Q40.0)

K31.2   Hourglass stricture and stenosis of stomach

> **Excludes1**   congenital hourglass stomach (Q40.2)
>   hourglass contraction of stomach (K31.89)

K31.3   Pylorospasm, not elsewhere classified

> **Excludes1**   congenital or infantile pylorospasm (Q40.0)
>   neurotic pylorospasm (F45.8)
>   psychogenic pylorospasm (F45.8)

K31.4   Gastric diverticulum

> **Excludes1**   congenital diverticulum of stomach (Q40.2)

Item 11–10 Achlorhydria, also known as gastric anacidity, is the absence of gastric acid.

K31.5 Obstruction of duodenum
    Constriction of duodenum
    Duodenal ileus (chronic)
    Stenosis of duodenum
        Narrowing
    Stricture of duodenum
        Narrowing
    Volvulus of duodenum
        Twisting/knotting
    Excludes1   congenital stenosis of duodenum (Q41.0)

K31.6 Fistula of stomach and duodenum
    Gastrocolic fistula
    Gastrojejunocolic fistula

K31.7 Polyp of stomach and duodenum
    Excludes1   adenomatous polyp of stomach (D13.1)

● **K31.8 Other specified diseases of stomach and duodenum**
  ● **K31.81 Angiodysplasia of stomach and duodenum**
      K31.811 Angiodysplasia of stomach and duodenum with bleeding
      K31.819 Angiodysplasia of stomach and duodenum without bleeding
         Angiodysplasia of stomach and duodenum NOS
    K31.82 Dieulafoy lesion (hemorrhagic) of stomach and duodenum
      Excludes2   Dieulafoy lesion of intestine (K63.81)
    K31.83 Achlorhydria
    K31.84 Gastroparesis
      Gastroparalysis
      Code first underlying disease, if known, such as:
        anorexia nervosa (F50.0-)
        diabetes mellitus (E08.43, E09.43, E10.43, E11.43, E13.43)
        scleroderma (M34.-)
    K31.89 Other diseases of stomach and duodenum
K31.9 Disease of stomach and duodenum, unspecified

DISEASES OF APPENDIX (K35-K38)

● **K35 Acute appendicitis**
  K35.2 Acute appendicitis with generalized peritonitis
    Appendicitis (acute) with generalized (diffuse) peritonitis following rupture or perforation of appendix
    Perforated appendix NOS
    Ruptured appendix NOS
  K35.3 Acute appendicitis with localized peritonitis
    Acute appendicitis with or without perforation or rupture NOS
    Acute appendicitis with or without perforation or rupture with localized peritonitis
    Acute appendicitis with peritoneal abscess
● **K35.8 Other and unspecified acute appendicitis**
  K35.80 Unspecified acute appendicitis
    Acute appendicitis NOS
    Acute appendicitis without (localized) (generalized) peritonitis
  K35.89 Other acute appendicitis

K36 Other appendicitis
    Chronic appendicitis
    Recurrent appendicitis

K37 Unspecified appendicitis
    Excludes1   -unspecified appendicitis with peritonitis (K35.2-K35.3)

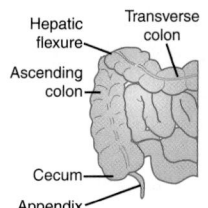

Figure 11-8 Acute appendicitis is the inflammation of the appendix, usually associated with obstruction. Most often this is a disease of adolescents and young adults.

● **K38 Other diseases of appendix**
  K38.0 Hyperplasia of appendix
  K38.1 Appendicular concretions
    Fecalith of appendix
    Stercolith of appendix
  K38.2 Diverticulum of appendix
  K38.3 Fistula of appendix
  K38.8 Other specified diseases of appendix
    Intussusception of appendix
  K38.9 Disease of appendix, unspecified

HERNIA (K40-K46)

Note: Hernia with both gangrene and obstruction is classified to hernia with gangrene.

Includes   acquired hernia
            congenital [except diaphragmatic or hiatus] hernia
            recurrent hernia

● **K40 Inguinal hernia**
  Includes   bubonocele
            direct inguinal hernia
            double inguinal hernia
            indirect inguinal hernia
            inguinal hernia NOS
            oblique inguinal hernia
            scrotal hernia
  ● **K40.0 Bilateral inguinal hernia, with obstruction, without gangrene**
    Inguinal hernia (bilateral) causing obstruction without gangrene
    Incarcerated inguinal hernia (bilateral) without gangrene
    Irreducible inguinal hernia (bilateral) without gangrene
    Strangulated inguinal hernia (bilateral) without gangrene
    K40.00 Bilateral inguinal hernia, with obstruction, without gangrene, not specified as recurrent
      Bilateral inguinal hernia, with obstruction, without gangrene NOS
    K40.01 Bilateral inguinal hernia, with obstruction, without gangrene, recurrent

Item 11–11 Hernias of the groin are the most common type, accounting for 80 percent of all hernias. There are two major types of inguinal hernias: indirect (oblique) affecting men only and direct. **Indirect inguinal hernias** result when the intestines emerge through the abdominal wall in an indirect fashion through the inguinal canal. **Direct inguinal hernias** penetrate through the abdominal wall in a direct fashion. **Femoral hernias** occur at the femoral ring where the femoral vessels enter the thigh and is most common in women. An abdominal wall hernia is also called a ventral or epigastric hernia and occurs in both sexes. Classification is based on location of the hernia and whether there is obstruction or gangrene.

Ventral, epigastric, or incisional hernia occurs on the abdominal surface caused by musculature weakness or a tear at a previous surgical site and is evidenced by a bulge that changes in size, becoming larger with exertion. An **incarcerated** hernia is one in which the intestines become trapped in the hernia. A **strangulated** hernia is one in which the blood supply to the intestines is lost. Hiatal hernia occurs when a loop of the stomach protrudes upward through the small opening in the diaphragm through which the esophagus passes, leaving the abdominal cavity and entering the chest. It occurs in both sexes.

CHAPTER 11 (K00-K95)

CHAPTER 11 (K00-K95)

Right Lumbar	Umbilical	Left Lumbar
RIGHT INGUINAL OR ILIAC	Hypogastric or pubic	LEFT INGUINAL OR ILIAC

Figure 11-9 Inguinal hernias are those that are located in the inguinal or iliac areas of the abdomen.

- **K40.1 Bilateral inguinal hernia, with gangrene**
  - **K40.10 Bilateral inguinal hernia, with gangrene, not specified as recurrent**
    Bilateral inguinal hernia, with gangrene NOS
  - **K40.11 Bilateral inguinal hernia, with gangrene, recurrent**
- **K40.2 Bilateral inguinal hernia, without obstruction or gangrene**
  - **K40.20 Bilateral inguinal hernia, without obstruction or gangrene, not specified as recurrent**
    Bilateral inguinal hernia NOS
  - **K40.21 Bilateral inguinal hernia, without obstruction or gangrene, recurrent**
- **K40.3 Unilateral inguinal hernia, with obstruction, without gangrene**
    Inguinal hernia (unilateral) causing obstruction without gangrene
    Incarcerated inguinal hernia (unilateral) without gangrene
    Irreducible inguinal hernia (unilateral) without gangrene
    Strangulated inguinal hernia (unilateral) without gangrene
  - **K40.30 Unilateral inguinal hernia, with obstruction, without gangrene, not specified as recurrent**
    Inguinal hernia, with obstruction NOS
    Unilateral inguinal hernia, with obstruction, without gangrene NOS
  - **K40.31 Unilateral inguinal hernia, with obstruction, without gangrene, recurrent**
- **K40.4 Unilateral inguinal hernia, with gangrene**
  - **K40.40 Unilateral inguinal hernia, with gangrene, not specified as recurrent**
    Inguinal hernia with gangrene NOS
    Unilateral inguinal hernia with gangrene NOS
  - **K40.41 Unilateral inguinal hernia, with gangrene, recurrent**
- **K40.9 Unilateral inguinal hernia, without obstruction or gangrene**
  - **K40.90 Unilateral inguinal hernia, without obstruction or gangrene, not specified as recurrent**
    Inguinal hernia NOS
    Unilateral inguinal hernia NOS
  - **K40.91 Unilateral inguinal hernia, without obstruction or gangrene, recurrent**

- **K41 Femoral hernia**
  - **K41.0 Bilateral femoral hernia, with obstruction, without gangrene**
    Femoral hernia (bilateral) causing obstruction, without gangrene
    Incarcerated femoral hernia (bilateral), without gangrene
    Irreducible femoral hernia (bilateral), without gangrene
    Strangulated femoral hernia (bilateral), without gangrene
    - **K41.00 Bilateral femoral hernia, with obstruction, without gangrene, not specified as recurrent**
      Bilateral femoral hernia, with obstruction, without gangrene NOS
    - **K41.01 Bilateral femoral hernia, with obstruction, without gangrene, recurrent**
  - **K41.1 Bilateral femoral hernia, with gangrene**
    - **K41.10 Bilateral femoral hernia, with gangrene, not specified as recurrent**
      Bilateral femoral hernia, with gangrene NOS
    - **K41.11 Bilateral femoral hernia, with gangrene, recurrent**
  - **K41.2 Bilateral femoral hernia, without obstruction or gangrene**
    - **K41.20 Bilateral femoral hernia, without obstruction or gangrene, not specified as recurrent**
      Bilateral femoral hernia NOS
    - **K41.21 Bilateral femoral hernia, without obstruction or gangrene, recurrent**
  - **K41.3 Unilateral femoral hernia, with obstruction, without gangrene**
    Femoral hernia (unilateral) causing obstruction, without gangrene
    Incarcerated femoral hernia (unilateral), without gangrene
    Irreducible femoral hernia (unilateral), without gangrene
    Strangulated femoral hernia (unilateral), without gangrene
    - **K41.30 Unilateral femoral hernia, with obstruction, without gangrene, not specified as recurrent**
      Femoral hernia, with obstruction NOS
      Unilateral femoral hernia, with obstruction NOS
    - **K41.31 Unilateral femoral hernia, with obstruction, without gangrene, recurrent**
  - **K41.4 Unilateral femoral hernia, with gangrene**
    - **K41.40 Unilateral femoral hernia, with gangrene, not specified as recurrent**
      Femoral hernia, with gangrene NOS
      Unilateral femoral hernia, with gangrene NOS
    - **K41.41 Unilateral femoral hernia, with gangrene, recurrent**
  - **K41.9 Unilateral femoral hernia, without obstruction or gangrene**
    - **K41.90 Unilateral femoral hernia, without obstruction or gangrene, not specified as recurrent**
      Femoral hernia NOS
      Unilateral femoral hernia NOS
    - **K41.91 Unilateral femoral hernia, without obstruction or gangrene, recurrent**

- **K42 Umbilical hernia**
  - **Includes**   paraumbilical hernia
  - **Excludes1**   omphalocele (Q79.2)
  - **K42.0 Umbilical hernia with obstruction, without gangrene**
    Umbilical hernia causing obstruction, without gangrene
    Incarcerated umbilical hernia, without gangrene
    Irreducible umbilical hernia, without gangrene
    Strangulated umbilical hernia, without gangrene

K42.1 **Umbilical hernia with gangrene**
Gangrenous umbilical hernia

K42.9 **Umbilical hernia without obstruction or gangrene**
Umbilical hernia NOS

● **K43 Ventral hernia**

K43.0 **Incisional hernia with obstruction, without gangrene**
Incisional hernia causing obstruction, without gangrene
Incarcerated incisional hernia, without gangrene
Irreducible incisional hernia, without gangrene
Strangulated incisional hernia, without gangrene

K43.1 **Incisional hernia with gangrene**
Gangrenous incisional hernia

K43.2 **Incisional hernia without obstruction or gangrene**
Incisional hernia NOS

K43.3 **Parastomal hernia with obstruction, without gangrene**
Incarcerated parastomal hernia, without gangrene
Irreducible parastomal hernia, without gangrene
Parastomal hernia causing obstruction, without gangrene
Strangulated parastomal hernia, without gangrene

K43.4 **Parastomal hernia with gangrene**
Gangrenous parastomal hernia

K43.5 **Parastomal hernia without obstruction or gangrene**
Parastomal hernia NOS

K43.6 **Other and unspecified ventral hernia with obstruction, without gangrene**
Epigastric hernia causing obstruction, without gangrene
Hypogastric hernia causing obstruction, without gangrene
Incarcerated epigastric hernia without gangrene
Incarcerated hypogastric hernia without gangrene
Incarcerated midline hernia without gangrene
Incarcerated spigelian hernia without gangrene
Incarcerated subxiphoid hernia without gangrene
Irreducible epigastric hernia without gangrene
Irreducible hypogastric hernia without gangrene
Irreducible midline hernia without gangrene
Irreducible spigelian hernia without gangrene
Irreducible subxiphoid hernia without gangrene
Midline hernia causing obstruction, without gangrene
Spigelian hernia causing obstruction, without gangrene
Strangulated epigastric hernia without gangrene
Strangulated hypogastric hernia without gangrene
Strangulated midline hernia without gangrene
Strangulated spigelian hernia without gangrene
Strangulated subxiphoid hernia without gangrene
Subxiphoid hernia causing obstruction, without gangrene

K43.7 **Other and unspecified ventral hernia with gangrene**
Any condition listed under K43.6 specified as gangrenous

K43.9 **Ventral hernia without obstruction or gangrene**
Epigastric hernia
Ventral hernia NOS

● **K44 Diaphragmatic hernia**

| **Includes** | hiatus hernia (esophageal) (sliding)
paraesophageal hernia |

| **Excludes1** | congenital diaphragmatic hernia (Q79.0)
congenital hiatus hernia (Q40.1) |

K44.0 **Diaphragmatic hernia with obstruction, without gangrene**
Diaphragmatic hernia causing obstruction
Incarcerated diaphragmatic hernia
Irreducible diaphragmatic hernia
Strangulated diaphragmatic hernia

K44.1 **Diaphragmatic hernia with gangrene**
Gangrenous diaphragmatic hernia

K44.9 **Diaphragmatic hernia without obstruction or gangrene**
Diaphragmatic hernia NOS

● **K45 Other abdominal hernia**

| **Includes** | abdominal hernia, specified site NEC
lumbar hernia
obturator hernia
pudendal hernia
retroperitoneal hernia
sciatic hernia |

K45.0 **Other specified abdominal hernia with obstruction, without gangrene**
Other specified abdominal hernia causing obstruction
Other specified incarcerated abdominal hernia
Other specified irreducible abdominal hernia
Other specified strangulated abdominal hernia

K45.1 **Other specified abdominal hernia with gangrene**
Any condition listed under K45 specified as gangrenous

K45.8 **Other specified abdominal hernia without obstruction or gangrene**

● **K46 Unspecified abdominal hernia**

| **Includes** | enterocele
epiplocele
hernia NOS
interstitial hernia
intestinal hernia
intra-abdominal hernia |

| **Excludes1** | vaginal enterocele (N81.5) |

K46.0 **Unspecified abdominal hernia with obstruction, without gangrene**
Unspecified abdominal hernia causing obstruction
Unspecified incarcerated abdominal hernia
Unspecified irreducible abdominal hernia
Unspecified strangulated abdominal hernia

K46.1 **Unspecified abdominal hernia with gangrene**
Any condition listed under K46 specified as gangrenous

K46.9 **Unspecified abdominal hernia without obstruction or gangrene**
Abdominal hernia NOS

(See Plate 284 on page NAP-29.)

NONINFECTIVE ENTERITIS AND COLITIS (K50-K52)

| **Includes** | noninfective inflammatory bowel disease |
| **Excludes1** | irritable bowel syndrome (K58.-)
megacolon (K59.3) |

● **K50 Crohn's disease [regional enteritis]**

| **Includes** | granulomatous enteritis |

Use additional code to identify manifestations, such as:
pyoderma gangrenosum (L88)

| **Excludes1** | ulcerative colitis (K51.-) |

● **K50.0 Crohn's disease of small intestine**
Crohn's disease [regional enteritis] of duodenum
Crohn's disease [regional enteritis] of ileum
Crohn's disease [regional enteritis] of jejunum
Regional ileitis
Terminal ileitis

| **Excludes1** | Crohn's disease of both small and large intestine (K50.8-) |

K50.00 **Crohn's disease of small intestine without complications**

◀ New   ◀|||| Revised   ~~deleted~~ Deleted   **OGCR** Official Guidelines   X Assign placeholder X   ● Use Additional Character(s)

| Excludes 1 | Excludes 2 | Includes | Use additional | Code first | Code also | Unspecified |

Item 11–12 Crohn's disease, also known as **regional enteritis,** is a chronic inflammatory disease of the intestines. Classification is based on location in the small (duodenum, ileum, jejunum) or large (cecum, colon, rectum, anal canal) intestine.

● K50.01   Crohn's disease of small intestine with complications
    K50.011   Crohn's disease of small intestine with rectal bleeding
    K50.012   Crohn's disease of small intestine with intestinal obstruction
    K50.013   Crohn's disease of small intestine with fistula
    K50.014   Crohn's disease of small intestine with abscess
    K50.018   Crohn's disease of small intestine with other complication
    K50.019   Crohn's disease of small intestine with unspecified complications

● K50.1   Crohn's disease of large intestine
    Crohn's disease [regional enteritis] of colon
    Crohn's disease [regional enteritis] of large bowel
    Crohn's disease [regional enteritis] of rectum
    Granulomatous colitis
    Regional colitis
    Excludes1   Crohn's disease of both small and large intestine (K50.8)

    K50.10   Crohn's disease of large intestine without complications
● K50.11   Crohn's disease of large intestine with complications
    K50.111   Crohn's disease of large intestine with rectal bleeding
    K50.112   Crohn's disease of large intestine with intestinal obstruction
    K50.113   Crohn's disease of large intestine with fistula
    K50.114   Crohn's disease of large intestine with abscess
    K50.118   Crohn's disease of large intestine with other complication
    K50.119   Crohn's disease of large intestine with unspecified complications

● K50.8   Crohn's disease of both small and large intestine
    K50.80   Crohn's disease of both small and large intestine without complications
● K50.81   Crohn's disease of both small and large intestine with complications
    K50.811   Crohn's disease of both small and large intestine with rectal bleeding
    K50.812   Crohn's disease of both small and large intestine with intestinal obstruction
    K50.813   Crohn's disease of both small and large intestine with fistula
    K50.814   Crohn's disease of both small and large intestine with abscess
    K50.818   Crohn's disease of both small and large intestine with other complication
    K50.819   Crohn's disease of both small and large intestine with unspecified complications

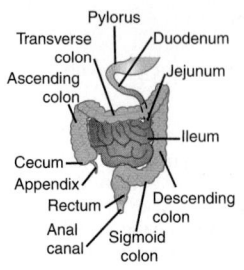

Figure 11-10   Small and large intestines.

Pylorus
Transverse colon
Duodenum
Ascending colon
Jejunum
Ileum
Cecum
Appendix
Rectum
Descending colon
Anal canal
Sigmoid colon

● K50.9   Crohn's disease, unspecified
    K50.90   Crohn's disease, unspecified, without complications
        Crohn's disease NOS
        Regional enteritis NOS
● K50.91   Crohn's disease, unspecified, with complications
    K50.911   Crohn's disease, unspecified, with rectal bleeding
    K50.912   Crohn's disease, unspecified, with intestinal obstruction
    K50.913   Crohn's disease, unspecified, with fistula
    K50.914   Crohn's disease, unspecified, with abscess
    K50.918   Crohn's disease, unspecified, with other complication
    K50.919   Crohn's disease, unspecified, with unspecified complications

● K51   **Ulcerative colitis**
    Use additional code to identify manifestations, such as: pyoderma gangrenosum (L88)
    Excludes1   Crohn's disease [regional enteritis] (K50.-)

● K51.0   Ulcerative (chronic) pancolitis
    Backwash ileitis
    K51.00   Ulcerative (chronic) pancolitis without complications
        Ulcerative (chronic) pancolitis NOS
● K51.01   Ulcerative (chronic) pancolitis with complications
    K51.011   Ulcerative (chronic) pancolitis with rectal bleeding
    K51.012   Ulcerative (chronic) pancolitis with intestinal obstruction
    K51.013   Ulcerative (chronic) pancolitis with fistula
    K51.014   Ulcerative (chronic) pancolitis with abscess
    K51.018   Ulcerative (chronic) pancolitis with other complication
    K51.019   Ulcerative (chronic) pancolitis with unspecified complications

Item 11–13 Ulcerative colitis attacks the colonic mucosa and forms abscesses. The disease involves the intestines. Classification is based on the location:
- Enterocolitis: large and small intestine
- Ileocolitis: ileum and colon
- Proctitis: rectum
- Proctosigmoiditis: sigmoid colon and rectum

◀ New   ◀▬ Revised   ~~deleted~~ Deleted   OGCR Official Guidelines   X Assign placeholder X   ● Use Additional Character(s)

Excludes 1   Excludes 2   Includes   Use additional   Code first   Code also   Unspecified

● **K51.2   Ulcerative (chronic) proctitis**
   K51.20   Ulcerative (chronic) proctitis without complications
      Ulcerative (chronic) proctitis NOS
● **K51.21   Ulcerative (chronic) proctitis with complications**
      K51.211   Ulcerative (chronic) proctitis with rectal bleeding
      K51.212   Ulcerative (chronic) proctitis with intestinal obstruction
      K51.213   Ulcerative (chronic) proctitis with fistula
      K51.214   Ulcerative (chronic) proctitis with abscess
      K51.218   Ulcerative (chronic) proctitis with other complication
      K51.219   Ulcerative (chronic) proctitis with unspecified complications
● **K51.3   Ulcerative (chronic) rectosigmoiditis**
   K51.30   Ulcerative (chronic) rectosigmoiditis without complications
      Ulcerative (chronic) rectosigmoiditis NOS
● **K51.31   Ulcerative (chronic) rectosigmoiditis with complications**
      K51.311   Ulcerative (chronic) rectosigmoiditis with rectal bleeding
      K51.312   Ulcerative (chronic) rectosigmoiditis with intestinal obstruction
      K51.313   Ulcerative (chronic) rectosigmoiditis with fistula
      K51.314   Ulcerative (chronic) rectosigmoiditis with abscess
      K51.318   Ulcerative (chronic) rectosigmoiditis with other complication
      K51.319   Ulcerative (chronic) rectosigmoiditis with unspecified complications
● **K51.4   Inflammatory polyps of colon**
   Excludes1   adenomatous polyp of colon (D12.6)
                    polyposis of colon (D12.6)
                    polyps of colon NOS (K63.5)
   K51.40   Inflammatory polyps of colon without complications
      Inflammatory polyps of colon NOS
● **K51.41   Inflammatory polyps of colon with complications**
      K51.411   Inflammatory polyps of colon with rectal bleeding
      K51.412   Inflammatory polyps of colon with intestinal obstruction
      K51.413   Inflammatory polyps of colon with fistula
      K51.414   Inflammatory polyps of colon with abscess
      K51.418   Inflammatory polyps of colon with other complication
      K51.419   Inflammatory polyps of colon with unspecified complications
● **K51.5   Left sided colitis**
      Left hemicolitis
   K51.50   Left sided colitis without complications
      Left sided colitis NOS
● **K51.51   Left sided colitis with complications**
      K51.511   Left sided colitis with rectal bleeding
      K51.512   Left sided colitis with intestinal obstruction
      K51.513   Left sided colitis with fistula
      K51.514   Left sided colitis with abscess
      K51.518   Left sided colitis with other complication
      K51.519   Left sided colitis with unspecified complications

● **K51.8   Other ulcerative colitis**
   K51.80   Other ulcerative colitis without complications
● **K51.81   Other ulcerative colitis with complications**
      K51.811   Other ulcerative colitis with rectal bleeding
      K51.812   Other ulcerative colitis with intestinal obstruction
      K51.813   Other ulcerative colitis with fistula
      K51.814   Other ulcerative colitis with abscess
      K51.818   Other ulcerative colitis with other complication
      K51.819   Other ulcerative colitis with unspecified complications
● **K51.9   Ulcerative colitis, unspecified**
   K51.90   Ulcerative colitis, unspecified, without complications
● **K51.91   Ulcerative colitis, unspecified, with complications**
      K51.911   Ulcerative colitis, unspecified with rectal bleeding
      K51.912   Ulcerative colitis, unspecified with intestinal obstruction
      K51.913   Ulcerative colitis, unspecified with fistula
      K51.914   Ulcerative colitis, unspecified with abscess
      K51.918   Ulcerative colitis, unspecified with other complication
      K51.919   Ulcerative colitis, unspecified with unspecified complications
● **K52   Other and unspecified noninfective gastroenteritis and colitis**
   K52.0   Gastroenteritis and colitis due to radiation
   K52.1   Toxic gastroenteritis and colitis
      Drug-induced gastroenteritis and colitis
      Code first (T51-T65) to identify toxic agent
      Use additional code for adverse effect, if applicable, to identify drug (T36-T50 with fifth or sixth character 5)
   K52.2   Allergic and dietetic gastroenteritis and colitis
      Food hypersensitivity gastroenteritis or colitis
      Use additional code to identify type of food allergy (Z91.01-, Z91.02-)
● **K52.8   Other specified noninfective gastroenteritis and colitis**
   K52.81   Eosinophilic gastritis or gastroenteritis
      Eosinophilic enteritis
      Excludes1   eosinophilic esophagitis (K20.0)
   K52.82   Eosinophilic colitis
   K52.89   Other specified noninfective gastroenteritis and colitis
      Collagenous colitis
      Lymphocytic colitis
      Microscopic colitis (collagenous or lymphocytic)
   K52.9   Noninfective gastroenteritis and colitis, unspecified
      Colitis NOS   Ileitis NOS
      Enteritis NOS   Jejunitis NOS
      Gastroenteritis NOS   Sigmoiditis NOS
      Excludes1   diarrhea NOS (R19.7)
                       functional diarrhea (K59.1)
                       infectious gastroenteritis and colitis NOS (A09)
                       neonatal diarrhea (noninfective) (P78.3)
                       psychogenic diarrhea (F45.8)

◄ New   ◄ Revised   deleted Deleted   OGCR Official Guidelines   X Assign placeholder X   ● Use Additional Character(s)
Excludes 1 | Excludes 2 | Includes | Use additional | Code first | Code also | Unspecified
979

CHAPTER 11 (K00-K95)

OTHER DISEASES OF INTESTINES (K55-K64)

● **K55   Vascular disorders of intestine**

> **Excludes1**   necrotizing enterocolitis of newborn (P77.-)

    K55.0   Acute vascular disorders of intestine
        Acute fulminant ischemic colitis
        Acute intestinal infarction
        Acute small intestine ischemia
        Infarction of appendices epiploicae
        Mesenteric (artery) (vein) embolism
        Mesenteric (artery) (vein) infarction
        Mesenteric (artery) (vein) thrombosis
        Necrosis of intestine
        Subacute ischemic colitis

    K55.1   Chronic vascular disorders of intestine
        Chronic ischemic colitis
        Chronic ischemic enteritis
        Chronic ischemic enterocolitis
        Ischemic stricture of intestine
        Mesenteric atherosclerosis
        Mesenteric vascular insufficiency

  ● **K55.2   Angiodysplasia of colon**
      K55.20   Angiodysplasia of colon without hemorrhage
      K55.21   Angiodysplasia of colon with hemorrhage

    K55.8   Other vascular disorders of intestine

    K55.9   Vascular disorder of intestine, unspecified
        Ischemic colitis
        Ischemic enteritis
        Ischemic enterocolitis

● **K56   Paralytic ileus and intestinal obstruction without hernia**

> **Excludes1**   congenital stricture or stenosis of intestine
>   (Q41-Q42)
>   cystic fibrosis with meconium ileus (E84.11)
>   ischemic stricture of intestine (K55.1)
>   meconium ileus NOS (P76.0)
>   neonatal intestinal obstructions classifiable
>   to P76.-
>   obstruction of duodenum (K31.5)
>   postprocedural intestinal obstruction (K91.3)
>   stenosis of anus or rectum (K62.4)
>   intestinal obstruction with hernia (K40-K46)

    K56.0   Paralytic ileus
        Paralysis of bowel
        Paralysis of colon
        Paralysis of intestine

> **Excludes1**   gallstone ileus (K56.3)
>   ileus NOS (K56.7)
>   obstructive ileus NOS (K56.69)

    K56.1   Intussusception
        Intussusception or invagination of bowel
        Intussusception or invagination of colon
        Intussusception or invagination of intestine
        Intussusception or invagination of rectum

> **Excludes2**   intussusception of appendix (K38.8)

SIMPLE TYPES   DOUBLE TYPES

Cecum and appendix

Ileum
Ileocecal valve

Ileum   Ileocecal
    valve

ILEOCOLIC

ILEOCECAL

Figure 11-11   Types of intussusception.

Item 11–14   Intussusception is the prolapse (telescoping) of a part of the intestine into another adjacent part of the intestine. Intussusception may be enteric (ileoileal, jejunoileal, jejunojejunal), colic (colocolic), or intracolic (ileocecal, ileocolic).

Item 11–15   Volvulus is the twisting of a segment of the intestine, resulting in obstruction. Paralytic ileus is paralysis of the intestine. It need not be a complete paralysis, but it must prohibit the passage of food through the intestine and lead to intestinal blockage. It is a common aftermath of some types of surgery.

    K56.2   Volvulus
        Strangulation of colon or intestine
        Torsion of colon or intestine
        Twist of colon or intestine

> **Excludes2**   volvulus of duodenum (K31.5)

    K56.3   Gallstone ileus
        Obstruction of intestine by gallstone

  ● **K56.4   Other impaction of intestine**
      K56.41   Fecal impaction

> **Excludes1**   constipation (K59.0-)
>   incomplete defecation (R15.0)

      K56.49   Other impaction of intestine

    K56.5   Intestinal adhesions [bands] with obstruction (postprocedural) (postinfection)
        Abdominal hernia due to adhesions with obstruction
        Peritoneal adhesions [bands] with intestinal obstruction
          (postprocedural) (postinfection)

  ● **K56.6   Other and unspecified intestinal obstruction**
      K56.60   Unspecified intestinal obstruction Intestinal obstruction NOS

> **Excludes1**   intestinal obstruction due to specified condition-code to condition

      K56.69   Other intestinal obstruction
          Enterostenosis NOS
          Obstructive ileus NOS
          Occlusion of colon or intestine NOS
          Stenosis of colon or intestine NOS
          Stricture of colon or intestine NOS

> **Excludes1**   intestinal obstruction due to specified condition-code to condition

    K56.7   Ileus, unspecified

> **Excludes1**   obstructive ileus (K56.69)

● **K57   Diverticular disease of intestine**

> **Excludes1**   congenital diverticulum of intestine (Q43.8)
>   Meckel's diverticulum (Q43.0)

> **Excludes2**   diverticulum of appendix (K38.2)

  ● **K57.0   Diverticulitis of small intestine with perforation and abscess**
        Diverticulitis of small intestine with peritonitis

> **Excludes1**   diverticulitis of both small and large intestine with perforation and abscess (K57.4-)

      K57.00   Diverticulitis of small intestine with perforation and abscess without bleeding
      K57.01   Diverticulitis of small intestine with perforation and abscess with bleeding

◄ New   ◄▥ Revised   ~~deleted~~ Deleted   **OGCR** Official Guidelines   X Assign placeholder X   ● Use Additional Character(s)

Excludes 1   Excludes 2   Includes   Use additional   Code first   Code also   Unspecified

Item 11–16   **Diverticula** of the intestines are acquired herniations of the mucosa. Diverticulum (singular): Pocket or pouch that bulges outward through a weak spot (herniation) in the colon. Diverticula (plural). **Diverticulosis** is the condition of having diverticula. **Diverticulitis** is inflammation of these pouches or herniations. Classification is based on location (small intestine or colon) and whether it occurs with or without hemorrhage.

● **K57.1**   **Diverticular disease of small intestine without perforation or abscess**
> **Excludes1**   diverticular disease of both small and large intestine without perforation or abscess (K57.5-)

     K57.10   **Diverticulosis of small intestine without perforation or abscess without bleeding**
> Diverticular disease of small intestine NOS

     K57.11   **Diverticulosis of small intestine without perforation or abscess with bleeding**

     K57.12   **Diverticulitis of small intestine without perforation or abscess without bleeding**

     K57.13   **Diverticulitis of small intestine without perforation or abscess with bleeding**

● **K57.2**   **Diverticulitis of large intestine with perforation and abscess**
> Diverticulitis of colon with peritonitis
> **Excludes1**   diverticulitis of both small and large intestine with perforation and abscess (K57.4-)

     K57.20   **Diverticulitis of large intestine with perforation and abscess without bleeding**

     K57.21   **Diverticulitis of large intestine with perforation and abscess with bleeding**

● **K57.3**   **Diverticular disease of large intestine without perforation or abscess**
> **Excludes1**   diverticular disease of both small and large intestine without perforation or abscess (K57.5-)

     K57.30   **Diverticulosis of large intestine without perforation or abscess without bleeding**
> Diverticular disease of colon NOS

     K57.31   **Diverticulosis of large intestine without perforation or abscess with bleeding**

     K57.32   **Diverticulitis of large intestine without perforation or abscess without bleeding**

     K57.33   **Diverticulitis of large intestine without perforation or abscess with bleeding**

● **K57.4**   **Diverticulitis of both small and large intestine with perforation and abscess**
> Diverticulitis of both small and large intestine with peritonitis

     K57.40   **Diverticulitis of both small and large intestine with perforation and abscess without bleeding**

     K57.41   **Diverticulitis of both small and large intestine with perforation and abscess with bleeding**

● **K57.5**   **Diverticular disease of both small and large intestine without perforation or abscess**

     K57.50   **Diverticulosis of both small and large intestine without perforation or abscess without bleeding**
> Diverticular disease of both small and large intestine NOS

     K57.51   **Diverticulosis of both small and large intestine without perforation or abscess with bleeding**

     K57.52   **Diverticulitis of both small and large intestine without perforation or abscess without bleeding**

     K57.53   **Diverticulitis of both small and large intestine without perforation or abscess with bleeding**

● **K57.8**   **Diverticulitis of intestine, part unspecified, with perforation and abscess**
> Diverticulitis of intestine NOS with peritonitis

     K57.80   **Diverticulitis of intestine, part unspecified, with perforation and abscess without bleeding**

     K57.81   **Diverticulitis of intestine, part unspecified, with perforation and abscess with bleeding**

● **K57.9**   **Diverticular disease of intestine, part unspecified, without perforation or abscess**

     K57.90   **Diverticulosis of intestine, part unspecified, without perforation or abscess without bleeding**
> Diverticular disease of intestine NOS

     K57.91   **Diverticulosis of intestine, part unspecified, without perforation or abscess with bleeding**

     K57.92   **Diverticulitis of intestine, part unspecified, without perforation or abscess without bleeding**

     K57.93   **Diverticulitis of intestine, part unspecified, without perforation or abscess with bleeding**

● **K58**   **Irritable bowel syndrome**
> **Includes**   irritable colon
> spastic colon

     K58.0   **Irritable bowel syndrome with diarrhea**

     K58.9   **Irritable bowel syndrome without diarrhea**
> Irritable bowel syndrome NOS

● **K59**   **Other functional intestinal disorders**
> **Excludes1**   change in bowel habit NOS (R19.4)
> intestinal malabsorption (K90.-)
> psychogenic intestinal disorders (F45.8)
> **Excludes2**   functional disorders of stomach (K31.-)

● **K59.0**   **Constipation**
> **Excludes1**   fecal impaction (K56.41)
> incomplete defecation (R15.0)

     K59.00   **Constipation, unspecified**

     K59.01   **Slow transit constipation**

     K59.02   **Outlet dysfunction constipation**

     K59.09   **Other constipation**

     K59.1   **Functional diarrhea**
> **Excludes1**   diarrhea NOS (R19.7)
> irritable bowel syndrome with diarrhea (K58.0)

     K59.2   **Neurogenic bowel, not elsewhere classified**

     K59.3   **Megacolon, not elsewhere classified**
> Dilatation of colon
> Toxic megacolon
> *Code first* (T51-T65) *to identify toxic agent*
> **Excludes1**   congenital megacolon (aganglionic) (Q43.1)
> megacolon (due to) (in) Chagas' disease (B57.32)
> megacolon (due to) (in) Clostridium difficile (A04.7)
> megacolon (due to) (in) Hirschsprung's disease (Q43.1)

     K59.4   **Anal spasm**
> Proctalgia fugax

     K59.8   **Other specified functional intestinal disorders**
> Atony of colon Pseudo-obstruction (acute) (chronic) of intestine

     K59.9   **Functional intestinal disorder, unspecified**

CHAPTER 11 (K00-K95)

Item 11–17 A **fissure** is a groove in the surface, whereas a **fistula** is an abnormal passage. An **abscess** is an accumulation of pus in a tissue cavity resulting from a bacterial or parasitic infection.

● **K60   Fissure and fistula of anal and rectal regions**

> **Excludes1**   fissure and fistula of anal and rectal regions with abscess or cellulitis (K61.-)
>
> **Excludes2**   anal sphincter tear (healed) (nontraumatic) (old) (K62.81)

    K60.0   Acute anal fissure

    K60.1   Chronic anal fissure

    K60.2   Anal fissure, unspecified

    K60.3   Anal fistula

    K60.4   Rectal fistula

> Fistula of rectum to skin
>
> **Excludes1**   rectovaginal fistula (N82.3)
> vesicorectal fistula (N32.1)

    K60.5   Anorectal fistula

● **K61   Abscess of anal and rectal regions**

> **Includes**   abscess of anal and rectal regions
> cellulitis of anal and rectal regions

    K61.0   Anal abscess

> Perianal abscess
>
> **Excludes1**   intrasphincteric abscess (K61.4)

    K61.1   Rectal abscess

> Perirectal abscess
>
> **Excludes1**   ischiorectal abscess (K61.3)

    K61.2   Anorectal abscess

    K61.3   Ischiorectal abscess

> Abscess of ischiorectal fossa

    K61.4   Intrasphincteric abscess

● **K62   Other diseases of anus and rectum**

> **Includes**   anal canal
>
> **Excludes2**   colostomy and enterostomy malfunction (K94.0-, K91.4-)
> fecal incontinence (R15.-)
> hemorrhoids (K64.-)

    K62.0   Anal polyp

    K62.1   Rectal polyp

> **Excludes1**   adenomatous polyp (D12.8)

    K62.2   Anal prolapse

> Prolapse of anal canal

    K62.3   Rectal prolapse

> Prolapse of rectal mucosa

    K62.4   Stenosis of anus and rectum

> Stricture of anus (sphincter)

    K62.5   Hemorrhage of anus and rectum

> **Excludes1**   gastrointestinal bleeding NOS (K92.2)
> melena (K92.1)
> neonatal rectal hemorrhage (P54.2)

    K62.6   Ulcer of anus and rectum

> Solitary ulcer of anus and rectum
> Stercoral ulcer of anus and rectum
>
> **Excludes1**   fissure and fistula of anus and rectum (K60.-)
> ulcerative colitis (K51.-)

    K62.7   Radiation proctitis

> Use additional code to identify the type of radiation (W90.-)

● **K62.8   Other specified diseases of anus and rectum**

> **Excludes2**   ulcerative proctitis (K51.2)

    K62.81   Anal sphincter tear (healed) (nontraumatic) (old)

> Tear of anus, nontraumatic
>
> Use additional code for any associated fecal incontinence (R15.-)
>
> **Excludes2**   anal fissure (K60.-)
> anal sphincter tear (healed) (old) complicating delivery (O34.7-)
> traumatic tear of anal sphincter (S31.831)

    K62.82   Dysplasia of anus

> Anal intraepithelial neoplasia I and II (AIN I and II) (histologically confirmed)
> Dysplasia of anus NOS
> Mild and moderate dysplasia of anus (histologically confirmed)
>
> **Excludes1**   abnormal results from anal cytologic examination without histologic confirmation (R85.61-)
> anal intraepithelial neoplasia III (D01.3)
> carcinoma in situ of anus (D01.3)
> HGSIL of anus (R85.613)
> severe dysplasia of anus (D01.3)

    K62.89   Other specified diseases of anus and rectum

> Proctitis NOS
>
> Use additional code for any associated fecal incontinence (R15.-)

    K62.9   Disease of anus and rectum, unspecified

● **K63   Other diseases of intestine**

    K63.0   Abscess of intestine

> **Excludes1**   abscess of intestine with Crohn's disease (K50.014, K50.114, K50.814, K50.914)
> abscess of intestine with diverticular disease (K57.0, K57.2, K57.4, K57.8)
> abscess of intestine with ulcerative colitis (K51.014, K51.214, K51.314, K51.414, K51.514, K51.814, K51.914)
>
> **Excludes2**   abscess of anal and rectal regions (K61.-)
> abscess of appendix (K35.3)

    K63.1   Perforation of intestine (nontraumatic)

> Perforation (nontraumatic) of rectum
>
> **Excludes1**   perforation (nontraumatic) of duodenum (K26.-)
> perforation (nontraumatic) of intestine with diverticular disease (K57.0, K57.2, K57.4, K57.8)
>
> **Excludes2**   perforation (nontraumatic) of appendix (K35.2, K35.3)

    K63.2   Fistula of intestine

> **Excludes1**   fistula of duodenum (K31.6)
> fistula of intestine with Crohn's disease (K50.013, K50.113, K50.813, K50.913)
> fistula of intestine with ulcerative colitis (K51.013, K51.213, K51.313, K51.413, K51.513, K51.813, K51.913)
>
> **Excludes2**   fistula of anal and rectal regions (K60.-)
> fistula of appendix (K38.3)
> intestinal-genital fistula, female (N82.2-N82.4)
> vesicointestinal fistula (N32.1)

K63.3   Ulcer of intestine
Primary ulcer of small intestine
> **Excludes1**   duodenal ulcer (K26.-)
> gastrointestinal ulcer (K28.-)
> gastrojejunal ulcer (K28.-)
> jejunal ulcer (K28.-)
> peptic ulcer, site unspecified (K27.-)
> ulcer of intestine with perforation (K63.1)
> ulcer of anus or rectum (K62.6)
> ulcerative colitis (K51.-)

K63.4   Enteroptosis

K63.5   Polyp of colon
> **Excludes1**   adenomatous polyp of colon (D12.6)
> inflammatory polyp of colon (K51.4-)
> polyposis of colon (D12.6)

● **K63.8   Other specified diseases of intestine**

     K63.81   Dieulafoy lesion of intestine
> **Excludes2**   Dieulafoy lesion of stomach and
> duodenum (K31.82)

     K63.89   Other specified diseases of intestine

K63.9   Disease of intestine, unspecified

● **K64   Hemorrhoids and perianal venous thrombosis**
> **Includes**   piles
> **Excludes1**   hemorrhoids complicating childbirth and the
> puerperium (O87.2)
> hemorrhoids complicating pregnancy (O22.4)

K64.0   First degree hemorrhoids
Grade/stage I hemorrhoids
Hemorrhoids (bleeding) without prolapse outside of
anal canal

K64.1   Second degree hemorrhoids
Grade/stage II hemorrhoids
Hemorrhoids (bleeding) that prolapse with straining,
but retract spontaneously

K64.2   Third degree hemorrhoids
Grade/stage III hemorrhoids
Hemorrhoids (bleeding) that prolapse with straining
and require manual replacement back inside anal
canal

K64.3   Fourth degree hemorrhoids
Grade/stage IV hemorrhoids
Hemorrhoids (bleeding) with prolapsed tissue that
cannot be manually replaced

K64.4   Residual hemorrhoidal skin tags
External hemorrhoids, NOS
Skin tags of anus

K64.5   Perianal venous thrombosis
External hemorrhoids with thrombosis
Perianal hematoma
Thrombosed hemorrhoids NOS

K64.8   Other hemorrhoids
Internal hemorrhoids, without mention of degree
Prolapsed hemorrhoids, degree not specified

K64.9   Unspecified hemorrhoids
Hemorrhoids (bleeding) NOS
Hemorrhoids (bleeding) without mention of degree

Item 11–18   Peritonitis is an inflammation of the lining (peritoneum) of the abdominal cavity and surface of the intestines.

Item 11-19   Retroperitoneal infections occur between the posterior parietal peritoneum and posterior abdominal wall where the kidneys, adrenal glands, ureters, duodenum, ascending colon, descending colon, pancreas, and the large vessels and nerves are located.

DISEASES OF PERITONEUM AND RETROPERITONEUM (K65-K68)

● **K65   Peritonitis**
> Use additional code (B95-B97), to identify infectious agent
> **Excludes1**   acute appendicitis with generalized peritonitis
> (K35.2)
> aseptic peritonitis (T81.6)
> benign paroxysmal peritonitis (E85.0)
> chemical peritonitis (T81.6)
> diverticulitis of both small and large intestine
> with peritonitis (K57.4-)
> diverticulitis of colon with peritonitis (K57.2-)
> diverticulitis of intestine, NOS, with peritonitis
> (K57.8-)
> diverticulitis of small intestine with peritonitis
> (K57.0-)
> gonococcal peritonitis (A54.85)
> neonatal peritonitis (P78.0-P78.1)
> pelvic peritonitis, female (N73.3-N73.5)
> periodic familial peritonitis (E85.0)
> peritonitis due to talc or other foreign substance
> (T81.6)
> peritonitis in chlamydia (A74.81)
> peritonitis in diphtheria (A36.89)
> peritonitis in syphilis (late) (A52.74)
> peritonitis in tuberculosis (A18.31)
> peritonitis with or following abortion or ectopic
> or molar pregnancy (O00-O07, O08.0)
> peritonitis with or following appendicitis (K35.-)
> peritonitis with or following diverticular disease
> of intestine (K57.-)
> puerperal peritonitis (O85)
> retroperitoneal infections (K68.-)

K65.0   Generalized (acute) peritonitis
Pelvic peritonitis (acute), male
Subphrenic peritonitis (acute)
Suppurative peritonitis (acute)

K65.1   Peritoneal abscess
Abdominopelvic abscess
Abscess (of) omentum
Abscess (of) peritoneum
Mesenteric abscess
Retrocecal abscess
Subdiaphragmatic abscess
Subhepatic abscess
Subphrenic abscess

K65.2   Spontaneous bacterial peritonitis
> **Excludes1**   bacterial peritonitis NOS (K65.9)

K65.3   Choleperitonitis
Peritonitis due to bile

K65.4   Sclerosing mesenteritis
Fat necrosis of peritoneum
(Idiopathic) sclerosing mesenteric fibrosis
Mesenteric lipodystrophy
Mesenteric panniculitis
Retractile mesenteritis

K65.8   Other peritonitis
Chronic proliferative peritonitis
Peritonitis due to urine

K65.9   Peritonitis, unspecified
Bacterial peritonitis NOS

CHAPTER 11 (K00-K95)

●K66 Other disorders of peritoneum

> Excludes2   ascites (R18.-)
> peritoneal effusion (chronic) (R18.8)

    K66.0 Peritoneal adhesions (postprocedural) (postinfection)
> Adhesions (of) abdominal (wall)
> Adhesions (of) diaphragm
> Adhesions (of) intestine
> Adhesions (of) male pelvis
> Adhesions (of) omentum
> Adhesions (of) stomach
> Adhesive bands
> Mesenteric adhesions
>> Excludes1   female pelvic adhesions [bands] (N73.6)
>> peritoneal adhesions with intestinal obstruction (K56.5)

    K66.1 Hemoperitoneum
> Excludes1   traumatic hemoperitoneum (S36.8-)

    K66.8 Other specified disorders of peritoneum

    K66.9 Disorder of peritoneum, unspecified

K67 Disorders of peritoneum in infectious diseases classified elsewhere
> *Code first underlying disease, such as:*
> congenital syphilis (A50.0)
> helminthiasis (B65.0-B83.9)
>> Excludes1   peritonitis in chlamydia (A74.81)
>> peritonitis in diphtheria (A36.89)
>> peritonitis in gonococcal (A54.85)
>> peritonitis in syphilis (late) (A52.74)
>> peritonitis in tuberculosis (A18.31)

●K68 Disorders of retroperitoneum

    ●K68.1 Retroperitoneal abscess

        K68.11 Postprocedural retroperitoneal abscess

        K68.12 Psoas muscle abscess

        K68.19 Other retroperitoneal abscess

    K68.9 Other disorders of retroperitoneum

DISEASES OF LIVER (K70-K77)

> Excludes1   jaundice NOS (R17)
> Excludes2   hemochromatosis (E83.11-)
> Reye's syndrome (G93.7)
> viral hepatitis (B15-B19)
> Wilson's disease (E83.0)

●K70 Alcoholic liver disease
> Use additional code to identify:
> alcohol abuse and dependence (F10.-)

    K70.0 Alcoholic fatty liver

    ●K70.1 Alcoholic hepatitis

        K70.10 Alcoholic hepatitis without ascites

        K70.11 Alcoholic hepatitis with ascites

    K70.2 Alcoholic fibrosis and sclerosis of liver

    ●K70.3 Alcoholic cirrhosis of liver
> Alcoholic cirrhosis NOS

        K70.30 Alcoholic cirrhosis of liver without ascites

        K70.31 Alcoholic cirrhosis of liver with ascites

    ●K70.4 Alcoholic hepatic failure
> Acute alcoholic hepatic failure
> Alcoholic hepatic failure NOS
> Chronic alcoholic hepatic failure
> Subacute alcoholic hepatic failure

        K70.40 Alcoholic hepatic failure without coma

        K70.41 Alcoholic hepatic failure with coma

    K70.9 Alcoholic liver disease, unspecified

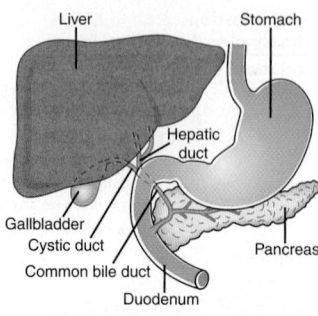

Figure 11-12   Liver and bile ducts.

●K71 Toxic liver disease

> Includes   drug-induced idiosyncratic (unpredictable) liver disease
> drug-induced toxic (predictable) liver disease

> *Code first poisoning due to drug or toxin, if applicable (T36-T65 with fifth or sixth character 1-4 or 6)*

> Use additional code for adverse effect, if applicable, to identify drug (T36-T50 with fifth or sixth character 5)

> Excludes2   alcoholic liver disease (K70.-)
> Budd-Chiari syndrome (I82.0)

    K71.0 Toxic liver disease with cholestasis
> Cholestasis with hepatocyte injury
> 'Pure' cholestasis

    ●K71.1 Toxic liver disease with hepatic necrosis
> Hepatic failure (acute) (chronic) due to drugs

        K71.10 Toxic liver disease with hepatic necrosis, without coma

        K71.11 Toxic liver disease with hepatic necrosis, with coma

    K71.2 Toxic liver disease with acute hepatitis

    K71.3 Toxic liver disease with chronic persistent hepatitis

    K71.4 Toxic liver disease with chronic lobular hepatitis

    ●K71.5 Toxic liver disease with chronic active hepatitis
> Toxic liver disease with lupoid hepatitis

        K71.50 Toxic liver disease with chronic active hepatitis without ascites

        K71.51 Toxic liver disease with chronic active hepatitis with ascites

    K71.6 Toxic liver disease with hepatitis, not elsewhere classified

    K71.7 Toxic liver disease with fibrosis and cirrhosis of liver

    K71.8 Toxic liver disease with other disorders of liver
> Toxic liver disease with focal nodular hyperplasia
> Toxic liver disease with hepatic granulomas
> Toxic liver disease with peliosis hepatis
> Toxic liver disease with veno-occlusive disease of liver

    K71.9 Toxic liver disease, unspecified

Item 11–20 Cirrhosis is the progressive fibrosis of the liver resulting in loss of liver function. The main causes of cirrhosis of the liver are alcohol abuse, chronic hepatitis (inflammation of the liver), biliary disease, and excessive amounts of iron. **Alcoholic cirrhosis of the liver** is also called portal, Laënnec's, or fatty nutritional cirrhosis.

◄ New   ⧯ Revised   ~~deleted~~ Deleted   OGCR Official Guidelines   X Assign placeholder X   ● Use Additional Character(s)

| Excludes 1 | Excludes 2 | Includes | Use additional | Code first | Code also | Unspecified |

● **K72   Hepatic failure, not elsewhere classified**

    Includes   acute hepatitis NEC, with hepatic failure
                fulminant hepatitis NEC, with hepatic failure
                hepatic encephalopathy NOS
                liver (cell) necrosis with hepatic failure
                malignant hepatitis NEC, with hepatic failure
                yellow liver atrophy or dystrophy

    Excludes1   alcoholic hepatic failure (K70.4)
                hepatic failure with toxic liver disease (K71.1-)
                icterus of newborn (P55-P59)
                postprocedural hepatic failure (K91.82)
                viral hepatitis with hepatic coma (B15-B19)

    Excludes2   hepatic failure complicating abortion or ectopic
                    or molar pregnancy (O00-O07, O08.8)
                hepatic failure complicating pregnancy, childbirth
                    and the puerperium (O26.6-)

  ● **K72.0   Acute and subacute hepatic failure**

      K72.00   Acute and subacute hepatic failure without coma

      K72.01   Acute and subacute hepatic failure with coma

  ● **K72.1   Chronic hepatic failure**

      K72.10   Chronic hepatic failure without coma

      K72.11   Chronic hepatic failure with coma

  ● **K72.9   Hepatic failure, unspecified**

      K72.90   Hepatic failure, unspecified without coma

      K72.91   Hepatic failure, unspecified with coma
             Hepatic coma NOS

● **K73   Chronic hepatitis, not elsewhere classified**

    Excludes1   alcoholic hepatitis (chronic) (K70.1-)
                drug-induced hepatitis (chronic) (K71.-)
                granulomatous hepatitis (chronic) NEC (K75.3)
                reactive, nonspecific hepatitis (chronic) (K75.2)
                viral hepatitis (chronic) (B15-B19)

  K73.0   Chronic persistent hepatitis, not elsewhere classified

  K73.1   Chronic lobular hepatitis, not elsewhere classified

  K73.2   Chronic active hepatitis, not elsewhere classified

  K73.8   Other chronic hepatitis, not elsewhere classified

  K73.9   Chronic hepatitis, unspecified

● **K74   Fibrosis and cirrhosis of liver**

    Code also, if applicable, viral hepatitis (acute) (chronic) (B15-B19)

    Excludes1   alcoholic cirrhosis (of liver) (K70.3)
                alcoholic fibrosis of liver (K70.2)
                cardiac sclerosis of liver (K76.1)
                cirrhosis (of liver) with toxic liver disease (K71.7)
                congenital cirrhosis (of liver) (P78.81)
                pigmentary cirrhosis (of liver) (E83.110)

  K74.0   Hepatic fibrosis

  K74.1   Hepatic sclerosis

  K74.2   Hepatic fibrosis with hepatic sclerosis

  K74.3   Primary biliary cirrhosis
      Chronic nonsuppurative destructive cholangitis

  K74.4   Secondary biliary cirrhosis

  K74.5   Biliary cirrhosis, unspecified

  ● **K74.6   Other and unspecified cirrhosis of liver**

      K74.60   Unspecified cirrhosis of liver
             Cirrhosis (of liver) NOS

      K74.69   Other cirrhosis of liver
             Cryptogenic cirrhosis (of liver)
             Macronodular cirrhosis (of liver)
              Micronodular cirrhosis (of liver)
              Mixed type cirrhosis (of liver)
              Portal cirrhosis (of liver)
              Postnecrotic cirrhosis (of liver)

● **K75   Other inflammatory liver diseases**

    Excludes2   toxic liver disease (K71.-)

  K75.0   Abscess of liver
      Cholangitic hepatic abscess
      Hematogenic hepatic abscess
      Hepatic abscess NOS
      Lymphogenic hepatic abscess
      Pylephlebitic hepatic abscess

      Excludes1   amebic liver abscess (A06.4)
                  cholangitis without liver abscess (K83.0)
                  pylephlebitis without liver abscess
                    (K75.1)

  K75.1   Phlebitis of portal vein
      Pylephlebitis

      Excludes1   pylephlebitic liver abscess (K75.0)

  K75.2   Nonspecific reactive hepatitis

      Excludes1   acute or subacute hepatitis (K72.0-)
                  chronic hepatitis NEC (K73.-)
                  viral hepatitis (B15-B19)

  K75.3   Granulomatous hepatitis, not elsewhere classified

      Excludes1   acute or subacute hepatitis (K72.0-)
                  chronic hepatitis NEC (K73.-)
                  viral hepatitis (B15-B19)

  K75.4   Autoimmune hepatitis
      Lupoid hepatitis NEC

  ● **K75.8   Other specified inflammatory liver diseases**

      K75.81   Nonalcoholic steatohepatitis (NASH)

      K75.89   Other specified inflammatory liver diseases

  K75.9   Inflammatory liver disease, unspecified
      Hepatitis NOS

      Excludes1   acute or subacute hepatitis (K72.0-)
                  chronic hepatitis NEC (K73.-)
                  viral hepatitis (B15-B19)

● **K76   Other diseases of liver**

    Excludes2   alcoholic liver disease (K70.-)
                amyloid degeneration of liver (E85.-)
                cystic disease of liver (congenital) (Q44.6)
                hepatic vein thrombosis (I82.0)
                hepatomegaly NOS (R16.0)
                pigmentary cirrhosis (of liver) (E83.110)
                portal vein thrombosis (I81)
                toxic liver disease (K71.-)

  K76.0   Fatty (change of) liver, not elsewhere classified
      Nonalcoholic fatty liver disease (NAFLD)

      Excludes1   nonalcoholic steatohepatitis (NASH)
                  (K75.81)

  K76.1   Chronic passive congestion of liver
      Cardiac cirrhosis
      Cardiac sclerosis

  K76.2   Central hemorrhagic necrosis of liver

      Excludes1   liver necrosis with hepatic failure (K72.-)

  K76.3   Infarction of liver

  K76.4   Peliosis hepatis
      Hepatic angiomatosis

  K76.5   Hepatic veno-occlusive disease

      Excludes1   Budd-Chiari syndrome (I82.0)

  K76.6   Portal hypertension
      Use additional code for any associated complications,
          such as:
          portal hypertensive gastropathy (K31.89)

  K76.7   Hepatorenal syndrome

      Excludes1   hepatorenal syndrome following labor
                  and delivery (O90.4)
                  postprocedural hepatorenal syndrome
                    (K91.82)

CHAPTER 11 (K00-K95)

● **K76.8**   **Other specified diseases of liver**

    K76.81   **Hepatopulmonary syndrome**

        Code first underlying liver disease, such as:
          alcoholic cirrhosis of liver (K70.3-)
          cirrhosis of liver without mention of alcohol
            (K74.6-)

    K76.89   **Other specified diseases of liver**
        Cyst (simple) of liver
        Focal nodular hyperplasia of liver
        Hepatoptosis

  K76.9   **Liver disease, unspecified**

K77   **Liver disorders in diseases classified elsewhere**

    Code first underlying disease, such as:
      amyloidosis (E85.-)
      congenital syphilis (A50.0, A50.5)
      congenital toxoplasmosis (P37.1)
      schistosomiasis (B65.0-B65.9)

      Excludes1   alcoholic hepatitis (K70.1-)
            alcoholic liver disease (K70.-)
            cytomegaloviral hepatitis (B25.1)
            herpesviral [herpes simplex] hepatitis (B00.81)
            infectious mononucleosis with liver disease
              (B27.0-B27.9 with .9)
            mumps hepatitis (B26.81)
            sarcoidosis with liver disease (D86.89)
            secondary syphilis with liver disease (A51.45)
            syphilis (late) with liver disease (A52.74)
            toxoplasmosis (acquired) hepatitis (B58.1)
            tuberculosis with liver disease (A18.83)

DISORDERS OF GALLBLADDER, BILIARY TRACT AND PANCREAS (K80–K87)

● **K80**   **Cholelithiasis**

  Presence or formation of gallstones

  Excludes1   retained cholelithiasis following cholecystectomy
          (K91.86)

  ● **K80.0**   **Calculus of gallbladder with acute cholecystitis**
      Any condition listed in K80.2 with acute cholecystitis
      Check documentation for acute/chronic gallbladder/common
      bile duct either with or without obstruction.

    K80.00   **Calculus of gallbladder with acute cholecystitis
         without obstruction**

    K80.01   **Calculus of gallbladder with acute cholecystitis
         with obstruction**

  ● **K80.1**   **Calculus of gallbladder with other cholecystitis**

    K80.10   **Calculus of gallbladder with chronic
         cholecystitis without obstruction**
         Cholelithiasis with cholecystitis NOS

    K80.11   **Calculus of gallbladder with chronic
         cholecystitis with obstruction**

    K80.12   **Calculus of gallbladder with acute and chronic
         cholecystitis without obstruction**

    K80.13   **Calculus of gallbladder with acute and chronic
         cholecystitis with obstruction**

    K80.18   **Calculus of gallbladder with other cholecystitis
         without obstruction**

    K80.19   **Calculus of gallbladder with other cholecystitis
         with obstruction**

● **K80.2**   **Calculus of gallbladder without cholecystitis**
    Cholecystolithiasis without cholecystitis
    Cholelithiasis (without cholecystitis)
    Colic (recurrent) of gallbladder (without cholecystitis)
    Gallstone (impacted) of cystic duct (without
      cholecystitis)
    Gallstone (impacted) of gallbladder (without
      cholecystitis)

    K80.20   **Calculus of gallbladder without cholecystitis
         without obstruction**

    K80.21   **Calculus of gallbladder without cholecystitis
         with obstruction**

● **K80.3**   **Calculus of bile duct with cholangitis**
    Any condition listed in K80.5 with cholangitis

    K80.30   **Calculus of bile duct with cholangitis,
         unspecified, without obstruction**

    K80.31   **Calculus of bile duct with cholangitis,
         unspecified, with obstruction**

    K80.32   **Calculus of bile duct with acute cholangitis
         without obstruction**

    K80.33   **Calculus of bile duct with acute cholangitis
         with obstruction**

    K80.34   **Calculus of bile duct with chronic cholangitis
         without obstruction**

    K80.35   **Calculus of bile duct with chronic cholangitis
         with obstruction**

    K80.36   **Calculus of bile duct with acute and chronic
         cholangitis without obstruction**

    K80.37   **Calculus of bile duct with acute and chronic
         cholangitis with obstruction**

● **K80.4**   **Calculus of bile duct with cholecystitis**
    Any condition listed in K80.5 with cholecystitis (with
      cholangitis)

    K80.40   **Calculus of bile duct with cholecystitis,
         unspecified, without obstruction**

    K80.41   **Calculus of bile duct with cholecystitis,
         unspecified, with obstruction**

    K80.42   **Calculus of bile duct with acute cholecystitis
         without obstruction**

    K80.43   **Calculus of bile duct with acute cholecystitis
         with obstruction**

    K80.44   **Calculus of bile duct with chronic cholecystitis
         without obstruction**

    K80.45   **Calculus of bile duct with chronic cholecystitis
         with obstruction**

    K80.46   **Calculus of bile duct with acute and chronic
         cholecystitis without obstruction**

    K80.47   **Calculus of bile duct with acute and chronic
         cholecystitis with obstruction**

● **K80.5**   **Calculus of bile duct without cholangitis or cholecystitis**
    Choledocholithiasis (without cholangitis or
      cholecystitis)
    Gallstone (impacted) of bile duct NOS (without
      cholangitis or cholecystitis)
    Gallstone (impacted) of common duct (without
      cholangitis or cholecystitis)
    Gallstone (impacted) of hepatic duct (without
      cholangitis or cholecystitis)
    Hepatic cholelithiasis (without cholangitis or
      cholecystitis)
    Hepatic colic (recurrent) (without cholangitis or
      cholecystitis)

    K80.50   **Calculus of bile duct without cholangitis or
         cholecystitis without obstruction**

    K80.51   **Calculus of bile duct without cholangitis or
         cholecystitis with obstruction**

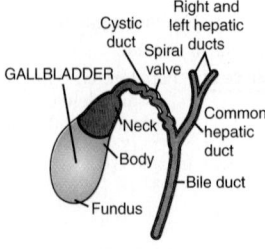

Figure 11-13   Gallbladder and bile ducts.

● **K80.6   Calculus of gallbladder and bile duct with cholecystitis**

     K80.60   Calculus of gallbladder and bile duct with cholecystitis unspecified, without obstruction

     K80.61   Calculus of gallbladder and bile duct with cholecystitis unspecified, with obstruction

     K80.62   Calculus of gallbladder and bile duct with acute cholecystitis without obstruction

     K80.63   Calculus of gallbladder and bile duct with acute cholecystitis with obstruction

     K80.64   Calculus of gallbladder and bile duct with chronic cholecystitis without obstruction

     K80.65   Calculus of gallbladder and bile duct with chronic cholecystitis with obstruction

     K80.66   Calculus of gallbladder and bile duct with acute and chronic cholecystitis without obstruction

     K80.67   Calculus of gallbladder and bile duct with acute and chronic cholecystitis with obstruction

● **K80.7   Calculus of gallbladder and bile duct without cholecystitis**

     K80.70   Calculus of gallbladder and bile duct without cholecystitis without obstruction

     K80.71   Calculus of gallbladder and bile duct without cholecystitis with obstruction

● **K80.8   Other cholelithiasis**

     K80.80   Other cholelithiasis without obstruction

     K80.81   Other cholelithiasis with obstruction

● **K81   Cholecystitis**

     Chronic or acute inflammation of the gallbladder.

     Excludes1   cholecystitis with cholelithiasis (K80.-)

     K81.0   Acute cholecystitis

         Abscess of gallbladder
         Angiocholecystitis
         Emphysematous (acute) cholecystitis
         Empyema of gallbladder
         Gangrene of gallbladder
         Gangrenous cholecystitis
         Suppurative cholecystitis

     K81.1   Chronic cholecystitis

     K81.2   Acute cholecystitis with chronic cholecystitis

     K81.9   Cholecystitis, unspecified

● **K82   Other diseases of gallbladder**

     Excludes1   nonvisualization of gallbladder (R93.2)
                postcholecystectomy syndrome (K91.5)

     K82.0   Obstruction of gallbladder

         Occlusion of cystic duct or gallbladder without cholelithiasis
         Stenosis of cystic duct or gallbladder without cholelithiasis
         Stricture of cystic duct or gallbladder without cholelithiasis

         Excludes1   obstruction of gallbladder with cholelithiasis (K80.-)

     K82.1   Hydrops of gallbladder

         Mucocele of gallbladder

     K82.2   Perforation of gallbladder

         Rupture of cystic duct or gallbladder

     K82.3   Fistula of gallbladder

         Cholecystocolic fistula
         Cholecystoduodenal fistula

     K82.4   Cholesterolosis of gallbladder

         Strawberry gallbladder

         Excludes1   cholesterolosis of gallbladder with cholecystitis (K81.-)
                     cholesterolosis of gallbladder with cholelithiasis (K80.-)

     K82.8   Other specified diseases of gallbladder

         Adhesions of cystic duct or gallbladder
         Atrophy of cystic duct or gallbladder
         Cyst of cystic duct or gallbladder
         Dyskinesia of cystic duct or gallbladder
         Hypertrophy of cystic duct or gallbladder
         Nonfunctioning of cystic duct or gallbladder
         Ulcer of cystic duct or gallbladder

     K82.9   Disease of gallbladder, unspecified

● **K83   Other diseases of biliary tract**

     Excludes1   postcholecystectomy syndrome (K91.5)

     Excludes2   conditions involving the gallbladder (K81-K82)
                conditions involving the cystic duct (K81-K82)

     K83.0   Cholangitis

         Ascending cholangitis   Sclerosing cholangitis
         Cholangitis NOS   Secondary cholangitis
         Primary cholangitis   Stenosing cholangitis
         Recurrent cholangitis   Suppurative cholangitis

         Excludes1   cholangitic liver abscess (K75.0)
                     cholangitis with choledocholithiasis (K80.3-, K80.4-)
                     chronic nonsuppurative destructive cholangitis (K74.3)

     K83.1   Obstruction of bile duct

         Occlusion of bile duct without cholelithiasis
         Stenosis of bile duct without cholelithiasis
         Stricture of bile duct without cholelithiasis

         Excludes1   congenital obstruction of bile duct (Q44.3)
                     obstruction of bile duct with cholelithiasis (K80.-)

     K83.2   Perforation of bile duct

         Rupture of bile duct

     K83.3   Fistula of bile duct

         Choledochoduodenal fistula

     K83.4   Spasm of sphincter of Oddi

     K83.5   Biliary cyst

     K83.8   Other specified diseases of biliary tract

         Adhesions of biliary tract
         Atrophy of biliary tract
         Hypertrophy of biliary tract
         Ulcer of biliary tract

     K83.9   Disease of biliary tract, unspecified

● **K85   Acute pancreatitis**

     Inflammatory process in which pancreatic enzymes autodigest the gland.

     Includes   abscess of pancreas
                acute necrosis of pancreas
                acute (recurrent) pancreatitis
                gangrene of (gangrenous) pancreas
                hemorrhagic pancreatitis
                infective necrosis of pancreas
                subacute pancreatitis
                suppurative pancreatitis

     K85.0   Idiopathic acute pancreatitis

     K85.1   Biliary acute pancreatitis

         Gallstone pancreatitis

     K85.2   Alcohol induced acute pancreatitis

         Excludes2   alcohol induced chronic pancreatitis (K86.0)

     K85.3   Drug induced acute pancreatitis

         Use additional code for adverse effect, if applicable, to identify drug (T36-T50 with fifth or sixth character 5)

         Use additional code to identify drug abuse and dependence (F11.-F17.-)

     K85.8   Other acute pancreatitis

     K85.9   Acute pancreatitis, unspecified

         Pancreatitis NOS

CHAPTER 11 (K00-K95)

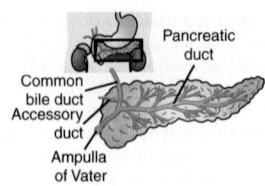

Figure 11-14   Pancreatic ductal system.

● **K86   Other diseases of pancreas**
> **Excludes2**   fibrocystic disease of pancreas (E84.-)
> islet cell tumor (of pancreas) (D13.7)
> pancreatic steatorrhea (K90.3)

K86.0   Alcohol-induced chronic pancreatitis
> Use additional code to identify:
> alcohol abuse and dependence (F10.-)
> > **Excludes2**   alcohol induced acute pancreatitis (K85.2)

K86.1   Other chronic pancreatitis
> Chronic pancreatitis NOS
> Infectious chronic pancreatitis
> Recurrent chronic pancreatitis
> Relapsing chronic pancreatitis

K86.2   Cyst of pancreas

K86.3   Pseudocyst of pancreas

K86.8   Other specified diseases of pancreas
> Aseptic pancreatic necrosis
> Atrophy of pancreas
> Calculus of pancreas
> Cirrhosis of pancreas
> Fibrosis of pancreas
> Pancreatic fat necrosis
> Pancreatic infantilism
> Pancreatic necrosis NOS

K86.9   Disease of pancreas, unspecified

K87   Disorders of gallbladder, biliary tract and pancreas in diseases classified elsewhere
> *Code first underlying disease*
> **Excludes1**   cytomegaloviral pancreatitis (B25.2)
> mumps pancreatitis (B26.3)
> syphilitic gallbladder (A52.74)
> syphilitic pancreas (A52.74)
> tuberculosis of gallbladder (A18.83)
> tuberculosis of pancreas (A18.83)

OTHER DISEASES OF THE DIGESTIVE SYSTEM (K90-K95)

● **K90   Intestinal malabsorption**
> **Excludes1**   intestinal malabsorption following gastrointestinal surgery (K91.2)

K90.0   Celiac disease
> Gluten-sensitive enteropathy
> Idiopathic steatorrhea
> Nontropical sprue
> Use additional code for associated disorders including:
> dermatitis herpetiformis (L13.0)
> gluten ataxia (G32.81)

K90.1   Tropical sprue
> Sprue NOS
> Tropical steatorrhea

K90.2   Blind loop syndrome, not elsewhere classified
> Blind loop syndrome NOS
> > **Excludes1**   congenital blind loop syndrome (Q43.8)
> > postsurgical blind loop syndrome (K91.2)

K90.3   Pancreatic steatorrhea

K90.4   Malabsorption due to intolerance, not elsewhere classified
> Malabsorption due to intolerance to carbohydrate
> Malabsorption due to intolerance to fat
> Malabsorption due to intolerance to protein
> Malabsorption due to intolerance to starch
> > **Excludes2**   gluten-sensitive enteropathy (K90.0)
> > lactose intolerance (E73.-)

● **K90.8   Other intestinal malabsorption**

K90.81   Whipple's disease

K90.89   Other intestinal malabsorption

K90.9   Intestinal malabsorption, unspecified

● **K91   Intraoperative and postprocedural complications and disorders of digestive system, not elsewhere classified**
> **Excludes2**   complications of artificial opening of digestive system (K94.-)
> complications of bariatric procedures (K95.-)
> gastrojejunal ulcer (K28.-)
> postprocedural (radiation) retroperitoneal abscess (K68.11)
> radiation colitis (K52.0)
> radiation gastroenteritis (K52.0)
> radiation proctitis (K62.7)

K91.0   Vomiting following gastrointestinal surgery

K91.1   Postgastric surgery syndromes
> Dumping syndrome
> Postgastrectomy syndrome
> Postvagotomy syndrome

K91.2   Postsurgical malabsorption, not elsewhere classified
> Postsurgical blind loop syndrome
> > **Excludes1**   malabsorption osteomalacia in adults (M83.2)
> > malabsorption osteoporosis, postsurgical (M80.8-, M81.8)

K91.3   Postprocedural intestinal obstruction

K91.5   Postcholecystectomy syndrome

● **K91.6   Intraoperative hemorrhage and hematoma of a digestive system organ or structure complicating a procedure**
> **Excludes1**   intraoperative hemorrhage and hematoma of a digestive system organ or structure due to accidental puncture and laceration during a procedure (K91.7-)

K91.61   Intraoperative hemorrhage and hematoma of a digestive system organ or structure complicating a digestive sytem procedure

K91.62   Intraoperative hemorrhage and hematoma of a digestive system organ or structure complicating other procedure

● **K91.7   Accidental puncture and laceration of a digestive system organ or structure during a procedure**

K91.71   Accidental puncture and laceration of a digestive system organ or structure during a digestive system procedure

K91.72   Accidental puncture and laceration of a digestive system organ or structure during other procedure

● **K91.8   Other intraoperative and postprocedural complications and disorders of digestive system**

K91.81   Other intraoperative complications of digestive system

K91.82   Postprocedural hepatic failure

K91.83   Postprocedural hepatorenal syndrome

● **K91.84** **Postprocedural hemorrhage and hematoma of a digestive system organ or structure following a procedure**

     K91.840 **Postprocedural hemorrhage and hematoma of a digestive system organ or structure following a digestive system procedure**

     K91.841 **Postprocedural hemorrhage and hematoma of a digestive system organ or structure following other procedure**

● **K91.85** **Complications of intestinal pouch**

     K91.850 **Pouchitis**
         Inflammation of internal ileoanal pouch

     K91.858 **Other complications of intestinal pouch**

K91.86 **Retained cholelithiasis following cholecystectomy**

K91.89 **Other postprocedural complications and disorders of digestive system**
     Use additional code, if applicable, to further specify disorder
     Excludes2   postprocedural retroperitoneal abscess (K68.11)

● **K92** **Other diseases of digestive system**
     Excludes1   neonatal gastrointestinal hemorrhage (P54.0-P54.3)

K92.0 **Hematemesis**

K92.1 **Melena**
     Excludes1   occult blood in feces (R19.5)

K92.2 **Gastrointestinal hemorrhage, unspecified**
     Gastric hemorrhage NOS
     Intestinal hemorrhage NOS
     Excludes1   acute hemorrhagic gastritis (K29.01)
         hemorrhage of anus and rectum (K62.5)
         angiodysplasia of stomach with hemorrhage (K31.811)
         diverticular disease with hemorrhage (K57.-)
         gastritis and duodenitis with hemorrhage (K29.-)
         peptic ulcer with hemorrhage (K25-K28)

● **K92.8** **Other specified diseases of the digestive system**

     K92.81 **Gastrointestinal mucositis (ulcerative)**
         Code also type of associated therapy, such as:
         antineoplastic and immunosuppressive drugs (T45.1X-)
         radiological procedure and radiotherapy (Y84.2)
         Excludes2   mucositis (ulcerative) of vagina and vulva (N76.81)
             nasal mucositis (ulcerative) (J34.81)
             oral mucositis (ulcerative) (K12.3-)

     K92.89 **Other specified diseases of the digestive system**

K92.9 **Disease of digestive system, unspecified**

● **K94** **Complications of artificial openings of the digestive system**

● **K94.0** **Colostomy complications**

     K94.00 **Colostomy complication, unspecified**

     K94.01 **Colostomy hemorrhage**

     K94.02 **Colostomy infection**
         Use additional code to specify type of infection, such as:
         cellulitis of abdominal wall (L03.311)
         sepsis (A40.-, A41.-)

     K94.03 **Colostomy malfunction**
         Mechanical complication of colostomy

     K94.09 **Other complications of colostomy**

● **K94.1** **Enterostomy complications**

     K94.10 **Enterostomy complication, unspecified**

     K94.11 **Enterostomy hemorrhage**

     K94.12 **Enterostomy infection**
         Use additional code to specify type of infection, such as:
         cellulitis of abdominal wall (L03.311)
         sepsis (A40.-, A41.-)

     K94.13 **Enterostomy malfunction**
         Mechanical complication of enterostomy

     K94.19 **Other complications of enterostomy**

● **K94.2** **Gastrostomy complications**

     K94.20 **Gastrostomy complication, unspecified**

     K94.21 **Gastrostomy hemorrhage**

     K94.22 **Gastrostomy infection**
         Use additional code to specify type of infection, such as:
         cellulitis of abdominal wall (L03.311)
         sepsis (A40.-, A41.-)

     K94.23 **Gastrostomy malfunction**
         Mechanical complication of gastrostomy

     K94.29 **Other complications of gastrostomy**

● **K94.3** **Esophagostomy complications**

     K94.30 **Esophagostomy complications, unspecified**

     K94.31 **Esophagostomy hemorrhage**

     K94.32 **Esophagostomy infection**
         Use additional code to identify the infection

     K94.33 **Esophagostomy malfunction**
         Mechanical complication of esophagostomy

     K94.39 **Other complications of esophagostomy**

● **K95** **Complications of bariatric procedures**

● **K95.0** **Complications of gastric band procedure**

     K95.01 **Infection due to gastric band procedure**
         Use additional code to specify type of infection or organism, such as:
         bacterial and viral infectious agents (B95.-, B96.-)
         cellulitis of abdominal wall (L03.311)
         sepsis (A40.-, A41.-)

     K95.09 **Other complications of gastric band procedure**
         Use additional code, if applicable, to further specify complication

● **K95.8** **Complications of other bariatric procedure**
     Excludes1   complications of gastric band surgery (K95.0-)

     K95.81 **Infection due to other bariatric procedure**
         Use additional code to specify type of infection or organism, such as:
         bacterial and viral infectious agents (B95.-, B96.-)
         cellulitis of abdominal wall (L03.311)
         sepsis (A40.-, A41.-)

     K95.89 **Other complications of other bariatric procedure**
         Use additional code, if applicable, to further specify complication

CHAPTER 11 (K00-K95)

◀ New   ⬅ Revised   ~~deleted~~ Deleted   OGCR Official Guidelines   X Assign placeholder X   ● Use Additional Character(s)

Excludes 1   Excludes 2   Includes   Use additional   Code first   Code also   Unspecified

Figure 12-1 Furuncle, also known as a boil, is a staphylococcal infection. The organism enters the body through a hair follicle and so furuncles usually appear in hairy areas of the body. A cluster of furuncles is known as a carbuncle and involves infection into the deep subcutaneous fascia. These usually appear on the back and neck. (**B** from Habif: Clinical Dermatology, ed 5, Mosby, 2009)

CHAPTER 12

DISEASES OF THE SKIN AND SUBCUTANEOUS TISSUE (L00-L99)

Excludes2   certain conditions originating in the perinatal period (P04-P96)
certain infectious and parasitic diseases (A00-B99)
complications of pregnancy, childbirth and the puerperium (O00-O9A)
congenital malformations, deformations, and chromosomal abnormalities (Q00-Q99)
endocrine, nutritional and metabolic diseases (E00-E88)
lipomelanotic reticulosis (I89.8)
neoplasms (C00-D49)
symptoms, signs and abnormal clinical and laboratory findings, not elsewhere classified (R00-R94)
systemic connective tissue disorders (M30-M36)
viral warts (B07.-)

This chapter contains the following blocks:

L00-L08	Infections of the skin and subcutaneous tissue
L10-L14	Bullous disorders
L20-L30	Dermatitis and eczema
L40-L45	Papulosquamous disorders
L49-L54	Urticaria and erythema
L55-L59	Radiation-related disorders of the skin and subcutaneous tissue
L60-L75	Disorders of skin appendages
L76	Intraoperative and postprocedural complications of skin and subcutaneous tissue
L80-L99	Other disorders of the skin and subcutaneous tissue

INFECTIONS OF THE SKIN AND SUBCUTANEOUS TISSUE (L00-L08)

Use additional code (B95-B97) to identify infectious agent.

Excludes2   hordeolum (H00.0)
infective dermatitis (L30.3)
local infections of skin classified in Chapter 1
lupus panniculitis (L93.2)
panniculitis NOS (M79.3)
panniculitis of neck and back (M54.0-)
Perlèche NOS (K13.0)
Perlèche due to candidiasis (B37.0)
Perlèche due to riboflavin deficiency (E53.0)
pyogenic granuloma (L98.0)
relapsing panniculitis [Weber-Christian] (M35.6)
viral warts (B07.-)
zoster (B02.-)

L00   **Staphylococcal scalded skin syndrome**
Ritter's disease
Use additional code to identify percentage of skin exfoliation (L49.-)
Excludes1   bullous impetigo (L01.03)
pemphigus neonatorum (L01.03)
toxic epidermal necrolysis [Lyell] (L51.2)

● **L01**   **Impetigo**
Contagious skin infection caused by a streptococcus or staphylococcus aureus, common skin infections among children.
Excludes1   impetigo herpetiformis (L40.1)
● **L01.0**   **Impetigo**
Impetigo contagiosa
Impetigo vulgaris
    L01.00   **Impetigo, unspecified**
Impetigo NOS
    L01.01   **Non-bullous impetigo**
    L01.02   **Bockhart's impetigo**
Impetigo follicularis
Perifolliculitis NOS
Superficial pustular perifolliculitis
    L01.03   **Bullous impetigo**
Impetigo neonatorum
Pemphigus neonatorum
Neonate = newborn
    L01.09   **Other impetigo**
Ulcerative impetigo
   L01.1   **Impetiginization of other dermatoses**

● **L02**   **Cutaneous abscess, furuncle and carbuncle**
Use additional code to identify organism (B95-B96)
Excludes2   abscess of anus and rectal regions (K61.-)
abscess of female genital organs (external) (N76.4)
abscess of male genital organs (external) (N48.2, N49.-)
● **L02.0**   **Cutaneous abscess, furuncle and carbuncle of face**
Excludes2   abscess of ear, external (H60.0)
abscess of eyelid (H00.0)
abscess of head [any part, except face] (L02.8)
abscess of lacrimal gland (H04.0)
abscess of lacrimal passages (H04.3)
abscess of mouth (K12.2)
abscess of nose (J34.0)
abscess of orbit (H05.0)
submandibular abscess (K12.2)
    L02.01   **Cutaneous abscess of face**
    L02.02   **Furuncle of face**
Boil of face
Folliculitis of face
    L02.03   **Carbuncle of face**
● **L02.1**   **Cutaneous abscess, furuncle and carbuncle of neck**
    L02.11   **Cutaneous abscess of neck**
    L02.12   **Furuncle of neck**
Boil of neck
Folliculitis of neck
    L02.13   **Carbuncle of neck**
● **L02.2**   **Cutaneous abscess, furuncle and carbuncle of trunk**
Excludes1   non-newborn omphalitis (L08.82)
omphalitis of newborn (P38.-)
Excludes2   abscess of breast (N61)
abscess of buttocks (L02.3)
abscess of female external genital organs (N76.4)
abscess of male external genital organs (N48.2, N49.-)
abscess of hip (L02.4)

● **L02.21**   **Cutaneous abscess of trunk**
- **L02.211**   Cutaneous abscess of abdominal wall
- **L02.212**   Cutaneous abscess of back [any part, except buttock]
- **L02.213**   Cutaneous abscess of chest wall
- **L02.214**   Cutaneous abscess of groin
- **L02.215**   Cutaneous abscess of perineum
- **L02.216**   Cutaneous abscess of umbilicus
- **L02.219**   Cutaneous abscess of trunk, unspecified

● **L02.22**   **Furuncle of trunk**
    Boil of trunk
    Folliculitis of trunk
- **L02.221**   Furuncle of abdominal wall
- **L02.222**   Furuncle of back [any part, except buttock]
- **L02.223**   Furuncle of chest wall
- **L02.224**   Furuncle of groin
- **L02.225**   Furuncle of perineum
- **L02.226**   Furuncle of umbilicus
- **L02.229**   Furuncle of trunk, unspecified

● **L02.23**   **Carbuncle of trunk**
- **L02.231**   Carbuncle of abdominal wall
- **L02.232**   Carbuncle of back [any part, except buttock]
- **L02.233**   Carbuncle of chest wall
- **L02.234**   Carbuncle of groin
- **L02.235**   Carbuncle of perineum
- **L02.236**   Carbuncle of umbilicus
- **L02.239**   Carbuncle of trunk, unspecified

● **L02.3**   **Cutaneous abscess, furuncle and carbuncle of buttock**
    | Excludes1 | pilonidal cyst with abscess (L05.01)
- **L02.31**   **Cutaneous abscess of buttock**
    Cutaneous abscess of gluteal region
- **L02.32**   **Furuncle of buttock**
    Boil of buttock
    Folliculitis of buttock
    Furuncle of gluteal region
- **L02.33**   **Carbuncle of buttock**
    Carbuncle of gluteal region

● **L02.4**   **Cutaneous abscess, furuncle and carbuncle of limb**
    | Excludes2 | Cutaneous abscess, furuncle and carbuncle of groin (L02.214, L02.224, L02.234)
    Cutaneous abscess, furuncle and carbuncle of hand (L02.5-)
    Cutaneous abscess, furuncle and carbuncle of foot (L02.6-)
- ● **L02.41**   **Cutaneous abscess of limb**
  - **L02.411**   Cutaneous abscess of right axilla
  - **L02.412**   Cutaneous abscess of left axilla
  - **L02.413**   Cutaneous abscess of right upper limb
  - **L02.414**   Cutaneous abscess of left upper limb
  - **L02.415**   Cutaneous abscess of right lower limb
  - **L02.416**   Cutaneous abscess of left lower limb
  - **L02.419**   Cutaneous abscess of limb, unspecified
- ● **L02.42**   **Furuncle of limb**
      Boil of limb
      Folliculitis of limb
  - **L02.421**   Furuncle of right axilla
  - **L02.422**   Furuncle of left axilla
  - **L02.423**   Furuncle of right upper limb

- **L02.424**   Furuncle of left upper limb
- **L02.425**   Furuncle of right lower limb
- **L02.426**   Furuncle of left lower limb
- **L02.429**   Furuncle of limb, unspecified

● **L02.43**   **Carbuncle of limb**
- **L02.431**   Carbuncle of right axilla
- **L02.432**   Carbuncle of left axilla
- **L02.433**   Carbuncle of right upper limb
- **L02.434**   Carbuncle of left upper limb
- **L02.435**   Carbuncle of right lower limb
- **L02.436**   Carbuncle of left lower limb
- **L02.439**   Carbuncle of limb, unspecified

● **L02.5**   **Cutaneous abscess, furuncle and carbuncle of hand**
- ● **L02.51**   **Cutaneous abscess of hand**
  - **L02.511**   Cutaneous abscess of right hand
  - **L02.512**   Cutaneous abscess of left hand
  - **L02.519**   Cutaneous abscess of unspecified hand
- ● **L02.52**   **Furuncle hand**
      Boil of hand
      Folliculitis of hand
  - **L02.521**   Furuncle right hand
  - **L02.522**   Furuncle left hand
  - **L02.529**   Furuncle unspecified hand
- ● **L02.53**   **Carbuncle of hand**
  - **L02.531**   Carbuncle of right hand
  - **L02.532**   Carbuncle of left hand
  - **L02.539**   Carbuncle of unspecified hand

● **L02.6**   **Cutaneous abscess, furuncle and carbuncle of foot**
- ● **L02.61**   **Cutaneous abscess of foot**
  - **L02.611**   Cutaneous abscess of right foot
  - **L02.612**   Cutaneous abscess of left foot
  - **L02.619**   Cutaneous abscess of unspecified foot
- ● **L02.62**   **Furuncle of foot**
      Boil of foot
      Folliculitis of foot
  - **L02.621**   Furuncle of right foot
  - **L02.622**   Furuncle of left foot
  - **L02.629**   Furuncle of unspecified foot
- ● **L02.63**   **Carbuncle of foot**
  - **L02.631**   Carbuncle of right foot
  - **L02.632**   Carbuncle of left foot
  - **L02.639**   Carbuncle of unspecified foot

● **L02.8**   **Cutaneous abscess, furuncle and carbuncle of other sites**
- ● **L02.81**   **Cutaneous abscess of other sites**
  - **L02.811**   Cutaneous abscess of head [any part, except face]
  - **L02.818**   Cutaneous abscess of other sites
- ● **L02.82**   **Furuncle of other sites**
      Boil of other sites
      Folliculitis of other sites
  - **L02.821**   Furuncle of head [any part, except face]
  - **L02.828**   Furuncle of other sites
- ● **L02.83**   **Carbuncle of other sites**
  - **L02.831**   Carbuncle of head [any part, except face]
  - **L02.838**   Carbuncle of other sites

● **L02.9**   **Cutaneous abscess, furuncle and carbuncle, unspecified**
- **L02.91**   **Cutaneous abscess, unspecified**
- **L02.92**   **Furuncle, unspecified**
      Boil NOS
      Furunculosis NOS
- **L02.93**   **Carbuncle, unspecified**

CHAPTER 12 (L00-L99)

Item 12-1 Onychia is an inflammation of the tissue surrounding the nail with pus accumulation and loss of the nail, resulting from microscopic pathogens entering through small wounds. **Paronychia** is a nail disease also known as felon or whitlow and is a bacterial or fungal infection.

● **L03 Cellulitis and acute lymphangitis**
     Excludes2   cellulitis of anal and rectal region (K61.-)
                   cellulitis of external auditory canal (H60.1)
                   cellulitis of eyelid (H00.0)
                   cellulitis of female external genital organs (N76.4)
                   cellulitis of lacrimal apparatus (H04.3)
                   cellulitis of male external genital organs (N48.2, N49.-)
                   cellulitis of mouth (K12.2)
                   cellulitis of nose (J34.0)
                   eosinophilic cellulitis [Wells] (L98.3)
                   febrile neutrophilic dermatosis [Sweet] (L98.2)
                   lymphangitis (chronic) (subacute) (I89.1)

   ● **L03.0 Cellulitis and acute lymphangitis of finger and toe**
       Infection of nail
       Onychia
       Paronychia
       Perionychia

     ● **L03.01 Cellulitis of finger**
         Felon
         Whitlow
         Excludes1   herpetic whitlow (B00.89)
         L03.011   **Cellulitis of right finger**
         L03.012   **Cellulitis of left finger**
         L03.019   **Cellulitis of unspecified finger**

     ● **L03.02 Acute lymphangitis of finger**
         Hangnail with lymphangitis of finger
         L03.021   **Acute lymphangitis of right finger**
         L03.022   **Acute lymphangitis of left finger**
         L03.029   **Acute lymphangitis of unspecified finger**

     ● **L03.03 Cellulitis of toe**
         L03.031   **Cellulitis of right toe**
         L03.032   **Cellulitis of left toe**
         L03.039   **Cellulitis of unspecified toe**

     ● **L03.04 Acute lymphangitis of toe**
         Hangnail with lymphangitis of toe
         L03.041   **Acute lymphangitis of right toe**
         L03.042   **Acute lymphangitis of left toe**
         L03.049   **Acute lymphangitis of unspecified toe**

   ● **L03.1 Cellulitis and acute lymphangitis of other parts of limb**
     ● **L03.11 Cellulitis of other parts of limb**
         Excludes2   cellulitis of fingers (L03.01-)
                       cellulitis of toes (L03.03-)
                       groin (L03.314)
         L03.111   **Cellulitis of right axilla**
         L03.112   **Cellulitis of left axilla**
         L03.113   **Cellulitis of right upper limb**
         L03.114   **Cellulitis of left upper limb**
         L03.115   **Cellulitis of right lower limb**
         L03.116   **Cellulitis of left lower limb**
         L03.119   **Cellulitis of unspecified part of limb**

     ● **L03.12 Acute lymphangitis of other parts of limb**
         Excludes2   acute lymphangitis of fingers (L03.2-)
                       acute lymphangitis of toes (L03.04-)
                       acute lymphangitis of groin (L03.324)
         L03.121   **Acute lymphangitis of right axilla**
         L03.122   **Acute lymphangitis of left axilla**

         L03.123   **Acute lymphangitis of right upper limb**
         L03.124   **Acute lymphangitis of left upper limb**
         L03.125   **Acute lymphangitis of right lower limb**
         L03.126   **Acute lymphangitis of left lower limb**
         L03.129   **Acute lymphangitis of unspecified part of limb**

   ● **L03.2 Cellulitis and acute lymphangitis of face and neck**
     ● **L03.21 Cellulitis and acute lymphangitis of face**
         L03.211   **Cellulitis of face**
             Excludes2   cellulitis of ear (H60.1-)
                         cellulitis of eyelid (H00.0-)
                         cellulitis of head (L03.81)
                         cellulitis of lacrimal apparatus (H04.3)
                         cellulitis of lip (K13.0)
                         cellulitis of mouth (K12.2)
                         cellulitis of nose (internal) (J34.0)
                         cellulitis of orbit (H05.0)
                         cellulitis of scalp (L03.81)

         L03.212   **Acute lymphangitis of face**
     ● **L03.22 Cellulitis and acute lymphangitis of neck**
         L03.221   **Cellulitis of neck**
         L03.222   **Acute lymphangitis of neck**

   ● **L03.3 Cellulitis and acute lymphangitis of trunk**
     ● **L03.31 Cellulitis of trunk**
         Excludes2   cellulitis of anal and rectal regions (K61.-)
                       cellulitis of breast NOS (N61)
                       cellulitis of female external genital organs (N76.4)
                       cellulitis of male external genital organs (N48.2, N49.-)
                       omphalitis of newborn (P38.-)
                       puerperal cellulitis of breast (O91.2)

         L03.311   **Cellulitis of abdominal wall**
             Excludes2   cellulitis of umbilicus (L03.316)
                         cellulitis of groin (L03.314)
         L03.312   **Cellulitis of back [any part except buttock]**
         L03.313   **Cellulitis of chest wall**
         L03.314   **Cellulitis of groin**
         L03.315   **Cellulitis of perineum**
         L03.316   **Cellulitis of umbilicus**
         L03.317   **Cellulitis of buttock**
         L03.319   **Cellulitis of trunk, unspecified**

Item 12–2 Cellulitis is an acute spreading bacterial infection below the surface of the skin characterized by redness (erythema), warmth, swelling, pain, fever, chills, and enlarged lymph nodes ("swollen glands").

L03.32   Acute lymphangitis of trunk
    L03.321   Acute lymphangitis of abdominal wall
    L03.322   Acute lymphangitis of back [any part except buttock]
    L03.323   Acute lymphangitis of chest wall
    L03.324   Acute lymphangitis of groin
    L03.325   Acute lymphangitis of perineum
    L03.326   Acute lymphangitis of umbilicus
    L03.327   Acute lymphangitis of buttock
    L03.329   Acute lymphangitis of trunk, unspecified

L03.8   Cellulitis and acute lymphangitis of other sites
  L03.81   Cellulitis of other sites
    L03.811   Cellulitis of head [any part, except face]
      Cellulitis of scalp
      Excludes2   cellulitis of face (L03.211)
    L03.818   Cellulitis of other sites
  L03.89   Acute lymphangitis of other sites
    L03.891   Acute lymphangitis of head [any part, except face]
    L03.898   Acute lymphangitis of other sites

L03.9   Cellulitis and acute lymphangitis, unspecified
  L03.90   Cellulitis, unspecified
  L03.91   Acute lymphangitis, unspecified
    Excludes1   lymphangitis NOS (I89.1)

L04   Acute lymphadenitis
    Short-term inflammation of lymph nodes which can be regionalized to involve a given area of the lymph system or systemic involving much of the body
    Includes   abscess (acute) of lymph nodes, except mesenteric
        acute lymphadenitis, except mesenteric
    Excludes1   chronic or subacute lymphadenitis, except mesenteric (I88.1)
        enlarged lymph nodes (R59.-)
        human immunodeficiency virus [HIV] disease resulting in generalized lymphadenopathy (B20)
        lymphadenitis NOS (I88.9)
        nonspecific mesenteric lymphadenitis (I88.0)
  L04.0   Acute lymphadenitis of face, head and neck
  L04.1   Acute lymphadenitis of trunk
  L04.2   Acute lymphadenitis of upper limb
    Acute lymphadenitis of axilla
    Acute lymphadenitis of shoulder
  L04.3   Acute lymphadenitis of lower limb
    Acute lymphadenitis of hip
    Excludes2   acute lymphadenitis of groin (L04.1)
  L04.8   Acute lymphadenitis of other sites
  L04.9   Acute lymphadenitis, unspecified

L05   Pilonidal cyst and sinus
  L05.0   Pilonidal cyst and sinus with abscess
    L05.01   Pilonidal cyst with abscess
      Parasacral dimple with abscess
      Pilonidal abscess
      Pilonidal dimple with abscess
      Postanal dimple with abscess
    L05.02   Pilonidal sinus with abscess
      Coccygeal fistula with abscess
      Coccygeal sinus with abscess
      Pilonidal fistula with abscess

Figure 12-2 Impetigo. A thick, honey-yellow adherent crust covers the entire eroded surface. (From Habif: Clinical Dermatology, ed 4, Mosby, Inc., 2004)

Item 12–3   Abscess is a localized collection of pus in tissues or organs and is a sign of infection resulting in swelling and inflammation.

Item 12–4   Pilonidal cyst, also called a coccygeal cyst, is the result of a disorder called pilonidal disease. The cyst usually contains hair and pus.

L05.9   Pilonidal cyst and sinus without abscess
  L05.91   Pilonidal cyst without abscess
    Parasacral dimple
    Pilonidal dimple
    Postanal dimple
    Pilonidal cyst NOS
  L05.92   Pilonidal sinus without abscess
    Coccygeal fistula
    Coccygeal sinus without abscess
    Pilonidal fistula

L08   Other local infections of skin and subcutaneous tissue
  L08.0   Pyoderma
    Dermatitis gangrenosa
    Purulent dermatitis
    Septic dermatitis
    Suppurative dermatitis
    Excludes1   pyoderma gangrenosum (L88)
        pyoderma vegetans (L08.81)
  L08.1   Erythrasma
  L08.8   Other specified local infections of the skin and subcutaneous tissue
    L08.81   Pyoderma vegetans
      Excludes1   pyoderma gangrenosum (L88)
        pyoderma NOS (L08.0)
    L08.82   Omphalitis not of newborn
      Excludes1   omphalitis of newborn (P38.-)
    L08.89   Other specified local infections of the skin and subcutaneous tissue
  L08.9   Local infection of the skin and subcutaneous tissue, unspecified

BULLOUS DISORDERS (L10-L14)

  Excludes1   benign familial pemphigus [Hailey-Hailey] (Q82.8)
    staphylococcal scalded skin syndrome (L00)
    toxic epidermal necrolysis [Lyell] (L51.2)

L10   Pemphigus
  Excludes1   pemphigus neonatorum (L01.03)
  L10.0   Pemphigus vulgaris
  L10.1   Pemphigus vegetans
  L10.2   Pemphigus foliaceous
  L10.3   Brazilian pemphigus [fogo selvagem]
  L10.4   Pemphigus erythematosus
    Senear-Usher syndrome
  L10.5   Drug-induced pemphigus
    Use additional code for adverse effect, if applicable, to identify drug (T36-T50 with fifth or sixth character 5)
  L10.8   Other pemphigus
    L10.81   Paraneoplastic pemphigus
    L10.89   Other pemphigus
  L10.9   Pemphigus, unspecified

CHAPTER 12 (L00-L99)

Item 12-5 Dermatitis herpetiformis, also known as Duhring's disease, is a systemic disease characterized by small blisters (3 to 5 mm) and occasionally large bullae (> 5 mm).

Figure 12-3 Dermatitis herpetiformis. (From Arnold HL, Odom RB, James WD: Andrews' Diseases of the Skin, Clinical Dermatology, ed 8, Philadelphia, WB Saunders, 1990)

● **L11 Other acantholytic disorders**

　　L11.0 Acquired keratosis follicularis
　　　　| **Excludes1** | keratosis follicularis (congenital) [Darier-White] (Q82.8) |

　　L11.1 Transient acantholytic dermatosis [Grover]

　　L11.8 Other specified acantholytic disorders

　　L11.9 Acantholytic disorder, unspecified

● **L12 Pemphigoid**
　　| **Excludes1** | herpes gestationis (O26.4-) |
　　| | impetigo herpetiformis (L40.1) |

　　L12.0 Bullous pemphigoid

　　L12.1 Cicatricial pemphigoid
　　　　Benign mucous membrane pemphigoid

　　L12.2 Chronic bullous disease of childhood
　　　　Juvenile dermatitis herpetiformis

　● **L12.3 Acquired epidermolysis bullosa**
　　　　| **Excludes1** | epidermolysis bullosa (congenital) (Q81.-) |

　　　　L12.30 Acquired epidermolysis bullosa, unspecified

　　　　L12.31 Epidermolysis bullosa due to drug
　　　　　　Use additional code for adverse effect, if applicable, to identify drug (T36-T50 with fifth or sixth character 5)

　　　　L12.35 Other acquired epidermolysis bullosa

　　L12.8 Other pemphigoid

　　L12.9 Pemphigoid, unspecified

● **L13 Other bullous disorders**

　　L13.0 Dermatitis herpetiformis
　　　　Duhring's disease
　　　　Hydroa herpetiformis
　　　　| **Excludes1** | juvenile dermatitis herpetiformis (L12.2) |
　　　　| | senile dermatitis herpetiformis (L12.0) |

　　L13.1 Subcorneal pustular dermatitis
　　　　Sneddon-Wilkinson disease

　　L13.8 Other specified bullous disorders

　　L13.9 Bullous disorder, unspecified

　L14 Bullous disorders in diseases classified elsewhere
　　　Code first underlying disease

Item 12-6 Seborrheic dermatitis is characterized by greasy, scaly, red patches and is associated with oily skin and scalp.

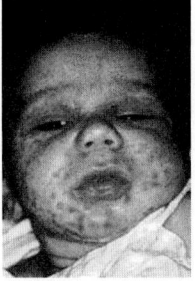

Figure 12-4 Seborrheic dermatitis. (From Cohen BA: Atlas of Pediatric Dermatology, St. Louis, Mosby, 1993)

Item 12-7 Atopic dermatitis, also known as atopic eczema, infantile eczema, disseminated neuro dermatitis, flexural eczema, and *prurigo diathesique* (Besnier), is characterized by intense itching and is often hereditary.

Figure 12-5 Atopic dermatitis. (From Moschella SL, Hurley HJ: Dermatology, ed 3, Philadelphia, WB Saunders, 1993)

DERMATITIS AND ECZEMA (L20-L30)

Note: In this block the terms dermatitis and eczema are used synonymously and interchangeably.

Excludes2	chronic (childhood) granulomatous disease (D71)
	dermatitis gangrenosa (L08.0)
	dermatitis herpetiformis (L13.0)
	dry skin dermatitis (L85.3)
	factitial dermatitis (L98.1)
	perioral dermatitis (L71.0)
	radiation-related disorders of the skin and subcutaneous tissue (L55-L59)
	stasis dermatitis (I83.1-I83.2)

● **L20 Atopic dermatitis**

　　L20.0 Besnier's prurigo

　● **L20.8 Other atopic dermatitis**
　　　　| **Excludes2** | circumscribed neurodermatitis (L28.0) |

　　　　L20.81 Atopic neurodermatitis
　　　　　　Diffuse neurodermatitis

　　　　L20.82 Flexural eczema

　　　　L20.83 Infantile (acute) (chronic) eczema

　　　　L20.84 Intrinsic (allergic) eczema

　　　　L20.89 Other atopic dermatitis

　　L20.9 Atopic dermatitis, unspecified

● **L21 Seborrheic dermatitis**
　　| **Excludes2** | infective dermatitis (L30.3) |
　　| | seborrheic keratosis (L82.-) |

　　L21.0 Seborrhea capitis
　　　　Cradle cap

　　L21.1 Seborrheic infantile dermatitis

　　L21.8 Other seborrheic dermatitis

　　L21.9 Seborrheic dermatitis, unspecified
　　　　Seborrhea NOS

　L22 Diaper dermatitis
　　　Diaper erythema
　　　Diaper rash
　　　Psoriasiform diaper rash

◄ New　　◄ Revised　　~~deleted~~ Deleted　　OGCR Official Guidelines　　X Assign placeholder X　　● Use Additional Character(s)

| Excludes 1 | | Excludes 2 | | Includes | | Use additional | | Code first | | Code also | | Unspecified |

● **L23   Allergic contact dermatitis**
> **Excludes1**   allergy NOS (T78.40)
>> contact dermatitis NOS (L25.9)
>> dermatitis NOS (L30.9)
>
> **Excludes2**   dermatitis due to substances taken internally
>> (L27.-)
>> dermatitis of eyelid (H01.1-)
>> diaper dermatitis (L22)
>> eczema of external ear (H60.5-)
>> irritant contact dermatitis (L24.-)
>> perioral dermatitis (L71.0)
>> radiation-related disorders of the skin and
>> subcutaneous tissue (L55-L59)

L23.0   Allergic contact dermatitis due to metals
> Allergic contact dermatitis due to chromium
> Allergic contact dermatitis due to nickel

L23.1   Allergic contact dermatitis due to adhesives

L23.2   Allergic contact dermatitis due to cosmetics

L23.3   Allergic contact dermatitis due to drugs in contact with skin
> Use additional code for adverse effect, if applicable,
> to identify drug (T36-T50 with fifth or sixth
> character 5)
>
> **Excludes2**   dermatitis due to ingested drugs and
>> medicaments (L27.0-L27.1)

L23.4   Allergic contact dermatitis due to dyes

L23.5   Allergic contact dermatitis due to other chemical products
> Allergic contact dermatitis due to cement
> Allergic contact dermatitis due to insecticide
> Allergic contact dermatitis due to plastic
> Allergic contact dermatitis due to rubber

L23.6   Allergic contact dermatitis due to food in contact with the skin
> **Excludes2**   dermatitis due to ingested food (L27.2)

L23.7   Allergic contact dermatitis due to plants, except food
> **Excludes2**   allergy NOS due to pollen (J30.1)

● **L23.8   Allergic contact dermatitis due to other agents**

L23.81   Allergic contact dermatitis due to animal (cat) (dog) dander
> Allergic contact dermatitis due to animal (cat) (dog) hair

L23.89   Allergic contact dermatitis due to other agents

L23.9   Allergic contact dermatitis, unspecified cause
> Allergic contact eczema NOS

● **L24   Irritant contact dermatitis**
> **Excludes1**   allergy NOS (T78.40)
>> contact dermatitis NOS (L25.9)
>> dermatitis NOS (L30.9)
>
> **Excludes2**   allergic contact dermatitis (L23.-)
>> dermatitis due to substances taken internally
>> (L27.-)
>> dermatitis of eyelid (H01.1-)
>> diaper dermatitis (L22)
>> eczema of external ear (H60.5-)
>> perioral dermatitis (L71.0)
>> radiation-related disorders of the skin and
>> subcutaneous tissue (L55-L59)

L24.0   Irritant contact dermatitis due to detergents

L24.1   Irritant contact dermatitis due to oils and greases

L24.2   Irritant contact dermatitis due to solvents
> Irritant contact dermatitis due to chlorocompound
> Irritant contact dermatitis due to cyclohexane
> Irritant contact dermatitis due to ester
> Irritant contact dermatitis due to glycol
> Irritant contact dermatitis due to hydrocarbon
> Irritant contact dermatitis due to ketone

L24.3   Irritant contact dermatitis due to cosmetics

L24.4   Irritant contact dermatitis due to drugs in contact with skin
> Use additional code for adverse effect, if applicable,
> to identify drug (T36-T50 with fifth or sixth
> character 5)

L24.5   Irritant contact dermatitis due to other chemical products
> Irritant contact dermatitis due to cement
> Irritant contact dermatitis due to insecticide
> Irritant contact dermatitis due to plastic
> Irritant contact dermatitis due to rubber

L24.6   Irritant contact dermatitis due to food in contact with skin
> **Excludes2**   dermatitis due to ingested food (L27.2)

L24.7   Irritant contact dermatitis due to plants, except food
> **Excludes2**   allergy NOS to pollen (J30.1)

● **L24.8   Irritant contact dermatitis due to other agents**

L24.81   Irritant contact dermatitis due to metals
> Irritant contact dermatitis due to chromium
> Irritant contact dermatitis due to nickel

L24.89   Irritant contact dermatitis due to other agents
> Irritant contact dermatitis due to dyes

L24.9   Irritant contact dermatitis, unspecified cause
> Irritant contact eczema NOS

● **L25   Unspecified contact dermatitis**
> **Excludes1**   allergic contact dermatitis (L23.-)
>> allergy NOS (T78.40)
>> dermatitis NOS (L30.9)
>> irritant contact dermatitis (L24.-)
>
> **Excludes2**   dermatitis due to ingested substances (L27.-)
>> dermatitis of eyelid (H01.1-)
>> eczema of external ear (H60.5-)
>> perioral dermatitis (L71.0)
>> radiation-related disorders of the skin and
>> subcutaneous tissue (L55-L59)

L25.0   Unspecified contact dermatitis due to cosmetics

L25.1   Unspecified contact dermatitis due to drugs in contact with skin
> Use additional code for adverse effect, if applicable,
> to identify drug (T36-T50 with fifth or sixth
> character 5)
>
> **Excludes2**   dermatitis due to ingested drugs and
>> medicaments (L27.0-L27.1)

L25.2   Unspecified contact dermatitis due to dyes

L25.3   Unspecified contact dermatitis due to other chemical products
> Unspecified contact dermatitis due to cement
> Unspecified contact dermatitis due to insecticide

L25.4   Unspecified contact dermatitis due to food in contact with skin
> **Excludes2**   dermatitis due to ingested food (L27.2)

L25.5   Unspecified contact dermatitis due to plants, except food
> **Excludes1**   nettle rash (L50.9)
> **Excludes2**   allergy NOS due to pollen (J30.1)

L25.8   Unspecified contact dermatitis due to other agents

L25.9   Unspecified contact dermatitis, unspecified cause
> Contact dermatitis (occupational) NOS
> Contact eczema (occupational) NOS

L26   Exfoliative dermatitis
> Hebra's pityriasis
> **Excludes1**   Ritter's disease (L00)

◀ New   ◀▥ Revised   ~~deleted~~ Deleted   OGCR Official Guidelines   X Assign placeholder X   ● Use Additional Character(s)

| Excludes 1 | Excludes 2 | Includes | Use additional | Code first | Code also | Unspecified |

● **L27 Dermatitis due to substances taken internally**
> **Excludes1**   allergy NOS (T78.40)
> **Excludes2**   adverse food reaction, except dermatitis
>   (T78.0-T78.1)
>   contact dermatitis (L23-L25)
>   drug photoallergic response (L56.1)
>   drug phototoxic response (L56.0)
>   urticaria (L50.-)

L27.0   **Generalized skin eruption due to drugs and medicaments taken internally**
> Use additional code for adverse effect, if applicable, to identify drug (T36-T50 with fifth or sixth character 5)

L27.1   **Localized skin eruption due to drugs and medicaments taken internally**
> Use additional code for adverse effect, if applicable, to identify drug (T36-T50 with fifth or sixth character 5)

L27.2   **Dermatitis due to ingested food**
> **Excludes2**   dermatitis due to food in contact with skin (L23.6, L24.6, L25.4)

L27.8   **Dermatitis due to other substances taken internally**

L27.9   **Dermatitis due to unspecified substance taken internally**

● **L28 Lichen simplex chronicus and prurigo**

L28.0   **Lichen simplex chronicus**
> Circumscribed neurodermatitis
> Lichen NOS

L28.1   **Prurigo nodularis**

L28.2   **Other prurigo**
> Prurigo NOS   Prurigo mitis
> Prurigo Hebra   Urticaria papulosa

● **L29 Pruritus**
> **Excludes1**   neurotic excoriation (L98.1)
>   psychogenic pruritus (F45.8)

L29.0   **Pruritus ani**

L29.1   **Pruritus scroti**

L29.2   **Pruritus vulvae**

L29.3   **Anogenital pruritus, unspecified**

L29.8   **Other pruritus**

L29.9   **Pruritus, unspecified**
> Itch NOS

● **L30 Other and unspecified dermatitis**
> **Excludes2**   contact dermatitis (L23-L25)
>   dry skin dermatitis (L85.3)
>   small plaque parapsoriasis (L41.3)
>   stasis dermatitis (I83.1-.2)

L30.0   **Nummular dermatitis**

L30.1   **Dyshidrosis [pompholyx]**

L30.2   **Cutaneous autosensitization**
> Candidid [levurid]   Eczematid
> Dermatophytid

L30.3   **Infective dermatitis**
> Infectious eczematoid dermatitis

L30.4   **Erythema intertrigo**

L30.5   **Pityriasis alba**

L30.8   **Other specified dermatitis**

L30.9   **Dermatitis, unspecified**
> Eczema NOS

Item 12–8 Psoriasis is a chronic, recurrent inflammatory skin disease characterized by small patches covered with thick silvery scales. **Parapsoriasis** is a treatment-resistant erythroderma. **Pityriasis rosea** is characterized by a herald patch that is a single large lesion and that usually appears on the trunk and is followed by scattered, smaller lesions.

PAPULOSQUAMOUS DISORDERS (L40-L45)

● **L40 Psoriasis**

L40.0   **Psoriasis vulgaris**
> Nummular psoriasis   Plaque psoriasis

L40.1   **Generalized pustular psoriasis**
> Impetigo herpetiformis
> Von Zumbusch's disease

L40.2   **Acrodermatitis continua**

L40.3   **Pustulosis palmaris et plantaris**

L40.4   **Guttate psoriasis**

● L40.5   **Arthropathic psoriasis**

    L40.50   **Arthropathic psoriasis, unspecified**

    L40.51   **Distal interphalangeal psoriatic arthropathy**

    L40.52   **Psoriatic arthritis mutilans**

    L40.53   **Psoriatic spondylitis**

    L40.54   **Psoriatic juvenile arthropathy**

    L40.59   **Other psoriatic arthropathy**

L40.8   **Other psoriasis**
> Flexural psoriasis

L40.9   **Psoriasis, unspecified**

● **L41 Parapsoriasis**
> **Excludes1**   poikiloderma vasculare atrophicans (L94.5)

L41.0   **Pityriasis lichenoides et varioliformis acuta**
> Mucha-Habermann disease

L41.1   **Pityriasis lichenoides chronica**

L41.3   **Small plaque parapsoriasis**

L41.4   **Large plaque parapsoriasis**

L41.5   **Retiform parapsoriasis**

L41.8   **Other parapsoriasis**

L41.9   **Parapsoriasis, unspecified**

L42   **Pityriasis rosea**

● **L43 Lichen planus**
> **Excludes1**   lichen planopilaris (L66.1)

L43.0   **Hypertrophic lichen planus**

L43.1   **Bullous lichen planus**

L43.2   **Lichenoid drug reaction**
> Use additional code for adverse effect, if applicable, to identify drug (T36-T50 with fifth or sixth character 5)

L43.3   **Subacute (active) lichen planus**
> Lichen planus tropicus

L43.8   **Other lichen planus**

L43.9   **Lichen planus, unspecified**

● **L44 Other papulosquamous disorders**

L44.0   **Pityriasis rubra pilaris**

L44.1   **Lichen nitidus**

L44.2   **Lichen striatus**

L44.3   **Lichen ruber moniliformis**

L44.4   **Infantile papular acrodermatitis [Gianotti-Crosti]**

L44.8   **Other specified papulosquamous disorders**

L44.9   **Papulosquamous disorder, unspecified**

L45   **Papulosquamous disorders in diseases classified elsewhere**
> *Code first underlying disease*

Figure 12-6 Erythematous plaques with silvery scales in a patient with psoriasis. (From Goldman: Cecil Textbook of Medicine, ed 22, Saunders, 2004)

Figure 12-7 Urticaria (hives). *(Courtesy of David Effron, MD.)* (From Marx: Rosen's Emergency Medicine: Concepts and Clinical Practice, ed 6, Mosby, Inc., 2006)

Item 12–9 **Urticaria** is a vascular reaction in which wheals surrounded by a red halo appear and cause severe itching. The causes of urticaria or hives are extensive and varied (e.g., food, heat, cold, drugs, stress, infections).

URTICARIA AND ERYTHEMA (L49-L54)

Excludes1   Lyme disease (A69.2-)
             rosacea (L71.-)

● **L49**   **Exfoliation due to erythematous conditions according to extent of body surface involved**

Code first erythematous condition causing exfoliation, such as:
    Ritter's disease (L00)
    (Staphylococcal) scalded skin syndrome (L00)
    Stevens-Johnson syndrome (L51.1)
    Stevens-Johnson syndrome-toxic epidermal necrolysis overlap syndrome (L51.3)
    Toxic epidermal necrolysis (L51.2)

L49.0   **Exfoliation due to erythematous condition involving less than 10 percent of body surface**
     Exfoliation due to erythematous condition NOS

L49.1   **Exfoliation due to erythematous condition involving 10-19 percent of body surface**

L49.2   **Exfoliation due to erythematous condition involving 20-29 percent of body surface**

L49.3   **Exfoliation due to erythematous condition involving 30-39 percent of body surface**

L49.4   **Exfoliation due to erythematous condition involving 40-49 percent of body surface**

L49.5   **Exfoliation due to erythematous condition involving 50-59 percent of body surface**

L49.6   **Exfoliation due to erythematous condition involving 60-69 percent of body surface**

L49.7   **Exfoliation due to erythematous condition involving 70-79 percent of body surface**

L49.8   **Exfoliation due to erythematous condition involving 80-89 percent of body surface**

L49.9   **Exfoliation due to erythematous condition involving 90 or more percent of body surface**

● **L50**   **Urticaria**

Excludes1   allergic contact dermatitis (L23.-)
             angioneurotic edema (T78.3)
             giant urticaria (T78.3)
             hereditary angio-edema (D84.1)
             Quincke's edema (T78.3)
             serum urticaria (T80.6-)
             solar urticaria (L56.3)
             urticaria neonatorum (P83.8)
             urticaria papulosa (L28.2)
             urticaria pigmentosa (Q82.2)

L50.0   **Allergic urticaria**

L50.1   **Idiopathic urticaria**

L50.2   **Urticaria due to cold and heat**

L50.3   **Dermatographic urticaria**

L50.4   **Vibratory urticaria**

L50.5   **Cholinergic urticaria**

L50.6   **Contact urticaria**

L50.8   **Other urticaria**
     Chronic urticaria
     Recurrent periodic urticaria

L50.9   **Urticaria, unspecified**

● **L51**   **Erythema multiforme**

Use additional code for adverse effect, if applicable, to identify drug (T36-T50 with fifth or sixth character 5)

Use additional code to identify associated manifestations, such as:
    arthropathy associated with dermatological disorders (M14.8-)
    conjunctival edema (H11.42)
    conjunctivitis (H10.22-)
    corneal scars and opacities (H17.-)
    corneal ulcer (H16.0-)
    edema of eyelid (H02.84)
    inflammation of eyelid (H01.8)
    keratoconjunctivitis sicca (H16.22-)
    mechanical lagophthalmos (H02.22-)
    stomatitis (K12.-)
    symblepharon (H11.23-)

Use additional code to identify percentage of skin exfoliation (L49.-)

Excludes1   staphylococcal scalded skin syndrome (L00)
             Ritter's disease (L00)

L51.0   **Nonbullous erythema multiforme**

L51.1   **Stevens-Johnson syndrome**

L51.2   **Toxic epidermal necrolysis [Lyell]**

L51.3   **Stevens-Johnson syndrome-toxic epidermal necrolysis overlap syndrome**
     SJS-TEN overlap syndrome

L51.8   **Other erythema multiforme**

L51.9   **Erythema multiforme, unspecified**
     Erythema iris
     Erythema multiforme major NOS
     Erythema multiforme minor NOS
     Herpes iris

L52   **Erythema nodosum**

Excludes1   tuberculous erythema nodosum (A18.4)

● **L53**   **Other erythematous conditions**

Excludes1   erythema ab igne (L59.0)
             erythema due to external agents in contact with skin (L23-L25)
             erythema intertrigo (L30.4)

L53.0   **Toxic erythema**

Code first poisoning due to drug or toxin, if applicable (T36-T65 with fifth or sixth character 1-4 or 6)

Use additional code for adverse effect, if applicable, to identify drug (T36-T50 with fifth or sixth character 5)

Excludes1   neonatal erythema toxicum (P83.1)

L53.1   **Erythema annulare centrifugum**

L53.2   **Erythema marginatum**

L53.3   **Other chronic figurate erythema**

◀ New   ⬛ Revised   ~~deleted~~ Deleted   OGCR Official Guidelines   X Assign placeholder X   ● Use Additional Character(s)

Excludes 1   Excludes 2   Includes   Use additional   Code first   Code also   Unspecified

L53.8   Other specified erythematous conditions

L53.9   Erythematous condition, **unspecified**
     Erythema NOS
     Erythroderma NOS

L54   Erythema in diseases classified elsewhere
     Code first underlying disease

RADIATION-RELATED DISORDERS OF THE SKIN AND SUBCUTANEOUS TISSUE (L55-L59)

● L55   Sunburn

L55.0   Sunburn of first degree

L55.1   Sunburn of second degree

L55.2   Sunburn of third degree

L55.9   Sunburn, **unspecified**

● L56   Other acute skin changes due to ultraviolet radiation
     Use additional code to identify the source of the ultraviolet radiation (W89, X32)

L56.0   Drug phototoxic response
     Use additional code for adverse effect, if applicable, to identify drug (T36-T50 with fifth or sixth character 5)

L56.1   Drug photoallergic response
     Use additional code for adverse effect, if applicable, to identify drug (T36-T50 with fifth or sixth character 5)

L56.2   Photocontact dermatitis [berloque dermatitis]

L56.3   Solar urticaria

L56.4   Polymorphous light eruption

L56.5   Disseminated superficial actinic porokeratosis (DSAP)

L56.8   Other specified acute skin changes due to ultraviolet radiation

L56.9   Acute skin change due to ultraviolet radiation, **unspecified**

● L57   Skin changes due to chronic exposure to nonionizing radiation
     Use additional code to identify the source of the ultraviolet radiation (W89, X32)

L57.0   Actinic keratosis
     Keratosis NOS   Solar keratosis
     Senile keratosis

L57.1   Actinic reticuloid

L57.2   Cutis rhomboidalis nuchae

L57.3   Poikiloderma of Civatte

L57.4   Cutis laxa senilis
     Elastosis senilis

L57.5   Actinic granuloma

L57.8   Other skin changes due to chronic exposure to nonionizing radiation
     Farmer's skin   Solar dermatitis
     Sailor's skin

L57.9   Skin changes due to chronic exposure to nonionizing radiation, **unspecified**

● L58   Radiodermatitis
     Use additional code to identify the source of the radiation (W88, W90)

L58.0   Acute radiodermatitis

L58.1   Chronic radiodermatitis

L58.9   Radiodermatitis, **unspecified**

● L59   Other disorders of skin and subcutaneous tissue related to radiation

L59.0   Erythema ab igne [dermatitis ab igne]

L59.8   Other specified disorders of the skin and subcutaneous tissue related to radiation

L59.9   Disorder of the skin and subcutaneous tissue related to radiation, **unspecified**

Item 12–10 Alopecia is lack of hair and takes many forms. The most common is male pattern alopecia, also known as **androgenetic alopecia. Telogen effluvium** is early and excessive loss of hair resulting from a trauma to the hair follicle (fever, drugs, surgery, etc.).

Figure 12-8   Male pattern alopecia.

DISORDERS OF SKIN APPENDAGES (L60-L75)

Excludes1   congenital malformations of integument (Q84.-)

● L60   Nail disorders

     Excludes2   clubbing of nails (R68.3)
                 onychia and paronychia (L03.0-)

L60.0   Ingrowing nail

L60.1   Onycholysis

L60.2   Onychogryphosis

L60.3   Nail dystrophy

L60.4   Beau's lines

L60.5   Yellow nail syndrome

L60.8   Other nail disorders

L60.9   Nail disorder, **unspecified**

L62   Nail disorders in diseases classified elsewhere
     Code first underlying disease, such as:
     pachydermoperiostosis (M89.4-)

● L63   Alopecia areata

L63.0   Alopecia (capitis) totalis

L63.1   Alopecia universalis

L63.2   Ophiasis

L63.8   Other alopecia areata

L63.9   Alopecia areata, **unspecified**

● L64   Androgenic alopecia

     Includes   male-pattern baldness

L64.0   Drug-induced androgenic alopecia
     Use additional code for adverse effect, if applicable, to identify drug (T36-T50 with fifth or sixth character 5)

L64.8   Other androgenic alopecia

L64.9   Androgenic alopecia, **unspecified**

● L65   Other nonscarring hair loss
     Use additional code for adverse effect, if applicable, to identify drug (T36-T50 with fifth or sixth character 5)

     Excludes1   trichotillomania (F63.3)

L65.0   Telogen effluvium

L65.1   Anagen effluvium

L65.2   Alopecia mucinosa

L65.8   Other specified nonscarring hair loss

L65.9   Nonscarring hair loss, **unspecified**
     Alopecia NOS

● **L66   Cicatricial alopecia [scarring hair loss]**
   L66.0   Pseudopelade
   L66.1   Lichen planopilaris
       Follicular lichen planus
   L66.2   Folliculitis decalvans
   L66.3   Perifolliculitis capitis abscedens
   L66.4   Folliculitis ulerythematosa reticulata
   L66.8   Other cicatricial alopecia
   L66.9   Cicatricial alopecia, unspecified

● **L67   Hair color and hair shaft abnormalities**
   | Excludes1 | monilethrix (Q84.1)
               pili annulati (Q84.1)
               telogen effluvium (L65.0)
   L67.0   Trichorrhexis nodosa
   L67.1   Variations in hair color
       Canities
       Greyness, hair (premature)
       Heterochromia of hair
       Poliosis circumscripta, acquired
       Poliosis NOS
   L67.8   Other hair color and hair shaft abnormalities
       Fragilitas crinium
   L67.9   Hair color and hair shaft abnormality, unspecified

● **L68   Hypertrichosis**
   | Includes | excess hair
   | Excludes1 | congenital hypertrichosis (Q84.2)
               persistent lanugo (Q84.2)
   L68.0   Hirsutism
       Excessive growth of hair
   L68.1   Acquired hypertrichosis lanuginosa
   L68.2   Localized hypertrichosis
   L68.3   Polytrichia
   L68.8   Other hypertrichosis
   L68.9   Hypertrichosis, unspecified

● **L70   Acne**
   | Excludes2 | acne keloid (L73.0)
   L70.0   Acne vulgaris
   L70.1   Acne conglobata
   L70.2   Acne varioliformis
       Acne necrotica miliaris
   L70.3   Acne tropica
   L70.4   Infantile acne
   L70.5   Acné excoriée des jeunes filles
       Picker's acne
   L70.8   Other acne
   L70.9   Acne, unspecified

● **L71   Rosacea**
   Use additional code for adverse effect, if applicable, to identify drug (T36-T50 with fifth or sixth character 5)
   L71.0   Perioral dermatitis
   L71.1   Rhinophyma
   L71.8   Other rosacea
   L71.9   Rosacea, unspecified

● **L72   Follicular cysts of skin and subcutaneous tissue**
   L72.0   Epidermal cyst
 ● **L72.1   Pilar and trichodermal cyst**
     L72.11   Pilar cyst
     L72.12   Trichodermal cyst
         Trichilemmal (proliferating) cyst
   L72.3   Sebaceous cyst
     | Excludes2 | pilar cyst (L72.11)
               trichilemmal (proliferating) cyst (L72.12)
   L72.2   Steatocystoma multiplex

   L72.8   Other follicular cysts of the skin and subcutaneous tissue
   L72.9   Follicular cyst of the skin and subcutaneous tissue, unspecified

● **L73   Other follicular disorders**
   L73.0   Acne keloid
   L73.1   Pseudofolliculitis barbae
   L73.2   Hidradenitis suppurativa
   L73.8   Other specified follicular disorders
       Sycosis barbae
   L73.9   Follicular disorder, unspecified

● **L74   Eccrine sweat disorders**
   | Excludes2 | generalized hyperhidrosis (R61)
   L74.0   Miliaria rubra
   L74.1   Miliaria crystallina
   L74.2   Miliaria profunda
       Miliaria tropicalis
   L74.3   Miliaria, unspecified
   L74.4   Anhidrosis
       Hypohidrosis
 ● **L74.5   Focal hyperhidrosis**
  ● **L74.51   Primary focal hyperhidrosis**
       L74.510   Primary focal hyperhidrosis, axilla
       L74.511   Primary focal hyperhidrosis, face
       L74.512   Primary focal hyperhidrosis, palms
       L74.513   Primary focal hyperhidrosis, soles
       L74.519   Primary focal hyperhidrosis, unspecified
     L74.52   Secondary focal hyperhidrosis
       Frey's syndrome
   L74.8   Other eccrine sweat disorders
   L74.9   Eccrine sweat disorder, unspecified
       Sweat gland disorder NOS

● **L75   Apocrine sweat disorders**
   | Excludes1 | dyshidrosis (L30.1)
               hidradenitis suppurativa (L73.2)
   L75.0   Bromhidrosis
   L75.1   Chromhidrosis
   L75.2   Apocrine miliaria
       Fox-Fordyce disease
   L75.8   Other apocrine sweat disorders
   L75.9   Apocrine sweat disorder, unspecified
       Intraoperative and postprocedural complications of skin and subcutaneous tissue (L76)

INTRAOPERATIVE AND POSTPROCEDURAL COMPLICATIONS OF SKIN AND SUBCUTANEOUS TISSUE (L76)

● **L76   Intraoperative and postprocedural complications of skin and subcutaneous tissue**
 ● **L76.0   Intraoperative hemorrhage and hematoma of skin and subcutaneous tissue complicating a procedure**
   | Excludes1 | intraoperative hemorrhage and hematoma of skin and subcutaneous tissue due to accidental puncture and laceration during a procedure (L76.1-)
     L76.01   Intraoperative hemorrhage and hematoma of skin and subcutaneous tissue complicating a dermatologic procedure
     L76.02   Intraoperative hemorrhage and hematoma of skin and subcutaneous tissue complicating other procedure

CHAPTER 12 (L00-L99)

◀ New   ◀◀ Revised   ~~deleted~~ Deleted   OGCR Official Guidelines   X Assign placeholder X   ● Use Additional Character(s)

| Excludes 1 | | Excludes 2 | | Includes | Use additional | Code first | Code also | Unspecified |

● **L76.1** **Accidental puncture and laceration of skin and subcutaneous tissue during a procedure**

    L76.11 Accidental puncture and laceration of skin and subcutaneous tissue during a dermatologic procedure

    L76.12 Accidental puncture and laceration of skin and subcutaneous tissue during other procedure

● **L76.2** **Postprocedural hemorrhage and hematoma of skin and subcutaneous tissue following a procedure**

    L76.21 Postprocedural hemorrhage and hematoma of skin and subcutaneous tissue following a dermatologic procedure

    L76.22 Postprocedural hemorrhage and hematoma of skin and subcutaneous tissue following other procedure

● **L76.8** **Other intraoperative and postprocedural complications of skin and subcutaneous tissue**

    Use additional code, if applicable, to further specify disorder

    L76.81 Other intraoperative complications of skin and subcutaneous tissue

    L76.82 Other postprocedural complications of skin and subcutaneous tissue

OTHER DISORDERS OF THE SKIN AND SUBCUTANEOUS TISSUE (L80-L99)

L80 **Vitiligo**

    Excludes2 vitiligo of eyelids (H02.73-)
               vitiligo of vulva (N90.89)

● **L81** **Other disorders of pigmentation**

    Excludes1 birthmark NOS (Q82.5)
               Peutz-Jeghers syndrome (Q85.8)

    Excludes2 nevus - see Alphabetical Index

    L81.0 **Postinflammatory hyperpigmentation**

    L81.1 **Chloasma**

    L81.2 **Freckles**

    L81.3 **Café au lait spots**

    L81.4 **Other melanin hyperpigmentation**
         Lentigo

    L81.5 **Leukoderma, not elsewhere classified**

    L81.6 **Other disorders of diminished melanin formation**

    L81.7 **Pigmented purpuric dermatosis**
         Angioma serpiginosum

    L81.8 **Other specified disorders of pigmentation**
         Iron pigmentation
         Tattoo pigmentation

    L81.9 **Disorder of pigmentation, unspecified**

● **L82** **Seborrheic keratosis**

    Includes dermatosis papulosa nigra
               Leser-Trélat disease

    Excludes2 seborrheic dermatitis (L21.-)

    L82.0 **Inflamed seborrheic keratosis**

    L82.1 **Other seborrheic keratosis**
         Seborrheic keratosis NOS

L83 **Acanthosis nigricans**
     Confluent and reticulated papillomatosis

L84 **Corns and callosities**
     Callus
     Clavus

● **L85** **Other epidermal thickening**

    Excludes2 hypertrophic disorders of the skin (L91.-)

    L85.0 **Acquired ichthyosis**
        Excludes1 congenital ichthyosis (Q80.-)

    L85.1 **Acquired keratosis [keratoderma] palmaris et plantaris**
        Excludes1 inherited keratosis palmaris et plantaris (Q82.8)

    L85.2 **Keratosis punctata (palmaris et plantaris) L85.3**
         Xerosis cutis
         Dry skin dermatitis

    L85.8 **Other specified epidermal thickening**
         Cutaneous horn

    L85.9 **Epidermal thickening, unspecified**

L86 **Keratoderma in diseases classified elsewhere**
     Firm horny papules that have a cobblestone appearance.

     Code first underlying disease, such as:
         Reiter's disease (M02.3-)

    Excludes1 gonococcal keratoderma (A54.89)
               gonococcal keratosis (A54.89)
               keratoderma due to vitamin A deficiency (E50.8)
               keratosis due to vitamin A deficiency (E50.8)
               xeroderma due to vitamin A deficiency (E50.8)

● **L87** **Transepidermal elimination disorders**
    Excludes1 granuloma annulare (perforating) (L92.0)

    L87.0 **Keratosis follicularis et parafollicularis in cutem penetrans**
         Kyrle disease
         Hyperkeratosis follicularis penetrans

    L87.1 **Reactive perforating collagenosis**

    L87.2 **Elastosis perforans serpiginosa**

    L87.8 **Other transepidermal elimination disorders**

    L87.9 **Transepidermal elimination disorder, unspecified**

L88 **Pyoderma gangrenosum**
     Phagedenic pyoderma

    Excludes1 dermatitis gangrenosa (L08.0)

OGCR Section I.B.14.

General Coding Guidelines

14. Documentation for BMI, Non-pressure ulcers and Pressure Ulcer Stages

For the Body Mass Index (BMI), depth of non-pressure chronic ulcers and pressure ulcer stage codes, code assignment may be based on medical record documentation from clinicians who are not the patient's provider (i.e., physician or other qualified healthcare practitioner legally accountable for establishing the patient's diagnosis), since this information is typically documented by other clinicians involved in the care of the patient (e.g., a dietitian often documents the BMI and nurses often documents the pressure ulcer stages). However, the associated diagnosis (such as overweight, obesity, or pressure ulcer) must be documented by the patient's provider. If there is conflicting medical record documentation, either from the same clinician or different clinicians, the patient's attending provider should be queried for clarification.

● **L89** **Pressure ulcer**

    Includes bed sore   pressure area
               decubitus ulcer   pressure sore
               plaster ulcer

     Code first any associated gangrene (I96)

    Excludes2 decubitus (trophic) ulcer of cervix (uteri) (N86)
               diabetic ulcers (E08.621, E08.622, E09.621, E09.622, E10.621, E10.622, E11.621, E11.622, E13.621, E13.622)
               non-pressure chronic ulcer of skin (L97.-)
               skin infections (L00-L08)
               varicose ulcer (I83.0, I83.2)

● **L89.0** **Pressure ulcer of elbow**

    ● **L89.00** **Pressure ulcer of unspecified elbow**

        L89.000 **Pressure ulcer of unspecified elbow, unstageable**

        L89.001 **Pressure ulcer of unspecified elbow, stage 1**
             Healing pressure ulcer of unspecified elbow, stage 1
             Pressure pre-ulcer skin changes limited to persistent focal edema, unspecified elbow

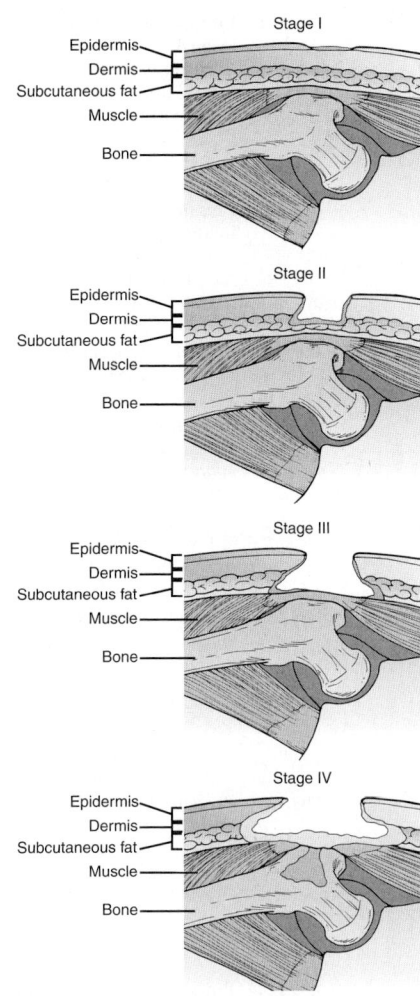

Figure 12-9 Stage I, II, III, and IV of pressure ulcers.

L89.002   **Pressure ulcer of unspecified elbow, stage 2**
Healing pressure ulcer of unspecified elbow, stage 2
Pressure ulcer with abrasion, blister, partial thickness skin loss involving epidermis and/or dermis, unspecified elbow

L89.003   **Pressure ulcer of unspecified elbow, stage 3**
Healing pressure ulcer of unspecified elbow, stage 3
Pressure ulcer with full thickness skin loss involving damage or necrosis of subcutaneous tissue, unspecified elbow

L89.004   **Pressure ulcer of unspecified elbow, stage 4**
Healing pressure ulcer of unspecified elbow, stage 4
Pressure ulcer with necrosis of soft tissues through to underlying muscle, tendon, or bone, unspecified elbow

L89.009   **Pressure ulcer of unspecified elbow, unspecified stage**
Healing pressure ulcer of elbow NOS
Healing pressure ulcer of unspecified elbow, unspecified stage

● **L89.01   Pressure ulcer of right elbow**
L89.010   **Pressure ulcer of right elbow, unstageable**
L89.011   **Pressure ulcer of right elbow, stage 1**
Healing pressure ulcer of right elbow, stage 1
Pressure pre-ulcer skin changes limited to persistent focal edema, right elbow

L89.012   **Pressure ulcer of right elbow, stage 2**
Healing pressure ulcer of right elbow, stage 2
Pressure ulcer with abrasion, blister, partial thickness skin loss involving epidermis and/or dermis, right elbow

L89.013   **Pressure ulcer of right elbow, stage 3**
Healing pressure ulcer of right elbow, stage 3
Pressure ulcer with full thickness skin loss involving damage or necrosis of subcutaneous tissue, right elbow

L89.014   **Pressure ulcer of right elbow, stage 4**
Healing pressure ulcer of right elbow, stage 4
Pressure ulcer with necrosis of soft tissues through to underlying muscle, tendon, or bone, right elbow

L89.019   **Pressure ulcer of right elbow, unspecified stage**
Healing pressure right of elbow NOS
Healing pressure ulcer of unspecified elbow, unspecified stage

● **L89.02   Pressure ulcer of left elbow**
L89.020   **Pressure ulcer of left elbow, unstageable**
L89.021   **Pressure ulcer of left elbow, stage 1**
Healing pressure ulcer of left elbow, stage 1
Pressure pre-ulcer skin changes limited to persistent focal edema, left elbow

L89.022   **Pressure ulcer of left elbow, stage 2**
Healing pressure ulcer of left elbow, stage 2
Pressure ulcer with abrasion, blister, partial thickness skin loss involving epidermis and/or dermis, left elbow

L89.023   **Pressure ulcer of left elbow, stage 3**
Healing pressure ulcer of left elbow, stage 3
Pressure ulcer with full thickness skin loss involving damage or necrosis of subcutaneous tissue, left elbow

L89.024   **Pressure ulcer of left elbow, stage 4**
Healing pressure ulcer of left elbow, stage 4
Pressure ulcer with necrosis of soft tissues through to underlying muscle, tendon, or bone, left elbow

L89.029   **Pressure ulcer of left elbow, unspecified stage**
Healing pressure ulcer of left of elbow NOS
Healing pressure ulcer of unspecified elbow, unspecified stage

CHAPTER 12 (L00-L99)

◀ New   ⬅ Revised   deleted Deleted   OGCR Official Guidelines   X Assign placeholder X   ● Use Additional Character(s)
Excludes 1   Excludes 2   Includes   Use additional   Code first   Code also   Unspecified

1001

● **L89.1   Pressure ulcer of back**
   ● **L89.10   Pressure ulcer of unspecified part of back**
      L89.100   Pressure ulcer of unspecified part of back, unstageable
      L89.101   Pressure ulcer of unspecified part of back, stage 1
        Healing pressure ulcer of unspecified part of back, stage 1
        Pressure pre-ulcer skin changes limited to persistent focal edema, unspecified part of back
      L89.102   Pressure ulcer of unspecified part of back, stage 2
        Healing pressure ulcer of unspecified part of back, stage 2
        Pressure ulcer with abrasion, blister, partial thickness skin loss involving epidermis and/or dermis, unspecified part of back
      L89.103   Pressure ulcer of unspecified part of back, stage 3
        Healing pressure ulcer of unspecified part of back, stage 3
        Pressure ulcer with full thickness skin loss involving damage or necrosis of subcutaneous tissue, unspecified part of back
      L89.104   Pressure ulcer of unspecified part of back, stage 4
        Healing pressure ulcer of unspecified part of back, stage 4
        Pressure ulcer with necrosis of soft tissues through to underlying muscle, tendon, or bone, unspecified part of back
      L89.109   Pressure ulcer of unspecified part of back, unspecified stage
        Healing pressure ulcer of unspecified part of back NOS
        Healing pressure ulcer of unspecified part of back, unspecified stage
   ● **L89.11   Pressure ulcer of right upper back**
      Pressure ulcer of right shoulder blade
      L89.110   Pressure ulcer of right upper back, unstageable
      L89.111   Pressure ulcer of right upper back, stage 1
        Healing pressure ulcer of right upper back, stage 1
        Pressure pre-ulcer skin changes limited to persistent focal edema, right upper back
      L89.112   Pressure ulcer of right upper back, stage 2
        Healing pressure ulcer of right upper back, stage 2
        Pressure ulcer with abrasion, blister, partial thickness skin loss involving epidermis and/or dermis, right upper back
      L89.113   Pressure ulcer of right upper back, stage 3
        Healing pressure ulcer of right upper back, stage 3
        Pressure ulcer with full thickness skin loss involving damage or necrosis of subcutaneous tissue, right upper back

      L89.114   Pressure ulcer of right upper back, stage 4
        Healing pressure ulcer of right upper back, stage 4
        Pressure ulcer with necrosis of soft tissues through to underlying muscle, tendon, or bone, right upper back
      L89.119   Pressure ulcer of right upper back, unspecified stage
        Healing pressure ulcer of right upper back NOS
        Healing pressure ulcer of right upper back, unspecified stage
   ● **L89.12   Pressure ulcer of left upper back**
      Pressure ulcer of left shoulder blade
      L89.120   Pressure ulcer of left upper back, unstageable
      L89.121   Pressure ulcer of left upper back, stage 1
        Healing pressure ulcer of left upper back, stage 1
        Pressure pre-ulcer skin changes limited to persistent focal edema, left upper back
      L89.122   Pressure ulcer of left upper back, stage 2
        Healing pressure ulcer of left upper back, stage 2
        Pressure ulcer with abrasion, blister, partial thickness skin loss involving epidermis and/or dermis, left upper back
      L89.123   Pressure ulcer of left upper back, stage 3
        Healing pressure ulcer of left upper back, stage 3
        Pressure ulcer with full thickness skin loss involving damage or necrosis of subcutaneous tissue, left upper back
      L89.124   Pressure ulcer of left upper back, stage 4
        Healing pressure ulcer of left upper back, stage 4
        Pressure ulcer with necrosis of soft tissues through to underlying muscle, tendon, or bone, left upper back
      L89.129   Pressure ulcer of left upper back, unspecified stage
        Healing pressure ulcer of left upper back NOS
        Healing pressure ulcer of left upper back, unspecified stage
   ● **L89.13   Pressure ulcer of right lower back**
      L89.130   Pressure ulcer of right lower back, unstageable
      L89.131   Pressure ulcer of right lower back, stage 1
        Healing pressure ulcer of right lower back, stage 1
        Pressure pre-ulcer skin changes limited to persistent focal edema, right lower back
      L89.132   Pressure ulcer of right lower back, stage 2
        Healing pressure ulcer of right lower back, stage 2
        Pressure ulcer with abrasion, blister, partial thickness skin loss involving epidermis and/or dermis, right lower back

CHAPTER 12 (L00-L99)

◀ New   ◀▥▥ Revised   ~~deleted~~ Deleted   OGCR Official Guidelines   X Assign placeholder X   ● Use Additional Character(s)

Excludes 1   Excludes 2   Includes   Use additional   Code first   Code also   Unspecified

L89.133   **Pressure ulcer of right lower back, stage 3**
> Healing pressure ulcer of right lower back, stage 3
> Pressure ulcer with full thickness skin loss involving damage or necrosis of subcutaneous tissue, right lower back

L89.134   **Pressure ulcer of right lower back, stage 4**
> Healing pressure ulcer of right lower back, stage 4
> Pressure ulcer with necrosis of soft tissues through to underlying muscle, tendon, or bone, right lower back

L89.139   **Pressure ulcer of right lower back, unspecified stage**
> Healing pressure ulcer of right lower back NOS
> Healing pressure ulcer of right lower back, unspecified stage

● **L89.14**   **Pressure ulcer of left lower back**

L89.140   **Pressure ulcer of left lower back, unstageable**

L89.141   **Pressure ulcer of left lower back, stage 1**
> Healing pressure ulcer of left lower back, stage 1
> Pressure pre-ulcer skin changes limited to persistent focal edema, left lower back

L89.142   **Pressure ulcer of left lower back, stage 2**
> Healing pressure ulcer of left lower back, stage 2
> Pressure ulcer with abrasion, blister, partial thickness skin loss involving epidermis and/or dermis, left lower back

L89.143   **Pressure ulcer of left lower back, stage 3**
> Healing pressure ulcer of left lower back, stage 3
> Pressure ulcer with full thickness skin loss involving damage or necrosis of subcutaneous tissue, left lower back

L89.144   **Pressure ulcer of left lower back, stage 4**
> Healing pressure ulcer of left lower back, stage 4
> Pressure ulcer with necrosis of soft tissues through to underlying muscle, tendon, or bone, left lower back

L89.149   **Pressure ulcer of left lower back, unspecified stage**
> Healing pressure ulcer of left lower back NOS
> Healing pressure ulcer of left lower back, unspecified stage

● **L89.15**   **Pressure ulcer of sacral region**
> Pressure ulcer of coccyx
> Pressure ulcer of tailbone

L89.150   **Pressure ulcer of sacral region, unstageable**

L89.151   **Pressure ulcer of sacral region, stage 1**
> Healing pressure ulcer of sacral region, stage 1
> Pressure pre-ulcer skin changes limited to persistent focal edema, sacral region

L89.152   **Pressure ulcer of sacral region, stage 2**
> Healing pressure ulcer of sacral region, stage 2
> Pressure ulcer with abrasion, blister, partial thickness skin loss involving epidermis and/or dermis, sacral region

L89.153   **Pressure ulcer of sacral region, stage 3**
> Healing pressure ulcer of sacral region, stage 3
> Pressure ulcer with full thickness skin loss involving damage or necrosis of subcutaneous tissue, sacral region

L89.154   **Pressure ulcer of sacral region, stage 4**
> Healing pressure ulcer of sacral region, stage 4
> Pressure ulcer with necrosis of soft tissues through to underlying muscle, tendon, or bone, sacral region

L89.159   **Pressure ulcer of sacral region, unspecified stage**
> Healing pressure ulcer of sacral region NOS
> Healing pressure ulcer of sacral region, unspecified stage

● **L89.2**   **Pressure ulcer of hip**

  ● **L89.20**   **Pressure ulcer of unspecified hip**

L89.200   **Pressure ulcer of unspecified hip, unstageable**

L89.201   **Pressure ulcer of unspecified hip, stage 1**
> Healing pressure ulcer of unspecified hip back, stage 1
> Pressure pre-ulcer skin changes limited to persistent focal edema, unspecified hip

L89.202   **Pressure ulcer of unspecified hip, stage 2**
> Healing pressure ulcer of unspecified hip, stage 2
> Pressure ulcer with abrasion, blister, partial thickness skin loss involving epidermis and/or dermis, unspecified hip

L89.203   **Pressure ulcer of unspecified hip, stage 3**
> Healing pressure ulcer of unspecified hip, stage 3
> Pressure ulcer with full thickness skin loss involving damage or necrosis of subcutaneous tissue, unspecified hip

L89.204   **Pressure ulcer of unspecified hip, stage 4**
> Healing pressure ulcer of unspecified hip, stage 4
> Pressure ulcer with necrosis of soft tissues through to underlying muscle, tendon, or bone, unspecified hip

L89.209   **Pressure ulcer of unspecified hip, unspecified stage**
> Healing pressure ulcer of unspecified hip NOS
> Healing pressure ulcer of unspecified hip, unspecified stage

CHAPTER 12 (L00-L99)

CHAPTER 12 (L00-L99)

● **L89.21**   **Pressure ulcer of right hip**

     L89.210   **Pressure ulcer of right hip, unstageable**

     L89.211   **Pressure ulcer of right hip, stage 1**
             Healing pressure ulcer of right hip back, stage 1
             Pressure pre-ulcer skin changes limited to persistent focal edema, right hip

     L89.212   **Pressure ulcer of right hip, stage 2**
             Healing pressure ulcer of right hip, stage 2
             Pressure ulcer with abrasion, blister, partial thickness skin loss involving epidermis and/or dermis, right hip

     L89.213   **Pressure ulcer of right hip, stage 3**
             Healing pressure ulcer of right hip, stage 3
             Pressure ulcer with full thickness skin loss involving damage or necrosis of subcutaneous tissue, right hip

     L89.214   **Pressure ulcer of right hip, stage 4**
             Healing pressure ulcer of right hip, stage 4
             Pressure ulcer with necrosis of soft tissues through to underlying muscle, tendon, or bone, right hip

     L89.219   **Pressure ulcer of right hip, unspecified stage**
             Healing pressure ulcer of right hip NOS
             Healing pressure ulcer of right hip, unspecified stage

● **L89.22**   **Pressure ulcer of left hip**

     L89.220   **Pressure ulcer of left hip, unstageable**

     L89.221   **Pressure ulcer of left hip, stage 1**
             Healing pressure ulcer of left hip back, stage 1
             Pressure pre-ulcer skin changes limited to persistent focal edema, left hip

     L89.222   **Pressure ulcer of left hip, stage 2**
             Healing pressure ulcer of left hip, stage 2
             Pressure ulcer with abrasion, blister, partial thickness skin loss involving epidermis and/or dermis, left hip

     L89.223   **Pressure ulcer of left hip, stage 3**
             Healing pressure ulcer of left hip, stage 3
             Pressure ulcer with full thickness skin loss involving damage or necrosis of subcutaneous tissue, left hip

     L89.224   **Pressure ulcer of left hip, stage 4**
             Healing pressure ulcer of left hip, stage 4
             Pressure ulcer with necrosis of soft tissues through to underlying muscle, tendon, or bone, left hip

     L89.229   **Pressure ulcer of left hip, unspecified stage**
             Healing pressure ulcer of left hip NOS
             Healing pressure ulcer of left hip, unspecified stage

● **L89.3**   **Pressure ulcer of buttock**

   ● **L89.30**   **Pressure ulcer of unspecified buttock**

     L89.300   **Pressure ulcer of unspecified buttock, unstageable**

     L89.301   **Pressure ulcer of unspecified buttock, stage 1**
             Healing pressure ulcer of unspecified buttock, stage 1
             Pressure pre-ulcer skin changes limited to persistent focal edema, unspecified buttock

     L89.302   **Pressure ulcer of unspecified buttock, stage 2**
             Healing pressure ulcer of unspecified buttock, stage 2
             Pressure ulcer with abrasion, blister, partial thickness skin loss involving epidermis and/or dermis, unspecified buttock

     L89.303   **Pressure ulcer of unspecified buttock, stage 3**
             Healing pressure ulcer of unspecified buttock, stage 3
             Pressure ulcer with full thickness skin loss involving damage or necrosis of subcutaneous tissue, unspecified buttock

     L89.304   **Pressure ulcer of unspecified buttock, stage 4**
             Healing pressure ulcer of unspecified buttock, stage 4
             Pressure ulcer with necrosis of soft tissues through to underlying muscle, tendon, or bone, unspecified buttock

     L89.309   **Pressure ulcer of unspecified buttock, unspecified stage**
             Healing pressure ulcer of unspecified buttock NOS
             Healing pressure ulcer of unspecified buttock, unspecified stage

   ● **L89.31**   **Pressure ulcer of right buttock**

     L89.310   **Pressure ulcer of right buttock, unstageable**

     L89.311   **Pressure ulcer of right buttock, stage 1**
             Healing pressure ulcer of right buttock, stage 1
             Pressure pre-ulcer skin changes limited to persistent focal edema, right buttock

     L89.312   **Pressure ulcer of right buttock, stage 2**
             Healing pressure ulcer of right buttock, stage 2
             Pressure ulcer with abrasion, blister, partial thickness skin loss involving epidermis and/or dermis, right buttock

     L89.313   **Pressure ulcer of right buttock, stage 3**
             Healing pressure ulcer of right buttock, stage 3
             Pressure ulcer with full thickness skin loss involving damage or necrosis of subcutaneous tissue, right buttock

     L89.314   **Pressure ulcer of right buttock, stage 4**
             Healing pressure ulcer of right buttock, stage 4
             Pressure ulcer with necrosis of soft tissues through to underlying muscle, tendon, or bone, right buttock

◀ New   ◀▥ Revised   ~~deleted~~ Deleted   OGCR Official Guidelines   X Assign placeholder X   ● Use Additional Character(s)

Excludes 1   Excludes 2   Includes   Use additional   Code first   Code also   Unspecified

    L89.319   **Pressure ulcer of right buttock, unspecified stage**
         Healing pressure ulcer of right buttock NOS
         Healing pressure ulcer of right buttock, unspecified stage

 ● **L89.32**   **Pressure ulcer of left buttock**

    L89.320   **Pressure ulcer of left buttock, unstageable**

    L89.321   **Pressure ulcer of left buttock, stage 1**
         Healing pressure ulcer of left buttock, stage 1
         Pressure pre-ulcer skin changes limited to persistent focal edema, left buttock

    L89.322   **Pressure ulcer of left buttock, stage 2**
         Healing pressure ulcer of left buttock, stage 2
         Pressure ulcer with abrasion, blister, partial thickness skin loss involving epidermis and/or dermis, left buttock

    L89.323   **Pressure ulcer of left buttock, stage 3**
         Healing pressure ulcer of left buttock, stage 3
         Pressure ulcer with full thickness skin loss involving damage or necrosis of subcutaneous tissue, left buttock

    L89.324   **Pressure ulcer of left buttock, stage 4**
         Healing pressure ulcer of left buttock, stage 4
         Pressure ulcer with necrosis of soft tissues through to underlying muscle, tendon, or bone, left buttock

    L89.329   **Pressure ulcer of left buttock, unspecified stage**
         Healing pressure ulcer of left buttock NOS
         Healing pressure ulcer of left buttock, unspecified stage

● **L89.4**   **Pressure ulcer of contiguous site of back, buttock and hip**

    L89.40   **Pressure ulcer of contiguous site of back, buttock and hip, unspecified stage**
         Healing pressure ulcer of contiguous site of back, buttock and hip NOS
         Healing pressure ulcer of contiguous site of back, buttock and hip, unspecified stage

    L89.41   **Pressure ulcer of contiguous site of back, buttock and hip, stage 1**
         Healing pressure ulcer of contiguous site of back, buttock and hip, stage 1
         Pressure pre-ulcer skin changes limited to persistent focal edema, contiguous site of back, buttock and hip

    L89.42   **Pressure ulcer of contiguous site of back, buttock and hip, stage 2**
         Healing pressure ulcer of contiguous site of back, buttock and hip, stage 2
         Pressure ulcer with abrasion, blister, partial thickness skin loss involving epidermis and/or dermis, contiguous site of back, buttock and hip

    L89.43   **Pressure ulcer of contiguous site of back, buttock and hip, stage 3**
         Healing pressure ulcer of contiguous site of back, buttock and hip, stage 3
         Pressure ulcer with full thickness skin loss involving damage or necrosis of subcutaneous tissue, contiguous site of back, buttock and hip

    L89.44   **Pressure ulcer of contiguous site of back, buttock and hip, stage 4**
         Healing pressure ulcer of contiguous site of back, buttock and hip, stage 4
         Pressure ulcer with necrosis of soft tissues through to underlying muscle, tendon, or bone, contiguous site of back, buttock and hip

    L89.45   **Pressure ulcer of contiguous site of back, buttock and hip, unstageable**

● **L89.5**   **Pressure ulcer of ankle**

 ● **L89.50**   **Pressure ulcer of unspecified ankle**

    L89.500   **Pressure ulcer of unspecified ankle, unstageable**

    L89.501   **Pressure ulcer of unspecified ankle, stage 1**
         Healing pressure ulcer of unspecified ankle, stage 1
         Pressure pre-ulcer skin changes limited to persistent focal edema, unspecified ankle

    L89.502   **Pressure ulcer of unspecified ankle, stage 2**
         Healing pressure ulcer of unspecified ankle, stage 2
         Pressure ulcer with abrasion, blister, partial thickness skin loss involving epidermis and/or dermis, unspecified ankle

    L89.503   **Pressure ulcer of unspecified ankle, stage 3**
         Healing pressure ulcer of unspecified ankle, stage 3
         Pressure ulcer with full thickness skin loss involving damage or necrosis of subcutaneous tissue, unspecified ankle

    L89.504   **Pressure ulcer of unspecified ankle, stage 4**
         Healing pressure ulcer of unspecified ankle, stage 4
         Pressure ulcer with necrosis of soft tissues through to underlying muscle, tendon, or bone, unspecified ankle

    L89.509   **Pressure ulcer of unspecified ankle, unspecified stage**
         Healing pressure ulcer of unspecified ankle NOS
         Healing pressure ulcer of unspecified ankle, unspecified stage

 ● **L89.51**   **Pressure ulcer of right ankle**

    L89.510   **Pressure ulcer of right ankle, unstageable**

    L89.511   **Pressure ulcer of right ankle, stage 1**
         Healing pressure ulcer of right ankle, stage 1
         Pressure pre-ulcer skin changes limited to persistent focal edema, right ankle

    L89.512   **Pressure ulcer of right ankle, stage 2**
         Healing pressure ulcer of right ankle, stage 2
         Pressure ulcer with abrasion, blister, partial thickness skin loss involving epidermis and/or dermis, right ankle

L89.513   **Pressure ulcer of right ankle, stage 3**
      Healing pressure ulcer of right ankle, stage 3
      Pressure ulcer with full thickness skin loss involving damage or necrosis of subcutaneous tissue, right ankle

L89.514   **Pressure ulcer of right ankle, stage 4**
      Healing pressure ulcer of right ankle, stage 4
      Pressure ulcer with necrosis of soft tissues through to underlying muscle, tendon, or bone, right ankle

L89.519   **Pressure ulcer of right ankle, unspecified stage**
      Healing pressure ulcer of right ankle NOS
      Healing pressure ulcer of right ankle, unspecified stage

● **L89.52**   **Pressure ulcer of left ankle**

L89.520   **Pressure ulcer of left ankle, unstageable**

L89.521   **Pressure ulcer of left ankle, stage 1**
      Healing pressure ulcer of left ankle, stage 1
      Pressure pre-ulcer skin changes limited to persistent focal edema, left ankle

L89.522   **Pressure ulcer of left ankle, stage 2**
      Healing pressure ulcer of left ankle, stage 2
      Pressure ulcer with abrasion, blister, partial thickness skin loss involving epidermis and/or dermis, left ankle

L89.523   **Pressure ulcer of left ankle, stage 3**
      Healing pressure ulcer of left ankle, stage 3
      Pressure ulcer with full thickness skin loss involving damage or necrosis of subcutaneous tissue, left ankle

L89.524   **Pressure ulcer of left ankle, stage 4**
      Healing pressure ulcer of left ankle, stage 4
      Pressure ulcer with necrosis of soft tissues through to underlying muscle, tendon, or bone, left ankle

L89.529   **Pressure ulcer of left ankle, unspecified stage**
      Healing pressure ulcer of left ankle NOS
      Healing pressure ulcer of left ankle, unspecified stage

● **L89.6**   **Pressure ulcer of heel**

   ● **L89.60**   **Pressure ulcer of unspecified heel**

L89.600   **Pressure ulcer of unspecified heel, unstageable**

L89.601   **Pressure ulcer of unspecified heel, stage 1**
      Healing pressure ulcer of unspecified heel, stage 1
      Pressure pre-ulcer skin changes limited to persistent focal edema, unspecified heel

L89.602   **Pressure ulcer of unspecified heel, stage 2**
      Healing pressure ulcer of unspecified heel, stage 2
      Pressure ulcer with abrasion, blister, partial thickness skin loss involving epidermis and/or dermis, unspecified heel

L89.603   **Pressure ulcer of unspecified heel, stage 3**
      Healing pressure ulcer of unspecified heel, stage 3
      Pressure ulcer with full thickness skin loss involving damage or necrosis of subcutaneous tissue, unspecified heel

L89.604   **Pressure ulcer of unspecified heel, stage 4**
      Healing pressure ulcer of unspecified heel, stage 4
      Pressure ulcer with necrosis of soft tissues through to underlying muscle, tendon, or bone, unspecified heel

L89.609   **Pressure ulcer of unspecified heel, unspecified stage**
      Healing pressure ulcer of unspecified heel NOS
      Healing pressure ulcer of unspecified heel, unspecified stage

● **L89.61**   **Pressure ulcer of right heel**

L89.610   **Pressure ulcer of right heel, unstageable**

L89.611   **Pressure ulcer of right heel, stage 1**
      Healing pressure ulcer of right heel, stage 1
      Pressure pre-ulcer skin changes limited to persistent focal edema, right heel

L89.612   **Pressure ulcer of right heel, stage 2**
      Healing pressure ulcer of right heel, stage 2
      Pressure ulcer with abrasion, blister, partial thickness skin loss involving epidermis and/or dermis, right heel

L89.613   **Pressure ulcer of right heel, stage 3**
      Healing pressure ulcer of right heel, stage 3
      Pressure ulcer with full thickness skin loss involving damage or necrosis of subcutaneous tissue, right heel

L89.614   **Pressure ulcer of right heel, stage 4**
      Healing pressure ulcer of right heel, stage 4
      Pressure ulcer with necrosis of soft tissues through to underlying muscle, tendon, or bone, right heel

L89.619   **Pressure ulcer of right heel, unspecified stage**
      Healing pressure ulcer of right heel NOS
      Healing pressure ulcer of unspecified heel, right stage

● **L89.62**   **Pressure ulcer of left heel**

L89.620   **Pressure ulcer of left heel, unstageable**

L89.621   **Pressure ulcer of left heel, stage 1**
      Healing pressure ulcer of left heel, stage 1
      Pressure pre-ulcer skin changes limited to persistent focal edema, left heel

L89.622   **Pressure ulcer of left heel, stage 2**
      Healing pressure ulcer of left heel, stage 2
      Pressure ulcer with abrasion, blister, partial thickness skin loss involving epidermis and/or dermis, left heel

CHAPTER 12 (L00-L99)

L89.623   **Pressure ulcer of left heel, stage 3**
Healing pressure ulcer of left heel,
stage 3
Pressure ulcer with full thickness
skin loss involving damage or
necrosis of subcutaneous tissue,
left heel

L89.624   **Pressure ulcer of left heel, stage 4**
Healing pressure ulcer of left heel,
stage 4
Pressure ulcer with necrosis of soft
tissues through to underlying
muscle, tendon, or bone, left
heel

L89.629   **Pressure ulcer of left heel, unspecified
stage**
Healing pressure ulcer of left heel
NOS
Healing pressure ulcer of left heel,
unspecified stage

● **L89.8   Pressure ulcer of other site**

   ● **L89.81   Pressure ulcer of head**
Pressure ulcer of face

L89.810   **Pressure ulcer of head, unstageable**

L89.811   **Pressure ulcer of head, stage 1**
Healing pressure ulcer of head,
stage 1
Pressure pre-ulcer skin changes
limited to persistent focal
edema, head

L89.812   **Pressure ulcer of head, stage 2**
Healing pressure ulcer of head,
stage 2
Pressure ulcer with abrasion, blister,
partial thickness skin loss
involving epidermis and/or
dermis, head

L89.813   **Pressure ulcer of head, stage 3**
Healing pressure ulcer of head,
stage 3
Pressure ulcer with full thickness
skin loss involving damage or
necrosis of subcutaneous tissue,
head

L89.814   **Pressure ulcer of head, stage 4**
Healing pressure ulcer of head,
stage 4
Pressure ulcer with necrosis of soft
tissues through to underlying
muscle, tendon, or bone, head

L89.819   **Pressure ulcer of head, unspecified
stage**
Healing pressure ulcer of head NOS
Healing pressure ulcer of head,
unspecified stage

   ● **L89.89   Pressure ulcer of other site**

L89.890   **Pressure ulcer of other site,
unstageable**

L89.891   **Pressure ulcer of other site, stage 1**
Healing pressure ulcer of other site,
stage 1
Pressure pre-ulcer skin changes
limited to persistent focal
edema, other site

L89.892   **Pressure ulcer of other site, stage 2**
Healing pressure ulcer of other site,
stage 2
Pressure ulcer with abrasion, blister,
partial thickness skin loss
involving epidermis and/or
dermis, other site

L89.893   **Pressure ulcer of other site, stage 3**
Healing pressure ulcer of other site,
stage 3
Pressure ulcer with full thickness
skin loss involving damage or
necrosis of subcutaneous tissue,
other site

L89.894   **Pressure ulcer of other site, stage 4**
Healing pressure ulcer of other site,
stage 4
Pressure ulcer with necrosis of soft
tissues through to underlying
muscle, tendon, or bone, other
site

L89.899   **Pressure ulcer of other site,
unspecified stage**
Healing pressure ulcer of other site
NOS
Healing pressure ulcer of other site,
unspecified stage

● **L89.9   Pressure ulcer of unspecified site**

L89.90   **Pressure ulcer of unspecified site, unspecified
stage**
Healing pressure ulcer of unspecified site NOS
Healing pressure ulcer of unspecified site,
unspecified stage

L89.91   **Pressure ulcer of unspecified site, stage 1**
Healing pressure ulcer of unspecified site,
stage 1
Pressure pre-ulcer skin changes limited to
persistent focal edema, unspecified site

L89.92   **Pressure ulcer of unspecified site, stage 2**
Healing pressure ulcer of unspecified site,
stage 2
Pressure ulcer with abrasion, blister, partial
thickness skin loss involving epidermis
and/or dermis, unspecified site

L89.93   **Pressure ulcer of unspecified site, stage 3**
Healing pressure ulcer of unspecified site,
stage 3
Pressure ulcer with full thickness skin
loss involving damage or necrosis of
subcutaneous tissue, unspecified site

L89.94   **Pressure ulcer of unspecified site, stage 4**
Healing pressure ulcer of unspecified site,
stage 4
Pressure ulcer with necrosis of soft tissues
through to underlying muscle, tendon, or
bone, unspecified site

L89.95   **Pressure ulcer of unspecified site, unstageable**

● **L90   Atrophic disorders of skin**

L90.0   **Lichen sclerosus et atrophicus**

| **Excludes2** | lichen sclerosus of external female genital
organs (N90.4)
lichen sclerosus of external male genital
organs (N48.0) |

L90.1   **Anetoderma of Schweninger-Buzzi**

L90.2   **Anetoderma of Jadassohn-Pellizzari**

L90.3   **Atrophoderma of Pasini and Pierini**

L90.4   **Acrodermatitis chronica atrophicans**

L90.5   **Scar conditions and fibrosis of skin**
Adherent scar (skin)
Cicatrix
Disfigurement of skin due to scar
Fibrosis of skin NOS
Scar NOS

| **Excludes2** | hypertrophic scar (L91.0)
keloid scar (L91.0) |

L90.6   **Striae atrophicae**

L90.8   **Other atrophic disorders of skin**

L90.9   **Atrophic disorder of skin, unspecified**

CHAPTER 12 (L00-L99)

● **L91**   **Hypertrophic disorders of skin**

   L91.0   **Keloid scar**
   Hypertrophic scar
   Keloid
   Excludes2   acne keloid (L73.0)
   scar NOS (L90.5)

   L91.8   **Other hypertrophic disorders of the skin**
   L91.9   **Hypertrophic disorder of the skin, unspecified**

● **L92**   **Granulomatous disorders of skin and subcutaneous tissue**
   Excludes2   actinic granuloma (L57.5)

   L92.0   **Granuloma annulare**
   Perforating granuloma annulare

   L92.1   **Necrobiosis lipoidica, not elsewhere classified**
   Excludes1   necrobiosis lipoidica associated with
   diabetes mellitus (E08-E13 with .620)

   L92.2   **Granuloma faciale [eosinophilic granuloma of skin]**

   L92.3   **Foreign body granuloma of the skin and subcutaneous tissue**
   Use additional code to identify the type of retained
   foreign body (Z18.-)

   L92.8   **Other granulomatous disorders of the skin and subcutaneous tissue**

   L92.9   **Granulomatous disorder of the skin and subcutaneous tissue, unspecified**

● **L93**   **Lupus erythematosus**
   Use additional code for adverse effect, if applicable, to identify
   drug (T36-T50 with fifth or sixth character 5)
   Excludes1   lupus exedens (A18.4)
   lupus vulgaris (A18.4)
   scleroderma (M34.-)
   systemic lupus erythematosus (M32.-)

   L93.0   **Discoid lupus erythematosus**
   Lupus erythematosus NOS

   L93.1   **Subacute cutaneous lupus erythematosus**

   L93.2   **Other local lupus erythematosus**
   Lupus erythematosus profundus
   Lupus panniculitis

● **L94**   **Other localized connective tissue disorders**
   Excludes1   systemic connective tissue disorders (M30-M36)

   L94.0   **Localized scleroderma [morphea]**
   Circumscribed scleroderma

   L94.1   **Linear scleroderma**
   En coup de sabre lesion

   L94.2   **Calcinosis cutis**
   L94.3   **Sclerodactyly**
   L94.4   **Gottron's papules**
   L94.5   **Poikiloderma vasculare atrophicans**
   L94.6   **Ainhum**
   L94.8   **Other specified localized connective tissue disorders**
   L94.9   **Localized connective tissue disorder, unspecified**

● **L95**   **Vasculitis limited to skin, not elsewhere classified**
   Excludes1   angioma serpiginosum (L81.7)
   Henoch(-Schönlein) purpura (D69.0)
   hypersensitivity angiitis (M31.0)
   lupus panniculitis (L93.2)
   panniculitis NOS (M79.3)
   panniculitis of neck and back (M54.0-)
   polyarteritis nodosa (M30.0)
   relapsing panniculitis (M35.6)
   rheumatoid vasculitis (M05.2)
   serum sickness (T80.6-)
   urticaria (L50.-)
   Wegener's granulomatosis (M31.3-)

   L95.0   **Livedoid vasculitis**
   Atrophie blanche (en plaque)

   L95.1   **Erythema elevatum diutinum**
   L95.8   **Other vasculitis limited to the skin**
   L95.9   **Vasculitis limited to the skin, unspecified**

● **L97**   **Non-pressure chronic ulcer of lower limb, not elsewhere classified**
   Includes   chronic ulcer of skin of lower limb NOS
   non-healing ulcer of skin
   non-infected sinus of skin
   trophic ulcer NOS
   tropical ulcer NOS
   ulcer of skin of lower limb NOS

   Code first any associated underlying condition, such as:
   any associated gangrene (I96)
   atherosclerosis of the lower extremities (I70.23-, I70.24-,
   I70.33-, I70.34-, I70.43-, I70.44-, I70.53-, I70.54-, I70.63-,
   I70.64-, I70.73-, I70.74-)
   chronic venous hypertension (I87.31-, I87.33-)
   diabetic ulcers (E08.621, E08.622, E09.621, E09.622, E10.621,
   E10.622, E11.621, E11.622, E13.621, E13.622)
   postphlebitic syndrome (I87.01-, I87.03-)
   postthrombotic syndrome (I87.01-, I87.03-)
   varicose ulcer (I83.0-, I83.2-)
   Excludes2   pressure ulcer (pressure area) (L89.-)
   skin infections (L00-L08)
   specific infections classified to A00-B99

● **L97.1**   **Non-pressure chronic ulcer of thigh**
   ● **L97.10**   **Non-pressure chronic ulcer of unspecified thigh**
   L97.101   **Non-pressure chronic ulcer of unspecified thigh limited to breakdown of skin**
   L97.102   **Non-pressure chronic ulcer of unspecified thigh with fat layer exposed**
   L97.103   **Non-pressure chronic ulcer of unspecified thigh with necrosis of muscle**
   L97.104   **Non-pressure chronic ulcer of unspecified thigh with necrosis of bone**
   L97.109   **Non-pressure chronic ulcer of unspecified thigh with unspecified severity**

   ● **L97.11**   **Non-pressure chronic ulcer of right thigh**
   L97.111   **Non-pressure chronic ulcer of right thigh limited to breakdown of skin**
   L97.112   **Non-pressure chronic ulcer of right thigh with fat layer exposed**
   L97.113   **Non-pressure chronic ulcer of right thigh with necrosis of muscle**
   L97.114   **Non-pressure chronic ulcer of right thigh with necrosis of bone**
   L97.119   **Non-pressure chronic ulcer of right thigh with unspecified severity**

Item 12–11   Scleroderma means hard skin. It is a group of diseases that
causes abnormal growth of connective tissues that support the skin and organs.
There are two types: localized scleroderma affecting the skin and systemic
scleroderma affecting blood vessels and internal organs and the skin.

◄ New   ⬅ Revised   ~~deleted~~ Deleted   OGCR Official Guidelines   X Assign placeholder X   ● Use Additional Character(s)

Excludes 1   Excludes 2   Includes   Use additional   Code first   Code also   Unspecified

● **L97.12**   Non-pressure chronic ulcer of left thigh

     L97.121   Non-pressure chronic ulcer of left thigh limited to breakdown of skin

     L97.122   Non-pressure chronic ulcer of left thigh with fat layer exposed

     L97.123   Non-pressure chronic ulcer of left thigh with necrosis of muscle

     L97.124   Non-pressure chronic ulcer of left thigh with necrosis of bone

     L97.129   Non-pressure chronic ulcer of left thigh with unspecified severity

● **L97.2**   Non-pressure chronic ulcer of calf

   ● **L97.20**   Non-pressure chronic ulcer of unspecified calf

     L97.201   Non-pressure chronic ulcer of unspecified calf limited to breakdown of skin

     L97.202   Non-pressure chronic ulcer of unspecified calf with fat layer exposed

     L97.203   Non-pressure chronic ulcer of unspecified calf with necrosis of muscle

     L97.204   Non-pressure chronic ulcer of unspecified calf with necrosis of bone

     L97.209   Non-pressure chronic ulcer of unspecified calf with unspecified severity

   ● **L97.21**   Non-pressure chronic ulcer of right calf

     L97.211   Non-pressure chronic ulcer of right calf limited to breakdown of skin

     L97.212   Non-pressure chronic ulcer of right calf with fat layer exposed

     L97.213   Non-pressure chronic ulcer of right calf with necrosis of muscle

     L97.214   Non-pressure chronic ulcer of right calf with necrosis of bone

     L97.219   Non-pressure chronic ulcer of right calf with unspecified severity

   ● **L97.22**   Non-pressure chronic ulcer of left calf

     L97.221   Non-pressure chronic ulcer of left calf limited to breakdown of skin

     L97.222   Non-pressure chronic ulcer of left calf with fat layer exposed

     L97.223   Non-pressure chronic ulcer of left calf with necrosis of muscle

     L97.224   Non-pressure chronic ulcer of left calf with necrosis of bone

     L97.229   Non-pressure chronic ulcer of left calf with unspecified severity

● **L97.3**   Non-pressure chronic ulcer of ankle

   ● **L97.30**   Non-pressure chronic ulcer of unspecified ankle

     L97.301   Non-pressure chronic ulcer of unspecified ankle limited to breakdown of skin

     L97.302   Non-pressure chronic ulcer of unspecified ankle with fat layer exposed

     L97.303   Non-pressure chronic ulcer of unspecified ankle with necrosis of muscle

     L97.304   Non-pressure chronic ulcer of unspecified ankle with necrosis of bone

     L97.309   Non-pressure chronic ulcer of unspecified ankle with unspecified severity

● **L97.31**   Non-pressure chronic ulcer of right ankle

     L97.311   Non-pressure chronic ulcer of right ankle limited to breakdown of skin

     L97.312   Non-pressure chronic ulcer of right ankle with fat layer exposed

     L97.313   Non-pressure chronic ulcer of right ankle with necrosis of muscle

     L97.314   Non-pressure chronic ulcer of right ankle with necrosis of bone

     L97.319   Non-pressure chronic ulcer of right ankle with unspecified severity

● **L97.32**   Non-pressure chronic ulcer of left ankle

     L97.321   Non-pressure chronic ulcer of left ankle limited to breakdown of skin

     L97.322   Non-pressure chronic ulcer of left ankle with fat layer exposed

     L97.323   Non-pressure chronic ulcer of left ankle with necrosis of muscle

     L97.324   Non-pressure chronic ulcer of left ankle with necrosis of bone

     L97.329   Non-pressure chronic ulcer of left ankle with unspecified severity

● **L97.4**   Non-pressure chronic ulcer of heel and midfoot
     Non-pressure chronic ulcer of plantar surface of midfoot

   ● **L97.40**   Non-pressure chronic ulcer of unspecified heel and midfoot

     L97.401   Non-pressure chronic ulcer of unspecified heel and midfoot limited to breakdown of skin

     L97.402   Non-pressure chronic ulcer of unspecified heel and midfoot with fat layer exposed

     L97.403   Non-pressure chronic ulcer of unspecified heel and midfoot with necrosis of muscle

     L97.404   Non-pressure chronic ulcer of unspecified heel and midfoot with necrosis of bone

     L97.409   Non-pressure chronic ulcer of unspecified heel and midfoot with unspecified severity

   ● **L97.41**   Non-pressure chronic ulcer of right heel and midfoot

     L97.411   Non-pressure chronic ulcer of right heel and midfoot limited to breakdown of skin

     L97.412   Non-pressure chronic ulcer of right heel and midfoot with fat layer exposed

     L97.413   Non-pressure chronic ulcer of right heel and midfoot with necrosis of muscle

     L97.414   Non-pressure chronic ulcer of right heel and midfoot with necrosis of bone

     L97.419   Non-pressure chronic ulcer of right heel and midfoot with unspecified severity

CHAPTER 12 (L00-L99)

● **L97.42　Non-pressure chronic ulcer of left heel and midfoot**

　　L97.421　Non-pressure chronic ulcer of left heel and midfoot limited to breakdown of skin

　　L97.422　Non-pressure chronic ulcer of left heel and midfoot with fat layer exposed

　　L97.423　Non-pressure chronic ulcer of left heel and midfoot with necrosis of muscle

　　L97.424　Non-pressure chronic ulcer of left heel and midfoot with necrosis of bone

　　L97.429　Non-pressure chronic ulcer of left heel and midfoot with unspecified severity

● **L97.5　Non-pressure chronic ulcer of other part of foot**
　　Non-pressure chronic ulcer of toe

● **L97.50　Non-pressure chronic ulcer of other part of unspecified foot**

　　L97.501　Non-pressure chronic ulcer of other part of unspecified foot limited to breakdown of skin

　　L97.502　Non-pressure chronic ulcer of other part of unspecified foot with fat layer exposed

　　L97.503　Non-pressure chronic ulcer of other part of unspecified foot with necrosis of muscle

　　L97.504　Non-pressure chronic ulcer of other part of unspecified foot with necrosis of bone

　　L97.509　Non-pressure chronic ulcer of other part of unspecified foot with unspecified severity

● **L97.51　Non-pressure chronic ulcer of other part of right foot**

　　L97.511　Non-pressure chronic ulcer of other part of right foot limited to breakdown of skin

　　L97.512　Non-pressure chronic ulcer of other part of right foot with fat layer exposed

　　L97.513　Non-pressure chronic ulcer of other part of right foot with necrosis of muscle

　　L97.514　Non-pressure chronic ulcer of other part of right foot with necrosis of bone

　　L97.519　Non-pressure chronic ulcer of other part of right foot with unspecified severity

● **L97.52　Non-pressure chronic ulcer of other part of left foot**

　　L97.521　Non-pressure chronic ulcer of other part of left foot limited to breakdown of skin

　　L97.522　Non-pressure chronic ulcer of other part of left foot with fat layer exposed

　　L97.523　Non-pressure chronic ulcer of other part of left foot with necrosis of muscle

　　L97.524　Non-pressure chronic ulcer of other part of left foot with necrosis of bone

　　L97.529　Non-pressure chronic ulcer of other part of left foot with unspecified severity

● **L97.8　Non-pressure chronic ulcer of other part of lower leg**

● **L97.80　Non-pressure chronic ulcer of other part of unspecified lower leg**

　　L97.801　Non-pressure chronic ulcer of other part of unspecified lower leg limited to breakdown of skin

　　L97.802　Non-pressure chronic ulcer of other part of unspecified lower leg with fat layer exposed

　　L97.803　Non-pressure chronic ulcer of other part of unspecified lower leg with necrosis of muscle

　　L97.804　Non-pressure chronic ulcer of other part of unspecified lower leg with necrosis of bone

　　L97.809　Non-pressure chronic ulcer of other part of unspecified lower leg with unspecified severity

● **L97.81　Non-pressure chronic ulcer of other part of right lower leg**

　　L97.811　Non-pressure chronic ulcer of other part of right lower leg limited to breakdown of skin

　　L97.812　Non-pressure chronic ulcer of other part of right lower leg with fat layer exposed

　　L97.813　Non-pressure chronic ulcer of other part of right lower leg with necrosis of muscle

　　L97.814　Non-pressure chronic ulcer of other part of right lower leg with necrosis of bone

　　L97.819　Non-pressure chronic ulcer of other part of right lower leg with unspecified severity

● **L97.82　Non-pressure chronic ulcer of other part of left lower leg**

　　L97.821　Non-pressure chronic ulcer of other part of left lower leg limited to breakdown of skin

　　L97.822　Non-pressure chronic ulcer of other part of left lower leg with fat layer exposed

　　L97.823　Non-pressure chronic ulcer of other part of left lower leg with necrosis of muscle

　　L97.824　Non-pressure chronic ulcer of other part of left lower leg with necrosis of bone

　　L97.829　Non-pressure chronic ulcer of other part of left lower leg with unspecified severity

● **L97.9　Non-pressure chronic ulcer of unspecified part of lower leg**

● **L97.90　Non-pressure chronic ulcer of unspecified part of unspecified lower leg**

　　L97.901　Non-pressure chronic ulcer of unspecified part of unspecified lower leg limited to breakdown of skin

　　L97.902　Non-pressure chronic ulcer of unspecified part of unspecified lower leg with fat layer exposed

　　L97.903　Non-pressure chronic ulcer of unspecified part of unspecified lower leg with necrosis of muscle

　　L97.904　Non-pressure chronic ulcer of unspecified part of unspecified lower leg with necrosis of bone

　　L97.909　Non-pressure chronic ulcer of unspecified part of unspecified lower leg with unspecified severity

● **L97.91**   **Non-pressure chronic ulcer of unspecified part of right lower leg**

    L97.911   Non-pressure chronic ulcer of unspecified part of right lower leg limited to breakdown of skin

    L97.912   Non-pressure chronic ulcer of unspecified part of right lower leg with fat layer exposed

    L97.913   Non-pressure chronic ulcer of unspecified part of right lower leg with necrosis of muscle

    L97.914   Non-pressure chronic ulcer of unspecified part of right lower leg with necrosis of bone

    L97.919   Non-pressure chronic ulcer of unspecified part of right lower leg with unspecified severity

● **L97.92**   **Non-pressure chronic ulcer of unspecified part of left lower leg**

    L97.921   Non-pressure chronic ulcer of unspecified part of left lower leg limited to breakdown of skin

    L97.922   Non-pressure chronic ulcer of unspecified part of left lower leg with fat layer exposed

    L97.923   Non-pressure chronic ulcer of unspecified part of left lower leg with necrosis of muscle

    L97.924   Non-pressure chronic ulcer of unspecified part of left lower leg with necrosis of bone

    L97.929   Non-pressure chronic ulcer of unspecified part of left lower leg with unspecified severity

● **L98**   **Other disorders of skin and subcutaneous tissue, not elsewhere classified**

   L98.0   **Pyogenic granuloma**

     | **Excludes2** | pyogenic granuloma of gingiva (K06.8)
     pyogenic granuloma of maxillary alveolar ridge (K04.5)
     pyogenic granuloma of oral mucosa (K13.4)

   L98.1   **Factitial dermatitis**
     Neurotic excoriation

   L98.2   **Febrile neutrophilic dermatosis [Sweet]**

   L98.3   **Eosinophilic cellulitis [Wells]**

● **L98.4**   **Non-pressure chronic ulcer of skin, not elsewhere classified**
     Chronic ulcer of skin NOS
     Tropical ulcer NOS
     Ulcer of skin NOS

     | **Excludes2** | pressure ulcer (pressure area) (L89.-)
     gangrene (I96)
     skin infections (L00-L08)
     specific infections classified to A00-B99
     ulcer of lower limb NEC (L97.-)
     varicose ulcer (I83.0-I82.2)

● **L98.41**   **Non-pressure chronic ulcer of buttock**

    L98.411   Non-pressure chronic ulcer of buttock limited to breakdown of skin

    L98.412   Non-pressure chronic ulcer of buttock with fat layer exposed

    L98.413   Non-pressure chronic ulcer of buttock with necrosis of muscle

    L98.414   Non-pressure chronic ulcer of buttock with necrosis of bone

    L98.419   Non-pressure chronic ulcer of buttock with unspecified severity

● **L98.42**   **Non-pressure chronic ulcer of back**

    L98.421   Non-pressure chronic ulcer of back limited to breakdown of skin

    L98.422   Non-pressure chronic ulcer of back with fat layer exposed

    L98.423   Non-pressure chronic ulcer of back with necrosis of muscle

    L98.424   Non-pressure chronic ulcer of back with necrosis of bone

    L98.429   Non-pressure chronic ulcer of back with unspecified severity

● **L98.49**   **Non-pressure chronic ulcer of skin of other sites**
     Non-pressure chronic ulcer of skin NOS

    L98.491   Non-pressure chronic ulcer of skin of other sites limited to breakdown of skin

    L98.492   Non-pressure chronic ulcer of skin of other sites with fat layer exposed

    L98.493   Non-pressure chronic ulcer of skin of other sites with necrosis of muscle

    L98.494   Non-pressure chronic ulcer of skin of other sites with necrosis of bone

    L98.499   Non-pressure chronic ulcer of skin of other sites with unspecified severity

   L98.5   **Mucinosis of the skin**
     Focal mucinosis
     Lichen myxedematosus
     Reticular erythematous mucinosis

     | **Excludes1** | focal oral mucinosis (K13.79)
     myxedema (E03.9)

   L98.6   **Other infiltrative disorders of the skin and subcutaneous tissue**

     | **Excludes1** | hyalinosis cutis et mucosae (E78.89)

   L98.8   **Other specified disorders of the skin and subcutaneous tissue**

   L98.9   **Disorder of the skin and subcutaneous tissue, unspecified**

  L99   **Other disorders of skin and subcutaneous tissue in diseases classified elsewhere**

     Code first underlying disease, such as:
     amyloidosis (E85.-)

     | **Excludes1** | skin disorders in diabetes (E08-E13 with .62)
     skin disorders in gonorrhea (A54.89)
     skin disorders in syphilis (A51.31, A52.79)

CHAPTER 12 (L00-L99)

OGCR Section I.C.a.-c.

a. Site and laterality

Most of the codes within Chapter 13 have site and laterality designations. The site represents the bone, joint or the muscle involved. For some conditions where more than one bone, joint or muscle is usually involved, such as osteoarthritis, there is a "multiple sites" code available. For categories where no multiple site code is provided and more than one bone, joint or muscle is involved, multiple codes should be used to indicate the different sites involved.

1) Bone versus joint

For certain conditions, the bone may be affected at the upper or lower end, (e.g., avascular necrosis of bone, M87, Osteoporosis, M80, M81). Though the portion of the bone affected may be at the joint, the site designation will be the bone, not the joint.

b. Acute traumatic versus chronic or recurrent musculoskeletal conditions

Many musculoskeletal conditions are a result of previous injury or trauma to a site, or are recurrent conditions. Bone, joint or muscle conditions that are the result of a healed injury are usually found in chapter 13. Recurrent bone, joint or muscle conditions are also usually found in chapter 13. Any current, acute injury should be coded to the appropriate injury code from chapter 19. Chronic or recurrent conditions should generally be coded with a code from chapter 13. If it is difficult to determine from the documentation in the record which code is best to describe a condition, query the provider.

c. Coding of Pathologic Fractures

7th character A is for use as long as the patient is receiving active treatment for the fracture. Examples of active treatment are: surgical treatment, emergency department encounter, evaluation and continuing treatment by the same or a different physician. While the patient may be seen by a new or different provider over the course of treatment for a pathological fracture, assignment of the 7th character is based on whether the patient is undergoing active treatment and not whether the provider is seeing the patient for the first time.

7th character, D is to be used for encounters after the patient has completed active treatment. The other 7th characters, listed under each subcategory in the Tabular List, are to be used for subsequent encounters for treatment of problems associated with the healing, such as malunions and nonunions, and sequelae. Care for complications of surgical treatment for fracture repairs during the healing or recovery phase should be coded with the appropriate complication codes.

See Section I.C.19. Coding of traumatic fractures.

CHAPTER 13

DISEASES OF THE MUSCULOSKELETAL SYSTEM AND CONNECTIVE TISSUE (M00-M99)

Note: Use an external cause code following the code for the musculoskeletal condition, if applicable, to identify the cause of the musculoskeletal condition

Excludes2 arthropathic psoriasis (L40.5-)
certain conditions originating in the perinatal period (P04-P96)
certain infectious and parasitic diseases (A00-B99)
compartment syndrome (traumatic) (T79.A-)
complications of pregnancy, childbirth and the puerperium (O00-O9A)
congenital malformations, deformations, and chromosomal abnormalities (Q00-Q99)
endocrine, nutritional and metabolic diseases (E00-E88)
injury, poisoning and certain other consequences of external causes (S00-T88)
neoplasms (C00-D49)
symptoms, signs and abnormal clinical and laboratory findings, not elsewhere classified (R00-R94)

This chapter contains the following blocks:

M00-M02	Infectious arthropathies
M05-M14	Inflammatory polyarthropathies
M15-M19	Osteoarthritis
M20-M25	Other joint disorders
M26-M27	Dentofacial anomalies [including malocclusion] and other disorders of jaw
M30-M36	Systemic connective tissue disorders
M40-M43	Deforming dorsopathies
M45-M49	Spondylopathies
M50-M54	Other dorsopathies
M60-M63	Disorders of muscles
M65-M67	Disorders of synovium and tendon
M70-M79	Other soft tissue disorders
M80-M85	Disorders of bone density and structure
M86-M90	Other osteopathies
M91-M94	Chondropathies
M95	Other disorders of the musculoskeletal system and connective tissue
M96	Intraoperative and postprocedural complications and disorders of musculoskeletal system, not elsewhere classified
M99	Biomechanical lesions, not elsewhere classified

ARTHROPATHIES (M00-M25)

Includes Disorders affecting predominantly peripheral (limb) joints

INFECTIOUS ARTHROPATHIES (M00-M02)

Note: This block comprises arthropathies due to microbiological agents.

Distinction is made between the following types of etiological relationship:

a) direct infection of joint, where organisms invade synovial tissue and microbial antigen is present in the joint;

b) indirect infection, which may be of two types: a reactive arthropathy, where microbial infection of the body is established but neither organisms nor antigens can be identified in the joint, and a postinfective arthropathy, where microbial antigen is present but recovery of an organism is inconstant and evidence of local multiplication is lacking.

● **M00 Pyogenic arthritis**

  ● **M00.0 Staphylococcal arthritis and polyarthritis**

    Use additional code (B95.61-B95.8) to identify bacterial agent

    Excludes2 infection and inflammatory reaction due to internal joint prosthesis (T84.5-)

    M00.00 **Staphylococcal arthritis, unspecified joint**

    ● M00.01 **Staphylococcal arthritis, shoulder**

      M00.011 **Staphylococcal arthritis, right shoulder**

      M00.012 **Staphylococcal arthritis, left shoulder**

      M00.019 **Staphylococcal arthritis, unspecified shoulder**

    ● M00.02 **Staphylococcal arthritis, elbow**

      M00.021 **Staphylococcal arthritis, right elbow**

      M00.022 **Staphylococcal arthritis, left elbow**

      M00.029 **Staphylococcal arthritis, unspecified elbow**

    ● M00.03 **Staphylococcal arthritis, wrist**
      Staphylococcal arthritis of carpal bones

      M00.031 **Staphylococcal arthritis, right wrist**

      M00.032 **Staphylococcal arthritis, left wrist**

      M00.039 **Staphylococcal arthritis, unspecified wrist**

◀ New   ⬅ Revised   ~~deleted~~ Deleted   OGCR Official Guidelines   X Assign placeholder X   ● Use Additional Character(s)

Excludes 1   Excludes 2   Includes   Use additional   Code first   Code also   Unspecified

● M00.04 **Staphylococcal arthritis, hand**
           Staphylococcal arthritis of metacarpus and
           phalanges
       M00.041 **Staphylococcal arthritis, right hand**
       M00.042 **Staphylococcal arthritis, left hand**
       M00.049 **Staphylococcal arthritis, unspecified
                 hand**
● M00.05 **Staphylococcal arthritis, hip**
       M00.051 **Staphylococcal arthritis, right hip**
       M00.052 **Staphylococcal arthritis, left hip**
       M00.059 **Staphylococcal arthritis, unspecified
                 hip**
● M00.06 **Staphylococcal arthritis, knee**
       M00.061 **Staphylococcal arthritis, right knee**
       M00.062 **Staphylococcal arthritis, left knee**
       M00.069 **Staphylococcal arthritis, unspecified
                 knee**
● M00.07 **Staphylococcal arthritis, ankle and foot**
           Staphylococcal arthritis, tarsus, metatarsus and
           phalanges
       M00.071 **Staphylococcal arthritis, right ankle
                 and foot**
       M00.072 **Staphylococcal arthritis, left ankle
                 and foot**
       M00.079 **Staphylococcal arthritis, unspecified
                 ankle and foot**
   M00.08 **Staphylococcal arthritis, vertebrae**
   M00.09 **Staphylococcal polyarthritis**
● M00.1 **Pneumococcal arthritis and polyarthritis**
   M00.10 **Pneumococcal arthritis, unspecified joint**
● M00.11 **Pneumococcal arthritis, shoulder**
       M00.111 **Pneumococcal arthritis, right shoulder**
       M00.112 **Pneumococcal arthritis, left shoulder**
       M00.119 **Pneumococcal arthritis, unspecified
                 shoulder**
● M00.12 **Pneumococcal arthritis, elbow**
       M00.121 **Pneumococcal arthritis, right elbow**
       M00.122 **Pneumococcal arthritis, left elbow**
       M00.129 **Pneumococcal arthritis, unspecified
                 elbow**
● M00.13 **Pneumococcal arthritis, wrist**
           Pneumococcal arthritis of carpal bones
       M00.131 **Pneumococcal arthritis, right wrist**
       M00.132 **Pneumococcal arthritis, left wrist**
       M00.139 **Pneumococcal arthritis, unspecified
                 wrist**
● M00.14 **Pneumococcal arthritis, hand**
           Pneumococcal arthritis of metacarpus and
           phalanges
       M00.141 **Pneumococcal arthritis, right hand**
       M00.142 **Pneumococcal arthritis, left hand**
       M00.149 **Pneumococcal arthritis, unspecified
                 hand**
● M00.15 **Pneumococcal arthritis, hip**
       M00.151 **Pneumococcal arthritis, right hip**
       M00.152 **Pneumococcal arthritis, left hip**
       M00.159 **Pneumococcal arthritis, unspecified
                 hip**
● M00.16 **Pneumococcal arthritis, knee**
       M00.161 **Pneumococcal arthritis, right knee**
       M00.162 **Pneumococcal arthritis, left knee**
       M00.169 **Pneumococcal arthritis, unspecified
                 knee**

● M00.17 **Pneumococcal arthritis, ankle and foot**
           Pneumococcal arthritis, tarsus, metatarsus and
           phalanges
       M00.171 **Pneumococcal arthritis, right ankle
                 and foot**
       M00.172 **Pneumococcal arthritis, left ankle and
                 foot**
       M00.179 **Pneumococcal arthritis, unspecified
                 ankle and foot**
   M00.18 **Pneumococcal arthritis, vertebrae**
   M00.19 **Pneumococcal polyarthritis**
● M00.2 **Other streptococcal arthritis and polyarthritis**
           Use additional code (B95.0-B95.2, B95.4-B95.5) to
           identify bacterial agent
   M00.20 **Other streptococcal arthritis, unspecified joint**
● M00.21 **Other streptococcal arthritis, shoulder**
       M00.211 **Other streptococcal arthritis, right
                 shoulder**
       M00.212 **Other streptococcal arthritis, left
                 shoulder**
       M00.219 **Other streptococcal arthritis,
                 unspecified shoulder**
● M00.22 **Other streptococcal arthritis, elbow**
       M00.221 **Other streptococcal arthritis, right
                 elbow**
       M00.222 **Other streptococcal arthritis, left
                 elbow**
       M00.229 **Other streptococcal arthritis,
                 unspecified elbow**
● M00.23 **Other streptococcal arthritis, wrist**
           Other streptococcal arthritis of carpal bones
       M00.231 **Other streptococcal arthritis, right
                 wrist**
       M00.232 **Other streptococcal arthritis, left wrist**
       M00.239 **Other streptococcal arthritis,
                 unspecified wrist**
● M00.24 **Other streptococcal arthritis, hand**
           Other streptococcal arthritis metacarpus and
           phalanges
       M00.241 **Other streptococcal arthritis, right
                 hand**
       M00.242 **Other streptococcal arthritis, left hand**
       M00.249 **Other streptococcal arthritis,
                 unspecified hand**
● M00.25 **Other streptococcal arthritis, hip**
       M00.251 **Other streptococcal arthritis, right hip**
       M00.252 **Other streptococcal arthritis, left hip**
       M00.259 **Other streptococcal arthritis,
                 unspecified hip**
● M00.26 **Other streptococcal arthritis, knee**
       M00.261 **Other streptococcal arthritis, right
                 knee**
       M00.262 **Other streptococcal arthritis, left knee**
       M00.269 **Other streptococcal arthritis,
                 unspecified knee**
● M00.27 **Other streptococcal arthritis, ankle and foot**
           Other streptococcal arthritis, tarsus, metatarsus
           and phalanges
       M00.271 **Other streptococcal arthritis, right
                 ankle and foot**
       M00.272 **Other streptococcal arthritis, left
                 ankle and foot**
       M00.279 **Other streptococcal arthritis,
                 unspecified ankle and foot**
   M00.28 **Other streptococcal arthritis, vertebrae**
   M00.29 **Other streptococcal polyarthritis**

CHAPTER 13 (M00-M99)

◀ New   ◀▥ Revised   ~~deleted~~ Deleted   OGCR Official Guidelines   X Assign placeholder X   ● Use Additional Character(s)

| Excludes 1 | Excludes 2 | Includes | Use additional | Code first | Code also | Unspecified |

● **M00.8** **Arthritis and polyarthritis due to other bacteria**
  Use additional code (B96) to identify bacteria
  M00.80 Arthritis due to other bacteria, unspecified joint
● **M00.81** Arthritis due to other bacteria, shoulder
    M00.811 Arthritis due to other bacteria, right shoulder
    M00.812 Arthritis due to other bacteria, left shoulder
    M00.819 Arthritis due to other bacteria, unspecified shoulder
● **M00.82** Arthritis due to other bacteria, elbow
    M00.821 Arthritis due to other bacteria, right elbow
    M00.822 Arthritis due to other bacteria, left elbow
    M00.829 Arthritis due to other bacteria, unspecified elbow
● **M00.83** Arthritis due to other bacteria, wrist
    Arthritis due to other bacteria, carpal bones
    M00.831 Arthritis due to other bacteria, right wrist
    M00.832 Arthritis due to other bacteria, left wrist
    M00.839 Arthritis due to other bacteria, unspecified wrist
● **M00.84** Arthritis due to other bacteria, hand
    Arthritis due to other bacteria, metacarpus and phalanges
    M00.841 Arthritis due to other bacteria, right hand
    M00.842 Arthritis due to other bacteria, left hand
    M00.849 Arthritis due to other bacteria, unspecified hand
● **M00.85** Arthritis due to other bacteria, hip
    M00.851 Arthritis due to other bacteria, right hip
    M00.852 Arthritis due to other bacteria, left hip
    M00.859 Arthritis due to other bacteria, unspecified hip
● **M00.86** Arthritis due to other bacteria, knee
    M00.861 Arthritis due to other bacteria, right knee
    M00.862 Arthritis due to other bacteria, left knee
    M00.869 Arthritis due to other bacteria, unspecified knee
● **M00.87** Arthritis due to other bacteria, ankle and foot
    Arthritis due to other bacteria, tarsus, metatarsus, and phalanges
    M00.871 Arthritis due to other bacteria, right ankle and foot
    M00.872 Arthritis due to other bacteria, left ankle and foot
    M00.879 Arthritis due to other bacteria, unspecified ankle and foot
  M00.88 Arthritis due to other bacteria, vertebrae
  M00.89 Polyarthritis due to other bacteria
M00.9 Pyogenic arthritis, unspecified
  Infective arthritis NOS

● **M01** **Direct infections of joint in infectious and parasitic diseases classified elsewhere**
  Code first underlying disease, such as:
    leprosy [Hansen's disease] (A30.-)
    mycoses (B35-B49)
    O'nyong-nyong fever (A92.1)
    paratyphoid fever (A01.1-A01.4)
  Excludes1 arthropathy in Lyme disease (A69.23)
    gonococcal arthritis (A54.42)
    meningococcal arthritis (A39.83)
    mumps arthritis (B26.85)
    postinfective arthropathy (M02.-)
    postmeningococcal arthritis (A39.84)
    reactive arthritis (M02.3)
    rubella arthritis (B06.82)
    sarcoidosis arthritis (D86.86)
    typhoid fever arthritis (A01.04)
    tuberculosis arthritis (A18.01-A18.02)
● **M01.X** Direct infection of joint in infectious and parasitic diseases classified elsewhere
    M01.X0 Direct infection of unspecified joint in infectious and parasitic diseases classified elsewhere
  ● **M01.X1** Direct infection of shoulder joint in infectious and parasitic diseases classified elsewhere
      M01.X11 Direct infection of right shoulder in infectious and parasitic diseases classified elsewhere
      M01.X12 Direct infection of left shoulder in infectious and parasitic diseases classified elsewhere
      M01.X19 Direct infection of unspecified shoulder in infectious and parasitic diseases classified elsewhere
  ● **M01.X2** Direct infection of elbow in infectious and parasitic diseases classified elsewhere
      M01.X21 Direct infection of right elbow in infectious and parasitic diseases classified elsewhere
      M01.X22 Direct infection of left elbow in infectious and parasitic diseases classified elsewhere
      M01.X29 Direct infection of unspecified elbow in infectious and parasitic diseases classified elsewhere
  ● **M01.X3** Direct infection of wrist in infectious and parasitic diseases classified elsewhere
      Direct infection of carpal bones in infectious and parasitic diseases classified elsewhere
      M01.X31 Direct infection of right wrist in infectious and parasitic diseases classified elsewhere
      M01.X32 Direct infection of left wrist in infectious and parasitic diseases classified elsewhere
      M01.X39 Direct infection of unspecified wrist in infectious and parasitic diseases classified elsewhere
  ● **M01.X4** Direct infection of hand in infectious and parasitic diseases classified elsewhere
      Direct infection of metacarpus and phalanges in infectious and parasitic diseases classified elsewhere
      M01.X41 Direct infection of right hand in infectious and parasitic diseases classified elsewhere
      M01.X42 Direct infection of left hand in infectious and parasitic diseases classified elsewhere
      M01.X49 Direct infection of unspecified hand in infectious and parasitic diseases classified elsewhere

● M01.X5 Direct infection of hip in infectious and parasitic diseases classified elsewhere

   M01.X51 Direct infection of right hip in infectious and parasitic diseases classified elsewhere

   M01.X52 Direct infection of left hip in infectious and parasitic diseases classified elsewhere

   M01.X59 Direct infection of unspecified hip in infectious and parasitic diseases classified elsewhere

● M01.X6 Direct infection of knee in infectious and parasitic diseases classified elsewhere

   M01.X61 Direct infection of right knee in infectious and parasitic diseases classified elsewhere

   M01.X62 Direct infection of left knee in infectious and parasitic diseases classified elsewhere

   M01.X69 Direct infection of unspecified knee in infectious and parasitic diseases classified elsewhere

● M01.X7 Direct infection of ankle and foot in infectious and parasitic diseases classified elsewhere
   Direct infection of tarsus, metatarsus and phalanges in infectious and parasitic diseases classified elsewhere

   M01.X71 Direct infection of right ankle and foot in infectious and parasitic diseases classified elsewhere

   M01.X72 Direct infection of left ankle and foot in infectious and parasitic diseases classified elsewhere

   M01.X79 Direct infection of unspecified ankle and foot in infectious and parasitic diseases classified elsewhere

   M01.X8 Direct infection of vertebrae in infectious and parasitic diseases classified elsewhere

   M01.X9 Direct infection of multiple joints in infectious and parasitic diseases classified elsewhere

● M02 Postinfective and reactive arthropathies

   Code first underlying disease, such as:
   congenital syphilis [Clutton's joints] (A50.5)
   enteritis due to Yersinia enterocolitica (A04.6)
   infective endocarditis (I33.0)
   viral hepatitis (B15-B19)

   | Excludes1 | Behçet's disease (M35.2) |

   direct infections of joint in infectious and parasitic diseases classified elsewhere (M01.-)
   postmeningococcal arthritis (A39.84)
   mumps arthritis (B26.85)
   rubella arthritis (B06.82)
   syphilis arthritis (late) (A52.77)
   rheumatic fever (I00)
   tabetic arthropathy [Charcôt's] (A52.16)

● M02.0 Arthropathy following intestinal bypass

   M02.00 Arthropathy following intestinal bypass, unspecified site

● M02.01 Arthropathy following intestinal bypass, shoulder

   M02.011 Arthropathy following intestinal bypass, right shoulder

   M02.012 Arthropathy following intestinal bypass, left shoulder

   M02.019 Arthropathy following intestinal bypass, unspecified shoulder

● M02.02 Arthropathy following intestinal bypass, elbow

   M02.021 Arthropathy following intestinal bypass, right elbow

   M02.022 Arthropathy following intestinal bypass, left elbow

   M02.029 Arthropathy following intestinal bypass, unspecified elbow

● M02.03 Arthropathy following intestinal bypass, wrist
   Arthropathy following intestinal bypass, carpal bones

   M02.031 Arthropathy following intestinal bypass, right wrist

   M02.032 Arthropathy following intestinal bypass, left wrist

   M02.039 Arthropathy following intestinal bypass, unspecified wrist

● M02.04 Arthropathy following intestinal bypass, hand
   Arthropathy following intestinal bypass, metacarpals and phalanges

   M02.041 Arthropathy following intestinal bypass, right hand

   M02.042 Arthropathy following intestinal bypass, left hand

   M02.049 Arthropathy following intestinal bypass, unspecified hand

● M02.05 Arthropathy following intestinal bypass, hip

   M02.051 Arthropathy following intestinal bypass, right hip

   M02.052 Arthropathy following intestinal bypass, left hip

   M02.059 Arthropathy following intestinal bypass, unspecified hip

● M02.06 Arthropathy following intestinal bypass, knee

   M02.061 Arthropathy following intestinal bypass, right knee

   M02.062 Arthropathy following intestinal bypass, left knee

   M02.069 Arthropathy following intestinal bypass, unspecified knee

● M02.07 Arthropathy following intestinal bypass, ankle and foot
   Arthropathy following intestinal bypass, tarsus, metatarsus and phalanges

   M02.071 Arthropathy following intestinal bypass, right ankle and foot

   M02.072 Arthropathy following intestinal bypass, left ankle and foot

   M02.079 Arthropathy following intestinal bypass, unspecified ankle and foot

   M02.08 Arthropathy following intestinal bypass, vertebrae

   M02.09 Arthropathy following intestinal bypass, multiple sites

● M02.1 Postdysenteric arthropathy

   M02.10 Postdysenteric arthropathy, unspecified site

● M02.11 Postdysenteric arthropathy, shoulder

   M02.111 Postdysenteric arthropathy, right shoulder

   M02.112 Postdysenteric arthropathy, left shoulder

   M02.119 Postdysenteric arthropathy, unspecified shoulder

CHAPTER 13 (M00-M99)

● M02.12   Postdysenteric arthropathy, elbow
    M02.121   Postdysenteric arthropathy, right elbow
    M02.122   Postdysenteric arthropathy, left elbow
    M02.129   Postdysenteric arthropathy, unspecified elbow

● M02.13   Postdysenteric arthropathy, wrist
    Postdysenteric arthropathy, carpal bones
    M02.131   Postdysenteric arthropathy, right wrist
    M02.132   Postdysenteric arthropathy, left wrist
    M02.139   Postdysenteric arthropathy, unspecified wrist

● M02.14   Postdysenteric arthropathy, hand
    Postdysenteric arthropathy, metacarpus and phalanges
    M02.141   Postdysenteric arthropathy, right hand
    M02.142   Postdysenteric arthropathy, left hand
    M02.149   Postdysenteric arthropathy, unspecified hand

● M02.15   Postdysenteric arthropathy, hip
    M02.151   Postdysenteric arthropathy, right hip
    M02.152   Postdysenteric arthropathy, left hip
    M02.159   Postdysenteric arthropathy, unspecified hip

● M02.16   Postdysenteric arthropathy, knee
    M02.161   Postdysenteric arthropathy, right knee
    M02.162   Postdysenteric arthropathy, left knee
    M02.169   Postdysenteric arthropathy, unspecified knee

● M02.17   Postdysenteric arthropathy, ankle and foot
    Postdysenteric arthropathy, tarsus, metatarsus and phalanges
    M02.171   Postdysenteric arthropathy, right ankle and foot
    M02.172   Postdysenteric arthropathy, left ankle and foot
    M02.179   Postdysenteric arthropathy, unspecified ankle and foot

    M02.18   Postdysenteric arthropathy, vertebrae
    M02.19   Postdysenteric arthropathy, multiple sites

● M02.2   Postimmunization arthropathy
    M02.20   Postimmunization arthropathy, unspecified site

● M02.21   Postimmunization arthropathy, shoulder
    M02.211   Postimmunization arthropathy, right shoulder
    M02.212   Postimmunization arthropathy, left shoulder
    M02.219   Postimmunization arthropathy, unspecified shoulder

● M02.22   Postimmunization arthropathy, elbow
    M02.221   Postimmunization arthropathy, right elbow
    M02.222   Postimmunization arthropathy, left elbow
    M02.229   Postimmunization arthropathy, unspecified elbow

● M02.23   Postimmunization arthropathy, wrist
    Postimmunization arthropathy, carpal bones
    M02.231   Postimmunization arthropathy, right wrist
    M02.232   Postimmunization arthropathy, left wrist
    M02.239   Postimmunization arthropathy, unspecified wrist

● M02.24   Postimmunization arthropathy, hand
    Postimmunization arthropathy, metacarpus and phalanges
    M02.241   Postimmunization arthropathy, right hand
    M02.242   Postimmunization arthropathy, left hand
    M02.249   Postimmunization arthropathy, unspecified hand

● M02.25   Postimmunization arthropathy, hip
    M02.251   Postimmunization arthropathy, right hip
    M02.252   Postimmunization arthropathy, left hip
    M02.259   Postimmunization arthropathy, unspecified hip

● M02.26   Postimmunization arthropathy, knee
    M02.261   Postimmunization arthropathy, right knee
    M02.262   Postimmunization arthropathy, left knee
    M02.269   Postimmunization arthropathy, unspecified knee

● M02.27   Postimmunization arthropathy, ankle and foot
    Postimmunization arthropathy, tarsus, metatarsus and phalanges
    M02.271   Postimmunization arthropathy, right ankle and foot
    M02.272   Postimmunization arthropathy, left ankle and foot
    M02.279   Postimmunization arthropathy, unspecified ankle and foot

    M02.28   Postimmunization arthropathy, vertebrae
    M02.29   Postimmunization arthropathy, multiple sites

● M02.3   Reiter's disease
    Reactive arthritis
    M02.30   Reiter's disease, unspecified site

● M02.31   Reiter's disease, shoulder
    M02.311   Reiter's disease, right shoulder
    M02.312   Reiter's disease, left shoulder
    M02.319   Reiter's disease, unspecified shoulder

● M02.32   Reiter's disease, elbow
    M02.321   Reiter's disease, right elbow
    M02.322   Reiter's disease, left elbow
    M02.329   Reiter's disease, unspecified elbow

● M02.33   Reiter's disease, wrist
    Reiter's disease, carpal bones
    M02.331   Reiter's disease, right wrist
    M02.332   Reiter's disease, left wrist
    M02.339   Reiter's disease, unspecified wrist

● M02.34   Reiter's disease, hand
    Reiter's disease, metacarpus and phalanges
    M02.341   Reiter's disease, right hand
    M02.342   Reiter's disease, left hand
    M02.349   Reiter's disease, unspecified hand

● M02.35   Reiter's disease, hip
    M02.351   Reiter's disease, right hip
    M02.352   Reiter's disease, left hip
    M02.359   Reiter's disease, unspecified hip

● M02.36   Reiter's disease, knee
    M02.361   Reiter's disease, right knee
    M02.362   Reiter's disease, left knee
    M02.369   Reiter's disease, unspecified knee

◄ New   ⬅ Revised   ~~deleted~~ Deleted   OGCR Official Guidelines   X Assign placeholder X   ● Use Additional Character(s)

Excludes 1   Excludes 2   Includes   Use additional   Code first   Code also   Unspecified

● M02.37 Reiter's disease, ankle and foot
        Reiter's disease, tarsus, metatarsus and
           phalanges
     M02.371 Reiter's disease, right ankle and foot
     M02.372 Reiter's disease, left ankle and foot
     M02.379 Reiter's disease, unspecified ankle
              and foot
  M02.38 Reiter's disease, vertebrae
  M02.39 Reiter's disease, multiple sites
● M02.8 Other reactive arthropathies
  M02.80 Other reactive arthropathies, unspecified site
● M02.81 Other reactive arthropathies, shoulder
     M02.811 Other reactive arthropathies, right
              shoulder
     M02.812 Other reactive arthropathies, left
              shoulder
     M02.819 Other reactive arthropathies,
              unspecified shoulder
● M02.82 Other reactive arthropathies, elbow
     M02.821 Other reactive arthropathies, right
              elbow
     M02.822 Other reactive arthropathies, left
              elbow
     M02.829 Other reactive arthropathies,
              unspecified elbow
● M02.83 Other reactive arthropathies, wrist
        Other reactive arthropathies, carpal bones
     M02.831 Other reactive arthropathies, right
              wrist
     M02.832 Other reactive arthropathies, left
              wrist
     M02.839 Other reactive arthropathies,
              unspecified wrist
● M02.84 Other reactive arthropathies, hand
        Other reactive arthropathies, metacarpus and
           phalanges
     M02.841 Other reactive arthropathies, right
              hand
     M02.842 Other reactive arthropathies, left
              hand
     M02.849 Other reactive arthropathies,
              unspecified hand
● M02.85 Other reactive arthropathies, hip
     M02.851 Other reactive arthropathies, right hip
     M02.852 Other reactive arthropathies, left hip
     M02.859 Other reactive arthropathies,
              unspecified hip
● M02.86 Other reactive arthropathies, knee
     M02.861 Other reactive arthropathies, right
              knee
     M02.862 Other reactive arthropathies, left knee
     M02.869 Other reactive arthropathies,
              unspecified knee
● M02.87 Other reactive arthropathies, ankle and foot
        Other reactive arthropathies, tarsus,
           metatarsus and phalanges
     M02.871 Other reactive arthropathies, right
              ankle and foot
     M02.872 Other reactive arthropathies, left
              ankle and foot
     M02.879 Other reactive arthropathies,
              unspecified ankle and foot
  M02.88 Other reactive arthropathies, vertebrae
  M02.89 Other reactive arthropathies, multiple sites
M02.9 Reactive arthropathy, unspecified

Item 13–1 Rheumatoid arthritis (RA) is a chronic systemic inflammatory autoimmune disease of undetermined etiology involving primarily the synovial membranes and articular structures of multiple joints. It can also affect other organs, including the eyes, blood vessels, heart, and lungs. The disease is often progressive. In late stages, deformity, ankylosis, and other **inflammatory polyarthropathies** develop.

INFLAMMATORY POLYARTHROPATHIES (M05-M14)

● M05 Rheumatoid arthritis with rheumatoid factor
    Excludes1 rheumatic fever (I00)
                juvenile rheumatoid arthritis (M08.-)
                rheumatoid arthritis of spine (M45.-)
● M05.0 Felty's syndrome
       Rheumatoid arthritis with splenoadenomegaly and
          leukopenia
  M05.00 Felty's syndrome, unspecified site
● M05.01 Felty's syndrome, shoulder
     M05.011 Felty's syndrome, right shoulder
     M05.012 Felty's syndrome, left shoulder
     M05.019 Felty's syndrome, unspecified
              shoulder
● M05.02 Felty's syndrome, elbow
     M05.021 Felty's syndrome, right elbow
     M05.022 Felty's syndrome, left elbow
     M05.029 Felty's syndrome, unspecified elbow
● M05.03 Felty's syndrome, wrist
       Felty's syndrome, carpal bones
     M05.031 Felty's syndrome, right wrist
     M05.032 Felty's syndrome, left wrist
     M05.039 Felty's syndrome, unspecified wrist
● M05.04 Felty's syndrome, hand
       Felty's syndrome, metacarpus and phalanges
     M05.041 Felty's syndrome, right hand
     M05.042 Felty's syndrome, left hand
     M05.049 Felty's syndrome, unspecified hand
● M05.05 Felty's syndrome, hip
     M05.051 Felty's syndrome, right hip
     M05.052 Felty's syndrome, left hip
     M05.059 Felty's syndrome, unspecified hip
● M05.06 Felty's syndrome, knee
     M05.061 Felty's syndrome, right knee
     M05.062 Felty's syndrome, left knee
     M05.069 Felty's syndrome, unspecified knee
● M05.07 Felty's syndrome, ankle and foot
       Felty's syndrome, tarsus, metatarsus and
          phalanges
     M05.071 Felty's syndrome, right ankle and foot
     M05.072 Felty's syndrome, left ankle and foot
     M05.079 Felty's syndrome, unspecified ankle
              and foot
  M05.09 Felty's syndrome, multiple sites
● M05.1 Rheumatoid lung disease with rheumatoid arthritis
  M05.10 Rheumatoid lung disease with rheumatoid
         arthritis of unspecified site
● M05.11 Rheumatoid lung disease with rheumatoid
         arthritis of shoulder
     M05.111 Rheumatoid lung disease with
              rheumatoid arthritis of right shoulder
     M05.112 Rheumatoid lung disease with
              rheumatoid arthritis of left shoulder
     M05.119 Rheumatoid lung disease with
              rheumatoid arthritis of unspecified
              shoulder

● M05.12 Rheumatoid lung disease with rheumatoid arthritis of elbow
   M05.121 Rheumatoid lung disease with rheumatoid arthritis of right elbow
   M05.122 Rheumatoid lung disease with rheumatoid arthritis of left elbow
   M05.129 Rheumatoid lung disease with rheumatoid arthritis of unspecified elbow

● M05.13 Rheumatoid lung disease with rheumatoid arthritis of wrist
   Rheumatoid lung disease with rheumatoid arthritis, carpal bones
   M05.131 Rheumatoid lung disease with rheumatoid arthritis of right wrist
   M05.132 Rheumatoid lung disease with rheumatoid arthritis of left wrist
   M05.139 Rheumatoid lung disease with rheumatoid arthritis of unspecified wrist

● M05.14 Rheumatoid lung disease with rheumatoid arthritis of hand
   Rheumatoid lung disease with rheumatoid arthritis, metacarpus and phalanges
   M05.141 Rheumatoid lung disease with rheumatoid arthritis of right hand
   M05.142 Rheumatoid lung disease with rheumatoid arthritis of left hand
   M05.149 Rheumatoid lung disease with rheumatoid arthritis of unspecified hand

● M05.15 Rheumatoid lung disease with rheumatoid arthritis of hip
   M05.151 Rheumatoid lung disease with rheumatoid arthritis of right hip
   M05.152 Rheumatoid lung disease with rheumatoid arthritis of left hip
   M05.159 Rheumatoid lung disease with rheumatoid arthritis of unspecified hip

● M05.16 Rheumatoid lung disease with rheumatoid arthritis of knee
   M05.161 Rheumatoid lung disease with rheumatoid arthritis of right knee
   M05.162 Rheumatoid lung disease with rheumatoid arthritis of left knee
   M05.169 Rheumatoid lung disease with rheumatoid arthritis of unspecified knee

● M05.17 Rheumatoid lung disease with rheumatoid arthritis of ankle and foot
   Rheumatoid lung disease with rheumatoid arthritis, tarsus, metatarsus and phalanges
   M05.171 Rheumatoid lung disease with rheumatoid arthritis of right ankle and foot
   M05.172 Rheumatoid lung disease with rheumatoid arthritis of left ankle and foot
   M05.179 Rheumatoid lung disease with rheumatoid arthritis of unspecified ankle and foot

M05.19 Rheumatoid lung disease with rheumatoid arthritis of multiple sites

● M05.2 Rheumatoid vasculitis with rheumatoid arthritis
  M05.20 Rheumatoid vasculitis with rheumatoid arthritis of unspecified site
● M05.21 Rheumatoid vasculitis with rheumatoid arthritis of shoulder
   M05.211 Rheumatoid vasculitis with rheumatoid arthritis of right shoulder
   M05.212 Rheumatoid vasculitis with rheumatoid arthritis of left shoulder
   M05.219 Rheumatoid vasculitis with rheumatoid arthritis of unspecified shoulder

● M05.22 Rheumatoid vasculitis with rheumatoid arthritis of elbow
   M05.221 Rheumatoid vasculitis with rheumatoid arthritis of right elbow
   M05.222 Rheumatoid vasculitis with rheumatoid arthritis of left elbow
   M05.229 Rheumatoid vasculitis with rheumatoid arthritis of unspecified elbow

● M05.23 Rheumatoid vasculitis with rheumatoid arthritis of wrist
   Rheumatoid vasculitis with rheumatoid arthritis, carpal bones
   M05.231 Rheumatoid vasculitis with rheumatoid arthritis of right wrist
   M05.232 Rheumatoid vasculitis with rheumatoid arthritis of left wrist
   M05.239 Rheumatoid vasculitis with rheumatoid arthritis of unspecified wrist

● M05.24 Rheumatoid vasculitis with rheumatoid arthritis of hand
   Rheumatoid vasculitis with rheumatoid arthritis, metacarpus and phalanges
   M05.241 Rheumatoid vasculitis with rheumatoid arthritis of right hand
   M05.242 Rheumatoid vasculitis with rheumatoid arthritis of left hand
   M05.249 Rheumatoid vasculitis with rheumatoid arthritis of unspecified hand

● M05.25 Rheumatoid vasculitis with rheumatoid arthritis of hip
   M05.251 Rheumatoid vasculitis with rheumatoid arthritis of right hip
   M05.252 Rheumatoid vasculitis with rheumatoid arthritis of left hip
   M05.259 Rheumatoid vasculitis with rheumatoid arthritis of unspecified hip

● M05.26 Rheumatoid vasculitis with rheumatoid arthritis of knee
   M05.261 Rheumatoid vasculitis with rheumatoid arthritis of right knee
   M05.262 Rheumatoid vasculitis with rheumatoid arthritis of left knee
   M05.269 Rheumatoid vasculitis with rheumatoid arthritis of unspecified knee

◀ New   ◀▦ Revised   ~~deleted~~ Deleted   OGCR Official Guidelines   X Assign placeholder X   ● Use Additional Character(s)
Excludes 1   Excludes 2   Includes   Use additional   Code first   Code also   Unspecified

● M05.27   **Rheumatoid vasculitis with rheumatoid arthritis of ankle and foot**
     Rheumatoid vasculitis with rheumatoid arthritis, tarsus, metatarsus and phalanges

     M05.271   **Rheumatoid vasculitis with rheumatoid arthritis of right ankle and foot**

     M05.272   **Rheumatoid vasculitis with rheumatoid arthritis of left ankle and foot**

     M05.279   **Rheumatoid vasculitis with rheumatoid arthritis of** unspecified **ankle and foot**

   M05.29   **Rheumatoid vasculitis with rheumatoid arthritis of multiple sites**

● M05.3   **Rheumatoid heart disease with rheumatoid arthritis**
     Rheumatoid carditis
     Rheumatoid endocarditis
     Rheumatoid myocarditis
     Rheumatoid pericarditis

   M05.30   **Rheumatoid heart disease with rheumatoid arthritis of** unspecified **site**

● M05.31   **Rheumatoid heart disease with rheumatoid arthritis of shoulder**

     M05.311   **Rheumatoid heart disease with rheumatoid arthritis of right shoulder**

     M05.312   **Rheumatoid heart disease with rheumatoid arthritis of left shoulder**

     M05.319   **Rheumatoid heart disease with rheumatoid arthritis of** unspecified **shoulder**

● M05.32   **Rheumatoid heart disease with rheumatoid arthritis of elbow**

     M05.321   **Rheumatoid heart disease with rheumatoid arthritis of right elbow**

     M05.322   **Rheumatoid heart disease with rheumatoid arthritis of left elbow**

     M05.329   **Rheumatoid heart disease with rheumatoid arthritis of** unspecified **elbow**

● M05.33   **Rheumatoid heart disease with rheumatoid arthritis of wrist**
     Rheumatoid heart disease with rheumatoid arthritis, carpal bones

     M05.331   **Rheumatoid heart disease with rheumatoid arthritis of right wrist**

     M05.332   **Rheumatoid heart disease with rheumatoid arthritis of left wrist**

     M05.339   **Rheumatoid heart disease with rheumatoid arthritis of** unspecified **wrist**

● M05.34   **Rheumatoid heart disease with rheumatoid arthritis of hand**
     Rheumatoid heart disease with rheumatoid arthritis, metacarpus and phalanges

     M05.341   **Rheumatoid heart disease with rheumatoid arthritis of right hand**

     M05.342   **Rheumatoid heart disease with rheumatoid arthritis of left hand**

     M05.349   **Rheumatoid heart disease with rheumatoid arthritis of** unspecified **hand**

● M05.35   **Rheumatoid heart disease with rheumatoid arthritis of hip**

     M05.351   **Rheumatoid heart disease with rheumatoid arthritis of right hip**

     M05.352   **Rheumatoid heart disease with rheumatoid arthritis of left hip**

     M05.359   **Rheumatoid heart disease with rheumatoid arthritis of** unspecified **hip**

● M05.36   **Rheumatoid heart disease with rheumatoid arthritis of knee**

     M05.361   **Rheumatoid heart disease with rheumatoid arthritis of right knee**

     M05.362   **Rheumatoid heart disease with rheumatoid arthritis of left knee**

     M05.369   **Rheumatoid heart disease with rheumatoid arthritis of** unspecified **knee**

● M05.37   **Rheumatoid heart disease with rheumatoid arthritis of ankle and foot**
     Rheumatoid heart disease with rheumatoid arthritis, tarsus, metatarsus and phalanges

     M05.371   **Rheumatoid heart disease with rheumatoid arthritis of right ankle and foot**

     M05.372   **Rheumatoid heart disease with rheumatoid arthritis of left ankle and foot**

     M05.379   **Rheumatoid heart disease with rheumatoid arthritis of** unspecified **ankle and foot**

   M05.39   **Rheumatoid heart disease with rheumatoid arthritis of multiple sites**

● M05.4   **Rheumatoid myopathy with rheumatoid arthritis**

   M05.40   **Rheumatoid myopathy with rheumatoid arthritis of** unspecified **site**

● M05.41   **Rheumatoid myopathy with rheumatoid arthritis of shoulder**

     M05.411   **Rheumatoid myopathy with rheumatoid arthritis of right shoulder**

     M05.412   **Rheumatoid myopathy with rheumatoid arthritis of left shoulder**

     M05.419   **Rheumatoid myopathy with rheumatoid arthritis of** unspecified **shoulder**

● M05.42   **Rheumatoid myopathy with rheumatoid arthritis of elbow**

     M05.421   **Rheumatoid myopathy with rheumatoid arthritis of right elbow**

     M05.422   **Rheumatoid myopathy with rheumatoid arthritis of left elbow**

     M05.429   **Rheumatoid myopathy with rheumatoid arthritis of** unspecified **elbow**

● M05.43   **Rheumatoid myopathy with rheumatoid arthritis of wrist**
     Rheumatoid myopathy with rheumatoid arthritis, carpal bones

     M05.431   **Rheumatoid myopathy with rheumatoid arthritis of right wrist**

     M05.432   **Rheumatoid myopathy with rheumatoid arthritis of left wrist**

     M05.439   **Rheumatoid myopathy with rheumatoid arthritis of** unspecified **wrist**

● M05.44   **Rheumatoid myopathy with rheumatoid arthritis of hand**
     Rheumatoid myopathy with rheumatoid arthritis, metacarpus and phalanges

     M05.441   **Rheumatoid myopathy with rheumatoid arthritis of right hand**

     M05.442   **Rheumatoid myopathy with rheumatoid arthritis of left hand**

     M05.449   **Rheumatoid myopathy with rheumatoid arthritis of** unspecified **hand**

◀ New   ◀◀◀ Revised   ~~deleted~~ Deleted   **OGCR** Official Guidelines   X Assign placeholder X   ● Use Additional Character(s)

Excludes 1   Excludes 2   Includes   Use additional   Code first   Code also   Unspecified

● M05.45   **Rheumatoid myopathy with rheumatoid arthritis of hip**

    M05.451   **Rheumatoid myopathy with rheumatoid arthritis of right hip**

    M05.452   **Rheumatoid myopathy with rheumatoid arthritis of left hip**

    M05.459   **Rheumatoid myopathy with rheumatoid arthritis of unspecified hip**

● M05.46   **Rheumatoid myopathy with rheumatoid arthritis of knee**

    M05.461   **Rheumatoid myopathy with rheumatoid arthritis of right knee**

    M05.462   **Rheumatoid myopathy with rheumatoid arthritis of left knee**

    M05.469   **Rheumatoid myopathy with rheumatoid arthritis of unspecified knee**

● M05.47   **Rheumatoid myopathy with rheumatoid arthritis of ankle and foot**

    Rheumatoid myopathy with rheumatoid arthritis, tarsus, metatarsus and phalanges

    M05.471   **Rheumatoid myopathy with rheumatoid arthritis of right ankle and foot**

    M05.472   **Rheumatoid myopathy with rheumatoid arthritis of left ankle and foot**

    M05.479   **Rheumatoid myopathy with rheumatoid arthritis of unspecified ankle and foot**

    M05.49   **Rheumatoid myopathy with rheumatoid arthritis of multiple sites**

● M05.5   **Rheumatoid polyneuropathy with rheumatoid arthritis**

    M05.50   **Rheumatoid polyneuropathy with rheumatoid arthritis of unspecified site**

● M05.51   **Rheumatoid polyneuropathy with rheumatoid arthritis of shoulder**

    M05.511   **Rheumatoid polyneuropathy with rheumatoid arthritis of right shoulder**

    M05.512   **Rheumatoid polyneuropathy with rheumatoid arthritis of left shoulder**

    M05.519   **Rheumatoid polyneuropathy with rheumatoid arthritis of unspecified shoulder**

● M05.52   **Rheumatoid polyneuropathy with rheumatoid arthritis of elbow**

    M05.521   **Rheumatoid polyneuropathy with rheumatoid arthritis of right elbow**

    M05.522   **Rheumatoid polyneuropathy with rheumatoid arthritis of left elbow**

    M05.529   **Rheumatoid polyneuropathy with rheumatoid arthritis of unspecified elbow**

● M05.53   **Rheumatoid polyneuropathy with rheumatoid arthritis of wrist**

    Rheumatoid polyneuropathy with rheumatoid arthritis, carpal bones

    M05.531   **Rheumatoid polyneuropathy with rheumatoid arthritis of right wrist**

    M05.532   **Rheumatoid polyneuropathy with rheumatoid arthritis of left wrist**

    M05.539   **Rheumatoid polyneuropathy with rheumatoid arthritis of unspecified wrist**

● M05.54   **Rheumatoid polyneuropathy with rheumatoid arthritis of hand**

    Rheumatoid polyneuropathy with rheumatoid arthritis, metacarpus and phalanges

    M05.541   **Rheumatoid polyneuropathy with rheumatoid arthritis of right hand**

    M05.542   **Rheumatoid polyneuropathy with rheumatoid arthritis of left hand**

    M05.549   **Rheumatoid polyneuropathy with rheumatoid arthritis of unspecified hand**

● M05.55   **Rheumatoid polyneuropathy with rheumatoid arthritis of hip**

    M05.551   **Rheumatoid polyneuropathy with rheumatoid arthritis of right hip**

    M05.552   **Rheumatoid polyneuropathy with rheumatoid arthritis of left hip**

    M05.559   **Rheumatoid polyneuropathy with rheumatoid arthritis of unspecified hip**

● M05.56   **Rheumatoid polyneuropathy with rheumatoid arthritis of knee**

    M05.561   **Rheumatoid polyneuropathy with rheumatoid arthritis of right knee**

    M05.562   **Rheumatoid polyneuropathy with rheumatoid arthritis of left knee**

    M05.569   **Rheumatoid polyneuropathy with rheumatoid arthritis of unspecified knee**

● M05.57   **Rheumatoid polyneuropathy with rheumatoid arthritis of ankle and foot**

    Rheumatoid polyneuropathy with rheumatoid arthritis, tarsus, metatarsus and phalanges

    M05.571   **Rheumatoid polyneuropathy with rheumatoid arthritis of right ankle and foot**

    M05.572   **Rheumatoid polyneuropathy with rheumatoid arthritis of left ankle and foot**

    M05.579   **Rheumatoid polyneuropathy with rheumatoid arthritis of unspecified ankle and foot**

    M05.59   **Rheumatoid polyneuropathy with rheumatoid arthritis of multiple sites**

● M05.6   **Rheumatoid arthritis with involvement of other organs and systems**

    M05.60   **Rheumatoid arthritis of unspecified site with involvement of other organs and systems**

● M05.61   **Rheumatoid arthritis of shoulder with involvement of other organs and systems**

    M05.611   **Rheumatoid arthritis of right shoulder with involvement of other organs and systems**

    M05.612   **Rheumatoid arthritis of left shoulder with involvement of other organs and systems**

    M05.619   **Rheumatoid arthritis of unspecified shoulder with involvement of other organs and systems**

● M05.62   **Rheumatoid arthritis of elbow with involvement of other organs and systems**

    M05.621   **Rheumatoid arthritis of right elbow with involvement of other organs and systems**

    M05.622   **Rheumatoid arthritis of left elbow with involvement of other organs and systems**

    M05.629   **Rheumatoid arthritis of unspecified elbow with involvement of other organs and systems**

◀ New   ◀▥▥ Revised   ~~deleted~~ Deleted   OGCR Official Guidelines   X Assign placeholder X   ● Use Additional Character(s)

Excludes 1   Excludes 2   Includes   Use additional   Code first   Code also   Unspecified

● M05.63 **Rheumatoid arthritis of wrist with involvement of other organs and systems**
    Rheumatoid arthritis of carpal bones with involvement of other organs and systems

  M05.631 **Rheumatoid arthritis of right wrist with involvement of other organs and systems**

  M05.632 **Rheumatoid arthritis of left wrist with involvement of other organs and systems**

  M05.639 **Rheumatoid arthritis of unspecified wrist with involvement of other organs and systems**

● M05.64 **Rheumatoid arthritis of hand with involvement of other organs and systems**
    Rheumatoid arthritis of metacarpus and phalanges with involvement of other organs and systems

  M05.641 **Rheumatoid arthritis of right hand with involvement of other organs and systems**

  M05.642 **Rheumatoid arthritis of left hand with involvement of other organs and systems**

  M05.649 **Rheumatoid arthritis of unspecified hand with involvement of other organs and systems**

● M05.65 **Rheumatoid arthritis of hip with involvement of other organs and systems**

  M05.651 **Rheumatoid arthritis of right hip with involvement of other organs and systems**

  M05.652 **Rheumatoid arthritis of left hip with involvement of other organs and systems**

  M05.659 **Rheumatoid arthritis of unspecified hip with involvement of other organs and systems**

● M05.66 **Rheumatoid arthritis of knee with involvement of other organs and systems**

  M05.661 **Rheumatoid arthritis of right knee with involvement of other organs and systems**

  M05.662 **Rheumatoid arthritis of left knee with involvement of other organs and systems**

  M05.669 **Rheumatoid arthritis of unspecified knee with involvement of other organs and systems**

● M05.67 **Rheumatoid arthritis of ankle and foot with involvement of other organs and systems**
    Rheumatoid arthritis of tarsus, metatarsus and phalanges with involvement of other organs and systems

  M05.671 **Rheumatoid arthritis of right ankle and foot with involvement of other organs and systems**

  M05.672 **Rheumatoid arthritis of left ankle and foot with involvement of other organs and systems**

  M05.679 **Rheumatoid arthritis of unspecified ankle and foot with involvement of other organs and systems**

  M05.69 **Rheumatoid arthritis of multiple sites with involvement of other organs and systems**

● M05.7 **Rheumatoid arthritis with rheumatoid factor without organ or systems involvement**

  M05.70 **Rheumatoid arthritis with rheumatoid factor of unspecified site without organ or systems involvement**

● M05.71 **Rheumatoid arthritis with rheumatoid factor of shoulder without organ or systems involvement**

  M05.711 **Rheumatoid arthritis with rheumatoid factor of right shoulder without organ or systems involvement**

  M05.712 **Rheumatoid arthritis with rheumatoid factor of left shoulder without organ or systems involvement**

  M05.719 **Rheumatoid arthritis with rheumatoid factor of unspecified shoulder without organ or systems involvement**

● M05.72 **Rheumatoid arthritis with rheumatoid factor of elbow without organ or systems involvement**

  M05.721 **Rheumatoid arthritis with rheumatoid factor of right elbow without organ or systems involvement**

  M05.722 **Rheumatoid arthritis with rheumatoid factor of left elbow without organ or systems involvement**

  M05.729 **Rheumatoid arthritis with rheumatoid factor of unspecified elbow without organ or systems involvement**

● M05.73 **Rheumatoid arthritis with rheumatoid factor of wrist without organ or systems involvement**

  M05.731 **Rheumatoid arthritis with rheumatoid factor of right wrist without organ or systems involvement**

  M05.732 **Rheumatoid arthritis with rheumatoid factor of left wrist without organ or systems involvement**

  M05.739 **Rheumatoid arthritis with rheumatoid factor of unspecified wrist without organ or systems involvement**

● M05.74 **Rheumatoid arthritis with rheumatoid factor of hand without organ or systems involvement**

  M05.741 **Rheumatoid arthritis with rheumatoid factor of right hand without organ or systems involvement**

  M05.742 **Rheumatoid arthritis with rheumatoid factor of left hand without organ or systems involvement**

  M05.749 **Rheumatoid arthritis with rheumatoid factor of unspecified hand without organ or systems involvement**

● M05.75 **Rheumatoid arthritis with rheumatoid factor of hip without organ or systems involvement**

  M05.751 **Rheumatoid arthritis with rheumatoid factor of right hip without organ or systems involvement**

  M05.752 **Rheumatoid arthritis with rheumatoid factor of left hip without organ or systems involvement**

  M05.759 **Rheumatoid arthritis with rheumatoid factor of unspecified hip without organ or systems involvement**

● M05.76 Rheumatoid arthritis with rheumatoid factor of knee without organ or systems involvement
   M05.761 Rheumatoid arthritis with rheumatoid factor of right knee without organ or systems involvement
   M05.762 Rheumatoid arthritis with rheumatoid factor of left knee without organ or systems involvement
   M05.769 Rheumatoid arthritis with rheumatoid factor of unspecified knee without organ or systems involvement
● M05.77 Rheumatoid arthritis with rheumatoid factor of ankle and foot without organ or systems involvement
   M05.771 Rheumatoid arthritis with rheumatoid factor of right ankle and foot without organ or systems involvement
   M05.772 Rheumatoid arthritis with rheumatoid factor of left ankle and foot without organ or systems involvement
   M05.779 Rheumatoid arthritis with rheumatoid factor of unspecified ankle and foot without organ or systems involvement
M05.79 Rheumatoid arthritis with rheumatoid factor of multiple sites without organ or systems involvement
● M05.8 Other rheumatoid arthritis with rheumatoid factor
M05.80 Other rheumatoid arthritis with rheumatoid factor of unspecified site
● M05.81 Other rheumatoid arthritis with rheumatoid factor of shoulder
   M05.811 Other rheumatoid arthritis with rheumatoid factor of right shoulder
   M05.812 Other rheumatoid arthritis with rheumatoid factor of left shoulder
   M05.819 Other rheumatoid arthritis with rheumatoid factor of unspecified shoulder
● M05.82 Other rheumatoid arthritis with rheumatoid factor of elbow
   M05.821 Other rheumatoid arthritis with rheumatoid factor of right elbow
   M05.822 Other rheumatoid arthritis with rheumatoid factor of left elbow
   M05.829 Other rheumatoid arthritis with rheumatoid factor of unspecified elbow
● M05.83 Other rheumatoid arthritis with rheumatoid factor of wrist
   M05.831 Other rheumatoid arthritis with rheumatoid factor of right wrist
   M05.832 Other rheumatoid arthritis with rheumatoid factor of left wrist
   M05.839 Other rheumatoid arthritis with rheumatoid factor of unspecified wrist
● M05.84 Other rheumatoid arthritis with rheumatoid factor of hand
   M05.841 Other rheumatoid arthritis with rheumatoid factor of right hand
   M05.842 Other rheumatoid arthritis with rheumatoid factor of left hand
   M05.849 Other rheumatoid arthritis with rheumatoid factor of unspecified hand

● M05.85 Other rheumatoid arthritis with rheumatoid factor of hip
   M05.851 Other rheumatoid arthritis with rheumatoid factor of right hip
   M05.852 Other rheumatoid arthritis with rheumatoid factor of left hip
   M05.859 Other rheumatoid arthritis with rheumatoid factor of unspecified hip
● M05.86 Other rheumatoid arthritis with rheumatoid factor of knee
   M05.861 Other rheumatoid arthritis with rheumatoid factor of right knee
   M05.862 Other rheumatoid arthritis with rheumatoid factor of left knee
   M05.869 Other rheumatoid arthritis with rheumatoid factor of unspecified knee
● M05.87 Other rheumatoid arthritis with rheumatoid factor of ankle and foot
   M05.871 Other rheumatoid arthritis with rheumatoid factor of right ankle and foot
   M05.872 Other rheumatoid arthritis with rheumatoid factor of left ankle and foot
   M05.879 Other rheumatoid arthritis with rheumatoid factor of unspecified ankle and foot
M05.89 Other rheumatoid arthritis with rheumatoid factor of multiple sites
M05.9 Rheumatoid arthritis with rheumatoid factor, unspecified
● M06 Other rheumatoid arthritis
● M06.0 Rheumatoid arthritis without rheumatoid factor
M06.00 Rheumatoid arthritis without rheumatoid factor, unspecified site
● M06.01 Rheumatoid arthritis without rheumatoid factor, shoulder
   M06.011 Rheumatoid arthritis without rheumatoid factor, right shoulder
   M06.012 Rheumatoid arthritis without rheumatoid factor, left shoulder
   M06.019 Rheumatoid arthritis without rheumatoid factor, unspecified shoulder
● M06.02 Rheumatoid arthritis without rheumatoid factor, elbow
   M06.021 Rheumatoid arthritis without rheumatoid factor, right elbow
   M06.022 Rheumatoid arthritis without rheumatoid factor, left elbow
   M06.029 Rheumatoid arthritis without rheumatoid factor, unspecified elbow
● M06.03 Rheumatoid arthritis without rheumatoid factor, wrist
   M06.031 Rheumatoid arthritis without rheumatoid factor, right wrist
   M06.032 Rheumatoid arthritis without rheumatoid factor, left wrist
   M06.039 Rheumatoid arthritis without rheumatoid factor, unspecified wrist
● M06.04 Rheumatoid arthritis without rheumatoid factor, hand
   M06.041 Rheumatoid arthritis without rheumatoid factor, right hand
   M06.042 Rheumatoid arthritis without rheumatoid factor, left hand
   M06.049 Rheumatoid arthritis without rheumatoid factor, unspecified hand

- M06.05 Rheumatoid arthritis without rheumatoid factor, hip
  - M06.051 Rheumatoid arthritis without rheumatoid factor, right hip
  - M06.052 Rheumatoid arthritis without rheumatoid factor, left hip
  - M06.059 Rheumatoid arthritis without rheumatoid factor, unspecified hip
- M06.06 Rheumatoid arthritis without rheumatoid factor, knee
  - M06.061 Rheumatoid arthritis without rheumatoid factor, right knee
  - M06.062 Rheumatoid arthritis without rheumatoid factor, left knee
  - M06.069 Rheumatoid arthritis without rheumatoid factor, unspecified knee
- M06.07 Rheumatoid arthritis without rheumatoid factor, ankle and foot
  - M06.071 Rheumatoid arthritis without rheumatoid factor, right ankle and foot
  - M06.072 Rheumatoid arthritis without rheumatoid factor, left ankle and foot
  - M06.079 Rheumatoid arthritis without rheumatoid factor, unspecified ankle and foot
  - M06.08 Rheumatoid arthritis without rheumatoid factor, vertebrae
  - M06.09 Rheumatoid arthritis without rheumatoid factor, multiple sites
- M06.1 **Adult-onset Still's disease**
  - **Excludes1** Still's disease NOS (M08.2-)
- M06.2 **Rheumatoid bursitis**
  - M06.20 Rheumatoid bursitis, unspecified site
- M06.21 Rheumatoid bursitis, shoulder
  - M06.211 Rheumatoid bursitis, right shoulder
  - M06.212 Rheumatoid bursitis, left shoulder
  - M06.219 Rheumatoid bursitis, unspecified shoulder
- M06.22 Rheumatoid bursitis, elbow
  - M06.221 Rheumatoid bursitis, right elbow
  - M06.222 Rheumatoid bursitis, left elbow
  - M06.229 Rheumatoid bursitis, unspecified elbow
- M06.23 Rheumatoid bursitis, wrist
  - M06.231 Rheumatoid bursitis, right wrist
  - M06.232 Rheumatoid bursitis, left wrist
  - M06.239 Rheumatoid bursitis, unspecified wrist
- M06.24 Rheumatoid bursitis, hand
  - M06.241 Rheumatoid bursitis, right hand
  - M06.242 Rheumatoid bursitis, left hand
  - M06.249 Rheumatoid bursitis, unspecified hand
- M06.25 Rheumatoid bursitis, hip
  - M06.251 Rheumatoid bursitis, right hip
  - M06.252 Rheumatoid bursitis, left hip
  - M06.259 Rheumatoid bursitis, unspecified hip
- M06.26 Rheumatoid bursitis, knee
  - M06.261 Rheumatoid bursitis, right knee
  - M06.262 Rheumatoid bursitis, left knee
  - M06.269 Rheumatoid bursitis, unspecified knee

- M06.27 Rheumatoid bursitis, ankle and foot
  - M06.271 Rheumatoid bursitis, right ankle and foot
  - M06.272 Rheumatoid bursitis, left ankle and foot
  - M06.279 Rheumatoid bursitis, unspecified ankle and foot
  - M06.28 Rheumatoid bursitis, vertebrae
  - M06.29 Rheumatoid bursitis, multiple sites
- M06.3 Rheumatoid nodule
  - M06.30 Rheumatoid nodule, unspecified site
- M06.31 Rheumatoid nodule, shoulder
  - M06.311 Rheumatoid nodule, right shoulder
  - M06.312 Rheumatoid nodule, left shoulder
  - M06.319 Rheumatoid nodule, unspecified shoulder
- M06.32 Rheumatoid nodule, elbow
  - M06.321 Rheumatoid nodule, right elbow
  - M06.322 Rheumatoid nodule, left elbow
  - M06.329 Rheumatoid nodule, unspecified elbow
- M06.33 Rheumatoid nodule, wrist
  - M06.331 Rheumatoid nodule, right wrist
  - M06.332 Rheumatoid nodule, left wrist
  - M06.339 Rheumatoid nodule, unspecified wrist
- M06.34 Rheumatoid nodule, hand
  - M06.341 Rheumatoid nodule, right hand
  - M06.342 Rheumatoid nodule, left hand
  - M06.349 Rheumatoid nodule, unspecified hand
- M06.35 Rheumatoid nodule, hip
  - M06.351 Rheumatoid nodule, right hip
  - M06.352 Rheumatoid nodule, left hip
  - M06.359 Rheumatoid nodule, unspecified hip
- M06.36 Rheumatoid nodule, knee
  - M06.361 Rheumatoid nodule, right knee
  - M06.362 Rheumatoid nodule, left knee
  - M06.369 Rheumatoid nodule, unspecified knee
- M06.37 Rheumatoid nodule, ankle and foot
  - M06.371 Rheumatoid nodule, right ankle and foot
  - M06.372 Rheumatoid nodule, left ankle and foot
  - M06.379 Rheumatoid nodule, unspecified ankle and foot
  - M06.38 Rheumatoid nodule, vertebrae
  - M06.39 Rheumatoid nodule, multiple sites
- M06.4 **Inflammatory polyarthropathy**
  - **Excludes1** polyarthritis NOS (M13.0)
- M06.8 Other specified rheumatoid arthritis
  - M06.80 Other specified rheumatoid arthritis, unspecified site
- M06.81 Other specified rheumatoid arthritis, shoulder
  - M06.811 Other specified rheumatoid arthritis, right shoulder
  - M06.812 Other specified rheumatoid arthritis, left shoulder
  - M06.819 Other specified rheumatoid arthritis, unspecified shoulder

◀ New　◀━ Revised　~~deleted~~ Deleted　OGCR Official Guidelines　X Assign placeholder X　● Use Additional Character(s)

| Excludes 1 | Excludes 2 | Includes | Use additional | Code first | Code also | Unspecified |

M06.82 Other specified rheumatoid arthritis, elbow
  M06.821 Other specified rheumatoid arthritis, right elbow
  M06.822 Other specified rheumatoid arthritis, left elbow
  M06.829 Other specified rheumatoid arthritis, unspecified elbow
M06.83 Other specified rheumatoid arthritis, wrist
  M06.831 Other specified rheumatoid arthritis, right wrist
  M06.832 Other specified rheumatoid arthritis, left wrist
  M06.839 Other specified rheumatoid arthritis, unspecified wrist
M06.84 Other specified rheumatoid arthritis, hand
  M06.841 Other specified rheumatoid arthritis, right hand
  M06.842 Other specified rheumatoid arthritis, left hand
  M06.849 Other specified rheumatoid arthritis, unspecified hand
M06.85 Other specified rheumatoid arthritis, hip
  M06.851 Other specified rheumatoid arthritis, right hip
  M06.852 Other specified rheumatoid arthritis, left hip
  M06.859 Other specified rheumatoid arthritis, unspecified hip
M06.86 Other specified rheumatoid arthritis, knee
  M06.861 Other specified rheumatoid arthritis, right knee
  M06.862 Other specified rheumatoid arthritis, left knee
  M06.869 Other specified rheumatoid arthritis, unspecified knee
M06.87 Other specified rheumatoid arthritis, ankle and foot
  M06.871 Other specified rheumatoid arthritis, right ankle and foot
  M06.872 Other specified rheumatoid arthritis, left ankle and foot
  M06.879 Other specified rheumatoid arthritis, unspecified ankle and foot
M06.88 Other specified rheumatoid arthritis, vertebrae
M06.89 Other specified rheumatoid arthritis, multiple sites
M06.9 Rheumatoid arthritis, unspecified

M07 Enteropathic arthropathies
Code also associated enteropathy, such as:
  regional enteritis [Crohn's disease] (K50.-)
  ulcerative colitis (K51.-)
Excludes1 psoriatic arthropathies (L40.5-)
M07.6 Enteropathic arthropathies
  M07.60 Enteropathic arthropathies, unspecified site
  M07.61 Enteropathic arthropathies, shoulder
    M07.611 Enteropathic arthropathies, right shoulder
    M07.612 Enteropathic arthropathies, left shoulder
    M07.619 Enteropathic arthropathies, unspecified shoulder
  M07.62 Enteropathic arthropathies, elbow
    M07.621 Enteropathic arthropathies, right elbow
    M07.622 Enteropathic arthropathies, left elbow
    M07.629 Enteropathic arthropathies, unspecified elbow

M07.63 Enteropathic arthropathies, wrist
  M07.631 Enteropathic arthropathies, right wrist
  M07.632 Enteropathic arthropathies, left wrist
  M07.639 Enteropathic arthropathies, unspecified wrist
M07.64 Enteropathic arthropathies, hand
  M07.641 Enteropathic arthropathies, right hand
  M07.642 Enteropathic arthropathies, left hand
  M07.649 Enteropathic arthropathies, unspecified hand
M07.65 Enteropathic arthropathies, hip
  M07.651 Enteropathic arthropathies, right hip
  M07.652 Enteropathic arthropathies, left hip
  M07.659 Enteropathic arthropathies, unspecified hip
M07.66 Enteropathic arthropathies, knee
  M07.661 Enteropathic arthropathies, right knee
  M07.662 Enteropathic arthropathies, left knee
  M07.669 Enteropathic arthropathies, unspecified knee
M07.67 Enteropathic arthropathies, ankle and foot
  M07.671 Enteropathic arthropathies, right ankle and foot
  M07.672 Enteropathic arthropathies, left ankle and foot
  M07.679 Enteropathic arthropathies, unspecified ankle and foot
M07.68 Enteropathic arthropathies, vertebrae
M07.69 Enteropathic arthropathies, multiple sites

M08 Juvenile arthritis
Code also any associated underlying condition, such as:
  regional enteritis [Crohn's disease] (K50.-)
  ulcerative colitis (K51.-)
Excludes1 arthropathy in Whipple's disease (M14.8)
  Felty's syndrome (M05.0)
  juvenile dermatomyositis (M33.0-)
  psoriatic juvenile arthropathy (L40.54)
M08.0 Unspecified juvenile rheumatoid arthritis
Juvenile rheumatoid arthritis with or without rheumatoid factor
  M08.00 Unspecified juvenile rheumatoid arthritis of unspecified site
  M08.01 Unspecified juvenile rheumatoid arthritis, shoulder
    M08.011 Unspecified juvenile rheumatoid arthritis, right shoulder
    M08.012 Unspecified juvenile rheumatoid arthritis, left shoulder
    M08.019 Unspecified juvenile rheumatoid arthritis, unspecified shoulder
  M08.02 Unspecified juvenile rheumatoid arthritis of elbow
    M08.021 Unspecified juvenile rheumatoid arthritis, right elbow
    M08.022 Unspecified juvenile rheumatoid arthritis, left elbow
    M08.029 Unspecified juvenile rheumatoid arthritis, unspecified elbow
  M08.03 Unspecified juvenile rheumatoid arthritis, wrist
    M08.031 Unspecified juvenile rheumatoid arthritis, right wrist
    M08.032 Unspecified juvenile rheumatoid arthritis, left wrist
    M08.039 Unspecified juvenile rheumatoid arthritis, unspecified wrist

◀ New   ◀ Revised   deleted Deleted   OGCR Official Guidelines   X Assign placeholder X   ● Use Additional Character(s)
Excludes 1   Excludes 2   Includes   Use additional   Code first   Code also   Unspecified

● M08.04   Unspecified juvenile rheumatoid arthritis, hand

    M08.041   Unspecified juvenile rheumatoid arthritis, right hand

    M08.042   Unspecified juvenile rheumatoid arthritis, left hand

    M08.049   Unspecified juvenile rheumatoid arthritis, unspecified hand

● M08.05   Unspecified juvenile rheumatoid arthritis, hip

    M08.051   Unspecified juvenile rheumatoid arthritis, right hip

    M08.052   Unspecified juvenile rheumatoid arthritis, left hip

    M08.059   Unspecified juvenile rheumatoid arthritis, unspecified hip

● M08.06   Unspecified juvenile rheumatoid arthritis, knee

    M08.061   Unspecified juvenile rheumatoid arthritis, right knee

    M08.062   Unspecified juvenile rheumatoid arthritis, left knee

    M08.069   Unspecified juvenile rheumatoid arthritis, unspecified knee

● M08.07   Unspecified juvenile rheumatoid arthritis, ankle and foot

    M08.071   Unspecified juvenile rheumatoid arthritis, right ankle and foot

    M08.072   Unspecified juvenile rheumatoid arthritis, left ankle and foot

    M08.079   Unspecified juvenile rheumatoid arthritis, unspecified ankle and foot

   M08.08   Unspecified juvenile rheumatoid arthritis, vertebrae

   M08.09   Unspecified juvenile rheumatoid arthritis, multiple sites

M08.1   Juvenile ankylosing spondylitis

   Excludes1   ankylosing spondylitis in adults (M45.0-)

● M08.2   Juvenile rheumatoid arthritis with systemic onset

   Still's disease NOS

   Excludes1   adult-onset Still's disease (M06.1-)

   M08.20   Juvenile rheumatoid arthritis with systemic onset, unspecified site

● M08.21   Juvenile rheumatoid arthritis with systemic onset, shoulder

    M08.211   Juvenile rheumatoid arthritis with systemic onset, right shoulder

    M08.212   Juvenile rheumatoid arthritis with systemic onset, left shoulder

    M08.219   Juvenile rheumatoid arthritis with systemic onset, unspecified shoulder

● M08.22   Juvenile rheumatoid arthritis with systemic onset, elbow

    M08.221   Juvenile rheumatoid arthritis with systemic onset, right elbow

    M08.222   Juvenile rheumatoid arthritis with systemic onset, left elbow

    M08.229   Juvenile rheumatoid arthritis with systemic onset, unspecified elbow

● M08.23   Juvenile rheumatoid arthritis with systemic onset, wrist

    M08.231   Juvenile rheumatoid arthritis with systemic onset, right wrist

    M08.232   Juvenile rheumatoid arthritis with systemic onset, left wrist

    M08.239   Juvenile rheumatoid arthritis with systemic onset, unspecified wrist

● M08.24   Juvenile rheumatoid arthritis with systemic onset, hand

    M08.241   Juvenile rheumatoid arthritis with systemic onset, right hand

    M08.242   Juvenile rheumatoid arthritis with systemic onset, left hand

    M08.249   Juvenile rheumatoid arthritis with systemic onset, unspecified hand

● M08.25   Juvenile rheumatoid arthritis with systemic onset, hip

    M08.251   Juvenile rheumatoid arthritis with systemic onset, right hip

    M08.252   Juvenile rheumatoid arthritis with systemic onset, left hip

    M08.259   Juvenile rheumatoid arthritis with systemic onset, unspecified hip

● M08.26   Juvenile rheumatoid arthritis with systemic onset, knee

    M08.261   Juvenile rheumatoid arthritis with systemic onset, right knee

    M08.262   Juvenile rheumatoid arthritis with systemic onset, left knee

    M08.269   Juvenile rheumatoid arthritis with systemic onset, unspecified knee

● M08.27   Juvenile rheumatoid arthritis with systemic onset, ankle and foot

    M08.271   Juvenile rheumatoid arthritis with systemic onset, right ankle and foot

    M08.272   Juvenile rheumatoid arthritis with systemic onset, left ankle and foot

    M08.279   Juvenile rheumatoid arthritis with systemic onset, unspecified ankle and foot

   M08.28   Juvenile rheumatoid arthritis with systemic onset, vertebrae

   M08.29   Juvenile rheumatoid arthritis with systemic onset, multiple sites

M08.3   Juvenile rheumatoid polyarthritis (seronegative)

● M08.4   Pauciarticular juvenile rheumatoid arthritis

   M08.40   Pauciarticular juvenile rheumatoid arthritis, unspecified site

● M08.41   Pauciarticular juvenile rheumatoid arthritis, shoulder

    M08.411   Pauciarticular juvenile rheumatoid arthritis, right shoulder

    M08.412   Pauciarticular juvenile rheumatoid arthritis, left shoulder

    M08.419   Pauciarticular juvenile rheumatoid arthritis, unspecified shoulder

● M08.42   Pauciarticular juvenile rheumatoid arthritis, elbow

    M08.421   Pauciarticular juvenile rheumatoid arthritis, right elbow

    M08.422   Pauciarticular juvenile rheumatoid arthritis, left elbow

    M08.429   Pauciarticular juvenile rheumatoid arthritis, unspecified elbow

● M08.43   Pauciarticular juvenile rheumatoid arthritis, wrist

    M08.431   Pauciarticular juvenile rheumatoid arthritis, right wrist

    M08.432   Pauciarticular juvenile rheumatoid arthritis, left wrist

    M08.439   Pauciarticular juvenile rheumatoid arthritis, unspecified wrist

CHAPTER 13 (M00-M99)

● **M08.44 Pauciarticular juvenile rheumatoid arthritis, hand**
   M08.441 Pauciarticular juvenile rheumatoid arthritis, right hand
   M08.442 Pauciarticular juvenile rheumatoid arthritis, left hand
   M08.449 Pauciarticular juvenile rheumatoid arthritis, unspecified hand

● **M08.45 Pauciarticular juvenile rheumatoid arthritis, hip**
   M08.451 Pauciarticular juvenile rheumatoid arthritis, right hip
   M08.452 Pauciarticular juvenile rheumatoid arthritis, left hip
   M08.459 Pauciarticular juvenile rheumatoid arthritis, unspecified hip

● **M08.46 Pauciarticular juvenile rheumatoid arthritis, knee**
   M08.461 Pauciarticular juvenile rheumatoid arthritis, right knee
   M08.462 Pauciarticular juvenile rheumatoid arthritis, left knee
   M08.469 Pauciarticular juvenile rheumatoid arthritis, unspecified knee

● **M08.47 Pauciarticular juvenile rheumatoid arthritis, ankle and foot**
   M08.471 Pauciarticular juvenile rheumatoid arthritis, right ankle and foot
   M08.472 Pauciarticular juvenile rheumatoid arthritis, left ankle and foot
   M08.479 Pauciarticular juvenile rheumatoid arthritis, unspecified ankle and foot

  M08.48 Pauciarticular juvenile rheumatoid arthritis, vertebrae

● **M08.8 Other juvenile arthritis**
  M08.80 Other juvenile arthritis, unspecified site

● **M08.81 Other juvenile arthritis, shoulder**
   M08.811 Other juvenile arthritis, right shoulder
   M08.812 Other juvenile arthritis, left shoulder
   M08.819 Other juvenile arthritis, unspecified shoulder

● **M08.82 Other juvenile arthritis, elbow**
   M08.821 Other juvenile arthritis, right elbow
   M08.822 Other juvenile arthritis, left elbow
   M08.829 Other juvenile arthritis, unspecified elbow

● **M08.83 Other juvenile arthritis, wrist**
   M08.831 Other juvenile arthritis, right wrist
   M08.832 Other juvenile arthritis, left wrist
   M08.839 Other juvenile arthritis, unspecified wrist

● **M08.84 Other juvenile arthritis, hand**
   M08.841 Other juvenile arthritis, right hand
   M08.842 Other juvenile arthritis, left hand
   M08.849 Other juvenile arthritis, unspecified hand

● **M08.85 Other juvenile arthritis, hip**
   M08.851 Other juvenile arthritis, right hip
   M08.852 Other juvenile arthritis, left hip
   M08.859 Other juvenile arthritis, unspecified hip

● **M08.86 Other juvenile arthritis, knee**
   M08.861 Other juvenile arthritis, right knee
   M08.862 Other juvenile arthritis, left knee
   M08.869 Other juvenile arthritis, unspecified knee

● **M08.87 Other juvenile arthritis, ankle and foot**
   M08.871 Other juvenile arthritis, right ankle and foot
   M08.872 Other juvenile arthritis, left ankle and foot
   M08.879 Other juvenile arthritis, unspecified ankle and foot

  M08.88 Other juvenile arthritis, other specified site
   Other juvenile arthritis, vertebrae

  M08.89 Other juvenile arthritis, multiple sites

● **M08.9 Juvenile arthritis, unspecified**
   Excludes1 juvenile rheumatoid arthritis, unspecified (M08.0-)

  M08.90 Juvenile arthritis, unspecified, unspecified site

● **M08.91 Juvenile arthritis, unspecified, shoulder**
   M08.911 Juvenile arthritis, unspecified, right shoulder
   M08.912 Juvenile arthritis, unspecified, left shoulder
   M08.919 Juvenile arthritis, unspecified, unspecified shoulder

● **M08.92 Juvenile arthritis, unspecified, elbow**
   M08.921 Juvenile arthritis, unspecified, right elbow
   M08.922 Juvenile arthritis, unspecified, left elbow
   M08.929 Juvenile arthritis, unspecified, unspecified elbow

● **M08.93 Juvenile arthritis, unspecified, wrist**
   M08.931 Juvenile arthritis, unspecified, right wrist
   M08.932 Juvenile arthritis, unspecified, left wrist
   M08.939 Juvenile arthritis, unspecified, unspecified wrist

● **M08.94 Juvenile arthritis, unspecified, hand**
   M08.941 Juvenile arthritis, unspecified, right hand
   M08.942 Juvenile arthritis, unspecified, left hand
   M08.949 Juvenile arthritis, unspecified, unspecified hand

● **M08.95 Juvenile arthritis, unspecified, hip**
   M08.951 Juvenile arthritis, unspecified, right hip
   M08.952 Juvenile arthritis, unspecified, left hip
   M08.959 Juvenile arthritis, unspecified, unspecified hip

● **M08.96 Juvenile arthritis, unspecified, knee**
   M08.961 Juvenile arthritis, unspecified, right knee
   M08.962 Juvenile arthritis, unspecified, left knee
   M08.969 Juvenile arthritis, unspecified, unspecified knee

● **M08.97 Juvenile arthritis, unspecified, ankle and foot**
   M08.971 Juvenile arthritis, unspecified, right ankle and foot
   M08.972 Juvenile arthritis, unspecified, left ankle and foot
   M08.979 Juvenile arthritis, unspecified, unspecified ankle and foot

  M08.98 Juvenile arthritis, unspecified, vertebrae
  M08.99 Juvenile arthritis, unspecified, multiple sites

◀ New   ◀≡ Revised   ~~deleted~~ Deleted   OGCR Official Guidelines   X Assign placeholder X   ● Use Additional Character(s)

Excludes 1   Excludes 2   Includes   Use additional   Code first   Code also   Unspecified

● **M1A Chronic gout**

Use additional code to identify:

Autonomic neuropathy in diseases classified elsewhere (G99.0)

Calculus of urinary tract in diseases classified elsewhere (N22)

Cardiomyopathy in diseases classified elsewhere (I43)

Disorders of external ear in diseases classified elsewhere (H61.1-, H62.8-)

Disorders of iris and ciliary body in diseases classified elsewhere (H22)

Glomerular disorders in diseases classified elsewhere (N08)

Excludes1 acute gout (M10.-)
gout NOS (M10.-)

The appropriate 7th character is to be added to each code from category M1A

0	without tophus (tophi)
1	with tophus (tophi)

● **M1A.0 Idiopathic chronic gout**

Chronic gouty bursitis
Primary chronic gout

X ● **M1A.00 Idiopathic chronic gout, unspecified site**

● **M1A.01 Idiopathic chronic gout, shoulder**

● **M1A.011 Idiopathic chronic gout, right shoulder**

● **M1A.012 Idiopathic chronic gout, left shoulder**

● **M1A.019 Idiopathic chronic gout, unspecified shoulder**

● **M1A.02 Idiopathic chronic gout, elbow**

● **M1A.021 Idiopathic chronic gout, right elbow**

● **M1A.022 Idiopathic chronic gout, left elbow**

● **M1A.029 Idiopathic chronic gout, unspecified elbow**

● **M1A.03 Idiopathic chronic gout, wrist**

● **M1A.031 Idiopathic chronic gout, right wrist**

● **M1A.032 Idiopathic chronic gout, left wrist**

● **M1A.039 Idiopathic chronic gout, unspecified wrist**

● **M1A.04 Idiopathic chronic gout, hand**

● **M1A.041 Idiopathic chronic gout, right hand**

● **M1A.042 Idiopathic chronic gout, left hand**

● **M1A.049 Idiopathic chronic gout, unspecified hand**

● **M1A.05 Idiopathic chronic gout, hip**

● **M1A.051 Idiopathic chronic gout, right hip**

● **M1A.052 Idiopathic chronic gout, left hip**

● **M1A.059 Idiopathic chronic gout, unspecified hip**

● **M1A.06 Idiopathic chronic gout, knee**

● **M1A.061 Idiopathic chronic gout, right knee**

● **M1A.062 Idiopathic chronic gout, left knee**

● **M1A.069 Idiopathic chronic gout, unspecified knee**

● **M1A.07 Idiopathic chronic gout, ankle and foot**

● **M1A.071 Idiopathic chronic gout, right ankle and foot**

● **M1A.072 Idiopathic chronic gout, left ankle and foot**

● **M1A.079 Idiopathic chronic gout, unspecified ankle and foot**

X ● **M1A.08 Idiopathic chronic gout, vertebrae**

X ● **M1A.09 Idiopathic chronic gout, multiple sites**

● **M1A.1 Lead-induced chronic gout**

Code first toxic effects of lead and its compounds (T56.0-)

X ● **M1A.10 Lead-induced chronic gout, unspecified site**

● **M1A.11 Lead-induced chronic gout, shoulder**

● **M1A.111 Lead-induced chronic gout, right shoulder**

● **M1A.112 Lead-induced chronic gout, left shoulder**

● **M1A.119 Lead-induced chronic gout, unspecified shoulder**

● **M1A.12 Lead-induced chronic gout, elbow**

● **M1A.121 Lead-induced chronic gout, right elbow**

● **M1A.122 Lead-induced chronic gout, left elbow**

● **M1A.129 Lead-induced chronic gout, unspecified elbow**

● **M1A.13 Lead-induced chronic gout, wrist**

● **M1A.131 Lead-induced chronic gout, right wrist**

● **M1A.132 Lead-induced chronic gout, left wrist**

● **M1A.139 Lead-induced chronic gout, unspecified wrist**

● **M1A.14 Lead-induced chronic gout, hand**

● **M1A.141 Lead-induced chronic gout, right hand**

● **M1A.142 Lead-induced chronic gout, left hand**

● **M1A.149 Lead-induced chronic gout, unspecified hand**

● **M1A.15 Lead-induced chronic gout, hip**

● **M1A.151 Lead-induced chronic gout, right hip**

● **M1A.152 Lead-induced chronic gout, left hip**

● **M1A.159 Lead-induced chronic gout, unspecified hip**

● **M1A.16 Lead-induced chronic gout, knee**

● **M1A.161 Lead-induced chronic gout, right knee**

● **M1A.162 Lead-induced chronic gout, left knee**

● **M1A.169 Lead-induced chronic gout, unspecified knee**

● **M1A.17 Lead-induced chronic gout, ankle and foot**

● **M1A.171 Lead-induced chronic gout, right ankle and foot**

● **M1A.172 Lead-induced chronic gout, left ankle and foot**

● **M1A.179 Lead-induced chronic gout, unspecified ankle and foot**

X ● **M1A.18 Lead-induced chronic gout, vertebrae**

X ● **M1A.19 Lead-induced chronic gout, multiple sites**

● **M1A.2 Drug-induced chronic gout**

Use additional code for adverse effect, if applicable, to identify drug (T36-T50 with fifth or sixth character 5)

X ● **M1A.20 Drug-induced chronic gout, unspecified site**

● **M1A.21 Drug-induced chronic gout, shoulder**

● **M1A.211 Drug-induced chronic gout, right shoulder**

● **M1A.212 Drug-induced chronic gout, left shoulder**

● **M1A.219 Drug-induced chronic gout, unspecified shoulder**

● **M1A.22 Drug-induced chronic gout, elbow**

● **M1A.221 Drug-induced chronic gout, right elbow**

● **M1A.222 Drug-induced chronic gout, left elbow**

● **M1A.229 Drug-induced chronic gout, unspecified elbow**

CHAPTER 13 (M00–M99)

CHAPTER 13 (M00-M99)

● M1A.23   Drug-induced chronic gout, wrist
- ● M1A.231   Drug-induced chronic gout, right wrist
- ● M1A.232   Drug-induced chronic gout, left wrist
- ● M1A.239   Drug-induced chronic gout, unspecified wrist

● M1A.24   Drug-induced chronic gout, hand
- ● M1A.241   Drug-induced chronic gout, right hand
- ● M1A.242   Drug-induced chronic gout, left hand
- ● M1A.249   Drug-induced chronic gout, unspecified hand

● M1A.25   Drug-induced chronic gout, hip
- ● M1A.251   Drug-induced chronic gout, right hip
- ● M1A.252   Drug-induced chronic gout, left hip
- ● M1A.259   Drug-induced chronic gout, unspecified hip

● M1A.26   Drug-induced chronic gout, knee
- ● M1A.261   Drug-induced chronic gout, right knee
- ● M1A.262   Drug-induced chronic gout, left knee
- ● M1A.269   Drug-induced chronic gout, unspecified knee

● M1A.27   Drug-induced chronic gout, ankle and foot
- ● M1A.271   Drug-induced chronic gout, right ankle and foot
- ● M1A.272   Drug-induced chronic gout, left ankle and foot
- ● M1A.279   Drug-induced chronic gout, unspecified ankle and foot

X ● M1A.28   Drug-induced chronic gout, vertebrae

X ● M1A.29   Drug-induced chronic gout, multiple sites

● M1A.3   Chronic gout due to renal impairment
Code first associated renal disease

X ● M1A.30   Chronic gout due to renal impairment, unspecified site

● M1A.31   Chronic gout due to renal impairment, shoulder
- ● M1A.311   Chronic gout due to renal impairment, right shoulder
- ● M1A.312   Chronic gout due to renal impairment, left shoulder
- ● M1A.319   Chronic gout due to renal impairment, unspecified shoulder

● M1A.32   Chronic gout due to renal impairment, elbow
- ● M1A.321   Chronic gout due to renal impairment, right elbow
- ● M1A.322   Chronic gout due to renal impairment, left elbow
- ● M1A.329   Chronic gout due to renal impairment, unspecified elbow

● M1A.33   Chronic gout due to renal impairment, wrist
- ● M1A.331   Chronic gout due to renal impairment, right wrist
- ● M1A.332   Chronic gout due to renal impairment, left wrist
- ● M1A.339   Chronic gout due to renal impairment, unspecified wrist

● M1A.34   Chronic gout due to renal impairment, hand
- ● M1A.341   Chronic gout due to renal impairment, right hand
- ● M1A.342   Chronic gout due to renal impairment, left hand
- ● M1A.349   Chronic gout due to renal impairment, unspecified hand

● M1A.35   Chronic gout due to renal impairment, hip
- ● M1A.351   Chronic gout due to renal impairment, right hip
- ● M1A.352   Chronic gout due to renal impairment, left hip
- ● M1A.359   Chronic gout due to renal impairment, unspecified hip

● M1A.36   Chronic gout due to renal impairment, knee
- ● M1A.361   Chronic gout due to renal impairment, right knee
- ● M1A.362   Chronic gout due to renal impairment, left knee
- ● M1A.369   Chronic gout due to renal impairment, unspecified knee

● M1A.37   Chronic gout due to renal impairment, ankle and foot
- ● M1A.371   Chronic gout due to renal impairment, right ankle and foot
- ● M1A.372   Chronic gout due to renal impairment, left ankle and foot
- ● M1A.379   Chronic gout due to renal impairment, unspecified ankle and foot

X ● M1A.38   Chronic gout due to renal impairment, vertebrae

X ● M1A.39   Chronic gout due to renal impairment, multiple sites

● M1A.4   Other secondary chronic gout
Code first associated condition

X ● M1A.40   Other secondary chronic gout, unspecified site

● M1A.41   Other secondary chronic gout, shoulder
- ● M1A.411   Other secondary chronic gout, right shoulder
- ● M1A.412   Other secondary chronic gout, left shoulder
- ● M1A.419   Other secondary chronic gout, unspecified shoulder

● M1A.42   Other secondary chronic gout, elbow
- ● M1A.421   Other secondary chronic gout, right elbow
- ● M1A.422   Other secondary chronic gout, left elbow
- ● M1A.429   Other secondary chronic gout, unspecified elbow

● M1A.43   Other secondary chronic gout, wrist
- ● M1A.431   Other secondary chronic gout, right wrist
- ● M1A.432   Other secondary chronic gout, left wrist
- ● M1A.439   Other secondary chronic gout, unspecified wrist

● M1A.44   Other secondary chronic gout, hand
- ● M1A.441   Other secondary chronic gout, right hand
- ● M1A.442   Other secondary chronic gout, left hand
- ● M1A.449   Other secondary chronic gout, unspecified hand

● M1A.45   Other secondary chronic gout, hip
- ● M1A.451   Other secondary chronic gout, right hip
- ● M1A.452   Other secondary chronic gout, left hip
- ● M1A.459   Other secondary chronic gout, unspecified hip

◀ New   ◀▥ Revised   ~~deleted~~ Deleted   OGCR Official Guidelines   X Assign placeholder X   ● Use Additional Character(s)

Excludes 1   Excludes 2   Includes   Use additional   Code first   Code also   Unspecified

- **M1A.46 Other secondary chronic gout, knee**
  - **M1A.461 Other secondary chronic gout, right knee**
  - **M1A.462 Other secondary chronic gout, left knee**
  - **M1A.469 Other secondary chronic gout, unspecified knee**
- **M1A.47 Other secondary chronic gout, ankle and foot**
  - **M1A.471 Other secondary chronic gout, right ankle and foot**
  - **M1A.472 Other secondary chronic gout, left ankle and foot**
  - **M1A.479 Other secondary chronic gout, unspecified ankle and foot**
- X **M1A.48 Other secondary chronic gout, vertebrae**
- X **M1A.49 Other secondary chronic gout, multiple sites**
- X **M1A.9 Chronic gout, unspecified**

- **M10 Gout**

  Accumulation of uric acid that results in swollen, red, hot, painful, stiff joints.

  Acute gout
  Gout attack
  Gout flare
  Gout NOS
  Podagra

  Use additional code to identify:
      Autonomic neuropathy in diseases classified elsewhere (G99.0)
      Calculus of urinary tract in diseases classified elsewhere (N22)
      Cardiomyopathy in diseases classified elsewhere (I43)
      Disorders of external ear in diseases classified elsewhere (H61.1-, H62.8-)
      Disorders of iris and ciliary body in diseases classified elsewhere (H22)
      Glomerular disorders in diseases classified elsewhere (N08)

  Excludes1   chronic gout (M1A.-)

  - **M10.0 Idiopathic gout**
    Gouty bursitis
    Primary gout
    - **M10.00 Idiopathic gout, unspecified site**
    - **M10.01 Idiopathic gout, shoulder**
      - M10.011 Idiopathic gout, right shoulder
      - M10.012 Idiopathic gout, left shoulder
      - M10.019 Idiopathic gout, unspecified shoulder
    - **M10.02 Idiopathic gout, elbow**
      - M10.021 Idiopathic gout, right elbow
      - M10.022 Idiopathic gout, left elbow
      - M10.029 Idiopathic gout, unspecified elbow
    - **M10.03 Idiopathic gout, wrist**
      - M10.031 Idiopathic gout, right wrist
      - M10.032 Idiopathic gout, left wrist
      - M10.039 Idiopathic gout, unspecified wrist
    - **M10.04 Idiopathic gout, hand**
      - M10.041 Idiopathic gout, right hand
      - M10.042 Idiopathic gout, left hand
      - M10.049 Idiopathic gout, unspecified hand
    - **M10.05 Idiopathic gout, hip**
      - M10.051 Idiopathic gout, right hip
      - M10.052 Idiopathic gout, left hip
      - M10.059 Idiopathic gout, unspecified hip
    - **M10.06 Idiopathic gout, knee**
      - M10.061 Idiopathic gout, right knee
      - M10.062 Idiopathic gout, left knee
      - M10.069 Idiopathic gout, unspecified knee

- **M10.07 Idiopathic gout, ankle and foot**
  - M10.071 Idiopathic gout, right ankle and foot
  - M10.072 Idiopathic gout, left ankle and foot
  - M10.079 Idiopathic gout, unspecified ankle and foot
- M10.08 Idiopathic gout, vertebrae
- M10.09 Idiopathic gout, multiple sites
- **M10.1 Lead-induced gout**
  Code first toxic effects of lead and its compounds (T56.0-)
  - M10.10 Lead-induced gout, unspecified site
  - **M10.11 Lead-induced gout, shoulder**
    - M10.111 Lead-induced gout, right shoulder
    - M10.112 Lead-induced gout, left shoulder
    - M10.119 Lead-induced gout, unspecified shoulder
  - **M10.12 Lead-induced gout, elbow**
    - M10.121 Lead-induced gout, right elbow
    - M10.122 Lead-induced gout, left elbow
    - M10.129 Lead-induced gout, unspecified elbow
  - **M10.13 Lead-induced gout, wrist**
    - M10.131 Lead-induced gout, right wrist
    - M10.132 Lead-induced gout, left wrist
    - M10.139 Lead-induced gout, unspecified wrist
  - **M10.14 Lead-induced gout, hand**
    - M10.141 Lead-induced gout, right hand
    - M10.142 Lead-induced gout, left hand
    - M10.149 Lead-induced gout, unspecified hand
  - **M10.15 Lead-induced gout, hip**
    - M10.151 Lead-induced gout, right hip
    - M10.152 Lead-induced gout, left hip
    - M10.159 Lead-induced gout, unspecified hip
  - **M10.16 Lead-induced gout, knee**
    - M10.161 Lead-induced gout, right knee
    - M10.162 Lead-induced gout, left knee
    - M10.169 Lead-induced gout, unspecified knee
  - **M10.17 Lead-induced gout, ankle and foot**
    - M10.171 Lead-induced gout, right ankle and foot
    - M10.172 Lead-induced gout, left ankle and foot
    - M10.179 Lead-induced gout, unspecified ankle and foot
  - M10.18 Lead-induced gout, vertebrae
  - M10.19 Lead-induced gout, multiple sites
- **M10.2 Drug-induced gout**
  Use additional code for adverse effect, if applicable, to identify drug (T36-T50 with fifth or sixth character 5)
  - **M10.20 Drug-induced gout, unspecified site**
  - **M10.21 Drug-induced gout, shoulder**
    - M10.211 Drug-induced gout, right shoulder
    - M10.212 Drug-induced gout, left shoulder
    - M10.219 Drug-induced gout, unspecified shoulder
  - **M10.22 Drug-induced gout, elbow**
    - M10.221 Drug-induced gout, right elbow
    - M10.222 Drug-induced gout, left elbow
    - M10.229 Drug-induced gout, unspecified elbow
  - **M10.23 Drug-induced gout, wrist**
    - M10.231 Drug-induced gout, right wrist
    - M10.232 Drug-induced gout, left wrist
    - M10.239 Drug-induced gout, unspecified wrist

CHAPTER 13 (M00-M99)

● M10.24 Drug-induced gout, hand
    M10.241 Drug-induced gout, right hand
    M10.242 Drug-induced gout, left hand
    M10.249 Drug-induced gout, unspecified hand
● M10.25 Drug-induced gout, hip
    M10.251 Drug-induced gout, right hip
    M10.252 Drug-induced gout, left hip
    M10.259 Drug-induced gout, unspecified hip
● M10.26 Drug-induced gout, knee
    M10.261 Drug-induced gout, right knee
    M10.262 Drug-induced gout, left knee
    M10.269 Drug-induced gout, unspecified knee
● M10.27 Drug-induced gout, ankle and foot
    M10.271 Drug-induced gout, right ankle and foot
    M10.272 Drug-induced gout, left ankle and foot
    M10.279 Drug-induced gout, unspecified ankle and foot
    M10.28 Drug-induced gout, vertebrae
    M10.29 Drug-induced gout, multiple sites
● M10.3 Gout due to renal impairment
    Code also associated renal disease
    M10.30 Gout due to renal impairment, unspecified site
● M10.31 Gout due to renal impairment, shoulder
    M10.311 Gout due to renal impairment, right shoulder
    M10.312 Gout due to renal impairment, left shoulder
    M10.319 Gout due to renal impairment, unspecified shoulder
● M10.32 Gout due to renal impairment, elbow
    M10.321 Gout due to renal impairment, right elbow
    M10.322 Gout due to renal impairment, left elbow
    M10.329 Gout due to renal impairment, unspecified elbow
● M10.33 Gout due to renal impairment, wrist
    M10.331 Gout due to renal impairment, right wrist
    M10.332 Gout due to renal impairment, left wrist
    M10.339 Gout due to renal impairment, unspecified wrist
● M10.34 Gout due to renal impairment, hand
    M10.341 Gout due to renal impairment, right hand
    M10.342 Gout due to renal impairment, left hand
    M10.349 Gout due to renal impairment, unspecified hand
● M10.35 Gout due to renal impairment, hip
    M10.351 Gout due to renal impairment, right hip
    M10.352 Gout due to renal impairment, left hip
    M10.359 Gout due to renal impairment, unspecified hip
● M10.36 Gout due to renal impairment, knee
    M10.361 Gout due to renal impairment, right knee
    M10.362 Gout due to renal impairment, left knee
    M10.369 Gout due to renal impairment, unspecified knee

● M10.37 Gout due to renal impairment, ankle and foot
    M10.371 Gout due to renal impairment, right ankle and foot
    M10.372 Gout due to renal impairment, left ankle and foot
    M10.379 Gout due to renal impairment, unspecified ankle and foot
    M10.38 Gout due to renal impairment, vertebrae
    M10.39 Gout due to renal impairment, multiple sites
● M10.4 Other secondary gout
    Code first associated condition
    M10.40 Other secondary gout, unspecified site
● M10.41 Other secondary gout, shoulder
    M10.411 Other secondary gout, right shoulder
    M10.412 Other secondary gout, left shoulder
    M10.419 Other secondary gout, unspecified shoulder
● M10.42 Other secondary gout, elbow
    M10.421 Other secondary gout, right elbow
    M10.422 Other secondary gout, left elbow
    M10.429 Other secondary gout, unspecified elbow
● M10.43 Other secondary gout, wrist
    M10.431 Other secondary gout, right wrist
    M10.432 Other secondary gout, left wrist
    M10.439 Other secondary gout, unspecified wrist
● M10.44 Other secondary gout, hand
    M10.441 Other secondary gout, right hand
    M10.442 Other secondary gout, left hand
    M10.449 Other secondary gout, unspecified hand
● M10.45 Other secondary gout, hip
    M10.451 Other secondary gout, right hip
    M10.452 Other secondary gout, left hip
    M10.459 Other secondary gout, unspecified hip
● M10.46 Other secondary gout, knee
    M10.461 Other secondary gout, right knee
    M10.462 Other secondary gout, left knee
    M10.469 Other secondary gout, unspecified knee
● M10.47 Other secondary gout, ankle and foot
    M10.471 Other secondary gout, right ankle and foot
    M10.472 Other secondary gout, left ankle and foot
    M10.479 Other secondary gout, unspecified ankle and foot
    M10.48 Other secondary gout, vertebrae
    M10.49 Other secondary gout, multiple sites
    M10.9 Gout, unspecified
        Gout NOS

● M11 Other crystal arthropathies
● M11.0 Hydroxyapatite deposition disease
    M11.00 Hydroxyapatite deposition disease, unspecified site
● M11.01 Hydroxyapatite deposition disease, shoulder
    M11.011 Hydroxyapatite deposition disease, right shoulder
    M11.012 Hydroxyapatite deposition disease, left shoulder
    M11.019 Hydroxyapatite deposition disease, unspecified shoulder

● M11.02   Hydroxyapatite deposition disease, elbow
  M11.021   Hydroxyapatite deposition disease, right elbow
  M11.022   Hydroxyapatite deposition disease, left elbow
  M11.029   Hydroxyapatite deposition disease, unspecified elbow
● M11.03   Hydroxyapatite deposition disease, wrist
  M11.031   Hydroxyapatite deposition disease, right wrist
  M11.032   Hydroxyapatite deposition disease, left wrist
  M11.039   Hydroxyapatite deposition disease, unspecified wrist
● M11.04   Hydroxyapatite deposition disease, hand
  M11.041   Hydroxyapatite deposition disease, right hand
  M11.042   Hydroxyapatite deposition disease, left hand
  M11.049   Hydroxyapatite deposition disease, unspecified hand
● M11.05   Hydroxyapatite deposition disease, hip
  M11.051   Hydroxyapatite deposition disease, right hip
  M11.052   Hydroxyapatite deposition disease, left hip
  M11.059   Hydroxyapatite deposition disease, unspecified hip
● M11.06   Hydroxyapatite deposition disease, knee
  M11.061   Hydroxyapatite deposition disease, right knee
  M11.062   Hydroxyapatite deposition disease, left knee
  M11.069   Hydroxyapatite deposition disease, unspecified knee
● M11.07   Hydroxyapatite deposition disease, ankle and foot
  M11.071   Hydroxyapatite deposition disease, right ankle and foot
  M11.072   Hydroxyapatite deposition disease, left ankle and foot
  M11.079   Hydroxyapatite deposition disease, unspecified ankle and foot
  M11.08   Hydroxyapatite deposition disease, vertebrae
  M11.09   Hydroxyapatite deposition disease, multiple sites
● M11.1   Familial chondrocalcinosis
  M11.10   Familial chondrocalcinosis, unspecified site
● M11.11   Familial chondrocalcinosis, shoulder
  M11.111   Familial chondrocalcinosis, right shoulder
  M11.112   Familial chondrocalcinosis, left shoulder
  M11.119   Familial chondrocalcinosis, unspecified shoulder
● M11.12   Familial chondrocalcinosis, elbow
  M11.121   Familial chondrocalcinosis, right elbow
  M11.122   Familial chondrocalcinosis, left elbow
  M11.129   Familial chondrocalcinosis, unspecified elbow
● M11.13   Familial chondrocalcinosis, wrist
  M11.131   Familial chondrocalcinosis, right wrist
  M11.132   Familial chondrocalcinosis, left wrist
  M11.139   Familial chondrocalcinosis, unspecified wrist

● M11.14   Familial chondrocalcinosis, hand
  M11.141   Familial chondrocalcinosis, right hand
  M11.142   Familial chondrocalcinosis, left hand
  M11.149   Familial chondrocalcinosis, unspecified hand
● M11.15   Familial chondrocalcinosis, hip
  M11.151   Familial chondrocalcinosis, right hip
  M11.152   Familial chondrocalcinosis, left hip
  M11.159   Familial chondrocalcinosis, unspecified hip
● M11.16   Familial chondrocalcinosis, knee
  M11.161   Familial chondrocalcinosis, right knee
  M11.162   Familial chondrocalcinosis, left knee
  M11.169   Familial chondrocalcinosis, unspecified knee
● M11.17   Familial chondrocalcinosis, ankle and foot
  M11.171   Familial chondrocalcinosis, right ankle and foot
  M11.172   Familial chondrocalcinosis, left ankle and foot
  M11.179   Familial chondrocalcinosis, unspecified ankle and foot
  M11.18   Familial chondrocalcinosis, vertebrae
  M11.19   Familial chondrocalcinosis, multiple sites
● M11.2   Other chondrocalcinosis
  Chondrocalcinosis NOS
  M11.20   Other chondrocalcinosis, unspecified site
● M11.21   Other chondrocalcinosis, shoulder
  M11.211   Other chondrocalcinosis, right shoulder
  M11.212   Other chondrocalcinosis, left shoulder
  M11.219   Other chondrocalcinosis, unspecified shoulder
● M11.22   Other chondrocalcinosis, elbow
  M11.221   Other chondrocalcinosis, right elbow
  M11.222   Other chondrocalcinosis, left elbow
  M11.229   Other chondrocalcinosis, unspecified elbow
● M11.23   Other chondrocalcinosis, wrist
  M11.231   Other chondrocalcinosis, right wrist
  M11.232   Other chondrocalcinosis, left wrist
  M11.239   Other chondrocalcinosis, unspecified wrist
● M11.24   Other chondrocalcinosis, hand
  M11.241   Other chondrocalcinosis, right hand
  M11.242   Other chondrocalcinosis, left hand
  M11.249   Other chondrocalcinosis, unspecified hand
● M11.25   Other chondrocalcinosis, hip
  M11.251   Other chondrocalcinosis, right hip
  M11.252   Other chondrocalcinosis, left hip
  M11.259   Other chondrocalcinosis, unspecified hip
● M11.26   Other chondrocalcinosis, knee
  M11.261   Other chondrocalcinosis, right knee
  M11.262   Other chondrocalcinosis, left knee
  M11.269   Other chondrocalcinosis, unspecified knee

CHAPTER 13 (M00-M99)

● M11.27   Other chondrocalcinosis, ankle and foot
    M11.271   Other chondrocalcinosis, right ankle and foot
    M11.272   Other chondrocalcinosis, left ankle and foot
    M11.279   Other chondrocalcinosis, unspecified ankle and foot
   M11.28   Other chondrocalcinosis, vertebrae
   M11.29   Other chondrocalcinosis, multiple sites
● M11.8   Other specified crystal arthropathies
   M11.80   Other specified crystal arthropathies, unspecified site
● M11.81   Other specified crystal arthropathies, shoulder
    M11.811   Other specified crystal arthropathies, right shoulder
    M11.812   Other specified crystal arthropathies, left shoulder
    M11.819   Other specified crystal arthropathies, unspecified shoulder
● M11.82   Other specified crystal arthropathies, elbow
    M11.821   Other specified crystal arthropathies, right elbow
    M11.822   Other specified crystal arthropathies, left elbow
    M11.829   Other specified crystal arthropathies, unspecified elbow
● M11.83   Other specified crystal arthropathies, wrist
    M11.831   Other specified crystal arthropathies, right wrist
    M11.832   Other specified crystal arthropathies, left wrist
    M11.839   Other specified crystal arthropathies, unspecified wrist
● M11.84   Other specified crystal arthropathies, hand
    M11.841   Other specified crystal arthropathies, right hand
    M11.842   Other specified crystal arthropathies, left hand
    M11.849   Other specified crystal arthropathies, unspecified hand
● M11.85   Other specified crystal arthropathies, hip
    M11.851   Other specified crystal arthropathies, right hip
    M11.852   Other specified crystal arthropathies, left hip
    M11.859   Other specified crystal arthropathies, unspecified hip
● M11.86   Other specified crystal arthropathies, knee
    M11.861   Other specified crystal arthropathies, right knee
    M11.862   Other specified crystal arthropathies, left knee
    M11.869   Other specified crystal arthropathies, unspecified knee
● M11.87   Other specified crystal arthropathies, ankle and foot
    M11.871   Other specified crystal arthropathies, right ankle and foot
    M11.872   Other specified crystal arthropathies, left ankle and foot
    M11.879   Other specified crystal arthropathies, unspecified ankle and foot
   M11.88   Other specified crystal arthropathies, vertebrae
   M11.89   Other specified crystal arthropathies, multiple sites
  M11.9   Crystal arthropathy, unspecified

● M12   Other and unspecified arthropathy
   Excludes1   arthrosis (M15-M19)
            cricoarytenoid arthropathy (J38.7)
● M12.0   Chronic postrheumatic arthropathy [Jaccoud]
   M12.00   Chronic postrheumatic arthropathy [Jaccoud], unspecified site
● M12.01   Chronic postrheumatic arthropathy [Jaccoud], shoulder
    M12.011   Chronic postrheumatic arthropathy [Jaccoud], right shoulder
    M12.012   Chronic postrheumatic arthropathy [Jaccoud], left shoulder
    M12.019   Chronic postrheumatic arthropathy [Jaccoud], unspecified shoulder
● M12.02   Chronic postrheumatic arthropathy [Jaccoud], elbow
    M12.021   Chronic postrheumatic arthropathy [Jaccoud], right elbow
    M12.022   Chronic postrheumatic arthropathy [Jaccoud], left elbow
    M12.029   Chronic postrheumatic arthropathy [Jaccoud], unspecified elbow
● M12.03   Chronic postrheumatic arthropathy [Jaccoud], wrist
    M12.031   Chronic postrheumatic arthropathy [Jaccoud], right wrist
    M12.032   Chronic postrheumatic arthropathy [Jaccoud], left wrist
    M12.039   Chronic postrheumatic arthropathy [Jaccoud], unspecified wrist
● M12.04   Chronic postrheumatic arthropathy [Jaccoud], hand
    M12.041   Chronic postrheumatic arthropathy [Jaccoud], right hand
    M12.042   Chronic postrheumatic arthropathy [Jaccoud], left hand
    M12.049   Chronic postrheumatic arthropathy [Jaccoud], unspecified hand
● M12.05   Chronic postrheumatic arthropathy [Jaccoud], hip
    M12.051   Chronic postrheumatic arthropathy [Jaccoud], right hip
    M12.052   Chronic postrheumatic arthropathy [Jaccoud], left hip
    M12.059   Chronic postrheumatic arthropathy [Jaccoud], unspecified hip
● M12.06   Chronic postrheumatic arthropathy [Jaccoud], knee
    M12.061   Chronic postrheumatic arthropathy [Jaccoud], right knee
    M12.062   Chronic postrheumatic arthropathy [Jaccoud], left knee
    M12.069   Chronic postrheumatic arthropathy [Jaccoud], unspecified knee
● M12.07   Chronic postrheumatic arthropathy [Jaccoud], ankle and foot
    M12.071   Chronic postrheumatic arthropathy [Jaccoud], right ankle and foot
    M12.072   Chronic postrheumatic arthropathy [Jaccoud], left ankle and foot
    M12.079   Chronic postrheumatic arthropathy [Jaccoud], unspecified ankle and foot
   M12.08   Chronic postrheumatic arthropathy [Jaccoud], other specified site
      Chronic postrheumatic arthropathy [Jaccoud], vertebrae
   M12.09   Chronic postrheumatic arthropathy [Jaccoud], multiple sites

- M12.1   Kaschin-Beck disease
         Osteochondroarthrosis deformans endemica
    M12.10   Kaschin-Beck disease, unspecified site
- M12.11   Kaschin-Beck disease, shoulder
     M12.111   Kaschin-Beck disease, right shoulder
     M12.112   Kaschin-Beck disease, left shoulder
     M12.119   Kaschin-Beck disease, unspecified shoulder
- M12.12   Kaschin-Beck disease, elbow
     M12.121   Kaschin-Beck disease, right elbow
     M12.122   Kaschin-Beck disease, left elbow
     M12.129   Kaschin-Beck disease, unspecified elbow
- M12.13   Kaschin-Beck disease, wrist
     M12.131   Kaschin-Beck disease, right wrist
     M12.132   Kaschin-Beck disease, left wrist
     M12.139   Kaschin-Beck disease, unspecified wrist
- M12.14   Kaschin-Beck disease, hand
     M12.141   Kaschin-Beck disease, right hand
     M12.142   Kaschin-Beck disease, left hand
     M12.149   Kaschin-Beck disease, unspecified hand
- M12.15   Kaschin-Beck disease, hip
     M12.151   Kaschin-Beck disease, right hip
     M12.152   Kaschin-Beck disease, left hip
     M12.159   Kaschin-Beck disease, unspecified hip
- M12.16   Kaschin-Beck disease, knee
     M12.161   Kaschin-Beck disease, right knee
     M12.162   Kaschin-Beck disease, left knee
     M12.169   Kaschin-Beck disease, unspecified knee
- M12.17   Kaschin-Beck disease, ankle and foot
     M12.171   Kaschin-Beck disease, right ankle and foot
     M12.172   Kaschin-Beck disease, left ankle and foot
     M12.179   Kaschin-Beck disease, unspecified ankle and foot
    M12.18   Kaschin-Beck disease, vertebrae
    M12.19   Kaschin-Beck disease, multiple sites
- M12.2   Villonodular synovitis (pigmented)
    M12.20   Villonodular synovitis (pigmented), unspecified site
- M12.21   Villonodular synovitis (pigmented), shoulder
     M12.211   Villonodular synovitis (pigmented), right shoulder
     M12.212   Villonodular synovitis (pigmented), left shoulder
     M12.219   Villonodular synovitis (pigmented), unspecified shoulder
- M12.22   Villonodular synovitis (pigmented), elbow
     M12.221   Villonodular synovitis (pigmented), right elbow
     M12.222   Villonodular synovitis (pigmented), left elbow
     M12.229   Villonodular synovitis (pigmented), unspecified elbow
- M12.23   Villonodular synovitis (pigmented), wrist
     M12.231   Villonodular synovitis (pigmented), right wrist
     M12.232   Villonodular synovitis (pigmented), left wrist
     M12.239   Villonodular synovitis (pigmented), unspecified wrist

- M12.24   Villonodular synovitis (pigmented), hand
     M12.241   Villonodular synovitis (pigmented), right hand
     M12.242   Villonodular synovitis (pigmented), left hand
     M12.249   Villonodular synovitis (pigmented), unspecified hand
- M12.25   Villonodular synovitis (pigmented), hip
     M12.251   Villonodular synovitis (pigmented), right hip
     M12.252   Villonodular synovitis (pigmented), left hip
     M12.259   Villonodular synovitis (pigmented), unspecified hip
- M12.26   Villonodular synovitis (pigmented), knee
     M12.261   Villonodular synovitis (pigmented), right knee
     M12.262   Villonodular synovitis (pigmented), left knee
     M12.269   Villonodular synovitis (pigmented), unspecified knee
- M12.27   Villonodular synovitis (pigmented), ankle and foot
     M12.271   Villonodular synovitis (pigmented), right ankle and foot
     M12.272   Villonodular synovitis (pigmented), left ankle and foot
     M12.279   Villonodular synovitis (pigmented), unspecified ankle and foot
    M12.28   Villonodular synovitis (pigmented), other specified site
             Villonodular synovitis (pigmented), vertebrae
    M12.29   Villonodular synovitis (pigmented), multiple sites
- M12.3   Palindromic rheumatism
    M12.30   Palindromic rheumatism, unspecified site
- M12.31   Palindromic rheumatism, shoulder
     M12.311   Palindromic rheumatism, right shoulder
     M12.312   Palindromic rheumatism, left shoulder
     M12.319   Palindromic rheumatism, unspecified shoulder
- M12.32   Palindromic rheumatism, elbow
     M12.321   Palindromic rheumatism, right elbow
     M12.322   Palindromic rheumatism, left elbow
     M12.329   Palindromic rheumatism, unspecified elbow
- M12.33   Palindromic rheumatism, wrist
     M12.331   Palindromic rheumatism, right wrist
     M12.332   Palindromic rheumatism, left wrist
     M12.339   Palindromic rheumatism, unspecified wrist
- M12.34   Palindromic rheumatism, hand
     M12.341   Palindromic rheumatism, right hand
     M12.342   Palindromic rheumatism, left hand
     M12.349   Palindromic rheumatism, unspecified hand
- M12.35   Palindromic rheumatism, hip
     M12.351   Palindromic rheumatism, right hip
     M12.352   Palindromic rheumatism, left hip
     M12.359   Palindromic rheumatism, unspecified hip

CHAPTER 13 (M00-M99)

CHAPTER 13 (M00-M99)

● M12.36 Palindromic rheumatism, knee
      M12.361 Palindromic rheumatism, right knee
      M12.362 Palindromic rheumatism, left knee
      M12.369 Palindromic rheumatism, unspecified knee
● M12.37 Palindromic rheumatism, ankle and foot
      M12.371 Palindromic rheumatism, right ankle and foot
      M12.372 Palindromic rheumatism, left ankle and foot
      M12.379 Palindromic rheumatism, unspecified ankle and foot
   M12.38 Palindromic rheumatism, other specified site
            Palindromic rheumatism, vertebrae
   M12.39 Palindromic rheumatism, multiple sites
● M12.4 Intermittent hydrarthrosis
   M12.40 Intermittent hydrarthrosis, unspecified site
● M12.41 Intermittent hydrarthrosis, shoulder
      M12.411 Intermittent hydrarthrosis, right shoulder
      M12.412 Intermittent hydrarthrosis, left shoulder
      M12.419 Intermittent hydrarthrosis, unspecified shoulder
● M12.42 Intermittent hydrarthrosis, elbow
      M12.421 Intermittent hydrarthrosis, right elbow
      M12.422 Intermittent hydrarthrosis, left elbow
      M12.429 Intermittent hydrarthrosis, unspecified elbow
● M12.43 Intermittent hydrarthrosis, wrist
      M12.431 Intermittent hydrarthrosis, right wrist
      M12.432 Intermittent hydrarthrosis, left wrist
      M12.439 Intermittent hydrarthrosis, unspecified wrist
● M12.44 Intermittent hydrarthrosis, hand
      M12.441 Intermittent hydrarthrosis, right hand
      M12.442 Intermittent hydrarthrosis, left hand
      M12.449 Intermittent hydrarthrosis, unspecified hand
● M12.45 Intermittent hydrarthrosis, hip
      M12.451 Intermittent hydrarthrosis, right hip
      M12.452 Intermittent hydrarthrosis, left hip
      M12.459 Intermittent hydrarthrosis, unspecified hip
● M12.46 Intermittent hydrarthrosis, knee
      M12.461 Intermittent hydrarthrosis, right knee
      M12.462 Intermittent hydrarthrosis, left knee
      M12.469 Intermittent hydrarthrosis, unspecified knee
● M12.47 Intermittent hydrarthrosis, ankle and foot
      M12.471 Intermittent hydrarthrosis, right ankle and foot
      M12.472 Intermittent hydrarthrosis, left ankle and foot
      M12.479 Intermittent hydrarthrosis, unspecified ankle and foot
   M12.48 Intermittent hydrarthrosis, other site
   M12.49 Intermittent hydrarthrosis, multiple sites

● M12.5 Traumatic arthropathy
      Excludes1 current injury-see Alphabetic Index
                 post-traumatic osteoarthritis of first carpometacarpal joint (M18.2-M18.3)
                 post-traumatic osteoarthritis of hip (M16.4-M16.5)
                 post-traumatic osteoarthritis of knee (M17.2-M17.3)
                 post-traumatic osteoarthritis NOS (M19.1-)
                 post-traumatic osteoarthritis of other single joints (M19.1-)
   M12.50 Traumatic arthropathy, unspecified site
● M12.51 Traumatic arthropathy, shoulder
      M12.511 Traumatic arthropathy, right shoulder
      M12.512 Traumatic arthropathy, left shoulder
      M12.519 Traumatic arthropathy, unspecified shoulder
● M12.52 Traumatic arthropathy, elbow
      M12.521 Traumatic arthropathy, right elbow
      M12.522 Traumatic arthropathy, left elbow
      M12.529 Traumatic arthropathy, unspecified elbow
● M12.53 Traumatic arthropathy, wrist
      M12.531 Traumatic arthropathy, right wrist
      M12.532 Traumatic arthropathy, left wrist
      M12.539 Traumatic arthropathy, unspecified wrist
● M12.54 Traumatic arthropathy, hand
      M12.541 Traumatic arthropathy, right hand
      M12.542 Traumatic arthropathy, left hand
      M12.549 Traumatic arthropathy, unspecified hand
● M12.55 Traumatic arthropathy, hip
      M12.551 Traumatic arthropathy, right hip
      M12.552 Traumatic arthropathy, left hip
      M12.559 Traumatic arthropathy, unspecified hip
● M12.56 Traumatic arthropathy, knee
      M12.561 Traumatic arthropathy, right knee
      M12.562 Traumatic arthropathy, left knee
      M12.569 Traumatic arthropathy, unspecified knee
● M12.57 Traumatic arthropathy, ankle and foot
      M12.571 Traumatic arthropathy, right ankle and foot
      M12.572 Traumatic arthropathy, left ankle and foot
      M12.579 Traumatic arthropathy, unspecified ankle and foot
   M12.58 Traumatic arthropathy, other specified site
            Traumatic arthropathy, vertebrae
   M12.59 Traumatic arthropathy, multiple sites
● M12.8 Other specific arthropathies, not elsewhere classified
         Transient arthropathy
   M12.80 Other specific arthropathies, not elsewhere classified, unspecified site
● M12.81 Other specific arthropathies, not elsewhere classified, shoulder
      M12.811 Other specific arthropathies, not elsewhere classified, right shoulder
      M12.812 Other specific arthropathies, not elsewhere classified, left shoulder
      M12.819 Other specific arthropathies, not elsewhere classified, unspecified shoulder

◀ New   ◀◀ Revised   ~~deleted~~ Deleted   OGCR Official Guidelines   X Assign placeholder X   ● Use Additional Character(s)

Excludes 1   Excludes 2   Includes   Use additional   Code first   Code also   Unspecified

● **M12.82   Other specific arthropathies, not elsewhere classified, elbow**
    M12.821   Other specific arthropathies, not elsewhere classified, right elbow
    M12.822   Other specific arthropathies, not elsewhere classified, left elbow
    M12.829   Other specific arthropathies, not elsewhere classified, unspecified elbow

● **M12.83   Other specific arthropathies, not elsewhere classified, wrist**
    M12.831   Other specific arthropathies, not elsewhere classified, right wrist
    M12.832   Other specific arthropathies, not elsewhere classified, left wrist
    M12.839   Other specific arthropathies, not elsewhere classified, unspecified wrist

● **M12.84   Other specific arthropathies, not elsewhere classified, hand**
    M12.841   Other specific arthropathies, not elsewhere classified, right hand
    M12.842   Other specific arthropathies, not elsewhere classified, left hand
    M12.849   Other specific arthropathies, not elsewhere classified, unspecified hand

● **M12.85   Other specific arthropathies, not elsewhere classified, hip**
    M12.851   Other specific arthropathies, not elsewhere classified, right hip
    M12.852   Other specific arthropathies, not elsewhere classified, left hip
    M12.859   Other specific arthropathies, not elsewhere classified, unspecified hip

● **M12.86   Other specific arthropathies, not elsewhere classified, knee**
    M12.861   Other specific arthropathies, not elsewhere classified, right knee
    M12.862   Other specific arthropathies, not elsewhere classified, left knee
    M12.869   Other specific arthropathies, not elsewhere classified, unspecified knee

● **M12.87   Other specific arthropathies, not elsewhere classified, ankle and foot**
    M12.871   Other specific arthropathies, not elsewhere classified, right ankle and foot
    M12.872   Other specific arthropathies, not elsewhere classified, left ankle and foot
    M12.879   Other specific arthropathies, not elsewhere classified, unspecified ankle and foot

   M12.88   Other specific arthropathies, not elsewhere classified, other specified site
       Other specific arthropathies, not elsewhere classified, vertebrae

   M12.89   Other specific arthropathies, not elsewhere classified, multiple sites

M12.9   Arthropathy, unspecified

● **M13   Other arthritis**
   [Excludes1]   arthrosis (M15-M19)
            osteoarthritis (M15-M19)

   M13.0   Polyarthritis, unspecified

●   M13.1   Monoarthritis, not elsewhere classified
     M13.10   Monoarthritis, not elsewhere classified, unspecified site

●   M13.11   Monoarthritis, not elsewhere classified, shoulder
       M13.111   Monoarthritis, not elsewhere classified, right shoulder
       M13.112   Monoarthritis, not elsewhere classified, left shoulder
       M13.119   Monoarthritis, not elsewhere classified, unspecified shoulder

●   M13.12   Monoarthritis, not elsewhere classified, elbow
       M13.121   Monoarthritis, not elsewhere classified, right elbow
       M13.122   Monoarthritis, not elsewhere classified, left elbow
       M13.129   Monoarthritis, not elsewhere classified, unspecified elbow

●   M13.13   Monoarthritis, not elsewhere classified, wrist
       M13.131   Monoarthritis, not elsewhere classified, right wrist
       M13.132   Monoarthritis, not elsewhere classified, left wrist
       M13.139   Monoarthritis, not elsewhere classified, unspecified wrist

●   M13.14   Monoarthritis, not elsewhere classified, hand
       M13.141   Monoarthritis, not elsewhere classified, right hand
       M13.142   Monoarthritis, not elsewhere classified, left hand
       M13.149   Monoarthritis, not elsewhere classified, unspecified hand

●   M13.15   Monoarthritis, not elsewhere classified, hip
       M13.151   Monoarthritis, not elsewhere classified, right hip
       M13.152   Monoarthritis, not elsewhere classified, left hip
       M13.159   Monoarthritis, not elsewhere classified, unspecified hip

●   M13.16   Monoarthritis, not elsewhere classified, knee
       M13.161   Monoarthritis, not elsewhere classified, right knee
       M13.162   Monoarthritis, not elsewhere classified, left knee
       M13.169   Monoarthritis, not elsewhere classified, unspecified knee

●   M13.17   Monoarthritis, not elsewhere classified, ankle and foot
       M13.171   Monoarthritis, not elsewhere classified, right ankle and foot
       M13.172   Monoarthritis, not elsewhere classified, left ankle and foot
       M13.179   Monoarthritis, not elsewhere classified, unspecified ankle and foot

● **M13.8   Other specified arthritis**
   Allergic arthritis
   Excludes1   osteoarthritis (M15-M19)
   M13.80   Other specified arthritis, unspecified site
● M13.81   Other specified arthritis, shoulder
      M13.811   Other specified arthritis, right shoulder
      M13.812   Other specified arthritis, left shoulder
      M13.819   Other specified arthritis, unspecified shoulder
● M13.82   Other specified arthritis, elbow
      M13.821   Other specified arthritis, right elbow
      M13.822   Other specified arthritis, left elbow
      M13.829   Other specified arthritis, unspecified elbow
● M13.83   Other specified arthritis, wrist
      M13.831   Other specified arthritis, right wrist
      M13.832   Other specified arthritis, left wrist
      M13.839   Other specified arthritis, unspecified wrist
● M13.84   Other specified arthritis, hand
      M13.841   Other specified arthritis, right hand
      M13.842   Other specified arthritis, left hand
      M13.849   Other specified arthritis, unspecified hand
● M13.85   Other specified arthritis, hip
      M13.851   Other specified arthritis, right hip
      M13.852   Other specified arthritis, left hip
      M13.859   Other specified arthritis, unspecified hip
● M13.86   Other specified arthritis, knee
      M13.861   Other specified arthritis, right knee
      M13.862   Other specified arthritis, left knee
      M13.869   Other specified arthritis, unspecified knee
● M13.87   Other specified arthritis, ankle and foot
      M13.871   Other specified arthritis, right ankle and foot
      M13.872   Other specified arthritis, left ankle and foot
      M13.879   Other specified arthritis, unspecified ankle and foot
   M13.88   Other specified arthritis, other site
   M13.89   Other specified arthritis, multiple sites

● **M14   Arthropathies in other diseases classified elsewhere**
   Excludes1   arthropathy in:
         diabetes mellitus (E08-E13 with .61-)
         hematological disorders (M36.2-M36.3)
         hypersensitivity reactions (M36.4)
         neoplastic disease (M36.1)
         neurosyphillis (A52.16)
         sarcoidosis (D86.86)
      enteropathic arthropathies (M07.0-)
      juvenile psoriatic arthropathy (L40.54)
      lipoid dermatoarthritis (E78.81)
● M14.6   Charcôt's joint
      Neuropathic arthropathy
      Excludes1   Charcôt's joint in diabetes mellitus (E08-E13 with .610)
                  Charcôt's joint in tabes dorsalis (A52.16)
   M14.60   Charcôt's joint, unspecified site
● M14.61   Charcôt's joint, shoulder
      M14.611   Charcôt's joint, right shoulder
      M14.612   Charcôt's joint, left shoulder
      M14.619   Charcôt's joint, unspecified shoulder

● M14.62   Charcôt's joint, elbow
      M14.621   Charcôt's joint, right elbow
      M14.622   Charcôt's joint, left elbow
      M14.629   Charcôt's joint, unspecified elbow
● M14.63   Charcôt's joint, wrist
      M14.631   Charcôt's joint, right wrist
      M14.632   Charcôt's joint, left wrist
      M14.639   Charcôt's joint, unspecified wrist
● M14.64   Charcôt's joint, hand
      M14.641   Charcôt's joint, right hand
      M14.642   Charcôt's joint, left hand
      M14.649   Charcôt's joint, unspecified hand
● M14.65   Charcôt's joint, hip
      M14.651   Charcôt's joint, right hip
      M14.652   Charcôt's joint, left hip
      M14.659   Charcôt's joint, unspecified hip
● M14.66   Charcôt's joint, knee
      M14.661   Charcôt's joint, right knee
      M14.662   Charcôt's joint, left knee
      M14.669   Charcôt's joint, unspecified knee
● M14.67   Charcôt's joint, ankle and foot
      M14.671   Charcôt's joint, right ankle and foot
      M14.672   Charcôt's joint, left ankle and foot
      M14.679   Charcôt's joint, unspecified ankle and foot
   M14.68   Charcôt's joint, vertebrae
   M14.69   Charcôt's joint, multiple sites
● **M14.8   Arthropathies in other specified diseases classified elsewhere**
      Code first underlying disease, such as:
         amyloidosis (E85.-)
         erythema multiforme (L51.-)
         erythema nodosum (L52)
         hemochromatosis (E83.11-)
         hyperparathyroidism (E21.-)
         hypothyroidism (E00-E03)
         sickle-cell disorders (D57.-)
         thyrotoxicosis [hyperthyroidism] (E05.-)
         Whipple's disease (K90.81)
   M14.80   Arthropathies in other specified diseases classified elsewhere, unspecified site
● M14.81   Arthropathies in other specified diseases classified elsewhere, shoulder
      M14.811   Arthropathies in other specified diseases classified elsewhere, right shoulder
      M14.812   Arthropathies in other specified diseases classified elsewhere, left shoulder
      M14.819   Arthropathies in other specified diseases classified elsewhere, unspecified shoulder
● M14.82   Arthropathies in other specified diseases classified elsewhere, elbow
      M14.821   Arthropathies in other specified diseases classified elsewhere, right elbow
      M14.822   Arthropathies in other specified diseases classified elsewhere, left elbow
      M14.829   Arthropathies in other specified diseases classified elsewhere, unspecified elbow

● **M14.83 Arthropathies in other specified diseases classified elsewhere, wrist**
   M14.831 Arthropathies in other specified diseases classified elsewhere, right wrist
   M14.832 Arthropathies in other specified diseases classified elsewhere, left wrist
   M14.839 Arthropathies in other specified diseases classified elsewhere, unspecified wrist

● **M14.84 Arthropathies in other specified diseases classified elsewhere, hand**
   M14.841 Arthropathies in other specified diseases classified elsewhere, right hand
   M14.842 Arthropathies in other specified diseases classified elsewhere, left hand
   M14.849 Arthropathies in other specified diseases classified elsewhere, unspecified hand

● **M14.85 Arthropathies in other specified diseases classified elsewhere, hip**
   M14.851 Arthropathies in other specified diseases classified elsewhere, right hip
   M14.852 Arthropathies in other specified diseases classified elsewhere, left hip
   M14.859 Arthropathies in other specified diseases classified elsewhere, unspecified hip

● **M14.86 Arthropathies in other specified diseases classified elsewhere, knee**
   M14.861 Arthropathies in other specified diseases classified elsewhere, right knee
   M14.862 Arthropathies in other specified diseases classified elsewhere, left knee
   M14.869 Arthropathies in other specified diseases classified elsewhere, unspecified knee

● **M14.87 Arthropathies in other specified diseases classified elsewhere, ankle and foot**
   M14.871 Arthropathies in other specified diseases classified elsewhere, right ankle and foot
   M14.872 Arthropathies in other specified diseases classified elsewhere, left ankle and foot
   M14.879 Arthropathies in other specified diseases classified elsewhere, unspecified ankle and foot

M14.88 Arthropathies in other specified diseases classified elsewhere, vertebrae

M14.89 Arthropathies in other specified diseases classified elsewhere, multiple sites

---

OSTEOARTHRITIS (M15-M19)

Osteoarthritis is the most common degenerative joint disease and form of arthritis that breaks down the cartilage causing pain, swelling, and reduced motion in the joints.

Excludes2   osteoarthritis of spine (M47.-)

● **M15 Polyosteoarthritis**
   Includes   arthritis of multiple sites
   Excludes1   bilateral involvement of single joint (M16-M19)

M15.0 Primary generalized (osteo)arthritis

M15.1 Heberden's nodes (with arthropathy)
   Interphalangeal distal osteoarthritis

M15.2 Bouchard's nodes (with arthropathy)
   Juxtaphalangeal distal osteoarthritis

M15.3 Secondary multiple arthritis
   Post-traumatic polyosteoarthritis

M15.4 Erosive (osteo)arthritis

M15.8 Other polyosteoarthritis

M15.9 Polyosteoarthritis, unspecified
   Generalized osteoarthritis NOS

● **M16 Osteoarthritis of hip**

M16.0 Bilateral primary osteoarthritis of hip

● **M16.1 Unilateral primary osteoarthritis of hip**
   Primary osteoarthritis of hip NOS
   M16.10 Unilateral primary osteoarthritis, unspecified hip
   M16.11 Unilateral primary osteoarthritis, right hip
   M16.12 Unilateral primary osteoarthritis, left hip

M16.2 Bilateral osteoarthritis resulting from hip dysplasia

● **M16.3 Unilateral osteoarthritis resulting from hip dysplasia**
   Dysplastic osteoarthritis of hip NOS
   M16.30 Unilateral osteoarthritis resulting from hip dysplasia, unspecified hip
   M16.31 Unilateral osteoarthritis resulting from hip dysplasia, right hip
   M16.32 Unilateral osteoarthritis resulting from hip dysplasia, left hip

M16.4 Bilateral post-traumatic osteoarthritis of hip

● **M16.5 Unilateral post-traumatic osteoarthritis of hip**
   Post-traumatic osteoarthritis of hip NOS
   M16.50 Unilateral post-traumatic osteoarthritis, unspecified hip
   M16.51 Unilateral post-traumatic osteoarthritis, right hip
   M16.52 Unilateral post-traumatic osteoarthritis, left hip

M16.6 Other bilateral secondary osteoarthritis of hip

M16.7 Other unilateral secondary osteoarthritis of hip
   Secondary osteoarthritis of hip NOS

M16.9 Osteoarthritis of hip, unspecified

● **M17 Osteoarthritis of knee**

M17.0 Bilateral primary osteoarthritis of knee

● **M17.1 Unilateral primary osteoarthritis of knee**
   Primary osteoarthritis of knee NOS
   M17.10 Unilateral primary osteoarthritis, unspecified knee
   M17.11 Unilateral primary osteoarthritis, right knee
   M17.12 Unilateral primary osteoarthritis, left knee

M17.2 Bilateral post-traumatic osteoarthritis of knee

● **M17.3 Unilateral post-traumatic osteoarthritis of knee**
   Post-traumatic osteoarthritis of knee NOS
   M17.30 Unilateral post-traumatic osteoarthritis, unspecified knee
   M17.31 Unilateral post-traumatic osteoarthritis, right knee
   M17.32 Unilateral post-traumatic osteoarthritis, left knee

M17.4 Other bilateral secondary osteoarthritis of knee

M17.5 Other unilateral secondary osteoarthritis of knee
   Secondary osteoarthritis of knee NOS

M17.9 Osteoarthritis of knee, unspecified

● **M18 Osteoarthritis of first carpometacarpal joint**

M18.0 Bilateral primary osteoarthritis of first carpometacarpal joints

● **M18.1 Unilateral primary osteoarthritis of first carpometacarpal joint**
   Primary osteoarthritis of first carpometacarpal joint NOS
   M18.10 Unilateral primary osteoarthritis of first carpometacarpal joint, unspecified hand
   M18.11 Unilateral primary osteoarthritis of first carpometacarpal joint, right hand
   M18.12 Unilateral primary osteoarthritis of first carpometacarpal joint, left hand

CHAPTER 13 (M00-M99)

M18.2 Bilateral post-traumatic osteoarthritis of first carpometacarpal joints

● M18.3 Unilateral post-traumatic osteoarthritis of first carpometacarpal joint
Post-traumatic osteoarthritis of first carpometacarpal joint NOS

    M18.30 Unilateral post-traumatic osteoarthritis of first carpometacarpal joint, unspecified hand

    M18.31 Unilateral post-traumatic osteoarthritis of first carpometacarpal joint, right hand

    M18.32 Unilateral post-traumatic osteoarthritis of first carpometacarpal joint, left hand

M18.4 Other bilateral secondary osteoarthritis of first carpometacarpal joints

● M18.5 Other unilateral secondary osteoarthritis of first carpometacarpal joint
Secondary osteoarthritis of first carpometacarpal joint NOS

    M18.50 Other unilateral secondary osteoarthritis of first carpometacarpal joint, unspecified hand

    M18.51 Other unilateral secondary osteoarthritis of first carpometacarpal joint, right hand

    M18.52 Other unilateral secondary osteoarthritis of first carpometacarpal joint, left hand

M18.9 Osteoarthritis of first carpometacarpal joint, unspecified

● M19 Other and unspecified osteoarthritis
Excludes1 polyarthritis (M15.-)
Excludes2 arthrosis of spine (M47.-)
hallux rigidus (M20.2)
osteoarthritis of spine (M47.-)

● M19.0 Primary osteoarthritis of other joints

  ● M19.01 Primary osteoarthritis, shoulder
    M19.011 Primary osteoarthritis, right shoulder
    M19.012 Primary osteoarthritis, left shoulder
    M19.019 Primary osteoarthritis, unspecified shoulder

  ● M19.02 Primary osteoarthritis, elbow
    M19.021 Primary osteoarthritis, right elbow
    M19.022 Primary osteoarthritis, left elbow
    M19.029 Primary osteoarthritis, unspecified elbow

  ● M19.03 Primary osteoarthritis, wrist
    M19.031 Primary osteoarthritis, right wrist
    M19.032 Primary osteoarthritis, left wrist
    M19.039 Primary osteoarthritis, unspecified wrist

  ● M19.04 Primary osteoarthritis, hand
    Excludes2 primary osteoarthritis of first carpometacarpal joint (M18.0-, M18.1-)
    M19.041 Primary osteoarthritis, right hand
    M19.042 Primary osteoarthritis, left hand
    M19.049 Primary osteoarthritis, unspecified hand

  ● M19.07 Primary osteoarthritis ankle and foot
    M19.071 Primary osteoarthritis, right ankle and foot
    M19.072 Primary osteoarthritis, left ankle and foot
    M19.079 Primary osteoarthritis, unspecified ankle and foot

● M19.1 Post-traumatic osteoarthritis of other joints

  ● M19.11 Post-traumatic osteoarthritis, shoulder
    M19.111 Post-traumatic osteoarthritis, right shoulder
    M19.112 Post-traumatic osteoarthritis, left shoulder
    M19.119 Post-traumatic osteoarthritis, unspecified shoulder

  ● M19.12 Post-traumatic osteoarthritis, elbow
    M19.121 Post-traumatic osteoarthritis, right elbow
    M19.122 Post-traumatic osteoarthritis, left elbow
    M19.129 Post-traumatic osteoarthritis, unspecified elbow

  ● M19.13 Post-traumatic osteoarthritis, wrist
    M19.131 Post-traumatic osteoarthritis, right wrist
    M19.132 Post-traumatic osteoarthritis, left wrist
    M19.139 Post-traumatic osteoarthritis, unspecified wrist

  ● M19.14 Post-traumatic osteoarthritis, hand
    Excludes2 post-traumatic osteoarthritis of first carpometacarpal joint (M18.2-, M18.3-)
    M19.141 Post-traumatic osteoarthritis, right hand
    M19.142 Post-traumatic osteoarthritis, left hand
    M19.149 Post-traumatic osteoarthritis, unspecified hand

  ● M19.17 Post-traumatic osteoarthritis, ankle and foot
    M19.171 Post-traumatic osteoarthritis, right ankle and foot
    M19.172 Post-traumatic osteoarthritis, left ankle and foot
    M19.179 Post-traumatic osteoarthritis, unspecified ankle and foot

● M19.2 Secondary osteoarthritis of other joints

  ● M19.21 Secondary osteoarthritis, shoulder
    M19.211 Secondary osteoarthritis, right shoulder
    M19.212 Secondary osteoarthritis, left shoulder
    M19.219 Secondary osteoarthritis, unspecified shoulder

  ● M19.22 Secondary osteoarthritis, elbow
    M19.221 Secondary osteoarthritis, right elbow
    M19.222 Secondary osteoarthritis, left elbow
    M19.229 Secondary osteoarthritis, unspecified elbow

  ● M19.23 Secondary osteoarthritis, wrist
    M19.231 Secondary osteoarthritis, right wrist
    M19.232 Secondary osteoarthritis, left wrist
    M19.239 Secondary osteoarthritis, unspecified wrist

  ● M19.24 Secondary osteoarthritis, hand
    M19.241 Secondary osteoarthritis, right hand
    M19.242 Secondary osteoarthritis, left hand
    M19.249 Secondary osteoarthritis, unspecified hand

  ● M19.27 Secondary osteoarthritis, ankle and foot
    M19.271 Secondary osteoarthritis, right ankle and foot
    M19.272 Secondary osteoarthritis, left ankle and foot
    M19.279 Secondary osteoarthritis, unspecified ankle and foot

◀ New ◀ Revised ~~deleted~~ Deleted OGCR Official Guidelines X Assign placeholder X ● Use Additional Character(s)
Excludes 1   Excludes 2   Includes   Use additional   Code first   Code also   Unspecified

M19.9 Osteoarthritis, unspecified site

    M19.90 **Unspecified osteoarthritis,** unspecified site
        Arthrosis NOS
        Arthritis NOS
        Osteoarthritis NOS

    M19.91 **Primary osteoarthritis,** unspecified site
        Primary osteoarthritis NOS

    M19.92 **Post-traumatic osteoarthritis,** unspecified site
        Post-traumatic osteoarthritis NOS

    M19.93 **Secondary osteoarthritis,** unspecified site
        Secondary osteoarthritis NOS

OTHER JOINT DISORDERS (M20-M25)

  Excludes2 joints of the spine (M40-M54)

● M20 **Acquired deformities of fingers and toes**
    Excludes1 acquired absence of fingers and toes (Z89.-)
          congenital absence of fingers and toes (Q71.3-, Q72.3-)
          congenital deformities and malformations of fingers and toes (Q66.-, Q68-Q70, Q74.-)

● M20.0 **Deformity of finger(s)**
    Excludes1 clubbing of fingers (R68.3)
          palmar fascial fibromatosis [Dupuytren] (M72.0)
          trigger finger (M65.3)

  ● M20.00 **Unspecified deformity of finger(s)**
    M20.001 **Unspecified** deformity of right finger(s)
    M20.002 **Unspecified** deformity of left finger(s)
    M20.009 **Unspecified** deformity of unspecified finger(s)

  ● M20.01 **Mallet finger**
    M20.011 **Mallet finger of right finger(s)**
    M20.012 **Mallet finger of left finger(s)**
    M20.019 **Mallet finger of** unspecified **finger(s)**

  ● M20.02 **Boutonnière deformity**
    M20.021 **Boutonnière deformity of right finger(s)**
    M20.022 **Boutonnière deformity of left finger(s)**
    M20.029 **Boutonnière deformity of** unspecified **finger(s)**

  ● M20.03 **Swan-neck deformity**
    M20.031 **Swan-neck deformity of right finger(s)**
    M20.032 **Swan-neck deformity of left finger(s)**
    M20.039 **Swan-neck deformity of** unspecified **finger(s)**

  ● M20.09 **Other deformity of finger(s)**
    M20.091 **Other deformity of right finger(s)**
    M20.092 **Other deformity of left finger(s)**
    M20.099 **Other deformity of finger(s),** unspecified **finger(s)**

● M20.1 **Hallux valgus (acquired)**
    Bunion
    M20.10 **Hallux valgus (acquired),** unspecified **foot**
    M20.11 **Hallux valgus (acquired), right foot**
    M20.12 **Hallux valgus (acquired), left foot**

● M20.2 **Hallux rigidus**
    M20.20 **Hallux rigidus,** unspecified **foot**
    M20.21 **Hallux rigidus, right foot**
    M20.22 **Hallux rigidus, left foot**

● M20.3 **Hallux varus (acquired)**
    M20.30 **Hallux varus (acquired),** unspecified **foot**
    M20.31 **Hallux varus (acquired), right foot**
    M20.32 **Hallux varus (acquired), left foot**

Figure 13-1 Hallux valgus or bunion.

Item 13-2 Hallux valgus or bunion is a sometimes painful structural deformity caused by an inflammation of the bursal sac at the base of the metatarsophalangeal joint (big toe). **Hallus varus** is a deviation of the great toe to the inner side of the foot or away from the next toe.

Item 13-3 Cubitus valgus is a deformity of the elbow resulting in an increased carrying angle in which the arm extends at the side and the palm faces forward, which results in the forearm and hand extended at a greater than 15 degrees.

● M20.4 **Other hammer toe(s) (acquired)**
    M20.40 **Other hammer toe(s) (acquired),** unspecified **foot**
    M20.41 **Other hammer toe(s) (acquired), right foot**
    M20.42 **Other hammer toe(s) (acquired), left foot**

● M20.5 **Other deformities of toe(s) (acquired)**
  ● M20.5X **Other deformities of toe(s) (acquired)**
    M20.5X1 **Other deformities of toe(s) (acquired), right foot**
    M20.5X2 **Other deformities of toe(s) (acquired), left foot**
    M20.5X9 **Other deformities of toe(s) (acquired),** unspecified **foot**

● M20.6 **Acquired deformities of toe(s), unspecified**
    M20.60 **Acquired deformities of toe(s), unspecified,** unspecified **foot**
    M20.61 **Acquired deformities of toe(s),** unspecified, **right foot**
    M20.62 **Acquired deformities of toe(s),** unspecified, **left foot**

● M21 **Other acquired deformities of limbs**
    Excludes1 acquired absence of limb (Z89.-)
          congenital absence of limbs (Q71-Q73)
          congenital deformities and malformations of limbs (Q65-Q66, Q68-Q74)
    Excludes2 acquired deformities of fingers or toes (M20.-)
          coxa plana (M91.2)

  ● M21.0 **Valgus deformity, not elsewhere classified**
    Excludes1 metatarsus valgus (Q66.6)
          talipes calcaneovalgus (Q66.4)
    M21.00 **Valgus deformity, not elsewhere classified,** unspecified **site**

◀ New ◀▬ Revised ̶d̶e̶l̶e̶t̶e̶d̶ Deleted **OGCR** Official Guidelines X Assign placeholder X ● Use Additional Character(s)

  Excludes 1   Excludes 2   Includes   Use additional   Code first   Code also   Unspecified

Item 13–4 Cubitus varus is a deformity of the elbow resulting in the arm extended at the side and the palm facing forward so that the forearm and hand are held at less than 5 degrees, decreasing the carrying angle.

● M21.02 Valgus deformity, not elsewhere classified, elbow
        Cubitus valgus
  M21.021 Valgus deformity, not elsewhere classified, right elbow
  M21.022 Valgus deformity, not elsewhere classified, left elbow
  M21.029 Valgus deformity, not elsewhere classified, unspecified elbow

● M21.05 Valgus deformity, not elsewhere classified, hip
  M21.051 Valgus deformity, not elsewhere classified, right hip
  M21.052 Valgus deformity, not elsewhere classified, left hip
  M21.059 Valgus deformity, not elsewhere classified, unspecified hip

● M21.06 Valgus deformity, not elsewhere classified, knee
        Genu valgum
        Knock knee
  M21.061 Valgus deformity, not elsewhere classified, right knee
  M21.062 Valgus deformity, not elsewhere classified, left knee
  M21.069 Valgus deformity, not elsewhere classified, unspecified knee

● M21.07 Valgus deformity, not elsewhere classified, ankle
  M21.071 Valgus deformity, not elsewhere classified, right ankle
  M21.072 Valgus deformity, not elsewhere classified, left ankle
  M21.079 Valgus deformity, not elsewhere classified, unspecified ankle

● M21.1 Varus deformity, not elsewhere classified
  Excludes1   metatarsus varus (Q66.2)
           tibia vara (M92.5)
  M21.10 Varus deformity, not elsewhere classified, unspecified site

● M21.12 Varus deformity, not elsewhere classified, elbow
        Cubitus varus, elbow
  M21.121 Varus deformity, not elsewhere classified, right elbow
  M21.122 Varus deformity, not elsewhere classified, left elbow
  M21.129 Varus deformity, not elsewhere classified, unspecified elbow

● M21.15 Varus deformity, not elsewhere classified, hip
  M21.151 Varus deformity, not elsewhere classified, right hip
  M21.152 Varus deformity, not elsewhere classified, left hip
  M21.159 Varus deformity, not elsewhere classified, unspecified

● M21.16 Varus deformity, not elsewhere classified, knee
        Bow leg
        Genu varum
  M21.161 Varus deformity, not elsewhere classified, right knee
  M21.162 Varus deformity, not elsewhere classified, left knee
  M21.169 Varus deformity, not elsewhere classified, unspecified knee

● M21.17 Varus deformity, not elsewhere classified, ankle
  M21.171 Varus deformity, not elsewhere classified, right ankle
  M21.172 Varus deformity, not elsewhere classified, left ankle
  M21.179 Varus deformity, not elsewhere classified, unspecified ankle

● M21.2 Flexion deformity
  M21.20 Flexion deformity, unspecified site

● M21.21 Flexion deformity, shoulder
  M21.211 Flexion deformity, right shoulder
  M21.212 Flexion deformity, left shoulder
  M21.219 Flexion deformity, unspecified shoulder

● M21.22 Flexion deformity, elbow
  M21.221 Flexion deformity, right elbow
  M21.222 Flexion deformity, left elbow
  M21.229 Flexion deformity, unspecified elbow

● M21.23 Flexion deformity, wrist
  M21.231 Flexion deformity, right wrist
  M21.232 Flexion deformity, left wrist
  M21.239 Flexion deformity, unspecified wrist

● M21.24 Flexion deformity, finger joints
  M21.241 Flexion deformity, right finger joints
  M21.242 Flexion deformity, left finger joints
  M21.249 Flexion deformity, unspecified finger joints

● M21.25 Flexion deformity, hip
  M21.251 Flexion deformity, right hip
  M21.252 Flexion deformity, left hip
  M21.259 Flexion deformity, unspecified hip

● M21.26 Flexion deformity, knee
  M21.261 Flexion deformity, right knee
  M21.262 Flexion deformity, left knee
  M21.269 Flexion deformity, unspecified knee

● M21.27 Flexion deformity, ankle and toes
  M21.271 Flexion deformity, right ankle and toes
  M21.272 Flexion deformity, left ankle and toes
  M21.279 Flexion deformity, unspecified ankle and toes

● M21.3 Wrist or foot drop (acquired)
● M21.33 Wrist drop (acquired)
  M21.331 Wrist drop, right wrist
  M21.332 Wrist drop, left wrist
  M21.339 Wrist drop, unspecified wrist

● M21.37 Foot drop (acquired)
  M21.371 Foot drop, right foot
  M21.372 Foot drop, left foot
  M21.379 Foot drop, unspecified foot

● M21.4 Flat foot [pes planus] (acquired)
  Excludes1   congenital pes planus (Q66.5-)
  M21.40 Flat foot [pes planus] (acquired), unspecified foot
  M21.41 Flat foot [pes planus] (acquired), right foot
  M21.42 Flat foot [pes planus] (acquired), left foot

● M21.5 Acquired clawhand, clubhand, clawfoot and clubfoot
  Excludes1   clubfoot, not specified as acquired (Q66.89)

● M21.51 Acquired clawhand
  M21.511 Acquired clawhand, right hand
  M21.512 Acquired clawhand, left hand
  M21.519 Acquired clawhand, unspecified hand

◄ New   ◄▪▪ Revised   ~~deleted~~ Deleted   OGCR Official Guidelines   X Assign placeholder X   ● Use Additional Character(s)

Excludes 1   Excludes 2   Includes   Use additional   Code first   Code also   Unspecified

● **M21.52 Acquired clubhand**
     M21.521   Acquired clubhand, right hand
     M21.522   Acquired clubhand, left hand
     M21.529   Acquired clubhand, unspecified hand

● **M21.53 Acquired clawfoot**
     M21.531   Acquired clawfoot, right foot
     M21.532   Acquired clawfoot, left foot
     M21.539   Acquired clawfoot, unspecified foot

● **M21.54 Acquired clubfoot**
     M21.541   Acquired clubfoot, right foot
     M21.542   Acquired clubfoot, left foot
     M21.549   Acquired clubfoot, unspecified foot

● **M21.6 Other acquired deformities of foot**
     Excludes2   deformities of toe (acquired) (M20.1-M20.6)

● **M21.6X Other acquired deformities of foot**
     M21.6X1   Other acquired deformities of right foot
     M21.6X2   Other acquired deformities of left foot
     M21.6X9   Other acquired deformities of unspecified foot

● **M21.7 Unequal limb length (acquired)**
     Note: The site used should correspond to the shorter limb.
     M21.70   Unequal limb length (acquired), unspecified site

● **M21.72 Unequal limb length (acquired), humerus**
     M21.721   Unequal limb length (acquired), right humerus
     M21.722   Unequal limb length (acquired), left humerus
     M21.729   Unequal limb length (acquired), unspecified humerus

● **M21.73 Unequal limb length (acquired), ulna and radius**
     M21.731   Unequal limb length (acquired), right ulna
     M21.732   Unequal limb length (acquired), left ulna
     M21.733   Unequal limb length (acquired), right radius
     M21.734   Unequal limb length (acquired), left radius
     M21.739   Unequal limb length (acquired), unspecified ulna and radius

● **M21.75 Unequal limb length (acquired), femur**
     M21.751   Unequal limb length (acquired), right femur
     M21.752   Unequal limb length (acquired), left femur
     M21.759   Unequal limb length (acquired), unspecified femur

● **M21.76 Unequal limb length (acquired), tibia and fibula**
     M21.761   Unequal limb length (acquired), right tibia
     M21.762   Unequal limb length (acquired), left tibia
     M21.763   Unequal limb length (acquired), right fibula
     M21.764   Unequal limb length (acquired), left fibula
     M21.769   Unequal limb length (acquired), unspecified tibia and fibula

● **M21.8 Other specified acquired deformities of limbs**
     Excludes2   coxa plana (M91.2)
     M21.80   Other specified acquired deformities of unspecified limb

● **M21.82 Other specified acquired deformities of upper arm**
     M21.821   Other specified acquired deformities of right upper arm
     M21.822   Other specified acquired deformities of left upper arm
     M21.829   Other specified acquired deformities of unspecified upper arm

● **M21.83 Other specified acquired deformities of forearm**
     M21.831   Other specified acquired deformities of right forearm
     M21.832   Other specified acquired deformities of left forearm
     M21.839   Other specified acquired deformities of unspecified forearm

● **M21.85 Other specified acquired deformities of thigh**
     M21.851   Other specified acquired deformities of right thigh
     M21.852   Other specified acquired deformities of left thigh
     M21.859   Other specified acquired deformities of unspecified thigh

● **M21.86 Other specified acquired deformities of lower leg**
     M21.861   Other specified acquired deformities of right lower leg
     M21.862   Other specified acquired deformities of left lower leg
     M21.869   Other specified acquired deformities of unspecified lower leg

● **M21.9 Unspecified acquired deformity of limb and hand**
     M21.90   Unspecified acquired deformity of unspecified limb

● **M21.92 Unspecified acquired deformity of upper arm**
     M21.921   Unspecified acquired deformity of right upper arm
     M21.922   Unspecified acquired deformity of left upper arm
     M21.929   Unspecified acquired deformity of unspecified upper arm

● **M21.93 Unspecified acquired deformity of forearm**
     M21.931   Unspecified acquired deformity of right forearm
     M21.932   Unspecified acquired deformity of left forearm
     M21.939   Unspecified acquired deformity of unspecified forearm

● **M21.94 Unspecified acquired deformity of hand**
     M21.941   Unspecified acquired deformity of hand, right hand
     M21.942   Unspecified acquired deformity of hand, left hand
     M21.949   Unspecified acquired deformity of hand, unspecified hand

● **M21.95 Unspecified acquired deformity of thigh**
     M21.951   Unspecified acquired deformity of right thigh
     M21.952   Unspecified acquired deformity of left thigh
     M21.959   Unspecified acquired deformity of unspecified thigh

CHAPTER 13 (M00-M99)

◀ New   ◀◀◀ Revised   ~~deleted~~ Deleted   **OGCR** Official Guidelines   X Assign placeholder X   ● Use Additional Character(s)

| Excludes 1 | Excludes 2 | Includes | Use additional | Code first | Code also | Unspecified |

● M21.96   Unspecified acquired deformity of lower leg
     M21.961   Unspecified acquired deformity of right lower leg
     M21.962   Unspecified acquired deformity of left lower leg
     M21.969   Unspecified acquired deformity of unspecified lower leg

● M22   Disorder of patella
   Excludes1   traumatic dislocation of patella (S83.0-)
   ● M22.0   Recurrent dislocation of patella
     M22.00   Recurrent dislocation of patella, unspecified knee
     M22.01   Recurrent dislocation of patella, right knee
     M22.02   Recurrent dislocation of patella, left knee
   ● M22.1   Recurrent subluxation of patella
     Incomplete dislocation of patella
     M22.10   Recurrent subluxation of patella, unspecified knee
     M22.11   Recurrent subluxation of patella, right knee
     M22.12   Recurrent subluxation of patella, left knee
   ● M22.2   Patellofemoral disorders
    ● M22.2X   Patellofemoral disorders
     M22.2X1   Patellofemoral disorders, right knee
     M22.2X2   Patellofemoral disorders, left knee
     M22.2X9   Patellofemoral disorders, unspecified knee
   ● M22.3   Other derangements of patella
    ● M22.3X   Other derangements of patella
     M22.3X1   Other derangements of patella, right knee
     M22.3X2   Other derangements of patella, left knee
     M22.3X9   Other derangements of patella, unspecified knee
   ● M22.4   Chondromalacia patellae
     M22.40   Chondromalacia patellae, unspecified knee
     M22.41   Chondromalacia patellae, right knee
     M22.42   Chondromalacia patellae, left knee
   ● M22.8   Other disorders of patella
    ● M22.8X   Other disorders of patella
     M22.8X1   Other disorders of patella, right knee
     M22.8X2   Other disorders of patella, left knee
     M22.8X9   Other disorders of patella, unspecified knee
   ● M22.9   Unspecified disorder of patella
     M22.90   Unspecified disorder of patella, unspecified knee
     M22.91   Unspecified disorder of patella, right knee
     M22.92   Unspecified disorder of patella, left knee

● M23   Internal derangement of knee
   Excludes1   ankylosis (M24.66)
           current injury - see injury of knee and lower leg (S80-S89)
           deformity of knee (M21.-)
           osteochondritis dissecans (M93.2)
           recurrent dislocation or subluxation of joints (M24.4)
           recurrent dislocation or subluxation of patella (M22.0-M22.1)
   ● M23.0   Cystic meniscus
    ● M23.00   Cystic meniscus, unspecified meniscus
     Cystic meniscus, unspecified lateral meniscus
     Cystic meniscus, unspecified medial meniscus
     M23.000   Cystic meniscus, unspecified lateral meniscus, right knee
     M23.001   Cystic meniscus, unspecified lateral meniscus, left knee

     M23.002   Cystic meniscus, unspecified lateral meniscus, unspecified knee
     M23.003   Cystic meniscus, unspecified medial meniscus, right knee
     M23.004   Cystic meniscus, unspecified medial meniscus, left knee
     M23.005   Cystic meniscus, unspecified medial meniscus, unspecified knee
     M23.006   Cystic meniscus, unspecified meniscus, right knee
     M23.007   Cystic meniscus, unspecified meniscus, left knee
     M23.009   Cystic meniscus, unspecified meniscus, unspecified knee
   ● M23.01   Cystic meniscus, anterior horn of medial meniscus
     M23.011   Cystic meniscus, anterior horn of medial meniscus, right knee
     M23.012   Cystic meniscus, anterior horn of medial meniscus, left knee
     M23.019   Cystic meniscus, anterior horn of medial meniscus, unspecified knee
   ● M23.02   Cystic meniscus, posterior horn of medial meniscus
     M23.021   Cystic meniscus, posterior horn of medial meniscus, right knee
     M23.022   Cystic meniscus, posterior horn of medial meniscus, left knee
     M23.029   Cystic meniscus, posterior horn of medial meniscus, unspecified knee
   ● M23.03   Cystic meniscus, other medial meniscus
     M23.031   Cystic meniscus, other medial meniscus, right knee
     M23.032   Cystic meniscus, other medial meniscus, left knee
     M23.039   Cystic meniscus, other medial meniscus, unspecified knee
   ● M23.04   Cystic meniscus, anterior horn of lateral meniscus
     M23.041   Cystic meniscus, anterior horn of lateral meniscus, right knee
     M23.042   Cystic meniscus, anterior horn of lateral meniscus, left knee
     M23.049   Cystic meniscus, anterior horn of lateral meniscus, unspecified knee
   ● M23.05   Cystic meniscus, posterior horn of lateral meniscus
     M23.051   Cystic meniscus, posterior horn of lateral meniscus, right knee
     M23.052   Cystic meniscus, posterior horn of lateral meniscus, left knee
     M23.059   Cystic meniscus, posterior horn of lateral meniscus, unspecified knee
   ● M23.06   Cystic meniscus, other lateral meniscus
     M23.061   Cystic meniscus, other lateral meniscus, right knee
     M23.062   Cystic meniscus, other lateral meniscus, left knee
     M23.069   Cystic meniscus, other lateral meniscus, unspecified knee

---

◀ New   ⬅ Revised   ~~deleted~~ Deleted   OGCR Official Guidelines   X Assign placeholder X   ● Use Additional Character(s)

Excludes 1   Excludes 2   Includes   Use additional   Code first   Code also   Unspecified

(See Plate 509 on page NAP-31.)

● **M23.2**   **Derangement of meniscus due to old tear or injury**
     Old bucket-handle tear

  ● **M23.20**   **Derangement of unspecified meniscus due to old tear or injury**
      Derangement of unspecified lateral meniscus due to old tear or injury
      Derangement of unspecified medial meniscus due to old tear or injury

     M23.200   Derangement of unspecified lateral meniscus due to old tear or injury, right knee

     M23.201   Derangement of unspecified lateral meniscus due to old tear or injury, left knee

     M23.202   Derangement of unspecified lateral meniscus due to old tear or injury, unspecified knee

     M23.203   Derangement of unspecified medial meniscus due to old tear or injury, right knee

     M23.204   Derangement of unspecified medial meniscus due to old tear or injury, left knee

     M23.205   Derangement of unspecified medial meniscus due to old tear or injury, unspecified knee

     M23.206   Derangement of unspecified meniscus due to old tear or injury, right knee

     M23.207   Derangement of unspecified meniscus due to old tear or injury, left knee

     M23.209   Derangement of unspecified meniscus due to old tear or injury, unspecified knee

  ● **M23.21**   **Derangement of anterior horn of medial meniscus due to old tear or injury**

     M23.211   Derangement of anterior horn of medial meniscus due to old tear or injury, right knee

     M23.212   Derangement of anterior horn of medial meniscus due to old tear or injury, left knee

     M23.219   Derangement of anterior horn of medial meniscus due to old tear or injury, unspecified knee

  ● **M23.22**   **Derangement of posterior horn of medial meniscus due to old tear or injury**

     M23.221   Derangement of posterior horn of medial meniscus due to old tear or injury, right knee

     M23.222   Derangement of posterior horn of medial meniscus due to old tear or injury, left knee

     M23.229   Derangement of posterior horn of medial meniscus due to old tear or injury, unspecified knee

  ● **M23.23**   **Derangement of other medial meniscus due to old tear or injury**

     M23.231   Derangement of other medial meniscus due to old tear or injury, right knee

     M23.232   Derangement of other medial meniscus due to old tear or injury, left knee

     M23.239   Derangement of other medial meniscus due to old tear or injury, unspecified knee

  ● **M23.24**   **Derangement of anterior horn of lateral meniscus due to old tear or injury**

     M23.241   Derangement of anterior horn of lateral meniscus due to old tear or injury, right knee

     M23.242   Derangement of anterior horn of lateral meniscus due to old tear or injury, left knee

     M23.249   Derangement of anterior horn of lateral meniscus due to old tear or injury, unspecified knee

  ● **M23.25**   **Derangement of posterior horn of lateral meniscus due to old tear or injury**

     M23.251   Derangement of posterior horn of lateral meniscus due to old tear or injury, right knee

     M23.252   Derangement of posterior horn of lateral meniscus due to old tear or injury, left knee

     M23.259   Derangement of posterior horn of lateral meniscus due to old tear or injury, unspecified knee

  ● **M23.26**   **Derangement of other lateral meniscus due to old tear or injury**

     M23.261   Derangement of other lateral meniscus due to old tear or injury, right knee

     M23.262   Derangement of other lateral meniscus due to old tear or injury, left knee

     M23.269   Derangement of other lateral meniscus due to old tear or injury, unspecified knee

● **M23.3**   **Other meniscus derangements**
     Degenerate meniscus
     Detached meniscus
     Retained meniscus

  ● **M23.30**   **Other meniscus derangements, unspecified meniscus**
      Other meniscus derangements, unspecified lateral meniscus
      Other meniscus derangements, unspecified medial meniscus

     M23.300   Other meniscus derangements, unspecified lateral meniscus, right knee

     M23.301   Other meniscus derangements, unspecified lateral meniscus, left knee

     M23.302   Other meniscus derangements, unspecified lateral meniscus, unspecified knee

     M23.303   Other meniscus derangements, unspecified medial meniscus, right knee

     M23.304   Other meniscus derangements, unspecified medial meniscus, left knee

     M23.305   Other meniscus derangements, unspecified medial meniscus, unspecified knee

     M23.306   Other meniscus derangements, unspecified meniscus, right knee

     M23.307   Other meniscus derangements, unspecified meniscus, left knee

     M23.309   Other meniscus derangements, unspecified meniscus, unspecified knee

● **M23.31** Other meniscus derangements, anterior horn of
medial meniscus

    M23.311 Other meniscus derangements,
anterior horn of medial meniscus,
right knee

    M23.312 Other meniscus derangements,
anterior horn of medial meniscus, left
knee

    M23.319 Other meniscus derangements,
anterior horn of medial meniscus,
unspecified knee

● **M23.32** Other meniscus derangements, posterior horn
of medial meniscus

    M23.321 Other meniscus derangements,
posterior horn of medial meniscus,
right knee

    M23.322 Other meniscus derangements,
posterior horn of medial meniscus,
left knee

    M23.329 Other meniscus derangements,
posterior horn of medial meniscus,
unspecified knee

● **M23.33** Other meniscus derangements, other medial
meniscus

    M23.331 Other meniscus derangements, other
medial meniscus, right knee

    M23.332 Other meniscus derangements, other
medial meniscus, left knee

    M23.339 Other meniscus derangements, other
medial meniscus, unspecified knee

● **M23.34** Other meniscus derangements, anterior horn of
lateral meniscus

    M23.341 Other meniscus derangements,
anterior horn of lateral meniscus,
right knee

    M23.342 Other meniscus derangements,
anterior horn of lateral meniscus, left
knee

    M23.349 Other meniscus derangements,
anterior horn of lateral meniscus,
unspecified knee

● **M23.35** Other meniscus derangements, posterior horn
of lateral meniscus

    M23.351 Other meniscus derangements,
posterior horn of lateral meniscus,
right knee

    M23.352 Other meniscus derangements,
posterior horn of lateral meniscus, left
knee

    M23.359 Other meniscus derangements,
posterior horn of lateral meniscus,
unspecified knee

● **M23.36** Other meniscus derangements, other lateral
meniscus

    M23.361 Other meniscus derangements, other
lateral meniscus, right knee

    M23.362 Other meniscus derangements, other
lateral meniscus, left knee

    M23.369 Other meniscus derangements, other
lateral meniscus, unspecified knee

● **M23.4** Loose body in knee

    M23.40 Loose body in knee, unspecified knee

    M23.41 Loose body in knee, right knee

    M23.42 Loose body in knee, left knee

● **M23.5** Chronic instability of knee

    M23.50 Chronic instability of knee, unspecified knee

    M23.51 Chronic instability of knee, right knee

    M23.52 Chronic instability of knee, left knee

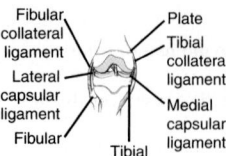

Figure 13-2 Collateral and cruciate
ligament of knee. (From DeLee: DeLee and
Drez's Orthopaedic Sports Medicine, ed 3,
Saunders, 2009)

● **M23.6** Other spontaneous disruption of ligament(s) of knee

  ● **M23.60** Other spontaneous disruption of unspecified
ligament of knee

    M23.601 Other spontaneous disruption of
unspecified ligament of right knee

    M23.602 Other spontaneous disruption of
unspecified ligament of left knee

    M23.609 Other spontaneous disruption of
unspecified ligament of unspecified
knee

  ● **M23.61** Other spontaneous disruption of anterior
cruciate ligament of knee

    M23.611 Other spontaneous disruption of
anterior cruciate ligament of right
knee

    M23.612 Other spontaneous disruption of
anterior cruciate ligament of left knee

    M23.619 Other spontaneous disruption
of anterior cruciate ligament of
unspecified knee

  ● **M23.62** Other spontaneous disruption of posterior
cruciate ligament of knee

    M23.621 Other spontaneous disruption of
posterior cruciate ligament of right
knee

    M23.622 Other spontaneous disruption of
posterior cruciate ligament of left
knee

    M23.629 Other spontaneous disruption
of posterior cruciate ligament of
unspecified knee

  ● **M23.63** Other spontaneous disruption of medial
collateral ligament of knee

    M23.631 Other spontaneous disruption of
medial collateral ligament of right
knee

    M23.632 Other spontaneous disruption of
medial collateral ligament of left knee

    M23.639 Other spontaneous disruption
of medial collateral ligament of
unspecified knee

  ● **M23.64** Other spontaneous disruption of lateral
collateral ligament of knee

    M23.641 Other spontaneous disruption of
lateral collateral ligament of right
knee

    M23.642 Other spontaneous disruption of
lateral collateral ligament of left knee

    M23.649 Other spontaneous disruption
of lateral collateral ligament of
unspecified knee

  ● **M23.67** Other spontaneous disruption of capsular
ligament of knee

    M23.671 Other spontaneous disruption of
capsular ligament of right knee

    M23.672 Other spontaneous disruption of
capsular ligament of left knee

    M23.679 Other spontaneous disruption of
capsular ligament of unspecified knee

● **M23.8**   **Other internal derangements of knee**
    Laxity of ligament of knee
    Snapping knee
  ● **M23.8X**   **Other internal derangements of knee**
      M23.8X1   **Other internal derangements of right knee**
      M23.8X2   **Other internal derangements of left knee**
      M23.8X9   **Other internal derangements of unspecified knee**

● **M23.9**   **Unspecified internal derangement of knee**
    M23.90   Unspecified internal derangement of unspecified knee
    M23.91   Unspecified internal derangement of right knee
    M23.92   Unspecified internal derangement of left knee

● **M24**   **Other specific joint derangements**
   Excludes1   current injury - see injury of joint by body region
   Excludes2   ganglion (M67.4)
                snapping knee (M23.8-)
                temporomandibular joint disorders (M26.6-)

● **M24.0**   **Loose body in joint**
   Excludes2   loose body in knee (M23.4)
    M24.00   Loose body in unspecified joint
  ● **M24.01**   **Loose body in shoulder**
      M24.011   Loose body in right shoulder
      M24.012   Loose body in left shoulder
      M24.019   Loose body in unspecified shoulder
  ● **M24.02**   **Loose body in elbow**
      M24.021   Loose body in right elbow
      M24.022   Loose body in left elbow
      M24.029   Loose body in unspecified elbow
  ● **M24.03**   **Loose body in wrist**
      M24.031   Loose body in right wrist
      M24.032   Loose body in left wrist
      M24.039   Loose body in unspecified wrist
  ● **M24.04**   **Loose body in finger joints**
      M24.041   Loose body in right finger joint(s)
      M24.042   Loose body in left finger joint(s)
      M24.049   Loose body in unspecified finger joint(s)
  ● **M24.05**   **Loose body in hip**
      M24.051   Loose body in right hip
      M24.052   Loose body in left hip
      M24.059   Loose body in unspecified hip
  ● **M24.07**   **Loose body in ankle and toe joints**
      M24.071   Loose body in right ankle
      M24.072   Loose body in left ankle
      M24.073   Loose body in unspecified ankle
      M24.074   Loose body in right toe joint(s)
      M24.075   Loose body in left toe joint(s)
      M24.076   Loose body in unspecified toe joints
    M24.08   Loose body, other site

● **M24.1**   **Other articular cartilage disorders**
   Excludes2   chondrocalcinosis (M11.1, M11.2-)
                internal derangement of knee (M23.-)
                metastatic calcification (E83.5)
                ochronosis (E70.2)
    M24.10   Other articular cartilage disorders, unspecified site
  ● **M24.11**   **Other articular cartilage disorders, shoulder**
      M24.111   Other articular cartilage disorders, right shoulder
      M24.112   Other articular cartilage disorders, left shoulder
      M24.119   Other articular cartilage disorders, unspecified shoulder

● **M24.12**   **Other articular cartilage disorders, elbow**
      M24.121   Other articular cartilage disorders, right elbow
      M24.122   Other articular cartilage disorders, left elbow
      M24.129   Other articular cartilage disorders, unspecified elbow
● **M24.13**   **Other articular cartilage disorders, wrist**
      M24.131   Other articular cartilage disorders, right wrist
      M24.132   Other articular cartilage disorders, left wrist
      M24.139   Other articular cartilage disorders, unspecified wrist
● **M24.14**   **Other articular cartilage disorders, hand**
      M24.141   Other articular cartilage disorders, right hand
      M24.142   Other articular cartilage disorders, left hand
      M24.149   Other articular cartilage disorders, unspecified hand
● **M24.15**   **Other articular cartilage disorders, hip**
      M24.151   Other articular cartilage disorders, right hip
      M24.152   Other articular cartilage disorders, left hip
      M24.159   Other articular cartilage disorders, unspecified hip
● **M24.17**   **Other articular cartilage disorders, ankle and foot**
      M24.171   Other articular cartilage disorders, right ankle
      M24.172   Other articular cartilage disorders, left ankle
      M24.173   Other articular cartilage disorders, unspecified ankle
      M24.174   Other articular cartilage disorders, right foot
      M24.175   Other articular cartilage disorders, left foot
      M24.176   Other articular cartilage disorders, unspecified foot

● **M24.2**   **Disorder of ligament**
    Instability secondary to old ligament injury
    Ligamentous laxity NOS
   Excludes1   familial ligamentous laxity (M35.7)
   Excludes2   internal derangement of knee (M23.5-M23.89)
    M24.20   Disorder of ligament, unspecified site
  ● **M24.21**   **Disorder of ligament, shoulder**
      M24.211   Disorder of ligament, right shoulder
      M24.212   Disorder of ligament, left shoulder
      M24.219   Disorder of ligament, unspecified shoulder
  ● **M24.22**   **Disorder of ligament, elbow**
      M24.221   Disorder of ligament, right elbow
      M24.222   Disorder of ligament, left elbow
      M24.229   Disorder of ligament, unspecified elbow
  ● **M24.23**   **Disorder of ligament, wrist**
      M24.231   Disorder of ligament, right wrist
      M24.232   Disorder of ligament, left wrist
      M24.239   Disorder of ligament, unspecified wrist
  ● **M24.24**   **Disorder of ligament, hand**
      M24.241   Disorder of ligament, right hand
      M24.242   Disorder of ligament, left hand
      M24.249   Disorder of ligament, unspecified hand

◄ New   ◀◀ Revised   ~~deleted~~ Deleted   OGCR Official Guidelines   X Assign placeholder X   ● Use Additional Character(s)

Excludes 1   Excludes 2   Includes   Use additional   Code first   Code also   Unspecified

● M24.25   Disorder of ligament, hip
-    M24.251   Disorder of ligament, right hip
-    M24.252   Disorder of ligament, left hip
-    M24.259   Disorder of ligament, unspecified hip

● M24.27   Disorder of ligament, ankle and foot
-    M24.271   Disorder of ligament, right ankle
-    M24.272   Disorder of ligament, left ankle
-    M24.273   Disorder of ligament, unspecified ankle
-    M24.274   Disorder of ligament, right foot
-    M24.275   Disorder of ligament, left foot
-    M24.276   Disorder of ligament, unspecified foot

   M24.28   Disorder of ligament, vertebrae

● M24.3   Pathological dislocation of joint, not elsewhere classified

> **Excludes1**   congenital dislocation or displacement of joint - see congenital malformations and deformations of the musculoskeletal system (Q65-Q79)
> current injury - see injury of joints and ligaments by body region
> recurrent dislocation of joint (M24.4-)

   M24.30   Pathological dislocation of unspecified joint, not elsewhere classified

● M24.31   Pathological dislocation of shoulder, not elsewhere classified
-    M24.311   Pathological dislocation of right shoulder, not elsewhere classified
-    M24.312   Pathological dislocation of left shoulder, not elsewhere classified
-    M24.319   Pathological dislocation of unspecified shoulder, not elsewhere classified

● M24.32   Pathological dislocation of elbow, not elsewhere classified
-    M24.321   Pathological dislocation of right elbow, not elsewhere classified
-    M24.322   Pathological dislocation of left elbow, not elsewhere classified
-    M24.329   Pathological dislocation of unspecified elbow, not elsewhere classified

● M24.33   Pathological dislocation of wrist, not elsewhere classified
-    M24.331   Pathological dislocation of right wrist, not elsewhere classified
-    M24.332   Pathological dislocation of left wrist, not elsewhere classified
-    M24.339   Pathological dislocation of unspecified wrist, not elsewhere classified

● M24.34   Pathological dislocation of hand, not elsewhere classified
-    M24.341   Pathological dislocation of right hand, not elsewhere classified
-    M24.342   Pathological dislocation of left hand, not elsewhere classified
-    M24.349   Pathological dislocation of unspecified hand, not elsewhere classified

● M24.35   Pathological dislocation of hip, not elsewhere classified
-    M24.351   Pathological dislocation of right hip, not elsewhere classified
-    M24.352   Pathological dislocation of left hip, not elsewhere classified
-    M24.359   Pathological dislocation of unspecified hip, not elsewhere classified

● M24.36   Pathological dislocation of knee, not elsewhere classified
-    M24.361   Pathological dislocation of right knee, not elsewhere classified
-    M24.362   Pathological dislocation of left knee, not elsewhere classified
-    M24.369   Pathological dislocation of unspecified knee, not elsewhere classified

● M24.37   Pathological dislocation of ankle and foot, not elsewhere classified
-    M24.371   Pathological dislocation of right ankle, not elsewhere classified
-    M24.372   Pathological dislocation of left ankle, not elsewhere classified
-    M24.373   Pathological dislocation of unspecified ankle, not elsewhere classified
-    M24.374   Pathological dislocation of right foot, not elsewhere classified
-    M24.375   Pathological dislocation of left foot, not elsewhere classified
-    M24.376   Pathological dislocation of unspecified foot, not elsewhere classified

● M24.4   Recurrent dislocation of joint

Recurrent subluxation of joint

> **Excludes2**   recurrent dislocation of patella (M22.0-M22.1)
> recurrent vertebral dislocation (M43.3-, M43.4, M43.5-)

   M24.40   Recurrent dislocation, unspecified joint

● M24.41   Recurrent dislocation, shoulder
-    M24.411   Recurrent dislocation, right shoulder
-    M24.412   Recurrent dislocation, left shoulder
-    M24.419   Recurrent dislocation, unspecified shoulder

● M24.42   Recurrent dislocation, elbow
-    M24.421   Recurrent dislocation, right elbow
-    M24.422   Recurrent dislocation, left elbow
-    M24.429   Recurrent dislocation, unspecified elbow

● M24.43   Recurrent dislocation, wrist
-    M24.431   Recurrent dislocation, right wrist
-    M24.432   Recurrent dislocation, left wrist
-    M24.439   Recurrent dislocation, unspecified wrist

● M24.44   Recurrent dislocation, hand and finger(s)
-    M24.441   Recurrent dislocation, right hand
-    M24.442   Recurrent dislocation, left hand
-    M24.443   Recurrent dislocation, unspecified hand
-    M24.444   Recurrent dislocation, right finger
-    M24.445   Recurrent dislocation, left finger
-    M24.446   Recurrent dislocation, unspecified finger

● M24.45   Recurrent dislocation, hip
-    M24.451   Recurrent dislocation, right hip
-    M24.452   Recurrent dislocation, left hip
-    M24.459   Recurrent dislocation, unspecified hip

● M24.46   Recurrent dislocation, knee
-    M24.461   Recurrent dislocation, right knee
-    M24.462   Recurrent dislocation, left knee
-    M24.469   Recurrent dislocation, unspecified knee

● **M24.47 Recurrent dislocation, ankle, foot and toes**
     M24.471   Recurrent dislocation, right ankle
     M24.472   Recurrent dislocation, left ankle
     M24.473   Recurrent dislocation, unspecified ankle
     M24.474   Recurrent dislocation, right foot
     M24.475   Recurrent dislocation, left foot
     M24.476   Recurrent dislocation, unspecified foot
     M24.477   Recurrent dislocation, right toe(s)
     M24.478   Recurrent dislocation, left toe(s)
     M24.479   Recurrent dislocation, unspecified toe(s)

● **M24.5 Contracture of joint**
     Excludes1   contracture of muscle without contracture of joint (M62.4-)
                     contracture of tendon (sheath) without contracture of joint (M62.4-)
                       Dupuytren's contracture (M72.0)
     Excludes2   acquired deformities of limbs (M20-M21)
     M24.50   Contracture, unspecified joint
●   M24.51   Contracture, shoulder
     M24.511   Contracture, right shoulder
     M24.512   Contracture, left shoulder
     M24.519   Contracture, unspecified shoulder
●   M24.52   Contracture, elbow
     M24.521   Contracture, right elbow
     M24.522   Contracture, left elbow
     M24.529   Contracture, unspecified elbow
●   M24.53   Contracture, wrist
     M24.531   Contracture, right wrist
     M24.532   Contracture, left wrist
     M24.539   Contracture, unspecified wrist
●   M24.54   Contracture, hand
     M24.541   Contracture, right hand
     M24.542   Contracture, left hand
     M24.549   Contracture, unspecified hand
●   M24.55   Contracture, hip
     M24.551   Contracture, right hip
     M24.552   Contracture, left hip
     M24.559   Contracture, unspecified hip
●   M24.56   Contracture, knee
     M24.561   Contracture, right knee
     M24.562   Contracture, left knee
     M24.569   Contracture, unspecified knee
●   M24.57   Contracture, ankle and foot
     M24.571   Contracture, right ankle
     M24.572   Contracture, left ankle
     M24.573   Contracture, unspecified ankle
     M24.574   Contracture, right foot
     M24.575   Contracture, left foot
     M24.576   Contracture, unspecified foot

● **M24.6 Ankylosis of joint**
     Excludes1   stiffness of joint without ankylosis (M25.6-)
     Excludes2   spine (M43.2-)
     M24.60   Ankylosis, unspecified joint
●   M24.61   Ankylosis, shoulder
     M24.611   Ankylosis, right shoulder
     M24.612   Ankylosis, left shoulder
     M24.619   Ankylosis, unspecified shoulder
●   M24.62   Ankylosis, elbow
     M24.621   Ankylosis, right elbow
     M24.622   Ankylosis, left elbow
     M24.629   Ankylosis, unspecified elbow

Item 13–5 Ankylosis or arthrokleisis is a consolidation of a joint due to disease, injury, or surgical procedure. Spondylosis is the degeneration of the vertebral processes and formation of osteophytes and commonly occurs with age. **Spondylitis** or ankylosing spondylitis is a type of arthritis that affects the spine or backbone causing back pain and stiffness.

●   M24.63   Ankylosis, wrist
     M24.631   Ankylosis, right wrist
     M24.632   Ankylosis, left wrist
     M24.639   Ankylosis, unspecified wrist
●   M24.64   Ankylosis, hand
     M24.641   Ankylosis, right hand
     M24.642   Ankylosis, left hand
     M24.649   Ankylosis, unspecified hand
●   M24.65   Ankylosis, hip
     M24.651   Ankylosis, right hip
     M24.652   Ankylosis, left hip
     M24.659   Ankylosis, unspecified hip
●   M24.66   Ankylosis, knee
     M24.661   Ankylosis, right knee
     M24.662   Ankylosis, left knee
     M24.669   Ankylosis, unspecified knee
●   M24.67   Ankylosis, ankle and foot
     M24.671   Ankylosis, right ankle
     M24.672   Ankylosis, left ankle
     M24.673   Ankylosis, unspecified ankle
     M24.674   Ankylosis, right foot
     M24.675   Ankylosis, left foot
     M24.676   Ankylosis, unspecified foot

  M24.7   Protrusio acetabuli
●   M24.8   Other specific joint derangements, not elsewhere classified
     Excludes2   iliotibial band syndrome (M76.3)
     M24.80   Other specific joint derangements of unspecified joint, not elsewhere classified
●   M24.81   Other specific joint derangements of shoulder, not elsewhere classified
     M24.811   Other specific joint derangements of right shoulder, not elsewhere classified
     M24.812   Other specific joint derangements of left shoulder, not elsewhere classified
     M24.819   Other specific joint derangements of unspecified shoulder, not elsewhere classified
●   M24.82   Other specific joint derangements of elbow, not elsewhere classified
     M24.821   Other specific joint derangements of right elbow, not elsewhere classified
     M24.822   Other specific joint derangements of left elbow, not elsewhere classified
     M24.829   Other specific joint derangements of unspecified elbow, not elsewhere classified
●   M24.83   Other specific joint derangements of wrist, not elsewhere classified
     M24.831   Other specific joint derangements of right wrist, not elsewhere classified
     M24.832   Other specific joint derangements of left wrist, not elsewhere classified
     M24.839   Other specific joint derangements of unspecified wrist, not elsewhere classified

CHAPTER 13 (M00-M99)

● **M24.84** Other specific joint derangements of hand, not elsewhere classified
    M24.841 Other specific joint derangements of right hand, not elsewhere classified
    M24.842 Other specific joint derangements of left hand, not elsewhere classified
    M24.849 Other specific joint derangements of unspecified hand, not elsewhere classified

● **M24.85** Other specific joint derangements of hip, not elsewhere classified
    Irritable hip
    M24.851 Other specific joint derangements of right hip, not elsewhere classified
    M24.852 Other specific joint derangements of left hip, not elsewhere classified
    M24.859 Other specific joint derangements of unspecified hip, not elsewhere classified

● **M24.87** Other specific joint derangements of ankle and foot, not elsewhere classified
    M24.871 Other specific joint derangements of right ankle, not elsewhere classified
    M24.872 Other specific joint derangements of left ankle, not elsewhere classified
    M24.873 Other specific joint derangements of unspecified ankle, not elsewhere classified
    M24.874 Other specific joint derangements of right foot, not elsewhere classified
    M24.875 Other specific joint derangements left foot, not elsewhere classified
    M24.876 Other specific joint derangements of unspecified foot, not elsewhere classified

M24.9 Joint derangement, unspecified

● **M25** Other joint disorder, not elsewhere classified
    Excludes2 abnormality of gait and mobility (R26.-)
            acquired deformities of limb (M20-M21)
            calcification of bursa (M71.4-)
            calcification of shoulder (joint) (M75.3)
            calcification of tendon (M65.2-)
            difficulty in walking (R26.2)
            temporomandibular joint disorder (M26.6-)

● **M25.0** Hemarthrosis
    Excludes1 current injury - see injury of joint by body region
            hemophilic arthropathy (M36.2)
    M25.00 Hemarthrosis, unspecified joint
  ● **M25.01** Hemarthrosis, shoulder
    M25.011 Hemarthrosis, right shoulder
    M25.012 Hemarthrosis, left shoulder
    M25.019 Hemarthrosis, unspecified shoulder
  ● **M25.02** Hemarthrosis, elbow
    M25.021 Hemarthrosis, right elbow
    M25.022 Hemarthrosis, left elbow
    M25.029 Hemarthrosis, unspecified elbow
  ● **M25.03** Hemarthrosis, wrist
    M25.031 Hemarthrosis, right wrist
    M25.032 Hemarthrosis, left wrist
    M25.039 Hemarthrosis, unspecified wrist
  ● **M25.04** Hemarthrosis, hand
    M25.041 Hemarthrosis, right hand
    M25.042 Hemarthrosis, left hand
    M25.049 Hemarthrosis, unspecified hand
  ● **M25.05** Hemarthrosis, hip
    M25.051 Hemarthrosis, right hip
    M25.052 Hemarthrosis, left hip
    M25.059 Hemarthrosis, unspecified hip

● **M25.06** Hemarthrosis, knee
    M25.061 Hemarthrosis, right knee
    M25.062 Hemarthrosis, left knee
    M25.069 Hemarthrosis, unspecified knee
● **M25.07** Hemarthrosis, ankle and foot
    M25.071 Hemarthrosis, right ankle
    M25.072 Hemarthrosis, left ankle
    M25.073 Hemarthrosis, unspecified ankle
    M25.074 Hemarthrosis, right foot
    M25.075 Hemarthrosis, left foot
    M25.076 Hemarthrosis, unspecified foot
  M25.08 Hemarthrosis, other specified site
    Hemarthrosis, vertebrae
● **M25.1** Fistula of joint
    M25.10 Fistula, unspecified joint
  ● **M25.11** Fistula, shoulder
    M25.111 Fistula, right shoulder
    M25.112 Fistula, left shoulder
    M25.119 Fistula, unspecified shoulder
  ● **M25.12** Fistula, elbow
    M25.121 Fistula, right elbow
    M25.122 Fistula, left elbow
    M25.129 Fistula, unspecified elbow
  ● **M25.13** Fistula, wrist
    M25.131 Fistula, right wrist
    M25.132 Fistula, left wrist
    M25.139 Fistula, unspecified wrist
  ● **M25.14** Fistula, hand
    M25.141 Fistula, right hand
    M25.142 Fistula, left hand
    M25.149 Fistula, unspecified hand
  ● **M25.15** Fistula, hip
    M25.151 Fistula, right hip
    M25.152 Fistula, left hip
    M25.159 Fistula, unspecified hip
  ● **M25.16** Fistula, knee
    M25.161 Fistula, right knee
    M25.162 Fistula, left knee
    M25.169 Fistula, unspecified knee
  ● **M25.17** Fistula, ankle and foot
    M25.171 Fistula, right ankle
    M25.172 Fistula, left ankle
    M25.173 Fistula, unspecified ankle
    M25.174 Fistula, right foot
    M25.175 Fistula, left foot
    M25.176 Fistula, unspecified foot
  M25.18 Fistula, other specified site
    Fistula, vertebrae
● **M25.2** Flail joint
    M25.20 Flail joint, unspecified joint
  ● **M25.21** Flail joint, shoulder
    M25.211 Flail joint, right shoulder
    M25.212 Flail joint, left shoulder
    M25.219 Flail joint, unspecified shoulder
  ● **M25.22** Flail joint, elbow
    M25.221 Flail joint, right elbow
    M25.222 Flail joint, left elbow
    M25.229 Flail joint, unspecified elbow
  ● **M25.23** Flail joint, wrist
    M25.231 Flail joint, right wrist
    M25.232 Flail joint, left wrist
    M25.239 Flail joint, unspecified wrist

◀ New   ◀ Revised   ~~deleted~~ Deleted   OGCR Official Guidelines   X Assign placeholder X   ● Use Additional Character(s)

Excludes 1   Excludes 2   Includes   Use additional   Code first   Code also   Unspecified

● M25.24 Flail joint, hand
    M25.241 Flail joint, right hand
    M25.242 Flail joint, left hand
    M25.249 Flail joint, unspecified hand
● M25.25 Flail joint, hip
    M25.251 Flail joint, right hip
    M25.252 Flail joint, left hip
    M25.259 Flail joint, unspecified hip
● M25.26 Flail joint, knee
    M25.261 Flail joint, right knee
    M25.262 Flail joint, left knee
    M25.269 Flail joint, unspecified knee
● M25.27 Flail joint, ankle and foot
    M25.271 Flail joint, right ankle and foot
    M25.272 Flail joint, left ankle and foot
    M25.279 Flail joint, unspecified ankle and foot
    M25.28 Flail joint, other site
● M25.3 Other instability of joint
    Excludes1 instability of joint secondary to old
                ligament injury (M24.2-)
              instability of joint secondary to removal
                 of joint prosthesis (M96.8-)
    Excludes2 spinal instabilities (M53.2-)
    M25.30 Other instability, unspecified joint
● M25.31 Other instability, shoulder
    M25.311 Other instability, right shoulder
    M25.312 Other instability, left shoulder
    M25.319 Other instability, unspecified
             shoulder
● M25.32 Other instability, elbow
    M25.321 Other instability, right elbow
    M25.322 Other instability, left elbow
    M25.329 Other instability, unspecified elbow
● M25.33 Other instability, wrist
    M25.331 Other instability, right wrist
    M25.332 Other instability, left wrist
    M25.339 Other instability, unspecified wrist
● M25.34 Other instability, hand
    M25.341 Other instability, right hand
    M25.342 Other instability, left hand
    M25.349 Other instability, unspecified hand
● M25.35 Other instability, hip
    M25.351 Other instability, right hip
    M25.352 Other instability, left hip
    M25.359 Other instability, unspecified hip
● M25.36 Other instability, knee
    M25.361 Other instability, right knee
    M25.362 Other instability, left knee
    M25.369 Other instability, unspecified knee
● M25.37 Other instability, ankle and foot
    M25.371 Other instability, right ankle
    M25.372 Other instability, left ankle
    M25.373 Other instability, unspecified ankle
    M25.374 Other instability, right foot
    M25.375 Other instability, left foot
    M25.376 Other instability, unspecified foot
● M25.4 Effusion of joint
    Excludes1 hydrarthrosis in yaws (A66.6)
              intermittent hydrarthrosis (M12.4-)
              other infective (teno)synovitis (M65.1-)
    M25.40 Effusion, unspecified joint
● M25.41 Effusion, shoulder
    M25.411 Effusion, right shoulder
    M25.412 Effusion, left shoulder
    M25.419 Effusion, unspecified shoulder

● M25.42 Effusion, elbow
    M25.421 Effusion, right elbow
    M25.422 Effusion, left elbow
    M25.429 Effusion, unspecified elbow
● M25.43 Effusion, wrist
    M25.431 Effusion, right wrist
    M25.432 Effusion, left wrist
    M25.439 Effusion, unspecified wrist
● M25.44 Effusion, hand
    M25.441 Effusion, right hand
    M25.442 Effusion, left hand
    M25.449 Effusion, unspecified hand
● M25.45 Effusion, hip
    M25.451 Effusion, right hip
    M25.452 Effusion, left hip
    M25.459 Effusion, unspecified hip
● M25.46 Effusion, knee
    M25.461 Effusion, right knee
    M25.462 Effusion, left knee
    M25.469 Effusion, unspecified knee
● M25.47 Effusion, ankle and foot
    M25.471 Effusion, right ankle
    M25.472 Effusion, left ankle
    M25.473 Effusion, unspecified ankle
    M25.474 Effusion, right foot
    M25.475 Effusion, left foot
    M25.476 Effusion, unspecified foot
    M25.48 Effusion, other site
● M25.5 Pain in joint
    Excludes2 pain in hand (M79.64-)
              pain in fingers (M79.64-)
              pain in foot (M79.67-)
              pain in limb (M79.6-)
              pain in toes (M79.67-)
    M25.50 Pain in unspecified joint
● M25.51 Pain in shoulder
    M25.511 Pain in right shoulder
    M25.512 Pain in left shoulder
    M25.519 Pain in unspecified shoulder
● M25.52 Pain in elbow
    M25.521 Pain in right elbow
    M25.522 Pain in left elbow
    M25.529 Pain in unspecified elbow
● M25.53 Pain in wrist
    M25.531 Pain in right wrist
    M25.532 Pain in left wrist
    M25.539 Pain in unspecified wrist
● M25.55 Pain in hip
    M25.551 Pain in right hip
    M25.552 Pain in left hip
    M25.559 Pain in unspecified hip
● M25.56 Pain in knee
    M25.561 Pain in right knee
    M25.562 Pain in left knee
    M25.569 Pain in unspecified knee
● M25.57 Pain in ankle and joints of foot
    M25.571 Pain in right ankle and joints of right
             foot
    M25.572 Pain in left ankle and joints of left
             foot
    M25.579 Pain in unspecified ankle and joints
             of unspecified foot

CHAPTER 13 (M00-M99)

◄ New   ◄▥ Revised   ~~deleted~~ Deleted   OGCR Official Guidelines   X Assign placeholder X   ● Use Additional Character(s)

 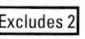 Excludes 1   Excludes 2   Includes   Use additional   Code first   Code also   Unspecified

● **M25.6 Stiffness of joint, not elsewhere classified**

> | Excludes1 | ankylosis of joint (M24.6-)
> contracture of joint (M24.5-)

M25.60   Stiffness of unspecified joint, not elsewhere classified

● M25.61   Stiffness of shoulder, not elsewhere classified

    M25.611   Stiffness of right shoulder, not elsewhere classified

    M25.612   Stiffness of left shoulder, not elsewhere classified

    M25.619   Stiffness of unspecified shoulder, not elsewhere classified

● M25.62   Stiffness of elbow, not elsewhere classified

    M25.621   Stiffness of right elbow, not elsewhere classified

    M25.622   Stiffness of left elbow, not elsewhere classified

    M25.629   Stiffness of unspecified elbow, not elsewhere classified

● M25.63   Stiffness of wrist, not elsewhere classified

    M25.631   Stiffness of right wrist, not elsewhere classified

    M25.632   Stiffness of left wrist, not elsewhere classified

    M25.639   Stiffness of unspecified wrist, not elsewhere classified

● M25.64   Stiffness of hand, not elsewhere classified

    M25.641   Stiffness of right hand, not elsewhere classified

    M25.642   Stiffness of left hand, not elsewhere classified

    M25.649   Stiffness of unspecified hand, not elsewhere classified

● M25.65   Stiffness of hip, not elsewhere classified

    M25.651   Stiffness of right hip, not elsewhere classified

    M25.652   Stiffness of left hip, not elsewhere classified

    M25.659   Stiffness of unspecified hip, not elsewhere classified

● M25.66   Stiffness of knee, not elsewhere classified

    M25.661   Stiffness of right knee, not elsewhere classified

    M25.662   Stiffness of left knee, not elsewhere classified

    M25.669   Stiffness of unspecified knee, not elsewhere classified

● M25.67   Stiffness of ankle and foot, not elsewhere classified

    M25.671   Stiffness of right ankle, not elsewhere classified

    M25.672   Stiffness of left ankle, not elsewhere classified

    M25.673   Stiffness of unspecified ankle, not elsewhere classified

    M25.674   Stiffness of right foot, not elsewhere classified

    M25.675   Stiffness of left foot, not elsewhere classified

    M25.676   Stiffness of unspecified foot, not elsewhere classified

● **M25.7 Osteophyte**

M25.70   Osteophyte, unspecified joint

● M25.71   Osteophyte, shoulder

    M25.711   Osteophyte, right shoulder

    M25.712   Osteophyte, left shoulder

    M25.719   Osteophyte, unspecified shoulder

● M25.72   Osteophyte, elbow

    M25.721   Osteophyte, right elbow

    M25.722   Osteophyte, left elbow

    M25.729   Osteophyte, unspecified elbow

● M25.73   Osteophyte, wrist

    M25.731   Osteophyte, right wrist

    M25.732   Osteophyte, left wrist

    M25.739   Osteophyte, unspecified wrist

● M25.74   Osteophyte, hand

    M25.741   Osteophyte, right hand

    M25.742   Osteophyte, left hand

    M25.749   Osteophyte, unspecified hand

● M25.75   Osteophyte, hip

    M25.751   Osteophyte, right hip

    M25.752   Osteophyte, left hip

    M25.759   Osteophyte, unspecified hip

● M25.76   Osteophyte, knee

    M25.761   Osteophyte, right knee

    M25.762   Osteophyte, left knee

    M25.769   Osteophyte, unspecified knee

● M25.77   Osteophyte, ankle and foot

    M25.771   Osteophyte, right ankle

    M25.772   Osteophyte, left ankle

    M25.773   Osteophyte, unspecified ankle

    M25.774   Osteophyte, right foot

    M25.775   Osteophyte, left foot

    M25.776   Osteophyte, unspecified foot

M25.78   Osteophyte, vertebrae

● **M25.8 Other specified joint disorders**

M25.80   Other specified joint disorders, unspecified joint

● M25.81   Other specified joint disorders, shoulder

    M25.811   Other specified joint disorders, right shoulder

    M25.812   Other specified joint disorders, left shoulder

    M25.819   Other specified joint disorders, unspecified shoulder

● M25.82   Other specified joint disorders, elbow

    M25.821   Other specified joint disorders, right elbow

    M25.822   Other specified joint disorders, left elbow

    M25.829   Other specified joint disorders, unspecified elbow

● M25.83   Other specified joint disorders, wrist

    M25.831   Other specified joint disorders, right wrist

    M25.832   Other specified joint disorders, left wrist

    M25.839   Other specified joint disorders, unspecified wrist

● M25.84   Other specified joint disorders, hand

    M25.841   Other specified joint disorders, right hand

    M25.842   Other specified joint disorders, left hand

    M25.849   Other specified joint disorders, unspecified hand

● M25.85   Other specified joint disorders, hip

    M25.851   Other specified joint disorders, right hip

    M25.852   Other specified joint disorders, left hip

    M25.859   Other specified joint disorders, unspecified hip

CHAPTER 13 (M00-M99)

◀ New   ◀▥ Revised   ~~deleted~~ Deleted   OGCR Official Guidelines   X Assign placeholder X   ● Use Additional Character(s)

Excludes 1   Excludes 2   Includes   Use additional   Code first   Code also   Unspecified

●M25.86   Other specified joint disorders, knee

    M25.861   Other specified joint disorders, right knee

    M25.862   Other specified joint disorders, left knee

    M25.869   Other specified joint disorders, unspecified knee

●M25.87   Other specified joint disorders, ankle and foot

    M25.871   Other specified joint disorders, right ankle and foot

    M25.872   Other specified joint disorders, left ankle and foot

    M25.879   Other specified joint disorders, unspecified ankle and foot

M25.9   Joint disorder, unspecified

DENTOFACIAL ANOMALIES [INCLUDING MALOCCLUSION] AND OTHER DISORDERS OF JAW (M26-M27)

| Excludes1 | hemifacial atrophy or hypertrophy (Q67.4) |
| | unilateral condylar hyperplasia or hypoplasia (M27.8) |

●M26   Dentofacial anomalies [including malocclusion]

●M26.0   Major anomalies of jaw size

| Excludes1 | acromegaly (E22.0) |
| | Robin's syndrome (Q87.0) |

    M26.00   Unspecified anomaly of jaw size

    M26.01   Maxillary hyperplasia

    M26.02   Maxillary hypoplasia

    M26.03   Mandibular hyperplasia

    M26.04   Mandibular hypoplasia

    M26.05   Macrogenia

    M26.06   Microgenia

    M26.07   Excessive tuberosity of jaw
         Entire maxillary tuberosity

    M26.09   Other specified anomalies of jaw size

●M26.1   Anomalies of jaw-cranial base relationship

    M26.10   Unspecified anomaly of jaw-cranial base relationship

    M26.11   Maxillary asymmetry

    M26.12   Other jaw asymmetry

    M26.19   Other specified anomalies of jaw-cranial base relationship

●M26.2   Anomalies of dental arch relationship

    M26.20   Unspecified anomaly of dental arch relationship

●M26.21   Malocclusion, Angle's class

    M26.211   Malocclusion, Angle's class I
         Neutro-occlusion

    M26.212   Malocclusion, Angle's class II
         Disto-occlusion Division I
         Disto-occlusion Division II

    M26.213   Malocclusion, Angle's class III
         Mesio-occlusion

    M26.219   Malocclusion, Angle's class, unspecified

Figure 13-3   Dentofacial malocclusion.

●M26.22   Open occlusal relationship

    M26.220   Open anterior occlusal relationship
         Anterior openbite

    M26.221   Open posterior occlusal relationship
         Posterior openbite

    M26.23   Excessive horizontal overlap
         Excessive horizontal overjet

    M26.24   Reverse articulation
         Crossbite (anterior) (posterior)

    M26.25   Anomalies of interarch distance

    M26.29   Other anomalies of dental arch relationship
         Midline deviation of dental arch
         Overbite (excessive) deep
         Overbite (excessive) horizontal
         Overbite (excessive) vertical
         Posterior lingual occlusion of mandibular teeth

●M26.3   Anomalies of tooth position of fully erupted tooth or teeth

| Excludes2 | embedded and impacted teeth (K01.-) |

    M26.30   Unspecified anomaly of tooth position of fully erupted tooth or teeth
         Abnormal spacing of fully erupted tooth or teeth NOS
         Displacement of fully erupted tooth or teeth NOS
         Transposition of fully erupted tooth or teeth NOS

    M26.31   Crowding of fully erupted teeth

    M26.32   Excessive spacing of fully erupted teeth
         Diastema of fully erupted tooth or teeth NOS

    M26.33   Horizontal displacement of fully erupted tooth or teeth
         Tipped tooth or teeth
         Tipping of fully erupted tooth

    M26.34   Vertical displacement of fully erupted tooth or teeth
         Extruded tooth
         Infraeruption of tooth or teeth
         Supraeruption of tooth or teeth

    M26.35   Rotation of fully erupted tooth or teeth

    M26.36   Insufficient interocclusal distance of fully erupted teeth (ridge)
         Lack of adequate intermaxillary vertical dimension of fully erupted teeth

    M26.37   Excessive interocclusal distance of fully erupted teeth
         Excessive intermaxillary vertical dimension of fully erupted teeth
         Loss of occlusal vertical dimension of fully erupted teeth

    M26.39   Other anomalies of tooth position of fully erupted tooth or teeth

M26.4   Malocclusion, unspecified

●M26.5   Dentofacial functional abnormalities

| Excludes1 | bruxism (F45.8) |
| | teeth-grinding NOS (F45.8) |

    M26.50   Dentofacial functional abnormalities, unspecified

    M26.51   Abnormal jaw closure

    M26.52   Limited mandibular range of motion

    M26.53   Deviation in opening and closing of the mandible

    M26.54   Insufficient anterior guidance
         Insufficient anterior occlusal guidance

    M26.55   Centric occlusion maximum intercuspation discrepancy

| Excludes1 | centric occlusion NOS (M26.59) |

    M26.56   Non-working side interference
         Balancing side interference

    M26.57   Lack of posterior occlusal support

Item 13–6   **Hyperplasia** is a condition of overdevelopment, whereas **hypoplasia** is a condition of underdevelopment. **Macrogenia** is overdevelopment of the chin, whereas **microgenia** is underdevelopment of the chin.

◀ New   ◀‖‖ Revised   ~~deleted~~ Deleted   **OGCR** Official Guidelines   X Assign placeholder X   ● Use Additional Character(s)

| Excludes 1 | Excludes 2 | Includes | Use additional | Code first | Code also | Unspecified |

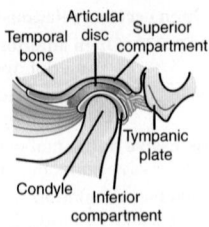

Figure 13-4 Temporomandibular joint.

Item 13-7 Dysfunction of the temporomandibular joint is termed **temporomandibular joint (TMJ) syndrome** and is characterized by pain and tenderness/spasm of the muscles of mastication, joint noise, and in the later stages, limited mandibular movement.

M26.59 **Other dentofacial functional abnormalities**
Centric occlusion (of teeth) NOS
Malocclusion due to abnormal swallowing
Malocclusion due to mouth breathing
Malocclusion due to tongue, lip or finger
habits

● M26.6 **Temporomandibular joint disorders**
Excludes2 current temporomandibular joint
dislocation (S03.0)
current temporomandibular joint sprain
(S03.4)
M26.60 **Temporomandibular joint disorder, unspecified**
M26.61 **Adhesions and ankylosis of
temporomandibular joint**
M26.62 **Arthralgia of temporomandibular joint**
M26.63 **Articular disc disorder of temporomandibular
joint**
M26.69 **Other specified disorders of
temporomandibular joint**

● M26.7 **Dental alveolar anomalies**
M26.70 **Unspecified alveolar anomaly**
M26.71 **Alveolar maxillary hyperplasia**
M26.72 **Alveolar mandibular hyperplasia**
M26.73 **Alveolar maxillary hypoplasia**
M26.74 **Alveolar mandibular hypoplasia**
M26.79 **Other specified alveolar anomalies**

● M26.8 **Other dentofacial anomalies**
M26.81 **Anterior soft tissue impingement**
Anterior soft tissue impingement on teeth
M26.82 **Posterior soft tissue impingement**
Posterior soft tissue impingement on teeth
M26.89 **Other dentofacial anomalies**

M26.9 **Dentofacial anomaly, unspecified**

● M27 **Other diseases of jaws**
M27.0 **Developmental disorders of jaws**
Latent bone cyst of jaw
Stafne's cyst
Torus mandibularis
Torus palatinus

M27.1 **Giant cell granuloma, central**
Giant cell granuloma NOS
Excludes1 peripheral giant cell granuloma (K06.8)

M27.2 **Inflammatory conditions of jaws**
Osteitis of jaw(s)
Osteomyelitis (neonatal) jaw(s)
Osteoradionecrosis jaw(s)
Periostitis jaw(s)
Sequestrum of jaw bone
Use additional code (W88-W90, X39.0) to identify
radiation, if radiation-induced
Excludes2 osteonecrosis of jaw due to drug
(M87.180)

M27.3 **Alveolitis of jaws**
Alveolar osteitis
Dry socket

● M27.4 **Other and unspecified cysts of jaw**
Excludes1 cysts of oral region (K09.-)
latent bone cyst of jaw (M27.0)
Stafne's cyst (M27.0)
M27.40 **Unspecified cyst of jaw**
Cyst of jaw NOS
M27.49 **Other cysts of jaw**
Aneurysmal cyst of jaw
Hemorrhagic cyst of jaw
Traumatic cyst of jaw

● M27.5 **Periradicular pathology associated with previous
endodontic treatment**
M27.51 **Perforation of root canal space due to
endodontic treatment**
M27.52 **Endodontic overfill**
M27.53 **Endodontic underfill**
M27.59 **Other periradicular pathology associated with
previous endodontic treatment**

● M27.6 **Endosseous dental implant failure**
M27.61 **Osseointegration failure of dental implant**
Hemorrhagic complications of dental implant
placement
Iatrogenic osseointegration failure of dental
implant
Osseointegration failure of dental implant due
to complications of systemic disease
Osseointegration failure of dental implant due
to poor bone quality
Pre-integration failure of dental implant NOS
Pre-osseointegration failure of dental implant
M27.62 **Post-osseointegration biological failure of
dental implant**
Failure of dental implant due to lack of
attached gingiva
Failure of dental implant due to occlusal
trauma (caused by poor prosthetic design)
Failure of dental implant due to parafunctional
habits
Failure of dental implant due to periodontal
infection (peri–implantitis)
Failure of dental implant due to poor oral
hygiene
Iatrogenic post-osseointegration failure of
dental implant
Post-osseointegration failure of dental implant
due to complications of systemic disease
M27.63 **Post-osseointegration mechanical failure of
dental implant**
Failure of dental prosthesis causing loss of
dental implant
Fracture of dental implant
Excludes2 cracked tooth (K03.81)
fractured dental restorative
material with loss of
material (K08.531)
fractured dental restorative
material without loss of
material (K08.530)
fractured tooth (S02.5)
M27.69 **Other endosseous dental implant failure**
Dental implant failure NOS

M27.8 **Other specified diseases of jaws**
Cherubism
Exostosis
Fibrous dysplasia
Unilateral condylar hyperplasia
Unilateral condylar hypoplasia
Excludes1 jaw pain (R68.84)

M27.9 **Disease of jaws, unspecified**

SYSTEMIC CONNECTIVE TISSUE DISORDERS (M30-M36)

Includes   autoimmune disease NOS
     collagen (vascular) disease NOS
     systemic autoimmune disease
     systemic collagen (vascular) disease

Excludes1   autoimmune disease, single organ or single cell-type - code to relevant condition category

● **M30 Polyarteritis nodosa and related conditions**
     Excludes1   microscopic polyarteritis (M31.7)

   M30.0 Polyarteritis nodosa

   M30.1 Polyarteritis with lung involvement [Churg-Strauss]
     Allergic granulomatous angiitis

   M30.2 Juvenile polyarteritis

   M30.3 Mucocutaneous lymph node syndrome [Kawasaki]

   M30.8 Other conditions related to polyarteritis nodosa
     Polyangiitis overlap syndrome

● **M31 Other necrotizing vasculopathies**

   M31.0 Hypersensitivity angiitis
     Goodpasture's syndrome

   M31.1 Thrombotic microangiopathy
     Thrombotic thrombocytopenic purpura

   M31.2 Lethal midline granuloma

   M31.3 Wegener's granulomatosis
     Necrotizing respiratory granulomatosis

     M31.30 Wegener's granulomatosis without renal involvement
       Wegener's granulomatosis NOS

     M31.31 Wegener's granulomatosis with renal involvement

   M31.4 Aortic arch syndrome [Takayasu]

   M31.5 Giant cell arteritis with polymyalgia rheumatica

   M31.6 Other giant cell arteritis

   M31.7 Microscopic polyangiitis
     Microscopic polyarteritis
     Excludes1   polyarteritis nodosa (M30.0)

   M31.8 Other specified necrotizing vasculopathies
     Hypocomplementemic vasculitis
     Septic vasculitis

   M31.9 Necrotizing vasculopathy, unspecified

● **M32 Systemic lupus erythematosus (SLE)**
   Autoimmune inflammatory connective tissue disease of unknown cause that occurs most often in women.
     Excludes1   lupus erythematosus (discoid) (NOS) (L93.0)

   M32.0 Drug-induced systemic lupus erythematosus
     Use additional code for adverse effect, if applicable, to identify drug (T36-T50 with fifth or sixth character 5)

●   **M32.1 Systemic lupus erythematosus with organ or system involvement**

     M32.10 Systemic lupus erythematosus, organ or system involvement unspecified

     M32.11 Endocarditis in systemic lupus erythematosus
       Libman-Sacks disease

     M32.12 Pericarditis in systemic lupus erythematosus
       Lupus pericarditis

     M32.13 Lung involvement in systemic lupus erythematosus
       Pleural effusion due to systemic lupus erythematosus

     M32.14 Glomerular disease in systemic lupus erythematosus
       Lupus renal disease NOS

     M32.15 Tubulo-interstitial nephropathy in systemic lupus erythematosus

     M32.19 Other organ or system involvement in systemic lupus erythematosus

   M32.8 Other forms of systemic lupus erythematosus

   M32.9 Systemic lupus erythematosus, unspecified
     SLE NOS
     Systemic lupus erythematosus NOS
     Systemic lupus erythematosus without organ involvement

● **M33 Dermatopolymyositis**

●   **M33.0 Juvenile dermatopolymyositis**

     M33.00 Juvenile dermatopolymyositis, organ involvement unspecified

     M33.01 Juvenile dermatopolymyositis with respiratory involvement

     M33.02 Juvenile dermatopolymyositis with myopathy

     M33.09 Juvenile dermatopolymyositis with other organ involvement

●   **M33.1 Other dermatopolymyositis**

     M33.10 Other dermatopolymyositis, organ involvement unspecified

     M33.11 Other dermatopolymyositis with respiratory involvement

     M33.12 Other dermatopolymyositis with myopathy

     M33.19 Other dermatopolymyositis with other organ involvement

●   **M33.2 Polymyositis**

     M33.20 Polymyositis, organ involvement unspecified

     M33.21 Polymyositis with respiratory involvement

     M33.22 Polymyositis with myopathy

     M33.29 Polymyositis with other organ involvement

●   **M33.9 Dermatopolymyositis, unspecified**

     M33.90 Dermatopolymyositis, unspecified, organ involvement unspecified

     M33.91 Dermatopolymyositis, unspecified with respiratory involvement

     M33.92 Dermatopolymyositis, unspecified with myopathy

     M33.99 Dermatopolymyositis, unspecified with other organ involvement

● **M34 Systemic sclerosis [scleroderma]**
     Excludes1   circumscribed scleroderma (L94.0)
         neonatal scleroderma (P83.8)

   M34.0 Progressive systemic sclerosis

   M34.1 CR(E)ST syndrome
     Combination of calcinosis, Raynaud's phenomenon, esophageal dysfunction, sclerodactyly, telangiectasia

   M34.2 Systemic sclerosis induced by drug and chemical
     Code first poisoning due to drug or toxin, if applicable (T36-T65 with fifth or sixth character 1-4 or 6)
     Use additional code for adverse effect, if applicable, to identify drug (T36-T50 with fifth or sixth character 5)

●   **M34.8 Other forms of systemic sclerosis**

     M34.81 Systemic sclerosis with lung involvement

     M34.82 Systemic sclerosis with myopathy

     M34.83 Systemic sclerosis with polyneuropathy

     M34.89 Other systemic sclerosis

   M34.9 Systemic sclerosis, unspecified

● **M35 Other systemic involvement of connective tissue**
     Excludes1   reactive perforating collagenosis (L87.1)

●   **M35.0 Sicca syndrome [Sjögren]**

     M35.00 Sicca syndrome, unspecified

     M35.01 Sicca syndrome with keratoconjunctivitis

     M35.02 Sicca syndrome with lung involvement

     M35.03 Sicca syndrome with myopathy

     M35.04 Sicca syndrome with tubulo-interstitial nephropathy
       Renal tubular acidosis in sicca syndrome

     M35.09 Sicca syndrome with other organ involvement

CHAPTER 13 (M00-M99)

◀ New   ◀▬ Revised   ~~deleted~~ Deleted   **OGCR** Official Guidelines   **X** Assign placeholder X   ● Use Additional Character(s)

Excludes 1   Excludes 2   Includes   Use additional   Code first   Code also   Unspecified

1053

Item 13–8   **Polymyalgia rheumatica** is a syndrome characterized by aching and morning stiffness and is related to aging and hereditary predisposition.

M35.1   **Other overlap syndromes**
Mixed connective tissue disease
Excludes1   polyangiitis overlap syndrome (M30.8)

M35.2   **Behçet's disease**

M35.3   **Polymyalgia rheumatica**
Excludes1   polymyalgia rheumatica with giant cell arteritis (M31.5)

M35.4   **Diffuse (eosinophilic) fasciitis**

M35.5   **Multifocal fibrosclerosis**

M35.6   **Relapsing panniculitis [Weber-Christian]**
Excludes1   lupus panniculitis (L93.2)
panniculitis NOS (M79.3-)

M35.7   **Hypermobility syndrome**
Familial ligamentous laxity
Excludes1   Ehlers-Danlos syndrome (Q79.6)
ligamentous laxity, NOS (M24.2-)

M35.8   **Other specified systemic involvement of connective tissue**

M35.9   **Systemic involvement of connective tissue, unspecified**
Autoimmune disease (systemic) NOS
Collagen (vascular) disease NOS

● M36   **Systemic disorders of connective tissue in diseases classified elsewhere**
Excludes2   arthropathies in diseases classified elsewhere (M14.-)

M36.0   **Dermato(poly)myositis in neoplastic disease**
Code first underlying neoplasm (C00-D49)

M36.1   **Arthropathy in neoplastic disease**
Code first underlying neoplasm, such as:
leukemia (C91-C95)
malignant histiocytosis (C96.A)
multiple myeloma (C90.0)

M36.2   **Hemophilic arthropathy**
Hemarthrosis in hemophilic arthropathy
Code first underlying disease, such as:
factor VIII deficiency (D66)
with vascular defect (D68.0)
factor IX deficiency (D67)
hemophilia (classical) (D66)
hemophilia B (D67)
hemophilia C (D68.1)

M36.3   **Arthropathy in other blood disorders**

M36.4   **Arthropathy in hypersensitivity reactions classified elsewhere**
Code first underlying disease, such as:
Henoch (-Schönlein) purpura (D69.0)
serum sickness (T80.6-)

M36.8   **Systemic disorders of connective tissue in other diseases classified elsewhere**
Code first underlying disease, such as:
alkaptonuria (E70.2)
hypogammaglobulinemia (D80.-)
ochronosis (E70.2)

Item 13–9   **Kyphosis** is an abnormal curvature of the spine. **Senile kyphosis** is a result of disc degeneration causing ossification (turning to bone). **Adolescent** or **juvenile** kyphosis is also known as **Scheuermann's disease,** a condition in which the discs of the lower thoracic spine herniate, causing the disc space to narrow and the spine to tilt forward. This condition is attributed to poor posture. Lordosis or swayback is an abnormal curvature of the spine resulting in an inward curve of the lumbar spine just above the buttocks. Scoliosis causes a sideways curve to the spine. The curves are S- or C-shaped, and it is most commonly acquired in late childhood and early teen years, when growth is fast.

DORSOPATHIES (M40-M54)

DEFORMING DORSOPATHIES (M40-M43)

● M40   **Kyphosis and lordosis**
Excludes1   congenital kyphosis and lordosis (Q76.4)
kyphoscoliosis (M41.-)
postprocedural kyphosis and lordosis (M96.-)

● M40.0   **Postural kyphosis**
Excludes1   osteochondrosis of spine (M42.-)
M40.00   Postural kyphosis, site unspecified
M40.03   Postural kyphosis, cervicothoracic region
M40.04   Postural kyphosis, thoracic region
M40.05   Postural kyphosis, thoracolumbar region

● M40.1   **Other secondary kyphosis**
M40.10   Other secondary kyphosis, site unspecified
M40.12   Other secondary kyphosis, cervical region
M40.13   Other secondary kyphosis, cervicothoracic region
M40.14   Other secondary kyphosis, thoracic region
M40.15   Other secondary kyphosis, thoracolumbar region

● M40.2   **Other and unspecified kyphosis**
● M40.20   Unspecified kyphosis
M40.202   Unspecified kyphosis, cervical region
M40.203   Unspecified kyphosis, cervicothoracic region
M40.204   Unspecified kyphosis, thoracic region
M40.205   Unspecified kyphosis, thoracolumbar region
M40.209   Unspecified kyphosis, site unspecified
● M40.29   Other kyphosis
M40.292   Other kyphosis, cervical region
M40.293   Other kyphosis, cervicothoracic region
M40.294   Other kyphosis, thoracic region
M40.295   Other kyphosis, thoracolumbar region
M40.299   Other kyphosis, site unspecified

● M40.3   **Flatback syndrome**
M40.30   Flatback syndrome, site unspecified
M40.35   Flatback syndrome, thoracolumbar region
M40.36   Flatback syndrome, lumbar region
M40.37   Flatback syndrome, lumbosacral region

● M40.4   **Postural lordosis**
Abnormal increase in the normal curvature of the lumbar spine (sway back)
Acquired lordosis
M40.40   Postural lordosis, site unspecified
M40.45   Postural lordosis, thoracolumbar region
M40.46   Postural lordosis, lumbar region
M40.47   Postural lordosis, lumbosacral region

◀ New   ◀▌▌▌ Revised   ~~deleted~~ Deleted   OGCR Official Guidelines   X Assign placeholder X   ● Use Additional Character(s)

| Excludes 1 | Excludes 2 | Includes | Use additional | Code first | Code also | Unspecified |

● M40.5 **Lordosis, unspecified**
     M40.50 **Lordosis, unspecified, site unspecified**
     M40.55 **Lordosis, unspecified, thoracolumbar region**
     M40.56 **Lordosis, unspecified, lumbar region**
     M40.57 **Lordosis, unspecified, lumbosacral region**

● M41 **Scoliosis**
     Includes   kyphoscoliosis
     Excludes1   congenital scoliosis NOS (Q67.5)
                 congenital scoliosis due to bony malformation (Q76.3)
                 postural congenital scoliosis (Q67.5)
                 kyphoscoliotic heart disease (I27.1)
                 postprocedural scoliosis (M96.-)

● M41.0 **Infantile idiopathic scoliosis**
     M41.00 **Infantile idiopathic scoliosis, site unspecified**
     M41.02 **Infantile idiopathic scoliosis, cervical region**
     M41.03 **Infantile idiopathic scoliosis, cervicothoracic region**
     M41.04 **Infantile idiopathic scoliosis, thoracic region**
     M41.05 **Infantile idiopathic scoliosis, thoracolumbar region**
     M41.06 **Infantile idiopathic scoliosis, lumbar region**
     M41.07 **Infantile idiopathic scoliosis, lumbosacral region**
     M41.08 **Infantile idiopathic scoliosis, sacral and sacrococcygeal region**

● M41.1 **Juvenile and adolescent idiopathic scoliosis**
     ● M41.11 **Juvenile idiopathic scoliosis**
         M41.112 **Juvenile idiopathic scoliosis, cervical region**
         M41.113 **Juvenile idiopathic scoliosis, cervicothoracic region**
         M41.114 **Juvenile idiopathic scoliosis, thoracic region**
         M41.115 **Juvenile idiopathic scoliosis, thoracolumbar region**
         M41.116 **Juvenile idiopathic scoliosis, lumbar region**
         M41.117 **Juvenile idiopathic scoliosis, lumbosacral region**
         M41.119 **Juvenile idiopathic scoliosis, site unspecified**
     ● M41.12 **Adolescent scoliosis**
         M41.122 **Adolescent idiopathic scoliosis, cervical region**
         M41.123 **Adolescent idiopathic scoliosis, cervicothoracic region**
         M41.124 **Adolescent idiopathic scoliosis, thoracic region**
         M41.125 **Adolescent idiopathic scoliosis, thoracolumbar region**
         M41.126 **Adolescent idiopathic scoliosis, lumbar region**
         M41.127 **Adolescent idiopathic scoliosis, lumbosacral region**
         M41.129 **Adolescent idiopathic scoliosis, site unspecified**

● M41.2 **Other idiopathic scoliosis**
     M41.20 **Other idiopathic scoliosis, site unspecified**
     M41.22 **Other idiopathic scoliosis, cervical region**
     M41.23 **Other idiopathic scoliosis, cervicothoracic region**
     M41.24 **Other idiopathic scoliosis, thoracic region**
     M41.25 **Other idiopathic scoliosis, thoracolumbar region**
     M41.26 **Other idiopathic scoliosis, lumbar region**
     M41.27 **Other idiopathic scoliosis, lumbosacral region**

● M41.3 **Thoracogenic scoliosis**
     M41.30 **Thoracogenic scoliosis, site unspecified**
     M41.34 **Thoracogenic scoliosis, thoracic region**
     M41.35 **Thoracogenic scoliosis, thoracolumbar region**

● M41.4 **Neuromuscular scoliosis**
     Scoliosis secondary to cerebral palsy, Friedreich's ataxia, poliomyelitis and other neuromuscular disorders
     Code also underlying condition
     M41.40 **Neuromuscular scoliosis, site unspecified**
     M41.41 **Neuromuscular scoliosis, occipito-atlanto-axial region**
     M41.42 **Neuromuscular scoliosis, cervical region**
     M41.43 **Neuromuscular scoliosis, cervicothoracic region**
     M41.44 **Neuromuscular scoliosis, thoracic region**
     M41.45 **Neuromuscular scoliosis, thoracolumbar region**
     M41.46 **Neuromuscular scoliosis, lumbar region**
     M41.47 **Neuromuscular scoliosis, lumbosacral region**

● M41.5 **Other secondary scoliosis**
     M41.50 **Other secondary scoliosis, site unspecified**
     M41.52 **Other secondary scoliosis, cervical region**
     M41.53 **Other secondary scoliosis, cervicothoracic region**
     M41.54 **Other secondary scoliosis, thoracic region**
     M41.55 **Other secondary scoliosis, thoracolumbar region**
     M41.56 **Other secondary scoliosis, lumbar region**
     M41.57 **Other secondary scoliosis, lumbosacral region**

● M41.8 **Other forms of scoliosis**
     M41.80 **Other forms of scoliosis, site unspecified**
     M41.82 **Other forms of scoliosis, cervical region**
     M41.83 **Other forms of scoliosis, cervicothoracic region**
     M41.84 **Other forms of scoliosis, thoracic region**
     M41.85 **Other forms of scoliosis, thoracolumbar region**
     M41.86 **Other forms of scoliosis, lumbar region**
     M41.87 **Other forms of scoliosis, lumbosacral region**

     M41.9 **Scoliosis, unspecified**

● M42 **Spinal osteochondrosis**
     ● M42.0 **Juvenile osteochondrosis of spine**
         Calvé's disease
         Scheuermann's disease
         Excludes1   postural kyphosis (M40.0)
         M42.00 **Juvenile osteochondrosis of spine, site unspecified**
         M42.01 **Juvenile osteochondrosis of spine, occipito-atlanto-axial region**
         M42.02 **Juvenile osteochondrosis of spine, cervical region**
         M42.03 **Juvenile osteochondrosis of spine, cervicothoracic region**
         M42.04 **Juvenile osteochondrosis of spine, thoracic region**
         M42.05 **Juvenile osteochondrosis of spine, thoracolumbar region**
         M42.06 **Juvenile osteochondrosis of spine, lumbar region**
         M42.07 **Juvenile osteochondrosis of spine, lumbosacral region**
         M42.08 **Juvenile osteochondrosis of spine, sacral and sacrococcygeal region**
         M42.09 **Juvenile osteochondrosis of spine, multiple sites in spine**

CHAPTER 13 (M00–M99)

● **M42.1　Adult osteochondrosis of spine**

　M42.10　Adult osteochondrosis of spine, site unspecified

　M42.11　Adult osteochondrosis of spine, occipitoatlanto-axial region

　M42.12　Adult osteochondrosis of spine, cervical region

　M42.13　Adult osteochondrosis of spine, cervicothoracic region

　M42.14　Adult osteochondrosis of spine, thoracic region

　M42.15　Adult osteochondrosis of spine, thoracolumbar region

　M42.16　Adult osteochondrosis of spine, lumbar region

　M42.17　Adult osteochondrosis of spine, lumbosacral region

　M42.18　Adult osteochondrosis of spine, sacral and sacrococcygeal region

　M42.19　Adult osteochondrosis of spine, multiple sites in spine

M42.9　Spinal osteochondrosis, unspecified

● **M43　Other deforming dorsopathies**

　Excludes1　congenital spondylolysis and spondylolisthesis (Q76.2)
　　　　　hemivertebra (Q76.3-Q76.4)
　　　　　Klippel-Feil syndrome (Q76.1)
　　　　　lumbarization and sacralization (Q76.4)
　　　　　platyspondylisis (Q76.4)
　　　　　spina bifida occulta (Q76.0)
　　　　　spinal curvature in osteoporosis (M80.-)
　　　　　spinal curvature in Paget's disease of bone [osteitis deformans] (M88.-)

● **M43.0　Spondylolysis**

　Excludes1　congenital spondylolysis (Q76.2)
　　　　　spondylolisthesis (M43.1)

　M43.00　Spondylolysis, site unspecified
　M43.01　Spondylolysis, occipito-atlanto-axial region
　M43.02　Spondylolysis, cervical region
　M43.03　Spondylolysis, cervicothoracic region
　M43.04　Spondylolysis, thoracic region
　M43.05　Spondylolysis, thoracolumbar region
　M43.06　Spondylolysis, lumbar region
　M43.07　Spondylolysis, lumbosacral region
　M43.08　Spondylolysis, sacral and sacrococcygeal region
　M43.09　Spondylolysis, multiple sites in spine

● **M43.1　Spondylolisthesis**

　Excludes1　acute traumatic of lumbosacral region (S33.1)
　　　　　acute traumatic of sites other than lumbosacral - code to Fracture, vertebra, by region
　　　　　congenital spondylolisthesis (Q76.2)

　M43.10　Spondylolisthesis, site unspecified
　M43.11　Spondylolisthesis, occipito-atlanto-axial region
　M43.12　Spondylolisthesis, cervical region
　M43.13　Spondylolisthesis, cervicothoracic region
　M43.14　Spondylolisthesis, thoracic region
　M43.15　Spondylolisthesis, thoracolumbar region
　M43.16　Spondylolisthesis, lumbar region
　M43.17　Spondylolisthesis, lumbosacral region
　M43.18　Spondylolisthesis, sacral and sacrococcygeal region
　M43.19　Spondylolisthesis, multiple sites in spine

● **M43.2　Fusion of spine**
　Ankylosis of spinal joint

　Excludes1　ankylosing spondylitis (M45.0-)
　　　　　congenital fusion of spine (Q76.4)

　Excludes2　arthrodesis status (Z98.1)
　　　　　pseudoarthrosis after fusion or arthrodesis (M96.0)

　M43.20　Fusion of spine, site unspecified
　M43.21　Fusion of spine, occipito-atlanto-axial region
　M43.22　Fusion of spine, cervical region
　M43.23　Fusion of spine, cervicothoracic region
　M43.24　Fusion of spine, thoracic region
　M43.25　Fusion of spine, thoracolumbar region
　M43.26　Fusion of spine, lumbar region
　M43.27　Fusion of spine, lumbosacral region
　M43.28　Fusion of spine, sacral and sacrococcygeal region

M43.3　Recurrent atlantoaxial dislocation with myelopathy

M43.4　Other recurrent atlantoaxial dislocation

● **M43.5　Other recurrent vertebral dislocation**

　Excludes1　biomechanical lesions NEC (M99.-)

● M43.5X　Other recurrent vertebral dislocation

　M43.5X2　Other recurrent vertebral dislocation, cervical region
　M43.5X3　Other recurrent vertebral dislocation, cervicothoracic region
　M43.5X4　Other recurrent vertebral dislocation, thoracic region
　M43.5X5　Other recurrent vertebral dislocation, thoracolumbar region
　M43.5X6　Other recurrent vertebral dislocation, lumbar region
　M43.5X7　Other recurrent vertebral dislocation, lumbosacral region
　M43.5X8　Other recurrent vertebral dislocation, sacral and sacrococcygeal region
　M43.5X9　Other recurrent vertebral dislocation, site unspecified

M43.6　Torticollis

　Excludes1　congenital (sternomastoid) torticollis (Q68.0)
　　　　　current injury - see Injury, of spine, by body region ocular torticollis (R29.891)
　　　　　psychogenic torticollis (F45.8)
　　　　　spasmodic torticollis (G24.3)
　　　　　torticollis due to birth injury (P15.2)

● **M43.8　Other specified deforming dorsopathies**

　Excludes2　kyphosis and lordosis (M40.-)
　　　　　scoliosis (M41.-)

● M43.8X　Other specified deforming dorsopathies

　M43.8X1　Other specified deforming dorsopathies, occipito-atlanto-axial region
　M43.8X2　Other specified deforming dorsopathies, cervical region
　M43.8X3　Other specified deforming dorsopathies, cervicothoracic region
　M43.8X4　Other specified deforming dorsopathies, thoracic region
　M43.8X5　Other specified deforming dorsopathies, thoracolumbar region
　M43.8X6　Other specified deforming dorsopathies, lumbar region
　M43.8X7　Other specified deforming dorsopathies, lumbosacral region

Item 13–10　Spondylolisthesis is a condition caused by the slipping forward of one disc over another.

M43.8X8 Other specified deforming dorsopathies, sacral and sacrococcygeal region

M43.8X9 Other specified deforming dorsopathies, site unspecified

M43.9 Deforming dorsopathy, unspecified
Curvature of spine NOS

SPONDYLOPATHIES (M45-M49)

● M45 Ankylosing spondylitis
Rheumatoid arthritis of spine

Excludes1 arthropathy in Reiter's disease (M02.3-)
juvenile (ankylosing) spondylitis (M08.1)

Excludes2 Behçet's disease (M35.2)

M45.0 Ankylosing spondylitis of multiple sites in spine

M45.1 Ankylosing spondylitis of occipito-atlanto-axial region

M45.2 Ankylosing spondylitis of cervical region

M45.3 Ankylosing spondylitis of cervicothoracic region

M45.4 Ankylosing spondylitis of thoracic region

M45.5 Ankylosing spondylitis of thoracolumbar region

M45.6 Ankylosing spondylitis lumbar region

M45.7 Ankylosing spondylitis of lumbosacral region

M45.8 Ankylosing spondylitis sacral and sacrococcygeal region

M45.9 Ankylosing spondylitis of unspecified sites in spine

● M46 Other inflammatory spondylopathies

● M46.0 Spinal enthesopathy
Disorder of ligamentous or muscular attachments of spine

M46.00 Spinal enthesopathy, site unspecified

M46.01 Spinal enthesopathy, occipito-atlanto-axial region

M46.02 Spinal enthesopathy, cervical region

M46.03 Spinal enthesopathy, cervicothoracic region

M46.04 Spinal enthesopathy, thoracic region

M46.05 Spinal enthesopathy, thoracolumbar region

M46.06 Spinal enthesopathy, lumbar region

M46.07 Spinal enthesopathy, lumbosacral region

M46.08 Spinal enthesopathy, sacral and sacrococcygeal region

M46.09 Spinal enthesopathy, multiple sites in spine

M46.1 Sacroiliitis, not elsewhere classified

● M46.2 Osteomyelitis of vertebra

M46.20 Osteomyelitis of vertebra, site unspecified

M46.21 Osteomyelitis of vertebra, occipito-atlanto-axial region

M46.22 Osteomyelitis of vertebra, cervical region

M46.23 Osteomyelitis of vertebra, cervicothoracic region

M46.24 Osteomyelitis of vertebra, thoracic region

M46.25 Osteomyelitis of vertebra, thoracolumbar region

M46.26 Osteomyelitis of vertebra, lumbar region

M46.27 Osteomyelitis of vertebra, lumbosacral region

M46.28 Osteomyelitis of vertebra, sacral and sacrococcygeal region

● M46.3 Infection of intervertebral disc (pyogenic)
Use additional code (B95-B97) to identify infectious agent

M46.30 Infection of intervertebral disc (pyogenic), site unspecified

M46.31 Infection of intervertebral disc (pyogenic), occipito-atlanto-axial region

M46.32 Infection of intervertebral disc (pyogenic), cervical region

M46.33 Infection of intervertebral disc (pyogenic), cervicothoracic region

M46.34 Infection of intervertebral disc (pyogenic), thoracic region

M46.35 Infection of intervertebral disc (pyogenic), thoracolumbar region

M46.36 Infection of intervertebral disc (pyogenic), lumbar region

M46.37 Infection of intervertebral disc (pyogenic), lumbosacral region

M46.38 Infection of intervertebral disc (pyogenic), sacral and sacrococcygeal region

M46.39 Infection of intervertebral disc (pyogenic), multiple sites in spine

● M46.4 Discitis, unspecified

M46.40 Discitis, unspecified, site unspecified

M46.41 Discitis, unspecified, occipito-atlanto-axial region

M46.42 Discitis, unspecified, cervical region

M46.43 Discitis, unspecified, cervicothoracic region

M46.44 Discitis, unspecified, thoracic region

M46.45 Discitis, unspecified, thoracolumbar region

M46.46 Discitis, unspecified, lumbar region

M46.47 Discitis, unspecified, lumbosacral region

M46.48 Discitis, unspecified, sacral and sacrococcygeal region

M46.49 Discitis, unspecified, multiple sites in spine

● M46.5 Other infective spondylopathies

M46.50 Other infective spondylopathies, site unspecified

M46.51 Other infective spondylopathies, occipitoatlanto-axial region

M46.52 Other infective spondylopathies, cervical region

M46.53 Other infective spondylopathies, cervicothoracic region

M46.54 Other infective spondylopathies, thoracic region

M46.55 Other infective spondylopathies, thoracolumbar region

M46.56 Other infective spondylopathies, lumbar region

M46.57 Other infective spondylopathies, lumbosacral region

M46.58 Other infective spondylopathies, sacral and sacrococcygeal region

M46.59 Other infective spondylopathies, multiple sites in spine

● M46.8 Other specified inflammatory spondylopathies

M46.80 Other specified inflammatory spondylopathies, site unspecified

M46.81 Other specified inflammatory spondylopathies, occipito-atlanto-axial region

M46.82 Other specified inflammatory spondylopathies, cervical region

M46.83 Other specified inflammatory spondylopathies, cervicothoracic region

M46.84 Other specified inflammatory spondylopathies, thoracic region

M46.85 Other specified inflammatory spondylopathies, thoracolumbar region

M46.86 Other specified inflammatory spondylopathies, lumbar region

M46.87 Other specified inflammatory spondylopathies, lumbosacral region

M46.88 Other specified inflammatory spondylopathies, sacral and sacrococcygeal region

M46.89 Other specified inflammatory spondylopathies, multiple sites in spine

CHAPTER 13 (M00-M99)

● **M46.9** **Unspecified inflammatory spondylopathy**
   M46.90 Unspecified inflammatory spondylopathy, site unspecified
   M46.91 Unspecified inflammatory spondylopathy, occipito-atlanto-axial region
   M46.92 Unspecified inflammatory spondylopathy, cervical region
   M46.93 Unspecified inflammatory spondylopathy, cervicothoracic region
   M46.94 Unspecified inflammatory spondylopathy, thoracic region
   M46.95 Unspecified inflammatory spondylopathy, thoracolumbar region
   M46.96 Unspecified inflammatory spondylopathy, lumbar region
   M46.97 Unspecified inflammatory spondylopathy, lumbosacral region
   M46.98 Unspecified inflammatory spondylopathy, sacral and sacrococcygeal region
   M46.99 Unspecified inflammatory spondylopathy, multiple sites in spine

● **M47** **Spondylosis**

   Includes   arthrosis or osteoarthritis of spine
                   degeneration of facet joints

  ● **M47.0** **Anterior spinal and vertebral artery compression syndromes**
    ● **M47.01** Anterior spinal artery compression syndromes
      M47.011 Anterior spinal artery compression syndromes, occipito-atlanto-axial region
      M47.012 Anterior spinal artery compression syndromes, cervical region
      M47.013 Anterior spinal artery compression syndromes, cervicothoracic region
      M47.014 Anterior spinal artery compression syndromes, thoracic region
      M47.015 Anterior spinal artery compression syndromes, thoracolumbar region
      M47.016 Anterior spinal artery compression syndromes, lumbar region
      M47.019 Anterior spinal artery compression syndromes, site unspecified
    ● **M47.02** Vertebral artery compression syndromes
      M47.021 Vertebral artery compression syndromes, occipito-atlanto-axial region
      M47.022 Vertebral artery compression syndromes, cervical region
      M47.029 Vertebral artery compression syndromes, site unspecified

  ● **M47.1** **Other spondylosis with myelopathy**
     Spondylogenic compression of spinal cord
     Excludes1   vertebral subluxation (M43.3-M43.59)
   M47.10 Other spondylosis with myelopathy, site unspecified
   M47.11 Other spondylosis with myelopathy, occipito-atlanto-axial region
   M47.12 Other spondylosis with myelopathy, cervical region
   M47.13 Other spondylosis with myelopathy, cervicothoracic region
   M47.14 Other spondylosis with myelopathy, thoracic region
   M47.15 Other spondylosis with myelopathy, thoracolumbar region
   M47.16 Other spondylosis with myelopathy, lumbar region

  ● **M47.2** **Other spondylosis with radiculopathy**
   M47.20 Other spondylosis with radiculopathy, site unspecified
   M47.21 Other spondylosis with radiculopathy, occipito-atlanto-axial region
   M47.22 Other spondylosis with radiculopathy, cervical region
   M47.23 Other spondylosis with radiculopathy, cervicothoracic region
   M47.24 Other spondylosis with radiculopathy, thoracic region
   M47.25 Other spondylosis with radiculopathy, thoracolumbar region
   M47.26 Other spondylosis with radiculopathy, lumbar region
   M47.27 Other spondylosis with radiculopathy, lumbosacral region
   M47.28 Other spondylosis with radiculopathy, sacral and sacrococcygeal region

  ● **M47.8** **Other spondylosis**
    ● **M47.81** Spondylosis without myelopathy or radiculopathy
      M47.811 Spondylosis without myelopathy or radiculopathy, occipito-atlanto-axial region
      M47.812 Spondylosis without myelopathy or radiculopathy, cervical region
      M47.813 Spondylosis without myelopathy or radiculopathy, cervicothoracic region
      M47.814 Spondylosis without myelopathy or radiculopathy, thoracic region
      M47.815 Spondylosis without myelopathy or radiculopathy, thoracolumbar region
      M47.816 Spondylosis without myelopathy or radiculopathy, lumbar region
      M47.817 Spondylosis without myelopathy or radiculopathy, lumbosacral region
      M47.818 Spondylosis without myelopathy or radiculopathy, sacral and sacrococcygeal region
      M47.819 Spondylosis without myelopathy or radiculopathy, site unspecified
    ● **M47.89** Other spondylosis
      M47.891 Other spondylosis, occipito-atlanto-axial region
      M47.892 Other spondylosis, cervical region
      M47.893 Other spondylosis, cervicothoracic region
      M47.894 Other spondylosis, thoracic region
      M47.895 Other spondylosis, thoracolumbar region
      M47.896 Other spondylosis, lumbar region
      M47.897 Other spondylosis, lumbosacral region
      M47.898 Other spondylosis, sacral and sacrococcygeal region
      M47.899 Other spondylosis, site unspecified

  M47.9 **Spondylosis, unspecified**

◀ New   ◀|||| Revised   deleted Deleted   **OGCR** Official Guidelines   X Assign placeholder X   ● Use Additional Character(s)

Excludes 1   Excludes 2   Includes   Use additional   Code first   Code also   Unspecified

● **M48   Other spondylopathies**

  ● **M48.0   Spinal stenosis**
       Caudal stenosis
       M48.00   Spinal stenosis, site unspecified
       M48.01   Spinal stenosis, occipito-atlanto-axial region
       M48.02   Spinal stenosis, cervical region
       M48.03   Spinal stenosis, cervicothoracic region
       M48.04   Spinal stenosis, thoracic region
       M48.05   Spinal stenosis, thoracolumbar region
       M48.06   Spinal stenosis, lumbar region
       M48.07   Spinal stenosis, lumbosacral region
       M48.08   Spinal stenosis, sacral and sacrococcygeal region

  ● **M48.1   Ankylosing hyperostosis [Forestier]**
       Diffuse idiopathic skeletal hyperostosis [DISH]
       M48.10   Ankylosing hyperostosis [Forestier], site unspecified
       M48.11   Ankylosing hyperostosis [Forestier], occipito-atlanto-axial region
       M48.12   Ankylosing hyperostosis [Forestier], cervical region
       M48.13   Ankylosing hyperostosis [Forestier], cervicothoracic region
       M48.14   Ankylosing hyperostosis [Forestier], thoracic region
       M48.15   Ankylosing hyperostosis [Forestier], thoracolumbar region
       M48.16   Ankylosing hyperostosis [Forestier], lumbar region
       M48.17   Ankylosing hyperostosis [Forestier], lumbosacral region
       M48.18   Ankylosing hyperostosis [Forestier], sacral and sacrococcygeal region
       M48.19   Ankylosing hyperostosis [Forestier], multiple sites in spine

  ● **M48.2   Kissing spine**
       M48.20   Kissing spine, site unspecified
       M48.21   Kissing spine, occipito-atlanto-axial region
       M48.22   Kissing spine, cervical region
       M48.23   Kissing spine, cervicothoracic region
       M48.24   Kissing spine, thoracic region
       M48.25   Kissing spine, thoracolumbar region
       M48.26   Kissing spine, lumbar region
       M48.27   Kissing spine, lumbosacral region

  ● **M48.3   Traumatic spondylopathy**
       M48.30   Traumatic spondylopathy, site unspecified
       M48.31   Traumatic spondylopathy, occipito-atlanto-axial region
       M48.32   Traumatic spondylopathy, cervical region
       M48.33   Traumatic spondylopathy, cervicothoracic region
       M48.34   Traumatic spondylopathy, thoracic region
       M48.35   Traumatic spondylopathy, thoracolumbar region
       M48.36   Traumatic spondylopathy, lumbar region
       M48.37   Traumatic spondylopathy, lumbosacral region
       M48.38   Traumatic spondylopathy, sacral and sacrococcygeal region

  ● **M48.4   Fatigue fracture of vertebra**
       Stress fracture of vertebra

       Excludes1   pathological fracture NOS (M84.4-)
                    pathological fracture of vertebra due to neoplasm (M84.58)
                    pathological fracture of vertebra due to other diagnosis (M84.68)
                    pathological fracture of vertebra due to osteoporosis (M80.-)
                    traumatic fracture of vertebrae (S12.0-S12.3-, S22.0-, S32.0-)

       The appropriate 7th character is to be added to each code from subcategory M48.4:

       A   initial encounter for fracture
       D   subsequent encounter for fracture with routine healing
       G   subsequent encounter for fracture with delayed healing
       S   sequela of fracture

     X ● M48.40   Fatigue fracture of vertebra, site unspecified
     X ● M48.41   Fatigue fracture of vertebra, occipitoatlanto-axial region
     X ● M48.42   Fatigue fracture of vertebra, cervical region
     X ● M48.43   Fatigue fracture of vertebra, cervicothoracic region
     X ● M48.44   Fatigue fracture of vertebra, thoracic region
     X ● M48.45   Fatigue fracture of vertebra, thoracolumbar region
     X ● M48.46   Fatigue fracture of vertebra, lumbar region
     X ● M48.47   Fatigue fracture of vertebra, lumbosacral region
     X ● M48.48   Fatigue fracture of vertebra, sacral and sacrococcygeal region

  ● **M48.5   Collapsed vertebra, not elsewhere classified**
       Collapsed vertebra NOS
       Wedging of vertebra NOS

       Excludes1   current injury - see Injury of spine, by body region
                    fatigue fracture of vertebra (M48.4)
                    pathological fracture of vertebra due to neoplasm (M84.58)
                    pathological fracture of vertebra due to other diagnosis (M84.68)
                    pathological fracture of vertebra due to osteoporosis (M80.-)
                    pathological fracture NOS (M84.4-)
                    stress fracture of vertebra (M48.4-)
                    traumatic fracture of vertebra (S12.-, S22.-, S32.-)

       The appropriate 7th character is to be added to each code from subcategory M48.5:

       A   initial encounter for fracture
       D   subsequent encounter for fracture with routine healing
       G   subsequent encounter for fracture with delayed healing
       S   sequela of fracture

     X ● M48.50   Collapsed vertebra, not elsewhere classified, site unspecified
     X ● M48.51   Collapsed vertebra, not elsewhere classified, occipito-atlanto-axial region
     X ● M48.52   Collapsed vertebra, not elsewhere classified, cervical region
     X ● M48.53   Collapsed vertebra, not elsewhere classified, cervicothoracic region

CHAPTER 13 (M00-M99)

X ● **M48.54 Collapsed vertebra, not elsewhere classified, thoracic region**

X ● **M48.55 Collapsed vertebra, not elsewhere classified, thoracolumbar region**

X ● **M48.56 Collapsed vertebra, not elsewhere classified, lumbar region**

X ● **M48.57 Collapsed vertebra, not elsewhere classified, lumbosacral region**

X ● **M48.58 Collapsed vertebra, not elsewhere classified, sacral and sacrococcygeal region**

● **M48.8 Other specified spondylopathies**
Ossification of posterior longitudinal ligament

● **M48.8X Other specified spondylopathies**

M48.8X1 Other specified spondylopathies, occipito-atlanto-axial region

M48.8X2 Other specified spondylopathies, cervical region

M48.8X3 Other specified spondylopathies, cervicothoracic region

M48.8X4 Other specified spondylopathies, thoracic region

M48.8X5 Other specified spondylopathies, thoracolumbar region

M48.8X6 Other specified spondylopathies, lumbar region

M48.8X7 Other specified spondylopathies, lumbosacral region

M48.8X8 Other specified spondylopathies, sacral and sacrococcygeal region

M48.8X9 Other specified spondylopathies, site unspecified

M48.9 Spondylopathy, unspecified

● **M49 Spondylopathies in diseases classified elsewhere**

Includes curvature of spine in diseases classified elsewhere
deformity of spine in diseases classified elsewhere
kyphosis in diseases classified elsewhere
scoliosis in diseases classified elsewhere
spondylopathy in diseases classified elsewhere

Code first underlying disease, such as:
brucellosis (A23.-)
Charcot-Marie-Tooth disease (G60.0)
enterobacterial infections (A01-A04)
osteitis fibrosa cystica (E21.0)

Excludes1 curvature of spine in tuberculosis [Pott's] (A18.01)
enteropathic arthropathies (M07.-)
gonococcal spondylitis (A54.41)
neuropathic [tabes dorsalis] spondylitis (A52.11)
neuropathic spondylopathy in syringomyelia (G95.0)
neuropathic spondylopathy in tabes dorsalis (A52.11)
nonsyphilitic neuropathic spondylopathy NEC (G98.0)
spondylitis in syphilis (acquired) (A52.77)
tuberculous spondylitis (A18.01)
typhoid fever spondylitis (A01.05)

● **M49.8 Spondylopathy in diseases classified elsewhere**

M49.80 Spondylopathy in diseases classified elsewhere, site unspecified

M49.81 Spondylopathy in diseases classified elsewhere, occipito-atlanto-axial region

M49.82 Spondylopathy in diseases classified elsewhere, cervical region

M49.83 Spondylopathy in diseases classified elsewhere, cervicothoracic region

M49.84 Spondylopathy in diseases classified elsewhere, thoracic region

M49.85 Spondylopathy in diseases classified elsewhere, thoracolumbar region

M49.86 Spondylopathy in diseases classified elsewhere, lumbar region

M49.87 Spondylopathy in diseases classified elsewhere, lumbosacral region

M49.88 Spondylopathy in diseases classified elsewhere, sacral and sacrococcygeal region

M49.89 Spondylopathy in diseases classified elsewhere, multiple sites in spine

---

OTHER DORSOPATHIES (M50-M54)

Excludes1 current injury - see injury of spine by body region
discitis NOS (M46.4-)

● **M50 Cervical disc disorders**
Note: Code to the most superior level of disorder.

Includes cervicothoracic disc disorders with cervicalgia
cervicothoracic disc disorders

● **M50.0 Cervical disc disorder with myelopathy**

M50.00 Cervical disc disorder with myelopathy, unspecified cervical region

M50.01 Cervical disc disorder with myelopathy, high cervical region
C2-C3 disc disorder with myelopathy
C3-C4 disc disorder with myelopathy

M50.02 Cervical disc disorder with myelopathy, mid-cervical region
C4-C5 disc disorder with myelopathy
C5-C6 disc disorder with myelopathy
C6-C7 disc disorder with myelopathy

M50.03 Cervical disc disorder with myelopathy, cervicothoracic region
C7-T1 disc disorder with myelopathy

● **M50.1 Cervical disc disorder with radiculopathy**
Excludes2 brachial radiculitis NOS (M54.13)

M50.10 Cervical disc disorder with radiculopathy, unspecified cervical region

M50.11 Cervical disc disorder with radiculopathy, high cervical region
C2-C3 disc disorder with radiculopathy
C3 radiculopathy due to disc disorder
C3-C4 disc disorder with radiculopathy
C4 radiculopathy due to disc disorder

M50.12 Cervical disc disorder with radiculopathy, mid-cervical region
C4-C5 disc disorder with radiculopathy
C5 radiculopathy due to disc disorder
C5-C6 disc disorder with radiculopathy
C6 radiculopathy due to disc disorder
C6-C7 disc disorder with radiculopathy
C7 radiculopathy due to disc disorder

M50.13 Cervical disc disorder with radiculopathy, cervicothoracic region
C7-T1 disc disorder with radiculopathy
C8 radiculopathy due to disc disorder

● **M50.2 Other cervical disc displacement**

M50.20 Other cervical disc displacement, unspecified cervical region

M50.21 Other cervical disc displacement, high cervical region
Other C2-C3 cervical disc displacement
Other C3-C4 cervical disc displacement

M50.22 Other cervical disc displacement, mid-cervical region
Other C4-C5 cervical disc displacement
Other C5-C6 cervical disc displacement
Other C6-C7 cervical disc displacement

M50.23 Other cervical disc displacement, cervicothoracic region
Other C7-T1 cervical disc displacement

◄ New   ◄ Revised   ~~deleted~~ Deleted   OGCR Official Guidelines   X Assign placeholder X   ● Use Additional Character(s)

Excludes 1   Excludes 2   Includes   Use additional   Code first   Code also   Unspecified

● **M50.3 Other cervical disc degeneration**

    M50.30 Other cervical disc degeneration, unspecified cervical region

    M50.31 Other cervical disc degeneration, high cervical region
        Other C2-C3 cervical disc degeneration
        Other C3-C4 cervical disc degeneration

    M50.32 Other cervical disc degeneration, mid-cervical region
        Other C4-C5 cervical disc degeneration
        Other C5-C6 cervical disc degeneration
        Other C6-C7 cervical disc degeneration

    M50.33 Other cervical disc degeneration, cervicothoracic region
        Other C7-T1 cervical disc degeneration

● **M50.8 Other cervical disc disorders**

    M50.80 Other cervical disc disorders, unspecified cervical region

    M50.81 Other cervical disc disorders, high cervical region
        Other C2-C3 cervical disc disorders
        Other C3-C4 cervical disc disorders

    M50.82 Other cervical disc disorders, mid-cervical region
        Other C4-C5 cervical disc disorders
        Other C5-C6 cervical disc disorders
        Other C6-C7 cervical disc disorders

    M50.83 Other cervical disc disorders, cervicothoracic region
        Other C7-T1 cervical disc disorders

● **M50.9 Cervical disc disorder, unspecified**

    M50.90 Cervical disc disorder, unspecified, unspecified cervical region

    M50.91 Cervical disc disorder, unspecified, high cervical region
        C2-C3 cervical disc disorder, unspecified
        C3-C4 cervical disc disorder, unspecified

    M50.92 Cervical disc disorder, unspecified, mid-cervical region
        C4-C5 cervical disc disorder, unspecified
        C5-C6 cervical disc disorder, unspecified
        C6-C7 cervical disc disorder, unspecified

    M50.93 Cervical disc disorder, unspecified, cervicothoracic region
        C7-T1 cervical disc disorder, unspecified

● **M51 Thoracic, thoracolumbar, and lumbosacral intervertebral disc disorders**

    Excludes2   cervical and cervicothoracic disc disorders (M50.-)
              sacral and sacrococcygeal disorders (M53.3)

● **M51.0 Thoracic, thoracolumbar and lumbosacral intervertebral disc disorders with myelopathy**

    M51.04 Intervertebral disc disorders with myelopathy, thoracic region

    M51.05 Intervertebral disc disorders with myelopathy, thoracolumbar region

    M51.06 Intervertebral disc disorders with myelopathy, lumbar region

● **M51.1 Thoracic, thoracolumbar and lumbosacral intervertebral disc disorders with radiculopathy**
    Sciatica due to intervertebral disc disorder

    Excludes1   lumbar radiculitis NOS (M54.16)
              sciatica NOS (M54.3)

    M51.14 Intervertebral disc disorders with radiculopathy, thoracic region

    M51.15 Intervertebral disc disorders with radiculopathy, thoracolumbar region

    M51.16 Intervertebral disc disorders with radiculopathy, lumbar region

    M51.17 Intervertebral disc disorders with radiculopathy, lumbosacral region

● **M51.2 Other thoracic, thoracolumbar and lumbosacral intervertebral disc displacement**
    Lumbago due to displacement of intervertebral disc

    M51.24 Other intervertebral disc displacement, thoracic region

    M51.25 Other intervertebral disc displacement, thoracolumbar region

    M51.26 Other intervertebral disc displacement, lumbar region

    M51.27 Other intervertebral disc displacement, lumbosacral region

● **M51.3 Other thoracic, thoracolumbar and lumbosacral intervertebral disc degeneration**

    M51.34 Other intervertebral disc degeneration, thoracic region

    M51.35 Other intervertebral disc degeneration, thoracolumbar region

    M51.36 Other intervertebral disc degeneration, lumbar region

    M51.37 Other intervertebral disc degeneration, lumbosacral region

● **M51.4 Schmorl's nodes**

    M51.44 Schmorl's nodes, thoracic region

    M51.45 Schmorl's nodes, thoracolumbar region

    M51.46 Schmorl's nodes, lumbar region

    M51.47 Schmorl's nodes, lumbosacral region

● **M51.8 Other thoracic, thoracolumbar and lumbosacral intervertebral disc disorders**

    M51.84 Other intervertebral disc disorders, thoracic region

    M51.85 Other intervertebral disc disorders, thoracolumbar region

    M51.86 Other intervertebral disc disorders, lumbar region

    M51.87 Other intervertebral disc disorders, lumbosacral region

    M51.9 Unspecified thoracic, thoracolumbar and lumbosacral intervertebral disc disorder

● **M53 Other and unspecified dorsopathies, not elsewhere classified**

    M53.0 Cervicocranial syndrome
        Posterior cervical sympathetic syndrome

    M53.1 Cervicobrachial syndrome

        Excludes2   cervical disc disorder (M50.-)
                  thoracic outlet syndrome (G54.0)

● **M53.2 Spinal instabilities**

    ● **M53.2X Spinal instabilities**

        M53.2X1 Spinal instabilities, occipito-atlanto-axial region

        M53.2X2 Spinal instabilities, cervical region

        M53.2X3 Spinal instabilities, cervicothoracic region

        M53.2X4 Spinal instabilities, thoracic region

        M53.2X5 Spinal instabilities, thoracolumbar region

        M53.2X6 Spinal instabilities, lumbar region

        M53.2X7 Spinal instabilities, lumbosacral region

        M53.2X8 Spinal instabilities, sacral and sacrococcygeal region

        M53.2X9 Spinal instabilities, site unspecified

    M53.3 Sacrococcygeal disorders, not elsewhere classified
        Coccygodynia

● **M53.8 Other specified dorsopathies**

    M53.80 Other specified dorsopathies, site unspecified

    M53.81 Other specified dorsopathies, occipito-atlanto-axial region

    M53.82 Other specified dorsopathies, cervical region

◀ New   ⬛ Revised   ~~deleted~~ Deleted   OGCR Official Guidelines   X Assign placeholder X   ● Use Additional Character(s)

Excludes 1   Excludes 2   Includes   Use additional   Code first   Code also   Unspecified

M53.83　Other specified dorsopathies, cervicothoracic region

M53.84　Other specified dorsopathies, thoracic region

M53.85　Other specified dorsopathies, thoracolumbar region

M53.86　Other specified dorsopathies, lumbar region

M53.87　Other specified dorsopathies, lumbosacral region

M53.88　Other specified dorsopathies, sacral and sacrococcygeal region

M53.9　Dorsopathy, unspecified

● M54　Dorsalgia

> Excludes1　psychogenic dorsalgia (F45.41)

● M54.0　Panniculitis affecting regions of neck and back

> Excludes1　lupus panniculitis (L93.2)
> panniculitis NOS (M79.3)
> relapsing [Weber-Christian] panniculitis (M35.6)

M54.00　Panniculitis affecting regions of neck and back, site unspecified

M54.01　Panniculitis affecting regions of neck and back, occipito-atlanto-axial region

M54.02　Panniculitis affecting regions of neck and back, cervical region

M54.03　Panniculitis affecting regions of neck and back, cervicothoracic region

M54.04　Panniculitis affecting regions of neck and back, thoracic region

M54.05　Panniculitis affecting regions of neck and back, thoracolumbar region

M54.06　Panniculitis affecting regions of neck and back, lumbar region

M54.07　Panniculitis affecting regions of neck and back, lumbosacral region

M54.08　Panniculitis affecting regions of neck and back, sacral and sacrococcygeal region

M54.09　Panniculitis affecting regions, neck and back, multiple sites in spine

● M54.1　Radiculopathy

Brachial neuritis or radiculitis NOS
Lumbar neuritis or radiculitis NOS
Lumbosacral neuritis or radiculitis NOS
Thoracic neuritis or radiculitis NOS
Radiculitis NOS

> Excludes1　neuralgia and neuritis NOS (M79.2)
> radiculopathy with cervical disc disorder (M50.1)
> radiculopathy with lumbar and other intervertebral disc disorder (M51.1-)
> radiculopathy with spondylosis (M47.2-)

M54.10　Radiculopathy, site unspecified

M54.11　Radiculopathy, occipito-atlanto-axial region

M54.12　Radiculopathy, cervical region

M54.13　Radiculopathy, cervicothoracic region

M54.14　Radiculopathy, thoracic region

M54.15　Radiculopathy, thoracolumbar region

M54.16　Radiculopathy, lumbar region

M54.17　Radiculopathy, lumbosacral region

M54.18　Radiculopathy, sacral and sacrococcygeal region

M54.2　Cervicalgia

> Excludes1　cervicalgia due to intervertebral cervical disc disorder (M50.-)

● M54.3　Sciatica

> Excludes1　lesion of sciatic nerve (G57.0)
> sciatica due to intervertebral disc disorder (M51.1-)
> sciatica with lumbago (M54.4-)

M54.30　Sciatica, unspecified side

M54.31　Sciatica, right side

M54.32　Sciatica, left side

● M54.4　Lumbago with sciatica

> Excludes1　lumbago with sciatica due to intervertebral disc disorder (M51.1-)

M54.40　Lumbago with sciatica, unspecified side

M54.41　Lumbago with sciatica, right side

M54.42　Lumbago with sciatica, left side

M54.5　Low back pain

Loin pain
Lumbago NOS

> Excludes1　low back strain (S39.012)
> lumbago due to intervertebral disc displacement (M51.2-)
> lumbago with sciatica (M54.4-)

M54.6　Pain in thoracic spine

> Excludes1　pain in thoracic spine due to intervertebral disc disorder (M51.)

● M54.8　Other dorsalgia

> Excludes1　dorsalgia in thoracic region (M54.6)
> low back pain (M54.5)

M54.81　Occipital neuralgia

M54.89　Other dorsalgia

M54.9　Dorsalgia, unspecified

Backache NOS
Back pain NOS

SOFT TISSUE DISORDERS (M60-M79)

DISORDERS OF MUSCLES (M60-M63)

> Excludes1　dermatopolymyositis (M33.-)
> muscular dystrophies and myopathies (G71-G72)
> myopathy in amyloidosis (E85.-)
> myopathy in polyarteritis nodosa (M30.0)
> myopathy in rheumatoid arthritis (M05.32)
> myopathy in scleroderma (M34.-)
> myopathy in Sjögren's syndrome (M35.03)
> myopathy in systemic lupus erythematosus (M32.-)

● M60　Myositis

> Excludes2　inclusion body myositis [IBM] (G72.41)

● M60.0　Infective myositis

Tropical pyomyositis

Use additional code (B95-B97) to identify infectious agent

● M60.00　Infective myositis, unspecified site

M60.000　Infective myositis, unspecified right arm

Infective myositis, right upper limb NOS

M60.001　Infective myositis, unspecified left arm

Infective myositis, left upper limb NOS

M60.002　Infective myositis, unspecified arm

Infective myositis, upper limb NOS

M60.003　Infective myositis, unspecified right leg

Infective myositis, right lower limb NOS

M60.004　Infective myositis, unspecified left leg

Infective myositis, left lower limb NOS

M60.005　Infective myositis, unspecified leg

Infective myositis, lower limb NOS

M60.009　Infective myositis, unspecified site

● M60.01　Infective myositis, shoulder

M60.011　Infective myositis, right shoulder

M60.012　Infective myositis, left shoulder

M60.019　Infective myositis, unspecified shoulder

◀ New　　◀▥ Revised　　~~deleted~~ Deleted　　OGCR Official Guidelines　　X Assign placeholder X　　● Use Additional Character(s)

Excludes 1　　Excludes 2　　Includes　　Use additional　　Code first　　Code also　　Unspecified

● M60.02 Infective myositis, upper arm
    M60.021 Infective myositis, right upper arm
    M60.022 Infective myositis, left upper arm
    M60.029 Infective myositis, unspecified upper
            arm
● M60.03 Infective myositis, forearm
    M60.031 Infective myositis, right forearm
    M60.032 Infective myositis, left forearm
    M60.039 Infective myositis, unspecified
            forearm
● M60.04 Infective myositis, hand and fingers
    M60.041 Infective myositis, right hand
    M60.042 Infective myositis, left hand
    M60.043 Infective myositis, unspecified hand
    M60.044 Infective myositis, right finger(s)
    M60.045 Infective myositis, left finger(s)
    M60.046 Infective myositis, unspecified
            finger(s)
● M60.05 Infective myositis, thigh
    M60.051 Infective myositis, right thigh
    M60.052 Infective myositis, left thigh
    M60.059 Infective myositis, unspecified thigh
● M60.06 Infective myositis, lower leg
    M60.061 Infective myositis, right lower leg
    M60.062 Infective myositis, left lower leg
    M60.069 Infective myositis, unspecified lower
            leg
● M60.07 Infective myositis, ankle, foot and toes
    M60.070 Infective myositis, right ankle
    M60.071 Infective myositis, left ankle
    M60.072 Infective myositis, unspecified ankle
    M60.073 Infective myositis, right foot
    M60.074 Infective myositis, left foot
    M60.075 Infective myositis, unspecified foot
    M60.076 Infective myositis, right toe(s)
    M60.077 Infective myositis, left toe(s)
    M60.078 Infective myositis, unspecified toe(s)
    M60.08 Infective myositis, other site
    M60.09 Infective myositis, multiple sites
● M60.1 Interstitial myositis
    M60.10 Interstitial myositis of unspecified site
● M60.11 Interstitial myositis, shoulder
    M60.111 Interstitial myositis, right shoulder
    M60.112 Interstitial myositis, left shoulder
    M60.119 Interstitial myositis, unspecified
            shoulder
● M60.12 Interstitial myositis, upper arm
    M60.121 Interstitial myositis, right upper arm
    M60.122 Interstitial myositis, left upper arm
    M60.129 Interstitial myositis, unspecified
            upper arm
● M60.13 Interstitial myositis, forearm
    M60.131 Interstitial myositis, right forearm
    M60.132 Interstitial myositis, left forearm
    M60.139 Interstitial myositis, unspecified
            forearm
● M60.14 Interstitial myositis, hand
    M60.141 Interstitial myositis, right hand
    M60.142 Interstitial myositis, left hand
    M60.149 Interstitial myositis, unspecified hand
● M60.15 Interstitial myositis, thigh
    M60.151 Interstitial myositis, right thigh
    M60.152 Interstitial myositis, left thigh
    M60.159 Interstitial myositis, unspecified thigh

● M60.16 Interstitial myositis, lower leg
    M60.161 Interstitial myositis, right lower leg
    M60.162 Interstitial myositis, left lower leg
    M60.169 Interstitial myositis, unspecified
            lower leg
● M60.17 Interstitial myositis, ankle and foot
    M60.171 Interstitial myositis, right ankle and
            foot
    M60.172 Interstitial myositis, left ankle and
            foot
    M60.179 Interstitial myositis, unspecified
            ankle and foot
    M60.18 Interstitial myositis, other site
    M60.19 Interstitial myositis, multiple sites
● M60.2 Foreign body granuloma of soft tissue, not elsewhere
        classified
        Use additional code to identify the type of retained
        foreign body (Z18.-)
        Excludes1   foreign body granuloma of skin and
                    subcutaneous tissue (L92.3)
    M60.20 Foreign body granuloma of soft tissue, not
            elsewhere classified, unspecified site
● M60.21 Foreign body granuloma of soft tissue, not
        elsewhere classified, shoulder
    M60.211 Foreign body granuloma of soft
            tissue, not elsewhere classified, right
            shoulder
    M60.212 Foreign body granuloma of soft
            tissue, not elsewhere classified, left
            shoulder
    M60.219 Foreign body granuloma of soft
            tissue, not elsewhere classified,
            unspecified shoulder
● M60.22 Foreign body granuloma of soft tissue, not
        elsewhere classified, upper arm
    M60.221 Foreign body granuloma of soft
            tissue, not elsewhere classified, right
            upper arm
    M60.222 Foreign body granuloma of soft
            tissue, not elsewhere classified, left
            upper arm
    M60.229 Foreign body granuloma of soft
            tissue, not elsewhere classified,
            unspecified upper arm
● M60.23 Foreign body granuloma of soft tissue, not
        elsewhere classified, forearm
    M60.231 Foreign body granuloma of soft
            tissue, not elsewhere classified, right
            forearm
    M60.232 Foreign body granuloma of soft
            tissue, not elsewhere classified, left
            forearm
    M60.239 Foreign body granuloma of soft
            tissue, not elsewhere classified,
            unspecified forearm
● M60.24 Foreign body granuloma of soft tissue, not
        elsewhere classified, hand
    M60.241 Foreign body granuloma of soft tissue,
            not elsewhere classified, right hand
    M60.242 Foreign body granuloma of soft
            tissue, not elsewhere classified, left
            hand
    M60.249 Foreign body granuloma of soft
            tissue, not elsewhere classified,
            unspecified hand

● M60.25   Foreign body granuloma of soft tissue, not elsewhere classified, thigh

     M60.251   Foreign body granuloma of soft tissue, not elsewhere classified, right thigh

     M60.252   Foreign body granuloma of soft tissue, not elsewhere classified, left thigh

     M60.259   Foreign body granuloma of soft tissue, not elsewhere classified, unspecified thigh

● M60.26   Foreign body granuloma of soft tissue, not elsewhere classified, lower leg

     M60.261   Foreign body granuloma of soft tissue, not elsewhere classified, right lower leg

     M60.262   Foreign body granuloma of soft tissue, not elsewhere classified, left lower leg

     M60.269   Foreign body granuloma of soft tissue, not elsewhere classified, unspecified lower leg

● M60.27   Foreign body granuloma of soft tissue, not elsewhere classified, ankle and foot

     M60.271   Foreign body granuloma of soft tissue, not elsewhere classified, right ankle and foot

     M60.272   Foreign body granuloma of soft tissue, not elsewhere classified, left ankle and foot

     M60.279   Foreign body granuloma of soft tissue, not elsewhere classified, unspecified ankle and foot

   M60.28   Foreign body granuloma of soft tissue, not elsewhere classified, other site

● M60.8   Other myositis

   M60.80   Other myositis, unspecified site

● M60.81   Other myositis shoulder

     M60.811   Other myositis, right shoulder

     M60.812   Other myositis, left shoulder

     M60.819   Other myositis, unspecified shoulder

● M60.82   Other myositis, upper arm

     M60.821   Other myositis, right upper arm

     M60.822   Other myositis, left upper arm

     M60.829   Other myositis, unspecified upper arm

● M60.83   Other myositis, forearm

     M60.831   Other myositis, right forearm

     M60.832   Other myositis, left forearm

     M60.839   Other myositis, unspecified forearm

● M60.84   Other myositis, hand

     M60.841   Other myositis, right hand

     M60.842   Other myositis, left hand

     M60.849   Other myositis, unspecified hand

● M60.85   Other myositis, thigh

     M60.851   Other myositis, right thigh

     M60.852   Other myositis, left thigh

     M60.859   Other myositis, unspecified thigh

● M60.86   Other myositis, lower leg

     M60.861   Other myositis, right lower leg

     M60.862   Other myositis, left lower leg

     M60.869   Other myositis, unspecified lower leg

● M60.87   Other myositis, ankle and foot

     M60.871   Other myositis, right ankle and foot

     M60.872   Other myositis, left ankle and foot

     M60.879   Other myositis, unspecified ankle and foot

   M60.88   Other myositis, other site

   M60.89   Other myositis, multiple sites

  M60.9   Myositis, unspecified

● M61   Calcification and ossification of muscle

  ● M61.0   Myositis ossificans traumatica

     M61.00   Myositis ossificans traumatica, unspecified site

   ● M61.01   Myositis ossificans traumatica, shoulder

     M61.011   Myositis ossificans traumatica, right shoulder

     M61.012   Myositis ossificans traumatica, left shoulder

     M61.019   Myositis ossificans traumatica, unspecified shoulder

   ● M61.02   Myositis ossificans traumatica, upper arm

     M61.021   Myositis ossificans traumatica, right upper arm

     M61.022   Myositis ossificans traumatica, left upper arm

     M61.029   Myositis ossificans traumatica, unspecified upper arm

   ● M61.03   Myositis ossificans traumatica, forearm

     M61.031   Myositis ossificans traumatica, right forearm

     M61.032   Myositis ossificans traumatica, left forearm

     M61.039   Myositis ossificans traumatica, unspecified forearm

   ● M61.04   Myositis ossificans traumatica, hand

     M61.041   Myositis ossificans traumatica, right hand

     M61.042   Myositis ossificans traumatica, left hand

     M61.049   Myositis ossificans traumatica, unspecified hand

   ● M61.05   Myositis ossificans traumatica, thigh

     M61.051   Myositis ossificans traumatica, right thigh

     M61.052   Myositis ossificans traumatica, left thigh

     M61.059   Myositis ossificans traumatica, unspecified thigh

   ● M61.06   Myositis ossificans traumatica, lower leg

     M61.061   Myositis ossificans traumatica, right lower leg

     M61.062   Myositis ossificans traumatica, left lower leg

     M61.069   Myositis ossificans traumatica, unspecified lower leg

   ● M61.07   Myositis ossificans traumatica, ankle and foot

     M61.071   Myositis ossificans traumatica, right ankle and foot

     M61.072   Myositis ossificans traumatica, left ankle and foot

     M61.079   Myositis ossificans traumatica, unspecified ankle and foot

     M61.08   Myositis ossificans traumatica, other site

     M61.09   Myositis ossificans traumatica, multiple sites

● M61.1　Myositis ossificans progressiva
　　　　Fibrodysplasia ossificans progressiva
　　M61.10　Myositis ossificans progressiva, unspecified site
● M61.11　Myositis ossificans progressiva, shoulder
　　　　M61.111　Myositis ossificans progressiva, right shoulder
　　　　M61.112　Myositis ossificans progressiva, left shoulder
　　　　M61.119　Myositis ossificans progressiva, unspecified shoulder
● M61.12　Myositis ossificans progressiva, upper arm
　　　　M61.121　Myositis ossificans progressiva, right upper arm
　　　　M61.122　Myositis ossificans progressiva, left upper arm
　　　　M61.129　Myositis ossificans progressiva, unspecified arm
● M61.13　Myositis ossificans progressiva, forearm
　　　　M61.131　Myositis ossificans progressiva, right forearm
　　　　M61.132　Myositis ossificans progressiva, left forearm
　　　　M61.139　Myositis ossificans progressiva, unspecified forearm
● M61.14　Myositis ossificans progressiva, hand and finger(s)
　　　　M61.141　Myositis ossificans progressiva, right hand
　　　　M61.142　Myositis ossificans progressiva, left hand
　　　　M61.143　Myositis ossificans progressiva, unspecified hand
　　　　M61.144　Myositis ossificans progressiva, right finger(s)
　　　　M61.145　Myositis ossificans progressiva, left finger(s)
　　　　M61.146　Myositis ossificans progressiva, unspecified finger(s)
● M61.15　Myositis ossificans progressiva, thigh
　　　　M61.151　Myositis ossificans progressiva, right thigh
　　　　M61.152　Myositis ossificans progressiva, left thigh
　　　　M61.159　Myositis ossificans progressiva, unspecified thigh
● M61.16　Myositis ossificans progressiva, lower leg
　　　　M61.161　Myositis ossificans progressiva, right lower leg
　　　　M61.162　Myositis ossificans progressiva, left lower leg
　　　　M61.169　Myositis ossificans progressiva, unspecified lower leg
● M61.17　Myositis ossificans progressiva, ankle, foot and toe(s)
　　　　M61.171　Myositis ossificans progressiva, right ankle
　　　　M61.172　Myositis ossificans progressiva, left ankle
　　　　M61.173　Myositis ossificans progressiva, unspecified ankle
　　　　M61.174　Myositis ossificans progressiva, right foot
　　　　M61.175　Myositis ossificans progressiva, left foot
　　　　M61.176　Myositis ossificans progressiva, unspecified foot
　　　　M61.177　Myositis ossificans progressiva, right toe(s)

　　　　M61.178　Myositis ossificans progressiva, left toe(s)
　　　　M61.179　Myositis ossificans progressiva, unspecified toe(s)
　　M61.18　Myositis ossificans progressiva, other site
　　M61.19　Myositis ossificans progressiva, multiple sites
● M61.2　Paralytic calcification and ossification of muscle
　　　　Myositis ossificans associated with quadriplegia or paraplegia
　　M61.20　Paralytic calcification and ossification of muscle, unspecified site
● M61.21　Paralytic calcification and ossification of muscle, shoulder
　　　　M61.211　Paralytic calcification and ossification of muscle, right shoulder
　　　　M61.212　Paralytic calcification and ossification of muscle, left shoulder
　　　　M61.219　Paralytic calcification and ossification of muscle, unspecified shoulder
● M61.22　Paralytic calcification and ossification of muscle, upper arm
　　　　M61.221　Paralytic calcification and ossification of muscle, right upper arm
　　　　M61.222　Paralytic calcification and ossification of muscle, left upper arm
　　　　M61.229　Paralytic calcification and ossification of muscle, unspecified upper arm
● M61.23　Paralytic calcification and ossification of muscle, forearm
　　　　M61.231　Paralytic calcification and ossification of muscle, right forearm
　　　　M61.232　Paralytic calcification and ossification of muscle, left forearm
　　　　M61.239　Paralytic calcification and ossification of muscle, unspecified forearm
● M61.24　Paralytic calcification and ossification of muscle, hand
　　　　M61.241　Paralytic calcification and ossification of muscle, right hand
　　　　M61.242　Paralytic calcification and ossification of muscle, left hand
　　　　M61.249　Paralytic calcification and ossification of muscle, unspecified hand
● M61.25　Paralytic calcification and ossification of muscle, thigh
　　　　M61.251　Paralytic calcification and ossification of muscle, right thigh
　　　　M61.252　Paralytic calcification and ossification of muscle, left thigh
　　　　M61.259　Paralytic calcification and ossification of muscle, unspecified thigh
● M61.26　Paralytic calcification and ossification of muscle, lower leg
　　　　M61.261　Paralytic calcification and ossification of muscle, right lower leg
　　　　M61.262　Paralytic calcification and ossification of muscle, left lower leg
　　　　M61.269　Paralytic calcification and ossification of muscle, unspecified lower leg
● M61.27　Paralytic calcification and ossification of muscle, ankle and foot
　　　　M61.271　Paralytic calcification and ossification of muscle, right ankle and foot
　　　　M61.272　Paralytic calcification and ossification of muscle, left ankle and foot
　　　　M61.279　Paralytic calcification and ossification of muscle, unspecified ankle and foot
　　M61.28　Paralytic calcification and ossification of muscle, other site
　　M61.29　Paralytic calcification and ossification of muscle, multiple sites

● M61.3   Calcification and ossification of muscles associated with burns

     Myositis ossificans associated with burns

   M61.30   Calcification and ossification of muscles associated with burns, unspecified site

● M61.31   Calcification and ossification of muscles associated with burns, shoulder

     M61.311   Calcification and ossification of muscles associated with burns, right shoulder

     M61.312   Calcification and ossification of muscles associated with burns, left shoulder

     M61.319   Calcification and ossification of muscles associated with burns, unspecified shoulder

● M61.32   Calcification and ossification of muscles associated with burns, upper arm

     M61.321   Calcification and ossification of muscles associated with burns, right upper arm

     M61.322   Calcification and ossification of muscles associated with burns, left upper arm

     M61.329   Calcification and ossification of muscles associated with burns, unspecified upper arm

● M61.33   Calcification and ossification of muscles associated with burns, forearm

     M61.331   Calcification and ossification of muscles associated with burns, right forearm

     M61.332   Calcification and ossification of muscles associated with burns, left forearm

     M61.339   Calcification and ossification of muscles associated with burns, unspecified forearm

● M61.34   Calcification and ossification of muscles associated with burns, hand

     M61.341   Calcification and ossification of muscles associated with burns, right hand

     M61.342   Calcification and ossification of muscles associated with burns, left hand

     M61.349   Calcification and ossification of muscles associated with burns, unspecified hand

● M61.35   Calcification and ossification of muscles associated with burns, thigh

     M61.351   Calcification and ossification of muscles associated with burns, right thigh

     M61.352   Calcification and ossification of muscles associated with burns, left thigh

     M61.359   Calcification and ossification of muscles associated with burns, unspecified thigh

● M61.36   Calcification and ossification of muscles associated with burns, lower leg

     M61.361   Calcification and ossification of muscles associated with burns, right lower leg

     M61.362   Calcification and ossification of muscles associated with burns, left lower leg

     M61.369   Calcification and ossification of muscles associated with burns, unspecified lower leg

● M61.37   Calcification and ossification of muscles associated with burns, ankle and foot

     M61.371   Calcification and ossification of muscles associated with burns, right ankle and foot

     M61.372   Calcification and ossification of muscles associated with burns, left ankle and foot

     M61.379   Calcification and ossification of muscles associated with burns, unspecified ankle and foot

   M61.38   Calcification and ossification of muscles associated with burns, other site

   M61.39   Calcification and ossification of muscles associated with burns, multiple sites

● M61.4   Other calcification of muscle

     | Excludes1 | calcific tendinitis NOS (M65.2-)

                  calcific tendinitis of shoulder (M75.3)

   M61.40   Other calcification of muscle, unspecified site

● M61.41   Other calcification of muscle, shoulder

     M61.411   Other calcification of muscle, right shoulder

     M61.412   Other calcification of muscle, left shoulder

     M61.419   Other calcification of muscle, unspecified shoulder

● M61.42   Other calcification of muscle, upper arm

     M61.421   Other calcification of muscle, right upper arm

     M61.422   Other calcification of muscle, left upper arm

     M61.429   Other calcification of muscle, unspecified upper arm

● M61.43   Other calcification of muscle, forearm

     M61.431   Other calcification of muscle, right forearm

     M61.432   Other calcification of muscle, left forearm

     M61.439   Other calcification of muscle, unspecified forearm

● M61.44   Other calcification of muscle, hand

     M61.441   Other calcification of muscle, right hand

     M61.442   Other calcification of muscle, left hand

     M61.449   Other calcification of muscle, unspecified hand

● M61.45   Other calcification of muscle, thigh

     M61.451   Other calcification of muscle, right thigh

     M61.452   Other calcification of muscle, left thigh

     M61.459   Other calcification of muscle, unspecified thigh

● M61.46   Other calcification of muscle, lower leg

     M61.461   Other calcification of muscle, right lower leg

     M61.462   Other calcification of muscle, left lower leg

     M61.469   Other calcification of muscle, unspecified lower leg

● M61.47   Other calcification of muscle, ankle and foot

     M61.471   Other calcification of muscle, right ankle and foot

     M61.472   Other calcification of muscle, left ankle and foot

     M61.479   Other calcification of muscle, unspecified ankle and foot

   M61.48   Other calcification of muscle, other site

   M61.49   Other calcification of muscle, multiple sites

● M61.5   Other ossification of muscle

     M61.50   Other ossification of muscle, unspecified site

     ● M61.51   Other ossification of muscle, shoulder

         M61.511   Other ossification of muscle, right shoulder

         M61.512   Other ossification of muscle, left shoulder

         M61.519   Other ossification of muscle, unspecified shoulder

     ● M61.52   Other ossification of muscle, upper arm

         M61.521   Other ossification of muscle, right upper arm

         M61.522   Other ossification of muscle, left upper arm

         M61.529   Other ossification of muscle, unspecified upper arm

     ● M61.53   Other ossification of muscle, forearm

         M61.531   Other ossification of muscle, right forearm

         M61.532   Other ossification of muscle, left forearm

         M61.539   Other ossification of muscle, unspecified forearm

     ● M61.54   Other ossification of muscle, hand

         M61.541   Other ossification of muscle, right hand

         M61.542   Other ossification of muscle, left hand

         M61.549   Other ossification of muscle, unspecified hand

     ● M61.55   Other ossification of muscle, thigh

         M61.551   Other ossification of muscle, right thigh

         M61.552   Other ossification of muscle, left thigh

         M61.559   Other ossification of muscle, unspecified thigh

     ● M61.56   Other ossification of muscle, lower leg

         M61.561   Other ossification of muscle, right lower leg

         M61.562   Other ossification of muscle, left lower leg

         M61.569   Other ossification of muscle, unspecified lower leg

     ● M61.57   Other ossification of muscle, ankle and foot

         M61.571   Other ossification of muscle, right ankle and foot

         M61.572   Other ossification of muscle, left ankle and foot

         M61.579   Other ossification of muscle, unspecified ankle and foot

     M61.58   Other ossification of muscle, other site

     M61.59   Other ossification of muscle, multiple sites

     M61.9   Calcification and ossification of muscle, unspecified

● M62   Other disorders of muscle

     Excludes1   alcoholic myopathy (G72.1)
              cramp and spasm (R25.2)
              drug-induced myopathy (G72.0)
              myalgia (M79.1)
              stiff-man syndrome (G25.82)

     Excludes2   nontraumatic hematoma of muscle (M79.81)

     ● M62.0   Separation of muscle (nontraumatic)

         Diastasis of muscle

         Excludes1   diastasis recti complicating pregnancy, labor and delivery (O71.8)
                  traumatic separation of muscle - see strain of muscle by body region

         M62.00   Separation of muscle (nontraumatic), unspecified site

● M62.01   Separation of muscle (nontraumatic), shoulder

     M62.011   Separation of muscle (nontraumatic), right shoulder

     M62.012   Separation of muscle (nontraumatic), left shoulder

     M62.019   Separation of muscle (nontraumatic), unspecified shoulder

● M62.02   Separation of muscle (nontraumatic), upper arm

     M62.021   Separation of muscle (nontraumatic), right upper arm

     M62.022   Separation of muscle (nontraumatic), left upper arm

     M62.029   Separation of muscle (nontraumatic), unspecified upper arm

● M62.03   Separation of muscle (nontraumatic), forearm

     M62.031   Separation of muscle (nontraumatic), right forearm

     M62.032   Separation of muscle (nontraumatic), left forearm

     M62.039   Separation of muscle (nontraumatic), unspecified forearm

● M62.04   Separation of muscle (nontraumatic), hand

     M62.041   Separation of muscle (nontraumatic), right hand

     M62.042   Separation of muscle (nontraumatic), left hand

     M62.049   Separation of muscle (nontraumatic), unspecified hand

● M62.05   Separation of muscle (nontraumatic), thigh

     M62.051   Separation of muscle (nontraumatic), right thigh

     M62.052   Separation of muscle (nontraumatic), left thigh

     M62.059   Separation of muscle (nontraumatic), unspecified thigh

● M62.06   Separation of muscle (nontraumatic), lower leg

     M62.061   Separation of muscle (nontraumatic), right lower leg

     M62.062   Separation of muscle (nontraumatic), left lower leg

     M62.069   Separation of muscle (nontraumatic), unspecified lower leg

● M62.07   Separation of muscle (nontraumatic), ankle and foot

     M62.071   Separation of muscle (nontraumatic), right ankle and foot

     M62.072   Separation of muscle (nontraumatic), left ankle and foot

     M62.079   Separation of muscle (nontraumatic), unspecified ankle and foot

     M62.08   Separation of muscle (nontraumatic), other site

● M62.1   Other rupture of muscle (nontraumatic)

     Excludes1   traumatic rupture of muscle - see strain of muscle by body region

     Excludes2   rupture of tendon (M66.-)

     M62.10   Other rupture of muscle (nontraumatic), unspecified site

     ● M62.11   Other rupture of muscle (nontraumatic), shoulder

         M62.111   Other rupture of muscle (nontraumatic), right shoulder

         M62.112   Other rupture of muscle (nontraumatic), left shoulder

         M62.119   Other rupture of muscle (nontraumatic), unspecified shoulder

● M62.12   Other rupture of muscle (nontraumatic), upper arm
- M62.121   Other rupture of muscle (nontraumatic), right upper arm
- M62.122   Other rupture of muscle (nontraumatic), left upper arm
- M62.129   Other rupture of muscle (nontraumatic), unspecified upper arm

● M62.13   Other rupture of muscle (nontraumatic), forearm
- M62.131   Other rupture of muscle (nontraumatic), right forearm
- M62.132   Other rupture of muscle (nontraumatic), left forearm
- M62.139   Other rupture of muscle (nontraumatic), unspecified forearm

● M62.14   Other rupture of muscle (nontraumatic), hand
- M62.141   Other rupture of muscle (nontraumatic), right hand
- M62.142   Other rupture of muscle (nontraumatic), left hand
- M62.149   Other rupture of muscle (nontraumatic), unspecified hand

● M62.15   Other rupture of muscle (nontraumatic), thigh
- M62.151   Other rupture of muscle (nontraumatic), right thigh
- M62.152   Other rupture of muscle (nontraumatic), left thigh
- M62.159   Other rupture of muscle (nontraumatic), unspecified thigh

● M62.16   Other rupture of muscle (nontraumatic), lower leg
- M62.161   Other rupture of muscle (nontraumatic), right lower leg
- M62.162   Other rupture of muscle (nontraumatic), left lower leg
- M62.169   Other rupture of muscle (nontraumatic), unspecified lower leg

● M62.17   Other rupture of muscle (nontraumatic), ankle and foot
- M62.171   Other rupture of muscle (nontraumatic), right ankle and foot
- M62.172   Other rupture of muscle (nontraumatic), left ankle and foot
- M62.179   Other rupture of muscle (nontraumatic), unspecified ankle and foot

M62.18   Other rupture of muscle (nontraumatic), other site

● M62.2   Nontraumatic ischemic infarction of muscle

Excludes1   compartment syndrome (traumatic) (T79.A-)
nontraumatic compartment syndrome (M79.A-)
traumatic ischemia of muscle (T79.6)
rhabdomyolysis (M62.82)
Volkmann's ischemic contracture (T79.6)

M62.20   Nontraumatic ischemic infarction of muscle, unspecified site

● M62.21   Nontraumatic ischemic infarction of muscle, shoulder
- M62.211   Nontraumatic ischemic infarction of muscle, right shoulder
- M62.212   Nontraumatic ischemic infarction of muscle, left shoulder
- M62.219   Nontraumatic ischemic infarction of muscle, unspecified shoulder

● M62.22   Nontraumatic ischemic infarction of muscle, upper arm
- M62.221   Nontraumatic ischemic infarction of muscle, right upper arm
- M62.222   Nontraumatic ischemic infarction of muscle, left upper arm
- M62.229   Nontraumatic ischemic infarction of muscle, unspecified upper arm

● M62.23   Nontraumatic ischemic infarction of muscle, forearm
- M62.231   Nontraumatic ischemic infarction of muscle, right forearm
- M62.232   Nontraumatic ischemic infarction of muscle, left forearm
- M62.239   Nontraumatic ischemic infarction of muscle, unspecified forearm

● M62.24   Nontraumatic ischemic infarction of muscle, hand
- M62.241   Nontraumatic ischemic infarction of muscle, right hand
- M62.242   Nontraumatic ischemic infarction of muscle, left hand
- M62.249   Nontraumatic ischemic infarction of muscle, unspecified hand

● M62.25   Nontraumatic ischemic infarction of muscle, thigh
- M62.251   Nontraumatic ischemic infarction of muscle, right thigh
- M62.252   Nontraumatic ischemic infarction of muscle, left thigh
- M62.259   Nontraumatic ischemic infarction of muscle, unspecified thigh

● M62.26   Nontraumatic ischemic infarction of muscle, lower leg
- M62.261   Nontraumatic ischemic infarction of muscle, right lower leg
- M62.262   Nontraumatic ischemic infarction of muscle, left lower leg
- M62.269   Nontraumatic ischemic infarction of muscle, unspecified lower leg

● M62.27   Nontraumatic ischemic infarction of muscle, ankle and foot
- M62.271   Nontraumatic ischemic infarction of muscle, right ankle and foot
- M62.272   Nontraumatic ischemic infarction of muscle, left ankle and foot
- M62.279   Nontraumatic ischemic infarction of muscle, unspecified ankle and foot

M62.28   Nontraumatic ischemic infarction of muscle, other site

M62.3   Immobility syndrome (paraplegic)

M62.4   Contracture of muscle

CONTRACTURE OF TENDON (SHEATH)

Excludes1   contracture of joint (M24.5-)

M62.40   Contracture of muscle, unspecified site

● M62.41   Contracture of muscle, shoulder
- M62.411   Contracture of muscle, right shoulder
- M62.412   Contracture of muscle, left shoulder
- M62.419   Contracture of muscle, unspecified shoulder

● M62.42   Contracture of muscle, upper arm
- M62.421   Contracture of muscle, right upper arm
- M62.422   Contracture of muscle, left upper arm
- M62.429   Contracture of muscle, unspecified upper arm

● M62.43   Contracture of muscle, forearm
     M62.431   Contracture of muscle, right forearm
     M62.432   Contracture of muscle, left forearm
     M62.439   Contracture of muscle, unspecified forearm

● M62.44   Contracture of muscle, hand
     M62.441   Contracture of muscle, right hand
     M62.442   Contracture of muscle, left hand
     M62.449   Contracture of muscle, unspecified hand

● M62.45   Contracture of muscle, thigh
     M62.451   Contracture of muscle, right thigh
     M62.452   Contracture of muscle, left thigh
     M62.459   Contracture of muscle, unspecified thigh

● M62.46   Contracture of muscle, lower leg
     M62.461   Contracture of muscle, right lower leg
     M62.462   Contracture of muscle, left lower leg
     M62.469   Contracture of muscle, unspecified lower leg

● M62.47   Contracture of muscle, ankle and foot
     M62.471   Contracture of muscle, right ankle and foot
     M62.472   Contracture of muscle, left ankle and foot
     M62.479   Contracture of muscle, unspecified ankle and foot

   M62.48   Contracture of muscle, other site

   M62.49   Contracture of muscle, multiple sites

● M62.5   Muscle wasting and atrophy, not elsewhere classified
     Disuse atrophy NEC

     Excludes1   neuralgic amyotrophy (G54.5)
                 progressive muscular atrophy (G12.29)

     Excludes2   pelvic muscle wasting (N81.84)

   M62.50   Muscle wasting and atrophy, not elsewhere classified, unspecified site

● M62.51   Muscle wasting and atrophy, not elsewhere classified, shoulder
     M62.511   Muscle wasting and atrophy, not elsewhere classified, right shoulder
     M62.512   Muscle wasting and atrophy, not elsewhere classified, left shoulder
     M62.519   Muscle wasting and atrophy, not elsewhere classified, unspecified shoulder

● M62.52   Muscle wasting and atrophy, not elsewhere classified, upper arm
     M62.521   Muscle wasting and atrophy, not elsewhere classified, right upper arm
     M62.522   Muscle wasting and atrophy, not elsewhere classified, left upper arm
     M62.529   Muscle wasting and atrophy, not elsewhere classified, unspecified upper arm

● M62.53   Muscle wasting and atrophy, not elsewhere classified, forearm
     M62.531   Muscle wasting and atrophy, not elsewhere classified, right forearm
     M62.532   Muscle wasting and atrophy, not elsewhere classified, left forearm
     M62.539   Muscle wasting and atrophy, not elsewhere classified, unspecified forearm

● M62.54   Muscle wasting and atrophy, not elsewhere classified, hand
     M62.541   Muscle wasting and atrophy, not elsewhere classified, right hand
     M62.542   Muscle wasting and atrophy, not elsewhere classified, left hand
     M62.549   Muscle wasting and atrophy, not elsewhere classified, unspecified hand

● M62.55   Muscle wasting and atrophy, not elsewhere classified, thigh
     M62.551   Muscle wasting and atrophy, not elsewhere classified, right thigh
     M62.552   Muscle wasting and atrophy, not elsewhere classified, left thigh
     M62.559   Muscle wasting and atrophy, not elsewhere classified, unspecified thigh

● M62.56   Muscle wasting and atrophy, not elsewhere classified, lower leg
     M62.561   Muscle wasting and atrophy, not elsewhere classified, right lower leg
     M62.562   Muscle wasting and atrophy, not elsewhere classified, left lower leg
     M62.569   Muscle wasting and atrophy, not elsewhere classified, unspecified lower leg

● M62.57   Muscle wasting and atrophy, not elsewhere classified, ankle and foot
     M62.571   Muscle wasting and atrophy, not elsewhere classified, right ankle and foot
     M62.572   Muscle wasting and atrophy, not elsewhere classified, left ankle and foot
     M62.579   Muscle wasting and atrophy, not elsewhere classified, unspecified ankle and foot

   M62.58   Muscle wasting and atrophy, not elsewhere classified, other site

   M62.59   Muscle wasting and atrophy, not elsewhere classified, multiple sites

● M62.8   Other specified disorders of muscle

     Excludes2   nontraumatic hematoma of muscle (M79.81)

   M62.81   Muscle weakness (generalized)

   M62.82   Rhabdomyolysis

     Excludes1   traumatic rhabdomyolysis (T79.6)

● M62.83   Muscle spasm
     M62.830   Muscle spasm of back
     M62.831   Muscle spasm of calf
               Charley-horse
     M62.838   Other muscle spasm

   M62.89   Other specified disorders of muscle
     Muscle (sheath) hernia

   M62.9   Disorder of muscle, unspecified

● **M63** **Disorders of muscle in diseases classified elsewhere**

Code first underlying disease, such as:
leprosy (A30.-)
neoplasm (C49.-, C79.89, D21.-, D48.1)
schistosomiasis (B65.-)
trichinellosis (B75)

| Excludes1 | myopathy in cysticercosis (B69.81)
myopathy in endocrine diseases (G73.7)
myopathy in metabolic diseases (G73.7)
myopathy in sarcoidosis (D86.87)
myopathy in secondary syphilis (A51.49)
myopathy in syphilis (late) (A52.78)
myopathy in toxoplasmosis (B58.82)
myopathy in tuberculosis (A18.09)

● **M63.8** **Disorders of muscle in diseases classified elsewhere**

M63.80 Disorders of muscle in diseases classified elsewhere, unspecified site

● **M63.81** Disorders of muscle in diseases classified elsewhere, shoulder

M63.811 Disorders of muscle in diseases classified elsewhere, right shoulder

M63.812 Disorders of muscle in diseases classified elsewhere, left shoulder

M63.819 Disorders of muscle in diseases classified elsewhere, unspecified shoulder

● **M63.82** Disorders of muscle in diseases classified elsewhere, upper arm

M63.821 Disorders of muscle in diseases classified elsewhere, right upper arm

M63.822 Disorders of muscle in diseases classified elsewhere, left upper arm

M63.829 Disorders of muscle in diseases classified elsewhere, unspecified upper arm

● **M63.83** Disorders of muscle in diseases classified elsewhere, forearm

M63.831 Disorders of muscle in diseases classified elsewhere, right forearm

M63.832 Disorders of muscle in diseases classified elsewhere, left forearm

M63.839 Disorders of muscle in diseases classified elsewhere, unspecified forearm

● **M63.84** Disorders of muscle in diseases classified elsewhere, hand

M63.841 Disorders of muscle in diseases classified elsewhere, right hand

M63.842 Disorders of muscle in diseases classified elsewhere, left hand

M63.849 Disorders of muscle in diseases classified elsewhere, unspecified hand

● **M63.85** Disorders of muscle in diseases classified elsewhere, thigh

M63.851 Disorders of muscle in diseases classified elsewhere, right thigh

M63.852 Disorders of muscle in diseases classified elsewhere, left thigh

M63.859 Disorders of muscle in diseases classified elsewhere, unspecified thigh

● **M63.86** Disorders of muscle in diseases classified elsewhere, lower leg

M63.861 Disorders of muscle in diseases classified elsewhere, right lower leg

M63.862 Disorders of muscle in diseases classified elsewhere, left lower leg

M63.869 Disorders of muscle in diseases classified elsewhere, unspecified lower leg

● **M63.87** Disorders of muscle in diseases classified elsewhere, ankle and foot

M63.871 Disorders of muscle in diseases classified elsewhere, right ankle and foot

M63.872 Disorders of muscle in diseases classified elsewhere, left ankle and foot

M63.879 Disorders of muscle in diseases classified elsewhere, unspecified ankle and foot

M63.88 Disorders of muscle in diseases classified elsewhere, other site

M63.89 Disorders of muscle in diseases classified elsewhere, multiple sites

DISORDERS OF SYNOVIUM AND TENDON (M65-M67)

● **M65** **Synovitis and tenosynovitis**

| Excludes1 | chronic crepitant synovitis of hand and wrist (M70.0-)
current injury - see injury of ligament or tendon by body region
soft tissue disorders related to use, overuse and pressure (M70.-)

● **M65.0** **Abscess of tendon sheath**

Use additional code (B95-B96) to identify bacterial agent

M65.00 Abscess of tendon sheath, unspecified site

● **M65.01** Abscess of tendon sheath, shoulder

M65.011 Abscess of tendon sheath, right shoulder

M65.012 Abscess of tendon sheath, left shoulder

M65.019 Abscess of tendon sheath, unspecified shoulder

● **M65.02** Abscess of tendon sheath, upper arm

M65.021 Abscess of tendon sheath, right upper arm

M65.022 Abscess of tendon sheath, left upper arm

M65.029 Abscess of tendon sheath, unspecified upper arm

● **M65.03** Abscess of tendon sheath, forearm

M65.031 Abscess of tendon sheath, right forearm

M65.032 Abscess of tendon sheath, left forearm

M65.039 Abscess of tendon sheath, unspecified forearm

● **M65.04** Abscess of tendon sheath, hand

M65.041 Abscess of tendon sheath, right hand

M65.042 Abscess of tendon sheath, left hand

M65.049 Abscess of tendon sheath, unspecified hand

● **M65.05** Abscess of tendon sheath, thigh

M65.051 Abscess of tendon sheath, right thigh

M65.052 Abscess of tendon sheath, left thigh

M65.059 Abscess of tendon sheath, unspecified thigh

Item 13–11 Synovitis is an inflammation of a synovial membrane resulting in pain on motion and is characterized by fluctuating swelling due to effusion in a synovial sac. **Tenosynovitis** is an inflammation of a tendon sheath and occurs most commonly in the wrists, hands, and feet. Bursitis is inflammation of a bursa (fluid filled sac) caused by repetitive use, trauma, infection, or systemic inflammatory disease. Bursae act as protectors and facilitate movement between bones and overlapping muscles (deep bursae) or between bones and tendons/skin (superficial bursae).

◀ New   ◀|||| Revised   ~~deleted~~ Deleted   OGCR Official Guidelines   X Assign placeholder X   ● Use Additional Character(s)

| Excludes 1 | | Excludes 2 | Includes   Use additional   Code first   Code also   Unspecified

● M65.06   Abscess of tendon sheath, lower leg

    M65.061   Abscess of tendon sheath, right lower leg

    M65.062   Abscess of tendon sheath, left lower leg

    M65.069   Abscess of tendon sheath, unspecified lower leg

● M65.07   Abscess of tendon sheath, ankle and foot

    M65.071   Abscess of tendon sheath, right ankle and foot

    M65.072   Abscess of tendon sheath, left ankle and foot

    M65.079   Abscess of tendon sheath, unspecified ankle and foot

   M65.08   Abscess of tendon sheath, other site

● M65.1   Other infective (teno)synovitis

   M65.10   Other infective (teno)synovitis, unspecified site

● M65.11   Other infective (teno)synovitis, shoulder

    M65.111   Other infective (teno)synovitis, right shoulder

    M65.112   Other infective (teno)synovitis, left shoulder

    M65.119   Other infective (teno)synovitis, unspecified shoulder

● M65.12   Other infective (teno)synovitis, elbow

    M65.121   Other infective (teno)synovitis, right elbow

    M65.122   Other infective (teno)synovitis, left elbow

    M65.129   Other infective (teno)synovitis, unspecified elbow

● M65.13   Other infective (teno)synovitis, wrist

    M65.131   Other infective (teno)synovitis, right wrist

    M65.132   Other infective (teno)synovitis, left wrist

    M65.139   Other infective (teno)synovitis, unspecified wrist

● M65.14   Other infective (teno)synovitis, hand

    M65.141   Other infective (teno)synovitis, right hand

    M65.142   Other infective (teno)synovitis, left hand

    M65.149   Other infective (teno)synovitis, unspecified hand

● M65.15   Other infective (teno)synovitis, hip

    M65.151   Other infective (teno)synovitis, right hip

    M65.152   Other infective (teno)synovitis, left hip

    M65.159   Other infective (teno)synovitis, unspecified hip

● M65.16   Other infective (teno)synovitis, knee

    M65.161   Other infective (teno)synovitis, right knee

    M65.162   Other infective (teno)synovitis, left knee

    M65.169   Other infective (teno)synovitis, unspecified knee

● M65.17   Other infective (teno)synovitis, ankle and foot

    M65.171   Other infective (teno)synovitis, right ankle and foot

    M65.172   Other infective (teno)synovitis, left ankle and foot

    M65.179   Other infective (teno)synovitis, unspecified ankle and foot

   M65.18   Other infective (teno)synovitis, other site

   M65.19   Other infective (teno)synovitis, multiple sites

● M65.2   Calcific tendinitis

   Excludes1   tendinitis as classified in M75-M77 calcified tendinitis of shoulder (M75.3)

   M65.20   Calcific tendinitis, unspecified site

● M65.22   Calcific tendinitis, upper arm

    M65.221   Calcific tendinitis, right upper arm

    M65.222   Calcific tendinitis, left upper arm

    M65.229   Calcific tendinitis, unspecified upper arm

● M65.23   Calcific tendinitis, forearm

    M65.231   Calcific tendinitis, right forearm

    M65.232   Calcific tendinitis, left forearm

    M65.239   Calcific tendinitis, unspecified forearm

● M65.24   Calcific tendinitis, hand

    M65.241   Calcific tendinitis, right hand

    M65.242   Calcific tendinitis, left hand

    M65.249   Calcific tendinitis, unspecified hand

● M65.25   Calcific tendinitis, thigh

    M65.251   Calcific tendinitis, right thigh

    M65.252   Calcific tendinitis, left thigh

    M65.259   Calcific tendinitis, unspecified thigh

● M65.26   Calcific tendinitis, lower leg

    M65.261   Calcific tendinitis, right lower leg

    M65.262   Calcific tendinitis, left lower leg

    M65.269   Calcific tendinitis, unspecified lower leg

● M65.27   Calcific tendinitis, ankle and foot

    M65.271   Calcific tendinitis, right ankle and foot

    M65.272   Calcific tendinitis, left ankle and foot

    M65.279   Calcific tendinitis, unspecified ankle and foot

   M65.28   Calcific tendinitis, other site

   M65.29   Calcific tendinitis, multiple sites

● M65.3   Trigger finger

   Nodular tendinous disease

   M65.30   Trigger finger, unspecified finger

● M65.31   Trigger thumb

    M65.311   Trigger thumb, right thumb

    M65.312   Trigger thumb, left thumb

    M65.319   Trigger thumb, unspecified thumb

● M65.32   Trigger finger, index finger

    M65.321   Trigger finger, right index finger

    M65.322   Trigger finger, left index finger

    M65.329   Trigger finger, unspecified index finger

● M65.33   Trigger finger, middle finger

    M65.331   Trigger finger, right middle finger

    M65.332   Trigger finger, left middle finger

    M65.339   Trigger finger, unspecified middle finger

● M65.34   Trigger finger, ring finger

    M65.341   Trigger finger, right ring finger

    M65.342   Trigger finger, left ring finger

    M65.349   Trigger finger, unspecified ring finger

● M65.35   Trigger finger, little finger

    M65.351   Trigger finger, right little finger

    M65.352   Trigger finger, left little finger

    M65.359   Trigger finger, unspecified little finger

   M65.4   Radial styloid tenosynovitis [de Quervain]

● **M65.8 Other synovitis and tenosynovitis**

    M65.80 Other synovitis and tenosynovitis, unspecified site

  ● M65.81 Other synovitis and tenosynovitis, shoulder

      M65.811 Other synovitis and tenosynovitis, right shoulder

      M65.812 Other synovitis and tenosynovitis, left shoulder

      M65.819 Other synovitis and tenosynovitis, unspecified shoulder

  ● M65.82 Other synovitis and tenosynovitis, upper arm

      M65.821 Other synovitis and tenosynovitis, right upper arm

      M65.822 Other synovitis and tenosynovitis, left upper arm

      M65.829 Other synovitis and tenosynovitis, unspecified upper arm

  ● M65.83 Other synovitis and tenosynovitis, forearm

      M65.831 Other synovitis and tenosynovitis, right forearm

      M65.832 Other synovitis and tenosynovitis, left forearm

      M65.839 Other synovitis and tenosynovitis, unspecified forearm

  ● M65.84 Other synovitis and tenosynovitis, hand

      M65.841 Other synovitis and tenosynovitis, right hand

      M65.842 Other synovitis and tenosynovitis, left hand

      M65.849 Other synovitis and tenosynovitis, unspecified hand

  ● M65.85 Other synovitis and tenosynovitis, thigh

      M65.851 Other synovitis and tenosynovitis, right thigh

      M65.852 Other synovitis and tenosynovitis, left thigh

      M65.859 Other synovitis and tenosynovitis, unspecified thigh

  ● M65.86 Other synovitis and tenosynovitis, lower leg

      M65.861 Other synovitis and tenosynovitis, right lower leg

      M65.862 Other synovitis and tenosynovitis, left lower leg

      M65.869 Other synovitis and tenosynovitis, unspecified lower leg

  ● M65.87 Other synovitis and tenosynovitis, ankle and foot

      M65.871 Other synovitis and tenosynovitis, right ankle and foot

      M65.872 Other synovitis and tenosynovitis, left ankle and foot

      M65.879 Other synovitis and tenosynovitis, unspecified ankle and foot

    M65.88 Other synovitis and tenosynovitis, other site

    M65.89 Other synovitis and tenosynovitis, multiple sites

M65.9 Synovitis and tenosynovitis, unspecified

● **M66 Spontaneous rupture of synovium and tendon**

   Includes   rupture that occurs when a normal force is applied to tissues that are inferred to have less than normal strength

   Excludes2   rotator cuff syndrome (M75.1-)

                rupture where an abnormal force is applied to normal tissue - see injury of tendon by body region

  M66.0 Rupture of popliteal cyst

● M66.1 **Rupture of synovium**

    Rupture of synovial cyst

    Excludes2   rupture of popliteal cyst (M66.0)

    M66.10 Rupture of synovium, unspecified joint

  ● M66.11 Rupture of synovium, shoulder

      M66.111 Rupture of synovium, right shoulder

      M66.112 Rupture of synovium, left shoulder

      M66.119 Rupture of synovium, unspecified shoulder

  ● M66.12 Rupture of synovium, elbow

      M66.121 Rupture of synovium, right elbow

      M66.122 Rupture of synovium, left elbow

      M66.129 Rupture of synovium, unspecified elbow

  ● M66.13 Rupture of synovium, wrist

      M66.131 Rupture of synovium, right wrist

      M66.132 Rupture of synovium, left wrist

      M66.139 Rupture of synovium, unspecified wrist

  ● M66.14 Rupture of synovium, hand and fingers

      M66.141 Rupture of synovium, right hand

      M66.142 Rupture of synovium, left hand

      M66.143 Rupture of synovium, unspecified hand

      M66.144 Rupture of synovium, right finger(s)

      M66.145 Rupture of synovium, left finger(s)

      M66.146 Rupture of synovium, unspecified finger(s)

  ● M66.15 Rupture of synovium, hip

      M66.151 Rupture of synovium, right hip

      M66.152 Rupture of synovium, left hip

      M66.159 Rupture of synovium, unspecified hip

  ● M66.17 Rupture of synovium, ankle, foot and toes

      M66.171 Rupture of synovium, right ankle

      M66.172 Rupture of synovium, left ankle

      M66.173 Rupture of synovium, unspecified ankle

      M66.174 Rupture of synovium, right foot

      M66.175 Rupture of synovium, left foot

      M66.176 Rupture of synovium, unspecified foot

      M66.177 Rupture of synovium, right toe(s)

      M66.178 Rupture of synovium, left toe(s)

      M66.179 Rupture of synovium, unspecified toe(s)

    M66.18 Rupture of synovium, other site

◀ New   ◀▥ Revised   ~~deleted~~ Deleted   OGCR Official Guidelines   X Assign placeholder X   ● Use Additional Character(s)

Excludes 1   Excludes 2   Includes   Use additional   Code first   Code also   Unspecified

● **M66.2   Spontaneous rupture of extensor tendons**

    M66.20   Spontaneous rupture of extensor tendons, unspecified site

●   M66.21   Spontaneous rupture of extensor tendons, shoulder

        M66.211   Spontaneous rupture of extensor tendons, right shoulder

        M66.212   Spontaneous rupture of extensor tendons, left shoulder

        M66.219   Spontaneous rupture of extensor tendons, unspecified shoulder

●   M66.22   Spontaneous rupture of extensor tendons, upper arm

        M66.221   Spontaneous rupture of extensor tendons, right upper arm

        M66.222   Spontaneous rupture of extensor tendons, left upper arm

        M66.229   Spontaneous rupture of extensor tendons, unspecified upper arm

●   M66.23   Spontaneous rupture of extensor tendons, forearm

        M66.231   Spontaneous rupture of extensor tendons, right forearm

        M66.232   Spontaneous rupture of extensor tendons, left forearm

        M66.239   Spontaneous rupture of extensor tendons, unspecified forearm

●   M66.24   Spontaneous rupture of extensor tendons, hand

        M66.241   Spontaneous rupture of extensor tendons, right hand

        M66.242   Spontaneous rupture of extensor tendons, left hand

        M66.249   Spontaneous rupture of extensor tendons, unspecified hand

●   M66.25   Spontaneous rupture of extensor tendons, thigh

        M66.251   Spontaneous rupture of extensor tendons, right thigh

        M66.252   Spontaneous rupture of extensor tendons, left thigh

        M66.259   Spontaneous rupture of extensor tendons, unspecified thigh

●   M66.26   Spontaneous rupture of extensor tendons, lower leg

        M66.261   Spontaneous rupture of extensor tendons, right lower leg

        M66.262   Spontaneous rupture of extensor tendons, left lower leg

        M66.269   Spontaneous rupture of extensor tendons, unspecified lower leg

●   M66.27   Spontaneous rupture of extensor tendons, ankle and foot

        M66.271   Spontaneous rupture of extensor tendons, right ankle and foot

        M66.272   Spontaneous rupture of extensor tendons, left ankle and foot

        M66.279   Spontaneous rupture of extensor tendons, unspecified ankle and foot

    M66.28   Spontaneous rupture of extensor tendons, other site

    M66.29   Spontaneous rupture of extensor tendons, multiple sites

● **M66.3   Spontaneous rupture of flexor tendons**

    M66.30   Spontaneous rupture of flexor tendons, unspecified site

●   M66.31   Spontaneous rupture of flexor tendons, shoulder

        M66.311   Spontaneous rupture of flexor tendons, right shoulder

        M66.312   Spontaneous rupture of flexor tendons, left shoulder

        M66.319   Spontaneous rupture of flexor tendons, unspecified shoulder

●   M66.32   Spontaneous rupture of flexor tendons, upper arm

        M66.321   Spontaneous rupture of flexor tendons, right upper arm

        M66.322   Spontaneous rupture of flexor tendons, left upper arm

        M66.329   Spontaneous rupture of flexor tendons, unspecified upper arm

●   M66.33   Spontaneous rupture of flexor tendons, forearm

        M66.331   Spontaneous rupture of flexor tendons, right forearm

        M66.332   Spontaneous rupture of flexor tendons, left forearm

        M66.339   Spontaneous rupture of flexor tendons, unspecified forearm

●   M66.34   Spontaneous rupture of flexor tendons, hand

        M66.341   Spontaneous rupture of flexor tendons, right hand

        M66.342   Spontaneous rupture of flexor tendons, left hand

        M66.349   Spontaneous rupture of flexor tendons, unspecified hand

●   M66.35   Spontaneous rupture of flexor tendons, thigh

        M66.351   Spontaneous rupture of flexor tendons, right thigh

        M66.352   Spontaneous rupture of flexor tendons, left thigh

        M66.359   Spontaneous rupture of flexor tendons, unspecified thigh

●   M66.36   Spontaneous rupture of flexor tendons, lower leg

        M66.361   Spontaneous rupture of flexor tendons, right lower leg

        M66.362   Spontaneous rupture of flexor tendons, left lower leg

        M66.369   Spontaneous rupture of flexor tendons, unspecified lower leg

●   M66.37   Spontaneous rupture of flexor tendons, ankle and foot

        M66.371   Spontaneous rupture of flexor tendons, right ankle and foot

        M66.372   Spontaneous rupture of flexor tendons, left ankle and foot

        M66.379   Spontaneous rupture of flexor tendons, unspecified ankle and foot

    M66.38   Spontaneous rupture of flexor tendons, other site

    M66.39   Spontaneous rupture of flexor tendons, multiple sites

CHAPTER 13 (M00-M99)

● **M66.8**   **Spontaneous rupture of other tendons**

     M66.80   Spontaneous rupture of other tendons, unspecified site

     ● **M66.81**   Spontaneous rupture of other tendons, shoulder

         M66.811   Spontaneous rupture of other tendons, right shoulder

         M66.812   Spontaneous rupture of other tendons, left shoulder

         M66.819   Spontaneous rupture of other tendons, unspecified shoulder

     ● **M66.82**   Spontaneous rupture of other tendons, upper arm

         M66.821   Spontaneous rupture of other tendons, right upper arm

         M66.822   Spontaneous rupture of other tendons, left upper arm

         M66.829   Spontaneous rupture of other tendons, unspecified upper arm

     ● **M66.83**   Spontaneous rupture of other tendons, forearm

         M66.831   Spontaneous rupture of other tendons, right forearm

         M66.832   Spontaneous rupture of other tendons, left forearm

         M66.839   Spontaneous rupture of other tendons, unspecified forearm

     ● **M66.84**   Spontaneous rupture of other tendons, hand

         M66.841   Spontaneous rupture of other tendons, right hand

         M66.842   Spontaneous rupture of other tendons, left hand

         M66.849   Spontaneous rupture of other tendons, unspecified hand

     ● **M66.85**   Spontaneous rupture of other tendons, thigh

         M66.851   Spontaneous rupture of other tendons, right thigh

         M66.852   Spontaneous rupture of other tendons, left thigh

         M66.859   Spontaneous rupture of other tendons, unspecified thigh

     ● **M66.86**   Spontaneous rupture of other tendons, lower leg

         M66.861   Spontaneous rupture of other tendons, right lower leg

         M66.862   Spontaneous rupture of other tendons, left lower leg

         M66.869   Spontaneous rupture of other tendons, unspecified lower leg

     ● **M66.87**   Spontaneous rupture of other tendons, ankle and foot

         M66.871   Spontaneous rupture of other tendons, right ankle and foot

         M66.872   Spontaneous rupture of other tendons, left ankle and foot

         M66.879   Spontaneous rupture of other tendons, unspecified ankle and foot

     M66.88   Spontaneous rupture of other tendons, other

     M66.89   Spontaneous rupture of other tendons, multiple sites

M66.9   **Spontaneous rupture of unspecified tendon**

     Rupture at musculotendinous junction, nontraumatic

● **M67**   **Other disorders of synovium and tendon**

     Excludes1   palmar fascial fibromatosis [Dupuytren] (M72.0)

         tendinitis NOS (M77.9-)

         xanthomatosis localized to tendons (E78.2)

     ● **M67.0**   Short Achilles tendon (acquired)

         M67.00   Short Achilles tendon (acquired), unspecified ankle

         M67.01   Short Achilles tendon (acquired), right ankle

         M67.02   Short Achilles tendon (acquired), left ankle

     ● **M67.2**   Synovial hypertrophy, not elsewhere classified

         Excludes1   villonodular synovitis (pigmented) (M12.2-)

         M67.20   Synovial hypertrophy, not elsewhere classified, unspecified site

     ● **M67.21**   Synovial hypertrophy, not elsewhere classified, shoulder

         M67.211   Synovial hypertrophy, not elsewhere classified, right shoulder

         M67.212   Synovial hypertrophy, not elsewhere classified, left shoulder

         M67.219   Synovial hypertrophy, not elsewhere classified, unspecified shoulder

     ● **M67.22**   Synovial hypertrophy, not elsewhere classified, upper arm

         M67.221   Synovial hypertrophy, not elsewhere classified, right upper arm

         M67.222   Synovial hypertrophy, not elsewhere classified, left upper arm

         M67.229   Synovial hypertrophy, not elsewhere classified, unspecified upper arm

     ● **M67.23**   Synovial hypertrophy, not elsewhere classified, forearm

         M67.231   Synovial hypertrophy, not elsewhere classified, right forearm

         M67.232   Synovial hypertrophy, not elsewhere classified, left forearm

         M67.239   Synovial hypertrophy, not elsewhere classified, unspecified forearm

     ● **M67.24**   Synovial hypertrophy, not elsewhere classified, hand

         M67.241   Synovial hypertrophy, not elsewhere classified, right hand

         M67.242   Synovial hypertrophy, not elsewhere classified, left hand

         M67.249   Synovial hypertrophy, not elsewhere classified, unspecified hand

     ● **M67.25**   Synovial hypertrophy, not elsewhere classified, thigh

         M67.251   Synovial hypertrophy, not elsewhere classified, right thigh

         M67.252   Synovial hypertrophy, not elsewhere classified, left thigh

         M67.259   Synovial hypertrophy, not elsewhere classified, unspecified thigh

     ● **M67.26**   Synovial hypertrophy, not elsewhere classified, lower leg

         M67.261   Synovial hypertrophy, not elsewhere classified, right lower leg

         M67.262   Synovial hypertrophy, not elsewhere classified, left lower leg

         M67.269   Synovial hypertrophy, not elsewhere classified, unspecified lower leg

◀ New   ◀▥ Revised   ~~deleted~~ Deleted   OGCR Official Guidelines   X Assign placeholder X   ● Use Additional Character(s)

Excludes 1   Excludes 2   Includes   Use additional   Code first   Code also   Unspecified

● M67.27   Synovial hypertrophy, not elsewhere classified, ankle and foot
     M67.271   Synovial hypertrophy, not elsewhere classified, right ankle and foot
     M67.272   Synovial hypertrophy, not elsewhere classified, left ankle and foot
     M67.279   Synovial hypertrophy, not elsewhere classified, unspecified ankle and foot
   M67.28   Synovial hypertrophy, not elsewhere classified, other site
   M67.29   Synovial hypertrophy, not elsewhere classified, multiple sites

● M67.3   Transient synovitis
     Toxic synovitis
     Excludes1   palindromic rheumatism (M12.3-)
   M67.30   Transient synovitis, unspecified site
● M67.31   Transient synovitis, shoulder
     M67.311   Transient synovitis, right shoulder
     M67.312   Transient synovitis, left shoulder
     M67.319   Transient synovitis, unspecified shoulder
● M67.32   Transient synovitis, elbow
     M67.321   Transient synovitis, right elbow
     M67.322   Transient synovitis, left elbow
     M67.329   Transient synovitis, unspecified elbow
● M67.33   Transient synovitis, wrist
     M67.331   Transient synovitis, right wrist
     M67.332   Transient synovitis, left wrist
     M67.339   Transient synovitis, unspecified wrist
● M67.34   Transient synovitis, hand
     M67.341   Transient synovitis, right hand
     M67.342   Transient synovitis, left hand
     M67.349   Transient synovitis, unspecified hand
● M67.35   Transient synovitis, hip
     M67.351   Transient synovitis, right hip
     M67.352   Transient synovitis, left hip
     M67.359   Transient synovitis, unspecified hip
● M67.36   Transient synovitis, knee
     M67.361   Transient synovitis, right knee
     M67.362   Transient synovitis, left knee
     M67.369   Transient synovitis, unspecified knee
● M67.37   Transient synovitis, ankle and foot
     M67.371   Transient synovitis, right ankle and foot
     M67.372   Transient synovitis, left ankle and foot
     M67.379   Transient synovitis, unspecified ankle and foot
   M67.38   Transient synovitis, other site
   M67.39   Transient synovitis, multiple sites

● M67.4   Ganglion
     Ganglion of joint or tendon (sheath)
     Excludes1   ganglion in yaws (A66.6)
     Excludes2   cyst of bursa (M71.2-M71.3)
                 cyst of synovium (M71.2-M71.3)
   M67.40   Ganglion, unspecified site
● M67.41   Ganglion, shoulder
     M67.411   Ganglion, right shoulder
     M67.412   Ganglion, left shoulder
     M67.419   Ganglion, unspecified shoulder

● M67.42   Ganglion, elbow
     M67.421   Ganglion, right elbow
     M67.422   Ganglion, left elbow
     M67.429   Ganglion, unspecified elbow
● M67.43   Ganglion, wrist
     M67.431   Ganglion, right wrist
     M67.432   Ganglion, left wrist
     M67.439   Ganglion, unspecified wrist
● M67.44   Ganglion, hand
     M67.441   Ganglion, right hand
     M67.442   Ganglion, left hand
     M67.449   Ganglion, unspecified hand
● M67.45   Ganglion, hip
     M67.451   Ganglion, right hip
     M67.452   Ganglion, left hip
     M67.459   Ganglion, unspecified hip
● M67.46   Ganglion, knee
     M67.461   Ganglion, right knee
     M67.462   Ganglion, left knee
     M67.469   Ganglion, unspecified knee
● M67.47   Ganglion, ankle and foot
     M67.471   Ganglion, right ankle and foot
     M67.472   Ganglion, left ankle and foot
     M67.479   Ganglion, unspecified ankle and foot
   M67.48   Ganglion, other site
   M67.49   Ganglion, multiple sites

● M67.5   Plica syndrome
     Plica knee
   M67.50   Plica syndrome, unspecified knee
   M67.51   Plica syndrome, right knee
   M67.52   Plica syndrome, left knee

● M67.8   Other specified disorders of synovium and tendon
   M67.80   Other specified disorders of synovium and tendon, unspecified site
● M67.81   Other specified disorders of synovium and tendon, shoulder
     M67.811   Other specified disorders of synovium, right shoulder
     M67.812   Other specified disorders of synovium, left shoulder
     M67.813   Other specified disorders of tendon, right shoulder
     M67.814   Other specified disorders of tendon, left shoulder
     M67.819   Other specified disorders of synovium and tendon, unspecified shoulder
● M67.82   Other specified disorders of synovium and tendon, elbow
     M67.821   Other specified disorders of synovium, right elbow
     M67.822   Other specified disorders of synovium, left elbow
     M67.823   Other specified disorders of tendon, right elbow
     M67.824   Other specified disorders of tendon, left elbow
     M67.829   Other specified disorders of synovium and tendon, unspecified elbow

CHAPTER 13 (M00-M99)

● M67.83   Other specified disorders of synovium and tendon, wrist

     M67.831   Other specified disorders of synovium, right wrist

     M67.832   Other specified disorders of synovium, left wrist

     M67.833   Other specified disorders of tendon, right wrist

     M67.834   Other specified disorders of tendon, left wrist

     M67.839   Other specified disorders of synovium and tendon, unspecified forearm

● M67.84   Other specified disorders of synovium and tendon, hand

     M67.841   Other specified disorders of synovium, right hand

     M67.842   Other specified disorders of synovium, left hand

     M67.843   Other specified disorders of tendon, right hand

     M67.844   Other specified disorders of tendon, left hand

     M67.849   Other specified disorders of synovium and tendon, unspecified hand

● M67.85   Other specified disorders of synovium and tendon, hip

     M67.851   Other specified disorders of synovium, right hip

     M67.852   Other specified disorders of synovium, left hip

     M67.853   Other specified disorders of tendon, right hip

     M67.854   Other specified disorders of tendon, left hip

     M67.859   Other specified disorders of synovium and tendon, unspecified hip

● M67.86   Other specified disorders of synovium and tendon, knee

     M67.861   Other specified disorders of synovium, right knee

     M67.862   Other specified disorders of synovium, left knee

     M67.863   Other specified disorders of tendon, right knee

     M67.864   Other specified disorders of tendon, left knee

     M67.869   Other specified disorders of synovium and tendon, unspecified knee

● M67.87   Other specified disorders of synovium and tendon, ankle and foot

     M67.871   Other specified disorders of synovium, right ankle and foot

     M67.872   Other specified disorders of synovium, left ankle and foot

     M67.873   Other specified disorders of tendon, right ankle and foot

     M67.874   Other specified disorders of tendon, left ankle and foot

     M67.879   Other specified disorders of synovium and tendon, unspecified ankle and foot

   M67.88   Other specified disorders of synovium and tendon, other site

   M67.89   Other specified disorders of synovium and tendon, multiple sites

● M67.9   Unspecified disorder of synovium and tendon

   M67.90   Unspecified disorder of synovium and tendon, unspecified site

● M67.91   Unspecified disorder of synovium and tendon, shoulder

     M67.911   Unspecified disorder of synovium and tendon, right shoulder

     M67.912   Unspecified disorder of synovium and tendon, left shoulder

     M67.919   Unspecified disorder of synovium and tendon, unspecified shoulder

● M67.92   Unspecified disorder of synovium and tendon, upper arm

     M67.921   Unspecified disorder of synovium and tendon, right upper arm

     M67.922   Unspecified disorder of synovium and tendon, left upper arm

     M67.929   Unspecified disorder of synovium and tendon, unspecified upper arm

● M67.93   Unspecified disorder of synovium and tendon, forearm

     M67.931   Unspecified disorder of synovium and tendon, right forearm

     M67.932   Unspecified disorder of synovium and tendon, left forearm

     M67.939   Unspecified disorder of synovium and tendon, unspecified forearm

● M67.94   Unspecified disorder of synovium and tendon, hand

     M67.941   Unspecified disorder of synovium and tendon, right hand

     M67.942   Unspecified disorder of synovium and tendon, left hand

     M67.949   Unspecified disorder of synovium and tendon, unspecified hand

● M67.95   Unspecified disorder of synovium and tendon, thigh

     M67.951   Unspecified disorder of synovium and tendon, right thigh

     M67.952   Unspecified disorder of synovium and tendon, left thigh

     M67.959   Unspecified disorder of synovium and tendon, unspecified thigh

● M67.96   Unspecified disorder of synovium and tendon, lower leg

     M67.961   Unspecified disorder of synovium and tendon, right lower leg

     M67.962   Unspecified disorder of synovium and tendon, left lower leg

     M67.969   Unspecified disorder of synovium and tendon, unspecified lower leg

● M67.97   Unspecified disorder of synovium and tendon, ankle and foot

     M67.971   Unspecified disorder of synovium and tendon, right ankle and foot

     M67.972   Unspecified disorder of synovium and tendon, left ankle and foot

     M67.979   Unspecified disorder of synovium and tendon, unspecified ankle and foot

   M67.98   Unspecified disorder of synovium and tendon, other site

   M67.99   Unspecified disorder of synovium and tendon, multiple sites

◀ New   ◀▓ Revised   ~~deleted~~ Deleted   OGCR Official Guidelines   X Assign placeholder X   ● Use Additional Character(s)

 Excludes 1   Excludes 2   Includes   Use additional   Code first   Code also   Unspecified

OTHER SOFT TISSUE DISORDERS (M70-M79)

● **M70   Soft tissue disorders related to use, overuse and pressure**

     Includes   soft tissue disorders of occupational origin

     Use additional external cause code to identify activity causing disorder (Y93.-)

     Excludes1   bursitis NOS (M71.9-)

     Excludes2   bursitis of shoulder (M75.5)

                     enthesopathies (M76-M77)

                     pressure ulcer (pressure area) (L89.-)

● **M70.0   Crepitant synovitis (acute) (chronic) of hand and wrist**

   ● **M70.03   Crepitant synovitis (acute) (chronic), wrist**

       M70.031   Crepitant synovitis (acute) (chronic), right wrist

       M70.032   Crepitant synovitis (acute) (chronic), left wrist

       M70.039   Crepitant synovitis (acute) (chronic), unspecified wrist

   ● **M70.04   Crepitant synovitis (acute) (chronic), hand**

       M70.041   Crepitant synovitis (acute) (chronic), right hand

       M70.042   Crepitant synovitis (acute) (chronic), left hand

       M70.049   Crepitant synovitis (acute) (chronic), unspecified hand

● **M70.1   Bursitis of hand**

     M70.10   Bursitis, unspecified hand

     M70.11   Bursitis, right hand

     M70.12   Bursitis, left hand

● **M70.2   Olecranon bursitis**

     M70.20   Olecranon bursitis, unspecified elbow

     M70.21   Olecranon bursitis, right elbow

     M70.22   Olecranon bursitis, left elbow

● **M70.3   Other bursitis of elbow**

     M70.30   Other bursitis of elbow, unspecified elbow

     M70.31   Other bursitis of elbow, right elbow

     M70.32   Other bursitis of elbow, left elbow

● **M70.4   Prepatellar bursitis**

     M70.40   Prepatellar bursitis, unspecified knee

     M70.41   Prepatellar bursitis, right knee

     M70.42   Prepatellar bursitis, left knee

● **M70.5   Other bursitis of knee**

     M70.50   Other bursitis of knee, unspecified knee

     M70.51   Other bursitis of knee, right knee

     M70.52   Other bursitis of knee, left knee

● **M70.6   Trochanteric bursitis**

     Trochanteric tendinitis

     M70.60   Trochanteric bursitis, unspecified hip

     M70.61   Trochanteric bursitis, right hip

     M70.62   Trochanteric bursitis, left hip

● **M70.7   Other bursitis of hip**

     Ischial bursitis

     M70.70   Other bursitis of hip, unspecified hip

     M70.71   Other bursitis of hip, right hip

     M70.72   Other bursitis of hip, left hip

● **M70.8   Other soft tissue disorders related to use, overuse and pressure**

     M70.80   Other soft tissue disorders related to use, overuse and pressure of unspecified site

   ● **M70.81   Other soft tissue disorders related to use, overuse and pressure of shoulder**

       M70.811   Other soft tissue disorders related to use, overuse and pressure, right shoulder

       M70.812   Other soft tissue disorders related to use, overuse and pressure, left shoulder

       M70.819   Other soft tissue disorders related to use, overuse and pressure, unspecified shoulder

   ● **M70.82   Other soft tissue disorders related to use, overuse and pressure of upper arm**

       M70.821   Other soft tissue disorders related to use, overuse and pressure, right upper arm

       M70.822   Other soft tissue disorders related to use, overuse and pressure, left upper arm

       M70.829   Other soft tissue disorders related to use, overuse and pressure, unspecified upper arms

   ● **M70.83   Other soft tissue disorders related to use, overuse and pressure of forearm**

       M70.831   Other soft tissue disorders related to use, overuse and pressure, right forearm

       M70.832   Other soft tissue disorders related to use, overuse and pressure, left forearm

       M70.839   Other soft tissue disorders related to use, overuse and pressure, unspecified forearm

   ● **M70.84   Other soft tissue disorders related to use, overuse and pressure of hand**

       M70.841   Other soft tissue disorders related to use, overuse and pressure, right hand

       M70.842   Other soft tissue disorders related to use, overuse and pressure, left hand

       M70.849   Other soft tissue disorders related to use, overuse and pressure, unspecified hand

   ● **M70.85   Other soft tissue disorders related to use, overuse and pressure of thigh**

       M70.851   Other soft tissue disorders related to use, overuse and pressure, right thigh

       M70.852   Other soft tissue disorders related to use, overuse and pressure, left thigh

       M70.859   Other soft tissue disorders related to use, overuse and pressure, unspecified thigh

   ● **M70.86   Other soft tissue disorders related to use, overuse and pressure lower leg**

       M70.861   Other soft tissue disorders related to use, overuse and pressure, right lower leg

       M70.862   Other soft tissue disorders related to use, overuse and pressure, left lower leg

       M70.869   Other soft tissue disorders related to use, overuse and pressure, unspecified leg

CHAPTER 13 (M00-M99)

● M70.87   Other soft tissue disorders related to use, overuse and pressure of ankle and foot

    M70.871   Other soft tissue disorders related to use, overuse and pressure, right ankle and foot

    M70.872   Other soft tissue disorders related to use, overuse and pressure, left ankle and foot

    M70.879   Other soft tissue disorders related to use, overuse and pressure, unspecified ankle and foot

   M70.88   Other soft tissue disorders related to use, overuse and pressure other site

   M70.89   Other soft tissue disorders related to use, overuse and pressure multiple sites

● M70.9   Unspecified soft tissue disorder related to use, overuse and pressure

   M70.90   Unspecified soft tissue disorder related to use, overuse and pressure of unspecified site

● M70.91   Unspecified soft tissue disorder related to use, overuse and pressure of shoulder

    M70.911   Unspecified soft tissue disorder related to use, overuse and pressure, right shoulder

    M70.912   Unspecified soft tissue disorder related to use, overuse and pressure, left shoulder

    M70.919   Unspecified soft tissue disorder related to use, overuse and pressure, unspecified shoulder

● M70.92   Unspecified soft tissue disorder related to use, overuse and pressure of upper arm

    M70.921   Unspecified soft tissue disorder related to use, overuse and pressure, right upper arm

    M70.922   Unspecified soft tissue disorder related to use, overuse and pressure, left upper arm

    M70.929   Unspecified soft tissue disorder related to use, overuse and pressure, unspecified upper arm

● M70.93   Unspecified soft tissue disorder related to use, overuse and pressure of forearm

    M70.931   Unspecified soft tissue disorder related to use, overuse and pressure, right forearm

    M70.932   Unspecified soft tissue disorder related to use, overuse and pressure, left forearm

    M70.939   Unspecified soft tissue disorder related to use, overuse and pressure, unspecified forearm

● M70.94   Unspecified soft tissue disorder related to use, overuse and pressure of hand

    M70.941   Unspecified soft tissue disorder related to use, overuse and pressure, right hand

    M70.942   Unspecified soft tissue disorder related to use, overuse and pressure, left hand

    M70.949   Unspecified soft tissue disorder related to use, overuse and pressure, unspecified hand

● M70.95   Unspecified soft tissue disorder related to use, overuse and pressure of thigh

    M70.951   Unspecified soft tissue disorder related to use, overuse and pressure, right thigh

    M70.952   Unspecified soft tissue disorder related to use, overuse and pressure, left thigh

    M70.959   Unspecified soft tissue disorder related to use, overuse and pressure, unspecified thigh

● M70.96   Unspecified soft tissue disorder related to use, overuse and pressure lower leg

    M70.961   Unspecified soft tissue disorder related to use, overuse and pressure, right lower leg

    M70.962   Unspecified soft tissue disorder related to use, overuse and pressure, left lower leg

    M70.969   Unspecified soft tissue disorder related to use, overuse and pressure, unspecified lower leg

● M70.97   Unspecified soft tissue disorder related to use, overuse and pressure of ankle and foot

    M70.971   Unspecified soft tissue disorder related to use, overuse and pressure, right ankle and foot

    M70.972   Unspecified soft tissue disorder related to use, overuse and pressure, left ankle and foot

    M70.979   Unspecified soft tissue disorder related to use, overuse and pressure, unspecified ankle and foot

   M70.98   Unspecified soft tissue disorder related to use, overuse and pressure other

   M70.99   Unspecified soft tissue disorder related to use, overuse and pressure multiple sites

● M71   Other bursopathies

   Excludes1   bunion (M20.1)
         bursitis related to use, overuse or pressure (M70.-)
         enthesopathies (M76-M77)

● M71.0   Abscess of bursa

   Use additional code (B95.-, B96.-) to identify causative organism

   M71.00   Abscess of bursa, unspecified site

● M71.01   Abscess of bursa, shoulder

    M71.011   Abscess of bursa, right shoulder

    M71.012   Abscess of bursa, left shoulder

    M71.019   Abscess of bursa, unspecified shoulder

● M71.02   Abscess of bursa, elbow

    M71.021   Abscess of bursa, right elbow

    M71.022   Abscess of bursa, left elbow

    M71.029   Abscess of bursa, unspecified elbow

● M71.03   Abscess of bursa, wrist

    M71.031   Abscess of bursa, right wrist

    M71.032   Abscess of bursa, left wrist

    M71.039   Abscess of bursa, unspecified wrist

● M71.04   Abscess of bursa, hand

    M71.041   Abscess of bursa, right hand

    M71.042   Abscess of bursa, left hand

    M71.049   Abscess of bursa, unspecified hand

◀ New   ◀▪▪ Revised   ~~deleted~~ Deleted   OGCR Official Guidelines   X Assign placeholder X   ● Use Additional Character(s)

Excludes 1   Excludes 2   Includes   Use additional   Code first   Code also   Unspecified

- M71.05 Abscess of bursa, hip
  - M71.051 Abscess of bursa, right hip
  - M71.052 Abscess of bursa, left hip
  - M71.059 Abscess of bursa, unspecified hip
- M71.06 Abscess of bursa, knee
  - M71.061 Abscess of bursa, right knee
  - M71.062 Abscess of bursa, left knee
  - M71.069 Abscess of bursa, unspecified knee
- M71.07 Abscess of bursa, ankle and foot
  - M71.071 Abscess of bursa, right ankle and foot
  - M71.072 Abscess of bursa, left ankle and foot
  - M71.079 Abscess of bursa, unspecified ankle and foot
  - M71.08 Abscess of bursa, other site
  - M71.09 Abscess of bursa, multiple sites
- M71.1 Other infective bursitis
  - Use additional code (B95.-, B96.-) to identify causative organism
  - M71.10 Other infective bursitis, unspecified site
- M71.11 Other infective bursitis, shoulder
  - M71.111 Other infective bursitis, right shoulder
  - M71.112 Other infective bursitis, left shoulder
  - M71.119 Other infective bursitis, unspecified shoulder
- M71.12 Other infective bursitis, elbow
  - M71.121 Other infective bursitis, right elbow
  - M71.122 Other infective bursitis, left elbow
  - M71.129 Other infective bursitis, unspecified elbow
- M71.13 Other infective bursitis, wrist
  - M71.131 Other infective bursitis, right wrist
  - M71.132 Other infective bursitis, left wrist
  - M71.139 Other infective bursitis, unspecified wrist
- M71.14 Other infective bursitis, hand
  - M71.141 Other infective bursitis, right hand
  - M71.142 Other infective bursitis, left hand
  - M71.149 Other infective bursitis, unspecified hand
- M71.15 Other infective bursitis, hip
  - M71.151 Other infective bursitis, right hip
  - M71.152 Other infective bursitis, left hip
  - M71.159 Other infective bursitis, unspecified hip
- M71.16 Other infective bursitis, knee
  - M71.161 Other infective bursitis, right knee
  - M71.162 Other infective bursitis, left knee
  - M71.169 Other infective bursitis, unspecified knee
- M71.17 Other infective bursitis, ankle and foot
  - M71.171 Other infective bursitis, right ankle and foot
  - M71.172 Other infective bursitis, left ankle and foot
  - M71.179 Other infective bursitis, unspecified ankle and foot
  - M71.18 Other infective bursitis, other site
  - M71.19 Other infective bursitis, multiple sites

- M71.2 Synovial cyst of popliteal space [Baker]
  - *Popliteal space = popliteal cavity, popliteal fossa. Depression in the posterior aspect of the knee (behind the knee).*
  - **Excludes1** synovial cyst of popliteal space with rupture (M66.0)
  - M71.20 Synovial cyst of popliteal space [Baker], unspecified knee
  - M71.21 Synovial cyst of popliteal space [Baker], right knee
  - M71.22 Synovial cyst of popliteal space [Baker], left knee
- M71.3 Other bursal cyst
  - Synovial cyst NOS
  - **Excludes1** synovial cyst with rupture (M66.1-)
  - M71.30 Other bursal cyst, unspecified site
- M71.31 Other bursal cyst, shoulder
  - M71.311 Other bursal cyst, right shoulder
  - M71.312 Other bursal cyst, left shoulder
  - M71.319 Other bursal cyst, unspecified shoulder
- M71.32 Other bursal cyst, elbow
  - M71.321 Other bursal cyst, right elbow
  - M71.322 Other bursal cyst, left elbow
  - M71.329 Other bursal cyst, unspecified elbow
- M71.33 Other bursal cyst, wrist
  - M71.331 Other bursal cyst, right wrist
  - M71.332 Other bursal cyst, left wrist
  - M71.339 Other bursal cyst, unspecified wrist
- M71.34 Other bursal cyst, hand
  - M71.341 Other bursal cyst, right hand
  - M71.342 Other bursal cyst, left hand
  - M71.349 Other bursal cyst, unspecified hand
- M71.35 Other bursal cyst, hip
  - M71.351 Other bursal cyst, right hip
  - M71.352 Other bursal cyst, left hip
  - M71.359 Other bursal cyst, unspecified hip
- M71.37 Other bursal cyst, ankle and foot
  - M71.371 Other bursal cyst, right ankle and foot
  - M71.372 Other bursal cyst, left ankle and foot
  - M71.379 Other bursal cyst, unspecified ankle and foot
  - M71.38 Other bursal cyst, other site
  - M71.39 Other bursal cyst, multiple sites
- M71.4 Calcium deposit in bursa
  - **Excludes2** calcium deposit in bursa of shoulder (M75.3)
  - M71.40 Calcium deposit in bursa, unspecified site
- M71.42 Calcium deposit in bursa, elbow
  - M71.421 Calcium deposit in bursa, right elbow
  - M71.422 Calcium deposit in bursa, left elbow
  - M71.429 Calcium deposit in bursa, unspecified elbow
- M71.43 Calcium deposit in bursa, wrist
  - M71.431 Calcium deposit in bursa, right wrist
  - M71.432 Calcium deposit in bursa, left wrist
  - M71.439 Calcium deposit in bursa, unspecified wrist
- M71.44 Calcium deposit in bursa, hand
  - M71.441 Calcium deposit in bursa, right hand
  - M71.442 Calcium deposit in bursa, left hand
  - M71.449 Calcium deposit in bursa, unspecified hand

● M71.45   Calcium deposit in bursa, hip
     M71.451   Calcium deposit in bursa, right hip
     M71.452   Calcium deposit in bursa, left hip
     M71.459   Calcium deposit in bursa, unspecified hip

● M71.46   Calcium deposit in bursa, knee
     M71.461   Calcium deposit in bursa, right knee
     M71.462   Calcium deposit in bursa, left knee
     M71.469   Calcium deposit in bursa, unspecified knee

● M71.47   Calcium deposit in bursa, ankle and foot
     M71.471   Calcium deposit in bursa, right ankle and foot
     M71.472   Calcium deposit in bursa, left ankle and foot
     M71.479   Calcium deposit in bursa, unspecified ankle and foot

   M71.48   Calcium deposit in bursa, other site
   M71.49   Calcium deposit in bursa, multiple sites

● M71.5   Other bursitis, not elsewhere classified

> **Excludes1**   bursitis NOS (M71.9-)
>
> **Excludes2**   bursitis of shoulder (M75.5)
>   bursitis of tibial collateral [Pellegrini-Stieda] (M76.4)

   M71.50   Other bursitis, not elsewhere classified, unspecified site

● M71.52   Other bursitis, not elsewhere classified, elbow
     M71.521   Other bursitis, not elsewhere classified, right elbow
     M71.522   Other bursitis, not elsewhere classified, left elbow
     M71.529   Other bursitis, not elsewhere classified, unspecified elbow

● M71.53   Other bursitis, not elsewhere classified, wrist
     M71.531   Other bursitis, not elsewhere classified, right wrist
     M71.532   Other bursitis, not elsewhere classified, left wrist
     M71.539   Other bursitis, not elsewhere classified, unspecified wrist

● M71.54   Other bursitis, not elsewhere classified, hand
     M71.541   Other bursitis, not elsewhere classified, right hand
     M71.542   Other bursitis, not elsewhere classified, left hand
     M71.549   Other bursitis, not elsewhere classified, unspecified hand

● M71.55   Other bursitis, not elsewhere classified, hip
     M71.551   Other bursitis, not elsewhere classified, right hip
     M71.552   Other bursitis, not elsewhere classified, left hip
     M71.559   Other bursitis, not elsewhere classified, unspecified hip

● M71.56   Other bursitis, not elsewhere classified, knee
     M71.561   Other bursitis, not elsewhere classified, right knee
     M71.562   Other bursitis, not elsewhere classified, left knee
     M71.569   Other bursitis, not elsewhere classified, unspecified knee

● M71.57   Other bursitis, not elsewhere classified, ankle and foot
     M71.571   Other bursitis, not elsewhere classified, right ankle and foot
     M71.572   Other bursitis, not elsewhere classified, left ankle and foot
     M71.579   Other bursitis, not elsewhere classified, unspecified ankle and foot

   M71.58   Other bursitis, not elsewhere classified, other site

● M71.8   Other specified bursopathies
   M71.80   Other specified bursopathies, unspecified site

● M71.81   Other specified bursopathies, shoulder
     M71.811   Other specified bursopathies, right shoulder
     M71.812   Other specified bursopathies, left shoulder
     M71.819   Other specified bursopathies, unspecified shoulder

● M71.82   Other specified bursopathies, elbow
     M71.821   Other specified bursopathies, right elbow
     M71.822   Other specified bursopathies, left elbow
     M71.829   Other specified bursopathies, unspecified elbow

● M71.83   Other specified bursopathies, wrist
     M71.831   Other specified bursopathies, right wrist
     M71.832   Other specified bursopathies, left wrist
     M71.839   Other specified bursopathies, unspecified wrist

● M71.84   Other specified bursopathies, hand
     M71.841   Other specified bursopathies, right hand
     M71.842   Other specified bursopathies, left hand
     M71.849   Other specified bursopathies, unspecified hand

● M71.85   Other specified bursopathies, hip
     M71.851   Other specified bursopathies, right hip
     M71.852   Other specified bursopathies, left hip
     M71.859   Other specified bursopathies, unspecified hip

● M71.86   Other specified bursopathies, knee
     M71.861   Other specified bursopathies, right knee
     M71.862   Other specified bursopathies, left knee
     M71.869   Other specified bursopathies, unspecified knee

● M71.87   Other specified bursopathies, ankle and foot
     M71.871   Other specified bursopathies, right ankle and foot
     M71.872   Other specified bursopathies, left ankle and foot
     M71.879   Other specified bursopathies, unspecified ankle and foot

   M71.88   Other specified bursopathies, other site
   M71.89   Other specified bursopathies, multiple sites

M71.9   Bursopathy, unspecified
     Bursitis NOS

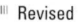

● M72 **Fibroblastic disorders**

  $\boxed{\text{Excludes2}}$ retroperitoneal fibromatosis (D48.3)

  M72.0 **Palmar fascial fibromatosis [Dupuytren]**

  M72.1 **Knuckle pads**

  M72.2 **Plantar fascial fibromatosis**
       Plantar fasciitis

  M72.4 **Pseudosarcomatous fibromatosis**
       Nodular fasciitis

  M72.6 **Necrotizing fasciitis**
       Use additional code (B95.-, B96.-) to identify causative
         organism

  M72.8 **Other fibroblastic disorders**
       Abscess of fascia
       Fasciitis NEC
       Other infective fasciitis
       Use additional code to (B95.-, B96.-) identify causative
         organism
       $\boxed{\text{Excludes1}}$ diffuse (eosinophilic) fasciitis (M35.4)
                 necrotizing fasciitis (M72.6)
                 nodular fasciitis (M72.4)
                 perirenal fasciitis NOS (N13.5)
                 perirenal fasciitis with infection (N13.6)
                 plantar fasciitis (M72.2)

  M72.9 **Fibroblastic disorder, unspecified**
       Fasciitis NOS
       Fibromatosis NOS

● M75 **Shoulder lesions**

  $\boxed{\text{Excludes2}}$ shoulder-hand syndrome (M89.0-)

  ● M75.0 **Adhesive capsulitis of shoulder**
       Frozen shoulder
       Periarthritis of shoulder
    M75.00 **Adhesive capsulitis of unspecified shoulder**
    M75.01 **Adhesive capsulitis of right shoulder**
    M75.02 **Adhesive capsulitis of left shoulder**

  ● M75.1 **Rotator cuff tear or rupture, not specified as traumatic**
       Rotator cuff syndrome
       Supraspinatus syndrome
       Supraspinatus tear or rupture, not specified as
         traumatic
       $\boxed{\text{Excludes1}}$ tear of rotator cuff, traumatic (S46.01-)
       Gradual onset due to repetitive stress to rotator cuff
    ● M75.10 **Unspecified rotator cuff tear or rupture, not
             specified as traumatic**
       M75.100 **Unspecified rotator cuff tear or
                 rupture of unspecified shoulder, not
                 specified as traumatic**
       M75.101 **Unspecified rotator cuff tear or
                 rupture of right shoulder, not
                 specified as traumatic**
       M75.102 **Unspecified rotator cuff tear or
                 rupture of left shoulder, not specified
                 as traumatic**
    ● M75.11 **Incomplete rotator cuff tear or rupture not
             specified as traumatic**
       M75.110 **Incomplete rotator cuff tear or rupture
                 of unspecified shoulder, not specified
                 as traumatic**
       M75.111 **Incomplete rotator cuff tear or rupture
                 of right shoulder, not specified as
                 traumatic**
       M75.112 **Incomplete rotator cuff tear or rupture
                 of left shoulder, not specified as
                 traumatic**

  ● M75.12 **Complete rotator cuff tear or rupture not
           specified as traumatic**
     M75.120 **Complete rotator cuff tear or rupture
               of unspecified shoulder, not specified
               as traumatic**
     M75.121 **Complete rotator cuff tear or rupture
               of right shoulder, not specified as
               traumatic**
     M75.122 **Complete rotator cuff tear or rupture
               of left shoulder, not specified as
               traumatic**

  ● M75.2 **Bicipital tendinitis**
    M75.20 **Bicipital tendinitis, unspecified shoulder**
    M75.21 **Bicipital tendinitis, right shoulder**
    M75.22 **Bicipital tendinitis, left shoulder**

  ● M75.3 **Calcific tendinitis of shoulder**
       Calcified bursa of shoulder
    M75.30 **Calcific tendinitis of unspecified shoulder**
    M75.31 **Calcific tendinitis of right shoulder**
    M75.32 **Calcific tendinitis of left shoulder**

  ● M75.4 **Impingement syndrome of shoulder**
    M75.40 **Impingement syndrome of unspecified
             shoulder**
    M75.41 **Impingement syndrome of right shoulder**
    M75.42 **Impingement syndrome of left shoulder**

  ● M75.5 **Bursitis of shoulder**
    M75.50 **Bursitis of unspecified shoulder**
    M75.51 **Bursitis of right shoulder**
    M75.52 **Bursitis of left shoulder**

  ● M75.8 **Other shoulder lesions**
    M75.80 **Other shoulder lesions, unspecified shoulder**
    M75.81 **Other shoulder lesions, right shoulder**
    M75.82 **Other shoulder lesions, left shoulder**

  ● M75.9 **Shoulder lesion, unspecified**
    M75.90 **Shoulder lesion, unspecified, unspecified
             shoulder**
    M75.91 **Shoulder lesion, unspecified, right shoulder**
    M75.92 **Shoulder lesion, unspecified, left shoulder**

● M76 **Enthesopathies, lower limb, excluding foot**

  $\boxed{\text{Excludes2}}$ bursitis due to use, overuse and pressure (M70.-)
             enthesopathies of ankle and foot (M77.5-)

  ● M76.0 **Gluteal tendinitis**
    M76.00 **Gluteal tendinitis, unspecified hip**
    M76.01 **Gluteal tendinitis, right hip**
    M76.02 **Gluteal tendinitis, left hip**

  ● M76.1 **Psoas tendinitis**
    M76.10 **Psoas tendinitis, unspecified hip**
    M76.11 **Psoas tendinitis, right hip**
    M76.12 **Psoas tendinitis, left hip**

  ● M76.2 **Iliac crest spur**
    M76.20 **Iliac crest spur, unspecified hip**
    M76.21 **Iliac crest spur, right hip**
    M76.22 **Iliac crest spur, left hip**

  ● M76.3 **Iliotibial band syndrome**
    M76.30 **Iliotibial band syndrome, unspecified leg**
    M76.31 **Iliotibial band syndrome, right leg**
    M76.32 **Iliotibial band syndrome, left leg**

  ● M76.4 **Tibial collateral bursitis [Pellegrini-Stieda]**
    M76.40 **Tibial collateral bursitis [Pellegrini-Stieda],
             unspecified leg**
    M76.41 **Tibial collateral bursitis [Pellegrini-Stieda],
             right leg**
    M76.42 **Tibial collateral bursitis [Pellegrini-Stieda], left
             leg**

CHAPTER 13 (M00-M99)

- **M76.5 Patellar tendinitis**
  - M76.50 Patellar tendinitis, unspecified knee
  - M76.51 Patellar tendinitis, right knee
  - M76.52 Patellar tendinitis, left knee
- **M76.6 Achilles tendinitis**
  - Achilles bursitis
  - M76.60 Achilles tendinitis, unspecified leg
  - M76.61 Achilles tendinitis, right leg
  - M76.62 Achilles tendinitis, left leg
- **M76.7 Peroneal tendinitis**
  - M76.70 Peroneal tendinitis, unspecified leg
  - M76.71 Peroneal tendinitis, right leg
  - M76.72 Peroneal tendinitis, left leg
- **M76.8 Other specified enthesopathies of lower limb, excluding foot**
  - **M76.81 Anterior tibial syndrome**
    - M76.811 Anterior tibial syndrome, right leg
    - M76.812 Anterior tibial syndrome, left leg
    - M76.819 Anterior tibial syndrome, unspecified leg
  - **M76.82 Posterior tibial tendinitis**
    - M76.821 Posterior tibial tendinitis, right leg
    - M76.822 Posterior tibial tendinitis, left leg
    - M76.829 Posterior tibial tendinitis, unspecified leg
  - **M76.89 Other specified enthesopathies of lower limb, excluding foot**
    - M76.891 Other specified enthesopathies of right lower limb, excluding foot
    - M76.892 Other specified enthesopathies of left lower limb, excluding foot
    - M76.899 Other specified enthesopathies of unspecified lower limb, excluding foot
- **M76.9 Unspecified enthesopathy, lower limb, excluding foot**

- **M77 Other enthesopathies**
  - **Excludes1** bursitis NOS (M71.9-)
  - **Excludes2** bursitis due to use, overuse and pressure (M70.-)
    - osteophyte (M25.7)
    - spinal enthesopathy (M46.0-)
  - **M77.0 Medial epicondylitis**
    - M77.00 Medial epicondylitis, unspecified elbow
    - M77.01 Medial epicondylitis, right elbow
    - M77.02 Medial epicondylitis, left elbow
  - **M77.1 Lateral epicondylitis**
    - Tennis elbow
    - M77.10 Lateral epicondylitis, unspecified elbow
    - M77.11 Lateral epicondylitis, right elbow
    - M77.12 Lateral epicondylitis, left elbow
  - **M77.2 Periarthritis of wrist**
    - M77.20 Periarthritis, unspecified wrist
    - M77.21 Periarthritis, right wrist
    - M77.22 Periarthritis, left wrist
  - **M77.3 Calcaneal spur**
    - M77.30 Calcaneal spur, unspecified foot
    - M77.31 Calcaneal spur, right foot
    - M77.32 Calcaneal spur, left foot
  - **M77.4 Metatarsalgia**
    - **Excludes1** Morton's metatarsalgia (G57.6)
    - M77.40 Metatarsalgia, unspecified foot
    - M77.41 Metatarsalgia, right foot
    - M77.42 Metatarsalgia, left foot

- **M77.5 Other enthesopathy of foot**
  - M77.50 Other enthesopathy of unspecified foot
  - M77.51 Other enthesopathy of right foot
  - M77.52 Other enthesopathy of left foot
- **M77.8 Other enthesopathies, not elsewhere classified**
- **M77.9 Enthesopathy, unspecified**
  - Bone spur NOS
  - Capsulitis NOS
  - Periarthritis NOS
  - Tendinitis NOS

- **M79 Other and unspecified soft tissue disorders, not elsewhere classified**
  - **Excludes1** psychogenic rheumatism (F45.8)
    - soft tissue pain, psychogenic (F45.41)
  - **M79.0 Rheumatism, unspecified**
    - **Excludes1** fibromyalgia (M79.7)
      - palindromic rheumatism (M12.3-)
  - **M79.1 Myalgia**
    - Myofascial pain syndrome
    - **Excludes1** fibromyalgia (M79.7)
      - myositis (M60.-)
  - **M79.2 Neuralgia and neuritis, unspecified**
    - **Excludes1** brachial radiculitis NOS (M54.1)
      - lumbosacral radiculitis NOS (M54.1)
      - mononeuropathies (G56-G58)
      - radiculitis NOS (M54.1)
      - sciatica (M54.3-M54.4)
  - **M79.3 Panniculitis, unspecified**
    - **Excludes1** lupus panniculitis (L93.2)
      - neck and back panniculitis (M54.0-)
      - relapsing [Weber-Christian] panniculitis (M35.6)
  - **M79.4 Hypertrophy of (infrapatellar) fat pad**
  - **M79.5 Residual foreign body in soft tissue**
    - **Excludes1** foreign body granuloma of skin and subcutaneous tissue (L92.3)
      - foreign body granuloma of soft tissue (M60.2-)
  - **M79.6 Pain in limb, hand, foot, fingers and toes**
    - **Excludes2** pain in joint (M25.5-)
    - **M79.60 Pain in limb, unspecified**
      - M79.601 Pain in right arm
        - Pain in right upper limb NOS
      - M79.602 Pain in left arm
        - Pain in left upper limb NOS
      - M79.603 Pain in arm, unspecified
        - Pain in upper limb NOS
      - M79.604 Pain in right leg
        - Pain in right lower limb NOS
      - M79.605 Pain in left leg
        - Pain in left lower limb NOS
      - M79.606 Pain in leg, unspecified
        - Pain in lower limb NOS
      - M79.609 Pain in unspecified limb
        - Pain in limb NOS
    - **M79.62 Pain in upper arm**
      - Pain in axillary region
      - M79.621 Pain in right upper arm
      - M79.622 Pain in left upper arm
      - M79.629 Pain in unspecified upper arm
    - **M79.63 Pain in forearm**
      - M79.631 Pain in right forearm
      - M79.632 Pain in left forearm
      - M79.639 Pain in unspecified forearm

◀ New   ⬅ Revised   ~~deleted~~ Deleted   **OGCR** Official Guidelines   X Assign placeholder X   ● Use Additional Character(s)

Excludes 1   Excludes 2   Includes   Use additional   Code first   Code also   Unspecified

● **M79.64 Pain in hand and fingers**
    M79.641 Pain in right hand
    M79.642 Pain in left hand
    M79.643 Pain in unspecified hand
    M79.644 Pain in right finger(s)
    M79.645 Pain in left finger(s)
    M79.646 Pain in unspecified finger(s)
● **M79.65 Pain in thigh**
    M79.651 Pain in right thigh
    M79.652 Pain in left thigh
    M79.659 Pain in unspecified thigh
● **M79.66 Pain in lower leg**
    M79.661 Pain in right lower leg
    M79.662 Pain in left lower leg
    M79.669 Pain in unspecified lower leg
● **M79.67 Pain in foot and toes**
    M79.671 Pain in right foot
    M79.672 Pain in left foot
    M79.673 Pain in unspecified foot
    M79.674 Pain in right toe(s)
    M79.675 Pain in left toe(s)
    M79.676 Pain in unspecified toe(s)

M79.7 Fibromyalgia
    Fibromyositis
    Fibrositis
    Myofibrositis

● **M79.A Nontraumatic compartment syndrome**
    Code first, if applicable, associated postprocedural
    complication

    Excludes1   compartment syndrome NOS (T79.A-)
         fibromyalgia (M79.7) nontraumatic
         ischemic infarction of muscle
         (M62.2-)
         traumatic compartment syndrome
         (T79.A-)

● **M79.A1 Nontraumatic compartment syndrome of upper extremity**
    Nontraumatic compartment syndrome of
    shoulder, arm, forearm, wrist, hand, and
    fingers
    M79.A11 Nontraumatic compartment syndrome of right upper extremity
    M79.A12 Nontraumatic compartment syndrome of left upper extremity
    M79.A19 Nontraumatic compartment syndrome of unspecified upper extremity

● **M79.A2 Nontraumatic compartment syndrome of lower extremity**
    Nontraumatic compartment syndrome of hip,
    buttock, thigh, leg, foot, and toes
    M79.A21 Nontraumatic compartment syndrome of right lower extremity
    M79.A22 Nontraumatic compartment syndrome of left lower extremity
    M79.A29 Nontraumatic compartment syndrome of unspecified lower extremity

    M79.A3 Nontraumatic compartment syndrome of abdomen

    M79.A9 Nontraumatic compartment syndrome of other sites

● **M79.8 Other specified soft tissue disorders**
    M79.81 Nontraumatic hematoma of soft tissue
       Nontraumatic hematoma of muscle
       Nontraumatic seroma of muscle and soft tissue

    M79.89 Other specified soft tissue disorders
       Polyalgia

M79.9 Soft tissue disorder, unspecified

OGCR See Section I.C., Chapter 13.d.
Osteoporosis

OSTEOPATHIES AND CHONDROPATHIES (M80-M94)

DISORDERS OF BONE DENSITY AND STRUCTURE (M80-M85)

M80 Osteoporosis with current pathological fracture
Excessive skeletal fragility (porous bone) resulting in bone fractures

    Includes   osteoporosis with current fragility fracture

    Use additional code to identify major osseous defect, if applicable (M89.7-)

    Excludes1   collapsed vertebra NOS (M48.5)
           pathological fracture NOS (M84.4)
           wedging of vertebra NOS (M48.5)

    Excludes2   personal history of (healed) osteoporosis fracture
           (Z87.310)

The appropriate 7th character is to be added to each code from category M80:

A	initial encounter for fracture
	All encounters involving diagnosis and treatment
D	subsequent encounter for fracture with routine healing
G	subsequent encounter for fracture with delayed healing
	Encounters for attention to casting or fixation devices, medication, and follow-up visits during the healing phase
K	subsequent encounter for fracture with nonunion
	Total failure of fracture healing
P	subsequent encounter for fracture with malunion
	Fracture ends do not heal together correctly.
S	sequela

● **M80.0 Age-related osteoporosis with current pathological fracture**
    Involutional osteoporosis with current pathological fracture
    Osteoporosis NOS with current pathological fracture
    Postmenopausal osteoporosis with current pathological fracture
    Senile osteoporosis with current pathological fracture

    X● **M80.00 Age-related osteoporosis with current pathological fracture, unspecified site**

    ● **M80.01 Age-related osteoporosis with current pathological fracture, shoulder**
       ● **M80.011 Age-related osteoporosis with current pathological fracture, right shoulder**
       ● **M80.012 Age-related osteoporosis with current pathological fracture, left shoulder**
       ● **M80.019 Age-related osteoporosis with current pathological fracture, unspecified shoulder**

    ● **M80.02 Age-related osteoporosis with current pathological fracture, humerus**
       ● **M80.021 Age-related osteoporosis with current pathological fracture, right humerus**
       ● **M80.022 Age-related osteoporosis with current pathological fracture, left humerus**
       ● **M80.029 Age-related osteoporosis with current pathological fracture, unspecified humerus**

    ● **M80.03 Age-related osteoporosis with current pathological fracture, forearm**
       Age-related osteoporosis with current pathological fracture of wrist
       ● **M80.031 Age-related osteoporosis with current pathological fracture, right forearm**
       ● **M80.032 Age-related osteoporosis with current pathological fracture, left forearm**
       ● **M80.039 Age-related osteoporosis with current pathological fracture, unspecified forearm**

◀ New   ◀|||| Revised   ~~deleted~~ Deleted   **OGCR** Official Guidelines   X Assign placeholder X   ● Use Additional Character(s)

Excludes 1   Excludes 2   Includes   Use additional   Code first   Code also   Unspecified

1083

CHAPTER 13 (M00-M99)

● **M80.04**   **Age-related osteoporosis with current pathological fracture, hand**
- ● **M80.041**   Age-related osteoporosis with current pathological fracture, right hand
- ● **M80.042**   Age-related osteoporosis with current pathological fracture, left hand
- ● **M80.049**   Age-related osteoporosis with current pathological fracture, unspecified hand

● **M80.05**   **Age-related osteoporosis with current pathological fracture, femur**
Age-related osteoporosis with current pathological fracture of hip
- ● **M80.051**   Age-related osteoporosis with current pathological fracture, right femur
- ● **M80.052**   Age-related osteoporosis with current pathological fracture, left femur
- ● **M80.059**   Age-related osteoporosis with current pathological fracture, unspecified femur

● **M80.06**   **Age-related osteoporosis with current pathological fracture, lower leg**
- ● **M80.061**   Age-related osteoporosis with current pathological fracture, right lower leg
- ● **M80.062**   Age-related osteoporosis with current pathological fracture, left lower leg
- ● **M80.069**   Age-related osteoporosis with current pathological fracture, unspecified lower leg

● **M80.07**   **Age-related osteoporosis with current pathological fracture, ankle and foot**
- ● **M80.071**   Age-related osteoporosis with current pathological fracture, right ankle and foot
- ● **M80.072**   Age-related osteoporosis with current pathological fracture, left ankle and foot
- ● **M80.079**   Age-related osteoporosis with current pathological fracture, unspecified ankle and foot

X ● **M80.08**   **Age-related osteoporosis with current pathological fracture, vertebra(e)**

● **M80.8**   **Other osteoporosis with current pathological fracture**
Drug-induced osteoporosis with current pathological fracture
Idiopathic osteoporosis with current pathological fracture
Osteoporosis of disuse with current pathological fracture
Postoophorectomy osteoporosis with current pathological fracture
Postsurgical malabsorption osteoporosis with current pathological fracture
Post-traumatic osteoporosis with current pathological fracture

Use additional code for adverse effect, if applicable, to identify drug (T36-T50 with fifth or sixth character 5)

X ● **M80.80**   **Other osteoporosis with current pathological fracture, unspecified site**

● **M80.81**   **Other osteoporosis with pathological fracture, shoulder**
- ● **M80.811**   Other osteoporosis with current pathological fracture, right shoulder
- ● **M80.812**   Other osteoporosis with current pathological fracture, left shoulder
- ● **M80.819**   Other osteoporosis with current pathological fracture, unspecified shoulder

● **M80.82**   **Other osteoporosis with current pathological fracture, humerus**
- ● **M80.821**   Other osteoporosis with current pathological fracture, right humerus
- ● **M80.822**   Other osteoporosis with current pathological fracture, left humerus
- ● **M80.829**   Other osteoporosis with current pathological fracture, unspecified humerus

● **M80.83**   **Other osteoporosis with current pathological fracture, forearm**
Other osteoporosis with current pathological fracture of wrist
- ● **M80.831**   Other osteoporosis with current pathological fracture, right forearm
- ● **M80.832**   Other osteoporosis with current pathological fracture, left forearm
- ● **M80.839**   Other osteoporosis with current pathological fracture, unspecified forearm

● **M80.84**   **Other osteoporosis with current pathological fracture, hand**
- ● **M80.841**   Other osteoporosis with current pathological fracture, right hand
- ● **M80.842**   Other osteoporosis with current pathological fracture, left hand
- ● **M80.849**   Other osteoporosis with current pathological fracture, unspecified hand

● **M80.85**   **Other osteoporosis with current pathological fracture, femur**
Other osteoporosis with current pathological fracture of hip
- ● **M80.851**   Other osteoporosis with current pathological fracture, right femur
- ● **M80.852**   Other osteoporosis with current pathological fracture, left femur
- ● **M80.859**   Other osteoporosis with current pathological fracture, unspecified femur

● **M80.86**   **Other osteoporosis with current pathological fracture, lower leg**
- ● **M80.861**   Other osteoporosis with current pathological fracture, right lower leg
- ● **M80.862**   Other osteoporosis with current pathological fracture, left lower leg
- ● **M80.869**   Other osteoporosis with current pathological fracture, unspecified lower leg

● **M80.87**   **Other osteoporosis with current pathological fracture, ankle and foot**
- ● **M80.871**   Other osteoporosis with current pathological fracture, right ankle and foot
- ● **M80.872**   Other osteoporosis with current pathological fracture, left ankle and foot
- ● **M80.879**   Other osteoporosis with current pathological fracture, unspecified ankle and foot

X ● **M80.88**   **Other osteoporosis with current pathological fracture, vertebra(e)**

● **M81   Osteoporosis without current pathological fracture**
     Use additional code to identify:
        major osseous defect, if applicable (M89.7-)
        personal history of (healed) osteoporosis fracture, if
          applicable (Z87.310)
     Excludes1   osteoporosis with current pathological fracture
                (M80.-)
               Sudeck's atrophy (M89.0)

   M81.0   Age-related osteoporosis without current pathological
         fracture
         Involutional osteoporosis without current pathological
            fracture
         Osteoporosis NOS
         Postmenopausal osteoporosis without current
            pathological fracture
         Senile osteoporosis without current pathological
            fracture

   M81.6   Localized osteoporosis [Lequesne]
     Excludes1   Sudeck's atrophy (M89.0)

   M81.8   Other osteoporosis without current pathological fracture
         Drug-induced osteoporosis without current
            pathological fracture
         Idiopathic osteoporosis without current pathological
            fracture
         Osteoporosis of disuse without current pathological
            fracture
         Postoophorectomy osteoporosis without current
            pathological fracture
         Postsurgical malabsorption osteoporosis without
            current pathological fracture
         Post-traumatic osteoporosis without current
            pathological fracture
     Use additional code for adverse effect, if applicable,
        to identify drug (T36-T50 with fifth or sixth
        character 5)

● **M83   Adult osteomalacia**
     Excludes1   infantile and juvenile osteomalacia (E55.0)
             renal osteodystrophy (N25.0)
             rickets (active) (E55.0)
             rickets (active) sequelae (E64.3)
             vitamin D-resistant osteomalacia (E83.3)
             vitamin D-resistant rickets (active) (E83.3)

   M83.0   Puerperal osteomalacia
   M83.1   Senile osteomalacia
   M83.2   Adult osteomalacia due to malabsorption
         Postsurgical malabsorption osteomalacia in adults
   M83.3   Adult osteomalacia due to malnutrition
   M83.4   Aluminum bone disease
   M83.5   Other drug-induced osteomalacia in adults
     Use additional code for adverse effect, if applicable,
        to identify drug (T36-T50 with fifth or sixth
        character 5)
   M83.8   Other adult osteomalacia
   M83.9   Adult osteomalacia, unspecified

● **M84   Disorder of continuity of bone**
     Excludes2   traumatic fracture of bone-see fracture, by site

   ● **M84.3   Stress fracture**
         Fatigue fracture
         March fracture
         Stress fracture NOS
         Stress reaction
     Use additional external cause code(s) to identify the
        cause of the stress fracture
     Excludes1   pathological fracture NOS (M84.4.-)
             pathological fracture due to osteoporosis
                (M80.-)
             traumatic fracture (S12.-, S22.-, S32.-,
                S42.-, S52.-, S62.-, S72.-, S82.-, S92.-)
     Excludes2   personal history of (healed) stress
             (fatigue) fracture (Z87.312)
             stress fracture of vertebra (M48.4-)
     The appropriate 7th character is to be added to each
        code from subcategory M84.3:

> A   initial encounter for fracture
> D   subsequent encounter for fracture
>   with routine healing
> G   subsequent encounter for fracture
>   with delayed healing
> K   subsequent encounter for fracture
>   with nonunion
> P   subsequent encounter for fracture
>   with malunion
> S   sequela

X ● **M84.30   Stress fracture, unspecified site**
   ● **M84.31   Stress fracture, shoulder**
     ● **M84.311   Stress fracture, right shoulder**
     ● **M84.312   Stress fracture, left shoulder**
     ● **M84.319   Stress fracture, unspecified shoulder**
   ● **M84.32   Stress fracture, humerus**
     ● **M84.321   Stress fracture, right humerus**
     ● **M84.322   Stress fracture, left humerus**
     ● **M84.329   Stress fracture, unspecified humerus**
   ● **M84.33   Stress fracture, ulna and radius**
     ● **M84.331   Stress fracture, right ulna**
     ● **M84.332   Stress fracture, left ulna**
     ● **M84.333   Stress fracture, right radius**
     ● **M84.334   Stress fracture, left radius**
     ● **M84.339   Stress fracture, unspecified ulna and**
                radius
   ● **M84.34   Stress fracture, hand and fingers**
     ● **M84.341   Stress fracture, right hand**
     ● **M84.342   Stress fracture, left hand**
     ● **M84.343   Stress fracture, unspecified hand**
     ● **M84.344   Stress fracture, right finger(s)**
     ● **M84.345   Stress fracture, left finger(s)**
     ● **M84.346   Stress fracture, unspecified finger(s)**
   ● **M84.35   Stress fracture, pelvis and femur**
         Stress fracture, hip
     ● **M84.350   Stress fracture, pelvis**
     ● **M84.351   Stress fracture, right femur**
     ● **M84.352   Stress fracture, left femur**
     ● **M84.353   Stress fracture, unspecified femur**
     ● **M84.359   Stress fracture, hip, unspecified**

CHAPTER 13 (M00-M99)

CHAPTER 13 (M00-M99)

● M84.36 Stress fracture, tibia and fibula
    ● M84.361 Stress fracture, right tibia
    ● M84.362 Stress fracture, left tibia
    ● M84.363 Stress fracture, right fibula
    ● M84.364 Stress fracture, left fibula
    ● M84.369 Stress fracture, unspecified tibia and fibula
● M84.37 Stress fracture, ankle, foot and toes
    ● M84.371 Stress fracture, right ankle
    ● M84.372 Stress fracture, left ankle
    ● M84.373 Stress fracture, unspecified ankle
    ● M84.374 Stress fracture, right foot
    ● M84.375 Stress fracture, left foot
    ● M84.376 Stress fracture, unspecified foot
    ● M84.377 Stress fracture, right toe(s)
    ● M84.378 Stress fracture, left toe(s)
    ● M84.379 Stress fracture, unspecified toe(s)
X ● M84.38 Stress fracture, other site

Excludes2 stress fracture of vertebra (M48.4-)

● M84.4 Pathological fracture, not elsewhere classified
    Chronic fracture
    Pathological fracture NOS

Excludes1 collapsed vertebra NEC (M48.5)
    pathological fracture in neoplastic disease (M84.5-)
    pathological fracture in osteoporosis (M80.-)
    pathological fracture in other disease (M84.6-)
    stress fracture (M84.3-)
    traumatic fracture (S12.-, S22.-, S32.-, S42.-, S52.-, S62.-, S72.-, S82.-, S92.-)

Excludes2 personal history of (healed) pathological fracture (Z87.311)

The appropriate 7th character is to be added to each code from subcategory M84.4:

A	initial encounter for fracture
D	subsequent encounter for fracture with routine healing
G	subsequent encounter for fracture with delayed healing
K	subsequent encounter for fracture with nonunion
P	subsequent encounter for fracture with malunion
S	sequela

X ● M84.40 Pathological fracture, unspecified site
● M84.41 Pathological fracture, shoulder
    ● M84.411 Pathological fracture, right shoulder
    ● M84.412 Pathological fracture, left shoulder
    ● M84.419 Pathological fracture, unspecified shoulder

● M84.42 Pathological fracture, humerus
    ● M84.421 Pathological fracture, right humerus
    ● M84.422 Pathological fracture, left humerus
    ● M84.429 Pathological fracture, unspecified humerus
● M84.43 Pathological fracture, ulna and radius
    ● M84.431 Pathological fracture, right ulna
    ● M84.432 Pathological fracture, left ulna
    ● M84.433 Pathological fracture, right radius
    ● M84.434 Pathological fracture, left radius
    ● M84.439 Pathological fracture, unspecified ulna and radius
● M84.44 Pathological fracture, hand and fingers
    ● M84.441 Pathological fracture, right hand
    ● M84.442 Pathological fracture, left hand
    ● M84.443 Pathological fracture, unspecified hand
    ● M84.444 Pathological fracture, right finger(s)
    ● M84.445 Pathological fracture, left finger(s)
    ● M84.446 Pathological fracture, unspecified finger(s)
● M84.45 Pathological fracture, femur and pelvis
    ● M84.451 Pathological fracture, right femur
    ● M84.452 Pathological fracture, left femur
    ● M84.453 Pathological fracture, unspecified femur
    ● M84.454 Pathological fracture, pelvis
    ● M84.459 Pathological fracture, hip, unspecified
● M84.46 Pathological fracture, tibia and fibula
    ● M84.461 Pathological fracture, right tibia
    ● M84.462 Pathological fracture, left tibia
    ● M84.463 Pathological fracture, right fibula
    ● M84.464 Pathological fracture, left fibula
    ● M84.469 Pathological fracture, unspecified tibia and fibula
● M84.47 Pathological fracture, ankle, foot and toes
    ● M84.471 Pathological fracture, right ankle
    ● M84.472 Pathological fracture, left ankle
    ● M84.473 Pathological fracture, unspecified ankle
    ● M84.474 Pathological fracture, right foot
    ● M84.475 Pathological fracture, left foot
    ● M84.476 Pathological fracture, unspecified foot
    ● M84.477 Pathological fracture, right toe(s)
    ● M84.478 Pathological fracture, left toe(s)
    ● M84.479 Pathological fracture, unspecified toe(s)
X ● M84.48 Pathological fracture, other site

OGCR Section I.a, Chapter 13.C.

Coding of Pathologic Fractures

7th character A is for use as long as the patient is receiving active treatment for the fracture. Examples of active treatment are: surgical treatment, emergency department encounter, evaluation and continuing treatment by the same or a different physician. While the patient may be seen by a new or different provider over the course of treatment for a pathological fracture, assignment of the 7th character is based on whether the patient is undergoing active treatment and not whether the provider is seeing the patient for the first time.3. 7th character, D is to be used for encounters after the patient has completed active treatment. The other 7th characters, listed under each subcategory in the Tabular List, are to be used for subsequent encounters for treatment of problems associated with the healing, such as malunions, nonunions, and sequelae.

Care for complications of surgical treatment for fracture repairs during the healing or recovery phase should be coded with the appropriate complication codes.

See Section I.C.19. Coding of traumatic fractures.

● **M84.5 Pathological fracture in neoplastic disease**
> Code also underlying neoplasm
> The appropriate 7th character is to be added to each code from subcategory M84.5:

> | | |
> |---|---|
> | A | initial encounter for fracture |
> | D | subsequent encounter for fracture with routine healing |
> | G | subsequent encounter for fracture with delayed healing |
> | K | subsequent encounter for fracture with nonunion |
> | P | subsequent encounter for fracture with malunion |
> | S | sequela |

X ● **M84.50 Pathological fracture in neoplastic disease, unspecified site**

● **M84.51 Pathological fracture in neoplastic disease, shoulder**
   ● M84.511 Pathological fracture in neoplastic disease, right shoulder
   ● M84.512 Pathological fracture in neoplastic disease, left shoulder
   ● M84.519 Pathological fracture in neoplastic disease, unspecified shoulder

● **M84.52 Pathological fracture in neoplastic disease, humerus**
   ● M84.521 Pathological fracture in neoplastic disease, right humerus
   ● M84.522 Pathological fracture in neoplastic disease, left humerus
   ● M84.529 Pathological fracture in neoplastic disease, unspecified humerus

● **M84.53 Pathological fracture in neoplastic disease, ulna and radius**
   ● M84.531 Pathological fracture in neoplastic disease, right ulna
   ● M84.532 Pathological fracture in neoplastic disease, left ulna
   ● M84.533 Pathological fracture in neoplastic disease, right radius
   ● M84.534 Pathological fracture in neoplastic disease, left radius
   ● M84.539 Pathological fracture in neoplastic disease, unspecified ulna and radius

● **M84.54 Pathological fracture in neoplastic disease, hand**
   ● M84.541 Pathological fracture in neoplastic disease, right hand
   ● M84.542 Pathological fracture in neoplastic disease, left hand
   ● M84.549 Pathological fracture in neoplastic disease, unspecified hand

● **M84.55 Pathological fracture in neoplastic disease, pelvis and femur**
   ● M84.550 Pathological fracture in neoplastic disease, pelvis
   ● M84.551 Pathological fracture in neoplastic disease, right femur
   ● M84.552 Pathological fracture in neoplastic disease, left femur
   ● M84.553 Pathological fracture in neoplastic disease, unspecified femur
   ● M84.559 Pathological fracture in neoplastic disease, hip, unspecified

● **M84.56 Pathological fracture in neoplastic disease, tibia and fibula**
   ● M84.561 Pathological fracture in neoplastic disease, right tibia
   ● M84.562 Pathological fracture in neoplastic disease, left tibia
   ● M84.563 Pathological fracture in neoplastic disease, right fibula
   ● M84.564 Pathological fracture in neoplastic disease, left fibula
   ● M84.569 Pathological fracture in neoplastic disease, unspecified tibia and fibula

● **M84.57 Pathological fracture in neoplastic disease, ankle and foot**
   ● M84.571 Pathological fracture in neoplastic disease, right ankle
   ● M84.572 Pathological fracture in neoplastic disease, left ankle
   ● M84.573 Pathological fracture in neoplastic disease, unspecified ankle
   ● M84.574 Pathological fracture in neoplastic disease, right foot
   ● M84.575 Pathological fracture in neoplastic disease, left foot
   ● M84.576 Pathological fracture in neoplastic disease, unspecified foot

X ● **M84.58 Pathological fracture in neoplastic disease, other specified site**
> Pathological fracture in neoplastic disease, vertebrae

● **M84.6 Pathological fracture in other disease**
> Code also underlying condition
> **Excludes1** pathological fracture in osteoporosis (M80.-)
> The appropriate 7th character is to be added to each code from subcategory M84.6:

> | | |
> |---|---|
> | A | initial encounter for fracture |
> | D | subsequent encounter for fracture with routine healing |
> | G | subsequent encounter for fracture with delayed healing |
> | K | subsequent encounter for fracture with nonunion |
> | P | subsequent encounter for fracture with malunion |
> | S | sequela |

X ● **M84.60 Pathological fracture in other disease, unspecified site**

● **M84.61 Pathological fracture in other disease, shoulder**
   ● M84.611 Pathological fracture in other disease, right shoulder
   ● M84.612 Pathological fracture in other disease, left shoulder
   ● M84.619 Pathological fracture in other disease, unspecified shoulder

◀ New   ◀▥ Revised   d̶e̶l̶e̶t̶e̶d̶ Deleted   **OGCR** Official Guidelines   X Assign placeholder X   ● Use Additional Character(s)

| Excludes 1 | Excludes 2 | Includes | Use additional | Code first | Code also | Unspecified |

● M84.62   Pathological fracture in other disease, humerus
- ● M84.621   Pathological fracture in other disease, right humerus
- ● M84.622   Pathological fracture in other disease, left humerus
- ● M84.629   Pathological fracture in other disease, unspecified humerus

● M84.63   Pathological fracture in other disease, ulna and radius
- ● M84.631   Pathological fracture in other disease, right ulna
- ● M84.632   Pathological fracture in other disease, left ulna
- ● M84.633   Pathological fracture in other disease, right radius
- ● M84.634   Pathological fracture in other disease, left radius
- ● M84.639   Pathological fracture in other disease, unspecified ulna and radius

● M84.64   Pathological fracture in other disease, hand
- ● M84.641   Pathological fracture in other disease, right hand
- ● M84.642   Pathological fracture in other disease, left hand
- ● M84.649   Pathological fracture in other disease, unspecified hand

● M84.65   Pathological fracture in other disease, pelvis and femur
- ● M84.650   Pathological fracture in other disease, pelvis
- ● M84.651   Pathological fracture in other disease, right femur
- ● M84.652   Pathological fracture in other disease, left femur
- ● M84.653   Pathological fracture in other disease, unspecified femur
- ● M84.659   Pathological fracture in other disease, hip, unspecified

● M84.66   Pathological fracture in other disease, tibia and fibula
- ● M84.661   Pathological fracture in other disease, right tibia
- ● M84.662   Pathological fracture in other disease, left tibia
- ● M84.663   Pathological fracture in other disease, right fibula
- ● M84.664   Pathological fracture in other disease, left fibula
- ● M84.669   Pathological fracture in other disease, unspecified tibia and fibula

● M84.67   Pathological fracture in other disease, ankle and foot
- ● M84.671   Pathological fracture in other disease, right ankle
- ● M84.672   Pathological fracture in other disease, left ankle
- ● M84.673   Pathological fracture in other disease, unspecified ankle
- ● M84.674   Pathological fracture in other disease, right foot
- ● M84.675   Pathological fracture in other disease, left foot
- ● M84.676   Pathological fracture in other disease, unspecified foot

X ● M84.68   Pathological fracture in other disease, other site

● M84.8   Other disorders of continuity of bone
- M84.80   Other disorders of continuity of bone, unspecified site
- ● M84.81   Other disorders of continuity of bone, shoulder
  - M84.811   Other disorders of continuity of bone, right shoulder
  - M84.812   Other disorders of continuity of bone, left shoulder
  - M84.819   Other disorders of continuity of bone, unspecified shoulder
- ● M84.82   Other disorders of continuity of bone, humerus
  - M84.821   Other disorders of continuity of bone, right humerus
  - M84.822   Other disorders of continuity of bone, left humerus
  - M84.829   Other disorders of continuity of bone, unspecified humerus
- ● M84.83   Other disorders of continuity of bone, ulna and radius
  - M84.831   Other disorders of continuity of bone, right ulna
  - M84.832   Other disorders of continuity of bone, left ulna
  - M84.833   Other disorders of continuity of bone, right radius
  - M84.834   Other disorders of continuity of bone, left radius
  - M84.839   Other disorders of continuity of bone, unspecified ulna and radius
- ● M84.84   Other disorders of continuity of bone, hand
  - M84.841   Other disorders of continuity of bone, right hand
  - M84.842   Other disorders of continuity of bone, left hand
  - M84.849   Other disorders of continuity of bone, unspecified hand
- ● M84.85   Other disorders of continuity of bone, pelvic region and thigh
  - M84.851   Other disorders of continuity of bone, right pelvic region and thigh
  - M84.852   Other disorders of continuity of bone, left pelvic region and thigh
  - M84.859   Other disorders of continuity of bone, unspecified pelvic region and thigh
- ● M84.86   Other disorders of continuity of bone, tibia and fibula
  - M84.861   Other disorders of continuity of bone, right tibia
  - M84.862   Other disorders of continuity of bone, left tibia
  - M84.863   Other disorders of continuity of bone, right fibula
  - M84.864   Other disorders of continuity of bone, left fibula
  - M84.869   Other disorders of continuity of bone, unspecified tibia and fibula
- ● M84.87   Other disorders of continuity of bone, ankle and foot
  - M84.871   Other disorders of continuity of bone, right ankle and foot
  - M84.872   Other disorders of continuity of bone, left ankle and foot
  - M84.879   Other disorders of continuity of bone, unspecified ankle and foot
- M84.88   Other disorders of continuity of bone, other site

M84.9   Disorder of continuity of bone, unspecified

● **M85**   **Other disorders of bone density and structure**

    Excludes1   osteogenesis imperfecta (Q78.0)
                 osteopetrosis (Q78.2)
                 osteopoikilosis (Q78.8)
                 polyostotic fibrous dysplasia (Q78.1)

● **M85.0**   **Fibrous dysplasia (monostotic)**

    Excludes2   fibrous dysplasia of jaw (M27.8)

      M85.00   Fibrous dysplasia (monostotic), unspecified site

●   **M85.01**   Fibrous dysplasia (monostotic), shoulder

         M85.011   Fibrous dysplasia (monostotic), right shoulder

         M85.012   Fibrous dysplasia (monostotic), left shoulder

         M85.019   Fibrous dysplasia (monostotic), unspecified shoulder

●   **M85.02**   Fibrous dysplasia (monostotic), upper arm

         M85.021   Fibrous dysplasia (monostotic), right upper arm

         M85.022   Fibrous dysplasia (monostotic), left upper arm

         M85.029   Fibrous dysplasia (monostotic), unspecified upper arm

●   **M85.03**   Fibrous dysplasia (monostotic), forearm

         M85.031   Fibrous dysplasia (monostotic), right forearm

         M85.032   Fibrous dysplasia (monostotic), left forearm

         M85.039   Fibrous dysplasia (monostotic), unspecified forearm

●   **M85.04**   Fibrous dysplasia (monostotic), hand

         M85.041   Fibrous dysplasia (monostotic), right hand

         M85.042   Fibrous dysplasia (monostotic), left hand

         M85.049   Fibrous dysplasia (monostotic), unspecified hand

●   **M85.05**   Fibrous dysplasia (monostotic), thigh

         M85.051   Fibrous dysplasia (monostotic), right thigh

         M85.052   Fibrous dysplasia (monostotic), left thigh

         M85.059   Fibrous dysplasia (monostotic), unspecified thigh

●   **M85.06**   Fibrous dysplasia (monostotic), lower leg

         M85.061   Fibrous dysplasia (monostotic), right lower leg

         M85.062   Fibrous dysplasia (monostotic), left lower leg

         M85.069   Fibrous dysplasia (monostotic), unspecified lower leg

●   **M85.07**   Fibrous dysplasia (monostotic), ankle and foot

         M85.071   Fibrous dysplasia (monostotic), right ankle and foot

         M85.072   Fibrous dysplasia (monostotic), left ankle and foot

         M85.079   Fibrous dysplasia (monostotic), unspecified ankle and foot

      M85.08   Fibrous dysplasia (monostotic), other site

      M85.09   Fibrous dysplasia (monostotic), multiple sites

● **M85.1**   **Skeletal fluorosis**

      M85.10   Skeletal fluorosis, unspecified site

●   **M85.11**   Skeletal fluorosis, shoulder

         M85.111   Skeletal fluorosis, right shoulder

         M85.112   Skeletal fluorosis, left shoulder

         M85.119   Skeletal fluorosis, unspecified shoulder

●   **M85.12**   Skeletal fluorosis, upper arm

         M85.121   Skeletal fluorosis, right upper arm

         M85.122   Skeletal fluorosis, left upper arm

         M85.129   Skeletal fluorosis, unspecified upper arm

●   **M85.13**   Skeletal fluorosis, forearm

         M85.131   Skeletal fluorosis, right forearm

         M85.132   Skeletal fluorosis, left forearm

         M85.139   Skeletal fluorosis, unspecified forearm

●   **M85.14**   Skeletal fluorosis, hand

         M85.141   Skeletal fluorosis, right hand

         M85.142   Skeletal fluorosis, left hand

         M85.149   Skeletal fluorosis, unspecified hand

●   **M85.15**   Skeletal fluorosis, thigh

         M85.151   Skeletal fluorosis, right thigh

         M85.152   Skeletal fluorosis, left thigh

         M85.159   Skeletal fluorosis, unspecified thigh

●   **M85.16**   Skeletal fluorosis, lower leg

         M85.161   Skeletal fluorosis, right lower leg

         M85.162   Skeletal fluorosis, left lower leg

         M85.169   Skeletal fluorosis, unspecified lower leg

●   **M85.17**   Skeletal fluorosis, ankle and foot

         M85.171   Skeletal fluorosis, right ankle and foot

         M85.172   Skeletal fluorosis, left ankle and foot

         M85.179   Skeletal fluorosis, unspecified ankle and foot

      M85.18   Skeletal fluorosis, other site

      M85.19   Skeletal fluorosis, multiple sites

   M85.2   **Hyperostosis of skull**

● **M85.3**   **Osteitis condensans**

      M85.30   Osteitis condensans, unspecified site

●   **M85.31**   Osteitis condensans, shoulder

         M85.311   Osteitis condensans, right shoulder

         M85.312   Osteitis condensans, left shoulder

         M85.319   Osteitis condensans, unspecified shoulder

●   **M85.32**   Osteitis condensans, upper arm

         M85.321   Osteitis condensans, right upper arm

         M85.322   Osteitis condensans, left upper arm

         M85.329   Osteitis condensans, unspecified upper arm

●   **M85.33**   Osteitis condensans, forearm

         M85.331   Osteitis condensans, right forearm

         M85.332   Osteitis condensans, left forearm

         M85.339   Osteitis condensans, unspecified forearm

●   **M85.34**   Osteitis condensans, hand

         M85.341   Osteitis condensans, right hand

         M85.342   Osteitis condensans, left hand

         M85.349   Osteitis condensans, unspecified hand

●   **M85.35**   Osteitis condensans, thigh

         M85.351   Osteitis condensans, right thigh

         M85.352   Osteitis condensans, left thigh

         M85.359   Osteitis condensans, unspecified thigh

●   **M85.36**   Osteitis condensans, lower leg

         M85.361   Osteitis condensans, right lower leg

         M85.362   Osteitis condensans, left lower leg

         M85.369   Osteitis condensans, unspecified lower leg

CHAPTER 13 (M00-M99)

◀ New   ◀▥ Revised   ~~deleted~~ Deleted   **OGCR** Official Guidelines   X Assign placeholder X   ● Use Additional Character(s)

Excludes 1   Excludes 2   Includes   Use additional   Code first   Code also   Unspecified

- M85.37 Osteitis condensans, ankle and foot
  - M85.371 Osteitis condensans, right ankle and foot
  - M85.372 Osteitis condensans, left ankle and foot
  - M85.379 Osteitis condensans, unspecified ankle and foot
  - M85.38 Osteitis condensans, other site
  - M85.39 Osteitis condensans, multiple sites
- M85.4 Solitary bone cyst
  - **Excludes2** solitary cyst of jaw (M27.4)
  - M85.40 Solitary bone cyst, unspecified site
- M85.41 Solitary bone cyst, shoulder
  - M85.411 Solitary bone cyst, right shoulder
  - M85.412 Solitary bone cyst, left shoulder
  - M85.419 Solitary bone cyst, unspecified shoulder
- M85.42 Solitary bone cyst, humerus
  - M85.421 Solitary bone cyst, right humerus
  - M85.422 Solitary bone cyst, left humerus
  - M85.429 Solitary bone cyst, unspecified humerus
- M85.43 Solitary bone cyst, ulna and radius
  - M85.431 Solitary bone cyst, right ulna and radius
  - M85.432 Solitary bone cyst, left ulna and radius
  - M85.439 Solitary bone cyst, unspecified ulna and radius
- M85.44 Solitary bone cyst, hand
  - M85.441 Solitary bone cyst, right hand
  - M85.442 Solitary bone cyst, left hand
  - M85.449 Solitary bone cyst, unspecified hand
- M85.45 Solitary bone cyst, pelvis
  - M85.451 Solitary bone cyst, right pelvis
  - M85.452 Solitary bone cyst, left pelvis
  - M85.459 Solitary bone cyst, unspecified pelvis
- M85.46 Solitary bone cyst, tibia and fibula
  - M85.461 Solitary bone cyst, right tibia and fibula
  - M85.462 Solitary bone cyst, left tibia and fibula
  - M85.469 Solitary bone cyst, unspecified tibia and fibula
- M85.47 Solitary bone cyst, ankle and foot
  - M85.471 Solitary bone cyst, right ankle and foot
  - M85.472 Solitary bone cyst, left ankle and foot
  - M85.479 Solitary bone cyst, unspecified ankle and foot
  - M85.48 Solitary bone cyst, other site
- M85.5 Aneurysmal bone cyst
  - **Excludes2** aneurysmal cyst of jaw (M27.4)
  - M85.50 Aneurysmal bone cyst, unspecified site
- M85.51 Aneurysmal bone cyst, shoulder
  - M85.511 Aneurysmal bone cyst, right shoulder
  - M85.512 Aneurysmal bone cyst, left shoulder
  - M85.519 Aneurysmal bone cyst, unspecified shoulder
- M85.52 Aneurysmal bone cyst, upper arm
  - M85.521 Aneurysmal bone cyst, right upper arm
  - M85.522 Aneurysmal bone cyst, left upper arm
  - M85.529 Aneurysmal bone cyst, unspecified upper arm

- M85.53 Aneurysmal bone cyst, forearm
  - M85.531 Aneurysmal bone cyst, right forearm
  - M85.532 Aneurysmal bone cyst, left forearm
  - M85.539 Aneurysmal bone cyst, unspecified forearm
- M85.54 Aneurysmal bone cyst, hand
  - M85.541 Aneurysmal bone cyst, right hand
  - M85.542 Aneurysmal bone cyst, left hand
  - M85.549 Aneurysmal bone cyst, unspecified hand
- M85.55 Aneurysmal bone cyst, thigh
  - M85.551 Aneurysmal bone cyst, right thigh
  - M85.552 Aneurysmal bone cyst, left thigh
  - M85.559 Aneurysmal bone cyst, unspecified thigh
- M85.56 Aneurysmal bone cyst, lower leg
  - M85.561 Aneurysmal bone cyst, right lower leg
  - M85.562 Aneurysmal bone cyst, left lower leg
  - M85.569 Aneurysmal bone cyst, unspecified lower leg
- M85.57 Aneurysmal bone cyst, ankle and foot
  - M85.571 Aneurysmal bone cyst, right ankle and foot
  - M85.572 Aneurysmal bone cyst, left ankle and foot
  - M85.579 Aneurysmal bone cyst, unspecified ankle and foot
  - M85.58 Aneurysmal bone cyst, other site
  - M85.59 Aneurysmal bone cyst, multiple sites
- M85.6 Other cyst of bone
  - **Excludes1** cyst of jaw NEC (M27.4)
    osteitis fibrosa cystica generalisata [von Recklinghausen's disease of bone] (E21.0)
  - M85.60 Other cyst of bone, unspecified site
- M85.61 Other cyst of bone, shoulder
  - M85.611 Other cyst of bone, right shoulder
  - M85.612 Other cyst of bone, left shoulder
  - M85.619 Other cyst of bone, unspecified shoulder
- M85.62 Other cyst of bone, upper arm
  - M85.621 Other cyst of bone, right upper arm
  - M85.622 Other cyst of bone, left upper arm
  - M85.629 Other cyst of bone, unspecified upper arm
- M85.63 Other cyst of bone, forearm
  - M85.631 Other cyst of bone, right forearm
  - M85.632 Other cyst of bone, left forearm
  - M85.639 Other cyst of bone, unspecified forearm
- M85.64 Other cyst of bone, hand
  - M85.641 Other cyst of bone, right hand
  - M85.642 Other cyst of bone, left hand
  - M85.649 Other cyst of bone, unspecified hand
- M85.65 Other cyst of bone, thigh
  - M85.651 Other cyst of bone, right thigh
  - M85.652 Other cyst of bone, left thigh
  - M85.659 Other cyst of bone, unspecified thigh
- M85.66 Other cyst of bone, lower leg
  - M85.661 Other cyst of bone, right lower leg
  - M85.662 Other cyst of bone, left lower leg
  - M85.669 Other cyst of bone, unspecified lower leg

◀ New   ⬅ Revised   ~~deleted~~ Deleted   OGCR Official Guidelines   X Assign placeholder X   ● Use Additional Character(s)

| Excludes 1 | Excludes 2 | Includes | Use additional | Code first | Code also | Unspecified |

● M85.67   Other cyst of bone, ankle and foot

    M85.671   Other cyst of bone, right ankle and foot

    M85.672   Other cyst of bone, left ankle and foot

    M85.679   Other cyst of bone, unspecified ankle and foot

   M85.68   Other cyst of bone, other site

   M85.69   Other cyst of bone, multiple sites

● M85.8   Other specified disorders of bone density and structure

    Hyperostosis of bones, except skull

    Osteosclerosis, acquired

> **Excludes1**   diffuse idiopathic skeletal hyperostosis [DISH] (M48.1)
> osteosclerosis congenita (Q77.4)
> osteosclerosis fragilitas (generalista) (Q78.2)
> osteosclerosis myelofibrosis (D75.81)

   M85.80   Other specified disorders of bone density and structure, unspecified site

● M85.81   Other specified disorders of bone density and structure, shoulder

    M85.811   Other specified disorders of bone density and structure, right shoulder

    M85.812   Other specified disorders of bone density and structure, left shoulder

    M85.819   Other specified disorders of bone density and structure, unspecified shoulder

● M85.82   Other specified disorders of bone density and structure, upper arm

    M85.821   Other specified disorders of bone density and structure, right upper arm

    M85.822   Other specified disorders of bone density and structure, left upper arm

    M85.829   Other specified disorders of bone density and structure, unspecified upper arm

● M85.83   Other specified disorders of bone density and structure, forearm

    M85.831   Other specified disorders of bone density and structure, right forearm

    M85.832   Other specified disorders of bone density and structure, left forearm

    M85.839   Other specified disorders of bone density and structure, unspecified forearm

● M85.84   Other specified disorders of bone density and structure, hand

    M85.841   Other specified disorders of bone density and structure, right hand

    M85.842   Other specified disorders of bone density and structure, left hand

    M85.849   Other specified disorders of bone density and structure, unspecified hand

● M85.85   Other specified disorders of bone density and structure, thigh

    M85.851   Other specified disorders of bone density and structure, right thigh

    M85.852   Other specified disorders of bone density and structure, left thigh

    M85.859   Other specified disorders of bone density and structure, unspecified thigh

● M85.86   Other specified disorders of bone density and structure, lower leg

    M85.861   Other specified disorders of bone density and structure, right lower leg

    M85.862   Other specified disorders of bone density and structure, left lower leg

    M85.869   Other specified disorders of bone density and structure, unspecified lower leg

● M85.87   Other specified disorders of bone density and structure, ankle and foot

    M85.871   Other specified disorders of bone density and structure, right ankle and foot

    M85.872   Other specified disorders of bone density and structure, left ankle and foot

    M85.879   Other specified disorders of bone density and structure, unspecified ankle and foot

   M85.88   Other specified disorders of bone density and structure, other site

   M85.89   Other specified disorders of bone density and structure, multiple sites

  M85.9   Disorder of bone density and structure, unspecified

OTHER OSTEOPATHIES (M86-M90)

> **Excludes1**   postprocedural osteopathies (M96.-)

● M86   Osteomyelitis

    Use additional code (B95-B97) to identify infectious agent

    Use additional code to identify major osseous defect, if applicable (M89.7-)

> **Excludes1**   osteomyelitis due to:
> echinococcus (B67.2)
> gonococcus (A54.43)
> salmonella (A02.24)

> **Excludes2**   ostemyelitis of:
> orbit (H05.0-)
> petrous bone (H70.2-)
> vertebra (M46.2-)

● M86.0   Acute hematogenous osteomyelitis

   M86.00   Acute hematogenous osteomyelitis, unspecified site

   ● M86.01   Acute hematogenous osteomyelitis, shoulder

    M86.011   Acute hematogenous osteomyelitis, right shoulder

    M86.012   Acute hematogenous osteomyelitis, left shoulder

    M86.019   Acute hematogenous osteomyelitis, unspecified shoulder

   ● M86.02   Acute hematogenous osteomyelitis, humerus

    M86.021   Acute hematogenous osteomyelitis, right humerus

    M86.022   Acute hematogenous osteomyelitis, left humerus

    M86.029   Acute hematogenous osteomyelitis, unspecified humerus

   ● M86.03   Acute hematogenous osteomyelitis, radius and ulna

    M86.031   Acute hematogenous osteomyelitis, right radius and ulna

    M86.032   Acute hematogenous osteomyelitis, left radius and ulna

    M86.039   Acute hematogenous osteomyelitis, unspecified radius and ulna

CHAPTER 13 (M00-M99)

Figure 13-5 Osteomyelitis of the spine. A lateral view of the lower thoracic spine demonstrates destruction of the disk space *(arrow)* as well as destruction of the adjoining vertebral bodies. (From Mettler: Essentials of Radiology, ed 2, Saunders, An Imprint of Elsevier, 2005)

Item 13–12 Osteomyelitis is an inflammation of the bone. **Acute osteomyelitis** is a rapidly destructive, pus-producing infection capable of causing severe bone destruction. **Chronic osteomyelitis** can remain long after the initial acute episode has passed and may lead to a recurrence of the acute phase. **Brodie's abscess** is an encapsulated focal abscess that must be surgically drained. Periostitis is an inflammation of the periosteum, a dense membrane composed of fibrous connective tissue that closely wraps all bone, except those with articulating surfaces in joints, which are covered by synovial membranes.

● M86.04 Acute hematogenous osteomyelitis, hand
    M86.041 Acute hematogenous osteomyelitis, right hand
    M86.042 Acute hematogenous osteomyelitis, left hand
    M86.049 Acute hematogenous osteomyelitis, unspecified hand
● M86.05 Acute hematogenous osteomyelitis, femur
    M86.051 Acute hematogenous osteomyelitis, right femur
    M86.052 Acute hematogenous osteomyelitis, left femur
    M86.059 Acute hematogenous osteomyelitis, unspecified femur
● M86.06 Acute hematogenous osteomyelitis, tibia and fibula
    M86.061 Acute hematogenous osteomyelitis, right tibia and fibula
    M86.062 Acute hematogenous osteomyelitis, left tibia and fibula
    M86.069 Acute hematogenous osteomyelitis, unspecified tibia and fibula
● M86.07 Acute hematogenous osteomyelitis, ankle and foot
    M86.071 Acute hematogenous osteomyelitis, right ankle and foot
    M86.072 Acute hematogenous osteomyelitis, left ankle and foot
    M86.079 Acute hematogenous osteomyelitis, unspecified ankle and foot
    M86.08 Acute hematogenous osteomyelitis, other sites
    M86.09 Acute hematogenous osteomyelitis, multiple sites
● M86.1 Other acute osteomyelitis
    M86.10 Other acute osteomyelitis, unspecified site
● M86.11 Other acute osteomyelitis, shoulder
    M86.111 Other acute osteomyelitis, right shoulder
    M86.112 Other acute osteomyelitis, left shoulder
    M86.119 Other acute osteomyelitis, unspecified shoulder

● M86.12 Other acute osteomyelitis, humerus
    M86.121 Other acute osteomyelitis, right humerus
    M86.122 Other acute osteomyelitis, left humerus
    M86.129 Other acute osteomyelitis, unspecified humerus
● M86.13 Other acute osteomyelitis, radius and ulna
    M86.131 Other acute osteomyelitis, right radius and ulna
    M86.132 Other acute osteomyelitis, left radius and ulna
    M86.139 Other acute osteomyelitis, unspecified radius and ulna
● M86.14 Other acute osteomyelitis, hand
    M86.141 Other acute osteomyelitis, right hand
    M86.142 Other acute osteomyelitis, left hand
    M86.149 Other acute osteomyelitis, unspecified hand
● M86.15 Other acute osteomyelitis, femur
    M86.151 Other acute osteomyelitis, right femur
    M86.152 Other acute osteomyelitis, left femur
    M86.159 Other acute osteomyelitis, unspecified femur
● M86.16 Other acute osteomyelitis, tibia and fibula
    M86.161 Other acute osteomyelitis, right tibia and fibula
    M86.162 Other acute osteomyelitis, left tibia and fibula
    M86.169 Other acute osteomyelitis, unspecified tibia and fibula
● M86.17 Other acute osteomyelitis, ankle and foot
    M86.171 Other acute osteomyelitis, right ankle and foot
    M86.172 Other acute osteomyelitis, left ankle and foot
    M86.179 Other acute osteomyelitis, unspecified ankle and foot
    M86.18 Other acute osteomyelitis, other site
    M86.19 Other acute osteomyelitis, multiple sites
● M86.2 Subacute osteomyelitis
    M86.20 Subacute osteomyelitis, unspecified site
● M86.21 Subacute osteomyelitis, shoulder
    M86.211 Subacute osteomyelitis, right shoulder
    M86.212 Subacute osteomyelitis, left shoulder
    M86.219 Subacute osteomyelitis, unspecified shoulder
● M86.22 Subacute osteomyelitis, humerus
    M86.221 Subacute osteomyelitis, right humerus
    M86.222 Subacute osteomyelitis, left humerus
    M86.229 Subacute osteomyelitis, unspecified humerus
● M86.23 Subacute osteomyelitis, radius and ulna
    M86.231 Subacute osteomyelitis, right radius and ulna
    M86.232 Subacute osteomyelitis, left radius and ulna
    M86.239 Subacute osteomyelitis, unspecified radius and ulna
● M86.24 Subacute osteomyelitis, hand
    M86.241 Subacute osteomyelitis, right hand
    M86.242 Subacute osteomyelitis, left hand
    M86.249 Subacute osteomyelitis, unspecified hand

● M86.25   Subacute osteomyelitis, femur
    M86.251   Subacute osteomyelitis, right femur
    M86.252   Subacute osteomyelitis, left femur
    M86.259   Subacute osteomyelitis, unspecified femur
● M86.26   Subacute osteomyelitis, tibia and fibula
    M86.261   Subacute osteomyelitis, right tibia and fibula
    M86.262   Subacute osteomyelitis, left tibia and fibula
    M86.269   Subacute osteomyelitis, unspecified tibia and fibula
● M86.27   Subacute osteomyelitis, ankle and foot
    M86.271   Subacute osteomyelitis, right ankle and foot
    M86.272   Subacute osteomyelitis, left ankle and foot
    M86.279   Subacute osteomyelitis, unspecified ankle and foot
   M86.28   Subacute osteomyelitis, other site
   M86.29   Subacute osteomyelitis, multiple sites
● M86.3   Chronic multifocal osteomyelitis
   M86.30   Chronic multifocal osteomyelitis, unspecified site
● M86.31   Chronic multifocal osteomyelitis, shoulder
    M86.311   Chronic multifocal osteomyelitis, right shoulder
    M86.312   Chronic multifocal osteomyelitis, left shoulder
    M86.319   Chronic multifocal osteomyelitis, unspecified shoulder
● M86.32   Chronic multifocal osteomyelitis, humerus
    M86.321   Chronic multifocal osteomyelitis, right humerus
    M86.322   Chronic multifocal osteomyelitis, left humerus
    M86.329   Chronic multifocal osteomyelitis, unspecified humerus
● M86.33   Chronic multifocal osteomyelitis, radius and ulna
    M86.331   Chronic multifocal osteomyelitis, right radius and ulna
    M86.332   Chronic multifocal osteomyelitis, left radius and ulna
    M86.339   Chronic multifocal osteomyelitis, unspecified radius and ulna
● M86.34   Chronic multifocal osteomyelitis, hand
    M86.341   Chronic multifocal osteomyelitis, right hand
    M86.342   Chronic multifocal osteomyelitis, left hand
    M86.349   Chronic multifocal osteomyelitis, unspecified hand
● M86.35   Chronic multifocal osteomyelitis, femur
    M86.351   Chronic multifocal osteomyelitis, right femur
    M86.352   Chronic multifocal osteomyelitis, left femur
    M86.359   Chronic multifocal osteomyelitis, unspecified femur
● M86.36   Chronic multifocal osteomyelitis, tibia and fibula
    M86.361   Chronic multifocal osteomyelitis, right tibia and fibula
    M86.362   Chronic multifocal osteomyelitis, left tibia and fibula
    M86.369   Chronic multifocal osteomyelitis, unspecified tibia and fibula

● M86.37   Chronic multifocal osteomyelitis, ankle and foot
    M86.371   Chronic multifocal osteomyelitis, right ankle and foot
    M86.372   Chronic multifocal osteomyelitis, left ankle and foot
    M86.379   Chronic multifocal osteomyelitis, unspecified ankle and foot
   M86.38   Chronic multifocal osteomyelitis, other site
   M86.39   Chronic multifocal osteomyelitis, multiple sites
● M86.4   Chronic osteomyelitis with draining sinus
   M86.40   Chronic osteomyelitis with draining sinus, unspecified site
● M86.41   Chronic osteomyelitis with draining sinus, shoulder
    M86.411   Chronic osteomyelitis with draining sinus, right shoulder
    M86.412   Chronic osteomyelitis with draining sinus, left shoulder
    M86.419   Chronic osteomyelitis with draining sinus, unspecified shoulder
● M86.42   Chronic osteomyelitis with draining sinus, humerus
    M86.421   Chronic osteomyelitis with draining sinus, right humerus
    M86.422   Chronic osteomyelitis with draining sinus, left humerus
    M86.429   Chronic osteomyelitis with draining sinus, unspecified humerus
● M86.43   Chronic osteomyelitis with draining sinus, radius and ulna
    M86.431   Chronic osteomyelitis with draining sinus, right radius and ulna
    M86.432   Chronic osteomyelitis with draining sinus, left radius and ulna
    M86.439   Chronic osteomyelitis with draining sinus, unspecified radius and ulna
● M86.44   Chronic osteomyelitis with draining sinus, hand
    M86.441   Chronic osteomyelitis with draining sinus, right hand
    M86.442   Chronic osteomyelitis with draining sinus, left hand
    M86.449   Chronic osteomyelitis with draining sinus, unspecified hand
● M86.45   Chronic osteomyelitis with draining sinus, femur
    M86.451   Chronic osteomyelitis with draining sinus, right femur
    M86.452   Chronic osteomyelitis with draining sinus, left femur
    M86.459   Chronic osteomyelitis with draining sinus, unspecified femur
● M86.46   Chronic osteomyelitis with draining sinus, tibia and fibula
    M86.461   Chronic osteomyelitis with draining sinus, right tibia and fibula
    M86.462   Chronic osteomyelitis with draining sinus, left tibia and fibula
    M86.469   Chronic osteomyelitis with draining sinus, unspecified tibia and fibula
● M86.47   Chronic osteomyelitis with draining sinus, ankle and foot
    M86.471   Chronic osteomyelitis with draining sinus, right ankle and foot
    M86.472   Chronic osteomyelitis with draining sinus, left ankle and foot
    M86.479   Chronic osteomyelitis with draining sinus, unspecified ankle and foot

M86.48 Chronic osteomyelitis with draining sinus, other site

M86.49 Chronic osteomyelitis with draining sinus, multiple sites

● M86.5 Other chronic hematogenous osteomyelitis

    M86.50 Other chronic hematogenous osteomyelitis, unspecified site

    ● M86.51 Other chronic hematogenous osteomyelitis, shoulder

        M86.511 Other chronic hematogenous osteomyelitis, right shoulder

        M86.512 Other chronic hematogenous osteomyelitis, left shoulder

        M86.519 Other chronic hematogenous osteomyelitis, unspecified shoulder

    ● M86.52 Other chronic hematogenous osteomyelitis, humerus

        M86.521 Other chronic hematogenous osteomyelitis, right humerus

        M86.522 Other chronic hematogenous osteomyelitis, left humerus

        M86.529 Other chronic hematogenous osteomyelitis, unspecified humerus

    ● M86.53 Other chronic hematogenous osteomyelitis, radius and ulna

        M86.531 Other chronic hematogenous osteomyelitis, right radius and ulna

        M86.532 Other chronic hematogenous osteomyelitis, left radius and ulna

        M86.539 Other chronic hematogenous osteomyelitis, unspecified radius and ulna

    ● M86.54 Other chronic hematogenous osteomyelitis, hand

        M86.541 Other chronic hematogenous osteomyelitis, right hand

        M86.542 Other chronic hematogenous osteomyelitis, left hand

        M86.549 Other chronic hematogenous osteomyelitis, unspecified hand

    ● M86.55 Other chronic hematogenous osteomyelitis, femur

        M86.551 Other chronic hematogenous osteomyelitis, right femur

        M86.552 Other chronic hematogenous osteomyelitis, left femur

        M86.559 Other chronic hematogenous osteomyelitis, unspecified femur

    ● M86.56 Other chronic hematogenous osteomyelitis, tibia and fibula

        M86.561 Other chronic hematogenous osteomyelitis, right tibia and fibula

        M86.562 Other chronic hematogenous osteomyelitis, left tibia and fibula

        M86.569 Other chronic hematogenous osteomyelitis, unspecified tibia and fibula

    ● M86.57 Other chronic hematogenous osteomyelitis, ankle and foot

        M86.571 Other chronic hematogenous osteomyelitis, right ankle and foot

        M86.572 Other chronic hematogenous osteomyelitis, left ankle and foot

        M86.579 Other chronic hematogenous osteomyelitis, unspecified ankle and foot

    M86.58 Other chronic hematogenous osteomyelitis, other site

    M86.59 Other chronic hematogenous osteomyelitis, multiple sites

● M86.6 Other chronic osteomyelitis

    M86.60 Other chronic osteomyelitis, unspecified site

    ● M86.61 Other chronic osteomyelitis, shoulder

        M86.611 Other chronic osteomyelitis, right shoulder

        M86.612 Other chronic osteomyelitis, left shoulder

        M86.619 Other chronic osteomyelitis, unspecified shoulder

    ● M86.62 Other chronic osteomyelitis, humerus

        M86.621 Other chronic osteomyelitis, right humerus

        M86.622 Other chronic osteomyelitis, left humerus

        M86.629 Other chronic osteomyelitis, unspecified humerus

    ● M86.63 Other chronic osteomyelitis, radius and ulna

        M86.631 Other chronic osteomyelitis, right radius and ulna

        M86.632 Other chronic osteomyelitis, left radius and ulna

        M86.639 Other chronic osteomyelitis, unspecified radius and ulna

    ● M86.64 Other chronic osteomyelitis, hand

        M86.641 Other chronic osteomyelitis, right hand

        M86.642 Other chronic osteomyelitis, left hand

        M86.649 Other chronic osteomyelitis, unspecified hand

    ● M86.65 Other chronic osteomyelitis, thigh

        M86.651 Other chronic osteomyelitis, right thigh

        M86.652 Other chronic osteomyelitis, left thigh

        M86.659 Other chronic osteomyelitis, unspecified thigh

    ● M86.66 Other chronic osteomyelitis, tibia and fibula

        M86.661 Other chronic osteomyelitis, right tibia and fibula

        M86.662 Other chronic osteomyelitis, left tibia and fibula

        M86.669 Other chronic osteomyelitis, unspecified tibia and fibula

    ● M86.67 Other chronic osteomyelitis, ankle and foot

        M86.671 Other chronic osteomyelitis, right ankle and foot

        M86.672 Other chronic osteomyelitis, left ankle and foot

        M86.679 Other chronic osteomyelitis, unspecified ankle and foot

    M86.68 Other chronic osteomyelitis, other site

    M86.69 Other chronic osteomyelitis, multiple sites

● M86.8 Other osteomyelitis
    Brodie's abscess

    ● M86.8X Other osteomyelitis

        M86.8X0 Other osteomyelitis, multiple sites

        M86.8X1 Other osteomyelitis, shoulder

        M86.8X2 Other osteomyelitis, upper arm

        M86.8X3 Other osteomyelitis, forearm

        M86.8X4 Other osteomyelitis, hand

        M86.8X5 Other osteomyelitis, thigh

        M86.8X6 Other osteomyelitis, lower leg

        M86.8X7 Other osteomyelitis, ankle and foot

        M86.8X8 Other osteomyelitis, other site

        M86.8X9 Other osteomyelitis, unspecified sites

M86.9 Osteomyelitis, unspecified
    Infection of bone NOS
    Periostitis without osteomyelitis

CHAPTER 13 (M00-M99)

◄ New   ◄▥ Revised   ~~deleted~~ Deleted   OGCR Official Guidelines   X Assign placeholder X   ● Use Additional Character(s)
Excludes 1   Excludes 2   Includes   Use additional   Code first   Code also   Unspecified

1094

● M87 Osteonecrosis
   Includes   avascular necrosis of bone
   Use additional code to identify major osseous defect, if
      applicable (M89.7-)
   Excludes1   juvenile osteonecrosis (M91-M92)
               osteochondropathies (M90-M93)

● M87.0 Idiopathic aseptic necrosis of bone
   M87.00 Idiopathic aseptic necrosis of unspecified bone
   ● M87.01 Idiopathic aseptic necrosis of shoulder
         Idiopathic aseptic necrosis of clavicle and
            scapula
      M87.011 Idiopathic aseptic necrosis of right
                  shoulder
      M87.012 Idiopathic aseptic necrosis of left
                  shoulder
      M87.019 Idiopathic aseptic necrosis of
                  unspecified shoulder
   ● M87.02 Idiopathic aseptic necrosis of humerus
      M87.021 Idiopathic aseptic necrosis of right
                  humerus
      M87.022 Idiopathic aseptic necrosis of left
                  humerus
      M87.029 Idiopathic aseptic necrosis of
                  unspecified humerus
   ● M87.03 Idiopathic aseptic necrosis of radius, ulna and
            carpus
      M87.031 Idiopathic aseptic necrosis of right
                  radius
      M87.032 Idiopathic aseptic necrosis of left
                  radius
      M87.033 Idiopathic aseptic necrosis of
                  unspecified radius
      M87.034 Idiopathic aseptic necrosis of right
                  ulna
      M87.035 Idiopathic aseptic necrosis of left ulna
      M87.036 Idiopathic aseptic necrosis of
                  unspecified ulna
      M87.037 Idiopathic aseptic necrosis of right
                  carpus
      M87.038 Idiopathic aseptic necrosis of left
                  carpus
      M87.039 Idiopathic aseptic necrosis of
                  unspecified carpus
   ● M87.04 Idiopathic aseptic necrosis of hand and fingers
         Idiopathic aseptic necrosis of metacarpals and
            phalanges of hands
      M87.041 Idiopathic aseptic necrosis of right
                  hand
      M87.042 Idiopathic aseptic necrosis of left
                  hand
      M87.043 Idiopathic aseptic necrosis of
                  unspecified hand
      M87.044 Idiopathic aseptic necrosis of right
                  finger(s)
      M87.045 Idiopathic aseptic necrosis of left
                  finger(s)
      M87.046 Idiopathic aseptic necrosis of
                  unspecified finger(s)
   ● M87.05 Idiopathic aseptic necrosis of pelvis and femur
      M87.050 Idiopathic aseptic necrosis of pelvis
      M87.051 Idiopathic aseptic necrosis of right
                  femur
      M87.052 Idiopathic aseptic necrosis of left
                  femur
      M87.059 Idiopathic aseptic necrosis of
                  unspecified femur
            Idiopathic aseptic necrosis of hip
               NOS

● M87.06 Idiopathic aseptic necrosis of tibia and fibula
      M87.061 Idiopathic aseptic necrosis of right
                  tibia
      M87.062 Idiopathic aseptic necrosis of left
                  tibia
      M87.063 Idiopathic aseptic necrosis of
                  unspecified tibia
      M87.064 Idiopathic aseptic necrosis of right
                  fibula
      M87.065 Idiopathic aseptic necrosis of left
                  fibula
      M87.066 Idiopathic aseptic necrosis of
                  unspecified fibula
   ● M87.07 Idiopathic aseptic necrosis of ankle, foot and
            toes
         Idiopathic aseptic necrosis of metatarsus,
            tarsus, and phalanges of toes
      M87.071 Idiopathic aseptic necrosis of right
                  ankle
      M87.072 Idiopathic aseptic necrosis of left
                  ankle
      M87.073 Idiopathic aseptic necrosis of
                  unspecified ankle
      M87.074 Idiopathic aseptic necrosis of right
                  foot
      M87.075 Idiopathic aseptic necrosis of left foot
      M87.076 Idiopathic aseptic necrosis of
                  unspecified foot
      M87.077 Idiopathic aseptic necrosis of right
                  toe(s)
      M87.078 Idiopathic aseptic necrosis of left
                  toe(s)
      M87.079 Idiopathic aseptic necrosis of
                  unspecified toe(s)
   M87.08 Idiopathic aseptic necrosis of bone, other site
   M87.09 Idiopathic aseptic necrosis of bone, multiple
            sites
● M87.1 Osteonecrosis due to drugs
   Use additional code for adverse effect, if applicable,
      to identify drug (T36-T50 with fifth or sixth
      character 5)
   M87.10 Osteonecrosis due to drugs, unspecified bone
   ● M87.11 Osteonecrosis due to drugs, shoulder
      M87.111 Osteonecrosis due to drugs, right
                  shoulder
      M87.112 Osteonecrosis due to drugs, left
                  shoulder
      M87.119 Osteonecrosis due to drugs,
                  unspecified shoulder
   ● M87.12 Osteonecrosis due to drugs, humerus
      M87.121 Osteonecrosis due to drugs, right
                  humerus
      M87.122 Osteonecrosis due to drugs, left
                  humerus
      M87.129 Osteonecrosis due to drugs,
                  unspecified humerus
   ● M87.13 Osteonecrosis due to drugs of radius, ulna and
            carpus
      M87.131 Osteonecrosis due to drugs of right
                  radius
      M87.132 Osteonecrosis due to drugs of left
                  radius
      M87.133 Osteonecrosis due to drugs of
                  unspecified radius
      M87.134 Osteonecrosis due to drugs of right
                  ulna
      M87.135 Osteonecrosis due to drugs of left
                  ulna

M87.136 Osteonecrosis due to drugs of unspecified ulna

M87.137 Osteonecrosis due to drugs of right carpus

M87.138 Osteonecrosis due to drugs of left carpus

M87.139 Osteonecrosis due to drugs of unspecified carpus

● M87.14 Osteonecrosis due to drugs, hand and fingers

M87.141 Osteonecrosis due to drugs, right hand

M87.142 Osteonecrosis due to drugs, left hand

M87.143 Osteonecrosis due to drugs, unspecified hand

M87.144 Osteonecrosis due to drugs, right finger(s)

M87.145 Osteonecrosis due to drugs, left finger(s)

M87.146 Osteonecrosis due to drugs, unspecified finger(s)

● M87.15 Osteonecrosis due to drugs, pelvis and femur

M87.150 Osteonecrosis due to drugs, pelvis

M87.151 Osteonecrosis due to drugs, right femur

M87.152 Osteonecrosis due to drugs, left femur

M87.159 Osteonecrosis due to drugs, unspecified femur

● M87.16 Osteonecrosis due to drugs, tibia and fibula

M87.161 Osteonecrosis due to drugs, right tibia

M87.162 Osteonecrosis due to drugs, left tibia

M87.163 Osteonecrosis due to drugs, unspecified tibia

M87.164 Osteonecrosis due to drugs, right fibula

M87.165 Osteonecrosis due to drugs, left fibula

M87.166 Osteonecrosis due to drugs, unspecified fibula

● M87.17 Osteonecrosis due to drugs, ankle, foot and toes

M87.171 Osteonecrosis due to drugs, right ankle

M87.172 Osteonecrosis due to drugs, left ankle

M87.173 Osteonecrosis due to drugs, unspecified ankle

M87.174 Osteonecrosis due to drugs, right foot

M87.175 Osteonecrosis due to drugs, left foot

M87.176 Osteonecrosis due to drugs, unspecified foot

M87.177 Osteonecrosis due to drugs, right toe(s)

M87.178 Osteonecrosis due to drugs, left toe(s)

M87.179 Osteonecrosis due to drugs, unspecified toe(s)

● M87.18 Osteonecrosis due to drugs, other site

M87.180 Osteonecrosis due to drugs, jaw

M87.188 Osteonecrosis due to drugs, other site

M87.19 Osteonecrosis due to drugs, multiple sites

● M87.2 Osteonecrosis due to previous trauma

M87.20 Osteonecrosis due to previous trauma, unspecified bone

● M87.21 Osteonecrosis due to previous trauma, shoulder

M87.211 Osteonecrosis due to previous trauma, right shoulder

M87.212 Osteonecrosis due to previous trauma, left shoulder

M87.219 Osteonecrosis due to previous trauma, unspecified shoulder

● M87.22 Osteonecrosis due to previous trauma, humerus

M87.221 Osteonecrosis due to previous trauma, right humerus

M87.222 Osteonecrosis due to previous trauma, left humerus

M87.229 Osteonecrosis due to previous trauma, unspecified humerus

● M87.23 Osteonecrosis due to previous trauma of radius, ulna and carpus

M87.231 Osteonecrosis due to previous trauma of right radius

M87.232 Osteonecrosis due to previous trauma of left radius

M87.233 Osteonecrosis due to previous trauma of unspecified radius

M87.234 Osteonecrosis due to previous trauma of right ulna

M87.235 Osteonecrosis due to previous trauma of left ulna

M87.236 Osteonecrosis due to previous trauma of unspecified ulna

M87.237 Osteonecrosis due to previous trauma of right carpus

M87.238 Osteonecrosis due to previous trauma of left carpus

M87.239 Osteonecrosis due to previous trauma of unspecified carpus

● M87.24 Osteonecrosis due to previous trauma, hand and fingers

M87.241 Osteonecrosis due to previous trauma, right hand

M87.242 Osteonecrosis due to previous trauma, left hand

M87.243 Osteonecrosis due to previous trauma, unspecified hand

M87.244 Osteonecrosis due to previous trauma, right finger(s)

M87.245 Osteonecrosis due to previous trauma, left finger(s)

M87.246 Osteonecrosis due to previous trauma, unspecified finger(s)

● M87.25 Osteonecrosis due to previous trauma, pelvis and femur

M87.250 Osteonecrosis due to previous trauma, pelvis

M87.251 Osteonecrosis due to previous trauma, right femur

M87.252 Osteonecrosis due to previous trauma, left femur

M87.256 Osteonecrosis due to previous trauma, unspecified femur

● M87.26 Osteonecrosis due to previous trauma, tibia and fibula

M87.261 Osteonecrosis due to previous trauma, right tibia

M87.262 Osteonecrosis due to previous trauma, left tibia

M87.263 Osteonecrosis due to previous trauma, unspecified tibia

M87.264 Osteonecrosis due to previous trauma, right fibula

M87.265 Osteonecrosis due to previous trauma, left fibula

M87.266 Osteonecrosis due to previous trauma, unspecified fibula

● M87.27 Osteonecrosis due to previous trauma, ankle, foot and toes
   M87.271 Osteonecrosis due to previous trauma, right ankle
   M87.272 Osteonecrosis due to previous trauma, left ankle
   M87.273 Osteonecrosis due to previous trauma, unspecified ankle
   M87.274 Osteonecrosis due to previous trauma, right foot
   M87.275 Osteonecrosis due to previous trauma, left foot
   M87.276 Osteonecrosis due to previous trauma, unspecified foot
   M87.277 Osteonecrosis due to previous trauma, right toe(s)
   M87.278 Osteonecrosis due to previous trauma, left toe(s)
   M87.279 Osteonecrosis due to previous trauma, unspecified toe(s)
M87.28 Osteonecrosis due to previous trauma, other site
M87.29 Osteonecrosis due to previous trauma, multiple sites
● M87.3 Other secondary osteonecrosis
  M87.30 Other secondary osteonecrosis, unspecified bone
● M87.31 Other secondary osteonecrosis, shoulder
   M87.311 Other secondary osteonecrosis, right shoulder
   M87.312 Other secondary osteonecrosis, left shoulder
   M87.319 Other secondary osteonecrosis, unspecified shoulder
● M87.32 Other secondary osteonecrosis, humerus
   M87.321 Other secondary osteonecrosis, right humerus
   M87.322 Other secondary osteonecrosis, left humerus
   M87.329 Other secondary osteonecrosis, unspecified humerus
● M87.33 Other secondary osteonecrosis of radius, ulna and carpus
   M87.331 Other secondary osteonecrosis of right radius
   M87.332 Other secondary osteonecrosis of left radius
   M87.333 Other secondary osteonecrosis of unspecified radius
   M87.334 Other secondary osteonecrosis of right ulna
   M87.335 Other secondary osteonecrosis of left ulna
   M87.336 Other secondary osteonecrosis of unspecified ulna
   M87.337 Other secondary osteonecrosis of right carpus
   M87.338 Other secondary osteonecrosis of left carpus
   M87.339 Other secondary osteonecrosis of unspecified carpus

● M87.34 Other secondary osteonecrosis, hand and fingers
   M87.341 Other secondary osteonecrosis, right hand
   M87.342 Other secondary osteonecrosis, left hand
   M87.343 Other secondary osteonecrosis, unspecified hand
   M87.344 Other secondary osteonecrosis, right finger(s)
   M87.345 Other secondary osteonecrosis, left finger(s)
   M87.346 Other secondary osteonecrosis, unspecified finger(s)
● M87.35 Other secondary osteonecrosis, pelvis and femur
   M87.350 Other secondary osteonecrosis, pelvis
   M87.351 Other secondary osteonecrosis, right femur
   M87.352 Other secondary osteonecrosis, left femur
   M87.353 Other secondary osteonecrosis, unspecified femur
● M87.36 Other secondary osteonecrosis, tibia and fibula
   M87.361 Other secondary osteonecrosis, right tibia
   M87.362 Other secondary osteonecrosis, left tibia
   M87.363 Other secondary osteonecrosis, unspecified tibia
   M87.364 Other secondary osteonecrosis, right fibula
   M87.365 Other secondary osteonecrosis, left fibula
   M87.366 Other secondary osteonecrosis, unspecified fibula
● M87.37 Other secondary osteonecrosis, ankle and foot
   M87.371 Other secondary osteonecrosis, right ankle
   M87.372 Other secondary osteonecrosis, left ankle
   M87.373 Other secondary osteonecrosis, unspecified ankle
   M87.374 Other secondary osteonecrosis, right foot
   M87.375 Other secondary osteonecrosis, left foot
   M87.376 Other secondary osteonecrosis, unspecified foot
   M87.377 Other secondary osteonecrosis, right toe(s)
   M87.378 Other secondary osteonecrosis, left toe(s)
   M87.379 Other secondary osteonecrosis, unspecified toe(s)
M87.38 Other secondary osteonecrosis, other site
M87.39 Other secondary osteonecrosis, multiple sites
● M87.8 Other osteonecrosis
  M87.80 Other osteonecrosis, unspecified bone
● M87.81 Other osteonecrosis, shoulder
   M87.811 Other osteonecrosis, right shoulder
   M87.812 Other osteonecrosis, left shoulder
   M87.819 Other osteonecrosis, unspecified shoulder

◄ New ◄ Revised ~~deleted~~ Deleted OGCR Official Guidelines X Assign placeholder X ● Use Additional Character(s)
Excludes 1 Excludes 2 Includes Use additional Code first Code also Unspecified

CHAPTER 13 (M00-M99)

● M87.82   Other osteonecrosis, humerus
    M87.821   Other osteonecrosis, right humerus
    M87.822   Other osteonecrosis, left humerus
    M87.829   Other osteonecrosis, unspecified humerus

● M87.83   Other osteonecrosis of radius, ulna and carpus
    M87.831   Other osteonecrosis of right radius
    M87.832   Other osteonecrosis of left radius
    M87.833   Other osteonecrosis of unspecified radius
    M87.834   Other osteonecrosis of right ulna
    M87.835   Other osteonecrosis of left ulna
    M87.836   Other osteonecrosis of unspecified ulna
    M87.837   Other osteonecrosis of right carpus
    M87.838   Other osteonecrosis of left carpus
    M87.839   Other osteonecrosis of unspecified carpus

● M87.84   Other osteonecrosis, hand and fingers
    M87.841   Other osteonecrosis, right hand
    M87.842   Other osteonecrosis, left hand
    M87.843   Other osteonecrosis, unspecified hand
    M87.844   Other osteonecrosis, right finger(s)
    M87.845   Other osteonecrosis, left finger(s)
    M87.849   Other osteonecrosis, unspecified finger(s)

● M87.85   Other osteonecrosis, pelvis and femur
    M87.850   Other osteonecrosis, pelvis
    M87.851   Other osteonecrosis, right femur
    M87.852   Other osteonecrosis, left femur
    M87.859   Other osteonecrosis, unspecified femur

● M87.86   Other osteonecrosis, tibia and fibula
    M87.861   Other osteonecrosis, right tibia
    M87.862   Other osteonecrosis, left tibia
    M87.863   Other osteonecrosis, unspecified tibia
    M87.864   Other osteonecrosis, right fibula
    M87.865   Other osteonecrosis, left fibula
    M87.869   Other osteonecrosis, unspecified fibula

● M87.87   Other osteonecrosis, ankle, foot and toes
    M87.871   Other osteonecrosis, right ankle
    M87.872   Other osteonecrosis, left ankle
    M87.873   Other osteonecrosis, unspecified ankle
    M87.874   Other osteonecrosis, right foot
    M87.875   Other osteonecrosis, left foot
    M87.876   Other osteonecrosis, unspecified foot
    M87.877   Other osteonecrosis, right toe(s)
    M87.878   Other osteonecrosis, left toe(s)
    M87.879   Other osteonecrosis, unspecified toe(s)

    M87.88   Other osteonecrosis, other site
    M87.89   Other osteonecrosis, multiple sites
M87.9   Osteonecrosis, unspecified
    Necrosis of bone NOS

● M88   **Osteitis deformans [Paget's disease of bone]**
    Chronic disorder that results in enlarged and deformed bones. The excessive breakdown and formation of bone tissue causes bones to weaken and results in bone pain, arthritis, deformities, and fractures.
    Excludes1   osteitis deformans in neoplastic disease (M90.6)
M88.0   Osteitis deformans of skull
M88.1   Osteitis deformans of vertebrae
● M88.8   Osteitis deformans of other bones
   ● M88.81   Osteitis deformans of shoulder
     M88.811   Osteitis deformans of right shoulder
     M88.812   Osteitis deformans of left shoulder
     M88.819   Osteitis deformans of unspecified shoulder
   ● M88.82   Osteitis deformans of upper arm
     M88.821   Osteitis deformans of right upper arm
     M88.822   Osteitis deformans of left upper arm
     M88.829   Osteitis deformans of unspecified upper arm
   ● M88.83   Osteitis deformans of forearm
     M88.831   Osteitis deformans of right forearm
     M88.832   Osteitis deformans of left forearm
     M88.839   Osteitis deformans of unspecified forearm
   ● M88.84   Osteitis deformans of hand
     M88.841   Osteitis deformans of right hand
     M88.842   Osteitis deformans of left hand
     M88.849   Osteitis deformans of unspecified hand
   ● M88.85   Osteitis deformans of thigh
     M88.851   Osteitis deformans of right thigh
     M88.852   Osteitis deformans of left thigh
     M88.859   Osteitis deformans of unspecified thigh
   ● M88.86   Osteitis deformans of lower leg
     M88.861   Osteitis deformans of right lower leg
     M88.862   Osteitis deformans of left lower leg
     M88.869   Osteitis deformans of unspecified lower leg
   ● M88.87   Osteitis deformans of ankle and foot
     M88.871   Osteitis deformans of right ankle and foot
     M88.872   Osteitis deformans of left ankle and foot
     M88.879   Osteitis deformans of unspecified ankle and foot
    M88.88   Osteitis deformans of other bones
     Excludes2   osteitis deformans of skull (M88.0)
         osteitis deformans of vertebrae (M88.1)
    M88.89   Osteitis deformans of multiple sites
M88.9   Osteitis deformans of unspecified bone

● M89   **Other disorders of bone**
   ● M89.0   **Algoneurodystrophy**
       Shoulder-hand syndrome
       Sudeck's atrophy
       Excludes1   causalgia, lower limb (G57.7-)
                  causalgia, upper limb (G56.4-)
                  complex regional pain syndrome II, lower
                    limb (G57.7-)
                  complex regional pain syndrome II,
                    upper limb (G56.4-)
                  reflex sympathetic dystrophy (G90.5-)
       M89.00   Algoneurodystrophy, unspecified site
     ● M89.01   Algoneurodystrophy, shoulder
         M89.011   Algoneurodystrophy, right shoulder
         M89.012   Algoneurodystrophy, left shoulder
         M89.019   Algoneurodystrophy, unspecified
                 shoulder
     ● M89.02   Algoneurodystrophy, upper arm
         M89.021   Algoneurodystrophy, right upper arm
         M89.022   Algoneurodystrophy, left upper arm
         M89.029   Algoneurodystrophy, unspecified
                 upper arm
     ● M89.03   Algoneurodystrophy, forearm
         M89.031   Algoneurodystrophy, right forearm
         M89.032   Algoneurodystrophy, left forearm
         M89.039   Algoneurodystrophy, unspecified
                 forearm
     ● M89.04   Algoneurodystrophy, hand
         M89.041   Algoneurodystrophy, right hand
         M89.042   Algoneurodystrophy, left hand
         M89.049   Algoneurodystrophy, unspecified
                 hand
     ● M89.05   Algoneurodystrophy, thigh
         M89.051   Algoneurodystrophy, right thigh
         M89.052   Algoneurodystrophy, left thigh
         M89.059   Algoneurodystrophy, unspecified
                 thigh
     ● M89.06   Algoneurodystrophy, lower leg
         M89.061   Algoneurodystrophy, right lower leg
         M89.062   Algoneurodystrophy, left lower leg
         M89.069   Algoneurodystrophy, unspecified
                 lower leg
     ● M89.07   Algoneurodystrophy, ankle and foot
         M89.071   Algoneurodystrophy, right ankle and
                 foot
         M89.072   Algoneurodystrophy, left ankle and
                 foot
         M89.079   Algoneurodystrophy, unspecified
                 ankle and foot
       M89.08   Algoneurodystrophy, other site
       M89.09   Algoneurodystrophy, multiple sites
   ● M89.1   **Physeal arrest**
       Arrest of growth plate
       Epiphyseal arrest
       Growth plate arrest
     ● M89.12   Physeal arrest, humerus
         M89.121   Complete physeal arrest, right
                 proximal humerus
         M89.122   Complete physeal arrest, left proximal
                 humerus
         M89.123   Partial physeal arrest, right proximal
                 humerus
         M89.124   Partial physeal arrest, left proximal
                 humerus
         M89.125   Complete physeal arrest, right distal
                 humerus

         M89.126   Complete physeal arrest, left distal
                 humerus
         M89.127   Partial physeal arrest, right distal
                 humerus
         M89.128   Partial physeal arrest, left distal
                 humerus
         M89.129   Physeal arrest, humerus, unspecified
     ● M89.13   Physeal arrest, forearm
         M89.131   Complete physeal arrest, right distal
                 radius
         M89.132   Complete physeal arrest, left distal
                 radius
         M89.133   Partial physeal arrest, right distal
                 radius
         M89.134   Partial physeal arrest, left distal
                 radius
         M89.138   Other physeal arrest of forearm
         M89.139   Physeal arrest, forearm, unspecified
     ● M89.15   Physeal arrest, femur
         M89.151   Complete physeal arrest, right
                 proximal femur
         M89.152   Complete physeal arrest, left proximal
                 femur
         M89.153   Partial physeal arrest, right proximal
                 femur
         M89.154   Partial physeal arrest, left proximal
                 femur
         M89.155   Complete physeal arrest, right distal
                 femur
         M89.156   Complete physeal arrest, left distal
                 femur
         M89.157   Partial physeal arrest, right distal
                 femur
         M89.158   Partial physeal arrest, left distal
                 femur
         M89.159   Physeal arrest, femur, unspecified
     ● M89.16   Physeal arrest, lower leg
         M89.160   Complete physeal arrest, right
                 proximal tibia
         M89.161   Complete physeal arrest, left proximal
                 tibia
         M89.162   Partial physeal arrest, right proximal
                 tibia
         M89.163   Partial physeal arrest, left proximal
                 tibia
         M89.164   Complete physeal arrest, right distal
                 tibia
         M89.165   Complete physeal arrest, left distal
                 tibia
         M89.166   Partial physeal arrest, right distal
                 tibia
         M89.167   Partial physeal arrest, left distal tibia
         M89.168   Other physeal arrest of lower leg
         M89.169   Physeal arrest, lower leg, unspecified
       M89.18   Physeal arrest, other site
   ● M89.2   **Other disorders of bone development and growth**
       M89.20   Other disorders of bone development and
              growth, unspecified site
     ● M89.21   Other disorders of bone development and
              growth, shoulder
         M89.211   Other disorders of bone development
                 and growth, right shoulder
         M89.212   Other disorders of bone development
                 and growth, left shoulder
         M89.219   Other disorders of bone development
                 and growth, unspecified shoulder

CHAPTER 13 (M00-M99)

◀ New   ◀▮▮▮ Revised   ~~deleted~~ Deleted   **OGCR** Official Guidelines   X Assign placeholder X   ● Use Additional Character(s)

Excludes 1   Excludes 2   Includes   Use additional   Code first   Code also   Unspecified

1099

CHAPTER 13 (M00-M99)

● M89.22　Other disorders of bone development and growth, humerus
　　　M89.221　Other disorders of bone development and growth, right humerus
　　　M89.222　Other disorders of bone development and growth, left humerus
　　　M89.229　Other disorders of bone development and growth, unspecified humerus

● M89.23　Other disorders of bone development and growth, ulna and radius
　　　M89.231　Other disorders of bone development and growth, right ulna
　　　M89.232　Other disorders of bone development and growth, left ulna
　　　M89.233　Other disorders of bone development and growth, right radius
　　　M89.234　Other disorders of bone development and growth, left radius
　　　M89.239　Other disorders of bone development and growth, unspecified ulna and radius

● M89.24　Other disorders of bone development and growth, hand
　　　M89.241　Other disorders of bone development and growth, right hand
　　　M89.242　Other disorders of bone development and growth, left hand
　　　M89.249　Other disorders of bone development and growth, unspecified hand

● M89.25　Other disorders of bone development and growth, femur
　　　M89.251　Other disorders of bone development and growth, right femur
　　　M89.252　Other disorders of bone development and growth, left femur
　　　M89.259　Other disorders of bone development and growth, unspecified femur

● M89.26　Other disorders of bone development and growth, tibia and fibula
　　　M89.261　Other disorders of bone development and growth, right tibia
　　　M89.262　Other disorders of bone development and growth, left tibia
　　　M89.263　Other disorders of bone development and growth, right fibula
　　　M89.264　Other disorders of bone development and growth, left fibula
　　　M89.269　Other disorders of bone development and growth, unspecified lower leg

● M89.27　Other disorders of bone development and growth, ankle and foot
　　　M89.271　Other disorders of bone development and growth, right ankle and foot
　　　M89.272　Other disorders of bone development and growth, left ankle and foot
　　　M89.279　Other disorders of bone development and growth, unspecified ankle and foot

　　M89.28　Other disorders of bone development and growth, other site

　　M89.29　Other disorders of bone development and growth, multiple sites

● M89.3　Hypertrophy of bone
　　M89.30　Hypertrophy of bone, unspecified site
● M89.31　Hypertrophy of bone, shoulder
　　　M89.311　Hypertrophy of bone, right shoulder
　　　M89.312　Hypertrophy of bone, left shoulder
　　　M89.319　Hypertrophy of bone, unspecified shoulder

● M89.32　Hypertrophy of bone, humerus
　　　M89.321　Hypertrophy of bone, right humerus
　　　M89.322　Hypertrophy of bone, left humerus
　　　M89.329　Hypertrophy of bone, unspecified humerus

● M89.33　Hypertrophy of bone, ulna and radius
　　　M89.331　Hypertrophy of bone, right ulna
　　　M89.332　Hypertrophy of bone, left ulna
　　　M89.333　Hypertrophy of bone, right radius
　　　M89.334　Hypertrophy of bone, left radius
　　　M89.339　Hypertrophy of bone, unspecified ulna and radius

● M89.34　Hypertrophy of bone, hand
　　　M89.341　Hypertrophy of bone, right hand
　　　M89.342　Hypertrophy of bone, left hand
　　　M89.349　Hypertrophy of bone, unspecified hand

● M89.35　Hypertrophy of bone, femur
　　　M89.351　Hypertrophy of bone, right femur
　　　M89.352　Hypertrophy of bone, left femur
　　　M89.359　Hypertrophy of bone, unspecified femur

● M89.36　Hypertrophy of bone, tibia and fibula
　　　M89.361　Hypertrophy of bone, right tibia
　　　M89.362　Hypertrophy of bone, left tibia
　　　M89.363　Hypertrophy of bone, right fibula
　　　M89.364　Hypertrophy of bone, left fibula
　　　M89.369　Hypertrophy of bone, unspecified tibia and fibula

● M89.37　Hypertrophy of bone, ankle and foot
　　　M89.371　Hypertrophy of bone, right ankle and foot
　　　M89.372　Hypertrophy of bone, left ankle and foot
　　　M89.379　Hypertrophy of bone, unspecified ankle and foot

　　M89.38　Hypertrophy of bone, other site

　　M89.39　Hypertrophy of bone, multiple sites

● M89.4　Other hypertrophic osteoarthropathy
　　　Marie-Bamberger disease
　　　Pachydermoperiostosis
　　M89.40　Other hypertrophic osteoarthropathy, unspecified site
● M89.41　Other hypertrophic osteoarthropathy, shoulder
　　　M89.411　Other hypertrophic osteoarthropathy, right shoulder
　　　M89.412　Other hypertrophic osteoarthropathy, left shoulder
　　　M89.419　Other hypertrophic osteoarthropathy, unspecified shoulder

● M89.42　Other hypertrophic osteoarthropathy, upper arm
　　　M89.421　Other hypertrophic osteoarthropathy, right upper arm
　　　M89.422　Other hypertrophic osteoarthropathy, left upper arm
　　　M89.429　Other hypertrophic osteoarthropathy, unspecified upper arm

● M89.43　Other hypertrophic osteoarthropathy, forearm
　　　M89.431　Other hypertrophic osteoarthropathy, right forearm
　　　M89.432　Other hypertrophic osteoarthropathy, left forearm
　　　M89.439　Other hypertrophic osteoarthropathy, unspecified forearm

● M89.44　Other hypertrophic osteoarthropathy, hand
　　　M89.441　Other hypertrophic osteoarthropathy, right hand
　　　M89.442　Other hypertrophic osteoarthropathy, left hand
　　　M89.449　Other hypertrophic osteoarthropathy, unspecified hand
● M89.45　Other hypertrophic osteoarthropathy, thigh
　　　M89.451　Other hypertrophic osteoarthropathy, right thigh
　　　M89.452　Other hypertrophic osteoarthropathy, left thigh
　　　M89.459　Other hypertrophic osteoarthropathy, unspecified thigh
● M89.46　Other hypertrophic osteoarthropathy, lower leg
　　　M89.461　Other hypertrophic osteoarthropathy, right lower leg
　　　M89.462　Other hypertrophic osteoarthropathy, left lower leg
　　　M89.469　Other hypertrophic osteoarthropathy, unspecified lower leg
● M89.47　Other hypertrophic osteoarthropathy, ankle and foot
　　　M89.471　Other hypertrophic osteoarthropathy, right ankle and foot
　　　M89.472　Other hypertrophic osteoarthropathy, left ankle and foot
　　　M89.479　Other hypertrophic osteoarthropathy, unspecified ankle and foot
　　M89.48　Other hypertrophic osteoarthropathy, other site
　　M89.49　Other hypertrophic osteoarthropathy, multiple sites
● M89.5　Osteolysis
　　　Use additional code to identify major osseous defect, if applicable (M89.7-)
　　　Excludes2　periprosthetic osteolysis of internal prosthetic joint (T84.05-)
　　M89.50　Osteolysis, unspecified site
● M89.51　Osteolysis, shoulder
　　　M89.511　Osteolysis, right shoulder
　　　M89.512　Osteolysis, left shoulder
　　　M89.519　Osteolysis, unspecified shoulder
● M89.52　Osteolysis, upper arm
　　　M89.521　Osteolysis, right upper arm
　　　M89.522　Osteolysis, left upper arm
　　　M89.529　Osteolysis, unspecified upper arm
● M89.53　Osteolysis, forearm
　　　M89.531　Osteolysis, right forearm
　　　M89.532　Osteolysis, left forearm
　　　M89.539　Osteolysis, unspecified forearm
● M89.54　Osteolysis, hand
　　　M89.541　Osteolysis, right hand
　　　M89.542　Osteolysis, left hand
　　　M89.549　Osteolysis, unspecified hand
● M89.55　Osteolysis, thigh
　　　M89.551　Osteolysis, right thigh
　　　M89.552　Osteolysis, left thigh
　　　M89.559　Osteolysis, unspecified thigh
● M89.56　Osteolysis, lower leg
　　　M89.561　Osteolysis, right lower leg
　　　M89.562　Osteolysis, left lower leg
　　　M89.569　Osteolysis, unspecified lower leg

● M89.57　Osteolysis, ankle and foot
　　　M89.571　Osteolysis, right ankle and foot
　　　M89.572　Osteolysis, left ankle and foot
　　　M89.579　Osteolysis, unspecified ankle and foot
　　M89.58　Osteolysis, other site
　　M89.59　Osteolysis, multiple sites
● M89.6　Osteopathy after poliomyelitis
　　　Use additional code (B91) to identify previous poliomyelitis
　　　Excludes1　postpolio syndrome (G14)
　　M89.60　Osteopathy after poliomyelitis, unspecified site
● M89.61　Osteopathy after poliomyelitis, shoulder
　　　M89.611　Osteopathy after poliomyelitis, right shoulder
　　　M89.612　Osteopathy after poliomyelitis, left shoulder
　　　M89.619　Osteopathy after poliomyelitis, unspecified shoulder
● M89.62　Osteopathy after poliomyelitis, upper arm
　　　M89.621　Osteopathy after poliomyelitis, right upper arm
　　　M89.622　Osteopathy after poliomyelitis, left upper arm
　　　M89.629　Osteopathy after poliomyelitis, unspecified upper arm
● M89.63　Osteopathy after poliomyelitis, forearm
　　　M89.631　Osteopathy after poliomyelitis, right forearm
　　　M89.632　Osteopathy after poliomyelitis, left forearm
　　　M89.639　Osteopathy after poliomyelitis, unspecified forearm
● M89.64　Osteopathy after poliomyelitis, hand
　　　M89.641　Osteopathy after poliomyelitis, right hand
　　　M89.642　Osteopathy after poliomyelitis, left hand
　　　M89.649　Osteopathy after poliomyelitis, unspecified hand
● M89.65　Osteopathy after poliomyelitis, thigh
　　　M89.651　Osteopathy after poliomyelitis, right thigh
　　　M89.652　Osteopathy after poliomyelitis, left thigh
　　　M89.659　Osteopathy after poliomyelitis, unspecified thigh
● M89.66　Osteopathy after poliomyelitis, lower leg
　　　M89.661　Osteopathy after poliomyelitis, right lower leg
　　　M89.662　Osteopathy after poliomyelitis, left lower leg
　　　M89.669　Osteopathy after poliomyelitis, unspecified lower leg
● M89.67　Osteopathy after poliomyelitis, ankle and foot
　　　M89.671　Osteopathy after poliomyelitis, right ankle and foot
　　　M89.672　Osteopathy after poliomyelitis, left ankle and foot
　　　M89.679　Osteopathy after poliomyelitis, unspecified ankle and foot
　　M89.68　Osteopathy after poliomyelitis, other site
　　M89.69　Osteopathy after poliomyelitis, multiple sites

CHAPTER 13 (M00-M99)

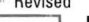

● **M89.7 Major osseous defect**
> *Code first underlying disease, if known, such as:*
> aseptic necrosis of bone (M87.-)
> malignant neoplasm of bone (C40.-)
> osteolysis (M89.5)
> osteomyelitis (M86.-)
> osteonecrosis (M87.-)
> osteoporosis (M80.-, M81.-)
> periprosthetic osteolysis (T84.05-)

   M89.70 Major osseous defect, unspecified site

● M89.71 Major osseous defect, shoulder region
> Major osseous defect clavicle or scapula

     M89.711 Major osseous defect, right shoulder region
     M89.712 Major osseous defect, left shoulder region
     M89.719 Major osseous defect, unspecified shoulder region

● M89.72 Major osseous defect, humerus
     M89.721 Major osseous defect, right humerus
     M89.722 Major osseous defect, left humerus
     M89.729 Major osseous defect, unspecified humerus

● M89.73 Major osseous defect, forearm
> Major osseous defect of radius and ulna

     M89.731 Major osseous defect, right forearm
     M89.732 Major osseous defect, left forearm
     M89.739 Major osseous defect, unspecified forearm

● M89.74 Major osseous defect, hand
> Major osseous defect of carpus, fingers, metacarpus

     M89.741 Major osseous defect, right hand
     M89.742 Major osseous defect, left hand
     M89.749 Major osseous defect, unspecified hand

● M89.75 Major osseous defect, pelvic region and thigh
> Major osseous defect of femur and pelvis

     M89.751 Major osseous defect, right pelvic region and thigh
     M89.752 Major osseous defect, left pelvic region and thigh
     M89.759 Major osseous defect, unspecified pelvic region and thigh

● M89.76 Major osseous defect, lower leg
> Major osseous defect of fibula and tibia

     M89.761 Major osseous defect, right lower leg
     M89.762 Major osseous defect, left lower leg
     M89.769 Major osseous defect, unspecified lower leg

● M89.77 Major osseous defect, ankle and foot
> Major osseous defect of metatarsus, tarsus, toes

     M89.771 Major osseous defect, right ankle and foot
     M89.772 Major osseous defect, left ankle and foot
     M89.779 Major osseous defect, unspecified ankle and foot

   M89.78 Major osseous defect, other site
   M89.79 Major osseous defect, multiple sites

● M89.8 Other specified disorders of bone
> Infantile cortical hyperostoses
> Post-traumatic subperiosteal ossification

● M89.8X Other specified disorders of bone
     M89.8X0 Other specified disorders of bone, multiple sites
     M89.8X1 Other specified disorders of bone, shoulder
     M89.8X2 Other specified disorders of bone, upper arm
     M89.8X3 Other specified disorders of bone, forearm
     M89.8X4 Other specified disorders of bone, hand
     M89.8X5 Other specified disorders of bone, thigh
     M89.8X6 Other specified disorders of bone, lower leg
     M89.8X7 Other specified disorders of bone, ankle and foot
     M89.8X8 Other specified disorders of bone, other site
     M89.8X9 Other specified disorders of bone, unspecified site

   M89.9 Disorder of bone, unspecified

● M90 Osteopathies in diseases classified elsewhere
> **Excludes1** osteochondritis, osteomyelitis, and osteopathy (in):
> cryptococcosis (B45.3)
> diabetes mellitus (E08-E13 with .61-)
> gonococcal (A54.43)
> neurogenic syphilis (A52.11)
> renal osteodystrophy (N25.0)
> salmoncllosis (A02.24)
> secondary syphilis (A51.46)
> syphilis (late) (A52.77)

● M90.5 Osteonecrosis in diseases classified elsewhere
> *Code first underlying disease, such as:*
> caisson disease (T70.3)
> hemoglobinopathy (D50-D64)

   M90.50 Osteonecrosis in diseases classified elsewhere, unspecified site

● M90.51 Osteonecrosis in diseases classified elsewhere, shoulder
     M90.511 Osteonecrosis in diseases classified elsewhere, right shoulder
     M90.512 Osteonecrosis in diseases classified elsewhere, left shoulder
     M90.519 Osteonecrosis in diseases classified elsewhere, unspecified shoulder

● M90.52 Osteonecrosis in diseases classified elsewhere, upper arm
     M90.521 Osteonecrosis in diseases classified elsewhere, right upper arm
     M90.522 Osteonecrosis in diseases classified elsewhere, left upper arm
     M90.529 Osteonecrosis in diseases classified elsewhere, unspecified upper arm

● M90.53 Osteonecrosis in diseases classified elsewhere, forearm
     M90.531 Osteonecrosis in diseases classified elsewhere, right forearm
     M90.532 Osteonecrosis in diseases classified elsewhere, left forearm
     M90.539 Osteonecrosis in diseases classified elsewhere, unspecified forearm

● **M90.54**   Osteonecrosis in diseases classified elsewhere, hand

     M90.541   Osteonecrosis in diseases classified elsewhere, right hand

     M90.542   Osteonecrosis in diseases classified elsewhere, left hand

     M90.549   Osteonecrosis in diseases classified elsewhere, unspecified hand

● **M90.55**   Osteonecrosis in diseases classified elsewhere, thigh

     M90.551   Osteonecrosis in diseases classified elsewhere, right thigh

     M90.552   Osteonecrosis in diseases classified elsewhere, left thigh

     M90.559   Osteonecrosis in diseases classified elsewhere, unspecified thigh

● **M90.56**   Osteonecrosis in diseases classified elsewhere, lower leg

     M90.561   Osteonecrosis in diseases classified elsewhere, right lower leg

     M90.562   Osteonecrosis in diseases classified elsewhere, left lower leg

     M90.569   Osteonecrosis in diseases classified elsewhere, unspecified lower leg

● **M90.57**   Osteonecrosis in diseases classified elsewhere, ankle and foot

     M90.571   Osteonecrosis in diseases classified elsewhere, right ankle and foot

     M90.572   Osteonecrosis in diseases classified elsewhere, left ankle and foot

     M90.579   Osteonecrosis in diseases classified elsewhere, unspecified ankle and foot

     M90.58   Osteonecrosis in diseases classified elsewhere, other site

     M90.59   Osteonecrosis in diseases classified elsewhere, multiple sites

● **M90.6**   Osteitis deformans in neoplastic diseases

     Osteitis deformans in malignant neoplasm of bone

     Code first the neoplasm (C40.-, C41.-)

     Excludes1   osteitis deformans [Paget's disease of bone] (M88.-)

     M90.60   Osteitis deformans in neoplastic diseases, unspecified site

● **M90.61**   Osteitis deformans in neoplastic diseases, shoulder

     M90.611   Osteitis deformans in neoplastic diseases, right shoulder

     M90.612   Osteitis deformans in neoplastic diseases, left shoulder

     M90.619   Osteitis deformans in neoplastic diseases, unspecified shoulder

● **M90.62**   Osteitis deformans in neoplastic diseases, upper arm

     M90.621   Osteitis deformans in neoplastic diseases, right upper arm

     M90.622   Osteitis deformans in neoplastic diseases, left upper arm

     M90.629   Osteitis deformans in neoplastic diseases, unspecified upper arm

● **M90.63**   Osteitis deformans in neoplastic diseases, forearm

     M90.631   Osteitis deformans in neoplastic diseases, right forearm

     M90.632   Osteitis deformans in neoplastic diseases, left forearm

     M90.639   Osteitis deformans in neoplastic diseases, unspecified forearm

● **M90.64**   Osteitis deformans in neoplastic diseases, hand

     M90.641   Osteitis deformans in neoplastic diseases, right hand

     M90.642   Osteitis deformans in neoplastic diseases, left hand

     M90.649   Osteitis deformans in neoplastic diseases, unspecified hand

● **M90.65**   Osteitis deformans in neoplastic diseases, thigh

     M90.651   Osteitis deformans in neoplastic diseases, right thigh

     M90.652   Osteitis deformans in neoplastic diseases, left thigh

     M90.659   Osteitis deformans in neoplastic diseases, unspecified thigh

● **M90.66**   Osteitis deformans in neoplastic diseases, lower leg

     M90.661   Osteitis deformans in neoplastic diseases, right lower leg

     M90.662   Osteitis deformans in neoplastic diseases, left lower leg

     M90.669   Osteitis deformans in neoplastic diseases, unspecified lower leg

● **M90.67**   Osteitis deformans in neoplastic diseases, ankle and foot

     M90.671   Osteitis deformans in neoplastic diseases, right ankle and foot

     M90.672   Osteitis deformans in neoplastic diseases, left ankle and foot

     M90.679   Osteitis deformans in neoplastic diseases, unspecified ankle and foot

     M90.68   Osteitis deformans in neoplastic diseases, other site

     M90.69   Osteitis deformans in neoplastic diseases, multiple sites

● **M90.8**   Osteopathy in diseases classified elsewhere

     Code first underlying disease, such as:

     rickets (E55.0)

     vitamin-D-resistant rickets (E83.3)

     M90.80   Osteopathy in diseases classified elsewhere, unspecified site

● **M90.81**   Osteopathy in diseases classified elsewhere, shoulder

     M90.811   Osteopathy in diseases classified elsewhere, right shoulder

     M90.812   Osteopathy in diseases classified elsewhere, left shoulder

     M90.819   Osteopathy in diseases classified elsewhere, unspecified shoulder

● **M90.82**   Osteopathy in diseases classified elsewhere, upper arm

     M90.821   Osteopathy in diseases classified elsewhere, right upper arm

     M90.822   Osteopathy in diseases classified elsewhere, left upper arm

     M90.829   Osteopathy in diseases classified elsewhere, unspecified upper arm

● **M90.83**   Osteopathy in diseases classified elsewhere, forearm

     M90.831   Osteopathy in diseases classified elsewhere, right forearm

     M90.832   Osteopathy in diseases classified elsewhere, left forearm

     M90.839   Osteopathy in diseases classified elsewhere, unspecified forearm

CHAPTER 13 (M00-M99)

●M90.84 Osteopathy in diseases classified elsewhere, hand

   M90.841 Osteopathy in diseases classified elsewhere, right hand

   M90.842 Osteopathy in diseases classified elsewhere, left hand

   M90.849 Osteopathy in diseases classified elsewhere, unspecified hand

●M90.85 Osteopathy in diseases classified elsewhere, thigh

   M90.851 Osteopathy in diseases classified elsewhere, right thigh

   M90.852 Osteopathy in diseases classified elsewhere, left thigh

   M90.859 Osteopathy in diseases classified elsewhere, unspecified thigh

●M90.86 Osteopathy in diseases classified elsewhere, lower leg

   M90.861 Osteopathy in diseases classified elsewhere, right lower leg

   M90.862 Osteopathy in diseases classified elsewhere, left lower leg

   M90.869 Osteopathy in diseases classified elsewhere, unspecified lower leg

●M90.87 Osteopathy in diseases classified elsewhere, ankle and foot

   M90.871 Osteopathy in diseases classified elsewhere, right ankle and foot

   M90.872 Osteopathy in diseases classified elsewhere, left ankle and foot

   M90.879 Osteopathy in diseases classified elsewhere, unspecified ankle and foot

  M90.88 Osteopathy in diseases classified elsewhere, other site

  M90.89 Osteopathy in diseases classified elsewhere, multiple sites

CHONDROPATHIES (M91-M94)

Excludes1 postprocedural chondropathies (M96.-)

●M91 Juvenile osteochondrosis of hip and pelvis

Excludes1 slipped upper femoral epiphysis (nontraumatic) (M93.0)

  M91.0 Juvenile osteochondrosis of pelvis

    Osteochondrosis (juvenile) of acetabulum
    Osteochondrosis (juvenile) of iliac crest [Buchanan]
    Osteochondrosis (juvenile) of ischiopubic synchondrosis [van Neck]
    Osteochondrosis (juvenile) of symphysis pubis [Pierson]

●M91.1 Juvenile osteochondrosis of head of femur [Legg-Calvé-Perthes]

   M91.10 Juvenile osteochondrosis of head of femur [Legg-Calvé-Perthes], unspecified leg

   M91.11 Juvenile osteochondrosis of head of femur [Legg-Calvé-Perthes], right leg

   M91.12 Juvenile osteochondrosis of head of femur [Legg-Calvé-Perthes], left leg

●M91.2 Coxa plana

    Hip deformity due to previous juvenile osteochondrosis

   M91.20 Coxa plana, unspecified hip

   M91.21 Coxa plana, right hip

   M91.22 Coxa plana, left hip

●M91.3 Pseudocoxalgia

   M91.30 Pseudocoxalgia, unspecified hip

   M91.31 Pseudocoxalgia, right hip

   M91.32 Pseudocoxalgia, left hip

●M91.4 Coxa magna

   M91.40 Coxa magna, unspecified hip

   M91.41 Coxa magna, right hip

   M91.42 Coxa magna, left hip

●M91.8 Other juvenile osteochondrosis of hip and pelvis

    Juvenile osteochondrosis after reduction of congenital dislocation of hip

   M91.80 Other juvenile osteochondrosis of hip and pelvis, unspecified leg

   M91.81 Other juvenile osteochondrosis of hip and pelvis, right leg

   M91.82 Other juvenile osteochondrosis of hip and pelvis, left leg

●M91.9 Juvenile osteochondrosis of hip and pelvis, unspecified

   M91.90 Juvenile osteochondrosis of hip and pelvis, unspecified, unspecified leg

   M91.91 Juvenile osteochondrosis of hip and pelvis, unspecified, right leg

   M91.92 Juvenile osteochondrosis of hip and pelvis, unspecified, left leg

●M92 Other juvenile osteochondrosis

●M92.0 Juvenile osteochondrosis of humerus

    Osteochondrosis (juvenile) of capitulum of humerus [Panner]
    Osteochondrosis (juvenile) of head of humerus [Haas]

   M92.00 Juvenile osteochondrosis of humerus, unspecified arm

   M92.01 Juvenile osteochondrosis of humerus, right arm

   M92.02 Juvenile osteochondrosis of humerus, left arm

●M92.1 Juvenile osteochondrosis of radius and ulna

    Osteochondrosis (juvenile) of lower ulna [Burns]
    Osteochondrosis (juvenile) of radial head [Brailsford]

   M92.10 Juvenile osteochondrosis of radius and ulna, unspecified arm

   M92.11 Juvenile osteochondrosis of radius and ulna, right arm

   M92.12 Juvenile osteochondrosis of radius and ulna, left arm

●M92.2 Juvenile osteochondrosis, hand

●M92.20 Unspecified juvenile osteochondrosis, hand

   M92.201 Unspecified juvenile osteochondrosis, right hand

   M92.202 Unspecified juvenile osteochondrosis, left hand

   M92.209 Unspecified juvenile osteochondrosis, unspecified hand

●M92.21 Osteochondrosis (juvenile) of carpal lunate [Kienböck]

   M92.211 Osteochondrosis (juvenile) of carpal lunate [Kienböck], right hand

   M92.212 Osteochondrosis (juvenile) of carpal lunate [Kienböck], left hand

   M92.219 Osteochondrosis (juvenile) of carpal lunate [Kienböck], unspecified hand

●M92.22 Osteochondrosis (juvenile) of metacarpal heads [Mauclaire]

   M92.221 Osteochondrosis (juvenile) of metacarpal heads [Mauclaire], right hand

   M92.222 Osteochondrosis (juvenile) of metacarpal heads [Mauclaire], left hand

   M92.229 Osteochondrosis (juvenile) of metacarpal heads [Mauclaire], unspecified hand

◀ New   ◀━ Revised   ~~deleted~~ Deleted   OGCR Official Guidelines   X Assign placeholder X   ● Use Additional Character(s)

Excludes 1   Excludes 2   Includes   Use additional   Code first   Code also   Unspecified

● M92.29   Other juvenile osteochondrosis, hand

     M92.291   Other juvenile osteochondrosis, right hand

     M92.292   Other juvenile osteochondrosis, left hand

     M92.299   Other juvenile osteochondrosis, unspecified hand

● M92.3   Other juvenile osteochondrosis, upper limb

     M92.30   Other juvenile osteochondrosis, unspecified upper limb

     M92.31   Other juvenile osteochondrosis, right upper limb

     M92.32   Other juvenile osteochondrosis, left upper limb

● M92.4   Juvenile osteochondrosis of patella

     Osteochondrosis (juvenile) of primary patellar center [Köhler]

     Osteochondrosis (juvenile) of secondary patellar center [Sinding Larsen]

     M92.40   Juvenile osteochondrosis of patella, unspecified knee

     M92.41   Juvenile osteochondrosis of patella, right knee

     M92.42   Juvenile osteochondrosis of patella, left knee

● M92.5   Juvenile osteochondrosis of tibia and fibula

     Osteochondrosis (juvenile) of proximal tibia [Blount]

     Osteochondrosis (juvenile) of tibial tubercle [Osgood-Schlatter]

     Tibia vara

     M92.50   Juvenile osteochondrosis of tibia and fibula, unspecified leg

     M92.51   Juvenile osteochondrosis of tibia and fibula, right leg

     M92.52   Juvenile osteochondrosis of tibia and fibula, left leg

● M92.6   Juvenile osteochondrosis of tarsus

     Osteochondrosis (juvenile) of calcaneum [Sever]

     Osteochondrosis (juvenile) of os tibiale externum [Haglund]

     Osteochondrosis (juvenile) of talus [Diaz]

     Osteochondrosis (juvenile) of tarsal navicular [Köhler]

     M92.60   Juvenile osteochondrosis of tarsus, unspecified ankle

     M92.61   Juvenile osteochondrosis of tarsus, right ankle

     M92.62   Juvenile osteochondrosis of tarsus, left ankle

● M92.7   Juvenile osteochondrosis of metatarsus

     Osteochondrosis (juvenile) of fifth metatarsus [Iselin]

     Osteochondrosis (juvenile) of second metatarsus [Freiberg]

     M92.70   Juvenile osteochondrosis of metatarsus, unspecified foot

     M92.71   Juvenile osteochondrosis of metatarsus, right foot

     M92.72   Juvenile osteochondrosis of metatarsus, left foot

M92.8   Other specified juvenile osteochondrosis

     Calcaneal apophysitis

M92.9   Juvenile osteochondrosis, unspecified

     Juvenile apophysitis NOS

     Juvenile epiphysitis NOS

     Juvenile osteochondritis NOS

     Juvenile osteochondrosis NOS

● M93   Other osteochondropathies

     Excludes2   osteochondrosis of spine (M42.-)

● M93.0   Slipped upper femoral epiphysis (nontraumatic)

     Use additional code for associated chondrolysis (M94.3)

     ● M93.00   Unspecified slipped upper femoral epiphysis (nontraumatic)

         M93.001   Unspecified slipped upper femoral epiphysis (nontraumatic), right hip

         M93.002   Unspecified slipped upper femoral epiphysis (nontraumatic), left hip

         M93.003   Unspecified slipped upper femoral epiphysis (nontraumatic), unspecified hip

     ● M93.01   Acute slipped upper femoral epiphysis (nontraumatic)

         M93.011   Acute slipped upper femoral epiphysis (nontraumatic), right hip

         M93.012   Acute slipped upper femoral epiphysis (nontraumatic), left hip

         M93.013   Acute slipped upper femoral epiphysis (nontraumatic), unspecified hip

     ● M93.02   Chronic slipped upper femoral epiphysis (nontraumatic)

         M93.021   Chronic slipped upper femoral epiphysis (nontraumatic), right hip

         M93.022   Chronic slipped upper femoral epiphysis (nontraumatic), left hip

         M93.023   Chronic slipped upper femoral epiphysis (nontraumatic), unspecified hip

     ● M93.03   Acute on chronic slipped upper femoral epiphysis (nontraumatic)

         M93.031   Acute on chronic slipped upper femoral epiphysis (nontraumatic), right hip

         M93.032   Acute on chronic slipped upper femoral epiphysis (nontraumatic), left hip

         M93.033   Acute on chronic slipped upper femoral epiphysis (nontraumatic), unspecified hip

M93.1   Kienböck's disease of adults

     Adult osteochondrosis of carpal lunates

● M93.2   Osteochondritis dissecans

     M93.20   Osteochondritis dissecans of unspecified site

     ● M93.21   Osteochondritis dissecans of shoulder

         M93.211   Osteochondritis dissecans, right shoulder

         M93.212   Osteochondritis dissecans, left shoulder

         M93.219   Osteochondritis dissecans, unspecified shoulder

     ● M93.22   Osteochondritis dissecans of elbow

         M93.221   Osteochondritis dissecans, right elbow

         M93.222   Osteochondritis dissecans, left elbow

         M93.229   Osteochondritis dissecans, unspecified elbow

     ● M93.23   Osteochondritis dissecans of wrist

         M93.231   Osteochondritis dissecans, right wrist

         M93.232   Osteochondritis dissecans, left wrist

         M93.239   Osteochondritis dissecans, unspecified wrist

CHAPTER 13 (M00-M99)

● M93.24 Osteochondritis dissecans of joints of hand
    M93.241 Osteochondritis dissecans, joints of right hand
    M93.242 Osteochondritis dissecans, joints of left hand
    M93.249 Osteochondritis dissecans, joints of unspecified hand

● M93.25 Osteochondritis dissecans of hip
    M93.251 Osteochondritis dissecans, right hip
    M93.252 Osteochondritis dissecans, left hip
    M93.259 Osteochondritis dissecans, unspecified hip

● M93.26 Osteochondritis dissecans knee
    M93.261 Osteochondritis dissecans, right knee
    M93.262 Osteochondritis dissecans, left knee
    M93.269 Osteochondritis dissecans, unspecified knee

● M93.27 Osteochondritis dissecans of ankle and joints of foot
    M93.271 Osteochondritis dissecans, right ankle and joints of right foot
    M93.272 Osteochondritis dissecans, left ankle and joints of left foot
    M93.279 Osteochondritis dissecans, unspecified ankle and joints of foot

  M93.28 Osteochondritis dissecans other site

  M93.29 Osteochondritis dissecans multiple sites

● M93.8 Other specified osteochondropathies
  M93.80 Other specified osteochondropathies of unspecified site

● M93.81 Other specified osteochondropathies of shoulder
    M93.811 Other specified osteochondropathies, right shoulder
    M93.812 Other specified osteochondropathies, left shoulder
    M93.819 Other specified osteochondropathies, unspecified shoulder

● M93.82 Other specified osteochondropathies of upper arm
    M93.821 Other specified osteochondropathies, right upper arm
    M93.822 Other specified osteochondropathies, left upper arm
    M93.829 Other specified osteochondropathies, unspecified upper arm

● M93.83 Other specified osteochondropathies of forearm
    M93.831 Other specified osteochondropathies, right forearm
    M93.832 Other specified osteochondropathies, left forearm
    M93.839 Other specified osteochondropathies, unspecified forearm

● M93.84 Other specified osteochondropathies of hand
    M93.841 Other specified osteochondropathies, right hand
    M93.842 Other specified osteochondropathies, left hand
    M93.849 Other specified osteochondropathies, unspecified hand

● M93.85 Other specified osteochondropathies of thigh
    M93.851 Other specified osteochondropathies, right thigh
    M93.852 Other specified osteochondropathies, left thigh
    M93.859 Other specified osteochondropathies, unspecified thigh

● M93.86 Other specified osteochondropathies lower leg
    M93.861 Other specified osteochondropathies, right lower leg
    M93.862 Other specified osteochondropathies, left lower leg
    M93.869 Other specified osteochondropathies, unspecified lower leg

● M93.87 Other specified osteochondropathies of ankle and foot
    M93.871 Other specified osteochondropathies, right ankle and foot
    M93.872 Other specified osteochondropathies, left ankle and foot
    M93.879 Other specified osteochondropathies, unspecified ankle and foot

  M93.88 Other specified osteochondropathies other

  M93.89 Other specified osteochondropathies multiple sites

M93.9 Osteochondropathy, unspecified
  Apophysitis NOS
  Epiphysitis NOS
  Osteochondritis NOS
  Osteochondrosis NOS

  M93.90 Osteochondropathy, unspecified of unspecified site

● M93.91 Osteochondropathy, unspecified of shoulder
    M93.911 Osteochondropathy, unspecified, right shoulder
    M93.912 Osteochondropathy, unspecified, left shoulder
    M93.919 Osteochondropathy, unspecified, unspecified shoulder

● M93.92 Osteochondropathy, unspecified of upper arm
    M93.921 Osteochondropathy, unspecified, right upper arm
    M93.922 Osteochondropathy, unspecified, left upper arm
    M93.929 Osteochondropathy, unspecified, unspecified upper arm

● M93.93 Osteochondropathy, unspecified of forearm
    M93.931 Osteochondropathy, unspecified, right forearm
    M93.932 Osteochondropathy, unspecified, left forearm
    M93.939 Osteochondropathy, unspecified, unspecified forearm

● M93.94 Osteochondropathy, unspecified of hand
    M93.941 Osteochondropathy, unspecified, right hand
    M93.942 Osteochondropathy, unspecified, left hand
    M93.949 Osteochondropathy, unspecified, unspecified hand

● M93.95 Osteochondropathy, unspecified of thigh
    M93.951 Osteochondropathy, unspecified, right thigh
    M93.952 Osteochondropathy, unspecified, left thigh
    M93.959 Osteochondropathy, unspecified, unspecified thigh

● M93.96 Osteochondropathy, unspecified lower leg
    M93.961 Osteochondropathy, unspecified, right lower leg
    M93.962 Osteochondropathy, unspecified, left lower leg
    M93.969 Osteochondropathy, unspecified, unspecified lower leg

● M93.97   Osteochondropathy, unspecified of ankle and foot

     M93.971   Osteochondropathy, unspecified, right ankle and foot

     M93.972   Osteochondropathy, unspecified, left ankle and foot

     M93.979   Osteochondropathy, unspecified, unspecified ankle and foot

   M93.98   Osteochondropathy, unspecified other

   M93.99   Osteochondropathy, unspecified multiple sites

● M94   Other disorders of cartilage

   M94.0   Chondrocostal junction syndrome [Tietze]
           Costochondritis

   M94.1   Relapsing polychondritis

● M94.2   Chondromalacia

     Excludes1   chondromalacia patellae (M22.4)

     M94.20   Chondromalacia, unspecified site

● M94.21   Chondromalacia, shoulder

     M94.211   Chondromalacia, right shoulder

     M94.212   Chondromalacia, left shoulder

     M94.219   Chondromalacia, unspecified shoulder

● M94.22   Chondromalacia, elbow

     M94.221   Chondromalacia, right elbow

     M94.222   Chondromalacia, left elbow

     M94.229   Chondromalacia, unspecified elbow

● M94.23   Chondromalacia, wrist

     M94.231   Chondromalacia, right wrist

     M94.232   Chondromalacia, left wrist

     M94.239   Chondromalacia, unspecified wrist

● M94.24   Chondromalacia, joints of hand

     M94.241   Chondromalacia, joints of right hand

     M94.242   Chondromalacia, joints of left hand

     M94.249   Chondromalacia, joints of unspecified hand

● M94.25   Chondromalacia, hip

     M94.251   Chondromalacia, right hip

     M94.252   Chondromalacia, left hip

     M94.259   Chondromalacia, unspecified hip

● M94.26   Chondromalacia, knee

     M94.261   Chondromalacia, right knee

     M94.262   Chondromalacia, left knee

     M94.269   Chondromalacia, unspecified knee

● M94.27   Chondromalacia, ankle and joints of foot

     M94.271   Chondromalacia, right ankle and joints of right foot

     M94.272   Chondromalacia, left ankle and joints of left foot

     M94.279   Chondromalacia, unspecified ankle and joints of foot

     M94.28   Chondromalacia, other site

     M94.29   Chondromalacia, multiple sites

● M94.3   Chondrolysis

     Code first any associated slipped upper femoral epiphysis (nontraumatic) (M93.0-)

● M94.35   Chondrolysis, hip

     M94.351   Chondrolysis, right hip

     M94.352   Chondrolysis, left hip

     M94.359   Chondrolysis, unspecified hip

● M94.8   Other specified disorders of cartilage

   ● M94.8X   Other specified disorders of cartilage

     M94.8X0   Other specified disorders of cartilage, multiple sites

     M94.8X1   Other specified disorders of cartilage, shoulder

     M94.8X2   Other specified disorders of cartilage, upper arm

     M94.8X3   Other specified disorders of cartilage, forearm

     M94.8X4   Other specified disorders of cartilage, hand

     M94.8X5   Other specified disorders of cartilage, thigh

     M94.8X6   Other specified disorders of cartilage, lower leg

     M94.8X7   Other specified disorders of cartilage, ankle and foot

     M94.8X8   Other specified disorders of cartilage, other site

     M94.8X9   Other specified disorders of cartilage, unspecified sites

   M94.9   Disorder of cartilage, unspecified

OTHER DISORDERS OF THE MUSCULOSKELETAL SYSTEM AND CONNECTIVE TISSUE (M95)

● M95   Other acquired deformities of musculoskeletal system and connective tissue

     Excludes2   acquired absence of limbs and organs (Z89-Z90)
           acquired deformities of limbs (M20-M21)
           congenital malformations and deformations of the musculoskeletal system (Q65-Q79)
           deforming dorsopathies (M40-M43)
           dentofacial anomalies [including malocclusion] (M26.-)
           postprocedural musculoskeletal disorders (M96.-)

   M95.0   Acquired deformity of nose

     Excludes2   deviated nasal septum (J34.2)

● M95.1   Cauliflower ear

     Excludes2   other acquired deformities of ear (H61.1)

     M95.10   Cauliflower ear, unspecified ear

     M95.11   Cauliflower ear, right ear

     M95.12   Cauliflower ear, left ear

   M95.2   Other acquired deformity of head

   M95.3   Acquired deformity of neck

   M95.4   Acquired deformity of chest and rib

   M95.5   Acquired deformity of pelvis

     Excludes1   maternal care for known or suspected disproportion (O33.-)

   M95.8   Other specified acquired deformities of musculoskeletal system

   M95.9   Acquired deformity of musculoskeletal system, unspecified

INTRAOPERATIVE AND POSTPROCEDURAL COMPLICATIONS AND DISORDERS OF MUSCULOSKELETAL SYSTEM, NOT ELSEWHERE CLASSIFIED (M96)

● M96   Intraoperative and postprocedural complications and disorders of musculoskeletal system, not elsewhere classified

     Excludes2   arthropathy following intestinal bypass (M02.0-)
           complications of internal orthopedic prosthetic devices, implants and grafts (T84.-)
           disorders associated with osteoporosis (M80)
           presence of functional implants and other devices (Z96-Z97)

   M96.0   Pseudarthrosis after fusion or arthrodesis

   M96.1   Postlaminectomy syndrome, not elsewhere classified

M96.2   Postradiation kyphosis

M96.3   Postlaminectomy kyphosis

M96.4   Postsurgical lordosis

M96.5   Postradiation scoliosis

● M96.6   Fracture of bone following insertion of orthopedic implant, joint prosthesis, or bone plate
            Intraoperative fracture of bone during insertion of orthopedic implant, joint prosthesis, or bone plate
            Excludes2   complication of internal orthopedic devices, implants or grafts (T84.-)

● M96.62   Fracture of humerus following insertion of orthopedic implant, joint prosthesis, or bone plate

M96.621   Fracture of humerus following insertion of orthopedic implant, joint prosthesis, or bone plate, right arm

M96.622   Fracture of humerus following insertion of orthopedic implant, joint prosthesis, or bone plate, left arm

M96.629   Fracture of humerus following insertion of orthopedic implant, joint prosthesis, or bone plate, unspecified arm

● M96.63   Fracture of radius or ulna following insertion of orthopedic implant, joint prosthesis, or bone plate

M96.631   Fracture of radius or ulna following insertion of orthopedic implant, joint prosthesis, or bone plate, right arm

M96.632   Fracture of radius or ulna following insertion of orthopedic implant, joint prosthesis, or bone plate, left arm

M96.639   Fracture of radius or ulna following insertion of orthopedic implant, joint prosthesis, or bone plate, unspecified arm

M96.65   Fracture of pelvis following insertion of orthopedic implant, joint prosthesis, or bone plate

● M96.66   Fracture of femur following insertion of orthopedic implant, joint prosthesis, or bone plate

M96.661   Fracture of femur following insertion of orthopedic implant, joint prosthesis, or bone plate, right leg

M96.662   Fracture of femur following insertion of orthopedic implant, joint prosthesis, or bone plate, left leg

M96.669   Fracture of femur following insertion of orthopedic implant, joint prosthesis, or bone plate, unspecified leg

● M96.67   Fracture of tibia or fibula following insertion of orthopedic implant, joint prosthesis, or bone plate

M96.671   Fracture of tibia or fibula following insertion of orthopedic implant, joint prosthesis, or bone plate, right leg

M96.672   Fracture of tibia or fibula following insertion of orthopedic implant, joint prosthesis, or bone plate, left leg

M96.679   Fracture of tibia or fibula following insertion of orthopedic implant, joint prosthesis, or bone plate, unspecified leg

M96.69   Fracture of other bone following insertion of orthopedic implant, joint prosthesis, or bone plate

● M96.8   Other intraoperative and postprocedural complications and disorders of musculoskeletal system, not elsewhere classified

● M96.81   Intraoperative hemorrhage and hematoma of a musculoskeletal structure complicating a procedure
            Excludes1   intraoperative hemorrhage and hematoma of a musculoskeletal structure due to accidental puncture and laceration during a procedure (M96.82-)

M96.810   Intraoperative hemorrhage and hematoma of a musculoskeletal structure complicating a musculoskeletal system procedure

M96.811   Intraoperative hemorrhage and hematoma of a musculoskeletal structure complicating other procedure

● M96.82   Accidental puncture and laceration of a musculoskeletal structure during a procedure

M96.820   Accidental puncture and laceration of a musculoskeletal structure during a musculoskeletal system procedure

M96.821   Accidental puncture and laceration of a musculoskeletal structure during other procedure

● M96.83   Postprocedural hemorrhage and hematoma of a musculoskeletal structure following a procedure

M96.830   Postprocedural hemorrhage and hematoma of a musculoskeletal structure following a musculoskeletal system procedure

M96.831   Postprocedural hemorrhage and hematoma of a musculoskeletal structure following other procedure

M96.89   Other intraoperative and postprocedural complications and disorders of the musculoskeletal system
            Instability of joint secondary to removal of joint prosthesis
            Use additional code, if applicable, to further specify disorder

---

BIOMECHANICAL LESIONS, NOT ELSEWHERE CLASSIFIED (M99)

● M99   Biomechanical lesions, not elsewhere classified
            Note: This category should not be used if the condition can be classified elsewhere.

● M99.0   Segmental and somatic dysfunction

M99.00   Segmental and somatic dysfunction of head region

M99.01   Segmental and somatic dysfunction of cervical region

M99.02   Segmental and somatic dysfunction of thoracic region

M99.03   Segmental and somatic dysfunction of lumbar region

M99.04   Segmental and somatic dysfunction of sacral region

M99.05   Segmental and somatic dysfunction of pelvic region

M99.06   Segmental and somatic dysfunction of lower extremity

M99.07   Segmental and somatic dysfunction of upper extremity

M99.08   Segmental and somatic dysfunction of rib cage

M99.09   Segmental and somatic dysfunction of abdomen and other regions

● M99.1   Subluxation complex (vertebral)

    M99.10   Subluxation complex (vertebral) of head region

    M99.11   Subluxation complex (vertebral) of cervical region

    M99.12   Subluxation complex (vertebral) of thoracic region

    M99.13   Subluxation complex (vertebral) of lumbar region

    M99.14   Subluxation complex (vertebral) of sacral region

    M99.15   Subluxation complex (vertebral) of pelvic region

    M99.16   Subluxation complex (vertebral) of lower extremity

    M99.17   Subluxation complex (vertebral) of upper extremity

    M99.18   Subluxation complex (vertebral) of rib cage

    M99.19   Subluxation complex (vertebral) of abdomen and other regions

● M99.2   Subluxation stenosis of neural canal

    M99.20   Subluxation stenosis of neural canal of head region

    M99.21   Subluxation stenosis of neural canal of cervical region

    M99.22   Subluxation stenosis of neural canal of thoracic region

    M99.23   Subluxation stenosis of neural canal of lumbar region

    M99.24   Subluxation stenosis of neural canal of sacral region

    M99.25   Subluxation stenosis of neural canal of pelvic region

    M99.26   Subluxation stenosis of neural canal of lower extremity

    M99.27   Subluxation stenosis of neural canal of upper extremity

    M99.28   Subluxation stenosis of neural canal of rib cage

    M99.29   Subluxation stenosis of neural canal of abdomen and other regions

● M99.3   Osseous stenosis of neural canal

    M99.30   Osseous stenosis of neural canal of head region

    M99.31   Osseous stenosis of neural canal of cervical region

    M99.32   Osseous stenosis of neural canal of thoracic region

    M99.33   Osseous stenosis of neural canal of lumbar region

    M99.34   Osseous stenosis of neural canal of sacral region

    M99.35   Osseous stenosis of neural canal of pelvic region

    M99.36   Osseous stenosis of neural canal of lower extremity

    M99.37   Osseous stenosis of neural canal of upper extremity

    M99.38   Osseous stenosis of neural canal of rib cage

    M99.39   Osseous stenosis of neural canal of abdomen and other regions

● M99.4   Connective tissue stenosis of neural canal

    M99.40   Connective tissue stenosis of neural canal of head region

    M99.41   Connective tissue stenosis of neural canal of cervical region

    M99.42   Connective tissue stenosis of neural canal of thoracic region

    M99.43   Connective tissue stenosis of neural canal of lumbar region

    M99.44   Connective tissue stenosis of neural canal of sacral region

    M99.45   Connective tissue stenosis of neural canal of pelvic region

    M99.46   Connective tissue stenosis of neural canal of lower extremity

    M99.47   Connective tissue stenosis of neural canal of upper extremity

    M99.48   Connective tissue stenosis of neural canal of rib cage

    M99.49   Connective tissue stenosis of neural canal of abdomen and other regions

● M99.5   Intervertebral disc stenosis of neural canal

    M99.50   Intervertebral disc stenosis of neural canal of head region

    M99.51   Intervertebral disc stenosis of neural canal of cervical region

    M99.52   Intervertebral disc stenosis of neural canal of thoracic region

    M99.53   Intervertebral disc stenosis of neural canal of lumbar region

    M99.54   Intervertebral disc stenosis of neural canal of sacral region

    M99.55   Intervertebral disc stenosis of neural canal of pelvic region

    M99.56   Intervertebral disc stenosis of neural canal of lower extremity

    M99.57   Intervertebral disc stenosis of neural canal of upper extremity

    M99.58   Intervertebral disc stenosis of neural canal of rib cage

    M99.59   Intervertebral disc stenosis of neural canal of abdomen and other regions

● M99.6   Osseous and subluxation stenosis of intervertebral foramina

    M99.60   Osseous and subluxation stenosis of intervertebral foramina of head region

    M99.61   Osseous and subluxation stenosis of intervertebral foramina of cervical region

    M99.62   Osseous and subluxation stenosis of intervertebral foramina of thoracic region

    M99.63   Osseous and subluxation stenosis of intervertebral foramina of lumbar region

    M99.64   Osseous and subluxation stenosis of intervertebral foramina of sacral region

    M99.65   Osseous and subluxation stenosis of intervertebral foramina of pelvic region

    M99.66   Osseous and subluxation stenosis of intervertebral foramina of lower extremity

    M99.67   Osseous and subluxation stenosis of intervertebral foramina of upper extremity

    M99.68   Osseous and subluxation stenosis of intervertebral foramina of rib cage

    M99.69   Osseous and subluxation stenosis of intervertebral foramina of abdomen and other regions

CHAPTER 13 (M00-M99)

● M99.7   Connective tissue and disc stenosis of intervertebral
         foramina
   M99.70   Connective tissue and disc stenosis of
            intervertebral foramina of head region
   M99.71   Connective tissue and disc stenosis of
            intervertebral foramina of cervical region
   M99.72   Connective tissue and disc stenosis of
            intervertebral foramina of thoracic region
   M99.73   Connective tissue and disc stenosis of
            intervertebral foramina of lumbar region
   M99.74   Connective tissue and disc stenosis of
            intervertebral foramina of sacral region
   M99.75   Connective tissue and disc stenosis of
            intervertebral foramina of pelvic region
   M99.76   Connective tissue and disc stenosis of
            intervertebral foramina of lower extremity
   M99.77   Connective tissue and disc stenosis of
            intervertebral foramina of upper extremity
   M99.78   Connective tissue and disc stenosis of
            intervertebral foramina of rib cage
   M99.79   Connective tissue and disc stenosis of
            intervertebral foramina of abdomen and other
            regions

● M99.8   Other biomechanical lesions
   M99.80   Other biomechanical lesions of head region
   M99.81   Other biomechanical lesions of cervical region
   M99.82   Other biomechanical lesions of thoracic region
   M99.83   Other biomechanical lesions of lumbar region
   M99.84   Other biomechanical lesions of sacral region
   M99.85   Other biomechanical lesions of pelvic region
   M99.86   Other biomechanical lesions of lower extremity
   M99.87   Other biomechanical lesions of upper extremity
   M99.88   Other biomechanical lesions of rib cage
   M99.89   Other biomechanical lesions of abdomen and
            other regions
   M99.9   Biomechanical lesion, unspecified

◀ New   ◀▥ Revised   deleted Deleted   OGCR Official Guidelines   X Assign placeholder X   ● Use Additional Character(s)
          Excludes 1   Excludes 2   Includes   Use additional   Code first   Code also   Unspecified

Item 14–1 Nephritis (inflammation) or **nephropathy** (disease) **with lesion of proliferative glomerulonephritis** results from a streptococcal infection.

   Nephritis (inflammation) or **nephropathy** (disease) **with lesion of membranous glomerulonephritis** is characterized by deposits along the epithelial side of the basement membrane.

   Nephritis (inflammation) or **nephropathy** (disease) **with lesion of membranoproliferative glomerulonephritis** is characterized by alterations in the basement membranes of the kidney and the glomerular cells.

   Nephritis (inflammation) or **nephropathy** (disease) **with lesion of rapidly progressive glomerulonephritis** is characterized by rapid and progressive decline in renal function.

   Nephritis (inflammation) or **nephropathy** (disease) **with lesion of renal cortical necrosis** is characterized by death of the cortical tissues.

   Nephritis (inflammation) or **nephropathy** (disease) **with lesion of renal medullary necrosis** is characterized by death of the tissues that collect urine.

Figure 14-1   Kidneys within the urinary system.

Item 14–2 Glomerulonephritis is nephritis accompanied by inflammation of the glomeruli of the kidney, resulting in the degeneration of the glomeruli and the nephrons.

   Acute glomerulonephritis primarily affects children and young adults and is usually a result of a streptococcal infection.

   Proliferative glomerulonephritis is the acute form of the disease resulting from a streptococcal infection.

   Rapidly progressive glomerulonephritis, also known as **crescentic** or **malignant glomerulonephritis**, is the acute form of the disease, which leads quickly to rapid and progressive decline in renal function.

CHAPTER 14

DISEASES OF THE GENITOURINARY SYSTEM (N00-N99)

Excludes2	certain conditions originating in the perinatal period (P04-P96)
	certain infectious and parasitic diseases (A00-B99)
	complications of pregnancy, childbirth and the puerperium (O00-O9A)
	congenital malformations, deformations and chromosomal abnormalities (Q00-Q99)
	endocrine, nutritional and metabolic diseases (E00-E88)
	injury, poisoning and certain other consequences of external causes (S00-T88)
	neoplasms (C00-D49)
	symptoms, signs and abnormal clinical and laboratory findings, not elsewhere classified (R00-R94)

This chapter contains the following blocks:

N00-N08	Glomerular diseases
N10-N16	Renal tubulo-interstitial diseases
N17-N19	Acute kidney failure and chronic kidney disease
N20-N23	Urolithiasis
N25-N29	Other disorders of kidney and ureter
N30-N39	Other diseases of the urinary system
N40-N53	Diseases of male genital organs
N60-N65	Disorders of breast
N70-N77	Inflammatory diseases of female pelvic organs
N80-N98	Noninflammatory disorders of female genital tract
N99	Intraoperative and postprocedural complications and disorders of genitourinary system, not elsewhere classified

GLOMERULAR DISEASES (N00-N08)

Code also any associated kidney failure (N17-N19)

Excludes1	hypertensive chronic kidney disease (I12.-)

● **N00**   **Acute nephritic syndrome**

Includes	acute glomerular disease
	acute glomerulonephritis
	acute nephritis

Excludes1	acute tubulo-interstitial nephritis (N10)
	nephritic syndrome NOS (N05.-)

   N00.0   **Acute nephritic syndrome with minor glomerular abnormality**
       Acute nephritic syndrome with minimal change lesion

   N00.1   **Acute nephritic syndrome with focal and segmental glomerular lesions**
       Acute nephritic syndrome with focal and segmental hyalinosis
       Acute nephritic syndrome with focal and segmental sclerosis
       Acute nephritic syndrome with focal glomerulonephritis

   N00.2   **Acute nephritic syndrome with diffuse membranous glomerulonephritis**

   N00.3   **Acute nephritic syndrome with diffuse mesangial proliferative glomerulonephritis**

   N00.4   **Acute nephritic syndrome with diffuse endocapillary proliferative glomerulonephritis**

   N00.5   **Acute nephritic syndrome with diffuse mesangiocapillary glomerulonephritis**
       Acute nephritic syndrome with membranoproliferative glomerulonephritis, types 1 and 3, or NOS

   N00.6   **Acute nephritic syndrome with dense deposit disease**
       Acute nephritic syndrome with membranoproliferative glomerulonephritis, type 2

   N00.7   **Acute nephritic syndrome with diffuse crescentic glomerulonephritis**
       Acute nephritic syndrome with extracapillary glomerulonephritis

   N00.8   **Acute nephritic syndrome with other morphologic changes**
       Acute nephritic syndrome with proliferative glomerulonephritis NOS

   N00.9   **Acute nephritic syndrome with unspecified morphologic changes**

◀ New   ◀⁞⁞⁞ Revised   ~~deleted~~ Deleted   **OGCR** Official Guidelines   X Assign placeholder X   ● Use Additional Character(s)

Excludes 1   Excludes 2   Includes   Use additional   Code first   Code also   Unspecified

1111

CHAPTER 14 (N00-N99)

● **N01   Rapidly progressive nephritic syndrome**

> **Includes**   rapidly progressive glomerular disease
> rapidly progressive glomerulonephritis
> rapidly progressive nephritis

> **Excludes1**   nephritic syndrome NOS (N05.-)

N01.0   Rapidly progressive nephritic syndrome with minor glomerular abnormality
> Rapidly progressive nephritic syndrome with minimal change lesion

N01.1   Rapidly progressive nephritic syndrome with focal and segmental glomerular lesions
> Rapidly progressive nephritic syndrome with focal and segmental hyalinosis
> Rapidly progressive nephritic syndrome with focal and segmental sclerosis
> Rapidly progressive nephritic syndrome with focal glomerulonephritis

N01.2   Rapidly progressive nephritic syndrome with diffuse membranous glomerulonephritis

N01.3   Rapidly progressive nephritic syndrome with diffuse mesangial proliferative glomerulonephritis

N01.4   Rapidly progressive nephritic syndrome with diffuse endocapillary proliferative glomerulonephritis

N01.5   Rapidly progressive nephritic syndrome with diffuse mesangiocapillary glomerulonephritis
> Rapidly progressive nephritic syndrome with membranoproliferative glomerulonephritis, types 1 and 3, or NOS

N01.6   Rapidly progressive nephritic syndrome with dense deposit disease
> Rapidly progressive nephritic syndrome with membranoproliferative glomerulonephritis, type 2

N01.7   Rapidly progressive nephritic syndrome with diffuse crescentic glomerulonephritis
> Rapidly progressive nephritic syndrome with extracapillary glomerulonephritis

N01.8   Rapidly progressive nephritic syndrome with other morphologic changes
> Rapidly progressive nephritic syndrome with proliferative glomerulonephritis NOS

N01.9   Rapidly progressive nephritic syndrome with unspecified morphologic changes

● **N02   Recurrent and persistent hematuria**

> **Excludes1**   acute cystitis with hematuria (N30.01)
> hematuria NOS (R31.9)
> hematuria not associated with specified morphologic lesions (R31.-)

N02.0   Recurrent and persistent hematuria with minor glomerular abnormality
> Recurrent and persistent hematuria with minimal change lesion

N02.1   Recurrent and persistent hematuria with focal and segmental glomerular lesions
> Recurrent and persistent hematuria with focal and segmental hyalinosis
> Recurrent and persistent hematuria with focal and segmental sclerosis
> Recurrent and persistent hematuria with focal glomerulonephritis

N02.2   Recurrent and persistent hematuria with diffuse membranous glomerulonephritis

N02.3   Recurrent and persistent hematuria with diffuse mesangial proliferative glomerulonephritis

N02.4   Recurrent and persistent hematuria with diffuse endocapillary proliferative glomerulonephritis

N02.5   Recurrent and persistent hematuria with diffuse mesangiocapillary glomerulonephritis
> Recurrent and persistent hematuria with membranoproliferative glomerulonephritis, types 1 and 3, or NOS

Item 14–3 Chronic glomerulonephritis (GN) persists over a period of years, with remissions and exacerbation.

Chronic GN with lesion of proliferative glomerulonephritis results from a streptococcal infection.

Chronic GN with lesion of membranous glomerulonephritis, also known as membranous nephropathy, is characterized by deposits along the epithelial side of the basement membrane.

Chronic GN with lesion of membrano-proliferative glomerulonephritis (MPGN) is a group of disorders characterized by alterations in the basement membranes of the kidney and the glomerular cells.

Chronic GN with lesion of rapidly progressive glomerulonephritis is characterized by necrosis, endothelial proliferation, and mesangial proliferation. The condition is marked by rapid and progressive decline in renal function.

N02.6   Recurrent and persistent hematuria with dense deposit disease
> Recurrent and persistent hematuria with membranoproliferative glomerulonephritis, type 2

N02.7   Recurrent and persistent hematuria with diffuse crescentic glomerulonephritis
> Recurrent and persistent hematuria with extracapillary glomerulonephritis

N02.8   Recurrent and persistent hematuria with other morphologic changes
> Recurrent and persistent hematuria with proliferative glomerulonephritis NOS

N02.9   Recurrent and persistent hematuria with unspecified morphologic changes

● **N03   Chronic nephritic syndrome**

> **Includes**   chronic glomerular disease
> chronic glomerulonephritis
> chronic nephritis

> **Excludes1**   chronic tubulo-interstitial nephritis (N11.-)
> diffuse sclerosing glomeruloncephritis (N05.8-)
> nephritic syndrome NOS (N05.-)

N03.0   Chronic nephritic syndrome with minor glomerular abnormality
> Chronic nephritic syndrome with minimal change lesion

N03.1   Chronic nephritic syndrome with focal and segmental glomerular lesions
> Chronic nephritic syndrome with focal and segmental hyalinosis
> Chronic nephritic syndrome with focal and segmental sclerosis
> Chronic nephritic syndrome with focal glomerulonephritis

N03.2   Chronic nephritic syndrome with diffuse membranous glomerulonephritis

N03.3   Chronic nephritic syndrome with diffuse mesangial proliferative glomerulonephritis

N03.4   Chronic nephritic syndrome with diffuse endocapillary proliferative glomerulonephritis

N03.5   Chronic nephritic syndrome with diffuse mesangiocapillary glomerulonephritis
> Chronic nephritic syndrome with membranoproliferative glomerulonephritis, types 1 and 3, or NOS

N03.6   Chronic nephritic syndrome with dense deposit disease
> Chronic nephritic syndrome with membranoproliferative glomerulonephritis, type 2

N03.7   Chronic nephritic syndrome with diffuse crescentic glomerulonephritis
> Chronic nephritic syndrome with extracapillary glomerulonephritis

N03.8   Chronic nephritic syndrome with other morphologic changes
> Chronic nephritic syndrome with proliferative glomerulonephritis NOS

N03.9   Chronic nephritic syndrome with unspecified morphologic changes

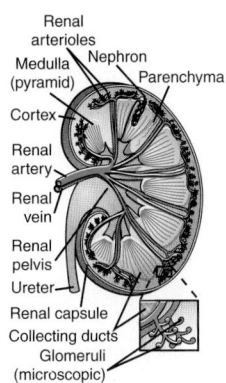

Renal
arterioles
Medulla   Nephron
(pyramid)   Parenchyma
Cortex
Renal
artery
Renal
vein
Renal
pelvis
Ureter
Renal capsule
Collecting ducts
Glomeruli
(microscopic)

Figure 14-2   Kidney cross section.

Item 14–4 Nephrotic syndrome (NS) is marked by massive proteinuria (protein in the urine) and water retention. Patients with NS are particularly vulnerable to staphylococcal and pneumococcal infections. NS with lesion of proliferative glomerulonephritis results from a streptococcal infection. NS with lesion of membranous glomerulonephritis results in thickening of the capillary walls. NS with lesion of minimal change glomerulonephritis is usually a benign disorder that occurs mostly in children and requires electron microscopy (biopsy) to verify changes in the glomeruli.

● **N04   Nephrotic syndrome**

     Includes   congenital nephrotic syndrome
                      lipoid nephrosis

   N04.0   **Nephrotic syndrome with minor glomerular abnormality**
          Nephrotic syndrome with minimal change lesion

   N04.1   **Nephrotic syndrome with focal and segmental glomerular lesions**
          Nephrotic syndrome with focal and segmental hyalinosis
          Nephrotic syndrome with focal and segmental sclerosis
          Nephrotic syndrome with focal glomerulonephritis

   N04.2   **Nephrotic syndrome with diffuse membranous glomerulonephritis**

   N04.3   **Nephrotic syndrome with diffuse mesangial proliferative glomerulonephritis**

   N04.4   **Nephrotic syndrome with diffuse endocapillary proliferative glomerulonephritis**

   N04.5   **Nephrotic syndrome with diffuse mesangiocapillary glomerulonephritis**
          Nephrotic syndrome with membranoproliferative glomerulonephritis, types 1 and 3, or NOS

   N04.6   **Nephrotic syndrome with dense deposit disease**
          Nephrotic syndrome with membranoproliferative glomerulonephritis, type 2

   N04.7   **Nephrotic syndrome with diffuse crescentic glomerulonephritis**
          Nephrotic syndrome with extracapillary glomerulonephritis

   N04.8   **Nephrotic syndrome with other morphologic changes**
          Nephrotic syndrome with proliferative glomerulonephritis NOS

   N04.9   **Nephrotic syndrome with unspecified morphologic changes**

● **N05   Unspecified nephritic syndrome**

     Includes   glomerular disease NOS
                      glomerulonephritis NOS
                      nephritis NOS
                      nephropathy NOS and renal disease NOS with morphological lesion specified in .0-.8

     Excludes1   nephropathy NOS with no stated morphological lesion (N28.9)
                      renal disease NOS with no stated morphological lesion (N28.9)
                      tubulo-interstitial nephritis NOS (N12)

   N05.0   **Unspecified nephritic syndrome with minor glomerular abnormality**
          Unspecified nephritic syndrome with minimal change lesion

   N05.1   **Unspecified nephritic syndrome with focal and segmental glomerular lesions**
          Unspecified nephritic syndrome with focal and segmental hyalinosis
          Unspecified nephritic syndrome with focal and segmental sclerosis
          Unspecified nephritic syndrome with focal glomerulonephritis

   N05.2   **Unspecified nephritic syndrome with diffuse membranous glomerulonephritis**

   N05.3   **Unspecified nephritic syndrome with diffuse mesangial proliferative glomerulonephritis**

   N05.4   **Unspecified nephritic syndrome with diffuse endocapillary proliferative glomerulonephritis**

   N05.5   **Unspecified nephritic syndrome with diffuse mesangiocapillary glomerulonephritis**
          Unspecified nephritic syndrome with membranoproliferative glomerulonephritis, types 1 and 3, or NOS

   N05.6   **Unspecified nephritic syndrome with dense deposit disease**
          Unspecified nephritic syndrome with membranoproliferative glomerulonephritis, type 2

   N05.7   **Unspecified nephritic syndrome with diffuse crescentic glomerulonephritis**
          Unspecified nephritic syndrome with extracapillary glomerulonephritis

   N05.8   **Unspecified nephritic syndrome with other morphologic changes**
          Unspecified nephritic syndrome with proliferative glomerulonephritis NOS

   N05.9   **Unspecified nephritic syndrome with unspecified morphologic changes**

● **N06   Isolated proteinuria with specified morphological lesion**

     Excludes1   proteinuria not associated with specific morphologic lesions (R80.0)

   N06.0   **Isolated proteinuria with minor glomerular abnormality**
          Isolated proteinuria with minimal change lesion

   N06.1   **Isolated proteinuria with focal and segmental glomerular lesions**
          Isolated proteinuria with focal and segmental hyalinosis
          Isolated proteinuria with focal and segmental sclerosis
          Isolated proteinuria with focal glomerulonephritis

   N06.2   **Isolated proteinuria with diffuse membranous glomerulonephritis**

   N06.3   **Isolated proteinuria with diffuse mesangial proliferative glomerulonephritis**

CHAPTER 14 (N00-N99)

◀ New   ◀▦ Revised   ~~deleted~~ Deleted   OGCR Official Guidelines   X Assign placeholder X   ● Use Additional Character(s)

Excludes 1   Excludes 2   Includes   Use additional   Code first   Code also   Unspecified

N06.4   Isolated proteinuria with diffuse endocapillary proliferative glomerulonephritis

N06.5   Isolated proteinuria with diffuse mesangiocapillary glomerulonephritis

Isolated proteinuria with membranoproliferative glomerulonephritis, types 1 and 3, or NOS

N06.6   Isolated proteinuria with dense deposit disease

Isolated proteinuria with membranoproliferative glomerulonephritis, type 2

N06.7   Isolated proteinuria with diffuse crescentic glomerulonephritis

Isolated proteinuria with extracapillary glomerulonephritis

N06.8   Isolated proteinuria with other morphologic lesion

Isolated proteinuria with proliferative glomerulonephritis NOS

N06.9   Isolated proteinuria with unspecified morphologic lesion

● **N07   Hereditary nephropathy, not elsewhere classified**

> **Excludes2**   Alport's syndrome (Q87.81-)
> hereditary amyloid nephropathy (E85.-)
> nail patella syndrome (Q87.2)
> non-neuropathic heredofamilial amyloidosis (E85.-)

N07.0   Hereditary nephropathy, not elsewhere classified with minor glomerular abnormality

Hereditary nephropathy, not elsewhere classified with minimal change lesion

N07.1   Hereditary nephropathy, not elsewhere classified with focal and segmental glomerular lesions

Hereditary nephropathy, not elsewhere classified with focal and segmental hyalinosis
Hereditary nephropathy, not elsewhere classified with focal and segmental sclerosis
Hereditary nephropathy, not elsewhere classified with focal glomeruloncphritis

N07.2   Hereditary nephropathy, not elsewhere classified with diffuse membranous glomerulonephritis

N07.3   Hereditary nephropathy, not elsewhere classified with diffuse mesangial proliferative glomerulonephritis

N07.4   Hereditary nephropathy, not elsewhere classified with diffuse endocapillary proliferative glomerulonephritis

N07.5   Hereditary nephropathy, not elsewhere classified with diffuse mesangiocapillary glomerulonephritis

Hereditary nephropathy, not elsewhere classified with membranoproliferative glomerulonephritis, types 1 and 3, or NOS

N07.6   Hereditary nephropathy, not elsewhere classified with dense deposit disease

Hereditary nephropathy, not elsewhere classified with membranoproliferative glomerulonephritis, type 2

N07.7   Hereditary nephropathy, not elsewhere classified with diffuse crescentic glomerulonephritis

Hereditary nephropathy, not elsewhere classified with extracapillary glomerulonephritis

N07.8   Hereditary nephropathy, not elsewhere classified with other morphologic lesions

Hereditary nephropathy, not elsewhere classified with proliferative glomerulonephritis NOS

N07.9   Hereditary nephropathy, not elsewhere classified with unspecified morphologic lesions

N08   Glomerular disorders in diseases classified elsewhere

Glomerulonephritis
Nephritis
Nephropathy

Code first underlying disease, such as:
amyloidosis (E85.-)
congenital syphilis (A50.5)
cryoglobulinemia (D89.1)
disseminated intravascular coagulation (D65)
gout (M1A.-, M10.-)
microscopic polyangiitis (M31.7)
multiple myeloma (C90.0-)
sepsis (A40.0-A41.9)
sickle-cell disease (D57.0-D57.8)

> **Excludes1**   glomerulonephritis, nephritis and nephropathy (in):
> antiglomerular basement membrane disease (M31.0)
> diabetes (E08-E13 with .21)
> gonococcal (A54.21)
> Goodpasture's syndrome (M31.0)
> hemolytic-uremic syndrome (D59.3)
> lupus (M32.14)
> mumps (B26.83)
> syphilis (A52.75)
> systemic lupus erythematosus (M32.14)
> Wegener's granulomatosis (M31.31)
> pyelonephritis in diseases classified elsewhere (N16)
> renal tubulo-interstitial disorders classified elsewhere (N16)

RENAL TUBULO-INTERSTITIAL DISEASES (N10-N16)

> **Includes**   pyelonephritis
> **Excludes1**   pyeloureteritis cystica (N28.85)

N10   Acute tubulo-interstitial ncphritis

Acute infectious interstitial nephritis
Acute pyelitis
Acute pyelonephritis
Hemoglobin nephrosis
Myoglobin nephrosis

Use additional code (B95-B97), to identify infectious agent

● **N11   Chronic tubulo-interstitial nephritis**

> **Includes**   chronic infectious interstitial nephritis
> chronic pyelitis
> chronic pyelonephritis

Use additional code (B95-B97), to identify infectious agent

N11.0   Nonobstructive reflux-associated chronic pyelonephritis

Pyelonephritis (chronic) associated with (vesicoureteral) reflux

> **Excludes1**   vesicoureteral reflux NOS (N13.70)

N11.1   Chronic obstructive pyelonephritis

Pyelonephritis (chronic) associated with anomaly of pelviureteric junction
Pyelonephritis (chronic) associated with anomaly of pyeloureteric junction
Pyelonephritis (chronic) associated with crossing of vessel
Pyelonephritis (chronic) associated with kinking of ureter
Pyelonephritis (chronic) associated with obstruction of ureter
Pyelonephritis (chronic) associated with stricture of pelviureteric junction
Pyelonephritis (chronic) associated with stricture of ureter

> **Excludes1**   calculous pyelonephritis (N20.9)
> obstructive uropathy (N13.-)

CHAPTER 14 (N00-N99)

Figure 14-3 Acute pyelonephritis. Cortical surface exhibits grayish white areas of inflammation and abscess formation. (From Kumar: Robbins and Cotran: Pathologic Basis of Disease, ed 8, Saunders, An Imprint of Elsevier, 2009)

Figure 14-4 Hydronephrosis of the kidney, with marked dilatation of pelvis and calyces and thinning of renal parenchyma. (From Kumar: Robbins and Cotran: Pathologic Basis of Disease, ed 8, Saunders, An Imprint of Elsevier, 2009)

Item 14–5 Pyelonephritis is an infection of the kidneys and ureters and may be chronic or acute in one or both kidneys.

N11.8 Other chronic tubulo-interstitial nephritis
  Nonobstructive chronic pyelonephritis NOS

N11.9 Chronic tubulo-interstitial nephritis, unspecified
  Chronic interstitial nephritis NOS
  Chronic pyelitis NOS
  Chronic pyelonephritis NOS

N12 Tubulo-interstitial nephritis, not specified as acute or chronic
  Interstitial nephritis NOS
  Pyelitis NOS
  Pyelonephritis NOS
  Excludes1 calculous pyelonephritis (N20.9)

●**N13 Obstructive and reflux uropathy**
  Excludes2 calculus of kidney and ureter without
    hydronephrosis (N20.-)
  congenital obstructive defects of renal pelvis and
    ureter (Q62.0-Q62.3)
  hydronephrosis with ureteropelvic junction
    obstruction (Q62.1)
  obstructive pyelonephritis (N11.1)

N13.1 Hydronephrosis with ureteral stricture, not elsewhere classified
  Excludes1 hydronephrosis with ureteral stricture
    with infection (N13.6)

N13.2 Hydronephrosis with renal and ureteral calculous obstruction
  Excludes1 hydronephrosis with renal and ureteral
    calculous obstruction with infection
    (N13.6)

●**N13.3 Other and unspecified hydronephrosis**
  Excludes1 hydronephrosis with infection (N13.6)
  N13.30 Unspecified hydronephrosis
  N13.39 Other hydronephrosis

N13.4 Hydroureter
  Excludes1 congenital hydroureter (Q62.3-)
    hydroureter with infection (N13.6)
    vesicoureteral-reflux with hydroureter
    (N13.73-)

N13.5 Crossing vessel and stricture of ureter without hydronephrosis
  Kinking and stricture of ureter without hydronephrosis
  Excludes1 crossing vessel and stricture of ureter
    without hydronephrosis with
    infection (N13.6)

N13.6 Pyonephrosis
  Conditions in N13.1-N13.5 with infection
  Obstructive uropathy with infection
  Use additional code (B95-B97), to identify infectious
    agent

●**N13.7 Vesicoureteral-reflux**
  Excludes1 reflux-associated pyelonephritis (N11.0)
  N13.70 Vesicoureteral-reflux, unspecified
    Occurs when urine flows from bladder back into
    ureters
    Vesicoureteral-reflux NOS
  N13.71 Vesicoureteral-reflux without reflux nephropathy
  ●**N13.72 Vesicoureteral-reflux with reflux nephropathy without hydroureter**
    N13.721 Vesicoureteral-reflux with reflux nephropathy without hydroureter, unilateral
    N13.722 Vesicoureteral-reflux with reflux nephropathy without hydroureter, bilateral
    N13.729 Vesicoureteral-reflux with reflux nephropathy without hydroureter, unspecified
  ●**N13.73 Vesicoureteral-reflux with reflux nephropathy with hydroureter**
    N13.731 Vesicoureteral-reflux with reflux nephropathy with hydroureter, unilateral
    N13.732 Vesicoureteral-reflux with reflux nephropathy with hydroureter, bilateral
    N13.739 Vesicoureteral-reflux with reflux nephropathy with hydroureter, unspecified

N13.8 Other obstructive and reflux uropathy
  Urinary tract obstruction due to specified cause
  Code first, if applicable, any causal condition first, such as:
    enlarged prostate (N40.1)

N13.9 Obstructive and reflux uropathy, unspecified
  Urinary tract obstruction NOS

●**N14 Drug- and heavy-metal-induced tubulo-interstitial and tubular conditions**
  Code first poisoning due to drug or toxin, if applicable (T36-T65 with
    fifth or sixth character 1-4 or 6)
  Use additional code for adverse effect, if applicable, to identify
    drug (T36-T50 with fifth or sixth character 5)

N14.0 Analgesic nephropathy

N14.1 Nephropathy induced by other drugs, medicaments and biological substances

N14.2 Nephropathy induced by unspecified drug, medicament or biological substance

N14.3 Nephropathy induced by heavy metals

N14.4 Toxic nephropathy, not elsewhere classified

●**N15 Other renal tubulo-interstitial diseases**

N15.0 Balkan nephropathy
  Balkan endemic nephropathy

N15.1 Renal and perinephric abscess

N15.8 Other specified renal tubulo-interstitial diseases

N15.9 Renal tubulo-interstitial disease, unspecified
  Infection of kidney NOS
  Excludes1 urinary tract infection NOS (N39.0)

Item 14–6 Decreased blood flow is the usual cause of **acute renal failure** that offers a good prognosis for recovery.

   Chronic renal failure is usually the result of long-standing kidney disease and is a very serious condition that generally results in death.

N16   Renal tubulo-interstitial disorders in diseases classified elsewhere

Pyelonephritis
Tubulo-interstitial nephritis

Code first underlying disease, such as:
brucellosis (A23.0-A23.9)
cryoglobulinemia (D89.1)
glycogen storage disease (E74.0)
leukemia (C91-C95)
lymphoma (C81.0-C85.9, C96.0-C96.9)
multiple myeloma (C90.0-)
sepsis (A40.0-A41.9)
Wilson's disease (E83.0)

Excludes1   diphtheritic pyelonephritis and tubulo-interstitial nephritis (A36.84)
pyelonephritis and tubulo-interstitial nephritis in candidiasis (B37.49)
pyelonephritis and tubulo-interstitial nephritis in cystinosis (E72.04)
pyelonephritis and tubulo-interstitial nephritis in salmonella infection (A02.25)
pyelonephritis and tubulo-interstitial nephritis in sarcoidosis (D86.84)
pyelonephritis and tubulo-interstitial nephritis in sicca syndrome [Sjogren's] (M35.04)
pyelonephritis and tubulo-interstitial nephritis in systemic lupus erythematosus (M32.15)
pyelonephritis and tubulo-interstitial nephritis in toxoplasmosis (B58.83)
renal tubular degeneration in diabetes (E08-E13 with .29)
syphilitic pyelonephritis and tubulo-interstitial nephritis (A52.75)

ACUTE KIDNEY FAILURE AND CHRONIC KIDNEY DISEASE (N17-N19)

Excludes2   congenital renal failure (P96.0)
drug- and heavy-metal-induced tubulo-interstitial and tubular conditions (N14.-)
extrarenal uremia (R39.2)
hemolytic-uremic syndrome (D59.3)
hepatorenal syndrome (K76.7)
postpartum hepatorenal syndrome (O90.4)
posttraumatic renal failure (T79.5)
prerenal uremia (R39.2)
renal failure complicating abortion or ectopic or molar pregnancy (O00-O07, O08.4)
renal failure following labor and delivery (O90.4)
renal failure postprocedural (N99.0)

● N17   Acute kidney failure

Code also associated underlying condition

Excludes1   posttraumatic renal failure (T79.5)

N17.0   Acute kidney failure with tubular necrosis
Acute tubular necrosis
Renal tubular necrosis
Tubular necrosis NOS

N17.1   Acute kidney failure with acute cortical necrosis
Acute cortical necrosis
Cortical necrosis NOS
Renal cortical necrosis

N17.2   Acute kidney failure with medullary necrosis
Medullary [papillary] necrosis NOS
Acute medullary [papillary] necrosis
Renal medullary [papillary] necrosis

N17.8   Other acute kidney failure

N17.9   Acute kidney failure, unspecified
Acute kidney injury (nontraumatic)

Excludes2   traumatic kidney injury (S37.0-)

● N18   Chronic kidney disease (CKD)

Code first any associated:
diabetic chronic kidney disease (E08.22, E09.22, E10.22, E11.22, E13.22)
hypertensive chronic kidney disease (I12.-, I13.-)

Use additional code to identify kidney transplant status, if applicable, (Z94.0)

N18.1   Chronic kidney disease, stage 1
N18.2   Chronic kidney disease, stage 2 (mild)
N18.3   Chronic kidney disease, stage 3 (moderate)
N18.4   Chronic kidney disease, stage 4 (severe)
N18.5   Chronic kidney disease, stage 5

Excludes1   chronic kidney disease, stage 5 requiring chronic dialysis (N18.6)

N18.6   End stage renal disease
Chronic kidney disease requiring chronic dialysis

Use additional code to identify dialysis status (Z99.2)

N18.9   Chronic kidney disease, unspecified
Chronic renal disease
Chronic renal failure NOS
Chronic renal insufficiency
Chronic uremia

N19   Unspecified kidney failure

Uremia NOS

Excludes1   acute kidney failure (N17.-)
chronic kidney disease (N18.-)
chronic uremia (N18.9)
extrarenal uremia (R39.2)
prerenal uremia (R39.2)
renal insufficiency (acute) (N28.9)
uremia of newborn (P96.0)

UROLITHIASIS (N20-N23)

● N20   Calculus of kidney and ureter

Calculous pyelonephritis

Excludes1   nephrocalcinosis (E83.5)
that with hydronephrosis (N13.2)

N20.0   Calculus of kidney
Nephrolithiasis NOS   Staghorn calculus
Renal calculus   Stone in kidney
Renal stone

N20.1   Calculus of ureter
Ureteric stone

N20.2   Calculus of kidney with calculus of ureter

N20.9   Urinary calculus, unspecified

● N21   Calculus of lower urinary tract

Includes   calculus of lower urinary tract with cystitis and urethritis

N21.0   Calculus in bladder
Calculus in diverticulum of bladder
Urinary bladder stone

Excludes2   staghorn calculus (N20.0)

N21.1   Calculus in urethra

Excludes2   calculus of prostate (N42.0)

N21.8   Other lower urinary tract calculus

N21.9   Calculus of lower urinary tract, unspecified

Excludes1   calculus of urinary tract NOS (N20.9)

N22   Calculus of urinary tract in diseases classified elsewhere

Code first underlying disease, such as:
gout (M1A.-, M10.-)
schistosomiasis (B65.0-B65.9)

N23   Unspecified renal colic

◄ New   ◄ Revised   deleted Deleted   OGCR Official Guidelines   X Assign placeholder X   ● Use Additional Character(s)

Excludes 1   Excludes 2   Includes   Use additional   Code first   Code also   Unspecified

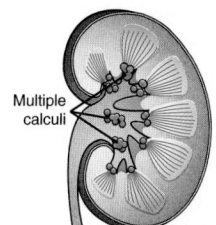

Figure 14-5 Multiple urinary calculi.

Multiple calculi

OTHER DISORDERS OF KIDNEY AND URETER (N25-N29)

Excludes2 disorders of kidney and ureter with urolithiasis (N20-N23)

● N25 **Disorders resulting from impaired renal tubular function**
    Excludes1 metabolic disorders classifiable to E70-E88
    N25.0 **Renal osteodystrophy**
        Azotemic osteodystrophy
        Phosphate-losing tubular disorders
        Renal rickets
        Renal short stature
    N25.1 **Nephrogenic diabetes insipidus**
        Excludes1 diabetes insipidus NOS (E23.2)
    ● N25.8 **Other disorders resulting from impaired renal tubular function**
        N25.81 **Secondary hyperparathyroidism of renal origin**
            Excludes1 secondary hyperparathyroidism, non-renal (E21.1)
        N25.89 **Other disorders resulting from impaired renal tubular function**
            Hypokalemic nephropathy
            Lightwood-Albright syndrome
            Renal tubular acidosis NOS
    N25.9 **Disorder resulting from impaired renal tubular function, unspecified**

● N26 **Unspecified contracted kidney**
    Excludes1 contracted kidney due to hypertension (I12.-)
        diffuse sclerosing glomerulonephritis (N05.8.-)
        hypertensive nephrosclerosis (arteriolar) (arteriosclerotic) (I12.-)
        small kidney of unknown cause (N27.-)
    N26.1 **Atrophy of kidney (terminal)**
    N26.2 **Page kidney**
    N26.9 **Renal sclerosis, unspecified**

● N27 **Small kidney of unknown cause**
    Includes oligonephronia
    N27.0 **Small kidney, unilateral**
    N27.1 **Small kidney, bilateral**
    N27.9 **Small kidney, unspecified**

● N28 **Other disorders of kidney and ureter, not elsewhere classified**
    N28.0 **Ischemia and infarction of kidney**
        Renal artery embolism
        Renal artery obstruction
        Renal artery occlusion
        Renal artery thrombosis
        Renal infarct
        Excludes1 atherosclerosis of renal artery (extrarenal part) (I70.1)
            congenital stenosis of renal artery (Q27.1)
            Goldblatt's kidney (I70.1)
    N28.1 **Cyst of kidney, acquired**
        Cyst (multiple)(solitary) of kidney, acquired
        Excludes1 cystic kidney disease (congenital) (Q61.-)

● N28.8 **Other specified disorders of kidney and ureter**
        Excludes1 hydroureter (N13.4)
            ureteric stricture with hydronephrosis (N13.1)
            ureteric stricture without hydronephrosis (N13.5)
    N28.81 **Hypertrophy of kidney**
    N28.82 **Megaloureter**
    N28.83 **Nephroptosis**
    N28.84 **Pyelitis cystica**
    N28.85 **Pyeloureteritis cystica**
    N28.86 **Ureteritis cystica**
    N28.89 **Other specified disorders of kidney and ureter**
    N28.9 **Disorder of kidney and ureter, unspecified**
        Nephropathy NOS
        Renal disease (acute) NOS
        Renal insufficiency (acute)
        Excludes1 chronic renal insufficiency (N18.9)
            unspecified nephritic syndrome (N05.-)

N29 **Other disorders of kidney and ureter in diseases classified elsewhere**
    Code first underlying disease, such as:
        amyloidosis (E85.-)
        nephrocalcinosis (E83.5)
        schistosomiasis (B65.0-B65.9)
    Excludes1 disorders of kidney and ureter in:
        cystinosis (E72.0)
        gonorrhea (A54.21)
        syphilis (A52.75)
        tuberculosis (A18.11)

OTHER DISEASES OF THE URINARY SYSTEM (N30-N39)

Excludes1 urinary infection (complicating):
    abortion or ectopic or molar pregnancy (O00-O07, O08.8)
    pregnancy, childbirth and the puerperium (O23.-, O75.3, O86.2-)

● N30 **Cystitis**
    Infection of bladder and irritation in lower urinary tract
    Use additional code to identify infectious agent (B95-B97)
    Excludes1 prostatocystitis (N41.3)
    ● N30.0 **Acute cystitis**
        Excludes1 irradiation cystitis (N30.4-)
            trigonitis (N30.3-)
        N30.00 **Acute cystitis without hematuria**
        N30.01 **Acute cystitis with hematuria**
    ● N30.1 **Interstitial cystitis (chronic)**
        Ongoing infection of kidney glomeruli and tubules
        N30.10 **Interstitial cystitis (chronic) without hematuria**
        N30.11 **Interstitial cystitis (chronic) with hematuria**
    ● N30.2 **Other chronic cystitis**
        N30.20 **Other chronic cystitis without hematuria**
        N30.21 **Other chronic cystitis with hematuria**
    ● N30.3 **Trigonitis**
        Inflammation of triangular area of bladder (where the ureters and urethra come together)
        Urethrotrigonitis
        N30.30 **Trigonitis without hematuria**
        N30.31 **Trigonitis with hematuria**
    ● N30.4 **Irradiation cystitis**
        N30.40 **Irradiation cystitis without hematuria**
        N30.41 **Irradiation cystitis with hematuria**
    ● N30.8 **Other cystitis**
        Abscess of bladder
        N30.80 **Other cystitis without hematuria**
        N30.81 **Other cystitis with hematuria**

CHAPTER 14 (N00-N99)

◀ New   ◀||||| Revised   ~~deleted~~ Deleted   OGCR Official Guidelines   X Assign placeholder X   ● Use Additional Character(s)
Excludes 1   Excludes 2   Includes   Use additional   Code first   Code also   Unspecified
1117

● **N30.9 Cystitis, unspecified**

    N30.90 Cystitis, unspecified without hematuria

    N30.91 Cystitis, unspecified with hematuria

● **N31 Neuromuscular dysfunction of bladder, not elsewhere classified**

    Use additional code to identify any associated urinary incontinence (N39.3-N39.4-)

    Excludes1 cord bladder NOS (G95.89)
        neurogenic bladder due to cauda equina syndrome (G83.4)
        neuromuscular dysfunction due to spinal cord lesion (G95.89)

    N31.0 Uninhibited neuropathic bladder, not elsewhere classified

    N31.1 Reflex neuropathic bladder, not elsewhere classified

    N31.2 Flaccid neuropathic bladder, not elsewhere classified
        Atonic (motor) (sensory) neuropathic bladder
        Diminished tone of bladder muscle
        Autonomous neuropathic bladder
        Nonreflex neuropathic bladder

    N31.8 Other neuromuscular dysfunction of bladder

    N31.9 Neuromuscular dysfunction of bladder, unspecified
        Neurogenic bladder dysfunction NOS

● **N32 Other disorders of bladder**

    Excludes2 calculus of bladder (N21.0)
        cystocele (N81.1-)
        hernia or prolapse of bladder, female (N81.1-)

    N32.0 Bladder-neck obstruction
        Bladder-neck stenosis (acquired)
        Excludes1 congenital bladder-neck obstruction (Q64.3-)

    N32.1 Vesicointestinal fistula
        Vesicorectal fistula

    N32.2 Vesical fistula, not elsewhere classified
        Excludes1 fistula between bladder and female genital tract (N82.0-N82.1)

    N32.3 Diverticulum of bladder
        Formation of sac from a herniation of wall of bladder
        Excludes1 congenital diverticulum of bladder (Q64.6)
        diverticulitis of bladder (N30.8-)

●   **N32.8 Other specified disorders of bladder**

        N32.81 Overactive bladder
            Detrusor muscle hyperactivity
            Excludes1 frequent urination due to specified bladder condition- code to condition

        N32.89 Other specified disorders of bladder
            Bladder hemorrhage
            Bladder hypertrophy
            Calcified bladder
            Contracted bladder

    N32.9 Bladder disorder, unspecified

   N33 Bladder disorders in diseases classified elsewhere

    Code first underlying disease, such as:
    schistosomiasis (B65.0-B65.9)

    Excludes1 bladder disorder in syphilis (A52.76)
        bladder disorder in tuberculosis (A18.12)
        candidal cystitis (B37.41)
        chlamydial cystitis(A56.01)
        cystitis in gonorrhea (A54.01)
        cystitis in neurogenic bladder (N31.-)
        diphtheritic cystitis (A36.85)
        syphilitic cystitis (A52.76)
        trichomonal cystitis (A59.03)

● **N34 Urethritis and urethral syndrome**

    Use additional code (B95-B97), to identify infectious agent

    Excludes2 Reiter's disease (M02.3-)
        urethritis in diseases with a predominantly sexual mode of transmission (A50-A64)
        urethrotrigonitis (N30.3-)

    N34.0 Urethral abscess
        Abscess (of) Cowper's gland
        Abscess (of) Littré's gland
        Abscess (of) urethral (gland)
        Periurethral abscess
        Excludes1 urethral caruncle (N36.2)

    N34.1 Nonspecific urethritis
        Nongonococcal urethritis
        Nonvenereal urethritis

    N34.2 Other urethritis
        Inflammation of urethra
        Meatitis, urethral
        Postmenopausal urethritis
        Ulcer of urethra (meatus)
        Urethritis NOS

    N34.3 Urethral syndrome, unspecified

● **N35 Urethral stricture**

    Narrowing of lumen of urethra caused by scarring due to infection or injury

    Excludes1 congenital urethral stricture (Q64.3-)
        postprocedural urethral stricture (N99.1-)

●   **N35.0 Post-traumatic urethral stricture**
    Urethral stricture due to injury

    Excludes1 postprocedural urethral stricture (N99.1-)

   ● **N35.01 Post-traumatic urethral stricture, male**
        N35.010 Post-traumatic urethral stricture, male, meatal
        N35.011 Post-traumatic bulbous urethral stricture
        N35.012 Post-traumatic membranous urethral stricture
        N35.013 Post-traumatic anterior urethral stricture
        N35.014 Post-traumatic urethral stricture, male, unspecified

   ● **N35.02 Post-traumatic urethral stricture, female**
        N35.021 Urethral stricture due to childbirth
        N35.028 Other post-traumatic stricture, female

●   **N35.1 Postinfective urethral stricture, not elsewhere classified**

    Excludes1 urethral stricture associated with schistosomiasis (B65.-, N29)
        gonococcal urethral stricture (A54.01)
        syphilitic urethral stricture (A52.76)

   ● **N35.11 Postinfective urethral stricture, not elsewhere classified, male**
        N35.111 Postinfective urethral stricture, not elsewhere classified, male, meatal
        N35.112 Postinfective bulbous urethral stricture, not elsewhere classified
        N35.113 Postinfective membranous urethral stricture, not elsewhere classified
        N35.114 Postinfective anterior urethral stricture, not elsewhere classified
        N35.119 Postinfective urethral stricture, not elsewhere classified, male, unspecified

    N35.12 Postinfective urethral stricture, not elsewhere classified, female

    N35.8 Other urethral stricture
        Excludes1 postprocedural urethral stricture (N99.1-)

    N35.9 Urethral stricture, unspecified

◀ New ⬅ Revised ~~deleted~~ Deleted OGCR Official Guidelines X Assign placeholder X ● Use Additional Character(s)

Excludes 1 Excludes 2 Includes Use additional Code first Code also Unspecified

● **N36   Other disorders of urethra**

    N36.0   Urethral fistula
       Urethroperineal fistula
       Urethrorectal fistula
       Urinary fistula NOS
       | Excludes1 | urethroscrotal fistula (N50.8)
                      urethrovaginal fistula (N82.1)
                      urethrovesicovaginal fistula (N82.1)

    N36.1   Urethral diverticulum

    N36.2   Urethral caruncle

●   **N36.4   Urethral functional and muscular disorders**
       Use additional code to identify associated urinary stress
           incontinence (N39.3)

       N36.41   Hypermobility of urethra

       N36.42   Intrinsic sphincter deficiency (ISD)

       **N36.43   Combined hypermobility of urethra and
              intrinsic sphincter deficiency**

       N36.44   Muscular disorders of urethra
           Bladder sphincter dyssynergy

    N36.5   Urethral false passage

    N36.8   Other specified disorders of urethra

    N36.9   Urethral disorder, unspecified

N37   Urethral disorders in diseases classified elsewhere
      Code first underlying disease
      | Excludes1 | urethritis (in):
                   candidal infection (B37.41)
                   chlamydial (A56.01)
                   gonorrhea (A54.01)
                   syphilis (A52.76)
                   trichomonal infection (A59.03)
                   tuberculosis (A18.13)

● **N39   Other disorders of urinary system**
      | Excludes2 | hematuria NOS (R31.-)
                   recurrent or persistent hematuria (N02.-)
                   recurrent or persistent hematuria with specified
                       morphological lesion (N02.-)
                   proteinuria NOS (R80.-)

    N39.0   Urinary tract infection, site not specified
       Use additional code (B95-B97), to identify infectious
           agent
       | Excludes1 | candidiasis of urinary tract (B37.4-)
                   neonatal urinary tract infection (P39.3)
                   urinary tract infection of specified site,
                     such as:
                     cystitis (N30.-)
                     urethritis (N34.-)

    N39.3   Stress incontinence (female) (male)
       Code also any associated overactive bladder (N32.81)
       | Excludes1 | mixed incontinence (N39.46)

●   **N39.4   Other specified urinary incontinence**
       Code also any associated overactive bladder (N32.81)
       | Excludes1 | enuresis NOS (R32)
                   functional urinary incontinence (R39.81)
                   urinary incontinence associated with
                     cognitive impairment (R39.81)
                   urinary incontinence NOS (R32)
                   urinary incontinence of nonorganic origin
                     (F98.0)

       N39.41   Urge incontinence
           | Excludes1 | mixed incontinence (N39.46)

       N39.42   Incontinence without sensory awareness

       N39.43   Post-void dribbling

       N39.44   Nocturnal enuresis

       N39.45   Continuous leakage

       N39.46   Mixed incontinence
           Urge and stress incontinence

● **N39.49   Other specified urinary incontinence**

       N39.490   Overflow incontinence

       N39.498   Other specified urinary incontinence
           Reflex incontinence
           Total incontinence

    N39.8   Other specified disorders of urinary system

    N39.9   Disorder of urinary system, unspecified

DISEASES OF MALE GENITAL ORGANS (N40-N53)

(See Plate 387 on page NAP-5.)

● **N40   Enlarged prostate**
      | Includes | adenofibromatous hypertrophy of prostate
                 benign hypertrophy of the prostate
                 *Enlargement of prostate gland usually occurring
                     with age and causing obstructed urine flow*
                 benign prostatic hyperplasia
                 benign prostatic hypertrophy
                 BPH
                 nodular prostate
                 polyp of prostate
      | Excludes1 | benign neoplasms of prostate (adenoma, benign)
                 (fibroadenoma) (fibroma) (myoma) (D29.1)
                 malignant neoplasm of prostate (C61)

    N40.0   Enlarged prostate without lower urinary tract symptoms
       Enlarged prostate without LUTS
       Enlarged prostate NOS

    **N40.1   Enlarged prostate with lower urinary tract symptoms
        (LUTS)**
       Enlarged prostate with LUTS
       Use additional code for associated symptoms, when
           specified:
           incomplete bladder emptying (R39.14)
           nocturia (R35.1)
           straining on urination (R39.16)
           urinary frequency (R35.0)
           urinary hesitancy (R39.11)
           urinary incontinence (N39.4-)
           urinary obstruction (N13.8)
           urinary retention (R33.8)
           urinary urgency (R39.15)
           weak urinary stream (R39.12)

    N40.2   Nodular prostate without lower urinary tract symptoms
       Nodular prostate without LUTS

    N40.3   Nodular prostate with lower urinary tract symptoms
       Use additional code for associated symptoms, when
           specified:
           incomplete bladder emptying (R39.14)
           nocturia (R35.1)
           straining on urination (R39.16)
           urinary frequency (R35.0)
           urinary hesitancy (R39.11)
           urinary incontinence (N39.4-)
           urinary obstruction (N13.8)
           urinary retention (R33.8)
           urinary urgency (R39.15)
           weak urinary stream (R39.12)

● **N41   Inflammatory diseases of prostate**
      Use additional code (B95-B97), to identify infectious agent

    N41.0   Acute prostatitis

    N41.1   Chronic prostatitis

    N41.2   Abscess of prostate

    N41.3   Prostatocystitis

    N41.4   Granulomatous prostatitis

    N41.8   Other inflammatory diseases of prostate

    N41.9   Inflammatory disease of prostate, unspecified
       Prostatitis NOS

CHAPTER 14 (N00-N99)

Item 14-7 **Hydrocele** is a sac of fluid accumulating in the testes membrane.

Blood
vessels
Vas
deferens
Epididymis
Testis
A   Hydrocele   B

Figure 14-6 **A.** Hydrocele. **B.** Newborn with large right hydrocele. (**B** from Behrman: Nelson Textbook of Pediatrics, ed 18, Saunders, An Imprint of Elsevier, 2007)

● N42 **Other and unspecified disorders of prostate**

N42.0 **Calculus of prostate**
Prostatic stone

N42.1 **Congestion and hemorrhage of prostate**
Excludes1 enlarged prostate (N40.-)
hematuria (R31.-)
hyperplasia of prostate (N40.-)
inflammatory diseases of prostate (N41.-)

N42.3 **Dysplasia of prostate**
Prostatic intraepithelial neoplasia I (PIN I)
Prostatic intraepithelial neoplasia II (PIN II)
Excludes1 prostatic intraepithelial neoplasia III (PIN III) (D07.5)

● N42.8 **Other specified disorders of prostate**
N42.81 **Prostatodynia syndrome**
Painful prostate syndrome
N42.82 **Prostatosis syndrome**
N42.83 **Cyst of prostate**
N42.89 **Other specified disorders of prostate**

N42.9 **Disorder of prostate, unspecified**

● N43 **Hydrocele and spermatocele**
Includes hydrocele of spermatic cord, testis or tunica vaginalis
Excludes1 congenital hydrocele (P83.5)
N43.0 **Encysted hydrocele**
N43.1 **Infected hydrocele**
Use additional code (B95-B97), to identify infectious agent
N43.2 **Other hydrocele**
N43.3 **Hydrocele, unspecified**
● N43.4 **Spermatocele of epididymis**
Spermatic cyst
N43.40 **Spermatocele of epididymis, unspecified**
N43.41 **Spermatocele of epididymis, single**
N43.42 **Spermatocele of epididymis, multiple**

● N44 **Noninflammatory disorders of testis**
● N44.0 **Torsion of testis**
N44.00 **Torsion of testis, unspecified**
N44.01 **Extravaginal torsion of spermatic cord**
N44.02 **Intravaginal torsion of spermatic cord**
Torsion of spermatic cord NOS
N44.03 **Torsion of appendix testis**
N44.04 **Torsion of appendix epididymis**
N44.1 **Cyst of tunica albuginea testis**
N44.2 **Benign cyst of testis**
N44.8 **Other noninflammatory disorders of the testis**

Item 14-8 Male infertility is the inability of the female sex partner to conceive after one year of unprotected intercourse.
Azoospermia is no sperm ejaculated and **oligospermia** is few sperm ejaculated—both resulting in infertility. Extratesticular causes such as injury, infections, radiation, and chemotherapy may also cause male infertility.

● N45 **Orchitis and epididymitis**
*Orchitis is inflammation of one or both of the testes as a result of mumps or other infection, trauma, or metastasis. **Epididymitis** is inflammation of the tubular structure that connects the testicle with the vas deferens.*
Use additional code (B95-B97), to identify infectious agent
N45.1 **Epididymitis**
N45.2 **Orchitis**
N45.3 **Epididymo-orchitis**
N45.4 **Abscess of epididymis or testis**

● N46 **Male infertility**
Excludes1 vasectomy status (Z98.52)
● N46.0 **Azoospermia**
Absolute male infertility
Male infertility due to germinal (cell) aplasia
Male infertility due to spermatogenic arrest (complete)
N46.01 **Organic azoospermia**
Azoospermia NOS
● N46.02 **Azoospermia due to extratesticular causes**
Code also associated cause
N46.021 **Azoospermia due to drug therapy**
N46.022 **Azoospermia due to infection**
N46.023 **Azoospermia due to obstruction of efferent ducts**
N46.024 **Azoospermia due to radiation**
N46.025 **Azoospermia due to systemic disease**
N46.029 **Azoospermia due to other extratesticular causes**
● N46.1 **Oligospermia**
Male infertility due to germinal cell desquamation
Male infertility due to hypospermatogenesis
Male infertility due to incomplete spermatogenic arrest
N46.11 **Organic oligospermia**
Oligospermia NOS
● N46.12 **Oligospermia due to extratesticular causes**
Code also associated cause
N46.121 **Oligospermia due to drug therapy**
N46.122 **Oligospermia due to infection**
N46.123 **Oligospermia due to obstruction of efferent ducts**
N46.124 **Oligospermia due to radiation**
N46.125 **Oligospermia due to systemic disease**
N46.129 **Oligospermia due to other extratesticular causes**
N46.8 **Other male infertility**
N46.9 **Male infertility, unspecified**

● N47 **Disorders of prepuce**
N47.0 **Adherent prepuce, newborn**
N47.1 **Phimosis**
N47.2 **Paraphimosis**
N47.3 **Deficient foreskin**
N47.4 **Benign cyst of prepuce**
N47.5 **Adhesions of prepuce and glans penis**

◀ New   ◀━ Revised   ~~deleted~~ Deleted   **OGCR** Official Guidelines   X Assign placeholder X   ● Use Additional Character(s)

Excludes 1   Excludes 2   Includes   Use additional   Code first   Code also   Unspecified

N47.6 Balanoposthitis

Use additional code (B95-B97), to identify infectious agent

Excludes1 balanitis (N48.1)

N47.7 Other inflammatory diseases of prepuce

Use additional code (B95-B97), to identify infectious agent

N47.8 Other disorders of prepuce

● **N48 Other disorders of penis**

N48.0 Leukoplakia of penis

Balanitis xerotica obliterans
Kraurosis of penis
Lichen sclerosus of external male genital organs

Excludes1 carcinoma in situ of penis (D07.4)

N48.1 Balanitis

Use additional code (B95-B97), to identify infectious agent

Excludes1 amebic balanitis (A06.8)
balanitis xerotica obliterans (N48.0)
candidal balanitis (B37.42)
gonococcal balanitis (A54.23)
herpesviral [herpes simplex] balanitis (A60.01)

● **N48.2 Other inflammatory disorders of penis**

Use additional code (B95-B97), to identify infectious agent

Excludes1 balanitis (N48.1)
balanitis xerotica obliterans (N48.0)
balanoposthitis (N47.6)

N48.21 Abscess of corpus cavernosum and penis

N48.22 Cellulitis of corpus cavernosum and penis

N48.29 Other inflammatory disorders of penis

● **N48.3 Priapism**

Painful erection

Code first underlying cause

N48.30 Priapism, unspecified

N48.31 Priapism due to trauma

N48.32 Priapism due to disease classified elsewhere

N48.33 Priapism, drug-induced

N48.39 Other priapism

N48.5 Ulcer of penis

N48.6 Induration penis plastica

Peyronie's disease
Plastic induration of penis

● **N48.8 Other specified disorders of penis**

N48.81 Thrombosis of superficial vein of penis

N48.82 Acquired torsion of penis

Acquired torsion of penis NOS

Excludes1 congenital torsion of penis (Q55.63)

N48.83 Acquired buried penis

Excludes1 congenital hidden penis (Q55.64)

N48.89 Other specified disorders of penis

N48.9 Disorder of penis, unspecified

● **N49 Inflammatory disorders of male genital organs, not elsewhere classified**

Use additional code (B95-B97), to identify infectious agent

Excludes1 inflammation of penis (N48.1, N48.2-)
orchitis and epididymitis (N45.-)

N49.0 Inflammatory disorders of seminal vesicle

Vesiculitis NOS

N49.1 Inflammatory disorders of spermatic cord, tunica vaginalis and vas deferens

Vasitis

N49.2 Inflammatory disorders of scrotum

N49.3 Fournier gangrene

Item 14–9 Seminal vesiculitis is an inflammation of the seminal vesicle. Spermatocele is a benign cystic accumulation of sperm arising from the head of the epididymis. Torsion of the testis is a medical emergency occurring most commonly in boys 7 to 12 years of age and results from a congenital abnormality of the covering of the testis allowing the testis to twist within its sac and cutting off the blood supply to the testis.

Figure 14-7 **A.** Torsion of testis. **B.** Torsion of the testis. (**B** from Kumar: Robbins and Cotran: Pathologic Basis of Disease, ed 8, Saunders, An Imprint of Elsevier, 2009)

N49.8 Inflammatory disorders of other specified male genital organs

Inflammation of multiple sites in male genital organs

N49.9 Inflammatory disorder of unspecified male genital organ

Abscess of unspecified male genital organ
Boil of unspecified male genital organ
Carbuncle of unspecified male genital organ
Cellulitis of unspecified male genital organ

● **N50 Other and unspecified disorders of male genital organs**

Excludes2 torsion of testis (N44.0-)

N50.0 Atrophy of testis

N50.1 Vascular disorders of male genital organs

Hematocele, NOS, of male genital organs
Hemorrhage of male genital organs
Thrombosis of male genital organs

N50.3 Cyst of epididymis

N50.8 Other specified disorders of male genital organs

Atrophy of scrotum, seminal vesicle, spermatic cord, tunica vaginalis and vas deferens
Edema of scrotum, seminal vesicle, spermatic cord, testis, tunica vaginalis and vas deferens
Hypertrophy of scrotum, seminal vesicle, spermatic cord, testis, tunica vaginalis and vas deferens
Ulcer of scrotum, seminal vesicle, spermatic cord, testis, tunica vaginalis and vas deferens
Chylocele, tunica vaginalis (nonfilarial) NOS
Urethroscrotal fistula
Stricture of spermatic cord, tunica vaginalis, and vas deferens

N50.9 Disorder of male genital organs, unspecified

N51 Disorders of male genital organs in diseases classified elsewhere

Code first underlying disease, such as:
filariasis (B74.0-B74.9)

Excludes1 amebic balanitis (A06.8)
candidal balanitis (B37.42)
gonococcal balanitis (A54.23)
gonococcal prostatitis (A54.22)
herpesviral [herpes simplex] balanitis (A60.01)
trichomonal prostatitis (A59.02)
tuberculous prostatitis (A18.14)

◀ New   ⬅ Revised   ~~deleted~~ Deleted   **OGCR** Official Guidelines   X Assign placeholder X   ● Use Additional Character(s)

Excludes 1   Excludes 2   Includes   Use additional   Code first   Code also   Unspecified

CHAPTER 14 (N00-N99)

● N52   **Male erectile dysfunction**
>> **Excludes1**   psychogenic impotence (F52.21)
● N52.0   **Vasculogenic erectile dysfunction**
>> N52.01   **Erectile dysfunction due to arterial insufficiency**
>> N52.02   **Corporo-venous occlusive erectile dysfunction**
>> N52.03   **Combined arterial insufficiency and corporo-venous occlusive erectile dysfunction**

   N52.1   **Erectile dysfunction due to diseases classified elsewhere**
>> *Code first underlying disease*

   N52.2   **Drug-induced erectile dysfunction**
● N52.3   **Post-surgical erectile dysfunction**
>> N52.31   **Erectile dysfunction following radical prostatectomy**
>> N52.32   **Erectile dysfunction following radical cystectomy**
>> N52.33   **Erectile dysfunction following urethral surgery**
>> N52.34   **Erectile dysfunction following simple prostatectomy**
>> N52.39   **Other post-surgical erectile dysfunction**

   N52.8   **Other male erectile dysfunction**
   N52.9   **Male erectile dysfunction, unspecified**
>> Impotence NOS

● N53   **Other male sexual dysfunction**
>> **Excludes1**   psychogenic sexual dysfunction (F52.-)
● N53.1   **Ejaculatory dysfunction**
>>> **Excludes1**   premature ejaculation (F52.4)
>> N53.11   **Retarded ejaculation**
>> N53.12   **Painful ejaculation**
>> N53.13   **Anejaculatory orgasm**
>> N53.14   **Retrograde ejaculation**
>> N53.19   **Other ejaculatory dysfunction**
>>> Ejaculatory dysfunction NOS

   N53.8   **Other male sexual dysfunction**
   N53.9   **Unspecified male sexual dysfunction**

DISORDERS OF BREAST (N60-N65)

> **Excludes1**   disorders of breast associated with childbirth (O91-O92)

● N60   **Benign mammary dysplasia**
> *Benign lumpiness of breast*
>> **Includes**   fibrocystic mastopathy
● N60.0   **Solitary cyst of breast**
>> Cyst of breast
>> N60.01   **Solitary cyst of right breast**
>> N60.02   **Solitary cyst of left breast**
>> N60.09   **Solitary cyst of unspecified breast**
● N60.1   **Diffuse cystic mastopathy**
>> Cystic breast
>> Fibrocystic disease of breast
>>> **Excludes1**   diffuse cystic mastopathy with epithelial proliferation (N60.3-)
>> N60.11   **Diffuse cystic mastopathy of right breast**
>> N60.12   **Diffuse cystic mastopathy of left breast**
>> N60.19   **Diffuse cystic mastopathy of unspecified breast**
● N60.2   **Fibroadenosis of breast**
>> Adenofibrosis of breast
>>> **Excludes2**   fibroadenoma of breast (D24.-)
>> N60.21   **Fibroadenosis of right breast**
>> N60.22   **Fibroadenosis of left breast**
>> N60.29   **Fibroadenosis of unspecified breast**

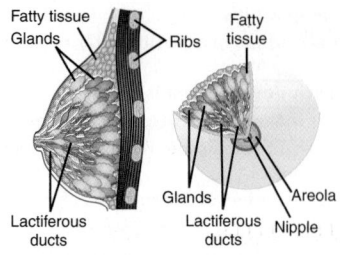

Figure 14-8   Breast.

● N60.3   **Fibrosclerosis of breast**
>> Cystic mastopathy with epithelial proliferation
>> N60.31   **Fibrosclerosis of right breast**
>> N60.32   **Fibrosclerosis of left breast**
>> N60.39   **Fibrosclerosis of unspecified breast**
● N60.4   **Mammary duct ectasia**
>> N60.41   **Mammary duct ectasia of right breast**
>> N60.42   **Mammary duct ectasia of left breast**
>> N60.49   **Mammary duct ectasia of unspecified breast**
● N60.8   **Other benign mammary dysplasias**
>> N60.81   **Other benign mammary dysplasias of right breast**
>> N60.82   **Other benign mammary dysplasias of left breast**
>> N60.89   **Other benign mammary dysplasias of unspecified breast**
● N60.9   **Unspecified benign mammary dysplasia**
>> N60.91   **Unspecified benign mammary dysplasia of right breast**
>> N60.92   **Unspecified benign mammary dysplasia of left breast**
>> N60.99   **Unspecified benign mammary dysplasia of unspecified breast**

  N61   **Inflammatory disorders of breast**
> Abscess (acute) (chronic) (nonpuerperal) of areola
> Abscess (acute) (chronic) (nonpuerperal) of breast
> Carbuncle of breast
> Infective mastitis (acute) (subacute) (nonpuerperal)
> Mastitis (acute) (subacute) (nonpuerperal) NOS
>> **Excludes1**   inflammatory carcinoma of breast (C50.9)
>> inflammatory disorder of breast associated with childbirth (O91.-)
>> neonatal infective mastitis (P39.0)
>> thrombophlebitis of breast [Mondor's disease] (I80.8)

  N62   **Hypertrophy of breast**
> Gynecomastia
> Hypertrophy of breast NOS
> Massive pubertal hypertrophy of breast
>> **Excludes1**   breast engorgement of newborn (P83.4)
>> disproportion of reconstructed breast (N65.1)

  N63   **Unspecified lump in breast**
> Nodule(s) NOS in breast

● N64   **Other disorders of breast**
>> **Excludes2**   mechanical complication of breast prosthesis and implant (T85.4-)
   N64.0   **Fissure and fistula of nipple**
   N64.1   **Fat necrosis of breast**
>> Fat necrosis (segmental) of breast
>> *Code first breast necrosis due to breast graft (T85.89)*
   N64.2   **Atrophy of breast**
   N64.3   **Galactorrhea not associated with childbirth**
>> *Excessive or spontaneous flow of milk*
   N64.4   **Mastodynia**

● **N64.5** **Other signs and symptoms in breast**

     Excludes2   abnormal findings on diagnostic imaging of breast (R92.-)

     N64.51   **Induration of breast**

     N64.52   **Nipple discharge**

         Excludes1   abnormal findings in nipple discharge (R89.-)

     N64.53   **Retraction of nipple**

     N64.59   **Other signs and symptoms in breast**

● **N64.8** **Other specified disorders of breast**

     N64.81   **Ptosis of breast**

         Excludes1   ptosis of native breast in relation to reconstructed breast (N65.1)

     N64.82   **Hypoplasia of breast**

         Micromastia

         Excludes1   congenital absence of breast (Q83.0)

                 hypoplasia of native breast in relation to reconstructed breast (N65.1)

     N64.89   **Other specified disorders of breast**

         Galactocele

         Subinvolution of breast (postlactational)

     N64.9   **Disorder of breast, unspecified**

● **N65** **Deformity and disproportion of reconstructed breast**

     N65.0   **Deformity of reconstructed breast**

         Contour irregularity in reconstructed breast

         Excess tissue in reconstructed breast

         Misshapen reconstructed breast

     N65.1   **Disproportion of reconstructed breast**

         Breast asymmetry between native breast and reconstructed breast

         Disproportion between native breast and reconstructed breast

---

INFLAMMATORY DISEASES OF FEMALE PELVIC ORGANS (N70-N77)

     Excludes1   inflammatory diseases of female pelvic organs complicating:

         abortion or ectopic or molar pregnancy (O00-O07, O08.0)

         pregnancy, childbirth and the puerperium (O23.-, O75.3, O85, O86.-)

(See Plate 360 on page NAP-32.)

● **N70** **Salpingitis and oophoritis**

     Oophoritis = inflammation of ovary

     Salpingitis = inflammation of falloplan tube

     Includes   abscess (of) fallopian tube

         abscess (of) ovary

         pyosalpinx

         salpingo-oophoritis

         tubo-ovarian abscess

         tubo-ovarian inflammatory disease

     Use additional code (B95-B97), to identify infectious agent

     Excludes1   gonococcal infection (A54.24)

                 tuberculous infection (A18.17)

● **N70.0** **Acute salpingitis and oophoritis**

     N70.01   **Acute salpingitis**

     N70.02   **Acute oophoritis**

     N70.03   **Acute salpingitis and oophoritis**

● **N70.1** **Chronic salpingitis and oophoritis**

     Hydrosalpinx

     N70.11   **Chronic salpingitis**

     N70.12   **Chronic oophoritis**

     N70.13   **Chronic salpingitis and oophoritis**

● **N70.9** **Salpingitis and oophoritis, unspecified**

     N70.91   **Salpingitis, unspecified**

     N70.92   **Oophoritis, unspecified**

     N70.93   **Salpingitis and oophoritis, unspecified**

Figure 14-9   **A.** Female genital system. **B.** External female genital system. (From Buck CJ: Step-by-Step Medical Coding, ed 2011, Philadelphia, WB Saunders, 2011)

Item 14–10 Salpingitis is an infection of one or both fallopian tubes. **Oophoritis** is an infection of one or both ovaries.

● **N71** **Inflammatory disease of uterus, except cervix**

     Includes   endo (myo) metritis

         metritis

         myometritis

         pyometra

         uterine abscess

     Use additional code (B95-B97), to identify infectious agent

     Excludes1   hyperplastic endometritis (N85.0-)

                 infection of uterus following delivery (O85, O86.-)

     N71.0   **Acute inflammatory disease of uterus**

     N71.1   **Chronic inflammatory disease of uterus**

     N71.9   **Inflammatory disease of uterus, unspecified**

  N72 **Inflammatory disease of cervix uteri**

     Includes   cervicitis (with or without erosion or ectropion)

         endocervicitis (with or without erosion or ectropion)

         exocervicitis (with or without erosion or ectropion)

     Use additional code (B95-B97), to identify infectious agent

     Excludes1   erosion and ectropion of cervix without cervicitis (N86)

● **N73** **Other female pelvic inflammatory diseases**

     Use additional code (B95-B97), to identify infectious agent

     N73.0   **Acute parametritis and pelvic cellulitis**

         Abscess of broad ligament

         Abscess of parametrium

         Pelvic cellulitis, female

     N73.1   **Chronic parametritis and pelvic cellulitis**

         Any condition in N73.0 specified as chronic

         Excludes1   tuberculous parametritis and pelvic cellultis (A18.17)

     N73.2   **Unspecified parametritis and pelvic cellulitis**

         Any condition in N73.0 unspecified whether acute or chronic

     N73.3   **Female acute pelvic peritonitis**

     N73.4   **Female chronic pelvic peritonitis**

         Excludes1   tuberculous pelvic (female) peritonitis (A18.17)

     N73.5   **Female pelvic peritonitis, unspecified**

     N73.6   **Female pelvic peritoneal adhesions (postinfective)**

         Excludes2   postprocedural pelvic peritoneal adhesions (N99.4)

     N73.8   **Other specified female pelvic inflammatory diseases**

     N73.9   **Female pelvic inflammatory disease, unspecified**

         Female pelvic infection or inflammation NOS

N74　Female pelvic inflammatory disorders in diseases classified elsewhere

　　Code first underlying disease

　　Excludes1　chlamydial cervicitis (A56.02)
　　　　　　　chlamydial pelvic inflammatory disease (A56.11)
　　　　　　　gonococcal cervicitis (A54.03)
　　　　　　　gonococcal pelvic inflammatory disease (A54.24)
　　　　　　　herpesviral [herpes simplex] cervicitis (A60.03)
　　　　　　　herpesviral [herpes simplex] pelvic inflammatory disease (A60.09)
　　　　　　　syphilitic cervicitis (A52.76)
　　　　　　　syphilitic pelvic inflammatory disease (A52.76)
　　　　　　　trichomonal cervicitis (A59.09)
　　　　　　　tuberculous cervicitis (A18.16)
　　　　　　　tuberculous pelvic inflammatory disease (A18.17)

● **N75　Diseases of Bartholin's gland**

　　N75.0　Cyst of Bartholin's gland
　　　　　Cysts filled with liquid or semisolid material.

　　N75.1　Abscess of Bartholin's gland
　　　　　Localized collection of pus

　　N75.8　Other diseases of Bartholin's gland
　　　　　Bartholinitis

　　N75.9　Disease of Bartholin's gland, unspecified

● **N76　Other inflammation of vagina and vulva**

　　Use additional code (B95-B97), to identify infectious agent

　　Excludes2　senile (atrophic) vaginitis (N95.2)
　　　　　　　vulvar vestibulitis (N94.810)

　　N76.0　Acute vaginitis
　　　　　Acute vulvovaginitis
　　　　　Vaginitis NOS
　　　　　Vulvovaginitis NOS

　　N76.1　Subacute and chronic vaginitis
　　　　　Chronic vulvovaginitis
　　　　　Subacute vulvovaginitis

　　N76.2　Acute vulvitis
　　　　　Vulvitis NOS

　　N76.3　Subacute and chronic vulvitis

　　N76.4　Abscess of vulva
　　　　　Furuncle of vulva

　　N76.5　Ulceration of vagina

　　N76.6　Ulceration of vulva

● **N76.8　Other specified inflammation of vagina and vulva**

　　N76.81　Mucositis (ulcerative) of vagina and vulva

　　　　　Code also type of associated therapy, such as:
　　　　　　antineoplastic and immunosuppressive drugs (T45.1X-)
　　　　　　radiological procedure and radiotherapy (Y84.2)

　　　　　Excludes2　gastrointestinal mucositis (ulcerative) (K92.81)
　　　　　　　　　　nasal mucositis (ulcerative) (J34.81)
　　　　　　　　　　oral mucositis (ulcerative) (K12.3-)

　　N76.89　Other specified inflammation of vagina and vulva

● **N77　Vulvovaginal ulceration and inflammation in diseases classified elsewhere**

　　N77.0　Ulceration of vulva in diseases classified elsewhere

　　　　　Code first underlying disease, such as:
　　　　　　Behçet's disease (M35.2)

　　　　　Excludes1　ulceration of vulva in gonococcal infection (A54.02)
　　　　　　　　　　ulceration of vulva in herpesviral [herpes simplex] infection (A60.04)
　　　　　　　　　　ulceration of vulva in syphilis (A51.0)
　　　　　　　　　　ulceration of vulva in tuberculosis (A18.18)

　　N77.1　Vaginitis, vulvitis and vulvovaginitis in diseases classified elsewhere

　　　　　Code first underlying disease, such as:
　　　　　　pinworm (B80)

　　　　　Excludes1　candidial vulvovaginitis (B37.3)
　　　　　　　　　　chlamydial vulvovaginitis (A56.02)
　　　　　　　　　　gonococcal vulvovaginitis (A54.02)
　　　　　　　　　　herpesviral [herpes simplex] vulvovaginitis (A60.04)
　　　　　　　　　　trichomonal vulvovaginitis (A59.01)
　　　　　　　　　　tuberculous vulvovaginitis (A18.18)
　　　　　　　　　　vulvovaginitis in early syphilis (A51.0)
　　　　　　　　　　vulvovaginitis in late syphilis (A52.76)

NONINFLAMMATORY DISORDERS OF FEMALE GENITAL TRACT (N80-N98)

● **N80　Endometriosis**

　　N80.0　Endometriosis of uterus
　　　　　Adenomyosis

　　　　　Excludes1　stromal endometriosis (D39.0)

　　N80.1　Endometriosis of ovary

　　N80.2　Endometriosis of fallopian tube

　　N80.3　Endometriosis of pelvic peritoneum

　　N80.4　Endometriosis of rectovaginal septum and vagina

　　N80.5　Endometriosis of intestine

　　N80.6　Endometriosis in cutaneous scar

　　N80.8　Other endometriosis

　　N80.9　Endometriosis, unspecified

● **N81　Female genital prolapse**

　　Excludes1　genital prolapse complicating pregnancy, labor or delivery (O34.5-)
　　　　　　　prolapse and hernia of ovary and fallopian tube (N83.4)
　　　　　　　prolapse of vaginal vault after hysterectomy (N99.3)

　　N81.0　Urethrocele

　　　　　Excludes1　urethrocele with cystocele (N81.1-)
　　　　　　　　　　urethrocele with prolapse of uterus (N81.2-N81.4)

● **N81.1　Cystocele**
　　　　　Cystocele with urethrocele
　　　　　Cystourethrocele

　　　　　Excludes1　cystocele with prolapse of uterus (N81.2-N81.4)

　　N81.10　Cystocele, unspecified
　　　　　Prolapse of (anterior) vaginal wall NOS

　　N81.11　Cystocele, midline

　　N81.12　Cystocele, lateral
　　　　　Paravaginal cystocele

Item 14–11 Endometriosis is a condition for which no clear cause has been identified. Endometrial tissue is expelled from the uterus into the abdominal cavity and can implant onto a variety of organs. Classification is based on the site of implant of the endometrial tissue.

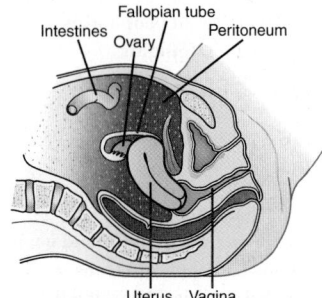

Figure 14-10 Sites of potential endometrial implants.

◀ New　◀▥ Revised　deleted Deleted　OGCR Official Guidelines　X Assign placeholder X　● Use Additional Character(s)

　　Excludes 1　Excludes 2　Includes　Use additional　Code first　Code also　Unspecified

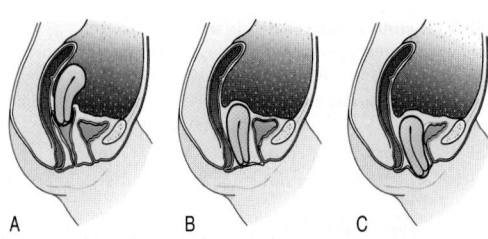

Figure 14-11   Three stages of uterine prolapse. **A.** Uterus is prolapsed. **B.** Vagina and uterus are prolapsed (incomplete uterovaginal prolapse). **C.** Vagina and uterus are completely prolapsed and are exposed through the external genitalia (complete uterovaginal prolapse).

N81.2   **Incomplete uterovaginal prolapse**
    First degree uterine prolapse
    Prolapse of cervix NOS
    Second degree uterine prolapse
    Excludes1   cervical stump prolaspe (N81.85)

N81.3   **Complete uterovaginal prolapse**
    Procidentia (uteri) NOS
    Third degree uterine prolapse

N81.4   **Uterovaginal prolapse, unspecified**
    Prolapse of uterus NOS

N81.5   **Vaginal enterocele**
    Excludes1   enterocele with prolapse of uterus
        (N81.2-N81.4)

N81.6   **Rectocele**
    Prolapse of posterior vaginal wall
    Use additional code for any associated fecal
       incontinence, if applicable (R15.-)
    Excludes2   perineocele (N81.81)
        rectal prolapse (K62.3)
        rectocele with prolapse of uterus
        (N81.2-N81.4)

● N81.8   **Other female genital prolapse**

    N81.81   **Perineocele**

    N81.82   **Incompetence or weakening of pubocervical tissue**

    N81.83   **Incompetence or weakening of rectovaginal tissue**

    N81.84   **Pelvic muscle wasting**
        Disuse atrophy of pelvic muscles and anal
          sphincter

    N81.85   **Cervical stump prolapse**

    N81.89   **Other female genital prolapse**
        Deficient perineum
        Old laceration of muscles of pelvic floor

N81.9   **Female genital prolapse, unspecified**

● N82   **Fistulae involving female genital tract**
    Excludes1   vesicointestinal fistulae (N32.1)

N82.0   **Vesicovaginal fistula**

N82.1   **Other female urinary-genital tract fistulae**
    Cervicovesical fistula
    Ureterovaginal fistula
    Urethrovaginal fistula
    Uteroureteric fistula
    Uterovesical fistula

N82.2   **Fistula of vagina to small intestine**

N82.3   **Fistula of vagina to large intestine**
    Rectovaginal fistula

N82.4   **Other female intestinal-genital tract fistulae**
    Intestinouterine fistula

N82.5   **Female genital tract-skin fistulae**
    Uterus to abdominal wall fistula
    Vaginoperineal fistula

N82.8   **Other female genital tract fistulae**

N82.9   **Female genital tract fistula, unspecified**

● N83   **Noninflammatory disorders of ovary, fallopian tube and broad ligament**
    Excludes2   hydrosalpinx (N70.1-)

N83.0   **Follicular cyst of ovary**
    Cyst of graafian follicle
    Hemorrhagic follicular cyst (of ovary)

N83.1   **Corpus luteum cyst**
    Hemorrhagic corpus luteum cyst

● N83.2   **Other and unspecified ovarian cysts**
    Excludes1   developmental ovarian cyst (Q50.1)
        neoplastic ovarian cyst (D27.-)
        polycystic ovarian syndrome (E28.2)
        Stein-Leventhal syndrome (E28.2)

    N83.20   **Unspecified ovarian cysts**

    N83.29   **Other ovarian cysts**
        Retention cyst of ovary
        Simple cyst of ovary

● N83.3   **Acquired atrophy of ovary and fallopian tube**

    N83.31   **Acquired atrophy of ovary**

    N83.32   **Acquired atrophy of fallopian tube**

    N83.33   **Acquired atrophy of ovary and fallopian tube**

N83.4   **Prolapse and hernia of ovary and fallopian tube**

● N83.5   **Torsion of ovary, ovarian pedicle and fallopian tube**
    Torsion of accessory tube

    N83.51   **Torsion of ovary and ovarian pedicle**

    N83.52   **Torsion of fallopian tube**
        Torsion of hydatid of Morgagni

    N83.53   **Torsion of ovary, ovarian pedicle and fallopian tube**

N83.6   **Hematosalpinx**
    Excludes1   hematosalpinx (with) (in):
        hematocolpos (N89.7)
        hematometra (N85.7)
        tubal pregnancy (O00.1)

N83.7   **Hematoma of broad ligament**

N83.8   **Other noninflammatory disorders of ovary, fallopian tube and broad ligament**
    Broad ligament laceration syndrome [Allen-Masters]

N83.9   **Noninflammatory disorder of ovary, fallopian tube and broad ligament, unspecified**

● N84   **Polyp of female genital tract**
    Excludes1   adenomatous polyp (D28.-)
        placental polyp (O90.89)

N84.0   **Polyp of corpus uteri**
    Polyp of endometrium
    Polyp of uterus NOS
    Excludes1   polypoid endometrial hyperplasia
        (N85.0-)

N84.1   **Polyp of cervix uteri**
    Mucous polyp of cervix

N84.2   **Polyp of vagina**

N84.3   **Polyp of vulva**
    Polyp of labia

N84.8   **Polyp of other parts of female genital tract**

N84.9   **Polyp of female genital tract, unspecified**

● N85   **Other noninflammatory disorders of uterus, except cervix**
    Excludes1   endometriosis (N80.-)
        inflammatory diseases of uterus (N71.-)
        noninflammatory disorders of cervix, except
          malposition (N86-N88)
        polyp of corpus uteri (N84.0)
        uterine prolapse (N81.-)

● N85.0   **Endometrial hyperplasia**

    N85.00   **Endometrial hyperplasia, unspecified**
        Hyperplasia (adenomatous) (cystic)
          (glandular) of endometrium
        Hyperplastic endometritis

◄ New   ◄▦ Revised   ~~deleted~~ Deleted   **OGCR** Official Guidelines   X Assign placeholder X   ● Use Additional Character(s)

Excludes 1 | Excludes 2 | Includes | Use additional | Code first | Code also | Unspecified

CHAPTER 14 (N00-N99)

N85.01   **Benign endometrial hyperplasia**
Endometrial hyperplasia (complex) (simple) without atypia

N85.02   **Endometrial intraepithelial neoplasia [EIN]**
Endometrial hyperplasia with atypia

> **Excludes1**   malignant neoplasm of endometrium (with endometrial intraepithelial neoplasia [EIN]) (C54.1)

N85.2   **Hypertrophy of uterus**
Bulky or enlarged uterus

> **Excludes1**   puerperal hypertrophy of uterus (O90.89)

N85.3   **Subinvolution of uterus**

> **Excludes1**   puerperal subinvolution of uterus (O90.89)

N85.4   **Malposition of uterus**
Anteversion of uterus
Retroflexion of uterus
Retroversion of uterus

> **Excludes1**   malposition of uterus complicating pregnancy, labor or delivery (O34.5-, O65.5)

N85.5   **Inversion of uterus**

> **Excludes1**   current obstetric trauma (O71.2)
> postpartum inversion of uterus (O71.2)

N85.6   **Intrauterine synechiae**

N85.7   **Hematometra**
Hematosalpinx with hematometra

> **Excludes1**   hematometra with hematocolpos (N89.7)

N85.8   **Other specified noninflammatory disorders of uterus**
Atrophy of uterus, acquired
Fibrosis of uterus NOS

N85.9   **Noninflammatory disorder of uterus, unspecified**
Disorder of uterus NOS

N86   **Erosion and ectropion of cervix uteri**
Decubitus (trophic) ulcer of cervix
Eversion of cervix

> **Excludes1**   erosion and ectropion of cervix with cervicitis (N72)

● **N87**   **Dysplasia of cervix uteri**

> **Excludes1**   abnormal results from cervical cytologic examination without histologic confirmation (R87.61-)
> carcinoma in situ of cervix uteri (D06.-)
> cervical intraepithelial neoplasia III [CIN III] (D06.-)
> HGSIL of cervix (R87.613)
> severe dysplasia of cervix uteri (D06.-)

N87.0   **Mild cervical dysplasia**
Cervical intraepithelial neoplasia I [CIN I]

N87.1   **Moderate cervical dysplasia**
Cervical intraepithelial neoplasia II [CIN II]

N87.9   **Dysplasia of cervix uteri, unspecified**
Anaplasia of cervix
Cervical atypism
Cervical dysplasia NOS

● **N88**   **Other noninflammatory disorders of cervix uteri**

> **Excludes2**   inflammatory disease of cervix (N72)
> polyp of cervix (N84.1)

N88.0   **Leukoplakia of cervix uteri**

N88.1   **Old laceration of cervix uteri**
Adhesions of cervix

> **Excludes1**   current obstetric trauma (O71.3)

N88.2   **Stricture and stenosis of cervix uteri**

> **Excludes1**   stricture and stenosis of cervix uteri complicating labor (O65.5)

N88.3   **Incompetence of cervix uteri**
Investigation and management of (suspected) cervical incompetence in a nonpregnant woman

> **Excludes1**   cervical incompetence complicating pregnancy (O34.3-)

N88.4   **Hypertrophic elongation of cervix uteri**

N88.8   **Other specified noninflammatory disorders of cervix uteri**

> **Excludes1**   current obstetric trauma (O71.3)

N88.9   **Noninflammatory disorder of cervix uteri, unspecified**

● **N89**   **Other noninflammatory disorders of vagina**

> **Excludes1**   abnormal results from vaginal cytologic examination without histologic confirmation (R87.62-)
> carcinoma in situ of vagina (D07.2)
> HGSIL of vagina (R87.623)
> inflammation of vagina (N76.-)
> senile (atrophic) vaginitis (N95.2)
> severe dysplasia of vagina (D07.2)
> trichomonal leukorrhea (A59.00)
> vaginal intraepithelial neoplasia [VAIN], grade III (D07.2)

N89.0   **Mild vaginal dysplasia**
Vaginal intraepithelial neoplasia [VAIN], grade I

N89.1   **Moderate vaginal dysplasia**
Vaginal intraepithelial neoplasia [VAIN], grade II

N89.3   **Dysplasia of vagina, unspecified**

N89.4   **Leukoplakia of vagina**

N89.5   **Stricture and atresia of vagina**
Vaginal adhesions   Vaginal stenosis

> **Excludes1**   congenital atresia or stricture (Q52.4)
> postprocedural adhesions of vagina (N99.2)

N89.6   **Tight hymenal ring**
Rigid hymen   Tight introitus

> **Excludes1**   imperforate hymen (Q52.3)

N89.7   **Hematocolpos**
Hematocolpos with hematometra or hematosalpinx

N89.8   **Other specified noninflammatory disorders of vagina**
Leukorrhea NOS
Old vaginal laceration
Pessary ulcer of vagina

> **Excludes1**   current obstetric trauma (O70.-, O71.4, O71.7-O71.8)
> old laceration involving muscles of pelvic floor (N81.8)

N89.9   **Noninflammatory disorder of vagina, unspecified**

● **N90**   **Other noninflammatory disorders of vulva and perineum**

> **Excludes1**   anogenital (venereal) warts (A63.0)
> carcinoma in situ of vulva (D07.1)
> condyloma acuminatum (A63.0)
> current obstetric trauma (O70.-, O71.7-O71.8)
> inflammation of vulva (N76.-)
> severe dysplasia of vulva (D07.1)
> vulvar intraepithelial neoplasm III [VIN III] (D07.1)

N90.0   **Mild vulvar dysplasia**
Vulvar intraepithelial neoplasia [VIN], grade I

N90.1   **Moderate vulvar dysplasia**
Vulvar intraepithelial neoplasia [VIN], grade II

N90.3   **Dysplasia of vulva, unspecified**

N90.4   **Leukoplakia of vulva**
Dystrophy of vulva
Kraurosis of vulva
Lichen sclerosus of external female genital organs

N90.5   **Atrophy of vulva**
Stenosis of vulva

N90.6   **Hypertrophy of vulva**
Hypertrophy of labia

N90.7   **Vulvar cyst**

◀ New   ◀▦ Revised   ~~deleted~~ Deleted   OGCR Official Guidelines   X Assign placeholder X   ● Use Additional Character(s)

Excludes 1   Excludes 2   Includes   Use additional   Code first   Code also   Unspecified

● **N90.8 Other specified noninflammatory disorders of vulva and perineum**
  ● **N90.81 Female genital mutilation status**
     Female genital cutting status
     N90.810 Female genital mutilation status, unspecified
       Female genital cutting status, unspecified
       Female genital mutilation status NOS
     N90.811 Female genital mutilation Type I status
       Clitorectomy status
       Female genital cutting Type I status
     N90.812 Female genital mutilation Type II status
       Clitorectomy with excision of labia minora status
       Female genital cutting Type II status
     N90.813 Female genital mutilation Type III status
       Female genital cutting Type III status
       Infibulation status
     N90.818 Other female genital mutilation status
       Female genital cutting Type IV status
       Female genital mutilation Type IV status
       Other female genital cutting status
   N90.89 Other specified noninflammatory disorders of vulva and perineum
     Adhesions of vulva
     Hypertrophy of clitoris
  N90.9 Noninflammatory disorder of vulva and perineum, unspecified

● **N91 Absent, scanty and rare menstruation**
   Excludes1   ovarian dysfunction (E28.-)
  N91.0 Primary amenorrhea
  N91.1 Secondary amenorrhea
  N91.2 Amenorrhea, unspecified
  N91.3 Primary oligomenorrhea
  N91.4 Secondary oligomenorrhea
  N91.5 Oligomenorrhea, unspecified
    Hypomenorrhea NOS

● **N92 Excessive, frequent and irregular menstruation**
   Excludes1   postmenopausal bleeding (N95.0)
      precocious puberty (menstruation) (E30.1)
  N92.0 Excessive and frequent menstruation with regular cycle
    Heavy periods NOS   Polymenorrhea
    Menorrhagia NOS
  N92.1 Excessive and frequent menstruation with irregular cycle
    Irregular intermenstrual bleeding
    Irregular, shortened intervals between menstrual bleeding
    Menometrorrhagia
    Metrorrhagia
  N92.2 Excessive menstruation at puberty
    Excessive bleeding associated with onset of menstrual periods
    Pubertal menorrhagia
    Puberty bleeding

  N92.3 Ovulation bleeding
    Regular intermenstrual bleeding
  N92.4 Excessive bleeding in the premenopausal period
    Climacteric menorrhagia or metrorrhagia
    Menopausal menorrhagia or metrorrhagia
    Preclimacteric menorrhagia or metrorrhagia
    Premenopausal menorrhagia or metrorrhagia
  N92.5 Other specified irregular menstruation
  N92.6 Irregular menstruation, unspecified
    Irregular bleeding NOS
    Irregular periods NOS
    Excludes1   irregular menstruation with:
       lengthened intervals or scanty bleeding (N91.3-N91.5)
       shortened intervals or excessive bleeding (N92.1)

● **N93 Other abnormal uterine and vaginal bleeding**
   Excludes1   neonatal vaginal hemorrhage (P54.6)
      precocious puberty (menstruation) (E30.1)
      pseudomenses (P54.6)
  N93.0 Postcoital and contact bleeding
  N93.8 Other specified abnormal uterine and vaginal bleeding
    Dysfunctional or functional uterine or vaginal bleeding NOS
  N93.9 Abnormal uterine and vaginal bleeding, unspecified

● **N94 Pain and other conditions associated with female genital organs and menstrual cycle**
  N94.0 Mittelschmerz
    Ovulation pain
  N94.1 Dyspareunia
    Painful intercourse/coitus
    Excludes1   psychogenic dyspareunia (F52.6)
  N94.2 Vaginismus
    Vagina tightness
    Excludes1   psychogenic vaginismus (F52.5)
  N94.3 Premenstrual tension syndrome
    AKA: PMS
    Premenstrual dysphoric disorder
    Code also associated menstrual migraine (G43.82-, G43.83-)
  N94.4 Primary dysmenorrhea
    Lifelong painful menstruation
  N94.5 Secondary dysmenorrhea
    Later onset of painful menstruation
  N94.6 Dysmenorrhea, unspecified
    Excludes1   psychogenic dysmenorrhea (F45.8)
● **N94.8 Other specified conditions associated with female genital organs and menstrual cycle**
  ● **N94.81 Vulvodynia**
     N94.810 Vulvar vestibulitis
     N94.818 Other vulvodynia
     N94.819 Vulvodynia, unspecified
       Vulvodynia NOS
   N94.89 Other specified conditions associated with female genital organs and menstrual cycle
  N94.9 Unspecified condition associated with female genital organs and menstrual cycle

◀ New   ◀ Revised   ~~deleted~~ Deleted   OGCR Official Guidelines   X Assign placeholder X   ● Use Additional Character(s)
Excludes 1   Excludes 2   Includes   Use additional   Code first   Code also   Unspecified
1127

CHAPTER 14 (N00-N99)

● N95   **Menopausal and other perimenopausal disorders**
         Menopausal and other perimenopausal disorders due to
              naturally occurring (age-related) menopause and
              perimenopause
         | Excludes1 | excessive bleeding in the premenopausal period
                          (N92.4)
                       menopausal and perimenopausal disorders due
                          to artificial or premature menopause (E89.4-,
                          E28.31-)
                       premature menopause (E28.31-)
         | Excludes2 | postmenopausal osteoporosis (M81.0-)
                       postmenopausal osteoporosis with current
                          pathological fracture (M80.0-)
                       postmenopausal urethritis (N34.2)

   N95.0   **Postmenopausal bleeding**
   N95.1   **Menopausal and female climacteric states**
            Symptoms such as flushing, sleeplessness, headache,
                lack of concentration, associated with natural (age-
                related) menopause
            Use additional code for associated symptoms
            | Excludes1 | asymptomatic menopausal state (Z78.0)
                           symptoms associated with artificial
                              menopause (E89.41)
                           symptoms associated with premature
                              menopause (E28.310)
   N95.2   **Postmenopausal atrophic vaginitis**
            Senile (atrophic) vaginitis
   N95.8   **Other specified menopausal and perimenopausal
            disorders**
   N95.9   **Unspecified menopausal and perimenopausal disorder**

● N96   **Recurrent pregnancy loss**
         Investigation or care in a nonpregnant woman with history of
              recurrent pregnancy loss
         | Excludes1 | recurrent pregnancy loss with current pregnancy
                          (O26.2-)

● N97   **Female infertility**
         | Includes | inability to achieve a pregnancy
                      sterility, female NOS
         | Excludes1 | female infertility associated with:
                          hypopituitarism (E23.0)
                          Stein-Leventhal syndrome (E28.2)
         | Excludes2 | incompetence of cervix uteri (N88.3)
   N97.0   **Female infertility associated with anovulation**
   N97.1   **Female infertility of tubal origin**
            Female infertility associated with congenital anomaly
                of tube
            Female infertility due to tubal block
            Female infertility due to tubal occlusion
            Female infertility due to tubal stenosis
   N97.2   **Female infertility of uterine origin**
            Female infertility associated with congenital anomaly
                of uterus
            Female infertility due to nonimplantation of ovum
   N97.8   **Female infertility of other origin**
   N97.9   **Female infertility, unspecified**

● N98   **Complications associated with artificial fertilization**
   N98.0   **Infection associated with artificial insemination**
   N98.1   **Hyperstimulation of ovaries**
            Hyperstimulation of ovaries NOS
            Hyperstimulation of ovaries associated with induced
                ovulation
   N98.2   **Complications of attempted introduction of fertilized
            ovum following in vitro fertilization**
   N98.3   **Complications of attempted introduction of embryo in
            embryo transfer**
   N98.8   **Other complications associated with artificial
            fertilization**
   N98.9   **Complication associated with artificial fertilization,
            unspecified**

**INTRAOPERATIVE AND POSTPROCEDURAL COMPLICATIONS AND DISORDERS
OF GENITOURINARY SYSTEM, NOT ELSEWHERE CLASSIFIED (N99)**

● N99   **Intraoperative and postprocedural complications and disorders
         of genitourinary system, not elsewhere classified**
         | Excludes2 | irradiation cystitis (N30.4-)
                       postoophorectomy osteoporosis with current
                          pathological fracture (M80.8-)
                       postoophorectomy osteoporosis without current
                          pathological fracture (M81.8)
   N99.0   **Postprocedural (acute) (chronic) kidney failure**
            Use additional code to type of kidney disease
● N99.1   **Postprocedural urethral stricture**
            Postcatheterization urethral stricture
     ● N99.11   **Postprocedural urethral stricture, male**
           N99.110   **Postprocedural urethral stricture,
                      male, meatal**
           N99.111   **Postprocedural bulbous urethral
                      stricture**
           N99.112   **Postprocedural membranous urethral
                      stricture**
           N99.113   **Postprocedural anterior urethral
                      stricture**
           N99.114   **Postprocedural urethral stricture,
                      male, unspecified**
       N99.12   **Postprocedural urethral stricture, female**
   N99.2   **Postprocedural adhesions of vagina**
   N99.3   **Prolapse of vaginal vault after hysterectomy**
   N99.4   **Postprocedural pelvic peritoneal adhesions**
            | Excludes2 | pelvic peritoneal adhesions NOS (N73.6)
                          postinfective pelvic peritoneal adhesions
                             (N73.6)
● N99.5   **Complications of stoma of urinary tract**
            | Excludes2 | mechanical complication of urinary
                          (indwelling) catheter (T83.0-)
     ● N99.51   **Complication of cystostomy**
           N99.510   **Cystostomy hemorrhage**
           N99.511   **Cystostomy infection**
           N99.512   **Cystostomy malfunction**
           N99.518   **Other cystostomy complication**
     ● N99.52   **Complication of other external stoma of urinary
                tract**
           N99.520   **Hemorrhage of other external stoma
                      of urinary tract**
           N99.521   **Infection of other external stoma of
                      urinary tract**
           N99.522   **Malfunction of other external stoma
                      of urinary tract**
           N99.528   **Other complication of other external
                      stoma of urinary tract**
     ● N99.53   **Complication of other stoma of urinary tract**
           N99.530   **Hemorrhage of other stoma of urinary
                      tract**
           N99.531   **Infection of other stoma of urinary
                      tract**
           N99.532   **Malfunction of other stoma of urinary
                      tract**
           N99.538   **Other complication of other stoma of
                      urinary tract**

CHAPTER 14 (N00-N99)

◀ New   ◀▥ Revised   deleted Deleted   OGCR Official Guidelines   X Assign placeholder X   ● Use Additional Character(s)
            | Excludes 1 | | Excludes 2 | Includes   Use additional   Code first   Code also   Unspecified

1128

● **N99.6** **Intraoperative hemorrhage and hematoma of a genitourinary system organ or structure complicating a procedure**

Excludes1　intraoperative hemorrhage and hematoma of a genitourinary system organ or structure due to accidental puncture or laceration during a procedure (N99.7-)

　　N99.61　**Intraoperative hemorrhage and hematoma of a genitourinary system organ or structure complicating a genitourinary system procedure**

　　N99.62　**Intraoperative hemorrhage and hematoma of a genitourinary system organ or structure complicating other procedure**

● **N99.7** **Accidental puncture and laceration of a genitourinary system organ or structure during a procedure**

　　N99.71　**Accidental puncture and laceration of a genitourinary system organ or structure during a genitourinary system procedure**

　　N99.72　**Accidental puncture and laceration of a genitourinary system organ or structure during other procedure**

● **N99.8** **Other intraoperative and postprocedural complications and disorders of genitourinary system**

　　N99.81　**Other intraoperative complications of genitourinary system**

● 　　N99.82　**Postprocedural hemorrhage and hematoma of a genitourinary system organ or structure following a procedure**

　　　　N99.820　Postprocedural hemorrhage and hematoma of a genitourinary system organ or structure following a genitourinary system procedure

　　　　N99.821　Postprocedural hemorrhage and hematoma of a genitourinary system organ or structure following other procedure

　　N99.83　**Residual ovary syndrome**

　　N99.89　**Other postprocedural complications and disorders of genitourinary system**

CHAPTER 14 (N00-N99)

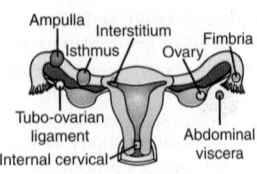

Figure 15-1 Implantation sites of ectopic pregnancy.

Item 15-1 Ectopic pregnancy most often occurs in the fallopian tube. Pregnancy outside the uterus may end in a lifethreatening rupture.

OGCR See Section I.C., Chapter 15
Pregnancy, Childbirth, and the Puerperium

(See Plate 375 on page NAP-4.)

CHAPTER 15

PREGNANCY, CHILDBIRTH AND THE PUERPERIUM (O00-O9A)

Note: CODES FROM THIS CHAPTER ARE FOR USE ONLY ON MATERNAL RECORDS, NEVER ON NEWBORN RECORDS

Codes from this chapter are for use for conditions related to or aggravated by the pregnancy, childbirth, or by the puerperium (maternal causes or obstetric causes)

Trimesters are counted from the first day of the last menstrual period. They are defined as follows:

1st trimester - less than 14 weeks 0 days

2nd trimester - 14 weeks 0 days to less than 28 weeks 0 days

3rd trimester - 28 weeks 0 days until delivery

Use additional code from category Z3A, Weeks of gestation, to identify the specific week of the pregnancy

Excludes1   supervision of normal pregnancy (Z34.-)

Excludes2   mental and behavioral disorders associated with the puerperium (F53)
obstetrical tetanus (A34)
postpartum necrosis of pituitary gland (E23.0)
puerperal osteomalacia (M83.0)

This chapter contains the following blocks:

O00-O08	Pregnancy with abortive outcome
O09	Supervision of high risk pregnancy
O10-O16	Edema, proteinuria and hypertensive disorders in pregnancy, childbirth and the puerperium
O20-O29	Other maternal disorders predominantly related to pregnancy
O30-O48	Maternal care related to the fetus and amniotic cavity and possible delivery problems
O60-O77	Complications of labor and delivery
O80, O82	Encounter for delivery
O85-O92	Complications predominantly related to the puerperium
O94-O9A	Other obstetric conditions, not elsewhere classified

Item 15-2 A **hydatidiform** mole is an overproduction of placental tissue. The tumor secretes a hormone, chorionic gonadotropic hormone (CGH), that indicates a positive pregnancy test. There is no viable fetus. More than 80% of hydatidiform moles are noncancerous.

PREGNANCY WITH ABORTIVE OUTCOME (O00-O08)

Excludes1   continuing pregnancy in multiple gestation after abortion of one fetus or more (O31.1-, O31.3-)

● **O00   Ectopic pregnancy**

Includes   ruptured ectopic pregnancy

Use additional code from category O08 to identify any associated complication

O00.0   Abdominal pregnancy

Excludes1   maternal care for viable fetus in abdominal pregnancy (O36.7-)

O00.1   Tubal pregnancy
Fallopian pregnancy
Rupture of (fallopian) tube due to pregnancy
Tubal abortion

O00.2   Ovarian pregnancy

O00.8   Other ectopic pregnancy
Cervical pregnancy
Cornual pregnancy
Intraligamentous pregnancy
Mural pregnancy

O00.9   Ectopic pregnancy, unspecified

● **O01   Hydatidiform mole**

Use additional code from category O08 to identify any associated complication

Excludes1   chorioadenoma (destruens) (D39.2)
malignant hydatidiform mole (D39.2)

O01.0   Classical hydatidiform mole
Complete hydatidiform mole

O01.1   Incomplete and partial hydatidiform mole

O01.9   Hydatidiform mole, unspecified
Trophoblastic disease NOS
Vesicular mole NOS

● **O02   Other abnormal products of conception**

Use additional code from category O08 to identify any associated complication

Excludes1   papyraceous fetus (O31.0-)

O02.0   Blighted ovum and nonhydatidiform mole
Carneous mole   Molar pregnancy NEC
Fleshy mole   Pathological ovum
Intrauterine mole NOS

O02.1   Missed abortion
Early fetal death, before completion of 20 weeks of gestation, with retention of dead fetus

Excludes1   failed induced abortion (O07.-)
fetal death (intrauterine) (late) (O36.4)
missed abortion with blighted ovum (O02.0)
missed abortion with hydatidiform mole (O01.-)
missed abortion with nonhydatidiform (O02.0)
missed abortion with other abnormal products of conception (O02.8-)
missed delivery (O36.4)
stillbirth (P95)

● **O02.8   Other specified abnormal products of conception**

> | Excludes1 | abnormal products of conception with blighted ovum (O02.0)
> abnormal products of conception with hydatidiform mole (O01.-)
> abnormal products of conception with nonhydatidiform mole (O02.0)

    O02.81   Inappropriate change in quantitative human chorionic gonadotropin (hCG) in early pregnancy

> Biochemical pregnancy
> Chemical pregnancy
> Inappropriate level of quantitative human chorionic gonadotropin (hCG) for gestational age in early pregnancy

    O02.89   Other abnormal products of conception

   O02.9   Abnormal product of conception, unspecified

● **O03   Spontaneous abortion**

Note: Incomplete abortion includes retained products of conception following spontaneous abortion.

> | Includes | miscarriage

   O03.0   Genital tract and pelvic infection following incomplete spontaneous abortion

> Endometritis following incomplete spontaneous abortion
> Oophoritis following incomplete spontaneous abortion
> Parametritis following incomplete spontaneous abortion
> Pelvic peritonitis following incomplete spontaneous abortion
> Salpingitis following incomplete spontaneous abortion
> Salpingo-oophoritis following incomplete spontaneous abortion

> | Excludes1 | sepsis following incomplete spontaneous abortion (O03.37)
> urinary tract infection following incomplete spontaneous abortion (O03.38)

   O03.1   Delayed or excessive hemorrhage following incomplete spontaneous abortion

> Afibrinogenemia following incomplete spontaneous abortion
> Defibrination syndrome following incomplete spontaneous abortion
> Hemolysis following incomplete spontaneous abortion
> Intravascular coagulation following incomplete spontaneous abortion

   O03.2   Embolism following incomplete spontaneous abortion

> Air embolism following incomplete spontaneous abortion
> Amniotic fluid embolism following incomplete spontaneous abortion
> Blood-clot embolism following incomplete spontaneous abortion
> Embolism NOS following incomplete spontaneous abortion
> Fat embolism following incomplete spontaneous abortion
> Pulmonary embolism following incomplete spontaneous abortion
> Pyemic embolism following incomplete spontaneous abortion
> Septic or septicopyemic embolism following incomplete spontaneous abortion
> Soap embolism following incomplete spontaneous abortion

● **O03.3   Other and unspecified complications following incomplete spontaneous abortion**

    O03.30   Unspecified complication following incomplete spontaneous abortion

    O03.31   Shock following incomplete spontaneous abortion

> Circulatory collapse following incomplete spontaneous abortion
> Shock (postprocedural) following incomplete spontaneous abortion

> | Excludes1 | shock due to infection following incomplete spontaneous abortion (O03.37)

    O03.32   Renal failure following incomplete spontaneous abortion

> Kidney failure (acute) following incomplete spontaneous abortion
> Oliguria following incomplete spontaneous abortion
> Renal shutdown following incomplete spontaneous abortion
> Renal tubular necrosis following incomplete spontaneous abortion
> Uremia following incomplete spontaneous abortion

    O03.33   Metabolic disorder following incomplete spontaneous abortion

    O03.34   Damage to pelvic organs following incomplete spontaneous abortion

> Laceration, perforation, tear or chemical damage of bladder following incomplete spontaneous abortion
> Laceration, perforation, tear or chemical damage of bowel following incomplete spontaneous abortion
> Laceration, perforation, tear or chemical damage of broad ligament following incomplete spontaneous abortion
> Laceration, perforation, tear or chemical damage of cervix following incomplete spontaneous abortion
> Laceration, perforation, tear or chemical damage of periurethral tissue following incomplete spontaneous abortion
> Laceration, perforation, tear or chemical damage of uterus following incomplete spontaneous abortion
> Laceration, perforation, tear or chemical damage of vagina following incomplete spontaneous abortion

    O03.35   Other venous complications following incomplete spontaneous abortion

    O03.36   Cardiac arrest following incomplete spontaneous abortion

    O03.37   Sepsis following incomplete spontaneous abortion

> Use additional code to identify infectious agent (B95-B97)
> Use additional code to identify severe sepsis, if applicable (R65.2-)

> | Excludes1 | septic or septicopyemic embolism following incomplete spontaneous abortion (O03.2)

    O03.38   Urinary tract infection following incomplete spontaneous abortion

> Cystitis following incomplete spontaneous abortion

    O03.39   Incomplete spontaneous abortion with other complications

CHAPTER 15 (O00-O9A)

O03.4 Incomplete spontaneous abortion without complication

O03.5 Genital tract and pelvic infection following complete or unspecified spontaneous abortion

Endometritis following complete or unspecified spontaneous abortion

Oophoritis following complete or unspecified spontaneous abortion

Parametritis following complete or unspecified spontaneous abortion

Pelvic peritonitis following complete or unspecified spontaneous abortion

Salpingitis following complete or unspecified spontaneous abortion

Salpingo-oophoritis following complete or unspecified spontaneous abortion

> **Excludes1**   sepsis following complete or unspecified spontaneous abortion (O03.87)
> urinary tract infection following complete or unspecified spontaneous abortion (O03.88)

O03.6 Delayed or excessive hemorrhage following complete or unspecified spontaneous abortion

Afibrinogenemia following complete or unspecified spontaneous abortion

Defibrination syndrome following complete or unspecified spontaneous abortion

Hemolysis following complete or unspecified spontaneous abortion

Intravascular coagulation following complete or unspecified spontaneous abortion

O03.7 Embolism following complete or unspecified spontaneous abortion

Air embolism following complete or unspecified spontaneous abortion

Amniotic fluid embolism following complete or unspecified spontaneous abortion

Blood-clot embolism following complete or unspecified spontaneous abortion

Embolism NOS following complete or unspecified spontaneous abortion

Fat embolism following complete or unspecified spontaneous abortion

Pulmonary embolism following complete or unspecified spontaneous abortion

Pyemic embolism following complete or unspecified spontaneous abortion

Septic or septicopyemic embolism following complete or unspecified spontaneous abortion

Soap embolism following complete or unspecified spontaneous abortion

● **O03.8 Other and unspecified complications following complete or unspecified spontaneous abortion**

O03.80 Unspecified complication following complete or unspecified spontaneous abortion

O03.81 Shock following complete or unspecified spontaneous abortion

Circulatory collapse following complete or unspecified spontaneous abortion

Shock (postprocedural) following complete or unspecified spontaneous abortion

> **Excludes1**   shock due to infection following complete or unspecified spontaneous abortion (O03.87)

O03.82 Renal failure following complete or unspecified spontaneous abortion

Kidney failure (acute) following complete or unspecified spontaneous abortion

Oliguria following complete or unspecified spontaneous abortion

Renal shutdown following complete or unspecified spontaneous abortion

Renal tubular necrosis following complete or unspecified spontaneous abortion

Uremia following complete or unspecified spontaneous abortion

O03.83 Metabolic disorder following complete or unspecified spontaneous abortion

O03.84 Damage to pelvic organs following complete or unspecified spontaneous abortion

Laceration, perforation, tear or chemical damage of bladder following complete or unspecified spontaneous abortion

Laceration, perforation, tear or chemical damage of bowel following complete or unspecified spontaneous abortion

Laceration, perforation, tear or chemical damage of broad ligament following complete or unspecified spontaneous abortion

Laceration, perforation, tear or chemical damage of cervix following complete or unspecified spontaneous abortion

Laceration, perforation, tear or chemical damage of periurethral tissue following complete or unspecified spontaneous abortion

Laceration, perforation, tear or chemical damage of uterus following complete or unspecified spontaneous abortion

Laceration, perforation, tear or chemical damage of vagina following complete or unspecified spontaneous abortion

O03.85 Other venous complications following complete or unspecified spontaneous abortion

O03.86 Cardiac arrest following complete or unspecified spontaneous abortion

O03.87 Sepsis following complete or unspecified spontaneous abortion

Use additional code to identify infectious agent (B95-B97)

Use additional code to identify severe sepsis, if applicable (R65.2-)

> **Excludes1**   septic or septicopyemic embolism following complete or unspecified spontaneous abortion (O03.7)

O03.88 Urinary tract infection following complete or unspecified spontaneous abortion

Cystitis following complete or unspecified spontaneous abortion

O03.89 Complete or unspecified spontaneous abortion with other complications

O03.9 Complete or unspecified spontaneous abortion without complication

Miscarriage NOS

Spontaneous abortion NOS

● **O04**   **Complications following (induced) termination of pregnancy**

     Includes   complications following (induced) termination of pregnancy

     Excludes1   encounter for elective termination of pregnancy, uncomplicated (Z33.2)

                    failed attempted termination of pregnancy (O07.-)

   O04.5   **Genital tract and pelvic infection following (induced) termination of pregnancy**

       Endometritis following (induced) termination of pregnancy

       Oophoritis following (induced) termination of pregnancy

       Parametritis following (induced) termination of pregnancy

       Pelvic peritonitis following (induced) termination of pregnancy

       Salpingitis following (induced) termination of pregnancy

       Salpingo-oophoritis following (induced) termination of pregnancy

       Excludes1   sepsis following (induced) termination of pregnancy (O04.87)

                  urinary tract infection following (induced) termination of pregnancy (O04.88)

   O04.6   **Delayed or excessive hemorrhage following (induced) termination of pregnancy**

       Afibrinogenemia following (induced) termination of pregnancy

       Defibrination syndrome following (induced) termination of pregnancy

       Hemolysis following (induced) termination of pregnancy

       Intravascular coagulation following (induced) termination of pregnancy

   O04.7   **Embolism following (induced) termination of pregnancy**

       Air embolism following (induced) termination of pregnancy

       Amniotic fluid embolism following (induced) termination of pregnancy

       Blood-clot embolism following (induced) termination of pregnancy

       Embolism NOS following (induced) termination of pregnancy

       Fat embolism following (induced) termination of pregnancy

       Pulmonary embolism following (induced) termination of pregnancy

       Pyemic embolism following (induced) termination of pregnancy

       Septic or septicopyemic embolism following (induced) termination of pregnancy

       Soap embolism following (induced) termination of pregnancy

● **O04.8**   **(Induced) termination of pregnancy with other and unspecified complications**

   O04.80   **(Induced) termination of pregnancy with unspecified complications**

   O04.81   **Shock following (induced) termination of pregnancy**

       Circulatory collapse following (induced) termination of pregnancy

       Shock (postprocedural) following (induced) termination of pregnancy

       Excludes1   shock due to infection following (induced) termination of pregnancy (O04.87)

   O04.82   **Renal failure following (induced) termination of pregnancy**

       Kidney failure (acute) following (induced) termination of pregnancy

       Oliguria following (induced) termination of pregnancy

       Renal shutdown following (induced) termination of pregnancy

       Renal tubular necrosis following (induced) termination of pregnancy

       Uremia following (induced) termination of pregnancy

   O04.83   **Metabolic disorder following (induced) termination of pregnancy**

   O04.84   **Damage to pelvic organs following (induced) termination of pregnancy**

       Laceration, perforation, tear or chemical damage of bladder following (induced) termination of pregnancy

       Laceration, perforation, tear or chemical damage of bowel following (induced) termination of pregnancy

       Laceration, perforation, tear or chemical damage of broad ligament following (induced) termination of pregnancy

       Laceration, perforation, tear or chemical damage of cervix following (induced) termination of pregnancy

       Laceration, perforation, tear or chemical damage of periurethral tissue following (induced) termination of pregnancy

       Laceration, perforation, tear or chemical damage of uterus following (induced) termination of pregnancy

       Laceration, perforation, tear or chemical damage of vagina following (induced) termination of pregnancy

   O04.85   **Other venous complications following (induced) termination of pregnancy**

   O04.86   **Cardiac arrest following (induced) termination of pregnancy**

   O04.87   **Sepsis following (induced) termination of pregnancy**

       Use additional code to identify infectious agent (B95-B97)

       Use additional code to identify severe sepsis, if applicable (R65.2-)

       Excludes1   septic or septicopyemic embolism following (induced) termination of pregnancy (O04.7)

   O04.88   **Urinary tract infection following (induced) termination of pregnancy**

       Cystitis following (induced) termination of pregnancy

   O04.89   **(Induced) termination of pregnancy with other complications**

CHAPTER 15 (O00-O9A)

● **O07   Failed attempted termination of pregnancy**

> **Includes**   failure of attempted induction of termination of pregnancy
> incomplete elective abortion
>
> **Excludes1**   incomplete spontaneous abortion (O03.0-)

O07.0   Genital tract and pelvic infection following failed attempted termination of pregnancy

> Endometritis following failed attempted termination of pregnancy
> Oophoritis following failed attempted termination of pregnancy
> Parametritis following failed attempted termination of pregnancy
> Pelvic peritonitis following failed attempted termination of pregnancy
> Salpingitis following failed attempted termination of pregnancy
> Salpingo-oophoritis following failed attempted termination of pregnancy
>
> > **Excludes1**   sepsis following failed attempted termination of pregnancy (O07.37)
> > urinary tract infection following failed attempted termination of pregnancy (O07.38)

O07.1   Delayed or excessive hemorrhage following failed attempted termination of pregnancy

> Afibrinogenemia following failed attempted termination of pregnancy
> Defibrination syndrome following failed attempted termination of pregnancy
> Hemolysis following failed attempted termination of pregnancy
> Intravascular coagulation following failed attempted termination of pregnancy

O07.2   Embolism following failed attempted termination of pregnancy

> Air embolism following failed attempted termination of pregnancy
> Amniotic fluid embolism following failed attempted termination of pregnancy
> Blood-clot embolism following failed attempted termination of pregnancy
> Embolism NOS following failed attempted termination of pregnancy
> Fat embolism following failed attempted termination of pregnancy
> Pulmonary embolism following failed attempted termination of pregnancy
> Pyemic embolism following failed attempted termination of pregnancy
> Septic or septicopyemic embolism following failed attempted termination of pregnancy
> Soap embolism following failed attempted termination of pregnancy

● **O07.3   Failed attempted termination of pregnancy with other and unspecified complications**

O07.30   Failed attempted termination of pregnancy with unspecified complications

O07.31   Shock following failed attempted termination of pregnancy

> Circulatory collapse following failed attempted termination of pregnancy
> Shock (postprocedural) following failed attempted termination of pregnancy
>
> > **Excludes1**   shock due to infection following failed attempted termination of pregnancy (O07.37)

O07.32   Renal failure following failed attempted termination of pregnancy

> Kidney failure (acute) following failed attempted termination of pregnancy
> Oliguria following failed attempted termination of pregnancy
> Renal shutdown following failed attempted termination of pregnancy
> Renal tubular necrosis following failed attempted termination of pregnancy
> Uremia following failed attempted termination of pregnancy

O07.33   Metabolic disorder following failed attempted termination of pregnancy

O07.34   Damage to pelvic organs following failed attempted termination of pregnancy

> Laceration, perforation, tear or chemical damage of bladder following failed attempted termination of pregnancy
> Laceration, perforation, tear or chemical damage of bowel following failed attempted termination of pregnancy
> Laceration, perforation, tear or chemical damage of broad ligament following failed attempted termination of pregnancy
> Laceration, perforation, tear or chemical damage of cervix following failed attempted termination of pregnancy
> Laceration, perforation, tear or chemical damage of periurethral tissue following failed attempted termination of pregnancy
> Laceration, perforation, tear or chemical damage of uterus following failed attempted termination of pregnancy
> Laceration, perforation, tear or chemical damage of vagina following failed attempted termination of pregnancy

O07.35   Other venous complications following failed attempted termination of pregnancy

O07.36   Cardiac arrest following failed attempted termination of pregnancy

O07.37   Sepsis following failed attempted termination of pregnancy

> Use additional code (B95-B97), to identify infectious agent
>
> Use additional code (R65.2-) to identify severe sepsis, if applicable
>
> > **Excludes1**   septic or septicopyemic embolism following failed attempted termination of pregnancy (O07.2)

O07.38   Urinary tract infection following failed attempted termination of pregnancy

> Cystitis following failed attempted termination of pregnancy

O07.39   Failed attempted termination of pregnancy with other complications

O07.4   Failed attempted termination of pregnancy without complication

● **O08   Complications following ectopic and molar pregnancy**

> This category is for use with categories O00-O02 to identify any associated complications.

O08.0   Genital tract and pelvic infection following ectopic and molar pregnancy

> Endometritis following ectopic and molar pregnancy
> Oophoritis following ectopic and molar pregnancy
> Parametritis following ectopic and molar pregnancy
> Pelvic peritonitis following ectopic and molar pregnancy
> Salpingitis following ectopic and molar pregnancy
> Salpingo-oophoritis following ectopic and molar pregnancy
>
> > **Excludes1**   sepsis following ectopic and molar pregnancy (O08.82)
> > urinary tract infection (O08.83)

O08.1   Delayed or excessive hemorrhage following ectopic and molar pregnancy
     Afibrinogenemia following ectopic and molar pregnancy
     Defibrination syndrome following ectopic and molar pregnancy
     Hemolysis following ectopic and molar pregnancy
     Intravascular coagulation following ectopic and molar pregnancy

> **Excludes1**   delayed or excessive hemorrhage due to incomplete abortion (O03.1)

O08.2   Embolism following ectopic and molar pregnancy
     Air embolism following ectopic and molar pregnancy
     Amniotic fluid embolism following ectopic and molar pregnancy
     Blood-clot embolism following ectopic and molar pregnancy
     Embolism NOS following ectopic and molar pregnancy
     Fat embolism following ectopic and molar pregnancy
     Pulmonary embolism following ectopic and molar pregnancy
     Pyemic embolism following ectopic and molar pregnancy
     Septic or septicopyemic embolism following ectopic and molar pregnancy
     Soap embolism following ectopic and molar pregnancy

O08.3   Shock following ectopic and molar pregnancy
     Circulatory collapse following ectopic and molar pregnancy
     Shock (postprocedural) following ectopic and molar pregnancy

> **Excludes1**   shock due to infection following ectopic and molar pregnancy (O08.82)

O08.4   Renal failure following ectopic and molar pregnancy
     Kidney failure (acute) following ectopic and molar pregnancy
     Oliguria following ectopic and molar pregnancy
     Renal shutdown following ectopic and molar pregnancy
     Renal tubular necrosis following ectopic and molar pregnancy
     Uremia following ectopic and molar pregnancy

O08.5   Metabolic disorders following an ectopic and molar pregnancy

O08.6   Damage to pelvic organs and tissues following an ectopic and molar pregnancy
     Laceration, perforation, tear or chemical damage of bladder following an ectopic and molar pregnancy
     Laceration, perforation, tear or chemical damage of bowel following an ectopic and molar pregnancy
     Laceration, perforation, tear or chemical damage of broad ligament following an ectopic and molar pregnancy
     Laceration, perforation, tear or chemical damage of cervix following an ectopic and molar pregnancy
     Laceration, perforation, tear or chemical damage of periurethral tissue following an ectopic and molar pregnancy
     Laceration, perforation, tear or chemical damage of uterus following an ectopic and molar pregnancy
     Laceration, perforation, tear or chemical damage of vagina following an ectopic and molar pregnancy

O08.7   Other venous complications following an ectopic and molar pregnancy

● **O08.8   Other complications following an ectopic and molar pregnancy**

   O08.81   Cardiac arrest following an ectopic and molar pregnancy

   O08.82   Sepsis following ectopic and molar pregnancy
     Use additional code (B95-B97), to identify infectious agent
     Use additional code (R65.2-) to identify severe sepsis, if applicable

> **Excludes1**   septic or septicopyemic embolism following ectopic and molar pregnancy (O08.2)

   O08.83   Urinary tract infection following an ectopic and molar pregnancy
     Cystitis following an ectopic and molar pregnancy

   O08.89   Other complications following an ectopic and molar pregnancy

O08.9   Unspecified complication following an ectopic and molar pregnancy

---

SUPERVISION OF HIGH RISK PREGNANCY (O09)

● **O09   Supervision of high risk pregnancy**

   ● **O09.0   Supervision of pregnancy with history of infertility**

     O09.00   Supervision of pregnancy with history of infertility, unspecified trimester

     O09.01   Supervision of pregnancy with history of infertility, first trimester

     O09.02   Supervision of pregnancy with history of infertility, second trimester

     O09.03   Supervision of pregnancy with history of infertility, third trimester

   ● **O09.1   Supervision of pregnancy with history of ectopic or molar pregnancy**

     O09.10   Supervision of pregnancy with history of ectopic or molar pregnancy, unspecified trimester

     O09.11   Supervision of pregnancy with history of ectopic or molar pregnancy, first trimester

     O09.12   Supervision of pregnancy with history of ectopic or molar pregnancy, second trimester

     O09.13   Supervision of pregnancy with history of ectopic or molar pregnancy, third trimester

   ● **O09.2   Supervision of pregnancy with other poor reproductive or obstetric history**

> **Excludes2**   pregnancy care for patient with history of recurrent pregnancy loss (O26.2-)

     ● **O09.21   Supervision of pregnancy with history of pre-term labor**

       O09.211   Supervision of pregnancy with history of pre-term labor, first trimester

       O09.212   Supervision of pregnancy with history of pre-term labor, second trimester

       O09.213   Supervision of pregnancy with history of pre-term labor, third trimester

       O09.219   Supervision of pregnancy with history of pre-term labor, unspecified trimester

● **O09.29** **Supervision of pregnancy with other poor reproductive or obstetric history**
Supervision of pregnancy with history of neonatal death
Supervision of pregnancy with history of stillbirth

     O09.291 Supervision of pregnancy with other poor reproductive or obstetric history, first trimester

     O09.292 Supervision of pregnancy with other poor reproductive or obstetric history, second trimester

     O09.293 Supervision of pregnancy with other poor reproductive or obstetric history, third trimester

     O09.299 Supervision of pregnancy with other poor reproductive or obstetric history, unspecified trimester

● **O09.3** **Supervision of pregnancy with insufficient antenatal care**
Supervision of concealed pregnancy
Supervision of hidden pregnancy

     O09.30 Supervision of pregnancy with insufficient antenatal care, unspecified trimester

     O09.31 Supervision of pregnancy with insufficient antenatal care, first trimester

     O09.32 Supervision of pregnancy with insufficient antenatal care, second trimester

     O09.33 Supervision of pregnancy with insufficient antenatal care, third trimester

● **O09.4** **Supervision of pregnancy with grand multiparity**

     O09.40 Supervision of pregnancy with grand multiparity, unspecified trimester

     O09.41 Supervision of pregnancy with grand multiparity, first trimester

     O09.42 Supervision of pregnancy with grand multiparity, second trimester

     O09.43 Supervision of pregnancy with grand multiparity, third trimester

● **O09.5** **Supervision of elderly primigravida and multigravida**
Pregnancy for a female 35 years and older at expected date of delivery

     ● **O09.51** **Supervision of elderly primigravida**

        O09.511 Supervision of elderly primigravida, first trimester

        O09.512 Supervision of elderly primigravida, second trimester

        O09.513 Supervision of elderly primigravida, third trimester

        O09.519 Supervision of elderly primigravida, unspecified trimester

     ● **O09.52** **Supervision of elderly multigravida**

        O09.521 Supervision of elderly multigravida, first trimester

        O09.522 Supervision of elderly multigravida, second trimester

        O09.523 Supervision of elderly multigravida, third trimester

        O09.529 Supervision of elderly multigravida, unspecified trimester

● **O09.6** **Supervision of young primigravida and multigravida**
Supervision of pregnancy for a female less than 16 years old at expected date of delivery

     ● **O09.61** **Supervision of young primigravida**

        O09.611 Supervision of young primigravida, first trimester

        O09.612 Supervision of young primigravida, second trimester

        O09.613 Supervision of young primigravida, third trimester

        O09.619 Supervision of young primigravida, unspecified trimester

     ● **O09.62** **Supervision of young multigravida**

        O09.621 Supervision of young multigravida, first trimester

        O09.622 Supervision of young multigravida, second trimester

        O09.623 Supervision of young multigravida, third trimester

        O09.629 Supervision of young multigravida, unspecified trimester

● **O09.7** **Supervision of high risk pregnancy due to social problems**

     O09.70 Supervision of high risk pregnancy due to social problems, unspecified trimester

     O09.71 Supervision of high risk pregnancy due to social problems, first trimester

     O09.72 Supervision of high risk pregnancy due to social problems, second trimester

     O09.73 Supervision of high risk pregnancy due to social problems, third trimester

● **O09.8** **Supervision of other high risk pregnancies**

     ● **O09.81** **Supervision of pregnancy resulting from assisted reproductive technology**
Supervision of pregnancy resulting from in-vitro fertilization

        O09.811 Supervision of pregnancy resulting from assisted reproductive technology, first trimester

        O09.812 Supervision of pregnancy resulting from assisted reproductive technology, second trimester

        O09.813 Supervision of pregnancy resulting from assisted reproductive technology, third trimester

        O09.819 Supervision of pregnancy resulting from assisted reproductive technology, unspecified trimester

     ● **O09.82** **Supervision of pregnancy with history of in utero procedure during previous pregnancy**

        O09.821 Supervision of pregnancy with history of in utero procedure during previous pregnancy, first trimester

        O09.822 Supervision of pregnancy with history of in utero procedure during previous pregnancy, second trimester

        O09.823 Supervision of pregnancy with history of in utero procedure during previous pregnancy, third trimester

        O09.829 Supervision of pregnancy with history of in utero procedure during previous pregnancy, unspecified trimester

          Excludes1 supervision of pregnancy affected by in utero procedure during current pregnancy (O35.7)

     ● **O09.89** **Supervision of other high risk pregnancies**

        O09.891 Supervision of other high risk pregnancies, first trimester

        O09.892 Supervision of other high risk pregnancies, second trimester

        O09.893 Supervision of other high risk pregnancies, third trimester

        O09.899 Supervision of other high risk pregnancies, unspecified trimester

● **O09.9 Supervision of high risk pregnancy, unspecified**

    O09.90 Supervision of high risk pregnancy, unspecified, unspecified trimester

    O09.91 Supervision of high risk pregnancy, unspecified, first trimester

    O09.92 Supervision of high risk pregnancy, unspecified, second trimester

    O09.93 Supervision of high risk pregnancy, unspecified, third trimester

---

EDEMA, PROTEINURIA AND HYPERTENSIVE DISORDERS IN PREGNANCY, CHILDBIRTH AND THE PUERPERIUM (O10-O16)

● **O10 Pre-existing hypertension complicating pregnancy, childbirth and the puerperium**

    Includes   pre-existing hypertension with pre-existing proteinuria complicating pregnancy, childbirth and the puerperium

    Excludes2   pre-existing hypertension with superimposed pre-eclampsia complicating pregnancy, childbirth and the puerperium (O11.-)

● **O10.0 Pre-existing essential hypertension complicating pregnancy, childbirth and the puerperium**

    Any condition in I10 specified as a reason for obstetric care during pregnancy, childbirth or the puerperium

    ● **O10.01 Pre-existing essential hypertension complicating pregnancy**

        O10.011 Pre-existing essential hypertension complicating pregnancy, first trimester

        O10.012 Pre-existing essential hypertension complicating pregnancy, second trimester

        O10.013 Pre-existing essential hypertension complicating pregnancy, third trimester

        O10.019 Pre-existing essential hypertension complicating pregnancy, unspecified trimester

    O10.02 Pre-existing essential hypertension complicating childbirth

    O10.03 Pre-existing essential hypertension complicating the puerperium

● **O10.1 Pre-existing hypertensive heart disease complicating pregnancy, childbirth and the puerperium**

    Any condition in I11 specified as a reason for obstetric care during pregnancy, childbirth or the puerperium

    Use additional code from I11 to identify the type of hypertensive heart disease

    ● **O10.11 Pre-existing hypertensive heart disease complicating pregnancy**

        O10.111 Pre-existing hypertensive heart disease complicating pregnancy, first trimester

        O10.112 Pre-existing hypertensive heart disease complicating pregnancy, second trimester

        O10.113 Pre-existing hypertensive heart disease complicating pregnancy, third trimester

        O10.119 Pre-existing hypertensive heart disease complicating pregnancy, unspecified trimester

    O10.12 Pre-existing hypertensive heart disease complicating childbirth

    O10.13 Pre-existing hypertensive heart disease complicating the puerperium

● **O10.2 Pre-existing hypertensive chronic kidney disease complicating pregnancy, childbirth and the puerperium**

    Any condition in I12 specified as a reason for obstetric care during pregnancy, childbirth or the puerperium

    Use additional code from I12 to identify the type of hypertensive chronic kidney disease

    ● **O10.21 Pre-existing hypertensive chronic kidney disease complicating pregnancy**

        O10.211 Pre-existing hypertensive chronic kidney disease complicating pregnancy, first trimester

        O10.212 Pre-existing hypertensive chronic kidney disease complicating pregnancy, second trimester

        O10.213 Pre-existing hypertensive chronic kidney disease complicating pregnancy, third trimester

        O10.219 Pre-existing hypertensive chronic kidney disease complicating pregnancy, unspecified trimester

    O10.22 Pre-existing hypertensive chronic kidney disease complicating childbirth

    O10.23 Pre-existing hypertensive chronic kidney disease complicating the puerperium

● **O10.3 Pre-existing hypertensive heart and chronic kidney disease complicating pregnancy, childbirth and the puerperium**

    Any condition in I13 specified as a reason for obstetric care during pregnancy, childbirth or the puerperium

    Use additional code from I13 to identify the type of hypertensive heart and chronic kidney disease

    ● **O10.31 Pre-existing hypertensive heart and chronic kidney disease complicating pregnancy**

        O10.311 Pre-existing hypertensive heart and chronic kidney disease complicating pregnancy, first trimester

        O10.312 Pre-existing hypertensive heart and chronic kidney disease complicating pregnancy, second trimester

        O10.313 Pre-existing hypertensive heart and chronic kidney disease complicating pregnancy, third trimester

        O10.319 Pre-existing hypertensive heart and chronic kidney disease complicating pregnancy, unspecified trimester

    O10.32 Pre-existing hypertensive heart and chronic kidney disease complicating childbirth

    O10.33 Pre-existing hypertensive heart and chronic kidney disease complicating the puerperium

● **O10.4 Pre-existing secondary hypertension complicating pregnancy, childbirth and the puerperium**

    Any condition in I15 specified as a reason for obstetric care during pregnancy, childbirth or the puerperium

    Use additional code from I15 to identify the type of secondary hypertension

    ● **O10.41 Pre-existing secondary hypertension complicating pregnancy**

        O10.411 Pre-existing secondary hypertension complicating pregnancy, first trimester

        O10.412 Pre-existing secondary hypertension complicating pregnancy, second trimester

        O10.413 Pre-existing secondary hypertension complicating pregnancy, third trimester

        O10.419 Pre-existing secondary hypertension complicating pregnancy, unspecified trimester

---

O10.42　Pre-existing secondary hypertension complicating childbirth

O10.43　Pre-existing secondary hypertension complicating the puerperium

● O10.9　Unspecified pre-existing hypertension complicating pregnancy, childbirth and the puerperium

　● O10.91　Unspecified pre-existing hypertension complicating pregnancy

　　　O10.911　Unspecified pre-existing hypertension complicating pregnancy, first trimester

　　　O10.912　Unspecified pre-existing hypertension complicating pregnancy, second trimester

　　　O10.913　Unspecified pre-existing hypertension complicating pregnancy, third trimester

　　　O10.919　Unspecified pre-existing hypertension complicating pregnancy, unspecified trimester

　　O10.92　Unspecified pre-existing hypertension complicating childbirth

　　O10.93　Unspecified pre-existing hypertension complicating the puerperium

● O11　Pre-existing hypertension with pre-eclampsia

　Includes　conditions in O10 complicated by pre-eclampsia pre-eclampsia superimposed pre-existing hypertension

　Use additional code from O10 to identify the type of hypertension

　O11.1　Pre-existing hypertension with pre-eclampsia, first trimester

　O11.2　Pre-existing hypertension with pre-eclampsia, second trimester

　O11.3　Pre-existing hypertension with pre-eclampsia, third trimester

　O11.9　Pre-existing hypertension with pre-eclampsia, unspecified trimester

● O12　Gestational [pregnancy-induced] edema and proteinuria without hypertension

　● O12.0　Gestational edema

　　　O12.00　Gestational edema, unspecified trimester

　　　O12.01　Gestational edema, first trimester

　　　O12.02　Gestational edema, second trimester

　　　O12.03　Gestational edema, third trimester

　● O12.1　Gestational proteinuria

　　　O12.10　Gestational proteinuria, unspecified trimester

　　　O12.11　Gestational proteinuria, first trimester

　　　O12.12　Gestational proteinuria, second trimester

　　　O12.13　Gestational proteinuria, third trimester

　● O12.2　Gestational edema with proteinuria

　　　O12.20　Gestational edema with proteinuria, unspecified trimester

　　　O12.21　Gestational edema with proteinuria, first trimester

　　　O12.22　Gestational edema with proteinuria, second trimester

　　　O12.23　Gestational edema with proteinuria, third trimester

● O13　Gestational [pregnancy-induced] hypertension without significant proteinuria

　Includes　gestational hypertension NOS

　O13.1　Gestational [pregnancy-induced] hypertension without significant proteinuria, first trimester

　O13.2　Gestational [pregnancy-induced] hypertension without significant proteinuria, second trimester

　O13.3　Gestational [pregnancy-induced] hypertension without significant proteinuria, third trimester

　O13.9　Gestational [pregnancy-induced] hypertension without significant proteinuria, unspecified trimester

● O14　Pre-eclampsia

　Excludes1　pre-existing hypertension with pre-eclampsia (O11)

　● O14.0　Mild to moderate pre-eclampsia

　　　O14.00　Mild to moderate pre-eclampsia, unspecified trimester

　　　O14.02　Mild to moderate pre-eclampsia, second trimester

　　　O14.03　Mild to moderate pre-eclampsia, third trimester

　● O14.1　Severe pre-eclampsia

　　　Excludes1　HELLP syndrome (O14.2-)

　　　H=hemolysis, EL=elevated liver enzymes, LP=low platelet count

　　　O14.10　Severe pre-eclampsia, unspecified trimester

　　　O14.12　Severe pre-eclampsia, second trimester

　　　O14.13　Severe pre-eclampsia, third trimester

　● O14.2　HELLP syndrome

　　　Severe pre-eclampsia with hemolysis, elevated liver enzymes and low platelet count (HELLP)

　　　O14.20　HELLP syndrome (HELLP), unspecified trimester

　　　O14.22　HELLP syndrome (HELLP), second trimester

　　　O14.23　HELLP syndrome (HELLP), third trimester

　● O14.9　Unspecified pre-eclampsia

　　　O14.90　Unspecified pre-eclampsia, unspecified trimester

　　　O14.92　Unspecified pre-eclampsia, second trimester

　　　O14.93　Unspecified pre-eclampsia, third trimester

● O15　Eclampsia

　Includes　convulsions following conditions in O10-O14 and O16

　● O15.0　Eclampsia in pregnancy

　　　O15.00　Eclampsia in pregnancy, unspecified trimester

　　　O15.02　Eclampsia in pregnancy, second trimester

　　　O15.03　Eclampsia in pregnancy, third trimester

　O15.1　Eclampsia in labor

　O15.2　Eclampsia in the puerperium

　O15.9　Eclampsia, unspecified as to time period
　　　Eclampsia NOS

● O16　Unspecified maternal hypertension

　O16.1　Unspecified maternal hypertension, first trimester

　O16.2　Unspecified maternal hypertension, second trimester

　O16.3　Unspecified maternal hypertension, third trimester

　O16.9　Unspecified maternal hypertension, unspecified trimester

OTHER MATERNAL DISORDERS PREDOMINANTLY RELATED TO PREGNANCY (O20-O29)

> **Excludes2**   maternal care related to the fetus and amniotic cavity and possible delivery problems (O30-O48)
> maternal diseases classifiable elsewhere but complicating pregnancy, labor and delivery, and the puerperium (O98-O99)

● **O20** **Hemorrhage in early pregnancy**

> **Includes**   hemorrhage before completion of 20 weeks gestation

> **Excludes1**   pregnancy with abortive outcome (O00-O08)

    O20.0 **Threatened abortion**
        Hemorrhage specified as due to threatened abortion

    O20.8 **Other hemorrhage in early pregnancy**

    O20.9 **Hemorrhage in early pregnancy, unspecified**

● **O21** **Excessive vomiting in pregnancy**

    O21.0 **Mild hyperemesis gravidarum**
        Hyperemesis gravidarum, mild or unspecified, starting before the end of the 20th week of gestation

    O21.1 **Hyperemesis gravidarum with metabolic disturbance**
        Hyperemesis gravidarum, starting before the end of the 20th week of gestation, with metabolic disturbance such as carbohydrate depletion
        Hyperemesis gravidarum, starting before the end of the 20th week of gestation, with metabolic disturbance such as dehydration
        Hyperemesis gravidarum, starting before the end of the 20th week of gestation, with metabolic disturbance such as electrolyte imbalance

    O21.2 **Late vomiting of pregnancy**
        Excessive vomiting starting after 20 completed weeks of gestation

    O21.8 **Other vomiting complicating pregnancy**
        Vomiting due to diseases classified elsewhere, complicating pregnancy

>   Use additional code, to identify cause

    O21.9 **Vomiting of pregnancy, unspecified**

● **O22** **Venous complications and hemorrhoids in pregnancy**

> **Excludes1**   venous complications of:
>   abortion NOS (O03.9)
>   ectopic or molar pregnancy (O08.7)
>   failed attempted abortion (O07.35)
>   induced abortion (O04.85)
>   spontaneous abortion (O03.89)

> **Excludes2**   obstetric pulmonary embolism (O88.-)
> venous complications and hemorrhoids of childbirth and the puerperium (O87.-)

  ● **O22.0** **Varicose veins of lower extremity in pregnancy**
        Varicose veins NOS in pregnancy

        O22.00 **Varicose veins of lower extremity in pregnancy, unspecified trimester**

        O22.01 **Varicose veins of lower extremity in pregnancy, first trimester**

        O22.02 **Varicose veins of lower extremity in pregnancy, second trimester**

        O22.03 **Varicose veins of lower extremity in pregnancy, third trimester**

● **O22.1** **Genital varices in pregnancy**
    Perineal varices in pregnancy
    Vaginal varices in pregnancy
    Vulval varices in pregnancy

    O22.10 **Genital varices in pregnancy, unspecified trimester**

    O22.11 **Genital varices in pregnancy, first trimester**

    O22.12 **Genital varices in pregnancy, second trimester**

    O22.13 **Genital varices in pregnancy, third trimester**

● **O22.2** **Superficial thrombophlebitis in pregnancy**
    Phlebitis in pregnancy NOS
    Thrombophlebitis of legs in pregnancy
    Thrombosis in pregnancy NOS

>   Use additional code to identify the superficial thrombophlebitis (I80.0-)

    O22.20 **Superficial thrombophlebitis in pregnancy, unspecified trimester**

    O22.21 **Superficial thrombophlebitis in pregnancy, first trimester**

    O22.22 **Superficial thrombophlebitis in pregnancy, second trimester**

    O22.23 **Superficial thrombophlebitis in pregnancy, third trimester**

● **O22.3** **Deep phlebothrombosis in pregnancy**
    Deep vein thrombosis, antepartum

>   Use additional code to identify the deep vein thrombosis (I82.4-, I82.5-, I82.62-. I82.72-)

>   Use additional code, if applicable, for associated long-term (current) use of anticoagulants (Z79.01)

    O22.30 **Deep phlebothrombosis in pregnancy, unspecified trimester**

    O22.31 **Deep phlebothrombosis in pregnancy, first trimester**

    O22.32 **Deep phlebothrombosis in pregnancy, second trimester**

    O22.33 **Deep phlebothrombosis in pregnancy, third trimester**

● **O22.4** **Hemorrhoids in pregnancy**

    O22.40 **Hemorrhoids in pregnancy, unspecified trimester**

    O22.41 **Hemorrhoids in pregnancy, first trimester**

    O22.42 **Hemorrhoids in pregnancy, second trimester**

    O22.43 **Hemorrhoids in pregnancy, third trimester**

● **O22.5** **Cerebral venous thrombosis in pregnancy**
    Cerebrovenous sinus thrombosis in pregnancy

    O22.50 **Cerebral venous thrombosis in pregnancy, unspecified trimester**

    O22.51 **Cerebral venous thrombosis in pregnancy, first trimester**

    O22.52 **Cerebral venous thrombosis in pregnancy, second trimester**

    O22.53 **Cerebral venous thrombosis in pregnancy, third trimester**

● **O22.8** **Other venous complications in pregnancy**

  ● **O22.8X** **Other venous complications in pregnancy**

        O22.8X1 **Other venous complications in pregnancy, first trimester**

        O22.8X2 **Other venous complications in pregnancy, second trimester**

        O22.8X3 **Other venous complications in pregnancy, third trimester**

        O22.8X9 **Other venous complications in pregnancy, unspecified trimester**

CHAPTER 15 (O00-O9A)

● **O22.9**   **Venous complication in pregnancy, unspecified**
      Gestational phlebitis NOS
      Gestational phlebopathy NOS
      Gestational thrombosis NOS

    O22.90   Venous complication in pregnancy, unspecified, unspecified trimester

    O22.91   Venous complication in pregnancy, unspecified, first trimester

    O22.92   Venous complication in pregnancy, unspecified, second trimester

    O22.93   Venous complication in pregnancy, unspecified, third trimester

● **O23**   **Infections of genitourinary tract in pregnancy**
    Use additional code to identify organism (B95.-, B96.-)

    Excludes2   gonococcal infections complicating pregnancy, childbirth and the puerperium (O98.2)
                 infections with a predominantly sexual mode of transmission NOS complicating pregnancy, childbirth and the puerperium (O98.3)
                 syphilis complicating pregnancy, childbirth and the puerperium (O98.1)
                 tuberculosis of genitourinary system complicating pregnancy, childbirth and the puerperium (O98.0)
                 venereal disease NOS complicating pregnancy, childbirth and the puerperium (O98.3)

● **O23.0**   **Infections of kidney in pregnancy**
    Pyelonephritis in pregnancy

    O23.00   Infections of kidney in pregnancy, unspecified trimester

    O23.01   Infections of kidney in pregnancy, first trimester

    O23.02   Infections of kidney in pregnancy, second trimester

    O23.03   Infections of kidney in pregnancy, third trimester

● **O23.1**   **Infections of bladder in pregnancy**

    O23.10   Infections of bladder in pregnancy, unspecified trimester

    O23.11   Infections of bladder in pregnancy, first trimester

    O23.12   Infections of bladder in pregnancy, second trimester

    O23.13   Infections of bladder in pregnancy, third trimester

● **O23.2**   **Infections of urethra in pregnancy**

    O23.20   Infections of urethra in pregnancy, unspecified trimester

    O23.21   Infections of urethra in pregnancy, first trimester

    O23.22   Infections of urethra in pregnancy, second trimester

    O23.23   Infections of urethra in pregnancy, third trimester

● **O23.3**   **Infections of other parts of urinary tract in pregnancy**

    O23.30   Infections of other parts of urinary tract in pregnancy, unspecified trimester

    O23.31   Infections of other parts of urinary tract in pregnancy, first trimester

    O23.32   Infections of other parts of urinary tract in pregnancy, second trimester

    O23.33   Infections of other parts of urinary tract in pregnancy, third trimester

● **O23.4**   **Unspecified infection of urinary tract in pregnancy**

    O23.40   Unspecified infection of urinary tract in pregnancy, unspecified trimester

    O23.41   Unspecified infection of urinary tract in pregnancy, first trimester

    O23.42   Unspecified infection of urinary tract in pregnancy, second trimester

    O23.43   Unspecified infection of urinary tract in pregnancy, third trimester

● **O23.5**   **Infections of the genital tract in pregnancy**

  ● **O23.51**   **Infection of cervix in pregnancy**

    O23.511   Infections of cervix in pregnancy, first trimester

    O23.512   Infections of cervix in pregnancy, second trimester

    O23.513   Infections of cervix in pregnancy, third trimester

    O23.519   Infections of cervix in pregnancy, unspecified trimester

  ● **O23.52**   **Salpingo-oophoritis in pregnancy**
    Oophoritis = inflammation of ovary
    Salpingitis = inflammation of fallopian tube
    Oophoritis in pregnancy
    Salpingitis in pregnancy

    O23.521   Salpingo-oophoritis in pregnancy, first trimester

    O23.522   Salpingo-oophoritis in pregnancy, second trimester

    O23.523   Salpingo-oophoritis in pregnancy, third trimester

    O23.529   Salpingo-oophoritis in pregnancy, unspecified trimester

  ● **O23.59**   **Infection of other part of genital tract in pregnancy**

    O23.591   Infection of other part of genital tract in pregnancy, first trimester

    O23.592   Infection of other part of genital tract in pregnancy, second trimester

    O23.593   Infection of other part of genital tract in pregnancy, third trimester

    O23.599   Infection of other part of genital tract in pregnancy, unspecified trimester

● **O23.9**   **Unspecified genitourinary tract infection in pregnancy**
    Genitourinary tract infection in pregnancy NOS

    O23.90   Unspecified genitourinary tract infection in pregnancy, unspecified trimester

    O23.91   Unspecified genitourinary tract infection in pregnancy, first trimester

    O23.92   Unspecified genitourinary tract infection in pregnancy, second trimester

    O23.93   Unspecified genitourinary tract infection in pregnancy, third trimester

CHAPTER 15 (O00-O9A)

OGCR Section I.C.15.g.

g. Diabetes mellitus in pregnancy

Diabetes mellitus is a significant complicating factor in pregnancy. Pregnant women who are diabetic should be assigned a code from category O24, Diabetes mellitus in pregnancy, childbirth, and the puerperium, first, followed by the appropriate diabetes code(s) (E08-E13) from Chapter 4.

OGCR Section I.C.15.i.

i. Gestational (pregnancy induced) diabetes

Gestational (pregnancy induced) diabetes can occur during the second and third trimester of pregnancy in women who were not diabetic prior to pregnancy. Gestational diabetes can cause complications in the pregnancy similar to those of pre-existing diabetes mellitus. It also puts the woman at greater risk of developing diabetes after the pregnancy. Codes for gestational diabetes are in subcategory O24.4, Gestational diabetes mellitus. No other code from category O24, Diabetes mellitus in pregnancy, childbirth, and the puerperium, should be used with a code from O24.4

The codes under subcategory O24.4 include diet controlled and insulin controlled. If a patient with gestational diabetes is treated with both diet and insulin is treated with both diet and insulin, only the code for insulin-controlled is required. Code Z79.4, Long-term (current) use of insulin, should not be assigned with codes from subcategory O24.4.

An abnormal glucose tolerance in pregnancy is assigned a code from subcategory O99.81, Abnormal glucose complicating pregnancy, childbirth, and the puerperium.

- ● **O24   Diabetes mellitus in pregnancy, childbirth, and the puerperium**
  - ● **O24.0   Pre-existing diabetes mellitus, type 1, in pregnancy, childbirth and the puerperium**
    Juvenile onset diabetes mellitus, in pregnancy, childbirth and the puerperium
    Ketosis-prone diabetes mellitus in pregnancy, childbirth and the puerperium
    Use additional code from category E10 to further identify any manifestations
    - ● **O24.01   Pre-existing diabetes mellitus, type 1, in pregnancy**
      - **O24.011   Pre-existing diabetes mellitus, type 1, in pregnancy, first trimester**
      - **O24.012   Pre-existing diabetes mellitus, type 1, in pregnancy, second trimester**
      - **O24.013   Pre-existing diabetes mellitus, type 1, in pregnancy, third trimester**
      - **O24.019   Pre-existing diabetes mellitus, type 1, in pregnancy, unspecified trimester**
    - **O24.02   Pre-existing diabetes mellitus, type 1, in childbirth**
    - **O24.03   Pre-existing diabetes mellitus, type 1, in the puerperium**
  - ● **O24.1   Pre-existing diabetes mellitus, type 2, in pregnancy, childbirth and the puerperium**
    Insulin-resistant diabetes mellitus in pregnancy, childbirth and the puerperium
    Use additional code (for):
    from category E11 to further identify any manifestations
    long-term (current) use of insulin (Z79.4)
    - ● **O24.11   Pre-existing diabetes mellitus, type 2, in pregnancy**
      - **O24.111   Pre-existing diabetes mellitus, type 2, in pregnancy, first trimester**
      - **O24.112   Pre-existing diabetes mellitus, type 2, in pregnancy, second trimester**
      - **O24.113   Pre-existing diabetes mellitus, type 2, in pregnancy, third trimester**
      - **O24.119   Pre-existing diabetes mellitus, type 2, in pregnancy, unspecified trimester**

  - **O24.12   Pre-existing diabetes mellitus, type 2, in childbirth**
  - **O24.13   Pre-existing diabetes mellitus, type 2, in the puerperium**
  - ● **O24.3   Unspecified pre-existing diabetes mellitus in pregnancy, childbirth and the puerperium**
    Use additional code (for):
    from category E11 to further identify any manifestation
    long-term (current) use of insulin (Z79.4)
    - ● **O24.31   Unspecified pre-existing diabetes mellitus in pregnancy**
      - **O24.311   Unspecified pre-existing diabetes mellitus in pregnancy, first trimester**
      - **O24.312   Unspecified pre-existing diabetes mellitus in pregnancy, second trimester**
      - **O24.313   Unspecified pre-existing diabetes mellitus in pregnancy, third trimester**
      - **O24.319   Unspecified pre-existing diabetes mellitus in pregnancy, unspecified trimester**
    - **O24.32   Unspecified pre-existing diabetes mellitus in childbirth**
    - **O24.33   Unspecified pre-existing diabetes mellitus in the puerperium**
  - ● **O24.4   Gestational diabetes mellitus**
    Diabetes mellitus arising in pregnancy
    Gestational diabetes mellitus NOS
    - ● **O24.41   Gestational diabetes mellitus in pregnancy**
      - **O24.410   Gestational diabetes mellitus in pregnancy, diet controlled**
      - **O24.414   Gestational diabetes mellitus in pregnancy, insulin controlled**
      - **O24.419   Gestational diabetes mellitus in pregnancy, unspecified control**
    - ● **O24.42   Gestational diabetes mellitus in childbirth**
      - **O24.420   Gestational diabetes mellitus in childbirth, diet controlled**
      - **O24.424   Gestational diabetes mellitus in childbirth, insulin controlled**
      - **O24.429   Gestational diabetes mellitus in childbirth, unspecified control**
    - ● **O24.43   Gestational diabetes mellitus in the puerperium**
      - **O24.430   Gestational diabetes mellitus in the puerperium, diet controlled**
      - **O24.434   Gestational diabetes mellitus in the puerperium, insulin controlled**
      - **O24.439   Gestational diabetes mellitus in the puerperium, unspecified control**
  - ● **O24.8   Other pre-existing diabetes mellitus in pregnancy, childbirth, and the puerperium**
    Use additional code (for):
    from categories E08, E09 and E13 to further identify any manifestation
    long-term (current) use of insulin (Z79.4)
    - ● **O24.81   Other pre-existing diabetes mellitus in pregnancy**
      - **O24.811   Other pre-existing diabetes mellitus in pregnancy, first trimester**
      - **O24.812   Other pre-existing diabetes mellitus in pregnancy, second trimester**
      - **O24.813   Other pre-existing diabetes mellitus in pregnancy, third trimester**
      - **O24.819   Other pre-existing diabetes mellitus in pregnancy, unspecified trimester**

◀ New   ◀▥ Revised   ~~deleted~~ Deleted   **OGCR** Official Guidelines   X Assign placeholder X   ● Use Additional Character(s)

Excludes 1   Excludes 2   Includes   Use additional   Code first   Code also   Unspecified

O24.82   Other pre-existing diabetes mellitus in childbirth

O24.83   Other pre-existing diabetes mellitus in the puerperium

● O24.9   Unspecified diabetes mellitus in pregnancy, childbirth and the puerperium

> Use additional code for long-term (current) use of insulin (Z79.4)
>
> *Unknown whether patient was diabetic before pregnancy occurred*

   ● O24.91   Unspecified diabetes mellitus in pregnancy

     O24.911   Unspecified diabetes mellitus in pregnancy, first trimester

     O24.912   Unspecified diabetes mellitus in pregnancy, second trimester

     O24.913   Unspecified diabetes mellitus in pregnancy, third trimester

     O24.919   Unspecified diabetes mellitus in pregnancy, unspecified trimester

   O24.92   Unspecified diabetes mellitus in childbirth

   O24.93   Unspecified diabetes mellitus in the puerperium

● O25   Malnutrition in pregnancy, childbirth and the puerperium

   ● O25.1   Malnutrition in pregnancy

     O25.10   Malnutrition in pregnancy, unspecified trimester

     O25.11   Malnutrition in pregnancy, first trimester

     O25.12   Malnutrition in pregnancy, second trimester

     O25.13   Malnutrition in pregnancy, third trimester

   O25.2   Malnutrition in childbirth

   O25.3   Malnutrition in the puerperium

● O26   Maternal care for other conditions predominantly related to pregnancy

   ● O26.0   Excessive weight gain in pregnancy

> Excludes2   gestational edema (O12.0, O12.2)

     O26.00   Excessive weight gain in pregnancy, unspecified trimester

     O26.01   Excessive weight gain in pregnancy, first trimester

     O26.02   Excessive weight gain in pregnancy, second trimester

     O26.03   Excessive weight gain in pregnancy, third trimester

   ● O26.1   Low weight gain in pregnancy

     O26.10   Low weight gain in pregnancy, unspecified trimester

     O26.11   Low weight gain in pregnancy, first trimester

     O26.12   Low weight gain in pregnancy, second trimester

     O26.13   Low weight gain in pregnancy, third trimester

   ● O26.2   Pregnancy care for patient with recurrent pregnancy loss

     O26.20   Pregnancy care for patient with recurrent pregnancy loss, unspecified trimester

     O26.21   Pregnancy care for patient with recurrent pregnancy loss, first trimester

     O26.22   Pregnancy care for patient with recurrent pregnancy loss, second trimester

     O26.23   Pregnancy care for patient with recurrent pregnancy loss, third trimester

● O26.3   Retained intrauterine contraceptive device in pregnancy

   O26.30   Retained intrauterine contraceptive device in pregnancy, unspecified trimester

   O26.31   Retained intrauterine contraceptive device in pregnancy, first trimester

   O26.32   Retained intrauterine contraceptive device in pregnancy, second trimester

   O26.33   Retained intrauterine contraceptive device in pregnancy, third trimester

● O26.4   Herpes gestationis

   O26.40   Herpes gestationis, unspecified trimester

   O26.41   Herpes gestationis, first trimester

   O26.42   Herpes gestationis, second trimester

   O26.43   Herpes gestationis, third trimester

● O26.5   Maternal hypotension syndrome

   Supine hypotensive syndrome

   O26.50   Maternal hypotension syndrome, unspecified trimester

   O26.51   Maternal hypotension syndrome, first trimester

   O26.52   Maternal hypotension syndrome, second trimester

   O26.53   Maternal hypotension syndrome, third trimester

● O26.6   Liver and biliary tract disorders in pregnancy, childbirth and the puerperium

> Use additional code to identify the specific disorder
>
> Excludes2   hepatorenal syndrome following labor and delivery (O90.4)

   ● O26.61   Liver and biliary tract disorders in pregnancy

     O26.611   Liver and biliary tract disorders in pregnancy, first trimester

     O26.612   Liver and biliary tract disorders in pregnancy, second trimester

     O26.613   Liver and biliary tract disorders in pregnancy, third trimester

     O26.619   Liver and biliary tract disorders in pregnancy, unspecified trimester

   O26.62   Liver and biliary tract disorders in childbirth

   O26.63   Liver and biliary tract disorders in the puerperium

● O26.7   Subluxation of symphysis (pubis) in pregnancy, childbirth and the puerperium

> Excludes1   traumatic separation of symphysis (pubis) during childbirth (O71.6)

   ● O26.71   Subluxation of symphysis (pubis) in pregnancy

     O26.711   Subluxation of symphysis (pubis) in pregnancy, first trimester

     O26.712   Subluxation of symphysis (pubis) in pregnancy, second trimester

     O26.713   Subluxation of symphysis (pubis) in pregnancy, third trimester

     O26.719   Subluxation of symphysis (pubis) in pregnancy, unspecified trimester

   O26.72   Subluxation of symphysis (pubis) in childbirth

   O26.73   Subluxation of symphysis (pubis) in the puerperium

● O26.8   Other specified pregnancy related conditions

   ● O26.81   Pregnancy related exhaustion and fatigue

     O26.811   Pregnancy related exhaustion and fatigue, first trimester

     O26.812   Pregnancy related exhaustion and fatigue, second trimester

     O26.813   Pregnancy related exhaustion and fatigue, third trimester

     O26.819   Pregnancy related exhaustion and fatigue, unspecified trimester

● **O26.82 Pregnancy related peripheral neuritis**

    O26.821 Pregnancy related peripheral neuritis, first trimester

    O26.822 Pregnancy related peripheral neuritis, second trimester

    O26.823 Pregnancy related peripheral neuritis, third trimester

    O26.829 Pregnancy related peripheral neuritis, unspecified trimester

● **O26.83 Pregnancy related renal disease**

    Use additional code to identify the specific disorder

    O26.831 Pregnancy related renal disease, first trimester

    O26.832 Pregnancy related renal disease, second trimester

    O26.833 Pregnancy related renal disease, third trimester

    O26.839 Pregnancy related renal disease, unspecified trimester

● **O26.84 Uterine size-date discrepancy complicating pregnancy**

    Excludes1 encounter for suspected problem with fetal growth ruled out (Z03.74)

    O26.841 Uterine size-date discrepancy, first trimester

    O26.842 Uterine size-date discrepancy, second trimester

    O26.843 Uterine size-date discrepancy, third trimester

    O26.849 Uterine size-date discrepancy, unspecified trimester

● **O26.85 Spotting complicating pregnancy**

    O26.851 Spotting complicating pregnancy, first trimester

    O26.852 Spotting complicating pregnancy, second trimester

    O26.853 Spotting complicating pregnancy, third trimester

    O26.859 Spotting complicating pregnancy, unspecified trimester

O26.86 Pruritic urticarial papules and plaques of pregnancy (PUPPP)

    Polymorphic eruption of pregnancy

● **O26.87 Cervical shortening**

    Excludes1 encounter for suspected cervical shortening ruled out (Z03.75)

    O26.872 Cervical shortening, second trimester

    O26.873 Cervical shortening, third trimester

    O26.879 Cervical shortening, unspecified trimester

● **O26.89 Other specified pregnancy related conditions**

    O26.891 Other specified pregnancy related conditions, first trimester

    O26.892 Other specified pregnancy related conditions, second trimester

    O26.893 Other specified pregnancy related conditions, third trimester

    O26.899 Other specified pregnancy related conditions, unspecified trimester

● **O26.9 Pregnancy related conditions, unspecified**

    O26.90 Pregnancy related conditions, unspecified, unspecified trimester

    O26.91 Pregnancy related conditions, unspecified, first trimester

    O26.92 Pregnancy related conditions, unspecified, second trimester

    O26.93 Pregnancy related conditions, unspecified, third trimester

● **O28 Abnormal findings on antenatal screening of mother**

    Excludes1 diagnostic findings classified elsewhere - see Alphabetical Index

    O28.0 Abnormal hematological finding on antenatal screening of mother

    O28.1 Abnormal biochemical finding on antenatal screening of mother

    O28.2 Abnormal cytological finding on antenatal screening of mother

    O28.3 Abnormal ultrasonic finding on antenatal screening of mother

    O28.4 Abnormal radiological finding on antenatal screening of mother

    O28.5 Abnormal chromosomal and genetic finding on antenatal screening of mother

    O28.8 Other abnormal findings on antenatal screening of mother

    O28.9 Unspecified abnormal findings on antenatal screening of mother

● **O29 Complications of anesthesia during pregnancy**

    Includes maternal complications arising from the administration of a general, regional or local anesthetic, analgesic or other sedation during pregnancy

    Use additional code, if necessary, to identify the complication

    Excludes2 complications of anesthesia during labor and delivery (O74.-)

    complications of anesthesia during the puerperium (O89.-)

  ● **O29.0 Pulmonary complications of anesthesia during pregnancy**

    ● **O29.01 Aspiration pneumonitis due to anesthesia during pregnancy**

      Inhalation of stomach contents or secretions NOS due to anesthesia during pregnancy

      Mendelson's syndrome due to anesthesia during pregnancy

      O29.011 Aspiration pneumonitis due to anesthesia during pregnancy, first trimester

      O29.012 Aspiration pneumonitis due to anesthesia during pregnancy, second trimester

      O29.013 Aspiration pneumonitis due to anesthesia during pregnancy, third trimester

      O29.019 Aspiration pneumonitis due to anesthesia during pregnancy, unspecified trimester

CHAPTER 15 (O00-O9A)

● O29.02   Pressure collapse of lung due to anesthesia during pregnancy

     O29.021   Pressure collapse of lung due to anesthesia during pregnancy, first trimester

     O29.022   Pressure collapse of lung due to anesthesia during pregnancy, second trimester

     O29.023   Pressure collapse of lung due to anesthesia during pregnancy, third trimester

     O29.029   Pressure collapse of lung due to anesthesia during pregnancy, unspecified trimester

● O29.09   Other pulmonary complications of anesthesia during pregnancy

     O29.091   Other pulmonary complications of anesthesia during pregnancy, first trimester

     O29.092   Other pulmonary complications of anesthesia during pregnancy, second trimester

     O29.093   Other pulmonary complications of anesthesia during pregnancy, third trimester

     O29.099   Other pulmonary complications of anesthesia during pregnancy, unspecified trimester

● O29.1   Cardiac complications of anesthesia during pregnancy

   ● O29.11   Cardiac arrest due to anesthesia during pregnancy

     O29.111   Cardiac arrest due to anesthesia during pregnancy, first trimester

     O29.112   Cardiac arrest due to anesthesia during pregnancy, second trimester

     O29.113   Cardiac arrest due to anesthesia during pregnancy, third trimester

     O29.119   Cardiac arrest due to anesthesia during pregnancy, unspecified trimester

   ● O29.12   Cardiac failure due to anesthesia during pregnancy

     O29.121   Cardiac failure due to anesthesia during pregnancy, first trimester

     O29.122   Cardiac failure due to anesthesia during pregnancy, second trimester

     O29.123   Cardiac failure due to anesthesia during pregnancy, third trimester

     O29.129   Cardiac failure due to anesthesia during pregnancy, unspecified trimester

   ● O29.19   Other cardiac complications of anesthesia during pregnancy

     O29.191   Other cardiac complications of anesthesia during pregnancy, first trimester

     O29.192   Other cardiac complications of anesthesia during pregnancy, second trimester

     O29.193   Other cardiac complications of anesthesia during pregnancy, third trimester

     O29.199   Other cardiac complications of anesthesia during pregnancy, unspecified trimester

● O29.2   Central nervous system complications of anesthesia during pregnancy

   ● O29.21   Cerebral anoxia due to anesthesia during pregnancy

     O29.211   Cerebral anoxia due to anesthesia during pregnancy, first trimester

     O29.212   Cerebral anoxia due to anesthesia during pregnancy, second trimester

     O29.213   Cerebral anoxia due to anesthesia during pregnancy, third trimester

     O29.219   Cerebral anoxia due to anesthesia during pregnancy, unspecified trimester

   ● O29.29   Other central nervous system complications of anesthesia during pregnancy

     O29.291   Other central nervous system complications of anesthesia during pregnancy, first trimester

     O29.292   Other central nervous system complications of anesthesia during pregnancy, second trimester

     O29.293   Other central nervous system complications of anesthesia during pregnancy, third trimester

     O29.299   Other central nervous system complications of anesthesia during pregnancy, unspecified trimester

● O29.3   Toxic reaction to local anesthesia during pregnancy

   ● O29.3X   Toxic reaction to local anesthesia during pregnancy

     O29.3X1   Toxic reaction to local anesthesia during pregnancy, first trimester

     O29.3X2   Toxic reaction to local anesthesia during pregnancy, second trimester

     O29.3X3   Toxic reaction to local anesthesia during pregnancy, third trimester

     O29.3X9   Toxic reaction to local anesthesia during pregnancy, unspecified trimester

● O29.4   Spinal and epidural anesthesia induced headache during pregnancy

     O29.40   Spinal and epidural anesthesia induced headache during pregnancy, unspecified trimester

     O29.41   Spinal and epidural anesthesia induced headache during pregnancy, first trimester

     O29.42   Spinal and epidural anesthesia induced headache during pregnancy, second trimester

     O29.43   Spinal and epidural anesthesia induced headache during pregnancy, third trimester

● O29.5   Other complications of spinal and epidural anesthesia during pregnancy

   ● O29.5X   Other complications of spinal and epidural anesthesia during pregnancy

     O29.5X1   Other complications of spinal and epidural anesthesia during pregnancy, first trimester

     O29.5X2   Other complications of spinal and epidural anesthesia during pregnancy, second trimester

     O29.5X3   Other complications of spinal and epidural anesthesia during pregnancy, third trimester

     O29.5X9   Other complications of spinal and epidural anesthesia during pregnancy, unspecified trimester

◀ New   ◀▥ Revised   ~~deleted~~ Deleted   **OGCR** Official Guidelines   X Assign placeholder X   ● Use Additional Character(s)

Excludes 1   Excludes 2   Includes   Use additional   Code first   Code also   Unspecified

● O29.6   Failed or difficult intubation for anesthesia during pregnancy

     O29.60   Failed or difficult intubation for anesthesia during pregnancy, unspecified trimester

     O29.61   Failed or difficult intubation for anesthesia during pregnancy, first trimester

     O29.62   Failed or difficult intubation for anesthesia during pregnancy, second trimester

     O29.63   Failed or difficult intubation for anesthesia during pregnancy, third trimester

● O29.8   Other complications of anesthesia during pregnancy

    ● O29.8X   Other complications of anesthesia during pregnancy

     O29.8X1   Other complications of anesthesia during pregnancy, first trimester

     O29.8X2   Other complications of anesthesia during pregnancy, second trimester

     O29.8X3   Other complications of anesthesia during pregnancy, third trimester

     O29.8X9   Other complications of anesthesia during pregnancy, unspecified trimester

● O29.9   Unspecified complication of anesthesia during pregnancy

     O29.90   Unspecified complication of anesthesia during pregnancy, unspecified trimester

     O29.91   Unspecified complication of anesthesia during pregnancy, first trimester

     O29.92   Unspecified complication of anesthesia during pregnancy, second trimester

     O29.93   Unspecified complication of anesthesia during pregnancy, third trimester

---

MATERNAL CARE RELATED TO THE FETUS AND AMNIOTIC CAVITY AND POSSIBLE DELIVERY PROBLEMS (O30-O48)

● O30   Multiple gestation

    Code also any complications specific to multiple gestation

    ● O30.0   Twin pregnancy

     ● O30.00   Twin pregnancy, unspecified number of placenta and unspecified number of amniotic sacs

     O30.001   Twin pregnancy, unspecified number of placenta and unspecified number of amniotic sacs, first trimester

     O30.002   Twin pregnancy, unspecified number of placenta and unspecified number of amniotic sacs, second trimester

     O30.003   Twin pregnancy, unspecified number of placenta and unspecified number of amniotic sacs, third trimester

     O30.009   Twin pregnancy, unspecified number of placenta and unspecified number of amniotic sacs, unspecified trimester

     ● O30.01   Twin pregnancy, monochorionic/monoamniotic

     Twin pregnancy, one placenta, one amniotic sac

     | **Excludes1** | conjoined twins (O30.02-) |

     O30.011   Twin pregnancy, monochorionic/monoamniotic, first trimester

     O30.012   Twin pregnancy, monochorionic/monoamniotic, second trimester

     O30.013   Twin pregnancy, monochorionic/monoamniotic, third trimester

     O30.019   Twin pregnancy, monochorionic/monoamniotic, unspecified trimester

● O30.02   Conjoined twin pregnancy

     O30.021   Conjoined twin pregnancy, first trimester

     O30.022   Conjoined twin pregnancy, second trimester

     O30.023   Conjoined twin pregnancy, third trimester

     O30.029   Conjoined twin pregnancy, unspecified trimester

● O30.03   Twin pregnancy, monochorionic/diamniotic

     Twin pregnancy, one placenta, two amniotic sacs

     O30.031   Twin pregnancy, monochorionic/diamniotic, first trimester

     O30.032   Twin pregnancy, monochorionic/diamniotic, second trimester

     O30.033   Twin pregnancy, monochorionic/diamniotic, third trimester

     O30.039   Twin pregnancy, monochorionic/diamniotic, unspecified trimester

● O30.04   Twin pregnancy, dichorionic/diamniotic

     Twin pregnancy, two placentae, two amniotic sacs

     O30.041   Twin pregnancy, dichorionic/diamniotic, first trimester

     O30.042   Twin pregnancy, dichorionic/diamniotic, second trimester

     O30.043   Twin pregnancy, dichorionic/diamniotic, third trimester

     O30.049   Twin pregnancy, dichorionic/diamniotic, unspecified trimester

● O30.09   Twin pregnancy, unable to determine number of placenta and number of amniotic sacs

     O30.091   Twin pregnancy, unable to determine number of placenta and number of amniotic sacs, first trimester

     O30.092   Twin pregnancy, unable to determine number of placenta and number of amniotic sacs, second trimester

     O30.093   Twin pregnancy, unable to determine number of placenta and number of amniotic sacs, third trimester

     O30.099   Twin pregnancy, unable to determine number of placenta and number of amniotic sacs, unspecified trimester

● O30.1   Triplet pregnancy

    ● O30.10   Triplet pregnancy, unspecified number of placenta and unspecified number of amniotic sacs

     O30.101   Triplet pregnancy, unspecified number of placenta and unspecified number of amniotic sacs, first trimester

     O30.102   Triplet pregnancy, unspecified number of placenta and unspecified number of amniotic sacs, second trimester

     O30.103   Triplet pregnancy, unspecified number of placenta and unspecified number of amniotic sacs, third trimester

     O30.109   Triplet pregnancy, unspecified number of placenta and unspecified number of amniotic sacs, unspecified trimester

---

CHAPTER 15 (O00-O9A)

- ● **O30.11**   Triplet pregnancy with two or more monochorionic fetuses
  - **O30.111**   Triplet pregnancy with two or more monochorionic fetuses, first trimester
  - **O30.112**   Triplet pregnancy with two or more monochorionic fetuses, second trimester
  - **O30.113**   Triplet pregnancy with two or more monochorionic fetuses, third trimester
  - **O30.119**   Triplet pregnancy with two or more monochorionic fetuses, unspecified trimester
- ● **O30.12**   Triplet pregnancy with two or more monoamniotic fetuses
  - **O30.121**   Triplet pregnancy with two or more monoamniotic fetuses, first trimester
  - **O30.122**   Triplet pregnancy with two or more monoamniotic fetuses, second trimester
  - **O30.123**   Triplet pregnancy with two or more monoamniotic fetuses, third trimester
  - **O30.129**   Triplet pregnancy with two or more monoamniotic fetuses, unspecified trimester
- ● **O30.19**   Triplet pregnancy, unable to determine number of placenta and number of amniotic sacs
  - **O30.191**   Triplet pregnancy, unable to determine number of placenta and number of amniotic sacs, first trimester
  - **O30.192**   Triplet pregnancy, unable to determine number of placenta and number of amniotic sacs, second trimester
  - **O30.193**   Triplet pregnancy, unable to determine number of placenta and number of amniotic sacs, third trimester
  - **O30.199**   Triplet pregnancy, unable to determine number of placenta and number of amniotic sacs, unspecified trimester
- ● **O30.2**   Quadruplet pregnancy
  - ● **O30.20**   Quadruplet pregnancy, unspecified number of placenta and unspecified number of amniotic sacs
    - **O30.201**   Quadruplet pregnancy, unspecified number of placenta and unspecified number of amniotic sacs, first trimester
    - **O30.202**   Quadruplet pregnancy, unspecified number of placenta and unspecified number of amniotic sacs, second trimester
    - **O30.203**   Quadruplet pregnancy, unspecified number of placenta and unspecified number of amniotic sacs, third trimester
    - **O30.209**   Quadruplet pregnancy, unspecified number of placenta and unspecified number of amniotic sacs, unspecified trimester

- ● **O30.21**   Quadruplet pregnancy with two or more monochorionic fetuses
  - **O30.211**   Quadruplet pregnancy with two or more monochorionic fetuses, first trimester
  - **O30.212**   Quadruplet pregnancy with two or more monochorionic fetuses, second trimester
  - **O30.213**   Quadruplet pregnancy with two or more monochorionic fetuses, third trimester
  - **O30.219**   Quadruplet pregnancy with two or more monochorionic fetuses, unspecified trimester
- ● **O30.22**   Quadruplet pregnancy with two or more monoamniotic fetuses
  - **O30.221**   Quadruplet pregnancy with two or more monoamniotic fetuses, first trimester
  - **O30.222**   Quadruplet pregnancy with two or more monoamniotic fetuses, second trimester
  - **O30.223**   Quadruplet pregnancy with two or more monoamniotic fetuses, third trimester
  - **O30.229**   Quadruplet pregnancy with two or more monoamniotic fetuses, unspecified trimester
- ● **O30.29**   Quadruplet pregnancy, unable to determine number of placenta and number of amniotic sacs
  - **O30.291**   Quadruplet pregnancy, unable to determine number of placenta and number of amniotic sacs, first trimester
  - **O30.292**   Quadruplet pregnancy, unable to determine number of placenta and number of amniotic sacs, second trimester
  - **O30.293**   Quadruplet pregnancy, unable to determine number of placenta and number of amniotic sacs, third trimester
  - **O30.299**   Quadruplet pregnancy, unable to determine number of placenta and number of amniotic sacs, unspecified trimester
- ● **O30.8**   Other specified multiple gestation
  Multiple gestation pregnancy greater then quadruplets
  - ● **O30.80**   Other specified multiple gestation, unspecified number of placenta and unspecified number of amniotic sacs
    - **O30.801**   Other specified multiple gestation, unspecified number of placenta and unspecified number of amniotic sacs, first trimester
    - **O30.802**   Other specified multiple gestation, unspecified number of placenta and unspecified number of amniotic sacs, second trimester
    - **O30.803**   Other specified multiple gestation, unspecified number of placenta and unspecified number of amniotic sacs, third trimester
    - **O30.809**   Other specified multiple gestation, unspecified number of placenta and unspecified number of amniotic sacs, unspecified trimester

◀ New   ◀ Revised   ~~deleted~~ Deleted   OGCR Official Guidelines   X Assign placeholder X   ● Use Additional Character(s)

Excludes 1   Excludes 2   Includes   Use additional   Code first   Code also   Unspecified

● O30.81　Other specified multiple gestation with two or more monochorionic fetuses

　　　O30.811　Other specified multiple gestation with two or more monochorionic fetuses, first trimester

　　　O30.812　Other specified multiple gestation with two or more monochorionic fetuses, second trimester

　　　O30.813　Other specified multiple gestation with two or more monochorionic fetuses, third trimester

　　　O30.819　Other specified multiple gestation with two or more monochorionic fetuses, unspecified trimester

● O30.82　Other specified multiple gestation with two or more monoamniotic fetuses

　　　O30.821　Other specified multiple gestation with two or more monoamniotic fetuses, first trimester

　　　O30.822　Other specified multiple gestation with two or more monoamniotic fetuses, second trimester

　　　O30.823　Other specified multiple gestation with two or more monoamniotic fetuses, third trimester

　　　O30.829　Other specified multiple gestation with two or more monoamniotic fetuses, unspecified trimester

● O30.89　Other specified multiple gestation, unable to determine number of placenta and number of amniotic sacs

　　　O30.891　Other specified multiple gestation, unable to determine number of placenta and number of amniotic sacs, first trimester

　　　O30.892　Other specified multiple gestation, unable to determine number of placenta and number of amniotic sacs, second trimester

　　　O30.893　Other specified multiple gestation, unable to determine number of placenta and number of amniotic sacs, third trimester

　　　O30.899　Other specified multiple gestation, unable to determine number of placenta and number of amniotic sacs, unspecified trimester

● O30.9　Multiple gestation, unspecified
　　　Multiple pregnancy NOS

　　　O30.90　Multiple gestation, unspecified, unspecified trimester

　　　O30.91　Multiple gestation, unspecified, first trimester

　　　O30.92　Multiple gestation, unspecified, second trimester

　　　O30.93　Multiple gestation, unspecified, third trimester

● O31　Complications specific to multiple gestation

　Excludes2　delayed delivery of second twin, triplet, etc. (O63.2)
　　　　　　malpresentation of one fetus or more (O32.9)
　　　　　　placental transfusion syndromes (O43.0-)

One of the following 7th characters is to be assigned to each code under category O31. 7th character 0 is for single gestations and multiple gestations where the fetus is unspecified. 7th characters 1 through 9 are for cases of multiple gestations to identify the fetus for which the code applies. The appropriate code from category O30, Multiple gestation, must also be assigned when assigning a code from category O31 that has a 7th character of 1 through 9.

0	not applicable or unspecified
1	fetus 1
2	fetus 2
3	fetus 3
4	fetus 4
5	fetus 5
9	other fetus

● O31.0　Papyraceous fetus
　　　Fetus compressus

　X ● O31.00　Papyraceous fetus, unspecified trimester

　X ● O31.01　Papyraceous fetus, first trimester

　X ● O31.02　Papyraceous fetus, second trimester

　X ● O31.03　Papyraceous fetus, third trimester

● O31.1　Continuing pregnancy after spontaneous abortion of one fetus or more

　X ● O31.10　Continuing pregnancy after spontaneous abortion of one fetus or more, unspecified trimester

　X ● O31.11　Continuing pregnancy after spontaneous abortion of one fetus or more, first trimester

　X ● O31.12　Continuing pregnancy after spontaneous abortion of one fetus or more, second trimester

　X ● O31.13　Continuing pregnancy after spontaneous abortion of one fetus or more, third trimester

● O31.2　Continuing pregnancy after intrauterine death of one fetus or more

　X ● O31.20　Continuing pregnancy after intrauterine death of one fetus or more, unspecified trimester

　X ● O31.21　Continuing pregnancy after intrauterine death of one fetus or more, first trimester

　X ● O31.22　Continuing pregnancy after intrauterine death of one fetus or more, second trimester

　X ● O31.23　Continuing pregnancy after intrauterine death of one fetus or more, third trimester

● O31.3　Continuing pregnancy after elective fetal reduction of one fetus or more
　　　Continuing pregnancy after selective termination of one fetus or more

　X ● O31.30　Continuing pregnancy after elective fetal reduction of one fetus or more, unspecified trimester

　X ● O31.31　Continuing pregnancy after elective fetal reduction of one fetus or more, first trimester

　X ● O31.32　Continuing pregnancy after elective fetal reduction of one fetus or more, second trimester

　X ● O31.33　Continuing pregnancy after elective fetal reduction of one fetus or more, third trimester

CHAPTER 15 (O00-O9A)

● **O31.8 Other complications specific to multiple gestation**
  ● **O31.8X Other complications specific to multiple gestation**
      ● **O31.8X1 Other complications specific to multiple gestation, first trimester**
      ● **O31.8X2 Other complications specific to multiple gestation, second trimester**
      ● **O31.8X3 Other complications specific to multiple gestation, third trimester**
      ● **O31.8X9 Other complications specific to multiple gestation, unspecified trimester**

● **O32 Maternal care for malpresentation of fetus**

Includes the listed conditions as a reason for observation, hospitalization or other obstetric care of the mother, or for cesarean delivery before onset of labor

Excludes1 malpresentation of fetus with obstructed labor (O64.-)

One of the following 7th characters is to be assigned to each code under category O32. 7th character 0 is for single gestations and multiple gestations where the fetus is unspecified. 7th characters 1 through 9 are for cases of multiple gestations to identify the fetus for which the code applies. The appropriate code from category O30, Multiple gestation, must also be assigned when assigning a code from category O32 that has a 7th character of 1 through 9.

0	not applicable or unspecified
1	fetus 1
2	fetus 2
3	fetus 3
4	fetus 4
5	fetus 5
9	other fetus

X● **O32.0 Maternal care for unstable lie**
X● **O32.1 Maternal care for breech presentation**
      Maternal care for buttocks presentation
      Maternal care for complete breech
      Maternal care for frank breech

Excludes1 footling presentation (O32.8)
              incomplete breech (O32.8)

X● **O32.2 Maternal care for transverse and oblique lie**
      Maternal care for oblique presentation
      Maternal care for transverse presentation
X● **O32.3 Maternal care for face, brow and chin presentation**
X● **O32.4 Maternal care for high head at term**
      Maternal care for failure of head to enter pelvic brim
X● **O32.6 Maternal care for compound presentation**
X● **O32.8 Maternal care for other malpresentation of fetus**
      Maternal care for footling presentation
      Maternal care for incomplete breech
X● **O32.9 Maternal care for malpresentation of fetus, unspecified**

● **O33 Maternal care for disproportion**

Includes the listed conditions as a reason for observation, hospitalization or other obstetric care of the mother, or for cesarean delivery before onset of labor

Excludes1 disproportion with obstructed labor (O65-O66)

O33.0 Maternal care for disproportion due to deformity of maternal pelvic bones
      Maternal care for disproportion due to pelvic deformity causing disproportion NOS
O33.1 Maternal care for disproportion due to generally contracted pelvis
      Maternal care for disproportion due to contracted pelvis NOS causing disproportion
O33.2 Maternal care for disproportion due to inlet contraction of pelvis
      Maternal care for disproportion due to inlet contraction (pelvis) causing disproportion
X● **O33.3 Maternal care for disproportion due to outlet contraction of pelvis**
      Maternal care for disproportion due to mid-cavity contraction (pelvis)
      Maternal care for disproportion due to outlet contraction (pelvis)

One of the following 7th characters is to be assigned to code O33.3. 7th character 0 is for single gestations and multiple gestations where the fetus is unspecified. 7th characters 1 through 9 are for cases of multiple gestations to identify the fetus for which the code applies. The appropriate code from category O30, Multiple gestation, must also be assigned when assigning code O33.3 with a 7th character of 1 through 9.

0	not applicable or unspecified
1	fetus 1
2	fetus 2
3	fetus 3
4	fetus 4
5	fetus 5
9	other fetus

X● **O33.4 Maternal care for disproportion of mixed maternal and fetal origin**

One of the following 7th characters is to be assigned to code O33.4. 7th character 0 is for single gestations and multiple gestations where the fetus is unspecified. 7th characters 1 through 9 are for cases of multiple gestations to identify the fetus for which the code applies. The appropriate code from category O30, Multiple gestation, must also be assigned when assigning code O33.4 with a 7th character of 1 through 9.

0	not applicable or unspecified
1	fetus 1
2	fetus 2
3	fetus 3
4	fetus 4
5	fetus 5
9	other fetus

X ● **O33.5** **Maternal care for disproportion due to unusually large fetus**

    Maternal care for disproportion due to disproportion of fetal origin with normally formed fetus

    Maternal care for disproportion due to fetal disproportion NOS

    One of the following 7th characters is to be assigned to code O33.5. 7th character 0 is for single gestations and multiple gestations where the fetus is unspecified. 7th characters 1 through 9 are for cases of multiple gestations to identify the fetus for which the code applies. The appropriate code from category O30, Multiple gestation, must also be assigned when assigning code O33.5 with a 7th character of 1 through 9.

0	not applicable or unspecified
1	fetus 1
2	fetus 2
3	fetus 3
4	fetus 4
5	fetus 5
9	other fetus

X ● **O33.6** **Maternal care for disproportion due to hydrocephalic fetus**

    One of the following 7th characters is to be assigned to code O33.6. 7th character 0 is for single gestations and multiple gestations where the fetus is unspecified. 7th characters 1 through 9 are for cases of multiple gestations to identify the fetus for which the code applies. The appropriate code from category O30, Multiple gestation, must also be assigned when assigning code O33.6 with a 7th character of 1 through 9.

0	not applicable or unspecified
1	fetus 1
2	fetus 2
3	fetus 3
4	fetus 4
5	fetus 5
9	other fetus

O33.7 **Maternal care for disproportion due to other fetal deformities**

    Maternal care for disproportion due to fetal ascites

    Maternal care for disproportion due to fetal hydrops

    Maternal care for disproportion due to fetal meningomyelocele

    Maternal care for disproportion due to fetal sacral teratoma

    Maternal care for disproportion due to fetal tumor

    Excludes1   obstructed labor due to other fetal deformities (O66.3)

O33.8 **Maternal care for disproportion of other origin**

O33.9 **Maternal care for disproportion, unspecified**

    Maternal care for disproportion due to cephalopelvic disproportion NOS

    Maternal care for disproportion due to fetopelvic disproportion NOS

● **O34** **Maternal care for abnormality of pelvic organs**

    Includes   the listed conditions as a reason for hospitalization or other obstetric care of the mother, or for cesarean delivery before onset of labor

    Code first any associated obstructed labor (O65.5)

    Use additional code for specific condition

● **O34.0** **Maternal care for congenital malformation of uterus**

    O34.00 **Maternal care for unspecified congenital malformation of uterus, unspecified trimester**

    O34.01 **Maternal care for unspecified congenital malformation of uterus, first trimester**

    O34.02 **Maternal care for unspecified congenital malformation of uterus, second trimester**

    O34.03 **Maternal care for unspecified congenital malformation of uterus, third trimester**

● **O34.1** **Maternal care for benign tumor of corpus uteri**

    Excludes2   maternal care for benign tumor of cervix (O34.4-)

         maternal care for malignant neoplasm of uterus (O9A.1-)

    O34.10 **Maternal care for benign tumor of corpus uteri, unspecified trimester**

    O34.11 **Maternal care for benign tumor of corpus uteri, first trimester**

    O34.12 **Maternal care for benign tumor of corpus uteri, second trimester**

    O34.13 **Maternal care for benign tumor of corpus uteri, third trimester**

● **O34.2** **Maternal care due to uterine scar from previous surgery**

    O34.21 **Maternal care for scar from previous cesarean delivery**

    O34.29 **Maternal care due to uterine scar from other previous surgery**

● **O34.3** **Maternal care for cervical incompetence**

    Maternal care for cerclage with or without cervical incompetence

    Maternal care for Shirodkar suture with or without cervical incompetence

    O34.30 **Maternal care for cervical incompetence, unspecified trimester**

    O34.31 **Maternal care for cervical incompetence, first trimester**

    O34.32 **Maternal care for cervical incompetence, second trimester**

    O34.33 **Maternal care for cervical incompetence, third trimester**

● **O34.4** **Maternal care for other abnormalities of cervix**

    O34.40 **Maternal care for other abnormalities of cervix, unspecified trimester**

    O34.41 **Maternal care for other abnormalities of cervix, first trimester**

    O34.42 **Maternal care for other abnormalities of cervix, second trimester**

    O34.43 **Maternal care for other abnormalities of cervix, third trimester**

CHAPTER 15 (O00-O9A)

● **O34.5   Maternal care for other abnormalities of gravid uterus**
  ● **O34.51   Maternal care for incarceration of gravid uterus**
    O34.511   Maternal care for incarceration of gravid uterus, first trimester
    O34.512   Maternal care for incarceration of gravid uterus, second trimester
    O34.513   Maternal care for incarceration of gravid uterus, third trimester
    O34.519   Maternal care for incarceration of gravid uterus, unspecified trimester
  ● **O34.52   Maternal care for prolapse of gravid uterus**
    O34.521   Maternal care for prolapse of gravid uterus, first trimester
    O34.522   Maternal care for prolapse of gravid uterus, second trimester
    O34.523   Maternal care for prolapse of gravid uterus, third trimester
    O34.529   Maternal care for prolapse of gravid uterus, unspecified trimester
  ● **O34.53   Maternal care for retroversion of gravid uterus**
    O34.531   Maternal care for retroversion of gravid uterus, first trimester
    O34.532   Maternal care for retroversion of gravid uterus, second trimester
    O34.533   Maternal care for retroversion of gravid uterus, third trimester
    O34.539   Maternal care for retroversion of gravid uterus, unspecified trimester
  ● **O34.59   Maternal care for other abnormalities of gravid uterus**
    O34.591   Maternal care for other abnormalities of gravid uterus, first trimester
    O34.592   Maternal care for other abnormalities of gravid uterus, second trimester
    O34.593   Maternal care for other abnormalities of gravid uterus, third trimester
    O34.599   Maternal care for other abnormalities of gravid uterus, unspecified trimester
● **O34.6   Maternal care for abnormality of vagina**
    Excludes2   maternal care for vaginal varices in pregnancy (O22.1-)
  O34.60   Maternal care for abnormality of vagina, unspecified trimester
  O34.61   Maternal care for abnormality of vagina, first trimester
  O34.62   Maternal care for abnormality of vagina, second trimester
  O34.63   Maternal care for abnormality of vagina, third trimester
● **O34.7   Maternal care for abnormality of vulva and perineum**
    Excludes2   maternal care for perineal and vulval varices in pregnancy (O22.1-)
  O34.70   Maternal care for abnormality of vulva and perineum, unspecified trimester
  O34.71   Maternal care for abnormality of vulva and perineum, first trimester
  O34.72   Maternal care for abnormality of vulva and perineum, second trimester
  O34.73   Maternal care for abnormality of vulva and perineum, third trimester

● **O34.8   Maternal care for other abnormalities of pelvic organs**
  O34.80   Maternal care for other abnormalities of pelvic organs, unspecified trimester
  O34.81   Maternal care for other abnormalities of pelvic organs, first trimester
  O34.82   Maternal care for other abnormalities of pelvic organs, second trimester
  O34.83   Maternal care for other abnormalities of pelvic organs, third trimester
● **O34.9   Maternal care for abnormality of pelvic organ, unspecified**
  O34.90   Maternal care for abnormality of pelvic organ, unspecified, unspecified trimester
  O34.91   Maternal care for abnormality of pelvic organ, unspecified, first trimester
  O34.92   Maternal care for abnormality of pelvic organ, unspecified, second trimester
  O34.93   Maternal care for abnormality of pelvic organ, unspecified, third trimester

OGCR Section I.C.15.e.l.

Fetal Conditions Affecting the Management of the Mother

1) Code from categories O35 and O36

Codes from categories O35, Maternal care for known or suspected fetal abnormality and damage, and O36, Maternal care for other fetal problems, are assigned only when the fetal condition is actually responsible for modifying the management of the mother, i.e., by requiring diagnostic studies, additional observation, special care, or termination of pregnancy. The fact that the fetal condition exists does not justify assigning a code from this series to the mother's record.

2) In utero surgery

In cases when surgery is performed on the fetus, a diagnosis code from category O35, Maternal care for known or suspected fetal abnormality and damage, should be assigned identifying the fetal condition. Assign the appropriate procedure code for the procedure performed.

No code from Chapter 16, the perinatal codes, should be used on the mother's record to identify fetal conditions. Surgery performed in utero on a fetus is still to be coded as an obstetric encounter.

● **O35   Maternal care for known or suspected fetal abnormality and damage**
  Includes   the listed conditions in the fetus as a reason for hospitalization or other obstetric care to the mother, or for termination of pregnancy
  Code also any associated maternal condition
  Excludes1   encounter for suspected maternal and fetal conditions ruled out (Z03.7-)

One of the following 7th characters is to be assigned to each code under category O35. 7th character 0 is for single gestations and multiple gestations where the fetus is unspecified. 7th characters 1 through 9 are for cases of multiple gestations to identify the fetus for which the code applies. The appropriate code from category O30, Multiple gestation, must also be assigned when assigning a code from category O35 that has a 7th character of 1 through 9.

0	not applicable or unspecified
1	fetus 1
2	fetus 2
3	fetus 3
4	fetus 4
5	fetus 5
9	other fetus

X ● **O35.0   Maternal care for (suspected) central nervous system malformation in fetus**
    Maternal care for fetal anencephaly
    Maternal care for fetal hydrocephalus
    Maternal care for fetal spina bifida
    Excludes2   chromosomal abnormality in fetus (O35.1)

X ● **O35.1   Maternal care for (suspected) chromosomal abnormality in fetus**

X ● **O35.2   Maternal care for (suspected) hereditary disease in fetus**

> Excludes2   chromosomal abnormality in fetus (O35.1)

X ● **O35.3   Maternal care for (suspected) damage to fetus from viral disease in mother**

> Maternal care for damage to fetus from maternal cytomegalovirus infection
> Maternal care for damage to fetus from maternal rubella

X ● **O35.4   Maternal care for (suspected) damage to fetus from alcohol**

X ● **O35.5   Maternal care for (suspected) damage to fetus by drugs**

> Maternal care for damage to fetus from drug addiction

X ● **O35.6   Maternal care for (suspected) damage to fetus by radiation**

X ● **O35.7   Maternal care for (suspected) damage to fetus by other medical procedures**

> Maternal care for damage to fetus by amniocentesis
> Maternal care for damage to fetus by biopsy procedures
> Maternal care for damage to fetus by hematological investigation
> Maternal care for damage to fetus by intrauterine contraceptive device
> Maternal care for damage to fetus by intrauterine surgery

X ● **O35.8   Maternal care for other (suspected) fetal abnormality and damage**

> Maternal care for damage to fetus from maternal listeriosis
> Maternal care for damage to fetus from maternal toxoplasmosis

X ● **O35.9   Maternal care for (suspected) fetal abnormality and damage, unspecified**

● **O36   Maternal care for other fetal problems**

> Includes   the listed conditions in the fetus as a reason for hospitalization or other obstetric care of the mother, or for termination of pregnancy

> Excludes1   encounter for suspected maternal and fetal conditions ruled out (Z03.7-)
> placental transfusion syndromes (O43.0-)

> Excludes2   labor and delivery complicated by fetal stress (O77.-)

One of the following 7th characters is to be assigned to each code under category O36. 7th character 0 is for single gestations and multiple gestations where the fetus is unspecified. 7th characters 1 through 9 are for cases of multiple gestations to identify the fetus for which the code applies. The appropriate code from category O30, Multiple gestation, must also be assigned when assigning a code from category O36 that has a 7th character of 1 through 9.

0	not applicable or unspecified
1	fetus 1
2	fetus 2
3	fetus 3
4	fetus 4
5	fetus 5
9	other fetus

● **O36.0   Maternal care for rhesus isoimmunization**

> Maternal care for Rh incompatibility (with hydrops fetalis)

> ● **O36.01   Maternal care for anti-D [Rh] antibodies**

> > ● **O36.011   Maternal care for anti-D [Rh] antibodies, first trimester**

> > ● **O36.012   Maternal care for anti-D [Rh] antibodies, second trimester**

> > ● **O36.013   Maternal care for anti-D [Rh] antibodies, third trimester**

> > ● **O36.019   Maternal care for anti-D [Rh] antibodies, unspecified trimester**

> ● **O36.09   Maternal care for other rhesus isoimmunization**

> > ● **O36.091   Maternal care for other rhesus isoimmunization, first trimester**

> > ● **O36.092   Maternal care for other rhesus isoimmunization, second trimester**

> > ● **O36.093   Maternal care for other rhesus isoimmunization, third trimester**

> > ● **O36.099   Maternal care for other rhesus isoimmunization, unspecified trimester**

● **O36.1   Maternal care for other isoimmunization**

> Maternal care for ABO isoimmunization

> ● **O36.11   Maternal care for Anti-A sensitization**

> > Maternal care for isoimmunization NOS (with hydrops fetalis)

> > ● **O36.111   Maternal care for Anti-A sensitization, first trimester**

> > ● **O36.112   Maternal care for Anti-A sensitization, second trimester**

> > ● **O36.113   Maternal care for Anti-A sensitization, third trimester**

> > ● **O36.119   Maternal care for Anti-A sensitization, unspecified trimester**

> ● **O36.19   Maternal care for other isoimmunization**

> > Maternal care for Anti-B sensitization

> > ● **O36.191   Maternal care for other isoimmunization, first trimester**

> > ● **O36.192   Maternal care for other isoimmunization, second trimester**

> > ● **O36.193   Maternal care for other isoimmunization, third trimester**

> > ● **O36.199   Maternal care for other isoimmunization, unspecified trimester**

● **O36.2   Maternal care for hydrops fetalis**

> Maternal care for hydrops fetalis NOS
> Maternal care for hydrops fetalis not associated with isoimmunization

> Excludes1   hydrops fetalis associated with ABO isoimmunization (O36.1-)
> hydrops fetalis associated with rhesus isoimmunization (O36.0-)

> ● **O36.20   Maternal care for hydrops fetalis, unspecified trimester**

> ● **O36.21   Maternal care for hydrops fetalis, first trimester**

> ● **O36.22   Maternal care for hydrops fetalis, second trimester**

> ● **O36.23   Maternal care for hydrops fetalis, third trimester**

● **O36.4   Maternal care for intrauterine death**

> Maternal care for intrauterine fetal death NOS
> Maternal care for intrauterine fetal death after completion of 20 weeks of gestation
> Maternal care for late fetal death
> Maternal care for missed delivery

> Excludes1   missed abortion (O02.1)
> stillbirth (P95)

● **O36.5   Maternal care for known or suspected poor fetal growth**

> ● **O36.51   Maternal care for known or suspected placental insufficiency**

> > ● **O36.511   Maternal care for known or suspected placental insufficiency, first trimester**

> > ● **O36.512   Maternal care for known or suspected placental insufficiency, second trimester**

CHAPTER 15 (O00-O9A)

● **O36.513**   Maternal care for known or suspected placental insufficiency, third trimester

● **O36.519**   Maternal care for known or suspected placental insufficiency, unspecified trimester

● **O36.59**   **Maternal care for other known or suspected poor fetal growth**
Maternal care for known or suspected light-for-dates NOS
Maternal care for known or suspected small-for-dates NOS

● **O36.591**   Maternal care for other known or suspected poor fetal growth, first trimester

● **O36.592**   Maternal care for other known or suspected poor fetal growth, second trimester

● **O36.593**   Maternal care for other known or suspected poor fetal growth, third trimester

● **O36.599**   Maternal care for other known or suspected poor fetal growth, unspecified trimester

● **O36.6**   **Maternal care for excessive fetal growth**
Maternal care for known or suspected large-for-dates

X● **O36.60**   Maternal care for excessive fetal growth, unspecified trimester

X● **O36.61**   Maternal care for excessive fetal growth, first trimester

X● **O36.62**   Maternal care for excessive fetal growth, second trimester

X● **O36.63**   Maternal care for excessive fetal growth, third trimester

● **O36.7**   **Maternal care for viable fetus in abdominal pregnancy**

X● **O36.70**   Maternal care for viable fetus in abdominal pregnancy, unspecified trimester

X● **O36.71**   Maternal care for viable fetus in abdominal pregnancy, first trimester

X● **O36.72**   Maternal care for viable fetus in abdominal pregnancy, second trimester

X● **O36.73**   Maternal care for viable fetus in abdominal pregnancy, third trimester

● **O36.8**   **Maternal care for other specified fetal problems**

X● **O36.80**   Pregnancy with inconclusive fetal viability
Encounter to determine fetal viability of pregnancy

● **O36.81**   Decreased fetal movements

  ● **O36.812**   Decreased fetal movements, second trimester

  ● **O36.813**   Decreased fetal movements, third trimester

  ● **O36.819**   Decreased fetal movements, unspecified trimester

● **O36.82**   Fetal anemia and thrombocytopenia

  ● **O36.821**   Fetal anemia and thrombocytopenia, first trimester

  ● **O36.822**   Fetal anemia and thrombocytopenia, second trimester

  ● **O36.823**   Fetal anemia and thrombocytopenia, third trimester

  ● **O36.829**   Fetal anemia and thrombocytopenia, unspecified trimester

● **O36.89**   Maternal care for other specified fetal problems

  ● **O36.891**   Maternal care for other specified fetal problems, first trimester

  ● **O36.892**   Maternal care for other specified fetal problems, second trimester

  ● **O36.893**   Maternal care for other specified fetal problems, third trimester

  ● **O36.899**   Maternal care for other specified fetal problems, unspecified trimester

● **O36.9**   Maternal care for fetal problem, unspecified

X● **O36.90**   Maternal care for fetal problem, unspecified, unspecified trimester

X● **O36.91**   Maternal care for fetal problem, unspecified, first trimester

X● **O36.92**   Maternal care for fetal problem, unspecified, second trimester

X● **O36.93**   Maternal care for fetal problem, unspecified, third trimester

● **O40**   **Polyhydramnios**
Overabundance of amniotic fluid

Includes	hydramnios
Excludes1	encounter for suspected maternal and fetal conditions ruled out (Z03.7-)

One of the following 7th characters is to be assigned to each code under category O40. 7th character 0 is for single gestations and multiple gestations where the fetus is unspecified. 7th characters 1 through 9 are for cases of multiple gestations to identify the fetus for which the code applies. The appropriate code from category O30, Multiple gestation, must also be assigned when assigning a code from category O40 that has a 7th character of 1 through 9.

0	not applicable or unspecified
1	fetus 1
2	fetus 2
3	fetus 3
4	fetus 4
5	fetus 5
9	other fetus

X● **O40.1**   Polyhydramnios, first trimester
X● **O40.2**   Polyhydramnios, second trimester
X● **O40.3**   Polyhydramnios, third trimester
X● **O40.9**   Polyhydramnios, unspecified trimester

● **O41**   **Other disorders of amniotic fluid and membranes**

Excludes1	encounter for suspected maternal and fetal conditions ruled out (Z03.7-)

One of the following 7th characters is to be assigned to each code under category O41. 7th character 0 is for single gestations and multiple gestations where the fetus is unspecified. 7th characters 1 through 9 are for cases of multiple gestations to identify the fetus for which the code applies. The appropriate code from category O30, Multiple gestation, must also be assigned when assigning a code from category O41 that has a 7th character of 1 through 9.

0	not applicable or unspecified
1	fetus 1
2	fetus 2
3	fetus 3
4	fetus 4
5	fetus 5
9	other fetus

● **O41.0**   Oligohydramnios
Scant volume of amniotic fluid
Oligohydramnios without rupture of membranes

X● **O41.00**   Oligohydramnios, unspecified trimester
X● **O41.01**   Oligohydramnios, first trimester
X● **O41.02**   Oligohydramnios, second trimester
X● **O41.03**   Oligohydramnios, third trimester

◀ New   ⬅ Revised   ~~deleted~~ Deleted   **OGCR** Official Guidelines   X Assign placeholder X   ● Use Additional Character(s)

Excludes 1   Excludes 2   Includes   Use additional   Code first   Code also   Unspecified

● O41.1   Infection of amniotic sac and membranes
    ● O41.10   Infection of amniotic sac and membranes, unspecified
       ● O41.101   Infection of amniotic sac and membranes, unspecified, first trimester
       ● O41.102   Infection of amniotic sac and membranes, unspecified, second trimester
       ● O41.103   Infection of amniotic sac and membranes, unspecified, third trimester
       ● O41.109   Infection of amniotic sac and membranes, unspecified, unspecified trimester
    ● O41.12   Chorioamnionitis
       ● O41.121   Chorioamnionitis, first trimester
       ● O41.122   Chorioamnionitis, second trimester
       ● O41.123   Chorioamnionitis, third trimester
       ● O41.129   Chorioamnionitis, unspecified trimester
    ● O41.14   Placentitis
       ● O41.141   Placentitis, first trimester
       ● O41.142   Placentitis, second trimester
       ● O41.143   Placentitis, third trimester
       ● O41.149   Placentitis, unspecified trimester
● O41.8   Other specified disorders of amniotic fluid and membranes
    ● O41.8X   Other specified disorders of amniotic fluid and membranes
       ● O41.8X1   Other specified disorders of amniotic fluid and membranes, first trimester
       ● O41.8X2   Other specified disorders of amniotic fluid and membranes, second trimester
       ● O41.8X3   Other specified disorders of amniotic fluid and membranes, third trimester
       ● O41.8X9   Other specified disorders of amniotic fluid and membranes, unspecified trimester
● O41.9   Disorder of amniotic fluid and membranes, unspecified
    X ● O41.90   Disorder of amniotic fluid and membranes, unspecified, unspecified trimester
    X ● O41.91   Disorder of amniotic fluid and membranes, unspecified, first trimester
    X ● O41.92   Disorder of amniotic fluid and membranes, unspecified, second trimester
    X ● O41.93   Disorder of amniotic fluid and membranes, unspecified, third trimester

● O42   Premature rupture of membranes
    ● O42.0   Premature rupture of membranes, onset of labor within 24 hours of rupture
       O42.00   Premature rupture of membranes, onset of labor within 24 hours of rupture, unspecified weeks of gestation
       ● O42.01   Preterm premature rupture of membranes, onset of labor within 24 hours of rupture
         Premature rupture of membranes before 37 completed weeks of gestation
         O42.011   Preterm premature rupture of membranes, onset of labor within 24 hours of rupture, first trimester
         O42.012   Preterm premature rupture of membranes, onset of labor within 24 hours of rupture, second trimester

         O42.013   Preterm premature rupture of membranes, onset of labor within 24 hours of rupture, third trimester
         O42.019   Preterm premature rupture of membranes, onset of labor within 24 hours of rupture, unspecified trimester
       O42.02   Full-term premature rupture of membranes, onset of labor within 24 hours of rupture
         Premature rupture of membranes after 37 completed weeks of gestation
    ● O42.1   Premature rupture of membranes, onset of labor more than 24 hours following rupture
       O42.10   Premature rupture of membranes, onset of labor more than 24 hours following rupture, unspecified weeks of gestation
       ● O42.11   Preterm premature rupture of membranes, onset of labor more than 24 hours following rupture
         Premature rupture of membranes before 37 completed weeks of gestation
         O42.111   Preterm premature rupture of membranes, onset of labor more than 24 hours following rupture, first trimester
         O42.112   Preterm premature rupture of membranes, onset of labor more than 24 hours following rupture, second trimester
         O42.113   Preterm premature rupture of membranes, onset of labor more than 24 hours following rupture, third trimester
         O42.119   Preterm premature rupture of membranes, onset of labor more than 24 hours following rupture, unspecified trimester
       O42.12   Full-term premature rupture of membranes, onset of labor more than 24 hours following rupture
         Premature rupture of membranes after 37 completed weeks of gestation
    ● O42.9   Premature rupture of membranes, unspecified as to length of time between rupture and onset of labor
       O42.90   Premature rupture of membranes, unspecified as to length of time between rupture and onset of labor, unspecified weeks of gestation
       ● O42.91   Preterm premature rupture of membranes, unspecified as to length of time between rupture and onset of labor
         Premature rupture of membranes before 37 completed weeks of gestation
         O42.911   Preterm premature rupture of membranes, unspecified as to length of time between rupture and onset of labor, first trimester
         O42.912   Preterm premature rupture of membranes, unspecified as to length of time between rupture and onset of labor, second trimester
         O42.913   Preterm premature rupture of membranes, unspecified as to length of time between rupture and onset of labor, third trimester
         O42.919   Preterm premature rupture of membranes, unspecified as to length of time between rupture and onset of labor, unspecified trimester
       O42.92   Full-term premature rupture of membranes, unspecified as to length of time between rupture and onset of labor
         Premature rupture of membranes after 37 completed weeks of gestation

CHAPTER 15 (O00–O9A)

● **O43   Placental disorders**

Excludes2   maternal care for poor fetal growth due to placental insufficiency (O36.5-)
placenta previa (O44.-)
placental polyp (O90.89)
placentitis (O41.14-)
premature separation of placenta [abruptio placentae] (O45.-)

● **O43.0   Placental transfusion syndromes**

● **O43.01   Fetomaternal placental transfusion syndrome**
Maternofetal placental transfusion syndrome

O43.011   Fetomaternal placental transfusion syndrome, first trimester

O43.012   Fetomaternal placental transfusion syndrome, second trimester

O43.013   Fetomaternal placental transfusion syndrome, third trimester

O43.019   Fetomaternal placental transfusion syndrome, unspecified trimester

● **O43.02   Fetus-to-fetus placental transfusion syndrome**

O43.021   Fetus-to-fetus placental transfusion syndrome, first trimester

O43.022   Fetus-to-fetus placental transfusion syndrome, second trimester

O43.023   Fetus-to-fetus placental transfusion syndrome, third trimester

O43.029   Fetus-to-fetus placental transfusion syndrome, unspecified trimester

● **O43.1   Malformation of placenta**

● **O43.10   Malformation of placenta, unspecified**
Abnormal placenta NOS

O43.101   Malformation of placenta, unspecified, first trimester

O43.102   Malformation of placenta, unspecified, second trimester

O43.103   Malformation of placenta, unspecified, third trimester

O43.109   Malformation of placenta, unspecified, unspecified trimester

● **O43.11   Circumvallate placenta**

O43.111   Circumvallate placenta, first trimester

O43.112   Circumvallate placenta, second trimester

O43.113   Circumvallate placenta, third trimester

O43.119   Circumvallate placenta, unspecified trimester

● **O43.12   Velamentous insertion of umbilical cord**

O43.121   Velamentous insertion of umbilical cord, first trimester

O43.122   Velamentous insertion of umbilical cord, second trimester

O43.123   Velamentous insertion of umbilical cord, third trimester

O43.129   Velamentous insertion of umbilical cord, unspecified trimester

● **O43.19   Other malformation of placenta**

O43.191   Other malformation of placenta, first trimester

O43.192   Other malformation of placenta, second trimester

O43.193   Other malformation of placenta, third trimester

O43.199   Other malformation of placenta, unspecified trimester

● **O43.2   Morbidly adherent placenta**

Code also associated third stage postpartum hemorrhage, if applicable (O72.0)

Excludes1   retained placenta (O73.-)

● **O43.21   Placenta accreta**

O43.211   Placenta accreta, first trimester

O43.212   Placenta accreta, second trimester

O43.213   Placenta accreta, third trimester

O43.219   Placenta accreta, unspecified trimester

● **O43.22   Placenta increta**

O43.221   Placenta increta, first trimester

O43.222   Placenta increta, second trimester

O43.223   Placenta increta, third trimester

O43.229   Placenta increta, unspecified trimester

● **O43.23   Placenta percreta**

O43.231   Placenta percreta, first trimester

O43.232   Placenta percreta, second trimester

O43.233   Placenta percreta, third trimester

O43.239   Placenta percreta, unspecified trimester

● **O43.8   Other placental disorders**

● **O43.81   Placental infarction**

O43.811   Placental infarction, first trimester

O43.812   Placental infarction, second trimester

O43.813   Placental infarction, third trimester

O43.819   Placental infarction, unspecified trimester

● **O43.89   Other placental disorders**
Placental dysfunction

O43.891   Other placental disorders, first trimester

O43.892   Other placental disorders, second trimester

O43.893   Other placental disorders, third trimester

O43.899   Other placental disorders, unspecified trimester

● **O43.9   Unspecified placental disorder**

O43.90   Unspecified placental disorder, unspecified trimester

O43.91   Unspecified placental disorder, first trimester

O43.92   Unspecified placental disorder, second trimester

O43.93   Unspecified placental disorder, third trimester

● **O44   Placenta previa**

● **O44.0   Placenta previa specified as without hemorrhage**
Low implantation of placenta specified as without hemorrhage

O44.00   Placenta previa specified as without hemorrhage, unspecified trimester

O44.01   Placenta previa specified as without hemorrhage, first trimester

O44.02   Placenta previa specified as without hemorrhage, second trimester

O44.03   Placenta previa specified as without hemorrhage, third trimester

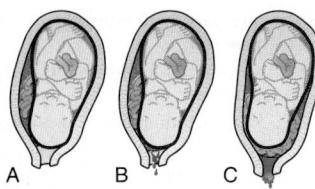

Figure 15-2 A. Marginal placento previa. **B.** Partial placenta previa. **C.** Total placento previa.

Item 15–3 Placenta previa is a condition in which the opening of the cervix is obstructed by the displaced placenta. The three types, marginal, partial, and total, are varying degrees of placenta displacement. Placenta abruption is the premature breaking away of the placenta from the site of the uterine implant before the delivery of the fetus.

- ● **O44.1 Placenta previa with hemorrhage**
  Low implantation of placenta, NOS or with hemorrhage
  Marginal placenta previa, NOS or with hemorrhage
  Partial placenta previa, NOS or with hemorrhage
  Total placenta previa, NOS or with hemorrhage
  > **Excludes1**   labor and delivery complicated by hemorrhage from vasa previa (O69.4)
  - O44.10 Placenta previa with hemorrhage, **unspecified** trimester
  - O44.11 Placenta previa with hemorrhage, first trimester
  - O44.12 Placenta previa with hemorrhage, second trimester
  - O44.13 Placenta previa with hemorrhage, third trimester

- ● **O45 Premature separation of placenta [abruptio placentae]**
  - ● **O45.0 Premature separation of placenta with coagulation defect**
    - ● O45.00 Premature separation of placenta with coagulation defect, unspecified
      - O45.001 Premature separation of placenta with coagulation defect, **unspecified**, first trimester
      - O45.002 Premature separation of placenta with coagulation defect, **unspecified**, second trimester
      - O45.003 Premature separation of placenta with coagulation defect, **unspecified**, third trimester
      - O45.009 Premature separation of placenta with coagulation defect, **unspecified**, unspecified trimester
    - ● O45.01 Premature separation of placenta with afibrinogenemia
      Premature separation of placenta with hypofibrinogenemia
      - O45.011 Premature separation of placenta with afibrinogenemia, first trimester
      - O45.012 Premature separation of placenta with afibrinogenemia, second trimester
      - O45.013 Premature separation of placenta with afibrinogenemia, third trimester
      - O45.019 Premature separation of placenta with afibrinogenemia, **unspecified** trimester

Figure 15-3 Abruptio placentae is classified according to the grade of separation of the placenta from the uterine wall. **A.** Mild separation in which hemorrhage is internal. **B.** Moderate separation in which there is external hemorrhage. **C.** Severe separation in which there is external hemorrhage and extreme separation.

- ● O45.02 Premature separation of placenta with disseminated intravascular coagulation
  - O45.021 Premature separation of placenta with disseminated intravascular coagulation, first trimester
  - O45.022 Premature separation of placenta with disseminated intravascular coagulation, second trimester
  - O45.023 Premature separation of placenta with disseminated intravascular coagulation, third trimester
  - O45.029 Premature separation of placenta with disseminated intravascular coagulation, **unspecified** trimester
- ● O45.09 Premature separation of placenta with other coagulation defect
  - O45.091 Premature separation of placenta with other coagulation defect, first trimester
  - O45.092 Premature separation of placenta with other coagulation defect, second trimester
  - O45.093 Premature separation of placenta with other coagulation defect, third trimester
  - O45.099 Premature separation of placenta with other coagulation defect, **unspecified** trimester
- ● O45.8 Other premature separation of placenta
  - ● O45.8X Other premature separation of placenta
    - O45.8X1 Other premature separation of placenta, first trimester
    - O45.8X2 Other premature separation of placenta, second trimester
    - O45.8X3 Other premature separation of placenta, third trimester
    - O45.8X9 Other premature separation of placenta, **unspecified** trimester
- ● O45.9 Premature separation of placenta, unspecified
  Abruptio placentae NOS
  - O45.90 Premature separation of placenta, **unspecified**, unspecified trimester
  - O45.91 Premature separation of placenta, **unspecified**, first trimester
  - O45.92 Premature separation of placenta, **unspecified**, second trimester
  - O45.93 Premature separation of placenta, **unspecified**, third trimester

◀ New   ◀◀◀ Revised   ~~deleted~~ Deleted   **OGCR** Official Guidelines   X Assign placeholder X   ● Use Additional Character(s)

| Excludes 1 | Excludes 2 | Includes | Use additional | Code first | Code also | Unspecified |

● **O46 Antepartum hemorrhage, not elsewhere classified**

> **Excludes1**   hemorrhage in early pregnancy (O20.-)
> intrapartum hemorrhage NEC (O67.-)
> placenta previa (O44.-)
> premature separation of placenta [abruptio placentae] (O45.-)

● **O46.0 Antepartum hemorrhage with coagulation defect**

  ● **O46.00 Antepartum hemorrhage with coagulation defect, unspecified**

     O46.001   Antepartum hemorrhage with coagulation defect, unspecified, first trimester

     O46.002   Antepartum hemorrhage with coagulation defect, unspecified, second trimester

     O46.003   Antepartum hemorrhage with coagulation defect, unspecified, third trimester

     O46.009   Antepartum hemorrhage with coagulation defect, unspecified, unspecified trimester

  ● **O46.01 Antepartum hemorrhage with afibrinogenemia**
     Antepartum hemorrhage with hypofibrinogenemia

     O46.011   Antepartum hemorrhage with afibrinogenemia, first trimester

     O46.012   Antepartum hemorrhage with afibrinogenemia, second trimester

     O46.013   Antepartum hemorrhage with afibrinogenemia, third trimester

     O46.019   Antepartum hemorrhage with afibrinogenemia, unspecified trimester

  ● **O46.02 Antepartum hemorrhage with disseminated intravascular coagulation**

     O46.021   Antepartum hemorrhage with disseminated intravascular coagulation, first trimester

     O46.022   Antepartum hemorrhage with disseminated intravascular coagulation, second trimester

     O46.023   Antepartum hemorrhage with disseminated intravascular coagulation, third trimester

     O46.029   Antepartum hemorrhage with disseminated intravascular coagulation, unspecified trimester

  ● **O46.09 Antepartum hemorrhage with other coagulation defect**

     O46.091   Antepartum hemorrhage with other coagulation defect, first trimester

     O46.092   Antepartum hemorrhage with other coagulation defect, second trimester

     O46.093   Antepartum hemorrhage with other coagulation defect, third trimester

     O46.099   Antepartum hemorrhage with other coagulation defect, unspecified trimester

● **O46.8 Other antepartum hemorrhage**

  ● **O46.8x Other antepartum hemorrhage**

     O46.8x1   Other antepartum hemorrhage, first trimester

     O46.8x2   Other antepartum hemorrhage, second trimester

     O46.8x3   Other antepartum hemorrhage, third trimester

     O46.8x9   Other antepartum hemorrhage, unspecified trimester

● **O46.9 Antepartum hemorrhage, unspecified**

     O46.90   Antepartum hemorrhage, unspecified, unspecified trimester

     O46.91   Antepartum hemorrhage, unspecified, first trimester

     O46.92   Antepartum hemorrhage, unspecified, second trimester

     O46.93   Antepartum hemorrhage, unspecified, third trimester

● **O47 False labor**

> **Includes**   Braxton Hicks contractions
> threatened labor

> **Excludes1**   preterm labor (O60.-)

● **O47.0 False labor before 37 completed weeks of gestation**

     O47.00   False labor before 37 completed weeks of gestation, unspecified trimester

     O47.02   False labor before 37 completed weeks of gestation, second trimester

     O47.03   False labor before 37 completed weeks of gestation, third trimester

   O47.1   False labor at or after 37 completed weeks of gestation

   O47.9   False labor, unspecified

● **O48 Late pregnancy**

   O48.0   **Post-term pregnancy**
     Pregnancy over 40 completed weeks to 42 completed weeks gestation

   O48.1   **Prolonged pregnancy**
     Pregnancy which has advanced beyond 42 completed weeks gestation

---

COMPLICATIONS OF LABOR AND DELIVERY (O60-O77)

● **O60 Preterm labor**

> **Includes**   onset (spontaneous) of labor before 37 completed weeks of gestation

> **Excludes1**   false labor (O47.0-)
> threatened labor NOS (O47.0-)

● **O60.0 Preterm labor without delivery**

     O60.00   Preterm labor without delivery, unspecified trimester

     O60.02   Preterm labor without delivery, second trimester

     O60.03   Preterm labor without delivery, third trimester

● **O60.1 Preterm labor with preterm delivery**

     One of the following 7th characters is to be assigned to each code under subcategory O60.1. 7th character 0 is for single gestations and multiple gestations where the fetus is unspecified. 7th characters 1 through 9 are for cases of multiple gestations to identify the fetus for which the code applies. The appropriate code from category O30, Multiple gestation, must also be assigned when assigning a code from subcategory O60.1 that has a 7th character of 1 through 9.

0	not applicable or unspecified
1	fetus 1
2	fetus 2
3	fetus 3
4	fetus 4
5	fetus 5
9	other fetus

X ● O60.10   Preterm labor with preterm delivery, unspecified trimester
     Preterm labor with delivery NOS

X ● O60.12   Preterm labor second trimester with preterm delivery second trimester

X ● O60.13   Preterm labor second trimester with preterm delivery third trimester

X ● O60.14   Preterm labor third trimester with preterm delivery third trimester

● **O60.2   Term delivery with preterm labor**

One of the following 7th characters is to be assigned to each code under subcategory O60.2. 7th character 0 is for single gestations and multiple gestations where the fetus is unspecified. 7th characters 1 through 9 are for cases of multiple gestations to identify the fetus for which the code applies. The appropriate code from category O30, Multiple gestation, must also be assigned when assigning a code from subcategory O60.2 that has a 7th character of 1 through 9.

0	not applicable or unspecified
1	fetus 1
2	fetus 2
3	fetus 3
4	fetus 4
5	fetus 5
9	other fetus

X ● **O60.20   Term delivery with preterm labor, unspecified trimester**

X ● **O60.22   Term delivery with preterm labor, second trimester**

X ● **O60.23   Term delivery with preterm labor, third trimester**

● **O61   Failed induction of labor**

O61.0   Failed medical induction of labor
    Failed induction (of labor) by oxytocin
    Failed induction (of labor) by prostaglandins

O61.1   Failed instrumental induction of labor
    Failed mechanical induction (of labor)
    Failed surgical induction (of labor)

O61.8   Other failed induction of labor

O61.9   Failed induction of labor, unspecified

● **O62   Abnormalities of forces of labor**

O62.0   Primary inadequate contractions
    Failure of cervical dilatation
    Primary hypotonic uterine dysfunction
    Uterine inertia during latent phase of labor

O62.1   Secondary uterine inertia
    Arrested active phase of labor
    Secondary hypotonic uterine dysfunction

O62.2   Other uterine inertia
    Atony of uterus without hemorrhage
    Atony of uterus NOS
    Desultory labor
    Hypotonic uterine dysfunction NOS
    Irregular labor
    Poor contractions
    Slow slope active phase of labor
    Uterine inertia NOS

> **Excludes1**   atony of uterus with hemorrhage (postpartum) (O72.1)
> postpartum atony of uterus without hemorrhage (O75.89)

O62.3   Precipitate labor

O62.4   Hypertonic, incoordinate, and prolonged uterine contractions
    Cervical spasm
    Contraction ring dystocia
    Dyscoordinate labor
    Hour-glass contraction of uterus
    Hypertonic uterine dysfunction
    Incoordinate uterine action
    Tetanic contractions
    Uterine dystocia NOS
    Uterine spasm

> **Excludes1**   dystocia (fetal) (maternal) NOS (O66.9)

O62.8   Other abnormalities of forces of labor

O62.9   Abnormality of forces of labor, unspecified

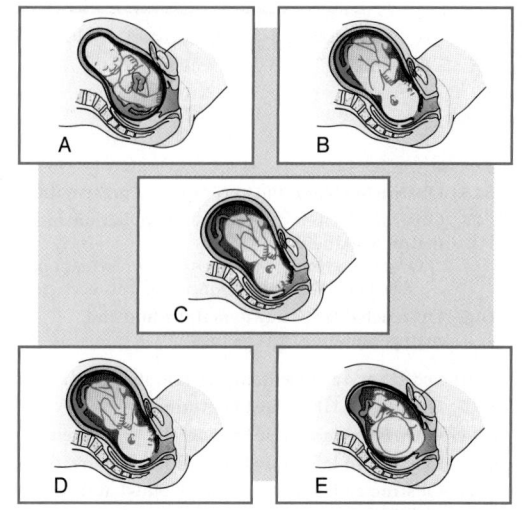

Figure 15-4   Five types of malposition and malpresentation of the fetus: **A.** Breech. **B.** Vertex. **C.** Face. **D.** Brow. **E.** Shoulder.

● **O63   Long labor**

O63.0   Prolonged first stage (of labor)

O63.1   Prolonged second stage (of labor)

O63.2   Delayed delivery of second twin, triplet, etc.

O63.9   Long labor, unspecified
    Prolonged labor NOS

● **O64   Obstructed labor due to malposition and malpresentation of fetus**

One of the following 7th characters is to be assigned to each code under category O64. 7th character 0 is for single gestations and multiple gestations where the fetus is unspecified. 7th characters 1 through 9 are for cases of multiple gestations to identify the fetus for which the code applies. The appropriate code from category O30, Multiple gestation, must also be assigned when assigning a code from category O64 that has a 7th character of 1 through 9.

0	not applicable or unspecified
1	fetus 1
2	fetus 2
3	fetus 3
4	fetus 4
5	fetus 5
9	other fetus

X ● **O64.0   Obstructed labor due to incomplete rotation of fetal head**
    Deep transverse arrest
    Obstructed labor due to persistent occipitoiliac (position)
    Obstructed labor due to persistent occipitoposterior (position)
    Obstructed labor due to persistent occipitosacral (position)
    Obstructed labor due to persistent occipitotransverse (position)

X ● **O64.1   Obstructed labor due to breech presentation**
    Obstructed labor due to buttocks presentation
    Obstructed labor due to complete breech presentation
    Obstructed labor due to frank breech presentation

X ● **O64.2   Obstructed labor due to face presentation**
    Obstructed labor due to chin presentation

X ● **O64.3   Obstructed labor due to brow presentation**

X ● **O64.4   Obstructed labor due to shoulder presentation**
    Prolapsed arm

> **Excludes1**   impacted shoulders (O66.0)
> shoulder dystocia (O66.0)

CHAPTER 15 (O00-O9A)

◀ New   ⬅ Revised   ~~deleted~~ Deleted   **OGCR** Official Guidelines   X Assign placeholder X   ● Use Additional Character(s)

| Excludes 1 | Excludes 2 | Includes | Use additional | Code first | Code also | Unspecified |

Figure 15-5 Hydrocephalic fetus causing disproportion.

X ● **O64.5 Obstructed labor due to compound presentation**
X ● **O64.8 Obstructed labor due to other malposition and malpresentation**
    Obstructed labor due to footling presentation
    Obstructed labor due to incomplete breech presentation
X ● **O64.9 Obstructed labor due to malposition and malpresentation, unspecified**

● **O65 Obstructed labor due to maternal pelvic abnormality**
  O65.0 Obstructed labor due to deformed pelvis
  O65.1 Obstructed labor due to generally contracted pelvis
  O65.2 Obstructed labor due to pelvic inlet contraction
  O65.3 Obstructed labor due to pelvic outlet and mid-cavity contraction
  O65.4 Obstructed labor due to fetopelvic disproportion, unspecified
      | Excludes1 | dystocia due to abnormality of fetus (O66.2-O66.3)
  O65.5 Obstructed labor due to abnormality of maternal pelvic organs
      Obstructed labor due to conditions listed in O34.-
      Use additional code to identify abnormality of pelvic organs O34.-
  O65.8 Obstructed labor due to other maternal pelvic abnormalities
  O65.9 Obstructed labor due to maternal pelvic abnormality, unspecified

● **O66 Other obstructed labor**
  O66.0 Obstructed labor due to shoulder dystocia
      Impacted shoulders
  O66.1 Obstructed labor due to locked twins
  O66.2 Obstructed labor due to unusually large fetus
  O66.3 Obstructed labor due to other abnormalities of fetus
      Dystocia due to fetal ascites
      Dystocia due to fetal hydrops
      Dystocia due to fetal meningomyelocele
      Dystocia due to fetal sacral teratoma
      Dystocia due to fetal tumor
      Dystocia due to hydrocephalic fetus
      Use additional code to identify cause of obstruction
● **O66.4 Failed trial of labor**
    O66.40 Failed trial of labor, unspecified
    O66.41 Failed attempted vaginal birth after previous cesarean delivery
        Code first rupture of uterus, if applicable (O71.0-, O71.1)
  O66.5 Attempted application of vacuum extractor and forceps
      Attempted application of vacuum or forceps, with subsequent delivery by forceps or cesarean delivery
  O66.6 Obstructed labor due to other multiple fetuses
  O66.8 Other specified obstructed labor
      Use additional code to identify cause of obstruction
  O66.9 Obstructed labor, unspecified
      Dystocia NOS
      Fetal dystocia NOS
      Maternal dystocia NOS

● **O67 Labor and delivery complicated by intrapartum hemorrhage, not elsewhere classified**
    | Excludes1 | antepartum hemorrhage NEC (O46.-)
                   placenta previa (O44.-)
                   premature separation of placenta [abruptio placentae] (O45.-)
    | Excludes2 | postpartum hemorrhage (O72.-)
  O67.0 Intrapartum hemorrhage with coagulation defect
      Intrapartum hemorrhage (excessive) associated with afibrinogenemia
      Intrapartum hemorrhage (excessive) associated with disseminated intravascular coagulation
      Intrapartum hemorrhage (excessive) associated with hyperfibrinolysis
      Intrapartum hemorrhage (excessive) associated with hypofibrinogenemia
  O67.8 Other intrapartum hemorrhage
      Excessive intrapartum hemorrhage
  O67.9 Intrapartum hemorrhage, unspecified

  O68 Labor and delivery complicated by abnormality of fetal acid-base balance
      Fetal acidemia complicating labor and delivery
      Fetal acidosis complicating labor and delivery
      Fetal alkalosis complicating labor and delivery
      Fetal metabolic acidemia complicating labor and delivery
    | Excludes1 | fetal stress NOS (O77.9)
                   labor and delivery complicated by electrocardiographic evidence of fetal stress (O77.8)
                   labor and delivery complicated by ultrasonic evidence of fetal stress (O77.8)
    | Excludes2 | abnormality in fetal heart rate or rhythm (O76)
                   labor and delivery complicated by meconium in amniotic fluid (O77.0)

● **O69 Labor and delivery complicated by umbilical cord complications**
    One of the following 7th characters is to be assigned to each code under category O69. 7th character 0 is for single gestations and multiple gestations where the fetus is unspecified. 7th characters 1 through 9 are for cases of multiple gestations to identify the fetus for which the code applies. The appropriate code from category O30, Multiple gestation, must also be assigned when assigning a code from category O69 that has a 7th character of 1 through 9.

0	not applicable or unspecified
1	fetus 1
2	fetus 2
3	fetus 3
4	fetus 4
5	fetus 5
9	other fetus

X ● **O69.0 Labor and delivery complicated by prolapse of cord**
X ● **O69.1 Labor and delivery complicated by cord around neck, with compression**
    | Excludes1 | labor and delivery complicated by cord around neck, without compression (O69.81)
X ● **O69.2 Labor and delivery complicated by other cord entanglement, with compression**
      Labor and delivery complicated by compression of cord NOS
      Labor and delivery complicated by entanglement of cords of twins in monoamniotic sac
      Labor and delivery complicated by knot in cord
    | Excludes1 | labor and delivery complicated by other cord entanglement, without compression (O69.82)

X● **O69.3　Labor and delivery complicated by short cord**

X● **O69.4　Labor and delivery complicated by vasa previa**
　　　Labor and delivery complicated by hemorrhage from vasa previa

X● **O69.5　Labor and delivery complicated by vascular lesion of cord**
　　　Labor and delivery complicated by cord bruising
　　　Labor and delivery complicated by cord hematoma
　　　Labor and delivery complicated by thrombosis of umbilical vessels

● **O69.8　Labor and delivery complicated by other cord complications**

　X● **O69.81　Labor and delivery complicated by cord around neck, without compression**

　X● **O69.82　Labor and delivery complicated by other cord entanglement, without compression**

　X● **O69.89　Labor and delivery complicated by other cord complications**

X● **O69.9　Labor and delivery complicated by cord complication, unspecified**

● **O70　Perineal laceration during delivery**
　　Includes　episiotomy extended by laceration
　　Excludes1　obstetric high vaginal laceration alone (O71.4)

　O70.0　First degree perineal laceration during delivery
　　　Perineal laceration, rupture or tear involving fourchette during delivery
　　　Perineal laceration, rupture or tear involving labia during delivery
　　　Perineal laceration, rupture or tear involving skin during delivery
　　　Perineal laceration, rupture or tear involving vagina during delivery
　　　Perineal laceration, rupture or tear involving vulva during delivery
　　　Slight perineal laceration, rupture or tear during delivery

　O70.1　Second degree perineal laceration during delivery
　　　Perineal laceration, rupture or tear during delivery as in O70.0, also involving pelvic floor
　　　Perineal laceration, rupture or tear during delivery as in O70.0, also involving perineal muscles
　　　Perineal laceration, rupture or tear during delivery as in O70.0, also involving vaginal muscles
　　　Excludes1　perineal laceration involving anal sphincter (O70.2)

　O70.2　Third degree perineal laceration during delivery
　　　Perineal laceration, rupture or tear during delivery as in O70.1, also involving anal sphincter
　　　Perineal laceration, rupture or tear during delivery as in O70.1, also involving rectovaginal septum
　　　Perineal laceration, rupture or tear during delivery as in O70.1, also involving sphincter NOS
　　　Excludes1　anal sphincter tear during delivery without third degree perineal laceration (O70.4)
　　　　　perineal laceration involving anal or rectal mucosa (O70.3)

　O70.3　Fourth degree perineal laceration during delivery
　　　Perineal laceration, rupture or tear during delivery as in O70.2, also involving anal mucosa
　　　Perineal laceration, rupture or tear during delivery as in O70.2, also involving rectal mucosa

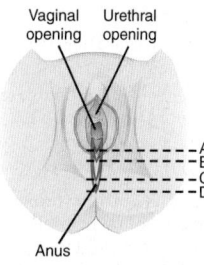

Figure 15-6　Perineal lacerations: **A.** First-degree is laceration of superficial tissues. **B.** Second-degree is limited to the pelvic floor and may involve the perineal or vaginal muscles. **C.** Third-degree involves the anal sphincter. **D.** Fourth-degree involves anal or rectal mucosa.

　O70.4　Anal sphincter tear complicating delivery, not associated with third degree laceration
　　　Excludes1　anal sphincter tear with third degree perineal laceration (O70.2)

　O70.9　Perineal laceration during delivery, unspecified

● **O71　Other obstetric trauma**
　　Includes　obstetric damage from instruments

　● **O71.0　Rupture of uterus (spontaneous) before onset of labor**
　　　Excludes1　disruption of (current) cesarean delivery wound (O90.0)
　　　　　laceration of uterus, NEC (O71.81)

　　O71.00　Rupture of uterus before onset of labor, unspecified trimester

　　O71.02　Rupture of uterus before onset of labor, second trimester

　　O71.03　Rupture of uterus before onset of labor, third trimester

　O71.1　Rupture of uterus during labor
　　　Rupture of uterus not stated as occurring before onset of labor
　　　Excludes1　disruption of cesarean delivery wound (O90.0)
　　　　　laceration of uterus, NEC (O71.81)

　O71.2　Postpartum inversion of uterus

　O71.3　Obstetric laceration of cervix
　　　Annular detachment of cervix

　O71.4　Obstetric high vaginal laceration alone
　　　Laceration of vaginal wall without perineal laceration
　　　Excludes1　obstetric high vaginal laceration with perineal laceration (O70.-)

　O71.5　Other obstetric injury to pelvic organs
　　　Obstetric injury to bladder
　　　Obstetric injury to urethra
　　　Excludes2　obstetric periurethral trauma (O71.82)

　O71.6　Obstetric damage to pelvic joints and ligaments
　　　Obstetric avulsion of inner symphyseal cartilage
　　　Obstetric damage to coccyx
　　　Obstetric traumatic separation of symphysis (pubis)

　O71.7　Obstetric hematoma of pelvis
　　　Obstetric hematoma of perineum
　　　Obstetric hematoma of vagina
　　　Obstetric hematoma of vulva

　● **O71.8　Other specified obstetric trauma**

　　O71.81　Laceration of uterus, not elsewhere classified

　　O71.82　Other specified trauma to perineum and vulva
　　　　Obstetric periurethral trauma

　　O71.89　Other specified obstetric trauma

　O71.9　Obstetric trauma, unspecified

CHAPTER 15 (O00-O9A)

● O72 Postpartum hemorrhage

> **Includes** hemorrhage after delivery of fetus or infant

    O72.0 Third-stage hemorrhage
> Hemorrhage associated with retained, trapped or adherent placenta
> Retained placenta NOS
>
> Code also type of adherent placenta (O43.2-)

    O72.1 Other immediate postpartum hemorrhage
> Hemorrhage following delivery of placenta
> Postpartum hemorrhage (atonic) NOS
> Uterine atony with hemorrhage
>
> > **Excludes1** uterine atony NOS (O62.2)
> > uterine atony without hemorrhage (O62.2)
> > postpartum atony of uterus without hemorrhage (O75.89)

    O72.2 Delayed and secondary postpartum hemorrhage
> Hemorrhage associated with retained portions of placenta or membranes after the first 24 hours following delivery of placenta
> Retained products of conception NOS, following delivery

    O72.3 Postpartum coagulation defects
> Postpartum afibrinogenemia
> Postpartum fibrinolysis

● O73 Retained placenta and membranes, without hemorrhage

> **Excludes1** placenta accreta (O43.21-)
> placenta increta (O43.22-)
> placenta percreta (O43.23-)

    O73.0 Retained placenta without hemorrhage
> Adherent placenta, without hemorrhage
> Trapped placenta without hemorrhage

    O73.1 Retained portions of placenta and membranes, without hemorrhage
> Retained products of conception following delivery, without hemorrhage

● O74 Complications of anesthesia during labor and delivery

> **Includes** maternal complications arising from the administration of a general, regional or local anesthetic, analgesic or other sedation during labor and delivery

> Use additional code, if applicable, to identify specific complication

    O74.0 Aspiration pneumonitis due to anesthesia during labor and delivery
> Inhalation of stomach contents or secretions NOS due to anesthesia during labor and delivery
> Mendelson's syndrome due to anesthesia during labor and delivery

    O74.1 Other pulmonary complications of anesthesia during labor and delivery

    O74.2 Cardiac complications of anesthesia during labor and delivery

    O74.3 Central nervous system complications of anesthesia during labor and delivery

    O74.4 Toxic reaction to local anesthesia during labor and delivery

    O74.5 Spinal and epidural anesthesia-induced headache during labor and delivery

    O74.6 Other complications of spinal and epidural anesthesia during labor and delivery

    O74.7 Failed or difficult intubation for anesthesia during labor and delivery

    O74.8 Other complications of anesthesia during labor and delivery

    O74.9 Complication of anesthesia during labor and delivery, unspecified

● O75 Other complications of labor and delivery, not elsewhere classified

> **Excludes2** puerperal (postpartum) infection (O86.-)
> puerperal (postpartum) sepsis (O85)

    O75.0 Maternal distress during labor and delivery

    O75.1 Shock during or following labor and delivery
> Obstetric shock following labor and delivery

    O75.2 Pyrexia during labor, not elsewhere classified

    O75.3 Other infection during labor
> Sepsis during labor
>
> Use additional code (B95-B97), to identify infectious agent

    O75.4 Other complications of obstetric surgery and procedures
> Cardiac arrest following obstetric surgery or procedures
> Cardiac failure following obstetric surgery or procedures
> Cerebral anoxia following obstetric surgery or procedures
> Pulmonary edema following obstetric surgery or procedures
>
> Use additional code to identify specific complication
>
> > **Excludes2** complications of anesthesia during labor and delivery (O74.-)
> > disruption of obstetrical (surgical) wound (O90.0-O90.1)
> > hematoma of obstetrical (surgical) wound (O90.2)
> > infection of obstetrical (surgical) wound (O86.0)

    O75.5 Delayed delivery after artificial rupture of membranes

    ● O75.8 Other specified complications of labor and delivery

        O75.81 Maternal exhaustion complicating labor and delivery

        O75.82 Onset (spontaneous) of labor after 37 completed weeks of gestation but before 39 completed weeks gestation, with delivery by (planned) cesarean section
> Delivery by (planned) cesarean section occurring after 37 completed weeks of gestation but before 39 completed weeks gestation due to (spontaneous) onset of labor
>
> Code first to specify reason for planned cesarean section such as:
> cephalopelvic disproportion (normally formed fetus) (O33.9)
> previous cesarean delivery (O34.21)

        O75.89 Other specified complications of labor and delivery

    O75.9 Complication of labor and delivery, unspecified

O76 Abnormality in fetal heart rate and rhythm complicating labor and delivery
> Depressed fetal heart rate tones complicating labor and delivery
> Fetal bradycardia complicating labor and delivery
> Fetal heart rate decelerations complicating labor and delivery
> Fetal heart rate irregularity complicating labor and delivery
> Fetal heart rate abnormal variability complicating labor and delivery
> Fetal tachycardia complicating labor and delivery
> Non-reassuring fetal heart rate or rhythm complicating labor and delivery
>
> > **Excludes1** fetal stress NOS (O77.9)
> > labor and delivery complicated by electrocardiographic evidence of fetal stress (O77.8)
> > labor and delivery complicated by ultrasonic evidence of fetal stress (O77.8)
>
> > **Excludes2** fetal metabolic acidemia (O68)
> > other fetal stress (O77.0-O77.1)

● **O77   Other fetal stress complicating labor and delivery**

    O77.0   Labor and delivery complicated by meconium in amniotic fluid

    O77.1   Fetal stress in labor or delivery due to drug administration

    O77.8   Labor and delivery complicated by other evidence of fetal stress

        Labor and delivery complicated by electrocardiographic evidence of fetal stress

        Labor and delivery complicated by ultrasonic evidence of fetal stress

        | Excludes1 | abnormality of fetal acid-base balance (O68) |

                abnormality in fetal heart rate or rhythm (O76)

                fetal metabolic acidemia (O68)

    O77.9   Labor and delivery complicated by fetal stress, unspecified

        | Excludes1 | abnormality of fetal acid-base balance (O68) |

                abnormality in fetal heart rate or rhythm (O76)

                fetal metabolic acidemia (O68)

OGCR Section I.C., Chapter 15.m.

Normal Delivery, Code O80

1) Encounter for full term uncomplicated delivery

Code O80 should be assigned when a woman is admitted for a full-term normal delivery and delivers a single, healthy infant without any complications antepartum, during the delivery, or postpartum during the delivery episode. Code O80 is always a principal diagnosis. It is not to be used if any other code from chapter 15 is needed to describe a current complication of the antenatal, delivery, or perinatal period. Additional codes from other chapters may be used with code O80 if they are not related to or are in any way complicating the pregnancy.

2) Uncomplicated delivery with resolved antepartum complication

Code O80 may be used if the patient had a complication at some point during the pregnancy, but the complication is not present at the time of the admission for delivery.

3) Outcome of delivery for O80

Z37.0, Single live brith, is the only outcome of delivery code appropriate for use with O80.

Figure 15-7 The four stages of normal delivery: **I.** Lightening, which occurs 2 to 4 weeks before birth, at which time the fetus turns with head toward the vagina. **II.** Regular contractions begin, the amniotic sac ruptures, and dilation is complete. **III.** Delivery of the head and rotation. **IV.** Expulsion of placenta.

ENCOUNTER FOR DELIVERY (O80-O82)

O80   Encounter for full-term uncomplicated delivery

    Delivery requiring minimal or no assistance, with or without episiotomy, without fetal manipulation [e.g., rotation version] or instrumentation [forceps] of a spontaneous, cephalic, vaginal, full-term, single, live-born infant. This code is for use as a single diagnosis code and is not to be used with any other code from chapter 15.

    Use additional code to indicate outcome of delivery (Z37.0)

O82   Encounter for cesarean delivery without indication

    Use additional code to indicate outcome of delivery (Z37.0)

COMPLICATIONS PREDOMINANTLY RELATED TO THE PUERPERIUM (O85-O92)

    | Excludes2 | mental and behavioral disorders associated with the puerperium (F53) |

                obstetrical tetanus (A34)

                puerperal osteomalacia (M83.0)

O85   Puerperal sepsis

    Postpartum sepsis

    Puerperal peritonitis

    Puerperal pyemia

    Use additional code (B95-B97), to identify infectious agent

    Use additional code (R65.2-) to identify severe sepsis, if applicable

    | Excludes1 | fever of unknown origin following delivery (O86.4) |

                genital tract infection following delivery (O86.1-)

                obstetric pyemic and septic embolism (O88.3-)

                puerperal septic thrombophlebitis (O86.81)

                urinary tract infection following delivery (O86.2-)

    | Excludes2 | sepsis during labor (O75.3) |

● **O86   Other puerperal infections**

    Use additional code (B95-B97), to identify infectious agent

    | Excludes2 | infection during labor (O75.3) |

                obstetrical tetanus (A34)

    O86.0   Infection of obstetric surgical wound

        Infected cesarean delivery wound following delivery

        Infected perineal repair following delivery

   ● **O86.1   Other infection of genital tract following delivery**

        O86.11   Cervicitis following delivery

        O86.12   Endometritis following delivery

        O86.13   Vaginitis following delivery

        O86.19   Other infection of genital tract following delivery

   ● **O86.2   Urinary tract infection following delivery**

        O86.20   Urinary tract infection following delivery, unspecified

            Puerperal urinary tract infection NOS

        O86.21   Infection of kidney following delivery

        O86.22   Infection of bladder following delivery

            Infection of urethra following delivery

        O86.29   Other urinary tract infection following delivery

    O86.4   Pyrexia of unknown origin following delivery

        Puerperal infection NOS following delivery

        Puerperal pyrexia NOS following delivery

        | Excludes2 | pyrexia during labor (O75.2) |

   ● **O86.8   Other specified puerperal infections**

        O86.81   Puerperal septic thrombophlebitis

        O86.89   Other specified puerperal infections

CHAPTER 15 (O00-O9A)

◀ New   ◀▦ Revised   ~~deleted~~ Deleted   **OGCR** Official Guidelines   X Assign placeholder X   ● Use Additional Character(s)

| Excludes 1 | | Excludes 2 | | Includes | | Use additional | | Code first | | Code also | | Unspecified |

● **O90 Complications of the puerperium, not elsewhere classified**

    O90.0 Disruption of cesarean delivery wound
        Dehiscence of cesarean delivery wound
        Excludes1   rupture of uterus (spontaneous) before
                     onset of labor (O71.0-)
                     rupture of uterus during labor (O71.1)

    O90.1 Disruption of perineal obstetric wound
        Disruption of wound of episiotomy
        Disruption of wound of perineal laceration
        Secondary perineal tear

    O90.2 Hematoma of obstetric wound

    O90.3 Peripartum cardiomyopathy
        Conditions in I42.- arising during pregnancy and the
           puerperium
        Excludes1   pre-existing heart disease complicating
                     pregnancy and the puerperium
                     (O99.4-)

    O90.4 Postpartum acute kidney failure
        Hepatorenal syndrome following labor and delivery

    O90.5 Postpartum thyroiditis

    O90.6 Postpartum mood disturbance
        Postpartum blues   Postpartum sadness
        Postpartum dysphoria
        Excludes1   postpartum depression (F53)
                     puerperal psychosis (F53)

● **O90.8 Other complications of the puerperium, not elsewhere
         classified**
    O90.81 Anemia of the puerperium
        Postpartum anemia NOS
        Excludes1   pre-existing anemia complicating
                     the puerperium (O99.03)

    **O90.89 Other complications of the puerperium, not
             elsewhere classified**
        Placental polyp

    O90.9 Complication of the puerperium, unspecified

● **O91 Infections of breast associated with pregnancy, the puerperium
   and lactation**
    Use additional code to identify infection

● **O91.0 Infection of nipple associated with pregnancy, the
       puerperium and lactation**
    ● **O91.01 Infection of nipple associated with pregnancy**
        Gestational abscess of nipple
        **O91.011 Infection of nipple associated with
              pregnancy, first trimester**
        **O91.012 Infection of nipple associated with
              pregnancy, second trimester**
        **O91.013 Infection of nipple associated with
              pregnancy, third trimester**
        **O91.019 Infection of nipple associated with
              pregnancy, unspecified trimester**

    **O91.02 Infection of nipple associated with the
            puerperium**
        Puerperal abscess of nipple

    O91.03 Infection of nipple associated with lactation
        Abscess of nipple associated with lactation

● **O91.1 Abscess of breast associated with pregnancy, the
       puerperium and lactation**
    ● **O91.11 Abscess of breast associated with pregnancy**
        Gestational mammary abscess
        Gestational purulent mastitis
        Gestational subareolar abscess
        **O91.111 Abscess of breast associated with
              pregnancy, first trimester**
        **O91.112 Abscess of breast associated with
              pregnancy, second trimester**
        **O91.113 Abscess of breast associated with
              pregnancy, third trimester**
        **O91.119 Abscess of breast associated with
              pregnancy, unspecified trimester**

    **O91.12 Abscess of breast associated with the
            puerperium**
        Puerperal mammary abscess
        Puerperal purulent mastitis
        Puerperal subareolar abscess

    O91.13 Abscess of breast associated with lactation
        Mammary abscess associated with lactation
        Purulent mastitis associated with lactation
        Subareolar abscess associated with lactation

● **O91.2 Nonpurulent mastitis associated with pregnancy, the
       puerperium and lactation**
    ● **O91.21 Nonpurulent mastitis associated with
          pregnancy**
        Gestational interstitial mastitis
        Gestational lymphangitis of breast
        Gestational mastitis NOS
        Gestational parenchymatous mastitis
        **O91.211 Nonpurulent mastitis associated with
              pregnancy, first trimester**
        **O91.212 Nonpurulent mastitis associated with
              pregnancy, second trimester**
        **O91.213 Nonpurulent mastitis associated with
              pregnancy, third trimester**
        **O91.219 Nonpurulent mastitis associated with
              pregnancy, unspecified trimester**

    **O91.22 Nonpurulent mastitis associated with the
            puerperium**
        Puerperal interstitial mastitis
        Puerperal lymphangitis of breast
        Puerperal mastitis NOS
        Puerperal parenchymatous mastitis

    O91.23 Nonpurulent mastitis associated with lactation
        Interstitial mastitis associated with lactation
        Lymphangitis of breast associated with
          lactation
        Mastitis NOS associated with lactation
        Parenchymatous mastitis associated with
          lactation

● **O92 Other disorders of breast and disorders of lactation associated
   with pregnancy and the puerperium**

● **O92.0 Retracted nipple associated with pregnancy, the
       puerperium, and lactation**
    ● **O92.01 Retracted nipple associated with pregnancy**
        **O92.011 Retracted nipple associated with
              pregnancy, first trimester**
        **O92.012 Retracted nipple associated with
              pregnancy, second trimester**
        **O92.013 Retracted nipple associated with
              pregnancy, third trimester**
        **O92.019 Retracted nipple associated with
              pregnancy, unspecified trimester**

    **O92.02 Retracted nipple associated with the
            puerperium**

    O92.03 Retracted nipple associated with lactation

● **O92.1 Cracked nipple associated with pregnancy, the
       puerperium, and lactation**
        Fissure of nipple, gestational or puerperal
    ● **O92.11 Cracked nipple associated with pregnancy**
        **O92.111 Cracked nipple associated with
              pregnancy, first trimester**
        **O92.112 Cracked nipple associated with
              pregnancy, second trimester**
        **O92.113 Cracked nipple associated with
              pregnancy, third trimester**
        **O92.119 Cracked nipple associated with
              pregnancy, unspecified trimester**

    O92.12 Cracked nipple associated with the puerperium

    O92.13 Cracked nipple associated with lactation

● O92.2　**Other and unspecified disorders of breast associated with pregnancy and the puerperium**
　O92.20　Unspecified disorder of breast associated with pregnancy and the puerperium
　O92.29　Other disorders of breast associated with pregnancy and the puerperium

O92.3　**Agalactia**
　Primary agalactia
　Excludes1　elective agalactia (O92.5)
　　　　　　secondary agalactia (O92.5)
　　　　　　therapeutic agalactia (O92.5)

O92.4　**Hypogalactia**

O92.5　**Suppressed lactation**
　Elective agalactia　　　　Therapeutic agalactia
　Secondary agalactia
　Excludes1　primary agalactia (O92.3)

O92.6　**Galactorrhea**

● O92.7　**Other and unspecified disorders of lactation**
　O92.70　Unspecified disorders of lactation
　O92.79　Other disorders of lactation
　　　　　Puerperal galactocele

OGCR Section I.C.2.l.3.

Malignant neoplasm in a pregnant patient

When a pregnant woman has a malignant neoplasm, a code from subcategory O9A.1-, Malignant neoplasm complicating pregnancy, childbirth, and the puerperium, should be sequenced first, followed by the appropriate code from Chapter 2 to indicate the type of neoplasm.

OTHER OBSTETRIC CONDITIONS, NOT ELSEWHERE CLASSIFIED (O94-O9A)

O94　**Sequelae of complication of pregnancy, childbirth, and the puerperium**
　Note: This category is to be used to indicate conditions in O00-O77.-, O85-O94 and O98-O9A.- as the cause of late effects. The 'sequelae' include conditions specified as such, or as late effects, which may occur at any time after the puerperium.
　Code first condition resulting from (sequela) of complication of pregnancy, childbirth, and the puerperium

O98　**Maternal infectious and parasitic diseases classifiable elsewhere but complicating pregnancy, childbirth and the puerperium**
　Includes　the listed conditions when complicating the pregnant state, when aggravated by the pregnancy, or as a reason for obstetric care
　Use additional code (Chapter 1), to identify specific infectious or parasitic disease
　Excludes2　herpes gestationis (O26.4-)
　　　　　　infectious carrier state (O99.82-, O99.83-)
　　　　　　obstetrical tetanus (A34)
　　　　　　puerperal infection (O86.-)
　　　　　　puerperal sepsis (O85)
　　　　　　when the reason for maternal care is that the disease is known or suspected to have affected the fetus (O35-O36)

● O98.0　**Tuberculosis complicating pregnancy, childbirth and the puerperium**
　Conditions in A15-A19
　● O98.01　Tuberculosis complicating pregnancy
　　O98.011　Tuberculosis complicating pregnancy, first trimester
　　O98.012　Tuberculosis complicating pregnancy, second trimester
　　O98.013　Tuberculosis complicating pregnancy, third trimester
　　O98.019　Tuberculosis complicating pregnancy, unspecified trimester
　O98.02　Tuberculosis complicating childbirth
　O98.03　Tuberculosis complicating the puerperium

● O98.1　**Syphilis complicating pregnancy, childbirth and the puerperium**
　Conditions in A50-A53
　● O98.11　Syphilis complicating pregnancy
　　O98.111　Syphilis complicating pregnancy, first trimester
　　O98.112　Syphilis complicating pregnancy, second trimester
　　O98.113　Syphilis complicating pregnancy, third trimester
　　O98.119　Syphilis complicating pregnancy, unspecified trimester
　O98.12　Syphilis complicating childbirth
　O98.13　Syphilis complicating the puerperium

● O98.2　**Gonorrhea complicating pregnancy, childbirth and the puerperium**
　Conditions in A54.-
　● O98.21　Gonorrhea complicating pregnancy
　　O98.211　Gonorrhea complicating pregnancy, first trimester
　　O98.212　Gonorrhea complicating pregnancy, second trimester
　　O98.213　Gonorrhea complicating pregnancy, third trimester
　　O98.219　Gonorrhea complicating pregnancy, unspecified trimester
　O98.22　Gonorrhea complicating childbirth
　O98.23　Gonorrhea complicating the puerperium

● O98.3　**Other infections with a predominantly sexual mode of transmission complicating pregnancy, childbirth and the puerperium**
　Conditions in A55-A64
　● O98.31　Other infections with a predominantly sexual mode of transmission complicating pregnancy
　　O98.311　Other infections with a predominantly sexual mode of transmission complicating pregnancy, first trimester
　　O98.312　Other infections with a predominantly sexual mode of transmission complicating pregnancy, second trimester
　　O98.313　Other infections with a predominantly sexual mode of transmission complicating pregnancy, third trimester
　　O98.319　Other infections with a predominantly sexual mode of transmission complicating pregnancy, unspecified trimester
　O98.32　Other infections with a predominantly sexual mode of transmission complicating childbirth
　O98.33　Other infections with a predominantly sexual mode of transmission complicating the puerperium

● O98.4　**Viral hepatitis complicating pregnancy, childbirth and the puerperium**
　Conditions in B15-B19
　● O98.41　Viral hepatitis complicating pregnancy
　　O98.411　Viral hepatitis complicating pregnancy, first trimester
　　O98.412　Viral hepatitis complicating pregnancy, second trimester
　　O98.413　Viral hepatitis complicating pregnancy, third trimester
　　O98.419　Viral hepatitis complicating pregnancy, unspecified trimester
　O98.42　Viral hepatitis complicating childbirth
　O98.43　Viral hepatitis complicating the puerperium

◄ New　◄⁞ Revised　~~deleted~~ Deleted　OGCR Official Guidelines　X Assign placeholder X　● Use Additional Character(s)

Excludes 1　Excludes 2　Includes　Use additional　Code first　Code also　Unspecified

● **O98.5** **Other viral diseases complicating pregnancy, childbirth and the puerperium**
    Conditions in A80-B09, B25-B34, R87.81-, R87.82-
    Excludes:1   human immunodeficiency virus [HIV] disease complicating pregnancy, childbirth and the puerperium (O98.7-)

  ● **O98.51** Other viral diseases complicating pregnancy
      O98.511   Other viral diseases complicating pregnancy, first trimester
      O98.512   Other viral diseases complicating pregnancy, second trimester
      O98.513   Other viral diseases complicating pregnancy, third trimester
      O98.519   Other viral diseases complicating pregnancy, unspecified trimester

    O98.52 Other viral diseases complicating childbirth
    O98.53 Other viral diseases complicating the puerperium

● **O98.6** **Protozoal diseases complicating pregnancy, childbirth and the puerperium**
    Conditions in B50-B64

  ● **O98.61** Protozoal diseases complicating pregnancy
      O98.611   Protozoal diseases complicating pregnancy, first trimester
      O98.612   Protozoal diseases complicating pregnancy, second trimester
      O98.613   Protozoal diseases complicating pregnancy, third trimester
      O98.619   Protozoal diseases complicating pregnancy, unspecified trimester

    O98.62 Protozoal diseases complicating childbirth
    O98.63 Protozoal diseases complicating the puerperium

● **O98.7** **Human immunodeficiency virus [HIV] disease complicating pregnancy, childbirth and the puerperium**
    Use additional code to identify the type of HIV disease:
      Acquired immune deficiency syndrome (AIDS) (B20)
      Asymptomatic HIV status (Z21)
      HIV positive NOS (Z21)
      Symptomatic HIV disease (B20)

    OGCR Section I.C.15.f.

    HIV Infection in Pregnancy, Childbirth and the Puerperium

    During pregnancy, childbirth or the puerperium, a patient admitted because of an HIV-related illness should receive a principal diagnosis from subcategory O98.7-. Human immunodeficiency [HIV] disease complicating pregnancy, childbirth and the puerperium, followed by the code(s) for the HIV-related illness(es).

    Patients with asymptomatic HIV infection status admitted during pregnancy, childbirth, or the puerperium should receive codes of O98.7- and Z21, Asymptomatic human immunodeficiency virus [HIV] infection status.

  ● **O98.71** Human immunodeficiency virus [HIV] disease complicating pregnancy
      O98.711   Human immunodeficiency virus [HIV] disease complicating pregnancy, first trimester
      O98.712   Human immunodeficiency virus [HIV] disease complicating pregnancy, second trimester
      O98.713   Human immunodeficiency virus [HIV] disease complicating pregnancy, third trimester
      O98.719   Human immunodeficiency virus [HIV] disease complicating pregnancy, unspecified trimester

    O98.72 Human immunodeficiency virus [HIV] disease complicating childbirth
    O98.73 Human immunodeficiency virus [HIV] disease complicating the puerperium

● **O98.8** **Other maternal infectious and parasitic diseases complicating pregnancy, childbirth and the puerperium**

  ● **O98.81** Other maternal infectious and parasitic diseases complicating pregnancy
      O98.811   Other maternal infectious and parasitic diseases complicating pregnancy, first trimester
      O98.812   Other maternal infectious and parasitic diseases complicating pregnancy, second trimester
      O98.813   Other maternal infectious and parasitic diseases complicating pregnancy, third trimester
      O98.819   Other maternal infectious and parasitic diseases complicating pregnancy, unspecified trimester

    O98.82 Other maternal infectious and parasitic diseases complicating childbirth
    O98.83 Other maternal infectious and parasitic diseases complicating the puerperium

● **O98.9** **Unspecified maternal infectious and parasitic disease complicating pregnancy, childbirth and the puerperium**

  ● **O98.91** Unspecified maternal infectious and parasitic disease complicating pregnancy
      O98.911   Unspecified maternal infectious and parasitic disease complicating pregnancy, first trimester
      O98.912   Unspecified maternal infectious and parasitic disease complicating pregnancy, second trimester
      O98.913   Unspecified maternal infectious and parasitic disease complicating pregnancy, third trimester
      O98.919   Unspecified maternal infectious and parasitic disease complicating pregnancy, unspecified trimester

    O98.92 Unspecified maternal infectious and parasitic disease complicating childbirth
    O98.93 Unspecified maternal infectious and parasitic disease complicating the puerperium

● **O99** **Other maternal diseases classifiable elsewhere but complicating pregnancy, childbirth and the puerperium**
    Includes: conditions which complicate the pregnant state, are aggravated by the pregnancy or are a main reason for obstetric care

    Use additional code to identify specific condition
    Excludes2   when the reason for maternal care is that the condition is known or suspected to have affected the fetus (O35-O36)

● **O99.0** **Anemia complicating pregnancy, childbirth and the puerperium**
    Conditions in D50-D64
    Excludes1   anemia arising in the puerperium (O90.81)
                postpartum anemia NOS (O90.81)

  ● **O99.01** Anemia complicating pregnancy
      O99.011   Anemia complicating pregnancy, first trimester
      O99.012   Anemia complicating pregnancy, second trimester
      O99.013   Anemia complicating pregnancy, third trimester
      O99.019   Anemia complicating pregnancy, unspecified trimester

CHAPTER 15 (O00-O9A)

CHAPTER 15 (O00-O9A)

O99.02   Anemia complicating childbirth

O99.03   Anemia complicating the puerperium

> **Excludes1**   postpartum anemia not pre-existing prior to delivery (O90.81)

● **O99.1**   Other diseases of the blood and blood-forming organs and certain disorders involving the immune mechanism complicating pregnancy, childbirth and the puerperium
Conditions in D65-D89

> **Excludes2**   hemorrhage with coagulation defects (O45.-, O46.0-, O67.0, O72.3)

● **O99.11**   Other diseases of the blood and blood-forming organs and certain disorders involving the immune mechanism complicating pregnancy

     O99.111   Other diseases of the blood and blood-forming organs and certain disorders involving the immune mechanism complicating pregnancy, first trimester

     O99.112   Other diseases of the blood and blood-forming organs and certain disorders involving the immune mechanism complicating pregnancy, second trimester

     O99.113   Other diseases of the blood and blood-forming organs and certain disorders involving the immune mechanism complicating pregnancy, third trimester

     O99.119   Other diseases of the blood and blood-forming organs and certain disorders involving the immune mechanism complicating pregnancy, unspecified trimester

O99.12   Other diseases of the blood and blood-forming organs and certain disorders involving the immune mechanism complicating childbirth

O99.13   Other diseases of the blood and blood-forming organs and certain disorders involving the immune mechanism complicating the puerperium

● **O99.2**   Endocrine, nutritional and metabolic diseases complicating pregnancy, childbirth and the puerperium
Conditions in E00-E88

> **Excludes2**   diabetes mellitus (O24.-)
> malnutrition (O25.-)
> postpartum thyroiditis (O90.5)

● **O99.21**   Obesity complicating pregnancy, childbirth, and the puerperium

> Use additional code to identify the type of obesity (E66.-)

     O99.210   Obesity complicating pregnancy, unspecified trimester

     O99.211   Obesity complicating pregnancy, first trimester

     O99.212   Obesity complicating pregnancy, second trimester

     O99.213   Obesity complicating pregnancy, third trimester

     O99.214   Obesity complicating childbirth

     O99.215   Obesity complicating the puerperium

● **O99.28**   Other endocrine, nutritional and metabolic diseases complicating pregnancy, childbirth and the puerperium

     O99.280   Endocrine, nutritional and metabolic diseases complicating pregnancy, unspecified trimester

     O99.281   Endocrine, nutritional and metabolic diseases complicating pregnancy, first trimester

     O99.282   Endocrine, nutritional and metabolic diseases complicating pregnancy, second trimester

     O99.283   Endocrine, nutritional and metabolic diseases complicating pregnancy, third trimester

     O99.284   Endocrine, nutritional and metabolic diseases complicating childbirth

     O99.285   Endocrine, nutritional and metabolic diseases complicating the puerperium

● **O99.3**   Mental disorders and diseases of the nervous system complicating pregnancy, childbirth and the puerperium

● **O99.31**   Alcohol use complicating pregnancy, childbirth, and the puerperium

> Use additional code(s) from F10 to identify manifestations of the alcohol use

     O99.310   Alcohol use complicating pregnancy, unspecified trimester

     O99.311   Alcohol use complicating pregnancy, first trimester

     O99.312   Alcohol use complicating pregnancy, second trimester

     O99.313   Alcohol use complicating pregnancy, third trimester

     O99.314   Alcohol use complicating childbirth

     O99.315   Alcohol use complicating the puerperium

● **O99.32**   Drug use complicating pregnancy, childbirth, and the puerperium

> Use additional code(s) from F11-F16 and F18-F19 to identify manifestations of the drug use

     O99.320   Drug use complicating pregnancy, unspecified trimester

     O99.321   Drug use complicating pregnancy, first trimester

     O99.322   Drug use complicating pregnancy, second trimester

     O99.323   Drug use complicating pregnancy, third trimester

     O99.324   Drug use complicating childbirth

     O99.325   Drug use complicating the puerperium

● **O99.33**   Smoking (tobacco) complicating pregnancy, childbirth, and the puerperium

> Use additional code from F17 to identify type of tobacco

     O99.330   Smoking (tobacco) complicating pregnancy, unspecified trimester

     O99.331   Smoking (tobacco) complicating pregnancy, first trimester

     O99.332   Smoking (tobacco) complicating pregnancy, second trimester

     O99.333   Smoking (tobacco) complicating pregnancy, third trimester

     O99.334   Smoking (tobacco) complicating childbirth

     O99.335   Smoking (tobacco) complicating the puerperium

◀ New   ◀▥ Revised   ~~deleted~~ Deleted   OGCR Official Guidelines   X Assign placeholder X   ● Use Additional Character(s)

Excludes 1   Excludes 2   Includes   Use additional   Code first   Code also   Unspecified

● O99.34 **Other mental disorders complicating pregnancy, childbirth, and the puerperium**
Conditions in F01-F09 and F20-F99

| Excludes2 | postpartum mood disturbance (O90.6)
postnatal psychosis (F53)
puerperal psychosis (F53) |

O99.340 Other mental disorders complicating pregnancy, unspecified trimester

O99.341 Other mental disorders complicating pregnancy, first trimester

O99.342 Other mental disorders complicating pregnancy, second trimester

O99.343 Other mental disorders complicating pregnancy, third trimester

O99.344 Other mental disorders complicating childbirth

O99.345 Other mental disorders complicating the puerperium

● O99.35 **Diseases of the nervous system complicating pregnancy, childbirth, and the puerperium**
Conditions in G00-G99

| Excludes2 | pregnancy related peripheral neuritis (O26.8-) |

O99.350 Diseases of the nervous system complicating pregnancy, unspecified trimester

O99.351 Diseases of the nervous system complicating pregnancy, first trimester

O99.352 Diseases of the nervous system complicating pregnancy, second trimester

O99.353 Diseases of the nervous system complicating pregnancy, third trimester

O99.354 Diseases of the nervous system complicating childbirth

O99.355 Diseases of the nervous system complicating the puerperium

● O99.4 **Diseases of the circulatory system complicating pregnancy, childbirth and the puerperium**
Conditions in I00-I99

| Excludes1 | peripartum cardiomyopathy (O90.3) |
| Excludes2 | hypertensive disorders (O10-O16)
obstetric embolism (O88.-)
venous complications and cerebrovenous sinus thrombosis in labor, childbirth and the puerperium (O87.-)
venous complications and cerebrovenous sinus thrombosis in pregnancy (O22.-) |

● O99.41 Diseases of the circulatory system complicating pregnancy

O99.411 Diseases of the circulatory system complicating pregnancy, first trimester

O99.412 Diseases of the circulatory system complicating pregnancy, second trimester

O99.413 Diseases of the circulatory system complicating pregnancy, third trimester

O99.419 Diseases of the circulatory system complicating pregnancy, unspecified trimester

O99.42 Diseases of the circulatory system complicating childbirth

O99.43 Diseases of the circulatory system complicating the puerperium

● O99.5 **Diseases of the respiratory system complicating pregnancy, childbirth and the puerperium**
Conditions in J00-J99

● O99.51 Diseases of the respiratory system complicating pregnancy

O99.511 Diseases of the respiratory system complicating pregnancy, first trimester

O99.512 Diseases of the respiratory system complicating pregnancy, second trimester

O99.513 Diseases of the respiratory system complicating pregnancy, third trimester

O99.519 Diseases of the respiratory system complicating pregnancy, unspecified trimester

O99.52 Diseases of the respiratory system complicating childbirth

O99.53 Diseases of the respiratory system complicating the puerperium

● O99.6 **Diseases of the digestive system complicating pregnancy, childbirth and the puerperium**
Conditions in K00-K93

| Excludes2 | liver and biliary tract disorders in pregnancy, childbirth and the puerperium (O26.6-) |

● O99.61 Diseases of the digestive system complicating pregnancy

O99.611 Diseases of the digestive system complicating pregnancy, first trimester

O99.612 Diseases of the digestive system complicating pregnancy, second trimester

O99.613 Diseases of the digestive system complicating pregnancy, third trimester

O99.619 Diseases of the digestive system complicating pregnancy, unspecified trimester

O99.62 Diseases of the digestive system complicating childbirth

O99.63 Diseases of the digestive system complicating the puerperium

● O99.7 **Diseases of the skin and subcutaneous tissue complicating pregnancy, childbirth and the puerperium**
Conditions in L00-L99

| Excludes2 | herpes gestationis (O26.4)
pruritic urticarial papules and plaques of pregnancy (PUPPP) (O26.86) |

● O99.71 Diseases of the skin and subcutaneous tissue complicating pregnancy

O99.711 Diseases of the skin and subcutaneous tissue complicating pregnancy, first trimester

O99.712 Diseases of the skin and subcutaneous tissue complicating pregnancy, second trimester

O99.713 Diseases of the skin and subcutaneous tissue complicating pregnancy, third trimester

O99.719 Diseases of the skin and subcutaneous tissue complicating pregnancy, unspecified trimester

O99.72 Diseases of the skin and subcutaneous tissue complicating childbirth

O99.73 Diseases of the skin and subcutaneous tissue complicating the puerperium

CHAPTER 15 (O00-O9A)

◄ New   ◄▥ Revised   ~~deleted~~ Deleted   **OGCR** Official Guidelines   X Assign placeholder X   ● Use Additional Character(s)

| Excludes 1 | Excludes 2 | Includes | Use additional | Code first | Code also | Unspecified |

● **O99.8 Other specified diseases and conditions complicating pregnancy, childbirth and the puerperium**
Conditions in D00-D48, H00-H95, M00-N99, and Q00-Q99
Use additional code to identify condition
Excludes2   genitourinary infections in pregnancy (O23.-)
infection of genitourinary tract following delivery (O86.1-O86.3)
malignant neoplasm complicating pregnancy, childbirth and the puerperium (O9A.1-)
maternal care for known or suspected abnormality of maternal pelvic organs (O34.-)
postpartum acute kidney failure (O90.4)
traumatic injuries in pregnancy (O9A.2-)

● **O99.81 Abnormal glucose complicating pregnancy, childbirth and the puerperium**
Excludes1   gestational diabetes (O24.4-)
O99.810 Abnormal glucose complicating pregnancy
O99.814 Abnormal glucose complicating childbirth
O99.815 Abnormal glucose complicating the puerperium

● **O99.82 Streptococcus B carrier state complicating pregnancy, childbirth and the puerperium**
O99.820 Streptococcus B carrier state complicating pregnancy
O99.824 Streptococcus B carrier state complicating childbirth
O99.825 Streptococcus B carrier state complicating the puerperium

● **O99.83 Other infection carrier state complicating pregnancy, childbirth and the puerperium**
Use additional code to identify the carrier state (Z22.-)
O99.830 Other infection carrier state complicating pregnancy
O99.834 Other infection carrier state complicating childbirth
O99.835 Other infection carrier state complicating the puerperium

● **O99.84 Bariatric surgery status complicating pregnancy, childbirth and the puerperium**
Gastric banding status complicating pregnancy, childbirth and the puerperium
Gastric bypass status for obesity complicating pregnancy, childbirth and the puerperium
Obesity surgery status complicating pregnancy, childbirth and the puerperium
O99.840 Bariatric surgery status complicating pregnancy, unspecified trimester
O99.841 Bariatric surgery status complicating pregnancy, first trimester
O99.842 Bariatric surgery status complicating pregnancy, second trimester
O99.843 Bariatric surgery status complicating pregnancy, third trimester
O99.844 Bariatric surgery status complicating childbirth
O99.845 Bariatric surgery status complicating the puerperium

O99.89 Other specified diseases and conditions complicating pregnancy, childbirth and the puerperium

● **O9A Maternal malignant neoplasms, traumatic injuries and abuse classifiable elsewhere but complicating pregnancy, childbirth and the puerperium**

● **O9A.1 Malignant neoplasm complicating pregnancy, childbirth and the puerperium**
Conditions in C00-C96
Use additional code to identify neoplasm
Excludes2   maternal care for benign tumor of corpus uteri (O34.1-)
maternal care for benign tumor of cervix (O34.4-)

● **O9A.11 Malignant neoplasm complicating pregnancy**
O9A.111 Malignant neoplasm complicating pregnancy, first trimester
O9A.112 Malignant neoplasm complicating pregnancy, second trimester
O9A.113 Malignant neoplasm complicating pregnancy, third trimester
O9A.119 Malignant neoplasm complicating pregnancy, unspecified trimester

O9A.12 Malignant neoplasm complicating childbirth

O9A.13 Malignant neoplasm complicating the puerperium

● **O9A.2 Injury, poisoning and certain other consequences of external causes complicating pregnancy, childbirth and the puerperium**
Conditions in S00-T88, except T74 and T76
Use additional code(s) to identify the injury or poisoning
Excludes2   physical, sexual and psychological abuse complicating pregnancy, childbirth and the puerperium (O9A.3-, O9A.4-, O9A.5-)

● **O9A.21 Injury, poisoning and certain other consequences of external causes complicating pregnancy**
O9A.211 Injury, poisoning and certain other consequences of external causes complicating pregnancy, first trimester
O9A.212 Injury, poisoning and certain other consequences of external causes complicating pregnancy, second trimester
O9A.213 Injury, poisoning and certain other consequences of external causes complicating pregnancy, third trimester
O9A.219 Injury, poisoning and certain other consequences of external causes complicating pregnancy, unspecified trimester

O9A.22 Injury, poisoning and certain other consequences of external causes complicating childbirth

O9A.23 Injury, poisoning and certain other consequences of external causes complicating the puerperium

◀ New   ◀▦ Revised   ~~deleted~~ Deleted   OGCR Official Guidelines   X Assign placeholder X   ● Use Additional Character(s)
Excludes 1   Excludes 2   Includes   Use additional   Code first   Code also   Unspecified

● **O9A.3   Physical abuse complicating pregnancy, childbirth and the puerperium**
     Conditions in T74.11 or T76.11
     Use additional code (if applicable):
       to identify any associated current injury due to physical abuse
       to identify the perpetrator of abuse (Y07.-)
     Excludes2   sexual abuse complicating pregnancy, childbirth and the puerperium (O9A.4)

  ● **O9A.31   Physical abuse complicating pregnancy**
       O9A.311   Physical abuse complicating pregnancy, first trimester
       O9A.312   Physical abuse complicating pregnancy, second trimester
       O9A.313   Physical abuse complicating pregnancy, third trimester
       O9A.319   Physical abuse complicating pregnancy, unspecified trimester
     O9A.32   Physical abuse complicating childbirth
     O9A.33   Physical abuse complicating the puerperium

● **O9A.4   Sexual abuse complicating pregnancy, childbirth and the puerperium**
     Conditions in T74.21 or T76.21
     Use additional code (if applicable):
       to identify any associated current injury due to sexual abuse
       to identify the perpetrator of abuse (Y07.-)

  ● **O9A.41   Sexual abuse complicating pregnancy**
       O9A.411   Sexual abuse complicating pregnancy, first trimester
       O9A.412   Sexual abuse complicating pregnancy, second trimester
       O9A.413   Sexual abuse complicating pregnancy, third trimester
       O9A.419   Sexual abuse complicating pregnancy, unspecified trimester
     O9A.42   Sexual abuse complicating childbirth
     O9A.43   Sexual abuse complicating the puerperium

● **O9A.5   Psychological abuse complicating pregnancy, childbirth and the puerperium**
     Conditions in T74.31 or T76.31
     Use additional code to identify the perpetrator of abuse (Y07.-)

  ● **O9A.51   Psychological abuse complicating pregnancy**
       O9A.511   Psychological abuse complicating pregnancy, first trimester
       O9A.512   Psychological abuse complicating pregnancy, second trimester
       O9A.513   Psychological abuse complicating pregnancy, third trimester
       O9A.519   Psychological abuse complicating pregnancy, unspecified trimester
     O9A.52   Psychological abuse complicating childbirth
     O9A.53   Psychological abuse complicating the puerperium

OGCR See Section I.C., Chapter 16
Newborn (Perinatal) Guidelines

CHAPTER 16

CERTAIN CONDITIONS ORIGINATING IN THE PERINATAL PERIOD (P00-P96)

Note: Codes from this chapter are for use on newborn records only, never on maternal records.

Includes   conditions that have their origin in the fetal or perinatal period (before birth through the first 28 days after birth) even if morbidity occurs later

Excludes2   congenital malformations, deformations and chromosomal abnormalities (Q00-Q99)
endocrine, nutritional and metabolic diseases (E00-E88)
injury, poisoning and certain other consequences of external causes (S00-T88)
neoplasms (C00-D49)
tetanus neonatorum (A33)

This chapter contains the following blocks:

P00-P04	Newborn affected by maternal factors and by complications of pregnancy, labor, and delivery
P05-P08	Disorders of newborns related to length of gestation and fetal growth
P09	Abnormal findings on neonatal screening
P10-P15	Birth trauma
P19-P29	Respiratory and cardiovascular disorders specific to the perinatal period
P35-P39	Infections specific to the perinatal period
P50-P61	Hemorrhagic and hematological disorders of newborn
P70-P74	Transitory endocrine and metabolic disorders specific to newborn
P76-P78	Digestive system disorders of newborn
P80-P83	Conditions involving the integument and temperature regulation of newborn
P84	Other problems with newborn
P90-P96	Other disorders originating in the perinatal period

NEWBORN AFFECTED BY MATERNAL FACTORS AND BY COMPLICATIONS OF PREGNANCY, LABOR, AND DELIVERY (P00–P04)

Note: These codes are for use when the listed maternal conditions are specified as the cause of confirmed morbidity or potential morbidity which have their origin in the perinatal period (before birth through the first 28 days after birth). Codes from these categories are also for use for newborns who are suspected of having an abnormal condition resulting from exposure from the mother or the birth process, but without signs or symptoms, and, which after examination and observation, is found not to exist. These codes may be used even if treatment is begun for a suspected condition that is ruled out.

● **P00**   **Newborn (suspected to be) affected by maternal conditions that may be unrelated to present pregnancy**

Code first any current condition in newborn

Excludes2   newborn (suspected to be) affected by maternal complications of pregnancy (P01.-)
newborn affected by maternal endocrine and metabolic disorders (P70–P74)
newborn affected by noxious substances transmitted via placenta or breast milk (P04.-)

P00.0   **Newborn (suspected to be) affected by maternal hypertensive disorders**
Newborn (suspected to be) affected by maternal conditions classifiable to O10-O11, O13-O16

P00.1   **Newborn (suspected to be) affected by maternal renal and urinary tract diseases**
Newborn (suspected to be) affected by maternal conditions classifiable to N00-N39

P00.2   **Newborn (suspected to be) affected by maternal infectious and parasitic diseases**
Newborn (suspected to be) affected by maternal infectious disease classifiable to A00-B99, J09 and J10

Excludes1   infections specific to the perinatal period (P35-P39)
maternal genital tract or other localized infections (P00.8)

P00.3   **Newborn (suspected to be) affected by other maternal circulatory and respiratory diseases**
Newborn (suspected to be) affected by maternal conditions classifiable to I00-I99, J00-J99, Q20-Q34 and not included in P00.0, P00.2

P00.4   **Newborn (suspected to be) affected by maternal nutritional disorders**
Newborn (suspected to be) affected by maternal disorders classifiable to E40-E64
Maternal malnutrition NOS

P00.5   **Newborn (suspected to be) affected by maternal injury**
Newborn (suspected to be) affected by maternal conditions classifiable to O9A.2-

P00.6   **Newborn (suspected to be) affected by surgical procedure on mother**
Newborn (suspected to be) affected by amniocentesis

Excludes1   Cesarean delivery for present delivery (P03.4)
damage to placenta from amniocentesis, cesarean delivery or surgical induction (P02.1)
previous surgery to uterus or pelvic organs (P03.89)

Excludes2   newborn affected by complication of (fetal) intrauterine procedure (P96.5)

P00.7   **Newborn (suspected to be) affected by other medical procedures on mother, not elsewhere classified**
Newborn (suspected to be) affected by radiation to mother

Excludes1   damage to placenta from amniocentesis, cesarean delivery or surgical induction (P02.1)
newborn affected by other complications of labor and delivery (P03.-)

● **P00.8**   **Newborn (suspected to be) affected by other maternal conditions**

P00.81   **Newborn (suspected to be) affected by periodontal disease in mother**

P00.89   **Newborn (suspected to be) affected by other maternal conditions**
Newborn (suspected to be) affected by conditions classifiable to T80-T88
Newborn (suspected to be) affected by maternal genital tract or other localized infections
Newborn (suspected to be) affected by maternal systemic lupus erythematosus

P00.9   **Newborn (suspected to be) affected by unspecified maternal condition**

● **P01**   **Newborn (suspected to be) affected by maternal complications of pregnancy**

Code first any current condition in newborn

P01.0   **Newborn (suspected to be) affected by incompetent cervix**

P01.1   **Newborn (suspected to be) affected by premature rupture of membranes**

P01.2   **Newborn (suspected to be) affected by oligohydramnios**

Excludes1   oligohydramnios due to premature rupture of membranes (P01.1)

P01.3   **Newborn (suspected to be) affected by polyhydramnios**
Excess of amniotic fluid, usually > 2000 mL
Newborn (suspected to be) affected by hydramnios

P01.4   **Newborn (suspected to be) affected by ectopic pregnancy**
> Newborn (suspected to be) affected by abdominal pregnancy

P01.5   **Newborn (suspected to be) affected by multiple pregnancy**
> Newborn (suspected to be) affected by triplet (pregnancy)
> Newborn (suspected to be) affected by twin (pregnancy)

P01.6   **Newborn (suspected to be) affected by maternal death**

P01.7   **Newborn (suspected to be) affected by malpresentation before labor**
> Newborn (suspected to be) affected by breech presentation before labor
> Newborn (suspected to be) affected by external version before labor
> Newborn (suspected to be) affected by face presentation before labor
> Newborn (suspected to be) affected by transverse lie before labor
> Newborn (suspected to be) affected by unstable lie before labor

P01.8   **Newborn (suspected to be) affected by other maternal complications of pregnancy**

P01.9   **Newborn (suspected to be) affected by maternal complication of pregnancy, unspecified**

● **P02**   **Newborn (suspected to be) affected by complications of placenta, cord and membranes**
> *Code first any current condition in newborn*

P02.0   **Newborn (suspected to be) affected by placenta previa**

P02.1   **Newborn (suspected to be) affected by other forms of placental separation and hemorrhage**
> Newborn (suspected to be) affected by abruptio placenta
> Newborn (suspected to be) affected by accidental hemorrhage
> Newborn (suspected to be) affected by antepartum hemorrhage
> Newborn (suspected to be) affected by damage to placenta from amniocentesis, cesarean delivery or surgical induction
> Newborn (suspected to be) affected by maternal blood loss
> Newborn (suspected to be) affected by premature separation of placenta

● **P02.2**   **Newborn (suspected to be) affected by other and unspecified morphological and functional abnormalities of placenta**

    P02.20   **Newborn (suspected to be) affected by unspecified morphological and functional abnormalities of placenta**

    P02.29   **Newborn (suspected to be) affected by other morphological and functional abnormalities of placenta**
> Newborn (suspected to be) affected by placental dysfunction
> Newborn (suspected to be) affected by placental infarction
> Newborn (suspected to be) affected by placental insufficiency

P02.3   **Newborn (suspected to be) affected by placental transfusion syndromes**
> Newborn (suspected to be) affected by placental and cord abnormalities resulting in twin-to-twin or other transplacental transfusion

P02.4   **Newborn (suspected to be) affected by prolapsed cord**

P02.5   **Newborn (suspected to be) affected by other compression of umbilical cord**
> Newborn (suspected to be) affected by umbilical cord (tightly) around neck
> Newborn (suspected to be) affected by entanglement of umbilical cord
> Newborn (suspected to be) affected by knot in umbilical cord

● **P02.6**   **Newborn (suspected to be) affected by other and unspecified conditions of umbilical cord**

    P02.60   **Newborn (suspected to be) affected by unspecified conditions of umbilical cord**

    P02.69   **Newborn (suspected to be) affected by other conditions of umbilical cord**
> Newborn (suspected to be) affected by short umbilical cord
> Newborn (suspected to be) affected by vasa previa

      Excludes1   newborn affected by single umbilical artery (Q27.0)

P02.7   **Newborn (suspected to be) affected by chorioamnionitis**
> *Inflammation of chorion and amnion*
> Newborn (suspected to be) affected by amnionitis
> Newborn (suspected to be) affected by membranitis
> Newborn (suspected to be) affected by placentitis

P02.8   **Newborn (suspected to be) affected by other abnormalities of membranes**

P02.9   **Newborn (suspected to be) affected by abnormality of membranes, unspecified**

● **P03**   **Newborn (suspected to be) affected by other complications of labor and delivery**
> *Code first any current condition in newborn*

P03.0   **Newborn (suspected to be) affected by breech delivery and extraction**

P03.1   **Newborn (suspected to be) affected by other malpresentation, malposition and disproportion during labor and delivery**
> Newborn (suspected to be) affected by contracted pelvis
> Newborn (suspected to be) affected by conditions classifiable to O64-O66
> Newborn (suspected to be) affected by persistent occipitoposterior
> Newborn (suspected to be) affected by transverse lie

P03.2   **Newborn (suspected to be) affected by forceps delivery**

P03.3   **Newborn (suspected to be) affected by delivery by vacuum extractor [ventouse]**

P03.4   **Newborn (suspected to be) affected by Cesarean delivery**

P03.5   **Newborn (suspected to be) affected by precipitate delivery**
> Newborn (suspected to be) affected by rapid second stage

P03.6   **Newborn (suspected to be) affected by abnormal uterine contractions**
> Newborn (suspected to be) affected by conditions classifiable to O62.-, except O62.3
> Newborn (suspected to be) affected by hypertonic labor
> Newborn (suspected to be) affected by uterine inertia

● **P03.8**   **Newborn (suspected to be) affected by other specified complications of labor and delivery**

  ● **P03.81**   **Newborn (suspected to be) affected by abnormality in fetal (intrauterine) heart rate or rhythm**

      Excludes1   neonatal cardiac dysrhythmia (P29.1-)

    P03.810   **Newborn (suspected to be) affected by abnormality in fetal (intrauterine) heart rate or rhythm before the onset of labor**

    P03.811   **Newborn (suspected to be) affected by abnormality in fetal (intrauterine) heart rate or rhythm during labor**

    P03.819   **Newborn (suspected to be) affected by abnormality in fetal (intrauterine) heart rate or rhythm, unspecified as to time of onset**

    P03.82   **Meconium passage during delivery**

      Excludes1   meconium aspiration (P24.00, P24.01)
> meconium staining (P96.83)

P03.89   **Newborn (suspected to be) affected by other specified complications of labor and delivery**
Newborn (suspected to be) affected by abnormality of maternal soft tissues
Newborn (suspected to be) affected by conditions classifiable to O60-O75 and by procedures used in labor and delivery not included in P02.- and P03.0-P03.6
Newborn (suspected to be) affected by induction of labor

P03.9   **Newborn (suspected to be) affected by complication of labor and delivery, unspecified**

● P04   **Newborn (suspected to be) affected by noxious substances transmitted via placenta or breast milk**

Includes   nonteratogenic effects of substances transmitted via placenta

Excludes2   congenital malformations (Q00-Q99)
neonatal jaundice from excessive hemolysis due to drugs or toxins transmitted from mother (P58.4)
newborn in contact with and (suspected) exposures hazardous to health not transmitted via placenta or breast milk (Z77.-)

P04.0   **Newborn (suspected to be) affected by maternal anesthesia and analgesia in pregnancy, labor and delivery**
Newborn (suspected to be) affected by reactions and intoxications from maternal opiates and tranquilizers administered during labor and delivery

P04.1   **Newborn (suspected to be) affected by other maternal medication**
Newborn (suspected to be) affected by cancer chemotherapy
Newborn (suspected to be) affected by cytotoxic drugs

Excludes1   dysmorphism due to warfarin (Q86.2)
fetal hydantoin syndrome (Q86.1)
maternal use of drugs of addiction (P04.4-)

P04.2   **Newborn (suspected to be) affected by maternal use of tobacco**
Newborn (suspected to be) affected by exposure in utero to tobacco smoke

Excludes2   newborn exposure to environmental tobacco smoke (P96.81)

P04.3   **Newborn (suspected to be) affected by maternal use of alcohol**

Excludes1   fetal alcohol syndrome (Q86.0)

● P04.4   **Newborn (suspected to be) affected by maternal use of drugs of addiction**

P04.41   **Newborn (suspected to be) affected by maternal use of cocaine**
'Crack baby'

P04.49   **Newborn (suspected to be) affected by maternal use of other drugs of addiction**

Excludes2   newborn (suspected to be) affected by maternal anesthesia and analgesia (P04.0)
withdrawal symptoms from maternal use of drugs of addiction (P96.1)

P04.5   **Newborn (suspected to be) affected by maternal use of nutritional chemical substances**

P04.6   **Newborn (suspected to be) affected by maternal exposure to environmental chemical substances**

P04.8   **Newborn (suspected to be) affected by other maternal noxious substances**

P04.9   **Newborn (suspected to be) affected by maternal noxious substance, unspecified**

OGCR Section I.C.16.d.

Prematurity and Fetal Growth Retardation
Providers utilize different criteria in determining prematurity. A code for prematurity should not be assigned unless it is documented. Assignment of codes in categories P05, Disorders of newborn related to slow fetal growth and fetal malnutrition, and P07, Disorders of newborn related to short gestation and low birth weight, not elsewhere classified, should be based on the recorded birth weight and estimated gestational age. Codes from category P05 should not be assigned with codes from category P07.

When both birth weight and gestational age are available, two codes from category P07 should be assigned, with the code for birth weight sequenced before the code for gestational age.

A code from P05 and codes from P07.2 and P07.3 may be used to specify weeks of gestation as documented by the provider in the record.

DISORDERS OF NEWBORN RELATED TO LENGTH OF GESTATION AND FETAL GROWTH (P05-P08)

● P05   **Disorders of newborn related to slow fetal growth and fetal malnutrition**

● P05.0   **Newborn light for gestational age**
Newborn light-for-dates

P05.00   **Newborn light for gestational age, unspecified weight**

P05.01   **Newborn light for gestational age, less than 500 grams**

P05.02   **Newborn light for gestational age, 500-749 grams**

P05.03   **Newborn light for gestational age, 750-999 grams**

P05.04   **Newborn light for gestational age, 1000-1249 grams**

P05.05   **Newborn light for gestational age, 1250-1499 grams**

P05.06   **Newborn light for gestational age, 1500-1749 grams**

P05.07   **Newborn light for gestational age, 1750-1999 grams**

P05.08   **Newborn light for gestational age, 2000-2499 grams**

● P05.1   **Newborn small for gestational age**
Newborn small-and-light-for-dates
Newborn small-for-dates

P05.10   **Newborn small for gestational age, unspecified weight**

P05.11   **Newborn small for gestational age, less than 500 grams**

P05.12   **Newborn small for gestational age, 500-749 grams**

P05.13   **Newborn small for gestational age, 750-999 grams**

P05.14   **Newborn small for gestational age, 1000-1249 grams**

P05.15   **Newborn small for gestational age, 1250-1499 grams**

P05.16   **Newborn small for gestational age, 1500-1749 grams**

P05.17   **Newborn small for gestational age, 1750-1999 grams**

P05.18   **Newborn small for gestational age, 2000-2499 grams**

◀ New   ◀▓ Revised   ~~deleted~~ Deleted   **OGCR** Official Guidelines   X Assign placeholder X   ● Use Additional Character(s)

Excludes 1   Excludes 2   Includes   Use additional   Code first   Code also   Unspecified

P05.2   **Newborn affected by fetal (intrauterine) malnutrition not light or small for gestational age**
Infant, not light or small for gestational age, showing signs of fetal malnutrition, such as dry, peeling skin and loss of subcutaneous tissue
> **Excludes1**   newborn affected by fetal malnutrition with light for gestational age (P05.0-)
> newborn affected by fetal malnutrition with small for gestational age (P05.1-)

P05.9   **Newborn affected by slow intrauterine growth, unspecified**
Newborn affected by fetal growth retardation NOS

● **P07**   **Disorders of newborn related to short gestation and low birth weight, not elsewhere classified**
Note: When both birth weight and gestational age of the newborn are available, both should be coded with birth weight sequenced before gestational age.
> **Includes** the listed conditions, without further specification, as the cause of morbidity or additional care, in newborn
> **Excludes1** low birth weight due to slow fetal growth and fetal malnutrition (P05.-)

● **P07.0**   **Extremely low birth weight newborn**
Newborn birth weight 999 g. or less

   P07.00   **Extremely low birth weight newborn, unspecified weight**

   P07.01   **Extremely low birth weight newborn, less than 500 grams**

   P07.02   **Extremely low birth weight newborn, 500-749 grams**

   P07.03   **Extremely low birth weight newborn, 750-999 grams**

● **P07.1**   **Other low birth weight newborn**
Newborn birth weight 1000-2499 g.

   P07.10   **Other low birth weight newborn, unspecified weight**

   P07.14   **Other low birth weight newborn, 1000-1249 grams**

   P07.15   **Other low birth weight newborn, 1250-1499 grams**

   P07.16   **Other low birth weight newborn, 1500-1749 grams**

   P07.17   **Other low birth weight newborn, 1750-1999 grams**

   P07.18   **Other low birth weight newborn, 2000-2499 grams**

● **P07.2**   **Extreme immaturity of newborn**
Less than 28 completed weeks (less than 196 completed days) of gestation

   P07.20   **Extreme immaturity of newborn, unspecified weeks of gestation**
Gestational age less than 28 completed weeks NOS

   P07.21   **Extreme immaturity of newborn, gestational age less than 23 completed weeks**
Extreme immaturity of newborn, gestational age less than 23 weeks, 0 days

   P07.22   **Extreme immaturity of newborn, gestational age 23 completed weeks**
Extreme immaturity of newborn, gestational age 23 weeks, 0 days through 23 weeks, 6 days

   P07.23   **Extreme immaturity of newborn, gestational age 24 completed weeks**
Extreme immaturity of newborn, gestational age 24 weeks, 0 days through 24 weeks, 6 days

   P07.24   **Extreme immaturity of newborn, gestational age 25 completed weeks**
Extreme immaturity of newborn, gestational age 25 weeks, 0 days through 25 weeks, 6 days

   P07.25   **Extreme immaturity of newborn, gestational age 26 completed weeks**
Extreme immaturity of newborn, gestational age 26 weeks, 0 days through 26 weeks, 6 days

   P07.26   **Extreme immaturity of newborn, gestational age 27 completed weeks**
Extreme immaturity of newborn, gestational age 27 weeks, 0 days through 27 weeks, 6 days

● **P07.3**   **Preterm [premature] newborn [other]**
28 completed weeks or more but less than 37 completed weeks (196 completed days but less than 259 completed days) of gestation
Prematurity NOS

   P07.30   **Preterm newborn, unspecified weeks of gestation**

   P07.31   **Preterm newborn, gestational age 28 completed weeks**
Preterm newborn, gestational age 28 weeks, 0 days through 28 weeks, 6 days

   P07.32   **Preterm newborn, gestational age 29 completed weeks**
Preterm newborn, gestational age 29 weeks, 0 days through 29 weeks, 6 days

   P07.33   **Preterm newborn, gestational age 30 completed weeks**
Preterm newborn, gestational age 30 weeks, 0 days through 30 weeks, 6 days

   P07.34   **Preterm newborn, gestational age 31 completed weeks**
Preterm newborn, gestational age 31 weeks, 0 days through 31 weeks, 6 days

   P07.35   **Preterm newborn, gestational age 32 completed weeks**
Preterm newborn, gestational age 32 weeks, 0 days through 32 weeks, 6 days

   P07.36   **Preterm newborn, gestational age 33 completed weeks**
Preterm newborn, gestational age 33 weeks, 0 days through 33 weeks, 6 days

   P07.37   **Preterm newborn, gestational age 34 completed weeks**
Preterm newborn, gestational age 34 weeks, 0 days through 34 weeks, 6 days

   P07.38   **Preterm newborn, gestational age 35 completed weeks**
Preterm newborn, gestational age 35 weeks, 0 days through 35 weeks, 6 days

   P07.39   **Preterm newborn, gestational age 36 completed weeks**
Preterm newborn, gestational age 36 weeks, 0 days through 36 weeks, 6 days

● **P08**   **Disorders of newborn related to long gestation and high birth weight**

    Note: When both birth weight and gestational age of the newborn are available, priority of assignment should be given to birth weight.

    Includes   the listed conditions, without further specification, as causes of morbidity or additional care, in newborn

  P08.0   **Exceptionally large newborn baby**
    Usually implies a birth weight of 4500 g. or more

    Excludes1   syndrome of infant of diabetic mother (P70.1)
            syndrome of infant of mother with gestational diabetes (P70.0)

  P08.1   **Other heavy for gestational age newborn**
    Other newborn heavy- or large-for-dates regardless of period of gestation
    Usually implies a birth weight of 4000 g. to 4499 g.

    Excludes1   newborn with a birth weight of 4500 or more (P08.0)
            syndrome of infant of diabetic mother (P70.1)
            syndrome of infant of mother with gestational diabetes (P70.0)

● **P08.2**   **Late newborn, not heavy for gestational age**

  P08.21   **Post-term newborn**
    Newborn with gestation period over 40 completed weeks to 42 completed weeks

  P08.22   **Prolonged gestation of newborn**
    Newborn with gestation period over 42 completed weeks (294 days or more), not heavy- or large-for-dates
    Postmaturity NOS

ABNORMAL FINDINGS ON NEONATAL SCREENING (P09)

  P09   **Abnormal findings on neonatal screening**

    Use additional code to identify signs, symptoms and conditions associated with the screening

    Excludes2   nonspecific serologic evidence of human immunodeficiency virus [HIV] (R75)

BIRTH TRAUMA (P10-P15)

● **P10**   **Intracranial laceration and hemorrhage due to birth injury**

    Excludes1   intracranial hemorrhage of newborn NOS (P52.9)
            intracranial hemorrhage of newborn due to anoxia or hypoxia (P52.-)
            nontraumatic intracranial hemorrhage of newborn (P52.-)

  P10.0   **Subdural hemorrhage due to birth injury**
    Subdural hematoma (localized) due to birth injury

    Excludes1   subdural hemorrhage accompanying tentorial tear (P10.4)

  P10.1   **Cerebral hemorrhage due to birth injury**

  P10.2   **Intraventricular hemorrhage due to birth injury**

  P10.3   **Subarachnoid hemorrhage due to birth injury**

  P10.4   **Tentorial tear due to birth injury**
    Pertaining to tentorium of cerebellum (extension of dura mater that separates cerebellum from inferior portion of occipital lobes)

  P10.8   **Other intracranial lacerations and hemorrhages due to birth injury**

  P10.9   **Unspecified intracranial laceration and hemorrhage due to birth injury**

● **P11**   **Other birth injuries to central nervous system**

  P11.0   **Cerebral edema due to birth injury**

  P11.1   **Other specified brain damage due to birth injury**

  P11.2   **Unspecified brain damage due to birth injury**

  P11.3   **Birth injury to facial nerve**
    Facial palsy due to birth injury

  P11.4   **Birth injury to other cranial nerves**

Item 16–1   The **peripheral nervous system** consists of 31 pairs of spinal nerves, 12 pairs of cranial nerves, and the autonomic nerves, which are divided into the parasympathetic and sympathetic nerves. The cranial nerves are: olfactory (I), optic (II), oculomotor (III), trochlear (IV), trigeminal (V), abducens (VI), facial (VII), vestibulocochlear (VIII), glossopharyngeal (IX), vagus (X), accessory (XI), and hypoglossal (XII).

Figure 16-1 **A.** Parasympathetic nervous system. **B.** Sympathetic nervous system. (From Buck CJ: Step-by-Step Medical Coding, Philadelphia, WB Saunders, 1998)

◀ New   ◀▥ Revised   ~~deleted~~ Deleted   **OGCR** Official Guidelines   X Assign placeholder X   ● Use Additional Character(s)

Excludes 1   Excludes 2   Includes   Use additional   Code first   Code also   Unspecified

P11.5   Birth injury to spine and spinal cord
    Fracture of spine due to birth injury
P11.9   Birth injury to central nervous system, unspecified

● **P12   Birth injury to scalp**
   P12.0   Cephalhematoma due to birth injury
   P12.1   Chignon (from vacuum extraction) due to birth injury
   P12.2   Epicranial subaponeurotic hemorrhage due to birth injury
     Subgaleal hemorrhage
   P12.3   Bruising of scalp due to birth injury
   P12.4   Injury of scalp of newborn due to monitoring equipment
     Sampling incision of scalp of newborn
     Scalp clip (electrode) injury of newborn
  ● **P12.8   Other birth injuries to scalp**
     P12.81   Caput succedaneum
     P12.89   Other birth injuries to scalp
   P12.9   Birth injury to scalp, unspecified

● **P13   Birth injury to skeleton**
   Excludes2   birth injury to spine (P11.5)
   P13.0   Fracture of skull due to birth injury
   P13.1   Other birth injuries to skull
     Excludes1   cephalhematoma (P12.0)
   P13.2   Birth injury to femur
   P13.3   Birth injury to other long bones
   P13.4   Fracture of clavicle due to birth injury
   P13.8   Birth injuries to other parts of skeleton
   P13.9   Birth injury to skeleton, unspecified

● **P14   Birth injury to peripheral nervous system**
   P14.0   Erb's paralysis due to birth injury
   P14.1   Klumpke's paralysis due to birth injury
   P14.2   Phrenic nerve paralysis due to birth injury
   P14.3   Other brachial plexus birth injuries
   P14.8   Birth injuries to other parts of peripheral nervous system
   P14.9   Birth injury to peripheral nervous system, unspecified

● **P15   Other birth injuries**
   P15.0   Birth injury to liver
     Rupture of liver due to birth injury
   P15.1   Birth injury to spleen
     Rupture of spleen due to birth injury
   P15.2   Sternomastoid injury due to birth injury
   P15.3   Birth injury to eye
     Subconjunctival hemorrhage due to birth injury
     Traumatic glaucoma due to birth injury
   P15.4   Birth injury to face
     Facial congestion due to birth injury
   P15.5   Birth injury to external genitalia
   P15.6   Subcutaneous fat necrosis due to birth injury
   P15.8   Other specified birth injuries
   P15.9   Birth injury, unspecified

RESPIRATORY AND CARDIOVASCULAR DISORDERS SPECIFIC TO THE PERINATAL PERIOD (P19-P29)

● **P19   Metabolic acidemia in newborn**
   Includes   metabolic acidemia in newborn
   P19.0   Metabolic acidemia in newborn first noted before onset of labor
   P19.1   Metabolic acidemia in newborn first noted during labor
   P19.2   Metabolic acidemia noted at birth
   P19.9   Metabolic acidemia, unspecified

● **P22   Respiratory distress of newborn**
   Excludes1   respiratory arrest of newborn (P28.81)
     respiratory failure of newborn NOS (P28.5)
   P22.0   Respiratory distress syndrome of newborn
     Cardiorespiratory distress syndrome of newborn
     Hyaline membrane disease
     Idiopathic respiratory distress syndrome [IRDS or RDS] of newborn
     Pulmonary hypoperfusion syndrome
     Respiratory distress syndrome, type I
   P22.1   Transient tachypnea of newborn
     Idiopathic tachypnea of newborn
     Respiratory distress syndrome, type II
     Wet lung syndrome
   P22.8   Other respiratory distress of newborn
   P22.9   Respiratory distress of newborn, unspecified

● **P23   Congenital pneumonia**
   Includes   infective pneumonia acquired in utero or during birth
   Excludes1   neonatal pneumonia resulting from aspiration (P24.-)
   P23.0   Congenital pneumonia due to viral agent
     Use additional code (B97) to identify organism
     Excludes1   congenital rubella pneumonitis (P35.0)
   P23.1   Congenital pneumonia due to Chlamydia
   P23.2   Congenital pneumonia due to staphylococcus
   P23.3   Congenital pneumonia due to streptococcus, group B
   P23.4   Congenital pneumonia due to Escherichia coli
   P23.5   Congenital pneumonia due to Pseudomonas
   P23.6   Congenital pneumonia due to other bacterial agents
     Congenital pneumonia due to Hemophilus influenzae
     Congenital pneumonia due to Klebsiella pneumoniae
     Congenital pneumonia due to Mycoplasma
     Congenital pneumonia due to Streptococcus, except group B
     Use additional code (B95-B96) to identify organism
   P23.8   Congenital pneumonia due to other organisms
   P23.9   Congenital pneumonia, unspecified

● **P24   Neonatal aspiration**
   Includes   aspiration in utero and during delivery
  ● **P24.0   Meconium aspiration**
     Excludes1   meconium passage (without aspiration) during delivery (P03.82)
     meconium staining (P96.83)
     P24.00   Meconium aspiration without respiratory symptoms
       Meconium aspiration NOS
     P24.01   Meconium aspiration with respiratory symptoms
       Meconium aspiration pneumonia
       Meconium aspiration pneumonitis
       Meconium aspiration syndrome NOS
       Use additional code to identify any secondary pulmonary hypertension, if applicable (I27.2)
  ● **P24.1   Neonatal aspiration of (clear) amniotic fluid and mucus**
     Neonatal aspiration of liquor (amnii)
     P24.10   Neonatal aspiration of (clear) amniotic fluid and mucus without respiratory symptoms
       Neonatal aspiration of amniotic fluid and mucus NOS
     P24.11   Neonatal aspiration of (clear) amniotic fluid and mucus with respiratory symptoms
       Neonatal aspiration of amniotic fluid and mucus with pneumonia
       Neonatal aspiration of amniotic fluid and mucus with pneumonitis
       Use additional code to identify any secondary pulmonary hypertension, if applicable (I27.2)

CHAPTER 16 (P00-P96)

● **P24.2**   Neonatal aspiration of blood
     P24.20   **Neonatal aspiration of blood without respiratory symptoms**
         Neonatal aspiration of blood NOS
     P24.21   **Neonatal aspiration of blood with respiratory symptoms**
         Neonatal aspiration of blood with pneumonia
         Neonatal aspiration of blood with pneumonitis
         Use additional code to identify any secondary pulmonary hypertension, if applicable (I27.2)

● **P24.3**   Neonatal aspiration of milk and regurgitated food
     Neonatal aspiration of stomach contents
     P24.30   **Neonatal aspiration of milk and regurgitated food without respiratory symptoms**
         Neonatal aspiration of milk and regurgitated food NOS
     P24.31   **Neonatal aspiration of milk and regurgitated food with respiratory symptoms**
         Neonatal aspiration of milk and regurgitated food with pneumonia
         Neonatal aspiration of milk and regurgitated food with pneumonitis
         Use additional code to identify any secondary pulmonary hypertension, if applicable (I27.2)

● **P24.8**   Other neonatal aspiration
     P24.80   **Other neonatal aspiration without respiratory symptoms**
         Neonatal aspiration NEC
     P24.81   **Other neonatal aspiration with respiratory symptoms**
         Neonatal aspiration pneumonia NEC
         Neonatal aspiration with pneumonitis NEC
         Neonatal aspiration with pneumonia NOS
         Neonatal aspiration with pneumonitis NOS
         Use additional code to identify any secondary pulmonary hypertension, if applicable (I27.2)

     P24.9   Neonatal aspiration, **unspecified**

● **P25**   Interstitial emphysema and related conditions originating in the perinatal period
     P25.0   **Interstitial emphysema originating in the perinatal period**
     P25.1   **Pneumothorax originating in the perinatal period**
     P25.2   **Pneumomediastinum originating in the perinatal period**
     P25.3   **Pneumopericardium originating in the perinatal period**
     P25.8   **Other conditions related to interstitial emphysema originating in the perinatal period**

● **P26**   Pulmonary hemorrhage originating in the perinatal period
     Excludes1   acute idiopathic hemorrhage in infants over 28 days old (R04.81)
     P26.0   **Tracheobronchial hemorrhage originating in the perinatal period**
     P26.1   **Massive pulmonary hemorrhage originating in the perinatal period**
     P26.8   **Other pulmonary hemorrhages originating in the perinatal period**
     P26.9   Unspecified pulmonary hemorrhage originating in the perinatal period

● **P27**   Chronic respiratory disease originating in the perinatal period
     Excludes1   respiratory distress of newborn (P22.0-P22.9)
     P27.0   **Wilson-Mikity syndrome**
     Pulmonary dysmaturity
     P27.1   **Bronchopulmonary dysplasia originating in the perinatal period**

P27.8   **Other chronic respiratory diseases originating in the perinatal period**
     Congenital pulmonary fibrosis
     Ventilator lung in newborn
P27.9   Unspecified chronic respiratory disease originating in the perinatal period

● **P28**   Other respiratory conditions originating in the perinatal period
     Excludes1   congenital malformations of the respiratory system (Q30-Q34)
     P28.0   **Primary atelectasis of newborn**
     Failure of lungs to expand properly at birth
     Primary failure to expand terminal respiratory units
     Pulmonary hypoplasia associated with short gestation
     Pulmonary immaturity NOS
   ● **P28.1**   **Other and unspecified atelectasis of newborn**
     P28.10   Unspecified atelectasis of newborn
         Atelectasis of newborn NOS
     P28.11   **Resorption atelectasis without respiratory distress syndrome**
         Excludes1   resorption atelectasis with respiratory distress syndrome (P22.0)
     P28.19   **Other atelectasis of newborn**
         Partial atelectasis of newborn
         Secondary atelectasis of newborn
     P28.2   **Cyanotic attacks of newborn**
         Excludes1   apnea of newborn (P28.3-P28.4)
     P28.3   **Primary sleep apnea of newborn**
     Central sleep apnea of newborn
     Obstructive sleep apnea of newborn
     Sleep apnea of newborn NOS
     P28.4   **Other apnea of newborn**
     Apnea of prematurity
     Obstructive apnea of newborn
         Excludes1   obstructive sleep apnea of newborn (P28.3)
     P28.5   **Respiratory failure of newborn**
         Excludes1   respiratory arrest of newborn (P28.81)
                 respiratory distress of newborn (P22.0-)
   ● **P28.8**   **Other specified respiratory conditions of newborn**
     P28.81   **Respiratory arrest of newborn**
     P28.89   **Other specified respiratory conditions of newborn**
         Congenital laryngeal stridor
         Sniffles in newborn
         Snuffles in newborn
         Excludes1   early congenital syphilitic rhinitis (A50.05)
     P28.9   **Respiratory condition of newborn, unspecified**
     Respiratory depression in newborn

● **P29**   Cardiovascular disorders originating in the perinatal period
     Excludes1   congenital malformations of the circulatory system (Q20-Q28)
     P29.0   **Neonatal cardiac failure**
   ● **P29.1**   **Neonatal cardiac dysrhythmia**
     P29.11   **Neonatal tachycardia**
     P29.12   **Neonatal bradycardia**
     P29.2   **Neonatal hypertension**
     P29.3   **Persistent fetal circulation**
     Delayed closure of ductus arteriosus
     (Persistent) pulmonary hypertension of newborn
     P29.4   **Transient myocardial ischemia in newborn**
   ● **P29.8**   **Other cardiovascular disorders originating in the perinatal period**
     P29.81   **Cardiac arrest of newborn**
     P29.89   **Other cardiovascular disorders originating in the perinatal period**
     P29.9   **Cardiovascular disorder originating in the perinatal period, unspecified**

◀ New   ◀═ Revised   ~~deleted~~ Deleted   OGCR Official Guidelines   X Assign placeholder X   ● Use Additional Character(s)

Excludes 1   Excludes 2   Includes   Use additional   Code first   Code also   Unspecified

INFECTIONS SPECIFIC TO THE PERINATAL PERIOD (P35-P39)

Infections acquired in utero, during birth via the umbilicus, or during the first 28 days after birth

Excludes2 asymptomatic human immunodeficiency virus [HIV] infection status (Z21)
congenital gonococcal infection (A54.-)
congenital pneumonia (P23.-)
congenital syphilis (A50.-)
human immunodeficiency virus [HIV] disease (B20)
infant botulism (A48.51)
infectious diseases not specific to the perinatal period (A00-B99, J09, J10.-)
intestinal infectious disease (A00-A09)
laboratory evidence of human immunodeficiency virus [HIV] (R75)
tetanus neonatorum (A33)

● **P35 Congenital viral diseases**

Includes infections acquired in utero or during birth

P35.0 Congenital rubella syndrome
Congenital rubella pneumonitis

P35.1 Congenital cytomegalovirus infection
Viruses transmitted by multiple routes that cause mild/subclinical infection

P35.2 Congenital herpesviral [herpes simplex] infection

P35.3 Congenital viral hepatitis

P35.8 Other congenital viral diseases
Congenital varicella [chickenpox]

P35.9 Congenital viral disease, unspecified

● **P36 Bacterial sepsis of newborn**

Includes congenital sepsis

Use additional code(s), if applicable, to identify severe sepsis (R65.2-) and associated acute organ dysfunction(s)

P36.0 Sepsis of newborn due to streptococcus, group B

● **P36.1 Sepsis of newborn due to other and unspecified streptococci**

  P36.10 Sepsis of newborn due to unspecified streptococci

  P36.19 Sepsis of newborn due to other streptococci

P36.2 Sepsis of newborn due to Staphylococcus aureus

● **P36.3 Sepsis of newborn due to other and unspecified staphylococci**

  P36.30 Sepsis of newborn due to unspecified staphylococci

  P36.39 Sepsis of newborn due to other staphylococci

P36.4 Sepsis of newborn due to Escherichia coli

P36.5 Sepsis of newborn due to anaerobes

P36.8 Other bacterial sepsis of newborn
Use additional code from category B96 to identify organism

P36.9 Bacterial sepsis of newborn, unspecified

● **P37 Other congenital infectious and parasitic diseases**

Excludes2 congenital syphilis (A50.-)
infectious neonatal diarrhea (A00-A09)
necrotizing enterocolitis in newborn (P77.-)
noninfectious neonatal diarrhea (P78.3)
ophthalmia neonatorum due to gonococcus (A54.31)
tetanus neonatorum (A33)

P37.0 Congenital tuberculosis

P37.1 Congenital toxoplasmosis
Parasitic infection, often causing mild flu-like illness
Hydrocephalus due to congenital toxoplasmosis

P37.2 Neonatal (disseminated) listeriosis
Acquired transplacentally or during/after parturition in which symptoms are those of sepsis

P37.3 Congenital falciparum malaria

P37.4 Other congenital malaria

P37.5 Neonatal candidiasis

P37.8 Other specified congenital infectious and parasitic diseases

P37.9 Congenital infectious or parasitic disease, unspecified

● **P38 Omphalitis of newborn**
Inflammation of umbilicus

Excludes1 omphalitis not of newborn (L08.82)
tetanus omphalitis (A33)
umbilical hemorrhage of newborn (P51.-)

P38.1 Omphalitis with mild hemorrhage

P38.9 Omphalitis without hemorrhage
Omphalitis of newborn NOS

● **P39 Other infections specific to the perinatal period**
Use additional code to identify organism or specific infection

P39.0 Neonatal infective mastitis

Excludes1 breast engorgement of newborn (P83.4)
noninfective mastitis of newborn (P83.4)

P39.1 Neonatal conjunctivitis and dacryocystitis
Neonatal chlamydial conjunctivitis
Ophthalmia neonatorum NOS
Neonate = newborn

Excludes1 gonococcal conjunctivitis (A54.31)

P39.2 Intra-amniotic infection affecting newborn, not elsewhere classified

P39.3 Neonatal urinary tract infection

P39.4 Neonatal skin infection
Neonatal pyoderma

Excludes1 pemphigus neonatorum (L00)
staphylococcal scalded skin syndrome (L00)

P39.8 Other specified infections specific to the perinatal period

P39.9 Infection specific to the perinatal period, unspecified

HEMORRHAGIC AND HEMATOLOGICAL DISORDERS OF NEWBORN (P50-P61)

Excludes1 congenital stenosis and stricture of bile ducts (Q44.3)
Crigler-Najjar syndrome (E80.5)
Dubin-Johnson syndrome (E80.6)
Gilbert syndrome (E80.4)
hereditary hemolytic anemias (D55-D58)

● **P50 Newborn affected by intrauterine (fetal) blood loss**

Excludes1 congenital anemia from intrauterine (fetal) blood loss (P61.3)

P50.0 Newborn affected by intrauterine (fetal) blood loss from vasa previa

P50.1 Newborn affected by intrauterine (fetal) blood loss from ruptured cord

P50.2 Newborn affected by intrauterine (fetal) blood loss from placenta

P50.3 Newborn affected by hemorrhage into co-twin

P50.4 Newborn affected by hemorrhage into maternal circulation

P50.5 Newborn affected by intrauterine (fetal) blood loss from cut end of co-twin's cord

P50.8 Newborn affected by other intrauterine (fetal) blood loss

P50.9 Newborn affected by intrauterine (fetal) blood loss, unspecified
Newborn affected by fetal hemorrhage NOS

● **P51** **Umbilical hemorrhage of newborn**

> **Excludes1** omphalitis with mild hemorrhage (P38.1)
> umbilical hemorrhage from cut end of co-twins
> cord (P50.5)

    P51.0 **Massive umbilical hemorrhage of newborn**

    P51.8 **Other umbilical hemorrhages of newborn**
        Slipped umbilical ligature NOS

    P51.9 **Umbilical hemorrhage of newborn, unspecified**

● **P52** **Intracranial nontraumatic hemorrhage of newborn**

> **Includes** intracranial hemorrhage due to anoxia or hypoxia
> **Excludes1** intracranial hemorrhage due to birth injury
> (P10.-)
> intracranial hemorrhage due to other injury
> (S06.-)

    P52.0 **Intraventricular (nontraumatic) hemorrhage, grade 1, of newborn**
        Subependymal hemorrhage (without intraventricular extension)
        Bleeding into germinal matrix

    P52.1 **Intraventricular (nontraumatic) hemorrhage, grade 2, of newborn**
        Subependymal hemorrhage with intraventricular extension
        Bleeding into ventricle

● **P52.2** **Intraventricular (nontraumatic) hemorrhage, grade 3 and grade 4, of newborn**

        P52.21 **Intraventricular (nontraumatic) hemorrhage, grade 3, of newborn**
            Subependymal hemorrhage with intraventricular extension with enlargement of ventricle

        P52.22 **Intraventricular (nontraumatic) hemorrhage, grade 4, of newborn**
            Bleeding into cerebral cortex
            Subependymal hemorrhage with intracerebral extension

    P52.3 **Unspecified intraventricular (nontraumatic) hemorrhage of newborn**

    P52.4 **Intracerebral (nontraumatic) hemorrhage of newborn**

    P52.5 **Subarachnoid (nontraumatic) hemorrhage of newborn**

    P52.6 **Cerebellar (nontraumatic) and posterior fossa hemorrhage of newborn**

    P52.8 **Other intracranial (nontraumatic) hemorrhages of newborn**

    P52.9 **Intracranial (nontraumatic) hemorrhage of newborn, unspecified**

  P53 **Hemorrhagic disease of newborn**
    Vitamin K deficiency of newborn

● **P54** **Other neonatal hemorrhages**

> **Excludes1** newborn affected by (intrauterine) blood loss
> (P50.-)
> pulmonary hemorrhage originating in the
> perinatal period (P26.-)

    P54.0 **Neonatal hematemesis**
        Vomiting of blood
        > **Excludes1** neonatal hematemesis due to swallowed maternal blood (P78.2)

    P54.1 **Neonatal melena**
        Dark-colored feces stained with blood pigments
        > **Excludes1** neonatal melena due to swallowed maternal blood (P78.2)

    P54.2 **Neonatal rectal hemorrhage**

    P54.3 **Other neonatal gastrointestinal hemorrhage**

    P54.4 **Neonatal adrenal hemorrhage**

    P54.5 **Neonatal cutaneous hemorrhage**
        Neonatal bruising
        Neonatal ecchymoses
        Neonatal petechiae
        Neonatal superficial hematomata
        > **Excludes2** bruising of scalp due to birth injury
        > (P12.3)
        > cephalhematoma due to birth injury
        > (P12.0)

    P54.6 **Neonatal vaginal hemorrhage**
        Neonatal pseudomenses

    P54.8 **Other specified neonatal hemorrhages**

    P54.9 **Neonatal hemorrhage, unspecified**

● **P55** **Hemolytic disease of newborn**
    AKA erythroblastosis fetalis and is due to Rh isoimmunization, result of Rh blood factor incompatibilities between mother (Rh negative) and fetus (Rh positive)

    P55.0 **Rh isoimmunization of newborn**

    P55.1 **ABO isoimmunization of newborn**

    P55.8 **Other hemolytic diseases of newborn**

    P55.9 **Hemolytic disease of newborn, unspecified**

● **P56** **Hydrops fetalis due to hemolytic disease**
    Caused by maternal sensitization to fetal blood group antigen
    > **Excludes1** hydrops fetalis NOS (P83.2)

    P56.0 **Hydrops fetalis due to isoimmunization**

● **P56.9** **Hydrops fetalis due to other and unspecified hemolytic disease**

        P56.90 **Hydrops fetalis due to unspecified hemolytic disease**

        P56.99 **Hydrops fetalis due to other hemolytic disease**

● **P57** **Kernicterus**
    High levels of bilirubin in blood, with severe neural symptoms

    P57.0 **Kernicterus due to isoimmunization**

    P57.8 **Other specified kernicterus**
        > **Excludes1** Crigler-Najjar syndrome (E80.5)

    P57.9 **Kernicterus, unspecified**

● **P58** **Neonatal jaundice due to other excessive hemolysis**
    > **Excludes1** jaundice due to isoimmunization (P55-P57)

    P58.0 **Neonatal jaundice due to bruising**

    P58.1 **Neonatal jaundice due to bleeding**

    P58.2 **Neonatal jaundice due to infection**

    P58.3 **Neonatal jaundice due to polycythemia**

● **P58.4** **Neonatal jaundice due to drugs or toxins transmitted from mother or given to newborn**

        Code first poisoning due to drug or toxin, if applicable (T36-T65 with fifth or sixth character 1-4 or 6)

        Use additional code for adverse effect, if applicable, to identify drug (T36-T50 with fifth or sixth character 5)

        P58.41 **Neonatal jaundice due to drugs or toxins transmitted from mother**

        P58.42 **Neonatal jaundice due to drugs or toxins given to newborn**

    P58.5 **Neonatal jaundice due to swallowed maternal blood**

    P58.8 **Neonatal jaundice due to other specified excessive hemolysis**

    P58.9 **Neonatal jaundice due to excessive hemolysis, unspecified**

◀ New   ◀▥ Revised   ~~deleted~~ Deleted   OGCR Official Guidelines   X Assign placeholder X   ● Use Additional Character(s)

Excludes 1   Excludes 2   Includes   Use additional   Code first   Code also   Unspecified

● **P59　Neonatal jaundice from other and unspecified causes**

> **Excludes1**　jaundice due to inborn errors of metabolism
> (E70-E88)
> kernicterus (P57.-)

　　P59.0　Neonatal jaundice associated with preterm delivery
　　　　　Hyperbilirubinemia of prematurity
　　　　　Jaundice due to delayed conjugation associated with
　　　　　　preterm delivery

　　P59.1　Inspissated bile syndrome

● **P59.2　Neonatal jaundice from other and unspecified
　　　　　hepatocellular damage**

> **Excludes1**　congenital viral hepatitis (P35.3)

　　　　**P59.20　Neonatal jaundice from unspecified
　　　　　　　hepatocellular damage**

　　　　**P59.29　Neonatal jaundice from other hepatocellular
　　　　　　　damage**
　　　　　　　Neonatal giant cell hepatitis
　　　　　　　Neonatal (idiopathic) hepatitis

　　P59.3　Neonatal jaundice from breast milk inhibitor

　　P59.8　Neonatal jaundice from other specified causes

　　P59.9　Neonatal jaundice, unspecified
　　　　　Neonatal physiological jaundice (intense)(prolonged)
　　　　　NOS

P60　Disseminated intravascular coagulation of newborn
　　　Defibrination syndrome of newborn

● **P61　Other perinatal hematological disorders**

> **Excludes1**　transient hypogammaglobulinemia of infancy
> (D80.7)

　　P61.0　Transient neonatal thrombocytopenia
　　　　　*Lack of sufficient numbers of circulating thrombocytes
　　　　　　(platelets)*
　　　　　Neonatal thrombocytopenia due to exchange
　　　　　　transfusion
　　　　　Neonatal thrombocytopenia due to idiopathic maternal
　　　　　　thrombocytopenia
　　　　　Neonatal thrombocytopenia due to isoimmunization

　　P61.1　Polycythemia neonatorum
　　　　　Neonate = newborn

　　P61.2　Anemia of prematurity

　　P61.3　Congenital anemia from fetal blood loss

　　P61.4　Other congenital anemias, not elsewhere classified
　　　　　Congenital anemia NOS

　　P61.5　Transient neonatal neutropenia
　　　　　Low levels of granulocytic neutrophilic white blood cells

> **Excludes1**　congenital neutropenia (nontransient)
> (D70.0)

　　P61.6　Other transient neonatal disorders of coagulation

　　P61.8　Other specified perinatal hematological disorders

　　P61.9　Perinatal hematological disorder, unspecified

TRANSITORY ENDOCRINE AND METABOLIC DISORDERS
SPECIFIC TO NEWBORN (P70-P74)

> **Includes**　transitory endocrine and metabolic disturbances
> caused by the infant's response to maternal
> endocrine and metabolic factors, or its
> adjustment to extrauterine environment

● **P70　Transitory disorders of carbohydrate metabolism specific to
　　　newborn**

　　**P70.0　Syndrome of infant of mother with gestational
　　　　　diabetes**
　　　　　Newborn (with hypoglycemia) affected by maternal
　　　　　　gestational diabetes

> **Excludes1**　newborn (with hypoglycemia) affected
> by maternal (pre-existing) diabetes
> mellitus (P70.1)
> syndrome of infant of a diabetic mother
> (P70.1)

　　P70.1　Syndrome of infant of a diabetic mother
　　　　　Newborn (with hypoglycemia) affected by maternal
　　　　　　(pre-existing) diabetes mellitus

> **Excludes1**　newborn (with hypoglycemia) affected by
> maternal gestational diabetes (P70.0)
> syndrome of infant of mother with
> gestational diabetes (P70.0)

　　P70.2　Neonatal diabetes mellitus

　　P70.3　Iatrogenic neonatal hypoglycemia

　　P70.4　Other neonatal hypoglycemia
　　　　　Transitory neonatal hypoglycemia

　　**P70.8　Other transitory disorders of carbohydrate metabolism
　　　　　of newborn**

　　**P70.9　Transitory disorder of carbohydrate metabolism of
　　　　　newborn, unspecified**

● **P71　Transitory neonatal disorders of calcium and magnesium
　　　metabolism**

　　P71.0　Cow's milk hypocalcemia in newborn

　　P71.1　Other neonatal hypocalcemia

> **Excludes1**　neonatal hypoparathyroidism (P71.4)

　　P71.2　Neonatal hypomagnesemia

　　**P71.3　Neonatal tetany without calcium or magnesium
　　　　　deficiency**
　　　　　Neonatal tetany NOS

　　P71.4　Transitory neonatal hypoparathyroidism

　　**P71.8　Other transitory neonatal disorders of calcium and
　　　　　magnesium metabolism**

　　**P71.9　Transitory neonatal disorder of calcium and magnesium
　　　　　metabolism, unspecified**

● **P72　Other transitory neonatal endocrine disorders**

> **Excludes1**　congenital hypothyroidism with or without goiter
> (E03.0-E03.1)
> dyshormogenetic goiter (E07.1)
> Pendred's syndrome (E07.1)

　　P72.0　Neonatal goiter, not elsewhere classified
　　　　　Transitory congenital goiter with normal functioning

　　P72.1　Transitory neonatal hyperthyroidism
　　　　　Neonatal thyrotoxicosis

　　**P72.2　Other transitory neonatal disorders of thyroid function,
　　　　　not elsewhere classified**
　　　　　Transitory neonatal hypothyroidism

　　P72.8　Other specified transitory neonatal endocrine disorders

　　P72.9　Transitory neonatal endocrine disorder, unspecified

● **P74　Other transitory neonatal electrolyte and metabolic disturbances**

　　P74.0　Late metabolic acidosis of newborn

> **Excludes1**　(fetal) metabolic acidosis of newborn (P19)

　　P74.1　Dehydration of newborn

　　P74.2　Disturbances of sodium balance of newborn

　　P74.3　Disturbances of potassium balance of newborn

　　P74.4　Other transitory electrolyte disturbances of newborn

　　P74.5　Transitory tyrosinemia of newborn

　　P74.6　Transitory hyperammonemia of newborn

　　P74.8　Other transitory metabolic disturbances of newborn
　　　　　Amino-acid metabolic disorders described as transitory

　　**P74.9　Transitory metabolic disturbance of newborn,
　　　　　unspecified**

DIGESTIVE SYSTEM DISORDERS OF NEWBORN (P76-P78)

● **P76   Other intestinal obstruction of newborn**

P76.0   **Meconium plug syndrome**
Fetal stool obstruction in large intestine, present at birth; may be symptom of organic disease.
Meconium ileus NOS

Excludes1   meconium ileus in cystic fibrosis (E84.11)

P76.1   **Transitory ileus of newborn**
Temporary obstruction of ileus (small intestine)

Excludes1   Hirschsprung's disease (Q43.1)

P76.2   **Intestinal obstruction due to inspissated milk**
Being thickened, dried, or made less fluid

P76.8   **Other specified intestinal obstruction of newborn**

Excludes1   intestinal obstruction classifiable to K56.-

P76.9   **Intestinal obstruction of newborn, unspecified**

● **P77   Necrotizing enterocolitis of newborn**

P77.1   **Stage 1 necrotizing enterocolitis in newborn**
Necrotizing enterocolitis without pneumatosis, without perforation

P77.2   **Stage 2 necrotizing enterocolitis in newborn**
Necrotizing enterocolitis with pneumatosis, without perforation

P77.3   **Stage 3 necrotizing enterocolitis in newborn**
Necrotizing enterocolitis with perforation
Necrotizing enterocolitis with pneumatosis and perforation

P77.9   **Necrotizing enterocolitis in newborn, unspecified**
Necrotizing enterocolitis in newborn, NOS

● **P78   Other perinatal digestive system disorders**

Excludes1   cystic fibrosis (E84.0-E84.9)
neonatal gastrointestinal hemorrhages (P54.0-P54.3)

P78.0   **Perinatal intestinal perforation**
Meconium peritonitis

P78.1   **Other neonatal peritonitis**
Neonatal peritonitis NOS

P78.2   **Neonatal hematemesis and melena due to swallowed maternal blood**

P78.3   **Noninfective neonatal diarrhea**
Neonatal diarrhea NOS

● P78.8   **Other specified perinatal digestive system disorders**

P78.81   **Congenital cirrhosis (of liver)**

P78.82   **Peptic ulcer of newborn**

P78.83   **Newborn esophageal reflux**
Neonatal esophageal reflux

P78.89   **Other specified perinatal digestive system disorders**

P78.9   **Perinatal digestive system disorder, unspecified**

CONDITIONS INVOLVING THE INTEGUMENT AND TEMPERATURE REGULATION OF NEWBORN (P80-P83)

● **P80   Hypothermia of newborn**

P80.0   **Cold injury syndrome**
Severe and usually chronic hypothermia associated with a pink flushed appearance, edema and neurological and biochemical abnormalities.

Excludes1   mild hypothermia of newborn (P80.8)

P80.8   **Other hypothermia of newborn**
Mild hypothermia of newborn

P80.9   **Hypothermia of newborn, unspecified**

● **P81   Other disturbances of temperature regulation of newborn**

P81.0   **Environmental hyperthermia of newborn**

P81.8   **Other specified disturbances of temperature regulation of newborn**

P81.9   **Disturbance of temperature regulation of newborn, unspecified**
Fever of newborn NOS

● **P83   Other conditions of integument specific to newborn**

Excludes1   congenital malformations of skin and integument (Q80-Q84)
hydrops fetalis due to hemolytic disease (P56.-)
neonatal skin infection (P39.4)
staphylococcal scalded skin syndrome (L00)

Excludes2   cradle cap (L21.0)
diaper [napkin] dermatitis (L22)

P83.0   **Sclerema neonatorum**
Neonate = newborn

P83.1   **Neonatal erythema toxicum**
Benign, generalized, transient pustules that become firm vesicles

P83.2   **Hydrops fetalis not due to hemolytic disease**
Severe, life-threatening problem of severe edema (swelling) as result of too much fluid leaving blood and entering tissue
Hydrops fetalis NOS

● P83.3   **Other and unspecified edema specific to newborn**

P83.30   **Unspecified edema specific to newborn**

P83.39   **Other edema specific to newborn**

P83.4   **Breast engorgement of newborn**
Noninfective mastitis of newborn

P83.5   **Congenital hydrocele**

P83.6   **Umbilical polyp of newborn**

P83.8   **Other specified conditions of integument specific to newborn**
Bronze baby syndrome
Neonatal scleroderma
Urticaria neonatorum

P83.9   **Condition of the integument specific to newborn, unspecified**

OTHER PROBLEMS WITH NEWBORN (P84)

P84   **Other problems with newborn**
Acidemia of newborn
Acidosis of newborn
Anoxia of newborn NOS
Asphyxia of newborn NOS
Hypercapnia of newborn
Hypoxemia of newborn
Hypoxia of newborn NOS
Mixed metabolic and respiratory acidosis of newborn

Excludes1   intracranial hemorrhage due to anoxia or hypoxia (P52.-)
hypoxic ischemic encephalopathy [HIE] (P91.6-)
late metabolic acidosis of newborn (P74.0)

OTHER DISORDERS ORIGINATING IN THE PERINATAL PERIOD (P90-P96)

P90   **Convulsions of newborn**

Excludes1   benign myoclonic epilepsy in infancy (G40.3-)
benign neonatal convulsions (familial) (G40.3-)

● **P91   Other disturbances of cerebral status of newborn**

P91.0   **Neonatal cerebral ischemia**

P91.1   **Acquired periventricular cysts of newborn**

P91.2   **Neonatal cerebral leukomalacia**
Degeneration of white matter adjacent to cerebral ventricles following cerebral hypoxia or brain ischemia in neonates
Periventricular leukomalacia

P91.3   **Neonatal cerebral irritability**

P91.4   **Neonatal cerebral depression**

P91.5   **Neonatal coma**

● **P91.6**   **Hypoxic ischemic encephalopathy [HIE]**

    P91.60   **Hypoxic ischemic encephalopathy [HIE], unspecified**

    P91.61   **Mild hypoxic ischemic encephalopathy [HIE]**

    P91.62   **Moderate hypoxic ischemic encephalopathy [HIE]**

    P91.63   **Severe hypoxic ischemic encephalopathy [HIE]**

   P91.8   **Other specified disturbances of cerebral status of newborn**

   P91.9   **Disturbance of cerebral status of newborn, unspecified**

● **P92**   **Feeding problems of newborn**

    Excludes1   feeding problems in child over 28 days old (R63.3)

 ● **P92.0**   **Vomiting of newborn**

    Excludes1   vomiting of child over 28 days old (R11.-)

    P92.01   **Bilious vomiting of newborn**

       Excludes1   bilious vomiting in child over 28 days old (R11.14)

    P92.09   **Other vomiting of newborn**

       Excludes1   regurgitation of food in newborn (P92.1)

   P92.1   **Regurgitation and rumination of newborn**

   P92.2   **Slow feeding of newborn**

   P92.3   **Underfeeding of newborn**

   P92.4   **Overfeeding of newborn**

   P92.5   **Neonatal difficulty in feeding at breast**

   P92.6   **Failure to thrive in newborn**

    Excludes1   failure to thrive in child over 28 days old (R62.51)

   P92.8   **Other feeding problems of newborn**

   P92.9   **Feeding problem of newborn, unspecified**

● **P93**   **Reactions and intoxications due to drugs administered to newborn**

    Includes   reactions and intoxications due to drugs administered to fetus affecting newborn

    Excludes1   jaundice due to drugs or toxins transmitted from mother or given to newborn (P58.4-)
       reactions and intoxications from maternal opiates, tranquilizers and other medication (P04.0-P04.1, P04.4)
       withdrawal symptoms from maternal use of drugs of addiction (P96.1)
       withdrawal symptoms from therapeutic use of drugs in newborn (P96.2)

   P93.0   **Grey baby syndrome**
      Grey syndrome from chloramphenicol administration in newborn

   P93.8   **Other reactions and intoxications due to drugs administered to newborn**

      Use additional code for adverse effect, if applicable, to identify drug (T36-T50 with fifth or sixth character 5)

● **P94**   **Disorders of muscle tone of newborn**

   P94.0   **Transient neonatal myasthenia gravis**

    Excludes1   myasthenia gravis (G70.0)

   P94.1   **Congenital hypertonia**

   P94.2   **Congenital hypotonia**
      Floppy baby syndrome, unspecified

   P94.8   **Other disorders of muscle tone of newborn**

   P94.9   **Disorder of muscle tone of newborn, unspecified**

P95   **Stillbirth**
     Deadborn fetus NOS
     Fetal death of unspecified cause
     Stillbirth NOS

    Excludes1   maternal care for intrauterine death (O36.4)
       missed abortion (O02.1)
       outcome of delivery, stillbirth (Z37.1, Z37.3, Z37.4, Z37.7)

OGCR Section I.C.16.g.

Stillbirth

Code P95, Stillbirth, is only for use for institutions that maintain separate records for stillbirths. No other code should be used with P95. Code P95 should not be used on the mother's record.

● **P96**   **Other conditions originating in the perinatal period**

   P96.0   **Congenital renal failure**
      Uremia of newborn

   P96.1   **Neonatal withdrawal symptoms from maternal use of drugs of addiction**
      Drug withdrawal syndrome in infant of dependent mother
      Neonatal abstinence syndrome

    Excludes1   reactions and intoxications from maternal opiates and tranquilizers administered during labor and delivery (P04.0)

   P96.2   **Withdrawal symptoms from therapeutic use of drugs in newborn**

   P96.3   **Wide cranial sutures of newborn**
      Neonatal craniotabes

   P96.5   **Complication to newborn due to (fetal) intrauterine procedure**

    Excludes2   newborn (suspected to be) affected by amniocentesis (P00.6)

 ● **P96.8**   **Other specified conditions originating in the perinatal period**

    P96.81   **Exposure to (parental) (environmental) tobacco smoke in the perinatal period**

       Excludes2   newborn affected by in utero exposure to tobacco (P04.2)
         exposure to environmental tobacco smoke after the perinatal period (Z77.22)

    P96.82   **Delayed separation of umbilical cord**

    P96.83   **Meconium staining**

       Excludes1   meconium aspiration (P24.00, P24.01)
         meconium passage during delivery (P03.82)

    P96.89   **Other specified conditions originating in the perinatal period**

       Use additional code to specify condition

   P96.9   **Condition originating in the perinatal period, unspecified**
      Congenital debility NOS

CHAPTER 16 (P00-P96)

◀ New   ◀◀◀ Revised   ~~deleted~~ Deleted   **OGCR** Official Guidelines   X Assign placeholder X   ● Use Additional Character(s)

Excludes 1   Excludes 2   Includes   Use additional   Code first   Code also   Unspecified

OGCR See Section I.C., Chapter 17
Congenital malformations, deformations, and chromosomal
abnormalities

CHAPTER 17

CONGENITAL MALFORMATIONS, DEFORMATIONS AND CHROMOSOMAL ABNORMALITIES (Q00-Q99)

Note: Codes from this chapter are not for use on maternal or
fetal records

Excludes2 inborn errors of metabolism (E70-E88)

This chapter contains the following blocks:

Q00-Q07	Congenital malformations of the nervous system
Q10-Q18	Congenital malformations of eye, ear, face and neck
Q20-Q28	Congenital malformations of the circulatory system
Q30-Q34	Congenital malformations of the respiratory system
Q35-Q37	Cleft lip and cleft palate
Q38-Q45	Other congenital malformations of the digestive system
Q50-Q56	Congenital malformations of genital organs
Q60-Q64	Congenital malformations of the urinary system
Q65-Q79	Congenital malformations and deformations of the musculoskeletal system
Q80-Q89	Other congenital malformations
Q90-Q99	Chromosomal abnormalities, not elsewhere classified

CONGENITAL MALFORMATIONS OF THE NERVOUS SYSTEM (Q00–Q07)

● **Q00   Anencephaly and similar malformations**
   Q00.0   Anencephaly
         *Absence of skull with cerebral hemispheres missing or
            reduced to small masses attached to base of cranium*
         Acephaly
         Acrania
         Amyelencephaly
         Hemianencephaly
         Hemicephaly
   Q00.1   Craniorachischisis
         *Developmental anomaly consisting of fissure of cranium and
            vertebral column*
   Q00.2   Iniencephaly
         *Developmental anomaly characterized by enlargement of
            foramen magnum and absence of laminae and spinous
            processes of cervical, dorsal*

● **Q01   Encephalocele**
      *Sac-like protrusions of brain and membranes visible through an
         opening in skull*
      Includes   Arnold-Chiari syndrome, type III
                  encephalocystocele
                  encephalomyelocele
                  hydroencephalocele
                  hydromeningocele, cranial
                  meningocele, cerebral
                  meningoencephalocele
      Excludes1   Meckel-Gruber syndrome (Q61.9)
   Q01.0   Frontal encephalocele
   Q01.1   Nasofrontal encephalocele

Figure 17-1 An infant with a large occipital
encephalocele. The large skin-covered
encephalocele is visible. (From Townsend:
Sabiston Textbook of Surgery, ed 19, Saunders,
An Imprint of Elsevier, 2012)

   Q01.2   Occipital encephalocele
   Q01.8   Encephalocele of other sites
   Q01.9   Encephalocele, unspecified

● **Q02   Microcephaly**
      *Head size measures significantly below normal based on standardized
         charts*
      Includes   hydromicrocephaly
                  micrencephalon
      Excludes1   Meckel-Gruber syndrome (Q61.9)

● **Q03   Congenital hydrocephalus**
      *Accumulation of cerebrospinal fluid in ventricles resulting in swelling
         and enlargement*
      Includes   hydrocephalus in newborn
      Excludes1   Arnold-Chiari syndrome, type II (Q07.0-)
                  acquired hydrocephalus (G91.-)
                  hydrocephalus due to congenital toxoplasmosis
                     (P37.1)
                  hydrocephalus with spina bifida (Q05.0-Q05.4)
   Q03.0   Malformations of aqueduct of Sylvius
         Anomaly of aqueduct of Sylvius
         Obstruction of aqueduct of Sylvius, congenital
         Stenosis of aqueduct of Sylvius
   Q03.1   Atresia of foramina of Magendie and Luschka
         Dandy-Walker syndrome
   Q03.8   Other congenital hydrocephalus
   Q03.9   Congenital hydrocephalus, unspecified

● **Q04   Other congenital malformations of brain**
      Excludes1   cyclopia (Q87.0)
                  macrocephaly (Q75.3)
   Q04.0   Congenital malformations of corpus callosum
         Agenesis of corpus callosum
   Q04.1   Arhinencephaly
         Congenital absence of olfactory bulbs, tract, or nerves
   Q04.2   Holoprosencephaly
         *Failure of cleavage of forebrain (prosencephalon) resulting in
            incomplete or absent cortical separation and deficits in
            midline facial development*
   Q04.3   Other reduction deformities of brain
         Absence of part of brain   Agyria
         Agenesis of part of brain
            *Cerebral cortex are not fully formed, brain surface is
               smooth*
         Aplasia of part of brain
         Hydranencephaly
         Hypoplasia of part of brain
         Lissencephaly
            *Congenital malformation or absence of convolutions of
               cerebral cortex*
         Microgyria
            *Malformation of brain characterized by excessive number
               of small convolutions (gyri) on surface*
         Pachygyria
            Reduction in number of sulci of cerebrum
         Excludes1   congenital malformations of corpus
                     callosum (Q04.0)
   Q04.4   Septo-optic dysplasia of brain
   Q04.5   Megalencephaly
         Abnormally large brain
   Q04.6   Congenital cerebral cysts
         Porencephaly   Schizencephaly
         Excludes1   acquired porencephalic cyst (G93.0)
   Q04.8   Other specified congenital malformations of brain
         Arnold-Chiari syndrome, type IV
         Macrogyria
   Q04.9   Congenital malformation of brain, unspecified
         Congenital anomaly NOS of brain
         Congenital deformity NOS of brain
         Congenital disease or lesion NOS of brain
         Multiple anomalies NOS of brain, congenital

● **Q05   Spina bifida**

Developmental anomaly characterized by defective closure of vertebral arch, through which spinal cord and meninges may protrude

    Includes   hydromeningocele (spinal)
                meningocele (spinal)
                meningomyelocele
                myelocele
                myelomeningocele
                rachischisis
                spina bifida (aperta)(cystica)
                syringomyelocele

    Use additional code for any associated paraplegia (paraparesis) (G82.2-)

    Excludes1   Arnold-Chiari syndrome, type II (Q07.0-)
                  spina bifida occulta (Q76.0)

   Q05.0   Cervical spina bifida with hydrocephalus

   Q05.1   Thoracic spina bifida with hydrocephalus
        Dorsal spina bifida with hydrocephalus
        Thoracolumbar spina bifida with hydrocephalus

   Q05.2   Lumbar spina bifida with hydrocephalus
        Lumbosacral spina bifida with hydrocephalus

   Q05.3   Sacral spina bifida with hydrocephalus

   Q05.4   Unspecified spina bifida with hydrocephalus

   Q05.5   Cervical spina bifida without hydrocephalus

   Q05.6   Thoracic spina bifida without hydrocephalus
        Dorsal spina bifida NOS
        Thoracolumbar spina bifida NOS

   Q05.7   Lumbar spina bifida without hydrocephalus
        Lumbosacral spina bifida NOS

   Q05.8   Sacral spina bifida without hydrocephalus

   Q05.9   Spina bifida, unspecified

● **Q06   Other congenital malformations of spinal cord**

   Q06.0   Amyelia
        Congenital absence of spinal cord

   Q06.1   Hypoplasia and dysplasia of spinal cord
        Underdevelopment of spinal cord
        Atelomyelia
          Congenitally incomplete development of spinal cord
        Myelatelia
        Myelodysplasia of spinal cord
          Defective development of spinal cord, especially lower segments

   Q06.2   Diastematomyelia
        Congenital anomaly, associated with spina bifida, in which spinal cord is split into halves and surrounded by dural sac

   Q06.3   Other congenital cauda equina malformations

   Q06.4   Hydromyelia
        Dilation of central canal of spinal cord with increased fluid accumulation
        Hydrorachis

   Q06.8   Other specified congenital malformations of spinal cord

   Q06.9   Congenital malformation of spinal cord, unspecified
        Congenital anomaly NOS of spinal cord
        Congenital deformity NOS of spinal cord
        Congenital disease or lesion NOS of spinal cord

● **Q07   Other congenital malformations of nervous system**

    Excludes2   congenital central alveolar hypoventilation syndrome (G47.35)
                  familial dysautonomia [Riley-Day] (G90.1)
                  neurofibromatosis (nonmalignant) (Q85.0-)

   Q07.0   Arnold-Chiari syndrome
        Herniation of cerebellar tonsils and vermis through foramen magnum into spinal canal
        Arnold-Chiari syndrome, type II

      Excludes1   Arnold-Chiari syndrome, type III (Q01.-)
                    Arnold-Chiari syndrome, type IV (Q04.8)

     Q07.00   Arnold-Chiari syndrome without spina bifida or hydrocephalus

     Q07.01   Arnold-Chiari syndrome with spina bifida

Figure 17-2   Bilateral congenital **hydrophthalmia,** in which the eyes are very large in comparison to the other facial features due to glaucoma.

     Q07.02   Arnold-Chiari syndrome with hydrocephalus

     Q07.03   Arnold-Chiari syndrome with spina bifida and hydrocephalus

   Q07.8   Other specified congenital malformations of nervous system
        Agenesis of nerve
        Displacement of brachial plexus
        Jaw-winking syndrome
        Marcus Gunn's syndrome

   Q07.9   Congenital malformation of nervous system, unspecified
        Congenital anomaly NOS of nervous system
        Congenital deformity NOS of nervous system
        Congenital disease or lesion NOS of nervous system

CONGENITAL MALFORMATIONS OF EYE, EAR, FACE AND NECK (Q10-Q18)

    Excludes2   cleft lip and cleft palate (Q35-Q37)
                  congenital malformation of cervical spine (Q05.0, Q05.5, Q67.5, Q76.0-Q76.4)
                  congenital malformation of larynx (Q31.-)
                  congenital malformation of lip NEC (Q38.0)
                  congenital malformation of nose (Q30.-)
                  congenital malformation of parathyroid gland (Q89.2)
                  congenital malformation of thyroid gland (Q89.2)

● **Q10   Congenital malformations of eyelid, lacrimal apparatus and orbit**

    Excludes1   cryptophthalmos NOS (Q11.2)
                  cryptophthalmos syndrome (Q87.0)

   Q10.0   Congenital ptosis
        Prolapse or drooping of upper eyelid from paralysis of third nerve or from sympathetic innervations

   Q10.1   Congenital ectropion
        Outward turning of eyelid

   Q10.2   Congenital entropion
        Inward turning of eyelid

   Q10.3   Other congenital malformations of eyelid
        Ablepharon
        Blepharophimosis, congenital
        Coloboma of eyelid
        Congenital absence or agenesis of cilia
        Congenital absence or agenesis of eyelid
        Congenital accessory eyelid
        Congenital accessory eye muscle
        Congenital malformation of eyelid NOS

   Q10.4   Absence and agenesis of lacrimal apparatus
        Congenital absence of punctum lacrimale

   Q10.5   Congenital stenosis and stricture of lacrimal duct

   Q10.6   Other congenital malformations of lacrimal apparatus
        Congenital malformation of lacrimal apparatus NOS

   Q10.7   Congenital malformation of orbit

● **Q11   Anophthalmos, microphthalmos and macrophthalmos**
     Absence of eye and optic pit

   Q11.0   Cystic eyeball

   Q11.1   Other anophthalmos
        Anophthalmos NOS
        Agenesis of eye
          Absence of eye
        Aplasia of eye

Q11.2   **Microphthalmos**
Partial absence of eye and optic pit
Cryptophthalmos NOS
Dysplasia of eye
Hypoplasia of eye
Rudimentary eye
Excludes1   cryptophthalmos syndrome (Q87.0)

Q11.3   **Macrophthalmos**
Congenital enlargement of eyes
Excludes1   macrophthalmos in congenital glaucoma
(Q15.0)

● Q12   **Congenital lens malformations**
Q12.0   **Congenital cataract**
Q12.1   **Congenital displaced lens**
Q12.2   **Coloboma of lens**
Q12.3   **Congenital aphakia**
Q12.4   **Spherophakia**
Smaller, more spherical optic lens than normal
Q12.8   **Other congenital lens malformations**
Microphakia
Q12.9   **Congenital lens malformation, unspecified**

● Q13   **Congenital malformations of anterior segment of eye**
Q13.0   **Coloboma of iris**
Coloboma NOS
Q13.1   **Absence of iris**
Aniridia
Use additional code for associated glaucoma (H42)
Q13.2   **Other congenital malformations of iris**
Anisocoria, congenital
Atresia of pupil
Congenital malformation of iris NOS
Corectopia
Q13.3   **Congenital corneal opacity**
Q13.4   **Other congenital corneal malformations**
Congenital malformation of cornea NOS
Microcornea
Peter's anomaly
Q13.5   **Blue sclera**
Condition of unusual blueness of sclera; not harmful
● Q13.8   **Other congenital malformations of anterior segment of eye**
Q13.81   **Rieger's anomaly**
Use additional code for associated glaucoma (H42)
Q13.89   **Other congenital malformations of anterior segment of eye**
Q13.9   **Congenital malformation of anterior segment of eye, unspecified**

● Q14   **Congenital malformations of posterior segment of eye**
Excludes2   optic nerve hypoplasia (H47.03-)
Q14.0   **Congenital malformation of vitreous humor**
Congenital vitreous opacity
Q14.1   **Congenital malformation of retina**
Congenital retinal aneurysm
Q14.2   **Congenital malformation of optic disc**
Coloboma of optic disc
Q14.3   **Congenital malformation of choroid**
Q14.8   **Other congenital malformations of posterior segment of eye**
Coloboma of the fundus
Q14.9   **Congenital malformation of posterior segment of eye, unspecified**

● Q15   **Other congenital malformations of eye**
Excludes1   congenital nystagmus (H55.01)
ocular albinism (E70.31-)
optic nerve hypoplasia (H47.03-)
retinitis pigmentosa (H35.52)
Q15.0   **Congenital glaucoma**
Axenfeld's anomaly
Buphthalmos
Congenital syndrome characterized by port-wine nevus covering portions of face and cranium
Glaucoma of childhood
Glaucoma of newborn
Hydrophthalmos
Keratoglobus, congenital, with glaucoma
Macrocornea with glaucoma
Macrophthalmos in congenital glaucoma
Megalocornea with glaucoma
Q15.8   **Other specified congenital malformations of eye**
Q15.9   **Congenital malformation of eye, unspecified**
Congenital anomaly of eye
Congenital deformity of eye

● Q16   **Congenital malformations of ear causing impairment of hearing**
Excludes1   congenital deafness (H90.-)
Q16.0   **Congenital absence of (ear) auricle**
Q16.1   **Congenital absence, atresia and stricture of auditory canal (external)**
Congenital atresia or stricture of osseous meatus
Q16.2   **Absence of eustachian tube**
Q16.3   **Congenital malformation of ear ossicles**
Congenital fusion of ear ossicles
Q16.4   **Other congenital malformations of middle ear**
Congenital malformation of middle ear NOS
Q16.5   **Congenital malformation of inner ear**
Congenital anomaly of membranous labyrinth
Congenital anomaly of organ of Corti
Q16.9   **Congenital malformation of ear causing impairment of hearing, unspecified**
Congenital absence of ear NOS

● Q17   **Other congenital malformations of ear**
Excludes1   congenital malformations of ear with impairment of hearing (Q16.0-Q16.9)
preauricular sinus (Q18.1)
Q17.0   **Accessory auricle**
Accessory tragus
Polyotia
Preauricular appendage or tag
Supernumerary ear
Supernumerary lobule
Q17.1   **Macrotia**
Enlarged ears
Q17.2   **Microtia**
An abnormally small or underdeveloped external ear
Q17.3   **Other misshapen ear**
Pointed ear
Q17.4   **Misplaced ear**
Low-set ears
Excludes1   cervical auricle (Q18.2)
Q17.5   **Prominent ear**
Bat ear
Q17.8   **Other specified congenital malformations of ear**
Congenital absence of lobe of ear
Q17.9   **Congenital malformation of ear, unspecified**
Congenital anomaly of ear NOS

◀ New   ⇐ Revised   deleted Deleted   OGCR Official Guidelines   X Assign placeholder X   ● Use Additional Character(s)
Excludes 1   Excludes 2   Includes   Use additional   Code first   Code also   Unspecified
1184

● **Q18**   **Other congenital malformations of face and neck**

> **Excludes1**   cleft lip and cleft palate (Q35-Q37)
> conditions classified to Q67.0-Q67.4
> congenital malformations of skull and face bones
>   (Q75.-)
> cyclopia (Q87.0)
> dentofacial anomalies [including malocclusion]
>   (M26.-)
> malformation syndromes affecting facial
>   appearance (Q87.0)
> persistent thyroglossal duct (Q89.2)

Q18.0   **Sinus, fistula and cyst of branchial cleft**
Branchial vestige
*Brachial remnants (cysts, fistula, skin tags) that are
developmental anomalies*

Q18.1   **Preauricular sinus and cyst**
Fistula of auricle, congenital
Cervicoaural fistula
*Abnormal passage in neck originating from first branchial
cleft*

Q18.2   **Other branchial cleft malformations**
Branchial cleft malformation NOS
Cervical auricle
Otocephaly

Q18.3   **Webbing of neck**
Pterygium colli
Thick fold of skin on side of neck

Q18.4   **Macrostomia**
*Results from failure of union of maxillary and mandibular
processes, results in abnormally large mouth*

Q18.5   **Microstomia**

Q18.6   **Macrocheilia**
Excessive size of lips
Hypertrophy of lip, congenital

Q18.7   **Microcheilia**
Abnormal smallness of lips

Q18.8   **Other specified congenital malformations of face and
neck**
Medial cyst of face and neck
Medial fistula of face and neck
Medial sinus of face and neck

Q18.9   **Congenital malformation of face and neck, unspecified**
Congenital anomaly NOS of face and neck

CONGENITAL MALFORMATIONS OF THE CIRCULATORY SYSTEM (Q20-Q28)

● **Q20**   **Congenital malformations of cardiac chambers and connections**

> **Excludes1**   dextrocardia with situs inversus (Q89.3)
> mirror-image atrial arrangement with situs
>   inversus (Q89.3)

Q20.0   **Common arterial trunk**
Persistent truncus arteriosus

> **Excludes1**   aortic septal defect (Q21.4)

Q20.1   **Double outlet right ventricle**
Taussig-Bing syndrome

Q20.2   **Double outlet left ventricle**

Q20.3   **Discordant ventriculoarterial connection**
Dextrotransposition of aorta
Transposition of great vessels (complete)

Q20.4   **Double inlet ventricle**
Common ventricle
Cor triloculare biatriatum
Single ventricle

Q20.5   **Discordant atrioventricular connection**
Corrected transposition
Levotransposition
Ventricular inversion

Q20.6   **Isomerism of atrial appendages**
Isomerism of atrial appendages with asplenia or
polysplenia

Q20.8   **Other congenital malformations of cardiac chambers
and connections**
Cor binoculare

Q20.9   **Congenital malformation of cardiac chambers and
connections, unspecified**

● **Q21**   **Congenital malformations of cardiac septa**

> **Excludes1**   acquired cardiac septal defect (I51.0)

Q21.0   **Ventricular septal defect**
Roger's disease

Q21.1   **Atrial septal defect**
Coronary sinus defect
Patent or persistent foramen ovale
Patent or persistent ostium secundum defect (type II)
Patent or persistent sinus venosus defect

Q21.2   **Atrioventricular septal defect**
Common atrioventricular canal
Endocardial cushion defect
Ostium primum atrial septal defect (type I)

Q21.3   **Tetralogy of Fallot**
Ventricular septal defect with pulmonary stenosis or
atresia, dextroposition of aorta and hypertrophy of
right ventricle.

Q21.4   **Aortopulmonary septal defect**
Aortic septal defect
Aortopulmonary window

Q21.8   **Other congenital malformations of cardiac septa**
Eisenmenger's defect
Pentalogy of Fallot

> **Excludes1**   Eisenmenger's complex (I27.8)
> Eisenmenger's syndrome (I27.8)

Q21.9   **Congenital malformation of cardiac septum, unspecified**
Septal (heart) defect NOS

● **Q22**   **Congenital malformations of pulmonary and tricuspid valves**

Q22.0   **Pulmonary valve atresia**

Q22.1   **Congenital pulmonary valve stenosis**

Q22.2   **Congenital pulmonary valve insufficiency**
Congenital pulmonary valve regurgitation

Q22.3   **Other congenital malformations of pulmonary valve**
Congenital malformation of pulmonary valve NOS
Supernumerary cusps of pulmonary valve

Q22.4   **Congenital tricuspid stenosis**
Congenital tricuspid atresia

Q22.5   **Ebstein's anomaly**
Malformation of tricuspid valve

Q22.6   **Hypoplastic right heart syndrome**

Q22.8   **Other congenital malformations of tricuspid valve**

Q22.9   **Congenital malformation of tricuspid valve, unspecified**

● **Q23**   **Congenital malformations of aortic and mitral valves**

Q23.0   **Congenital stenosis of aortic valve**
Congenital aortic atresia
Congenital aortic stenosis NOS

> **Excludes1**   congenital stenosis of aortic valve in
> hypoplastic left heart syndrome
> (Q23.4)
> congenital subaortic stenosis (Q24.4)
> supravalvular aortic stenosis (congenital)
> (Q25.3)

Q23.1   **Congenital insufficiency of aortic valve**
Bicuspid aortic valve
Congenital aortic insufficiency

Q23.2   **Congenital mitral stenosis**
Congenital mitral atresia

Q23.3   **Congenital mitral insufficiency**

Q23.4   **Hypoplastic left heart syndrome**

Q23.8   **Other congenital malformations of aortic and mitral
valves**

Q23.9   **Congenital malformation of aortic and mitral valves,
unspecified**

CHAPTER 17 (Q00-Q99)

● **Q24   Other congenital malformations of heart**
> **Excludes1**   endocardial fibroelastosis (I42.4)

Q24.0   Dextrocardia
Heart is located in right hemithorax
> **Excludes1**   dextrocardia with situs inversus (Q89.3)
> isomerism of atrial appendages (with asplenia or polysplenia) (Q20.6)
> mirror-image atrial arrangement with situs inversus (Q89.3)

Q24.1   Levocardia
Normal position of heart but related structures on wrong side

Q24.2   Cor triatriatum
Congenital heart defect; left atrium is subdivided

Q24.3   Pulmonary infundibular stenosis
Subvalvular pulmonic stenosis

Q24.4   Congenital subaortic stenosis

Q24.5   Malformation of coronary vessels
Congenital coronary (artery) aneurysm

Q24.6   Congenital heart block

Q24.8   Other specified congenital malformations of heart
Congenital diverticulum of left ventricle
Congenital malformation of myocardium
Congenital malformation of pericardium
Malposition of heart
Uhl's disease

Q24.9   Congenital malformation of heart, unspecified
Congenital anomaly of heart
Congenital disease of heart

● **Q25   Congenital malformations of great arteries**

Q25.0   Patent ductus arteriosus
Fetal blood vessel connecting left pulmonary artery directly to descending aorta
Patent ductus Botallo
Persistent ductus arteriosus

Q25.1   Coarctation of aorta
Coarctation of aorta (preductal) (postductal)

Q25.2   Atresia of aorta

Q25.3   Supravalvular aortic stenosis
> **Excludes1**   congenital aortic stenosis NOS (Q23.0)
> congenital stenosis of aortic valve (Q23.0)

Q25.4   Other congenital malformations of aorta
Absence of aorta
Aneurysm of sinus of Valsalva (ruptured)
Aplasia of aorta
Congenital aneurysm of aorta
Congenital malformations of aorta
Congenital dilatation of aorta
Double aortic arch [vascular ring of aorta]
Hypoplasia of aorta
Persistent convolutions of aortic arch
Persistent right aortic arch
> **Excludes1**   hypoplasia of aorta in hypoplastic left heart syndrome (Q23.4)

Q25.5   Atresia of pulmonary artery

Q25.6   Stenosis of pulmonary artery
Supravalvular pulmonary stenosis

● **Q25.7   Other congenital malformations of pulmonary artery**

Q25.71   Coarctation of pulmonary artery

Q25.72   Congenital pulmonary arteriovenous malformation
Congenital pulmonary arteriovenous aneurysm

Q25.79   Other congenital malformations of pulmonary artery
Aberrant pulmonary artery
Agenesis of pulmonary artery
Congenital aneurysm of pulmonary artery
Congenital anomaly of pulmonary artery
Hypoplasia of pulmonary artery

Q25.8   Other congenital malformations of other great arteries

Q25.9   Congenital malformation of great arteries, unspecified

● **Q26   Congenital malformations of great veins**

Q26.0   Congenital stenosis of vena cava
Congenital stenosis of vena cava (inferior)(superior)

Q26.1   Persistent left superior vena cava

Q26.2   Total anomalous pulmonary venous connection
Total anomalous pulmonary venous return [TAPVR], subdiaphragmatic
Total anomalous pulmonary venous return [TAPVR], supradiaphragmatic

Q26.3   Partial anomalous pulmonary venous connection
Partial anomalous pulmonary venous return

Q26.4   Anomalous pulmonary venous connection, unspecified

Q26.5   Anomalous portal venous connection

Q26.6   Portal vein-hepatic artery fistula

Q26.8   Other congenital malformations of great veins
Absence of vena cava (inferior) (superior)
Azygos continuation of inferior vena cava
Persistent left posterior cardinal vein
Scimitar syndrome

Q26.9   Congenital malformation of great vein, unspecified
Congenital anomaly of vena cava (inferior) (superior) NOS

● **Q27   Other congenital malformations of peripheral vascular system**
> **Excludes2**   anomalies of cerebral and precerebral vessels (Q28.0-Q28.3)
> anomalies of coronary vessels (Q24.5)
> anomalies of pulmonary artery (Q25.5-Q25.7)
> congenital retinal aneurysm (Q14.1)
> hemangioma and lymphangioma (D18.-)

Q27.0   Congenital absence and hypoplasia of umbilical artery
Single umbilical artery

Q27.1   Congenital renal artery stenosis

Q27.2   Other congenital malformations of renal artery
Congenital malformation of renal artery NOS
Multiple renal arteries

● **Q27.3   Arteriovenous malformation (peripheral)**
Arteriovenous aneurysm
> **Excludes1**   acquired arteriovenous aneurysm (I77.0)
> **Excludes2**   arteriovenous malformation of cerebral vessels (Q28.2)
> arteriovenous malformation of precerebral vessels (Q28.0)

Q27.30   Arteriovenous malformation, site unspecified

Q27.31   Arteriovenous malformation of vessel of upper limb

Q27.32   Arteriovenous malformation of vessel of lower limb

Q27.33   Arteriovenous malformation of digestive system vessel

Q27.34   Arteriovenous malformation of renal vessel

Q27.39   Arteriovenous malformation, other site

Q27.4   Congenital phlebectasia

Q27.8   Other specified congenital malformations of peripheral vascular system
Absence of peripheral vascular system
Atresia of peripheral vascular system
Congenital aneurysm (peripheral)
Congenital stricture, artery
Congenital varix
> **Excludes1**   arteriovenous malformation (Q27.3-)

Q27.9   Congenital malformation of peripheral vascular system, unspecified
Anomaly of artery or vein NOS

● Q28   Other congenital malformations of circulatory system

> Excludes1   congenital aneurysm NOS (Q27.8)
> congenital coronary aneurysm (Q24.5)
> ruptured cerebral arteriovenous malformation
> (I60.8)
> ruptured malformation of precerebral vessels
> (I72.0)

> Excludes2   congenital peripheral aneurysm (Q27.8)
> congenital pulmonary aneurysm (Q25.79)
> congenital retinal aneurysm (Q14.1)

Q28.0   **Arteriovenous malformation of precerebral vessels**
Congenital arteriovenous precerebral aneurysm
(nonruptured)

Q28.1   **Other malformations of precerebral vessels**
Congenital malformation of precerebral vessels NOS
Congenital precerebral aneurysm (nonruptured)

Q28.2   **Arteriovenous malformation of cerebral vessels**
Arteriovenous malformation of brain NOS
Congenital arteriovenous cerebral aneurysm
(nonruptured)

Q28.3   **Other malformations of cerebral vessels**
Congenital cerebral aneurysm (nonruptured)
Congenital malformation of cerebral vessels NOS
Developmental venous anomaly

Q28.8   **Other specified congenital malformations of circulatory system**
Congenital aneurysm, specified site NEC
Spinal vessel anomaly

Q28.9   **Congenital malformation of circulatory system, unspecified**

CONGENITAL MALFORMATIONS OF THE RESPIRATORY SYSTEM (Q30-Q34)

● Q30   Congenital malformations of nose

> Excludes1   congenital deviation of nasal septum (Q67.4)

Q30.0   **Choanal atresia**
Atresia of nares (anterior) (posterior)
Congenital stenosis of nares (anterior) (posterior)

Q30.1   **Agenesis and underdevelopment of nose**
Congenital absent of nose

Q30.2   **Fissured, notched and cleft nose**

Q30.3   **Congenital perforated nasal septum**

Q30.8   **Other congenital malformations of nose**
Accessory nose
Congenital anomaly of nasal sinus wall

Q30.9   **Congenital malformation of nose, unspecified**

● Q31   Congenital malformations of larynx

> Excludes1   congenital laryngeal stridor NOS (P28.89)

Q31.0   **Web of larynx**
Glottic web of larynx
Subglottic web of larynx
Web of larynx NOS

Q31.1   **Congenital subglottic stenosis**

Q31.2   **Laryngeal hypoplasia**

Q31.3   **Laryngocele**

Q31.5   **Congenital laryngomalacia**

Q31.8   **Other congenital malformations of larynx**
Absence of larynx
Agenesis of larynx
Atresia of larynx
Congenital cleft thyroid cartilage
Congenital fissure of epiglottis
Congenital stenosis of larynx NEC
Posterior cleft of cricoid cartilage

Q31.9   **Congenital malformation of larynx, unspecified**

● Q32   Congenital malformations of trachea and bronchus

> Excludes1   congenital bronchiectasis (Q33.4)

Q32.0   **Congenital tracheomalacia**

Q32.1   **Other congenital malformations of trachea**
Atresia of trachea
Congenital anomaly of tracheal cartilage
Congenital dilatation of trachea
Congenital malformation of trachea
Congenital stenosis of trachea
Congenital tracheocele

Q32.2   **Congenital bronchomalacia**

Q32.3   **Congenital stenosis of bronchus**

Q32.4   **Other congenital malformations of bronchus**
Absence of bronchus
Agenesis of bronchus
Atresia of bronchus
Congenital diverticulum of bronchus
Congenital malformation of bronchus NOS

● Q33   Congenital malformations of lung

Q33.0   **Congenital cystic lung**
Congenital cystic lung disease
Congenital honeycomb lung
Congenital polycystic lung disease

> Excludes1   cystic fibrosis (E84.0)
> cystic lung disease, acquired or
> unspecified (J98.4)

Q33.1   **Accessory lobe of lung**
Azygos lobe (fissured), lung

Q33.2   **Sequestration of lung**

Q33.3   **Agenesis of lung**
Congenital absence of lung (lobe)

Q33.4   **Congenital bronchiectasis**

Q33.5   **Ectopic tissue in lung**

Q33.6   **Congenital hypoplasia and dysplasia of lung**

> Excludes1   pulmonary hypoplasia associated with
> short gestation (P28.0)

Q33.8   **Other congenital malformations of lung**

Q33.9   **Congenital malformation of lung, unspecified**

● Q34   Other congenital malformations of respiratory system

> Excludes2   congenital central alveolar hypoventilation
> syndrome (G47.35)

Q34.0   **Anomaly of pleura**

Q34.1   **Congenital cyst of mediastinum**

Q34.8   **Other specified congenital malformations of respiratory system**
Atresia of nasopharynx

Q34.9   **Congenital malformation of respiratory system, unspecified**
Congenital absence of respiratory system
Congenital anomaly of respiratory system NOS

CLEFT LIP AND CLEFT PALATE (Q35-Q37)

Use additional code to identify associated malformation of the
nose (Q30.2)

> Excludes1   Robin's syndrome (Q87.0)

● Q35   Cleft palate

> Includes   fissure of palate
> palatoschisis

> Excludes1   cleft palate with cleft lip (Q37.-)

Q35.1   **Cleft hard palate**

Q35.3   **Cleft soft palate**

Figure 17-3 Cleft palate.

Q35.5   Cleft hard palate with cleft soft palate

Q35.7   Cleft uvula

Q35.9   Cleft palate, unspecified
    Cleft palate NOS

● **Q36   Cleft lip**

   Includes   cheiloschisis
               congenital fissure of lip
               harelip
               labium leporinum

    &boxed{**Excludes1**}   cleft lip with cleft palate (Q37.-)

Q36.0   Cleft lip, bilateral

Q36.1   Cleft lip, median

Q36.9   Cleft lip, unilateral
    Cleft lip NOS

● **Q37   Cleft palate with cleft lip**

   Includes   cheilopalatoschisis

Q37.0   Cleft hard palate with bilateral cleft lip

Q37.1   Cleft hard palate with unilateral cleft lip
    Cleft hard palate with cleft lip NOS

Q37.2   Cleft soft palate with bilateral cleft lip

Q37.3   Cleft soft palate with unilateral cleft lip
    Cleft soft palate with cleft lip NOS

Q37.4   Cleft hard and soft palate with bilateral cleft lip

Q37.5   Cleft hard and soft palate with unilateral cleft lip
    Cleft hard and soft palate with cleft lip NOS

Q37.8   Unspecified cleft palate with bilateral cleft lip

Q37.9   Unspecified cleft palate with unilateral cleft lip
    Cleft palate with cleft lip NOS

OTHER CONGENITAL MALFORMATIONS OF THE DIGESTIVE SYSTEM (Q38-Q45)

● **Q38   Other congenital malformations of tongue, mouth and pharynx**

   Excludes1   dentofacial anomalies (M26.-)
             macrostomia (Q18.4)
             microstomia (Q18.5)

Q38.0   Congenital malformations of lips, not elsewhere classified
    Congenital fistula of lip
    Congenital malformation of lip NOS
    Van der Woude's syndrome

    Excludes1   cleft lip (Q36.-)
             cleft lip with cleft palate (Q37.-)
             macrocheilia (Q18.6)
             microcheilia (Q18.7)

Q38.1   Ankyloglossia
    Restricted movement of tongue resulting in speech difficulty
    Tongue tie

Q38.2   Macroglossia
    Excessive size of tongue
    Congenital hypertrophy of tongue

Q38.3   Other congenital malformations of tongue
    Aglossia
    Bifid tongue
    Congenital adhesion of tongue
    Congenital fissure of tongue
    Congenital malformation of tongue NOS
    Double tongue
    Hypoglossia
    Hypoplasia of tongue
    Microglossia

Q38.4   Congenital malformations of salivary glands and ducts
    Atresia of salivary glands and ducts
    Congenital absence of salivary glands and ducts
    Congenital accessory salivary glands and ducts
    Congenital fistula of salivary gland

Q38.5   Congenital malformations of palate, not elsewhere classified
    Congenital absence of uvula
    Congenital malformation of palate NOS
    Congenital high arched palate

    Excludes1   cleft palate (Q35.-)
             cleft palate with cleft lip (Q37.-)

Q38.6   Other congenital malformations of mouth
    Congenital malformation of mouth NOS

Q38.7   Congenital pharyngeal pouch
    Congenital diverticulum of pharynx

    Excludes1   pharyngeal pouch syndrome (D82.1)

Q38.8   Other congenital malformations of pharynx
    Congenital malformation of pharynx NOS
    Imperforate pharynx

● **Q39   Congenital malformations of esophagus**

Q39.0   Atresia of esophagus without fistula
    Atresia of esophagus NOS

Q39.1   Atresia of esophagus with tracheo-esophageal fistula
    Atresia of esophagus with broncho-esophageal fistula

Q39.2   Congenital tracheo-esophageal fistula without atresia
    Congenital tracheo-esophageal fistula NOS

Q39.3   Congenital stenosis and stricture of esophagus

Q39.4   Esophageal web

Q39.5   Congenital dilatation of esophagus
    Congenital cardiospasm

Q39.6   Congenital diverticulum of esophagus
    Congenital esophageal pouch

Q39.8   Other congenital malformations of esophagus
    Congenital absence of esophagus
    Congenital displacement of esophagus
    Congenital duplication of esophagus

Q39.9   Congenital malformation of esophagus, unspecified

● **Q40   Other congenital malformations of upper alimentary tract**

Q40.0   Congenital hypertrophic pyloric stenosis
    Congenital or infantile constriction
    Congenital or infantile hypertrophy
    Congenital or infantile spasm
    Congenital or infantile stenosis
    Congenital or infantile stricture

Q40.1   Congenital hiatus hernia
    Congenital displacement of cardia through esophageal hiatus

    Excludes1   congenital diaphragmatic hernia (Q79.0)

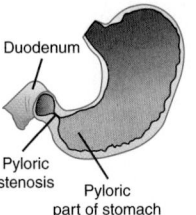

Figure 17-4 Pyloric stenosis.

Duodenum

Pyloric stenosis

Pyloric part of stomach

◀ New   ◀▥ Revised   ~~deleted~~ Deleted   OGCR Official Guidelines   X Assign placeholder X   ● Use Additional Character(s)

Excludes 1   Excludes 2   Includes   Use additional   Code first   Code also   Unspecified

Q40.2   **Other specified congenital malformations of stomach**
     Congenital displacement of stomach
     Congenital diverticulum of stomach
     Congenital hourglass stomach
     Congenital duplication of stomach
     Megalogastria
     Microgastria

Q40.3   **Congenital malformation of stomach, unspecified**

Q40.8   **Other specified congenital malformations of upper alimentary tract**

Q40.9   **Congenital malformation of upper alimentary tract, unspecified**
     Congenital anomaly of upper alimentary tract
     Congenital deformity of upper alimentary tract

● **Q41**   **Congenital absence, atresia and stenosis of small intestine**
     Includes   congenital obstruction, occlusion or stricture of small intestine or intestine NOS
     Excludes1   cystic fibrosis with intestinal manifestation (E84.11)
                     meconium ileus NOS (without cystic fibrosis) (P76.0)

Q41.0   **Congenital absence, atresia and stenosis of duodenum**

Q41.1   **Congenital absence, atresia and stenosis of jejunum**
     Apple peel syndrome
     Imperforate jejunum

Q41.2   **Congenital absence, atresia and stenosis of ileum**

Q41.8   **Congenital absence, atresia and stenosis of other specified parts of small intestine**

Q41.9   **Congenital absence, atresia and stenosis of small intestine, part unspecified**
     Congenital absence, atresia and stenosis of intestine NOS

● **Q42**   **Congenital absence, atresia and stenosis of large intestine**
     Includes   congenital obstruction, occlusion and stricture of large intestine

Q42.0   **Congenital absence, atresia and stenosis of rectum with fistula**

Q42.1   **Congenital absence, atresia and stenosis of rectum without fistula**
     Imperforate rectum

Q42.2   **Congenital absence, atresia and stenosis of anus with fistula**

Q42.3   **Congenital absence, atresia and stenosis of anus without fistula**
     Imperforate anus

Q42.8   **Congenital absence, atresia and stenosis of other parts of large intestine**

Q42.9   **Congenital absence, atresia and stenosis of large intestine, part unspecified**

● **Q43**   **Other congenital malformations of intestine**

Q43.0   **Meckel's diverticulum (displaced) (hypertrophic)**
     Congenital abnormality in which a pouch remains on the lower end of the small intestine
     Persistent omphalomesenteric duct
     Persistent vitelline duct

Q43.1   **Hirschsprung's disease**
     Developmental disorder of enteric nervous system characterized by absence of ganglion cells in distal colon resulting in functional obstruction.
     Aganglionosis
     Congenital (aganglionic) megacolon

Q43.2   **Other congenital functional disorders of colon**
     Congenital dilatation of colon

Q43.3   **Congenital malformations of intestinal fixation**
     Congenital omental, anomalous adhesions [bands]
     Congenital peritoneal adhesions [bands]
     Incomplete rotation of cecum and colon
     Insufficient rotation of cecum and colon
     Jackson's membrane
     Malrotation of colon
     Rotation failure of cecum and colon
     Universal mesentery

Q43.4   **Duplication of intestine**

Q43.5   **Ectopic anus**
     Anal opening in abnormal location

Q43.6   **Congenital fistula of rectum and anus**
     Excludes1   congenital fistula of anus with absence, atresia and stenosis (Q42.2)
                   congenital fistula of rectum with absence, atresia and stenosis (Q42.0)
                   congenital rectovaginal fistula (Q52.2)
                   congenital urethrorectal fistula (Q64.73)
                   pilonidal fistula or sinus (L05.-)

Q43.7   **Persistent cloaca**
     Malformation in which rectum, vagina, and urinary tract form one channel AKA congenital cloaca
     Cloaca NOS

Q43.8   **Other specified congenital malformations of intestine**
     Congenital blind loop syndrome
     Congenital diverticulitis, colon
     Congenital diverticulum, intestine
     Dolichocolon
     Megaloappendix
     Megaloduodenum
     Microcolon
     Transposition of appendix
     Transposition of colon
     Transposition of intestine

Q43.9   **Congenital malformation of intestine, unspecified**

● **Q44**   **Congenital malformations of gallbladder, bile ducts and liver**

Q44.0   **Agenesis, aplasia and hypoplasia of gallbladder**
     Congenital absence of gallbladder

Q44.1   **Other congenital malformations of gallbladder**
     Congenital malformation of gallbladder NOS
     Intrahepatic gallbladder

Q44.2   **Atresia of bile ducts**

Q44.3   **Congenital stenosis and stricture of bile ducts**

Q44.4   **Choledochal cyst**

Q44.5   **Other congenital malformations of bile ducts**
     Accessory hepatic duct
     Biliary duct duplication
     Congenital malformation of bile duct NOS
     Cystic duct duplication

Q44.6   **Cystic disease of liver**
     Fibrocystic disease of liver

Q44.7   **Other congenital malformations of liver**
     Accessory liver
     Alagille's syndrome
     Congenital absence of liver
     Congenital hepatomegaly
     Congenital malformation of liver NOS

● **Q45**   **Other congenital malformations of digestive system**
     Excludes2   congenital diaphragmatic hernia (Q79.0)
                   congenital hiatus hernia (Q40.1)

Q45.0   **Agenesis, aplasia and hypoplasia of pancreas**
     Congenital absence of pancreas

Q45.1   **Annular pancreas**

Q45.2   **Congenital pancreatic cyst**

CHAPTER 17 (Q00-Q99)

Q45.3　Other congenital malformations of pancreas and pancreatic duct
　　Accessory pancreas
　　Congenital malformation of pancreas or pancreatic duct NOS
　　　Excludes1　congenital diabetes mellitus (E10.-)
　　　　　cystic fibrosis (E84.0-E84.9)
　　　　　fibrocystic disease of pancreas (E84.-)
　　　　　neonatal diabetes mellitus (P70.2)

Q45.8　Other specified congenital malformations of digestive system
　　Absence (complete) (partial) of alimentary tract NOS
　　Duplication of digestive system
　　Malposition, congenital of digestive system

Q45.9　Congenital malformation of digestive system, unspecified
　　Congenital anomaly of digestive system
　　Congenital deformity of digestive system

CONGENITAL MALFORMATIONS OF GENITAL ORGANS (Q50-Q56)
　Excludes1　androgen insensitivity syndrome (E34.5-)
　　　syndromes associated with anomalies in the number and form of chromosomes (Q90-Q99)

Q50　Congenital malformations of ovaries, fallopian tubes and broad ligaments
　Q50.0　Congenital absence of ovary
　　　Excludes1　Turner's syndrome (Q96.-)
　　　Q50.01　Congenital absence of ovary, unilateral
　　　Q50.02　Congenital absence of ovary, bilateral
　Q50.1　Developmental ovarian cyst
　Q50.2　Congenital torsion of ovary
　Q50.3　Other congenital malformations of ovary
　　　Q50.31　Accessory ovary
　　　Q50.32　Ovarian streak
　　　　　Inadequate ovaries with absent follicular and hormonal function
　　　　　46, XX with streak gonads
　　　Q50.39　Other congenital malformation of ovary
　　　　　Congenital malformation of ovary NOS
　Q50.4　Embryonic cyst of fallopian tube
　　　Fimbrial cyst
　Q50.5　Embryonic cyst of broad ligament
　　　Epoophoron cyst
　　　Parovarian cyst
　Q50.6　Other congenital malformations of fallopian tube and broad ligament
　　　Absence of fallopian tube and broad ligament
　　　Accessory fallopian tube and broad ligament
　　　Atresia of fallopian tube and broad ligament
　　　Congenital malformation of fallopian tube or broad ligament NOS

Q51　Congenital malformations of uterus and cervix
　Q51.0　Agenesis and aplasia of uterus
　　　Congenital absence of uterus
　Q51.1　Doubling of uterus with doubling of cervix and vagina
　　　Q51.10　Doubling of uterus with doubling of cervix and vagina without obstruction
　　　　　Doubling of uterus with doubling of cervix and vagina NOS
　　　Q51.11　Doubling of uterus with doubling of cervix and vagina with obstruction
　Q51.2　Other doubling of uterus
　　　Doubling of uterus NOS
　　　Septate uterus, complete or partial
　Q51.3　Bicornate uterus
　　　Bicornate uterus, complete or partial
　　　Birth defect in which uterus has two separate 'horns' that form top of uterus

Q51.4　Unicornate uterus
　　Unicornate uterus with or without a separate uterine horn
　　Uterus with only one functioning horn
　　Uterus with half being undeveloped

Q51.5　Agenesis and aplasia of cervix
　　Congenital absence of cervix

Q51.6　Embryonic cyst of cervix

Q51.7　Congenital fistulae between uterus and digestive and urinary tracts

Q51.8　Other congenital malformations of uterus and cervix
　Q51.81　Other congenital malformations of uterus
　　　Q51.810　Arcuate uterus
　　　　　Arcuatus uterus
　　　Q51.811　Hypoplasia of uterus
　　　Q51.818　Other congenital malformations of uterus
　　　　　Müllerian anomaly of uterus NEC
　Q51.82　Other congenital malformations of cervix
　　　Q51.820　Cervical duplication
　　　Q51.821　Hypoplasia of cervix
　　　Q51.828　Other congenital malformations of cervix

Q51.9　Congenital malformation of uterus and cervix, unspecified

Q52　Other congenital malformations of female genitalia
　Q52.0　Congenital absence of vagina
　　　Vaginal agenesis, total or partial
　Q52.1　Doubling of vagina
　　　Excludes1　doubling of vagina with doubling of uterus and cervix (Q51.1-)
　　　Q52.10　Doubling of vagina, unspecified
　　　　　Septate vagina NOS
　　　Q52.11　Transverse vaginal septum
　　　Q52.12　Longitudinal vaginal septum
　　　　　Longitudinal vaginal septum with or without obstruction
　Q52.2　Congenital rectovaginal fistula
　　　Excludes1　cloaca (Q43.7)
　Q52.3　Imperforate hymen
　　　Membrane (hymen) completely closes vaginal orifice
　Q52.4　Other congenital malformations of vagina
　　　Canal of Nuck cyst, congenital
　　　Congenital malformation of vagina NOS
　　　Embryonic vaginal cyst
　　　Gartner's duct cyst
　Q52.5　Fusion of labia
　Q52.6　Congenital malformation of clitoris
　Q52.7　Other and unspecified congenital malformations of vulva
　　　Q52.70　Unspecified congenital malformations of vulva
　　　　　Congenital malformation of vulva NOS
　　　Q52.71　Congenital absence of vulva
　　　Q52.79　Other congenital malformations of vulva
　　　　　Congenital cyst of vulva
　Q52.8　Other specified congenital malformations of female genitalia
　Q52.9　Congenital malformation of female genitalia, unspecified

Item 17-1 Testes form in the abdomen of the male and only descend into the scrotum during normal embryonic development. "Ectopic" testes are out of their normal place or "retained" (left behind) in the abdomen. Crypto (hidden) orchism (testicle) is a major risk factor for testicular cancer.

ECTOPIC TESTES	CRYPTORCHID TESTES
Penile	Abdominal
Superficial inguinal	Inguinal
(most common)	Prepubic
Femoral	(most common)

Figure 17-5 Undescended testes and the positions of the testes in various types of cryptorchidism or abnormal paths of descent.

● **Q53   Undescended and ectopic testicle**
- ● **Q53.0   Ectopic testis**
  - **Q53.00   Ectopic testis, unspecified**
  - **Q53.01   Ectopic testis, unilateral**
  - **Q53.02   Ectopic testes, bilateral**
- ● **Q53.1   Undescended testicle, unilateral**
  - **Q53.10   Unspecified undescended testicle, unilateral**
  - **Q53.11   Abdominal testis, unilateral**
  - **Q53.12   Ectopic perineal testis, unilateral**
- ● **Q53.2   Undescended testicle, bilateral**
  - **Q53.20   Undescended testicle, unspecified, bilateral**
  - **Q53.21   Abdominal testis, bilateral**
  - **Q53.22   Ectopic perineal testis, bilateral**
- **Q53.9   Undescended testicle, unspecified**
  - Cryptorchism NOS

● **Q54   Hypospadias**
  - *Birth defect of male; urethra opens in abnormal location on shaft*
  - **Excludes1**   epispadias (Q64.0)
- **Q54.0   Hypospadias, balanic**
  - Hypospadias, coronal
  - Hypospadias, glandular
- **Q54.1   Hypospadias, penile**
- **Q54.2   Hypospadias, penoscrotal**
- **Q54.3   Hypospadias, perineal**
- **Q54.4   Congenital chordee**
  - Chordee without hypospadias
- **Q54.8   Other hypospadias**
  - Hypospadias with intersex state
- **Q54.9   Hypospadias, unspecified**

● **Q55   Other congenital malformations of male genital organs**
  - **Excludes1**   congenital hydrocele (P83.5)
  - hypospadias (Q54.-)
- **Q55.0   Absence and aplasia of testis**
  - Monorchism
- **Q55.1   Hypoplasia of testis and scrotum**
  - Fusion of testes
- ● **Q55.2   Other and unspecified congenital malformations of testis and scrotum**
  - **Q55.20   Unspecified congenital malformations of testis and scrotum**
    - Congenital malformation of testis or scrotum NOS

- **Q55.21   Polyorchism**
  - *Developmental anomaly characterized by presence of more than two testes*
- **Q55.22   Retractile testis**
- **Q55.23   Scrotal transposition**
- **Q55.29   Other congenital malformations of testis and scrotum**
- **Q55.3   Atresia of vas deferens**
  - *Code first any associated cystic fibrosis (E84.-)*
- **Q55.4   Other congenital malformations of vas deferens, epididymis, seminal vesicles and prostate**
  - Absence or aplasia of prostate
  - Absence or aplasia of spermatic cord
  - Congenital malformation of vas deferens, epididymis, seminal vesicles or prostate NOS
- **Q55.5   Congenital absence and aplasia of penis**
- ● **Q55.6   Other congenital malformations of penis**
  - **Q55.61   Curvature of penis (lateral)**
  - **Q55.62   Hypoplasia of penis**
    - *Underdevelopment penis*
    - Micropenis
  - **Q55.63   Congenital torsion of penis**
    - **Excludes1**   acquired torsion of penis (N48.82)
  - **Q55.64   Hidden penis**
    - Buried penis
    - Concealed penis
    - **Excludes1**   acquired buried penis (N48.83)
  - **Q55.69   Other congenital malformation of penis**
    - Congenital malformation of penis NOS
- **Q55.7   Congenital vasocutaneous fistula**
  - *Abnormal opening between vas deferens and skin*
- **Q55.8   Other specified congenital malformations of male genital organs**
- **Q55.9   Congenital malformation of male genital organ, unspecified**
  - Congenital anomaly of male genital organ
  - Congenital deformity of male genital organ

● **Q56   Indeterminate sex and pseudohermaphroditism**
  - *Internal reproductive organs are opposite external physical characteristics.*
  - **Excludes1**   46,XX true hermaphrodite (Q99.1)
    - androgen insensitivity syndrome (E34.5-)
    - chimera 46,XX/46,XY true hermaphrodite (Q99.0)
    - female pseudohermaphroditism with adrenocortical disorder (E25.-)
    - pseudohermaphroditism with specified chromosomal anomaly (Q96-Q99)
    - pure gonadal dysgenesis (Q99.1)
- **Q56.0   Hermaphroditism, not elsewhere classified**
  - Ovotestis
- **Q56.1   Male pseudohermaphroditism, not elsewhere classified**
  - 46, XY with streak gonads
  - Male pseudohermaphroditism NOS
- **Q56.2   Female pseudohermaphroditism, not elsewhere classified**
  - Female pseudohermaphroditism NOS
- **Q56.3   Pseudohermaphroditism, unspecified**
- **Q56.4   Indeterminate sex, unspecified**
  - Ambiguous genitalia

CHAPTER 17 (Q00-Q99)

◀ New   ◀▥ Revised   ~~deleted~~ Deleted   **OGCR** Official Guidelines   X Assign placeholder X   ● Use Additional Character(s)

| Excludes 1 | Excludes 2 | Includes | Use additional | Code first | Code also | Unspecified |

CONGENITAL MALFORMATIONS OF THE URINARY SYSTEM (Q60-Q64)

● Q60 **Renal agenesis and other reduction defects of kidney**

    Includes   congenital absence of kidney
            congenital atrophy of kidney
            infantile atrophy of kidney

    Q60.0 **Renal agenesis, unilateral**

    Q60.1 **Renal agenesis, bilateral**

    Q60.2 **Renal agenesis, unspecified**

    Q60.3 **Renal hypoplasia, unilateral**

    Q60.4 **Renal hypoplasia, bilateral**

    Q60.5 **Renal hypoplasia, unspecified**

    Q60.6 **Potter's syndrome**

● Q61 **Cystic kidney disease**

    Cysts that develop in failing kidney due to end-stage renal disease

    Excludes1   acquired cyst of kidney (N28.1)
                  Potter's syndrome (Q60.6)

   ● Q61.0 **Congenital renal cyst**

        Q61.00 **Congenital renal cyst, unspecified**
               Cyst of kidney NOS (congenital)

        Q61.01 **Congenital single renal cyst**

        Q61.02 **Congenital multiple renal cysts**

   ● Q61.1 **Polycystic kidney, infantile type**
        Polycystic kidney, autosomal recessive

        Q61.11 **Cystic dilatation of collecting ducts**

        Q61.19 **Other polycystic kidney, infantile type**

    Q61.2 **Polycystic kidney, adult type**
        Polycystic kidney, autosomal dominant

    Q61.3 **Polycystic kidney, unspecified**

    Q61.4 **Renal dysplasia**
        Multicystic dysplastic kidney
        Multicystic kidney (development)
        Multicystic kidney disease
        Multicystic renal dysplasia

        Excludes1   polycystic kidney disease (Q61.11-Q61.3)

    Q61.5 **Medullary cystic kidney**
        Nephronopthisis
        Sponge kidney NOS

    Q61.8 **Other cystic kidney diseases**
        Fibrocystic kidney
        Fibrocystic renal degeneration or disease

    Q61.9 **Cystic kidney disease, unspecified**
        Meckel-Gruber syndrome

● Q62 **Congenital obstructive defects of renal pelvis and congenital malformations of ureter**

    Q62.0 **Congenital hydronephrosis**

   ● Q62.1 **Congenital occlusion of ureter**
        Atresia and stenosis of ureter

        Q62.10 **Congenital occlusion of ureter, unspecified**

        Q62.11 **Congenital occlusion of ureteropelvic junction**

        Q62.12 **Congenital occlusion of ureterovesical orifice**

    Q62.2 **Congenital megaureter**
        Congenital dilatation of ureter

   ● Q62.3 **Other obstructive defects of renal pelvis and ureter**

        Q62.31 **Congenital ureterocele, orthotopic**

        Q62.32 **Cecoureterocele**
               Ectopic ureterocele

        Q62.39 **Other obstructive defects of renal pelvis and ureter**
               Ureteropelvic junction obstruction NOS

    Q62.4 **Agenesis of ureter**
        Congenital absence ureter

    Q62.5 **Duplication of ureter**
        Accessory ureter
        Double ureter

● Q62.6 **Malposition of ureter**

    Q62.60 **Malposition of ureter, unspecified**

    Q62.61 **Deviation of ureter**

    Q62.62 **Displacement of ureter**

    Q62.63 **Anomalous implantation of ureter**
        Ectopia of ureter
        Ectopic ureter

    Q62.69 **Other malposition of ureter**

   Q62.7 **Congenital vesico-uretero-renal reflux**

   Q62.8 **Other congenital malformations of ureter**
        Anomaly of ureter NOS

● Q63 **Other congenital malformations of kidney**

    Excludes1   congenital nephrotic syndrome (N04.-)

   Q63.0 **Accessory kidney**

   Q63.1 **Lobulated, fused and horseshoe kidney**

   Q63.2 **Ectopic kidney**
        Congenital displaced kidney
        Malrotation of kidney

   Q63.3 **Hyperplastic and giant kidney**
        Compensatory hypertrophy of kidney

   Q63.8 **Other specified congenital malformations of kidney**
        Congenital renal calculi

   Q63.9 **Congenital malformation of kidney, unspecified**

● Q64 **Other congenital malformations of urinary system**

   Q64.0 **Epispadias**
        Urethral opening somewhere on dorsum of penis

        Excludes1   hypospadias (Q54.-)

   ● Q64.1 **Exstrophy of urinary bladder**
        Bladder is exposed, inside out, and protrudes through abdominal wall

        Q64.10 **Exstrophy of urinary bladder, unspecified**
               Ectopia vesicae

        Q64.11 **Supravesical fissure of urinary bladder**

        Q64.12 **Cloacal extrophy of urinary bladder**

        Q64.19 **Other exstrophy of urinary bladder**
               Extroversion of bladder

   Q64.2 **Congenital posterior urethral valves**

   ● Q64.3 **Other atresia and stenosis of urethra and bladder neck**

        Q64.31 **Congenital bladder neck obstruction**
               Congenital obstruction of vesicourethral orifice

        Q64.32 **Congenital stricture of urethra**

        Q64.33 **Congenital stricture of urinary meatus**

        Q64.39 **Other atresia and stenosis of urethra and bladder neck**
               Atresia and stenosis of urethra and bladder neck NOS

   Q64.4 **Malformation of urachus**
        Cyst of urachus
        Patent urachus
        Prolapse of urachus

   Q64.5 **Congenital absence of bladder and urethra**

   Q64.6 **Congenital diverticulum of bladder**

   ● Q64.7 **Other and unspecified congenital malformations of bladder and urethra**

        Excludes1   congenital prolapse of bladder (mucosa) (Q79.4)

        Q64.70 **Unspecified congenital malformation of bladder and urethra**
               Malformation of bladder or urethra NOS

        Q64.71 **Congenital prolapse of urethra**

        Q64.72 **Congenital prolapse of urinary meatus**

        Q64.73 **Congenital urethrorectal fistula**

        Q64.74 **Double urethra**

        Q64.75 **Double urinary meatus**

        Q64.79 **Other congenital malformations of bladder and urethra**

Q64.8   Other specified congenital malformations of urinary system

Q64.9   Congenital malformation of urinary system, unspecified
Congenital anomaly NOS of urinary system
Congenital deformity NOS of urinary system

CONGENITAL MALFORMATIONS AND DEFORMATIONS OF THE MUSCULOSKELETAL SYSTEM (Q65-Q79)

● Q65   Congenital deformities of hip
Excludes1   clicking hip (R29.4)

● Q65.0   Congenital dislocation of hip, unilateral
Q65.00   Congenital dislocation of unspecified hip, unilateral
Q65.01   Congenital dislocation of right hip, unilateral
Q65.02   Congenital dislocation of left hip, unilateral

Q65.1   Congenital dislocation of hip, bilateral

Q65.2   Congenital dislocation of hip, unspecified

● Q65.3   Congenital partial dislocation of hip, unilateral
Q65.30   Congenital partial dislocation of unspecified hip, unilateral
Q65.31   Congenital partial dislocation of right hip, unilateral
Q65.32   Congenital partial dislocation of left hip, unilateral

Q65.4   Congenital partial dislocation of hip, bilateral

Q65.5   Congenital partial dislocation of hip, unspecified

Q65.6   Congenital unstable hip
Congenital dislocatable hip

● Q65.8   Other congenital deformities of hip
Q65.81   Congenital coxa valga
Q65.82   Congenital coxa vara
Q65.89   Other specified congenital deformities of hip
Anteversion of femoral neck
Congenital acetabular dysplasia

Q65.9   Congenital deformity of hip, unspecified

● Q66   Congenital deformities of feet
Excludes1   reduction defects of feet (Q72.-)
valgus deformities (acquired) (M21.0-)
varus deformities (acquired) (M21.1-)

Q66.0   Congenital talipes equinovarus
Heel is turned inward from midline and foot is plantar flexed; AKA clubfoot

Q66.1   Congenital talipes calcaneovarus
Deformity of foot in which heel is turned toward midline of body and anterior of foot is elevated

Q66.2   Congenital metatarsus (primus) varus
Angulation of first metatarsal bone toward midline of body

Q66.3   Other congenital varus deformities of feet
Hallux varus, congenital

Q66.4   Congenital talipes calcaneovalgus

Figure 17-7   Talipes. (From Dorland: Dorland's Illustrated Medical Dictionary, ed 31, Saunders, 2007, p 1893)

● Q66.5   Congenital pes planus
Congenital flat foot
Congenital rigid flat foot
Congenital spastic (everted) flat foot
Excludes1   pes planus, acquired (M21.4)
Q66.50   Congenital pes planus, unspecified foot
Q66.51   Congenital pes planus, right foot
Q66.52   Congenital pes planus, left foot

Q66.6   Other congenital valgus deformities of feet
Inward angulation
Congenital metatarsus valgus

Q66.7   Congenital pes cavus

● Q66.8   Other congenital deformities of feet
Q66.80   Congenital vertical talus deformity, unspecified foot
Q66.81   Congenital vertical talus deformity, right foot
Q66.82   Congenital vertical talus deformity, left foot
Q66.89   Other specified congenital deformities of feet
Congenital asymmetric talipes
Congenital clubfoot NOS
Congenital talipes NOS
Congenital tarsal coalition
Hammer toe, congenital

Q66.9   Congenital deformity of feet, unspecified

● Q67   Congenital musculoskeletal deformities of head, face, spine and chest
Excludes1   congenital malformation syndromes classified to Q87.-
Potter's syndrome (Q60.6)

Q67.0   Congenital facial asymmetry

Q67.1   Congenital compression facies

Q67.2   Dolichocephaly
Long head dimension

Q67.3   Plagiocephaly
Asymmetric shape of head resulting from irregular closure of cranial sutures

Q67.4   Other congenital deformities of skull, face and jaw
Congenital depressions in skull
Congenital hemifacial atrophy or hypertrophy
Deviation of nasal septum, congenital
Squashed or bent nose, congenital
Excludes1   dentofacial anomalies [including malocclusion] (M26.-)
syphilitic saddle nose (A50.5)

Item 17-2   Equinus foot is a term referring to the hoof of a horse. The deformity is usually congenital or spastic. Talipes equinovarus is referred to as clubfoot. The foot tends to be smaller than normal, with the heel pointing downward and the forefoot turning inward. The heel cord (Achilles tendon) is tight, causing the heel to be drawn up toward the leg.

Figure 17-6   Supination and cavus deformity of forefoot. *(Courtesy Jay Cummings, MD.)* (From Canale: Campbell's Operative Orthopaedics, ed 11, Mosby, Inc., 2007)

◀ New   ◀= Revised   ~~deleted~~ Deleted   **OGCR** Official Guidelines   X Assign placeholder X   ● Use Additional Character(s)

Excludes 1   Excludes 2   Includes   Use additional   Code first   Code also   Unspecified

Figure 17-8   Mild to moderate inbowing of the lower leg. (From Jones KL: Smith's Recognizable Patterns of Human Malformation, ed 6, Philadelphia, Saunders, 2005)

Figure 17-9   Polydactyly, congenital duplicated thumb. (From DeLee: DeLee and Drez's Orthopaedic Sports Medicine, ed 3, Saunders, An Imprint of Elsevier, 2009)

Q67.5   **Congenital deformity of spine**
Congenital postural scoliosis
Congenital scoliosis NOS
> **Excludes1**   infantile idiopathic scoliosis (M41.0)
> scoliosis due to congenital bony
> malformation (Q76.3)

Q67.6   **Pectus excavatum**
Congenital funnel chest
Funnel-shaped chest depression

Q67.7   **Pectus carinatum**
Congenital pigeon chest

Q67.8   **Other congenital deformities of chest**
Congenital deformity of chest wall NOS

● Q68   **Other congenital musculoskeletal deformities**
> **Excludes1**   reduction defects of limb(s) (Q71-Q73)
> **Excludes2**   congenital myotonic chondrodystrophy (G71.13)

Q68.0   **Congenital deformity of sternocleidomastoid muscle**
Congenital contracture of sternocleidomastoid (muscle)
Congenital (sternomastoid) torticollis
Sternomastoid tumor (congenital)

Q68.1   **Congenital deformity of finger(s) and hand**
Congenital clubfinger
Spade-like hand (congenital)

Q68.2   **Congenital deformity of knee**
Congenital dislocation of knee
Congenital genu recurvatum
Hyperextension of knee resulting from hypermobility

Q68.3   **Congenital bowing of femur**
> **Excludes1**   anteversion of femur (neck) (Q65.89)

Q68.4   **Congenital bowing of tibia and fibula**

Q68.5   **Congenital bowing of long bones of leg, unspecified**

Q68.6   **Discoid meniscus**

Q68.8   **Other specified congenital musculoskeletal deformities**
Congenital deformity of clavicle
Congenital deformity of elbow
Congenital deformity of forearm
Congenital deformity of scapula
Congenital deformity of wrist
Congenital dislocation of elbow
Congenital dislocation of shoulder
Congenital dislocation of wrist

● Q69   **Polydactyly**
AKA hyperdactyly, consists of supernumerary fingers or toes

Q69.0   **Accessory finger(s)**

Q69.1   **Accessory thumb(s)**

Q69.2   **Accessory toe(s)**
Accessory hallux

Q69.9   **Polydactyly, unspecified**
Supernumerary digit(s) NOS

● Q70   **Syndactyly**
Webbing between distal phalanges of adjacent digits

● Q70.0   **Fused fingers**
Complex syndactyly of fingers with synostosis
Q70.00   **Fused fingers, unspecified hand**
Q70.01   **Fused fingers, right hand**
Q70.02   **Fused fingers, left hand**
Q70.03   **Fused fingers, bilateral**

● Q70.1   **Webbed fingers**
Simple syndactyly of fingers without synostosis
Q70.10   **Webbed fingers, unspecified hand**
Q70.11   **Webbed fingers, right hand**
Q70.12   **Webbed fingers, left hand**
Q70.13   **Webbed fingers, bilateral**

● Q70.2   **Fused toes**
Complex syndactyly of toes with synostosis
Q70.20   **Fused toes, unspecified foot**
Q70.21   **Fused toes, right foot**
Q70.22   **Fused toes, left foot**
Q70.23   **Fused toes, bilateral**

● Q70.3   **Webbed toes**
Simple syndactyly of toes without synostosis
Q70.30   **Webbed toes, unspecified foot**
Q70.31   **Webbed toes, right foot**
Q70.32   **Webbed toes, left foot**
Q70.33   **Webbed toes, bilateral**

Q70.4   **Polysyndactyly, unspecified**
> **Excludes1**   specified syndactyly of hand and
> feet - code to specified conditions
> (Q70.0- -Q70.3-)
Extra and webbed digits

Q70.9   **Syndactyly, unspecified**
Symphalangy NOS

● Q71   **Reduction defects of upper limb**
● Q71.0   **Congenital complete absence of upper limb**
Q71.00   **Congenital complete absence of unspecified upper limb**
Q71.01   **Congenital complete absence of right upper limb**
Q71.02   **Congenital complete absence of left upper limb**
Q71.03   **Congenital complete absence of upper limb, bilateral**

● Q71.1   **Congenital absence of upper arm and forearm with hand present**
Q71.10   **Congenital absence of unspecified upper arm and forearm with hand present**
Q71.11   **Congenital absence of right upper arm and forearm with hand present**
Q71.12   **Congenital absence of left upper arm and forearm with hand present**
Q71.13   **Congenital absence of upper arm and forearm with hand present, bilateral**

● Q71.2   **Congenital absence of both forearm and hand**
Q71.20   **Congenital absence of both forearm and hand, unspecified upper limb**
Q71.21   **Congenital absence of both forearm and hand, right upper limb**
Q71.22   **Congenital absence of both forearm and hand, left upper limb**
Q71.23   **Congenital absence of both forearm and hand, bilateral**

● Q71.3   **Congenital absence of hand and finger**
Q71.30   **Congenital absence of unspecified hand and finger**
Q71.31   **Congenital absence of right hand and finger**
Q71.32   **Congenital absence of left hand and finger**
Q71.33   **Congenital absence of hand and finger, bilateral**

● Q71.4   Longitudinal reduction defect of radius
            Clubhand (congenital)
            Radial clubhand
       Q71.40   Longitudinal reduction defect of unspecified
                 radius
       Q71.41   Longitudinal reduction defect of right radius
       Q71.42   Longitudinal reduction defect of left radius
       Q71.43   Longitudinal reduction defect of radius,
                 bilateral
● Q71.5   Longitudinal reduction defect of ulna
       Q71.50   Longitudinal reduction defect of unspecified
                 ulna
       Q71.51   Longitudinal reduction defect of right ulna
       Q71.52   Longitudinal reduction defect of left ulna
       Q71.53   Longitudinal reduction defect of ulna, bilateral
● Q71.6   Lobster-claw hand
       Q71.60   Lobster-claw hand, unspecified hand
       Q71.61   Lobster-claw right hand
       Q71.62   Lobster-claw left hand
       Q71.63   Lobster-claw hand, bilateral
● Q71.8   Other reduction defects of upper limb
     ● Q71.81   Congenital shortening of upper limb
            Q71.811   Congenital shortening of right upper
                       limb
            Q71.812   Congenital shortening of left upper
                       limb
            Q71.813   Congenital shortening of upper limb,
                       bilateral
            Q71.819   Congenital shortening of unspecified
                       upper limb
     ● Q71.89 Other reduction defects of upper limb
            Q71.891   Other reduction defects of right upper
                       limb
            Q71.892   Other reduction defects of left upper
                       limb
            Q71.893   Other reduction defects of upper
                       limb, bilateral
            Q71.899   Other reduction defects of
                       unspecified upper limb
● Q71.9   Unspecified reduction defect of upper limb
       Q71.90   Unspecified reduction defect of unspecified
                 upper limb
       Q71.91   Unspecified reduction defect of right upper
                 limb
       Q71.92   Unspecified reduction defect of left upper limb
       Q71.93   Unspecified reduction defect of upper limb,
                 bilateral

● Q72   Reduction defects of lower limb
   ● Q72.0   Congenital complete absence of lower limb
       Q72.00   Congenital complete absence of unspecified
                 lower limb
       Q72.01   Congenital complete absence of right lower
                 limb
       Q72.02   Congenital complete absence of left lower limb
       Q72.03   Congenital complete absence of lower limb,
                 bilateral
   ● Q72.1   Congenital absence of thigh and lower leg with foot
             present
       Q72.10   Congenital absence of unspecified thigh and
                 lower leg with foot present
       Q72.11   Congenital absence of right thigh and lower leg
                 with foot present
       Q72.12   Congenital absence of left thigh and lower leg
                 with foot present
       Q72.13   Congenital absence of thigh and lower leg with
                 foot present, bilateral

● Q72.2   Congenital absence of both lower leg and foot
       Q72.20   Congenital absence of both lower leg and foot,
                 unspecified lower limb
       Q72.21   Congenital absence of both lower leg and foot,
                 right lower limb
       Q72.22   Congenital absence of both left lower leg and
                 foot, left lower limb
       Q72.23   Congenital absence of both lower leg and foot,
                 bilateral
● Q72.3   Congenital absence of foot and toe(s)
       Q72.30   Congenital absence of unspecified foot and
                 toe(s)
       Q72.31   Congenital absence of right foot and toe(s)
       Q72.32   Congenital absence of left foot and toe(s)
       Q72.33   Congenital absence of foot and toe(s), bilateral
● Q72.4   Longitudinal reduction defect of femur
            Proximal femoral focal deficiency
       Q72.40   Longitudinal reduction defect of unspecified
                 femur
       Q72.41   Longitudinal reduction defect of right femur
       Q72.42   Longitudinal reduction defect of left femur
       Q72.43   Longitudinal reduction defect of femur,
                 bilateral
● Q72.5   Longitudinal reduction defect of tibia
       Q72.50   Longitudinal reduction defect of unspecified
                 tibia
       Q72.51   Longitudinal reduction defect of right tibia
       Q72.52   Longitudinal reduction defect of left tibia
       Q72.53   Longitudinal reduction defect of tibia, bilateral
● Q72.6   Longitudinal reduction defect of fibula
       Q72.60   Longitudinal reduction defect of unspecified
                 fibula
       Q72.61   Longitudinal reduction defect of right fibula
       Q72.62   Longitudinal reduction defect of left fibula
       Q72.63   Longitudinal reduction defect of fibula,
                 bilateral
● Q72.7   Split foot
       Q72.70   Split foot, unspecified lower limb
       Q72.71   Split foot, right lower limb
       Q72.72   Split foot, left lower limb
       Q72.73   Split foot, bilateral
● Q72.8   Other reduction defects of lower limb
     ● Q72.81   Congenital shortening of lower limb
            Q72.811   Congenital shortening of right lower
                       limb
            Q72.812   Congenital shortening of left lower
                       limb
            Q72.813   Congenital shortening of lower limb,
                       bilateral
            Q72.819   Congenital shortening of unspecified
                       lower limb
     ● Q72.89   Other reduction defects of lower limb
            Q72.891   Other reduction defects of right lower
                       limb
            Q72.892   Other reduction defects of left lower
                       limb
            Q72.893   Other reduction defects of lower
                       limb, bilateral
            Q72.899   Other reduction defects of
                       unspecified lower limb
● Q72.9   Unspecified reduction defect of lower limb
       Q72.90   Unspecified reduction defect of unspecified
                 lower limb
       Q72.91   Unspecified reduction defect of right lower
                 limb
       Q72.92   Unspecified reduction defect of left lower limb
       Q72.93   Unspecified reduction defect of lower limb,
                 bilateral

CHAPTER 17 (Q00-Q99)

● **Q73**   **Reduction defects of unspecified limb**

    Q73.0   **Congenital absence of unspecified limb(s)**
        Amelia NOS

    Q73.1   **Phocomelia, unspecified limb(s)**
        Phocomelia NOS
          Absence/shortening of long bones primarily as a result of thalidomide

    Q73.8   **Other reduction defects of unspecified limb(s)**
        Longitudinal reduction deformity of unspecified limb(s)
        Ectromelia of limb NOS
          Gross hypoplasia or aplasia of one or more long bones of limb(s)
        Hemimelia of limb NOS
          Absence of one-half of long bone
        Reduction defect of limb NOS

● **Q74**   **Other congenital malformations of limb(s)**
      | Excludes1 | polydactyly (Q69.-)
                reduction defect of limb (Q71-Q73)
                syndactyly (Q70.-)

    Q74.0   **Other congenital malformations of upper limb(s), including shoulder girdle**
        Accessory carpal bones
        Cleidocranial dysostosis
        Congenital pseudarthrosis of clavicle
        Macrodactylia (fingers)
        Madelung's deformity
        Radioulnar synostosis
        Sprengel's deformity
        Triphalangeal thumb

    Q74.1   **Congenital malformation of knee**
        Congenital absence of patella
        Congenital dislocation of patella
        Congenital genu valgum
        Congenital genu varum
        Rudimentary patella
      | Excludes1 | congenital dislocation of knee (Q68.2)
                congenital genu recurvatum (Q68.2)
                nail patella syndrome (Q87.2)

    Q74.2   **Other congenital malformations of lower limb(s), including pelvic girdle**
        Congenital fusion of sacroiliac joint
        Congenital malformation of ankle joint
        Congenital malformation of sacroiliac joint
      | Excludes1 | anteversion of femur (neck) (Q65.89)

    Q74.3   **Arthrogryposis multiplex congenita**

    Q74.8   **Other specified congenital malformations of limb(s)**

    Q74.9   **Unspecified congenital malformation of limb(s)**
        Congenital anomaly of limb(s) NOS

● **Q75**   **Other congenital malformations of skull and face bones**
      | Excludes1 | congenital malformation of face NOS (Q18.-)
                congenital malformation syndromes classified to Q87.-
                dentofacial anomalies [including malocclusion] (M26.-)
                musculoskeletal deformities of head and face (Q67.0-Q67.4)
                skull defects associated with congenital anomalies of brain such as:
                anencephaly (Q00.0)
                encephalocele (Q01.-)
                hydrocephalus (Q03.-)
                microcephaly (Q02)

    Q75.0   **Craniosynostosis**
        Premature closure of sutures of skull
        Acrocephaly
        Imperfect fusion of skull
        Oxycephaly
        Trigonocephaly

    Q75.1   **Craniofacial dysostosis**
        Congenital deformity of head
        Crouzon's disease

Item 17–3 **Anencephalus** is a congenital deformity of the cranial vault. **Craniosynostosis,** also known as craniostenosis and stenocephaly, signifies any form of congenital deformity of the skull that results from the premature closing of the sutures of the skull. **Iniencephaly** is a deformity in which the head and neck are flexed backward to a great extent and the head is very large in comparison to the shortened body.

Figure 17-10 Generalized craniosynostosis in a 4-year-old girl without symptoms or signs of increased intracranial pressure. (From Bell WE, McCormick WF: Increased Intracranial Pressure in Children, ed 2, Philadelphia, WB Saunders, 1978, p 116)

    Q75.2   **Hypertelorism**

    Q75.3   **Macrocephaly**
        Unusually large size of head; AKA megalocephaly

    Q75.4   **Mandibulofacial dysostosis**
        Franceschetti syndrome
        Treacher Collins syndrome

    Q75.5   **Oculomandibular dysostosis**
        Ossification of occular and mandibular bones

    Q75.8   **Other specified congenital malformations of skull and face bones**
        Absence of skull bone, congenital
        Congenital deformity of forehead
        Platybasia

    Q75.9   **Congenital malformation of skull and face bones, unspecified**
        Congenital anomaly of face bones NOS
        Congenital anomaly of skull NOS

● **Q76**   **Congenital malformations of spine and bony thorax**
      | Excludes1 | congenital musculoskeletal deformities of spine and chest (Q67.5-Q67.8)

    Q76.0   **Spina bifida occulta**
      | Excludes1 | meningocele (spinal) (Q05.-)
                spina bifida (aperta) (cystica) (Q05.-)

    Q76.1   **Klippel-Feil syndrome**
        Cervical fusion syndrome

    Q76.2   **Congenital spondylolisthesis**
        Congenital spondylolysis
      | Excludes1 | spondylolisthesis (acquired) (M43.1-)
                spondylolysis (acquired) (M43.0-)

    Q76.3   **Congenital scoliosis due to congenital bony malformation**
        Hemivertebra fusion or failure of segmentation with scoliosis

● **Q76.4**   **Other congenital malformations of spine, not associated with scoliosis**
    ● **Q76.41**   **Congenital kyphosis**
        Abnormal increase in convexity curvature of thoracic spinal column; AKA humpback

        Q76.411   **Congenital kyphosis, occipito-atlanto-axial region**
        Q76.412   **Congenital kyphosis, cervical region**
        Q76.413   **Congenital kyphosis, cervicothoracic region**
        Q76.414   **Congenital kyphosis, thoracic region**
        Q76.415   **Congenital kyphosis, thoracolumbar region**
        Q76.419   **Congenital kyphosis, unspecified region**

◄ New   ◄▥ Revised   ~~deleted~~ Deleted   **OGCR** Official Guidelines   X Assign placeholder X   ● Use Additional Character(s)

| Excludes 1 | | Excludes 2 | Includes   Use additional   Code first   Code also   Unspecified

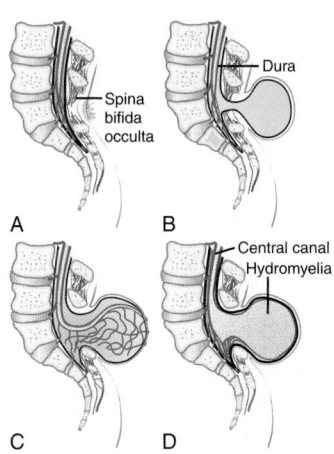

Spina bifida occulta

Dura

A   B

Central canal
Hydromyelia

C   D

Figure 17-11 **A.** Spina bifida occulta. **B.** Meningocele.
C. Myelomeningocele. **D.** Myelocystocele (syringomyelocele)
or hydromyelia.

Item 17–4 **Spina bifida** is a midline spinal defect in which one or more vertebrae fail to fuse, leaving an opening in the vertebral canal. When the defect is not visible, it is called spina bifida occulta, and when it is visible, it is called spina bifida cystica.

● **Q76.42 Congenital lordosis**
An abnormal increase in curvature of lumbar spine (sway back)

Q76.425 Congenital lordosis, thoracolumbar region

Q76.426 Congenital lordosis, lumbar region

Q76.427 Congenital lordosis, lumbosacral region

Q76.428 Congenital lordosis, sacral and sacrococcygeal region

Q76.429 Congenital lordosis, unspecified region

Q76.49 Other congenital malformations of spine, not associated with scoliosis
Congenital absence of vertebra NOS
Congenital fusion of spine NOS
Congenital malformation of lumbosacral (joint) (region) NOS
Congenital malformation of spine NOS
Hemivertebra NOS
Malformation of spine NOS
Platyspondylisis NOS
Supernumerary vertebra NOS

Q76.5 Cervical rib
Supernumerary rib in cervical region

Q76.6 Other congenital malformations of ribs
Accessory rib
Congenital absence of rib
Congenital fusion of ribs
Congenital malformation of ribs NOS
Excludes1 short rib syndrome (Q77.2)

Q76.7 Congenital malformation of sternum
Congenital absence of sternum
Sternum bifidum

Q76.8 Other congenital malformations of bony thorax

Q76.9 Congenital malformation of bony thorax, unspecified

● **Q77 Osteochondrodysplasia with defects of growth of tubular bones and spine**
Excludes1 mucopolysaccharidosis (E76.0-E76.3)
Excludes2 congenital myotonic chondrodystrophy (G71.13)

Q77.0 Achondrogenesis
Hypochondrogenesis

Q77.1 Thanatophoric short stature

Q77.2 Short rib syndrome
Asphyxiating thoracic dysplasia [Jeune]

Q77.3 Chondrodysplasia punctata
Benign cartilaginous neoplasms
Excludes1 rhizomelic chondrodysplasia punctata (E71.43)

Q77.4 Achondroplasia
Disturbance of epiphyseal chondroblastic growth and maturation, results in dwarfism
Hypochondroplasia
Osteosclerosis congenita

Q77.5 Diastrophic dysplasia

Q77.6 Chondroectodermal dysplasia
Defective development of skin, hair, teeth, with polydactyly and defect of cardiac septum
Ellis-van Creveld syndrome

Q77.7 Spondyloepiphyseal dysplasia

Q77.8 Other osteochondrodysplasia with defects of growth of tubular bones and spine

Q77.9 Osteochondrodysplasia with defects of growth of tubular bones and spine, unspecified

● **Q78 Other osteochondrodysplasias**
Disorder of development of bone and cartilage; common cause of dwarfism
Excludes2 congenital myotonic chondrodystrophy (G71.13)

Q78.0 Osteogenesis imperfecta
Fragilitas ossium
Osteopsathyrosis

Q78.1 Polyostotic fibrous dysplasia
Albright(-McCune)(-Sternberg) syndrome

Q78.2 Osteopetrosis
Abnormally dense bone; AKA marble bones disease, ivory bones
Albers-Schönberg syndrome
Osteosclerosis NOS

Q78.3 Progressive diaphyseal dysplasia
Camurati-Engelmann syndrome

Q78.4 Enchondromatosis
Thinning of overlying cortex of bone and distorted length
Maffucci's syndrome
Ollier's disease

Q78.5 Metaphyseal dysplasia
Disturbance in enchondral bone growth, causing ends of shafts to remain larger than normal in circumference
Pyle's syndrome

Q78.6 Multiple congenital exostoses
Diaphyseal aclasis

Q78.8 Other specified osteochondrodysplasias
Osteopoikilosis

Q78.9 Osteochondrodysplasia, unspecified
Chondrodystrophy NOS
AKA skeletal dysplasia (dwarfism) caused by genetic mutations affecting hyaline cartilage capping long bones and vertebrae
Osteodystrophy NOS

CHAPTER 17 (Q00-Q99)

● **Q79   Congenital malformations of musculoskeletal system, not elsewhere classified**

     Excludes2   congenital (sternomastoid) torticollis (Q68.0)

   Q79.0   Congenital diaphragmatic hernia

       Excludes1   congenital hiatus hernia (Q40.1)

   Q79.1   Other congenital malformations of diaphragm
       Absence of diaphragm
       Congenital malformation of diaphragm NOS
       Eventration of diaphragm

   Q79.2   Exomphalos
       Abdominal hernia in which part of intestine protrudes at umbilicus; AKA exomphalos and exumbilication
       Omphalocele

       Excludes1   umbilical hernia (K42.-)

   Q79.3   Gastroschisis
       Congenital fissure of anterior abdominal wall often with protrusion of small/large intestine

   Q79.4   Prune belly syndrome
       Congenital prolapse of bladder mucosa
       Eagle-Barrett syndrome

●   **Q79.5   Other congenital malformations of abdominal wall**

       Excludes1   umbilical hernia (K42.-)

      Q79.51   Congenital hernia of bladder

      Q79.59   Other congenital malformations of abdominal wall

   Q79.6   Ehlers-Danlos syndrome
       Group of inherited disorders of connective tissue; AKA cutis hyperelastica

   Q79.8   Other congenital malformations of musculoskeletal system
       Absence of muscle
       Absence of tendon
       Accessory muscle
       Amyotrophia congenita
       Congenital constricting bands
       Congenital shortening of tendon
       Poland syndrome

   Q79.9   Congenital malformation of musculoskeletal system, unspecified
       Congenital anomaly of musculoskeletal system NOS
       Congenital deformity of musculoskeletal system NOS

OTHER CONGENITAL MALFORMATIONS (Q80-Q89)

● **Q80   Congenital ichthyosis**
     Characterized by increased keratinization, resulting in noninflammatory scaling of skin

     Excludes1   Refsum's disease (G60.1)

   Q80.0   Ichthyosis vulgaris

   Q80.1   X-linked ichthyosis

   Q80.2   Lamellar ichthyosis
       Collodion baby

   Q80.3   Congenital bullous ichthyosiform erythroderma

   Q80.4   Harlequin fetus

   Q80.8   Other congenital ichthyosis

   Q80.9   Congenital ichthyosis, unspecified

● **Q81   Epidermolysis bullosa**
     Loosening of epidermis

   Q81.0   Epidermolysis bullosa simplex

       Excludes1   Cockayne's syndrome (Q87.1)

   Q81.1   Epidermolysis bullosa letalis
       Herlitz' syndrome

   Q81.2   Epidermolysis bullosa dystrophica

   Q81.8   Other epidermolysis bullosa

   Q81.9   Epidermolysis bullosa, unspecified

● **Q82   Other congenital malformations of skin**

     Excludes1   acrodermatitis enteropathica (E83.2)
         congenital erythropoietic porphyria (E80.0)
         pilonidal cyst or sinus (L05.-)
         Sturge-Weber (-Dimitri) syndrome (Q85.8)

   Q82.0   Hereditary lymphedema
       Characterized by swelling of subcutaneous tissue caused by obstruction of lymphatic vessels and resulting edema of lymph fluid

   Q82.1   Xeroderma pigmentosum
       Dry, rough, discolored state of skin, and formation of scaly desquamation

   Q82.2   Mastocytosis
       Characterized by infiltrates of mast cells in tissues/organs
       Urticaria pigmentosa

       Excludes1   malignant mastocytosis (C96.2)

   Q82.3   Incontinentia pigmenti
       Characterized by hyperpigmented cutaneous

   Q82.4   Ectodermal dysplasia (anhidrotic)
       Absence/deficiency of tissues/structures, including teeth, hair, nails, and certain glands

       Excludes1   Ellis-van Creveld syndrome (Q77.6)

   Q82.5   Congenital non-neoplastic nevus
       Birthmark NOS
       Flammeus Nevus
       Portwine Nevus
       Sanguineous Nevus
       Strawberry Nevus
       Vascular Nevus NOS
       Verrucous Nevus

       Excludes2   Café au lait spots (L81.3)
         lentigo (L81.4)
         nevus NOS (D22.-)
         araneus nevus (I78.1)
         melanocytic nevus (D22.-)
         pigmented nevus (D22.-)
         spider nevus (I78.1)
         stellar nevus (I78.1)

   Q82.8   Other specified congenital malformations of skin
       Abnormal palmar creases
       Accessory skin tags
       Benign familial pemphigus [Hailey-Hailey]
       Congenital poikiloderma
       Cutis laxa (hyperelastica)
       Dermatoglyphic anomalies
       Inherited keratosis palmaris et plantaris
       Keratosis follicularis [Darier-White]

       Excludes1   Ehlers-Danlos syndrome (Q79.6)

   Q82.9   Congenital malformation of skin, unspecified

● **Q83   Congenital malformations of breast**

     Excludes2   absence of pectoral muscle (Q79.8)
         hypoplasia of breast (N64.82)
         micromastia (N64.82)

   Q83.0   Congenital absence of breast with absent nipple

   Q83.1   Accessory breast
       Supernumerary breast

   Q83.2   Absent nipple

   Q83.3   Accessory nipple
       Supernumerary nipple

   Q83.8   Other congenital malformations of breast

   Q83.9   Congenital malformation of breast, unspecified

● **Q84　Other congenital malformations of integument**

Q84.0　Congenital alopecia
　　　Congenital atrichosis

Q84.1　Congenital morphological disturbances of hair, not elsewhere classified
　　　Beaded hair
　　　Monilethrix
　　　Pili annulati
　　　Excludes1　Menkes' kinky hair syndrome (E83.0)

Q84.2　Other congenital malformations of hair
　　　Congenital hypertrichosis
　　　Congenital malformation of hair NOS
　　　Persistent lanugo

Q84.3　Anonychia
　　　Absence of nail
　　　Excludes1　nail patella syndrome (Q87.2)

Q84.4　Congenital leukonychia
　　　Opaque, whitish discoloration of nails; AKA leukopathia unguium

Q84.5　Enlarged and hypertrophic nails
　　　Congenital onychauxis
　　　Pachyonychia

Q84.6　Other congenital malformations of nails
　　　Congenital clubnail
　　　Congenital koilonychia
　　　Congenital malformation of nail NOS

Q84.8　Other specified congenital malformations of integument
　　　Aplasia cutis congenita

Q84.9　Congenital malformation of integument, unspecified
　　　Congenital anomaly of integument NOS
　　　Congenital deformity of integument NOS

● **Q85　Phakomatoses, not elsewhere classified**
　　　Excludes1　ataxia telangiectasia [Louis-Bar] (G11.3)
　　　　　　　familial dysautonomia [Riley-Day] (G90.1)

● **Q85.0　Neurofibromatosis (nonmalignant)**
　　　Developmental changes in nervous system and other structures, with formation of neurofibromas

　　　Q85.00　Neurofibromatosis, unspecified

　　　Q85.01　Neurofibromatosis, type 1
　　　　　　Von Recklinghausen disease

　　　Q85.02　Neurofibromatosis, type 2
　　　　　　Acoustic neurofibromatosis

　　　Q85.03　Schwannomatosis

　　　Q85.09　Other neurofibromatosis

Q85.1　Tuberous sclerosis
　　　Bourneville's disease
　　　Epiloia

Q85.8　Other phakomatoses, not elsewhere classified
　　　Peutz-Jeghers Syndrome
　　　Sturge-Weber(-Dimitri) syndrome
　　　von Hippel-Lindau syndrome
　　　Excludes1　Meckel-Gruber syndrome (Q61.9)

Q85.9　Phakomatosis, unspecified
　　　Hamartosis NOS

● **Q86　Congenital malformation syndromes due to known exogenous causes, not elsewhere classified**
　　　Excludes2　iodine-deficiency-related hypothyroidism (E00-E02)
　　　　　　　nonteratogenic effects of substances transmitted via placenta or breast milk (P04.-)

Q86.0　Fetal alcohol syndrome (dysmorphic)

Q86.1　Fetal hydantoin syndrome
　　　Meadow's syndrome

Q86.2　Dysmorphism due to warfarin

Q86.8　Other congenital malformation syndromes due to known exogenous causes

● **Q87　Other specified congenital malformation syndromes affecting multiple systems**
　　　Use additional code(s) to identify all associated manifestations

Q87.0　Congenital malformation syndromes predominantly affecting facial appearance
　　　Acrocephalopolysyndactyly
　　　Acrocephalosyndactyly [Apert]
　　　Cryptophthalmos syndrome
　　　Cyclopia
　　　Goldenhar syndrome
　　　Moebius syndrome
　　　Oro-facial-digital syndrome
　　　Robin syndrome
　　　Whistling face

Q87.1　Congenital malformation syndromes predominantly associated with short stature
　　　Aarskog syndrome
　　　Cockayne syndrome
　　　De Lange syndrome
　　　Dubowitz syndrome
　　　Noonan syndrome
　　　Prader-Willi syndrome
　　　Robinow-Silverman-Smith syndrome
　　　Russell-Silver syndrome
　　　Seckel syndrome
　　　Excludes1　Ellis-van Creveld syndrome (Q77.6)
　　　　　　　Smith-Lemli-Opitz syndrome (E78.72)

Q87.2　Congenital malformation syndromes predominantly involving limbs
　　　Holt-Oram syndrome
　　　Klippel-Trenaunay-Weber syndrome
　　　Nail patella syndrome
　　　Rubinstein-Taybi syndrome
　　　Sirenomelia syndrome
　　　Thrombocytopenia with absent radius [TAR] syndrome
　　　VATER syndrome

Q87.3　Congenital malformation syndromes involving early overgrowth
　　　Beckwith-Wiedemann syndrome
　　　Sotos' syndrome
　　　Weaver syndrome

● **Q87.4　Marfan's syndrome**

　　　Q87.40　Marfan's syndrome, unspecified

　● **Q87.41　Marfan's syndrome with cardiovascular manifestations**

　　　　　Q87.410　Marfan's syndrome with aortic dilation

　　　　　Q87.418　Marfan's syndrome with other cardiovascular manifestations

　　　Q87.42　Marfan's syndrome with ocular manifestations

　　　Q87.43　Marfan's syndrome with skeletal manifestation

Q87.5　Other congenital malformation syndromes with other skeletal changes

● **Q87.8　Other specified congenital malformation syndromes, not elsewhere classified**
　　　Excludes1　Zellweger syndrome (E71.510)

　　　Q87.81　Alport syndrome
　　　　　Progressive sensorineural hearing loss, progressive pyelonephritis or glomerulonephritis, and ocular defects
　　　　　Use additional code to identify stage of chronic kidney disease (N18.1-N18.6)

　　　Q87.89　Other specified congenital malformation syndromes, not elsewhere classified
　　　　　Laurence-Moon (-Bardet)-Biedl syndrome

CHAPTER 17 (Q00-Q99)

● **Q89   Other congenital malformations, not elsewhere classified**

   ● **Q89.0   Congenital absence and malformations of spleen**

     Excludes1   isomerism of atrial appendages (with asplenia or polysplenia) (Q20.6)

     Q89.01   Asplenia (congenital)

     Q89.09   Congenital malformations of spleen
       Congenital splenomegaly

   Q89.1   Congenital malformations of adrenal gland

     Excludes1   adrenogenital disorders (E25.-)
       congenital adrenal hyperplasia (E25.0)

   Q89.2   Congenital malformations of other endocrine glands
     Congenital malformation of parathyroid or thyroid gland
     Persistent thyroglossal duct
     Thyroglossal cyst

     Excludes1   congenital goiter (E03.0)
       congenital hypothyroidism (E03.1)

   Q89.3   Situs inversus
     Lateral transposition of viscera of thorax and abdomen
     Dextrocardia with situs inversus
     Mirror-image atrial arrangement with situs inversus
     Situs inversus or transversus abdominalis
     Situs inversus or transversus thoracis
     Transposition of abdominal viscera
     Transposition of thoracic viscera

     Excludes1   dextrocardia NOS (Q24.0)

   Q89.4   Conjoined twins
     Craniopagus
     Dicephaly
     Pygopagus
     Thoracopagus

   Q89.7   Multiple congenital malformations, not elsewhere classified
     Multiple congenital anomalies NOS
     Multiple congenital deformities NOS

     Excludes1   congenital malformation syndromes affecting multiple systems (Q87.-)

   Q89.8   Other specified congenital malformations
     Use additional code(s) to identify all associated manifestations

   Q89.9   Congenital malformation, unspecified
     Congenital anomaly NOS
     Congenital deformity NOS

CHROMOSOMAL ABNORMALITIES, NOT ELSEWHERE CLASSIFIED (Q90-Q99)

   Excludes2   mitochondrial metabolic disorders (E88.4-)

● **Q90   Down syndrome**
   Use additional code(s) to identify any associated physical conditions and degree of intellectual disabilities (F70-F79)

   Q90.0   Trisomy 21, nonmosaicism (meiotic nondisjunction)
     Trisomy 21, nondisjunction, accounts for 95% of Downs syndrome cases

   Q90.1   Trisomy 21, mosaicism (mitotic nondisjunction)

   Q90.2   Trisomy 21, translocation

   Q90.9   Down syndrome, unspecified
     Trisomy 21 NOS

● **Q91   Trisomy 18 and Trisomy 13**

   Q91.0   Trisomy 18, nonmosaicism (meiotic nondisjunction)

   Q91.1   Trisomy 18, mosaicism (mitotic nondisjunction)

   Q91.2   Trisomy 18, translocation

   Q91.3   Trisomy 18, unspecified

   Q91.4   Trisomy 13, nonmosaicism (meiotic nondisjunction)

   Q91.5   Trisomy 13, mosaicism (mitotic nondisjunction)

   Q91.6   Trisomy 13, translocation

   Q91.7   Trisomy 13, unspecified

● **Q92   Other trisomies and partial trisomies of the autosomes, not elsewhere classified**

   Includes   unbalanced translocations and insertions

   Excludes1   trisomies of chromosomes 13, 18, 21 (Q90-Q91)

   Q92.0   Whole chromosome trisomy, nonmosaicism (meiotic nondisjunction)

   Q92.1   Whole chromosome trisomy, mosaicism (mitotic nondisjunction)

   Q92.2   Partial trisomy
     Less than whole arm duplicated
     Whole arm or more duplicated

     Excludes1   partial trisomy due to unbalanced translocation (Q92.5)

   Q92.5   Duplications with other complex rearrangements
     Partial trisomy due to unbalanced translocations

     Code also any associated deletions due to unbalanced translocations, inversions and insertions (Q93.7)

   ● **Q92.6   Marker chromosomes**
     Trisomies due to dicentrics
     Trisomies due to extra rings
     Trisomies due to isochromosomes
     Individual with marker heterochromatin

     Q92.61   Marker chromosomes in normal individual

     Q92.62   Marker chromosomes in abnormal individual

   Q92.7   Triploidy and polyploidy

   Q92.8   Other specified trisomies and partial trisomies of autosomes
     Duplications identified by fluorescence in situ hybridization (FISH)
     Duplications identified by in situ hybridization (ISH)
     Duplications seen only at prometaphase

   Q92.9   Trisomy and partial trisomy of autosomes, unspecified

● **Q93   Monosomies and deletions from the autosomes, not elsewhere classified**

   Q93.0   Whole chromosome monosomy, nonmosaicism (meiotic nondisjunction)

   Q93.1   Whole chromosome monosomy, mosaicism (mitotic nondisjunction)

   Q93.2   Chromosome replaced with ring, dicentric or isochromosome

   Q93.3   Deletion of short arm of chromosome 4
     Wolff-Hirschorn syndrome

   Q93.4   Deletion of short arm of chromosome 5
     Cri-du-chat syndrome

   Q93.5   Other deletions of part of a chromosome
     Angelman syndrome

   Q93.7   Deletions with other complex rearrangements
     Deletions due to unbalanced translocations, inversions and insertions

     Code also any associated duplications due to unbalanced translocations, inversions and insertions (Q92.5)

   ● **Q93.8   Other deletions from the autosomes**

     Q93.81   Velo-cardio-facial syndrome
       Deletion 22q11.2

     Q93.88   Other microdeletions Miller-Dieker syndrome
       Smith-Magenis syndrome

     Q93.89   Other deletions from the autosomes
       Deletions identified by fluorescence in situ hybridization (FISH)
       Deletions identified by in situ hybridization (ISH)
       Deletions seen only at prometaphase

   Q93.9   Deletion from autosomes, unspecified

● **Q95　Balanced rearrangements and structural markers, not elsewhere classified**

> **Includes**　　Robertsonian and balanced reciprocal translocations and insertions

　　Q95.0　Balanced translocation and insertion in normal individual

　　Q95.1　Chromosome inversion in normal individual

　　Q95.2　Balanced autosomal rearrangement in abnormal individual

　　Q95.3　Balanced sex/autosomal rearrangement in abnormal individual

　　Q95.5　Individual with autosomal fragile site

　　Q95.8　Other balanced rearrangements and structural markers

　　Q95.9　Balanced rearrangement and structural marker, unspecified

● **Q96　Turner's syndrome**

> *Caused by missing or incomplete X chromosome affecting growth and sexual development*

> **Excludes1**　Noonan syndrome (Q87.1)

　　Q96.0　Karyotype 45, X

　　Q96.1　Karyotype 46, X iso (Xq)
　　　　　　Karyotype 46, isochromosome Xq

　　Q96.2　Karyotype 46, X with abnormal sex chromosome, except iso (Xq)
　　　　　　Karyotype 46, X with abnormal sex chromosome, except isochromosome Xq

　　Q96.3　Mosaicism, 45, X/46, XX or XY

　　Q96.4　Mosaicism, 45, X/other cell line(s) with abnormal sex chromosome

　　Q96.8　Other variants of Turner's syndrome

　　Q96.9　Turner's syndrome, unspecified

● **Q97　Other sex chromosome abnormalities, female phenotype, not elsewhere classified**

> **Excludes1**　Turner's syndrome (Q96.-)

　　Q97.0　Karyotype 47, XXX

　　Q97.1　Female with more than three X chromosomes

　　Q97.2　Mosaicism, lines with various numbers of X chromosomes

　　Q97.3　Female with 46, XY karyotype

　　Q97.8　Other specified sex chromosome abnormalities, female phenotype

　　Q97.9　Sex chromosome abnormality, female phenotype, unspecified

● **Q98　Other sex chromosome abnormalities, male phenotype, not elsewhere classified**

　　Q98.0　Klinefelter syndrome karyotype 47, XXY

　　Q98.1　Klinefelter syndrome, male with more than two X chromosomes

　　Q98.3　Other male with 46, XX karyotype

　　Q98.4　Klinefelter syndrome, unspecified

　　Q98.5　Karyotype 47, XYY

　　Q98.6　Male with structurally abnormal sex chromosome

　　Q98.7　Male with sex chromosome mosaicism

　　Q98.8　Other specified sex chromosome abnormalities, male phenotype

　　Q98.9　Sex chromosome abnormality, male phenotype, unspecified

● **Q99　Other chromosome abnormalities, not elsewhere classified**

　　Q99.0　Chimera 46, XX/46, XY
　　　　　　Chimera 46, XX/46, XY true hermaphrodite

　　Q99.1　46, XX true hermaphrodite
　　　　　　46, XX with streak gonads
　　　　　　46, XY with streak gonads
　　　　　　Pure gonadal dysgenesis

　　Q99.2　Fragile X chromosome
　　　　　　Fragile X syndrome

　　Q99.8　Other specified chromosome abnormalities

　　Q99.9　Chromosomal abnormality, unspecified

CHAPTER 17 (Q00-Q99)

OGCR Section I.B.4.

Signs and symptoms

Codes that describe symptoms and signs, as opposed to diagnoses, are acceptable for reporting purposes when a related definitive diagnosis has not been established (confirmed) by the provider. Chapter 18 of ICD-10-CM, Symptoms, Signs, and Abnormal Clinical and Laboratory Findings, Not Elsewhere Classified (codes R00.0-R99) contains many, but not all codes for symptoms.

Section I.C.18.a. to c.

Symptoms, signs, and abnormal clinical and laboratory findings, not elsewhere classified.

Chapter 18 includes symptoms, signs, abnormal results of clinical or other investigative procedures, and ill-defined conditions regarding which no diagnosis classifiable elsewhere is recorded. Signs and symptoms that point to a specific diagnosis have been assigned to a category in other chapters of the classification.

a. Use of symptom codes

Codes that describe symptoms and signs are acceptable for reporting purposes when a related definitive diagnosis has not been established (confirmed) by the provider.

b. Use of a symptom code with a definitive diagnosis code

Codes for signs and symptoms may be reported in addition to a related definitive diagnosis when the sign or symptom is not routinely associated with that diagnosis, such as the various signs and symptoms associated with complex syndromes. The definitive diagnosis code should be sequenced before the symptom code.

Signs or symptoms that are associated routinely with a disease process should not be assigned as additional codes, unless otherwise instructed by the classification.

c. Combination codes that include symptoms

ICD-10-CM contains a number of combination codes that identify both the definitive diagnosis and common symptoms of that diagnosis. When using one of these combination codes, an additional code should not be assigned for the symptom.

CHAPTER 18

SYMPTOMS, SIGNS AND ABNORMAL CLINICAL AND LABORATORY FINDINGS, NOT ELSEWHERE CLASSIFIED (R00-R99)

Note: This chapter includes symptoms, signs, abnormal results of clinical or other investigative procedures, and ill-defined conditions regarding which no diagnosis classifiable elsewhere is recorded.

Signs and symptoms that point rather definitely to a given diagnosis have been assigned to a category in other chapters of the classification. In general, categories in this chapter include the less well-defined conditions and symptoms that, without the necessary study of the case to establish a final diagnosis, point perhaps equally to two or more diseases or to two or more systems of the body. Practically all categories in the chapter could be designated 'not otherwise specified', 'unknown etiology' or 'transient'. The Alphabetical Index should be consulted to determine which symptoms and signs are to be allocated here and which to other chapters. The residual subcategories, numbered .8, are generally provided for other relevant symptoms that cannot be allocated elsewhere in the classification.

The conditions and signs or symptoms included in categories R00-R94 consist of:
(a) cases for which no more specific diagnosis can be made even after all the facts bearing on the case have been investigated;
(b) signs or symptoms existing at the time of initial encounter that proved to be transient and whose causes could not be determined;
(c) provisional diagnosis in a patient who failed to return for further investigation or care;

(d) cases referred elsewhere for investigation or treatment before the diagnosis was made;
(e) cases in which a more precise diagnosis was not available for any other reason;
(f) certain symptoms, for which supplementary information is provided, that represent important problems in medical care in their own right.

Excludes2	abnormal findings on antenatal screening of mother (O28.-)
	certain conditions originating in the perinatal period (P04-P96)
	signs and symptoms classified in the body system chapters
	signs and symptoms of breast (N63, N64.5)

This chapter contains the following blocks:

R00-R09	Symptoms and signs involving the circulatory and respiratory systems
R10-R19	Symptoms and signs involving the digestive system and abdomen
R20-R23	Symptoms and signs involving the skin and subcutaneous tissue
R25-R29	Symptoms and signs involving the nervous and musculoskeletal systems
R30-R39	Symptoms and signs involving the genitourinary system
R40-R46	Symptoms and signs involving cognition, perception, emotional state and behavior
R47-R49	Symptoms and signs involving speech and voice
R50-R69	General symptoms and signs
R70-R79	Abnormal findings on examination of blood, without diagnosis
R80-R82	Abnormal findings on examination of urine, without diagnosis
R83-R89	Abnormal findings on examination of other body fluids, substances and tissues, without diagnosis
R90-R94	Abnormal findings on diagnostic imaging and in function studies, without diagnosis
R97	Abnormal tumor markers
R99	Ill-defined and unknown cause of mortality

SYMPTOMS AND SIGNS INVOLVING THE CIRCULATORY AND RESPIRATORY SYSTEMS (R00-R09)

● **R00** **Abnormalities of heart beat**

| Excludes1 | abnormalities originating in the perinatal period (P29.1-) |
| | specified arrhythmias (I47-I49) |

R00.0 **Tachycardia, unspecified**
Rapid heart rate >100 beats
Rapid heart beat
Sinoauricular tachycardia NOS
Sinus [sinusal] tachycardia NOS

| Excludes1 | neonatal tachycardia (P29.11) |
| | paroxysmal tachycardia (I47.-) |

R00.1 **Bradycardia, unspecified**
Slow heart rate, <60
Sinoatrial bradycardia
Sinus bradycardia
Slow heart beat
Vagal bradycardia

Use additional code for adverse effect, if applicable, to identify drug (T36-T50 with fifth or sixth character 5)

| Excludes1 | neonatal bradycardia (P29.12) |

R00.2 **Palpitations**
Awareness of heart beat

R00.8 **Other abnormalities of heart beat**

R00.9 **Unspecified abnormalities of heart beat**

◀ New   ◀▥ Revised   ~~deleted~~ Deleted   **OGCR** Official Guidelines   X Assign placeholder X   ● Use Additional Character(s)

| Excludes 1 | Excludes 2 | Includes | Use additional | Code first | Code also | Unspecified |

R01   Cardiac murmurs and other cardiac sounds
> **Excludes1**   cardiac murmurs and sounds originating in the perinatal period (P29.8)

R01.0   Benign and innocent cardiac murmurs
> Functional cardiac murmur

R01.1   Cardiac murmur, unspecified
> Cardiac bruit NOS
> Heart murmur NOS

R01.2   Other cardiac sounds
> Cardiac dullness, increased or decreased
> Precordial friction

OGCR Section I.C.9.a.7.

Hypertension, Transient
Assign code R03.0, Elevated blood pressure reading without diagnosis of hypertension, unless patient has an established diagnosis of hypertension. Assign code O13.-, Gestational [pregnancy-induced] hypertension with significant proteinuria, or O14.-, Pre-eclampsia, for transient hypertension of pregnancy.

R03   Abnormal blood-pressure reading, without diagnosis

R03.0   Elevated blood-pressure reading, without diagnosis of hypertension
> **Note:** This category is to be used to record an episode of elevated blood pressure in a patient in whom no formal diagnosis of hypertension has been made, or as an isolated incidental finding.

R03.1   Nonspecific low blood-pressure reading
> **Excludes1**   hypotension (I95.-)
> maternal hypotension syndrome (O26.5-)
> neurogenic orthostatic hypotension (G90.3)

R04   Hemorrhage from respiratory passages

R04.0   Epistaxis
> Hemorrhage from nose
> Nosebleed

R04.1   Hemorrhage from throat
> **Excludes2**   hemoptysis (R04.2)

R04.2   Hemoptysis
> Blood-stained sputum
> Cough with hemorrhage

R04.8   Hemorrhage from other sites in respiratory passages

R04.81   Acute idiopathic pulmonary hemorrhage in infants
> AIPHI
> Acute idiopathic hemorrhage in infants over 28 days old
> > **Excludes1**   perinatal pulmonary hemorrhage (P26.-)
> > von Willebrand's disease (D68.0)

R04.89   Hemorrhage from other sites in respiratory passages
> Pulmonary hemorrhage NOS

R04.9   Hemorrhage from respiratory passages, unspecified

R05   Cough
> **Excludes1**   cough with hemorrhage (R04.2)
> smoker's cough (J41.0)

R06   Abnormalities of breathing
> **Excludes1**   acute respiratory distress syndrome (J80)
> respiratory arrest (R09.2)
> respiratory arrest of newborn (P28.81)
> respiratory distress syndrome of newborn (P22.-)
> respiratory failure (J96.-)
> respiratory failure of newborn (P28.5)

R06.0   Dyspnea
> **Excludes1**   tachypnea NOS (R06.82)
> transient tachypnea of newborn (P22.1)

R06.00   Dyspnea, unspecified
R06.01   Orthopnea
R06.02   Shortness of breath
R06.09   Other forms of dyspnea

R06.1   Stridor
> *Harsh, high-pitched breath sound*
> **Excludes1**   congenital laryngeal stridor (P28.89)
> laryngismus (stridulus) (J38.5)

R06.2   Wheezing
> **Excludes1**   Asthma (J45.-)

R06.3   Periodic breathing
> Cheyne-Stokes breathing
> *An abnormal pattern of breathing with gradually increasing and decreasing tidal volume with some periods of apnea*

R06.4   Hyperventilation
> **Excludes1**   psychogenic hyperventilation (F45.8)

R06.5   Mouth breathing
> **Excludes2**   dry mouth NOS (R68.2)

R06.6   Hiccough
> **Excludes1**   psychogenic hiccough (F45.8)

R06.7   Sneezing

R06.8   Other abnormalities of breathing

R06.81   Apnea, not elsewhere classified
> Apnea NOS
> > **Excludes1**   apnea (of) newborn (P28.4)
> > sleep apnea (G47.3-)
> > sleep apnea of newborn (primary) (P28.3)

R06.82   Tachypnea, not elsewhere classified
> Tachypnea NOS
> > **Excludes1**   transitory tachypnea of newborn (P22.1)

R06.83   Snoring
R06.89   Other abnormalities of breathing
> Breath-holding (spells)
> Sighing

R06.9   Unspecified abnormalities of breathing

R07   Pain in throat and chest
> **Excludes1**   epidemic myalgia (B33.0)
> **Excludes2**   jaw pain R68.84
> pain in breast (N64.4)

R07.0   Pain in throat
> **Excludes1**   chronic sore throat (J31.2)
> sore throat (acute) NOS (J02.9)
> **Excludes2**   dysphagia (R13.1-)
> pain in neck (M54.2)

R07.1   Chest pain on breathing
> Painful respiration

R07.2   Precordial pain

R07.8   Other chest pain

R07.81   Pleurodynia
> Pleurodynia NOS
> > **Excludes1**   epidemic pleurodynia (B33.0)

R07.82   Intercostal pain
R07.89   Other chest pain
> Anterior chest-wall pain NOS

R07.9   Chest pain, unspecified

◀ New   ◀▥ Revised   ~~deleted~~ Deleted   **OGCR** Official Guidelines   X Assign placeholder X   ● Use Additional Character(s)
Excludes 1   Excludes 2   Includes   Use additional   Code first   Code also   Unspecified
CHAPTER 18 (R00-R99)   1203

● R09   **Other symptoms and signs involving the circulatory and respiratory system**
> Excludes1   acute respiratory distress syndrome (J80)
> respiratory arrest of newborn (P28.81)
> respiratory distress syndrome of newborn (P22.0)
> respiratory failure (J96.-)
> respiratory failure of newborn (P28.5)

● R09.0   **Asphyxia and hypoxemia**
> Excludes1   asphyxia due to carbon monoxide (T58.-)
> asphyxia due to foreign body in respiratory tract (T17.-)
> birth (intrauterine) asphyxia (P84)
> hypercapnia (R06.4)
> hyperventilation (R06.4)
> traumatic asphyxia (T71.-)

R09.01   **Asphyxia**

R09.02   **Hypoxemia**

R09.1   **Pleurisy**
> *Occurs when double membrane (pleura) lining chest cavity and lung surface becomes inflamed causing sharp pain on inspiration/expiration.*
> Excludes1   pleurisy with effusion (J90)

R09.2   **Respiratory arrest**
> Cardiorespiratory failure
> Excludes1   cardiac arrest (I46.-)
> respiratory arrest of newborn (P28.81)
> respiratory distress of newborn (P22.0)
> respiratory failure (J96.-)
> respiratory failure of newborn (P28.5)
> respiratory insufficiency (R06.89)
> respiratory insufficiency of newborn (P28.5)

R09.3   **Abnormal sputum**
> Abnormal amount of sputum
> Abnormal color of sputum
> Abnormal odor of sputum
> Excessive sputum
> Excludes1   blood-stained sputum (R04.2)

● R09.8   **Other specified symptoms and signs involving the circulatory and respiratory systems**

R09.81   **Nasal congestion**

R09.82   **Postnasal drip**

R09.89   **Other specified symptoms and signs involving the circulatory and respiratory systems**
> Bruit (arterial)
> Abnormal chest percussion
> Feeling of foreign body in throat
> Friction sounds in chest
> Chest tympany
> Choking sensation
> Rales
> > *Wet rattling, clicking, crackling sounds on auscultation*
> Weak pulse
> Excludes2   foreign body in throat (T17.2-)
> wheezing (R06.2)

SYMPTOMS AND SIGNS INVOLVING THE DIGESTIVE SYSTEM AND ABDOMEN (R10-R19)

> Excludes1   congenital or infantile pylorospasm (Q40.0)
> gastrointestinal hemorrhage (K92.0-K92.2)
> intestinal obstruction (K56.-)
> newborn gastrointestinal hemorrhage (P54.0-P54.3)
> newborn intestinal obstruction (P76.-)
> pylorospasm (K31.3)
> signs and symptoms involving the urinary system (R30-R39)
> symptoms referable to female genital organs (N94.-)
> symptoms referable to male genital organs male (N48-N50)

● R10   **Abdominal and pelvic pain**
> Excludes1   renal colic (N23)
> Excludes2   dorsalgia (M54.-)
> flatulence and related conditions (R14.-)

R10.0   **Acute abdomen**
> Severe abdominal pain (generalized) (with abdominal rigidity)
> Excludes1   abdominal rigidity NOS (R19.3)
> generalized abdominal pain NOS (R10.84)
> localized abdominal pain (R10.1-R10.3-)

● R10.1   **Pain localized to upper abdomen**

R10.10   **Upper abdominal pain, unspecified**

R10.11   **Right upper quadrant pain**

R10.12   **Left upper quadrant pain**

R10.13   **Epigastric pain**
> Dyspepsia
> Excludes1   functional dyspepsia (K30)

R10.2   **Pelvic and perineal pain**
> Excludes1   vulvodynia (N94.81)

● R10.3   **Pain localized to other parts of lower abdomen**

R10.30   **Lower abdominal pain, unspecified**

R10.31   **Right lower quadrant pain**

R10.32   **Left lower quadrant pain**

R10.33   **Periumbilical pain**

● R10.8   **Other abdominal pain**

● R10.81   **Abdominal tenderness**
> Abdominal tenderness NOS

R10.811   **Right upper quadrant abdominal tenderness**

R10.812   **Left upper quadrant abdominal tenderness**

R10.813   **Right lower quadrant abdominal tenderness**

R10.814   **Left lower quadrant abdominal tenderness**

R10.815   **Periumbilic abdominal tenderness**

R10.816   **Epigastric abdominal tenderness**

R10.817   **Generalized abdominal tenderness**

R10.819   **Abdominal tenderness, unspecified site**

● R10.82   **Rebound abdominal tenderness**

R10.821   **Right upper quadrant rebound abdominal tenderness**

R10.822   **Left upper quadrant rebound abdominal tenderness**

R10.823   **Right lower quadrant rebound abdominal tenderness**

R10.824   **Left lower quadrant rebound abdominal tenderness**

R10.825   **Periumbilic rebound abdominal tenderness**

R10.826   **Epigastric rebound abdominal tenderness**

R10.827   **Generalized rebound abdominal tenderness**

R10.829   **Rebound abdominal tenderness, unspecified site**

R10.83   **Colic**
> Colic NOS
> Infantile colic
> Excludes1   colic in adult and child over 12 months old (R10.84)

R10.84   **Generalized abdominal pain**
> Excludes1   generalized abdominal pain associated with acute abdomen (R10.0)

R10.9   **Unspecified abdominal pain**

● R11   **Nausea and vomiting**
> **Excludes1**   cyclical vomiting associated with migraine (G43.A-)
> excessive vomiting in pregnancy (O21.-)
> hematemesis (K92.0)
> neonatal hematemesis (P54.0)
> newborn vomiting (P92.0-)
> psychogenic vomiting (F50.8)
> vomiting associated with bulimia nervosa (F50.2)
> vomiting following gastrointestinal surgery (K91.0)

● R11.0   **Nausea**
> Nausea NOS
> Nausea without vomiting

● R11.1   **Vomiting**

     R11.10   **Vomiting, unspecified**
> Vomiting NOS

     R11.11   **Vomiting without nausea**

     R11.12   **Projectile vomiting**

     R11.13   **Vomiting of fecal matter**

     R11.14   **Bilious vomiting**
> Bilious emesis

   R11.2   **Nausea with vomiting, unspecified**
> Persistent nausea with vomiting NOS

R12   **Heartburn**
> **Excludes1**   dyspepsia NOS (R10.13)
> functional dyspepsia (K30)

● R13   **Aphagia and dysphagia**

   R13.0   **Aphagia**
> Inability to swallow
> **Excludes1**   psychogenic aphagia (F50.9)

● R13.1   **Dysphagia**
> *Difficulty swallowing*
> *Code first, if applicable, dysphagia following cerebrovascular disease (I69. with final characters -91)*
> **Excludes1**   psychogenic dysphagia (F45.8)

     R13.10   **Dysphagia, unspecified**
> Difficulty in swallowing NOS

     R13.11   **Dysphagia, oral phase**

     R13.12   **Dysphagia, oropharyngeal phase**

     R13.13   **Dysphagia, pharyngeal phase**

     R13.14   **Dysphagia, pharyngoesophageal phase**

     R13.19   **Other dysphagia**
> Cervical dysphagia
> Neurogenic dysphagia

● R14   **Flatulence and related conditions**
> **Excludes1**   psychogenic aerophagy (F45.8)

   R14.0   **Abdominal distension (gaseous)**
> Bloating
> Tympanites (abdominal) (intestinal)

   R14.1   **Gas pain**

   R14.2   **Eructation**
> *Belching air from stomach through mouth*

   R14.3   **Flatulence**

● R15   **Fecal incontinence**
> **Includes**   encopresis NOS
> **Excludes1**   fecal incontinence of nonorganic origin (F98.1)

   R15.0   **Incomplete defecation**
> **Excludes1**   constipation (K59.0-)
> fecal impaction (K56.41)

   R15.1   **Fecal smearing**
> Fecal soiling

   R15.2   **Fecal urgency**

   R15.9   **Full incontinence of feces**
> Fecal incontinence NOS

● R16   **Hepatomegaly and splenomegaly, not elsewhere classified**
> *Enlargement of liver or spleen*

   R16.0   **Hepatomegaly, not elsewhere classified**
> Hepatomegaly NOS

   R16.1   **Splenomegaly, not elsewhere classified**
> Splenomegaly NOS

   R16.2   **Hepatomegaly with splenomegaly, not elsewhere classified**
> Hepatosplenomegaly NOS

R17   **Unspecified jaundice**
> **Excludes1**   neonatal jaundice (P55, P57-P59)

● R18   **Ascites**
> **Includes**   fluid in peritoneal cavity
> **Excludes1**   ascites in alcoholic cirrhosis (K70.31)
> ascites in alcoholic hepatitis (K70.11)
> ascites in toxic liver disease with chronic active hepatitis (K71.51)

   R18.0   **Malignant ascites**
> *Code first malignancy, such as:*
> malignant neoplasm of ovary (C56.-)
> secondary malignant neoplasm of retroperitoneum and peritoneum (C78.6)

   R18.8   **Other ascites**
> Ascites NOS
> Peritoneal effusion (chronic)

● R19   **Other symptoms and signs involving the digestive system and abdomen**
> **Excludes1**   acute abdomen (R10.0)

● R19.0   **Intra-abdominal and pelvic swelling, mass and lump**
> **Excludes1**   abdominal distension (gaseous) (R14.-)
> ascites (R18.-)

     R19.00   **Intra-abdominal and pelvic swelling, mass and lump, unspecified site**

     R19.01   **Right upper quadrant abdominal swelling, mass and lump**

     R19.02   **Left upper quadrant abdominal swelling, mass and lump**

     R19.03   **Right lower quadrant abdominal swelling, mass and lump**

     R19.04   **Left lower quadrant abdominal swelling, mass and lump**

     R19.05   **Periumbilic swelling, mass or lump**
> Diffuse or generalized umbilical swelling or mass

     R19.06   **Epigastric swelling, mass or lump**

     R19.07   **Generalized intra-abdominal and pelvic swelling, mass and lump**
> Diffuse or generalized intra-abdominal swelling or mass NOS
> Diffuse or generalized pelvic swelling or mass NOS

     R19.09   **Other intra-abdominal and pelvic swelling, mass and lump**

● R19.1   **Abnormal bowel sounds**

     R19.11   **Absent bowel sounds**

     R19.12   **Hyperactive bowel sounds**

     R19.15   **Other abnormal bowel sounds**
> Abnormal bowel sounds NOS

   R19.2   **Visible peristalsis**
> Hyperperistalsis

● R19.3   **Abdominal rigidity**
> **Excludes1**   abdominal rigidity with severe abdominal pain (R10.0)

     R19.30   **Abdominal rigidity, unspecified site**

     R19.31   **Right upper quadrant abdominal rigidity**

CHAPTER 18 (R00-R99)

◄ New   ◄▬ Revised   ~~deleted~~ Deleted   **OGCR** Official Guidelines   X Assign placeholder X   ● Use Additional Character(s)

Excludes 1   Excludes 2   Includes   Use additional   Code first   Code also   Unspecified

CHAPTER 18 (R00-R99)

R19.32   Left upper quadrant abdominal rigidity

R19.33   Right lower quadrant abdominal rigidity

R19.34   Left lower quadrant abdominal rigidity

R19.35   Periumbilic abdominal rigidity

R19.36   Epigastric abdominal rigidity

R19.37   Generalized abdominal rigidity

R19.4   **Change in bowel habit**

> **Excludes1**   constipation (K59.0-)
> functional diarrhea (K59.1)

R19.5   **Other fecal abnormalities**

> Abnormal stool color
> Bulky stools
> Mucus in stools
> Occult blood in feces
> Occult blood in stools
>
> **Excludes1**   melena (K92.1)
> neonatal melena (P54.1)

R19.6   **Halitosis**

R19.7   **Diarrhea, unspecified**

> Diarrhea NOS
>
> **Excludes1**   functional diarrhea (K59.1)
> neonatal diarrhea (P78.3)
> psychogenic diarrhea (F45.8)

R19.8   **Other specified symptoms and signs involving the digestive system and abdomen**

SYMPTOMS AND SIGNS INVOLVING THE SKIN AND SUBCUTANEOUS TISSUE (R20-R23)

> **Excludes2**   symptoms relating to breast (N64.4-N64.5)

● R20   **Disturbances of skin sensation**

> **Excludes1**   dissociative anesthesia and sensory loss (F44.6)
> psychogenic disturbances (F45.8)

R20.0   **Anesthesia of skin**

> *Loss of sensation*

R20.1   **Hypoesthesia of skin**

> *Unpleasant abnormal sensation*

R20.2   **Paresthesia of skin**

> *Abnormal touch sensation, including burning, prickling, often in absence of external stimulus*
> Formication   Tingling skin
> Pins and needles
>
> **Excludes1**   acroparesthesia (I73.8)

R20.3   **Hyperesthesia**

R20.8   **Other disturbances of skin sensation**

R20.9   **Unspecified disturbances of skin sensation**

R21   **Rash and other nonspecific skin eruption**

> **Includes**   rash NOS
>
> **Excludes1**   specified type of rash- code to condition
> vesicular eruption (R23.8)

● R22   **Localized swelling, mass and lump of skin and subcutaneous tissue**

> **Includes**   subcutaneous nodules (localized) (superficial)
>
> **Excludes1**   abnormal findings on diagnostic imaging (R90-R93)
> edema (R60.-)
> enlarged lymph nodes (R59.-)
> localized adiposity (E65)
> swelling of joint (M25.4-)

R22.0   **Localized swelling, mass and lump, head**

R22.1   **Localized swelling, mass and lump, neck**

R22.2   **Localized swelling, mass and lump, trunk**

> **Excludes1**   intra-abdominal or pelvic mass and lump (R19.0-)
> intra-abdominal or pelvic swelling (R19.0-)
>
> **Excludes2**   breast mass and lump (N63)

● R22.3   **Localized swelling, mass and lump, upper limb**

R22.30   Localized swelling, mass and lump, unspecified upper limb

R22.31   Localized swelling, mass and lump, right upper limb

R22.32   Localized swelling, mass and lump, left upper limb

R22.33   Localized swelling, mass and lump, upper limb, bilateral

● R22.4   **Localized swelling, mass and lump, lower limb**

R22.40   Localized swelling, mass and lump, unspecified lower limb

R22.41   Localized swelling, mass and lump, right lower limb

R22.42   Localized swelling, mass and lump, left lower limb

R22.43   Localized swelling, mass and lump, lower limb, bilateral

R22.9   **Localized swelling, mass and lump, unspecified**

● R23   **Other skin changes**

R23.0   **Cyanosis**

> **Excludes1**   acrocyanosis (I73.8)
> cyanotic attacks of newborn (P28.2)

R23.1   **Pallor**

> Clammy skin

R23.2   **Flushing**

> Excessive blushing
>
> *Code first, if applicable, menopausal and female climacteric states (N95.1)*

R23.3   **Spontaneous ecchymoses**

> *Small hemorrhagic spot of skin; AKA black and blue spot*
> Petechiae
>
> **Excludes1**   ecchymoses of newborn (P54.5)
> purpura (D69.-)

R23.4   **Changes in skin texture**

> Desquamation of skin   Scaling of skin
> Induration of skin
>
> **Excludes1**   epidermal thickening NOS (L85.9)

R23.8   **Other skin changes**

R23.9   **Unspecified skin changes**

SYMPTOMS AND SIGNS INVOLVING THE NERVOUS AND MUSCULOSKELETAL SYSTEMS (R25-R29)

● R25   **Abnormal involuntary movements**

> **Excludes1**   specific movement disorders (G20-G26)
> stereotyped movement disorders (F98.4)
> tic disorders (F95.-)

R25.0   **Abnormal head movements**

R25.1   **Tremor, unspecified**

> **Excludes1**   chorea NOS (G25.5)
> essential tremor (G25.0)
> hysterical tremor (F44.4)
> intention tremor (G25.2)

R25.2   **Cramp and spasm**

> **Excludes2**   carpopedal spasm (R29.0)
> charley-horse (M62.831)
> infantile spasms (G40.4-)
> muscle spasm of back (M62.830)
> muscle spasm of calf (M62.831)

R25.3   **Fasciculation**

> Twitching NOS

R25.8   **Other abnormal involuntary movements**

R25.9   **Unspecified abnormal involuntary movements**

● **R26   Abnormalities of gait and mobility**
> **Excludes1**   ataxia NOS (R27.0)
>> hereditary ataxia (G11.-)
>> locomotor (syphilitic) ataxia (A52.11)
>> immobility syndrome (paraplegic) (M62.3)

     R26.0   Ataxic gait
>> Staggering gait

     R26.1   Paralytic gait
>> Spastic gait

     R26.2   Difficulty in walking, not elsewhere classified
> **Excludes1**   falling (R29.6)
>> unsteadiness on feet (R26.81)

●   **R26.8   Other abnormalities of gait and mobility**
         R26.81   Unsteadiness on feet
         R26.89   Other abnormalities of gait and mobility
     R26.9   Unspecified abnormalities of gait and mobility

● **R27   Other lack of coordination**
> **Excludes1**   ataxic gait (R26.0)
>> hereditary ataxia (G11.-)
>> vertigo NOS (R42)

     R27.0   Ataxia, unspecified
> **Excludes1**   ataxia following cerebrovascular disease
>> (I69. with final characters -93)

     R27.8   Other lack of coordination
     R27.9   Unspecified lack of coordination

● **R29   Other symptoms and signs involving the nervous and musculoskeletal systems**
     R29.0   Tetany
>> *Hyperexcitability of nerves and muscles characterized by spasm, twitching, and cramps*
>> Carpopedal spasm
> **Excludes1**   hysterical tetany (F44.5)
>> neonatal tetany (P71.3)
>> parathyroid tetany (E20.9)
>> post-thyroidectomy tetany (E89.2)

     R29.1   Meningismus
     R29.2   Abnormal reflex
> **Excludes2**   abnormal pupillary reflex (H57.0)
>> hyperactive gag reflex (J39.2)
>> vasovagal reaction or syncope (R55)

     R29.3   Abnormal posture
     R29.4   Clicking hip
> **Excludes1**   congenital deformities of hip (Q65.-)

     R29.5   Transient paralysis
>> *Code first any associated spinal cord injury (S14.0, S14.1-, S24.0, S24.1-, S34.0-, S34.1-)*
> **Excludes1**   transient ischemic attack (G45.9)

     R29.6   Repeated falls
>> Falling
>> Tendency to fall
> **Excludes2**   at risk for falling (Z91.81)
>> history of falling (Z91.81)

     OGCR Section I.C.18.d.

> Repeated falls
>
> Code R29.6, Repeated falls, is for use for encounters when a patient has recently fallen and the reason for the fall is being investigated.
>
> Code Z91.81, History of falling, is for use when a patient has fallen in the past and is at risk for future falls. When appropriate, both codes R29.6 and Z91.81 may be assigned together.

●   **R29.8   Other symptoms and signs involving the nervous and musculoskeletal systems**
●   **R29.81   Other symptoms and signs involving the nervous system**
         R29.810   Facial weakness
>>> Facial droop
>> **Excludes1**   Bell's palsy (G51.0)
>>> facial weakness following cerebrovascular disease (I69. with final characters -92)

         R29.818   Other symptoms and signs involving the nervous system

●   **R29.89   Other symptoms and signs involving the musculoskeletal system**
>> **Excludes2**   pain in limb (M79.6-)
         R29.890   Loss of height
>> **Excludes1**   osteoporosis (M80-M81)

         R29.891   Ocular torticollis
>> **Excludes1**   congenital (sterno-mastoid) torticollis Q68.0
>>> psychogenic torticollis (F45.8)
>>> spasmodic torticollis (G24.3)
>>> torticollis due to birth injury (P15.8)
>>> torticollis NOS M43.6

         R29.898   Other symptoms and signs involving the musculoskeletal system

●   **R29.9   Unspecified symptoms and signs involving the nervous and musculoskeletal systems**
       R29.90   Unspecified symptoms and signs involving the nervous system
       R29.91   Unspecified symptoms and signs involving the musculoskeletal system

---

SYMPTOMS AND SIGNS INVOLVING THE GENITOURINARY SYSTEM (R30-R39)

● **R30   Pain associated with micturition**
> **Excludes1**   psychogenic pain associated with micturition (F45.8)

     R30.0   Dysuria
>> *Painful urination*
>> Strangury

     R30.1   Vesical tenesmus
>> *Straining to urinate*

     R30.9   Painful micturition, unspecified
>> Painful urination NOS

● **R31   Hematuria**
> **Excludes1**   hematuria included with underlying conditions, such as:
>> acute cystitis with hematuria (N30.01)
>> recurrent and persistent hematuria in glomerular diseases (N02.-)

     R31.0   Gross hematuria
     R31.1   Benign essential microscopic hematuria
     R31.2   Other microscopic hematuria
     R31.9   Hematuria, unspecified

CHAPTER 18 (R00-R99)

R32   Unspecified urinary incontinence
Enuresis NOS

Excludes1	functional urinary incontinence (R39.81)
	nonorganic enuresis (F98.0)
	stress incontinence and other specified urinary incontinence (N39.3-N39.4-)
	urinary incontinence associated with cognitive impairment (R39.81)

●**R33   Retention of urine**

| Excludes1 | psychogenic retention of urine (F45.8) |

R33.0   Drug induced retention of urine
Use additional code for adverse effect, if applicable, to identify drug (T36-T50 with fifth or sixth character 5)

R33.8   Other retention of urine
Code first, if applicable, any causal condition, such as:
enlarged prostate (N40.1)

R33.9   Retention of urine, unspecified

R34   Anuria and oliguria

Excludes1	anuria and oliguria complicating abortion or ectopic or molar pregnancy (O00-O07, O08.4)
	anuria and oliguria complicating pregnancy (O26.83-)
	anuria and oliguria complicating the puerperium (O90.4)

●**R35   Polyuria**
Passage of excessive volume of urine

Code first, if applicable, any causal condition, such as:
enlarged prostate (N40.1)

| Excludes1 | psychogenic polyuria (F45.8) |

R35.0   Frequency of micturition
Discharge or passage of urine; AKA uresis

R35.1   Nocturia
Urinary frequency at night

R35.8   Other polyuria
Polyuria NOS

●**R36   Urethral discharge**

R36.0   Urethral discharge without blood

R36.1   Hematospermia
Presence of blood in semen

R36.9   Urethral discharge, unspecified
Penile discharge NOS
Urethrorrhea

R37   Sexual dysfunction, unspecified

●**R39   Other and unspecified symptoms and signs involving the genitourinary system**

R39.0   Extravasation of urine
Leakage, discharge

●**R39.1   Other difficulties with micturition**
Code first, if applicable, any causal condition, such as:
enlarged prostate (N40.1)

R39.11   Hesitancy of micturition

R39.12   Poor urinary stream
Weak urinary steam

R39.13   Splitting of urinary stream

R39.14   Feeling of incomplete bladder emptying

R39.15   Urgency of urination

| Excludes1 | urge incontinence (N39.41, N39.46) |

R39.16   Straining to void

R39.19   Other difficulties with micturition

R39.2   Extrarenal uremia
Prerenal uremia

| Excludes1 | uremia NOS (N19) |

●**R39.8   Other symptoms and signs involving the genitourinary system**

R39.81   Functional urinary incontinence
Urinary incontinence due to cognitive impairment, or severe physical disability or immobility

| Excludes1 | stress incontinence and other specified urinary incontinence (N39.3-N39.4-) |
| | urinary incontinence NOS (R32) |

R39.89   Other symptoms and signs involving the genitourinary system

R39.9   Unspecified symptoms and signs involving the genitourinary system

---

SYMPTOMS AND SIGNS INVOLVING COGNITION, PERCEPTION, EMOTIONAL STATE AND BEHAVIOR (R40-R46)

| Excludes1 | symptoms and signs constituting part of a pattern of mental disorder (F01-F99) |

●**R40   Somnolence, stupor and coma**

Excludes1	neonatal coma (P91.5)
	somnolence, stupor and coma in diabetes (E08-E13)
	somnolence, stupor and coma in hepatic failure (K72.-)
	somnolence, stupor and coma in hypoglycemia (nondiabetic) (E15)

R40.0   Somnolence
Drowsiness

| Excludes1 | coma (R40.2-) |

R40.1   Stupor
Lowered level of consciousness
Catatonic stupor
Semicoma

Excludes1	catatonic schizophrenia (F20.2)
	coma (R40.2-)
	depressive stupor (F31-F33)
	dissociative stupor (F44.2)
	manic stupor (F30.2)

OGCR Section I.C.18.e.

Coma scale

The coma scale codes (R40.2-) can be used in conjunction with traumatic brain injury codes, acute cerebrovascular disease or sequelae of cerebrovascular disease codes. These codes are primarily for use by trauma registries, but they may be used in any setting where this information is collected. The coma scale codes should be sequenced after the diagnosis code(s).

These codes, one from each subcategory, are needed to complete the scale. The 7th character indicates when the scale was recorded. The 7th character should match for all three codes.

At a minimum, report the initial score documented on presentation at your facility. This may be a score from the emergency medicine technician (EMT) or in the emergency department. If desired, a facility may choose to capture multiple coma scale scores.

Assign code R40.24, Glasgow coma scale, total score, when only the total score is documented in the medical record and not the individual score(s).

●**R40.2   Coma**
Code first any associated:
fracture of skull (S02.-)
intracranial injury (S06.-)

Note: One code from subcategories R40.21-R40-23 is required to complete the coma scale

R40.20   Unspecified coma
Coma NOS
Unconsciousness NOS

● R40.21   **Coma scale, eyes open**

> The following appropriate 7th character is to be added to subcategory R40.21-:
>
> | | |
> |---|---|
> | 0 | unspecified time |
> | 1 | in the field [EMT or ambulance] |
> | 2 | at arrival to emergency department |
> | 3 | at hospital admission |
> | 4 | 24 hours or more after hospital admission |

     ● R40.211   **Coma scale, eyes open, never**

     ● R40.212   **Coma scale, eyes open, to pain**

     ● R40.213   **Coma scale, eyes open, to sound**

     ● R40.214   **Coma scale, eyes open, spontaneous**

● R40.22   **Coma scale, best verbal response**

> The following appropriate 7th character is to be added to subcategory R40.22-:
>
> | | |
> |---|---|
> | 0 | unspecified time |
> | 1 | in the field [EMT or ambulance] |
> | 2 | at arrival to emergency department |
> | 3 | at hospital admission |
> | 4 | 24 hours or more after hospital admission |

     ● R40.221   **Coma scale, best verbal response, none**

     ● R40.222   **Coma scale, best verbal response, incomprehensible words**

     ● R40.223   **Coma scale, best verbal response, inappropriate words**

     ● R40.224   **Coma scale, best verbal response, confused conversation**

     ● R40.225   **Coma scale, best verbal response, oriented**

Glasgow Coma Scale

Eye Opening Response	
• Spontaneous--open with blinking at baseline	4 points
• To verbal stimuli, command, speech	3 points
• To pain only (not applied to face)	2 points
• No response	1 point
Verbal Response	
• Oriented	5 points
• Confused conversation, but able to answer questions	4 points
• Inappropriate words	3 points
• Incomprehensible speech	2 points
• No response	1 point
Motor Response	
• Obeys commands for movement	6 points
• Purposeful movement to painful stimulus	5 points
• Withdraws in response to pain	4 points
• Flexion in response to pain (decorticate posturing)	3 points
• Extension response in response to pain (decerebrate posturing)	2 points
• No response	1 point
Categorization:	
Coma: No eye opening, no ability to follow commands, no word verbalizations (3-8)	
Head Injury Classification:	
Severe Head Injury--GCS score of 8 or less	
Moderate Head Injury--GCS score of 9 to 12	
Mild head injury--GCS score of 13 to 15	
(Adapted from: Advanced Trauma Life Support: Course for Physicians, American College of Surgeons, 1993). http://www.bt.cdc.gov/masscasulatires/gscale.asp	

Figure 18-1

● R40.23   **Coma scale, best motor response**

> The following appropriate 7th character is to be added to subcategory R40.23-:
>
> | | |
> |---|---|
> | 0 | unspecified time |
> | 1 | in the field [EMT or ambulance] |
> | 2 | at arrival to emergency department |
> | 3 | at hospital admission |
> | 4 | 24 hours or more after hospital admission |

     ● R40.231   **Coma scale, best motor response, none**

     ● R40.232   **Coma scale, best motor response, extension**

     ● R40.233   **Coma scale, best motor response, abnormal**

     ● R40.234   **Coma scale, best motor response, flexion withdrawal**

     ● R40.235   **Coma scale, best motor response, localizes pain**

     ● R40.236   **Coma scale, best motor response, obeys commands**

● R40.24   **Glasgow coma scale, total score**

> Use codes R40.21- through R40.23- only when the individual score(s) are documented

     R40.241   **Glasgow coma scale score 13-15**

     R40.242   **Glasgow coma scale score 9-12**

     R40.243   **Glasgow coma scale score 3-8**

     R40.244   **Other coma, without documented Glasgow coma scale score, or with partial score reported**

R40.3   **Persistent vegetative state**

R40.4   **Transient alteration of awareness**

● R41   **Other symptoms and signs involving cognitive functions and awareness**

> | Excludes1 | dissociative [conversion] disorders (F44.-) |
> |---|---|
> | | mild cognitive impairment, so stated (G31.84) |

R41.0   **Disorientation, unspecified**
> Confusion NOS   Delirium NOS

R41.1   **Anterograde amnesia**

R41.2   **Retrograde amnesia**

R41.3   **Other amnesia**
> Amnesia NOS
> Memory loss NOS

> | Excludes1 | amnestic disorder due to known physiologic condition (F04) |
> |---|---|
> | | amnestic syndrome due to psychoactive substance use (F10-F19 with 5th character .6) |
> | | mild memory disturbance due to known physiological condition (F06.8) |
> | | transient global amnesia (G45.4) |

R41.4   **Neurologic neglect syndrome**
> | Asomatognosia | Left-sided neglect |
> |---|---|
> | Hemi-akinesia | Sensory neglect |
> | Hemi-inattention | Visuospatial neglect |
> | Hemispatial neglect | |

> | Excludes1 | visuospatial deficit (R41.842) |
> |---|---|

● R41.8   **Other symptoms and signs involving cognitive functions and awareness**

     R41.81   **Age-related cognitive decline**
> Senility NOS

     R41.82   **Altered mental status, unspecified**
> Change in mental status NOS

> | Excludes1 | altered level of consciousness (R40.-) |
> |---|---|
> | | altered mental status due to known condition - code to condition |
> | | delirium NOS (R41.0) |

R41.83 **Borderline intellectual functioning**
IQ level 71 to 84
> **Excludes1** intellectual disabilities (F70-F79)

● R41.84 **Other specified cognitive deficit**
R41.840 **Attention and concentration deficit**
> **Excludes1** attention-deficit hyperactivity disorders (F90.-)

R41.841 **Cognitive communication deficit**
R41.842 **Visuospatial deficit**
R41.843 **Psychomotor deficit**
R41.844 **Frontal lobe and executive function deficit**

R41.89 **Other symptoms and signs involving cognitive functions and awareness**
Anosognosia

R41.9 **Unspecified symptoms and signs involving cognitive functions and awareness**

R42 **Dizziness and giddiness**
Light-headedness
Vertigo NOS
> **Excludes1** vertiginous syndromes (H81.-)
> vertigo from infrasound (T75.23)

● R43 **Disturbances of smell and taste**
R43.0 **Anosmia**
Absence of sense of smell; AKA anosphresia and olfactory anesthesia

R43.1 **Parosmia**
R43.2 **Parageusia**
Perversion of sense of taste or bad taste in mouth; AKA dysgeusia

R43.8 **Other disturbances of smell and taste**
Mixed disturbance of smell and taste

R43.9 **Unspecified disturbances of smell and taste**

● R44 **Other symptoms and signs involving general sensations and perceptions**
> **Excludes1** alcoholic hallucinations (F1.5)
> hallucinations in drug psychosis (F11-F19 with .5)
> hallucinations in mood disorders with psychotic symptoms (F30.2, F31.5, F32.3, F33.3)
> hallucinations in schizophrenia, schizotypal and delusional disorders (F20-F29)

> **Excludes2** disturbances of skin sensation (R20.-)

R44.0 **Auditory hallucinations**
R44.1 **Visual hallucinations**
R44.2 **Other hallucinations**
R44.3 **Hallucinations, unspecified**
R44.8 **Other symptoms and signs involving general sensations and perceptions**
R44.9 **Unspecified symptoms and signs involving general sensations and perceptions**

● R45 **Symptoms and signs involving emotional state**
R45.0 **Nervousness**
Nervous tension

R45.1 **Restlessness and agitation**
R45.2 **Unhappiness**
R45.3 **Demoralization and apathy**
> **Excludes1** anhedonia (R45.84)

R45.4 **Irritability and anger**
R45.5 **Hostility**
R45.6 **Violent behavior**
R45.7 **State of emotional shock and stress, unspecified**

● R45.8 **Other symptoms and signs involving emotional state**
R45.81 **Low self-esteem**
R45.82 **Worries**
R45.83 **Excessive crying of child, adolescent or adult**
> **Excludes1** excessive crying of infant (baby) R68.11

R45.84 **Anhedonia**
Total loss of feeling of pleasure in pleasurable acts

● R45.85 **Homicidal and suicidal ideations**
> **Excludes1** suicide attempt (T14.91)
R45.850 **Homicidal ideations**
R45.851 **Suicidal ideations**

R45.86 **Emotional lability**
R45.87 **Impulsiveness**
R45.89 **Other symptoms and signs involving emotional state**

● R46 **Symptoms and signs involving appearance and behavior**
> **Excludes1** appearance and behavior in schizophrenia, schizotypal and delusional disorders (F20-F29)
> mental and behavioral disorders (F01-F99)

R46.0 **Very low level of personal hygiene**
R46.1 **Bizarre personal appearance**
R46.2 **Strange and inexplicable behavior**
R46.3 **Overactivity**
R46.4 **Slowness and poor responsiveness**
> **Excludes1** stupor (R40.1)

R46.5 **Suspiciousness and marked evasiveness**
R46.6 **Undue concern and preoccupation with stressful events**
R46.7 **Verbosity and circumstantial detail obscuring reason for contact**

● R46.8 **Other symptoms and signs involving appearance and behavior**
R46.81 **Obsessive-compulsive behavior**
> **Excludes1** obsessive-compulsive disorder (F42)

R46.89 **Other symptoms and signs involving appearance and behavior**

SYMPTOMS AND SIGNS INVOLVING SPEECH AND VOICE (R47-R49)

● R47 **Speech disturbances, not elsewhere classified**
> **Excludes1** autism (F84.0)
> cluttering (F80.81)
> specific developmental disorders of speech and language (F80.-)
> stuttering (F80.81)

● R47.0 **Dysphasia and aphasia**
R47.01 **Aphasia**
> **Excludes1** aphasia following cerebrovascular disease (I69. with final characters -20)
> progressive isolated aphasia (G31.01)

R47.02 **Dysphasia**
Impairment in comprehension of speech, caused by left-sided brain damage
> **Excludes1** dysphasia following cerebrovascular disease (I69. with final characters -21)

R47.1 **Dysarthria and anarthria**
Motor speech disorder
> **Excludes1** dysarthria following cerebrovascular disease (I69. with final characters -22)

◀ New ◀═ Revised ~~deleted~~ Deleted **OGCR** Official Guidelines X Assign placeholder X ● Use Additional Character(s)

Excludes 1 | Excludes 2 | Includes | Use additional | Code first | Code also | Unspecified

● **R47.8   Other speech disturbances**

     | Excludes1 | dysarthria following cerebrovascular disease (I69. with final characters -28)

    R47.81   Slurred speech

    R47.82   Fluency disorder in conditions classified elsewhere

       Stuttering in conditions classified elsewhere

       Code first underlying disease or condition, such as:
       Parkinson's disease (G20)

       | Excludes1 | adult onset fluency disorder (F98.5)

               childhood onset fluency disorder (F80.81)

               fluency disorder (stuttering) following cerebrovascular disease (I69. with final characters -23)

    R47.89   Other speech disturbances

   R47.9   Unspecified speech disturbances

● **R48   Dyslexia and other symbolic dysfunctions, not elsewhere classified**

     | Excludes1 | specific developmental disorders of scholastic skills (F81.-)

   R48.0   Dyslexia and alexia

   R48.1   Agnosia

       Loss of ability to recognize objects, persons, sounds, shapes, or smells

       Astereognosia (astereognosis)

       Autotopagnosia

       | Excludes1 | visual object agnosia (R48.3)

   R48.2   Apraxia

       Loss of ability to execute or carry out learned purposeful movements

       | Excludes1 | apraxia following cerebrovascular disease (I69. with final characters -90)

   R48.3   Visual agnosia

       Prosopagnosia

       Simultanagnosia (asimultagnosia)

   R48.8   Other symbolic dysfunctions

       Acalculia

       Difficulty performing simple mathematical tasks resulting from neurological injury

       Agraphia

   R48.9   Unspecified symbolic dysfunctions

● **R49   Voice and resonance disorders**

     | Excludes1 | psychogenic voice and resonance disorders (F44.4)

   R49.0   Dysphonia

       Hoarseness

   R49.1   Aphonia

       Loss of voice

● **R49.2   Hypernasality and hyponasality**

    R49.21   Hypernasality

    R49.22   Hyponasality

   R49.8   Other voice and resonance disorders

   R49.9   Unspecified voice and resonance disorder

       Change in voice NOS

       Resonance disorder NOS

GENERAL SYMPTOMS AND SIGNS (R50-R69)

● **R50   Fever of other and unknown origin**

     | Excludes1 | chills without fever (R68.83)

               febrile convulsions (R56.0-)

               fever of unknown origin during labor (O75.2)

               fever of unknown origin in newborn (P81.9)

               hypothermia due to illness (R68.0)

               malignant hyperthermia due to anesthesia (T88.3)

               puerperal pyrexia NOS (O86.4)

   R50.2   Drug induced fever

       Use additional code for adverse effect, if applicable, to identify drug (T36-T50 with fifth or sixth character 5)

       | Excludes1 | postvaccination (postimmunization) fever (R50.83)

● **R50.8   Other specified fever**

    R50.81   Fever presenting with conditions classified elsewhere

       Code first underlying condition when associated fever is present, such as with:

       leukemia (C91-C95)

       neutropenia (D70.-)

       sickle-cell disease (D57.-)

    R50.82   Postprocedural fever

       | Excludes1 | postprocedural infection (T81.4)

               posttransfusion fever (R50.84)

               postvaccination (postimmunization) fever (R50.83)

    R50.83   Postvaccination fever

       Postimmunization fever

    R50.84   Febrile nonhemolytic transfusion reaction

       FNHTR

       Posttransfusion fever

   R50.9   Fever, unspecified

       Fever NOS

       Fever of unknown origin [FUO]

       Fever with chills

       Fever with rigors

       Hyperpyrexia NOS

       Persistent fever

       Pyrexia NOS

R51   Headache

       Facial pain NOS

     | Excludes1 | atypical face pain (G50.1)

               migraine and other headache syndromes (G43-G44)

               trigeminal neuralgia (G50.0)

R52   Pain, unspecified

       Acute pain NOS   Pain NOS

       Generalized pain NOS

     | Excludes1 | acute and chronic pain, not elsewhere classified (G89.-)

               localized pain, unspecified type - code to pain by site, such as:

               abdomen pain (R10.-)

               back pain (M54.9)

               breast pain (N64.4)

               chest pain (R07.1-R07.9)

               ear pain (H92.0-)

               eye pain (H57.1)

               headache (R51)

               joint pain (M25.5-)

               limb pain (M79.6-)

               lumbar region pain (M54.5)

               pelvic and perineal pain (R10.2)

               shoulder pain (M25.51-)

               spine pain (M54.-)

               throat pain (R07.0)

               tongue pain (K14.6)

               tooth pain (K08.8)

               renal colic (N23)

              pain disorders exclusively related to psychological factors (F45.41)

CHAPTER 18 (R00-R99)

◀ New   ◀▥ Revised   ~~deleted~~ Deleted   **OGCR** Official Guidelines   X Assign placeholder X   ● Use Additional Character(s)

| Excludes 1 | | Excludes 2 | Includes   Use additional   Code first   Code also   Unspecified

CHAPTER 18 (R00-R99)

● **R53   Malaise and fatigue**

    R53.0   Neoplastic (malignant) related fatigue
        Code first associated neoplasm

    R53.1   Weakness
        Asthenia NOS
        Excludes1   age-related weakness (R54)
                muscle weakness (M62.8-)
                senile asthenia (R54)

    R53.2   Functional quadriplegia
        Complete immobility due to severe physical disability
           or frailty
        Excludes1   frailty NOS (R54)
                hysterical paralysis (F44.4)
                immobility syndrome (M62.3)
                neurologic quadriplegia (G82.5-)
                quadriplegia (G82.50)

  ● **R53.8   Other malaise and fatigue**
        Excludes1   combat exhaustion and fatigue (F43.0)
                congenital debility (P96.9)
                exhaustion and fatigue due to depressive
                    episode (F32.-)
                exhaustion and fatigue due to excessive
                    exertion (T73.3)
                exhaustion and fatigue due to exposure
                    (T73.2)
                exhaustion and fatigue due to heat (T67.-)
                exhaustion and fatigue due to pregnancy
                    (O26.8-)
                exhaustion and fatigue due to recurrent
                    depressive episode (F33)
                exhaustion and fatigue due to senile
                    debility (R54)

        R53.81   Other malaise
            Chronic debility
            Debility NOS
            General physical deterioration
            Malaise NOS
            Nervous debility
            Excludes1   age-related physical debility
                    (R54)

        R53.82   Chronic fatigue, unspecified
            Chronic fatigue syndrome NOS
            Excludes1   postviral fatigue syndrome
                    (G93.3)

        R53.83   Other fatigue
            Fatigue NOS   Lethargy
            Lack of energy   Tiredness

R54   Age-related physical debility
    Frailty   Senile asthenia
    Old age   Senile debility
    Senescence
    Excludes1   age-related cognitive decline (R41.81)
                senile psychosis (F03)
                senility NOS (R41.81)

R55   Syncope and collapse
    Blackout
    Fainting
    Vasovagal attack
    Excludes1   cardiogenic shock (R57.0)
                carotid sinus syncope (G90.01)
                heat syncope (T67.1)
                neurocirculatory asthenia (F45.8)
                neurogenic orthostatic hypotension (G90.3)
                orthostatic hypotension (I95.1)
                postprocedural shock (T81.1-)
                psychogenic syncope (F48.8)
                shock NOS (R57.9)
                shock complicating or following abortion or
                    ectopic or molar pregnancy (O00-O07, O08.3)
                shock complicating or following labor and
                    delivery (O75.1)
                Stokes-Adams attack (I45.9)
                unconsciousness NOS (R40.2-)

● **R56   Convulsions, not elsewhere classified**
    Excludes1   dissociative convulsions and seizures (F44.5)
                epileptic convulsions and seizures (G40.-)
                newborn convulsions and seizures (P90)

  ● **R56.0   Febrile convulsions**

        R56.00   Simple febrile convulsions
            Febrile convulsion NOS
            Febrile seizure NOS

        R56.01   Complex febrile convulsions
            Atypical febrile seizure
            Complex febrile seizure
            Complicated febrile seizure
            Excludes1   status epilepticus (G40.901)

    R56.1   Post traumatic seizures
        Excludes1   post traumatic epilepsy (G40.-)

    R56.9   Unspecified convulsions
        Convulsion disorder   Recurrent convulsions
        Fit NOS   Seizure(s) (convulsive) NOS

● **R57   Shock, not elsewhere classified**
    Excludes1   anaphylactic shock NOS (T78.2)
                anaphylactic reaction or shock due to adverse
                    food reaction (T78.0-)
                anaphylactic shock due to adverse effect of
                    correct drug or medicament properly
                    administered (T88.6)
                anaphylactic shock due to serum (T80.5-)
                anesthetic shock (T88.3)
                electric shock (T75.4)
                obstetric shock (O75.1)
                postprocedural shock (T81.1-)
                psychic shock (F43.0)
                septic shock (R65.21)
                shock complicating or following ectopic or molar
                    pregnancy (O00-O07, O08.3)
                shock due to lightning (T75.01)
                traumatic shock (T79.4)
                toxic shock syndrome (A48.3)

    R57.0   Cardiogenic shock

    R57.1   Hypovolemic shock
        Decreased blood volume (loss)

    R57.8   Other shock

    R57.9   Shock, unspecified
        Failure of peripheral circulation NOS
        Resulting in significant blood pressure drop

R58   Hemorrhage, not elsewhere classified
    Hemorrhage NOS
    Excludes1   hemorrhage included with underlying
                    conditions, such as:
                    acute duodenal ulcer with hemorrhage (K26.0)
                    acute gastritis with bleeding (K29.01)
                    ulcerative enterocolitis with rectal bleeding
                      (K51.01)

● **R59   Enlarged lymph nodes**
    Includes   swollen glands
    Excludes1   lymphadenitis NOS (I88.9)
                acute lymphadenitis (L04.-)
                chronic lymphadenitis (I88.1)
                mesenteric (acute) (chronic) lymphadenitis (I88.0)

    R59.0   Localized enlarged lymph nodes

    R59.1   Generalized enlarged lymph nodes
        Lymphadenopathy NOS

    R59.9   Enlarged lymph nodes, unspecified

● R60　**Edema, not elsewhere classified**

Excludes1　angioneurotic edema (T78.3)
　　　　　　ascites (R18.-)
　　　　　　cerebral edema (G93.6)
　　　　　　cerebral edema due to birth injury (P11.0)
　　　　　　edema of larynx (J38.4)
　　　　　　edema of nasopharynx (J39.2)
　　　　　　edema of pharynx (J39.2)
　　　　　　gestational edema (O12.0-)
　　　　　　hereditary edema (Q82.0)
　　　　　　hydrops fetalis NOS (P83.2)
　　　　　　hydrothorax (J94.8)
　　　　　　nutritional edema (E40-E46)
　　　　　　hydrops fetalis NOS (P83.2)
　　　　　　newborn edema (P83.3)
　　　　　　pulmonary edema (J81.-)

R60.0　**Localized edema**

R60.1　**Generalized edema**

R60.9　**Edema, unspecified**
　　　　Fluid retention NOS

R61　**Generalized hyperhidrosis**
　　　Excessive sweating
　　　Night sweats
　　　Secondary hyperhidrosis

　　　Code first, if applicable, menopausal and female climacteric states (N95.1)

　　　Excludes1　focal (primary) (secondary) hyperhidrosis (L74.5-)
　　　　　　　　Frey's syndrome (L74.52)
　　　　　　　　localized (primary) (secondary) hyperhidrosis (L74.5-)

● R62　**Lack of expected normal physiological development in childhood and adults**

　　　Excludes1　delayed puberty (E30.0)
　　　　　　　　gonadal dysgenesis (Q99.1)
　　　　　　　　hypopituitarism (E23.0)

R62.0　**Delayed milestone in childhood**
　　　　Delayed attainment of expected physiological developmental stage
　　　　Late talker
　　　　Late walker

● R62.5　**Other and unspecified lack of expected normal physiological development in childhood**
　　　　Excludes1　HIV disease resulting in failure to thrive (B20)
　　　　　　　　　physical retardation due to malnutrition (E45)

　　R62.50　**Unspecified lack of expected normal physiological development in childhood**
　　　　　　Infantilism NOS

　　R62.51　**Failure to thrive (child)**
　　　　　　Failure to gain weight
　　　　　　Excludes1　failure to thrive in child under 28 days old (P92.6)

　　R62.52　**Short stature (child)**
　　　　　　Lack of growth　　　　Short stature NOS
　　　　　　Physical retardation
　　　　　　Excludes1　short stature due to endocrine disorder (E34.3)

　　R62.59　**Other lack of expected normal physiological development in childhood**

R62.7　**Adult failure to thrive**

● R63　**Symptoms and signs concerning food and fluid intake**

　　　Excludes1　bulimia NOS (F50.2)
　　　　　　　　eating disorders of nonorganic origin (F50.-)
　　　　　　　　malnutrition (E40-E46)

R63.0　**Anorexia**
　　　　Loss of appetite
　　　　Excludes1　anorexia nervosa (F50.0-)
　　　　　　　　　loss of appetite of nonorganic origin (F50.8)

R63.1　**Polydipsia**
　　　　Excessive thirst

R63.2　**Polyphagia**
　　　　Excessive eating　　　　Hyperalimentation NOS

R63.3　**Feeding difficulties**
　　　　Feeding problem (elderly) (infant) NOS
　　　　Excludes1　feeding problems of newborn (P92.-)
　　　　　　　　　infant feeding disorder of nonorganic origin (F98.2-)

R63.4　**Abnormal weight loss**

R63.5　**Abnormal weight gain**
　　　　Excludes1　excessive weight gain in pregnancy (O26.0-)
　　　　　　　　　obesity (E66.-)

R63.6　**Underweight**
　　　　Use additional code to identify body mass index (BMI), if known (Z68.-)
　　　　Excludes1　abnormal weight loss (R63.4)
　　　　　　　　　anorexia nervosa (F50.0-)
　　　　　　　　　malnutrition (E40-E46)

R63.8　**Other symptoms and signs concerning food and fluid intake**

R64　**Cachexia**
　　　Wasting syndrome
　　　Code first underlying condition, if known
　　　Excludes1　abnormal weight loss (R63.4)
　　　　　　　　nutritional marasmus (E41)

OGCR Section I.C.18.g.

SIRS due to Non-Infectious Process

The systemic inflammatory response syndrome (SIRS) can develop as a result of certain non-infectious disease processes, such as trauma, malignant neoplasm, or pancreatitis. When SIRS is documented with a noninfectious condition, and no subsequent infection is documented, the code for the underlying condition, such as an injury, should be assigned, followed by code R65.10, Systemic inflammatory response syndrome (SIRS) of non-infectious origin without acute organ dysfunction, or code R65.11, Systemic inflammatory response syndrome (SIRS) of non-infectious origin with acute organ dysfunction. If an associated acute organ dysfunction is documented, the appropriate code(s) for the specific type of organ dysfunction(s) should be assigned in addition to code R65.11. If acute organ dysfunction is documented, but it cannot be determined if the acute organ dysfunction is associated with SIRS or due to another condition (e.g., directly due to the trauma), the provider should be queried.

● R65　**Symptoms and signs specifically associated with systemic inflammation and infection**

● R65.1　**Systemic inflammatory response syndrome (SIRS) of non-infectious origin**
　　　Code first underlying condition, such as:
　　　　heatstroke (T67.0)
　　　　injury and trauma (S00-T88)
　　　Excludes1　sepsis - code to infection
　　　　　　　　severe sepsis (R65.2)

　　R65.10　**Systemic inflammatory response syndrome (SIRS) of non-infectious origin without acute organ dysfunction**
　　　　　　Systemic inflammatory response syndrome (SIRS) NOS

R65.11 **Systemic inflammatory response syndrome (SIRS) of non-infectious origin with acute organ dysfunction**

Use additional code to identify specific acute organ dysfunction, such as:
acute kidney failure (N17.-)
acute respiratory failure (J96.0-)
critical illness myopathy (G72.81)
critical illness polyneuropathy (G62.81)
disseminated intravascular coagulopathy [DIC] (D65)
encephalopathy (metabolic) (septic) (G93.41)
hepatic failure (K72.0-)

● **R65.2** **Severe sepsis**

Infection with associated acute organ dysfunction
Sepsis with acute organ dysfunction
Sepsis with multiple organ dysfunction
Systemic inflammatory response syndrome due to infectious process with acute organ dysfunction

Code first underlying infection, such as:
infection following a procedure (T81.4)
infections following infusion, transfusion and therapeutic injection (T80.2-)
puerperal sepsis (O85)
sepsis following complete or unspecified spontaneous abortion (O03.87)
sepsis following ectopic and molar pregnancy (O08.82)
sepsis following incomplete spontaneous abortion (O03.37)
sepsis following (induced) termination of pregnancy (O04.87)
sepsis NOS (A41.9)

Use additional code to identify specific acute organ dysfunction, such as:
acute kidney failure (N17.-)
acute respiratory failure (J96.0-)
critical illness myopathy (G72.81)
critical illness polyneuropathy (G62.81)
disseminated intravascular coagulopathy [DIC] (D65)
encephalopathy (metabolic) (septic) (G93.41)
hepatic failure (K72.0-)

R65.20 **Severe sepsis without septic shock**
Severe sepsis NOS

R65.21 **Severe sepsis with septic shock**

● **R68** **Other general symptoms and signs**

R68.0 **Hypothermia, not associated with low environmental temperature**

Excludes1   hypothermia NOS (accidental) (T68)
hypothermia due to anesthesia (T88.51)
hypothermia due to low environmental temperature (T68)
newborn hypothermia (P80.-)

● **R68.1** **Nonspecific symptoms peculiar to infancy**

Excludes1   colic, infantile (R10.83)
neonatal cerebral irritability (P91.3)
teething syndrome (K00.7)

R68.11 **Excessive crying of infant (baby)**

Excludes1   excessive crying of child, adolescent, or adult (R45.83)

R68.12 **Fussy infant (baby)**
Irritable infant

R68.13 **Apparent life threatening event in infant (ALTE)**

Apparent life threatening event in newborn

Code first confirmed diagnosis, if known

Use additional code(s) for associated signs and symptoms if no confirmed diagnosis established, or if signs and symptoms are not associated routinely with confirmed diagnosis, or provide additional information for cause of ALTE

R68.19 **Other nonspecific symptoms peculiar to infancy**

R68.2 **Dry mouth, unspecified**

Excludes1   dry mouth due to dehydration (E86.0)
dry mouth due to sicca syndrome [Sjögren] (M35.0-)
salivary gland hyposecretion (K11.7)

R68.3 **Clubbing of fingers**
Clubbing of nails

Excludes1   congenital clubfinger (Q68.1)

● **R68.8** **Other general symptoms and signs**

R68.81 **Early satiety**

R68.82 **Decreased libido**
Decreased sexual desire

R68.83 **Chills (without fever)**
Chills NOS

Excludes1   chills with fever (R50.9)

R68.84 **Jaw pain**
Mandibular pain
Maxilla pain

Excludes1   temporomandibular joint arthralgia (M26.62)

R68.89 **Other general symptoms and signs**

R69 **Illness, unspecified**
Unknown and unspecified cases of morbidity

ABNORMAL FINDINGS ON EXAMINATION OF BLOOD, WITHOUT DIAGNOSIS (R70-R79)

Excludes1   abnormalities (of)(on):
abnormal findings on antenatal screening of mother (O28.-)
coagulation hemorrhagic disorders (D65-D68)
lipids (E78.-)
platelets and thrombocytes (D69.-)
white blood cells classified elsewhere (D70-D72)
diagnostic abnormal findings classified elsewhere - see Alphabetical Index
hemorrhagic and hematological disorders of newborn (P50-P61)

● **R70** **Elevated erythrocyte sedimentation rate and abnormality of plasma viscosity**

R70.0 **Elevated erythrocyte sedimentation rate**

R70.1 **Abnormal plasma viscosity**

● **R71**   **Abnormality of red blood cells**
> **Excludes1**   anemias (D50-D64)
> anemia of premature infant (P61.2)
> benign (familial) polycythemia (D75.0)
> congenital anemias (P61.2-P61.4)
> newborn anemia due to isoimmunization (P55.-)
> polycythemia neonatorum (P61.1)
> polycythemia NOS (D75.1)
> polycythemia vera (D45)
> secondary polycythemia (D75.1)

   R71.0   **Precipitous drop in hematocrit**
> Drop (precipitous) in hemoglobin
> Drop in hematocrit
> *Blood volume that is red blood cells*

   R71.8   **Other abnormality of red blood cells**
> Abnormal red-cell morphology NOS
> Abnormal red-cell volume NOS
> Anisocytosis
> *Red blood cells of unequal size*
> Poikilocytosis
> *Red blood cells of abnormal shape*

● **R73**   **Elevated blood glucose level**
> **Excludes1**   diabetes mellitus (E08-E13)
> diabetes mellitus in pregnancy, childbirth and the
>   puerperium (O24.-)
> neonatal disorders (P70.0-P70.2)
> postsurgical hypoinsulinemia (E89.1)

   ● **R73.0**   **Abnormal glucose**
> **Excludes1**   abnormal glucose in pregnancy (O99.81-)
> diabetes mellitus (E08-E13)
> dysmetabolic syndrome X (E88.81)
> gestational diabetes (O24.4-)
> glycosuria (R81)
> hypoglycemia (E16.2)

     R73.01   **Impaired fasting glucose**
> Elevated fasting glucose

     R73.02   **Impaired glucose tolerance (oral)**
> Elevated glucose tolerance

     R73.09   **Other abnormal glucose**
> Abnormal glucose NOS
> Abnormal non-fasting glucose tolerance
> Latent diabetes
> Prediabetes

   R73.9   **Hyperglycemia, unspecified**

● **R74**   **Abnormal serum enzyme levels**
   R74.0   **Nonspecific elevation of levels of transaminase and lactic acid dehydrogenase [LDH]**
   R74.8   **Abnormal levels of other serum enzymes**
> Abnormal level of acid phosphatase
> Abnormal level of alkaline phosphatase
> Abnormal level of amylase
> Abnormal level of lipase [triacylglycerol lipase]

   R74.9   **Abnormal serum enzyme level, unspecified**

OGCR Section I.C.1.2.e and f.

Patients with inconclusive HIV serology

e. Patients with inconclusive HIV serology, but no definitive diagnosis or manifestations of the illness, may be assigned code R75, Inconclusive laboratory evidence of human immunodeficiency virus [HIV].

f. Previously diagnosed HIV-related illness

Patients with any known prior diagnosis of an HIV-related illness should be coded to B20. Once a patient has developed an HIV-related illness, the patient should always be assigned code B20 on every subsequent admission/encounter. Patients previously diagnosed with any HIV illness (B20) should never be assigned to R75 or Z21, Asymptomatic human immunodeficiency virus [HIV] infection status.

R75   **Inconclusive laboratory evidence of human immunodeficiency virus [HIV]**
> Nonconclusive HIV-test finding in infants
> **Excludes1**   asymptomatic human immunodeficiency virus [HIV] infection status (Z21)
> human immunodeficiency virus [HIV] disease (B20)

● **R76**   **Other abnormal immunological findings in serum**
   R76.0   **Raised antibody titer**
> **Excludes1**   isoimmunization in pregnancy (O36.0-O36.1)
> isoimmunization affecting newborn (P55.-)

   ● **R76.1**   **Nonspecific reaction to test for tuberculosis**
     R76.11   **Nonspecific reaction to tuberculin skin test without active tuberculosis**
> Abnormal result of Mantoux test
> PPD positive
> Tuberculin (skin test) positive
> Tuberculin (skin test) reactor
> **Excludes1**   nonspecific reaction to cell mediated immunity measurement of gamma interferon antigen response without active tuberculosis (R76.12)

     R76.12   **Nonspecific reaction to cell mediated immunity measurement of gamma interferon antigen response without active tuberculosis**
> Nonspecific reaction to QuantiFERON-TB test (QFT) without active tuberculosis
> **Excludes1**   nonspecific reaction to tuberculin skin test without active tuberculosis (R76.11)
> positive tuberculin skin test (R76.11)

   R76.8   **Other specified abnormal immunological findings in serum**
> Raised level of immunoglobulins NOS

   R76.9   **Abnormal immunological finding in serum, unspecified**

● **R77**   **Other abnormalities of plasma proteins**
> **Excludes1**   disorders of plasma-protein metabolism (E88.0)
   R77.0   **Abnormality of albumin**
   R77.1   **Abnormality of globulin**
> Hyperglobulinemia NOS
   R77.2   **Abnormality of alphafetoprotein**
   R77.8   **Other specified abnormalities of plasma proteins**
   R77.9   **Abnormality of plasma protein, unspecified**

● R78   Findings of drugs and other substances, not normally found in blood

Use additional code to identify any retained foreign body, if applicable (Z18.-)

Excludes1   mental or behavioral disorders due to psychoactive substance use (F10-F19)

R78.0   Finding of alcohol in blood

Use additional external cause code (Y90.-), for detail regarding alcohol level.

R78.1   Finding of opiate drug in blood

R78.2   Finding of cocaine in blood

R78.3   Finding of hallucinogen in blood

R78.4   Finding of other drugs of addictive potential in blood

R78.5   Finding of other psychotropic drug in blood

R78.6   Finding of steroid agent in blood

● R78.7   Finding of abnormal level of heavy metals in blood

R78.71   Abnormal lead level in blood

Excludes1   lead poisoning (T56.0-)

R78.79   Finding of abnormal level of heavy metals in blood

● R78.8   Finding of other specified substances, not normally found in blood

R78.81   Bacteremia

Blood poisoning/bacteremia

Excludes1   sepsis-code to specified infection (A00-B99)

R78.89   Finding of other specified substances, not normally found in blood

Finding of abnormal level of lithium in blood

R78.9   Finding of unspecified substance, not normally found in blood

● R79   Other abnormal findings of blood chemistry

Use additional code to identify any retained foreign body, if applicable (Z18.-)

Excludes1   abnormality of fluid, electrolyte or acid-base balance (E86-E87)

asymptomatic hyperuricemia (E79.0)
hyperglycemia NOS (R73.9)
hypoglycemia NOS (E16.2)
neonatal hypoglycemia (P70.3-P70.4)
specific findings indicating disorder of amino-acid metabolism (E70-E72)
specific findings indicating disorder of carbohydrate metabolism (E73-E74)
specific findings indicating disorder of lipid metabolism (E75.-)

R79.0   Abnormal level of blood mineral

Abnormal blood level of cobalt
Abnormal blood level of copper
Abnormal blood level of iron
Abnormal blood level of magnesium
Abnormal blood level of mineral NEC
Abnormal blood level of zinc

Excludes1   abnormal level of lithium (R78.89)
disorders of mineral metabolism (E83.-)
neonatal hypomagnesemia (P71.2)
nutritional mineral deficiency (E58-E61)

R79.1   Abnormal coagulation profile

Abnormal or prolonged bleeding time
Abnormal or prolonged coagulation time
Abnormal or prolonged partial thromboplastin time [PTT]
Abnormal or prolonged prothrombin time [PT]

Excludes1   coagulation defects (D68.-)

● R79.8   Other specified abnormal findings of blood chemistry

R79.81   Abnormal blood-gas level

R79.82   Elevated C-reactive protein (CRP)

R79.89   Other specified abnormal findings of blood chemistry

R79.9   Abnormal finding of blood chemistry, unspecified

ABNORMAL FINDINGS ON EXAMINATION OF URINE, WITHOUT DIAGNOSIS (R80-R82)

Excludes1   abnormal findings on antenatal screening of mother (O28.-)
diagnostic abnormal findings classified elsewhere - see Alphabetical Index
specific findings indicating disorder of amino-acid metabolism (E70-E72)
specific findings indicating disorder of carbohydrate metabolism (E73-E74)

● R80   Proteinuria

Excludes1   gestational proteinuria (O12.1-)

R80.0   Isolated proteinuria

Idiopathic proteinuria

Excludes1   isolated proteinuria with specific morphological lesion (N06.-)

R80.1   Persistent proteinuria, unspecified

R80.2   Orthostatic proteinuria, unspecified

Postural proteinuria

R80.3   Bence Jones proteinuria

R80.8   Other proteinuria

R80.9   Proteinuria, unspecified

Albuminuria NOS

R81   Glycosuria

Excludes1   renal glycosuria (E74.8)

● R82   Other and unspecified abnormal findings in urine

Includes   chromoabnormalities in urine

Use additional code to identify any retained foreign body, if applicable (Z18.-)

Excludes2   hematuria (R31.-)

R82.0   Chyluria

White milky urine

Excludes1   filarial chyluria (B74.-)

R82.1   Myoglobinuria

Presence of myoglobin (iron containing protein) in urine

R82.2   Biliuria

Presence of bile pigments/salts in urine

R82.3   Hemoglobinuria

Presence of hemoglobin in urine

Excludes1   hemoglobinuria due to hemolysis from external causes NEC (D59.6)
hemoglobinuria due to paroxysmal nocturnal [Marchiafava-Micheli] (D59.5)

R82.4   Acetonuria

Ketonuria

R82.5   Elevated urine levels of drugs, medicaments and biological substances

Elevated urine levels of catecholamines
Elevated urine levels of indoleacetic acid
Elevated urine levels of 17-ketosteroids
Elevated urine levels of steroids

R82.6   Abnormal urine levels of substances chiefly nonmedicinal as to source

Abnormal urine level of heavy metals

R82.7   Abnormal findings on microbiological examination of urine

Positive culture findings of urine

Excludes1   colonization status (Z22.-)

R82.8   Abnormal findings on cytological and histological examination of urine

◀ New   ◀▥ Revised   ~~deleted~~ Deleted   OGCR Official Guidelines   X Assign placeholder X   ● Use Additional Character(s)

Excludes 1   Excludes 2   Includes   Use additional   Code first   Code also   Unspecified

● R82.9   Other and unspecified abnormal findings in urine

    R82.90   Unspecified abnormal findings in urine

    R82.91   Other chromoabnormalities of urine
       Chromoconversion (dipstick)
       Idiopathic dipstick converts positive for blood with no cellular forms in sediment

       | Excludes1 | hemoglobinuria (R82.3)
                           myoglobinuria (R82.1)

    R82.99   Other abnormal findings in urine
       Cells and casts in urine
       Crystalluria
       Melanuria

ABNORMAL FINDINGS ON EXAMINATION OF OTHER BODY FLUIDS, SUBSTANCES AND TISSUES, WITHOUT DIAGNOSIS (R83-R89)

    | Excludes1 | abnormal findings on antenatal screening of mother (O28.-)
                 diagnostic abnormal findings classified elsewhere - see Alphabetical Index

    | Excludes2 | abnormal findings on examination of blood, without diagnosis (R70-R79)
                 abnormal findings on examination of urine, without diagnosis (R80-R82)
                 abnormal tumor markers (R97.-)

● R83   Abnormal findings in cerebrospinal fluid

    R83.0   Abnormal level of enzymes in cerebrospinal fluid

    R83.1   Abnormal level of hormones in cerebrospinal fluid

    R83.2   Abnormal level of other drugs, medicaments and biological substances in cerebrospinal fluid

    R83.3   Abnormal level of substances chiefly nonmedicinal as to source in cerebrospinal fluid

    R83.4   Abnormal immunological findings in cerebrospinal fluid

    R83.5   Abnormal microbiological findings in cerebrospinal fluid
       Positive culture findings in cerebrospinal fluid

       | Excludes1 | colonization status (Z22.-)

    R83.6   Abnormal cytological findings in cerebrospinal fluid

    R83.8   Other abnormal findings in cerebrospinal fluid
       Abnormal chromosomal findings in cerebrospinal fluid

    R83.9   Unspecified abnormal finding in cerebrospinal fluid

● R84   Abnormal findings in specimens from respiratory organs and thorax

    | Includes | abnormal findings in bronchial washings
              abnormal findings in nasal secretions
              abnormal findings in pleural fluid
              abnormal findings in sputum
              abnormal findings in throat scrapings

    | Excludes1 | blood-stained sputum (R04.2)

    R84.0   Abnormal level of enzymes in specimens from respiratory organs and thorax

    R84.1   Abnormal level of hormones in specimens from respiratory organs and thorax

    R84.2   Abnormal level of other drugs, medicaments and biological substances in specimens from respiratory organs and thorax

    R84.3   Abnormal level of substances chiefly nonmedicinal as to source in specimens from respiratory organs and thorax

    R84.4   Abnormal immunological findings in specimens from respiratory organs and thorax

    R84.5   Abnormal microbiological findings in specimens from respiratory organs and thorax
       Positive culture findings in specimens from respiratory organs and thorax

       | Excludes1 | colonization status (Z22.-)

    R84.6   Abnormal cytological findings in specimens from respiratory organs and thorax

    R84.7   Abnormal histological findings in specimens from respiratory organs and thorax

    R84.8   Other abnormal findings in specimens from respiratory organs and thorax
       Abnormal chromosomal findings in specimens from respiratory organs and thorax

    R84.9   Unspecified abnormal finding in specimens from respiratory organs and thorax

● R85   Abnormal findings in specimens from digestive organs and abdominal cavity

    | Includes | abnormal findings in peritoneal fluid
              abnormal findings in saliva

    | Excludes1 | cloudy peritoneal dialysis effluent (R88.0)
                 fecal abnormalities (R19.5)

    R85.0   Abnormal level of enzymes in specimens from digestive organs and abdominal cavity

    R85.1   Abnormal level of hormones in specimens from digestive organs and abdominal cavity

    R85.2   Abnormal level of other drugs, medicaments and biological substances in specimens from digestive organs and abdominal cavity

    R85.3   Abnormal level of substances chiefly nonmedicinal as to source in specimens from digestive organs and abdominal cavity

    R85.4   Abnormal immunological findings in specimens from digestive organs and abdominal cavity

    R85.5   Abnormal microbiological findings in specimens from digestive organs and abdominal cavity
       Positive culture findings in specimens from digestive organs and abdominal cavity

       | Excludes1 | colonization status (Z22.-)

●   R85.6   Abnormal cytological findings in specimens from digestive organs and abdominal cavity

    ● R85.61   Abnormal cytologic smear of anus

       | Excludes1 | abnormal cytological findings in specimens from other digestive organs and abdominal cavity (R85.69)
                 carcinoma in situ of anus (histologically confirmed) (D01.3)
                 anal intraepithelial neoplasia I [AIN I] (K62.82)
                 anal intraepithelial neoplasia II [AIN II] (K62.82)
                 anal intraepithelial neoplasia III [AIN III] (D01.3)
                 dysplasia (mild) (moderate) of anus (histologically confirmed) (K62.82)
                 severe dysplasia of anus (histologically confirmed) (D01.3)

       | Excludes2 | anal high risk human papillomavirus (HPV) DNA test positive (R85.81)
                 anal low risk human papillomavirus (HPV) DNA test positive (R85.82)

       R85.610   Atypical squamous cells of undetermined significance on cytologic smear of anus (ASC-US)

       R85.611   Atypical squamous cells cannot exclude high grade squamous intraepithelial lesion on cytologic smear of anus (ASC-H)

       R85.612   Low grade squamous intraepithelial lesion on cytologic smear of anus (LGSIL)

       R85.613   High grade squamous intraepithelial lesion on cytologic smear of anus (HGSIL)

    R85.614   **Cytologic evidence of malignancy on smear of anus**

    R85.615   **Unsatisfactory cytologic smear of anus**
              Inadequate sample of cytologic smear of anus

    R85.616   **Satisfactory anal smear but lacking transformation zone**

    R85.618   **Other abnormal cytological findings on specimens from anus**

    R85.619   **Unspecified abnormal cytological findings in specimens from anus**
              Abnormal anal cytology NOS
              Atypical glandular cells of anus NOS

  R85.69   **Abnormal cytological findings in specimens from other digestive organs and abdominal cavity**

R85.7   **Abnormal histological findings in specimens from digestive organs and abdominal cavity**

● R85.8   **Other abnormal findings in specimens from digestive organs and abdominal cavity**

  R85.81   **Anal high risk human papillomavirus (HPV) DNA test positive**
        Excludes1   anogenital warts due to human papillomavirus (HPV) (A63.0)
                 condyloma acuminatum (A63.0)

  R85.82   **Anal low risk human papillomavirus (HPV) DNA test positive**
        Use additional code for associated human papillomavirus (B97.7)

  R85.89   **Other abnormal findings in specimens from digestive organs and abdominal cavity**
        Abnormal chromosomal findings in specimens from digestive organs and abdominal cavity

R85.9   **Unspecified abnormal finding in specimens from digestive organs and abdominal cavity**

● R86   **Abnormal findings in specimens from male genital organs**
    Includes   abnormal findings in prostatic secretions
              abnormal findings in semen, seminal fluid
              abnormal spermatozoa
    Excludes1   azoospermia (N46.0-)
              oligospermia (N46.1-)

R86.0   **Abnormal level of enzymes in specimens from male genital organs**

R86.1   **Abnormal level of hormones in specimens from male genital organs**

R86.2   **Abnormal level of other drugs, medicaments and biological substances in specimens from male genital organs**

R86.3   **Abnormal level of substances chiefly nonmedicinal as to source in specimens from male genital organs**

R86.4   **Abnormal immunological findings in specimens from male genital organs**

R86.5   **Abnormal microbiological findings in specimens from male genital organs**
    Positive culture findings in specimens from male genital organs
    Excludes1   colonization status (Z22.-)

R86.6   **Abnormal cytological findings in specimens from male genital organs**

R86.7   **Abnormal histological findings in specimens from male genital organs**

R86.8   **Other abnormal findings in specimens from male genital organs**
    Abnormal chromosomal findings in specimens from male genital organs

R86.9   **Unspecified abnormal finding in specimens from male genital organs**

● R87   **Abnormal findings in specimens from female genital organs**
    Includes   abnormal findings in secretion and smears from cervix uteri
              abnormal findings in secretion and smears from vagina
              abnormal findings in secretion and smears from vulva

R87.0   **Abnormal level of enzymes in specimens from female genital organs**

R87.1   **Abnormal level of hormones in specimens from female genital organs**

R87.2   **Abnormal level of other drugs, medicaments and biological substances in specimens from female genital organs**

R87.3   **Abnormal level of substances chiefly nonmedicinal as to source in specimens from female genital organs**

R87.4   **Abnormal immunological findings in specimens from female genital organs**

R87.5   **Abnormal microbiological findings in specimens from female genital organs**
    Positive culture findings in specimens from female genital organs
    Excludes1   colonization status (Z22.-)

● R87.6   **Abnormal cytological findings in specimens from female genital organs**

  ● R87.61   **Abnormal cytological findings in specimens from cervix uteri**
        Excludes1   abnormal cytological findings in specimens from other female genital organs (R87.69)
                 abnormal cytological findings in specimens from vagina (R87.62-)
                 carcinoma in situ of cervix uteri (histologically confirmed) (D06.-)
                 cervical intraepithelial neoplasia I [CIN I] (N87.0)
                 cervical intraepithelial neoplasia II [CIN II] (N87.1)
                 cervical intraepithelial neoplasia III [CIN III] (D06.-)
                 dysplasia (mild) (moderate) of cervix uteri (histologically confirmed) (N87.-)
                 severe dysplasia of cervix uteri (histologically confirmed) (D06.-)
        Excludes2   cervical high risk human papillomavirus (HPV) DNA test positive (R87.810)
                 cervical low risk human papillomavirus (HPV) DNA test positive (R87.820)

    R87.610   **Atypical squamous cells of undetermined significance on cytologic smear of cervix (ASC-US)**

    R87.611   **Atypical squamous cells cannot exclude high grade squamous intraepithelial lesion on cytologic smear of cervix (ASC-H)**

    R87.612   **Low grade squamous intraepithelial lesion on cytologic smear of cervix (LGSIL)**

    R87.613   **High grade squamous intraepithelial lesion on cytologic smear of cervix (HGSIL)**

    R87.614   **Cytologic evidence of malignancy on smear of cervix**

R87.615   **Unsatisfactory cytologic smear of cervix**
       Inadequate sample of cytologic smear of cervix

R87.616   **Satisfactory cervical smear but lacking transformation zone**

R87.618   **Other abnormal cytological findings on specimens from cervix uteri**

R87.619   **Unspecified abnormal cytological findings in specimens from cervix uteri**
       Abnormal cervical cytology NOS
       Abnormal Papanicolaou smear of cervix NOS
       Abnormal thin preparation smear of cervix NOS
       Atypical endocervical cells of cervix NOS
       Atypical endometrial cells of cervix NOS
       Atypical glandular cells of cervix NOS

● R87.62   **Abnormal cytological findings in specimens from vagina**
     Use additional code to identify acquired absence of uterus and cervix, if applicable (Z90.71-)

     Excludes1   abnormal cytological findings in specimens from cervix uteri (R87.61-)
       abnormal cytological findings in specimens from other female genital organs (R87.69)
       carcinoma in situ of vagina (histologically confirmed) (D07.2)
       vaginal intraepithelial neoplasia I [VAIN I] (N89.0)
       vaginal intraepithelial neoplasia II [VAIN II] (N89.1)
       vaginal intraepithelial neoplasia III [VAIN III] (D07.2)
       dysplasia (mild) (moderate) of vagina (histologically confirmed) (N89.-)
       severe dysplasia of vagina (histologically confirmed) (D07.2)

     Excludes2   vaginal high risk human papillomavirus (HPV) DNA test positive (R87.811)
       vaginal low risk human papillomavirus (HPV) DNA test positive (R87.821)

R87.620   **Atypical squamous cells of undetermined significance on cytologic smear of vagina (ASC-US)**

R87.621   **Atypical squamous cells cannot exclude high grade squamous intraepithelial lesion on cytologic smear of vagina (ASC-H)**

R87.622   **Low grade squamous intraepithelial lesion on cytologic smear of vagina (LGSIL)**

R87.623   **High grade squamous intraepithelial lesion on cytologic smear of vagina (HGSIL)**

R87.624   **Cytologic evidence of malignancy on smear of vagina**

R87.625   **Unsatisfactory cytologic smear of vagina**
       Inadequate sample of cytologic smear of vagina

R87.628   **Other abnormal cytological findings on specimens from vagina**

R87.629   **Unspecified abnormal cytological findings in specimens from vagina**
       Abnormal Papanicolaou smear of vagina NOS
       Abnormal thin preparation smear of vagina NOS
       Abnormal vaginal cytology NOS
       Atypical endocervical cells of vagina NOS
       Atypical endometrial cells of vagina NOS
       Atypical glandular cells of vagina NOS

R87.69   **Abnormal cytological findings in specimens from other female genital organs**
       Abnormal cytological findings in specimens from female genital organs NOS
     Excludes1   dysplasia of vulva (histologically confirmed) (N90.0-N90.3)

R87.7   **Abnormal histological findings in specimens from female genital organs**
     Excludes1   carcinoma in situ (histologically confirmed) of female genital organs (D06-D07.3)
       cervical intraepithelial neoplasia I [CIN I] (N87.0)
       cervical intraepithelial neoplasia II [CIN II] (N87.1)
       cervical intraepithelial neoplasia III [CIN III] (D06.-)
       dysplasia (mild) (moderate) of cervix uteri (histologically confirmed) (N87.-)
       dysplasia (mild) (moderate) of vagina (histologically confirmed) (N89.-)
       vaginal intraepithelial neoplasia I [VAIN I] (N89.0)
       vaginal intraepithelial neoplasia II [VAIN II] (N89.1)
       vaginal intraepithelial neoplasia III [VAIN III] (D07.2)
       severe dysplasia of cervix uteri (histologically confirmed) (D06.-)
       severe dysplasia of vagina (histologically confirmed) (D07.2)

● R87.8   **Other abnormal findings in specimens from female genital organs**

● R87.81   **High risk human papillomavirus (HPV) DNA test positive from female genital organs**
     Excludes1   anogenital warts due to human papillomavirus (HPV) (A63.0)
       condyloma acuminatum (A63.0)

R87.810   **Cervical high risk human papillomavirus (HPV) DNA test positive**

R87.811   **Vaginal high risk human papillomavirus (HPV) DNA test positive**

● R87.82   **Low risk human papillomavirus (HPV) DNA test positive from female genital organs**
     Use additional code for associated human papillomavirus (B97.7)

R87.820   **Cervical low risk human papillomavirus (HPV) DNA test positive**

R87.821   **Vaginal low risk human papillomavirus (HPV) DNA test positive**

R87.89   **Other abnormal findings in specimens from female genital organs**
       Abnormal chromosomal findings in specimens from female genital organs

R87.9   **Unspecified abnormal finding in specimens from female genital organs**

● **R88   Abnormal findings in other body fluids and substances**

    R88.0   Cloudy (hemodialysis) (peritoneal) dialysis effluent

    R88.8   Abnormal findings in other body fluids and substances

● **R89   Abnormal findings in specimens from other organs, systems and tissues**

> **Includes**   abnormal findings in nipple discharge
> abnormal findings in synovial fluid
> abnormal findings in wound secretions

    R89.0   **Abnormal level of enzymes in specimens from other organs, systems and tissues**

    R89.1   **Abnormal level of hormones in specimens from other organs, systems and tissues**

    R89.2   **Abnormal level of other drugs, medicaments and biological substances in specimens from other organs, systems and tissues**

    R89.3   **Abnormal level of substances chiefly nonmedicinal as to source in specimens from other organs, systems and tissues**

    R89.4   **Abnormal immunological findings in specimens from other organs, systems and tissues**

    R89.5   **Abnormal microbiological findings in specimens from other organs, systems and tissues**

> Positive culture findings in specimens from other organs, systems and tissues

> **Excludes1**   colonization status (Z22.-)

    R89.6   **Abnormal cytological findings in specimens from other organs, systems and tissues**

    R89.7   **Abnormal histological findings in specimens from other organs, systems and tissues**

    R89.8   **Other abnormal findings in specimens from other organs, systems and tissues**

> Abnormal chromosomal findings in specimens from other organs, systems and tissues

    R89.9   **Unspecified abnormal finding in specimens from other organs, systems and tissues**

ABNORMAL FINDINGS ON DIAGNOSTIC IMAGING AND IN FUNCTION STUDIES, WITHOUT DIAGNOSIS (R90-R94)

> **Includes**   nonspecific abnormal findings on diagnostic imaging by computerized axial tomography [CAT scan]
> nonspecific abnormal findings on diagnostic imaging by magnetic resonance imaging [MRI][NMR]
> nonspecific abnormal findings on diagnostic imaging by positron emission tomography [PET scan]
> nonspecific abnormal findings on diagnostic imaging by thermography
> nonspecific abnormal findings on diagnostic imaging by ultrasound [echogram]
> nonspecific abnormal findings on diagnostic imaging by X-ray examination

> **Excludes1**   abnormal findings on antenatal screening of mother (O28.-)
> diagnostic abnormal findings classified elsewhere - see Alphabetical Index

● **R90   Abnormal findings on diagnostic imaging of central nervous system**

    R90.0   **Intracranial space-occupying lesion found on diagnostic imaging of central nervous system**

  ● R90.8   **Other abnormal findings on diagnostic imaging of central nervous system**

        R90.81   **Abnormal echoencephalogram**

        R90.82   **White matter disease, unspecified**

        R90.89   **Other abnormal findings on diagnostic imaging of central nervous system**

> Other cerebrovascular abnormality found on diagnostic imaging of central nervous system

● **R91   Abnormal findings on diagnostic imaging of lung**

    R91.1   **Solitary pulmonary nodule**

> Coin lesion lung
> Solitary pulmonary nodule, subsegmental branch of the bronchial tree

    R91.8   **Other nonspecific abnormal finding of lung field**

> Lung mass NOS found on diagnostic imaging of lung
> Pulmonary infiltrate NOS
> Shadow, lung

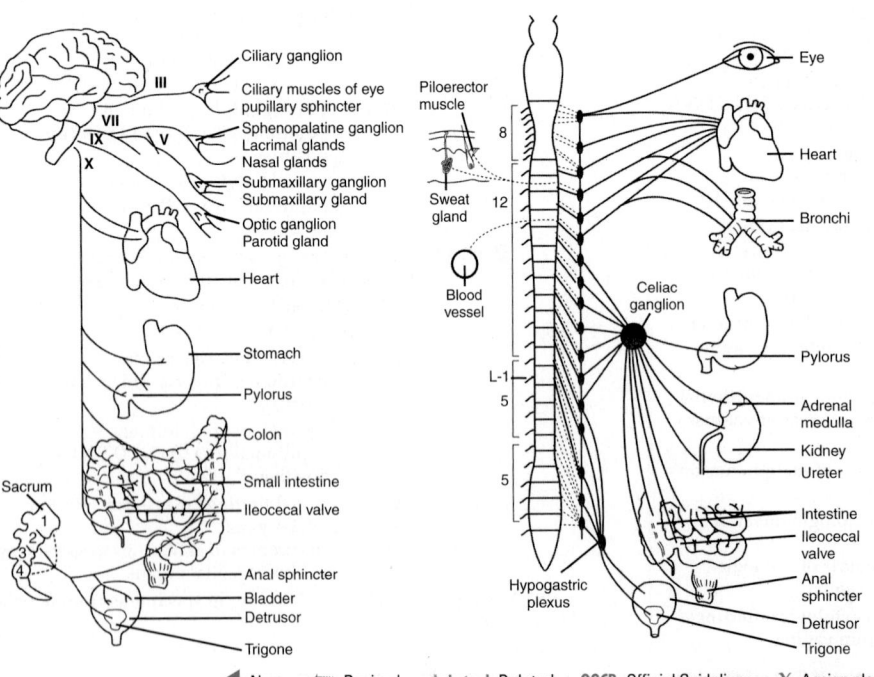

Figure 18-2 A. Parasympathetic nervous system. **B.** Sympathetic nervous system. (From Buck CJ: Step-by-Step Medical Coding, Philadelphia, WB Saunders, 1998)

◀ New   ◀▥ Revised   ~~deleted~~ Deleted   **OGCR** Official Guidelines   X Assign placeholder X   ● Use Additional Character(s)

Excludes 1   Excludes 2   Includes   Use additional   Code first   Code also   Unspecified

● **R92   Abnormal and inconclusive findings on diagnostic imaging of breast**

    R92.0   Mammographic microcalcification found on diagnostic imaging of breast

        Excludes2 mammographic calcification (calculus) found on diagnostic imaging of breast (R92.1)

    R92.1   Mammographic calcification found on diagnostic imaging of breast

        Mammographic calculus found on diagnostic imaging of breast

    R92.2   Inconclusive mammogram

        Dense breasts NOS
        Inconclusive mammogram NEC
        Inconclusive mammography due to dense breasts
        Inconclusive mammography NEC

    R92.8   Other abnormal and inconclusive findings on diagnostic imaging of breast

● **R93   Abnormal findings on diagnostic imaging of other body structures**

    R93.0   Abnormal findings on diagnostic imaging of skull and head, not elsewhere classified

        Excludes1 intracranial space-occupying lesion found on diagnostic imaging (R90.0)

    R93.1   Abnormal findings on diagnostic imaging of heart and coronary circulation

        Abnormal echocardiogram NOS
        Abnormal heart shadow

    R93.2   Abnormal findings on diagnostic imaging of liver and biliary tract

        Nonvisualization of gallbladder

    R93.3   Abnormal findings on diagnostic imaging of other parts of digestive tract

    R93.4   Abnormal findings on diagnostic imaging of urinary organs

        Filling defect of bladder found on diagnostic imaging
        Filling defect of kidney found on diagnostic imaging
        Filling defect of ureter found on diagnostic imaging

        Excludes1 hypertrophy of kidney (N28.81)

    R93.5   Abnormal findings on diagnostic imaging of other abdominal regions, including retroperitoneum

    R93.6   Abnormal findings on diagnostic imaging of limbs

        Excludes2 abnormal finding in skin and subcutaneous tissue (R93.8)

    R93.7   Abnormal findings on diagnostic imaging of other parts of musculoskeletal system

        Excludes2 abnormal findings on diagnostic imaging of skull (R93.0)

    R93.8   Abnormal findings on diagnostic imaging of other specified body structures

        Abnormal finding by radioisotope localization of placenta
        Abnormal radiological finding in skin and subcutaneous tissue
        Mediastinal shift

    R93.9   Diagnostic imaging inconclusive due to excess body fat of patient

---

Item 18–1 The **peripheral nervous system** consists of 31 pairs of spinal nerves, 12 pairs of cranial nerves, and the autonomic nerves, which are divided into the parasympathetic and sympathetic nerves. The cranial nerves are: olfactory (I), optic (II), oculomotor (III), trochlear (IV), trigeminal (V), abducens (VI), facial (VII), vestibulocochlear (VIII), glossopharyngeal (IX), vagus (X), accessory (XI), and hypoglossal (XII).

● **R94   Abnormal results of function studies**

    Includes abnormal results of radionuclide [radioisotope] uptake studies
        abnormal results of scintigraphy

  ● **R94.0   Abnormal results of function studies of central nervous system**

    R94.01   Abnormal electroencephalogram [EEG]

    R94.02   Abnormal brain scan

    R94.09   Abnormal results of other function studies of central nervous system

  ● **R94.1   Abnormal results of function studies of peripheral nervous system and special senses**

    ● **R94.11   Abnormal results of function studies of eye**

        R94.110   Abnormal electro-oculogram [EOG]

        R94.111   Abnormal electroretinogram [ERG]
            Abnormal retinal function study

        R94.112   Abnormal visually evoked potential [VEP]

        R94.113   Abnormal oculomotor study

        R94.118   Abnormal results of other function studies of eye

    ● **R94.12   Abnormal results of function studies of ear and other special senses**

        R94.120   Abnormal auditory function study

        R94.121   Abnormal vestibular function study

        R94.128   Abnormal results of other function studies of ear and other special senses

    ● **R94.13   Abnormal results of function studies of peripheral nervous system**

        R94.130   Abnormal response to nerve stimulation, unspecified

        R94.131   Abnormal electromyogram [EMG]

            Excludes1 electromyogram of eye (R94.113)

        R94.138   Abnormal results of other function studies of peripheral nervous system

    R94.2   Abnormal results of pulmonary function studies

        Reduced ventilatory capacity
        Reduced vital capacity

  ● **R94.3   Abnormal results of cardiovascular function studies**

    R94.30   Abnormal result of cardiovascular function study, unspecified

    R94.31   Abnormal electrocardiogram [ECG] [EKG]

        Excludes1 long QT syndrome (I45.81)

    R94.39   Abnormal result of other cardiovascular function study

        Abnormal electrophysiological intracardiac studies
        Abnormal phonocardiogram
        Abnormal vectorcardiogram

    R94.4   Abnormal results of kidney function studies

        Abnormal renal function test

    R94.5   Abnormal results of liver function studies

    R94.6   Abnormal results of thyroid function studies

    R94.7   Abnormal results of other endocrine function studies

        Excludes2 abnormal glucose (R73.0-)

    R94.8   Abnormal results of function studies of other organs and systems

        Abnormal basal metabolic rate [BMR]
        Abnormal bladder function test
        Abnormal splenic function test

CHAPTER 18 (R00-R99)

ABNORMAL TUMOR MARKERS (R97)

● **R97   Abnormal tumor markers**
          Elevated tumor associated antigens [TAA]
          Elevated tumor specific antigens [TSA]

   R97.0   Elevated carcinoembryonic antigen [CEA]

   R97.1   Elevated cancer antigen 125 [CA 125]

   R97.2   Elevated prostate specific antigen [PSA]

   R97.8   Other abnormal tumor markers

ILL-DEFINED AND UNKNOWN CAUSE OF MORTALITY (R99)

R99   Ill-defined and unknown cause of mortality
        Death (unexplained) NOS
        Unspecified cause of mortality

OGCR Section I.C.18.h.

18.6 Death NOS

Code R99, Ill-defined and unknown cause of mortality, is only for
use in the very limited circumstance when a patient who has already
died is brought into the emergency department or other healthcare
facility and is pronounced dead upon arrival. It does not represent the
discharge disposition of death.

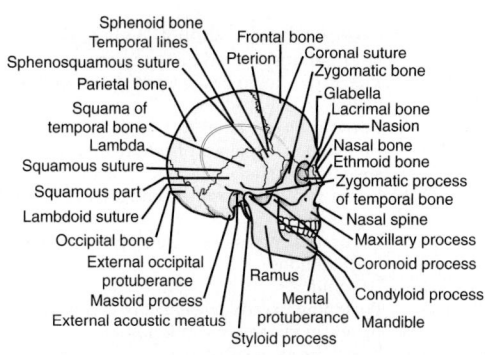

Figure 19-1 Lateral view of skull.

Figure 19-2 Frontal view of skull.

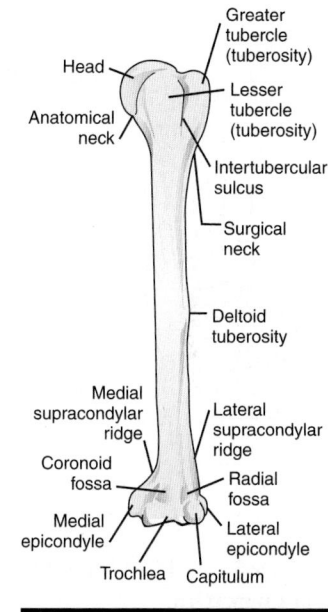

Figure 19-3 Anterior view of vertebral column.

Figure 19-4 Vertebra viewed from above.

Figure 19-5 Anterior view of rib cage.

Figure 19-6 Anterior aspect of left humerus.

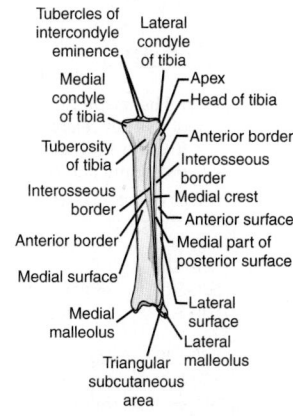

Figure 19-7 Anterior aspect of left radius and ulna.

Figure 19-8 Right hand and wrist: **A.** Dorsal surface. **B.** Palmar surface.

Figure 19-9 Anterior aspect of right femur.

Figure 19-10 Anterior aspect of left tibia and fibula.

◀ New ⬅ Revised ~~deleted~~ Deleted **OGCR** Official Guidelines X Assign placeholder X ● Use Additional Character(s)

Excludes 1   Excludes 2   Includes   Use additional   Code first   Code also   Unspecified

CHAPTER 19 (S00-T88)

1223

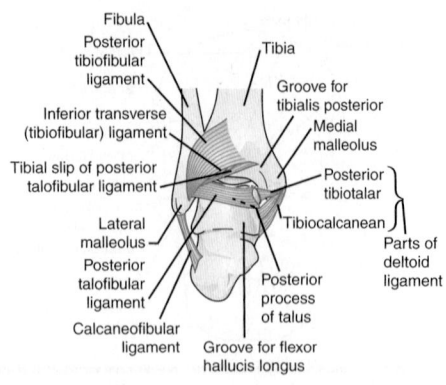

Figure 19-11 Posterior aspect of the left ankle joint.

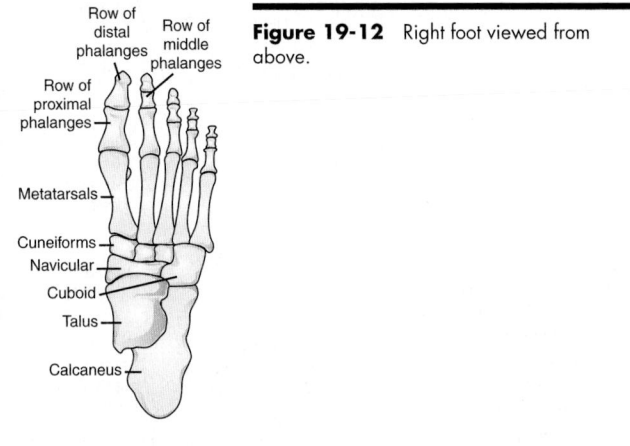

Figure 19-12 Right foot viewed from above.

OGCR See Section I.C., Chapter 19

CHAPTER 19

INJURY, POISONING AND CERTAIN OTHER CONSEQUENCES OF EXTERNAL CAUSES (S00-T88)

Note: Use secondary code(s) from Chapter 20, External causes of morbidity, to indicate cause of injury. Codes within the T section that include the external cause do not require an additional external cause code.

Use additional code to identify any retained foreign body, if applicable (Z18.-)

Excludes1 birth trauma (P10-P15)
obstetric trauma (O70-O71)

Note: The chapter uses the S-section for coding different types of injuries related to single body regions and the T-section to cover injuries to unspecified body regions as well as poisoning and certain other consequences of external causes.

This chapter contains the following blocks:

S00-S09	Injuries to the head
S10-S19	Injuries to the neck
S20-S29	Injuries to the thorax
S30-S39	Injuries to the abdomen, lower back, lumbar spine, pelvis and external genitals
S40-S49	Injuries to the shoulder and upper arm
S50-S59	Injuries to the elbow and forearm
S60-S69	Injuries to the wrist, hand, and fingers
S70-S79	Injuries to the hip and thigh
S80-S89	Injuries to the knee and lower leg
S90-S99	Injuries to the ankle and foot

T07	Injuries involving multiple body regions
T14	Injury of unspecified body region
T15-T19	Effects of foreign body entering through natural orifice
T20-T32	Burns and corrosions
T20-T25	Burns and corrosions of external body surface, specified by site
T26-T28	Burns and corrosions confined to eye and internal organs
T30-T32	Burns and corrosions of multiple and unspecified body regions
T33-T34	Frostbite
T36-T50	Poisoning by, adverse effect of and underdosing of drugs, medicaments and biological substances
T51-T65	Toxic effects of substances chiefly nonmedicinal as to source
T66-T78	Other and unspecified effects of external causes
T79	Certain early complications of trauma
T80-T88	Complications of surgical and medical care, not elsewhere classified

INJURIES TO THE HEAD (S00-S09)

Includes injuries of ear
injuries of eye
injuries of face [any part]
injuries of gum
injuries of jaw
injuries of oral cavity
injuries of palate
injuries of periocular area
injuries of scalp
injuries of temporomandibular joint area
injuries of tongue
injuries of tooth

Code also for any associated infection

Excludes2 burns and corrosions (T20-T32)
effects of foreign body in ear (T16)
effects of foreign body in larynx (T17.3)
effects of foreign body in mouth NOS (T18.0)
effects of foreign body in nose (T17.0-T17.1)
effects of foreign body in pharynx (T17.2)
effects of foreign body on external eye (T15.-)
frostbite (T33-T34)
insect bite or sting, venomous (T63.4)

● **S00 Superficial injury of head**

Excludes1 diffuse cerebral contusion (S06.2-)
focal cerebral contusion (S06.3-)
injury of eye and orbit (S05.-)
open wound of head (S01.-)

The appropriate 7th character is to be added to each code from category S00

A	initial encounter
	All encounters involving diagnosis and treatment
D	subsequent encounter
	Encounters during the healing phase
S	sequela

● **S00.0 Superficial injury of scalp**

X● **S00.00 Unspecified superficial injury of scalp**

X● **S00.01 Abrasion of scalp**

X● **S00.02 Blister (nonthermal) of scalp**

X● **S00.03 Contusion of scalp**
Bruise of scalp
Hematoma of scalp

X● **S00.04 External constriction of part of scalp**

X● **S00.05 Superficial foreign body of scalp**
Splinter in the scalp

X● **S00.06 Insect bite (nonvenomous) of scalp**

X● **S00.07 Other superficial bite of scalp**
Excludes1 open bite of scalp (S01.05)

◀ New   ◀▥ Revised   ~~deleted~~ Deleted   **OGCR** Official Guidelines   X Assign placeholder X   ● Use Additional Character(s)

Excludes 1   Excludes 2   Includes   Use additional   Code first   Code also   Unspecified

CHAPTER 19 (S00-T88)

● S00.1　Contusion of eyelid and periocular area
　　　　Black eye
　　　　Excludes2　contusion of eyeball and orbital tissues
　　　　　　　　　　　(S05.1)
X ● S00.10　Contusion of unspecified eyelid and periocular
　　　　　　area
X ● S00.11　Contusion of right eyelid and periocular area
X ● S00.12　Contusion of left eyelid and periocular area
● S00.2　Other and unspecified superficial injuries of eyelid and
　　　　periocular area
　　　　Excludes2　superficial injury of conjunctiva and
　　　　　　　　　　　cornea (S05.0-)
　● S00.20　Unspecified superficial injury of eyelid and
　　　　　　periocular area
　　　● S00.201　Unspecified superficial injury of right
　　　　　　　　eyelid and periocular area
　　　● S00.202　Unspecified superficial injury of left
　　　　　　　　eyelid and periocular area
　　　● S00.209　Unspecified superficial injury of
　　　　　　　　unspecified eyelid and periocular area
　● S00.21　Abrasion of eyelid and periocular area
　　　● S00.211　Abrasion of right eyelid and
　　　　　　　　periocular area
　　　● S00.212　Abrasion of left eyelid and periocular
　　　　　　　　area
　　　● S00.219　Abrasion of unspecified eyelid and
　　　　　　　　periocular area
　● S00.22　Blister (nonthermal) of eyelid and periocular
　　　　　　area
　　　● S00.221　Blister (nonthermal) of right eyelid
　　　　　　　　and periocular area
　　　● S00.222　Blister (nonthermal) of left eyelid and
　　　　　　　　periocular area
　　　● S00.229　Blister (nonthermal) of unspecified
　　　　　　　　eyelid and periocular area
　● S00.24　External constriction of eyelid and periocular
　　　　　　area
　　　● S00.241　External constriction of right eyelid
　　　　　　　　and periocular area
　　　● S00.242　External constriction of left eyelid
　　　　　　　　and periocular area
　　　● S00.249　External constriction of unspecified
　　　　　　　　eyelid and periocular area
　● S00.25　Superficial foreign body of eyelid and
　　　　　　periocular area
　　　　　　Splinter of eyelid and periocular area
　　　　　　Excludes2　retained foreign body in eyelid
　　　　　　　　　　　　(H02.81-)
　　　● S00.251　Superficial foreign body of right
　　　　　　　　eyelid and periocular area
　　　● S00.252　Superficial foreign body of left eyelid
　　　　　　　　and periocular area
　　　● S00.259　Superficial foreign body of
　　　　　　　　unspecified eyelid and periocular area
　● S00.26　Insect bite (nonvenomous) of eyelid and
　　　　　　periocular area
　　　● S00.261　Insect bite (nonvenomous) of right
　　　　　　　　eyelid and periocular area
　　　● S00.262　Insect bite (nonvenomous) of left
　　　　　　　　eyelid and periocular area
　　　● S00.269　Insect bite (nonvenomous) of
　　　　　　　　unspecified eyelid and periocular area

● S00.27　Other superficial bite of eyelid and periocular
　　　　area
　　　　Excludes1　open bite of eyelid and
　　　　　　　　　　　periocular area (S01.15)
　● S00.271　Other superficial bite of right eyelid
　　　　　　　and periocular area
　● S00.272　Other superficial bite of left eyelid
　　　　　　　and periocular area
　● S00.279　Other superficial bite of unspecified
　　　　　　　eyelid and periocular area
● S00.3　Superficial injury of nose
X ● S00.30　Unspecified superficial injury of nose
X ● S00.31　Abrasion of nose
X ● S00.32　Blister (nonthermal) of nose
X ● S00.33　Contusion of nose
　　　　　Bruise of nose
　　　　　Hematoma of nose
X ● S00.34　External constriction of nose
X ● S00.35　Superficial foreign body of nose
　　　　　Splinter in the nose
X ● S00.36　Insect bite (nonvenomous) of nose
X ● S00.37　Other superficial bite of nose
　　　　　Excludes1　open bite of nose (S01.25)
● S00.4　Superficial injury of ear
　● S00.40　Unspecified superficial injury of ear
　　　● S00.401　Unspecified superficial injury of right
　　　　　　　　ear
　　　● S00.402　Unspecified superficial injury of left
　　　　　　　　ear
　　　● S00.409　Unspecified superficial injury of
　　　　　　　　unspecified ear
　● S00.41　Abrasion of ear
　　　● S00.411　Abrasion of right ear
　　　● S00.412　Abrasion of left ear
　　　● S00.419　Abrasion of unspecified ear
　● S00.42　Blister (nonthermal) of ear
　　　● S00.421　Blister (nonthermal) of right ear
　　　● S00.422　Blister (nonthermal) of left ear
　　　● S00.429　Blister (nonthermal) of unspecified
　　　　　　　　ear
　● S00.43　Contusion of ear
　　　　　Bruise of ear
　　　　　Hematoma of ear
　　　● S00.431　Contusion of right ear
　　　● S00.432　Contusion of left ear
　　　● S00.439　Contusion of unspecified ear
　● S00.44　External constriction of ear
　　　● S00.441　External constriction of right ear
　　　● S00.442　External constriction of left ear
　　　● S00.449　External constriction of unspecified
　　　　　　　　ear
　● S00.45　Superficial foreign body of ear
　　　　　Splinter in the ear
　　　● S00.451　Superficial foreign body of right ear
　　　● S00.452　Superficial foreign body of left ear
　　　● S00.459　Superficial foreign body of
　　　　　　　　unspecified ear
　● S00.46　Insect bite (nonvenomous) of ear
　　　● S00.461　Insect bite (nonvenomous) of right
　　　　　　　　ear
　　　● S00.462　Insect bite (nonvenomous) of left ear
　　　● S00.469　Insect bite (nonvenomous) of
　　　　　　　　unspecified ear

● S00.47   Other superficial bite of ear
    Excludes1   open bite of ear (S01.35)
    ● S00.471   Other superficial bite of right ear
    ● S00.472   Other superficial bite of left ear
    ● S00.479   Other superficial bite of unspecified ear
● S00.5   Superficial injury of lip and oral cavity
  ● S00.50   Unspecified superficial injury of lip and oral cavity
    ● S00.501   Unspecified superficial injury of lip
    ● S00.502   Unspecified superficial injury of oral cavity
  ● S00.51   Abrasion of lip and oral cavity
    ● S00.511   Abrasion of lip
    ● S00.512   Abrasion of oral cavity
  ● S00.52   Blister (nonthermal) of lip and oral cavity
    ● S00.521   Blister (nonthermal) of lip
    ● S00.522   Blister (nonthermal) of oral cavity
  ● S00.53   Contusion of lip and oral cavity
    ● S00.531   Contusion of lip
      Bruise of lip
      Hematoma of oral cavity
    ● S00.532   Contusion of oral cavity
      Bruise of lip
      Hematoma of oral cavity
  ● S00.54   External constriction of lip and oral cavity
    ● S00.541   External constriction of lip
    ● S00.542   External constriction of oral cavity
  ● S00.55   Superficial foreign body of lip and oral cavity
    ● S00.551   Superficial foreign body of lip
      Splinter of lip and oral cavity
    ● S00.552   Superficial foreign body of oral cavity
      Splinter of lip and oral cavity
  ● S00.56   Insect bite (nonvenomous) of lip and oral cavity
    ● S00.561   Insect bite (nonvenomous) of lip
    ● S00.562   Insect bite (nonvenomous) of oral cavity
  ● S00.57   Other superficial bite of lip and oral cavity
    ● S00.571   Other superficial bite of lip
      Excludes1   open bite of lip (S01.551)
    ● S00.572   Other superficial bite of oral cavity
      Excludes1   open bite of oral cavity (S01.552)
● S00.8   Superficial injury of other parts of head
  X ● S00.80   Unspecified superficial injury of other part of head
  X ● S00.81   Abrasion of other part of head
  X ● S00.82   Blister (nonthermal) of other part of head
  X ● S00.83   Contusion of other part of head
    Bruise of other part of head
    Hematoma of other part of head
  X ● S00.84   External constriction of other part of head
  X ● S00.85   Superficial foreign body of other part of head
    Splinter in other part of head
  X ● S00.86   Insect bite (nonvenomous) of other part of head
  X ● S00.87   Other superficial bite of other part of head
    Excludes1   open bite of other part of head (S01.85)
● S00.9   Superficial injury of unspecified part of head
  X ● S00.90   Unspecified superficial injury of unspecified part of head
  X ● S00.91   Abrasion of unspecified part of head
  X ● S00.92   Blister (nonthermal) of unspecified part of head
  X ● S00.93   Contusion of unspecified part of head
    Bruise of head
    Hematoma of head

X ● S00.94   External constriction of unspecified part of head
X ● S00.95   Superficial foreign body of unspecified part of head
    Splinter of head
X ● S00.96   Insect bite (nonvenomous) of unspecified part of head
X ● S00.97   Other superficial bite of unspecified part of head
    Excludes1   open bite of head (S01.95)

● S01   Open wound of head
  Code also any associated:
    injury of cranial nerve (S04.-)
    injury of muscle and tendon of head (S09.1-)
    intracranial injury (S06.-)
    wound infection
    Excludes1   open skull fracture (S02.- with 7th character B)
    Excludes2   injury of eye and orbit (S05.-)
      traumatic amputation of part of head (S08.-)
  The appropriate 7th character is to be added to each code from category S01

    A   initial encounter
    D   subsequent encounter
    S   sequela

  ● S01.0   Open wound of scalp
    Excludes1   avulsion of scalp (S08.0)
    X ● S01.00   Unspecified open wound of scalp
    X ● S01.01   Laceration without foreign body of scalp
    X ● S01.02   Laceration with foreign body of scalp
    X ● S01.03   Puncture wound without foreign body of scalp
    X ● S01.04   Puncture wound with foreign body of scalp
    X ● S01.05   Open bite of scalp
      Bite of scalp NOS
      Excludes1   superficial bite of scalp (S00.06, S00.07-)

  ● S01.1   Open wound of eyelid and periocular area
    Open wound of eyelid and periocular area with or without involvement of lacrimal passages
    ● S01.10   Unspecified open wound of eyelid and periocular area
      ● S01.101   Unspecified open wound of right eyelid and periocular area
      ● S01.102   Unspecified open wound of left eyelid and periocular area
      ● S01.109   Unspecified open wound of unspecified eyelid and periocular area
    ● S01.11   Laceration without foreign body of eyelid and periocular area
      ● S01.111   Laceration without foreign body of right eyelid and periocular area
      ● S01.112   Laceration without foreign body of left eyelid and periocular area
      ● S01.119   Laceration without foreign body of unspecified eyelid and periocular area
    ● S01.12   Laceration with foreign body of eyelid and periocular area
      ● S01.121   Laceration with foreign body of right eyelid and periocular area
      ● S01.122   Laceration with foreign body of left eyelid and periocular area
      ● S01.129   Laceration with foreign body of unspecified eyelid and periocular area

◀ New   ◀▥ Revised   ~~deleted~~ Deleted   **OGCR** Official Guidelines   X Assign placeholder X   ● Use Additional Character(s)
Excludes 1   Excludes 2   Includes   Use additional   Code first   Code also   Unspecified

● **S01.13**   Puncture wound without foreign body of eyelid and periocular area

     ● **S01.131**   Puncture wound without foreign body of right eyelid and periocular area

     ● **S01.132**   Puncture wound without foreign body of left eyelid and periocular area

     ● **S01.139**   Puncture wound without foreign body of unspecified eyelid and periocular area

● **S01.14**   Puncture wound with foreign body of eyelid and periocular area

     ● **S01.141**   Puncture wound with foreign body of right eyelid and periocular area

     ● **S01.142**   Puncture wound with foreign body of left eyelid and periocular area

     ● **S01.149**   Puncture wound with foreign body of unspecified eyelid and periocular area

● **S01.15**   Open bite of eyelid and periocular area

     Bite of eyelid and periocular area NOS

     | **Excludes1** | superficial bite of eyelid and periocular area (S00.26, S00.27)

     ● **S01.151**   Open bite of right eyelid and periocular area

     ● **S01.152**   Open bite of left eyelid and periocular area

     ● **S01.159**   Open bite of unspecified eyelid and periocular area

● **S01.2**   Open wound of nose

  X ● **S01.20**   Unspecified open wound of nose

  X ● **S01.21**   Laceration without foreign body of nose

  X ● **S01.22**   Laceration with foreign body of nose

  X ● **S01.23**   Puncture wound without foreign body of nose

  X ● **S01.24**   Puncture wound with foreign body of nose

  X ● **S01.25**   Open bite of nose

     Bite of nose NOS

     | **Excludes1** | superficial bite of nose (S00.36, S00.37)

● **S01.3**   Open wound of ear

     ● **S01.30**   Unspecified open wound of ear

       ● **S01.301**   Unspecified open wound of right ear

       ● **S01.302**   Unspecified open wound of left ear

       ● **S01.309**   Unspecified open wound of unspecified ear

     ● **S01.31**   Laceration without foreign body of ear

       ● **S01.311**   Laceration without foreign body of right ear

       ● **S01.312**   Laceration without foreign body of left ear

       ● **S01.319**   Laceration without foreign body of unspecified ear

     ● **S01.32**   Laceration with foreign body of ear

       ● **S01.321**   Laceration with foreign body of right ear

       ● **S01.322**   Laceration with foreign body of left ear

       ● **S01.329**   Laceration with foreign body of unspecified ear

     ● **S01.33**   Puncture wound without foreign body of ear

       ● **S01.331**   Puncture wound without foreign body of right ear

       ● **S01.332**   Puncture wound without foreign body of left ear

       ● **S01.339**   Puncture wound without foreign body of unspecified ear

● **S01.34**   Puncture wound with foreign body of ear

     ● **S01.341**   Puncture wound with foreign body of right ear

     ● **S01.342**   Puncture wound with foreign body of left ear

     ● **S01.349**   Puncture wound with foreign body of unspecified ear

● **S01.35**   Open bite of ear

     Bite of ear NOS

     | **Excludes1** | superficial bite of ear (S00.46, S00.47)

     ● **S01.351**   Open bite of right ear

     ● **S01.352**   Open bite of left ear

     ● **S01.359**   Open bite of unspecified ear

● **S01.4**   Open wound of cheek and temporomandibular area

     ● **S01.40**   Unspecified open wound of cheek and temporomandibular area

       ● **S01.401**   Unspecified open wound of right cheek and temporomandibular area

       ● **S01.402**   Unspecified open wound of left cheek and temporomandibular area

       ● **S01.409**   Unspecified open wound of unspecified cheek and temporomandibular area

     ● **S01.41**   Laceration without foreign body of cheek and temporomandibular area

       ● **S01.411**   Laceration without foreign body of right cheek and temporomandibular area

       ● **S01.412**   Laceration without foreign body of left cheek and temporomandibular area

       ● **S01.419**   Laceration without foreign body of unspecified cheek and temporomandibular area

     ● **S01.42**   Laceration with foreign body of cheek and temporomandibular area

       ● **S01.421**   Laceration with foreign body of right cheek and temporomandibular area

       ● **S01.422**   Laceration with foreign body of left cheek and temporomandibular area

       ● **S01.429**   Laceration with foreign body of unspecified cheek and temporomandibular area

     ● **S01.43**   Puncture wound without foreign body of cheek and temporomandibular area

       ● **S01.431**   Puncture wound without foreign body of right cheek and temporomandibular area

       ● **S01.432**   Puncture wound without foreign body of left cheek and temporomandibular area

       ● **S01.439**   Puncture wound without foreign body of unspecified cheek and temporomandibular area

     ● **S01.44**   Puncture wound with foreign body of cheek and temporomandibular area

       ● **S01.441**   Puncture wound with foreign body of right cheek and temporomandibular area

       ● **S01.442**   Puncture wound with foreign body of left cheek and temporomandibular area

       ● **S01.449**   Puncture wound with foreign body of unspecified cheek and temporomandibular area

● **S01.45**   **Open bite of cheek and temporomandibular area**
     Bite of cheek and temporomandibular area NOS
     | **Excludes2** | superficial bite of cheek and temporomandibular area (S00.86, S00.87) |

    ● **S01.451**   Open bite of right cheek and temporomandibular area
    ● **S01.452**   Open bite of left cheek and temporomandibular area
    ● **S01.459**   Open bite of unspecified cheek and temporomandibular area

● **S01.5**   **Open wound of lip and oral cavity**
     | **Excludes2** | tooth dislocation (S03.2) |
     | | tooth fracture (S02.5) |

   ● **S01.50**   Unspecified open wound of lip and oral cavity
    ● **S01.501**   Unspecified open wound of lip
    ● **S01.502**   Unspecified open wound of oral cavity

   ● **S01.51**   Laceration of lip and oral cavity without foreign body
    ● **S01.511**   Laceration without foreign body of lip
    ● **S01.512**   Laceration without foreign body of oral cavity

   ● **S01.52**   Laceration of lip and oral cavity with foreign body
    ● **S01.521**   Laceration with foreign body of lip
    ● **S01.522**   Laceration with foreign body of oral cavity

   ● **S01.53**   Puncture wound of lip and oral cavity without foreign body
    ● **S01.531**   Puncture wound without foreign body of lip
    ● **S01.532**   Puncture wound without foreign body of oral cavity

   ● **S01.54**   Puncture wound of lip and oral cavity with foreign body
    ● **S01.541**   Puncture wound with foreign body of lip
    ● **S01.542**   Puncture wound with foreign body of oral cavity

   ● **S01.55**   Open bite of lip and oral cavity
    ● **S01.551**   Open bite of lip
      Bite of lip NOS
      | **Excludes1** | superficial bite of lip (S00.571) |
    ● **S01.552**   Open bite of oral cavity
      Bite of oral cavity NOS
      | **Excludes1** | superficial bite of oral cavity (S00.572) |

● **S01.8**   **Open wound of other parts of head**
   X ● **S01.80**   Unspecified open wound of other part of head
   X ● **S01.81**   Laceration without foreign body of other part of head
   X ● **S01.82**   Laceration with foreign body of other part of head
   X ● **S01.83**   Puncture wound without foreign body of other part of head
   X ● **S01.84**   Puncture wound with foreign body of other part of head
   X ● **S01.85**   Open bite of other part of head
     Bite of other part of head NOS
     | **Excludes1** | superficial bite of other part of head (S00.85) |

● **S01.9**   **Open wound of unspecified part of head**
   X ● **S01.90**   Unspecified open wound of unspecified part of head
   X ● **S01.91**   Laceration without foreign body of unspecified part of head
   X ● **S01.92**   Laceration with foreign body of unspecified part of head
   X ● **S01.93**   Puncture wound without foreign body of unspecified part of head
   X ● **S01.94**   Puncture wound with foreign body of unspecified part of head
   X ● **S01.95**   Open bite of unspecified part of head
     Bite of head NOS
     | **Excludes1** | superficial bite of head NOS (S00.97) |

● **S02**   **Fracture of skull and facial bones**
   Note: A fracture not indicated as open or closed should be coded to closed
     The appropriate 7th character is to be added to each code from category S02

A	initial encounter for closed fracture
B	initial encounter for open fracture
D	subsequent encounter for fracture with routine healing
G	subsequent encounter for fracture with delayed healing
K	subsequent encounter for fracture with nonunion
S	sequela

   Code also any associated intracranial injury (S06.-)

   X ● **S02.0**   **Fracture of vault of skull**
     Fracture of frontal bone
     Fracture of parietal bone

   ● **S02.1**   **Fracture of base of skull**
     | **Excludes1** | orbit NOS (S02.8) |
     | **Excludes2** | orbital floor (S02.3-) |

    X ● **S02.10**   Unspecified fracture of base of skull
    ● **S02.11**   Fracture of occiput
     ● **S02.110**   Type I occipital condyle fracture
     ● **S02.111**   Type II occipital condyle fracture
     ● **S02.112**   Type III occipital condyle fracture
     ● **S02.113**   Unspecified occipital condyle fracture
     ● **S02.118**   Other fracture of occiput
     ● **S02.119**   Unspecified fracture of occiput
    X ● **S02.19**   Other fracture of base of skull
     Fracture of anterior fossa of base of skull
     Fracture of ethmoid sinus
     Fracture of frontal sinus
     Fracture of middle fossa of base of skull
     Fracture of orbital roof
     Fracture of posterior fossa of base of skull
     Fracture of sphenoid
     Fracture of temporal bone

   X ● **S02.2**   **Fracture of nasal bones**
   X ● **S02.3**   **Fracture of orbital floor**
     | **Excludes1** | orbit NOS (S02.8) |
     | **Excludes2** | orbital roof (S02.1-) |

   ● **S02.4**   **Fracture of malar, maxillary and zygoma bones**
     Fracture of superior maxilla
     Fracture of upper jaw (bone)
     Fracture of zygomatic process of temporal bone

    ● **S02.40**   Fracture of malar, maxillary and zygoma bones, unspecified
     ● **S02.400**   Malar fracture unspecified
     ● **S02.401**   Maxillary fracture, unspecified
     ● **S02.402**   Zygomatic fracture, unspecified

● **S02.41**   **LeFort fracture**
   ● **S02.411**   **LeFort I fracture**
   ● **S02.412**   **LeFort II fracture**
   ● **S02.413**   **LeFort III fracture**
X● **S02.42**   **Fracture of alveolus of maxilla**
X● **S02.5**   **Fracture of tooth (traumatic) Broken tooth**
    Excludes1   cracked tooth (nontraumatic) (K03.81)

● **S02.6**   **Fracture of mandible**
    Fracture of lower jaw (bone)
  ● **S02.60**   **Fracture of mandible of unspecified site**
   ● **S02.600**   **Fracture of unspecified part of body of mandible**
   ● **S02.609**   **Fracture of mandible, unspecified**
  X● **S02.61**   **Fracture of condylar process of mandible**
  X● **S02.62**   **Fracture of subcondylar process of mandible**
  X● **S02.63**   **Fracture of coronoid process of mandible**
  X● **S02.64**   **Fracture of ramus of mandible**
  X● **S02.65**   **Fracture of angle of mandible**
  X● **S02.66**   **Fracture of symphysis of mandible**
  X● **S02.67**   **Fracture of alveolus of mandible**
  X● **S02.69**   **Fracture of mandible of other specified site**
X● **S02.8**   **Fractures of other specified skull and facial bones**
    Fracture of orbit NOS
    Fracture of palate
    Excludes1   fracture of orbital floor (S02.3-)
              fracture of orbital roof (S02.1-)
● **S02.9**   **Fracture of unspecified skull and facial bones**
  X● **S02.91**   **Unspecified fracture of skull**
  X● **S02.92**   **Unspecified fracture of facial bones**

● **S03**   **Dislocation and sprain of joints and ligaments of head**
    Includes   avulsion of joint (capsule) or ligament of head
              laceration of cartilage, joint (capsule) or ligament of head
              sprain of cartilage, joint (capsule) or ligament of head
              traumatic hemarthrosis of joint or ligament of head
              traumatic rupture of joint or ligament of head
              traumatic subluxation of joint or ligament of head
              traumatic tear of joint or ligament of head
    Code also any associated open wound
    Excludes2   Strain of muscle or tendon of head (S09.1)
    The appropriate 7th character is to be added to each code from category S03

    A   initial encounter
    D   subsequent encounter
    S   sequela

  X● **S03.0**   **Dislocation of jaw**
      Dislocation of jaw (cartilage) (meniscus)
      Dislocation of mandible
      Dislocation of temporomandibular (joint)
  X● **S03.1**   **Dislocation of septal cartilage of nose**
  X● **S03.2**   **Dislocation of tooth**
  X● **S03.4**   **Sprain of jaw**
      Sprain of temporomandibular (joint) (ligament)
  X● **S03.8**   **Sprain of joints and ligaments of other parts of head**
  X● **S03.9**   **Sprain of joints and ligaments of unspecified parts of head**

● **S04**   **Injury of cranial nerve**
    The selection of side should be based on the side of the body being affected
    Code first any associated intracranial injury (S06.-)
    Code also any associated:
      open wound of head (S01.-)
      skull fracture (S02.-)
    The appropriate 7th character is to be added to each code from category S04

    A   initial encounter
    D   subsequent encounter
    S   sequela

● **S04.0**   **Injury of optic nerve and pathways**
    Use additional code to identify any visual field defect or blindness (H53.4-, H54)
  ● **S04.01**   **Injury of optic nerve**
      Injury of 2nd cranial nerve
   ● **S04.011**   **Injury of optic nerve, right eye**
   ● **S04.012**   **Injury of optic nerve, left eye**
   ● **S04.019**   **Injury of optic nerve, unspecified eye**
       Injury of optic nerve NOS
  X● **S04.02**   **Injury of optic chiasm**
  ● **S04.03**   **Injury of optic tract and pathways**
      Injury of optic radiation
   ● **S04.031**   **Injury of optic tract and pathways, right eye**
   ● **S04.032**   **Injury of optic tract and pathways, left eye**
   ● **S04.039**   **Injury of optic tract and pathways, unspecified eye**
       Injury of optic tract and pathways NOS
  ● **S04.04**   **Injury of visual cortex**
   ● **S04.041**   **Injury of visual cortex, right eye**
   ● **S04.042**   **Injury of visual cortex, left eye**
   ● **S04.049**   **Injury of visual cortex, unspecified eye**
       Injury of visual cortex NOS
● **S04.1**   **Injury of oculomotor nerve**
    Injury of 3rd cranial nerve
  X● **S04.10**   **Injury of oculomotor nerve, unspecified side**
  X● **S04.11**   **Injury of oculomotor nerve, right side**
  X● **S04.12**   **Injury of oculomotor nerve, left side**
● **S04.2**   **Injury of trochlear nerve**
    Injury of 4th cranial nerve
  X● **S04.20**   **Injury of trochlear nerve, unspecified side**
  X● **S04.21**   **Injury of trochlear nerve, right side**
  X● **S04.22**   **Injury of trochlear nerve, left side**
● **S04.3**   **Injury of trigeminal nerve**
    Injury of 5th cranial nerve
  X● **S04.30**   **Injury of trigeminal nerve, unspecified side**
  X● **S04.31**   **Injury of trigeminal nerve, right side**
  X● **S04.32**   **Injury of trigeminal nerve, left side**
● **S04.4**   **Injury of abducent nerve**
    Injury of 6th cranial nerve
  X● **S04.40**   **Injury of abducent nerve, unspecified side**
  X● **S04.41**   **Injury of abducent nerve, right side**
  X● **S04.42**   **Injury of abducent nerve, left side**
● **S04.5**   **Injury of facial nerve**
    Injury of 7th cranial nerve
  X● **S04.50**   **Injury of facial nerve, unspecified side**
  X● **S04.51**   **Injury of facial nerve, right side**
  X● **S04.52**   **Injury of facial nerve, left side**

CHAPTER 19 (S00-T88)

● **S04.6**   **Injury of acoustic nerve**
     Injury of auditory nerve
     Injury of 8th cranial nerve
   X● **S04.60**   Injury of acoustic nerve, unspecified side
   X● **S04.61**   Injury of acoustic nerve, right side
   X● **S04.62**   Injury of acoustic nerve, left side

● **S04.7**   **Injury of accessory nerve**
     Injury of 11th cranial nerve
   X● **S04.70**   Injury of accessory nerve, unspecified side
   X● **S04.71**   Injury of accessory nerve, right side
   X● **S04.72**   Injury of accessory nerve, left side

● **S04.8**   **Injury of other cranial nerves**
   ● **S04.81**   **Injury of olfactory [1st] nerve**
     ● S04.811   Injury of olfactory [1st] nerve, right side
     ● S04.812   Injury of olfactory [1st] nerve, left side
     ● S04.819   Injury of olfactory [1st] nerve, unspecified side
   ● **S04.89**   **Injury of other cranial nerves**
     Injury of vagus [10th] nerve
     ● S04.891   Injury of other cranial nerves, right side
     ● S04.892   Injury of other cranial nerves, left side
     ● S04.899   Injury of other cranial nerves, unspecified side

   X● **S04.9**   **Injury of unspecified cranial nerve**

● **S05**   **Injury of eye and orbit**
   Includes   open wound of eye and orbit
   Excludes2   2nd cranial [optic] nerve injury (S04.0-)
        3rd cranial [oculomotor] nerve injury (S04.1-)
        open wound of eyelid and periocular area (S01.1-)
        orbital bone fracture (S02.1-, S02.3-, S02.8-)
        superficial injury of eyelid (S00.1-S00.2)

   The appropriate 7th character is to be added to each code from category S05

     A   initial encounter
     D   subsequent encounter
     S   sequela

   ● **S05.0**   **Injury of conjunctiva and corneal abrasion without foreign body**
     Excludes1   foreign body in conjunctival sac (T15.1)
         foreign body in cornea (T15.0)
     X● **S05.00**   Injury of conjunctiva and corneal abrasion without foreign body, unspecified eye
     X● **S05.01**   Injury of conjunctiva and corneal abrasion without foreign body, right eye
     X● **S05.02**   Injury of conjunctiva and corneal abrasion without foreign body, left eye

   ● **S05.1**   **Contusion of eyeball and orbital tissues**
     Traumatic hyphema
     Excludes2   black eye NOS (S00.1)
         contusion of eyelid and periocular area (S00.1)
     X● **S05.10**   Contusion of eyeball and orbital tissues, unspecified eye
     X● **S05.11**   Contusion of eyeball and orbital tissues, right eye
     X● **S05.12**   Contusion of eyeball and orbital tissues, left eye

● **S05.2**   **Ocular laceration and rupture with prolapse or loss of intraocular tissue**
   X● **S05.20**   Ocular laceration and rupture with prolapse or loss of intraocular tissue, unspecified eye
   X● **S05.21**   Ocular laceration and rupture with prolapse or loss of intraocular tissue, right eye
   X● **S05.22**   Ocular laceration and rupture with prolapse or loss of intraocular tissue, left eye

● **S05.3**   **Ocular laceration without prolapse or loss of intraocular tissue**
   Laceration of eye NOS
   X● **S05.30**   Ocular laceration without prolapse or loss of intraocular tissue, unspecified eye
   X● **S05.31**   Ocular laceration without prolapse or loss of intraocular tissue, right eye
   X● **S05.32**   Ocular laceration without prolapse or loss of intraocular tissue, left eye

● **S05.4**   **Penetrating wound of orbit with or without foreign body**
   Excludes2   retained (old) foreign body following penetrating wound in orbit (H05.5-)
   X● **S05.40**   Penetrating wound of orbit with or without foreign body, unspecified eye
   X● **S05.41**   Penetrating wound of orbit with or without foreign body, right eye
   X● **S05.42**   Penetrating wound of orbit with or without foreign body, left eye

● **S05.5**   **Penetrating wound with foreign body of eyeball**
   Excludes2   retained (old) intraocular foreign body (H44.6-, H44.7)
   X● **S05.50**   Penetrating wound with foreign body of unspecified eyeball
   X● **S05.51**   Penetrating wound with foreign body of right eyeball
   X● **S05.52**   Penetrating wound with foreign body of left eyeball

● **S05.6**   **Penetrating wound without foreign body of eyeball**
   Ocular penetration NOS
   X● **S05.60**   Penetrating wound without foreign body of unspecified eyeball
   X● **S05.61**   Penetrating wound without foreign body of right eyeball
   X● **S05.62**   Penetrating wound without foreign body of left eyeball

● **S05.7**   **Avulsion of eye**
   Traumatic enucleation
   X● **S05.70**   Avulsion of unspecified eye
   X● **S05.71**   Avulsion of right eye
   X● **S05.72**   Avulsion of left eye

● **S05.8**   **Other injuries of eye and orbit**
   Lacrimal duct injury
   ● **S05.8X**   **Other injuries of eye and orbit**
     ● S05.8X1   Other injuries of right eye and orbit
     ● S05.8X2   Other injuries of left eye and orbit
     ● S05.8X9   Other injuries of unspecified eye and orbit

● **S05.9**   **Unspecified injury of eye and orbit**
   Injury of eye NOS
   X● **S05.90**   Unspecified injury of unspecified eye and orbit
   X● **S05.91**   Unspecified injury of right eye and orbit
   X● **S05.92**   Unspecified injury of left eye and orbit

● S06   **Intracranial injury**

Includes   traumatic brain injury

Code also any associated:
open wound of head (S01.-)
skull fracture (S02.-)

Excludes1   head injury NOS (S09.90)

The appropriate 7th character is to be added to each code from category S06

A   initial encounter
D   subsequent encounter
S   sequela

● **S06.0   Concussion**
Commotio cerebri

Excludes1   concussion with other intracranial injuries classified in category S06- code to specified intracranial injury

● **S06.0X   Concussion**

● **S06.0X0   Concussion without loss of consciousness**

● **S06.0X1   Concussion with loss of consciousness of 30 minutes or less**

● **S06.0X2   Concussion with loss of consciousness of 31 minutes to 59 minutes**

● **S06.0X3   Concussion with loss of consciousness of 1 hour to 5 hours 59 minutes**

● **S06.0X4   Concussion with loss of consciousness of 6 hours to 24 hours**

● **S06.0X5   Concussion with loss of consciousness greater than 24 hours with return to pre-existing conscious level**

● **S06.0X6   Concussion with loss of consciousness greater than 24 hours without return to pre-existing conscious level with patient surviving**

● **S06.0X7   Concussion with loss of consciousness of any duration with death due to brain injury prior to regaining consciousness**

● **S06.0X8   Concussion with loss of consciousness of any duration with death due to other cause prior to regaining consciousness**

● **S06.0X9   Concussion with loss of consciousness of unspecified duration**
Concussion NOS

● **S06.1   Traumatic cerebral edema**
Diffuse traumatic cerebral edema
Focal traumatic cerebral edema

● **S06.1X   Traumatic cerebral edema**

● **S06.1X0   Traumatic cerebral edema without loss of consciousness**

● **S06.1X1   Traumatic cerebral edema with loss of consciousness of 30 minutes or less**

● **S06.1X2   Traumatic cerebral edema with loss of consciousness of 31 minutes to 59 minutes**

● **S06.1X3   Traumatic cerebral edema with loss of consciousness of 1 hour to 5 hours 59 minutes**

● **S06.1X4   Traumatic cerebral edema with loss of consciousness of 6 hours to 24 hours**

● **S06.1X5   Traumatic cerebral edema with loss of consciousness greater than 24 hours with return to pre-existing conscious level**

● **S06.1X6   Traumatic cerebral edema with loss of consciousness greater than 24 hours without return to pre-existing conscious level with patient surviving**

● **S06.1X7   Traumatic cerebral edema with loss of consciousness of any duration with death due to brain injury prior to regaining consciousness**

● **S06.1X8   Traumatic cerebral edema with loss of consciousness of any duration with death due to other cause prior to regaining consciousness**

● **S06.1X9   Traumatic cerebral edema with loss of consciousness of unspecified duration**
Traumatic cerebral edema NOS

● **S06.2   Diffuse traumatic brain injury**
Diffuse axonal brain injury

Excludes1   traumatic diffuse cerebral edema (S06.1X-)

● **S06.2X   Diffuse traumatic brain injury**

● **S06.2X0   Diffuse traumatic brain injury without loss of consciousness**

● **S06.2X1   Diffuse traumatic brain injury with loss of consciousness of 30 minutes or less**

● **S06.2X2   Diffuse traumatic brain injury with loss of consciousness of 31 minutes to 59 minutes**

● **S06.2X3   Diffuse traumatic brain injury with loss of consciousness of 1 hour to 5 hours 59 minutes**

● **S06.2X4   Diffuse traumatic brain injury with loss of consciousness of 6 hours to 24 hours**

● **S06.2X5   Diffuse traumatic brain injury with loss of consciousness greater than 24 hours with return to pre-existing conscious levels**

● **S06.2X6   Diffuse traumatic brain injury with loss of consciousness greater than 24 hours without return to pre-existing conscious level with patient surviving**

● **S06.2X7   Diffuse traumatic brain injury with loss of consciousness of any duration with death due to brain injury prior to regaining consciousness**

● **S06.2X8   Diffuse traumatic brain injury with loss of consciousness of any duration with death due to other cause prior to regaining consciousness**

● **S06.2X9   Diffuse traumatic brain injury with loss of consciousness of unspecified duration**
Diffuse traumatic brain injury NOS

● **S06.3   Focal traumatic brain injury**

Excludes1   any condition classifiable to S06.4-S06.6 focal cerebral edema (S06.1)

● **S06.30   Unspecified focal traumatic brain injury**

● **S06.300   Unspecified focal traumatic brain injury without loss of consciousness**

● **S06.301   Unspecified focal traumatic brain injury with loss of consciousness of 30 minutes or less**

● **S06.302   Unspecified focal traumatic brain injury with loss of consciousness of 31 minutes to 59 minutes**

● **S06.303   Unspecified focal traumatic brain injury with loss of consciousness of 1 hour to 5 hours 59 minutes**

● S06.304　Unspecified focal traumatic brain injury with loss of consciousness of 6 hours to 24 hours

● S06.305　Unspecified focal traumatic brain injury with loss of consciousness greater than 24 hours with return to pre-existing conscious level

● S06.306　Unspecified focal traumatic brain injury with loss of consciousness greater than 24 hours without return to pre-existing conscious level with patient surviving

● S06.307　Unspecified focal traumatic brain injury with loss of consciousness of any duration with death due to brain injury prior to regaining consciousness

● S06.308　Unspecified focal traumatic brain injury with loss of consciousness of any duration with death due to other cause prior to regaining consciousness

● S06.309　Unspecified focal traumatic brain injury with loss of consciousness of unspecified duration
　　　　　Unspecified focal traumatic brain injury NOS

● S06.31　Contusion and laceration of right cerebrum

● S06.310　Contusion and laceration of right cerebrum without loss of consciousness

● S06.311　Contusion and laceration of right cerebrum with loss of consciousness of 30 minutes or less

● S06.312　Contusion and laceration of right cerebrum with loss of consciousness of 31 minutes to 59 minutes

● S06.313　Contusion and laceration of right cerebrum with loss of consciousness of 1 hour to 5 hours 59 minutes

● S06.314　Contusion and laceration of right cerebrum with loss of consciousness of 6 hours to 24 hours

● S06.315　Contusion and laceration of right cerebrum with loss of consciousness greater than 24 hours with return to pre-existing conscious level

● S06.316　Contusion and laceration of right cerebrum with loss of consciousness greater than 24 hours without return to pre-existing conscious level with patient surviving

● S06.317　Contusion and laceration of right cerebrum with loss of consciousness of any duration with death due to brain injury prior to regaining consciousness

● S06.318　Contusion and laceration of right cerebrum with loss of consciousness of any duration with death due to other cause prior to regaining consciousness

● S06.319　Contusion and laceration of right cerebrum with loss of consciousness of unspecified duration
　　　　　Contusion and laceration of right cerebrum NOS

● S06.32　Contusion and laceration of left cerebrum

● S06.320　Contusion and laceration of left cerebrum without loss of consciousness

● S06.321　Contusion and laceration of left cerebrum with loss of consciousness of 30 minutes or less

● S06.322　Contusion and laceration of left cerebrum with loss of consciousness of 31 minutes to 59 minutes

● S06.323　Contusion and laceration of left cerebrum with loss of consciousness of 1 hour to 5 hours 59 minutes

● S06.324　Contusion and laceration of left cerebrum with loss of consciousness of 6 hours to 24 hours

● S06.325　Contusion and laceration of left cerebrum with loss of consciousness greater than 24 hours with return to pre-existing conscious level

● S06.326　Contusion and laceration of left cerebrum with loss of consciousness greater than 24 hours without return to pre-existing conscious level with patient surviving

● S06.327　Contusion and laceration of left cerebrum with loss of consciousness of any duration with death due to brain injury prior to regaining consciousness

● S06.328　Contusion and laceration of left cerebrum with loss of consciousness of any duration with death due to other cause prior to regaining consciousness

● S06.329　Contusion and laceration of left cerebrum with loss of consciousness of unspecified duration
　　　　　Contusion and laceration of left cerebrum NOS

● S06.33　Contusion and laceration of cerebrum, unspecified

● S06.330　Contusion and laceration of cerebrum, unspecified, without loss of consciousness

● S06.331　Contusion and laceration of cerebrum, unspecified, with loss of consciousness of 30 minutes or less

● S06.332　Contusion and laceration of cerebrum, unspecified, with loss of consciousness of 31 minutes to 59 minutes

● S06.333　Contusion and laceration of cerebrum, unspecified, with loss of consciousness of 1 hour to 5 hours 59 minutes

● S06.334　Contusion and laceration of cerebrum, unspecified, with loss of consciousness of 6 hours to 24 hours

● S06.335　Contusion and laceration of cerebrum, unspecified, with loss of consciousness greater than 24 hours with return to pre-existing conscious level

● S06.336　Contusion and laceration of cerebrum, unspecified, with loss of consciousness greater than 24 hours without return to pre-existing conscious level with patient surviving

◀ New　◀▥ Revised　~~deleted~~ Deleted　OGCR Official Guidelines　X Assign placeholder X　● Use Additional Character(s)

Excludes 1　Excludes 2　Includes　Use additional　Code first　Code also　Unspecified

● S06.337 Contusion and laceration of cerebrum, unspecified, with loss of consciousness of any duration with death due to brain injury prior to regaining consciousness

● S06.338 Contusion and laceration of cerebrum, unspecified, with loss of consciousness of any duration with death due to other cause prior to regaining consciousness

● S06.339 Contusion and laceration of cerebrum, unspecified, with loss of consciousness of unspecified duration
   Contusion and laceration of cerebrum NOS

● S06.34 Traumatic hemorrhage of right cerebrum
   Traumatic intracerebral hemorrhage and hematoma of right cerebrum

● S06.340 Traumatic hemorrhage of right cerebrum without loss of consciousness

● S06.341 Traumatic hemorrhage of right cerebrum with loss of consciousness of 30 minutes or less

● S06.342 Traumatic hemorrhage of right cerebrum with loss of consciousness of 31 minutes to 59 minutes

● S06.343 Traumatic hemorrhage of right cerebrum with loss of consciousness of 1 hours to 5 hours 59 minutes

● S06.344 Traumatic hemorrhage of right cerebrum with loss of consciousness of 6 hours to 24 hours

● S06.345 Traumatic hemorrhage of right cerebrum with loss of consciousness greater than 24 hours with return to pre-existing conscious level

● S06.346 Traumatic hemorrhage of right cerebrum with loss of consciousness greater than 24 hours without return to pre-existing conscious level with patient surviving

● S06.347 Traumatic hemorrhage of right cerebrum with loss of consciousness of any duration with death due to brain injury prior to regaining consciousness

● S06.348 Traumatic hemorrhage of right cerebrum with loss of consciousness of any duration with death due to other cause prior to regaining consciousness

● S06.349 Traumatic hemorrhage of right cerebrum with loss of consciousness of unspecified duration
   Traumatic hemorrhage of right cerebrum NOS

● S06.35 Traumatic hemorrhage of left cerebrum
   Traumatic intracerebral hemorrhage and hematoma of left cerebrum

● S06.350 Traumatic hemorrhage of left cerebrum without loss of consciousness

● S06.351 Traumatic hemorrhage of left cerebrum with loss of consciousness of 30 minutes or less

● S06.352 Traumatic hemorrhage of left cerebrum with loss of consciousness of 31 minutes to 59 minutes

● S06.353 Traumatic hemorrhage of left cerebrum with loss of consciousness of 1 hours to 5 hours 59 minutes

● S06.354 Traumatic hemorrhage of left cerebrum with loss of consciousness of 6 hours to 24 hours

● S06.355 Traumatic hemorrhage of left cerebrum with loss of consciousness greater than 24 hours with return to pre-existing conscious level

● S06.356 Traumatic hemorrhage of left cerebrum with loss of consciousness greater than 24 hours without return to pre-existing conscious level with patient surviving

● S06.357 Traumatic hemorrhage of left cerebrum with loss of consciousness of any duration with death due to brain injury prior to regaining consciousness

● S06.358 Traumatic hemorrhage of left cerebrum with loss of consciousness of any duration with death due to other cause prior to regaining consciousness

● S06.359 Traumatic hemorrhage of left cerebrum with loss of consciousness of unspecified duration
   Traumatic hemorrhage of left cerebrum NOS

● S06.36 Traumatic hemorrhage of cerebrum, unspecified
   Traumatic intracerebral hemorrhage and hematoma, unspecified

● S06.360 Traumatic hemorrhage of cerebrum, unspecified, without loss of consciousness

● S06.361 Traumatic hemorrhage of cerebrum, unspecified, with loss of consciousness of 30 minutes or less

● S06.362 Traumatic hemorrhage of cerebrum, unspecified, with loss of consciousness of 31 minutes to 59 minutes

● S06.363 Traumatic hemorrhage of cerebrum, unspecified, with loss of consciousness of 1 hours to 5 hours 59 minutes

● S06.364 Traumatic hemorrhage of cerebrum, unspecified, with loss of consciousness of 6 hours to 24 hours

● S06.365 Traumatic hemorrhage of cerebrum, unspecified, with loss of consciousness greater than 24 hours with return to pre-existing conscious level

● S06.366 Traumatic hemorrhage of cerebrum, unspecified, with loss of consciousness greater than 24 hours without return to pre-existing conscious level with patient surviving

● S06.367 Traumatic hemorrhage of cerebrum, unspecified, with loss of consciousness of any duration with death due to brain injury prior to regaining consciousness

● S06.368 Traumatic hemorrhage of cerebrum, unspecified, with loss of consciousness of any duration with death due to other cause prior to regaining consciousness

● S06.369 Traumatic hemorrhage of cerebrum, unspecified, with loss of consciousness of unspecified duration
   Traumatic hemorrhage of cerebrum NOS

◀ New   ◀▥ Revised   ~~deleted~~ Deleted   **OGCR** Official Guidelines   X Assign placeholder X   ● Use Additional Character(s)

| Excludes 1 | Excludes 2 | Includes | Use additional | Code first | Code also | Unspecified |

● **S06.37**   Contusion, laceration, and hemorrhage of cerebellum

  ● **S06.370**   Contusion, laceration, and hemorrhage of cerebellum without loss of consciousness

  ● **S06.371**   Contusion, laceration, and hemorrhage of cerebellum with loss of consciousness of 30 minutes or less

  ● **S06.372**   Contusion, laceration, and hemorrhage of cerebellum with loss of consciousness of 31 minutes to 59 minutes

  ● **S06.373**   Contusion, laceration, and hemorrhage of cerebellum with loss of consciousness of 1 hour to 5 hours 59 minutes

  ● **S06.374**   Contusion, laceration, and hemorrhage of cerebellum with loss of consciousness of 6 hours to 24 hours

  ● **S06.375**   Contusion, laceration, and hemorrhage of cerebellum with loss of consciousness greater than 24 hours with return to pre-existing conscious level

  ● **S06.376**   Contusion, laceration, and hemorrhage of cerebellum with loss of consciousness greater than 24 hours without return to pre-existing conscious level with patient surviving

  ● **S06.377**   Contusion, laceration, and hemorrhage of cerebellum with loss of consciousness of any duration with death due to brain injury prior to regaining consciousness

  ● **S06.378**   Contusion, laceration, and hemorrhage of cerebellum with loss of consciousness of any duration with death due to other cause prior to regaining consciousness

  ● **S06.379**   Contusion, laceration, and hemorrhage of cerebellum with loss of consciousness of unspecified duration

       Contusion, laceration, and hemorrhage of cerebellum NOS

● **S06.38**   Contusion, laceration, and hemorrhage of brainstem

  ● **S06.380**   Contusion, laceration, and hemorrhage of brainstem without loss of consciousness

  ● **S06.381**   Contusion, laceration, and hemorrhage of brainstem with loss of consciousness of 30 minutes or less

  ● **S06.382**   Contusion, laceration, and hemorrhage of brainstem with loss of consciousness of 31 minutes to 59 minutes

  ● **S06.383**   Contusion, laceration, and hemorrhage of brainstem with loss of consciousness of 1 hour to 5 hours 59 minutes

  ● **S06.384**   Contusion, laceration, and hemorrhage of brainstem with loss of consciousness of 6 hours to 24 hours

  ● **S06.385**   Contusion, laceration, and hemorrhage of brainstem with loss of consciousness greater than 24 hours with return to pre-existing conscious level

  ● **S06.386**   Contusion, laceration, and hemorrhage of brainstem with loss of consciousness greater than 24 hours without return to pre-existing conscious level with patient surviving

  ● **S06.387**   Contusion, laceration, and hemorrhage of brainstem with loss of consciousness of any duration with death due to brain injury prior to regaining consciousness

  ● **S06.388**   Contusion, laceration, and hemorrhage of brainstem with loss of consciousness of any duration with death due to other cause prior to regaining consciousness

  ● **S06.389**   Contusion, laceration, and hemorrhage of brainstem with loss of consciousness of unspecified duration

       Contusion, laceration, and hemorrhage of brainstem NOS

● **S06.4**   Epidural hemorrhage

    Situated outside dura mater

    Extradural hemorrhage NOS

      Intracranial hemorrhage due to trauma

    Extradural hemorrhage (traumatic)

  ● **S06.4X**   Epidural hemorrhage

    ● **S06.4X0**   Epidural hemorrhage without loss of consciousness

    ● **S06.4X1**   Epidural hemorrhage with loss of consciousness of 30 minutes or less

    ● **S06.4X2**   Epidural hemorrhage with loss of consciousness of 31 minutes to 59 minutes

    ● **S06.4X3**   Epidural hemorrhage with loss of consciousness of 1 hour to 5 hours 59 minutes

    ● **S06.4X4**   Epidural hemorrhage with loss of consciousness of 6 hours to 24 hours

    ● **S06.4X5**   Epidural hemorrhage with loss of consciousness greater than 24 hours with return to pre-existing conscious level

    ● **S06.4X6**   Epidural hemorrhage with loss of consciousness greater than 24 hours without return to pre-existing conscious level with patient surviving

    ● **S06.4X7**   Epidural hemorrhage with loss of consciousness of any duration with death due to brain injury prior to regaining consciousness

    ● **S06.4X8**   Epidural hemorrhage with loss of consciousness of any duration with death due to other causes prior to regaining consciousness

    ● **S06.4X9**   Epidural hemorrhage with loss of consciousness of unspecified duration

        Epidural hemorrhage NOS

● **S06.5**   Traumatic subdural hemorrhage

  ● **S06.5X**   Traumatic subdural hemorrhage

    ● **S06.5X0**   Traumatic subdural hemorrhage without loss of consciousness

    ● **S06.5X1**   Traumatic subdural hemorrhage with loss of consciousness of 30 minutes or less

    ● **S06.5X2**   Traumatic subdural hemorrhage with loss of consciousness of 31 minutes to 59 minutes

◄ New   ◄█ Revised   ~~deleted~~ Deleted   **OGCR** Official Guidelines   X Assign placeholder X   ● Use Additional Character(s)

Excludes 1   Excludes 2   Includes   Use additional   Code first   Code also   Unspecified

● S06.5X3   Traumatic subdural hemorrhage with loss of consciousness of 1 hour to 5 hours 59 minutes

● S06.5X4   Traumatic subdural hemorrhage with loss of consciousness of 6 hours to 24 hours

● S06.5X5   Traumatic subdural hemorrhage with loss of consciousness greater than 24 hours with return to pre-existing conscious level

● S06.5X6   Traumatic subdural hemorrhage with loss of consciousness greater than 24 hours without return to pre-existing conscious level with patient surviving

● S06.5X7   Traumatic subdural hemorrhage with loss of consciousness of any duration with death due to brain injury before regaining consciousness

● S06.5X8   Traumatic subdural hemorrhage with loss of consciousness of any duration with death due to other cause before regaining consciousness

● S06.5X9   Traumatic subdural hemorrhage with loss of consciousness of unspecified duration
     Traumatic subdural hemorrhage NOS

● S06.6   **Traumatic subarachnoid hemorrhage**
     Between arachnoid and pia mater

    ● S06.6X   Traumatic subarachnoid hemorrhage

        ● S06.6X0   Traumatic subarachnoid hemorrhage without loss of consciousness

        ● S06.6X1   Traumatic subarachnoid hemorrhage with loss of consciousness of 30 minutes or less

        ● S06.6X2   Traumatic subarachnoid hemorrhage with loss of consciousness of 31 minutes to 59 minutes

        ● S06.6X3   Traumatic subarachnoid hemorrhage with loss of consciousness of 1 hour to 5 hours 59 minutes

        ● S06.6X4   Traumatic subarachnoid hemorrhage with loss of consciousness of 6 hours to 24 hours

        ● S06.6X5   Traumatic subarachnoid hemorrhage with loss of consciousness greater than 24 hours with return to pre-existing conscious level

        ● S06.6X6   Traumatic subarachnoid hemorrhage with loss of consciousness greater than 24 hours without return to pre-existing conscious level with patient surviving

        ● S06.6X7   Traumatic subarachnoid hemorrhage with loss of consciousness of any duration with death due to brain injury prior to regaining consciousness

        ● S06.6X8   Traumatic subarachnoid hemorrhage with loss of consciousness of any duration with death due to other cause prior to regaining consciousness

        ● S06.6X9   Traumatic subarachnoid hemorrhage with loss of consciousness of unspecified duration
           Traumatic subarachnoid hemorrhage NOS

● S06.8   **Other specified intracranial injuries**

    ● S06.81   Injury of right internal carotid artery, intracranial portion, not elsewhere classified

        ● S06.810   Injury of right internal carotid artery, intracranial portion, not elsewhere classified without loss of consciousness

        ● S06.811   Injury of right internal carotid artery, intracranial portion, not elsewhere classified with loss of consciousness of 30 minutes or less

        ● S06.812   Injury of right internal carotid artery, intracranial portion, not elsewhere classified with loss of consciousness of 31 minutes to 59 minutes

        ● S06.813   Injury of right internal carotid artery, intracranial portion, not elsewhere classified with loss of consciousness of 1 hour to 5 hours 59 minutes

        ● S06.814   Injury of right internal carotid artery, intracranial portion, not elsewhere classified with loss of consciousness of 6 hours to 24 hours

        ● S06.815   Injury of right internal carotid artery, intracranial portion, not elsewhere classified with loss of consciousness greater than 24 hours with return to pre-existing conscious level

        ● S06.816   Injury of right internal carotid artery, intracranial portion, not elsewhere classified with loss of consciousness greater than 24 hours without return to pre-existing conscious level with patient surviving

        ● S06.817   Injury of right internal carotid artery, intracranial portion, not elsewhere classified with loss of consciousness of any duration with death due to brain injury prior to regaining consciousness

        ● S06.818   Injury of right internal carotid artery, intracranial portion, not elsewhere classified with loss of consciousness of any duration with death due to other cause prior to regaining consciousness

        ● S06.819   Injury of right internal carotid artery, intracranial portion, not elsewhere classified with loss of consciousness of unspecified duration
           Injury of right internal carotid artery, intracranial portion, not elsewhere classified NOS

    ● S06.82   Injury of left internal carotid artery, intracranial portion, not elsewhere classified

        ● S06.820   Injury of left internal carotid artery, intracranial portion, not elsewhere classified without loss of consciousness

        ● S06.821   Injury of left internal carotid artery, intracranial portion, not elsewhere classified with loss of consciousness of 30 minutes or less

        ● S06.822   Injury of left internal carotid artery, intracranial portion, not elsewhere classified with loss of consciousness of 31 minutes to 59 minutes

CHAPTER 19 (S00-T88)

● S06.823   Injury of left internal carotid artery, intracranial portion, not elsewhere classified with loss of consciousness of 1 hour to 5 hours 59 minutes

● S06.824   Injury of left internal carotid artery, intracranial portion, not elsewhere classified with loss of consciousness of 6 hours to 24 hours

● S06.825   Injury of left internal carotid artery, intracranial portion, not elsewhere classified with loss of consciousness greater than 24 hours with return to pre-existing conscious level

● S06.826   Injury of left internal carotid artery, intracranial portion, not elsewhere classified with loss of consciousness greater than 24 hours without return to pre-existing conscious level with patient surviving

● S06.827   Injury of left internal carotid artery, intracranial portion, not elsewhere classified with loss of consciousness of any duration with death due to brain injury prior to regaining consciousness

● S06.828   Injury of left internal carotid artery, intracranial portion, not elsewhere classified with loss of consciousness of any duration with death due to other cause prior to regaining consciousness

● S06.829   Injury of left internal carotid artery, intracranial portion, not elsewhere classified with loss of consciousness of unspecified duration

     Injury of left internal carotid artery, intracranial portion, not elsewhere classified NOS

● S06.89   Other specified intracranial injury

● S06.890   Other specified intracranial injury without loss of consciousness

● S06.891   Other specified intracranial injury with loss of consciousness of 30 minutes or less

● S06.892   Other specified intracranial injury with loss of consciousness of 31 minutes to 59 minutes

● S06.893   Other specified intracranial injury with loss of consciousness of 1 hour to 5 hours 59 minutes

● S06.894   Other specified intracranial injury with loss of consciousness of 6 hours to 24 hours

● S06.895   Other specified intracranial injury with loss of consciousness greater than 24 hours with return to pre-existing conscious level

● S06.896   Other specified intracranial injury with loss of consciousness greater than 24 hours without return to pre-existing conscious level with patient surviving

● S06.897   Other specified intracranial injury with loss of consciousness of any duration with death due to brain injury prior to regaining consciousness

● S06.898   Other specified intracranial injury with loss of consciousness of any duration with death due to other cause prior to regaining consciousness

● S06.899   Other specified intracranial injury with loss of consciousness of unspecified duration

● S06.9   Unspecified intracranial injury
     Brain injury NOS
     Head injury NOS with loss of consciousness
     Excludes1   head injury NOS (S09.90)

● S06.9X   Unspecified intracranial injury

● S06.9X0   Unspecified intracranial injury without loss of consciousness

● S06.9X1   Unspecified intracranial injury with loss of consciousness of 30 minutes or less

● S06.9X2   Unspecified intracranial injury with loss of consciousness of 31 minutes to 59 minutes

● S06.9X3   Unspecified intracranial injury with loss of consciousness of 1 hour to 5 hours 59 minutes

● S06.9X4   Unspecified intracranial injury with loss of consciousness of 6 hours to 24 hours

● S06.9X5   Unspecified intracranial injury with loss of consciousness greater than 24 hours with return to pre-existing conscious level

● S06.9X6   Unspecified intracranial injury with loss of consciousness greater than 24 hours without return to pre-existing conscious level with patient surviving

● S06.9X7   Unspecified intracranial injury with loss of consciousness of any duration with death due to brain injury prior to regaining consciousness

● S06.9X8   Unspecified intracranial injury with loss of consciousness of any duration with death due to other cause prior to regaining consciousness

● S06.9X9   Unspecified intracranial injury with loss of consciousness of unspecified duration

● S07   Crushing injury of head
     Use additional code for all associated injuries, such as:
       intracranial injuries (S06.-)
       skull fractures (S02.-)

     The appropriate 7th character is to be added to each code from category S07

A	initial encounter
D	subsequent encounter
S	sequela

X ● S07.0   Crushing injury of face

X ● S07.1   Crushing injury of skull

X ● S07.8   Crushing injury of other parts of head

X ● S07.9   Crushing injury of head, part unspecified

◀ New   ◀▦ Revised   deleted Deleted   OGCR Official Guidelines   X Assign placeholder X   ● Use Additional Character(s)

Excludes 1   Excludes 2   Includes   Use additional   Code first   Code also   Unspecified

- **S08　Avulsion and traumatic amputation of part of head**

  An amputation not identified as partial or complete should be coded to complete

  The appropriate 7th character is to be added to each code from category S08

  > A　initial encounter
  > D　subsequent encounter
  > S　sequela

  - X ● **S08.0　Avulsion of scalp**
  - ● **S08.1　Traumatic amputation of ear**
    - ● **S08.11　Complete traumatic amputation of ear**
      - ● **S08.111　Complete traumatic amputation of right ear**
      - ● **S08.112　Complete traumatic amputation of left ear**
      - ● **S08.119　Complete traumatic amputation of** unspecified **ear**
    - ● **S08.12　Partial traumatic amputation of ear**
      - ● **S08.121　Partial traumatic amputation of right ear**
      - ● **S08.122　Partial traumatic amputation of left ear**
      - ● **S08.129　Partial traumatic amputation of** unspecified **ear**
  - ● **S08.8　Traumatic amputation of other parts of head**
    - ● **S08.81　Traumatic amputation of nose**
      - ● **S08.811　Complete traumatic amputation of nose**
      - ● **S08.812　Partial traumatic amputation of nose**
    - X ● **S08.89　Traumatic amputation of other parts of head**

- **S09　Other and unspecified injuries of head**

  The appropriate 7th character is to be added to each code from category S09

  > A　initial encounter
  > D　subsequent encounter
  > S　sequela

  - X ● **S09.0　Injury of blood vessels of head, not elsewhere classified**
    - **Excludes1**　injury of cerebral blood vessels (S06.-)
      injury of precerebral blood vessels (S15.-)
  - ● **S09.1　Injury of muscle and tendon of head**
    - Code also any associated open wound (S01.-)
    - **Excludes2**　sprain to joints and ligament of head (S03.9)
    - X ● **S09.10　Unspecified injury of muscle and tendon of head**
      Injury of muscle and tendon of head NOS
    - X ● **S09.11　Strain of muscle and tendon of head**
    - X ● **S09.12　Laceration of muscle and tendon of head**
    - X ● **S09.19　Other specified injury of muscle and tendon of head**
  - ● **S09.2　Traumatic rupture of ear drum**
    - **Excludes1**　traumatic rupture of ear drum due to blast injury (S09.31-)
    - X ● **S09.20　Traumatic rupture of** unspecified **ear drum**
    - X ● **S09.21　Traumatic rupture of right ear drum**
    - X ● **S09.22　Traumatic rupture of left ear drum**

- ● **S09.3　Other specified and unspecified injury of middle and inner ear**
  - **Excludes1**　injury to ear NOS (S09.91-)
  - **Excludes2**　injury to external ear (S00.4-, S01.3-, S08.1-)
  - ● **S09.30　Unspecified injury of middle and inner ear**
    - ● **S09.301　**Unspecified **injury of right middle and inner ear**
    - ● **S09.302　**Unspecified **injury of left middle and inner ear**
    - ● **S09.309　**Unspecified **injury of unspecified middle and inner ear**
  - ● **S09.31　Primary blast injury of ear**
    Blast injury of ear NOS
    - ● **S09.311　Primary blast injury of right ear**
    - ● **S09.312　Primary blast injury of left ear**
    - ● **S09.313　Primary blast injury of ear, bilateral**
    - ● **S09.319　Primary blast injury of** unspecified **ear**
  - ● **S09.39　Other specified injury of middle and inner ear**
    Secondary blast injury to ear
    - ● **S09.391　Other specified injury of right middle and inner ear**
    - ● **S09.392　Other specified injury of left middle and inner ear**
    - ● **S09.399　Other specified injury of** unspecified **middle and inner ear**
- X ● **S09.8　Other specified injuries of head**
- ● **S09.9　Unspecified injury of face and head**
  - X ● **S09.90　Unspecified injury of head**
    Head injury NOS
    - **Excludes1**　brain injury NOS (S06.9-)
      head injury NOS with loss of consciousness (S06.9-)
      intracranial injury NOS (S06.9-)
  - X ● **S09.91　Unspecified injury of ear**
    Injury of ear NOS
  - X ● **S09.92　Unspecified injury of nose**
    Injury of nose NOS
  - X ● **S09.93　Unspecified injury of face**
    Injury of face NOS

INJURIES TO THE NECK (S10-S19)

> **Includes**　injuries of nape
> injuries of supraclavicular region
> injuries of throat

> **Excludes2**　burns and corrosions (T20-T32)
> effects of foreign body in esophagus (T18.1)
> effects of foreign body in larynx (T17.3)
> effects of foreign body in pharynx (T17.2)
> effects of foreign body in trachea (T17.4)
> frostbite (T33-T34)
> insect bite or sting, venomous (T63.4)

- ● **S10　Superficial injury of neck**

  The appropriate 7th character is to be added to each code from category S10

  > A　initial encounter
  > D　subsequent encounter
  > S　sequela

  - X ● **S10.0　Contusion of throat**
    Contusion of cervical esophagus
    Contusion of larynx
    Contusion of pharynx
    Contusion of trachea

◀ New　　◀▥▥ Revised　　d̶e̶l̶e̶t̶e̶d̶ Deleted　　**OGCR** Official Guidelines　　X Assign placeholder X　　● Use Additional Character(s)

| Excludes 1 | Excludes 2 | Includes | Use additional | Code first | Code also | Unspecified |

1237

● **S10.1**   Other and unspecified superficial injuries of throat
- X● **S10.10**   Unspecified superficial injuries of throat
- X● **S10.11**   Abrasion of throat
- X● **S10.12**   Blister (nonthermal) of throat
- X● **S10.14**   External constriction of part of throat
- X● **S10.15**   Superficial foreign body of throat
  - Splinter in the throat
- X● **S10.16**   Insect bite (nonvenomous) of throat
- X● **S10.17**   Other superficial bite of throat
  - **Excludes1**   open bite of throat (S11.85)

● **S10.8**   Superficial injury of other specified parts of neck
- X● **S10.80**   Unspecified superficial injury of other specified part of neck
- X● **S10.81**   Abrasion of other specified part of neck
- X● **S10.82**   Blister (nonthermal) of other specified part of neck
- X● **S10.83**   Contusion of other specified part of neck
- X● **S10.84**   External constriction of other specified part of neck
- X● **S10.85**   Superficial foreign body of other specified part of neck
  - Splinter in other part of neck
- X● **S10.86**   Insect bite of other specified part of neck
- X● **S10.87**   Other superficial bite of other specified part of neck
  - **Excludes1**   open bite of other specified parts of neck (S11.85)

● **S10.9**   Superficial injury of unspecified part of neck
- X● **S10.90**   Unspecified superficial injury of unspecified part of neck
- X● **S10.91**   Abrasion of unspecified part of neck
- X● **S10.92**   Blister (nonthermal) of unspecified part of neck
- X● **S10.93**   Contusion of unspecified part of neck
- X● **S10.94**   External constriction of unspecified part of neck
- X● **S10.95**   Superficial foreign body of unspecified part of neck
- X● **S10.96**   Insect bite of unspecified part of neck
- X● **S10.97**   Other superficial bite of unspecified part of neck

● **S11**   Open wound of neck

Code also any associated:
spinal cord injury (S14.0, S14.1-)
wound infection

   Excludes2   open fracture of vertebra (S12.- with 7th character B)

The appropriate 7th character is to be added to each code from category S11

A	initial encounter
D	subsequent encounter
S	sequela

● **S11.0**   Open wound of larynx and trachea
- ● **S11.01**   Open wound of larynx
  - **Excludes2**   open wound of vocal cord (S11.03)
  - ● **S11.011**   Laceration without foreign body of larynx
  - ● **S11.012**   Laceration with foreign body of larynx
  - ● **S11.013**   Puncture wound without foreign body of larynx
  - ● **S11.014**   Puncture wound with foreign body of larynx
  - ● **S11.015**   Open bite of larynx
    - Bite of larynx NOS
  - ● **S11.019**   Unspecified open wound of larynx

● **S11.02**   Open wound of trachea
- Open wound of cervical trachea
- Open wound of trachea NOS
  - **Excludes2**   open wound of thoracic trachea (S27.5-)
  - ● **S11.021**   Laceration without foreign body of trachea
  - ● **S11.022**   Laceration with foreign body of trachea
  - ● **S11.023**   Puncture wound without foreign body of trachea
  - ● **S11.024**   Puncture wound with foreign body of trachea
  - ● **S11.025**   Open bite of trachea
    - Bite of trachea NOS
  - ● **S11.029**   Unspecified open wound of trachea
- ● **S11.03**   Open wound of vocal cord
  - ● **S11.031**   Laceration without foreign body of vocal cord
  - ● **S11.032**   Laceration with foreign body of vocal cord
  - ● **S11.033**   Puncture wound without foreign body of vocal cord
  - ● **S11.034**   Puncture wound with foreign body of vocal cord
  - ● **S11.035**   Open bite of vocal cord
    - Bite of vocal cord NOS
  - ● **S11.039**   Unspecified open wound of vocal cord

● **S11.1**   Open wound of thyroid gland
- X● **S11.10**   Unspecified open wound of thyroid gland
- X● **S11.11**   Laceration without foreign body of thyroid gland
- X● **S11.12**   Laceration with foreign body of thyroid gland
- X● **S11.13**   Puncture wound without foreign body of thyroid gland
- X● **S11.14**   Puncture wound with foreign body of thyroid gland
- X● **S11.15**   Open bite of thyroid gland
  - Bite of thyroid gland NOS

● **S11.2**   Open wound of pharynx and cervical esophagus
  - **Excludes1**   open wound of esophagus NOS (S27.8-)
- X● **S11.20**   Unspecified open wound of pharynx and cervical esophagus
- X● **S11.21**   Laceration without foreign body of pharynx and cervical esophagus
- X● **S11.22**   Laceration with foreign body of pharynx and cervical esophagus
- X● **S11.23**   Puncture wound without foreign body of pharynx and cervical esophagus
- X● **S11.24**   Puncture wound with foreign body of pharynx and cervical esophagus
- X● **S11.25**   Open bite of pharynx and cervical esophagus
  - Bite of pharynx and cervical esophagus NOS

● **S11.8**   Open wound of other specified parts of neck
- X● **S11.80**   Unspecified open specified wound of other part of neck
- X● **S11.81**   Laceration without foreign body of other specified part of neck
- X● **S11.82**   Laceration with foreign body of other specified part of neck
- X● **S11.83**   Puncture wound without foreign body of other specified part of neck
- X● **S11.84**   Puncture wound with foreign body of other specified part of neck
- X● **S11.85**   Open bite of other specified part of neck
  - Bite of other part of neck NOS
  - **Excludes1**   superficial bite of other specified part of neck (S10.87)
- X● **S11.89**   Other open wound of other part of neck

● **S11.9   Open wound of unspecified part of neck**

   X● **S11.90   Unspecified** open wound of **unspecified** part of neck

   X● **S11.91   Laceration without foreign body of unspecified** part of neck

   X● **S11.92   Laceration with foreign body of unspecified** part of neck

   X● **S11.93   Puncture wound without foreign body of unspecified** part of neck

   X● **S11.94   Puncture wound with foreign body of unspecified** part of neck

   X● **S11.95   Open bite of unspecified** part of neck
                Bite of neck NOS

                Excludes1   superficial bite of neck (S10.97)

● **S12   Fracture of cervical vertebra and other parts of neck**

   Note: A fracture not indicated as displaced or nondisplaced should be coded to displaced

   A fracture not indicated as open or closed should be coded to closed

   Includes   fracture of cervical neural arch
                fracture of cervical spine
                fracture of cervical spinous process
                fracture of cervical transverse process
                fracture of cervical vertebral arch
                fracture of neck

   Code first any associated cervical spinal cord injury (S14.0, S14.1-)

   The appropriate 7th character is to be added to all codes from subcategories S12.0-S12.6

A	initial encounter for closed fracture
B	initial encounter for open fracture
D	subsequent encounter for fracture with routine healing
G	subsequent encounter for fracture with delayed healing
K	subsequent encounter for fracture with nonunion
S	sequela

● **S12.0   Fracture of first cervical vertebra**
            Atlas

   ● **S12.00   Unspecified fracture of first cervical vertebra**

      ● **S12.000   Unspecified** displaced fracture of first cervical vertebra

      ● **S12.001   Unspecified** nondisplaced fracture of first cervical vertebra

   X● **S12.01   Stable burst fracture of first cervical vertebra**

   X● **S12.02   Unstable burst fracture of first cervical vertebra**

   ● **S12.03   Posterior arch fracture of first cervical vertebra**

      ● **S12.030   Displaced posterior arch fracture of first cervical vertebra**

      ● **S12.031   Nondisplaced posterior arch fracture of first cervical vertebra**

   ● **S12.04   Lateral mass fracture of first cervical vertebra**

      ● **S12.040   Displaced lateral mass fracture of first cervical vertebra**

      ● **S12.041   Nondisplaced lateral mass fracture of first cervical vertebra**

   ● **S12.09   Other fracture of first cervical vertebra**

      ● **S12.090   Other displaced fracture of first cervical vertebra**

      ● **S12.091   Other nondisplaced fracture of first cervical vertebra**

● **S12.1   Fracture of second cervical vertebra**
            Axis

   ● **S12.10   Unspecified fracture of second cervical vertebra**

      ● **S12.100   Unspecified** displaced fracture of second cervical vertebra

      ● **S12.101   Unspecified** nondisplaced fracture of second cervical vertebra

● **S12.11   Type II dens fracture**

   ● **S12.110   Anterior displaced Type II dens fracture**

   ● **S12.111   Posterior displaced Type II dens fracture**

   ● **S12.112   Nondisplaced Type II dens fracture**

● **S12.12   Other dens fracture**

   ● **S12.120   Other displaced dens fracture**

   ● **S12.121   Other nondisplaced dens fracture**

● **S12.13   Unspecified traumatic spondylolisthesis of second cervical vertebra**

   ● **S12.130   Unspecified** traumatic displaced spondylolisthesis of second cervical vertebra

   ● **S12.131   Unspecified** traumatic nondisplaced spondylolisthesis of second cervical vertebra

X● **S12.14   Type III traumatic spondylolisthesis of second cervical vertebra**

● **S12.15   Other traumatic spondylolisthesis of second cervical vertebra**

   ● **S12.150   Other traumatic displaced spondylolisthesis of second cervical vertebra**

   ● **S12.151   Other traumatic nondisplaced spondylolisthesis of second cervical vertebra**

● **S12.19   Other fracture of second cervical vertebra**

   ● **S12.190   Other displaced fracture of second cervical vertebra**

   ● **S12.191   Other nondisplaced fracture of second cervical vertebra**

● **S12.2   Fracture of third cervical vertebra**

   ● **S12.20   Unspecified fracture of third cervical vertebra**

      ● **S12.200   Unspecified** displaced fracture of third cervical vertebra

      ● **S12.201   Unspecified** nondisplaced fracture of third cervical vertebra

   ● **S12.23   Unspecified traumatic spondylolisthesis of third cervical vertebra**

      ● **S12.230   Unspecified** traumatic displaced spondylolisthesis of third cervical vertebra

      ● **S12.231   Unspecified** traumatic nondisplaced spondylolisthesis of third cervical vertebra

   X● **S12.24   Type III traumatic spondylolisthesis of third cervical vertebra**

   ● **S12.25   Other traumatic spondylolisthesis of third cervical vertebra**

      ● **S12.250   Other traumatic displaced spondylolisthesis of third cervical vertebra**

      ● **S12.251   Other traumatic nondisplaced spondylolisthesis of third cervical vertebra**

   ● **S12.29   Other fracture of third cervical vertebra**

      ● **S12.290   Other displaced fracture of third cervical vertebra**

      ● **S12.291   Other nondisplaced fracture of third cervical vertebra**

● **S12.3   Fracture of fourth cervical vertebra**

   ● **S12.30   Unspecified fracture of fourth cervical vertebra**

      ● **S12.300   Unspecified** displaced fracture of fourth cervical vertebra

      ● **S12.301   Unspecified** nondisplaced fracture of fourth cervical vertebra

CHAPTER 19 (S00-T88)

- ● S12.33   Unspecified traumatic spondylolisthesis of fourth cervical vertebra
  - ● S12.330   Unspecified traumatic displaced spondylolisthesis of fourth cervical vertebra
  - ● S12.331   Unspecified traumatic nondisplaced spondylolisthesis of fourth cervical vertebra
- X ● S12.34   Type III traumatic spondylolisthesis of fourth cervical vertebra
- ● S12.35   Other traumatic spondylolisthesis of fourth cervical vertebra
  - ● S12.350   Other traumatic displaced spondylolisthesis of fourth cervical vertebra
  - ● S12.351   Other traumatic nondisplaced spondylolisthesis of fourth cervical vertebra
- ● S12.39   Other fracture of fourth cervical vertebra
  - ● S12.390   Other displaced fracture of fourth cervical vertebra
  - ● S12.391   Other nondisplaced fracture of fourth cervical vertebra
- ● S12.4   Fracture of fifth cervical vertebra
  - ● S12.40   Unspecified fracture of fifth cervical vertebra
    - ● S12.400   Unspecified displaced fracture of fifth cervical vertebra
    - ● S12.401   Unspecified nondisplaced fracture of fifth cervical vertebra
  - ● S12.43   Unspecified traumatic spondylolisthesis of fifth cervical vertebra
    - ● S12.430   Unspecified traumatic displaced spondylolisthesis of fifth cervical vertebra
    - ● S12.431   Unspecified traumatic nondisplaced spondylolisthesis of fifth cervical vertebra
  - X ● S12.44   Type III traumatic spondylolisthesis of fifth cervical vertebra
  - ● S12.45   Other traumatic spondylolisthesis of fifth cervical vertebra
    - ● S12.450   Other traumatic displaced spondylolisthesis of fifth cervical vertebra
    - ● S12.451   Other traumatic nondisplaced spondylolisthesis of fifth cervical vertebra
  - ● S12.49   Other fracture of fifth cervical vertebra
    - ● S12.490   Other displaced fracture of fifth cervical vertebra
    - ● S12.491   Other nondisplaced fracture of fifth cervical vertebra
- ● S12.5   Fracture of sixth cervical vertebra
  - ● S12.50   Unspecified fracture of sixth cervical vertebra
    - ● S12.500   Unspecified displaced fracture of sixth cervical vertebra
    - ● S12.501   Unspecified nondisplaced fracture of sixth cervical vertebra
  - ● S12.53   Unspecified traumatic spondylolisthesis of sixth cervical vertebra
    - ● S12.530   Unspecified traumatic displaced spondylolisthesis of sixth cervical vertebra
    - ● S12.531   Unspecified traumatic nondisplaced spondylolisthesis of sixth cervical vertebra
  - X ● S12.54   Type III traumatic spondylolisthesis of sixth cervical vertebra

- ● S12.55   Other traumatic spondylolisthesis of sixth cervical vertebra
  - ● S12.550   Other traumatic displaced spondylolisthesis of sixth cervical vertebra
  - ● S12.551   Other traumatic nondisplaced spondylolisthesis of sixth cervical vertebra
- ● S12.59   Other fracture of sixth cervical vertebra
  - ● S12.590   Other displaced fracture of sixth cervical vertebra
  - ● S12.591   Other nondisplaced fracture of sixth cervical vertebra
- ● S12.6   Fracture of seventh cervical vertebra
  - S12.60   Unspecified fracture of seventh cervical vertebra
    - ● S12.600   Unspecified displaced fracture of seventh cervical vertebra
    - ● S12.601   Unspecified nondisplaced fracture of seventh cervical vertebra
  - ● S12.63   Unspecified traumatic spondylolisthesis of seventh cervical vertebra
    - ● S12.630   Unspecified traumatic displaced spondylolisthesis of seventh cervical vertebra
    - ● S12.631   Unspecified traumatic nondisplaced spondylolisthesis of seventh cervical vertebra
  - X ● S12.64   Type III traumatic spondylolisthesis of seventh cervical vertebra
  - ● S12.65   Other traumatic spondylolisthesis of seventh cervical vertebra
    - ● S12.650   Other traumatic displaced spondylolisthesis of seventh cervical vertebra
    - ● S12.651   Other traumatic nondisplaced spondylolisthesis of seventh cervical vertebra
  - ● S12.69   Other fracture of seventh cervical vertebra
    - ● S12.690   Other displaced fracture of seventh cervical vertebra
    - ● S12.691   Other nondisplaced fracture of seventh cervical vertebra
- X ● S12.8   Fracture of other parts of neck

  Hyoid bone   Thyroid cartilage
  Larynx   Trachea

  The appropriate 7th character is to be added to code S12.8

A	initial encounter
D	subsequent encounter
S	sequela

- X ● S12.9   Fracture of neck, unspecified

  Fracture of neck NOS
  Fracture of cervical spine NOS
  Fracture of cervical vertebra NOS

  The appropriate 7th character is to be added to code S12.9

A	initial encounter
D	subsequent encounter
S	sequela

● **S13**   **Dislocation and sprain of joints and ligaments at neck level**

> **Includes**   avulsion of joint or ligament at neck level
>> laceration of cartilage, joint or ligament at neck level
>> sprain of cartilage, joint or ligament at neck level
>> traumatic hemarthrosis of joint or ligament at neck level
>> traumatic rupture of joint or ligament at neck level
>> traumatic subluxation of joint or ligament at neck level
>> traumatic tear of joint or ligament at neck level

> Code also any associated open wound

> **Excludes2**   strain of muscle or tendon at neck level (S16.1)

> The appropriate 7th character is to be added to each code from category S13

> | | |
> |---|---|
> | A | initial encounter |
> | D | subsequent encounter |
> | S | sequela |

X ● **S13.0**   **Traumatic rupture of cervical intervertebral disc**

> **Excludes1**   rupture or displacement (nontraumatic) of cervical intervertebral disc NOS (M50.-)

● **S13.1**   **Subluxation and dislocation of cervical vertebrae**

> Code also any associated:
>> open wound of neck (S11.-)
>> spinal cord injury (S14.1-)

> **Excludes2**   fracture of cervical vertebrae (S12.0-S12.3-)

> ● **S13.10**   **Subluxation and dislocation of unspecified cervical vertebrae**
>> ● **S13.100**   **Subluxation of unspecified cervical vertebrae**
>> ● **S13.101**   **Dislocation of unspecified cervical vertebrae**

> ● **S13.11**   **Subluxation and dislocation of C_0/C_1 cervical vertebrae**
>> Subluxation and dislocation of atlantooccipital joint
>> Subluxation and dislocation of atloidooccipital joint
>> Subluxation and dislocation of occipitoatloid joint
>> ● **S13.110**   **Subluxation of C_0/C_1 cervical vertebrae**
>> ● **S13.111**   **Dislocation of C_0/C_1 cervical vertebrae**

> ● **S13.12**   **Subluxation and dislocation of C_1/C_2 cervical vertebrae**
>> Subluxation and dislocation of atlantoaxial joint
>> ● **S13.120**   **Subluxation of C_1/C_2 cervical vertebrae**
>> ● **S13.121**   **Dislocation of C_1/C_2 cervical vertebrae**

> ● **S13.13**   **Subluxation and dislocation of C_2/C_3 cervical vertebrae**
>> ● **S13.130**   **Subluxation of C_2/C_3 cervical vertebrae**
>> ● **S13.131**   **Dislocation of C_2/C_3 cervical vertebrae**

> ● **S13.14**   **Subluxation and dislocation of C_3/C_4 cervical vertebrae**
>> ● **S13.140**   **Subluxation of C_3/C_4 cervical vertebrae**
>> ● **S13.141**   **Dislocation of C_3/C_4 cervical vertebrae**

> ● **S13.15**   **Subluxation and dislocation of C_4/C_5 cervical vertebrae**
>> ● **S13.150**   **Subluxation of C_4/C_5 cervical vertebrae**
>> ● **S13.151**   **Dislocation of C_4/C_5 cervical vertebrae**

> ● **S13.16**   **Subluxation and dislocation of C_5/C_6 cervical vertebrae**
>> ● **S13.160**   **Subluxation of C_5/C_6 cervical vertebrae**
>> ● **S13.161**   **Dislocation of C_5/C_6 cervical vertebrae**

> ● **S13.17**   **Subluxation and dislocation of C_6/C_7 cervical vertebrae**
>> ● **S13.170**   **Subluxation of C_6/C_7 cervical vertebrae**
>> ● **S13.171**   **Dislocation of C_6/C_7 cervical vertebrae**

> ● **S13.18**   **Subluxation and dislocation of C_7/T_1 cervical vertebrae**
>> ● **S13.180**   **Subluxation of C_7/T_1 cervical vertebrae**
>> ● **S13.181**   **Dislocation of C_7/T_1 cervical vertebrae**

● **S13.2**   **Dislocation of other and unspecified parts of neck**
> X ● **S13.20**   **Dislocation of unspecified parts of neck**
> X ● **S13.29**   **Dislocation of other parts of neck**

X ● **S13.4**   **Sprain of ligaments of cervical spine**
> Sprain of anterior longitudinal (ligament), cervical
> Sprain of atlanto-axial (joints)
> Sprain of atlanto-occipital (joints)
> Whiplash injury of cervical spine

X ● **S13.5**   **Sprain of thyroid region**
> Sprain of cricoarytenoid (joint) (ligament)
> Sprain of cricothyroid (joint) (ligament)
> Sprain of thyroid cartilage

X ● **S13.8**   **Sprain of joints and ligaments of other parts of neck**

X ● **S13.9**   **Sprain of joints and ligaments of unspecified parts of neck**

● **S14**   **Injury of nerves and spinal cord at neck level**

> **Note:** Code to highest level of cervical cord injury

> Code also any associated:
>> fracture of cervical vertebra (S12.0--S12.6.-)
>> open wound of neck (S11.-)
>> transient paralysis (R29.5)

> The appropriate 7th character is to be added to each code from category S14

> | | |
> |---|---|
> | A | initial encounter |
> | D | subsequent encounter |
> | S | sequela |

X ● **S14.0**   **Concussion and edema of cervical spinal cord**

● **S14.1**   **Other and unspecified injuries of cervical spinal cord**
> ● **S14.10**   **Unspecified injury of cervical spinal cord**
>> ● **S14.101**   **Unspecified injury at C_1 level of cervical spinal cord**
>> ● **S14.102**   **Unspecified injury at C_2 level of cervical spinal cord**
>> ● **S14.103**   **Unspecified injury at C_3 level of cervical spinal cord**
>> ● **S14.104**   **Unspecified injury at C_4 level of cervical spinal cord**
>> ● **S14.105**   **Unspecified injury at C_5 level of cervical spinal cord**
>> ● **S14.106**   **Unspecified injury at C_6 level of cervical spinal cord**
>> ● **S14.107**   **Unspecified injury at C_7 level of cervical spinal cord**
>> ● **S14.108**   **Unspecified injury at C_8 level of cervical spinal cord**
>> ● **S14.109**   **Unspecified injury at unspecified level of cervical spinal cord**
>>> Injury of cervical spinal cord NOS

CHAPTER 19 (S00-T88)

● **S14.11**   Complete lesion of cervical spinal cord
    ● **S14.111**   Complete lesion at C_1 level of cervical spinal cord
    ● **S14.112**   Complete lesion at C_2 level of cervical spinal cord
    ● **S14.113**   Complete lesion at C_3 level of cervical spinal cord
    ● **S14.114**   Complete lesion at C_4 level of cervical spinal cord
    ● **S14.115**   Complete lesion at C_5 level of cervical spinal cord
    ● **S14.116**   Complete lesion at C_6 level of cervical spinal cord
    ● **S14.117**   Complete lesion at C_7 level of cervical spinal cord
    ● **S14.118**   Complete lesion at C_8 level of cervical spinal cord
    ● **S14.119**   Complete lesion at unspecified level of cervical spinal cord

● **S14.12**   Central cord syndrome of cervical spinal cord
    ● **S14.121**   Central cord syndrome at C_1 level of cervical spinal cord
    ● **S14.122**   Central cord syndrome at C_2 level of cervical spinal cord
    ● **S14.123**   Central cord syndrome at C_3 level of cervical spinal cord
    ● **S14.124**   Central cord syndrome at C_4 level of cervical spinal cord
    ● **S14.125**   Central cord syndrome at C_5 level of cervical spinal cord
    ● **S14.126**   Central cord syndrome at C_6 level of cervical spinal cord
    ● **S14.127**   Central cord syndrome at C_7 level of cervical spinal cord
    ● **S14.128**   Central cord syndrome at C_8 level of cervical spinal cord
    ● **S14.129**   Central cord syndrome at unspecified level of cervical spinal cord

● **S14.13**   Anterior cord syndrome of cervical spinal cord
    ● **S14.131**   Anterior cord syndrome at C_1 level of cervical spinal cord
    ● **S14.132**   Anterior cord syndrome at C_2 level of cervical spinal cord
    ● **S14.133**   Anterior cord syndrome at C_3 level of cervical spinal cord
    ● **S14.134**   Anterior cord syndrome at C_4 level of cervical spinal cord
    ● **S14.135**   Anterior cord syndrome at C_5 level of cervical spinal cord
    ● **S14.136**   Anterior cord syndrome at C_6 level of cervical spinal cord
    ● **S14.137**   Anterior cord syndrome at C_7 level of cervical spinal cord
    ● **S14.138**   Anterior cord syndrome at C_8 level of cervical spinal cord
    ● **S14.139**   Anterior cord syndrome at unspecified level of cervical spinal cord

● **S14.14**   Brown-Séquard syndrome of cervical spinal cord
    ● **S14.141**   Brown-Séquard syndrome at C_1 level of cervical spinal cord
    ● **S14.142**   Brown-Séquard syndrome at C_2 level of cervical spinal cord
    ● **S14.143**   Brown-Séquard syndrome at C_3 level of cervical spinal cord
    ● **S14.144**   Brown-Séquard syndrome at C_4 level of cervical spinal cord
    ● **S14.145**   Brown-Séquard syndrome at C_5 level of cervical spinal cord

    ● **S14.146**   Brown-Séquard syndrome at C_6 level of cervical spinal cord
    ● **S14.147**   Brown-Séquard syndrome at C_7 level of cervical spinal cord
    ● **S14.148**   Brown-Séquard syndrome at C_8 level of cervical spinal cord
    ● **S14.149**   Brown-Séquard syndrome at unspecified level of cervical spinal cord

● **S14.15**   Other incomplete lesions of cervical spinal cord
     Incomplete lesion of cervical spinal cord NOS
     Posterior cord syndrome of cervical spinal cord
    ● **S14.151**   Other incomplete lesion at C_1 level of cervical spinal cord
    ● **S14.152**   Other incomplete lesion at C_2 level of cervical spinal cord
    ● **S14.153**   Other incomplete lesion at C_3 level of cervical spinal cord
    ● **S14.154**   Other incomplete lesion at C_4 level of cervical spinal cord
    ● **S14.155**   Other incomplete lesion at C_5 level of cervical spinal cord
    ● **S14.156**   Other incomplete lesion at C_6 level of cervical spinal cord
    ● **S14.157**   Other incomplete lesion at C_7 level of cervical spinal cord
    ● **S14.158**   Other incomplete lesion at C_8 level of cervical spinal cord
    ● **S14.159**   Other incomplete lesion at unspecified level of cervical spinal cord

X ● **S14.2**   Injury of nerve root of cervical spine
X ● **S14.3**   Injury of brachial plexus
X ● **S14.4**   Injury of peripheral nerves of neck
X ● **S14.5**   Injury of cervical sympathetic nerves
X ● **S14.8**   Injury of other specified nerves of neck
X ● **S14.9**   Injury of unspecified nerves of neck

● **S15**   **Injury of blood vessels at neck level**
     Code also any associated open wound (S11.-)
     The appropriate 7th character is to be added to each code from category S15

> A   initial encounter
> D   subsequent encounter
> S   sequela

● **S15.0**   Injury of carotid artery of neck
     Injury of carotid artery (common) (external) (internal, extracranial portion)
     Injury of carotid artery NOS
     Excludes1   injury of internal carotid artery, intracranial portion (S06.8)
    ● **S15.00**   Unspecified injury of carotid artery
       ● **S15.001**   Unspecified injury of right carotid artery
       ● **S15.002**   Unspecified injury of left carotid artery
       ● **S15.009**   Unspecified injury of unspecified carotid artery
    ● **S15.01**   Minor laceration of carotid artery
      Incomplete transection of carotid artery
      Laceration of carotid artery NOS
      Superficial laceration of carotid artery
       ● **S15.011**   Minor laceration of right carotid artery
       ● **S15.012**   Minor laceration of left carotid artery
       ● **S15.019**   Minor laceration of unspecified carotid artery

- ● **S15.02   Major laceration of carotid artery**
  Complete transection of carotid artery
  Traumatic rupture of carotid artery
  - ● **S15.021   Major laceration of right carotid artery**
  - ● **S15.022   Major laceration of left carotid artery**
  - ● **S15.029   Major laceration of unspecified carotid artery**
- ● **S15.09   Other specified injury of carotid artery**
  - ● **S15.091   Other specified injury of right carotid artery**
  - ● **S15.092   Other specified injury of left carotid artery**
  - ● **S15.099   Other specified injury of unspecified carotid artery**
- ● **S15.1   Injury of vertebral artery**
  - ● **S15.10   Unspecified injury of vertebral artery**
    - ● **S15.101   Unspecified injury of right vertebral artery**
    - ● **S15.102   Unspecified injury of left vertebral artery**
    - ● **S15.109   Unspecified injury of unspecified vertebral artery**
  - ● **S15.11   Minor laceration of vertebral artery**
    Incomplete transection of vertebral artery
    Laceration of vertebral artery NOS
    Superficial laceration of vertebral artery
    - ● **S15.111   Minor laceration of right vertebral artery**
    - ● **S15.112   Minor laceration of left vertebral artery**
    - ● **S15.119   Minor laceration of unspecified vertebral artery**
  - ● **S15.12   Major laceration of vertebral artery**
    Complete transection of vertebral artery
    Traumatic rupture of vertebral artery
    - ● **S15.121   Major laceration of right vertebral artery**
    - ● **S15.122   Major laceration of left vertebral artery**
    - ● **S15.129   Major laceration of unspecified vertebral artery**
  - ● **S15.19   Other specified injury of vertebral artery**
    - ● **S15.191   Other specified injury of right vertebral artery**
    - ● **S15.192   Other specified injury of left vertebral artery**
    - ● **S15.199   Other specified injury of unspecified vertebral artery**
- ● **S15.2   Injury of external jugular vein**
  - ● **S15.20   Unspecified injury of external jugular vein**
    - ● **S15.201   Unspecified injury of right external jugular vein**
    - ● **S15.202   Unspecified injury of left external jugular vein**
    - ● **S15.209   Unspecified injury of unspecified external jugular vein**
  - ● **S15.21   Minor laceration of external jugular vein**
    Incomplete transection of external jugular vein
    Laceration of external jugular vein NOS
    Superficial laceration of external jugular vein
    - ● **S15.211   Minor laceration of right external jugular vein**
    - ● **S15.212   Minor laceration of left external jugular vein**
    - ● **S15.219   Minor laceration of unspecified external jugular vein**

- ● **S15.22   Major laceration of external jugular vein**
  Complete transection of external jugular vein
  Traumatic rupture of external jugular vein
  - ● **S15.221   Major laceration of right external jugular vein**
  - ● **S15.222   Major laceration of left external jugular vein**
  - ● **S15.229   Major laceration of unspecified external jugular vein**
- ● **S15.29   Other specified injury of external jugular vein**
  - ● **S15.291   Other specified injury of right external jugular vein**
  - ● **S15.292   Other specified injury of left external jugular vein**
  - ● **S15.299   Other specified injury of unspecified external jugular vein**
- ● **S15.3   Injury of internal jugular vein**
  - ● **S15.30   Unspecified injury of internal jugular vein**
    - ● **S15.301   Unspecified injury of right internal jugular vein**
    - ● **S15.302   Unspecified injury of left internal jugular vein**
    - ● **S15.309   Unspecified injury of unspecified internal jugular vein**
  - ● **S15.31   Minor laceration of internal jugular vein**
    Incomplete transection of internal jugular vein
    Laceration of internal jugular vein NOS
    Superficial laceration of internal jugular vein
    - ● **S15.311   Minor laceration of right internal jugular vein**
    - ● **S15.312   Minor laceration of left internal jugular vein**
    - ● **S15.319   Minor laceration of unspecified internal jugular vein**
  - ● **S15.32   Major laceration of internal jugular vein**
    Complete transection of internal jugular vein
    Traumatic rupture of internal jugular vein
    - ● **S15.321   Major laceration of right internal jugular vein**
    - ● **S15.322   Major laceration of left internal jugular vein**
    - ● **S15.329   Major laceration of unspecified internal jugular vein**
  - ● **S15.39   Other specified injury of internal jugular vein**
    - ● **S15.391   Other specified injury of right internal jugular vein**
    - ● **S15.392   Other specified injury of left internal jugular vein**
    - ● **S15.399   Other specified injury of unspecified internal jugular vein**
- X ● **S15.8   Injury of other specified blood vessels at neck level**
- X ● **S15.9   Injury of unspecified blood vessel at neck level**
- ● **S16   Injury of muscle, fascia and tendon at neck level**
  Code also any associated open wound (S11.-)
  Excludes2   sprain of joint or ligament at neck level (S13.9)
  The appropriate 7th character is to be added to each code from category S16

A	initial encounter
D	subsequent encounter
S	sequela

- X ● **S16.1   Strain of muscle, fascia and tendon at neck level**
- X ● **S16.2   Laceration of muscle, fascia and tendon at neck level**
- X ● **S16.8   Other specified injury of muscle, fascia and tendon at neck level**
- X ● **S16.9   Unspecified injury of muscle, fascia and tendon at neck level**

CHAPTER 19 (S00-T88)

● **S17   Crushing injury of neck**
> Use additional code for all associated injuries, such as:
>> injury of blood vessels (S15.-)
>> open wound of neck (S11.-)
>> spinal cord injury (S14.0, S14.1-)
>> vertebral fracture (S12.0--S12.3-)
>
> The appropriate 7th character is to be added to each code from category S17

A	initial encounter
D	subsequent encounter
S	sequela

X ● **S17.0   Crushing injury of larynx and trachea**
X ● **S17.8   Crushing injury of other specified parts of neck**
X ● **S17.9   Crushing injury of neck, part unspecified**

● **S19   Other and unspecified injuries of neck**
> The appropriate 7th character is to be added to each code from category S19

A	initial encounter
D	subsequent encounter
S	sequela

  ● **S19.8   Other specified injuries of neck**
    X ● **S19.80   Other specified injuries of unspecified part of neck**
    X ● **S19.81   Other specified injuries of larynx**
    X ● **S19.82   Other specified injuries of cervical trachea**
    > **Excludes2**   other specified injury of thoracic trachea (S27.5-)
    X ● **S19.83   Other specified injuries of vocal cord**
    X ● **S19.84   Other specified injuries of thyroid gland**
    X ● **S19.85   Other specified injuries of pharynx and cervical esophagus**
    X ● **S19.89   Other specified injuries of other specified part of neck**
  X ● **S19.9   Unspecified injury of neck**

INJURIES TO THE THORAX (S20-S29)

Includes   injuries of breast
                injuries of chest (wall)
                injuries of interscapular area

Excludes2   burns and corrosions (T20-T32)
                effects of foreign body in bronchus (T17.5)
                effects of foreign body in esophagus (T18.1)
                effects of foreign body in lung (T17.8)
                effects of foreign body in trachea (T17.4)
                frostbite (T33-T34)
                injuries of axilla
                injuries of clavicle
                injuries of scapular region
                injuries of shoulder
                insect bite or sting, venomous (T63.4)

● **S20   Superficial injury of thorax**
> The appropriate 7th character is to be added to each code from category S20

A	initial encounter
D	subsequent encounter
S	sequela

  ● **S20.0   Contusion of breast**
    X ● **S20.00   Contusion of breast, unspecified breast**
    X ● **S20.01   Contusion of right breast**
    X ● **S20.02   Contusion of left breast**

● **S20.1   Other and unspecified superficial injuries of breast**
  ● **S20.10   Unspecified superficial injuries of breast**
    ● **S20.101   Unspecified superficial injuries of breast, right breast**
    ● **S20.102   Unspecified superficial injuries of breast, left breast**
    ● **S20.109   Unspecified superficial injuries of breast, unspecified breast**
  ● **S20.11   Abrasion of breast**
    ● **S20.111   Abrasion of breast, right breast**
    ● **S20.112   Abrasion of breast, left breast**
    ● **S20.119   Abrasion of breast, unspecified breast**
  ● **S20.12   Blister (nonthermal) of breast**
    ● **S20.121   Blister (nonthermal) of breast, right breast**
    ● **S20.122   Blister (nonthermal) of breast, left breast**
    ● **S20.129   Blister (nonthermal) of breast, unspecified breast**
  ● **S20.14   External constriction of part of breast**
    ● **S20.141   External constriction of part of breast, right breast**
    ● **S20.142   External constriction of part of breast, left breast**
    ● **S20.149   External constriction of part of breast, unspecified breast**
  ● **S20.15   Superficial foreign body of breast**
    > Splinter in the breast
    ● **S20.151   Superficial foreign body of breast, right breast**
    ● **S20.152   Superficial foreign body of breast, left breast**
    ● **S20.159   Superficial foreign body of breast, unspecified breast**
  ● **S20.16   Insect bite (nonvenomous) of breast**
    ● **S20.161   Insect bite (nonvenomous) of breast, right breast**
    ● **S20.162   Insect bite (nonvenomous) of breast, left breast**
    ● **S20.169   Insect bite (nonvenomous) of breast, unspecified breast**
  ● **S20.17   Other superficial bite of breast**
    > **Excludes1**   open bite of breast (S21.05-)
    ● **S20.171   Other superficial bite of breast, right breast**
    ● **S20.172   Other superficial bite of breast, left breast**
    ● **S20.179   Other superficial bite of breast, unspecified breast**
● **S20.2   Contusion of thorax**
  X ● **S20.20   Contusion of thorax, unspecified**
  ● **S20.21   Contusion of front wall of thorax**
    ● **S20.211   Contusion of right front wall of thorax**
    ● **S20.212   Contusion of left front wall of thorax**
    ● **S20.219   Contusion of unspecified front wall of thorax**
  ● **S20.22   Contusion of back wall of thorax**
    ● **S20.221   Contusion of right back wall of thorax**
    ● **S20.222   Contusion of left back wall of thorax**
    ● **S20.229   Contusion of unspecified back wall of thorax**

◀ New   ◀⁞⁞⁞ Revised   ~~deleted~~ Deleted   OGCR Official Guidelines   X Assign placeholder X   ● Use Additional Character(s)

Excludes 1   Excludes 2   Includes   Use additional   Code first   Code also   Unspecified

● **S20.3**   **Other and unspecified superficial injuries of front wall of thorax**

    ● **S20.30**   Unspecified superficial injuries of front wall of thorax

       ● **S20.301**   Unspecified superficial injuries of right front wall of thorax

       ● **S20.302**   Unspecified superficial injuries of left front wall of thorax

       ● **S20.309**   Unspecified superficial injuries of unspecified front wall of thorax

    ● **S20.31**   Abrasion of front wall of thorax

       ● **S20.311**   Abrasion of right front wall of thorax

       ● **S20.312**   Abrasion of left front wall of thorax

       ● **S20.319**   Abrasion of unspecified front wall of thorax

    ● **S20.32**   Blister (nonthermal) of front wall of thorax

       ● **S20.321**   Blister (nonthermal) of right front wall of thorax

       ● **S20.322**   Blister (nonthermal) of left front wall of thorax

       ● **S20.329**   Blister (nonthermal) of unspecified front wall of thorax

    ● **S20.34**   External constriction of front wall of thorax

       ● **S20.341**   External constriction of right front wall of thorax

       ● **S20.342**   External constriction of left front wall of thorax

       ● **S20.349**   External constriction of unspecified front wall of thorax

    ● **S20.35**   Superficial foreign body of front wall of thorax
         Splinter in front wall of thorax

       ● **S20.351**   Superficial foreign body of right front wall of thorax

       ● **S20.352**   Superficial foreign body of left front wall of thorax

       ● **S20.359**   Superficial foreign body of unspecified front wall of thorax

    ● **S20.36**   Insect bite (nonvenomous) of front wall of thorax

       ● **S20.361**   Insect bite (nonvenomous) of right front wall of thorax

       ● **S20.362**   Insect bite (nonvenomous) of left front wall of thorax

       ● **S20.369**   Insect bite (nonvenomous) of unspecified front wall of thorax

    ● **S20.37**   Other superficial bite of front wall of thorax

       | **Excludes1** | open bite of front wall of thorax (S21.14) |

       ● **S20.371**   Other superficial bite of right front wall of thorax

       ● **S20.372**   Other superficial bite of left front wall of thorax

       ● **S20.379**   Other superficial bite of unspecified front wall of thorax

● **S20.4**   **Other and unspecified superficial injuries of back wall of thorax**

    ● **S20.40**   Unspecified superficial injuries of back wall of thorax

       ● **S20.401**   Unspecified superficial injuries of right back wall of thorax

       ● **S20.402**   Unspecified superficial injuries of left back wall of thorax

       ● **S20.409**   Unspecified superficial injuries of unspecified back wall of thorax

    ● **S20.41**   Abrasion of back wall of thorax

       ● **S20.411**   Abrasion of right back wall of thorax

       ● **S20.412**   Abrasion of left back wall of thorax

       ● **S20.419**   Abrasion of unspecified back wall of thorax

Item 19-1   **Pneumothorax** is a collection of gas (positive air pressure) in the pleural space resulting in the lung collapsing. A tension pneumothorax is life-threatening and is a result of air in the pleural space causing a displacement in the mediastinal structures and cardiopulmonary function compromise. A traumatic pneumothorax results from blunt or penetrating injury that disrupts the parietal/visceral pleura. **Hemothorax** is blood or bloody fluid in the pleural cavity as a result of traumatic blood vessel rupture or inflammation of the lungs from pneumonia.

    ● **S20.42**   Blister (nonthermal) of back wall of thorax

       ● **S20.421**   Blister (nonthermal) of right back wall of thorax

       ● **S20.422**   Blister (nonthermal) of left back wall of thorax

       ● **S20.429**   Blister (nonthermal) of unspecified back wall of thorax

    ● **S20.44**   External constriction of back wall of thorax

       ● **S20.441**   External constriction of right back wall of thorax

       ● **S20.442**   External constriction of left back wall of thorax

       ● **S20.449**   External constriction of unspecified back wall of thorax

    ● **S20.45**   Superficial foreign body of back wall of thorax
         Splinter of back wall of thorax

       ● **S20.451**   Superficial foreign body of right back wall of thorax

       ● **S20.452**   Superficial foreign body of left back wall of thorax

       ● **S20.459**   Superficial foreign body of unspecified back wall of thorax

    ● **S20.46**   Insect bite (nonvenomous) of back wall of thorax

       ● **S20.461**   Insect bite (nonvenomous) of right back wall of thorax

       ● **S20.462**   Insect bite (nonvenomous) of left back wall of thorax

       ● **S20.469**   Insect bite (nonvenomous) of unspecified back wall of thorax

    ● **S20.47**   Other superficial bite of back wall of thorax

       | **Excludes1** | open bite of back wall of thorax (S21.24) |

       ● **S20.471**   Other superficial bite of right back wall of thorax

       ● **S20.472**   Other superficial bite of left back wall of thorax

       ● **S20.479**   Other superficial bite of unspecified back wall of thorax

● **S20.9**   **Superficial injury of unspecified parts of thorax**

    | **Excludes1** | contusion of thorax NOS (S20.20) |

   X ● **S20.90**   Unspecified superficial injury of unspecified parts of thorax
         Superficial injury of thoracic wall NOS

   X ● **S20.91**   Abrasion of unspecified parts of thorax

   X ● **S20.92**   Blister (nonthermal) of unspecified parts of thorax

   X ● **S20.94**   External constriction of unspecified parts of thorax

   X ● **S20.95**   Superficial foreign body of unspecified parts of thorax
         Splinter in thorax NOS

   X ● **S20.96**   Insect bite (nonvenomous) of unspecified parts of thorax

   X ● **S20.97**   Other superficial bite of unspecified parts of thorax

       | **Excludes1** | open bite of thorax NOS (S21.95) |

◀ New   ◀═ Revised   ~~deleted~~ Deleted   **OGCR** Official Guidelines   X Assign placeholder X   ● Use Additional Character(s)

| Excludes 1 | | Excludes 2 | | Includes | Use additional | | Code first | Code also | Unspecified |

● **S21   Open wound of thorax**

Code also any associated injury such as:
  injury of heart (S26.-)
  injury of intrathoracic organs (S27.-)
  rib fracture (S22.3-, S22.4-)
  spinal cord injury (S24.0-, S24.1-)
  traumatic hemothorax (S27.1)
  traumatic hemopneumothorax (S27.3)
  traumatic pneumothorax (S27.0)
  wound infection

  | **Excludes1** | traumatic amputation (partial) of thorax (S28.1) |

The appropriate 7th character is to be added to each code from
  category S21

A	initial encounter
D	subsequent encounter
S	sequela

● **S21.0   Open wound of breast**
  ● **S21.00   Unspecified open wound of breast**
    ● **S21.001   Unspecified open wound of right breast**
    ● **S21.002   Unspecified open wound of left breast**
    ● **S21.009   Unspecified open wound of unspecified breast**
  ● **S21.01   Laceration without foreign body of breast**
    ● **S21.011   Laceration without foreign body of right breast**
    ● **S21.012   Laceration without foreign body of left breast**
    ● **S21.019   Laceration without foreign body of unspecified breast**
  ● **S21.02   Laceration with foreign body of breast**
    ● **S21.021   Laceration with foreign body of right breast**
    ● **S21.022   Laceration with foreign body of left breast**
    ● **S21.029   Laceration with foreign body of unspecified breast**
  ● **S21.03   Puncture wound without foreign body of breast**
    ● **S21.031   Puncture wound without foreign body of right breast**
    ● **S21.032   Puncture wound without foreign body of left breast**
    ● **S21.039   Puncture wound without foreign body of unspecified breast**
  ● **S21.04   Puncture wound with foreign body of breast**
    ● **S21.041   Puncture wound with foreign body of right breast**
    ● **S21.042   Puncture wound with foreign body of left breast**
    ● **S21.049   Puncture wound with foreign body of unspecified breast**
  ● **S21.05   Open bite of breast**
      Bite of breast NOS

    | **Excludes1** | superficial bite of breast (S20.17) |

    ● **S21.051   Open bite of right breast**
    ● **S21.052   Open bite of left breast**
    ● **S21.059   Open bite of unspecified breast**

● **S21.1   Open wound of front wall of thorax without penetration into thoracic cavity**
    Open wound of chest without penetration into thoracic cavity
  ● **S21.10   Unspecified open wound of front wall of thorax without penetration into thoracic cavity**
    ● **S21.101   Unspecified open wound of right front wall of thorax without penetration into thoracic cavity**
    ● **S21.102   Unspecified open wound of left front wall of thorax without penetration into thoracic cavity**
    ● **S21.109   Unspecified open wound of unspecified front wall of thorax without penetration into thoracic cavity**
  ● **S21.11   Laceration without foreign body of front wall of thorax without penetration into thoracic cavity**
    ● **S21.111   Laceration without foreign body of right front wall of thorax without penetration into thoracic cavity**
    ● **S21.112   Laceration without foreign body of left front wall of thorax without penetration into thoracic cavity**
    ● **S21.119   Laceration without foreign body of unspecified front wall of thorax without penetration into thoracic cavity**
  ● **S21.12   Laceration with foreign body of front wall of thorax without penetration into thoracic cavity**
    ● **S21.121   Laceration with foreign body of right front wall of thorax without penetration into thoracic cavity**
    ● **S21.122   Laceration with foreign body of left front wall of thorax without penetration into thoracic cavity**
    ● **S21.129   Laceration with foreign body of unspecified front wall of thorax without penetration into thoracic cavity**
  ● **S21.13   Puncture wound without foreign body of front wall of thorax without penetration into thoracic cavity**
    ● **S21.131   Puncture wound without foreign body of right front wall of thorax without penetration into thoracic cavity**
    ● **S21.132   Puncture wound without foreign body of left front wall of thorax without penetration into thoracic cavity**
    ● **S21.139   Puncture wound without foreign body of unspecified front wall of thorax without penetration into thoracic cavity**
  ● **S21.14   Puncture wound with foreign body of front wall of thorax without penetration into thoracic cavity**
    ● **S21.141   Puncture wound with foreign body of right front wall of thorax without penetration into thoracic cavity**
    ● **S21.142   Puncture wound with foreign body of left front wall of thorax without penetration into thoracic cavity**
    ● **S21.149   Puncture wound with foreign body of unspecified front wall of thorax without penetration into thoracic cavity**

● **S21.15**   **Open bite of front wall of thorax without penetration into thoracic cavity**
    Bite of front wall of thorax NOS
    | Excludes1 | superficial bite of front wall of thorax (S20.37)

    ● **S21.151**   **Open bite of right front wall of thorax without penetration into thoracic cavity**

    ● **S21.152**   **Open bite of left front wall of thorax without penetration into thoracic cavity**

    ● **S21.159**   **Open bite of unspecified front wall of thorax without penetration into thoracic cavity**

● **S21.2**   **Open wound of back wall of thorax without penetration into thoracic cavity**

    ● **S21.20**   **Unspecified open wound of back wall of thorax without penetration into thoracic cavity**

      ● **S21.201**   **Unspecified open wound of right back wall of thorax without penetration into thoracic cavity**

      ● **S21.202**   **Unspecified open wound of left back wall of thorax without penetration into thoracic cavity**

      ● **S21.209**   **Unspecified open wound of unspecified back wall of thorax without penetration into thoracic cavity**

    ● **S21.21**   **Laceration without foreign body of back wall of thorax without penetration into thoracic cavity**

      ● **S21.211**   **Laceration without foreign body of right back wall of thorax without penetration into thoracic cavity**

      ● **S21.212**   **Laceration without foreign body of left back wall of thorax without penetration into thoracic cavity**

      ● **S21.219**   **Laceration without foreign body of unspecified back wall of thorax without penetration into thoracic cavity**

    ● **S21.22**   **Laceration with foreign body of back wall of thorax without penetration into thoracic cavity**

      ● **S21.221**   **Laceration with foreign body of right back wall of thorax without penetration into thoracic cavity**

      ● **S21.222**   **Laceration with foreign body of left back wall of thorax without penetration into thoracic cavity**

      ● **S21.229**   **Laceration with foreign body of unspecified back wall of thorax without penetration into thoracic cavity**

    ● **S21.23**   **Puncture wound without foreign body of back wall of thorax without penetration into thoracic cavity**

      ● **S21.231**   **Puncture wound without foreign body of right back wall of thorax without penetration into thoracic cavity**

      ● **S21.232**   **Puncture wound without foreign body of left back wall of thorax without penetration into thoracic cavity**

      ● **S21.239**   **Puncture wound without foreign body of unspecified back wall of thorax without penetration into thoracic cavity**

● **S21.24**   **Puncture wound with foreign body of back wall of thorax without penetration into thoracic cavity**

    ● **S21.241**   **Puncture wound with foreign body of right back wall of thorax without penetration into thoracic cavity**

    ● **S21.242**   **Puncture wound with foreign body of left back wall of thorax without penetration into thoracic cavity**

    ● **S21.249**   **Puncture wound with foreign body of unspecified back wall of thorax without penetration into thoracic cavity**

● **S21.25**   **Open bite of back wall of thorax without penetration into thoracic cavity**
    Bite of back wall of thorax NOS
    | Excludes1 | superficial bite of back wall of thorax (S20.47)

    ● **S21.251**   **Open bite of right back wall of thorax without penetration into thoracic cavity**

    ● **S21.252**   **Open bite of left back wall of thorax without penetration into thoracic cavity**

    ● **S21.259**   **Open bite of unspecified back wall of thorax without penetration into thoracic cavity**

● **S21.3**   **Open wound of front wall of thorax with penetration into thoracic cavity**
    Open wound of chest with penetration into thoracic cavity

    ● **S21.30**   **Unspecified open wound of front wall of thorax with penetration into thoracic cavity**

      ● **S21.301**   **Unspecified open wound of right front wall of thorax with penetration into thoracic cavity**

      ● **S21.302**   **Unspecified open wound of left front wall of thorax with penetration into thoracic cavity**

      ● **S21.309**   **Unspecified open wound of unspecified front wall of thorax with penetration into thoracic cavity**

    ● **S21.31**   **Laceration without foreign body of front wall of thorax with penetration into thoracic cavity**

      ● **S21.311**   **Laceration without foreign body of right front wall of thorax with penetration into thoracic cavity**

      ● **S21.312**   **Laceration without foreign body of left front wall of thorax with penetration into thoracic cavity**

      ● **S21.319**   **Laceration without foreign body of unspecified front wall of thorax with penetration into thoracic cavity**

    ● **S21.32**   **Laceration with foreign body of front wall of thorax with penetration into thoracic cavity**

      ● **S21.321**   **Laceration with foreign body of right front wall of thorax with penetration into thoracic cavity**

      ● **S21.322**   **Laceration with foreign body of left front wall of thorax with penetration into thoracic cavity**

      ● **S21.329**   **Laceration with foreign body of unspecified front wall of thorax with penetration into thoracic cavity**

● S21.33 **Puncture wound without foreign body of front wall of thorax with penetration into thoracic cavity**
  ● S21.331 **Puncture wound without foreign body of right front wall of thorax with penetration into thoracic cavity**
  ● S21.332 **Puncture wound without foreign body of left front wall of thorax with penetration into thoracic cavity**
  ● S21.339 **Puncture wound without foreign body of unspecified front wall of thorax with penetration into thoracic cavity**

● S21.34 **Puncture wound with foreign body of front wall of thorax with penetration into thoracic cavity**
  ● S21.341 **Puncture wound with foreign body of right front wall of thorax with penetration into thoracic cavity**
  ● S21.342 **Puncture wound with foreign body of left front wall of thorax with penetration into thoracic cavity**
  ● S21.349 **Puncture wound with foreign body of unspecified front wall of thorax with penetration into thoracic cavity**

● S21.35 **Open bite of front wall of thorax with penetration into thoracic cavity**
  Excludes1 superficial bite of front wall of thorax (S20.37)
  ● S21.351 **Open bite of right front wall of thorax with penetration into thoracic cavity**
  ● S21.352 **Open bite of left front wall of thorax with penetration into thoracic cavity**
  ● S21.359 **Open bite of unspecified front wall of thorax with penetration into thoracic cavity**

● S21.4 **Open wound of back wall of thorax with penetration into thoracic cavity**
  ● S21.40 **Unspecified open wound of back wall of thorax with penetration into thoracic cavity**
    ● S21.401 **Unspecified open wound of right back wall of thorax with penetration into thoracic cavity**
    ● S21.402 **Unspecified open wound of left back wall of thorax with penetration into thoracic cavity**
    ● S21.409 **Unspecified open wound of unspecified back wall of thorax with penetration into thoracic cavity**
  ● S21.41 **Laceration without foreign body of back wall of thorax with penetration into thoracic cavity**
    ● S21.411 **Laceration without foreign body of right back wall of thorax with penetration into thoracic cavity**
    ● S21.412 **Laceration without foreign body of left back wall of thorax with penetration into thoracic cavity**
    ● S21.419 **Laceration without foreign body of unspecified back wall of thorax with penetration into thoracic cavity**

● S21.42 **Laceration with foreign body of back wall of thorax with penetration into thoracic cavity**
  ● S21.421 **Laceration with foreign body of right back wall of thorax with penetration into thoracic cavity**
  ● S21.422 **Laceration with foreign body of left back wall of thorax with penetration into thoracic cavity**
  ● S21.429 **Laceration with foreign body of unspecified back wall of thorax with penetration into thoracic cavity**

● S21.43 **Puncture wound without foreign body of back wall of thorax with penetration into thoracic cavity**
  ● S21.431 **Puncture wound without foreign body of right back wall of thorax with penetration into thoracic cavity**
  ● S21.432 **Puncture wound without foreign body of left back wall of thorax with penetration into thoracic cavity**
  ● S21.439 **Puncture wound without foreign body of unspecified back wall of thorax with penetration into thoracic cavity**

● S21.44 **Puncture wound with foreign body of back wall of thorax with penetration into thoracic cavity**
  ● S21.441 **Puncture wound with foreign body of right back wall of thorax with penetration into thoracic cavity**
  ● S21.442 **Puncture wound with foreign body of left back wall of thorax with penetration into thoracic cavity**
  ● S21.449 **Puncture wound with foreign body of unspecified back wall of thorax with penetration into thoracic cavity**

● S21.45 **Open bite of back wall of thorax with penetration into thoracic cavity**
  Bite of back wall of thorax NOS
  Excludes1 superficial bite of back wall of thorax (S20.47)
  ● S21.451 **Open bite of right back wall of thorax with penetration into thoracic cavity**
  ● S21.452 **Open bite of left back wall of thorax with penetration into thoracic cavity**
  ● S21.459 **Open bite of unspecified back wall of thorax with penetration into thoracic cavity**

● S21.9 **Open wound of unspecified part of thorax**
  Open wound of thoracic wall NOS
  X ● S21.90 **Unspecified open wound of unspecified part of thorax**
  X ● S21.91 **Laceration without foreign body of unspecified part of thorax**
  X ● S21.92 **Laceration with foreign body of unspecified part of thorax**
  X ● S21.93 **Puncture wound without foreign body of unspecified part of thorax**
  X ● S21.94 **Puncture wound with foreign body of unspecified part of thorax**
  X ● S21.95 **Open bite of unspecified part of thorax**
    Excludes1 superficial bite of thorax (S20.97)

● **S22   Fracture of rib(s), sternum and thoracic spine**

Note: A fracture not indicated as displaced or nondisplaced should be coded to displaced

A fracture not indicated as open or closed should be coded to closed

Includes	fracture of thoracic neural arch
	fracture of thoracic spinous process
	fracture of thoracic transverse process
	fracture of thoracic vertebra
	fracture of thoracic vertebral arch

Code first any associated:
injury of intrathoracic organ (S27.-)
spinal cord injury (S24.0-, S24.1-)

Excludes1	transection of thorax (S28.1)
Excludes2	fracture of clavicle (S42.0-)
	fracture of scapula (S42.1-)

The appropriate 7th character is to be added to each code from category S22

A	initial encounter for closed fracture
B	initial encounter for open fracture
D	subsequent encounter for fracture with routine healing
G	subsequent encounter for fracture with delayed healing
K	subsequent encounter for fracture with nonunion
S	sequela

● **S22.0   Fracture of thoracic vertebra**

  ● **S22.00   Fracture of unspecified thoracic vertebra**

   ● S22.000   Wedge compression fracture of unspecified thoracic vertebra
   ● S22.001   Stable burst fracture of unspecified thoracic vertebra
   ● S22.002   Unstable burst fracture of unspecified thoracic vertebra
   ● S22.008   Other fracture of unspecified thoracic vertebra
   ● S22.009   Unspecified fracture of unspecified thoracic vertebra

  ● **S22.01   Fracture of first thoracic vertebra**

   ● S22.010   Wedge compression fracture of first thoracic vertebra
   ● S22.011   Stable burst fracture of first thoracic vertebra
   ● S22.012   Unstable burst fracture of first thoracic vertebra
   ● S22.018   Other fracture of first thoracic vertebra
   ● S22.019   Unspecified fracture of first thoracic vertebra

  ● **S22.02   Fracture of second thoracic vertebra**

   ● S22.020   Wedge compression fracture of second thoracic vertebra
   ● S22.021   Stable burst fracture of second thoracic vertebra
   ● S22.022   Unstable burst fracture of second thoracic vertebra
   ● S22.028   Other fracture of second thoracic vertebra
   ● S22.029   Unspecified fracture of second thoracic vertebra

  ● **S22.03   Fracture of third thoracic vertebra**

   ● S22.030   Wedge compression fracture of third thoracic vertebra
   ● S22.031   Stable burst fracture of third thoracic vertebra
   ● S22.032   Unstable burst fracture of third thoracic vertebra
   ● S22.038   Other fracture of third thoracic vertebra
   ● S22.039   Unspecified fracture of third thoracic vertebra

● **S22.04   Fracture of fourth thoracic vertebra**

   ● S22.040   Wedge compression fracture of fourth thoracic vertebra
   ● S22.041   Stable burst fracture of fourth thoracic vertebra
   ● S22.042   Unstable burst fracture of fourth thoracic vertebra
   ● S22.048   Other fracture of fourth thoracic vertebra
   ● S22.049   Unspecified fracture of fourth thoracic vertebra

● **S22.05   Fracture of T_5-T_6 vertebra**

   ● S22.050   Wedge compression fracture of T_5-T_6 vertebra
   ● S22.051   Stable burst fracture of T_5-T_6 vertebra
   ● S22.052   Unstable burst fracture of T_5-T_6 vertebra
   ● S22.058   Other fracture of T_5-T_6 vertebra
   ● S22.059   Unspecified fracture of T_5-T_6 vertebra

● **S22.06   Fracture of T_7-T_8 vertebra**

   ● S22.060   Wedge compression fracture of T_7-T_8 vertebra
   ● S22.061   Stable burst fracture of T_7-T_8 vertebra
   ● S22.062   Unstable burst fracture of T_7-T_8 vertebra
   ● S22.068   Other fracture of T_7-T_8 thoracic vertebra
   ● S22.069   Unspecified fracture of T_7-T_8 vertebra

● **S22.07   Fracture of T_9-T_{10} vertebra**

   ● S22.070   Wedge compression fracture of T_9-T_{10} vertebra
   ● S22.071   Stable burst fracture of T_9-T_{10} vertebra
   ● S22.072   Unstable burst fracture of T_9-T_{10} vertebra
   ● S22.078   Other fracture of T_9-T_{10} vertebra
   ● S22.079   Unspecified fracture of T_9-T_{10} vertebra

● **S22.08   Fracture of T_{11}-T_{12} vertebra**

   ● S22.080   Wedge compression fracture of T_{11}-T_{12} vertebra
   ● S22.081   Stable burst fracture of T_{11}-T_{12} vertebra
   ● S22.082   Unstable burst fracture of T_{11}-T_{12} vertebra
   ● S22.088   Other fracture of T_{11}-T_{12} vertebra
   ● S22.089   Unspecified fracture of T_{11}-T_{12} vertebra

● **S22.2   Fracture of sternum**

   X ● S22.20   Unspecified fracture of sternum
   X ● S22.21   Fracture of manubrium
   X ● S22.22   Fracture of body of sternum
   X ● S22.23   Sternal manubrial dissociation
   X ● S22.24   Fracture of xiphoid process

● **S22.3 Fracture of one rib**

   X ● S22.31   Fracture of one rib, right side
   X ● S22.32   Fracture of one rib, left side
   X ● S22.39   Fracture of one rib, unspecified side

● **S22.4   Multiple fractures of ribs**

Fractures of two or more ribs

Excludes1	flail chest (S22.5-)

   X ● S22.41   Multiple fractures of ribs, right side
   X ● S22.42   Multiple fractures of ribs, left side
   X ● S22.43   Multiple fractures of ribs, bilateral
   X ● S22.49   Multiple fractures of ribs, unspecified side

X ● **S22.5   Flail chest**

Unstable chest due to sternum and/or rib fracture

X ● **S22.9   Fracture of bony thorax, part unspecified**

CHAPTER 19 (S00-T88)

CHAPTER 19 (S00-T88)

● **S23**   **Dislocation and sprain of joints and ligaments of thorax**

Includes   avulsion of joint or ligament of thorax
laceration of cartilage, joint or ligament of thorax
sprain of cartilage, joint or ligament of thorax
traumatic hemarthrosis of joint or ligament of thorax
traumatic rupture of joint or ligament of thorax
traumatic subluxation of joint or ligament of thorax
traumatic tear of joint or ligament of thorax

Code also any associated open wound

Excludes2   dislocation, sprain of sternoclavicular joint (S43.2, S43.6)
strain of muscle or tendon of thorax (S29.01-)

The appropriate 7th character is to be added to each code from category S23

> A   initial encounter
> D   subsequent encounter
> S   sequela

X ● **S23.0**   **Traumatic rupture of thoracic intervertebral disc**

Excludes1   rupture or displacement (nontraumatic) of thoracic intervertebral disc NOS (M51.- with fifth character 4)

● **S23.1**   **Subluxation and dislocation of thoracic vertebra**

Code also any associated
open wound of thorax (S21.-)
spinal cord injury (S24.0-, S24.1-)

Excludes2   fracture of thoracic vertebrae (S22.0-)

● **S23.10**   **Subluxation and dislocation of unspecified thoracic vertebra**

     ● **S23.100**   **Subluxation of unspecified thoracic vertebra**

     ● **S23.101**   **Dislocation of unspecified thoracic vertebra**

● **S23.11**   **Subluxation and dislocation of T_1/T_2 thoracic vertebra**

     ● **S23.110**   **Subluxation of T_1/T_2 thoracic vertebra**

     ● **S23.111**   **Dislocation of T_1/T_2 thoracic vertebra**

● **S23.12**   **Subluxation and dislocation of T_2/T_3-T_3/T_4 thoracic vertebra**

     ● **S23.120**   **Subluxation of T_2/T_3 thoracic vertebra**

     ● **S23.121**   **Dislocation of T_2/T_3 thoracic vertebra**

     ● **S23.122**   **Subluxation of T_3/T_4 thoracic vertebra**

     ● **S23.123**   **Dislocation of T_3/T_4 thoracic vertebra**

● **S23.13**   **Subluxation and dislocation of T_4/T_5-T_5/T_6 thoracic vertebra**

     ● **S23.130**   **Subluxation of T_4/T_5 thoracic vertebra**

     ● **S23.131**   **Dislocation of T_4/T_5 thoracic vertebra**

     ● **S23.132**   **Subluxation of T_5/T_6 thoracic vertebra**

     ● **S23.133**   **Dislocation of T_5/T_6 thoracic vertebra**

● **S23.14**   **Subluxation and dislocation of T_6/T_7-T_7/T_8 thoracic vertebra**

     ● **S23.140**   **Subluxation of T_6/T_7 thoracic vertebra**

     ● **S23.141**   **Dislocation of T_6/T_7 thoracic vertebra**

     ● **S23.142**   **Subluxation of T_7/T_8 thoracic vertebra**

     ● **S23.143**   **Dislocation of T_7/T_8 thoracic vertebra**

● **S23.15**   **Subluxation and dislocation of T_8/T_9-T_9/T_{10} thoracic vertebra**

     ● **S23.150**   **Subluxation of T_8/T_9 thoracic vertebra**

     ● **S23.151**   **Dislocation of T_8/T_9 thoracic vertebra**

     ● **S23.152**   **Subluxation of T_9/T_{10} thoracic vertebra**

     ● **S23.153**   **Dislocation of T_9/T_{10} thoracic vertebra**

● **S23.16**   **Subluxation and dislocation of T_{10}/T_{11}-T_{11}/T_{12} thoracic vertebra**

     ● **S23.160**   **Subluxation of T_{10}/T_{11} thoracic vertebra**

     ● **S23.161**   **Dislocation of T_{10}/T_{11} thoracic vertebra**

     ● **S23.162**   **Subluxation of T_{11}/T_{12} thoracic vertebra**

     ● **S23.163**   **Dislocation of T_{11}/T_{12} thoracic vertebra**

● **S23.17**   **Subluxation and dislocation of T_{12}/L_1 thoracic vertebra**

     ● **S23.170**   **Subluxation of T_{12}/L_1 thoracic vertebra**

     ● **S23.171**   **Dislocation of T_{12}/L_1 thoracic vertebra**

● **S23.2**   **Dislocation of other and unspecified parts of thorax**

X ● **S23.20**   **Dislocation of unspecified part of thorax**

X ● **S23.29**   **Dislocation of other parts of thorax**

X ● **S23.3**   **Sprain of ligaments of thoracic spine**

● **S23.4**   **Sprain of ribs and sternum**

X ● **S23.41**   **Sprain of ribs**

● **S23.42**   **Sprain of sternum**

     ● **S23.420**   **Sprain of sternoclavicular (joint) (ligament)**

     ● **S23.421**   **Sprain of chondrosternal joint**

     ● **S23.428**   **Other sprain of sternum**

     ● **S23.429**   **Unspecified sprain of sternum**

X ● **S23.8**   **Sprain of other specified parts of thorax**

X ● **S23.9**   **Sprain of unspecified parts of thorax**

● **S24**   **Injury of nerves and spinal cord at thorax level**

Note: Code to highest level of thoracic spinal cord injury.

Injuries to the spinal cord (S24.0 and S24.1) refer to the cord level and not bone level injury, and can affect nerve roots at and below the level given.

Code also any associated:
fracture of thoracic vertebra (S22.0-)
open wound of thorax (S21.-)
transient paralysis (R29.5)

Excludes2   injury of brachial plexus (S14.3)

The appropriate 7th character is to be added to each code from category S24

> A   initial encounter
> D   subsequent encounter
> S   sequela

X ● **S24.0**   **Concussion and edema of thoracic spinal cord**

● **S24.1**   **Other and unspecified injuries of thoracic spinal cord**

● **S24.10**   **Unspecified injury of thoracic spinal cord**

     ● **S24.101**   **Unspecified injury at T_1 level of thoracic spinal cord**

     ● **S24.102**   **Unspecified injury at T_2-T_6 level of thoracic spinal cord**

     ● **S24.103**   **Unspecified injury at T_7-T_{10} level of thoracic spinal cord**

     ● **S24.104**   **Unspecified injury at T_{11}-T_{12} level of thoracic spinal cord**

     ● **S24.109**   **Unspecified injury at unspecified level of thoracic spinal cord**
Injury of thoracic spinal cord NOS

● **S24.11**   **Complete lesion of thoracic spinal cord**

     ● **S24.111**   **Complete lesion at T_1 level of thoracic spinal cord**

     ● **S24.112**   **Complete lesion at T_2-T_6 level of thoracic spinal cord**

     ● **S24.113**   **Complete lesion at T_7-T_{10} level of thoracic spinal cord**

     ● **S24.114**   **Complete lesion at T_{11}-T_{12} level of thoracic spinal cord**

     ● **S24.119**   **Complete lesion at unspecified level of thoracic spinal cord**

◀ New   ◀|||| Revised   ~~deleted~~ Deleted   **OGCR** Official Guidelines   X Assign placeholder X   ● Use Additional Character(s)

Excludes 1   Excludes 2   Includes   Use additional   Code first   Code also   Unspecified

1250

● **S24.13**   **Anterior cord syndrome of thoracic spinal cord**
    ● **S24.131**   Anterior cord syndrome at T_1 level of thoracic spinal cord
    ● **S24.132**   Anterior cord syndrome at T_2-T_6 level of thoracic spinal cord
    ● **S24.133**   Anterior cord syndrome at T_7-T_{10} level of thoracic spinal cord
    ● **S24.134**   Anterior cord syndrome at T_{11}-T_{12} level of thoracic spinal cord
    ● **S24.139**   Anterior cord syndrome at unspecified level of thoracic spinal cord

● **S24.14**   **Brown-Séquard syndrome of thoracic spinal cord**
    ● **S24.141**   Brown-Séquard syndrome at T_1 level of thoracic spinal cord
    ● **S24.142**   Brown-Séquard syndrome at T_2-T_6 level of thoracic spinal cord
    ● **S24.143**   Brown-Séquard syndrome at T_7-T_{10} level of thoracic spinal cord
    ● **S24.144**   Brown-Séquard syndrome at T_{11}-T_{12} level of thoracic spinal cord
    ● **S24.149**   Brown-Séquard syndrome at unspecified level of thoracic spinal cord

● **S24.15**   **Other incomplete lesions of thoracic spinal cord**
    Incomplete lesion of thoracic spinal cord NOS
    Posterior cord syndrome of thoracic spinal cord
    ● **S24.151**   Other incomplete lesion at T_1 level of thoracic spinal cord
    ● **S24.152**   Other incomplete lesion at T_2-T_6 level of thoracic spinal cord
    ● **S24.153**   Other incomplete lesion at T_7-T_{10} level of thoracic spinal cord
    ● **S24.154**   Other incomplete lesion at T_{11}-T_{12} level of thoracic spinal cord
    ● **S24.159**   Other incomplete lesion at unspecified level of thoracic spinal cord

X ● **S24.2**   **Injury of nerve root of thoracic spine**
X ● **S24.3**   **Injury of peripheral nerves of thorax**
X ● **S24.4**   **Injury of thoracic sympathetic nervous system**
    Injury of cardiac plexus
    Injury of esophageal plexus
    Injury of pulmonary plexus
    Injury of stellate ganglion
    Injury of thoracic sympathetic ganglion
X ● **S24.8**   **Injury of other specified nerves of thorax**
X ● **S24.9**   **Injury of unspecified nerve of thorax**

● **S25**   **Injury of blood vessels of thorax**
    The appropriate 7th character is to be added to each code from category S25

> A   initial encounter
> D   subsequent encounter
> S   sequela

    Code also any associated open wound (S21.-)

● **S25.0**   **Injury of thoracic aorta**
    Injury of aorta NOS
    X ● **S25.00**   Unspecified injury of thoracic aorta
    X ● **S25.01**   Minor laceration of thoracic aorta
      Incomplete transection of thoracic aorta
      Laceration of thoracic aorta NOS
      Superficial laceration of thoracic aorta
    X ● **S25.02**   Major laceration of thoracic aorta
      Complete transection of thoracic aorta
      Traumatic rupture of thoracic aorta
    X ● **S25.09**   Other specified injury of thoracic aorta

● **S25.1**   **Injury of innominate or subclavian artery**
    ● **S25.10**   Unspecified injury of innominate or subclavian artery
      ● **S25.101**   Unspecified injury of right innominate or subclavian artery
      ● **S25.102**   Unspecified injury of left innominate or subclavian artery
      ● **S25.109**   Unspecified injury of unspecified innominate or subclavian artery
    ● **S25.11**   Minor laceration of innominate or subclavian artery
      Incomplete transection of innominate or subclavian artery
      Laceration of innominate or subclavian artery NOS
      Superficial laceration of innominate or subclavian artery
      ● **S25.111**   Minor laceration of right innominate or subclavian artery
      ● **S25.112**   Minor laceration of left innominate or subclavian artery
      ● **S25.119**   Minor laceration of unspecified innominate or subclavian artery
    ● **S25.12**   Major laceration of innominate or subclavian artery
      Complete transection of innominate or subclavian artery
      Traumatic rupture of innominate or subclavian artery
      ● **S25.121**   Major laceration of right innominate or subclavian artery
      ● **S25.122**   Major laceration of left innominate or subclavian artery
      ● **S25.129**   Major laceration of unspecified innominate or subclavian artery
    ● **S25.19**   Other specified injury of innominate or subclavian artery
      ● **S25.191**   Other specified injury of right innominate or subclavian artery
      ● **S25.192**   Other specified injury of left innominate or subclavian artery
      ● **S25.199**   Other specified injury of unspecified innominate or subclavian artery

● **S25.2**   **Injury of superior vena cava**
    Injury of vena cava NOS
    X ● **S25.20**   Unspecified injury of superior vena cava
    X ● **S25.21**   Minor laceration of superior vena cava
      Incomplete transection of superior vena cava
      Laceration of superior vena cava NOS
      Superficial laceration of superior vena cava
    X ● **S25.22**   Major laceration of superior vena cava
      Complete transection of superior vena cava
      Traumatic rupture of superior vena cava
    X ● **S25.29**   Other specified injury of superior vena cava

● **S25.3**   **Injury of innominate or subclavian vein**
    ● **S25.30**   Unspecified injury of innominate or subclavian vein
      ● **S25.301**   Unspecified injury of right innominate or subclavian vein
      ● **S25.302**   Unspecified injury of left innominate or subclavian vein
      ● **S25.309**   Unspecified injury of unspecified innominate or subclavian vein

---

◀ New   ⬅ Revised   ~~deleted~~ Deleted   **OGCR** Official Guidelines   X Assign placeholder X   ● Use Additional Character(s)

Excludes 1   Excludes 2   Includes   Use additional   Code first   Code also   Unspecified

● **S25.31**   **Minor laceration of innominate or subclavian vein**
Incomplete transection of innominate or subclavian vein
Laceration of innominate or subclavian vein NOS
Superficial laceration of innominate or subclavian vein

    ● **S25.311**   **Minor laceration of right innominate or subclavian vein**

    ● **S25.312**   **Minor laceration of left innominate or subclavian vein**

    ● **S25.319**   **Minor laceration of unspecified innominate or subclavian vein**

    ● **S25.32**   **Major laceration of innominate or subclavian vein**
Complete transection of innominate or subclavian vein
Traumatic rupture of innominate or subclavian vein

    ● **S25.321**   **Major laceration of right innominate or subclavian vein**

    ● **S25.322**   **Major laceration of left innominate or subclavian vein**

    ● **S25.329**   **Major laceration of unspecified innominate or subclavian vein**

● **S25.39**   **Other specified injury of innominate or subclavian vein**

    ● **S25.391**   **Other specified injury of right innominate or subclavian vein**

    ● **S25.392**   **Other specified injury of left innominate or subclavian vein**

    ● **S25.399**   **Other specified injury of unspecified innominate or subclavian vein**

● **S25.4**   **Injury of pulmonary blood vessels**

  ● **S25.40**   **Unspecified injury of pulmonary blood vessels**

    ● **S25.401**   **Unspecified injury of right pulmonary blood vessels**

    ● **S25.402**   **Unspecified injury of left pulmonary blood vessels**

    ● **S25.409**   **Unspecified injury of unspecified pulmonary blood vessels**

  ● **S25.41**   **Minor laceration of pulmonary blood vessels**
Incomplete transection of pulmonary blood vessels
Laceration of pulmonary blood vessels NOS
Superficial laceration of pulmonary blood vessels

    ● **S25.411**   **Minor laceration of right pulmonary blood vessels**

    ● **S25.412**   **Minor laceration of left pulmonary blood vessels**

    ● **S25.419**   **Minor laceration of unspecified pulmonary blood vessels**

  ● **S25.42**   **Major laceration of pulmonary blood vessels**
Complete transection of pulmonary blood vessels
Traumatic rupture of pulmonary blood vessels

    ● **S25.421**   **Major laceration of right pulmonary blood vessels**

    ● **S25.422**   **Major laceration of left pulmonary blood vessels**

    ● **S25.429**   **Major laceration of unspecified pulmonary blood vessels**

● **S25.49**   **Other specified injury of pulmonary blood vessels**

    ● **S25.491**   **Other specified injury of right pulmonary blood vessels**

    ● **S25.492**   **Other specified injury of left pulmonary blood vessels**

    ● **S25.499**   **Other specified injury of unspecified pulmonary blood vessels**

● **S25.5**   **Injury of intercostal blood vessels**

  ● **S25.50**   **Unspecified injury of intercostal blood vessels**

    ● **S25.501**   **Unspecified injury of intercostal blood vessels, right side**

    ● **S25.502**   **Unspecified injury of intercostal blood vessels, left side**

    ● **S25.509**   **Unspecified injury of intercostal blood vessels, unspecified side**

  ● **S25.51**   **Laceration of intercostal blood vessels**

    ● **S25.511**   **Laceration of intercostal blood vessels, right side**

    ● **S25.512**   **Laceration of intercostal blood vessels, left side**

    ● **S25.519**   **Laceration of intercostal blood vessels, unspecified side**

  ● **S25.59**   **Other specified injury of intercostal blood vessels**

    ● **S25.591**   **Other specified injury of intercostal blood vessels, right side**

    ● **S25.592**   **Other specified injury of intercostal blood vessels, left side**

    ● **S25.599**   **Other specified injury of intercostal blood vessels, unspecified side**

● **S25.8**   **Injury of other blood vessels of thorax**
Injury of azygos vein
Injury of mammary artery or vein

  ● **S25.80**   **Unspecified injury of other blood vessels of thorax**

    ● **S25.801**   **Unspecified injury of other blood vessels of thorax, right side**

    ● **S25.802**   **Unspecified injury of other blood vessels of thorax, left side**

    ● **S25.809**   **Unspecified injury of other blood vessels of thorax, unspecified side**

  ● **S25.81**   **Laceration of other blood vessels of thorax**

    ● **S25.811**   **Laceration of other blood vessels of thorax, right side**

    ● **S25.812**   **Laceration of other blood vessels of thorax, left side**

    ● **S25.819**   **Laceration of other blood vessels of thorax, unspecified side**

  ● **S25.89**   **Other specified injury of other blood vessels of thorax**

    ● **S25.891**   **Other specified injury of other blood vessels of thorax, right side**

    ● **S25.892**   **Other specified injury of other blood vessels of thorax, left side**

    ● **S25.899**   **Other specified injury of other blood vessels of thorax, unspecified side**

● **S25.9**   **Injury of unspecified blood vessel of thorax**

  X ● **S25.90**   **Unspecified injury of unspecified blood vessel of thorax**

  X ● **S25.91**   **Laceration of unspecified blood vessel of thorax**

  X ● **S25.99**   **Other specified injury of unspecified blood vessel of thorax**

◀ New   ◀▥ Revised   ~~deleted~~ Deleted   OGCR Official Guidelines   X Assign placeholder X   ● Use Additional Character(s)

Excludes 1   Excludes 2   Includes   Use additional   Code first   Code also   Unspecified

Item 19–2 Pneumothorax is a collection of gas (positive air pressure) in the pleural space resulting in the lung collapsing. A tension pneumothorax is life-threatening and is a result of air in the pleural space causing a displacement in the mediastinal structures and cardiopulmonary function compromise. A traumatic pneumothorax results from blunt or penetrating injury that disrupts the parietal/visceral pleura. **Hemothorax** is blood or bloody fluid in the pleural cavity as a result of traumatic blood vessel rupture or inflammation of the lungs from pneumonia.

● **S26 Injury of heart**

> The appropriate 7th character is to be added to each code from category S26

> | | |
> |---|---|
> | A | initial encounter |
> | D | subsequent encounter |
> | S | sequela |

> Code also any associated:
> open wound of thorax (S21.-)
> traumatic hemopneumothorax (S27.2)
> traumatic hemothorax (S27.1)
> traumatic pneumothorax (S27.0)

● **S26.0 Injury of heart with hemopericardium**
> *Hemopericardium: effusion of blood within pericardium*

  X● **S26.00 Unspecified injury of heart with hemopericardium**

  X● **S26.01 Contusion of heart with hemopericardium**

  ● **S26.02 Laceration of heart with hemopericardium**

    ● **S26.020 Mild laceration of heart with hemopericardium**
> Laceration of heart without penetration of heart chamber

    ● **S26.021 Moderate laceration of heart with hemopericardium**
> Laceration of heart with penetration of heart chamber

    ● **S26.022 Major laceration of heart with hemopericardium**
> Laceration of heart with penetration of multiple heart chambers

  X● **S26.09 Other injury of heart with hemopericardium**

● **S26.1 Injury of heart without hemopericardium**
> *Hemopericardium: effusion of blood within pericardium*

  X● **S26.10 Unspecified injury of heart without hemopericardium**

  X● **S26.11 Contusion of heart without hemopericardium**

  X● **S26.12 Laceration of heart without hemopericardium**

  X● **S26.19 Other injury of heart without hemopericardium**

● **S26.9 Injury of heart, unspecified with or without hemopericardium**
> *Hemopericardium: effusion of blood within pericardium*

  X● **S26.90 Unspecified injury of heart, unspecified with or without hemopericardium**

  X● **S26.91 Contusion of heart, unspecified with or without hemopericardium**

  X● **S26.92 Laceration of heart, unspecified with or without hemopericardium**
> Laceration of heart NOS

  X● **S26.99 Other injury of heart, unspecified with or without hemopericardium**

● **S27 Injury of other and unspecified intrathoracic organs**

> Code also any associated open wound of thorax (S21.-)
> **Excludes2** injury of cervical esophagus (S10-S19)
> injury of trachea (cervical) (S10-S19)

> The appropriate 7th character is to be added to each code from category S27

> | | |
> |---|---|
> | A | initial encounter |
> | D | subsequent encounter |
> | S | sequela |

X● **S27.0 Traumatic pneumothorax**
> **Excludes1** spontaneous pneumothorax (J93.-)

X● **S27.1 Traumatic hemothorax**

X● **S27.2 Traumatic hemopneumothorax**

● **S27.3 Other and unspecified injuries of lung**

  ● **S27.30 Unspecified injury of lung**

    ● **S27.301 Unspecified injury of lung, unilateral**

    ● **S27.302 Unspecified injury of lung, bilateral**

    ● **S27.309 Unspecified injury of lung, unspecified**

  ● **S27.31 Primary blast injury of lung**
> Blast injury of lung NOS

    ● **S27.311 Primary blast injury of lung, unilateral**

    ● **S27.312 Primary blast injury of lung, bilateral**

    ● **S27.319 Primary blast injury of lung, unspecified**

  ● **S27.32 Contusion of lung**

    ● **S27.321 Contusion of lung, unilateral**

    ● **S27.322 Contusion of lung, bilateral**

    ● **S27.329 Contusion of lung, unspecified**

  ● **S27.33 Laceration of lung**

    ● **S27.331 Laceration of lung, unilateral**

    ● **S27.332 Laceration of lung, bilateral**

    ● **S27.339 Laceration of lung, unspecified**

  ● **S27.39 Other injuries of lung**
> Secondary blast injury of lung

    ● **S27.391 Other injuries of lung, unilateral**

    ● **S27.392 Other injuries of lung, bilateral**

    ● **S27.399 Other injuries of lung, unspecified**

● **S27.4 Injury of bronchus**

  ● **S27.40 Unspecified injury of bronchus**

    ● **S27.401 Unspecified injury of bronchus, unilateral**

    ● **S27.402 Unspecified injury of bronchus, bilateral**

    ● **S27.409 Unspecified injury of bronchus, unspecified**

  ● **S27.41 Primary blast injury of bronchus**
> Blast injury of bronchus NOS

    ● **S27.411 Primary blast injury of bronchus, unilateral**

    ● **S27.412 Primary blast injury of bronchus, bilateral**

    ● **S27.419 Primary blast injury of bronchus, unspecified**

  ● **S27.42 Contusion of bronchus**

    ● **S27.421 Contusion of bronchus, unilateral**

    ● **S27.422 Contusion of bronchus, bilateral**

    ● **S27.429 Contusion of bronchus, unspecified**

CHAPTER 19 (S00-T88)

● S27.43   Laceration of bronchus
   ● S27.431   Laceration of bronchus, unilateral
   ● S27.432   Laceration of bronchus, bilateral
   ● S27.439   Laceration of bronchus, unspecified
● S27.49   Other injury of bronchus
               Secondary blast injury of bronchus
   ● S27.491   Other injury of bronchus, unilateral
   ● S27.492   Other injury of bronchus, bilateral
   ● S27.499   Other injury of bronchus, unspecified
● S27.5   Injury of thoracic trachea
   X ● S27.50   Unspecified injury of thoracic trachea
   X ● S27.51   Primary blast injury of thoracic trachea
                  Blast injury of thoracic trachea NOS
   X ● S27.52   Contusion of thoracic trachea
   X ● S27.53   Laceration of thoracic trachea
   X ● S27.59   Other injury of thoracic trachea
                  Secondary blast injury of thoracic trachea
● S27.6   Injury of pleura
   X ● S27.60   Unspecified injury of pleura
   X ● S27.63   Laceration of pleura
   X ● S27.69   Other injury of pleura
● S27.8   Injury of other specified intrathoracic organs
   ● S27.80   Injury of diaphragm
      ● S27.802   Contusion of diaphragm
      ● S27.803   Laceration of diaphragm
      ● S27.808   Other injury of diaphragm
      ● S27.809   Unspecified injury of diaphragm
   ● S27.81   Injury of esophagus (thoracic part)
      ● S27.812   Contusion of esophagus (thoracic part)
      ● S27.813   Laceration of esophagus (thoracic part)
      ● S27.818   Other injury of esophagus (thoracic part)
      ● S27.819   Unspecified injury of esophagus (thoracic part)
   ● S27.89   Injury of other specified intrathoracic organs
                  Injury of lymphatic thoracic duct
                  Injury of thymus gland
      ● S27.892   Contusion of other specified intrathoracic organs
      ● S27.893   Laceration of other specified intrathoracic organs
      ● S27.898   Other injury of other specified intrathoracic organs
      ● S27.899   Unspecified injury of other specified intrathoracic organs
   X ● S27.9   Injury of unspecified intrathoracic organ
● S28   Crushing injury of thorax, and traumatic amputation of part of thorax
            The appropriate 7th character is to be added to each code from category S28

            | A | initial encounter |
            | D | subsequent encounter |
            | S | sequela |

   X ● S28.0   Crushed chest
                  Use additional code for all associated injuries
                  Excludes1   flail chest (S22.5)
   X ● S28.1   Traumatic amputation (partial) of part of thorax, except breast

● S28.2   Traumatic amputation of breast
   ● S28.21   Complete traumatic amputation of breast
                  Traumatic amputation of breast NOS
      ● S28.211   Complete traumatic amputation of right breast
      ● S28.212   Complete traumatic amputation of left breast
      ● S28.219   Complete traumatic amputation of unspecified breast
   ● S28.22   Partial traumatic amputation of breast
      ● S28.221   Partial traumatic amputation of right breast
      ● S28.222   Partial traumatic amputation of left breast
      ● S28.229   Partial traumatic amputation of unspecified breast
● S29   Other and unspecified injuries of thorax
            Code also any associated open wound (S21.-)
            The appropriate 7th character is to be added to each code from category S29

            | A | initial encounter |
            | D | subsequent encounter |
            | S | sequela |

   ● S29.0   Injury of muscle and tendon at thorax level
      ● S29.00   Unspecified injury of muscle and tendon of thorax
         ● S29.001   Unspecified injury of muscle and tendon of front wall of thorax
         ● S29.002   Unspecified injury of muscle and tendon of back wall of thorax
         ● S29.009   Unspecified injury of muscle and tendon of unspecified wall of thorax
      ● S29.01   Strain of muscle and tendon of thorax
         ● S29.011   Strain of muscle and tendon of front wall of thorax
         ● S29.012   Strain of muscle and tendon of back wall of thorax
         ● S29.019   Strain of muscle and tendon of unspecified wall of thorax
      ● S29.02   Laceration of muscle and tendon of thorax
         ● S29.021   Laceration of muscle and tendon of front wall of thorax
         ● S29.022   Laceration of muscle and tendon of back wall of thorax
         ● S29.029   Laceration of muscle and tendon of unspecified wall of thorax
      ● S29.09   Other injury of muscle and tendon of thorax
         ● S29.091   Other injury of muscle and tendon of front wall of thorax
         ● S29.092   Other injury of muscle and tendon of back wall of thorax
         ● S29.099   Other injury of muscle and tendon of unspecified wall of thorax
   X ● S29.8   Other specified injuries of thorax
   X ● S29.9   Unspecified injury of thorax

INJURIES TO THE ABDOMEN, LOWER BACK, LUMBAR SPINE, PELVIS AND EXTERNAL GENITALS (S30-S39)

Includes	injuries to the abdominal wall
	injuries to the anus
	injuries to the buttock
	injuries to the external genitalia
	injuries to the flank
	injuries to the groin

Excludes2	burns and corrosions (T20-T32)
	effects of foreign body in anus and rectum (T18.5)
	effects of foreign body in genitourinary tract (T19.-)
	effects of foreign body in stomach, small intestine and colon (T18.2-T18.4)
	frostbite (T33-T34)
	insect bite or sting, venomous (T63.4)

● **S30   Superficial injury of abdomen, lower back, pelvis and external genitals**

Excludes2	superficial injury of hip (S70.-)

The appropriate 7th character is to be added to each code from category S30

A	initial encounter
D	subsequent encounter
S	sequela

X ● **S30.0   Contusion of lower back and pelvis**
Contusion of buttock

X ● **S30.1   Contusion of abdominal wall**
Contusion of flank
Contusion of groin

● **S30.2   Contusion of external genital organs**

● **S30.20   Contusion of unspecified external genital organ**

● **S30.201   Contusion of unspecified external genital organ, male**

● **S30.202   Contusion of unspecified external genital organ, female**

X ● **S30.21   Contusion of penis**

X ● **S30.22   Contusion of scrotum and testes**

X ● **S30.23   Contusion of vagina and vulva**

X ● **S30.3   Contusion of anus**

● **S30.8   Other superficial injuries of abdomen, lower back, pelvis and external genitals**

● **S30.81   Abrasion of abdomen, lower back, pelvis and external genitals**

● **S30.810   Abrasion of lower back and pelvis**

● **S30.811   Abrasion of abdominal wall**

● **S30.812   Abrasion of penis**

● **S30.813   Abrasion of scrotum and testes**

● **S30.814   Abrasion of vagina and vulva**

● **S30.815   Abrasion of unspecified external genital organs, male**

● **S30.816   Abrasion of unspecified external genital organs, female**

● **S30.817   Abrasion of anus**

● **S30.82   Blister (nonthermal) of abdomen, lower back, pelvis and external genitals**

● **S30.820   Blister (nonthermal) of lower back and pelvis**

● **S30.821   Blister (nonthermal) of abdominal wall**

● **S30.822   Blister (nonthermal) of penis**

● **S30.823   Blister (nonthermal) of scrotum and testes**

● **S30.824   Blister (nonthermal) of vagina and vulva**

● **S30.825   Blister (nonthermal) of unspecified external genital organs, male**

● **S30.826   Blister (nonthermal) of unspecified external genital organs, female**

● **S30.827   Blister (nonthermal) of anus**

● **S30.84   External constriction of abdomen, lower back, pelvis and external genitals**

● **S30.840   External constriction of lower back and pelvis**

● **S30.841   External constriction of abdominal wall**

● **S30.842   External constriction of penis**
Hair tourniquet syndrome of penis
Use additional cause code to identify the constricting item (W49.0-)

● **S30.843   External constriction of scrotum and testes**

● **S30.844   External constriction of vagina and vulva**

● **S30.845   External constriction of unspecified external genital organs, male**

● **S30.846   External constriction of unspecified external genital organs, female**

● **S30.85   Superficial foreign body of abdomen, lower back, pelvis and external genitals**
Splinter in the abdomen, lower back, pelvis and external genitals

● **S30.850   Superficial foreign body of lower back and pelvis**

● **S30.851   Superficial foreign body of abdominal wall**

● **S30.852   Superficial foreign body of penis**

● **S30.853   Superficial foreign body of scrotum and testes**

● **S30.854   Superficial foreign body of vagina and vulva**

● **S30.855   Superficial foreign body of unspecified external genital organs, male**

● **S30.856   Superficial foreign body of unspecified external genital organs, female**

● **S30.857   Superficial foreign body of anus**

● **S30.86   Insect bite (nonvenomous) of abdomen, lower back, pelvis and external genitals**

● **S30.860   Insect bite (nonvenomous) of lower back and pelvis**

● **S30.861   Insect bite (nonvenomous) of abdominal wall**

● **S30.862   Insect bite (nonvenomous) of penis**

● **S30.863   Insect bite (nonvenomous) of scrotum and testes**

● **S30.864   Insect bite (nonvenomous) of vagina and vulva**

● **S30.865   Insect bite (nonvenomous) of unspecified external genital organs, male**

● **S30.866   Insect bite (nonvenomous) of unspecified external genital organs, female**

● **S30.867   Insect bite (nonvenomous) of anus**

CHAPTER 19 (S00-T88)

◀ New	◀▥ Revised	~~deleted~~ Deleted	**OGCR** Official Guidelines	X Assign placeholder X	● Use Additional Character(s)

Excludes 1	Excludes 2	Includes	Use additional	Code first	Code also	Unspecified

● **S30.87**   **Other superficial bite of abdomen, lower back, pelvis and external genitals**

> **Excludes1**   open bite of abdomen, lower back, pelvis and external genitals (S31.05, S31.15, S31.25, S31.35, S31.45, S31.55)

● **S30.870**   **Other superficial bite of lower back and pelvis**

● **S30.871**   **Other superficial bite of abdominal wall**

● **S30.872**   **Other superficial bite of penis**

● **S30.873**   **Other superficial bite of scrotum and testes**

● **S30.874**   **Other superficial bite of vagina and vulva**

● **S30.875**   **Other superficial bite of unspecified external genital organs, male**

● **S30.876**   **Other superficial bite of unspecified external genital organs, female**

● **S30.877**   **Other superficial bite of anus**

● **S30.9**   **Unspecified superficial injury of abdomen, lower back, pelvis and external genitals**

X ● **S30.91**   **Unspecified superficial injury of lower back and pelvis**

X ● **S30.92**   **Unspecified superficial injury of abdominal wall**

X ● **S30.93**   **Unspecified superficial injury of penis**

X ● **S30.94**   **Unspecified superficial injury of scrotum and testes**

X ● **S30.95**   **Unspecified superficial injury of vagina and vulva**

X ● **S30.96**   **Unspecified superficial injury of unspecified external genital organs, male**

X ● **S30.97**   **Unspecified superficial injury of unspecified external genital organs, female**

X ● **S30.98**   **Unspecified superficial injury of anus**

● **S31**   **Open wound of abdomen, lower back, pelvis and external genitals**

> **Code also** any associated:
> spinal cord injury (S24.0, S24.1-, S34.0-, S34.1-)
> wound infection

> **Excludes1**   traumatic amputation of part of abdomen, lower back and pelvis (S38.2-, S38.3)

> **Excludes2**   open wound of hip (S71.00-S71.02)
> open fracture of pelvis (S32.1--S32.9 with 7th character B)

> The appropriate 7th character is to be added to each code from category S31

> | | |
> |---|---|
> | A | initial encounter |
> | D | subsequent encounter |
> | S | sequela |

● **S31.0**   **Open wound of lower back and pelvis**

● **S31.00**   **Unspecified open wound of lower back and pelvis**

● **S31.000**   **Unspecified open wound of lower back and pelvis without penetration into retroperitoneum**
> Unspecified open wound of lower back and pelvis NOS

● **S31.001**   **Unspecified open wound of lower back and pelvis with penetration into retroperitoneum**

● **S31.01**   **Laceration without foreign body of lower back and pelvis**

● **S31.010**   **Laceration without foreign body of lower back and pelvis without penetration into retroperitoneum**
> Laceration without foreign body of lower back and pelvis NOS

● **S31.011**   **Laceration without foreign body of lower back and pelvis with penetration into retroperitoneum**

● **S31.02**   **Laceration with foreign body of lower back and pelvis**

● **S31.020**   **Laceration with foreign body of lower back and pelvis without penetration into retroperitoneum**
> Laceration with foreign body of lower back and pelvis NOS

● **S31.021**   **Laceration with foreign body of lower back and pelvis with penetration into retroperitoneum**

● **S31.03**   **Puncture wound without foreign body of lower back and pelvis**

● **S31.030**   **Puncture wound without foreign body of lower back and pelvis without penetration into retroperitoneum**
> Puncture wound without foreign body of lower back and pelvis NOS

● **S31.031**   **Puncture wound without foreign body of lower back and pelvis with penetration into retroperitoneum**

● **S31.04**   **Puncture wound with foreign body of lower back and pelvis**

● **S31.040**   **Puncture wound with foreign body of lower back and pelvis without penetration into retroperitoneum**
> Puncture wound with foreign body of lower back and pelvis NOS

● **S31.041**   **Puncture wound with foreign body of lower back and pelvis with penetration into retroperitoneum**

● **S31.05**   **Open bite of lower back and pelvis**
> Bite of lower back and pelvis NOS

> **Excludes1**   superficial bite of lower back and pelvis (S30.860, S30.870)

● **S31.050**   **Open bite of lower back and pelvis without penetration into retroperitoneum**
> Open bite of lower back and pelvis NOS

● **S31.051**   **Open bite of lower back and pelvis with penetration into retroperitoneum**

● **S31.1**   **Open wound of abdominal wall without penetration into peritoneal cavity**
> Open wound of abdominal wall NOS

> **Excludes2**   open wound of abdominal wall with penetration into peritoneal cavity (S31.6-)

● **S31.10**   **Unspecified open wound of abdominal wall without penetration into peritoneal cavity**

● **S31.100**   **Unspecified open wound of abdominal wall, right upper quadrant without penetration into peritoneal cavity**

● **S31.101**   **Unspecified open wound of abdominal wall, left upper quadrant without penetration into peritoneal cavity**

◄ New   ◀▥▥ Revised   ~~deleted~~ Deleted   **OGCR** Official Guidelines   X Assign placeholder X   ● Use Additional Character(s)

Excludes 1   Excludes 2   Includes   Use additional   Code first   Code also   Unspecified

● S31.102   Unspecified open wound of abdominal wall, epigastric region without penetration into peritoneal cavity

● S31.103   Unspecified open wound of abdominal wall, right lower quadrant without penetration into peritoneal cavity

● S31.104   Unspecified open wound of abdominal wall, left lower quadrant without penetration into peritoneal cavity

● S31.105   Unspecified open wound of abdominal wall, periumbilic region without penetration into peritoneal cavity

● S31.109   Unspecified open wound of abdominal wall, unspecified quadrant without penetration into peritoneal cavity

     Unspecified open wound of abdominal wall NOS

● S31.11   Laceration without foreign body of abdominal wall without penetration into peritoneal cavity

● S31.110   Laceration without foreign body of abdominal wall, right upper quadrant without penetration into peritoneal cavity

● S31.111   Laceration without foreign body of abdominal wall, left upper quadrant without penetration into peritoneal cavity

● S31.112   Laceration without foreign body of abdominal wall, epigastric region without penetration into peritoneal cavity

● S31.113   Laceration without foreign body of abdominal wall, right lower quadrant without penetration into peritoneal cavity

● S31.114   Laceration without foreign body of abdominal wall, left lower quadrant without penetration into peritoneal cavity

● S31.115   Laceration without foreign body of abdominal wall, periumbilic region without penetration into peritoneal cavity

● S31.119   Laceration without foreign body of abdominal wall, unspecified quadrant without penetration into peritoneal cavity

● S31.12   Laceration with foreign body of abdominal wall without penetration into peritoneal cavity

● S31.120   Laceration of abdominal wall with foreign body, right upper quadrant without penetration into peritoneal cavity

● S31.121   Laceration of abdominal wall with foreign body, left upper quadrant without penetration into peritoneal cavity

● S31.122   Laceration of abdominal wall with foreign body, epigastric region without penetration into peritoneal cavity

● S31.123   Laceration of abdominal wall with foreign body, right lower quadrant without penetration into peritoneal cavity

● S31.124   Laceration of abdominal wall with foreign body, left lower quadrant without penetration into peritoneal cavity

● S31.125   Laceration of abdominal wall with foreign body, periumbilic region without penetration into peritoneal cavity

● S31.129   Laceration of abdominal wall with foreign body, unspecified quadrant without penetration into peritoneal cavity

● S31.13   Puncture wound of abdominal wall without foreign body without penetration into peritoneal cavity

● S31.130   Puncture wound of abdominal wall without foreign body, right upper quadrant without penetration into peritoneal cavity

● S31.131   Puncture wound of abdominal wall without foreign body, left upper quadrant without penetration into peritoneal cavity

● S31.132   Puncture wound of abdominal wall without foreign body, epigastric region without penetration into peritoneal cavity

● S31.133   Puncture wound of abdominal wall without foreign body, right lower quadrant without penetration into peritoneal cavity

● S31.134   Puncture wound of abdominal wall without foreign body, left lower quadrant without penetration into peritoneal cavity

● S31.135   Puncture wound of abdominal wall without foreign body, periumbilic region without penetration into peritoneal cavity

● S31.139   Puncture wound of abdominal wall without foreign body, unspecified quadrant without penetration into peritoneal cavity

● S31.14   Puncture wound of abdominal wall with foreign body without penetration into peritoneal cavity

● S31.140   Puncture wound of abdominal wall with foreign body, right upper quadrant without penetration into peritoneal cavity

● S31.141   Puncture wound of abdominal wall with foreign body, left upper quadrant without penetration into peritoneal cavity

● S31.142   Puncture wound of abdominal wall with foreign body, epigastric region without penetration into peritoneal cavity

● S31.143   Puncture wound of abdominal wall with foreign body, right lower quadrant without penetration into peritoneal cavity

● S31.144   Puncture wound of abdominal wall with foreign body, left lower quadrant without penetration into peritoneal cavity

● S31.145   Puncture wound of abdominal wall with foreign body, periumbilic region without penetration into peritoneal cavity

● S31.149   Puncture wound of abdominal wall with foreign body, unspecified quadrant without penetration into peritoneal cavity

● **S31.15**   **Open bite of abdominal wall without penetration into peritoneal cavity**
Bite of abdominal wall NOS

> **Excludes1**   superficial bite of abdominal wall (S30.871)

  ● **S31.150**   Open bite of abdominal wall, right upper quadrant without penetration into peritoneal cavity

  ● **S31.151**   Open bite of abdominal wall, left upper quadrant without penetration into peritoneal cavity

  ● **S31.152**   Open bite of abdominal wall, epigastric region without penetration into peritoneal cavity

  ● **S31.153**   Open bite of abdominal wall, right lower quadrant without penetration into peritoneal cavity

  ● **S31.154**   Open bite of abdominal wall, left lower quadrant without penetration into peritoneal cavity

  ● **S31.155**   Open bite of abdominal wall, periumbilic region without penetration into peritoneal cavity

  ● **S31.159**   Open bite of abdominal wall, unspecified quadrant without penetration into peritoneal cavity

● **S31.2**   **Open wound of penis**

X ● **S31.20**   Unspecified open wound of penis

X ● **S31.21**   Laceration without foreign body of penis

X ● **S31.22**   Laceration with foreign body of penis

X ● **S31.23**   Puncture wound without foreign body of penis

X ● **S31.24**   Puncture wound with foreign body of penis

X ● **S31.25**   Open bite of penis
Bite of penis NOS

> **Excludes1**   superficial bite of penis (S30.862, S30.872)

● **S31.3**   **Open wound of scrotum and testes**

X ● **S31.30**   Unspecified open wound of scrotum and testes

X ● **S31.31**   Laceration without foreign body of scrotum and testes

X ● **S31.32**   Laceration with foreign body of scrotum and testes

X ● **S31.33**   Puncture wound without foreign body of scrotum and testes

X ● **S31.34**   Puncture wound with foreign body of scrotum and testes

X ● **S31.35**   Open bite of scrotum and testes
Bite of scrotum and testes NOS

> **Excludes1**   superficial bite of scrotum and testes (S30.863, S30.873)

● **S31.4**   **Open wound of vagina and vulva**

> **Excludes1**   injury to vagina and vulva during delivery (O70.-, O71.4)

X ● **S31.40**   Unspecified open wound of vagina and vulva

X ● **S31.41**   Laceration without foreign body of vagina and vulva

X ● **S31.42**   Laceration with foreign body of vagina and vulva

X ● **S31.43**   Puncture wound without foreign body of vagina and vulva

X ● **S31.44**   Puncture wound with foreign body of vagina and vulva

X ● **S31.45**   Open bite of vagina and vulva
Bite of vagina and vulva NOS

> **Excludes1**   superficial bite of vagina and vulva (S30.864, S30.874)

● **S31.5**   **Open wound of unspecified external genital organs**

> **Excludes1**   traumatic amputation of external genital organs (S38.21, S38.22)

  ● **S31.50**   Unspecified open wound of unspecified external genital organs

    ● **S31.501**   Unspecified open wound of unspecified external genital organs, male

    ● **S31.502**   Unspecified open wound of unspecified external genital organs, female

  ● **S31.51**   Laceration without foreign body of unspecified external genital organs

    ● **S31.511**   Laceration without foreign body of unspecified external genital organs, male

    ● **S31.512**   Laceration without foreign body of unspecified external genital organs, female

  ● **S31.52**   Laceration with foreign body of unspecified external genital organs

    ● **S31.521**   Laceration with foreign body of unspecified external genital organs, male

    ● **S31.522**   Laceration with foreign body of unspecified external genital organs, female

  ● **S31.53**   Puncture wound without foreign body of unspecified external genital organs

    ● **S31.531**   Puncture wound without foreign body of unspecified external genital organs, male

    ● **S31.532**   Puncture wound without foreign body of unspecified external genital organs, female

  ● **S31.54**   Puncture wound with foreign body of unspecified external genital organs

    ● **S31.541**   Puncture wound with foreign body of unspecified external genital organs, male

    ● **S31.542**   Puncture wound with foreign body of unspecified external genital organs, female

  ● **S31.55**   Open bite of unspecified external genital organs
Bite of unspecified external genital organs NOS

> **Excludes1**   superficial bite of unspecified external genital organs (S30.865, S30.866, S30.875, S30.876)

    ● **S31.551**   Open bite of unspecified external genital organs, male

    ● **S31.552**   Open bite of unspecified external genital organs, female

● **S31.6**   **Open wound of abdominal wall with penetration into peritoneal cavity**

  ● **S31.60**   Unspecified open wound of abdominal wall with penetration into peritoneal cavity

    ● **S31.600**   Unspecified open wound of abdominal wall, right upper quadrant with penetration into peritoneal cavity

    ● **S31.601**   Unspecified open wound of abdominal wall, left upper quadrant with penetration into peritoneal cavity

● S31.602   Unspecified open wound of abdominal wall, epigastric region with penetration into peritoneal cavity

● S31.603   Unspecified open wound of abdominal wall, right lower quadrant with penetration into peritoneal cavity

● S31.604   Unspecified open wound of abdominal wall, left lower quadrant with penetration into peritoneal cavity

● S31.605   Unspecified open wound of abdominal wall, periumbilic region with penetration into peritoneal cavity

● S31.609   Unspecified open wound of abdominal wall, unspecified quadrant with penetration into peritoneal cavity

● S31.61   Laceration without foreign body of abdominal wall with penetration into peritoneal cavity

● S31.610   Laceration without foreign body of abdominal wall, right upper quadrant with penetration into peritoneal cavity

● S31.611   Laceration without foreign body of abdominal wall, left upper quadrant with penetration into peritoneal cavity

● S31.612   Laceration without foreign body of abdominal wall, epigastric region with penetration into peritoneal cavity

● S31.613   Laceration without foreign body of abdominal wall, right lower quadrant with penetration into peritoneal cavity

● S31.614   Laceration without foreign body of abdominal wall, left lower quadrant with penetration into peritoneal cavity

● S31.615   Laceration without foreign body of abdominal wall, periumbilic region with penetration into peritoneal cavity

● S31.619   Laceration without foreign body of abdominal wall, unspecified quadrant with penetration into peritoneal cavity

● S31.62   Laceration with foreign body of abdominal wall with penetration into peritoneal cavity

● S31.620   Laceration with foreign body of abdominal wall, right upper quadrant with penetration into peritoneal cavity

● S31.621   Laceration with foreign body of abdominal wall, left upper quadrant with penetration into peritoneal cavity

● S31.622   Laceration with foreign body of abdominal wall, epigastric region with penetration into peritoneal cavity

● S31.623   Laceration with foreign body of abdominal wall, right lower quadrant with penetration into peritoneal cavity

● S31.624   Laceration with foreign body of abdominal wall, left lower quadrant with penetration into peritoneal cavity

● S31.625   Laceration with foreign body of abdominal wall, periumbilic region with penetration into peritoneal cavity

● S31.629   Laceration with foreign body of abdominal wall, unspecified quadrant with penetration into peritoneal cavity

● S31.63   Puncture wound without foreign body of abdominal wall with penetration into peritoneal cavity

● S31.630   Puncture wound without foreign body of abdominal wall, right upper quadrant with penetration into peritoneal cavity

● S31.631   Puncture wound without foreign body of abdominal wall, left upper quadrant with penetration into peritoneal cavity

● S31.632   Puncture wound without foreign body of abdominal wall, epigastric region with penetration into peritoneal cavity

● S31.633   Puncture wound without foreign body of abdominal wall, right lower quadrant with penetration into peritoneal cavity

● S31.634   Puncture wound without foreign body of abdominal wall, left lower quadrant with penetration into peritoneal cavity

● S31.635   Puncture wound without foreign body of abdominal wall, periumbilic region with penetration into peritoneal cavity

● S31.639   Puncture wound without foreign body of abdominal wall, unspecified quadrant with penetration into peritoneal cavity

● S31.64   Puncture wound with foreign body of abdominal wall with penetration into peritoneal cavity

● S31.640   Puncture wound with foreign body of abdominal wall, right upper quadrant with penetration into peritoneal cavity

● S31.641   Puncture wound with foreign body of abdominal wall, left upper quadrant with penetration into peritoneal cavity

● S31.642   Puncture wound with foreign body of abdominal wall, epigastric region with penetration into peritoneal cavity

● S31.643   Puncture wound with foreign body of abdominal wall, right lower quadrant with penetration into peritoneal cavity

● S31.644   Puncture wound with foreign body of abdominal wall, left lower quadrant with penetration into peritoneal cavity

● S31.645   Puncture wound with foreign body of abdominal wall, periumbilic region with penetration into peritoneal cavity

● S31.649   Puncture wound with foreign body of abdominal wall, unspecified quadrant with penetration into peritoneal cavity

CHAPTER 19 (S00-T88)

◀ New   ◀▥ Revised   d̶e̶l̶e̶t̶e̶d̶ Deleted   **OGCR** Official Guidelines   X Assign placeholder X   ● Use Additional Character(s)

Excludes 1   Excludes 2   Includes   Use additional   Code first   Code also   Unspecified

1259

CHAPTER 19 (S00-T88)

● **S31.65**   **Open bite of abdominal wall with penetration into peritoneal cavity**
> **Excludes1**   superficial bite of abdominal wall (S30.861, S30.871)

● **S31.650**   Open bite of abdominal wall, right upper quadrant with penetration into peritoneal cavity

● **S31.651**   Open bite of abdominal wall, left upper quadrant with penetration into peritoneal cavity

● **S31.652**   Open bite of abdominal wall, epigastric region with penetration into peritoneal cavity

● **S31.653**   Open bite of abdominal wall, right lower quadrant with penetration into peritoneal cavity

● **S31.654**   Open bite of abdominal wall, left lower quadrant with penetration into peritoneal cavity

● **S31.655**   Open bite of abdominal wall, periumbilic region with penetration into peritoneal cavity

● **S31.659**   Open bite of abdominal wall, unspecified quadrant with penetration into peritoneal cavity

● **S31.8**   **Open wound of other parts of abdomen, lower back and pelvis**

● **S31.80**   **Open wound of unspecified buttock**

● **S31.801**   Laceration without foreign body of unspecified buttock

● **S31.802**   Laceration with foreign body of unspecified buttock

● **S31.803**   Puncture wound without foreign body of unspecified buttock

● **S31.804**   Puncture wound with foreign body of unspecified buttock

● **S31.805**   Open bite of unspecified buttock
Bite of buttock NOS
> **Excludes1**   superficial bite of buttock (S30.870)

● **S31.809**   Unspecified open wound of unspecified buttock

● **S31.81**   **Open wound of right buttock**

● **S31.811**   Laceration without foreign body of right buttock

● **S31.812**   Laceration with foreign body of right buttock

● **S31.813**   Puncture wound without foreign body of right buttock

● **S31.814**   Puncture wound with foreign body of right buttock

● **S31.815**   Open bite of right buttock
Bite of right buttock NOS
> **Excludes1**   superficial bite of buttock (S30.870)

● **S31.819**   Unspecified open wound of right buttock

● **S31.82**   **Open wound of left buttock**

● **S31.821**   Laceration without foreign body of left buttock

● **S31.822**   Laceration with foreign body of left buttock

● **S31.823**   Puncture wound without foreign body of left buttock

● **S31.824**   Puncture wound with foreign body of left buttock

● **S31.825**   Open bite of left buttock
Bite of left buttock NOS
> **Excludes1**   superficial bite of buttock (S30.870)

● **S31.829**   Unspecified open wound of left buttock

● **S31.83**   **Open wound of anus**

● **S31.831**   Laceration without foreign body of anus

● **S31.832**   Laceration with foreign body of anus

● **S31.833**   Puncture wound without foreign body of anus

● **S31.834**   Puncture wound with foreign body of anus

● **S31.835**   Open bite of anus
Bite of anus NOS
> **Excludes1**   superficial bite of anus (S30.877)

● **S31.839**   Unspecified open wound of anus

● **S32**   **Fracture of lumbar spine and pelvis**
Note: A fracture not indicated as displaced or nondisplaced should be coded to displaced
A fracture not indicated as opened or closed should be coded to closed

> **Includes**   fracture of lumbosacral neural arch
> fracture of lumbosacral spinous process
> fracture of lumbosacral transverse process
> fracture of lumbosacral vertebra
> fracture of lumbosacral vertebral arch

Code first any associated spinal cord and spinal nerve injury (S34.-)
> **Excludes1**   transection of abdomen (S38.3)
> **Excludes2**   fracture of hip NOS (S72.0-)

The appropriate 7th character is to be added to each code from category S32

A	initial encounter for closed fracture
B	initial encounter for open fracture
D	subsequent encounter for fracture with routine healing
G	subsequent encounter for fracture with delayed healing
K	subsequent encounter for fracture with nonunion
S	sequela

● **S32.0**   **Fracture of lumbar vertebra**
Fracture of lumbar spine NOS

● **S32.00**   **Fracture of unspecified lumbar vertebra**

● **S32.000**   Wedge compression fracture of unspecified lumbar vertebra

● **S32.001**   Stable burst fracture of unspecified lumbar vertebra

● **S32.002**   Unstable burst fracture of unspecified lumbar vertebra

● **S32.008**   Other fracture of unspecified lumbar vertebra

● **S32.009**   Unspecified fracture of unspecified lumbar vertebra

● **S32.01**   **Fracture of first lumbar vertebra**

● **S32.010**   Wedge compression fracture of first lumbar vertebra

● **S32.011**   Stable burst fracture of first lumbar vertebra

● **S32.012**   Unstable burst fracture of first lumbar vertebra

● **S32.018**   Other fracture of first lumbar vertebra

● **S32.019**   Unspecified fracture of first lumbar vertebra

● **S32.02**   Fracture of second lumbar vertebra
  ● **S32.020**   Wedge compression fracture of second lumbar vertebra
  ● **S32.021**   Stable burst fracture of second lumbar vertebra
  ● **S32.022**   Unstable burst fracture of second lumbar vertebra
  ● **S32.028**   Other fracture of second lumbar vertebra
  ● **S32.029**   Unspecified fracture of second lumbar vertebra

● **S32.03**   Fracture of third lumbar vertebra
  ● **S32.030**   Wedge compression fracture of third lumbar vertebra
  ● **S32.031**   Stable burst fracture of third lumbar vertebra
  ● **S32.032**   Unstable burst fracture of third lumbar vertebra
  ● **S32.038**   Other fracture of third lumbar vertebra
  ● **S32.039**   Unspecified fracture of third lumbar vertebra

● **S32.04**   Fracture of fourth lumbar vertebra
  ● **S32.040**   Wedge compression fracture of fourth lumbar vertebra
  ● **S32.041**   Stable burst fracture of fourth lumbar vertebra
  ● **S32.042**   Unstable burst fracture of fourth lumbar vertebra
  ● **S32.048**   Other fracture of fourth lumbar vertebra
  ● **S32.049**   Unspecified fracture of fourth lumbar vertebra

● **S32.05**   Fracture of fifth lumbar vertebra
  ● **S32.050**   Wedge compression fracture of fifth lumbar vertebra
  ● **S32.051**   Stable burst fracture of fifth lumbar vertebra
  ● **S32.052**   Unstable burst fracture of fifth lumbar vertebra
  ● **S32.058**   Other fracture of fifth lumbar vertebra
  ● **S32.059**   Unspecified fracture of fifth lumbar vertebra

● **S32.1**   Fracture of sacrum
  For vertical fractures, code to most medial fracture extension
  Use two codes if both a vertical and transverse fracture are present
  Code also any associated fracture of pelvic ring (S32.8-)

X ● **S32.10**   Unspecified fracture of sacrum
● **S32.11**   Zone I fracture of sacrum
  Vertical sacral ala fracture of sacrum
  ● **S32.110**   Nondisplaced Zone I fracture of sacrum
  ● **S32.111**   Minimally displaced Zone I fracture of sacrum
  ● **S32.112**   Severely displaced Zone I fracture of sacrum
  ● **S32.119**   Unspecified Zone I fracture of sacrum
● **S32.12**   Zone II fracture of sacrum
  Vertical foraminal region fracture of sacrum
  ● **S32.120**   Nondisplaced Zone II fracture of sacrum
  ● **S32.121**   Minimally displaced Zone II fracture of sacrum

  ● **S32.122**   Severely displaced Zone II fracture of sacrum
  ● **S32.129**   Unspecified Zone II fracture of sacrum
● **S32.13**   Zone III fracture of sacrum
  Vertical fracture into spinal canal region of sacrum
  ● **S32.130**   Nondisplaced Zone III fracture of sacrum
  ● **S32.131**   Minimally displaced Zone III fracture of sacrum
  ● **S32.132**   Severely displaced Zone III fracture of sacrum
  ● **S32.139**   Unspecified Zone III fracture of sacrum
X ● **S32.14**   Type 1 fracture of sacrum
  Transverse flexion fracture of sacrum without displacement
X ● **S32.15**   Type 2 fracture of sacrum
  Transverse flexion fracture of sacrum with posterior displacement
X ● **S32.16**   Type 3 fracture of sacrum
  Transverse extension fracture of sacrum with anterior displacement
X ● **S32.17**   Type 4 fracture of sacrum
  Transverse segmental comminution of upper sacrum
X ● **S32.19**   Other fracture of sacrum
X ● **S32.2**   Fracture of coccyx
● **S32.3**   Fracture of ilium
  Excludes1   fracture of ilium with associated disruption of pelvic ring (S32.8-)
  ● **S32.30**   Unspecified fracture of ilium
    ● **S32.301**   Unspecified fracture of right ilium
    ● **S32.302**   Unspecified fracture of left ilium
    ● **S32.309**   Unspecified fracture of unspecified ilium
  ● **S32.31**   Avulsion fracture of ilium
    ● **S32.311**   Displaced avulsion fracture of right ilium
    ● **S32.312**   Displaced avulsion fracture of left ilium
    ● **S32.313**   Displaced avulsion fracture of unspecified ilium
    ● **S32.314**   Nondisplaced avulsion fracture of right ilium
    ● **S32.315**   Nondisplaced avulsion fracture of left ilium
    ● **S32.316**   Nondisplaced avulsion fracture of unspecified ilium
  ● **S32.39**   Other fracture of ilium
    ● **S32.391**   Other fracture of right ilium
    ● **S32.392**   Other fracture of left ilium
    ● **S32.399**   Other fracture of unspecified ilium
● **S32.4**   Fracture of acetabulum
  Code also any associated fracture of pelvic ring (S32.8-)
  ● **S32.40**   Unspecified fracture of acetabulum
    ● **S32.401**   Unspecified fracture of right acetabulum
    ● **S32.402**   Unspecified fracture of left acetabulum
    ● **S32.409**   Unspecified fracture of unspecified acetabulum

CHAPTER 19 (S00–T88)

- ● S32.41   Fracture of anterior wall of acetabulum
  - ● S32.411   Displaced fracture of anterior wall of right acetabulum
  - ● S32.412   Displaced fracture of anterior wall of left acetabulum
  - ● S32.413   Displaced fracture of anterior wall of unspecified acetabulum
  - ● S32.414   Nondisplaced fracture of anterior wall of right acetabulum
  - ● S32.415   Nondisplaced fracture of anterior wall of left acetabulum
  - ● S32.416   Nondisplaced fracture of anterior wall of unspecified acetabulum
- ● S32.42   Fracture of posterior wall of acetabulum
  - ● S32.421   Displaced fracture of posterior wall of right acetabulum
  - ● S32.422   Displaced fracture of posterior wall of left acetabulum
  - ● S32.423   Displaced fracture of posterior wall of unspecified acetabulum
  - ● S32.424   Nondisplaced fracture of posterior wall of right acetabulum
  - ● S32.425   Nondisplaced fracture of posterior wall of left acetabulum
  - ● S32.426   Nondisplaced fracture of posterior wall of unspecified acetabulum
- ● S32.43   Fracture of anterior column [iliopubic] of acetabulum
  - ● S32.431   Displaced fracture of anterior column [iliopubic] of right acetabulum
  - ● S32.432   Displaced fracture of anterior column [iliopubic] of left acetabulum
  - ● S32.433   Displaced fracture of anterior column [iliopubic] of unspecified acetabulum
  - ● S32.434   Nondisplaced fracture of anterior column [iliopubic] of right acetabulum
  - ● S32.435   Nondisplaced fracture of anterior column [iliopubic] of left acetabulum
  - ● S32.436   Nondisplaced fracture of anterior column [iliopubic] of unspecified acetabulum
- ● S32.44   Fracture of posterior column [ilioischial] of acetabulum
  - ● S32.441   Displaced fracture of posterior column [ilioischial] of right acetabulum
  - ● S32.442   Displaced fracture of posterior column [ilioischial] of left acetabulum
  - ● S32.443   Displaced fracture of posterior column [ilioischial] of unspecified acetabulum
  - ● S32.444   Nondisplaced fracture of posterior column [ilioischial] of right acetabulum
  - ● S32.445   Nondisplaced fracture of posterior column [ilioischial] of left acetabulum
  - ● S32.446   Nondisplaced fracture of posterior column [ilioischial] of unspecified acetabulum
- ● S32.45   Transverse fracture of acetabulum
  - ● S32.451   Displaced transverse fracture of right acetabulum
  - ● S32.452   Displaced transverse fracture of left acetabulum
  - ● S32.453   Displaced transverse fracture of unspecified acetabulum
  - ● S32.454   Nondisplaced transverse fracture of right acetabulum
  - ● S32.455   Nondisplaced transverse fracture of left acetabulum
  - ● S32.456   Nondisplaced transverse fracture of unspecified acetabulum
- ● S32.46   Associated transverse-posterior fracture of acetabulum
  - ● S32.461   Displaced associated transverse-posterior fracture of right acetabulum
  - ● S32.462   Displaced associated transverse-posterior fracture of left acetabulum
  - ● S32.463   Displaced associated transverse-posterior fracture of unspecified acetabulum
  - ● S32.464   Nondisplaced associated transverse-posterior fracture of right acetabulum
  - ● S32.465   Nondisplaced associated transverse-posterior fracture of left acetabulum
  - ● S32.466   Nondisplaced associated transverse-posterior fracture of unspecified acetabulum
- ● S32.47   Fracture of medial wall of acetabulum
  - ● S32.471   Displaced fracture of medial wall of right acetabulum
  - ● S32.472   Displaced fracture of medial wall of left acetabulum
  - ● S32.473   Displaced fracture of medial wall of unspecified acetabulum
  - ● S32.474   Nondisplaced fracture of medial wall of right acetabulum
  - ● S32.475   Nondisplaced fracture of medial wall of left acetabulum
  - ● S32.476   Nondisplaced fracture of medial wall of unspecified acetabulum
- ● S32.48   Dome fracture of acetabulum
  - ● S32.481   Displaced dome fracture of right acetabulum
  - ● S32.482   Displaced dome fracture of left acetabulum
  - ● S32.483   Displaced dome fracture of unspecified acetabulum
  - ● S32.484   Nondisplaced dome fracture of right acetabulum
  - ● S32.485   Nondisplaced dome fracture of left acetabulum
  - ● S32.486   Nondisplaced dome fracture of unspecified acetabulum
- ● S32.49   Other fracture of acetabulum
  - ● S32.491   Other fracture of right acetabulum
  - ● S32.492   Other fracture of left acetabulum
  - ● S32.499   Other fracture of unspecified acetabulum
- ● S32.5   Fracture of pubis

  > Excludes1   fracture of pubis with associated disruption of pelvic ring (S32.8-)

  - ● S32.50   Unspecified fracture of pubis
    - ● S32.501   Unspecified fracture of right pubis
    - ● S32.502   Unspecified fracture of left pubis
    - ● S32.509   Unspecified fracture of unspecified pubis
  - ● S32.51   Fracture of superior rim of pubis
    - ● S32.511   Fracture of superior rim of right pubis
    - ● S32.512   Fracture of superior rim of left pubis
    - ● S32.519   Fracture of superior rim of unspecified pubis

S32.59   Other specified fracture of pubis
- S32.591   Other specified fracture of right pubis
- S32.592   Other specified fracture of left pubis
- S32.599   Other specified fracture of unspecified pubis

S32.6   Fracture of ischium
Excludes1   fracture of ischium with associated disruption of pelvic ring (S32.8-)

S32.60   Unspecified fracture of ischium
- S32.601   Unspecified fracture of right ischium
- S32.602   Unspecified fracture of left ischium
- S32.609   Unspecified fracture of unspecified ischium

S32.61   Avulsion fracture of ischium
- S32.611   Displaced avulsion fracture of right ischium
- S32.612   Displaced avulsion fracture of left ischium
- S32.613   Displaced avulsion fracture of unspecified ischium
- S32.614   Nondisplaced avulsion fracture of right ischium
- S32.615   Nondisplaced avulsion fracture of left ischium
- S32.616   Nondisplaced avulsion fracture of unspecified ischium

S32.69   Other specified fracture of ischium
- S32.691   Other specified fracture of right ischium
- S32.692   Other specified fracture of left ischium
- S32.699   Other specified fracture of unspecified ischium

S32.8   Fracture of other parts of pelvis
Code also any associated:
fracture of acetabulum (S32.4-)
sacral fracture (S32.1-)

S32.81   Multiple fractures of pelvis with disruption of pelvic ring
Multiple pelvic fractures with disruption of pelvic circle
- S32.810   Multiple fractures of pelvis with stable disruption of pelvic ring
- S32.811   Multiple fractures of pelvis with unstable disruption of pelvic ring

X S32.82   Multiple fractures of pelvis without disruption of pelvic ring
Multiple pelvic fractures without disruption of pelvic circle

X S32.89   Fracture of other parts of pelvis

X S32.9   Fracture of unspecified parts of lumbosacral spine and pelvis
Fracture of lumbosacral spine NOS
Fracture of pelvis NOS

S33   Dislocation and sprain of joints and ligaments of lumbar spine and pelvis
Includes   avulsion of joint or ligament of lumbar spine and pelvis
laceration of cartilage, joint or ligament of lumbar spine and pelvis
sprain of cartilage, joint or ligament of lumbar spine and pelvis
traumatic hemarthrosis of joint or ligament of lumbar spine and pelvis
traumatic rupture of joint or ligament of lumbar spine and pelvis
traumatic subluxation of joint or ligament of lumbar spine and pelvis
traumatic tear of joint or ligament of lumbar spine and pelvis
Code also any associated open wound
Excludes1   nontraumatic rupture or displacement of lumbar intervertebral disc NOS (M51.-)
obstetric damage to pelvic joints and ligaments (O71.6)
Excludes2   dislocation and sprain of joints and ligaments of hip (S73.-)
strain of muscle of lower back and pelvis (S39.01-)

The appropriate 7th character is to be added to each code from category S33

A	initial encounter
D	subsequent encounter
S	sequela

X S33.0   Traumatic rupture of lumbar intervertebral disc
Excludes1   rupture or displacement (nontraumatic) of lumbar intervertebral disc NOS (M51.- with fifth character 6)

S33.1   Subluxation and dislocation of lumbar vertebra
Code also any associated:
open wound of abdomen, lower back and pelvis (S31)
spinal cord injury (S24.0, S24.1-, S34.0-, S34.1-)
Excludes2   fracture of lumbar vertebrae (S32.0-)

S33.10   Subluxation and dislocation of unspecified lumbar vertebra
- S33.100   Subluxation of unspecified lumbar vertebra
- S33.101   Dislocation of unspecified lumbar vertebra

S33.11   Subluxation and dislocation of L_1/L_2 lumbar vertebra
- S33.110   Subluxation of L_1/L_2 lumbar vertebra
- S33.111   Dislocation of L_1/L_2 lumbar vertebra

S33.12   Subluxation and dislocation of L_2/L_3 lumbar vertebra
- S33.120   Subluxation of L_2/L_3 lumbar vertebra
- S33.121   Dislocation of L_2/L_3 lumbar vertebra

S33.13   Subluxation and dislocation of L_3/L_4 lumbar vertebra
- S33.130   Subluxation of L_3/L_4 lumbar vertebra
- S33.131   Dislocation of L_3/L_4 lumbar vertebra

S33.14   Subluxation and dislocation of L_4/L_5 lumbar vertebra
- S33.140   Subluxation of L_4/L_5 lumbar vertebra
- S33.141   Dislocation of L_4/L_5 lumbar vertebra

CHAPTER 19 (S00-T88)

◄ New   ◄▥ Revised   deleted Deleted   OGCR Official Guidelines   X Assign placeholder X   ● Use Additional Character(s)
Excludes 1   Excludes 2   Includes   Use additional   Code first   Code also   Unspecified
1263

X ● S33.2   **Dislocation of sacroiliac and sacrococcygeal joint**

● S33.3   **Dislocation of other and unspecified parts of lumbar spine and pelvis**

    X ● S33.30   Dislocation of unspecified parts of lumbar spine and pelvis

    X ● S33.39   Dislocation of other parts of lumbar spine and pelvis

X ● S33.4   **Traumatic rupture of symphysis pubis**

X ● S33.5   **Sprain of ligaments of lumbar spine**

X ● S33.6   **Sprain of sacroiliac joint**

X ● S33.8   **Sprain of other parts of lumbar spine and pelvis**

X ● S33.9   **Sprain of unspecified parts of lumbar spine and pelvis**

● S34   **Injury of lumbar and sacral spinal cord and nerves at abdomen, lower back and pelvis level**

    Note: Code to highest level of lumbar cord injury

       Injuries to the spinal cord (S34.0 and S34.1) refer to the cord level and not bone level injury, and can affect nerve roots at and below the level given.

       The appropriate 7th character is to be added to each code from category S34

A	initial encounter
D	subsequent encounter
S	sequela

       Code also any associated:
         fracture of vertebra (S22.0-, S32.0-)
         open wound of abdomen, lower back and pelvis (S31.-)
         transient paralysis (R29.5)

● S34.0   **Concussion and edema of lumbar and sacral spinal cord**

    X ● S34.01   Concussion and edema of lumbar spinal cord

    X ● S34.02   Concussion and edema of sacral spinal cord
            Concussion and edema of conus medullaris

● S34.1   **Other and unspecified injury of lumbar and sacral spinal cord**

    ● S34.10   Unspecified injury to lumbar spinal cord

       ● S34.101   Unspecified injury to L_1 level of lumbar spinal cord

       ● S34.102   Unspecified injury to L_2 level of lumbar spinal cord

       ● S34.103   Unspecified injury to L_3 level of lumbar spinal cord

       ● S34.104   Unspecified injury to L_4 level of lumbar spinal cord

       ● S34.105   Unspecified injury to L_5 level of lumbar spinal cord

       ● S34.109   Unspecified injury to unspecified level of lumbar spinal cord

    ● S34.11   Complete lesion of lumbar spinal cord

       ● S34.111   Complete lesion of L_1 level of lumbar spinal cord

       ● S34.112   Complete lesion of L_2 level of lumbar spinal cord

       ● S34.113   Complete lesion of L_3 level of lumbar spinal cord

       ● S34.114   Complete lesion of L_4 level of lumbar spinal cord

       ● S34.115   Complete lesion of L_5 level of lumbar spinal cord

       ● S34.119   Complete lesion of unspecified level of lumbar spinal cord

    ● S34.12   Incomplete lesion of lumbar spinal cord

       ● S34.121   Incomplete lesion of L_1 level of lumbar spinal cord

       ● S34.122   Incomplete lesion of L_2 level of lumbar spinal cord

       ● S34.123   Incomplete lesion of L_3 level of lumbar spinal cord

       ● S34.124   Incomplete lesion of L_4 level of lumbar spinal cord

       ● S34.125   Incomplete lesion of L_5 level of lumbar spinal cord

       ● S34.129   Incomplete lesion of unspecified level of lumbar spinal cord

    ● S34.13   Other and unspecified injury to sacral spinal cord
            Other injury to conus medullaris

       ● S34.131   Complete lesion of sacral spinal cord
            Complete lesion of conus medullaris

       ● S34.132   Incomplete lesion of sacral spinal cord
            Incomplete lesion of conus medullaris

       ● S34.139   Unspecified injury to sacral spinal cord
            Unspecified injury of conus medullaris

● S34.2   **Injury of nerve root of lumbar and sacral spine**

    X ● S34.21   Injury of nerve root of lumbar spine

    X ● S34.22   Injury of nerve root of sacral spine

X ● S34.3   **Injury of cauda equina**

X ● S34.4   **Injury of lumbosacral plexus**

X ● S34.5   **Injury of lumbar, sacral and pelvic sympathetic nerves**
       Injury of celiac ganglion or plexus
       Injury of hypogastric plexus
       Injury of mesenteric plexus (inferior) (superior)
       Injury of splanchnic nerve

X ● S34.6   **Injury of peripheral nerve(s) at abdomen, lower back and pelvis level**

X ● S34.8   **Injury of other nerves at abdomen, lower back and pelvis level**

X ● S34.9   **Injury of unspecified nerves at abdomen, lower back and pelvis level**

● S35   **Injury of blood vessels at abdomen, lower back and pelvis level**

    The appropriate 7th character is to be added to each code from category S35

A	initial encounter
D	subsequent encounter
S	sequela

    Code also any associated open wound (S31.-)

● S35.0   **Injury of abdominal aorta**
    Excludes1   injury of aorta NOS (S25.0)

    X ● S35.00   Unspecified injury of abdominal aorta

    X ● S35.01   Minor laceration of abdominal aorta
       Incomplete transection of abdominal aorta
       Laceration of abdominal aorta NOS
       Superficial laceration of abdominal aorta

    X ● S35.02   Major laceration of abdominal aorta
       Complete transection of abdominal aorta
       Traumatic rupture of abdominal aorta

    X ● S35.09   Other injury of abdominal aorta

● S35.1   **Injury of inferior vena cava**
       Injury of hepatic vein
    Excludes1   injury of vena cava NOS (S25.2)

    X ● S35.10   Unspecified injury of inferior vena cava

    X ● S35.11   Minor laceration of inferior vena cava
       Incomplete transection of inferior vena cava
       Laceration of inferior vena cava NOS
       Superficial laceration of inferior vena cava

    X ● S35.12   Major laceration of inferior vena cava
       Complete transection of inferior vena cava
       Traumatic rupture of inferior vena cava

    X ● S35.19   Other injury of inferior vena cava

- ● S35.2   Injury of celiac or mesenteric artery and branches
  - ● S35.21   Injury of celiac artery
    - ● S35.211   **Minor laceration of celiac artery**
      Incomplete transection of celiac artery
      Laceration of celiac artery NOS
      Superficial laceration of celiac artery
    - ● S35.212   **Major laceration of celiac artery**
      Complete transection of celiac artery
      Traumatic rupture of celiac artery
    - ● S35.218   **Other injury of celiac artery**
    - ● S35.219   **Unspecified injury of celiac artery**
  - ● S35.22   Injury of superior mesenteric artery
    - ● S35.221   **Minor laceration of superior mesenteric artery**
      Incomplete transection of superior mesenteric artery
      Laceration of superior mesenteric artery NOS
      Superficial laceration of superior mesenteric artery
    - ● S35.222   **Major laceration of superior mesenteric artery**
      Complete transection of superior mesenteric artery
      Traumatic rupture of superior mesenteric artery
    - ● S35.228   **Other injury of superior mesenteric artery**
    - ● S35.229   **Unspecified injury of superior mesenteric artery**
  - ● S35.23   Injury of inferior mesenteric artery
    - ● S35.231   **Minor laceration of inferior mesenteric artery**
      Incomplete transection of inferior mesenteric artery
      Laceration of inferior mesenteric artery NOS
      Superficial laceration of inferior mesenteric artery
    - ● S35.232   **Major laceration of inferior mesenteric artery**
      Complete transection of inferior mesenteric artery
      Traumatic rupture of inferior mesenteric artery
    - ● S35.238   **Other injury of inferior mesenteric artery**
    - ● S35.239   **Unspecified injury of inferior mesenteric artery**
  - ● S35.29   Injury of branches of celiac and mesenteric artery
    Injury of gastric artery
    Injury of gastroduodenal artery
    Injury of hepatic artery
    Injury of splenic artery
    - ● S35.291   **Minor laceration of branches of celiac and mesenteric artery**
      Incomplete transection of branches of celiac and mesenteric artery
      Laceration of branches of celiac and mesenteric artery NOS
      Superficial laceration of branches of celiac and mesenteric artery
    - ● S35.292   **Major laceration of branches of celiac and mesenteric artery**
      Complete transection of branches of celiac and mesenteric artery
      Traumatic rupture of branches of celiac and mesenteric artery
    - ● S35.298   **Other injury of branches of celiac and mesenteric artery**
    - ● S35.299   **Unspecified injury of branches of celiac and mesenteric artery**

- ● S35.3   Injury of portal or splenic vein and branches
  - ● S35.31   Injury of portal vein
    - ● S35.311   **Laceration of portal vein**
    - ● S35.318   **Other specified injury of portal vein**
    - ● S35.319   **Unspecified injury of portal vein**
  - ● S35.32   Injury of splenic vein
    - ● S35.321   **Laceration of splenic vein**
    - ● S35.328   **Other specified injury of splenic vein**
    - ● S35.329   **Unspecified injury of splenic vein**
  - ● S35.33   Injury of superior mesenteric vein
    - ● S35.331   **Laceration of superior mesenteric vein**
    - ● S35.338   **Other specified injury of superior mesenteric vein**
    - ● S35.339   **Unspecified injury of superior mesenteric vein**
  - ● S35.34   Injury of inferior mesenteric vein
    - ● S35.341   **Laceration of inferior mesenteric vein**
    - ● S35.348   **Other specified injury of inferior mesenteric vein**
    - ● S35.349   **Unspecified injury of inferior mesenteric vein**
- ● S35.4   Injury of renal blood vessels
  - ● S35.40   Unspecified injury of renal blood vessel
    - ● S35.401   **Unspecified injury of right renal artery**
    - ● S35.402   **Unspecified injury of left renal artery**
    - ● S35.403   **Unspecified injury of unspecified renal artery**
    - ● S35.404   **Unspecified injury of right renal vein**
    - ● S35.405   **Unspecified injury of left renal vein**
    - ● S35.406   **Unspecified injury of unspecified renal vein**
  - ● S35.41   Laceration of renal blood vessel
    - ● S35.411   **Laceration of right renal artery**
    - ● S35.412   **Laceration of left renal artery**
    - ● S35.413   **Laceration of unspecified renal artery**
    - ● S35.414   **Laceration of right renal vein**
    - ● S35.415   **Laceration of left renal vein**
    - ● S35.416   **Laceration of unspecified renal vein**
  - ● S35.49   Other specified injury of renal blood vessel
    - ● S35.491   **Other specified injury of right renal artery**
    - ● S35.492   **Other specified injury of left renal artery**
    - ● S35.493   **Other specified injury of unspecified renal artery**
    - ● S35.494   **Other specified injury of right renal vein**
    - ● S35.495   **Other specified injury of left renal vein**
    - ● S35.496   **Other specified injury of unspecified renal vein**
- ● S35.5   Injury of iliac blood vessels
  - X ● S35.50   **Injury of unspecified iliac blood vessel(s)**
  - ● S35.51   Injury of iliac artery or vein
    Injury of hypogastric artery or vein
    - ● S35.511   **Injury of right iliac artery**
    - ● S35.512   **Injury of left iliac artery**
    - ● S35.513   **Injury of unspecified iliac artery**
    - ● S35.514   **Injury of right iliac vein**
    - ● S35.515   **Injury of left iliac vein**
    - ● S35.516   **Injury of unspecified iliac vein**

● S35.53   Injury of uterine artery or vein
    ● S35.531   Injury of right uterine artery
    ● S35.532   Injury of left uterine artery
    ● S35.533   Injury of unspecified uterine artery
    ● S35.534   Injury of right uterine vein
    ● S35.535   Injury of left uterine vein
    ● S35.536   Injury of unspecified uterine vein
X ● S35.59   Injury of other iliac blood vessels
● S35.8   Injury of other blood vessels at abdomen, lower back and pelvis level
    Injury of ovarian artery or vein
  ● S35.8X   Injury of other blood vessels at abdomen, lower back and pelvis level
    ● S35.8X1   Laceration of other blood vessels at abdomen, lower back and pelvis level
    ● S35.8X8   Other specified injury of other blood vessels at abdomen, lower back and pelvis level
    ● S35.8X9   Unspecified injury of other blood vessels at abdomen, lower back and pelvis level
● S35.9   Injury of unspecified blood vessel at abdomen, lower back and pelvis level
X ● S35.90   Unspecified injury of unspecified blood vessel at abdomen, lower back and pelvis level
X ● S35.91   Laceration of unspecified blood vessel at abdomen, lower back and pelvis level
X ● S35.99   Other specified injury of unspecified blood vessel at abdomen, lower back and pelvis level

● S36   Injury of intra-abdominal organs
    The appropriate 7th character is to be added to each code from category S36

    | A | initial encounter |
    | D | subsequent encounter |
    | S | sequela |

    Code also any associated open wound (S31.-)
● S36.0   Injury of spleen
X ● S36.00   Unspecified injury of spleen
  ● S36.02   Contusion of spleen
    ● S36.020   Minor contusion of spleen
        Contusion of spleen less than 2 cm
    ● S36.021   Major contusion of spleen
        Contusion of spleen greater than 2 cm
    ● S36.029   Unspecified contusion of spleen
  ● S36.03   Laceration of spleen
    ● S36.030   Superficial (capsular) laceration of spleen
        Laceration of spleen less than 1 cm
        Minor laceration of spleen
    ● S36.031   Moderate laceration of spleen
        Laceration of spleen 1 to 3 cm
    ● S36.032   Major laceration of spleen
        Avulsion of spleen
        Laceration of spleen greater than 3 cm
        Massive laceration of spleen
        Multiple moderate lacerations of spleen
        Stellate laceration of spleen
    ● S36.039   Unspecified laceration of spleen
X ● S36.09   Other injury of spleen

● S36.1   Injury of liver and gallbladder and bile duct
  ● S36.11   Injury of liver
    ● S36.112   Contusion of liver
    ● S36.113   Laceration of liver, unspecified degree
    ● S36.114   Minor laceration of liver
        Laceration involving capsule only, or, without significant involvement of hepatic parenchyma [i.e., less than 1 cm deep]
    ● S36.115   Moderate laceration of liver
        Laceration involving parenchyma but without major disruption of parenchyma [i.e., less than 10 cm long and less than 3 cm deep]
    ● S36.116   Major laceration of liver
        Laceration with significant disruption of hepatic parenchyma [i.e., greater than 10 cm long and 3 cm deep]
        Multiple moderate lacerations, with or without hematoma
        Stellate laceration of liver
    ● S36.118   Other injury of liver
    ● S36.119   Unspecified injury of liver
  ● S36.12   Injury of gallbladder
    ● S36.122   Contusion of gallbladder
    ● S36.123   Laceration of gallbladder
    ● S36.128   Other injury of gallbladder
    ● S36.129   Unspecified injury of gallbladder
X ● S36.13   Injury of bile duct
● S36.2   Injury of pancreas
  ● S36.20   Unspecified injury of pancreas
    ● S36.200   Unspecified injury of head of pancreas
    ● S36.201   Unspecified injury of body of pancreas
    ● S36.202   Unspecified injury of tail of pancreas
    ● S36.209   Unspecified injury of unspecified part of pancreas
  ● S36.22   Contusion of pancreas
    ● S36.220   Contusion of head of pancreas
    ● S36.221   Contusion of body of pancreas
    ● S36.222   Contusion of tail of pancreas
    ● S36.229   Contusion of unspecified part of pancreas
  ● S36.23   Laceration of pancreas, unspecified degree
    ● S36.230   Laceration of head of pancreas, unspecified degree
    ● S36.231   Laceration of body of pancreas, unspecified degree
    ● S36.232   Laceration of tail of pancreas, unspecified degree
    ● S36.239   Laceration of unspecified part of pancreas, unspecified degree
  ● S36.24   Minor laceration of pancreas
    ● S36.240   Minor laceration of head of pancreas
    ● S36.241   Minor laceration of body of pancreas
    ● S36.242   Minor laceration of tail of pancreas
    ● S36.249   Minor laceration of unspecified part of pancreas

● S36.25   Moderate laceration of pancreas
   ● S36.250   Moderate laceration of head of pancreas
   ● S36.251   Moderate laceration of body of pancreas
   ● S36.252   Moderate laceration of tail of pancreas
   ● S36.259   Moderate laceration of unspecified part of pancreas
● S36.26   Major laceration of pancreas
   ● S36.260   Major laceration of head of pancreas
   ● S36.261   Major laceration of body of pancreas
   ● S36.262   Major laceration of tail of pancreas
   ● S36.269   Major laceration of unspecified part of pancreas
● S36.29   Other injury of pancreas
   ● S36.290   Other injury of head of pancreas
   ● S36.291   Other injury of body of pancreas
   ● S36.292   Other injury of tail of pancreas
   ● S36.299   Other injury of unspecified part of pancreas
● S36.3   Injury of stomach
  X ● S36.30   Unspecified injury of stomach
  X ● S36.32   Contusion of stomach
  X ● S36.33   Laceration of stomach
  X ● S36.39   Other injury of stomach
● S36.4   Injury of small intestine
   ● S36.40   Unspecified injury of small intestine
      ● S36.400   Unspecified injury of duodenum
      ● S36.408   Unspecified injury of other part of small intestine
      ● S36.409   Unspecified injury of unspecified part of small intestine
   ● S36.41   Primary blast injury of small intestine
      Blast injury of small intestine NOS
      ● S36.410   Primary blast injury of duodenum
      ● S36.418   Primary blast injury of other part of small intestine
      ● S36.419   Primary blast injury of unspecified part of small intestine
   ● S36.42   Contusion of small intestine
      ● S36.420   Contusion of duodenum
      ● S36.428   Contusion of other part of small intestine
      ● S36.429   Contusion of unspecified part of small intestine
   ● S36.43   Laceration of small intestine
      ● S36.430   Laceration of duodenum
      ● S36.438   Laceration of other part of small intestine
      ● S36.439   Laceration of unspecified part of small intestine
   ● S36.49   Other injury of small intestine
      ● S36.490   Other injury of duodenum
      ● S36.498   Other injury of other part of small intestine
      ● S36.499   Other injury of unspecified part of small intestine
● S36.5   Injury of colon
   Excludes2   injury of rectum (S36.6-)
   ● S36.50   Unspecified injury of colon
      ● S36.500   Unspecified injury of ascending [right] colon
      ● S36.501   Unspecified injury of transverse colon
      ● S36.502   Unspecified injury of descending [left] colon

      ● S36.503   Unspecified injury of sigmoid colon
      ● S36.508   Unspecified injury of other part of colon
      ● S36.509   Unspecified injury of unspecified part of colon
   ● S36.51   Primary blast injury of colon
      Blast injury of colon NOS
      ● S36.510   Primary blast injury of ascending [right] colon
      ● S36.511   Primary blast injury of transverse colon
      ● S36.512   Primary blast injury of descending [left] colon
      ● S36.513   Primary blast injury of sigmoid colon
      ● S36.518   Primary blast injury of other part of colon
      ● S36.519   Primary blast injury of unspecified part of colon
   ● S36.52   Contusion of colon
      ● S36.520   Contusion of ascending [right] colon
      ● S36.521   Contusion of transverse colon
      ● S36.522   Contusion of descending [left] colon
      ● S36.523   Contusion of sigmoid colon
      ● S36.528   Contusion of other part of colon
      ● S36.529   Contusion of unspecified part of colon
   ● S36.53   Laceration of colon
      ● S36.530   Laceration of ascending [right] colon
      ● S36.531   Laceration of transverse colon
      ● S36.532   Laceration of descending [left] colon
      ● S36.533   Laceration of sigmoid colon
      ● S36.538   Laceration of other part of colon
      S36.539   Laceration of unspecified part of colon
   ● S36.59   Other injury of colon
      Secondary blast injury of colon
      ● S36.590   Other injury of ascending [right] colon
      ● S36.591   Other injury of transverse colon
      ● S36.592   Other injury of descending [left] colon
      ● S36.593   Other injury of sigmoid colon
      ● S36.598   Other injury of other part of colon
      ● S36.599   Other injury of unspecified part of colon
● S36.6   Injury of rectum
  X ● S36.60   Unspecified injury of rectum
  X ● S36.61   Primary blast injury of rectum
      Blast injury of rectum NOS
  X ● S36.62   Contusion of rectum
  X ● S36.63   Laceration of rectum
  X ● S36.69   Other injury of rectum
      Secondary blast injury of rectum
● S36.8   Injury of other intra-abdominal organs
  X ● S36.81   Injury of peritoneum
   ● S36.89   Injury of other intra-abdominal organs
      Injury of retroperitoneum
      ● S36.892   Contusion of other intra-abdominal organs
      ● S36.893   Laceration of other intra-abdominal organs
      ● S36.898   Other injury of other intra-abdominal organs
      S36.899   Unspecified injury of other intra-abdominal organs

CHAPTER 19 (S00-T88)

◀ New   ◀▥ Revised   ~~deleted~~ Deleted   **OGCR** Official Guidelines   X Assign placeholder X   ● Use Additional Character(s)

   Excludes 1   Excludes 2   Includes   Use additional   Code first   Code also   Unspecified

● **S36.9**　**Injury of unspecified intra-abdominal organ**
　　X● **S36.90**　**Unspecified injury of unspecified intra-abdominal organ**
　　X● **S36.92**　**Contusion of unspecified intra-abdominal organ**
　　X● **S36.93**　**Laceration of unspecified intra-abdominal organ**
　　X● **S36.99**　**Other injury of unspecified intra-abdominal organ**

● **S37**　**Injury of urinary and pelvic organs**
　　Code also any associated open wound (S31.-)
　　Excludes1　obstetric trauma to pelvic organs (O71.-)
　　Excludes2　injury of peritoneum (S36.81)
　　　　　　　injury of retroperitoneum (S36.89-)

　　The appropriate 7th character is to be added to each code from category S37

　　A　initial encounter
　　D　subsequent encounter
　　S　sequela

● **S37.0**　**Injury of kidney**
　　Excludes2　acute kidney injury (nontraumatic) (N17.9)
　　● **S37.00**　**Unspecified injury of kidney**
　　　　● **S37.001**　**Unspecified injury of right kidney**
　　　　● **S37.002**　**Unspecified injury of left kidney**
　　　　● **S37.009**　**Unspecified injury of unspecified kidney**
　　● **S37.01**　**Minor contusion of kidney**
　　　　Contusion of kidney less than 2 cm
　　　　Contusion of kidney NOS
　　　　● **S37.011**　**Minor contusion of right kidney**
　　　　● **S37.012**　**Minor contusion of left kidney**
　　　　● **S37.019**　**Minor contusion of unspecified kidney**
　　● **S37.02**　**Major contusion of kidney**
　　　　Contusion of kidney greater than 2 cm
　　　　● **S37.021**　**Major contusion of right kidney**
　　　　● **S37.022**　**Major contusion of left kidney**
　　　　● **S37.029**　**Major contusion of unspecified kidney**
　　● **S37.03**　**Laceration of kidney, unspecified degree**
　　　　● **S37.031**　**Laceration of right kidney, unspecified degree**
　　　　● **S37.032**　**Laceration of left kidney, unspecified degree**
　　　　● **S37.039**　**Laceration of unspecified kidney, unspecified degree**
　　● **S37.04**　**Minor laceration of kidney**
　　　　Laceration of kidney less than 1 cm
　　　　● **S37.041**　**Minor laceration of right kidney**
　　　　● **S37.042**　**Minor laceration of left kidney**
　　　　● **S37.049**　**Minor laceration of unspecified kidney**
　　● **S37.05**　**Moderate laceration of kidney**
　　　　Laceration of kidney 1 to 3 cm
　　　　● **S37.051**　**Moderate laceration of right kidney**
　　　　● **S37.052**　**Moderate laceration of left kidney**
　　　　● **S37.059**　**Moderate laceration of unspecified kidney**

● **S37.06**　**Major laceration of kidney**
　　Avulsion of kidney
　　Laceration of kidney greater than 3 cm
　　Massive laceration of kidney
　　Multiple moderate lacerations of kidney
　　Stellate laceration of kidney
　　● **S37.061**　**Major laceration of right kidney**
　　● **S37.062**　**Major laceration of left kidney**
　　● **S37.069**　**Major laceration of unspecified kidney**
● **S37.09**　**Other injury of kidney**
　　● **S37.091**　**Other injury of right kidney**
　　● **S37.092**　**Other injury of left kidney**
　　● **S37.099**　**Other injury of unspecified kidney**
● **S37.1**　**Injury of ureter**
　　X● **S37.10**　**Unspecified injury of ureter**
　　X● **S37.12**　**Contusion of ureter**
　　X● **S37.13**　**Laceration of ureter**
　　X● **S37.19**　**Other injury of ureter**
● **S37.2**　**Injury of bladder**
　　X● **S37.20**　**Unspecified injury of bladder**
　　X● **S37.22**　**Contusion of bladder**
　　X● **S37.23**　**Laceration of bladder**
　　X● **S37.29**　**Other injury of bladder**
● **S37.3**　**Injury of urethra**
　　X● **S37.30**　**Unspecified injury of urethra**
　　X● **S37.32**　**Contusion of urethra**
　　X● **S37.33**　**Laceration of urethra**
　　X● **S37.39**　**Other injury of urethra**
● **S37.4**　**Injury of ovary**
　　● **S37.40**　**Unspecified injury of ovary**
　　　　● **S37.401**　**Unspecified injury of ovary, unilateral**
　　　　● **S37.402**　**Unspecified injury of ovary, bilateral**
　　　　● **S37.409**　**Unspecified injury of ovary, unspecified**
　　● **S37.42**　**Contusion of ovary**
　　　　● **S37.421**　**Contusion of ovary, unilateral**
　　　　● **S37.422**　**Contusion of ovary, bilateral**
　　　　● **S37.429**　**Contusion of ovary, unspecified**
　　● **S37.43**　**Laceration of ovary**
　　　　● **S37.431**　**Laceration of ovary, unilateral**
　　　　● **S37.432**　**Laceration of ovary, bilateral**
　　　　● **S37.439**　**Laceration of ovary, unspecified**
　　● **S37.49**　**Other injury of ovary**
　　　　● **S37.491**　**Other injury of ovary, unilateral**
　　　　● **S37.492**　**Other injury of ovary, bilateral**
　　　　● **S37.499**　**Other injury of ovary, unspecified**
● **S37.5**　**Injury of fallopian tube**
　　● **S37.50**　**Unspecified injury of fallopian tube**
　　　　● **S37.501**　**Unspecified injury of fallopian tube, unilateral**
　　　　● **S37.502**　**Unspecified injury of fallopian tube, bilateral**
　　　　● **S37.509**　**Unspecified injury of fallopian tube, unspecified**
　　● **S37.51**　**Primary blast injury of fallopian tube**
　　　　Blast injury of fallopian tube NOS
　　　　● **S37.511**　**Primary blast injury of fallopian tube, unilateral**
　　　　● **S37.512**　**Primary blast injury of fallopian tube, bilateral**
　　　　● **S37.519**　**Primary blast injury of fallopian tube, unspecified**

◀ New　　◀⃓ Revised　　deleted Deleted　　OGCR Official Guidelines　　X Assign placeholder X　　● Use Additional Character(s)
Excludes 1　Excludes 2　Includes　Use additional　Code first　Code also　Unspecified

● S37.52 Contusion of fallopian tube
   ● S37.521 Contusion of fallopian tube, unilateral
   ● S37.522 Contusion of fallopian tube, bilateral
   ● S37.529 Contusion of fallopian tube, unspecified

● S37.53 Laceration of fallopian tube
   ● S37.531 Laceration of fallopian tube, unilateral
   ● S37.532 Laceration of fallopian tube, bilateral
   ● S37.539 Laceration of fallopian tube, unspecified

● S37.59 Other injury of fallopian tube
   Secondary blast injury of fallopian tube
   ● S37.591 Other injury of fallopian tube, unilateral
   ● S37.592 Other injury of fallopian tube, bilateral
   ● S37.599 Other injury of fallopian tube, unspecified

● S37.6 Injury of uterus
   Excludes1 injury to gravid uterus (O9A.2-)
              injury to uterus during delivery (O71.-)
   X ● S37.60 Unspecified injury of uterus
   X ● S37.62 Contusion of uterus
   X ● S37.63 Laceration of uterus
   X ● S37.69 Other injury of uterus

● S37.8 Injury of other urinary and pelvic organs
   ● S37.81 Injury of adrenal gland
      ● S37.812 Contusion of adrenal gland
      ● S37.813 Laceration of adrenal gland
      ● S37.818 Other injury of adrenal gland
      ● S37.819 Unspecified injury of adrenal gland
   ● S37.82 Injury of prostate
      ● S37.822 Contusion of prostate
      ● S37.823 Laceration of prostate
      ● S37.828 Other injury of prostate
      ● S37.829 Unspecified injury of prostate
   ● S37.89 Injury of other urinary and pelvic organ
      ● S37.892 Contusion of other urinary and pelvic organ
      ● S37.893 Laceration of other urinary and pelvic organ
      ● S37.898 Other injury of other urinary and pelvic organ
      ● S37.899 Unspecified injury of other urinary and pelvic organ

● S37.9 Injury of unspecified urinary and pelvic organ
   X ● S37.90 Unspecified injury of unspecified urinary and pelvic organ
   X ● S37.92 Contusion of unspecified urinary and pelvic organ
   X ● S37.93 Laceration of unspecified urinary and pelvic organ
   X ● S37.99 Other injury of unspecified urinary and pelvic organ

● S38 Crushing injury and traumatic amputation of abdomen, lower back, pelvis and external genitals
   An amputation not identified as partial or complete should be coded to complete
   The appropriate 7th character is to be added to each code from category S38

A	initial encounter
D	subsequent encounter
S	sequela

● S38.0 Crushing injury of external genital organs
   Use additional code for any associated injuries
   ● S38.00 Crushing injury of unspecified external genital organs
      ● S38.001 Crushing injury of unspecified external genital organs, male
      ● S38.002 Crushing injury of unspecified external genital organs, female
   X ● S38.01 Crushing injury of penis
   X ● S38.02 Crushing injury of scrotum and testis
   X ● S38.03 Crushing injury of vulva

X ● S38.1 Crushing injury of abdomen, lower back, and pelvis
   Use additional code for all associated injuries, such as:
      fracture of thoracic or lumbar spine and pelvis (S22.0-, S32.-)
      injury to intra-abdominal organs (S36.-)
      injury to urinary and pelvic organs (S37.-)
      open wound of abdominal wall (S31.-)
      spinal cord injury (S34.0, S34.1-)
   Excludes2 crushing injury of external genital organs (S38.0-)

● S38.2 Traumatic amputation of external genital organs
   ● S38.21 Traumatic amputation of female external genital organs
      Traumatic amputation of clitoris
      Traumatic amputation of labium (majus) (minus)
      Traumatic amputation of vulva
      ● S38.211 Complete traumatic amputation of female external genital organs
      ● S38.212 Partial traumatic amputation of female external genital organs
   ● S38.22 Traumatic amputation of penis
      ● S38.221 Complete traumatic amputation of penis
      ● S38.222 Partial traumatic amputation of penis
   ● S38.23 Traumatic amputation of scrotum and testis
      ● S38.231 Complete traumatic amputation of scrotum and testis
      ● S38.232 Partial traumatic amputation of scrotum and testis

X ● S38.3 Transection (partial) of abdomen

◀ New   ◀▥ Revised   ~~deleted~~ Deleted   **OGCR** Official Guidelines   X Assign placeholder X   ● Use Additional Character(s)

Excludes 1   Excludes 2   Includes   Use additional   Code first   Code also   Unspecified

● **S39** **Other and unspecified injuries of abdomen, lower back, pelvis and external genitals**

Code also any associated open wound (S31.-)

Excludes2　sprain of joints and ligaments of lumbar spine and pelvis (S33.-)

The appropriate 7th character is to be added to each code from category S39

> A　initial encounter
> D　subsequent encounter
> S　sequela

● **S39.0** **Injury of muscle, fascia and tendon of abdomen, lower back and pelvis**

● **S39.00** Unspecified injury of muscle, fascia and tendon of abdomen, lower back and pelvis

● S39.001　Unspecified injury of muscle, fascia and tendon of abdomen

● S39.002　Unspecified injury of muscle, fascia and tendon of lower back

● S39.003　Unspecified injury of muscle, fascia and tendon of pelvis

● **S39.01** Strain of muscle, fascia and tendon of abdomen, lower back and pelvis

● S39.011　Strain of muscle, fascia and tendon of abdomen

● S39.012　Strain of muscle, fascia and tendon of lower back

● S39.013　Strain of muscle, fascia and tendon of pelvis

● **S39.02** Laceration of muscle, fascia and tendon of abdomen, lower back and pelvis

● S39.021　Laceration of muscle, fascia and tendon of abdomen

● S39.022　Laceration of muscle, fascia and tendon of lower back

● S39.023　Laceration of muscle, fascia and tendon of pelvis

● **S39.09** Other injury of muscle, fascia and tendon of abdomen, lower back and pelvis

● S39.091　Other injury of muscle, fascia and tendon of abdomen

● S39.092　Other injury of muscle, fascia and tendon of lower back

● S39.093　Other injury of muscle, fascia and tendon of pelvis

● **S39.8** **Other specified injuries of abdomen, lower back, pelvis and external genitals**

X ● S39.81　Other specified injuries of abdomen

X ● S39.82　Other specified injuries of lower back

X ● S39.83　Other specified injuries of pelvis

● S39.84　Other specified injuries of external genitals

● S39.840　Fracture of corpus cavernosum penis

● S39.848　Other specified injuries of external genitals

● **S39.9** **Unspecified injury of abdomen, lower back, pelvis and external genitals**

X ● S39.91　Unspecified injury of abdomen

X ● S39.92　Unspecified injury of lower back

X ● S39.93　Unspecified injury of pelvis

X ● S39.94　Unspecified injury of external genitals

INJURIES TO THE SHOULDER AND UPPER ARM (S40-S49)

Includes　injuries of axilla injuries of scapular region

Excludes2　burns and corrosions (T20-T32)
frostbite (T33-T34)
injuries of elbow (S50-S59)
insect bite or sting, venomous (T63.4)

● **S40** **Superficial injury of shoulder and upper arm**

The appropriate 7th character is to be added to each code from category S40

> A　initial encounter
> D　subsequent encounter
> S　sequela

● **S40.0** **Contusion of shoulder and upper arm**

● **S40.01** Contusion of shoulder

● S40.011　Contusion of right shoulder

● S40.012　Contusion of left shoulder

● S40.019　Contusion of unspecified shoulder

● **S40.02** Contusion of upper arm

● S40.021　Contusion of right upper arm

● S40.022　Contusion of left upper arm

● S40.029　Contusion of unspecified upper arm

● **S40.2** **Other superficial injuries of shoulder**

● **S40.21** Abrasion of shoulder

● S40.211　Abrasion of right shoulder

● S40.212　Abrasion of left shoulder

● S40.219　Abrasion of unspecified shoulder

● **S40.22** Blister (nonthermal) of shoulder

● S40.221　Blister (nonthermal) of right shoulder

● S40.222　Blister (nonthermal) of left shoulder

● S40.229　Blister (nonthermal) of unspecified shoulder

● **S40.24** External constriction of shoulder

● S40.241　External constriction of right shoulder

● S40.242　External constriction of left shoulder

● S40.249　External constriction of unspecified shoulder

● **S40.25** Superficial foreign body of shoulder
Splinter in the shoulder

● S40.251　Superficial foreign body of right shoulder

● S40.252　Superficial foreign body of left shoulder

● S40.259　Superficial foreign body of unspecified shoulder

● **S40.26** Insect bite (nonvenomous) of shoulder

● S40.261　Insect bite (nonvenomous) of right shoulder

● S40.262　Insect bite (nonvenomous) of left shoulder

● S40.269　Insect bite (nonvenomous) of unspecified shoulder

● **S40.27** Other superficial bite of shoulder

Excludes1　open bite of shoulder (S41.05)

● S40.271　Other superficial bite of right shoulder

● S40.272　Other superficial bite of left shoulder

● S40.279　Other superficial bite of unspecified shoulder

● **S40.8   Other superficial injuries of upper arm**
  ● **S40.81   Abrasion of upper arm**
    ● **S40.811   Abrasion of right upper arm**
    ● **S40.812   Abrasion of left upper arm**
    ● **S40.819   Abrasion of unspecified upper arm**
  ● **S40.82   Blister (nonthermal) of upper arm**
    ● **S40.821   Blister (nonthermal) of right upper arm**
    ● **S40.822   Blister (nonthermal) of left upper arm**
    ● **S40.829   Blister (nonthermal) of unspecified upper arm**
  ● **S40.84   External constriction of upper arm**
    ● **S40.841   External constriction of right upper arm**
    ● **S40.842   External constriction of left upper arm**
    ● **S40.849   External constriction of unspecified upper arm**
  ● **S40.85   Superficial foreign body of upper arm**
    Splinter in the upper arm
    ● **S40.851   Superficial foreign body of right upper arm**
    ● **S40.852   Superficial foreign body of left upper arm**
    ● **S40.859   Superficial foreign body of unspecified upper arm**
  ● **S40.86   Insect bite (nonvenomous) of upper arm**
    ● **S40.861   Insect bite (nonvenomous) of right upper arm**
    ● **S40.862   Insect bite (nonvenomous) of left upper arm**
    ● **S40.869   Insect bite (nonvenomous) of unspecified upper arm**
  ● **S40.87   Other superficial bite of upper arm**
    | **Excludes1** | open bite of upper arm (S41.14) |
    | **Excludes2** | other superficial bite of shoulder (S40.27-) |
    ● **S40.871   Other superficial bite of right upper arm**
    ● **S40.872   Other superficial bite of left upper arm**
    ● **S40.879   Other superficial bite of unspecified upper arm**
● **S40.9   Unspecified superficial injury of shoulder and upper arm**
  ● **S40.91   Unspecified superficial injury of shoulder**
    ● **S40.911   Unspecified superficial injury of right shoulder**
    ● **S40.912   Unspecified superficial injury of left shoulder**
    ● **S40.919   Unspecified superficial injury of unspecified shoulder**
  ● **S40.92   Unspecified superficial injury of upper arm**
    ● **S40.921   Unspecified superficial injury of right upper arm**
    ● **S40.922   Unspecified superficial injury of left upper arm**
    ● **S40.929   Unspecified superficial injury of unspecified upper arm**

● **S41   Open wound of shoulder and upper arm**
  Code also any associated wound infection
  | **Excludes1** | traumatic amputation of shoulder and upper arm (S48.-) |
  | **Excludes2** | open fracture of shoulder and upper arm (S42.- with 7th character B or C) |
  The appropriate 7th character is to be added to each code from category S41

A	initial encounter
D	subsequent encounter
S	sequela

  ● **S41.0   Open wound of shoulder**
    ● **S41.00   Unspecified open wound of shoulder**
      ● **S41.001   Unspecified open wound of right shoulder**
      ● **S41.002   Unspecified open wound of left shoulder**
      ● **S41.009   Unspecified open wound of unspecified shoulder**
    ● **S41.01   Laceration without foreign body of shoulder**
      ● **S41.011   Laceration without foreign body of right shoulder**
      ● **S41.012   Laceration without foreign body of left shoulder**
      ● **S41.019   Laceration without foreign body of unspecified shoulder**
    ● **S41.02   Laceration with foreign body of shoulder**
      ● **S41.021   Laceration with foreign body of right shoulder**
      ● **S41.022   Laceration with foreign body of left shoulder**
      ● **S41.029   Laceration with foreign body of unspecified shoulder**
    ● **S41.03   Puncture wound without foreign body of shoulder**
      ● **S41.031   Puncture wound without foreign body of right shoulder**
      ● **S41.032   Puncture wound without foreign body of left shoulder**
      ● **S41.039   Puncture wound without foreign body of unspecified shoulder**
    ● **S41.04   Puncture wound with foreign body of shoulder**
      ● **S41.041   Puncture wound with foreign body of right shoulder**
      ● **S41.042   Puncture wound with foreign body of left shoulder**
      ● **S41.049   Puncture wound with foreign body of unspecified shoulder**
    ● **S41.05   Open bite of shoulder**
      Bite of shoulder NOS
      | **Excludes1** | superficial bite of shoulder (S40.27) |
      ● **S41.051   Open bite of right shoulder**
      ● **S41.052   Open bite of left shoulder**
      ● **S41.059   Open bite of unspecified shoulder**
  ● **S41.1   Open wound of upper arm**
    ● **S41.10   Unspecified open wound of upper arm**
      ● **S41.101   Unspecified open wound of right upper arm**
      ● **S41.102   Unspecified open wound of left upper arm**
      ● **S41.109   Unspecified open wound of unspecified upper arm**

- S41.11 Laceration without foreign body of upper arm
  - S41.111 Laceration without foreign body of right upper arm
  - S41.112 Laceration without foreign body of left upper arm
  - S41.119 Laceration without foreign body of unspecified upper arm
- S41.12 Laceration with foreign body of upper arm
  - S41.121 Laceration with foreign body of right upper arm
  - S41.122 Laceration with foreign body of left upper arm
  - S41.129 Laceration with foreign body of unspecified upper arm
- S41.13 Puncture wound without foreign body of upper arm
  - S41.131 Puncture wound without foreign body of right upper arm
  - S41.132 Puncture wound without foreign body of left upper arm
  - S41.139 Puncture wound without foreign body of unspecified upper arm
- S41.14 Puncture wound with foreign body of upper arm
  - S41.141 Puncture wound with foreign body of right upper arm
  - S41.142 Puncture wound with foreign body of left upper arm
  - S41.149 Puncture wound with foreign body of unspecified upper arm
- S41.15 Open bite of upper arm
  Bite of upper arm NOS
  > **Excludes1** superficial bite of upper arm (S40.87)
  - S41.151 Open bite of right upper arm
  - S41.152 Open bite of left upper arm
  - S41.159 Open bite of unspecified upper arm

- S42 Fracture of shoulder and upper arm
  Note: A fracture not indicated as displaced or nondisplaced should be coded to displaced

  A fracture not indicated as open or closed should be coded to closed

  > **Excludes1** traumatic amputation of shoulder and upper arm (S48.-)

  The appropriate 7th character is to be added to all codes from category S42

A	initial encounter for closed fracture
B	initial encounter for open fracture
D	subsequent encounter for fracture with routine healing
G	subsequent encounter for fracture with delayed healing
K	subsequent encounter for fracture with nonunion
P	subsequent encounter for fracture with malunion
S	sequela

- S42.0 Fracture of clavicle
  - S42.00 Fracture of unspecified part of clavicle
    - S42.001 Fracture of unspecified part of right clavicle
    - S42.002 Fracture of unspecified part of left clavicle
    - S42.009 Fracture of unspecified part of unspecified clavicle

- S42.01 Fracture of sternal end of clavicle
  - S42.011 Anterior displaced fracture of sternal end of right clavicle
  - S42.012 Anterior displaced fracture of sternal end of left clavicle
  - S42.013 Anterior displaced fracture of sternal end of unspecified clavicle
    Displaced fracture of sternal end of clavicle NOS
  - S42.014 Posterior displaced fracture of sternal end of right clavicle
  - S42.015 Posterior displaced fracture of sternal end of left clavicle
  - S42.016 Posterior displaced fracture of sternal end of unspecified clavicle
  - S42.017 Nondisplaced fracture of sternal end of right clavicle
  - S42.018 Nondisplaced fracture of sternal end of left clavicle
  - S42.019 Nondisplaced fracture of sternal end of unspecified clavicle
- S42.02 Fracture of shaft of clavicle
  - S42.021 Displaced fracture of shaft of right clavicle
  - S42.022 Displaced fracture of shaft of left clavicle
  - S42.023 Displaced fracture of shaft of unspecified clavicle
  - S42.024 Nondisplaced fracture of shaft of right clavicle
  - S42.025 Nondisplaced fracture of shaft of left clavicle
  - S42.026 Nondisplaced fracture of shaft of unspecified clavicle
- S42.03 Fracture of lateral end of clavicle
  Fracture of acromial end of clavicle
  - S42.031 Displaced fracture of lateral end of right clavicle
  - S42.032 Displaced fracture of lateral end of left clavicle
  - S42.033 Displaced fracture of lateral end of unspecified clavicle
  - S42.034 Nondisplaced fracture of lateral end of right clavicle
  - S42.035 Nondisplaced fracture of lateral end of left clavicle
  - S42.036 Nondisplaced fracture of lateral end of unspecified clavicle
- S42.1 Fracture of scapula
  - S42.10 Fracture of unspecified part of scapula
    - S42.101 Fracture of unspecified part of scapula, right shoulder
    - S42.102 Fracture of unspecified part of scapula, left shoulder
    - S42.109 Fracture of unspecified part of scapula, unspecified shoulder
  - S42.11 Fracture of body of scapula
    - S42.111 Displaced fracture of body of scapula, right shoulder
    - S42.112 Displaced fracture of body of scapula, left shoulder
    - S42.113 Displaced fracture of body of scapula, unspecified shoulder
    - S42.114 Nondisplaced fracture of body of scapula, right shoulder
    - S42.115 Nondisplaced fracture of body of scapula, left shoulder
    - S42.116 Nondisplaced fracture of body of scapula, unspecified shoulder

◄ New ◄◄ Revised ~~deleted~~ Deleted **OGCR** Official Guidelines X Assign placeholder X ● Use Additional Character(s)

| Excludes 1 | Excludes 2 | Includes | Use additional | Code first | Code also | Unspecified |

● **S42.12**   **Fracture of acromial process**
   ● **S42.121**   Displaced fracture of acromial process, right shoulder
   ● **S42.122**   Displaced fracture of acromial process, left shoulder
   ● **S42.123**   Displaced fracture of acromial process, unspecified shoulder
   ● **S42.124**   Nondisplaced fracture of acromial process, right shoulder
   ● **S42.125**   Nondisplaced fracture of acromial process, left shoulder
   ● **S42.126**   Nondisplaced fracture, of acromial process, unspecified shoulder

● **S42.13**   **Fracture of coracoid process**
   ● **S42.131**   Displaced fracture of coracoid process, right shoulder
   ● **S42.132**   Displaced fracture of coracoid process, left shoulder
   ● **S42.133**   Displaced fracture of coracoid process, unspecified shoulder
   ● **S42.134**   Nondisplaced fracture of coracoid process, right shoulder
   ● **S42.135**   Nondisplaced fracture of coracoid process, left shoulder
   ● **S42.136**   Nondisplaced fracture of coracoid process, unspecified shoulder

● **S42.14**   **Fracture of glenoid cavity of scapula**
   ● **S42.141**   Displaced fracture of glenoid cavity of scapula, right shoulder
   ● **S42.142**   Displaced fracture of glenoid cavity of scapula, left shoulder
   ● **S42.143**   Displaced fracture of glenoid cavity of scapula, unspecified shoulder
   ● **S42.144**   Nondisplaced fracture of glenoid cavity of scapula, right shoulder
   ● **S42.145**   Nondisplaced fracture of glenoid cavity of scapula, left shoulder
   ● **S42.146**   Nondisplaced fracture of glenoid cavity of scapula, unspecified shoulder

● **S42.15**   **Fracture of neck of scapula**
   ● **S42.151**   Displaced fracture of neck of scapula, right shoulder
   ● **S42.152**   Displaced fracture of neck of scapula, left shoulder
   ● **S42.153**   Displaced fracture of neck of scapula, unspecified shoulder
   ● **S42.154**   Nondisplaced fracture of neck of scapula, right shoulder
   ● **S42.155**   Nondisplaced fracture of neck of scapula, left shoulder
   ● **S42.156**   Nondisplaced fracture of neck of scapula, unspecified shoulder

● **S42.19**   **Fracture of other part of scapula**
   ● **S42.191**   Fracture of other part of scapula, right shoulder
   ● **S42.192**   Fracture of other part of scapula, left shoulder
   ● **S42.199**   Fracture of other part of scapula, unspecified shoulder

● **S42.2**   **Fracture of upper end of humerus**
   Fracture of proximal end of humerus
   Excludes2   fracture of shaft of humerus (S42.3-)
               physeal fracture of upper end of humerus (S49.0-)
  ● **S42.20**   Unspecified fracture of upper end of humerus
    ● **S42.201**   Unspecified fracture of upper end of right humerus
    ● **S42.202**   Unspecified fracture of upper end of left humerus
    ● **S42.209**   Unspecified fracture of upper end of unspecified humerus
  ● **S42.21**   Unspecified fracture of surgical neck of humerus
    Fracture of neck of humerus NOS
    ● **S42.211**   Unspecified displaced fracture of surgical neck of right humerus
    ● **S42.212**   Unspecified displaced fracture of surgical neck of left humerus
    ● **S42.213**   Unspecified displaced fracture of surgical neck of unspecified humerus
    ● **S42.214**   Unspecified nondisplaced fracture of surgical neck of right humerus
    ● **S42.215**   Unspecified nondisplaced fracture of surgical neck of left humerus
    ● **S42.216**   Unspecified nondisplaced fracture of surgical neck of unspecified humerus
  ● **S42.22**   2-part fracture of surgical neck of humerus
    ● **S42.221**   2-part displaced fracture of surgical neck of right humerus
    ● **S42.222**   2-part displaced fracture of surgical neck of left humerus
    ● **S42.223**   2-part displaced fracture of surgical neck of unspecified humerus
    ● **S42.224**   2-part nondisplaced fracture of surgical neck of right humerus
    ● **S42.225**   2-part nondisplaced fracture of surgical neck of left humerus
    ● **S42.226**   2-part nondisplaced fracture of surgical neck of unspecified humerus
  ● **S42.23**   3-part fracture of surgical neck of humerus
    ● **S42.231**   3-part fracture of surgical neck of right humerus
    ● **S42.232**   3-part fracture of surgical neck of left humerus
    ● **S42.239**   3-part fracture of surgical neck of unspecified humerus
  ● **S42.24**   4-part fracture of surgical neck of humerus
    ● **S42.241**   4-part fracture of surgical neck of right humerus
    ● **S42.242**   4-part fracture of surgical neck of left humerus
    ● **S42.249**   4-part fracture of surgical neck of unspecified humerus
  ● **S42.25**   Fracture of greater tuberosity of humerus
    ● **S42.251**   Displaced fracture of greater tuberosity of right humerus
    ● **S42.252**   Displaced fracture of greater tuberosity of left humerus
    ● **S42.253**   Displaced fracture of greater tuberosity of unspecified humerus
    ● **S42.254**   Nondisplaced fracture of greater tuberosity of right humerus
    ● **S42.255**   Nondisplaced fracture of greater tuberosity of left humerus
    ● **S42.256**   Nondisplaced fracture of greater tuberosity of unspecified humerus

CHAPTER 19 (S00-T88)

● **S42.26**   **Fracture of lesser tuberosity of humerus**
    ● **S42.261**   Displaced fracture of lesser tuberosity of right humerus
    ● **S42.262**   Displaced fracture of lesser tuberosity of left humerus
    ● **S42.263**   Displaced fracture of lesser tuberosity of unspecified humerus
    ● **S42.264**   Nondisplaced fracture of lesser tuberosity of right humerus
    ● **S42.265**   Nondisplaced fracture of lesser tuberosity of left humerus
    ● **S42.266**   Nondisplaced fracture of lesser tuberosity of unspecified humerus

● **S42.27**   **Torus fracture of upper end of humerus**
    The appropriate 7th character is to be added to all codes in subcategory S42.27

> A   initial encounter for closed fracture
> D   subsequent encounter for fracture with routine healing
> G   subsequent encounter for fracture with delayed healing
> K   subsequent encounter for fracture with nonunion
> P   subsequent encounter for fracture with malunion
> S   sequela

    ● **S42.271**   Torus fracture of upper end of right humerus
    ● **S42.272**   Torus fracture of upper end of left humerus
    ● **S42.279**   Torus fracture of upper end of unspecified humerus

● **S42.29**   **Other fracture of upper end of humerus**
    Fracture of anatomical neck of humerus
    Fracture of articular head of humerus
    ● **S42.291**   Other displaced fracture of upper end of right humerus
    ● **S42.292**   Other displaced fracture of upper end of left humerus
    ● **S42.293**   Other displaced fracture of upper end of unspecified humerus
    ● **S42.294**   Other nondisplaced fracture of upper end of right humerus
    ● **S42.295**   Other nondisplaced fracture of upper end of left humerus
    ● **S42.296**   Other nondisplaced fracture of upper end of unspecified humerus

● **S42.3**   **Fracture of shaft of humerus**
    Fracture of humerus NOS
    Fracture of upper arm NOS
    Excludes2   physeal fractures of upper end of humerus (S49.0-)
              physeal fractures of lower end of humerus (S49.1-)

   ● **S42.30**   **Unspecified fracture of shaft of humerus**
    ● **S42.301**   Unspecified fracture of shaft of humerus, right arm
    ● **S42.302**   Unspecified fracture of shaft of humerus, left arm
    ● **S42.309**   Unspecified fracture of shaft of humerus, unspecified arm

● **S42.31**   **Greenstick fracture of shaft of humerus**
    The appropriate 7th character is to be added to all codes in subcategory S42.31

> A   initial encounter for closed fracture
> D   subsequent encounter for fracture with routine healing
> G   subsequent encounter for fracture with delayed healing
> K   subsequent encounter for fracture with nonunion
> P   subsequent encounter for fracture with malunion
> S   sequela

    ● **S42.311**   Greenstick fracture of shaft of humerus, right arm
    ● **S42.312**   Greenstick fracture of shaft of humerus, left arm
    ● **S42.319**   Greenstick fracture of shaft of humerus, unspecified arm

● **S42.32**   **Transverse fracture of shaft of humerus**
    ● **S42.321**   Displaced transverse fracture of shaft of humerus, right arm
    ● **S42.322**   Displaced transverse fracture of shaft of humerus, left arm
    ● **S42.323**   Displaced transverse fracture of shaft of humerus, unspecified arm
    ● **S42.324**   Nondisplaced transverse fracture of shaft of humerus, right arm
    ● **S42.325**   Nondisplaced transverse fracture of shaft of humerus, left arm
    ● **S42.326**   Nondisplaced transverse fracture of shaft of humerus, unspecified arm

● **S42.33**   **Oblique fracture of shaft of humerus**
    ● **S42.331**   Displaced oblique fracture of shaft of humerus, right arm
    ● **S42.332**   Displaced oblique fracture of shaft of humerus, left arm
    ● **S42.333**   Displaced oblique fracture of shaft of humerus, unspecified arm
    ● **S42.334**   Nondisplaced oblique fracture of shaft of humerus, right arm
    ● **S42.335**   Nondisplaced oblique fracture of shaft of humerus, left arm
    ● **S42.336**   Nondisplaced oblique fracture of shaft of humerus, unspecified arm

● **S42.34**   **Spiral fracture of shaft of humerus**
    ● **S42.341**   Displaced spiral fracture of shaft of humerus, right arm
    ● **S42.342**   Displaced spiral fracture of shaft of humerus, left arm
    ● **S42.343**   Displaced spiral fracture of shaft of humerus, unspecified arm
    ● **S42.344**   Nondisplaced spiral fracture of shaft of humerus, right arm
    ● **S42.345**   Nondisplaced spiral fracture of shaft of humerus, left arm
    ● **S42.346**   Nondisplaced spiral fracture of shaft of humerus, unspecified arm

◀ New   ⬅ Revised   ~~deleted~~ Deleted   **OGCR** Official Guidelines   X Assign placeholder X   ● Use Additional Character(s)

Excludes 1   Excludes 2   Includes   Use additional   Code first   Code also   Unspecified

● S42.35   Comminuted fracture of shaft of humerus
    ● S42.351   Displaced comminuted fracture of shaft of humerus, right arm
    ● S42.352   Displaced comminuted fracture of shaft of humerus, left arm
    ● S42.353   Displaced comminuted fracture of shaft of humerus, unspecified arm
    ● S42.354   Nondisplaced comminuted fracture of shaft of humerus, right arm
    ● S42.355   Nondisplaced comminuted fracture of shaft of humerus, left arm
    ● S42.356   Nondisplaced comminuted fracture of shaft of humerus, unspecified arm

● S42.36   Segmental fracture of shaft of humerus
    ● S42.361   Displaced segmental fracture of shaft of humerus, right arm
    ● S42.362   Displaced segmental fracture of shaft of humerus, left arm
    ● S42.363   Displaced segmental fracture of shaft of humerus, unspecified arm
    ● S42.364   Nondisplaced segmental fracture of shaft of humerus, right arm
    ● S42.365   Nondisplaced segmental fracture of shaft of humerus, left arm
    ● S42.366   Nondisplaced segmental fracture of shaft of humerus, unspecified arm

● S42.39   Other fracture of shaft of humerus
    ● S42.391   Other fracture of shaft of right humerus
    ● S42.392   Other fracture of shaft of left humerus
    ● S42.399   Other fracture of shaft of unspecified humerus

● S42.4   Fracture of lower end of humerus
    Fracture of distal end of humerus
    Excludes2   fracture of shaft of humerus (S42.3-)
               physeal fracture of lower end of humerus (S49.1-)

    ● S42.40   Unspecified fracture of lower end of humerus
        Fracture of elbow NOS
      ● S42.401   Unspecified fracture of lower end of right humerus
      ● S42.402   Unspecified fracture of lower end of left humerus
      ● S42.409   Unspecified fracture of lower end of unspecified humerus

    ● S42.41   Simple supracondylar fracture without intercondylar fracture of humerus
      ● S42.411   Displaced simple supracondylar fracture without intercondylar fracture of right humerus
      ● S42.412   Displaced simple supracondylar fracture without intercondylar fracture of left humerus
      ● S42.413   Displaced simple supracondylar fracture without intercondylar fracture of unspecified humerus
      ● S42.414   Nondisplaced simple supracondylar fracture without intercondylar fracture of right humerus
      ● S42.415   Nondisplaced simple supracondylar fracture without intercondylar fracture of left humerus
      ● S42.416   Nondisplaced simple supracondylar fracture without intercondylar fracture of unspecified humerus

● S42.42   Comminuted supracondylar fracture without intercondylar fracture of humerus
    ● S42.421   Displaced comminuted supracondylar fracture without intercondylar fracture of right humerus
    ● S42.422   Displaced comminuted supracondylar fracture without intercondylar fracture of left humerus
    ● S42.423   Displaced comminuted supracondylar fracture without intercondylar fracture of unspecified humerus
    ● S42.424   Nondisplaced comminuted supracondylar fracture without intercondylar fracture of right humerus
    ● S42.425   Nondisplaced comminuted supracondylar fracture without intercondylar fracture of left humerus
    ● S42.426   Nondisplaced comminuted supracondylar fracture without intercondylar fracture of unspecified humerus

● S42.43   Fracture (avulsion) of lateral epicondyle of humerus
    ● S42.431   Displaced fracture (avulsion) of lateral epicondyle of right humerus
    ● S42.432   Displaced fracture (avulsion) of lateral epicondyle of left humerus
    ● S42.433   Displaced fracture (avulsion) of lateral epicondyle of unspecified humerus
    ● S42.434   Nondisplaced fracture (avulsion) of lateral epicondyle of right humerus
    ● S42.435   Nondisplaced fracture (avulsion) of lateral epicondyle of left humerus
    ● S42.436   Nondisplaced fracture (avulsion) of lateral epicondyle of unspecified humerus

● S42.44   Fracture (avulsion) of medial epicondyle of humerus
    ● S42.441   Displaced fracture (avulsion) of medial epicondyle of right humerus
    ● S42.442   Displaced fracture (avulsion) of medial epicondyle of left humerus
    ● S42.443   Displaced fracture (avulsion) of medial epicondyle of unspecified humerus
    ● S42.444   Nondisplaced fracture (avulsion) of medial epicondyle of right humerus
    ● S42.445   Nondisplaced fracture (avulsion) of medial epicondyle of left humerus
    ● S42.446   Nondisplaced fracture (avulsion) of medial epicondyle of unspecified humerus
    ● S42.447   Incarcerated fracture (avulsion) of medial epicondyle of right humerus
    ● S42.448   Incarcerated fracture (avulsion) of medial epicondyle of left humerus
    ● S42.449   Incarcerated fracture (avulsion) of medial epicondyle of unspecified humerus

● S42.45   Fracture of lateral condyle of humerus
    Fracture of capitellum of humerus
    ● S42.451   Displaced fracture of lateral condyle of right humerus
    ● S42.452   Displaced fracture of lateral condyle of left humerus
    ● S42.453   Displaced fracture of lateral condyle of unspecified humerus

S42.454 **Nondisplaced fracture of lateral condyle of right humerus**

S42.455 **Nondisplaced fracture of lateral condyle of left humerus**

S42.456 **Nondisplaced fracture of lateral condyle of unspecified humerus**

S42.46 **Fracture of medial condyle of humerus**
Trochlea fracture of humerus

S42.461 **Displaced fracture of medial condyle of right humerus**

S42.462 **Displaced fracture of medial condyle of left humerus**

S42.463 **Displaced fracture of medial condyle of unspecified humerus**

S42.464 **Nondisplaced fracture of medial condyle of right humerus**

S42.465 **Nondisplaced fracture of medial condyle of left humerus**

S42.466 **Nondisplaced fracture of medial condyle of unspecified humerus**

S42.47 **Transcondylar fracture of humerus**

S42.471 **Displaced transcondylar fracture of right humerus**

S42.472 **Displaced transcondylar fracture of left humerus**

S42.473 **Displaced transcondylar fracture of unspecified humerus**

S42.474 **Nondisplaced transcondylar fracture of right humerus**

S42.475 **Nondisplaced transcondylar fracture of left humerus**

S42.476 **Nondisplaced transcondylar fracture of unspecified humerus**

S42.48 **Torus fracture of lower end of humerus**

The appropriate 7th character is to be added to all codes in subcategory S42.48

A	initial encounter for closed fracture
D	subsequent encounter for fracture with routine healing
G	subsequent encounter for fracture with delayed healing
K	subsequent encounter for fracture with nonunion
P	subsequent encounter for fracture with malunion
S	sequela

S42.481 **Torus fracture of lower end of right humerus**

S42.482 **Torus fracture of lower end of left humerus**

S42.489 **Torus fracture of lower end of unspecified humerus**

S42.49 **Other fracture of lower end of humerus**

S42.491 **Other displaced fracture of lower end of right humerus**

S42.492 **Other displaced fracture of lower end of left humerus**

S42.493 **Other displaced fracture of lower end of unspecified humerus**

S42.494 **Other nondisplaced fracture of lower end of right humerus**

S42.495 **Other nondisplaced fracture of lower end of left humerus**

S42.496 **Other nondisplaced fracture of lower end of unspecified humerus**

S42.9 **Fracture of shoulder girdle, part unspecified**
Fracture of shoulder NOS

X S42.90 **Fracture of unspecified shoulder girdle, part unspecified**

X S42.91 **Fracture of right shoulder girdle, part unspecified**

X S42.92 **Fracture of left shoulder girdle, part unspecified**

S43 **Dislocation and sprain of joints and ligaments of shoulder girdle**

Includes   avulsion of joint or ligament of shoulder girdle
laceration of cartilage, joint or ligament of shoulder girdle
sprain of cartilage, joint or ligament of shoulder girdle
traumatic hemarthrosis of joint or ligament of shoulder girdle
traumatic rupture of joint or ligament of shoulder girdle
traumatic subluxation of joint or ligament of shoulder girdle
traumatic tear of joint or ligament of shoulder girdle

Code also any associated open wound

Excludes2   strain of muscle, fascia and tendon of shoulder and upper arm (S46.-)

The appropriate 7th character is to be added to each code from category S43

A	initial encounter
D	subsequent encounter
S	sequela

S43.0 **Subluxation and dislocation of shoulder joint**
Dislocation of glenohumeral joint
Subluxation of glenohumeral joint

S43.00 **Unspecified subluxation and dislocation of shoulder joint**
Dislocation of humerus NOS
Subluxation of humerus NOS

S43.001 **Unspecified subluxation of right shoulder joint**

S43.002 **Unspecified subluxation of left shoulder joint**

S43.003 **Unspecified subluxation of unspecified shoulder joint**

S43.004 **Unspecified dislocation of right shoulder joint**

S43.005 **Unspecified dislocation of left shoulder joint**

S43.006 **Unspecified dislocation of unspecified shoulder joint**

S43.01 **Anterior subluxation and dislocation of humerus**

S43.011 **Anterior subluxation of right humerus**

S43.012 **Anterior subluxation of left humerus**

S43.013 **Anterior subluxation of unspecified humerus**

S43.014 **Anterior dislocation of right humerus**

S43.015 **Anterior dislocation of left humerus**

S43.016 **Anterior dislocation of unspecified humerus**

● S43.02   Posterior subluxation and dislocation of humerus
   ● S43.021   Posterior subluxation of right humerus
   ● S43.022   Posterior subluxation of left humerus
   ● S43.023   Posterior subluxation of unspecified humerus
   ● S43.024   Posterior dislocation of right humerus
   ● S43.025   Posterior dislocation of left humerus
   ● S43.026   Posterior dislocation of unspecified humerus

● S43.03   Inferior subluxation and dislocation of humerus
   ● S43.031   Inferior subluxation of right humerus
   ● S43.032   Inferior subluxation of left humerus
   ● S43.033   Inferior subluxation of unspecified humerus
   ● S43.034   Inferior dislocation of right humerus
   ● S43.035   Inferior dislocation of left humerus
   ● S43.036   Inferior dislocation of unspecified humerus

● S43.08   Other subluxation and dislocation of shoulder joint
   ● S43.081   Other subluxation of right shoulder joint
   ● S43.082   Other subluxation of left shoulder joint
   ● S43.083   Other subluxation of unspecified shoulder joint
   ● S43.084   Other dislocation of right shoulder joint
   ● S43.085   Other dislocation of left shoulder joint
   ● S43.086   Other dislocation of unspecified shoulder joint

● S43.1   Subluxation and dislocation of acromioclavicular joint
   ● S43.10   Unspecified dislocation of acromioclavicular joint
     ● S43.101   Unspecified dislocation of right acromioclavicular joint
     ● S43.102   Unspecified dislocation of left acromioclavicular joint
     ● S43.109   Unspecified dislocation of unspecified acromioclavicular joint
   ● S43.11   Subluxation of acromioclavicular joint
     ● S43.111   Subluxation of right acromioclavicular joint
     ● S43.112   Subluxation of left acromioclavicular joint
     ● S43.119   Subluxation of unspecified acromioclavicular joint
   ● S43.12   Dislocation of acromioclavicular joint, 100%-200% displacement
     ● S43.121   Dislocation of right acromioclavicular joint, 100%-200% displacement
     ● S43.122   Dislocation of left acromioclavicular joint, 100%-200% displacement
     ● S43.129   Dislocation of unspecified acromioclavicular joint, 100%-200% displacement
   ● S43.13   Dislocation of acromioclavicular joint, greater than 200% displacement
     ● S43.131   Dislocation of right acromioclavicular joint, greater than 200% displacement
     ● S43.132   Dislocation of left acromioclavicular joint, greater than 200% displacement
     ● S43.139   Dislocation of unspecified acromioclavicular joint, greater than 200% displacement

● S43.14   Inferior dislocation of acromioclavicular joint
   ● S43.141   Inferior dislocation of right acromioclavicular joint
   ● S43.142   Inferior dislocation of left acromioclavicular joint
   ● S43.149   Inferior dislocation of unspecified acromioclavicular joint
● S43.15   Posterior dislocation of acromioclavicular joint
   ● S43.151   Posterior dislocation of right acromioclavicular joint
   ● S43.152   Posterior dislocation of left acromioclavicular joint
   ● S43.159   Posterior dislocation of unspecified acromioclavicular joint

● S43.2   Subluxation and dislocation of sternoclavicular joint
   ● S43.20   Unspecified subluxation and dislocation of sternoclavicular joint
     ● S43.201   Unspecified subluxation of right sternoclavicular joint
     ● S43.202   Unspecified subluxation of left sternoclavicular joint
     ● S43.203   Unspecified subluxation of unspecified sternoclavicular joint
     ● S43.204   Unspecified dislocation of right sternoclavicular joint
     ● S43.205   Unspecified dislocation of left sternoclavicular joint
     ● S43.206   Unspecified dislocation of unspecified sternoclavicular joint
   ● S43.21   Anterior subluxation and dislocation of sternoclavicular joint
     ● S43.211   Anterior subluxation of right sternoclavicular joint
     ● S43.212   Anterior subluxation of left sternoclavicular joint
     ● S43.213   Anterior subluxation of unspecified sternoclavicular joint
     ● S43.214   Anterior dislocation of right sternoclavicular joint
     ● S43.215   Anterior dislocation of left sternoclavicular joint
     ● S43.216   Anterior dislocation of unspecified sternoclavicular joint
   ● S43.22   Posterior subluxation and dislocation of sternoclavicular joint
     ● S43.221   Posterior subluxation of right sternoclavicular joint
     ● S43.222   Posterior subluxation of left sternoclavicular joint
     ● S43.223   Posterior subluxation of unspecified sternoclavicular joint
     ● S43.224   Posterior dislocation of right sternoclavicular joint
     ● S43.225   Posterior dislocation of left sternoclavicular joint
     ● S43.226   Posterior dislocation of unspecified sternoclavicular joint

● S43.3   Subluxation and dislocation of other and unspecified parts of shoulder girdle
   ● S43.30   Subluxation and dislocation of unspecified parts of shoulder girdle
     Dislocation of shoulder girdle NOS
     Subluxation of shoulder girdle NOS
     ● S43.301   Subluxation of unspecified parts of right shoulder girdle
     ● S43.302   Subluxation of unspecified parts of left shoulder girdle

CHAPTER 19 (S00-T88)

CHAPTER 19 (S00-T88)

● S43.303   Subluxation of unspecified parts of unspecified shoulder girdle

● S43.304   Dislocation of unspecified parts of right shoulder girdle

● S43.305   Dislocation of unspecified parts of left shoulder girdle

● S43.306   Dislocation of unspecified parts of unspecified shoulder girdle

● S43.31   Subluxation and dislocation of scapula

● S43.311   Subluxation of right scapula

● S43.312   Subluxation of left scapula

● S43.313   Subluxation of unspecified scapula

● S43.314   Dislocation of right scapula

● S43.315   Dislocation of left scapula

● S43.316   Dislocation of unspecified scapula

● S43.39   Subluxation and dislocation of other parts of shoulder girdle

● S43.391   Subluxation of other parts of right shoulder girdle

● S43.392   Subluxation of other parts of left shoulder girdle

● S43.393   Subluxation of other parts of unspecified shoulder girdle

● S43.394   Dislocation of other parts of right shoulder girdle

● S43.395   Dislocation of other parts of left shoulder girdle

● S43.396   Dislocation of other parts of unspecified shoulder girdle

● S43.4   Sprain of shoulder joint

● S43.40   Unspecified sprain of shoulder joint

● S43.401   Unspecified sprain of right shoulder joint

● S43.402   Unspecified sprain of left shoulder joint

● S43.409   Unspecified sprain of unspecified shoulder joint

● S43.41   Sprain of coracohumeral (ligament)

● S43.411   Sprain of right coracohumeral (ligament)

● S43.412   Sprain of left coracohumeral (ligament)

● S43.419   Sprain of unspecified coracohumeral (ligament)

● S43.42   Sprain of rotator cuff capsule

> **Excludes1**   rotator cuff syndrome (complete) (incomplete), not specified as traumatic (M75.1-)

> **Excludes2**   injury of tendon of rotator cuff (S46.0-)

Encounters during the healing phase

● S43.421   Sprain of right rotator cuff capsule

● S43.422   Sprain of left rotator cuff capsule

● S43.429   Sprain of unspecified rotator cuff capsule

● S43.43   Superior glenoid labrum lesion
SLAP lesion

● S43.431   Superior glenoid labrum lesion of right shoulder

● S43.432   Superior glenoid labrum lesion of left shoulder

● S43.439   Superior glenoid labrum lesion of unspecified shoulder

● S43.49   Other sprain of shoulder joint

● S43.491   Other sprain of right shoulder joint

● S43.492   Other sprain of left shoulder joint

● S43.499   Other sprain of unspecified shoulder joint

● S43.5   Sprain of acromioclavicular joint
Sprain of acromioclavicular ligament

X ● S43.50   Sprain of unspecified acromioclavicular joint

X ● S43.51   Sprain of right acromioclavicular joint

X ● S43.52   Sprain of left acromioclavicular joint

● S43.6   Sprain of sternoclavicular joint

X ● S43.60   Sprain of unspecified sternoclavicular joint

X ● S43.61   Sprain of right sternoclavicular joint

X ● S43.62   Sprain of left sternoclavicular joint

● S43.8   Sprain of other specified parts of shoulder girdle

X ● S43.80   Sprain of other specified parts of unspecified shoulder girdle

X ● S43.81   Sprain of other specified parts of right shoulder girdle

X ● S43.82   Sprain of other specified parts of left shoulder girdle

● S43.9   Sprain of unspecified parts of shoulder girdle

X ● S43.90   Sprain of unspecified parts of unspecified shoulder girdle
Sprain of shoulder girdle NOS

X ● S43.91   Sprain of unspecified parts of right shoulder girdle

X ● S43.92   Sprain of unspecified parts of left shoulder girdle

● S44   Injury of nerves at shoulder and upper arm level

Code also any associated open wound (S41.-)

> **Excludes2**   injury of brachial plexus (S14.3-)

The appropriate 7th character is to be added to each code from category S44

A	initial encounter
D	subsequent encounter
S	sequela

● S44.0   Injury of ulnar nerve at upper arm level

> **Excludes1**   ulnar nerve NOS (S54.0)

X ● S44.00   Injury of ulnar nerve at upper arm level, unspecified arm

X ● S44.01   Injury of ulnar nerve at upper arm level, right arm

X ● S44.02   Injury of ulnar nerve at upper arm level, left arm

● S44.1   Injury of median nerve at upper arm level

> **Excludes1**   median nerve NOS (S54.1)

X ● S44.10   Injury of median nerve at upper arm level, unspecified arm

X ● S44.11   Injury of median nerve at upper arm level, right arm

X ● S44.12   Injury of median nerve at upper arm level, left arm

● S44.2   Injury of radial nerve at upper arm level

> **Excludes1**   radial nerve NOS (S54.2)

X ● S44.20   Injury of radial nerve at upper arm level, unspecified arm

X ● S44.21   Injury of radial nerve at upper arm level, right arm

X ● S44.22   Injury of radial nerve at upper arm level, left arm

◀ New   ⬅ Revised   ~~deleted~~ Deleted   OGCR Official Guidelines   X Assign placeholder X   ● Use Additional Character(s)

Excludes 1   Excludes 2   Includes   Use additional   Code first   Code also   Unspecified

● **S44.3   Injury of axillary nerve**
   X● **S44.30**   Injury of axillary nerve, unspecified arm
   X● **S44.31**   Injury of axillary nerve, right arm
   X● **S44.32**   Injury of axillary nerve, left arm

● **S44.4   Injury of musculocutaneous nerve**
   X● **S44.40**   Injury of musculocutaneous nerve, unspecified arm
   X● **S44.41**   Injury of musculocutaneous nerve, right arm
   X● **S44.42**   Injury of musculocutaneous nerve, left arm

● **S44.5   Injury of cutaneous sensory nerve at shoulder and upper arm level**
   X● **S44.50**   Injury of cutaneous sensory nerve at shoulder and upper arm level, unspecified arm
   X● **S44.51**   Injury of cutaneous sensory nerve at shoulder and upper arm level, right arm
   X● **S44.52**   Injury of cutaneous sensory nerve at shoulder and upper arm level, left arm

● **S44.8   Injury of other nerves at shoulder and upper arm level**
   ● **S44.8X**   Injury of other nerves at shoulder and upper arm level
     ● **S44.8X1**   Injury of other nerves at shoulder and upper arm level, right arm
     ● **S44.8X2**   Injury of other nerves at shoulder and upper arm level, left arm
     ● **S44.8X9**   Injury of other nerves at shoulder and upper arm level, unspecified arm

● **S44.9   Injury of unspecified nerve at shoulder and upper arm level**
   X● **S44.90**   Injury of unspecified nerve at shoulder and upper arm level, unspecified arm
   X● **S44.91**   Injury of unspecified nerve at shoulder and upper arm level, right arm
   X● **S44.92**   Injury of unspecified nerve at shoulder and upper arm level, left arm

● **S45   Injury of blood vessels at shoulder and upper arm level**
   Code also any associated open wound (S41.-)
   Excludes2   injury of subclavian artery (S25.1)
            injury of subclavian vein (S25.3)
   The appropriate 7th character is to be added to each code from category S45

> A   initial encounter
> D   subsequent encounter
> S   sequela

● **S45.0   Injury of axillary artery**
   ● **S45.00**   Unspecified injury of axillary artery
     ● **S45.001**   Unspecified injury of axillary artery, right side
     ● **S45.002**   Unspecified injury of axillary artery, left side
     ● **S45.009**   Unspecified injury of axillary artery, unspecified side
   ● **S45.01**   Laceration of axillary artery
     ● **S45.011**   Laceration of axillary artery, right side
     ● **S45.012**   Laceration of axillary artery, left side
     ● **S45.019**   Laceration of axillary artery, unspecified side
   ● **S45.09**   Other specified injury of axillary artery
     ● **S45.091**   Other specified injury of axillary artery, right side
     ● **S45.092**   Other specified injury of axillary artery, left side
     ● **S45.099**   Other specified injury of axillary artery, unspecified side

● **S45.1   Injury of brachial artery**
   ● **S45.10**   Unspecified injury of brachial artery
     ● **S45.101**   Unspecified injury of brachial artery, right side
     ● **S45.102**   Unspecified injury of brachial artery, left side
     ● **S45.109**   Unspecified injury of brachial artery, unspecified side
   ● **S45.11**   Laceration of brachial artery
     ● **S45.111**   Laceration of brachial artery, right side
     ● **S45.112**   Laceration of brachial artery, left side
     ● **S45.119**   Laceration of brachial artery, unspecified side
   ● **S45.19**   Other specified injury of brachial artery
     ● **S45.191**   Other specified injury of brachial artery, right side
     ● **S45.192**   Other specified injury of brachial artery, left side
     ● **S45.199**   Other specified injury of brachial artery, unspecified side

● **S45.2   Injury of axillary or brachial vein**
   ● **S45.20**   Unspecified injury of axillary or brachial vein
     ● **S45.201**   Unspecified injury of axillary or brachial vein, right side
     ● **S45.202**   Unspecified injury of axillary or brachial vein, left side
     ● **S45.209**   Unspecified injury of axillary or brachial vein, unspecified side
   ● **S45.21**   Laceration of axillary or brachial vein
     ● **S45.211**   Laceration of axillary or brachial vein, right side
     ● **S45.212**   Laceration of axillary or brachial vein, left side
     ● **S45.219**   Laceration of axillary or brachial vein, unspecified side
   ● **S45.29**   Other specified injury of axillary or brachial vein
     ● **S45.291**   Other specified injury of axillary or brachial vein, right side
     ● **S45.292**   Other specified injury of axillary or brachial vein, left side
     ● **S45.299**   Other specified injury of axillary or brachial vein, unspecified side

● **S45.3   Injury of superficial vein at shoulder and upper arm level**
   ● **S45.30**   Unspecified injury of superficial vein at shoulder and upper arm level
     ● **S45.301**   Unspecified injury of superficial vein at shoulder and upper arm level, right arm
     ● **S45.302**   Unspecified injury of superficial vein at shoulder and upper arm level, left arm
     ● **S45.309**   Unspecified injury of superficial vein at shoulder and upper arm level, unspecified arm
   ● **S45.31**   Laceration of superficial vein at shoulder and upper arm level
     ● **S45.311**   Laceration of superficial vein at shoulder and upper arm level, right arm
     ● **S45.312**   Laceration of superficial vein at shoulder and upper arm level, left arm
     ● **S45.319**   Laceration of superficial vein at shoulder and upper arm level, unspecified arm

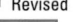

● S45.39   Other specified injury of superficial vein at shoulder and upper arm level
- ● S45.391   Other specified injury of superficial vein at shoulder and upper arm level, right arm
- ● S45.392   Other specified injury of superficial vein at shoulder and upper arm level, left arm
- ● S45.399   Other specified injury of superficial vein at shoulder and upper arm level, unspecified arm

● S45.8   Injury of other specified blood vessels at shoulder and upper arm level
- ● S45.80   Unspecified injury of other specified blood vessels at shoulder and upper arm level
  - ● S45.801   Unspecified injury of other specified blood vessels at shoulder and upper arm level, right arm
  - ● S45.802   Unspecified injury of other specified blood vessels at shoulder and upper arm level, left arm
  - ● S45.809   Unspecified injury of other specified blood vessels at shoulder and upper arm level, unspecified arm
- ● S45.81   Laceration of other specified blood vessels at shoulder and upper arm level
  - ● S45.811   Laceration of other specified blood vessels at shoulder and upper arm level, right arm
  - ● S45.812   Laceration of other specified blood vessels at shoulder and upper arm level, left arm
  - ● S45.819   Laceration of other specified blood vessels at shoulder and upper arm level, unspecified arm
- ● S45.89   Other specified injury of other specified blood vessels at shoulder and upper arm level
  - ● S45.891   Other specified injury of other specified blood vessels at shoulder and upper arm level, right arm
  - ● S45.892   Other specified injury of other specified blood vessels at shoulder and upper arm level, left arm
  - ● S45.899   Other specified injury of other specified blood vessels at shoulder and upper arm level, unspecified arm

● S45.9   Injury of unspecified blood vessel at shoulder and upper arm level
- ● S45.90   Unspecified injury of unspecified blood vessel at shoulder and upper arm level
  - ● S45.901   Unspecified injury of unspecified blood vessel at shoulder and upper arm level, right arm
  - ● S45.902   Unspecified injury of unspecified blood vessel at shoulder and upper arm level, left arm
  - ● S45.909   Unspecified injury of unspecified blood vessel at shoulder and upper arm level, unspecified arm
- ● S45.91   Laceration of unspecified blood vessel at shoulder and upper arm level
  - ● S45.911   Laceration of unspecified blood vessel at shoulder and upper arm level, right arm
  - ● S45.912   Laceration of unspecified blood vessel at shoulder and upper arm level, left arm
  - ● S45.919   Laceration of unspecified blood vessel at shoulder and upper arm level, unspecified arm

● S45.99   Other specified injury of unspecified blood vessel at shoulder and upper arm level
- ● S45.991   Other specified injury of unspecified blood vessel at shoulder and upper arm level, right arm
- ● S45.992   Other specified injury of unspecified blood vessel at shoulder and upper arm level, left arm
- ● S45.999   Other specified injury of unspecified blood vessel at shoulder and upper arm level, unspecified arm

● S46   Injury of muscle, fascia and tendon at shoulder and upper arm level

     Code also any associated open wound (S41.-)

     Excludes2   injury of muscle, fascia and tendon at elbow (S56.-)
         sprain of joints and ligaments of shoulder girdle (S43.9)

     The appropriate 7th character is to be added to each code from category S46

A	initial encounter
D	subsequent encounter
S	sequela

● S46.0   Injury of muscle(s) and tendon(s) of the rotator cuff of shoulder
- ● S46.00   Unspecified injury of muscle(s) and tendon(s) of the rotator cuff of shoulder
  - ● S46.001   Unspecified injury of muscle(s) and tendon(s) of the rotator cuff of right shoulder
  - ● S46.002   Unspecified injury of muscle(s) and tendon(s) of the rotator cuff of left shoulder
  - ● S46.009   Unspecified injury of muscle(s) and tendon(s) of the rotator cuff of unspecified shoulder
- ● S46.01   Strain of muscle(s) and tendon(s) of the rotator cuff of shoulder
  - *Acute onset due to trauma to rotator cuff muscle/tendon*
  - ● S46.011   Strain of muscle(s) and tendon(s) of the rotator cuff of right shoulder
  - ● S46.012   Strain of muscle(s) and tendon(s) of the rotator cuff of left shoulder
  - ● S46.019   Strain of muscle(s) and tendon(s) of the rotator cuff of unspecified shoulder
- ● S46.02   Laceration of muscle(s) and tendon(s) of the rotator cuff of shoulder
  - ● S46.021   Laceration of muscle(s) and tendon(s) of the rotator cuff of right shoulder
  - ● S46.022   Laceration of muscle(s) and tendon(s) of the rotator cuff of left shoulder
  - ● S46.029   Laceration of muscle(s) and tendon(s) of the rotator cuff of unspecified shoulder
- ● S46.09   Other injury of muscle(s) and tendon(s) of the rotator cuff of shoulder
  - ● S46.091   Other injury of muscle(s) and tendon(s) of the rotator cuff of right shoulder
  - ● S46.092   Other injury of muscle(s) and tendon(s) of the rotator cuff of left shoulder
  - ● S46.099   Other injury of muscle(s) and tendon(s) of the rotator cuff of unspecified shoulder

● S46.1 Injury of muscle, fascia and tendon of long head of biceps
- ● S46.10 Unspecified injury of muscle, fascia and tendon of long head of biceps
  - ● S46.101 Unspecified injury of muscle, fascia and tendon of long head of biceps, right arm
  - ● S46.102 Unspecified injury of muscle, fascia and tendon of long head of biceps, left arm
  - ● S46.109 Unspecified injury of muscle, fascia and tendon of long head of biceps, unspecified arm
- ● S46.11 Strain of muscle, fascia and tendon of long head of biceps
  - ● S46.111 Strain of muscle, fascia and tendon of long head of biceps, right arm
  - ● S46.112 Strain of muscle, fascia and tendon of long head of biceps, left arm
  - ● S46.119 Strain of muscle, fascia and tendon of long head of biceps, unspecified arm
- ● S46.12 Laceration of muscle, fascia and tendon of long head of biceps
  - ● S46.121 Laceration of muscle, fascia and tendon of long head of biceps, right arm
  - ● S46.122 Laceration of muscle, fascia and tendon of long head of biceps, left arm
  - ● S46.129 Laceration of muscle, fascia and tendon of long head of biceps, unspecified arm
- ● S46.19 Other injury of muscle, fascia and tendon of long head of biceps
  - ● S46.191 Other injury of muscle, fascia and tendon of long head of biceps, right arm
  - ● S46.192 Other injury of muscle, fascia and tendon of long head of biceps, left arm
  - ● S46.199 Other injury of muscle, fascia and tendon of long head of biceps, unspecified arm

● S46.2 Injury of muscle, fascia and tendon of other parts of biceps
- ● S46.20 Unspecified injury of muscle, fascia and tendon of other parts of biceps
  - ● S46.201 Unspecified injury of muscle, fascia and tendon of other parts of biceps, right arm
  - ● S46.202 Unspecified injury of muscle, fascia and tendon of other parts of biceps, left arm
  - ● S46.209 Unspecified injury of muscle, fascia and tendon of other parts of biceps, unspecified arm
- ● S46.21 Strain of muscle, fascia and tendon of other parts of biceps
  - ● S46.211 Strain of muscle, fascia and tendon of other parts of biceps, right arm
  - ● S46.212 Strain of muscle, fascia and tendon of other parts of biceps, left arm
  - ● S46.219 Strain of muscle, fascia and tendon of other parts of biceps, unspecified arm

● S46.22 Laceration of muscle, fascia and tendon of other parts of biceps
- ● S46.221 Laceration of muscle, fascia and tendon of other parts of biceps, right arm
- ● S46.222 Laceration of muscle, fascia and tendon of other parts of biceps, left arm
- ● S46.229 Laceration of muscle, fascia and tendon of other parts of biceps, unspecified arm

● S46.29 Other injury of muscle, fascia and tendon of other parts of biceps
- ● S46.291 Other injury of muscle, fascia and tendon of other parts of biceps, right arm
- ● S46.292 Other injury of muscle, fascia and tendon of other parts of biceps, left arm
- ● S46.299 Other injury of muscle, fascia and tendon of other parts of biceps, unspecified arm

● S46.3 Injury of muscle, fascia and tendon of triceps
- ● S46.30 Unspecified injury of muscle, fascia and tendon of triceps
  - ● S46.301 Unspecified injury of muscle, fascia and tendon of triceps, right arm
  - ● S46.302 Unspecified injury of muscle, fascia and tendon of triceps, left arm
  - ● S46.309 Unspecified injury of muscle, fascia and tendon of triceps, unspecified arm
- ● S46.31 Strain of muscle, fascia and tendon of triceps
  - ● S46.311 Strain of muscle, fascia and tendon of triceps, right arm
  - ● S46.312 Strain of muscle, fascia and tendon of triceps, left arm
  - ● S46.319 Strain of muscle, fascia and tendon of triceps, unspecified arm
- ● S46.32 Laceration of muscle, fascia and tendon of triceps
  - ● S46.321 Laceration of muscle, fascia and tendon of triceps, right arm
  - ● S46.322 Laceration of muscle, fascia and tendon of triceps, left arm
  - ● S46.329 Laceration of muscle, fascia and tendon of triceps, unspecified arm
- ● S46.39 Other injury of muscle, fascia and tendon of triceps
  - ● S46.391 Other injury of muscle, fascia and tendon of triceps, right arm
  - ● S46.392 Other injury of muscle, fascia and tendon of triceps, left arm
  - ● S46.399 Other injury of muscle, fascia and tendon of triceps, unspecified arm

● S46.8 Injury of other muscles, fascia and tendons at shoulder and upper arm level
- ● S46.80 Unspecified injury of other muscles, fascia and tendons at shoulder and upper arm level
  - ● S46.801 Unspecified injury of other muscles, fascia and tendons at shoulder and upper arm level, right arm
  - ● S46.802 Unspecified injury of other muscles, fascia and tendons at shoulder and upper arm level, left arm
  - ● S46.809 Unspecified injury of other muscles, fascia and tendons at shoulder and upper arm level, unspecified arm

CHAPTER 19 (S00-T88)

● S46.81   Strain of other muscles, fascia and tendons at shoulder and upper arm level

  ● S46.811   Strain of other muscles, fascia and tendons at shoulder and upper arm level, right arm

  ● S46.812   Strain of other muscles, fascia and tendons at shoulder and upper arm level, left arm

  ● S46.819   Strain of other muscles, fascia and tendons at shoulder and upper arm level, unspecified arm

● S46.82   Laceration of other muscles, fascia and tendons at shoulder and upper arm level

  ● S46.821   Laceration of other muscles, fascia and tendons at shoulder and upper arm level, right arm

  ● S46.822   Laceration of other muscles, fascia and tendons at shoulder and upper arm level, left arm

  ● S46.829   Laceration of other muscles, fascia and tendons at shoulder and upper arm level, unspecified arm

● S46.89   Other injury of other muscles, fascia and tendons at shoulder and upper arm level

  ● S46.891   Other injury of other muscles, fascia and tendons at shoulder and upper arm level, right arm

  ● S46.892   Other injury of other muscles, fascia and tendons at shoulder and upper arm level, left arm

  ● S46.899   Other injury of other muscles, fascia and tendons at shoulder and upper arm level, unspecified arm

● S46.9   Injury of unspecified muscle, fascia and tendon at shoulder and upper arm level

  ● S46.90   Unspecified injury of unspecified muscle, fascia and tendon at shoulder and upper arm level

    ● S46.901   Unspecified injury of unspecified muscle, fascia and tendon at shoulder and upper arm level, right arm

    ● S46.902   Unspecified injury of unspecified muscle, fascia and tendon at shoulder and upper arm level, left arm

    ● S46.909   Unspecified injury of unspecified muscle, fascia and tendon at shoulder and upper arm level, unspecified arm

  ● S46.91   Strain of unspecified muscle, fascia and tendon at shoulder and upper arm level

    ● S46.911   Strain of unspecified muscle, fascia and tendon at shoulder and upper arm level, right arm

    ● S46.912   Strain of unspecified muscle, fascia and tendon at shoulder and upper arm level, left arm

    ● S46.919   Strain of unspecified muscle, fascia and tendon at shoulder and upper arm level, unspecified arm

  ● S46.92   Laceration of unspecified muscle, fascia and tendon at shoulder and upper arm level

    ● S46.921   Laceration of unspecified muscle, fascia and tendon at shoulder and upper arm level, right arm

    ● S46.922   Laceration of unspecified muscle, fascia and tendon at shoulder and upper arm level, left arm

    ● S46.929   Laceration of unspecified muscle, fascia and tendon at shoulder and upper arm level, unspecified arm

● S46.99   Other injury of unspecified muscle, fascia and tendon at shoulder and upper arm level

  ● S46.991   Other injury of unspecified muscle, fascia and tendon at shoulder and upper arm level, right arm

  ● S46.992   Other injury of unspecified muscle, fascia and tendon at shoulder and upper arm level, left arm

  ● S46.999   Other injury of unspecified muscle, fascia and tendon at shoulder and upper arm level, unspecified arm

● S47   Crushing injury of shoulder and upper arm

Use additional code for all associated injuries

Excludes2   crushing injury of elbow (S57.0-)

The appropriate 7th character is to be added to each code from category S47

A	initial encounter
D	subsequent encounter
S	sequela

X ● S47.1   Crushing injury of right shoulder and upper arm

X ● S47.2   Crushing injury of left shoulder and upper arm

X ● S47.9   Crushing injury of shoulder and upper arm, unspecified arm

● S48   Traumatic amputation of shoulder and upper arm

An amputation not identified as partial or complete should be coded to complete

Excludes1   traumatic amputation at elbow level (S58.0)

The appropriate 7th character is to be added to each code from category S48

A	initial encounter
D	subsequent encounter
S	sequela

● S48.0   Traumatic amputation at shoulder joint

  ● S48.01   Complete traumatic amputation at shoulder joint

    ● S48.011   Complete traumatic amputation at right shoulder joint

    ● S48.012   Complete traumatic amputation at left shoulder joint

    ● S48.019   Complete traumatic amputation at unspecified shoulder joint

  ● S48.02   Partial traumatic amputation at shoulder joint

    ● S48.021   Partial traumatic amputation at right shoulder joint

    ● S48.022   Partial traumatic amputation at left shoulder joint

    ● S48.029   Partial traumatic amputation at unspecified shoulder joint

● S48.1   Traumatic amputation at level between shoulder and elbow

  ● S48.11   Complete traumatic amputation at level between shoulder and elbow

    ● S48.111   Complete traumatic amputation at level between right shoulder and elbow

    ● S48.112   Complete traumatic amputation at level between left shoulder and elbow

    ● S48.119   Complete traumatic amputation at level between unspecified shoulder and elbow

● S48.12   Partial traumatic amputation at level between shoulder and elbow
  ● S48.121   Partial traumatic amputation at level between right shoulder and elbow
  ● S48.122   Partial traumatic amputation at level between left shoulder and elbow
  ● S48.129   Partial traumatic amputation at level between unspecified shoulder and elbow
● S48.9   Traumatic amputation of shoulder and upper arm, level unspecified
  ● S48.91   Complete traumatic amputation of shoulder and upper arm, level unspecified
    ● S48.911   Complete traumatic amputation of right shoulder and upper arm, level unspecified
    ● S48.912   Complete traumatic amputation of left shoulder and upper arm, level unspecified
    ● S48.919   Complete traumatic amputation of unspecified shoulder and upper arm, level unspecified
  ● S48.92   Partial traumatic amputation of shoulder and upper arm, level unspecified
    ● S48.921   Partial traumatic amputation of right shoulder and upper arm, level unspecified
    ● S48.922   Partial traumatic amputation of left shoulder and upper arm, level unspecified
    ● S48.929   Partial traumatic amputation of unspecified shoulder and upper arm, level unspecified

● S49   Other and unspecified injuries of shoulder and upper arm

The appropriate 7th character is to be added to each code from subcategories S49.0 and S49.1

A	initial encounter for closed fracture
D	subsequent encounter for fracture with routine healing
G	subsequent encounter for fracture with delayed healing
K	subsequent encounter for fracture with nonunion
P	subsequent encounter for fracture with malunion
S	sequela

● S49.0   Physeal fracture of upper end of humerus
  ● S49.00   Unspecified physeal fracture of upper end of humerus
    ● S49.001   Unspecified physeal fracture of upper end of humerus, right arm
    ● S49.002   Unspecified physeal fracture of upper end of humerus, left arm
    ● S49.009   Unspecified physeal fracture of upper end of humerus, unspecified arm
  ● S49.01   Salter-Harris Type I physeal fracture of upper end of humerus
    ● S49.011   Salter-Harris Type I physeal fracture of upper end of humerus, right arm
    ● S49.012   Salter-Harris Type I physeal fracture of upper end of humerus, left arm
    ● S49.019   Salter-Harris Type I physeal fracture of upper end of humerus, unspecified arm

Item 19-3 SALTER-HARRIS TYPE 1: epiphysis is completely separated from end of bone, or metaphysic growth plate remains attached to epiphysis

SALTER-HARRIS TYPE 2: epiphysis and growth plate are partially separated from metaphysis, which is cracked—most common type

SALTER-HARRIS TYPE 3: fracture occurring through epiphysis and separates part of epiphysis and growth plate from metaphysis fracture, usually at distal end of tibia

SALTER-HARRIS TYPE 4: fracture runs through epiphysis, across growth plate, into metaphysic, surgery is required to restore joint surface to normal and align growth plate

● S49.02   Salter-Harris Type II physeal fracture of upper end of humerus
  ● S49.021   Salter-Harris Type II physeal fracture of upper end of humerus, right arm
  ● S49.022   Salter-Harris Type II physeal fracture of upper end of humerus, left arm
  ● S49.029   Salter-Harris Type II physeal fracture of upper end of humerus, unspecified arm
● S49.03   Salter-Harris Type III physeal fracture of upper end of humerus
  ● S49.031   Salter Harris Type III physeal fracture of upper end of humerus, right arm
  ● S49.032   Salter Harris Type III physeal fracture of upper end of humerus, left arm
  ● S49.039   Salter Harris Type III physeal fracture of upper end of humerus, unspecified arm
● S49.04   Salter-Harris Type IV physeal fracture of upper end of humerus
  ● S49.041   Salter-Harris Type IV physeal fracture of upper end of humerus, right arm
  ● S49.042   Salter-Harris Type IV physeal fracture of upper end of humerus, left arm
  ● S49.049   Salter-Harris Type IV physeal fracture of upper end of humerus, unspecified arm
● S49.09   Other physeal fracture of upper end of humerus
  ● S49.091   Other physeal fracture of upper end of humerus, right arm
  ● S49.092   Other physeal fracture of upper end of humerus, left arm
  ● S49.099   Other physeal fracture of upper end of humerus, unspecified arm
● S49.1   Physeal fracture of lower end of humerus
  ● S49.10   Unspecified physeal fracture of lower end of humerus
    ● S49.101   Unspecified physeal fracture of lower end of humerus, right arm
    ● S49.102   Unspecified physeal fracture of lower end of humerus, left arm
    ● S49.109   Unspecified physeal fracture of lower end of humerus, unspecified arm
  ● S49.11   Salter-Harris Type I physeal fracture of lower end of humerus
    ● S49.111   Salter-Harris Type I physeal fracture of lower end of humerus, right arm
    ● S49.112   Salter-Harris Type I physeal fracture of lower end of humerus, left arm
    ● S49.119   Salter-Harris Type I physeal fracture of lower end of humerus, unspecified arm

● **S49.12**   **Salter-Harris Type II physeal fracture of lower end of humerus**
     ● S49.121   Salter-Harris Type II physeal fracture of lower end of humerus, right arm
     ● S49.122   Salter-Harris Type II physeal fracture of lower end of humerus, left arm
     ● S49.129   Salter-Harris Type II physeal fracture of lower end of humerus, unspecified arm

● **S49.13**   **Salter Harris Type III physeal fracture of lower end of humerus**
     ● S49.131   Salter Harris Type III physeal fracture of lower end of humerus, right arm
     ● S49.132   Salter Harris Type III physeal fracture of lower end of humerus, left arm
     ● S49.139   Salter Harris Type III physeal fracture of lower end of humerus, unspecified arm

● **S49.14**   **Salter-Harris Type IV physeal fracture of lower end of humerus**
     ● S49.141   Salter-Harris Type IV physeal fracture of lower end of humerus, right arm
     ● S49.142   Salter-Harris Type IV physeal fracture of lower end of humerus, left arm
     ● S49.149   Salter-Harris Type IV physeal fracture of lower end of humerus, unspecified arm

● **S49.19**   **Other physeal fracture of lower end of humerus**
     ● S49.191   Other physeal fracture of lower end of humerus, right arm
     ● S49.192   Other physeal fracture of lower end of humerus, left arm
     ● S49.199   Other physeal fracture of lower end of humerus, unspecified arm

● **S49.8**   **Other specified injuries of shoulder and upper arm**
The appropriate 7th character is to be added to each code in subcategory S49.8

A	initial encounter
D	subsequent encounter
S	sequela

   X ● **S49.80**   **Other specified injuries of shoulder and upper arm, unspecified arm**
   X ● **S49.81**   **Other specified injuries of right shoulder and upper arm**
   X ● **S49.82**   **Other specified injuries of left shoulder and upper arm**

● **S49.9**   **Unspecified injury of shoulder and upper arm**
The appropriate 7th character is to be added to each code in subcategory S49.9

A	initial encounter
D	subsequent encounter
S	sequela

   X ● **S49.90**   **Unspecified injury of shoulder and upper arm, unspecified arm**
   X ● **S49.91**   **Unspecified injury of right shoulder and upper arm**
   X ● **S49.92**   **Unspecified injury of left shoulder and upper arm**

INJURIES TO THE ELBOW AND FOREARM (S50-S59)

Excludes2	burns and corrosions (T20-T32)
	frostbite (T33-T34)
	injuries of wrist and hand (S60-S69)
	insect bite or sting, venomous (T63.4)

● **S50**   **Superficial injury of elbow and forearm**

Excludes2	superficial injury of wrist and hand (S60.-)

The appropriate 7th character is to be added to each code from category S50

A	initial encounter
D	subsequent encounter
S	sequela

● **S50.0**   **Contusion of elbow**
   X ● S50.00   Contusion of unspecified elbow
   X ● S50.01   Contusion of right elbow
   X ● S50.02   Contusion of left elbow

● **S50.1**   **Contusion of forearm**
   X ● S50.10   Contusion of unspecified forearm
   X ● S50.11   Contusion of right forearm
   X ● S50.12   Contusion of left forearm

● **S50.3**   **Other superficial injuries of elbow**
   ● **S50.31**   **Abrasion of elbow**
     ● S50.311   Abrasion of right elbow
     ● S50.312   Abrasion of left elbow
     ● S50.319   Abrasion of unspecified elbow
   ● **S50.32**   **Blister (nonthermal) of elbow**
     ● S50.321   Blister (nonthermal) of right elbow
     ● S50.322   Blister (nonthermal) of left elbow
     ● S50.329   Blister (nonthermal) of unspecified elbow
   ● **S50.34**   **External constriction of elbow**
     ● S50.341   External constriction of right elbow
     ● S50.342   External constriction of left elbow
     ● S50.349   External constriction of unspecified elbow
   ● **S50.35**   **Superficial foreign body of elbow**
     Splinter in the elbow
     ● S50.351   Superficial foreign body of right elbow
     ● S50.352   Superficial foreign body of left elbow
     ● S50.359   Superficial foreign body of unspecified elbow
   ● **S50.36**   **Insect bite (nonvenomous) of elbow**
     ● S50.361   Insect bite (nonvenomous) of right elbow
     ● S50.362   Insect bite (nonvenomous) of left elbow
     ● S50.369   Insect bite (nonvenomous) of unspecified elbow
   ● **S50.37**   **Other superficial bite of elbow**

Excludes1	open bite of elbow (S51.04)

     ● S50.371   Other superficial bite of right elbow
     ● S50.372   Other superficial bite of left elbow
     ● S50.379   Other superficial bite of unspecified elbow

● **S50.8**   **Other superficial injuries of forearm**
   ● **S50.81**   **Abrasion of forearm**
     ● S50.811   Abrasion of right forearm
     ● S50.812   Abrasion of left forearm
     ● S50.819   Abrasion of unspecified forearm

◄ New   ◄▥ Revised   ~~deleted~~ Deleted   **OGCR** Official Guidelines   X Assign placeholder X   ● Use Additional Character(s)

Excludes 1	Excludes 2	Includes	Use additional	Code first	Code also	Unspecified

- ● S50.82   **Blister (nonthermal) of forearm**
  - ● S50.821   Blister (nonthermal) of right forearm
  - ● S50.822   Blister (nonthermal) of left forearm
  - ● S50.829   Blister (nonthermal) of unspecified forearm
- ● S50.84   **External constriction of forearm**
  - ● S50.841   External constriction of right forearm
  - ● S50.842   External constriction of left forearm
  - ● S50.849   External constriction of unspecified forearm
- ● S50.85   **Superficial foreign body of forearm**
  Splinter in the forearm
  - ● S50.851   Superficial foreign body of right forearm
  - ● S50.852   Superficial foreign body of left forearm
  - ● S50.859   Superficial foreign body of unspecified forearm
- ● S50.86   **Insect bite (nonvenomous) of forearm**
  - ● S50.861   Insect bite (nonvenomous) of right forearm
  - ● S50.862   Insect bite (nonvenomous) of left forearm
  - ● S50.869   Insect bite (nonvenomous) of unspecified forearm
- ● S50.87   **Other superficial bite of forearm**
  | **Excludes1** | open bite of forearm (S51.84) |
  - ● S50.871   Other superficial bite of right forearm
  - ● S50.872   Other superficial bite of left forearm
  - ● S50.879   Other superficial bite of unspecified forearm
- ● S50.9   **Unspecified superficial injury of elbow and forearm**
  - ● S50.90   **Unspecified superficial injury of elbow**
    - ● S50.901   Unspecified superficial injury of right elbow
    - ● S50.902   Unspecified superficial injury of left elbow
    - ● S50.909   Unspecified superficial injury of unspecified elbow
  - ● S50.91   **Unspecified superficial injury of forearm**
    - ● S50.911   Unspecified superficial injury of right forearm
    - ● S50.912   Unspecified superficial injury of left forearm
    - ● S50.919   Unspecified superficial injury of unspecified forearm
- ● S51   **Open wound of elbow and forearm**
  Code also any associated wound infection
Excludes1	open fracture of elbow and forearm (S52.- with open fracture 7th character)
	traumatic amputation of elbow and forearm (S58.-)
Excludes2	open wound of wrist and hand (S61.-)
  The appropriate 7th character is to be added to each code from category S51

A	initial encounter
D	subsequent encounter
S	sequela

  - ● S51.0   **Open wound of elbow**
    - ● S51.00   **Unspecified open wound of elbow**
      - ● S51.001   Unspecified open wound of right elbow
      - ● S51.002   Unspecified open wound of left elbow
      - ● S51.009   Unspecified open wound of unspecified elbow
        Open wound of elbow NOS

- ● S51.01   **Laceration without foreign body of elbow**
  - ● S51.011   Laceration without foreign body of right elbow
  - ● S51.012   Laceration without foreign body of left elbow
  - ● S51.019   Laceration without foreign body of unspecified elbow
- ● S51.02   **Laceration with foreign body of elbow**
  - ● S51.021   Laceration with foreign body of right elbow
  - ● S51.022   Laceration with foreign body of left elbow
  - ● S51.029   Laceration with foreign body of unspecified elbow
- ● S51.03   **Puncture wound without foreign body of elbow**
  - ● S51.031   Puncture wound without foreign body of right elbow
  - ● S51.032   Puncture wound without foreign body of left elbow
  - ● S51.039   Puncture wound without foreign body of unspecified elbow
- ● S51.04   **Puncture wound with foreign body of elbow**
  - ● S51.041   Puncture wound with foreign body of right elbow
  - ● S51.042   Puncture wound with foreign body of left elbow
  - ● S51.049   Puncture wound with foreign body of unspecified elbow
- ● S51.05   **Open bite of elbow**
  Bite of elbow NOS
  | **Excludes1** | superficial bite of elbow (S50.36, S50.37) |
  - ● S51.051   Open bite, right elbow
  - ● S51.052   Open bite, left elbow
  - ● S51.059   Open bite, unspecified elbow
- ● S51.8   **Open wound of forearm**
  | **Excludes2** | open wound of elbow (S51.0-) |
  - ● S51.80   **Unspecified open wound of forearm**
    - ● S51.801   Unspecified open wound of right forearm
    - ● S51.802   Unspecified open wound of left forearm
    - ● S51.809   Unspecified open wound of unspecified forearm
      Open wound of forearm NOS
  - ● S51.81   **Laceration without foreign body of forearm**
    - ● S51.811   Laceration without foreign body of right forearm
    - ● S51.812   Laceration without foreign body of left forearm
    - ● S51.819   Laceration without foreign body of unspecified forearm
  - ● S51.82   **Laceration with foreign body of forearm**
    - ● S51.821   Laceration with foreign body of right forearm
    - ● S51.822   Laceration with foreign body of left forearm
    - ● S51.829   Laceration with foreign body of unspecified forearm
  - ● S51.83   **Puncture wound without foreign body of forearm**
    - ● S51.831   Puncture wound without foreign body of right forearm
    - ● S51.832   Puncture wound without foreign body of left forearm
    - ● S51.839   Puncture wound without foreign body of unspecified forearm

● **S51.84   Puncture wound with foreign body of forearm**
    ● **S51.841   Puncture wound with foreign body of right forearm**
    ● **S51.842   Puncture wound with foreign body of left forearm**
    ● **S51.849   Puncture wound with foreign body of unspecified forearm**
● **S51.85   Open bite of forearm**
    Bite of forearm NOS
    | Excludes1 | superficial bite of forearm (S50.86, S50.87)
    ● **S51.851   Open bite of right forearm**
    ● **S51.852   Open bite of left forearm**
    ● **S51.859   Open bite of unspecified forearm**

● **S52   Fracture of forearm**
    Note: A fracture not identified as displaced or nondisplaced should be coded to displaced
    A fracture not designated as open or closed should be coded to closed
    The open fracture designations are based on the Gustilo open fracture classification
    | Excludes1 | traumatic amputation of forearm (S58.-)
    | Excludes2 | fracture at wrist and hand level (S62.-)
    The appropriate 7th character is to be added to all codes from category S52

A	initial encounter for closed fracture
B	initial encounter for open fracture type I or II
	initial encounter for open fracture NOS
C	initial encounter for open fracture type IIIA, IIIB, or IIIC
D	subsequent encounter for closed fracture with routine healing
E	subsequent encounter for open fracture type I or II with routine healing
F	subsequent encounter for open fracture type IIIA, IIIB, or IIIC with routine healing
G	subsequent encounter for closed fracture with delayed healing
H	subsequent encounter for open fracture type I or II with delayed healing
J	subsequent encounter for open fracture type IIIA, IIIB, or IIIC with delayed healing
K	subsequent encounter for closed fracture with nonunion
M	subsequent encounter for open fracture type I or II with nonunion
N	subsequent encounter for open fracture type IIIA, IIIB, or IIIC with nonunion
P	subsequent encounter for closed fracture with malunion
Q	subsequent encounter for open fracture type I or II with malunion
R	subsequent encounter for open fracture type IIIA, IIIB, or IIIC with malunion
S	sequela

● **S52.0   Fracture of upper end of ulna**
    Fracture of proximal end of ulna
    | Excludes2 | fracture of elbow NOS (S42.40-)
               fractures of shaft of ulna (S52.2-)
   ● **S52.00   Unspecified fracture of upper end of ulna**
     ● **S52.001   Unspecified fracture of upper end of right ulna**
     ● **S52.002   Unspecified fracture of upper end of left ulna**
     ● **S52.009   Unspecified fracture of upper end of unspecified ulna**

● **S52.01   Torus fracture of upper end of ulna**
    The appropriate 7th character is to be added to all codes in subcategory S52.01

A	initial encounter for closed fracture
D	subsequent encounter for fracture with routine healing
G	subsequent encounter for fracture with delayed healing
K	subsequent encounter for fracture with nonunion
P	subsequent encounter for fracture with malunion
S	sequela

   ● **S52.011   Torus fracture of upper end of right ulna**
   ● **S52.012   Torus fracture of upper end of left ulna**
   ● **S52.019   Torus fracture of upper end of unspecified ulna**
● **S52.02   Fracture of olecranon process without intraarticular extension of ulna**
   ● **S52.021   Displaced fracture of olecranon process without intraarticular extension of right ulna**
   ● **S52.022   Displaced fracture of olecranon process without intraarticular extension of left ulna**
   ● **S52.023   Displaced fracture of olecranon process without intraarticular extension of unspecified ulna**
   ● **S52.024   Nondisplaced fracture of olecranon process without intraarticular extension of right ulna**
   ● **S52.025   Nondisplaced fracture of olecranon process without intraarticular extension of left ulna**
   ● **S52.026   Nondisplaced fracture of olecranon process without intraarticular extension of unspecified ulna**
● **S52.03   Fracture of olecranon process with intraarticular extension of ulna**
   ● **S52.031   Displaced fracture of olecranon process with intraarticular extension of right ulna**
   ● **S52.032   Displaced fracture of olecranon process with intraarticular extension of left ulna**
   ● **S52.033   Displaced fracture of olecranon process with intraarticular extension of unspecified ulna**
   ● **S52.034   Nondisplaced fracture of olecranon process with intraarticular extension of right ulna**
   ● **S52.035   Nondisplaced fracture of olecranon process with intraarticular extension of left ulna**
   ● **S52.036   Nondisplaced fracture of olecranon process with intraarticular extension of unspecified ulna**
● **S52.04   Fracture of coronoid process of ulna**
   ● **S52.041   Displaced fracture of coronoid process of right ulna**
   ● **S52.042   Displaced fracture of coronoid process of left ulna**
   ● **S52.043   Displaced fracture of coronoid process of unspecified ulna**
   ● **S52.044   Nondisplaced fracture of coronoid process of right ulna**
   ● **S52.045   Nondisplaced fracture of coronoid process of left ulna**
   ● **S52.046   Nondisplaced fracture of coronoid process of unspecified ulna**

- S52.09   Other fracture of upper end of ulna
  - S52.091   Other fracture of upper end of right ulna
  - S52.092   Other fracture of upper end of left ulna
  - S52.099   Other fracture of upper end of unspecified ulna
- S52.1   Fracture of upper end of radius
  Fracture of proximal end of radius
  Excludes2   physeal fractures of upper end of radius (S59.2-)
  fracture of shaft of radius (S52.3-)
  - S52.10   Unspecified fracture of upper end of radius
    - S52.101   Unspecified fracture of upper end of right radius
    - S52.102   Unspecified fracture of upper end of left radius
    - S52.109   Unspecified fracture of upper end of unspecified radius
  - S52.11   Torus fracture of upper end of radius
    The appropriate 7th character is to be added to all codes in subcategory S52.11

A	initial encounter for closed fracture
D	subsequent encounter for fracture with routine healing
G	subsequent encounter for fracture with delayed healing
K	subsequent encounter for fracture with nonunion
P	subsequent encounter for fracture with malunion
S	sequela

    - S52.111   Torus fracture of upper end of right radius
    - S52.112   Torus fracture of upper end of left radius
    - S52.119   Torus fracture of upper end of unspecified radius
  - S52.12   Fracture of head of radius
    - S52.121   Displaced fracture of head of right radius
    - S52.122   Displaced fracture of head of left radius
    - S52.123   Displaced fracture of head of unspecified radius
    - S52.124   Nondisplaced fracture of head of right radius
    - S52.125   Nondisplaced fracture of head of left radius
    - S52.126   Nondisplaced fracture of head of unspecified radius
  - S52.13   Fracture of neck of radius
    - S52.131   Displaced fracture of neck of right radius
    - S52.132   Displaced fracture of neck of left radius
    - S52.133   Displaced fracture of neck of unspecified radius
    - S52.134   Nondisplaced fracture of neck of right radius
    - S52.135   Nondisplaced fracture of neck of left radius
    - S52.136   Nondisplaced fracture of neck of unspecified radius

- S52.18   Other fracture of upper end of radius
  - S52.181   Other fracture of upper end of right radius
  - S52.182   Other fracture of upper end of left radius
  - S52.189   Other fracture of upper end of unspecified radius
- S52.2   Fracture of shaft of ulna
  - S52.20   Unspecified fracture of shaft of ulna
    Fracture of ulna NOS
    - S52.201   Unspecified fracture of shaft of right ulna
    - S52.202   Unspecified fracture of shaft of left ulna
    - S52.209   Unspecified fracture of shaft of unspecified ulna
  - S52.21   Greenstick fracture of shaft of ulna
    The appropriate 7th character is to be added to all codes in subcategory S52.21

A	initial encounter for closed fracture
D	subsequent encounter for fracture with routine healing
G	subsequent encounter for fracture with delayed healing
K	subsequent encounter for fracture with nonunion
P	subsequent encounter for fracture with malunion
S	sequela

    - S52.211   Greenstick fracture of shaft of right ulna
    - S52.212   Greenstick fracture of shaft of left ulna
    - S52.219   Greenstick fracture of shaft of unspecified ulna
  - S52.22   Transverse fracture of shaft of ulna
    - S52.221   Displaced transverse fracture of shaft of right ulna
    - S52.222   Displaced transverse fracture of shaft of left ulna
    - S52.223   Displaced transverse fracture of shaft of unspecified ulna
    - S52.224   Nondisplaced transverse fracture of shaft of right ulna
    - S52.225   Nondisplaced transverse fracture of shaft of left ulna
    - S52.226   Nondisplaced transverse fracture of shaft of unspecified ulna
  - S52.23   Oblique fracture of shaft of ulna
    - S52.231   Displaced oblique fracture of shaft of right ulna
    - S52.232   Displaced oblique fracture of shaft of left ulna
    - S52.233   Displaced oblique fracture of shaft of unspecified ulna
    - S52.234   Nondisplaced oblique fracture of shaft of right ulna
    - S52.235   Nondisplaced oblique fracture of shaft of left ulna
    - S52.236   Nondisplaced oblique fracture of shaft of unspecified ulna

CHAPTER 19 (S00–T88)

● S52.24   Spiral fracture of shaft of ulna
   ● S52.241   Displaced spiral fracture of shaft of ulna, right arm
   ● S52.242   Displaced spiral fracture of shaft of ulna, left arm
   ● S52.243   Displaced spiral fracture of shaft of ulna, unspecified arm
   ● S52.244   Nondisplaced spiral fracture of shaft of ulna, right arm
   ● S52.245   Nondisplaced spiral fracture of shaft of ulna, left arm
   ● S52.246   Nondisplaced spiral fracture of shaft of ulna, unspecified arm
● S52.25   Comminuted fracture of shaft of ulna
   ● S52.251   Displaced comminuted fracture of shaft of ulna, right arm
   ● S52.252   Displaced comminuted fracture of shaft of ulna, left arm
   ● S52.253   Displaced comminuted fracture of shaft of ulna, unspecified arm
   ● S52.254   Nondisplaced comminuted fracture of shaft of ulna, right arm
   ● S52.255   Nondisplaced comminuted fracture of shaft of ulna, left arm
   ● S52.256   Nondisplaced comminuted fracture of shaft of ulna, unspecified arm
● S52.26   Segmental fracture of shaft of ulna
   ● S52.261   Displaced segmental fracture of shaft of ulna, right arm
   ● S52.262   Displaced segmental fracture of shaft of ulna, left arm
   ● S52.263   Displaced segmental fracture of shaft of ulna, unspecified arm
   ● S52.264   Nondisplaced segmental fracture of shaft of ulna, right arm
   ● S52.265   Nondisplaced segmental fracture of shaft of ulna, left arm
   ● S52.266   Nondisplaced segmental fracture of shaft of ulna, unspecified arm
● S52.27   Monteggia's fracture of ulna
            Fracture of upper shaft of ulna with dislocation of radial head
   ● S52.271   Monteggia's fracture of right ulna
   ● S52.272   Monteggia's fracture of left ulna
   ● S52.279   Monteggia's fracture of unspecified ulna
● S52.28   Bent bone of ulna
   ● S52.281   Bent bone of right ulna
   ● S52.282   Bent bone of left ulna
   ● S52.283   Bent bone of unspecified ulna
● S52.29   Other fracture of shaft of ulna
   ● S52.291   Other fracture of shaft of right ulna
   ● S52.292   Other fracture of shaft of left ulna
   ● S52.299   Other fracture of shaft of unspecified ulna
● S52.3   Fracture of shaft of radius
   ● S52.30   Unspecified fracture of shaft of radius
      ● S52.301   Unspecified fracture of shaft of right radius
      ● S52.302   Unspecified fracture of shaft of left radius
      ● S52.309   Unspecified fracture of shaft of unspecified radius

● S52.31   Greenstick fracture of shaft of radius
            The appropriate 7th character is to be added to all codes in subcategory S52.31

┌───┐
│ A   initial encounter for closed fracture   │
│ D   subsequent encounter for fracture with   │
│   routine healing   │
│ G   subsequent encounter for fracture with   │
│   delayed healing   │
│ K   subsequent encounter for fracture with   │
│   nonunion   │
│ P   subsequent encounter for fracture with   │
│   malunion   │
│ S   sequela   │
└───┘

   ● S52.311   Greenstick fracture of shaft of radius, right arm
   ● S52.312   Greenstick fracture of shaft of radius, left arm
   ● S52.319   Greenstick fracture of shaft of radius, unspecified arm
● S52.32   Transverse fracture of shaft of radius
   ● S52.321   Displaced transverse fracture of shaft of right radius
   ● S52.322   Displaced transverse fracture of shaft of left radius
   ● S52.323   Displaced transverse fracture of shaft of unspecified radius
   ● S52.324   Nondisplaced transverse fracture of shaft of right radius
   ● S52.325   Nondisplaced transverse fracture of shaft of left radius
   ● S52.326   Nondisplaced transverse fracture of shaft of unspecified radius
● S52.33   Oblique fracture of shaft of radius
   ● S52.331   Displaced oblique fracture of shaft of right radius
   ● S52.332   Displaced oblique fracture of shaft of left radius
   ● S52.333   Displaced oblique fracture of shaft of unspecified radius
   ● S52.334   Nondisplaced oblique fracture of shaft of right radius
   ● S52.335   Nondisplaced oblique fracture of shaft of left radius
   ● S52.336   Nondisplaced oblique fracture of shaft of unspecified radius
● S52.34   Spiral fracture of shaft of radius
   ● S52.341   Displaced spiral fracture of shaft of radius, right arm
   ● S52.342   Displaced spiral fracture of shaft of radius, left arm
   ● S52.343   Displaced spiral fracture of shaft of radius, unspecified arm
   ● S52.344   Nondisplaced spiral fracture of shaft of radius, right arm
   ● S52.345   Nondisplaced spiral fracture of shaft of radius, left arm
   ● S52.346   Nondisplaced spiral fracture of shaft of radius, unspecified arm

●S52.35   Comminuted fracture of shaft of radius
   ●S52.351   Displaced comminuted fracture of shaft of radius, right arm
   ●S52.352   Displaced comminuted fracture of shaft of radius, left arm
   ●S52.353   Displaced comminuted fracture of shaft of radius, unspecified arm
   ●S52.354   Nondisplaced comminuted fracture of shaft of radius, right arm
   ●S52.355   Nondisplaced comminuted fracture of shaft of radius, left arm
   ●S52.356   Nondisplaced comminuted fracture of shaft of radius, unspecified arm

●S52.36   Segmental fracture of shaft of radius
   ●S52.361   Displaced segmental fracture of shaft of radius, right arm
   ●S52.362   Displaced segmental fracture of shaft of radius, left arm
   ●S52.363   Displaced segmental fracture of shaft of radius, unspecified arm
   ●S52.364   Nondisplaced segmental fracture of shaft of radius, right arm
   ●S52.365   Nondisplaced segmental fracture of shaft of radius, left arm
   ●S52.366   Nondisplaced segmental fracture of shaft of radius, unspecified arm

●S52.37   Galeazzi's fracture
      Fracture of lower shaft of radius with radioulnar joint dislocation
   ●S52.371   Galeazzi's fracture of right radius
   ●S52.372   Galeazzi's fracture of left radius
   ●S52.379   Galeazzi's fracture of unspecified radius

●S52.38   Bent bone of radius
   ●S52.381   Bent bone of right radius
   ●S52.382   Bent bone of left radius
   ●S52.389   Bent bone of unspecified radius

●S52.39   Other fracture of shaft of radius
   ●S52.391   Other fracture of shaft of radius, right arm
   ●S52.392   Other fracture of shaft of radius, left arm
   ●S52.399   Other fracture of shaft of radius, unspecified arm

●S52.5   Fracture of lower end of radius
      Fracture of distal end of radius
    Excludes2   physeal fractures of lower end of radius (S59.2-)

●S52.50   Unspecified fracture of the lower end of radius
   ●S52.501   Unspecified fracture of the lower end of right radius
   ●S52.502   Unspecified fracture of the lower end of left radius
   ●S52.509   Unspecified fracture of the lower end of unspecified radius

●S52.51   Fracture of radial styloid process
   ●S52.511   Displaced fracture of right radial styloid process
   ●S52.512   Displaced fracture of left radial styloid process
   ●S52.513   Displaced fracture of unspecified radial styloid process
   ●S52.514   Nondisplaced fracture of right radial styloid process
   ●S52.515   Nondisplaced fracture of left radial styloid process
   ●S52.516   Nondisplaced fracture of unspecified radial styloid process

●S52.52   Torus fracture of lower end of radius
      The appropriate 7th character is to be added to all codes in subcategory S52.52

A	initial encounter for closed fracture
D	subsequent encounter for fracture with routine healing
G	subsequent encounter for fracture with delayed healing
K	subsequent encounter for fracture with nonunion
P	subsequent encounter for fracture with malunion
S	sequela

   ●S52.521   Torus fracture of lower end of right radius
   ●S52.522   Torus fracture of lower end of left radius
   ●S52.529   Torus fracture of lower end of unspecified radius

●S52.53   Colles' fracture
   ●S52.531   Colles' fracture of right radius
   ●S52.532   Colles' fracture of left radius
   ●S52.539   Colles' fracture of unspecified radius

●S52.54   Smith's fracture
   ●S52.541   Smith's fracture of right radius
   ●S52.542   Smith's fracture of left radius
   ●S52.549   Smith's fracture of unspecified radius

●S52.55   Other extraarticular fracture of lower end of radius
   ●S52.551   Other extraarticular fracture of lower end of right radius
   ●S52.552   Other extraarticular fracture of lower end of left radius
   ●S52.559   Other extraarticular fracture of lower end of unspecified radius

●S52.56   Barton's fracture
   ●S52.561   Barton's fracture of right radius
   ●S52.562   Barton's fracture of left radius
   ●S52.569   Barton's fracture of unspecified radius

●S52.57   Other intraarticular fracture of lower end of radius
   ●S52.571   Other intraarticular fracture of lower end of right radius
   ●S52.572   Other intraarticular fracture of lower end of left radius
   ●S52.579   Other intraarticular fracture of lower end of unspecified radius

●S52.59   Other fractures of lower end of radius
   ●S52.591   Other fractures of lower end of right radius
   ●S52.592   Other fractures of lower end of left radius
   ●S52.599   Other fractures of lower end of unspecified radius

●S52.6   Fracture of lower end of ulna
●S52.60   Unspecified fracture of lower end of ulna
   ●S52.601   Unspecified fracture of lower end of right ulna
   ●S52.602   Unspecified fracture of lower end of left ulna
   ●S52.609   Unspecified fracture of lower end of unspecified ulna

●S52.61   Fracture of ulna styloid process
   ●S52.611   Displaced fracture of right ulna styloid process
   ●S52.612   Displaced fracture of left ulna styloid process

CHAPTER 19 (S00-T88)

● S52.613　Displaced fracture of unspecified ulna styloid process

● S52.614　Nondisplaced fracture of right ulna styloid process

● S52.615　Nondisplaced fracture of left ulna styloid process

● S52.616　Nondisplaced fracture of unspecified ulna styloid process

● S52.62　Torus fracture of lower end of ulna

The appropriate 7th character is to be added to all codes in subcategory S52.62

> A　initial encounter for closed fracture
> D　subsequent encounter for fracture with routine healing
> G　subsequent encounter for fracture with delayed healing
> K　subsequent encounter for fracture with nonunion
> P　subsequent encounter for fracture with malunion
> S　sequela

● S52.621　Torus fracture of lower end of right ulna

● S52.622　Torus fracture of lower end of left ulna

● S52.629　Torus fracture of lower end of unspecified ulna

● S52.69　Other fracture of lower end of ulna

● S52.691　Other fracture of lower end of right ulna

● S52.692　Other fracture of lower end of left ulna

● S52.699　Other fracture of lower end of unspecified ulna

● S52.9　Unspecified fracture of forearm

X ● S52.90　Unspecified fracture of unspecified forearm

X ● S52.91　Unspecified fracture of right forearm

X ● S52.92　Unspecified fracture of left forearm

● S53　Dislocation and sprain of joints and ligaments of elbow

Includes　avulsion of joint or ligament of elbow
laceration of cartilage, joint or ligament of elbow
sprain of cartilage, joint or ligament of elbow
traumatic hemarthrosis of joint or ligament of elbow
traumatic rupture of joint or ligament of elbow
traumatic subluxation of joint or ligament of elbow
traumatic tear of joint or ligament of elbow

Code also any associated open wound

Excludes2　strain of muscle, fascia and tendon at forearm level (S56.-)

The appropriate 7th character is to be added to each code from category S53

> A　initial encounter
> D　subsequent encounter
> S　sequela

● S53.0　Subluxation and dislocation of radial head
Dislocation of radiohumeral joint
Subluxation of radiohumeral joint

Excludes1　Monteggia's fracture-dislocation (S52.27-)

● S53.00　Unspecified subluxation and dislocation of radial head

● S53.001　Unspecified subluxation of right radial head

● S53.002　Unspecified subluxation of left radial head

● S53.003　Unspecified subluxation of unspecified radial head

● S53.004　Unspecified dislocation of right radial head

● S53.005　Unspecified dislocation of left radial head

● S53.006　Unspecified dislocation of unspecified radial head

● S53.01　Anterior subluxation and dislocation of radial head
Anteriomedial subluxation and dislocation of radial head

● S53.011　Anterior subluxation of right radial head

● S53.012　Anterior subluxation of left radial head

● S53.013　Anterior subluxation of unspecified radial head

● S53.014　Anterior dislocation of right radial head

● S53.015　Anterior dislocation of left radial head

● S53.016　Anterior dislocation of unspecified radial head

● S53.02　Posterior subluxation and dislocation of radial head
Posteriolateral subluxation and dislocation of radial head

● S53.021　Posterior subluxation of right radial head

● S53.022　Posterior subluxation of left radial head

● S53.023　Posterior subluxation of unspecified radial head

● S53.024　Posterior dislocation of right radial head

● S53.025　Posterior dislocation of left radial head

● S53.026　Posterior dislocation of unspecified radial head

● S53.03　Nursemaid's elbow

● S53.031　Nursemaid's elbow, right elbow

● S53.032　Nursemaid's elbow, left elbow

● S53.033　Nursemaid's elbow, unspecified elbow

● S53.09　Other subluxation and dislocation of radial head

● S53.091　Other subluxation of right radial head

● S53.092　Other subluxation of left radial head

● S53.093　Other subluxation of unspecified radial head

● S53.094　Other dislocation of right radial head

● S53.095　Other dislocation of left radial head

● S53.096　Other dislocation of unspecified radial head

● S53.1　Subluxation and dislocation of ulnohumeral joint
Subluxation and dislocation of elbow NOS

Excludes1　dislocation of radial head alone (S53.0-)

● S53.10　Unspecified subluxation and dislocation of ulnohumeral joint

● S53.101　Unspecified subluxation of right ulnohumeral joint

● S53.102　Unspecified subluxation of left ulnohumeral joint

● S53.103　Unspecified subluxation of unspecified ulnohumeral joint

● S53.104　Unspecified dislocation of right ulnohumeral joint

● S53.105　Unspecified dislocation of left ulnohumeral joint

● S53.106　Unspecified dislocation of unspecified ulnohumeral joint

- ● S53.11 Anterior subluxation and dislocation of ulnohumeral joint
  - ● S53.111 Anterior subluxation of right ulnohumeral joint
  - ● S53.112 Anterior subluxation of left ulnohumeral joint
  - ● S53.113 Anterior subluxation of unspecified ulnohumeral joint
  - ● S53.114 Anterior dislocation of right ulnohumeral joint
  - ● S53.115 Anterior dislocation of left ulnohumeral joint
  - ● S53.116 Anterior dislocation of unspecified ulnohumeral joint
- ● S53.12 Posterior subluxation and dislocation of ulnohumeral joint
  - ● S53.121 Posterior subluxation of right ulnohumeral joint
  - ● S53.122 Posterior subluxation of left ulnohumeral joint
  - ● S53.123 Posterior subluxation of unspecified ulnohumeral joint
  - ● S53.124 Posterior dislocation of right ulnohumeral joint
  - ● S53.125 Posterior dislocation of left ulnohumeral joint
  - ● S53.126 Posterior dislocation of unspecified ulnohumeral joint
- ● S53.13 Medial subluxation and dislocation of ulnohumeral joint
  - ● S53.131 Medial subluxation of right ulnohumeral joint
  - ● S53.132 Medial subluxation of left ulnohumeral joint
  - ● S53.133 Medial subluxation of unspecified ulnohumeral joint
  - ● S53.134 Medial dislocation of right ulnohumeral joint
  - ● S53.135 Medial dislocation of left ulnohumeral joint
  - ● S53.136 Medial dislocation of unspecified ulnohumeral joint
- ● S53.14 Lateral subluxation and dislocation of ulnohumeral joint
  - ● S53.141 Lateral subluxation of right ulnohumeral joint
  - ● S53.142 Lateral subluxation of left ulnohumeral joint
  - ● S53.143 Lateral subluxation of unspecified ulnohumeral joint
  - ● S53.144 Lateral dislocation of right ulnohumeral joint
  - ● S53.145 Lateral dislocation of left ulnohumeral joint
  - ● S53.146 Lateral dislocation of unspecified ulnohumeral joint
- ● S53.19 Other subluxation and dislocation of ulnohumeral joint
  - ● S53.191 Other subluxation of right ulnohumeral joint
  - ● S53.192 Other subluxation of left ulnohumeral joint

- ● S53.193 Other subluxation of unspecified ulnohumeral joint
- ● S53.194 Other dislocation of right ulnohumeral joint
- ● S53.195 Other dislocation of left ulnohumeral joint
- ● S53.196 Other dislocation of unspecified ulnohumeral joint
- ● S53.2 Traumatic rupture of radial collateral ligament
  - Excludes1 sprain of radial collateral ligament NOS (S53.43-)
  - X ● S53.20 Traumatic rupture of unspecified radial collateral ligament
  - X ● S53.21 Traumatic rupture of right radial collateral ligament
  - X ● S53.22 Traumatic rupture of left radial collateral ligament
- ● S53.3 Traumatic rupture of ulnar collateral ligament
  - Excludes1 sprain of ulnar collateral ligament (S53.44-)
  - X ● S53.30 Traumatic rupture of unspecified ulnar collateral ligament
  - X ● S53.31 Traumatic rupture of right ulnar collateral ligament
  - X ● S53.32 Traumatic rupture of left ulnar collateral ligament
- ● S53.4 Sprain of elbow
  - Excludes2 traumatic rupture of radial collateral ligament (S53.2-)
    traumatic rupture of ulnar collateral ligament (S53.3-)
  - ● S53.40 Unspecified sprain of elbow
    - ● S53.401 Unspecified sprain of right elbow
    - ● S53.402 Unspecified sprain of left elbow
    - ● S53.409 Unspecified sprain of unspecified elbow
      Sprain of elbow NOS
  - ● S53.41 Radiohumeral (joint) sprain
    - ● S53.411 Radiohumeral (joint) sprain of right elbow
    - ● S53.412 Radiohumeral (joint) sprain of left elbow
    - ● S53.419 Radiohumeral (joint) sprain of unspecified elbow
  - ● S53.42 Ulnohumeral (joint) sprain
    - ● S53.421 Ulnohumeral (joint) sprain of right elbow
    - ● S53.422 Ulnohumeral (joint) sprain of left elbow
    - ● S53.429 Ulnohumeral (joint) sprain of unspecified elbow
  - ● S53.43 Radial collateral ligament sprain
    - ● S53.431 Radial collateral ligament sprain of right elbow
    - ● S53.432 Radial collateral ligament sprain of left elbow
    - ● S53.439 Radial collateral ligament sprain of unspecified elbow
  - ● S53.44 Ulnar collateral ligament sprain
    - ● S53.441 Ulnar collateral ligament sprain of right elbow
    - ● S53.442 Ulnar collateral ligament sprain of left elbow
    - ● S53.449 Ulnar collateral ligament sprain of unspecified elbow

CHAPTER 19 (S00-T88)

● S53.49   Other sprain of elbow
    ● S53.491   Other sprain of right elbow
    ● S53.492   Other sprain of left elbow
    ● S53.499   Other sprain of unspecified elbow

● S54   Injury of nerves at forearm level
    Code also any associated open wound (S51.-)
    Excludes2   injury of nerves at wrist and hand level (S64.-)
    The appropriate 7th character is to be added to each code from category S54

A	initial encounter
D	subsequent encounter
S	sequela

  ● S54.0   Injury of ulnar nerve at forearm level
      Injury of ulnar nerve NOS
    X ● S54.00   Injury of ulnar nerve at forearm level, unspecified arm
    X ● S54.01   Injury of ulnar nerve at forearm level, right arm
    X ● S54.02   Injury of ulnar nerve at forearm level, left arm

  ● S54.1   Injury of median nerve at forearm level
      Injury of median nerve NOS
    X ● S54.10   Injury of median nerve at forearm level, unspecified arm
    X ● S54.11   Injury of median nerve at forearm level, right arm
    X ● S54.12   Injury of median nerve at forearm level, left arm

  ● S54.2   Injury of radial nerve at forearm level
      Injury of radial nerve NOS
    X ● S54.20   Injury of radial nerve at forearm level, unspecified arm
    X ● S54.21   Injury of radial nerve at forearm level, right arm
    X ● S54.22   Injury of radial nerve at forearm level, left arm

  ● S54.3   Injury of cutaneous sensory nerve at forearm level
    X ● S54.30   Injury of cutaneous sensory nerve at forearm level, unspecified arm
    X ● S54.31   Injury of cutaneous sensory nerve at forearm level, right arm
    X ● S54.32   Injury of cutaneous sensory nerve at forearm level, left arm

  ● S54.8   Injury of other nerves at forearm level
    ● S54.8X   Unspecified injury of other nerves at forearm level
      ● S54.8X1   Unspecified injury of other nerves at forearm level, right arm
      ● S54.8X2   Unspecified injury of other nerves at forearm level, left arm
      ● S54.8X9   Unspecified injury of other nerves at forearm level, unspecified arm

  ● S54.9   Injury of unspecified nerve at forearm level
    X ● S54.90   Injury of unspecified nerve at forearm level, unspecified arm
    X ● S54.91   Injury of unspecified nerve at forearm level, right arm
    X ● S54.92   Injury of unspecified nerve at forearm level, left arm

● S55   Injury of blood vessels at forearm level
    Code also any associated open wound (S51.-)
    Excludes2   injury of blood vessels at wrist and hand level (S65.-)
          injury of brachial vessels (S45.1-S45.2)
    The appropriate 7th character is to be added to each code from category S55

A	initial encounter
D	subsequent encounter
S	sequela

  ● S55.0   Injury of ulnar artery at forearm level
    ● S55.00   Unspecified injury of ulnar artery at forearm level
      ● S55.001   Unspecified injury of ulnar artery at forearm level, right arm
      ● S55.002   Unspecified injury of ulnar artery at forearm level, left arm
      ● S55.009   Unspecified injury of ulnar artery at forearm level, unspecified arm

    ● S55.01   Laceration of ulnar artery at forearm level
      ● S55.011   Laceration of ulnar artery at forearm level, right arm
      ● S55.012   Laceration of ulnar artery at forearm level, left arm
      ● S55.019   Laceration of ulnar artery at forearm level, unspecified arm

    ● S55.09   Other specified injury of ulnar artery at forearm level
      ● S55.091   Other specified injury of ulnar artery at forearm level, right arm
      ● S55.092   Other specified injury of ulnar artery at forearm level, left arm
      ● S55.099   Other specified injury of ulnar artery at forearm level, unspecified arm

  ● S55.1   Injury of radial artery at forearm level
    ● S55.10   Unspecified injury of radial artery at forearm level
      ● S55.101   Unspecified injury of radial artery at forearm level, right arm
      ● S55.102   Unspecified injury of radial artery at forearm level, left arm
      ● S55.109   Unspecified injury of radial artery at forearm level, unspecified arm

    ● S55.11   Laceration of radial artery at forearm level
      ● S55.111   Laceration of radial artery at forearm level, right arm
      ● S55.112   Laceration of radial artery at forearm level, left arm
      ● S55.119   Laceration of radial artery at forearm level, unspecified arm

    ● S55.19   Other specified injury of radial artery at forearm level
      ● S55.191   Other specified injury of radial artery at forearm level, right arm
      ● S55.192   Other specified injury of radial artery at forearm level, left arm
      ● S55.199   Other specified injury of radial artery at forearm level, unspecified arm

  ● S55.2   Injury of vein at forearm level
    ● S55.20   Unspecified injury of vein at forearm level
      ● S55.201   Unspecified injury of vein at forearm level, right arm
      ● S55.202   Unspecified injury of vein at forearm level, left arm
      ● S55.209   Unspecified injury of vein at forearm level, unspecified arm

◀ New   ◀▥ Revised   ~~deleted~~ Deleted   OGCR Official Guidelines   X Assign placeholder X   ● Use Additional Character(s)

Excludes 1   Excludes 2   Includes   Use additional   Code first   Code also   Unspecified

● S55.21   Laceration of vein at forearm level
    ● S55.211   Laceration of vein at forearm level, right arm
    ● S55.212   Laceration of vein at forearm level, left arm
    ● S55.219   Laceration of vein at forearm level, unspecified arm

● S55.29   Other specified injury of vein at forearm level
    ● S55.291   Other specified injury of vein at forearm level, right arm
    ● S55.292   Other specified injury of vein at forearm level, left arm
    ● S55.299   Other specified injury of vein at forearm level, unspecified arm

● S55.8   Injury of other blood vessels at forearm level
    ● S55.80   Unspecified injury of other blood vessels at forearm level
      ● S55.801   Unspecified injury of other blood vessels at forearm level, right arm
      ● S55.802   Unspecified injury of other blood vessels at forearm level, left arm
      ● S55.809   Unspecified injury of other blood vessels at forearm level, unspecified arm

    ● S55.81   Laceration of other blood vessels at forearm level
      ● S55.811   Laceration of other blood vessels at forearm level, right arm
      ● S55.812   Laceration of other blood vessels at forearm level, left arm
      ● S55.819   Laceration of other blood vessels at forearm level, unspecified arm

    ● S55.89   Other specified injury of other blood vessels at forearm level
      ● S55.891   Other specified injury of other blood vessels at forearm level, right arm
      ● S55.892   Other specified injury of other blood vessels at forearm level, left arm
      ● S55.899   Other specified injury of other blood vessels at forearm level, unspecified arm

● S55.9   Injury of unspecified blood vessel at forearm level
    ● S55.90   Unspecified injury of unspecified blood vessel at forearm level
      ● S55.901   Unspecified injury of unspecified blood vessel at forearm level, right arm
      ● S55.902   Unspecified injury of unspecified blood vessel at forearm level, left arm
      ● S55.909   Unspecified injury of unspecified blood vessel at forearm level, unspecified arm

    ● S55.91   Laceration of unspecified blood vessel at forearm level
      ● S55.911   Laceration of unspecified blood vessel at forearm level, right arm
      ● S55.912   Laceration of unspecified blood vessel at forearm level, left arm
      ● S55.919   Laceration of unspecified blood vessel at forearm level, unspecified arm

    ● S55.99   Other specified injury of unspecified blood vessel at forearm level
      ● S55.991   Other specified injury of unspecified blood vessel at forearm level, right arm
      ● S55.992   Other specified injury of unspecified blood vessel at forearm level, left arm
      ● S55.999   Other specified injury of unspecified blood vessel at forearm level, unspecified arm

● S56   Injury of muscle, fascia and tendon at forearm level

    Code also any associated open wound (S51.-)

    Excludes2   injury of muscle, fascia and tendon at or below wrist (S66.-)
              sprain of joints and ligaments of elbow (S53.4-)

    The appropriate 7th character is to be added to each code from category S56

A	initial encounter
D	subsequent encounter
S	sequela

● S56.0   Injury of flexor muscle, fascia and tendon of thumb at forearm level
    ● S56.00   Unspecified injury of flexor muscle, fascia and tendon of thumb at forearm level
      ● S56.001   Unspecified injury of flexor muscle, fascia and tendon of right thumb at forearm level
      ● S56.002   Unspecified injury of flexor muscle, fascia and tendon of left thumb at forearm level
      ● S56.009   Unspecified injury of flexor muscle, fascia and tendon of unspecified thumb at forearm level

    ● S56.01   Strain of flexor muscle, fascia and tendon of thumb at forearm level
      ● S56.011   Strain of flexor muscle, fascia and tendon of right thumb at forearm level
      ● S56.012   Strain of flexor muscle, fascia and tendon of left thumb at forearm level
      ● S56.019   Strain of flexor muscle, fascia and tendon of unspecified thumb at forearm level

    ● S56.02   Laceration of flexor muscle, fascia and tendon of thumb at forearm level
      ● S56.021   Laceration of flexor muscle, fascia and tendon of right thumb at forearm level
      ● S56.022   Laceration of flexor muscle, fascia and tendon of left thumb at forearm level
      ● S56.029   Laceration of flexor muscle, fascia and tendon of unspecified thumb at forearm level

    ● S56.09   Other injury of flexor muscle, fascia and tendon of thumb at forearm level
      ● S56.091   Other injury of flexor muscle, fascia and tendon of right thumb at forearm level
      ● S56.092   Other injury of flexor muscle, fascia and tendon of left thumb at forearm level
      ● S56.099   Other injury of flexor muscle, fascia and tendon of unspecified thumb at forearm level

● S56.1   Injury of flexor muscle, fascia and tendon of other and unspecified finger at forearm level
    ● S56.10   Unspecified injury of flexor muscle, fascia and tendon of other and unspecified finger at forearm level
      ● S56.101   Unspecified injury of flexor muscle, fascia and tendon of right index finger at forearm level
      ● S56.102   Unspecified injury of flexor muscle, fascia and tendon of left index finger at forearm level
      ● S56.103   Unspecified injury of flexor muscle, fascia and tendon of right middle finger at forearm level

◀ New   ◀||| Revised   ~~deleted~~ Deleted   **OGCR** Official Guidelines   X Assign placeholder X   ● Use Additional Character(s)

Excludes 1   Excludes 2   Includes   Use additional   Code first   Code also   Unspecified

1293

CHAPTER 19 (S00–T88)

CHAPTER 19 (S00-T88)

● S56.104   Unspecified injury of flexor muscle, fascia and tendon of left middle finger at forearm level

● S56.105   Unspecified injury of flexor muscle, fascia and tendon of right ring finger at forearm level

● S56.106   Unspecified injury of flexor muscle, fascia and tendon of left ring finger at forearm level

● S56.107   Unspecified injury of flexor muscle, fascia and tendon of right little finger at forearm level

● S56.108   Unspecified injury of flexor muscle, fascia and tendon of left little finger at forearm level

● S56.109   Unspecified injury of flexor muscle, fascia and tendon of unspecified finger at forearm level

● S56.11   Strain of flexor muscle, fascia and tendon of other and unspecified finger at forearm level

● S56.111   Strain of flexor muscle, fascia and tendon of right index finger at forearm level

● S56.112   Strain of flexor muscle, fascia and tendon of left index finger at forearm level

● S56.113   Strain of flexor muscle, fascia and tendon of right middle finger at forearm level

● S56.114   Strain of flexor muscle, fascia and tendon of left middle finger at forearm level

● S56.115   Strain of flexor muscle, fascia and tendon of right ring finger at forearm level

● S56.116   Strain of flexor muscle, fascia and tendon of left ring finger at forearm level

● S56.117   Strain of flexor muscle, fascia and tendon of right little finger at forearm level

● S56.118   Strain of flexor muscle, fascia and tendon of left little finger at forearm level

● S56.119   Strain of flexor muscle, fascia and tendon of finger of unspecified finger at forearm level

● S56.12   Laceration of flexor muscle, fascia and tendon of other and unspecified finger at forearm level

● S56.121   Laceration of flexor muscle, fascia and tendon of right index finger at forearm level

● S56.122   Laceration of flexor muscle, fascia and tendon of left index finger at forearm level

● S56.123   Laceration of flexor muscle, fascia and tendon of right middle finger at forearm level

● S56.124   Laceration of flexor muscle, fascia and tendon of left middle finger at forearm level

● S56.125   Laceration of flexor muscle, fascia and tendon of right ring finger at forearm level

● S56.126   Laceration of flexor muscle, fascia and tendon of left ring finger at forearm level

● S56.127   Laceration of flexor muscle, fascia and tendon of right little finger at forearm level

● S56.128   Laceration of flexor muscle, fascia and tendon of left little finger at forearm level

● S56.129   Laceration of flexor muscle, fascia and tendon of unspecified finger at forearm level

● S56.19   Other injury of flexor muscle, fascia and tendon of other and unspecified finger at forearm level

● S56.191   Other injury of flexor muscle, fascia and tendon of right index finger at forearm level

● S56.192   Other injury of flexor muscle, fascia and tendon of left index finger at forearm level

● S56.193   Other injury of flexor muscle, fascia and tendon of right middle finger at forearm level

● S56.194   Other injury of flexor muscle, fascia and tendon of left middle finger at forearm level

● S56.195   Other injury of flexor muscle, fascia and tendon of right ring finger at forearm level

● S56.196   Other injury of flexor muscle, fascia and tendon of left ring finger at forearm level

● S56.197   Other injury of flexor muscle, fascia and tendon of right little finger at forearm level

● S56.198   Other injury of flexor muscle, fascia and tendon of left little finger at forearm level

● S56.199   Other injury of flexor muscle, fascia and tendon of unspecified finger at forearm level

● S56.2   Injury of other flexor muscle, fascia and tendon at forearm level

● S56.20   Unspecified injury of other flexor muscle, fascia and tendon at forearm level

● S56.201   Unspecified injury of other flexor muscle, fascia and tendon at forearm level, right arm

● S56.202   Unspecified injury of other flexor muscle, fascia and tendon at forearm level, left arm

● S56.209   Unspecified injury of other flexor muscle, fascia and tendon at forearm level, unspecified arm

● S56.21   Strain of other flexor muscle, fascia and tendon at forearm level

● S56.211   Strain of other flexor muscle, fascia and tendon at forearm level, right arm

● S56.212   Strain of other flexor muscle, fascia and tendon at forearm level, left arm

● S56.219   Strain of other flexor muscle, fascia and tendon at forearm level, unspecified arm

● S56.22   Laceration of other flexor muscle, fascia and tendon at forearm level

● S56.221   Laceration of other flexor muscle, fascia and tendon at forearm level, right arm

● S56.222   Laceration of other flexor muscle, fascia and tendon at forearm level, left arm

● S56.229   Laceration of other flexor muscle, fascia and tendon at forearm level, unspecified arm

◀ New   ◀∥∥ Revised   ~~deleted~~ Deleted   OGCR Official Guidelines   X Assign placeholder X   ● Use Additional Character(s)

Excludes 1   Excludes 2   Includes   Use additional   Code first   Code also   Unspecified

●S56.29   Other injury of other flexor muscle, fascia and tendon at forearm level
- ●S56.291   Other injury of other flexor muscle, fascia and tendon at forearm level, right arm
- ●S56.292   Other injury of other flexor muscle, fascia and tendon at forearm level, left arm
- ●S56.299   Other injury of other flexor muscle, fascia and tendon at forearm level, unspecified arm

●S56.3   Injury of extensor or abductor muscles, fascia and tendons of thumb at forearm level
- ●S56.30   Unspecified injury of extensor or abductor muscles, fascia and tendons of thumb at forearm level
  - ●S56.301   Unspecified injury of extensor or abductor muscles, fascia and tendons of right thumb at forearm level
  - ●S56.302   Unspecified injury of extensor or abductor muscles, fascia and tendons of left thumb at forearm level
  - ●S56.309   Unspecified injury of extensor or abductor muscles, fascia and tendons of unspecified thumb at forearm level
- ●S56.31   Strain of extensor or abductor muscles, fascia and tendons of thumb at forearm level
  - ●S56.311   Strain of extensor or abductor muscles, fascia and tendons of right thumb at forearm level
  - ●S56.312   Strain of extensor or abductor muscles, fascia and tendons of left thumb at forearm level
  - ●S56.319   Strain of extensor or abductor muscles, fascia and tendons of unspecified thumb at forearm level
- ●S56.32   Laceration of extensor or abductor muscles, fascia and tendons of thumb at forearm level
  - ●S56.321   Laceration of extensor or abductor muscles, fascia and tendons of right thumb at forearm level
  - ●S56.322   Laceration of extensor or abductor muscles, fascia and tendons of left thumb at forearm level
  - ●S56.329   Laceration of extensor or abductor muscles, fascia and tendons of unspecified thumb at forearm level
- ●S56.39   Other injury of extensor or abductor muscles, fascia and tendons of thumb at forearm level
  - ●S56.391   Other injury of extensor or abductor muscles, fascia and tendons of right thumb at forearm level
  - ●S56.392   Other injury of extensor or abductor muscles, fascia and tendons of left thumb at forearm level
  - ●S56.399   Other injury of extensor or abductor muscles, fascia and tendons of unspecified thumb at forearm level

●S56.4   Injury of extensor muscle, fascia and tendon of other and unspecified finger at forearm level
- ●S56.40   Unspecified injury of extensor muscle, fascia and tendon of other and unspecified finger at forearm level
  - ●S56.401   Unspecified injury of extensor muscle, fascia and tendon of right index finger at forearm level
  - ●S56.402   Unspecified injury of extensor muscle, fascia and tendon of left index finger at forearm level

●S56.403   Unspecified injury of extensor muscle, fascia and tendon of right middle finger at forearm level
●S56.404   Unspecified injury of extensor muscle, fascia and tendon of left middle finger at forearm level
●S56.405   Unspecified injury of extensor muscle, fascia and tendon of right ring finger at forearm level
●S56.406   Unspecified injury of extensor muscle, fascia and tendon of left ring finger at forearm level
●S56.407   Unspecified injury of extensor muscle, fascia and tendon of right little finger at forearm level
●S56.408   Unspecified injury of extensor muscle, fascia and tendon of left little finger at forearm level
●S56.409   Unspecified injury of extensor muscle, fascia and tendon of unspecified finger at forearm level

●S56.41   Strain of extensor muscle, fascia and tendon of other and unspecified finger at forearm level
- ●S56.411   Strain of extensor muscle, fascia and tendon of right index finger at forearm level
- ●S56.412   Strain of extensor muscle, fascia and tendon of left index finger at forearm level
- ●S56.413   Strain of extensor muscle, fascia and tendon of right middle finger at forearm level
- ●S56.414   Strain of extensor muscle, fascia and tendon of left middle finger at forearm level
- ●S56.415   Strain of extensor muscle, fascia and tendon of right ring finger at forearm level
- ●S56.416   Strain of extensor muscle, fascia and tendon of left ring finger at forearm level
- ●S56.417   Strain of extensor muscle, fascia and tendon of right little finger at forearm level
- ●S56.418   Strain of extensor muscle, fascia and tendon of left little finger at forearm level
- ●S56.419   Strain of extensor muscle, fascia and tendon of finger, unspecified finger at forearm level

●S56.42   Laceration of extensor muscle, fascia and tendon of other and unspecified finger at forearm level
- ●S56.421   Laceration of extensor muscle, fascia and tendon of right index finger at forearm level
- ●S56.422   Laceration of extensor muscle, fascia and tendon of left index finger at forearm level
- ●S56.423   Laceration of extensor muscle, fascia and tendon of right middle finger at forearm level
- ●S56.424   Laceration of extensor muscle, fascia and tendon of left middle finger at forearm level
- ●S56.425   Laceration of extensor muscle, fascia and tendon of right ring finger at forearm level

◀ New   ◀▥ Revised   ~~deleted~~ Deleted   OGCR Official Guidelines   X Assign placeholder X   ● Use Additional Character(s)

| Excludes 1 | Excludes 2 | Includes | Use additional | Code first | Code also | Unspecified |

● S56.426   Laceration of extensor muscle, fascia
            and tendon of left ring finger at
            forearm level
● S56.427   Laceration of extensor muscle, fascia
            and tendon of right little finger at
            forearm level
● S56.428   Laceration of extensor muscle, fascia
            and tendon of left little finger at
            forearm level
● S56.429   Laceration of extensor muscle, fascia
            and tendon of unspecified finger at
            forearm level
● S56.49   Other injury of extensor muscle, fascia and
           tendon of other and unspecified finger at
           forearm level
    ● S56.491   Other injury of extensor muscle,
                fascia and tendon of right index finger
                at forearm level
    ● S56.492   Other injury of extensor muscle,
                fascia and tendon of left index finger
                at forearm level
    ● S56.493   Other injury of extensor muscle,
                fascia and tendon of right middle
                finger at forearm level
    ● S56.494   Other injury of extensor muscle,
                fascia and tendon of left middle
                finger at forearm level
    ● S56.495   Other injury of extensor muscle,
                fascia and tendon of right ring finger
                at forearm level
    ● S56.496   Other injury of extensor muscle,
                fascia and tendon of left ring finger at
                forearm level
    ● S56.497   Other injury of extensor muscle,
                fascia and tendon of right little finger
                at forearm level
    ● S56.498   Other injury of extensor muscle,
                fascia and tendon of left little finger
                at forearm level
    ● S56.499   Other injury of extensor muscle,
                fascia and tendon of unspecified
                finger at forearm level
● S56.5   Injury of other extensor muscle, fascia and tendon at
          forearm level
    ● S56.50   Unspecified injury of other extensor muscle,
               fascia and tendon at forearm level
        ● S56.501   Unspecified injury of other extensor
                    muscle, fascia and tendon at forearm
                    level, right arm
        ● S56.502   Unspecified injury of other extensor
                    muscle, fascia and tendon at forearm
                    level, left arm
        ● S56.509   Unspecified injury of other extensor
                    muscle, fascia and tendon at forearm
                    level, unspecified arm
    ● S56.51   Strain of other extensor muscle, fascia and
               tendon at forearm level
        ● S56.511   Strain of other extensor muscle, fascia
                    and tendon at forearm level, right arm
        ● S56.512   Strain of other extensor muscle, fascia
                    and tendon at forearm level, left arm
        ● S56.519   Strain of other extensor muscle,
                    fascia and tendon at forearm level,
                    unspecified arm

● S56.52   Laceration of other extensor muscle, fascia and
           tendon at forearm level
    ● S56.521   Laceration of other extensor muscle,
                fascia and tendon at forearm level,
                right arm
    ● S56.522   Laceration of other extensor muscle,
                fascia and tendon at forearm level,
                left arm
    ● S56.529   Laceration of other extensor muscle,
                fascia and tendon at forearm level,
                unspecified arm
● S56.59   Other injury of other extensor muscle, fascia
           and tendon at forearm level
    ● S56.591   Other injury of other extensor muscle,
                fascia and tendon at forearm level,
                right arm
    ● S56.592   Other injury of other extensor muscle,
                fascia and tendon at forearm level,
                left arm
    ● S56.599   Other injury of other extensor muscle,
                fascia and tendon at forearm level,
                unspecified arm
● S56.8   Injury of other muscles, fascia and tendons at forearm
          level
    ● S56.80   Unspecified injury of other muscles, fascia and
               tendons at forearm level
        ● S56.801   Unspecified injury of other muscles,
                    fascia and tendons at forearm level,
                    right arm
        ● S56.802   Unspecified injury of other muscles,
                    fascia and tendons at forearm level,
                    left arm
        ● S56.809   Unspecified injury of other muscles,
                    fascia and tendons at forearm level,
                    unspecified arm
    ● S56.81   Strain of other muscles, fascia and tendons at
               forearm level
        ● S56.811   Strain of other muscles, fascia and
                    tendons at forearm level, right arm
        ● S56.812   Strain of other muscles, fascia and
                    tendons at forearm level, left arm
        ● S56.819   Strain of other muscles, fascia and
                    tendons at forearm level, unspecified
                    arm
    ● S56.82   Laceration of other muscles, fascia and tendons
               at forearm level
        ● S56.821   Laceration of other muscles, fascia
                    and tendons at forearm level, right
                    arm
        ● S56.822   Laceration of other muscles, fascia
                    and tendons at forearm level, left arm
        ● S56.829   Laceration of other muscles, fascia
                    and tendons at forearm level,
                    unspecified arm
    ● S56.89   Other injury of other muscles, fascia and
               tendons at forearm level
        ● S56.891   Other injury of other muscles, fascia
                    and tendons at forearm level, right
                    arm
        ● S56.892   Other injury of other muscles, fascia
                    and tendons at forearm level, left arm
        ● S56.899   Other injury of other muscles,
                    fascia and tendons at forearm level,
                    unspecified arm

- ● **S56.9**   **Injury of unspecified muscles, fascia and tendons at forearm level**
  - ● **S56.90**   Unspecified injury of unspecified muscles, fascia and tendons at forearm level
    - ● **S56.901**   Unspecified injury of unspecified muscles, fascia and tendons at forearm level, right arm
    - ● **S56.902**   Unspecified injury of unspecified muscles, fascia and tendons at forearm level, left arm
    - ● **S56.909**   Unspecified injury of unspecified muscles, fascia and tendons at forearm level, unspecified arm
  - ● **S56.91**   Strain of unspecified muscles, fascia and tendons at forearm level
    - ● **S56.911**   Strain of unspecified muscles, fascia and tendons at forearm level, right arm
    - ● **S56.912**   Strain of unspecified muscles, fascia and tendons at forearm level, left arm
    - ● **S56.919**   Strain of unspecified muscles, fascia and tendons at forearm level, unspecified arm
  - ● **S56.92**   Laceration of unspecified muscles, fascia and tendons at forearm level
    - ● **S56.921**   Laceration of unspecified muscles, fascia and tendons at forearm level, right arm
    - ● **S56.922**   Laceration of unspecified muscles, fascia and tendons at forearm level, left arm
    - ● **S56.929**   Laceration of unspecified muscles, fascia and tendons at forearm level, unspecified arm
  - ● **S56.99**   Other injury of unspecified muscles, fascia and tendons at forearm level
    - ● **S56.991**   Other injury of unspecified muscles, fascia and tendons at forearm level, right arm
    - ● **S56.992**   Other injury of unspecified muscles, fascia and tendons at forearm level, left arm
    - ● **S56.999**   Other injury of unspecified muscles, fascia and tendons at forearm level, unspecified arm

- ● **S57**   **Crushing injury of elbow and forearm**
  Use additional code(s) for all associated injuries

  Excludes2   crushing injury of wrist and hand (S67.-)

  The appropriate 7th character is to be added to each code from category S57

A	initial encounter
D	subsequent encounter
S	sequela

  - ● **S57.0**   Crushing injury of elbow
    - X ● **S57.00**   Crushing injury of unspecified elbow
    - X ● **S57.01**   Crushing injury of right elbow
    - X ● **S57.02**   Crushing injury of left elbow
  - ● **S57.8**   Crushing injury of forearm
    - X ● **S57.80**   Crushing injury of unspecified forearm
    - X ● **S57.81**   Crushing injury of right forearm
    - X ● **S57.82**   Crushing injury of left forearm

- ● **S58**   **Traumatic amputation of elbow and forearm**
  An amputation not identified as partial or complete should be coded to complete

  Excludes1   traumatic amputation of wrist and hand (S68.-)

  The appropriate 7th character is to be added to each code from category S58

A	initial encounter
D	subsequent encounter
S	sequela

  - ● **S58.0**   Traumatic amputation at elbow level
    - ● **S58.01**   Complete traumatic amputation at elbow level
      - ● **S58.011**   Complete traumatic amputation at elbow level, right arm
      - ● **S58.012**   Complete traumatic amputation at elbow level, left arm
      - ● **S58.019**   Complete traumatic amputation at elbow level, unspecified arm
    - ● **S58.02**   Partial traumatic amputation at elbow level
      - ● **S58.021**   Partial traumatic amputation at elbow level, right arm
      - ● **S58.022**   Partial traumatic amputation at elbow level, left arm
      - ● **S58.029**   Partial traumatic amputation at elbow level, unspecified arm
  - ● **S58.1**   Traumatic amputation at level between elbow and wrist
    - ● **S58.11**   Complete traumatic amputation at level between elbow and wrist
      - ● **S58.111**   Complete traumatic amputation at level between elbow and wrist, right arm
      - ● **S58.112**   Complete traumatic amputation at level between elbow and wrist, left arm
      - ● **S58.119**   Complete traumatic amputation at level between elbow and wrist, unspecified arm
    - ● **S58.12**   Partial traumatic amputation at level between elbow and wrist
      - ● **S58.121**   Partial traumatic amputation at level between elbow and wrist, right arm
      - ● **S58.122**   Partial traumatic amputation at level between elbow and wrist, left arm
      - ● **S58.129**   Partial traumatic amputation at level between elbow and wrist, unspecified arm
  - ● **S58.9**   Traumatic amputation of forearm, level unspecified

    Excludes1   traumatic amputation of wrist (S68.-)
    - ● **S58.91**   Complete traumatic amputation of forearm, level unspecified
      - ● **S58.911**   Complete traumatic amputation of right forearm, level unspecified
      - ● **S58.912**   Complete traumatic amputation of left forearm, level unspecified
      - ● **S58.919**   Complete traumatic amputation of unspecified forearm, level unspecified
    - ● **S58.92**   Partial traumatic amputation of forearm, level unspecified
      - ● **S58.921**   Partial traumatic amputation of right forearm, level unspecified
      - ● **S58.922**   Partial traumatic amputation of left forearm, level unspecified
      - ● **S58.929**   Partial traumatic amputation of unspecified forearm, level unspecified

Item 19-4 SALTER-HARRIS TYPE 1: epiphysis is completely separated from end of bone, or metaphysic growth plate remains attached to epiphysis

SALTER-HARRIS TYPE 2: epiphysis and growth plate are partially separated from metaphysis, which is cracked—most common type

SALTER-HARRIS TYPE 3: fracture occurring through epiphysis and separates part of epiphysis and growth plate from metaphysis fracture, usually at distal end of tibia

SALTER-HARRIS TYPE 4: fracture runs through epiphysis, across growth plate, into metaphysic, surgery is required to restore joint surface to normal and align growth plate

- S59　Other and unspecified injuries of elbow and forearm

  Excludes2　other and unspecified injuries of wrist and hand (S69.-)

  The appropriate 7th character is to be added to each code from subcategories S59.0, S59.1, and S59.2

A	initial encounter for closed fracture
D	subsequent encounter for fracture with routine healing
G	subsequent encounter for fracture with delayed healing
K	subsequent encounter for fracture with nonunion
P	subsequent encounter for fracture with malunion
S	sequela

  - S59.0　Physeal fracture of lower end of ulna
    - S59.00　Unspecified physeal fracture of lower end of ulna
      - S59.001　Unspecified physeal fracture of lower end of ulna, right arm
      - S59.002　Unspecified physeal fracture of lower end of ulna, left arm
      - S59.009　Unspecified physeal fracture of lower end of ulna, unspecified arm
    - S59.01　Salter-Harris Type I physeal fracture of lower end of ulna
      - S59.011　Salter-Harris Type I physeal fracture of lower end of ulna, right arm
      - S59.012　Salter-Harris Type I physeal fracture of lower end of ulna, left arm
      - S59.019　Salter-Harris Type I physeal fracture of lower end of ulna, unspecified arm
    - S59.02　Salter-Harris Type II physeal fracture of lower end of ulna
      - S59.021　Salter-Harris Type II physeal fracture of lower end of ulna, right arm
      - S59.022　Salter-Harris Type II physeal fracture of lower end of ulna, left arm
      - S59.029　Salter-Harris Type II physeal fracture of lower end of ulna, unspecified arm
    - S59.03　Salter-Harris Type III physeal fracture of lower end of ulna
      - S59.031　Salter-Harris Type III physeal fracture of lower end of ulna, right arm
      - S59.032　Salter-Harris Type III physeal fracture of lower end of ulna, left arm
      - S59.039　Salter-Harris Type III physeal fracture of lower end of ulna, unspecified arm
    - S59.04　Salter-Harris Type IV physeal fracture of lower end of ulna
      - S59.041　Salter-Harris Type IV physeal fracture of lower end of ulna, right arm
      - S59.042　Salter-Harris Type IV physeal fracture of lower end of ulna, left arm
      - S59.049　Salter-Harris Type IV physeal fracture of lower end of ulna, unspecified arm

  - S59.09　Other physeal fracture of lower end of ulna
    - S59.091　Other physeal fracture of lower end of ulna, right arm
    - S59.092　Other physeal fracture of lower end of ulna, left arm
    - S59.099　Other physeal fracture of lower end of ulna, unspecified arm
  - S59.1　Physeal fracture of upper end of radius
    - S59.10　Unspecified physeal fracture of upper end of radius
      - S59.101　Unspecified physeal fracture of upper end of radius, right arm
      - S59.102　Unspecified physeal fracture of upper end of radius, left arm
      - S59.109　Unspecified physeal fracture of upper end of radius, unspecified arm
    - S59.11　Salter-Harris Type I physeal fracture of upper end of radius
      - S59.111　Salter-Harris Type I physeal fracture of upper end of radius, right arm
      - S59.112　Salter-Harris Type I physeal fracture of upper end of radius, left arm
      - S59.119　Salter-Harris Type I physeal fracture of upper end of radius, unspecified arm
    - S59.12　Salter-Harris Type II physeal fracture of upper end of radius
      - S59.121　Salter-Harris Type II physeal fracture of upper end of radius, right arm
      - S59.122　Salter-Harris Type II physeal fracture of upper end of radius, left arm
      - S59.129　Salter-Harris Type II physeal fracture of upper end of radius, unspecified arm
    - S59.13　Salter-Harris Type III physeal fracture of upper end of radius
      - S59.131　Salter-Harris Type III physeal fracture of upper end of radius, right arm
      - S59.132　Salter-Harris Type III physeal fracture of upper end of radius, left arm
      - S59.139　Salter-Harris Type III physeal fracture of upper end of radius, unspecified arm
    - S59.14　Salter-Harris Type IV physeal fracture of upper end of radius
      - S59.141　Salter-Harris Type IV physeal fracture of upper end of radius, right arm
      - S59.142　Salter-Harris Type IV physeal fracture of upper end of radius, left arm
      - S59.149　Salter-Harris Type IV physeal fracture of upper end of radius, unspecified arm
    - S59.19　Other physeal fracture of upper end of radius
      - S59.191　Other physeal fracture of upper end of radius, right arm
      - S59.192　Other physeal fracture of upper end of radius, left arm
      - S59.199　Other physeal fracture of upper end of radius, unspecified arm
  - S59.2　Physeal fracture of lower end of radius
    - S59.20　Unspecified physeal fracture of lower end of radius
      - S59.201　Unspecified physeal fracture of lower end of radius, right arm
      - S59.202　Unspecified physeal fracture of lower end of radius, left arm
      - S59.209　Unspecified physeal fracture of lower end of radius, unspecified arm

◀ New　　◀▥▥ Revised　　deleted Deleted　　OGCR Official Guidelines　　X Assign placeholder X　　● Use Additional Character(s)

Excludes 1　　Excludes 2　　Includes　　Use additional　　Code first　　Code also　　Unspecified

● S59.21 **Salter-Harris Type I physeal fracture of lower end of radius**
  ● S59.211 **Salter-Harris Type I physeal fracture of lower end of radius, right arm**
  ● S59.212 **Salter-Harris Type I physeal fracture of lower end of radius, left arm**
  ● S59.219 **Salter-Harris Type I physeal fracture of lower end of radius, unspecified arm**

● S59.22 **Salter-Harris Type II physeal fracture of lower end of radius**
  ● S59.221 **Salter-Harris Type II physeal fracture of lower end of radius, right arm**
  ● S59.222 **Salter-Harris Type II physeal fracture of lower end of radius, left arm**
  ● S59.229 **Salter-Harris Type II physeal fracture of lower end of radius, unspecified arm**

● S59.23 **Salter-Harris Type III physeal fracture of lower end of radius**
  ● S59.231 **Salter-Harris Type III physeal fracture of lower end of radius, right arm**
  ● S59.232 **Salter-Harris Type III physeal fracture of lower end of radius, left arm**
  ● S59.239 **Salter-Harris Type III physeal fracture of lower end of radius, unspecified arm**

● S59.24 **Salter-Harris Type IV physeal fracture of lower end of radius**
  ● S59.241 **Salter-Harris Type IV physeal fracture of lower end of radius, right arm**
  ● S59.242 **Salter-Harris Type IV physeal fracture of lower end of radius, left arm**
  ● S59.249 **Salter-Harris Type IV physeal fracture of lower end of radius, unspecified arm**

● S59.29 **Other physeal fracture of lower end of radius**
  ● S59.291 **Other physeal fracture of lower end of radius, right arm**
  ● S59.292 **Other physeal fracture of lower end of radius, left arm**
  ● S59.299 **Other physeal fracture of lower end of radius, unspecified arm**

● S59.8 **Other specified injuries of elbow and forearm**
The appropriate 7th character is to be added to each code in subcategory S59.8

A	initial encounter
D	subsequent encounter
S	sequela

  ● S59.80 **Other specified injuries of elbow**
    ● S59.801 **Other specified injuries of right elbow**
    ● S59.802 **Other specified injuries of left elbow**
    ● S59.809 **Other specified injuries of unspecified elbow**
  ● S59.81 **Other specified injuries of forearm**
    ● S59.811 **Other specified injuries right forearm**
    ● S59.812 **Other specified injuries left forearm**
    ● S59.819 **Other specified injuries unspecified forearm**

● S59.9 **Unspecified injury of elbow and forearm**
The appropriate 7th character is to be added to each code in subcategory S59.9

A	initial encounter
D	subsequent encounter
S	sequela

  ● S59.90 **Unspecified injury of elbow**
    ● S59.901 **Unspecified injury of right elbow**
    ● S59.902 **Unspecified injury of left elbow**
    ● S59.909 **Unspecified injury of unspecified elbow**
  ● S59.91 **Unspecified injury of forearm**
    ● S59.911 **Unspecified injury of right forearm**
    ● S59.912 **Unspecified injury of left forearm**
    ● S59.919 **Unspecified injury of unspecified forearm**

INJURIES TO THE WRIST, HAND AND FINGERS (S60-S69)

Excludes2   burns and corrosions (T20-T32)
frostbite (T33-T34)
insect bite or sting, venomous (T63.4)

● S60 **Superficial injury of wrist, hand and fingers**
The appropriate 7th character is to be added to each code from category S60

A	initial encounter
D	subsequent encounter
S	sequela

  ● S60.0 **Contusion of finger without damage to nail**
    Excludes1   contusion involving nail (matrix) (S60.1)
  X ● S60.00 **Contusion of unspecified finger without damage to nail**
    Contusion of finger(s) NOS
  ● S60.01 **Contusion of thumb without damage to nail**
    ● S60.011 **Contusion of right thumb without damage to nail**
    ● S60.012 **Contusion of left thumb without damage to nail**
    ● S60.019 **Contusion of unspecified thumb without damage to nail**
  ● S60.02 **Contusion of index finger without damage to nail**
    ● S60.021 **Contusion of right index finger without damage to nail**
    ● S60.022 **Contusion of left index finger without damage to nail**
    ● S60.029 **Contusion of unspecified index finger without damage to nail**
  ● S60.03 **Contusion of middle finger without damage to nail**
    ● S60.031 **Contusion of right middle finger without damage to nail**
    ● S60.032 **Contusion of left middle finger without damage to nail**
    ● S60.039 **Contusion of unspecified middle finger without damage to nail**
  ● S60.04 **Contusion of ring finger without damage to nail**
    ● S60.041 **Contusion of right ring finger without damage to nail**
    ● S60.042 **Contusion of left ring finger without damage to nail**
    ● S60.049 **Contusion of unspecified ring finger without damage to nail**

CHAPTER 19 (S00-T88)

● **S60.05**   Contusion of little finger without damage to nail
- ● **S60.051**   Contusion of right little finger without damage to nail
- ● **S60.052**   Contusion of left little finger without damage to nail
- ● **S60.059**   Contusion of unspecified little finger without damage to nail

● **S60.1**   Contusion of finger with damage to nail
- X ● **S60.10**   Contusion of unspecified finger with damage to nail
- ● **S60.11**   Contusion of thumb with damage to nail
  - ● **S60.111**   Contusion of right thumb with damage to nail
  - ● **S60.112**   Contusion of left thumb with damage to nail
  - ● **S60.119**   Contusion of unspecified thumb with damage to nail
- ● **S60.12**   Contusion of index finger with damage to nail
  - ● **S60.121**   Contusion of right index finger with damage to nail
  - ● **S60.122**   Contusion of left index finger with damage to nail
  - ● **S60.129**   Contusion of unspecified index finger with damage to nail
- ● **S60.13**   Contusion of middle finger with damage to nail
  - ● **S60.131**   Contusion of right middle finger with damage to nail
  - ● **S60.132**   Contusion of left middle finger with damage to nail
  - ● **S60.139**   Contusion of unspecified middle finger with damage to nail
- ● **S60.14**   Contusion of ring finger with damage to nail
  - ● **S60.141**   Contusion of right ring finger with damage to nail
  - ● **S60.142**   Contusion of left ring finger with damage to nail
  - ● **S60.149**   Contusion of unspecified ring finger with damage to nail
- ● **S60.15**   Contusion of little finger with damage to nail
  - ● **S60.151**   Contusion of right little finger with damage to nail
  - ● **S60.152**   Contusion of left little finger with damage to nail
  - ● **S60.159**   Contusion of unspecified little finger with damage to nail

● **S60.2**   Contusion of wrist and hand
> **Excludes2**   contusion of fingers (S60.0-, S60.1-)
- ● **S60.21**   Contusion of wrist
  - ● **S60.211**   Contusion of right wrist
  - ● **S60.212**   Contusion of left wrist
  - ● **S60.219**   Contusion of unspecified wrist
- ● **S60.22**   Contusion of hand
  - ● **S60.221**   Contusion of right hand
  - ● **S60.222**   Contusion of left hand
  - ● **S60.229**   Contusion of unspecified hand

● **S60.3**   Other superficial injuries of thumb
- ● **S60.31**   Abrasion of thumb
  - ● **S60.311**   Abrasion of right thumb
  - ● **S60.312**   Abrasion of left thumb
  - ● **S60.319**   Abrasion of unspecified thumb
- ● **S60.32**   Blister (nonthermal) of thumb
  - ● **S60.321**   Blister (nonthermal) of right thumb
  - ● **S60.322**   Blister (nonthermal) of left thumb
  - ● **S60.329**   Blister (nonthermal) of unspecified thumb
- ● **S60.34**   External constriction of thumb
  - Hair tourniquet syndrome of thumb
  - Use additional cause code to identify the constricting item (W49.0-)
  - ● **S60.341**   External constriction of right thumb
  - ● **S60.342**   External constriction of left thumb
  - ● **S60.349**   External constriction of unspecified thumb
- ● **S60.35**   Superficial foreign body of thumb
  - Splinter in the thumb
  - ● **S60.351**   Superficial foreign body of right thumb
  - ● **S60.352**   Superficial foreign body of left thumb
  - ● **S60.359**   Superficial foreign body of unspecified thumb
- ● **S60.36**   Insect bite (nonvenomous) of thumb
  - ● **S60.361**   Insect bite (nonvenomous) of right thumb
  - ● **S60.362**   Insect bite (nonvenomous) of left thumb
  - ● **S60.369**   Insect bite (nonvenomous) of unspecified thumb
- ● **S60.37**   Other superficial bite of thumb
  > **Excludes1**   open bite of thumb (S61.05-, S61.15-)
  - ● **S60.371**   Other superficial bite of right thumb
  - ● **S60.372**   Other superficial bite of left thumb
  - ● **S60.379**   Other superficial bite of unspecified thumb
- ● **S60.39**   Other superficial injuries of thumb
  - ● **S60.391**   Other superficial injuries of right thumb
  - ● **S60.392**   Other superficial injuries of left thumb
  - ● **S60.399**   Other superficial injuries of unspecified thumb

● **S60.4**   Other superficial injuries of other fingers
- ● **S60.41**   Abrasion of fingers
  - ● **S60.410**   Abrasion of right index finger
  - ● **S60.411**   Abrasion of left index finger
  - ● **S60.412**   Abrasion of right middle finger
  - ● **S60.413**   Abrasion of left middle finger
  - ● **S60.414**   Abrasion of right ring finger
  - ● **S60.415**   Abrasion of left ring finger
  - ● **S60.416**   Abrasion of right little finger
  - ● **S60.417**   Abrasion of left little finger
  - ● **S60.418**   Abrasion of other finger
    - Abrasion of specified finger with unspecified laterality
  - ● **S60.419**   Abrasion of unspecified finger

◀ New   ◀▥ Revised   ~~deleted~~ Deleted   OGCR Official Guidelines   X Assign placeholder X   ● Use Additional Character(s)

| Excludes 1 | Excludes 2 | Includes | Use additional | Code first | Code also | Unspecified |

● S60.42   Blister (nonthermal) of fingers
    ● S60.420   Blister (nonthermal) of right index finger
    ● S60.421   Blister (nonthermal) of left index finger
    ● S60.422   Blister (nonthermal) of right middle finger
    ● S60.423   Blister (nonthermal) of left middle finger
    ● S60.424   Blister (nonthermal) of right ring finger
    ● S60.425   Blister (nonthermal) of left ring finger
    ● S60.426   Blister (nonthermal) of right little finger
    ● S60.427   Blister (nonthermal) of left little finger
    ● S60.428   Blister (nonthermal) of other finger
        Blister (nonthermal) of specified finger with unspecified laterality
    ● S60.429   Blister (nonthermal) of unspecified finger

● S60.44   External constriction of fingers
    Hair tourniquet syndrome of finger
    Use additional cause code to identify the constricting item (W49.0-)
    ● S60.440   External constriction of right index finger
    ● S60.441   External constriction of left index finger
    ● S60.442   External constriction of right middle finger
    ● S60.443   External constriction of left middle finger
    ● S60.444   External constriction of right ring finger
    ● S60.445   External constriction of left ring finger
    ● S60.446   External constriction of right little finger
    ● S60.447   External constriction of left little finger
    ● S60.448   External constriction of other finger
        External constriction of specified finger with unspecified laterality
    ● S60.449   External constriction of unspecified finger

● S60.45   Superficial foreign body of fingers
    Splinter in the finger(s)
    ● S60.450   Superficial foreign body of right index finger
    ● S60.451   Superficial foreign body of left index finger
    ● S60.452   Superficial foreign body of right middle finger
    ● S60.453   Superficial foreign body of left middle finger
    ● S60.454   Superficial foreign body of right ring finger
    ● S60.455   Superficial foreign body of left ring finger
    ● S60.456   Superficial foreign body of right little finger

    ● S60.457   Superficial foreign body of left little finger
    ● S60.458   Superficial foreign body of other finger
        Superficial foreign body of specified finger with unspecified laterality
    ● S60.459   Superficial foreign body of unspecified finger

● S60.46   Insect bite (nonvenomous) of fingers
    ● S60.460   Insect bite (nonvenomous) of right index finger
    ● S60.461   Insect bite (nonvenomous) of left index finger
    ● S60.462   Insect bite (nonvenomous) of right middle finger
    ● S60.463   Insect bite (nonvenomous) of left middle finger
    ● S60.464   Insect bite (nonvenomous) of right ring finger
    ● S60.465   Insect bite (nonvenomous) of left ring finger
    ● S60.466   Insect bite (nonvenomous) of right little finger
    ● S60.467   Insect bite (nonvenomous) of left little finger
    ● S60.468   Insect bite (nonvenomous) of other finger
        Insect bite (nonvenomous) of specified finger with unspecified laterality
    ● S60.469   Insect bite (nonvenomous) of unspecified finger

● S60.47   Other superficial bite of fingers
    Excludes1   open bite of fingers (S61.25-, S61.35-)
    ● S60.470   Other superficial bite of right index finger
    ● S60.471   Other superficial bite of left index finger
    ● S60.472   Other superficial bite of right middle finger
    ● S60.473   Other superficial bite of left middle finger
    ● S60.474   Other superficial bite of right ring finger
    ● S60.475   Other superficial bite of left ring finger
    ● S60.476   Other superficial bite of right little finger
    ● S60.477   Other superficial bite of left little finger
    ● S60.478   Other superficial bite of other finger
        Other superficial bite of specified finger with unspecified laterality
    ● S60.479   Other superficial bite of unspecified finger

● S60.5   Other superficial injuries of hand
    Excludes2   superficial injuries of fingers (S60.3-, S60.4-)
  ● S60.51   Abrasion of hand
    ● S60.511   Abrasion of right hand
    ● S60.512   Abrasion of left hand
    ● S60.519   Abrasion of unspecified hand

◄ New   ◄▥ Revised   ~~deleted~~ Deleted   OGCR Official Guidelines   X Assign placeholder X   ● Use Additional Character(s)

Excludes 1   Excludes 2   Includes   Use additional   Code first   Code also   Unspecified

CHAPTER 19 (S00-T88)

- S60.52 Blister (nonthermal) of hand
  - S60.521 Blister (nonthermal) of right hand
  - S60.522 Blister (nonthermal) of left hand
  - S60.529 Blister (nonthermal) of unspecified hand
- S60.54 External constriction of hand
  - S60.541 External constriction of right hand
  - S60.542 External constriction of left hand
  - S60.549 External constriction of unspecified hand
- S60.55 Superficial foreign body of hand
  Splinter in the hand
  - S60.551 Superficial foreign body of right hand
  - S60.552 Superficial foreign body of left hand
  - S60.559 Superficial foreign body of unspecified hand
- S60.56 Insect bite (nonvenomous) of hand
  - S60.561 Insect bite (nonvenomous) of right hand
  - S60.562 Insect bite (nonvenomous) of left hand
  - S60.569 Insect bite (nonvenomous) of unspecified hand
- S60.57 Other superficial bite of hand
  Excludes1 open bite of hand (S61.45-)
  - S60.571 Other superficial bite of hand of right hand
  - S60.572 Other superficial bite of hand of left hand
  - S60.579 Other superficial bite of hand of unspecified hand
- S60.8 Other superficial injuries of wrist
  - S60.81 Abrasion of wrist
    - S60.811 Abrasion of right wrist
    - S60.812 Abrasion of left wrist
    - S60.819 Abrasion of unspecified wrist
  - S60.82 Blister (nonthermal) of wrist
    - S60.821 Blister (nonthermal) of right wrist
    - S60.822 Blister (nonthermal) of left wrist
    - S60.829 Blister (nonthermal) of unspecified wrist
  - S60.84 External constriction of wrist
    - S60.841 External constriction of right wrist
    - S60.842 External constriction of left wrist
    - S60.849 External constriction of unspecified wrist
  - S60.85 Superficial foreign body of wrist
    Splinter in the wrist
    - S60.851 Superficial foreign body of right wrist
    - S60.852 Superficial foreign body of left wrist
    - S60.859 Superficial foreign body of unspecified wrist
  - S60.86 Insect bite (nonvenomous) of wrist
    - S60.861 Insect bite (nonvenomous) of right wrist
    - S60.862 Insect bite (nonvenomous) of left wrist
    - S60.869 Insect bite (nonvenomous) of unspecified wrist
  - S60.87 Other superficial bite of wrist
    Excludes1 open bite of wrist (S61.55)
    - S60.871 Other superficial bite of right wrist
    - S60.872 Other superficial bite of left wrist
    - S60.879 Other superficial bite of unspecified wrist

- S60.9 Unspecified superficial injury of wrist, hand and fingers
  - S60.91 Unspecified superficial injury of wrist
    - S60.911 Unspecified superficial injury of right wrist
    - S60.912 Unspecified superficial injury of left wrist
    - S60.919 Unspecified superficial injury of unspecified wrist
  - S60.92 Unspecified superficial injury of hand
    - S60.921 Unspecified superficial injury of right hand
    - S60.922 Unspecified superficial injury of left hand
    - S60.929 Unspecified superficial injury of unspecified hand
  - S60.93 Unspecified superficial injury of thumb
    - S60.931 Unspecified superficial injury of right thumb
    - S60.932 Unspecified superficial injury of left thumb
    - S60.939 Unspecified superficial injury of unspecified thumb
  - S60.94 Unspecified superficial injury of other fingers
    - S60.940 Unspecified superficial injury of right index finger
    - S60.941 Unspecified superficial injury of left index finger
    - S60.942 Unspecified superficial injury of right middle finger
    - S60.943 Unspecified superficial injury of left middle finger
    - S60.944 Unspecified superficial injury of right ring finger
    - S60.945 Unspecified superficial injury of left ring finger
    - S60.946 Unspecified superficial injury of right little finger
    - S60.947 Unspecified superficial injury of left little finger
    - S60.948 Unspecified superficial injury of other finger
      Unspecified superficial injury of specified finger with unspecified laterality
    - S60.949 Unspecified superficial injury of unspecified finger

- S61 Open wound of wrist, hand and fingers
  Code also any associated wound infection
  Excludes1 open fracture of wrist, hand and finger (S62.- with 7th character B)
  traumatic amputation of wrist and hand (S68.-)
  The appropriate 7th character is to be added to each code from category S61

A	initial encounter
D	subsequent encounter
S	sequela

  - S61.0 Open wound of thumb without damage to nail
    Excludes1 open wound of thumb with damage to nail (S61.1-)
    - S61.00 Unspecified open wound of thumb without damage to nail
      - S61.001 Unspecified open wound of right thumb without damage to nail
      - S61.002 Unspecified open wound of left thumb without damage to nail
      - S61.009 Unspecified open wound of unspecified thumb without damage to nail

◄ New   ◄┅ Revised   ~~deleted~~ Deleted   OGCR Official Guidelines   X Assign placeholder X   ● Use Additional Character(s)

Excludes 1   Excludes 2   Includes   Use additional   Code first   Code also   Unspecified

● **S61.01** Laceration without foreign body of thumb without damage to nail
     ● **S61.011** Laceration without foreign body of right thumb without damage to nail
     ● **S61.012** Laceration without foreign body of left thumb without damage to nail
     ● **S61.019** Laceration without foreign body of unspecified thumb without damage to nail

● **S61.02** Laceration with foreign body of thumb without damage to nail
     ● **S61.021** Laceration with foreign body of right thumb without damage to nail
     ● **S61.022** Laceration with foreign body of left thumb without damage to nail
     ● **S61.029** Laceration with foreign body of unspecified thumb without damage to nail

● **S61.03** Puncture wound without foreign body of thumb without damage to nail
     ● **S61.031** Puncture wound without foreign body of right thumb without damage to nail
     ● **S61.032** Puncture wound without foreign body of left thumb without damage to nail
     ● **S61.039** Puncture wound without foreign body of unspecified thumb without damage to nail

● **S61.04** Puncture wound with foreign body of thumb without damage to nail
     ● **S61.041** Puncture wound with foreign body of right thumb without damage to nail
     ● **S61.042** Puncture wound with foreign body of left thumb without damage to nail
     ● **S61.049** Puncture wound with foreign body of unspecified thumb without damage to nail

● **S61.05** Open bite of thumb without damage to nail
     Bite of thumb NOS
     Excludes1   superficial bite of thumb (S60.36-, S60.37-)
     ● **S61.051** Open bite of right thumb without damage to nail
     ● **S61.052** Open bite of left thumb without damage to nail
     ● **S61.059** Open bite of unspecified thumb without damage to nail

● **S61.1** Open wound of thumb with damage to nail
     ● **S61.10** Unspecified open wound of thumb with damage to nail
         ● **S61.101** Unspecified open wound of right thumb with damage to nail
         ● **S61.102** Unspecified open wound of left thumb with damage to nail
         ● **S61.109** Unspecified open wound of unspecified thumb with damage to nail
     ● **S61.11** Laceration without foreign body of thumb with damage to nail
         ● **S61.111** Laceration without foreign body of right thumb with damage to nail
         ● **S61.112** Laceration without foreign body of left thumb with damage to nail
         ● **S61.119** Laceration without foreign body of unspecified thumb with damage to nail

● **S61.12** Laceration with foreign body of thumb with damage to nail
     ● **S61.121** Laceration with foreign body of right thumb with damage to nail
     ● **S61.122** Laceration with foreign body of left thumb with damage to nail
     ● **S61.129** Laceration with foreign body of unspecified thumb with damage to nail

● **S61.13** Puncture wound without foreign body of thumb with damage to nail
     ● **S61.131** Puncture wound without foreign body of right thumb with damage to nail
     ● **S61.132** Puncture wound without foreign body of left thumb with damage to nail
     ● **S61.139** Puncture wound without foreign body of unspecified thumb with damage to nail

● **S61.14** Puncture wound with foreign body of thumb with damage to nail
     ● **S61.141** Puncture wound with foreign body of right thumb with damage to nail
     ● **S61.142** Puncture wound with foreign body of left thumb with damage to nail
     ● **S61.149** Puncture wound with foreign body of unspecified thumb with damage to nail

● **S61.15** Open bite of thumb with damage to nail
     Bite of thumb with damage to nail NOS
     Excludes1   superficial bite of thumb (S60.36-, S60.37-)
     ● **S61.151** Open bite of right thumb with damage to nail
     ● **S61.152** Open bite of left thumb with damage to nail
     ● **S61.159** Open bite of unspecified thumb with damage to nail

● **S61.2** Open wound of other finger without damage to nail
     Excludes1   open wound of finger involving nail (matrix) (S61.3-)
     Excludes2   open wound of thumb without damage to nail (S61.0-)
     ● **S61.20** Unspecified open wound of other finger without damage to nail
         ● **S61.200** Unspecified open wound of right index finger without damage to nail
         ● **S61.201** Unspecified open wound of left index finger without damage to nail
         ● **S61.202** Unspecified open wound of right middle finger without damage to nail
         ● **S61.203** Unspecified open wound of left middle finger without damage to nail
         ● **S61.204** Unspecified open wound of right ring finger without damage to nail
         ● **S61.205** Unspecified open wound of left ring finger without damage to nail
         ● **S61.206** Unspecified open wound of right little finger without damage to nail
         ● **S61.207** Unspecified open wound of left little finger without damage to nail
         ● **S61.208** Unspecified open wound of other finger without damage to nail
             Unspecified open wound of specified finger with unspecified laterality without damage to nail
         ● **S61.209** Unspecified open wound of unspecified finger without damage to nail

CHAPTER 19 (S00-T88)

● S61.21   Laceration without foreign body of finger
            without damage to nail
    ● S61.210   Laceration without foreign body of
                 right index finger without damage to
                 nail
    ● S61.211   Laceration without foreign body of
                 left index finger without damage to
                 nail
    ● S61.212   Laceration without foreign body of
                 right middle finger without damage
                 to nail
    ● S61.213   Laceration without foreign body of
                 left middle finger without damage to
                 nail
    ● S61.214   Laceration without foreign body of
                 right ring finger without damage to
                 nail
    ● S61.215   Laceration without foreign body of
                 left ring finger without damage to nail
    ● S61.216   Laceration without foreign body of
                 right little finger without damage to
                 nail
    ● S61.217   Laceration without foreign body of
                 left little finger without damage to
                 nail
    ● S61.218   Laceration without foreign body of
                 other finger without damage to nail
                     Laceration without foreign body
                         of specified finger with
                         unspecified laterality without
                         damage to nail
    ● S61.219   Laceration without foreign body of
                 unspecified finger without damage to
                 nail
● S61.22   Laceration with foreign body of finger without
            damage to nail
    ● S61.220   Laceration with foreign body of right
                 index finger without damage to nail
    ● S61.221   Laceration with foreign body of left
                 index finger without damage to nail
    ● S61.222   Laceration with foreign body of right
                 middle finger without damage to nail
    ● S61.223   Laceration with foreign body of left
                 middle finger without damage to nail
    ● S61.224   Laceration with foreign body of right
                 ring finger without damage to nail
    ● S61.225   Laceration with foreign body of left
                 ring finger without damage to nail
    ● S61.226   Laceration with foreign body of right
                 little finger without damage to nail
    ● S61.227   Laceration with foreign body of left
                 little finger without damage to nail
    ● S61.228   Laceration with foreign body of other
                 finger without damage to nail
                     Laceration with foreign body
                         of specified finger with
                         unspecified laterality without
                         damage to nail
    ● S61.229   Laceration with foreign body of
                 unspecified finger without damage to
                 nail

● S61.23   Puncture wound without foreign body of finger
            without damage to nail
    ● S61.230   Puncture wound without foreign
                 body of right index finger without
                 damage to nail
    ● S61.231   Puncture wound without foreign
                 body of left index finger without
                 damage to nail
    ● S61.232   Puncture wound without foreign
                 body of right middle finger without
                 damage to nail
    ● S61.233   Puncture wound without foreign
                 body of left middle finger without
                 damage to nail
    ● S61.234   Puncture wound without foreign
                 body of right ring finger without
                 damage to nail
    ● S61.235   Puncture wound without foreign
                 body of left ring finger without
                 damage to nail
    ● S61.236   Puncture wound without foreign
                 body of right little finger without
                 damage to nail
    ● S61.237   Puncture wound without foreign
                 body of left little finger without
                 damage to nail
    ● S61.238   Puncture wound without foreign
                 body of other finger without damage
                 to nail
                     Puncture wound without foreign
                         body of specified finger with
                         unspecified laterality without
                         damage to nail
    ● S61.239   Puncture wound without foreign
                 body of unspecified finger without
                 damage to nail
● S61.24   Puncture wound with foreign body of finger
            without damage to nail
    ● S61.240   Puncture wound with foreign body of
                 right index finger without damage to
                 nail
    ● S61.241   Puncture wound with foreign body
                 of left index finger without damage to
                 nail
    ● S61.242   Puncture wound with foreign body of
                 right middle finger without damage
                 to nail
    ● S61.243   Puncture wound with foreign body of
                 left middle finger without damage to
                 nail
    ● S61.244   Puncture wound with foreign body
                 of right ring finger without damage to
                 nail
    ● S61.245   Puncture wound with foreign body of
                 left ring finger without damage to nail
    ● S61.246   Puncture wound with foreign body of
                 right little finger without damage to
                 nail
    ● S61.247   Puncture wound with foreign body
                 of left little finger without damage to
                 nail
    ● S61.248   Puncture wound with foreign body of
                 other finger without damage to nail
                     Puncture wound with foreign
                         body of specified finger with
                         unspecified laterality without
                         damage to nail
    ● S61.249   Puncture wound with foreign body of
                 unspecified finger without damage to
                 nail

◄ New   ◄▥ Revised   ~~deleted~~ Deleted   OGCR Official Guidelines   X Assign placeholder X   ● Use Additional Character(s)

Excludes 1   Excludes 2   Includes   Use additional   Code first   Code also   Unspecified

● S61.25   **Open bite of finger without damage to nail**
            Bite of finger without damage to nail NOS
            Excludes1   superficial bite of finger (S60.46-, S60.47-)

● S61.250   **Open bite of right index finger without damage to nail**

● S61.251   **Open bite of left index finger without damage to nail**

● S61.252   **Open bite of right middle finger without damage to nail**

● S61.253   **Open bite of left middle finger without damage to nail**

● S61.254   **Open bite of right ring finger without damage to nail**

● S61.255   **Open bite of left ring finger without damage to nail**

● S61.256   **Open bite of right little finger without damage to nail**

● S61.257   **Open bite of left little finger without damage to nail**

● S61.258   **Open bite of other finger without damage to nail**
            Open bite of specified finger with unspecified laterality without damage to nail

● S61.259   **Open bite of unspecified finger without damage to nail**

● S61.3   **Open wound of other finger with damage to nail**

● S61.30   **Unspecified open wound of finger with damage to nail**

● S61.300   **Unspecified open wound of right index finger with damage to nail**

● S61.301   **Unspecified open wound of left index finger with damage to nail**

● S61.302   **Unspecified open wound of right middle finger with damage to nail**

● S61.303   **Unspecified open wound of left middle finger with damage to nail**

● S61.304   **Unspecified open wound of right ring finger with damage to nail**

● S61.305   **Unspecified open wound of left ring finger with damage to nail**

● S61.306   **Unspecified open wound of right little finger with damage to nail**

● S61.307   **Unspecified open wound of left little finger with damage to nail**

● S61.308   **Unspecified open wound of other finger with damage to nail**
            Unspecified open wound of specified finger with unspecified laterality with damage to nail

● S61.309   **Unspecified open wound of unspecified finger with damage to nail**

● S61.31   **Laceration without foreign body of finger with damage to nail**

● S61.310   **Laceration without foreign body of right index finger with damage to nail**

● S61.311   **Laceration without foreign body of left index finger with damage to nail**

● S61.312   **Laceration without foreign body of right middle finger with damage to nail**

● S61.313   **Laceration without foreign body of left middle finger with damage to nail**

● S61.314   **Laceration without foreign body of right ring finger with damage to nail**

● S61.315   **Laceration without foreign body of left ring finger with damage to nail**

● S61.316   **Laceration without foreign body of right little finger with damage to nail**

● S61.317   **Laceration without foreign body of left little finger with damage to nail**

● S61.318   **Laceration without foreign body of other finger with damage to nail**
            Laceration without foreign body of specified finger with unspecified laterality with damage to nail

● S61.319   **Laceration without foreign body of unspecified finger with damage to nail**

● S61.32   **Laceration with foreign body of finger with damage to nail**

● S61.320   **Laceration with foreign body of right index finger with damage to nail**

● S61.321   **Laceration with foreign body of left index finger with damage to nail**

● S61.322   **Laceration with foreign body of right middle finger with damage to nail**

● S61.323   **Laceration with foreign body of left middle finger with damage to nail**

● S61.324   **Laceration with foreign body of right ring finger with damage to nail**

● S61.325   **Laceration with foreign body of left ring finger with damage to nail**

● S61.326   **Laceration with foreign body of right little finger with damage to nail**

● S61.327   **Laceration with foreign body of left little finger with damage to nail**

● S61.328   **Laceration with foreign body of other finger with damage to nail**
            Laceration with foreign body of specified finger with unspecified laterality with damage to nail

● S61.329   **Laceration with foreign body of unspecified finger with damage to nail**

● S61.33   **Puncture wound without foreign body of finger with damage to nail**

● S61.330   **Puncture wound without foreign body of right index finger with damage to nail**

● S61.331   **Puncture wound without foreign body of left index finger with damage to nail**

● S61.332   **Puncture wound without foreign body of right middle finger with damage to nail**

● S61.333   **Puncture wound without foreign body of left middle finger with damage to nail**

● S61.334   **Puncture wound without foreign body of right ring finger with damage to nail**

● S61.335   **Puncture wound without foreign body of left ring finger with damage to nail**

● S61.336   **Puncture wound without foreign body of right little finger with damage to nail**

● S61.337   **Puncture wound without foreign body of left little finger with damage to nail**

- S61.338   **Puncture wound without foreign body of other finger with damage to nail**
  - Puncture wound without foreign body of specified finger with unspecified laterality with damage to nail
- S61.339   **Puncture wound without foreign body of unspecified finger with damage to nail**
- S61.34   **Puncture wound with foreign body of finger with damage to nail**
  - S61.340   **Puncture wound with foreign body of right index finger with damage to nail**
  - S61.341   **Puncture wound with foreign body of left index finger with damage to nail**
  - S61.342   **Puncture wound with foreign body of right middle finger with damage to nail**
  - S61.343   **Puncture wound with foreign body of left middle finger with damage to nail**
  - S61.344   **Puncture wound with foreign body of right ring finger with damage to nail**
  - S61.345   **Puncture wound with foreign body of left ring finger with damage to nail**
  - S61.346   **Puncture wound with foreign body of right little finger with damage to nail**
  - S61.347   **Puncture wound with foreign body of left little finger with damage to nail**
  - S61.348   **Puncture wound with foreign body of other finger with damage to nail**
    - Puncture wound with foreign body of specified finger with unspecified laterality with damage to nail
  - S61.349   **Puncture wound with foreign body of unspecified finger with damage to nail**
- S61.35   **Open bite of finger with damage to nail**
  - Bite of finger with damage to nail NOS
  - **Excludes1**   superficial bite of finger (S60.46-, S60.47-)
  - S61.350   **Open bite of right index finger with damage to nail**
  - S61.351   **Open bite of left index finger with damage to nail**
  - S61.352   **Open bite of right middle finger with damage to nail**
  - S61.353   **Open bite of left middle finger with damage to nail**
  - S61.354   **Open bite of right ring finger with damage to nail**
  - S61.355   **Open bite of left ring finger with damage to nail**
  - S61.356   **Open bite of right little finger with damage to nail**
  - S61.357   **Open bite of left little finger with damage to nail**
  - S61.358   **Open bite of other finger with damage to nail**
    - Open bite of specified finger with unspecified laterality with damage to nail
  - S61.359   **Open bite of unspecified finger with damage to nail**

- S61.4   **Open wound of hand**
  - S61.40   **Unspecified open wound of hand**
    - S61.401   **Unspecified open wound of right hand**
    - S61.402   **Unspecified open wound of left hand**
    - S61.409   **Unspecified open wound of unspecified hand**
  - S61.41   **Laceration without foreign body of hand**
    - S61.411   **Laceration without foreign body of right hand**
    - S61.412   **Laceration without foreign body of left hand**
    - S61.419   **Laceration without foreign body of unspecified hand**
  - S61.42   **Laceration with foreign body of hand**
    - S61.421   **Laceration with foreign body of right hand**
    - S61.422   **Laceration with foreign body of left hand**
    - S61.429   **Laceration with foreign body of unspecified hand**
  - S61.43   **Puncture wound without foreign body of hand**
    - S61.431   **Puncture wound without foreign body of right hand**
    - S61.432   **Puncture wound without foreign body of left hand**
    - S61.439   **Puncture wound without foreign body of unspecified hand**
  - S61.44   **Puncture wound with foreign body of hand**
    - S61.441   **Puncture wound with foreign body of right hand**
    - S61.442   **Puncture wound with foreign body of left hand**
    - S61.449   **Puncture wound with foreign body of unspecified hand**
  - S61.45   **Open bite of hand**
    - Bite of hand NOS
    - **Excludes1**   superficial bite of hand (S60.56-, S60.57-)
    - S61.451   **Open bite of right hand**
    - S61.452   **Open bite of left hand**
    - S61.459   **Open bite of unspecified hand**
- S61.5   **Open wound of wrist**
  - S61.50   **Unspecified open wound of wrist**
    - S61.501   **Unspecified open wound of right wrist**
    - S61.502   **Unspecified open wound of left wrist**
    - S61.509   **Unspecified open wound of unspecified wrist**
  - S61.51   **Laceration without foreign body of wrist**
    - S61.511   **Laceration without foreign body of right wrist**
    - S61.512   **Laceration without foreign body of left wrist**
    - S61.519   **Laceration without foreign body of unspecified wrist**
  - S61.52   **Laceration with foreign body of wrist**
    - S61.521   **Laceration with foreign body of right wrist**
    - S61.522   **Laceration with foreign body of left wrist**
    - S61.529   **Laceration with foreign body of unspecified wrist**

◀ New   ◀ Revised   ~~deleted~~ Deleted   OGCR Official Guidelines   X Assign placeholder X   ● Use Additional Character(s)

Excludes 1   Excludes 2   Includes   Use additional   Code first   Code also   Unspecified

● **S61.53**   **Puncture wound without foreign body of wrist**
    ● **S61.531**   **Puncture wound without foreign body of right wrist**
    ● **S61.532**   **Puncture wound without foreign body of left wrist**
    ● **S61.539**   **Puncture wound without foreign body of unspecified wrist**

● **S61.54**   **Puncture wound with foreign body of wrist**
    ● **S61.541**   **Puncture wound with foreign body of right wrist**
    ● **S61.542**   **Puncture wound with foreign body of left wrist**
    ● **S61.549**   **Puncture wound with foreign body of unspecified wrist**

● **S61.55**   **Open bite of wrist**
    Bite of wrist NOS
    Excludes1   superficial bite of wrist (S60.86-, S60.87-)
    ● **S61.551**   **Open bite of right wrist**
    ● **S61.552**   **Open bite of left wrist**
    ● **S61.559**   **Open bite of unspecified wrist**

● **S62**   **Fracture at wrist and hand level**
    Note: A fracture not indicated as displaced or nondisplaced should be coded to displaced

    A fracture not indicated as open or closed should be coded to closed

    Excludes1   traumatic amputation of wrist and hand (S68.-)
    Excludes2   fracture of distal parts of ulna and radius (S52.-)

    The appropriate 7th character is to be added to each code from category S62

    A   initial encounter for closed fracture
    B   initial encounter for open fracture
    D   subsequent encounter for fracture with routine healing
    G   subsequent encounter for fracture with delayed healing
    K   subsequent encounter for fracture with nonunion
    P   subsequent encounter for fracture with malunion
    S   sequela

● **S62.0**   **Fracture of navicular [scaphoid] bone of wrist**
    ● **S62.00**   **Unspecified fracture of navicular [scaphoid] bone of wrist**
      ● **S62.001**   **Unspecified fracture of navicular [scaphoid] bone of right wrist**
      ● **S62.002**   **Unspecified fracture of navicular [scaphoid] bone of left wrist**
      ● **S62.009**   **Unspecified fracture of navicular [scaphoid] bone of unspecified wrist**

    ● **S62.01**   **Fracture of distal pole of navicular [scaphoid] bone of wrist**
      Fracture of volar tuberosity of navicular [scaphoid] bone of wrist
      ● **S62.011**   **Displaced fracture of distal pole of navicular [scaphoid] bone of right wrist**
      ● **S62.012**   **Displaced fracture of distal pole of navicular [scaphoid] bone of left wrist**
      ● **S62.013**   **Displaced fracture of distal pole of navicular [scaphoid] bone of unspecified wrist**
      ● **S62.014**   **Nondisplaced fracture of distal pole of navicular [scaphoid] bone of right wrist**
      ● **S62.015**   **Nondisplaced fracture of distal pole of navicular [scaphoid] bone of left wrist**
      ● **S62.016**   **Nondisplaced fracture of distal pole of navicular [scaphoid] bone of unspecified wrist**

● **S62.02**   **Fracture of middle third of navicular [scaphoid] bone of wrist**
    ● **S62.021**   **Displaced fracture of middle third of navicular [scaphoid] bone of right wrist**
    ● **S62.022**   **Displaced fracture of middle third of navicular [scaphoid] bone of left wrist**
    ● **S62.023**   **Displaced fracture of middle third of navicular [scaphoid] bone of unspecified wrist**
    ● **S62.024**   **Nondisplaced fracture of middle third of navicular [scaphoid] bone of right wrist**
    ● **S62.025**   **Nondisplaced fracture of middle third of navicular [scaphoid] bone of left wrist**
    ● **S62.026**   **Nondisplaced fracture of middle third of navicular [scaphoid] bone of unspecified wrist**

● **S62.03**   **Fracture of proximal third of navicular [scaphoid] bone of wrist**
    ● **S62.031**   **Displaced fracture of proximal third of navicular [scaphoid] bone of right wrist**
    ● **S62.032**   **Displaced fracture of proximal third of navicular [scaphoid] bone of left wrist**
    ● **S62.033**   **Displaced fracture of proximal third of navicular [scaphoid] bone of unspecified wrist**
    ● **S62.034**   **Nondisplaced fracture of proximal third of navicular [scaphoid] bone of right wrist**
    ● **S62.035**   **Nondisplaced fracture of proximal third of navicular [scaphoid] bone of left wrist**
    ● **S62.036**   **Nondisplaced fracture of proximal third of navicular [scaphoid] bone of unspecified wrist**

● **S62.1**   **Fracture of other and unspecified carpal bone(s)**
    Excludes2   fracture of scaphoid of wrist (S62.0-)
    ● **S62.10**   **Fracture of unspecified carpal bone**
      Fracture of wrist NOS
      ● **S62.101**   **Fracture of unspecified carpal bone, right wrist**
      ● **S62.102**   **Fracture of unspecified carpal bone, left wrist**
      ● **S62.109**   **Fracture of unspecified carpal bone, unspecified wrist**

    ● **S62.11**   **Fracture of triquetrum [cuneiform] bone of wrist**
      ● **S62.111**   **Displaced fracture of triquetrum [cuneiform] bone, right wrist**
      ● **S62.112**   **Displaced fracture of triquetrum [cuneiform] bone, left wrist**
      ● **S62.113**   **Displaced fracture of triquetrum [cuneiform] bone, unspecified wrist**
      ● **S62.114**   **Nondisplaced fracture of triquetrum [cuneiform] bone, right wrist**
      ● **S62.115**   **Nondisplaced fracture of triquetrum [cuneiform] bone, left wrist**
      ● **S62.116**   **Nondisplaced fracture of triquetrum [cuneiform] bone, unspecified wrist**

    ● **S62.12**   **Fracture of lunate [semilunar]**
      ● **S62.121**   **Displaced fracture of lunate [semilunar], right wrist**
      ● **S62.122**   **Displaced fracture of lunate [semilunar], left wrist**

- **S62.123** Displaced fracture of lunate [semilunar], unspecified wrist
- **S62.124** Nondisplaced fracture of lunate [semilunar], right wrist
- **S62.125** Nondisplaced fracture of lunate [semilunar], left wrist
- **S62.126** Nondisplaced fracture of lunate [semilunar], unspecified wrist
- **S62.13** Fracture of capitate [os magnum] bone
  - **S62.131** Displaced fracture of capitate [os magnum] bone, right wrist
  - **S62.132** Displaced fracture of capitate [os magnum] bone, left wrist
  - **S62.133** Displaced fracture of capitate [os magnum] bone, unspecified wrist
  - **S62.134** Nondisplaced fracture of capitate [os magnum] bone, right wrist
  - **S62.135** Nondisplaced fracture of capitate [os magnum] bone, left wrist
  - **S62.136** Nondisplaced fracture of capitate [os magnum] bone, unspecified wrist
- **S62.14** Fracture of body of hamate [unciform] bone
  Fracture of hamate [unciform] bone NOS
  - **S62.141** Displaced fracture of body of hamate [unciform] bone, right wrist
  - **S62.142** Displaced fracture of body of hamate [unciform] bone, left wrist
  - **S62.143** Displaced fracture of body of hamate [unciform] bone, unspecified wrist
  - **S62.144** Nondisplaced fracture of body of hamate [unciform] bone, right wrist
  - **S62.145** Nondisplaced fracture of body of hamate [unciform] bone, left wrist
  - **S62.146** Nondisplaced fracture of body of hamate [unciform] bone, unspecified wrist
- **S62.15** Fracture of hook process of hamate [unciform] bone
  Fracture of unciform process of hamate [unciform] bone
  - **S62.151** Displaced fracture of hook process of hamate [unciform] bone, right wrist
  - **S62.152** Displaced fracture of hook process of hamate [unciform] bone, left wrist
  - **S62.153** Displaced fracture of hook process of hamate [unciform] bone, unspecified wrist
  - **S62.154** Nondisplaced fracture of hook process of hamate [unciform] bone, right wrist
  - **S62.155** Nondisplaced fracture of hook process of hamate [unciform] bone, left wrist
  - **S62.156** Nondisplaced fracture of hook process of hamate [unciform] bone, unspecified wrist
- **S62.16** Fracture of pisiform
  - **S62.161** Displaced fracture of pisiform, right wrist
  - **S62.162** Displaced fracture of pisiform, left wrist
  - **S62.163** Displaced fracture of pisiform, unspecified wrist
  - **S62.164** Nondisplaced fracture of pisiform, right wrist
  - **S62.165** Nondisplaced fracture of pisiform, left wrist
  - **S62.166** Nondisplaced fracture of pisiform, unspecified wrist

- **S62.17** Fracture of trapezium [larger multangular]
  - **S62.171** Displaced fracture of trapezium [larger multangular], right wrist
  - **S62.172** Displaced fracture of trapezium [larger multangular], left wrist
  - **S62.173** Displaced fracture of trapezium [larger multangular], unspecified wrist
  - **S62.174** Nondisplaced fracture of trapezium [larger multangular], right wrist
  - **S62.175** Nondisplaced fracture of trapezium [larger multangular], left wrist
  - **S62.176** Nondisplaced fracture of trapezium [larger multangular], unspecified wrist
- **S62.18** Fracture of trapezoid [smaller multangular]
  - **S62.181** Displaced fracture of trapezoid [smaller multangular], right wrist
  - **S62.182** Displaced fracture of trapezoid [smaller multangular], left wrist
  - **S62.183** Displaced fracture of trapezoid [smaller multangular], unspecified wrist
  - **S62.184** Nondisplaced fracture of trapezoid [smaller multangular], right wrist
  - **S62.185** Nondisplaced fracture of trapezoid [smaller multangular], left wrist
  - **S62.186** Nondisplaced fracture of trapezoid [smaller multangular], unspecified wrist
- **S62.2** Fracture of first metacarpal bone
  - **S62.20** Unspecified fracture of first metacarpal bone
    - **S62.201** Unspecified fracture of first metacarpal bone, right hand
    - **S62.202** Unspecified fracture of first metacarpal bone, left hand
    - **S62.209** Unspecified fracture of first metacarpal bone, unspecified hand
  - **S62.21** Bennett's fracture
    - **S62.211** Bennett's fracture, right hand
    - **S62.212** Bennett's fracture, left hand
    - **S62.213** Bennett's fracture, unspecified hand
  - **S62.22** Rolando's fracture
    - **S62.221** Displaced Rolando's fracture, right hand
    - **S62.222** Displaced Rolando's fracture, left hand
    - **S62.223** Displaced Rolando's fracture, unspecified hand
    - **S62.224** Nondisplaced Rolando's fracture, right hand
    - **S62.225** Nondisplaced Rolando's fracture, left hand
    - **S62.226** Nondisplaced Rolando's fracture, unspecified hand
  - **S62.23** Other fracture of base of first metacarpal bone
    - **S62.231** Other displaced fracture of base of first metacarpal bone, right hand
    - **S62.232** Other displaced fracture of base of first metacarpal bone, left hand
    - **S62.233** Other displaced fracture of base of first metacarpal bone, unspecified hand
    - **S62.234** Other nondisplaced fracture of base of first metacarpal bone, right hand
    - **S62.235** Other nondisplaced fracture of base of first metacarpal bone, left hand
    - **S62.236** Other nondisplaced fracture of base of first metacarpal bone, unspecified hand

● S62.24   Fracture of shaft of first metacarpal bone
- ● S62.241   Displaced fracture of shaft of first metacarpal bone, right hand
- ● S62.242   Displaced fracture of shaft of first metacarpal bone, left hand
- ● S62.243   Displaced fracture of shaft of first metacarpal bone, unspecified hand
- ● S62.244   Nondisplaced fracture of shaft of first metacarpal bone, right hand
- ● S62.245   Nondisplaced fracture of shaft of first metacarpal bone, left hand
- ● S62.246   Nondisplaced fracture of shaft of first metacarpal bone, unspecified hand

● S62.25   Fracture of neck of first metacarpal bone
- ● S62.251   Displaced fracture of neck of first metacarpal bone, right hand
- ● S62.252   Displaced fracture of neck of first metacarpal bone, left hand
- ● S62.253   Displaced fracture of neck of first metacarpal bone, unspecified hand
- ● S62.254   Nondisplaced fracture of neck of first metacarpal bone, right hand
- ● S62.255   Nondisplaced fracture of neck of first metacarpal bone, left hand
- ● S62.256   Nondisplaced fracture of neck of first metacarpal bone, unspecified hand

● S62.29   Other fracture of first metacarpal bone
- ● S62.291   Other fracture of first metacarpal bone, right hand
- ● S62.292   Other fracture of first metacarpal bone, left hand
- ● S62.299   Other fracture of first metacarpal bone, unspecified hand

● S62.3   Fracture of other and unspecified metacarpal bone
> **Excludes2**   fracture of first metacarpal bone (S62.2-)

● S62.30   Unspecified fracture of other metacarpal bone
- ● S62.300   Unspecified fracture of second metacarpal bone, right hand
- ● S62.301   Unspecified fracture of second metacarpal bone, left hand
- ● S62.302   Unspecified fracture of third metacarpal bone, right hand
- ● S62.303   Unspecified fracture of third metacarpal bone, left hand
- ● S62.304   Unspecified fracture of fourth metacarpal bone, right hand
- ● S62.305   Unspecified fracture of fourth metacarpal bone, left hand
- ● S62.306   Unspecified fracture of fifth metacarpal bone, right hand
- ● S62.307   Unspecified fracture of fifth metacarpal bone, left hand
- ● S62.308   Unspecified fracture of other metacarpal bone
  > Unspecified fracture of specified metacarpal bone with unspecified laterality
- ● S62.309   Unspecified fracture of unspecified metacarpal bone

● S62.31   Displaced fracture of base of other metacarpal bone
- ● S62.310   Displaced fracture of base of second metacarpal bone, right hand
- ● S62.311   Displaced fracture of base of second metacarpal bone, left hand
- ● S62.312   Displaced fracture of base of third metacarpal bone, right hand

- ● S62.313   Displaced fracture of base of third metacarpal bone, left hand
- ● S62.314   Displaced fracture of base of fourth metacarpal bone, right hand
- ● S62.315   Displaced fracture of base of fourth metacarpal bone, left hand
- ● S62.316   Displaced fracture of base of fifth metacarpal bone, right hand
- ● S62.317   Displaced fracture of base of fifth metacarpal bone, left hand
- ● S62.318   Displaced fracture of base of other metacarpal bone
  > Displaced fracture of base of specified metacarpal bone with unspecified laterality
- ● S62.319   Displaced fracture of base of unspecified metacarpal bone

● S62.32   Displaced fracture of shaft of other metacarpal bone
- ● S62.320   Displaced fracture of shaft of second metacarpal bone, right hand
- ● S62.321   Displaced fracture of shaft of second metacarpal bone, left hand
- ● S62.322   Displaced fracture of shaft of third metacarpal bone, right hand
- ● S62.323   Displaced fracture of shaft of third metacarpal bone, left hand
- ● S62.324   Displaced fracture of shaft of fourth metacarpal bone, right hand
- ● S62.325   Displaced fracture of shaft of fourth metacarpal bone, left hand
- ● S62.326   Displaced fracture of shaft of fifth metacarpal bone, right hand
- ● S62.327   Displaced fracture of shaft of fifth metacarpal bone, left hand
- ● S62.328   Displaced fracture of shaft of other metacarpal bone
  > Displaced fracture of shaft of specified metacarpal bone with unspecified laterality
- ● S62.329   Displaced fracture of shaft of unspecified metacarpal bone

● S62.33   Displaced fracture of neck of other metacarpal bone
- ● S62.330   Displaced fracture of neck of second metacarpal bone, right hand
- ● S62.331   Displaced fracture of neck of second metacarpal bone, left hand
- ● S62.332   Displaced fracture of neck of third metacarpal bone, right hand
- ● S62.333   Displaced fracture of neck of third metacarpal bone, left hand
- ● S62.334   Displaced fracture of neck of fourth metacarpal bone, right hand
- ● S62.335   Displaced fracture of neck of fourth metacarpal bone, left hand
- ● S62.336   Displaced fracture of neck of fifth metacarpal bone, right hand
- ● S62.337   Displaced fracture of neck of fifth metacarpal bone, left hand
- ● S62.338   Displaced fracture of neck of other metacarpal bone
  > Displaced fracture of neck of specified metacarpal bone with unspecified laterality
- ● S62.339   Displaced fracture of neck of unspecified metacarpal bone

◀ New   ◀|||| Revised   ~~deleted~~ Deleted   **OGCR** Official Guidelines   X Assign placeholder X   ● Use Additional Character(s)

Excludes 1   Excludes 2   Includes   Use additional   Code first   Code also   Unspecified

1309

● S62.34 Nondisplaced fracture of base of other metacarpal bone
  ● S62.340 Nondisplaced fracture of base of second metacarpal bone, right hand
  ● S62.341 Nondisplaced fracture of base of second metacarpal bone, left hand
  ● S62.342 Nondisplaced fracture of base of third metacarpal bone, right hand
  ● S62.343 Nondisplaced fracture of base of third metacarpal bone, left hand
  ● S62.344 Nondisplaced fracture of base of fourth metacarpal bone, right hand
  ● S62.345 Nondisplaced fracture of base of fourth metacarpal bone, left hand
  ● S62.346 Nondisplaced fracture of base of fifth metacarpal bone, right hand
  ● S62.347 Nondisplaced fracture of base of fifth metacarpal bone, left hand
  ● S62.348 Nondisplaced fracture of base of other metacarpal bone
    Nondisplaced fracture of base of specified metacarpal bone with unspecified laterality
  ● S62.349 Nondisplaced fracture of base of unspecified metacarpal bone

● S62.35 Nondisplaced fracture of shaft of other metacarpal bone
  ● S62.350 Nondisplaced fracture of shaft of second metacarpal bone, right hand
  ● S62.351 Nondisplaced fracture of shaft of second metacarpal bone, left hand
  ● S62.352 Nondisplaced fracture of shaft of third metacarpal bone, right hand
  ● S62.353 Nondisplaced fracture of shaft of third metacarpal bone, left hand
  ● S62.354 Nondisplaced fracture of shaft of fourth metacarpal bone, right hand
  ● S62.355 Nondisplaced fracture of shaft of fourth metacarpal bone, left hand
  ● S62.356 Nondisplaced fracture of shaft of fifth metacarpal bone, right hand
  ● S62.357 Nondisplaced fracture of shaft of fifth metacarpal bone, left hand
  ● S62.358 Nondisplaced fracture of shaft of other metacarpal bone
    Nondisplaced fracture of shaft of specified metacarpal bone with unspecified laterality
  ● S62.359 Nondisplaced fracture of shaft of unspecified metacarpal bone

● S62.36 Nondisplaced fracture of neck of other metacarpal bone
  ● S62.360 Nondisplaced fracture of neck of second metacarpal bone, right hand
  ● S62.361 Nondisplaced fracture of neck of second metacarpal bone, left hand
  ● S62.362 Nondisplaced fracture of neck of third metacarpal bone, right hand
  ● S62.363 Nondisplaced fracture of neck of third metacarpal bone, left hand
  ● S62.364 Nondisplaced fracture of neck of fourth metacarpal bone, right hand
  ● S62.365 Nondisplaced fracture of neck of fourth metacarpal bone, left hand
  ● S62.366 Nondisplaced fracture of neck of fifth metacarpal bone, right hand
  ● S62.367 Nondisplaced fracture of neck of fifth metacarpal bone, left hand

● S62.368 Nondisplaced fracture of neck of other metacarpal bone
    Nondisplaced fracture of neck of specified metacarpal bone with unspecified laterality
  ● S62.369 Nondisplaced fracture of neck of unspecified metacarpal bone

● S62.39 Other fracture of other metacarpal bone
  ● S62.390 Other fracture of second metacarpal bone, right hand
  ● S62.391 Other fracture of second metacarpal bone, left hand
  ● S62.392 Other fracture of third metacarpal bone, right hand
  ● S62.393 Other fracture of third metacarpal bone, left hand
  ● S62.394 Other fracture of fourth metacarpal bone, right hand
  ● S62.395 Other fracture of fourth metacarpal bone, left hand
  ● S62.396 Other fracture of fifth metacarpal bone, right hand
  ● S62.397 Other fracture of fifth metacarpal bone, left hand
  ● S62.398 Other fracture of other metacarpal bone
    Other fracture of specified metacarpal bone with unspecified laterality
  ● S62.399 Other fracture of unspecified metacarpal bone

● S62.5 Fracture of thumb
  ● S62.50 Fracture of unspecified phalanx of thumb
    ● S62.501 Fracture of unspecified phalanx of right thumb
    ● S62.502 Fracture of unspecified phalanx of left thumb
    ● S62.509 Fracture of unspecified phalanx of unspecified thumb
  ● S62.51 Fracture of proximal phalanx of thumb
    ● S62.511 Displaced fracture of proximal phalanx of right thumb
    ● S62.512 Displaced fracture of proximal phalanx of left thumb
    ● S62.513 Displaced fracture of proximal phalanx of unspecified thumb
    ● S62.514 Nondisplaced fracture of proximal phalanx of right thumb
    ● S62.515 Nondisplaced fracture of proximal phalanx of left thumb
    ● S62.516 Nondisplaced fracture of proximal phalanx of unspecified thumb
  ● S62.52 Fracture of distal phalanx of thumb
    ● S62.521 Displaced fracture of distal phalanx of right thumb
    ● S62.522 Displaced fracture of distal phalanx of left thumb
    ● S62.523 Displaced fracture of distal phalanx of unspecified thumb
    ● S62.524 Nondisplaced fracture of distal phalanx of right thumb
    ● S62.525 Nondisplaced fracture of distal phalanx of left thumb
    ● S62.526 Nondisplaced fracture of distal phalanx of unspecified thumb

◄ New   ◄▥ Revised   ~~deleted~~ Deleted   OGCR Official Guidelines   X Assign placeholder X   ● Use Additional Character(s)

Excludes 1   Excludes 2   Includes   Use additional   Code first   Code also   Unspecified

● **S62.6**   **Fracture of other and unspecified finger(s)**
   Excludes2   fracture of thumb (S62.5-)

   ● **S62.60**   **Fracture of unspecified phalanx of finger**

     ● **S62.600**   Fracture of unspecified phalanx of right index finger

     ● **S62.601**   Fracture of unspecified phalanx of left index finger

     ● **S62.602**   Fracture of unspecified phalanx of right middle finger

     ● **S62.603**   Fracture of unspecified phalanx of left middle finger

     ● **S62.604**   Fracture of unspecified phalanx of right ring finger

     ● **S62.605**   Fracture of unspecified phalanx of left ring finger

     ● **S62.606**   Fracture of unspecified phalanx of right little finger

     ● **S62.607**   Fracture of unspecified phalanx of left little finger

     ● **S62.608**   Fracture of unspecified phalanx of other finger
        Fracture of unspecified phalanx of specified finger with unspecified laterality

     ● **S62.609**   Fracture of unspecified phalanx of unspecified finger

   ● **S62.61**   **Displaced fracture of proximal phalanx of finger**

     ● **S62.610**   Displaced fracture of proximal phalanx of right index finger

     ● **S62.611**   Displaced fracture of proximal phalanx of left index finger

     ● **S62.612**   Displaced fracture of proximal phalanx of right middle finger

     ● **S62.613**   Displaced fracture of proximal phalanx of left middle finger

     ● **S62.614**   Displaced fracture of proximal phalanx of right ring finger

     ● **S62.615**   Displaced fracture of proximal phalanx of left ring finger

     ● **S62.616**   Displaced fracture of proximal phalanx of right little finger

     ● **S62.617**   Displaced fracture of proximal phalanx of left little finger

     ● **S62.618**   Displaced fracture of proximal phalanx of other finger
        Displaced fracture of proximal phalanx of specified finger with unspecified laterality

     ● **S62.619**   Displaced fracture of proximal phalanx of unspecified finger

   ● **S62.62**   **Displaced fracture of medial phalanx of finger**

     ● **S62.620**   Displaced fracture of medial phalanx of right index finger

     ● **S62.621**   Displaced fracture of medial phalanx of left index finger

     ● **S62.622**   Displaced fracture of medial phalanx of right middle finger

     ● **S62.623**   Displaced fracture of medial phalanx of left middle finger

     ● **S62.624**   Displaced fracture of medial phalanx of right ring finger

     ● **S62.625**   Displaced fracture of medial phalanx of left ring finger

     ● **S62.626**   Displaced fracture of medial phalanx of right little finger

     ● **S62.627**   Displaced fracture of medial phalanx of left little finger

     ● **S62.628**   Displaced fracture of medial phalanx of other finger
        Displaced fracture of medial phalanx of specified finger with unspecified laterality

     ● **S62.629**   Displaced fracture of medial phalanx of unspecified finger

   ● **S62.63**   **Displaced fracture of distal phalanx of finger**

     ● **S62.630**   Displaced fracture of distal phalanx of right index finger

     ● **S62.631**   Displaced fracture of distal phalanx of left index finger

     ● **S62.632**   Displaced fracture of distal phalanx of right middle finger

     ● **S62.633**   Displaced fracture of distal phalanx of left middle finger

     ● **S62.634**   Displaced fracture of distal phalanx of right ring finger

     ● **S62.635**   Displaced fracture of distal phalanx of left ring finger

     ● **S62.636**   Displaced fracture of distal phalanx of right little finger

     ● **S62.637**   Displaced fracture of distal phalanx of left little finger

     ● **S62.638**   Displaced fracture of distal phalanx of other finger
        Displaced fracture of distal phalanx of specified finger with unspecified laterality

     ● **S62.639**   Displaced fracture of distal phalanx of unspecified finger

   ● **S62.64**   **Nondisplaced fracture of proximal phalanx of finger**

     ● **S62.640**   Nondisplaced fracture of proximal phalanx of right index finger

     ● **S62.641**   Nondisplaced fracture of proximal phalanx of left index finger

     ● **S62.642**   Nondisplaced fracture of proximal phalanx of right middle finger

     ● **S62.643**   Nondisplaced fracture of proximal phalanx of left middle finger

     ● **S62.644**   Nondisplaced fracture of proximal phalanx of right ring finger

     ● **S62.645**   Nondisplaced fracture of proximal phalanx of left ring finger

     ● **S62.646**   Nondisplaced fracture of proximal phalanx of right little finger

     ● **S62.647**   Nondisplaced fracture of proximal phalanx of left little finger

     ● **S62.648**   Nondisplaced fracture of proximal phalanx of other finger
        Nondisplaced fracture of proximal phalanx of specified finger with unspecified laterality

     ● **S62.649**   Nondisplaced fracture of proximal phalanx of unspecified finger

   ● **S62.65**   **Nondisplaced fracture of medial phalanx of finger**

     ● **S62.650**   Nondisplaced fracture of medial phalanx of right index finger

     ● **S62.651**   Nondisplaced fracture of medial phalanx of left index finger

     ● **S62.652**   Nondisplaced fracture of medial phalanx of right middle finger

     ● **S62.653**   Nondisplaced fracture of medial phalanx of left middle finger

     ● **S62.654**   Nondisplaced fracture of medial phalanx of right ring finger

     ● **S62.655**   Nondisplaced fracture of medial phalanx of left ring finger

---

◀ New   ◀▥ Revised   ~~deleted~~ Deleted   OGCR Official Guidelines   X Assign placeholder X   ● Use Additional Character(s)

| Excludes 1 | Excludes 2 | Includes | Use additional | Code first | Code also | Unspecified |

S62.656 Nondisplaced fracture of medial phalanx of right little finger

S62.657 Nondisplaced fracture of medial phalanx of left little finger

S62.658 Nondisplaced fracture of medial phalanx of other finger
    Nondisplaced fracture of medial phalanx of specified finger with unspecified laterality

S62.659 Nondisplaced fracture of medial phalanx of unspecified finger

S62.66 Nondisplaced fracture of distal phalanx of finger

S62.660 Nondisplaced fracture of distal phalanx of right index finger

S62.661 Nondisplaced fracture of distal phalanx of left index finger

S62.662 Nondisplaced fracture of distal phalanx of right middle finger

S62.663 Nondisplaced fracture of distal phalanx of left middle finger

S62.664 Nondisplaced fracture of distal phalanx of right ring finger

S62.665 Nondisplaced fracture of distal phalanx of left ring finger

S62.666 Nondisplaced fracture of distal phalanx of right little finger

S62.667 Nondisplaced fracture of distal phalanx of left little finger

S62.668 Nondisplaced fracture of distal phalanx of other finger
    Nondisplaced fracture of distal phalanx of specified finger with unspecified laterality

S62.669 Nondisplaced fracture of distal phalanx of unspecified finger

S62.9 Unspecified fracture of wrist and hand

X ● S62.90 Unspecified fracture of unspecified wrist and hand

X ● S62.91 Unspecified fracture of right wrist and hand

X ● S62.92 Unspecified fracture of left wrist and hand

● S63 Dislocation and sprain of joints and ligaments at wrist and hand level

Includes avulsion of joint or ligament at wrist and hand level
laceration of cartilage, joint or ligament at wrist and hand level
sprain of cartilage, joint or ligament at wrist and hand level
traumatic hemarthrosis of joint or ligament at wrist and hand level
traumatic rupture of joint or ligament at wrist and hand level
traumatic subluxation of joint or ligament at wrist and hand level
traumatic tear of joint or ligament at wrist and hand level

Code also any associated open wound

Excludes2 strain of muscle, fascia and tendon of wrist and hand (S66.-)

The appropriate 7th character is to be added to each code from category S63

A initial encounter
D subsequent encounter
S sequela

● S63.0 Subluxation and dislocation of wrist and hand joints

● S63.00 Unspecified subluxation and dislocation of wrist and hand
Dislocation of carpal bone NOS
Dislocation of distal end of radius NOS
Subluxation of carpal bone NOS
Subluxation of distal end of radius NOS

A   B

Figure 19-13 Dislocation including displacement and subluxation. (From Grainger & Allison's Diagnostic Radiology: A Textbook of Medical Imaging, ed 4, Churchill Livingstone, 2001)

● S63.001 Unspecified subluxation of right wrist and hand

● S63.002 Unspecified subluxation of left wrist and hand

● S63.003 Unspecified subluxation of unspecified wrist and hand

● S63.004 Unspecified dislocation of right wrist and hand

● S63.005 Unspecified dislocation of left wrist and hand

● S63.006 Unspecified dislocation of unspecified wrist and hand

● S63.01 Subluxation and dislocation of distal radioulnar joint

● S63.011 Subluxation of distal radioulnar joint of right wrist

● S63.012 Subluxation of distal radioulnar joint of left wrist

● S63.013 Subluxation of distal radioulnar joint of unspecified wrist

● S63.014 Dislocation of distal radioulnar joint of right wrist

● S63.015 Dislocation of distal radioulnar joint of left wrist

● S63.016 Dislocation of distal radioulnar joint of unspecified wrist

● S63.02 Subluxation and dislocation of radiocarpal joint

● S63.021 Subluxation of radiocarpal joint of right wrist

● S63.022 Subluxation of radiocarpal joint of left wrist

● S63.023 Subluxation of radiocarpal joint of unspecified wrist

● S63.024 Dislocation of radiocarpal joint of right wrist

● S63.025 Dislocation of radiocarpal joint of left wrist

● S63.026 Dislocation of radiocarpal joint of unspecified wrist

● S63.03 Subluxation and dislocation of midcarpal joint

● S63.031 Subluxation of midcarpal joint of right wrist

● S63.032 Subluxation of midcarpal joint of left wrist

● S63.033 Subluxation of midcarpal joint of unspecified wrist

● S63.034 Dislocation of midcarpal joint of right wrist

● S63.035 Dislocation of midcarpal joint of left wrist

● S63.036 Dislocation of midcarpal joint of unspecified wrist

◀ New   ◀▦ Revised   ~~deleted~~ Deleted   OGCR Official Guidelines   X Assign placeholder X   ● Use Additional Character(s)

Excludes 1   Excludes 2   Includes   Use additional   Code first   Code also   Unspecified

● S63.04   Subluxation and dislocation of carpometacarpal joint of thumb

     Excludes2   interphalangeal subluxation and dislocation of thumb (S63.1-)

     ● S63.041   Subluxation of carpometacarpal joint of right thumb

     ● S63.042   Subluxation of carpometacarpal joint of left thumb

     ● S63.043   Subluxation of carpometacarpal joint of unspecified thumb

     ● S63.044   Dislocation of carpometacarpal joint of right thumb

     ● S63.045   Dislocation of carpometacarpal joint of left thumb

     ● S63.046   Dislocation of carpometacarpal joint of unspecified thumb

● S63.05   Subluxation and dislocation of other carpometacarpal joint

     Excludes2   subluxation and dislocation of carpometacarpal joint of thumb (S63.04-)

     ● S63.051   Subluxation of other carpometacarpal joint of right hand

     ● S63.052   Subluxation of other carpometacarpal joint of left hand

     ● S63.053   Subluxation of other carpometacarpal joint of unspecified hand

     ● S63.054   Dislocation of other carpometacarpal joint of right hand

     ● S63.055   Dislocation of other carpometacarpal joint of left hand

     ● S63.056   Dislocation of other carpometacarpal joint of unspecified hand

● S63.06   Subluxation and dislocation of metacarpal (bone), proximal end

     ● S63.061   Subluxation of metacarpal (bone), proximal end of right hand

     ● S63.062   Subluxation of metacarpal (bone), proximal end of left hand

     ● S63.063   Subluxation of metacarpal (bone), proximal end of unspecified hand

     ● S63.064   Dislocation of metacarpal (bone), proximal end of right hand

     ● S63.065   Dislocation of metacarpal (bone), proximal end of left hand

     ● S63.066   Dislocation of metacarpal (bone), proximal end of unspecified hand

● S63.07   Subluxation and dislocation of distal end of ulna

     ● S63.071   Subluxation of distal end of right ulna

     ● S63.072   Subluxation of distal end of left ulna

     ● S63.073   Subluxation of distal end of unspecified ulna

     ● S63.074   Dislocation of distal end of right ulna

     ● S63.075   Dislocation of distal end of left ulna

     ● S63.076   Dislocation of distal end of unspecified ulna

● S63.09   Other subluxation and dislocation of wrist and hand

     ● S63.091   Other subluxation of right wrist and hand

     ● S63.092   Other subluxation of left wrist and hand

     ● S63.093   Other subluxation of unspecified wrist and hand

     ● S63.094   Other dislocation of right wrist and hand

     ● S63.095   Other dislocation of left wrist and hand

     ● S63.096   Other dislocation of unspecified wrist and hand

● S63.1   Subluxation and dislocation of thumb

     ● S63.10   Unspecified subluxation and dislocation of thumb

         ● S63.101   Unspecified subluxation of right thumb

         ● S63.102   Unspecified subluxation of left thumb

         ● S63.103   Unspecified subluxation of unspecified thumb

         ● S63.104   Unspecified dislocation of right thumb

         ● S63.105   Unspecified dislocation of left thumb

         ● S63.106   Unspecified dislocation of unspecified thumb

     ● S63.11   Subluxation and dislocation of metacarpophalangeal joint of thumb

         ● S63.111   Subluxation of metacarpophalangeal joint of right thumb

         ● S63.112   Subluxation of metacarpophalangeal joint of left thumb

         ● S63.113   Subluxation of metacarpophalangeal joint of unspecified thumb

         ● S63.114   Dislocation of metacarpophalangeal joint of right thumb

         ● S63.115   Dislocation of metacarpophalangeal joint of left thumb

         ● S63.116   Dislocation of metacarpophalangeal joint of unspecified thumb

     ● S63.12   Subluxation and dislocation of unspecified interphalangeal joint of thumb

         ● S63.121   Subluxation of unspecified interphalangeal joint of right thumb

         ● S63.122   Subluxation of unspecified interphalangeal joint of left thumb

         ● S63.123   Subluxation of unspecified interphalangeal joint of unspecified thumb

         ● S63.124   Dislocation of unspecified interphalangeal joint of right thumb

         ● S63.125   Dislocation of unspecified interphalangeal joint of left thumb

         ● S63.126   Dislocation of unspecified interphalangeal joint of unspecified thumb

     ● S63.13   Subluxation and dislocation of proximal interphalangeal joint of thumb

         ● S63.131   Subluxation of proximal interphalangeal joint of right thumb

         ● S63.132   Subluxation of proximal interphalangeal joint of left thumb

         ● S63.133   Subluxation of proximal interphalangeal joint of unspecified thumb

         ● S63.134   Dislocation of proximal interphalangeal joint of right thumb

         ● S63.135   Dislocation of proximal interphalangeal joint of left thumb

         ● S63.136   Dislocation of proximal interphalangeal joint of unspecified thumb

CHAPTER 19 (S00–T88)

● **S63.14**   Subluxation and dislocation of distal interphalangeal joint of thumb
     ● **S63.141**   Subluxation of distal interphalangeal joint of right thumb
     ● **S63.142**   Subluxation of distal interphalangeal joint of left thumb
     ● **S63.143**   Subluxation of distal interphalangeal joint of unspecified thumb
     ● **S63.144**   Dislocation of distal interphalangeal joint of right thumb
     ● **S63.145**   Dislocation of distal interphalangeal joint of left thumb
     ● **S63.146**   Dislocation of distal interphalangeal joint of unspecified thumb

● **S63.2**   Subluxation and dislocation of other finger(s)
     Excludes2   subluxation and dislocation of thumb (S63.1-)
     ● **S63.20**   Unspecified subluxation of other finger
       ● **S63.200**   Unspecified subluxation of right index finger
       ● **S63.201**   Unspecified subluxation of left index finger
       ● **S63.202**   Unspecified subluxation of right middle finger
       ● **S63.203**   Unspecified subluxation of left middle finger
       ● **S63.204**   Unspecified subluxation of right ring finger
       ● **S63.205**   Unspecified subluxation of left ring finger
       ● **S63.206**   Unspecified subluxation of right little finger
       ● **S63.207**   Unspecified subluxation of left little finger
       ● **S63.208**   Unspecified subluxation of other finger
         Unspecified subluxation of specified finger with unspecified laterality
       ● **S63.209**   Unspecified subluxation of unspecified finger
     ● **S63.21**   Subluxation of metacarpophalangeal joint of finger
       ● **S63.210**   Subluxation of metacarpophalangeal joint of right index finger
       ● **S63.211**   Subluxation of metacarpophalangeal joint of left index finger
       ● **S63.212**   Subluxation of metacarpophalangeal joint of right middle finger
       ● **S63.213**   Subluxation of metacarpophalangeal joint of left middle finger
       ● **S63.214**   Subluxation of metacarpophalangeal joint of right ring finger
       ● **S63.215**   Subluxation of metacarpophalangeal joint of left ring finger
       ● **S63.216**   Subluxation of metacarpophalangeal joint of right little finger
       ● **S63.217**   Subluxation of metacarpophalangeal joint of left little finger
       ● **S63.218**   Subluxation of metacarpophalangeal joint of other finger
         Subluxation of metacarpophalangeal joint of specified finger with unspecified laterality
       ● **S63.219**   Subluxation of metacarpophalangeal joint of unspecified finger

● **S63.22**   Subluxation of unspecified interphalangeal joint of finger
     ● **S63.220**   Subluxation of unspecified interphalangeal joint of right index finger
     ● **S63.221**   Subluxation of unspecified interphalangeal joint of left index finger
     ● **S63.222**   Subluxation of unspecified interphalangeal joint of right middle finger
     ● **S63.223**   Subluxation of unspecified interphalangeal joint of left middle finger
     ● **S63.224**   Subluxation of unspecified interphalangeal joint of right ring finger
     ● **S63.225**   Subluxation of unspecified interphalangeal joint of left ring finger
     ● **S63.226**   Subluxation of unspecified interphalangeal joint of right little finger
     ● **S63.227**   Subluxation of unspecified interphalangeal joint of left little finger
     ● **S63.228**   Subluxation of unspecified interphalangeal joint of other finger
       Subluxation of unspecified interphalangeal joint of specified finger with unspecified laterality
     ● **S63.229**   Subluxation of unspecified interphalangeal joint of unspecified finger
● **S63.23**   Subluxation of proximal interphalangeal joint of finger
     ● **S63.230**   Subluxation of proximal interphalangeal joint of right index finger
     ● **S63.231**   Subluxation of proximal interphalangeal joint of left index finger
     ● **S63.232**   Subluxation of proximal interphalangeal joint of right middle finger
     ● **S63.233**   Subluxation of proximal interphalangeal joint of left middle finger
     ● **S63.234**   Subluxation of proximal interphalangeal joint of right ring finger
     ● **S63.235**   Subluxation of proximal interphalangeal joint of left ring finger
     ● **S63.236**   Subluxation of proximal interphalangeal joint of right little finger
     ● **S63.237**   Subluxation of proximal interphalangeal joint of left little finger
     ● **S63.238**   Subluxation of proximal interphalangeal joint of other finger
       Subluxation of proximal interphalangeal joint of specified finger with unspecified laterality
     ● **S63.239**   Subluxation of proximal interphalangeal joint of unspecified finger

● **S63.24** Subluxation of distal interphalangeal joint of finger
   ● **S63.240** Subluxation of distal interphalangeal joint of right index finger
   ● **S63.241** Subluxation of distal interphalangeal joint of left index finger
   ● **S63.242** Subluxation of distal interphalangeal joint of right middle finger
   ● **S63.243** Subluxation of distal interphalangeal joint of left middle finger
   ● **S63.244** Subluxation of distal interphalangeal joint of right ring finger
   ● **S63.245** Subluxation of distal interphalangeal joint of left ring finger
   ● **S63.246** Subluxation of distal interphalangeal joint of right little finger
   ● **S63.247** Subluxation of distal interphalangeal joint of left little finger
   ● **S63.248** Subluxation of distal interphalangeal joint of other finger
       Subluxation of distal interphalangeal joint of specified finger with unspecified laterality
   ● **S63.249** Subluxation of distal interphalangeal joint of unspecified finger

● **S63.25** Unspecified dislocation of other finger
   ● **S63.250** Unspecified dislocation of right index finger
   ● **S63.251** Unspecified dislocation of left index finger
   ● **S63.252** Unspecified dislocation of right middle finger
   ● **S63.253** Unspecified dislocation of left middle finger
   ● **S63.254** Unspecified dislocation of right ring finger
   ● **S63.255** Unspecified dislocation of left ring finger
   ● **S63.256** Unspecified dislocation of right little finger
   ● **S63.257** Unspecified dislocation of left little finger
   ● **S63.258** Unspecified dislocation of other finger
       Unspecified dislocation of specified finger with unspecified laterality
   ● **S63.259** Unspecified dislocation of unspecified finger
       Unspecified dislocation of specified finger with unspecified laterality

● **S63.26** Dislocation of metacarpophalangeal joint of finger
   ● **S63.260** Dislocation of metacarpophalangeal joint of right index finger
   ● **S63.261** Dislocation of metacarpophalangeal joint of left index finger
   ● **S63.262** Dislocation of metacarpophalangeal joint of right middle finger
   ● **S63.263** Dislocation of metacarpophalangeal joint of left middle finger
   ● **S63.264** Dislocation of metacarpophalangeal joint of right ring finger
   ● **S63.265** Dislocation of metacarpophalangeal joint of left ring finger

   ● **S63.266** Dislocation of metacarpophalangeal joint of right little finger
   ● **S63.267** Dislocation of metacarpophalangeal joint of left little finger
   ● **S63.268** Dislocation of metacarpophalangeal joint of other finger
       Dislocation of metacarpophalangeal joint of specified finger with unspecified laterality
   ● **S63.269** Dislocation of metacarpophalangeal joint of unspecified finger

● **S63.27** Dislocation of unspecified interphalangeal joint of finger
   ● **S63.270** Dislocation of unspecified interphalangeal joint of right index finger
   ● **S63.271** Dislocation of unspecified interphalangeal joint of left index finger
   ● **S63.272** Dislocation of unspecified interphalangeal joint of right middle finger
   ● **S63.273** Dislocation of unspecified interphalangeal joint of left middle finger
   ● **S63.274** Dislocation of unspecified interphalangeal joint of right ring finger
   ● **S63.275** Dislocation of unspecified interphalangeal joint of left ring finger
   ● **S63.276** Dislocation of unspecified interphalangeal joint of right little finger
   ● **S63.277** Dislocation of unspecified interphalangeal joint of left little finger
   ● **S63.278** Dislocation of unspecified interphalangeal joint of other finger
       Dislocation of unspecified interphalangeal joint of specified finger with unspecified laterality
   ● **S63.279** Dislocation of unspecified interphalangeal joint of unspecified finger
       Dislocation of unspecified interphalangeal joint of specified finger without specified laterality

● **S63.28** Dislocation of proximal interphalangeal joint of finger
   ● **S63.280** Dislocation of proximal interphalangeal joint of right index finger
   ● **S63.281** Dislocation of proximal interphalangeal joint of left index finger
   ● **S63.282** Dislocation of proximal interphalangeal joint of right middle finger
   ● **S63.283** Dislocation of proximal interphalangeal joint of left middle finger
   ● **S63.284** Dislocation of proximal interphalangeal joint of right ring finger

CHAPTER 19 (S00-T88)

● S63.285   Dislocation of proximal interphalangeal joint of left ring finger
● S63.286   Dislocation of proximal interphalangeal joint of right little finger
● S63.287   Dislocation of proximal interphalangeal joint of left little finger
● S63.288   Dislocation of proximal interphalangeal joint of other finger
            Dislocation of proximal interphalangeal joint of specified finger with unspecified laterality
● S63.289   Dislocation of proximal interphalangeal joint of unspecified finger
● S63.29   Dislocation of distal interphalangeal joint of finger
● S63.290   Dislocation of distal interphalangeal joint of right index finger
● S63.291   Dislocation of distal interphalangeal joint of left index finger
● S63.292   Dislocation of distal interphalangeal joint of right middle finger
● S63.293   Dislocation of distal interphalangeal joint of left middle finger
● S63.294   Dislocation of distal interphalangeal joint of right ring finger
● S63.295   Dislocation of distal interphalangeal joint of left ring finger
● S63.296   Dislocation of distal interphalangeal joint of right little finger
● S63.297   Dislocation of distal interphalangeal joint of left little finger
● S63.298   Dislocation of distal interphalangeal joint of other finger
            Dislocation of distal interphalangeal joint of specified finger with unspecified laterality
● S63.299   Dislocation of distal interphalangeal joint of unspecified finger
● S63.3   Traumatic rupture of ligament of wrist
● S63.30   Traumatic rupture of unspecified ligament of wrist
● S63.301   Traumatic rupture of unspecified ligament of right wrist
● S63.302   Traumatic rupture of unspecified ligament of left wrist
● S63.309   Traumatic rupture of unspecified ligament of unspecified wrist
● S63.31   Traumatic rupture of collateral ligament of wrist
● S63.311   Traumatic rupture of collateral ligament of right wrist
● S63.312   Traumatic rupture of collateral ligament of left wrist
● S63.319   Traumatic rupture of collateral ligament of unspecified wrist
● S63.32   Traumatic rupture of radiocarpal ligament
● S63.321   Traumatic rupture of right radiocarpal ligament
● S63.322   Traumatic rupture of left radiocarpal ligament
● S63.329   Traumatic rupture of unspecified radiocarpal ligament

● S63.33   Traumatic rupture of ulnocarpal (palmar) ligament
● S63.331   Traumatic rupture of right ulnocarpal (palmar) ligament
● S63.332   Traumatic rupture of left ulnocarpal (palmar) ligament
● S63.339   Traumatic rupture of unspecified ulnocarpal (palmar) ligament
● S63.39   Traumatic rupture of other ligament of wrist
● S63.391   Traumatic rupture of other ligament of right wrist
● S63.392   Traumatic rupture of other ligament of left wrist
● S63.399   Traumatic rupture of other ligament of unspecified wrist
● S63.4   Traumatic rupture of ligament of finger at metacarpophalangeal and interphalangeal joint(s)
● S63.40   Traumatic rupture of unspecified ligament of finger at metacarpophalangeal and interphalangeal joint
● S63.400   Traumatic rupture of unspecified ligament of right index finger at metacarpophalangeal and interphalangeal joint
● S63.401   Traumatic rupture of unspecified ligament of left index finger at metacarpophalangeal and interphalangeal joint
● S63.402   Traumatic rupture of unspecified ligament of right middle finger at metacarpophalangeal and interphalangeal joint
● S63.403   Traumatic rupture of unspecified ligament of left middle finger at metacarpophalangeal and interphalangeal joint
● S63.404   Traumatic rupture of unspecified ligament of right ring finger at metacarpophalangeal and interphalangeal joint
● S63.405   Traumatic rupture of unspecified ligament of left ring finger at metacarpophalangeal and interphalangeal joint
● S63.406   Traumatic rupture of unspecified ligament of right little finger at metacarpophalangeal and interphalangeal joint
● S63.407   Traumatic rupture of unspecified ligament of left little finger at metacarpophalangeal and interphalangeal joint
● S63.408   Traumatic rupture of unspecified ligament of other finger at metacarpophalangeal and interphalangeal joint
            Traumatic rupture of unspecified ligament of specified finger with unspecified laterality at metacarpophalangeal and interphalangeal joint
● S63.409   Traumatic rupture of unspecified ligament of unspecified finger at metacarpophalangeal and interphalangeal joint

● **S63.41   Traumatic rupture of collateral ligament of finger at metacarpophalangeal and interphalangeal joint**

● **S63.410   Traumatic rupture of collateral ligament of right index finger at metacarpophalangeal and interphalangeal joint**

● **S63.411   Traumatic rupture of collateral ligament of left index finger at metacarpophalangeal and interphalangeal joint**

● **S63.412   Traumatic rupture of collateral ligament of right middle finger at metacarpophalangeal and interphalangeal joint**

● **S63.413   Traumatic rupture of collateral ligament of left middle finger at metacarpophalangeal and interphalangeal joint**

● **S63.414   Traumatic rupture of collateral ligament of right ring finger at metacarpophalangeal and interphalangeal joint**

● **S63.415   Traumatic rupture of collateral ligament of left ring finger at metacarpophalangeal and interphalangeal joint**

● **S63.416   Traumatic rupture of collateral ligament of right little finger at metacarpophalangeal and interphalangeal joint**

● **S63.417   Traumatic rupture of collateral ligament of left little finger at metacarpophalangeal and interphalangeal joint**

● **S63.418   Traumatic rupture of collateral ligament of other finger at metacarpophalangeal and interphalangeal joint**
    Traumatic rupture of collateral ligament of specified finger with unspecified laterality at metacarpophalangeal and interphalangeal joint

● **S63.419   Traumatic rupture of collateral ligament of unspecified finger at metacarpophalangeal and interphalangeal joint**

● **S63.42   Traumatic rupture of palmar ligament of finger at metacarpophalangeal and interphalangeal joint**

● **S63.420   Traumatic rupture of palmar ligament of right index finger at metacarpophalangeal and interphalangeal joint**

● **S63.421   Traumatic rupture of palmar ligament of left index finger at metacarpophalangeal and interphalangeal joint**

● **S63.422   Traumatic rupture of palmar ligament of right middle finger at metacarpophalangeal and interphalangeal joint**

● **S63.423   Traumatic rupture of palmar ligament of left middle finger at metacarpophalangeal and interphalangeal joint**

● **S63.424   Traumatic rupture of palmar ligament of right ring finger at metacarpophalangeal and interphalangeal joint**

● **S63.425   Traumatic rupture of palmar ligament of left ring finger at metacarpophalangeal and interphalangeal joint**

● **S63.426   Traumatic rupture of palmar ligament of right little finger at metacarpophalangeal and interphalangeal joint**

● **S63.427   Traumatic rupture of palmar ligament of left little finger at metacarpophalangeal and interphalangeal joint**

● **S63.428   Traumatic rupture of palmar ligament of other finger at metacarpophalangeal and interphalangeal joint**
    Traumatic rupture of palmar ligament of specified finger with unspecified laterality at metacarpophalangeal and interphalangeal joint

● **S63.429   Traumatic rupture of palmar ligament of unspecified finger at metacarpophalangeal and interphalangeal joint**

● **S63.43   Traumatic rupture of volar plate of finger at metacarpophalangeal and interphalangeal joint**

● **S63.430   Traumatic rupture of volar plate of right index finger at metacarpophalangeal and interphalangeal joint**

● **S63.431   Traumatic rupture of volar plate of left index finger at metacarpophalangeal and interphalangeal joint**

● **S63.432   Traumatic rupture of volar plate of right middle finger at metacarpophalangeal and interphalangeal joint**

● **S63.433   Traumatic rupture of volar plate of left middle finger at metacarpophalangeal and interphalangeal joint**

● **S63.434   Traumatic rupture of volar plate of right ring finger at metacarpophalangeal and interphalangeal joint**

● **S63.435   Traumatic rupture of volar plate of left ring finger at metacarpophalangeal and interphalangeal joint**

● **S63.436   Traumatic rupture of volar plate of right little finger at metacarpophalangeal and interphalangeal joint**

● **S63.437   Traumatic rupture of volar plate of left little finger at metacarpophalangeal and interphalangeal joint**

● **S63.438   Traumatic rupture of volar plate of other finger at metacarpophalangeal and interphalangeal joint**
    Traumatic rupture of volar plate of specified finger with unspecified laterality at metacarpophalangeal and interphalangeal joint

● **S63.439   Traumatic rupture of volar plate of unspecified finger at metacarpophalangeal and interphalangeal joint**

CHAPTER 19 (S00-T88)

● **S63.49**   Traumatic rupture of other ligament of finger at metacarpophalangeal and interphalangeal joint

  ● **S63.490**   Traumatic rupture of other ligament of right index finger at metacarpophalangeal and interphalangeal joint

  ● **S63.491**   Traumatic rupture of other ligament of left index finger at metacarpophalangeal and interphalangeal joint

  ● **S63.492**   Traumatic rupture of other ligament of right middle finger at metacarpophalangeal and interphalangeal joint

  ● **S63.493**   Traumatic rupture of other ligament of left middle finger at metacarpophalangeal and interphalangeal joint

  ● **S63.494**   Traumatic rupture of other ligament of right ring finger at metacarpophalangeal and interphalangeal joint

  ● **S63.495**   Traumatic rupture of other ligament of left ring finger at metacarpophalangeal and interphalangeal joint

  ● **S63.496**   Traumatic rupture of other ligament of right little finger at metacarpophalangeal and interphalangeal joint

  ● **S63.497**   Traumatic rupture of other ligament of left little finger at metacarpophalangeal and interphalangeal joint

  ● **S63.498**   Traumatic rupture of other ligament of other finger at metacarpophalangeal and interphalangeal joint

     Traumatic rupture of ligament of specified finger with unspecified laterality at metacarpophalangeal and interphalangeal joint

  ● **S63.499**   Traumatic rupture of other ligament of unspecified finger at metacarpophalangeal and interphalangeal joint

● **S63.5**   Other and unspecified sprain of wrist

  ● **S63.50**   Unspecified sprain of wrist

    ● **S63.501**   Unspecified sprain of right wrist

    ● **S63.502**   Unspecified sprain of left wrist

    ● **S63.509**   Unspecified sprain of unspecified wrist

  ● **S63.51**   Sprain of carpal (joint)

    ● **S63.511**   Sprain of carpal joint of right wrist

    ● **S63.512**   Sprain of carpal joint of left wrist

    ● **S63.519**   Sprain of carpal joint of unspecified wrist

  ● **S63.52**   Sprain of radiocarpal joint

     Excludes1   traumatic rupture of radiocarpal ligament (S63.32-)

    ● **S63.521**   Sprain of radiocarpal joint of right wrist

    ● **S63.522**   Sprain of radiocarpal joint of left wrist

    ● **S63.529**   Sprain of radiocarpal joint of unspecified wrist

● **S63.59**   Other specified sprain of wrist

  ● **S63.591**   Other specified sprain of right wrist

  ● **S63.592**   Other specified sprain of left wrist

  ● **S63.599**   Other specified sprain of unspecified wrist

● **S63.6**   Other and unspecified sprain of finger(s)

     Excludes1   traumatic rupture of ligament of finger at metacarpophalangeal and interphalangeal joint(s) (S63.4-)

  ● **S63.60**   Unspecified sprain of thumb

    ● **S63.601**   Unspecified sprain of right thumb

    ● **S63.602**   Unspecified sprain of left thumb

    ● **S63.609**   Unspecified sprain of unspecified thumb

  ● **S63.61**   Unspecified sprain of other and unspecified finger(s)

    ● **S63.610**   Unspecified sprain of right index finger

    ● **S63.611**   Unspecified sprain of left index finger

    ● **S63.612**   Unspecified sprain of right middle finger

    ● **S63.613**   Unspecified sprain of left middle finger

    ● **S63.614**   Unspecified sprain of right ring finger

    ● **S63.615**   Unspecified sprain of left ring finger

    ● **S63.616**   Unspecified sprain of right little finger

    ● **S63.617**   Unspecified sprain of left little finger

    ● **S63.618**   Unspecified sprain of other finger

       Unspecified sprain of specified finger with unspecified laterality

    ● **S63.619**   Unspecified sprain of unspecified finger

  ● **S63.62**   Sprain of interphalangeal joint of thumb

    ● **S63.621**   Sprain of interphalangeal joint of right thumb

    ● **S63.622**   Sprain of interphalangeal joint of left thumb

    ● **S63.629**   Sprain of interphalangeal joint of unspecified thumb

  ● **S63.63**   Sprain of interphalangeal joint of other and unspecified finger(s)

    ● **S63.630**   Sprain of interphalangeal joint of right index finger

    ● **S63.631**   Sprain of interphalangeal joint of left index finger

    ● **S63.632**   Sprain of interphalangeal joint of right middle finger

    ● **S63.633**   Sprain of interphalangeal joint of left middle finger

    ● **S63.634**   Sprain of interphalangeal joint of right ring finger

    ● **S63.635**   Sprain of interphalangeal joint of left ring finger

    ● **S63.636**   Sprain of interphalangeal joint of right little finger

    ● **S63.637**   Sprain of interphalangeal joint of left little finger

    ● **S63.638**   Sprain of interphalangeal joint of other finger

    ● **S63.639**   Sprain of interphalangeal joint of unspecified finger

◀ New   ◀◀◀ Revised   ~~deleted~~ Deleted   **OGCR** Official Guidelines   X Assign placeholder X   ● Use Additional Character(s)

Excludes 1   Excludes 2   Includes   Use additional   Code first   Code also   Unspecified

● S63.64   Sprain of metacarpophalangeal joint of thumb
 ● S63.641   Sprain of metacarpophalangeal joint of right thumb
 ● S63.642   Sprain of metacarpophalangeal joint of left thumb
 ● S63.649   Sprain of metacarpophalangeal joint of unspecified thumb
● S63.65   Sprain of metacarpophalangeal joint of other and unspecified finger(s)
 ● S63.650   Sprain of metacarpophalangeal joint of right index finger
 ● S63.651   Sprain of metacarpophalangeal joint of left index finger
 ● S63.652   Sprain of metacarpophalangeal joint of right middle finger
 ● S63.653   Sprain of metacarpophalangeal joint of left middle finger
 ● S63.654   Sprain of metacarpophalangeal joint of right ring finger
 ● S63.655   Sprain of metacarpophalangeal joint of left ring finger
 ● S63.656   Sprain of metacarpophalangeal joint of right little finger
 ● S63.657   Sprain of metacarpophalangeal joint of left little finger
 ● S63.658   Sprain of metacarpophalangeal joint of other finger
  Sprain of metacarpophalangeal joint of specified finger with unspecified laterality
 ● S63.659   Sprain of metacarpophalangeal joint of unspecified finger
● S63.68   Other sprain of thumb
 ● S63.681   Other sprain of right thumb
 ● S63.682   Other sprain of left thumb
 ● S63.689   Other sprain of unspecified thumb
● S63.69   Other sprain of other and unspecified finger(s)
 ● S63.690   Other sprain of right index finger
 ● S63.691   Other sprain of left index finger
 ● S63.692   Other sprain of right middle finger
 ● S63.693   Other sprain of left middle finger
 ● S63.694   Other sprain of right ring finger
 ● S63.695   Other sprain of left ring finger
 ● S63.696   Other sprain of right little finger
 ● S63.697   Other sprain of left little finger
 ● S63.698   Other sprain of other finger
  Other sprain of specified finger with unspecified laterality
 ● S63.699   Other sprain of unspecified finger
● S63.8   Sprain of other part of wrist and hand
 ● S63.8X   Sprain of other part of wrist and hand
  ● S63.8X1   Sprain of other part of right wrist and hand
  ● S63.8X2   Sprain of other part of left wrist and hand
  ● S63.8X9   Sprain of other part of unspecified wrist and hand
● S63.9   Sprain of unspecified part of wrist and hand
 X● S63.90   Sprain of unspecified part of unspecified wrist and hand
 X● S63.91   Sprain of unspecified part of right wrist and hand
 X● S63.92   Sprain of unspecified part of left wrist and hand

● S64   Injury of nerves at wrist and hand level
The appropriate 7th character is to be added to each code from category S64

A	initial encounter
D	subsequent encounter
S	sequela

Code also any associated open wound (S61.-)
● S64.0   Injury of ulnar nerve at wrist and hand level
 X● S64.00   Injury of ulnar nerve at wrist and hand level of unspecified arm
 X● S64.01   Injury of ulnar nerve at wrist and hand level of right arm
 X● S64.02   Injury of ulnar nerve at wrist and hand level of left arm
● S64.1   Injury of median nerve at wrist and hand level
 X● S64.10   Injury of median nerve at wrist and hand level of unspecified arm
 X● S64.11   Injury of median nerve at wrist and hand level of right arm
 X● S64.12   Injury of median nerve at wrist and hand level of left arm
● S64.2   Injury of radial nerve at wrist and hand level
 X● S64.20   Injury of radial nerve at wrist and hand level of unspecified arm
 X● S64.21   Injury of radial nerve at wrist and hand level of right arm
 X● S64.22   Injury of radial nerve at wrist and hand level of left arm
● S64.3   Injury of digital nerve of thumb
 X● S64.30   Injury of digital nerve of unspecified thumb
 X● S64.31   Injury of digital nerve of right thumb
 X● S64.32   Injury of digital nerve of left thumb
● S64.4   Injury of digital nerve of other and unspecified finger
 X● S64.40   Injury of digital nerve of unspecified finger
 ● S64.49   Injury of digital nerve of other finger
  ● S64.490   Injury of digital nerve of right index finger
  ● S64.491   Injury of digital nerve of left index finger
  ● S64.492   Injury of digital nerve of right middle finger
  ● S64.493   Injury of digital nerve of left middle finger
  ● S64.494   Injury of digital nerve of right ring finger
  ● S64.495   Injury of digital nerve of left ring finger
  ● S64.496   Injury of digital nerve of right little finger
  ● S64.497   Injury of digital nerve of left little finger
  ● S64.498   Injury of digital nerve of other finger
   Injury of digital nerve of specified finger with unspecified laterality

◄ New ⇐ Revised deleted Deleted OGCR Official Guidelines X Assign placeholder X ● Use Additional Character(s)

Excludes 1 Excludes 2 Includes Use additional Code first Code also Unspecified

1319

● S64.8   Injury of other nerves at wrist and hand level
     ● S64.8X   Injury of other nerves at wrist and hand level
         ● S64.8X1   Injury of other nerves at wrist and hand level of right arm
         ● S64.8X2   Injury of other nerves at wrist and hand level of left arm
         ● S64.8X9   Injury of other nerves at wrist and hand level of unspecified arm

● S64.9   Injury of unspecified nerve at wrist and hand level
     X ● S64.90   Injury of unspecified nerve at wrist and hand level of unspecified arm
     X ● S64.91   Injury of unspecified nerve at wrist and hand level of right arm
     X ● S64.92   Injury of unspecified nerve at wrist and hand level of left arm

● S65   Injury of blood vessels at wrist and hand level
     The appropriate 7th character is to be added to each code from category S65

> A   initial encounter
> D   subsequent encounter
> S   sequela

     Code also any associated open wound (S61.-)

   ● S65.0   Injury of ulnar artery at wrist and hand level
     ● S65.00   Unspecified injury of ulnar artery at wrist and hand level
         ● S65.001   Unspecified injury of ulnar artery at wrist and hand level of right arm
         ● S65.002   Unspecified injury of ulnar artery at wrist and hand level of left arm
         ● S65.009   Unspecified injury of ulnar artery at wrist and hand level of unspecified arm
     ● S65.01   Laceration of ulnar artery at wrist and hand level
         ● S65.011   Laceration of ulnar artery at wrist and hand level of right arm
         ● S65.012   Laceration of ulnar artery at wrist and hand level of left arm
         ● S65.019   Laceration of ulnar artery at wrist and hand level of unspecified arm
     ● S65.09   Other specified injury of ulnar artery at wrist and hand level
         ● S65.091   Other specified injury of ulnar artery at wrist and hand level of right arm
         ● S65.092   Other specified injury of ulnar artery at wrist and hand level of left arm
         ● S65.099   Other specified injury of ulnar artery at wrist and hand level of unspecified arm

   ● S65.1   Injury of radial artery at wrist and hand level
     ● S65.10   Unspecified injury of radial artery at wrist and hand level
         ● S65.101   Unspecified injury of radial artery at wrist and hand level of right arm
         ● S65.102   Unspecified injury of radial artery at wrist and hand level of left arm
         ● S65.109   Unspecified injury of radial artery at wrist and hand level of unspecified arm
     ● S65.11   Laceration of radial artery at wrist and hand level
         ● S65.111   Laceration of radial artery at wrist and hand level of right arm
         ● S65.112   Laceration of radial artery at wrist and hand level of left arm
         ● S65.119   Laceration of radial artery at wrist and hand level of unspecified arm

● S65.19   Other specified injury of radial artery at wrist and hand level
     ● S65.191   Other specified injury of radial artery at wrist and hand level of right arm
     ● S65.192   Other specified injury of radial artery at wrist and hand level of left arm
     ● S65.199   Other specified injury of radial artery at wrist and hand level of unspecified arm

● S65.2   Injury of superficial palmar arch
   ● S65.20   Unspecified injury of superficial palmar arch
     ● S65.201   Unspecified injury of superficial palmar arch of right hand
     ● S65.202   Unspecified injury of superficial palmar arch of left hand
     ● S65.209   Unspecified injury of superficial palmar arch of unspecified hand
   ● S65.21   Laceration of superficial palmar arch
     ● S65.211   Laceration of superficial palmar arch of right hand
     ● S65.212   Laceration of superficial palmar arch of left hand
     ● S65.219   Laceration of superficial palmar arch of unspecified hand
   ● S65.29   Other specified injury of superficial palmar arch
     ● S65.291   Other specified injury of superficial palmar arch of right hand
     ● S65.292   Other specified injury of superficial palmar arch of left hand
     ● S65.299   Other specified injury of superficial palmar arch of unspecified hand

● S65.3   Injury of deep palmar arch
   ● S65.30   Unspecified injury of deep palmar arch
     ● S65.301   Unspecified injury of deep palmar arch of right hand
     ● S65.302   Unspecified injury of deep palmar arch of left hand
     ● S65.309   Unspecified injury of deep palmar arch of unspecified hand
   ● S65.31   Laceration of deep palmar arch
     ● S65.311   Laceration of deep palmar arch of right hand
     ● S65.312   Laceration of deep palmar arch of left hand
     ● S65.319   Laceration of deep palmar arch of unspecified hand
   ● S65.39   Other specified injury of deep palmar arch
     ● S65.391   Other specified injury of deep palmar arch of right hand
     ● S65.392   Other specified injury of deep palmar arch of left hand
     ● S65.399   Other specified injury of deep palmar arch of unspecified hand

● S65.4   Injury of blood vessel of thumb
   ● S65.40   Unspecified injury of blood vessel of thumb
     ● S65.401   Unspecified injury of blood vessel of right thumb
     ● S65.402   Unspecified injury of blood vessel of left thumb
     ● S65.409   Unspecified injury of blood vessel of unspecified thumb

● S65.41   Laceration of blood vessel of thumb
   ● S65.411   Laceration of blood vessel of right thumb
   ● S65.412   Laceration of blood vessel of left thumb
   ● S65.419   Laceration of blood vessel of unspecified thumb
● S65.49   Other specified injury of blood vessel of thumb
   ● S65.491   Other specified injury of blood vessel of right thumb
   ● S65.492   Other specified injury of blood vessel of left thumb
   ● S65.499   Other specified injury of blood vessel of unspecified thumb

● S65.5   Injury of blood vessel of other and unspecified finger
  ● S65.50   Unspecified injury of blood vessel of other and unspecified finger
   ● S65.500   Unspecified injury of blood vessel of right index finger
   ● S65.501   Unspecified injury of blood vessel of left index finger
   ● S65.502   Unspecified injury of blood vessel of right middle finger
   ● S65.503   Unspecified injury of blood vessel of left middle finger
   ● S65.504   Unspecified injury of blood vessel of right ring finger
   ● S65.505   Unspecified injury of blood vessel of left ring finger
   ● S65.506   Unspecified injury of blood vessel of right little finger
   ● S65.507   Unspecified injury of blood vessel of left little finger
   ● S65.508   Unspecified injury of blood vessel of other finger
       Unspecified injury of blood vessel of specified finger with unspecified laterality
   ● S65.509   Unspecified injury of blood vessel of unspecified finger
  ● S65.51   Laceration of blood vessel of other and unspecified finger
   ● S65.510   Laceration of blood vessel of right index finger
   ● S65.511   Laceration of blood vessel of left index finger
   ● S65.512   Laceration of blood vessel of right middle finger
   ● S65.513   Laceration of blood vessel of left middle finger
   ● S65.514   Laceration of blood vessel of right ring finger
   ● S65.515   Laceration of blood vessel of left ring finger
   ● S65.516   Laceration of blood vessel of right little finger
   ● S65.517   Laceration of blood vessel of left little finger
   ● S65.518   Laceration of blood vessel of other finger
       Laceration of blood vessel of specified finger with unspecified laterality
   ● S65.519   Laceration of blood vessel of unspecified finger

● S65.59   Other specified injury of blood vessel of other and unspecified finger
   ● S65.590   Other specified injury of blood vessel of right index finger
   ● S65.591   Other specified injury of blood vessel of left index finger
   ● S65.592   Other specified injury of blood vessel of right middle finger
   ● S65.593   Other specified injury of blood vessel of left middle finger
   ● S65.594   Other specified injury of blood vessel of right ring finger
   ● S65.595   Other specified injury of blood vessel of left ring finger
   ● S65.596   Other specified injury of blood vessel of right little finger
   ● S65.597   Other specified injury of blood vessel of left little finger
   ● S65.598   Other specified injury of blood vessel of other finger
       Other specified injury of blood vessel of specified finger with unspecified laterality
   ● S65.599   Other specified injury of blood vessel of unspecified finger

● S65.8   Injury of other blood vessels at wrist and hand level
  ● S65.80   Unspecified injury of other blood vessels at wrist and hand level
   ● S65.801   Unspecified injury of other blood vessels at wrist and hand level of right arm
   ● S65.802   Unspecified injury of other blood vessels at wrist and hand level of left arm
   ● S65.809   Unspecified injury of other blood vessels at wrist and hand level of unspecified arm
  ● S65.81   Laceration of other blood vessels at wrist and hand level
   ● S65.811   Laceration of other blood vessels at wrist and hand level of right arm
   ● S65.812   Laceration of other blood vessels at wrist and hand level of left arm
   ● S65.819   Laceration of other blood vessels at wrist and hand level of unspecified arm
  ● S65.89   Other specified injury of other blood vessels at wrist and hand level
   ● S65.891   Other specified injury of other blood vessels at wrist and hand level of right arm
   ● S65.892   Other specified injury of other blood vessels at wrist and hand level of left arm
   ● S65.899   Other specified injury of other blood vessels at wrist and hand level of unspecified arm

CHAPTER 19 (S00-T88)

◀ New   ◀■■ Revised   ~~deleted~~ Deleted   OGCR Official Guidelines   X Assign placeholder X   ● Use Additional Character(s)
Excludes 1   Excludes 2   Includes   Use additional   Code first   Code also   Unspecified
1321

- S65.9 **Injury of unspecified blood vessel at wrist and hand level**
  - S65.90 **Unspecified injury of unspecified blood vessel at wrist and hand level**
    - S65.901 Unspecified injury of unspecified blood vessel at wrist and hand level of right arm
    - S65.902 Unspecified injury of unspecified blood vessel at wrist and hand level of left arm
    - S65.909 Unspecified injury of unspecified blood vessel at wrist and hand level of unspecified arm
  - S65.91 **Laceration of unspecified blood vessel at wrist and hand level**
    - S65.911 Laceration of unspecified blood vessel at wrist and hand level of right arm
    - S65.912 Laceration of unspecified blood vessel at wrist and hand level of left arm
    - S65.919 Laceration of unspecified blood vessel at wrist and hand level of unspecified arm
  - S65.99 **Other specified injury of unspecified blood vessel at wrist and hand level**
    - S65.991 Other specified injury of unspecified blood vessel at wrist and hand of right arm
    - S65.992 Other specified injury of unspecified blood vessel at wrist and hand of left arm
    - S65.999 Other specified injury of unspecified blood vessel at wrist and hand of unspecified arm

- S66 **Injury of muscle, fascia and tendon at wrist and hand level**

  Code also any associated open wound (S61.-)

  Excludes2 sprain of joints and ligaments of wrist and hand (S63.-)

  The appropriate 7th character is to be added to each code from category S66

A	initial encounter
D	subsequent encounter
S	sequela

  - S66.0 **Injury of long flexor muscle, fascia and tendon of thumb at wrist and hand level**
    - S66.00 **Unspecified injury of long flexor muscle, fascia and tendon of thumb at wrist and hand level**
      - S66.001 Unspecified injury of long flexor muscle, fascia and tendon of right thumb at wrist and hand level
      - S66.002 Unspecified injury of long flexor muscle, fascia and tendon of left thumb at wrist and hand level
      - S66.009 Unspecified injury of long flexor muscle, fascia and tendon of unspecified thumb at wrist and hand level
    - S66.01 **Strain of long flexor muscle, fascia and tendon of thumb at wrist and hand level**
      - S66.011 Strain of long flexor muscle, fascia and tendon of right thumb at wrist and hand level
      - S66.012 Strain of long flexor muscle, fascia and tendon of left thumb at wrist and hand level
      - S66.019 Strain of long flexor muscle, fascia and tendon of unspecified thumb at wrist and hand level

  - S66.02 **Laceration of long flexor muscle, fascia and tendon of thumb at wrist and hand level**
    - S66.021 Laceration of long flexor muscle, fascia and tendon of right thumb at wrist and hand level
    - S66.022 Laceration of long flexor muscle, fascia and tendon of left thumb at wrist and hand level
    - S66.029 Laceration of long flexor muscle, fascia and tendon of unspecified thumb at wrist and hand level
  - S66.09 **Other specified injury of long flexor muscle, fascia and tendon of thumb at wrist and hand level**
    - S66.091 Other specified injury of long flexor muscle, fascia and tendon of right thumb at wrist and hand level
    - S66.092 Other specified injury of long flexor muscle, fascia and tendon of left thumb at wrist and hand level
    - S66.099 Other specified injury of long flexor muscle, fascia and tendon of unspecified thumb at wrist and hand level

  - S66.1 **Injury of flexor muscle, fascia and tendon of other and unspecified finger at wrist and hand level**

    Excludes2 injury of long flexor muscle, fascia and tendon of thumb at wrist and hand level (S66.0-)

    - S66.10 **Unspecified injury of flexor muscle, fascia and tendon of other and unspecified finger at wrist and hand level**
      - S66.100 Unspecified injury of flexor muscle, fascia and tendon of right index finger at wrist and hand level
      - S66.101 Unspecified injury of flexor muscle, fascia and tendon of left index finger at wrist and hand level
      - S66.102 Unspecified injury of flexor muscle, fascia and tendon of right middle finger at wrist and hand level
      - S66.103 Unspecified injury of flexor muscle, fascia and tendon of left middle finger at wrist and hand level
      - S66.104 Unspecified injury of flexor muscle, fascia and tendon of right ring finger at wrist and hand level
      - S66.105 Unspecified injury of flexor muscle, fascia and tendon of left ring finger at wrist and hand level
      - S66.106 Unspecified injury of flexor muscle, fascia and tendon of right little finger at wrist and hand level
      - S66.107 Unspecified injury of flexor muscle, fascia and tendon of left little finger at wrist and hand level
      - S66.108 Unspecified injury of flexor muscle, fascia and tendon of other finger at wrist and hand level

        Unspecified injury of flexor muscle, fascia and tendon of specified finger with unspecified laterality at wrist and hand level
      - S66.109 Unspecified injury of flexor muscle, fascia and tendon of unspecified finger at wrist and hand level

● S66.11   Strain of flexor muscle, fascia and tendon of other and unspecified finger at wrist and hand level

     ● S66.110   Strain of flexor muscle, fascia and tendon of right index finger at wrist and hand level

     ● S66.111   Strain of flexor muscle, fascia and tendon of left index finger at wrist and hand level

     ● S66.112   Strain of flexor muscle, fascia and tendon of right middle finger at wrist and hand level

     ● S66.113   Strain of flexor muscle, fascia and tendon of left middle finger at wrist and hand level

     ● S66.114   Strain of flexor muscle, fascia and tendon of right ring finger at wrist and hand level

     ● S66.115   Strain of flexor muscle, fascia and tendon of left ring finger at wrist and hand level

     ● S66.116   Strain of flexor muscle, fascia and tendon of right little finger at wrist and hand level

     ● S66.117   Strain of flexor muscle, fascia and tendon of left little finger at wrist and hand level

     ● S66.118   Strain of flexor muscle, fascia and tendon of other finger at wrist and hand level

         Strain of flexor muscle, fascia and tendon of specified finger with unspecified laterality at wrist and hand level

     ● S66.119   Strain of flexor muscle, fascia and tendon of unspecified finger at wrist and hand level

● S66.12   Laceration of flexor muscle, fascia and tendon of other and unspecified finger at wrist and hand level

     ● S66.120   Laceration of flexor muscle, fascia and tendon of right index finger at wrist and hand level

     ● S66.121   Laceration of flexor muscle, fascia and tendon of left index finger at wrist and hand level

     ● S66.122   Laceration of flexor muscle, fascia and tendon of right middle finger at wrist and hand level

     ● S66.123   Laceration of flexor muscle, fascia and tendon of left middle finger at wrist and hand level

     ● S66.124   Laceration of flexor muscle, fascia and tendon of right ring finger at wrist and hand level

     ● S66.125   Laceration of flexor muscle, fascia and tendon of left ring finger at wrist and hand level

     ● S66.126   Laceration of flexor muscle, fascia and tendon of right little finger at wrist and hand level

     ● S66.127   Laceration of flexor muscle, fascia and tendon of left little finger at wrist and hand level

● S66.128   Laceration of flexor muscle, fascia and tendon of other finger at wrist and hand level

         Laceration of flexor muscle, fascia and tendon of specified finger with unspecified laterality at wrist and hand level

     ● S66.129   Laceration of flexor muscle, fascia and tendon of unspecified finger at wrist and hand level

● S66.19   Other injury of flexor muscle, fascia and tendon of other and unspecified finger at wrist and hand level

     ● S66.190   Other injury of flexor muscle, fascia and tendon of right index finger at wrist and hand level

     ● S66.191   Other injury of flexor muscle, fascia and tendon of left index finger at wrist and hand level

     ● S66.192   Other injury of flexor muscle, fascia and tendon of right middle finger at wrist and hand level

     ● S66.193   Other injury of flexor muscle, fascia and tendon of left middle finger at wrist and hand level

     ● S66.194   Other injury of flexor muscle, fascia and tendon of right ring finger at wrist and hand level

     ● S66.195   Other injury of flexor muscle, fascia and tendon of left ring finger at wrist and hand level

     ● S66.196   Other injury of flexor muscle, fascia and tendon of right little finger at wrist and hand level

     ● S66.197   Other injury of flexor muscle, fascia and tendon of left little finger at wrist and hand level

     ● S66.198   Other injury of flexor muscle, fascia and tendon of other finger at wrist and hand level

         Other injury of flexor muscle, fascia and tendon of specified finger with unspecified laterality at wrist and hand level

     ● S66.199   Other injury of flexor muscle, fascia and tendon of unspecified finger at wrist and hand level

● S66.2   Injury of extensor muscle, fascia and tendon of thumb at wrist and hand level

     ● S66.20   Unspecified injury of extensor muscle, fascia and tendon of thumb at wrist and hand level

         ● S66.201   Unspecified injury of extensor muscle, fascia and tendon of right thumb at wrist and hand level

         ● S66.202   Unspecified injury of extensor muscle, fascia and tendon of left thumb at wrist and hand level

         ● S66.209   Unspecified injury of extensor muscle, fascia and tendon of unspecified thumb at wrist and hand level

     ● S66.21   Strain of extensor muscle, fascia and tendon of thumb at wrist and hand level

         ● S66.211   Strain of extensor muscle, fascia and tendon of right thumb at wrist and hand level

         ● S66.212   Strain of extensor muscle, fascia and tendon of left thumb at wrist and hand level

         ● S66.219   Strain of extensor muscle, fascia and tendon of unspecified thumb at wrist and hand level

● **S66.22**   **Laceration of extensor muscle, fascia and tendon of thumb at wrist and hand level**

     ● **S66.221**   Laceration of extensor muscle, fascia and tendon of right thumb at wrist and hand level

     ● **S66.222**   Laceration of extensor muscle, fascia and tendon of left thumb at wrist and hand level

     ● **S66.229**   Laceration of extensor muscle, fascia and tendon of unspecified thumb at wrist and hand level

● **S66.29**   **Other specified injury of extensor muscle, fascia and tendon of thumb at wrist and hand level**

     ● **S66.291**   Other specified injury of extensor muscle, fascia and tendon of right thumb at wrist and hand level

     ● **S66.292**   Other specified injury of extensor muscle, fascia and tendon of left thumb at wrist and hand level

     ● **S66.299**   Other specified injury of extensor muscle, fascia and tendon of unspecified thumb at wrist and hand level

● **S66.3**   **Injury of extensor muscle, fascia and tendon of other and unspecified finger at wrist and hand level**

     Excludes2   injury of extensor muscle, fascia and tendon of thumb at wrist and hand level (S66.2-)

     ● **S66.30**   **Unspecified injury of extensor muscle, fascia and tendon of other and unspecified finger at wrist and hand level**

         ● **S66.300**   Unspecified injury of extensor muscle, fascia and tendon of right index finger at wrist and hand level

         ● **S66.301**   Unspecified injury of extensor muscle, fascia and tendon of left index finger at wrist and hand level

         ● **S66.302**   Unspecified injury of extensor muscle, fascia and tendon of right middle finger at wrist and hand level

         ● **S66.303**   Unspecified injury of extensor muscle, fascia and tendon of left middle finger at wrist and hand level

         ● **S66.304**   Unspecified injury of extensor muscle, fascia and tendon of right ring finger at wrist and hand level

         ● **S66.305**   Unspecified injury of extensor muscle, fascia and tendon of left ring finger at wrist and hand level

         ● **S66.306**   Unspecified injury of extensor muscle, fascia and tendon of right little finger at wrist and hand level

         ● **S66.307**   Unspecified injury of extensor muscle, fascia and tendon of left little finger at wrist and hand level

         ● **S66.308**   Unspecified injury of extensor muscle, fascia and tendon of other finger at wrist and hand level

             Unspecified injury of extensor muscle, fascia and tendon of specified finger with unspecified laterality at wrist and hand level

         ● **S66.309**   Unspecified injury of extensor muscle, fascia and tendon of unspecified finger at wrist and hand level

● **S66.31**   **Strain of extensor muscle, fascia and tendon of other and unspecified finger at wrist and hand level**

     ● **S66.310**   Strain of extensor muscle, fascia and tendon of right index finger at wrist and hand level

     ● **S66.311**   Strain of extensor muscle, fascia and tendon of left index finger at wrist and hand level

     ● **S66.312**   Strain of extensor muscle, fascia and tendon of right middle finger at wrist and hand level

     ● **S66.313**   Strain of extensor muscle, fascia and tendon of left middle finger at wrist and hand level

     ● **S66.314**   Strain of extensor muscle, fascia and tendon of right ring finger at wrist and hand level

     ● **S66.315**   Strain of extensor muscle, fascia and tendon of left ring finger at wrist and hand level

     ● **S66.316**   Strain of extensor muscle, fascia and tendon of right little finger at wrist and hand level

     ● **S66.317**   Strain of extensor muscle, fascia and tendon of left little finger at wrist and hand level

     ● **S66.318**   Strain of extensor muscle, fascia and tendon of other finger at wrist and hand level

         Strain of extensor muscle, fascia and tendon of specified finger with unspecified laterality at wrist and hand level

     ● **S66.319**   Strain of extensor muscle, fascia and tendon of unspecified finger at wrist and hand level

● **S66.32**   **Laceration of extensor muscle, fascia and tendon of other and unspecified finger at wrist and hand level**

     ● **S66.320**   Laceration of extensor muscle, fascia and tendon of right index finger at wrist and hand level

     ● **S66.321**   Laceration of extensor muscle, fascia and tendon of left index finger at wrist and hand level

     ● **S66.322**   Laceration of extensor muscle, fascia and tendon of right middle finger at wrist and hand level

     ● **S66.323**   Laceration of extensor muscle, fascia and tendon of left middle finger at wrist and hand level

     ● **S66.324**   Laceration of extensor muscle, fascia and tendon of right ring finger at wrist and hand level

     ● **S66.325**   Laceration of extensor muscle, fascia and tendon of left ring finger at wrist and hand level

     ● **S66.326**   Laceration of extensor muscle, fascia and tendon of right little finger at wrist and hand level

     ● **S66.327**   Laceration of extensor muscle, fascia and tendon of left little finger at wrist and hand level

     ● **S66.328**   Laceration of extensor muscle, fascia and tendon of other finger at wrist and hand level

         Laceration of extensor muscle, fascia and tendon of specified finger with unspecified laterality at wrist and hand level

     ● **S66.329**   Laceration of extensor muscle, fascia and tendon of unspecified finger at wrist and hand level

CHAPTER 19 (S00-T88)

● S66.39   Other injury of extensor muscle, fascia and tendon of other and unspecified finger at wrist and hand level

   ● S66.390   Other injury of extensor muscle, fascia and tendon of right index finger at wrist and hand level

   ● S66.391   Other injury of extensor muscle, fascia and tendon of left index finger at wrist and hand level

   ● S66.392   Other injury of extensor muscle, fascia and tendon of right middle finger at wrist and hand level

   ● S66.393   Other injury of extensor muscle, fascia and tendon of left middle finger at wrist and hand level

   ● S66.394   Other injury of extensor muscle, fascia and tendon of right ring finger at wrist and hand level

   ● S66.395   Other injury of extensor muscle, fascia and tendon of left ring finger at wrist and hand level

   ● S66.396   Other injury of extensor muscle, fascia and tendon of right little finger at wrist and hand level

   ● S66.397   Other injury of extensor muscle, fascia and tendon of left little finger at wrist and hand level

   ● S66.398   Other injury of extensor muscle, fascia and tendon of other finger at wrist and hand level

         Other injury of extensor muscle, fascia and tendon of specified finger with unspecified laterality at wrist and hand level

   ● S66.399   Other injury of extensor muscle, fascia and tendon of unspecified finger at wrist and hand level

● S66.4   Injury of intrinsic muscle, fascia and tendon of thumb at wrist and hand level

   ● S66.40   Unspecified injury of intrinsic muscle, fascia and tendon of thumb at wrist and hand level

     ● S66.401   Unspecified injury of intrinsic muscle, fascia and tendon of right thumb at wrist and hand level

     ● S66.402   Unspecified injury of intrinsic muscle, fascia and tendon of left thumb at wrist and hand level

     ● S66.409   Unspecified injury of intrinsic muscle, fascia and tendon of unspecified thumb at wrist and hand level

   ● S66.41   Strain of intrinsic muscle, fascia and tendon of thumb at wrist and hand level

     ● S66.411   Strain of intrinsic muscle, fascia and tendon of right thumb at wrist and hand level

     ● S66.412   Strain of intrinsic muscle, fascia and tendon of left thumb at wrist and hand level

     ● S66.419   Strain of intrinsic muscle, fascia and tendon of unspecified thumb at wrist and hand level

● S66.42   Laceration of intrinsic muscle, fascia and tendon of thumb at wrist and hand level

   ● S66.421   Laceration of intrinsic muscle, fascia and tendon of right thumb at wrist and hand level

   ● S66.422   Laceration of intrinsic muscle, fascia and tendon of left thumb at wrist and hand level

   ● S66.429   Laceration of intrinsic muscle, fascia and tendon of unspecified thumb at wrist and hand level

● S66.49   Other specified injury of intrinsic muscle, fascia and tendon of thumb at wrist and hand level

   ● S66.491   Other specified injury of intrinsic muscle, fascia and tendon of right thumb at wrist and hand level

   ● S66.492   Other specified injury of intrinsic muscle, fascia and tendon of left thumb at wrist and hand level

   ● S66.499   Other specified injury of intrinsic muscle, fascia and tendon of unspecified thumb at wrist and hand level

● S66.5   Injury of intrinsic muscle, fascia and tendon of other and unspecified finger at wrist and hand level

    Excludes2   injury of intrinsic muscle, fascia and tendon of thumb at wrist and hand level (S66.4-)

   ● S66.50   Unspecified injury of intrinsic muscle, fascia and tendon of other and unspecified finger at wrist and hand level

     ● S66.500   Unspecified injury of intrinsic muscle, fascia and tendon of right index finger at wrist and hand level

     ● S66.501   Unspecified injury of intrinsic muscle, fascia and tendon of left index finger at wrist and hand level

     ● S66.502   Unspecified injury of intrinsic muscle, fascia and tendon of right middle finger at wrist and hand level

     ● S66.503   Unspecified injury of intrinsic muscle, fascia and tendon of left middle finger at wrist and hand level

     ● S66.504   Unspecified injury of intrinsic muscle, fascia and tendon of right ring finger at wrist and hand level

     ● S66.505   Unspecified injury of intrinsic muscle, fascia and tendon of left ring finger at wrist and hand level

     ● S66.506   Unspecified injury of intrinsic muscle, fascia and tendon of right little finger at wrist and hand level

     ● S66.507   Unspecified injury of intrinsic muscle, fascia and tendon of left little finger at wrist and hand level

     ● S66.508   Unspecified injury of intrinsic muscle, fascia and tendon of other finger at wrist and hand level

         Unspecified injury of intrinsic muscle, fascia and tendon of specified finger with unspecified laterality at wrist and hand level

     ● S66.509   Unspecified injury of intrinsic muscle, fascia and tendon of unspecified finger at wrist and hand level

S66.51 Strain of intrinsic muscle, fascia and tendon of other and unspecified finger at wrist and hand level

S66.510 Strain of intrinsic muscle, fascia and tendon of right index finger at wrist and hand level

S66.511 Strain of intrinsic muscle, fascia and tendon of left index finger at wrist and hand level

S66.512 Strain of intrinsic muscle, fascia and tendon of right middle finger at wrist and hand level

S66.513 Strain of intrinsic muscle, fascia and tendon of left middle finger at wrist and hand level

S66.514 Strain of intrinsic muscle, fascia and tendon of right ring finger at wrist and hand level

S66.515 Strain of intrinsic muscle, fascia and tendon of left ring finger at wrist and hand level

S66.516 Strain of intrinsic muscle, fascia and tendon of right little finger at wrist and hand level

S66.517 Strain of intrinsic muscle, fascia and tendon of left little finger at wrist and hand level

S66.518 Strain of intrinsic muscle, fascia and tendon of other finger at wrist and hand level
Strain of intrinsic muscle, fascia and tendon of specified finger with unspecified laterality at wrist and hand level

S66.519 Strain of intrinsic muscle, fascia and tendon of unspecified finger at wrist and hand level

S66.52 Laceration of intrinsic muscle, fascia and tendon of other and unspecified finger at wrist and hand level

S66.520 Laceration of intrinsic muscle, fascia and tendon of right index finger at wrist and hand level

S66.521 Laceration of intrinsic muscle, fascia and tendon of left index finger at wrist and hand level

S66.522 Laceration of intrinsic muscle, fascia and tendon of right middle finger at wrist and hand level

S66.523 Laceration of intrinsic muscle, fascia and tendon of left middle finger at wrist and hand level

S66.524 Laceration of intrinsic muscle, fascia and tendon of right ring finger at wrist and hand level

S66.525 Laceration of intrinsic muscle, fascia and tendon of left ring finger at wrist and hand level

S66.526 Laceration of intrinsic muscle, fascia and tendon of right little finger at wrist and hand level

S66.527 Laceration of intrinsic muscle, fascia and tendon of left little finger at wrist and hand level

S66.528 Laceration of intrinsic muscle, fascia and tendon of other finger at wrist and hand level
Laceration of intrinsic muscle, fascia and tendon of specified finger with unspecified laterality at wrist and hand level

S66.529 Laceration of intrinsic muscle, fascia and tendon of unspecified finger at wrist and hand level

S66.59 Other injury of intrinsic muscle, fascia and tendon of other and unspecified finger at wrist and hand level

S66.590 Other injury of intrinsic muscle, fascia and tendon of right index finger at wrist and hand level

S66.591 Other injury of intrinsic muscle, fascia and tendon of left index finger at wrist and hand level

S66.592 Other injury of intrinsic muscle, fascia and tendon of right middle finger at wrist and hand level

S66.593 Other injury of intrinsic muscle, fascia and tendon of left middle finger at wrist and hand level

S66.594 Other injury of intrinsic muscle, fascia and tendon of right ring finger at wrist and hand level

S66.595 Other injury of intrinsic muscle, fascia and tendon of left ring finger at wrist and hand level

S66.596 Other injury of intrinsic muscle, fascia and tendon of right little finger at wrist and hand level

S66.597 Other injury of intrinsic muscle, fascia and tendon of left little finger at wrist and hand level

S66.598 Other injury of intrinsic muscle, fascia and tendon of other finger at wrist and hand level
Other injury of intrinsic muscle, fascia and tendon of specified finger with unspecified laterality at wrist and hand level

S66.599 Other injury of intrinsic muscle, fascia and tendon of unspecified finger at wrist and hand level

S66.8 Injury of other specified muscles, fascia and tendons at wrist and hand level

S66.80 Unspecified injury of other specified muscles, fascia and tendons at wrist and hand level

S66.801 Unspecified injury of other specified muscles, fascia and tendons at wrist and hand level, right hand

S66.802 Unspecified injury of other specified muscles, fascia and tendons at wrist and hand level, left hand

S66.809 Unspecified injury of other specified muscles, fascia and tendons at wrist and hand level, unspecified hand

S66.81 Strain of other specified muscles, fascia and tendons at wrist and hand level

S66.811 Strain of other specified muscles, fascia and tendons at wrist and hand level, right hand

S66.812 Strain of other specified muscles, fascia and tendons at wrist and hand level, left hand

S66.819 Strain of other specified muscles, fascia and tendons at wrist and hand level, unspecified hand

S66.82 Laceration of other specified muscles, fascia and tendons at wrist and hand level

S66.821 Laceration of other specified muscles, fascia and tendons at wrist and hand level, right hand

S66.822 Laceration of other specified muscles, fascia and tendons at wrist and hand level, left hand

S66.829 Laceration of other specified muscles, fascia and tendons at wrist and hand level, unspecified hand

◄ New   ◄▥ Revised   ~~deleted~~ Deleted   OGCR Official Guidelines   X Assign placeholder X   ● Use Additional Character(s)

Excludes 1   Excludes 2   Includes   Use additional   Code first   Code also   Unspecified

- S66.89   Other injury of other specified muscles, fascia and tendons at wrist and hand level
  - S66.891   Other injury of other specified muscles, fascia and tendons at wrist and hand level, right hand
  - S66.892   Other injury of other specified muscles, fascia and tendons at wrist and hand level, left hand
  - S66.899   Other injury of other specified muscles, fascia and tendons at wrist and hand level, unspecified hand
- S66.9   Injury of unspecified muscle, fascia and tendon at wrist and hand level
  - S66.90   Unspecified injury of unspecified muscle, fascia and tendon at wrist and hand level
    - S66.901   Unspecified injury of unspecified muscle, fascia and tendon at wrist and hand level, right hand
    - S66.902   Unspecified injury of unspecified muscle, fascia and tendon at wrist and hand level, left hand
    - S66.909   Unspecified injury of unspecified muscle, fascia and tendon at wrist and hand level, unspecified hand
  - S66.91   Strain of unspecified muscle, fascia and tendon at wrist and hand level
    - S66.911   Strain of unspecified muscle, fascia and tendon at wrist and hand level, right hand
    - S66.912   Strain of unspecified muscle, fascia and tendon at wrist and hand level, left hand
    - S66.919   Strain of unspecified muscle, fascia and tendon at wrist and hand level, unspecified hand
  - S66.92   Laceration of unspecified muscle, fascia and tendon at wrist and hand level
    - S66.921   Laceration of unspecified muscle, fascia and tendon at wrist and hand level, right hand
    - S66.922   Laceration of unspecified muscle, fascia and tendon at wrist and hand level, left hand
    - S66.929   Laceration of unspecified muscle, fascia and tendon at wrist and hand level, unspecified hand
  - S66.99   Other injury of unspecified muscle, fascia and tendon at wrist and hand level
    - S66.991   Other injury of unspecified muscle, fascia and tendon at wrist and hand level, right hand
    - S66.992   Other injury of unspecified muscle, fascia and tendon at wrist and hand level, left hand
    - S66.999   Other injury of unspecified muscle, fascia and tendon at wrist and hand level, unspecified hand

- S67   **Crushing injury of wrist, hand and fingers**

  Use additional code for all associated injuries, such as:
  fracture of wrist and hand (S62.-)
  open wound of wrist and hand (S61.-)

  The appropriate 7th character is to be added to each code from category S67

A	initial encounter
D	subsequent encounter
S	sequela

  - S67.0   Crushing injury of thumb
    - X ● S67.00   Crushing injury of unspecified thumb
    - X ● S67.01   Crushing injury of right thumb
    - X ● S67.02   Crushing injury of left thumb

  - S67.1   Crushing injury of other and unspecified finger(s)

    Excludes2   crushing injury of thumb (S67.0-)
    - X ● S67.10   Crushing injury of unspecified finger(s)
    - ● S67.19   Crushing injury of other finger(s)
      - ● S67.190   Crushing injury of right index finger
      - ● S67.191   Crushing injury of left index finger
      - ● S67.192   Crushing injury of right middle finger
      - ● S67.193   Crushing injury of left middle finger
      - ● S67.194   Crushing injury of right ring finger
      - ● S67.195   Crushing injury of left ring finger
      - ● S67.196   Crushing injury of right little finger
      - ● S67.197   Crushing injury of left little finger
      - ● S67.198   Crushing injury of other finger
        Crushing injury of specified finger with unspecified laterality

  - S67.2   Crushing injury of hand

    Excludes2   crushing injury of fingers (S67.1-)
    crushing injury of thumb (S67.0-)
    - X ● S67.20   Crushing injury of unspecified hand
    - X ● S67.21   Crushing injury of right hand
    - X ● S67.22   Crushing injury of left hand

  - S67.3   Crushing injury of wrist
    - X ● S67.30   Crushing injury of unspecified wrist
    - X ● S67.31   Crushing injury of right wrist
    - X ● S67.32   Crushing injury of left wrist

  - S67.4   Crushing injury of wrist and hand

    Excludes1   crushing injury of hand alone (S67.2-)
    crushing injury of wrist alone (S67.3-)

    Excludes2   crushing injury of fingers (S67.1-)
    crushing injury of thumb (S67.0-)
    - X ● S67.40   Crushing injury of unspecified wrist and hand
    - X ● S67.41   Crushing injury of right wrist and hand
    - X ● S67.42   Crushing injury of left wrist and hand

  - S67.9   Crushing injury of unspecified part(s) of wrist, hand and fingers
    - X ● S67.90   Crushing injury of unspecified part(s) of unspecified wrist, hand and fingers
    - X ● S67.91   Crushing injury of unspecified part(s) of right wrist, hand and fingers
    - X ● S67.92   Crushing injury of unspecified part(s) of left wrist, hand and fingers

- S68   **Traumatic amputation of wrist, hand and fingers**

  An amputation not identified as partial or complete should be coded to complete

  The appropriate 7th character is to be added to each code from category S68

A	initial encounter
D	subsequent encounter
S	sequela

  - S68.0   Traumatic metacarpophalangeal amputation of thumb
    Traumatic amputation of thumb NOS
    - ● S68.01   Complete traumatic metacarpophalangeal amputation of thumb
      - ● S68.011   Complete traumatic metacarpophalangeal amputation of right thumb
      - ● S68.012   Complete traumatic metacarpophalangeal amputation of left thumb
      - ● S68.019   Complete traumatic metacarpophalangeal amputation of unspecified thumb

CHAPTER 19 (S00-T88)

◀ New   ◀▥ Revised   d̶e̶l̶e̶t̶e̶d̶ Deleted   **OGCR** Official Guidelines   X Assign placeholder X   ● Use Additional Character(s)

| Excludes 1 | Excludes 2 | Includes | Use additional | Code first | Code also | Unspecified |

1327

- S68.02 Partial traumatic metacarpophalangeal
  amputation of thumb
  - S68.021 Partial traumatic
    metacarpophalangeal amputation of
    right thumb
  - S68.022 Partial traumatic
    metacarpophalangeal amputation of
    left thumb
  - S68.029 Partial traumatic
    metacarpophalangeal amputation of
    unspecified thumb
- S68.1 Traumatic metacarpophalangeal amputation of other and
  unspecified finger
  Traumatic amputation of finger NOS
  Excludes2 traumatic metacarpophalangeal
            amputation of thumb (S68.0-)
  - S68.11 Complete traumatic metacarpophalangeal
    amputation of other and unspecified finger
    - S68.110 Complete traumatic
      metacarpophalangeal amputation of
      right index finger
    - S68.111 Complete traumatic
      metacarpophalangeal amputation of
      left index finger
    - S68.112 Complete traumatic
      metacarpophalangeal amputation of
      right middle finger
    - S68.113 Complete traumatic
      metacarpophalangeal amputation of
      left middle finger
    - S68.114 Complete traumatic
      metacarpophalangeal amputation of
      right ring finger
    - S68.115 Complete traumatic
      metacarpophalangeal amputation of
      left ring finger
    - S68.116 Complete traumatic
      metacarpophalangeal amputation of
      right little finger
    - S68.117 Complete traumatic
      metacarpophalangeal amputation of
      left little finger
    - S68.118 Complete traumatic
      metacarpophalangeal amputation of
      other finger
      Complete traumatic
        metacarpophalangeal
        amputation of specified finger
        with unspecified laterality
    - S68.119 Complete traumatic
      metacarpophalangeal amputation of
      unspecified finger
  - S68.12 Partial traumatic metacarpophalangeal
    amputation of other and unspecified finger
    - S68.120 Partial traumatic
      metacarpophalangeal amputation of
      right index finger
    - S68.121 Partial traumatic
      metacarpophalangeal amputation of
      left index finger
    - S68.122 Partial traumatic
      metacarpophalangeal amputation of
      right middle finger

- S68.123 Partial traumatic
  metacarpophalangeal amputation of
  left middle finger
- S68.124 Partial traumatic
  metacarpophalangeal amputation of
  right ring finger
- S68.125 Partial traumatic
  metacarpophalangeal amputation of
  left ring finger
- S68.126 Partial traumatic
  metacarpophalangeal amputation of
  right little finger
- S68.127 Partial traumatic
  metacarpophalangeal amputation of
  left little finger
- S68.128 Partial traumatic
  metacarpophalangeal amputation of
  other finger
  Partial traumatic
    metacarpophalangeal
    amputation of specified finger
    with unspecified laterality
- S68.129 Partial traumatic
  metacarpophalangeal amputation of
  unspecified finger
- S68.4 Traumatic amputation of hand at wrist level
  Traumatic amputation of hand NOS
  Traumatic amputation of wrist
  - S68.41 Complete traumatic amputation of hand at
    wrist level
    - S68.411 Complete traumatic amputation of
      right hand at wrist level
    - S68.412 Complete traumatic amputation of
      left hand at wrist level
    - S68.419 Complete traumatic amputation of
      unspecified hand at wrist level
  - S68.42 Partial traumatic amputation of hand at wrist
    level
    - S68.421 Partial traumatic amputation of right
      hand at wrist level
    - S68.422 Partial traumatic amputation of left
      hand at wrist level
    - S68.429 Partial traumatic amputation of
      unspecified hand at wrist level
- S68.5 Traumatic transphalangeal amputation of thumb
  Traumatic interphalangeal joint amputation of thumb
  - S68.51 Complete traumatic transphalangeal
    amputation of thumb
    - S68.511 Complete traumatic transphalangeal
      amputation of right thumb
    - S68.512 Complete traumatic transphalangeal
      amputation of left thumb
    - S68.519 Complete traumatic transphalangeal
      amputation of unspecified thumb
  - S68.52 Partial traumatic transphalangeal amputation of
    thumb
    - S68.521 Partial traumatic transphalangeal
      amputation of right thumb
    - S68.522 Partial traumatic transphalangeal
      amputation of left thumb
    - S68.529 Partial traumatic transphalangeal
      amputation of unspecified thumb

● **S68.6** Traumatic transphalangeal amputation of other and unspecified finger
  ● **S68.61** Complete traumatic transphalangeal amputation of other and unspecified finger(s)
    ● **S68.610** Complete traumatic transphalangeal amputation of right index finger
    ● **S68.611** Complete traumatic transphalangeal amputation of left index finger
    ● **S68.612** Complete traumatic transphalangeal amputation of right middle finger
    ● **S68.613** Complete traumatic transphalangeal amputation of left middle finger
    ● **S68.614** Complete traumatic transphalangeal amputation of right ring finger
    ● **S68.615** Complete traumatic transphalangeal amputation of left ring finger
    ● **S68.616** Complete traumatic transphalangeal amputation of right little finger
    ● **S68.617** Complete traumatic transphalangeal amputation of left little finger
    ● **S68.618** Complete traumatic transphalangeal amputation of other finger
       Complete traumatic transphalangeal amputation of specified finger with unspecified laterality
    ● **S68.619** Complete traumatic transphalangeal amputation of unspecified finger
  ● **S68.62** Partial traumatic transphalangeal amputation of other and unspecified finger
    ● **S68.620** Partial traumatic transphalangeal amputation of right index finger
    ● **S68.621** Partial traumatic transphalangeal amputation of left index finger
    ● **S68.622** Partial traumatic transphalangeal amputation of right middle finger
    ● **S68.623** Partial traumatic transphalangeal amputation of left middle finger
    ● **S68.624** Partial traumatic transphalangeal amputation of right ring finger
    ● **S68.625** Partial traumatic transphalangeal amputation of left ring finger
    ● **S68.626** Partial traumatic transphalangeal amputation of right little finger
    ● **S68.627** Partial traumatic transphalangeal amputation of left little finger
    ● **S68.628** Partial traumatic transphalangeal amputation of other finger
       Partial traumatic transphalangeal amputation of specified finger with unspecified laterality
    ● **S68.629** Partial traumatic transphalangeal amputation of unspecified finger
● **S68.7** Traumatic transmetacarpal amputation of hand
  ● **S68.71** Complete traumatic transmetacarpal amputation of hand
    ● **S68.711** Complete traumatic transmetacarpal amputation of right hand
    ● **S68.712** Complete traumatic transmetacarpal amputation of left hand
    ● **S68.719** Complete traumatic transmetacarpal amputation of unspecified hand
  ● **S68.72** Partial traumatic transmetacarpal amputation of hand
    ● **S68.721** Partial traumatic transmetacarpal amputation of right hand
    ● **S68.722** Partial traumatic transmetacarpal amputation of left hand
    ● **S68.729** Partial traumatic transmetacarpal amputation of unspecified hand

● **S69** Other and unspecified injuries of wrist, hand and finger(s)
The appropriate 7th character is to be added to each code from category S69

> A   initial encounter
> D   subsequent encounter
> S   sequela

  ● **S69.8** Other specified injuries of wrist, hand and finger(s)
   X● **S69.80** Other specified injuries of unspecified wrist, hand and finger(s)
   X● **S69.81** Other specified injuries of right wrist, hand and finger(s)
   X● **S69.82** Other specified injuries of left wrist, hand and finger(s)
  ● **S69.9** Unspecified injury of wrist, hand and finger(s)
   X● **S69.90** Unspecified injury of unspecified wrist, hand and finger(s)
   X● **S69.91** Unspecified injury of right wrist, hand and finger(s)
   X● **S69.92** Unspecified injury of left wrist, hand and finger(s)

INJURIES TO THE HIP AND THIGH (S70-S79)

Excludes2   burns and corrosions (T20-T32)
frostbite (T33-T34)
snake bite (T63.0-)
venomous insect bite or sting (T63.4-)

● **S70** Superficial injury of hip and thigh
The appropriate 7th character is to be added to each code from category S70

> A   initial encounter
> D   subsequent encounter
> S   sequela

  ● **S70.0** Contusion of hip
   X● **S70.00** Contusion of unspecified hip
   X● **S70.01** Contusion of right hip
   X● **S70.02** Contusion of left hip
  ● **S70.1** Contusion of thigh
   X● **S70.10** Contusion of unspecified thigh
   X● **S70.11** Contusion of right thigh
   X● **S70.12** Contusion of left thigh
  ● **S70.2** Other superficial injuries of hip
   ● **S70.21** Abrasion of hip
    ● **S70.211** Abrasion, right hip
    ● **S70.212** Abrasion, left hip
    ● **S70.219** Abrasion, unspecified hip
   ● **S70.22** Blister (nonthermal) of hip
    ● **S70.221** Blister (nonthermal), right hip
    ● **S70.222** Blister (nonthermal), left hip
    ● **S70.229** Blister (nonthermal), unspecified hip
   ● **S70.24** External constriction of hip
    ● **S70.241** External constriction, right hip
    ● **S70.242** External constriction, left hip
    ● **S70.249** External constriction, unspecified hip
   ● **S70.25** Superficial foreign body of hip
    Splinter in the hip
    ● **S70.251** Superficial foreign body, right hip
    ● **S70.252** Superficial foreign body, left hip
    ● **S70.259** Superficial foreign body, unspecified hip

CHAPTER 19 (S00-T88)

- S70.26 Insect bite (nonvenomous) of hip
  - S70.261 Insect bite (nonvenomous), right hip
  - S70.262 Insect bite (nonvenomous), left hip
  - S70.269 Insect bite (nonvenomous), unspecified hip
- S70.27 Other superficial bite of hip
  - **Excludes1** open bite of hip (S71.05-)
  - S70.271 Other superficial bite of hip, right hip
  - S70.272 Other superficial bite of hip, left hip
  - S70.279 Other superficial bite of hip, unspecified hip
- S70.3 Other superficial injuries of thigh
  - S70.31 Abrasion of thigh
    - S70.311 Abrasion, right thigh
    - S70.312 Abrasion, left thigh
    - S70.319 Abrasion, unspecified thigh
  - S70.32 Blister (nonthermal) of thigh
    - S70.321 Blister (nonthermal), right thigh
    - S70.322 Blister (nonthermal), left thigh
    - S70.329 Blister (nonthermal), unspecified thigh
  - S70.34 External constriction of thigh
    - S70.341 External constriction, right thigh
    - S70.342 External constriction, left thigh
    - S70.349 External constriction, unspecified thigh
  - S70.35 Superficial foreign body of thigh
    Splinter in the thigh
    - S70.351 Superficial foreign body, right thigh
    - S70.352 Superficial foreign body, left thigh
    - S70.359 Superficial foreign body, unspecified thigh
  - S70.36 Insect bite (nonvenomous) of thigh
    - S70.361 Insect bite (nonvenomous), right thigh
    - S70.362 Insect bite (nonvenomous), left thigh
    - S70.369 Insect bite (nonvenomous), unspecified thigh
  - S70.37 Other superficial bite of thigh
    - **Excludes1** open bite of thigh (S71.15)
    - S70.371 Other superficial bite of right thigh
    - S70.372 Other superficial bite of left thigh
    - S70.379 Other superficial bite of unspecified thigh
- S70.9 Unspecified superficial injury of hip and thigh
  - S70.91 Unspecified superficial injury of hip
    - S70.911 Unspecified superficial injury of right hip
    - S70.912 Unspecified superficial injury of left hip
    - S70.919 Unspecified superficial injury of unspecified hip
  - S70.92 Unspecified superficial injury of thigh
    - S70.921 Unspecified superficial injury of right thigh
    - S70.922 Unspecified superficial injury of left thigh
    - S70.929 Unspecified superficial injury of unspecified thigh

- S71 Open wound of hip and thigh
  Code also any associated wound infection
  - **Excludes1** open fracture of hip and thigh (S72.-)
    traumatic amputation of hip and thigh (S78.-)
  - **Excludes2** bite of venomous animal (T63.-)
    open wound of ankle, foot and toes (S91.-)
    open wound of knee and lower leg (S81.-)

  The appropriate 7th character is to be added to each code from category S71

A	initial encounter
D	subsequent encounter
S	sequela

  - S71.0 Open wound of hip
    - S71.00 Unspecified open wound of hip
      - S71.001 Unspecified open wound, right hip
      - S71.002 Unspecified open wound, left hip
      - S71.009 Unspecified open wound, unspecified hip
    - S71.01 Laceration without foreign body of hip
      - S71.011 Laceration without foreign body, right hip
      - S71.012 Laceration without foreign body, left hip
      - S71.019 Laceration without foreign body, unspecified hip
    - S71.02 Laceration with foreign body of hip
      - S71.021 Laceration with foreign body, right hip
      - S71.022 Laceration with foreign body, left hip
      - S71.029 Laceration with foreign body, unspecified hip
    - S71.03 Puncture wound without foreign body of hip
      - S71.031 Puncture wound without foreign body, right hip
      - S71.032 Puncture wound without foreign body, left hip
      - S71.039 Puncture wound without foreign body, unspecified hip
    - S71.04 Puncture wound with foreign body of hip
      - S71.041 Puncture wound with foreign body, right hip
      - S71.042 Puncture wound with foreign body, left hip
      - S71.049 Puncture wound with foreign body, unspecified hip
    - S71.05 Open bite of hip
      Bite of hip NOS
      - **Excludes1** superficial bite of hip (S70.26, S70.27)
      - S71.051 Open bite, right hip
      - S71.052 Open bite, left hip
      - S71.059 Open bite, unspecified hip
  - S71.1 Open wound of thigh
    - S71.10 Unspecified open wound of thigh
      - S71.101 Unspecified open wound, right thigh
      - S71.102 Unspecified open wound, left thigh
      - S71.109 Unspecified open wound, unspecified thigh
    - S71.11 Laceration without foreign body of thigh
      - S71.111 Laceration without foreign body, right thigh
      - S71.112 Laceration without foreign body, left thigh
      - S71.119 Laceration without foreign body, unspecified thigh

● **S71.12** **Laceration with foreign body of thigh**
　　● **S71.121** **Laceration with foreign body, right thigh**
　　● **S71.122** **Laceration with foreign body, left thigh**
　　● **S71.129** **Laceration with foreign body, unspecified thigh**
● **S71.13** **Puncture wound without foreign body of thigh**
　　● **S71.131** **Puncture wound without foreign body, right thigh**
　　● **S71.132** **Puncture wound without foreign body, left thigh**
　　● **S71.139** **Puncture wound without foreign body, unspecified thigh**
● **S71.14** **Puncture wound with foreign body of thigh**
　　● **S71.141** **Puncture wound with foreign body, right thigh**
　　● **S71.142** **Puncture wound with foreign body, left thigh**
　　● **S71.149** **Puncture wound with foreign body, unspecified thigh**
● **S71.15** **Open bite of thigh**
　　　Bite of thigh NOS
　　　Excludes1 superficial bite of thigh (S70.37-)
　　● **S71.151** **Open bite, right thigh** ✳
　　● **S71.152** **Open bite, left thigh**
　　● **S71.159** **Open bite, unspecified thigh**

● **S72** **Fracture of femur**
　　Note: A fracture not indicated as displaced or nondisplaced should be coded to displaced

　　　A fracture not indicated as open or closed should be coded to closed

　　　The open fracture designations are based on the Gustilo open fracture classification

　　Excludes1 traumatic amputation of hip and thigh (S78.-)
　　Excludes2 fracture of lower leg and ankle (S82.-)
　　　　　fracture of foot (S92.-)
　　　　　periprosthetic fracture of prosthetic implant of hip (T84.040, T84.041)

　　The appropriate 7th character is to be added to all codes from category S72

A	initial encounter for closed fracture
B	initial encounter for open fracture type I or II ✳ initial encounter for open fracture NOS
C	initial encounter for open fracture type IIIA, IIIB, or IIIC
D	subsequent encounter for closed fracture with routine healing
E	subsequent encounter for open fracture type I or II with routine healing
F	subsequent encounter for open fracture type IIIA, IIIB, or IIIC with routine healing
G	subsequent encounter for closed fracture with delayed healing
H	subsequent encounter for open fracture type I or II with delayed healing
J	subsequent encounter for open fracture type IIIA, IIIB, or IIIC with delayed healing
K	subsequent encounter for closed fracture with nonunion
M	subsequent encounter for open fracture type I or II with nonunion
N	subsequent encounter for open fracture type IIIA, IIIB, or IIIC with nonunion
P	subsequent encounter for closed fracture with malunion
Q	subsequent encounter for open fracture type I or II with malunion
R	subsequent encounter for open fracture type IIIA, IIIB, or IIIC with malunion
S	sequela

● **S72.0** **Fracture of head and neck of femur**
　　Excludes2 physeal fracture of upper end of femur (S79.0-)
● **S72.00** **Fracture of unspecified part of neck of femur**
　　　Fracture of hip NOS
　　　Fracture of neck of femur NOS
　　● **S72.001** **Fracture of unspecified part of neck of right femur**
　　● **S72.002** **Fracture of unspecified part of neck of left femur**
　　● **S72.009** **Fracture of unspecified part of neck of unspecified femur**
● **S72.01** **Unspecified intracapsular fracture of femur**
　　　Subcapital fracture of femur
　　● **S72.011** **Unspecified intracapsular fracture of right femur**
　　● **S72.012** **Unspecified intracapsular fracture of left femur**
　　● **S72.019** **Unspecified intracapsular fracture of unspecified femur**
● **S72.02** **Fracture of epiphysis (separation) (upper) of femur**
　　　Transepiphyseal fracture of femur
　　　Fracture and separation across growth plate
　　　Excludes1 capital femoral epiphyseal fracture (pediatric) of femur (S79.01-)
　　　　　Salter-Harris Type I physeal fracture of upper end of femur (S79.01-)
　　● **S72.021** **Displaced fracture of epiphysis (separation) (upper) of right femur**
　　✳ ● **S72.022** **Displaced fracture of epiphysis (separation) (upper) of left femur**
　　● **S72.023** **Displaced fracture of epiphysis (separation) (upper) of unspecified femur**
　　● **S72.024** **Nondisplaced fracture of epiphysis (separation) (upper) of right femur**
　　● **S72.025** **Nondisplaced fracture of epiphysis (separation) (upper) of left femur**
　　● **S72.026** **Nondisplaced fracture of epiphysis (separation) (upper) of unspecified femur**
● **S72.03** **Midcervical fracture of femur**
　　　Transcervical fracture of femur NOS
　　● **S72.031** **Displaced midcervical fracture of right femur**
　　● **S72.032** **Displaced midcervical fracture of left femur**
　　● **S72.033** **Displaced midcervical fracture of unspecified femur**
　　● **S72.034** **Nondisplaced midcervical fracture of right femur**
　　● **S72.035** **Nondisplaced midcervical fracture of left femur**
　　● **S72.036** **Nondisplaced midcervical fracture of unspecified femur**

CHAPTER 19 (S00-T88)

CHAPTER 19 (S00-T88)

● S72.04   Fracture of base of neck of femur
        Cervicotrochanteric fracture of femur
  ● S72.041   Displaced fracture of base of neck of right femur
  ● S72.042   Displaced fracture of base of neck of left femur
  ● S72.043   Displaced fracture of base of neck of unspecified femur
  ● S72.044   Nondisplaced fracture of base of neck of right femur
  ● S72.045   Nondisplaced fracture of base of neck of left femur
  ● S72.046   Nondisplaced fracture of base of neck of unspecified femur

● S72.05   Unspecified fracture of head of femur
        Fracture of head of femur NOS
  ● S72.051   Unspecified fracture of head of right femur
  ● S72.052   Unspecified fracture of head of left femur
  ● S72.059   Unspecified fracture of head of unspecified femur

● S72.06   Articular fracture of head of femur
  ● S72.061   Displaced articular fracture of head of right femur
  ● S72.062   Displaced articular fracture of head of left femur
  ● S72.063   Displaced articular fracture of head of unspecified femur
  ● S72.064   Nondisplaced articular fracture of head of right femur
  ● S72.065   Nondisplaced articular fracture of head of left femur
  ● S72.066   Nondisplaced articular fracture of head of unspecified femur

● S72.09   Other fracture of head and neck of femur
  ● S72.091   Other fracture of head and neck of right femur
  ● S72.092   Other fracture of head and neck of left femur
  ● S72.099   Other fracture of head and neck of unspecified femur

● S72.1   Pertrochanteric fracture
    Fracture extending close to, but not into, joint

● S72.10   Unspecified trochanteric fracture of femur
        Fracture of trochanter NOS
  ● S72.101   Unspecified trochanteric fracture of right femur
  ● S72.102   Unspecified trochanteric fracture of left femur
  ● S72.109   Unspecified trochanteric fracture of unspecified femur

● S72.11   Fracture of greater trochanter of femur
  ● S72.111   Displaced fracture of greater trochanter of right femur
  ● S72.112   Displaced fracture of greater trochanter of left femur
  ● S72.113   Displaced fracture of greater trochanter of unspecified femur
  ● S72.114   Nondisplaced fracture of greater trochanter of right femur
  ● S72.115   Nondisplaced fracture of greater trochanter of left femur
  ● S72.116   Nondisplaced fracture of greater trochanter of unspecified femur

● S72.12   Fracture of lesser trochanter of femur
  ● S72.121   Displaced fracture of lesser trochanter of right femur
  ● S72.122   Displaced fracture of lesser trochanter of left femur
  ● S72.123   Displaced fracture of lesser trochanter of unspecified femur
  ● S72.124   Nondisplaced fracture of lesser trochanter of right femur
  ● S72.125   Nondisplaced fracture of lesser trochanter of left femur
  ● S72.126   Nondisplaced fracture of lesser trochanter of unspecified femur

● S72.13   Apophyseal fracture of femur
    Pertaining to articulations between articular facets of adjacent vertebrae

    Excludes1   chronic (nontraumatic) slipped upper femoral epiphysis (M93.0-)

  ● S72.131   Displaced apophyseal fracture of right femur
  ● S72.132   Displaced apophyseal fracture of left femur
  ● S72.133   Displaced apophyseal fracture of unspecified femur
  ● S72.134   Nondisplaced apophyseal fracture of right femur
  ● S72.135   Nondisplaced apophyseal fracture of left femur
  ● S72.136   Nondisplaced apophyseal fracture of unspecified femur

● S72.14   Intertrochanteric fracture of femur
  ● S72.141   Displaced intertrochanteric fracture of right femur
  ● S72.142   Displaced intertrochanteric fracture of left femur
  ● S72.143   Displaced intertrochanteric fracture of unspecified femur
  ● S72.144   Nondisplaced intertrochanteric fracture of right femur
  ● S72.145   Nondisplaced intertrochanteric fracture of left femur
  ● S72.146   Nondisplaced intertrochanteric fracture of unspecified femur

● S72.2   Subtrochanteric fracture of femur
    Subtrochanteric: inferior to trochanter
  X ● S72.21   Displaced subtrochanteric fracture of right femur
  X ● S72.22   Displaced subtrochanteric fracture of left femur
  X ● S72.23   Displaced subtrochanteric fracture of unspecified femur
  X ● S72.24   Nondisplaced subtrochanteric fracture of right femur
  X ● S72.25   Nondisplaced subtrochanteric fracture of left femur
  X ● S72.26   Nondisplaced subtrochanteric fracture of unspecified femur

● S72.3   Fracture of shaft of femur
  ● S72.30   Unspecified fracture of shaft of femur
    ● S72.301   Unspecified fracture of shaft of right femur
    ● S72.302   Unspecified fracture of shaft of left femur
    ● S72.309   Unspecified fracture of shaft of unspecified femur

● S72.32   Transverse fracture of shaft of femur
 ● S72.321   Displaced transverse fracture of shaft of right femur
 ● S72.322   Displaced transverse fracture of shaft of left femur
 ● S72.323   Displaced transverse fracture of shaft of unspecified femur
 ● S72.324   Nondisplaced transverse fracture of shaft of right femur
 ● S72.325   Nondisplaced transverse fracture of shaft of left femur
 ● S72.326   Nondisplaced transverse fracture of shaft of unspecified femur

● S72.33   Oblique fracture of shaft of femur
 ● S72.331   Displaced oblique fracture of shaft of right femur
 ● S72.332   Displaced oblique fracture of shaft of left femur
 ● S72.333   Displaced oblique fracture of shaft of unspecified femur
 ● S72.334   Nondisplaced oblique fracture of shaft of right femur
 ● S72.335   Nondisplaced oblique fracture of shaft of left femur
 ● S72.336   Nondisplaced oblique fracture of shaft of unspecified femur

● S72.34   Spiral fracture of shaft of femur
 ● S72.341   Displaced spiral fracture of shaft of right femur
 ● S72.342   Displaced spiral fracture of shaft of left femur
 ● S72.343   Displaced spiral fracture of shaft of unspecified femur
 ● S72.344   Nondisplaced spiral fracture of shaft of right femur
 ● S72.345   Nondisplaced spiral fracture of shaft of left femur
 ● S72.346   Nondisplaced spiral fracture of shaft of unspecified femur

● S72.35   Comminuted fracture of shaft of femur
 ● S72.351   Displaced comminuted fracture of shaft of right femur
 ● S72.352   Displaced comminuted fracture of shaft of left femur
 ● S72.353   Displaced comminuted fracture of shaft of unspecified femur
 ● S72.354   Nondisplaced comminuted fracture of shaft of right femur
 ● S72.355   Nondisplaced comminuted fracture of shaft of left femur
 ● S72.356   Nondisplaced comminuted fracture of shaft of unspecified femur

● S72.36   Segmental fracture of shaft of femur
 ● S72.361   Displaced segmental fracture of shaft of right femur
 ● S72.362   Displaced segmental fracture of shaft of left femur
 ● S72.363   Displaced segmental fracture of shaft of unspecified femur

 ● S72.364   Nondisplaced segmental fracture of shaft of right femur
 ● S72.365   Nondisplaced segmental fracture of shaft of left femur
 ● S72.366   Nondisplaced segmental fracture of shaft of unspecified femur

● S72.39   Other fracture of shaft of femur
 ● S72.391   Other fracture of shaft of right femur
 ● S72.392   Other fracture of shaft of left femur
 ● S72.399   Other fracture of shaft of unspecified femur

● S72.4   Fracture of lower end of femur
 Fracture of distal end of femur
 | Excludes2 | fracture of shaft of femur (S72.3-)
      physeal fracture of lower end of femur (S79.1-)

 ● S72.40   Unspecified fracture of lower end of femur
  ● S72.401   Unspecified fracture of lower end of right femur
  ● S72.402   Unspecified fracture of lower end of left femur
  ● S72.409   Unspecified fracture of lower end of unspecified femur

 ● S72.41   Unspecified condyle fracture of lower end of femur
  Condyle fracture of femur NOS
  ● S72.411   Displaced unspecified condyle fracture of lower end of right femur
  ● S72.412   Displaced unspecified condyle fracture of lower end of left femur
  ● S72.413   Displaced unspecified condyle fracture of lower end of unspecified femur
  ● S72.414   Nondisplaced unspecified condyle fracture of lower end of right femur
  ● S72.415   Nondisplaced unspecified condyle fracture of lower end of left femur
  ● S72.416   Nondisplaced unspecified condyle fracture of lower end of unspecified femur

 ● S72.42   Fracture of lateral condyle of femur
  ● S72.421   Displaced fracture of lateral condyle of right femur
  ● S72.422   Displaced fracture of lateral condyle of left femur
  ● S72.423   Displaced fracture of lateral condyle of unspecified femur
  ● S72.424   Nondisplaced fracture of lateral condyle of right femur
  ● S72.425   Nondisplaced fracture of lateral condyle of left femur
  ● S72.426   Nondisplaced fracture of lateral condyle of unspecified femur

 ● S72.43   Fracture of medial condyle of femur
  ● S72.431   Displaced fracture of medial condyle of right femur
  ● S72.432   Displaced fracture of medial condyle of left femur
  ● S72.433   Displaced fracture of medial condyle of unspecified femur

● S72.434   Nondisplaced fracture of medial condyle of right femur

● S72.435   Nondisplaced fracture of medial condyle of left femur

● S72.436   Nondisplaced fracture of medial condyle of unspecified femur

● S72.44   Fracture of lower epiphysis (separation) of femur

> **Excludes1**   Salter-Harris Type I physeal fracture of lower end of femur (S79.11-)

● S72.441   Displaced fracture of lower epiphysis (separation) of right femur

● S72.442   Displaced fracture of lower epiphysis (separation) of left femur

● S72.443   Displaced fracture of lower epiphysis (separation) of unspecified femur

● S72.444   Nondisplaced fracture of lower epiphysis (separation) of right femur

● S72.445   Nondisplaced fracture of lower epiphysis (separation) of left femur

● S72.446   Nondisplaced fracture of lower epiphysis (separation) of unspecified femur

● S72.45   Supracondylar fracture without intracondylar extension of lower end of femur

> Supracondylar fracture of lower end of femur NOS
>
> **Excludes1**   supracondylar fracture with intracondylar extension of lower end of femur (S72.46-)

● S72.451   Displaced supracondylar fracture without intracondylar extension of lower end of right femur

● S72.452   Displaced supracondylar fracture without intracondylar extension of lower end of left femur

● S72.453   Displaced supracondylar fracture without intracondylar extension of lower end of unspecified femur

● S72.454   Nondisplaced supracondylar fracture without intracondylar extension of lower end of right femur

● S72.455   Nondisplaced supracondylar fracture without intracondylar extension of lower end of left femur

● S72.456   Nondisplaced supracondylar fracture without intracondylar extension of lower end of unspecified femur

● S72.46   Supracondylar fracture with intracondylar extension of lower end of femur

> **Excludes1**   supracondylar fracture without intracondylar extension of lower end of femur (S72.45-)

● S72.461   Displaced supracondylar fracture with intracondylar extension of lower end of right femur

● S72.462   Displaced supracondylar fracture with intracondylar extension of lower end of left femur

● S72.463   Displaced supracondylar fracture with intracondylar extension of lower end of unspecified femur

● S72.464   Nondisplaced supracondylar fracture with intracondylar extension of lower end of right femur

● S72.465   Nondisplaced supracondylar fracture with intracondylar extension of lower end of left femur

● S72.466   Nondisplaced supracondylar fracture with intracondylar extension of lower end of unspecified femur

● S72.47   Torus fracture of lower end of femur

> The appropriate 7th character is to be added to all codes in subcategory S72.47

A	initial encounter for closed fracture
D	subsequent encounter for fracture with routine healing
G	subsequent encounter for fracture with delayed healing
K	subsequent encounter for fracture with nonunion
P	subsequent encounter for fracture with malunion
S	sequela

● S72.471   Torus fracture of lower end of right femur

● S72.472   Torus fracture of lower end of left femur

● S72.479   Torus fracture of lower end of unspecified femur

● S72.49   Other fracture of lower end of femur

● S72.491   Other fracture of lower end of right femur

● S72.492   Other fracture of lower end of left femur

● S72.499   Other fracture of lower end of unspecified femur

● S72.8   Other fracture of femur

● S72.8X   Other fracture of femur

● S72.8X1   Other fracture of right femur

● S72.8X2   Other fracture of left femur

● S72.8X9   Other fracture of unspecified femur

● S72.9   Unspecified fracture of femur

> Fracture of thigh NOS
> Fracture of upper leg NOS
>
> **Excludes1**   fracture of hip NOS (S72.00-, S72.01-)

X ● S72.90   Unspecified fracture of unspecified femur

X ● S72.91   Unspecified fracture of right femur

X ● S72.92   Unspecified fracture of left femur

◀ New   ◀ Revised   ~~deleted~~ Deleted   OGCR Official Guidelines   X Assign placeholder X   ● Use Additional Character(s)

Excludes 1   Excludes 2   Includes   Use additional   Code first   Code also   Unspecified

● S73   Dislocation and sprain of joint and ligaments of hip
    Includes   avulsion of joint or ligament of hip
        laceration of cartilage, joint or ligament of hip
        sprain of cartilage, joint or ligament of hip
        traumatic hemarthrosis of joint or ligament of hip
        traumatic rupture of joint or ligament of hip
        traumatic subluxation of joint or ligament of hip
        traumatic tear of joint or ligament of hip

    Code also any associated open wound
    Excludes2   strain of muscle, fascia and tendon of hip and
            thigh (S76.-)

    The appropriate 7th character is to be added to each code from
    category S73

    | | |
    A   initial encounter
    D   subsequent encounter
    S   sequela

● S73.0   Subluxation and dislocation of hip
    Out of position
    Excludes2   dislocation and subluxation of hip
            prosthesis (T84.020, T84.021)

  ● S73.00   Unspecified subluxation and dislocation of hip
      Dislocation of hip NOS
      Subluxation of hip NOS
    ● S73.001   Unspecified subluxation of right hip
    ● S73.002   Unspecified subluxation of left hip
    ● S73.003   Unspecified subluxation of
           unspecified hip
    ● S73.004   Unspecified dislocation of right hip
    ● S73.005   Unspecified dislocation of left hip
    ● S73.006   Unspecified dislocation of unspecified
           hip

  ● S73.01   Posterior subluxation and dislocation of hip
    ● S73.011   Posterior subluxation of right hip
    ● S73.012   Posterior subluxation of left hip
    ● S73.013   Posterior subluxation of unspecified
           hip
    ● S73.014   Posterior dislocation of right hip
    ● S73.015   Posterior dislocation of left hip
    ● S73.016   Posterior dislocation of unspecified
           hip

  ● S73.02   Obturator subluxation and dislocation of hip
    ● S73.021   Obturator subluxation of right hip
    ● S73.022   Obturator subluxation of left hip
    ● S73.023   Obturator subluxation of unspecified
           hip
    ● S73.024   Obturator dislocation of right hip
    ● S73.025   Obturator dislocation of left hip
    ● S73.026   Obturator dislocation of unspecified
           hip

  ● S73.03   Other anterior dislocation of hip
    ● S73.031   Other anterior subluxation of right
           hip
    ● S73.032   Other anterior subluxation of left hip
    ● S73.033   Other anterior subluxation of
           unspecified hip
    ● S73.034   Other anterior dislocation of right hip
    ● S73.035   Other anterior dislocation of left hip
    ● S73.036   Other anterior dislocation of
           unspecified hip

● S73.04   Central dislocation of hip
  ● S73.041   Central subluxation of right hip
  ● S73.042   Central subluxation of left hip
  ● S73.043   Central subluxation of unspecified
        hip
  ● S73.044   Central dislocation of right hip
  ● S73.045   Central dislocation of left hip
  ● S73.046   Central dislocation of unspecified hip

● S73.1   Sprain of hip
  ● S73.10   Unspecified sprain of hip
    ● S73.101   Unspecified sprain of right hip
    ● S73.102   Unspecified sprain of left hip
    ● S73.109   Unspecified sprain of unspecified hip
  ● S73.11   Iliofemoral ligament sprain of hip
    ● S73.111   Iliofemoral ligament sprain of right
           hip
    ● S73.112   Iliofemoral ligament sprain of left hip
    ● S73.119   Iliofemoral ligament sprain of
           unspecified hip
  ● S73.12   Ischiocapsular (ligament) sprain of hip
    ● S73.121   Ischiocapsular ligament sprain of
           right hip
    ● S73.122   Ischiocapsular ligament sprain of left
           hip
    ● S73.129   Ischiocapsular ligament sprain of
           unspecified hip
  ● S73.19   Other sprain of hip
    ● S73.191   Other sprain of right hip
    ● S73.192   Other sprain of left hip
    ● S73.199   Other sprain of unspecified hip

● S74   Injury of nerves at hip and thigh level
    Code also any associated open wound (S71.-)
    Excludes2   injury of nerves at ankle and foot level (S94.-)
            injury of nerves at lower leg level (S84.-)
    The appropriate 7th character is to be added to each code from
    category S74

    A   initial encounter
    D   subsequent encounter
    S   sequela

● S74.0   Injury of sciatic nerve at hip and thigh level
  X ● S74.00   Injury of sciatic nerve at hip and thigh level,
          unspecified leg
  X ● S74.01   Injury of sciatic nerve at hip and thigh level,
          right leg
  X ● S74.02   Injury of sciatic nerve at hip and thigh level,
          left leg
● S74.1   Injury of femoral nerve at hip and thigh level
  X ● S74.10   Injury of femoral nerve at hip and thigh level,
          unspecified leg
  X ● S74.11   Injury of femoral nerve at hip and thigh level,
          right leg
  X ● S74.12   Injury of femoral nerve at hip and thigh level,
          left leg
● S74.2   Injury of cutaneous sensory nerve at hip and thigh level
  X ● S74.20   Injury of cutaneous sensory nerve at hip and
          thigh level, unspecified leg
  X ● S74.21   Injury of cutaneous sensory nerve at hip and
          high level, right leg
  X ● S74.22   Injury of cutaneous sensory nerve at hip and
          thigh level, left leg

CHAPTER 19 (S00-T88)

- ● S74.8 Injury of other nerves at hip and thigh level
  - ● S74.8X Injury of other nerves at hip and thigh level
    - ● S74.8X1 Injury of other nerves at hip and thigh level, right leg
    - ● S74.8X2 Injury of other nerves at hip and thigh level, left leg
    - ● S74.8X9 Injury of other nerves at hip and thigh level, unspecified leg
- ● S74.9 Injury of unspecified nerve at hip and thigh level
  - X ● S74.90 Injury of unspecified nerve at hip and thigh level, unspecified leg
  - X ● S74.91 Injury of unspecified nerve at hip and thigh level, right leg
  - X ● S74.92 Injury of unspecified nerve at hip and thigh level, left leg
- ● S75 Injury of blood vessels at hip and thigh level

  Code also any associated open wound (S71.-)

  Excludes2 injury of blood vessels at lower leg level (S85.-)
  injury of popliteal artery (S85.0)

  The appropriate 7th character is to be added to each code from category S75

A	initial encounter
D	subsequent encounter
S	sequela

  - ● S75.0 Injury of femoral artery
    - ● S75.00 Unspecified injury of femoral artery
      - ● S75.001 Unspecified injury of femoral artery, right leg
      - ● S75.002 Unspecified injury of femoral artery, left leg
      - ● S75.009 Unspecified injury of femoral artery, unspecified leg
    - ● S75.01 Minor laceration of femoral artery
      Incomplete transection of femoral artery
      Laceration of femoral artery NOS
      Superficial laceration of femoral artery
      - ● S75.011 Minor laceration of femoral artery, right leg
      - ● S75.012 Minor laceration of femoral artery, left leg
      - ● S75.019 Minor laceration of femoral artery, unspecified leg
    - ● S75.02 Major laceration of femoral artery
      Complete transection of femoral artery
      Traumatic rupture of femoral artery
      - ● S75.021 Major laceration of femoral artery, right leg
      - ● S75.022 Major laceration of femoral artery, left leg
      - ● S75.029 Major laceration of femoral artery, unspecified leg
    - ● S75.09 Other specified injury of femoral artery
      - ● S75.091 Other specified injury of femoral artery, right leg
      - ● S75.092 Other specified injury of femoral artery, left leg
      - ● S75.099 Other specified injury of femoral artery, unspecified leg

- ● S75.1 Injury of femoral vein at hip and thigh level
  - ● S75.10 Unspecified injury of femoral vein at hip and thigh level
    - ● S75.101 Unspecified injury of femoral vein at hip and thigh level, right leg
    - ● S75.102 Unspecified injury of femoral vein at hip and thigh level, left leg
    - ● S75.109 Unspecified injury of femoral vein at hip and thigh level, unspecified leg
  - ● S75.11 Minor laceration of femoral vein at hip and thigh level
    Incomplete transection of femoral vein at hip and thigh level
    Laceration of femoral vein at hip and thigh level NOS
    Superficial laceration of femoral vein at hip and thigh level
    - ● S75.111 Minor laceration of femoral vein at hip and thigh level, right leg
    - ● S75.112 Minor laceration of femoral vein at hip and thigh level, left leg
    - ● S75.119 Minor laceration of femoral vein at hip and thigh level, unspecified leg
  - ● S75.12 Major laceration of femoral vein at hip and thigh level
    Complete transection of femoral vein at hip and thigh level
    Traumatic rupture of femoral vein at hip and thigh level
    - ● S75.121 Major laceration of femoral vein at hip and thigh level, right leg
    - ● S75.122 Major laceration of femoral vein at hip and thigh level, left leg
    - ● S75.129 Major laceration of femoral vein at hip and thigh level, unspecified leg
  - ● S75.19 Other specified injury of femoral vein at hip and thigh level
    - ● S75.191 Other specified injury of femoral vein at hip and thigh level, right leg
    - ● S75.192 Other specified injury of femoral vein at hip and thigh level, left leg
    - ● S75.199 Other specified injury of femoral vein at hip and thigh level, unspecified leg
- ● S75.2 Injury of greater saphenous vein at hip and thigh level

  Excludes1 greater saphenous vein NOS (S85.3)

  - ● S75.20 Unspecified injury of greater saphenous vein at hip and thigh level
    - ● S75.201 Unspecified injury of greater saphenous vein at hip and thigh level, right leg
    - ● S75.202 Unspecified injury of greater saphenous vein at hip and thigh level, left leg
    - ● S75.209 Unspecified injury of greater saphenous vein at hip and thigh level, unspecified leg
  - ● S75.21 Minor laceration of greater saphenous vein at hip and thigh level
    Incomplete transection of greater saphenous vein at hip and thigh level
    Laceration of greater saphenous vein at hip and thigh level NOS
    Superficial laceration of greater saphenous vein at hip and thigh level
    - ● S75.211 Minor laceration of greater saphenous vein at hip and thigh level, right leg
    - ● S75.212 Minor laceration of greater saphenous vein at hip and thigh level, left leg
    - ● S75.219 Minor laceration of greater saphenous vein at hip and thigh level, unspecified leg

◀ New   ◀▦ Revised   ~~deleted~~ Deleted   **OGCR** Official Guidelines   X Assign placeholder X   ● Use Additional Character(s)

[Excludes 1]   [Excludes 2]   Includes   Use additional   Code first   Code also   Unspecified

● **S75.22**   **Major laceration of greater saphenous vein at hip and thigh level**
> Complete transection of greater saphenous vein at hip and thigh level
> Traumatic rupture of greater saphenous vein at hip and thigh level

     ● **S75.221**   Major laceration of greater saphenous vein at hip and thigh level, right leg

     ● **S75.222**   Major laceration of greater saphenous vein at hip and thigh level, left leg

     ● **S75.229**   Major laceration of greater saphenous vein at hip and thigh level, unspecified leg

● **S75.29**   **Other specified injury of greater saphenous vein at hip and thigh level**

     ● **S75.291**   Other specified injury of greater saphenous vein at hip and thigh level, right leg

     ● **S75.292**   Other specified injury of greater saphenous vein at hip and thigh level, left leg

     ● **S75.299**   Other specified injury of greater saphenous vein at hip and thigh level, unspecified leg

● **S75.8**   **Injury of other blood vessels at hip and thigh level**

   ● **S75.80**   **Unspecified injury of other blood vessels at hip and thigh level**

     ● **S75.801**   Unspecified injury of other blood vessels at hip and thigh level, right leg

     ● **S75.802**   Unspecified injury of other blood vessels at hip and thigh level, left leg

     ● **S75.809**   Unspecified injury of other blood vessels at hip and thigh level, unspecified leg

   ● **S75.81**   **Laceration of other blood vessels at hip and thigh level**

     ● **S75.811**   Laceration of other blood vessels at hip and thigh level, right leg

     ● **S75.812**   Laceration of other blood vessels at hip and thigh level, left leg

     ● **S75.819**   Laceration of other blood vessels at hip and thigh level, unspecified leg

   ● **S75.89**   **Other specified injury of other blood vessels at hip and thigh level**

     ● **S75.891**   Other specified injury of other blood vessels at hip and thigh level, right leg

     ● **S75.892**   Other specified injury of other blood vessels at hip and thigh level, left leg

     ● **S75.899**   Other specified injury of other blood vessels at hip and thigh level, unspecified leg

● **S75.9**   **Injury of unspecified blood vessel at hip and thigh level**

   ● **S75.90**   **Unspecified injury of unspecified blood vessel at hip and thigh level**

     ● **S75.901**   Unspecified injury of unspecified blood vessel at hip and thigh level, right leg

     ● **S75.902**   Unspecified injury of unspecified blood vessel at hip and thigh level, left leg

     ● **S75.909**   Unspecified injury of unspecified blood vessel at hip and thigh level, unspecified leg

   ● **S75.91**   **Laceration of unspecified blood vessel at hip and thigh level**

     ● **S75.911**   Laceration of unspecified blood vessel at hip and thigh level, right leg

     ● **S75.912**   Laceration of unspecified blood vessel at hip and thigh level, left leg

     ● **S75.919**   Laceration of unspecified blood vessel at hip and thigh level, unspecified leg

   ● **S75.99**   **Other specified injury of unspecified blood vessel at hip and thigh level**

     ● **S75.991**   Other specified injury of unspecified blood vessel at hip and thigh level, right leg

     ● **S75.992**   Other specified injury of unspecified blood vessel at hip and thigh level, left leg

     ● **S75.999**   Other specified injury of unspecified blood vessel at hip and thigh level, unspecified leg

● **S76**   **Injury of muscle, fascia and tendon at hip and thigh level**
> Code also any associated open wound (S71.-)

> | Excludes2 | injury of muscle, fascia and tendon at lower leg level (S86) |
> |---|---|
> | | sprain of joint and ligament of hip (S73.1) |

> The appropriate 7th character is to be added to each code from category S76

> | | |
> |---|---|
> | A | initial encounter |
> | D | subsequent encounter |
> | S | sequela |

   ● **S76.0**   **Injury of muscle, fascia and tendon of hip**

     ● **S76.00**   **Unspecified injury of muscle, fascia and tendon of hip**

      ● **S76.001**   Unspecified injury of muscle, fascia and tendon of right hip

      ● **S76.002**   Unspecified injury of muscle, fascia and tendon of left hip

      ● **S76.009**   Unspecified injury of muscle, fascia and tendon of unspecified hip

     ● **S76.01**   **Strain of muscle, fascia and tendon of hip**

      ● **S76.011**   Strain of muscle, fascia and tendon of right hip

      ● **S76.012**   Strain of muscle, fascia and tendon of left hip

      ● **S76.019**   Strain of muscle, fascia and tendon of unspecified hip

     ● **S76.02**   **Laceration of muscle, fascia and tendon of hip**

      ● **S76.021**   Laceration of muscle, fascia and tendon of right hip

      ● **S76.022**   Laceration of muscle, fascia and tendon of left hip

      ● **S76.029**   Laceration of muscle, fascia and tendon of unspecified hip

     ● **S76.09**   **Other specified injury of muscle, fascia and tendon of hip**

      ● **S76.091**   Other specified injury of muscle, fascia and tendon of right hip

      ● **S76.092**   Other specified injury of muscle, fascia and tendon of left hip

      ● **S76.099**   Other specified injury of muscle, fascia and tendon of unspecified hip

CHAPTER 19 (S00-T88)

● **S76.1**   **Injury of quadriceps muscle, fascia and tendon**
  Injury of patellar ligament (tendon)

  ● **S76.10**   Unspecified injury of quadriceps muscle, fascia and tendon

    ● S76.101   Unspecified injury of right quadriceps muscle, fascia and tendon

    ● S76.102   Unspecified injury of left quadriceps muscle, fascia and tendon

    ● S76.109   Unspecified injury of unspecified quadriceps muscle, fascia and tendon

  ● **S76.11**   Strain of quadriceps muscle, fascia and tendon

    ● S76.111   Strain of right quadriceps muscle, fascia and tendon

    ● S76.112   Strain of left quadriceps muscle, fascia and tendon

    ● S76.119   Strain of unspecified quadriceps muscle, fascia and tendon

  ● **S76.12**   Laceration of quadriceps muscle, fascia and tendon

    ● S76.121   Laceration of right quadriceps muscle, fascia and tendon

    ● S76.122   Laceration of left quadriceps muscle, fascia and tendon

    ● S76.129   Laceration of unspecified quadriceps muscle, fascia and tendon

  ● **S76.19**   Other specified injury of quadriceps muscle, fascia and tendon

    ● S76.191   Other specified injury of right quadriceps muscle, fascia and tendon

    ● S76.192   Other specified injury of left quadriceps muscle, fascia and tendon

    ● S76.199   Other specified injury of unspecified quadriceps muscle, fascia and tendon

● **S76.2**   **Injury of adductor muscle, fascia and tendon of thigh**

  ● **S76.20**   Unspecified injury of adductor muscle, fascia and tendon of thigh

    ● S76.201   Unspecified injury of adductor muscle, fascia and tendon of right thigh

    ● S76.202   Unspecified injury of adductor muscle, fascia and tendon of left thigh

    ● S76.209   Unspecified injury of adductor muscle, fascia and tendon of unspecified thigh

  ● **S76.21**   Strain of adductor muscle, fascia and tendon of thigh

    ● S76.211   Strain of adductor muscle, fascia and tendon of right thigh

    ● S76.212   Strain of adductor muscle, fascia and tendon of left thigh

    ● S76.219   Strain of adductor muscle, fascia and tendon of unspecified thigh

  ● **S76.22**   Laceration of adductor muscle, fascia and tendon of thigh

    ● S76.221   Laceration of adductor muscle, fascia and tendon of right thigh

    ● S76.222   Laceration of adductor muscle, fascia and tendon of left thigh

    ● S76.229   Laceration of adductor muscle, fascia and tendon of unspecified thigh

  ● **S76.29**   Other injury of adductor muscle, fascia and tendon of thigh

    ● S76.291   Other injury of adductor muscle, fascia and tendon of right thigh

    ● S76.292   Other injury of adductor muscle, fascia and tendon of left thigh

    ● S76.299   Other injury of adductor muscle, fascia and tendon of unspecified thigh

● **S76.3**   **Injury of muscle, fascia and tendon of the posterior muscle group at thigh level**

  ● **S76.30**   Unspecified injury of muscle, fascia and tendon of the posterior muscle group at thigh level

    ● S76.301   Unspecified injury of muscle, fascia and tendon of the posterior muscle group at thigh level, right thigh

    ● S76.302   Unspecified injury of muscle, fascia and tendon of the posterior muscle group at thigh level, left thigh

    ● S76.309   Unspecified injury of muscle, fascia and tendon of the posterior muscle group at thigh level, unspecified thigh

  ● **S76.31**   Strain of muscle, fascia and tendon of the posterior muscle group at thigh level

    ● S76.311   Strain of muscle, fascia and tendon of the posterior muscle group at thigh level, right thigh

    ● S76.312   Strain of muscle, fascia and tendon of the posterior muscle group at thigh level, left thigh

    ● S76.319   Strain of muscle, fascia and tendon of the posterior muscle group at thigh level, unspecified thigh

  ● **S76.32**   Laceration of muscle, fascia and tendon of the posterior muscle group at thigh level

    ● S76.321   Laceration of muscle, fascia and tendon of the posterior muscle group at thigh level, right thigh

    ● S76.322   Laceration of muscle, fascia and tendon of the posterior muscle group at thigh level, left thigh

    ● S76.329   Laceration of muscle, fascia and tendon of the posterior muscle group at thigh level, unspecified thigh

  ● **S76.39**   Other specified injury of muscle, fascia and tendon of the posterior muscle group at thigh level

    ● S76.391   Other specified injury of muscle, fascia and tendon of the posterior muscle group at thigh level, right thigh

    ● S76.392   Other specified injury of muscle, fascia and tendon of the posterior muscle group at thigh level, left thigh

    ● S76.399   Other specified injury of muscle, fascia and tendon of the posterior muscle group at thigh level, unspecified thigh

◀ New   ◀▥ Revised   ~~deleted~~ Deleted   OGCR Official Guidelines   X Assign placeholder X   ● Use Additional Character(s)

Excludes 1   Excludes 2   Includes   Use additional   Code first   Code also   Unspecified

● S76.8   Injury of other specified muscles, fascia and tendons at thigh level
    ● S76.80   Unspecified injury of other specified muscles, fascia and tendons at thigh level
      ● S76.801   Unspecified injury of other specified muscles, fascia and tendons at thigh level, right thigh
      ● S76.802   Unspecified injury of other specified muscles, fascia and tendons at thigh level, left thigh
      ● S76.809   Unspecified injury of other specified muscles, fascia and tendons at thigh level, unspecified thigh
    ● S76.81   Strain of other specified specified muscles, fascia and tendons at thigh level
      ● S76.811   Strain of other specified muscles, fascia and tendons at thigh level, right thigh
      ● S76.812   Strain of other specified muscles, fascia and tendons at thigh level, left thigh
      ● S76.819   Strain of other specified muscles, fascia and tendons at thigh level, unspecified thigh
    ● S76.82   Laceration of other specified muscles, fascia and tendons at thigh level
      ● S76.821   Laceration of other specified muscles, fascia and tendons at thigh level, right thigh
      ● S76.822   Laceration of other specified muscles, fascia and tendons at thigh level, left thigh
      ● S76.829   Laceration of other specified muscles, fascia and tendons at thigh level, unspecified thigh
    ● S76.89   Other injury of other specified muscles, fascia and tendons at thigh level
      ● S76.891   Other injury of other specified muscles, fascia and tendons at thigh level, right thigh
      ● S76.892   Other injury of other specified muscles, fascia and tendons at thigh level, left thigh
      ● S76.899   Other injury of other specified muscles, fascia and tendons at thigh level, unspecified thigh
● S76.9   Injury of unspecified muscles, fascia and tendons at thigh level
    ● S76.90   Unspecified injury of unspecified muscles, fascia and tendons at thigh level
      ● S76.901   Unspecified injury of unspecified muscles, fascia and tendons at thigh level, right thigh
      ● S76.902   Unspecified injury of unspecified muscles, fascia and tendons at thigh level, left thigh
      ● S76.909   Unspecified injury of unspecified muscles, fascia and tendons at thigh level, unspecified thigh
    ● S76.91   Strain of unspecified muscles, fascia and tendons at thigh level
      ● S76.911   Strain of unspecified muscles, fascia and tendons at thigh level, right thigh
      ● S76.912   Strain of unspecified muscles, fascia and tendons at thigh level, left thigh
      ● S76.919   Strain of unspecified muscles, fascia and tendons at thigh level, unspecified thigh

● S76.92   Laceration of unspecified muscles, fascia and tendons at thigh level
      ● S76.921   Laceration of unspecified muscles, fascia and tendons at thigh level, right thigh
      ● S76.922   Laceration of unspecified muscles, fascia and tendons at thigh level, left thigh
      ● S76.929   Laceration of unspecified muscles, fascia and tendons at thigh level, unspecified thigh
    ● S76.99   Other specified injury of unspecified muscles, fascia and tendons at thigh level
      ● S76.991   Other specified injury of unspecified muscles, fascia and tendons at thigh level, right thigh
      ● S76.992   Other specified injury of unspecified muscles, fascia and tendons at thigh level, left thigh
      ● S76.999   Other specified injury of unspecified muscles, fascia and tendons at thigh level, unspecified thigh

● S77   Crushing injury of hip and thigh
    Use additional code(s) for all associated injuries
    Excludes2   crushing injury of ankle and foot (S97.-)
               crushing injury of lower leg (S87.-)
    The appropriate 7th character is to be added to each code from category S77

    A   initial encounter
    D   subsequent encounter
    S   sequela

    ● S77.0   Crushing injury of hip
      X ● S77.00   Crushing injury of unspecified hip
      X ● S77.01   Crushing injury of right hip
      X ● S77.02   Crushing injury of left hip
    ● S77.1   Crushing injury of thigh
      X ● S77.10   Crushing injury of unspecified thigh
      X ● S77.11   Crushing injury of right thigh
      X ● S77.12   Crushing injury of left thigh
    ● S77.2   Crushing injury of hip with thigh
      X ● S77.20   Crushing injury of unspecified hip with thigh
      X ● S77.21   Crushing injury of right hip with thigh
      X ● S77.22   Crushing injury of left hip with thigh

● S78   Traumatic amputation of hip and thigh
    An amputation not identified as partial or complete should be coded to complete
    Excludes1   traumatic amputation of knee (S88.0-)
    The appropriate 7th character is to be added to each code from category S78

    A   initial encounter
    D   subsequent encounter
    S   sequela

    ● S78.0   Traumatic amputation at hip joint
      ● S78.01   Complete traumatic amputation at hip joint
        ● S78.011   Complete traumatic amputation at right hip joint
        ● S78.012   Complete traumatic amputation at left hip joint
        ● S78.019   Complete traumatic amputation at unspecified hip joint

CHAPTER 19 (S00-T88)

● S78.02   Partial traumatic amputation at hip joint
    ● S78.021   Partial traumatic amputation at right hip joint
    ● S78.022   Partial traumatic amputation at left hip joint
    ● S78.029   Partial traumatic amputation at unspecified hip joint

● S78.1   Traumatic amputation at level between hip and knee
    Excludes1   traumatic amputation of knee (S88.0-)

  ● S78.11   Complete traumatic amputation at level between hip and knee
    ● S78.111   Complete traumatic amputation at level between right hip and knee
    ● S78.112   Complete traumatic amputation at level between left hip and knee
    ● S78.119   Complete traumatic amputation at level between unspecified hip and knee

  ● S78.12   Partial traumatic amputation at level between hip and knee
    ● S78.121   Partial traumatic amputation at level between right hip and knee
    ● S78.122   Partial traumatic amputation at level between left hip and knee
    ● S78.129   Partial traumatic amputation at level between unspecified hip and knee

● S78.9   Traumatic amputation of hip and thigh, level unspecified
  ● S78.91   Complete traumatic amputation of hip and thigh, level unspecified
    ● S78.911   Complete traumatic amputation of right hip and thigh, level unspecified
    ● S78.912   Complete traumatic amputation of left hip and thigh, level unspecified
    ● S78.919   Complete traumatic amputation of unspecified hip and thigh, level unspecified

  ● S78.92   Partial traumatic amputation of hip and thigh, level unspecified
    ● S78.921   Partial traumatic amputation of right hip and thigh, level unspecified
    ● S78.922   Partial traumatic amputation of left hip and thigh, level unspecified
    ● S78.929   Partial traumatic amputation of unspecified hip and thigh, level unspecified

● S79   **Other and unspecified injuries of hip and thigh**
    Note: A fracture not indicated as open or closed should be coded to closed
    The appropriate 7th character is to be added to each code from subcategories S79.0 and S79.1

> A   initial encounter for closed fracture
> D   subsequent encounter for fracture with routine healing
> G   subsequent encounter for fracture with delayed healing
> K   subsequent encounter for fracture with nonunion
> P   subsequent encounter for fracture with malunion
> S   sequela

  ● S79.0   Physeal fracture of upper end of femur
    Excludes1   apophyseal fracture of upper end of femur (S72.13-)
         nontraumatic slipped upper femoral epiphysis (M93.0-)

    ● S79.00   Unspecified physeal fracture of upper end of femur
      ● S79.001   Unspecified physeal fracture of upper end of right femur
      ● S79.002   Unspecified physeal fracture of upper end of left femur
      ● S79.009   Unspecified physeal fracture of upper end of unspecified femur

Item 19–5   SALTER-HARRIS TYPE 1: epiphysis is completely separated from end of bone, or metaphysic growth plate remains attached to epiphysis

SALTER-HARRIS TYPE 2: epiphysis and growth plate are partially separated from metaphysis, which is cracked—most common type

SALTER-HARRIS TYPE 3: fracture occurring through epiphysis and separates part of epiphysis and growth plate from metaphysis fracture, usually at distal end of tibia

SALTER-HARRIS TYPE 4: fracture runs through epiphysis, across growth plate, into metaphysic, surgery is required to restore joint surface to normal and align growth plate

  ● S79.01   Salter-Harris Type I physeal fracture of upper end of femur
    Acute on chronic slipped capital femoral epiphysis (traumatic)
    Acute slipped capital femoral epiphysis (traumatic)
    Capital femoral epiphyseal fracture
    Excludes1   chronic slipped upper femoral epiphysis (nontraumatic) (M93.02-)

    ● S79.011   Salter-Harris Type I physeal fracture of upper end of right femur
    ● S79.012   Salter-Harris Type I physeal fracture of upper end of left femur
    ● S79.019   Salter-Harris Type I physeal fracture of upper end of unspecified femur

  ● S79.09   Other physeal fracture of upper end of femur
    ● S79.091   Other physeal fracture of upper end of right femur
    ● S79.092   Other physeal fracture of upper end of left femur
    ● S79.099   Other physeal fracture of upper end of unspecified femur

● S79.1   Physeal fracture of lower end of femur
  ● S79.10   Unspecified physeal fracture of lower end of femur
    ● S79.101   Unspecified physeal fracture of lower end of right femur
    ● S79.102   Unspecified physeal fracture of lower end of left femur
    ● S79.109   Unspecified physeal fracture of lower end of unspecified femur

  ● S79.11   Salter-Harris Type I physeal fracture of lower end of femur
    ● S79.111   Salter-Harris Type I physeal fracture of lower end of right femur
    ● S79.112   Salter-Harris Type I physeal fracture of lower end of left femur
    ● S79.119   Salter-Harris Type I physeal fracture of lower end of unspecified femur

  ● S79.12   Salter-Harris Type II physeal fracture of lower end of femur
    ● S79.121   Salter-Harris Type II physeal fracture of lower end of right femur
    ● S79.122   Salter-Harris Type II physeal fracture of lower end of left femur
    ● S79.129   Salter-Harris Type II physeal fracture of lower end of unspecified femur

  ● S79.13   Salter-Harris Type III physeal fracture of lower end of femur
    ● S79.131   Salter-Harris Type III physeal fracture of lower end of right femur
    ● S79.132   Salter-Harris Type III physeal fracture of lower end of left femur
    ● S79.139   Salter-Harris Type III physeal fracture of lower end of unspecified femur

---

◀ New   ◀ Revised   ~~deleted~~ Deleted   OGCR Official Guidelines   X Assign placeholder X   ● Use Additional Character(s)

Excludes 1   Excludes 2   Includes   Use additional   Code first   Code also   Unspecified

● S79.14 Salter-Harris Type IV physeal fracture of lower end of femur
   ● S79.141 Salter-Harris Type IV physeal fracture of lower end of right femur
   ● S79.142 Salter-Harris Type IV physeal fracture of lower end of left femur
   ● S79.149 Salter-Harris Type IV physeal fracture of lower end of unspecified femur
● S79.19 Other physeal fracture of lower end of femur
   ● S79.191 Other physeal fracture of lower end of right femur
   ● S79.192 Other physeal fracture of lower end of left femur
   ● S79.199 Other physeal fracture of lower end of unspecified femur

● S79.8 Other specified injuries of hip and thigh

The appropriate 7th character is to be added to each code in subcategory S79.8

> A   initial encounter
> D   subsequent encounter
> S   sequela

  ● S79.81 Other specified injuries of hip
    ● S79.811 Other specified injuries of right hip
    ● S79.812 Other specified injuries of left hip
    ● S79.819 Other specified injuries of unspecified hip
  ● S79.82 Other specified injuries of thigh
    ● S79.821 Other specified injuries of right thigh
    ● S79.822 Other specified injuries of left thigh
    ● S79.829 Other specified injuries of unspecified thigh

● S79.9 Unspecified injury of hip and thigh

The appropriate 7th character is to be added to each code in subcategory S79.9

> A   initial encounter
> D   subsequent encounter
> S   sequela

  ● S79.91 Unspecified injury of hip
    ● S79.911 Unspecified injury of right hip
    ● S79.912 Unspecified injury of left hip
    ● S79.919 Unspecified injury of unspecified hip
  ● S79.92 Unspecified injury of thigh
    ● S79.921 Unspecified injury of right thigh
    ● S79.922 Unspecified injury of left thigh
    ● S79.929 Unspecified injury of unspecified thigh

INJURIES TO THE KNEE AND LOWER LEG (S80-S89)

Excludes2	burns and corrosions (T20-T32)
	frostbite (T33-T34)
	injuries of ankle and foot, except fracture of ankle and malleolus (S90-S99)
	insect bite or sting, venomous (T63.4)

● S80 Superficial injury of knee and lower leg

Excludes2	superficial injury of ankle and foot (S90.-)

The appropriate 7th character is to be added to each code from category S80

> A   initial encounter
> D   subsequent encounter
> S   sequela

  ● S80.0 Contusion of knee
   X ● S80.00 Contusion of unspecified knee
   X ● S80.01 Contusion of right knee
   X ● S80.02 Contusion of left knee

  ● S80.1 Contusion of lower leg
   X ● S80.10 Contusion of unspecified lower leg
   X ● S80.11 Contusion of right lower leg
   X ● S80.12 Contusion of left lower leg
  ● S80.2 Other superficial injuries of knee
    ● S80.21 Abrasion of knee
     ● S80.211 Abrasion, right knee
     ● S80.212 Abrasion, left knee
     ● S80.219 Abrasion, unspecified knee
    ● S80.22 Blister (nonthermal) of knee
     ● S80.221 Blister (nonthermal), right knee
     ● S80.222 Blister (nonthermal), left knee
     ● S80.229 Blister (nonthermal), unspecified knee
    ● S80.24 External constriction of knee
     ● S80.241 External constriction, right knee
     ● S80.242 External constriction, left knee
     ● S80.249 External constriction, unspecified knee
    ● S80.25 Superficial foreign body of knee
     Splinter in the knee
     ● S80.251 Superficial foreign body, right knee
     ● S80.252 Superficial foreign body, left knee
     ● S80.259 Superficial foreign body, unspecified knee
    ● S80.26 Insect bite (nonvenomous) of knee
     ● S80.261 Insect bite (nonvenomous), right knee
     ● S80.262 Insect bite (nonvenomous), left knee
     ● S80.269 Insect bite (nonvenomous), unspecified knee
    ● S80.27 Other superficial bite of knee

Excludes1	open bite of knee (S81.05-)

     ● S80.271 Other superficial bite of right knee
     ● S80.272 Other superficial bite of left knee
     ● S80.279 Other superficial bite of unspecified knee
  ● S80.8 Other superficial injuries of lower leg
    ● S80.81 Abrasion of lower leg
     ● S80.811 Abrasion, right lower leg
     ● S80.812 Abrasion, left lower leg
     ● S80.819 Abrasion, unspecified lower leg
    ● S80.82 Blister (nonthermal) of lower leg
     ● S80.821 Blister (nonthermal), right lower leg
     ● S80.822 Blister (nonthermal), left lower leg
     ● S80.829 Blister (nonthermal), unspecified lower leg
    ● S80.84 External constriction of lower leg
     ● S80.841 External constriction, right lower leg
     ● S80.842 External constriction, left lower leg
     ● S80.849 External constriction, unspecified lower leg
    ● S80.85 Superficial foreign body of lower leg
     Splinter in the lower leg
     ● S80.851 Superficial foreign body, right lower leg
     ● S80.852 Superficial foreign body, left lower leg
     ● S80.859 Superficial foreign body, unspecified lower leg

CHAPTER 19 (S00-T88)

CHAPTER 19 (S00-T88)

- S80.86   Insect bite (nonvenomous) of lower leg
  - S80.861   Insect bite (nonvenomous), right lower leg
  - S80.862   Insect bite (nonvenomous), left lower leg
  - S80.869   Insect bite (nonvenomous), unspecified lower leg
- S80.87   Other superficial bite of lower leg
  > **Excludes1**   open bite of lower leg (S81.85-)
  - S80.871   Other superficial bite, right lower leg
  - S80.872   Other superficial bite, left lower leg
  - S80.879   Other superficial bite, unspecified lower leg
- S80.9   Unspecified superficial injury of knee and lower leg
  - S80.91   Unspecified superficial injury of knee
    - S80.911   Unspecified superficial injury of right knee
    - S80.912   Unspecified superficial injury of left knee
    - S80.919   Unspecified superficial injury of unspecified knee
  - S80.92   Unspecified superficial injury of lower leg
    - S80.921   Unspecified superficial injury of right lower leg
    - S80.922   Unspecified superficial injury of left lower leg
    - S80.929   Unspecified superficial injury of unspecified lower leg

- S81   Open wound of knee and lower leg
  Code also any associated wound infection
  > **Excludes1**   open fracture of knee and lower leg (S82.-)
  > traumatic amputation of lower leg (S88.-)

  > **Excludes2**   open wound of ankle and foot (S91.-)

  The appropriate 7th character is to be added to each code from category S81

A	initial encounter
D	subsequent encounter
S	sequela

  - S81.0   Open wound of knee
    - S81.00   Unspecified open wound of knee
      - S81.001   Unspecified open wound, right knee
      - S81.002   Unspecified open wound, left knee
      - S81.009   Unspecified open wound, unspecified knee
    - S81.01   Laceration without foreign body of knee
      - S81.011   Laceration without foreign body, right knee
      - S81.012   Laceration without foreign body, left knee
      - S81.019   Laceration without foreign body, unspecified knee
    - S81.02   Laceration with foreign body of knee
      - S81.021   Laceration with foreign body, right knee
      - S81.022   Laceration with foreign body, left knee
      - S81.029   Laceration with foreign body, unspecified knee

- S81.03   Puncture wound without foreign body of knee
  - S81.031   Puncture wound without foreign body, right knee
  - S81.032   Puncture wound without foreign body, left knee
  - S81.039   Puncture wound without foreign body, unspecified knee
- S81.04   Puncture wound with foreign body of knee
  - S81.041   Puncture wound with foreign body, right knee
  - S81.042   Puncture wound with foreign body, left knee
  - S81.049   Puncture wound with foreign body, unspecified knee
- S81.05   Open bite of knee
  Bite of knee NOS
  > **Excludes1**   superficial bite of knee (S80.27-)
  - S81.051   Open bite, right knee
  - S81.052   Open bite, left knee
  - S81.059   Open bite, unspecified knee
- S81.8   Open wound of lower leg
  - S81.80   Unspecified open wound of lower leg
    - S81.801   Unspecified open wound, right lower leg
    - S81.802   Unspecified open wound, left lower leg
    - S81.809   Unspecified open wound, unspecified lower leg
  - S81.81   Laceration without foreign body of lower leg
    - S81.811   Laceration without foreign body, right lower leg
    - S81.812   Laceration without foreign body, left lower leg
    - S81.819   Laceration without foreign body, unspecified lower leg
  - S81.82   Laceration with foreign body of lower leg
    - S81.821   Laceration with foreign body, right lower leg
    - S81.822   Laceration with foreign body, left lower leg
    - S81.829   Laceration with foreign body, unspecified lower leg
  - S81.83   Puncture wound without foreign body of lower leg
    - S81.831   Puncture wound without foreign body, right lower leg
    - S81.832   Puncture wound without foreign body, left lower leg
    - S81.839   Puncture wound without foreign body, unspecified lower leg
  - S81.84   Puncture wound with foreign body of lower leg
    - S81.841   Puncture wound with foreign body, right lower leg
    - S81.842   Puncture wound with foreign body, left lower leg
    - S81.849   Puncture wound with foreign body, unspecified lower leg
  - S81.85   Open bite of lower leg
    Bite of lower leg NOS
    > **Excludes1**   superficial bite of lower leg (S80.86-, S80.87-)
    - S81.851   Open bite, right lower leg
    - S81.852   Open bite, left lower leg
    - S81.859   Open bite, unspecified lower leg

● **S82 Fracture of lower leg, including ankle**

> **Note:** A fracture not indicated as displaced or nondisplaced should be coded to displaced
>
> A fracture not indicated as open or closed should be coded to closed
>
> The open fracture designations are based on the Gustilo open fracture classification

Includes	fracture of malleolus
Excludes1	traumatic amputation of lower leg (S88.-)
Excludes2	fracture of foot, except ankle (S92.-)
	periprosthetic fracture of prosthetic implant of knee (T84.042, T84.043)

> The appropriate 7th character is to be added to all codes from category S82

A	initial encounter for closed fracture
B	initial encounter for open fracture type I or II initial encounter for open fracture NOS
C	initial encounter for open fracture type IIIA, IIIB, or IIIC
D	subsequent encounter for closed fracture with routine healing
E	subsequent encounter for open fracture type I or II with routine healing
F	subsequent encounter for open fracture type IIIA, IIIB, or IIIC with routine healing
G	subsequent encounter for closed fracture with delayed healing
H	subsequent encounter for open fracture type I or II with delayed healing
J	subsequent encounter for open fracture type IIIA, IIIB, or IIIC with delayed healing
K	subsequent encounter for closed fracture with nonunion
M	subsequent encounter for open fracture type I or II with nonunion
N	subsequent encounter for open fracture type IIIA, IIIB, or IIIC with nonunion
P	subsequent encounter for closed fracture with malunion
Q	subsequent encounter for open fracture type I or II with malunion
R	subsequent encounter for open fracture type IIIA, IIIB, or IIIC with malunion
S	sequela

● **S82.0 Fracture of patella**
> *Knee cap*

  ● **S82.00 Unspecified fracture of patella**

    ● S82.001 Unspecified fracture of right patella

    ● S82.002 Unspecified fracture of left patella

    ● S82.009 Unspecified fracture of unspecified patella

  ● **S82.01 Osteochondral fracture of patella**

    ● S82.011 Displaced osteochondral fracture of right patella

    ● S82.012 Displaced osteochondral fracture of left patella

    ● S82.013 Displaced osteochondral fracture of unspecified patella

    ● S82.014 Nondisplaced osteochondral fracture of right patella

    ● S82.015 Nondisplaced osteochondral fracture of left patella

    ● S82.016 Nondisplaced osteochondral fracture of unspecified patella

● **S82.02 Longitudinal fracture of patella**

  ● S82.021 Displaced longitudinal fracture of right patella

  ● S82.022 Displaced longitudinal fracture of left patella

  ● S82.023 Displaced longitudinal fracture of unspecified patella

  ● S82.024 Nondisplaced longitudinal fracture of right patella

  ● S82.025 Nondisplaced longitudinal fracture of left patella

  ● S82.026 Nondisplaced longitudinal fracture of unspecified patella

● **S82.03 Transverse fracture of patella**

  ● S82.031 Displaced transverse fracture of right patella

  ● S82.032 Displaced transverse fracture of left patella

  ● S82.033 Displaced transverse fracture of unspecified patella

  ● S82.034 Nondisplaced transverse fracture of right patella

  ● S82.035 Nondisplaced transverse fracture of left patella

  ● S82.036 Nondisplaced transverse fracture of unspecified patella

● **S82.04 Comminuted fracture of patella**

  ● S82.041 Displaced comminuted fracture of right patella

  ● S82.042 Displaced comminuted fracture of left patella

  ● S82.043 Displaced comminuted fracture of unspecified patella

  ● S82.044 Nondisplaced comminuted fracture of right patella

  ● S82.045 Nondisplaced comminuted fracture of left patella

  ● S82.046 Nondisplaced comminuted fracture of unspecified patella

● **S82.09 Other fracture of patella**

  ● S82.091 Other fracture of right patella

  ● S82.092 Other fracture of left patella

  ● S82.099 Other fracture of unspecified patella

● **S82.1 Fracture of upper end of tibia**
> Fracture of proximal end of tibia

Excludes2	fracture of shaft of tibia (S82.2-)
	physeal fracture of upper end of tibia (S89.0-)

  ● **S82.10 Unspecified fracture of upper end of tibia**

    ● S82.101 Unspecified fracture of upper end of right tibia

    ● S82.102 Unspecified fracture of upper end of left tibia

    ● S82.109 Unspecified fracture of upper end of unspecified tibia

  ● **S82.11 Fracture of tibial spine**

    ● S82.111 Displaced fracture of right tibial spine

    ● S82.112 Displaced fracture of left tibial spine

    ● S82.113 Displaced fracture of unspecified tibial spine

CHAPTER 19 (S00-T88)

● S82.114   Nondisplaced fracture of right tibial spine
● S82.115   Nondisplaced fracture of left tibial spine
● S82.116   Nondisplaced fracture of unspecified tibial spine

● S82.12   Fracture of lateral condyle of tibia
● S82.121   Displaced fracture of lateral condyle of right tibia
● S82.122   Displaced fracture of lateral condyle of left tibia
● S82.123   Displaced fracture of lateral condyle of unspecified tibia
● S82.124   Nondisplaced fracture of lateral condyle of right tibia
● S82.125   Nondisplaced fracture of lateral condyle of left tibia
● S82.126   Nondisplaced fracture of lateral condyle of unspecified tibia

● S82.13   Fracture of medial condyle of tibia
● S82.131   Displaced fracture of medial condyle of right tibia
● S82.132   Displaced fracture of medial condyle of left tibia
● S82.133   Displaced fracture of medial condyle of unspecified tibia
● S82.134   Nondisplaced fracture of medial condyle of right tibia
● S82.135   Nondisplaced fracture of medial condyle of left tibia
● S82.136   Nondisplaced fracture of medial condyle of unspecified tibia

● S82.14   Bicondylar fracture of tibia
         Fracture of tibial plateau NOS
● S82.141   Displaced bicondylar fracture of right tibia
● S82.142   Displaced bicondylar fracture of left tibia
● S82.143   Displaced bicondylar fracture of unspecified tibia
● S82.144   Nondisplaced bicondylar fracture of right tibia
● S82.145   Nondisplaced bicondylar fracture of left tibia
● S82.146   Nondisplaced bicondylar fracture of unspecified tibia

● S82.15   Fracture of tibial tuberosity
● S82.151   Displaced fracture of right tibial tuberosity
● S82.152   Displaced fracture of left tibial tuberosity
● S82.153   Displaced fracture of unspecified tibial tuberosity
● S82.154   Nondisplaced fracture of right tibial tuberosity
● S82.155   Nondisplaced fracture of left tibial tuberosity
● S82.156   Nondisplaced fracture of unspecified tibial tuberosity

● S82.16   Torus fracture of upper end of tibia
         The appropriate 7th character is to be added to all codes in subcategory S82.16

A	initial encounter for closed fracture
D	subsequent encounter for fracture with routine healing
G	subsequent encounter for fracture with delayed healing
K	subsequent encounter for fracture with nonunion
P	subsequent encounter for fracture with malunion
S	sequela

● S82.161   Torus fracture of upper end of right tibia
● S82.162   Torus fracture of upper end of left tibia
● S82.169   Torus fracture of upper end of unspecified tibia

● S82.19   Other fracture of upper end of tibia
● S82.191   Other fracture of upper end of right tibia
● S82.192   Other fracture of upper end of left tibia
● S82.199   Other fracture of upper end of unspecified tibia

● S82.2   Fracture of shaft of tibia
● S82.20   Unspecified fracture of shaft of tibia
         Fracture of tibia NOS
● S82.201   Unspecified fracture of shaft of right tibia
● S82.202   Unspecified fracture of shaft of left tibia
● S82.209   Unspecified fracture of shaft of unspecified tibia

● S82.22   Transverse fracture of shaft of tibia
● S82.221   Displaced transverse fracture of shaft of right tibia
● S82.222   Displaced transverse fracture of shaft of left tibia
● S82.223   Displaced transverse fracture of shaft of unspecified tibia
● S82.224   Nondisplaced transverse fracture of shaft of right tibia
● S82.225   Nondisplaced transverse fracture of shaft of left tibia
● S82.226   Nondisplaced transverse fracture of shaft of unspecified tibia

● S82.23   Oblique fracture of shaft of tibia
● S82.231   Displaced oblique fracture of shaft of right tibia
● S82.232   Displaced oblique fracture of shaft of left tibia
● S82.233   Displaced oblique fracture of shaft of unspecified tibia
● S82.234   Nondisplaced oblique fracture of shaft of right tibia
● S82.235   Nondisplaced oblique fracture of shaft of left tibia
● S82.236   Nondisplaced oblique fracture of shaft of unspecified tibia

● S82.24   Spiral fracture of shaft of tibia
　　　　　　Toddler fracture
　● S82.241   Displaced spiral fracture of shaft of right tibia
　● S82.242   Displaced spiral fracture of shaft of left tibia
　● S82.243   Displaced spiral fracture of shaft of unspecified tibia
　● S82.244   Nondisplaced spiral fracture of shaft of right tibia
　● S82.245   Nondisplaced spiral fracture of shaft of left tibia
　● S82.246   Nondisplaced spiral fracture of shaft of unspecified tibia
● S82.25   Comminuted fracture of shaft of tibia
　● S82.251   Displaced comminuted fracture of shaft of right tibia
　● S82.252   Displaced comminuted fracture of shaft of left tibia
　● S82.253   Displaced comminuted fracture of shaft of unspecified tibia
　● S82.254   Nondisplaced comminuted fracture of shaft of right tibia
　● S82.255   Nondisplaced comminuted fracture of shaft of left tibia
　● S82.256   Nondisplaced comminuted fracture of shaft of unspecified tibia
● S82.26   Segmental fracture of shaft of tibia
　● S82.261   Displaced segmental fracture of shaft of right tibia
　● S82.262   Displaced segmental fracture of shaft of left tibia
　● S82.263   Displaced segmental fracture of shaft of unspecified tibia
　● S82.264   Nondisplaced segmental fracture of shaft of right tibia
　● S82.265   Nondisplaced segmental fracture of shaft of left tibia
　● S82.266   Nondisplaced segmental fracture of shaft of unspecified tibia
● S82.29   Other fracture of shaft of tibia
　● S82.291   Other fracture of shaft of right tibia
　● S82.292   Other fracture of shaft of left tibia
　● S82.299   Other fracture of shaft of unspecified tibia
● S82.3   Fracture of lower end of tibia
　　Excludes1   bimalleolar fracture of lower leg (S82.84-)
　　　　　　　　fracture of medial malleolus alone (S82.5-)
　　　　　　　　Maisonneuve's fracture (S82.86-)
　　　　　　　　pilon fracture of distal tibia (S82.87-)
　　　　　　　　trimalleolar fractures of lower leg (S82.85-)
　● S82.30   Unspecified fracture of lower end of tibia
　　● S82.301   Unspecified fracture of lower end of right tibia
　　● S82.302   Unspecified fracture of lower end of left tibia
　　● S82.309   Unspecified fracture of lower end of unspecified tibia

● S82.31   Torus fracture of lower end of tibia
　　The appropriate 7th character is to be added to all codes in subcategory S82.31

A	initial encounter for closed fracture
D	subsequent encounter for fracture with routine healing
G	subsequent encounter for fracture with delayed healing
K	subsequent encounter for fracture with nonunion
P	subsequent encounter for fracture with malunion
S	sequela

　● S82.311   Torus fracture of lower end of right tibia
　● S82.312   Torus fracture of lower end of left tibia
　● S82.319   Torus fracture of lower end of unspecified tibia
● S82.39   Other fracture of lower end of tibia
　● S82.391   Other fracture of lower end of right tibia
　● S82.392   Other fracture of lower end of left tibia
　● S82.399   Other fracture of lower end of unspecified tibia
● S82.4   Fracture of shaft of fibula
　　Excludes2   fracture of lateral malleolus alone (S82.6-)
　● S82.40   Unspecified fracture of shaft of fibula
　　● S82.401   Unspecified fracture of shaft of right fibula
　　● S82.402   Unspecified fracture of shaft of left fibula
　　● S82.409   Unspecified fracture of shaft of unspecified fibula
　● S82.42   Transverse fracture of shaft of fibula
　　● S82.421   Displaced transverse fracture of shaft of right fibula
　　● S82.422   Displaced transverse fracture of shaft of left fibula
　　● S82.423   Displaced transverse fracture of shaft of unspecified fibula
　　● S82.424   Nondisplaced transverse fracture of shaft of right fibula
　　● S82.425   Nondisplaced transverse fracture of shaft of left fibula
　　● S82.426   Nondisplaced transverse fracture of shaft of unspecified fibula
　● S82.43   Oblique fracture of shaft of fibula
　　● S82.431   Displaced oblique fracture of shaft of right fibula
　　● S82.432   Displaced oblique fracture of shaft of left fibula
　　● S82.433   Displaced oblique fracture of shaft of unspecified fibula
　　● S82.434   Nondisplaced oblique fracture of shaft of right fibula
　　● S82.435   Nondisplaced oblique fracture of shaft of left fibula
　　● S82.436   Nondisplaced oblique fracture of shaft of unspecified fibula

CHAPTER 19 (S00-T88)

● **S82.44**   **Spiral fracture of shaft of fibula**
  ● **S82.441**   Displaced spiral fracture of shaft of right fibula
  ● **S82.442**   Displaced spiral fracture of shaft of left fibula
  ● **S82.443**   Displaced spiral fracture of shaft of unspecified fibula
  ● **S82.444**   Nondisplaced spiral fracture of shaft of right fibula
  ● **S82.445**   Nondisplaced spiral fracture of shaft of left fibula
  ● **S82.446**   Nondisplaced spiral fracture of shaft of unspecified fibula
● **S82.45**   **Comminuted fracture of shaft of fibula**
  ● **S82.451**   Displaced comminuted fracture of shaft of right fibula
  ● **S82.452**   Displaced comminuted fracture of shaft of left fibula
  ● **S82.453**   Displaced comminuted fracture of shaft of unspecified fibula
  ● **S82.454**   Nondisplaced comminuted fracture of shaft of right fibula
  ● **S82.455**   Nondisplaced comminuted fracture of shaft of left fibula
  ● **S82.456**   Nondisplaced comminuted fracture of shaft of unspecified fibula
● **S82.46**   **Segmental fracture of shaft of fibula**
  ● **S82.461**   Displaced segmental fracture of shaft of right fibula
  ● **S82.462**   Displaced segmental fracture of shaft of left fibula
  ● **S82.463**   Displaced segmental fracture of shaft of unspecified fibula
  ● **S82.464**   Nondisplaced segmental fracture of shaft of right fibula
  ● **S82.465**   Nondisplaced segmental fracture of shaft of left fibula
  ● **S82.466**   Nondisplaced segmental fracture of shaft of unspecified fibula
● **S82.49**   **Other fracture of shaft of fibula**
  ● **S82.491**   Other fracture of shaft of right fibula
  ● **S82.492**   Other fracture of shaft of left fibula
  ● **S82.499**   Other fracture of shaft of unspecified fibula
● **S82.5**   **Fracture of medial malleolus**
  Excludes1   pilon fracture of distal tibia (S82.87-)
             Salter-Harris type III of lower end of tibia (S89.13-)
             Salter-Harris type IV of lower end of tibia (S89.14-)
  X ● **S82.51**   Displaced fracture of medial malleolus of right tibia
  X ● **S82.52**   Displaced fracture of medial malleolus of left tibia
  X ● **S82.53**   Displaced fracture of medial malleolus of unspecified tibia
  X ● **S82.54**   Nondisplaced fracture of medial malleolus of right tibia
  X ● **S82.55**   Nondisplaced fracture of medial malleolus of left tibia
  X ● **S82.56**   Nondisplaced fracture of medial malleolus of unspecified tibia

● **S82.6**   **Fracture of lateral malleolus**
  Excludes1   pilon fracture of distal tibia (S82.87-)
  X ● **S82.61**   Displaced fracture of lateral malleolus of right fibula
  X ● **S82.62**   Displaced fracture of lateral malleolus of left fibula
  X ● **S82.63**   Displaced fracture of lateral malleolus of unspecified fibula
  X ● **S82.64**   Nondisplaced fracture of lateral malleolus of right fibula
  X ● **S82.65**   Nondisplaced fracture of lateral malleolus of left fibula
  X ● **S82.66**   Nondisplaced fracture of lateral malleolus of unspecified fibula
● **S82.8**   **Other fractures of lower leg**
  ● **S82.81**   **Torus fracture of upper end of fibula**
    The appropriate 7th character is to be added to all codes in subcategory S82.81

A	initial encounter for closed fracture
D	subsequent encounter for fracture with routine healing
G	subsequent encounter for fracture with delayed healing
K	subsequent encounter for fracture with nonunion
P	subsequent encounter for fracture with malunion
S	sequela

    ● **S82.811**   Torus fracture of upper end of right fibula
    ● **S82.812**   Torus fracture of upper end of left fibula
    ● **S82.819**   Torus fracture of upper end of unspecified fibula
  ● **S82.82**   **Torus fracture of lower end of fibula**
    The appropriate 7th character is to be added to all codes in subcategory S82.82

A	initial encounter for closed fracture
D	subsequent encounter for fracture with routine healing
G	subsequent encounter for fracture with delayed healing
K	subsequent encounter for fracture with nonunion
P	subsequent encounter for fracture with malunion
S	sequela

    ● **S82.821**   Torus fracture of lower end of right fibula
    ● **S82.822**   Torus fracture of lower end of left fibula
    ● **S82.829**   Torus fracture of lower end of unspecified fibula
  ● **S82.83**   **Other fracture of upper and lower end of fibula**
    ● **S82.831**   Other fracture of upper and lower end of right fibula
    ● **S82.832**   Other fracture of upper and lower end of left fibula
    ● **S82.839**   Other fracture of upper and lower end of unspecified fibula

● S82.84   **Bimalleolar fracture of lower leg**
　　● S82.841   Displaced bimalleolar fracture of right lower leg
　　● S82.842   Displaced bimalleolar fracture of left lower leg
　　● S82.843   Displaced bimalleolar fracture of unspecified lower leg
　　● S82.844   Nondisplaced bimalleolar fracture of right lower leg
　　● S82.845   Nondisplaced bimalleolar fracture of left lower leg
　　● S82.846   Nondisplaced bimalleolar fracture of unspecified lower leg
● S82.85   **Trimalleolar fracture of lower leg**
　　● S82.851   Displaced trimalleolar fracture of right lower leg
　　● S82.852   Displaced trimalleolar fracture of left lower leg
　　● S82.853   Displaced trimalleolar fracture of unspecified lower leg
　　● S82.854   Nondisplaced trimalleolar fracture of right lower leg
　　● S82.855   Nondisplaced trimalleolar fracture of left lower leg
　　● S82.856   Nondisplaced trimalleolar fracture of unspecified lower leg
● S82.86   **Maisonneuve's fracture**
　　● S82.861   Displaced Maisonneuve's fracture of right leg
　　● S82.862   Displaced Maisonneuve's fracture of left leg
　　● S82.863   Displaced Maisonneuve's fracture of unspecified leg
　　● S82.864   Nondisplaced Maisonneuve's fracture of right leg
　　● S82.865   Nondisplaced Maisonneuve's fracture of left leg
　　● S82.866   Nondisplaced Maisonneuve's fracture of unspecified leg
● S82.87   **Pilon fracture of tibia**
　　● S82.871   Displaced pilon fracture of right tibia
　　● S82.872   Displaced pilon fracture of left tibia
　　● S82.873   Displaced pilon fracture of unspecified tibia
　　● S82.874   Nondisplaced pilon fracture of right tibia
　　● S82.875   Nondisplaced pilon fracture of left tibia
　　● S82.876   Nondisplaced pilon fracture of unspecified tibia
● S82.89   **Other fractures of lower leg**
　　　　Fracture of ankle NOS
　　● S82.891   Other fracture of right lower leg
　　● S82.892   Other fracture of left lower leg
　　● S82.899   Other fracture of unspecified lower leg
● S82.9   **Unspecified fracture of lower leg**
　X ● S82.90   Unspecified fracture of unspecified lower leg
　X ● S82.91   Unspecified fracture of right lower leg
　X ● S82.92   Unspecified fracture of left lower leg

● S83   **Dislocation and sprain of joints and ligaments of knee**
　　Includes　avulsion of joint or ligament of knee
　　　　laceration of cartilage, joint or ligament of knee
　　　　sprain of cartilage, joint or ligament of knee
　　　　traumatic hemarthrosis of joint or ligament of knee
　　　　traumatic rupture of joint or ligament of knee
　　　　traumatic subluxation of joint or ligament of knee
　　　　traumatic tear of joint or ligament of knee
　　Code also any associated open wound
　　Excludes1　derangement of patella (M22.0-M22.3)
　　　　injury of patellar ligament (tendon) (S76.1-)
　　　　internal derangement of knee (M23.-)
　　　　old dislocation of knee (M24.36)
　　　　pathological dislocation of knee (M24.36)
　　　　recurrent dislocation of knee (M22.0)
　　Excludes2　strain of muscle, fascia and tendon of lower leg (S86.-)

　　The appropriate 7th character is to be added to each code from category S83

　　　A　initial encounter
　　　D　subsequent encounter
　　　S　sequela

● S83.0   **Subluxation and dislocation of patella**
　● S83.00   **Unspecified subluxation and dislocation of patella**
　　● S83.001   Unspecified subluxation of right patella
　　● S83.002   Unspecified subluxation of left patella
　　● S83.003   Unspecified subluxation of unspecified patella
　　● S83.004   Unspecified dislocation of right patella
　　● S83.005   Unspecified dislocation of left patella
　　● S83.006   Unspecified dislocation of unspecified patella
　● S83.01   **Lateral subluxation and dislocation of patella**
　　● S83.011   Lateral subluxation of right patella
　　● S83.012   Lateral subluxation of left patella
　　● S83.013   Lateral subluxation of unspecified patella
　　● S83.014   Lateral dislocation of right patella
　　● S83.015   Lateral dislocation of left patella
　　● S83.016   Lateral dislocation of unspecified patella
　● S83.09   **Other subluxation and dislocation of patella**
　　● S83.091   Other subluxation of right patella
　　● S83.092   Other subluxation of left patella
　　● S83.093   Other subluxation of unspecified patella
　　● S83.094   Other dislocation of right patella
　　● S83.095   Other dislocation of left patella
　　● S83.096   Other dislocation of unspecified patella
● S83.1   **Subluxation and dislocation of knee**
　　Excludes2　instability of knee prosthesis (T84.022, T84.023)
　● S83.10   **Unspecified subluxation and dislocation of knee**
　　● S83.101   Unspecified subluxation of right knee
　　● S83.102   Unspecified subluxation of left knee
　　● S83.103   Unspecified subluxation of unspecified knee

CHAPTER 19 (S00-T88)

- S83.104 Unspecified dislocation of right knee
- S83.105 Unspecified dislocation of left knee
- S83.106 Unspecified dislocation of unspecified knee
- S83.11 **Anterior subluxation and dislocation of proximal end of tibia**
  Posterior subluxation and dislocation of distal end of femur
  - S83.111 Anterior subluxation of proximal end of tibia, right knee
  - S83.112 Anterior subluxation of proximal end of tibia, left knee
  - S83.113 Anterior subluxation of proximal end of tibia, unspecified knee
  - S83.114 Anterior dislocation of proximal end of tibia, right knee
  - S83.115 Anterior dislocation of proximal end of tibia, left knee
  - S83.116 Anterior dislocation of proximal end of tibia, unspecified knee
- S83.12 **Posterior subluxation and dislocation of proximal end of tibia**
  Anterior dislocation of distal end of femur
  - S83.121 Posterior subluxation of proximal end of tibia, right knee
  - S83.122 Posterior subluxation of proximal end of tibia, left knee
  - S83.123 Posterior subluxation of proximal end of tibia, unspecified knee
  - S83.124 Posterior dislocation of proximal end of tibia, right knee
  - S83.125 Posterior dislocation of proximal end of tibia, left knee
  - S83.126 Posterior dislocation of proximal end of tibia, unspecified knee
- S83.13 **Medial subluxation and dislocation of proximal end of tibia**
  - S83.131 Medial subluxation of proximal end of tibia, right knee
  - S83.132 Medial subluxation of proximal end of tibia, left knee
  - S83.133 Medial subluxation of proximal end of tibia, unspecified knee
  - S83.134 Medial dislocation of proximal end of tibia, right knee
  - S83.135 Medial dislocation of proximal end of tibia, left knee
  - S83.136 Medial dislocation of proximal end of tibia, unspecified knee
- S83.14 **Lateral subluxation and dislocation of proximal end of tibia**
  - S83.141 Lateral subluxation of proximal end of tibia, right knee
  - S83.142 Lateral subluxation of proximal end of tibia, left knee
  - S83.143 Lateral subluxation of proximal end of tibia, unspecified knee
  - S83.144 Lateral dislocation of proximal end of tibia, right knee
  - S83.145 Lateral dislocation of proximal end of tibia, left knee
  - S83.146 Lateral dislocation of proximal end of tibia, unspecified knee

- S83.19 **Other subluxation and dislocation of knee**
  - S83.191 Other subluxation of right knee
  - S83.192 Other subluxation of left knee
  - S83.193 Other subluxation of unspecified knee
  - S83.194 Other dislocation of right knee
  - S83.195 Other dislocation of left knee
  - S83.196 Other dislocation of unspecified knee
- S83.2 **Tear of meniscus, current injury**
  Excludes1 old bucket-handle tear (M23.2)
  - S83.20 **Tear of unspecified meniscus, current injury**
    Tear of meniscus of knee NOS
    - S83.200 Bucket-handle tear of unspecified meniscus, current injury, right knee
    - S83.201 Bucket-handle tear of unspecified meniscus, current injury, left knee
    - S83.202 Bucket-handle tear of unspecified meniscus, current injury, unspecified knee
    - S83.203 Other tear of unspecified meniscus, current injury, right knee
    - S83.204 Other tear of unspecified meniscus, current injury, left knee
    - S83.205 Other tear of unspecified meniscus, current injury, unspecified knee
    - S83.206 Unspecified tear of unspecified meniscus, current injury, right knee
    - S83.207 Unspecified tear of unspecified meniscus, current injury, left knee
    - S83.209 Unspecified tear of unspecified meniscus, current injury, unspecified knee
  - S83.21 **Bucket-handle tear of medial meniscus, current injury**
    - S83.211 Bucket-handle tear of medial meniscus, current injury, right knee
    - S83.212 Bucket-handle tear of medial meniscus, current injury, left knee
    - S83.219 Bucket-handle tear of medial meniscus, current injury, unspecified knee
  - S83.22 **Peripheral tear of medial meniscus, current injury**
    - S83.221 Peripheral tear of medial meniscus, current injury, right knee
    - S83.222 Peripheral tear of medial meniscus, current injury, left knee
    - S83.229 Peripheral tear of medial meniscus, current injury, unspecified knee
  - S83.23 **Complex tear of medial meniscus, current injury**
    - S83.231 Complex tear of medial meniscus, current injury, right knee
    - S83.232 Complex tear of medial meniscus, current injury, left knee
    - S83.239 Complex tear of medial meniscus, current injury, unspecified knee
  - S83.24 **Other tear of medial meniscus, current injury**
    - S83.241 Other tear of medial meniscus, current injury, right knee
    - S83.242 Other tear of medial meniscus, current injury, left knee
    - S83.249 Other tear of medial meniscus, current injury, unspecified knee

● S83.25　Bucket-handle tear of lateral meniscus, current injury
- ● S83.251　Bucket-handle tear of lateral meniscus, current injury, right knee
- ● S83.252　Bucket-handle tear of lateral meniscus, current injury, left knee
- ● S83.259　Bucket-handle tear of lateral meniscus, current injury, unspecified knee

● S83.26　Peripheral tear of lateral meniscus, current injury
- ● S83.261　Peripheral tear of lateral meniscus, current injury, right knee
- ● S83.262　Peripheral tear of lateral meniscus, current injury, left knee
- ● S83.269　Peripheral tear of lateral meniscus, current injury, unspecified knee

● S83.27　Complex tear of lateral meniscus, current injury
- ● S83.271　Complex tear of lateral meniscus, current injury, right knee
- ● S83.272　Complex tear of lateral meniscus, current injury, left knee
- ● S83.279　Complex tear of lateral meniscus, current injury, unspecified knee

● S83.28　Other tear of lateral meniscus, current injury
- ● S83.281　Other tear of lateral meniscus, current injury, right knee
- ● S83.282　Other tear of lateral meniscus, current injury, left knee
- ● S83.289　Other tear of lateral meniscus, current injury, unspecified knee

● S83.3　Tear of articular cartilage of knee, current
- X ● S83.30　Tear of articular cartilage of unspecified knee, current
- X ● S83.31　Tear of articular cartilage of right knee, current
- X ● S83.32　Tear of articular cartilage of left knee, current

● S83.4　Sprain of collateral ligament of knee
- ● S83.40　Sprain of unspecified collateral ligament of knee
  - ● S83.401　Sprain of unspecified collateral ligament of right knee
  - ● S83.402　Sprain of unspecified collateral ligament of left knee
  - ● S83.409　Sprain of unspecified collateral ligament of unspecified knee
- ● S83.41　Sprain of medial collateral ligament of knee
  Sprain of tibial collateral ligament
  - ● S83.411　Sprain of medial collateral ligament of right knee
  - ● S83.412　Sprain of medial collateral ligament of left knee
  - ● S83.419　Sprain of medial collateral ligament of unspecified knee
- ● S83.42　Sprain of lateral collateral ligament of knee
  Sprain of fibular collateral ligament
  - ● S83.421　Sprain of lateral collateral ligament of right knee
  - ● S83.422　Sprain of lateral collateral ligament of left knee
  - ● S83.429　Sprain of lateral collateral ligament of unspecified knee

● S83.5　Sprain of cruciate ligament of knee
- ● S83.50　Sprain of unspecified cruciate ligament of knee
  - ● S83.501　Sprain of unspecified cruciate ligament of right knee
  - ● S83.502　Sprain of unspecified cruciate ligament of left knee
  - ● S83.509　Sprain of unspecified cruciate ligament of unspecified knee

● S83.51　Sprain of anterior cruciate ligament of knee
- ● S83.511　Sprain of anterior cruciate ligament of right knee
- ● S83.512　Sprain of anterior cruciate ligament of left knee
- ● S83.519　Sprain of anterior cruciate ligament of unspecified knee

● S83.52　Sprain of posterior cruciate ligament of knee
- ● S83.521　Sprain of posterior cruciate ligament of right knee
- ● S83.522　Sprain of posterior cruciate ligament of left knee
- ● S83.529　Sprain of posterior cruciate ligament of unspecified knee

● S83.6　Sprain of the superior tibiofibular joint and ligament
- X ● S83.60　Sprain of the superior tibiofibular joint and ligament, unspecified knee
- X ● S83.61　Sprain of the superior tibiofibular joint and ligament, right knee
- X ● S83.62　Sprain of the superior tibiofibular joint and ligament, left knee

● S83.8　Sprain of other specified parts of knee
- ● S83.8X　Sprain of other specified parts of knee
  - ● S83.8X1　Sprain of other specified parts of right knee
  - ● S83.8X2　Sprain of other specified parts of left knee
  - ● S83.8X9　Sprain of other specified parts of unspecified knee

● S83.9　Sprain of unspecified site of knee
- X ● S83.90　Sprain of unspecified site of unspecified knee
- X ● S83.91　Sprain of unspecified site of right knee
- X ● S83.92　Sprain of unspecified site of left knee

● S84　Injury of nerves at lower leg level
Code also any associated open wound (S81.-)

Excludes2　injury of nerves at ankle and foot level (S94.-)

The appropriate 7th character is to be added to each code from category S84

A	initial encounter
D	subsequent encounter
S	sequela

● S84.0　Injury of tibial nerve at lower leg level
- X ● S84.00　Injury of tibial nerve at lower leg level, unspecified leg
- X ● S84.01　Injury of tibial nerve at lower leg level, right leg
- X ● S84.02　Injury of tibial nerve at lower leg level, left leg

● S84.1　Injury of peroneal nerve at lower leg level
- X ● S84.10　Injury of peroneal nerve at lower leg level, unspecified leg
- X ● S84.11　Injury of peroneal nerve at lower leg level, right leg
- X ● S84.12　Injury of peroneal nerve at lower leg level, left leg

● S84.2　Injury of cutaneous sensory nerve at lower leg level
- X ● S84.20　Injury of cutaneous sensory nerve at lower leg level, unspecified leg
- X ● S84.21　Injury of cutaneous sensory nerve at lower leg level, right leg
- X ● S84.22　Injury of cutaneous sensory nerve at lower leg level, left leg

● S84.8　Injury of other nerves at lower leg level
- ● S84.80　Injury of other nerves at lower leg level
  - ● S84.801　Injury of other nerves at lower leg level, right leg
  - ● S84.802　Injury of other nerves at lower leg level, left leg
  - ● S84.809　Injury of other nerves at lower leg level, unspecified leg

● S84.9   Injury of unspecified nerve at lower leg level
  X● S84.90   Injury of unspecified nerve at lower leg level, unspecified leg
  X● S84.91   Injury of unspecified nerve at lower leg level, right leg
  X● S84.92   Injury of unspecified nerve at lower leg level, left leg

● S85   Injury of blood vessels at lower leg level
    Code also any associated open wound (S81.-)
    Excludes2   injury of blood vessels at ankle and foot level (S95.-)

    The appropriate 7th character is to be added to each code from category S85

    A   initial encounter
    D   subsequent encounter
    S   sequela

  ● S85.0   Injury of popliteal artery
    ● S85.00   Unspecified injury of popliteal artery
      ● S85.001   Unspecified injury of popliteal artery, right leg
      ● S85.002   Unspecified injury of popliteal artery, left leg
      ● S85.009   Unspecified injury of popliteal artery, unspecified leg
    ● S85.01   Laceration of popliteal artery
      ● S85.011   Laceration of popliteal artery, right leg
      ● S85.012   Laceration of popliteal artery, left leg
      ● S85.019   Laceration of popliteal artery, unspecified leg
    ● S85.09   Other specified injury of popliteal artery
      ● S85.091   Other specified injury of popliteal artery, right leg
      ● S85.092   Other specified injury of popliteal artery, left leg
      ● S85.099   Other specified injury of popliteal artery, unspecified leg
  ● S85.1   Injury of tibial artery
    ● S85.10   Unspecified injury of unspecified tibial artery
        Injury of tibial artery NOS
      ● S85.101   Unspecified injury of unspecified tibial artery, right leg
      ● S85.102   Unspecified injury of unspecified tibial artery, left leg
      ● S85.109   Unspecified injury of unspecified tibial artery, unspecified leg
    ● S85.11   Laceration of unspecified tibial artery
      ● S85.111   Laceration of unspecified tibial artery, right leg
      ● S85.112   Laceration of unspecified tibial artery, left leg
      ● S85.119   Laceration of unspecified tibial artery, unspecified leg
    ● S85.12   Other specified injury of unspecified tibial artery
      ● S85.121   Other specified injury of unspecified tibial artery, right leg
      ● S85.122   Other specified injury of unspecified tibial artery, left leg
      ● S85.129   Other specified injury of unspecified tibial artery, unspecified leg
    ● S85.13   Unspecified injury of anterior tibial artery
      ● S85.131   Unspecified injury of anterior tibial artery, right leg
      ● S85.132   Unspecified injury of anterior tibial artery, left leg
      ● S85.139   Unspecified injury of anterior tibial artery, unspecified leg

● S85.14   Laceration of anterior tibial artery
  ● S85.141   Laceration of anterior tibial artery, right leg
  ● S85.142   Laceration of anterior tibial artery, left leg
  ● S85.149   Laceration of anterior tibial artery, unspecified leg
● S85.15   Other specified injury of anterior tibial artery
  ● S85.151   Other specified injury of anterior tibial artery, right leg
  ● S85.152   Other specified injury of anterior tibial artery, left leg
  ● S85.159   Other specified injury of anterior tibial artery, unspecified leg
● S85.16   Unspecified injury of posterior tibial artery
  ● S85.161   Unspecified injury of posterior tibial artery, right leg
  ● S85.162   Unspecified injury of posterior tibial artery, left leg
  ● S85.169   Unspecified injury of posterior tibial artery, unspecified leg
● S85.17   Laceration of posterior tibial artery
  ● S85.171   Laceration of posterior tibial artery, right leg
  ● S85.172   Laceration of posterior tibial artery, left leg
  ● S85.179   Laceration of posterior tibial artery, unspecified leg
● S85.18   Other specified injury of posterior tibial artery
  ● S85.181   Other specified injury of posterior tibial artery, right leg
  ● S85.182   Other specified injury of posterior tibial artery, left leg
  ● S85.189   Other specified injury of posterior tibial artery, unspecified leg
● S85.2   Injury of peroneal artery
  ● S85.20   Unspecified injury of peroneal artery
    ● S85.201   Unspecified injury of peroneal artery, right leg
    ● S85.202   Unspecified injury of peroneal artery, left leg
    ● S85.209   Unspecified injury of peroneal artery, unspecified leg
  ● S85.21   Laceration of peroneal artery
    ● S85.211   Laceration of peroneal artery, right leg
    ● S85.212   Laceration of peroneal artery, left leg
    ● S85.219   Laceration of peroneal artery, unspecified leg
  ● S85.29   Other specified injury of peroneal artery
    ● S85.291   Other specified injury of peroneal artery, right leg
    ● S85.292   Other specified injury of peroneal artery, left leg
    ● S85.299   Other specified injury of peroneal artery, unspecified leg
● S85.3   Injury of greater saphenous vein at lower leg level
      Injury of greater saphenous vein NOS
      Injury of saphenous vein NOS
  ● S85.30   Unspecified injury of greater saphenous vein at lower leg level
    ● S85.301   Unspecified injury of greater saphenous vein at lower leg level, right leg
    ● S85.302   Unspecified injury of greater saphenous vein at lower leg level, left leg
    ● S85.309   Unspecified injury of greater saphenous vein at lower leg level, unspecified leg

- S85.31   Laceration of greater saphenous vein at lower leg level
  - S85.311   Laceration of greater saphenous vein at lower leg level, right leg
  - S85.312   Laceration of greater saphenous vein at lower leg level, left leg
  - S85.319   Laceration of greater saphenous vein at lower leg level, unspecified leg
- S85.39   Other specified injury of greater saphenous vein at lower leg level
  - S85.391   Other specified injury of greater saphenous vein at lower leg level, right leg
  - S85.392   Other specified injury of greater saphenous vein at lower leg level, left leg
  - S85.399   Other specified injury of greater saphenous vein at lower leg level, unspecified leg
- S85.4   Injury of lesser saphenous vein at lower leg level
  - S85.40   Unspecified injury of lesser saphenous vein at lower leg level
    - S85.401   Unspecified injury of lesser saphenous vein at lower leg level, right leg
    - S85.402   Unspecified injury of lesser saphenous vein at lower leg level, left leg
    - S85.409   Unspecified injury of lesser saphenous vein at lower leg level, unspecified leg
  - S85.41   Laceration of lesser saphenous vein at lower leg level
    - S85.411   Laceration of lesser saphenous vein at lower leg level, right leg
    - S85.412   Laceration of lesser saphenous vein at lower leg level, left leg
    - S85.419   Laceration of lesser saphenous vein at lower leg level, unspecified leg
  - S85.49   Other specified injury of lesser saphenous vein at lower leg level
    - S85.491   Other specified injury of lesser saphenous vein at lower leg level, right leg
    - S85.492   Other specified injury of lesser saphenous vein at lower leg level, left leg
    - S85.499   Other specified injury of lesser saphenous vein at lower leg level, unspecified leg
- S85.5   Injury of popliteal vein
  - S85.50   Unspecified injury of popliteal vein
    - S85.501   Unspecified injury of popliteal vein, right leg
    - S85.502   Unspecified injury of popliteal vein, left leg
    - S85.509   Unspecified injury of popliteal vein, unspecified leg
  - S85.51   Laceration of popliteal vein
    - S85.511   Laceration of popliteal vein, right leg
    - S85.512   Laceration of popliteal vein, left leg
    - S85.519   Laceration of popliteal vein, unspecified leg

- S85.59   Other specified injury of popliteal vein
  - S85.591   Other specified injury of popliteal vein, right leg
  - S85.592   Other specified injury of popliteal vein, left leg
  - S85.599   Other specified injury of popliteal vein, unspecified leg
- S85.8   Injury of other blood vessels at lower leg level
  - S85.80   Unspecified injury of other blood vessels at lower leg level
    - S85.801   Unspecified injury of other blood vessels at lower leg level, right leg
    - S85.802   Unspecified injury of other blood vessels at lower leg level, left leg
    - S85.809   Unspecified injury of other blood vessels at lower leg level, unspecified leg
  - S85.81   Laceration of other blood vessels at lower leg level
    - S85.811   Laceration of other blood vessels at lower leg level, right leg
    - S85.812   Laceration of other blood vessels at lower leg level, left leg
    - S85.819   Laceration of other blood vessels at lower leg level, unspecified leg
  - S85.89   Other specified injury of other blood vessels at lower leg level
    - S85.891   Other specified injury of other blood vessels at lower leg level, right leg
    - S85.892   Other specified injury of other blood vessels at lower leg level, left leg
    - S85.899   Other specified injury of other blood vessels at lower leg level, unspecified leg
- S85.9   Injury of unspecified blood vessel at lower leg level
  - S85.90   Unspecified injury of unspecified blood vessel at lower leg level
    - S85.901   Unspecified injury of unspecified blood vessel at lower leg level, right leg
    - S85.902   Unspecified injury of unspecified blood vessel at lower leg level, left leg
    - S85.909   Unspecified injury of unspecified blood vessel at lower leg level, unspecified leg
  - S85.91   Laceration of unspecified blood vessel at lower leg level
    - S85.911   Laceration of unspecified blood vessel at lower leg level, right leg
    - S85.912   Laceration of unspecified blood vessel at lower leg level, left leg
    - S85.919   Laceration of unspecified blood vessel at lower leg level, unspecified leg
  - S85.99   Other specified injury of unspecified blood vessel at lower leg level
    - S85.991   Other specified injury of unspecified blood vessel at lower leg level, right leg
    - S85.992   Other specified injury of unspecified blood vessel at lower leg level, left leg
    - S85.999   Other specified injury of unspecified blood vessel at lower leg level, unspecified leg

● **S86　Injury of muscle, fascia and tendon at lower leg level**

　　Code also any associated open wound (S81.-)

　　　Excludes2　injury of muscle, fascia and tendon at ankle (S96.-)

　　　　　　injury of patellar ligament (tendon) (S76.1-)

　　　　　　sprain of joints and ligaments of knee (S83.-)

　　The appropriate 7th character is to be added to each code from category S86

　　　A　initial encounter
　　　D　subsequent encounter
　　　S　sequela

　● **S86.0　Injury of Achilles tendon**

　　● **S86.00　Unspecified injury of Achilles tendon**

　　　● S86.001　Unspecified injury of right Achilles tendon

　　　● S86.002　Unspecified injury of left Achilles tendon

　　　● S86.009　Unspecified injury of unspecified Achilles tendon

　　● **S86.01　Strain of Achilles tendon**

　　　● S86.011　Strain of right Achilles tendon

　　　● S86.012　Strain of left Achilles tendon

　　　● S86.019　Strain of unspecified Achilles tendon

　　● **S86.02　Laceration of Achilles tendon**

　　　● S86.021　Laceration of right Achilles tendon

　　　● S86.022　Laceration of left Achilles tendon

　　　● S86.029　Laceration of unspecified Achilles tendon

　　● **S86.09　Other specified injury of Achilles tendon**

　　　● S86.091　Other specified injury of right Achilles tendon

　　　● S86.092　Other specified injury of left Achilles tendon

　　　● S86.099　Other specified injury of unspecified Achilles tendon

　● **S86.1　Injury of other muscle(s) and tendon(s) of posterior muscle group at lower leg level**

　　● **S86.10　Unspecified injury of other muscle(s) and tendon(s) of posterior muscle group at lower leg level**

　　　● S86.101　Unspecified injury of other muscle(s) and tendon(s) of posterior muscle group at lower leg level, right leg

　　　● S86.102　Unspecified injury of other muscle(s) and tendon(s) of posterior muscle group at lower leg level, left leg

　　　● S86.109　Unspecified injury of other muscle(s) and tendon(s) of posterior muscle group at lower leg level, unspecified leg

　　● **S86.11　Strain of other muscle(s) and tendon(s) of posterior muscle group at lower leg level**

　　　● S86.111　Strain of other muscle(s) and tendon(s) of posterior muscle group at lower leg level, right leg

　　　● S86.112　Strain of other muscle(s) and tendon(s) of posterior muscle group at lower leg level, left leg

　　　● S86.119　Strain of other muscle(s) and tendon(s) of posterior muscle group at lower leg level, unspecified leg

　　● **S86.12　Laceration of other muscle(s) and tendon(s) of posterior muscle group at lower leg level**

　　　● S86.121　Laceration of other muscle(s) and tendon(s) of posterior muscle group at lower leg level, right leg

　　　● S86.122　Laceration of other muscle(s) and tendon(s) of posterior muscle group at lower leg level, left leg

　　　● S86.129　Laceration of other muscle(s) and tendon(s) of posterior muscle group at lower leg level, unspecified leg

　　● **S86.19　Other injury of other muscle(s) and tendon(s) of posterior muscle group at lower leg level**

　　　● S86.191　Other injury of other muscle(s) and tendon(s) of posterior muscle group at lower leg level, right leg

　　　● S86.192　Other injury of other muscle(s) and tendon(s) of posterior muscle group at lower leg level, left leg

　　　● S86.199　Other injury of other muscle(s) and tendon(s) of posterior muscle group at lower leg level, unspecified leg

　● **S86.2　Injury of muscle(s) and tendon(s) of anterior muscle group at lower leg level**

　　● **S86.20　Unspecified injury of muscle(s) and tendon(s) of anterior muscle group at lower leg level**

　　　● S86.201　Unspecified injury of muscle(s) and tendon(s) of anterior muscle group at lower leg level, right leg

　　　● S86.202　Unspecified injury of muscle(s) and tendon(s) of anterior muscle group at lower leg level, left leg

　　　● S86.209　Unspecified injury of muscle(s) and tendon(s) of anterior muscle group at lower leg level, unspecified leg

　　● **S86.21　Strain of muscle(s) and tendon(s) of anterior muscle group at lower leg level**

　　　● S86.211　Strain of muscle(s) and tendon(s) of anterior muscle group at lower leg level, right leg

　　　● S86.212　Strain of muscle(s) and tendon(s) of anterior muscle group at lower leg level, left leg

　　　● S86.219　Strain of muscle(s) and tendon(s) of anterior muscle group at lower leg level, unspecified leg

　　● **S86.22　Laceration of muscle(s) and tendon(s) of anterior muscle group at lower leg level**

　　　● S86.221　Laceration of muscle(s) and tendon(s) of anterior muscle group at lower leg level, right leg

　　　● S86.222　Laceration of muscle(s) and tendon(s) of anterior muscle group at lower leg level, left leg

　　　● S86.229　Laceration of muscle(s) and tendon(s) of anterior muscle group at lower leg level, unspecified leg

　　● **S86.29　Other injury of muscle(s) and tendon(s) of anterior muscle group at lower leg level**

　　　● S86.291　Other injury of muscle(s) and tendon(s) of anterior muscle group at lower leg level, right leg

　　　● S86.292　Other injury of muscle(s) and tendon(s) of anterior muscle group at lower leg level, left leg

　　　● S86.299　Other injury of muscle(s) and tendon(s) of anterior muscle group at lower leg level, unspecified leg

S86.3 Injury of muscle(s) and tendon(s) of peroneal muscle group at lower leg level
- S86.30 Unspecified injury of muscle(s) and tendon(s) of peroneal muscle group at lower leg level
  - S86.301 Unspecified injury of muscle(s) and tendon(s) of peroneal muscle group at lower leg level, right leg
  - S86.302 Unspecified injury of muscle(s) and tendon(s) of peroneal muscle group at lower leg level, left leg
  - S86.309 Unspecified injury of muscle(s) and tendon(s) of peroneal muscle group at lower leg level, unspecified leg
- S86.31 Strain of muscle(s) and tendon(s) of peroneal muscle group at lower leg level
  - S86.311 Strain of muscle(s) and tendon(s) of peroneal muscle group at lower leg level, right leg
  - S86.312 Strain of muscle(s) and tendon(s) of peroneal muscle group at lower leg level, left leg
  - S86.319 Strain of muscle(s) and tendon(s) of peroneal muscle group at lower leg level, unspecified leg
- S86.32 Laceration of muscle(s) and tendon(s) of peroneal muscle group at lower leg level
  - S86.321 Laceration of muscle(s) and tendon(s) of peroneal muscle group at lower leg level, right leg
  - S86.322 Laceration of muscle(s) and tendon(s) of peroneal muscle group at lower leg level, left leg
  - S86.329 Laceration of muscle(s) and tendon(s) of peroneal muscle group at lower leg level, unspecified leg
- S86.39 Other injury of muscle(s) and tendon(s) of peroneal muscle group at lower leg level
  - S86.391 Other injury of muscle(s) and tendon(s) of peroneal muscle group at lower leg level, right leg
  - S86.392 Other injury of muscle(s) and tendon(s) of peroneal muscle group at lower leg level, left leg
  - S86.399 Other injury of muscle(s) and tendon(s) of peroneal muscle group at lower leg level, unspecified leg

S86.8 Injury of other muscles and tendons at lower leg level
- S86.80 Unspecified injury of other muscles and tendons at lower leg level
  - S86.801 Unspecified injury of other muscle(s) and tendon(s) at lower leg level, right leg
  - S86.802 Unspecified injury of other muscle(s) and tendon(s) at lower leg level, left leg
  - S86.809 Unspecified injury of other muscle(s) and tendon(s) at lower leg level, unspecified leg
- S86.81 Strain of other muscles and tendons at lower leg level
  - S86.811 Strain of other muscle(s) and tendon(s) at lower leg level, right leg
  - S86.812 Strain of other muscle(s) and tendon(s) at lower leg level, left leg
  - S86.819 Strain of other muscle(s) and tendon(s) at lower leg level, unspecified leg
- S86.82 Laceration of other muscles and tendons at lower leg level
  - S86.821 Laceration of other muscle(s) and tendon(s) at lower leg level, right leg
  - S86.822 Laceration of other muscle(s) and tendon(s) at lower leg level, left leg
  - S86.829 Laceration of other muscle(s) and tendon(s) at lower leg level, unspecified leg
- S86.89 Other injury of other muscles and tendons at lower leg level
  - S86.891 Other injury of other muscle(s) and tendon(s) at lower leg level, right leg
  - S86.892 Other injury of other muscle(s) and tendon(s) at lower leg level, left leg
  - S86.899 Other injury of other muscle(s) and tendon(s) at lower leg level, unspecified leg

S86.9 Injury of unspecified muscle and tendon at lower leg level
- S86.90 Unspecified injury of unspecified muscle and tendon at lower leg level
  - S86.901 Unspecified injury of unspecified muscle(s) and tendon(s) at lower leg level, right leg
  - S86.902 Unspecified injury of unspecified muscle(s) and tendon(s) at lower leg level, left leg
  - S86.909 Unspecified injury of unspecified muscle(s) and tendon(s) at lower leg level, unspecified leg
- S86.91 Strain of unspecified muscle and tendon at lower leg level
  - S86.911 Strain of unspecified muscle(s) and tendon(s) at lower leg level, right leg
  - S86.912 Strain of unspecified muscle(s) and tendon(s) at lower leg level, left leg
  - S86.919 Strain of unspecified muscle(s) and tendon(s) at lower leg level, unspecified leg
- S86.92 Laceration of unspecified muscle and tendon at lower leg level
  - S86.921 Laceration of unspecified muscle(s) and tendon(s) at lower leg level, right leg
  - S86.922 Laceration of unspecified muscle(s) and tendon(s) at lower leg level, left leg
  - S86.929 Laceration of unspecified muscle(s) and tendon(s) at lower leg level, unspecified leg
- S86.99 Other injury of unspecified muscle and tendon at lower leg level
  - S86.991 Other injury of unspecified muscle(s) and tendon(s) at lower leg level, right leg
  - S86.992 Other injury of unspecified muscle(s) and tendon(s) at lower leg level, left leg
  - S86.999 Other injury of unspecified muscle(s) and tendon(s) at lower leg level, unspecified leg

● **S87　Crushing injury of lower leg**
Use additional code(s) for all associated injuries
Excludes2　crushing injury of ankle and foot (S97.-)
The appropriate 7th character is to be added to each code from category S87

> A　initial encounter
> D　subsequent encounter
> S　sequela

● **S87.0　Crushing injury of knee**
　X● S87.00　Crushing injury of unspecified knee
　X● S87.01　Crushing injury of right knee
　X● S87.02　Crushing injury of left knee
● **S87.8　Crushing injury of lower leg**
　X● S87.80　Crushing injury of unspecified lower leg
　X● S87.81　Crushing injury of right lower leg
　X● S87.82　Crushing injury of left lower leg

● **S88　Traumatic amputation of lower leg**
An amputation not identified as partial or complete should be coded to complete
Excludes1　traumatic amputation of ankle and foot (S98.-)
The appropriate 7th character is to be added to each code from category S88

> A　initial encounter
> D　subsequent encounter
> S　sequela

● **S88.0　Traumatic amputation at knee level**
● S88.01　Complete traumatic amputation at knee level
　● S88.011　Complete traumatic amputation at knee level, right lower leg
　● S88.012　Complete traumatic amputation at knee level, left lower leg
　● S88.019　Complete traumatic amputation at knee level, unspecified lower leg
● S88.02　Partial traumatic amputation at knee level
　● S88.021　Partial traumatic amputation at knee level, right lower leg
　● S88.022　Partial traumatic amputation at knee level, left lower leg
　● S88.029　Partial traumatic amputation at knee level, unspecified lower leg
● **S88.1　Traumatic amputation at level between knee and ankle**
● S88.11　Complete traumatic amputation at level between knee and ankle
　● S88.111　Complete traumatic amputation at level between knee and ankle, right lower leg
　● S88.112　Complete traumatic amputation at level between knee and ankle, left lower leg
　● S88.119　Complete traumatic amputation at level between knee and ankle, unspecified lower leg
● S88.12　Partial traumatic amputation at level between knee and ankle
　● S88.121　Partial traumatic amputation at level between knee and ankle, right lower leg
　● S88.122　Partial traumatic amputation at level between knee and ankle, left lower leg
　● S88.129　Partial traumatic amputation at level between knee and ankle, unspecified lower leg

● **S88.9　Traumatic amputation of lower leg, level unspecified**
● S88.91　Complete traumatic amputation of lower leg, level unspecified
　● S88.911　Complete traumatic amputation of right lower leg, level unspecified
　● S88.912　Complete traumatic amputation of left lower leg, level unspecified
　● S88.919　Complete traumatic amputation of unspecified lower leg, level unspecified
● S88.92　Partial traumatic amputation of lower leg, level unspecified
　● S88.921　Partial traumatic amputation of right lower leg, level unspecified
　● S88.922　Partial traumatic amputation of left lower leg, level unspecified
　● S88.929　Partial traumatic amputation of unspecified lower leg, level unspecified

● **S89　Other and unspecified injuries of lower leg**
Note: A fracture not indicated as open or closed should be coded to closed
Excludes2　other and unspecified injuries of ankle and foot (S99.-)
The appropriate 7th character is to be added to each code from subcategories S89.0, S89.1, S89.2, and S89.3

> A　initial encounter for closed fracture
> D　subsequent encounter for fracture with routine healing
> G　subsequent encounter for fracture with delayed healing
> K　subsequent encounter for fracture with nonunion
> P　subsequent encounter for fracture with malunion
> S　sequela

● **S89.0　Physeal fracture of upper end of tibia**
● S89.00　Unspecified physeal fracture of upper end of tibia
　● S89.001　Unspecified physeal fracture of upper end of right tibia
　● S89.002　Unspecified physeal fracture of upper end of left tibia
　● S89.009　Unspecified physeal fracture of upper end of unspecified tibia
● S89.01　Salter-Harris Type I physeal fracture of upper end of tibia
　● S89.011　Salter-Harris Type I physeal fracture of upper end of right tibia
　● S89.012　Salter-Harris Type I physeal fracture of upper end of left tibia
　● S89.019　Salter-Harris Type I physeal fracture of upper end of unspecified tibia
● S89.02　Salter-Harris Type II physeal fracture of upper end of tibia
　● S89.021　Salter-Harris Type II physeal fracture of upper end of right tibia
　● S89.022　Salter-Harris Type II physeal fracture of upper end of left tibia
　● S89.029　Salter-Harris Type II physeal fracture of upper end of unspecified tibia
● S89.03　Salter-Harris Type III physeal fracture of upper end of tibia
　● S89.031　Salter-Harris Type III physeal fracture of upper end of right tibia
　● S89.032　Salter-Harris Type III physeal fracture of upper end of left tibia
　● S89.039　Salter-Harris Type III physeal fracture of upper end of unspecified tibia

◀ New　◀║║ Revised　~~deleted~~ Deleted　OGCR Official Guidelines　X Assign placeholder X　● Use Additional Character(s)
Excludes 1　Excludes 2　Includes　Use additional　Code first　Code also　Unspecified

- S89.04 Salter-Harris Type IV physeal fracture of upper end of tibia
  - S89.041 Salter-Harris Type IV physeal fracture of upper end of right tibia
  - S89.042 Salter-Harris Type IV physeal fracture of upper end of left tibia
  - S89.049 Salter-Harris Type IV physeal fracture of upper end of unspecified tibia
- S89.09 Other physeal fracture of upper end of tibia
  - S89.091 Other physeal fracture of upper end of right tibia
  - S89.092 Other physeal fracture of upper end of left tibia
  - S89.099 Other physeal fracture of upper end of unspecified tibia
- S89.1 Physeal fracture of lower end of tibia
  - S89.10 Unspecified physeal fracture of lower end of tibia
    - S89.101 Unspecified physeal fracture of lower end of right tibia
    - S89.102 Unspecified physeal fracture of lower end of left tibia
    - S89.109 Unspecified physeal fracture of lower end of unspecified tibia
  - S89.11 Salter-Harris Type I physeal fracture of lower end of tibia
    - S89.111 Salter-Harris Type I physeal fracture of lower end of right tibia
    - S89.112 Salter-Harris Type I physeal fracture of lower end of left tibia
    - S89.119 Salter-Harris Type I physeal fracture of lower end of unspecified tibia
  - S89.12 Salter-Harris Type II physeal fracture of lower end of tibia
    - S89.121 Salter-Harris Type II physeal fracture of lower end of right tibia
    - S89.122 Salter-Harris Type II physeal fracture of lower end of left tibia
    - S89.129 Salter-Harris Type II physeal fracture of lower end of unspecified tibia
  - S89.13 Salter-Harris Type III physeal fracture of lower end of tibia
    - **Excludes1**   fracture of medial malleolus (adult) (S82.5-)
    - S89.131 Salter-Harris Type III physeal fracture of lower end of right tibia
    - S89.132 Salter-Harris Type III physeal fracture of lower end of left tibia
    - S89.139 Salter-Harris Type III physeal fracture of lower end of unspecified tibia
  - S89.14 Salter-Harris Type IV physeal fracture of lower end of tibia
    - **Excludes1**   fracture of medial malleolus (adult) (S82.5-)
    - S89.141 Salter-Harris Type IV physeal fracture of lower end of right tibia
    - S89.142 Salter-Harris Type IV physeal fracture of lower end of left tibia
    - S89.149 Salter-Harris Type IV physeal fracture of lower end of unspecified tibia
  - S89.19 Other physeal fracture of lower end of tibia
    - S89.191 Other physeal fracture of lower end of right tibia
    - S89.192 Other physeal fracture of lower end of left tibia
    - S89.199 Other physeal fracture of lower end of unspecified tibia

- S89.2 Physeal fracture of upper end of fibula
  - S89.20 Unspecified physeal fracture of upper end of fibula
    - S89.201 Unspecified physeal fracture of upper end of right fibula
    - S89.202 Unspecified physeal fracture of upper end of left fibula
    - S89.209 Unspecified physeal fracture of upper end of unspecified fibula
  - S89.21 Salter-Harris Type I physeal fracture of upper end of fibula
    - S89.211 Salter-Harris Type I physeal fracture of upper end of right fibula
    - S89.212 Salter-Harris Type I physeal fracture of upper end of left fibula
    - S89.219 Salter-Harris Type I physeal fracture of upper end of unspecified fibula
  - S89.22 Salter-Harris Type II physeal fracture of upper end of fibula
    - S89.221 Salter-Harris Type II physeal fracture of upper end of right fibula
    - S89.222 Salter-Harris Type II physeal fracture of upper end of left fibula
    - S89.229 Salter-Harris Type II physeal fracture of upper end of unspecified fibula
  - S89.29 Other physeal fracture of upper end of fibula
    - S89.291 Other physeal fracture of upper end of right fibula
    - S89.292 Other physeal fracture of upper end of left fibula
    - S89.299 Other physeal fracture of upper end of unspecified fibula
- S89.3 Physeal fracture of lower end of fibula
  - S89.30 Unspecified physeal fracture of lower end of fibula
    - S89.301 Unspecified physeal fracture of lower end of right fibula
    - S89.302 Unspecified physeal fracture of lower end of left fibula
    - S89.309 Unspecified physeal fracture of lower end of unspecified fibula
  - S89.31 Salter-Harris Type I physeal fracture of lower end of fibula
    - S89.311 Salter-Harris Type I physeal fracture of lower end of right fibula
    - S89.312 Salter-Harris Type I physeal fracture of lower end of left fibula
    - S89.319 Salter-Harris Type I physeal fracture of lower end of unspecified fibula
  - S89.32 Salter-Harris Type II physeal fracture of lower end of fibula
    - S89.321 Salter-Harris Type II physeal fracture of lower end of right fibula
    - S89.322 Salter-Harris Type II physeal fracture of lower end of left fibula
    - S89.329 Salter-Harris Type II physeal fracture of lower end of unspecified fibula
  - S89.39 Other physeal fracture of lower end of fibula
    - S89.391 Other physeal fracture of lower end of right fibula
    - S89.392 Other physeal fracture of lower end of left fibula
    - S89.399 Other physeal fracture of lower end of unspecified fibula

CHAPTER 19 (S00-T88)

● **S89.8 Other specified injuries of lower leg**

The appropriate 7th character is to be added to each code in subcategory S89.8

A	initial encounter
D	subsequent encounter
S	sequela

X● **S89.80 Other specified injuries of unspecified lower leg**

X● **S89.81 Other specified injuries of right lower leg**

X● **S89.82 Other specified injuries of left lower leg**

● **S89.9 Unspecified injury of lower leg**

The appropriate 7th character is to be added to each code in subcategory S89.9

A	initial encounter
D	subsequent encounter
S	sequela

X● **S89.90 Unspecified injury of unspecified lower leg**

X● **S89.91 Unspecified injury of right lower leg**

X● **S89.92 Unspecified injury of left lower leg**

INJURIES TO THE ANKLE AND FOOT (S90-S99)

Excludes2   burns and corrosions (T20-T32)
          fracture of ankle and malleolus (S82.-)
          frostbite (T33-T34)
          insect bite or sting, venomous (T63.4)

● **S90 Superficial injury of ankle, foot and toes**

The appropriate 7th character is to be added to each code from category S90

A	initial encounter
D	subsequent encounter
S	sequela

● **S90.0 Contusion of ankle**

X● **S90.00 Contusion of unspecified ankle**

X● **S90.01 Contusion of right ankle**

X● **S90.02 Contusion of left ankle**

● **S90.1 Contusion of toe without damage to nail**

● **S90.11 Contusion of great toe without damage to nail**

● **S90.111 Contusion of right great toe without damage to nail**

● **S90.112 Contusion of left great toe without damage to nail**

● **S90.119 Contusion of unspecified great toe without damage to nail**

● **S90.12 Contusion of lesser toe without damage to nail**

● **S90.121 Contusion of right lesser toe(s) without damage to nail**

● **S90.122 Contusion of left lesser toe(s) without damage to nail**

● **S90.129 Contusion of unspecified lesser toe(s) without damage to nail**
Contusion of toe NOS

● **S90.2 Contusion of toe with damage to nail**

● **S90.21 Contusion of great toe with damage to nail**

● **S90.211 Contusion of right great toe with damage to nail**

● **S90.212 Contusion of left great toe with damage to nail**

● **S90.219 Contusion of unspecified great toe with damage to nail**

● **S90.22 Contusion of lesser toe with damage to nail**

● **S90.221 Contusion of right lesser toe(s) with damage to nail**

● **S90.222 Contusion of left lesser toe(s) with damage to nail**

● **S90.229 Contusion of unspecified lesser toe(s) with damage to nail**

● **S90.3 Contusion of foot**

Excludes2   contusion of toes (S90.1-, S90.2-)

X● **S90.30 Contusion of unspecified foot**
Contusion of foot NOS

X● **S90.31 Contusion of right foot**

X● **S90.32 Contusion of left foot**

● **S90.4 Other superficial injuries of toe**

● **S90.41 Abrasion of toe**

● **S90.411 Abrasion, right great toe**

● **S90.412 Abrasion, left great toe**

● **S90.413 Abrasion, unspecified great toe**

● **S90.414 Abrasion, right lesser toe(s)**

● **S90.415 Abrasion, left lesser toe(s)**

● **S90.416 Abrasion, unspecified lesser toe(s)**

● **S90.42 Blister (nonthermal) of toe**

● **S90.421 Blister (nonthermal), right great toe**

● **S90.422 Blister (nonthermal), left great toe**

● **S90.423 Blister (nonthermal), unspecified great toe**

● **S90.424 Blister (nonthermal), right lesser toe(s)**

● **S90.425 Blister (nonthermal), left lesser toe(s)**

● **S90.426 Blister (nonthermal), unspecified lesser toe(s)**

● **S90.44 External constriction of toe**
Hair tourniquet syndrome of toe

● **S90.441 External constriction, right great toe**

● **S90.442 External constriction, left great toe**

● **S90.443 External constriction, unspecified great toe**

● **S90.444 External constriction, right lesser toe(s)**

● **S90.445 External constriction, left lesser toe(s)**

● **S90.446 External constriction, unspecified lesser toe(s)**

● **S90.45 Superficial foreign body of toe**
Splinter in the toe

● **S90.451 Superficial foreign body, right great toe**

● **S90.452 Superficial foreign body, left great toe**

● **S90.453 Superficial foreign body, unspecified great toe**

● **S90.454 Superficial foreign body, right lesser toe(s)**

● **S90.455 Superficial foreign body, left lesser toe(s)**

● **S90.456 Superficial foreign body, unspecified lesser toe(s)**

● **S90.46 Insect bite (nonvenomous) of toe**

● **S90.461 Insect bite (nonvenomous), right great toe**

● **S90.462 Insect bite (nonvenomous), left great toe**

● **S90.463 Insect bite (nonvenomous), unspecified great toe**

● **S90.464 Insect bite (nonvenomous), right lesser toe(s)**

● **S90.465 Insect bite (nonvenomous), left lesser toe(s)**

● **S90.466 Insect bite (nonvenomous), unspecified lesser toe(s)**

◀ New   ◀▥ Revised   ~~deleted~~ Deleted   OGCR Official Guidelines   X Assign placeholder X   ● Use Additional Character(s)

Excludes 1   Excludes 2   Includes   Use additional   Code first   Code also   Unspecified

● S90.47　Other superficial bite of toe
　　　　Excludes1　open bite of toe (S91.15-, S91.25-)
　　● S90.471　Other superficial bite of right great toe
　　● S90.472　Other superficial bite of left great toe
　　● S90.473　Other superficial bite of unspecified great toe
　　● S90.474　Other superficial bite of right lesser toe(s)
　　● S90.475　Other superficial bite of left lesser toe(s)
　　● S90.476　Other superficial bite of unspecified lesser toe(s)
● S90.5　Other superficial injuries of ankle
　● S90.51　Abrasion of ankle
　　● S90.511　Abrasion, right ankle
　　● S90.512　Abrasion, left ankle
　　● S90.519　Abrasion, unspecified ankle
　● S90.52　Blister (nonthermal) of ankle
　　● S90.521　Blister (nonthermal), right ankle
　　● S90.522　Blister (nonthermal), left ankle
　　● S90.529　Blister (nonthermal), unspecified ankle
　● S90.54　External constriction of ankle
　　● S90.541　External constriction, right ankle
　　● S90.542　External constriction, left ankle
　　● S90.549　External constriction, unspecified ankle
　● S90.55　Superficial foreign body of ankle
　　　　Splinter in the ankle
　　● S90.551　Superficial foreign body, right ankle
　　● S90.552　Superficial foreign body, left ankle
　　● S90.559　Superficial foreign body, unspecified ankle
　● S90.56　Insect bite (nonvenomous) of ankle
　　● S90.561　Insect bite (nonvenomous), right ankle
　　● S90.562　Insect bite (nonvenomous), left ankle
　　● S90.569　Insect bite (nonvenomous), unspecified ankle
　● S90.57　Other superficial bite of ankle
　　　　Excludes1　open bite of ankle (S91.05-)
　　● S90.571　Other superficial bite of ankle, right ankle
　　● S90.572　Other superficial bite of ankle, left ankle
　　● S90.579　Other superficial bite of ankle, unspecified ankle
● S90.8　Other superficial injuries of foot
　● S90.81　Abrasion of foot
　　● S90.811　Abrasion, right foot
　　● S90.812　Abrasion, left foot
　　● S90.819　Abrasion, unspecified foot
　● S90.82　Blister (nonthermal) of foot
　　● S90.821　Blister (nonthermal), right foot
　　● S90.822　Blister (nonthermal), left foot
　　● S90.829　Blister (nonthermal), unspecified foot
　● S90.84　External constriction of foot
　　● S90.841　External constriction, right foot
　　● S90.842　External constriction, left foot
　　● S90.849　External constriction, unspecified foot

● S90.85　Superficial foreign body of foot
　　　　Splinter in the foot
　　● S90.851　Superficial foreign body, right foot
　　● S90.852　Superficial foreign body, left foot
　　● S90.859　Superficial foreign body, unspecified foot
● S90.86　Insect bite (nonvenomous) of foot
　　● S90.861　Insect bite (nonvenomous), right foot
　　● S90.862　Insect bite (nonvenomous), left foot
　　● S90.869　Insect bite (nonvenomous), unspecified foot
● S90.87　Other superficial bite of foot
　　　　Excludes1　open bite of foot (S91.35-)
　　● S90.871　Other superficial bite of right foot
　　● S90.872　Other superficial bite of left foot
　　● S90.879　Other superficial bite of unspecified foot
● S90.9　Unspecified superficial injury of ankle, foot and toe
　● S90.91　Unspecified superficial injury of ankle
　　● S90.911　Unspecified superficial injury of right ankle
　　● S90.912　Unspecified superficial injury of left ankle
　　● S90.919　Unspecified superficial injury of unspecified ankle
　● S90.92　Unspecified superficial injury of foot
　　● S90.921　Unspecified superficial injury of right foot
　　● S90.922　Unspecified superficial injury of left foot
　　● S90.929　Unspecified superficial injury of unspecified foot
　　S90.93　Unspecified superficial injury of toes
　　● S90.931　Unspecified superficial injury of right great toe
　　● S90.932　Unspecified superficial injury of left great toe
　　● S90.933　Unspecified superficial injury of unspecified great toe
　　● S90.934　Unspecified superficial injury of right lesser toe(s)
　　● S90.935　Unspecified superficial injury of left lesser toe(s)
　　● S90.936　Unspecified superficial injury of unspecified lesser toe(s)

● S91　Open wound of ankle, foot and toes
　　Code also any associated wound infection
　　Excludes1　open fracture of ankle, foot and toes (S92.-with 7th character B)
　　　　　　　　traumatic amputation of ankle and foot (S98.-)
　　The appropriate 7th character is to be added to each code from category S91

A	initial encounter
D	subsequent encounter
S	sequela

● S91.0　Open wound of ankle
　● S91.00　Unspecified open wound of ankle
　　● S91.001　Unspecified open wound, right ankle
　　● S91.002　Unspecified open wound, left ankle
　　● S91.009　Unspecified open wound, unspecified ankle

● S91.01   Laceration without foreign body of ankle
   ● S91.011   Laceration without foreign body, right ankle
   ● S91.012   Laceration without foreign body, left ankle
   ● S91.019   Laceration without foreign body, unspecified ankle
● S91.02   Laceration with foreign body of ankle
   ● S91.021   Laceration with foreign body, right ankle
   ● S91.022   Laceration with foreign body, left ankle
   ● S91.029   Laceration with foreign body, unspecified ankle
● S91.03   Puncture wound without foreign body of ankle
   ● S91.031   Puncture wound without foreign body, right ankle
   ● S91.032   Puncture wound without foreign body, left ankle
   ● S91.039   Puncture wound without foreign body, unspecified ankle
● S91.04   Puncture wound with foreign body of ankle
   ● S91.041   Puncture wound with foreign body, right ankle
   ● S91.042   Puncture wound with foreign body, left ankle
   ● S91.049   Puncture wound with foreign body, unspecified ankle
● S91.05   Open bite of ankle
       | Excludes1 | superficial bite of ankle (S90.56-, S90.57-)
   ● S91.051   Open bite, right ankle
   ● S91.052   Open bite, left ankle
   ● S91.059   Open bite, unspecified ankle
● S91.1   Open wound of toe without damage to nail
   ● S91.10   Unspecified open wound of toe without damage to nail
     ● S91.101   Unspecified open wound of right great toe without damage to nail
     ● S91.102   Unspecified open wound of left great toe without damage to nail
     ● S91.103   Unspecified open wound of unspecified great toe without damage to nail
     ● S91.104   Unspecified open wound of right lesser toe(s) without damage to nail
     ● S91.105   Unspecified open wound of left lesser toe(s) without damage to nail
     ● S91.106   Unspecified open wound of unspecified lesser toe(s) without damage to nail
     ● S91.109   Unspecified open wound of unspecified toe(s) without damage to nail
   ● S91.11   Laceration without foreign body of toe without damage to nail
     ● S91.111   Laceration without foreign body of right great toe without damage to nail
     ● S91.112   Laceration without foreign body of left great toe without damage to nail
     ● S91.113   Laceration without foreign body of unspecified great toe without damage to nail
     ● S91.114   Laceration without foreign body of right lesser toe(s) without damage to nail
     ● S91.115   Laceration without foreign body of left lesser toe(s) without damage to nail

● S91.116   Laceration without foreign body of unspecified lesser toe(s) without damage to nail
● S91.119   Laceration without foreign body of unspecified toe without damage to nail
● S91.12   Laceration with foreign body of toe without damage to nail
   ● S91.121   Laceration with foreign body of right great toe without damage to nail
   ● S91.122   Laceration with foreign body of left great toe without damage to nail
   ● S91.123   Laceration with foreign body of unspecified great toe without damage to nail
   ● S91.124   Laceration with foreign body of right lesser toe(s) without damage to nail
   ● S91.125   Laceration with foreign body of left lesser toe(s) without damage to nail
   ● S91.126   Laceration with foreign body of unspecified lesser toe(s) without damage to nail
   ● S91.129   Laceration with foreign body of unspecified toe(s) without damage to nail
● S91.13   Puncture wound without foreign body of toe without damage to nail
   ● S91.131   Puncture wound without foreign body of right great toe without damage to nail
   ● S91.132   Puncture wound without foreign body of left great toe without damage to nail
   ● S91.133   Puncture wound without foreign body of unspecified great toe without damage to nail
   ● S91.134   Puncture wound without foreign body of right lesser toe(s) without damage to nail
   ● S91.135   Puncture wound without foreign body of left lesser toe(s) without damage to nail
   ● S91.136   Puncture wound without foreign body of unspecified lesser toe(s) without damage to nail
   ● S91.139   Puncture wound without foreign body of unspecified toe(s) without damage to nail
● S91.14   Puncture wound with foreign body of toe without damage to nail
   ● S91.141   Puncture wound with foreign body of right great toe without damage to nail
   ● S91.142   Puncture wound with foreign body of left great toe without damage to nail
   ● S91.143   Puncture wound with foreign body of unspecified great toe without damage to nail
   ● S91.144   Puncture wound with foreign body of right lesser toe(s) without damage to nail
   ● S91.145   Puncture wound with foreign body of left lesser toe(s) without damage to nail
   ● S91.146   Puncture wound with foreign body of unspecified lesser toe(s) without damage to nail
   ● S91.149   Puncture wound with foreign body of unspecified toe(s) without damage to nail

◀ New   ◀ Revised   deleted Deleted   OGCR Official Guidelines   X Assign placeholder X   ● Use Additional Character(s)

| Excludes 1 | | Excludes 2 | Includes   Use additional   Code first   Code also   Unspecified

● S91.15   **Open bite of toe without damage to nail**
    Bite of toe NOS

    Excludes1   superficial bite of toe (S90.46-, S90.47-)

    ● S91.151   **Open bite of right great toe without damage to nail**

    ● S91.152   **Open bite of left great toe without damage to nail**

    ● S91.153   **Open bite of unspecified great toe without damage to nail**

    ● S91.154   **Open bite of right lesser toe(s) without damage to nail**

    ● S91.155   **Open bite of left lesser toe(s) without damage to nail**

    ● S91.156   **Open bite of unspecified lesser toe(s) without damage to nail**

    ● S91.159   **Open bite of unspecified toe(s) without damage to nail**

● S91.2   **Open wound of toe with damage to nail**

    ● S91.20   **Unspecified open wound of toe with damage to nail**

      ● S91.201   **Unspecified open wound of right great toe with damage to nail**

      ● S91.202   **Unspecified open wound of left great toe with damage to nail**

      ● S91.203   **Unspecified open wound of unspecified great toe with damage to nail**

      ● S91.204   **Unspecified open wound of right lesser toe(s) with damage to nail**

      ● S91.205   **Unspecified open wound of left lesser toe(s) with damage to nail**

      ● S91.206   **Unspecified open wound of unspecified lesser toe(s) with damage to nail**

      ● S91.209   **Unspecified open wound of unspecified toe(s) with damage to nail**

    ● S91.21   **Laceration without foreign body of toe with damage to nail**

      ● S91.211   **Laceration without foreign body of right great toe with damage to nail**

      ● S91.212   **Laceration without foreign body of left great toe with damage to nail**

      ● S91.213   **Laceration without foreign body of unspecified great toe with damage to nail**

      ● S91.214   **Laceration without foreign body of right lesser toe(s) with damage to nail**

      ● S91.215   **Laceration without foreign body of left lesser toe(s) with damage to nail**

      ● S91.216   **Laceration without foreign body of unspecified lesser toe(s) with damage to nail**

      ● S91.219   **Laceration without foreign body of unspecified toe(s) with damage to nail**

    ● S91.22   **Laceration with foreign body of toe with damage to nail**

      ● S91.221   **Laceration with foreign body of right great toe with damage to nail**

      ● S91.222   **Laceration with foreign body of left great toe with damage to nail**

      ● S91.223   **Laceration with foreign body of unspecified great toe with damage to nail**

      ● S91.224   **Laceration with foreign body of right lesser toe(s) with damage to nail**

      ● S91.225   **Laceration with foreign body of left lesser toe(s) with damage to nail**

      ● S91.226   **Laceration with foreign body of unspecified lesser toe(s) with damage to nail**

      ● S91.229   **Laceration with foreign body of unspecified toe(s) with damage to nail**

    ● S91.23   **Puncture wound without foreign body of toe with damage to nail**

      ● S91.231   **Puncture wound without foreign body of right great toe with damage to nail**

      ● S91.232   **Puncture wound without foreign body of left great toe with damage to nail**

      ● S91.233   **Puncture wound without foreign body of unspecified great toe with damage to nail**

      ● S91.234   **Puncture wound without foreign body of right lesser toe(s) with damage to nail**

      ● S91.235   **Puncture wound without foreign body of left lesser toe(s) with damage to nail**

      ● S91.236   **Puncture wound without foreign body of unspecified lesser toe(s) with damage to nail**

      ● S91.239   **Puncture wound without foreign body of unspecified toe(s) with damage to nail**

    ● S91.24   **Puncture wound with foreign body of toe with damage to nail**

      ● S91.241   **Puncture wound with foreign body of right great toe with damage to nail**

      ● S91.242   **Puncture wound with foreign body of left great toe with damage to nail**

      ● S91.243   **Puncture wound with foreign body of unspecified great toe with damage to nail**

      ● S91.244   **Puncture wound with foreign body of right lesser toe(s) with damage to nail**

      ● S91.245   **Puncture wound with foreign body of left lesser toe(s) with damage to nail**

      ● S91.246   **Puncture wound with foreign body of unspecified lesser toe(s) with damage to nail**

      ● S91.249   **Puncture wound with foreign body of unspecified toe(s) with damage to nail**

    ● S91.25   **Open bite of toe with damage to nail**
      Bite of toe with damage to nail NOS

      Excludes1   superficial bite of toe (S90.46-, S90.47-)

      ● S91.251   **Open bite of right great toe with damage to nail**

      ● S91.252   **Open bite of left great toe with damage to nail**

      ● S91.253   **Open bite of unspecified great toe with damage to nail**

      ● S91.254   **Open bite of right lesser toe(s) with damage to nail**

      ● S91.255   **Open bite of left lesser toe(s) with damage to nail**

      ● S91.256   **Open bite of unspecified lesser toe(s) with damage to nail**

      ● S91.259   **Open bite of unspecified toe(s) with damage to nail**

CHAPTER 19 (S00-T88)

CHAPTER 19 (S00-T88)

- **S91.3**   Open wound of foot
  - **S91.30**   Unspecified open wound of foot
    - **S91.301**   Unspecified open wound, right foot
    - **S91.302**   Unspecified open wound, left foot
    - **S91.309**   Unspecified open wound, unspecified foot
  - **S91.31**   Laceration without foreign body of foot
    - **S91.311**   Laceration without foreign body, right foot
    - **S91.312**   Laceration without foreign body, left foot
    - **S91.319**   Laceration without foreign body, unspecified foot
  - **S91.32**   Laceration with foreign body of foot
    - **S91.321**   Laceration with foreign body, right foot
    - **S91.322**   Laceration with foreign body, left foot
    - **S91.329**   Laceration with foreign body, unspecified foot
  - **S91.33**   Puncture wound without foreign body of foot
    - **S91.331**   Puncture wound without foreign body, right foot
    - **S91.332**   Puncture wound without foreign body, left foot
    - **S91.339**   Puncture wound without foreign body, unspecified foot
  - **S91.34**   Puncture wound with foreign body of foot
    - **S91.341**   Puncture wound with foreign body, right foot
    - **S91.342**   Puncture wound with foreign body, left foot
    - **S91.349**   Puncture wound with foreign body, unspecified foot
  - **S91.35**   Open bite of foot
    - **Excludes1**   superficial bite of foot (S90.86-, S90.87-)
    - **S91.351**   Open bite, right foot
    - **S91.352**   Open bite, left foot
    - **S91.359**   Open bite, unspecified foot
- **S92**   Fracture of foot and toe, except ankle

  Note: A fracture not indicated as displaced or nondisplaced should be coded to displaced

  A fracture not indicated as open or closed should be coded to closed

  Excludes1   traumatic amputation of ankle and foot (S98.-)
  Excludes2   fracture of ankle (S82.-)
           fracture of malleolus (S82.-)

  The appropriate 7th character is to be added to each code from category S92

A	initial encounter for closed fracture
B	initial encounter for open fracture
D	subsequent encounter for fracture with routine healing
G	subsequent encounter for fracture with delayed healing
K	subsequent encounter for fracture with nonunion
P	subsequent encounter for fracture with malunion
S	sequela

  - **S92.0**   Fracture of calcaneus
        Heel bone   Os calcis
    - **S92.00**   Unspecified fracture of calcaneus
      - **S92.001**   Unspecified fracture of right calcaneus
      - **S92.002**   Unspecified fracture of left calcaneus
      - **S92.009**   Unspecified fracture of unspecified calcaneus

- **S92.01**   Fracture of body of calcaneus
  - **S92.011**   Displaced fracture of body of right calcaneus
  - **S92.012**   Displaced fracture of body of left calcaneus
  - **S92.013**   Displaced fracture of body of unspecified calcaneus
  - **S92.014**   Nondisplaced fracture of body of right calcaneus
  - **S92.015**   Nondisplaced fracture of body of left calcaneus
  - **S92.016**   Nondisplaced fracture of body of unspecified calcaneus
- **S92.02**   Fracture of anterior process of calcaneus
  - **S92.021**   Displaced fracture of anterior process of right calcaneus
  - **S92.022**   Displaced fracture of anterior process of left calcaneus
  - **S92.023**   Displaced fracture of anterior process of unspecified calcaneus
  - **S92.024**   Nondisplaced fracture of anterior process of right calcaneus
  - **S92.025**   Nondisplaced fracture of anterior process of left calcaneus
  - **S92.026**   Nondisplaced fracture of anterior process of unspecified calcaneus
- **S92.03**   Avulsion fracture of tuberosity of calcaneus
  - **S92.031**   Displaced avulsion fracture of tuberosity of right calcaneus
  - **S92.032**   Displaced avulsion fracture of tuberosity of left calcaneus
  - **S92.033**   Displaced avulsion fracture of tuberosity of unspecified calcaneus
  - **S92.034**   Nondisplaced avulsion fracture of tuberosity of right calcaneus
  - **S92.035**   Nondisplaced avulsion fracture of tuberosity of left calcaneus
  - **S92.036**   Nondisplaced avulsion fracture of tuberosity of unspecified calcaneus
- **S92.04**   Other fracture of tuberosity of calcaneus
  - **S92.041**   Displaced other fracture of tuberosity of right calcaneus
  - **S92.042**   Displaced other fracture of tuberosity of left calcaneus
  - **S92.043**   Displaced other fracture of tuberosity of unspecified calcaneus
  - **S92.044**   Nondisplaced other fracture of tuberosity of right calcaneus
  - **S92.045**   Nondisplaced other fracture of tuberosity of left calcaneus
  - **S92.046**   Nondisplaced other fracture of tuberosity of unspecified calcaneus
- **S92.05**   Other extraarticular fracture of calcaneus
  - **S92.051**   Displaced other extraarticular fracture of right calcaneus
  - **S92.052**   Displaced other extraarticular fracture of left calcaneus
  - **S92.053**   Displaced other extraarticular fracture of unspecified calcaneus
  - **S92.054**   Nondisplaced other extraarticular fracture of right calcaneus
  - **S92.055**   Nondisplaced other extraarticular fracture of left calcaneus
  - **S92.056**   Nondisplaced other extraarticular fracture of unspecified calcaneus

- S92.06   Intraarticular fracture of calcaneus
  - S92.061   Displaced intraarticular fracture of right calcaneus
  - S92.062   Displaced intraarticular fracture of left calcaneus
  - S92.063   Displaced intraarticular fracture of unspecified calcaneus
  - S92.064   Nondisplaced intraarticular fracture of right calcaneus
  - S92.065   Nondisplaced intraarticular fracture of left calcaneus
  - S92.066   Nondisplaced intraarticular fracture of unspecified calcaneus
- S92.1   Fracture of talus
  - Astragalus
  - S92.10   Unspecified fracture of talus
    - S92.101   Unspecified fracture of right talus
    - S92.102   Unspecified fracture of left talus
    - S92.109   Unspecified fracture of unspecified talus
  - S92.11   Fracture of neck of talus
    - S92.111   Displaced fracture of neck of right talus
    - S92.112   Displaced fracture of neck of left talus
    - S92.113   Displaced fracture of neck of unspecified talus
    - S92.114   Nondisplaced fracture of neck of right talus
    - S92.115   Nondisplaced fracture of neck of left talus
    - S92.116   Nondisplaced fracture of neck of unspecified talus
  - S92.12   Fracture of body of talus
    - S92.121   Displaced fracture of body of right talus
    - S92.122   Displaced fracture of body of left talus
    - S92.123   Displaced fracture of body of unspecified talus
    - S92.124   Nondisplaced fracture of body of right talus
    - S92.125   Nondisplaced fracture of body of left talus
    - S92.126   Nondisplaced fracture of body of unspecified talus
  - S92.13   Fracture of posterior process of talus
    - S92.131   Displaced fracture of posterior process of right talus
    - S92.132   Displaced fracture of posterior process of left talus
    - S92.133   Displaced fracture of posterior process of unspecified talus
    - S92.134   Nondisplaced fracture of posterior process of right talus
    - S92.135   Nondisplaced fracture of posterior process of left talus
    - S92.136   Nondisplaced fracture of posterior process of unspecified talus
  - S92.14   Dome fracture of talus
    - **Excludes1**   osteochondritis dissecans (M93.2)
    - S92.141   Displaced dome fracture of right talus
    - S92.142   Displaced dome fracture of left talus
    - S92.143   Displaced dome fracture of unspecified talus
    - S92.144   Nondisplaced dome fracture of right talus

- S92.145   Nondisplaced dome fracture of left talus
- S92.146   Nondisplaced dome fracture of unspecified talus
- S92.15   Avulsion fracture (chip fracture) of talus
  - S92.151   Displaced avulsion fracture (chip fracture) of right talus
  - S92.152   Displaced avulsion fracture (chip fracture) of left talus
  - S92.153   Displaced avulsion fracture (chip fracture) of unspecified talus
  - S92.154   Nondisplaced avulsion fracture (chip fracture) of right talus
  - S92.155   Nondisplaced avulsion fracture (chip fracture) of left talus
  - S92.156   Nondisplaced avulsion fracture (chip fracture) of unspecified talus
- S92.19   Other fracture of talus
  - S92.191   Other fracture of right talus
  - S92.192   Other fracture of left talus
  - S92.199   Other fracture of unspecified talus
- S92.2   Fracture of other and unspecified tarsal bone(s)
  - S92.20   Fracture of unspecified tarsal bone(s)
    - S92.201   Fracture of unspecified tarsal bone(s) of right foot
    - S92.202   Fracture of unspecified tarsal bone(s) of left foot
    - S92.209   Fracture of unspecified tarsal bone(s) of unspecified foot
  - S92.21   Fracture of cuboid bone
    - S92.211   Displaced fracture of cuboid bone of right foot
    - S92.212   Displaced fracture of cuboid bone of left foot
    - S92.213   Displaced fracture of cuboid bone of unspecified foot
    - S92.214   Nondisplaced fracture of cuboid bone of right foot
    - S92.215   Nondisplaced fracture of cuboid bone of left foot
    - S92.216   Nondisplaced fracture of cuboid bone of unspecified foot
  - S92.22   Fracture of lateral cuneiform
    - S92.221   Displaced fracture of lateral cuneiform of right foot
    - S92.222   Displaced fracture of lateral cuneiform of left foot
    - S92.223   Displaced fracture of lateral cuneiform of unspecified foot
    - S92.224   Nondisplaced fracture of lateral cuneiform of right foot
    - S92.225   Nondisplaced fracture of lateral cuneiform of left foot
    - S92.226   Nondisplaced fracture of lateral cuneiform of unspecified foot
  - S92.23   Fracture of intermediate cuneiform
    - S92.231   Displaced fracture of intermediate cuneiform of right foot
    - S92.232   Displaced fracture of intermediate cuneiform of left foot
    - S92.233   Displaced fracture of intermediate cuneiform of unspecified foot
    - S92.234   Nondisplaced fracture of intermediate cuneiform of right foot
    - S92.235   Nondisplaced fracture of intermediate cuneiform of left foot
    - S92.236   Nondisplaced fracture of intermediate cuneiform of unspecified foot

CHAPTER 19 (S00–T88)

● S92.24   **Fracture of medial cuneiform**
  ● S92.241   Displaced fracture of medial cuneiform of right foot
  ● S92.242   Displaced fracture of medial cuneiform of left foot
  ● S92.243   Displaced fracture of medial cuneiform of unspecified foot
  ● S92.244   Nondisplaced fracture of medial cuneiform of right foot
  ● S92.245   Nondisplaced fracture of medial cuneiform of left foot
  ● S92.246   Nondisplaced fracture of medial cuneiform of unspecified foot

● S92.25   **Fracture of navicular [scaphoid] of foot**
  ● S92.251   Displaced fracture of navicular [scaphoid] of right foot
  ● S92.252   Displaced fracture of navicular [scaphoid] of left foot
  ● S92.253   Displaced fracture of navicular [scaphoid] of unspecified foot
  ● S92.254   Nondisplaced fracture of navicular [scaphoid] of right foot
  ● S92.255   Nondisplaced fracture of navicular [scaphoid] of left foot
  ● S92.256   Nondisplaced fracture of navicular [scaphoid] of unspecified foot

● S92.3   **Fracture of metatarsal bone(s)**
  ● S92.30   Fracture of unspecified metatarsal bone(s)
    ● S92.301   Fracture of unspecified metatarsal bone(s), right foot
    ● S92.302   Fracture of unspecified metatarsal bone(s), left foot
    ● S92.309   Fracture of unspecified metatarsal bone(s), unspecified foot

  ● S92.31   Fracture of first metatarsal bone
    ● S92.311   Displaced fracture of first metatarsal bone, right foot
    ● S92.312   Displaced fracture of first metatarsal bone, left foot
    ● S92.313   Displaced fracture of first metatarsal bone, unspecified foot
    ● S92.314   Nondisplaced fracture of first metatarsal bone, right foot
    ● S92.315   Nondisplaced fracture of first metatarsal bone, left foot
    ● S92.316   Nondisplaced fracture of first metatarsal bone, unspecified foot

  ● S92.32   Fracture of second metatarsal bone
    ● S92.321   Displaced fracture of second metatarsal bone, right foot
    ● S92.322   Displaced fracture of second metatarsal bone, left foot
    ● S92.323   Displaced fracture of second metatarsal bone, unspecified foot
    ● S92.324   Nondisplaced fracture of second metatarsal bone, right foot
    ● S92.325   Nondisplaced fracture of second metatarsal bone, left foot
    ● S92.326   Nondisplaced fracture of second metatarsal bone, unspecified foot

  ● S92.33   Fracture of third metatarsal bone
    ● S92.331   Displaced fracture of third metatarsal bone, right foot
    ● S92.332   Displaced fracture of third metatarsal bone, left foot
    ● S92.333   Displaced fracture of third metatarsal bone, unspecified foot
    ● S92.334   Nondisplaced fracture of third metatarsal bone, right foot

● S92.335   Nondisplaced fracture of third metatarsal bone, left foot
● S92.336   Nondisplaced fracture of third metatarsal bone, unspecified foot

● S92.34   **Fracture of fourth metatarsal bone**
  ● S92.341   Displaced fracture of fourth metatarsal bone, right foot
  ● S92.342   Displaced fracture of fourth metatarsal bone, left foot
  ● S92.343   Displaced fracture of fourth metatarsal bone, unspecified foot
  ● S92.344   Nondisplaced fracture of fourth metatarsal bone, right foot
  ● S92.345   Nondisplaced fracture of fourth metatarsal bone, left foot
  ● S92.346   Nondisplaced fracture of fourth metatarsal bone, unspecified foot

● S92.35   **Fracture of fifth metatarsal bone**
  ● S92.351   Displaced fracture of fifth metatarsal bone, right foot
  ● S92.352   Displaced fracture of fifth metatarsal bone, left foot
  ● S92.353   Displaced fracture of fifth metatarsal bone, unspecified foot
  ● S92.354   Nondisplaced fracture of fifth metatarsal bone, right foot
  ● S92.355   Nondisplaced fracture of fifth metatarsal bone, left foot
  ● S92.356   Nondisplaced fracture of fifth metatarsal bone, unspecified foot

● S92.4   **Fracture of great toe**
  ● S92.40   Unspecified fracture of great toe
    ● S92.401   Displaced unspecified fracture of right great toe
    ● S92.402   Displaced unspecified fracture of left great toe
    ● S92.403   Displaced unspecified fracture of unspecified great toe
    ● S92.404   Nondisplaced unspecified fracture of right great toe
    ● S92.405   Nondisplaced unspecified fracture of left great toe
    ● S92.406   Nondisplaced unspecified fracture of unspecified great toe

  ● S92.41   Fracture of proximal phalanx of great toe
    ● S92.411   Displaced fracture of proximal phalanx of right great toe
    ● S92.412   Displaced fracture of proximal phalanx of left great toe
    ● S92.413   Displaced fracture of proximal phalanx of unspecified great toe
    ● S92.414   Nondisplaced fracture of proximal phalanx of right great toe
    ● S92.415   Nondisplaced fracture of proximal phalanx of left great toe
    ● S92.416   Nondisplaced fracture of proximal phalanx of unspecified great toe

  ● S92.42   Fracture of distal phalanx of great toe
    ● S92.421   Displaced fracture of distal phalanx of right great toe
    ● S92.422   Displaced fracture of distal phalanx of left great toe
    ● S92.423   Displaced fracture of distal phalanx of unspecified great toe
    ● S92.424   Nondisplaced fracture of distal phalanx of right great toe
    ● S92.425   Nondisplaced fracture of distal phalanx of left great toe
    ● S92.426   Nondisplaced fracture of distal phalanx of unspecified great toe

◄ New   ◄ Revised   ~~deleted~~ Deleted   OGCR Official Guidelines   X Assign placeholder X   ● Use Additional Character(s)

Excludes 1   Excludes 2   Includes   Use additional   Code first   Code also   Unspecified

● **S92.49**   **Other fracture of great toe**
    ● **S92.491**   Other fracture of right great toe
    ● **S92.492**   Other fracture of left great toe
    ● **S92.499**   Other fracture of unspecified great toe

● **S92.5**   **Fracture of lesser toe(s)**
   ● **S92.50**   **Unspecified fracture of lesser toe(s)**
    ● **S92.501**   Displaced unspecified fracture of right lesser toe(s)
    ● **S92.502**   Displaced unspecified fracture of left lesser toe(s)
    ● **S92.503**   Displaced unspecified fracture of unspecified lesser toe(s)
    ● **S92.504**   Nondisplaced unspecified fracture of right lesser toe(s)
    ● **S92.505**   Nondisplaced unspecified fracture of left lesser toe(s)
    ● **S92.506**   Nondisplaced unspecified fracture of unspecified lesser toe(s)

   ● **S92.51**   **Fracture of proximal phalanx of lesser toe(s)**
    ● **S92.511**   Displaced fracture of proximal phalanx of right lesser toe(s)
    ● **S92.512**   Displaced fracture of proximal phalanx of left lesser toe(s)
    ● **S92.513**   Displaced fracture of proximal phalanx of unspecified lesser toe(s)
    ● **S92.514**   Nondisplaced fracture of proximal phalanx of right lesser toe(s)
    ● **S92.515**   Nondisplaced fracture of proximal phalanx of left lesser toe(s)
    ● **S92.516**   Nondisplaced fracture of proximal phalanx of unspecified lesser toe(s)

   ● **S92.52**   **Fracture of medial phalanx of lesser toe(s)**
    ● **S92.521**   Displaced fracture of medial phalanx of right lesser toe(s)
    ● **S92.522**   Displaced fracture of medial phalanx of left lesser toe(s)
    ● **S92.523**   Displaced fracture of medial phalanx of unspecified lesser toe(s)
    ● **S92.524**   Nondisplaced fracture of medial phalanx of right lesser toe(s)
    ● **S92.525**   Nondisplaced fracture of medial phalanx of left lesser toe(s)
    ● **S92.526**   Nondisplaced fracture of medial phalanx of unspecified lesser toe(s)

   ● **S92.53**   **Fracture of distal phalanx of lesser toe(s)**
    ● **S92.531**   Displaced fracture of distal phalanx of right lesser toe(s)
    ● **S92.532**   Displaced fracture of distal phalanx of left lesser toe(s)
    ● **S92.533**   Displaced fracture of distal phalanx of unspecified lesser toe(s)
    ● **S92.534**   Nondisplaced fracture of distal phalanx of right lesser toe(s)
    ● **S92.535**   Nondisplaced fracture of distal phalanx of left lesser toe(s)
    ● **S92.536**   Nondisplaced fracture of distal phalanx of unspecified lesser toe(s)

   ● **S92.59**   **Other fracture of lesser toe(s)**
    ● **S92.591**   Other fracture of right lesser toe(s)
    ● **S92.592**   Other fracture of left lesser toe(s)
    ● **S92.599**   Other fracture of unspecified lesser toe(s)

● **S92.9**   **Unspecified fracture of foot and toe**
   ● **S92.90**   **Unspecified fracture of foot**
    ● **S92.901**   Unspecified fracture of right foot
    ● **S92.902**   Unspecified fracture of left foot
    ● **S92.909**   Unspecified fracture of unspecified foot

   ● **S92.91**   **Unspecified fracture of toe**
    ● **S92.911**   Unspecified fracture of right toe(s)
    ● **S92.912**   Unspecified fracture of left toe(s)
    ● **S92.919**   Unspecified fracture of unspecified toe(s)

● **S93**   **Dislocation and sprain of joints and ligaments at ankle, foot and toe level**

   Includes   avulsion of joint or ligament of ankle, foot and toe
      laceration of cartilage, joint or ligament of ankle, foot and toe
      sprain of cartilage, joint or ligament of ankle, foot and toe
      traumatic hemarthrosis of joint or ligament of ankle, foot and toe
      traumatic rupture of joint or ligament of ankle, foot and toe
      traumatic subluxation of joint or ligament of ankle, foot and toe
      traumatic tear of joint or ligament of ankle, foot and toe

   Code also any associated open wound

   Excludes2   strain of muscle and tendon of ankle and foot (S96.-)

   The appropriate 7th character is to be added to each code from category S93

A	initial encounter
D	subsequent encounter
S	sequela

   ● **S93.0**   **Subluxation and dislocation of ankle joint**
      Subluxation and dislocation of astragalus
      Subluxation and dislocation of fibula, lower end
      Subluxation and dislocation of talus
      Subluxation and dislocation of tibia, lower end
    X ● **S93.01**   Subluxation of right ankle joint
    X ● **S93.02**   Subluxation of left ankle joint
    X ● **S93.03**   Subluxation of unspecified ankle joint
    X ● **S93.04**   Dislocation of right ankle joint
    X ● **S93.05**   Dislocation of left ankle joint
    X ● **S93.06**   Dislocation of unspecified ankle joint

   ● **S93.1**   **Subluxation and dislocation of toe**
    ● **S93.10**   **Unspecified subluxation and dislocation of toe**
      Dislocation of toe NOS
      Subluxation of toe NOS
     ● **S93.101**   Unspecified subluxation of right toe(s)
     ● **S93.102**   Unspecified subluxation of left toe(s)
     ● **S93.103**   Unspecified subluxation of unspecified toe(s)
     ● **S93.104**   Unspecified dislocation of right toe(s)
     ● **S93.105**   Unspecified dislocation of left toe(s)
     ● **S93.106**   Unspecified dislocation of unspecified toe(s)

    ● **S93.11**   **Dislocation of interphalangeal joint**
     ● **S93.111**   Dislocation of interphalangeal joint of right great toe
     ● **S93.112**   Dislocation of interphalangeal joint of left great toe
     ● **S93.113**   Dislocation of interphalangeal joint of unspecified great toe
     ● **S93.114**   Dislocation of interphalangeal joint of right lesser toe(s)
     ● **S93.115**   Dislocation of interphalangeal joint of left lesser toe(s)
     ● **S93.116**   Dislocation of interphalangeal joint of unspecified lesser toe(s)
     ● **S93.119**   Dislocation of interphalangeal joint of unspecified toe(s)

CHAPTER 19 (S00-T88)

● S93.12   Dislocation of metatarsophalangeal joint
- ● S93.121   Dislocation of metatarsophalangeal joint of right great toe
- ● S93.122   Dislocation of metatarsophalangeal joint of left great toe
- ● S93.123   Dislocation of metatarsophalangeal joint of unspecified great toe
- ● S93.124   Dislocation of metatarsophalangeal joint of right lesser toe(s)
- ● S93.125   Dislocation of metatarsophalangeal joint of left lesser toe(s)
- ● S93.126   Dislocation of metatarsophalangeal joint of unspecified lesser toe(s)
- ● S93.129   Dislocation of metatarsophalangeal joint of unspecified toe(s)

● S93.13   Subluxation of interphalangeal joint
- ● S93.131   Subluxation of interphalangeal joint of right great toe
- ● S93.132   Subluxation of interphalangeal joint of left great toe
- ● S93.133   Subluxation of interphalangeal joint of unspecified great toe
- ● S93.134   Subluxation of interphalangeal joint of right lesser toe(s)
- ● S93.135   Subluxation of interphalangeal joint of left lesser toe(s)
- ● S93.136   Subluxation of interphalangeal joint of unspecified lesser toe(s)
- ● S93.139   Subluxation of interphalangeal joint of unspecified toe(s)

● S93.14   Subluxation of metatarsophalangeal joint
- ● S93.141   Subluxation of metatarsophalangeal joint of right great toe
- ● S93.142   Subluxation of metatarsophalangeal joint of left great toe
- ● S93.143   Subluxation of metatarsophalangeal joint of unspecified great toe
- ● S93.144   Subluxation of metatarsophalangeal joint of right lesser toe(s)
- ● S93.145   Subluxation of metatarsophalangeal joint of left lesser toe(s)
- ● S93.146   Subluxation of metatarsophalangeal joint of unspecified lesser toe(s)
- ● S93.149   Subluxation of metatarsophalangeal joint of unspecified toe(s)

● S93.3   Subluxation and dislocation of foot

> **Excludes2**   dislocation of toe (S93.1-)

● S93.30   Unspecified subluxation and dislocation of foot
Dislocation of foot NOS
Subluxation of foot NOS
- ● S93.301   Unspecified subluxation of right foot
- ● S93.302   Unspecified subluxation of left foot
- ● S93.303   Unspecified subluxation of unspecified foot
- ● S93.304   Unspecified dislocation of right foot
- ● S93.305   Unspecified dislocation of left foot
- ● S93.306   Unspecified dislocation of unspecified foot

● S93.31   Subluxation and dislocation of tarsal joint
- ● S93.311   Subluxation of tarsal joint of right foot
- ● S93.312   Subluxation of tarsal joint of left foot
- ● S93.313   Subluxation of tarsal joint of unspecified foot
- ● S93.314   Dislocation of tarsal joint of right foot
- ● S93.315   Dislocation of tarsal joint of left foot
- ● S93.316   Dislocation of tarsal joint of unspecified foot

● S93.32   Subluxation and dislocation of tarsometatarsal joint
- ● S93.321   Subluxation of tarsometatarsal joint of right foot
- ● S93.322   Subluxation of tarsometatarsal joint of left foot
- ● S93.323   Subluxation of tarsometatarsal joint of unspecified foot
- ● S93.324   Dislocation of tarsometatarsal joint of right foot
- ● S93.325   Dislocation of tarsometatarsal joint of left foot
- ● S93.326   Dislocation of tarsometatarsal joint of unspecified foot

● S93.33   Other subluxation and dislocation of foot
- ● S93.331   Other subluxation of right foot
- ● S93.332   Other subluxation of left foot
- ● S93.333   Other subluxation of unspecified foot
- ● S93.334   Other dislocation of right foot
- ● S93.335   Other dislocation of left foot
- ● S93.336   Other dislocation of unspecified foot

● S93.4   Sprain of ankle
Injury to ligaments when one or more is stretched/torn

> **Excludes2**   injury of Achilles tendon (S86.0-)

● S93.40   Sprain of unspecified ligament of ankle
Sprain of ankle NOS
Sprained ankle NOS
- ● S93.401   Sprain of unspecified ligament of right ankle
- ● S93.402   Sprain of unspecified ligament of left ankle
- ● S93.409   Sprain of unspecified ligament of unspecified ankle

● S93.41   Sprain of calcaneofibular ligament
- ● S93.411   Sprain of calcaneofibular ligament of right ankle
- ● S93.412   Sprain of calcaneofibular ligament of left ankle
- ● S93.419   Sprain of calcaneofibular ligament of unspecified ankle

● S93.42   Sprain of deltoid ligament
- ● S93.421   Sprain of deltoid ligament of right ankle
- ● S93.422   Sprain of deltoid ligament of left ankle
- ● S93.429   Sprain of deltoid ligament of unspecified ankle

● S93.43   Sprain of tibiofibular ligament
- ● S93.431   Sprain of tibiofibular ligament of right ankle
- ● S93.432   Sprain of tibiofibular ligament of left ankle
- ● S93.439   Sprain of tibiofibular ligament of unspecified ankle

● S93.49   Sprain of other ligament of ankle
Sprain of internal collateral ligament
Sprain of talofibular ligament
- ● S93.491   Sprain of other ligament of right ankle
- ● S93.492   Sprain of other ligament of left ankle
- ● S93.499   Sprain of other ligament of unspecified ankle

◀ New   ◀◀◀ Revised   ~~deleted~~ Deleted   OGCR Official Guidelines   X Assign placeholder X   ● Use Additional Character(s)

| Excludes 1 | Excludes 2 | Includes | Use additional | Code first | Code also | Unspecified |

● **S93.5**   **Sprain of toe**
   ● **S93.50**   **Unspecified sprain of toe**
     ● **S93.501**   Unspecified sprain of right great toe
     ● **S93.502**   Unspecified sprain of left great toe
     ● **S93.503**   Unspecified sprain of unspecified great toe
     ● **S93.504**   Unspecified sprain of right lesser toe(s)
     ● **S93.505**   Unspecified sprain of left lesser toe(s)
     ● **S93.506**   Unspecified sprain of unspecified lesser toe(s)
     ● **S93.509**   Unspecified sprain of unspecified toe(s)
   ● **S93.51**   **Sprain of interphalangeal joint of toe**
     ● **S93.511**   Sprain of interphalangeal joint of right great toe
     ● **S93.512**   Sprain of interphalangeal joint of left great toe
     ● **S93.513**   Sprain of interphalangeal joint of unspecified great toe
     ● **S93.514**   Sprain of interphalangeal joint of right lesser toe(s)
     ● **S93.515**   Sprain of interphalangeal joint of left lesser toe(s)
     ● **S93.516**   Sprain of interphalangeal joint of unspecified lesser toe(s)
     ● **S93.519**   Sprain of interphalangeal joint of unspecified toe(s)
   ● **S93.52**   **Sprain of metatarsophalangeal joint of toe**
     ● **S93.521**   Sprain of metatarsophalangeal joint of right great toe
     ● **S93.522**   Sprain of metatarsophalangeal joint of left great toe
     ● **S93.523**   Sprain of metatarsophalangeal joint of unspecified great toe
     ● **S93.524**   Sprain of metatarsophalangeal joint of right lesser toe(s)
     ● **S93.525**   Sprain of metatarsophalangeal joint of left lesser toe(s)
     ● **S93.526**   Sprain of metatarsophalangeal joint of unspecified lesser toe(s)
     ● **S93.529**   Sprain of metatarsophalangeal joint of unspecified toe(s)
● **S93.6**   **Sprain of foot**
    Excludes2   sprain of metatarsophalangeal joint of toe (S93.52-)
               sprain of toe (S93.5-)
   ● **S93.60**   **Unspecified sprain of foot**
     ● **S93.601**   Unspecified sprain of right foot
     ● **S93.602**   Unspecified sprain of left foot
     ● **S93.609**   Unspecified sprain of unspecified foot
   ● **S93.61**   **Sprain of tarsal ligament of foot**
     ● **S93.611**   Sprain of tarsal ligament of right foot
     ● **S93.612**   Sprain of tarsal ligament of left foot
     ● **S93.619**   Sprain of tarsal ligament of unspecified foot
   ● **S93.62**   **Sprain of tarsometatarsal ligament of foot**
     ● **S93.621**   Sprain of tarsometatarsal ligament of right foot
     ● **S93.622**   Sprain of tarsometatarsal ligament of left foot
     ● **S93.629**   Sprain of tarsometatarsal ligament of unspecified foot
   ● **S93.69**   **Other sprain of foot**
     ● **S93.691**   Other sprain of right foot
     ● **S93.692**   Other sprain of left foot
     ● **S93.699**   Other sprain of unspecified foot

● **S94**   **Injury of nerves at ankle and foot level**
   The appropriate 7th character is to be added to each code from category S94

A	initial encounter
D	subsequent encounter
S	sequela

   Code also any associated open wound (S91.-)
  ● **S94.0**   **Injury of lateral plantar nerve**
   X ● **S94.00**   Injury of lateral plantar nerve, unspecified leg
   X ● **S94.01**   Injury of lateral plantar nerve, right leg
   X ● **S94.02**   Injury of lateral plantar nerve, left leg
  ● **S94.1**   **Injury of medial plantar nerve**
   X ● **S94.10**   Injury of medial plantar nerve, unspecified leg
   X ● **S94.11**   Injury of medial plantar nerve, right leg
   X ● **S94.12**   Injury of medial plantar nerve, left leg
  ● **S94.2**   **Injury of deep peroneal nerve at ankle and foot level**
     Injury of terminal, lateral branch of deep peroneal nerve
   X ● **S94.20**   Injury of deep peroneal nerve at ankle and foot level, unspecified leg
   X ● **S94.21**   Injury of deep peroneal nerve at ankle and foot level, right leg
   X ● **S94.22**   Injury of deep peroneal nerve at ankle and foot level, left leg
  ● **S94.3**   **Injury of cutaneous sensory nerve at ankle and foot level**
   X ● **S94.30**   Injury of cutaneous sensory nerve at ankle and foot level, unspecified leg
   X ● **S94.31**   Injury of cutaneous sensory nerve at ankle and foot level, right leg
   X ● **S94.32**   Injury of cutaneous sensory nerve at ankle and foot level, left leg
  ● **S94.8**   **Injury of other nerves at ankle and foot level**
   ● **S94.8X**   **Injury of other nerves at ankle and foot level**
     ● **S94.8X1**   Injury of other nerves at ankle and foot level, right leg
     ● **S94.8X2**   Injury of other nerves at ankle and foot level, left leg
     ● **S94.8X9**   Injury of other nerves at ankle and foot level, unspecified leg
  ● **S94.9**   **Injury of unspecified nerve at ankle and foot level**
   X ● **S94.90**   Injury of unspecified nerve at ankle and foot level, unspecified leg
   X ● **S94.91**   Injury of unspecified nerve at ankle and foot level, right leg
   X ● **S94.92**   Injury of unspecified nerve at ankle and foot level, left leg

● **S95**   **Injury of blood vessels at ankle and foot level**
   Code also any associated open wound (S91.-)
    Excludes2   injury of posterior tibial artery and vein (S85.1-, S85.8-)
   The appropriate 7th character is to be added to each code from category S95

A	initial encounter
D	subsequent encounter
S	sequela

  ● **S95.0**   **Injury of dorsal artery of foot**
   ● **S95.00**   **Unspecified injury of dorsal artery of foot**
     ● **S95.001**   Unspecified injury of dorsal artery of right foot
     ● **S95.002**   Unspecified injury of dorsal artery of left foot
     ● **S95.009**   Unspecified injury of dorsal artery of unspecified foot

- S95.01   Laceration of dorsal artery of foot
  - S95.011   Laceration of dorsal artery of right foot
  - S95.012   Laceration of dorsal artery of left foot
  - S95.019   Laceration of dorsal artery of unspecified foot
- S95.09   Other specified injury of dorsal artery of foot
  - S95.091   Other specified injury of dorsal artery of right foot
  - S95.092   Other specified injury of dorsal artery of left foot
  - S95.099   Other specified injury of dorsal artery of unspecified foot
- S95.1   Injury of plantar artery of foot
  - S95.10   Unspecified injury of plantar artery of foot
    - S95.101   Unspecified injury of plantar artery of right foot
    - S95.102   Unspecified injury of plantar artery of left foot
    - S95.109   Unspecified injury of plantar artery of unspecified foot
  - S95.11   Laceration of plantar artery of foot
    - S95.111   Laceration of plantar artery of right foot
    - S95.112   Laceration of plantar artery of left foot
    - S95.119   Laceration of plantar artery of unspecified foot
  - S95.19   Other specified injury of plantar artery of foot
    - S95.191   Other specified injury of plantar artery of right foot
    - S95.192   Other specified injury of plantar artery of left foot
    - S95.199   Other specified injury of plantar artery of unspecified foot
- S95.2   Injury of dorsal vein of foot
  - S95.20   Unspecified injury of dorsal vein of foot
    - S95.201   Unspecified injury of dorsal vein of right foot
    - S95.202   Unspecified injury of dorsal vein of left foot
    - S95.209   Unspecified injury of dorsal vein of unspecified foot
  - S95.21   Laceration of dorsal vein of foot
    - S95.211   Laceration of dorsal vein of right foot
    - S95.212   Laceration of dorsal vein of left foot
    - S95.219   Laceration of dorsal vein of unspecified foot
  - S95.29   Other specified injury of dorsal vein of foot
    - S95.291   Other specified injury of dorsal vein of right foot
    - S95.292   Other specified injury of dorsal vein of left foot
    - S95.299   Other specified injury of dorsal vein of unspecified foot

- S95.8   Injury of other blood vessels at ankle and foot level
  - S95.80   Unspecified injury of other blood vessels at ankle and foot level
    - S95.801   Unspecified injury of other blood vessels at ankle and foot level, right leg
    - S95.802   Unspecified injury of other blood vessels at ankle and foot level, left leg
    - S95.809   Unspecified injury of other blood vessels at ankle and foot level, unspecified leg
  - S95.81   Laceration of other blood vessels at ankle and foot level
    - S95.811   Laceration of other blood vessels at ankle and foot level, right leg
    - S95.812   Laceration of other blood vessels at ankle and foot level, left leg
    - S95.819   Laceration of other blood vessels at ankle and foot level, unspecified leg
  - S95.89   Other specified injury of other blood vessels at ankle and foot level
    - S95.891   Other specified injury of other blood vessels at ankle and foot level, right leg
    - S95.892   Other specified injury of other blood vessels at ankle and foot level, left leg
    - S95.899   Other specified injury of other blood vessels at ankle and foot level, unspecified leg
- S95.9   Injury of unspecified blood vessel at ankle and foot level
  - S95.90   Unspecified injury of unspecified blood vessel at ankle and foot level
    - S95.901   Unspecified injury of unspecified blood vessel at ankle and foot level, right leg
    - S95.902   Unspecified injury of unspecified blood vessel at ankle and foot level, left leg
    - S95.909   Unspecified injury of unspecified blood vessel at ankle and foot level, unspecified leg
  - S95.91   Laceration of unspecified blood vessel at ankle and foot level
    - S95.911   Laceration of unspecified blood vessel at ankle and foot level, right leg
    - S95.912   Laceration of unspecified blood vessel at ankle and foot level, left leg
    - S95.919   Laceration of unspecified blood vessel at ankle and foot level, unspecified leg
  - S95.99   Other specified injury of unspecified blood vessel at ankle and foot level
    - S95.991   Other specified injury of unspecified blood vessel at ankle and foot level, right leg
    - S95.992   Other specified injury of unspecified blood vessel at ankle and foot level, left leg
    - S95.999   Other specified injury of unspecified blood vessel at ankle and foot level, unspecified leg

◀ New   ◀≡ Revised   ~~deleted~~ Deleted   OGCR Official Guidelines   X Assign placeholder X   ● Use Additional Character(s)

Excludes 1   Excludes 2   Includes   Use additional   Code first   Code also   Unspecified

● **S96   Injury of muscle and tendon at ankle and foot level**

Code also any associated open wound (S91.-)

Excludes2	injury of Achilles tendon (S86.0-)
	sprain of joints and ligaments of ankle and foot (S93.-)

The appropriate 7th character is to be added to each code from category S96

A	initial encounter
D	subsequent encounter
S	sequela

● **S96.0   Injury of muscle and tendon of long flexor muscle of toe at ankle and foot level**

● **S96.00   Unspecified injury of muscle and tendon of long flexor muscle of toe at ankle and foot level**

● S96.001   Unspecified injury of muscle and tendon of long flexor muscle of toe at ankle and foot level, right foot

● S96.002   Unspecified injury of muscle and tendon of long flexor muscle of toe at ankle and foot level, left foot

● S96.009   Unspecified injury of muscle and tendon of long flexor muscle of toe at ankle and foot level, unspecified foot

● **S96.01   Strain of muscle and tendon of long flexor muscle of toe at ankle and foot level**

● S96.011   Strain of muscle and tendon of long flexor muscle of toe at ankle and foot level, right foot

● S96.012   Strain of muscle and tendon of long flexor muscle of toe at ankle and foot level, left foot

● S96.019   Strain of muscle and tendon of long flexor muscle of toe at ankle and foot level, unspecified foot

● **S96.02   Laceration of muscle and tendon of long flexor muscle of toe at ankle and foot level**

● S96.021   Laceration of muscle and tendon of long flexor muscle of toe at ankle and foot level, right foot

● S96.022   Laceration of muscle and tendon of long flexor muscle of toe at ankle and foot level, left foot

● S96.029   Laceration of muscle and tendon of long flexor muscle of toe at ankle and foot level, unspecified foot

● **S96.09   Other injury of muscle and tendon of long flexor muscle of toe at ankle and foot level**

● S96.091   Other injury of muscle and tendon of long flexor muscle of toe at ankle and foot level, right foot

● S96.092   Other injury of muscle and tendon of long flexor muscle of toe at ankle and foot level, left foot

● S96.099   Other injury of muscle and tendon of long flexor muscle of toe at ankle and foot level, unspecified foot

● **S96.1   Injury of muscle and tendon of long extensor muscle of toe at ankle and foot level**

● **S96.10   Unspecified injury of muscle and tendon of long extensor muscle of toe at ankle and foot level**

● S96.101   Unspecified injury of muscle and tendon of long extensor muscle of toe at ankle and foot level, right foot

● S96.102   Unspecified injury of muscle and tendon of long extensor muscle of toe at ankle and foot level, left foot

● S96.109   Unspecified injury of muscle and tendon of long extensor muscle of toe at ankle and foot level, unspecified foot

● **S96.11   Strain of muscle and tendon of long extensor muscle of toe at ankle and foot level**

● S96.111   Strain of muscle and tendon of long extensor muscle of toe at ankle and foot level, right foot

● S96.112   Strain of muscle and tendon of long extensor muscle of toe at ankle and foot level, left foot

● S96.119   Strain of muscle and tendon of long extensor muscle of toe at ankle and foot level, unspecified foot

● **S96.12   Laceration of muscle and tendon of long extensor muscle of toe at ankle and foot level**

● S96.121   Laceration of muscle and tendon of long extensor muscle of toe at ankle and foot level, right foot

● S96.122   Laceration of muscle and tendon of long extensor muscle of toe at ankle and foot level, left foot

● S96.129   Laceration of muscle and tendon of long extensor muscle of toe at ankle and foot level, unspecified foot

● **S96.19   Other specified injury of muscle and tendon of long extensor muscle of toe at ankle and foot level**

● S96.191   Other specified injury of muscle and tendon of long extensor muscle of toe at ankle and foot level, right foot

● S96.192   Other specified injury of muscle and tendon of long extensor muscle of toe at ankle and foot level, left foot

● S96.199   Other specified injury of muscle and tendon of long extensor muscle of toe at ankle and foot level, unspecified foot

● **S96.2   Injury of intrinsic muscle and tendon at ankle and foot level**

● **S96.20   Unspecified injury of intrinsic muscle and tendon at ankle and foot level**

● S96.201   Unspecified injury of intrinsic muscle and tendon at ankle and foot level, right foot

● S96.202   Unspecified injury of intrinsic muscle and tendon at ankle and foot level, left foot

● S96.209   Unspecified injury of intrinsic muscle and tendon at ankle and foot level, unspecified foot

● **S96.21   Strain of intrinsic muscle and tendon at ankle and foot level**

● S96.211   Strain of intrinsic muscle and tendon at ankle and foot level, right foot

● S96.212   Strain of intrinsic muscle and tendon at ankle and foot level, left foot

● S96.219   Strain of intrinsic muscle and tendon at ankle and foot level, unspecified foot

● **S96.22   Laceration of intrinsic muscle and tendon at ankle and foot level**

● S96.221   Laceration of intrinsic muscle and tendon at ankle and foot level, right foot

● S96.222   Laceration of intrinsic muscle and tendon at left ankle and foot level, left foot

● S96.229   Laceration of intrinsic muscle and tendon at ankle and foot level, unspecified foot

◀ New	◀━ Revised	~~deleted~~ Deleted	**OGCR** Official Guidelines	X Assign placeholder X	● Use Additional Character(s)

Excludes 1	Excludes 2	Includes	Use additional	Code first	Code also	Unspecified

● **S96.29**   Other specified injury of intrinsic muscle and tendon at ankle and foot level
- ● **S96.291**   Other specified injury of intrinsic muscle and tendon at ankle and foot level, right foot
- ● **S96.292**   Other specified injury of intrinsic muscle and tendon at ankle and foot level, left foot
- ● **S96.299**   Other specified injury of intrinsic muscle and tendon at ankle and foot level, unspecified foot

● **S96.8**   Injury of other specified muscles and tendons at ankle and foot level
- ● **S96.80**   Unspecified injury of other specified muscles and tendons at ankle and foot level
  - ● **S96.801**   Unspecified injury of other specified muscles and tendons at ankle and foot level, right foot
  - ● **S96.802**   Unspecified injury of other specified muscles and tendons at ankle and foot level, left foot
  - ● **S96.809**   Unspecified injury of other specified muscles and tendons at ankle and foot level, unspecified foot
- ● **S96.81**   Strain of other specified muscles and tendons at ankle and foot level
  - ● **S96.811**   Strain of other specified muscles and tendons at ankle and foot level, right foot
  - ● **S96.812**   Strain of other specified muscles and tendons at ankle and foot level, left foot
  - ● **S96.819**   Strain of other specified muscles and tendons at ankle and foot level, unspecified foot
- ● **S96.82**   Laceration of other specified muscles and tendons at ankle and foot level
  - ● **S96.821**   Laceration of other specified muscles and tendons at ankle and foot level, right foot
  - ● **S96.822**   Laceration of other specified muscles and tendons at ankle and foot level, left foot
  - ● **S96.829**   Laceration of other specified muscles and tendons at ankle and foot level, unspecified foot
- ● **S96.89**   Other specified injury of other specified muscles and tendons at ankle and foot level
  - ● **S96.891**   Other specified injury of other specified muscles and tendons at ankle and foot level, right foot
  - ● **S96.892**   Other specified injury of other specified muscles and tendons at ankle and foot level, left foot
  - ● **S96.899**   Other specified injury of other specified muscles and tendons at ankle and foot level, unspecified foot

● **S96.9**   Injury of unspecified muscle and tendon at ankle and foot level
- ● **S96.90**   Unspecified injury of unspecified muscle and tendon at ankle and foot level
  - ● **S96.901**   Unspecified injury of unspecified muscle and tendon at ankle and foot level, right foot
  - ● **S96.902**   Unspecified injury of unspecified muscle and tendon at ankle and foot level, left foot
  - ● **S96.909**   Unspecified injury of unspecified muscle and tendon at ankle and foot level, unspecified foot

● **S96.91**   Strain of unspecified muscle and tendon at ankle and foot level
- ● **S96.911**   Strain of unspecified muscle and tendon at ankle and foot level, right foot
- ● **S96.912**   Strain of unspecified muscle and tendon at ankle and foot level, left foot
- ● **S96.919**   Strain of unspecified muscle and tendon at ankle and foot level, unspecified foot

● **S96.92**   Laceration of unspecified muscle and tendon at ankle and foot level
- ● **S96.921**   Laceration of unspecified muscle and tendon at ankle and foot level, right foot
- ● **S96.922**   Laceration of unspecified muscle and tendon at ankle and foot level, left foot
- ● **S96.929**   Laceration of unspecified muscle and tendon at ankle and foot level, unspecified foot

● **S96.99**   Other specified injury of unspecified muscle and tendon at ankle and foot level
- ● **S96.991**   Other specified injury of unspecified muscle and tendon at ankle and foot level, right foot
- ● **S96.992**   Other specified injury of unspecified muscle and tendon at ankle and foot level, left foot
- ● **S96.999**   Other specified injury of unspecified muscle and tendon at ankle and foot level, unspecified foot

● **S97**   **Crushing injury of ankle and foot**

Use additional code(s) for all associated injuries

The appropriate 7th character is to be added to each code from category S97

A	initial encounter
D	subsequent encounter
S	sequela

● **S97.0**   Crushing injury of ankle
- X ● **S97.00**   Crushing injury of unspecified ankle
- X ● **S97.01**   Crushing injury of right ankle
- X ● **S97.02**   Crushing injury of left ankle

● **S97.1**   Crushing injury of toe
- ● **S97.10**   Crushing injury of unspecified toe(s)
  - ● **S97.101**   Crushing injury of unspecified right toe(s)
  - ● **S97.102**   Crushing injury of unspecified left toe(s)
  - ● **S97.109**   Crushing injury of unspecified toe(s)
    Crushing injury of toe NOS
- ● **S97.11**   Crushing injury of great toe
  - ● **S97.111**   Crushing injury of right great toe
  - ● **S97.112**   Crushing injury of left great toe
  - ● **S97.119**   Crushing injury of unspecified great toe
- ● **S97.12**   Crushing injury of lesser toe(s)
  - ● **S97.121**   Crushing injury of right lesser toe(s)
  - ● **S97.122**   Crushing injury of left lesser toe(s)
  - ● **S97.129**   Crushing injury of lesser toe(s), unspecified toe(s)

● **S97.8**   Crushing injury of foot
- X ● **S97.80**   Crushing injury of foot, unspecified side
  Crushing injury of foot NOS
- X ● **S97.81**   Crushing injury of right foot
- X ● **S97.82**   Crushing injury of left foot

◀ New   ◀|||| Revised   ~~deleted~~ Deleted   **OGCR** Official Guidelines   X Assign placeholder X   ● Use Additional Character(s)

Excludes 1   Excludes 2   Includes   Use additional   Code first   Code also   Unspecified

- ● **S98   Traumatic amputation of ankle and foot**

  An amputation not identified as partial or complete should be coded to complete

  The appropriate 7th character is to be added to each code from category S98

A	initial encounter
D	subsequent encounter
S	sequela

  - ● **S98.0   Traumatic amputation of foot at ankle level**
    - ● S98.01   Complete traumatic amputation of foot at ankle level
      - ● S98.011   Complete traumatic amputation of right foot at ankle level
      - ● S98.012   Complete traumatic amputation of left foot at ankle level
      - ● S98.019   Complete traumatic amputation of unspecified foot at ankle level
    - ● S98.02   Partial traumatic amputation of foot at ankle level
      - ● S98.021   Partial traumatic amputation of right foot at ankle level
      - ● S98.022   Partial traumatic amputation of left foot at ankle level
      - ● S98.029   Partial traumatic amputation of unspecified foot at ankle level
  - ● **S98.1   Traumatic amputation of one toe**
    - ● S98.11   Complete traumatic amputation of great toe
      - ● S98.111   Complete traumatic amputation of right great toe
      - ● S98.112   Complete traumatic amputation of left great toe
      - ● S98.119   Complete traumatic amputation of unspecified great toe
    - ● S98.12   Partial traumatic amputation of great toe
      - ● S98.121   Partial traumatic amputation of right great toe
      - ● S98.122   Partial traumatic amputation of left great toe
      - ● S98.129   Partial traumatic amputation of unspecified great toe
    - ● S98.13   Complete traumatic amputation of one lesser toe

      Traumatic amputation of toe NOS
      - ● S98.131   Complete traumatic amputation of one right lesser toe
      - ● S98.132   Complete traumatic amputation of one left lesser toe
      - ● S98.139   Complete traumatic amputation of one unspecified lesser toe
    - ● S98.14   Partial traumatic amputation of one lesser toe
      - ● S98.141   Partial traumatic amputation of one right lesser toe
      - ● S98.142   Partial traumatic amputation of one left lesser toe
      - ● S98.149   Partial traumatic amputation of one unspecified lesser toe
  - ● **S98.2   Traumatic amputation of two or more lesser toes**
    - ● S98.21   Complete traumatic amputation of two or more lesser toes
      - ● S98.211   Complete traumatic amputation of two or more right lesser toes
      - ● S98.212   Complete traumatic amputation of two or more left lesser toes
      - ● S98.219   Complete traumatic amputation of two or more unspecified lesser toes

    - ● S98.22   Partial traumatic amputation of two or more lesser toes
      - ● S98.221   Partial traumatic amputation of two or more right lesser toes
      - ● S98.222   Partial traumatic amputation of two or more left lesser toes
      - ● S98.229   Partial traumatic amputation of two or more unspecified lesser toes
  - ● **S98.3   Traumatic amputation of midfoot**
    - ● S98.31   Complete traumatic amputation of midfoot
      - ● S98.311   Complete traumatic amputation of right midfoot
      - ● S98.312   Complete traumatic amputation of left midfoot
      - ● S98.319   Complete traumatic amputation of unspecified midfoot
    - ● S98.32   Partial traumatic amputation of midfoot
      - ● S98.321   Partial traumatic amputation of right midfoot
      - ● S98.322   Partial traumatic amputation of left midfoot
      - ● S98.329   Partial traumatic amputation of unspecified midfoot
  - ● **S98.9   Traumatic amputation of foot, level unspecified**
    - ● S98.91   Complete traumatic amputation of foot, level unspecified
      - ● S98.911   Complete traumatic amputation of right foot, level unspecified
      - ● S98.912   Complete traumatic amputation of left foot, level unspecified
      - ● S98.919   Complete traumatic amputation of unspecified foot, level unspecified
    - ● S98.92   Partial traumatic amputation of foot, level unspecified
      - ● S98.921   Partial traumatic amputation of right foot, level unspecified
      - ● S98.922   Partial traumatic amputation of left foot, level unspecified
      - ● S98.929   Partial traumatic amputation of unspecified foot, level unspecified

- ● **S99   Other and unspecified injuries of ankle and foot**

  The appropriate 7th character is to be added to each code from category S99

A	initial encounter
D	subsequent encounter
S	sequela

  - ● **S99.8   Other specified injuries of ankle and foot**
    - ● S99.81   Other specified injuries of ankle
      - ● S99.811   Other specified injuries of right ankle
      - ● S99.812   Other specified injuries of left ankle
      - ● S99.819   Other specified injuries of unspecified ankle
    - ● S99.82   Other specified injuries of foot
      - ● S99.821   Other specified injuries of right foot
      - ● S99.822   Other specified injuries of left foot
      - ● S99.829   Other specified injuries of unspecified foot
  - ● **S99.9   Unspecified injury of ankle and foot**
    - ● S99.91   Unspecified injury of ankle
      - ● S99.911   Unspecified injury of right ankle
      - ● S99.912   Unspecified injury of left ankle
      - ● S99.919   Unspecified injury of unspecified ankle
    - ● S99.92   Unspecified injury of foot
      - ● S99.921   Unspecified injury of right foot
      - ● S99.922   Unspecified injury of left foot
      - ● S99.929   Unspecified injury of unspecified foot

CHAPTER 19 (S00–T88)

◀ New   ◀▥ Revised   ~~deleted~~ Deleted   **OGCR** Official Guidelines   X Assign placeholder X   ● Use Additional Character(s)

| Excludes 1 | Excludes 2 | Includes | Use additional | Code first | Code also | Unspecified |

INJURY, POISONING AND CERTAIN OTHER CONSEQUENCES OF EXTERNAL CAUSES (T07-T88)

INJURIES INVOLVING MULTIPLE BODY REGIONS (T07)

Excludes1   burns and corrosions (T20-T32)
frostbite (T33-T34)
insect bite or sting, venomous (T63.4)
sunburn (L55.-)

T07   Unspecified multiple injuries

Excludes1   injury NOS (T14)

INJURY OF UNSPECIFIED BODY REGION (T14)

● T14   Injury of unspecified body region

Excludes1   multiple unspecified injuries (T07)

T14.8   Other injury of unspecified body region
Abrasion NOS   Fracture NOS
Contusion NOS   Skin injury NOS
Crush injury NOS   Vascular injury NOS

● T14.9   Unspecified injury

T14.90   Injury, unspecified
Injury NOS

T14.91   Suicide attempt
Attempted suicide NOS

EFFECTS OF FOREIGN BODY ENTERING THROUGH NATURAL ORIFICE (T15-T19)

Excludes2   foreign body accidentally left in operation wound (T81.5-)
foreign body in penetrating wound - see open wound by body region
residual foreign body in soft tissue (M79.5)
splinter, without open wound - see superficial injury by body region

● T15   Foreign body on external eye

Excludes2   foreign body in penetrating wound of orbit and eye ball (S05.4-, S05.5-)
open wound of eyelid and periocular area (S01.1-)
retained foreign body in eyelid (H02.8-)
retained (old) foreign body in penetrating wound of orbit and eye ball (H05.5-, H44.6-, H44.7-)
superficial foreign body of eyelid and periocular area (S00.25-)

The appropriate 7th character is to be added to each code from category T15

A	initial encounter
D	subsequent encounter
S	sequela

● T15.0   Foreign body in cornea
X ● T15.00   Foreign body in cornea, unspecified eye
X ● T15.01   Foreign body in cornea, right eye
X ● T15.02   Foreign body in cornea, left eye
● T15.1   Foreign body in conjunctival sac
X ● T15.10   Foreign body in conjunctival sac, unspecified eye
X ● T15.11   Foreign body in conjunctival sac, right eye
X ● T15.12   Foreign body in conjunctival sac, left eye
● T15.8   Foreign body in other and multiple parts of external eye
Foreign body in lacrimal punctum
X ● T15.80   Foreign body in other and multiple parts of external eye, unspecified eye
X ● T15.81   Foreign body in other and multiple parts of external eye, right eye
X ● T15.82   Foreign body in other and multiple parts of external eye, left eye

● T15.9   Foreign body on external eye, part unspecified
X ● T15.90   Foreign body on external eye, part unspecified, unspecified eye
X ● T15.91   Foreign body on external eye, part unspecified, right eye
X ● T15.92   Foreign body on external eye, part unspecified, left eye

● T16   Foreign body in ear

Includes   foreign body in auditory canal

The appropriate 7th character is to be added to each code from category T16

A	initial encounter
D	subsequent encounter
S	sequela

X ● T16.1   Foreign body in right ear
X ● T16.2   Foreign body in left ear
X ● T16.9   Foreign body in ear, unspecified ear

● T17   Foreign body in respiratory tract

The appropriate 7th character is to be added to each code from category T17

A	initial encounter
D	subsequent encounter
S	sequela

X ● T17.0   Foreign body in nasal sinus
X ● T17.1   Foreign body in nostril
Foreign body in nose NOS
● T17.2   Foreign body in pharynx
Foreign body in nasopharynx
Foreign body in throat NOS
● T17.20   Unspecified foreign body in pharynx
● T17.200   Unspecified foreign body in pharynx causing asphyxiation
● T17.208   Unspecified foreign body in pharynx causing other injury
● T17.21   Gastric contents in pharynx
Aspiration of gastric contents into pharynx
Vomitus in pharynx
● T17.210   Gastric contents in pharynx causing asphyxiation
● T17.218   Gastric contents in pharynx causing other injury
● T17.22   Food in pharynx
Bones in pharynx
Seeds in pharynx
● T17.220   Food in pharynx causing asphyxiation
● T17.228   Food in pharynx causing other injury
● T17.29   Other foreign object in pharynx
● T17.290   Other foreign object in pharynx causing asphyxiation
● T17.298   Other foreign object in pharynx causing other injury
● T17.3   Foreign body in larynx
● T17.30   Unspecified foreign body in larynx
● T17.300   Unspecified foreign body in larynx causing asphyxiation
● T17.308   Unspecified foreign body in larynx causing other injury
● T17.31   Gastric contents in larynx
Aspiration of gastric contents into larynx
Vomitus in larynx
● T17.310   Gastric contents in larynx causing asphyxiation
● T17.318   Gastric contents in larynx causing other injury

◄ New   ◄≡ Revised   ~~deleted~~ Deleted   OGCR Official Guidelines   X Assign placeholder X   ● Use Additional Character(s)

Excludes 1   Excludes 2   Includes   Use additional   Code first   Code also   Unspecified

CHAPTER 19 (S00-T88)

- **T17.32**   **Food in larynx**
  Bones in larynx
  Seeds in larynx
  - **T17.320**   Food in larynx causing asphyxiation
  - **T17.328**   Food in larynx causing other injury
- **T17.39**   **Other foreign object in larynx**
  - **T17.390**   Other foreign object in larynx causing asphyxiation
  - **T17.398**   Other foreign object in larynx causing other injury
- **T17.4**   **Foreign body in trachea**
  - **T17.40**   Unspecified foreign body in trachea
    - **T17.400**   Unspecified foreign body in trachea causing asphyxiation
    - **T17.408**   Unspecified foreign body in trachea causing other injury
  - **T17.41**   Gastric contents in trachea
    Aspiration of gastric contents into trachea
    Vomitus in trachea
    - **T17.410**   Gastric contents in trachea causing asphyxiation
    - **T17.418**   Gastric contents in trachea causing other injury
  - **T17.42**   Food in trachea
    Bones in trachea
    Seeds in trachea
    - **T17.420**   Food in trachea causing asphyxiation
    - **T17.428**   Food in trachea causing other injury
  - **T17.49**   Other foreign object in trachea
    - **T17.490**   Other foreign object in trachea causing asphyxiation
    - **T17.498**   Other foreign object in trachea causing other injury
- **T17.5**   **Foreign body in bronchus**
  - **T17.50**   Unspecified foreign body in bronchus
    - **T17.500**   Unspecified foreign body in bronchus causing asphyxiation
    - **T17.508**   Unspecified foreign body in bronchus causing other injury
  - **T17.51**   Gastric contents in bronchus
    Aspiration of gastric contents into bronchus
    Vomitus in bronchus
    - **T17.510**   Gastric contents in bronchus causing asphyxiation
    - **T17.518**   Gastric contents in bronchus causing other injury
  - **T17.52**   Food in bronchus
    Bones in bronchus
    Seeds in bronchus
    - **T17.520**   Food in bronchus causing asphyxiation
    - **T17.528**   Food in bronchus causing other injury
  - **T17.59**   Other foreign object in bronchus
    - **T17.590**   Other foreign object in bronchus causing asphyxiation
    - **T17.598**   Other foreign object in bronchus causing other injury

- **T17.8**   **Foreign body in other parts of respiratory tract**
  Foreign body in bronchioles
  Foreign body in lung
  - **T17.80**   Unspecified foreign body in other parts of respiratory tract
    - **T17.800**   Unspecified foreign body in other parts of respiratory tract causing asphyxiation
    - **T17.808**   Unspecified foreign body in other parts of respiratory tract causing other injury
  - **T17.81**   Gastric contents in other parts of respiratory tract
    Aspiration of gastric contents into other parts of respiratory tract
    Vomitus in other parts of respiratory tract
    - **T17.810**   Gastric contents in other parts of respiratory tract causing asphyxiation
    - **T17.818**   Gastric contents in other parts of respiratory tract causing other injury
  - **T17.82**   Food in other parts of respiratory tract
    Bones in other parts of respiratory tract
    Seeds in other parts of respiratory tract
    - **T17.820**   Food in other parts of respiratory tract causing asphyxiation
    - **T17.828**   Food in other parts of respiratory tract causing other injury
  - **T17.89**   Other foreign object in other parts of respiratory tract
    - **T17.890**   Other foreign object in other parts of respiratory tract causing asphyxiation
    - **T17.898**   Other foreign object in other parts of respiratory tract causing other injury
- **T17.9**   **Foreign body in respiratory tract, part unspecified**
  - **T17.90**   Unspecified foreign body in respiratory tract, part unspecified
    - **T17.900**   Unspecified foreign body in respiratory tract, part unspecified causing asphyxiation
    - **T17.908**   Unspecified foreign body in respiratory tract, part unspecified causing other injury
  - **T17.91**   Gastric contents in respiratory tract, part unspecified
    Aspiration of gastric contents into respiratory tract, part unspecified
    Vomitus in trachea respiratory tract, part unspecified
    - **T17.910**   Gastric contents in respiratory tract, part unspecified causing asphyxiation
    - **T17.918**   Gastric contents in respiratory tract, part unspecified causing other injury
  - **T17.92**   Food in respiratory tract, part unspecified
    Bones in respiratory tract, part unspecified
    Seeds in respiratory tract, part unspecified
    - **T17.920**   Food in respiratory tract, part unspecified causing asphyxiation
    - **T17.928**   Food in respiratory tract, part unspecified causing other injury
  - **T17.99**   Other foreign object in respiratory tract, part unspecified
    - **T17.990**   Other foreign object in respiratory tract, part unspecified in causing asphyxiation
    - **T17.998**   Other foreign object in respiratory tract, part unspecified causing other injury

---

◀ New   ◀▥ Revised   ~~deleted~~ Deleted   **OGCR** Official Guidelines   X Assign placeholder X   ● Use Additional Character(s)

| Excludes 1 | Excludes 2 | Includes | Use additional | Code first | Code also | Unspecified |

CHAPTER 19 (S00-T88)

● **T18**   **Foreign body in alimentary tract**

> Excludes2   foreign body in pharynx (T17.2-)

The appropriate 7th character is to be added to each code from category T18

> A   initial encounter
> D   subsequent encounter
> S   sequela

X ● **T18.0**   **Foreign body in mouth**

X ● **T18.1**   **Foreign body in esophagus**

> Excludes2   foreign body in respiratory tract (T17.-)

  ● **T18.10**   **Unspecified foreign body in esophagus**

    ● **T18.100**   **Unspecified foreign body in esophagus causing compression of trachea**
        Unspecified foreign body in esophagus causing obstruction of respiration

    ● **T18.108**   **Unspecified foreign body in esophagus causing other injury**

  ● **T18.11**   **Gastric contents in esophagus**
    Vomitus in esophagus

    ● **T18.110**   **Gastric contents in esophagus causing compression of trachea**
        Gastric contents in esophagus causing obstruction of respiration

    ● **T18.118**   **Gastric contents in esophagus causing other injury**

  ● **T18.12**   **Food in esophagus**
    Bones in esophagus
    Seeds in esophagus

    ● **T18.120**   **Food in esophagus causing compression of trachea**
        Food in esophagus causing obstruction of respiration

    ● **T18.128**   **Food in esophagus causing other injury**

  ● **T18.19**   **Other foreign object in esophagus**

    ● **T18.190**   **Other foreign object in esophagus causing compression of trachea**
        Other foreign body in esophagus causing obstruction of respiration

    ● **T18.198**   **Other foreign object in esophagus causing other injury**

X ● **T18.2**   **Foreign body in stomach**

X ● **T18.3**   **Foreign body in small intestine**

X ● **T18.4**   **Foreign body in colon**

X ● **T18.5**   **Foreign body in anus and rectum**
    Foreign body in rectosigmoid (junction)

X ● **T18.8**   **Foreign body in other parts of alimentary tract**

X ● **T18.9**   **Foreign body of alimentary tract, part unspecified**
    Foreign body in digestive system NOS
    Swallowed foreign body NOS

● **T19**   **Foreign body in genitourinary tract**

> Excludes2   complications due to implanted mesh (T83.7-)
> mechanical complications of contraceptive device (intrauterine) (vaginal) (T83.3-)
> presence of contraceptive device (intrauterine) (vaginal) (Z97.5)

The appropriate 7th character is to be added to each code from category T19

> A   initial encounter
> D   subsequent encounter
> S   sequela

X ● **T19.0**   **Foreign body in urethra**

X ● **T19.1**   **Foreign body in bladder**

X ● **T19.2**   **Foreign body in vulva and vagina**

X ● **T19.3**   **Foreign body in uterus**

X ● **T19.4**   **Foreign body in penis**

X ● **T19.8**   **Foreign body in other parts of genitourinary tract**

X ● **T19.9**   **Foreign body in genitourinary tract, part unspecified**

BURNS AND CORROSIONS (T20-T32)

> Includes   burns (thermal) from electrical heating appliances
> burns (thermal) from electricity
> burns (thermal) from flame
> burns (thermal) from friction
> burns (thermal) from hot air and hot gases
> burns (thermal) from hot objects
> burns (thermal) from lightning
> burns (thermal) from radiation chemical
> burn [corrosion] (external) (internal) scalds

> Excludes2   erythema [dermatitis] ab igne (L59.0)
> radiation-related disorders of the skin and subcutaneous tissue (L55-L59)
> sunburn (L55.-)

OGCR Section I.C.19.d.

Burns and Corrosions

The ICD-10-CM makes a distinction between burn and corrosions. The burn codes are for thermal burns, except sunburns, that come from a heat source, such as a fire or hot appliance. The burn codes are also for burns resulting from electricity and radiation. Corrosions are burns due to chemicals. The guidelines for burns and corrosions are the same.

Current burns (T20-T25) are classified by depth, extent and by agent (X code). Burns are classified by depth as first degree (erythema), second degree (blistering), and third degree (full-thickness involvement). Burns of the eye and internal organs (T26-T28) are classified by site, but not by degree.

1) Sequencing of burn and related condition codes

Sequence first the code that reflects the highest degree of burn when more than one burn is present.

a. When the reason for the admission or encounter is for treatment of external multiple burns, sequence first the code that reflects the burn of the highest degree.

b. When a patient has both internal and external burns, the circumstances of admission govern the selection of the principal diagnosis or first-listed diagnosis.

c. When a patient is admitted for burn injuries and other related conditions such as smoke inhalation and/or respiratory failure, the circumstances of admission govern the selection of the principal or first-listed diagnosis.

2) Burns of the same local site

Classify burns of the same local site (three-character category level, T20-T28) but of different degrees to the subcategory identifying the highest degree recorded in the diagnosis.

Figure 19-14 **A.** Second-degree burn. **B.** Third-degree burn. (From Cummings: Otolaryngology: Head & Neck Surgery, ed 4, Mosby, 2005)

BURNS AND CORROSIONS OF EXTERNAL BODY SURFACE, SPECIFIED BY SITE (T20-T25)

Includes   burns and corrosions of first degree [erythema]
burns and corrosions of second degree [blisters] [epidermal loss]
burns and corrosions of third degree [deep necrosis of underlying tissue] [full-thickness skin loss]

Use additional code from category T31 or T32 to identify extent of body surface involved

● **T20**   **Burn and corrosion of head, face, and neck**

Excludes2   burn and corrosion of ear drum (T28.41, T28.91)
burn and corrosion of eye and adnexa (T26.-)
burn and corrosion of mouth and pharynx (T28.0)

The appropriate 7th character is to be added to each code from category T20

     A   initial encounter
     D   subsequent encounter
     S   sequela

● **T20.0**   **Burn of unspecified degree of head, face, and neck**

Use additional external cause code to identify the source, place and intent of the burn (X00-X19, X75-X77, X96-X98, Y92)

X ● **T20.00**   Burn of unspecified degree of head, face, and neck, unspecified site

● **T20.01**   Burn of unspecified degree of ear [any part, except ear drum]

Excludes2   burn of ear drum (T28.41-)

● **T20.011**   Burn of unspecified degree of right ear [any part, except ear drum]

● **T20.012**   Burn of unspecified degree of left ear [any part, except ear drum]

● **T20.019**   Burn of unspecified degree of unspecified ear [any part, except ear drum]

X ● **T20.02**   Burn of unspecified degree of lip(s)

X ● **T20.03**   Burn of unspecified degree of chin

X ● **T20.04**   Burn of unspecified degree of nose (septum)

X ● **T20.05**   Burn of unspecified degree of scalp [any part]

X ● **T20.06**   Burn of unspecified degree of forehead and cheek

X ● **T20.07**   Burn of unspecified degree of neck

X ● **T20.09**   Burn of unspecified degree of multiple sites of head, face, and neck

● **T20.1**   **Burn of first degree of head, face, and neck**

Use additional external cause code to identify the source, place and intent of the burn (X00-X19, X75-X77, X96-X98, Y92)

X ● **T20.10**   Burn of first degree of head, face, and neck, unspecified site

● **T20.11**   Burn of first degree of ear [any part, except ear drum]

Excludes2   burn of ear drum (T28.41-)

● **T20.111**   Burn of first degree of right ear [any part, except ear drum]

● **T20.112**   Burn of first degree of left ear [any part, except ear drum]

● **T20.119**   Burn of first degree of unspecified ear [any part, except ear drum]

X ● **T20.12**   Burn of first degree of lip(s)

X ● **T20.13**   Burn of first degree of chin

X ● **T20.14**   Burn of first degree of nose (septum)

X ● **T20.15**   Burn of first degree of scalp [any part]

X ● **T20.16**   Burn of first degree of forehead and cheek

X ● **T20.17**   Burn of first degree of neck

X ● **T20.19**   Burn of first degree of multiple sites of head, face, and neck

● **T20.2**   **Burn of second degree of head, face, and neck**

Use additional external cause code to identify the source, place and intent of the burn (X00-X19, X75-X77, X96-X98, Y92)

X ● **T20.20**   Burn of second degree of head, face, and neck, unspecified site

● **T20.21**   Burn of second degree of ear [any part, except ear drum]

Excludes2   burn of ear drum (T28.41-)

● **T20.211**   Burn of second degree of right ear [any part, except ear drum]

● **T20.212**   Burn of second degree of left ear [any part, except ear drum]

● **T20.219**   Burn of second degree of unspecified ear [any part, except ear drum]

X ● **T20.22**   Burn of second degree of lip(s)

X ● **T20.23**   Burn of second degree of chin

X ● **T20.24**   Burn of second degree of nose (septum)

X ● **T20.25**   Burn of second degree of scalp [any part]

X ● **T20.26**   Burn of second degree of forehead and cheek

X ● **T20.27**   Burn of second degree of neck

X ● **T20.29**   Burn of second degree of multiple sites of head, face, and neck

● **T20.3**   **Burn of third degree of head, face, and neck**

Use additional external cause code to identify the source, place and intent of the burn (X00-X19, X75-X77, X96-X98, Y92)

X ● **T20.30**   Burn of third degree of head, face, and neck, unspecified site

● **T20.31**   Burn of third degree of ear [any part, except ear drum]

Excludes2   burn of ear drum (T28.41-)

● **T20.311**   Burn of third degree of right ear [any part, except ear drum]

● **T20.312**   Burn of third degree of left ear [any part, except ear drum]

● **T20.319**   Burn of third degree of unspecified ear [any part, except ear drum]

X ● **T20.32**　Burn of third degree of lip(s)

X ● **T20.33**　Burn of third degree of chin

X ● **T20.34**　Burn of third degree of nose (septum)

X ● **T20.35**　Burn of third degree of scalp [any part]

X ● **T20.36**　Burn of third degree of forehead and cheek

X ● **T20.37**　Burn of third degree of neck

X ● **T20.39**　Burn of third degree of multiple sites of head, face, and neck

● **T20.4**　Corrosion of unspecified degree of head, face, and neck

Code first (T51-T65) to identify chemical and intent

Use additional external cause code to identify place (Y92)

X ● **T20.40**　Corrosion of unspecified degree of head, face, and neck, unspecified site

● **T20.41**　Corrosion of unspecified degree of ear [any part, except ear drum]

Excludes2　corrosion of ear drum (T28.91-)

● **T20.411**　Corrosion of unspecified degree of right ear [any part, except ear drum]

● **T20.412**　Corrosion of unspecified degree of left ear [any part, except ear drum]

● **T20.419**　Corrosion of unspecified degree of unspecified ear [any part, except ear drum]

X ● **T20.42**　Corrosion of unspecified degree of lip(s)

X ● **T20.43**　Corrosion of unspecified degree of chin

X ● **T20.44**　Corrosion of unspecified degree of nose (septum)

X ● **T20.45**　Corrosion of unspecified degree of scalp [any part]

X ● **T20.46**　Corrosion of unspecified degree of forehead and cheek

X ● **T20.47**　Corrosion of unspecified degree of neck

X ● **T20.49**　Corrosion of unspecified degree of multiple sites of head, face, and neck

● **T20.5**　Corrosion of first degree of head, face, and neck

Code first (T51-T65) to identify chemical and intent

Use additional external cause code to identify place (Y92)

X ● **T20.50**　Corrosion of first degree of head, face, and neck, unspecified site

● **T20.51**　Corrosion of first degree of ear [any part, except ear drum]

Excludes2　corrosion of ear drum (T28.91-)

● **T20.511**　Corrosion of first degree of right ear [any part, except ear drum]

● **T20.512**　Corrosion of first degree of left ear [any part, except ear drum]

● **T20.519**　Corrosion of first degree of unspecified ear [any part, except ear drum]

X ● **T20.52**　Corrosion of first degree of lip(s)

X ● **T20.53**　Corrosion of first degree of chin

X ● **T20.54**　Corrosion of first degree of nose (septum)

X ● **T20.55**　Corrosion of first degree of scalp [any part]

X ● **T20.56**　Corrosion of first degree of forehead and cheek

X ● **T20.57**　Corrosion of first degree of neck

X ● **T20.59**　Corrosion of first degree of multiple sites of head, face, and neck

● **T20.6**　Corrosion of second degree of head, face, and neck

Code first (T51-T65) to identify chemical and intent

Use additional external cause code to identify place (Y92)

X ● **T20.60**　Corrosion of second degree of head, face, and neck, unspecified site

● **T20.61**　Corrosion of second degree of ear [any part, except ear drum]

Excludes2　corrosion of ear drum (T28.91-)

● **T20.611**　Corrosion of second degree of right ear [any part, except ear drum]

● **T20.612**　Corrosion of second degree of left ear [any part, except ear drum]

● **T20.619**　Corrosion of second degree of unspecified ear [any part, except ear drum]

X ● **T20.62**　Corrosion of second degree of lip(s)

X ● **T20.63**　Corrosion of second degree of chin

X ● **T20.64**　Corrosion of second degree of nose (septum)

X ● **T20.65**　Corrosion of second degree of scalp [any part]

X ● **T20.66**　Corrosion of second degree of forehead and cheek

X ● **T20.67**　Corrosion of second degree of neck

X ● **T20.69**　Corrosion of second degree of multiple sites of head, face, and neck

● **T20.7**　Corrosion of third degree of head, face, and neck

Code first (T51-T65) to identify chemical and intent

Use additional external cause code to identify place (Y92)

X ● **T20.70**　Corrosion of third degree of head, face, and neck, unspecified site

● **T20.71**　Corrosion of third degree of ear [any part, except ear drum]

Excludes2　corrosion of ear drum (T28.91-)

● **T20.711**　Corrosion of third degree of right ear [any part, except ear drum]

● **T20.712**　Corrosion of third degree of left ear [any part, except ear drum]

● **T20.719**　Corrosion of third degree of unspecified ear [any part, except ear drum]

X ● **T20.72**　Corrosion of third degree of lip(s)

X ● **T20.73**　Corrosion of third degree of chin

X ● **T20.74**　Corrosion of third degree of nose (septum)

X ● **T20.75**　Corrosion of third degree of scalp [any part]

X ● **T20.76**　Corrosion of third degree of forehead and cheek

X ● **T20.77**　Corrosion of third degree of neck

X ● **T20.79**　Corrosion of third degree of multiple sites of head, face, and neck

● **T21** **Burn and corrosion of trunk**

 ⬛ Includes burns and corrosion of hip region

 ☐ Excludes2 burns and corrosion of axilla (T22.- with fifth
 character 4)
 burns and corrosion of scapular region
 (T22.- with fifth character 6)
 burns and corrosion of shoulder (T22.- with fifth
 character 5)

 The appropriate 7th character is to be added to each code from
 category T21

 > A initial encounter
 > D subsequent encounter
 > S sequela

● **T21.0** **Burn of unspecified degree of trunk**

 Use additional external cause code to identify the
 source, place and intent of the burn (X00-X19,
 X75-X77, X96-X98, Y92)

 X● **T21.00** **Burn of unspecified degree of trunk,
 unspecified site**

 X● **T21.01** **Burn of unspecified degree of chest wall**
 Burn of of unspecified degree of breast

 X● **T21.02** **Burn of unspecified degree of abdominal wall**
 Burn of unspecified degree of flank
 Burn of unspecified degree of groin

 X● **T21.03** **Burn of unspecified degree of upper back**
 Burn of unspecified degree of interscapular
 region

 X● **T21.04** **Burn of unspecified degree of lower back**

 X● **T21.05** **Burn of unspecified degree of buttock**
 Burn of unspecified degree of anus

 X● **T21.06** **Burn of unspecified degree of male genital
 region**
 Burn of unspecified degree of penis
 Burn of unspecified degree of scrotum
 Burn of unspecified degree of testis

 X● **T21.07** **Burn of unspecified degree of female genital
 region**
 Burn of unspecified degree of labium (majus)
 (minus)
 Burn of unspecified degree of perineum
 Burn of unspecified degree of vulva

 ☐ Excludes2 burn of vagina (T28.3)

 X● **T21.09** **Burn of unspecified degree of other site of
 trunk**

● **T21.1** **Burn of first degree of trunk**

 Use additional external cause code to identify the
 source, place and intent of the burn (X00-X19,
 X75-X77, X96-X98, Y92)

 X● **T21.10** **Burn of first degree of trunk, unspecified site**

 X● **T21.11** **Burn of first degree of chest wall**
 Burn of first degree of breast

 X● **T21.12** **Burn of first degree of abdominal wall**
 Burn of first degree of flank
 Burn of first degree of groin

 X● **T21.13** **Burn of first degree of upper back**
 Burn of first degree of interscapular region

 X● **T21.14** **Burn of first degree of lower back**

 X● **T21.15** **Burn of first degree of buttock**
 Burn of first degree of anus

 X● **T21.16** **Burn of first degree of male genital region**
 Burn of first degree of penis
 Burn of first degree of scrotum
 Burn of first degree of testis

 X● **T21.17** **Burn of first degree of female genital region**
 Burn of first degree of labium (majus) (minus)
 Burn of first degree of perineum
 Burn of first degree of vulva

 ☐ Excludes2 burn of vagina (T28.3)

 X● **T21.19** **Burn of first degree of other site of trunk**

● **T21.2** **Burn of second degree of trunk**

 Use additional external cause code to identify the
 source, place and intent of the burn (X00-X19,
 X75-X77, X96-X98, Y92)

 X● **T21.20** **Burn of second degree of trunk, unspecified site**

 X● **T21.21** **Burn of second degree of chest wall**
 Burn of second degree of breast

 X● **T21.22** **Burn of second degree of abdominal wall**
 Burn of second degree of flank
 Burn of second degree of groin

 X● **T21.23** **Burn of second degree of upper back**
 Burn of second degree of interscapular region

 X● **T21.24** **Burn of second degree of lower back**

 X● **T21.25** **Burn of second degree of buttock**
 Burn of second degree of anus

 X● **T21.26** **Burn of second degree of male genital region**
 Burn of second degree of penis
 Burn of second degree of scrotum
 Burn of second degree of testis

 X● **T21.27** **Burn of second degree of female genital region**
 Burn of second degree of labium (majus)
 (minus)
 Burn of second degree of perineum
 Burn of second degree of vulva

 ☐ Excludes2 burn of vagina (T28.3)

 X● **T21.29** **Burn of second degree of other site of trunk**

● **T21.3** **Burn of third degree of trunk**

 Use additional external cause code to identify the
 source, place and intent of the burn (X00-X19,
 X75-X77, X96-X98, Y92)

 X● **T21.30** **Burn of third degree of trunk, unspecified site**

 X● **T21.31** **Burn of third degree of chest wall**
 Burn of third degree of breast

 X● **T21.32** **Burn of third degree of abdominal wall**
 Burn of third degree of flank
 Burn of third degree of groin

 X● **T21.33** **Burn of third degree of upper back**
 Burn of third degree of interscapular region

 X● **T21.34** **Burn of third degree of lower back**

 X● **T21.35** **Burn of third degree of buttock**
 Burn of third degree of anus

 X● **T21.36** **Burn of third degree of male genital region**
 Burn of third degree of penis
 Burn of third degree of scrotum
 Burn of third degree of testis

 X● **T21.37** **Burn of third degree of female genital region**
 Burn of third degree of labium (majus) (minus)
 Burn of third degree of perineum
 Burn of third degree of vulva

 ☐ Excludes2 burn of vagina (T28.3)

 X● **T21.39** **Burn of third degree of other site of trunk**

● **T21.4** **Corrosion of unspecified degree of trunk**

 Code first (T51-T65) to identify chemical and intent
 Use additional external cause code to identify
 place (Y92)

 X● **T21.40** **Corrosion of unspecified degree of trunk,
 unspecified site**

 X● **T21.41** **Corrosion of unspecified degree of chest wall**
 Corrosion of unspecified degree of breast

 X● **T21.42** **Corrosion of unspecified degree of abdominal
 wall**
 Corrosion of unspecified degree of flank
 Corrosion of unspecified degree of groin

 X● **T21.43** **Corrosion of unspecified degree of upper back**
 Corrosion of unspecified degree of
 interscapular region

◀ New ◀▥ Revised ~~deleted~~ Deleted **OGCR** Official Guidelines X Assign placeholder X ● Use Additional Character(s)

☐ Excludes 1 ☐ Excludes 2 ⬛ Includes ⬛ Use additional ⬛ Code first ⬛ Code also ⬛ Unspecified

CHAPTER 19 (S00-T88)

X● **T21.44**   **Corrosion of** unspecified **degree of lower back**

X● **T21.45**   **Corrosion of** unspecified **degree of buttock**
      Corrosion of unspecified degree of anus

X● **T21.46**   **Corrosion of** unspecified **degree of male genital region**
      Corrosion of unspecified degree of penis
      Corrosion of unspecified degree of scrotum
      Corrosion of unspecified degree of testis

X● **T21.47**   **Corrosion of** unspecified **degree of female genital region**
      Corrosion of unspecified degree of labium (majus) (minus)
      Corrosion of unspecified degree of perineum
      Corrosion of unspecified degree of vulva
      Excludes2   corrosion of vagina (T28.8)

X● **T21.49**   **Corrosion of** unspecified **degree of other site of trunk**

● **T21.5**   **Corrosion of first degree of trunk**
      Code first (T51-T65) to identify chemical and intent
      Use additional external cause code to identify place (Y92)

X● **T21.50**   **Corrosion of first degree of trunk,** unspecified **site**

X● **T21.51**   **Corrosion of first degree of chest wall**
      Corrosion of first degree of breast

X● **T21.52**   **Corrosion of first degree of abdominal wall**
      Corrosion of first degree of flank
      Corrosion of first degree of groin

X● **T21.53**   **Corrosion of first degree of upper back**
      Corrosion of first degree of interscapular region

X● **T21.54**   **Corrosion of first degree of lower back**

X● **T21.55**   **Corrosion of first degree of buttock**
      Corrosion of first degree of anus

X● **T21.56**   **Corrosion of first degree of male genital region**
      Corrosion of first degree of penis
      Corrosion of first degree of scrotum
      Corrosion of first degree of testis

X● **T21.57**   **Corrosion of first degree of female genital region**
      Corrosion of first degree of labium (majus) (minus)
      Corrosion of first degree of perineum
      Corrosion of first degree of vulva
      Excludes2   corrosion of vagina (T28.8)

X● **T21.59**   **Corrosion of first degree of other site of trunk**

● **T21.6**   **Corrosion of second degree of trunk**
      Code first (T51-T65) to identify chemical and intent
      Use additional external cause code to identify place (Y92)

X● **T21.60**   **Corrosion of second degree of trunk,** unspecified **site**

X● **T21.61**   **Corrosion of second degree of chest wall**
      Corrosion of second degree of breast

X● **T21.62**   **Corrosion of second degree of abdominal wall**
      Corrosion of second degree of flank
      Corrosion of second degree of groin

X● **T21.63**   **Corrosion of second degree of upper back**
      Corrosion of second degree of interscapular region

X● **T21.64**   **Corrosion of second degree of lower back**

X● **T21.65**   **Corrosion of second degree of buttock**
      Corrosion of second degree of anus

X● **T21.66**   **Corrosion of second degree of male genital region**
      Corrosion of second degree of penis
      Corrosion of second degree of scrotum
      Corrosion of second degree of testis

X● **T21.67**   **Corrosion of second degree of female genital region**
      Corrosion of second degree of labium (majus) (minus)
      Corrosion of second degree of perineum
      Corrosion of second degree of vulva
      Excludes2   corrosion of vagina (T28.8)

X● **T21.69**   **Corrosion of second degree of other site of trunk**

● **T21.7**   **Corrosion of third degree of trunk**
      Code first (T51-T65) to identify chemical and intent
      Use additional external cause code to identify place (Y92)

X● **T21.70**   **Corrosion of third degree of trunk,** unspecified **site**

X● **T21.71**   **Corrosion of third degree of chest wall**
      Corrosion of third degree of breast

X● **T21.72**   **Corrosion of third degree of abdominal wall**
      Corrosion of third degree of flank
      Corrosion of third degree of groin

X● **T21.73**   **Corrosion of third degree of upper back**
      Corrosion of third degree of interscapular region

X● **T21.74**   **Corrosion of third degree of lower back**

X● **T21.75**   **Corrosion of third degree of buttock**
      Corrosion of third degree of anus

X● **T21.76**   **Corrosion of third degree of male genital region**
      Corrosion of third degree of penis
      Corrosion of third degree of scrotum
      Corrosion of third degree of testis

X● **T21.77**   **Corrosion of third degree of female genital region**
      Corrosion of third degree of labium (majus) (minus)
      Corrosion of third degree of perineum
      Corrosion of third degree of vulva
      Excludes2   corrosion of vagina (T28.8)

X● **T21.79**   **Corrosion of third degree of other site of trunk**

● **T22**   **Burn and corrosion of shoulder and upper limb, except wrist and hand**
      Excludes2   burn and corrosion of interscapular region (T21.-)
                  burn and corrosion of wrist and hand (T23.-)

      The appropriate 7th character is to be added to each code from category T22

A	initial encounter
D	subsequent encounter
S	sequela

● **T22.0**   **Burn of unspecified degree of shoulder and upper limb, except wrist and hand**
      Use additional external cause code to identify the source, place and intent of the burn (X00-X19, X75-X77, X96-X98, Y92)

X● **T22.00**   **Burn of** unspecified **degree of shoulder and upper limb, except wrist and hand, unspecified site**

● **T22.01**   **Burn of unspecified degree of forearm**

● **T22.011**   **Burn of** unspecified **degree of right forearm**

● **T22.012**   **Burn of** unspecified **degree of left forearm**

● **T22.019**   **Burn of** unspecified **degree of unspecified forearm**

● **T22.02**   **Burn of unspecified degree of elbow**

● **T22.021**   **Burn of** unspecified **degree of right elbow**

● **T22.022**   **Burn of** unspecified **degree of left elbow**

● **T22.029**   **Burn of** unspecified **degree of unspecified elbow**

◀ New   ◀️ Revised   ~~deleted~~ Deleted   **OGCR** Official Guidelines   X Assign placeholder X   ● Use Additional Character(s)

Excludes 1   Excludes 2   Includes   Use additional   Code first   Code also   Unspecified

● T22.03   Burn of unspecified degree of upper arm
    ● T22.031   Burn of unspecified degree of right upper arm
    ● T22.032   Burn of unspecified degree of left upper arm
    ● T22.039   Burn of unspecified degree of unspecified upper arm
● T22.04   Burn of unspecified degree of axilla
    ● T22.041   Burn of unspecified degree of right axilla
    ● T22.042   Burn of unspecified degree of left axilla
    ● T22.049   Burn of unspecified degree of unspecified axilla
● T22.05   Burn of unspecified degree of shoulder
    ● T22.051   Burn of unspecified degree of right shoulder
    ● T22.052   Burn of unspecified degree of left shoulder
    ● T22.059   Burn of unspecified degree of unspecified shoulder
● T22.06   Burn of unspecified degree of scapular region
    ● T22.061   Burn of unspecified degree of right scapular region
    ● T22.062   Burn of unspecified degree of left scapular region
    ● T22.069   Burn of unspecified degree of unspecified scapular region
● T22.09   Burn of unspecified degree of multiple sites of shoulder and upper limb, except wrist and hand
    ● T22.091   Burn of unspecified degree of multiple sites of right shoulder and upper limb, except wrist and hand
    ● T22.092   Burn of unspecified degree of multiple sites of left shoulder and upper limb, except wrist and hand
    ● T22.099   Burn of unspecified degree of multiple sites of unspecified shoulder and upper limb, except wrist and hand
● T22.1   Burn of first degree of shoulder and upper limb, except wrist and hand
    Use additional external cause code to identify the source, place and intent of the burn (X00-X19, X75-X77, X96-X98, Y92)
X ● T22.10   Burn of first degree of shoulder and upper limb, except wrist and hand, unspecified site
● T22.11   Burn of first degree of forearm
    ● T22.111   Burn of first degree of right forearm
    ● T22.112   Burn of first degree of left forearm
    ● T22.119   Burn of first degree of unspecified forearm
● T22.12   Burn of first degree of elbow
    ● T22.121   Burn of first degree of right elbow
    ● T22.122   Burn of first degree of left elbow
    ● T22.129   Burn of first degree of unspecified elbow
● T22.13   Burn of first degree of upper arm
    ● T22.131   Burn of first degree of right upper arm
    ● T22.132   Burn of first degree of left upper arm
    ● T22.139   Burn of first degree of unspecified upper arm
● T22.14   Burn of first degree of axilla
    ● T22.141   Burn of first degree of right axilla
    ● T22.142   Burn of first degree of left axilla
    ● T22.149   Burn of first degree of unspecified axilla

● T22.15   Burn of first degree of shoulder
    ● T22.151   Burn of first degree of right shoulder
    ● T22.152   Burn of first degree of left shoulder
    ● T22.159   Burn of first degree of unspecified shoulder
● T22.16   Burn of first degree of scapular region
    ● T22.161   Burn of first degree of right scapular region
    ● T22.162   Burn of first degree of left scapular region
    ● T22.169   Burn of first degree of unspecified scapular region
● T22.19   Burn of first degree of multiple sites of shoulder and upper limb, except wrist and hand
    ● T22.191   Burn of first degree of multiple sites of right shoulder and upper limb, except wrist and hand
    ● T22.192   Burn of first degree of multiple sites of left shoulder and upper limb, except wrist and hand
    ● T22.199   Burn of first degree of multiple sites of unspecified shoulder and upper limb, except wrist and hand
● T22.2   Burn of second degree of shoulder and upper limb, except wrist and hand
    Use additional external cause code to identify the source, place and intent of the burn (X00-X19, X75-X77, X96-X98, Y92)
X ● T22.20   Burn of second degree of shoulder and upper limb, except wrist and hand, unspecified site
● T22.21   Burn of second degree of forearm
    ● T22.211   Burn of second degree of right forearm
    ● T22.212   Burn of second degree of left forearm
    ● T22.219   Burn of second degree of unspecified forearm
● T22.22   Burn of second degree of elbow
    ● T22.221   Burn of second degree of right elbow
    ● T22.222   Burn of second degree of left elbow
    ● T22.229   Burn of second degree of unspecified elbow
● T22.23   Burn of second degree of upper arm
    ● T22.231   Burn of second degree of right upper arm
    ● T22.232   Burn of second degree of left upper arm
    ● T22.239   Burn of second degree of unspecified upper arm
● T22.24   Burn of second degree of axilla
    ● T22.241   Burn of second degree of right axilla
    ● T22.242   Burn of second degree of left axilla
    ● T22.249   Burn of second degree of unspecified axilla
● T22.25   Burn of second degree of shoulder
    ● T22.251   Burn of second degree of right shoulder
    ● T22.252   Burn of second degree of left shoulder
    ● T22.259   Burn of second degree of unspecified shoulder
● T22.26   Burn of second degree of scapular region
    ● T22.261   Burn of second degree of right scapular region
    ● T22.262   Burn of second degree of left scapular region
    ● T22.269   Burn of second degree of unspecified scapular region

CHAPTER 19 (S00-T88)

◀ New   ◀⁞⁞ Revised   ~~deleted~~ Deleted   **OGCR** Official Guidelines   X Assign placeholder X   ● Use Additional Character(s)

Excludes 1   Excludes 2   Includes   Use additional   Code first   Code also   Unspecified

● **T22.29** Burn of second degree of multiple sites of shoulder and upper limb, except wrist and hand
- ● **T22.291** Burn of second degree of multiple sites of right shoulder and upper limb, except wrist and hand
- ● **T22.292** Burn of second degree of multiple sites of left shoulder and upper limb, except wrist and hand
- ● **T22.299** Burn of second degree of multiple sites of unspecified shoulder and upper limb, except wrist and hand

● **T22.3** Burn of third degree of shoulder and upper limb, except wrist and hand

Use additional external cause code to identify the source, place and intent of the burn (X00-X19, X75-X77, X96-X98, Y92)

X ● **T22.30** Burn of third degree of shoulder and upper limb, except wrist and hand, unspecified site

● **T22.31** Burn of third degree of forearm
- ● **T22.311** Burn of third degree of right forearm
- ● **T22.312** Burn of third degree of left forearm
- ● **T22.319** Burn of third degree of unspecified forearm

● **T22.32** Burn of third degree of elbow
- ● **T22.321** Burn of third degree of right elbow
- ● **T22.322** Burn of third degree of left elbow
- ● **T22.329** Burn of third degree of unspecified elbow

● **T22.33** Burn of third degree of upper arm
- ● **T22.331** Burn of third degree of right upper arm
- ● **T22.332** Burn of third degree of left upper arm
- ● **T22.339** Burn of third degree of unspecified upper arm

● **T22.34** Burn of third degree of axilla
- ● **T22.341** Burn of third degree of right axilla
- ● **T22.342** Burn of third degree of left axilla
- ● **T22.349** Burn of third degree of unspecified axilla

● **T22.35** Burn of third degree of shoulder
- ● **T22.351** Burn of third degree of right shoulder
- ● **T22.352** Burn of third degree of left shoulder
- ● **T22.359** Burn of third degree of unspecified shoulder

● **T22.36** Burn of third degree of scapular region
- ● **T22.361** Burn of third degree of right scapular region
- ● **T22.362** Burn of third degree of left scapular region
- ● **T22.369** Burn of third degree of unspecified scapular region

● **T22.39** Burn of third degree of multiple sites of shoulder and upper limb, except wrist and hand
- ● **T22.391** Burn of third degree of multiple sites of right shoulder and upper limb, except wrist and hand
- ● **T22.392** Burn of third degree of multiple sites of left shoulder and upper limb, except wrist and hand
- ● **T22.399** Burn of third degree of multiple sites of unspecified shoulder and upper limb, except wrist and hand

● **T22.4** Corrosion of unspecified degree of shoulder and upper limb, except wrist and hand

Code first (T51-T65) to identify chemical and intent

Use additional external cause code to identify place (Y92)

X ● **T22.40** Corrosion of unspecified degree of shoulder and upper limb, except wrist and hand, unspecified site

● **T22.41** Corrosion of unspecified degree of forearm
- ● **T22.411** Corrosion of unspecified degree of right forearm
- ● **T22.412** Corrosion of unspecified degree of left forearm
- ● **T22.419** Corrosion of unspecified degree of unspecified forearm

● **T22.42** Corrosion of unspecified degree of elbow
- ● **T22.421** Corrosion of unspecified degree of right elbow
- ● **T22.422** Corrosion of unspecified degree of left elbow
- ● **T22.429** Corrosion of unspecified degree of unspecified elbow

● **T22.43** Corrosion of unspecified degree of upper arm
- ● **T22.431** Corrosion of unspecified degree of right upper arm
- ● **T22.432** Corrosion of unspecified degree of left upper arm
- ● **T22.439** Corrosion of unspecified degree of unspecified upper arm

● **T22.44** Corrosion of unspecified degree of axilla
- ● **T22.441** Corrosion of unspecified degree of right axilla
- ● **T22.442** Corrosion of unspecified degree of left axilla
- ● **T22.449** Corrosion of unspecified degree of unspecified axilla

● **T22.45** Corrosion of unspecified degree of shoulder
- ● **T22.451** Corrosion of unspecified degree of right shoulder
- ● **T22.452** Corrosion of unspecified degree of left shoulder
- ● **T22.459** Corrosion of unspecified degree of unspecified shoulder

● **T22.46** Corrosion of unspecified degree of scapular region
- ● **T22.461** Corrosion of unspecified degree of right scapular region
- ● **T22.462** Corrosion of unspecified degree of left scapular region
- ● **T22.469** Corrosion of unspecified degree of unspecified scapular region

● **T22.49** Corrosion of unspecified degree of multiple sites of shoulder and upper limb, except wrist and hand
- ● **T22.491** Corrosion of unspecified degree of multiple sites of right shoulder and upper limb, except wrist and hand
- ● **T22.492** Corrosion of unspecified degree of multiple sites of left shoulder and upper limb, except wrist and hand
- ● **T22.499** Corrosion of unspecified degree of multiple sites of unspecified shoulder and upper limb, except wrist and hand

◀ New   ⬅ Revised   ~~deleted~~ Deleted   **OGCR** Official Guidelines   X Assign placeholder X   ● Use Additional Character(s)

Excludes 1   Excludes 2   Includes   Use additional   Code first   Code also   Unspecified

● **T22.5**   Corrosion of first degree of shoulder and upper limb, except wrist and hand

     Code first (T51-T65) to identify chemical and intent

     Use additional external cause code to identify place (Y92)

X ● **T22.50**   Corrosion of first degree of shoulder and upper limb, except wrist and hand unspecified site

● **T22.51**   Corrosion of first degree of forearm

     ● **T22.511**   Corrosion of first degree of right forearm

     ● **T22.512**   Corrosion of first degree of left forearm

     ● **T22.519**   Corrosion of first degree of unspecified forearm

● **T22.52**   Corrosion of first degree of elbow

     ● **T22.521**   Corrosion of first degree of right elbow

     ● **T22.522**   Corrosion of first degree of left elbow

     ● **T22.529**   Corrosion of first degree of unspecified elbow

● **T22.53**   Corrosion of first degree of upper arm

     ● **T22.531**   Corrosion of first degree of right upper arm

     ● **T22.532**   Corrosion of first degree of left upper arm

     ● **T22.539**   Corrosion of first degree of unspecified upper arm

● **T22.54**   Corrosion of first degree of axilla

     ● **T22.541**   Corrosion of first degree of right axilla

     ● **T22.542**   Corrosion of first degree of left axilla

     ● **T22.549**   Corrosion of first degree of unspecified axilla

● **T22.55**   Corrosion of first degree of shoulder

     ● **T22.551**   Corrosion of first degree of right shoulder

     ● **T22.552**   Corrosion of first degree of left shoulder

     ● **T22.559**   Corrosion of first degree of unspecified shoulder

● **T22.56**   Corrosion of first degree of scapular region

     ● **T22.561**   Corrosion of first degree of right scapular region

     ● **T22.562**   Corrosion of first degree of left scapular region

     ● **T22.569**   Corrosion of first degree of unspecified scapular region

● **T22.59**   Corrosion of first degree of multiple sites of shoulder and upper limb, except wrist and hand

     ● **T22.591**   Corrosion of first degree of multiple sites of right shoulder and upper limb, except wrist and hand

     ● **T22.592**   Corrosion of first degree of multiple sites of left shoulder and upper limb, except wrist and hand

     ● **T22.599**   Corrosion of first degree of multiple sites of unspecified shoulder and upper limb, except wrist and hand

● **T22.6**   Corrosion of second degree of shoulder and upper limb, except wrist and hand

     Code first (T51-T65) to identify chemical and intent

     Use additional external cause code to identify place (Y92)

X ● **T22.60**   Corrosion of second degree of shoulder and upper limb, except wrist and hand, unspecified site

● **T22.61**   Corrosion of second degree of forearm

     ● **T22.611**   Corrosion of second degree of right forearm

     ● **T22.612**   Corrosion of second degree of left forearm

     ● **T22.619**   Corrosion of second degree of unspecified forearm

● **T22.62**   Corrosion of second degree of elbow

     ● **T22.621**   Corrosion of second degree of right elbow

     ● **T22.622**   Corrosion of second degree of left elbow

     ● **T22.629**   Corrosion of second degree of unspecified elbow

● **T22.63**   Corrosion of second degree of upper arm

     ● **T22.631**   Corrosion of second degree of right upper arm

     ● **T22.632**   Corrosion of second degree of left upper arm

     ● **T22.639**   Corrosion of second degree of unspecified upper arm

● **T22.64**   Corrosion of second degree of axilla

     ● **T22.641**   Corrosion of second degree of right axilla

     ● **T22.642**   Corrosion of second degree of left axilla

     ● **T22.649**   Corrosion of second degree of unspecified axilla

● **T22.65**   Corrosion of second degree of shoulder

     ● **T22.651**   Corrosion of second degree of right shoulder

     ● **T22.652**   Corrosion of second degree of left shoulder

     ● **T22.659**   Corrosion of second degree of unspecified shoulder

● **T22.66**   Corrosion of second degree of scapular region

     ● **T22.661**   Corrosion of second degree of right scapular region

     ● **T22.662**   Corrosion of second degree of left scapular region

     ● **T22.669**   Corrosion of second degree of unspecified scapular region

● **T22.69**   Corrosion of second degree of multiple sites of shoulder and upper limb, except wrist and hand

     ● **T22.691**   Corrosion of second degree of multiple sites of right shoulder and upper limb, except wrist and hand

     ● **T22.692**   Corrosion of second degree of multiple sites of left shoulder and upper limb, except wrist and hand

     ● **T22.699**   Corrosion of second degree of multiple sites of unspecified shoulder and upper limb, except wrist and hand

CHAPTER 19 (S00-T88)

◀ New   ◀▥ Revised   ~~deleted~~ Deleted   OGCR Official Guidelines   X Assign placeholder X   ● Use Additional Character(s)

Excludes 1   Excludes 2   Includes   Use additional   Code first   Code also   Unspecified

● T22.7　Corrosion of third degree of shoulder and upper limb, except wrist and hand

> *Code first (T51-T65) to identify chemical and intent*
> Use additional external cause code to identify place (Y92)

X ● T22.70　Corrosion of third degree of shoulder and upper limb, except wrist and hand, unspecified site

● T22.71　Corrosion of third degree of forearm
- ● T22.711　Corrosion of third degree of right forearm
- ● T22.712　Corrosion of third degree of left forearm
- ● T22.719　Corrosion of third degree of unspecified forearm

● T22.72　Corrosion of third degree of elbow
- ● T22.721　Corrosion of third degree of right elbow
- ● T22.722　Corrosion of third degree of left elbow
- ● T22.729　Corrosion of third degree of unspecified elbow

● T22.73　Corrosion of third degree of upper arm
- ● T22.731　Corrosion of third degree of right upper arm
- ● T22.732　Corrosion of third degree of left upper arm
- ● T22.739　Corrosion of third degree of unspecified upper arm

● T22.74　Corrosion of third degree of axilla
- ● T22.741　Corrosion of third degree of right axilla
- ● T22.742　Corrosion of third degree of left axilla
- ● T22.749　Corrosion of third degree of unspecified axilla

● T22.75　Corrosion of third degree of shoulder
- ● T22.751　Corrosion of third degree of right shoulder
- ● T22.752　Corrosion of third degree of left shoulder
- ● T22.759　Corrosion of third degree of unspecified shoulder

● T22.76　Corrosion of third degree of scapular region
- ● T22.761　Corrosion of third degree of right scapular region
- ● T22.762　Corrosion of third degree of left scapular region
- ● T22.769　Corrosion of third degree of unspecified scapular region

● T22.79　Corrosion of third degree of multiple sites of shoulder and upper limb, except wrist and hand
- ● T22.791　Corrosion of third degree of multiple sites of right shoulder and upper limb, except wrist and hand
- ● T22.792　Corrosion of third degree of multiple sites of left shoulder and upper limb, except wrist and hand
- ● T22.799　Corrosion of third degree of multiple sites of unspecified shoulder and upper limb, except wrist and hand

● T23　Burn and corrosion of wrist and hand

> The appropriate 7th character is to be added to each code from category T23

A	initial encounter
D	subsequent encounter
S	sequela

● T23.0　Burn of unspecified degree of wrist and hand

> Use additional external cause code to identify the source, place and intent of the burn (X00-X19, X75-X77, X96-X98, Y92)

● T23.00　Burn of unspecified degree of hand, unspecified site
- ● T23.001　Burn of unspecified degree of right hand, unspecified site
- ● T23.002　Burn of unspecified degree of left hand, unspecified site
- ● T23.009　Burn of unspecified degree of unspecified hand, unspecified site

● T23.01　Burn of unspecified degree of thumb (nail)
- ● T23.011　Burn of unspecified degree of right thumb (nail)
- ● T23.012　Burn of unspecified degree of left thumb (nail)
- ● T23.019　Burn of unspecified degree of unspecified thumb (nail)

● T23.02　Burn of unspecified degree of single finger (nail) except thumb
- ● T23.021　Burn of unspecified degree of single right finger (nail) except thumb
- ● T23.022　Burn of unspecified degree of single left finger (nail) except thumb
- ● T23.029　Burn of unspecified degree of unspecified single finger (nail) except thumb

● T23.03　Burn of unspecified degree of multiple fingers (nail), not including thumb
- ● T23.031　Burn of unspecified degree of multiple right fingers (nail), not including thumb
- ● T23.032　Burn of unspecified degree of multiple left fingers (nail), not including thumb
- ● T23.039　Burn of unspecified degree of unspecified multiple fingers (nail), not including thumb

● T23.04　Burn of unspecified degree of multiple fingers (nail), including thumb
- ● T23.041　Burn of unspecified degree of multiple right fingers (nail), including thumb
- ● T23.042　Burn of unspecified degree of multiple left fingers (nail), including thumb
- ● T23.049　Burn of unspecified degree of unspecified multiple fingers (nail), including thumb

● T23.05　Burn of unspecified degree of palm
- ● T23.051　Burn of unspecified degree of right palm
- ● T23.052　Burn of unspecified degree of left palm
- ● T23.059　Burn of unspecified degree of unspecified palm

● **T23.06**   Burn of unspecified degree of back of hand
     ● **T23.061**   Burn of unspecified degree of back of right hand
     ● **T23.062**   Burn of unspecified degree of back of left hand
     ● **T23.069**   Burn of unspecified degree of back of unspecified hand

● **T23.07**   Burn of unspecified degree of wrist
     ● **T23.071**   Burn of unspecified degree of right wrist
     ● **T23.072**   Burn of unspecified degree of left wrist
     ● **T23.079**   Burn of unspecified degree of unspecified wrist

● **T23.09**   Burn of unspecified degree of multiple sites of wrist and hand
     ● **T23.091**   Burn of unspecified degree of multiple sites of right wrist and hand
     ● **T23.092**   Burn of unspecified degree of multiple sites of left wrist and hand
     ● **T23.099**   Burn of unspecified degree of multiple sites of unspecified wrist and hand

● **T23.1**   Burn of first degree of wrist and hand
     Use additional external cause code to identify the source, place and intent of the burn (X00-X19, X75-X77, X96-X98, Y92)
     ● **T23.10**   Burn of first degree of hand, unspecified site
         ● **T23.101**   Burn of first degree of right hand, unspecified site
         ● **T23.102**   Burn of first degree of left hand, unspecified site
         ● **T23.109**   Burn of first degree of unspecified hand, unspecified site
     ● **T23.11**   Burn of first degree of thumb (nail)
         ● **T23.111**   Burn of first degree of right thumb (nail)
         ● **T23.112**   Burn of first degree of left thumb (nail)
         ● **T23.119**   Burn of first degree of unspecified thumb (nail)
     ● **T23.12**   Burn of first degree of single finger (nail) except thumb
         ● **T23.121**   Burn of first degree of single right finger (nail) except thumb
         ● **T23.122**   Burn of first degree of single left finger (nail) except thumb
         ● **T23.129**   Burn of first degree of unspecified single finger (nail) except thumb
     ● **T23.13**   Burn of first degree of multiple fingers (nail), not including thumb
         ● **T23.131**   Burn of first degree of multiple right fingers (nail), not including thumb
         ● **T23.132**   Burn of first degree of multiple left fingers (nail), not including thumb
         ● **T23.139**   Burn of first degree of unspecified multiple fingers (nail), not including thumb
     ● **T23.14**   Burn of first degree of multiple fingers (nail), including thumb
         ● **T23.141**   Burn of first degree of multiple right fingers (nail), including thumb
         ● **T23.142**   Burn of first degree of multiple left fingers (nail), including thumb
         ● **T23.149**   Burn of first degree of unspecified multiple fingers (nail), including thumb

● **T23.15**   Burn of first degree of palm
     ● **T23.151**   Burn of first degree of right palm
     ● **T23.152**   Burn of first degree of left palm
     ● **T23.159**   Burn of first degree of unspecified palm

● **T23.16**   Burn of first degree of back of hand
     ● **T23.161**   Burn of first degree of back of right hand
     ● **T23.162**   Burn of first degree of back of left hand
     ● **T23.169**   Burn of first degree of back of unspecified hand

● **T23.17**   Burn of first degree of wrist
     ● **T23.171**   Burn of first degree of right wrist
     ● **T23.172**   Burn of first degree of left wrist
     ● **T23.179**   Burn of first degree of unspecified wrist

● **T23.19**   Burn of first degree of multiple sites of wrist and hand
     ● **T23.191**   Burn of first degree of multiple sites of right wrist and hand
     ● **T23.192**   Burn of first degree of multiple sites of left wrist and hand
     ● **T23.199**   Burn of first degree of multiple sites of unspecified wrist and hand

● **T23.2**   Burn of second degree of wrist and hand
     Use additional external cause code to identify the source, place and intent of the burn (X00-X19, X75-X77, X96-X98, Y92)
     ● **T23.20**   Burn of second degree of hand, unspecified site
         ● **T23.201**   Burn of second degree of right hand, unspecified site
         ● **T23.202**   Burn of second degree of left hand, unspecified site
         ● **T23.209**   Burn of second degree of unspecified hand, unspecified site
     ● **T23.21**   Burn of second degree of thumb (nail)
         ● **T23.211**   Burn of second degree of right thumb (nail)
         ● **T23.212**   Burn of second degree of left thumb (nail)
         ● **T23.219**   Burn of second degree of unspecified thumb (nail)
     ● **T23.22**   Burn of second degree of single finger (nail) except thumb
         ● **T23.221**   Burn of second degree of single right finger (nail) except thumb
         ● **T23.222**   Burn of second degree of single left finger (nail) except thumb
         ● **T23.229**   Burn of second degree of unspecified single finger (nail) except thumb
     ● **T23.23**   Burn of second degree of multiple fingers (nail), not including thumb
         ● **T23.231**   Burn of second degree of multiple right fingers (nail), not including thumb
         ● **T23.232**   Burn of second degree of multiple left fingers (nail), not including thumb
         ● **T23.239**   Burn of second degree of unspecified multiple fingers (nail), not including thumb
     ● **T23.24**   Burn of second degree of multiple fingers (nail), including thumb
         ● **T23.241**   Burn of second degree of multiple right fingers (nail), including thumb
         ● **T23.242**   Burn of second degree of multiple left fingers (nail), including thumb
         ● **T23.249**   Burn of second degree of unspecified multiple fingers (nail), including thumb

◀ New   ◀▏▏▏ Revised   ~~deleted~~ Deleted   **OGCR** Official Guidelines   X Assign placeholder X   ● Use Additional Character(s)

| Excludes 1 | Excludes 2 | Includes | Use additional | Code first | Code also | Unspecified |

● T23.25   Burn of second degree of palm
- ● T23.251   Burn of second degree of right palm
- ● T23.252   Burn of second degree of left palm
- ● T23.259   Burn of second degree of unspecified palm

● T23.26   Burn of second degree of back of hand
- ● T23.261   Burn of second degree of back of right hand
- ● T23.262   Burn of second degree of back of left hand
- ● T23.269   Burn of second degree of back of unspecified hand

● T23.27   Burn of second degree of wrist
- ● T23.271   Burn of second degree of right wrist
- ● T23.272   Burn of second degree of left wrist
- ● T23.279   Burn of second degree of unspecified wrist

● T23.29   Burn of second degree of multiple sites of wrist and hand
- ● T23.291   Burn of second degree of multiple sites of right wrist and hand
- ● T23.292   Burn of second degree of multiple sites of left wrist and hand
- ● T23.299   Burn of second degree of multiple sites of unspecified wrist and hand

● T23.3   Burn of third degree of wrist and hand

    Use additional external cause code to identify the source, place and intent of the burn (X00-X19, X75-X77, X96-X98, Y92)

● T23.30   Burn of third degree of hand, unspecified site
- ● T23.301   Burn of third degree of right hand, unspecified site
- ● T23.302   Burn of third degree of left hand, unspecified site
- ● T23.309   Burn of third degree of unspecified hand, unspecified site

● T23.31   Burn of third degree of thumb (nail)
- ● T23.311   Burn of third degree of right thumb (nail)
- ● T23.312   Burn of third degree of left thumb (nail)
- ● T23.319   Burn of third degree of unspecified thumb (nail)

● T23.32   Burn of third degree of single finger (nail) except thumb
- ● T23.321   Burn of third degree of single right finger (nail) except thumb
- ● T23.322   Burn of third degree of single left finger (nail) except thumb
- ● T23.329   Burn of third degree of unspecified single finger (nail) except thumb

● T23.33   Burn of third degree of multiple fingers (nail), not including thumb
- ● T23.331   Burn of third degree of multiple right fingers (nail), not including thumb
- ● T23.332   Burn of third degree of multiple left fingers (nail), not including thumb
- ● T23.339   Burn of third degree of unspecified multiple fingers (nail), not including thumb

● T23.34   Burn of third degree of multiple fingers (nail), including thumb
- ● T23.341   Burn of third degree of multiple right fingers (nail), including thumb
- ● T23.342   Burn of third degree of multiple left fingers (nail), including thumb
- ● T23.349   Burn of third degree of unspecified multiple fingers (nail), including thumb

● T23.35   Burn of third degree of palm
- ● T23.351   Burn of third degree of right palm
- ● T23.352   Burn of third degree of left palm
- ● T23.359   Burn of third degree of unspecified palm

● T23.36   Burn of third degree of back of hand
- ● T23.361   Burn of third degree of back of right hand
- ● T23.362   Burn of third degree of back of left hand
- ● T23.369   Burn of third degree of back of unspecified hand

● T23.37   Burn of third degree of wrist
- ● T23.371   Burn of third degree of right wrist
- ● T23.372   Burn of third degree of left wrist
- ● T23.379   Burn of third degree of unspecified wrist

● T23.39   Burn of third degree of multiple sites of wrist and hand
- ● T23.391   Burn of third degree of multiple sites of right wrist and hand
- ● T23.392   Burn of third degree of multiple sites of left wrist and hand
- ● T23.399   Burn of third degree of multiple sites of unspecified wrist and hand

● T23.4   Corrosion of unspecified degree of wrist and hand

    Code first (T51-T65) to identify chemical and intent

    Use additional external cause code to identify place (Y92)

● T23.40   Corrosion of unspecified degree of hand, unspecified site
- ● T23.401   Corrosion of unspecified degree of right hand, unspecified site
- ● T23.402   Corrosion of unspecified degree of left hand, unspecified site
- ● T23.409   Corrosion of unspecified degree of unspecified hand, unspecified site

● T23.41   Corrosion of unspecified degree of thumb (nail)
- ● T23.411   Corrosion of unspecified degree of right thumb (nail)
- ● T23.412   Corrosion of unspecified degree of left thumb (nail)
- ● T23.419   Corrosion of unspecified degree of unspecified thumb (nail)

● T23.42   Corrosion of unspecified degree of single finger (nail) except thumb
- ● T23.421   Corrosion of unspecified degree of single right finger (nail) except thumb
- ● T23.422   Corrosion of unspecified degree of single left finger (nail) except thumb
- ● T23.429   Corrosion of unspecified degree of unspecified single finger (nail) except thumb

● T23.43   Corrosion of unspecified degree of multiple fingers (nail), not including thumb
- ● T23.431   Corrosion of unspecified degree of multiple right fingers (nail), not including thumb
- ● T23.432   Corrosion of unspecified degree of multiple left fingers (nail), not including thumb
- ● T23.439   Corrosion of unspecified degree of unspecified multiple fingers (nail), not including thumb

---

● **T23.44** Corrosion of unspecified degree of multiple fingers (nail), including thumb
  ● **T23.441** Corrosion of unspecified degree of multiple right fingers (nail), including thumb
  ● **T23.442** Corrosion of unspecified degree of multiple left fingers (nail), including thumb
  ● **T23.449** Corrosion of unspecified degree of unspecified multiple fingers (nail), including thumb
● **T23.45** Corrosion of unspecified degree of palm
  ● **T23.451** Corrosion of unspecified degree of right palm
  ● **T23.452** Corrosion of unspecified degree of left palm
  ● **T23.459** Corrosion of unspecified degree of unspecified palm
● **T23.46** Corrosion of unspecified degree of back of hand
  ● **T23.461** Corrosion of unspecified degree of back of right hand
  ● **T23.462** Corrosion of unspecified degree of back of left hand
  ● **T23.469** Corrosion of unspecified degree of back of unspecified hand
● **T23.47** Corrosion of unspecified degree of wrist
  ● **T23.471** Corrosion of unspecified degree of right wrist
  ● **T23.472** Corrosion of unspecified degree of left wrist
  ● **T23.479** Corrosion of unspecified degree of unspecified wrist
● **T23.49** Corrosion of unspecified degree of multiple sites of wrist and hand
  ● **T23.491** Corrosion of unspecified degree of multiple sites of right wrist and hand
  ● **T23.492** Corrosion of unspecified degree of multiple sites of left wrist and hand
  ● **T23.499** Corrosion of unspecified degree of multiple sites of unspecified wrist and hand
● **T23.5** Corrosion of first degree of wrist and hand
  Code first (T51-T65) to identify chemical and intent
  Use additional external cause code to identify place (Y92)
  ● **T23.50** Corrosion of first degree of hand, unspecified site
    ● **T23.501** Corrosion of first degree of right hand, unspecified site
    ● **T23.502** Corrosion of first degree of left hand, unspecified site
    ● **T23.509** Corrosion of first degree of unspecified hand, unspecified site
  ● **T23.51** Corrosion of first degree of thumb (nail)
    ● **T23.511** Corrosion of first degree of right thumb (nail)
    ● **T23.512** Corrosion of first degree of left thumb (nail)
    ● **T23.519** Corrosion of first degree of unspecified thumb (nail)
  ● **T23.52** Corrosion of first degree of single finger (nail) except thumb
    ● **T23.521** Corrosion of first degree of single right finger (nail) except thumb
    ● **T23.522** Corrosion of first degree of single left finger (nail) except thumb
    ● **T23.529** Corrosion of first degree of unspecified single finger (nail) except thumb

● **T23.53** Corrosion of first degree of multiple fingers (nail), not including thumb
  ● **T23.531** Corrosion of first degree of multiple right fingers (nail), not including thumb
  ● **T23.532** Corrosion of first degree of multiple left fingers (nail), not including thumb
  ● **T23.539** Corrosion of first degree of unspecified multiple fingers (nail), not including thumb
● **T23.54** Corrosion of first degree of multiple fingers (nail), including thumb
  ● **T23.541** Corrosion of first degree of multiple right fingers (nail), including thumb
  ● **T23.542** Corrosion of first degree of multiple left fingers (nail), including thumb
  ● **T23.549** Corrosion of first degree of unspecified multiple fingers (nail), including thumb
● **T23.55** Corrosion of first degree of palm
  ● **T23.551** Corrosion of first degree of right palm
  ● **T23.552** Corrosion of first degree of left palm
  ● **T23.559** Corrosion of first degree of unspecified palm
● **T23.56** Corrosion of first degree of back of hand
  ● **T23.561** Corrosion of first degree of back of right hand
  ● **T23.562** Corrosion of first degree of back of left hand
  ● **T23.569** Corrosion of first degree of back of unspecified hand
● **T23.57** Corrosion of first degree of wrist
  ● **T23.571** Corrosion of first degree of right wrist
  ● **T23.572** Corrosion of first degree of left wrist
  ● **T23.579** Corrosion of first degree of unspecified wrist
● **T23.59** Corrosion of first degree of multiple sites of wrist and hand
  ● **T23.591** Corrosion of first degree of multiple sites of right wrist and hand
  ● **T23.592** Corrosion of first degree of multiple sites of left wrist and hand
  ● **T23.599** Corrosion of first degree of multiple sites of unspecified wrist and hand
● **T23.6** Corrosion of second degree of wrist and hand
  Code first (T51-T65) to identify chemical and intent
  Use additional external cause code to identify place (Y92)
  ● **T23.60** Corrosion of second degree of hand, unspecified site
    ● **T23.601** Corrosion of second degree of right hand, unspecified site
    ● **T23.602** Corrosion of second degree of left hand, unspecified site
    ● **T23.609** Corrosion of second degree of unspecified hand, unspecified site
  ● **T23.61** Corrosion of second degree of thumb (nail)
    ● **T23.611** Corrosion of second degree of right thumb (nail)
    ● **T23.612** Corrosion of second degree of left thumb (nail)
    ● **T23.619** Corrosion of second degree of unspecified thumb (nail)
  ● **T23.62** Corrosion of second degree of single finger (nail) except thumb
    ● **T23.621** Corrosion of second degree of single right finger (nail) except thumb
    ● **T23.622** Corrosion of second degree of single left finger (nail) except thumb
    ● **T23.629** Corrosion of second degree of unspecified single finger (nail) except thumb

CHAPTER 19 (S00-T88)

● T23.63   Corrosion of second degree of multiple fingers (nail), not including thumb
  ● T23.631   Corrosion of second degree of multiple right fingers (nail), not including thumb
  ● T23.632   Corrosion of second degree of multiple left fingers (nail), not including thumb
  ● T23.639   Corrosion of second degree of unspecified multiple fingers (nail), not including thumb

● T23.64   Corrosion of second degree of multiple fingers (nail), including thumb
  ● T23.641   Corrosion of second degree of multiple right fingers (nail), including thumb
  ● T23.642   Corrosion of second degree of multiple left fingers (nail), including thumb
  ● T23.649   Corrosion of second degree of unspecified multiple fingers (nail), including thumb

● T23.65   Corrosion of second degree of palm
  ● T23.651   Corrosion of second degree of right palm
  ● T23.652   Corrosion of second degree of left palm
  ● T23.659   Corrosion of second degree of unspecified palm

● T23.66   Corrosion of second degree of back of hand
  ● T23.661   Corrosion of second degree back of right hand
  ● T23.662   Corrosion of second degree back of left hand
  ● T23.669   Corrosion of second degree back of unspecified hand

● T23.67   Corrosion of second degree of wrist
  ● T23.671   Corrosion of second degree of right wrist
  ● T23.672   Corrosion of second degree of left wrist
  ● T23.679   Corrosion of second degree of unspecified wrist

● T23.69   Corrosion of second degree of multiple sites of wrist and hand
  ● T23.691   Corrosion of second degree of multiple sites of right wrist and hand
  ● T23.692   Corrosion of second degree of multiple sites of left wrist and hand
  ● T23.699   Corrosion of second degree of multiple sites of unspecified wrist and hand

● T23.7   Corrosion of third degree of wrist and hand
  Code first (T51-T65) *to identify chemical and intent*
  Use additional external cause code to identify place (Y92)

● T23.70   Corrosion of third degree of hand, unspecified site
  ● T23.701   Corrosion of third degree of right hand, unspecified site
  ● T23.702   Corrosion of third degree of left hand, unspecified site
  ● T23.709   Corrosion of third degree of unspecified hand, unspecified site

● T23.71   Corrosion of third degree of thumb (nail)
  ● T23.711   Corrosion of third degree of right thumb (nail)
  ● T23.712   Corrosion of third degree of left thumb (nail)
  ● T23.719   Corrosion of third degree of unspecified thumb (nail)

● T23.72   Corrosion of third degree of single finger (nail) except thumb
  ● T23.721   Corrosion of third degree of single right finger (nail) except thumb
  ● T23.722   Corrosion of third degree of single left finger (nail) except thumb
  ● T23.729   Corrosion of third degree of unspecified single finger (nail) except thumb

● T23.73   Corrosion of third degree of multiple fingers (nail), not including thumb
  ● T23.731   Corrosion of third degree of multiple right fingers (nail), not including thumb
  ● T23.732   Corrosion of third degree of multiple left fingers (nail), not including thumb
  ● T23.739   Corrosion of third degree of unspecified multiple fingers (nail), not including thumb

● T23.74   Corrosion of third degree of multiple fingers (nail), including thumb
  ● T23.741   Corrosion of third degree of multiple right fingers (nail), including thumb
  ● T23.742   Corrosion of third degree of multiple left fingers (nail), including thumb
  ● T23.749   Corrosion of third degree of unspecified multiple fingers (nail), including thumb

● T23.75   Corrosion of third degree of palm
  ● T23.751   Corrosion of third degree of right palm
  ● T23.752   Corrosion of third degree of left palm
  ● T23.759   Corrosion of third degree of unspecified palm

● T23.76   Corrosion of third degree of back of hand
  ● T23.761   Corrosion of third degree of back of right hand
  ● T23.762   Corrosion of third degree of back of left hand
  ● T23.769   Corrosion of third degree of back of unspecified hand

● T23.77   Corrosion of third degree of wrist
  ● T23.771   Corrosion of third degree of right wrist
  ● T23.772   Corrosion of third degree of left wrist
  ● T23.779   Corrosion of third degree of unspecified wrist

● T23.79   Corrosion of third degree of multiple sites of wrist and hand
  ● T23.791   Corrosion of third degree of multiple sites of right wrist and hand
  ● T23.792   Corrosion of third degree of multiple sites of left wrist and hand
  ● T23.799   Corrosion of third degree of multiple sites of unspecified wrist and hand

● **T24   Burn and corrosion of lower limb, except ankle and foot**

> **Excludes2**   burn and corrosion of ankle and foot (T25.-)
> burn and corrosion of hip region (T21.-)

The appropriate 7th character is to be added to each code from category T24

> A   initial encounter
> D   subsequent encounter
> S   sequela

● **T24.0   Burn of unspecified degree of lower limb, except ankle and foot**

> Use additional external cause code to identify the source, place and intent of the burn (X00-X19, X75-X77, X96-X98, Y92)

● **T24.00   Burn of unspecified degree of unspecified site of lower limb, except ankle and foot**

● **T24.001   Burn of unspecified degree of unspecified site of right lower limb, except ankle and foot**

● **T24.002   Burn of unspecified degree of unspecified site of left lower limb, except ankle and foot**

● **T24.009   Burn of unspecified degree of unspecified site of unspecified lower limb, except ankle and foot**

● **T24.01   Burn of unspecified degree of thigh**

● **T24.011   Burn of unspecified degree of right thigh**

● **T24.012   Burn of unspecified degree of left thigh**

● **T24.019   Burn of unspecified degree of unspecified thigh**

● **T24.02   Burn of unspecified degree of knee**

● **T24.021   Burn of unspecified degree of right knee**

● **T24.022   Burn of unspecified degree of left knee**

● **T24.029   Burn of unspecified degree of unspecified knee**

● **T24.03   Burn of unspecified degree of lower leg**

● **T24.031   Burn of unspecified degree of right lower leg**

● **T24.032   Burn of unspecified degree of left lower leg**

● **T24.039   Burn of unspecified degree of unspecified lower leg**

● **T24.09   Burn of unspecified degree of multiple sites of lower limb, except ankle and foot**

● **T24.091   Burn of unspecified degree of multiple sites of right lower limb, except ankle and foot**

● **T24.092   Burn of unspecified degree of multiple sites of left lower limb, except ankle and foot**

● **T24.099   Burn of unspecified degree of multiple sites of unspecified lower limb, except ankle and foot**

● **T24.1   Burn of first degree of lower limb, except ankle and foot**

> Use additional external cause code to identify the source, place and intent of the burn (X00-X19, X75-X77, X96-X98, Y92)

● **T24.10   Burn of first degree of unspecified site of lower limb, except ankle and foot**

● **T24.101   Burn of first degree of unspecified site of right lower limb, except ankle and foot**

● **T24.102   Burn of first degree of unspecified site of left lower limb, except ankle and foot**

● **T24.109   Burn of first degree of unspecified site of unspecified lower limb, except ankle and foot**

● **T24.11   Burn of first degree of thigh**

● **T24.111   Burn of first degree of right thigh**

● **T24.112   Burn of first degree of left thigh**

● **T24.119   Burn of first degree of unspecified thigh**

● **T24.12   Burn of first degree of knee**

● **T24.121   Burn of first degree of right knee**

● **T24.122   Burn of first degree of left knee**

● **T24.129   Burn of first degree of unspecified knee**

● **T24.13   Burn of first degree of lower leg**

● **T24.131   Burn of first degree of right lower leg**

● **T24.132   Burn of first degree of left lower leg**

● **T24.139   Burn of first degree of unspecified lower leg**

● **T24.19   Burn of first degree of multiple sites of lower limb, except ankle and foot**

● **T24.191   Burn of first degree of multiple sites of right lower limb, except ankle and foot**

● **T24.192   Burn of first degree of multiple sites of left lower limb, except ankle and foot**

● **T24.199   Burn of first degree of multiple sites of unspecified lower limb, except ankle and foot**

● **T24.2   Burn of second degree of lower limb, except ankle and foot**

> Use additional external cause code to identify the source, place and intent of the burn (X00-X19, X75-X77, X96-X98, Y92)

● **T24.20   Burn of second degree of unspecified site of lower limb, except ankle and foot**

● **T24.201   Burn of second degree of unspecified site of right lower limb, except ankle and foot**

● **T24.202   Burn of second degree of unspecified site of left lower limb, except ankle and foot**

● **T24.209   Burn of second degree of unspecified site of unspecified lower limb, except ankle and foot**

● **T24.21   Burn of second degree of thigh**

● **T24.211   Burn of second degree of right thigh**

● **T24.212   Burn of second degree of left thigh**

● **T24.219   Burn of second degree of unspecified thigh**

● **T24.22   Burn of second degree of knee**

● **T24.221   Burn of second degree of right knee**

● **T24.222   Burn of second degree of left knee**

● **T24.229   Burn of second degree of unspecified knee**

● **T24.23   Burn of second degree of lower leg**

● **T24.231   Burn of second degree of right lower leg**

● **T24.232   Burn of second degree of left lower leg**

● **T24.239   Burn of second degree of unspecified lower leg**

● **T24.29   Burn of second degree of multiple sites of lower limb, except ankle and foot**

● **T24.291   Burn of second degree of multiple sites of right lower limb, except ankle and foot**

● **T24.292   Burn of second degree of multiple sites of left lower limb, except ankle and foot**

● **T24.299   Burn of second degree of multiple sites of unspecified lower limb, except ankle and foot**

CHAPTER 19 (S00-T88)

CHAPTER 19 (S00-T88)

● **T24.3**   Burn of third degree of lower limb, except ankle and foot

Use additional external cause code to identify the source, place and intent of the burn (X00-X19, X75-X77, X96-X98, Y92)

    ● **T24.30**   Burn of third degree of unspecified site of lower limb, except ankle and foot

       ● **T24.301**   Burn of third degree of unspecified site of right lower limb, except ankle and foot

       ● **T24.302**   Burn of third degree of unspecified site of left lower limb, except ankle and foot

       ● **T24.309**   Burn of third degree of unspecified site of unspecified lower limb, except ankle and foot

    ● **T24.31**   Burn of third degree of thigh

       ● **T24.311**   Burn of third degree of right thigh

       ● **T24.312**   Burn of third degree of left thigh

       ● **T24.319**   Burn of third degree of unspecified thigh

    ● **T24.32**   Burn of third degree of knee

       ● **T24.321**   Burn of third degree of right knee

       ● **T24.322**   Burn of third degree of left knee

       ● **T24.329**   Burn of third degree of unspecified knee

    ● **T24.33**   Burn of third degree of lower leg

       ● **T24.331**   Burn of third degree of right lower leg

       ● **T24.332**   Burn of third degree of left lower leg

       ● **T24.339**   Burn of third degree of unspecified lower leg

    ● **T24.39**   Burn of third degree of multiple sites of lower limb, except ankle and foot

       ● **T24.391**   Burn of third degree of multiple sites of right lower limb, except ankle and foot

       ● **T24.392**   Burn of third degree of multiple sites of left lower limb, except ankle and foot

       ● **T24.399**   Burn of third degree of multiple sites of unspecified lower limb, except ankle and foot

● **T24.4**   Corrosion of unspecified degree of lower limb, except ankle and foot

Code first (T51-T65) to identify chemical and intent

Use additional external cause code to identify place (Y92)

    ● **T24.40**   Corrosion of unspecified degree of unspecified site of lower limb, except ankle and foot

       ● **T24.401**   Corrosion of unspecified degree of unspecified site of right lower limb, except ankle and foot

       ● **T24.402**   Corrosion of unspecified degree of unspecified site of left lower limb, except ankle and foot

       ● **T24.409**   Corrosion of unspecified degree of unspecified site of unspecified lower limb, except ankle and foot

    ● **T24.41**   Corrosion of unspecified degree of thigh

       ● **T24.411**   Corrosion of unspecified degree of right thigh

       ● **T24.412**   Corrosion of unspecified degree of left thigh

       ● **T24.419**   Corrosion of unspecified degree of unspecified thigh

    ● **T24.42**   Corrosion of unspecified degree of knee

       ● **T24.421**   Corrosion of unspecified degree of right knee

       ● **T24.422**   Corrosion of unspecified degree of left knee

       ● **T24.429**   Corrosion of unspecified degree of unspecified knee

    ● **T24.43**   Corrosion of unspecified degree of lower leg

       ● **T24.431**   Corrosion of unspecified degree of right lower leg

       ● **T24.432**   Corrosion of unspecified degree of left lower leg

       ● **T24.439**   Corrosion of unspecified degree of unspecified lower leg

    ● **T24.49**   Corrosion of unspecified degree of multiple sites of lower limb, except ankle and foot

       ● **T24.491**   Corrosion of unspecified degree of multiple sites of right lower limb, except ankle and foot

       ● **T24.492**   Corrosion of unspecified degree of multiple sites of left lower limb, except ankle and foot

       ● **T24.499**   Corrosion of unspecified degree of multiple sites of unspecified lower limb, except ankle and foot

● **T24.5**   Corrosion of first degree of lower limb, except ankle and foot

Code first (T51-T65) to identify chemical and intent

Use additional external cause code to identify place (Y92)

    ● **T24.50**   Corrosion of first degree of unspecified site of lower limb, except ankle and foot

       ● **T24.501**   Corrosion of first degree of unspecified site of right lower limb, except ankle and foot

       ● **T24.502**   Corrosion of first degree of unspecified site of left lower limb, except ankle and foot

       ● **T24.509**   Corrosion of first degree of unspecified site of unspecified lower limb, except ankle and foot

    ● **T24.51**   Corrosion of first degree of thigh

       ● **T24.511**   Corrosion of first degree of right thigh

       ● **T24.512**   Corrosion of first degree of left thigh

       ● **T24.519**   Corrosion of first degree of unspecified thigh

    ● **T24.52**   Corrosion of first degree of knee

       ● **T24.521**   Corrosion of first degree of right knee

       ● **T24.522**   Corrosion of first degree of left knee

       ● **T24.529**   Corrosion of first degree of unspecified knee

    ● **T24.53**   Corrosion of first degree of lower leg

       ● **T24.531**   Corrosion of first degree of right lower leg

       ● **T24.532**   Corrosion of first degree of left lower leg

       ● **T24.539**   Corrosion of first degree of unspecified lower leg

    ● **T24.59**   Corrosion of first degree of multiple sites of lower limb, except ankle and foot

       ● **T24.591**   Corrosion of first degree of multiple sites of right lower limb, except ankle and foot

       ● **T24.592**   Corrosion of first degree of multiple sites of left lower limb, except ankle and foot

       ● **T24.599**   Corrosion of first degree of multiple sites of unspecified lower limb, except ankle and foot

◀ New   ◀▥ Revised   ~~deleted~~ Deleted   **OGCR** Official Guidelines   X Assign placeholder X   ● Use Additional Character(s)

Excludes 1   Excludes 2   Includes   Use additional   Code first   Code also   Unspecified

● **T24.6**   **Corrosion of second degree of lower limb, except ankle and foot**
    Code first (T51-T65) to identify chemical and intent
    Use additional external cause code to identify place (Y92)
  ● **T24.60**   Corrosion of second degree of unspecified site of lower limb, except ankle and foot
    ● **T24.601**   Corrosion of second degree of unspecified site of right lower limb, except ankle and foot
    ● **T24.602**   Corrosion of second degree of unspecified site of left lower limb, except ankle and foot
    ● **T24.609**   Corrosion of second degree of unspecified site of unspecified lower limb, except ankle and foot
  ● **T24.61**   Corrosion of second degree of thigh
    ● **T24.611**   Corrosion of second degree of right thigh
    ● **T24.612**   Corrosion of second degree of left thigh
    ● **T24.619**   Corrosion of second degree of unspecified thigh
  ● **T24.62**   Corrosion of second degree of knee
    ● **T24.621**   Corrosion of second degree of right knee
    ● **T24.622**   Corrosion of second degree of left knee
    ● **T24.629**   Corrosion of second degree of unspecified knee
  ● **T24.63**   Corrosion of second degree of lower leg
    ● **T24.631**   Corrosion of second degree of right lower leg
    ● **T24.632**   Corrosion of second degree of left lower leg
    ● **T24.639**   Corrosion of second degree of unspecified lower leg
  ● **T24.69**   Corrosion of second degree of multiple sites of lower limb, except ankle and foot
    ● **T24.691**   Corrosion of second degree of multiple sites of right lower limb, except ankle and foot
    ● **T24.692**   Corrosion of second degree of multiple sites of left lower limb, except ankle and foot
    ● **T24.699**   Corrosion of second degree of multiple sites of unspecified lower limb, except ankle and foot

● **T24.7**   **Corrosion of third degree of lower limb, except ankle and foot**
    Code first (T51-T65) to identify chemical and intent
    Use additional external cause code to identify place (Y92)
  ● **T24.70**   Corrosion of third degree of unspecified site of lower limb, except ankle and foot
    ● **T24.701**   Corrosion of third degree of unspecified site of right lower limb, except ankle and foot
    ● **T24.702**   Corrosion of third degree of unspecified site of left lower limb, except ankle and foot
    ● **T24.709**   Corrosion of third degree of unspecified site of unspecified lower limb, except ankle and foot

  ● **T24.71**   Corrosion of third degree of thigh
    ● **T24.711**   Corrosion of third degree of right thigh
    ● **T24.712**   Corrosion of third degree of left thigh
    ● **T24.719**   Corrosion of third degree of unspecified thigh
  ● **T24.72**   Corrosion of third degree of knee
    ● **T24.721**   Corrosion of third degree of right knee
    ● **T24.722**   Corrosion of third degree of left knee
    ● **T24.729**   Corrosion of third degree of unspecified knee
  ● **T24.73**   Corrosion of third degree of lower leg
    ● **T24.731**   Corrosion of third degree of right lower leg
    ● **T24.732**   Corrosion of third degree of left lower leg
    ● **T24.739**   Corrosion of third degree of unspecified lower leg
  ● **T24.79**   Corrosion of third degree of multiple sites of lower limb, except ankle and foot
    ● **T24.791**   Corrosion of third degree of multiple sites of right lower limb, except ankle and foot
    ● **T24.792**   Corrosion of third degree of multiple sites of left lower limb, except ankle and foot
    ● **T24.799**   Corrosion of third degree of multiple sites of unspecified lower limb, except ankle and foot

● **T25**   **Burn and corrosion of ankle and foot**
    The appropriate 7th character is to be added to each code from category T25

> A   initial encounter
> D   subsequent encounter
> S   sequela

● **T25.0**   **Burn of unspecified degree of ankle and foot**
    Use additional external cause code to identify the source, place and intent of the burn (X00-X19, X75-X77, X96-X98, Y92)
  ● **T25.01**   Burn of unspecified degree of ankle
    ● **T25.011**   Burn of unspecified degree of right ankle
    ● **T25.012**   Burn of unspecified degree of left ankle
    ● **T25.019**   Burn of unspecified degree of unspecified ankle
  ● **T25.02**   Burn of unspecified degree of foot
    Excludes2   burn of unspecified degree of toe(s) (nail) (T25.03-)
    ● **T25.021**   Burn of unspecified degree of right foot
    ● **T25.022**   Burn of unspecified degree of left foot
    ● **T25.029**   Burn of unspecified degree of unspecified foot
  ● **T25.03**   Burn of unspecified degree of toe(s) (nail)
    ● **T25.031**   Burn of unspecified degree of right toe(s) (nail)
    ● **T25.032**   Burn of unspecified degree of left toe(s) (nail)
    ● **T25.039**   Burn of unspecified degree of unspecified toe(s) (nail)

● **T25.09**   Burn of unspecified degree of multiple sites of ankle and foot
  ● **T25.091**   Burn of unspecified degree of multiple sites of right ankle and foot
  ● **T25.092**   Burn of unspecified degree of multiple sites of left ankle and foot
  ● **T25.099**   Burn of unspecified degree of multiple sites of unspecified ankle and foot

● **T25.1**   **Burn of first degree of ankle and foot**
  Use additional external cause code to identify the source, place and intent of the burn (X00-X19, X75-X77, X96-X98, Y92)
  ● **T25.11**   Burn of first degree of ankle
    ● **T25.111**   Burn of first degree of right ankle
    ● **T25.112**   Burn of first degree of left ankle
    ● **T25.119**   Burn of first degree of unspecified ankle
  ● **T25.12**   Burn of first degree of foot
    Excludes2   burn of first degree of toe(s) (nail) (T25.13-)
    ● **T25.121**   Burn of first degree of right foot
    ● **T25.122**   Burn of first degree of left foot
    ● **T25.129**   Burn of first degree of unspecified foot
  ● **T25.13**   Burn of first degree of toe(s) (nail)
    ● **T25.131**   Burn of first degree of right toe(s) (nail)
    ● **T25.132**   Burn of first degree of left toe(s) (nail)
    ● **T25.139**   Burn of first degree of unspecified toe(s) (nail)
  ● **T25.19**   Burn of first degree of multiple sites of ankle and foot
    ● **T25.191**   Burn of first degree of multiple sites of right ankle and foot
    ● **T25.192**   Burn of first degree of multiple sites of left ankle and foot
    ● **T25.199**   Burn of first degree of multiple sites of unspecified ankle and foot

● **T25.2**   **Burn of second degree of ankle and foot**
  Use additional external cause code to identify the source, place and intent of the burn (X00-X19, X75-X77, X96-X98, Y92)
  ● **T25.21**   Burn of second degree of ankle
    ● **T25.211**   Burn of second degree of right ankle
    ● **T25.212**   Burn of second degree of left ankle
    ● **T25.219**   Burn of second degree of unspecified ankle
  ● **T25.22**   Burn of second degree of foot
    Excludes2   burn of second degree of toe(s) (nail) (T25.23-)
    ● **T25.221**   Burn of second degree of right foot
    ● **T25.222**   Burn of second degree of left foot
    ● **T25.229**   Burn of second degree of unspecified foot
  ● **T25.23**   Burn of second degree of toe(s) (nail)
    ● **T25.231**   Burn of second degree of right toe(s) (nail)
    ● **T25.232**   Burn of second degree of left toe(s) (nail)
    ● **T25.239**   Burn of second degree of unspecified toe(s) (nail)

● **T25.29**   Burn of second degree of multiple sites of ankle and foot
  ● **T25.291**   Burn of second degree of multiple sites of right ankle and foot
  ● **T25.292**   Burn of second degree of multiple sites of left ankle and foot
  ● **T25.299**   Burn of second degree of multiple sites of unspecified ankle and foot

● **T25.3**   **Burn of third degree of ankle and foot**
  Use additional external cause code to identify the source, place and intent of the burn (X00-X19, X75-X77, X96-X98, Y92)
  ● **T25.31**   Burn of third degree of ankle
    ● **T25.311**   Burn of third degree of right ankle
    ● **T25.312**   Burn of third degree of left ankle
    ● **T25.319**   Burn of third degree of unspecified ankle
  ● **T25.32**   Burn of third degree of foot
    Excludes2   burn of third degree of toe(s) (nail) (T25.33-)
    ● **T25.321**   Burn of third degree of right foot
    ● **T25.322**   Burn of third degree of left foot
    ● **T25.329**   Burn of third degree of unspecified foot
  ● **T25.33**   Burn of third degree of toe(s) (nail)
    ● **T25.331**   Burn of third degree of right toe(s) (nail)
    ● **T25.332**   Burn of third degree of left toe(s) (nail)
    ● **T25.339**   Burn of third degree of unspecified toe(s) (nail)
  ● **T25.39**   Burn of third degree of multiple sites of ankle and foot
    ● **T25.391**   Burn of third degree of multiple sites of right ankle and foot
    ● **T25.392**   Burn of third degree of multiple sites of left ankle and foot
    ● **T25.399**   Burn of third degree of multiple sites of unspecified ankle and foot

● **T25.4**   **Corrosion of unspecified degree of ankle and foot**
  Code first (T51-T65) to identify chemical and intent
  Use additional external cause code to identify place (Y92)
  ● **T25.41**   Corrosion of unspecified degree of ankle
    ● **T25.411**   Corrosion of unspecified degree of right ankle
    ● **T25.412**   Corrosion of unspecified degree of left ankle
    ● **T25.419**   Corrosion of unspecified degree of unspecified ankle
  ● **T25.42**   Corrosion of unspecified degree of foot
    Excludes2   corrosion of unspecified degree of toe(s) (nail) (T25.43-)
    ● **T25.421**   Corrosion of unspecified degree of right foot
    ● **T25.422**   Corrosion of unspecified degree of left foot
    ● **T25.429**   Corrosion of unspecified degree of unspecified foot
  ● **T25.43**   Corrosion of unspecified degree of toe(s) (nail)
    ● **T25.431**   Corrosion of unspecified degree of right toe(s) (nail)
    ● **T25.432**   Corrosion of unspecified degree of left toe(s) (nail)
    ● **T25.439**   Corrosion of unspecified degree of unspecified toe(s) (nail)

◄ New   ◄|||| Revised   deleted Deleted   OGCR Official Guidelines   X Assign placeholder X   ● Use Additional Character(s)
Excludes 1   Excludes 2   Includes   Use additional   Code first   Code also   Unspecified
1388

● **T25.49**   Corrosion of unspecified degree of multiple sites of ankle and foot
  ● **T25.491**   Corrosion of unspecified degree of multiple sites of right ankle and foot
  ● **T25.492**   Corrosion of unspecified degree of multiple sites of left ankle and foot
  ● **T25.499**   Corrosion of unspecified degree of multiple sites of unspecified ankle and foot

● **T25.5**   Corrosion of first degree of ankle and foot
  Code first (T51-T65) to identify chemical and intent
  Use additional external cause code to identify place (Y92)
  ● **T25.51**   Corrosion of first degree of ankle
    ● **T25.511**   Corrosion of first degree of right ankle
    ● **T25.512**   Corrosion of first degree of left ankle
    ● **T25.519**   Corrosion of first degree of unspecified ankle
  ● **T25.52**   Corrosion of first degree of foot
    | Excludes2 | corrosion of first degree of toe(s) (nail) (T25.53-)
    ● **T25.521**   Corrosion of first degree of right foot
    ● **T25.522**   Corrosion of first degree of left foot
    ● **T25.529**   Corrosion of first degree of unspecified foot
  ● **T25.53**   Corrosion of first degree of toe(s) (nail)
    ● **T25.531**   Corrosion of first degree of right toe(s) (nail)
    ● **T25.532**   Corrosion of first degree of left toe(s) (nail)
    ● **T25.539**   Corrosion of first degree of unspecified toe(s) (nail)
  ● **T25.59**   Corrosion of first degree of multiple sites of ankle and foot
    ● **T25.591**   Corrosion of first degree of multiple sites of right ankle and foot
    ● **T25.592**   Corrosion of first degree of multiple sites of left ankle and foot
    ● **T25.599**   Corrosion of first degree of multiple sites of unspecified ankle and foot

● **T25.6**   Corrosion of second degree of ankle and foot
  Code first (T51-T65) to identify chemical and intent
  Use additional external cause code to identify place (Y92)
  ● **T25.61**   Corrosion of second degree of ankle
    ● **T25.611**   Corrosion of second degree of right ankle
    ● **T25.612**   Corrosion of second degree of left ankle
    ● **T25.619**   Corrosion of second degree of unspecified ankle
  ● **T25.62**   Corrosion of second degree of foot
    | Excludes2 | corrosion of second degree of toe(s) (nail) (T25.63-)
    ● **T25.621**   Corrosion of second degree of right foot
    ● **T25.622**   Corrosion of second degree of left foot
    ● **T25.629**   Corrosion of second degree of unspecified foot
  ● **T25.63**   Corrosion of second degree of toe(s) (nail)
    ● **T25.631**   Corrosion of second degree of right toe(s) (nail)
    ● **T25.632**   Corrosion of second degree of left toe(s) (nail)
    ● **T25.639**   Corrosion of second degree of unspecified toe(s) (nail)

● **T25.69**   Corrosion of second degree of multiple sites of ankle and foot
  ● **T25.691**   Corrosion of second degree of right ankle and foot
  ● **T25.692**   Corrosion of second degree of left ankle and foot
  ● **T25.699**   Corrosion of second degree of unspecified ankle and foot

● **T25.7**   Corrosion of third degree of ankle and foot
  Code first (T51-T65) to identify chemical and intent
  Use additional external cause code to identify place (Y92)
  ● **T25.71**   Corrosion of third degree of ankle
    ● **T25.711**   Corrosion of third degree of right ankle
    ● **T25.712**   Corrosion of third degree of left ankle
    ● **T25.719**   Corrosion of third degree of unspecified ankle
  ● **T25.72**   Corrosion of third degree of foot
    | Excludes2 | corrosion of third degree of toe(s) (nail) (T25.73-)
    ● **T25.721**   Corrosion of third degree of right foot
    ● **T25.722**   Corrosion of third degree of left foot
    ● **T25.729**   Corrosion of third degree of unspecified foot
  ● **T25.73**   Corrosion of third degree of toe(s) (nail)
    ● **T25.731**   Corrosion of third degree of right toe(s) (nail)
    ● **T25.732**   Corrosion of third degree of left toe(s) (nail)
    ● **T25.739**   Corrosion of third degree of unspecified toe(s) (nail)
  ● **T25.79**   Corrosion of third degree of multiple sites of ankle and foot
    ● **T25.791**   Corrosion of third degree of multiple sites of right ankle and foot
    ● **T25.792**   Corrosion of third degree of multiple sites of left ankle and foot
    ● **T25.799**   Corrosion of third degree of multiple sites of unspecified ankle and foot

---

BURNS AND CORROSIONS CONFINED TO EYE AND INTERNAL ORGANS (T26-T28)

● **T26**   Burn and corrosion confined to eye and adnexa
  The appropriate 7th character is to be added to each code from category T26

A	initial encounter
D	subsequent encounter
S	sequela

  ● **T26.0**   Burn of eyelid and periocular area
    Use additional external cause code to identify the source, place and intent of the burn (X00-X19, X75-X77, X96-X98, Y92)
    X ● **T26.00**   Burn of unspecified eyelid and periocular area
    X ● **T26.01**   Burn of right eyelid and periocular area
    X ● **T26.02**   Burn of left eyelid and periocular area
  ● **T26.1**   Burn of cornea and conjunctival sac
    Use additional external cause code to identify the source, place and intent of the burn (X00-X19, X75-X77, X96-X98, Y92)
    X ● **T26.10**   Burn of cornea and conjunctival sac, unspecified eye
    X ● **T26.11**   Burn of cornea and conjunctival sac, right eye
    X ● **T26.12**   Burn of cornea and conjunctival sac, left eye

CHAPTER 19 (S00-T88)

● **T26.2　Burn with resulting rupture and destruction of eyeball**

　　Use additional external cause code to identify the source, place and intent of the burn (X00-X19, X75-X77, X96-X98, Y92)

　X● **T26.20　Burn with resulting rupture and destruction of unspecified eyeball**

　X● **T26.21　Burn with resulting rupture and destruction of right eyeball**

　X● **T26.22　Burn with resulting rupture and destruction of left eyeball**

● **T26.3　Burns of other specified parts of eye and adnexa**

　　Use additional external cause code to identify the source, place and intent of the burn (X00-X19, X75-X77, X96-X98, Y92)

　X● **T26.30　Burns of other specified parts of unspecified eye and adnexa**

　X● **T26.31　Burns of other specified parts of right eye and adnexa**

　X● **T26.32　Burns of other specified parts of left eye and adnexa**

● **T26.4　Burn of eye and adnexa, part unspecified**

　　Use additional external cause code to identify the source, place and intent of the burn (X00-X19, X75-X77, X96-X98, Y92)

　X● **T26.40　Burn of unspecified eye and adnexa, part unspecified**

　X● **T26.41　Burn of right eye and adnexa, part unspecified**

　X● **T26.42　Burn of left eye and adnexa, part unspecified**

● **T26.5　Corrosion of eyelid and periocular area**

　　Code first (T51-T65) to identify chemical and intent

　　Use additional external cause code to identify place (Y92)

　X● **T26.50　Corrosion of unspecified eyelid and periocular area**

　X● **T26.51　Corrosion of right eyelid and periocular area**

　X● **T26.52　Corrosion of left eyelid and periocular area**

● **T26.6　Corrosion of cornea and conjunctival sac**

　　Code first (T51-T65) to identify chemical and intent

　　Use additional external cause code to identify place (Y92)

　X● **T26.60　Corrosion of cornea and conjunctival sac, unspecified eye**

　X● **T26.61　Corrosion of cornea and conjunctival sac, right eye**

　X● **T26.62　Corrosion of cornea and conjunctival sac, left eye**

● **T26.7　Corrosion with resulting rupture and destruction of eyeball**

　　Code first (T51-T65) to identify chemical and intent

　　Use additional external cause code to identify place (Y92)

　X● **T26.70　Corrosion with resulting rupture and destruction of unspecified eyeball**

　X● **T26.71　Corrosion with resulting rupture and destruction of right eyeball**

　X● **T26.72　Corrosion with resulting rupture and destruction of left eyeball**

● **T26.8　Corrosions of other specified parts of eye and adnexa**

　　Code first (T51-T65) to identify chemical and intent

　　Use additional external cause code to identify place (Y92)

　X● **T26.80　Corrosions of other specified parts of unspecified eye and adnexa**

　X● **T26.81　Corrosions of other specified parts of right eye and adnexa**

　X● **T26.82　Corrosions of other specified parts of left eye and adnexa**

● **T26.9　Corrosion of eye and adnexa, part unspecified**

　　Code first (T51-T65) to identify chemical and intent

　　Use additional external cause code to identify place (Y92)

　X● **T26.90　Corrosion of unspecified eye and adnexa, part unspecified**

　X● **T26.91　Corrosion of right eye and adnexa, part unspecified**

　X● **T26.92　Corrosion of left eye and adnexa, part unspecified**

● **T27　Burn and corrosion of respiratory tract**

　　Use additional external cause code to identify the source and intent of the burn (X00-X19, X75-X77, X96-X98)

　　Use additional external cause code to identify place (Y92)

　　The appropriate 7th character is to be added to each code from category T27

A	initial encounter
D	subsequent encounter
S	sequela

　X● **T27.0　Burn of larynx and trachea**

　X● **T27.1　Burn involving larynx and trachea with lung**

　X● **T27.2　Burn of other parts of respiratory tract**

　　　Burn of thoracic cavity

　X● **T27.3　Burn of respiratory tract, part unspecified**

　　　Code first (T51-T65) to identify chemical and intent for codes T27.4-T27.7

　X● **T27.4　Corrosion of larynx and trachea**

　X● **T27.5　Corrosion involving larynx and trachea with lung**

　X● **T27.6　Corrosion of other parts of respiratory tract**

　X● **T27.7　Corrosion of respiratory tract, part unspecified**

● **T28　Burn and corrosion of other internal organs**

　　Use additional external cause code to identify the source and intent of the burn (X00-X19, X75-X77, X96-X98)

　　Use additional external cause code to identify place (Y92)

　　The appropriate 7th character is to be added to each code from category T28

A	initial encounter
D	subsequent encounter
S	sequela

　X● **T28.0　Burn of mouth and pharynx**

　X● **T28.1　Burn of esophagus**

　X● **T28.2　Burn of other parts of alimentary tract**

　X● **T28.3　Burn of internal genitourinary organs**

　X● **T28.4　Burns of other and unspecified internal organs**

　　X● **T28.40　Burn of unspecified internal organ**

　　● **T28.41　Burn of ear drum**

　　　● **T28.411　Burn of right ear drum**

　　　● **T28.412　Burn of left ear drum**

　　　● **T28.419　Burn of unspecified ear drum**

　　X● **T28.49　Burn of other internal organ**

　　　Code first (T51-T65) to identify chemical and intent for T28.5-T28.9-

　X● **T28.5　Corrosion of mouth and pharynx**

　X● **T28.6　Corrosion of esophagus**

　X● **T28.7　Corrosion of other parts of alimentary tract**

　X● **T28.8　Corrosion of internal genitourinary organs**

　● **T28.9　Corrosions of other and unspecified internal organs**

　　X● **T28.90　Corrosions of unspecified internal organs**

　　● **T28.91　Corrosions of ear drum**

　　　● **T28.911　Corrosions of right ear drum**

　　　● **T28.912　Corrosions of left ear drum**

　　　● **T28.919　Corrosions of unspecified ear drum**

　　X● **T28.99　Corrosions of other internal organs**

◀ New　◀▥ Revised　~~deleted~~ Deleted　OGCR Official Guidelines　X Assign placeholder X　● Use Additional Character(s)

| Excludes 1 | Excludes 2 | Includes | Use additional | Code first | Code also | Unspecified |

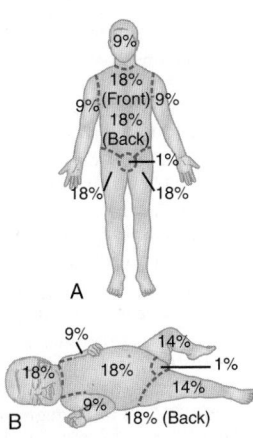

Figure 19-15 Rule of nines: percentages of total body area. (From Marx: Rosen's Emergency Medicine: Concepts and Clinical Practice, ed 6, Mosby, 2006)

OGCR Section I.C.19.d.5.

Assign separate code for each burn site

When coding burns, assign separate codes for each burn site. Category T30, Burn and corrosion, body region unspecified is extremely vague and should rarely be used.

OGCR See Section I.C.19.d.

BURNS AND CORROSIONS OF MULTIPLE AND UNSPECIFIED BODY REGIONS (T30-T32)

● **T30   Burn and corrosion, body region unspecified**

    T30.0   Burn of unspecified **body region, unspecified degree**
        This code is not for inpatient use. Code to specified site and degree of burns
        Burn NOS
        Multiple burns NOS

    T30.4   Corrosion of unspecified **body region, unspecified degree**
        This code is not for inpatient use. Code to specified site and degree of corrosion
        Corrosion NOS
        Multiple corrosion NOS

● **T31   Burns classified according to extent of body surface involved**

    Note: This category is to be used as the primary code only when the site of the burn is unspecified. It should be used as a supplementary code with categories T20-T25 when the site is specified.

    T31.0   Burns involving less than 10% of body surface

●   **T31.1   Burns involving 10-19% of body surface**

        T31.10   Burns involving 10-19% of body surface with 0% to 9% third degree burns
            Burns involving 10-19% of body surface NOS

        T31.11   Burns involving 10-19% of body surface with 10-19% third degree burns

●   **T31.2   Burns involving 20-29% of body surface**

        T31.20   Burns involving 20-29% of body surface with 0% to 9% third degree burns
            Burns involving 20-29% of body surface NOS

        T31.21   Burns involving 20-29% of body surface with 10-19% third degree burns

        T31.22   Burns involving 20-29% of body surface with 20-29% third degree burns

● **T31.3   Burns involving 30-39% of body surface**

    T31.30   Burns involving 30-39% of body surface with 0% to 9% third degree burns
        Burns involving 30-39% of body surface NOS

    T31.31   Burns involving 30-39% of body surface with 10-19% third degree burns

    T31.32   Burns involving 30-39% of body surface with 20-29% third degree burns

    T31.33   Burns involving 30-39% of body surface with 30-39% third degree burns

● **T31.4   Burns involving 40-49% of body surface**

    T31.40   Burns involving 40-49% of body surface with 0% to 9% third degree burns
        Burns involving 40-49% of body surface NOS

    T31.41   Burns involving 40-49% of body surface with 10-19% third degree burns

    T31.42   Burns involving 40-49% of body surface with 20-29% third degree burns

    T31.43   Burns involving 40-49% of body surface with 30-39% third degree burns

    T31.44   Burns involving 40-49% of body surface with 40-49% third degree burns

● **T31.5   Burns involving 50-59% of body surface**

    T31.50   Burns involving 50-59% of body surface with 0% to 9% third degree burns
        Burns involving 50-59% of body surface NOS

    T31.51   Burns involving 50-59% of body surface with 10-19% third degree burns

    T31.52   Burns involving 50-59% of body surface with 20-29% third degree burns

    T31.53   Burns involving 50-59% of body surface with 30-39% third degree burns

    T31.54   Burns involving 50-59% of body surface with 40-49% third degree burns

    T31.55   Burns involving 50-59% of body surface with 50-59% third degree burns

● **T31.6   Burns involving 60-69% of body surface**

    T31.60   Burns involving 60-69% of body surface with 0% to 9% third degree burns
        Burns involving 60-69% of body surface NOS

    T31.61   Burns involving 60-69% of body surface with 10-19% third degree burns

    T31.62   Burns involving 60-69% of body surface with 20-29% third degree burns

    T31.63   Burns involving 60-69% of body surface with 30-39% third degree burns

    T31.64   Burns involving 60-69% of body surface with 40-49% third degree burns

    T31.65   Burns involving 60-69% of body surface with 50-59% third degree burns

    T31.66   Burns involving 60-69% of body surface with 60-69% third degree burns

● **T31.7   Burns involving 70-79% of body surface**

    T31.70   Burns involving 70-79% of body surface with 0% to 9% third degree burns
        Burns involving 70-79% of body surface NOS

    T31.71   Burns involving 70-79% of body surface with 10-19% third degree burns

    T31.72   Burns involving 70-79% of body surface with 20-29% third degree burns

    T31.73   Burns involving 70-79% of body surface with 30-39% third degree burns

    T31.74   Burns involving 70-79% of body surface with 40-49% third degree burns

    T31.75   Burns involving 70-79% of body surface with 50-59% third degree burns

    T31.76   Burns involving 70-79% of body surface with 60-69% third degree burns

    T31.77   Burns involving 70-79% of body surface with 70-79% third degree burns

◀ New   ◀▦ Revised   ~~deleted~~ Deleted   **OGCR** Official Guidelines   X Assign placeholder X   ● Use Additional Character(s)

Excludes 1   Excludes 2   Includes   Use additional   Code first   Code also   Unspecified

● **T31.8**　**Burns involving 80-89% of body surface**

T31.80　Burns involving 80-89% of body surface with 0% to 9% third degree burns
　　　　　Burns involving 80-89% of body surface NOS

T31.81　Burns involving 80-89% of body surface with 10-19% third degree burns

T31.82　Burns involving 80-89% of body surface with 20-29% third degree burns

T31.83　Burns involving 80-89% of body surface with 30-39% third degree burns

T31.84　Burns involving 80-89% of body surface with 40-49% third degree burns

T31.85　Burns involving 80-89% of body surface with 50-59% third degree burns

T31.86　Burns involving 80-89% of body surface with 60-69% third degree burns

T31.87　Burns involving 80-89% of body surface with 70-79% third degree burns

T31.88　Burns involving 80-89% of body surface with 80-89% third degree burns

● **T31.9**　**Burns involving 90% or more of body surface**

T31.90　Burns involving 90% or more of body surface with 0% to 9% third degree burns
　　　　　Burns involving 90% or more of body surface NOS

T31.91　Burns involving 90% or more of body surface with 10-19% third degree burns

T31.92　Burns involving 90% or more of body surface with 20-29% third degree burns

T31.93　Burns involving 90% or more of body surface with 30-39% third degree burns

T31.94　Burns involving 90% or more of body surface with 40-49% third degree burns

T31.95　Burns involving 90% or more of body surface with 50-59% third degree burns

T31.96　Burns involving 90% or more of body surface with 60-69% third degree burns

T31.97　Burns involving 90% or more of body surface with 70-79% third degree burns

T31.98　Burns involving 90% or more of body surface with 80-89% third degree burns

T31.99　Burns involving 90% or more of body surface with 90% or more third degree burns

● **T32**　**Corrosions classified according to extent of body surface involved**

Note: This category is to be used as the primary code only when the site of the corrosion is unspecified. It may be used as a supplementary code with categories T20-T25 when the site is specified.

T32.0　**Corrosions involving less than 10% of body surface**

● **T32.1**　**Corrosions involving 10-19% of body surface**

T32.10　Corrosions involving 10-19% of body surface with 0% to 9% third degree corrosion
　　　　　Corrosions involving 10-19% of body surface NOS

T32.11　Corrosions involving 10-19% of body surface with 10-19% third degree corrosion

● **T32.2**　**Corrosions involving 20-29% of body surface**

T32.20　Corrosions involving 20-29% of body surface with 0% to 9% third degree corrosion

T32.21　Corrosions involving 20-29% of body surface with 10-19% third degree corrosion

T32.22　Corrosions involving 20-29% of body surface with 20-29% third degree corrosion

● **T32.3**　**Corrosions involving 30-39% of body surface**

T32.30　Corrosions involving 30-39% of body surface with 0% to 9% third degree corrosion

T32.31　Corrosions involving 30-39% of body surface with 10-19% third degree corrosion

T32.32　Corrosions involving 30-39% of body surface with 20-29% third degree corrosion

T32.33　Corrosions involving 30-39% of body surface with 30-39% third degree corrosion

● **T32.4**　**Corrosions involving 40-49% of body surface**

T32.40　Corrosions involving 40-49% of body surface with 0% to 9% third degree corrosion

T32.41　Corrosions involving 40-49% of body surface with 10-19% third degree corrosion

T32.42　Corrosions involving 40-49% of body surface with 20-29% third degree corrosion

T32.43　Corrosions involving 40-49% of body surface with 30-39% third degree corrosion

T32.44　Corrosions involving 40-49% of body surface with 40-49% third degree corrosion

● **T32.5**　**Corrosions involving 50-59% of body surface**

T32.50　Corrosions involving 50-59% of body surface with 0% to 9% third degree corrosion

T32.51　Corrosions involving 50-59% of body surface with 10-19% third degree corrosion

T32.52　Corrosions involving 50-59% of body surface with 20-29% third degree corrosion

T32.53　Corrosions involving 50-59% of body surface with 30-39% third degree corrosion

T32.54　Corrosions involving 50-59% of body surface with 40-49% third degree corrosion

T32.55　Corrosions involving 50-59% of body surface with 50-59% third degree corrosion

● **T32.6**　**Corrosions involving 60-69% of body surface**

T32.60　Corrosions involving 60-69% of body surface with 0% to 9% third degree corrosion

T32.61　Corrosions involving 60-69% of body surface with 10-19% third degree corrosion

T32.62　Corrosions involving 60-69% of body surface with 20-29% third degree corrosion

T32.63　Corrosions involving 60-69% of body surface with 30-39% third degree corrosion

T32.64　Corrosions involving 60-69% of body surface with 40-49% third degree corrosion

T32.65　Corrosions involving 60-69% of body surface with 50-59% third degree corrosion

T32.66　Corrosions involving 60-69% of body surface with 60-69% third degree corrosion

● **T32.7**　**Corrosions involving 70-79% of body surface**

T32.70　Corrosions involving 70-79% of body surface with 0% to 9% third degree corrosion

T32.71　Corrosions involving 70-79% of body surface with 10-19% third degree corrosion

T32.72　Corrosions involving 70-79% of body surface with 20-29% third degree corrosion

T32.73　Corrosions involving 70-79% of body surface with 30-39% third degree corrosion

T32.74　Corrosions involving 70-79% of body surface with 40-49% third degree corrosion

T32.75　Corrosions involving 70-79% of body surface with 50-59% third degree corrosion

T32.76　Corrosions involving 70-79% of body surface with 60-69% third degree corrosion

T32.77　Corrosions involving 70-79% of body surface with 70-79% third degree corrosion

◄ New　◄▥ Revised　~~deleted~~ Deleted　**OGCR** Official Guidelines　X Assign placeholder X　● Use Additional Character(s)

Excludes 1　Excludes 2　Includes　Use additional　Code first　Code also　Unspecified

●T32.8   Corrosions involving 80-89% of body surface

    T32.80   Corrosions involving 80-89% of body surface with 0% to 9% third degree corrosion

    T32.81   Corrosions involving 80-89% of body surface with 10-19% third degree corrosion

    T32.82   Corrosions involving 80-89% of body surface with 20-29% third degree corrosion

    T32.83   Corrosions involving 80-89% of body surface with 30-39% third degree corrosion

    T32.84   Corrosions involving 80-89% of body surface with 40-49% third degree corrosion

    T32.85   Corrosions involving 80-89% of body surface with 50-59% third degree corrosion

    T32.86   Corrosions involving 80-89% of body surface with 60-69% third degree corrosion

    T32.87   Corrosions involving 80-89% of body surface with 70-79% third degree corrosion

    T32.88   Corrosions involving 80-89% of body surface with 80-89% third degree corrosion

●T32.9   Corrosions involving 90% or more of body surface

    T32.90   Corrosions involving 90% or more of body surface with 0% to 9% third degree corrosion

    T32.91   Corrosions involving 90% or more of body surface with 10-19% third degree corrosion

    T32.92   Corrosions involving 90% or more of body surface with 20-29% third degree corrosion

    T32.93   Corrosions involving 90% or more of body surface with 30-39% third degree corrosion

    T32.94   Corrosions involving 90% or more of body surface with 40-49% third degree corrosion

    T32.95   Corrosions involving 90% or more of body surface with 50-59% third degree corrosion

    T32.96   Corrosions involving 90% or more of body surface with 60-69% third degree corrosion

    T32.97   Corrosions involving 90% or more of body surface with 70-79% third degree corrosion

    T32.98   Corrosions involving 90% or more of body surface with 80-89% third degree corrosion

    T32.99   Corrosions involving 90% or more of body surface with 90% or more third degree corrosion

FROSTBITE (T33-T34)

Excludes2   hypothermia and other effects of reduced temperature (T68, T69.-)

●T33   **Superficial frostbite**

    Includes   frostbite with partial thickness skin loss

    The appropriate 7th character is to be added to each code from category T33

> A   initial encounter
> D   subsequent encounter
> S   sequela

●T33.0   Superficial frostbite of head

    ●T33.01   Superficial frostbite of ear

      ●T33.011   Superficial frostbite of right ear

      ●T33.012   Superficial frostbite of left ear

      ●T33.019   Superficial frostbite of unspecified ear

    X●T33.02   Superficial frostbite of nose

    X●T33.09   Superficial frostbite of other part of head

X●T33.1   Superficial frostbite of neck

X●T33.2   Superficial frostbite of thorax

X●T33.3   Superficial frostbite of abdominal wall, lower back and pelvis

●T33.4   Superficial frostbite of arm

    Excludes2   superficial frostbite of wrist and hand (T33.5-)

    X●T33.40   Superficial frostbite of unspecified arm

    X●T33.41   Superficial frostbite of right arm

    X●T33.42   Superficial frostbite of left arm

●T33.5   Superficial frostbite of wrist, hand, and fingers

    ●T33.51   Superficial frostbite of wrist

      ●T33.511   Superficial frostbite of right wrist

      ●T33.512   Superficial frostbite of left wrist

      ●T33.519   Superficial frostbite of unspecified wrist

    ●T33.52   Superficial frostbite of hand

      Excludes2   superficial frostbite of fingers (T33.53-)

      ●T33.521   Superficial frostbite of right hand

      ●T33.522   Superficial frostbite of left hand

      ●T33.529   Superficial frostbite of unspecified hand

    ●T33.53   Superficial frostbite of finger(s)

      ●T33.531   Superficial frostbite of right finger(s)

      ●T33.532   Superficial frostbite of left finger(s)

      ●T33.539   Superficial frostbite of unspecified finger(s)

●T33.6   Superficial frostbite of hip and thigh

    X●T33.60   Superficial frostbite of unspecified hip and thigh

    X●T33.61   Superficial frostbite of right hip and thigh

    X●T33.62   Superficial frostbite of left hip and thigh

●T33.7   Superficial frostbite of knee and lower leg

    Excludes2   superficial frostbite of ankle and foot (T33.8-)

    X●T33.70   Superficial frostbite of unspecified knee and lower leg

    X●T33.71   Superficial frostbite of right knee and lower leg

    X●T33.72   Superficial frostbite of left knee and lower leg

●T33.8   Superficial frostbite of ankle, foot, and toe(s)

    ●T33.81   Superficial frostbite of ankle

      ●T33.811   Superficial frostbite of right ankle

      ●T33.812   Superficial frostbite of left ankle

      ●T33.819   Superficial frostbite of unspecified ankle

    ●T33.82   Superficial frostbite of foot

      ●T33.821   Superficial frostbite of right foot

      ●T33.822   Superficial frostbite of left foot

      ●T33.829   Superficial frostbite of unspecified foot

    ●T33.83   Superficial frostbite of toe(s)

      ●T33.831   Superficial frostbite of right toe(s)

      ●T33.832   Superficial frostbite of left toe(s)

      ●T33.839   Superficial frostbite of unspecified toe(s)

●T33.9   Superficial frostbite of other and unspecified sites

    X●T33.90   Superficial frostbite of unspecified sites
      Superficial frostbite NOS

    X●T33.99   Superficial frostbite of other sites
      Superficial frostbite of leg NOS
      Superficial frostbite of trunk NOS

●T34   Frostbite with tissue necrosis

    The appropriate 7th character is to be added to each code from category T34

> A   initial encounter
> D   subsequent encounter
> S   sequela

●T34.0   Frostbite with tissue necrosis of head

    ●T34.01   Frostbite with tissue necrosis of ear

      ●T34.011   Frostbite with tissue necrosis of right ear

      ●T34.012   Frostbite with tissue necrosis of left ear

      ●T34.019   Frostbite with tissue necrosis of unspecified ear

CHAPTER 19 (S00-T88)

X ● **T34.02** Frostbite with tissue necrosis of nose

X ● **T34.09** Frostbite with tissue necrosis of other part of head

X ● **T34.1** Frostbite with tissue necrosis of neck

X ● **T34.2** Frostbite with tissue necrosis of thorax

X ● **T34.3** Frostbite with tissue necrosis of abdominal wall, lower back and pelvis

● **T34.4** Frostbite with tissue necrosis of arm

> **Excludes2** frostbite with tissue necrosis of wrist and hand (T34.5-)

X ● **T34.40** Frostbite with tissue necrosis of unspecified arm

X ● **T34.41** Frostbite with tissue necrosis of right arm

X ● **T34.42** Frostbite with tissue necrosis of left arm

● **T34.5** Frostbite with tissue necrosis of wrist, hand, and finger(s)

● **T34.51** Frostbite with tissue necrosis of wrist

● **T34.511** Frostbite with tissue necrosis of right wrist

● **T34.512** Frostbite with tissue necrosis of left wrist

● **T34.519** Frostbite with tissue necrosis of unspecified wrist

● **T34.52** Frostbite with tissue necrosis of hand

> **Excludes2** frostbite with tissue necrosis of finger(s) (T34.53-)

● **T34.521** Frostbite with tissue necrosis of right hand

● **T34.522** Frostbite with tissue necrosis of left hand

● **T34.529** Frostbite with tissue necrosis of unspecified hand

● **T34.53** Frostbite with tissue necrosis of finger(s)

● **T34.531** Frostbite with tissue necrosis of right finger(s)

● **T34.532** Frostbite with tissue necrosis of left finger(s)

● **T34.539** Frostbite with tissue necrosis of unspecified finger(s)

● **T34.6** Frostbite with tissue necrosis of hip and thigh

X ● **T34.60** Frostbite with tissue necrosis of unspecified hip and thigh

X ● **T34.61** Frostbite with tissue necrosis of right hip and thigh

X ● **T34.62** Frostbite with tissue necrosis of left hip and thigh

● **T34.7** Frostbite with tissue necrosis of knee and lower leg

> **Excludes2** frostbite with tissue necrosis of ankle and foot (T34.8-)

X ● **T34.70** Frostbite with tissue necrosis of unspecified knee and lower leg

X ● **T34.71** Frostbite with tissue necrosis of right knee and lower leg

X ● **T34.72** Frostbite with tissue necrosis of left knee and lower leg

● **T34.8** Frostbite with tissue necrosis of ankle, foot, and toe(s)

● **T34.81** Frostbite with tissue necrosis of ankle

● **T34.811** Frostbite with tissue necrosis of right ankle

● **T34.812** Frostbite with tissue necrosis of left ankle

● **T34.819** Frostbite with tissue necrosis of unspecified ankle

● **T34.82** Frostbite with tissue necrosis of foot

● **T34.821** Frostbite with tissue necrosis of right foot

● **T34.822** Frostbite with tissue necrosis of left foot

● **T34.829** Frostbite with tissue necrosis of unspecified foot

● **T34.83** Frostbite with tissue necrosis of toe(s)

● **T34.831** Frostbite with tissue necrosis of right toe(s)

● **T34.832** Frostbite with tissue necrosis of left toe(s)

● **T34.839** Frostbite with tissue necrosis of unspecified toe(s)

● **T34.9** Frostbite with tissue necrosis of other and unspecified sites

X ● **T34.90** Frostbite with tissue necrosis of unspecified sites

Frostbite with tissue necrosis NOS

X ● **T34.99** Frostbite with tissue necrosis of other sites

Frostbite with tissue necrosis of leg NOS

Frostbite with tissue necrosis of trunk NOS

OGCR See Section I.C.19.e.

Adverse Effects, Poisoning, Underdosing and Toxic Effects

POISONING BY, ADVERSE EFFECTS OF AND UNDERDOSING OF DRUGS, MEDICAMENTS AND BIOLOGICAL SUBSTANCES (T36-T50)

Includes adverse effect of correct substance properly administered

poisoning by overdose of substance

poisoning by wrong substance given or taken in error

underdosing by (inadvertently) (deliberately) taking less substance than prescribed or instructed

Code first, for adverse effects, the nature of the adverse effect, such as:

adverse effect NOS (T88.7)

aspirin gastritis (K29.-)

blood disorders (D56-D76)

contact dermatitis (L23-L25)

dermatitis due to substances taken internally (L27.-)

nephropathy (N14.0-N14.2)

Note: The drug giving rise to the adverse effect should be identified by use of codes from categories T36-T50 with fifth or sixth character 5.

Use additional code(s) to specify:

manifestations of poisoning

underdosing or failure in dosage during medical and surgical care (Y63.6, Y63.8-Y63.9)

underdosing of medication regimen (Z91.12-, Z91.13-)

> **Excludes1** toxic reaction to local anesthesia in pregnancy (O29.3-)

> **Excludes2** abuse and dependence of psychoactive substances (F10-F19)

abuse of non-dependence-producing substances (F55.-)

drug reaction and poisoning affecting newborn (P00-P96)

pathological drug intoxication (inebriation) (F10-F19)

● **T36** Poisoning by, adverse effect of and underdosing of systemic antibiotics

> **Excludes1** antineoplastic antibiotics (T45.1-)

locally applied antibiotic NEC (T49.0)

topically used antibiotic for ear, nose and throat (T49.6)

topically used antibiotic for eye (T49.5)

The appropriate 7th character is to be added to each code from category T36

A	initial encounter
D	subsequent encounter
S	sequela

● **T36.0** Poisoning by, adverse effect of and underdosing of penicillins

● **T36.0X** Poisoning by, adverse effect of and underdosing of penicillins

● **T36.0X1** Poisoning by penicillins, accidental (unintentional)

Poisoning by penicillins NOS

◄ New ◄|||| Revised ~~deleted~~ Deleted **OGCR** Official Guidelines X Assign placeholder X ● Use Additional Character(s)

Excludes 1 Excludes 2 Includes Use additional Code first Code also Unspecified

- ● T36.0X2 Poisoning by penicillins, intentional self-harm
- ● T36.0X3 Poisoning by penicillins, assault
- ● T36.0X4 Poisoning by penicillins, undetermined
- ● T36.0X5 Adverse effect of penicillins
- ● T36.0X6 Underdosing of penicillins
- ● T36.1 Poisoning by, adverse effect of and underdosing of cephalosporins and other betalactam antibiotics
  - ● T36.1X Poisoning by, adverse effect of and underdosing of cephalosporins and other beta-lactam antibiotics
    - ● T36.1X1 Poisoning by cephalosporins and other beta-lactam antibiotics, accidental (unintentional)
      Poisoning by cephalosporins and other beta-lactam antibiotics NOS
    - ● T36.1X2 Poisoning by cephalosporins and other beta-lactam antibiotics, intentional self-harm
    - ● T36.1X3 Poisoning by cephalosporins and other beta-lactam antibiotics, assault
    - ● T36.1X4 Poisoning by cephalosporins and other beta-lactam antibiotics, undetermined
    - ● T36.1X5 Adverse effect of cephalosporins and other beta-lactam antibiotics
    - ● T36.1X6 Underdosing of cephalosporins and other beta-lactam antibiotics
- ● T36.2 Poisoning by, adverse effect of and underdosing of chloramphenicol group
  - ● T36.2X Poisoning by, adverse effect of and underdosing of chloramphenicol group
    - ● T36.2X1 Poisoning by chloramphenicol group, accidental (unintentional)
      Poisoning by chloramphenicol group NOS
    - ● T36.2X2 Poisoning by chloramphenicol group, intentional self-harm
    - ● T36.2X3 Poisoning by chloramphenicol group, assault
    - ● T36.2X4 Poisoning by chloramphenicol group, undetermined
    - ● T36.2X5 Adverse effect of chloramphenicol group
    - ● T36.2X6 Underdosing of chloramphenicol group
- ● T36.3 Poisoning by, adverse effect of and underdosing of macrolides
  - ● T36.3X Poisoning by, adverse effect of and underdosing of macrolides
    - ● T36.3X1 Poisoning by macrolides, accidental (unintentional)
      Poisoning by macrolides NOS
    - ● T36.3X2 Poisoning by macrolides, intentional self-harm
    - ● T36.3X3 Poisoning by macrolides, assault
    - ● T36.3X4 Poisoning by macrolides, undetermined
    - ● T36.3X5 Adverse effect of macrolides
    - ● T36.3X6 Underdosing of macrolides

- ● T36.4 Poisoning by, adverse effect of and underdosing of tetracyclines
  - ● T36.4X Poisoning by, adverse effect of and underdosing of tetracyclines
    - ● T36.4X1 Poisoning by tetracyclines, accidental (unintentional)
      Poisoning by tetracyclines NOS
    - ● T36.4X2 Poisoning by tetracyclines, intentional self-harm
    - ● T36.4X3 Poisoning by tetracyclines, assault
    - ● T36.4X4 Poisoning by tetracyclines, undetermined
    - ● T36.4X5 Adverse effect of tetracyclines
    - ● T36.4X6 Underdosing of tetracyclines
- ● T36.5 Poisoning by, adverse effect of and underdosing of aminoglycosides
  Poisoning by, adverse effect of and underdosing of streptomycin
  - ● T36.5X Poisoning by, adverse effect of and underdosing of aminoglycosides
    - ● T36.5X1 Poisoning by aminoglycosides, accidental (unintentional)
      Poisoning by aminoglycosides NOS
    - ● T36.5X2 Poisoning by aminoglycosides, intentional self-harm
    - ● T36.5X3 Poisoning by aminoglycosides, assault
    - ● T36.5X4 Poisoning by aminoglycosides, undetermined
    - ● T36.5X5 Adverse effect of aminoglycosides
    - ● T36.5X6 Underdosing of aminoglycosides
- ● T36.6 Poisoning by, adverse effect of and underdosing of rifampicins
  - ● T36.6X Poisoning by, adverse effect of and underdosing of rifampicins
    - ● T36.6X1 Poisoning by rifampicins, accidental (unintentional)
      Poisoning by rifampicins NOS
    - ● T36.6X2 Poisoning by rifampicins, intentional self-harm
    - ● T36.6X3 Poisoning by rifampicins, assault
    - ● T36.6X4 Poisoning by rifampicins, undetermined
    - ● T36.6X5 Adverse effect of rifampicins
    - ● T36.6X6 Underdosing of rifampicins
- ● T36.7 Poisoning by, adverse effect of and underdosing of antifungal antibiotics, systemically used
  - ● T36.7X Poisoning by, adverse effect of and underdosing of antifungal antibiotics, systemically used
    - ● T36.7X1 Poisoning by antifungal antibiotics, systemically used, accidental (unintentional)
      Poisoning by antifungal antibiotics, systemically used NOS
    - ● T36.7X2 Poisoning by antifungal antibiotics, systemically used, intentional self-harm
    - ● T36.7X3 Poisoning by antifungal antibiotics, systemically used, assault
    - ● T36.7X4 Poisoning by antifungal antibiotics, systemically used, undetermined
    - ● T36.7X5 Adverse effect of antifungal antibiotics, systemically used
    - ● T36.7X6 Underdosing of antifungal antibiotics, systemically used

● T36.8   Poisoning by, adverse effect of and underdosing of other systemic antibiotics
  ● T36.8X   Poisoning by, adverse effect of and underdosing of other systemic antibiotics
    ● T36.8X1   Poisoning by other systemic antibiotics, accidental (unintentional)
                Poisoning by other systemic antibiotics NOS
    ● T36.8X2   Poisoning by other systemic antibiotics, intentional self-harm
    ● T36.8X3   Poisoning by other systemic antibiotics, assault
    ● T36.8X4   Poisoning by other systemic antibiotics, undetermined
    ● T36.8X5   Adverse effect of other systemic antibiotics
    ● T36.8X6   Underdosing of other systemic antibiotics
● T36.9   Poisoning by, adverse effect of and underdosing of unspecified systemic antibiotic
  X ● T36.91   Poisoning by unspecified systemic antibiotic, accidental (unintentional)
              Poisoning by systemic antibiotic NOS
  X ● T36.92   Poisoning by unspecified systemic antibiotic, intentional self-harm
  X ● T36.93   Poisoning by unspecified systemic antibiotic, assault
  X ● T36.94   Poisoning by unspecified systemic antibiotic, undetermined
  X ● T36.95   Adverse effect of unspecified systemic antibiotic
  X ● T36.96   Underdosing of unspecified systemic antibiotic

● T37   Poisoning by, adverse effect of and underdosing of other systemic anti-infectives and antiparasitics

  Excludes1   anti-infectives topically used for ear, nose and throat (T49.6-)
               anti-infectives topically used for eye (T49.5-)
               locally applied anti-infectives NEC (T49.0-)

  The appropriate 7th character is to be added to each code from category T37

A	initial encounter
D	subsequent encounter
S	sequela

● T37.0   Poisoning by, adverse effect of and underdosing of sulfonamides
  ● T37.0X   Poisoning by, adverse effect of and underdosing of sulfonamides
    ● T37.0X1   Poisoning by sulfonamides, accidental (unintentional)
                Poisoning by sulfonamides NOS
    ● T37.0X2   Poisoning by sulfonamides, intentional self-harm
    ● T37.0X3   Poisoning by sulfonamides, assault
    ● T37.0X4   Poisoning by sulfonamides, undetermined
    ● T37.0X5   Adverse effect of sulfonamides
    ● T37.0X6   Underdosing of sulfonamides
● T37.1   Poisoning by, adverse effect of and underdosing of antimycobacterial drugs
    Excludes1   rifampicins (T36.6-) streptomycin (T36.5-)
  ● T37.1X   Poisoning by, adverse effect of and underdosing of antimycobacterial drugs
    ● T37.1X1   Poisoning by antimycobacterial drugs, accidental (unintentional)
                Poisoning by antimycobacterial drugs NOS
    ● T37.1X2   Poisoning by antimycobacterial drugs, intentional self-harm

    ● T37.1X3   Poisoning by antimycobacterial drugs, assault
    ● T37.1X4   Poisoning by antimycobacterial drugs, undetermined
    ● T37.1X5   Adverse effect of antimycobacterial drugs
    ● T37.1X6   Underdosing of antimycobacterial drugs
● T37.2   Poisoning by, adverse effect of and underdosing of antimalarials and drugs acting on other blood protozoa
    Excludes1   hydroxyquinoline derivatives (T37.8-)
  ● T37.2X   Poisoning by, adverse effect of and underdosing of antimalarials and drugs acting on other blood protozoa
    ● T37.2X1   Poisoning by antimalarials and drugs acting on other blood protozoa, accidental (unintentional)
                Poisoning by antimalarials and drugs acting on other blood protozoa NOS
    ● T37.2X2   Poisoning by antimalarials and drugs acting on other blood protozoa, intentional self-harm
    ● T37.2X3   Poisoning by antimalarials and drugs acting on other blood protozoa, assault
    ● T37.2X4   Poisoning by antimalarials and drugs acting on other blood protozoa, undetermined
    ● T37.2X5   Adverse effect of antimalarials and drugs acting on other blood protozoa
    ● T37.2X6   Underdosing of antimalarials and drugs acting on other blood protozoa
● T37.3   Poisoning by, adverse effect of and underdosing of other antiprotozoal drugs
  ● T37.3X   Poisoning by, adverse effect of and underdosing of other antiprotozoal drugs
    ● T37.3X1   Poisoning by other antiprotozoal drugs, accidental (unintentional)
                Poisoning by other antiprotozoal drugs NOS
    ● T37.3X2   Poisoning by other antiprotozoal drugs, intentional self-harm
    ● T37.3X3   Poisoning by other antiprotozoal drugs, assault
    ● T37.3X4   Poisoning by other antiprotozoal drugs, undetermined
    ● T37.3X5   Adverse effect of other antiprotozoal drugs
    ● T37.3X6   Underdosing of other antiprotozoal drugs
● T37.4   Poisoning by, adverse effect of and underdosing of anthelminthics
  ● T37.4X   Poisoning by, adverse effect of and underdosing of anthelminthics
    ● T37.4X1   Poisoning by anthelminthics, accidental (unintentional)
                Poisoning by anthelminthics NOS
    ● T37.4X2   Poisoning by anthelminthics, intentional self-harm
    ● T37.4X3   Poisoning by anthelminthics, assault
    ● T37.4X4   Poisoning by anthelminthics, undetermined
    ● T37.4X5   Adverse effect of anthelminthics
    ● T37.4X6   Underdosing of anthelminthics

● **T37.5** Poisoning by, adverse effect of and underdosing of antiviral drugs

> Excludes1 amantadine (T42.8-)
> cytarabine (T45.1-)

● **T37.5X** Poisoning by, adverse effect of and underdosing of antiviral drugs

   ● **T37.5X1** Poisoning by antiviral drugs, accidental (unintentional)
      Poisoning by antiviral drugs NOS

   ● **T37.5X2** Poisoning by antiviral drugs, intentional self-harm

   ● **T37.5X3** Poisoning by antiviral drugs, assault

   ● **T37.5X4** Poisoning by antiviral drugs, undetermined

   ● **T37.5X5** Adverse effect of antiviral drugs

   ● **T37.5X6** Underdosing of antiviral drugs

● **T37.8** Poisoning by, adverse effect of and underdosing of other specified systemic anti-infectives and antiparasitics

> Poisoning by, adverse effect of and underdosing of hydroxyquinoline derivatives

> Excludes1 antimalarial drugs (T37.2-)

● **T37.8X** Poisoning by, adverse effect of and underdosing of other specified systemic anti-infectives and antiparasitics

   ● **T37.8X1** Poisoning by other specified systemic anti-infectives and antiparasitics, accidental (unintentional)
      Poisoning by other specified systemic anti-infectives and antiparasitics NOS

   ● **T37.8X2** Poisoning by other specified systemic anti-infectives and antiparasitics, intentional self-harm

   ● **T37.8X3** Poisoning by other specified systemic anti-infectives and antiparasitics, assault

   ● **T37.8X4** Poisoning by other specified systemic anti-infectives and antiparasitics, undetermined

   ● **T37.8X5** Adverse effect of other specified systemic anti-infectives and antiparasitics

   ● **T37.8X6** Underdosing of other specified systemic anti-infectives and antiparasitics

● **T37.9** Poisoning by, adverse effect of and underdosing of unspecified systemic anti-infective and antiparasitics

X ● **T37.91** Poisoning by unspecified systemic anti-infective and antiparasitics, accidental (unintentional)
      Poisoning by, adverse effect of and underdosing of systemic anti-infective and antiparasitics NOS

X ● **T37.92** Poisoning by unspecified systemic anti-infective and antiparasitics, intentional self-harm

X ● **T37.93** Poisoning by unspecified systemic anti-infective and antiparasitics, assault

X ● **T37.94** Poisoning by unspecified systemic anti-infective and antiparasitics, undetermined

X ● **T37.95** Adverse effect of unspecified systemic anti-infective and antiparasitic

X ● **T37.96** Underdosing of unspecified systemic anti-infectives and antiparasitics

● **T38** Poisoning by, adverse effect of and underdosing of hormones and their synthetic substitutes and antagonists, not elsewhere classified

> Excludes1 mineralocorticoids and their antagonists (T50.0-)
> oxytocic hormones (T48.0-)
> parathyroid hormones and derivatives (T50.9-)

The appropriate 7th character is to be added to each code from category T38

> A   initial encounter
> D   subsequent encounter
> S   sequela

● **T38.0** Poisoning by, adverse effect of and underdosing of glucocorticoids and synthetic analogues

> Excludes1 glucocorticoids, topically used (T49.-)

● **T38.0X** Poisoning by, adverse effect of and underdosing of glucocorticoids and synthetic analogues

   ● **T38.0X1** Poisoning by glucocorticoids and synthetic analogues, accidental (unintentional)
      Poisoning by glucocorticoids and synthetic analogues NOS

   ● **T38.0X2** Poisoning by glucocorticoids and synthetic analogues, intentional self-harm

   ● **T38.0X3** Poisoning by glucocorticoids and synthetic analogues, assault

   ● **T38.0X4** Poisoning by glucocorticoids and synthetic analogues, undetermined

   ● **T38.0X5** Adverse effect of glucocorticoids and synthetic analogues

   ● **T38.0X6** Underdosing of glucocorticoids and synthetic analogues

● **T38.1** Poisoning by, adverse effect of and underdosing of thyroid hormones and substitutes

● **T38.1X** Poisoning by, adverse effect of and underdosing of thyroid hormones and substitutes

   ● **T38.1X1** Poisoning by thyroid hormones and substitutes, accidental (unintentional)
      Poisoning by thyroid hormones and substitutes NOS

   ● **T38.1X2** Poisoning by thyroid hormones and substitutes, intentional self-harm

   ● **T38.1X3** Poisoning by thyroid hormones and substitutes, assault

   ● **T38.1X4** Poisoning by thyroid hormones and substitutes, undetermined

   ● **T38.1X5** Adverse effect of thyroid hormones and substitutes

   ● **T38.1X6** Underdosing of thyroid hormones and substitutes

● **T38.2** Poisoning by, adverse effect of and underdosing of antithyroid drugs

● **T38.2X** Poisoning by, adverse effect of and underdosing of antithyroid drugs

   ● **T38.2X1** Poisoning by antithyroid drugs, accidental (unintentional)
      Poisoning by antithyroid drugs NOS

   ● **T38.2X2** Poisoning by antithyroid drugs, intentional self-harm

   ● **T38.2X3** Poisoning by antithyroid drugs, assault

   ● **T38.2X4** Poisoning by antithyroid drugs, undetermined

   ● **T38.2X5** Adverse effect of antithyroid drugs

   ● **T38.2X6** Underdosing of antithyroid drugs

● **T38.3**   Poisoning by, adverse effect of and underdosing of insulin and oral hypoglycemic [antidiabetic] drugs
  ● **T38.3X**   Poisoning by, adverse effect of and underdosing of insulin and oral hypoglycemic [antidiabetic] drugs
    ● **T38.3X1**   Poisoning by insulin and oral hypoglycemic [antidiabetic] drugs, accidental (unintentional)
      Poisoning by insulin and oral hypoglycemic [antidiabetic] drugs NOS
    ● **T38.3X2**   Poisoning by insulin and oral hypoglycemic [antidiabetic] drugs, intentional self-harm
    ● **T38.3X3**   Poisoning by insulin and oral hypoglycemic [antidiabetic] drugs, assault
    ● **T38.3X4**   Poisoning by insulin and oral hypoglycemic [antidiabetic] drugs, undetermined
    ● **T38.3X5**   Adverse effect of insulin and oral hypoglycemic [antidiabetic] drugs
    ● **T38.3X6**   Underdosing of insulin and oral hypoglycemic [antidiabetic] drugs

● **T38.4**   Poisoning by, adverse effect of and underdosing of oral contraceptives
  Poisoning by, adverse effect of and underdosing of multiple- and single-ingredient oral contraceptive preparations
  ● **T38.4X**   Poisoning by, adverse effect of and underdosing of oral contraceptives
    ● **T38.4X1**   Poisoning by oral contraceptives, accidental (unintentional)
      Poisoning by oral contraceptives NOS
    ● **T38.4X2**   Poisoning by oral contraceptives, intentional self-harm
    ● **T38.4X3**   Poisoning by oral contraceptives, assault
    ● **T38.4X4**   Poisoning by oral contraceptives, undetermined
    ● **T38.4X5**   Adverse effect of oral contraceptives
    ● **T38.4X6**   Underdosing of oral contraceptives

● **T38.5**   Poisoning by, adverse effect of and underdosing of other estrogens and progestogens
  Poisoning by, adverse effect of and underdosing of estrogens and progestogens mixtures and substitutes
  ● **T38.5X**   Poisoning by, adverse effect of and underdosing of other estrogens and progestogens
    ● **T38.5X1**   Poisoning by other estrogens and progestogens, accidental (unintentional)
      Poisoning by other estrogens and progestogens NOS
    ● **T38.5X2**   Poisoning by other estrogens and progestogens, intentional self-harm
    ● **T38.5X3**   Poisoning by other estrogens and progestogens, assault
    ● **T38.5X4**   Poisoning by other estrogens and progestogens, undetermined
    ● **T38.5X5**   Adverse effect of other estrogens and progestogens
    ● **T38.5X6**   Underdosing of other estrogens and progestogens

● **T38.6**   Poisoning by, adverse effect of and underdosing of antigonadotrophins, antiestrogens, antiandrogens, not elsewhere classified
  Poisoning by, adverse effect of and underdosing of tamoxifen
  ● **T38.6X**   Poisoning by, adverse effect of and underdosing of antigonadotrophins, antiestrogens, antiandrogens, not elsewhere classified
    ● **T38.6X1**   Poisoning by antigonadotrophins, antiestrogens, antiandrogens, not elsewhere classified, accidental (unintentional)
      Poisoning by antigonadotrophins, antiestrogens, antiandrogens, not elsewhere classified NOS
    ● **T38.6X2**   Poisoning by antigonadotrophins, antiestrogens, antiandrogens, not elsewhere classified, intentional self-harm
    ● **T38.6X3**   Poisoning by antigonadotrophins, antiestrogens, antiandrogens, not elsewhere classified, assault
    ● **T38.6X4**   Poisoning by antigonadotrophins, antiestrogens, antiandrogens, not elsewhere classified, undetermined
    ● **T38.6X5**   Adverse effect of antigonadotrophins, antiestrogens, antiandrogens, not elsewhere classified
    ● **T38.6X6**   Underdosing of antigonadotrophins, antiestrogens, antiandrogens, not elsewhere classified

● **T38.7**   Poisoning by, adverse effect of and underdosing of androgens and anabolic congeners
  ● **T38.7X**   Poisoning by, adverse effect of and underdosing of androgens and anabolic congeners
    ● **T38.7X1**   Poisoning by androgens and anabolic congeners, accidental (unintentional)
      Poisoning by androgens and anabolic congeners NOS
    ● **T38.7X2**   Poisoning by androgens and anabolic congeners, intentional self-harm
    ● **T38.7X3**   Poisoning by androgens and anabolic congeners, assault
    ● **T38.7X4**   Poisoning by androgens and anabolic congeners, undetermined
    ● **T38.7X5**   Adverse effect of androgens and anabolic congeners
    ● **T38.7X6**   Underdosing of androgens and anabolic congeners

● **T38.8**   Poisoning by, adverse effect of and underdosing of other and unspecified hormones and synthetic substitutes
  ● **T38.80**   Poisoning by, adverse effect of and underdosing of unspecified hormones and synthetic substitutes
    ● **T38.801**   Poisoning by unspecified hormones and synthetic substitutes, accidental (unintentional)
      Poisoning by unspecified hormones and synthetic substitutes NOS
    ● **T38.802**   Poisoning by unspecified hormones and synthetic substitutes, intentional self-harm
    ● **T38.803**   Poisoning by unspecified hormones and synthetic substitutes, assault
    ● **T38.804**   Poisoning by unspecified hormones and synthetic substitutes, undetermined
    ● **T38.805**   Adverse effect of unspecified hormones and synthetic substitutes
    ● **T38.806**   Underdosing of unspecified hormones and synthetic substitutes

◀ New   ◀▬ Revised   ~~deleted~~ Deleted   **OGCR** Official Guidelines   X Assign placeholder X   ● Use Additional Character(s)

| Excludes 1 | Excludes 2 | Includes | Use additional | Code first | Code also | Unspecified |

● **T38.81** **Poisoning by, adverse effect of and underdosing of anterior pituitary [adenohypophyseal] hormones**

● **T38.811** **Poisoning by anterior pituitary [adenohypophyseal] hormones, accidental (unintentional)**
Poisoning by anterior pituitary [adenohypophyseal] hormones NOS

● **T38.812** **Poisoning by anterior pituitary [adenohypophyseal] hormones, intentional self-harm**

● **T38.813** **Poisoning by anterior pituitary [adenohypophyseal] hormones, assault**

● **T38.814** **Poisoning by anterior pituitary [adenohypophyseal] hormones, undetermined**

● **T38.815** **Adverse effect of anterior pituitary [adenohypophyseal] hormones**

● **T38.816** **Underdosing of anterior pituitary [adenohypophyseal] hormones**

● **T38.89** **Poisoning by, adverse effect of and underdosing of other hormones and synthetic substitutes**

● **T38.891** **Poisoning by other hormones and synthetic substitutes, accidental (unintentional)**
Poisoning by other hormones and synthetic substitutes NOS

● **T38.892** **Poisoning by other hormones and synthetic substitutes, intentional self-harm**

● **T38.893** **Poisoning by other hormones and synthetic substitutes, assault**

● **T38.894** **Poisoning by other hormones and synthetic substitutes, undetermined**

● **T38.895** **Adverse effect of other hormones and synthetic substitutes**

● **T38.896** **Underdosing of other hormones and synthetic substitutes**

● **T38.9** **Poisoning by, adverse effect of and underdosing of other and unspecified hormone antagonists**

● **T38.90** **Poisoning by, adverse effect of and underdosing of unspecified hormone antagonists**

● **T38.901** **Poisoning by unspecified hormone antagonists, accidental (unintentional)**
Poisoning by unspecified hormone antagonists NOS

● **T38.902** **Poisoning by unspecified hormone antagonists, intentional self-harm**

● **T38.903** **Poisoning by unspecified hormone antagonists, assault**

● **T38.904** **Poisoning by unspecified hormone antagonists, undetermined**

● **T38.905** **Adverse effect of unspecified hormone antagonists**

● **T38.906** **Underdosing of unspecified hormone antagonists**

● **T38.99** **Poisoning by, adverse effect of and underdosing of other hormone antagonists**

● **T38.991** **Poisoning by other hormone antagonists, accidental (unintentional)**
Poisoning by other hormone antagonists NOS

● **T38.992** **Poisoning by other hormone antagonists, intentional self-harm**

● **T38.993** **Poisoning by other hormone antagonists, assault**

● **T38.994** **Poisoning by other hormone antagonists, undetermined**

● **T38.995** **Adverse effect of other hormone antagonists**

● **T38.996** **Underdosing of other hormone antagonists**

● **T39** **Poisoning by, adverse effect of and underdosing of nonopioid analgesics, antipyretics and antirheumatics**
The appropriate 7th character is to be added to each code from category T39

A	initial encounter
D	subsequent encounter
S	sequela

● **T39.0** **Poisoning by, adverse effect of and underdosing of salicylates**

● **T39.01** **Poisoning by, adverse effect of and underdosing of aspirin**
Poisoning by, adverse effect of and underdosing of acetylsalicylic acid

● **T39.011** **Poisoning by aspirin, accidental (unintentional)**

● **T39.012** **Poisoning by aspirin, intentional self-harm**

● **T39.013** **Poisoning by aspirin, assault**

● **T39.014** **Poisoning by aspirin, undetermined**

● **T39.015** **Adverse effect of aspirin**

● **T39.016** **Underdosing of aspirin**

● **T39.09** **Poisoning by, adverse effect of and underdosing of other salicylates**

● **T39.091** **Poisoning by salicylates, accidental (unintentional)**
Poisoning by salicylates NOS

● **T39.092** **Poisoning by salicylates, intentional self-harm**

● **T39.093** **Poisoning by salicylates, assault**

● **T39.094** **Poisoning by salicylates, undetermined**

● **T39.095** **Adverse effect of salicylates**

● **T39.096** **Underdosing of salicylates**

● **T39.1** **Poisoning by, adverse effect of and underdosing of 4-Aminophenol derivatives**

● **T39.1X** **Poisoning by, adverse effect of and underdosing of 4-Aminophenol derivatives**

● **T39.1X1** **Poisoning by 4-Aminophenol derivatives, accidental (unintentional)**
Poisoning by 4-Aminophenol derivatives NOS

● **T39.1X2** **Poisoning by 4-Aminophenol derivatives, intentional self-harm**

● **T39.1X3** **Poisoning by 4-Aminophenol derivatives, assault**

● **T39.1X4** **Poisoning by 4-Aminophenol derivatives, undetermined**

● **T39.1X5** **Adverse effect of 4-Aminophenol derivatives**

● **T39.1X6** **Underdosing of 4-Aminophenol derivatives**

CHAPTER 19 (S00-T88)

●T39.2   Poisoning by, adverse effect of and underdosing of pyrazolone derivatives

   ●T39.2X   Poisoning by, adverse effect of and underdosing of pyrazolone derivatives

      ●T39.2X1   Poisoning by pyrazolone derivatives, accidental (unintentional)
                     Poisoning by pyrazolone derivatives NOS

      ●T39.2X2   Poisoning by pyrazolone derivatives, intentional self-harm

      ●T39.2X3   Poisoning by pyrazolone derivatives, assault

      ●T39.2X4   Poisoning by pyrazolone derivatives, undetermined

      ●T39.2X5   Adverse effect of pyrazolone derivatives

      ●T39.2X6   Underdosing of pyrazolone derivatives

●T39.3   Poisoning by, adverse effect of and underdosing of other nonsteroidal anti-inflammatory drugs [NSAID]

   ●T39.31   Poisoning by, adverse effect of and underdosing of propionic acid derivatives
                Poisoning by, adverse effect of and underdosing of fenoprofen
                Poisoning by, adverse effect of and underdosing of flurbiprofen
                Poisoning by, adverse effect of and underdosing of ibuprofen
                Poisoning by, adverse effect of and underdosing of ketoprofen
                Poisoning by, adverse effect of and underdosing of naproxen
                Poisoning by, adverse effect of and underdosing of oxaprozin

      ●T39.311   Poisoning by propionic acid derivatives, accidental (unintentional)

      ●T39.312   Poisoning by propionic acid derivatives, intentional self-harm

      ●T39.313   Poisoning by propionic acid derivatives, assault

      ●T39.314   Poisoning by propionic acid derivatives, undetermined

      ●T39.315   Adverse effect of propionic acid derivatives

      ●T39.316   Underdosing of propionic acid derivatives

   ●T39.39   Poisoning by, adverse effect of and underdosing of other nonsteroidal anti-inflammatory drugs [NSAID]

      ●T39.391   Poisoning by other nonsteroidal anti-inflammatory drugs [NSAID], accidental (unintentional)
                     Poisoning by other nonsteroidal anti-inflammatory drugs NOS

      ●T39.392   Poisoning by other nonsteroidal anti-inflammatory drugs [NSAID], intentional self-harm

      ●T39.393   Poisoning by other nonsteroidal anti-inflammatory drugs [NSAID], assault

      ●T39.394   Poisoning by other nonsteroidal anti-inflammatory drugs [NSAID], undetermined

      ●T39.395   Adverse effect of other nonsteroidal anti-inflammatory drugs [NSAID]

      ●T39.396   Underdosing of other nonsteroidal anti-inflammatory drugs [NSAID]

●T39.4   Poisoning by, adverse effect of and underdosing of antirheumatics, not elsewhere classified

   Excludes1   poisoning by, adverse effect of and underdosing of glucocorticoids (T38.0-)
               poisoning by, adverse effect of and underdosing of salicylates (T39.0-)

   ●T39.4X   Poisoning by, adverse effect of and underdosing of antirheumatics, not elsewhere classified

      ●T39.4X1   Poisoning by antirheumatics, not elsewhere classified, accidental (unintentional)
                     Poisoning by antirheumatics, not elsewhere classified NOS

      ●T39.4X2   Poisoning by antirheumatics, not elsewhere classified, intentional self-harm

      ●T39.4X3   Poisoning by antirheumatics, not elsewhere classified, assault

      ●T39.4X4   Poisoning by antirheumatics, not elsewhere classified, undetermined

      ●T39.4X5   Adverse effect of antirheumatics, not elsewhere classified

      ●T39.4X6   Underdosing of antirheumatics, not elsewhere classified

●T39.8   Poisoning by, adverse effect of and underdosing of other nonopioid analgesics and antipyretics, not elsewhere classified

   ●T39.8X   Poisoning by, adverse effect of and underdosing of other nonopioid analgesics and antipyretics, not elsewhere classified

      ●T39.8X1   Poisoning by other nonopioid analgesics and antipyretics, not elsewhere classified, accidental (unintentional)
                     Poisoning by other nonopioid analgesics and antipyretics, not elsewhere classified NOS

      ●T39.8X2   Poisoning by other nonopioid analgesics and antipyretics, not elsewhere classified, intentional self-harm

      ●T39.8X3   Poisoning by other nonopioid analgesics and antipyretics, not elsewhere classified, assault

      ●T39.8X4   Poisoning by other nonopioid analgesics and antipyretics, not elsewhere classified, undetermined

      ●T39.8X5   Adverse effect of other nonopioid analgesics and antipyretics, not elsewhere classified

      ●T39.8X6   Underdosing of other nonopioid analgesics and antipyretics, not elsewhere classified

●T39.9   Poisoning by, adverse effect of and underdosing of unspecified nonopioid analgesic, antipyretic and antirheumatic

   X●T39.91   Poisoning by unspecified nonopioid analgesic, antipyretic and antirheumatic, accidental (unintentional)
                 Poisoning by nonopioid analgesic, antipyretic and antirheumatic NOS

   X●T39.92   Poisoning by unspecified nonopioid analgesic, antipyretic and antirheumatic, intentional self-harm

   X●T39.93   Poisoning by unspecified nonopioid analgesic, antipyretic and antirheumatic, assault

   X●T39.94   Poisoning by unspecified nonopioid analgesic, antipyretic and antirheumatic, undetermined

   X●T39.95   Adverse effect of unspecified nonopioid analgesic, antipyretic and antirheumatic

   X●T39.96   Underdosing of unspecified nonopioid analgesic, antipyretic and antirheumatic

◀ New   ◀▥ Revised   ~~deleted~~ Deleted   OGCR Official Guidelines   X Assign placeholder X   ● Use Additional Character(s)

Excludes 1   Excludes 2   Includes   Use additional   Code first   Code also   Unspecified

● T40 **Poisoning by, adverse effect of and underdosing of narcotics and psychodysleptics [hallucinogens]**

Excludes2 drug dependence and related mental and behavioral disorders due to psychoactive substance use (F10.-F19.-)

The appropriate 7th character is to be added to each code from category T40

> A   initial encounter
> D   subsequent encounter
> S   sequela

● T40.0 **Poisoning by, adverse effect of and underdosing of opium**

● T40.0X **Poisoning by, adverse effect of and underdosing of opium**

● T40.0X1 **Poisoning by opium, accidental (unintentional)**
Poisoning by opium NOS

● T40.0X2 **Poisoning by opium, intentional self-harm**

● T40.0X3 **Poisoning by opium, assault**

● T40.0X4 **Poisoning by opium, undetermined**

● T40.0X5 **Adverse effect of opium**

● T40.0X6 **Underdosing of opium**

● T40.1 **Poisoning by and adverse effect of heroin**

● T40.1X **Poisoning by and adverse effect of heroin**

● T40.1X1 **Poisoning by heroin, accidental (unintentional)**
Poisoning by heroin NOS

● T40.1X2 **Poisoning by heroin, intentional self-harm**

● T40.1X3 **Poisoning by heroin, assault**

● T40.1X4 **Poisoning by heroin, undetermined**

● T40.2 **Poisoning by, adverse effect of and underdosing of other opioids**

● T40.2X **Poisoning by, adverse effect of and underdosing of other opioids**

● T40.2X1 **Poisoning by other opioids, accidental (unintentional)**
Poisoning by other opioids NOS

● T40.2X2 **Poisoning by other opioids, intentional self-harm**

● T40.2X3 **Poisoning by other opioids, assault**

● T40.2X4 **Poisoning by other opioids, undetermined**

● T40.2X5 **Adverse effect of other opioids**

● T40.2X6 **Underdosing of other opioids**

● T40.3 **Poisoning by, adverse effect of and underdosing of methadone**

● T40.3X **Poisoning by, adverse effect of and underdosing of methadone**

● T40.3X1 **Poisoning by methadone, accidental (unintentional)**
Poisoning by methadone NOS

● T40.3X2 **Poisoning by methadone, intentional self-harm**

● T40.3X3 **Poisoning by methadone, assault**

● T40.3X4 **Poisoning by methadone, undetermined**

● T40.3X5 **Adverse effect of methadone**

● T40.3X6 **Underdosing of methadone**

● T40.4 **Poisoning by, adverse effect of and underdosing of other synthetic narcotics**

● T40.4X **Poisoning by, adverse effect of and underdosing of other synthetic narcotics**

● T40.4X1 **Poisoning by other synthetic narcotics, accidental (unintentional)**
Poisoning by other synthetic narcotics NOS

● T40.4X2 **Poisoning by other synthetic narcotics, intentional self-harm**

● T40.4X3 **Poisoning by other synthetic narcotics, assault**

● T40.4X4 **Poisoning by other synthetic narcotics, undetermined**

● T40.4X5 **Adverse effect of other synthetic narcotics**

● T40.4X6 **Underdosing of other synthetic narcotics**

● T40.5 **Poisoning by, adverse effect of and underdosing of cocaine**

● T40.5X **Poisoning by, adverse effect of and underdosing of cocaine**

● T40.5X1 **Poisoning by cocaine, accidental (unintentional)**
Poisoning by cocaine NOS

● T40.5X2 **Poisoning by cocaine, intentional self-harm**

● T40.5X3 **Poisoning by cocaine, assault**

● T40.5X4 **Poisoning by cocaine, undetermined**

● T40.5X5 **Adverse effect of cocaine**

● T40.5X6 **Underdosing of cocaine**

● T40.6 **Poisoning by, adverse effect of and underdosing of other and unspecified narcotics**

● T40.60 **Poisoning by, adverse effect of and underdosing of unspecified narcotics**

● T40.601 **Poisoning by unspecified narcotics, accidental (unintentional)**
Poisoning by narcotics NOS

● T40.602 **Poisoning by unspecified narcotics, intentional self-harm**

● T40.603 **Poisoning by unspecified narcotics, assault**

● T40.604 **Poisoning by unspecified narcotics, undetermined**

● T40.605 **Adverse effect of unspecified narcotics**

● T40.606 **Underdosing of unspecified narcotics**

● T40.69 **Poisoning by, adverse effect of and underdosing of other narcotics**

● T40.691 **Poisoning by other narcotics, accidental (unintentional)**
Poisoning by other narcotics NOS

● T40.692 **Poisoning by other narcotics, intentional self-harm**

● T40.693 **Poisoning by other narcotics, assault**

● T40.694 **Poisoning by other narcotics, undetermined**

● T40.695 **Adverse effect of other narcotics**

● T40.696 **Underdosing of other narcotics**

● **T40.7** Poisoning by, adverse effect of and underdosing of cannabis (derivatives)

  ● **T40.7X** Poisoning by, adverse effect of and underdosing of cannabis (derivatives)

    ● **T40.7X1** Poisoning by cannabis (derivatives), accidental (unintentional)
      Poisoning by cannabis NOS

    ● **T40.7X2** Poisoning by cannabis (derivatives), intentional self-harm

    ● **T40.7X3** Poisoning by cannabis (derivatives), assault

    ● **T40.7X4** Poisoning by cannabis (derivatives), undetermined

    ● **T40.7X5** Adverse effect of cannabis (derivatives)

    ● **T40.7X6** Underdosing of cannabis (derivatives)

● **T40.8** Poisoning by and adverse effect of lysergide [LSD]

  ● **T40.8X** Poisoning by and adverse effect of lysergide [LSD]

    ● **T40.8X1** Poisoning by lysergide [LSD], accidental (unintentional)
      Poisoning by lysergide [LSD] NOS

    ● **T40.8X2** Poisoning by lysergide [LSD], intentional self-harm

    ● **T40.8X3** Poisoning by lysergide [LSD], assault

    ● **T40.8X4** Poisoning by lysergide [LSD], undetermined

● **T40.9** Poisoning by, adverse effect of and underdosing of other and unspecified psychodysleptics [hallucinogens]

  ● **T40.90** Poisoning by, adverse effect of and underdosing of unspecified psychodysleptics [hallucinogens]

    ● **T40.901** Poisoning by unspecified psychodysleptics [hallucinogens], accidental (unintentional)

    ● **T40.902** Poisoning by unspecified psychodysleptics [hallucinogens], intentional self-harm

    ● **T40.903** Poisoning by unspecified psychodysleptics [hallucinogens], assault

    ● **T40.904** Poisoning by unspecified psychodysleptics [hallucinogens], undetermined

    ● **T40.905** Adverse effect of unspecified psychodysleptics [hallucinogens]

    ● **T40.906** Underdosing of unspecified psychodysleptics

  ● **T40.99** Poisoning by, adverse effect of and underdosing of other psychodysleptics [hallucinogens]

    ● **T40.991** Poisoning by other psychodysleptics [hallucinogens], accidental (unintentional)
      Poisoning by other psychodysleptics [hallucinogens] NOS

    ● **T40.992** Poisoning by other psychodysleptics [hallucinogens], intentional self-harm

    ● **T40.993** Poisoning by other psychodysleptics [hallucinogens], assault

    ● **T40.994** Poisoning by other psychodysleptics [hallucinogens], undetermined

    ● **T40.995** Adverse effect of other psychodysleptics [hallucinogens]

    ● **T40.996** Underdosing of other psychodysleptics

● **T41** Poisoning by, adverse effect of and underdosing of anesthetics and therapeutic gases

  | Excludes1 | benzodiazepines (T42.4-)
  cocaine (T40.5-)
  complications of anesthesia during pregnancy (O29.-)
  complications of anesthesia during labor and delivery (O74.-)
  complications of anesthesia during the puerperium (O89.-) opioids (T40.0-T40.2-)

The appropriate 7th character is to be added to each code from category T41

  A initial encounter
  D subsequent encounter
  S sequela

● **T41.0** Poisoning by, adverse effect of and underdosing of inhaled anesthetics

  | Excludes1 | oxygen (T41.5-)

  ● **T41.0X** Poisoning by, adverse effect of and underdosing of inhaled anesthetics

    ● **T41.0X1** Poisoning by inhaled anesthetics, accidental (unintentional)
      Poisoning by inhaled anesthetics NOS

    ● **T41.0X2** Poisoning by inhaled anesthetics, intentional self-harm

    ● **T41.0X3** Poisoning by inhaled anesthetics, assault

    ● **T41.0X4** Poisoning by inhaled anesthetics, undetermined

    ● **T41.0X5** Adverse effect of inhaled anesthetics

    ● **T41.0X6** Underdosing of inhaled anesthetics

● **T41.1** Poisoning by, adverse effect of and underdosing of intravenous anesthetics
  Poisoning by, adverse effect of and underdosing of thiobarbiturates

  ● **T41.1X** Poisoning by, adverse effect of and underdosing of intravenous anesthetics

    ● **T41.1X1** Poisoning by intravenous anesthetics, accidental (unintentional)
      Poisoning by intravenous anesthetics NOS

    ● **T41.1X2** Poisoning by intravenous anesthetics, intentional self-harm

    ● **T41.1X3** Poisoning by intravenous anesthetics, assault

    ● **T41.1X4** Poisoning by intravenous anesthetics, undetermined

    ● **T41.1X5** Adverse effect of intravenous anesthetics

    ● **T41.1X6** Underdosing of intravenous anesthetics

● **T41.2** Poisoning by, adverse effect of and underdosing of other and unspecified general anesthetics

  ● **T41.20** Poisoning by, adverse effect of and underdosing of unspecified general anesthetics

    ● **T41.201** Poisoning by unspecified general anesthetics, accidental (unintentional)
      Poisoning by general anesthetics NOS

    ● **T41.202** Poisoning by unspecified general anesthetics, intentional self-harm

    ● **T41.203** Poisoning by unspecified general anesthetics, assault

    ● **T41.204** Poisoning by unspecified general anesthetics, undetermined

    ● **T41.205** Adverse effect of unspecified general anesthetics

    ● **T41.206** Underdosing of unspecified general anesthetics

◄ New   ◄▥ Revised   ~~deleted~~ Deleted   **OGCR** Official Guidelines   X Assign placeholder X   ● Use Additional Character(s)

| Excludes 1 | | Excludes 2 | | Includes | | Use additional | | Code first | | Code also | | Unspecified |

● T41.29   Poisoning by, adverse effect of and
           underdosing of other general anesthetics
    ● T41.291   Poisoning by other general anesthetics,
               accidental (unintentional)
                   Poisoning by other general
                   anesthetics NOS
    ● T41.292   Poisoning by other general anesthetics,
               intentional self-harm
    ● T41.293   Poisoning by other general
               anesthetics, assault
    ● T41.294   Poisoning by other general
               anesthetics, undetermined
    ● T41.295   Adverse effect of other general
               anesthetics
    ● T41.296   Underdosing of other general
               anesthetics
● T41.3   Poisoning by, adverse effect of and underdosing of local
          anesthetics
             Cocaine (topical)
          Excludes2   poisoning by cocaine used as a central
                      nervous system stimulant (T40.5X1-
                      T40.5X4)
    ● T41.3X   Poisoning by, adverse effect of and
              underdosing of local anesthetics
        ● T41.3X1   Poisoning by local anesthetics,
                   accidental (unintentional)
                       Poisoning by local anesthetics NOS
        ● T41.3X2   Poisoning by local anesthetics,
                   intentional self-harm
        ● T41.3X3   Poisoning by local anesthetics, assault
        ● T41.3X4   Poisoning by local anesthetics,
                   undetermined
        ● T41.3X5   Adverse effect of local anesthetics
        ● T41.3X6   Underdosing of local anesthetics
● T41.4   Poisoning by, adverse effect of and underdosing of
          unspecified anesthetic
    X ● T41.41   Poisoning by unspecified anesthetic, accidental
               (unintentional)
                   Poisoning by anesthetic NOS
    X ● T41.42   Poisoning by unspecified anesthetic,
               intentional self-harm
    X ● T41.43   Poisoning by unspecified anesthetic, assault
    X ● T41.44   Poisoning by unspecified anesthetic,
               undetermined
    X ● T41.45   Adverse effect of unspecified anesthetic
    X ● T41.46   Underdosing of unspecified anesthetics
● T41.5   Poisoning by, adverse effect of and underdosing of
          therapeutic gases
    ● T41.5X   Poisoning by, adverse effect of and
              underdosing of therapeutic gases
        ● T41.5X1   Poisoning by therapeutic gases,
                   accidental (unintentional)
                       Poisoning by therapeutic gases NOS
        ● T41.5X2   Poisoning by therapeutic gases,
                   intentional self-harm
        ● T41.5X3   Poisoning by therapeutic gases,
                   assault
        ● T41.5X4   Poisoning by therapeutic gases,
                   undetermined
        ● T41.5X5   Adverse effect of therapeutic gases
        ● T41.5X6   Underdosing of therapeutic gases

● T42   Poisoning by, adverse effect of and underdosing of
        antiepileptic, sedative-hypnotic and antiparkinsonism drugs
        Excludes2   drug dependence and related mental and
                    behavioral disorders due to psychoactive
                    substance use (F10.--F19.-)
        The appropriate 7th character is to be added to each code from
        category T42

        | A | initial encounter |
        | D | subsequent encounter |
        | S | sequela |

    ● T42.0   Poisoning by, adverse effect of and underdosing of
              hydantoin derivatives
        ● T42.0X   Poisoning by, adverse effect of and
                  underdosing of hydantoin derivatives
            ● T42.0X1   Poisoning by hydantoin derivatives,
                       accidental (unintentional)
                           Poisoning by hydantoin derivatives
                           NOS
            ● T42.0X2   Poisoning by hydantoin derivatives,
                       intentional self-harm
            ● T42.0X3   Poisoning by hydantoin derivatives,
                       assault
            ● T42.0X4   Poisoning by hydantoin derivatives,
                       undetermined
            ● T42.0X5   Adverse effect of hydantoin
                       derivatives
            ● T42.0X6   Underdosing of hydantoin derivatives
    ● T42.1   Poisoning by, adverse effect of and underdosing of
              iminostilbenes
                 Poisoning by, adverse effect of and underdosing of
                 carbamazepine
        ● T42.1X   Poisoning by, adverse effect of and
                  underdosing of iminostilbenes
            ● T42.1X1   Poisoning by iminostilbenes,
                       accidental (unintentional)
                           Poisoning by iminostilbenes NOS
            ● T42.1X2   Poisoning by iminostilbenes,
                       intentional self-harm
            ● T42.1X3   Poisoning by iminostilbenes, assault
            ● T42.1X4   Poisoning by iminostilbenes,
                       undetermined
            ● T42.1X5   Adverse effect of iminostilbenes
            ● T42.1X6   Underdosing of iminostilbenes
    ● T42.2   Poisoning by, adverse effect of and underdosing of
              succinimides and oxazolidinediones
        ● T42.2X   Poisoning by, adverse effect of and underdosing
                  of succinimides and oxazolidinediones
            ● T42.2X1   Poisoning by succinimides and
                       oxazolidinediones, accidental
                       (unintentional)
                           Poisoning by succinimides and
                           oxazolidinediones NOS
            ● T42.2X2   Poisoning by succinimides and
                       oxazolidinediones, intentional self-
                       harm
            ● T42.2X3   Poisoning by succinimides and
                       oxazolidinediones, assault
            ● T42.2X4   Poisoning by succinimides and
                       oxazolidinediones, undetermined
            ● T42.2X5   Adverse effect of succinimides and
                       oxazolidinediones
            ● T42.2X6   Underdosing of succinimides and
                       oxazolidinediones

- ● T42.3   Poisoning by, adverse effect of and underdosing of barbiturates
  - **Excludes1**   poisoning by, adverse effect of and underdosing of thiobarbiturates (T41.1-)
  - ● T42.3X   Poisoning by, adverse effect of and underdosing of barbiturates
    - ● T42.3X1   Poisoning by barbiturates, accidental (unintentional)
      - Poisoning by barbiturates NOS
    - ● T42.3X2   Poisoning by barbiturates, intentional self-harm
    - ● T42.3X3   Poisoning by barbiturates, assault
    - ● T42.3X4   Poisoning by barbiturates, undetermined
    - ● T42.3X5   Adverse effect of barbiturates
    - ● T42.3X6   Underdosing of barbiturates
- ● T42.4   Poisoning by, adverse effect of and underdosing of benzodiazepines
  - ● T42.4X   Poisoning by, adverse effect of and underdosing of benzodiazepines
    - ● T42.4X1   Poisoning by benzodiazepines, accidental (unintentional)
      - Poisoning by benzodiazepines NOS
    - ● T42.4X2   Poisoning by benzodiazepines, intentional self-harm
    - ● T42.4X3   Poisoning by benzodiazepines, assault
    - ● T42.4X4   Poisoning by benzodiazepines, undetermined
    - ● T42.4X5   Adverse effect of benzodiazepines
    - ● T42.4X6   Underdosing of benzodiazepines
- ● T42.5   Poisoning by, adverse effect of and underdosing of mixed antiepileptics
  - ● T42.5X   Poisoning by, adverse effect of and underdosing of antiepileptics
    - ● T42.5X1   Poisoning by mixed antiepileptics, accidental (unintentional)
      - Poisoning by mixed antiepileptics NOS
    - ● T42.5X2   Poisoning by mixed antiepileptics, intentional self-harm
    - ● T42.5X3   Poisoning by mixed antiepileptics, assault
    - ● T42.5X4   Poisoning by mixed antiepileptics, undetermined
    - ● T42.5X5   Adverse effect of mixed antiepileptics
    - ● T42.5X6   Underdosing of mixed antiepileptics
- ● T42.6   Poisoning by, adverse effect of and underdosing of other antiepileptic and sedative-hypnotic drugs
  - Poisoning by, adverse effect of and underdosing of methaqualone
  - Poisoning by, adverse effect of and underdosing of valproic acid
  - **Excludes1**   poisoning by, adverse effect of and underdosing of carbamazepine (T42.1-)
  - ● T42.6X   Poisoning by, adverse effect of and underdosing of other antiepileptic and sedative-hypnotic drugs
    - ● T42.6X1   Poisoning by other antiepileptic and sedative-hypnotic drugs, accidental (unintentional)
      - Poisoning by other antiepileptic and sedative-hypnotic drugs NOS

- ● T42.6X2   Poisoning by other antiepileptic and sedative-hypnotic drugs, intentional self-harm
- ● T42.6X3   Poisoning by other antiepileptic and sedative-hypnotic drugs, assault
- ● T42.6X4   Poisoning by other antiepileptic and sedative-hypnotic drugs, undetermined
- ● T42.6X5   Adverse effect of other antiepileptic and sedative-hypnotic drugs
- ● T42.6X6   Underdosing of other antiepileptic and sedative-hypnotic drugs
- ● T42.7   Poisoning by, adverse effect of and underdosing of unspecified antiepileptic and sedative-hypnotic drugs
  - X ● T42.71   Poisoning by unspecified antiepileptic and sedative-hypnotic drugs, accidental (unintentional)
    - Poisoning by antiepileptic and sedative-hypnotic drugs NOS
  - X ● T42.72   Poisoning by unspecified antiepileptic and sedative-hypnotic drugs, intentional self-harm
  - X ● T42.73   Poisoning by unspecified antiepileptic and sedative-hypnotic drugs, assault
  - X ● T42.74   Poisoning by unspecified antiepileptic and sedative-hypnotic drugs, undetermined
  - X ● T42.75   Adverse effect of unspecified antiepileptic and sedative-hypnotic drugs
  - X ● T42.76   Underdosing of unspecified antiepileptic and sedative-hypnotic drugs
- ● T42.8   Poisoning by, adverse effect of and underdosing of antiparkinsonism drugs and other central muscle-tone depressants
  - Poisoning by, adverse effect of and underdosing of amantadine
  - ● T42.8X   Poisoning by, adverse effect of and underdosing of antiparkinsonism drugs and other central muscle-tone depressants
    - ● T42.8X1   Poisoning by antiparkinsonism drugs and other central muscle-tone depressants, accidental (unintentional)
      - Poisoning by antiparkinsonism drugs and other central muscle-tone depressants NOS
    - ● T42.8X2   Poisoning by antiparkinsonism drugs and other central muscle-tone depressants, intentional self-harm
    - ● T42.8X3   Poisoning by antiparkinsonism drugs and other central muscle-tone depressants, assault
    - ● T42.8X4   Poisoning by antiparkinsonism drugs and other central muscle-tone depressants, undetermined
    - ● T42.8X5   Adverse effect of antiparkinsonism drugs and other central muscle-tone depressants
    - ● T42.8X6   Underdosing of antiparkinsonism drugs and other central muscle-tone depressants

- **T43** Poisoning by, adverse effect of and underdosing of psychotropic drugs, not elsewhere classified

  Excludes1   appetite depressants (T50.5-)
  barbiturates (T42.3-)
  benzodiazepines (T42.4-)
  methaqualone (T42.6-)
  psychodysleptics [hallucinogens] (T40.7-T40.9-)

  Excludes2   drug dependence and related mental and behavioral disorders due to psychoactive substance use (F10.--F19.-)

  The appropriate 7th character is to be added to each code from category T43

  A   initial encounter
  D   subsequent encounter
  S   sequela

- **T43.0** Poisoning by, adverse effect of and underdosing of tricyclic and tetracyclic antidepressants
  - **T43.01** Poisoning by, adverse effect of and underdosing of tricyclic antidepressants
    - **T43.011** Poisoning by tricyclic antidepressants, accidental (unintentional)
      Poisoning by tricyclic antidepressants NOS
    - **T43.012** Poisoning by tricyclic antidepressants, intentional self-harm
    - **T43.013** Poisoning by tricyclic antidepressants, assault
    - **T43.014** Poisoning by tricyclic antidepressants, undetermined
    - **T43.015** Adverse effect of tricyclic antidepressants
    - **T43.016** Underdosing of tricyclic antidepressants
  - **T43.02** Poisoning by, adverse effect of and underdosing of tetracyclic antidepressants
    - **T43.021** Poisoning by tetracyclic antidepressants, accidental (unintentional)
      Poisoning by tetracyclic antidepressants NOS
    - **T43.022** Poisoning by tetracyclic antidepressants, intentional self-harm
    - **T43.023** Poisoning by tetracyclic antidepressants, assault
    - **T43.024** Poisoning by tetracyclic antidepressants, undetermined
    - **T43.025** Adverse effect of tetracyclic antidepressants
    - **T43.026** Underdosing of tetracyclic antidepressants
- **T43.1** Poisoning by, adverse effect of and underdosing of monoamine-oxidase-inhibitor antidepressants
  - **T43.1X** Poisoning by, adverse effect of and underdosing of monoamine-oxidase-inhibitor antidepressants
    - **T43.1X1** Poisoning by monoamine-oxidase-inhibitor antidepressants, accidental (unintentional)
      Poisoning by monoamine-oxidase-inhibitor antidepressants NOS
    - **T43.1X2** Poisoning by monoamine-oxidase-inhibitor antidepressants, intentional self-harm
    - **T43.1X3** Poisoning by monoamine-oxidase-inhibitor antidepressants, assault

- **T43.1X4** Poisoning by monoamine-oxidase-inhibitor antidepressants, undetermined
- **T43.1X5** Adverse effect of monoamine-oxidase-inhibitor antidepressants
- **T43.1X6** Underdosing of monoamine-oxidase-inhibitor antidepressants
- **T43.2** Poisoning by, adverse effect of and underdosing of other and unspecified antidepressants
  - **T43.20** Poisoning by, adverse effect of and underdosing of unspecified antidepressants
    - **T43.201** Poisoning by unspecified antidepressants, accidental (unintentional)
      Poisoning by antidepressants NOS
    - **T43.202** Poisoning by unspecified antidepressants, intentional self-harm
    - **T43.203** Poisoning by unspecified antidepressants, assault
    - **T43.204** Poisoning by unspecified antidepressants, undetermined
    - **T43.205** Adverse effect of unspecified antidepressants
    - **T43.206** Underdosing of unspecified antidepressants
  - **T43.21** Poisoning by, adverse effect of and underdosing of selective serotonin and norepinephrine reuptake inhibitors
    Poisoning by, adverse effect of and underdosing of SSNRI antidepressants
    - **T43.211** Poisoning by selective serotonin and norepinephrine reuptake inhibitors, accidental (unintentional)
    - **T43.212** Poisoning by selective serotonin and norepinephrine reuptake inhibitors, intentional self-harm
    - **T43.213** Poisoning by selective serotonin and norepinephrine reuptake inhibitors, assault
    - **T43.214** Poisoning by selective serotonin and norepinephrine reuptake inhibitors, undetermined
    - **T43.215** Adverse effect of selective serotonin and norepinephrine reuptake inhibitors
    - **T43.216** Underdosing of selective serotonin and norepinephrine reuptake inhibitors
  - **T43.22** Poisoning by, adverse effect of and underdosing of selective serotonin reuptake inhibitors
    Poisoning by, adverse effect of and underdosing of SSRI antidepressants
    - **T43.221** Poisoning by selective serotonin reuptake inhibitors, accidental (unintentional)
    - **T43.222** Poisoning by selective serotonin reuptake inhibitors, intentional self-harm
    - **T43.223** Poisoning by selective serotonin reuptake inhibitors, assault
    - **T43.224** Poisoning by selective serotonin reuptake inhibitors, undetermined
    - **T43.225** Adverse effect of selective serotonin reuptake inhibitors
    - **T43.226** Underdosing of selective serotonin reuptake inhibitors

● T43.29   Poisoning by, adverse effect of and underdosing of other antidepressants

  ● T43.291   Poisoning by other antidepressants, accidental (unintentional)
     Poisoning by other antidepressants NOS

  ● T43.292   Poisoning by other antidepressants, intentional self-harm

  ● T43.293   Poisoning by other antidepressants, assault

  ● T43.294   Poisoning by other antidepressants, undetermined

  ● T43.295   Adverse effect of other antidepressants

  ● T43.296   Underdosing of other antidepressants

● T43.3   Poisoning by, adverse effect of and underdosing of phenothiazine antipsychotics and neuroleptics

  ● T43.3X   Poisoning by, adverse effect of and underdosing of phenothiazine antipsychotics and neuroleptics

    ● T43.3X1   Poisoning by phenothiazine antipsychotics and neuroleptics, accidental (unintentional)
      Poisoning by phenothiazine antipsychotics and neuroleptics NOS

    ● T43.3X2   Poisoning by phenothiazine antipsychotics and neuroleptics, intentional self-harm

    ● T43.3X3   Poisoning by phenothiazine antipsychotics and neuroleptics, assault

    ● T43.3X4   Poisoning by phenothiazine antipsychotics and neuroleptics, undetermined

    ● T43.3X5   Adverse effect of phenothiazine antipsychotics and neuroleptics

    ● T43.3X6   Underdosing of phenothiazine antipsychotics and neuroleptics

● T43.4   Poisoning by, adverse effect of and underdosing of butyrophenone and thiothixene neuroleptics

  ● T43.4X   Poisoning by, adverse effect of and underdosing of butyrophenone and thiothixene neuroleptics

    ● T43.4X1   Poisoning by butyrophenone and thiothixene neuroleptics, accidental (unintentional)
      Poisoning by butyrophenone and thiothixene neuroleptics NOS

    ● T43.4X2   Poisoning by butyrophenone and thiothixene neuroleptics, intentional self-harm

    ● T43.4X3   Poisoning by butyrophenone and thiothixene neuroleptics, assault

    ● T43.4X4   Poisoning by butyrophenone and thiothixene neuroleptics, undetermined

    ● T43.4X5   Adverse effect of butyrophenone and thiothixene neuroleptics

    ● T43.4X6   Underdosing of butyrophenone and thiothixene neuroleptics

● T43.5   Poisoning by, adverse effect of and underdosing of other and unspecified antipsychotics and neuroleptics

  Excludes1   poisoning by, adverse effect of and underdosing of rauwolfia (T46.5-)

  ● T43.50   Poisoning by, adverse effect of and underdosing of unspecified antipsychotics and neuroleptics

    ● T43.501   Poisoning by unspecified antipsychotics and neuroleptics, accidental (unintentional)
      Poisoning by antipsychotics and neuroleptics NOS

    ● T43.502   Poisoning by unspecified antipsychotics and neuroleptics, intentional self-harm

    ● T43.503   Poisoning by unspecified antipsychotics and neuroleptics, assault

    ● T43.504   Poisoning by unspecified antipsychotics and neuroleptics, undetermined

    ● T43.505   Adverse effect of unspecified antipsychotics and neuroleptics

    ● T43.506   Underdosing of unspecified antipsychotics and neuroleptics

  ● T43.59   Poisoning by, adverse effect of and underdosing of other antipsychotics and neuroleptics

    ● T43.591   Poisoning by other antipsychotics and neuroleptics, accidental (unintentional)
      Poisoning by other antipsychotics and neuroleptics NOS

    ● T43.592   Poisoning by other antipsychotics and neuroleptics, intentional self-harm

    ● T43.593   Poisoning by other antipsychotics and neuroleptics, assault

    ● T43.594   Poisoning by other antipsychotics and neuroleptics, undetermined

    ● T43.595   Adverse effect of other antipsychotics and neuroleptics

    ● T43.596   Underdosing of other antipsychotics and neuroleptics

● T43.6   Poisoning by, adverse effect of and underdosing of psychostimulants

  Excludes1   poisoning by, adverse effect of and underdosing of cocaine (T40.5-)

  ● T43.60   Poisoning by, adverse effect of and underdosing of unspecified psychostimulant

    ● T43.601   Poisoning by unspecified psychostimulants, accidental (unintentional)
      Poisoning by psychostimulants NOS

    ● T43.602   Poisoning by unspecified psychostimulants, intentional self-harm

    ● T43.603   Poisoning by unspecified psychostimulants, assault

    ● T43.604   Poisoning by unspecified psychostimulants, undetermined

    ● T43.605   Adverse effect of unspecified psychostimulants

    ● T43.606   Underdosing of unspecified psychostimulants

- ● T43.61   Poisoning by, adverse effect of and underdosing of caffeine
  - ● T43.611   Poisoning by caffeine, accidental (unintentional)
    Poisoning by caffeine NOS
  - ● T43.612   Poisoning by caffeine, intentional self-harm
  - ● T43.613   Poisoning by caffeine, assault
  - ● T43.614   Poisoning by caffeine, undetermined
  - ● T43.615   Adverse effect of caffeine
  - ● T43.616   Underdosing of caffeine
- ● T43.62   Poisoning by, adverse effect of and underdosing of amphetamines
  Poisoning by, adverse effect of and underdosing of methamphetamines
  - ● T43.621   Poisoning by amphetamines, accidental (unintentional)
    Poisoning by amphetamines NOS
  - ● T43.622   Poisoning by amphetamines, intentional self-harm
  - ● T43.623   Poisoning by amphetamines, assault
  - ● T43.624   Poisoning by amphetamines, undetermined
  - ● T43.625   Adverse effect of amphetamines
  - ● T43.626   Underdosing of amphetamines
- ● T43.63   Poisoning by, adverse effect of and underdosing of methylphenidate
  - ● T43.631   Poisoning by methylphenidate, accidental (unintentional)
    Poisoning by methylphenidate NOS
  - ● T43.632   Poisoning by methylphenidate, intentional self-harm
  - ● T43.633   Poisoning by methylphenidate, assault
  - ● T43.634   Poisoning by methylphenidate, undetermined
  - ● T43.635   Adverse effect of methylphenidate
  - ● T43.636   Underdosing of methylphenidate
- ● T43.69   Poisoning by, adverse effect of and underdosing of other psychostimulants
  - ● T43.691   Poisoning by other psychostimulants, accidental (unintentional)
    Poisoning by other psychostimulants NOS
  - ● T43.692   Poisoning by other psychostimulants, intentional self-harm
  - ● T43.693   Poisoning by other psychostimulants, assault
  - ● T43.694   Poisoning by other psychostimulants, undetermined
  - ● T43.695   Adverse effect of other psychostimulants
  - ● T43.696   Underdosing of other psychostimulants
- ● T43.8   Poisoning by, adverse effect of and underdosing of other psychotropic drugs
  - ● T43.8X   Poisoning by, adverse effect of and underdosing of other psychotropic drugs
    - ● T43.8X1   Poisoning by other psychotropic drugs, accidental (unintentional)
      Poisoning by other psychotropic drugs NOS
    - ● T43.8X2   Poisoning by other psychotropic drugs, intentional self-harm
    - ● T43.8X3   Poisoning by other psychotropic drugs, assault
    - ● T43.8X4   Poisoning by other psychotropic drugs, undetermined

- ● T43.8X5   Adverse effect of other psychotropic drugs
- ● T43.8X6   Underdosing of other psychotropic drugs
- ● T43.9   Poisoning by, adverse effect of and underdosing of unspecified psychotropic drug
  - X ● T43.91   Poisoning by unspecified psychotropic drug, accidental (unintentional)
    Poisoning by psychotropic drug NOS
  - X ● T43.92   Poisoning by unspecified psychotropic drug, intentional self-harm
  - X ● T43.93   Poisoning by unspecified psychotropic drug, assault
  - X ● T43.94   Poisoning by unspecified psychotropic drug, undetermined
  - X ● T43.95   Adverse effect of unspecified psychotropic drug
  - X ● T43.96   Underdosing of unspecified psychotropic drug
- ● T44   Poisoning by, adverse effect of and underdosing of drugs primarily affecting the autonomic nervous system

  The appropriate 7th character is to be added to each code from category T44

A	initial encounter
D	subsequent encounter
S	sequela

  - ● T44.0   Poisoning by, adverse effect of and underdosing of anticholinesterase agents
    - ● T44.0X   Poisoning by, adverse effect of and underdosing of anticholinesterase agents
      - ● T44.0X1   Poisoning by anticholinesterase agents, accidental (unintentional)
        Poisoning by anticholinesterase agents NOS
      - ● T44.0X2   Poisoning by anticholinesterase agents, intentional self-harm
      - ● T44.0X3   Poisoning by anticholinesterase agents, assault
      - ● T44.0X4   Poisoning by anticholinesterase agents, undetermined
      - ● T44.0X5   Adverse effect of anticholinesterase agents
      - ● T44.0X6   Underdosing of anticholinesterase agents
  - ● T44.1   Poisoning by, adverse effect of and underdosing of other parasympathomimetics [cholinergics]
    - ● T44.1X   Poisoning by, adverse effect of and underdosing of other parasympathomimetics [cholinergics]
      - ● T44.1X1   Poisoning by other parasympathomimetics [cholinergics], accidental (unintentional)
        Poisoning by other parasympathomimetics [cholinergics] NOS
      - ● T44.1X2   Poisoning by other parasympathomimetics [cholinergics], intentional self-harm
      - ● T44.1X3   Poisoning by other parasympathomimetics [cholinergics], assault
      - ● T44.1X4   Poisoning by other parasympathomimetics [cholinergics], undetermined
      - ● T44.1X5   Adverse effect of other parasympathomimetics [cholinergics]
      - ● T44.1X6   Underdosing of other parasympathomimetics

CHAPTER 19 (S00-T88)

● **T44.2** Poisoning by, adverse effect of and underdosing of ganglionic blocking drugs

  ● **T44.2X** Poisoning by, adverse effect of and underdosing of ganglionic blocking drugs

    ● **T44.2X1** Poisoning by ganglionic blocking drugs, accidental (unintentional)
        Poisoning by ganglionic blocking drugs NOS

    ● **T44.2X2** Poisoning by ganglionic blocking drugs, intentional self-harm

    ● **T44.2X3** Poisoning by ganglionic blocking drugs, assault

    ● **T44.2X4** Poisoning by ganglionic blocking drugs, undetermined

    ● **T44.2X5** Adverse effect of ganglionic blocking drugs

    ● **T44.2X6** Underdosing of ganglionic blocking drugs

● **T44.3** Poisoning by, adverse effect of and underdosing of other parasympatholytics [anticholinergics and antimuscarinics] and spasmolytics
    Poisoning by, adverse effect of and underdosing of papaverine

  ● **T44.3X** Poisoning by, adverse effect of and underdosing of other parasympatholytics [anticholinergics and antimuscarinics] and spasmolytics

    ● **T44.3X1** Poisoning by other parasympatholytics [anticholinergics and antimuscarinics] and spasmolytics, accidental (unintentional)
        Poisoning by other parasympatholytics [anticholinergics and antimuscarinics] and spasmolytics NOS

    ● **T44.3X2** Poisoning by other parasympatholytics [anticholinergics and antimuscarinics] and spasmolytics, intentional self-harm

    ● **T44.3X3** Poisoning by other parasympatholytics [anticholinergics and antimuscarinics] and spasmolytics, assault

    ● **T44.3X4** Poisoning by other parasympatholytics [anticholinergics and antimuscarinics] and spasmolytics, undetermined

    ● **T44.3X5** Adverse effect of other parasympatholytics [anticholinergics and antimuscarinics] and spasmolytics

    ● **T44.3X6** Underdosing of other parasympatholytics [anticholinergics and antimuscarinics] and spasmolytics

● **T44.4** Poisoning by, adverse effect of and underdosing of predominantly alpha-adrenoreceptor agonists
    Poisoning by, adverse effect of and underdosing of metaraminol

  ● **T44.4X** Poisoning by, adverse effect of and underdosing of predominantly alpha-adrenoreceptor agonists

    ● **T44.4X1** Poisoning by predominantly alpha-adrenoreceptor agonists, accidental (unintentional)
        Poisoning by predominantly alpha-adrenoreceptor agonists NOS

    ● **T44.4X2** Poisoning by predominantly alpha-adrenoreceptor agonists, intentional self-harm

    ● **T44.4X3** Poisoning by predominantly alpha-adrenoreceptor agonists, assault

    ● **T44.4X4** Poisoning by predominantly alpha-adrenoreceptor agonists, undetermined

    ● **T44.4X5** Adverse effect of predominantly alpha-adrenoreceptor agonists

    ● **T44.4X6** Underdosing of predominantly alpha-adrenoreceptor agonists

● **T44.5** Poisoning by, adverse effect of and underdosing of predominantly beta-adrenoreceptor agonists

    Excludes1　poisoning by, adverse effect of and underdosing of beta-adrenoreceptor agonists used in asthma therapy (T48.6-)

  ● **T44.5X** Poisoning by, adverse effect of and underdosing of predominantly beta-adrenoreceptor agonists

    ● **T44.5X1** Poisoning by predominantly beta-adrenoreceptor agonists, accidental (unintentional)
        Poisoning by predominantly beta-adrenoreceptor agonists NOS

    ● **T44.5X2** Poisoning by predominantly beta-adrenoreceptor agonists, intentional self-harm

    ● **T44.5X3** Poisoning by predominantly beta-adrenoreceptor agonists, assault

    ● **T44.5X4** Poisoning by predominantly beta-adrenoreceptor agonists, undetermined

    ● **T44.5X5** Adverse effect of predominantly beta-adrenoreceptor agonists

    ● **T44.5X6** Underdosing of predominantly beta-adrenoreceptor agonists

● **T44.6** Poisoning by, adverse effect of and underdosing of alpha-adrenoreceptor antagonists

    Excludes1　poisoning by, adverse effect of and underdosing of ergot alkaloids (T48.0)

  ● **T44.6X** Poisoning by, adverse effect of and underdosing of alpha-adrenoreceptor antagonists

    ● **T44.6X1** Poisoning by alpha-adrenoreceptor antagonists, accidental (unintentional)
        Poisoning by alpha-adrenoreceptor antagonists NOS

    ● **T44.6X2** Poisoning by alpha-adrenoreceptor antagonists, intentional self-harm

    ● **T44.6X3** Poisoning by alpha-adrenoreceptor antagonists, assault

    ● **T44.6X4** Poisoning by alpha-adrenoreceptor antagonists, undetermined

    ● **T44.6X5** Adverse effect of alpha-adrenoreceptor antagonists

    ● **T44.6X6** Underdosing of alpha-adrenoreceptor antagonists

● **T44.7** Poisoning by, adverse effect of and underdosing of beta-adrenoreceptor antagonists

  ● **T44.7X** Poisoning by, adverse effect of and underdosing of beta-adrenoreceptor antagonists

    ● **T44.7X1** Poisoning by beta-adrenoreceptor antagonists, accidental (unintentional)
        Poisoning by beta-adrenoreceptor antagonists NOS

    ● **T44.7X2** Poisoning by beta-adrenoreceptor antagonists, intentional self-harm

    ● **T44.7X3** Poisoning by beta-adrenoreceptor antagonists, assault

    ● **T44.7X4** Poisoning by beta-adrenoreceptor antagonists, undetermined

    ● **T44.7X5** Adverse effect of beta-adrenoreceptor antagonists

    ● **T44.7X6** Underdosing of beta-adrenoreceptor antagonists

◀ New　◀▥ Revised　deleted Deleted　**OGCR** Official Guidelines　X Assign placeholder X　● Use Additional Character(s)

Excludes 1　Excludes 2　Includes　Use additional　Code first　Code also　Unspecified

● **T44.8** **Poisoning by, adverse effect of and underdosing of centrally-acting and adrenergic-neuron-blocking agents**

> **Excludes1**   poisoning by, adverse effect of and underdosing of clonidine (T46.5)
> poisoning by, adverse effect of and underdosing of guanethidine (T46.5)

● **T44.8X** **Poisoning by, adverse effect of and underdosing of centrally-acting and adrenergic-neuron-blocking agents**

● **T44.8X1** **Poisoning by centrally-acting and adrenergic-neuron-blocking agents, accidental (unintentional)**
> Poisoning by centrally-acting and adrenergic-neuron-blocking agents NOS

● **T44.8X2** **Poisoning by centrally-acting and adrenergic-neuron-blocking agents, intentional self-harm**

● **T44.8X3** **Poisoning by centrally-acting and adrenergic-neuron-blocking agents, assault**

● **T44.8X4** **Poisoning by centrally-acting and adrenergic-neuron-blocking agents, undetermined**

● **T44.8X5** **Adverse effect of centrally-acting and adrenergic-neuron-blocking agents**

● **T44.8X6** **Underdosing of centrally-acting and adrenergic-neuron-blocking agents**

● **T44.9** **Poisoning by, adverse effect of and underdosing of other and unspecified drugs primarily affecting the autonomic nervous system**
> Poisoning by, adverse effect of and underdosing of drug stimulating both alpha and beta-adrenoreceptors

● **T44.90** **Poisoning by, adverse effect of and underdosing of unspecified drugs primarily affecting the autonomic nervous system**

● **T44.901** **Poisoning by unspecified drugs primarily affecting the autonomic nervous system, accidental (unintentional)**
> Poisoning by unspecified drugs primarily affecting the autonomic nervous system NOS

● **T44.902** **Poisoning by unspecified drugs primarily affecting the autonomic nervous system, intentional self-harm**

● **T44.903** **Poisoning by unspecified drugs primarily affecting the autonomic nervous system, assault**

● **T44.904** **Poisoning by unspecified drugs primarily affecting the autonomic nervous system, undetermined**

● **T44.905** **Adverse effect of unspecified drugs primarily affecting the autonomic nervous system**

● **T44.906** **Underdosing of unspecified drugs primarily affecting the autonomic nervous system**

● **T44.99** **Poisoning by, adverse effect of and underdosing of other drugs primarily affecting the autonomic nervous system**

● **T44.991** **Poisoning by other drug primarily affecting the autonomic nervous system, accidental (unintentional)**
> Poisoning by other drugs primarily affecting the autonomic nervous system NOS

● **T44.992** **Poisoning by other drug primarily affecting the autonomic nervous system, intentional self-harm**

● **T44.993** **Poisoning by other drug primarily affecting the autonomic nervous system, assault**

● **T44.994** **Poisoning by other drug primarily affecting the autonomic nervous system, undetermined**

● **T44.995** **Adverse effect of other drug primarily affecting the autonomic nervous system**

● **T44.996** **Underdosing of other drug primarily affecting the autonomic nervous system**

● **T45** **Poisoning by, adverse effect of and underdosing of primarily systemic and hematological agents, not elsewhere classified**

> The appropriate 7th character is to be added to each code from category T45

> | A | initial encounter |
> |---|---|
> | D | subsequent encounter |
> | S | sequela |

● **T45.0** **Poisoning by, adverse effect of and underdosing of antiallergic and antiemetic drugs**

> **Excludes1**   poisoning by, adverse effect of and underdosing of phenothiazine-based neuroleptics (T43.3)

● **T45.0X** **Poisoning by, adverse effect of and underdosing of antiallergic and antiemetic drugs**

● **T45.0X1** **Poisoning by antiallergic and antiemetic drugs, accidental (unintentional)**
> Poisoning by antiallergic and antiemetic drugs NOS

● **T45.0X2** **Poisoning by antiallergic and antiemetic drugs, intentional self-harm**

● **T45.0X3** **Poisoning by antiallergic and antiemetic drugs, assault**

● **T45.0X4** **Poisoning by antiallergic and antiemetic drugs, undetermined**

● **T45.0X5** **Adverse effect of antiallergic and antiemetic drugs**

● **T45.0X6** **Underdosing of antiallergic and antiemetic drugs**

● **T45.1** **Poisoning by, adverse effect of and underdosing of antineoplastic and immunosuppressive drugs**

> **Excludes1**   poisoning by, adverse effect of and underdosing of tamoxifen (T38.6)

● **T45.1X** **Poisoning by, adverse effect of and underdosing of antineoplastic and immunosuppressive drugs**

● **T45.1X1** **Poisoning by antineoplastic and immunosuppressive drugs, accidental (unintentional)**
> Poisoning by antineoplastic and immunosuppressive drugs NOS

● **T45.1X2** **Poisoning by antineoplastic and immunosuppressive drugs, intentional self-harm**

● **T45.1X3** **Poisoning by antineoplastic and immunosuppressive drugs, assault**

● **T45.1X4** **Poisoning by antineoplastic and immunosuppressive drugs, undetermined**

● **T45.1X5** **Adverse effect of antineoplastic and immunosuppressive drugs**

● **T45.1X6** **Underdosing of antineoplastic and immunosuppressive drugs**

CHAPTER 19 (S00-T88)

CHAPTER 19 (S00-T88)

● **T45.2**   **Poisoning by, adverse effect of and underdosing of vitamins**

     Excludes2   poisoning by, adverse effect of and underdosing of nicotinic acid (derivatives) (T46.7)

                poisoning by, adverse effect of and underdosing of iron (T45.4)

                poisoning by, adverse effect of and underdosing of vitamin K (T45.7)

   ● **T45.2X**   **Poisoning by, adverse effect of and underdosing of vitamins**

     ● **T45.2X1**   **Poisoning by vitamins, accidental (unintentional)**

         Poisoning by vitamins NOS

     ● **T45.2X2**   **Poisoning by vitamins, intentional self-harm**

     ● **T45.2X3**   **Poisoning by vitamins, assault**

     ● **T45.2X4**   **Poisoning by vitamins, undetermined**

     ● **T45.2X5**   **Adverse effect of vitamins**

     ● **T45.2X6**   **Underdosing of vitamins**

         Excludes1   vitamin deficiencies (E50-E56)

● **T45.3**   **Poisoning by, adverse effect of and underdosing of enzymes**

   ● **T45.3X**   **Poisoning by, adverse effect of and underdosing of enzymes**

     ● **T45.3X1**   **Poisoning by enzymes, accidental (unintentional)**

         Poisoning by enzymes NOS

     ● **T45.3X2**   **Poisoning by enzymes, intentional self-harm**

     ● **T45.3X3**   **Poisoning by enzymes, assault**

     ● **T45.3X4**   **Poisoning by enzymes, undetermined**

     ● **T45.3X5**   **Adverse effect of enzymes**

     ● **T45.3X6**   **Underdosing of enzymes**

● **T45.4**   **Poisoning by, adverse effect of and underdosing of iron and its compounds**

   ● **T45.4X**   **Poisoning by, adverse effect of and underdosing of iron and its compounds**

     ● **T45.4X1**   **Poisoning by iron and its compounds, accidental (unintentional)**

         Poisoning by iron and its compounds NOS

     ● **T45.4X2**   **Poisoning by iron and its compounds, intentional self-harm**

     ● **T45.4X3**   **Poisoning by iron and its compounds, assault**

     ● **T45.4X4**   **Poisoning by iron and its compounds, undetermined**

     ● **T45.4X5**   **Adverse effect of iron and its compounds**

     ● **T45.4X6**   **Underdosing of iron and its compounds**

         Excludes1   iron deficiency (E61.1)

● **T45.5**   **Poisoning by, adverse effect of and underdosing of anticoagulants and antithrombotic drugs**

   ● **T45.51**   **Poisoning by, adverse effect of and underdosing of anticoagulants**

     T45.511   **Poisoning by anticoagulants, accidental (unintentional)**

         Poisoning by anticoagulants NOS

     ● **T45.512**   **Poisoning by anticoagulants, intentional self-harm**

     ● **T45.513**   **Poisoning by anticoagulants, assault**

     ● **T45.514**   **Poisoning by anticoagulants, undetermined**

     ● **T45.515**   **Adverse effect of anticoagulants**

     ● **T45.516**   **Underdosing of anticoagulants**

● **T45.52**   **Poisoning by, adverse effect of and underdosing of antithrombotic drugs**

     Poisoning by, adverse effect of and underdosing of antiplatelet drugs

     Excludes2   poisoning by, adverse effect of and underdosing of aspirin (T39.01-)

                poisoning by, adverse effect of and underdosing of acetylsalicylic acid (T39.01-)

   ● **T45.521**   **Poisoning by antithrombotic drugs, accidental (unintentional)**

         Poisoning by antithrombotic drug NOS

   ● **T45.522**   **Poisoning by antithrombotic drugs, intentional self-harm**

   ● **T45.523**   **Poisoning by antithrombotic drugs, assault**

   ● **T45.524**   **Poisoning by antithrombotic drugs, undetermined**

   ● **T45.525**   **Adverse effect of antithrombotic drugs**

   ● **T45.526**   **Underdosing of antithrombotic drugs**

● **T45.6**   **Poisoning by, adverse effect of and underdosing of fibrinolysis-affecting drugs**

   ● **T45.60**   **Poisoning by, adverse effect of and underdosing of unspecified fibrinolysis-affecting drugs**

     ● **T45.601**   **Poisoning by unspecified fibrinolysis-affecting drugs, accidental (unintentional)**

         Poisoning by fibrinolysis-affecting drug NOS

     ● **T45.602**   **Poisoning by unspecified fibrinolysis-affecting drugs, intentional self-harm**

     ● **T45.603**   **Poisoning by unspecified fibrinolysis-affecting drugs, assault**

     ● **T45.604**   **Poisoning by unspecified fibrinolysis-affecting drugs, undetermined**

     ● **T45.605**   **Adverse effect of unspecified fibrinolysis-affecting drugs**

     ● **T45.606**   **Underdosing of unspecified fibrinolysis-affecting drugs**

   ● **T45.61**   **Poisoning by, adverse effect of and underdosing of thrombolytic drugs**

     ● **T45.611**   **Poisoning by thrombolytic drug, accidental (unintentional)**

         Poisoning by thrombolytic drug NOS

     ● **T45.612**   **Poisoning by thrombolytic drug, intentional self-harm**

     ● **T45.613**   **Poisoning by thrombolytic drug, assault**

     ● **T45.614**   **Poisoning by thrombolytic drug, undetermined**

     ● **T45.615**   **Adverse effect of thrombolytic drugs**

     ● **T45.616**   **Underdosing of thrombolytic drugs**

   ● **T45.62**   **Poisoning by, adverse effect of and underdosing of hemostatic drugs**

     ● **T45.621**   **Poisoning by hemostatic drug, accidental (unintentional)**

         Poisoning by hemostatic drug NOS

     ● **T45.622**   **Poisoning by hemostatic drug, intentional self-harm**

     ● **T45.623**   **Poisoning by hemostatic drug, assault**

     ● **T45.624**   **Poisoning by hemostatic drug, undetermined**

     ● **T45.625**   **Adverse effect of hemostatic drug**

     ● **T45.626**   **Underdosing of hemostatic drugs**

- ● T45.69   Poisoning by, adverse effect of and underdosing of other fibrinolysis-affecting drugs
  - ● T45.691   Poisoning by other fibrinolysis-affecting drugs, accidental (unintentional)
    Poisoning by other fibrinolysis-affecting drug NOS
  - ● T45.692   Poisoning by other fibrinolysis-affecting drugs, intentional self-harm
  - ● T45.693   Poisoning by other fibrinolysis-affecting drugs, assault
  - ● T45.694   Poisoning by other fibrinolysis-affecting drugs, undetermined
  - ● T45.695   Adverse effect of other fibrinolysis-affecting drugs
  - ● T45.696   Underdosing of other fibrinolysis-affecting drugs
- ● T45.7   Poisoning by, adverse effect of and underdosing of anticoagulant antagonists, vitamin K and other coagulants
  - ● T45.7X   Poisoning by, adverse effect of and underdosing of anticoagulant antagonists, vitamin K and other coagulants
    - ● T45.7X1   Poisoning by anticoagulant antagonists, vitamin K and other coagulants, accidental (unintentional)
      Poisoning by anticoagulant antagonists, vitamin K and other coagulants NOS
    - ● T45.7X2   Poisoning by anticoagulant antagonists, vitamin K and other coagulants, intentional self-harm
    - ● T45.7X3   Poisoning by anticoagulant antagonists, vitamin K and other coagulants, assault
    - ● T45.7X4   Poisoning by anticoagulant antagonists, vitamin K and other coagulants, undetermined
    - ● T45.7X5   Adverse effect of anticoagulant antagonists, vitamin K and other coagulants
    - ● T45.7X6   Underdosing of anticoagulant antagonist, vitamin K and other coagulants
      | Excludes1 | vitamin K deficiency (E56.1)
- ● T45.8   Poisoning by, adverse effect of and underdosing of other primarily systemic and hematological agents
    Poisoning by, adverse effect of and underdosing of liver preparations and other antianemic agents
    Poisoning by, adverse effect of and underdosing of natural blood and blood products
    Poisoning by, adverse effect of and underdosing of plasma substitute
    | Excludes2 | poisoning by, adverse effect of and underdosing of immunoglobulin (T50.Z1)
        poisoning by, adverse effect of and underdosing of iron (T45.4)
        transfusion reactions (T80.-)
  - ● T45.8X   Poisoning by, adverse effect of and underdosing of other primarily systemic and hematological agents
    - ● T45.8X1   Poisoning by other primarily systemic and hematological agents, accidental (unintentional)
      Poisoning by other primarily systemic and hematological agents NOS
    - ● T45.8X2   Poisoning by other primarily systemic and hematological agents, intentional self-harm

- ● T45.8X3   Poisoning by other primarily systemic and hematological agents, assault
- ● T45.8X4   Poisoning by other primarily systemic and hematological agents, undetermined
- ● T45.8X5   Adverse effect of other primarily systemic and hematological agents
- ● T45.8X6   Underdosing of other primarily systemic and hematological agents
- ● T45.9   Poisoning by, adverse effect of and underdosing of unspecified primarily systemic and hematological agent
  - X ● T45.91   Poisoning by unspecified primarily systemic and hematological agent, accidental (unintentional)
    Poisoning by primarily systemic and hematological agent NOS
  - X ● T45.92   Poisoning by unspecified primarily systemic and hematological agent, intentional self-harm
  - X ● T45.93   Poisoning by unspecified primarily systemic and hematological agent, assault
  - X ● T45.94   Poisoning by unspecified primarily systemic and hematological agent, undetermined
  - X ● T45.95   Adverse effect of unspecified primarily systemic and hematological agent
  - X ● T45.96   Underdosing of unspecified primarily systemic and hematological agent
- ● T46   Poisoning by, adverse effect of and underdosing of agents primarily affecting the cardiovascular system
  | Excludes1 | poisoning by, adverse effect of and underdosing of metaraminol (T44.4)

  The appropriate 7th character is to be added to each code from category T46

A	initial encounter
D	subsequent encounter
S	sequela

  - ● T46.0   Poisoning by, adverse effect of and underdosing of cardiac-stimulant glycosides and drugs of similar action
    - ● T46.0X   Poisoning by, adverse effect of and underdosing of cardiac-stimulant glycosides and drugs of similar action
      - ● T46.0X1   Poisoning by cardiac-stimulant glycosides and drugs of similar action, accidental (unintentional)
        Poisoning by cardiac-stimulant glycosides and drugs of similar action NOS
      - ● T46.0X2   Poisoning by cardiac-stimulant glycosides and drugs of similar action, intentional self-harm
      - ● T46.0X3   Poisoning by cardiac-stimulant glycosides and drugs of similar action, assault
      - ● T46.0X4   Poisoning by cardiac-stimulant glycosides and drugs of similar action, undetermined
      - ● T46.0X5   Adverse effect of cardiac-stimulant glycosides and drugs of similar action
      - ● T46.0X6   Underdosing of cardiac-stimulant glycosides and drugs of similar action
  - ● T46.1   Poisoning by, adverse effect of and underdosing of calcium-channel blockers
    - ● T46.1X   Poisoning by, adverse effect of and underdosing of calcium-channel blockers
      - ● T46.1X1   Poisoning by calcium-channel blockers, accidental (unintentional)
        Poisoning by calcium-channel blockers NOS
      - ● T46.1X2   Poisoning by calcium-channel blockers, intentional self-harm
      - ● T46.1X3   Poisoning by calcium-channel blockers, assault

◀ New   ⬅ Revised   d̶e̶l̶e̶t̶e̶d̶ Deleted   **OGCR** Official Guidelines   X Assign placeholder X   ● Use Additional Character(s)

| Excludes 1 | | Excludes 2 | Includes   Use additional   Code first   Code also   Unspecified

1411

● T46.1X4   Poisoning by calcium-channel blockers, undetermined

● T46.1X5   Adverse effect of calcium-channel blockers

● T46.1X6   Underdosing of calcium-channel blockers

● T46.2   Poisoning by, adverse effect of and underdosing of other antidysrhythmic drugs, not elsewhere classified

    Excludes1   poisoning by, adverse effect of and underdosing of beta-adrenoreceptor antagonists (T44.7-)

● T46.2X   Poisoning by, adverse effect of and underdosing of other antidysrhythmic drugs

    ● T46.2X1   Poisoning by other antidysrhythmic drugs, accidental (unintentional)
      Poisoning by other antidysrhythmic drugs NOS

    ● T46.2X2   Poisoning by other antidysrhythmic drugs, intentional self-harm

    ● T46.2X3   Poisoning by other antidysrhythmic drugs, assault

    ● T46.2X4   Poisoning by other antidysrhythmic drugs, undetermined

    ● T46.2X5   Adverse effect of other antidysrhythmic drugs

    ● T46.2X6   Underdosing of other antidysrhythmic drugs

● T46.3   Poisoning by, adverse effect of and underdosing of coronary vasodilators
   Poisoning by, adverse effect of and underdosing of dipyridamole

    Excludes1   poisoning by, adverse effect of and underdosing of calcium-channel blockers (T46.1)

● T46.3X   Poisoning by, adverse effect of and underdosing of coronary vasodilators

    ● T46.3X1   Poisoning by coronary vasodilators, accidental (unintentional)
      Poisoning by coronary vasodilators NOS

    ● T46.3X2   Poisoning by coronary vasodilators, intentional self-harm

    ● T46.3X3   Poisoning by coronary vasodilators, assault

    ● T46.3X4   Poisoning by coronary vasodilators, undetermined

    ● T46.3X5   Adverse effect of coronary vasodilators

    ● T46.3X6   Underdosing of coronary vasodilators

● T46.4   Poisoning by, adverse effect of and underdosing of angiotensin-converting-enzyme inhibitors

● T46.4X   Poisoning by, adverse effect of and underdosing of angiotensin-converting-enzyme inhibitors

    ● T46.4X1   Poisoning by angiotensin-converting-enzyme inhibitors, accidental (unintentional)
      Poisoning by angiotensin-converting-enzyme inhibitors NOS

    ● T46.4X2   Poisoning by angiotensin-converting-enzyme inhibitors, intentional self-harm

    ● T46.4X3   Poisoning by angiotensin-converting-enzyme inhibitors, assault

    ● T46.4X4   Poisoning by angiotensin-converting-enzyme inhibitors, undetermined

    ● T46.4X5   Adverse effect of angiotensin-converting-enzyme inhibitors

    ● T46.4X6   Underdosing of angiotensin-converting-enzyme inhibitors

● T46.5   Poisoning by, adverse effect of and underdosing of other antihypertensive drugs

    Excludes2   poisoning by, adverse effect of and underdosing of beta-adrenoreceptor antagonists (T44.7)
      poisoning by, adverse effect of and underdosing of calcium-channel blockers (T46.1)
      poisoning by, adverse effect of and underdosing of diuretics (T50.0-T50.2)

● T46.5X   Poisoning by, adverse effect of and underdosing of other antihypertensive drugs

    ● T46.5X1   Poisoning by other antihypertensive drugs, accidental (unintentional)
      Poisoning by other antihypertensive drugs NOS

    ● T46.5X2   Poisoning by other antihypertensive drugs, intentional self-harm

    ● T46.5X3   Poisoning by other antihypertensive drugs, assault

    ● T46.5X4   Poisoning by other antihypertensive drugs, undetermined

    ● T46.5X5   Adverse effect of other antihypertensive drugs

    ● T46.5X6   Underdosing of other antihypertensive drugs

● T46.6   Poisoning by, adverse effect of and underdosing of antihyperlipidemic and antiarteriosclerotic drugs

● T46.6X   Poisoning by, adverse effect of and underdosing of antihyperlipidemic and antiarteriosclerotic drugs

    ● T46.6X1   Poisoning by antihyperlipidemic and antiarteriosclerotic drugs, accidental (unintentional)
      Poisoning by antihyperlipidemic and antiarteriosclerotic drugs NOS

    ● T46.6X2   Poisoning by antihyperlipidemic and antiarteriosclerotic drugs, intentional self-harm

    ● T46.6X3   Poisoning by antihyperlipidemic and antiarteriosclerotic drugs, assault

    ● T46.6X4   Poisoning by antihyperlipidemic and antiarteriosclerotic drugs, undetermined

    ● T46.6X5   Adverse effect of antihyperlipidemic and antiarteriosclerotic drugs

    ● T46.6X6   Underdosing of antihyperlipidemic and antiarteriosclerotic drugs

● T46.7   Poisoning by, adverse effect of and underdosing of peripheral vasodilators
   Poisoning by, adverse effect of and underdosing of nicotinic acid (derivatives)

    Excludes1   poisoning by, adverse effect of and underdosing of papaverine (T44.3)

● T46.7X   Poisoning by, adverse effect of and underdosing of peripheral vasodilators

    ● T46.7X1   Poisoning by peripheral vasodilators, accidental (unintentional)
      Poisoning by peripheral vasodilators NOS

    ● T46.7X2   Poisoning by peripheral vasodilators, intentional self-harm

    ● T46.7X3   Poisoning by peripheral vasodilators, assault

    ● T46.7X4   Poisoning by peripheral vasodilators, undetermined

    ● T46.7X5   Adverse effect of peripheral vasodilators

    ● T46.7X6   Underdosing of peripheral vasodilators

◄ New   ◄▒ Revised   ~~deleted~~ Deleted   **OGCR** Official Guidelines   X Assign placeholder X   ● Use Additional Character(s)

Excludes 1   Excludes 2   Includes   Use additional   Code first   Code also   Unspecified

● **T46.8**   Poisoning by, adverse effect of and underdosing of antivaricose drugs, including sclerosing agents

  ● **T46.8X**   Poisoning by, adverse effect of and underdosing of antivaricose drugs, including sclerosing agents

    ● **T46.8X1**   Poisoning by antivaricose drugs, including sclerosing agents, accidental (unintentional)
        Poisoning by antivaricose drugs, including sclerosing agents NOS

    ● **T46.8X2**   Poisoning by antivaricose drugs, including sclerosing agents, intentional self-harm

    ● **T46.8X3**   Poisoning by antivaricose drugs, including sclerosing agents, assault

    ● **T46.8X4**   Poisoning by antivaricose drugs, including sclerosing agents, undetermined

    ● **T46.8X5**   Adverse effect of antivaricose drugs, including sclerosing agents

    ● **T46.8X6**   Underdosing of antivaricose drugs, including sclerosing agents

● **T46.9**   Poisoning by, adverse effect of and underdosing of other and unspecified agents primarily affecting the cardiovascular system

  ● **T46.90**   Poisoning by, adverse effect of and underdosing of unspecified agents primarily affecting the cardiovascular system

    ● **T46.901**   Poisoning by unspecified agents primarily affecting the cardiovascular system, accidental (unintentional)

    ● **T46.902**   Poisoning by unspecified agents primarily affecting the cardiovascular system, intentional self-harm

    ● **T46.903**   Poisoning by unspecified agents primarily affecting the cardiovascular system, assault

    ● **T46.904**   Poisoning by unspecified agents primarily affecting the cardiovascular system, undetermined

    ● **T46.905**   Adverse effect of unspecified agents primarily affecting the cardiovascular system

    ● **T46.906**   Underdosing of unspecified agents primarily affecting the cardiovascular system

  ● **T46.99**   Poisoning by, adverse effect of and underdosing of other agents primarily affecting the cardiovascular system

    ● **T46.991**   Poisoning by other agents primarily affecting the cardiovascular system, accidental (unintentional)

    ● **T46.992**   Poisoning by other agents primarily affecting the cardiovascular system, intentional self-harm

    ● **T46.993**   Poisoning by other agents primarily affecting the cardiovascular system, assault

    ● **T46.994**   Poisoning by other agents primarily affecting the cardiovascular system, undetermined

    ● **T46.995**   Adverse effect of other agents primarily affecting the cardiovascular system

    ● **T46.996**   Underdosing of other agents primarily affecting the cardiovascular system

● **T47**   Poisoning by, adverse effect of and underdosing of agents primarily affecting the gastrointestinal system

    The appropriate 7th character is to be added to each code from category T47

A	initial encounter
D	subsequent encounter
S	sequela

● **T47.0**   Poisoning by, adverse effect of and underdosing of histamine H2-receptor blockers

  ● **T47.0X**   Poisoning by, adverse effect of and underdosing of histamine H2-receptor blockers

    ● **T47.0X1**   Poisoning by histamine H2-receptor blockers, accidental (unintentional)
        Poisoning by histamine H2-receptor blockers NOS

    ● **T47.0X2**   Poisoning by histamine H2-receptor blockers, intentional self-harm

    ● **T47.0X3**   Poisoning by histamine H2-receptor blockers, assault

    ● **T47.0X4**   Poisoning by histamine H2-receptor blockers, undetermined

    ● **T47.0X5**   Adverse effect of histamine H2-receptor blockers

    ● **T47.0X6**   Underdosing of histamine H2-receptor blockers

● **T47.1**   Poisoning by, adverse effect of and underdosing of other antacids and anti-gastric-secretion drugs

  ● **T47.1X**   Poisoning by, adverse effect of and underdosing of other antacids and anti-gastric-secretion drugs

    ● **T47.1X1**   Poisoning by other antacids and anti-gastric-secretion drugs, accidental (unintentional)
        Poisoning by other antacids and anti-gastric-secretion drugs NOS

    ● **T47.1X2**   Poisoning by other antacids and anti-gastric-secretion drugs, intentional self-harm

    ● **T47.1X3**   Poisoning by other antacids and anti-gastric-secretion drugs, assault

    ● **T47.1X4**   Poisoning by other antacids and anti-gastric-secretion drugs, undetermined

    ● **T47.1X5**   Adverse effect of other antacids and anti-gastric-secretion drugs

    ● **T47.1X6**   Underdosing of other antacids and anti-gastric-secretion drugs

● **T47.2**   Poisoning by, adverse effect of and underdosing of stimulant laxatives

  ● **T47.2X**   Poisoning by, adverse effect of and underdosing of stimulant laxatives

    ● **T47.2X1**   Poisoning by stimulant laxatives, accidental (unintentional)
        Poisoning by stimulant laxatives NOS

    ● **T47.2X2**   Poisoning by stimulant laxatives, intentional self-harm

    ● **T47.2X3**   Poisoning by stimulant laxatives, assault

    ● **T47.2X4**   Poisoning by stimulant laxatives, undetermined

    ● **T47.2X5**   Adverse effect of stimulant laxatives

    ● **T47.2X6**   Underdosing of stimulant laxatives

CHAPTER 19 (S00-T88)

- T47.3 Poisoning by, adverse effect of and underdosing of saline and osmotic laxatives
  - T47.3X Poisoning by and adverse effect of saline and osmotic laxatives
    - T47.3X1 Poisoning by saline and osmotic laxatives, accidental (unintentional)
      Poisoning by saline and osmotic laxatives NOS
    - T47.3X2 Poisoning by saline and osmotic laxatives, intentional self-harm
    - T47.3X3 Poisoning by saline and osmotic laxatives, assault
    - T47.3X4 Poisoning by saline and osmotic laxatives, undetermined
    - T47.3X5 Adverse effect of saline and osmotic laxatives
    - T47.3X6 Underdosing of saline and osmotic laxatives
- T47.4 Poisoning by, adverse effect of and underdosing of other laxatives
  - T47.4X Poisoning by, adverse effect of and underdosing of other laxatives
    - T47.4X1 Poisoning by other laxatives, accidental (unintentional)
      Poisoning by other laxatives NOS
    - T47.4X2 Poisoning by other laxatives, intentional self-harm
    - T47.4X3 Poisoning by other laxatives, assault
    - T47.4X4 Poisoning by other laxatives, undetermined
    - T47.4X5 Adverse effect of other laxatives
    - T47.4X6 Underdosing of other laxatives
- T47.5 Poisoning by, adverse effect of and underdosing of digestants
  - T47.5X Poisoning by, adverse effect of and underdosing of digestants
    - T47.5X1 Poisoning by digestants, accidental (unintentional)
      Poisoning by digestants NOS
    - T47.5X2 Poisoning by digestants, intentional self-harm
    - T47.5X3 Poisoning by digestants, assault
    - T47.5X4 Poisoning by digestants, undetermined
    - T47.5X5 Adverse effect of digestants
    - T47.5X6 Underdosing of digestants
- T47.6 Poisoning by, adverse effect of and underdosing of antidiarrheal drugs

  Excludes2 poisoning by, adverse effect of and underdosing of systemic antibiotics and other anti-infectives (T36-T37)

  - T47.6X Poisoning by, adverse effect of and underdosing of antidiarrheal drugs
    - T47.6X1 Poisoning by antidiarrheal drugs, accidental (unintentional)
      Poisoning by antidiarrheal drugs NOS
    - T47.6X2 Poisoning by antidiarrheal drugs, intentional self-harm
    - T47.6X3 Poisoning by antidiarrheal drugs, assault
    - T47.6X4 Poisoning by antidiarrheal drugs, undetermined
    - T47.6X5 Adverse effect of antidiarrheal drugs
    - T47.6X6 Underdosing of antidiarrheal drugs

- T47.7 Poisoning by, adverse effect of and underdosing of emetics
  - T47.7X Poisoning by, adverse effect of and underdosing of emetics
    - T47.7X1 Poisoning by emetics, accidental (unintentional)
      Poisoning by emetics NOS
    - T47.7X2 Poisoning by emetics, intentional self-harm
    - T47.7X3 Poisoning by emetics, assault
    - T47.7X4 Poisoning by emetics, undetermined
    - T47.7X5 Adverse effect of emetics
    - T47.7X6 Underdosing of emetics
- T47.8 Poisoning by, adverse effect of and underdosing of other agents primarily affecting gastrointestinal system
  - T47.8X Poisoning by, adverse effect of and underdosing of other agents primarily affecting gastrointestinal system
    - T47.8X1 Poisoning by other agents primarily affecting gastrointestinal system, accidental (unintentional)
      Poisoning by other agents primarily affecting gastrointestinal system NOS
    - T47.8X2 Poisoning by other agents primarily affecting gastrointestinal system, intentional self-harm
    - T47.8X3 Poisoning by other agents primarily affecting gastrointestinal system, assault
    - T47.8X4 Poisoning by other agents primarily affecting gastrointestinal system, undetermined
    - T47.8X5 Adverse effect of other agents primarily affecting gastrointestinal system
    - T47.8X6 Underdosing of other agents primarily affecting gastrointestinal system
- T47.9 Poisoning by, adverse effect of and underdosing of unspecified agents primarily affecting the gastrointestinal system
  - X ● T47.91 Poisoning by unspecified agents primarily affecting the gastrointestinal system, accidental (unintentional)
    Poisoning by agents primarily affecting the gastrointestinal system NOS
  - X ● T47.92 Poisoning by unspecified agents primarily affecting the gastrointestinal system, intentional self-harm
  - X ● T47.93 Poisoning by unspecified agents primarily affecting the gastrointestinal system, assault
  - X ● T47.94 Poisoning by unspecified agents primarily affecting the gastrointestinal system, undetermined
  - X ● T47.95 Adverse effect of unspecified agents primarily affecting the gastrointestinal system
  - X ● T47.96 Underdosing of unspecified agents primarily affecting the gastrointestinal system

● **T48   Poisoning by, adverse effect of and underdosing of agents primarily acting on smooth and skeletal muscles and the respiratory system**

> The appropriate 7th character is to be added to each code from category T48

> | | | |
> |---|---|---|
> | A | initial encounter | |
> | D | subsequent encounter | |
> | S | sequela | |

● **T48.0   Poisoning by, adverse effect of and underdosing of oxytocic drugs**

> **Excludes1**   poisoning by, adverse effect of and underdosing of estrogens, progestogens and antagonists (T38.4-T38.6)

> ● **T48.0X   Poisoning by, adverse effect of and underdosing of oxytocic drugs**

>> ● **T48.0X1   Poisoning by oxytocic drugs, accidental (unintentional)**
>> Poisoning by oxytocic drugs NOS

>> ● **T48.0X2   Poisoning by oxytocic drugs, intentional self-harm**

>> ● **T48.0X3   Poisoning by oxytocic drugs, assault**

>> ● **T48.0X4   Poisoning by oxytocic drugs, undetermined**

>> ● **T48.0X5   Adverse effect of oxytocic drugs**

>> ● **T48.0X6   Underdosing of oxytocic drugs**

● **T48.1   Poisoning by, adverse effect of and underdosing of skeletal muscle relaxants [neuromuscular blocking agents]**

> ● **T48.1X   Poisoning by, adverse effect of and underdosing of skeletal muscle relaxants [neuromuscular blocking agents]**

>> ● **T48.1X1   Poisoning by skeletal muscle relaxants [neuromuscular blocking agents], accidental (unintentional)**
>> Poisoning by skeletal muscle relaxants [neuromuscular blocking agents] NOS

>> ● **T48.1X2   Poisoning by skeletal muscle relaxants [neuromuscular blocking agents], intentional self-harm**

>> ● **T48.1X3   Poisoning by skeletal muscle relaxants [neuromuscular blocking agents], assault**

>> ● **T48.1X4   Poisoning by skeletal muscle relaxants [neuromuscular blocking agents], undetermined**

>> ● **T48.1X5   Adverse effect of skeletal muscle relaxants [neuromuscular blocking agents]**

>> ● **T48.1X6   Underdosing of skeletal muscle relaxants [neuromuscular blocking agents]**

● **T48.2   Poisoning by, adverse effect of and underdosing of other and unspecified drugs acting on muscles**

> ● **T48.20   Poisoning by, adverse effect of and underdosing of unspecified drugs acting on muscles**

>> ● **T48.201   Poisoning by unspecified drugs acting on muscles, accidental (unintentional)**
>> Poisoning by unspecified drugs acting on muscles NOS

>> ● **T48.202   Poisoning by unspecified drugs acting on muscles, intentional self-harm**

>> ● **T48.203   Poisoning by unspecified drugs acting on muscles, assault**

>> ● **T48.204   Poisoning by unspecified drugs acting on muscles, undetermined**

>> ● **T48.205   Adverse effect of unspecified drugs acting on muscles**

>> ● **T48.206   Underdosing of unspecified drugs acting on muscles**

● **T48.29   Poisoning by, adverse effect of and underdosing of other drugs acting on muscles**

>> ● **T48.291   Poisoning by other drugs acting on muscles, accidental (unintentional)**
>> Poisoning by other drugs acting on muscles NOS

>> ● **T48.292   Poisoning by other drugs acting on muscles, intentional self-harm**

>> ● **T48.293   Poisoning by other drugs acting on muscles, assault**

>> ● **T48.294   Poisoning by other drugs acting on muscles, undetermined**

>> ● **T48.295   Adverse effect of other drugs acting on muscles**

>> ● **T48.296   Underdosing of other drugs acting on muscles**

● **T48.3   Poisoning by, adverse effect of and underdosing of antitussives**

> ● **T48.3X   Poisoning by, adverse effect of and underdosing of antitussives**

>> ● **T48.3X1   Poisoning by antitussives, accidental (unintentional)**
>> Poisoning by antitussives NOS

>> ● **T48.3X2   Poisoning by antitussives, intentional self-harm**

>> ● **T48.3X3   Poisoning by antitussives, assault**

>> ● **T48.3X4   Poisoning by antitussives, undetermined**

>> ● **T48.3X5   Adverse effect of antitussives**

>> ● **T48.3X6   Underdosing of antitussives**

● **T48.4   Poisoning by, adverse effect of and underdosing of expectorants**

> ● **T48.4X   Poisoning by, adverse effect of and underdosing of expectorants**

>> ● **T48.4X1   Poisoning by expectorants, accidental (unintentional)**
>> Poisoning by expectorants NOS

>> ● **T48.4X2   Poisoning by expectorants, intentional self-harm**

>> ● **T48.4X3   Poisoning by expectorants, assault**

>> ● **T48.4X4   Poisoning by expectorants, undetermined**

>> ● **T48.4X5   Adverse effect of expectorants**

>> ● **T48.4X6   Underdosing of expectorants**

● **T48.5   Poisoning by, adverse effect of and underdosing of other anti-common-cold drugs**

> Poisoning by, adverse effect of and underdosing of decongestants

> **Excludes2**   poisoning by, adverse effect of and underdosing of antipyretics, NEC (T39.9-)
> poisoning by, adverse effect of and underdosing of non-steroidal antiinflammatory drugs (T39.3-)
> poisoning by, adverse effect of and underdosing of salicylates (T39.0-)

> ● **T48.5X   Poisoning by, adverse effect of and underdosing of other anti-common-cold drugs**

>> ● **T48.5X1   Poisoning by other anti-common-cold drugs, accidental (unintentional)**
>> Poisoning by other anti-common-cold drugs NOS

>> ● **T48.5X2   Poisoning by other anti-common-cold drugs, intentional self-harm**

>> ● **T48.5X3   Poisoning by other anti-common-cold drugs, assault**

>> ● **T48.5X4   Poisoning by other anti-common-cold drugs, undetermined**

>> ● **T48.5X5   Adverse effect of other anti-common-cold drugs**

>> ● **T48.5X6   Underdosing of other anti-common-cold drugs**

● **T48.6** **Poisoning by, adverse effect of and underdosing of antiasthmatics, not elsewhere classified**
Poisoning by, adverse effect of and underdosing of beta-adrenoreceptor agonists used in asthma therapy

Excludes1   poisoning by, adverse effect of and underdosing of beta-adrenoreceptor agonists not used in asthma therapy (T44.5)
poisoning by, adverse effect of and underdosing of anterior pituitary [adenohypophyseal] hormones (T38.8)

● **T48.6X** **Poisoning by, adverse effect of and underdosing of antiasthmatics**

● **T48.6X1** **Poisoning by antiasthmatics, accidental (unintentional)**
Poisoning by antiasthmatics NOS

● **T48.6X2** **Poisoning by antiasthmatics, intentional self-harm**

● **T48.6X3** **Poisoning by antiasthmatics, assault**

● **T48.6X4** **Poisoning by antiasthmatics, undetermined**

● **T48.6X5** **Adverse effect of antiasthmatics**

● **T48.6X6** **Underdosing of antiasthmatics**

● **T48.9** **Poisoning by, adverse effect of and underdosing of other and unspecified agents primarily acting on the respiratory system**

● **T48.90** **Poisoning by, adverse effect of and underdosing of unspecified agents primarily acting on the respiratory system**

● **T48.901** **Poisoning by unspecified agents primarily acting on the respiratory system, accidental (unintentional)**

● **T48.902** **Poisoning by unspecified agents primarily acting on the respiratory system, intentional self-harm**

● **T48.903** **Poisoning by unspecified agents primarily acting on the respiratory system, assault**

● **T48.904** **Poisoning by unspecified agents primarily acting on the respiratory system, undetermined**

● **T48.905** **Adverse effect of unspecified agents primarily acting on the respiratory system**

● **T48.906** **Underdosing of unspecified agents primarily acting on the respiratory system**

● **T48.99** **Poisoning by, adverse effect of and underdosing of other agents primarily acting on the respiratory system**

● **T48.991** **Poisoning by other agents primarily acting on the respiratory system, accidental (unintentional)**

● **T48.992** **Poisoning by other agents primarily acting on the respiratory system, intentional self-harm**

● **T48.993** **Poisoning by other agents primarily acting on the respiratory system, assault**

● **T48.994** **Poisoning by other agents primarily acting on the respiratory system, undetermined**

● **T48.995** **Adverse effect of other agents primarily acting on the respiratory system**

● **T48.996** **Underdosing of other agents primarily acting on the respiratory system**

● **T49** **Poisoning by, adverse effect of and underdosing of topical agents primarily affecting skin and mucous membrane and by ophthalmological, otorhinorlaryngological and dental drugs**

Includes   poisoning by, adverse effect of and underdosing of glucocorticoids, topically used

The appropriate 7th character is to be added to each code from category T49

A   initial encounter
D   subsequent encounter
S   sequela

● **T49.0** **Poisoning by, adverse effect of and underdosing of local antifungal, anti-infective and anti-inflammatory drugs**

● **T49.0X** **Poisoning by, adverse effect of and underdosing of local antifungal, anti-infective and anti-inflammatory drugs**

● **T49.0X1** **Poisoning by local antifungal, anti-infective and anti-inflammatory drugs, accidental (unintentional)**
Poisoning by local antifungal, anti-infective and anti-inflammatory drugs NOS

● **T49.0X2** **Poisoning by local antifungal, anti-infective and anti-inflammatory drugs, intentional self-harm**

● **T49.0X3** **Poisoning by local antifungal, anti-infective and anti-inflammatory drugs, assault**

● **T49.0X4** **Poisoning by local antifungal, anti-infective and anti-inflammatory drugs, undetermined**

● **T49.0X5** **Adverse effect of local antifungal, anti-infective and anti-inflammatory drugs**

● **T49.0X6** **Underdosing of local antifungal, anti-infective and anti-inflammatory drugs**

● **T49.1** **Poisoning by, adverse effect of and underdosing of antipruritics**

● **T49.1X** **Poisoning by, adverse effect of and underdosing of antipruritics**

● **T49.1X1** **Poisoning by antipruritics, accidental (unintentional)**
Poisoning by antipruritics NOS

● **T49.1X2** **Poisoning by antipruritics, intentional self-harm**

● **T49.1X3** **Poisoning by antipruritics, assault**

● **T49.1X4** **Poisoning by antipruritics, undetermined**

● **T49.1X5** **Adverse effect of antipruritics**

● **T49.1X6** **Underdosing of antipruritics**

● **T49.2** **Poisoning by, adverse effect of and underdosing of local astringents and local detergents**

● **T49.2X** **Poisoning by, adverse effect of and underdosing of local astringents and local detergents**

● **T49.2X1** **Poisoning by local astringents and local detergents, accidental (unintentional)**
Poisoning by local astringents and local detergents NOS

● **T49.2X2** **Poisoning by local astringents and local detergents, intentional self-harm**

● **T49.2X3** **Poisoning by local astringents and local detergents, assault**

● **T49.2X4** **Poisoning by local astringents and local detergents, undetermined**

● **T49.2X5** **Adverse effect of local astringents and local detergents**

● **T49.2X6** **Underdosing of local astringents and local detergents**

- ● T49.3   Poisoning by, adverse effect of and underdosing of emollients, demulcents and protectants
  - ● T49.3X   Poisoning by, adverse effect of and underdosing of emollients, demulcents and protectants
    - ● T49.3X1   Poisoning by emollients, demulcents and protectants, accidental (unintentional)
      Poisoning by emollients, demulcents and protectants NOS
    - ● T49.3X2   Poisoning by emollients, demulcents and protectants, intentional self-harm
    - ● T49.3X3   Poisoning by emollients, demulcents and protectants, assault
    - ● T49.3X4   Poisoning by emollients, demulcents and protectants, undetermined
    - ● T49.3X5   Adverse effect of emollients, demulcents and protectants
    - ● T49.3X6   Underdosing of emollients, demulcents and protectants
- ● T49.4   Poisoning by, adverse effect of and underdosing of keratolytics, keratoplastics, and other hair treatment drugs and preparations
  - ● T49.4X   Poisoning by, adverse effect of and underdosing of keratolytics, keratoplastics, and other hair treatment drugs and preparations
    - ● T49.4X1   Poisoning by keratolytics, keratoplastics, and other hair treatment drugs and preparations, accidental (unintentional)
      Poisoning by keratolytics, keratoplastics, and other hair treatment drugs and preparations NOS
    - ● T49.4X2   Poisoning by keratolytics, keratoplastics, and other hair treatment drugs and preparations, intentional self-harm
    - ● T49.4X3   Poisoning by keratolytics, keratoplastics, and other hair treatment drugs and preparations, assault
    - ● T49.4X4   Poisoning by keratolytics, keratoplastics, and other hair treatment drugs and preparations, undetermined
    - ● T49.4X5   Adverse effect of keratolytics, keratoplastics, and other hair treatment drugs and preparations
    - ● T49.4X6   Underdosing of keratolytics, keratoplastics, and other hair treatment drugs and preparations
- ● T49.5   Poisoning by, adverse effect of and underdosing of ophthalmological drugs and preparations
  - ● T49.5X   Poisoning by, adverse effect of and underdosing of ophthalmological drugs and preparations
    - ● T49.5X1   Poisoning by ophthalmological drugs and preparations, accidental (unintentional)
      Poisoning by ophthalmological drugs and preparations NOS
    - ● T49.5X2   Poisoning by ophthalmological drugs and preparations, intentional self-harm
    - ● T49.5X3   Poisoning by ophthalmological drugs and preparations, assault
    - ● T49.5X4   Poisoning by ophthalmological drugs and preparations, undetermined
    - ● T49.5X5   Adverse effect of ophthalmological drugs and preparations
    - ● T49.5X6   Underdosing of ophthalmological drugs and preparations

- ● T49.6   Poisoning by, adverse effect of and underdosing of otorhinolaryngological drugs and preparations
  - ● T49.6X   Poisoning by, adverse effect of and underdosing of otorhinolaryngological drugs and preparations
    - ● T49.6X1   Poisoning by otorhinolaryngological drugs and preparations, accidental (unintentional)
      Poisoning by otorhinolaryngological drugs and preparations NOS
    - ● T49.6X2   Poisoning by otorhinolaryngological drugs and preparations, intentional self-harm
    - ● T49.6X3   Poisoning by otorhinolaryngological drugs and preparations, assault
    - ● T49.6X4   Poisoning by otorhinolaryngological drugs and preparations, undetermined
    - ● T49.6X5   Adverse effect of otorhinolaryngological drugs and preparations
    - ● T49.6X6   Underdosing of otorhinolaryngological drugs and preparations
- ● T49.7   Poisoning by, adverse effect of and underdosing of dental drugs, topically applied
  - ● T49.7X   Poisoning by, adverse effect of and underdosing of dental drugs, topically applied
    - ● T49.7X1   Poisoning by dental drugs, topically applied, accidental (unintentional)
      Poisoning by dental drugs, topically applied NOS
    - ● T49.7X2   Poisoning by dental drugs, topically applied, intentional self-harm
    - ● T49.7X3   Poisoning by dental drugs, topically applied, assault
    - ● T49.7X4   Poisoning by dental drugs, topically applied, undetermined
    - ● T49.7X5   Adverse effect of dental drugs, topically applied
    - ● T49.7X6   Underdosing of dental drugs, topically applied
- ● T49.8   Poisoning by, adverse effect of and underdosing of other topical agents
  Poisoning by, adverse effect of and underdosing of spermicides
  - ● T49.8X   Poisoning by, adverse effect of and underdosing of other topical agents
    - ● T49.8X1   Poisoning by other topical agents, accidental (unintentional)
      Poisoning by other topical agents NOS
    - ● T49.8X2   Poisoning by other topical agents, intentional self-harm
    - ● T49.8X3   Poisoning by other topical agents, assault
    - ● T49.8X4   Poisoning by other topical agents, undetermined
    - ● T49.8X5   Adverse effect of other topical agents
    - ● T49.8X6   Underdosing of other topical agents
- ● T49.9   Poisoning by, adverse effect of and underdosing of unspecified topical agent
  - X ● T49.91   Poisoning by unspecified topical agent, accidental (unintentional)
  - X ● T49.92   Poisoning by unspecified topical agent, intentional self-harm
  - X ● T49.93   Poisoning by unspecified topical agent, assault
  - X ● T49.94   Poisoning by unspecified topical agent, undetermined
  - X ● T49.95   Adverse effect of unspecified topical agent
  - X ● T49.96   Underdosing of unspecified topical agent

CHAPTER 19 (S00-T88)

● **T50   Poisoning by, adverse effect of and underdosing of diuretics and other and unspecified drugs, medicaments and biological substances**

> The appropriate 7th character is to be added to each code from category T50

> | | |
> |---|---|
> | A | initial encounter |
> | D | subsequent encounter |
> | S | sequela |

● **T50.0   Poisoning by, adverse effect of and underdosing of mineralocorticoids and their antagonists**

● **T50.0X   Poisoning by, adverse effect of and underdosing of mineralocorticoids and their antagonists**

● **T50.0X1   Poisoning by mineralocorticoids and their antagonists, accidental (unintentional)**
> Poisoning by mineralocorticoids and their antagonists NOS

● **T50.0X2   Poisoning by mineralocorticoids and their antagonists, intentional self-harm**

● **T50.0X3   Poisoning by mineralocorticoids and their antagonists, assault**

● **T50.0X4   Poisoning by mineralocorticoids and their antagonists, undetermined**

● **T50.0X5   Adverse effect of mineralocorticoids and their antagonists**

● **T50.0X6   Underdosing of mineralocorticoids and their antagonists**

● **T50.1   Poisoning by, adverse effect of and underdosing of loop [high-ceiling] diuretics**

● **T50.1X   Poisoning by, adverse effect of and underdosing of loop [high-ceiling] diuretics**

● **T50.1X1   Poisoning by loop [high-ceiling] diuretics, accidental (unintentional)**
> Poisoning by loop [high-ceiling] diuretics NOS

● **T50.1X2   Poisoning by loop [high-ceiling] diuretics, intentional self-harm**

● **T50.1X3   Poisoning by loop [high-ceiling] diuretics, assault**

● **T50.1X4   Poisoning by loop [high-ceiling] diuretics, undetermined**

● **T50.1X5   Adverse effect of loop [high-ceiling] diuretics**

● **T50.1X6   Underdosing of loop [high-ceiling] diuretics**

● **T50.2   Poisoning by, adverse effect of and underdosing of carbonic-anhydrase inhibitors, benzothiadiazides and other diuretics**
> Poisoning by, adverse effect of and underdosing of acetazolamide

● **T50.2X   Poisoning by, adverse effect of and underdosing of carbonic-anhydrase inhibitors, benzothiadiazides and other diuretics**

● **T50.2X1   Poisoning by carbonic-anhydrase inhibitors, benzothiadiazides and other diuretics, accidental (unintentional)**
> Poisoning by carbonic-anhydrase inhibitors, benzothiadiazides and other diuretics NOS

● **T50.2X2   Poisoning by carbonic-anhydrase inhibitors, benzothiadiazides and other diuretics, intentional self-harm**

● **T50.2X3   Poisoning by carbonic-anhydrase inhibitors, benzothiadiazides and other diuretics, assault**

● **T50.2X4   Poisoning by carbonic-anhydrase inhibitors, benzothiadiazides and other diuretics, undetermined**

● **T50.2X5   Adverse effect of carbonic-anhydrase inhibitors, benzothiadiazides and other diuretics**

● **T50.2X6   Underdosing of carbonic-anhydrase inhibitors, benzothiadiazides and other diuretics**

● **T50.3   Poisoning by, adverse effect of and underdosing of electrolytic, caloric and water-balance agents**
> Poisoning by, adverse effect of and underdosing of oral rehydration salts

● **T50.3X   Poisoning by, adverse effect of and underdosing of electrolytic, caloric and water-balance agents**

● **T50.3X1   Poisoning by electrolytic, caloric and water-balance agents, accidental (unintentional)**
> Poisoning by electrolytic, caloric and water-balance agents NOS

● **T50.3X2   Poisoning by electrolytic, caloric and water-balance agents, intentional self-harm**

● **T50.3X3   Poisoning by electrolytic, caloric and water-balance agents, assault**

● **T50.3X4   Poisoning by electrolytic, caloric and water-balance agents, undetermined**

● **T50.3X5   Adverse effect of electrolytic, caloric and water-balance agents**

● **T50.3X6   Underdosing of electrolytic, caloric and water-balance agents**

● **T50.4   Poisoning by, adverse effect of and underdosing of drugs affecting uric acid metabolism**

● **T50.4X   Poisoning by, adverse effect of and underdosing of drugs affecting uric acid metabolism**

● **T50.4X1   Poisoning by drugs affecting uric acid metabolism, accidental (unintentional)**
> Poisoning by drugs affecting uric acid metabolism NOS

● **T50.4X2   Poisoning by drugs affecting uric acid metabolism, intentional self-harm**

● **T50.4X3   Poisoning by drugs affecting uric acid metabolism, assault**

● **T50.4X4   Poisoning by drugs affecting uric acid metabolism, undetermined**

● **T50.4X5   Adverse effect of drugs affecting uric acid metabolism**

● **T50.4X6   Underdosing of drugs affecting uric acid metabolism**

● **T50.5   Poisoning by, adverse effect of and underdosing of appetite depressants**

● **T50.5X   Poisoning by, adverse effect of and underdosing of appetite depressants**

● **T50.5X1   Poisoning by appetite depressants, accidental (unintentional)**
> Poisoning by appetite depressants NOS

● **T50.5X2   Poisoning by appetite depressants, intentional self-harm**

● **T50.5X3   Poisoning by appetite depressants, assault**

● **T50.5X4   Poisoning by appetite depressants, undetermined**

● **T50.5X5   Adverse effect of appetite depressants**

● **T50.5X6   Underdosing of appetite depressants**

◀ New   ◀▥ Revised   ~~deleted~~ Deleted   **OGCR** Official Guidelines   X Assign placeholder X   ● Use Additional Character(s)

Excludes 1   Excludes 2   Includes   Use additional   Code first   Code also   Unspecified

● **T50.6 Poisoning by, adverse effect of and underdosing of antidotes and chelating agents**

Poisoning by, adverse effect of and underdosing of alcohol deterrents

● **T50.6X Poisoning by, adverse effect of and underdosing of antidotes and chelating agents**

● T50.6X1 Poisoning by antidotes and chelating agents, accidental (unintentional)

Poisoning by antidotes and chelating agents NOS

● T50.6X2 Poisoning by antidotes and chelating agents, intentional self-harm

● T50.6X3 Poisoning by antidotes and chelating agents, assault

● T50.6X4 Poisoning by antidotes and chelating agents, undetermined

● T50.6X5 Adverse effect of antidotes and chelating agents

● T50.6X6 Underdosing of antidotes and chelating agents

● **T50.7 Poisoning by, adverse effect of and underdosing of analeptics and opioid receptor antagonists**

● **T50.7X Poisoning by, adverse effect of and underdosing of analeptics and opioid receptor antagonists**

● T50.7X1 Poisoning by analeptics and opioid receptor antagonists, accidental (unintentional)

Poisoning by analeptics and opioid receptor antagonists NOS

● T50.7X2 Poisoning by analeptics and opioid receptor antagonists, intentional self-harm

● T50.7X3 Poisoning by analeptics and opioid receptor antagonists, assault

● T50.7X4 Poisoning by analeptics and opioid receptor antagonists, undetermined

● T50.7X5 Adverse effect of analeptics and opioid receptor antagonists

● T50.7X6 Underdosing of analeptics and opioid receptor antagonists

● **T50.8 Poisoning by, adverse effect of and underdosing of diagnostic agents**

● **T50.8X Poisoning by, adverse effect of and underdosing of diagnostic agents**

● T50.8X1 Poisoning by diagnostic agents, accidental (unintentional)

Poisoning by diagnostic agents NOS

● T50.8X2 Poisoning by diagnostic agents, intentional self-harm

● T50.8X3 Poisoning by diagnostic agents, assault

● T50.8X4 Poisoning by diagnostic agents, undetermined

● T50.8X5 Adverse effect of diagnostic agents

● T50.8X6 Underdosing of diagnostic agents

● **T50.A Poisoning by, adverse effect of and underdosing of bacterial vaccines**

● **T50.A1 Poisoning by, adverse effect of and underdosing of pertussis vaccine, including combinations with a pertussis component**

● T50.A11 Poisoning by pertussis vaccine, including combinations with a pertussis component, accidental (unintentional)

● T50.A12 Poisoning by pertussis vaccine, including combinations with a pertussis component, intentional self-harm

● T50.A13 Poisoning by pertussis vaccine, including combinations with a pertussis component, assault

● T50.A14 Poisoning by pertussis vaccine, including combinations with a pertussis component, undetermined

● T50.A15 Adverse effect of pertussis vaccine, including combinations with a pertussis component

● T50.A16 Underdosing of pertussis vaccine, including combinations with a pertussis component

● **T50.A2 Poisoning by, adverse effect of and underdosing of mixed bacterial vaccines without a pertussis component**

● T50.A21 Poisoning by mixed bacterial vaccines without a pertussis component, accidental (unintentional)

● T50.A22 Poisoning by mixed bacterial vaccines without a pertussis component, intentional self-harm

● T50.A23 Poisoning by mixed bacterial vaccines without a pertussis component, assault

● T50.A24 Poisoning by mixed bacterial vaccines without a pertussis component, undetermined

● T50.A25 Adverse effect of mixed bacterial vaccines without a pertussis component

● T50.A26 Underdosing of mixed bacterial vaccines without a pertussis component

● **T50.A9 Poisoning by, adverse effect of and underdosing of other bacterial vaccines**

● T50.A91 Poisoning by other bacterial vaccines, accidental (unintentional)

● T50.A92 Poisoning by other bacterial vaccines, intentional self-harm

● T50.A93 Poisoning by other bacterial vaccines, assault

● T50.A94 Poisoning by other bacterial vaccines, undetermined

● T50.A95 Adverse effect of other bacterial vaccines

● T50.A96 Underdosing of other bacterial vaccines

● **T50.B Poisoning by, adverse effect of and underdosing of viral vaccines**

● **T50.B1 Poisoning by, adverse effect of and underdosing of smallpox vaccines**

● T50.B11 Poisoning by smallpox vaccines, accidental (unintentional)

● T50.B12 Poisoning by smallpox vaccines, intentional self-harm

● T50.B13 Poisoning by smallpox vaccines, assault

● T50.B14 Poisoning by smallpox vaccines, undetermined

● T50.B15 Adverse effect of smallpox vaccines

● T50.B16 Underdosing of smallpox vaccines

● **T50.B9 Poisoning by, adverse effect of and underdosing of other viral vaccines**

● T50.B91 Poisoning by other viral vaccines, accidental (unintentional)

● T50.B92 Poisoning by other viral vaccines, intentional self-harm

● T50.B93 Poisoning by other viral vaccines, assault

● T50.B94   Poisoning by other viral vaccines, undetermined
● T50.B95   Adverse effect of other viral vaccines
● T50.B96   Underdosing of other viral vaccines

● T50.Z   Poisoning by, adverse effect of and underdosing of other vaccines and biological substances
  ● T50.Z1   Poisoning by, adverse effect of and underdosing of immunoglobulin
    ● T50.Z11   Poisoning by immunoglobulin, accidental (unintentional)
    ● T50.Z12   Poisoning by immunoglobulin, intentional self-harm
    ● T50.Z13   Poisoning by immunoglobulin, assault
    ● T50.Z14   Poisoning by immunoglobulin, undetermined
    ● T50.Z15   Adverse effect of immunoglobulin
    ● T50.Z16   Underdosing of immunoglobulin
  ● T50.Z9   Poisoning by, adverse effect of and underdosing of other vaccines and biological substances
    ● T50.Z91   Poisoning by other vaccines and biological substances, accidental (unintentional)
    ● T50.Z92   Poisoning by other vaccines and biological substances, intentional self-harm
    ● T50.Z93   Poisoning by other vaccines and biological substances, assault
    ● T50.Z94   Poisoning by other vaccines and biological substances, undetermined
    ● T50.Z95   Adverse effect of other vaccines and biological substances
    ● T50.Z96   Underdosing of other vaccines and biological substances

● T50.9   Poisoning by, adverse effect of and underdosing of other and unspecified drugs, medicaments and biological substances
  ● T50.90   Poisoning by, adverse effect of and underdosing of unspecified drugs, medicaments and biological substances
    ● T50.901   Poisoning by unspecified drugs, medicaments and biological substances, accidental (unintentional)
    ● T50.902   Poisoning by unspecified drugs, medicaments and biological substances, intentional self-harm
    ● T50.903   Poisoning by unspecified drugs, medicaments and biological substances, assault
    ● T50.904   Poisoning by unspecified drugs, medicaments and biological substances, undetermined
    ● T50.905   Adverse effect of unspecified drugs, medicaments and biological substances
    ● T50.906   Underdosing of unspecified drugs, medicaments and biological substances
  ● T50.99   Poisoning by, adverse effect of and underdosing of other drugs, medicaments and biological substances
    ● T50.991   Poisoning by other drugs, medicaments and biological substances, accidental (unintentional)
    ● T50.992   Poisoning by other drugs, medicaments and biological substances, intentional self-harm

● T50.993   Poisoning by other drugs, medicaments and biological substances, assault
● T50.994   Poisoning by other drugs, medicaments and biological substances, undetermined
● T50.995   Adverse effect of other drugs, medicaments and biological substances
● T50.996   Underdosing of other drugs, medicaments and biological substances

TOXIC EFFECTS OF SUBSTANCES CHIEFLY NONMEDICINAL AS TO SOURCE (T51-T65)

Note: When no intent is indicated code to accidental. Undetermined intent is only for use when there is specific documentation in the record that the intent of the toxic effect cannot be determined.

Use additional code(s): for all associated manifestations of toxic effect, such as:
respiratory conditions due to external agents (J60-J70)
personal history of foreign body fully removed (Z87.821)
to identify any retained foreign body, if applicable (Z18.-)

Excludes1   contact with and (suspected) exposure to toxic substances (Z77.-)

● T51   Toxic effect of alcohol
  The appropriate 7th character is to be added to each code from category T51

A	initial encounter
D	subsequent encounter
S	sequela

  ● T51.0   Toxic effect of ethanol
    Toxic effect of ethyl alcohol
    Excludes2   acute alcohol intoxication or 'hangover' effects (F10.129, F10.229, F10.929)
    drunkenness (F10.129, F10.229, F10.929)
    pathological alcohol intoxication (F10.129, F10.229, F10.929)
    ● T51.0X   Toxic effect of ethanol
      ● T51.0X1   Toxic effect of ethanol, accidental (unintentional)
        Toxic effect of ethanol NOS
      ● T51.0X2   Toxic effect of ethanol, intentional self-harm
      ● T51.0X3   Toxic effect of ethanol, assault
      ● T51.0X4   Toxic effect of ethanol, undetermined
  ● T51.1   Toxic effect of methanol
    Toxic effect of methyl alcohol
    ● T51.1X   Toxic effect of methanol
      ● T51.1X1   Toxic effect of methanol, accidental (unintentional)
        Toxic effect of methanol NOS
      ● T51.1X2   Toxic effect of methanol, intentional self-harm
      ● T51.1X3   Toxic effect of methanol, assault
      ● T51.1X4   Toxic effect of methanol, undetermined
  ● T51.2   Toxic effect of 2-Propanol
    Toxic effect of isopropyl alcohol
    ● T51.2X   Toxic effect of 2-Propanol
      ● T51.2X1   Toxic effect of 2-Propanol, accidental (unintentional)
        Toxic effect of 2-Propanol NOS
      ● T51.2X2   Toxic effect of 2-Propanol, intentional self-harm
      ● T51.2X3   Toxic effect of 2-Propanol, assault
      ● T51.2X4   Toxic effect of 2-Propanol, undetermined

● **T51.3   Toxic effect of fusel oil**
      Toxic effect of amyl alcohol
      Toxic effect of butyl [1-butanol] alcohol
      Toxic effect of propyl [1-propanol] alcohol
   ● **T51.3X Toxic effect of fusel oil**
      ● **T51.3X1 Toxic effect of fusel oil, accidental (unintentional)**
           Toxic effect of fusel oil NOS
      ● **T51.3X2 Toxic effect of fusel oil, intentional self-harm**
      ● **T51.3X3 Toxic effect of fusel oil, assault**
      ● **T51.3X4 Toxic effect of fusel oil, undetermined**

● **T51.8   Toxic effect of other alcohols**
   ● **T51.8X Toxic effect of other alcohols**
      ● **T51.8X1 Toxic effect of other alcohols, accidental (unintentional)**
           Toxic effect of other alcohols NOS
      ● **T51.8X2 Toxic effect of other alcohols, intentional self-harm**
      ● **T51.8X3 Toxic effect of other alcohols, assault**
      ● **T51.8X4 Toxic effect of other alcohols, undetermined**

● **T51.9   Toxic effect of unspecified alcohol**
  X ● **T51.91 Toxic effect of unspecified alcohol, accidental (unintentional)**
  X ● **T51.92 Toxic effect of unspecified alcohol, intentional self-harm**
  X ● **T51.93 Toxic effect of unspecified alcohol, assault**
  X ● **T51.94 Toxic effect of unspecified alcohol, undetermined**

● **T52   Toxic effect of organic solvents**
    Excludes1 halogen derivatives of aliphatic and aromatic hydrocarbons (T53.-)
    The appropriate 7th character is to be added to each code from category T52

A	initial encounter
D	subsequent encounter
S	sequela

● **T52.0   Toxic effects of petroleum products**
      Toxic effects of gasoline [petrol]
      Toxic effects of kerosene [paraffin oil]
      Toxic effects of paraffin wax
      Toxic effects of ether petroleum
      Toxic effects of naphtha petroleum
      Toxic effects of spirit petroleum
   ● **T52.0X Toxic effects of petroleum products**
      ● **T52.0X1 Toxic effect of petroleum products, accidental (unintentional)**
           Toxic effects of petroleum products NOS
      ● **T52.0X2 Toxic effect of petroleum products, intentional self-harm**
      ● **T52.0X3 Toxic effect of petroleum products, assault**
      ● **T52.0X4 Toxic effect of petroleum products, undetermined**

● **T52.1   Toxic effects of benzene**
    Excludes1 homologues of benzene (T52.2)
           nitroderivatives and aminoderivatives of benzene and its homologues (T65.3)
   ● **T52.1X Toxic effects of benzene**
      ● **T52.1X1 Toxic effect of benzene, accidental (unintentional)**
           Toxic effects of benzene NOS
      ● **T52.1X2 Toxic effect of benzene, intentional self-harm**
      ● **T52.1X3 Toxic effect of benzene, assault**
      ● **T52.1X4 Toxic effect of benzene, undetermined**

● **T52.2   Toxic effects of homologues of benzene**
      Toxic effects of toluene [methylbenzene]
      Toxic effects of xylene [dimethylbenzene]
   ● **T52.2X Toxic effects of homologues of benzene**
      ● **T52.2X1 Toxic effect of homologues of benzene, accidental (unintentional)**
           Toxic effects of homologues of benzene NOS
      ● **T52.2X2 Toxic effect of homologues of benzene, intentional self-harm**
      ● **T52.2X3 Toxic effect of homologues of benzene, assault**
      ● **T52.2X4 Toxic effect of homologues of benzene, undetermined**

● **T52.3   Toxic effects of glycols**
   ● **T52.3X Toxic effects of glycols**
      ● **T52.3X1 Toxic effect of glycols, accidental (unintentional)**
           Toxic effects of glycols NOS
      ● **T52.3X2 Toxic effect of glycols, intentional self-harm**
      ● **T52.3X3 Toxic effect of glycols, assault**
      ● **T52.3X4 Toxic effect of glycols, undetermined**

● **T52.4   Toxic effects of ketones**
   ● **T52.4X Toxic effects of ketones**
      ● **T52.4X1 Toxic effect of ketones, accidental (unintentional)**
           Toxic effects of ketones NOS
      ● **T52.4X2 Toxic effect of ketones, intentional self-harm**
      ● **T52.4X3 Toxic effect of ketones, assault**
      ● **T52.4X4 Toxic effect of ketones, undetermined**

● **T52.8   Toxic effects of other organic solvents**
   ● **T52.8X Toxic effects of other organic solvents**
      ● **T52.8X1 Toxic effect of other organic solvents, accidental (unintentional)**
           Toxic effects of other organic solvents NOS
      ● **T52.8X2 Toxic effect of other organic solvents, intentional self-harm**
      ● **T52.8X3 Toxic effect of other organic solvents, assault**
      ● **T52.8X4 Toxic effect of other organic solvents, undetermined**

● **T52.9   Toxic effects of unspecified organic solvent**
  X ● **T52.91 Toxic effect of unspecified organic solvent, accidental (unintentional)**
  X ● **T52.92 Toxic effect of unspecified organic solvent, intentional self-harm**
  X ● **T52.93 Toxic effect of unspecified organic solvent, assault**
  X ● **T52.94 Toxic effect of unspecified organic solvent, undetermined**

● **T53   Toxic effect of halogen derivatives of aliphatic and aromatic hydrocarbons**
    The appropriate 7th character is to be added to each code from category T53

A	initial encounter
D	subsequent encounter
S	sequela

● **T53.0   Toxic effects of carbon tetrachloride**
      Toxic effects of tetrachloromethane
   ● **T53.0X Toxic effects of carbon tetrachloride**
      ● **T53.0X1 Toxic effect of carbon tetrachloride, accidental (unintentional)**
           Toxic effects of carbon tetrachloride NOS
      ● **T53.0X2 Toxic effect of carbon tetrachloride, intentional self-harm**

CHAPTER 19 (S00-T88)

● **T53.0X3**   Toxic effect of carbon tetrachloride, assault

● **T53.0X4**   Toxic effect of carbon tetrachloride, undetermined

● **T53.1**   **Toxic effects of chloroform**
Toxic effects of trichloromethane

● **T53.1X**   **Toxic effects of chloroform**

● **T53.1X1**   Toxic effect of chloroform, accidental (unintentional)
Toxic effects of chloroform NOS

● **T53.1X2**   Toxic effect of chloroform, intentional self-harm

● **T53.1X3**   Toxic effect of chloroform, assault

● **T53.1X4**   Toxic effect of chloroform, undetermined

● **T53.2**   **Toxic effects of trichloroethylene**
Toxic effects of trichloroethene

● **T53.2X**   **Toxic effects of trichloroethylene**

● **T53.2X1**   Toxic effect of trichloroethylene, accidental (unintentional)
Toxic effects of trichloroethylene NOS

● **T53.2X2**   Toxic effect of trichloroethylene, intentional self-harm

● **T53.2X3**   Toxic effect of trichloroethylene, assault

● **T53.2X4**   Toxic effect of trichloroethylene, undetermined

● **T53.3**   **Toxic effects of tetrachloroethylene**
Toxic effects of perchloroethylene
Toxic effect of tetrachloroethene

● **T53.3X**   **Toxic effects of tetrachloroethylene**

● **T53.3X1**   Toxic effect of tetrachloroethylene, accidental (unintentional)
Toxic effects of tetrachloroethylene NOS

● **T53.3X2**   Toxic effect of tetrachloroethylene, intentional self-harm

● **T53.3X3**   Toxic effect of tetrachloroethylene, assault

● **T53.3X4**   Toxic effect of tetrachloroethylene, undetermined

● **T53.4**   **Toxic effects of dichloromethane**
Toxic effects of methylene chloride

● **T53.4X**   **Toxic effects of dichloromethane**

● **T53.4X1**   Toxic effect of dichloromethane, accidental (unintentional)
Toxic effects of dichloromethane NOS

● **T53.4X2**   Toxic effect of dichloromethane, intentional self-harm

● **T53.4X3**   Toxic effect of dichloromethane, assault

● **T53.4X4**   Toxic effect of dichloromethane, undetermined

● **T53.5**   **Toxic effects of chlorofluorocarbons**

● **T53.5X**   **Toxic effects of chlorofluorocarbons**

● **T53.5X1**   Toxic effect of chlorofluorocarbons, accidental (unintentional)
Toxic effects of chlorofluorocarbons NOS

● **T53.5X2**   Toxic effect of chlorofluorocarbons, intentional self-harm

● **T53.5X3**   Toxic effect of chlorofluorocarbons, assault

● **T53.5X4**   Toxic effect of chlorofluorocarbons, undetermined

● **T53.6**   **Toxic effects of other halogen derivatives of aliphatic hydrocarbons**

● **T53.6X**   **Toxic effects of other halogen derivatives of aliphatic hydrocarbons**

● **T53.6X1**   Toxic effect of other halogen derivatives of aliphatic hydrocarbons, accidental (unintentional)
Toxic effects of other halogen derivatives of aliphatic hydrocarbons NOS

● **T53.6X2**   Toxic effect of other halogen derivatives of aliphatic hydrocarbons, intentional self-harm

● **T53.6X3**   Toxic effect of other halogen derivatives of aliphatic hydrocarbons, assault

● **T53.6X4**   Toxic effect of other halogen derivatives of aliphatic hydrocarbons, undetermined

● **T53.7**   **Toxic effects of other halogen derivatives of aromatic hydrocarbons**

● **T53.7X**   **Toxic effects of other halogen derivatives of aromatic hydrocarbons**

● **T53.7X1**   Toxic effect of other halogen derivatives of aromatic hydrocarbons, accidental (unintentional)
Toxic effects of other halogen derivatives of aromatic hydrocarbons NOS

● **T53.7X2**   Toxic effect of other halogen derivatives of aromatic hydrocarbons, intentional self-harm

● **T53.7X3**   Toxic effect of other halogen derivatives of aromatic hydrocarbons, assault

● **T53.7X4**   Toxic effect of other halogen derivatives of aromatic hydrocarbons, undetermined

● **T53.9**   **Toxic effects of unspecified halogen derivatives of aliphatic and aromatic hydrocarbons**

X ● **T53.91**   Toxic effect of unspecified halogen derivatives of aliphatic and aromatic hydrocarbons, accidental (unintentional)

X ● **T53.92**   Toxic effect of unspecified halogen derivatives of aliphatic and aromatic hydrocarbons, intentional self-harm

X ● **T53.93**   Toxic effect of unspecified halogen derivatives of aliphatic and aromatic hydrocarbons, assault

X ● **T53.94**   Toxic effect of unspecified halogen derivatives of aliphatic and aromatic hydrocarbons, undetermined

● **T54**   **Toxic effect of corrosive substances**
The appropriate 7th character is to be added to each code from category T54

A	initial encounter
D	subsequent encounter
S	sequela

● **T54.0**   **Toxic effects of phenol and phenol homologues**

● **T54.0X**   **Toxic effects of phenol and phenol homologues**

● **T54.0X1**   Toxic effect of phenol and phenol homologues, accidental (unintentional)
Toxic effects of phenol and phenol homologues NOS

● **T54.0X2**   Toxic effect of phenol and phenol homologues, intentional self-harm

● **T54.0X3**   Toxic effect of phenol and phenol homologues, assault

● **T54.0X4**   Toxic effect of phenol and phenol homologues, undetermined

● **T54.1**   **Toxic effects of other corrosive organic compounds**
- ● **T54.1X**   **Toxic effects of other corrosive organic compounds**
  - ● **T54.1X1**   **Toxic effect of other corrosive organic compounds, accidental (unintentional)**
    Toxic effects of other corrosive organic compounds NOS
  - ● **T54.1X2**   **Toxic effect of other corrosive organic compounds, intentional self-harm**
  - ● **T54.1X3**   **Toxic effect of other corrosive organic compounds, assault**
  - ● **T54.1X4**   **Toxic effect of other corrosive organic compounds, undetermined**

● **T54.2**   **Toxic effects of corrosive acids and acid-like substances**
Toxic effects of hydrochloric acid
Toxic effects of sulfuric acid
- ● **T54.2X**   **Toxic effects of corrosive acids and acid-like substances**
  - ● **T54.2X1**   **Toxic effect of corrosive acids and acid-like substances, accidental (unintentional)**
    Toxic effects of corrosive acids and acid-like substances NOS
  - ● **T54.2X2**   **Toxic effect of corrosive acids and acid-like substances, intentional self-harm**
  - ● **T54.2X3**   **Toxic effect of corrosive acids and acid-like substances, assault**
  - ● **T54.2X4**   **Toxic effect of corrosive acids and acid-like substances, undetermined**

● **T54.3**   **Toxic effects of corrosive alkalis and alkali-like substances**
Toxic effects of potassium hydroxide
Toxic effects of sodium hydroxide
- ● **T54.3X**   **Toxic effects of corrosive alkalis and alkali-like substances**
  - ● **T54.3X1**   **Toxic effect of corrosive alkalis and alkali-like substances, accidental (unintentional)**
    Toxic effects of corrosive alkalis and alkali-like substances NOS
  - ● **T54.3X2**   **Toxic effect of corrosive alkalis and alkali-like substances, intentional self-harm**
  - ● **T54.3X3**   **Toxic effect of corrosive alkalis and alkali-like substances, assault**
  - ● **T54.3X4**   **Toxic effect of corrosive alkalis and alkali-like substances, undetermined**

● **T54.9**   **Toxic effects of unspecified corrosive substance**
- X ● **T54.91**   **Toxic effect of unspecified corrosive substance, accidental (unintentional)**
- X ● **T54.92**   **Toxic effect of unspecified corrosive substance, intentional self-harm**
- X ● **T54.93**   **Toxic effect of unspecified corrosive substance, assault**
- X ● **T54.94**   **Toxic effect of unspecified corrosive substance, undetermined**

● **T55**   **Toxic effect of soaps and detergents**
The appropriate 7th character is to be added to each code from category T55

A	initial encounter
D	subsequent encounter
S	sequela

● **T55.0**   **Toxic effect of soaps**
- ● **T55.0X**   **Toxic effect of soaps**
  - ● **T55.0X1**   **Toxic effect of soaps, accidental (unintentional)**
    Toxic effect of soaps NOS
  - ● **T55.0X2**   **Toxic effect of soaps, intentional self-harm**
  - ● **T55.0X3**   **Toxic effect of soaps, assault**
  - ● **T55.0X4**   **Toxic effect of soaps, undetermined**

● **T55.1**   **Toxic effect of detergents**
- ● **T55.1X**   **Toxic effect of detergents**
  - ● **T55.1X1**   **Toxic effect of detergents, accidental (unintentional)**
    Toxic effect of detergents NOS
  - ● **T55.1X2**   **Toxic effect of detergents, intentional self-harm**
  - ● **T55.1X3**   **Toxic effect of detergents, assault**
  - ● **T55.1X4**   **Toxic effect of detergents, undetermined**

● **T56**   **Toxic effect of metals**

> **Includes**   toxic effects of fumes and vapors of metals
> toxic effects of metals from all sources, except medicinal substances

Use additional code to identify any retained metal foreign body, if applicable (Z18.0-, T18.1-)

> **Excludes1**   arsenic and its compounds (T57.0)
> manganese and its compounds (T57.2)

The appropriate 7th character is to be added to each code from category T56

A	initial encounter
D	subsequent encounter
S	sequela

● **T56.0**   **Toxic effects of lead and its compounds**
- ● **T56.0X**   **Toxic effects of lead and its compounds**
  - ● **T56.0X1**   **Toxic effect of lead and its compounds, accidental (unintentional)**
    Toxic effects of lead and its compounds NOS
  - ● **T56.0X2**   **Toxic effect of lead and its compounds, intentional self-harm**
  - ● **T56.0X3**   **Toxic effect of lead and its compounds, assault**
  - ● **T56.0X4**   **Toxic effect of lead and its compounds, undetermined**

● **T56.1**   **Toxic effects of mercury and its compounds**
- ● **T56.1X**   **Toxic effects of mercury and its compounds**
  - ● **T56.1X1**   **Toxic effect of mercury and its compounds, accidental (unintentional)**
    Toxic effects of mercury and its compounds NOS
  - ● **T56.1X2**   **Toxic effect of mercury and its compounds, intentional self-harm**
  - ● **T56.1X3**   **Toxic effect of mercury and its compounds, assault**
  - ● **T56.1X4**   **Toxic effect of mercury and its compounds, undetermined**

CHAPTER 19 (S00-T88)

- ● T56.2   Toxic effects of chromium and its compounds
  - ● T56.2X   Toxic effects of chromium and its compounds
    - ● T56.2X1   Toxic effect of chromium and its compounds, accidental (unintentional)
      Toxic effects of chromium and its compounds NOS
    - ● T56.2X2   Toxic effect of chromium and its compounds, intentional self-harm
    - ● T56.2X3   Toxic effect of chromium and its compounds, assault
    - ● T56.2X4   Toxic effect of chromium and its compounds, undetermined
- ● T56.3   Toxic effects of cadmium and its compounds
  - ● T56.3X   Toxic effects of cadmium and its compounds
    - ● T56.3X1   Toxic effect of cadmium and its compounds, accidental (unintentional)
      Toxic effects of cadmium and its compounds NOS
    - ● T56.3X2   Toxic effect of cadmium and its compounds, intentional self-harm
    - ● T56.3X3   Toxic effect of cadmium and its compounds, assault
    - ● T56.3X4   Toxic effect of cadmium and its compounds, undetermined
- ● T56.4   Toxic effects of copper and its compounds
  - ● T56.4X   Toxic effects of copper and its compounds
    - ● T56.4X1   Toxic effect of copper and its compounds, accidental (unintentional)
      Toxic effects of copper and its compounds NOS
    - ● T56.4X2   Toxic effect of copper and its compounds, intentional self-harm
    - ● T56.4X3   Toxic effect of copper and its compounds, assault
    - ● T56.4X4   Toxic effect of copper and its compounds, undetermined
- ● T56.5   Toxic effects of zinc and its compounds
  - ● T56.5X   Toxic effects of zinc and its compounds
    - ● T56.5X1   Toxic effect of zinc and its compounds, accidental (unintentional)
      Toxic effects of zinc and its compounds NOS
    - ● T56.5X2   Toxic effect of zinc and its compounds, intentional self-harm
    - ● T56.5X3   Toxic effect of zinc and its compounds, assault
    - ● T56.5X4   Toxic effect of zinc and its compounds, undetermined
- ● T56.6   Toxic effects of tin and its compounds
  - ● T56.6X   Toxic effects of tin and its compounds
    - ● T56.6X1   Toxic effect of tin and its compounds, accidental (unintentional)
      Toxic effects of tin and its compounds NOS
    - ● T56.6X2   Toxic effect of tin and its compounds, intentional self-harm
    - ● T56.6X3   Toxic effect of tin and its compounds, assault
    - ● T56.6X4   Toxic effect of tin and its compounds, undetermined

- ● T56.7   Toxic effects of beryllium and its compounds
  - ● T56.7X   Toxic effects of beryllium and its compounds
    - ● T56.7X1   Toxic effect of beryllium and its compounds, accidental (unintentional)
      Toxic effects of beryllium and its compounds NOS
    - ● T56.7X2   Toxic effect of beryllium and its compounds, intentional self-harm
    - ● T56.7X3   Toxic effect of beryllium and its compounds, assault
    - ● T56.7X4   Toxic effect of beryllium and its compounds, undetermined
- ● T56.8   Toxic effects of other metals
  - ● T56.81   Toxic effect of thallium
    - ● T56.811   Toxic effect of thallium, accidental (unintentional)
      Toxic effect of thallium NOS
    - ● T56.812   Toxic effect of thallium, intentional self-harm
    - ● T56.813   Toxic effect of thallium, assault
    - ● T56.814   Toxic effect of thallium, undetermined
  - ● T56.89   Toxic effects of other metals
    - ● T56.891   Toxic effect of other metals, accidental (unintentional)
      Toxic effects of other metals NOS
    - ● T56.892   Toxic effect of other metals, intentional self-harm
    - ● T56.893   Toxic effect of other metals, assault
    - ● T56.894   Toxic effect of other metals, undetermined
- ● T56.9   Toxic effects of unspecified metal
  - X ● T56.91   Toxic effect of unspecified metal, accidental (unintentional)
  - X ● T56.92   Toxic effect of unspecified metal, intentional self-harm
  - X ● T56.93   Toxic effect of unspecified metal, assault
  - X ● T56.94   Toxic effect of unspecified metal, undetermined
- ● T57   Toxic effect of other inorganic substances
  The appropriate 7th character is to be added to each code from category T57

A	initial encounter
D	subsequent encounter
S	sequela

  - ● T57.0   Toxic effect of arsenic and its compounds
    - ● T57.0X   Toxic effect of arsenic and its compounds
      - ● T57.0X1   Toxic effect of arsenic and its compounds, accidental (unintentional)
        Toxic effect of arsenic and its compounds NOS
      - ● T57.0X2   Toxic effect of arsenic and its compounds, intentional self-harm
      - ● T57.0X3   Toxic effect of arsenic and its compounds, assault
      - ● T57.0X4   Toxic effect of arsenic and its compounds, undetermined

● **T57.1**   **Toxic effect of phosphorus and its compounds**
    Excludes1   organophosphate insecticides (T60.0)
   ● **T57.1X**   Toxic effect of phosphorus and its compounds
     ● **T57.1X1**   Toxic effect of phosphorus and its compounds, accidental (unintentional)
       Toxic effect of phosphorus and its compounds NOS
     ● **T57.1X2**   Toxic effect of phosphorus and its compounds, intentional self-harm
     ● **T57.1X3**   Toxic effect of phosphorus and its compounds, assault
     ● **T57.1X4**   Toxic effect of phosphorus and its compounds, undetermined

● **T57.2**   **Toxic effect of manganese and its compounds**
   ● **T57.2X**   Toxic effect of manganese and its compounds
     ● **T57.2X1**   Toxic effect of manganese and its compounds, accidental (unintentional)
       Toxic effect of manganese and its compounds NOS
     ● **T57.2X2**   Toxic effect of manganese and its compounds, intentional self-harm
     ● **T57.2X3**   Toxic effect of manganese and its compounds, assault
     ● **T57.2X4**   Toxic effect of manganese and its compounds, undetermined

● **T57.3**   **Toxic effect of hydrogen cyanide**
   ● **T57.3X**   Toxic effect of hydrogen cyanide
     ● **T57.3X1**   Toxic effect of hydrogen cyanide, accidental (unintentional)
       Toxic effect of hydrogen cyanide NOS
     ● **T57.3X2**   Toxic effect of hydrogen cyanide, intentional self-harm
     ● **T57.3X3**   Toxic effect of hydrogen cyanide, assault
     ● **T57.3X4**   Toxic effect of hydrogen cyanide, undetermined

● **T57.8**   **Toxic effect of other specified inorganic substances**
   ● **T57.8X**   Toxic effect of other specified inorganic substances
     ● **T57.8X1**   Toxic effect of other specified inorganic substances, accidental (unintentional)
       Toxic effect of other specified inorganic substances NOS
     ● **T57.8X2**   Toxic effect of other specified inorganic substances, intentional self-harm
     ● **T57.8X3**   Toxic effect of other specified inorganic substances, assault
     ● **T57.8X4**   Toxic effect of other specified inorganic substances, undetermined

● **T57.9**   **Toxic effect of unspecified inorganic substance**
   X ● **T57.91**   Toxic effect of unspecified inorganic substance, accidental (unintentional)
   X ● **T57.92**   Toxic effect of unspecified inorganic substance, intentional self-harm
   X ● **T57.93**   Toxic effect of unspecified inorganic substance, assault
   X ● **T57.94**   Toxic effect of unspecified inorganic substance, undetermined

● **T58**   **Toxic effect of carbon monoxide**
    Includes   asphyxiation from carbon monoxide
       toxic effect of carbon monoxide from all sources
   The appropriate 7th character is to be added to each code from category T58

    A   initial encounter
    D   subsequent encounter
    S   sequela

● **T58.0**   **Toxic effect of carbon monoxide from motor vehicle exhaust**
     Toxic effect of exhaust gas from gas engine
     Toxic effect of exhaust gas from motor pump
   X ● **T58.01**   Toxic effect of carbon monoxide from motor vehicle exhaust, accidental (unintentional)
   X ● **T58.02**   Toxic effect of carbon monoxide from motor vehicle exhaust, intentional self-harm
   X ● **T58.03**   Toxic effect of carbon monoxide from motor vehicle exhaust, assault
   X ● **T58.04**   Toxic effect of carbon monoxide from motor vehicle exhaust, undetermined

● **T58.1**   **Toxic effect of carbon monoxide from utility gas**
     Toxic effect of acetylene
     Toxic effect of gas NOS used for lighting, heating, cooking
     Toxic effect of water gas
   X ● **T58.11**   Toxic effect of carbon monoxide from utility gas, accidental (unintentional)
   X ● **T58.12**   Toxic effect of carbon monoxide from utility gas, intentional self-harm
   X ● **T58.13**   Toxic effect of carbon monoxide from utility gas, assault
   X ● **T58.14**   Toxic effect of carbon monoxide from utility gas, undetermined

● **T58.2**   **Toxic effect of carbon monoxide from incomplete combustion of other domestic fuels**
     Toxic effect of carbon monoxide from incomplete combustion of coal, coke, kerosene, wood
   ● **T58.2X**   Toxic effect of carbon monoxide from incomplete combustion of other domestic fuels
     ● **T58.2X1**   Toxic effect of carbon monoxide from incomplete combustion of other domestic fuels, accidental (unintentional)
     ● **T58.2X2**   Toxic effect of carbon monoxide from incomplete combustion of other domestic fuels, intentional self-harm
     ● **T58.2X3**   Toxic effect of carbon monoxide from incomplete combustion of other domestic fuels, assault
     ● **T58.2X4**   Toxic effect of carbon monoxide from incomplete combustion of other domestic fuels, undetermined

● **T58.8**   **Toxic effect of carbon monoxide from other source**
     Toxic effect of carbon monoxide from blast furnace gas
     Toxic effect of carbon monoxide from fuels in industrial use
     Toxic effect of carbon monoxide from kiln vapor
   ● **T58.8X**   Toxic effect of carbon monoxide from other source
     ● **T58.8X1**   Toxic effect of carbon monoxide from other source, accidental (unintentional)
     ● **T58.8X2**   Toxic effect of carbon monoxide from other source, intentional self-harm
     ● **T58.8X3**   Toxic effect of carbon monoxide from other source, assault
     ● **T58.8X4**   Toxic effect of carbon monoxide from other source, undetermined

CHAPTER 19 (S00-T88)

● **T58.9**   **Toxic effect of carbon monoxide from unspecified source**
   X ● **T58.91**   Toxic effect of carbon monoxide from unspecified source, accidental (unintentional)
   X ● **T58.92**   Toxic effect of carbon monoxide from unspecified source, intentional self-harm
   X ● **T58.93**   Toxic effect of carbon monoxide from unspecified source, assault
   X ● **T58.94**   Toxic effect of carbon monoxide from unspecified source, undetermined

● **T59**   **Toxic effect of other gases, fumes and vapors**

> **Includes**   aerosol propellants
> **Excludes1**   chlorofluorocarbons (T53.5)

> The appropriate 7th character is to be added to each code from category T59

> | A | initial encounter |
> |---|---|
> | D | subsequent encounter |
> | S | sequela |

● **T59.0**   **Toxic effect of nitrogen oxides**
   ● **T59.0X**   Toxic effect of nitrogen oxides
     ● **T59.0X1**   Toxic effect of nitrogen oxides, accidental (unintentional)
        Toxic effect of nitrogen oxides NOS
     ● **T59.0X2**   Toxic effect of nitrogen oxides, intentional self-harm
     ● **T59.0X3**   Toxic effect of nitrogen oxides, assault
     ● **T59.0X4**   Toxic effect of nitrogen oxides, undetermined

● **T59.1**   **Toxic effect of sulfur dioxide**
   ● **T59.1X**   Toxic effect of sulfur dioxide
     ● **T59.1X1**   Toxic effect of sulfur dioxide, accidental (unintentional)
        Toxic effect of sulfur dioxide NOS
     ● **T59.1X2**   Toxic effect of sulfur dioxide, intentional self-harm
     ● **T59.1X3**   Toxic effect of sulfur dioxide, assault
     ● **T59.1X4**   Toxic effect of sulfur dioxide, undetermined

● **T59.2**   **Toxic effect of formaldehyde**
   ● **T59.2X**   Toxic effect of formaldehyde
     ● **T59.2X1**   Toxic effect of formaldehyde, accidental (unintentional)
        Toxic effect of formaldehyde NOS
     ● **T59.2X2**   Toxic effect of formaldehyde, intentional self-harm
     ● **T59.2X3**   Toxic effect of formaldehyde, assault
     ● **T59.2X4**   Toxic effect of formaldehyde, undetermined

● **T59.3**   **Toxic effect of lacrimogenic gas**
     Toxic effect of tear gas
   ● **T59.3X**   Toxic effect of lacrimogenic gas
     ● **T59.3X1**   Toxic effect of lacrimogenic gas, accidental (unintentional)
        Toxic effect of lacrimogenic gas NOS
     ● **T59.3X2**   Toxic effect of lacrimogenic gas, intentional self-harm
     ● **T59.3X3**   Toxic effect of lacrimogenic gas, assault
     ● **T59.3X4**   Toxic effect of lacrimogenic gas, undetermined

● **T59.4**   **Toxic effect of chlorine gas**
   ● **T59.4X**   Toxic effect of chlorine gas
     ● **T59.4X1**   Toxic effect of chlorine gas, accidental (unintentional)
        Toxic effect of chlorine gas NOS
     ● **T59.4X2**   Toxic effect of chlorine gas, intentional self-harm
     ● **T59.4X3**   Toxic effect of chlorine gas, assault
     ● **T59.4X4**   Toxic effect of chlorine gas, undetermined

● **T59.5**   **Toxic effect of fluorine gas and hydrogen fluoride**
   ● **T59.5X**   Toxic effect of fluorine gas and hydrogen fluoride
     ● **T59.5X1**   Toxic effect of fluorine gas and hydrogen fluoride, accidental (unintentional)
        Toxic effect of fluorine gas and hydrogen fluoride NOS
     ● **T59.5X2**   Toxic effect of fluorine gas and hydrogen fluoride, intentional self-harm
     ● **T59.5X3**   Toxic effect of fluorine gas and hydrogen fluoride, assault
     ● **T59.5X4**   Toxic effect of fluorine gas and hydrogen fluoride, undetermined

● **T59.6**   **Toxic effect of hydrogen sulfide**
   ● **T59.6X**   Toxic effect of hydrogen sulfide
     ● **T59.6X1**   Toxic effect of hydrogen sulfide, accidental (unintentional)
        Toxic effect of hydrogen sulfide NOS
     ● **T59.6X2**   Toxic effect of hydrogen sulfide, intentional self-harm
     ● **T59.6X3**   Toxic effect of hydrogen sulfide, assault
     ● **T59.6X4**   Toxic effect of hydrogen sulfide, undetermined

● **T59.7**   **Toxic effect of carbon dioxide**
   ● **T59.7X**   Toxic effect of carbon dioxide
     ● **T59.7X1**   Toxic effect of carbon dioxide, accidental (unintentional)
        Toxic effect of carbon dioxide NOS
     ● **T59.7X2**   Toxic effect of carbon dioxide, intentional self-harm
     ● **T59.7X3**   Toxic effect of carbon dioxide, assault
     ● **T59.7X4**   Toxic effect of carbon dioxide, undetermined

● **T59.8**   **Toxic effect of other specified gases, fumes and vapors**
   ● **T59.81**   Toxic effect of smoke
     Smoke inhalation

> **Excludes2**   toxic effect of cigarette (tobacco) smoke (T65.22-)

     ● **T59.811**   Toxic effect of smoke, accidental (unintentional)
        Toxic effect of smoke NOS
     ● **T59.812**   Toxic effect of smoke, intentional self-harm
     ● **T59.813**   Toxic effect of smoke, assault
     ● **T59.814**   Toxic effect of smoke, undetermined
   ● **T59.89**   Toxic effect of other specified gases, fumes and vapors
     ● **T59.891**   Toxic effect of other specified gases, fumes and vapors, accidental (unintentional)
     ● **T59.892**   Toxic effect of other specified gases, fumes and vapors, intentional self-harm
     ● **T59.893**   Toxic effect of other specified gases, fumes and vapors, assault
     ● **T59.894**   Toxic effect of other specified gases, fumes and vapors, undetermined

◀ New   ◀◀ Revised   ~~deleted~~ Deleted   OGCR Official Guidelines   X Assign placeholder X   ● Use Additional Character(s)

Excludes 1   Excludes 2   Includes   Use additional   Code first   Code also   Unspecified

● **T59.9**   Toxic effect of unspecified gases, fumes and vapors
    X ● **T59.91**   Toxic effect of unspecified gases, fumes and vapors, accidental (unintentional)
    X ● **T59.92**   Toxic effect of unspecified gases, fumes and vapors, intentional self-harm
    X ● **T59.93**   Toxic effect of unspecified gases, fumes and vapors, assault
    X ● **T59.94**   Toxic effect of unspecified gases, fumes and vapors, undetermined

● **T60**   Toxic effect of pesticides

> **Includes**   toxic effect of wood preservatives

> The appropriate 7th character is to be added to each code from category T60

> | | |
> |---|---|
> | A | initial encounter |
> | D | subsequent encounter |
> | S | sequela |

● **T60.0**   Toxic effect of organophosphate and carbamate insecticides
   ● **T60.0X**   Toxic effect of organophosphate and carbamate insecticides
     ● **T60.0X1**   Toxic effect of organophosphate and carbamate insecticides, accidental (unintentional)
       Toxic effect of organophosphate and carbamate insecticides NOS
     ● **T60.0X2**   Toxic effect of organophosphate and carbamate insecticides, intentional self-harm
     ● **T60.0X3**   Toxic effect of organophosphate and carbamate insecticides, assault
     ● **T60.0X4**   Toxic effect of organophosphate and carbamate insecticides, undetermined

● **T60.1**   Toxic effect of halogenated insecticides

> **Excludes1**   chlorinated hydrocarbon (T53.-)

   ● **T60.1X**   Toxic effect of halogenated insecticides
     ● **T60.1X1**   Toxic effect of halogenated insecticides, accidental (unintentional)
       Toxic effect of halogenated insecticides NOS
     ● **T60.1X2**   Toxic effect of halogenated insecticides, intentional self-harm
     ● **T60.1X3**   Toxic effect of halogenated insecticides, assault
     ● **T60.1X4**   Toxic effect of halogenated insecticides, undetermined

● **T60.2**   Toxic effect of other insecticides
   ● **T60.2X**   Toxic effect of other insecticides
     ● **T60.2X1**   Toxic effect of other insecticides, accidental (unintentional)
       Toxic effect of other insecticides NOS
     ● **T60.2X2**   Toxic effect of other insecticides, intentional self-harm
     ● **T60.2X3**   Toxic effect of other insecticides, assault
     ● **T60.2X4**   Toxic effect of other insecticides, undetermined

● **T60.3**   Toxic effect of herbicides and fungicides
   ● **T60.3X**   Toxic effect of herbicides and fungicides
     ● **T60.3X1**   Toxic effect of herbicides and fungicides, accidental (unintentional)
       Toxic effect of herbicides and fungicides NOS
     ● **T60.3X2**   Toxic effect of herbicides and fungicides, intentional self-harm
     ● **T60.3X3**   Toxic effect of herbicides and fungicides, assault
     ● **T60.3X4**   Toxic effect of herbicides and fungicides, undetermined

● **T60.4**   Toxic effect of rodenticides

> **Excludes1**   strychnine and its salts (T65.1)
> thallium (T56.81-)

   ● **T60.4X**   Toxic effect of rodenticides
     ● **T60.4X1**   Toxic effect of rodenticides, accidental (unintentional)
       Toxic effect of rodenticides NOS
     ● **T60.4X2**   Toxic effect of rodenticides, intentional self-harm
     ● **T60.4X3**   Toxic effect of rodenticides, assault
     ● **T60.4X4**   Toxic effect of rodenticides, undetermined

● **T60.8**   Toxic effect of other pesticides
   ● **T60.8X**   Toxic effect of other pesticides
     ● **T60.8X1**   Toxic effect of other pesticides, accidental (unintentional)
       Toxic effect of other pesticides NOS
     ● **T60.8X2**   Toxic effect of other pesticides, intentional self-harm
     ● **T60.8X3**   Toxic effect of other pesticides, assault
     ● **T60.8X4**   Toxic effect of other pesticides, undetermined

● **T60.9**   Toxic effect of unspecified pesticide
    X ● **T60.91**   Toxic effect of unspecified pesticide, accidental (unintentional)
    X ● **T60.92**   Toxic effect of unspecified pesticide, intentional self-harm
    X ● **T60.93**   Toxic effect of unspecified pesticide, assault
    X ● **T60.94**   Toxic effect of unspecified pesticide, undetermined

● **T61**   Toxic effect of noxious substances eaten as seafood

> **Excludes1**   allergic reaction to food, such as:
> anaphylactic reaction or shock due to adverse food reaction (T78.0-)
> bacterial foodborne intoxications (A05.-)
> dermatitis (L23.6, L25.4, L27.2)
> gastroenteritis (noninfective) (K52.2)
> toxic effect of aflatoxin and other mycotoxins (T64)
> toxic effect of cyanides (T65.0-)
> toxic effect of harmful algae bloom (T65.82-)
> toxic effect of hydrogen cyanide (T57.3-)
> toxic effect of mercury (T56.1-)
> toxic effect of red tide (T65.82-)

> The appropriate 7th character is to be added to each code from category T61

> | | |
> |---|---|
> | A | initial encounter |
> | D | subsequent encounter |
> | S | sequela |

● **T61.0**   Ciguatera fish poisoning
    X ● **T61.01**   Ciguatera fish poisoning, accidental (unintentional)
    X ● **T61.02**   Ciguatera fish poisoning, intentional self-harm
    X ● **T61.03**   Ciguatera fish poisoning, assault
    X ● **T61.04**   Ciguatera fish poisoning, undetermined

● **T61.1**   Scombroid fish poisoning
    Histamine-like syndrome
    X ● **T61.11**   Scombroid fish poisoning, accidental (unintentional)
    X ● **T61.12**   Scombroid fish poisoning, intentional self-harm
    X ● **T61.13**   Scombroid fish poisoning, assault
    X ● **T61.14**   Scombroid fish poisoning, undetermined

CHAPTER 19 (S00-T88)

◀ New   ⇐ Revised   ~~deleted~~ Deleted   **OGCR** Official Guidelines   X Assign placeholder X   ● Use Additional Character(s)

Excludes 1	Excludes 2	Includes	Use additional	Code first	Code also	Unspecified

CHAPTER 19 (S00-T88)

● T61.7 Other fish and shellfish poisoning
  ● T61.77 Other fish poisoning
    ● T61.771 Other fish poisoning, accidental (unintentional)
    ● T61.772 Other fish poisoning, intentional self-harm
    ● T61.773 Other fish poisoning, assault
    ● T61.774 Other fish poisoning, undetermined
  ● T61.78 Other shellfish poisoning
    ● T61.781 Other shellfish poisoning, accidental (unintentional)
    ● T61.782 Other shellfish poisoning, intentional self-harm
    ● T61.783 Other shellfish poisoning, assault
    ● T61.784 Other shellfish poisoning, undetermined
● T61.8 Toxic effect of other seafood
  ● T61.8X Toxic effect of other seafood
    ● T61.8X1 Toxic effect of other seafood, accidental (unintentional)
    ● T61.8X2 Toxic effect of other seafood, intentional self-harm
    ● T61.8X3 Toxic effect of other seafood, assault
    ● T61.8X4 Toxic effect of other seafood, undetermined
● T61.9 Toxic effect of unspecified seafood
  X ● T61.91 Toxic effect of unspecified seafood, accidental (unintentional)
  X ● T61.92 Toxic effect of unspecified seafood, intentional self-harm
  X ● T61.93 Toxic effect of unspecified seafood, assault
  X ● T61.94 Toxic effect of unspecified seafood, undetermined

● T62 Toxic effect of other noxious substances eaten as food

  Excludes1 allergic reaction to food, such as:
  anaphylactic shock (reaction) due to adverse food reaction (T78.0-)
  dermatitis (L23.6, L25.4, L27.2)
  gastroenteritis (noninfective) (K52.2)
  bacterial food borne intoxications (A05.-)
  toxic effect of aflatoxin and other mycotoxins (T64)
  toxic effect of cyanides (T65.0-)
  toxic effect of hydrogen cyanide (T57.3-)
  toxic effect of mercury (T56.1-)

  The appropriate 7th character is to be added to each code from category T62

A	initial encounter
D	subsequent encounter
S	sequela

● T62.0 Toxic effect of ingested mushrooms
  ● T62.0X Toxic effect of ingested mushrooms
    ● T62.0X1 Toxic effect of ingested mushrooms, accidental (unintentional)
      Toxic effect of ingested mushrooms NOS
    ● T62.0X2 Toxic effect of ingested mushrooms, intentional self-harm
    ● T62.0X3 Toxic effect of ingested mushrooms, assault
    ● T62.0X4 Toxic effect of ingested mushrooms, undetermined

● T62.1 Toxic effect of ingested berries
  ● T62.1X Toxic effect of ingested berries
    ● T62.1X1 Toxic effect of ingested berries, accidental (unintentional)
      Toxic effect of ingested berries NOS
    ● T62.1X2 Toxic effect of ingested berries, intentional self-harm
    ● T62.1X3 Toxic effect of ingested berries, assault
    ● T62.1X4 Toxic effect of ingested berries, undetermined
● T62.2 Toxic effect of other ingested (parts of) plant(s)
  ● T62.2X Toxic effect of other ingested (parts of) plant(s)
    ● T62.2X1 Toxic effect of other ingested (parts of) plant(s), accidental (unintentional)
      Toxic effect of other ingested (parts of) plant(s) NOS
    ● T62.2X2 Toxic effect of other ingested (parts of) plant(s), intentional self-harm
    ● T62.2X3 Toxic effect of other ingested (parts of) plant(s), assault
    ● T62.2X4 Toxic effect of other ingested (parts of) plant(s), undetermined
● T62.8 Toxic effect of other specified noxious substances eaten as food
  ● T62.8X Toxic effect of other specified noxious substances eaten as food
    ● T62.8X1 Toxic effect of other specified noxious substances eaten as food, accidental (unintentional)
      Toxic effect of other specified noxious substances eaten as food NOS
    ● T62.8X2 Toxic effect of other specified noxious substances eaten as food, intentional self-harm
    ● T62.8X3 Toxic effect of other specified noxious substances eaten as food, assault
    ● T62.8X4 Toxic effect of other specified noxious substances eaten as food, undetermined
● T62.9 Toxic effect of unspecified noxious substance eaten as food
  X ● T62.91 Toxic effect of unspecified noxious substance eaten as food, accidental (unintentional)
    Toxic effect of unspecified noxious substance eaten as food NOS
  X ● T62.92 Toxic effect of unspecified noxious substance eaten as food, intentional self-harm
  X ● T62.93 Toxic effect of unspecified noxious substance eaten as food, assault
  X ● T62.94 Toxic effect of unspecified noxious substance eaten as food, undetermined

● T63 Toxic effect of contact with venomous animals and plants

  Includes bite or touch of venomous animal
  pricked or stuck by thorn or leaf

  Excludes2 ingestion of toxic animal or plant (T61.-, T62.-)

  The appropriate 7th character is to be added to each code from category T63

A	initial encounter
D	subsequent encounter
S	sequela

● T63.0 Toxic effect of snake venom
  ● T63.00 Toxic effect of unspecified snake venom
    ● T63.001 Toxic effect of unspecified snake venom, accidental (unintentional)
      Toxic effect of unspecified snake venom NOS
    ● T63.002 Toxic effect of unspecified snake venom, intentional self-harm
    ● T63.003 Toxic effect of unspecified snake venom, assault
    ● T63.004 Toxic effect of unspecified snake venom, undetermined

● **T63.01**   Toxic effect of rattlesnake venom
   ● **T63.011**   Toxic effect of rattlesnake venom, accidental (unintentional)
          Toxic effect of rattlesnake venom NOS
   ● **T63.012**   Toxic effect of rattlesnake venom, intentional self-harm
   ● **T63.013**   Toxic effect of rattlesnake venom, assault
   ● **T63.014**   Toxic effect of rattlesnake venom, undetermined

● **T63.02**   Toxic effect of coral snake venom
   ● **T63.021**   Toxic effect of coral snake venom, accidental (unintentional)
          Toxic effect of coral snake venom NOS
   ● **T63.022**   Toxic effect of coral snake venom, intentional self-harm
   ● **T63.023**   Toxic effect of coral snake venom, assault
   ● **T63.024**   Toxic effect of coral snake venom, undetermined

● **T63.03**   Toxic effect of taipan venom
   ● **T63.031**   Toxic effect of taipan venom, accidental (unintentional)
          Toxic effect of taipan venom NOS
   ● **T63.032**   Toxic effect of taipan venom, intentional self-harm
   ● **T63.033**   Toxic effect of taipan venom, assault
   ● **T63.034**   Toxic effect of taipan venom, undetermined

● **T63.04**   Toxic effect of cobra venom
   ● **T63.041**   Toxic effect of cobra venom, accidental (unintentional)
          Toxic effect of cobra venom NOS
   ● **T63.042**   Toxic effect of cobra venom, intentional self-harm
   ● **T63.043**   Toxic effect of cobra venom, assault
   ● **T63.044**   Toxic effect of cobra venom, undetermined

● **T63.06**   Toxic effect of venom of other North and South American snake
   ● **T63.061**   Toxic effect of venom of other North and South American snake, accidental (unintentional)
          Toxic effect of venom of other North and South American snake NOS
   ● **T63.062**   Toxic effect of venom of other North and South American snake, intentional self-harm
   ● **T63.063**   Toxic effect of venom of other North and South American snake, assault
   ● **T63.064**   Toxic effect of venom of other North and South American snake, undetermined

● **T63.07**   Toxic effect of venom of other Australian snake
   ● **T63.071**   Toxic effect of venom of other Australian snake, accidental (unintentional)
          Toxic effect of venom of other Australian snake NOS
   ● **T63.072**   Toxic effect of venom of other Australian snake, intentional self-harm
   ● **T63.073**   Toxic effect of venom of other Australian snake, assault
   ● **T63.074**   Toxic effect of venom of other Australian snake, undetermined

● **T63.08**   Toxic effect of venom of other African and Asian snake
   ● **T63.081**   Toxic effect of venom of other African and Asian snake, accidental (unintentional)
          Toxic effect of venom of other African and Asian snake NOS
   ● **T63.082**   Toxic effect of venom of other African and Asian snake, intentional self-harm
   ● **T63.083**   Toxic effect of venom of other African and Asian snake, assault
   ● **T63.084**   Toxic effect of venom of other African and Asian snake, undetermined

● **T63.09**   Toxic effect of venom of other snake
   ● **T63.091**   Toxic effect of venom of other snake, accidental (unintentional)
          Toxic effect of venom of other snake NOS
   ● **T63.092**   Toxic effect of venom of other snake, intentional self-harm
   ● **T63.093**   Toxic effect of venom of other snake, assault
   ● **T63.094**   Toxic effect of venom of other snake, undetermined

● **T63.1**   Toxic effect of venom of other reptiles
   ● **T63.11**   Toxic effect of venom of gila monster
      ● **T63.111**   Toxic effect of venom of gila monster, accidental (unintentional)
            Toxic effect of venom of gila monster NOS
      ● **T63.112**   Toxic effect of venom of gila monster, intentional self-harm
      ● **T63.113**   Toxic effect of venom of gila monster, assault
      ● **T63.114**   Toxic effect of venom of gila monster, undetermined

   ● **T63.12**   Toxic effect of venom of other venomous lizard
      ● **T63.121**   Toxic effect of venom of other venomous lizard, accidental (unintentional)
            Toxic effect of venom of other venomous lizard NOS
      ● **T63.122**   Toxic effect of venom of other venomous lizard, intentional self-harm
      ● **T63.123**   Toxic effect of venom of other venomous lizard, assault
      ● **T63.124**   Toxic effect of venom of other venomous lizard, undetermined

   ● **T63.19**   Toxic effect of venom of other reptiles
      ● **T63.191**   Toxic effect of venom of other reptiles, accidental (unintentional)
            Toxic effect of venom of other reptiles NOS
      ● **T63.192**   Toxic effect of venom of other reptiles, intentional self-harm
      ● **T63.193**   Toxic effect of venom of other reptiles, assault
      ● **T63.194**   Toxic effect of venom of other reptiles, undetermined

● **T63.2**   Toxic effect of venom of scorpion
   ● **T63.2X**   Toxic effect of venom of scorpion
      ● **T63.2X1**   Toxic effect of venom of scorpion, accidental (unintentional)
            Toxic effect of venom of scorpion NOS
      ● **T63.2X2**   Toxic effect of venom of scorpion, intentional self-harm
      ● **T63.2X3**   Toxic effect of venom of scorpion, assault
      ● **T63.2X4**   Toxic effect of venom of scorpion, undetermined

CHAPTER 19 (S00-T88)

CHAPTER 19 (S00-T88)

● T63.3   Toxic effect of venom of spider
   ● T63.30   Toxic effect of unspecified spider venom
      ● T63.301   Toxic effect of unspecified spider venom, accidental (unintentional)
      ● T63.302   Toxic effect of unspecified spider venom, intentional self-harm
      ● T63.303   Toxic effect of unspecified spider venom, assault
      ● T63.304   Toxic effect of unspecified spider venom, undetermined
   ● T63.31   Toxic effect of venom of black widow spider
      ● T63.311   Toxic effect of venom of black widow spider, accidental (unintentional)
      ● T63.312   Toxic effect of venom of black widow spider, intentional self-harm
      ● T63.313   Toxic effect of venom of black widow spider, assault
      ● T63.314   Toxic effect of venom of black widow spider, undetermined
   ● T63.32   Toxic effect of venom of tarantula
      ● T63.321   Toxic effect of venom of tarantula, accidental (unintentional)
      ● T63.322   Toxic effect of venom of tarantula, intentional self-harm
      ● T63.323   Toxic effect of venom of tarantula, assault
      ● T63.324   Toxic effect of venom of tarantula, undetermined
   ● T63.33   Toxic effect of venom of brown recluse spider
      ● T63.331   Toxic effect of venom of brown recluse spider, accidental (unintentional)
      ● T63.332   Toxic effect of venom of brown recluse spider, intentional self-harm
      ● T63.333   Toxic effect of venom of brown recluse spider, assault
      ● T63.334   Toxic effect of venom of brown recluse spider, undetermined
   ● T63.39   Toxic effect of venom of other spider
      ● T63.391   Toxic effect of venom of other spider, accidental (unintentional)
      ● T63.392   Toxic effect of venom of other spider, intentional self-harm
      ● T63.393   Toxic effect of venom of other spider, assault
      ● T63.394   Toxic effect of venom of other spider, undetermined
● T63.4   Toxic effect of venom of other arthropods
   ● T63.41   Toxic effect of venom of centipedes and venomous millipedes
      ● T63.411   Toxic effect of venom of centipedes and venomous millipedes, accidental (unintentional)
      ● T63.412   Toxic effect of venom of centipedes and venomous millipedes, intentional self-harm
      ● T63.413   Toxic effect of venom of centipedes and venomous millipedes, assault
      ● T63.414   Toxic effect of venom of centipedes and venomous millipedes, undetermined
   ● T63.42   Toxic effect of venom of ants
      ● T63.421   Toxic effect of venom of ants, accidental (unintentional)
      ● T63.422   Toxic effect of venom of ants, intentional self-harm
      ● T63.423   Toxic effect of venom of ants, assault
      ● T63.424   Toxic effect of venom of ants, undetermined

   ● T63.43   Toxic effect of venom of caterpillars
      ● T63.431   Toxic effect of venom of caterpillars, accidental (unintentional)
      ● T63.432   Toxic effect of venom of caterpillars, intentional self-harm
      ● T63.433   Toxic effect of venom of caterpillars, assault
      ● T63.434   Toxic effect of venom of caterpillars, undetermined
   ● T63.44   Toxic effect of venom of bees
      ● T63.441   Toxic effect of venom of bees, accidental (unintentional)
      ● T63.442   Toxic effect of venom of bees, intentional self-harm
      ● T63.443   Toxic effect of venom of bees, assault
      ● T63.444   Toxic effect of venom of bees, undetermined
   ● T63.45   Toxic effect of venom of hornets
      ● T63.451   Toxic effect of venom of hornets, accidental (unintentional)
      ● T63.452   Toxic effect of venom of hornets, intentional self-harm
      ● T63.453   Toxic effect of venom of hornets, assault
      ● T63.454   Toxic effect of venom of hornets, undetermined
   ● T63.46   Toxic effect of venom of wasps
                Toxic effect of yellow jacket
      ● T63.461   Toxic effect of venom of wasps, accidental (unintentional)
      ● T63.462   Toxic effect of venom of wasps, intentional self-harm
      ● T63.463   Toxic effect of venom of wasps, assault
      ● T63.464   Toxic effect of venom of wasps, undetermined
   ● T63.48   Toxic effect of venom of other arthropod
      ● T63.481   Toxic effect of venom of other arthropod, accidental (unintentional)
      ● T63.482   Toxic effect of venom of other arthropod, intentional self-harm
      ● T63.483   Toxic effect of venom of other arthropod, assault
      ● T63.484   Toxic effect of venom of other arthropod, undetermined
● T63.5   Toxic effect of contact with venomous fish
   Excludes2   poisoning by ingestion of fish (T61.-)
   ● T63.51   Toxic effect of contact with stingray
      ● T63.511   Toxic effect of contact with stingray, accidental (unintentional)
      ● T63.512   Toxic effect of contact with stingray, intentional self-harm
      ● T63.513   Toxic effect of contact with stingray, assault
      ● T63.514   Toxic effect of contact with stingray, undetermined
   ● T63.59   Toxic effect of contact with other venomous fish
      ● T63.591   Toxic effect of contact with other venomous fish, accidental (unintentional)
      ● T63.592   Toxic effect of contact with other venomous fish, intentional self-harm
      ● T63.593   Toxic effect of contact with other venomous fish, assault
      ● T63.594   Toxic effect of contact with other venomous fish, undetermined

● **T63.6**   **Toxic effect of contact with other venomous marine animals**
> **Excludes1**   sea-snake venom (T63.09)
> **Excludes2**   poisoning by ingestion of shellfish (T61.78-)

● **T63.61**   **Toxic effect of contact with Portugese Man-o-war**
> Toxic effect of contact with bluebottle

   ● **T63.611**   Toxic effect of contact with Portugese Man-o-war, accidental (unintentional)

   ● **T63.612**   Toxic effect of contact with Portugese Man-o-war, intentional self-harm

   ● **T63.613**   Toxic effect of contact with Portugese Man-o-war, assault

   ● **T63.614**   Toxic effect of contact with Portugese Man-o-war, undetermined

● **T63.62**   **Toxic effect of contact with other jellyfish**

   ● **T63.621**   Toxic effect of contact with other jellyfish, accidental (unintentional)

   ● **T63.622**   Toxic effect of contact with other jellyfish, intentional self-harm

   ● **T63.623**   Toxic effect of contact with other jellyfish, assault

   ● **T63.624**   Toxic effect of contact with other jellyfish, undetermined

● **T63.63**   **Toxic effect of contact with sea anemone**

   ● **T63.631**   Toxic effect of contact with sea anemone, accidental (unintentional)

   ● **T63.632**   Toxic effect of contact with sea anemone, intentional self-harm

   ● **T63.633**   Toxic effect of contact with sea anemone, assault

   ● **T63.634**   Toxic effect of contact with sea anemone, undetermined

● **T63.69**   **Toxic effect of contact with other venomous marine animals**

   ● **T63.691**   Toxic effect of contact with other venomous marine animals, accidental (unintentional)

   ● **T63.692**   Toxic effect of contact with other venomous marine animals, intentional self-harm

   ● **T63.693**   Toxic effect of contact with other venomous marine animals, assault

   ● **T63.694**   Toxic effect of contact with other venomous marine animals, undetermined

● **T63.7**   **Toxic effect of contact with venomous plant**

● **T63.71**   **Toxic effect of contact with venomous marine plant**

   ● **T63.711**   Toxic effect of contact with venomous marine plant, accidental (unintentional)

   ● **T63.712**   Toxic effect of contact with venomous marine plant, intentional self-harm

   ● **T63.713**   Toxic effect of contact with venomous marine plant, assault

   ● **T63.714**   Toxic effect of contact with venomous marine plant, undetermined

● **T63.79**   **Toxic effect of contact with other venomous plant**

   ● **T63.791**   Toxic effect of contact with other venomous plant, accidental (unintentional)

   ● **T63.792**   Toxic effect of contact with other venomous plant, intentional self-harm

   ● **T63.793**   Toxic effect of contact with other venomous plant, assault

   ● **T63.794**   Toxic effect of contact with other venomous plant, undetermined

● **T63.8**   **Toxic effect of contact with other venomous animals**

● **T63.81**   **Toxic effect of contact with venomous frog**
> **Excludes1**   contact with nonvenomous frog (W62.0)

   ● **T63.811**   Toxic effect of contact with venomous frog, accidental (unintentional)

   ● **T63.812**   Toxic effect of contact with venomous frog, intentional self-harm

   ● **T63.813**   Toxic effect of contact with venomous frog, assault

   ● **T63.814**   Toxic effect of contact with venomous frog, undetermined

● **T63.82**   **Toxic effect of contact with venomous toad**
> **Excludes1**   contact with nonvenomous toad (W62.1)

   ● **T63.821**   Toxic effect of contact with venomous toad, accidental (unintentional)

   ● **T63.822**   Toxic effect of contact with venomous toad, intentional self-harm

   ● **T63.823**   Toxic effect of contact with venomous toad, assault

   ● **T63.824**   Toxic effect of contact with venomous toad, undetermined

● **T63.83**   **Toxic effect of contact with other venomous amphibian**
> **Excludes1**   contact with nonvenomous amphibian (W62.9)

   ● **T63.831**   Toxic effect of contact with other venomous amphibian, accidental (unintentional)

   ● **T63.832**   Toxic effect of contact with other venomous amphibian, intentional self-harm

   ● **T63.833**   Toxic effect of contact with other venomous amphibian, assault

   ● **T63.834**   Toxic effect of contact with other venomous amphibian, undetermined

● **T63.89**   **Toxic effect of contact with other venomous animals**

   ● **T63.891**   Toxic effect of contact with other venomous animals, accidental (unintentional)

   ● **T63.892**   Toxic effect of contact with other venomous animals, intentional self-harm

   ● **T63.893**   Toxic effect of contact with other venomous animals, assault

   ● **T63.894**   Toxic effect of contact with other venomous animals, undetermined

● **T63.9**   **Toxic effect of contact with unspecified venomous animal**

   X ● **T63.91**   Toxic effect of contact with unspecified venomous animal, accidental (unintentional)

   X ● **T63.92**   Toxic effect of contact with unspecified venomous animal, intentional self-harm

   X ● **T63.93**   Toxic effect of contact with unspecified venomous animal, assault

   X ● **T63.94**   Toxic effect of contact with unspecified venomous animal, undetermined

CHAPTER 19 (S00-T88)

CHAPTER 19 (S00-T88)

● **T64**   **Toxic effect of aflatoxin and other mycotoxin food contaminants**

The appropriate 7th character is to be added to each code from category T64

> A   initial encounter
> D   subsequent encounter
> S   sequela

● **T64.0**   **Toxic effect of aflatoxin**

X● **T64.01**   **Toxic effect of aflatoxin, accidental (unintentional)**

X● **T64.02**   **Toxic effect of aflatoxin, intentional self-harm**

X● **T64.03**   **Toxic effect of aflatoxin, assault**

X● **T64.04**   **Toxic effect of aflatoxin, undetermined**

● **T64.8**   **Toxic effect of other mycotoxin food contaminants**

X● **T64.81**   **Toxic effect of other mycotoxin food contaminants, accidental (unintentional)**

X● **T64.82**   **Toxic effect of other mycotoxin food contaminants, intentional self-harm**

X● **T64.83**   **Toxic effect of other mycotoxin food contaminants, assault**

X● **T64.84**   **Toxic effect of other mycotoxin food contaminants, undetermined**

● **T65**   **Toxic effect of other and unspecified substances**

The appropriate 7th character is to be added to each code from category T65

> A   initial encounter
> D   subsequent encounter
> S   sequela

● **T65.0**   **Toxic effect of cyanides**

> **Excludes1**   hydrogen cyanide (T57.3-)

● **T65.0X**   **Toxic effect of cyanides**

● **T65.0X1**   **Toxic effect of cyanides, accidental (unintentional)**
Toxic effect of cyanides NOS

● **T65.0X2**   **Toxic effect of cyanides, intentional self-harm**

● **T65.0X3**   **Toxic effect of cyanides, assault**

● **T65.0X4**   **Toxic effect of cyanides, undetermined**

● **T65.1**   **Toxic effect of strychnine and its salts**

● **T65.1X**   **Toxic effect of strychnine and its salts**

● **T65.1X1**   **Toxic effect of strychnine and its salts, accidental (unintentional)**
Toxic effect of strychnine and its salts NOS

● **T65.1X2**   **Toxic effect of strychnine and its salts, intentional self-harm**

● **T65.1X3**   **Toxic effect of strychnine and its salts, assault**

● **T65.1X4**   **Toxic effect of strychnine and its salts, undetermined**

● **T65.2**   **Toxic effect of tobacco and nicotine**

> **Excludes2**   nicotine dependence (F17.-)

● **T65.21**   **Toxic effect of chewing tobacco**

● **T65.211**   **Toxic effect of chewing tobacco, accidental (unintentional)**
Toxic effect of chewing tobacco NOS

● **T65.212**   **Toxic effect of chewing tobacco, intentional self-harm**

● **T65.213**   **Toxic effect of chewing tobacco, assault**

● **T65.214**   **Toxic effect of chewing tobacco, undetermined**

● **T65.22**   **Toxic effect of tobacco cigarettes**
Toxic effect of tobacco smoke

Use additional code for exposure to second hand tobacco smoke (Z57.31, Z77.22)

● **T65.221**   **Toxic effect of tobacco cigarettes, accidental (unintentional)**
Toxic effect of tobacco cigarettes NOS

● **T65.222**   **Toxic effect of tobacco cigarettes, intentional self-harm**

● **T65.223**   **Toxic effect of tobacco cigarettes, assault**

● **T65.224**   **Toxic effect of tobacco cigarettes, undetermined**

● **T65.29**   **Toxic effect of other tobacco and nicotine**

● **T65.291**   **Toxic effect of other tobacco and nicotine, accidental (unintentional)**
Toxic effect of other tobacco and nicotine NOS

● **T65.292**   **Toxic effect of other tobacco and nicotine, intentional self-harm**

● **T65.293**   **Toxic effect of other tobacco and nicotine, assault**

● **T65.294**   **Toxic effect of other tobacco and nicotine, undetermined**

● **T65.3**   **Toxic effect of nitroderivatives and aminoderivatives of benzene and its homologues**
Toxic effect of anilin [benzenamine]
Toxic effect of nitrobenzene
Toxic effect of trinitrotoluene

● **T65.3X**   **Toxic effect of nitroderivatives and aminoderivatives of benzene and its homologues**

● **T65.3X1**   **Toxic effect of nitroderivatives and aminoderivatives of benzene and its homologues, accidental (unintentional)**
Toxic effect of nitroderivatives and aminoderivatives of benzene and its homologues NOS

● **T65.3X2**   **Toxic effect of nitroderivatives and aminoderivatives of benzene and its homologues, intentional self-harm**

● **T65.3X3**   **Toxic effect of nitroderivatives and aminoderivatives of benzene and its homologues, assault**

● **T65.3X4**   **Toxic effect of nitroderivatives and aminoderivatives of benzene and its homologues, undetermined**

● **T65.4**   **Toxic effect of carbon disulfide**

● **T65.4X**   **Toxic effect of carbon disulfide**

● **T65.4X1**   **Toxic effect of carbon disulfide, accidental (unintentional)**
Toxic effect of carbon disulfide NOS

● **T65.4X2**   **Toxic effect of carbon disulfide, intentional self-harm**

● **T65.4X3**   **Toxic effect of carbon disulfide, assault**

● **T65.4X4**   **Toxic effect of carbon disulfide, undetermined**

◄ New   ◄ Revised   ~~deleted~~ Deleted   **OGCR** Official Guidelines   X Assign placeholder X   ● Use Additional Character(s)

Excludes 1   Excludes 2   Includes   Use additional   Code first   Code also   Unspecified

● T65.5   Toxic effect of nitroglycerin and other nitric acids and esters
   Toxic effect of 1,2,3-Propanetriol trinitrate

 ● T65.5X   Toxic effect of nitroglycerin and other nitric acids and esters

  ● T65.5X1   Toxic effect of nitroglycerin and other nitric acids and esters, accidental (unintentional)
     Toxic effect of nitroglycerin and other nitric acids and esters NOS

  ● T65.5X2   Toxic effect of nitroglycerin and other nitric acids and esters, intentional self-harm

  ● T65.5X3   Toxic effect of nitroglycerin and other nitric acids and esters, assault

  ● T65.5X4   Toxic effect of nitroglycerin and other nitric acids and esters, undetermined

● T65.6   Toxic effect of paints and dyes, not elsewhere classified

 ● T65.6X   Toxic effect of paints and dyes, not elsewhere classified

  ● T65.6X1   Toxic effect of paints and dyes, not elsewhere classified, accidental (unintentional)
     Toxic effect of paints and dyes NOS

  ● T65.6X2   Toxic effect of paints and dyes, not elsewhere classified, intentional self-harm

  ● T65.6X3   Toxic effect of paints and dyes, not elsewhere classified, assault

  ● T65.6X4   Toxic effect of paints and dyes, not elsewhere classified, undetermined

● T65.8   Toxic effect of other specified substances

 ● T65.81   Toxic effect of latex

  ● T65.811   Toxic effect of latex, accidental (unintentional)
     Toxic effect of latex NOS

  ● T65.812   Toxic effect of latex, intentional self-harm

  ● T65.813   Toxic effect of latex, assault

  ● T65.814   Toxic effect of latex, undetermined

 ● T65.82   Toxic effect of harmful algae and algae toxins
   Toxic effect of (harmful) algae bloom NOS
   Toxic effect of blue-green algae bloom
   Toxic effect of brown tide
   Toxic effect of cyanobacteria bloom
   Toxic effect of Florida red tide
   Toxic effect of pfiesteria piscicida
   Toxic effect of red tide

  ● T65.821   Toxic effect of harmful algae and algae toxins, accidental (unintentional)
     Toxic effect of harmful algae and algae toxins NOS

  ● T65.822   Toxic effect of harmful algae and algae toxins, intentional self-harm

  ● T65.823   Toxic effect of harmful algae and algae toxins, assault

  ● T65.824   Toxic effect of harmful algae and algae toxins, undetermined

 ● T65.83   Toxic effect of fiberglass

  ● T65.831   Toxic effect of fiberglass, accidental (unintentional)
     Toxic effect of fiberglass NOS

  ● T65.832   Toxic effect of fiberglass, intentional self-harm

  ● T65.833   Toxic effect of fiberglass, assault

  ● T65.834   Toxic effect of fiberglass, undetermined

● T65.89   Toxic effect of other specified substances

  ● T65.891   Toxic effect of other specified substances, accidental (unintentional)
     Toxic effect of other specified substances NOS

  ● T65.892   Toxic effect of other specified substances, intentional self-harm

  ● T65.893   Toxic effect of other specified substances, assault

  ● T65.894   Toxic effect of other specified substances, undetermined

 ● T65.9   Toxic effect of unspecified substance

  X ● T65.91   Toxic effect of unspecified substance, accidental (unintentional)
     Poisoning NOS

  X ● T65.92   Toxic effect of unspecified substance, intentional self-harm

  X ● T65.93   Toxic effect of unspecified substance, assault

  X ● T65.94   Toxic effect of unspecified substance, undetermined

---

OTHER AND UNSPECIFIED EFFECTS OF EXTERNAL CAUSES (T66-T78)

● T66   Radiation sickness, unspecified

 | Excludes1 | specified adverse effects of radiation, such as:
    burns (T20-T31)
    leukemia (C91-C95)
    radiation gastroenteritis and colitis (K52.0)
    radiation pneumonitis (J70.0)
    radiation related disorders of the skin and subcutaneous tissue (L55-L59)
    sunburn (L55.-)

 The appropriate 7th character is to be added to code T66

  A   initial encounter
  D   subsequent encounter
  S   sequela

● T67   Effects of heat and light

 | Excludes1 | erythema [dermatitis] ab igne (L59.0)
    malignant hyperpyrexia due to anesthesia (T88.3)
    radiation-related disorders of the skin and subcutaneous tissue (L55-L59)

 | Excludes2 | burns (T20-T31)
    sunburn (L55.-)
    sweat disorder due to heat (L74-L75)

 The appropriate 7th character is to be added to each code from category T67

  A   initial encounter
  D   subsequent encounter
  S   sequela

 X ● T67.0   Heatstroke and sunstroke
   Heat apoplexy
   Heat pyrexia
   Siriasis
   Thermoplegia
   Use additional code(s) to identify any associated complications of heatstroke, such as:
    coma and stupor (R40.-)
    systemic inflammatory response syndrome (R65.1-)

 X ● T67.1   Heat syncope
   Heat collapse

 X ● T67.2   Heat cramp

 X ● T67.3   Heat exhaustion, anhydrotic
   Heat prostration due to water depletion
   | Excludes1 | heat exhaustion due to salt depletion (T67.4)

 X ● T67.4   Heat exhaustion due to salt depletion
   Heat prostration due to salt (and water) depletion

X● **T67.5**   **Heat exhaustion, unspecified**
         Heat prostration NOS

X● **T67.6**   **Heat fatigue, transient**

X● **T67.7**   **Heat edema**

X● **T67.8**   **Other effects of heat and light**

X● **T67.9**   **Effect of heat and light, unspecified**

● **T68**   **Hypothermia**
       Accidental hypothermia
       Hypothermia NOS

       Use additional code to identify source of exposure:
         Exposure to excessive cold of man-made origin (W93)
         Exposure to excessive cold of natural origin (X31)

       Excludes1   hypothermia following anesthesia (T88.51)
                   hypothermia not associated with low
                      environmental temperature (R68.0)
                   hypothermia of newborn (P80.-)

       Excludes2   frostbite (T33-T34)

       The appropriate 7th character is to be added to code T68

         A   initial encounter
         D   subsequent encounter
         S   sequela

● **T69**   **Other effects of reduced temperature**
       Use additional code to identify source of exposure:
         Exposure to excessive cold of man-made origin (W93)
         Exposure to excessive cold of natural origin (X31)

       Excludes2   frostbite (T33-T34)

       The appropriate 7th character is to be added to each code from
       category T69

         A   initial encounter
         D   subsequent encounter
         S   sequela

  ● **T69.0**   **Immersion hand and foot**

    ● **T69.01**   **Immersion hand**

      ● **T69.011**   **Immersion hand, right hand**

      ● **T69.012**   **Immersion hand, left hand**

      ● **T69.019**   **Immersion hand, unspecified hand**

    ● **T69.02**   **Immersion foot**
         Trench foot

      ● **T69.021**   **Immersion foot, right foot**

      ● **T69.022**   **Immersion foot, left foot**

      ● **T69.029**   **Immersion foot, unspecified foot**

X● **T69.1**   **Chilblains**

X● **T69.8**   **Other specified effects of reduced temperature**

X● **T69.9**   **Effect of reduced temperature, unspecified**

● **T70**   **Effects of air pressure and water pressure**
       The appropriate 7th character is to be added to each code from
       category T70

         A   initial encounter
         D   subsequent encounter
         S   sequela

X● **T70.0**   **Otitic barotrauma**
       Aero-otitis media
       Effects of change in ambient atmospheric pressure or
         water pressure on ears

X● **T70.1**   **Sinus barotrauma**
       Aerosinusitis
       Effects of change in ambient atmospheric pressure on
         sinuses

● **T70.2**   **Other and unspecified effects of high altitude**
       Excludes2   polycythemia due to high altitude (D75.1)

X● **T70.20**   **Unspecified effects of high altitude**

X● **T70.29**   **Other effects of high altitude**
       Alpine sickness
       Anoxia due to high altitude
       Barotrauma NOS
       Hypobaropathy
       Mountain sickness

X● **T70.3**   **Caisson disease [decompression sickness]**
       Compressed-air disease
       Diver's palsy or paralysis

X● **T70.4**   **Effects of high-pressure fluids**
       Hydraulic jet injection (industrial)
       Pneumatic jet injection (industrial)
       Traumatic jet injection (industrial)

X● **T70.8**   **Other effects of air pressure and water pressure**

X● **T70.9**   **Effect of air pressure and water pressure, unspecified**

● **T71**   **Asphyxiation**
       Mechanical suffocation
       Traumatic suffocation

       Excludes1   acute respiratory distress (syndrome) (J80)
                  anoxia due to high altitude (T70.2)
                  asphyxia NOS (R09.01)
                  asphyxia from carbon monoxide (T58.-)
                  asphyxia from inhalation of food or foreign body
                      (T17.-)
                  asphyxia from other gases, fumes and vapors
                      (T59.-)
                  respiratory distress (syndrome) in newborn
                      (P22.-)

       The appropriate 7th character is to be added to each code from
       category T71

         A   initial encounter
         D   subsequent encounter
         S   sequela

● **T71.1**   **Asphyxiation due to mechanical threat to breathing**
       Suffocation due to mechanical threat to breathing

  ● **T71.11**   **Asphyxiation due to smothering under pillow**

    ● **T71.111**   **Asphyxiation due to smothering
                         under pillow, accidental**
           Asphyxiation due to smothering
             under pillow NOS

    ● **T71.112**   **Asphyxiation due to smothering
                         under pillow, intentional self-harm**

    ● **T71.113**   **Asphyxiation due to smothering
                         under pillow, assault**

    ● **T71.114**   **Asphyxiation due to smothering
                         under pillow, undetermined**

  ● **T71.12**   **Asphyxiation due to plastic bag**

    ● **T71.121**   **Asphyxiation due to plastic bag,
                         accidental**
           Asphyxiation due to plastic bag
             NOS

    ● **T71.122**   **Asphyxiation due to plastic bag,
                         intentional self-harm**

    ● **T71.123**   **Asphyxiation due to plastic bag,
                         assault**

    ● **T71.124**   **Asphyxiation due to plastic bag,
                         undetermined**

● **T71.13**   **Asphyxiation due to being trapped in bed linens**

    ● **T71.131**   **Asphyxiation due to being trapped in bed linens, accidental**
          Asphyxiation due to being trapped in bed linens NOS

    ● **T71.132**   **Asphyxiation due to being trapped in bed linens, intentional self-harm**

    ● **T71.133**   **Asphyxiation due to being trapped in bed linens, assault**

    ● **T71.134**   **Asphyxiation due to being trapped in bed linens, undetermined**

● **T71.14**   **Asphyxiation due to smothering under another person's body (in bed)**

    ● **T71.141**   **Asphyxiation due to smothering under another person's body (in bed), accidental**
          Asphyxiation due to smothering under another person's body (in bed) NOS

    ● **T71.143**   **Asphyxiation due to smothering under another person's body (in bed), assault**

    ● **T71.144**   **Asphyxiation due to smothering under another person's body (in bed), undetermined**

● **T71.15**   **Asphyxiation due to smothering in furniture**

    ● **T71.151**   **Asphyxiation due to smothering in furniture, accidental**
          Asphyxiation due to smothering in furniture NOS

    ● **T71.152**   **Asphyxiation due to smothering in furniture, intentional self-harm**

    ● **T71.153**   **Asphyxiation due to smothering in furniture, assault**

    ● **T71.154**   **Asphyxiation due to smothering in furniture, undetermined**

● **T71.16**   **Asphyxiation due to hanging**
     Hanging by window shade cord
     Use additional code for any associated injuries, such as:
         crushing injury of neck (S17.-)
         fracture of cervical vertebrae (S12.0-S12.2-)
         open wound of neck (S11.-)

    ● **T71.161**   **Asphyxiation due to hanging, accidental**
          Asphyxiation due to hanging NOS
          Hanging NOS

    ● **T71.162**   **Asphyxiation due to hanging, intentional self-harm**

    ● **T71.163**   **Asphyxiation due to hanging, assault**

    ● **T71.164**   **Asphyxiation due to hanging, undetermined**

● **T71.19**   **Asphyxiation due to mechanical**
     Threat to breathing due to other causes

    ● **T71.191**   **Asphyxiation due to mechanical threat to breathing due to other causes, accidental**
          Asphyxiation due to other causes NOS

    ● **T71.192**   **Asphyxiation due to mechanical threat to breathing due to other causes, intentional self-harm**

    ● **T71.193**   **Asphyxiation due to mechanical threat to breathing due to other causes, assault**

    ● **T71.194**   **Asphyxiation due to mechanical threat to breathing due to other causes, undetermined**

● **T71.2**   **Asphyxiation due to systemic oxygen deficiency due to low oxygen content in ambient air**
     Suffocation due to systemic oxygen deficiency due to low oxygen content in ambient air

X ● **T71.20**   **Asphyxiation due to systemic oxygen deficiency due to low oxygen content in ambient air due to unspecified cause**

X ● **T71.21**   **Asphyxiation due to cave-in or falling earth**
         Use additional code for any associated cataclysm (X34-X38)

● **T71.22**   **Asphyxiation due to being trapped in a car trunk**

    ● **T71.221**   **Asphyxiation due to being trapped in a car trunk, accidental**

    ● **T71.222**   **Asphyxiation due to being trapped in a car trunk, intentional self-harm**

    ● **T71.223**   **Asphyxiation due to being trapped in a car trunk, assault**

    ● **T71.224**   **Asphyxiation due to being trapped in a car trunk, undetermined**

● **T71.23**   **Asphyxiation due to being trapped in a (discarded) refrigerator**

    ● **T71.231**   **Asphyxiation due to being trapped in a (discarded) refrigerator, accidental**

    ● **T71.232**   **Asphyxiation due to being trapped in a (discarded) refrigerator, intentional self-harm**

    ● **T71.233**   **Asphyxiation due to being trapped in a (discarded) refrigerator, assault**

    ● **T71.234**   **Asphyxiation due to being trapped in a (discarded) refrigerator, undetermined**

X ● **T71.29**   **Asphyxiation due to being trapped in other low oxygen environment**

X ● **T71.9**   **Asphyxiation due to unspecified cause**
     Suffocation (by strangulation) due to unspecified cause
     Suffocation NOS
     Systemic oxygen deficiency due to low oxygen content in ambient air due to unspecified cause
     Systemic oxygen deficiency due to mechanical threat to breathing due to unspecified cause
     Traumatic asphyxia NOS

● **T73**   **Effects of other deprivation**
     The appropriate 7th character is to be added to each code from category T73

A	initial encounter
D	subsequent encounter
S	sequela

X ● **T73.0**   **Starvation**
     Deprivation of food

X ● **T73.1**   **Deprivation of water**

X ● **T73.2**   **Exhaustion due to exposure**

X ● **T73.3**   **Exhaustion due to excessive exertion**
     Exhaustion due to overexertion

X ● **T73.8**   **Other effects of deprivation**

X ● **T73.9**   **Effect of deprivation, unspecified**

● **T74   Adult and child abuse, neglect and other maltreatment, confirmed**

> Use additional code, if applicable, to identify any associated current injury
>
> external cause code to identify perpetrator, if known (Y07.-)

> **Excludes1**   abuse and maltreatment in pregnancy (O9A.3-, O9A.4-, O9A.5-)
>
>   adult and child maltreatment, suspected (T76.-)

> The appropriate 7th character is to be added to each code from category T74

> | A | initial encounter |
> |---|---|
> | D | subsequent encounter |
> | S | sequela |

● **T74.0   Neglect or abandonment, confirmed**
   X● **T74.01   Adult neglect or abandonment, confirmed**
   X● **T74.02   Child neglect or abandonment, confirmed**
● **T74.1   Physical abuse, confirmed**
> **Excludes2**   sexual abuse (T74.2-)

   X● **T74.11   Adult physical abuse, confirmed**
   X● **T74.12   Child physical abuse, confirmed**
> **Excludes2**   shaken infant syndrome (T74.4)

● **T74.2   Sexual abuse, confirmed**
> Rape, confirmed
> Sexual assault, confirmed

   X● **T74.21   Adult sexual abuse, confirmed**
   X● **T74.22   Child sexual abuse, confirmed**
● **T74.3   Psychological abuse, confirmed**
   X● **T74.31   Adult psychological abuse, confirmed**
   X● **T74.32   Child psychological abuse, confirmed**
X● **T74.4   Shaken infant syndrome**
● **T74.9   Unspecified maltreatment, confirmed**
   X● **T74.91   Unspecified adult maltreatment, confirmed**
   X● **T74.92   Unspecified child maltreatment, confirmed**

● **T75   Other and unspecified effects of other external causes**
> **Excludes1**   adverse effects NEC (T78.-)
> **Excludes2**   burns (electric) (T20-T31)

> The appropriate 7th character is to be added to each code from category T75

> | A | initial encounter |
> |---|---|
> | D | subsequent encounter |
> | S | sequela |

● **T75.0   Effects of lightning**
> Struck by lightning

   X● **T75.00   Unspecified effects of lightning**
> Struck by lightning NOS

   X● **T75.01   Shock due to being struck by lightning**
   X● **T75.09   Other effects of lightning**
> Use additional code for other effects of lightning

X● **T75.1   Unspecified effects of drowning and nonfatal submersion**
> Immersion
> **Excludes1**   specified effects of drowning code to effects

● **T75.2   Effects of vibration**
   X● **T75.20   Unspecified effects of vibration**
   X● **T75.21   Pneumatic hammer syndrome**
   X● **T75.22   Traumatic vasospastic syndrome**
   X● **T75.23   Vertigo from infrasound**
> **Excludes1**   vertigo NOS (R42)

   X● **T75.29   Other effects of vibration**
X● **T75.3   Motion sickness**
> Airsickness   Travel sickness
> Seasickness
> Use additional external cause code to identify vehicle or type of motion (Y92.81-, Y93.5-)

X● **T75.4   Electrocution**
> Shock from electric current
> Shock from electroshock gun (taser)

● **T75.8   Other specified effects of external causes**
   X● **T75.81   Effects of abnormal gravitation [G] forces**
   X● **T75.82   Effects of weightlessness**
   X● **T75.89   Other specified effects of external causes**

● **T76   Adult and child abuse, neglect and other maltreatment, suspected**

> Use additional code, if applicable, to identify any associated current injury

> **Excludes1**   adult and child maltreatment, confirmed (T74.-)
>   suspected abuse and maltreatment in pregnancy (O9A.3-, O9A.4-, O9A.5-)
>   suspected adult physical abuse, ruled out (Z04.71)
>   suspected adult sexual abuse, ruled out (Z04.41)
>   suspected child physical abuse, ruled out (Z04.72)
>   suspected child sexual abuse, ruled out (Z04.42)

> The appropriate 7th character is to be added to each code from category T76

> | A | initial encounter |
> |---|---|
> | D | subsequent encounter |
> | S | sequela |

● **T76.0   Neglect or abandonment, suspected**
   X● **T76.01   Adult neglect or abandonment, suspected**
   X● **T76.02   Child neglect or abandonment, suspected**
● **T76.1   Physical abuse, suspected**
   X● **T76.11   Adult physical abuse, suspected**
   X● **T76.12   Child physical abuse, suspected**
● **T76.2   Sexual abuse, suspected**
> Rape, suspected
> Sexual abuse, suspected
> **Excludes1**   alleged abuse, ruled out (Z04.7)

   X● **T76.21   Adult sexual abuse, suspected**
   X● **T76.22   Child sexual abuse, suspected**
● **T76.3   Psychological abuse, suspected**
   X● **T76.31   Adult psychological abuse, suspected**
   X● **T76.32   Child psychological abuse, suspected**
● **T76.9   Unspecified maltreatment, suspected**
   X● **T76.91   Unspecified adult maltreatment, suspected**
   X● **T76.92   Unspecified child maltreatment, suspected**

● **T78 Adverse effects, not elsewhere classified**

> Excludes2 complications of surgical and medical care NEC (T80-T88)

The appropriate 7th character is to be added to each code from category T78

> A   initial encounter
> D   subsequent encounter
> S   sequela

● **T78.0 Anaphylactic reaction due to food**
> Anaphylactic reaction due to adverse food reaction
> Anaphylactic shock or reaction due to nonpoisonous foods
> Anaphylactoid reaction due to food

X● **T78.00 Anaphylactic reaction due to unspecified food**

X● **T78.01 Anaphylactic reaction due to peanuts**

X● **T78.02 Anaphylactic reaction due to shellfish (crustaceans)**

X● **T78.03 Anaphylactic reaction due to other fish**

X● **T78.04 Anaphylactic reaction due to fruits and vegetables**

X● **T78.05 Anaphylactic reaction due to tree nuts and seeds**
> Excludes1 anaphylactic reaction due to peanuts (T78.01)

X● **T78.06 Anaphylactic reaction due to food additives**

X● **T78.07 Anaphylactic reaction due to milk and dairy products**

X● **T78.08 Anaphylactic reaction due to eggs**

X● **T78.09 Anaphylactic reaction due to other food products**

X● **T78.1 Other adverse food reactions, not elsewhere classified**
> Use additional code to identify the type of reaction
> Excludes1 anaphylactic reaction or shock due to adverse food reaction (T78.0-)
> anaphylactic reaction due to food (T78.0-)
> bacterial food borne intoxications (A05.-)
> Excludes2 allergic and dietetic gastroenteritis and colitis (K52.2)
> allergic rhinitis due to food (J30.5)
> dermatitis due to food in contact with skin (L23.6, L24.6, L25.4)
> dermatitis due to ingested food (L27.2)

X● **T78.2 Anaphylactic shock, unspecified**
> *Occurs when allergic response triggers large quantities of histamines, prostaglandins, leukotrienes resulting in systemic vasodilation*
> Allergic shock
> Anaphylactic reaction
> Anaphylaxis
> Excludes1 anaphylactic reaction or shock due to adverse effect of correct medicinal substance properly administered (T88.6)
> anaphylactic reaction or shock due to adverse food reaction (T78.0-)
> anaphylactic reaction or shock due to serum (T80.5-)

X● **T78.3 Angioneurotic edema**
> Allergic angioedema
> Giant urticaria
> *Vascular disorder resulting from abnormalities of autonomic nervous system fibers supplying blood vessels*
> Quincke's edema
> Excludes1 serum urticaria (T80.6-)
> urticaria (L50.-)

● **T78.4 Other and unspecified allergy**
> Excludes1 specified types of allergic reaction such as:
> allergic diarrhea (K52.2)
> allergic gastroenteritis and colitis (K52.2)
> dermatitis (L23-L25, L27.-)
> hay fever (J30.1)

X● **T78.40 Allergy, unspecified**
> Allergic reaction NOS
> Hypersensitivity NOS

X● **T78.41 Arthus phenomenon**
> Arthus reaction

X● **T78.49 Other allergy**

X● **T78.8 Other adverse effects, not elsewhere classified**

CERTAIN EARLY COMPLICATIONS OF TRAUMA (T79)

● **T79 Certain early complications of trauma, not elsewhere classified**
> Excludes2 acute respiratory distress syndrome (J80)
> complications occurring during or following medical procedures (T80-T88)
> complications of surgical and medical care NEC (T80-T88)
> newborn respiratory distress syndrome (P22.0)

The appropriate 7th character is to be added to each code from category T79

> A   initial encounter
> D   subsequent encounter
> S   sequela

X● **T79.0 Air embolism (traumatic)**
> Excludes1 air embolism complicating abortion or ectopic or molar pregnancy (O00-O07, O08.2)
> air embolism complicating pregnancy, childbirth and the puerperium (O88.0)
> air embolism following infusion, transfusion, and therapeutic injection (T80.0)
> air embolism following procedure NEC (T81.7-)

X● **T79.1 Fat embolism (traumatic)**
> Excludes1 fat embolism complicating:
> abortion or ectopic or molar pregnancy (O00-O07, O08.2)
> pregnancy, childbirth and the puerperium (O88.8)

X● **T79.2 Traumatic secondary and recurrent hemorrhage and seroma**

X ● **T79.4 Traumatic shock**
Shock (immediate) (delayed) following injury

> **Excludes1** anaphylactic shock due to adverse food reaction (T78.0-)
> anaphylactic shock due to correct medicinal substance properly administered (T88.6)
> anaphylactic shock due to serum (T80.5-)
> anaphylactic shock NOS (T78.2)
> anesthetic shock (T88.2)
> electric shock (T75.4)
> nontraumatic shock NEC (R57.-)
> obstetric shock (O75.1)
> postprocedural shock (T81.1-)
> septic shock (R65.21)
> shock complicating abortion or ectopic or molar pregnancy (O00-O07, O08.3)
> shock due to lightning (T75.01)
> shock NOS (R57.9)

X ● **T79.5 Traumatic anuria**
Crush syndrome
Renal failure following crushing

X ● **T79.6 Traumatic ischemia of muscle**
Traumatic rhabdomyolysis
Volkmann's ischemic contracture

> **Excludes2** anterior tibial syndrome (M76.8)
> compartment syndrome (traumatic) (T79.A-)
> nontraumatic ischemia of muscle (M62.2-)

X ● **T79.7 Traumatic subcutaneous emphysema**

> **Excludes1** emphysema NOS (J43)
> emphysema (subcutaneous) resulting from a procedure (T81.82)

● **T79.A Traumatic compartment syndrome**

> **Excludes1** fibromyalgia (M79.7)
> nontraumatic compartment syndrome (M79.A-)
> traumatic ischemic infarction of muscle (T79.6)

X ● **T79.A0 Compartment syndrome, unspecified**
Compartment syndrome NOS

● **T79.A1 Traumatic compartment syndrome of upper extremity**
Traumatic compartment syndrome of shoulder, arm, forearm, wrist, hand, and fingers

> ● **T79.A11 Traumatic compartment syndrome of right upper extremity**
> ● **T79.A12 Traumatic compartment syndrome of left upper extremity**
> ● **T79.A19 Traumatic compartment syndrome of unspecified upper extremity**

● **T79.A2 Traumatic compartment syndrome of lower extremity**
Traumatic compartment syndrome of hip, buttock, thigh, leg, foot, and toes

> ● **T79.A21 Traumatic compartment syndrome of right lower extremity**
> ● **T79.A22 Traumatic compartment syndrome of left lower extremity**
> ● **T79.A29 Traumatic compartment syndrome of unspecified lower extremity**

X ● **T79.A3 Traumatic compartment syndrome of abdomen**
X ● **T79.A9 Traumatic compartment syndrome of other sites**

X ● **T79.8 Other early complications of trauma**
X ● **T79.9 Unspecified early complication of trauma**

COMPLICATIONS OF SURGICAL AND MEDICAL CARE, NOT ELSEWHERE CLASSIFIED (T80-T88)

Use additional code for adverse effect, if applicable, to identify drug (T36-T50 with fifth or sixth character 5)
Use additional code(s) to identify the specified condition resulting from the complication.
Use additional code to identify devices involved and details of circumstances (Y62-Y82)

> **Excludes2** any encounters with medical care for postprocedural conditions in which no complications are present, such as:
> artificial opening status (Z93.-)
> closure of external stoma (Z43.-)
> fitting and adjustment of external prosthetic device (Z44.-)
> burns and corrosions from local applications and irradiation (T20-T32)
> complications of surgical procedures during pregnancy, childbirth and the puerperium (O00-O9A)
> mechanical complication of respirator [ventilator] (J95.850)
> poisoning and toxic effects of drugs and chemicals (T36-T65 with fifth or sixth character 1-4 or 6)
> postprocedural fever (R50.82)
> specified complications classified elsewhere, such as:
> cerebrospinal fluid leak from spinal puncture (G97.0)
> colostomy malfunction (K94.0-)
> disorders of fluid and electrolyte imbalance (E86-E87)
> functional disturbances following cardiac surgery (I97.0-I97.1)
> intraoperative and postprocedural complications of specified body systems (D78.-, E36.-, E89.-, G97.3-, G97.4, H59.3-, H59.-, H95.2-, H95.3, I97.4-, I97.5, J95.6-, J95.7, K91.6-, L76.-, M96.-, N99.-)
> ostomy complications (J95.0-, K94.-, N99.5-)
> postgastric surgery syndromes (K91.1)
> postlaminectomy syndrome NEC (M96.1)
> postmastectomy lymphedema syndrome (I97.2)
> postsurgical blind-loop syndrome (K91.2)
> ventilator associated pneumonia (J95.851)

● **T80 Complications following infusion, transfusion and therapeutic injection**

> **Includes** complications following perfusion
> **Excludes2** bone marrow transplant rejection (T86.01)
> febrile nonhemolytic transfusion reaction (R50.84)
> fluid overload due to transfusion (E87.71)
> posttransfusion purpura (D69.51)
> transfusion associated circulatory overload (TACO) (E87.71)
> transfusion (red blood cell) associated hemochromatosis (E83.111)
> transfusion related acute lung injury (TRALI) (J95.84)

The appropriate 7th character is to be added to each code from category T80

A	initial encounter
D	subsequent encounter
S	sequela

X ● **T80.0 Air embolism following infusion, transfusion and therapeutic injection**

◀ New   ◀▥▥ Revised   deleted Deleted   OGCR Official Guidelines   X Assign placeholder X   ● Use Additional Character(s)

Excludes 1   Excludes 2   Includes   Use additional   Code first   Code also   Unspecified

X ● **T80.1** **Vascular complications following infusion, transfusion and therapeutic injection**

Use additional code to identify the vascular complication

Excludes2 extravasation of vesicant agent (T80.81-)
infiltration of vesicant agent (T80.81-)
vascular complications specified as due to prosthetic devices, implants and grafts (T82.8- T83.8, T84.8-, T85.8)
postprocedural vascular complications (T81.7-)

● **T80.2** **Infections following infusion, transfusion and therapeutic injection**

Use additional code to identify the specific infection, such as:
sepsis (A41.9)

Use additional code (R65.2-) to identify severe sepsis, if applicable

Excludes2 infections specified as due to prosthetic devices, implants and grafts (T82.6-T82.7, T83.5-T83.6, T84.5-T84.7, T85.7)
postprocedural infections (T81.4)

● **T80.21** **Infection due to central venous catheter**

● **T80.211** **Bloodstream infection due to central venous catheter**

Catheter-related bloodstream infection (CRBSI) NOS
Central line-associated bloodstream infection (CLABSI)
Bloodstream infection due to Hickman catheter
Bloodstream infection due to peripherally inserted central catheter (PICC)
Bloodstream infection due to portacath (port-a-cath)
Bloodstream infection due to triple lumen catheter
Bloodstream infection due to umbilical venous catheter

● **T80.212** **Local infection due to central venous catheter**

Exit or insertion site infection
Local infection due to Hickman catheter
Local infection due to peripherally inserted central catheter (PICC)
Local infection due to portacath (port-a-cath)
Local infection due to triple lumen catheter
Local infection due to umbilical venous catheter
Port or reservoir infection
Tunnel infection

● **T80.218** **Other infection due to central venous catheter**

Other central line-associated infection
Other infection due to Hickman catheter
Other infection due to peripherally inserted central catheter (PICC)
Other infection due to portacath (port-a-cath)
Other infection due to triple lumen catheter
Other infection due to umbilical venous catheter

● **T80.219** **Unspecified infection due to central venous catheter**

Central line-associated infection NOS
Unspecified infection due to Hickman catheter
Unspecified infection due to peripherally inserted central catheter (PICC)
Unspecified infection due to portacath (port-a-cath)
Unspecified infection due to triple lumen catheter
Unspecified infection due to umbilical venous catheter

X ● **T80.22** **Acute infection following transfusion, infusion, or injection of blood and blood products**

X ● **T80.29** **Infection following other infusion, transfusion and therapeutic injection**

● **T80.3** **ABO incompatibility reaction due to transfusion of blood or blood products**

Excludes1 minor blood group antigens reactions (Duffy) (E) (K(ell)) (Kidd) (Lewis) (M) (N) (P) (S) (T80.A)

X ● **T80.30** **ABO incompatibility reaction due to transfusion of blood or blood products, unspecified**

ABO incompatibility blood transfusion NOS
Reaction to ABO incompatibility from transfusion NOS

● **T80.31** **ABO incompatibility with hemolytic transfusion reaction**

● **T80.310** **ABO incompatibility with acute hemolytic transfusion reaction**

ABO incompatibility with hemolytic transfusion reaction less than 24 hours after transfusion
Acute hemolytic transfusion reaction (AHTR) due to ABO incompatibility

● **T80.311** **ABO incompatibility with delayed hemolytic transfusion reaction**

ABO incompatibility with hemolytic transfusion reaction 24 hours or more after transfusion
Delayed hemolytic transfusion reaction (DHTR) due to ABO incompatibility

● **T80.319** **ABO incompatibility with hemolytic transfusion reaction, unspecified**

ABO incompatibility with hemolytic transfusion reaction at unspecified time after transfusion
Hemolytic transfusion reaction (HTR) due to ABO incompatibility NOS

X ● **T80.39** **Other ABO incompatibility reaction due to transfusion of blood or blood products**

Delayed serologic transfusion reaction (DSTR) from ABO incompatibility
Other ABO incompatible blood transfusion
Other reaction to ABO incompatible blood transfusion

● **T80.4** **Rh incompatibility reaction due to transfusion of blood or blood products**

Reaction due to incompatibility of Rh antigens (C) (c) (D) (E) (e)

X ● **T80.40** **Rh incompatibility reaction due to transfusion of blood or blood products, unspecified**

Reaction due to Rh factor in transfusion NOS
Rh incompatible blood transfusion NOS

CHAPTER 19 (S00-T88)

◄ New   ◄▥ Revised   ~~deleted~~ Deleted   **OGCR** Official Guidelines   X Assign placeholder X   ● Use Additional Character(s)

| Excludes 1 | Excludes 2 | Includes | Use additional | Code first | Code also | Unspecified |

● **T80.41**   **Rh incompatibility with hemolytic transfusion reaction**

   ● **T80.410**   **Rh incompatibility with acute hemolytic transfusion reaction**
      Acute hemolytic transfusion reaction (AHTR) due to Rh incompatibility
      Rh incompatibility with hemolytic transfusion reaction less than 24 hours after transfusion

   ● **T80.411**   **Rh incompatibility with delayed hemolytic transfusion reaction**
      Delayed hemolytic transfusion reaction (DHTR) due to Rh incompatibility
      Rh incompatibility with hemolytic transfusion reaction 24 hours or more after transfusion

   ● **T80.419**   **Rh incompatibility with hemolytic transfusion reaction, unspecified**
      Rh incompatibility with hemolytic transfusion reaction at unspecified time after transfusion
      Hemolytic transfusion reaction (HTR) due to Rh incompatibility NOS

X● **T80.49**   **Other Rh incompatibility reaction due to transfusion of blood or blood products**
    Delayed serologic transfusion reaction (DSTR) from Rh incompatibility
    Other reaction to Rh incompatible blood transfusion

● **T80.A**   **Non-ABO incompatibility reaction due to transfusion of blood or blood products**
   Reaction due to incompatibility of minor antigens (Duffy) (Kell) (Kidd) (Lewis) (M) (N) (P) (S)

X● **T80.A0**   **Non-ABO incompatibility reaction due to transfusion of blood or blood products, unspecified**
    Non-ABO antigen incompatibility reaction from transfusion NOS

● **T80.A1**   **Non-ABO incompatibility with hemolytic transfusion reaction**

   ● **T80.A10**   **Non-ABO incompatibility with acute hemolytic transfusion reaction**
      Acute hemolytic transfusion reaction (AHTR) due to non-ABO incompatibility
      Non-ABO incompatibility with hemolytic transfusion reaction less than 24 hours after transfusion

   ● **T80.A11**   **Non-ABO incompatibility with delayed hemolytic transfusion reaction**
      Delayed hemolytic transfusion reaction (DHTR) due to non-ABO incompatibility
      Non-ABO incompatibility with hemolytic transfusion reaction 24 or more hours after transfusion

   ● **T80.A19**   **Non-ABO incompatibility with hemolytic transfusion reaction, unspecified**
      Hemolytic transfusion reaction (HTR) due to non-ABO incompatibility NOS
      Non-ABO incompatibility with hemolytic transfusion reaction at unspecified time after transfusion

X● **T80.A9**   **Other non-ABO incompatibility reaction due to transfusion of blood or blood products**
    Delayed serologic transfusion reaction (DSTR) from non-ABO incompatibility
    Other reaction to non-ABO incompatible blood transfusion

● **T80.5**   **Anaphylactic reaction due to serum**
   Allergic reaction due to serum
   Anaphylactic shock due to serum
   Anaphylactoid reaction due to serum
   Anaphylaxis due to serum

   Excludes1   ABO incompatibility reaction due to transfusion of blood or blood products (T80.3-)
      allergic reaction or shock NOS (T78.2)
      anaphylactic reaction or shock NOS (T78.2)
      anaphylactic reaction or shock due to adverse effect of correct medicinal substance properly administered (T88.6)
      other serum reaction (T80.6-)

X● **T80.51**   **Anaphylactic reaction due to administration of blood and blood products**

X● **T80.52**   **Anaphylactic reaction due to vaccination**

X● **T80.59**   **Anaphylactic reaction due to other serum**

● **T80.6**   **Other serum reactions**
   Intoxication by serum   Serum sickness
   Protein sickness   Serum urticaria
   Serum rash

   Excludes2   serum hepatitis (B16.-)

X● **T80.61**   **Other serum reaction due to administration of blood and blood products**

X● **T80.62**   **Other serum reaction due to vaccination**

X● **T80.69**   **Other serum reaction due to other serum**

● **T80.8**   **Other complications following infusion, transfusion and therapeutic injection**

   ● **T80.81**   **Extravasation of vesicant agent**
      Infiltration of vesicant agent

      ● **T80.810**   **Extravasation of vesicant antineoplastic chemotherapy**
        Infiltration of vesicant antineoplastic chemotherapy

      ● **T80.818**   **Extravasation of other vesicant agent**
        Infiltration of other vesicant agent

   X● **T80.89**   **Other complications following infusion, transfusion and therapeutic injection**
      Delayed serologic transfusion reaction (DSTR), unspecified incompatibility
      Use additional code to identify graft-versus-host reaction, if applicable, (D89.81-)

● **T80.9**   **Unspecified complication following infusion, transfusion and therapeutic injection**

   X● **T80.90**   **Unspecified complication following infusion and therapeutic injection**

   ● **T80.91**   **Hemolytic transfusion reaction, unspecified incompatibility**

      Excludes1   ABO incompatibility with hemolytic transfusion reaction (T80.31-)
        Non-ABO incompatibility with hemolytic transfusion reaction (T80.A1-)
        Rh incompatibility with hemolytic transfusion reaction (T80.41-)

      ● **T80.910**   **Acute hemolytic transfusion reaction, unspecified incompatibility**

      ● **T80.911**   **Delayed hemolytic transfusion reaction, unspecified incompatibility**

      ● **T80.919**   **Hemolytic transfusion reaction, unspecified incompatibility, unspecified as acute or delayed**
        Hemolytic transfusion reaction NOS

   X● **T80.92**   **Unspecified transfusion reaction**
      Transfusion reaction NOS

◀ New   ◀ Revised   deleted Deleted   **OGCR** Official Guidelines   X Assign placeholder X   ● Use Additional Character(s)

Excludes 1   Excludes 2   Includes   Use additional   Code first   Code also   Unspecified

● **T81**   **Complications of procedures, not elsewhere classified**

Use additional code for adverse effect, if applicable, to identify drug (T36-T50 with fifth or sixth character 5)

Excludes2   complications following immunization (T88.0-T88.1)

complications following infusion, transfusion and therapeutic injection (T80.-)

complications of transplanted organs and tissue (T86.-)

poisoning and toxic effects of drugs and chemicals (T36-T65 with fifth or sixth character 1-4 or 6)

specified complications classified elsewhere, such as:

     complication of prosthetic devices, implants and grafts (T82-T85)

     dermatitis due to drugs and medicaments (L23.3, L24.4, L25.1, L27.0-L27.1)

     endosseous dental implant failure (M27.6-)

     floppy iris syndrome (IFIS) (intraoperative) H21.81

     intraoperative and postprocedural complications of specific body system (D78.-, E36.-, E89.-, G97.3-, G97.4, H59.3-, H59.-, H95.2-, H95.3, I97.4-, I97.5, J95, K91.-, L76.-, M96.-, N99.-)

     ostomy complications (J95.0-, K94.-, N99.5-)

     plateau iris syndrome (post-iridectomy) (postprocedural) H21.82

The appropriate 7th character is to be added to each code from category T81

A	initial encounter
D	subsequent encounter
S	sequela

● **T81.1**   **Postprocedural shock**

Shock during or resulting from a procedure, not elsewhere classified

Excludes1   anaphylactic shock NOS (T78.2)

anaphylactic shock due to correct substance properly administered (T88.6)

anaphylactic shock due to serum (T80.5-)

anesthetic shock (T88.2)

electric shock (T75.4)

obstetric shock (O75.1)

septic shock (R65.21)

shock following abortion or ectopic or molar pregnancy (O00-O07, O08.3)

traumatic shock (T79.4)

X ● **T81.10**   **Postprocedural shock unspecified**

Collapse NOS during or resulting from a procedure, not elsewhere classified

Postprocedural failure of peripheral circulation

Postprocedural shock NOS

X ● **T81.11**   **Postprocedural cardiogenic shock**

X ● **T81.12**   **Postprocedural septic shock**

Postprocedural endotoxic shock during or resulting from a procedure, not elsewhere classified

Postprocedural gram-negative shock during or resulting from a procedure, not elsewhere classified

Code first underlying infection

Use additional code, to identify any associated acute organ dysfunction, if applicable

X ● **T81.19**   **Other postprocedural shock**

Postprocedural hypovolemic shock

● **T81.3**   **Disruption of wound, not elsewhere classified**

Disruption of any suture materials or other closure methods

Excludes1   breakdown (mechanical) of permanent sutures (T85.612)

displacement of permanent sutures (T85.622)

disruption of cesarean delivery wound (O90.0)

disruption of perineal obstetric wound (O90.1)

mechanical complication of permanent sutures NEC (T85.692)

X ● **T81.30**   **Disruption of wound, unspecified**

Disruption of wound NOS

X ● **T81.31**   **Disruption of external operation (surgical) wound, not elsewhere classified**

Excludes1   dehiscence of amputation stump (T87.81)

Dehiscence of operation wound NOS

Disruption of operation wound NOS

Disruption or dehiscence of closure of cornea

Disruption or dehiscence of closure of mucosa

Disruption or dehiscence of closure of skin and subcutaneous tissue

Full-thickness skin disruption or dehiscence

Superficial disruption or dehiscence of operation wound

X ● **T81.32**   **Disruption of internal operation (surgical) wound, not elsewhere classified**

Deep disruption or dehiscence of operation wound NOS

Disruption or dehiscence of closure of internal organ or other internal tissue

Disruption or dehiscence of closure of muscle or muscle flap

Disruption or dehiscence of closure of ribs or rib cage

Disruption or dehiscence of closure of skull or craniotomy

Disruption or dehiscence of closure of sternum or sternotomy

Disruption or dehiscence of closure of tendon or ligament

Disruption or dehiscence of closure of superficial or muscular fascia

X ● **T81.33**   **Disruption of traumatic injury wound repair**

Disruption or dehiscence of closure of traumatic laceration (external) (internal)

X ● **T81.4**   **Infection following a procedure**

Intra-abdominal abscess following a procedure

Postprocedural infection, not elsewhere classified

Sepsis following a procedure

Stitch abscess following a procedure

Subphrenic abscess following a procedure

Wound abscess following a procedure

Use additional code to identify infection

Use additional code (R65.2-) to identify severe sepsis, if applicable

Excludes1   obstetric surgical wound infection (O86.0)

postprocedural fever NOS (R50.82)

postprocedural retroperitoneal abscess (K68.11)

Excludes2   bleb associated endophthalmitis (H59.4-)

infection due to infusion, transfusion and therapeutic injection (T80.2-)

infection due to prosthetic devices, implants and grafts (T82.6-T82.7, T83.5-T83.6, T84.5-T84.7, T85.7)

CHAPTER 19 (S00-T88)

◀ New   ◀▦ Revised   ~~deleted~~ Deleted   **OGCR** Official Guidelines   X Assign placeholder X   ● Use Additional Character(s)

Excludes 1	Excludes 2	Includes	Use additional	Code first	Code also	Unspecified

1441

● T81.5 Complications of foreign body accidentally left in body following procedure
　● T81.50 Unspecified complication of foreign body accidentally left in body following procedure
　　● T81.500 Unspecified complication of foreign body accidentally left in body following surgical operation
　　● T81.501 Unspecified complication of foreign body accidentally left in body following infusion or transfusion
　　● T81.502 Unspecified complication of foreign body accidentally left in body following kidney dialysis
　　● T81.503 Unspecified complication of foreign body accidentally left in body following injection or immunization
　　● T81.504 Unspecified complication of foreign body accidentally left in body following endoscopic examination
　　● T81.505 Unspecified complication of foreign body accidentally left in body following heart catheterization
　　● T81.506 Unspecified complication of foreign body accidentally left in body following aspiration, puncture or other catheterization
　　● T81.507 Unspecified complication of foreign body accidentally left in body following removal of catheter or packing
　　● T81.508 Unspecified complication of foreign body accidentally left in body following other procedure
　　● T81.509 Unspecified complication of foreign body accidentally left in body following unspecified procedure
　● T81.51 Adhesions due to foreign body accidentally left in body following procedure
　　● T81.510 Adhesions due to foreign body accidentally left in body following surgical operation
　　● T81.511 Adhesions due to foreign body accidentally left in body following infusion or transfusion
　　● T81.512 Adhesions due to foreign body accidentally left in body following kidney dialysis
　　● T81.513 Adhesions due to foreign body accidentally left in body following injection or immunization
　　● T81.514 Adhesions due to foreign body accidentally left in body following endoscopic examination
　　● T81.515 Adhesions due to foreign body accidentally left in body following heart catheterization
　　● T81.516 Adhesions due to foreign body accidentally left in body following aspiration, puncture or other catheterization
　　● T81.517 Adhesions due to foreign body accidentally left in body following removal of catheter or packing
　　● T81.518 Adhesions due to foreign body accidentally left in body following other procedure
　　● T81.519 Adhesions due to foreign body accidentally left in body following unspecified procedure

● T81.52 Obstruction due to foreign body accidentally left in body following procedure
　● T81.520 Obstruction due to foreign body accidentally left in body following surgical operation
　● T81.521 Obstruction due to foreign body accidentally left in body following infusion or transfusion
　● T81.522 Obstruction due to foreign body accidentally left in body following kidney dialysis
　● T81.523 Obstruction due to foreign body accidentally left in body following injection or immunization
　● T81.524 Obstruction due to foreign body accidentally left in body following endoscopic examination
　● T81.525 Obstruction due to foreign body accidentally left in body following heart catheterization
　● T81.526 Obstruction due to foreign body accidentally left in body following aspiration, puncture or other catheterization
　● T81.527 Obstruction due to foreign body accidentally left in body following removal of catheter or packing
　● T81.528 Obstruction due to foreign body accidentally left in body following other procedure
　● T81.529 Obstruction due to foreign body accidentally left in body following unspecified procedure
● T81.53 Perforation due to foreign body accidentally left in body following procedure
　● T81.530 Perforation due to foreign body accidentally left in body following surgical operation
　● T81.531 Perforation due to foreign body accidentally left in body following infusion or transfusion
　● T81.532 Perforation due to foreign body accidentally left in body following kidney dialysis
　● T81.533 Perforation due to foreign body accidentally left in body following injection or immunization
　● T81.534 Perforation due to foreign body accidentally left in body following endoscopic examination
　● T81.535 Perforation due to foreign body accidentally left in body following heart catheterization
　● T81.536 Perforation due to foreign body accidentally left in body following aspiration, puncture or other catheterization
　● T81.537 Perforation due to foreign body accidentally left in body following removal of catheter or packing
　● T81.538 Perforation due to foreign body accidentally left in body following other procedure
　● T81.539 Perforation due to foreign body accidentally left in body following unspecified procedure

◀ New ◀▥ Revised deleted Deleted OGCR Official Guidelines X Assign placeholder X ● Use Additional Character(s) | Excludes 1 | Excludes 2 | Includes | Use additional | Code first | Code also | Unspecified

●**T81.59**   Other complications of foreign body accidentally left in body following procedure

> Excludes2   obstruction or perforation due to prosthetic devices and implants intentionally left in body (T82.0-T82.5, T83.0-T83.4, T83.7, T84.0-T84.4, T85.0-T85.6)

> ●**T81.590**   Other complications of foreign body accidentally left in body following surgical operation

> ●**T81.591**   Other complications of foreign body accidentally left in body following infusion or transfusion

> ●**T81.592**   Other complications of foreign body accidentally left in body following kidney dialysis

> ●**T81.593**   Other complications of foreign body accidentally left in body following injection or immunization

> ●**T81.594**   Other complications of foreign body accidentally left in body following endoscopic examination

> ●**T81.595**   Other complications of foreign body accidentally left in body following heart catheterization

> ●**T81.596**   Other complications of foreign body accidentally left in body following aspiration, puncture or other catheterization

> ●**T81.597**   Other complications of foreign body accidentally left in body following removal of catheter or packing

> ●**T81.598**   Other complications of foreign body accidentally left in body following other procedure

> ●**T81.599**   Other complications of foreign body accidentally left in body following unspecified procedure

●**T81.6**   Acute reaction to foreign substance accidentally left during a procedure

> Excludes2   complications of foreign body accidentally left in body cavity or operation wound following procedure (T81.5-)

> X ●**T81.60**   Unspecified acute reaction to foreign substance accidentally left during a procedure

> X ●**T81.61**   Aseptic peritonitis due to foreign substance accidentally left during a procedure
> > Chemical peritonitis

> X ●**T81.69**   Other acute reaction to foreign substance accidentally left during a procedure

●**T81.7**   Vascular complications following a procedure, not elsewhere classified

> Air embolism following procedure NEC
> Phlebitis or thrombophlebitis resulting from a procedure

> Excludes1   embolism complicating abortion or ectopic or molar pregnancy (O00-O07, O08.2)
> embolism complicating pregnancy, childbirth and the puerperium (O88.-)
> traumatic embolism (T79.0)

> Excludes2   embolism due to prosthetic devices, implants and grafts (T82.8, T83.8, T84.8-, T85.8)
> embolism following infusion, transfusion and therapeutic injection (T80.0)

●**T81.71**   Complication of artery following a procedure, not elsewhere classified

> ●**T81.710**   Complication of mesenteric artery following a procedure, not elsewhere classified

> ●**T81.711**   Complication of renal artery following a procedure, not elsewhere classified

> ●**T81.718**   Complication of other artery following a procedure, not elsewhere classified

> ●**T81.719**   Complication of unspecified artery following a procedure, not elsewhere classified

X ●**T81.72**   Complication of vein following a procedure, not elsewhere classified

●**T81.8**   Other complications of procedures, not elsewhere classified

> Excludes2   hypothermia following anesthesia (T88.51)
> malignant hyperpyrexia due to anesthesia (T88.3)

> X ●**T81.81**   Complication of inhalation therapy

> X ●**T81.82**   Emphysema (subcutaneous) resulting from a procedure

> X ●**T81.83**   Persistent postprocedural fistula

> X ●**T81.89**   Other complications of procedures, not elsewhere classified
> > Use additional code to specify complication, such as:
> > postprocedural delirium (F05)

X ●**T81.9**   Unspecified complication of procedure

●**T82**   Complications of cardiac and vascular prosthetic devices, implants and grafts

> Excludes2   failure and rejection of transplanted organs and tissue (T86.-)

> The appropriate 7th character is to be added to each code from category T82

> | | |
> |---|---|
> | A | initial encounter |
> | D | subsequent encounter |
> | S | sequela |

●**T82.0**   Mechanical complication of heart valve prosthesis
> Mechanical complication of artificial heart valve

> Excludes1   mechanical complication of biological heart valve graft (T82.22-)

> X ●**T82.01**   Breakdown (mechanical) of heart valve prosthesis

> X ●**T82.02**   Displacement of heart valve prosthesis
> > Malposition of heart valve prosthesis

> X ●**T82.03**   Leakage of heart valve prosthesis

> X ●**T82.09**   Other mechanical complication of heart valve prosthesis
> > Obstruction (mechanical) of heart valve prosthesis
> > Perforation of heart valve prosthesis
> > Protrusion of heart valve prosthesis

●**T82.1**   Mechanical complication of cardiac electronic device

> ●**T82.11**   Breakdown (mechanical) of cardiac electronic device

> > ●**T82.110**   Breakdown (mechanical) of cardiac electrode

> > ●**T82.111**   Breakdown (mechanical) of cardiac pulse generator (battery)

> > ●**T82.118**   Breakdown (mechanical) of other cardiac electronic device

> > ●**T82.119**   Breakdown (mechanical) of unspecified cardiac electronic device

◀ New   ◀⫶⫶⫶ Revised   ~~deleted~~ Deleted   **OGCR** Official Guidelines   X Assign placeholder X   ● Use Additional Character(s)

Excludes 1   Excludes 2   Includes   Use additional   Code first   Code also   Unspecified

1443

● **T82.12   Displacement of cardiac electronic device**
      Malposition of cardiac electronic device
  ● **T82.120   Displacement of cardiac electrode**
  ● **T82.121   Displacement of cardiac pulse generator (battery)**
  ● **T82.128   Displacement of other cardiac electronic device**
  ● **T82.129   Displacement of** unspecified **cardiac electronic device**
● **T82.19   Other mechanical complication of cardiac electronic device**
      Leakage of cardiac electronic device
      Obstruction of cardiac electronic device
      Perforation of cardiac electronic device
      Protrusion of cardiac electronic device
  ● **T82.190   Other mechanical complication of cardiac electrode**
  ● **T82.191   Other mechanical complication of cardiac pulse generator (battery)**
  ● **T82.198   Other mechanical complication of other cardiac electronic device**
  ● **T82.199   Other mechanical complication of** unspecified **cardiac device**
● **T82.2   Mechanical complication of coronary artery bypass graft and biological heart valve graft**
   | **Excludes1** | mechanical complication of artificial heart valve prosthesis (T82.0-) |
● **T82.21   Mechanical complication of coronary artery bypass graft**
  ● **T82.211   Breakdown (mechanical) of coronary artery bypass graft**
  ● **T82.212   Displacement of coronary artery bypass graft**
        Malposition of coronary artery bypass graft
  ● **T82.213   Leakage of coronary artery bypass graft**
  ● **T82.218   Other mechanical complication of coronary artery bypass graft**
        Obstruction, mechanical of coronary artery bypass graft
        Perforation of coronary artery bypass graft
        Protrusion of coronary artery bypass graft
● **T82.22   Mechanical complication of biological heart valve graft**
  ● **T82.221   Breakdown (mechanical) of biological heart valve graft**
  ● **T82.222   Displacement of biological heart valve graft**
        Malposition of biological heart valve graft
  ● **T82.223   Leakage of biological heart valve graft**
  ● **T82.228   Other mechanical complication of biological heart valve graft**
        Obstruction of biological heart valve graft
        Perforation of biological heart valve graft
        Protrusion of biological heart valve graft

● **T82.3   Mechanical complication of other vascular grafts**
● **T82.31   Breakdown (mechanical) of other vascular grafts**
  ● **T82.310   Breakdown (mechanical) of aortic (bifurcation) graft (replacement)**
  ● **T82.311   Breakdown (mechanical) of carotid arterial graft (bypass)**
  ● **T82.312   Breakdown (mechanical) of femoral arterial graft (bypass)**
  ● **T82.318   Breakdown (mechanical) of other vascular grafts**
  ● **T82.319   Breakdown (mechanical) of** unspecified **vascular grafts**
● **T82.32   Displacement of other vascular grafts**
      Malposition of other vascular grafts
  ● **T82.320   Displacement of aortic (bifurcation) graft (replacement)**
  ● **T82.321   Displacement of carotid arterial graft (bypass)**
  ● **T82.322   Displacement of femoral arterial graft (bypass)**
  ● **T82.328   Displacement of other vascular grafts**
  ● **T82.329   Displacement of** unspecified **vascular grafts**
● **T82.33   Leakage of other vascular grafts**
  ● **T82.330   Leakage of aortic (bifurcation) graft (replacement)**
  ● **T82.331   Leakage of carotid arterial graft (bypass)**
  ● **T82.332   Leakage of femoral arterial graft (bypass)**
  ● **T82.338   Leakage of other vascular grafts**
  ● **T82.339   Leakage of** unspecified **vascular graft**
● **T82.39   Other mechanical complication of other vascular grafts**
      Obstruction (mechanical) of other vascular grafts
      Perforation of other vascular grafts
      Protrusion of other vascular grafts
  ● **T82.390   Other mechanical complication of aortic (bifurcation) graft (replacement)**
  ● **T82.391   Other mechanical complication of carotid arterial graft (bypass)**
  ● **T82.392   Other mechanical complication of femoral arterial graft (bypass)**
  ● **T82.398   Other mechanical complication of other vascular grafts**
  ● **T82.399   Other mechanical complication of** unspecified **vascular grafts**
● **T82.4   Mechanical complication of vascular dialysis catheter**
      Mechanical complication of hemodialysis catheter
   | **Excludes1** | mechanical complication of intraperitoneal dialysis catheter (T85.62) |
X ● **T82.41   Breakdown (mechanical) of vascular dialysis catheter**
X ● **T82.42   Displacement of vascular dialysis catheter**
      Malposition of vascular dialysis catheter
X ● **T82.43   Leakage of vascular dialysis catheter**
X ● **T82.49   Other complication of vascular dialysis catheter**
      Obstruction (mechanical) of vascular dialysis catheter
      Perforation of vascular dialysis catheter
      Protrusion of vascular dialysis catheter

◀ New   ◀ Revised   ~~deleted~~ Deleted   **OGCR** Official Guidelines   X Assign placeholder X   ● Use Additional Character(s)

| Excludes 1 | Excludes 2 | Includes | Use additional | Code first | Code also | Unspecified |

● **T82.5**   Mechanical complication of other cardiac and vascular devices and implants
> 　 Excludes2   mechanical complication of epidural and subdural infusion catheter (T85.61)

● **T82.51**   Breakdown (mechanical) of other cardiac and vascular devices and implants

    ● **T82.510**   Breakdown (mechanical) of surgically created arteriovenous fistula

    ● **T82.511**   Breakdown (mechanical) of surgically created arteriovenous shunt

    ● **T82.512**   Breakdown (mechanical) of artificial heart

    ● **T82.513**   Breakdown (mechanical) of balloon (counterpulsation) device

    ● **T82.514**   Breakdown (mechanical) of infusion catheter

    ● **T82.515**   Breakdown (mechanical) of umbrella device

    ● **T82.518**   Breakdown (mechanical) of other cardiac and vascular devices and implants

    ● **T82.519**   Breakdown (mechanical) of unspecified cardiac and vascular devices and implants

● **T82.52**   Displacement of other cardiac and vascular devices and implants
> Malposition of other cardiac and vascular devices and implants

    ● **T82.520**   Displacement of surgically created arteriovenous fistula

    ● **T82.521**   Displacement of surgically created arteriovenous shunt

    ● **T82.522**   Displacement of artificial heart

    ● **T82.523**   Displacement of balloon (counterpulsation) device

    ● **T82.524**   Displacement of infusion catheter

    ● **T82.525**   Displacement of umbrella device

    ● **T82.528**   Displacement of other cardiac and vascular devices and implants

    ● **T82.529**   Displacement of unspecified cardiac and vascular devices and implants

● **T82.53**   Leakage of other cardiac and vascular devices and implants

    ● **T82.530**   Leakage of surgically created arteriovenous fistula

    ● **T82.531**   Leakage of surgically created arteriovenous shunt

    ● **T82.532**   Leakage of artificial heart

    ● **T82.533**   Leakage of balloon (counterpulsation) device

    ● **T82.534**   Leakage of infusion catheter

    ● **T82.535**   Leakage of umbrella device

    ● **T82.538**   Leakage of other cardiac and vascular devices and implants

    ● **T82.539**   Leakage of unspecified cardiac and vascular devices and implants

● **T82.59**   Other mechanical complication of other cardiac and vascular devices and implants
> Obstruction (mechanical) of other cardiac and vascular devices and implants
> Perforation of other cardiac and vascular devices and implants
> Protrusion of other cardiac and vascular devices and implants

    ● **T82.590**   Other mechanical complication of surgically created arteriovenous fistula

    ● **T82.591**   Other mechanical complication of surgically created arteriovenous shunt

    ● **T82.592**   Other mechanical complication of artificial heart

    ● **T82.593**   Other mechanical complication of balloon (counterpulsation) device

    ● **T82.594**   Other mechanical complication of infusion catheter

    ● **T82.595**   Other mechanical complication of umbrella device

    ● **T82.598**   Other mechanical complication of other cardiac and vascular devices and implants

    ● **T82.599**   Other mechanical complication of unspecified cardiac and vascular devices and implants

X ● **T82.6**   Infection and inflammatory reaction due to cardiac valve prosthesis
> Use additional code to identify infection

X ● **T82.7**   Infection and inflammatory reaction due to other cardiac and vascular devices, implants and grafts
> Use additional code to identify infection

● **T82.8**   Other specified complications of cardiac and vascular prosthetic devices, implants and grafts

● **T82.81**   Embolism of cardiac and vascular prosthetic devices, implants and grafts

    ● **T82.817**   Embolism of cardiac prosthetic devices, implants and grafts

    ● **T82.818**   Embolism of vascular prosthetic devices, implants and grafts

● **T82.82**   Fibrosis of cardiac and vascular prosthetic devices, implants and grafts

    ● **T82.827**   Fibrosis of cardiac prosthetic devices, implants and grafts

    ● **T82.828**   Fibrosis of vascular prosthetic devices, implants and grafts

● **T82.83**   Hemorrhage of cardiac and vascular prosthetic devices, implants and grafts

    ● **T82.837**   Hemorrhage of cardiac prosthetic devices, implants and grafts

    ● **T82.838**   Hemorrhage of vascular prosthetic devices, implants and grafts

● **T82.84**   Pain from cardiac and vascular prosthetic devices, implants and grafts

    ● **T82.847**   Pain from cardiac prosthetic devices, implants and grafts

    ● **T82.848**   Pain from vascular prosthetic devices, implants and grafts

● **T82.85**   Stenosis of cardiac and vascular prosthetic devices, implants and grafts

    ● **T82.857**   Stenosis of cardiac prosthetic devices, implants and grafts

    ● **T82.858**   Stenosis of vascular prosthetic devices, implants and grafts

● **T82.86**   Thrombosis of cardiac and vascular prosthetic devices, implants and grafts

    ● **T82.867**   Thrombosis of cardiac prosthetic devices, implants and grafts

    ● **T82.868**   Thrombosis of vascular prosthetic devices, implants and grafts

● **T82.89**   Other specified complication of cardiac and vascular prosthetic devices, implants and grafts

    ● **T82.897**   Other specified complication of cardiac prosthetic devices, implants and grafts

    ● **T82.898**   Other specified complication of vascular prosthetic devices, implants and grafts

X ● **T82.9**   Unspecified complication of cardiac and vascular prosthetic device, implant and graft

---

◀ New   ⬅ Revised   ~~deleted~~ Deleted   **OGCR** Official Guidelines   X Assign placeholder X   ● Use Additional Character(s)

Excludes 1   Excludes 2   Includes   Use additional   Code first   Code also   Unspecified

CHAPTER 19 (S00-T88)

● **T83   Complications of genitourinary prosthetic devices, implants and grafts**

> **Excludes2**   failure and rejection of transplanted organs and tissue (T86.-)

> The appropriate 7th character is to be added to each code from category T83

> A   initial encounter
> D   subsequent encounter
> S   sequela

● **T83.0   Mechanical complication of urinary (indwelling) catheter**

> **Excludes2**   complications of stoma of urinary tract (N99.5-)

   ● **T83.01   Breakdown (mechanical) of urinary (indwelling) catheter**

     ● **T83.010   Breakdown (mechanical) of cystostomy catheter**

     ● **T83.018   Breakdown (mechanical) of other indwelling urethral catheter**

   ● **T83.02   Displacement of urinary (indwelling) catheter**
     Malposition of urinary (indwelling) catheter

     ● **T83.020   Displacement of cystostomy catheter**

     ● **T83.028   Displacement of other indwelling urethral catheter**

   ● **T83.03   Leakage of urinary (indwelling) catheter**

     ● **T83.030   Leakage of cystostomy catheter**

     ● **T83.038   Leakage of other indwelling urethral catheter**

   ● **T83.09   Other mechanical complication of urinary (indwelling) catheter**
     Obstruction (mechanical) of urinary (indwelling) catheter
     Perforation of urinary (indwelling) catheter
     Protrusion of urinary (indwelling) catheter

     ● **T83.090   Other mechanical complication of cystostomy catheter**

     ● **T83.098   Other mechanical complication of other indwelling urethral catheter**

● **T83.1   Mechanical complication of other urinary devices and implants**

   ● **T83.11   Breakdown (mechanical) of other urinary devices and implants**

     ● **T83.110   Breakdown (mechanical) of urinary electronic stimulator device**

     ● **T83.111   Breakdown (mechanical) of urinary sphincter implant**

     ● **T83.112   Breakdown (mechanical) of urinary stent**

     ● **T83.118   Breakdown (mechanical) of other urinary devices and implants**

   ● **T83.12   Displacement of other urinary devices and implants**
     Malposition of other urinary devices and implants

     ● **T83.120   Displacement of urinary electronic stimulator device**

     ● **T83.121   Displacement of urinary sphincter implant**

     ● **T83.122   Displacement of urinary stent**

     ● **T83.128   Displacement of other urinary devices and implants**

● **T83.19   Other mechanical complication of other urinary devices and implants**
   Leakage of other urinary devices and implants
   Obstruction (mechanical) of other urinary devices and implants
   Perforation of other urinary devices and implants
   Protrusion of other urinary devices and implants

   ● **T83.190   Other mechanical complication of urinary electronic stimulator device**

   ● **T83.191   Other mechanical complication of urinary sphincter implant**

   ● **T83.192   Other mechanical complication of urinary stent**

   ● **T83.198   Other mechanical complication of other urinary devices and implants**

● **T83.2   Mechanical complication of graft of urinary organ**

   X ● **T83.21   Breakdown (mechanical) of graft of urinary organ**

   X ● **T83.22   Displacement of graft of urinary organ**
     Malposition of graft of urinary organ

   X ● **T83.23   Leakage of graft of urinary organ**

   X ● **T83.29   Other mechanical complication of graft of urinary organ**
     Obstruction (mechanical) of graft of urinary organ
     Perforation of graft of urinary organ
     Protrusion of graft of urinary organ

● **T83.3   Mechanical complication of intrauterine contraceptive device**

   X ● **T83.31   Breakdown (mechanical) of intrauterine contraceptive device**

   X ● **T83.32   Displacement of intrauterine contraceptive device**
     Malposition of intrauterine contraceptive device

   X ● **T83.39   Other mechanical complication of intrauterine contraceptive device**
     Leakage of intrauterine contraceptive device
     Obstruction (mechanical) of intrauterine contraceptive device
     Perforation of intrauterine contraceptive device
     Protrusion of intrauterine contraceptive device

● **T83.4   Mechanical complication of other prosthetic devices, implants and grafts of genital tract**

   ● **T83.41   Breakdown (mechanical) of other prosthetic devices, implants and grafts of genital tract**

     ● **T83.410   Breakdown (mechanical) of penile (implanted) prosthesis**

     ● **T83.418   Breakdown (mechanical) of other prosthetic devices, implants and grafts of genital tract**

   ● **T83.42   Displacement of other prosthetic devices, implants and grafts of genital tract**
     Malposition of other prosthetic devices, implants and grafts of genital tract

     ● **T83.420   Displacement of penile (implanted) prosthesis**

     ● **T83.428   Displacement of other prosthetic devices, implants and grafts of genital tract**

● **T83.49**   **Other mechanical complication of other prosthetic devices, implants and grafts of genital tract**
> Leakage of other prosthetic devices, implants and grafts of genital tract
> Obstruction, mechanical of other prosthetic devices, implants and grafts of genital tract
> Perforation of other prosthetic devices, implants and grafts of genital tract
> Protrusion of other prosthetic devices, implants and grafts of genital tract

> ● **T83.490**   **Other mechanical complication of penile (implanted) prosthesis**

> ● **T83.498**   **Other mechanical complication of other prosthetic devices, implants and grafts of genital tract**

● **T83.5**   **Infection and inflammatory reaction due to prosthetic device, implant and graft in urinary system**
> Use additional code to identify infection

> X ● **T83.51**   **Infection and inflammatory reaction due to indwelling urinary catheter**
>> Excludes2   complications of stoma of urinary tract (N99.5-)

> X ● **T83.59**   **Infection and inflammatory reaction due to prosthetic device, implant and graft in urinary system**

X ● **T83.6**   **Infection and inflammatory reaction due to prosthetic device, implant and graft in genital tract**
> Use additional code to identify infection

● **T83.7**   **Complications due to implanted mesh and other prosthetic materials**

> ● **T83.71**   **Erosion of implanted mesh and other prosthetic materials to surrounding organ or tissue**

>> ● **T83.711**   **Erosion of implanted vaginal mesh and other prosthetic materials to surrounding organ or tissue**
>>> Erosion of implanted vaginal mesh and other prosthetic materials into pelvic floor muscles

>> ● **T83.718**   **Erosion of other implanted mesh and other prosthetic materials to surrounding organ or tissue**

> ● **T83.72**   **Exposure of implanted mesh and other prosthetic materials into surrounding organ or tissue**

>> ● **T83.721**   **Exposure of implanted vaginal mesh and other prosthetic materials into vagina**
>>> Exposure of implanted vaginal mesh and other prosthetic materials through vaginal wall

>> ● **T83.728**   **Exposure of other implanted mesh and other prosthetic materials to surrounding organ or tissue**

● **T83.8**   **Other specified complications of genitourinary prosthetic devices, implants and grafts**

> X ● **T83.81**   **Embolism of genitourinary prosthetic devices, implants and grafts**

> X ● **T83.82**   **Fibrosis of genitourinary prosthetic devices, implants and grafts**

> X ● **T83.83**   **Hemorrhage of genitourinary prosthetic devices, implants and grafts**

> X ● **T83.84**   **Pain from genitourinary prosthetic devices, implants and grafts**

> X ● **T83.85**   **Stenosis of genitourinary prosthetic devices, implants and grafts**

> X ● **T83.86**   **Thrombosis of genitourinary prosthetic devices, implants and grafts**

> X ● **T83.89**   **Other specified complication of genitourinary prosthetic devices, implants and grafts**

X ● **T83.9**   **Unspecified complication of genitourinary prosthetic device, implant and graft**

● **T84**   **Complications of internal orthopedic prosthetic devices, implants and grafts**
> Excludes2   failure and rejection of transplanted organs and tissues (T86.-)
> fracture of bone following insertion of orthopedic implant, joint prosthesis or bone plate (M96.6)

> The appropriate 7th character is to be added to each code from category T84

> | | |
> |---|---|
> | A | initial encounter |
> | D | subsequent encounter |
> | S | sequela |

● **T84.0**   **Mechanical complication of internal joint prosthesis**

> ● **T84.01**   **Broken internal joint prosthesis**
>> Breakage (fracture) of prosthetic joint
>> Broken prosthetic joint implant
>> Excludes1   periprosthetic joint implant fracture (T84.04)

>> ● **T84.010**   **Broken internal right hip prosthesis**
>> ● **T84.011**   **Broken internal left hip prosthesis**
>> ● **T84.012**   **Broken internal right knee prosthesis**
>> ● **T84.013**   **Broken internal left knee prosthesis**
>> ● **T84.018**   **Broken internal joint prosthesis, other site**
>>> Use additional code to identify the joint (Z96.6-)

>> ● **T84.019**   **Broken internal joint prosthesis, unspecified site**

> ● **T84.02**   **Dislocation of internal joint prosthesis**
>> Instability of internal joint prosthesis
>> Subluxation of internal joint prosthesis

>> ● **T84.020**   **Dislocation of internal right hip prosthesis**
>> ● **T84.021**   **Dislocation of internal left hip prosthesis**
>> ● **T84.022**   **Instability of internal right knee prosthesis**
>> ● **T84.023**   **Instability of internal left knee prosthesis**
>> ● **T84.028**   **Dislocation of other internal joint prosthesis**
>>> Use additional code to identify the joint (Z96.6-)

>> ● **T84.029**   **Dislocation of unspecified internal joint prosthesis**

> ● **T84.03**   **Mechanical loosening of internal prosthetic joint**
>> Aseptic loosening of prosthetic joint

>> ● **T84.030**   **Mechanical loosening of internal right hip prosthetic joint**
>> ● **T84.031**   **Mechanical loosening of internal left hip prosthetic joint**
>> ● **T84.032**   **Mechanical loosening of internal right knee prosthetic joint**
>> ● **T84.033**   **Mechanical loosening of internal left knee prosthetic joint**
>> ● **T84.038**   **Mechanical loosening of other internal prosthetic joint**
>>> Use additional code to identify the joint (Z96.6-)

>> ● **T84.039**   **Mechanical loosening of unspecified internal prosthetic joint**

● **T84.04**   **Periprosthetic fracture around internal prosthetic joint**
    Excludes2   breakage (fracture) of prosthetic joint (T84.01)

- ● **T84.040**   Periprosthetic fracture around internal prosthetic right hip joint
- ● **T84.041**   Periprosthetic fracture around internal prosthetic left hip joint
- ● **T84.042**   Periprosthetic fracture around internal prosthetic right knee joint
- ● **T84.043**   Periprosthetic fracture around internal prosthetic left knee joint
- ● **T84.048**   Periprosthetic fracture around other internal prosthetic joint
      Use additional code to identify the joint (Z96.6-)
- ● **T84.049**   Periprosthetic fracture around unspecified internal prosthetic joint

● **T84.05**   **Periprosthetic osteolysis of internal prosthetic joint**
    Use additional code to identify major osseous defect, if applicable (M89.7-)

- ● **T84.050**   Periprosthetic osteolysis of internal prosthetic right hip joint
- ● **T84.051**   Periprosthetic osteolysis of internal prosthetic left hip joint
- ● **T84.052**   Periprosthetic osteolysis of internal prosthetic right knee joint
- ● **T84.053**   Periprosthetic osteolysis of internal prosthetic left knee joint
- ● **T84.058**   Periprosthetic osteolysis of other internal prosthetic joint
      Use additional code to identify the joint (Z96.6-)
- ● **T84.059**   Periprosthetic osteolysis of unspecified internal prosthetic joint

● **T84.06**   **Wear of articular bearing surface of internal prosthetic joint**

- ● **T84.060**   Wear of articular bearing surface of internal prosthetic right hip joint
- ● **T84.061**   Wear of articular bearing surface of internal prosthetic left hip joint
- ● **T84.062**   Wear of articular bearing surface of internal prosthetic right knee joint
- ● **T84.063**   Wear of articular bearing surface of internal prosthetic left knee joint
- ● **T84.068**   Wear of articular bearing surface of other internal prosthetic joint
      Use additional code to identify the joint (Z96.6-)
- ● **T84.069**   Wear of articular bearing surface of unspecified internal prosthetic joint

● **T84.09**   **Other mechanical complication of internal joint prosthesis**
    Prosthetic joint implant failure NOS

- ● **T84.090**   Other mechanical complication of internal right hip prosthesis
- ● **T84.091**   Other mechanical complication of internal left hip prosthesis
- ● **T84.092**   Other mechanical complication of internal right knee prosthesis
- ● **T84.093**   Other mechanical complication of internal left knee prosthesis
- ● **T84.098**   Other mechanical complication of other internal joint prosthesis
      Use additional code to identify the joint (Z96.6-)
- ● **T84.099**   Other mechanical complication of unspecified internal joint prosthesis

● **T84.1**   **Mechanical complication of internal fixation device of bones of limb**
    Excludes2   mechanical complication of internal fixation device of bones of feet (T84.2-)
        mechanical complication of internal fixation device of bones of fingers (T84.2-)
        mechanical complication of internal fixation device of bones of hands (T84.2-)
        mechanical complication of internal fixation device of bones of toes (T84.2-)

● **T84.11**   **Breakdown (mechanical) of internal fixation device of bones of limb**

- ● **T84.110**   Breakdown (mechanical) of internal fixation device of right humerus
- ● **T84.111**   Breakdown (mechanical) of internal fixation device of left humerus
- ● **T84.112**   Breakdown (mechanical) of internal fixation device of bone of right forearm
- ● **T84.113**   Breakdown (mechanical) of internal fixation device of bone of left forearm
- ● **T84.114**   Breakdown (mechanical) of internal fixation device of right femur
- ● **T84.115**   Breakdown (mechanical) of internal fixation device of left femur
- ● **T84.116**   Breakdown (mechanical) of internal fixation device of bone of right lower leg
- ● **T84.117**   Breakdown (mechanical) of internal fixation device of bone of left lower leg
- ● **T84.119**   Breakdown (mechanical) of internal fixation device of unspecified bone of limb

● **T84.12**   **Displacement of internal fixation device of bones of limb**
    Malposition of internal fixation device of bones of limb

- ● **T84.120**   Displacement of internal fixation device of right humerus
- ● **T84.121**   Displacement of internal fixation device of left humerus
- ● **T84.122**   Displacement of internal fixation device of bone of right forearm
- ● **T84.123**   Displacement of internal fixation device of bone of left forearm
- ● **T84.124**   Displacement of internal fixation device of right femur
- ● **T84.125**   Displacement of internal fixation device of left femur
- ● **T84.126**   Displacement of internal fixation device of bone of right lower leg
- ● **T84.127**   Displacement of internal fixation device of bone of left lower leg
- ● **T84.129**   Displacement of internal fixation device of unspecified bone of limb

● T84.19   Other mechanical complication of internal
fixation device of bones of limb
   Obstruction (mechanical) of internal fixation
     device of bones of limb
   Perforation of internal fixation device of bones
     of limb
   Protrusion of internal fixation device of bones
     of limb

  ● T84.190   Other mechanical complication
       of internal fixation device of right
       humerus

  ● T84.191   Other mechanical complication
       of internal fixation device of left
       humerus

  ● T84.192   Other mechanical complication of
       internal fixation device of bone of
       right forearm

  ● T84.193   Other mechanical complication of
       internal fixation device of bone of left
       forearm

  ● T84.194   Other mechanical complication of
       internal fixation device of right femur

  ● T84.195   Other mechanical complication of
       internal fixation device of left femur

  ● T84.196   Other mechanical complication of
       internal fixation device of bone of
       right lower leg

  ● T84.197   Other mechanical complication of
       internal fixation device of bone of left
       lower leg

  ● T84.199   Other mechanical complication of
       internal fixation device of unspecified
       bone of limb

● T84.2   Mechanical complication of internal fixation device of
other bones

  ● T84.21   Breakdown (mechanical) of internal fixation
     device of other bones

    ● T84.210   Breakdown (mechanical) of internal
         fixation device of bones of hand and
         fingers

    ● T84.213   Breakdown (mechanical) of internal
         fixation device of bones of foot and
         toes

    ● T84.216   Breakdown (mechanical) of internal
         fixation device of vertebrae

    ● T84.218   Breakdown (mechanical) of internal
         fixation device of other bones

  ● T84.22   Displacement of internal fixation device of
     other bones
      Malposition of internal fixation device of other
       bones

    ● T84.220   Displacement of internal fixation
         device of bones of hand and fingers

    ● T84.223   Displacement of internal fixation
         device of bones of foot and toes

    ● T84.226   Displacement of internal fixation
         device of vertebrae

    ● T84.228   Displacement of internal fixation
         device of other bones

  ● T84.29   Other mechanical complication of internal
     fixation device of other bones
      Obstruction (mechanical) of internal fixation
       device of other bones
      Perforation of internal fixation device of other
       bones
      Protrusion of internal fixation device of other
       bones

    ● T84.290   Other mechanical complication of
         internal fixation device of bones of
         hand and fingers

    ● T84.293   Other mechanical complication of
         internal fixation device of bones of
         foot and toes

  ● T84.296   Other mechanical complication of
       internal fixation device of vertebrae

  ● T84.298   Other mechanical complication of
       internal fixation device of other bones

● T84.3   Mechanical complication of other bone devices,
implants and grafts

   Excludes2   other complications of bone graft
        (T86.83-)

  ● T84.31   Breakdown (mechanical) of other bone devices,
     implants and grafts

    ● T84.310   Breakdown (mechanical) of electronic
         bone stimulator

    ● T84.318   Breakdown (mechanical) of other
         bone devices, implants and grafts

  ● T84.32   Displacement of other bone devices, implants
     and grafts
      Malposition of other bone devices, implants
       and grafts

    ● T84.320   Displacement of electronic bone
         stimulator

    ● T84.328   Displacement of other bone devices,
         implants and grafts

  ● T84.39   Other mechanical complication of other bone
     devices, implants and grafts
      Obstruction (mechanical) of other bone
       devices, implants and grafts
      Perforation of other bone devices, implants
       and grafts
      Protrusion of other bone devices, implants and
       grafts

    ● T84.390   Other mechanical complication of
         electronic bone stimulator

    ● T84.398   Other mechanical complication of
         other bone devices, implants and
         grafts

● T84.4   Mechanical complication of other internal orthopedic
devices, implants and grafts

  ● T84.41   Breakdown (mechanical) of other internal
     orthopedic devices, implants and grafts

    ● T84.410   Breakdown (mechanical) of muscle
         and tendon graft

    ● T84.418   Breakdown (mechanical) of other
         internal orthopedic devices, implants
         and grafts

  ● T84.42   Displacement of other internal orthopedic
     devices, implants and grafts
      Malposition of other internal orthopedic
       devices, implants and grafts

    ● T84.420   Displacement of muscle and tendon
         graft

    ● T84.428   Displacement of other internal
         orthopedic devices, implants and
         grafts

  ● T84.49   Other mechanical complication of other
     internal orthopedic devices, implants and grafts
      Mechanical complication of other internal
       orthopedic devices, implants and grafts
       NOS
      Obstruction (mechanical) of other internal
       orthopedic devices, implants and grafts
      Perforation of other internal orthopedic
       devices, implants and grafts
      Protrusion of other internal orthopedic devices,
       implants and grafts

    ● T84.490   Other mechanical complication of
         muscle and tendon graft

    ● T84.498   Other mechanical complication of
         other internal orthopedic devices,
         implants and grafts

CHAPTER 19 (S00-T88)

● **T84.5** Infection and inflammatory reaction due to internal joint prosthesis

Use additional code to identify infection

X ● **T84.50** Infection and inflammatory reaction due to unspecified internal joint prosthesis

X ● **T84.51** Infection and inflammatory reaction due to internal right hip prosthesis

X ● **T84.52** Infection and inflammatory reaction due to internal left hip prosthesis

X ● **T84.53** Infection and inflammatory reaction due to internal right knee prosthesis

X ● **T84.54** Infection and inflammatory reaction due to internal left knee prosthesis

X ● **T84.59** Infection and inflammatory reaction due to other internal joint prosthesis

● **T84.6** Infection and inflammatory reaction due to internal fixation device

Use additional code to identify infection

X ● **T84.60** Infection and inflammatory reaction due to internal fixation device of unspecified site

● **T84.61** Infection and inflammatory reaction due to internal fixation device of arm

● **T84.610** Infection and inflammatory reaction due to internal fixation device of right humerus

● **T84.611** Infection and inflammatory reaction due to internal fixation device of left humerus

● **T84.612** Infection and inflammatory reaction due to internal fixation device of right radius

● **T84.613** Infection and inflammatory reaction due to internal fixation device of left radius

● **T84.614** Infection and inflammatory reaction due to internal fixation device of right ulna

● **T84.615** Infection and inflammatory reaction due to internal fixation device of left ulna

● **T84.619** Infection and inflammatory reaction due to internal fixation device of unspecified bone of arm

● **T84.62** Infection and inflammatory reaction due to internal fixation device of leg

● **T84.620** Infection and inflammatory reaction due to internal fixation device of right femur

● **T84.621** Infection and inflammatory reaction due to internal fixation device of left femur

● **T84.622** Infection and inflammatory reaction due to internal fixation device of right tibia

● **T84.623** Infection and inflammatory reaction due to internal fixation device of left tibia

● **T84.624** Infection and inflammatory reaction due to internal fixation device of right fibula

● **T84.625** Infection and inflammatory reaction due to internal fixation device of left fibula

● **T84.629** Infection and inflammatory reaction due to internal fixation device of unspecified bone of leg

X ● **T84.63** Infection and inflammatory reaction due to internal fixation device of spine

X ● **T84.69** Infection and inflammatory reaction due to internal fixation device of other site

● **T84.7** Infection and inflammatory reaction due to other internal orthopedic prosthetic devices, implants and grafts

Use additional code to identify infection

● **T84.8** Other specified complications of internal orthopedic prosthetic devices, implants and grafts

X ● **T84.81** Embolism due to internal orthopedic prosthetic devices, implants and grafts

X ● **T84.82** Fibrosis due to internal orthopedic prosthetic devices, implants and grafts

X ● **T84.83** Hemorrhage due to internal orthopedic prosthetic devices, implants and grafts

X ● **T84.84** Pain due to internal orthopedic prosthetic devices, implants and grafts

X ● **T84.85** Stenosis due to internal orthopedic prosthetic devices, implants and grafts

X ● **T84.86** Thrombosis due to internal orthopedic prosthetic devices, implants and grafts

X ● **T84.89** Other specified complication of internal orthopedic prosthetic devices, implants and grafts

X ● **T84.9** Unspecified complication of internal orthopedic prosthetic device, implant and graft

● **T85** Complications of other internal prosthetic devices, implants and grafts

Excludes2 failure and rejection of transplanted organs and tissue (T86.-)

The appropriate 7th character is to be added to each code from category T85

A	initial encounter
D	subsequent encounter
S	sequela

● **T85.0** Mechanical complication of ventricular intracranial (communicating) shunt

X ● **T85.01** Breakdown (mechanical) of ventricular intracranial (communicating) shunt

X ● **T85.02** Displacement of ventricular intracranial (communicating) shunt

Malposition of ventricular intracranial (communicating) shunt

X ● **T85.03** Leakage of ventricular intracranial (communicating) shunt

X ● **T85.09** Other mechanical complication of ventricular intracranial (communicating) shunt

Obstruction (mechanical) of ventricular intracranial (communicating) shunt

Perforation of ventricular intracranial (communicating) shunt

Protrusion of ventricular intracranial (communicating) shunt

● **T85.1** Mechanical complication of implanted electronic stimulator of nervous system

● **T85.11** Breakdown (mechanical) of implanted electronic stimulator of nervous system

● **T85.110** Breakdown (mechanical) of implanted electronic neurostimulator (electrode) of brain

● **T85.111** Breakdown (mechanical) of implanted electronic neurostimulator (electrode) of peripheral nerve

● **T85.112** Breakdown (mechanical) of implanted electronic neurostimulator (electrode) of spinal cord

● **T85.118** Breakdown (mechanical) of other implanted electronic stimulator of nervous system

◄ New   ◄▥ Revised   ~~deleted~~ Deleted   OGCR Official Guidelines   X Assign placeholder X   ● Use Additional Character(s)

Excludes 1   Excludes 2   Includes   Use additional   Code first   Code also   Unspecified

● **T85.12 Displacement of implanted electronic stimulator of nervous system**
  Malposition of implanted electronic stimulator of nervous system

  ● **T85.120 Displacement of implanted electronic neurostimulator (electrode) of brain**

  ● **T85.121 Displacement of implanted electronic neurostimulator (electrode) of peripheral nerve**

  ● **T85.122 Displacement of implanted electronic neurostimulator (electrode) of spinal cord**

  ● **T85.128 Displacement of other implanted electronic stimulator of nervous system**

● **T85.19 Other mechanical complication of implanted electronic stimulator of nervous system**
  Leakage of implanted electronic stimulator of nervous system
  Obstruction (mechanical) of implanted electronic stimulator of nervous system
  Perforation of implanted electronic stimulator of nervous system
  Protrusion of implanted electronic stimulator of nervous system

  ● **T85.190 Other mechanical complication of implanted electronic neurostimulator (electrode) of brain**

  ● **T85.191 Other mechanical complication of implanted electronic neurostimulator (electrode) of peripheral nerve**

  ● **T85.192 Other mechanical complication of implanted electronic neurostimulator (electrode) of spinal cord**

  ● **T85.199 Other mechanical complication of other implanted electronic stimulator of nervous system**

● **T85.2 Mechanical complication of intraocular lens**

  X ● **T85.21 Breakdown (mechanical) of intraocular lens**

  X ● **T85.22 Displacement of intraocular lens**
  Malposition of intraocular lens

  X ● **T85.29 Other mechanical complication of intraocular lens**
  Obstruction (mechanical) of intraocular lens
  Perforation of intraocular lens
  Protrusion of intraocular lens

● **T85.3 Mechanical complication of other ocular prosthetic devices, implants and grafts**
  Excludes2   other complications of corneal graft (T86.84-)

  ● **T85.31 Breakdown (mechanical) of other ocular prosthetic devices, implants and grafts**

    ● **T85.310 Breakdown (mechanical) of prosthetic orbit of right eye**

    ● **T85.311 Breakdown (mechanical) of prosthetic orbit of left eye**

    ● **T85.318 Breakdown (mechanical) of other ocular prosthetic devices, implants and grafts**

  ● **T85.32 Displacement of other ocular prosthetic devices, implants and grafts**
  Malposition of other ocular prosthetic devices, implants and grafts

    ● **T85.320 Displacement of prosthetic orbit of right eye**

    ● **T85.321 Displacement of prosthetic orbit of left eye**

    ● **T85.328 Displacement of other ocular prosthetic devices, implants and grafts**

● **T85.39 Other mechanical complication of other ocular prosthetic devices, implants and grafts**
  Obstruction (mechanical) of other ocular prosthetic devices, implants and grafts
  Perforation of other ocular prosthetic devices, implants and grafts
  Protrusion of other ocular prosthetic devices, implants and grafts

  ● **T85.390 Other mechanical complication of prosthetic orbit of right eye**

  ● **T85.391 Other mechanical complication of prosthetic orbit of left eye**

  ● **T85.398 Other mechanical complication of other ocular prosthetic devices, implants and grafts**

● **T85.4 Mechanical complication of breast prosthesis and implant**

  X ● **T85.41 Breakdown (mechanical) of breast prosthesis and implant**

  X ● **T85.42 Displacement of breast prosthesis and implant**
  Malposition of breast prosthesis and implant

  X ● **T85.43 Leakage of breast prosthesis and implant**

  X ● **T85.44 Capsular contracture of breast implant**

  X ● **T85.49 Other mechanical complication of breast prosthesis and implant**
  Obstruction (mechanical) of breast prosthesis and implant
  Perforation of breast prosthesis and implant
  Protrusion of breast prosthesis and implant

● **T85.5 Mechanical complication of gastrointestinal prosthetic devices, implants and grafts**

  ● **T85.51 Breakdown (mechanical) of gastrointestinal prosthetic devices, implants and grafts**

    ● **T85.510 Breakdown (mechanical) of bile duct prosthesis**

    ● **T85.511 Breakdown (mechanical) of esophageal anti-reflux device**

    ● **T85.518 Breakdown (mechanical) of other gastrointestinal prosthetic devices, implants and grafts**

  ● **T85.52 Displacement of gastrointestinal prosthetic devices, implants and grafts**
  Malposition of gastrointestinal prosthetic devices, implants and grafts

    ● **T85.520 Displacement of bile duct prosthesis**

    ● **T85.521 Displacement of esophageal anti-reflux device**

    ● **T85.528 Displacement of other gastrointestinal prosthetic devices, implants and grafts**

  ● **T85.59 Other mechanical complication of gastrointestinal prosthetic devices, implants and**
  Obstruction, mechanical of gastrointestinal prosthetic devices, implants and grafts
  Perforation of gastrointestinal prosthetic devices, implants and grafts
  Protrusion of gastrointestinal prosthetic devices, implants and grafts

    ● **T85.590 Other mechanical complication of bile duct prosthesis**

    ● **T85.591 Other mechanical complication of esophageal anti-reflux device**

    ● **T85.598 Other mechanical complication of other gastrointestinal prosthetic devices, implants and grafts**

CHAPTER 19 (S00-T88)

● **T85.6**   **Mechanical complication of other specified internal and external prosthetic devices, implants and grafts**
   ● **T85.61**   **Breakdown (mechanical) of other specified internal prosthetic devices, implants and grafts**
     ● **T85.610**   **Breakdown (mechanical) of epidural and subdural infusion catheter**
     ● **T85.611**   **Breakdown (mechanical) of intraperitoneal dialysis catheter**
       Excludes1   mechanical complication of vascular dialysis catheter (T82.4-)
     ● **T85.612**   **Breakdown (mechanical) of permanent sutures**
       Excludes1   mechanical complication of permanent (wire) suture used in bone repair (T84.1-T84.2)
     ● **T85.613**   **Breakdown (mechanical) of artificial skin graft and decellularized allodermis**
       Failure of artificial skin graft and decellularized allodermis
       Non-adherence of artificial skin graft and decellularized allodermis
       Poor incorporation of artificial skin graft and decellularized allodermis
       Shearing of artificial skin graft and decellularized allodermis
     ● **T85.614**   **Breakdown (mechanical) of insulin pump**
     ● **T85.618**   **Breakdown (mechanical) of other specified internal prosthetic devices, implants and grafts**
   ● **T85.62**   **Displacement of other specified internal prosthetic devices, implants and grafts**
     Malposition of other specified internal prosthetic devices, implants and grafts
     ● **T85.620**   **Displacement of epidural and subdural infusion catheter**
     ● **T85.621**   **Displacement of intraperitoneal dialysis catheter**
       Excludes1   mechanical complication of vascular dialysis catheter (T82.4-)
     ● **T85.622**   **Displacement of permanent sutures**
       Excludes1   mechanical complication of permanent (wire) suture used in bone repair (T84.1-T84.2)
     ● **T85.623**   **Displacement of artificial skin graft and decellularized allodermis**
       Dislodgement of artificial skin graft and decellularized allodermis
       Displacement of artificial skin graft and decellularized allodermis
     ● **T85.624**   **Displacement of insulin pump**
     ● **T85.628**   **Displacement of other specified internal prosthetic devices, implants and grafts**

● **T85.63**   **Leakage of other specified internal prosthetic devices, implants and grafts**
     ● **T85.630**   **Leakage of epidural and subdural infusion catheter**
     ● **T85.631**   **Leakage of intraperitoneal dialysis catheter**
       Excludes1   mechanical complication of vascular dialysis catheter (T82.4)
     ● **T85.633**   **Leakage of insulin pump**
     ● **T85.638**   **Leakage of other specified internal prosthetic devices, implants and grafts**
   ● **T85.69**   **Other mechanical complication of other specified internal prosthetic devices, implants and grafts**
     Obstruction, mechanical of other specified internal prosthetic devices, implants and grafts
     Perforation of other specified internal prosthetic devices, implants and grafts
     Protrusion of other specified internal prosthetic devices, implants and grafts
     ● **T85.690**   **Other mechanical complication of epidural and subdural infusion catheter**
     ● **T85.691**   **Other mechanical complication of intraperitoneal dialysis catheter**
       Excludes1   mechanical complication of vascular dialysis catheter (T82.4)
     ● **T85.692**   **Other mechanical complication of permanent sutures**
       Excludes1   mechanical complication of permanent (wire) suture used in bone repair (T84.1-T84.2)
     ● **T85.693**   **Other mechanical complication of artificial skin graft and decellularized allodermis**
     ● **T85.694**   **Other mechanical complication of insulin pump**
     ● **T85.698**   **Other mechanical complication of other specified internal prosthetic devices, implants and grafts**
       Mechanical complication of nonabsorbable surgical material NOS
● **T85.7**   **Infection and inflammatory reaction due to other internal prosthetic devices, implants and grafts**
     Use additional code to identify infection
   X ● **T85.71**   **Infection and inflammatory reaction due to peritoneal dialysis catheter**
   X ● **T85.72**   **Infection and inflammatory reaction due to insulin pump**
   X ● **T85.79**   **Infection and inflammatory reaction due to other internal prosthetic devices, implants and grafts**

◀ New   ◀▦ Revised   ~~deleted~~ Deleted   OGCR Official Guidelines   X Assign placeholder X   ● Use Additional Character(s)

Excludes 1   Excludes 2   Includes   Use additional   Code first   Code also   Unspecified

● **T85.8**   **Other specified complications of internal prosthetic devices, implants and grafts, not elsewhere classified**

X ● **T85.81**   Embolism due to internal prosthetic devices, implants and grafts, not elsewhere classified

X ● **T85.82**   Fibrosis due to internal prosthetic devices, implants and grafts, not elsewhere classified

X ● **T85.83**   Hemorrhage due to internal prosthetic devices, implants and grafts, not elsewhere classified

X ● **T85.84**   Pain due to internal prosthetic devices, implants and grafts, not elsewhere classified

X ● **T85.85**   Stenosis due to internal prosthetic devices, implants and grafts, not elsewhere classified

X ● **T85.86**   Thrombosis due to internal prosthetic devices, implants and grafts, not elsewhere classified

X ● **T85.89**   Other specified complication of internal prosthetic devices, implants and grafts, not elsewhere classified

X ● **T85.9**   **Unspecified complication of internal prosthetic device, implant and graft**

> Complication of internal prosthetic device, implant and graft NOS

● **T86**   **Complications of transplanted organs and tissue**

> Use additional code to identify other transplant complications, such as:
> graft-versus-host disease (D89.81-)
> malignancy associated with organ transplant (C80.2)
> post-transplant lymphoproliferative disorders (PTLD) (D47.Z1)

● **T86.0**   **Complications of bone marrow transplant**

T86.00   Unspecified complication of bone marrow transplant

T86.01   Bone marrow transplant rejection

T86.02   Bone marrow transplant failure

T86.03   Bone marrow transplant infection

T86.09   Other complications of bone marrow transplant

● **T86.1**   **Complications of kidney transplant**

T86.10   Unspecified complication of kidney transplant

T86.11   Kidney transplant rejection

T86.12   Kidney transplant failure

T86.13   Kidney transplant infection

> Use additional code to specify infection

T86.19   Other complication of kidney transplant

● **T86.2**   **Complications of heart transplant**

> **Excludes1**   complication of:
> artificial heart device (T82.5)
> heart-lung transplant (T86.3)

T86.20   Unspecified complication of heart transplant

T86.21   Heart transplant rejection

T86.22   Heart transplant failure

T86.23   Heart transplant infection

> Use additional code to specify infection

● **T86.29**   Other complications of heart transplant

T86.290   Cardiac allograft vasculopathy

> **Excludes1**   atherosclerosis of coronary arteries (I25.75-, I25.76-, I25.81-)

T86.298   Other complications of heart transplant

● **T86.3**   **Complications of heart-lung transplant**

T86.30   Unspecified complication of heart-lung transplant

T86.31   Heart-lung transplant rejection

T86.32   Heart-lung transplant failure

T86.33   Heart-lung transplant infection

> Use additional code to specify infection

T86.39   Other complications of heart-lung transplant

● **T86.4**   **Complications of liver transplant**

T86.40   Unspecified complication of liver transplant

T86.41   Liver transplant rejection

T86.42   Liver transplant failure

T86.43   Liver transplant infection

> Use additional code to identify infection, such as:
> Cytomegalovirus (CMV) infection (B25.-)

T86.49   Other complications of liver transplant

● **T86.5**   **Complications of stem cell transplant**

> Complications from stem cells from peripheral blood
> Complications from stem cells from umbilical cord

● **T86.8**   **Complications of other transplanted organs and tissues**

● **T86.81**   Complications of lung transplant

> **Excludes1**   complication of heart-lung transplant (T86.3-)

T86.810   Lung transplant rejection

T86.811   Lung transplant failure

T86.812   Lung transplant infection

> Use additional code to specify infection

T86.818   Other complications of lung transplant

T86.819   Unspecified complication of lung transplant

● **T86.82**   Complications of skin graft (allograft) (autograft)

> **Excludes2**   complication of artificial skin graft (T85.693)

T86.820   Skin graft (allograft) rejection

T86.821   Skin graft (allograft) (autograft) failure

T86.822   Skin graft (allograft) (autograft) infection

> Use additional code to specify infection

T86.828   Other complications of skin graft (allograft) (autograft)

T86.829   Unspecified complication of skin graft (allograft) (autograft)

OGCR Section I.C.19.g.3.

Organ Transplant Complications

Transplant Complications

(a) Transplant complications other than kidney

Codes under category T86, Complications of transplanted organs and tissues, are for use for both complications and rejection of transplanted organs. A transplant complication code is only assigned if the complication affects the function of the transplanted organ. Two codes are required to fully describe a transplant complication: the appropriate code from category T86 and a secondary code that identifies the complication.

Pre-existing conditions or conditions that develop after the transplant are not coded as complications unless they affect the function of the transplanted organs.

See I.C.21 for transplant organ removal status

See I.C.2 for malignant neoplasm associated with transplanted organ.

CHAPTER 19 (S00-T88)

CHAPTER 19 (S00-T88)

● T86.83   Complications of bone graft
> **Excludes2**   mechanical complications of bone graft (T84.3-)

     T86.830   Bone graft rejection
     T86.831   Bone graft failure
     T86.832   Bone graft infection
> Use additional code to specify infection

     T86.838   Other complications of bone graft
     T86.839   Unspecified complication of bone graft

● T86.84   Complications of corneal transplant
> **Excludes2**   mechanical complications of corneal graft (T85.3-)

     T86.840   Corneal transplant rejection
     T86.841   Corneal transplant failure
     T86.842   Corneal transplant infection
> Use additional code to specify infection

     T86.848   Other complications of corneal transplant
     T86.849   Unspecified complication of corneal transplant

● T86.85   Complication of intestine transplant
     T86.850   Intestine transplant rejection
     T86.851   Intestine transplant failure
     T86.852   Intestine transplant infection
> Use additional code to specify infection

     T86.858   Other complications of intestine transplant
     T86.859   Unspecified complication of intestine transplant

● T86.89   Complications of other transplanted tissue
> Transplant failure or rejection of pancreas

     T86.890   Other transplanted tissue rejection
     T86.891   Other transplanted tissue failure
     T86.892   Other transplanted tissue infection
> Use additional code to specify infection

     T86.898   Other complications of other transplanted tissue
     T86.899   Unspecified complication of other transplanted tissue

● T86.9   Complication of unspecified transplanted organ and tissue
     T86.90   Unspecified complication of unspecified transplanted organ and tissue
     T86.91   Unspecified transplanted organ and tissue rejection
     T86.92   Unspecified transplanted organ and tissue failure
     T86.93   Unspecified transplanted organ and tissue infection
> Use additional code to specify infection

     T86.99   Other complications of unspecified transplanted organ and tissue

● T87   Complications peculiar to reattachment and amputation
● T87.0   Complications of reattached (part of) upper extremity
  ● T87.0X   Complications of reattached (part of) upper extremity
     T87.0X1   Complications of reattached (part of) right upper extremity
     T87.0X2   Complications of reattached (part of) left upper extremity
     T87.0X9   Complications of reattached (part of) unspecified upper extremity

● T87.1   Complications of reattached (part of) lower extremity
  ● T87.1X   Complications of reattached (part of) lower extremity
     T87.1X1   Complications of reattached (part of) right lower extremity
     T87.1X2   Complications of reattached (part of) left lower extremity
     T87.1X9   Complications of reattached (part of) unspecified lower extremity

T87.2   Complications of other reattached body part

● T87.3   Neuroma of amputation stump
     T87.30   Neuroma of amputation stump, unspecified extremity
     T87.31   Neuroma of amputation stump, right upper extremity
     T87.32   Neuroma of amputation stump, left upper extremity
     T87.33   Neuroma of amputation stump, right lower extremity
     T87.34   Neuroma of amputation stump, left lower extremity

● T87.4   Infection of amputation stump
     T87.40   Infection of amputation stump, unspecified extremity
     T87.41   Infection of amputation stump, right upper extremity
     T87.42   Infection of amputation stump, left upper extremity
     T87.43   Infection of amputation stump, right lower extremity
     T87.44   Infection of amputation stump, left lower extremity

● T87.5   Necrosis of amputation stump
     T87.50   Necrosis of amputation stump, unspecified extremity
     T87.51   Necrosis of amputation stump, right upper extremity
     T87.52   Necrosis of amputation stump, left upper extremity
     T87.53   Necrosis of amputation stump, right lower extremity
     T87.54   Necrosis of amputation stump, left lower extremity

● T87.8   Other complications of amputation stump
     T87.81   Dehiscence of amputation stump
     T87.89   Other complications of amputation stump
> Amputation stump contracture
> Amputation stump contracture of next proximal joint
> Amputation stump flexion
> Amputation stump edema
> Amputation stump hematoma
> **Excludes2**   phantom limb syndrome (G54.6-G54.7)

T87.9   Unspecified complications of amputation stump

◀ New   ◀▥ Revised   ~~deleted~~ Deleted   **OGCR** Official Guidelines   X Assign placeholder X   ● Use Additional Character(s)

Excludes 1   Excludes 2   Includes   Use additional   Code first   Code also   Unspecified

● **T88**   **Other complications of surgical and medical care, not elsewhere classified**

     Excludes2   complication following infusion, transfusion and therapeutic injection (T80.-)
           complication following procedure NEC (T81.-)
           complications of anesthesia in labor and delivery (O74.-)
           complications of anesthesia in pregnancy (O29.-)
           complications of anesthesia in puerperium (O89.-)
           complications of devices, implants and grafts (T82-T85)
           complications of obstetric surgery and procedure (O75.4)
           dermatitis due to drugs and medicaments (L23.3, L24.4, L25.1, L27.0-L27.1)
           poisoning and toxic effects of drugs and chemicals (T36-T65 with fifth or sixth character 1-4 or 6)
           specified complications classified elsewhere

     The appropriate 7th character is to be added to each code from category T88

       | | |
       A   initial encounter
       D   subsequent encounter
       S   sequela

X ● **T88.0**   **Infection following immunization**
      Sepsis following immunization

X ● **T88.1**   **Other complications following immunization, not elsewhere classified**
      Generalized vaccinia
      Rash following immunization

      Excludes1   vaccinia not from vaccine (B08.011)
      Excludes2   anaphylactic shock due to serum (T80.5-)
           other serum reactions (T80.6-)
           postimmunization arthropathy (M02.2)
           postimmunization encephalitis (G04.02)
           postimmunization fever (R50.83)

X ● **T88.2**   **Shock due to anesthesia**
      Use additional code for adverse effect, if applicable, to identify drug (T41.- with fifth or sixth character 5)

      Excludes1   complications of anesthesia (in):
           labor and delivery (O74.-)
           pregnancy (O29.-)
           puerperium (O89.-)
           postprocedural shock NOS (T81.1-)

X ● **T88.3**   **Malignant hyperthermia due to anesthesia**
      Use additional code for adverse effect, if applicable, to identify drug (T41.- with fifth or sixth character 5)

X ● **T88.4**   **Failed or difficult intubation**

X ● **T88.5**   **Other complications of anesthesia**
      Use additional code for adverse effect, if applicable, to identify drug (T41.- with fifth or sixth character 5)

X ● **T88.51**   **Hypothermia following anesthesia**

X ● **T88.52**   **Failed moderate sedation during procedure**
      Failed conscious sedation during procedure

      Excludes2   personal history of failed moderate sedation (Z92.83)

X ● **T88.59**   **Other complications of anesthesia**

X ● **T88.6**   **Anaphylactic reaction due to adverse effect of correct drug or medicament properly administered**
      Anaphylactic shock due to adverse effect of correct drug or medicament properly administered
      Anaphylactoid reaction NOS

      Use additional code for adverse effect, if applicable, to identify drug (T36-T50 with fifth or sixth character 5)

      Excludes1   anaphylactic reaction due to serum (T80.5-)
           anaphylactic shock or reaction due to adverse food reaction (T78.0-)

X ● **T88.7**   **Unspecified adverse effect of drug or medicament**
      Drug hypersensitivity NOS
      Drug reaction NOS

      Use additional code for adverse effect, if applicable, to identify drug (T36-T50 with fifth or sixth character 5)

      Excludes1   specified adverse effects of drugs and medicaments (A00-R94 and T80-T88.6, T88.8)

X ● **T88.8**   **Other specified complications of surgical and medical care, not elsewhere classified**
      Use additional code to identify the complication

X ● **T88.9**   **Complication of surgical and medical care, unspecified**

CHAPTER 19 (S00-T88)

OGCR See Section I.C.20.

CHAPTER 20

EXTERNAL CAUSES OF MORBIDITY (V00-Y99)

Note: This chapter permits the classification of environmental events and circumstances as the cause of injury, and other adverse effects. Where a code from this section is applicable, it is intended that it shall be used secondary to a code from another chapter of the Classification indicating the nature of the condition. Most often, the condition will be classifiable to Chapter 19, Injury, poisoning and certain other consequences of external causes (S00-T88). Other conditions that may be stated to be due to external causes are classified in Chapters I to XVIII. For these conditions, codes from Chapter 20 should be used to provide additional information as to the cause of the condition.

This chapter contains the following blocks:

V00-X58	Accidents
V00-V99	Transport accidents
V00-V09	Pedestrian injured in transport accident
V10-V19	Pedal cycle rider injured in transport accident
V20-V29	Motorcycle rider injured in transport accident
V30-V39	Occupant of three-wheeled motor vehicle injured in transport accident
V40-V49	Car occupant injured in transport accident
V50-V59	Occupant of pick-up truck or van injured in transport accident
V60-V69	Occupant of heavy transport vehicle injured in transport accident
V70-V79	Bus occupant injured in transport accident
V80-V89	Other land transport accidents
V90-V94	Water transport accidents
V95-V97	Air and space transport accidents
V98-V99	Other and unspecified transport accidents
W00-X58	Other external causes of accidental injury
W00-W19	Slipping, tripping, stumbling and falls
W20-W49	Exposure to inanimate mechanical forces
W50-W64	Exposure to animate mechanical forces
W65-W74	Accidental non-transport drowning and submersion
W85-W99	Exposure to electric current, radiation and extreme ambient air temperature and pressure
X00-X08	Exposure to smoke, fire and flames
X10-X19	Contact with heat and hot substances
X30-X39	Exposure to forces of nature
X52, X58	Accidental exposure to other specified factors
X71-X83	Intentional self-harm
X92-Y08	Assault
Y21-Y33	Event of undetermined intent
Y35-Y38	Legal intervention, operations of war, military operations, and terrorism
Y62-Y84	Complications of medical and surgical care
Y62-Y69	Misadventures to patients during surgical and medical care
Y70-Y82	Medical devices associated with adverse incidents in diagnostic and therapeutic use
Y83-Y84	Surgical and other medical procedures as the cause of abnormal reaction of the patient, or of later complication, without mention of misadventure at the time of the procedure
Y90-Y99	Supplementary factors related to causes of morbidity classified elsewhere

ACCIDENTS (V00-X58)

TRANSPORT ACCIDENTS (V00-V99)

Note: This section is structured in 12 groups. Those relating to land transport accidents (V01-V89) reflect the victim's mode of transport and are subdivided to identify the victim's 'counterpart' or the type of event. The vehicle of which the injured person is an occupant is identified in the first two characters since it is seen as the most important factor to identify for prevention purposes. A transport accident is one in which the vehicle involved must be moving or running or in use for transport purposes at the time of the accident.

Use additional code to identify:
Airbag injury (W22.1)
Type of street or road (Y92.4-)
Use of cellular telephone and other electronic equipment at the time of the transport accident (Y93.C-)

Excludes1 agricultural vehicles in stationary use or maintenance (W31.-)
assault by crashing of motor vehicle (Y03.-)
automobile or motor cycle in stationary use or maintenance - code to type of accident
crashing of motor vehicle, undetermined intent (Y32)
intentional self-harm by crashing of motor vehicle (X82)

Excludes2 transport accidents due to cataclysm (X34-X38)

Note: Definitions of transport vehicles:

(a) A transport accident is any accident involving a device designed primarily for, or used at the time primarily for, conveying persons or good from one place to another.

(b) A public highway [trafficway] or street is the entire width between property lines (or other boundary lines) of land open to the public as a matter of right or custom for purposes of moving persons or property from one place to another. A roadway is that part of the public highway designed, improved and customarily used for vehicular traffic.

(c) A traffic accident is any vehicle accident occurring on the public highway [i.e., originating on, terminating on, or involving a vehicle partially on the highway]. A vehicle accident is assumed to have occurred on the public highway unless another place is specified, except in the case of accidents involving only off-road motor vehicles, which are classified as nontraffic accidents unless the contrary is stated.

(d) A nontraffic accident is any vehicle accident that occurs entirely in any place other than a public highway.

(e) A pedestrian is any person involved in an accident who was not at the time of the accident riding in or on a motor vehicle, railway train, streetcar or animal-drawn or other vehicle, or on a pedal cycle or animal. This includes, a person changing a tire or working on a parked car. It also includes the use of a pedestrian conveyance such as a baby carriage, ice-skates, roller skates, a skateboard, nonmotorized or motorized wheelchair, motorized mobility scooter, or nonmotorized scooter.

(f) A driver is an occupant of a transport vehicle who is operating or intending to operate it.

(g) A passenger is any occupant of a transport vehicle other than the driver, except a person traveling on the outside of the vehicle.

(h) A person on the outside of a vehicle is any person being transported by a vehicle but not occupying the space normally reserved for the driver or passengers, or the space intended for the transport of property. This includes the body, bumper, fender, roof, running board or step of a vehicle.

◀ New ◀▥▥ Revised ~~deleted~~ Deleted **OGCR** Official Guidelines X Assign placeholder X ● Use Additional Character(s)

| Excludes 1 | Excludes 2 | Includes | Use additional | Code first | Code also | Unspecified |

(i)   A pedal cycle is any land transport vehicle operated solely by nonmotorized pedals including a bicycle or tricycle.

(j)   A pedal cyclist is any person riding a pedal cycle or in a sidecar or trailer attached to a pedal cycle.

(k)   A motorcycle is a two-wheeled motor vehicle with one or two riding saddles and sometimes with a third wheel for the support of a sidecar. The sidecar is considered part of the motorcycle.

(l)   A motorcycle rider is any person riding a motorcycle or in a sidecar or trailer attached to the motorcycle.

(m)   A three-wheeled motor vehicle is a motorized tricycle designed primarily for on-road use. This includes a motor-driven tricycle, a motorized rickshaw, or a three-wheeled motor car.

(n)   A car [automobile] is a four-wheeled motor vehicle designed primarily for carrying up to 7 persons. A trailer being towed by the car is considered part of the car.

(o)   A pick-up truck or van is a four or six-wheeled motor vehicle designed for carrying passengers as well as property or cargo weighing less than the local limit for classification as a heavy goods vehicle, and not requiring a special driver's license. This includes a minivan and a sport-utility vehicle (SUV).

(p)   A heavy transport vehicle is a motor vehicle designed primarily for carrying property, meeting local criteria for classification as a heavy goods vehicle in terms of weight and requiring a special driver's license.

(q)   A bus (coach) is a motor vehicle designed or adapted primarily for carrying more than 10 passengers, and requiring a special driver's license.

(r)   A railway train or railway vehicle is any device, with or without freight or passenger cars coupled to it, designed for traffic on a railway track. This includes subterranean (subways) or elevated trains.

(s)   A streetcar is a device designed and used primarily for transporting passengers within a municipality, running on rails, usually subject to normal traffic control signals, and operated principally on a right-of-way that forms part of the roadway. This includes a tram or trolley that runs on rails. A trailer being towed by a streetcar is considered part of the streetcar.

(t)   A special vehicle mainly used on industrial premises is a motor vehicle designed primarily for use within the buildings and premises of industrial or commercial establishments. This includes battery-powered trucks, forklifts, coal-cars in a coal mine, logging cars and trucks used in mines or quarries.

(u)   A special vehicle mainly used in agriculture is a motor vehicle designed specifically for use in farming and agriculture (horticulture), to work the land, tend and harvest crops and transport materials on the farm. This includes harvesters, farm machinery and tractor and trailers.

(v)   A special construction vehicle is a motor vehicle designed specifically for use on construction and demolition sites. This includes bulldozers, diggers, earth levellers, dump trucks, backhoes, front-end loaders, pavers, and mechanical shovels.

(w)   A special all-terrain vehicle is a motor vehicle of special design to enable it to negotiate over rough or soft terrain, snow or sand. This includes snow mobiles, all-terrain vehicles (ATV), and dune buggies. It does not include passenger vehicle designated as sport utility vehicles (SUV).

(x)   A watercraft is any device designed for transporting passengers or goods on water. This includes motor or sail boats, ships, and hovercraft.

(y)   An aircraft is any device for transporting passengers or goods in the air. This includes hot-air balloons, gliders, helicopters and airplanes.

(z)   A military vehicle is any motorized vehicle operating on a public roadway owned by the military and being operated by a member of the military.

PEDESTRIAN INJURED IN TRANSPORT ACCIDENT (V00-V09)

Includes   person changing tire on transport vehicle
     person examining engine of vehicle broken down in (on side of) road

Excludes1   fall due to non-transport collision with other person (W03)
     pedestrian on foot falling (slipping) on ice and snow (W00.-)
     struck or bumped by another person (W51)

● **V00   Pedestrian conveyance accident**

<u>Use additional</u> place of occurrence and activity external cause codes, if known (Y92.-, Y93.-)

Excludes1   collision with another person without fall (W51)
     fall due to person on foot colliding with another person on foot (W03)
     fall from non-moving wheelchair, nonmotorized scooter and motorized mobility scooter without collision (W05.-)
     pedestrian (conveyance) collision with other land transport vehicle (V01-V09)
     pedestrian on foot falling (slipping) on ice and snow (W00.-)

The appropriate 7th character is to be added to each code from category V00

A	initial encounter
D	subsequent encounter
S	sequela

● **V00.0   Pedestrian on foot injured in collision with pedestrian conveyance**

   X ● **V00.01   Pedestrian on foot injured in collision with roller-skater**

   X ● **V00.02   Pedestrian on foot injured in collision with skateboarder**

   X ● **V00.09   Pedestrian on foot injured in collision with other pedestrian conveyance**

● **V00.1   Rolling-type pedestrian conveyance accident**

   Excludes1   accident with babystroller (V00.82-)
       accident with wheelchair (powered) (V00.81-)
       accident with motorized mobility scooter (V00.83-)

   ● **V00.11   In-line roller-skate accident**

     ● **V00.111   Fall from in-line roller-skates**

     ● **V00.112   In-line roller-skater colliding with stationary object**

     ● **V00.118   Other in-line roller-skate accident**

       Excludes1   roller-skater collision with other land transport vehicle (V01-V09 with 5th character 1)

   ● **V00.12   Non-in-line roller-skate accident**

     ● **V00.121   Fall from non-in-line roller-skates**

     ● **V00.122   Non-in-line roller-skater colliding with stationary object**

     ● **V00.128   Other non-in-line roller-skating accident**

       Excludes1   roller-skater collision with other land transport vehicle (V01-V09 with 5th character 1)

● **V00.13   Skateboard accident**
  ● V00.131   Fall from skateboard
  ● V00.132   Skateboarder colliding with
               stationary object
  ● V00.138   Other skateboard accident
               | **Excludes1** | skateboarder collision
               with other land
               transport vehicle
               (V01-V09 with
               5th character 2) |

● **V00.14   Scooter (nonmotorized) accident**
             | **Excludes1** | motorscooter accident (V20-V29) |
  ● V00.141   Fall from scooter (nonmotorized)
  ● V00.142   Scooter (nonmotorized) colliding
               with stationary object
  ● V00.148   Other scooter (nonmotorized)
               accident
               | **Excludes1** | scooter (non-
               motorized)
               collision with
               other land
               transport vehicle
               (V01-V09 with
               fifth character 9) |

● **V00.15   Heelies accident**
             Rolling shoe
             Wheeled shoe
             Wheelies accident
  ● V00.151   Fall from heelies
  ● V00.152   Heelies colliding with stationary
               object
  ● V00.158   Other heelies accident

● **V00.18   Accident on other rolling-type pedestrian
             conveyance**
  ● V00.181   Fall from other rolling-type
               pedestrian conveyance
  ● V00.182   Pedestrian on other rolling-type
               pedestrian conveyance colliding with
               stationary object
  ● V00.188   Other accident on other rolling-type
               pedestrian conveyance

● **V00.2   Gliding-type pedestrian conveyance accident**
  ● **V00.21   Ice-skates accident**
    ● V00.211   Fall from ice-skates
    ● V00.212   Ice-skater colliding with stationary
                 object
    ● V00.218   Other ice-skates accident
                 | **Excludes1** | ice-skater collision
                 with other land
                 transport vehicle
                 (V01-V09 with
                 5th digit 9) |

  ● **V00.22   Sled accident**
    ● V00.221   Fall from sled
    ● V00.222   Sledder colliding with stationary
                 object
    ● V00.228   Other sled accident
                 | **Excludes1** | sled collision with
                 other land
                 transport vehicle
                 (V01-V09 with
                 5th digit 9) |

● **V00.28   Other gliding-type pedestrian conveyance
             accident**
  ● V00.281   Fall from other gliding-type
               pedestrian conveyance
  ● V00.282   Pedestrian on other gliding-type
               pedestrian conveyance colliding with
               stationary object
  ● V00.288   Other accident on other gliding-type
               pedestrian conveyance
               | **Excludes1** | gliding-type
               pedestrian
               conveyance
               collision with
               other land
               transport vehicle
               (V01-V09 with
               5th digit 9) |

● **V00.3   Flat-bottomed pedestrian conveyance accident**
  ● **V00.31   Snowboard accident**
    ● V00.311   Fall from snowboard
    ● V00.312   Snowboarder colliding with
                 stationary object
    ● V00.318   Other snowboard accident
                 | **Excludes1** | snowboarder collision
                 with other land
                 transport vehicle
                 (V01-V09 with
                 5th digit 9) |

  ● **V00.32   Snow-ski accident**
    ● V00.321   Fall from snow-skis
    ● V00.322   Snow-skier colliding with stationary
                 object
    ● V00.328   Other snow-ski accident
                 | **Excludes1** | snow-skier collision
                 with other land
                 transport vehicle
                 (V01-V09 with
                 5th digit 9) |

  ● **V00.38   Other flat-bottomed pedestrian conveyance
               accident**
    ● V00.381   Fall from other flat-bottomed
                 pedestrian conveyance
    ● V00.382   Pedestrian on other flat-bottomed
                 pedestrian conveyance colliding with
                 stationary object
    ● V00.388   Other accident on other flat-bottomed
                 pedestrian conveyance

● **V00.8   Accident on other pedestrian conveyance**
  ● **V00.81   Accident with wheelchair (powered)**
    ● V00.811   Fall from moving wheelchair
                 (powered)
                 | **Excludes1** | fall from non-moving
                 wheelchair
                 (W05.0) |
    ● V00.812   Wheelchair (powered) colliding with
                 stationary object
    ● V00.818   Other accident with wheelchair
                 (powered)
  ● **V00.82   Accident with babystroller**
    ● V00.821   Fall from babystroller
    ● V00.822   Babystroller colliding with stationary
                 object
    ● V00.828   Other accident with babystroller

● **V00.83   Accident with motorized mobility scooter**

   ● **V00.831   Fall from motorized mobility scooter**

       Excludes1   fall from non-moving motorized mobility scooter (W05.2)

   ● **V00.832   Motorized mobility scooter colliding with stationary object**

   ● **V00.838   Other accident with motorized mobility scooter**

● **V00.89   Accident on other pedestrian conveyance**

   ● **V00.891   Fall from other pedestrian conveyance**

   ● **V00.892   Pedestrian on other pedestrian conveyance colliding with stationary object**

   ● **V00.898   Other accident on other pedestrian conveyance**

       Excludes1   other pedestrian (conveyance) collision with other land transport vehicle (V01-V09 with 5th digit 9)

● **V01   Pedestrian injured in collision with pedal cycle**

The appropriate 7th character is to be added to each code from category V01

A	initial encounter
D	subsequent encounter
S	sequela

● **V01.0   Pedestrian injured in collision with pedal cycle in nontraffic accident**

   X● **V01.00   Pedestrian on foot injured in collision with pedal cycle in nontraffic accident**

       Pedestrian NOS injured in collision with pedal cycle in nontraffic accident

   X● **V01.01   Pedestrian on roller-skates injured in collision with pedal cycle in nontraffic accident**

   X● **V01.02   Pedestrian on skateboard injured in collision with pedal cycle in nontraffic accident**

   X● **V01.09   Pedestrian with other conveyance injured in collision with pedal cycle in nontraffic accident**

       Pedestrian with babystroller injured in collision with pedal cycle in nontraffic accident

       Pedestrian in wheelchair (powered) injured in collision with pedal cycle in nontraffic accident

       Pedestrian in motorized mobility scooter injured in collision with pedal cycle in nontraffic accident

       Pedestrian on ice-skates injured in collision with pedal cycle in nontraffic accident

       Pedestrian on nonmotorized scooter injured in collision with pedal cycle in nontraffic accident

       Pedestrian on sled injured in collision with pedal cycle in nontraffic accident

       Pedestrian on snowboard injured in collision with pedal cycle in nontraffic accident

       Pedestrian on snow-skis injured in collision with pedal cycle in nontraffic accident

● **V01.1   Pedestrian injured in collision with pedal cycle in traffic accident**

   X● **V01.10   Pedestrian on foot injured in collision with pedal cycle in traffic accident**

       Pedestrian NOS injured in collision with pedal cycle in traffic accident

   X● **V01.11   Pedestrian on roller-skates injured in collision with pedal cycle in traffic accident**

   X● **V01.12   Pedestrian on skateboard injured in collision with pedal cycle in traffic accident**

   X● **V01.19   Pedestrian with other conveyance injured in collision with pedal cycle in traffic accident**

       Pedestrian with babystroller injured in collision with pedal cycle in traffic accident

       Pedestrian in wheelchair (powered) injured in collision with pedal cycle in traffic accident

       Pedestrian in motorized mobility scooter injured in collision with pedal cycle in traffic accident

       Pedestrian on ice-skates injured in collision with pedal cycle in traffic accident

       Pedestrian on nonmotorized scooter injured in collision with pedal cycle in traffic accident

       Pedestrian on sled injured in collision with pedal cycle in traffic accident

       Pedestrian on snowboard injured in collision with pedal cycle in traffic accident

       Pedestrian on snow-skis injured in collision with pedal cycle in traffic accident

● **V01.9   Pedestrian injured in collision with pedal cycle, unspecified whether traffic or nontraffic accident**

   X● **V01.90   Pedestrian on foot injured in collision with pedal cycle, unspecified whether traffic or nontraffic accident**

       Pedestrian NOS injured in collision with pedal cycle, unspecified whether traffic or nontraffic accident

   X● **V01.91   Pedestrian on roller-skates injured in collision with pedal cycle, unspecified whether traffic or nontraffic accident**

   X● **V01.92   Pedestrian on skateboard injured in collision with pedal cycle, unspecified whether traffic or nontraffic accident**

   X● **V01.99   Pedestrian with other conveyance injured in collision with pedal cycle, unspecified whether traffic or nontraffic accident**

       Pedestrian with babystroller injured in collision with pedal cycle, unspecified whether traffic or nontraffic accident

       Pedestrian in wheelchair (powered) injured in collision with pedal cycle, unspecified whether traffic or nontraffic accident

       Pedestrian in motorized mobility scooter injured in collision with pedal cycle, unspecified whether traffic or nontraffic accident

       Pedestrian on ice-skates injured in collision with pedal cycle unspecified, whether traffic or nontraffic accident

       Pedestrian on nonmotorized scooter injured in collision with pedal cycle, unspecified whether traffic or nontraffic accident

       Pedestrian on sled injured in collision with pedal cycle unspecified, whether traffic or nontraffic accident

       Pedestrian on snowboard injured in collision with pedal cycle, unspecified whether traffic or nontraffic accident

       Pedestrian on snow-skis injured in collision with pedal cycle, unspecified whether traffic or nontraffic accident

---

◄ New   ⬅ Revised   ~~deleted~~ Deleted   **OGCR** Official Guidelines   X Assign placeholder X   ● Use Additional Character(s)

Excludes 1   Excludes 2   Includes   Use additional   Code first   Code also   Unspecified

● **V02　Pedestrian injured in collision with two- or three-wheeled motor vehicle**

The appropriate 7th character is to be added to each code from category V02

> A　initial encounter
> D　subsequent encounter
> S　sequela

● **V02.0　Pedestrian injured in collision with two- or three-wheeled motor vehicle in nontraffic accident**

X● **V02.00　Pedestrian on foot injured in collision with two- or three-wheeled motor vehicle in nontraffic accident**

Pedestrian NOS injured in collision with two- or three-wheeled motor vehicle in nontraffic accident

X● **V02.01　Pedestrian on roller-skates injured in collision with two- or three-wheeled motor vehicle in nontraffic accident**

X● **V02.02　Pedestrian on skateboard injured in collision with two- or three-wheeled motor vehicle in nontraffic accident**

X● **V02.09　Pedestrian with other conveyance injured in collision with two- or three-wheeled motor vehicle in nontraffic accident**

Pedestrian with babystroller injured in collision with two- or three-wheeled motor vehicle in nontraffic accident

Pedestrian on ice-skates injured in collision with two- or three-wheeled motor vehicle in nontraffic accident

Pedestrian in wheelchair (powered) injured in collision with two- or three-wheeled motor vehicle in nontraffic accident

Pedestrian in motorized mobility scooter injured in collision with two- or three-wheeled motor vehicle in nontraffic accident

Pedestrian on nonmotorized scooter injured in collision with two- or three-wheeled motor vehicle in nontraffic accident

Pedestrian on sled injured in collision with two- or three-wheeled motor vehicle in nontraffic accident

Pedestrian on snowboard injured in collision with two- or three-wheeled motor vehicle in nontraffic accident

Pedestrian on snow-skis injured in collision with two- or three-wheeled motor vehicle in nontraffic accident

● **V02.1　Pedestrian injured in collision with two- or three-wheeled motor vehicle in traffic accident**

X● **V02.10　Pedestrian on foot injured in collision with two- or three-wheeled motor vehicle in traffic accident**

Pedestrian NOS injured in collision with two- or three-wheeled motor vehicle in traffic accident

X● **V02.11　Pedestrian on roller-skates injured in collision with two- or three-wheeled motor vehicle in traffic accident**

X● **V02.12　Pedestrian on skateboard injured in collision with two- or three-wheeled motor vehicle in traffic accident**

X● **V02.19　Pedestrian with other conveyance injured in collision with two- or three-wheeled motor vehicle in traffic accident**

Pedestrian with babystroller injured in collision with two- or three-wheeled motor vehicle in traffic accident

Pedestrian in wheelchair (powered) injured in collision with two- or three-wheeled motor vehicle in traffic accident

Pedestrian in motorized mobility scooter injured in collision with two- or three-wheeled motor vehicle in traffic accident

Pedestrian on ice-skates injured in collision with two- or three-wheeled motor vehicle in traffic accident

Pedestrian on nonmotorized scooter injured in collision with two- or three-wheeled motor vehicle in traffic accident

Pedestrian on sled injured in collision with two- or three-wheeled motor vehicle in traffic accident

Pedestrian on snowboard injured in collision with two- or three-wheeled motor vehicle in traffic accident

Pedestrian on snow-skis injured in collision with two- or three-wheeled motor vehicle in traffic accident

● **V02.9　Pedestrian injured in collision with two- or three-wheeled motor vehicle, unspecified whether traffic or nontraffic accident**

X● **V02.90　Pedestrian on foot injured in collision with two- or three-wheeled motor vehicle, unspecified whether traffic or nontraffic accident**

Pedestrian NOS injured in collision with two- or three-wheeled motor vehicle, unspecified whether traffic or nontraffic accident

X● **V02.91　Pedestrian on roller-skates injured in collision with two- or three-wheeled motor vehicle, unspecified whether traffic or nontraffic accident**

X● **V02.92　Pedestrian on skateboard injured in collision with two- or three-wheeled motor vehicle, unspecified whether traffic or nontraffic accident**

X● **V02.99　Pedestrian with other conveyance injured in collision with two- or three-wheeled motor vehicle, unspecified whether traffic or nontraffic accident**

Pedestrian with babystroller injured in collision with two- or three-wheeled motor vehicle, unspecified whether traffic or nontraffic accident

Pedestrian in wheelchair (powered) injured in collision with two- or three-wheeled motor vehicle, unspecified whether traffic or nontraffic accident

Pedestrian in motorized mobility scooter injured in collision with two- or three-wheeled motor vehicle, unspecified whether traffic or nontraffic accident

Pedestrian on ice-skates injured in collision with two- or three-wheeled motor vehicle, unspecified whether traffic or nontraffic accident

Pedestrian on nonmotorized scooter injured in collision with two- or three-wheeled motor vehicle, unspecified whether traffic or nontraffic accident

Pedestrian on sled injured in collision with two- or three-wheeled motor vehicle, unspecified whether traffic or nontraffic accident

Pedestrian on snowboard injured in collision with two- or three-wheeled motor vehicle, unspecified whether traffic or nontraffic accident

Pedestrian on snow-skis injured in collision with two- or three-wheeled motor vehicle, unspecified whether traffic or nontraffic accident

● **V03 Pedestrian injured in collision with car, pick-up truck or van**

The appropriate 7th character is to be added to each code from category V03

A initial encounter
D subsequent encounter
S sequela

● **V03.0 Pedestrian injured in collision with car, pick-up truck or van in nontraffic accident**

X● **V03.00 Pedestrian on foot injured in collision with car, pick-up truck or van in nontraffic accident**
Pedestrian NOS injured in collision with car, pick-up truck or van in nontraffic accident

X● **V03.01 Pedestrian on roller-skates injured in collision with car, pick-up truck or van in nontraffic accident**

X● **V03.02 Pedestrian on skateboard injured in collision with car, pick-up truck or van in nontraffic accident**

X● **V03.09 Pedestrian with other conveyance injured in collision with car, pick-up truck or van in nontraffic accident**
Pedestrian with babystroller injured in collision with car, pick-up truck or van in nontraffic accident
Pedestrian in wheelchair (powered) injured in collision with car, pick-up truck or van in nontraffic accident
Pedestrian in motorized mobility scooter injured in collision with car, pick-up truck or van in nontraffic accident
Pedestrian on ice-skates injured in collision with car, pick-up truck or van in nontraffic accident
Pedestrian on nonmotorized scooter injured in collision with car, pick-up truck or van in nontraffic accident
Pedestrian on sled injured in collision with car, pick-up truck or van in nontraffic accident
Pedestrian on snowboard injured in collision with car, pick-up truck or van in nontraffic accident
Pedestrian on snow-skis injured in collision with car, pick-up truck or van in nontraffic accident

● **V03.1 Pedestrian injured in collision with car, pick-up truck or van in traffic accident**

X● **V03.10 Pedestrian on foot injured in collision with car, pick-up truck or van in traffic accident**
Pedestrian NOS injured in collision with car, pick-up truck or van in traffic accident

X● **V03.11 Pedestrian on roller-skates injured in collision with car, pick-up truck or van in traffic accident**

X● **V03.12 Pedestrian on skateboard injured in collision with car, pick-up truck or van in traffic accident**

X● **V03.19 Pedestrian with other conveyance injured in collision with car, pick-up truck or van in traffic accident**
Pedestrian with babystroller injured in collision with car, pick-up truck or van in traffic accident
Pedestrian in wheelchair (powered) injured in collision with car, pick-up truck or van in traffic accident
Pedestrian in motorized mobility scooter injured in collision with car, pick-up truck or van in traffic accident
Pedestrian on ice-skates injured in collision with car, pick-up truck or van in traffic accident
Pedestrian on nonmotorized scooter injured in collision with car, pick-up truck or van in traffic accident
Pedestrian on sled injured in collision with car, pick-up truck or van in traffic accident
Pedestrian on snowboard injured in collision with car, pick-up truck or van in traffic accident
Pedestrian on snow-skis injured in collision with car, pick-up truck or van in traffic accident

● **V03.9 Pedestrian injured in collision with car, pick-up truck or van, unspecified whether traffic or nontraffic accident**

X● **V03.90 Pedestrian on foot injured in collision with car, pick-up truck or van, unspecified whether traffic or nontraffic accident**
Pedestrian NOS injured in collision with car, pick-up truck or van, unspecified whether traffic or nontraffic accident

X● **V03.91 Pedestrian on roller-skates injured in collision with car, pick-up truck or van, unspecified whether traffic or nontraffic accident**

X● **V03.92 Pedestrian on skateboard injured in collision with car, pick-up truck or van, unspecified whether traffic or nontraffic accident**

X● **V03.99 Pedestrian with other conveyance injured in collision with car, pick-up truck or van, unspecified whether traffic or nontraffic accident**
Pedestrian with babystroller injured in collision with car, pick-up truck or van, unspecified whether traffic or nontraffic accident
Pedestrian in wheelchair (powered) injured in collision with car, pick-up truck or van, unspecified whether traffic or nontraffic accident
Pedestrian in motorized mobility scooter injured in collision with car, pick-up truck or van, unspecified whether traffic or nontraffic accident
Pedestrian on ice-skates injured in collision with car, pick-up truck or van, unspecified whether traffic or nontraffic accident
Pedestrian on nonmotorized scooter injured in collision with car, pick-up truck or van, unspecified whether traffic or nontraffic accident
Pedestrian on sled injured in collision with car, pick-up truck or van in nontraffic accident
Pedestrian on snowboard injured in collision with car, pick-up truck or van, unspecified whether traffic or nontraffic accident
Pedestrian on snow-skis injured in collision with car, pick-up truck or van, unspecified whether traffic or nontraffic accident

CHAPTER 20 (V01-Y99)

◄ New ◄▮▮ Revised deleted Deleted OGCR Official Guidelines X Assign placeholder X ● Use Additional Character(s)
Excludes 1 Excludes 2 Includes Use additional Code first Code also Unspecified

1461

● **V04 Pedestrian injured in collision with heavy transport vehicle or bus**

> **Excludes1** pedestrian injured in collision with military vehicle (V09.01, V09.21)

The appropriate 7th character is to be added to each code from category V04

> A initial encounter
> D subsequent encounter
> S sequela

● **V04.0 Pedestrian injured in collision with heavy transport vehicle or bus in nontraffic accident**

X● **V04.00 Pedestrian on foot injured in collision with heavy transport vehicle or bus in nontraffic accident**
> Pedestrian NOS injured in collision with heavy transport vehicle or bus in nontraffic accident

X● **V04.01 Pedestrian on roller-skates injured in collision with heavy transport vehicle or bus in nontraffic accident**

X● **V04.02 Pedestrian on skateboard injured in collision with heavy transport vehicle or bus in nontraffic accident**

X● **V04.09 Pedestrian with other conveyance injured in collision with heavy transport vehicle or bus in nontraffic accident**
> Pedestrian with babystroller injured in collision with heavy transport vehicle or bus in nontraffic accident
> Pedestrian in wheelchair (powered) injured in collision with heavy transport vehicle or bus in nontraffic accident
> Pedestrian in motorized mobility scooter injured in collision with heavy transport vehicle or bus in nontraffic accident
> Pedestrian on ice-skates injured in collision with heavy transport vehicle or bus in nontraffic accident
> Pedestrian on nonmotorized scooter injured in collision with heavy transport vehicle or bus in nontraffic accident
> Pedestrian on sled injured in collision with heavy transport vehicle or bus in nontraffic accident
> Pedestrian on snowboard injured in collision with heavy transport vehicle or bus in nontraffic accident
> Pedestrian on snow-skis injured in collision with heavy transport vehicle or bus in nontraffic accident

● **V04.1 Pedestrian injured in collision with heavy transport vehicle or bus in traffic accident**

X● **V04.10 Pedestrian on foot injured in collision with heavy transport vehicle or bus in traffic accident**
> Pedestrian NOS injured in collision with heavy transport vehicle or bus in traffic accident

X● **V04.11 Pedestrian on roller-skates injured in collision with heavy transport vehicle or bus in traffic accident**

X● **V04.12 Pedestrian on skateboard injured in collision with heavy transport vehicle or bus in traffic accident**

X● **V04.19 Pedestrian with other conveyance injured in collision with heavy transport vehicle or bus in traffic accident**
> Pedestrian with babystroller injured in collision with heavy transport vehicle or bus in traffic accident
> Pedestrian in wheelchair (powered) injured in collision with heavy transport vehicle or bus in traffic accident
> Pedestrian in motorized mobility scooter injured in collision with heavy transport vehicle or bus in traffic accident
> Pedestrian on ice-skates injured in collision with heavy transport vehicle or bus in traffic accident
> Pedestrian on nonmotorized scooter injured in collision with heavy transport vehicle or bus in traffic accident
> Pedestrian on sled injured in collision with heavy transport vehicle or bus in traffic accident
> Pedestrian on snowboard injured in collision with heavy transport vehicle or bus in traffic accident
> Pedestrian on snow-skis injured in collision with heavy transport vehicle or bus in traffic accident

● **V04.9 Pedestrian injured in collision with heavy transport vehicle or bus, unspecified whether traffic or nontraffic accident**

X● **V04.90 Pedestrian on foot injured in collision with heavy transport vehicle or bus, unspecified whether traffic or nontraffic accident**
> Pedestrian NOS injured in collision with heavy transport vehicle or bus, unspecified whether traffic or nontraffic accident

X● **V04.91 Pedestrian on roller-skates injured in collision with heavy transport vehicle or bus, unspecified whether traffic or nontraffic accident**

X● **V04.92 Pedestrian on skateboard injured in collision with heavy transport vehicle or bus, unspecified whether traffic or nontraffic accident**

X● **V04.99 Pedestrian with other conveyance injured in collision with heavy transport vehicle or bus, unspecified whether traffic or nontraffic accident**
> Pedestrian with babystroller injured in collision with heavy transport vehicle or bus, unspecified whether traffic or nontraffic accident
> Pedestrian in wheelchair (powered) injured in collision with heavy transport vehicle or bus, unspecified whether traffic or nontraffic accident
> Pedestrian in motorized mobility scooter injured in collision with heavy transport vehicle or bus, unspecified whether traffic or nontraffic accident
> Pedestrian on ice-skates injured in collision with heavy transport vehicle or bus, unspecified whether traffic or nontraffic accident
> Pedestrian on nonmotorized scooter injured in collision with heavy transport vehicle or bus, unspecified whether traffic or nontraffic accident
> Pedestrian on sled injured in collision with heavy transport vehicle or bus, unspecified whether traffic or nontraffic accident
> Pedestrian on snowboard injured in collision with heavy transport vehicle or bus, unspecified whether traffic or nontraffic accident
> Pedestrian on snow-skis injured in collision with heavy transport vehicle or bus, unspecified whether traffic or nontraffic accident

◀ New ◀ Revised ~~deleted~~ Deleted OGCR Official Guidelines X Assign placeholder X ● Use Additional Character(s)
1462
Excludes 1 Excludes 2 Includes Use additional Code first Code also Unspecified

● **V05   Pedestrian injured in collision with railway train or railway vehicle**

> The appropriate 7th character is to be added to each code from category V05

> | | |
> |---|---|
> | A | initial encounter |
> | D | subsequent encounter |
> | S | sequela |

● **V05.0   Pedestrian injured in collision with railway train or railway vehicle in nontraffic accident**

X ● **V05.00   Pedestrian on foot injured in collision with railway train or railway vehicle in nontraffic accident**
> Pedestrian NOS injured in collision with railway train or railway vehicle in nontraffic accident

X ● **V05.01   Pedestrian on roller-skates injured in collision with railway train or railway vehicle in nontraffic accident**

X ● **V05.02   Pedestrian on skateboard injured in collision with railway train or railway vehicle in nontraffic accident**

X ● **V05.09   Pedestrian with other conveyance injured in collision with railway train or railway vehicle in nontraffic accident**
> Pedestrian with babystroller injured in collision with railway train or railway vehicle in nontraffic accident
> Pedestrian in wheelchair (powered) injured in collision with railway train or railway vehicle in nontraffic accident
> Pedestrian in motorized mobility scooter injured in collision with railway train or railway vehicle in nontraffic accident
> Pedestrian on ice-skates injured in collision with railway train or railway vehicle in nontraffic accident
> Pedestrian on nonmotorized scooter injured in collision with railway train or railway vehicle in nontraffic accident
> Pedestrian on sled injured in collision with railway train or railway vehicle in nontraffic accident
> Pedestrian on snowboard injured in collision with railway train or railway vehicle in nontraffic accident
> Pedestrian on snow-skis injured in collision with railway train or railway vehicle in nontraffic accident

● **V05.1   Pedestrian injured in collision with railway train or railway vehicle in traffic accident**

X ● **V05.10   Pedestrian on foot injured in collision with railway train or railway vehicle in traffic accident**
> Pedestrian NOS injured in collision with railway train or railway vehicle in traffic accident

X ● **V05.11   Pedestrian on roller-skates injured in collision with railway train or railway vehicle in traffic accident**

X ● **V05.12   Pedestrian on skateboard injured in collision with railway train or railway vehicle in traffic accident**

X ● **V05.19   Pedestrian with other conveyance injured in collision with railway train or railway vehicle in traffic accident**
> Pedestrian with babystroller injured in collision with railway train or railway vehicle in traffic accident
> Pedestrian in wheelchair (powered) injured in collision with railway train or railway vehicle in traffic accident
> Pedestrian in motorized mobility scooter injured in collision with railway train or railway vehicle in traffic accident
> Pedestrian on ice-skates injured in collision with railway train or railway vehicle in traffic accident
> Pedestrian on nonmotorized scooter injured in collision with railway train or railway vehicle in traffic accident
> Pedestrian on sled injured in collision with railway train or railway vehicle in traffic accident
> Pedestrian on snowboard injured in collision with railway train or railway vehicle in traffic accident
> Pedestrian on snow-skis injured in collision with railway train or railway vehicle in traffic accident

● **V05.9   Pedestrian injured in collision with railway train or railway vehicle, unspecified whether traffic or nontraffic accident**

X ● **V05.90   Pedestrian on foot injured in collision with railway train or railway vehicle, unspecified whether traffic or nontraffic accident**
> Pedestrian NOS injured in collision with railway train or railway vehicle, unspecified whether traffic or nontraffic accident

X ● **V05.91   Pedestrian on roller-skates injured in collision with railway train or railway vehicle, unspecified whether traffic or nontraffic accident**

X ● **V05.92   Pedestrian on skateboard injured in collision with railway train or railway vehicle, unspecified whether traffic or nontraffic accident**

X ● **V05.99   Pedestrian with other conveyance injured in collision with railway train or railway vehicle, unspecified whether traffic or nontraffic accident**
> Pedestrian with babystroller injured in collision with railway train or railway vehicle, unspecified whether traffic or nontraffic
> Pedestrian in wheelchair (powered) injured in collision with railway train or railway vehicle, unspecified whether traffic or nontraffic
> Pedestrian in motorized mobility scooter injured in collision with railway train or railway vehicle, unspecified whether traffic or nontraffic
> Pedestrian on ice-skates injured in collision with railway train or railway vehicle, unspecified whether traffic or nontraffic
> Pedestrian on nonmotorized scooter injured in collision with railway train or railway vehicle, unspecified whether traffic or nontraffic
> Pedestrian on sled injured in collision with railway train or railway vehicle, unspecified whether traffic or nontraffic
> Pedestrian on snowboard injured in collision with railway train or railway vehicle, unspecified whether traffic or nontraffic
> Pedestrian on snow-skis injured in collision with railway train or railway vehicle, unspecified whether traffic or nontraffic

CHAPTER 20 (V01-Y99)

● **V06**   **Pedestrian injured in collision with other nonmotor vehicle**

> **Includes**   collision with animal-drawn vehicle, animal being ridden, nonpowered streetcar

> **Excludes1**   pedestrian injured in collision with pedestrian conveyance (V00.0-)

The appropriate 7th character is to be added to each code from category V06

> A   initial encounter
> D   subsequent encounter
> S   sequela

● **V06.0**   **Pedestrian injured in collision with other nonmotor vehicle in nontraffic accident**

   X ● **V06.00**   **Pedestrian on foot injured in collision with other nonmotor vehicle in nontraffic accident**
      Pedestrian NOS injured in collision with other nonmotor vehicle in nontraffic accident

   X ● **V06.01**   **Pedestrian on roller-skates injured in collision with other nonmotor vehicle in nontraffic accident**

   X ● **V06.02**   **Pedestrian on skateboard injured in collision with other nonmotor vehicle in nontraffic accident**

   X ● **V06.09**   **Pedestrian with other conveyance injured in collision with other nonmotor vehicle in nontraffic accident**
      Pedestrian with babystroller injured in collision with other nonmotor vehicle in nontraffic accident
      Pedestrian in wheelchair (powered) injured in collision with other nonmotor vehicle in nontraffic accident
      Pedestrian in motorized mobility scooter injured in collision with other nonmotor vehicle in nontraffic accident
      Pedestrian on ice-skates injured in collision with other nonmotor vehicle in nontraffic accident
      Pedestrian on nonmotorized scooter injured in collision with other nonmotor vehicle in nontraffic accident
      Pedestrian on sled injured in collision with other nonmotor vehicle in nontraffic accident
      Pedestrian on snowboard injured in collision with other nonmotor vehicle in nontraffic accident
      Pedestrian on snow-skis injured in collision with other nonmotor vehicle in nontraffic accident

● **V06.1**   **Pedestrian injured in collision with other nonmotor vehicle in traffic accident**

   X ● **V06.10**   **Pedestrian on foot injured in collision with other nonmotor vehicle in traffic accident**
      Pedestrian NOS injured in collision with other nonmotor vehicle in traffic accident

   X ● **V06.11**   **Pedestrian on roller-skates injured in collision with other nonmotor vehicle in traffic accident**

   X ● **V06.12**   **Pedestrian on skateboard injured in collision with other nonmotor vehicle in traffic accident**

   X ● **V06.19**   **Pedestrian with other conveyance injured in collision with other nonmotor vehicle in traffic accident**
      Pedestrian with babystroller injured in collision with other nonmotor vehicle in nontraffic accident
      Pedestrian in wheelchair (powered) injured in collision with other nonmotor vehicle in traffic accident
      Pedestrian in motorized mobility scooter injured in collision with other nonmotor vehicle in traffic accident
      Pedestrian on ice-skates injured in collision with other nonmotor vehicle in traffic accident
      Pedestrian on nonmotorized scooter injured in collision with other nonmotor vehicle in traffic accident
      Pedestrian on sled injured in collision with other nonmotor vehicle in traffic accident
      Pedestrian on snowboard injured in collision with other nonmotor vehicle in traffic accident
      Pedestrian on snow-skis injured in collision with other nonmotor vehicle in traffic accident

● **V06.9**   **Pedestrian injured in collision with other nonmotor vehicle, unspecified whether traffic or nontraffic accident**

   X ● **V06.90**   **Pedestrian on foot injured in collision with other nonmotor vehicle, unspecified whether traffic or nontraffic accident**
      Pedestrian NOS injured in collision with other nonmotor vehicle, unspecified whether traffic or nontraffic accident

   X ● **V06.91**   **Pedestrian on roller-skates injured in collision with other nonmotor vehicle, unspecified whether traffic or nontraffic accident**

   X ● **V06.92**   **Pedestrian on skateboard injured in collision with other nonmotor vehicle, unspecified whether traffic or nontraffic accident**

   X ● **V06.99**   **Pedestrian with other conveyance injured in collision with other nonmotor vehicle, unspecified whether traffic or nontraffic accident**
      Pedestrian with babystroller injured in collision with other nonmotor vehicle, unspecified whether traffic or nontraffic accident
      Pedestrian in wheelchair (powered) injured in collision with other nonmotor vehicle, unspecified whether traffic or nontraffic accident
      Pedestrian in motorized mobility scooter injured in collision with other nonmotor vehicle, unspecified whether traffic or nontraffic accident
      Pedestrian on ice-skates injured in collision with other nonmotor vehicle, unspecified whether traffic or nontraffic accident
      Pedestrian on nonmotorized scooter injured in collision with other nonmotor vehicle, unspecified whether traffic or nontraffic accident
      Pedestrian on sled injured in collision with other nonmotor vehicle, unspecified whether traffic or nontraffic accident
      Pedestrian on snowboard injured in collision with other nonmotor vehicle, unspecified whether traffic or nontraffic accident
      Pedestrian on snow-skis injured in collision with other nonmotor vehicle, unspecified whether traffic or nontraffic accident

● **V09** **Pedestrian injured in other and unspecified transport accidents**
> The appropriate 7th character is to be added to each code from category V09

> | A | initial encounter |
> |---|---|
> | D | subsequent encounter |
> | S | sequela |

- ● **V09.0** **Pedestrian injured in nontraffic accident involving other and unspecified motor vehicles**
  - X ● **V09.00** Pedestrian injured in nontraffic accident involving unspecified motor vehicles
  - X ● **V09.01** Pedestrian injured in nontraffic accident involving military vehicle
  - X ● **V09.09** Pedestrian injured in nontraffic accident involving other motor vehicles
    > Pedestrian injured in nontraffic accident by special vehicle
- X ● **V09.1** Pedestrian injured in unspecified nontraffic accident
- ● **V09.2** **Pedestrian injured in traffic accident involving other and unspecified motor vehicles**
  - X ● **V09.20** Pedestrian injured in traffic accident involving unspecified motor vehicles
  - X ● **V09.21** Pedestrian injured in traffic accident involving military vehicle
  - X ● **V09.29** Pedestrian injured in traffic accident involving other motor vehicles
- X ● **V09.3** Pedestrian injured in unspecified traffic accident
- X ● **V09.9** Pedestrian injured in unspecified transport accident

PEDAL CYCLE RIDER INJURED IN TRANSPORT ACCIDENT (V10-V19)

> | Includes | any non-motorized vehicle, excluding an animal-drawn vehicle, or a sidecar or trailer attached to the pedal cycle |
> |---|---|
> | Excludes2 | rupture of pedal cycle tire (W37.0) |

● **V10** **Pedal cycle rider injured in collision with pedestrian or animal**

> | Excludes1 | pedal cycle rider collision with animal-drawn vehicle or animal being ridden (V16.-) |
> |---|---|

> The appropriate 7th character is to be added to each code from category V10

> | A | initial encounter |
> |---|---|
> | D | subsequent encounter |
> | S | sequela |

- X ● **V10.0** Pedal cycle driver injured in collision with pedestrian or animal in nontraffic accident
- X ● **V10.1** Pedal cycle passenger injured in collision with pedestrian or animal in nontraffic accident
- X ● **V10.2** Unspecified pedal cyclist injured in collision with pedestrian or animal in nontraffic accident
- X ● **V10.3** Person boarding or alighting a pedal cycle injured in collision with pedestrian or animal
- X ● **V10.4** Pedal cycle driver injured in collision with pedestrian or animal in traffic accident
- X ● **V10.5** Pedal cycle passenger injured in collision with pedestrian or animal in traffic accident
- X ● **V10.9** Unspecified pedal cyclist injured in collision with pedestrian or animal in traffic accident

● **V11** **Pedal cycle rider injured in collision with other pedal cycle**
> The appropriate 7th character is to be added to each code from category V11

> | A | initial encounter |
> |---|---|
> | D | subsequent encounter |
> | S | sequela |

- X ● **V11.0** Pedal cycle driver injured in collision with other pedal cycle in nontraffic accident
- X ● **V11.1** Pedal cycle passenger injured in collision with other pedal cycle in nontraffic accident
- X ● **V11.2** Unspecified pedal cyclist injured in collision with other pedal cycle in nontraffic accident
- X ● **V11.3** Person boarding or alighting a pedal cycle injured in collision with other pedal cycle
- X ● **V11.4** Pedal cycle driver injured in collision with other pedal cycle in traffic accident
- X ● **V11.5** Pedal cycle passenger injured in collision with other pedal cycle in traffic accident
- X ● **V11.9** Unspecified pedal cyclist injured in collision with other pedal cycle in traffic accident

● **V12** **Pedal cycle rider injured in collision with two- or three-wheeled motor vehicle**
> The appropriate 7th character is to be added to each code from category V12

> | A | initial encounter |
> |---|---|
> | D | subsequent encounter |
> | S | sequela |

- X ● **V12.0** Pedal cycle driver injured in collision with two- or three-wheeled motor vehicle in nontraffic accident
- X ● **V12.1** Pedal cycle passenger injured in collision with two- or three-wheeled motor vehicle in nontraffic accident
- X ● **V12.2** Unspecified pedal cyclist injured in collision with two- or three-wheeled motor vehicle in nontraffic accident
- X ● **V12.3** Person boarding or alighting a pedal cycle injured in collision with two- or three-wheeled motor vehicle
- X ● **V12.4** Pedal cycle driver injured in collision with two- or three-wheeled motor vehicle in traffic accident
- X ● **V12.5** Pedal cycle passenger injured in collision with two- or three-wheeled motor vehicle in traffic accident
- X ● **V12.9** Unspecified pedal cyclist injured in collision with two- or three-wheeled motor vehicle in traffic accident

● **V13** **Pedal cycle rider injured in collision with car, pick-up truck or van**
> The appropriate 7th character is to be added to each code from category V13

> | A | initial encounter |
> |---|---|
> | D | subsequent encounter |
> | S | sequela |

- X ● **V13.0** Pedal cycle driver injured in collision with car, pick-up truck or van in nontraffic accident
- X ● **V13.1** Pedal cycle passenger injured in collision with car, pick-up truck or van in nontraffic accident
- X ● **V13.2** Unspecified pedal cyclist injured in collision with car, pick-up truck or van in nontraffic accident
- X ● **V13.3** Person boarding or alighting a pedal cycle injured in collision with car, pick-up truck or van
- X ● **V13.4** Pedal cycle driver injured in collision with car, pick-up truck or van in traffic accident
- X ● **V13.5** Pedal cycle passenger injured in collision with car, pick-up truck or van in traffic accident
- X ● **V13.9** Unspecified pedal cyclist injured in collision with car, pick-up truck or van in traffic accident

● **V14 Pedal cycle rider injured in collision with heavy transport vehicle or bus**

> **Excludes1** pedal cycle rider injured in collision with military vehicle (V19.81)

> The appropriate 7th character is to be added to each code from category V14

> | A | initial encounter |
> |---|---|
> | D | subsequent encounter |
> | S | sequela |

X ● **V14.0** Pedal cycle driver injured in collision with heavy transport vehicle or bus in nontraffic accident

X ● **V14.1** Pedal cycle passenger injured in collision with heavy transport vehicle or bus in nontraffic accident

X ● **V14.2** Unspecified pedal cyclist injured in collision with heavy transport vehicle or bus in nontraffic accident

X ● **V14.3** Person boarding or alighting a pedal cycle injured in collision with heavy transport vehicle or bus

X ● **V14.4** Pedal cycle driver injured in collision with heavy transport vehicle or bus in traffic accident

X ● **V14.5** Pedal cycle passenger injured in collision with heavy transport vehicle or bus in traffic accident

X ● **V14.9** Unspecified pedal cyclist injured in collision with heavy transport vehicle or bus in traffic accident

● **V15 Pedal cycle rider injured in collision with railway train or railway vehicle**

> The appropriate 7th character is to be added to each code from category V15

> | A | initial encounter |
> |---|---|
> | D | subsequent encounter |
> | S | sequela |

X ● **V15.0** Pedal cycle driver injured in collision with railway train or railway vehicle in nontraffic accident

X ● **V15.1** Pedal cycle passenger injured in collision with railway train or railway vehicle in nontraffic accident

X ● **V15.2** Unspecified pedal cyclist injured in collision with railway train or railway vehicle in nontraffic accident

X ● **V15.3** Person boarding or alighting a pedal cycle injured in collision with railway train or railway vehicle

X ● **V15.4** Pedal cycle driver injured in collision with railway train or railway vehicle in traffic accident

X ● **V15.5** Pedal cycle passenger injured in collision with railway train or railway vehicle in traffic accident

X ● **V15.9** Unspecified pedal cyclist injured in collision with railway train or railway vehicle in traffic accident

● **V16 Pedal cycle rider injured in collision with other nonmotor vehicle**

> **Includes** collision with animal-drawn vehicle, animal being ridden, streetcar

> The appropriate 7th character is to be added to each code from category V16

> | A | initial encounter |
> |---|---|
> | D | subsequent encounter |
> | S | sequela |

X ● **V16.0** Pedal cycle driver injured in collision with other nonmotor vehicle in nontraffic accident

X ● **V16.1** Pedal cycle passenger injured in collision with other nonmotor vehicle in nontraffic accident

X ● **V16.2** Unspecified pedal cyclist injured in collision with other nonmotor vehicle in nontraffic accident

X ● **V16.3** Person boarding or alighting a pedal cycle injured in collision with other nonmotor vehicle in nontraffic accident

X ● **V16.4** Pedal cycle driver injured in collision with other nonmotor vehicle in traffic accident

X ● **V16.5** Pedal cycle passenger injured in collision with other nonmotor vehicle in traffic accident

X ● **V16.9** Unspecified pedal cyclist injured in collision with other nonmotor vehicle in traffic accident

● **V17 Pedal cycle rider injured in collision with fixed or stationary object**

> The appropriate 7th character is to be added to each code from category V17

> | A | initial encounter |
> |---|---|
> | D | subsequent encounter |
> | S | sequela |

X ● **V17.0** Pedal cycle driver injured in collision with fixed or stationary object in nontraffic accident

X ● **V17.1** Pedal cycle passenger injured in collision with fixed or stationary object in nontraffic accident

X ● **V17.2** Unspecified pedal cyclist injured in collision with fixed or stationary object in nontraffic accident

X ● **V17.3** Person boarding or alighting a pedal cycle injured in collision with fixed or stationary object

X ● **V17.4** Pedal cycle driver injured in collision with fixed or stationary object in traffic accident

X ● **V17.5** Pedal cycle passenger injured in collision with fixed or stationary object in traffic accident

X ● **V17.9** Unspecified pedal cyclist injured in collision with fixed or stationary object in traffic accident

● **V18 Pedal cycle rider injured in noncollision transport accident**

> **Includes** fall or thrown from pedal cycle (without antecedent collision)
> overturning pedal cycle NOS
> overturning pedal cycle without collision

> The appropriate 7th character is to be added to each code from category V18

> | A | initial encounter |
> |---|---|
> | D | subsequent encounter |
> | S | sequela |

X ● **V18.0** Pedal cycle driver injured in noncollision transport accident in nontraffic accident

X ● **V18.1** Pedal cycle passenger injured in noncollision transport accident in nontraffic accident

X ● **V18.2** Unspecified pedal cyclist injured in noncollision transport accident in nontraffic accident

X ● **V18.3** Person boarding or alighting a pedal cycle injured in noncollision transport accident

X ● **V18.4** Pedal cycle driver injured in noncollision transport accident in traffic accident

X ● **V18.5** Pedal cycle passenger injured in noncollision transport accident in traffic accident

X ● **V18.9** Unspecified pedal cyclist injured in noncollision transport accident in traffic accident

● **V19 Pedal cycle rider injured in other and unspecified transport accidents**

> The appropriate 7th character is to be added to each code from category V19

> | A | initial encounter |
> |---|---|
> | D | subsequent encounter |
> | S | sequela |

● **V19.0** Pedal cycle driver injured in collision with other and unspecified motor vehicles in nontraffic accident

X ● **V19.00** Pedal cycle driver injured in collision with unspecified motor vehicles in nontraffic accident

X ● **V19.09** Pedal cycle driver injured in collision with other motor vehicles in nontraffic accident

◀ New   ◀▥ Revised   ~~deleted~~ Deleted   **OGCR** Official Guidelines   X Assign placeholder X   ● Use Additional Character(s)

Excludes 1   Excludes 2   Includes   Use additional   Code first   Code also   Unspecified

● **V19.1**   Pedal cycle passenger injured in collision with other and unspecified motor vehicles in nontraffic accident

X ● **V19.10**   Pedal cycle passenger injured in collision with unspecified motor vehicles in nontraffic accident

X ● **V19.19**   Pedal cycle passenger injured in collision with other motor vehicles in nontraffic accident

● **V19.2**   Unspecified pedal cyclist injured in collision with other and unspecified motor vehicles in nontraffic accident

X ● **V19.20**   Unspecified pedal cyclist injured in collision with unspecified motor vehicles in nontraffic accident

Pedal cycle collision NOS, nontraffic

X ● **V19.29**   Unspecified pedal cyclist injured in collision with other motor vehicles in nontraffic accident

X ● **V19.3**   Pedal cyclist (driver) (passenger) injured in unspecified nontraffic accident

Pedal cycle accident NOS, nontraffic
Pedal cyclist injured in nontraffic accident NOS

● **V19.4**   Pedal cycle driver injured in collision with other and unspecified motor vehicles in traffic accident

X ● **V19.40**   Pedal cycle driver injured in collision with unspecified motor vehicles in traffic accident

X ● **V19.49**   Pedal cycle driver injured in collision with other motor vehicles in traffic accident

● **V19.5**   Pedal cycle passenger injured in collision with other and unspecified motor vehicles in traffic accident

X ● **V19.50**   Pedal cycle passenger injured in collision with unspecified motor vehicles in traffic accident

X ● **V19.59**   Pedal cycle passenger injured in collision with other motor vehicles in traffic accident

● **V19.6**   Unspecified pedal cyclist injured in collision with other and unspecified motor vehicles in traffic accident

X ● **V19.60**   Unspecified pedal cyclist injured in collision with unspecified motor vehicles in traffic accident

Pedal cycle collision NOS (traffic)

X ● **V19.69**   Unspecified pedal cyclist injured in collision with other motor vehicles in traffic accident

● **V19.8**   Pedal cyclist (driver) (passenger) injured in other specified transport accidents

X ● **V19.81**   Pedal cyclist (driver) (passenger) injured in transport accident with military vehicle

X ● **V19.88**   Pedal cyclist (driver) (passenger) injured in other specified transport accidents

X ● **V19.9**   Pedal cyclist (driver) (passenger) injured in unspecified traffic accident

Pedal cycle accident NOS

MOTORCYCLE RIDER INJURED IN TRANSPORT ACCIDENT (V20-V29)

Includes	moped motorcycle with sidecar motorized bicycle motor scooter

Excludes1	three-wheeled motor vehicle (V30-V39)

● **V20**   Motorcycle rider injured in collision with pedestrian or animal

Excludes1	motorcycle rider collision with animal-drawn vehicle or animal being ridden (V26.-)

The appropriate 7th character is to be added to each code from category V20

A	initial encounter
D	subsequent encounter
S	sequela

X ● **V20.0**   Motorcycle driver injured in collision with pedestrian or animal in nontraffic accident

X ● **V20.1**   Motorcycle passenger injured in collision with pedestrian or animal in nontraffic accident

X ● **V20.2**   Unspecified motorcycle rider injured in collision with pedestrian or animal in nontraffic accident

X ● **V20.3**   Person boarding or alighting a motorcycle injured in collision with pedestrian or animal

X ● **V20.4**   Motorcycle driver injured in collision with pedestrian or animal in traffic accident

X ● **V20.5**   Motorcycle passenger injured in collision with pedestrian or animal in traffic accident

X ● **V20.9**   Unspecified motorcycle rider injured in collision with pedestrian or animal in traffic accident

● **V21**   Motorcycle rider injured in collision with pedal cycle

The appropriate 7th character is to be added to each code from category V21

A	initial encounter
D	subsequent encounter
S	sequela

X ● **V21.0**   Motorcycle driver injured in collision with pedal cycle in nontraffic accident

X ● **V21.1**   Motorcycle passenger injured in collision with pedal cycle in nontraffic accident

X ● **V21.2**   Unspecified motorcycle rider injured in collision with pedal cycle in nontraffic accident

X ● **V21.3**   Person boarding or alighting a motorcycle injured in collision with pedal cycle

X ● **V21.4**   Motorcycle driver injured in collision with pedal cycle in traffic accident

X ● **V21.5**   Motorcycle passenger injured in collision with pedal cycle in traffic accident

X ● **V21.9**   Unspecified motorcycle rider injured in collision with pedal cycle in traffic accident

● **V22**   Motorcycle rider injured in collision with two- or three-wheeled motor vehicle

The appropriate 7th character is to be added to each code from category V22

A	initial encounter
D	subsequent encounter
S	sequela

X ● **V22.0**   Motorcycle driver injured in collision with two- or three-wheeled motor vehicle in nontraffic accident

X ● **V22.1**   Motorcycle passenger injured in collision with two- or three-wheeled motor vehicle in nontraffic accident

X ● **V22.2**   Unspecified motorcycle rider injured in collision with two- or three-wheeled motor vehicle in nontraffic accident

X ● **V22.3**   Person boarding or alighting a motorcycle injured in collision with two- or three-wheeled motor vehicle

X ● **V22.4**   Motorcycle driver injured in collision with two- or three-wheeled motor vehicle in traffic accident

X ● **V22.5**   Motorcycle passenger injured in collision with two- or three-wheeled motor vehicle in traffic accident

X ● **V22.9**   Unspecified motorcycle rider injured in collision with two- or three-wheeled motor vehicle in traffic accident

● **V23**   Motorcycle rider injured in collision with car, pick-up truck or van

The appropriate 7th character is to be added to each code from category V23

A	initial encounter
D	subsequent encounter
S	sequela

X ● **V23.0**   Motorcycle driver injured in collision with car, pick-up truck or van in nontraffic accident

X ● **V23.1**   Motorcycle passenger injured in collision with car, pick-up truck or van in nontraffic accident

X ● **V23.2**   Unspecified motorcycle rider injured in collision with car, pick-up truck or van in nontraffic accident

X ● **V23.3**   Person boarding or alighting a motorcycle injured in collision with car, pick-up truck or van

X ● **V23.4**   Motorcycle driver injured in collision with car, pick-up truck or van in traffic accident

CHAPTER 20 (V01-Y99)

X ● **V23.5** Motorcycle passenger injured in collision with car, pick-up truck or van in traffic accident

X ● **V23.9** Unspecified motorcycle rider injured in collision with car, pick-up truck or van in traffic accident

● **V24** Motorcycle rider injured in collision with heavy transport vehicle or bus

> **Excludes1** motorcycle rider injured in collision with military vehicle (V29.81)

> The appropriate 7th character is to be added to each code from category V24

> | A | initial encounter |
> |---|---|
> | D | subsequent encounter |
> | S | sequela |

X ● **V24.0** Motorcycle driver injured in collision with heavy transport vehicle or bus in nontraffic accident

X ● **V24.1** Motorcycle passenger injured in collision with heavy transport vehicle or bus in nontraffic accident

X ● **V24.2** Unspecified motorcycle rider injured in collision with heavy transport vehicle or bus in nontraffic accident

X ● **V24.3** Person boarding or alighting a motorcycle injured in collision with heavy transport vehicle or bus

X ● **V24.4** Motorcycle driver injured in collision with heavy transport vehicle or bus in traffic accident

X ● **V24.5** Motorcycle passenger injured in collision with heavy transport vehicle or bus in traffic accident

X ● **V24.9** Unspecified motorcycle rider injured in collision with heavy transport vehicle or bus in traffic accident

● **V25** Motorcycle rider injured in collision with railway train or railway vehicle

> The appropriate 7th character is to be added to each code from category V25

> | A | initial encounter |
> |---|---|
> | D | subsequent encounter |
> | S | sequela |

X ● **V25.0** Motorcycle driver injured in collision with railway train or railway vehicle in nontraffic accident

X ● **V25.1** Motorcycle passenger injured in collision with railway train or railway vehicle in nontraffic accident

X ● **V25.2** Unspecified motorcycle rider injured in collision with railway train or railway vehicle in nontraffic accident

X ● **V25.3** Person boarding or alighting a motorcycle injured in collision with railway train or railway vehicle

X ● **V25.4** Motorcycle driver injured in collision with railway train or railway vehicle in traffic accident

X ● **V25.5** Motorcycle passenger injured in collision with railway train or railway vehicle in traffic accident

X ● **V25.9** Unspecified motorcycle rider injured in collision with railway train or railway vehicle in traffic accident

● **V26** Motorcycle rider injured in collision with other nonmotor vehicle

> **Includes** collision with animal-drawn vehicle, animal being ridden, streetcar

> The appropriate 7th character is to be added to each code from category V26

> | A | initial encounter |
> |---|---|
> | D | subsequent encounter |
> | S | sequela |

X ● **V26.0** Motorcycle driver injured in collision with other nonmotor vehicle in nontraffic accident

X ● **V26.1** Motorcycle passenger injured in collision with other nonmotor vehicle in nontraffic accident

X ● **V26.2** Unspecified motorcycle rider injured in collision with other nonmotor vehicle in nontraffic accident

X ● **V26.3** Person boarding or alighting a motorcycle injured in collision with other nonmotor vehicle

X ● **V26.4** Motorcycle driver injured in collision with other nonmotor vehicle in traffic accident

X ● **V26.5** Motorcycle passenger injured in collision with other nonmotor vehicle in traffic accident

X ● **V26.9** Unspecified motorcycle rider injured in collision with other nonmotor vehicle in traffic accident

● **V27** Motorcycle rider injured in collision with fixed or stationary object

> The appropriate 7th character is to be added to each code from category V27

> | A | initial encounter |
> |---|---|
> | D | subsequent encounter |
> | S | sequela |

X ● **V27.0** Motorcycle driver injured in collision with fixed or stationary object in nontraffic accident

X ● **V27.1** Motorcycle passenger injured in collision with fixed or stationary object in nontraffic accident

X ● **V27.2** Unspecified motorcycle rider injured in collision with fixed or stationary object in nontraffic accident

X ● **V27.3** Person boarding or alighting a motorcycle injured in collision with fixed or stationary object

X ● **V27.4** Motorcycle driver injured in collision with fixed or stationary object in traffic accident

X ● **V27.5** Motorcycle passenger injured in collision with fixed or stationary object in traffic accident

X ● **V27.9** Unspecified motorcycle rider injured in collision with fixed or stationary object in traffic accident

● **V28** Motorcycle rider injured in noncollision transport accident

> **Includes** fall or thrown from motorcycle (without antecedent collision)
> overturning motorcycle NOS
> overturning motorcycle without collision

> The appropriate 7th character is to be added to each code from category V28

> | A | initial encounter |
> |---|---|
> | D | subsequent encounter |
> | S | sequela |

X ● **V28.0** Motorcycle driver injured in noncollision transport accident in nontraffic accident

X ● **V28.1** Motorcycle passenger injured in noncollision transport accident in nontraffic accident

X ● **V28.2** Unspecified motorcycle rider injured in noncollision transport accident in nontraffic accident

X ● **V28.3** Person boarding or alighting a motorcycle injured in noncollision transport accident

X ● **V28.4** Motorcycle driver injured in noncollision transport accident in traffic accident

X ● **V28.5** Motorcycle passenger injured in noncollision transport accident in traffic accident

X ● **V28.9** Unspecified motorcycle rider injured in noncollision transport accident in traffic accident

● **V29** Motorcycle rider injured in other and unspecified transport accidents

> The appropriate 7th character is to be added to each code from category V29

> | A | initial encounter |
> |---|---|
> | D | subsequent encounter |
> | S | sequela |

● **V29.0** Motorcycle driver injured in collision with other and unspecified motor vehicles in nontraffic accident

X ● **V29.00** Motorcycle driver injured in collision with unspecified motor vehicles in nontraffic accident

X ● **V29.09** Motorcycle driver injured in collision with other motor vehicles in nontraffic accident

◄ New   ◄▦ Revised   ~~deleted~~ Deleted   **OGCR** Official Guidelines   X Assign placeholder X   ● Use Additional Character(s)

Excludes 1   Excludes 2   Includes   Use additional   Code first   Code also   Unspecified

● **V29.1**   Motorcycle passenger injured in collision with other and unspecified motor vehicles in nontraffic accident

    X ● **V29.10**   Motorcycle passenger injured in collision with unspecified motor vehicles in nontraffic accident

    X ● **V29.19**   Motorcycle passenger injured in collision with other motor vehicles in nontraffic accident

● **V29.2**   Unspecified motorcycle rider injured in collision with other and unspecified motor vehicles in nontraffic accident

    X ● **V29.20**   Unspecified motorcycle rider injured in collision with unspecified motor vehicles in nontraffic accident
          Motorcycle collision NOS, nontraffic

    X ● **V29.29**   Unspecified motorcycle rider injured in collision with other motor vehicles in nontraffic accident

X ● **V29.3**   Motorcycle rider (driver) (passenger) injured in unspecified nontraffic accident
       Motorcycle accident NOS, nontraffic
       Motorcycle rider injured in nontraffic accident NOS

● **V29.4**   Motorcycle driver injured in collision with other and unspecified motor vehicles in traffic accident

    X ● **V29.40**   Motorcycle driver injured in collision with unspecified motor vehicles in traffic accident

    X ● **V29.49**   Motorcycle driver injured in collision with other motor vehicles in traffic accident

● **V29.5**   Motorcycle passenger injured in collision with other and unspecified motor vehicles in traffic accident

    X ● **V29.50**   Motorcycle passenger injured in collision with unspecified motor vehicles in traffic accident

    X ● **V29.59**   Motorcycle passenger injured in collision with other motor vehicles in traffic accident

● **V29.6**   Unspecified motorcycle rider injured in collision with other and unspecified motor vehicles in traffic accident

    X ● **V29.60**   Unspecified motorcycle rider injured in collision with unspecified motor vehicles in traffic accident
          Motorcycle collision NOS (traffic)

    X ● **V29.69**   Unspecified motorcycle rider injured in collision with other motor vehicles in traffic accident

● **V29.8**   Motorcycle rider (driver) (passenger) injured in other specified transport accidents

    X ● **V29.81**   Motorcycle rider (driver) (passenger) injured in transport accident with military vehicle

    X ● **V29.88**   Motorcycle rider (driver) (passenger) injured in other specified transport accidents

X ● **V29.9**   Motorcycle rider (driver) (passenger) injured in unspecified traffic accident
       Motorcycle accident NOS

OCCUPANT OF THREE-WHEELED MOTOR VEHICLE INJURED IN TRANSPORT ACCIDENT (V30-V39)

Includes	motorized tricycle
	motorized rickshaw
	three-wheeled motor car

Excludes1	all-terrain vehicles (V86.-)
	motorcycle with sidecar (V20-V29)
	vehicle designed primarily for off-road use (V86.-)

● **V30**   Occupant of three-wheeled motor vehicle injured in collision with pedestrian or animal

Excludes1	three-wheeled motor vehicle collision with animal-drawn vehicle or animal being ridden (V36.-)

The appropriate 7th character is to be added to each code from category V30

A	initial encounter
D	subsequent encounter
S	sequela

    X ● **V30.0**   Driver of three-wheeled motor vehicle injured in collision with pedestrian or animal in nontraffic accident

    X ● **V30.1**   Passenger in three-wheeled motor vehicle injured in collision with pedestrian or animal in nontraffic accident

    X ● **V30.2**   Person on outside of three-wheeled motor vehicle injured in collision with pedestrian or animal in nontraffic accident

    X ● **V30.3**   Unspecified occupant of three-wheeled motor vehicle injured in collision with pedestrian or animal in nontraffic accident

    X ● **V30.4**   Person boarding or alighting a three-wheeled motor vehicle injured in collision with pedestrian or animal

    X ● **V30.5**   Driver of three-wheeled motor vehicle injured in collision with pedestrian or animal in traffic accident

    X ● **V30.6**   Passenger in three-wheeled motor vehicle injured in collision with pedestrian or animal in traffic accident

    X ● **V30.7**   Person on outside of three-wheeled motor vehicle injured in collision with pedestrian or animal in traffic accident

    X ● **V30.9**   Unspecified occupant of three-wheeled motor vehicle injured in collision with pedestrian or animal in traffic accident

● **V31**   Occupant of three-wheeled motor vehicle injured in collision with pedal cycle

The appropriate 7th character is to be added to each code from category V31

A	initial encounter
D	subsequent encounter
S	sequela

    X ● **V31.0**   Driver of three-wheeled motor vehicle injured in collision with pedal cycle in nontraffic accident

    X ● **V31.1**   Passenger in three-wheeled motor vehicle injured in collision with pedal cycle in nontraffic accident

    X ● **V31.2**   Person on outside of three-wheeled motor vehicle injured in collision with pedal cycle in nontraffic accident

    X ● **V31.3**   Unspecified occupant of three-wheeled motor vehicle injured in collision with pedal cycle in nontraffic accident

    X ● **V31.4**   Person boarding or alighting a three-wheeled motor vehicle injured in collision with pedal cycle

    X ● **V31.5**   Driver of three-wheeled motor vehicle injured in collision with pedal cycle in traffic accident

    X ● **V31.6**   Passenger in three-wheeled motor vehicle injured in collision with pedal cycle in traffic accident

    X ● **V31.7**   Person on outside of three-wheeled motor vehicle injured in collision with pedal cycle in traffic accident

    X ● **V31.9**   Unspecified occupant of three-wheeled motor vehicle injured in collision with pedal cycle in traffic accident

CHAPTER 20 (V01-Y99)

● V32   **Occupant of three-wheeled motor vehicle injured in collision with two- or three-wheeled motor vehicle**

> The appropriate 7th character is to be added to each code from category V32

> A   initial encounter
> D   subsequent encounter
> S   sequela

X ● V32.0   Driver of three-wheeled motor vehicle injured in collision with two- or three-wheeled motor vehicle in nontraffic accident

X ● V32.1   Passenger in three-wheeled motor vehicle injured in collision with two- or three-wheeled motor vehicle in nontraffic accident

X ● V32.2   Person on outside of three-wheeled motor vehicle injured in collision with two- or three-wheeled motor vehicle in nontraffic accident

X ● V32.3   Unspecified occupant of three-wheeled motor vehicle injured in collision with two- or three-wheeled motor vehicle in nontraffic accident

X ● V32.4   Person boarding or alighting a three-wheeled motor vehicle injured in collision with two- or three-wheeled motor vehicle

X ● V32.5   Driver of three-wheeled motor vehicle injured in collision with two- or three-wheeled motor vehicle in traffic accident

X ● V32.6   Passenger in three-wheeled motor vehicle injured in collision with two- or three-wheeled motor vehicle in traffic accident

X ● V32.7   Person on outside of three-wheeled motor vehicle injured in collision with two- or three-wheeled motor vehicle in traffic accident

X ● V32.9   Unspecified occupant of three-wheeled motor vehicle injured in collision with two- or three-wheeled motor vehicle in traffic accident

● V33   **Occupant of three-wheeled motor vehicle injured in collision with car, pick-up truck or van**

> The appropriate 7th character is to be added to each code from category V33

> A   initial encounter
> D   subsequent encounter
> S   sequela

X ● V33.0   Driver of three-wheeled motor vehicle injured in collision with car, pick-up truck or van in nontraffic accident

X ● V33.1   Passenger in three-wheeled motor vehicle injured in collision with car, pick-up truck or van in nontraffic accident

X ● V33.2   Person on outside of three-wheeled motor vehicle injured in collision with car, pick-up truck or van in nontraffic accident

X ● V33.3   Unspecified occupant of three-wheeled motor vehicle injured in collision with car, pick-up truck or van in nontraffic accident

X ● V33.4   Person boarding or alighting a three-wheeled motor vehicle injured in collision with car, pick-up truck or van

X ● V33.5   Driver of three-wheeled motor vehicle injured in collision with car, pick-up truck or van in traffic accident

X ● V33.6   Passenger in three-wheeled motor vehicle injured in collision with car, pick-up truck or van in traffic accident

X ● V33.7   Person on outside of three-wheeled motor vehicle injured in collision with car, pick-up truck or van in traffic accident

X ● V33.9   Unspecified occupant of three-wheeled motor vehicle injured in collision with car, pick-up truck or van in traffic accident

● V34   **Occupant of three-wheeled motor vehicle injured in collision with heavy transport vehicle or bus**

> **Excludes1**   occupant of three-wheeled motor vehicle injured in collision with military vehicle (V39.81)

> The appropriate 7th character is to be added to each code from category V34

> A   initial encounter
> D   subsequent encounter
> S   sequela

X ● V34.0   Driver of three-wheeled motor vehicle injured in collision with heavy transport vehicle or bus in nontraffic accident

X ● V34.1   Passenger in three-wheeled motor vehicle injured in collision with heavy transport vehicle or bus in nontraffic accident

X ● V34.2   Person on outside of three-wheeled motor vehicle injured in collision with heavy transport vehicle or bus in nontraffic accident

X ● V34.3   Unspecified occupant of three-wheeled motor vehicle injured in collision with heavy transport vehicle or bus in nontraffic accident

X ● V34.4   Person boarding or alighting a three-wheeled motor vehicle injured in collision with heavy transport vehicle or bus

X ● V34.5   Driver of three-wheeled motor vehicle injured in collision with heavy transport vehicle or bus in traffic accident

X ● V34.6   Passenger in three-wheeled motor vehicle injured in collision with heavy transport vehicle or bus in traffic accident

X ● V34.7   Person on outside of three-wheeled motor vehicle injured in collision with heavy transport vehicle or bus in traffic accident

X ● V34.9   Unspecified occupant of three-wheeled motor vehicle injured in collision with heavy transport vehicle or bus in traffic accident

● V35   **Occupant of three-wheeled motor vehicle injured in collision with railway train or railway vehicle**

> The appropriate 7th character is to be added to each code from category V35

> A   initial encounter
> D   subsequent encounter
> S   sequela

X ● V35.0   Driver of three-wheeled motor vehicle injured in collision with railway train or railway vehicle in nontraffic accident

X ● V35.1   Passenger in three-wheeled motor vehicle injured in collision with railway train or railway vehicle in nontraffic accident

X ● V35.2   Person on outside of three-wheeled motor vehicle injured in collision with railway train or railway vehicle in nontraffic accident

X ● V35.3   Unspecified occupant of three-wheeled motor vehicle injured in collision with railway train or railway vehicle in nontraffic accident

X ● V35.4   Person boarding or alighting a three-wheeled motor vehicle injured in collision with railway train or railway vehicle

X ● V35.5   Driver of three-wheeled motor vehicle injured in collision with railway train or railway vehicle in traffic accident

X ● V35.6   Passenger in three-wheeled motor vehicle injured in collision with railway train or railway vehicle in traffic accident

X ● V35.7   Person on outside of three-wheeled motor vehicle injured in collision with railway train or railway vehicle in traffic accident

X ● V35.9   Unspecified occupant of three-wheeled motor vehicle injured in collision with railway train or railway vehicle in traffic accident

◄ New   ◄▮▮▮ Revised   ~~deleted~~ Deleted   OGCR Official Guidelines   X Assign placeholder X   ● Use Additional Character(s)

Excludes 1   Excludes 2   Includes   Use additional   Code first   Code also   Unspecified

● V36   Occupant of three-wheeled motor vehicle injured in collision with other nonmotor vehicle

   Includes   collision with animal-drawn vehicle, animal being ridden, streetcar

   The appropriate 7th character is to be added to each code from category V36

A	initial encounter
D	subsequent encounter
S	sequela

X ● V36.0   Driver of three-wheeled motor vehicle injured in collision with other nonmotor vehicle in nontraffic accident

X ● V36.1   Passenger in three-wheeled motor vehicle injured in collision with other nonmotor vehicle in nontraffic accident

X ● V36.2   Person on outside of three-wheeled motor vehicle injured in collision with other nonmotor vehicle in nontraffic accident

X ● V36.3   Unspecified occupant of three-wheeled motor vehicle injured in collision with other nonmotor vehicle in nontraffic accident

X ● V36.4   Person boarding or alighting a three-wheeled motor vehicle injured in collision with other nonmotor vehicle

X ● V36.5   Driver of three-wheeled motor vehicle injured in collision with other nonmotor vehicle in traffic accident

X ● V36.6   Passenger in three-wheeled motor vehicle injured in collision with other nonmotor vehicle in traffic accident

X ● V36.7   Person on outside of three-wheeled motor vehicle injured in collision with other nonmotor vehicle in traffic accident

X ● V36.9   Unspecified occupant of three-wheeled motor vehicle injured in collision with other nonmotor vehicle in traffic accident

● V37   Occupant of three-wheeled motor vehicle injured in collision with fixed or stationary object

   The appropriate 7th character is to be added to each code from category V37

A	initial encounter
D	subsequent encounter
S	sequela

X ● V37.0   Driver of three-wheeled motor vehicle injured in collision with fixed or stationary object in nontraffic accident

X ● V37.1   Passenger in three-wheeled motor vehicle injured in collision with fixed or stationary object in nontraffic accident

X ● V37.2   Person on outside of three-wheeled motor vehicle injured in collision with fixed or stationary object in nontraffic accident

X ● V37.3   Unspecified occupant of three-wheeled motor vehicle injured in collision with fixed or stationary object in nontraffic accident

X ● V37.4   Person boarding or alighting a three-wheeled motor vehicle injured in collision with fixed or stationary object

X ● V37.5   Driver of three-wheeled motor vehicle injured in collision with fixed or stationary object in traffic accident

X ● V37.6   Passenger in three-wheeled motor vehicle injured in collision with fixed or stationary object in traffic accident

X ● V37.7   Person on outside of three-wheeled motor vehicle injured in collision with fixed or stationary object in traffic accident

X ● V37.9   Unspecified occupant of three-wheeled motor vehicle injured in collision with fixed or stationary object in traffic accident

● V38   Occupant of three-wheeled motor vehicle injured in noncollision transport accident

   Includes   fall or thrown from three-wheeled motor vehicle
   overturning of three-wheeled motor vehicle NOS
   overturning of three-wheeled motor vehicle without collision

   The appropriate 7th character is to be added to each code from category V38

A	initial encounter
D	subsequent encounter
S	sequela

X ● V38.0   Driver of three-wheeled motor vehicle injured in noncollision transport accident in nontraffic accident

X ● V38.1   Passenger in three-wheeled motor vehicle injured in noncollision transport accident in nontraffic accident

X ● V38.2   Person on outside of three-wheeled motor vehicle injured in noncollision transport accident in nontraffic accident

X ● V38.3   Unspecified occupant of three-wheeled motor vehicle injured in noncollision transport accident in nontraffic accident

X ● V38.4   Person boarding or alighting a three-wheeled motor vehicle injured in noncollision transport accident

X ● V38.5   Driver of three-wheeled motor vehicle injured in noncollision transport accident in traffic accident

X ● V38.6   Passenger in three-wheeled motor vehicle injured in noncollision transport accident in traffic accident

X ● V38.7   Person on outside of three-wheeled motor vehicle injured in noncollision transport accident in traffic accident

X ● V38.9   Unspecified occupant of three-wheeled motor vehicle injured in noncollision transport accident in traffic accident

● V39   Occupant of three-wheeled motor vehicle injured in other and unspecified transport accidents

   The appropriate 7th character is to be added to each code from category V39

A	initial encounter
D	subsequent encounter
S	sequela

● V39.0   Driver of three-wheeled motor vehicle injured in collision with other and unspecified motor vehicles in nontraffic accident

   X ● V39.00   Driver of three-wheeled motor vehicle injured in collision with unspecified motor vehicles in nontraffic accident

   X ● V39.09   Driver of three-wheeled motor vehicle injured in collision with other motor vehicles in nontraffic accident

● V39.1   Passenger in three-wheeled motor vehicle injured in collision with other and unspecified motor vehicles in nontraffic accident

   X ● V39.10   Passenger in three-wheeled motor vehicle injured in collision with unspecified motor vehicles in nontraffic accident

   X ● V39.19   Passenger in three-wheeled motor vehicle injured in collision with other motor vehicles in nontraffic accident

● V39.2   Unspecified occupant of three-wheeled motor vehicle injured in collision with other and unspecified motor vehicles in nontraffic accident

   X ● V39.20   Unspecified occupant of three-wheeled motor vehicle injured in collision with unspecified motor vehicles in nontraffic accident

      Collision NOS involving three-wheeled motor vehicle, nontraffic

   X ● V39.29   Unspecified occupant of three-wheeled motor vehicle injured in collision with other motor vehicles in nontraffic accident

CHAPTER 20 (V01-Y99)

X ● **V39.3** **Occupant (driver) (passenger) of three-wheeled motor vehicle injured in** unspecified **nontraffic accident**
> Accident NOS involving three-wheeled motor vehicle, nontraffic
> Occupant of three-wheeled motor vehicle injured in nontraffic accident NOS

● **V39.4** **Driver of three-wheeled motor vehicle injured in collision with other and unspecified motor vehicles in traffic accident**

X ● **V39.40** **Driver of three-wheeled motor vehicle injured in collision with** unspecified **motor vehicles in traffic accident**

X ● **V39.49** **Driver of three-wheeled motor vehicle injured in collision with other motor vehicles in traffic accident**

● **V39.5** **Passenger in three-wheeled motor vehicle injured in collision with other and unspecified motor vehicles in traffic accident**

X ● **V39.50** **Passenger in three-wheeled motor vehicle injured in collision with** unspecified **motor vehicles in traffic accident**

X ● **V39.59** **Passenger in three-wheeled motor vehicle injured in collision with other motor vehicles in traffic accident**

● **V39.6** **Unspecified occupant of three-wheeled motor vehicle injured in collision with other and unspecified motor vehicles in traffic accident**

X ● **V39.60** Unspecified **occupant of three-wheeled motor vehicle injured in collision with unspecified motor vehicles in traffic accident**
> Collision NOS involving three-wheeled motor vehicle (traffic)

X ● **V39.69** Unspecified **occupant of three-wheeled motor vehicle injured in collision with other motor vehicles in traffic accident**

● **V39.8** **Occupant (driver) (passenger) of three wheeled motor vehicle injured in other specified transport accidents**

X ● **V39.81** **Occupant (driver) (passenger) of three-wheeled motor vehicle injured in transport accident with military vehicle**

X ● **V39.89** **Occupant (driver) (passenger) of three-wheeled motor vehicle injured in other specified transport accidents**

X ● **V39.9** **Occupant (driver) (passenger) of three-wheeled motor vehicle injured in** unspecified **traffic accident**
> Accident NOS involving three-wheeled motor vehicle

CAR OCCUPANT INJURED IN TRANSPORT ACCIDENT (V40-V49)

Includes	a four-wheeled motor vehicle designed primarily for carrying passengers
	automobile (pulling a trailer or camper)

Excludes1	bus (V50-V59)
	minibus (V50-V59)
	minivan (V50-V59)
	motorcoach (V70-V79)
	pick-up truck (V50-V59)
	sport utility vehicle (SUV) (V50-V59)

● **V40** **Car occupant injured in collision with pedestrian or animal**

Excludes1	car collision with animal-drawn vehicle or animal being ridden (V46.-)

The appropriate 7th character is to be added to each code from category V40

A	initial encounter
D	subsequent encounter
S	sequela

X ● **V40.0** **Car driver injured in collision with pedestrian or animal in nontraffic accident**

X ● **V40.1** **Car passenger injured in collision with pedestrian or animal in nontraffic accident**

X ● **V40.2** **Person on outside of car injured in collision with pedestrian or animal in nontraffic accident**

X ● **V40.3** Unspecified **car occupant injured in collision with pedestrian or animal in nontraffic accident**

X ● **V40.4** **Person boarding or alighting a car injured in collision with pedestrian or animal**

X ● **V40.5** **Car driver injured in collision with pedestrian or animal in traffic accident**

X ● **V40.6** **Car passenger injured in collision with pedestrian or animal in traffic accident**

X ● **V40.7** **Person on outside of car injured in collision with pedestrian or animal in traffic accident**

X ● **V40.9** Unspecified **car occupant injured in collision with pedestrian or animal in traffic accident**

● **V41** **Car occupant injured in collision with pedal cycle**

The appropriate 7th character is to be added to each code from category V41

A	initial encounter
D	subsequent encounter
S	sequela

X ● **V41.0** **Car driver injured in collision with pedal cycle in nontraffic accident**

X ● **V41.1** **Car passenger injured in collision with pedal cycle in nontraffic accident**

X ● **V41.2** **Person on outside of car injured in collision with pedal cycle in nontraffic accident**

X ● **V41.3** Unspecified **car occupant injured in collision with pedal cycle in nontraffic accident**

X ● **V41.4** **Person boarding or alighting a car injured in collision with pedal cycle**

X ● **V41.5** **Car driver injured in collision with pedal cycle in traffic accident**

X ● **V41.6** **Car passenger injured in collision with pedal cycle in traffic accident**

X ● **V41.7** **Person on outside of car injured in collision with pedal cycle in traffic accident**

X ● **V41.9** Unspecified **car occupant injured in collision with pedal cycle in traffic accident**

● **V42** **Car occupant injured in collision with two- or three-wheeled motor vehicle**

The appropriate 7th character is to be added to each code from category V42

A	initial encounter
D	subsequent encounter
S	sequela

X ● **V42.0** **Car driver injured in collision with two- or three-wheeled motor vehicle in nontraffic accident**

X ● **V42.1** **Car passenger injured in collision with two- or three-wheeled motor vehicle in nontraffic accident**

X ● **V42.2** **Person on outside of car injured in collision with two- or three-wheeled motor vehicle in nontraffic accident**

X ● **V42.3** Unspecified **car occupant injured in collision with two- or three-wheeled motor vehicle in nontraffic accident**

X ● **V42.4** **Person boarding or alighting a car injured in collision with two- or three-wheeled motor vehicle**

X ● **V42.5** **Car driver injured in collision with two- or three-wheeled motor vehicle in traffic accident**

X ● **V42.6** **Car passenger injured in collision with two- or three-wheeled motor vehicle in traffic accident**

X ● **V42.7** **Person on outside of car injured in collision with two- or three-wheeled motor vehicle in traffic accident**

X ● **V42.9** Unspecified **car occupant injured in collision with two- or three-wheeled motor vehicle in traffic accident**

● **V43**   Car occupant injured in collision with car, pick-up truck or van

     The appropriate 7th character is to be added to each code from category V43

> A   initial encounter
> D   subsequent encounter
> S   sequela

   ● **V43.0**   Car driver injured in collision with car, pick-up truck or van in nontraffic accident

     X ● **V43.01**   Car driver injured in collision with sport utility vehicle in nontraffic accident

     X ● **V43.02**   Car driver injured in collision with other type car in nontraffic accident

     X ● **V43.03**   Car driver injured in collision with pick-up truck in nontraffic accident

     X ● **V43.04**   Car driver injured in collision with van in nontraffic accident

   ● **V43.1**   Car passenger injured in collision with car, pick-up truck or van in nontraffic accident

     X ● **V43.11**   Car passenger injured in collision with sport utility vehicle in nontraffic accident

     X ● **V43.12**   Car passenger injured in collision with other type car in nontraffic accident

     X ● **V43.13**   Car passenger injured in collision with pick-up in nontraffic accident

     X ● **V43.14**   Car passenger injured in collision with van in nontraffic accident

   ● **V43.2**   Person on outside of car injured in collision with car, pick-up truck or van in nontraffic accident

     X ● **V43.21**   Person on outside of car injured in collision with sport utility vehicle in nontraffic accident

     X ● **V43.22**   Person on outside of car injured in collision with other type car in nontraffic accident

     X ● **V43.23**   Person on outside of car injured in collision with pick-up truck in nontraffic accident

     X ● **V43.24**   Person on outside of car injured in collision with van in nontraffic accident

   ● **V43.3**   Unspecified car occupant injured in collision with car, pick-up truck or van in nontraffic accident

     X ● **V43.31**   Unspecified car occupant injured in collision with sport utility vehicle in nontraffic accident

     X ● **V43.32**   Unspecified car occupant injured in collision with other type car in nontraffic accident

     X ● **V43.33**   Unspecified car occupant injured in collision with pick-up truck in nontraffic accident

     X ● **V43.34**   Unspecified car occupant injured in collision with van in nontraffic accident

   ● **V43.4**   Person boarding or alighting a car injured in collision with car, pick-up truck or van

     X ● **V43.41**   Person boarding or alighting a car injured in collision with sport utility vehicle

     X ● **V43.42**   Person boarding or alighting a car injured in collision with other type car

     X ● **V43.43**   Person boarding or alighting a car injured in collision with pick-up truck

     X ● **V43.44**   Person boarding or alighting a car injured in collision with van

   ● **V43.5**   Car driver injured in collision with car, pick-up truck or van in traffic accident

     X ● **V43.51**   Car driver injured in collision with sport utility vehicle in traffic accident

     X ● **V43.52**   Car driver injured in collision with other type car in traffic accident

     X ● **V43.53**   Car driver injured in collision with pick-up truck in traffic accident

     X ● **V43.54**   Car driver injured in collision with van in traffic accident

   ● **V43.6**   Car passenger injured in collision with car, pick-up truck or van in traffic accident

     X ● **V43.61**   Car passenger injured in collision with sport utility vehicle in traffic accident

     X ● **V43.62**   Car passenger injured in collision with other type car in traffic accident

     X ● **V43.63**   Car passenger injured in collision with pick-up truck in traffic accident

     X ● **V43.64**   Car passenger injured in collision with van in traffic accident

   ● **V43.7**   Person on outside of car injured in collision with car, pick-up truck or van in traffic accident

     X ● **V43.71**   Person on outside of car injured in collision with sport utility vehicle in traffic accident

     X ● **V43.72**   Person on outside of car injured in collision with other type car in traffic accident

     X ● **V43.73**   Person on outside of car injured in collision with pick-up truck in traffic accident

     X ● **V43.74**   Person on outside of car injured in collision with van in traffic accident

   ● **V43.9**   Unspecified car occupant injured in collision with car, pick-up truck or van in traffic accident

     X ● **V43.91**   Unspecified car occupant injured in collision with sport utility vehicle in traffic accident

     X ● **V43.92**   Unspecified car occupant injured in collision with other type car in traffic accident

     X ● **V43.93**   Unspecified car occupant injured in collision with pick-up truck in traffic accident

     X ● **V43.94**   Unspecified car occupant injured in collision with van in traffic accident

● **V44**   Car occupant injured in collision with heavy transport vehicle or bus

> **Excludes1**   car occupant injured in collision with military vehicle (V49.81)

     The appropriate 7th character is to be added to each code from category V44

> A   initial encounter
> D   subsequent encounter
> S   sequela

   X ● **V44.0**   Car driver injured in collision with heavy transport vehicle or bus in nontraffic accident

   X ● **V44.1**   Car passenger injured in collision with heavy transport vehicle or bus in nontraffic accident

   X ● **V44.2**   Person on outside of car injured in collision with heavy transport vehicle or bus in nontraffic accident

   X ● **V44.3**   Unspecified car occupant injured in collision with heavy transport vehicle or bus in nontraffic accident

   X ● **V44.4**   Person boarding or alighting a car injured in collision with heavy transport vehicle or bus

   X ● **V44.5**   Car driver injured in collision with heavy transport vehicle or bus in traffic accident

   X ● **V44.6**   Car passenger injured in collision with heavy transport vehicle or bus in traffic accident

   X ● **V44.7**   Person on outside of car injured in collision with heavy transport vehicle or bus in traffic accident

   X ● **V44.9**   Unspecified car occupant injured in collision with heavy transport vehicle or bus in traffic accident

---

● **V45**   **Car occupant injured in collision with railway train or railway vehicle**

The appropriate 7th character is to be added to each code from category V45

> A   initial encounter
> D   subsequent encounter
> S   sequela

X ● **V45.0**   Car driver injured in collision with railway train or railway vehicle in nontraffic accident

X ● **V45.1**   Car passenger injured in collision with railway train or railway vehicle in nontraffic accident

X ● **V45.2**   Person on outside of car injured in collision with railway train or railway vehicle in nontraffic accident

X ● **V45.3**   Unspecified car occupant injured in collision with railway train or railway vehicle in nontraffic accident

X ● **V45.4**   Person boarding or alighting a car injured in collision with railway train or railway vehicle

X ● **V45.5**   Car driver injured in collision with railway train or railway vehicle in traffic accident

X ● **V45.6**   Car passenger injured in collision with railway train or railway vehicle in traffic accident

X ● **V45.7**   Person on outside of car injured in collision with railway train or railway vehicle in traffic accident

X ● **V45.9**   Unspecified car occupant injured in collision with railway train or railway vehicle in traffic accident

● **V46**   **Car occupant injured in collision with other nonmotor vehicle**

Includes   collision with animal-drawn vehicle, animal being ridden, streetcar

The appropriate 7th character is to be added to each code from category V46

> A   initial encounter
> D   subsequent encounter
> S   sequela

X ● **V46.0**   Car driver injured in collision with other nonmotor vehicle in nontraffic accident

X ● **V46.1**   Car passenger injured in collision with other nonmotor vehicle in nontraffic accident

X ● **V46.2**   Person on outside of car injured in collision with other nonmotor vehicle in nontraffic accident

X ● **V46.3**   Unspecified car occupant injured in collision with other nonmotor vehicle in nontraffic accident

X ● **V46.4**   Person boarding or alighting a car injured in collision with other nonmotor vehicle

X ● **V46.5**   Car driver injured in collision with other nonmotor vehicle in traffic accident

X ● **V46.6**   Car passenger injured in collision with other nonmotor vehicle in traffic accident

X ● **V46.7**   Person on outside of car injured in collision with other nonmotor vehicle in traffic accident

X ● **V46.9**   Unspecified car occupant injured in collision with other nonmotor vehicle in traffic accident

● **V47**   **Car occupant injured in collision with fixed or stationary object**

The appropriate 7th character is to be added to each code from category V47

> A   initial encounter
> D   subsequent encounter
> S   sequela

● **V47.0**   Car driver injured in collision with fixed or stationary object in nontraffic accident

   X ● **V47.01**   Driver of sport utility vehicle injured in collision with fixed or stationary object in nontraffic accident

   X ● **V47.02**   Driver of other type car injured in collision with fixed or stationary object in nontraffic accident

● **V47.1**   Car passenger injured in collision with fixed or stationary object in nontraffic accident

   X ● **V47.11**   Passenger of sport utility vehicle injured in collision with fixed or stationary object in nontraffic accident

   X ● **V47.12**   Passenger of other type car injured in collision with fixed or stationary object in nontraffic accident

X ● **V47.2**   Person on outside of car injured in collision with fixed or stationary object in nontraffic accident

● **V47.3**   Unspecified car occupant injured in collision with fixed or stationary object in nontraffic accident

   X ● **V47.31**   Unspecified occupant of sport utility vehicle injured in collision with fixed or stationary object in nontraffic accident

   X ● **V47.32**   Unspecified occupant of other type car injured in collision with fixed or stationary object in nontraffic accident

X ● **V47.4**   Person boarding or alighting a car injured in collision with fixed or stationary object

● **V47.5**   Car driver injured in collision with fixed or stationary object in traffic accident

   X ● **V47.51**   Driver of sport utility vehicle injured in collision with fixed or stationary object in traffic accident

   X ● **V47.52**   Driver of other type car injured in collision with fixed or stationary object in traffic accident

● **V47.6**   Car passenger injured in collision with fixed or stationary object in traffic accident

   X ● **V47.61**   Passenger of sport utility vehicle injured in collision with fixed or stationary object in traffic accident

   X ● **V47.62**   Passenger of other type car injured in collision with fixed or stationary object in traffic accident

X ● **V47.7**   Person on outside of car injured in collision with fixed or stationary object in traffic accident

● **V47.9**   Unspecified car occupant injured in collision with fixed or stationary object in traffic accident

   X ● **V47.91**   Unspecified occupant of sport utility vehicle injured in collision with fixed or stationary object in traffic accident

   X ● **V47.92**   Unspecified occupant of other type car injured in collision with fixed or stationary object in traffic accident

● **V48**   **Car occupant injured in noncollision transport accident**

Includes   overturning car NOS
overturning car without collision

The appropriate 7th character is to be added to each code from category V48

> A   initial encounter
> D   subsequent encounter
> S   sequela

X ● **V48.0**   Car driver injured in noncollision transport accident in nontraffic accident

X ● **V48.1**   Car passenger injured in noncollision transport accident in nontraffic accident

X ● **V48.2**   Person on outside of car injured in noncollision transport accident in nontraffic accident

X ● **V48.3**   Unspecified car occupant injured in noncollision transport accident in nontraffic accident

X ● **V48.4**   Person boarding or alighting a car injured in noncollision transport accident

X ● **V48.5**   Car driver injured in noncollision transport accident in traffic accident

X ● **V48.6**   Car passenger injured in noncollision transport accident in traffic accident

X ● **V48.7**   Person on outside of car injured in noncollision transport accident in traffic accident

X ● **V48.9**   Unspecified car occupant injured in noncollision transport accident in traffic accident

- **V49   Car occupant injured in other and unspecified transport accidents**

  The appropriate 7th character is to be added to each code from category V49

A	initial encounter
D	subsequent encounter
S	sequela

  - **V49.0   Driver injured in collision with other and unspecified motor vehicles in nontraffic accident**
    - X● **V49.00   Driver injured in collision with unspecified motor vehicles in nontraffic accident**
    - X● **V49.09   Driver injured in collision with other motor vehicles in nontraffic accident**
  - **V49.1   Passenger injured in collision with other and unspecified motor vehicles in nontraffic accident**
    - X● **V49.10   Passenger injured in collision with unspecified motor vehicles in nontraffic accident**
    - X● **V49.19   Passenger injured in collision with other motor vehicles in nontraffic accident**
  - **V49.2   Unspecified car occupant injured in collision with other and unspecified motor vehicles in nontraffic accident**
    - X● **V49.20   Unspecified car occupant injured in collision with unspecified motor vehicles in nontraffic accident**

      Car collision NOS, nontraffic
    - X● **V49.29   Unspecified car occupant injured in collision with other motor vehicles in nontraffic accident**
  - X● **V49.3   Car occupant (driver) (passenger) injured in unspecified nontraffic accident**

    Car accident NOS, nontraffic
    Car occupant injured in nontraffic accident NOS
  - **V49.4   Driver injured in collision with other and unspecified motor vehicles in traffic accident**
    - X● **V49.40   Driver injured in collision with unspecified motor vehicles in traffic accident**
    - X● **V49.49   Driver injured in collision with other motor vehicles in traffic accident**
  - **V49.5   Passenger injured in collision with other and unspecified motor vehicles in traffic accident**
    - X● **V49.50   Passenger injured in collision with unspecified motor vehicles in traffic accident**
    - X● **V49.59   Passenger injured in collision with other motor vehicles in traffic accident**
  - **V49.6   Unspecified car occupant injured in collision with other and unspecified motor vehicles in traffic accident**
    - X● **V49.60   Unspecified car occupant injured in collision with unspecified motor vehicles in traffic accident**

      Car collision NOS (traffic)
    - X● **V49.69   Unspecified car occupant injured in collision with other motor vehicles in traffic accident**
  - **V49.8   Car occupant (driver) (passenger) injured in other specified transport accidents**
    - X● **V49.81   Car occupant (driver) (passenger) injured in transport accident with military vehicle**
    - X● **V49.88   Car occupant (driver) (passenger) injured in other specified transport accidents**
  - X● **V49.9   Car occupant (driver) (passenger) injured in unspecified traffic accident**

    Car accident NOS

OCCUPANT OF PICK-UP TRUCK OR VAN INJURED IN TRANSPORT ACCIDENT (V50-V59)

Includes	a four- or six-wheel motor vehicle designed primarily for carrying passengers and property but weighing less than the local limit for classification as a heavy goods vehicle
	minibus
	minivan
	sport utility vehicle (SUV)
	truck
	van
Excludes1	heavy transport vehicle (V60-V69)

- **V50   Occupant of pick-up truck or van injured in collision with pedestrian or animal**

Excludes1	pick-up truck or van collision with animal-drawn vehicle or animal being ridden (V56.-)

  The appropriate 7th character is to be added to each code from category V50

A	initial encounter
D	subsequent encounter
S	sequela

  - X● **V50.0   Driver of pick-up truck or van injured in collision with pedestrian or animal in nontraffic accident**
  - X● **V50.1   Passenger in pick-up truck or van injured in collision with pedestrian or animal in nontraffic accident**
  - X● **V50.2   Person on outside of pick-up truck or van injured in collision with pedestrian or animal in nontraffic accident**
  - X● **V50.3   Unspecified occupant of pick-up truck or van injured in collision with pedestrian or animal in nontraffic accident**
  - X● **V50.4   Person boarding or alighting a pick-up truck or van injured in collision with pedestrian or animal**
  - X● **V50.5   Driver of pick-up truck or van injured in collision with pedestrian or animal in traffic accident**
  - X● **V50.6   Passenger in pick-up truck or van injured in collision with pedestrian or animal in traffic accident**
  - X● **V50.7   Person on outside of pick-up truck or van injured in collision with pedestrian or animal in traffic accident**
  - X● **V50.9   Unspecified occupant of pick-up truck or van injured in collision with pedestrian or animal in traffic accident**

- **V51   Occupant of pick-up truck or van injured in collision with pedal cycle**

  The appropriate 7th character is to be added to each code from category V51

A	initial encounter
D	subsequent encounter
S	sequela

  - X● **V51.0   Driver of pick-up truck or van injured in collision with pedal cycle in nontraffic accident**
  - X● **V51.1   Passenger in pick-up truck or van injured in collision with pedal cycle in nontraffic accident**
  - X● **V51.2   Person on outside of pick-up truck or van injured in collision with pedal cycle in nontraffic accident**
  - X● **V51.3   Unspecified occupant of pick-up truck or van injured in collision with pedal cycle in nontraffic accident**
  - X● **V51.4   Person boarding or alighting a pick-up truck or van injured in collision with pedal cycle**
  - X● **V51.5   Driver of pick-up truck or van injured in collision with pedal cycle in traffic accident**
  - X● **V51.6   Passenger in pick-up truck or van injured in collision with pedal cycle in traffic accident**
  - X● **V51.7   Person on outside of pick-up truck or van injured in collision with pedal cycle in traffic accident**
  - X● **V51.9   Unspecified occupant of pick-up truck or van injured in collision with pedal cycle in traffic accident**

◄ New   ◄▥ Revised   ̶d̶e̶l̶e̶t̶e̶d̶ Deleted   **OGCR** Official Guidelines   X Assign placeholder X   ● Use Additional Character(s)

Excludes 1   Excludes 2   Includes   Use additional   Code first   Code also   Unspecified

1475

● **V52** **Occupant of pick-up truck or van injured in collision with two- or three-wheeled motor vehicle**

The appropriate 7th character is to be added to each code from category V52

A	initial encounter
D	subsequent encounter
S	sequela

X ● **V52.0** Driver of pick-up truck or van injured in collision with two- or three-wheeled motor vehicle in nontraffic accident

X ● **V52.1** Passenger in pick-up truck or van injured in collision with two- or three-wheeled motor vehicle in nontraffic accident

X ● **V52.2** Person on outside of pick-up truck or van injured in collision with two- or three-wheeled motor vehicle in nontraffic accident

X ● **V52.3** Unspecified occupant of pick-up truck or van injured in collision with two- or three-wheeled motor vehicle in nontraffic accident

X ● **V52.4** Person boarding or alighting a pick-up truck or van injured in collision with two- or three-wheeled motor vehicle

X ● **V52.5** Driver of pick-up truck or van injured in collision with two- or three-wheeled motor vehicle in traffic accident

X ● **V52.6** Passenger in pick-up truck or van injured in collision with two- or three-wheeled motor vehicle in traffic accident

X ● **V52.7** Person on outside of pick-up truck or van injured in collision with two- or three-wheeled motor vehicle in traffic accident

X ● **V52.9** Unspecified occupant of pick-up truck or van injured in collision with two- or three-wheeled motor vehicle in traffic accident

● **V53** **Occupant of pick-up truck or van injured in collision with car, pick-up truck or van**

The appropriate 7th character is to be added to each code from category V53

A	initial encounter
D	subsequent encounter
S	sequela

X ● **V53.0** Driver of pick-up truck or van injured in collision with car, pick-up truck or van in nontraffic accident

X ● **V53.1** Passenger in pick-up truck or van injured in collision with car, pick-up truck or van in nontraffic accident

X ● **V53.2** Person on outside of pick-up truck or van injured in collision with car, pick-up truck or van in nontraffic accident

X ● **V53.3** Unspecified occupant of pick-up truck or van injured in collision with car, pick-up truck or van in nontraffic accident

X ● **V53.4** Person boarding or alighting a pick-up truck or van injured in collision with car, pick-up truck or van

X ● **V53.5** Driver of pick-up truck or van injured in collision with car, pick-up truck or van in traffic accident

X ● **V53.6** Passenger in pick-up truck or van injured in collision with car, pick-up truck or van in traffic accident

X ● **V53.7** Person on outside of pick-up truck or van injured in collision with car, pick-up truck or van in traffic accident

X ● **V53.9** Unspecified occupant of pick-up truck or van injured in collision with car, pick-up truck or van in traffic accident

● **V54** **Occupant of pick-up truck or van injured in collision with heavy transport vehicle or bus**

> **Excludes1** occupant of pick-up truck or van injured in collision with military vehicle (V59.81)

The appropriate 7th character is to be added to each code from category V54

A	initial encounter
D	subsequent encounter
S	sequela

X ● **V54.0** Driver of pick-up truck or van injured in collision with heavy transport vehicle or bus in nontraffic accident

X ● **V54.1** Passenger in pick-up truck or van injured in collision with heavy transport vehicle or bus in nontraffic accident

X ● **V54.2** Person on outside of pick-up truck or van injured in collision with heavy transport vehicle or bus in nontraffic accident

X ● **V54.3** Unspecified occupant of pick-up truck or van injured in collision with heavy transport vehicle or bus in nontraffic accident

X ● **V54.4** Person boarding or alighting a pick-up truck or van injured in collision with heavy transport vehicle or bus

X ● **V54.5** Driver of pick-up truck or van injured in collision with heavy transport vehicle or bus in traffic accident

X ● **V54.6** Passenger in pick-up truck or van injured in collision with heavy transport vehicle or bus in traffic accident

X ● **V54.7** Person on outside of pick-up truck or van injured in collision with heavy transport vehicle or bus in traffic accident

X ● **V54.9** Unspecified occupant of pick-up truck or van injured in collision with heavy transport vehicle or bus in traffic accident

● **V55** **Occupant of pick-up truck or van injured in collision with railway train or railway vehicle**

The appropriate 7th character is to be added to each code from category V55

A	initial encounter
D	subsequent encounter
S	sequela

X ● **V55.0** Driver of pick-up truck or van injured in collision with railway train or railway vehicle in nontraffic accident

X ● **V55.1** Passenger in pick-up truck or van injured in collision with railway train or railway vehicle in nontraffic accident

X ● **V55.2** Person on outside of pick-up truck or van injured in collision with railway train or railway vehicle in nontraffic accident

X ● **V55.3** Unspecified occupant of pick-up truck or van injured in collision with railway train or railway vehicle in nontraffic accident

X ● **V55.4** Person boarding or alighting a pick-up truck or van injured in collision with railway train or railway vehicle

X ● **V55.5** Driver of pick-up truck or van injured in collision with railway train or railway vehicle in traffic accident

X ● **V55.6** Passenger in pick-up truck or van injured in collision with railway train or railway vehicle in traffic accident

X ● **V55.7** Person on outside of pick-up truck or van injured in collision with railway train or railway vehicle in traffic accident

X ● **V55.9** Unspecified occupant of pick-up truck or van injured in collision with railway train or railway vehicle in traffic accident

● **V56** **Occupant of pick-up truck or van injured in collision with other nonmotor vehicle**

> **Includes**   collision with animal-drawn vehicle, animal being ridden, streetcar

> The appropriate 7th character is to be added to each code from category V56

> | | |
> |---|---|
> | A | initial encounter |
> | D | subsequent encounter |
> | S | sequela |

X ● **V56.0** Driver of pick-up truck or van injured in collision with other nonmotor vehicle in nontraffic accident

X ● **V56.1** Passenger in pick-up truck or van injured in collision with other nonmotor vehicle in nontraffic accident

X ● **V56.2** Person on outside of pick-up truck or van injured in collision with other nonmotor vehicle in nontraffic accident

X ● **V56.3** Unspecified occupant of pick-up truck or van injured in collision with other nonmotor vehicle in nontraffic accident

X ● **V56.4** Person boarding or alighting a pick-up truck or van injured in collision with other nonmotor vehicle

X ● **V56.5** Driver of pick-up truck or van injured in collision with other nonmotor vehicle in traffic accident

X ● **V56.6** Passenger in pick-up truck or van injured in collision with other nonmotor vehicle in traffic accident

X ● **V56.7** Person on outside of pick-up truck or van injured in collision with other nonmotor vehicle in traffic accident

X ● **V56.9** Unspecified occupant of pick-up truck or van injured in collision with other nonmotor vehicle in traffic accident

● **V57** **Occupant of pick-up truck or van injured in collision with fixed or stationary object**

> The appropriate 7th character is to be added to each code from category V57

> | | |
> |---|---|
> | A | initial encounter |
> | D | subsequent encounter |
> | S | sequela |

X ● **V57.0** Driver of pick-up truck or van injured in collision with fixed or stationary object in nontraffic accident

X ● **V57.1** Passenger in pick-up truck or van injured in collision with fixed or stationary object in nontraffic accident

X ● **V57.2** Person on outside of pick-up truck or van injured in collision with fixed or stationary object in nontraffic accident

X ● **V57.3** Unspecified occupant of pick-up truck or van injured in collision with fixed or stationary object in nontraffic accident

X ● **V57.4** Person boarding or alighting a pick-up truck or van injured in collision with fixed or stationary object

X ● **V57.5** Driver of pick-up truck or van injured in collision with fixed or stationary object in traffic accident

X ● **V57.6** Passenger in pick-up truck or van injured in collision with fixed or stationary object in traffic accident

X ● **V57.7** Person on outside of pick-up truck or van injured in collision with fixed or stationary object in traffic accident

X ● **V57.9** Unspecified occupant of pick-up truck or van injured in collision with fixed or stationary object in traffic accident

● **V58** **Occupant of pick-up truck or van injured in noncollision transport accident**

> **Includes**   overturning pick-up truck or van NOS
>   overturning pick-up truck or van without collision

> The appropriate 7th character is to be added to each code from category V58

> | | |
> |---|---|
> | A | initial encounter |
> | D | subsequent encounter |
> | S | sequela |

X ● **V58.0** Driver of pick-up truck or van injured in noncollision transport accident in nontraffic accident

X ● **V58.1** Passenger in pick-up truck or van injured in noncollision transport accident in nontraffic accident

X ● **V58.2** Person on outside of pick-up truck or van injured in noncollision transport accident in nontraffic accident

X ● **V58.3** Unspecified occupant of pick-up truck or van injured in noncollision transport accident in nontraffic accident

X ● **V58.4** Person boarding or alighting a pick-up truck or van injured in noncollision transport accident

X ● **V58.5** Driver of pick-up truck or van injured in noncollision transport accident in traffic accident

X ● **V58.6** Passenger in pick-up truck or van injured in noncollision transport accident in traffic accident

X ● **V58.7** Person on outside of pick-up truck or van injured in noncollision transport accident in traffic accident

X ● **V58.9** Unspecified occupant of pick-up truck or van injured in noncollision transport accident in traffic accident

● **V59** **Occupant of pick-up truck or van injured in other and unspecified transport accidents**

> The appropriate 7th character is to be added to each code from category V59

> | | |
> |---|---|
> | A | initial encounter |
> | D | subsequent encounter |
> | S | sequela |

● **V59.0** Driver of pick-up truck or van injured in collision with other and unspecified motor vehicles in nontraffic accident

X ● **V59.00** Driver of pick-up truck or van injured in collision with unspecified motor vehicles in nontraffic accident

X ● **V59.09** Driver of pick-up truck or van injured in collision with other motor vehicles in nontraffic accident

● **V59.1** Passenger in pick-up truck or van injured in collision with other and unspecified motor vehicles in nontraffic accident

X ● **V59.10** Passenger in pick-up truck or van injured in collision with unspecified motor vehicles in nontraffic accident

X ● **V59.19** Passenger in pick-up truck or van injured in collision with other motor vehicles in nontraffic accident

CHAPTER 20 (V01-Y99)

CHAPTER 20 (V01-Y99)

● **V59.2** Unspecified occupant of pick-up truck or van injured in collision with other and unspecified motor vehicles in nontraffic accident

   X ● **V59.20** Unspecified occupant of pick-up truck or van injured in collision with unspecified motor vehicles in nontraffic accident

         Collision NOS involving pick-up truck or van, nontraffic

   X ● **V59.29** Unspecified occupant of pick-up truck or van injured in collision with other motor vehicles in nontraffic accident

 X ● **V59.3** Occupant (driver) (passenger) of pick-up truck or van injured in unspecified nontraffic accident

      Accident NOS involving pick-up truck or van, nontraffic

      Occupant of pick-up truck or van injured in nontraffic accident NOS

● **V59.4** Driver of pick-up truck or van injured in collision with other and unspecified motor vehicles in traffic accident

   X ● **V59.40** Driver of pick-up truck or van injured in collision with unspecified motor vehicles in traffic accident

   X ● **V59.49** Driver of pick-up truck or van injured in collision with other motor vehicles in traffic accident

● **V59.5** Passenger in pick-up truck or van injured in collision with other and unspecified motor vehicles in traffic accident

   X ● **V59.50** Passenger in pick-up truck or van injured in collision with unspecified motor vehicles in traffic accident

   X ● **V59.59** Passenger in pick-up truck or van injured in collision with other motor vehicles in traffic accident

● **V59.6** Unspecified occupant of pick-up truck or van injured in collision with other and unspecified motor vehicles in traffic accident

   X ● **V59.60** Unspecified occupant of pick-up truck or van injured in collision with unspecified motor vehicles in traffic accident

         Collision NOS involving pick-up truck or van (traffic)

   X ● **V59.69** Unspecified occupant of pick-up truck or van injured in collision with other motor vehicles in traffic accident

● **V59.8** Occupant (driver) (passenger) of pick-up truck or van injured in other specified transport accidents

   X ● **V59.81** Occupant (driver) (passenger) of pick-up truck or van injured in transport accident with military vehicle

   X ● **V59.88** Occupant (driver) (passenger) of pick-up truck or van injured in other specified transport accidents

 X ● **V59.9** Occupant (driver) (passenger) of pick-up truck or van injured in unspecified traffic accident

      Accident NOS involving pick-up truck or van

OCCUPANT OF HEAVY TRANSPORT VEHICLE INJURED IN TRANSPORT ACCIDENT (V60-V69)

Includes	18 wheeler
	armored car
	panel truck
Excludes1	bus
	motorcoach

● **V60** Occupant of heavy transport vehicle injured in collision with pedestrian or animal

    Excludes1 heavy transport vehicle collision with animal-drawn vehicle or animal being ridden (V66.-)

   The appropriate 7th character is to be added to each code from category V60

     A   initial encounter
     D   subsequent encounter
     S   sequela

 X ● **V60.0** Driver of heavy transport vehicle injured in collision with pedestrian or animal in nontraffic accident

 X ● **V60.1** Passenger in heavy transport vehicle injured in collision with pedestrian or animal in nontraffic accident

 X ● **V60.2** Person on outside of heavy transport vehicle injured in collision with pedestrian or animal in nontraffic accident

 X ● **V60.3** Unspecified occupant of heavy transport vehicle injured in collision with pedestrian or animal in nontraffic accident

 X ● **V60.4** Person boarding or alighting a heavy transport vehicle injured in collision with pedestrian or animal

 X ● **V60.5** Driver of heavy transport vehicle injured in collision with pedestrian or animal in traffic accident

 X ● **V60.6** Passenger in heavy transport vehicle injured in collision with pedestrian or animal in traffic accident

 X ● **V60.7** Person on outside of heavy transport vehicle injured in collision with pedestrian or animal in traffic accident

 X ● **V60.9** Unspecified occupant of heavy transport vehicle injured in collision with pedestrian or animal in traffic accident

● **V61** Occupant of heavy transport vehicle injured in collision with pedal cycle

   The appropriate 7th character is to be added to each code from category V61

     A   initial encounter
     D   subsequent encounter
     S   sequela

 X ● **V61.0** Driver of heavy transport vehicle injured in collision with pedal cycle in nontraffic accident

 X ● **V61.1** Passenger in heavy transport vehicle injured in collision with pedal cycle in nontraffic accident

 X ● **V61.2** Person on outside of heavy transport vehicle injured in collision with pedal cycle in nontraffic accident

 X ● **V61.3** Unspecified occupant of heavy transport vehicle injured in collision with pedal cycle in nontraffic accident

 X ● **V61.4** Person boarding or alighting a heavy transport vehicle injured in collision with pedal cycle while boarding or alighting

 X ● **V61.5** Driver of heavy transport vehicle injured in collision with pedal cycle in traffic accident

 X ● **V61.6** Passenger in heavy transport vehicle injured in collision with pedal cycle in traffic accident

 X ● **V61.7** Person on outside of heavy transport vehicle injured in collision with pedal cycle in traffic accident

 X ● **V61.9** Unspecified occupant of heavy transport vehicle injured in collision with pedal cycle in traffic accident

---

◀ New   ◀▦ Revised   ~~deleted~~ Deleted   OGCR Official Guidelines   X Assign placeholder X   ● Use Additional Character(s)

Excludes 1   Excludes 2   Includes   Use additional   Code first   Code also   Unspecified

● **V62**   **Occupant of heavy transport vehicle injured in collision with two- or three-wheeled motor vehicle**

> The appropriate 7th character is to be added to each code from category V62

> | A | initial encounter |
> |---|---|
> | D | subsequent encounter |
> | S | sequela |

X ● **V62.0**   Driver of heavy transport vehicle injured in collision with two- or three-wheeled motor vehicle in nontraffic accident

X ● **V62.1**   Passenger in heavy transport vehicle injured in collision with two- or three-wheeled motor vehicle in nontraffic accident

X ● **V62.2**   Person on outside of heavy transport vehicle injured in collision with two- or three-wheeled motor vehicle in nontraffic accident

X ● **V62.3**   Unspecified occupant of heavy transport vehicle injured in collision with two- or three-wheeled motor vehicle in nontraffic accident

X ● **V62.4**   Person boarding or alighting a heavy transport vehicle injured in collision with two- or three-wheeled motor vehicle

X ● **V62.5**   Driver of heavy transport vehicle injured in collision with two- or three-wheeled motor vehicle in traffic accident

X ● **V62.6**   Passenger in heavy transport vehicle injured in collision with two- or three-wheeled motor vehicle in traffic accident

X ● **V62.7**   Person on outside of heavy transport vehicle injured in collision with two- or three-wheeled motor vehicle in traffic accident

X ● **V62.9**   Unspecified occupant of heavy transport vehicle injured in collision with two- or three-wheeled motor vehicle in traffic accident

● **V63**   **Occupant of heavy transport vehicle injured in collision with car, pick-up truck or van**

> The appropriate 7th character is to be added to each code from category V63

> | A | initial encounter |
> |---|---|
> | D | subsequent encounter |
> | S | sequela |

X ● **V63.0**   Driver of heavy transport vehicle injured in collision with car, pick-up truck or van in nontraffic accident

X ● **V63.1**   Passenger in heavy transport vehicle injured in collision with car, pick-up truck or van in nontraffic accident

X ● **V63.2**   Person on outside of heavy transport vehicle injured in collision with car, pick-up truck or van in nontraffic accident

X ● **V63.3**   Unspecified occupant of heavy transport vehicle injured in collision with car, pick-up truck or van in nontraffic accident

X ● **V63.4**   Person boarding or alighting a heavy transport vehicle injured in collision with car, pick-up truck or van

X ● **V63.5**   Driver of heavy transport vehicle injured in collision with car, pick-up truck or van in traffic accident

X ● **V63.6**   Passenger in heavy transport vehicle injured in collision with car, pick-up truck or van in traffic accident

X ● **V63.7**   Person on outside of heavy transport vehicle injured in collision with car, pick-up truck or van in traffic accident

X ● **V63.9**   Unspecified occupant of heavy transport vehicle injured in collision with car, pick-up truck or van in traffic accident

● **V64**   **Occupant of heavy transport vehicle injured in collision with heavy transport vehicle or bus**

> **Excludes1**   occupant of heavy transport vehicle injured in collision with military vehicle (V69.81)

> The appropriate 7th character is to be added to each code from category V64

> | A | initial encounter |
> |---|---|
> | D | subsequent encounter |
> | S | sequela |

X ● **V64.0**   Driver of heavy transport vehicle injured in collision with heavy transport vehicle or bus in nontraffic accident

X ● **V64.1**   Passenger in heavy transport vehicle injured in collision with heavy transport vehicle or bus in nontraffic accident

X ● **V64.2**   Person on outside of heavy transport vehicle injured in collision with heavy transport vehicle or bus in nontraffic accident

X ● **V64.3**   Unspecified occupant of heavy transport vehicle injured in collision with heavy transport vehicle or bus in nontraffic accident

X ● **V64.4**   Person boarding or alighting a heavy transport vehicle injured in collision with heavy transport vehicle or bus while boarding or alighting

X ● **V64.5**   Driver of heavy transport vehicle injured in collision with heavy transport vehicle or bus in traffic accident

X ● **V64.6**   Passenger in heavy transport vehicle injured in collision with heavy transport vehicle or bus in traffic accident

X ● **V64.7**   Person on outside of heavy transport vehicle injured in collision with heavy transport vehicle or bus in traffic accident

X ● **V64.9**   Unspecified occupant of heavy transport vehicle injured in collision with heavy transport vehicle or bus in traffic accident

● **V65**   **Occupant of heavy transport vehicle injured in collision with railway train or railway vehicle**

> The appropriate 7th character is to be added to each code from category V65

> | A | initial encounter |
> |---|---|
> | D | subsequent encounter |
> | S | sequela |

X ● **V65.0**   Driver of heavy transport vehicle injured in collision with railway train or railway vehicle in nontraffic accident

X ● **V65.1**   Passenger in heavy transport vehicle injured in collision with railway train or railway vehicle in nontraffic accident

X ● **V65.2**   Person on outside of heavy transport vehicle injured in collision with railway train or railway vehicle in nontraffic accident

X ● **V65.3**   Unspecified occupant of heavy transport vehicle injured in collision with railway train or railway vehicle in nontraffic accident

X ● **V65.4**   Person boarding or alighting a heavy transport vehicle injured in collision with railway train or railway vehicle

X ● **V65.5**   Driver of heavy transport vehicle injured in collision with railway train or railway vehicle in traffic accident

X ● **V65.6**   Passenger in heavy transport vehicle injured in collision with railway train or railway vehicle in traffic accident

X ● **V65.7**   Person on outside of heavy transport vehicle injured in collision with railway train or railway vehicle in traffic accident

X ● **V65.9**   Unspecified occupant of heavy transport vehicle injured in collision with railway train or railway vehicle in traffic accident

CHAPTER 20 (V01-Y99)

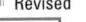

● **V66 Occupant of heavy transport vehicle injured in collision with other nonmotor vehicle**

> **Includes**   collision with animal-drawn vehicle, animal being ridden, streetcar

The appropriate 7th character is to be added to each code from category V66

> A   initial encounter
> D   subsequent encounter
> S   sequela

X● **V66.0** Driver of heavy transport vehicle injured in collision with other nonmotor vehicle in nontraffic accident

X● **V66.1** Passenger in heavy transport vehicle injured in collision with other nonmotor vehicle in nontraffic accident

X● **V66.2** Person on outside of heavy transport vehicle injured in collision with other nonmotor vehicle in nontraffic accident

X● **V66.3** Unspecified occupant of heavy transport vehicle injured in collision with other nonmotor vehicle in nontraffic accident

X● **V66.4** Person boarding or alighting a heavy transport vehicle injured in collision with other nonmotor vehicle

X● **V66.5** Driver of heavy transport vehicle injured in collision with other nonmotor vehicle in traffic accident

X● **V66.6** Passenger in heavy transport vehicle injured in collision with other nonmotor vehicle in traffic accident

X● **V66.7** Person on outside of heavy transport vehicle injured in collision with other nonmotor vehicle in traffic accident

X● **V66.9** Unspecified occupant of heavy transport vehicle injured in collision with other nonmotor vehicle in traffic accident

● **V67 Occupant of heavy transport vehicle injured in collision with fixed or stationary object**

The appropriate 7th character is to be added to each code from category V67

> A   initial encounter
> D   subsequent encounter
> S   sequela

X● **V67.0** Driver of heavy transport vehicle injured in collision with fixed or stationary object in nontraffic accident

X● **V67.1** Passenger in heavy transport vehicle injured in collision with fixed or stationary object in nontraffic accident

X● **V67.2** Person on outside of heavy transport vehicle injured in collision with fixed or stationary object in nontraffic accident

X● **V67.3** Unspecified occupant of heavy transport vehicle injured in collision with fixed or stationary object in nontraffic accident

X● **V67.4** Person boarding or alighting a heavy transport vehicle injured in collision with fixed or stationary object

X● **V67.5** Driver of heavy transport vehicle injured in collision with fixed or stationary object in traffic accident

X● **V67.6** Passenger in heavy transport vehicle injured in collision with fixed or stationary object in traffic accident

X● **V67.7** Person on outside of heavy transport vehicle injured in collision with fixed or stationary object in traffic accident

X● **V67.9** Unspecified occupant of heavy transport vehicle injured in collision with fixed or stationary object in traffic accident

● **V68 Occupant of heavy transport vehicle injured in noncollision transport accident**

> **Includes**   overturning heavy transport vehicle NOS
> overturning heavy transport vehicle without collision

The appropriate 7th character is to be added to each code from category V68

> A   initial encounter
> D   subsequent encounter
> S   sequela

X● **V68.0** Driver of heavy transport vehicle injured in noncollision transport accident in nontraffic accident

X● **V68.1** Passenger in heavy transport vehicle injured in noncollision transport accident in nontraffic accident

X● **V68.2** Person on outside of heavy transport vehicle injured in noncollision transport accident in nontraffic accident

X● **V68.3** Unspecified occupant of heavy transport vehicle injured in noncollision transport accident in nontraffic accident

X● **V68.4** Person boarding or alighting a heavy transport vehicle injured in noncollision transport accident

X● **V68.5** Driver of heavy transport vehicle injured in noncollision transport accident in traffic accident

X● **V68.6** Passenger in heavy transport vehicle injured in noncollision transport accident in traffic accident

X● **V68.7** Person on outside of heavy transport vehicle injured in noncollision transport accident in traffic accident

X● **V68.9** Unspecified occupant of heavy transport vehicle injured in noncollision transport accident in traffic accident

● **V69 Occupant of heavy transport vehicle injured in other and unspecified transport accidents**

The appropriate 7th character is to be added to each code from category V69

> A   initial encounter
> D   subsequent encounter
> S   sequela

● **V69.0** Driver of heavy transport vehicle injured in collision with other and unspecified motor vehicles in nontraffic accident

   X● **V69.00** Driver of heavy transport vehicle injured in collision with unspecified motor vehicles in nontraffic accident

   X● **V69.09** Driver of heavy transport vehicle injured in collision with other motor vehicles in nontraffic accident

● **V69.1** Passenger in heavy transport vehicle injured in collision with other and unspecified motor vehicles in nontraffic accident

   X● **V69.10** Passenger in heavy transport vehicle injured in collision with unspecified motor vehicles in nontraffic accident

   X● **V69.19** Passenger in heavy transport vehicle injured in collision with other motor vehicles in nontraffic accident

● **V69.2** Unspecified occupant of heavy transport vehicle injured in collision with other and unspecified motor vehicles in nontraffic accident

   X● **V69.20** Unspecified occupant of heavy transport vehicle injured in collision with unspecified motor vehicles in nontraffic accident
> Collision NOS involving heavy transport vehicle, nontraffic

   X● **V69.29** Unspecified occupant of heavy transport vehicle injured in collision with other motor vehicles in nontraffic accident

X● **V69.3** Occupant (driver) (passenger) of heavy transport vehicle injured in unspecified nontraffic accident

> Accident NOS involving heavy transport vehicle, nontraffic
>
> Occupant of heavy transport vehicle injured in nontraffic accident NOS

● **V69.4** Driver of heavy transport vehicle injured in collision with other and unspecified motor vehicles in traffic accident

X● **V69.40** Driver of heavy transport vehicle injured in collision with unspecified motor vehicles in traffic accident

X● **V69.49** Driver of heavy transport vehicle injured in collision with other motor vehicles in traffic accident

● **V69.5** Passenger in heavy transport vehicle injured in collision with other and unspecified motor vehicles in traffic accident

X● **V69.50** Passenger in heavy transport vehicle injured in collision with unspecified motor vehicles in traffic accident

X● **V69.59** Passenger in heavy transport vehicle injured in collision with other motor vehicles in traffic accident

● **V69.6** Unspecified occupant of heavy transport vehicle injured in collision with other and unspecified motor vehicles in traffic accident

X● **V69.60** Unspecified occupant of heavy transport vehicle injured in collision with unspecified motor vehicles in traffic accident

> Collision NOS involving heavy transport vehicle (traffic)

X● **V69.69** Unspecified occupant of heavy transport vehicle injured in collision with other motor vehicles in traffic accident

● **V69.8** Occupant (driver) (passenger) of heavy transport vehicle injured in other specified transport accidents

X● **V69.81** Occupant (driver) (passenger) of heavy transport vehicle injured in transport accidents with military vehicle

X● **V69.88** Occupant (driver) (passenger) of heavy transport vehicle injured in other specified transport accidents

X● **V69.9** Occupant (driver) (passenger) of heavy transport vehicle injured in unspecified traffic accident

> Accident NOS involving heavy transport vehicle

BUS OCCUPANT INJURED IN TRANSPORT ACCIDENT (V70-V79)

Includes	motorcoach
Excludes1	minibus (V50-V59)

● **V70** Bus occupant injured in collision with pedestrian or animal

Excludes1	bus collision with animal-drawn vehicle or animal being ridden (V76.-)

The appropriate 7th character is to be added to each code from category V70

> | A | initial encounter |
> |---|---|
> | D | subsequent encounter |
> | S | sequela |

X● **V70.0** Driver of bus injured in collision with pedestrian or animal in nontraffic accident

X● **V70.1** Passenger on bus injured in collision with pedestrian or animal in nontraffic accident

X● **V70.2** Person on outside of bus injured in collision with pedestrian or animal in nontraffic accident

X● **V70.3** Unspecified occupant of bus injured in collision with pedestrian or animal in nontraffic accident

X● **V70.4** Person boarding or alighting from bus injured in collision with pedestrian or animal

X● **V70.5** Driver of bus injured in collision with pedestrian or animal in traffic accident

X● **V70.6** Passenger on bus injured in collision with pedestrian or animal in traffic accident

X● **V70.7** Person on outside of bus injured in collision with pedestrian or animal in traffic accident

X● **V70.9** Unspecified occupant of bus injured in collision with pedestrian or animal in traffic accident

● **V71** Bus occupant injured in collision with pedal cycle

The appropriate 7th character is to be added to each code from category V71

> | A | initial encounter |
> |---|---|
> | D | subsequent encounter |
> | S | sequela |

X● **V71.0** Driver of bus injured in collision with pedal cycle in nontraffic accident

X● **V71.1** Passenger on bus injured in collision with pedal cycle in nontraffic accident

X● **V71.2** Person on outside of bus injured in collision with pedal cycle in nontraffic accident

X● **V71.3** Unspecified occupant of bus injured in collision with pedal cycle in nontraffic accident

X● **V71.4** Person boarding or alighting from bus injured in collision with pedal cycle

X● **V71.5** Driver of bus injured in collision with pedal cycle in traffic accident

X● **V71.6** Passenger on bus injured in collision with pedal cycle in traffic accident

X● **V71.7** Person on outside of bus injured in collision with pedal cycle in traffic accident

X● **V71.9** Unspecified occupant of bus injured in collision with pedal cycle in traffic accident

● **V72** Bus occupant injured in collision with two- or three-wheeled motor vehicle

The appropriate 7th character is to be added to each code from category V72

> | A | initial encounter |
> |---|---|
> | D | subsequent encounter |
> | S | sequela |

X● **V72.0** Driver of bus injured in collision with two- or three-wheeled motor vehicle in nontraffic accident

X● **V72.1** Passenger on bus injured in collision with two- or three-wheeled motor vehicle in nontraffic accident

X● **V72.2** Person on outside of bus injured in collision with two- or three-wheeled motor vehicle in nontraffic accident

X● **V72.3** Unspecified occupant of bus injured in collision with two- or three-wheeled motor vehicle in nontraffic accident

X● **V72.4** Person boarding or alighting from bus injured in collision with two- or three-wheeled motor vehicle

X● **V72.5** Driver of bus injured in collision with two- or three-wheeled motor vehicle in traffic accident

X● **V72.6** Passenger on bus injured in collision with two- or three-wheeled motor vehicle in traffic accident

X● **V72.7** Person on outside of bus injured in collision with two- or three-wheeled motor vehicle in traffic accident

X● **V72.9** Unspecified occupant of bus injured in collision with two- or three-wheeled motor vehicle in traffic accident

● **V73 Bus occupant injured in collision with car, pick-up truck or van**

The appropriate 7th character is to be added to each code from category V73

> A   initial encounter
> D   subsequent encounter
> S   sequela

X● **V73.0** Driver of bus injured in collision with car, pick-up truck or van in nontraffic accident

X● **V73.1** Passenger on bus injured in collision with car, pick-up truck or van in nontraffic accident

X● **V73.2** Person on outside of bus injured in collision with car, pick-up truck or van in nontraffic accident

X● **V73.3** Unspecified occupant of bus injured in collision with car, pick-up truck or van in nontraffic accident

X● **V73.4** Person boarding or alighting from bus injured in collision with car, pick-up truck or van

X● **V73.5** Driver of bus injured in collision with car, pick-up truck or van in traffic accident

X● **V73.6** Passenger on bus injured in collision with car, pick-up truck or van in traffic accident

X● **V73.7** Person on outside of bus injured in collision with car, pick-up truck or van in traffic accident

X● **V73.9** Unspecified occupant of bus injured in collision with car, pick-up truck or van in traffic accident

● **V74 Bus occupant injured in collision with heavy transport vehicle or bus**

> **Excludes1** bus occupant injured in collision with military vehicle (V79.81)

The appropriate 7th character is to be added to each code from category V74

> A   initial encounter
> D   subsequent encounter
> S   sequela

X● **V74.0** Driver of bus injured in collision with heavy transport vehicle or bus in nontraffic accident

X● **V74.1** Passenger on bus injured in collision with heavy transport vehicle or bus in nontraffic accident

X● **V74.2** Person on outside of bus injured in collision with heavy transport vehicle or bus in nontraffic accident

X● **V74.3** Unspecified occupant of bus injured in collision with heavy transport vehicle or bus in nontraffic accident

X● **V74.4** Person boarding or alighting from bus injured in collision with heavy transport vehicle or bus

X● **V74.5** Driver of bus injured in collision with heavy transport vehicle or bus in traffic accident

X● **V74.6** Passenger on bus injured in collision with heavy transport vehicle or bus in traffic accident

X● **V74.7** Person on outside of bus injured in collision with heavy transport vehicle or bus in traffic accident

X● **V74.9** Unspecified occupant of bus injured in collision with heavy transport vehicle or bus in traffic accident

● **V75 Bus occupant injured in collision with railway train or railway vehicle**

The appropriate 7th character is to be added to each code from category V75

> A   initial encounter
> D   subsequent encounter
> S   sequela

X● **V75.0** Driver of bus injured in collision with railway train or railway vehicle in nontraffic accident

X● **V75.1** Passenger on bus injured in collision with railway train or railway vehicle in nontraffic accident

X● **V75.2** Person on outside of bus injured in collision with railway train or railway vehicle in nontraffic accident

X● **V75.3** Unspecified occupant of bus injured in collision with railway train or railway vehicle in nontraffic accident

X● **V75.4** Person boarding or alighting from bus injured in collision with railway train or railway vehicle

X● **V75.5** Driver of bus injured in collision with railway train or railway vehicle in traffic accident

X● **V75.6** Passenger on bus injured in collision with railway train or railway vehicle in traffic accident

X● **V75.7** Person on outside of bus injured in collision with railway train or railway vehicle in traffic accident

X● **V75.9** Unspecified occupant of bus injured in collision with railway train or railway vehicle in traffic accident

● **V76 Bus occupant injured in collision with other nonmotor vehicle**

> **Includes** collision with animal-drawn vehicle, animal being ridden, streetcar

The appropriate 7th character is to be added to each code from category V76

> A   initial encounter
> D   subsequent encounter
> S   sequela

X● **V76.0** Driver of bus injured in collision with other nonmotor vehicle in nontraffic accident

X● **V76.1** Passenger on bus injured in collision with other nonmotor vehicle in nontraffic accident

X● **V76.2** Person on outside of bus injured in collision with other nonmotor vehicle in nontraffic accident

X● **V76.3** Unspecified occupant of bus injured in collision with other nonmotor vehicle in nontraffic accident

X● **V76.4** Person boarding or alighting from bus injured in collision with other nonmotor vehicle

X● **V76.5** Driver of bus injured in collision with other nonmotor vehicle in traffic accident

X● **V76.6** Passenger on bus injured in collision with other nonmotor vehicle in traffic accident

X● **V76.7** Person on outside of bus injured in collision with other nonmotor vehicle in traffic accident

X● **V76.9** Unspecified occupant of bus injured in collision with other nonmotor vehicle in traffic accident

● **V77 Bus occupant injured in collision with fixed or stationary object**

The appropriate 7th character is to be added to each code from category V77

> A   initial encounter
> D   subsequent encounter
> S   sequela

X● **V77.0** Driver of bus injured in collision with fixed or stationary object in nontraffic accident

X● **V77.1** Passenger on bus injured in collision with fixed or stationary object in nontraffic accident

X● **V77.2** Person on outside of bus injured in collision with fixed or stationary object in nontraffic accident

X● **V77.3** Unspecified occupant of bus injured in collision with fixed or stationary object in nontraffic accident

X● **V77.4** Person boarding or alighting from bus injured in collision with fixed or stationary object

X● **V77.5** Driver of bus injured in collision with fixed or stationary object in traffic accident

X● **V77.6** Passenger on bus injured in collision with fixed or stationary object in traffic accident

X● **V77.7** Person on outside of bus injured in collision with fixed or stationary object in traffic accident

X● **V77.9** Unspecified occupant of bus injured in collision with fixed or stationary object in traffic accident

● **V78   Bus occupant injured in noncollision transport accident**

    Includes   overturning bus NOS
                overturning bus without collision

    The appropriate 7th character is to be added to each code from category V78

A	initial encounter
D	subsequent encounter
S	sequela

X ● **V78.0** Driver of bus injured in noncollision transport accident in nontraffic accident

X ● **V78.1** Passenger on bus injured in noncollision transport accident in nontraffic accident

X ● **V78.2** Person on outside of bus injured in noncollision transport accident in nontraffic accident

X ● **V78.3** Unspecified occupant of bus injured in noncollision transport accident in nontraffic accident

X ● **V78.4** Person boarding or alighting from bus injured in noncollision transport accident

X ● **V78.5** Driver of bus injured in noncollision transport accident in traffic accident

X ● **V78.6** Passenger on bus injured in noncollision transport accident in traffic accident

X ● **V78.7** Person on outside of bus injured in noncollision transport accident in traffic accident

X ● **V78.9** Unspecified occupant of bus injured in noncollision transport accident in traffic accident

● **V79   Bus occupant injured in other and unspecified transport accidents**

    The appropriate 7th character is to be added to each code from category V79

A	initial encounter
D	subsequent encounter
S	sequela

● **V79.0** Driver of bus injured in collision with other and unspecified motor vehicles in nontraffic accident

  X ● **V79.00** Driver of bus injured in collision with unspecified motor vehicles in nontraffic accident

  X ● **V79.09** Driver of bus injured in collision with other motor vehicles in nontraffic accident

● **V79.1** Passenger on bus injured in collision with other and unspecified motor vehicles in nontraffic accident

  X ● **V79.10** Passenger on bus injured in collision with unspecified motor vehicles in nontraffic accident

  X ● **V79.19** Passenger on bus injured in collision with other motor vehicles in nontraffic accident

● **V79.2** Unspecified bus occupant injured in collision with other and unspecified motor vehicles in nontraffic accident

  X ● **V79.20** Unspecified bus occupant injured in collision with unspecified motor vehicles in nontraffic accident
        Bus collision NOS, nontraffic

  X ● **V79.29** Unspecified bus occupant injured in collision with other motor vehicles in nontraffic accident

X ● **V79.3** Bus occupant (driver) (passenger) injured in unspecified nontraffic accident
      Bus accident NOS, nontraffic
      Bus occupant injured in nontraffic accident NOS

● **V79.4** Driver of bus injured in collision with other and unspecified motor vehicles in traffic accident

  X ● **V79.40** Driver of bus injured in collision with unspecified motor vehicles in traffic accident

  X ● **V79.49** Driver of bus injured in collision with other motor vehicles in traffic accident

● **V79.5** Passenger on bus injured in collision with other and unspecified motor vehicles in traffic accident

  X ● **V79.50** Passenger on bus injured in collision with unspecified motor vehicles in traffic accident

  X ● **V79.59** Passenger on bus injured in collision with other motor vehicles in traffic accident

● **V79.6** Unspecified bus occupant injured in collision with other and unspecified motor vehicles in traffic accident

  X ● **V79.60** Unspecified bus occupant injured in collision with unspecified motor vehicles in traffic accident
        Bus collision NOS (traffic)

  X ● **V79.69** Unspecified bus occupant injured in collision with other motor vehicles in traffic accident

● **V79.8** Bus occupant (driver) (passenger) injured in other specified transport accidents

  X ● **V79.81** Bus occupant (driver) (passenger) injured in transport accidents with military vehicle

  X ● **V79.88** Bus occupant (driver) (passenger) injured in other specified transport accidents

X ● **V79.9** Bus occupant (driver) (passenger) injured in unspecified traffic accident
      Bus accident NOS

OTHER LAND TRANSPORT ACCIDENTS (V80-V89)

● **V80   Animal-rider or occupant of animal-drawn vehicle injured in transport accident**

    The appropriate 7th character is to be added to each code from category V80

A	initial encounter
D	subsequent encounter
S	sequela

● **V80.0** Animal-rider or occupant of animal drawn vehicle injured by fall from or being thrown from animal or animal-drawn vehicle in noncollision accident

  ● **V80.01** Animal-rider injured by fall from or being thrown from animal in noncollision accident

    ● **V80.010** Animal-rider injured by fall from or being thrown from horse in noncollision accident

    ● **V80.018** Animal-rider injured by fall from or being thrown from other animal in noncollision accident

  X ● **V80.02** Occupant of animal-drawn vehicle injured by fall from or being thrown from animal-drawn vehicle in noncollision accident
      Overturning animal-drawn vehicle NOS
      Overturning animal-drawn vehicle without collision

● **V80.1** Animal-rider or occupant of animal-drawn vehicle injured in collision with pedestrian or animal

    Excludes1   animal-rider or animal-drawn vehicle collision with animal-drawn vehicle or animal being ridden (V80.7)

  X ● **V80.11** Animal-rider injured in collision with pedestrian or animal

  X ● **V80.12** Occupant of animal-drawn vehicle injured in collision with pedestrian or animal

◀ New   ⬅ Revised ~~deleted~~ Deleted **OGCR** Official Guidelines X Assign placeholder X ● Use Additional Character(s)

Excludes 1	Excludes 2	Includes	Use additional	Code first	Code also	Unspecified

1483

● **V80.2 Animal-rider or occupant of animal-drawn vehicle injured in collision with pedal cycle**

X ● V80.21 Animal-rider injured in collision with pedal cycle

X ● V80.22 Occupant of animal-drawn vehicle injured in collision with pedal cycle

● **V80.3 Animal-rider or occupant of animal-drawn vehicle injured in collision with two- or three-wheeled motor vehicle**

X ● V80.31 Animal-rider injured in collision with two- or three-wheeled motor vehicle

X ● V80.32 Occupant of animal-drawn vehicle injured in collision with two- or three-wheeled motor vehicle

● **V80.4 Animal-rider or occupant of animal-drawn vehicle injured in collision with car, pick-up truck, van, heavy transport vehicle or bus**

> **Excludes1**   animal-rider injured in collision with military vehicle (V80.910)
> occupant of animal-drawn vehicle injured in collision with military vehicle (V80.920)

X ● V80.41 Animal-rider injured in collision with car, pick-up truck, van, heavy transport vehicle or bus

X ● V80.42 Occupant of animal-drawn vehicle injured in collision with car, pick-up truck, van, heavy transport vehicle or bus

● **V80.5 Animal-rider or occupant of animal-drawn vehicle injured in collision with other specified motor vehicle**

X ● V80.51 Animal-rider injured in collision with other specified motor vehicle

X ● V80.52 Occupant of animal-drawn vehicle injured in collision with other specified motor vehicle

● **V80.6 Animal-rider or occupant of animal-drawn vehicle injured in collision with railway train or railway vehicle**

X ● V80.61 Animal-rider injured in collision with railway train or railway vehicle

X ● V80.62 Occupant of animal-drawn vehicle injured in collision with railway train or railway vehicle

● **V80.7 Animal-rider or occupant of animal-drawn vehicle injured in collision with other nonmotor vehicles**

● V80.71 Animal-rider or occupant of animal-drawn vehicle injured in collision with animal being ridden

● V80.710 Animal-rider injured in collision with other animal being ridden

● V80.711 Occupant of animal-drawn vehicle injured in collision with animal being ridden

● V80.72 Animal-rider or occupant of animal-drawn vehicle injured in collision with other animal-drawn vehicle

● V80.720 Animal-rider injured in collision with animal-drawn vehicle

● V80.721 Occupant of animal-drawn vehicle injured in collision with other animal-drawn vehicle

● V80.73 Animal-rider or occupant of animal-drawn vehicle injured in collision with streetcar

● V80.730 Animal-rider injured in collision with streetcar

● V80.731 Occupant of animal-drawn vehicle injured in collision with streetcar

● V80.79 Animal-rider or occupant of animal-drawn vehicle injured in collision with other nonmotor vehicles

● V80.790 Animal-rider injured in collision with other nonmotor vehicles

● V80.791 Occupant of animal-drawn vehicle injured in collision with other nonmotor vehicles

● **V80.8 Animal-rider or occupant of animal-drawn vehicle injured in collision with fixed or stationary object**

X ● V80.81 Animal-rider injured in collision with fixed or stationary object

X ● V80.82 Occupant of animal-drawn vehicle injured in collision with fixed or stationary object

● **V80.9 Animal-rider or occupant of animal-drawn vehicle injured in other and unspecified transport accidents**

● V80.91 Animal-rider injured in other and unspecified transport accidents

● V80.910 Animal-rider injured in transport accident with military vehicle

● V80.918 Animal-rider injured in other transport accident

● V80.919 Animal-rider injured in unspecified transport accident
Animal rider accident NOS

● V80.92 Occupant of animal-drawn vehicle injured in other and unspecified transport accidents

● V80.920 Occupant of animal-drawn vehicle injured in transport accident with military vehicle

● V80.928 Occupant of animal-drawn vehicle injured in other transport accident

● V80.929 Occupant of animal drawn vehicle injured in unspecified transport accident
Animal-drawn vehicle accident NOS

● **V81 Occupant of railway train or railway vehicle injured in transport accident**

> **Includes**   derailment of railway train or railway vehicle
> person on outside of train

> **Excludes1**   streetcar (V82.-)

The appropriate 7th character is to be added to each code from category V81

A	initial encounter
D	subsequent encounter
S	sequela

X ● **V81.0 Occupant of railway train or railway vehicle injured in collision with motor vehicle in nontraffic accident**

> **Excludes1**   occupant of railway train or railway vehicle injured due to collision with military vehicle (V81.83)

X ● **V81.1 Occupant of railway train or railway vehicle injured in collision with motor vehicle in traffic accident**

> **Excludes1**   occupant of railway train or railway vehicle injured due to collision with military vehicle (V81.83)

X ● **V81.2 Occupant of railway train or railway vehicle injured in collision with or hit by rolling stock**

X ● **V81.3 Occupant of railway train or railway vehicle injured in collision with other object**
Railway collision NOS

X ● **V81.4 Person injured while boarding or alighting from railway train or railway vehicle**

X ● **V81.5 Occupant of railway train or railway vehicle injured by fall in railway train or railway vehicle**

X ● **V81.6 Occupant of railway train or railway vehicle injured by fall from railway train or railway vehicle**

◀ New   ◀▥ Revised   ~~deleted~~ Deleted   **OGCR** Official Guidelines   X Assign placeholder X   ● Use Additional Character(s)

Excludes 1   Excludes 2   Includes   Use additional   Code first   Code also   Unspecified

X● **V81.7   Occupant of railway train or railway vehicle injured in derailment without antecedent collision**

● **V81.8   Occupant of railway train or railway vehicle injured in other specified railway accidents**

X● **V81.81   Occupant of railway train or railway vehicle injured due to explosion or fire on train**

X● **V81.82   Occupant of railway train or railway vehicle injured due to object falling onto train**
Occupant of railway train or railway vehicle injured due to falling earth onto train
Occupant of railway train or railway vehicle injured due to falling rocks onto train
Occupant of railway train or railway vehicle injured due to falling snow onto train
Occupant of railway train or railway vehicle injured due to falling trees onto train

X● **V81.83   Occupant of railway train or railway vehicle injured due to collision with military vehicle**

X● **V81.89   Occupant of railway train or railway vehicle injured due to other specified railway accident**

X● **V81.9   Occupant of railway train or railway vehicle injured in unspecified railway accident**
Railway accident NOS

● **V82   Occupant of powered streetcar injured in transport accident**

    Includes   interurban electric car
person on outside of streetcar
tram (car)
trolley (car)

    Excludes1   bus (V70-V79)
motorcoach (V70-V79)
nonpowered streetcar (V76.-)
train (V81.-)

The appropriate 7th character is to be added to each code from category V82

A	initial encounter
D	subsequent encounter
S	sequela

X● **V82.0   Occupant of streetcar injured in collision with motor vehicle in nontraffic accident**

X● **V82.1   Occupant of streetcar injured in collision with motor vehicle in traffic accident**

X● **V82.2   Occupant of streetcar injured in collision with or hit by rolling stock**

X● **V82.3   Occupant of streetcar injured in collision with other object**
    Excludes1   collision with animal-drawn vehicle or animal being ridden (V82.8)

X● **V82.4   Person injured while boarding or alighting from streetcar**

X● **V82.5   Occupant of streetcar injured by fall in streetcar**
    Excludes1   fall in streetcar:
while boarding or alighting (V82.4)
with antecedent collision (V82.0-V82.3)

X● **V82.6   Occupant of streetcar injured by fall from streetcar**
    Excludes1   fall from streetcar:
while boarding or alighting (V82.4)
with antecedent collision (V82.0-V82.3)

X● **V82.7   Occupant of streetcar injured in derailment without antecedent collision**
    Excludes1   occupant of streetcar injured in derailment with antecedent collision (V82.0-V82.3)

X● **V82.8   Occupant of streetcar injured in other specified transport accidents**
Streetcar collision with military vehicle
Streetcar collision with train or nonmotor vehicles

X● **V82.9   Occupant of streetcar injured in unspecified traffic accident**
Streetcar accident NOS

● **V83   Occupant of special vehicle mainly used on industrial premises injured in transport accident**

    Includes   battery-powered airport passenger vehicle
battery-powered truck (baggage) (mail)
coal-car in mine
forklift (truck)
logging car
self-propelled industrial truck
station baggage truck (powered)
tram, truck, or tub (powered) in mine or quarry

    Excludes1   special construction vehicles (V85.-)
special industrial vehicle in stationary use or maintenance (W31.-)

The appropriate 7th character is to be added to each code from category V83

A	initial encounter
D	subsequent encounter
S	sequela

X● **V83.0   Driver of special industrial vehicle injured in traffic accident**

X● **V83.1   Passenger of special industrial vehicle injured in traffic accident**

X● **V83.2   Person on outside of special industrial vehicle injured in traffic accident**

X● **V83.3   Unspecified occupant of special industrial vehicle injured in traffic accident**

X● **V83.4   Person injured while boarding or alighting from special industrial vehicle**

X● **V83.5   Driver of special industrial vehicle injured in nontraffic accident**

X● **V83.6   Passenger of special industrial vehicle injured in nontraffic accident**

X● **V83.7   Person on outside of special industrial vehicle injured in nontraffic accident**

X● **V83.9   Unspecified occupant of special industrial vehicle injured in nontraffic accident**
Special-industrial-vehicle accident NOS

● **V84   Occupant of special vehicle mainly used in agriculture injured in transport accident**

    Includes   self-propelled farm machinery
tractor (and trailer)

    Excludes1   animal-powered farm machinery accident (W30.8-)
contact with combine harvester (W30.0)
special agricultural vehicle in stationary use or maintenance (W30.-)

The appropriate 7th character is to be added to each code from category V84

A	initial encounter
D	subsequent encounter
S	sequela

X● **V84.0   Driver of special agricultural vehicle injured in traffic accident**

X● **V84.1   Passenger of special agricultural vehicle injured in traffic accident**

X● **V84.2   Person on outside of special agricultural vehicle injured in traffic accident**

X● **V84.3   Unspecified occupant of special agricultural vehicle injured in traffic accident**

X● **V84.4   Person injured while boarding or alighting from special agricultural vehicle**

X● **V84.5   Driver of special agricultural vehicle injured in nontraffic accident**

X● **V84.6   Passenger of special agricultural vehicle injured in nontraffic accident**

X● **V84.7   Person on outside of special agricultural vehicle injured in nontraffic accident**

X● **V84.9   Unspecified occupant of special agricultural vehicle injured in nontraffic accident**
Special-agricultural vehicle accident NOS

◀ New   ◀━ Revised   ~~deleted~~ Deleted   OGCR Official Guidelines   X Assign placeholder X   ● Use Additional Character(s)

Excludes 1   Excludes 2   Includes   Use additional   Code first   Code also   Unspecified

● **V85** **Occupant of special construction vehicle injured in transport accident**

    Includes   bulldozer
                 digger
                 dump truck
                 earth-leveller
                 mechanical shovel
                 road-roller

    Excludes1   special industrial vehicle (V83.-)
                 special construction vehicle in stationary use or maintenance (W31.-)

The appropriate 7th character is to be added to each code from category V85

    A   initial encounter
    D   subsequent encounter
    S   sequela

X● **V85.0** Driver of special construction vehicle injured in traffic accident

X● **V85.1** Passenger of special construction vehicle injured in traffic accident

X● **V85.2** Person on outside of special construction vehicle injured in traffic accident

X● **V85.3** Unspecified occupant of special construction vehicle injured in traffic accident

X● **V85.4** Person injured while boarding or alighting from special construction vehicle

X● **V85.5** Driver of special construction vehicle injured in nontraffic accident

X● **V85.6** Passenger of special construction vehicle injured in nontraffic accident

X● **V85.7** Person on outside of special construction vehicle injured in nontraffic accident

X● **V85.9** Unspecified occupant of special construction vehicle injured in nontraffic accident
    Special-construction-vehicle accident NOS

● **V86** **Occupant of special all-terrain or other off-road motor vehicle, injured in transport accident**

    Excludes1   special all-terrain vehicle in stationary use or maintenance (W31.-)
                 sport-utility vehicle (V50-V59)
                 three-wheeled motor vehicle designed for on-road use (V30-V39)

The appropriate 7th character is to be added to each code from category V86

    A   initial encounter
    D   subsequent encounter
    S   sequela

● **V86.0** Driver of special all-terrain or other off-road motor vehicle injured in traffic accident

X● **V86.01** Driver of ambulance or fire engine injured in traffic accident

X● **V86.02** Driver of snowmobile injured in traffic accident

X● **V86.03** Driver of dune buggy injured in traffic accident

X● **V86.04** Driver of military vehicle injured in traffic accident

X● **V86.09** Driver of other off-road special all-terrain or other off-road vehicle injured in traffic accident
    Driver of dirt bike injured in traffic accident
    Driver of go cart injured in traffic accident
    Driver of golf cart injured in traffic accident

● **V86.1** Passenger of special all-terrain or other off-road motor vehicle injured in traffic accident

X● **V86.11** Passenger of ambulance or fire engine injured in traffic accident

X● **V86.12** Passenger of snowmobile injured in traffic accident

X● **V86.13** Passenger of dune buggy injured in traffic accident

X● **V86.14** Passenger of military vehicle injured in traffic accident

X● **V86.19** Passenger of other off-road special all-terrain or other off-road off-road motor vehicle injured in traffic accident
    Passenger of dirt bike injured in traffic accident
    Passenger of go cart injured in traffic accident
    Passenger of golf cart injured in traffic accident

● **V86.2** Person on outside of special all-terrain or other off-road motor vehicle injured in traffic accident

X● **V86.21** Person on outside of ambulance or fire engine injured in traffic accident

X● **V86.22** Person on outside of snowmobile injured in traffic accident

X● **V86.23** Person on outside of dune buggy injured in traffic accident

X● **V86.24** Person on outside of military vehicle injured in traffic accident

X● **V86.29** Person on outside of other special all-terrain or other off-road motor vehicle injured in traffic accident
    Person on outside of dirt bike injured in traffic accident
    Person on outside of go cart in traffic accident
    Person on outside of golf cart injured in traffic accident

● **V86.3** Unspecified occupant of special all-terrain or other off-road motor vehicle injured in traffic accident

X● **V86.31** Unspecified occupant of ambulance or fire engine injured in traffic accident

X● **V86.32** Unspecified occupant of snowmobile injured in traffic accident

X● **V86.33** Unspecified occupant of dune buggy injured in traffic accident

X● **V86.34** Unspecified occupant of military vehicle injured in traffic accident

X● **V86.39** Unspecified occupant of other special all-terrain or other off-road motor vehicle injured in traffic accident
    Unspecified occupant of dirt bike injured in traffic accident
    Unspecified occupant of go cart injured in traffic accident
    Unspecified occupant of golf cart injured in traffic accident

● **V86.4** Person injured while boarding or alighting from special all-terrain or other off-road motor vehicle

X● **V86.41** Person injured while boarding or alighting from ambulance or fire engine

X● **V86.42** Person injured while boarding or alighting from snowmobile

X● **V86.43** Person injured while boarding or alighting from dune buggy

X● **V86.44** Person injured while boarding or alighting from military vehicle

X● **V86.49** Person injured while boarding or alighting from other special all-terrain or other off-road motor vehicle
    Person injured while boarding or alighting from dirt bike
    Person injured while boarding or alighting from go cart
    Person injured while boarding or alighting from golf cart

◄ New   ◄▬▬ Revised   ~~deleted~~ Deleted   **OGCR** Official Guidelines   X Assign placeholder X   ● Use Additional Character(s)

Excludes 1   Excludes 2   Includes   Use additional   Code first   Code also   Unspecified

● **V86.5**   **Driver of special all-terrain or other off-road motor vehicle injured in nontraffic accident**

   X ● **V86.51**   Driver of ambulance or fire engine injured in nontraffic accident

   X ● **V86.52**   Driver of snowmobile injured in nontraffic accident

   X ● **V86.53**   Driver of dune buggy injured in nontraffic accident

   X ● **V86.54**   Driver of military vehicle injured in nontraffic accident

   X ● **V86.59**   Driver of other off-road special all-terrain or other off-road motor vehicle injured in nontraffic accident

      Driver of dirt bike injured in nontraffic accident

      Driver of go cart injured in nontraffic accident

      Driver of golf cart injured in nontraffic accident

● **V86.6**   **Passenger of special all-terrain or other off-road motor vehicle injured in nontraffic accident**

   X ● **V86.61**   Passenger of ambulance or fire engine injured in nontraffic accident

   X ● **V86.62**   Passenger of snowmobile injured in nontraffic accident

   X ● **V86.63**   Passenger of dune buggy injured in nontraffic accident

   X ● **V86.64**   Passenger of military vehicle injured in nontraffic accident

   X ● **V86.69**   Passenger of other special all-terrain or other off-road vehicle injured in nontraffic accident

      Passenger of dirt bike injured in nontraffic accident

      Passenger of go cart injured in nontraffic accident

      Passenger of golf cart injured in nontraffic accident

● **V86.7**   **Person on outside of special all-terrain or other off-road motor vehicle injured in nontraffic accident**

   X ● **V86.71**   Person on outside of ambulance or fire engine injured in nontraffic accident

   X ● **V86.72**   Person on outside of snowmobile injured in nontraffic accident

   X ● **V86.73**   Person on outside of dune buggy injured in nontraffic accident

   X ● **V86.74**   Person on outside of military vehicle injured in nontraffic accident

   X ● **V86.79**   Person on outside of other special all-terrain or other off-road motor vehicles injured in nontraffic accident

      Person on outside of dirt bike injured in nontraffic accident

      Person on outside of go cart injured in nontraffic accident

      Person on outside of golf cart injured in nontraffic accident

● **V86.9**   **Unspecified occupant of special all-terrain or other off-road motor vehicle injured in nontraffic accident**

   X ● **V86.91**   Unspecified occupant of ambulance or fire engine injured in nontraffic accident

   X ● **V86.92**   Unspecified occupant of snowmobile injured in nontraffic accident

   X ● **V86.93**   Unspecified occupant of dune buggy injured in nontraffic accident

   X ● **V86.94**   Unspecified occupant of military vehicle injured in nontraffic accident

   X ● **V86.99**   Unspecified occupant of other off-road special all-terrain or other off-road motor vehicle injured in nontraffic accident

      All-terrain motor-vehicle accident NOS

      Off-road motor-vehicle accident NOS

      Other motor-vehicle accident NOS

      Unspecified occupant of dirt bike injured in nontraffic accident

      Unspecified occupant of go cart injured in nontraffic accident

      Unspecified occupant of golf cart injured in nontraffic accident

      Unspecified occupant of race car injured in nontraffic accident

● **V87**   **Traffic accident of specified type but victim's mode of transport unknown**

   Excludes1   collision involving:
      pedal cycle (V10-V19)
      pedestrian (V01-V09)

   The appropriate 7th character is to be added to each code from category V87

A	initial encounter
D	subsequent encounter
S	sequela

   X ● **V87.0**   Person injured in collision between car and two- or three-wheeled powered vehicle (traffic)

   X ● **V87.1**   Person injured in collision between other motor vehicle and two- or three-wheeled motor vehicle (traffic)

   X ● **V87.2**   Person injured in collision between car and pick-up truck or van (traffic)

   X ● **V87.3**   Person injured in collision between car and bus (traffic)

   X ● **V87.4**   Person injured in collision between car and heavy transport vehicle (traffic)

   X ● **V87.5**   Person injured in collision between heavy transport vehicle and bus (traffic)

   X ● **V87.6**   Person injured in collision between railway train or railway vehicle and car (traffic)

   X ● **V87.7**   Person injured in collision between other specified motor vehicles (traffic)

   X ● **V87.8**   Person injured in other specified noncollision transport accidents involving motor vehicle (traffic)

   X ● **V87.9**   Person injured in other specified (collision) (noncollision) transport accidents involving nonmotor vehicle (traffic)

● **V88**   **Nontraffic accident of specified type but victim's mode of transport unknown**

   Excludes1   collision involving:
      pedal cycle (V10-V19)
      pedestrian (V01-V09)

   The appropriate 7th character is to be added to each code from category V88

A	initial encounter
D	subsequent encounter
S	sequela

   X ● **V88.0**   Person injured in collision between car and two- or three-wheeled motor vehicle, nontraffic

   X ● **V88.1**   Person injured in collision between other motor vehicle and two- or three-wheeled motor vehicle, nontraffic

   X ● **V88.2**   Person injured in collision between car and pick-up truck or van, nontraffic

CHAPTER 20 (V01-Y99)

CHAPTER 20 (V01-Y99)

X● **V88.3** Person injured in collision between car and bus, nontraffic

X● **V88.4** Person injured in collision between car and heavy transport vehicle, nontraffic

X● **V88.5** Person injured in collision between heavy transport vehicle and bus, nontraffic

X● **V88.6** Person injured in collision between railway train or railway vehicle and car, nontraffic

X● **V88.7** Person injured in collision between other specified motor vehicle, nontraffic

X● **V88.8** Person injured in other specified noncollision transport accidents involving motor vehicle, nontraffic

X● **V88.9** Person injured in other specified (collision) (noncollision) transport accidents involving nonmotor vehicle, nontraffic

● **V89** Motor- or nonmotor-vehicle accident, type of vehicle unspecified

The appropriate 7th character is to be added to each code from category V89

> A   initial encounter
> D   subsequent encounter
> S   sequela

X● **V89.0** Person injured in unspecified motor-vehicle accident, nontraffic
  Motor-vehicle accident NOS, nontraffic

X● **V89.1** Person injured in unspecified nonmotor-vehicle accident, nontraffic
  Nonmotor-vehicle accident NOS (nontraffic)

X● **V89.2** Person injured in unspecified motor-vehicle accident, traffic
  Motor-vehicle accident [MVA] NOS
  Road (traffic) accident [RTA] NOS

X● **V89.3** Person injured in unspecified nonmotor-vehicle accident, traffic
  Nonmotor-vehicle traffic accident NOS

X● **V89.9** Person injured in unspecified vehicle accident
  Collision NOS

WATER TRANSPORT ACCIDENTS (V90-V94)

● **V90** Drowning and submersion due to accident to watercraft

> **Excludes1** civilian water transport accident involving military watercraft (V94.81-)
> fall into water not from watercraft (W16.-)
> military watercraft accident in military or war operations (Y36.0-, Y37.0-)
> water-transport–related drowning or submersion without accident to watercraft (V92.-)

The appropriate 7th character is to be added to each code from category V90

> A   initial encounter
> D   subsequent encounter
> S   sequela

● **V90.0** Drowning and submersion due to watercraft overturning

X● **V90.00** Drowning and submersion due to merchant ship overturning

X● **V90.01** Drowning and submersion due to passenger ship overturning
  Drowning and submersion due to ferry-boat overturning
  Drowning and submersion due to liner overturning

X● **V90.02** Drowning and submersion due to fishing boat overturning

X● **V90.03** Drowning and submersion due to other powered watercraft overturning
  Drowning and submersion due to hovercraft (on open water) overturning
  Drowning and submersion due to jet ski overturning

X● **V90.04** Drowning and submersion due to sailboat overturning

X● **V90.05** Drowning and submersion due to canoe or kayak overturning

X● **V90.06** Drowning and submersion due to (nonpowered) inflatable craft overturning

X● **V90.08** Drowning and submersion due to other unpowered watercraft overturning
  Drowning and submersion due to windsurfer overturning

X● **V90.09** Drowning and submersion due to unspecified watercraft overturning
  Drowning and submersion due to boat NOS overturning
  Drowning and submersion due to ship NOS overturning
  Drowning and submersion due to watercraft NOS overturning

● **V90.1** Drowning and submersion due to watercraft sinking

X● **V90.10** Drowning and submersion due to merchant ship sinking

X● **V90.11** Drowning and submersion due to passenger ship sinking
  Drowning and submersion due to ferry-boat sinking
  Drowning and submersion due to liner sinking

X● **V90.12** Drowning and submersion due to fishing boat sinking

X● **V90.13** Drowning and submersion due to other powered watercraft sinking
  Drowning and submersion due to hovercraft (on open water) sinking
  Drowning and submersion due to jet ski sinking

X● **V90.14** Drowning and submersion due to sailboat sinking

X● **V90.15** Drowning and submersion due to canoe or kayak sinking

X● **V90.16** Drowning and submersion due to (nonpowered) inflatable craft sinking

X● **V90.18** Drowning and submersion due to other unpowered watercraft sinking

X● **V90.19** Drowning and submersion due to unspecified watercraft sinking
  Drowning and submersion due to boat NOS sinking
  Drowning and submersion due to ship NOS sinking
  Drowning and submersion due to watercraft NOS sinking

◀ New   ◀⁞⁞ Revised   ~~deleted~~ Deleted   OGCR Official Guidelines   X Assign placeholder X   ● Use Additional Character(s)

Excludes 1   Excludes 2   Includes   Use additional   Code first   Code also   Unspecified

● **V90.2   Drowning and submersion due to falling or jumping from burning watercraft**

   X ● **V90.20   Drowning and submersion due to falling or jumping from burning merchant ship**

   X ● **V90.21   Drowning and submersion due to falling or jumping from burning passenger ship**
       Drowning and submersion due to falling or jumping from burning ferry-boat
       Drowning and submersion due to falling or jumping from burning liner

   X ● **V90.22   Drowning and submersion due to falling or jumping from burning fishing boat**

   X ● **V90.23   Drowning and submersion due to falling or jumping from other burning powered watercraft**
       Drowning and submersion due to falling and jumping from burning hovercraft (on open water)
       Drowning and submersion due to falling and jumping from burning jet ski

   X ● **V90.24   Drowning and submersion due to falling or jumping from burning sailboat**

   X ● **V90.25   Drowning and submersion due to falling or jumping from burning canoe or kayak**

   X ● **V90.26   Drowning and submersion due to falling or jumping from burning (nonpowered) inflatable craft**

   X ● **V90.27   Drowning and submersion due to falling or jumping from burning water-skis**

   X ● **V90.28   Drowning and submersion due to falling or jumping from other burning unpowered watercraft**
       Drowning and submersion due to falling and jumping from burning surf-board
       Drowning and submersion due to falling and jumping from burning windsurfer

   X ● **V90.29   Drowning and submersion due to falling or jumping from unspecified burning watercraft**
       Drowning and submersion due to falling or jumping from burning boat NOS
       Drowning and submersion due to falling or jumping from burning ship NOS
       Drowning and submersion due to falling or jumping from burning watercraft NOS

● **V90.3   Drowning and submersion due to falling or jumping from crushed watercraft**

   X ● **V90.30   Drowning and submersion due to falling or jumping from crushed merchant ship**

   X ● **V90.31   Drowning and submersion due to falling or jumping from crushed passenger ship**
       Drowning and submersion due to falling and jumping from crushed ferry-boat
       Drowning and submersion due to falling and jumping from crushed liner

   X ● **V90.32   Drowning and submersion due to falling or jumping from crushed fishing boat**

   X ● **V90.33   Drowning and submersion due to falling or jumping from other crushed powered watercraft**
       Drowning and submersion due to falling and jumping from crushed hovercraft
       Drowning and submersion due to falling and jumping from crushed jet ski

   X ● **V90.34   Drowning and submersion due to falling or jumping from crushed sailboat**

   X ● **V90.35   Drowning and submersion due to falling or jumping from crushed canoe or kayak**

   X ● **V90.36   Drowning and submersion due to falling or jumping from crushed (nonpowered) inflatable craft**

   X ● **V90.37   Drowning and submersion due to falling or jumping from crushed water-skis**

   X ● **V90.38   Drowning and submersion due to falling or jumping from other crushed unpowered watercraft**
       Drowning and submersion due to falling and jumping from crushed surf-board
       Drowning and submersion due to falling and jumping from crushed windsurfer

   X ● **V90.39   Drowning and submersion due to falling or jumping from crushed unspecified watercraft**
       Drowning and submersion due to falling and jumping from crushed boat NOS
       Drowning and submersion due to falling and jumping from crushed ship NOS
       Drowning and submersion due to falling and jumping from crushed watercraft NOS

● **V90.8   Drowning and submersion due to other accident to watercraft**

   X ● **V90.80   Drowning and submersion due to other accident to merchant ship**

   X ● **V90.81   Drowning and submersion due to other accident to passenger ship**
       Drowning and submersion due to other accident to ferry-boat
       Drowning and submersion due to other accident to liner

   X ● **V90.82   Drowning and submersion due to other accident to fishing boat**

   X ● **V90.83   Drowning and submersion due to other accident to other powered watercraft**
       Drowning and submersion due to other accident to hovercraft (on open water)
       Drowning and submersion due to other accident to jet ski

   X ● **V90.84   Drowning and submersion due to other accident to sailboat**

   X ● **V90.85   Drowning and submersion due to other accident to canoe or kayak**

   X ● **V90.86   Drowning and submersion due to other accident to (nonpowered) inflatable craft**

   X ● **V90.87   Drowning and submersion due to other accident to water-skis**

   X ● **V90.88   Drowning and submersion due to other accident to other unpowered watercraft**
       Drowning and submersion due to other accident to surf-board
       Drowning and submersion due to other accident to windsurfer

   X ● **V90.89   Drowning and submersion due to other accident to unspecified watercraft**
       Drowning and submersion due to other accident to boat NOS
       Drowning and submersion due to other accident to ship NOS
       Drowning and submersion due to other accident to watercraft NOS

CHAPTER 20 (V01-Y99)

● **V91   Other injury due to accident to watercraft**

Includes   any injury except drowning and submersion as a result of an accident to watercraft

Excludes1   civilian water transport accident involving military watercraft (V94.81-)
military watercraft accident in military or war operations (Y36, Y37.-)

Excludes2   drowning and submersion due to accident to watercraft (V90.-)

The appropriate 7th character is to be added to each code from category V91

A   initial encounter
D   subsequent encounter
S   sequela

● **V91.0   Burn due to watercraft on fire**

Excludes1   burn from localized fire or explosion on board ship without accident to watercraft (V93.-)

X● **V91.00   Burn due to merchant ship on fire**

X● **V91.01   Burn due to passenger ship on fire**
Burn due to ferry-boat on fire
Burn due to liner on fire

X● **V91.02   Burn due to fishing boat on fire**

X● **V91.03   Burn due to other powered watercraft on fire**
Burn due to hovercraft (on open water) on fire
Burn due to jet ski on fire

X● **V91.04   Burn due to sailboat on fire**

X● **V91.05   Burn due to canoe or kayak on fire**

X● **V91.06   Burn due to (nonpowered) inflatable craft on fire**

X● **V91.07   Burn due to water-skis on fire**

X● **V91.08   Burn due to other unpowered watercraft on fire**

X● **V91.09   Burn due to unspecified watercraft on fire**
Burn due to boat NOS on fire
Burn due to ship NOS on fire
Burn due to watercraft NOS on fire

● **V91.1   Crushed between watercraft and other watercraft or other object due to collision**
Crushed by lifeboat after abandoning ship in a collision

Note: Select the specified type of watercraft that the victim was on at the time of the collision.

X● **V91.10   Crushed between merchant ship and other watercraft or other object due to collision**

X● **V91.11   Crushed between passenger ship and other watercraft or other object due to collision**
Crushed between ferry-boat and other watercraft or other object due to collision
Crushed between liner and other watercraft or other object due to collision

X● **V91.12   Crushed between fishing boat and other watercraft or other object due to collision**

X● **V91.13   Crushed between other powered watercraft and other watercraft or other object due to collision**
Crushed between hovercraft (on open water) and other watercraft or other object due to collision
Crushed between jet ski and other watercraft or other object due to collision

X● **V91.14   Crushed between sailboat and other watercraft or other object due to collision**

X● **V91.15   Crushed between canoe or kayak and other watercraft or other object due to collision**

X● **V91.16   Crushed between (nonpowered) inflatable craft and other watercraft or other object due to collision**

X● **V91.18   Crushed between other unpowered watercraft and other watercraft or other object due to collision**
Crushed between surfboard and other watercraft or other object due to collision
Crushed between windsurfer and other watercraft or other object due to collision

X● **V91.19   Crushed between unspecified watercraft and other watercraft or other object due to collision**
Crushed between boat NOS and other watercraft or other object due to collision
Crushed between ship NOS and other watercraft or other object due to collision
Crushed between watercraft NOS and other watercraft or other object due to collision

● **V91.2   Fall due to collision between watercraft and other watercraft or other object**
Fall while remaining on watercraft after collision

Note: Select the specified type of watercraft that the victim was on at the time of the collision.

Excludes1   crushed between watercraft and other watercraft and other object due to collision (V91.1-)
drowning and submersion due to falling from crushed watercraft (V90.3-)

X● **V91.20   Fall due to collision between merchant ship and other watercraft or other object**

X● **V91.21   Fall due to collision between passenger ship and other watercraft or other object**
Fall due to collision between ferry-boat and other watercraft or other object
Fall due to collision between liner and other watercraft or other object

X● **V91.22   Fall due to collision between fishing boat and other watercraft or other object**

X● **V91.23   Fall due to collision between other powered watercraft and other watercraft or other object**
Fall due to collision between hovercraft (on open water) and other watercraft or other object
Fall due to collision between jet ski and other watercraft or other object

X● **V91.24   Fall due to collision between sailboat and other watercraft or other object**

X● **V91.25   Fall due to collision between canoe or kayak and other watercraft or other object**

X● **V91.26   Fall due to collision between (nonpowered) inflatable craft and other watercraft or other object**

X● **V91.29   Fall due to collision between unspecified watercraft and other watercraft or other object**
Fall due to collision between boat NOS and other watercraft or other object
Fall due to collision between ship NOS and other watercraft or other object
Fall due to collision between watercraft NOS and other watercraft or other object

CHAPTER 20 (V01-Y99)

● **V91.3**   **Hit or struck by falling object due to accident to watercraft**
    Hit or struck by falling object (part of damaged watercraft or other object) after falling or jumping from damaged watercraft

Excludes2	drowning or submersion due to fall or jumping from damaged watercraft (V90.2-, V90.3-)

X ● **V91.30**   **Hit or struck by falling object due to accident to merchant ship**

X ● **V91.31**   **Hit or struck by falling object due to accident to passenger ship**
    Hit or struck by falling object due to accident to ferry-boat
    Hit or struck by falling object due to accident to liner

X ● **V91.32**   **Hit or struck by falling object due to accident to fishing boat**

X ● **V91.33**   **Hit or struck by falling object due to accident to other powered watercraft**
    Hit or struck by falling object due to accident to hovercraft (on open water)
    Hit or struck by falling object due to accident to jet ski

X ● **V91.34**   **Hit or struck by falling object due to accident to sailboat**

X ● **V91.35**   **Hit or struck by falling object due to accident to canoe or kayak**

X ● **V91.36**   **Hit or struck by falling object due to accident to (nonpowered) inflatable craft**

X ● **V91.37**   **Hit or struck by falling object due to accident to water-skis**
    Hit by water-skis after jumping off of waterskis

X ● **V91.38**   **Hit or struck by falling object due to accident to other unpowered watercraft**
    Hit or struck by surf-board after falling off damaged surf-board
    Hit or struck by object after falling off damaged windsurfer

X ● **V91.39**   **Hit or struck by falling object due to accident to** unspecified **watercraft**
    Hit or struck by falling object due to accident to boat NOS
    Hit or struck by falling object due to accident to ship NOS
    Hit or struck by falling object due to accident to watercraft NOS

● **V91.8**   **Other injury due to other accident to watercraft**

X ● **V91.80**   **Other injury due to other accident to merchant ship**

X ● **V91.81**   **Other injury due to other accident to passenger ship**
    Other injury due to other accident to ferry-boat
    Other injury due to other accident to liner

X ● **V91.82**   **Other injury due to other accident to fishing boat**

X ● **V91.83**   **Other injury due to other accident to other powered watercraft**
    Other injury due to other accident to hovercraft (on open water)
    Other injury due to other accident to jet ski

X ● **V91.84**   **Other injury due to other accident to sailboat**

X ● **V91.85**   **Other injury due to other accident to canoe or kayak**

X ● **V91.86**   **Other injury due to other accident to (nonpowered) inflatable craft**

X ● **V91.87**   **Other injury due to other accident to water-skis**

X ● **V91.88**   **Other injury due to other accident to other unpowered watercraft**
    Other injury due to other accident to surf-board
    Other injury due to other accident to windsurfer

X ● **V91.89**   **Other injury due to other accident to** unspecified **watercraft**
    Other injury due to other accident to boat NOS
    Other injury due to other accident to ship NOS
    Other injury due to other accident to watercraft NOS

● **V92**   **Drowning and submersion due to accident on board watercraft, without accident to watercraft**

Excludes1	civilian water transport accident involving military watercraft (V94.81-)
	drowning or submersion due to accident to watercraft (V90-V91)
	drowning or submersion of diver who voluntarily jumps from boat not involved in an accident (W16.711, W16.721)
	fall into water without watercraft (W16.-)
	military watercraft accident in military or war operations (Y36, Y37)

The appropriate 7th character is to be added to each code from category V92

A	initial encounter
D	subsequent encounter
S	sequela

● **V92.0**   **Drowning and submersion due to fall off watercraft**
    Drowning and submersion due to fall from gangplank of watercraft
    Drowning and submersion due to fall overboard watercraft

Excludes2	hitting head on object or bottom of body of water due to fall from watercraft (V94.0-)

X ● **V92.00**   **Drowning and submersion due to fall off merchant ship**

X ● **V92.01**   **Drowning and submersion due to fall off passenger ship**
    Drowning and submersion due to fall off ferry-boat
    Drowning and submersion due to fall off liner

X ● **V92.02**   **Drowning and submersion due to fall off fishing boat**

X ● **V92.03**   **Drowning and submersion due to fall off other powered watercraft**
    Drowning and submersion due to fall off hovercraft (on open water)
    Drowning and submersion due to fall off jet ski

X ● **V92.04**   **Drowning and submersion due to fall off sailboat**

X ● **V92.05**   **Drowning and submersion due to fall off canoe or kayak**

X ● **V92.06**   **Drowning and submersion due to fall off (nonpowered) inflatable craft**

◀ New   ◀━ Revised   ~~deleted~~ Deleted   **OGCR** Official Guidelines   X Assign placeholder X   ● Use Additional Character(s)

Excludes 1	Excludes 2	Includes	Use additional	Code first	Code also	Unspecified

1491

X ● **V92.07**   **Drowning and submersion due to fall off water-skis**

> **Excludes1**   drowning and submersion due to falling off burning water-skis (V90.27)
> drowning and submersion due to falling off crushed water-skis (V90.37)
> hit by boat while water-skiing NOS (V94.X)

X ● **V92.08**   **Drowning and submersion due to fall off other unpowered watercraft**

> Drowning and submersion due to fall off surf-board
> Drowning and submersion due to fall off windsurfer

> **Excludes1**   drowning and submersion due to fall off burning unpowered watercraft (V90.28)
> drowning and submersion due to fall off crushed unpowered watercraft (V90.38)
> drowning and submersion due to fall off damaged unpowered watercraft (V90.88)
> drowning and submersion due to rider of nonpowered watercraft being hit by other watercraft (V94.-)
> other injury due to rider of nonpowered watercraft being hit by other watercraft (V94.-)

X ● **V92.09**   **Drowning and submersion due to fall off unspecified watercraft**

> Drowning and submersion due to fall off boat NOS
> Drowning and submersion due to fall off ship
> Drowning and submersion due to fall off watercraft NOS

● **V92.1**   **Drowning and submersion due to being thrown overboard by motion of watercraft**

> **Excludes1**   drowning and submersion due to fall off surf-board (V92.08)
> drowning and submersion due to fall off water-skis (V92.07)
> drowning and submersion due to fall off windsurfer (V92.08)

X ● **V92.10**   **Drowning and submersion due to being thrown overboard by motion of merchant ship**

X ● **V92.11**   **Drowning and submersion due to being thrown overboard by motion of passenger ship**

> Drowning and submersion due to being thrown overboard by motion of ferry-boat
> Drowning and submersion due to being thrown overboard by motion of liner

X ● **V92.12**   **Drowning and submersion due to being thrown overboard by motion of fishing boat**

X ● **V92.13**   **Drowning and submersion due to being thrown overboard by motion of other powered watercraft**

> Drowning and submersion due to being thrown overboard by motion of hovercraft

X ● **V92.14**   **Drowning and submersion due to being thrown overboard by motion of sailboat**

X ● **V92.15**   **Drowning and submersion due to being thrown overboard by motion of canoe or kayak**

X ● **V92.16**   **Drowning and submersion due to being thrown overboard by motion of (nonpowered) inflatable craft**

X ● **V92.19**   **Drowning and submersion due to being thrown overboard by motion of unspecified watercraft**

> Drowning and submersion due to being thrown overboard by motion of boat NOS
> Drowning and submersion due to being thrown overboard by motion of ship NOS
> Drowning and submersion due to being thrown overboard by motion of watercraft NOS

● **V92.2**   **Drowning and submersion due to being washed overboard from watercraft**

> *Code first any associated cataclysm (X37.0-)*

X ● **V92.20**   **Drowning and submersion due to being washed overboard from merchant ship**

X ● **V92.21**   **Drowning and submersion due to being washed overboard from passenger ship**

> Drowning and submersion due to being washed overboard from ferry-boat
> Drowning and submersion due to being washed overboard from liner

X ● **V92.22**   **Drowning and submersion due to being washed overboard from fishing boat**

X ● **V92.23**   **Drowning and submersion due to being washed overboard from other powered watercraft**

> Drowning and submersion due to being washed overboard from hovercraft (on open water)
> Drowning and submersion due to being washed overboard from jet ski

X ● **V92.24**   **Drowning and submersion due to being washed overboard from sailboat**

X ● **V92.25**   **Drowning and submersion due to being washed overboard from canoe or kayak**

X ● **V92.26**   **Drowning and submersion due to being washed overboard from (nonpowered) inflatable craft**

X ● **V92.27**   **Drowning and submersion due to being washed overboard from water-skis**

> **Excludes1**   drowning and submersion due to fall off water-skis (V92.07)

X ● **V92.28**   **Drowning and submersion due to being washed overboard from other unpowered watercraft**

> Drowning and submersion due to being washed overboard from surf-board
> Drowning and submersion due to being washed overboard from windsurfer

X ● **V92.29**   **Drowning and submersion due to being washed overboard from unspecified watercraft**

> Drowning and submersion due to being washed overboard from boat NOS
> Drowning and submersion due to being washed overboard from ship NOS
> Drowning and submersion due to being washed overboard from watercraft NOS

CHAPTER 20 (V01-Y99)

◀ New   ◀═ Revised   ~~deleted~~ Deleted   **OGCR** Official Guidelines   X Assign placeholder X   ● Use Additional Character(s)

Excludes 1   Excludes 2   Includes   Use additional   Code first   Code also   Unspecified

● V93 **Other injury due to accident on board watercraft, without accident to watercraft**

> **Excludes1** civilian water transport accident involving military watercraft (V94.81-)
> other injury due to accident to watercraft (V91.-)
> military watercraft accident in military or war operations (Y36, Y37.-)

> **Excludes2** drowning and submersion due to accident on board watercraft, without accident to watercraft (V92.-)

The appropriate 7th character is to be added to each code from category V93

> A   initial encounter
> D   subsequent encounter
> S   sequela

● V93.0 **Burn due to localized fire on board watercraft**

> **Excludes1** burn due to watercraft on fire (V91.0-)

X ● V93.00 **Burn due to localized fire on board merchant vessel**

X ● V93.01 **Burn due to localized fire on board passenger vessel**
> Burn due to localized fire on board ferry-boat
> Burn due to localized fire on board liner

X ● V93.02 **Burn due to localized fire on board fishing boat**

X ● V93.03 **Burn due to localized fire on board other powered watercraft**
> Burn due to localized fire on board hovercraft
> Burn due to localized fire on board jet ski

X ● V93.04 **Burn due to localized fire on board sailboat**

X ● V93.09 **Burn due to localized fire on board unspecified watercraft**
> Burn due to localized fire on board boat NOS
> Burn due to localized fire on board ship NOS
> Burn due to localized fire on board watercraft NOS

● V93.1 **Other burn on board watercraft**
> Burn due to source other than fire on board watercraft

> **Excludes1** burn due to watercraft on fire (V91.0-)

X ● V93.10 **Other burn on board merchant vessel**

X ● V93.11 **Other burn on board passenger vessel**
> Other burn on board ferry-boat
> Other burn on board liner

X ● V93.12 **Other burn on board fishing boat**

X ● V93.13 **Other burn on board other powered watercraft**
> Other burn on board hovercraft
> Other burn on board jet ski

X ● V93.14 **Other burn on board sailboat**

X ● V93.19 **Other burn on board unspecified watercraft**
> Other burn on board boat NOS
> Other burn on board ship NOS
> Other burn on board watercraft NOS

● V93.2 **Heat exposure on board watercraft**

> **Excludes1** exposure to man-made heat not aboard watercraft (W92)
> exposure to natural heat while on board watercraft (X30)
> exposure to sunlight while on board watercraft (X32)

> **Excludes2** burn due to fire on board watercraft (V93.0-)

X ● V93.20 **Heat exposure on board merchant ship**

X ● V93.21 **Heat exposure on board passenger ship**
> Heat exposure on board ferry-boat
> Heat exposure on board liner

X ● V93.22 **Heat exposure on board fishing boat**

X ● V93.23 **Heat exposure on board other powered watercraft**
> Heat exposure on board hovercraft

X ● V93.24 **Heat exposure on board sailboat**

X ● V93.29 **Heat exposure on board unspecified watercraft**
> Heat exposure on board boat NOS
> Heat exposure on board ship NOS
> Heat exposure on board watercraft NOS

● V93.3 **Fall on board watercraft**

> **Excludes1** fall due to collision of watercraft (V91.2-)

X ● V93.30 **Fall on board merchant ship**

X ● V93.31 **Fall on board passenger ship**
> Fall on board ferry-boat
> Fall on board liner

X ● V93.32 **Fall on board fishing boat**

X ● V93.33 **Fall on board other powered watercraft**
> Fall on board hovercraft (on open water)
> Fall on board jet ski

X ● V93.34 **Fall on board sailboat**

X ● V93.35 **Fall on board canoe or kayak**

X ● V93.36 **Fall on board (nonpowered) inflatable craft**

X ● V93.38 **Fall on board other unpowered watercraft**

X ● V93.39 **Fall on board unspecified watercraft**
> Fall on board boat NOS
> Fall on board ship NOS
> Fall on board watercraft NOS

● V93.4 **Struck by falling object on board watercraft**
> Hit by falling object on board watercraft

> **Excludes1** struck by falling object due to accident to watercraft (V91.3)

X ● V93.40 **Struck by falling object on merchant ship**

X ● V93.41 **Struck by falling object on passenger ship**
> Struck by falling object on ferry-boat
> Struck by falling object on liner

X ● V93.42 **Struck by falling object on fishing boat**

X ● V93.43 **Struck by falling object on other powered watercraft**
> Struck by falling object on hovercraft

X ● V93.44 **Struck by falling object on sailboat**

X ● V93.48 **Struck by falling object on other unpowered watercraft**

X ● V93.49 **Struck by falling object on unspecified watercraft**

● V93.5 **Explosion on board watercraft**
> Boiler explosion on steamship

> **Excludes2** fire on board watercraft (V93.0-)

X ● V93.50 **Explosion on board merchant ship**

X ● V93.51 **Explosion on board passenger ship**
> Explosion on board ferry-boat
> Explosion on board liner

X ● V93.52 **Explosion on board fishing boat**

X ● V93.53 **Explosion on board other powered watercraft**
> Explosion on board hovercraft
> Explosion on board jet ski

X ● V93.54 **Explosion on board sailboat**

X ● V93.59 **Explosion on board unspecified watercraft**
> Explosion on board boat NOS
> Explosion on board ship NOS
> Explosion on board watercraft NOS

CHAPTER 20 (V01-Y99)

● **V93.6   Machinery accident on board watercraft**
       Excludes1   machinery explosion on board watercraft (V93.4-)
                 machinery fire on board watercraft (V93.0-)

X● **V93.60   Machinery accident on board merchant ship**

X● **V93.61   Machinery accident on board passenger ship**
         Machinery accident on board ferry-boat
         Machinery accident on board liner

X● **V93.62   Machinery accident on board fishing boat**

X● **V93.63   Machinery accident on board other powered watercraft**
         Machinery accident on board hovercraft

X● **V93.64   Machinery accident on board sailboat**

X● **V93.69   Machinery accident on board unspecified watercraft**
         Machinery accident on board boat NOS
         Machinery accident on board ship NOS
         Machinery accident on board watercraft NOS

● **V93.8   Other injury due to other accident on board watercraft**
         Accidental poisoning by gases or fumes on watercraft

X● **V93.80   Other injury due to other accident on board merchant ship**

X● **V93.81   Other injury due to other accident on board passenger ship**
         Other injury due to other accident on board ferry-boat
         Other injury due to other accident on board liner

X● **V93.82   Other injury due to other accident on board fishing boat**

X● **V93.83   Other injury due to other accident on board other powered watercraft**
         Other injury due to other accident on board hovercraft
         Other injury due to other accident on board jet ski

X● **V93.84   Other injury due to other accident on board sailboat**

X● **V93.85   Other injury due to other accident on board canoe or kayak**

X● **V93.86   Other injury due to other accident on board (nonpowered) inflatable craft**

X● **V93.87   Other injury due to other accident on board water-skis**
         Hit or struck by object while waterskiing

X● **V93.88   Other injury due to other accident on board other unpowered watercraft**
         Hit or struck by object while surfing
         Hit or struck by object while on board windsurfer

X● **V93.89   Other injury due to other accident on board unspecified watercraft**
         Other injury due to other accident on board boat NOS
         Other injury due to other accident on board ship NOS
         Other injury due to other accident on board watercraft NOS

● **V94   Other and unspecified water transport accidents**
       Excludes1   military watercraft accidents in military or war operations (Y36, Y37)

The appropriate 7th character is to be added to each code from category V94

A	initial encounter
D	subsequent encounter
S	sequela

X● **V94.0   Hitting object or bottom of body of water due to fall from watercraft**
       Excludes2   drowning and submersion due to fall from watercraft (V92.0-)

● **V94.1   Bather struck by watercraft**
         Swimmer hit by watercraft

X● **V94.11   Bather struck by powered watercraft**

X● **V94.12   Bather struck by nonpowered watercraft**

● **V94.2   Rider of nonpowered watercraft struck by other watercraft**

X● **V94.21   Rider of nonpowered watercraft struck by other nonpowered watercraft**
         Canoer hit by other nonpowered watercraft
         Surfer hit by other nonpowered watercraft
         Windsurfer hit by other nonpowered watercraft

X● **V94.22   Rider of nonpowered watercraft struck by powered watercraft**
         Canoer hit by motorboat
         Surfer hit by motorboat
         Windsurfer hit by motorboat

● **V94.3   Injury to rider of (inflatable) watercraft being pulled behind other watercraft**

X● **V94.31   Injury to rider of (inflatable) recreational watercraft being pulled behind other watercraft**
         Injury to rider of inner-tube pulled behind motor boat

X● **V94.32   Injury to rider of non-recreational watercraft being pulled behind other watercraft**
         Injury to occupant of dingy being pulled behind boat or ship
         Injury to occupant of life-raft being pulled behind boat or ship

X● **V94.4   Injury to barefoot water-skier**
         Injury to person being pulled behind boat or ship

● **V94.8   Other water transport accident**

● **V94.81   Water transport accident involving military watercraft**

● **V94.810   Civilian watercraft involved in water transport accident with military watercraft**
         Passenger on civilian watercraft injured due to accident with military watercraft

● **V94.811   Civilian in water injured by military watercraft**

● **V94.818   Other water transport accident involving military watercraft**

X● **V94.89   Other water transport accident**

X● **V94.9   Unspecified water transport accident**
         Water transport accident NOS

◀ New   ◀▦ Revised   ~~deleted~~ Deleted   **OGCR** Official Guidelines   X Assign placeholder X   ● Use Additional Character(s)

Excludes 1   Excludes 2   Includes   Use additional   Code first   Code also   Unspecified

AIR AND SPACE TRANSPORT ACCIDENTS (V95-V97)

> Excludes1   military aircraft accidents in military or war operations (Y36, Y37)

● **V95**   **Accident to powered aircraft causing injury to occupant**

> The appropriate 7th character is to be added to each code from category V95

> | | |
> |---|---|
> | A | initial encounter |
> | D | subsequent encounter |
> | S | sequela |

● **V95.0**   **Helicopter accident injuring occupant**

    X ● **V95.00**   Unspecified helicopter accident injuring occupant

    X ● **V95.01**   Helicopter crash injuring occupant

    X ● **V95.02**   Forced landing of helicopter injuring occupant

    X ● **V95.03**   Helicopter collision injuring occupant
> Helicopter collision with any object, fixed, movable or moving

    X ● **V95.04**   Helicopter fire injuring occupant

    X ● **V95.05**   Helicopter explosion injuring occupant

    X ● **V95.09**   Other helicopter accident injuring occupant

● **V95.1**   **Ultralight, microlight or powered-glider accident injuring occupant**

    X ● **V95.10**   Unspecified ultralight, microlight or powered-glider accident injuring occupant

    X ● **V95.11**   Ultralight, microlight or powered-glider crash injuring occupant

    X ● **V95.12**   Forced landing of ultralight, microlight or powered-glider injuring occupant

    X ● **V95.13**   Ultralight, microlight or powered-glider collision injuring occupant
> Ultralight, microlight or powered-glider collision with any object, fixed, movable or moving

    X ● **V95.14**   Ultralight, microlight or powered-glider fire injuring occupant

    X ● **V95.15**   Ultralight, microlight or powered-glider explosion injuring occupant

    X ● **V95.19**   Other ultralight, microlight or powered-glider accident injuring occupant

● **V95.2**   **Other private fixed-wing aircraft accident injuring occupant**

    X ● **V95.20**   Unspecified accident to other private fixed-wing aircraft, injuring occupant

    X ● **V95.21**   Other private fixed-wing aircraft crash injuring occupant

    X ● **V95.22**   Forced landing of other private fixed-wing aircraft injuring occupant

    X ● **V95.23**   Other private fixed-wing aircraft collision injuring occupant
> Other private fixed-wing aircraft collision with any object, fixed, movable or moving

    X ● **V95.24**   Other private fixed-wing aircraft fire injuring occupant

    X ● **V95.25**   Other private fixed-wing aircraft explosion injuring occupant

    X ● **V95.29**   Other accident to other private fixed-wing aircraft injuring occupant

● **V95.3**   **Commercial fixed-wing aircraft accident injuring occupant**

    X ● **V95.30**   Unspecified accident to commercial fixed-wing aircraft injuring occupant

    X ● **V95.31**   Commercial fixed-wing aircraft crash injuring occupant

    X ● **V95.32**   Forced landing of commercial fixed-wing aircraft injuring occupant

    X ● **V95.33**   Commercial fixed-wing aircraft collision injuring occupant
> Commercial fixed-wing aircraft collision with any object, fixed, movable or moving

    X ● **V95.34**   Commercial fixed-wing aircraft fire injuring occupant

    X ● **V95.35**   Commercial fixed-wing aircraft explosion injuring occupant

    X ● **V95.39**   Other accident to commercial fixed-wing aircraft injuring occupant

● **V95.4**   **Spacecraft accident injuring occupant**

    X ● **V95.40**   Unspecified spacecraft accident injuring occupant

    X ● **V95.41**   Spacecraft crash injuring occupant

    X ● **V95.42**   Forced landing of spacecraft injuring occupant

    X ● **V95.43**   Spacecraft collision injuring occupant
> Spacecraft collision with any object, fixed, moveable or moving

    X ● **V95.44**   Spacecraft fire injuring occupant

    X ● **V95.45**   Spacecraft explosion injuring occupant

    X ● **V95.49**   Other spacecraft accident injuring occupant

    X ● **V95.8**   Other powered aircraft accidents injuring occupant

    X ● **V95.9**   Unspecified aircraft accident injuring occupant
> Aircraft accident NOS
> Air transport accident NOS

● **V96**   **Accident to nonpowered aircraft causing injury to occupant**

> The appropriate 7th character is to be added to each code from category V96

> | | |
> |---|---|
> | A | initial encounter |
> | D | subsequent encounter |
> | S | sequela |

● **V96.0**   **Balloon accident injuring occupant**

    X ● **V96.00**   Unspecified balloon accident injuring occupant

    X ● **V96.01**   Balloon crash injuring occupant

    X ● **V96.02**   Forced landing of balloon injuring occupant

    X ● **V96.03**   Balloon collision injuring occupant
> Balloon collision with any object, fixed, moveable or moving

    X ● **V96.04**   Balloon fire injuring occupant

    X ● **V96.05**   Balloon explosion injuring occupant

    X ● **V96.09**   Other balloon accident injuring occupant

● **V96.1**   **Hang-glider accident injuring occupant**

    X ● **V96.10**   Unspecified hang-glider accident injuring occupant

    X ● **V96.11**   Hang-glider crash injuring occupant

    X ● **V96.12**   Forced landing of hang-glider injuring occupant

    X ● **V96.13**   Hang-glider collision injuring occupant
> Hang-glider collision with any object, fixed, moveable or moving

    X ● **V96.14**   Hang-glider fire injuring occupant

    X ● **V96.15**   Hang-glider explosion injuring occupant

    X ● **V96.19**   Other hang-glider accident injuring occupant

● V96.2 Glider (nonpowered) accident injuring occupant
X ● V96.20 Unspecified glider (nonpowered) accident injuring occupant
X ● V96.21 Glider (nonpowered) crash injuring occupant
X ● V96.22 Forced landing of glider (nonpowered) injuring occupant
X ● V96.23 Glider (nonpowered) collision injuring occupant
    Glider (nonpowered) collision with any object, fixed, moveable or moving
X ● V96.24 Glider (nonpowered) fire injuring occupant
X ● V96.25 Glider (nonpowered) explosion injuring occupant
X ● V96.29 Other glider (nonpowered) accident injuring occupant
X ● V96.8 Other nonpowered-aircraft accidents injuring occupant
    Kite carrying a person accident injuring occupant
X ● V96.9 Unspecified nonpowered-aircraft accident injuring occupant
    Nonpowered-aircraft accident NOS

● V97 Other specified air transport accidents
The appropriate 7th character is to be added to each code from category V97

A	initial encounter
D	subsequent encounter
S	sequela

X ● V97.0 Occupant of aircraft injured in other specified air transport accidents
    Fall in, on or from aircraft in air transport accident
    Excludes1   accident while boarding or alighting aircraft (V97.1)
X ● V97.1 Person injured while boarding or alighting from aircraft
● V97.2 Parachutist accident
X ● V97.21 Parachutist entangled in object
    Parachutist landing in tree
X ● V97.22 Parachutist injured on landing
X ● V97.29 Other parachutist accident
● V97.3 Person on ground injured in air transport accident
X ● V97.31 Hit by object falling from aircraft
    Hit by crashing aircraft
    Injured by aircraft hitting house
    Injured by aircraft hitting car
X ● V97.32 Injured by rotating propeller
X ● V97.33 Sucked into jet engine
X ● V97.39 Other injury to person on ground due to air transport accident
● V97.8 Other air transport accidents, not elsewhere classified
    Excludes1   aircraft accident NOS (V95.9)
        exposure to changes in air pressure during ascent or descent (W94.-)
● V97.81 Air transport accident involving military aircraft
● V97.810 Civilian aircraft involved in air transport accident with military aircraft
    Passenger in civilian aircraft injured due to accident with military aircraft
● V97.811 Civilian injured by military aircraft
● V97.818 Other air transport accident involving military aircraft
X ● V97.89 Other air transport accidents, not elsewhere classified
    Injury from machinery on aircraft

OTHER AND UNSPECIFIED TRANSPORT ACCIDENTS (V98-V99)

Excludes1   vehicle accident, type of vehicle unspecified (V89.-)

● V98 Other specified transport accidents
The appropriate 7th character is to be added to each code from category V98

A	initial encounter
D	subsequent encounter
S	sequela

X ● V98.0 Accident to, on or involving cable-car, not on rails
    Caught or dragged by cable-car, not on rails
    Fall or jump from cable-car, not on rails
    Object thrown from or in cable-car, not on rails
X ● V98.1 Accident to, on or involving land-yacht
X ● V98.2 Accident to, on or involving ice yacht
X ● V98.3 Accident to, on or involving ski lift
    Accident to, on or involving ski chair-lift
    Accident to, on or involving ski-lift with gondola
X ● V98.8 Other specified transport accidents

X ● V99 Unspecified transport accident
The appropriate 7th character is to be added to code V99

A	initial encounter
D	subsequent encounter
S	sequela

OTHER EXTERNAL CAUSES OF ACCIDENTAL INJURY (W00-X58)

SLIPPING, TRIPPING, STUMBLING AND FALLS (W00-W19)

Excludes1   assault involving a fall (Y01-Y02)
    fall from animal (V80.-)
    fall (in) (from) machinery (in operation) (W28-W31)
    fall (in) (from) transport vehicle (V01-V99)
    intentional self-harm involving a fall (X80-X81)
Excludes2   at risk for fall (history of fall) Z91.81
    fall (in) (from) burning building (X00.-)
    fall into fire (X00-X04, X08-X09)

● W00 Fall due to ice and snow
Includes   pedestrian on foot falling (slipping) on ice and snow
Excludes1   fall on (from) ice and snow involving pedestrian conveyance (V00.-)
    fall from stairs and steps not due to ice and snow (W10.-)
The appropriate 7th character is to be added to each code from category W00

A	initial encounter
D	subsequent encounter
S	sequela

X ● W00.0 Fall on same level due to ice and snow
X ● W00.1 Fall from stairs and steps due to ice and snow
X ● W00.2 Other fall from one level to another due to ice and snow
X ● W00.9 Unspecified fall due to ice and snow

◀ New   ◀ Revised   deleted Deleted   OGCR Official Guidelines   X Assign placeholder X   ● Use Additional Character(s)

Excludes 1   Excludes 2   Includes   Use additional   Code first   Code also   Unspecified

● **W01   Fall on same level from slipping, tripping and stumbling**

Includes	fall on moving sidewalk
Excludes1	fall due to bumping (striking) against object (W18.0-)
	fall in shower or bathtub (W18.2-)
	fall on same level NOS (W18.30)
	fall on same level from slipping, tripping and stumbling due to ice or snow (W00.0)
	fall off or from toilet (W18.1-)
	slipping, tripping and stumbling NOS (W18.40)
	slipping, tripping and stumbling without falling (W18.4-)

The appropriate 7th character is to be added to each code from category W01

A	initial encounter
D	subsequent encounter
S	sequela

X● **W01.0   Fall on same level from slipping, tripping and stumbling without subsequent striking against object**
     Falling over animal

● **W01.1   Fall on same level from slipping, tripping and stumbling with subsequent striking against object**

   X● **W01.10   Fall on same level from slipping, tripping and stumbling with subsequent striking against unspecified object**

   ● **W01.11   Fall on same level from slipping, tripping and stumbling with subsequent striking against sharp object**

     ● **W01.110   Fall on same level from slipping, tripping and stumbling with subsequent striking against sharp glass**

     ● **W01.111   Fall on same level from slipping, tripping and stumbling with subsequent striking against power tool or machine**

     ● **W01.118   Fall on same level from slipping, tripping and stumbling with subsequent striking against other sharp object**

     ● **W01.119   Fall on same level from slipping, tripping and stumbling with subsequent striking against unspecified sharp object**

   ● **W01.19   Fall on same level from slipping, tripping and stumbling with subsequent striking against other object**

     ● **W01.190   Fall on same level from slipping, tripping and stumbling with subsequent striking against furniture**

     ● **W01.198   Fall on same level from slipping, tripping and stumbling with subsequent striking against other object**

X● **W03   Other fall on same level due to collision with another person**
     Fall due to non-transport collision with other person

Excludes1	collision with another person without fall (W51)
	crushed or pushed by a crowd or human stampede (W52)
	fall involving pedestrian conveyance (V00-V09)
	fall due to ice or snow (W00)
	fall on same level NOS (W18.30)

The appropriate 7th character is to be added to code W03

A	initial encounter
D	subsequent encounter
S	sequela

X● **W04   Fall while being carried or supported by other persons**
     Accidentally dropped while being carried

The appropriate 7th character is to be added to code W04

A	initial encounter
D	subsequent encounter
S	sequel

● **W05   Fall from non-moving wheelchair, nonmotorized scooter and motorized mobility scooter**

Excludes1	fall from moving wheelchair (powered) (V00.811)
	fall from moving motorized mobility scooter (V00.831)
	fall from nonmotorized scooter (V00.141)

The appropriate 7th character is to be added to each code from category W05

A	initial encounter
D	subsequent encounter
S	sequela

   X● **W05.0   Fall from non-moving wheelchair**
   X● **W05.1   Fall from non-moving nonmotorized scooter**
   X● **W05.2   Fall from non-moving motorized mobility scooter**

X● **W06   Fall from bed**

The appropriate 7th character is to be added to code W06

A	initial encounter
D	subsequent encounter
S	sequela

X● **W07   Fall from chair**

The appropriate 7th character is to be added to code W07

A	initial encounter
D	subsequent encounter
S	sequela

X● **W08   Fall from other furniture**

The appropriate 7th character is to be added to code W08

A	initial encounter
D	subsequent encounter
S	sequela

CHAPTER 20 (V01-Y99)

◀ New   ◀▥ Revised   ~~deleted~~ Deleted   OGCR Official Guidelines   X Assign placeholder X   ● Use Additional Character(s)

| Excludes 1 | Excludes 2 | Includes | Use additional | Code first | Code also | Unspecified |

● **W09   Fall on and from playground equipment**

> **Excludes1**   fall involving recreational machinery (W31)

> The appropriate 7th character is to be added to each code from category W09

> | | |
> |---|---|
> | A | initial encounter |
> | D | subsequent encounter |
> | S | sequela |

X ● **W09.0   Fall on or from playground slide**
X ● **W09.1   Fall from playground swing**
X ● **W09.2   Fall on or from jungle gym**
X ● **W09.8   Fall on or from other playground equipment**

● **W10   Fall on and from stairs and steps**

> **Excludes1**   fall from stairs and steps due to ice and snow (W00.1)

> The appropriate 7th character is to be added to each code from category W10

> | | |
> |---|---|
> | A | initial encounter |
> | D | subsequent encounter |
> | S | sequela |

X ● **W10.0   Fall (on) (from) escalator**
X ● **W10.1   Fall (on) (from) sidewalk curb**
X ● **W10.2   Fall (on) (from) incline**
> Fall (on) (from) ramp
X ● **W10.8   Fall (on) (from) other stairs and steps**
X ● **W10.9   Fall (on) (from) unspecified stairs and steps**

X ● **W11   Fall on and from ladder**

> The appropriate 7th character is to be added to code W11

> | | |
> |---|---|
> | A | initial encounter |
> | D | subsequent encounter |
> | S | sequela |

X ● **W12   Fall on and from scaffolding**

> The appropriate 7th character is to be added to code W12

> | | |
> |---|---|
> | A | initial encounter |
> | D | subsequent encounter |
> | S | sequela |

● **W13   Fall from, out of or through building or structure**

> The appropriate 7th character is to be added to each code from category W13

> | | |
> |---|---|
> | A | initial encounter |
> | D | subsequent encounter |
> | S | sequela |

X ● **W13.0   Fall from, out of or through balcony**
> Fall from, out of or through railing
X ● **W13.1   Fall from, out of or through bridge**
X ● **W13.2   Fall from, out of or through roof**
X ● **W13.3   Fall through floor**
X ● **W13.4   Fall from, out of or through window**
> **Excludes2**   fall with subsequent striking against sharp glass (W01.110)
X ● **W13.8   Fall from, out of or through other building or structure**
> Fall from, out of or through viaduct
> Fall from, out of or through wall
> Fall from, out of or through flag-pole
X ● **W13.9   Fall from, out of or through building, not otherwise specified**
> **Excludes1**   collapse of a building or structure (W20.-)
> fall or jump from burning building or structure (X00.-)

X ● **W14   Fall from tree**

> The appropriate 7th character is to be added to code W14

> | | |
> |---|---|
> | A | initial encounter |
> | D | subsequent encounter |
> | S | sequela |

X ● **W15   Fall from cliff**

> The appropriate 7th character is to be added to code W15

> | | |
> |---|---|
> | A | initial encounter |
> | D | subsequent encounter |
> | S | sequela |

● **W16   Fall, jump or diving into water**

> **Excludes1**   accidental non-watercraft drowning and submersion not involving fall (W65-W74)
> effects of air pressure from diving (W94.-)
> fall into water from watercraft (V90-V94)
> hitting an object or against bottom when falling from watercraft (V94.0)

> **Excludes2**   striking or hitting diving board (W21.4)

> The appropriate 7th character is to be added to each code from category W16

> | | |
> |---|---|
> | A | initial encounter |
> | D | subsequent encounter |
> | S | sequela |

● **W16.0   Fall into swimming pool**
> Fall into swimming pool NOS
> **Excludes1**   fall into empty swimming pool (W17.3)
● **W16.01   Fall into swimming pool striking water surface**
● **W16.011   Fall into swimming pool striking water surface causing drowning and submersion**
> **Excludes1**   drowning and submersion while in swimming pool without fall (W67)
● **W16.012   Fall into swimming pool striking water surface causing other injury**
● **W16.02   Fall into swimming pool striking bottom**
● **W16.021   Fall into swimming pool striking bottom causing drowning and submersion**
> **Excludes1**   drowning and submersion while in swimming pool without fall (W67)
● **W16.022   Fall into swimming pool striking bottom causing other injury**
● **W16.03   Fall into swimming pool striking wall**
● **W16.031   Fall into swimming pool striking wall causing drowning and submersion**
> **Excludes1**   drowning and submersion while in swimming pool without fall (W67)
● **W16.032   Fall into swimming pool striking wall causing other injury**

◄ New   ◄ Revised   ~~deleted~~ Deleted   **OGCR** Official Guidelines   X Assign placeholder X   ● Use Additional Character(s)

Excludes 1	Excludes 2	Includes	Use additional	Code first	Code also	Unspecified

● **W16.1   Fall into natural body of water**
Fall into lake
Fall into open sea
Fall into river
Fall into stream

  ● **W16.11   Fall into natural body of water striking water surface**

    ● **W16.111   Fall into natural body of water striking water surface causing drowning and submersion**

       Excludes1   drowning and submersion while in natural body of water without fall (W69)

    ● **W16.112   Fall into natural body of water striking water surface causing other injury**

  ● **W16.12   Fall into natural body of water striking bottom**

    ● **W16.121   Fall into natural body of water striking bottom causing drowning and submersion**

       Excludes1   drowning and submersion while in natural body of water without fall (W69)

    ● **W16.122   Fall into natural body of water striking bottom causing other injury**

  ● **W16.13   Fall into natural body of water striking side**

    ● **W16.131   Fall into natural body of water striking side causing drowning and submersion**

       Excludes1   drowning and submersion while in natural body of water without fall (W69)

    ● **W16.132   Fall into natural body of water striking side causing other injury**

● **W16.2   Fall in (into) filled bathtub or bucket of water**

  ● **W16.21   Fall in (into) filled bathtub**

     Excludes1   fall into empty bathtub (W18.2)

    ● **W16.211   Fall in (into) filled bathtub causing drowning and submersion**

       Excludes1   drowning and submersion while in filled bathtub without fall (W65)

    ● **W16.212   Fall in (into) filled bathtub causing other injury**

  ● **W16.22   Fall in (into) bucket of water**

    ● **W16.221   Fall in (into) bucket of water causing drowning and submersion**

    ● **W16.222   Fall in (into) bucket of water causing other injury**

● **W16.3   Fall into other water**
Fall into fountain
Fall into reservoir

  ● **W16.31   Fall into other water striking water surface**

    ● **W16.311   Fall into other water striking water surface causing drowning and submersion**

       Excludes1   drowning and submersion while in other water without fall (W73)

    ● **W16.312   Fall into other water striking water surface causing other injury**

● **W16.32   Fall into other water striking bottom**

  ● **W16.321   Fall into other water striking bottom causing drowning and submersion**

     Excludes1   drowning and submersion while in other water without fall (W73)

  ● **W16.322   Fall into other water striking bottom causing other injury**

● **W16.33   Fall into other water striking wall**

  ● **W16.331   Fall into other water striking wall causing drowning and submersion**

     Excludes1   drowning and submersion while in other water without fall (W73)

  ● **W16.332   Fall into other water striking wall causing other injury**

● **W16.4   Fall into unspecified water**

   X ● **W16.41   Fall into unspecified water causing drowning and submersion**

   X ● **W16.42   Fall into unspecified water causing other injury**

● **W16.5   Jumping or diving into swimming pool**

  ● **W16.51   Jumping or diving into swimming pool striking water surface**

    ● **W16.511   Jumping or diving into swimming pool striking water surface causing drowning and submersion**

       Excludes1   drowning and submersion while in swimming pool without jumping or diving (W67)

    ● **W16.512   Jumping or diving into swimming pool striking water surface causing other injury**

  ● **W16.52   Jumping or diving into swimming pool striking bottom**

    ● **W16.521   Jumping or diving into swimming pool striking bottom causing drowning and submersion**

       Excludes1   drowning and submersion while in swimming pool without jumping or diving (W67)

    ● **W16.522   Jumping or diving into swimming pool striking bottom causing other injury**

  ● **W16.53   Jumping or diving into swimming pool striking wall**

    ● **W16.531   Jumping or diving into swimming pool striking wall causing drowning and submersion**

       Excludes1   drowning and submersion while in swimming pool without jumping or diving (W67)

    ● **W16.532   Jumping or diving into swimming pool striking wall causing other injury**

CHAPTER 20 (V01-Y99)

- ● W16.6   Jumping or diving into natural body of water
  Jumping or diving into lake
  Jumping or diving into open sea
  Jumping or diving into river
  Jumping or diving into stream
  - ● W16.61   Jumping or diving into natural body of water striking water surface
    - ● W16.611   Jumping or diving into natural body of water striking water surface causing drowning and submersion
      - **Excludes1**   drowning and submersion while in natural body of water without jumping or diving (W69)
    - ● W16.612   Jumping or diving into natural body of water striking water surface causing other injury
  - ● W16.62   Jumping or diving into natural body of water striking bottom
    - ● W16.621   Jumping or diving into natural body of water striking bottom causing drowning and submersion
      - **Excludes1**   drowning and submersion while in natural body of water without jumping or diving (W69)
    - ● W16.622   Jumping or diving into natural body of water striking bottom causing other injury
- ● W16.7   Jumping or diving from boat
  - **Excludes1**   fall from boat into water - see watercraft accident (V90-V94)
  - ● W16.71   Jumping or diving from boat striking water surface
    - ● W16.711   Jumping or diving from boat striking water surface causing drowning and submersion
    - ● W16.712   Jumping or diving from boat striking water surface causing other injury
  - ● W16.72   Jumping or diving from boat striking bottom
    - ● W16.721   Jumping or diving from boat striking bottom causing drowning and submersion
    - ● W16.722   Jumping or diving from boat striking bottom causing other injury
- ● W16.8   Jumping or diving into other water
  Jumping or diving into fountain
  Jumping or diving into reservoir
  - ● W16.81   Jumping or diving into other water striking water surface
    - ● W16.811   Jumping or diving into other water striking water surface causing drowning and submersion
      - **Excludes1**   drowning and submersion while in other water without jumping or diving (W73)
    - ● W16.812   Jumping or diving into other water striking water surface causing other injury

- ● W16.82   Jumping or diving into other water striking bottom
  - ● W16.821   Jumping or diving into other water striking bottom causing drowning and submersion
    - **Excludes1**   drowning and submersion while in other water without jumping or diving (W73)
  - ● W16.822   Jumping or diving into other water striking bottom causing other injury
- ● W16.83   Jumping or diving into other water striking wall
  - ● W16.831   Jumping or diving into other water striking wall causing drowning and submersion
    - **Excludes1**   drowning and submersion while in other water without jumping or diving (W73)
  - ● W16.832   Jumping or diving into other water striking wall causing other injury
- ● W16.9   Jumping or diving into unspecified water
  - X ● W16.91   Jumping or diving into unspecified water causing drowning and submersion
  - X ● W16.92   Jumping or diving into unspecified water causing other injury
- ● W17   Other fall from one level to another
  The appropriate 7th character is to be added to each code from category W17

A	initial encounter
D	subsequent encounter
S	sequela

  - X ● W17.0   Fall into well
  - X ● W17.1   Fall into storm drain or manhole
  - X ● W17.2   Fall into hole
    Fall into pit
  - X ● W17.3   Fall into empty swimming pool
    - **Excludes1**   fall into filled swimming pool (W16.0-)
  - X ● W17.4   Fall from dock
  - ● W17.8   Other fall from one level to another
    - X ● W17.81   Fall down embankment (hill)
    - X ● W17.82   Fall from (out of) grocery cart
      Fall due to grocery cart tipping over
    - X ● W17.89   Other fall from one level to another
      Fall from cherry picker
      Fall from lifting device
      Fall from mobile elevated work platform [MEWP]
      Fall from sky lift

● **W18   Other slipping, tripping and stumbling and falls**

The appropriate 7th character is to be added to each code from category W18

> A   initial encounter
> D   subsequent encounter
> S   sequela

● **W18.0   Fall due to bumping against object**
Striking against object with subsequent fall

> **Excludes1**   fall on same level due to slipping, tripping, or stumbling with subsequent striking against object (W01.1-)

X● **W18.00   Striking against unspecified object with subsequent fall**

X● **W18.01   Striking against sports equipment with subsequent fall**

X● **W18.02   Striking against glass with subsequent fall**

X● **W18.09   Striking against other object with subsequent fall**

● **W18.1   Fall from or off toilet**

X● **W18.11   Fall from or off toilet without subsequent striking against object**
Fall from (off) toilet NOS

X● **W18.12   Fall from or off toilet with subsequent striking against object**

X● **W18.2   Fall in (into) shower or empty bathtub**

> **Excludes1**   fall in full bathtub causing drowning or submersion (W16.21-)

● **W18.3   Other and unspecified fall on same level**

X● **W18.30   Fall on same level, unspecified**

X● **W18.31   Fall on same level due to stepping on an object**
Fall on same level due to stepping on an animal

> **Excludes1**   slipping, tripping and stumbling without fall due to stepping on animal (W18.41)

X● **W18.39   Other fall on same level**

● **W18.4   Slipping, tripping and stumbling without falling**

> **Excludes1**   collision with another person without fall (W51)

X● **W18.40   Slipping, tripping and stumbling without falling, unspecified**

X● **W18.41   Slipping, tripping and stumbling without falling due to stepping on object**
Slipping, tripping and stumbling without falling due to stepping on animal

> **Excludes1**   slipping, tripping and stumbling with fall due to stepping on animal (W18.31)

X● **W18.42   Slipping, tripping and stumbling without falling due to stepping into hole or opening**

X● **W18.43   Slipping, tripping and stumbling without falling due to stepping from one level to another**

X● **W18.49   Other slipping, tripping and stumbling without falling**

X● **W19   Unspecified fall**
Accidental fall NOS

The appropriate 7th character is to be added to code W19

> A   initial encounter
> D   subsequent encounter
> S   sequela

> **Excludes1**   assault (X92-Y08)
> contact or collision with animals or persons (W50-W64)
> exposure to inanimate mechanical forces involving military or war operations (Y36.-, Y37.-)
> intentional self-harm (X71-X83)

● **W20   Struck by thrown, projected or falling object**

Code first any associated:
cataclysm (X34-X39)
lightning strike (T75.00)

> **Excludes1**   falling object in machinery accident (W24, W28-W31)
> falling object in transport accident (V01-V99)
> object set in motion by explosion (W35-W40)
> object set in motion by firearm (W32-W34)
> struck by thrown sports equipment (W21.-)

The appropriate 7th character is to be added to each code from category W20

> A   initial encounter
> D   subsequent encounter
> S   sequela

X● **W20.0   Struck by falling object in cave-in**

> **Excludes2**   asphyxiation due to cave-in (T71.21)

X● **W20.1   Struck by object due to collapse of building**

> **Excludes1**   struck by object due to collapse of burning building (X00.2, X02.2)

X● **W20.8   Other cause of strike by thrown, projected or falling object**

> **Excludes1**   struck by thrown sports equipment (W21.-)

● **W21   Striking against or struck by sports equipment**

> **Excludes1**   assault with sports equipment (Y08.0-)
> striking against or struck by sports equipment with subsequent fall (W18.01)

The appropriate 7th character is to be added to each code from category W21

> A   initial encounter
> D   subsequent encounter
> S   sequela

● **W21.0   Struck by hit or thrown ball**

X● **W21.00   Struck by hit or thrown ball, unspecified type**

X● **W21.01   Struck by football**

X● **W21.02   Struck by soccer ball**

X● **W21.03   Struck by baseball**

X● **W21.04   Struck by golf ball**

X● **W21.05   Struck by basketball**

X● **W21.06   Struck by volleyball**

X● **W21.07   Struck by softball**

X● **W21.09   Struck by other hit or thrown ball**

● **W21.1   Struck by bat, racquet or club**

X● **W21.11   Struck by baseball bat**

X● **W21.12   Struck by tennis racquet**

X● **W21.13   Struck by golf club**

X● **W21.19   Struck by other bat, racquet or club**

● **W21.2   Struck by hockey stick or puck**

◀ New   ◀▥ Revised   ~~deleted~~ Deleted   **OGCR** Official Guidelines   X Assign placeholder X   ● Use Additional Character(s)
Excludes 1   Excludes 2   Includes   Use additional   Code first   Code also   Unspecified

● W21.21 **Struck by hockey stick**
  ● W21.210 **Struck by ice hockey stick**
  ● W21.211 **Struck by field hockey stick**
● W21.22 **Struck by hockey puck**
  ● W21.220 **Struck by ice hockey puck**
  ● W21.221 **Struck by field hockey puck**
● W21.3 **Struck by sports foot wear**
  X ● W21.31 **Struck by shoe cleats**
          Stepped on by shoe cleats
  X ● W21.32 **Struck by skate blades**
          Skated over by skate blades
  X ● W21.39 **Struck by other sports foot wear**
X ● W21.4 **Striking against diving board**
          Use additional code for subsequent falling into water, if
          applicable (W16.-)
● W21.8 **Striking against or struck by other sports equipment**
  X ● W21.81 **Striking against or struck by football helmet**
  X ● W21.89 **Striking against or struck by other sports
          equipment**
X ● W21.9 **Striking against or struck by unspecified sports
          equipment**

● W22 **Striking against or struck by other objects**
      | Excludes1 | striking against or struck by object with
                  subsequent fall (W18.09)

      The appropriate 7th character is to be added to each code from
          category W22

      | A | initial encounter |
      | D | subsequent encounter |
      | S | sequela |

● W22.0 **Striking against stationary object**
      | Excludes1 | striking against stationary sports
                  equipment (W21.8)
  X ● W22.01 **Walked into wall**
  X ● W22.02 **Walked into lamppost**
  X ● W22.03 **Walked into furniture**
  ● W22.04 **Striking against wall of swimming pool**
    ● W22.041 **Striking against wall of swimming
          pool causing drowning and
          submersion**
          | Excludes1 | drowning and
                      submersion
                      while swimming
                      without striking
                      against wall
                      (W67)
    ● W22.042 **Striking against wall of swimming
          pool causing other injury**
  X ● W22.09 **Striking against other stationary object**
● W22.1 **Striking against or struck by automobile airbag**
  X ● W22.10 **Striking against or struck by unspecified
          automobile airbag**
  X ● W22.11 **Striking against or struck by driver side
          automobile airbag**
  X ● W22.12 **Striking against or struck by front passenger
          side automobile airbag**
  X ● W22.19 **Striking against or struck by other automobile
          airbag**
X ● W22.8 **Striking against or struck by other objects**
          Striking against or struck by object NOS
          | Excludes1 | struck by thrown, projected or falling
                      object (W20.-)

● W23 **Caught, crushed, jammed or pinched in or between objects**
      | Excludes1 | injury caused by cutting or piercing instruments
                  (W25-W27)
                  injury caused by firearms malfunction (W32.1,
                      W33.1-, W34.1-)
                  injury caused by lifting and transmission devices
                      (W24.-)
                  injury caused by machinery (W28-W31)
                  injury caused by nonpowered hand tools (W27.-)
                  injury caused by transport vehicle being used as a
                      means of transportation (V01-V99)
                  injury caused by struck by thrown, projected or
                      falling object (W20.-)
      The appropriate 7th character is to be added to each code from
          category W23

      | A | initial encounter |
      | D | subsequent encounter |
      | S | sequela |

X ● W23.0 **Caught, crushed, jammed, or pinched between moving
          objects**
X ● W23.1 **Caught, crushed, jammed, or pinched between
          stationary objects**

● W24 **Contact with lifting and transmission devices, not elsewhere
      classified**
      | Excludes1 | transport accidents (V01-V99)
      The appropriate 7th character is to be added to each code from
          category W24

      | A | initial encounter |
      | D | subsequent encounter |
      | S | sequela |

X ● W24.0 **Contact with lifting devices, not elsewhere classified**
          Contact with chain hoist
          Contact with drive belt
          Contact with pulley (block)
X ● W24.1 **Contact with transmission devices, not elsewhere
          classified**
          Contact with transmission belt or cable

X ● W25 **Contact with sharp glass**
      Code first any associated:
          injury due to flying glass from explosion or firearm discharge
              (W32-W40)
          transport accident (V00-V99)
      | Excludes1 | fall on same level due to slipping, tripping and
                  stumbling with subsequent striking against
                  sharp glass (W01.10)
                  striking against sharp glass with subsequent fall
                  (W18.02)
      The appropriate 7th character is to be added to code W25

      | A | initial encounter |
      | D | subsequent encounter |
      | S | sequela |

● W26 **Contact with knife, sword or dagger**
      The appropriate 7th character is to be added to each code from
          category W26

      | A | initial encounter |
      | D | subsequent encounter |
      | S | sequela |

X ● W26.0 **Contact with knife**
          | Excludes1 | contact with electric knife (W29.1)
X ● W26.1 **Contact with sword or dagger**

● **W27　Contact with nonpowered hand tool**

> The appropriate 7th character is to be added to each code from category W27

> | | |
> |---|---|
> | A | initial encounter |
> | D | subsequent encounter |
> | S | sequela |

X ● **W27.0　Contact with workbench tool**
> Contact with auger
> Contact with axe
> Contact with chisel
> Contact with handsaw
> Contact with screwdriver

X ● **W27.1　Contact with garden tool**
> Contact with hoe
> Contact with nonpowered lawn mower
> Contact with pitchfork
> Contact with rake

X ● **W27.2　Contact with scissors**

X ● **W27.3　Contact with needle (sewing)**
> **Excludes1**　contact with hypodermic needle (W46.-)

X ● **W27.4　Contact with kitchen utensil**
> Contact with fork
> Contact with ice-pick
> Contact with can-opener NOS

X ● **W27.5　Contact with paper-cutter**

X ● **W27.8　Contact with other nonpowered hand tool**
> Contact with nonpowered sewing machine
> Contact with shovel

X ● **W28　Contact with powered lawn mower**
> Powered lawn mower (commercial) (residential)
> **Excludes1**　contact with nonpowered lawn mower (W27.1)
> **Excludes2**　exposure to electric current (W86.-)
> The appropriate 7th character is to be added to code W28

> | | |
> |---|---|
> | A | initial encounter |
> | D | subsequent encounter |
> | S | sequela |

● **W29　Contact with other powered hand tools and household machinery**
> **Excludes1**　contact with commercial machinery (W31.82)
> contact with hot household appliance (X15)
> contact with nonpowered hand tool (W27.-)
> exposure to electric current (W86)

> The appropriate 7th character is to be added to each code from category W29

> | | |
> |---|---|
> | A | initial encounter |
> | D | subsequent encounter |
> | S | sequela |

X ● **W29.0　Contact with powered kitchen appliance**
> Contact with blender
> Contact with can-opener
> Contact with garbage disposal
> Contact with mixer

X ● **W29.1　Contact with electric knife**

X ● **W29.2　Contact with other powered household machinery**
> Contact with electric fan
> Contact with powered dryer (clothes) (powered) (spin)
> Contact with washing-machine
> Contact with sewing machine

X ● **W29.3　Contact with powered garden and outdoor hand tools and machinery**
> Contact with chainsaw
> Contact with edger
> Contact with garden cultivator (tiller)
> Contact with hedge trimmer
> Contact with other powered garden tool
> **Excludes1**　contact with powered lawn mower (W28)

X ● **W29.4　Contact with nail gun**

X ● **W29.8　Contact with other powered powered hand tools and household machinery**
> Contact with do-it-yourself tool NOS

● **W30　Contact with agricultural machinery**
> **Includes**　animal-powered farm machine
> **Excludes1**　agricultural transport vehicle accident (V01-V99)
> explosion of grain store (W40.8)
> exposure to electric current (W86.-)

> The appropriate 7th character is to be added to each code from category W30

> | | |
> |---|---|
> | A | initial encounter |
> | D | subsequent encounter |
> | S | sequela |

X ● **W30.0　Contact with combine harvester**
> Contact with reaper
> Contact with thresher

X ● **W30.1　Contact with power take-off devices (PTO)**

X ● **W30.2　Contact with hay derrick**

X ● **W30.3　Contact with grain storage elevator**
> **Excludes1**　explosion of grain store (W40.8)

● **W30.8　Contact with other specified agricultural machinery**

X ● **W30.81　Contact with agricultural transport vehicle in stationary use**
> Contact with agricultural transport vehicle under repair, not on public roadway
> **Excludes1**　agricultural transport vehicle accident (V01-V99)

X ● **W30.89　Contact with other specified agricultural machinery**

X ● **W30.9　Contact with unspecified agricultural machinery**
> Contact with farm machinery NOS

● **W31　Contact with other and unspecified machinery**
> **Excludes1**　contact with agricultural machinery (W30.-)
> contact with machinery in transport under own power or being towed by a vehicle (V01-V99)
> exposure to electric current (W86)

> The appropriate 7th character is to be added to each code from category W31

> | | |
> |---|---|
> | A | initial encounter |
> | D | subsequent encounter |
> | S | sequela |

X ● **W31.0　Contact with mining and earth-drilling machinery**
> Contact with bore or drill (land) (seabed)
> Contact with shaft hoist
> Contact with shaft lift
> Contact with undercutter

X ● **W31.1　Contact with metalworking machines**
> Contact with abrasive wheel
> Contact with forging machine
> Contact with lathe
> Contact with mechanical shears
> Contact with metal drilling machine
> Contact with milling machine
> Contact with power press
> Contact with rolling-mill
> Contact with metal sawing machine

X ● **W31.2　Contact with powered woodworking and forming machines**
> Contact with band saw
> Contact with bench saw
> Contact with circular saw
> Contact with molding machine
> Contact with overhead plane
> Contact with powered saw
> Contact with radial saw
> Contact with sander
> **Excludes1**　nonpowered woodworking tools (W27.0)

 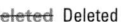

X● **W31.3   Contact with prime movers**
    Contact with gas turbine
    Contact with internal combustion engine
    Contact with steam engine
    Contact with water driven turbine

● **W31.8   Contact with other specified machinery**

X● **W31.81   Contact with recreational machinery**
    Contact with roller-coaster

X● **W31.82   Contact with other commercial machinery**
    Contact with commercial electric fan
    Contact with commercial kitchen appliances
    Contact with commercial powered dryer
        (clothes) (powered) (spin)
    Contact with commercial washing-machine
    Contact with commercial sewing machine

    | Excludes1 | contact with household machinery (W29.-) |
    contact with powered lawn mower (W28)

X● **W31.83   Contact with special construction vehicle in stationary use**
    Contact with special construction vehicle under repair, not on public roadway

    | Excludes1 | special construction vehicle accident (V01-V99) |

X● **W31.89   Contact with other specified machinery**

X● **W31.9   Contact with unspecified machinery**
    Contact with machinery NOS

● **W32   Accidental handgun discharge and malfunction**

    | Includes | accidental discharge and malfunction of gun for single hand use |
    accidental discharge and malfunction of pistol
    accidental discharge and malfunction of revolver
    handgun discharge and malfunction NOS

    | Excludes1 | accidental airgun discharge and malfunction (W34.010, W34.110) |
    accidental BB gun discharge and malfunction (W34.010, W34.110)
    accidental pellet gun discharge and malfunction (W34.010, W34.110)
    accidental shotgun discharge and malfunction (W33.01, W33.11)
    assault by handgun discharge (X93)
    handgun discharge involving legal intervention (Y35.0-)
    handgun discharge involving military or war operations (Y36.4-)
    intentional self-harm by handgun discharge (X72)
    Very pistol discharge and malfunction (W34.09, W34.19)

The appropriate 7th character is to be added to each code from category W32

    | A | initial encounter |
    | D | subsequent encounter |
    | S | sequela |

X● **W32.0   Accidental handgun discharge**
X● **W32.1   Accidental handgun malfunction**
    Injury due to explosion of handgun (parts)
    Injury due to malfunction of mechanism or component of handgun
    Injury due to recoil of handgun
    Powder burn from handgun

● **W33   Accidental rifle, shotgun and larger firearm discharge and malfunction**

    | Includes | rifle, shotgun and larger firearm discharge and malfunction NOS |

    | Excludes1 | accidental airgun discharge and malfunction (W34.010, W34.110) |
    accidental BB gun discharge and malfunction (W34.010, W34.110)
    accidental handgun discharge and malfunction (W32.-)
    accidental pellet gun discharge and malfunction (W34.010, W34.110)
    assault by rifle, shotgun and larger firearm discharge (X94)
    firearm discharge involving legal intervention (Y35.0-)
    firearm discharge involving military or war operations (Y36.4-)
    intentional self-harm by rifle, shotgun and larger firearm discharge (X73)

The appropriate 7th character is to be added to each code from category W33

    | A | initial encounter |
    | D | subsequent encounter |
    | S | sequela |

● **W33.0   Accidental rifle, shotgun and larger firearm discharge**

X● **W33.00   Accidental discharge of unspecified larger firearm**
    Discharge of unspecified larger firearm NOS

X● **W33.01   Accidental discharge of shotgun**
    Discharge of shotgun NOS

X● **W33.02   Accidental discharge of hunting rifle**
    Discharge of hunting rifle NOS

X● **W33.03   Accidental discharge of machine gun**
    Discharge of machine gun NOS

X● **W33.09   Accidental discharge of other larger firearm**
    Discharge of other larger firearm NOS

● **W33.1   Accidental rifle, shotgun and larger firearm malfunction**
    Injury due to explosion of rifle, shotgun and larger firearm (parts)
    Injury due to malfunction of mechanism or component of rifle, shotgun and larger firearm
    Injury due to piercing, cutting, crushing or pinching due to (by) slide trigger mechanism, scope or other gun part
    Injury due to recoil of rifle, shotgun and larger firearm
    Powder burn from rifle, shotgun and larger firearm

X● **W33.10   Accidental malfunction of unspecified larger firearm**
    Malfunction of unspecified larger firearm NOS

X● **W33.11   Accidental malfunction of shotgun**
    Malfunction of shotgun NOS

X● **W33.12   Accidental malfunction of hunting rifle**
    Malfunction of hunting rifle NOS

X● **W33.13   Accidental malfunction of machine gun**
    Malfunction of machine gun NOS

X● **W33.19   Accidental malfunction of other larger firearm**
    Malfunction of other larger firearm NOS

● **W34 Accidental discharge and malfunction from other and unspecified firearms and guns**

The appropriate 7th character is to be added to each code from category W34

A	initial encounter
D	subsequent encounter
S	sequela

  ● **W34.0 Accidental discharge from other and unspecified firearms and guns**

  X● **W34.00 Accidental discharge from unspecified firearms or gun**
      Discharge from firearm NOS
      Gunshot wound NOS
      Shot NOS

  ● **W34.01 Accidental discharge of gas, air or spring-operated guns**

    ● **W34.010 Accidental discharge of airgun**
        Accidental discharge of BB gun
        Accidental discharge of pellet gun

    ● **W34.011 Accidental discharge of paintball gun**
        Accidental injury due to paintball discharge

    ● **W34.018 Accidental discharge of other gas, air or spring-operated gun**

  X● **W34.09 Accidental discharge from other specified firearms**
      Accidental discharge from Very pistol [flare]

  ● **W34.1 Accidental malfunction from other and unspecified firearms and guns**

  X● **W34.10 Accidental malfunction from unspecified firearms or gun**
      Firearm malfunction NOS

  ● **W34.11 Accidental malfunction of gas, air or spring-operated guns**

    ● **W34.110 Accidental malfunction of airgun**
        Accidental malfunction of BB gun
        Accidental malfunction of pellet gun

    ● **W34.111 Accidental malfunction of paintball gun**
        Accidental injury due to paintball gun malfunction

    ● **W34.118 Accidental malfunction of other gas, air or spring-operated gun**

  X● **W34.19 Accidental malfunction from other specified firearms**
      Accidental malfunction from Very pistol [flare]

X● **W35 Explosion and rupture of boiler**
  Excludes1 explosion and rupture of boiler on watercraft (V93.4)

The appropriate 7th character is to be added to code W35

A	initial encounter
D	subsequent encounter
S	sequela

● **W36 Explosion and rupture of gas cylinder**

The appropriate 7th character is to be added to each code from category W36

A	initial encounter
D	subsequent encounter
S	sequela

  X● **W36.1 Explosion and rupture of aerosol can**
  X● **W36.2 Explosion and rupture of air tank**
  X● **W36.3 Explosion and rupture of pressurized-gas tank**
  X● **W36.8 Explosion and rupture of other gas cylinder**
  X● **W36.9 Explosion and rupture of unspecified gas cylinder**

● **W37 Explosion and rupture of pressurized tire, pipe or hose**

The appropriate 7th character is to be added to each code from category W37

A	initial encounter
D	subsequent encounter
S	sequela

  X● **W37.0 Explosion of bicycle tire**
  X● **W37.8 Explosion and rupture of other pressurized tire, pipe or hose**

X● **W38 Explosion and rupture of other specified pressurized devices**

The appropriate 7th character is to be added to code W38

A	initial encounter
D	subsequent encounter
S	sequela

X● **W39 Discharge of firework**

The appropriate 7th character is to be added to code W39

A	initial encounter
D	subsequent encounter
S	sequela

● **W40 Explosion of other materials**
  Excludes1 assault by explosive material (X96)
    explosion involving legal intervention (Y35.1-)
    explosion involving military or war operations (Y36.0-, Y36.2-)
    intentional self-harm by explosive material (X75)

The appropriate 7th character is to be added to each code from category W40

A	initial encounter
D	subsequent encounter
S	sequela

  X● **W40.0 Explosion of blasting material**
      Explosion of blasting cap
      Explosion of detonator
      Explosion of dynamite
      Explosion of explosive (any) used in blasting operations

  X● **W40.1 Explosion of explosive gases**
      Explosion of acetylene
      Explosion of butane
      Explosion of coal gas
      Explosion in mine NOS
      Explosion of explosive gas
      Explosion of fire damp
      Explosion of gasoline fumes
      Explosion of methane
      Explosion of propane

  X● **W40.8 Explosion of other specified explosive materials**
      Explosion in dump NOS
      Explosion in factory NOS
      Explosion in grain store
      Explosion in munitions
      Excludes1 explosion involving legal intervention (Y35.1-)
        explosion involving military or war operations (Y36.0-, Y36.2-)

  X● **W40.9 Explosion of unspecified explosive materials**
      Explosion NOS

● **W42 Exposure to noise**

The appropriate 7th character is to be added to each code from category W42

A	initial encounter
D	subsequent encounter
S	sequela

  X● **W42.0 Exposure to supersonic waves**
  X● **W42.9 Exposure to other noise**
      Exposure to sound waves NOS

CHAPTER 20 (V01-Y99)

● **W45   Foreign body or object entering through skin**

    Excludes2   contact with hand tools (nonpowered) (powered) (W27-W29)
           contact with knife, sword or dagger (W26.-)
           contact with sharp glass (W25.-)
           struck by objects (W20-W22)

    The appropriate 7th character is to be added to each code from category W45

A	initial encounter
D	subsequent encounter
S	sequela

X ● **W45.0   Nail entering through skin**

X ● **W45.1   Paper entering through skin**
       Paper cut

X ● **W45.2   Lid of can entering through skin**

X ● **W45.8   Other foreign body or object entering through skin**
       Splinter in skin NOS

● **W46   Contact with hypodermic needle**

    The appropriate 7th character is to be added to each code from category W46

A	initial encounter
D	subsequent encounter
S	sequela

X ● **W46.0   Contact with hypodermic needle**
       Hypodermic needle stick NOS

X ● **W46.1   Contact with contaminated hypodermic needle**

● **W49   Exposure to other inanimate mechanical forces**

    Includes   exposure to abnormal gravitational [G] forces
           exposure to inanimate mechanical forces NEC

    Excludes1   exposure to inanimate mechanical forces involving military or war operations (Y36.-, Y37.-)

    The appropriate 7th character is to be added to each code from category W49

A	initial encounter
D	subsequent encounter
S	sequela

   ● **W49.0   Item causing external constriction**

     X ● **W49.01   Hair causing external constriction**

     X ● **W49.02   String or thread causing external constriction**

     X ● **W49.03   Rubber band causing external constriction**

     X ● **W49.04   Ring or other jewelry causing external constriction**

     X ● **W49.09   Other item causing external constriction**

  X ● **W49.9   Exposure to other inanimate mechanical forces**

EXPOSURE TO ANIMATE MECHANICAL FORCES (W50-W64)

    Excludes1   toxic effect of contact with venomous animals and plants (T63.-)

● **W50   Accidental hit, strike, kick, twist, bite or scratch by another person**

    Includes   hit, strike, kick, twist, bite, or scratch by another person NOS

    Excludes1   assault by bodily force (Y04)
           struck by objects (W20-W22)

    The appropriate 7th character is to be added to each code from category W50

A	initial encounter
D	subsequent encounter
S	sequela

X ● **W50.0   Accidental hit or strike by another person**
       Hit or strike by another person NOS

X ● **W50.1   Accidental kick by another person**
       Kick by another person NOS

X ● **W50.2   Accidental twist by another person**
       Twist by another person NOS

X ● **W50.3   Accidental bite by another person**
       Human bite
       Bite by another person NOS

X ● **W50.4   Accidental scratch by another person**
       Scratch by another person NOS

X ● **W51   Accidental striking against or bumped into by another person**

    Excludes1   assault by striking against or bumping into by another person (Y04.2)
           fall due to collision with another person (W03)

    The appropriate 7th character is to be added to code W51

A	initial encounter
D	subsequent encounter
S	sequela

X ● **W52   Crushed, pushed or stepped on by crowd or human stampede**
       Crushed, pushed or stepped on by crowd or human stampede with or without fall

    The appropriate 7th character is to be added to code W52

A	initial encounter
D	subsequent encounter
S	sequela

● **W53   Contact with rodent**

    Includes   contact with saliva, feces or urine of rodent

    The appropriate 7th character is to be added to each code from category W53

A	initial encounter
D	subsequent encounter
S	sequela

   ● **W53.0   Contact with mouse**

     X ● **W53.01   Bitten by mouse**

     X ● **W53.09   Other contact with mouse**

   ● **W53.1   Contact with rat**

     X ● **W53.11   Bitten by rat**

     X ● **W53.19   Other contact with rat**

   ● **W53.2   Contact with squirrel**

     X ● **W53.21   Bitten by squirrel**

     X ● **W53.29   Other contact with squirrel**

   ● **W53.8   Contact with other rodent**

     X ● **W53.81   Bitten by other rodent**

     X ● **W53.89   Other contact with other rodent**

● **W54   Contact with dog**

    Includes   contact with saliva, feces or urine of dog

    The appropriate 7th character is to be added to each code from category W54

A	initial encounter
D	subsequent encounter
S	sequela

X ● **W54.0   Bitten by dog**

X ● **W54.1   Struck by dog**
       Knocked over by dog

X ● **W54.8   Other contact with dog**

◀ New   ◀▥ Revised   ~~deleted~~ Deleted   **OGCR** Official Guidelines   X Assign placeholder X   ● Use Additional Character(s)

Excludes 1   Excludes 2   Includes   Use additional   Code first   Code also   Unspecified

● **W55　Contact with other mammals**

> **Includes**　contact with saliva, feces or urine of mammal
>
> **Excludes1**　animal being ridden - see transport accidents
> bitten or struck by dog (W54)
> bitten or struck by rodent (W53.-)
> contact with marine mammals (W56.X-)

> The appropriate 7th character is to be added to each code from category W55

> | A | initial encounter |
> | D | subsequent encounter |
> | S | sequela |

● **W55.0　Contact with cat**
　X● **W55.01　Bitten by cat**
　X● **W55.03　Scratched by cat**
　X● **W55.09　Other contact with cat**

● **W55.1　Contact with horse**
　X● **W55.11　Bitten by horse**
　X● **W55.12　Struck by horse**
　X● **W55.19　Other contact with horse**

● **W55.2　Contact with cow**
　　　Contact with bull
　X● **W55.21　Bitten by cow**
　X● **W55.22　Struck by cow**
　　　　Gored by bull
　X● **W55.29　Other contact with cow**

● **W55.3　Contact with other hoof stock**
　　　Contact with goats
　　　Contact with sheep
　X● **W55.31　Bitten by other hoof stock**
　X● **W55.32　Struck by other hoof stock**
　　　　Gored by goat
　　　　Gored by ram
　X● **W55.39　Other contact with other hoof stock**

● **W55.4　Contact with pig**
　X● **W55.41　Bitten by pig**
　X● **W55.42　Struck by pig**
　X● **W55.49　Other contact with pig**

● **W55.5　Contact with raccoon**
　X● **W55.51　Bitten by raccoon**
　X● **W55.52　Struck by raccoon**
　X● **W55.59　Other contact with raccoon**

● **W55.8　Contact with other mammals**
　X● **W55.81　Bitten by other mammals**
　X● **W55.82　Struck by other mammals**
　X● **W55.89　Other contact with other mammals**

● **W56　Contact with nonvenomous marine animal**

> **Excludes1**　contact with venomous marine animal (T63.-)

> The appropriate 7th character is to be added to each code from category W56

> | A | initial encounter |
> | D | subsequent encounter |
> | S | sequela |

● **W56.0　Contact with dolphin**
　X● **W56.01　Bitten by dolphin**
　X● **W56.02　Struck by dolphin**
　X● **W56.09　Other contact with dolphin**

● **W56.1　Contact with sea lion**
　X● **W56.11　Bitten by sea lion**
　X● **W56.12　Struck by sea lion**
　X● **W56.19　Other contact with sea lion**

● **W56.2　Contact with orca**
　　　Contact with killer whale
　X● **W56.21　Bitten by orca**
　X● **W56.22　Struck by orca**
　X● **W56.29　Other contact with orca**

● **W56.3　Contact with other marine mammals**
　X● **W56.31　Bitten by other marine mammals**
　X● **W56.32　Struck by other marine mammals**
　X● **W56.39　Other contact with other marine mammals**

● **W56.4　Contact with shark**
　X● **W56.41　Bitten by shark**
　X● **W56.42　Struck by shark**
　X● **W56.49　Other contact with shark**

● **W56.5　Contact with other fish**
　X● **W56.51　Bitten by other fish**
　X● **W56.52　Struck by other fish**
　X● **W56.59　Other contact with other fish**

● **W56.8　Contact with other nonvenomous marine animals**
　X● **W56.81　Bitten by other nonvenomous marine animals**
　X● **W56.82　Struck by other nonvenomous marine animals**
　X● **W56.89　Other contact with other nonvenomous marine animals**

X● **W57　Bitten or stung by nonvenomous insect and other nonvenomous arthropods**

> **Excludes1**　contact with venomous insects and arthropods (T63.2-, T63.3-, T63.4-)

> The appropriate 7th character is to be added to code W57

> | A | initial encounter |
> | D | subsequent encounter |
> | S | sequela |

● **W58　Contact with crocodile or alligator**

> The appropriate 7th character is to be added to each code from category W58

> | A | initial encounter |
> | D | subsequent encounter |
> | S | sequela |

● **W58.0　Contact with alligator**
　X● **W58.01　Bitten by alligator**
　X● **W58.02　Struck by alligator**
　X● **W58.03　Crushed by alligator**
　X● **W58.09　Other contact with alligator**

● **W58.1　Contact with crocodile**
　X● **W58.11　Bitten by crocodile**
　X● **W58.12　Struck by crocodile**
　X● **W58.13　Crushed by crocodile**
　X● **W58.19　Other contact with crocodile**

● **W59　Contact with other nonvenomous reptiles**

> **Excludes1**　contact with venomous reptile (T63.0-, T63.1-)

> The appropriate 7th character is to be added to each code from category W59

> | A | initial encounter |
> | D | subsequent encounter |
> | S | sequela |

● **W59.0　Contact with nonvenomous lizards**
　X● **W59.01　Bitten by nonvenomous lizards**
　X● **W59.02　Struck by nonvenomous lizards**
　X● **W59.09　Other contact with nonvenomous lizards**
　　　Exposure to nonvenomous lizards

CHAPTER 20 (V01-Y99)

● **W59.1 Contact with nonvenomous snakes**
   X ● **W59.11 Bitten by nonvenomous snake**
   X ● **W59.12 Struck by nonvenomous snake**
   X ● **W59.13 Crushed by nonvenomous snake**
   X ● **W59.19 Other contact with nonvenomous snake**
● **W59.2 Contact with turtles**
   | Excludes1 | contact with tortoises (W59.8-)
   X ● **W59.21 Bitten by turtle**
   X ● **W59.22 Struck by turtle**
   X ● **W59.29 Other contact with turtle**
        Exposure to turtles
● **W59.8 Contact with other nonvenomous reptiles**
   X ● **W59.81 Bitten by other nonvenomous reptiles**
   X ● **W59.82 Struck by other nonvenomous reptiles**
   X ● **W59.83 Crushed by other nonvenomous reptiles**
   X ● **W59.89 Other contact with other nonvenomous reptiles**

X ● **W60 Contact with nonvenomous plant thorns and spines and sharp leaves**
   | Excludes1 | contact with venomous plants (T63.X7-)
   The appropriate 7th character is to be added to code W60

     A   initial encounter
     D   subsequent encounter
     S   sequela

● **W61 Contact with birds (domestic) (wild)**
   | Includes | contact with excreta of birds
   The appropriate 7th character is to be added to each code from category W61

     A   initial encounter
     D   subsequent encounter
     S   sequela

● **W61.0 Contact with parrot**
   X ● **W61.01 Bitten by parrot**
   X ● **W61.02 Struck by parrot**
   X ● **W61.09 Other contact with parrot**
        Exposure to parrots
● **W61.1 Contact with macaw**
   X ● **W61.11 Bitten by macaw**
   X ● **W61.12 Struck by macaw**
   X ● **W61.19 Other contact with macaw**
        Exposure to macaws
● **W61.2 Contact with other psittacines**
   X ● **W61.21 Bitten by other psittacines**
   X ● **W61.22 Struck by other psittacines**
   X ● **W61.29 Other contact with other psittacines**
        Exposure to other psittacines
● **W61.3 Contact with chicken**
   X ● **W61.32 Struck by chicken**
   X ● **W61.33 Pecked by chicken**
   X ● **W61.39 Other contact with chicken**
        Exposure to chickens
● **W61.4 Contact with turkey**
   X ● **W61.42 Struck by turkey**
   X ● **W61.43 Pecked by turkey**
   X ● **W61.49 Other contact with turkey**
● **W61.5 Contact with goose**
   X ● **W61.51 Bitten by goose**
   X ● **W61.52 Struck by goose**
   X ● **W61.59 Other contact with goose**

● **W61.6 Contact with duck**
   X ● **W61.61 Bitten by duck**
   X ● **W61.62 Struck by duck**
   X ● **W61.69 Other contact with duck**
● **W61.9 Contact with other birds**
   X ● **W61.91 Bitten by other birds**
   X ● **W61.92 Struck by other birds**
   X ● **W61.99 Other contact with other birds**
        Contact with bird NOS

● **W62 Contact with nonvenomous amphibians**
   | Excludes1 | contact with venomous amphibians (T63.81-R63.83)
   The appropriate 7th character is to be added to each code from category W62

     A   initial encounter
     D   subsequent encounter
     S   sequela

X ● **W62.0 Contact with nonvenomous frogs**
X ● **W62.1 Contact with nonvenomous toads**
X ● **W62.9 Contact with other nonvenomous amphibians**

X ● **W64 Exposure to other animate mechanical forces**
   | Includes | exposure to nonvenomous animal NOS
   | Excludes1 | contact with venomous animal (T63.-)
   The appropriate 7th character is to be added to code W64

     A   initial encounter
     D   subsequent encounter
     S   sequela

ACCIDENTAL NON-TRANSPORT DROWNING AND SUBMERSION (W65-W74)

   | Excludes1 | accidental drowning and submersion due to fall into water (W16.-)
        accidental drowning and submersion due to water transport accident (V90.-, V92.-)
   | Excludes2 | accidental drowning and submersion due to cataclysm (X34-X39)

X ● **W65 Accidental drowning and submersion while in bathtub**
   | Excludes1 | accidental drowning and submersion due to fall in (into) bathtub (W16.211)
   The appropriate 7th character is to be added to code W65

     A   initial encounter
     D   subsequent encounter
     S   sequela

X ● **W67 Accidental drowning and submersion while in swimming pool**
   | Excludes1 | accidental drowning and submersion due to fall into swimming pool (W16.011, W16.021, W16.031)
        accidental drowning and submersion due to striking into wall of swimming pool (W22.041)
   The appropriate 7th character is to be added to code W67

     A   initial encounter
     D   subsequent encounter
     S   sequela

X● **W69   Accidental drowning and submersion while in natural water**
Accidental drowning and submersion while in lake
Accidental drowning and submersion while in open sea
Accidental drowning and submersion while in river
Accidental drowning and submersion while in stream

   Excludes1   accidental drowning and submersion due to
               fall into natural body of water (W16.111,
               W16.121, W16.131)

The appropriate 7th character is to be added to code W69

A	initial encounter
D	subsequent encounter
S	sequela

X● **W73   Other specified cause of accidental non-transport drowning and submersion**
Accidental drowning and submersion while in quenching tank
Accidental drowning and submersion while in reservoir

   Excludes1   accidental drowning and submersion due to
               fall into other water (W16.311, W16.321,
               W16.331)

The appropriate 7th character is to be added to code W73

A	initial encounter
D	subsequent encounter
S	sequela

X● **W74   Unspecified cause of accidental drowning and submersion**
Drowning NOS

The appropriate 7th character is to be added to code W74

A	initial encounter
D	subsequent encounter
S	sequela

EXPOSURE TO ELECTRIC CURRENT, RADIATION AND EXTREME AMBIENT AIR TEMPERATURE AND PRESSURE (W85-W99)

   Excludes1   exposure to:
          failure in dosage of radiation or temperature
             during surgical and medical care
             (Y63.2-Y63.5)
          lightning (T75.0-)
          natural cold (X31)
          natural heat (X30)
          natural radiation NOS (X39)
          radiological procedure and radiotherapy
             (Y84.2)
          sunlight (X32)

X● **W85   Exposure to electric transmission lines**
Broken power line

The appropriate 7th character is to be added to code W85

A	initial encounter
D	subsequent encounter
S	sequela

● **W86   Exposure to other specified electric current**

The appropriate 7th character is to be added to each code from category W86

A	initial encounter
D	subsequent encounter
S	sequela

X● **W86.0   Exposure to domestic wiring and appliances**

X● **W86.1   Exposure to industrial wiring, appliances and electrical machinery**
Exposure to conductors
Exposure to control apparatus
Exposure to electrical equipment and machinery
Exposure to transformers

X● **W86.8   Exposure to other electric current**
Exposure to wiring and appliances in or on farm (not farmhouse)
Exposure to wiring and appliances outdoors
Exposure to wiring and appliances in or on public building
Exposure to wiring and appliances in or on residential institutions
Exposure to wiring and appliances in or on schools

● **W88   Exposure to ionizing radiation**

   Excludes1   exposure to sunlight (X32)

The appropriate 7th character is to be added to each code from category W88

A	initial encounter
D	subsequent encounter
S	sequela

X● **W88.0   Exposure to X-rays**
X● **W88.1   Exposure to radioactive isotopes**
X● **W88.8   Exposure to other ionizing radiation**

● **W89   Exposure to man-made visible and ultraviolet light**

   Includes   exposure to welding light (arc)
   Excludes2   exposure to sunlight (X32)

The appropriate 7th character is to be added to each code from category W89

A	initial encounter
D	subsequent encounter
S	sequela

X● **W89.0   Exposure to welding light (arc)**
X● **W89.1   Exposure to tanning bed**
X● **W89.8   Exposure to other man-made visible and ultraviolet light**
X● **W89.9   Exposure to unspecified man-made visible and ultraviolet light**

● **W90   Exposure to other nonionizing radiation**

   Excludes1   exposure to sunlight (X32)

The appropriate 7th character is to be added to each code from category W90

A	initial encounter
D	subsequent encounter
S	sequela

X● **W90.0   Exposure to radiofrequency**
X● **W90.1   Exposure to infrared radiation**
X● **W90.2   Exposure to laser radiation**
X● **W90.8   Exposure to other nonionizing radiation**

X● **W92   Exposure to excessive heat of man-made origin**

The appropriate 7th character is to be added to code W92

A	initial encounter
D	subsequent encounter
S	sequela

CHAPTER 20 (V01-Y99)

CHAPTER 20 (V01-Y99)

● W93 **Exposure to excessive cold of man-made origin**

The appropriate 7th character is to be added to each code from category W93

> A initial encounter
> D subsequent encounter
> S sequela

● W93.0 **Contact with or inhalation of dry ice**
   X ● W93.01 **Contact with dry ice**
   X ● W93.02 **Inhalation of dry ice**
● W93.1 **Contact with or inhalation of liquid air**
   X ● W93.11 **Contact with liquid air**
           Contact with liquid hydrogen
           Contact with liquid nitrogen
   X ● W93.12 **Inhalation of liquid air**
           Inhalation of liquid hydrogen
           Inhalation of liquid nitrogen
 X ● W93.2 **Prolonged exposure in deep freeze unit or refrigerator**
 X ● W93.8 **Exposure to other excessive cold of man-made origin**

● W94 **Exposure to high and low air pressure and changes in air pressure**

The appropriate 7th character is to be added to each code from category W94

> A initial encounter
> D subsequent encounter
> S sequela

 X ● W94.0 **Exposure to prolonged high air pressure**
● W94.1 **Exposure to prolonged low air pressure**
   X ● W94.11 **Exposure to residence or prolonged visit at high altitude**
   X ● W94.12 **Exposure to other prolonged low air pressure**
● W94.2 **Exposure to rapid changes in air pressure during ascent**
   X ● W94.21 **Exposure to reduction in atmospheric pressure while surfacing from deep-water diving**
   X ● W94.22 **Exposure to reduction in atmospheric pressure while surfacing from underground**
   X ● W94.23 **Exposure to sudden change in air pressure in aircraft during ascent**
   X ● W94.29 **Exposure to other rapid changes in air pressure during ascent**
● W94.3 **Exposure to rapid changes in air pressure during descent**
   X ● W94.31 **Exposure to sudden change in air pressure in aircraft during descent**
   X ● W94.32 **Exposure to high air pressure from rapid descent in water**
   X ● W94.39 **Exposure to other rapid changes in air pressure during descent**

X ● W99 **Exposure to other man-made environmental factors**

The appropriate 7th character is to be added to code W99

> A initial encounter
> D subsequent encounter
> S sequela

EXPOSURE TO SMOKE, FIRE AND FLAMES (X00-X08)

> **Excludes1** arson (X97)
> **Excludes2** explosions (W35-W40)
>   lightning (T75.0-)
>   transport accident (V01-V99)

● X00 **Exposure to uncontrolled fire in building or structure**

> **Includes** conflagration in building or structure

Code first any associated cataclysm

> **Excludes2** exposure to ignition or melting of nightwear (X05)
>   exposure to ignition or melting of other clothing and apparel (X06.-)
>   exposure to other specified smoke, fire and flames (X08.-)

The appropriate 7th character is to be added to each code from category X00

> A initial encounter
> D subsequent encounter
> S sequela

 X ● X00.0 **Exposure to flames in uncontrolled fire in building or structure**
 X ● X00.1 **Exposure to smoke in uncontrolled fire in building or structure**
 X ● X00.2 **Injury due to collapse of burning building or structure in uncontrolled fire**
> **Excludes1** injury due to collapse of building not on fire (W20.1)
 X ● X00.3 **Fall from burning building or structure in uncontrolled fire**
 X ● X00.4 **Hit by object from burning building or structure in uncontrolled fire**
 X ● X00.5 **Jump from burning building or structure in uncontrolled fire**
 X ● X00.8 **Other exposure to uncontrolled fire in building or structure**

● X01 **Exposure to uncontrolled fire, not in building or structure**

> **Includes** exposure to forest fire

The appropriate 7th character is to be added to each code from category X01

> A initial encounter
> D subsequent encounter
> S sequela

 X ● X01.0 **Exposure to flames in uncontrolled fire, not in building or structure**
 X ● X01.1 **Exposure to smoke in uncontrolled fire, not in building or structure**
 X ● X01.3 **Fall due to uncontrolled fire, not in building or structure**
 X ● X01.4 **Hit by object due to uncontrolled fire, not in building or structure**
 X ● X01.8 **Other exposure to uncontrolled fire, not in building or structure**

◀ New   ◀ Revised   deleted Deleted   **OGCR** Official Guidelines   X Assign placeholder X   ● Use Additional Character(s)

Excludes 1   Excludes 2   Includes   Use additional   Code first   Code also   Unspecified

● **X02**   **Exposure to controlled fire in building or structure**

    Includes   exposure to fire in fireplace exposure to fire in stove

    The appropriate 7th character is to be added to each code from category X02

A	initial encounter
D	subsequent encounter
S	sequela

X● **X02.0**   **Exposure to flames in controlled fire in building or structure**

X● **X02.1**   **Exposure to smoke in controlled fire in building or structure**

X● **X02.2**   **Injury due to collapse of burning building or structure in controlled fire**

     Excludes1   injury due to collapse of building not on fire (W20.1)

X● **X02.3**   **Fall from burning building or structure in controlled fire**

X● **X02.4**   **Hit by object from burning building or structure in controlled fire**

X● **X02.5**   **Jump from burning building or structure in controlled fire**

X● **X02.8**   **Other exposure to controlled fire in building or structure**

● **X03**   **Exposure to controlled fire, not in building or structure**

    Includes   exposure to bon fire exposure to camp fire exposure to trash fire

    The appropriate 7th character is to be added to each code from category X03

A	initial encounter
D	subsequent encounter
S	sequela

X● **X03.0**   **Exposure to flames in controlled fire, not in building or structure**

X● **X03.1**   **Exposure to smoke in controlled fire, not in building or structure**

X● **X03.3**   **Fall due to controlled fire, not in building or structure**

X● **X03.4**   **Hit by object due to controlled fire, not in building or structure**

X● **X03.8**   **Other exposure to controlled fire, not in building or structure**

X● **X04**   **Exposure to ignition of highly flammable material**

    Exposure to ignition of gasoline

    Exposure to ignition of kerosene

    Exposure to ignition of petrol

     Excludes2   exposure to ignition or melting of nightwear (X05)

          exposure to ignition or melting of other clothing and apparel (X06)

    The appropriate 7th character is to be added to code X04

A	initial encounter
D	subsequent encounter
S	sequela

X● **X05**   **Exposure to ignition or melting of nightwear**

     Excludes2   exposure to uncontrolled fire in building or structure (X00.-)

          exposure to uncontrolled fire, not in building or structure (X01.-)

          exposure to controlled fire in building or structure (X02.-)

          exposure to controlled fire, not in building or structure (X03.-)

          exposure to ignition of highly flammable materials (X04.-)

    The appropriate 7th character is to be added to code X05

A	initial encounter
D	subsequent encounter
S	sequela

● **X06**   **Exposure to ignition or melting of other clothing and apparel**

     Excludes2   exposure to uncontrolled fire in building or structure (X00.-)

          exposure to uncontrolled fire, not in building or structure (X01.-)

          exposure to controlled fire in building or structure (X02.-)

          exposure to controlled fire, not in building or structure (X03.-)

          exposure to ignition of highly flammable materials (X04.-)

    The appropriate 7th character is to be added to each code from category X06

A	initial encounter
D	subsequent encounter
S	sequela

X● **X06.0**   **Exposure to ignition of plastic jewelry**

X● **X06.1**   **Exposure to melting of plastic jewelry**

X● **X06.2**   **Exposure to ignition of other clothing and apparel**

X● **X06.3**   **Exposure to melting of other clothing and apparel**

● **X08**   **Exposure to other specified smoke, fire and flames**

    The appropriate 7th character is to be added to each code from category X08

A	initial encounter
D	subsequent encounter
S	sequela

● **X08.0**   **Exposure to bed fire**

    Exposure to mattress fire

X● **X08.00**   **Exposure to bed fire due to unspecified burning material**

X● **X08.01**   **Exposure to bed fire due to burning cigarette**

X● **X08.09**   **Exposure to bed fire due to other burning material**

● **X08.1**   **Exposure to sofa fire**

X● **X08.10**   **Exposure to sofa fire due to unspecified burning material**

X● **X08.11**   **Exposure to sofa fire due to burning cigarette**

X● **X08.19**   **Exposure to sofa fire due to other burning material**

● **X08.2**   **Exposure to other furniture fire**

X● **X08.20**   **Exposure to other furniture fire due to unspecified burning material**

X● **X08.21**   **Exposure to other furniture fire due to burning cigarette**

X● **X08.29**   **Exposure to other furniture fire due to other burning material**

X● **X08.8**   **Exposure to other specified smoke, fire and flames**

CHAPTER 20 (V01-Y99)

CONTACT WITH HEAT AND HOT SUBSTANCES (X10-X19)

Excludes1   exposure to excessive natural heat (X30)
exposure to fire and flames (X00-X09)

● **X10   Contact with hot drinks, food, fats and cooking oils**

The appropriate 7th character is to be added to each code from category X10

A	initial encounter
D	subsequent encounter
S	sequela

X● **X10.0   Contact with hot drinks**
X● **X10.1   Contact with hot food**
X● **X10.2   Contact with fats and cooking oils**

● **X11   Contact with hot tap-water**

Includes   contact with boiling tap-water
contact with boiling water NOS

Excludes1   contact with water heated on stove (X12)

The appropriate 7th character is to be added to each code from category X11

A	initial encounter
D	subsequent encounter
S	sequela

X● **X11.0   Contact with hot water in bath or tub**

Excludes1   contact with running hot water in bath or tub (X11.1)

X● **X11.1   Contact with running hot water**
Contact with hot water running out of hose
Contact with hot water running out of tap

X● **X11.8   Contact with other hot tap-water**
Contact with hot water in bucket
Contact with hot tap-water NOS

X● **X12   Contact with other hot fluids**
Contact with water heated on stove

Excludes1   hot (liquid) metals (X18)

The appropriate 7th character is to be added to code X12

A	initial encounter
D	subsequent encounter
S	sequela

● **X13   Contact with steam and other hot vapors**

The appropriate 7th character is to be added to each code from category X13

A	initial encounter
D	subsequent encounter
S	sequela

X● **X13.0   Inhalation of steam and other hot vapors**
X● **X13.1   Other contact with steam and other hot vapors**

● **X14   Contact with hot air and other hot gases**

The appropriate 7th character is to be added to each code from category X14

A	initial encounter
D	subsequent encounter
S	sequela

X● **X14.0   Inhalation of hot air and gases**
X● **X14.1   Other contact with hot air and other hot gases**

● **X15   Contact with hot household appliances**

Excludes1   contact with heating appliances (X16)
contact with powered household appliances (W29.-)
exposure to controlled fire in building or structure due to household appliance (X02.8)
exposure to household appliances electrical current (W86.0)

The appropriate 7th character is to be added to each code from category X15

A	initial encounter
D	subsequent encounter
S	sequela

X● **X15.0   Contact with hot stove (kitchen)**
X● **X15.1   Contact with hot toaster**
X● **X15.2   Contact with hotplate**
X● **X15.3   Contact with hot saucepan or skillet**
X● **X15.8   Contact with other hot household appliances**
Contact with cooker
Contact with kettle
Contact with light bulbs

X● **X16   Contact with hot heating appliances, radiators and pipes**

Excludes1   contact with powered appliances (W29.-)
exposure to controlled fire in building or structure due to appliance (X02.8)
exposure to industrial appliances electrical current (W86.1)

The appropriate 7th character is to be added to code X16

A	initial encounter
D	subsequent encounter
S	sequela

X● **X17   Contact with hot engines, machinery and tools**

Excludes1   contact with hot heating appliances, radiators and pipes (X16)
contact with hot household appliances (X15)

The appropriate 7th character is to be added to code X17

A	initial encounter
D	subsequent encounter
S	sequela

X● **X18   Contact with other hot metals**
Contact with liquid metal

The appropriate 7th character is to be added to code X18

A	initial encounter
D	subsequent encounter
S	sequela

X● **X19   Contact with other heat and hot substances**

Excludes1   objects that are not normally hot, e.g., an object made hot by a house fire (X00-X09)

The appropriate 7th character is to be added to code X19

A	initial encounter
D	subsequent encounter
S	sequela

◀ New   ◀▥ Revised   ~~deleted~~ Deleted   **OGCR** Official Guidelines   X Assign placeholder X   ● Use Additional Character(s)

Excludes 1   Excludes 2   Includes   Use additional   Code first   Code also   Unspecified

EXPOSURE TO FORCES OF NATURE (X30-X39)

X● **X30**   **Exposure to excessive natural heat**
Exposure to excessive heat as the cause of sunstroke
Exposure to heat NOS

Excludes1	excessive heat of man-made origin (W92)
	exposure to man-made radiation (W89)
	exposure to sunlight (X32)
	exposure to tanning bed (W89)

The appropriate 7th character is to be added to code X30

A	initial encounter
D	subsequent encounter
S	sequela

X● **X31**   **Exposure to excessive natural cold**
Excessive cold as the cause of chilblains NOS
Excessive cold as the cause of immersion foot or hand
Exposure to cold NOS
Exposure to weather conditions

Excludes1	cold of man-made origin (W93.-)
	contact with or inhalation of dry ice (W93.-)
	contact with or inhalation of liquefied gas (W93.-)

The appropriate 7th character is to be added to code X31

A	initial encounter
D	subsequent encounter
S	sequela

X● **X32**   **Exposure to sunlight**

| Excludes1 | radiation-related disorders of the skin and subcutaneous tissue (L55-L59) |
| | man-made radiation (tanning bed) (W89) |

The appropriate 7th character is to be added to code X32

A	initial encounter
D	subsequent encounter
S	sequela

X● **X34**   **Earthquake**

| Excludes2 | tidal wave (tsunami) due to earthquake (X37.41) |

The appropriate 7th character is to be added to code X34

A	initial encounter
D	subsequent encounter
S	sequela

X● **X35**   **Volcanic eruption**

| Excludes2 | tidal wave (tsunami) due to volcanic eruption (X37.41) |

The appropriate 7th character is to be added to code X35

A	initial encounter
D	subsequent encounter
S	sequela

● **X36**   **Avalanche, landslide and other earth movements**

Includes	victim of mudslide of cataclysmic nature
Excludes1	earthquake (X34)
Excludes2	transport accident involving collision with avalanche or landslide not in motion (V01-V99)

The appropriate 7th character is to be added to each code from category X36

A	initial encounter
D	subsequent encounter
S	sequela

X● **X36.0**   **Collapse of dam or man-made structure causing earth movement**
X● **X36.1**   **Avalanche, landslide, or mudslide**

● **X37**   **Cataclysmic storm**
The appropriate 7th character is to be added to each code from category X37

A	initial encounter
D	subsequent encounter
S	sequela

X● **X37.0**   **Hurricane**
    Storm surge   Typhoon
X● **X37.1**   **Tornado**
    Cyclone   Twister
X● **X37.2**   **Blizzard (snow) (ice)**
X● **X37.3**   **Dust storm**
● **X37.4**   **Tidalwave**

X● **X37.41**   **Tidal wave due to earthquake or volcanic eruption**
    Tidal wave NOS
    Tsunami

X● **X37.42**   **Tidal wave due to storm**
X● **X37.43**   **Tidal wave due to landslide**
X● **X37.8**   **Other cataclysmic storms**
    Cloudburst
    Torrential rain

| Excludes2 | flood (X38) |

X● **X37.9**   **Unspecified cataclysmic storm**
    Storm NOS

| Excludes1 | collapse of dam or man-made structure causing earth movement (X39.0) |

X● **X38**   **Flood**
Flood arising from remote storm
Flood of cataclysmic nature arising from melting snow
Flood resulting directly from storm

Excludes1	collapse of dam or man-made structure causing earth movement (X39.0)
	tidal wave NOS (X37.41)
	tidal wave caused by storm (X37.2)

The appropriate 7th character is to be added to code X38

A	initial encounter
D	subsequent encounter
S	sequela

● **X39**   **Exposure to other forces of nature**
The appropriate 7th character is to be added to each code from category X39

A	initial encounter
D	subsequent encounter
S	sequela

● **X39.0**   **Exposure to natural radiation**

Excludes1	contact with and (suspected) exposure to radon and other naturally occuring radiation (Z77.122)
	exposure to man-made radiation (W88-W90)
	exposure to sunlight (X32)

X● **X39.01**   **Exposure to radon**
X● **X39.08**   **Exposure to other natural radiation**
X● **X39.8**   **Other exposure to forces of nature**

CHAPTER 20 (V01-Y99)

ACCIDENTAL EXPOSURE TO OTHER SPECIFIED FACTORS (X52, X58)

X● **X52** **Prolonged stay in weightless environment**
Weightlessness in spacecraft (simulator)

The appropriate 7th character is to be added to code X52

A	initial encounter
D	subsequent encounter
S	sequela

X● **X58** **Exposure to other specified factors**
Accident NOS
Exposure NOS

The appropriate 7th character is to be added to code X58

A	initial encounter
D	subsequent encounter
S	sequela

INTENTIONAL SELF-HARM (X71-X83)

Purposely self-inflicted injury
Suicide (attempted)

● **X71** **Intentional self-harm by drowning and submersion**

The appropriate 7th character is to be added to each code from
category X71

A	initial encounter
D	subsequent encounter
S	sequela

X● **X71.0** **Intentional self-harm by drowning and submersion while in bathtub**
X● **X71.1** **Intentional self-harm by drowning and submersion while in swimming pool**
X● **X71.2** **Intentional self-harm by drowning and submersion after jump into swimming pool**
X● **X71.3** **Intentional self-harm by drowning and submersion in natural water**
X● **X71.8** **Other intentional self-harm by drowning and submersion**
X● **X71.9** **Intentional self-harm by drowning and submersion, unspecified**

X● **X72** **Intentional self-harm by handgun discharge**
Intentional self-harm by gun for single hand use
Intentional self-harm by pistol
Intentional self-harm by revolver

Excludes1 Very pistol (X74.8)

The appropriate 7th character is to be added to code X72

A	initial encounter
D	subsequent encounter
S	sequela

● **X73** **Intentional self-harm by rifle, shotgun and larger firearm discharge**

Excludes1 airgun (X74.01)

The appropriate 7th character is to be added to each code from
category X73

A	initial encounter
D	subsequent encounter
S	sequela

X● **X73.0** **Intentional self-harm by shotgun discharge**
X● **X73.1** **Intentional self-harm by hunting rifle discharge**
X● **X73.2** **Intentional self-harm by machine gun discharge**
X● **X73.8** **Intentional self-harm by other larger firearm discharge**
X● **X73.9** **Intentional self-harm by unspecified larger firearm discharge**

● **X74** **Intentional self-harm by other and unspecified firearm and gun discharge**

The appropriate 7th character is to be added to each code from
category X74

A	initial encounter
D	subsequent encounter
S	sequela

● **X74.0** **Intentional self-harm by gas, air or spring-operated guns**
X● **X74.01** **Intentional self-harm by airgun**
Intentional self-harm by BB gun discharge
Intentional self-harm by pellet gun discharge
X● **X74.02** **Intentional self-harm by paintball gun**
X● **X74.09** **Intentional self-harm by other gas, air or spring-operated gun**
X● **X74.8** **Intentional self-harm by other firearm discharge**
Intentional self-harm by Very pistol [flare] discharge
X● **X74.9** **Intentional self-harm by unspecified firearm discharge**

X● **X75** **Intentional self-harm by explosive material**

The appropriate 7th character is to be added to code X75

A	initial encounter
D	subsequent encounter
S	sequela

X● **X76** **Intentional self-harm by smoke, fire and flames**

The appropriate 7th character is to be added to code X76

A	initial encounter
D	subsequent encounter
S	sequela

● **X77** **Intentional self-harm by steam, hot vapors and hot objects**

The appropriate 7th character is to be added to each code from
category X77

A	initial encounter
D	subsequent encounter
S	sequela

X● **X77.0** **Intentional self-harm by steam or hot vapors**
X● **X77.1** **Intentional self-harm by hot tap water**
X● **X77.2** **Intentional self-harm by other hot fluids**
X● **X77.3** **Intentional self-harm by hot household appliances**
X● **X77.8** **Intentional self-harm by other hot objects**
X● **X77.9** **Intentional self-harm by unspecified hot objects**

● **X78** **Intentional self-harm by sharp object**

The appropriate 7th character is to be added to each code from
category X78

A	initial encounter
D	subsequent encounter
S	sequela

X● **X78.0** **Intentional self-harm by sharp glass**
X● **X78.1** **Intentional self-harm by knife**
X● **X78.2** **Intentional self-harm by sword or dagger**
X● **X78.8** **Intentional self-harm by other sharp object**
X● **X78.9** **Intentional self-harm by unspecified sharp object**

X● **X79** **Intentional self-harm by blunt object**

The appropriate 7th character is to be added to code X79

A	initial encounter
D	subsequent encounter
S	sequela

◀ New   ◀▥ Revised   ~~deleted~~ Deleted   OGCR Official Guidelines   X Assign placeholder X   ● Use Additional Character(s)

Excludes 1   Excludes 2   Includes   Use additional   Code first   Code also   Unspecified

X● **X80**   **Intentional self-harm by jumping from a high place**
     Intentional fall from one level to another

     The appropriate 7th character is to be added to code X80

A	initial encounter
D	subsequent encounter
S	sequela

●**X81**   **Intentional self-harm by jumping or lying in front of moving object**

     The appropriate 7th character is to be added to each code from category X81

A	initial encounter
D	subsequent encounter
S	sequela

   X● **X81.0**   **Intentional self-harm by jumping or lying in front of motor vehicle**

   X● **X81.1**   **Intentional self-harm by jumping or lying in front of (subway) train**

   X● **X81.8**   **Intentional self-harm by jumping or lying in front of other moving object**

●**X82**   **Intentional self-harm by crashing of motor vehicle**

     The appropriate 7th character is to be added to each code from category X82

A	initial encounter
D	subsequent encounter
S	sequela

   X● **X82.0**   **Intentional collision of motor vehicle with other motor vehicle**

   X● **X82.1**   **Intentional collision of motor vehicle with train**

   X● **X82.2**   **Intentional collision of motor vehicle with tree**

   X● **X82.8**   **Other intentional self-harm by crashing of motor vehicle**

●**X83**   **Intentional self-harm by other specified means**

     Excludes1   intentional self-harm by poisoning or contact with toxic substance - see Table of Drugs and Chemicals

     The appropriate 7th character is to be added to each code from category X83

A	initial encounter
D	subsequent encounter
S	sequela

   X● **X83.0**   **Intentional self-harm by crashing of aircraft**

   X● **X83.1**   **Intentional self-harm by electrocution**

   X● **X83.2**   **Intentional self-harm by exposure to extremes of cold**

   X● **X83.8**   **Intentional self-harm by other specified means**

ASSAULT (X92-Y08)

Includes	homicide injuries inflicted by another person with intent to injure or kill, by any means
Excludes1	injuries due to legal intervention (Y35.-) injuries due to operations of war (Y36.-) injuries due to terrorism (Y38.-)

●**X92**   **Assault by drowning and submersion**

     The appropriate 7th character is to be added to each code from category X92

A	initial encounter
D	subsequent encounter
S	sequela

   X● **X92.0**   **Assault by drowning and submersion while in bathtub**

   X● **X92.1**   **Assault by drowning and submersion while in swimming pool**

   X● **X92.2**   **Assault by drowning and submersion after push into swimming pool**

   X● **X92.3**   **Assault by drowning and submersion in natural water**

   X● **X92.8**   **Other assault by drowning and submersion**

   X● **X92.9**   **Assault by drowning and submersion, unspecified**

X● **X93**   **Assault by handgun discharge**
     Assault by discharge of gun for single hand use
     Assault by discharge of pistol
     Assault by discharge of revolver

     | **Excludes1** | Very pistol (X95.8) |

     The appropriate 7th character is to be added to code X93

A	initial encounter
D	subsequent encounter
S	sequela

●**X94**   **Assault by rifle, shotgun and larger firearm discharge**

     | **Excludes1** | airgun (X95.01) |

     The appropriate 7th character is to be added to each code from category X94

A	initial encounter
D	subsequent encounter
S	sequela

   X● **X94.0**   **Assault by shotgun**

   X● **X94.1**   **Assault by hunting rifle**

   X● **X94.2**   **Assault by machine gun**

   X● **X94.8**   **Assault by other larger firearm discharge**

   X● **X94.9**   **Assault by unspecified larger firearm discharge**

●**X95**   **Assault by other and unspecified firearm and gun discharge**

     The appropriate 7th character is to be added to each code from category X95

A	initial encounter
D	subsequent encounter
S	sequela

   ●**X95.0**   **Assault by gas, air or spring-operated guns**

     X● **X95.01**   **Assault by airgun discharge**
        Assault by BB gun discharge
        Assault by pellet gun discharge

     X● **X95.02**   **Assault by paintball gun discharge**

     X● **X95.09**   **Assault by other gas, air or spring-operated gun**

   X● **X95.8**   **Assault by other firearm discharge**
     Assault by very pistol [flare] discharge

   X● **X95.9**   **Assault by unspecified firearm discharge**

●**X96**   **Assault by explosive material**

     | **Excludes1** | incendiary device (X97)
terrorism involving explosive material (Y38.2-) |

     The appropriate 7th character is to be added to each code from category X96

A	initial encounter
D	subsequent encounter
S	sequela

   X● **X96.0**   **Assault by antipersonnel bomb**

     | **Excludes1** | antipersonnel bomb use in military or war (Y36.2-) |

   X● **X96.1**   **Assault by gasoline bomb**

   X● **X96.2**   **Assault by letter bomb**

   X● **X96.3**   **Assault by fertilizer bomb**

   X● **X96.4**   **Assault by pipe bomb**

   X● **X96.8**   **Assault by other specified explosive**

   X● **X96.9**   **Assault by unspecified explosive**

CHAPTER 20 (V01-Y99)

X ● **X97   Assault by smoke, fire and flames**
    Assault by arson
    Assault by cigarettes
    Assault by incendiary device
    The appropriate 7th character is to be added to code X97

A	initial encounter
D	subsequent encounter
S	sequela

● **X98   Assault by steam, hot vapors and hot objects**
    The appropriate 7th character is to be added to each code from
    category X98

A	initial encounter
D	subsequent encounter
S	sequela

X ● **X98.0   Assault by steam or hot vapors**
X ● **X98.1   Assault by hot tap water**
X ● **X98.2   Assault by hot fluids**
X ● **X98.3   Assault by hot household appliances**
X ● **X98.8   Assault by other hot objects**
X ● **X98.9   Assault by unspecified hot objects**

● **X99   Assault by sharp object**
    Excludes1   assault by strike by sports equipment (Y08.0-)
    The appropriate 7th character is to be added to each code from
    category X99

A	initial encounter
D	subsequent encounter
S	sequela

X ● **X99.0   Assault by sharp glass**
X ● **X99.1   Assault by knife**
X ● **X99.2   Assault by sword or dagger**
X ● **X99.8   Assault by other sharp object**
X ● **X99.9   Assault by unspecified sharp object**
        Assault by stabbing NOS

X ● **Y00   Assault by blunt object**
    Excludes1   assault by strike by sports equipment (Y08.0)
    The appropriate 7th character is to be added to code Y00

A	initial encounter
D	subsequent encounter
S	sequela

X ● **Y01   Assault by pushing from high place**
    The appropriate 7th character is to be added to code Y01

A	initial encounter
D	subsequent encounter
S	sequela

● **Y02   Assault by pushing or placing victim in front of moving object**
    The appropriate 7th character is to be added to each code from
    category Y02

A	initial encounter
D	subsequent encounter
S	sequela

X ● **Y02.0   Assault by pushing or placing victim in front of motor vehicle**
X ● **Y02.1   Assault by pushing or placing victim in front of (subway) train**
X ● **Y02.8   Assault by pushing or placing victim in front of other moving object**

● **Y03   Assault by crashing of motor vehicle**
    The appropriate 7th character is to be added to each code from
    category Y03

A	initial encounter
D	subsequent encounter
S	sequela

X ● **Y03.0   Assault by being hit or run over by motor vehicle**
X ● **Y03.8   Other assault by crashing of motor vehicle**

● **Y04   Assault by bodily force**
    Excludes1   assault by:
            submersion (X92.-)
            use of weapon (X93-X95, X99, Y00)
    The appropriate 7th character is to be added to each code from
    category Y04

A	initial encounter
D	subsequent encounter
S	sequela

X ● **Y04.0   Assault by unarmed brawl or fight**
X ● **Y04.1   Assault by human bite**
X ● **Y04.2   Assault by strike against or bumped into by another person**
X ● **Y04.8   Assault by other bodily force**
        Assault by bodily force NOS

OGCR Section I.C.19.f.

Adult and child abuse, neglect and other maltreatment

Sequence first the appropriate code from categories T74.- or T76.- for abuse, neglect and other maltreatment, followed by any accompanying mental health or injury code(s).

If the documentation in the medical record states abuse or neglect it is coded as confirmed. It is coded as suspected if it is documented as suspected.

For cases of confirmed abuse or neglect an external cause code from the assault section (X92-Y08) should be added to identify the cause of any physical injuries. A perpetrator code (Y07) should be added when the perpetrator of the abuse is known. For suspected cases of abuse or neglect, do not report external cause or perpetrator code.

If a suspected case of abuse, neglect or mistreatment is ruled out during an encounter code Z04.71, Encounter for examination and observation following alleged physical adult abuse, ruled out, or code Z04.72, Encounter for examination and observation following alleged child physical abuse, ruled out, should be used, not a code from T76.

If a suspected case of alleged rape or sexual abuse is ruled out during an encounter code Z04.41, Encounter for examination and observation following alleged physical adult abuse, ruled out, or code Z04.42, Encounter for examination and observation following alleged rape or sexual abuse, ruled out, should be used, not a code from T76.

● **Y07   Perpetrator of assault, maltreatment and neglect**
    Note: Codes from this category are for use only in cases of confirmed abuse (T74.-)

        Selection of the correct perpetrator code is based on the relationship between the perpetrator and the victim
        Includes   perpetrator of abandonment
                perpetrator of emotional neglect
                perpetrator of mental cruelty
                perpetrator of physical abuse
                perpetrator of physical neglect
                perpetrator of sexual abuse
                perpetrator of torture

● **Y07.0   Spouse or partner, perpetrator of maltreatment and neglect**
        Spouse or partner, perpetrator of maltreatment and neglect against spouse or partner

    Y07.01   Husband, perpetrator of maltreatment and neglect

    Y07.02   Wife, perpetrator of maltreatment and neglect

◀ New   ◀|||| Revised   ~~deleted~~ Deleted   **OGCR** Official Guidelines   X Assign placeholder X   ● Use Additional Character(s)

Excludes 1   Excludes 2   Includes   Use additional   Code first   Code also   Unspecified

Y07.03   Male partner, perpetrator of maltreatment and neglect

Y07.04   Female partner, perpetrator of maltreatment and neglect

● Y07.1   Parent (adoptive) (biological), perpetrator of maltreatment and neglect

Y07.11   Biological father, perpetrator of maltreatment and neglect

Y07.12   Biological mother, perpetrator of maltreatment and neglect

Y07.13   Adoptive father, perpetrator of maltreatment and neglect

Y07.14   Adoptive mother, perpetrator of maltreatment and neglect

● Y07.4   Other family member, perpetrator of maltreatment and neglect

● Y07.41   Sibling, perpetrator of maltreatment and neglect

> **Excludes 1**   stepsibling, perpetrator of maltreatment and neglect (Y07.435, Y07.436)

Y07.410   Brother, perpetrator of maltreatment and neglect

Y07.411   Sister, perpetrator of maltreatment and neglect

● Y07.42   Foster parent, perpetrator of maltreatment and neglect

Y07.420   Foster father, perpetrator of maltreatment and neglect

Y07.421   Foster mother, perpetrator of maltreatment and neglect

● Y07.43   Stepparent or stepsibling, perpetrator of maltreatment and neglect

Y07.430   Stepfather, perpetrator of maltreatment and neglect

Y07.432   Male friend of parent (co-residing in household), perpetrator of maltreatment and neglect

Y07.433   Stepmother, perpetrator of maltreatment and neglect

Y07.434   Female friend of parent (co-residing in household), perpetrator of maltreatment and neglect

Y07.435   Stepbrother, perpetrator or maltreatment and neglect

Y07.436   Stepsister, perpetrator of maltreatment and neglect

● Y07.49   Other family member, perpetrator of maltreatment and neglect

Y07.490   Male cousin, perpetrator of maltreatment and neglect

Y07.491   Female cousin, perpetrator of maltreatment and neglect

Y07.499   Other family member, perpetrator of maltreatment and neglect

● Y07.5   Non-family member, perpetrator of maltreatment and neglect

Y07.50   Unspecified non-family member, perpetrator of maltreatment and neglect

● Y07.51   Daycare provider, perpetrator of maltreatment and neglect

Y07.510   At-home childcare provider, perpetrator of maltreatment and neglect

Y07.511   Daycare center childcare provider, perpetrator of maltreatment and neglect

Y07.512   At-home adultcare provider, perpetrator of maltreatment and neglect

Y07.513   Adultcare center provider, perpetrator of maltreatment and neglect

Y07.519   Unspecified daycare provider, perpetrator of maltreatment and neglect

● Y07.52   Healthcare provider, perpetrator of maltreatment and neglect

Y07.521   Mental health provider, perpetrator of maltreatment and neglect

Y07.528   Other therapist or healthcare provider, perpetrator of maltreatment and neglect

> Nurse perpetrator of maltreatment and neglect
> Occupational therapist perpetrator of maltreatment and neglect
> Physical therapist perpetrator of maltreatment and neglect
> Speech therapist perpetrator of maltreatment and neglect

Y07.529   Unspecified healthcare provider, perpetrator of maltreatment and neglect

Y07.53   Teacher or instructor, perpetrator of maltreatment and neglect

> Coach, perpetrator of maltreatment and neglect

Y07.59   Other non-family member, perpetrator of maltreatment and neglect

● Y07.9   Unspecified perpetrator of maltreatment and neglect

● Y08   Assault by other specified means

The appropriate 7th character is to be added to each code from category Y08

> A   initial encounter
> D   subsequent encounter
> S   sequela

● Y08.0   Assault by strike by sport equipment

X ● Y08.01   Assault by strike by hockey stick

X ● Y08.02   Assault by strike by baseball bat

X ● Y08.09   Assault by strike by other specified type of sport equipment

● Y08.8   Assault by other specified means

X ● Y08.81   Assault by crashing of aircraft

X ● Y08.89   Assault by other specified means

● Y09   Assault by unspecified means

> Assassination (attempted) NOS
> Homicide (attempted) NOS
> Manslaughter (attempted) NOS
> Murder (attempted) NOS

EVENT OF UNDETERMINED INTENT (Y21-Y33)

Undetermined intent is only for use when there is specific documentation in the record that the intent of the injury cannot be determined. If no such documentation is present, code to accidental (unintentional)

● Y21   Drowning and submersion, undetermined intent

The appropriate 7th character is to be added to each code from category Y21

> A   initial encounter
> D   subsequent encounter
> S   sequela

X ● Y21.0   Drowning and submersion while in bathtub, undetermined intent

X ● Y21.1   Drowning and submersion after fall into bathtub, undetermined intent

CHAPTER 20 (V01-Y99)

X● **Y21.2** Drowning and submersion while in swimming pool, undetermined intent

X● **Y21.3** Drowning and submersion after fall into swimming pool, undetermined intent

X● **Y21.4** Drowning and submersion in natural water, undetermined intent

X● **Y21.8** Other drowning and submersion, undetermined intent

X● **Y21.9** Unspecified drowning and submersion, undetermined intent

X●**Y22** Handgun discharge, undetermined intent
Discharge of gun for single hand use, undetermined intent
Discharge of pistol, undetermined intent
Discharge of revolver, undetermined intent

Excludes2   very pistol (Y24.8)

The appropriate 7th character is to be added to code Y22

> A   initial encounter
> D   subsequent encounter
> S   sequela

●**Y23** Rifle, shotgun and larger firearm discharge, undetermined intent

Excludes2   airgun (Y24.0)

The appropriate 7th character is to be added to each code from category Y23

> A   initial encounter
> D   subsequent encounter
> S   sequela

X● **Y23.0** Shotgun discharge, undetermined intent

X● **Y23.1** Hunting rifle discharge, undetermined intent

X● **Y23.2** Military firearm discharge, undetermined intent

X● **Y23.3** Machine gun discharge, undetermined intent

X● **Y23.8** Other larger firearm discharge, undetermined intent

X● **Y23.9** Unspecified larger firearm discharge, undetermined intent

●**Y24** Other and unspecified firearm discharge, undetermined intent

The appropriate 7th character is to be added to each code from category Y24

> A   initial encounter
> D   subsequent encounter
> S   sequela

X● **Y24.0** Airgun discharge, undetermined intent
BB gun discharge, undetermined intent
Pellet gun discharge, undetermined intent

X● **Y24.8** Other firearm discharge, undetermined intent
Paintball gun discharge, undetermined intent
Very pistol [flare] discharge, undetermined intent

X● **Y24.9** Unspecified firearm discharge, undetermined intent

X●**Y25** Contact with explosive material, undetermined intent

The appropriate 7th character is to be added to code Y25

> A   initial encounter
> D   subsequent encounter
> S   sequela

X●**Y26** Exposure to smoke, fire and flames, undetermined intent

The appropriate 7th character is to be added to code Y26

> A   initial encounter
> D   subsequent encounter
> S   sequela

●**Y27** Contact with steam, hot vapors and hot objects, undetermined intent

The appropriate 7th character is to be added to each code from category Y27

> A   initial encounter
> D   subsequent encounter
> S   sequela

X● **Y27.0** Contact with steam and hot vapors, undetermined intent

X● **Y27.1** Contact with hot tap water, undetermined intent

X● **Y27.2** Contact with hot fluids, undetermined intent

X● **Y27.3** Contact with hot household appliance, undetermined intent

X● **Y27.8** Contact with other hot objects, undetermined intent

X● **Y27.9** Contact with unspecified hot objects, undetermined intent

●**Y28** Contact with sharp object, undetermined intent

The appropriate 7th character is to be added to each code from category Y28

> A   initial encounter
> D   subsequent encounter
> S   sequela

X● **Y28.0** Contact with sharp glass, undetermined intent

X● **Y28.1** Contact with knife, undetermined intent

X● **Y28.2** Contact with sword or dagger, undetermined intent

X● **Y28.8** Contact with other sharp object, undetermined intent

X● **Y28.9** Contact with unspecified sharp object, undetermined intent

X●**Y29** Contact with blunt object, undetermined intent

The appropriate 7th character is to be added to code Y29

> A   initial encounter
> D   subsequent encounter
> S   sequela

X●**Y30** Falling, jumping or pushed from a high place, undetermined intent
Victim falling from one level to another, undetermined intent

The appropriate 7th character is to be added to code Y30

> A   initial encounter
> D   subsequent encounter
> S   sequela

X●**Y31** Falling, lying or running before or into moving object, undetermined intent

The appropriate 7th character is to be added to code Y31

> A   initial encounter
> D   subsequent encounter
> S   sequela

X●**Y32** Crashing of motor vehicle, undetermined intent

The appropriate 7th character is to be added to code Y32

> A   initial encounter
> D   subsequent encounter
> S   sequela

X●**Y33** Other specified events, undetermined intent

The appropriate 7th character is to be added to code Y33

> A   initial encounter
> D   subsequent encounter
> S   sequela

LEGAL INTERVENTION, OPERATIONS OF WAR, MILITARY OPERATIONS, AND TERRORISM (Y35-Y38)

● Y35   **Legal intervention**

Includes   any injury sustained as a result of an encounter with any law enforcement official, serving in any capacity at the time of the encounter, whether on-duty or off-duty. Includes: injury to law enforcement official, suspect and bystander

The appropriate 7th character is to be added to each code from category Y35

A	initial encounter
D	subsequent encounter
S	sequela

● Y35.0   **Legal intervention involving firearm discharge**

● Y35.00   **Legal intervention involving unspecified firearm discharge**
Legal intervention involving gunshot wound
Legal intervention involving shot NOS

● Y35.001   **Legal intervention involving unspecified firearm discharge, law enforcement official injured**

● Y35.002   **Legal intervention involving unspecified firearm discharge, bystander injured**

● Y35.003   **Legal intervention involving unspecified firearm discharge, suspect injured**

● Y35.01   **Legal intervention involving injury by machine gun**

● Y35.011   **Legal intervention involving injury by machine gun, law enforcement official injured**

● Y35.012   **Legal intervention involving injury by machine gun, bystander injured**

● Y35.013   **Legal intervention involving injury by machine gun, suspect injured**

● Y35.02   **Legal intervention involving injury by handgun**

● Y35.021   **Legal intervention involving injury by handgun, law enforcement official injured**

● Y35.022   **Legal intervention involving injury by handgun, bystander injured**

● Y35.023   **Legal intervention involving injury by handgun, suspect injured**

● Y35.03   **Legal intervention involving injury by rifle pellet**

● Y35.031   **Legal intervention involving injury by rifle pellet, law enforcement official injured**

● Y35.032   **Legal intervention involving injury by rifle pellet, bystander injured**

● Y35.033   **Legal intervention involving injury by rifle pellet, suspect injured**

● Y35.04   **Legal intervention involving injury by rubber bullet**

● Y35.041   **Legal intervention involving injury by rubber bullet, law enforcement official injured**

● Y35.042   **Legal intervention involving injury by rubber bullet, bystander injured**

● Y35.043   **Legal intervention involving injury by rubber bullet, suspect injured**

● Y35.09   **Legal intervention involving other firearm discharge**

● Y35.091   **Legal intervention involving other firearm discharge, law enforcement official injured**

● Y35.092   **Legal intervention involving other firearm discharge, bystander injured**

● Y35.093   **Legal intervention involving other firearm discharge, suspect injured**

● Y35.1   **Legal intervention involving explosives**

● Y35.10   **Legal intervention involving unspecified explosives**

● Y35.101   **Legal intervention involving unspecified explosives, law enforcement official injured**

● Y35.102   **Legal intervention involving unspecified explosives, bystander injured**

● Y35.103   **Legal intervention involving unspecified explosives, suspect injured**

● Y35.11   **Legal intervention involving injury by dynamite**

● Y35.111   **Legal intervention involving injury by dynamite, law enforcement official injured**

● Y35.112   **Legal intervention involving injury by dynamite, bystander injured**

● Y35.113   **Legal intervention involving injury by dynamite, suspect injured**

● Y35.12   **Legal intervention involving injury by explosive shell**

● Y35.121   **Legal intervention involving injury by explosive shell, law enforcement official injured**

● Y35.122   **Legal intervention involving injury by explosive shell, bystander injured**

● Y35.123   **Legal intervention involving injury by explosive shell, suspect injured**

● Y35.19   **Legal intervention involving other explosives**
Legal intervention involving injury by grenade
Legal intervention involving injury by mortar bomb

● Y35.191   **Legal intervention involving other explosives, law enforcement official injured**

● Y35.192   **Legal intervention involving other explosives, bystander injured**

● Y35.193   **Legal intervention involving other explosives, suspect injured**

● Y35.2   **Legal intervention involving gas**
Legal intervention involving asphyxiation by gas
Legal intervention involving poisoning by gas

● Y35.20   **Legal intervention involving unspecified gas**

● Y35.201   **Legal intervention involving unspecified gas, law enforcement official injured**

● Y35.202   **Legal intervention involving unspecified gas, bystander injured**

● Y35.203   **Legal intervention involving unspecified gas, suspect injured**

● Y35.21   **Legal intervention involving injury by tear gas**

● Y35.211   **Legal intervention involving injury by tear gas, law enforcement official injured**

● Y35.212   **Legal intervention involving injury by tear gas, bystander injured**

● Y35.213   **Legal intervention involving injury by tear gas, suspect injured**

● Y35.29   Legal intervention involving other gas
  ● Y35.291   Legal intervention involving other gas, law enforcement official injured
  ● Y35.292   Legal intervention involving other gas, bystander injured
  ● Y35.293   Legal intervention involving other gas, suspect injured

● Y35.3   Legal intervention involving blunt objects
  Legal intervention involving being hit or struck by blunt object
  ● Y35.30   Legal intervention involving unspecified blunt objects
    ● Y35.301   Legal intervention involving unspecified blunt objects, law enforcement official injured
    ● Y35.302   Legal intervention involving unspecified blunt objects, bystander injured
    ● Y35.303   Legal intervention involving unspecified blunt objects, suspect injured
  ● Y35.31   Legal intervention involving baton
    ● Y35.311   Legal intervention involving baton, law enforcement official injured
    ● Y35.312   Legal intervention involving baton, bystander injured
    ● Y35.313   Legal intervention involving baton, suspect injured
  ● Y35.39   Legal intervention involving other blunt objects
    ● Y35.391   Legal intervention involving other blunt objects, law enforcement official injured
    ● Y35.392   Legal intervention involving other blunt objects, bystander injured
    ● Y35.393   Legal intervention involving other blunt objects, suspect injured

● Y35.4   Legal intervention involving sharp objects
  Legal intervention involving being cut by sharp objects
  Legal intervention involving being stabbed by sharp objects
  ● Y35.40   Legal intervention involving unspecified sharp objects
    ● Y35.401   Legal intervention involving unspecified sharp objects, law enforcement official injured
    ● Y35.402   Legal intervention involving unspecified sharp objects, bystander injured
    ● Y35.403   Legal intervention involving unspecified sharp objects, suspect injured
  ● Y35.41   Legal intervention involving bayonet
    ● Y35.411   Legal intervention involving bayonet, law enforcement official injured
    ● Y35.412   Legal intervention involving bayonet, bystander injured
    ● Y35.413   Legal intervention involving bayonet, suspect injured
  ● Y35.49   Legal intervention involving other sharp objects
    ● Y35.491   Legal intervention involving other sharp objects, law enforcement official injured
    ● Y35.492   Legal intervention involving other sharp objects, bystander injured
    ● Y35.493   Legal intervention involving other sharp objects, suspect injured

● Y35.8   Legal intervention involving other specified means
  ● Y35.81   Legal intervention involving manhandling
    ● Y35.811   Legal intervention involving manhandling, law enforcement official injured
    ● Y35.812   Legal intervention involving manhandling, bystander injured
    ● Y35.813   Legal intervention involving manhandling, suspect injured
  ● Y35.89   Legal intervention involving other specified means
    ● Y35.891   Legal intervention involving other specified means, law enforcement official injured
    ● Y35.892   Legal intervention involving other specified means, bystander injured
    ● Y35.893   Legal intervention involving other specified means, suspect injured

● Y35.9   Legal intervention, means unspecified
  X ● Y35.91   Legal intervention, means unspecified, law enforcement official injured
  X ● Y35.92   Legal intervention, means unspecified, bystander injured
  X ● Y35.93   Legal intervention, means unspecified, suspect injured

● Y36   Operations of war

Includes	injuries to military personnel and civilians caused by war, civil insurrection, and peacekeeping missions
Excludes1	injury to military personnel occurring during peacetime military operations (Y37.-) military vehicles involved in transport accidents with non-military vehicle during peacetime (V09.01, V09.21, V19.81, V29.81, V39.81, V49.81, V59.81, V69.81, V79.81)

The appropriate 7th character is to be added to each code from category Y36

A	initial encounter
D	subsequent encounter
S	sequela

● Y36.0   War operations involving explosion of marine weapons
  Weapons and military watercraft
  ● Y36.00   War operations involving explosion of unspecified marine weapon
    War operations involving underwater blast NOS
    ● Y36.000   War operations involving explosion of unspecified marine weapon, military personnel
    ● Y36.001   War operations involving explosion of unspecified marine weapon, civilian
  ● Y36.01   War operations involving explosion of depth-charge
    ● Y36.010   War operations involving explosion of depth-charge, military personnel
    ● Y36.011   War operations involving explosion of depth-charge, civilian
  ● Y36.02   War operations involving explosion of marine mine
    War operations involving explosion of marine mine, at sea or in harbor
    ● Y36.020   War operations involving explosion of marine mine, military personnel
    ● Y36.021   War operations involving explosion of marine mine, civilian

- Y36.03   War operations involving explosion of sea-based artillery shell
  - Y36.030   War operations involving explosion of sea-based artillery shell, military personnel
  - Y36.031   War operations involving explosion of sea-based artillery shell, civilian
- Y36.04   War operations involving explosion of torpedo
  - Y36.040   War operations involving explosion of torpedo, military personnel
  - Y36.041   War operations involving explosion of torpedo, civilian
- Y36.05   War operations involving accidental detonation of onboard marine weapons
  - Y36.050   War operations involving accidental detonation of onboard marine weapons, military personnel
  - Y36.051   War operations involving accidental detonation of onboard marine weapons, civilian
- Y36.09   War operations involving explosion of other marine weapons
  - Y36.090   War operations involving explosion of other marine weapons, military personnel
  - Y36.091   War operations involving explosion of other marine weapons, civilian
- Y36.1   War operations involving destruction of aircraft
  - Y36.10   War operations involving unspecified destruction of aircraft
    - Y36.100   War operations involving unspecified destruction of aircraft, military personnel
    - Y36.101   War operations involving unspecified destruction of aircraft, civilian
  - Y36.11   War operations involving destruction of aircraft due to enemy fire or explosives
    War operations involving destruction of aircraft due to air to air missile
    War operations involving destruction of aircraft due to explosive placed on aircraft
    War operations involving destruction of aircraft due to rocket propelled grenade [RPG]
    War operations involving destruction of aircraft due to small arms fire
    War operations involving destruction of aircraft due to surface to air missile
    - Y36.110   War operations involving destruction of aircraft due to enemy fire or explosives, military personnel
    - Y36.111   War operations involving destruction of aircraft due to enemy fire or explosives, civilian
  - Y36.12   War operations involving destruction of aircraft due to collision with other aircraft
    - Y36.120   War operations involving destruction of aircraft due to collision with other aircraft, military personnel
    - Y36.121   War operations involving destruction of aircraft due to collision with other aircraft, civilian
  - Y36.13   War operations involving destruction of aircraft due to onboard fire
    - Y36.130   War operations involving destruction of aircraft due to onboard fire, military personnel
    - Y36.131   War operations involving destruction of aircraft due to onboard fire, civilian

- Y36.14   War operations involving destruction of aircraft due to accidental detonation of onboard munitions and explosives
  - Y36.140   War operations involving destruction of aircraft due to accidental detonation of onboard munitions and explosives, military personnel
  - Y36.141   War operations involving destruction of aircraft due to accidental detonation of onboard munitions and explosives, civilian
- Y36.19   War operations involving other destruction of aircraft
  - Y36.190   War operations involving other destruction of aircraft, military personnel
  - Y36.191   War operations involving other destruction of aircraft, civilian
- Y36.2   War operations involving other explosions and fragments

  > Excludes1   war operations involving explosion of aircraft (Y36.1-)
  > war operations involving explosion of marine weapons (Y36.0-)
  > war operations involving explosion of nuclear weapons (Y36.5-)
  > war operations involving explosion occurring after cessation of hostilities (Y36.8-)

  - Y36.20   War operations involving unspecified explosion and fragments
    War operations involving air blast NOS
    War operations involving blast NOS
    War operations involving blast fragments NOS
    War operations involving blast wave NOS
    War operations involving blast wind NOS
    War operations involving explosion NOS
    War operations involving explosion of bomb NOS
    - Y36.200   War operations involving unspecified explosion and fragments, military personnel
    - Y36.201   War operations involving unspecified explosion and fragments, civilian
  - Y36.21   War operations involving explosion of aerial bomb
    - Y36.210   War operations involving explosion of aerial bomb, military personnel
    - Y36.211   War operations involving explosion of aerial bomb, civilian
  - Y36.22   War operations involving explosion of guided missile
    - Y36.220   War operations involving explosion of guided missile, military personnel
    - Y36.221   War operations involving explosion of guided missile, civilian
  - Y36.23   War operations involving explosion of improvised explosive device [IED]
    War operations involving explosion of person-borne improvised explosive device [IED]
    War operations involving explosion of vehicle-borne improvised explosive device [IED]
    War operations involving explosion of roadside improvised explosive device [IED]
    - Y36.230   War operations involving explosion of improvised explosive device [IED], military personnel
    - Y36.231   War operations involving explosion of improvised explosive device [IED], civilian

◀ New   ◀═ Revised   ~~deleted~~ Deleted   **OGCR** Official Guidelines   X Assign placeholder X   ● Use Additional Character(s)

Excludes 1   Excludes 2   Includes   Use additional   Code first   Code also   Unspecified

- Y36.24 **War operations involving explosion due to accidental detonation and discharge of own munitions or munitions launch device**
  - Y36.240 **War operations involving explosion due to accidental detonation and discharge of own munitions or munitions launch device, military personnel**
  - Y36.241 **War operations involving explosion due to accidental detonation and discharge of own munitions or munitions launch device, civilian**
- Y36.25 **War operations involving fragments from munitions**
  - Y36.250 **War operations involving fragments from munitions, military personnel**
  - Y36.251 **War operations involving fragments from munitions, civilian**
- Y36.26 **War operations involving fragments of improvised explosive device [IED]**
  War operations involving fragments of person-borne improvised explosive device [IED]
  War operations involving fragments of vehicle-borne improvised explosive device [IED]
  War operations involving fragments of roadside improvised explosive device [IED]
  - Y36.260 **War operations involving fragments of improvised explosive device [IED], military personnel**
  - Y36.261 **War operations involving fragments of improvised explosive device [IED], civilian**
- Y36.27 **War operations involving fragments from weapons**
  - Y36.270 **War operations involving fragments from weapons, military personnel**
  - Y36.271 **War operations involving fragments from weapons, civilian**
- Y36.29 **War operations involving other explosions and fragments**
  War operations involving explosion of grenade
  War operations involving explosions of land mine
  War operations involving shrapnel NOS
  - Y36.290 **War operations involving other explosions and fragments, military personnel**
  - Y36.291 **War operations involving other explosions and fragments, civilian**
- Y36.3 **War operations involving fires, conflagrations and hot substances**
  War operations involving smoke, fumes, and heat from fires, conflagrations and hot substances
  | Excludes1 | war operations involving fires and conflagrations aboard military aircraft (Y36.1-) |

  war operations involving fires and conflagrations aboard military watercraft (Y36.0-)
  war operations involving fires and conflagrations caused indirectly by conventional weapons (Y36.2-)
  war operations involving fires and thermal effects of nuclear weapons (Y36.53-)
  - Y36.30 **War operations involving unspecified fire, conflagration and hot substance**
    - Y36.300 **War operations involving unspecified fire, conflagration and hot substance, military personnel**
    - Y36.301 **War operations involving unspecified fire, conflagration and hot substance, civilian**

- Y36.31 **War operations involving gasoline bomb**
  War operations involving incendiary bomb
  War operations involving petrol bomb
  - Y36.310 **War operations involving gasoline bomb, military personnel**
  - Y36.311 **War operations involving gasoline bomb, civilian**
- Y36.32 **War operations involving incendiary bullet**
  - Y36.320 **War operations involving incendiary bullet, military personnel**
  - Y36.321 **War operations involving incendiary bullet, civilian**
- Y36.33 **War operations involving flamethrower**
  - Y36.330 **War operations involving flamethrower, military personnel**
  - Y36.331 **War operations involving flamethrower, civilian**
- Y36.39 **War operations involving other fires, conflagrations and hot substances**
  - Y36.390 **War operations involving other fires, conflagrations and hot substances, military personnel**
  - Y36.391 **War operations involving other fires, conflagrations and hot substances, civilian**
- Y36.4 **War operations involving firearm discharge and other forms of conventional warfare**
  - Y36.41 **War operations involving rubber bullets**
    - Y36.410 **War operations involving rubber bullets, military personnel**
    - Y36.411 **War operations involving rubber bullets, civilian**
  - Y36.42 **War operations involving firearms pellets**
    - Y36.420 **War operations involving firearms pellets, military personnel**
    - Y36.421 **War operations involving firearms pellets, civilian**
  - Y36.43 **War operations involving other firearms discharge**
    War operations involving bullets NOS
    | Excludes1 | war operations involving munitions fragments (Y36.25-) |

    war operations involving incendiary bullets (Y36.32-)
    - Y36.430 **War operations involving other firearms discharge, military personnel**
    - Y36.431 **War operations involving other firearms discharge, civilian**
  - Y36.44 **War operations involving unarmed hand to hand combat**
    | Excludes1 | war operations involving combat using blunt or piercing object (Y36.45-) |

    war operations involving intentional restriction of air and airway (Y36.46-)
    war operations involving unintentional restriction of air and airway (Y36.47-)
    - Y36.440 **War operations involving unarmed hand to hand combat, military personnel**
    - Y36.441 **War operations involving unarmed hand to hand combat, civilian**

◀ New   ◀|||| Revised   ~~deleted~~ Deleted   **OGCR** Official Guidelines   X Assign placeholder X   ● Use Additional Character(s)

| Excludes 1 | | Excludes 2 | | Includes | | Use additional | | Code first | | Code also | | Unspecified |

● Y36.45   War operations involving combat using blunt or piercing object
     ● Y36.450   War operations involving combat using blunt or piercing object, military personnel
     ● Y36.451   War operations involving combat using blunt or piercing object, civilian
● Y36.46   War operations involving intentional restriction of air and airway
     ● Y36.460   War operations involving intentional restriction of air and airway, military personnel
     ● Y36.461   War operations involving intentional restriction of air and airway, civilian
● Y36.47   War operations involving unintentional restriction of air and airway
     ● Y36.470   War operations involving unintentional restriction of air and airway, military personnel
     ● Y36.471   War operations involving unintentional restriction of air and airway, civilian
● Y36.49   War operations involving other forms of conventional warfare
     ● Y36.490   War operations involving other forms of conventional warfare, military personnel
     ● Y36.491   War operations involving other forms of conventional warfare, civilian
● Y36.5   War operations involving nuclear weapons
     War operations involving dirty bomb NOS
   ● Y36.50   War operations involving unspecified effect of nuclear weapon
     ● Y36.500   War operations involving unspecified effect of nuclear weapon, military personnel
     ● Y36.501   War operations involving unspecified effect of nuclear weapon, civilian
   ● Y36.51   War operations involving direct blast effect of nuclear weapon
     War operations involving blast pressure of nuclear weapon
     ● Y36.510   War operations involving direct blast effect of nuclear weapon, military personnel
     ● Y36.511   War operations involving direct blast effect of nuclear weapon, civilian
   ● Y36.52   War operations involving indirect blast effect of nuclear weapon
     War operations involving being thrown by blast of nuclear weapon
     War operations involving being struck or crushed by blast debris of nuclear weapon
     ● Y36.520   War operations involving indirect blast effect of nuclear weapon, military personnel
     ● Y36.521   War operations involving indirect blast effect of nuclear weapon, civilian
   ● Y36.53   War operations involving thermal radiation effect of nuclear weapon
     War operations involving direct heat from nuclear weapon
     War operation involving fireball effects from nuclear weapon
     ● Y36.530   War operations involving thermal radiation effect of nuclear weapon, military personnel
     ● Y36.531   War operations involving thermal radiation effect of nuclear weapon, civilian

● Y36.54   War operation involving nuclear radiation effects of nuclear weapon
     War operation involving acute radiation exposure from nuclear weapon
     War operation involving exposure to immediate ionizing radiation from nuclear weapon
     War operation involving fallout exposure from nuclear weapon
     War operation involving secondary effects of nuclear weapons
     ● Y36.540   War operation involving nuclear radiation effects of nuclear weapon, military personnel
     ● Y36.541   War operation involving nuclear radiation effects of nuclear weapon, civilian
● Y36.59   War operation involving other effects of nuclear weapons
     ● Y36.590   War operation involving other effects of nuclear weapons, military personnel
     ● Y36.591   War operation involving other effects of nuclear weapons, civilian
● Y36.6   War operations involving biological weapons
   ● Y36.6X   War operations involving biological weapons
     ● Y36.6X0   War operations involving biological weapons, military personnel
     ● Y36.6X1   War operations involving biological weapons, civilian
● Y36.7   War operations involving chemical weapons and other forms of unconventional warfare
     Excludes1   war operations involving incendiary devices (Y36.3-, Y36.5-)
   ● Y36.7X   War operations involving chemical weapons and other forms of unconventional warfare
     ● Y36.7X0   War operations involving chemical weapons and other forms of unconventional warfare, military personnel
     ● Y36.7X1   War operations involving chemical weapons and other forms of unconventional warfare, civilian
● Y36.8   War operations occurring after cessation of hostilities
     War operations classifiable to categories Y36.0-Y36.8 but occurring after cessation of hostilities
   ● Y36.81   Explosion of mine placed during war operations but exploding after cessation of hostilities
     ● Y36.810   Explosion of mine placed during war operations but exploding after cessation of hostilities, military personnel
     ● Y36.811   Explosion of mine placed during war operations but exploding after cessation of hostilities, civilian
   ● Y36.82   Explosion of bomb placed during war operations but exploding after cessation of hostilities
     ● Y36.820   Explosion of bomb placed during war operations but exploding after cessation of hostilities, military personnel
     ● Y36.821   Explosion of bomb placed during war operations but exploding after cessation of hostilities, civilian

● Y36.88   Other war operations occurring after cessation of hostilities
    ● Y36.880   Other war operations occurring after cessation of hostilities, military personnel
    ● Y36.881   Other war operations occurring after cessation of hostilities, civilian

● Y36.89   Unspecified war operations occurring after cessation of hostilities
    ● Y36.890   Unspecified war operations occurring after cessation of hostilities, military personnel
    ● Y36.891   Unspecified war operations occurring after cessation of hostilities, civilian

● Y36.9   Other and unspecified war operations
    X ● Y36.90   War operations, unspecified
    X ● Y36.91   War operations involving unspecified weapon of mass destruction [WMD]
    X ● Y36.92   War operations involving friendly fire

● Y37   Military operations
    Includes   Injuries to military personnel and civilians occurring during peacetime on military property and during routine military exercises and operations

    Excludes1   military aircraft involved in aircraft accident with civilian aircraft (V97.81-)
        military vehicles involved in transport accident with civilian vehicle (V09.01, V09.21, V19.81, V29.81, V39.81, V49.81, V59.81, V69.81, V79.81)
        military watercraft involved in water transport accident with civilian watercraft (V94.81-)
        war operations (Y36.-)

    The appropriate 7th character is to be added to each code from category Y37

    A   initial encounter
    D   subsequent encounter
    S   sequela

● Y37.0   Military operations involving explosion of marine weapons
    ● Y37.00   Military operations involving explosion of unspecified marine weapon
        Military operations involving underwater blast NOS
        ● Y37.000   Military operations involving explosion of unspecified marine weapon, military personnel
        ● Y37.001   Military operations involving explosion of unspecified marine weapon, civilian
    ● Y37.01   Military operations involving explosion of depth-charge
        ● Y37.010   Military operations involving explosion of depth-charge, military personnel
        ● Y37.011   Military operations involving explosion of depth-charge, civilian
    ● Y37.02   Military operations involving explosion of marine mine
        Military operations involving explosion of marine mine, at sea or in harbor
        ● Y37.020   Military operations involving explosion of marine mine, military personnel
        ● Y37.021   Military operations involving explosion of marine mine, civilian

● Y37.03   Military operations involving explosion of sea-based artillery shell
    ● Y37.030   Military operations involving explosion of sea-based artillery shell, military personnel
    ● Y37.031   Military operations involving explosion of sea-based artillery shell, civilian

● Y37.04   Military operations involving explosion of torpedo
    ● Y37.040   Military operations involving explosion of torpedo, military personnel
    ● Y37.041   Military operations involving explosion of torpedo, civilian

● Y37.05   Military operations involving accidental detonation of onboard marine weapons
    ● Y37.050   Military operations involving accidental detonation of onboard marine weapons, military personnel
    ● Y37.051   Military operations involving accidental detonation of onboard marine weapons, civilian

● Y37.09   Military operations involving explosion of other marine weapons
    ● Y37.090   Military operations involving explosion of other marine weapons, military personnel
    ● Y37.091   Military operations involving explosion of other marine weapons, civilian

● Y37.1   Military operations involving destruction of aircraft
    ● Y37.10   Military operations involving unspecified destruction of aircraft
        ● Y37.100   Military operations involving unspecified destruction of aircraft, military personnel
        ● Y37.101   Military operations involving unspecified destruction of aircraft, civilian
    ● Y37.11   Military operations involving destruction of aircraft due to enemy fire or explosives
        Military operations involving destruction of aircraft due to air to air missile
        Military operations involving destruction of aircraft due to explosive placed on aircraft
        Military operations involving destruction of aircraft due to rocket propelled grenade [RPG]
        Military operations involving destruction of aircraft due to small arms fire
        Military operations involving destruction of aircraft due to surface to air missile
        ● Y37.110   Military operations involving destruction of aircraft due to enemy fire or explosives, military personnel
        ● Y37.111   Military operations involving destruction of aircraft due to enemy fire or explosives, civilian
    ● Y37.12   Military operations involving destruction of aircraft due to collision with other aircraft
        ● Y37.120   Military operations involving destruction of aircraft due to collision with other aircraft, military personnel
        ● Y37.121   Military operations involving destruction of aircraft due to collision with other aircraft, civilian

◀ New   ◀ Revised   deleted Deleted   OGCR Official Guidelines   X Assign placeholder X   ● Use Additional Character(s)

Excludes 1   Excludes 2   Includes   Use additional   Code first   Code also   Unspecified

● **Y37.13** Military operations involving destruction of aircraft due to onboard fire
  ● **Y37.130** Military operations involving destruction of aircraft due to onboard fire, military personnel
  ● **Y37.131** Military operations involving destruction of aircraft due to onboard fire, civilian
● **Y37.14** Military operations involving destruction of aircraft due to accidental detonation of onboard munitions and explosives
  ● **Y37.140** Military operations involving destruction of aircraft due to accidental detonation of onboard munitions and explosives, military personnel
  ● **Y37.141** Military operations involving destruction of aircraft due to accidental detonation of onboard munitions and explosives, civilian
● **Y37.19** Military operations involving other destruction of aircraft
  ● **Y37.190** Military operations involving other destruction of aircraft, military personnel
  ● **Y37.191** Military operations involving other destruction of aircraft, civilian
● **Y37.2** Military operations involving other explosions and fragments

Excludes1: military operations involving explosion of aircraft (Y37.1-)
military operations involving explosion of marine weapons (Y37.0-)
military operations involving explosion of nuclear weapons (Y37.5-)

  ● **Y37.20** Military operations involving unspecified explosion and fragments
Military operations involving air blast NOS
Military operations involving blast NOS
Military operations involving blast fragments NOS
Military operations involving blast wave NOS
Military operations involving blast wind NOS
Military operations involving explosion NOS
Military operations involving explosion of bomb NOS
  ● **Y37.200** Military operations involving unspecified explosion and fragments, military personnel
  ● **Y37.201** Military operations involving unspecified explosion and fragments, civilian
  ● **Y37.21** Military operations involving explosion of aerial bomb
  ● **Y37.210** Military operations involving explosion of aerial bomb, military personnel
  ● **Y37.211** Military operations involving explosion of aerial bomb, civilian
  ● **Y37.22** Military operations involving explosion of guided missile
  ● **Y37.220** Military operations involving explosion of guided missile, military personnel
  ● **Y37.221** Military operations involving explosion of guided missile, civilian

● **Y37.23** Military operations involving explosion of improvised explosive device [IED]
Military operations involving explosion of person-borne improvised explosive device [IED]
Military operations involving explosion of vehicle-borne improvised explosive device [IED]
Military operations involving explosion of roadside improvised explosive device [IED]
  ● **Y37.230** Military operations involving explosion of improvised explosive device [IED], military personnel
  ● **Y37.231** Military operations involving explosion of improvised explosive device [IED], civilian
● **Y37.24** Military operations involving explosion due to accidental detonation and discharge of own munitions or munitions launch device
  ● **Y37.240** Military operations involving explosion due to accidental detonation and discharge of own munitions or munitions launch device, military personnel
  ● **Y37.241** Military operations involving explosion due to accidental detonation and discharge of own munitions or munitions launch device, civilian
● **Y37.25** Military operations involving fragments from munitions
  ● **Y37.250** Military operations involving fragments from munitions, military personnel
  ● **Y37.251** Military operations involving fragments from munitions, civilian
● **Y37.26** Military operations involving fragments of improvised explosive device [IED]
Military operations involving fragments of person-borne improvised explosive device [IED]
Military operations involving fragments of vehicle-borne improvised explosive device [IED]
Military operations involving fragments of roadside improvised explosive device [IED]
  ● **Y37.260** Military operations involving fragments of improvised explosive device [IED], military personnel
  ● **Y37.261** Military operations involving fragments of improvised explosive device [IED], civilian
● **Y37.27** Military operations involving fragments from weapons
  ● **Y37.270** Military operations involving fragments from weapons, military personnel
  ● **Y37.271** Military operations involving fragments from weapons, civilian
● **Y37.29** Military operations involving other explosions and fragments
Military operations involving explosion of grenade
Military operations involving explosions of land mine
Military operations involving shrapnel NOS
  ● **Y37.290** Military operations involving other explosions and fragments, military personnel
  ● **Y37.291** Military operations involving other explosions and fragments, civilian

CHAPTER 20 (V01-Y99)

◄ New ◄ Revised ~~deleted~~ Deleted OGCR Official Guidelines X Assign placeholder X ● Use Additional Character(s)
Excludes 1 | Excludes 2 | Includes | Use additional | Code first | Code also | Unspecified

● **Y37.3** **Military operations involving fires, conflagrations and hot substances**
  Military operations involving smoke, fumes, and heat from fires, conflagrations and hot substances
  Excludes1   military operations involving fires and conflagrations aboard military aircraft (Y37.1-)
  military operations involving fires and conflagrations aboard military watercraft (Y37.0-)
  military operations involving fires and conflagrations caused indirectly by conventional weapons (Y37.2-)
  military operations involving fires and thermal effects of nuclear weapons (Y36.53-)

  ● **Y37.30** **Military operations involving unspecified fire, conflagration and hot substance**
    ● **Y37.300** Military operations involving unspecified fire, conflagration and hot substance, military personnel
    ● **Y37.301** Military operations involving unspecified fire, conflagration and hot substance, civilian

  ● **Y37.31** **Military operations involving gasoline bomb**
    Military operations involving incendiary bomb
    Military operations involving petrol bomb
    ● **Y37.310** Military operations involving gasoline bomb, military personnel
    ● **Y37.311** Military operations involving gasoline bomb, civilian

  ● **Y37.32** **Military operations involving incendiary bullet**
    ● **Y37.320** Military operations involving incendiary bullet, military personnel
    ● **Y37.321** Military operations involving incendiary bullet, civilian

  ● **Y37.33** **Military operations involving flamethrower**
    ● **Y37.330** Military operations involving flamethrower, military personnel
    ● **Y37.331** Military operations involving flamethrower, civilian

  ● **Y37.39** **Military operations involving other fires, conflagrations and hot substances**
    ● **Y37.390** Military operations involving other fires, conflagrations and hot substances, military personnel
    ● **Y37.391** Military operations involving other fires, conflagrations and hot substances, civilian

● **Y37.4** **Military operations involving firearm discharge and other forms of conventional warfare**
  ● **Y37.41** **Military operations involving rubber bullets**
    ● **Y37.410** Military operations involving rubber bullets, military personnel
    ● **Y37.411** Military operations involving rubber bullets, civilian

  ● **Y37.42** **Military operations involving firearms pellets**
    ● **Y37.420** Military operations involving firearms pellets, military personnel
    ● **Y37.421** Military operations involving firearms pellets, civilian

● **Y37.43** **Military operations involving other firearms discharge**
  Military operations involving bullets NOS
  Excludes1   military operations involving munitions fragments (Y37.25-)
  military operations involving incendiary bullets (Y37.32-)
  ● **Y37.430** Military operations involving other firearms discharge, military personnel
  ● **Y37.431** Military operations involving other firearms discharge, civilian

● **Y37.44** **Military operations involving unarmed hand to hand combat**
  Excludes1   military operations involving combat using blunt or piercing object (Y37.45-)
  military operations involving intentional restriction of air and airway (Y37.46-)
  military operations involving unintentional restriction of air and airway (Y37.47-)
  ● **Y37.440** Military operations involving unarmed hand to hand combat, military personnel
  ● **Y37.441** Military operations involving unarmed hand to hand combat, civilian

● **Y37.45** **Military operations involving combat using blunt or piercing object**
  ● **Y37.450** Military operations involving combat using blunt or piercing object, military personnel
  ● **Y37.451** Military operations involving combat using blunt or piercing object, civilian

● **Y37.46** **Military operations involving intentional restriction of air and airway**
  ● **Y37.460** Military operations involving intentional restriction of air and airway, military personnel
  ● **Y37.461** Military operations involving intentional restriction of air and airway, civilian

● **Y37.47** **Military operations involving unintentional restriction of air and airway**
  ● **Y37.470** Military operations involving unintentional restriction of air and airway, military personnel
  ● **Y37.471** Military operations involving unintentional restriction of air and airway, civilian

● **Y37.49** **Military operations involving other forms of conventional warfare**
  ● **Y37.490** Military operations involving other forms of conventional warfare, military personnel
  ● **Y37.491** Military operations involving other forms of conventional warfare, civilian

◀ New   ◀▥ Revised   deleted Deleted   OGCR Official Guidelines   X Assign placeholder X   ● Use Additional Character(s)
Excludes 1   Excludes 2   Includes   Use additional   Code first   Code also   Unspecified

● **Y37.5**   **Military operations involving nuclear weapons**
Military operation involving dirty bomb NOS

● **Y37.50**   **Military operations involving unspecified effect of nuclear weapon**

    ● **Y37.500**   **Military operations involving unspecified effect of nuclear weapon, military personnel**

    ● **Y37.501**   **Military operations involving unspecified effect of nuclear weapon, civilian**

● **Y37.51**   **Military operations involving direct blast effect of nuclear weapon**
Military operations involving blast pressure of nuclear weapon

    ● **Y37.510**   **Military operations involving direct blast effect of nuclear weapon, military personnel**

    ● **Y37.511**   **Military operations involving direct blast effect of nuclear weapon, civilian**

● **Y37.52**   **Military operations involving indirect blast effect of nuclear weapon**
Military operations involving being thrown by blast of nuclear weapon
Military operations involving being struck or crushed by blast debris of nuclear weapon

    ● **Y37.520**   **Military operations involving indirect blast effect of nuclear weapon, military personnel**

    ● **Y37.521**   **Military operations involving indirect blast effect of nuclear weapon, civilian**

● **Y37.53**   **Military operations involving thermal radiation effect of nuclear weapon**
Military operations involving direct heat from nuclear weapon
Military operation involving fireball effects from nuclear weapon

    ● **Y37.530**   **Military operations involving thermal radiation effect of nuclear weapon, military personnel**

    ● **Y37.531**   **Military operations involving thermal radiation effect of nuclear weapon, civilian**

● **Y37.54**   **Military operation involving nuclear radiation effects of nuclear weapon**
Military operation involving acute radiation exposure from nuclear weapon
Military operation involving exposure to immediate ionizing radiation from nuclear weapon
Military operation involving fallout exposure from nuclear weapon
Military operation involving secondary effects of nuclear weapons

    ● **Y37.540**   **Military operation involving nuclear radiation effects of nuclear weapon, military personnel**

    ● **Y37.541**   **Military operation involving nuclear radiation effects of nuclear weapon, civilian**

● **Y37.59**   **Military operation involving other effects of nuclear weapons**

    ● **Y37.590**   **Military operation involving other effects of nuclear weapons, military personnel**

    ● **Y37.591**   **Military operation involving other effects of nuclear weapons, civilian**

● **Y37.6**   **Military operations involving biological weapons**

● **Y37.6X**   **Military operations involving biological weapons**

    ● **Y37.6X0**   **Military operations involving biological weapons, military personnel**

    ● **Y37.6X1**   **Military operations involving biological weapons, civilian**

● **Y37.7**   **Military operations involving chemical weapons and other forms of unconventional warfare**

    | **Excludes1** | military operations involving incendiary devices (Y36.3-, Y36.5-)

● **Y37.7X**   **Military operations involving chemical weapons and other forms of unconventional warfare**

    ● **Y37.7X0**   **Military operations involving chemical weapons and other forms of unconventional warfare, military personnel**

    ● **Y37.7X1**   **Military operations involving chemical weapons and other forms of unconventional warfare, civilian**

● **Y37.9**   **Other and unspecified military operations**

   X ● **Y37.90**   **Military operations, unspecified**

   X ● **Y37.91**   **Military operations involving unspecified weapon of mass destruction [WMD]**

   X ● **Y37.92**   **Military operations involving friendly fire**

● **Y38**   **Terrorism**
These codes are for use to identify injuries resulting from the unlawful use of force or violence against persons or property to intimidate or coerce a government, the civilian population, or any segment thereof, in furtherance of political or social objective

Use additional code for place of occurrence (Y92.-)

The appropriate 7th character is to be added to each code from category Y38

A	initial encounter
D	subsequent encounter
S	sequela

● **Y38.0**   **Terrorism involving explosion of marine weapons**
Terrorism involving depth-charge
Terrorism involving marine mine
Terrorism involving mine NOS, at sea or in harbor
Terrorism involving sea-based artillery shell
Terrorism involving torpedo
Terrorism involving underwater blast

● **Y38.0X**   **Terrorism involving explosion of marine weapons**

    ● **Y38.0X1**   **Terrorism involving explosion of marine weapons, public safety official injured**

    ● **Y38.0X2**   **Terrorism involving explosion of marine weapons, civilian injured**

    ● **Y38.0X3**   **Terrorism involving explosion of marine weapons, terrorist injured**

● **Y38.1**   **Terrorism involving destruction of aircraft**
Terrorism involving aircraft burned
Terrorism involving aircraft exploded
Terrorism involving aircraft being shot down
Terrorism involving aircraft used as a weapon

● **Y38.1X**   **Terrorism involving destruction of aircraft**

    ● **Y38.1X1**   **Terrorism involving destruction of aircraft, public safety official injured**

    ● **Y38.1X2**   **Terrorism involving destruction of aircraft, civilian injured**

    ● **Y38.1X3**   **Terrorism involving destruction of aircraft, terrorist injured**

CHAPTER 20 (V01-Y99)

● **Y38.2 Terrorism involving other explosions and fragments**
Terrorism involving antipersonnel (fragments) bomb
Terrorism involving blast NOS
Terrorism involving explosion NOS
Terrorism involving explosion of breech block
Terrorism involving explosion of cannon block
Terrorism involving explosion (fragments) of artillery shell
Terrorism involving explosion (fragments) of bomb
Terrorism involving explosion (fragments) of grenade
Terrorism involving explosion (fragments) of guided missile
Terrorism involving explosion (fragments) of land mine
Terrorism involving explosion of mortar bomb
Terrorism involving explosion of munitions
Terrorism involving explosion (fragments) of rocket
Terrorism involving explosion (fragments) of shell
Terrorism involving shrapnel
Terrorism involving mine NOS, on land

> **Excludes1**   terrorism involving explosion of nuclear weapon (Y38.5)
> terrorism involving suicide bomber (Y38.81)

● **Y38.2X Terrorism involving other explosions and fragments**

● **Y38.2X1 Terrorism involving other explosions and fragments, public safety official injured**

● **Y38.2X2 Terrorism involving other explosions and fragments, civilian injured**

● **Y38.2X3 Terrorism involving other explosions and fragments, terrorist injured**

● **Y38.3 Terrorism involving fires, conflagration and hot substances**
Terrorism involving conflagration NOS
Terrorism involving fire NOS
Terrorism involving petrol bomb

> **Excludes1**   terrorism involving fire or heat of nuclear weapon (Y38.5)

● **Y38.3X Terrorism involving fires, conflagration and hot substances**

● **Y38.3X1 Terrorism involving fires, conflagration and hot substances, public safety official injured**

● **Y38.3X2 Terrorism involving fires, conflagration and hot substances, civilian injured**

● **Y38.3X3 Terrorism involving fires, conflagration and hot substances, terrorist injured**

● **Y38.4 Terrorism involving firearms**
Terrorism involving carbine bullet
Terrorism involving machine gun bullet
Terrorism involving pellets (shotgun)
Terrorism involving pistol bullet
Terrorism involving rifle bullet
Terrorism involving rubber (rifle) bullet

● **Y38.4X Terrorism involving firearms**

● **Y38.4X1 Terrorism involving firearms, public safety official injured**

● **Y38.4X2 Terrorism involving firearms, civilian injured**

● **Y38.4X3 Terrorism involving firearms, terrorist injured**

● **Y38.5 Terrorism involving nuclear weapons**
Terrorism involving blast effects of nuclear weapon
Terrorism involving exposure to ionizing radiation from nuclear weapon
Terrorism involving fireball effect of nuclear weapon
Terrorism involving heat from nuclear weapon

● **Y38.5X Terrorism involving nuclear weapons**

● **Y38.5X1 Terrorism involving nuclear weapons, public safety official injured**

● **Y38.5X2 Terrorism involving nuclear weapons, civilian injured**

● **Y38.5X3 Terrorism involving nuclear weapons, terrorist injured**

● **Y38.6 Terrorism involving biological weapons**
Terrorism involving anthrax
Terrorism involving cholera
A serious, often deadly, infectious disease of small intestine
Terrorism involving smallpox

● **Y38.6X Terrorism involving biological weapons**

● **Y38.6X1 Terrorism involving biological weapons, public safety official injured**

● **Y38.6X2 Terrorism involving biological weapons, civilian injured**

● **Y38.6X3 Terrorism involving biological weapons, terrorist injured**

● **Y38.7 Terrorism involving chemical weapons**
Terrorism involving gases, fumes, chemicals
Terrorism involving hydrogen cyanide
Terrorism involving phosgene
Terrorism involving sarin

● **Y38.7X Terrorism involving chemical weapons**

● **Y38.7X1 Terrorism involving chemical weapons, public safety official injured**

● **Y38.7X2 Terrorism involving chemical weapons, civilian injured**

● **Y38.7X3 Terrorism involving chemical weapons, terrorist injured**

● **Y38.8 Terrorism involving other and unspecified means**

● **Y38.80 Terrorism involving unspecified means**
Terrorism NOS

● **Y38.81 Terrorism involving suicide bomber**

● **Y38.811 Terrorism involving suicide bomber, public safety official injured**

● **Y38.812 Terrorism involving suicide bomber, civilian injured**

● **Y38.89 Terrorism involving other means**
Terrorism involving drowning and submersion
Terrorism involving lasers
Terrorism involving piercing or stabbing instruments

● **Y38.891 Terrorism involving other means, public safety official injured**

● **Y38.892 Terrorism involving other means, civilian injured**

● **Y38.893 Terrorism involving other means, terrorist injured**

● **Y38.9 Terrorism, secondary effects**

> **Note:** This code is for use to identify conditions occurring subsequent to a terrorist attack not those that are due to the initial terrorist attack.

● **Y38.9X Terrorism, secondary effects**

● **Y38.9X1 Terrorism, secondary effects, public safety official injured**

● **Y38.9X2 Terrorism, secondary effects, civilian injured categories**

COMPLICATIONS OF MEDICAL AND SURGICAL CARE (Y62-Y84)

Includes complications of medical devices surgical and medical procedures as the cause of abnormal reaction of the patient, or of later complication, without mention of misadventure at the time of the procedure

MISADVENTURES TO PATIENTS DURING SURGICAL AND MEDICAL CARE (Y62-Y69)

Excludes2 breakdown or malfunctioning of medical device (during procedure) (after implantation) (ongoing use) (Y70-Y82)
surgical and medical procedures as the cause of abnormal reaction of the patient, without mention of misadventure at the time of the procedure (Y83-Y84)

● Y62　**Failure of sterile precautions during surgical and medical care**
　Y62.0　**Failure of sterile precautions during surgical operation**
　Y62.1　**Failure of sterile precautions during infusion or transfusion**
　Y62.2　**Failure of sterile precautions during kidney dialysis and other perfusion**
　Y62.3　**Failure of sterile precautions during injection or immunization**
　Y62.4　**Failure of sterile precautions during endoscopic examination**
　Y62.5　**Failure of sterile precautions during heart catheterization**
　Y62.6　**Failure of sterile precautions during aspiration, puncture and other catheterization**
　Y62.8　**Failure of sterile precautions during other surgical and medical care**
　Y62.9　**Failure of sterile precautions during unspecified surgical and medical care**

● Y63　**Failure in dosage during surgical and medical care**
　Excludes2 accidental overdose of drug or wrong drug given in error (T36-T50)
　Y63.0　**Excessive amount of blood or other fluid given during transfusion or infusion**
　Y63.1　**Incorrect dilution of fluid used during infusion**
　Y63.2　**Overdose of radiation given during therapy**
　Y63.3　**Inadvertent exposure of patient to radiation during medical care**
　Y63.4　**Failure in dosage in electroshock or insulin-shock therapy**
　Y63.5　**Inappropriate temperature in local application and packing**
　Y63.6　**Underdosing and nonadministration of necessary drug, medicament or biological substance**
　Y63.8　**Failure in dosage during other surgical and medical care**
　Y63.9　**Failure in dosage during unspecified surgical and medical care**

● Y64　**Contaminated medical or biological substances**
　Y64.0　**Contaminated medical or biological substance, transfused or infused**
　Y64.1　**Contaminated medical or biological substance, injected or used for immunization**
　Y64.8　**Contaminated medical or biological substance administered by other means**
　Y64.9　**Contaminated medical or biological substance administered by unspecified means**
　　Administered contaminated medical or biological substance NOS

● Y65　**Other misadventures during surgical and medical care**
　Y65.0　**Mismatched blood in transfusion**
　Y65.1　**Wrong fluid used in infusion**
　Y65.2　**Failure in suture or ligature during surgical operation**
　Y65.3　**Endotracheal tube wrongly placed during anesthetic procedure**
　Y65.4　**Failure to introduce or to remove other tube or instrument**
● Y65.5　**Performance of wrong procedure (operation)**
　● Y65.51　**Performance of wrong procedure (operation) on correct patient**
　　Wrong device implanted into correct surgical site
　　Excludes1 performance of correct procedure (operation) on wrong side or body part (Y65.53)
　● Y65.52　**Performance of procedure (operation) on patient not scheduled for surgery**
　　Performance of procedure (operation) intended for another patient
　　Performance of procedure (operation) on wrong patient
　● Y65.53　**Performance of correct procedure (operation) on wrong side or body part**
　　Performance of correct procedure (operation) on wrong side
　　Performance of correct procedure (operation) on wrong site
　Y65.8　**Other specified misadventures during surgical and medical care**

　Y66　**Nonadministration of surgical and medical care**
　　Premature cessation of surgical and medical care
　　Excludes1 DNR status (Z66)
　　　palliative care (Z51.5)

　Y69　**Unspecified misadventure during surgical and medical care**

MEDICAL DEVICES ASSOCIATED WITH ADVERSE INCIDENTS IN DIAGNOSTIC AND THERAPEUTIC USE (Y70-Y82)

Includes breakdown or malfunction of medical devices (during use) (after implantation) (ongoing use)

Excludes1 misadventure to patients during surgical and medical care, classifiable to (Y62-Y69)
later complications following use of medical devices without breakdown or malfunctioning of device (Y83-Y84)

● Y70　**Anesthesiology devices associated with adverse incidents**
　Y70.0　**Diagnostic and monitoring anesthesiology devices associated with adverse incidents**
　Y70.1　**Therapeutic (nonsurgical) and rehabilitative anesthesiology devices associated with adverse incidents**
　Y70.2　**Prosthetic and other implants, materials and accessory anesthesiology devices associated with adverse incidents**
　Y70.3　**Surgical instruments, materials and anesthesiology devices (including sutures) associated with adverse incidents**
　Y70.8　**Miscellaneous anesthesiology devices associated with adverse incidents, not elsewhere classified**

● Y71   **Cardiovascular devices associated with adverse incidents**

    Y71.0   Diagnostic and monitoring cardiovascular devices associated with adverse incidents

    Y71.1   Therapeutic (nonsurgical) and rehabilitative cardiovascular devices associated with adverse incidents

    Y71.2   Prosthetic and other implants, materials and accessory cardiovascular devices associated with adverse incidents

    Y71.3   Surgical instruments, materials and cardiovascular devices (including sutures) associated with adverse incidents

    Y71.8   Miscellaneous cardiovascular devices associated with adverse incidents, not elsewhere classified

● Y72   **Otorhinolaryngological devices associated with adverse incidents**

    Y72.0   Diagnostic and monitoring otorhinolaryngological devices associated with adverse incidents

    Y72.1   Therapeutic (nonsurgical) and rehabilitative otorhinolaryngological devices associated with adverse incidents

    Y72.2   Prosthetic and other implants, materials and accessory otorhinolaryngological devices associated with adverse incidents

    Y72.3   Surgical instruments, materials and otorhinolaryngological devices (including sutures) associated with adverse incidents

    Y72.8   Miscellaneous otorhinolaryngological devices associated with adverse incidents, not elsewhere classified

● Y73   **Gastroenterology and urology devices associated with adverse incidents**

    Y73.0   Diagnostic and monitoring gastroenterology and urology devices associated with adverse incidents

    Y73.1   Therapeutic (nonsurgical) and rehabilitative gastroenterology and urology devices associated with adverse incidents

    Y73.2   Prosthetic and other implants, materials and accessory gastroenterology and urology devices associated with adverse incidents

    Y73.3   Surgical instruments, materials and gastroenterology and urology devices (including sutures) associated with adverse incidents

    Y73.8   Miscellaneous gastroenterology and urology devices associated with adverse incidents, not elsewhere classified

● Y74   **General hospital and personal-use devices associated with adverse incidents**

    Y74.0   Diagnostic and monitoring general hospital and personal-use devices associated with adverse incidents

    Y74.1   Therapeutic (nonsurgical) and rehabilitative general hospital and personal-use devices associated with adverse incidents

    Y74.2   Prosthetic and other implants, materials and accessory general hospital and personal-use devices associated with adverse incidents

    Y74.3   Surgical instruments, materials and general hospital and personal-use devices (including sutures) associated with adverse incidents

    Y74.8   Miscellaneous general hospital and personal-use devices associated with adverse incidents, not elsewhere classified

● Y75   **Neurological devices associated with adverse incidents**

    Y75.0   Diagnostic and monitoring neurological devices associated with adverse incidents

    Y75.1   Therapeutic (nonsurgical) and rehabilitative neurological devices associated with adverse incidents

    Y75.2   Prosthetic and other implants, materials and neurological devices associated with adverse incidents

    Y75.3   Surgical instruments, materials and neurological devices (including sutures) associated with adverse incidents

    Y75.8   Miscellaneous neurological devices associated with adverse incidents, not elsewhere classified

● Y76   **Obstetric and gynecological devices associated with adverse incidents**

    Y76.0   Diagnostic and monitoring obstetric and gynecological devices associated with adverse incidents

    Y76.1   Therapeutic (nonsurgical) and rehabilitative obstetric and gynecological devices associated with adverse incidents

    Y76.2   Prosthetic and other implants, materials and accessory obstetric and gynecological devices associated with adverse incidents

    Y76.3   Surgical instruments, materials and obstetric and gynecological devices (including sutures) associated with adverse incidents

    Y76.8   Miscellaneous obstetric and gynecological devices associated with adverse incidents, not elsewhere classified

● Y77   **Ophthalmic devices associated with adverse incidents**

    Y77.0   Diagnostic and monitoring ophthalmic devices associated with adverse incidents

    Y77.1   Therapeutic (nonsurgical) and rehabilitative ophthalmic devices associated with adverse incidents

    Y77.2   Prosthetic and other implants, materials and accessory ophthalmic devices associated with adverse incidents

    Y77.3   Surgical instruments, materials and ophthalmic devices (including sutures) associated with adverse incidents

    Y77.8   Miscellaneous ophthalmic devices associated with adverse incidents, not elsewhere classified

● Y78   **Radiological devices associated with adverse incidents**

    Y78.0   Diagnostic and monitoring radiological devices associated with adverse incidents

    Y78.1   Therapeutic (nonsurgical) and rehabilitative radiological devices associated with adverse incidents

    Y78.2   Prosthetic and other implants, materials and accessory radiological devices associated with adverse incidents

    Y78.3   Surgical instruments, materials and radiological devices (including sutures) associated with adverse incidents

    Y78.8   Miscellaneous radiological devices associated with adverse incidents, not elsewhere classified

● Y79   **Orthopedic devices associated with adverse incidents**

    Y79.0   Diagnostic and monitoring orthopedic devices associated with adverse incidents

    Y79.1   Therapeutic (nonsurgical) and rehabilitative orthopedic devices associated with adverse incidents

    Y79.2   Prosthetic and other implants, materials and accessory orthopedic devices associated with adverse incidents

    Y79.3   Surgical instruments, materials and orthopedic devices (including sutures) associated with adverse incidents

    Y79.8   Miscellaneous orthopedic devices associated with adverse incidents, not elsewhere classified

◀ New   ◀▦ Revised   ~~deleted~~ Deleted   **OGCR** Official Guidelines   X Assign placeholder X   ● Use Additional Character(s)

Excludes 1   Excludes 2   Includes   Use additional   Code first   Code also   Unspecified

● Y80   Physical medicine devices associated with adverse incidents

    Y80.0   Diagnostic and monitoring physical medicine devices associated with adverse incidents

    Y80.1   Therapeutic (nonsurgical) and rehabilitative physical medicine devices associated with adverse incidents

    Y80.2   Prosthetic and other implants, materials and accessory physical medicine devices associated with adverse incidents

    Y80.3   Surgical instruments, materials and physical medicine devices (including sutures) associated with adverse incidents

    Y80.8   Miscellaneous physical medicine devices associated with adverse incidents, not elsewhere classified

● Y81   General- and plastic-surgery devices associated with adverse incidents

    Y81.0   Diagnostic and monitoring general- and plastic-surgery devices associated with adverse incidents

    Y81.1   Therapeutic (nonsurgical) and rehabilitative general- and plastic-surgery devices associated with adverse incidents

    Y81.2   Prosthetic and other implants, materials and accessory general- and plastic-surgery devices associated with adverse incidents

    Y81.3   Surgical instruments, materials and general- and plastic-surgery devices (including sutures) associated with adverse incidents

    Y81.8   Miscellaneous general- and plastic-surgery devices associated with adverse incidents, not elsewhere classified

● Y82   Other and unspecified medical devices associated with adverse incidents

    Y82.8   Other medical devices associated with adverse incidents

    Y82.9   Unspecified medical devices associated with adverse incidents

SURGICAL AND OTHER MEDICAL PROCEDURES AS THE CAUSE OF ABNORMAL REACTION OF THE PATIENT, OR OF LATER COMPLICATION, WITHOUT MENTION OF MISADVENTURE AT THE TIME OF THE PROCEDURE (Y83-Y84)

| Excludes1 | misadventures to patients during surgical and medical care, classifiable to (Y62-Y69) |

● Y83   Surgical operation and other surgical procedures as the cause of abnormal reaction of the patient, or of later complication, without mention of misadventure at the time of the procedure

    Y83.0   Surgical operation with transplant of whole organ as the cause of abnormal reaction of the patient, or of later complication, without mention of misadventure at the time of the procedure

    Y83.1   Surgical operation with implant of artificial internal device as the cause of abnormal reaction of the patient, or of later complication, without mention of misadventure at the time of the procedure

    Y83.2   Surgical operation with anastomosis, bypass or graft as the cause of abnormal reaction of the patient, or of later complication, without mention of misadventure at the time of the procedure

    Y83.3   Surgical operation with formation of external stoma as the cause of abnormal reaction of the patient, or of later complication, without mention of misadventure at the time of the procedure

    Y83.4   Other reconstructive surgery as the cause of abnormal reaction of the patient, or of later complication, without mention of misadventure at the time of the procedure

    Y83.5   Amputation of limb(s) as the cause of abnormal reaction of the patient, or of later complication, without mention of misadventure at the time of the procedure

    Y83.6   Removal of other organ (partial) (total) as the cause of abnormal reaction of the patient, or of later complication, without mention of misadventure at the time of the procedure

    Y83.8   Other surgical procedures as the cause of abnormal reaction of the patient, or of later complication, without mention of misadventure at the time of the procedure

    Y83.9   Surgical procedure, unspecified as the cause of abnormal reaction of the patient, or of later complication, without mention of misadventure at the time of the procedure

● Y84   Other medical procedures as the cause of abnormal reaction of the patient, or of later complication, without mention of misadventure at the time of the procedure

    Y84.0   Cardiac catheterization as the cause of abnormal reaction of the patient, or of later complication, without mention of misadventure at the time of the procedure

    Y84.1   Kidney dialysis as the cause of abnormal reaction of the patient, or of later complication, without mention of misadventure at the time of the procedure

    Y84.2   Radiological procedure and radiotherapy as the cause of abnormal reaction of the patient, or of later complication, without mention of misadventure at the time of the procedure

    Y84.3   Shock therapy as the cause of abnormal reaction of the patient, or of later complication, without mention of misadventure at the time of the procedure

    Y84.4   Aspiration of fluid as the cause of abnormal reaction of the patient, or of later complication, without mention of misadventure at the time of the procedure

    Y84.5   Insertion of gastric or duodenal sound as the cause of abnormal reaction of the patient, or of later complication, without mention of misadventure at the time of the procedure

    Y84.6   Urinary catheterization as the cause of abnormal reaction of the patient, or of later complication, without mention of misadventure at the time of the procedure

    Y84.7   Blood-sampling as the cause of abnormal reaction of the patient, or of later complication, without mention of misadventure at the time of the procedure

    Y84.8   Other medical procedures as the cause of abnormal reaction of the patient, or of later complication, without mention of misadventure at the time of the procedure

    Y84.9   Medical procedure, unspecified as the cause of abnormal reaction of the patient, or of later complication, without mention of misadventure at the time of the procedure

SUPPLEMENTARY FACTORS RELATED TO CAUSES OF MORBIDITY CLASSIFIED ELSEWHERE (Y90-Y99)

Note: These categories may be used to provide supplementary information concerning causes of morbidity. They are not to be used for single-condition coding.

● Y90   Evidence of alcohol involvement determined by blood alcohol level

    Code first any associated alcohol related disorders (F10)

    Y90.0   Blood alcohol level of less than 20 mg/100 ml

    Y90.1   Blood alcohol level of 20-39 mg/100 ml

    Y90.2   Blood alcohol level of 40-59 mg/100 ml

    Y90.3   Blood alcohol level of 60-79 mg/100 ml

    Y90.4   Blood alcohol level of 80-99 mg/100 ml

    Y90.5   Blood alcohol level of 100-119 mg/100 ml

    Y90.6   Blood alcohol level of 120-199 mg/100 ml

    Y90.7   Blood alcohol level of 200-239 mg/100 ml

    Y90.8   Blood alcohol level of 240 mg/100 ml or more

    Y90.9   Presence of alcohol in blood, level not specified

CHAPTER 20 (V01-Y99)

OGCR Section I.C.20.b.

20.9 Place of Occurrence

Place of Occurrence Guideline

Codes from category Y92, Place of occurrence of the external cause, are secondary codes for use after other external cause codes to identify the location of the patient at the time of injury or other condition.

Generally, a place of occurrence code is assigned only once, at the initial encounter for treatment. However, in the rare instance that a new injury occurs during hospitalization, an additional place of occurrence code may be assigned. No 7th characters are used for Y92. Only one code from Y92 should be recorded on a medical record. A place of occurrence code should be used in conjunction with an activity code, Y93.

Do not use place of occurrence code Y92.9 if the place is not stated or is not applicable.

● **Y92**   **Place of occurrence of the external cause**

The following category is for use, when relevant, to identify the place of occurrence of the external cause. Use in conjunction with an activity code.

Place of occurrence should be recorded only at the initial encounter for treatment

● **Y92.0**   **Non-institutional (private) residence as the place of occurrence of the external cause**

    Excludes1   abandoned or derelict house (Y92.89)
                     home under construction but not yet occupied (Y92.6-)
                     institutional place of residence (Y92.1-)

● **Y92.00**   **Unspecified non-institutional (private) residence as the place of occurrence of the external cause**

    Y92.000   Kitchen of unspecified non-institutional (private) residence as the place of occurrence of the external cause

    Y92.001   Dining room of unspecified non-institutional (private) residence as the place of occurrence of the external cause

    Y92.002   Bathroom of unspecified non-institutional (private) residence single-family (private) house as the place of occurrence of the external cause

    Y92.003   Bedroom of unspecified non-institutional (private) residence as the place of occurrence of the external cause

    Y92.007   Garden or yard of unspecified non-institutional (private) residence as the place of occurrence of the external cause

    Y92.008   Other place in unspecified non-institutional (private) residence as the place of occurrence of the external cause

    Y92.009   Unspecified place in unspecified non-institutional (private) residence as the place of occurrence of the external cause
                Home (NOS) as the place of occurrence of the external cause

● **Y92.01**   **Single-family non-institutional (private) house as the place of occurrence of the external cause**
    Farmhouse as the place of occurrence of the external cause

    Excludes1   barn (Y92.71)
                 chicken coop or hen house (Y92.72)
                 farm field (Y92.73)
                 orchard (Y92.74)
                 single family mobile home or trailer (Y92.02-)
                 slaughter house (Y92.86)

    Y92.010   Kitchen of single-family (private) house as the place of occurrence of the external cause

    Y92.011   Dining room of single-family (private) house as the place of occurrence of the external cause

    Y92.012   Bathroom of single-family (private) house as the place of occurrence of the external cause

    Y92.013   Bedroom of single-family (private) house as the place of occurrence of the external cause

    Y92.014   Private driveway to single-family (private) house as the place of occurrence of the external cause

    Y92.015   Private garage of single-family (private) house as the place of occurrence of the external cause

    Y92.016   Swimming pool in single-family (private) house or garden as the place of occurrence of the external cause

    Y92.017   Garden or yard in single-family (private) house as the place of occurrence of the external cause

    Y92.018   Other place in single-family (private) house as the place of occurrence of the external cause

    Y92.019   Unspecified place in single-family (private) house as the place of occurrence of the external cause

● **Y92.02**   **Mobile home as the place of occurrence of the external cause**

    Y92.020   Kitchen in mobile home as the place of occurrence of the external cause

    Y92.021   Dining room in mobile home as the place of occurrence of the external cause

    Y92.022   Bathroom in mobile home as the place of occurrence of the external cause

    Y92.023   Bedroom in mobile home as the place of occurrence of the external cause

    Y92.024   Driveway of mobile home as the place of occurrence of the external cause

    Y92.025   Garage of mobile home as the place of occurrence of the external cause

    Y92.026   Swimming pool of mobile home as the place of occurrence of the external cause

    Y92.027   Garden or yard of mobile home as the place of occurrence of the external cause

    Y92.028   Other place in mobile home as the place of occurrence of the external cause

    Y92.029   Unspecified place in mobile home as the place of occurrence of the external cause

◀ New   ◀▥ Revised   ~~deleted~~ Deleted   **OGCR** Official Guidelines   X Assign placeholder X   ● Use Additional Character(s)

Excludes 1   Excludes 2   Includes   Use additional   Code first   Code also   Unspecified

● Y92.03   **Apartment as the place of occurrence of the external cause**
Condominium as the place of occurrence of the external cause
Co-op apartment as the place of occurrence of the external cause

Y92.030   Kitchen in apartment as the place of occurrence of the external cause

Y92.031   Bathroom in apartment as the place of occurrence of the external cause

Y92.032   Bedroom in apartment as the place of occurrence of the external cause

Y92.038   Other place in apartment as the place of occurrence of the external cause

Y92.039   Unspecified place in apartment as the place of occurrence of the external cause

● Y92.04   Boarding-house as the place of occurrence of the external cause

Y92.040   Kitchen in boarding-house as the place of occurrence of the external cause

Y92.041   Bathroom in boarding-house as the place of occurrence of the external cause

Y92.042   Bedroom in boarding-house as the place of occurrence of the external cause

Y92.043   Driveway of boarding-house as the place of occurrence of the external cause

Y92.044   Garage of boarding-house as the place of occurrence of the external cause

Y92.045   Swimming pool of boarding-house as the place of occurrence of the external cause

Y92.046   Garden or yard of boarding-house as the place of occurrence of the external cause

Y92.048   Other place in boarding-house as the place of occurrence of the external cause

Y92.049   Unspecified place in boarding-house as the place of occurrence of the external cause

● Y92.09   Other non-institutional residence as the place of occurrence of the external cause

Y92.090   Kitchen in other non-institutional residence as the place of occurrence of the external cause

Y92.091   Bathroom in other non-institutional residence as the place of occurrence of the external cause

Y92.092   Bedroom in other non-institutional residence as the place of occurrence of the external cause

Y92.093   Driveway of other non-institutional residence as the place of occurrence of the external cause

Y92.094   Garage of other non-institutional residence as the place of occurrence of the external cause

Y92.095   Swimming pool of other non-institutional residence as the place of occurrence of the external cause

Y92.096   Garden or yard of other non-institutional residence as the place of occurrence of the external cause

Y92.098   Other place in other non-institutional residence as the place of occurrence of the external cause

Y92.099   Unspecified place in other non-institutional residence as the place of occurrence of the external cause

● Y92.1   Institutional (nonprivate) residence as the place of occurrence of the external cause

Y92.10   Unspecified residential institution as the place of occurrence of the external cause

● Y92.11   Children's home and orphanage as the place of occurrence of the external cause

Y92.110   Kitchen in children's home and orphanage as the place of occurrence of the external cause

Y92.111   Bathroom in children's home and orphanage as the place of occurrence of the external cause

Y92.112   Bedroom in children's home and orphanage as the place of occurrence of the external cause

Y92.113   Driveway of children's home and orphanage as the place of occurrence of the external cause

Y92.114   Garage of children's home and orphanage as the place of occurrence of the external cause

Y92.115   Swimming pool of children's home and orphanage as the place of occurrence of the external cause

Y92.116   Garden or yard of children's home and orphanage as the place of occurrence of the external cause

Y92.118   Other place in children's home and orphanage as the place of occurrence of the external cause

Y92.119   Unspecified place in children's home and orphanage as the place of occurrence of the external cause

● Y92.12   Nursing home as the place of occurrence of the external cause
Home for the sick as the place of occurrence of the external cause
Hospice as the place of occurrence of the external cause

Y92.120   Kitchen in nursing home as the place of occurrence of the external cause

Y92.121   Bathroom in nursing home as the place of occurrence of the external cause

Y92.122   Bedroom in nursing home as the place of occurrence of the external cause

Y92.123   Driveway of nursing home as the place of occurrence of the external cause

Y92.124   Garage of nursing home as the place of occurrence of the external cause

Y92.125   Swimming pool of nursing home as the place of occurrence of the external cause

Y92.126   Garden or yard of nursing home as the place of occurrence of the external cause

Y92.128   Other place in nursing home as the place of occurrence of the external cause

Y92.129   Unspecified place in nursing home as the place of occurrence of the external cause

◀ New   ◀▥ Revised   ~~deleted~~ Deleted   OGCR Official Guidelines   X Assign placeholder X   ● Use Additional Character(s)
Excludes 1   Excludes 2   Includes   Use additional   Code first   Code also   Unspecified

CHAPTER 20 (V01-Y99)

1533

CHAPTER 20 (V01-Y99)

● Y92.13   Military base as the place of occurrence of the external cause
            Excludes1   military training grounds (Y92.83)

    Y92.130   Kitchen on military base as the place of occurrence of the external cause

    Y92.131   Mess hall on military base as the place of occurrence of the external cause

    Y92.133   Barracks on military base as the place of occurrence of the external cause

    Y92.135   Garage on military base as the place of occurrence of the external cause

    Y92.136   Swimming pool on military base as the place of occurrence of the external cause

    Y92.137   Garden or yard on military base as the place of occurrence of the external cause

    Y92.138   Other place on military base as the place of occurrence of the external cause

    Y92.139   Unspecified place military base as the place of occurrence of the external cause

● Y92.14   Prison as the place of occurrence of the external cause

    Y92.140   Kitchen in prison as the place of occurrence of the external cause

    Y92.141   Dining room in prison as the place of occurrence of the external cause

    Y92.142   Bathroom in prison as the place of occurrence of the external cause

    Y92.143   Cell of prison as the place of occurrence of the external cause

    Y92.146   Swimming pool of prison as the place of occurrence of the external cause

    Y92.147   Courtyard of prison as the place of occurrence of the external cause

    Y92.148   Other place in prison as the place of occurrence of the external cause

    Y92.149   Unspecified place in prison as the place of occurrence of the external cause

● Y92.15   Reform school as the place of occurrence of the external cause

    Y92.150   Kitchen in reform school as the place of occurrence of the external cause

    Y92.151   Dining room in reform school as the place of occurrence of the external cause

    Y92.152   Bathroom in reform school as the place of occurrence of the external cause

    Y92.153   Bedroom in reform school as the place of occurrence of the external cause

    Y92.154   Driveway of reform school as the place of occurrence of the external cause

    Y92.155   Garage of reform school as the place of occurrence of the external cause

    Y92.156   Swimming pool of reform school as the place of occurrence of the external cause

    Y92.157   Garden or yard of reform school as the place of occurrence of the external cause

    Y92.158   Other place in reform school as the place of occurrence of the external cause

    Y92.159   Unspecified place in reform school as the place of occurrence of the external cause

● Y92.16   School dormitory as the place of occurrence of the external cause
            Excludes1   reform school as the place of occurrence of the external cause (Y92.15-)
            school buildings and grounds as the place of occurrence of the external cause (Y92.2-)
            school sports and athletic areas as the place of occurrence of the external cause (Y92.3-)

    Y92.160   Kitchen in school dormitory as the place of occurrence of the external cause

    Y92.161   Dining room in school dormitory as the place of occurrence of the external cause

    Y92.162   Bathroom in school dormitory as the place of occurrence of the external cause

    Y92.163   Bedroom in school dormitory as the place of occurrence of the external cause

    Y92.168   Other place in school dormitory as the place of occurrence of the external cause

    Y92.169   Unspecified place in school dormitory as the place of occurrence of the external cause

● Y92.19   Other specified residential institution as the place of occurrence of the external cause

    Y92.190   Kitchen in other specified residential institution as the place of occurrence of the external cause

    Y92.191   Dining room in other specified residential institution as the place of occurrence of the external cause

    Y92.192   Bathroom in other specified residential institution as the place of occurrence of the external cause

    Y92.193   Bedroom in other specified residential institution as the place of occurrence of the external cause

    Y92.194   Driveway of other specified residential institution as the place of occurrence of the external cause

    Y92.195   Garage of other specified residential institution as the place of occurrence of the external cause

    Y92.196   Pool of other specified residential institution as the place of occurrence of the external cause

    Y92.197   Garden or yard of other specified residential institution as the place of occurrence of the external cause

    Y92.198   Other place in other specified residential institution as the place of occurrence of the external cause

    Y92.199   Unspecified place in other specified residential institution as the place of occurrence of the external cause

● **Y92.2** **School, other institution and public administrative area as the place of occurrence of the external cause**
   Building and adjacent grounds used by the general public or by a particular group of the public

   | Excludes1 | building under construction as the place of occurrence of the external cause (Y92.6) |

   residential institution as the place of occurrence of the external cause (Y92.1)
   school dormitory as the place of occurrence of the external cause (Y92.16-)
   sports and athletics area of schools as the place of occurrence of the external cause (Y92.3-)

● **Y92.21** **School (private) (public) (state) as the place of occurrence of the external cause**

   Y92.210 Daycare center as the place of occurrence of the external cause

   Y92.211 Elementary school as the place of occurrence of the external cause
      Kindergarten as the place of occurrence of the external cause

   Y92.212 Middle school as the place of occurrence of the external cause

   Y92.213 High school as the place of occurrence of the external cause

   Y92.214 College as the place of occurrence of the external cause
      University as the place of occurrence of the external cause

   Y92.215 Trade school as the place of occurrence of the external cause

   Y92.218 Other school as the place of occurrence of the external cause

   Y92.219 Unspecified school as the place of occurrence of the external cause

Y92.22 **Religious institution as the place of occurrence of the external cause**
   Church as the place of occurrence of the external cause
   Mosque as the place of occurrence of the external cause
   Synagogue as the place of occurrence of the external cause

● **Y92.23** **Hospital as the place of occurrence of the external cause**

   | Excludes1 | ambulatory (outpatient) health services establishments (Y92.53-) |

   home for the sick as the place of occurrence of the external cause (Y92.12-)
   hospice as the place of occurrence of the external cause (Y92.12-)
   nursing home as the place of occurrence of the external cause (Y92.12-)

   Y92.230 Patient room in hospital as the place of occurrence of the external cause

   Y92.231 Patient bathroom in hospital as the place of occurrence of the external cause

   Y92.232 Corridor of hospital as the place of occurrence of the external cause

   Y92.233 Cafeteria of hospital as the place of occurrence of the external cause

   Y92.234 Operating room of hospital as the place of occurrence of the external cause

   Y92.238 Other place in hospital as the place of occurrence of the external cause

   Y92.239 Unspecified place in hospital as the place of occurrence of the external cause

● **Y92.24** **Public administrative building as the place of occurrence of the external cause**

   Y92.240 Courthouse as the place of occurrence of the external cause

   Y92.241 Library as the place of occurrence of the external cause

   Y92.242 Post office as the place of occurrence of the external cause

   Y92.243 City hall as the place of occurrence of the external cause

   Y92.248 Other public administrative building as the place of occurrence of the external cause

● **Y92.25** **Cultural building as the place of occurrence of the external cause**

   Y92.250 Art gallery as the place of occurrence of the external cause

   Y92.251 Museum as the place of occurrence of the external cause

   Y92.252 Music hall as the place of occurrence of the external cause

   Y92.253 Opera house as the place of occurrence of the external cause

   Y92.254 Theater (live) as the place of occurrence of the external cause

   Y92.258 Other cultural public building as the place of occurrence of the external cause

Y92.26 **Movie house or cinema as the place of occurrence of the external cause**

Y92.29 **Other specified public building as the place of occurrence of the external cause**
   Assembly hall as the place of occurrence of the external cause
   Clubhouse as the place of occurrence of the external cause

● **Y92.3** **Sports and athletics area as the place of occurrence of the external cause**

● **Y92.31** **Athletic court as the place of occurrence of the external cause**

   | Excludes1 | tennis court in private home or garden (Y92.09) |

   Y92.310 Basketball court as the place of occurrence of the external cause

   Y92.311 Squash court as the place of occurrence of the external cause

   Y92.312 Tennis court as the place of occurrence of the external cause

   Y92.318 Other athletic court as the place of occurrence of the external cause

● **Y92.32** **Athletic field as the place of occurrence of the external cause**

   Y92.320 Baseball field as the place of occurrence of the external cause

   Y92.321 Football field as the place of occurrence of the external cause

   Y92.322 Soccer field as the place of occurrence of the external cause

   Y92.328 Other athletic field as the place of occurrence of the external cause
      Cricket field as the place of occurrence of the external cause
      Hockey field as the place of occurrence of the external cause

● Y92.33   **Skating rink as the place of occurrence of the external cause**

   Y92.330   **Ice skating rink (indoor) (outdoor) as the place of occurrence of the external cause**

   Y92.331   **Roller skating rink as the place of occurrence of the external cause**

Y92.34   **Swimming pool (public) as the place of occurrence of the external cause**

   | Excludes1 | swimming pool in private home or garden (Y92.016)

Y92.39   **Other specified sports and athletic area as the place of occurrence of the external cause**

   Golf-course as the place of occurrence of the external cause

   Gymnasium as the place of occurrence of the external cause

   Riding-school as the place of occurrence of the external cause

   Stadium as the place of occurrence of the external cause

● Y92.4   **Street, highway and other paved roadways as the place of occurrence of the external cause**

   | Excludes1 | private driveway of residence (Y92.014, Y92.024, Y92.043, Y92.093, Y92.113, Y92.123, Y92.154, Y92.194)

● Y92.41   **Street and highway as the place of occurrence of the external cause**

   Y92.410   **Unspecified street and highway as the place of occurrence of the external cause**

     Road NOS as the place of occurrence of the external cause

   Y92.411   **Interstate highway as the place of occurrence of the external cause**

     Freeway as the place of occurrence of the external cause

     Motorway as the place of occurrence of the external cause

   Y92.412   **Parkway as the place of occurrence of the external cause**

   Y92.413   **State road as the place of occurrence of the external cause**

   Y92.414   **Local residential or business street as the place of occurrence of the external cause**

   Y92.415   **Exit ramp or entrance ramp of street or highway as the place of occurrence of the external cause**

● Y92.48   **Other paved roadways as the place of occurrence of the external cause**

   Y92.480   **Sidewalk as the place of occurrence of the external cause**

   Y92.481   **Parking lot as the place of occurrence of the external cause**

   Y92.482   **Bike path as the place of occurrence of the external cause**

   Y92.488   **Other paved roadways as the place of occurrence of the external cause**

● Y92.5   **Trade and service area as the place of occurrence of the external cause**

   | Excludes1 | garage in private home (Y92.015) schools and other public administration buildings (Y92.2-)

● Y92.51   **Private commercial establishments as the place of occurrence of the external cause**

   Y92.510   **Bank as the place of occurrence of the external cause**

   Y92.511   **Restaurant or café as the place of occurrence of the external cause**

   Y92.512   **Supermarket, store or market as the place of occurrence of the external cause**

   Y92.513   **Shop (commercial) as the place of occurrence of the external cause**

● Y92.52   **Service areas as the place of occurrence of the external cause**

   Y92.520   **Airport as the place of occurrence of the external cause**

   Y92.521   **Bus station as the place of occurrence of the external cause**

   Y92.522   **Railway station as the place of occurrence of the external cause**

   Y92.523   **Highway rest stop as the place of occurrence of the external cause**

   Y92.524   **Gas station as the place of occurrence of the external cause**

     Petroleum station as the place of occurrence of the external cause

     Service station as the place of occurrence of the external cause

● Y92.53   **Ambulatory health services establishments as the place of occurrence of the external cause**

   Y92.530   **Ambulatory surgery center as the place of occurrence of the external cause**

     Outpatient surgery center, including that connected with a hospital as the place of occurrence of the external cause

     Same day surgery center, including that connected with a hospital as the place of occurrence of the external cause

   Y92.531   **Health care provider office as the place of occurrence of the external cause**

     Physician office as the place of occurrence of the external cause

   Y92.532   **Urgent care center as the place of occurrence of the external cause**

   Y92.538   **Other ambulatory health services establishments as the place of occurrence of the external cause**

Y92.59   **Other trade areas as the place of occurrence of the external cause**

   Office building as the place of occurrence of the external cause

   Casino as the place of occurrence of the external cause

   Garage (commercial) as the place of occurrence of the external cause

   Hotel as the place of occurrence of the external cause

   Radio or television station as the place of occurrence of the external cause

   Shopping mall as the place of occurrence of the external cause

   Warehouse as the place of occurrence of the external cause

◄ New   ◄▥ Revised   ~~deleted~~ Deleted   OGCR Official Guidelines   X Assign placeholder X   ● Use Additional Character(s)

| Excludes 1 | | Excludes 2 | | Includes | | Use additional | | Code first | | Code also | | Unspecified |

● Y92.6 **Industrial and construction area as the place of occurrence of the external cause**

    Y92.61 **Building [any] under construction as the place of occurrence of the external cause**

    Y92.62 **Dock or shipyard as the place of occurrence of the external cause**
        Dockyard as the place of occurrence of the external cause
        Dry dock as the place of occurrence of the external cause
        Shipyard as the place of occurrence of the external cause

    Y92.63 **Factory as the place of occurrence of the external cause**
        Factory building as the place of occurrence of the external cause
        Factory premises as the place of occurrence of the external cause
        Industrial yard as the place of occurrence of the external cause

    Y92.64 **Mine or pit as the place of occurrence of the external cause**
        Mine as the place of occurrence of the external cause

    Y92.65 **Oil rig as the place of occurrence of the external cause**
        Pit (coal) (gravel) (sand) as the place of occurrence of the external cause

    Y92.69 **Other specified industrial and construction area as the place of occurrence of the external cause**
        Gasworks as the place of occurrence of the external cause
        Power-station (coal) (nuclear) (oil) as the place of occurrence of the external cause
        Tunnel under construction as the place of occurrence of the external cause
        Workshop as the place of occurrence of the external cause

● Y92.7 **Farm as the place of occurrence of the external cause**
    Ranch as the place of occurrence of the external cause
    Excludes1 farmhouse and home premises of farm (Y92.01-)

    Y92.71 **Barn as the place of occurrence of the external cause**

    Y92.72 **Chicken coop as the place of occurrence of the external cause**
        Hen house as the place of occurrence of the external cause

    Y92.73 **Farm field as the place of occurrence of the external cause**

    Y92.74 **Orchard as the place of occurrence of the external cause**

    Y92.79 **Other farm location as the place of occurrence of the external cause**

● Y92.8 **Other places as the place of occurrence of the external cause**

    ● Y92.81 **Transport vehicle as the place of occurrence of the external cause**
        Excludes1 transport accidents (V00-V99)

      Y92.810 **Car as the place of occurrence of the external cause**
      Y92.811 **Bus as the place of occurrence of the external cause**
      Y92.812 **Truck as the place of occurrence of the external cause**
      Y92.813 **Airplane as the place of occurrence of the external cause**
      Y92.814 **Boat as the place of occurrence of the external cause**
      Y92.815 **Train as the place of occurrence of the external cause**
      Y92.816 **Subway car as the place of occurrence of the external cause**
      Y92.818 **Other transport vehicle as the place of occurrence of the external cause**

    ● Y92.82 **Wilderness area**
      Y92.820 **Desert as the place of occurrence of the external cause**
      Y92.821 **Forest as the place of occurrence of the external cause**
      Y92.828 **Other wilderness area as the place of occurrence of the external cause**
        Swamp as the place of occurrence of the external cause
        Mountain as the place of occurrence of the external cause
        Marsh as the place of occurrence of the external cause
        Prairie as the place of occurrence of the external cause

    ● Y92.83 **Recreation area as the place of occurrence of the external cause**
      Y92.830 **Public park as the place of occurrence of the external cause**
      Y92.831 **Amusement park as the place of occurrence of the external cause**
      Y92.832 **Beach as the place of occurrence of the external cause**
        Seashore as the place of occurrence of the external cause
      Y92.833 **Campsite as the place of occurrence of the external cause**
      Y92.834 **Zoological garden (zoo) as the place of occurrence of the external cause**
      Y92.838 **Other recreation area as the place of occurrence of the external cause**

    Y92.84 **Military training ground as the place of occurrence of the external cause**

    Y92.85 **Railroad track as the place of occurrence of the external cause**

    Y92.86 **Slaughter house as the place of occurrence of the external cause**

    Y92.89 **Other specified places as the place of occurrence of the external cause**
        Derelict house as the place of occurrence of the external cause

Y92.9 **Unspecified place or not applicable**

OGCR See Section I.C.20.c.

Activity code

● **Y93   Activity codes**

> **Note:** Category Y93 is provided for use to indicate the activity of the person seeking healthcare for an injury or health condition, such as a heart attack while shoveling snow, which resulted from, or was contributed to, by the activity. These codes are appropriate for use for both acute injuries, such as those from chapter 19, and conditions that are due to the long-term, cumulative effects of an activity, such as those from chapter 13. They are also appropriate for use with external cause codes for cause and intent if identifying the activity provides additional information on the event. These codes should be used in conjunction with codes for external cause status (Y99) and place of occurrence (Y92).
>
> **This section contains the following broad activity categories:**
>
> Y93.0   Activities involving walking and running
>
> Y93.1   Activities involving water and water craft
>
> Y93.2   Activities involving ice and snow
>
> Y93.3   Activities involving climbing, rappelling, and jumping off
>
> Y93.4   Activities involving dancing and other rhythmic movement
>
> Y93.5   Activities involving other sports and athletics played individually
>
> Y93.6   Activities involving other sports and athletics played as a team or group
>
> Y93.7   Activities involving other specified sports and athletics
>
> Y93.A   Activities involving other cardiorespiratory exercise
>
> Y93.B   Activities involving other muscle strengthening exercises
>
> Y93.C   Activities involving computer technology and electronic devices
>
> Y93.D   Activities involving arts and handcrafts
>
> Y93.E   Activities involving personal hygiene and interior property and clothing maintenance
>
> Y93.F   Activities involving caregiving
>
> Y93.G   Activities involving food preparation, cooking and grilling
>
> Y93.H   Activities involving exterior property and land maintenance, building and construction
>
> Y93.I   Activities involving roller coasters and other types of external motion
>
> Y93.J   Activities involving playing musical instrument
>
> Y93.K   Activities involving animal care
>
> Y93.8   Activities, other specified
>
> Y93.9   Activity, unspecified

● **Y93.0   Activities involving walking and running**

> Excludes1   Activity, walking an animal (Y93.K1)
> Activity, walking or running on a treadmill (Y93.A1)

Y93.01   **Activity, walking, marching and hiking**
> Activity, walking, marching and hiking on level or elevated terrain
>
> Excludes1   activity, mountain climbing (Y93.31)

Y93.02   **Activity, running**

● **Y93.1   Activities involving water and water craft**

> Excludes1   activities involving ice (Y93.2-)

Y93.11   **Activity, swimming**

Y93.12   **Activity, springboard and platform diving**

Y93.13   **Activity, water polo**

Y93.14   **Activity, water aerobics and water exercise**

Y93.15   **Activity, underwater diving and snorkeling**
> Activity, SCUBA diving

Y93.16   **Activity, rowing, canoeing, kayaking, rafting and tubing**
> Activity, canoeing, kayaking, rafting and tubing in calm and turbulent water

Y93.17   **Activity, water skiing and wake boarding**

Y93.18   **Activity, surfing, windsurfing and boogie boarding**
> Activity, water sliding

Y93.19   **Activity, other involving water and watercraft**
> Activity involving water NOS
> Activity, parasailing
> Activity, water survival training and testing

● **Y93.2   Activities involving ice and snow**

> Excludes1   activity, shoveling ice and snow (Y93.H1)

Y93.21   **Activity, ice skating**
> Activity, figure skating (singles) (pairs)
> Activity, ice dancing
>
> Excludes1   activity, ice hockey (Y93.22)

Y93.22   **Activity, ice hockey**

Y93.23   **Activity, snow (alpine) (downhill) skiing, snow boarding, sledding, tobogganing and snow tubing**
> Excludes1   activity, cross country skiing (Y93.24)

Y93.24   **Activity, cross country skiing**
> Activity, nordic skiing

Y93.29   **Activity, other activity involving ice and snow**
> Activity, activity involving ice and snow NOS

● **Y93.3   Activities involving climbing, rappelling and jumping off**

> Excludes1   activity, hiking on level or elevated terrain (Y93.01)
> activity, jumping rope (Y93.56)
> activity, trampoline jumping (Y93.44)

Y93.31   **Activity, mountain climbing, rock climbing and wall climbing**

Y93.32   **Activity, rappelling**

Y93.33   **Activity, BASE jumping**
> Activity, building, Antenna, Span, Earth jumping

Y93.34   **Activity, bungee jumping**

Y93.35   **Activity, hang gliding**

Y93.39   **Activity, other activity involving climbing, rappelling and jumping off**

● **Y93.4   Activities involving dancing and other rhythmic movement**

> Excludes1   activity, martial arts (Y93.75)

Y93.41   **Activity, dancing**

Y93.42   **Activity, yoga**

Y93.43   **Activity, gymnastics**
> Activity, rhythmic gymnastics
>
> Excludes1   activity, trampolining (Y93.44)

Y93.44   **Activity, trampolining**

Y93.45   **Activity, cheerleading**

Y93.49   **Activity, other involving dancing and other rhythmic movements**

◄ New   ◄▥ Revised   ~~deleted~~ Deleted   OGCR Official Guidelines   X Assign placeholder X   ● Use Additional Character(s)

Excludes 1   Excludes 2   Includes   Use additional   Code first   Code also   Unspecified

● **Y93.5**   **Activities involving other sports and athletics played individually**

> Excludes1   activity, dancing (Y93.41)
> activity, gymnastic (Y93.43)
> activity, trampolining (Y93.44)
> activity, yoga (Y93.42)

Y93.51   **Activity, roller skating (inline) and skateboarding**

Y93.52   **Activity, horseback riding**

Y93.53   **Activity, golf**

Y93.54   **Activity, bowling**

Y93.55   **Activity, bike riding**

Y93.56   **Activity, jumping rope**

Y93.57   **Activity, non-running track and field events**

> Excludes1   activity, running (any form) (Y93.02)

Y93.59   **Activity, other involving other sports and athletics played individually**

> Excludes1   activities involving climbing, rappelling, and jumping (Y93.3-)
> activities involving ice and snow (Y93.2-)
> activities involving walking and running (Y93.0-)
> activities involving water and watercraft (Y93.1-)

● **Y93.6**   **Activities involving other sports and athletics played as a team or group**

> Excludes1   activity, ice hockey (Y93.22)
> activity, water polo (Y93.13)

Y93.61   **Activity, American tackle football**
     Activity, football NOS

Y93.62   **Activity, American flag or touch football**

Y93.63   **Activity, rugby**

Y93.64   **Activity, baseball**
     Activity, softball

Y93.65   **Activity, lacrosse and field hockey**

Y93.66   **Activity, soccer**

Y93.67   **Activity, basketball**

Y93.68   **Activity, volleyball (beach) (court)**

Y93.6A   **Activity, physical games generally associated with school recess, summer camp and children**
     Activity, capture the flag
     Activity, dodge ball
     Activity, four square
     Activity, kickball

Y93.69   **Activity, other involving other sports and athletics played as a team or group**
     Cricket

● **Y93.7**   **Activities involving other specified sports and athletics**

Y93.71   **Activity, boxing**

Y93.72   **Activity, wrestling**

Y93.73   **Activity, racquet and hand sports**
     Activity, handball
     Activity, racquetball
     Activity, squash
     Activity, tennis

Y93.74   **Activity, frisbee**
     Activity, ultimate frisbee

Y93.75   **Activity, martial arts**
     Activity, combatives

Y93.79   **Activity, other specified sports and athletics**

> Excludes1   sports and athletics activities specified in categories Y93.0-Y93.6

● **Y93.A**   **Activities involving other cardiorespiratory exercise**
     Activities involving physical training

Y93.A1   **Activity, exercise machines primarily for cardiorespiratory conditioning**
     Activity, elliptical and stepper machines
     Activity, stationary bike
     Activity, treadmill

Y93.A2   **Activity, calisthenics**
     Activity, jumping jacks
     Activity, warm up and cool down

Y93.A3   **Activity, aerobic and step exercise**

Y93.A4   **Activity, circuit training**

Y93.A5   **Activity, obstacle course**
     Activity, challenge course
     Activity, confidence course

Y93.A6   **Activity, grass drills**
     Activity, guerilla drills

Y93.A9   **Activity, other involving other cardiorespiratory exercise**

> Excludes1   activities involving cardiorespiratory exercise specified in categories Y93.0-Y93.7

● **Y93.B**   **Activity involving other muscle strengthening exercises**

Y93.B1   **Activity, exercise machines primarily for muscle strengthening**

Y93.B2   **Activity, push-ups, pull-ups, sit-ups**

Y93.B3   **Activity, free weights**
     Activity, barbells
     Activity, dumbbells

Y93.B4   **Activity, pilates**

Y93.B9   **Activity, other involving other muscle strengthening exercises**

> Excludes1   activities involving muscle strengthening specified in categories Y93.0-Y93.A

● **Y93.C**   **Activities involving computer technology and electronic devices**

> Excludes1   activity, electronic musical keyboard or instruments (Y93.J-)

Y93.C1   **Activity, computer keyboarding**
     Activity, electronic game playing using keyboard or other stationary device

Y93.C2   **Activity, hand held interactive electronic device**
     Activity, cellular telephone and communication device
     Activity, electronic game playing using interactive device

> Excludes1   activity, electronic game playing using keyboard or other stationary device (Y93.C1)

Y93.C9   **Activity, other involving computer technology and electronic devices**

● **Y93.D**   **Activities involving arts and handcrafts**

> Excludes1   activities involving playing musical instrument (Y93.J-)

Y93.D1   **Knitting and crocheting**

Y93.D2   **Sewing**

Y93.D3   **Furniture building and finishing**
     Furniture repair

Y93.D9   **Activity, other involving arts and handcrafts**

◀ New   ◀■■ Revised   ~~deleted~~ Deleted   **OGCR** Official Guidelines   X Assign placeholder X   ● Use Additional Character(s)

| Excludes 1 | Excludes 2 | Includes | Use additional | Code first | Code also | Unspecified |

● **Y93.E** **Activities involving personal hygiene and interior property and clothing maintenance**
> **Excludes1**   activities involving cooking and grilling (Y93.G-)
> activities involving exterior property and land maintenance, building and construction (Y93.H-)
> activity involving caregiving (Y93.F-)
> activity, dishwashing (Y93.G1)
> activity, food preparation (Y93.G1)
> activity, gardening (Y93.H2)

    Y93.E1   **Activity, personal bathing and showering**

    Y93.E2   **Activity, laundry**

    Y93.E3   **Activity, vacuuming**

    Y93.E4   **Activity, ironing**

    Y93.E5   **Activity, floor mopping and cleaning**

    Y93.E6   **Activity, residential relocation**
> Activity, packing up and unpacking involved in moving to a new residence

    Y93.E8   **Activity, other personal hygiene activity**

    Y93.E9   **Activity, other household maintenance**

● **Y93.F** **Activities involving person providing caregiving**
> Activity involving the provider of caregiving

    Y93.F1   **Activity, caregiving involving bathing**

    Y93.F2   **Activity, caregiving involving lifting**

    Y93.F9   **Activity, other caregiving**

● **Y93.G** **Activities involving food preparation, cooking and grilling**

    Y93.G1   **Activity, food preparation and clean up**
> Activity, dishwashing

    Y93.G2   **Activity, grilling and smoking food**

    Y93.G3   **Activity, cooking and baking**
> Activity, use of stove, oven and microwave oven

    Y93.G9   **Activity, other activity involving cooking and grilling**

● **Y93.H** **Activities involving property and land maintenance, building and construction**

    Y93.H1   **Activity, digging, shoveling and raking**
> Activity, dirt digging
> Activity, raking leaves
> Activity, snow shoveling

    Y93.H2   **Activity, gardening and landscaping**
> Activity, pruning, trimming shrubs, weeding

    Y93.H3   **Activity, building and construction**

    Y93.H9   **Activity, other activity involving property and land maintenance, building and construction**

● **Y93.I** **Activities involving roller coasters and other types of external motion**

    Y93.I1   **Activity, rollercoaster riding**

    Y93.I9   **Activity, other involving external motion**

● **Y93.J** **Activities involving playing musical instrument**
> Activity involving playing electric musical instrument

    Y93.J1   **Activity, piano playing**
> Activity, musical keyboard (electronic) playing

    Y93.J2   **Activity, drum and other percussion instrument playing**

    Y93.J3   **Activity, string instrument playing**

    Y93.J4   **Activity, winds and brass instrument playing**

● **Y93.K** **Activities involving animal care**
> **Excludes1**   activity, horseback riding (Y93.52)

    Y93.K1   **Activity, walking an animal**

    Y93.K2   **Activity, milking an animal**

    Y93.K3   **Activity, grooming and shearing an animal**

    Y93.K9   **Activity, other activity involving animal care**

● **Y93.8** **Other activity**

    Y93.81   **Activity, refereeing a sports activity**

    Y93.82   **Activity, spectator at an event**

    Y93.83   **Activity, rough housing and horseplay**

    Y93.84   **Activity, sleeping**

    Y93.89   **Activity, other specified**

● **Y93.9** **Activity, unspecified**

 Y95 **Nosocomial condition**

● **Y99** **External cause status**
> **Note:** A single code from category Y99 should be used in conjunction with the external cause code(s) assigned to a record to indicate the status of the person at the time the event occurred.

    Y99.0   **Civilian activity done for income or pay**
> Civilian activity done for financial or other compensation
> **Excludes1**   military activity (Y99.1)
> volunteer activity (Y99.2)

    Y99.1   **Military activity**
> **Excludes1**   activity of off duty military personnel (Y99.8)

    Y99.2   **Volunteer activity**
> **Excludes1**   activity of child or other family member assisting in compensated work of other family member (Y99.8)

    Y99.8   **Other external cause status**
> Activity NEC
> Activity of child or other family member assisting in compensated work of other family member
> Hobby not done for income
> Leisure activity
> Off-duty activity of military personnel
> Recreation or sport not for income or while a student
> Student activity
> **Excludes1**   civilian activity done for income or compensation (Y99.0)
> military activity (Y99.1)

    Y99.9   **Unspecified external cause status**

OGCR See Section I.C.21.

CHAPTER 21

FACTORS INFLUENCING HEALTH STATUS AND CONTACT WITH HEALTH SERVICES (Z00-Z99)

Note: Z codes represent reasons for encounters. A corresponding procedure code must accompany a Z code if a procedure is performed. Categories Z00-Z99 are provided for occasions when circumstances other than a disease, injury or external cause classifiable to categories A00-Y89 are recorded as 'diagnoses' or 'problems.' This can arise in two main ways:

(a) When a person who may or may not be sick encounters the health services for some specific purpose, such as to receive limited care or service for a current condition, to donate an organ or tissue, to receive prophylactic vaccination (immunization), or to discuss a problem which is in itself not a disease or injury.

(b) When some circumstance or problem is present which influences the person's health status but is not in itself a current illness or injury.

This chapter contains the following blocks:

Z00-Z13	Persons encountering health services for examination
Z14-Z15	Genetic carrier and genetic susceptibility to disease
Z16	Resistance to antimicrobial drugs
Z17	Estrogen receptor status
Z18	Retained foreign body fragments
Z20-Z28	Persons with potential health hazards related to communicable diseases
Z30-Z39	Persons encountering health services in circumstances related to reproduction
Z40-Z53	Encounters for other specific health care
Z55-Z65	Persons with potential health hazards related to socioeconomic and psychosocial circumstances
Z66	Do not resuscitate status
Z67	Blood type
Z68	Body mass index (BMI)
Z69-Z76	Persons encountering health services in other circumstances
Z77-Z99	Persons with potential health hazards related to family and personal history and certain conditions influencing health status

PERSONS ENCOUNTERING HEALTH SERVICES FOR EXAMINATIONS (Z00-Z13)

Note: Nonspecific abnormal findings disclosed at the time of these examinations are classified to categories R70-R94.

Excludes1 examinations related to pregnancy and reproduction (Z30-Z36, Z39.-)

● **Z00 Encounter for general examination without complaint, suspected or reported diagnosis**

Excludes1 encounter for examination for administrative purposes (Z02.-)

Excludes2 encounter for pre-procedural examinations (Z01.81-)
special screening examinations (Z11-Z13)

● **Z00.0 Encounter for general adult medical examination**
Encounter for adult periodic examination (annual) (physical) and any associated laboratory and radiologic examinations

Excludes1 encounter for examination of sign or symptom - code to sign or symptom
general health check-up of infant or child (Z00.12.-)

Z00.00 Encounter for general adult medical examination without abnormal findings
Encounter for adult health check-up NOS

Z00.01 Encounter for general adult medical examination with abnormal findings
Use additional code to identify abnormal findings

● **Z00.1 Encounter for newborn, infant and child health examinations**

● **Z00.11 Newborn health examination**
Health check for child under 29 days old
Use additional code to identify any abnormal findings

Excludes1 health check for child over 28 days old (Z00.12-)

Z00.110 Health examination for newborn under 8 days old
Health check for newborn under 8 days old

Z00.111 Health examination for newborn 8 to 28 days old
Health check for newborn 8 to 28 days old
Newborn weight check

● **Z00.12 Encounter for routine child health examination**
Encounter for development testing of infant or child
Health check (routine) for child over 28 days old

Excludes1 health check for child under 29 days old (Z00.11-)
health supervision of foundling or other healthy infant or child (Z76.1-Z76.2)
newborn health examination (Z00.11-)

Z00.121 Encounter for routine child health examination with abnormal findings
Use additional code to identify abnormal findings

Z00.129 Encounter for routine child health examination without abnormal findings
Encounter for routine child health examination NOS

Z00.2 Encounter for examination for period of rapid growth in childhood

Z00.3 Encounter for examination for adolescent development state
Encounter for puberty development state

Z00.5 Encounter for examination of potential donor of organ and tissue

Z00.6 Encounter for examination for normal comparison and control in clinical research program
Examination of participant or control in clinical research program

● **Z00.7 Encounter for examination for period of delayed growth in childhood**

Z00.70 Encounter for examination for period of delayed growth in childhood without abnormal findings

Z00.71 Encounter for examination for period of delayed growth in childhood with abnormal findings
Use additional code to identify abnormal findings

Z00.8 Encounter for other general examination
Encounter for health examination in population surveys

CHAPTER 21 (Z00-Z99)

◀ New	◀▥ Revised	~~deleted~~ Deleted	OGCR Official Guidelines	X Assign placeholder X ● Use Additional Character(s)
Excludes 1	Excludes 2	Includes	Use additional	Code first Code also Unspecified

● **Z01   Encounter for other special examination without complaint, suspected or reported diagnosis**

Includes   routine examination of specific system

Note: Codes from category Z01 represent the reason for the encounter. A separate procedure code is required to identify any examinations or procedures performed.

Excludes1   encounter for examination for administrative purposes (Z02.-)
encounter for examination for suspected conditions, proven not to exist (Z03.-)
encounter for laboratory and radiologic examinations as a component of general medical examinations (Z00.0-)
encounter for laboratory, radiologic and imaging examinations for sign(s) and symptom(s) - code to the sign(s) or symptom(s)

Excludes2   screening examinations (Z11-Z13)

● **Z01.0   Encounter for examination of eyes and vision**

Excludes1   examination for driving license (Z02.4)

Z01.00   Encounter for examination of eyes and vision without abnormal findings
Encounter for examination of eyes and vision NOS

Z01.01   Encounter for examination of eyes and vision with abnormal findings
Use additional code to identify abnormal findings

● **Z01.1   Encounter for examination of ears and hearing**

Z01.10   Encounter for examination of ears and hearing without abnormal findings
Encounter for examination of ears and hearing NOS

● **Z01.11   Encounter for examination of ears and hearing with abnormal findings**

Z01.110   Encounter for hearing examination following failed hearing screening

Z01.118   Encounter for examination of ears and hearing with other abnormal findings
Use additional code to identify abnormal findings

Z01.12   Encounter for hearing conservation and treatment

● **Z01.2   Encounter for dental examination and cleaning**

Z01.20   Encounter for dental examination and cleaning without abnormal findings
Encounter for dental examination and cleaning NOS

Z01.21   Encounter for dental examination and cleaning with abnormal findings
Use additional code to identify abnormal findings

● **Z01.3   Encounter for examination of blood pressure**

Z01.30   Encounter for examination of blood pressure without abnormal findings
Encounter for examination of blood pressure NOS

Z01.31   Encounter for examination of blood pressure with abnormal findings
Use additional code to identify abnormal findings

● **Z01.4   Encounter for gynecological examination**

Excludes2   pregnancy examination or test (Z32.0-)
routine examination for contraceptive maintenance (Z30.4-)

● **Z01.41   Encounter for routine gynecological examination**
Encounter for general gynecological examination with or without cervical smear
Encounter for gynecological examination (general) (routine) NOS
Encounter for pelvic examination (annual) (periodic)
Use additional code:
for screening for human papillomavirus, if applicable (Z11.51)
for screening vaginal pap smear, if applicable (Z12.72)
to identify acquired absence of uterus, if applicable (Z90.71-)

Excludes1   gynecologic examination status-post hysterectomy for malignant condition (Z08)
screening cervical pap smear not a part of a routine gynecological examination (Z12.4)

Z01.411   Encounter for gynecological examination (general) (routine) with abnormal findings

Z01.419   Encounter for gynecological examination (general) (routine) without abnormal findings
Use additional code to identify abnormal findings

Z01.42   Encounter for cervical smear to confirm findings of recent normal smear following initial abnormal smear

● **Z01.8   Encounter for other specified special examinations**

● **Z01.81   Encounter for preprocedural examinations**
Encounter for preoperative examinations
Encounter for radiological and imaging examinations as part of preprocedural examination

Z01.810   Encounter for preprocedural cardiovascular examination

Z01.811   Encounter for preprocedural respiratory examination

Z01.812   Encounter for preprocedural laboratory examination
Blood and urine tests prior to treatment or procedure

Z01.818   Encounter for other preprocedural examination
Encounter for preprocedural examination NOS
Encounter for examinations prior to antineoplastic chemotherapy

Z01.82   Encounter for allergy testing

Excludes1   encounter for antibody response examination (Z01.84)

Z01.83   Encounter for blood typing
Encounter for Rh typing

Z01.84   Encounter for antibody response examination
Encounter for immunity status testing

Excludes1   encounter for allergy testing (Z01.82)

Z01.89   Encounter for other specified special examinations

◀ New   ◀▦ Revised   ~~deleted~~ Deleted   **OGCR** Official Guidelines   X Assign placeholder X   ● Use Additional Character(s)

Excludes 1   Excludes 2   Includes   Use additional   Code first   Code also   Unspecified

● **Z02   Encounter for administrative examination**

     Z02.0   Encounter for examination for admission to educational institution
         Encounter for examination for admission to preschool (education)
         Encounter for examination for re-admission to school following illness or medical treatment

     Z02.1   Encounter for pre-employment examination

     Z02.2   Encounter for examination for admission to residential institution
         | **Excludes1** | examination for admission to prison (Z02.89) |

     Z02.3   Encounter for examination for recruitment to armed forces

     Z02.4   Encounter for examination for driving license

     Z02.5   Encounter for examination for participation in sport
         | **Excludes1** | blood-alcohol and blood-drug test (Z02.83) |

     Z02.6   Encounter for examination for insurance purposes

●   **Z02.7   Encounter for issue of medical certificate**
         | **Excludes1** | encounter for general medical examination (Z00-Z01, Z02.0-Z02.6, Z02.8-Z02.9) |

         Z02.71   Encounter for disability determination
            Encounter for issue of medical certificate of incapacity
            Encounter for issue of medical certificate of invalidity

         Z02.79   Encounter for issue of other medical certificate

●   **Z02.8   Encounter for other administrative examinations**

         Z02.81   Encounter for paternity testing

         Z02.82   Encounter for adoption services

         Z02.83   Encounter for blood-alcohol and blood-drug test
            | Use additional | code for findings of alcohol or drugs in blood (R78.-) |

         Z02.89   Encounter for other administrative examinations
            Encounter for examination for admission to prison
            Encounter for examination for admission to summer camp
            Encounter for immigration examination
            Encounter for naturalization examination
            Encounter for premarital examination
            | **Excludes1** | health supervision of foundling or other healthy infant or child (Z76.1-Z76.2) |

     Z02.9   Encounter for administrative examinations, unspecified

---

OGCR Section II.C.21.c.6.

21.2.2. Observation

There are two observation Z code categories. They are for use in very limited circumstances when a person is being observed for a suspected condition that is ruled out. The observation codes are not for use if an injury or illnesses or any signs or symptoms related to the suspected condition are present. In such cases the diagnosis/symptom code is used with the corresponding external cause code.

The observation codes are to be used as principal diagnosis only. Additional codes may be used in addition to the observation code but only if they are unrelated to the suspected condition being observed.

Codes from subcategory Z03.7 Encounter for suspected maternal and fetal conditions ruled out, may either be used as a first listed or as an additional code assignment depending on the case. They are for use in very limited circumstances on a maternal record when an encounter is for a suspected maternal or fetal condition that is ruled out during that encounter (for example, a maternal or fetal condition may be suspected due to an abnormal test result). These codes should not be used when the condition is confirmed. In those cases, the confirmed condition should be coded. In addition, these codes are not for use if an illness or any signs or symptoms related to the suspected condition or problem are present. In such cases the diagnosis/symptom code is used.

Additional codes may be used in addition to the code from subcategory Z03.7, but only if they are unrelated to the suspected condition being evaluated.

Codes from subcategory Z03.7 may not be used for encounters for antenatal screening of mother. *See Section I.C.21. Screening.*

For encounters for suspected fetal condition that are inconclusive following testing and evaluation, assign the appropriate code from category O35, O36, O40 or O41.

The observation Z code categories:

Z03   Encounter for medical observation for suspected diseases and conditions ruled out

Z04   Encounter for examination and observation for other reasons

Except: Z04.9, Encounter for examination and observation for unspecified reason

● **Z03   Encounter for medical observation for suspected diseases and conditions ruled out**
     This category is to be used when a person without a diagnosis is suspected of having an abnormal condition, without signs or symptoms, which requires study, but after examination and observation, is ruled out. This category is also for use for administrative and legal observation status.
     | **Excludes1** | contact with and (suspected) exposures hazardous to health (Z77.-) |
         newborn observation for suspected condition, ruled out (P00-P04)
         person with feared complaint in whom no diagnosis is made (Z71.1)
         signs or symptoms under study - code to signs or symptoms

     Z03.6   Encounter for observation for suspected toxic effect from ingested substance ruled out
         Encounter for observation for suspected adverse effect from drug
         Encounter for observation for suspected poisoning

CHAPTER 21 (Z00-Z99)

● Z03.7　Encounter for suspected maternal and fetal conditions ruled out

Encounter for suspected maternal and fetal conditions not found

> **Excludes1**　known or suspected fetal anomalies affecting management of mother, not ruled out (O26.-, O35.-, O36.-, O40.-, O41.-)

Z03.71　Encounter for suspected problem with amniotic cavity and membrane ruled out

Encounter for suspected oligohydramnios ruled out

Encounter for suspected polyhydramnios ruled out

Z03.72　Encounter for suspected placental problem ruled out

Z03.73　Encounter for suspected fetal anomaly ruled out

Z03.74　Encounter for suspected problem with fetal growth ruled out

Z03.75　Encounter for suspected cervical shortening ruled out

Z03.79　Encounter for other suspected maternal and fetal conditions ruled out

● Z03.8　Encounter for observation for other suspected diseases and conditions ruled out

● Z03.81　Encounter for observation for suspected exposure to biological agents ruled out

Z03.810　Encounter for observation for suspected exposure to anthrax ruled out

Z03.818　Encounter for observation for suspected exposure to other biological agents ruled out

Z03.89　Encounter for observation for other suspected diseases and conditions ruled out

● Z04　Encounter for examination and observation for other reasons

> **Includes**　encounter for examination for medicolegal reasons
>
> This category is to be used when a person without a diagnosis is suspected of having an abnormal condition, without signs or symptoms, which requires study, but after examination and observation, is ruled-out. This category is also for use for administrative and legal observation status.

Z04.1　Encounter for examination and observation following transport accident

> **Excludes1**　encounter for examination and observation following work accident (Z04.2)

Z04.2　Encounter for examination and observation following work accident

Z04.3　Encounter for examination and observation following other accident

● Z04.4　Encounter for examination and observation following alleged rape

Encounter for examination and observation of victim following alleged rape

Encounter for examination and observation of victim following alleged sexual abuse

Z04.41　Encounter for examination and observation following alleged adult rape

Suspected adult rape, ruled out

Suspected adult sexual abuse, ruled out

Z04.42　Encounter for examination and observation following alleged child rape

Suspected child rape, ruled out

Suspected child sexual abuse, ruled out

Z04.6　Encounter for general psychiatric examination, requested by authority

● Z04.7　Encounter for examination and observation following alleged physical abuse

Z04.71　Encounter for examination and observation following alleged adult physical abuse

Suspected adult physical abuse, ruled out

> **Excludes1**　confirmed case of adult physical abuse (T74.-)
>
> encounter for examination and observation following alleged adult sexual abuse (Z04.41)
>
> suspected case of adult physical abuse, not ruled out (T76.-)

Z04.72　Encounter for examination and observation following alleged child physical abuse

Suspected child physical abuse, ruled out

> **Excludes1**　confirmed case of child physical abuse (T74.-)
>
> encounter for examination and observation following alleged child sexual abuse (Z04.42)
>
> suspected case of child physical abuse, not ruled out (T76.-)

Z04.8　Encounter for examination and observation for other specified reasons

Encounter for examination and observation for request for expert evidence

Z04.9　Encounter for examination and observation for unspecified reason

Encounter for observation NOS

OGCR　See Section II.C.21.c.7.

> The follow-up codes are used to explain continuing surveillance following completed treatment of a disease, condition, or injury. They imply that the condition has been fully treated and no longer exists. They should not be confused with aftercare codes, or injury codes with 7th character "D," that explain ongoing care of a healing condition or its sequelae. Follow-up codes may be used in conjunction with history codes to provide the full picture of the healed condition and its treatment. The follow-up code is sequenced first, followed by the history code.
>
> A follow-up code may be used to explain multiple visits. Should a condition be found to have recurred on the follow-up visit, then the diagnosis code for the condition should be assigned in place of the follow-up code.
>
> The follow-up Z code categories:
>
> Z08　Encounter for follow-up examination after completed treatment for malignant neoplasm
>
> Z09　Encounter for follow-up examination after completed treatment for conditions other than malignant neoplasm
>
> Z39　Encounter for maternal postpartum care and examination

Z08　Encounter for follow-up examination after completed treatment for malignant neoplasm

Medical surveillance following completed treatment

> **Use additional** code to identify any acquired absence of organs (Z90.-)
>
> **Use additional** code to identify the personal history of malignant neoplasm (Z85.-)
>
> **Excludes1**　aftercare following medical care (Z43-Z49, Z51)

Z09　Encounter for follow-up examination after completed treatment for conditions other than malignant neoplasm

Medical surveillance following completed treatment

> **Use additional** code to identify any applicable history of disease code (Z86.-. Z87.-)
>
> **Excludes1**　aftercare following medical care (Z43-Z49, Z51)
>
> surveillance of contraception (Z30.4-)
>
> surveillance of prosthetic and other medical devices (Z44-Z46)

◀ New　　⬅ Revised　　deleted Deleted　　**OGCR** Official Guidelines　　X Assign placeholder X　　● Use Additional Character(s)

Excludes 1　　Excludes 2　　Includes　　Use additional　　Code first　　Code also　　Unspecified

- **Z11   Encounter for screening for infectious and parasitic diseases**

  Screening is the testing for disease or disease precursors in asymptomatic individuals so that early detection and treatment can be provided for those who test positive for the disease.

  > **Excludes1**   encounter for diagnostic examination - code to sign or symptom

  Z11.0   Encounter for screening for intestinal infectious diseases

  Z11.1   Encounter for screening for respiratory tuberculosis

  Z11.2   Encounter for screening for other bacterial diseases

  Z11.3   Encounter for screening for infections with a predominantly sexual mode of transmission

  > **Excludes2**   encounter for screening for human immunodeficiency virus [HIV] (Z11.4)
  > encounter for screening for human papillomavirus (Z11.51)

  Z11.4   Encounter for screening for human immunodeficiency virus [HIV]

- **Z11.5   Encounter for screening for other viral diseases**

  > **Excludes2**   encounter for screening for viral intestinal disease (Z11.0)

  Z11.51   Encounter for screening for human papillomavirus (HPV)

  Z11.59   Encounter for screening for other viral diseases

  Z11.6   Encounter for screening for other protozoal diseases and helminthiases

  Diseases or infestations caused by parasitic worms

  > **Excludes2**   encounter for screening for protozoal intestinal disease (Z11.0)

  Z11.8   Encounter for screening for other infectious and parasitic diseases

  Encounter for screening for chlamydia
  Encounter for screening for rickettsial
  Encounter for screening for spirochetal
  Encounter for screening for mycoses

  Z11.9   Encounter for screening for infectious and parasitic diseases, unspecified

- **Z12   Encounter for screening for malignant neoplasms**

  Screening is the testing for disease or disease precursors in asymptomatic individuals so that early detection and treatment can be provided for those who test positive for the disease.

  Use additional code to identify any family history of malignant neoplasm (Z80.-)

  > **Excludes1**   encounter for diagnostic examination - code to sign or symptom

  Z12.0   Encounter for screening for malignant neoplasm of stomach

- **Z12.1   Encounter for screening for malignant neoplasm of intestinal tract**

  Z12.10   Encounter for screening for malignant neoplasm of intestinal tract, unspecified

  Z12.11   Encounter for screening for malignant neoplasm of colon

  Encounter for screening colonoscopy NOS

  Z12.12   Encounter for screening for malignant neoplasm of rectum

  Z12.13   Encounter for screening for malignant neoplasm of small intestine

  Z12.2   Encounter for screening for malignant neoplasm of respiratory organs

- **Z12.3   Encounter for screening for malignant neoplasm of breast**

  Z12.31   Encounter for screening mammogram for malignant neoplasm of breast

  > **Excludes1**   inconclusive mammogram (R92.2)

  Z12.39   Encounter for other screening for malignant neoplasm of breast

  Z12.4   Encounter for screening for malignant neoplasm of cervix

  Encounter for screening pap smear for malignant neoplasm of cervix

  > **Excludes1**   encounter for screening for human papillomavirus (Z11.51)
  > when screening is part of general gynecological examination (Z01.4-)

  Z12.5   Encounter for screening for malignant neoplasm of prostate

  Z12.6   Encounter for screening for malignant neoplasm of bladder

- **Z12.7   Encounter for screening for malignant neoplasm of other genitourinary organs**

  Z12.71   Encounter for screening for malignant neoplasm of testis

  Z12.72   Encounter for screening for malignant neoplasm of vagina

  Vaginal pap smear status - post hysterectomy for non-malignant condition

  Use additional code to identify acquired absence of uterus (Z90.71-)

  > **Excludes1**   vaginal pap smear status - post hysterectomy for malignant conditions (Z08)

  Z12.73   Encounter for screening for malignant neoplasm of ovary

  Z12.79   Encounter for screening for malignant neoplasm of other genitourinary organs

- **Z12.8   Encounter for screening for malignant neoplasm of other sites**

  Z12.81   Encounter for screening for malignant neoplasm of oral cavity

  Z12.82   Encounter for screening for malignant neoplasm of nervous system

Z12.83   Encounter for screening for malignant neoplasm of skin

Z12.89   Encounter for screening for malignant neoplasm of other sites

Z12.9   Encounter for screening for malignant neoplasm, site unspecified

● Z13   Encounter for screening for other diseases and disorders
Screening is the testing for disease or disease precursors in asymptomatic individuals so that early detection and treatment can be provided for those who test positive for the disease.

Excludes1   encounter for diagnostic examination - code to sign or symptom

Z13.0   Encounter for screening for diseases of the blood and blood-forming organs and certain disorders involving the immune mechanism

Z13.1   Encounter for screening for diabetes mellitus

● Z13.2   Encounter for screening for nutritional, metabolic and other endocrine disorders

Z13.21   Encounter for screening for nutritional disorder

● Z13.22   Encounter for screening for metabolic disorder

Z13.220   Encounter for screening for lipid disorders
Encounter for screening for cholesterol level
Encounter for screening for hypercholesterolemia
Encounter for screening for hyperlipidemia

Z13.228   Encounter for screening for other metabolic disorders

Z13.29   Encounter for screening for other suspected endocrine disorder

Excludes1   encounter for screening for diabetes mellitus (Z13.1)

Z13.4   Encounter for screening for certain developmental disorders in childhood
Encounter for screening for developmental handicaps in early childhood

Excludes1   routine development testing of infant or child (Z00.1-)

Z13.5   Encounter for screening for eye and ear disorders

Excludes2   encounter for general hearing examination (Z01.1-)
encounter for general vision examination (Z01.0-)

Z13.6   Encounter for screening for cardiovascular disorders

● Z13.7   Encounter for screening for genetic and chromosomal anomalies

Excludes1   genetic testing for procreative management (Z31.4-)

Z13.71   Encounter for nonprocreative screening for genetic disease carrier status

Z13.79   Encounter for other screening for genetic and chromosomal anomalies

● Z13.8   Encounter for screening for other specified diseases and disorders

Excludes2   screening for malignant neoplasms (Z12.-)

● Z13.81   Encounter for screening for digestive system disorders

Z13.810   Encounter for screening for upper gastrointestinal disorder

Z13.811   Encounter for screening for lower gastrointestinal disorder

Excludes1   encounter for screening for intestinal infectious disease (Z11.0)

Z13.818   Encounter for screening for other digestive system disorders

● Z13.82   Encounter for screening for musculoskeletal disorder

Z13.820   Encounter for screening for osteoporosis

Z13.828   Encounter for screening for other musculoskeletal disorder

Z13.83   Encounter for screening for respiratory disorder NEC

Excludes1   encounter for screening for respiratory tuberculosis (Z11.1)

Z13.84   Encounter for screening for dental disorders

● Z13.85   Encounter for screening for nervous system disorders

Z13.850   Encounter for screening for traumatic brain injury

Z13.858   Encounter for screening for other nervous system disorders

Z13.88   Encounter for screening for disorder due to exposure to contaminants

Excludes1   those exposed to contaminants without suspected disorders (Z57-Z77.-)

Z13.89   Encounter for screening for other disorder
Encounter for screening for genitourinary disorders

Z13.9   Encounter for screening, unspecified

GENETIC CARRIER AND GENETIC SUSCEPTIBILITY TO DISEASE (Z14-Z15)

● Z14   Genetic carrier

● Z14.0   Hemophilia A carrier

Z14.01   Asymptomatic hemophilia A carrier

Z14.02   Symptomatic hemophilia A carrier

Z14.1   Cystic fibrosis carrier

Z14.8   Genetic carrier of other disease

● Z15   Genetic susceptibility to disease

Excludes1   chromosomal anomalies (Q90-Q99)

Includes   confirmed abnormal gene

Use additional code, if applicable, for any associated family history of the disease (Z80-Z84)

● Z15.0   Genetic susceptibility to malignant neoplasm

Code first if applicable, any current malignant neoplasm (C00-C75, C81-C96)

Use additional code, if applicable, for any personal history of malignant neoplasm (Z85.-)

Z15.01   Genetic susceptibility to malignant neoplasm of breast

Z15.02   Genetic susceptibility to malignant neoplasm of ovary

Z15.03   Genetic susceptibility to malignant neoplasm of prostate

Z15.04   Genetic susceptibility to malignant neoplasm of endometrium

Z15.09   Genetic susceptibility to other malignant neoplasm

● Z15.8   Genetic susceptibility to other disease

Z15.81   Genetic susceptibility to multiple endocrine neoplasia [MEN]

Excludes1   multiple endocrine neoplasia [MEN] syndromes (E31.2-)

Z15.89   Genetic susceptibility to other disease

◄ New   ◄▥ Revised   ~~deleted~~ Deleted   OGCR Official Guidelines   X Assign placeholder X   ● Use Additional Character(s)

Excludes 1   Excludes 2   Includes   Use additional   Code first   Code also   Unspecified

RESISTANCE TO ANTIMICROBIAL DRUGS (Z16)

● **Z16   Resistance to antimicrobial drugs**

Note: The codes in this category are provided for use as additional codes to identify the resistance and non-responsiveness of a condition to antimicrobial drugs.

Code first the infection

Excludes1   Methicillin resistant Staphylococcus aureus infection (A49.02)
Methicillin resistant Staphylococcus aureus infection in diseases classified elsewhere (B95.62)
Methicillin resistant Staphylococcus aureus pneumonia (J15.212)
Sepsis due to Methicillin resistant Staphylococcus aureus (A41.02)

● **Z16.1   Resistance to beta lactam antibiotics**

Z16.10   Resistance to unspecified beta lactam antibiotics

Z16.11   Resistance to penicillins
Resistance to amoxicillin
Resistance to ampicillin

Z16.12   Extended spectrum beta lactamase (ESBL) resistance

Z16.19   Resistance to other specified beta lactam antibiotics
Resistance to cephalosporins

● **Z16.2   Resistance to other antibiotics**

Z16.20   Resistance to unspecified antibiotic
Resistance to antibiotics NOS

Z16.21   Resistance to vancomycin

Z16.22   Resistance to vancomycin related antibiotics

Z16.23   Resistance to quinolones and fluoroquinolones

Z16.24   Resistance to multiple antibiotics

Z16.29   Resistance to other single specified antibiotic
Resistance to aminoglycosides
Resistance to macrolides
Resistance to sulfonamides
Resistance to tetracyclines

● **Z16.3   Resistance to other antimicrobial drugs**

Excludes1   resistance to antibiotics (Z16.1-, Z16.2-)

Z16.30   Resistance to unspecified antimicrobial drugs
Drug resistance NOS

Z16.31   Resistance to antiparasitic drug(s)
Resistance to quinine and related compounds

Z16.32   Resistance to antifungal drug(s)

Z16.33   Resistance to antiviral drug(s)

● **Z16.34   Resistance to antimycobacterial drug(s)**
Resistance to tuberculostatics

Z16.341   Resistance to single antimycobacterial drug
Resistance to antimycobacterial drug NOS

Z16.342   Resistance to multiple antimycobacterial drugs

Z16.35   Resistance to multiple antimicrobial drugs

Excludes1   Resistance to multiple antibiotics only (Z16.24)

Z16.39   Resistance to other specified antimicrobial drug

ESTROGEN RECEPTOR STATUS (Z17)

● **Z17   Estrogen receptor status**

Code first malignant neoplasm of breast (C50.-)

Z17.0   Estrogen receptor positive status [ER+]

Z17.1   Estrogen receptor negative status [ER-]

RETAINED FOREIGN BODY FRAGMENTS (Z18)

● **Z18   Retained foreign body fragments**

Includes   embedded fragment (status)
embedded splinter (status)
retained foreign body status

Excludes1   artificial joint prosthesis status (Z96.6-)
foreign body accidentally left during a procedure (T81.5-)
foreign body entering through orifice (T15-T19)
in situ cardiac device (Z95.-)
organ or tissue replaced by means other than transplant (Z96.-, Z97.-)
organ or tissue replaced by transplant (Z94.-)
personal history of retained foreign body fully removed Z87.821
superficial foreign body (non-embedded splinter) - code to superficial foreign body, by site

● **Z18.0   Retained radioactive fragments**

Z18.01   Retained depleted uranium fragments

Z18.09   Other retained radioactive fragments
Other retained depleted isotope fragments
Retained nontherapeutic radioactive fragments

● **Z18.1   Retained metal fragments**

Excludes1   retained radioactive metal fragments (Z18.01-Z18.09)

Z18.10   Retained metal fragments, unspecified
Retained metal fragment NOS

Z18.11   Retained magnetic metal fragments

Z18.12   Retained nonmagnetic metal fragments

Z18.2   Retained plastic fragments
Acrylics fragments
Diethylhexylphthalates fragments
Isocyanate fragments

● **Z18.3   Retained organic fragments**

Z18.31   Retained animal quills or spines

Z18.32   Retained tooth

Z18.33   Retained wood fragments

Z18.39   Other retained organic fragments

● **Z18.8   Other specified retained foreign body**

Z18.81   Retained glass fragments

Z18.83   Retained stone or crystalline fragments
Retained concrete or cement fragments

Z18.89   Other specified retained foreign body fragments

Z18.9   Retained foreign body fragments, unspecified material

PERSONS WITH POTENTIAL HEALTH HAZARDS RELATED TO COMMUNICABLE DISEASES (Z20-Z28)

● **Z20   Contact with and (suspected) exposure to communicable diseases**

Excludes1   carrier of infectious disease (Z22.-)
diagnosed current infectious or parasitic disease - see Alphabetic Index

Excludes2   personal history of infectious and parasitic diseases (Z86.1-)

● **Z20.0   Contact with and (suspected) exposure to intestinal infectious diseases**

Z20.01   Contact with and (suspected) exposure to intestinal infectious diseases due to Escherichia coli (E. coli)

Z20.09   Contact with and (suspected) exposure to other intestinal infectious diseases

Z20.1   Contact with and (suspected) exposure to tuberculosis

Z20.2   Contact with and (suspected) exposure to infections with a predominantly sexual mode of transmission

Z20.3   Contact with and (suspected) exposure to rabies

CHAPTER 21 (Z00-Z99)

CHAPTER 21 (Z00-Z99)

Z20.4　Contact with and (suspected) exposure to rubella

Z20.5　Contact with and (suspected) exposure to viral hepatitis

Z20.6　Contact with and (suspected) exposure to human immunodeficiency virus [HIV]

> **Excludes1**　asymptomatic human immunodeficiency virus [HIV] (Z21)
> HIV infection status (Z21)

Z20.7　Contact with and (suspected) exposure to pediculosis, acariasis and other infestations

● Z20.8　Contact with and (suspected) exposure to other communicable diseases

　● Z20.81　Contact with and (suspected) exposure to other bacterial communicable diseases

　　Z20.810　Contact with and (suspected) exposure to anthrax

　　Z20.811　Contact with and (suspected) exposure to meningococcus

　　Z20.818　Contact with and (suspected) exposure to other bacterial communicable diseases

　● Z20.82　Contact with and (suspected) exposure to other viral communicable diseases

　　Z20.820　Contact with and (suspected) exposure to varicella

　　Z20.828　Contact with and (suspected) exposure to other viral communicable diseases

　Z20.89　Contact with and (suspected) exposure to other communicable diseases

Z20.9　Contact with and (suspected) exposure to unspecified communicable disease

Z21　Asymptomatic human immunodeficiency virus [HIV] infection status

　HIV positive NOS

　Code first Human immunodeficiency virus [HIV] disease complicating pregnancy, childbirth and the puerperium, if applicable (O98.7-)

> **Excludes1**　acquired immunodeficiency syndrome (B20)
> contact with human immunodeficiency virus [HIV] (Z20.6)
> exposure to human immunodeficiency virus [HIV] (Z20.6)
> human immunodeficiency virus [HIV] disease (B20)
> inconclusive laboratory evidence of human immunodeficiency virus [HIV] (R75)

● Z22　Carrier of infectious disease

> **Includes**　colonization status
> suspected carrier

Z22.0　Carrier of typhoid

Z22.1　Carrier of other intestinal infectious diseases

Z22.2　Carrier of diphtheria

● Z22.3　Carrier of other specified bacterial diseases

　Z22.31　Carrier of bacterial disease due to meningococci

　● Z22.32　Carrier of bacterial disease due to staphylococci

　　Z22.321　Carrier or suspected carrier of Methicillin susceptible Staphylococcus aureus
　　　MSSA colonization

　　Z22.322　Carrier or suspected carrier of Methicillin resistant Staphylococcus aureus
　　　MRSA colonization

　Z22.33　Carrier of bacterial disease due to streptococci

　　Z22.330　Carrier of Group B streptococcus

　　Z22.338　Carrier of other streptococcus

　Z22.39　Carrier of other specified bacterial diseases

Z22.4　Carrier of infections with a predominantly sexual mode of transmission

● Z22.5　Carrier of viral hepatitis

　Z22.50　Carrier of unspecified viral hepatitis

　Z22.51　Carrier of viral hepatitis B
　　Hepatitis B surface antigen [HBsAg] carrier

　Z22.52　Carrier of viral hepatitis C

　Z22.59　Carrier of other viral hepatitis

Z22.6　Carrier of human T-lymphotropic virus type-1 [HTLV-1] infection

Z22.8　Carrier of other infectious diseases

Z22.9　Carrier of infectious disease, unspecified

Z23　Encounter for immunization

　Code first any routine childhood examination

　Note: Procedure codes are required to identify the types of immunizations given.

● Z28　Immunization not carried out and underimmunization status

> **Includes**　vaccination not carried out

● Z28.0　Immunization not carried out because of contraindication

　Z28.01　Immunization not carried out because of acute illness of patient

　Z28.02　Immunization not carried out because of chronic illness or condition of patient

　Z28.03　Immunization not carried out because of immune compromised state of patient

　Z28.04　Immunization not carried out because of patient allergy to vaccine or component

　Z28.09　Immunization not carried out because of other contraindication

Z28.1　Immunization not carried out because of patient decision for reasons of belief or group pressure
　Immunization not carried out because of religious belief

● Z28.2　Immunization not carried out because of patient decision for other and unspecified reason

　Z28.20　Immunization not carried out because of patient decision for unspecified reason

　Z28.21　Immunization not carried out because of patient refusal

　Z28.29　Immunization not carried out because of patient decision for other reason

Z28.3　Underimmunization status
　Delinquent immunization status
　Lapsed immunization schedule status

● Z28.8　Immunization not carried out for other reason

　Z28.81　Immunization not carried out due to patient having had the disease

　Z28.82　Immunization not carried out because of caregiver refusal
　　Immunization not carried out because of guardian refusal
　　Immunization not carried out because of parent refusal

> **Excludes1**　immunization not carried out because of caregiver refusal because of religious belief (Z28.1)

　Z28.89　Immunization not carried out for other reason

Z28.9　Immunization not carried out for unspecified reason

◀ New　⧏⧏⧏ Revised　d̶e̶l̶e̶t̶e̶d̶ Deleted　**OGCR** Official Guidelines　X Assign placeholder X　● Use Additional Character(s)

Excludes 1　Excludes 2　Includes　Use additional　Code first　Code also　Unspecified

PERSONS ENCOUNTERING HEALTH SERVICES IN CIRCUMSTANCES RELATED TO REPRODUCTION (Z30-Z39)

● **Z30   Encounter for contraceptive management**

  ● **Z30.0   Encounter for general counseling and advice on contraception**

    ● **Z30.01   Encounter for initial prescription of contraceptives**

       Excludes1   encounter for surveillance of contraceptives (Z30.4-)

       Z30.011   Encounter for initial prescription of contraceptive pills

       Z30.012   Encounter for prescription of emergency contraception

         Encounter for postcoital contraception

       Z30.013   Encounter for initial prescription of injectable contraceptive

       Z30.014   Encounter for initial prescription of intrauterine contraceptive device

         Excludes1   encounter for insertion of intrauterine contraceptive device (Z30.430, Z30.432)

       Z30.018   Encounter for initial prescription of other contraceptives

       Z30.019   Encounter for initial prescription of contraceptives, unspecified

     Z30.02   Counseling and instruction in natural family planning to avoid pregnancy

     Z30.09   Encounter for other general counseling and advice on contraception

       Encounter for family planning advice NOS

   Z30.2   Encounter for sterilization

  ● **Z30.4   Encounter for surveillance of contraceptives**

     Z30.40   Encounter for surveillance of contraceptives, unspecified

     Z30.41   Encounter for surveillance of contraceptive pills

       Encounter for repeat prescription for contraceptive pill

     Z30.42   Encounter for surveillance of injectable contraceptive

    ● **Z30.43   Encounter for surveillance of intrauterine contraceptive device**

       Z30.430   Encounter for insertion of intrauterine contraceptive device

       Z30.431   Encounter for routine checking of intrauterine contraceptive device

       Z30.432   Encounter for removal of intrauterine contraceptive device

       Z30.433   Encounter for removal and reinsertion of intrauterine contraceptive device

         Encounter for replacement of intrauterine contraceptive device

     Z30.49   Encounter for surveillance of other contraceptives

   Z30.8   Encounter for other contraceptive management

     Encounter for postvasectomy sperm count

     Encounter for routine examination for contraceptive maintenance

       Excludes1   sperm count following sterilization reversal (Z31.42)

         sperm count for fertility testing (Z31.41)

   Z30.9   Encounter for contraceptive management, unspecified

● **Z31   Encounter for procreative management**

     Excludes1   complications associated with artificial fertilization (N98.-)

       female infertility (N97.-)

       male infertility (N46.-)

   Z31.0   Encounter for reversal of previous sterilization

  ● **Z31.4   Encounter for procreative investigation and testing**

     Excludes1   postvasectomy sperm count (Z30.8)

     Z31.41   Encounter for fertility testing

       Encounter for fallopian tube patency testing

       Encounter for sperm count for fertility testing

     Z31.42   Aftercare following sterilization reversal

       Sperm count following sterilization reversal

    ● **Z31.43   Encounter for genetic testing of female for procreative management**

       Use additional code for recurrent pregnancy loss, if applicable (N96, O26.2-)

       Excludes1   nonprocreative genetic testing (Z13.7-)

       Z31.430   Encounter of female for testing for genetic disease carrier status for procreative management

       Z31.438   Encounter for other genetic testing of female for procreative management

    ● **Z31.44   Encounter for genetic testing of male for procreative management**

       Excludes1   nonprocreative genetic testing (Z13.7-)

       Z31.440   Encounter of male for testing for genetic disease carrier status for procreative management

       Z31.441   Encounter for testing of male partner of patient with recurrent pregnancy loss

       Z31.448   Encounter for other genetic testing of male for procreative management

     Z31.49   Encounter for other procreative investigation and testing

   Z31.5   Encounter for genetic counseling

  ● **Z31.6   Encounter for general counseling and advice on procreation**

     Z31.61   Procreative counseling and advice using natural family planning

     Z31.62   Encounter for fertility preservation counseling

       Encounter for fertility preservation counseling prior to cancer therapy

       Encounter for fertility preservation counseling prior to surgical removal of gonads

     Z31.69   Encounter for other general counseling and advice on procreation

  ● **Z31.8   Encounter for other procreative management**

     Z31.81   Encounter for male factor infertility in female patient

     Z31.82   Encounter for Rh incompatibility status

     Z31.83   Encounter for assisted reproductive fertility procedure cycle

       Patient undergoing in vitro fertilization cycle

       Use additional code to identify the type of infertility

       Excludes1   pre-cycle diagnosis and testing - code to reason for encounter

     Z31.84   Encounter for fertility preservation procedure

       Encounter for fertility preservation procedure prior to cancer therapy

       Encounter for fertility preservation procedure prior to surgical removal of gonads

     Z31.89   Encounter for other procreative management

   Z31.9   Encounter for procreative management, unspecified

CHAPTER 21 (Z00-Z99)

● **Z32 Encounter for pregnancy test and childbirth and childcare instruction**

  ● **Z32.0 Encounter for pregnancy test**

    Z32.00 Encounter for pregnancy test, result unknown
      Encounter for pregnancy test NOS

    Z32.01 Encounter for pregnancy test, result positive

    Z32.02 Encounter for pregnancy test, result negative

  Z32.2 Encounter for childbirth instruction

  Z32.3 Encounter for childcare instruction
    Encounter for prenatal or postpartum childcare instruction

● **Z33 Pregnant state**

  Z33.1 Pregnant state, incidental
    Pregnant state NOS
    Excludes1   complications of pregnancy (O00-O9A)

  Z33.2 Encounter for elective termination of pregnancy
    Excludes1   early fetal death with retention of dead fetus (O02.1)
      late fetal death (O36.4)
      spontaneous abortion (O03)

● **Z34 Encounter for supervision of normal pregnancy**

  Excludes1   any complication of pregnancy (O00-O9A)
    encounter for pregnancy test (Z32.0-)
    encounter for supervision of high risk pregnancy (O09.-)

  ● **Z34.0 Encounter for supervision of normal first pregnancy**

    Z34.00 Encounter for supervision of normal first pregnancy, unspecified trimester

    Z34.01 Encounter for supervision of normal first pregnancy, first trimester

    Z34.02 Encounter for supervision of normal first pregnancy, second trimester

    Z34.03 Encounter for supervision of normal first pregnancy, third trimester

  ● **Z34.8 Encounter for supervision of other normal pregnancy**

    Z34.80 Encounter for supervision of other normal pregnancy, unspecified trimester

    Z34.81 Encounter for supervision of other normal pregnancy, first trimester

    Z34.82 Encounter for supervision of other normal pregnancy, second trimester

    Z34.83 Encounter for supervision of other normal pregnancy, third trimester

  ● **Z34.9 Encounter for supervision of normal pregnancy, unspecified**

    Z34.90 Encounter for supervision of normal pregnancy, unspecified, unspecified trimester

    Z34.91 Encounter for supervision of normal pregnancy, unspecified, first trimester

    Z34.92 Encounter for supervision of normal pregnancy, unspecified, second trimester

    Z34.93 Encounter for supervision of normal pregnancy, unspecified, third trimester

● **Z36 Encounter for antenatal screening of mother**

  Excludes1   abnormal findings on antenatal screening of mother (O28.-)
    diagnostic examination - code to sign or symptom
    encounter for suspected maternal and fetal conditions ruled out (Z03.7-)
    suspected fetal condition affecting management of pregnancy - code to condition in Chapter 15

  Excludes2   genetic counseling and testing (Z31.43-, Z31.5)
    routine prenatal care (Z34)

● **Z3A Weeks of gestation**

  Note: Codes from category Z3A are for use, only on the maternal record, to indicate the weeks of gestation of the pregnancy.

  Code first complications of pregnancy, childbirth and the puerperium (O00-O9A)

  ● **Z3A.0 Weeks of gestation of pregnancy, unspecified or less than 10 weeks**

    Z3A.00 Weeks of gestation of pregnancy not specified

    Z3A.01 Less than 8 weeks gestation of pregnancy

    Z3A.08 8 weeks gestation of pregnancy

    Z3A.09 9 weeks gestation of pregnancy

  ● **Z3A.1 Weeks of gestation of pregnancy, weeks 10-19**

    Z3A.10 10 weeks gestation of pregnancy

    Z3A.11 11 weeks gestation of pregnancy

    Z3A.12 12 weeks gestation of pregnancy

    Z3A.13 13 weeks gestation of pregnancy

    Z3A.14 14 weeks gestation of pregnancy

    Z3A.15 15 weeks gestation of pregnancy

    Z3A.16 16 weeks gestation of pregnancy

    Z3A.17 17 weeks gestation of pregnancy

    Z3A.18 18 weeks gestation of pregnancy

    Z3A.19 19 weeks gestation of pregnancy

  ● **Z3A.2 Weeks of gestation of pregnancy, weeks 20-29**

    Z3A.20 20 weeks gestation of pregnancy

    Z3A.21 21 weeks gestation of pregnancy

    Z3A.22 22 weeks gestation of pregnancy

    Z3A.23 23 weeks gestation of pregnancy

    Z3A.24 24 weeks gestation of pregnancy

    Z3A.25 25 weeks gestation of pregnancy

    Z3A.26 26 weeks gestation of pregnancy

    Z3A.27 27 weeks gestation of pregnancy

    Z3A.28 28 weeks gestation of pregnancy

    Z3A.29 29 weeks gestation of pregnancy

  ● **Z3A.3 Weeks of gestation of pregnancy, weeks 30-39**

    Z3A.30 30 weeks gestation of pregnancy

    Z3A.31 31 weeks gestation of pregnancy

    Z3A.32 32 weeks gestation of pregnancy

    Z3A.33 33 weeks gestation of pregnancy

    Z3A.34 34 weeks gestation of pregnancy

    Z3A.35 35 weeks gestation of pregnancy

    Z3A.36 36 weeks gestation of pregnancy

    Z3A.37 37 weeks gestation of pregnancy

    Z3A.38 38 weeks gestation of pregnancy

    Z3A.39 39 weeks gestation of pregnancy

  ● **Z3A.4 Weeks of gestation of pregnancy, weeks 40 or greater**

    Z3A.40 40 weeks gestation of pregnancy

    Z3A.41 41 weeks gestation of pregnancy

    Z3A.42 42 weeks gestation of pregnancy

    Z3A.49 Greater than 42 weeks gestation of pregnancy

● **Z37**   **Outcome of delivery**
This category is intended for use as an additional code to identify the outcome of delivery on the mother's record. It is not for use on the newborn record.

> **Excludes1**   stillbirth (P95)

Z37.0   **Single live birth**

Z37.1   **Single stillbirth**

Z37.2   **Twins, both liveborn**

Z37.3   **Twins, one liveborn and one stillborn**

Z37.4   **Twins, both stillborn**

● Z37.5   **Other multiple births, all liveborn**

     Z37.50   **Multiple births, unspecified, all liveborn**

     Z37.51   **Triplets, all liveborn**

     Z37.52   **Quadruplets, all liveborn**

     Z37.53   **Quintuplets, all liveborn**

     Z37.54   **Sextuplets, all liveborn**

     Z37.59   **Other multiple births, all liveborn**

● Z37.6   **Other multiple births, some liveborn**

     Z37.60   **Multiple births, unspecified, some liveborn**

     Z37.61   **Triplets, some liveborn**

     Z37.62   **Quadruplets, some liveborn**

     Z37.63   **Quintuplets, some liveborn**

     Z37.64   **Sextuplets, some liveborn**

     Z37.69   **Other multiple births, some liveborn**

Z37.7   **Other multiple births, all stillborn**

Z37.9   **Outcome of delivery, unspecified**
     Multiple birth NOS
     Single birth NOS

● **Z38**   **Liveborn infants according to place of birth and type of delivery**
This category is for use as the principal code on the initial record of a newborn baby. It is to be used for the initial birth record only. It is not to be used on the mother's record.

● Z38.0   **Single liveborn infant, born in hospital**
     Single liveborn infant, born in birthing center or other health care facility

     Z38.00   **Single liveborn infant, delivered vaginally**

     Z38.01   **Single liveborn infant, delivered by cesarean**

Z38.1   **Single liveborn infant, born outside hospital**

Z38.2   **Single liveborn infant, unspecified as to place of birth**
     Single liveborn infant NOS

● Z38.3   **Twin liveborn infant, born in hospital**

     Z38.30   **Twin liveborn infant, delivered vaginally**

     Z38.31   **Twin liveborn infant, delivered by cesarean**

Z38.4   **Twin liveborn infant, born outside hospital**

Z38.5   **Twin liveborn infant, unspecified as to place of birth**

● Z38.6   **Other multiple liveborn infant, born in hospital**

     Z38.61   **Triplet liveborn infant, delivered vaginally**

     Z38.62   **Triplet liveborn infant, delivered by cesarean**

     Z38.63   **Quadruplet liveborn infant, delivered vaginally**

     Z38.64   **Quadruplet liveborn infant, delivered by cesarean**

     Z38.65   **Quintuplet liveborn infant, delivered vaginally**

     Z38.66   **Quintuplet liveborn infant, delivered by cesarean**

     Z38.68   **Other multiple liveborn infant, delivered vaginally**

     Z38.69   **Other multiple liveborn infant, delivered by cesarean**

Z38.7   **Other multiple liveborn infant, born outside hospital**

Z38.8   **Other multiple liveborn infant, unspecified as to place of birth**

● **Z39**   **Encounter for maternal postpartum care and examination**

Z39.0   **Encounter for care and examination of mother immediately after delivery**
     Care and observation in uncomplicated cases when the delivery occurs outside a healthcare facility

> **Excludes1**   care for postpartum complication - see Alphabetic index

Z39.1   **Encounter for care and examination of lactating mother**
     Encounter for supervision of lactation

> **Excludes1**   disorders of lactation (O92.-)

Z39.2   **Encounter for routine postpartum follow-up**

ENCOUNTERS FOR OTHER SPECIFIC HEALTH CARE (Z40-Z53)

Categories Z40-Z53 are intended for use to indicate a reason for care. They may be used for patients who have already been treated for a disease or injury, but who are receiving aftercare or prophylactic care, or care to consolidate the treatment, or to deal with a residual state

> **Excludes2**   follow-up examination for medical surveillance after treatment (Z08-Z09)

● **Z40**   **Encounter for prophylactic surgery**

> **Excludes1**   organ donations (Z52.-)
>   therapeutic organ removal - code to condition

● Z40.0   **Encounter for prophylactic surgery for risk factors related to malignant neoplasms**
     Admission for prophylactic organ removal
     Use additional code to identify risk factor

     Z40.00   **Encounter for prophylactic removal of unspecified organ**

     Z40.01   **Encounter for prophylactic removal of breast**

     Z40.02   **Encounter for prophylactic removal of ovary**

     Z40.09   **Encounter for prophylactic removal of other organ**

Z40.8   **Encounter for other prophylactic surgery**

Z40.9   **Encounter for prophylactic surgery, unspecified**

● **Z41**   **Encounter for procedures for purposes other than remedying health state**

Z41.1   **Encounter for cosmetic surgery**
     Encounter for cosmetic breast implant
     Encounter for cosmetic procedure

> **Excludes1**   encounter for plastic and reconstructive surgery following medical procedure or healed injury (Z42.-)
>   encounter for post-mastectomy breast implantation (Z42.1)

Z41.2   **Encounter for routine and ritual male circumcision**

Z41.3   **Encounter for ear piercing**

Z41.8   **Encounter for other procedures for purposes other than remedying health state**

Z41.9   **Encounter for procedure for purposes other than remedying health state, unspecified**

● **Z42**   **Encounter for plastic and reconstructive surgery following medical procedure or healed injury**

> **Excludes1**   encounter for cosmetic plastic surgery (Z41.1)
>   encounter for plastic surgery for treatment of current injury - code to relevent injury

Z42.1   **Encounter for breast reconstruction following mastectomy**

> **Excludes1**   deformity and disproportion of reconstructed breast (N65.1-)

Z42.8   **Encounter for other plastic and reconstructive surgery following medical procedure or healed injury**

CHAPTER 21 (Z00-Z99)

● **Z43   Encounter for attention to artificial openings**

   Includes   closure of artificial openings
              passage of sounds or bougies through artificial
                openings
              reforming artificial openings
              removal of catheter from artificial openings
              toilet or cleansing of artificial openings

   Excludes1   artificial opening status only, without need for
              care (Z93.-)
              complications of external stoma (J95.0-, K94.-,
              N99.5-)

   Excludes2   fitting and adjustment of prosthetic and other
              devices (Z44-Z46)

Z43.0   Encounter for attention to tracheostomy

Z43.1   Encounter for attention to gastrostomy

Z43.2   Encounter for attention to ileostomy

Z43.3   Encounter for attention to colostomy

**Z43.4   Encounter for attention to other artificial openings of
       digestive tract**

Z43.5   Encounter for attention to cystostomy

**Z43.6   Encounter for attention to other artificial openings of
       urinary tract**
       Encounter for attention to nephrostomy
       Encounter for attention to ureterostomy
       Encounter for attention to urethrostomy

Z43.7   Encounter for attention to artificial vagina

Z43.8   Encounter for attention to other artificial openings

Z43.9   Encounter for attention to unspecified artificial opening

● **Z44   Encounter for fitting and adjustment of external prosthetic
device**

   Includes   removal or replacement of external prosthetic
            device

   Excludes1   malfunction or other complications of device - see
              Alphabetical Index presence of prosthetic
              device (Z97.-)

● **Z44.0   Encounter for fitting and adjustment of artificial arm**

  ● **Z44.00   Encounter for fitting and adjustment of
           unspecified artificial arm**

     **Z44.001   Encounter for fitting and adjustment
             of unspecified right artificial arm**

     **Z44.002   Encounter for fitting and adjustment
             of unspecified left artificial arm**

     **Z44.009   Encounter for fitting and adjustment
             of unspecified artificial arm,
             unspecified arm**

  ● **Z44.01   Encounter for fitting and adjustment of
           complete artificial arm**

     **Z44.011   Encounter for fitting and adjustment
             of complete right artificial arm**

     **Z44.012   Encounter for fitting and adjustment
             of complete left artificial arm**

     **Z44.019   Encounter for fitting and adjustment
             of complete artificial arm, unspecified
             arm**

  ● **Z44.02   Encounter for fitting and adjustment of partial
           artificial arm**

     **Z44.021   Encounter for fitting and adjustment
             of partial artificial right arm**

     **Z44.022   Encounter for fitting and adjustment
             of partial artificial left arm**

     **Z44.029   Encounter for fitting and adjustment
             of partial artificial arm, unspecified
             arm**

● **Z44.1   Encounter for fitting and adjustment of artificial leg**

  ● **Z44.10   Encounter for fitting and adjustment of
           unspecified artificial leg**

     **Z44.101   Encounter for fitting and adjustment
             of unspecified right artificial leg**

     **Z44.102   Encounter for fitting and adjustment
             of unspecified left artificial leg**

     **Z44.109   Encounter for fitting and adjustment
             of unspecified artificial leg,
             unspecified leg**

  ● **Z44.11   Encounter for fitting and adjustment of
           complete artificial leg**

     **Z44.111   Encounter for fitting and adjustment
             of complete right artificial leg**

     **Z44.112   Encounter for fitting and adjustment
             of complete left artificial leg**

     **Z44.119   Encounter for fitting and adjustment
             of complete artificial leg, unspecified
             leg**

  ● **Z44.12   Encounter for fitting and adjustment of partial
           artificial leg**

     **Z44.121   Encounter for fitting and adjustment
             of partial artificial right leg**

     **Z44.122   Encounter for fitting and adjustment
             of partial artificial left leg**

     **Z44.129   Encounter for fitting and adjustment
             of partial artificial leg, unspecified leg**

● **Z44.2   Encounter for fitting and adjustment of artificial eye**

   Excludes1   mechanical complication of ocular
              prosthesis (T85.3)

  **Z44.20   Encounter for fitting and adjustment of artificial
           eye, unspecified**

  **Z44.21   Encounter for fitting and adjustment of artificial
           right eye**

  **Z44.22   Encounter for fitting and adjustment of artificial
           left eye**

● **Z44.3   Encounter for fitting and adjustment of external breast
prosthesis**

   Excludes1   complications of breast implant (T85.4-)
              encounter for adjustment or removal of
              breast implant (Z45.81-)
              encounter for initial breast implant
              insertion for cosmetic breast
              augmentation (Z41.1)
              encounter for breast reconstruction
              following mastectomy (Z42.1)

  **Z44.30   Encounter for fitting and adjustment of external
           breast prosthesis, unspecified breast**

  **Z44.31   Encounter for fitting and adjustment of external
           right breast prosthesis**

  **Z44.32   Encounter for fitting and adjustment of external
           left breast prosthesis**

**Z44.8   Encounter for fitting and adjustment of other external
       prosthetic devices**

**Z44.9   Encounter for fitting and adjustment of unspecified
       external prosthetic device**

◀ New   ◀▥ Revised   ~~deleted~~ Deleted   **OGCR** Official Guidelines   X Assign placeholder X   ● Use Additional Character(s)

Excludes 1   Excludes 2   Includes   Use additional   Code first   Code also   Unspecified

● **Z45** **Encounter for adjustment and management of implanted device**

> **Includes** removal or replacement of implanted device
>
> **Excludes1** malfunction or other complications of device - see Alphabetical Index
> presence of prosthetic and other devices (Z95-Z97)
>
> **Excludes2** encounter for fitting and adjustment of non-implanted device (Z46.-)

● **Z45.0** **Encounter for adjustment and management of cardiac device**

> ● **Z45.01** **Encounter for adjustment and management of cardiac pacemaker**
>
> > **Excludes1** encounter for adjustment and management of automatic implantable cardiac defibrillator with synchronous cardiac pacemaker (Z45.02)
> >
> > **Z45.010** **Encounter for checking and testing of cardiac pacemaker pulse generator [battery]**
> > Encounter for replacing cardiac pacemaker pulse generator [battery]
> >
> > **Z45.018** **Encounter for adjustment and management of other part of cardiac pacemaker**
>
> **Z45.02** **Encounter for adjustment and management of automatic implantable cardiac defibrillator**
> Encounter for adjustment and management of automatic implantable cardiac defibrillator with synchronous cardiac pacemaker
>
> **Z45.09** **Encounter for adjustment and management of other cardiac device**

Z45.1 **Encounter for adjustment and management of infusion pump**

Z45.2 **Encounter for adjustment and management of vascular access device**
Encounter for adjustment and management of vascular catheters

> **Excludes1** encounter for adjustment and management of renal dialysis catheter (Z49.01)

● **Z45.3** **Encounter for adjustment and management of implanted devices of the special senses**

> **Z45.31** **Encounter for adjustment and management of implanted visual substitution device**
>
> ● **Z45.32** **Encounter for adjustment and management of implanted hearing device**
>
> > **Excludes1** encounter for fitting and adjustment of hearing aide (Z46.1)
> >
> > **Z45.320** **Encounter for adjustment and management of bone conduction device**
> >
> > **Z45.321** **Encounter for adjustment and management of cochlear device**
> >
> > **Z45.328** **Encounter for adjustment and management of other implanted hearing device**

● **Z45.4** **Encounter for adjustment and management of implanted nervous system device**

> **Z45.41** **Encounter for adjustment and management of cerebrospinal fluid drainage device**
> Encounter for adjustment and management of cerebral ventricular (communicating) shunt
>
> **Z45.42** **Encounter for adjustment and management of neuropacemaker (brain) (peripheral nerve) (spinal cord)**
>
> **Z45.49** **Encounter for adjustment and management of other implanted nervous system device**

● **Z45.8** **Encounter for adjustment and management of other implanted devices**

> ● **Z45.81** **Encounter for adjustment or removal of breast implant**
> Encounter for elective implant exchange (different material) (different size)
> Encounter removal of tissue expander without synchronous insertion of permanent implant
>
> > **Excludes1** complications of breast implant (T85.4-)
> > encounter for initial breast implant insertion for cosmetic breast augmentation (Z41.1)
> > encounter for breast reconstruction following mastectomy (Z42.1)
> >
> > **Z45.811** **Encounter for adjustment or removal of right breast implant**
> >
> > **Z45.812** **Encounter for adjustment or removal of left breast implant**
> >
> > **Z45.819** **Encounter for adjustment or removal of unspecified breast implant**
>
> **Z45.82** **Encounter for adjustment or removal of myringotomy device (stent) (tube)**
>
> **Z45.89** **Encounter for adjustment and management of other implanted devices**

Z45.9 **Encounter for adjustment and management of unspecified implanted device**

● **Z46** **Encounter for fitting and adjustment of other devices**

> **Includes** removal or replacement of other device
>
> **Excludes1** malfunction or other complications of device - see Alphabetical Index
>
> **Excludes2** encounter for fitting and management of implanted devices (Z45.-)
> issue of repeat prescription only (Z76.0)
> presence of prosthetic and other devices (Z95-Z97)

Z46.0 **Encounter for fitting and adjustment of spectacles and contact lenses**

Z46.1 **Encounter for fitting and adjustment of hearing aid**

> **Excludes1** encounter for adjustment and management of implanted hearing device (Z45.32-)

Z46.2 **Encounter for fitting and adjustment of other devices related to nervous system and special senses**

> **Excludes2** encounter for adjustment and management of implanted nervous system device (Z45.4-)
> encounter for adjustment and management of implanted visual substitution device (Z45.31)

Z46.3 **Encounter for fitting and adjustment of dental prosthetic device**
Encounter for fitting and adjustment of dentures

Z46.4 **Encounter for fitting and adjustment of orthodontic device**

CHAPTER 21 (Z00-Z99)

CHAPTER 21 (Z00-Z99)

● **Z46.5 Encounter for fitting and adjustment of other gastrointestinal appliance and device**

    Excludes1   encounter for attention to artificial openings of digestive tract (Z43.1-Z43.4)

    Z46.51 Encounter for fitting and adjustment of gastric lap band

    Z46.59 Encounter for fitting and adjustment of other gastrointestinal appliance and device

Z46.6 Encounter for fitting and adjustment of urinary device

    Excludes2   attention to artificial openings of urinary tract (Z43.5, Z43.6)

● **Z46.8 Encounter for fitting and adjustment of other specified devices**

    Z46.81 Encounter for fitting and adjustment of insulin pump

         Encounter for insulin pump instruction and training

         Encounter for insulin pump titration

    Z46.82 Encounter for fitting and adjustment of non-vascular catheter

    Z46.89 Encounter for fitting and adjustment of other specified devices

         Encounter for fitting and adjustment of wheelchair

Z46.9 Encounter for fitting and adjustment of unspecified device

● **Z47 Orthopedic aftercare**

    Excludes1   aftercare for healing fracture - code to fracture with 7th character D

Z47.1 Aftercare following joint replacement surgery

     Use additional code to identify the joint (Z96.6-)

Z47.2 Encounter for removal of internal fixation device

    Excludes1   encounter for adjustment of internal fixation device for fracture treatment - code to fracture with appropriate 7th character

         encounter for removal of external fixation device - code to fracture with 7th character D

         infection or inflammatory reaction to internal fixation device (T84.6-)

         mechanical complication of internal fixation device (T84.1-)

● **Z47.3 Aftercare following explantation of joint prosthesis**

     Aftercare following explantation of joint prosthesis, staged procedure

     Encounter for joint prosthesis insertion following prior explantation of joint prosthesis

    Z47.31 Aftercare following explantation of shoulder joint prosthesis

        Excludes1   acquired absence of shoulder joint following prior explantation of shoulder joint prosthesis (Z89.23-)

             shoulder joint prosthesis explantation status (Z89.23-)

    Z47.32 Aftercare following explantation of hip joint prosthesis

        Excludes1   acquired absence of hip joint following prior explantation of hip joint prosthesis (Z89.62-)

             hip joint prosthesis explantation status (Z89.62-)

    Z47.33 Aftercare following explantation of knee joint prosthesis

        Excludes1   acquired absence of knee joint following prior explantation of knee prosthesis (Z89.52-)

             knee joint prosthesis explantation status (Z89.52-)

● **Z47.8 Encounter for other orthopedic aftercare**

    Z47.81 Encounter for orthopedic aftercare following surgical amputation

         Use additional code to identify the limb amputated (Z89.-)

    Z47.82 Encounter for orthopedic aftercare following scoliosis surgery

    Z47.89 Encounter for other orthopedic aftercare

● **Z48 Encounter for other postprocedural aftercare**

    Excludes1   encounter for follow-up examination after completed treatment (Z08-Z09)

    Excludes2   encounter for attention to artificial openings (Z43.-)

         encounter for fitting and adjustment of prosthetic and other devices (Z44-Z46)

● **Z48.0 Encounter for attention to dressings, sutures and drains**

    Excludes1   encounter for planned postprocedural wound closure (Z48.1)

    Z48.00 Encounter for change or removal of nonsurgical wound dressing

         Encounter for change or removal of wound dressing NOS

    Z48.01 Encounter for change or removal of surgical wound dressing

    Z48.02 Encounter for removal of sutures

         Encounter for removal of staples

    Z48.03 Encounter for change or removal of drains

Z48.1 Encounter for planned postprocedural wound closure

    Excludes1   encounter for attention to dressings and sutures (Z48.0-)

● **Z48.2 Encounter for aftercare following organ transplant**

    Z48.21 Encounter for aftercare following heart transplant

    Z48.22 Encounter for aftercare following kidney transplant

    Z48.23 Encounter for aftercare following liver transplant

    Z48.24 Encounter for aftercare following lung transplant

    ● **Z48.28 Encounter for aftercare following multiple organ transplant**

        Z48.280 Encounter for aftercare following heart-lung transplant

        Z48.288 Encounter for aftercare following multiple organ transplant

    ● **Z48.29 Encounter for aftercare following other organ transplant**

        Z48.290 Encounter for aftercare following bone marrow transplant

        Z48.298 Encounter for aftercare following other organ transplant

Z48.3 Aftercare following surgery for neoplasm

     Use additional code to identify the neoplasm

◄ New   ◄▦ Revised   ~~deleted~~ Deleted   **OGCR** Official Guidelines   X Assign placeholder X   ● Use Additional Character(s)

Excludes 1   Excludes 2   Includes   Use additional   Code first   Code also   Unspecified

● **Z48.8**   **Encounter for other specified postprocedural aftercare**
   ● **Z48.81**   **Encounter for surgical aftercare following surgery on specified body systems**
        These codes identify the body system requiring aftercare. They are for use in conjunction with other aftercare codes to fully explain the aftercare encounter. The condition treated should also be coded if still present.

         | **Excludes1** | aftercare for injury - code the injury with 7th character D
                 aftercare following surgery for neoplasm (Z48.3)

         | **Excludes2** | aftercare following organ transplant (Z48.2-)
                 orthopedic aftercare (Z47.-)

       Z48.810   Encounter for surgical aftercare following surgery on the sense organs
       Z48.811   Encounter for surgical aftercare following surgery on the nervous system

           | **Excludes2** | encounter for surgical aftercare following surgery on the sense organs (Z48.810)

       Z48.812   Encounter for surgical aftercare following surgery on the circulatory system
       Z48.813   Encounter for surgical aftercare following surgery on the respiratory system
       Z48.814   Encounter for surgical aftercare following surgery on the teeth or oral cavity
       Z48.815   Encounter for surgical aftercare following surgery on the digestive system
       Z48.816   Encounter for surgical aftercare following surgery on the genitourinary system

           | **Excludes1** | encounter for aftercare following sterilization reversal (Z31.42)

       Z48.817   Encounter for surgical aftercare following surgery on the skin and subcutaneous tissue
    Z48.89   Encounter for other specified surgical aftercare

● **Z49**   **Encounter for care involving renal dialysis**
   Code also associated end stage renal disease (N18.6)
   ● **Z49.0**   **Preparatory care for renal dialysis**
      Encounter for dialysis instruction and training
       Z49.01   **Encounter for fitting and adjustment of extracorporeal dialysis catheter**
          Removal or replacement of renal dialysis catheter
          Toilet or cleansing of renal dialysis catheter
       Z49.02   **Encounter for fitting and adjustment of peritoneal dialysis catheter**

● **Z49.3**   **Encounter for adequacy testing for dialysis**
       Z49.31   **Encounter for adequacy testing for hemodialysis**
       Z49.32   **Encounter for adequacy testing for peritoneal dialysis**
         Encounter for peritoneal equilibration test

● **Z51**   **Encounter for other aftercare**
   Code also condition requiring care

    | **Excludes1** | follow-up examination after treatment (Z08-Z09)

    Z51.0   Encounter for antineoplastic radiation therapy
   ● **Z51.1**   **Encounter for antineoplastic chemotherapy and immunotherapy**

       | **Excludes2** | encounter for chemotherapy and immunotherapy for nonneoplastic condition-code to condition

       Z51.11   Encounter for antineoplastic chemotherapy
       Z51.12   Encounter for antineoplastic immunotherapy
    Z51.5   Encounter for palliative care
   ● **Z51.8**   **Encounter for other specified aftercare**

       | **Excludes1** | holiday relief care (Z75.5)

       Z51.81   **Encounter for therapeutic drug level monitoring**
         Code also any long-term (current) drug therapy (Z79.-)

          | **Excludes1** | encounter for blood-drug test for administrative or medicolegal reasons (Z02.83)

       Z51.89   Encounter for other specified aftercare

● **Z52**   **Donors of organs and tissues**

    | **Includes** | autologous and other living donors
    | **Excludes1** | cadaveric donor - omit code
          examination of potential donor (Z00.5)

   ● **Z52.0**   **Blood donor**
      ● **Z52.00**   **Unspecified blood donor**
          Z52.000   Unspecified donor, whole blood
          Z52.001   Unspecified donor, stem cells
          Z52.008   Unspecified donor, other blood
      ● **Z52.01**   **Autologous blood donor**
          Z52.010   Autologous donor, whole blood
          Z52.011   Autologous donor, stem cells
          Z52.018   Autologous donor, other blood
      ● **Z52.09**   **Other blood donor**
         Volunteer donor
          Z52.090   Other blood donor, whole blood
          Z52.091   Other blood donor, stem cells
          Z52.098   Other blood donor, other blood
   ● **Z52.1**   **Skin donor**
       Z52.10   Skin donor, unspecified
       Z52.11   Skin donor, autologous
       Z52.19   Skin donor, other
   ● **Z52.2**   **Bone donor**
       Z52.20   Bone donor, unspecified
       Z52.21   Bone donor, autologous
       Z52.29   Bone donor, other
    Z52.3   Bone marrow donor
    Z52.4   Kidney donor
    Z52.5   Cornea donor
    Z52.6   Liver donor

CHAPTER 21 (Z00-Z99)

● Z52.8   Donor of other specified organs or tissues
    ● Z52.81   Egg (Oocyte) donor
        Z52.810   Egg (Oocyte) donor under age 35, anonymous recipient
            Egg donor under age 35 NOS
        Z52.811   Egg (Oocyte) donor under age 35, designated recipient
        Z52.812   Egg (Oocyte) donor age 35 and over, anonymous recipient
            Egg donor age 35 and over NOS
        Z52.813   Egg (Oocyte) donor age 35 and over, designated recipient
        Z52.819   Egg (Oocyte) donor, unspecified
    Z52.89   Donor of other specified organs or tissues
  Z52.9   Donor of unspecified organ or tissue
    Donor NOS

● Z53   Persons encountering health services for specific procedures and treatment, not carried out
  ● Z53.0   Procedure and treatment not carried out because of contraindication
    Z53.01   Procedure and treatment not carried out due to patient smoking
    Z53.09   Procedure and treatment not carried out because of other contraindication
  Z53.1   Procedure and treatment not carried out because of patient's decision for reasons of belief and group pressure
  ● Z53.2   Procedure and treatment not carried out because of patient's decision for other and unspecified reasons
    Z53.20   Procedure and treatment not carried out because of patient's decision for unspecified reasons
    Z53.21   Procedure and treatment not carried out due to patient leaving prior to being seen by health care provider
    Z53.29   Procedure and treatment not carried out because of patient's decision for other reasons
  Z53.8   Procedure and treatment not carried out for other reasons
  Z53.9   Procedure and treatment not carried out, unspecified reason

PERSONS WITH POTENTIAL HEALTH HAZARDS RELATED TO SOCIOECONOMIC AND PSYCHOSOCIAL CIRCUMSTANCES (Z55-Z65)

● Z55   Problems related to education and literacy
  Excludes1   disorders of psychological development (F80-F89)
  Z55.0   Illiteracy and low-level literacy
  Z55.1   Schooling unavailable and unattainable
  Z55.2   Failed school examinations
  Z55.3   Underachievement in school
  Z55.4   Educational maladjustment and discord with teachers and classmates
  Z55.8   Other problems related to education and literacy
    Problems related to inadequate teaching
  Z55.9   Problems related to education and literacy, unspecified
    Academic problems NOS

● Z56   Problems related to employment and unemployment
  Excludes2   occupational exposure to risk factors (Z57.-)
    problems related to housing and economic circumstances (Z59.-)
  Z56.0   Unemployment, unspecified
  Z56.1   Change of job
  Z56.2   Threat of job loss
  Z56.3   Stressful work schedule

  Z56.4   Discord with boss and workmates
  Z56.5   Uncongenial work environment
    Difficult conditions at work
  Z56.6   Other physical and mental strain related to work
  ● Z56.8   Other problems related to employment
    Z56.81   Sexual harassment on the job
    Z56.82   Military deployment status
        Individual (civilian or military) currently deployed in theater or in support of military war, peacekeeping and humanitarian operations
    Z56.89   Other problems related to employment
  Z56.9   Unspecified problems related to employment
    Occupational problems NOS

● Z57   Occupational exposure to risk factors
  Z57.0   Occupational exposure to noise
  Z57.1   Occupational exposure to radiation
  Z57.2   Occupational exposure to dust
  ● Z57.3   Occupational exposure to other air contaminants
    Z57.31   Occupational exposure to environmental tobacco smoke
      Excludes2   exposure to environmental tobacco smoke (Z77.22)
    Z57.39   Occupational exposure to other air contaminants
  Z57.4   Occupational exposure to toxic agents in agriculture
    Occupational exposure to solids, liquids, gases or vapors in agriculture
  Z57.5   Occupational exposure to toxic agents in other industries
    Occupational exposure to solids, liquids, gases or vapors in other industries
  Z57.6   Occupational exposure to extreme temperature
  Z57.7   Occupational exposure to vibration
  Z57.8   Occupational exposure to other risk factors
  Z57.9   Occupational exposure to unspecified risk factor

● Z59   Problems related to housing and economic circumstances
  Excludes2   problems related to upbringing (Z62.-)
  Z59.0   Homelessness
  Z59.1   Inadequate housing
    Lack of heating
    Restriction of space
    Technical defects in home preventing adequate care
    Unsatisfactory surroundings
    Excludes1   problems related to the natural and physical environment (Z77.1-)
  Z59.2   Discord with neighbors, lodgers and landlord
  Z59.3   Problems related to living in residential institution
    Boarding-school resident
    Excludes1   institutional upbringing (Z62.2)
  Z59.4   Lack of adequate food and safe drinking water
    Inadequate drinking water supply
    Excludes1   effects of hunger (T73.0)
        inappropriate diet or eating habits (Z72.4)
        malnutrition (E40-E46)
  Z59.5   Extreme poverty
  Z59.6   Low income
  Z59.7   Insufficient social insurance and welfare support
  Z59.8   Other problems related to housing and economic circumstances
    Foreclosure on loan
    Isolated dwelling
    Problems with creditors
  Z59.9   Problem related to housing and economic circumstances, unspecified

◀ New   ◀▦ Revised   ~~deleted~~ Deleted   OGCR Official Guidelines   X Assign placeholder X   ● Use Additional Character(s)

Excludes 1   Excludes 2   Includes   Use additional   Code first   Code also   Unspecified

● **Z60**   **Problems related to social environment**

     Z60.0   **Problems of adjustment to life-cycle transitions**
         Empty nest syndrome
         Phase of life problem
         Problem with adjustment to retirement [pension]

     Z60.2   **Problems related to living alone**

     Z60.3   **Acculturation difficulty**
         Problem with migration
         Problem with social transplantation

     Z60.4   **Social exclusion and rejection**
         Exclusion and rejection on the basis of personal characteristics, such as unusual physical appearance, illness or behavior.
         | **Excludes1** | target of adverse discrimination such as for racial or religious reasons (Z60.5) |

     Z60.5   **Target of (perceived) adverse discrimination and persecution**
         | **Excludes1** | social exclusion and rejection (Z60.4) |

     Z60.8   **Other problems related to social environment**

     Z60.9   **Problem related to social environment, unspecified**

● **Z62**   **Problems related to upbringing**
     | **Includes** | current and past negative life events in childhood <br> current and past problems of a child related to upbringing |
     | **Excludes2** | maltreatment syndrome (T74.-)
 problems related to housing and economic circumstances (Z59.-) |

     Z62.0   **Inadequate parental supervision and control**

     Z62.1   **Parental overprotection**

   ● **Z62.2**   **Upbringing away from parents**
     | **Excludes1** | problems with boarding school (Z59.3) |

       Z62.21   **Child in welfare custody**
          Child in care of non-parental family member
          Child in foster care
          | **Excludes2** | problem for parent due to child in welfare custody (Z63.5) |

       Z62.22   **Institutional upbringing**
          Child living in orphanage or group home

       Z62.29   **Other upbringing away from parents**

     Z62.3   **Hostility towards and scapegoating of child**

     Z62.6   **Inappropriate (excessive) parental pressure**

   ● **Z62.8**   **Other specified problems related to upbringing**

     ● **Z62.81**   **Personal history of abuse in childhood**

       Z62.810   **Personal history of physical and sexual abuse in childhood**
          | **Excludes1** | current child physical abuse (T74.12, T76.12)
 current child sexual abuse (T74.22, T76.22) |

       Z62.811   **Personal history of psychological abuse in childhood**
          | **Excludes1** | current child psychological abuse (T74.32, T76.32) |

       Z62.812   **Personal history of neglect in childhood**
          | **Excludes1** | current child neglect (T74.02, T76.02) |

       Z62.819   **Personal history of unspecified abuse in childhood**
          | **Excludes1** | current child abuse NOS (T74.92, T76.92) |

     ● **Z62.82**   **Parent-child conflict**

       Z62.820   **Parent-biological child conflict**
          Parent-child problem NOS

       Z62.821   **Parent-adopted child conflict**

       Z62.822   **Parent-foster child conflict**

     ● **Z62.89**   **Other specified problems related to upbringing**

       Z62.890   **Parent-child estrangement NEC**

       Z62.891   **Sibling rivalry**

       Z62.898   **Other specified problems related to upbringing**

     Z62.9   **Problem related to upbringing, unspecified**

● **Z63**   **Other problems related to primary support group, including family circumstances**
     | **Excludes2** | maltreatment syndrome (T74.-, T76)
 parent-child problems (Z62.-)
 problems related to negative life events in childhood (Z62.-)
 problems related to upbringing (Z62.-) |

     Z63.0   **Problems in relationship with spouse or partner**
     | **Excludes1** | counseling for spousal or partner abuse problems (Z69.1)
 counseling related to sexual attitude, behavior, and orientation (Z70.-) |

     Z63.1   **Problems in relationship with in-laws**

   ● **Z63.3**   **Absence of family member**
     | **Excludes1** | absence of family member due to disappearance and death (Z63.4)
 absence of family member due to separation and divorce (Z63.5) |

       Z63.31   **Absence of family member due to military deployment**
          Individual or family affected by other family member being on military deployment
          | **Excludes1** | family disruption due to return of family member from military deployment (Z63.71) |

       Z63.32   **Other absence of family member**

     Z63.4   **Disappearance and death of family member**
         Assumed death of family member
         Bereavement

     Z63.5   **Disruption of family by separation and divorce**
         Marital estrangement

     Z63.6   **Dependent relative needing care at home**

   ● **Z63.7**   **Other stressful life events affecting family and household**

       Z63.71   **Stress on family due to return of family member from military deployment**
          Individual or family affected by family member having returned from military deployment (current or past conflict)

       Z63.72   **Alcoholism and drug addiction in family**

       Z63.79   **Other stressful life events affecting family and household**
          Anxiety (normal) about sick person in family
          Health problems within family
          Ill or disturbed family member
          Isolated family

     Z63.8   **Other specified problems related to primary support group**
         Family discord NOS
         Family estrangement NOS
         High expressed emotional level within family
         Inadequate family support NOS
         Inadequate or distorted communication within family

     Z63.9   **Problem related to primary support group, unspecified**
         Relationship disorder NOS

CHAPTER 21 (Z00-Z99)

●Z64　Problems related to certain psychosocial circumstances
　　Z64.0　Problems related to unwanted pregnancy
　　Z64.1　Problems related to multiparity
　　Z64.4　Discord with counselors
　　　　　Discord with probation officer
　　　　　Discord with social worker

●Z65　Problems related to other psychosocial circumstances
　　Z65.0　Conviction in civil and criminal proceedings without imprisonment
　　Z65.1　Imprisonment and other incarceration
　　Z65.2　Problems related to release from prison
　　Z65.3　Problems related to other legal circumstances
　　　　　Arrest
　　　　　Child custody or support proceedings
　　　　　Litigation
　　　　　Prosecution
　　Z65.4　Victim of crime and terrorism
　　　　　Victim of torture
　　Z65.5　Exposure to disaster, war and other hostilities
　　　　　Excludes1　target of perceived discrimination or persecution (Z60.5)
　　Z65.8　Other specified problems related to psychosocial circumstances
　　Z65.9　Problem related to unspecified psychosocial circumstances

DO NOT RESUSCITATE STATUS (Z66)

Z66　Do not resuscitate
　　DNR status

BLOOD TYPE (Z67)

●Z67　Blood type
　●Z67.1　Type A blood
　　　Z67.10　Type A blood, Rh positive
　　　Z67.11　Type A blood, Rh negative
　●Z67.2　Type B blood
　　　Z67.20　Type B blood, Rh positive
　　　Z67.21　Type B blood, Rh negative
　●Z67.3　Type AB blood
　　　Z67.30　Type AB blood, Rh positive
　　　Z67.31　Type AB blood, Rh negative
　●Z67.4　Type O blood
　　　Z67.40　Type O blood, Rh positive
　　　Z67.41　Type O blood, Rh negative
　●Z67.9　Unspecified blood type
　　　Z67.90　Unspecified blood type, Rh positive
　　　Z67.91　Unspecified blood type, Rh negative

BODY MASS INDEX [BMI] (Z68)

OGCR Section I.B.14.

General Coding Guidelines

14. Documentation for BMI, Non-pressure ulcers and Pressure Ulcer Stages

For the Body Mass Index (BMI), depth of non-pressure chronic ulcers and pressure ulcer stage codes, code assignment may be based on medical record documentation from clinicians who are not the patient's provider (i.e., physician or other qualified healthcare practitioner legally accountable for establishing the patient's diagnosis), since this information is typically documented by other clinicians involved in the care of the patient (e.g., a dietitian often documents the BMI and nurses often documents the pressure ulcer stages). However, the associated diagnosis (such as overweight, obesity, or pressure ulcer) must be documented by the patient's provider. If there is conflicting medical record documentation, either from the same clinician or different clinicians, the patient's attending provider should be queried for clarification.

The BMI codes should only be reported as secondary diagnoses.

●Z68　Body mass index [BMI]
　　Kilograms per meters squared
　　Note: BMI adult codes are for use for persons 21 years of age or older.
　　　　BMI pediatric codes are for use for persons 2-20 years of age. These percentiles are based on the growth charts published by the Centers for Disease Control and Prevention (CDC)
　　Z68.1　Body mass index (BMI) 19 or less, adult
　●Z68.2　Body mass index (BMI) 20-29, adult
　　　Z68.20　Body mass index (BMI) 20.0-20.9, adult
　　　Z68.21　Body mass index (BMI) 21.0-21.9, adult
　　　Z68.22　Body mass index (BMI) 22.0-22.9, adult
　　　Z68.23　Body mass index (BMI) 23.0-23.9, adult
　　　Z68.24　Body mass index (BMI) 24.0-24.9, adult
　　　Z68.25　Body mass index (BMI) 25.0-25.9, adult
　　　Z68.26　Body mass index (BMI) 26.0-26.9, adult
　　　Z68.27　Body mass index (BMI) 27.0-27.9, adult
　　　Z68.28　Body mass index (BMI) 28.0-28.9, adult
　　　Z68.29　Body mass index (BMI) 29.0-29.9, adult
　●Z68.3　Body mass index (BMI) 30-39, adult
　　　Z68.30　Body mass index (BMI) 30.0-30.9, adult
　　　Z68.31　Body mass index (BMI) 31.0-31.9, adult
　　　Z68.32　Body mass index (BMI) 32.0-32.9, adult
　　　Z68.33　Body mass index (BMI) 33.0-33.9, adult
　　　Z68.34　Body mass index (BMI) 34.0-34.9, adult
　　　Z68.35　Body mass index (BMI) 35.0-35.9, adult
　　　Z68.36　Body mass index (BMI) 36.0-36.9, adult
　　　Z68.37　Body mass index (BMI) 37.0-37.9, adult
　　　Z68.38　Body mass index (BMI) 38.0-38.9, adult
　　　Z68.39　Body mass index (BMI) 39.0-39.9, adult
　●Z68.4　Body mass index (BMI) 40 or greater, adult
　　　Z68.41　Body mass index (BMI) 40.0-44.9, adult
　　　Z68.42　Body mass index (BMI) 45.0-49.9, adult
　　　Z68.43　Body mass index (BMI) 50-59.9, adult
　　　Z68.44　Body mass index (BMI) 60.0-69.9, adult
　　　Z68.45　Body mass index (BMI) 70 or greater, adult
　●Z68.5　Body mass index (BMI) pediatric
　　　Z68.51　Body mass index (BMI) pediatric, less than 5th percentile for age
　　　Z68.52　Body mass index (BMI) pediatric, 5th percentile to less than 85th percentile for age
　　　Z68.53　Body mass index (BMI) pediatric, 85th percentile to less than 95th percentile for age
　　　Z68.54　Body mass index (BMI) pediatric, greater than or equal to 95th percentile for age

PERSONS ENCOUNTERING HEALTH SERVICES IN OTHER CIRCUMSTANCES (Z69-Z76)

●Z69　Encounter for mental health services for victim and perpetrator of abuse
　　　Includes　counseling for victims and perpetrators of abuse
　●Z69.0　Encounter for mental health services for child abuse problems
　　●Z69.01　Encounter for mental health services for parental child abuse
　　　　Z69.010　Encounter for mental health services for victim of parental child abuse
　　　　Z69.011　Encounter for mental health services for perpetrator of parental child abuse
　　　　　Excludes1　encounter for mental health services for non-parental child abuse (Z69.02-)

◀ New　◀▥ Revised　~~deleted~~ Deleted　OGCR Official Guidelines　X Assign placeholder X　● Use Additional Character(s)
Excludes 1　Excludes 2　Includes　Use additional　Code first　Code also　Unspecified

● **Z69.02**   **Encounter for mental health services for non-parental child abuse**

     Z69.020   Encounter for mental health services for victim of non-parental child abuse

     Z69.021   Encounter for mental health services for perpetrator of non- parental child abuse

● **Z69.1**   **Encounter for mental health services for spousal or partner abuse problems**

     Z69.11   Encounter for mental health services for victim of spousal or partner abuse

     Z69.12   Encounter for mental health services for perpetrator of spousal or partner abuse

● **Z69.8**   **Encounter for mental health services for victim or perpetrator of other abuse**

     Z69.81   Encounter for mental health services for victim of other abuse
            Encounter for rape victim counseling

     Z69.82   Encounter for mental health services for perpetrator of other abuse

● **Z70**   **Counseling related to sexual attitude, behavior and orientation**

     Includes   encounter for mental health services for sexual attitude, behavior and orientation

     Excludes2   contraceptive or procreative counseling (Z30-Z31)

     Z70.0   **Counseling related to sexual attitude**

     Z70.1   **Counseling related to patient's sexual behavior and orientation**
            Patient concerned regarding impotence
            Patient concerned regarding non-responsiveness
            Patient concerned regarding promiscuity
            Patient concerned regarding sexual orientation

     Z70.2   **Counseling related to sexual behavior and orientation of third party**
            Advice sought regarding sexual behavior and orientation of child
            Advice sought regarding sexual behavior and orientation of partner
            Advice sought regarding sexual behavior and orientation of spouse

     Z70.3   **Counseling related to combined concerns regarding sexual attitude, behavior and orientation**

     Z70.8   **Other sex counseling**
            Encounter for sex education

     Z70.9   **Sex counseling, unspecified**

● **Z71**   **Persons encountering health services for other counseling and medical advice, not elsewhere classified**

     Excludes2   contraceptive or procreation counseling (Z30-Z31)
            sex counseling (Z70.-)

     Z71.0   **Person encountering health services to consult on behalf of another person**
            Person encountering health services to seek advice or treatment for non-attending third party

         Excludes2   anxiety (normal) about sick person in family (Z63.7)
                 expectant (adoptive) parent(s) pre-birth pediatrician visit (Z76.81)

     Z71.1   **Person with feared health complaint in whom no diagnosis is made**
            Person encountering health services with feared condition which was not demonstrated
            Person encountering health services in which problem was normal state
            'Worried well'

         Excludes1   medical observation for suspected diseases and conditions proven not to exist (Z03.-)

Z71.2   **Person consulting for explanation of examination or test findings**

Z71.3   **Dietary counseling and surveillance**
     Use additional code for any associated underlying medical condition
     Use additional code to identify body mass index (BMI), if known (Z68.-)

● **Z71.4**   **Alcohol abuse counseling and surveillance**
     Use additional code for alcohol abuse or dependence (F10.-)

     Z71.41   **Alcohol abuse counseling and surveillance of alcoholic**

     Z71.42   **Counseling for family member of alcoholic**
            Counseling for significant other, partner, or friend of alcoholic

● **Z71.5**   **Drug abuse counseling and surveillance**
     Use additional code for drug abuse or dependence (F11-F16, F18-F19)

     Z71.51   **Drug abuse counseling and surveillance of drug abuser**

     Z71.52   **Counseling for family member of drug abuser**
            Counseling for significant other, partner, or friend of drug abuser

Z71.6   **Tobacco abuse counseling**
     Use additional code for nicotine dependence (F17.-)

Z71.7   **Human immunodeficiency virus [HIV] counseling**

● **Z71.8**   **Other specified counseling**

     Excludes2   counseling for contraception (Z30.0-)
            counseling for genetics (Z31.5)
            counseling for procreative management (Z31.6-)

     Z71.81   **Spiritual or religious counseling**

     Z71.89   **Other specified counseling**

Z71.9   **Counseling, unspecified**
     Encounter for medical advice NOS

● **Z72**   **Problems related to lifestyle**

     Excludes2   problems related to life-management difficulty (Z73.-)
            problems related to socioeconomic and psychosocial circumstances (Z55-Z65)

     Z72.0   **Tobacco use**
            Tobacco use NOS

         Excludes1   history of tobacco dependence (Z87.891)
                 nicotine dependence (F17.2-)
                 tobacco dependence (F17.2-)
                 tobacco use during pregnancy (O99.33-)

     Z72.3   **Lack of physical exercise**

     Z72.4   **Inappropriate diet and eating habits**

         Excludes1   behavioral eating disorders of infancy or childhood (F98.2.-F98.3)
                 eating disorders (F50.-)
                 lack of adequate food (Z59.4)
                 malnutrition and other nutritional deficiencies (E40-E64)

● **Z72.5**   **High risk sexual behavior**
            Promiscuity

         Excludes1   paraphilias (F65)

     Z72.51   **High risk heterosexual behavior**

     Z72.52   **High risk homosexual behavior**

     Z72.53   **High risk bisexual behavior**

     Z72.6   **Gambling and betting**

         Excludes1   compulsive or pathological gambling (F63.0)

● Z72.8   **Other problems related to lifestyle**

  ● Z72.81   **Antisocial behavior**

     Excludes1   conduct disorders (F91.-)

     Z72.810   **Child and adolescent antisocial behavior**

       Antisocial behavior (child) (adolescent) without manifest psychiatric disorder

       Delinquency NOS

       Group delinquency

       Offenses in the context of gang membership

       Stealing in company with others

       Truancy from school

     Z72.811   **Adult antisocial behavior**

       Adult antisocial behavior without manifest psychiatric disorder

  ● Z72.82   **Problems related to sleep**

     Z72.820   **Sleep deprivation**

       Lack of adequate sleep

       Excludes1   insomnia (G47.0-)

     Z72.821   **Inadequate sleep hygiene**

       Bad sleep habits

       Irregular sleep habits

       Unhealthy sleep wake schedule

       Excludes1   insomnia (F51.0-, G47.0-)

     Z72.89   **Other problems related to lifestyle**

       Self-damaging behavior

   Z72.9   **Problem related to lifestyle, unspecified**

● Z73   **Problems related to life management difficulty**

   Excludes2   problems related to socioeconomic and psychosocial circumstances (Z55-Z65)

   Z73.0   **Burn-out**

   Z73.1   **Type A behavior pattern**

   Z73.2   **Lack of relaxation and leisure**

   Z73.3   **Stress, not elsewhere classified**

     Physical and mental strain NOS

     Excludes1   stress related to employment or unemployment (Z56.-)

   Z73.4   **Inadequate social skills, not elsewhere classified**

   Z73.5   **Social role conflict, not elsewhere classified**

   Z73.6   **Limitation of activities due to disability**

     Excludes1   care-provider dependency (Z74.-)

  ● Z73.8   **Other problems related to life management difficulty**

    ● Z73.81   **Behavioral insomnia of childhood**

       Z73.810   **Behavioral insomnia of childhood, sleep-onset association type**

       Z73.811   **Behavioral insomnia of childhood, limit setting type**

       Z73.812   **Behavioral insomnia of childhood, combined type**

       Z73.819   **Behavioral insomnia of childhood, unspecified type**

     Z73.82   **Dual sensory impairment**

     Z73.89   **Other problems related to life management difficulty**

   Z73.9   **Problem related to life management difficulty, unspecified**

● Z74   **Problems related to care provider dependency**

   Excludes2   dependence on enabling machines or devices NEC (Z99.-)

  ● Z74.0   **Reduced mobility**

     Z74.01   **Bed confinement status**

       Bedridden

     Z74.09   **Other reduced mobility**

       Chairridden

       Reduced mobility NOS

       Excludes2   wheelchair dependence (Z99.3)

Z74.1   **Need for assistance with personal care**

Z74.2   **Need for assistance at home and no other household member able to render care**

Z74.3   **Need for continuous supervision**

Z74.8   **Other problems related to care provider dependency**

Z74.9   **Problem related to care provider dependency, unspecified**

● Z75   **Problems related to medical facilities and other health care**

   Z75.0   **Medical services not available in home**

     Excludes1   no other household member able to render care (Z74.2)

   Z75.1   **Person awaiting admission to adequate facility elsewhere**

   Z75.2   **Other waiting period for investigation and treatment**

   Z75.3   **Unavailability and inaccessibility of health care facilities**

     Excludes1   bed unavailable (Z75.1)

   Z75.4   **Unavailability and inaccessibility of other helping agencies**

   Z75.5   **Holiday relief care**

   Z75.8   **Other problems related to medical facilities and other health care**

   Z75.9   **Unspecified problem related to medical facilities and other health care**

● Z76   **Persons encountering health services in other circumstances**

   Z76.0   **Encounter for issue of repeat prescription**

     Encounter for issue of repeat prescription for appliance

     Encounter for issue of repeat prescription for medicaments

     Encounter for issue of repeat prescription for spectacles

     Excludes2   issue of medical certificate (Z02.7)

       repeat prescription for contraceptive (Z30.4-)

   Z76.1   **Encounter for health supervision and care of foundling**

   Z76.2   **Encounter for health supervision and care of other healthy infant and child**

     Encounter for medical or nursing care or supervision of healthy infant under circumstances such as adverse socioeconomic conditions at home

     Encounter for medical or nursing care or supervision of healthy infant under circumstances such as awaiting foster or adoptive placement

     Encounter for medical or nursing care or supervision of healthy infant under circumstances such as maternal illness

     Encounter for medical or nursing care or supervision of healthy infant under circumstances such as number of children at home preventing or interfering with normal care

   Z76.3   **Healthy person accompanying sick person**

   Z76.4   **Other boarder to healthcare facility**

     Excludes1   homelessness (Z59.0)

   Z76.5   **Malingerer [conscious simulation]**

     Person feigning illness (with obvious motivation)

     Excludes1   factitious disorder (F68.1-)

       peregrinating patient (F68.1-)

  ● Z76.8   **Persons encountering health services in other specified circumstances**

     Z76.81   **Expectant parent(s) prebirth pediatrician visit**

       Pre-adoption pediatrician visit for adoptive parent(s)

     Z76.82   **Awaiting organ transplant status**

       Patient waiting for organ availability

     Z76.89   **Persons encountering health services in other specified circumstances**

       Persons encountering health services NOS

◀ New   ⬅ Revised   ~~deleted~~ Deleted   OGCR Official Guidelines   X Assign placeholder X   ● Use Additional Character(s)

Excludes 1   Excludes 2   Includes   Use additional   Code first   Code also   Unspecified

PERSONS WITH POTENTIAL HEALTH HAZARDS RELATED TO FAMILY AND PERSONAL HISTORY AND CERTAIN CONDITIONS INFLUENCING HEALTH STATUS (Z77-Z99)

Code also any follow-up examination (Z08-Z09)

● Z77   **Other contact with and (suspected) exposures hazardous to health**

Includes   contact with and (suspected) exposures to potential hazards to health

Excludes2   contact with and (suspected) exposure to communicable diseases (Z20.-)
exposure to (parental) (environmental) tobacco smoke in the perinatal period (P96.81)
newborn (suspected to be) affected by noxious substances transmitted via placenta or breast milk (P04.-)
occupational exposure to risk factors (Z57.-)
retained foreign body (Z18.-)
retained foreign body fully removed (Z87.821)
toxic effects of substances chiefly nonmedicinal as to source (T51-T65)

● Z77.0   **Contact with and (suspected) exposure to hazardous, chiefly nonmedicinal, chemicals**

● Z77.01   **Contact with and (suspected) exposure to hazardous metals**

Z77.010   **Contact with and (suspected) exposure to arsenic**

Z77.011   **Contact with and (suspected) exposure to lead**

Z77.012   **Contact with and (suspected) exposure to uranium**

Excludes1   retained depleted uranium fragments (Z18.01)

Z77.018   **Contact with and (suspected) exposure to other hazardous metals**
Contact with and (suspected) exposure to chromium compounds
Contact with and (suspected) exposure to nickel dust

● Z77.02   **Contact with and (suspected) exposure to hazardous aromatic compounds**

Z77.020   **Contact with and (suspected) exposure to aromatic amines**

Z77.021   **Contact with and (suspected) exposure to benzene**

Z77.028   **Contact with and (suspected) exposure to other hazardous aromatic compounds**
Aromatic dyes NOS
Polycyclic aromatic hydrocarbons

● Z77.09   **Contact with and (suspected) exposure to other hazardous, chiefly nonmedicinal, chemicals**

Z77.090   **Contact with and (suspected) exposure to asbestos**

Z77.098   **Contact with and (suspected) exposure to other hazardous, chiefly nonmedicinal, chemicals**
Dyes NOS

● Z77.1   **Contact with and (suspected) exposure to environmental pollution and hazards in the physical environment**

● Z77.11   **Contact with and (suspected) exposure to environmental pollution**

Z77.110   **Contact with and (suspected) exposure to air pollution**

Z77.111   **Contact with and (suspected) exposure to water pollution**

Z77.112   **Contact with and (suspected) exposure to soil pollution**

Z77.118   **Contact with and (suspected) exposure to other environmental pollution**

● Z77.12   **Contact with and (suspected) exposure to hazards in the physical environment**

Z77.120   **Contact with and (suspected) exposure to mold (toxic)**

Z77.121   **Contact with and (suspected) exposure to harmful algae and algae toxins**
Contact with and (suspected) exposure to (harmful) algae bloom NOS
Contact with and (suspected) exposure to blue-green algae bloom
Contact with and (suspected) exposure to brown tide
Contact with and (suspected) exposure to cyanobacteria bloom
Contact with and (suspected) exposure to Florida red tide
Contact with and (suspected) exposure to pfiesteria piscicida
Contact with and (suspected) exposure to red tide

Z77.122   **Contact with and (suspected) exposure to noise**

Z77.123   **Contact with and (suspected) exposure to radon and other naturally occuring radiation**

Excludes2   radiation exposure as the cause of a confirmed condition (W88-W90, X39.0-)
radiation sickness NOS (T66)

Z77.128   **Contact with and (suspected) exposure to other hazards in the physical environment**

● Z77.2   **Contact with and (suspected) exposure to other hazardous substances**

Z77.21   **Contact with and (suspected) exposure to potentially hazardous body fluids**

Z77.22   **Contact with and (suspected) exposure to environmental tobacco smoke (acute) (chronic)**
Exposure to second hand tobacco smoke (acute) (chronic)
Passive smoking (acute) (chronic)

Excludes1   nicotine dependence (F17.-)
tobacco use (Z72.0)

Excludes2   occupational exposure to environmental tobacco smoke (Z57.31)

Z77.29   **Contact with and (suspected) exposure to other hazardous substances**

Z77.9   **Other contact with and (suspected) exposures hazardous to health**

CHAPTER 21 (Z00-Z99)

● **Z78   Other specified health status**

     Excludes2   asymptomatic human immunodeficiency virus
                         [HIV] infection status (Z21)
                         postprocedural status (Z93-Z99)
                         sex reassignment status (Z87.890)

   Z78.0   Asymptomatic menopausal state
          Menopausal state NOS
          Postmenopausal status NOS

          Excludes2   symptomatic menopausal state (N95.1)

   Z78.1   Physical restraint status

          Excludes1   physical restraint due to a procedure -
                        omit code

   Z78.9   Other specified health status

● **Z79   Long term (current) drug therapy**

     Includes   long term (current) drug use for prophylactic
                   purposes

   Code also any therapeutic drug level monitoring (Z51.81)

     Excludes2   drug abuse and dependence (F11-F19)
                     drug use complicating pregnancy, childbirth, and
                       the puerperium (O99.32-)

 ● **Z79.0   Long term (current) use of anticoagulants and
            antithrombotics/antiplatelets**

        Excludes2   long term (current) use of aspirin (Z79.82)

     Z79.01   Long term (current) use of anticoagulants

     **Z79.02   Long term (current) use of antithrombotics/
              antiplatelets**

   **Z79.1   Long term (current) use of non-steroidal anti-
          inflammatories (NSAID)**

        Excludes2   long term (current) use of aspirin (Z79.82)

   Z79.2   Long term (current) use of antibiotics

   Z79.3   Long term (current) use of hormonal contraceptives
          Long term (current) use of birth control pill or patch

   Z79.4   Long term (current) use of insulin

 ● **Z79.5   Long term (current) use of steroids**

     Z79.51   Long term (current) use of inhaled steroids

     Z79.52   Long term (current) use of systemic steroids

 ● **Z79.8   Other long term (current) drug therapy**

  ● **Z79.81 Long term (current) use of agents affecting
             estrogen receptors and estrogen levels**

         Code first, if applicable:
          malignant neoplasm of breast (C50.-)
          malignant neoplasm of prostate (C61)

         Use additional code, if applicable, to identify:
          estrogen receptor positive status (Z17.0)
          family history of breast cancer (Z80.3)
          genetic susceptibility to malignant neoplasm
            (cancer) (Z15.0-)
          personal history of breast cancer (Z85.3)
          personal history of prostate cancer (Z85.46)
          postmenopausal status (Z78.0)

         Excludes1   hormone replacement therapy
                     (postmenopausal) (Z79.890)

     **Z79.810   Long term (current) use of selective
              estrogen receptor modulators
              (SERMs)**
               Long term (current) use of raloxifene
                  (Evista)
              Long term (current) use of tamoxifen
                  (Nolvadex)
              Long term (current) use of
                  toremifene (Fareston)

     **Z79.811   Long term (current) use of aromatase
              inhibitors**
              Long term (current) use of
                  anastrozole (Arimidex)
              Long term (current) use of
                  exemestane (Aromasin)
              Long term (current) use of letrozole
                  (Femara)

     **Z79.818   Long term (current) use of other
              agents affecting estrogen receptors
              and estrogen levels**
              Long term (current) use of estrogen
                  receptor downregulators
              Long term (current) use of
                  fulvestrant (Faslodex)
              Long term (current) use of
                  gonadotropin-releasing
                  hormone (GnRH) agonist
              Long term (current) use of goserelin
                  acetate (Zoladex)
              Long term (current) use of
                  leuprolide acetate (leuprorelin)
                  (Lupron)
              Long term (current) use of megestrol
                  acetate (Megace)

   Z79.82   Long term (current) use of aspirin

   Z79.83   Long term (current) use of bisphosphonates

 ● **Z79.89   Other long term (current) drug therapy**

     **Z79.890   Hormone replacement therapy
              (postmenopausal)**

     **Z79.891   Long term (current) use of opiate
              analgesic**
              Long term (current) use of
                  methadone for pain
                  management

              Excludes1   methadone use NOS
                        (F11.2-)
                        use of methodone
                            for treatment of
                            heroin addiction
                            (F11.2-)

     **Z79.899   Other long term (current) drug
              therapy**

● **Z80   Family history of primary malignant neoplasm**

   **Z80.0   Family history of malignant neoplasm of digestive
          organs**
          Conditions classifiable to C15-C26

   **Z80.1   Family history of malignant neoplasm of trachea,
          bronchus and lung**
          Conditions classifiable to C33-C34

   **Z80.2   Family history of malignant neoplasm of other
          respiratory and intrathoracic organs**
          Conditions classifiable to C30-C32, C37-C39

   Z80.3   Family history of malignant neoplasm of breast
          Conditions classifiable to C50.-

 ● **Z80.4   Family history of malignant neoplasm of genital organs**
          Conditions classifiable to C51-C63

     Z80.41   Family history of malignant neoplasm of ovary

     **Z80.42   Family history of malignant neoplasm of
              prostate**

     Z80.43   Family history of malignant neoplasm of testis

     **Z80.49   Family history of malignant neoplasm of other
              genital organs**

 ● **Z80.5   Family history of malignant neoplasm of urinary tract**
          Conditions classifiable to C64-C68

     **Z80.51   Family history of malignant neoplasm of
              kidney**

     **Z80.52   Family history of malignant neoplasm of
              bladder**

     **Z80.59   Family history of malignant neoplasm of other
              urinary tract organ**

   Z80.6   Family history of leukemia
          Conditions classifiable to C91-C95

◀ New   ⬅ Revised   ~~deleted~~ Deleted   **OGCR** Official Guidelines   X Assign placeholder X   ● Use Additional Character(s)

                 Excludes 1   Excludes 2   Includes   Use additional   Code first   Code also   Unspecified

Z80.7   **Family history of other malignant neoplasms of lymphoid, hematopoietic and related tissues**
Conditions classifiable to C81-C90, C96.-

Z80.8   **Family history of malignant neoplasm of other organs or systems**
Conditions classifiable to C00-C14, C40-C49, C69-C79

Z80.9   **Family history of malignant neoplasm, unspecified**
Conditions classifiable to C80.1

● Z81   **Family history of mental and behavioral disorders**

Z81.0   **Family history of intellectual disabilities**
Conditions classifiable to F70-F79

Z81.1   **Family history of alcohol abuse and dependence**
Conditions classifiable to F10.-

Z81.2   **Family history of tobacco abuse and dependence**
Conditions classifiable to F17.-

Z81.3   **Family history of other psychoactive substance abuse and dependence**
Conditions classifiable to F11-F16, F18-F19

Z81.4   **Family history of other substance abuse and dependence**
Conditions classifiable to F55

Z81.8   **Family history of other mental and behavioral disorders**
Conditions classifiable elsewhere in F01-F99

● Z82   **Family history of certain disabilities and chronic diseases (leading to disablement)**

Z82.0   **Family history of epilepsy and other diseases of the nervous system**
Conditions classifiable to G00-G99

Z82.1   **Family history of blindness and visual loss**
Conditions classifiable to H54.-

Z82.2   **Family history of deafness and hearing loss**
Conditions classifiable to H90-H91

Z82.3   **Family history of stroke**
Conditions classifiable to I60-I64

● Z82.4   **Family history of ischemic heart disease and other diseases of the circulatory system**
Conditions classifiable to I00-I52, I65-I99

Z82.41   **Family history of sudden cardiac death**

Z82.49   **Family history of ischemic heart disease and other diseases of the circulatory system**

Z82.5   **Family history of asthma and other chronic lower respiratory diseases**
Conditions classifiable to J40-J47

Excludes2   family history of other diseases of the respiratory system (Z83.6)

● Z82.6   **Family history of arthritis and other diseases of the musculoskeletal system and connective tissue**
Conditions classifiable to M00-M99

Z82.61   **Family history of arthritis**

Z82.62   **Family history of osteoporosis**

Z82.69   **Family history of other diseases of the musculoskeletal system and connective tissue**

● Z82.7   **Family history of congenital malformations, deformations and chromosomal abnormalities**
Conditions classifiable to Q00-Q99

Z82.71   **Family history of polycystic kidney**

Z82.79   **Family history of other congenital malformations, deformations and chromosomal abnormalities**

Z82.8   **Family history of other disabilities and chronic diseases leading to disablement, not elsewhere classified**

● Z83   **Family history of other specific disorders**

Excludes2   contact with and (suspected) exposure to communicable disease in the family (Z20.-)

Z83.0   **Family history of human immunodeficiency virus [HIV] disease**
Conditions classifiable to B20

Z83.1   **Family history of other infectious and parasitic diseases**
Conditions classifiable to A00-B19, B25-B94, B99

Z83.2   **Family history of diseases of the blood and blood-forming organs and certain disorders involving the immune mechanism**
Conditions classifiable to D50-D89

Z83.3   **Family history of diabetes mellitus**
Conditions classifiable to E08-E13

● Z83.4   **Family history of other endocrine, nutritional and metabolic diseases**
Conditions classifiable to E00-E07, E15-E88

Z83.41   **Family history of multiple endocrine neoplasia [MEN] syndrome**

Z83.49   **Family history of other endocrine, nutritional and metabolic diseases**

● Z83.5   **Family history of eye and ear disorders**

● Z83.51   **Family history of eye disorders**
Conditions classifiable to H00-H53, H55-H59

Excludes2   family history of blindness and visual loss (Z82.1)

Z83.511   **Family history of glaucoma**

Z83.518   **Family history of other specified eye disorder**

Z83.52   **Family history of ear disorders**
Conditions classifiable to H60-H83, H92-H95

Excludes2   family history of deafness and hearing loss (Z82.2)

Z83.6   **Family history of other diseases of the respiratory system**
Conditions classifiable to J00-J39, J60-J99

Excludes2   family history of asthma and other chronic lower respiratory diseases (Z82.5)

● Z83.7   **Family history of diseases of the digestive system**
Conditions classifiable to K00-K93

Z83.71   **Family history of colonic polyps**

Excludes1   family history of malignant neoplasm of digestive organs (Z80.0)

Z83.79   **Family history of other diseases of the digestive system**

● Z84   **Family history of other conditions**

Z84.0   **Family history of diseases of the skin and subcutaneous tissue**
Conditions classifiable to L00-L99

Z84.1   **Family history of disorders of kidney and ureter**
Conditions classifiable to N00-N29

Z84.2   **Family history of other diseases of the genitourinary system**
Conditions classifiable to N30-N99

Z84.3   **Family history of consanguinity**

● Z84.8   **Family history of other specified conditions**

Z84.81   **Family history of carrier of genetic disease**

Z84.89   **Family history of other specified conditions**

● **Z85   Personal history of malignant neoplasm**

Code first any follow-up examination after treatment of malignant neoplasm (Z08)

Use additional code to identify:
alcohol use and dependence (F10.-)
exposure to environmental tobacco smoke (Z77.22)
history of tobacco use (Z87.891)
occupational exposure to environmental tobacco smoke (Z57.31)
tobacco dependence (F17.-)
tobacco use (Z72.0)

Excludes2   personal history of benign neoplasm (Z86.01-)
personal history of carcinoma-in-situ (Z86.00-)

● **Z85.0   Personal history of malignant neoplasm of digestive organs**

Z85.00   Personal history of malignant neoplasm of unspecified digestive organ

Z85.01   Personal history of malignant neoplasm of esophagus
Conditions classifiable to C15

● **Z85.02   Personal history of malignant neoplasm of stomach**

Z85.020   Personal history of malignant carcinoid tumor of stomach
Conditions classifiable to C7A.092

Z85.028   Personal history of other malignant neoplasm of stomach
Conditions classifiable to C16

● **Z85.03   Personal history of malignant neoplasm of large intestine**

Z85.030   Personal history of malignant carcinoid tumor of large intestine
Conditions classifiable to C7A.022-C7A.025, C7A.029

Z85.038   Personal history of other malignant neoplasm of large intestine
Conditions classifiable to C18

● **Z85.04   Personal history of malignant neoplasm of rectum, rectosigmoid junction, and anus**

Z85.040   Personal history of malignant carcinoid tumor of rectum
Conditions classifiable to C7A.026

Z85.048   Personal history of other malignant neoplasm of rectum, rectosigmoid junction, and anus
Conditions classifiable to C19-C21

Z85.05   Personal history of malignant neoplasm of liver
Conditions classifiable to C22

● **Z85.06   Personal history of malignant neoplasm of small intestine**

Z85.060   Personal history of malignant carcinoid tumor of small intestine
Conditions classifiable to C7A.01-

Z85.068   Personal history of other malignant neoplasm of small intestine
Conditions classifiable to C17

Z85.07   Personal history of malignant neoplasm of pancreas
Conditions classifiable to C25

Z85.09   Personal history of malignant neoplasm of other digestive organs

● **Z85.1   Personal history of malignant neoplasm of trachea, bronchus and lung**

● **Z85.11   Personal history of malignant neoplasm of bronchus and lung**

Z85.110   Personal history of malignant carcinoid tumor of bronchus and lung
Conditions classifiable to C7A.090

Z85.118   Personal history of other malignant neoplasm of bronchus and lung
Conditions classifiable to C34

Z85.12   Personal history of malignant neoplasm of trachea
Conditions classifiable to C33

● **Z85.2   Personal history of malignant neoplasm of other respiratory and intrathoracic organs**

Z85.20   Personal history of malignant neoplasm of unspecified respiratory organ

Z85.21   Personal history of malignant neoplasm of larynx
Conditions classifiable to C32

Z85.22   Personal history of malignant neoplasm of nasal cavities, middle ear, and accessory sinuses
Conditions classifiable to C30-C31

● **Z85.23   Personal history of malignant neoplasm of thymus**

Z85.230   Personal history of malignant carcinoid tumor of thymus
Conditions classifiable to C7A.091

Z85.238   Personal history of other malignant neoplasm of thymus
Conditions classifiable to C37

Z85.29   Personal history of malignant neoplasm of other respiratory and intrathoracic organs

Z85.3   Personal history of malignant neoplasm of breast
Conditions classifiable to C50.-

● **Z85.4   Personal history of malignant neoplasm of genital organs**
Conditions classifiable to C51-C63

Z85.40   Personal history of malignant neoplasm of unspecified female genital organ

Z85.41   Personal history of malignant neoplasm of cervix uteri

Z85.42   Personal history of malignant neoplasm of other parts of uterus

Z85.43   Personal history of malignant neoplasm of ovary

Z85.44   Personal history of malignant neoplasm of other female genital organs

Z85.45   Personal history of malignant neoplasm of unspecified male genital organ

Z85.46   Personal history of malignant neoplasm of prostate

Z85.47   Personal history of malignant neoplasm of testis

Z85.48   Personal history of malignant neoplasm of epididymis

Z85.49   Personal history of malignant neoplasm of other male genital organs

◀ New   ◀▥ Revised   ~~deleted~~ Deleted   OGCR Official Guidelines   X Assign placeholder X   ● Use Additional Character(s)

Excludes 1   Excludes 2   Includes   Use additional   Code first   Code also   Unspecified

● **Z85.5**   **Personal history of malignant neoplasm of urinary tract**
Conditions classifiable to C64-C68

    Z85.50   Personal history of malignant neoplasm of unspecified urinary tract organ

    Z85.51   Personal history of malignant neoplasm of bladder

●   **Z85.52**   Personal history of malignant neoplasm of kidney
       Excludes1   personal history of malignant neoplasm of renal pelvis (Z85.53)

       Z85.520   Personal history of malignant carcinoid tumor of kidney
Conditions classifiable to C7A.093

       Z85.528   Personal history of other malignant neoplasm of kidney
Conditions classifiable to C64

    Z85.53   Personal history of malignant neoplasm of renal pelvis

    Z85.54   Personal history of malignant neoplasm of ureter

    Z85.59   Personal history of malignant neoplasm of other urinary tract organ

● **Z85.6**   **Personal history of leukemia**
Conditions classifiable to C91-C95
    Excludes1   leukemia in remission C91.0-C95.9 with 5th character 1

● **Z85.7**   **Personal history of other malignant neoplasms of lymphoid, hematopoietic and related tissues**

    Z85.71   Personal history of Hodgkin lymphoma
Conditions classifiable to C81

    Z85.72   Personal history of non-Hodgkin lymphomas
Conditions classifiable to C82-C85

    Z85.79   Personal history of other malignant neoplasms of lymphoid, hematopoietic and related tissues
Conditions classifiable to C88-C90, C96
      Excludes1   multiple myeloma in remission (C90.01)
plasma cell leukemia in remission (C90.11)
plasmacytoma in remission (C90.21)

● **Z85.8**   **Personal history of malignant neoplasms of other organs and systems**
Conditions classifiable to C00-C14, C40-C49, C69-C79, C7A.098

●   **Z85.81**   Personal history of malignant neoplasm of lip, oral cavity, and pharynx

      Z85.810   Personal history of malignant neoplasm of tongue

      Z85.818   Personal history of malignant neoplasm of other sites of lip, oral cavity, and pharynx

      Z85.819   Personal history of malignant neoplasm of unspecified site of lip, oral cavity, and pharynx

●   **Z85.82**   Personal history of malignant neoplasm of skin

      Z85.820   Personal history of malignant melanoma of skin
Conditions classifiable to C43

      Z85.821   Personal history of Merkel cell carcinoma
Conditions classifiable to C4A

      Z85.828   Personal history of other malignant neoplasm of skin
Conditions classifiable to C44

●   **Z85.83**   Personal history of malignant neoplasm of bone and soft tissue

      Z85.830   Personal history of malignant neoplasm of bone

      Z85.831   Personal history of malignant neoplasm of soft tissue
       Excludes2   personal history of malignant neoplasm of skin (Z85.82-)

●   **Z85.84**   Personal history of malignant neoplasm of eye and nervous tissue

      Z85.840   Personal history of malignant neoplasm of eye

      Z85.841   Personal history of malignant neoplasm of brain

      Z85.848   Personal history of malignant neoplasm of other parts of nervous tissue

●   **Z85.85**   Personal history of malignant neoplasm of endocrine glands

      Z85.850   Personal history of malignant neoplasm of thyroid

      Z85.858   Personal history of malignant neoplasm of other endocrine glands

    Z85.89   Personal history of malignant neoplasm of other organs and systems

    Z85.9   Personal history of malignant neoplasm, unspecified
Conditions classifiable to C7A.00, C80.1

● **Z86**   **Personal history of certain other diseases**
Code first any follow-up examination after treatment (Z09)

● **Z86.0**   **Personal history of in-situ and benign neoplasms and neoplasms of uncertain behavior**
    Excludes2   personal history of malignant neoplasms (Z85.-)

● **Z86.00**   Personal history of in-situ neoplasm

    Z86.000   Personal history of in-situ neoplasm of breast

    Z86.001   Personal history of in-situ neoplasm of cervix uteri

    Z86.008   Personal history of in-situ neoplasm of other site

● **Z86.01**   Personal history of benign neoplasm

    Z86.010   Personal history of colonic polyps

    Z86.011   Personal history of benign neoplasm of the brain

    Z86.012   Personal history of benign carcinoid tumor

    Z86.018   Personal history of other benign neoplasm

    Z86.03   Personal history of neoplasm of uncertain behavior

● **Z86.1**   **Personal history of infectious and parasitic diseases**
Conditions classifiable to A00-B89, B99
    Excludes1   personal history of infectious diseases specific to a body system sequelae of infectious and parasitic diseases (B90-B94)

    Z86.11   Personal history of tuberculosis

    Z86.12   Personal history of poliomyelitis

    Z86.13   Personal history of malaria

    Z86.14   Personal history of Methicillin resistant Staphylococcus aureus infection
Personal history of MRSA infection

    Z86.19   Personal history of other infectious and parasitic diseases

Z86.2 **Personal history of diseases of the blood and blood-forming organs and certain disorders involving the immune mechanism**
Conditions classifiable to D50-D89

● **Z86.3** **Personal history of endocrine, nutritional and metabolic diseases**
Conditions classifiable to E00-E88

Z86.31 **Personal history of diabetic foot ulcer**
Excludes2 current diabetic foot ulcer (E08.621, E09.621, E10.621, E11.621, E13.621)

Z86.32 **Personal history of gestational diabetes**
Personal history of conditions classifiable to O24.4-
Excludes1 gestational diabetes mellitus in current pregnancy (O24.4-)

Z86.39 **Personal history of other endocrine, nutritional and metabolic disease**

● **Z86.5** **Personal history of mental and behavioral disorders**
Conditions classifiable to F40-F59

Z86.51 **Personal history of combat and operational stress reaction**

Z86.59 **Personal history of other mental and behavioral disorders**

● **Z86.6** **Personal history of diseases of the nervous system and sense organs**
Conditions classifiable to G00-G99, H00-H95

Z86.61 **Personal history of infections of the central nervous system**
Personal history of encephalitis
Personal history of meningitis

Z86.69 **Personal history of other diseases of the nervous system and sense organs**

● **Z86.7** **Personal history of diseases of the circulatory system**
Conditions classifiable to I00-I99
Excludes2 old myocardial infarction (I25.2)
personal history of anaphylactic shock (Z87.892)
postmyocardial infarction syndrome (I24.1)

● **Z86.71** **Personal history of venous thrombosis and embolism**

Z86.711 **Personal history of pulmonary embolism**

Z86.718 **Personal history of other venous thrombosis and embolism**

Z86.72 **Personal history of thrombophlebitis**

Z86.73 **Personal history of transient ischemic attack (TIA), and cerebral infarction without residual deficits**
Personal history of prolonged reversible ischemic neurological deficit (PRIND)
Personal history of stroke NOS without residual deficits
Excludes1 personal history of traumatic brain injury (Z87.820)
sequelae of cerebrovascular disease (I69.-)

Z86.74 **Personal history of sudden cardiac arrest**
Personal history of sudden cardiac death successfully resuscitated

Z86.79 **Personal history of other diseases of the circulatory system**

● **Z87** **Personal history of other diseases and conditions**
Code first any follow-up examination after treatment (Z09)

● **Z87.0** **Personal history of diseases of the respiratory system**
Conditions classifiable to J00-J99

Z87.01 **Personal history of pneumonia (recurrent)**

Z87.09 **Personal history of other diseases of the respiratory system**

● **Z87.1** **Personal history of diseases of the digestive system**
Conditions classifiable to K00-K93

Z87.11 **Personal history of peptic ulcer disease**

Z87.19 **Personal history of other diseases of the digestive system**

Z87.2 **Personal history of diseases of the skin and subcutaneous tissue**
Conditions classifiable to L00-L99
Excludes2 personal history of diabetic foot ulcer (Z86.31)

● **Z87.3** **Personal history of diseases of the musculoskeletal system and connective tissue**
Conditions classifiable to M00-M99
Excludes2 personal history of (healed) traumatic fracture (Z87.81)

● **Z87.31** **Personal history of (healed) nontraumatic fracture**

Z87.310 **Personal history of (healed) osteoporosis fracture**
Personal history of (healed) fragility fracture
Personal history of (healed) collapsed vertebra due to osteoporosis

Z87.311 **Personal history of (healed) other pathological fracture**
Personal history of (healed) collapsed vertebra NOS
Excludes2 personal history of osteoporosis fracture (Z87.310)

Z87.312 **Personal history of (healed) stress fracture**
Personal history of (healed) fatigue fracture

Z87.39 **Personal history of other diseases of the musculoskeletal system and connective tissue**

● **Z87.4** **Personal history of diseases of genitourinary system**
Conditions classifiable to N00-N99

● **Z87.41** **Personal history of dysplasia of the female genital tract**
Excludes1 personal history of malignant neoplasm of female genital tract (Z85.40-Z85.44)

Z87.410 **Personal history of cervical dysplasia**

Z87.411 **Personal history of vaginal dysplasia**

Z87.412 **Personal history of vulvar dysplasia**

Z87.42 **Personal history of other diseases of the female genital tract**

CHAPTER 21 (Z00-Z99)

● **Z87.43   Personal history of diseases of male genital organs**

    Z87.430   **Personal history of prostatic dysplasia**

        Excludes1   personal history of malignant neoplasm of prostate (Z85.46)

    Z87.438   **Personal history of other diseases of male genital organs**

● **Z87.44   Personal history of diseases of urinary system**

    Excludes1   personal history of malignant neoplasm of cervix uteri (Z85.41)

    Z87.440   **Personal history of urinary (tract) infections**

    Z87.441   **Personal history of nephrotic syndrome**

    Z87.442   **Personal history of urinary calculi**

        Personal history of kidney stones

    Z87.448   **Personal history of other diseases of urinary system**

● **Z87.5   Personal history of complications of pregnancy, childbirth and the puerperium**

    Conditions classifiable to O00-O9A

    Excludes2   recurrent pregnancy loss (N96)

    Z87.51   **Personal history of pre-term labor**

        Excludes1   current pregnancy with history of pre-term labor (O09.21-)

    Z87.59   **Personal history of other complications of pregnancy, childbirth and the puerperium**

        Personal history of trophoblastic disease

● **Z87.7   Personal history of (corrected) congenital malformations**

    Conditions classifiable to Q00-Q89 that have been repaired or corrected

    Excludes1   congenital malformations that have been partially corrected or repair but which still require medical treatment - code to condition

    Excludes2   other postprocedural states (Z98.-)

        personal history of medical treatment (Z92.-)

        presence of cardiac and vascular implants and grafts (Z95.-)

        presence of other devices (Z97.-)

        presence of other functional implants (Z96.-)

        transplanted organ and tissue status (Z94.-)

● **Z87.71   Personal history of (corrected) congenital malformations of genitourinary system**

    Z87.710   **Personal history of (corrected) hypospadias**

    Z87.718   **Personal history of other specified (corrected) congenital malformations of genitourinary system**

● **Z87.72   Personal history of (corrected) congenital malformations of nervous system and sense organs**

    Z87.720   **Personal history of (corrected) congenital malformations of eye**

    Z87.721   **Personal history of (corrected) congenital malformations of ear**

    Z87.728   **Personal history of other specified (corrected) congenital malformations of nervous system and sense organs**

● **Z87.73   Personal history of (corrected) congenital malformations of digestive system**

    Z87.730   **Personal history of (corrected) cleft lip and palate**

    Z87.738   **Personal history of other specified (corrected) congenital malformations of digestive system**

  Z87.74   Personal history of (corrected) congenital malformations of heart and circulatory system

  Z87.75   Personal history of (corrected) congenital malformations of respiratory system

  Z87.76   Personal history of (corrected) congenital malformations of integument, limbs and musculoskeletal system

● **Z87.79   Personal history of other (corrected) congenital malformations**

    Z87.790   **Personal history of (corrected) congenital malformations of face and neck**

    Z87.798   **Personal history of other (corrected) congenital malformations**

● **Z87.8   Personal history of other specified conditions**

    Excludes2   personal history of self harm (Z91.5)

    Z87.81   **Personal history of (healed) traumatic fracture**

        Excludes2   personal history of (healed) nontraumatic fracture (Z87.31-)

● **Z87.82   Personal history of other (healed) physical injury and trauma**

    Conditions classifiable to S00-T88, except traumatic fractures

    Z87.820   **Personal history of traumatic brain injury**

        Excludes1   personal history of transient ischemic attack (TIA), and cerebral infarction without residual deficits (Z86.73)

    Z87.821   **Personal history of retained foreign body fully removed**

    Z87.828   **Personal history of other (healed) physical injury and trauma**

● **Z87.89   Personal history of other specified conditions**

    Z87.890   **Personal history of sex reassignment**

    Z87.891   **Personal history of nicotine dependence**

        Excludes1   current nicotine dependence (F17.2-)

    Z87.892   **Personal history of anaphylaxis**

        Code also allergy status such as: allergy status to drugs, medicaments and biological substances (Z88.-)

        allergy status, other than to drugs and biological substances (Z91.0-)

    Z87.898   **Personal history of other specified conditions**

CHAPTER 21 (Z00-Z99)

◄ New   ◄▥ Revised   ~~deleted~~ Deleted   **OGCR** Official Guidelines   X Assign placeholder X   ● Use Additional Character(s)

| Excludes 1 | Excludes 2 | Includes | Use additional | Code first | Code also | Unspecified |

●**Z88 Allergy status to drugs, medicaments and biological substances**
> Excludes2   allergy status, other than to drugs and biological substances (Z91.0-)

Z88.0   Allergy status to penicillin
Z88.1   Allergy status to other antibiotic agents status
Z88.2   Allergy status to sulfonamides status
Z88.3   Allergy status to other anti-infective agents status
Z88.4   Allergy status to anesthetic agent status
Z88.5   Allergy status to narcotic agent status
Z88.6   Allergy status to analgesic agent status
Z88.7   Allergy status to serum and vaccine status
Z88.8   Allergy status to other drugs, medicaments and biological substances status
Z88.9   Allergy status to unspecified drugs, medicaments and biological substances status

●**Z89 Acquired absence of limb**
> Includes   amputation status
> postprocedural loss of limb
> post-traumatic loss of limb
> Excludes1   acquired deformities of limbs (M20-M21)
> congenital absence of limbs (Q71-Q73)

●Z89.0   Acquired absence of thumb and other finger(s)
  ●Z89.01   Acquired absence of thumb
    Z89.011   Acquired absence of right thumb
    Z89.012   Acquired absence of left thumb
    Z89.019   Acquired absence of unspecified thumb
  ●Z89.02   Acquired absence of other finger(s)
> Excludes2   acquired absence of thumb (Z89.01-)

    Z89.021   Acquired absence of right finger(s)
    Z89.022   Acquired absence of left finger(s)
    Z89.029   Acquired absence of unspecified finger(s)
●Z89.1   Acquired absence of hand and wrist
  ●Z89.11   Acquired absence of hand
    Z89.111   Acquired absence of right hand
    Z89.112   Acquired absence of left hand
    Z89.119   Acquired absence of unspecified hand
  ●Z89.12   Acquired absence of wrist
> Disarticulation at wrist

    Z89.121   Acquired absence of right wrist
    Z89.122   Acquired absence of left wrist
    Z89.129   Acquired absence of unspecified wrist
●Z89.2   Acquired absence of upper limb above wrist
  ●Z89.20   Acquired absence of upper limb, unspecified level
    Z89.201   Acquired absence of right upper limb, unspecified level
    Z89.202   Acquired absence of left upper limb, unspecified level
    Z89.209   Acquired absence of unspecified upper limb, unspecified level
> Acquired absence of arm NOS
  ●Z89.21   Acquired absence of upper limb below elbow
    Z89.211   Acquired absence of right upper limb below elbow
    Z89.212   Acquired absence of left upper limb below elbow
    Z89.219   Acquired absence of unspecified upper limb below elbow

●Z89.22   Acquired absence of upper limb above elbow
> Disarticulation at elbow
    Z89.221   Acquired absence of right upper limb above elbow
    Z89.222   Acquired absence of left upper limb above elbow
    Z89.229   Acquired absence of unspecified upper limb above elbow
●Z89.23   Acquired absence of shoulder
> Acquired absence of shoulder joint following explantation of shoulder joint prosthesis, with or without presence of antibiotic-impregnated cement spacer
    Z89.231   Acquired absence of right shoulder
    Z89.232   Acquired absence of left shoulder
    Z89.239   Acquired absence of unspecified shoulder
●Z89.4   Acquired absence of toe(s), foot, and ankle
  ●Z89.41   Acquired absence of great toe
    Z89.411   Acquired absence of right great toe
    Z89.412   Acquired absence of left great toe
    Z89.419   Acquired absence of unspecified great toe
  ●Z89.42   Acquired absence of other toe(s)
> Excludes2   acquired absence of great toe (Z89.41-)
    Z89.421   Acquired absence of other right toe(s)
    Z89.422   Acquired absence of other left toe(s)
    Z89.429   Acquired absence of other toe(s), unspecified side
  ●Z89.43   Acquired absence of foot
    Z89.431   Acquired absence of right foot
    Z89.432   Acquired absence of left foot
    Z89.439   Acquired absence of unspecified foot
  ●Z89.44   Acquired absence of ankle
> Disarticulation of ankle
    Z89.441   Acquired absence of right ankle
    Z89.442   Acquired absence of left ankle
    Z89.449   Acquired absence of unspecified ankle
●Z89.5   Acquired absence of leg below knee
  ●Z89.51   Acquired absence of leg below knee
    Z89.511   Acquired absence of right leg below knee
    Z89.512   Acquired absence of left leg below knee
    Z89.519   Acquired absence of unspecified leg below knee
  ●Z89.52   Acquired absence of knee
> Acquired absence of knee joint following explantation of knee joint prosthesis, with or without presence of antibiotic-impregnated cement spacer
    Z89.521   Acquired absence of right knee
    Z89.522   Acquired absence of left knee
    Z89.529   Acquired absence of unspecified knee

◀ New   ◀▥ Revised   ~~deleted~~ Deleted   **OGCR** Official Guidelines   X Assign placeholder X   ● Use Additional Character(s)

Excludes 1   Excludes 2   Includes   Use additional   Code first   Code also   Unspecified

● **Z89.6 Acquired absence of leg above knee**
  ● **Z89.61 Acquired absence of leg above knee**
       Acquired absence of leg NOS
       Disarticulation at knee
       Z89.611 Acquired absence of right leg above knee
       Z89.612 Acquired absence of left leg above knee
       Z89.619 Acquired absence of unspecified leg above knee
  ● **Z89.62 Acquired absence of hip**
       Acquired absence of hip joint following explantation of hip joint prosthesis, with or without presence of antibiotic-impregnated cement spacer
       Disarticulation at hip
       Z89.621 Acquired absence of right hip joint
       Z89.622 Acquired absence of left hip joint
       Z89.629 Acquired absence of unspecified hip joint
  Z89.9 Acquired absence of limb, unspecified

● **Z90 Acquired absence of organs, not elsewhere classified**
Includes	postprocedural or post-traumatic loss of body part NEC
Excludes1	congenital absence - see Alphabetical Index
Excludes2	postprocedural absence of endocrine glands (E89.-)
  ● **Z90.0 Acquired absence of part of head and neck**
       Z90.01 Acquired absence of eye
       Z90.02 Acquired absence of larynx
       Z90.09 Acquired absence of other part of head and neck
            Acquired absence of nose
            | **Excludes2** | teeth (K08.1) |
  ● **Z90.1 Acquired absence of breast and nipple**
       Z90.10 Acquired absence of unspecified breast and nipple
       Z90.11 Acquired absence of right breast and nipple
       Z90.12 Acquired absence of left breast and nipple
       Z90.13 Acquired absence of bilateral breasts and nipples
  Z90.2 Acquired absence of lung [part of]
  Z90.3 Acquired absence of stomach [part of]
  ● **Z90.4 Acquired absence of other specified parts of digestive tract**
     ● **Z90.41 Acquired absence of pancreas**
          Use additional code to identify any associated:
            insulin use (Z79.4)
            diabetes mellitus, postpancreatectomy (E13.-)
          Z90.410 Acquired total absence of pancreas
               Acquired absence of pancreas NOS
          Z90.411 Acquired partial absence of pancreas
       Z90.49 Acquired absence of other specified parts of digestive tract
  Z90.5 Acquired absence of kidney
  Z90.6 Acquired absence of other parts of urinary tract
       Acquired absence of bladder

● **Z90.7 Acquired absence of genital organ(s)**
  | **Excludes1** | personal history of sex reassignment (Z87.890) |
  | **Excludes2** | female genital mutilation status (N90.81-) |
  ● **Z90.71 Acquired absence of cervix and uterus**
       Z90.710 Acquired absence of both cervix and uterus
            Acquired absence of uterus NOS
            Status post total hysterectomy
       Z90.711 Acquired absence of uterus with remaining cervical stump
            Status post partial hysterectomy with remaining cervical stump
       Z90.712 Acquired absence of cervix with remaining uterus
  ● **Z90.72 Acquired absence of ovaries**
       Z90.721 Acquired absence of ovaries, unilateral
       Z90.722 Acquired absence of ovaries, bilateral
  Z90.79 Acquired absence of other genital organ(s)
● **Z90.8 Acquired absence of other organs**
  Z90.81 Acquired absence of spleen
  Z90.89 Acquired absence of other organs

● **Z91 Personal risk factors, not elsewhere classified**
Excludes2	contact with and (suspected) exposures hazardous to health (Z77.-)
	exposure to pollution and other problems related to physical environment (Z77.1-)
	occupational exposure to risk factors (Z57.-)
	personal history of physical injury and trauma (Z87.81, Z87.82-)
  ● **Z91.0 Allergy status, other than to drugs and biological substances**
     | **Excludes2** | allergy status to drugs, medicaments, and biological substances (Z88.-) |
     ● **Z91.01 Food allergy status**
          | **Excludes2** | food additives allergy status (Z91.02) |
          Z91.010 Allergy to peanuts
          Z91.011 Allergy to milk products
               | **Excludes1** | lactose intolerance (E73.-) |
          Z91.012 Allergy to eggs
          Z91.013 Allergy to seafood
               Allergy to shellfish
               Allergy to octopus or squid ink
          Z91.018 Allergy to other foods
               Allergy to nuts other than peanuts
       Z91.02 Food additives allergy status
     ● **Z91.03 Insect allergy status**
          Z91.030 Bee allergy status
          Z91.038 Other insect allergy status
     ● **Z91.04 Nonmedicinal substance allergy status**
          Z91.040 Latex allergy status
               Latex sensitivity status
          Z91.041 Radiographic dye allergy status
               Allergy status to contrast media used for diagnostic X-ray procedure
          Z91.048 Other nonmedicinal substance allergy status
       Z91.09 Other allergy status, other than to drugs and biological substances

● **Z91.1   Patient's noncompliance with medical treatment and regimen**

     Z91.11   Patient's noncompliance with dietary regimen

     ● **Z91.12   Patient's intentional underdosing of medication regimen**

         Code first underdosing of medication (T36-T50) with fifth or sixth character 6

         Excludes1   adverse effect of prescribed drug taken as directed - code to adverse effect

                 poisoning (overdose) - code to poisoning

         Z91.120   Patient's intentional underdosing of medication regimen due to financial hardship

         Z91.128   Patient's intentional underdosing of medication regimen for other reason

     ● **Z91.13   Patient's unintentional underdosing of medication regimen**

         Code first underdosing of medication (T36-T50) with fifth or sixth character 6

         Excludes1   adverse effect of prescribed drug taken as directed - code to adverse effect

                 poisoning (overdose) - code to poisoning

         Z91.130   Patient's unintentional underdosing of medication regimen due to age-related debility

         Z91.138   Patient's unintentional underdosing of medication regimen for other reason

     Z91.14   Patient's other noncompliance with medication regimen

         Patient's underdosing of medication NOS

     Z91.15   Patient's noncompliance with renal dialysis

     Z91.19   Patient's noncompliance with other medical treatment and regimen

● **Z91.4   Personal history of psychological trauma, not elsewhere classified**

     ● **Z91.41   Personal history of adult abuse**

         Excludes2   personal history of abuse in childhood (Z62.81-)

         Z91.410   Personal history of adult physical and sexual abuse

            Excludes1   current adult physical abuse (T74.11, T76.11)

                     current adult sexual abuse (T74.21, T76.11)

         Z91.411   Personal history of adult psychological abuse

         Z91.412   Personal history of adult neglect

            Excludes1   current adult neglect (T74.01, T76.01)

         Z91.419   Personal history of unspecified adult abuse

     Z91.49   Other personal history of psychological trauma, not elsewhere classified

     Z91.5   Personal history of self-harm

         Personal history of parasuicide

         Personal history of self-poisoning

         Personal history of suicide attempt

● **Z91.8   Other specified personal risk factors, not elsewhere classified**

     Z91.81   History of falling

         At risk for falling

     Z91.82   Personal history of military deployment

         Individual (civilian or military) with past history of military war, peacekeeping and humanitarian deployment (current or past conflict)

         Returned from military deployment

     Z91.83   Wandering in diseases classified elsewhere

         Code first underlying disorder such as:

         Alzheimer's disease (G30.-)

         autism or pervasive developmental disorder (F84.-)

         intellectual disabilities (F70-F79)

         unspecified dementia with behavioral disturbance (F03.9-)

     Z91.89   Other specified personal risk factors, not elsewhere classified

● **Z92   Personal history of medical treatment**

     Excludes2   postprocedural states (Z98.-)

     Z92.0   Personal history of contraception

         Excludes1   counseling or management of current contraceptive practices (Z30.-)

                 long term (current) use of contraception (Z79.3)

                 presence of (intrauterine) contraceptive device (Z97.5)

     ● **Z92.2   Personal history of drug therapy**

         Excludes2   long term (current) drug therapy (Z79.-)

         Z92.21   Personal history of antineoplastic chemotherapy

         Z92.22   Personal history of monoclonal drug therapy

         Z92.23   Personal history of estrogen therapy

         ● **Z92.24   Personal history of steroid therapy**

            Z92.240   Personal history of inhaled steroid therapy

            Z92.241   Personal history of systemic steroid therapy

                Personal history of steroid therapy NOS

         Z92.25   Personal history of immunosupression therapy

            Excludes2   personal history of steroid therapy (Z92.24)

         Z92.29   Personal history of other drug therapy

     Z92.3   Personal history of irradiation

         Personal history of exposure to therapeutic radiation

         Excludes1   exposure to radiation in the physical environment (Z77.12)

                 occupational exposure to radiation (Z57.1)

     ● **Z92.8   Personal history of other medical treatment**

         Z92.81   Personal history of extracorporeal membrane oxygenation (ECMO)

         Z92.82   Status post administration of tPA (rtPA) in a different facility within the last 24 hours prior to admission to current facility

         Code first condition requiring tPA administration, such as:

         acute cerebral infarction (I63.-)

         acute myocardial infarction (I21.-, I22.-)

         Z92.83   Personal history of failed moderate sedation

         Personal history of failed conscious sedation

         Excludes2   failed moderate sedation during procedure (T88.52)

         Z92.89   Personal history of other medical treatment

◀ New   ◀▥ Revised   ~~deleted~~ Deleted   **OGCR** Official Guidelines   X Assign placeholder X   ● Use Additional Character(s)

Excludes 1   Excludes 2   Includes   Use additional   Code first   Code also   Unspecified

● **Z93 Artificial opening status**
> **Excludes1** artificial openings requiring attention or management (Z43.-)
> complications of external stoma (J95.0-, K94.-, N99.5-)

Z93.0 Tracheostomy status

Z93.1 Gastrostomy status

Z93.2 Ileostomy status

Z93.3 Colostomy status

Z93.4 Other artificial openings of gastrointestinal tract status

● Z93.5 **Cystostomy status**

    Z93.50 Unspecified cystostomy status

    Z93.51 Cutaneous-vesicostomy status

    Z93.52 Appendico-vesicostomy status

    Z93.59 Other cystostomy status

Z93.6 Other artificial openings of urinary tract status
> Nephrostomy status
> Ureterostomy status
> Urethrostomy status

Z93.8 Other artificial opening status

Z93.9 Artificial opening status, unspecified

● **Z94 Transplanted organ and tissue status**
> **Includes** organ or tissue replaced by heterogenous or homogenous transplant
> **Excludes1** complications of transplanted organ or tissue - see Alphabetical Index
> **Excludes2** presence of vascular grafts (Z95.-)

Z94.0 Kidney transplant status

Z94.1 Heart transplant status
> **Excludes1** artificial heart status (Z95.812)
> heart-valve replacement status (Z95.2-Z95.4)

Z94.2 Lung transplant status

Z94.3 Heart and lungs transplant status

Z94.4 Liver transplant status

Z94.5 Skin transplant status
> Autogenous skin transplant status

Z94.6 Bone transplant status

Z94.7 Corneal transplant status

● Z94.8 **Other transplanted organ and tissue status**

    Z94.81 Bone marrow transplant status

    Z94.82 Intestine transplant status

    Z94.83 Pancreas transplant status

    Z94.84 Stem cells transplant status

    Z94.89 Other transplanted organ and tissue status

Z94.9 Transplanted organ and tissue status, unspecified

● **Z95 Presence of cardiac and vascular implants and grafts**
> **Excludes1** complications of cardiac and vascular devices, implants and grafts (T82.-)

Z95.0 Presence of cardiac pacemaker
> **Excludes1** adjustment or management of cardiac pacemaker (Z45.0)
> presence of automatic (implantable) cardiac defibrillator with synchronous cardiac pacemaker (Z95.810)

Z95.1 Presence of aortocoronary bypass graft

Z95.2 Presence of prosthetic heart valve
> Presence of heart valve NOS

Z95.3 Presence of xenogenic heart valve

Z95.4 Presence of other heart-valve replacement

Z95.5 Presence of coronary angioplasty implant and graft
> **Excludes1** coronary angioplasty status without implant and graft (Z98.61)

● Z95.8 **Presence of other cardiac and vascular implants and grafts**

● Z95.81 **Presence of other cardiac implants and grafts**

    Z95.810 Presence of automatic (implantable) cardiac defibrillator
> Presence of automatic (implantable) cardiac defibrillator with synchronous cardiac pacemaker

    Z95.811 Presence of heart assist device

    Z95.812 Presence of fully implantable artificial heart

    Z95.818 Presence of other cardiac implants and grafts

● Z95.82 **Presence of other vascular implants and grafts**

    Z95.820 Peripheral vascular angioplasty status with implants and grafts
> **Excludes1** peripheral vascular angioplasty without implant and graft (Z98.62)

    Z95.828 Presence of other vascular implants and grafts
> Presence of intravascular prosthesis NEC

Z95.9 Presence of cardiac and vascular implant and graft, unspecified

● **Z96 Presence of other functional implants**
> **Excludes2** complications of internal prosthetic devices, implants and grafts (T82-T85)
> fitting and adjustment of prosthetic and other devices (Z44-Z46)

Z96.0 Presence of urogenital implants

Z96.1 Presence of intraocular lens
> Presence of pseudophakia

● Z96.2 **Presence of otological and audiological implants**

    Z96.20 Presence of otological and audiological implant, unspecified

    Z96.21 Cochlear implant status

    Z96.22 Myringotomy tube(s) status

    Z96.29 Presence of other otological and audiological implants
> Presence of bone-conduction hearing device
> Presence of eustachian tube stent
> Stapes replacement

Z96.3 Presence of artificial larynx

● Z96.4 **Presence of endocrine implants**

    Z96.41 Presence of insulin pump (external) (internal)

    Z96.49 Presence of other endocrine implants

Z96.5 Presence of tooth-root and mandibular implants

● Z96.6 **Presence of orthopedic joint implants**

    Z96.60 Presence of unspecified orthopedic joint implant

● Z96.61 **Presence of artificial shoulder joint**

    Z96.611 Presence of right artificial shoulder joint

    Z96.612 Presence of left artificial shoulder joint

    Z96.619 Presence of unspecified artificial shoulder joint

● **Z96.62 Presence of artificial elbow joint**
     Z96.621 Presence of right artificial elbow joint
     Z96.622 Presence of left artificial elbow joint
     Z96.629 Presence of unspecified artificial elbow joint

● **Z96.63 Presence of artificial wrist joint**
     Z96.631 Presence of right artificial wrist joint
     Z96.632 Presence of left artificial wrist joint
     Z96.639 Presence of unspecified artificial wrist joint

● **Z96.64 Presence of artificial hip joint**
     Hip-joint replacement (partial) (total)
     Z96.641 Presence of right artificial hip joint
     Z96.642 Presence of left artificial hip joint
     Z96.643 Presence of artificial hip joint, bilateral
     Z96.649 Presence of unspecified artificial hip joint

● **Z96.65 Presence of artificial knee joint**
     Z96.651 Presence of right artificial knee joint
     Z96.652 Presence of left artificial knee joint
     Z96.653 Presence of artificial knee joint, bilateral
     Z96.659 Presence of unspecified artificial knee joint

● **Z96.66 Presence of artificial ankle joint**
     Z96.661 Presence of right artificial ankle joint
     Z96.662 Presence of left artificial ankle joint
     Z96.669 Presence of unspecified artificial ankle joint

● **Z96.69 Presence of other orthopedic joint implants**
     Z96.691 Finger-joint replacement of right hand
     Z96.692 Finger-joint replacement of left hand
     Z96.693 Finger-joint replacement, bilateral
     Z96.698 Presence of other orthopedic joint implants

Z96.7 Presence of other bone and tendon implants
     Presence of skull plate

● **Z96.8 Presence of other specified functional implants**
     Z96.81 Presence of artificial skin
     Z96.89 Presence of other specified functional implants

Z96.9 Presence of functional implant, unspecified

● **Z97 Presence of other devices**
     Excludes1 complications of internal prosthetic devices, implants and grafts (T82-T85)
            fitting and adjustment of prosthetic and other devices (Z44-Z46)
     Excludes2 presence of cerebrospinal fluid drainage device (Z98.2)

Z97.0 Presence of artificial eye

● **Z97.1 Presence of artificial limb (complete) (partial)**
     Z97.10 Presence of artificial limb (complete) (partial), unspecified
     Z97.11 Presence of artificial right arm (complete) (partial)
     Z97.12 Presence of artificial left arm (complete) (partial)

     Z97.13 Presence of artificial right leg (complete) (partial)
     Z97.14 Presence of artificial left leg (complete) (partial)
     Z97.15 Presence of artificial arms, bilateral (complete) (partial)
     Z97.16 Presence of artificial legs, bilateral (complete) (partial)

Z97.2 Presence of dental prosthetic device (complete) (partial)
     Presence of dentures (complete) (partial)

Z97.3 Presence of spectacles and contact lenses

Z97.4 Presence of external hearing-aid

Z97.5 Presence of (intrauterine) contraceptive device
     Excludes1 checking, reinsertion or removal of contraceptive device (Z30.43)

Z97.8 Presence of other specified devices

● **Z98 Other postprocedural states**
     Excludes2 aftercare (Z43-Z49, Z51)
            follow-up medical care (Z08-Z09)
            postprocedural complication - see Alphabetical Index

Z98.0 Intestinal bypass and anastomosis status
     Excludes2 bariatric surgery status (Z98.84)
            gastric bypass status (Z98.84)
            obesity surgery status (Z98.84)

Z98.1 Arthrodesis status

Z98.2 Presence of cerebrospinal fluid drainage device
     Presence of CSF shunt

Z98.3 Post therapeutic collapse of lung status
     Code first underlying disease

● **Z98.4 Cataract extraction status**
     Use additional code to identify intraocular lens implant status (Z96.1)
     Excludes1 aphakia (H27.0)
     Z98.41 Cataract extraction status, right eye
     Z98.42 Cataract extraction status, left eye
     Z98.49 Cataract extraction status, unspecified eye

● **Z98.5 Sterilization status**
     Excludes1 female infertility (N97.-)
            male infertility (N46.-)
     Z98.51 Tubal ligation status
     Z98.52 Vasectomy status

● **Z98.6 Angioplasty status**
     Z98.61 Coronary angioplasty status
         Excludes1 coronary angioplasty status with implant and graft (Z95.5)
     Z98.62 Peripheral vascular angioplasty status
         Excludes1 peripheral vascular angioplasty status with implant and graft (Z95.820)

● **Z98.8 Other specified postprocedural states**
     ● Z98.81 Dental procedure status
         Z98.810 Dental sealant status
         Z98.811 Dental restoration status
            Dental crown status
            Dental fillings status
         Z98.818 Other dental procedure status
     Z98.82 Breast implant status
         Excludes1 breast implant removal status (Z98.86)

◀ New   ◀▥ Revised   ~~deleted~~ Deleted   **OGCR** Official Guidelines   X Assign placeholder X   ● Use Additional Character(s)
Excludes 1   Excludes 2   Includes   Use additional   Code first   Code also   Unspecified

Z98.83 **Filtering (vitreous) bleb after glaucoma surgery status**

> **Excludes1** inflammation (infection) of postprocedural bleb (H59.4-)

Z98.84 **Bariatric surgery status**
Gastric banding status
Gastric bypass status for obesity
Obesity surgery status

> **Excludes1** bariatric surgery status complicating pregnancy, childbirth, or the puerperium (O99.84)

> **Excludes2** intestinal bypass and anastomosis status (Z98.0)

Z98.85 **Transplanted organ removal status**
Transplanted organ previously removed due to complication, failure, rejection or infection

> **Excludes1** encounter for removal of transplanted organ -code to complication of transplanted organ (T86.-)

Z98.86 **Personal history of breast implant removal**

● Z98.87 **Personal history of in utero procedure**

Z98.870 **Personal history of in utero procedure during pregnancy**

> **Excludes2** complications from in utero procedure for current pregnancy (O35.7)
> supervision of current pregnancy with history of in utero procedure during previous pregnancy (O09.82-)

Z98.871 **Personal history of in utero procedure while a fetus**

Z98.89 **Other specified postprocedural states**
Personal history of surgery, not elsewhere classified

● Z99 **Dependence on enabling machines and devices, not elsewhere classified**

> **Excludes1** cardiac pacemaker status (Z95.0)

Z99.0 **Dependence on aspirator**

● Z99.1 **Dependence on respirator**
Dependence on ventilator

Z99.11 **Dependence on respirator [ventilator] status**

Z99.12 **Encounter for respirator [ventilator] dependence during power failure**

> **Excludes1** mechanical complication of respirator [ventilator] (J95.850)

Z99.2 **Dependence on renal dialysis**
Hemodialysis status
Peritoneal dialysis status
Presence of arteriovenous shunt for dialysis
Renal dialysis status NOS

> **Excludes1** encounter for fitting and adjustment of dialysis catheter (Z49.0-)
> noncompliance with renal dialysis (Z91.15)

Z99.3 **Dependence on wheelchair**
Wheelchair confinement status
Code first cause of dependence, such as:
muscular dystrophy (G71.0)
obesity (E66.-)

● Z99.8 **Dependence on other enabling machines and devices**

Z99.81 **Dependence on supplemental oxygen**
Dependence on long-term oxygen

Z99.89 **Dependence on other enabling machines and devices**
Dependence on machine or device NOS

CHAPTER 21 (Z00-Z99)

Trust Carol J. Buck and Elsevier
to take you through the levels
of coding success

Step 4:
Professional Resources

Step 3:
Certify

With the resources you need for every level of coding success, Carol J. Buck and Elsevier are with you every step of your coding career. From beginning to advanced, from the classroom to the workplace, from application to certification, the Step Series products are your guides to greater opportunities and successful career advancement.

Step 2:
Practice

Step 1:
Learn

Keep climbing with the most trusted names in medical coding.

Author and Educator
Carol J. Buck,
MS, CPC, CCS-P

Lead Technical Collaborator
Jackie L. Grass,
CPC

B-00

Trust Elsevier
to provide your complete curriculum solution!

Content

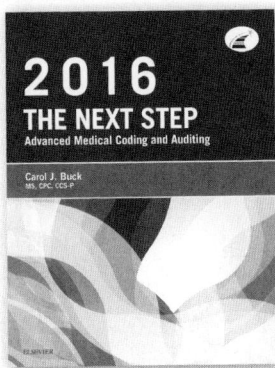

2016 STEP-BY-STEP Medical Coding — Carol J. Buck, MS, CPC, CCS-P
978-0-323-38919-8

2016 THE NEXT STEP Advanced Medical Coding and Auditing — Carol J. Buck, MS, CPC, CCS-P
978-0-323-38910-5

E/M AUDITING STEP Third Edition — CAROL J. BUCK, MS, CPC, CPC-H, CCS-P
978-1-4557-5199-0

Study Tools

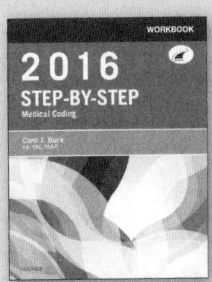

WORKBOOK **2016 STEP-BY-STEP** Medical Coding — Carol J. Buck
978-0-323-38921-1

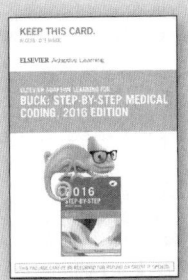

KEEP THIS CARD. ELSEVIER Adaptive Learning — BUCK: STEP-BY-STEP MEDICAL CODING, 2016 EDITION
978-0-323-40124-1

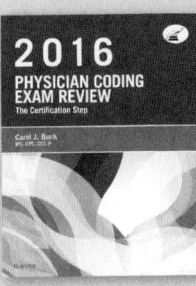

2016 PHYSICIAN CODING EXAM REVIEW The Certification Step — Carol J. Buck
978-0-323-22750-6

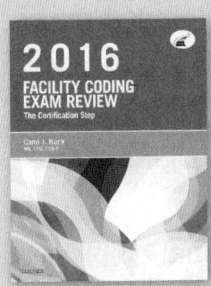

2016 FACILITY CODING EXAM REVIEW The Certification Step — Carol J. Buck
978-0-323-27982-6

evolve

More study tools available

Simulations

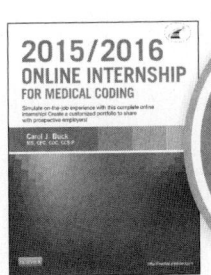

2015/2016 ONLINE INTERNSHIP FOR MEDICAL CODING — Carol J. Buck, MS, CPC, CGC, CCS-P
978-0-323-39250-1

Create a customized portfolio to show employers

Courses

SimChart for the medical office — LEARNING THE MEDICAL OFFICE WORKFLOW
978-0-323-39423-9

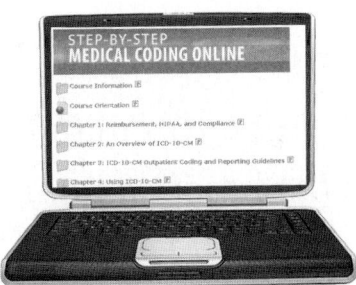

STEP-BY-STEP MEDICAL CODING ONLINE
978-0-323-38922-8

Learn more at Elsevieradvantage.com!

Make the most of your physician coding exam review!

1. Assess!
Take the Pre-Exam

Use the Pre-Exam located on the companion Evolve site to gauge your strengths and weaknesses, develop a plan for focused study, and gain a better understanding of the testing process.

2016
PHYSICIAN CODING
EXAM REVIEW
The Certification Step

Carol J. Buck
MS, CPC, CCS-P

ELSEVIER

ISBN: 978-0-323-22750-6

2. Study!

Use the quizzes in this book to sharpen your skills and build competency.

3. Apply!
Take the Post-Exam

After studying, apply your knowledge to the Post-Exam located on the companion Evolve site. When finished, you'll receive scores for both the Pre- and Post-Exams and a breakdown of incorrect answers to help you identify areas where you need more detailed study and review.

4. Test!
Take the Final Exam

Gauge your readiness for the actual physician coding exam with the Final Exam. Boost your test-taking confidence and ensure certification success.

Perfect your understanding and prepare for certification—start your review now!

Make the most of your facility coding exam review!

1. Assess!
Take the Pre-Exam

Use the Pre-Exam located on the companion Evolve site to gauge your strengths and weaknesses, develop a plan for focused study, and gain a better understanding of the testing process.

2. Study!

Use the quizzes in this book to sharpen your skills and build competency.

3. Apply!
Take the Post-Exam

After studying, apply your knowledge to the Post-Exam located on the companion Evolve site. You'll receive scores for both the Pre- and Post-Exams and a breakdown of incorrect answers to help you identify areas where you need more detailed study and review.

4. Test!
Take the Final Exam

Gauge your readiness for the actual facility coding exam with the Final Exam, also located on the companion Evolve site. Boost your test-taking confidence and ensure certification success.

2016
FACILITY CODING EXAM REVIEW
The Certification Step

Carol J. Buck
MS, CPC, CCS-P

ELSEVIER

ISBN: 978-0-323-27982-6

Perfect your understanding and prepare for certification— start your review now!